NEUROLOGICAL THERAPEUTICS: PRINCIPLES AND PRACTICE

Volume 2

NEUROLOGICAL THERAPEUTICS: PRINCIPLES AND PRACTICE

Volume 2

Editor-in-Chief

John H Noseworthy MD

Chair, Department of Neurology, Mayo Clinic; Professor of Neurology, Mayo Medical School; Rochester MN, USA.

With 345 contributing authors

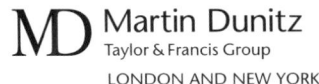
Martin Dunitz
Taylor & Francis Group
LONDON AND NEW YORK

© 2003 Mayo Foundation for Medical Education and Research
Published by
Martin Dunitz
Taylor and Francis Group
11 New Fetter Lane
London EC4P 4EE
UNITED KINGDOM

Distributed in the USA by
Fulfilment Center
Taylor & Francis
10650 Tobben Drive
Independence, KY 41051, USA
Toll Free Tel.: +1 800 634 7064
E-mail: taylorandfrancis@thomsonlearning.com

Distributed in Canada by
Taylor & Francis
74 Rolark Drive
Scarborough, Ontario M1R 4G2, Canada
Toll Free Tel.: +1 877 226 2237
E-mail: tal_fran@istar.ca

Distributed in the rest of the world by
Thomson Publishing Services
Cheriton House
North Way
Andover, Hampshire SP10 5BE, UK
Tel.: +44 (0)1264 332424
E-mail: salesorder.tandf@thomsonpublishingservices.co.uk

Composition and artwork by Wearset Ltd, Boldon, Tyne and Wear
Printed in Spain by Grafos S.A. Arte Sobre Papel

ISBN 1-85317-623-0

10 9 8 7 6 5 4 3 2 1

Care has been taken to confirm the accuracy of the information presented and to describe generally accepted practices. However, the authors, editors, publisher, and Mayo are not responsible for errors or omissions or for any consequences from application of the information in this book and make no warranty, expressed or implied, with respect to the currency, completeness, or accuracy of the contents of the publication. Application of this information in a particular situation remains the professional responsibility of the practitioner, who at all times must exercise independent clinical judgment. No endorsement of any company or product is implied or intended.

The authors, editors, and publisher have exerted every effort to ensure that drug selection and dosage set forth in this text are in accordance with current recommendations and practice at the time of publication. However, in view of ongoing research, changes in government regulations, and the constant flow of information relating to drug therapy and drug reactions, the reader is urged to check the package insert for each drug for any change in indications and dosage and for added warnings and precautions. This is particularly important when the recommended agent is a new or infrequently employed drug.

Some drugs and medical devices presented in this publication have Food and Drug Administration (FDA) clearance for limited use in restricted research settings. It is the responsibility of the health care provider to ascertain the FDA status of each drug or device planned for use in their clinical practice.

Contents

Section IV   Cerebrovascular Disease
Section editor: José Biller

Volume 2

List of Contributors

Nada G Abou-Fayssal MD
Assistant Professor of Neurology
Mount Sinai School of Medicine
New York NY, USA
Chapter 182 – Peripheral Neuropathy and HIV

Lauren E Abrey MD
Assistant Professor
Memorial Sloan-Kettering Cancer Center
New York NY, USA
Chapter 70 – Germ Cell Tumors and Primary Central
    Nervous System Lymphoma

Harold P Adams MD
Professor
Division of Cerebrovascular Disorders
Department of Neurology
University of Iowa
Iowa City IO, USA
Chapter 43 – Management of Patients with Acute
    Ischemic Stroke
Chapter 115 – Cardiac Tumors

Robert J Adams MD
Regents' Professor of Neurology
Department of Neurology
Medical College of Georgia
Augusta GA, USA
Chapter 125 – Hemoglobinopathies and Thalassemias:
    Treatment of Stroke and Other Neurological
    Complications

Allen J Aksamit MD
Consultant
Department of Neurology
Mayo Clinic
Associate Professor of Neurology
Mayo Medical School
Rochester MN, USA
Chapter 179 – Varicella Zoster Virus, Herpes Simplex
    Virus, Bell's Palsy
Chapter 180 – Peripheral Nervous System Lyme
    Disease
Chapter 181 – Diphtheritic Neuropathy

Ann W Alexander MD
Morris Center
Gainesville FL, USA
Chapter 261 – Treatment of Developmental Language
    Disorders

Michael P Alexander MD
Clinical Associate Professor of Neurology
Harvard Medical School
Department of Neurology
Beth Israel Deaconess Medical Center
Boston MA, USA
Chapter 267 – Executive Disorders

Ahmed S Aly MD
Resident
Department of Neurology
Boston Medical Center
Boston MA, USA
Chapter 47 – Treatment of Intracerebral Hemorrhage

Jeffrey M Anderson PhD
Research Fellow
Department of Radiology
Harvard Medical School
Nuclear Magnetic Resonance Center
Charlestown MA, USA
Department of Neurology
University of Florida College of Medicine
Center for Neuropsychological Studies and the
    Malcolm Randall Veterans Affairs Hospital
Gainesville FL, USA
Chapter 271 – Treatment of Emotional
    Communication Disorders

Joseph H Antin MD
Associate Professor of Medicine
Harvard Medical School
Chief
Adult Oncology Stem Cell Transplantation
Dana-Farber Cancer Institute and Brigham Women's
    Hospital
Boston MA, USA
Chapter 129 – Neurological Aspects of
    Transplantation

Ajay K Arora MD
Fellow
Department of Neurology
Grady Hospital
Atlanta GA, USA
Chapter 40 – Thrombolytic Therapy for Stroke

Tetsuo Ashizawa MD
Professor
Parkinson's Disease Center and Movement Disorders
    Clinic
Department of Neurology
Baylor College of Medicine
Houston TX, USA
Chapter 239 – Huntington's Disease

Neeraj Badjatia MD
Fellow
Department of Neurology
Grady Hospital
Atlanta GA, USA
Chapter 40 – Thrombolytic Therapy for Stroke

Jean-Paul Bahary MD FRCP(C)
Associate Professor
Centre Hospitalier de L'Université de Montréal
Montréal PQ, Canada
Chapter 65 – Radiotherapy for CNS Neoplasms:
    Principles, Technologies and Indications

Laura J Balcer MD MSCE
Assistant Professor
Departments of Neurology and Ophthalmology
University of Pennsylvania School of Medicine
Philadelphia PA, USA
Chapter 161 – Optic Neuropathies

James F Bale Jr MD
Professor
Division of Child Neurology
The Departments of Pediatrics and Neurology
The University of Utah School of Medicine
Salt Lake City UT, USA
Chapter 93 – Perinatal Infections

Martha J Bale MS MT (ASCP)
Group Manager
Infectious Diseases and Molecular Pathology
ARUP Laboratories
Division of Child Neurology
The Departments of Pediatrics and Neurology
The University of Utah School of Medicine
Salt Lake City UT, USA
Chapter 93 – Perinatal Infections

Robert W Baloh MD
Professor
UCLA Department of Neurology
Los Angeles CA, USA
Chapter 173 – Disorders of the Inner Ear

Brenda L Banwell MD
Assistant Professor of Pediatrics (Neurology)
The Hospital for Sick Children
University of Toronto
Toronto ON, Canada
Chapter 220 – Principles of Muscle Disorders
Chapter 222 – Muscular Dystrophies

Amilton Antunes Barreira MD PhD
Professor of Neurology
Medical School of Ribeirão Preto
Department of Neurology
University of São Paulo
Head of the Neuromuscular Division
University Hospital of Ribeirão Preto
Ribeirão Preto SP, Brazil
Chapter 184 – Peripheral Neuropathies in Chagas
    Disease

H Hunt Batjer MD
Michael J. Marchese Professor of Neurosurgery
Chairman
Department of Neurological Surgery
Northwestern University Medical School
Chicago IL, USA
Chapter 49 – Cerebral Aneurysms and Vascular
    Malformations

Glenn S Bauman
Associate Professor
Department of Oncology
University of Western Ontario and London Regional
    Cancer Centre
London ON, Canada
Chapter 65 – Radiotherapy for CNS Neoplasms:
    Principles, Technologies and Indications

Carl W Bazil MD PhD
Assistant Professor of Neurology
Director
Clinical Anticonvulsant Drug Trials
Columbia Comprehensive Epilepsy Center
New York-Presbyterian Medical Center
New York NY, USA
Chapter 29 – Antiseizure Drugs

Pelagie M Beeson PhD
Associate Professor
National Center for Neurogenic Communication
    Disorders and Department of Speech and Hearing
    Sciences
University of Arizona
Tucson AZ
Department of Neurology
University of Arizona
Tucson AZ, USA
Chapter 260 – Treatment of Alexia and Agraphia

Miles J Belgrade MD
Clinical Associate Professor
Medical Director
Fairview Pain Management Center
Fairview-University Medical Center
Clinical Associate
Department of Neurology
University of Minnesota Medical School
Minneapolis MN, USA
Chapter 18 – Radicular Limb Pain

Larry S Benardo MD PhD
Professor of Neurology,
    Physiology and Pharmacology
Vice Chairman of Neurology
SUNY Downstate Medical Center
Director SUNY Downstate Epilepsy Center
Brooklyn NY, USA
Chapter 27 – Pathophysiology of the Epilepsies

Eduardo E Benarroch MD
Consultant
Department of Neurology
Mayo Clinic
Professor of Neurology
Mayo Medical School
Rochester MN, USA
Chapter 1 – Basic Pharmaceutical Principles and the
    Blood–Brain Barrier
Chapter 219 – Treatment of Central Autonomic
    Disorders

Bernard R Bendok MD (BRB)
Chief Resident
Department of Neurological Surgery
Northwestern University Medical School
Chicago IL, USA
Chapter 49 – Cerebral Aneurysms and Vascular
    Malformations

Joseph R Berger MD
Professor and Chair
Department of Neurology
University of Kentucky Medical Center
Professor of Internal Medicine
Department of Internal Medicine
University of Kentucky Medical Center
Lexington KY, USA
Chapter 130 – Immunodeficiency Diseases

James L Bernat MD
Professor of Medicine (Neurology)
Dartmouth Medical School
Hanover NH, USA
Chapter 6 – Ethical Issues in Neurological Treatment
    and Clinical Trials

Bradley E Bernstein MD PhD
Resident
Department of Pathology
Brigham and Women's Hospital and Harvard
    Medical School
Boston MA, USA
Chapter 123 – Use of Therapeutic Plasma Exchange
    and Intravenous Immunoglobulin for the
    Treatment of Neurological Disease

Adil E Bharucha MD
Consultant
Division of Gastroenterology and Hepatology and
    Internal Medicine
Mayo Clinic
Associate Professor of Medicine
Mayo Medical School
Rochester MN, USA
Chapter 216 – Gastrointestinal Dysmotility and
    Sphincter Dysfunction

José Biller MD
Professor and Chairman
Department of Neurology
Indiana University School of Medicine
Indiana University Medical Center
Indianapolis IN, USA
Chapter 45 – Cerebral Complications after Cardiac
    Surgery and Cardiac Arrest
Chapter 61 – Stroke in Children
Chapter 62 – Stroke in Pregnancy

Jean-Pierre Bissonnette PhD
Physicist
Centre Hospitalier de L'Université de Montréal
Montréal PQ, Canada
Chapter 65 – Radiotherapy for CNS Neoplasms:
    Principles, Technologies and Indications

Kyra Blatt MD
Movement Disorders Fellow
Department of Neurology
Beth Israel Medical Center
New York NY, USA
Chapter 237 – Generalized Torsion Dystonia

John B Bodensteiner MD
Chief
Division of Child Neurology
Children's Health Center
St Joseph's Hospital and the Barrow Neurological
    Institute
Phoenix AZ, USA
Chapter 154 – Developmental Problems of the Brain,
    Skull, and Spine

Bradley F Boeve MD
Consultant
Department of Neurology
Consultant
Sleep Disorders Center
Mayo Clinic
Assistant Professor of Neurology
Mayo Medical School
Rochester MN, USA
Chapter 269 – Diagnosis and Management of the
    Non-Alzheimer Dementias

Charles F Bolton MD
Senior Associate Consultant
Department of Neurology
Mayo Clinic
Professor of Neurology
Mayo Medical School
Rochester MN, USA
Chapter 213 – Critical Illness Polyneuropathy

Cecil O Borel MD
Associate Professor Anesthesiology
Duke University
Medical Director
Neurosciences Critical Care Unit
Division Chief
Otolaryngology/Head/Neck and Neuroanesthesia
Durham NC, USA
Chapter 99 – Airway Management and Mechanical
    Ventilation

E Peter Bosch MD
Consultant
Department of Neurology
Mayo Clinic
Scottsdale AZ, USA
Professor of Neurology
Mayo Medical School
Rochester MN, USA
Chapter 190 – Neuropathies in Liver Disease and
    Chronic Renal Failure

Marie-Germaine Bousser MD
Professor and Chief
Service de Neurologie
Hôpital Lariboisière
Paris, France
Chapter 59 – Cerebral Autosomal Dominant
    Arteriopathy With Subcortical Infarcts and
    Leukoencephalopathy (CADASIL)

Paul W Brazis MD
Consultant
Department of Ophthalmology
Mayo Clinic
Jacksonville FL, USA
Associate Professor of Neurology and of
    Ophthalmology
Mayo Medical School
Rochester MN, USA
Chapter 163 – Chiasm and Retrochiasmal Disorders

Susan B Bressman MD
Professor
Department of Neurology
Albert Einstein College of Medicine
Yeshiva University
Chair
Department of Neurology
Beth Israel Medical Center
New York NY, USA
Chapter 237 – Generalized Torsion Dystonia
Chapter 238 – Dopa-Responsive Dystonia

Robin L Brey MD
Professor
University of Texas Health Science Center at San
    Antonio
San Antonio TX, USA
Chapter 56 – Antiphospholipid Antibodies and
    Variants

Robert D Brown Jr MD
Consultant
Department of Neurology
Mayo Clinic
Associate Professor of Neurology
Mayo Medical School
Rochester MN, USA
Chapter 41 – Asymptomatic Carotid Artery Stenosis

Askiel Bruno MD
Associate Professor
Department of Neurology
Indiana University
Indianapolis IN, USA
Chapter 42 – Transient Ischemic Attacks
Chapter 45 – Cerebral Complications after Cardiac
    Surgery and Cardiac Arrest

Jan C Buckner MD
Consultant
Division of Medical Oncology
Mayo Clinic
Professor of Oncology
Mayo Medical School
Rochester MN, USA
Chapter 68 – Diffuse Cerebral Gliomas in Adults

Ted M Burns MD
Assistant Professor of Neurology
University of Virginia
Charlottesville VA, USA
Chapter 205 – Inherited Neuropathies With Known
    Metabolic Derangement

Grant Butterbaugh PhD
Associate Professor of Psychiatry
Louisiana State University Health Science Center
New Orleans LA, USA
Chapter 155 – Mental Retardation and Cerebral Palsy

Laurel J Buxbaum MD
Research Associate Professor
Moss Rehabilitation Research Institute
Philadelphia PA, USA
Chapter 262 – Treatment of Neglect

J Gregory Cairncross MD
Professor and Chairman
Department of Oncology
Professor
Department of Clinical Neurological Sciences
University of Western Ontario
London Regional Cancer Centre
London ON, Canada
Chapter 63 – A Perspective on Neuro-oncology

Michael Camilleri MD
Consultant
Division of Gastroenterology and Hepatology and
    Internal Medicine
Mayo Clinic
Atherton and Winifred W Bean Professor
Professor of Medicine and Physiology
Mayo Medical School
Rochester MN, USA
Chapter 216 – Gastrointestinal Dysmotility and
    Sphincter Dysfunction

Stephen C Cannon MD PhD
Assistant Professor
Department of Neurobiology
Harvard Medical School
Department of Neurology
Massachusetts General Hospital
Boston MA, USA
Chapter 225 – Myotonia and Periodic Paralysis:
    Disorders of Voltage-Gated Ion Channels

David J Capobianco MD
Consultant
Department of Neurology
Mayo Clinic
Jacksonville FL
Assistant Professor of Neurology
Mayo Medical School
Rochester MN, USA
Chapter 10 – Cluster Headache

J Aidan Carney MD PhD FRCPI
Emeritus Member
Department of Laboratory Medicine and Pathology
Mayo Clinic
Emeritus Professor of Pathology
Mayo Medical School
Rochester MN, USA
Chapter 189 – Multiple Endocrine Neoplasia, Type 2B

Hugues Chabriat MD PhD
Professor
Service de Neurologie
Hôpital Lariboisière
Paris, France
Chapter 59 – Cerebral Autosomal Dominant
    Arteriopathy With Subcortical Infarcts and
    Leukoencephalopathy (CADASIL)

Colin Chalk MD
Associate Professor
Department of Neurology and Neurosurgery
McGill University
Montréal General Hospital
Division of Neurology
Montréal PQ, Canada
Chapter 175 – Disorders of the Glossopharyngeal,
    Vagus, Accessory, and Hypoglossal Nerves

Phillip F Chance MD FACMG
Chief
Division of Genetics and Development
Children's Hospital and Regional Medical Center
Professor of Pediatrics and Neurology
University of Washington School of Medicine
Seattle WA, USA
Chapter 209 – Hereditary Neuropathy With Liability
    to Pressure Palsy

Praful Chandarana MD ChB FRCPC ABPN
Associate Professor
Department of Psychiatry
University of Western Ontario
London ON, Canada
Chapter 25 – Pain Disorder

Michael E Charness MD
Associate Professor
Department of Neurology
VA Boston Healthcare System
Brigham and Women's Hospital Department of
    Neurology
Harvard Medical School
Boston MA, USA
Chapter 142 – Alcohol

Cathy Chuang MD
Fellow
Department of Neurology
Columbia College of Physicians and Surgeons
New York NY, USA
Chapter 241 – Sydenham Chorea

Winthrop H Churchill MD
Medical Director
Therapeutic Services
Brigham and Women's Hospital
Associate Professor of Medicine at Brigham and
    Women's Hospital
Harvard Medical School
Boston MA, USA
Chapter 123 – Use of Therapeutic Plasma Exchange
    and Intravenous Immunoglobulin for the
    Treatment of Neurological Disease

Roberto Ciordia MD
Fellow
Neuro-Oncology
Harvard Medical School
The Massachusetts General Hospital
Boston MA, USA
Chapter 126 – Therapy of the Neurological
    Complications of Lymphoma and Leukemia

Joe TR Clarke MD PhD FRCP(C)
Professor
Division of Clinical and Metabolic Genetics
Hospital for Sick Children
Toronto ON, Canada
Chapter 224 – Metabolic Myopathies

David B Clifford MD
Seay Professor of Clinical Neuropharmacology in
    Neurology
Department of Neurology
Washington University School of Medicine
St Louis MO, USA
Chapter 85 – Neurological Complications of HIV
    Infection

Bruce H Cohen MD
Section of Pediatric Neurology
Cleveland Clinic Foundation
Cleveland OH, USA
Chapter 152 – The Neurological Examination of the
    Infant and Child

Aaron A Cohen-Gadol MD
Resident in Neurosurgery
Mayo Graduate School of Medicine
Rochester MN, USA
Chapter 108 – Management of Head Trauma and
    Spinal Cord Injury in Adults

Michael P Collins MD
Assistant Professor of Neurology
The Ohio State University
Columbus OH, USA
Chapter 198 – Vasculitis of the Peripheral Nervous
    System

Cynthia Comella MD
Associate Professor
Department of Neurology
Rush Medical School
Chicago IL, USA
Chapter 236 – Focal Dystonias: Blepharospasm,
    Cervical Dystonia, Spasmodic Dysphonia, Writer's
    Cramp

Christopher Commichau MD
Assistant Clinical Professor of Medicine
John A Burns School of Medicine
Director
Neurosciences ICU
Associate Director
The Neurosciences Institute
The Queens Medical Center
Honolulu HI, USA
Chapter 46 – Hypoxic–Ischemic Encephalopathy

Paul Cooper MD FRCP
Associate Professor
Clinical Neurological Sciences
University of Western Ontario
London ON, Canada
Chapter 136 – Hypothalamus, Anterior and Posterior
    Pituitary and Adrenal (Including Disorders of
    Temperature Regulation)

David R Cornblath MD
Professor of Neurology
The Johns Hopkins University School of Medicine
Neurologist
The Johns Hopkins Hospital
Baltimore MD, USA
Chapter 192 – Acute Inflammatory Demyelinating
    Polyradiculoneuropathy, Acute Motor Axonal
    Neuropathy and Acute Motor and Sensory Axonal
    Neuropathy

H Branch Coslett MD
Professor of Neurology
University of Pennsylvania School of Medicine
Philadelphia PA, USA
Chapter 262 – Treatment of Neglect

Bruce Coull MD
Professor and Head
Department of Neurology
University of Arizona College of Medicine
Tucson AZ, USA
Chapter 55 – Disorders of Coagulation

Patricia H Davis MD
Associate Professor
Division of Cerebrovascular Disorders
Department of Neurology
University of Iowa
Iowa City IA, USA
Chapter 115 – Cardiac Tumors

Lisa M DeAngelis MD
Professor
Memorial Sloan-Kettering Cancer Center
New York NY, USA
Chapter 70 – Germ Cell Tumors and Primary Central
    Nervous System Lymphoma

Christopher M DeGiorgio MD
Associate Professor in Residence and Vice Chairman
UCLA Department of Neurology
Los Angeles CA, USA
Chapter 31 – Status Epilepticus

Oscar H Del Brutto MD
Coordinator
Stroke Unit
Department of Neurological Sciences
Hospital-Clinica Kennedy
Guayaquil, Ecuador
Chapter 90 – Helminthic Infections of the Central
    Nervous System

Franco DeMonte MD FRCSC FACS
Associate Professor
Department of Neurosurgery
MD Anderson Cancer Center
Houston TX, USA
Chapter 66 – Surgically Curable Brain Tumors of
    Adults

Lyle J Dennis MD
Fellow in Critical Care Neurology
Columbia University College of Physicians and
    Surgeons
New York NY, USA
Chapter 101 – Management of Increased Intracranial
    Pressure

Kapil Dev Sethi MD FRCP (UK)
Professor of Neurology
Medical College of Georgia
Augusta GA, USA
Chapter 242 – Ballism and Chorea

Michael N Diringer MD FCCM
Associate Professor of Neurology
Neurosurgery and Anesthesiology
Director
Neurology/Neurosurgery Intensive Care Unit
Department of Neurology
Washington University School of Medicine
St Louis MO, USA
Chapter 103 – Disturbances of Fluid and Electrolytes
    in Critically Ill Neurological Patients

Angela Dispenzieri MD
Consultant
Division of Hematology and Internal Medicine
Mayo Clinic
Assistant Professor of Medicine
Mayo Medical School
Rochester MN, USA
Chapter 202 – Amyloidosis

David W Dodick MD
Consultant
Department of Neurology
Mayo Clinic
Scottsdale, AZ, USA
Associate Professor of Neurology
Mayo Medical School
Rochester MN, USA
Chapter 10 – Cluster Headache
Chapter 14 – Indomethacin-Responsive Headache
    Syndromes
Chapter 15 – Giant Cell Arteritis

Colin Doherty MB MRCP(I)
Fellow
Department of Neurology
Partners Neurology Program
Brigham and Women's Hospital and Massachusetts
    General Hospital
Boston MA, USA
Chapter 137 – The Neurological Manifestations of
    Thyroid Disease

Rose M Dotson MD
Consultant
Department of Neurology
Mayo Clinic
Assistant Professor of Neurology
Mayo Medical School
Rochester MN, USA
Chapter 214 – Paresthesias and Pain

Richard L Doty MD
Professor and Director
Smell and Taste Center
University of Pennsylvania Medical Center
Philadelphia PA, USA
Chapter 160 – Disturbances of Smell and Taste

P James B Dyck MD
Consultant
Peripheral Nerve Research Center
Mayo Clinic
Assistant Professor of Neurology
Mayo Medical School
Rochester MN, USA
Chapter 187 – Diabetic Radiculoplexus Neuropathies
Chapter 196 – Nondiabetic Lumbosacral
    Radiculoplexus Neuropathy

Peter J Dyck MD
Head
Peripheral Neuropathy Research Center
Mayo Clinic
Roy E and Merle Meyer
    Professor of Neuroscience
Professor of Neurology
Mayo Medical School
Rochester MN, USA
Chapter 186 – Diabetic Polyneuropathy
Chapter 207 – Hereditary Sensory and Autonomic
    Neuropathies

John G Edmeads MD FRCPC
Professor
Division of Neurology
Department of Medicine
Sunnybrook and Women's Health Sciences Center
Toronto ON, Canada
Chapter 8 – Principles of Pain Management
Chapter 9 – Migraine
Chapter 20 – Complex Regional Pain Syndrome
    (Reflex Sympathetic Dystrophy, Causalgia,
    Shoulder–Hand Syndrome)

Benjamin H Eidelman MD
Senior Associate Consultant
Department of Neurology
Mayo Clinic
Jacksonville, FL, USA
Professor of Neurology
Mayo Medical School
Rochester MN, USA
Chapter 106 – Organ Transplant Complications in the
    Intensive Care Unit

Erin Elmore MD
Senior Resident, Neurology
Beth Israel Medical Center
New York NY, USA
Chapter 238 – Dopa-Responsive Dystonia

Andrew G Engel MD
Consultant
Department of Neurology
Mayo Clinic
William L McKnight-3M Professor of Neuroscience
Mayo Medical School
Rochester MN, USA
Chapter 226 – Myasthenia Gravis and Myasthenic
    Syndromes

Alberto Espay MD
Resident
Department of Neurology
Indiana University School of Medicine
Indiana University Hospital
Indianapolis IN, USA
Chapter 91 – Neurology of Arachnida (Spiders, Ticks,
    Scorpions) and Hymenoptera (Ants, Bees, Wasps)
    Envenomations

Stanley Fahn MD
H Houston Merritt Professor of Neurology
Columbia University
Neurological Institute
Columbia-Presbyterian Medical Center
New York NY, USA
Chapter 230 – Overview of Movement Disorders
Chapter 231 – Medical Treatment of Parkinson's
    Disease and its Complications
Chapter 247 – Tardive Dyskinesia and Related
    Disorders
Chapter 249 – Paroxysmal Dyskinesias
Chapter 254 – Psychogenic Movement Disorders

Adel G Fam MD FRCP(C) FACP
Professor of Medicine and Head
Division of Rheumatology
Sunnybrook Women's College Health Sciences Center
University of Toronto
Toronto ON, Canada
Chapter 24 – Fibromyalgia and Myofascial Pain
    Syndrome

Michael G Fehlings MD PhD FRCS(C)
Professor of Surgery
Robert O Lawson Chair in Neural Repair and
    Regeneration
Research Director
Division of Neurosurgery
University of Toronto, Canada
Head Spinal Program
Toronto Western Hospital
University Health Network
Toronto ON, Canada
Chapter 72 – Primary Tumors of the Spinal Cord,
    Root, Plexus, and Nerve Sheath

Robert G Feldman MD
Director
Environmental and Occupational Neurology Program
Professor of Neurology,
    Pharmacology and Environmental Health
Boston University Schools of Medicine and Public
    Health: Lecturer in Occupational Health
Harvard University Medical School
Boston MA, USA
Chapter 144 – Treatment of the Neurotoxic Effects of
    Organic Solvents
Chapter 145 – Treatment of the Neurotoxic Effects of
    Gases: Carbon Monoxide, Hydrogen Sulfide and
    the Nitrogen Oxides

Edward Feldmann MD
Professor
Brown University
School of Medicine
Department of Clinical Neurosciences
Providence RI, USA
Chapter 52 – Fibromuscular Dysplasia

Steven K Feske MD
Assistant Professor of Neurology
Harvard Medical School
Director
Stroke Division
Neurology Department
Brigham and Women's Hospital
Boston MA, USA
Chapter 147 – Toxemia of Pregnancy

John K Fink MD
Professor
Department of Neurology
University of Michigan and Geriatric Research
    Education and Care Center
Ann Arbor Veterans Affairs Medical Center
Ann Arbor MI, USA
Chapter 257 – Hereditary Spastic Paraplegia

Kelly D Flemming MD
Consultant
Department of Neurology
Mayo Clinic
Assistant Professor of Neurology
Mayo Medical School
Rochester MN, USA
Chapter 50 – Unruptured Intracranial Aneurysms

Robert B Fogel MD
Instructor in Medicine
Harvard Medical School
Division of Sleep Medicine
Associate Physician
Department of Medicine
Brigham and Women's Hospital
Boston MA, USA
Chapter 119 – Disorders of Excessive Sleepiness
Chapter 120 – Parasomnias

Blair Ford MD
Associate Professor of Clinical Neurology
Columbia University
Neurological Institute
Columbia-Presbyterian Medical Center
New York NY, USA
Chapter 231 – Medical Treatment of Parkinson's
    Disease and its Complications
Chapter 241 – Sydenham Chorea
Chapter 254 – Psychogenic Movement Disorders

Mariê-Andre Fortin MD FRCP(C)
Centre Hospitalier de L'Université de Montréal
Montréal PQ, Canada
Chapter 65 – Radiotherapy for CNS Neoplasms:
    Principles, Technologies and Indications

Michael R Frankel MD
Associate Professor
Chief of Neurology
Grady Hospital
Department of Neurology
Atlanta GA, USA
Chapter 40 – Thrombolytic Therapy for Stroke

Mark N Friedman MD
Instructor
Harvard Neuroendocrine Unit
Beth Israel Deaconess Medical Center
Boston MA, USA
Chapter 138 – Reproductive Endocrinology and
    Gender-Specific Issues in Neurology

Neil R Friedman MB ChB
Section of Pediatric Neurology
Cleveland Clinic Foundation
Cleveland OH, USA
Chapter 152 – The Neurological Examination of the
    Infant and Child

Steven J Frucht MD
Assistant Professor of Neurology
Columbia-Presbyterian Medical Center
New York NY, USA
Chapter 234 – The Diagnosis and Treatment of
    Normal Pressure Hydrocephalus
Chapter 245 – Myoclonus

Jimmy R Fulgham MD
Consultant
Department of Neurology
Mayo Clinic
Assistant Professor of Neurology
Mayo Medical School
Rochester MN, USA
Chapter 104 – Anticoagulation and Thrombolysis in
    the Intensive Care Unit

Evanthia Galanis MD
Consultant
Division of Medical Oncology
Mayo Clinic
Associate Professor of Oncology
Mayo Medical School
Rochester MN, USA
Chapter 68 – Diffuse Cerebral Gliomas in Adults

Steven L Galetta MD
Van Miter Professor of Neurology
Director
Neuro-Ophthalmology Program
Departments of Neurology and Ophthalmology
University of Pennsylvania School of Medicine
Philadelphia PA, USA
Chapter 161 – Optic Neuropathies

Bhargavi Gali MD
Consultant
Critical Care Service
Mayo Clinic
Instructor in Anesthesiology
Mayo Medical School
Rochester MN, USA
Chapter 102 – Management of Sedation and Pain in
    the Intensive Care Unit

Juan C Garcia-Monco MD
Associate Professor
Chief
Service of Neurology
Hospital de Galdacano
Galdacano
Vizcaya, Spain
Chapter 80 – Tuberculosis and Other Mycobacterial
    Infections

Bhuwan P Garg MB BS
Professor of Neurology
Department of Neurology
James Whitcomb Riley Hospital for Children
Indiana University School of Medicine
Indianapolis IN, USA
Chapter 61 – Stroke in Children

Christopher C Getch MD
Assistant Professor of Neurological Surgery
Northwestern University Medical School
Chicago IL, USA
Chapter 49 – Cerebral Aneurysms and Vascular
    Malformations

Frank Gilliam MD MPH
Associate Professor of Neurology
Washington University
St Louis MO, USA
Chapter 30 – Surgery and Non-pharmacological
    Therapies for Epilepsy

Christopher G Goetz MD
Harold L Klawans Professor of Neurological Sciences
    and Pharmacology
Director
Section of Movement Disorders
Department of Neurological Sciences
Rush-Presbyterian-St Luke's Medical Center
Chicago IL, USA
Chapter 146 – Pesticides

Robert R Goodman MD PhD
Associate Professor
Neurological Surgery
Columbia University College of Physicians and
    Surgeons
New York NY, USA
Chapter 234 – The Diagnosis and Treatment of
    Normal Pressure Hydrocephalus

Philip B Gorelick MD MPH FACP
Deborah R and Edgar D Jannotta Presidential
    Professor of Neurology
Director
Center for Stroke Research and Section of
    Cerebrovascular Disease and Neurologic Critical
    Care
Department of Neurologic Sciences
Rush Medical College
Chicago IL, USA
Chapter 38 – Stroke Prevention

John L Goudreau DO PhD
Resident in Neurology
Mayo Graduate School of Medicine
Rochester MN, USA
Chapter 210 – Hereditary Spinocerebellar
    Degeneration

IA Grant MD FRCP(C)
Assistant Professor
Dalhousie University
Staff Neurologist
Division of Neurology
QEII Health Sciences Centre
Halifax NS, Canada
Chapter 197 – Treatment of Nonmalignant Sensory
    Ganglionopathies

Harry Greenberg MD
Professor of Neurology and Neurosurgery
Department of Neurology
University of Michigan Medical Center
Taubman Center
Ann Arbor MI, USA
Chapter 73 – Metastases to the Spine Meninges and
    Plexus

Paul E Greene MD
Assistant Professor
Department of Neurology
Columbia Presbyterian Medical Center
Neurological Institute
New York NY, USA
Chapter 244 – Treatment of Orthostatic Tremor
Chapter 252 – Treatment of Hemifacial Spasm

James C Grotta MD
Professor
Roy M and Phyllis Gough Huffington Distinguished
    Chair in Neurology
Director Stroke Program
Professor of Neurology
University of Texas-Houston
Houston TX, USA
Chapter 60 – Moyamoya Disease

Michael A Grotzer MD
Assistant Professor of Pediatrics and Pediatric
    Oncology
Division of Oncology
University Children's Hospital
Zurich, Switzerland
Chapter 69 – Malignant Brain Tumors of Childhood

Thomas M Habermann MD
Consultant
Division of Hematology and Internal Medicine
Mayo Clinic
Professor of Medicine
Mayo Medical School
Rochester MN, USA
Chapter 203 – Peripheral Neuropathy in the
    Lymphomas and Leukemias

Angelika F Hahn MD FRCP(C)
Professor of Neurology
Department of Clinical Neurological Sciences
London Health Sciences Centre
The University of Western Ontario
London ON, Canada
Chapter 193 – Chronic Inflammatory Demyelinating
    Polyradiculoneuropathy

Christiana E Hall MD
Resident
Department of Neurology
Medical College of Georgia
Augusta GA, USA
Chapter 125 – Hemoglobinopathies and Thalassemias:
    Treatment of Stroke and Other Neurological
    Complications

Hamilton Hall MD
Professor
Department of Surgery
University of Toronto and Spine Services
Sunnybrook and Women's College Health Sciences
    Centre
Toronto ON, Canada
Chapter 19 – Back Pain

Mark Hallett MD
Chief
Medical Neurology Branch
NINDS
NIH
Bethesda MD, USA
Chapter 236 – Focal Dystonias: Blepharospasm,
    Cervical Dystonia, Spasmodic Dysphonia, Writer's
    Cramp

Daniel K Hall-Flavin MD
Consultant
Section of Adult Psychiatry
Mayo Clinic
Assistant Professor of Psychiatry
Mayo Medical School
Rochester MN, USA
Chapter 143 – Stimulants, Sedatives, and Opiates

C Michel Harper Jr MD
Consultant
Section of Electromyography
Mayo Clinic
Associate Professor of Neurology
Mayo Medical School
Rochester MN, USA
Chapter 229 – Cramps and Myalgias

Hans-Peter Hartung MD
Professor
Department of Neurology
Heinrich-Heine-University
Düsseldorf, Germany
Chapter 96 – Autoimmunity in the Nervous System
Chapter 97 – Multiple Sclerosis and Related
    Conditions

Julia H Hayes MD
Resident
Internal Medicine
New York Presbyterian Hospital
Columbia Campus
New York NY, USA
Chapter 122 – Acid–Base Disturbances and the
    Central Nervous System

Kenneth M Heilman MD
The James E Rooks Jr Distinguished Professor of
    Neurology and Program Director
University of Florida College of Medicine and Chief
    North Florida–South Georgia Veterans Affairs
    Health System
Gainsville FL, USA
Chapter 258 – Treatment of Disorders of Cognition:
    An Introduction
Chapter 261 – Treatment of Developmental Language
    Disorders
Chapter 271 – Treatment of Emotional
    Communication Disorders

Galen V Henderson MD
Instructor, Neurology
Director of Stroke and Critical Care Neurology
Brigham and Women's Hospital
Harvard Medical School
Boston MA, USA
Chapter 118 – Acute Respiratory Failure in
    Neurological Disease

Wayne A Hening MD
Assistant Clinical Professor, Neurology
University of Medicine and Dentistry of New Jersey
Robert Wood Johnson Medical School
New Brunswick NJ, USA
Chapter 251 – The Restless Legs Syndrome and
    Periodic Limb Movements

Robert C Hermann Jr MD
Consultant
Department of Neurology
Mayo Clinic
Assistant Professor of Neurology
Mayo Medical School
Rochester MN, USA
Chapter 178 – Mechanical Nerve Injuries

Andrew G Herzog MD
Associate Professor, Neurology
Harvard Neuroendocrine Unit
Beth Israel Deaconess Medical Center
Boston MA, USA
Chapter 138 – Reproductive Endocrinology and
    Gender-Specific Issues in Neurology

David C Hess MD
Professor of Neurology
Medical College of Georgia
VA Medical Center
Augusta GA, USA
Chapter 37 – Principles of Atherosclerosis and
    Atherogenesis

Alan Hill MD PhD
Head
Division of Neurology
Professor
Department of Pediatrics
University of British Columbia
British Columbia's Children's Hospital
Vancouver BC, Canada
Chapter 153 – Perinatal Neurology

Fred H Hochberg MD
Associate Professor of Neurology and Attending
    Neurologist
Harvard Medical School
Neuro-Oncology
The Massachusetts General Hospital
Boston MA, USA
Chapter 126 – Therapy of the Neurological
    Complications of Lymphoma and Leukemia

Virginia E Hofmann MD
Senior Associate Consultant
Section of Adult Psychiatry
Mayo Clinic
Assistant Professor of Psychiatry
Mayo Medical School
Rochester MN, USA
Chapter 143 – Stimulants, Sedatives, and Opiates

Robert G Holloway MD MPH
Associate Professor
Department of Neurology
University of Rochester
Rochester
New York NY, USA
Chapter 5 – Evidence-Based Medicine

Richard AC Hughes MD FRCP FMedSci
Professor of Neurology
Department of Clinical Neurosciences
Guy's, King's and St Thomas' School of Medicine
Consultant Neurologist
Guy's Hospital
London, UK
Chapter 192 – Acute Inflammatory Demyelinating
    Polyradiculoneuropathy, Acute Motor Axonal
    Neuropathy and Acute Motor and Sensory Axonal
    Neuropathy

Joseph Jankovic MD
Professor
Department of Neurology
Director of Parkinson's Disease Center and
    Movement Disorders Clinic
Baylor College of Medicine
Houston TX, USA
Chapter 232 – Parkinsonism Plus Disorders
Chapter 239 – Huntington's Disease
Chapter 240 – Neuroacanthocytosis

William J Jones MD
Assistant Professor, Department of Neurology
Indiana University School of Medicine
Indianapolis IN, USA
Chapter 45 – Cerebral Complications after Cardiac
    Surgery and Cardiac Arrest

Patrick S Kamath MD
Consultant
Division of Gastroenterology and Hepatology and
    Internal Medicine
Mayo Clinic
Professor of Medicine
Mayo Medical School
Rochester MN, USA
Chapter 117 – Hepatic Encephalopathy—Diagnosis
    and Management

Orhun H Kantarci MD
Research Fellow in Neurology
Mayo Graduate School of Medicine
Rochester MN, USA
Chapter 95 – Behçet Disease: Diagnosis and
    Management

Steven Karceski MD
Assistant Professor, Neurology
Columbia Comprehensive Epilepsy Center
The Neurological Institute of New York
The New York Presbyterian Hospital
New York NY, USA
Chapter 28 – Principles in Epilepsy: Diagnosis and
    Pharmacotherapy

Randy Kardon MD PhD
Associate Professor
Michigan State University
Department of Neurology and Ophthalmology
East Lansing MI, USA
Chapter 164 – Disturbances of the Pupil

George Karpati MD FRCP(C) FRS(C) OC
Professor
Montréal Neurological Institute and Hospital
Montréal PQ, Canada
Chapter 2 – Molecular Therapies for the Nervous
    System and Muscle

Carlos S Kase MD
Professor, Neurology
Boston University School of Medicine
Boston MA, USA
Attending Neurologist
Director
Stroke Center
Boston Medical Center
Boston MA, USA
Chapter 47 – Treatment of Intracerebral Hemorrhage

Stefan Kastenbauer MD
Resident
Department of Neurology
Ludwig-Maximilians University
Munich, Germany
Chapter 78 – Infectious Intracranial Mass Lesions

Russell Katz MD
Director of the Division of Neuropharmacological
    Drug Products
Center for Drug Evaluation and Research
Food and Drug Administration
Rockville MD, USA
Chapter 3 – Clinical Trial Methodology,
    FDA Terminology and Procedures

Horacio Kaufmann MD
Associate Professor of Neurology
Director
Autonomic Disorders Research and Treatment Center
Mount Sinai School of Medicine
New York NY, USA
Chapter 113 – Syncope

James R Keane MD
Professor of Neurology
University of Southern California
Los Angeles CA, USA
Chapter 177 – Functional Diseases Affecting the
    Cranial Nerves

Praful Kelkar MBBS MD
Associate Professor
University of Iowa
University of Iowa Hospitals
Iowa City IA, USA
Chapter 195 – Brachial Plexus Neuropathy

John J Kelly MD
Professor and Chairman
Department of Neurology
The George Washington University Medical Center
Washington DC, USA
Chapter 127 – Neurologic Disorders in Benign and
    Malignant Plasma Cell Dyscrasias

Samia J Khoury MD
Associate Professor of Neurology
Director
Clinical Immunology Laboratory
Center for Neurologic Diseases
Harvard Medical School
Boston MA, USA
Chapter 149 – Pregnancy and Multiple Sclerosis:
    Therapeutic Aspects

Bernd C Kieseier MD
Assistant Professor
Department of Neurology
Heinrich-Heine-University
Düsseldorf, Germany
Chapter 96 – Autoimmunity in the Nervous System

Laurence J Kinsella MD
Associate Professor
Chief
Department of Neurology
St Louis University
Forest Park Hospital
St Louis MO, USA
Chapter 124 – Megaloblastic Anemias—Vitamin B_{12},
    Folate

John T Kissel MD
Professor of Neurology
Department of Neurology
The Ohio State University
Columbus OH, USA
Chapter 198 – Vasculitis of the Peripheral Nervous
    System

Caroline M Klein MD PhD
Fellow in Neurology
Mayo Graduate School of Medicine
Rochester MN, USA
Chapter 128 – Neurological Manifestations of
    Systemic Disease: Cryoglobulinemia
Chapter 188 – Peripheral Neuropathy Associated
    With Hypothyroidism and Acromegaly
Chapter 200 – Sarcoidosis and Peripheral Neuropathy

Christopher J Klein MD
Mayo Foundation Scholar
Mayo Clinic
Rochester MN, USA
Chapter 207 – Hereditary Sensory and Autonomic
    Neuropathies

Galit Kleiner-Fisman MD FRCP(C)
Resident
Department of Neurology
University of Toronto
Toronto ON, Canada
Chapter 233 – Surgical Treatment of Parkinson's
    Disease

Thomas Klockgether MD
Professor
Department of Neurology
University of Bonn
Bonn, Germany
Chapter 255 – Hereditary Ataxias and other
    Cerebellar Degenerations

Martin E Kochevar RPh MS BCNSP
Hospital Pharmacy Services
Mayo Clinic
Rochester MN, USA
Chapter 109 – Management of Nutrition

William C Koller MD PhD
Professor of Neurology
National Research Director
National Parkinson Foundation
University of Miami School of Medicine
Miami FL, USA
Chapter 1 – Basic Pharmaceutical Principles and the
    Blood–Brain Barrier
Chapter 243 – Essential Tremor

Edwin H Kolodny MD
Bernard A and Charlotte Marden Professor and
    Chairman
Department of Neurology
New York University School of Medicine
New York NY, USA
Chapter 140 – Lysosomal Storage Diseases

Amos D Korczyn MD MSc
Professor
Sieratzki Chair of Neurology
Sackler School of Medicine
Tel-Aviv University
Ramat-Aviv, Israel
Chapter 256 – Therapy of Human Prion Diseases

William E Krauss MD
Consultant
Department of Neurologic Surgery
Mayo Clinic
Assistant Professor of Neurosurgery
Mayo Medical School
Rochester MN, USA
Chapter 235 – Syringomyelia

Allan Krumholz MD
Professor
Director
University of Maryland Epilepsy Center
Department of Neurology
University of Maryland School of Medicine
Baltimore MA, USA
Chapter 36 – Legal and Regulatory Issues for People
    with Epilepsy

Mark J Kupersmith MD
Professor of Ophthalmology and Neurology
New York University School of Medicine
Director of Neuro-ophthalmology
Hyman-Newman Institute of Neurology and
    Neurosurgery of Beth Israel Medical Center and
    New York Eye and Ear Infirmary
New York City NY, USA
Chapter 169 – Cavernous Sinus Disorders

Jerome E Kurent MD MPH
Associate Professor of Medicine,
    Neurology and Psychiatry
Medical University of South Carolina
Department of Medicine
Division of General Internal Medicine/Geriatrics
Charleston SC, USA
Chapter 131 – Vasculitis Involving the Nervous
    System

Roger Kurlan MD
Professor
Department of Neurology
University of Rochester Medical Center
Rochester NY, USA
Chapter 248 – Tourette's Syndrome and Tic Disorders

Robert A Kyle MD
Consultant
Division of Hematology and Internal Medicine
Mayo Clinic
Professor of Medicine and of Laboratory Medicine
Mayo Medical School
Rochester MN, USA
Chapter 201 – Neuropathy Associated with the
    Monoclonal Gammopathies
Chapter 202 – Amyloidosis

David Lacomis MD
Assistant Professor
Departments of Neurology and Pathology
University of Pittsburgh School of Medicine
Pittsburgh PA, USA
Chapter 105 – Management of Generalized Weakness
    in Medical and Surgical Intensive Care Units

Sumeer Lal MD FRCSC
Fellow
Department of Neurosurgery
MD Anderson Cancer Center
Houston TX, USA
Chapter 66 – Surgically Curable Brain Tumors of
    Adults

Anthony E Lang MD FRCPC
Professor of Neurology
Jack Clark Chair for Parkinson's Disease Research
Director
Movements Disorders Clinic
Toronto West Hospital
Toronto ON, Canada
Chapter 233 – Surgical Treatment of Parkinson's
    Disease
Chapter 250 – Painful Legs and Moving Toes

Robert Laureno MD
Associate Professor
Department of Neurology
Washington Hospital Center
Washington DC, USA
Chapter 121 – Disorders of Water and Sodium
    Balance

Paul Leber MD
Director
Neuro-Pharm Group LLC
Potomac MD, USA
Chapter 3 – Clinical Trial Methodology, FDA
    Terminology and Procedures

Andrew G Lee MD
Associate Professor of Ophthalmology,
    Neurology and Neurosurgery
The University of Iowa Hospitals and Clinics
Iowa City IA, USA
Chapter 163 – Chiasm and Retrochiasmal Disorders

Jay C Lee MD FRCS(C)
Clinical Lecturer
Department of Surgery
Division of Urology
Director
Sexual Dysfunction Clinic
University of Calgary
Calgary AB, Canada
Chapter 215 – Treatment of Sexual Dysfunction and
    Cystopathy in Peripheral Nerve Disorders

David S Lefkowitz MD
Associate Professor
Department of Neurology
Wake Forest University School of Medicine
Wake Forest University Baptist Medical Center
Winston-Salem NC, USA
Chapter 53 – Venous Disorders

Daniel R Lefton MD
Assistant Director of Neuroradiology
Beth Israel Medical Center
Assistant Professor of Radiology
Albert Einstein School of Medicine
New York NY, USA
Chapter 169 – Cavernous Sinus Disorders

Clarence W Legerton III MD
Associate Professor of Medicine
Medical University of South Carolina
Charleston SC, USA
Chapter 131 – Vasculitis Involving the Nervous
    System

Robert M Levin MD
Associate Professor of Medicine
Boston University School of Medicine
Boston MA, USA
Chapter 139 – Disorders of Bone and Mineral
    Metabolism

Donald W Lewis MD
Professor of Pediatrics and Neurology
Children's Hospital of the King's Daughter
Eastern Virginia Medical School
Norfolk VA, USA
Chapter 16 – Headache "Syndromes" in Children and
    Adolescents

Steven L Lewis MD
Associate Professor
Department of Neurological Sciences
Rush-Presbyterian-St Luke's Medical Center
Chicago IL, USA
Chapter 146 – Pesticides

Peter LeWitt MD
Professor
Departments of Neurology, Psychiatry and
    Behavioral Neuroscience
Wayne State University School of Medicine and the
    Clinical Neuroscience Center
Southfield MI, USA
Chapter 253 – Wilson's Disease

David S Liebeskind MD
Assistant Professor
Department of Neurology
Comprehensive Stroke Center
University of Pennsylvania
Pennsylvania PA, USA
Chapter 51 – Cervicocephalic Arterial Dissections

Michael J Link MD
Consultant
Department of Neurologic Surgery
Mayo Clinic
Assistant Professor of Neurosurgery
Mayo Medical School
Rochester MN, USA
Chapter 67 – Diagnosis and Treatment of Pituitary
    Tumors

Eric Logigian MD
Professor
Department of Neurology
University of Rochester
Rochester NY, USA
Chapter 128 – Neurological Manifestations of
    Systemic Disease: Cryoglobulinemia

Betsy B Love MD
Clinical Associate Professor
Department of Neurology
Indiana University School of Medicine
Indianapolis IN, USA
Chapter 54 – Spinal Cord Vascular Syndromes

Phillip A Low MD
Consultant
Department of Neurology
Mayo Clinic
Professor of Neurology
Mayo Medical School
Rochester MN, USA
Chapter 217 – Neurogenic Orthostatic Hypotension
Chapter 218 – Orthostatic Intolerance

Christy Ludlow MSc PhD
Medical Neurology Branch
NINDS
NIH
Bethesda MD, USA
Chapter 236 – Focal Dystonias: Blepharospasm,
    Cervical Dystonia, Spasmodic Dysphonia, Writer's
    Cramp

Linda M Luxon BSc MB BS FRCP
Professor
Department of Neuro-otology
The National Hospital for Neurology and
    Neurosurgery
London, UK
ICH Unit of Audiological Medicine
The Great Ormond Street Hospital for Children
London, UK
Chapter 174 – Tinnitus and Deafness

Lynn M Maher PhD
Associate Professor
Department of Physical Medicine and Rehabilitation
Baylor College of Medicine
Houston TX, USA
Chapter 259 – Aphasia

Karim Makhlouf MD
Research Fellow
Center for Neurologic Diseases
Harvard Medical School
Boston MA, USA
Chapter 149 – Pregnancy and Multiple Sclerosis:
    Therapeutic Aspects

Atul Malhotra MD FRCPC
Instructor in Medicine and Attending Physician
Pulmonary and Critical Care and Sleep Medicine
    Divisions
Brigham and Women's Hospital and Massachusetts
    General Hospital and Harvard Medical School
Boston MA, USA
Chapter 119 – Disorders of Excessive Sleepiness

Timothy Malisch MD
Associate Professor
Chief
Section of Interventional Neuroradiology
University of Illinois
Chicago IL, USA
Chapter 49 – Cerebral Aneurysms and Vascular
    Malformations

Edward M Manno MD
Senior Associate Consultant
Department of Neurology
Mayo Clinic
Assistant Professor of Neurology
Mayo Medical School
Rochester MN, USA
Chapter 108 – Management of Head Trauma and
    Spinal Cord Injury in Adults

Adriana R Marques MD
Laboratory of Clinical Investigation
National Institute of Allergy and Infectious Diseases
    (NIAID)
National Institute of Health (NIH)
Bethseda MD, USA
Chapter 82 – Lyme Disease

Roland Martin MD
Neuroimmunology Branch
National Institute of Neurological Disorders and
    Stroke (NINDS)
NIH
Bethseda MD, USA
Chapter 82 – Lyme Disease

Janice M Massey MD
Professor
Department of Medicine
Division of Neurology
Duke University Medical Center
Durham NC, USA
Chapter 7 – Domestic Violence in Neurological
    Practice

FL Mastaglia MD
Professor
Departments of Neurology and Clinical Immunology
Sir Charles Gairdner Hospital
Centre for Neuromuscular and Neurological
    Disorders
Australian Neuromuscular Research Institute
University of Western Australia
Perth, Australia
Chapter 223 – Inflammatory Myopathies

James A Mastrianni MD PhD
Assistant Professor of Neurology
Co-Director
Center for Comprehensive Care and Research on
    Memory Disorders
The University of Chicago
Department of Neurology
Chicago IL, USA
Chapter 92 – Prion Diseases: Transmissible
    Spongiform Encephalopathies

David M Masur PhD
Director
Neuropsychology
Montefiore Medical Center
Clinical Professor of Neurology
Albert Einstein College of Medicine
New York NY, USA
Chapter 13 – Post-Traumatic Headache

Ninan T Mathew MD FRCP(C)
Clinical Professor
Department of Neurology
University of Texas Medical School
Galveston TX
Director
Houston Headache Clinic
Houston TX, USA
Chapter 12 – Chronic Daily Headache

Stephan A Mayer MD
Assistant Professor of Neurology (in Neurological
    Surgery)
Columbia University College of Physicians and
    Surgeons
Director
Neurological Intensive Care Unit
Columbia-Presbyterian Center
New York Presbyterian Hospital
New York NY, USA
Chapter 101 – Management of Increased Intracranial
    Pressure

Kathleen M McEvoy MD
Consultant
Department of Neurology
Mayo Clinic
Assistant Professor of Medicine
Mayo Medical School
Rochester MN, USA
Chapter 228 – Stiff-Man Syndrome

M Molly McMahon MD
Consultant
Division of Endocrinology, Diabetes, Metabolism,
    Nutrition, and Internal Medicine
Mayo Clinic
Associate Professor of Medicine
Mayo Medical School
Rochester MN, USA
Chapter 109 – Management of Nutrition

Michel Melanson MD
Assistant Professor
Division of Neurology
Queens University
Kingston General Hospital
Kingston ON, Canada
Chapter 208 – Hereditary Motor Neuropathies

Kozhikade V Narayanan Menon MD
Senior Associate Consultant
Division of Gastroenterology and Hepatology and
    Internal Medicine
Mayo Clinic
Instructor in Medicine
Mayo Medical School
Rochester MN, USA
Chapter 117 – Hepatic Encephalopathy—Diagnosis
    and Management

Harold Merskey DM FRCP
Professor Emeritus
Department of Psychiatry
University of Western Ontario
London ON, Canada
Chapter 25 – Pain Disorder

Jan Meuleman PhD
Senior Fellow
Neurogenetics Laboratory
Division of Genetics and Development
University of Washington School of Medicine
Seattle WA, USA
Chapter 209 – Hereditary Neuropathy With Liability
    to Pressure Palsy

Alireza Minagar MD
Assistant Professor of Neurology
Department of Neurology
Louisiana State University
Shreveport LA, USA
Chapter 1 – Basic Pharmaceutical Principles and the
    Blood–Brain Barrier
Chapter 243 – Essential Tremor

Maria J Molnar MD PhD
Senior Researcher
Neurology and Psychiatry
Montréal Neurological Institute and Hospital
Montréal PQ, Canada
Chapter 2 – Molecular Therapies for the Nervous
    System and Muscle

Patricia M Moore MD
Associate Professor
Department of Neurology
University of Pittsburgh
Pittsburgh PA, USA
Chapter 57 – Systemic and Central Nervous System
    Vasculitides

Thomas J Moore MD
Assistant Provost for Clinical Research
Director
Office of Clinical Research
Boston University Medical Center
Boston MA, USA
Chapter 116 – Arterial Hypertension and
    Hypertensive Encephalopathy

Martha J Morrell MD
Professor
Department of Neurology
The Neurological Institute
Columbia University
New York NY, USA
Chapter 28 – Principles in Epilepsy: Diagnosis and
    Pharmacotherapy
Chapter 33 – Seizures and Epilepsy in Women

Mark J Morrow MD
Dizziness and Balance Disorders Clinic
Hattiesburg Clinic
Hattiesburg MS, USA
Chapter 171 – Disorders of the Facial Nerve

Mark Moster MD
Professor
Jefferson Medical College
Chairman
Department of Neurosensory Sciences
Albert Einstein Medical Center
Philadelphia PA, USA
Chapter 168 – Ocular Myasthenia Gravis

Dwight E Moulin MD
Associate Professor
Department of Clinical Neurological Sciences and
    Oncology
University of Western Ontario
Director
Pain and Symptom Management
Department of Oncology
London Regional Cancer Center
London ON, Canada
Chapter 22 – Peripheral (Neuropathic) Pain Disorders

Thomas P Moyer PhD
Consultant
Division of Clinical Biochemistry and Immunology
Mayo Clinic
Professor of Laboratory Medicine
Mayo Medical School
Rochester MN, USA
Chapter 212 – Neurotoxic Metals

Gilbert H Mudge MD
Associate Professor
Cardiology
Director of Cardiac Transplantation
Brigham and Women's Hospital
Boston MA, USA
Chapter 114 – Cardiomyopathy

Todd Mulderink BS
Feinberg Fellow
Feinberg Neuroscience Institute
Northwestern University Medical School
Chicago IL, USA
Chapter 49 – Cerebral Aneurysms and Vascular
    Malformations

Stephen E Nadeau MD
Professor of Neurology
University of Florida College of Medicine
Geriatric Research
Education and Clinical Center
Brain Rehabilitation Outcomes Research Center
Malcolm Randall DVA Medical Center
Gainesville FL, USA
Chapter 265 – Intentional Disorders

Osvaldo JM Nascimento MD PhD
Professor of Neurology
Head
Peripheral Neuropathy Section
Department of Neurology
Fluminense Federal University
Rio de Janeiro, Brazil
Chapter 184 – Peripheral Neuropathies in Chagas
    Disease

Anette V Nieves MD
Assistant Professor, Neurology
Morton and Gloria Shulman Movement Disorders
    Centre
Toronto Western Hospital
Toronto ON, Canada
Chapter 250 – Painful Legs and Moving Toes

Puiu Nisipeanu MD PhD
Department of Neurology
Hillel Yaffe Hospital
Hadera, Israel
Chapter 256 – Therapy of Human Prion Diseases

Kathryn N North MD
Associate Professor, Neurology
Neurogenetics Research Unit
Royal Alexandra Hospital for Children
Parramatta NSW, Australia
Chapter 221 – Congenital Myopathies

John H Noseworthy MD FRCPC
Chair
Department of Neurology
Mayo Clinic
Professor of Neurology
Mayo Medical School
Rochester MN, USA
Chapter 97 – Multiple Sclerosis and Related
    Conditions

Cynthia Ochipa PhD
Associate Professor
Speech Pathology Section Chief
James A. Haley Veterans' Hospital
Tampa FL, USA
Chapter 264 – Limb Apraxia

Margaret G O'Connor PhD
Assistant Professor of Neurology
Harvard Medical School
Director of Neuropsychology
Division of Behavioral Neurology
Beth Israel Deaconess Medical Center
Boston MA, USA
Memory Disorders Research Center
VA Boston Healthcare System
Boston MA, USA
Chapter 266 – Evaluation and Management of
    Amnesic Disorders

Gareth J Parry MB ChB FRACP
Professor
Department of Neurology
University of Minnesota
Minneapolis MN, USA
Chapter 195 – Brachial Plexus Neuropathy

Gregory M Pastores MD
Assistant Professor of Neurology and Pediatrics
New York University School of Medicine
New York NY, USA
Chapter 140 – Lysosomal Storage Diseases

Roy A Patchell MD
Chief of Neuro-oncology
Associate Professor of Neurosurgery and Neurology
University of Kentucky Medical Center
Lexington KY, USA
Chapter 71 – Brain Metastases

James R Perry MD DCE FRCPC
Assistant Professor
Department of Medicine
Division of Neurology
University of Toronto
Neuro-oncologist
Director
University of Toronto Neurology Residency Program
Sunnybrook and Women's College Health Sciences
    Centre
Toronto ON, Canada
Chapter 176 – Multiple Cranial Nerve Palsies

Alan Pestronk MD
Professor of Neurology and Pathology
Washington University in St Louis
Department of Neurology
St Louis MO, USA
Chapter 204 – Paraneoplastic Neuropathy Syndromes:
    Principles and Treatment

Ronald C Petersen MD PhD
Consultant
Department of Neurology
Mayo Clinic
Cora Kanow Professor of Alzheimer's Disease
    Research
Professor of Neurology
Mayo Medical School
Rochester MN, USA
Chapter 268 – Alzheimer Disease and Mild Cognitive
    Impairment

Hans-Walter Pfister MD
Professor
Department of Neurology
Klinikum Grossharden
Ludwig-Maximilians-University of Munich
Munich, Germany
Chapter 77 – Bacterial Meningitis

Thanh G Phan MD
Fellow in Neurology
Mayo Graduate School of Medicine
Rochester MN, USA
Chapter 41 – Asymptomatic Carotid Artery Stenosis

BA Phillips PhD
Senior Lecturer
Departments of Neurology and Clinical Immunology
Sir Charles Gairdner Hospital
Centre for Neuromuscular and Neurological
    Disorders
Australian Neuromuscular Research Institute
University of Western Australia
Perth, Australia
Chapter 223 – Inflammatory Myopathies

John P Phillips MD
Associate Professor
Departments of Pediatrics and Neurology
University of New Mexico School of Medicine
Director
Senior Lecturer
Pediatric Rehabilitation
Carrie Tingley Hospital
University of New Mexico Health Sciences Center
Albuquerque NM, USA
Chapter 159 – Pediatric Brain and Spinal Cord Injury

Peter C Phillips MD
Professor of Neurology and Oncology
Director of Neuro-Oncology Programs
Children's Hospital of Philadelphia
Philadelphia PA, USA
Chapter 69 – Malignant Brain Tumors of Childhood

Mark A Pichelmann MD
Resident in Neurosurgery
Mayo Graduate School of Medicine
Rochester MN, USA
Chapter 108 – Management of Head Trauma and
    Spinal Cord Injury in Adults

Monica L Piecyk MD
Instructor in Medicine
Division of Rheumatology and Immunology
Brigham and Women's Hospital
Boston MA, USA
Chapter 132 – Neurological Manifestations of
    Rheumatoid Arthritis

Samuel J Pleasure MD PhD
Professor
Neurodevelopmental Disorders Laboratory
Department of Neurology
UCSF
San Francisco CA, USA
Chapter 87 – Rabies

David J Plevak MD
Consultant
Critical Care Service
Mayo Clinic
Professor of Anesthesiology
Mayo Medical School
Rochester MN, USA
Chapter 102 – Management of Sedation and Pain in
    the Intensive Care Unit

Bruce E Pollock MD
Consultant
Department of Neurologic Surgery
Mayo Clinic
Assistant Professor of Neurosurgery
Mayo Medical School
Rochester MN, USA
Chapter 67 – Diagnosis and Treatment of Pituitary
    Tumors

David C Preston MD
Associate Professor of Neurology
Case Western Reserve University
Director
Neuromuscular Service
University Hospitals of Cleveland
Cleveland OH, USA
Chapter 148 – Therapy of Neurological Disorders:
    Neuropathies and Neuromuscular Junction
    Disorders of Pregnancy

Donald Price PhD
Professor
Department of Oral and Maxillofacial Surgery
University of Florida College of Dentistry
Gainesville FL, USA
Chapter 4 – Placebos

Michael B Pritz MD PhD
Professor
Section of Neurological Surgery
Indiana University School of Medicine
Indianapolis IN, USA
Chapter 48 – Subarachnoid Hemorrhage Due to
    Cerebral Aneurysms

Amy Pruitt MD
Hospital of the University of Pennsylvania
Associate Professor of Neurology
University of Pennsylvania School of Medicine
Philadelphia PA, USA
Chapter 112 – Endocarditis (Infective and Non-
    Infective)

Ewa Raglan MD DLO FRCS
Consultant Audiological Physician
Department of Audiological Medicine
The Great Ormond Street Hospital for Children
London, UK
Department of Audiology
St George's Hospital
London, UK
Chapter 174 – Tinnitus and Deafness

Didier Raoult MD
Professor
Director
Clinical Microbiology Department
Université de la Méditerranée
Faculté de Médecine
Unité des Rickettsies
Marseille, France
Chapter 84 – Rickettsial Infections

Steven Z Rapcsak MD
Associate Professor
Department of Neurology
University of Arizona
Neurology Section
VA Medical Center
Tucson AZ, USA
Chapter 260 – Treatment of Alexia and Agraphia

Marcia H Ratner BA
Project Manager
Environmental and Occupational Neurology Program
Research Associate
Department of Neurology
Boston MA, USA
Adjunct Instructor in Biochemistry
Program in Biomedical Laboratory and Clinical
  Sciences
Department of Biochemistry
Boston University School of Medicine
Boston MA, USA
Chapter 145 – Treatment of the Neurotoxic Effects of
  Gases: Carbon Monoxide, Hydrogen Sulfide and
  the Nitrogen Oxides

Anastasia M Raymer PhD
Associate Professor
Department of Early Childhood
Speech-Language Pathology and Special Education
Old Dominion University
Norfolk VA, USA
Chapter 259 – Aphasia

Daniel Rayson MD FRCP(C)
Assistant Professor
Division of Medical Oncology
Department of Medicine
Dalhousie University
Halifax NS, Canada
Chapter 75 – Metabolic and Nutritional
  Complications Associated with Cancer

Kevin I Reid DMD
Chair
Department of Dental Specialties
Mayo Clinic
Assistant Professor of Dentistry
Mayo Medical School
Rochester MN, USA
Chapter 17 – Diagnosis and Treatment of Common
  Orofacial Pain Conditions

Deborah L Renaud MD FRCP(C)
Clinical and Research Fellow
Division of Clinical and Metabolic Genetics
Hospital for Sick Children
Toronto ON, Canada
Chapter 224 – Metabolic Myopathies

Robert A Rizza MD
Consultant
Division of Endocrinology
Diabetes, Metabolism, Nutrition, and Internal
  Medicine
Mayo Clinic
Professor of Medicine
Mayo Medical School
Rochester MN, USA
Chapter 186 – Diabetic Polyneuropathy

Loran A Rolak MD
Department of Neurosciences
The Marshfield Clinic
Marshfield WI, USA
Associate Professor of Clinical Neurology
University of Wisconsin
Madison WI, USA
Adjunct Associate Professor of Neurology
Baylor College of Medicine
Houston TX, USA
Chapter 134 – Neurological Complications of
  Progressive Systemic Sclerosis

Gustavo C Román MD FACP FRSM (Lond)
Professor of Medicine/Neurology
University of Texas Health Science Center
San Antonio TX, USA
Chapter 86 – Neurological Complications of HTLV-I
  Infection

Michael Ronthal MBBCh FRCP FRCPE
Associate Professor of Neurology
Harvard Medical School
Beth Israel Deaconess Medical Center
Boston MA, USA
Chapter 133 – Cervical Spondylosis, Ankylosing
  Spondylitis, and Lumbar Disk Disease

Karen L Roos MD
John and Nancy Nelsen Professor of Neurology
Indiana University School of Medicine
Indianapolis IN, USA
Chapter 77 – Bacterial Meningitis
Chapter 79 – Viral Meningitis and Encephalitis
Chapter 81 – Neurosyphilis
Chapter 83 – Tetanus
Chapter 91 – Neurology of Arachnida (Spiders, Ticks, Scorpions) and Hymenoptera (Ants, Bees, Wasps) Envenomations
Chapter 94 – Infection in Solid Organ and Bone Marrow Transplant Recipients

Peter B Rosenberger MD
Assistant Professor of Neurology
Harvard Medical School
Neurologist and Associate Pediatrician and Director
Learning Disorders Unit
Massachusetts General Hospital
Boston MA, USA
Chapter 156 – Disorders of Learning and Behavior in Children

Leslie J Gonzalez Rothi PhD
Professor of Neurology
Program Director
Brain Rehabilitation Research Center
VA Medical Center
Gainesville FL, USA
Chapter 258 – Treatment of Disorders of Cognition: An Introduction

A James Rowan MD
Professor
Department of Neurology
Mount Sinai Hospital
New York NY, USA
Chapter 34 – Epilepsy in the Elderly

Robert S Rust MA MD
Thomas E. Worrall Jr. Professor of Epileptology and Neurology and Professor of Pediatrics
The University of Virginia School of Medicine
Charlottesville VA, USA
Chapter 158 – Neurocutaneous Disorders

Thomas D Sabin MD
Interim Chief of Neurology
New England Medical Center
Professor and Vice Chair of Neurology
Tufts University School of Medicine
New England Medical Center
Boston MA, USA
Chapter 183 – The Neuropathies of Leprosy

Paola Santalucia MD
Fellow
Brown University School of Medicine
Department of Clinical Neurosciences
Providence RI, USA
Chapter 52 – Fibromuscular Dysplasia

Jeffrey L Saver MD
Associate Professor
Neurology Director
UCLA Stroke Center
University of California
Los Angeles CA, USA
Chapter 51 – Cervicocephalic Arterial Dissections

Steven C Schachter MD
Professor of Neurology
Harvard Medical School
Medical Director
Office of Clinical Investigations
Beth Israel Deaconess Medical Center
Boston MA, USA
Chapter 35 – Imitators of Epilepsy

Jeremy D Schmahmann MD
Associate Professor of Neurology
Harvard Medical School
Director
Ataxia Unit
Cognitive/Behavioral Neurology Unit
Geriatric Neurobehavior Clinic
Department of Neurology
Massachusetts General Hospital
Boston MA, USA
Chapter 141 – Whipple Disease of the Nervous System

Erich Schmutzhard MD DTM&H (Liv.)
Professor
University-Hospital Innsbruck
Department of Neurology
Innsbruck, Austria
Chapter 88 – Fungal Infections
Chapter 89 – Protozoal Infections

Peter H Schur MD
Professor of Medicine
Brigham and Women's Hospital
Division of Rheumatology
Boston MA, USA
Chapter 132 – Neurological Manifestations of Rheumatoid Arthritis

Michael Schwarzschild MD PhD
Assistant Professor of Neurology
Harvard Medical School
Molecular Neurobiology Laboratory
Center for Aging
Genetics and Neurodegeneration
Massachusetts General Hospital
Boston MA, USA
Chapter 150 – Movement Disorders During Pregnancy

Thomas F Scott MD
Associate Professor of Neurology
Medical College of Pennsylvania and Hanemann
    University
Pittsburgh PA, USA
Chapter 135 – Treatment of Neurosarcoidosis

Julian L Seifter MD
Associate Professor of Nephrology
Renal Division
Brigham and Women's Hospital
Boston MA, USA
Chapter 122 – Acid–Base Disturbances and the
    Central Nervous System

Nutan Sharma MD PhD
Clinical and Research Fellow
Department of Neurology
Massachusetts General Hospital
Boston MA, USA
Chapter 150 – Movement Disorders During
    Pregnancy

James A Sharpe MD FRCPC
Professor of Neurology and Head
Division of Neurology
University of Toronto
Toronto ON, Canada
Chapter 166 – Nystagmus and Saccadic Oscillations
Chapter 167 – Gaze Disorders

Bennett A Shaywitz MD
Professor of Pediatrics and Neurology
Co-Director
NICHD-Yale Center for the Study of Learning and
    Attention
Department of Pediatrics
Yale University School of Medicine
New Haven CT, USA
Chapter 263 – Management of Attention-Deficit/
    Hyperactivity Disorder and Dyslexia (Specific
    Reading Disability)

Sally E Shaywitz MD
Professor of Pediatrics
Co-Director
NICHD-Yale Center for the Study of Learning and
    Attention
Department of Pediatrics
Yale University School of Medicine
New Haven CT, USA
Chapter 263 – Management of Attention-Deficit/
    Hyperactivity Disorder and Dyslexia (Specific
    Reading Disability)

Michael I Shevell MD CM FRCP
Associate Professor-Departments of
    Neurology/Neurosurgery and Pediatrics
Associate Member–Department of Human Genetics
McGill University
Division of Pediatric Neurology–Montréal Children's
    Hospital
Montréal PQ, Canada
Chapter 157 – Chromosomal Disorders, Inborn Errors
    of Metabolism and Degenerative Diseases

Cathy A Sila MD
Associate Medical Director
Cerebrovascular Center
Section of Stroke and Neurologic Intensive Care
Department of Neurology
Cleveland Clinic
Cleveland OH, USA
Chapter 44 – Cardioembolic Stroke
Chapter 110 – Neurological Complications of Cardiac
    Procedures: Catheterization, Interventional
    Procedures and Surgery

Stephen D Silberstein MD FACP
Director
Jefferson Headache Center
Professor of Neurology
Thomas Jefferson University Hospital
Philadelphia PA, USA
Chapter 11 – Tension-type Headache

David Simpson MD
Professor of Neurology
Mount Sinai School of Medicine
Director
Neuro-AIDS Research Program
Director
Clinical Neurophysiology Laboratories
Mount Sinai Medical Center
New York NY, USA
Chapter 182 – Peripheral Neuropathy and HIV

Aksel Siva MD
Professor
Department of Neurology
Istanbul University
Cerrahpasa Medical School
Istanbul, Turkey
Chapter 95 – Behçet Disease: Diagnosis and
    Management

Frank M Skidmore MD
Resident
Department of Neurology
Indiana University School of Medicine
Indianapolis IN, USA
Chapter 62 – Stroke in Pregnancy

PAE Sillevis Smitt MD PhD
Professor
Head, Neurology Department
Erasmus University Medical Center
Rotterdam, the Netherlands
Chapter 74 – Treatment of Paraneoplastic
    Neurological Syndromes
Chapter 76 – Neurological Complications of
    Antineoplastic Treatment

Elson L So MD
Consultant
Division of Epilepsy
Mayo Clinic
Professor of Neurology
Mayo Medical School
Rochester MN, USA
Chapter 26 – Classification and Epidemiology of
    Seizure Disorders: Therapeutic Implications and
    Importance

Seymour Solomon MD
Director
Headache Unit
Montefiore Medical Center
Professor of Neurology
Albert Einstein College of Medicine
New York NY, USA
Chapter 13 – Post-Traumatic Headache

Jayashree Srinivasan MD
Assistant Professor of Neurological Surgery
Department of Neurological Surgery
Northwestern University Medical School
Chicago IL, USA
Chapter 49 – Cerebral Aneurysms and Vascular
    Malformations

Christian L Stallworth BS
Research Assistant
University of Texas Health Science Center at San
    Antonio
San Antonio TX, USA
Chapter 56 – Antiphospholipid Antibodies and
    Variants

Andreas Stein MD
Professor
Université de la Méditerranée
Faculté de Médecine
Unité des Rickettsies
Marseille, France
Chapter 84 – Rickettsial Infections

Barney Stern MD
Professor of Neurology
Department of Neurology
Emory University
Atlanta GA, USA
Chapter 135 – Treatment of Neurosarcoidosis

Jonathan T Stewart MD
Professor in Psychiatry
University of South Florida College of Medicine
Chief
Geropsychiatry Section
Bay Pines
VA Medical Center
Tampa FL, USA
Chapter 270 – Behavioral and Emotional
    Complications of Neurological Disorders

Donald T Stuss PhD C Psych ABPP-CN, O Ont
Vice-President, Research
Baycrest Centre for Geriatric Care
Director
The Rotman Research Institute
Baycrest Centre
Reva James Leeds Chair in Neuroscience and
    Research Leadership
Baycrest Centre and University of Toronto
Professor of Medicine (Neurology Rehabilitation
    Science) and Psychology
University of Toronto
Toronto ON, Canada
Chapter 267 – Executive Disorders

Guillermo A Suarez MD
Consultant
Department of Neurology
Mayo Clinic
Assistant Professor of Neurology
Mayo Medical School
Rochester MN, USA
Chapter 128 – Neurological Manifestations of
    Systemic Disease: Cryoglobulinemia
Chapter 191 – Peripheral Neuropathy Associated with
    Alcoholism, Malnutrition, and Vitamin
    Deficiencies

Ann Sweeney MD
Fellow
Department of Medicine
Section of Endocrinology,
    Nutrition and Diabetes
Boston University School of Medicine
Boston MA, USA
Chapter 139 – Disorders of Bone and Mineral
    Metabolism

Thomas R Swift MD
Professor Emeritus of Neurology
Medical College of Georgia
Augusta GA, USA
Chapter 183 – The Neuropathies of Leprosy

Michele Tagliati MD
Assistant Professor of Neurology
Albert Einstein College of Medicine
Department of Neurology
Beth Israel Medical Center
New York NY, USA
Chapter 237 – Generalized Torsion Dystonia
Chapter 238 – Dopa-Responsive Dystonia

William T Talman MD
Professor of Neurology and Neuroscience
University of Iowa
Chief VAMC Neurology Service
Veterans Affairs Medical Center
Iowa City IA, USA
Chapter 111 – Cardiac Arrhythmias and Sudden
    Death

RR Tasker MD MA FRCS(C)
Professor Emeritus
Division of Neurosurgery
Western Division
The Toronto Hospital
Toronto ON, Canada
Chapter 21 – The Treatment of Central Pain

Bruce V Taylor MB BS MD FRACP
Clinical Senior Lecturer
University of Tasmania
Head
Department of Neurology
Royal Hobart Hospital
Hobart, Tasmania, Australia
Chapter 199 – The Treatment of Multifocal Motor
    Neuropathy with Conduction Block (MMN-CB)

Jeanne S Teitelbaum MD FRCP(C)
Associate Professor
Neurology and Critical Care
University of Montreal and McGill University of
    Quebec, Canada
Chapter 100 – Management of Blood Pressure in
    Acute Neurological Illnesses

Madhavi Thomas MD
Fellow in Neurology
Parkinson's Disease Center and Movement Disorders
    Clinic
Baylor College of Medicine
Houston TX, USA
Chapter 232 – Parkinsonism Plus Disorders
Chapter 240 – Neuroacanthocytosis

Dominic Thyagarajan MD FRACP
Associate Professor
Head of Neurology
Flinders Medical Center
South Australia
Chapter 151 – Mitochondrial Disease

Ann H Tilton MD
Associate Professor of Neurology and Pediatrics
Chief, Section of Child Neurology
Lousiana State University Health Science Center
New Orleans LA, USA
Chapter 155 – Mental Retardation and Cerebral Palsy

David M Treiman MD
Professor of Neurology
University of Medicine and Dentistry of New Jersey
Robert Wood Johnson Memorial School
New Brunswick NJ, USA
Chapter 31 – Status Epilepticus

Martha Trieschmann MD
Fellow
Department of Clinical Neurosciences
Brown University School of Medicine
Providence RI, USA
Chapter 39 – Anticoagulant Therapy and Antiplatelet
    Drugs

Jonathan D Trobe MD
Professor
Kellogg Eye Center
Departments of Ophthalmology and Neurology
University of Michigan
Ann Arbor MI, USA
Chapter 165 – Ocular Motor Nerve Palsies

Shoji Tsuji MD PhD
Professor
Department of Neurology
University of Tokyo
7-3-1 Hongo
Bunkyo-Ku
Tokyo 113-8655, Japan
Chapter 246 – Dentatorubral-pallidoluysian Atrophy
    (DRPLA)

Ronald J Tusa MD PhD
Research Professor
Dizziness and Balance Center
Yerkes Research Institute and Department of
    Neurology
Emory University
Atlanta GA, USA
Chapter 172 – Vertigo, Vestibular Nerve, and Central
    Vestibular Disorders

Joon H Uhm MD FRCP(C)
Consultant
Division of Neuro-Oncology
Mayo Clinic
Assistant Professor of Neurology
Mayo Medical School
Rochester MN, USA
Chapter 64 – Chemotherapy and Antineoplastic
    Agents

Taufik A Valiante MD PhD
Resident in Neurosurgery
Division of Neurosurgery
University of Toronto
Toronto Western Hospital
University Health Network
Toronto, Ontario, Canada
Chapter 72 – Primary Tumors of the Spinal Cord,
    Root, Plexus, and Nerve Sheath

Charles J Vecht MD PhD
Neuro-oncologist
Department of Neurology
Medical Center
The Hague, POB 432 the Netherlands
Chapter 74 – Treatment of Paraneoplastic
    Neurological Syndromes
Chapter 76 – Neurological Complications of
    Antineoplastic Treatment

Mieke Verfaellie PhD
Associate Professor of Psychiatry
Boston University School of Medicine
Director – Boston University Memory Disorders
    Research Center
VA Boston Healthcare System
Boston MA, USA
Chapter 266 – Evaluation and Management of
    Amnesic Disorders

Barbara G Vickrey MD MPH
Professor
Department of Neurology
University of California Los Angeles
Los Angeles CA, USA
Chapter 5 – Evidence-Based Medicine

Michael Wall MD
Professor of Neurology and Ophthalmology
University of Iowa College of Medicine
Iowa City IA, USA
Chapter 162 – Papilledema and Idiopathic Intracranial
    Hypertension (Pseudotumor Cerebri)

Christopher J Watling MD FRCPC
Assistant Professor
Department of Clinical Neurological Sciences
University of Western Ontario
London ON, Canada
Chapter 23 – Cancer Pain

C Peter N Watson MD FRCP(C)
Assistant Professor
Department of Medicine
University of Toronto
Toronto ON, Canada
Chapter 21 – The Treatment of Central Pain
Chapter 170 – Trigeminal Neuropathy and Neuralgia

Denise J Wedel MD
Consultant
Division of Multispecialty Anesthesia
Mayo Clinic
Professor of Anesthesiology
Mayo Medical School
Rochester MN, USA
Chapter 227 – Malignant Hyperthermia

Theodore H Wein MD FRCPC
Assistant Professor of Neurology and Neurosurgery
McGill University
Department of Neurology
St Mary's Hospital Center
Montréal PQ, Canada
Chapter 60 – Moyamoya Disease

Myron H Weinberger MD
Professor of Medicine
Director
Hypertension Research Center
Indiana University School of Medicine
Indianapolis IN, USA
Chapter 58 – Hypertensive Encephalopathy

David P White MD
Associate Professor
Divisions of Sleep Medicine and Pulmonary and
    Critical Care Medicine
Department of Medicine
Brigham and Women's Hospital and Harvard
    Medical School
Boston MA, USA
Chapter 119 – Disorders of Excessive Sleepiness

David O Wiebers MD
Consultant
Department of Neurology and of Health Sciences
    Research
Mayo Clinic
Professor of Neurology
Mayo Medical School
Rochester MN, USA
Chapter 41 – Asymptomatic Carotid Artery Stenosis
Chapter 50 – Unruptured Intracranial Aneurysms

Eelco FM Wijdicks MD
Consultant
Department of Neurology
Mayo Clinic
Professor of Neurology
Mayo Medical School
Rochester MN, USA
Chapter 98 – Therapy for Critically Ill Neurological
    Patients

Russell A Wilke MD PhD
Fellow in Preventive and Occupational Medicine
Mayo Clinic
Rochester MN, USA
Chapter 212 – Neurotoxic Metals

Daniel Williams MD
Clinical Professor of Psychiatry
Columbia Presbyterian
New York NY, USA
Chapter 254 – Psychogenic Movement Disorders

Linda S Williams MD
Assistant Professor
Department of Neurology
Indiana University School of Medicine
Indianapolis IN, USA
Chapter 62 – Stroke in Pregnancy

Hugh J Willison MB BS PhD FRCP
Professor of Neurology
Division of Clinical Neurosciences
University of Glasgow
Honorary Consultant Neurologist
South Glasgow University Hospitals NHS Trust
University Department of Neurology
Southern General Hospital
Glasgow, Scotland, UK
Chapter 194 – Miller Fisher Syndrome

Janet Wilterdink MD
Associate Professor
Department of Clinical Neurosciences
Brown University School of Medicine
Providence RI, USA
Chapter 39 – Anticoagulant Therapy and Antiplatelet
    Drugs

Anthony J Windebank MD
Consultant
Department of Neurology
Mayo Clinic
Professor of Neurology
Mayo Medical School
Rochester MN, USA
Chapter 185 – Late Effects of Polio
Chapter 206 – Porphyria
Chapter 211 – Motor Neuron Diseases

John W Winkelman MD PhD
Assistant Professor
Clinical Laboratories
Brigham and Women's Hospital
Department of Pathology
Harvard Medical School
Boston MA, USA
Chapter 120 – Parasomnias

Paul Winner DO
Co-Director
Palm Beach Headache Center
Palm Beach FL, USA
Chapter 16 – Headache "Syndromes" in Children and
    Adolescents

Claire C Yang MD
Assistant Professor of Urology
Adjunct Assistant Professor of Neurology
University of Washington
Staff Physician
VA-Puget Sound Health Care System
Seattle WA, USA
Chapter 215 – Treatment of Sexual Dysfunction and
    Cystopathy in Peripheral Nerve Disorders

G Bryan Young MD FRCPC
Professor
Department of Clinical Neurological Sciences
The University of Western Ontario
London ON, Canada
Chapter 107 – Aspects of Metabolic Coma in the
    Intensive Care Unit

PJ Zilko MB BS
Consultant Immunologist
Departments of Neurology and Clinical Immunology
Sir Charles Gairdner Hospital
Centre for Neuromuscular and Neurological
    Disorders
Australian Neuromuscular Research Institute
University of Western Australia
Perth, Australia
Chapter 223 – Inflammatory Myopathies

Mary L Zupanc MD
Associate Professor
Columbia University
Director
Pediatric Epilepsy Section
Babies and Children's Hospital
New York NY, USA
Chapter 32 – The Treatment of Epilepsy in Children
    and Infants

Preface

"Diagnose and dismiss." In the early years of my career, this was the often cited, yet misguided, summary of the role of the neurologist. Few predicted the rapid evolution of the field of neurological therapeutics. The "Decade of the Brain (1991–2000)" has recently passed but not the era of landmark advancements in the treatment of patients with neurological disorders. The number of treatment options available for our patients is growing. Many of them have been validated by proper randomized controlled clinical trials and supported by evidence-based medicine. The future looks even brighter.

Neurological Therapeutics: Principles and Practice was created to address the need for a comprehensive textbook focused primarily on therapeutics and directed to busy neurologists and students of neurology. In developing this text, we strove to provide a reference that would be both authoritative and accessible for daily use. Authors were asked to focus on the issues underlying treatment decisions not only for the most readily treated disorders but also for conditions with few existing, definitive therapeutic options. In all cases, authors were encouraged to provide their best estimate of the future direction of therapeutics for their topic.

In editing each chapter, I assumed my daily role as the office generalist and subspecialist, now 15 to 20 years removed from residency. I considered what might be needed to understand the treatment options for each topic. Authors created comprehensive summary tables and informative figures to guide treatment decisions in the busy clinic setting, supported by a thorough discussion of the reasons for these recommendations in the text. Without exception, these renowned experts exceeded what I imagined possible.

The book is organized to cover 13 major subspecialty groupings of neurological disorders, and an introductory section addresses selected topics relevant to the principles of therapeutics. The Section Editors are internationally recognized leaders in their fields. These colleagues successfully recruited authoritative authors to discuss the more than 270 major topics covering the vast patient mix primarily treated by adult and pediatric neurologists. Each chapter focuses principally on issues of treatment (past, current, and under development). The chapters are generously illustrated with summary tables and figures to assist in making immediate decisions about treatment. Each chapter also contains sufficient background information on the topic (clinical presentation, pathogenesis, classification, and so forth) to direct diagnostic decisions.

The scope of this project was immediately apparent but grew as the Section Editors and I decided to cover the widening array of topics facing contemporary clinicians. The publisher has done a splendid job creating a book that is well illustrated with more than *1,300* figures (more than *50* in color) and tables. The publisher acquiesced to my insistence that our experts should be permitted (within reason) to define the optimal chapter length to cover their assignment (hence the wide range in the length of chapters). The publisher similarly agreed not to use a smaller font (especially in the bibliography) to save pages and permit a single volume. A Selected Tables and Figures handbook containing many of the summary tables, algorithms, and figures supplements the text. The final product is a two-volume text that is admittedly larger and heavier than we initially imagined.

If we have achieved our aim, this text will be used as an important reference for treatment decisions in offices of neurological practice, in clinics, and in hospitals and will later be read in depth when time permits. Our authors have provided the information needed to guide the treatment of neurological disorders. We are most grateful for their efforts and their expertise. The editors are confident that this book will assist students, clinicians, and clinician-scientists in understanding the current status of neurological therapeutics and will help in planning the care of their patients.

John H. Noseworthy, MD, FRCPC
Editor-in-Chief

Dedication

This book is dedicated to our patients, for their dignity and courage when our answers fall short,
Dr HJM Barnett, for asking important questions, Dr GC Ebers, for demanding lasting answers,
my parents, for commitment to others, and Peter, Mark, and Pat, for everything.

Acknowledgements

Many persons contributed to bringing this book to completion. From the initial discussions to the final launch, Alan Burgess at Martin Dunitz Ltd has been an enthusiastic, flexible, creative, and supportive Senior Publisher. The fifteen Section Editors determined the content of their sections and used their international reputations to recruit a superb team of contributing authors. I owe my sincere appreciation to the chapter authors who are always essential to the success of any multi-authored book. Selected because they contribute new knowledge to their area of special interest, these experts shared their insights and responded willingly to requests for revisions and additions. I thank the staff of the Mayo Clinic Section of Scientific Publications, including Dr. O. Eugene Millhouse, editor, Roberta Schwartz, production editor, and Dianne Kemp, editorial assistant, for their help with the chapters written by my colleagues at Mayo Clinic. At Wearset Ltd, Sarah Coulson and Brian Tait did a marvelous job handling the editing of the non-Mayo-authored chapters and overseeing the final production of all the text. I would also like to thank several excellent secretaries, including Laura Irlbeck, Mary Bennett, and Melissa Fenske. My special thanks, as always, goes to my wonderful wife, Pat, who patiently accepted "the book" as a recurring companion for most of the last 4 years.

John H. Noseworthy, MD, FRCPC
Editor-in-Chief

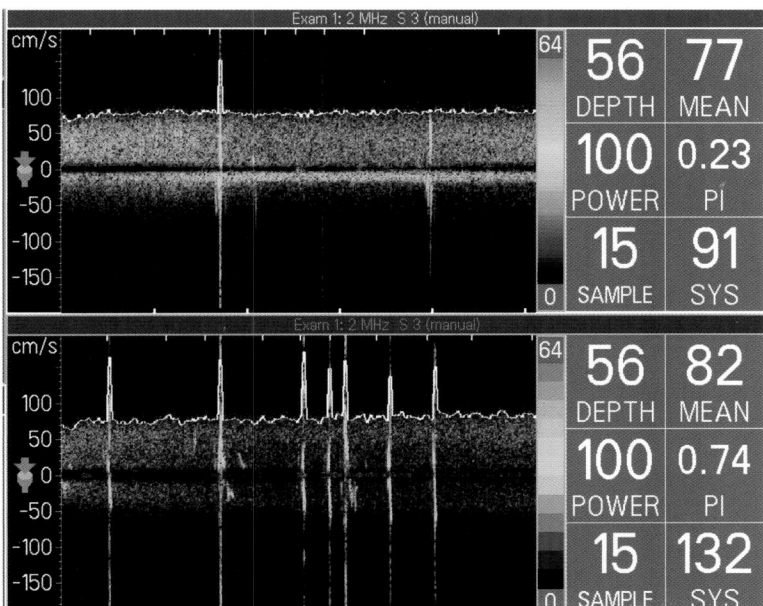

Figure 110.3 Embolus during bypass—transcranial Doppler.

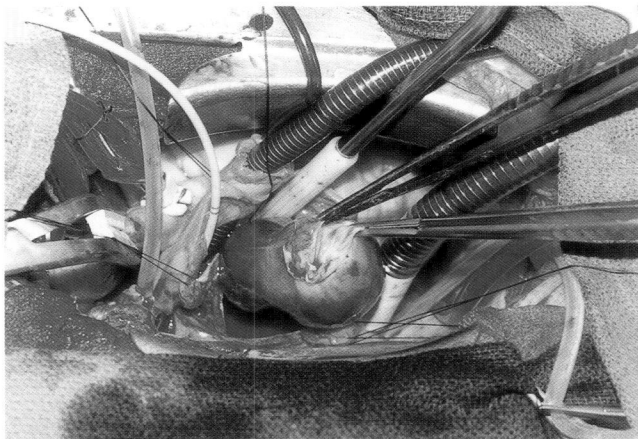

Figure 115.2 Intraoperative photograph demonstrating excision of a large left atrial myxoma.

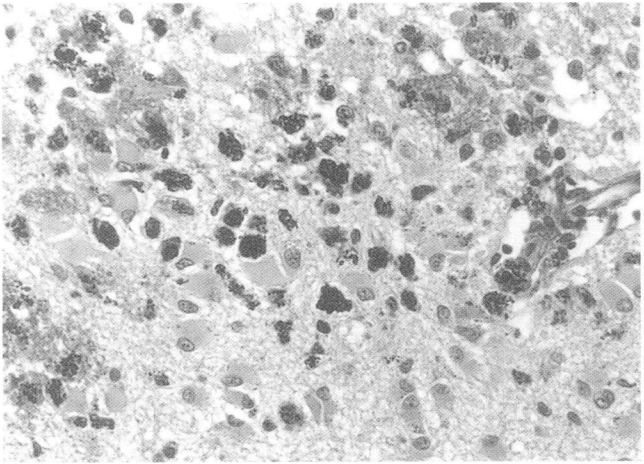

Figure 141.3 Light microscopic features characteristic of infection of the brain with *T. whippelii*, including foamy macrophages filled with PAS-positive and diastase-resistant material. Numerous reactive astrocytes are present. (Stain for periodic acid–Schiff reaction, 40× magnification. Courtesy of Massachusetts General Hospital Department of Neuropathology.)

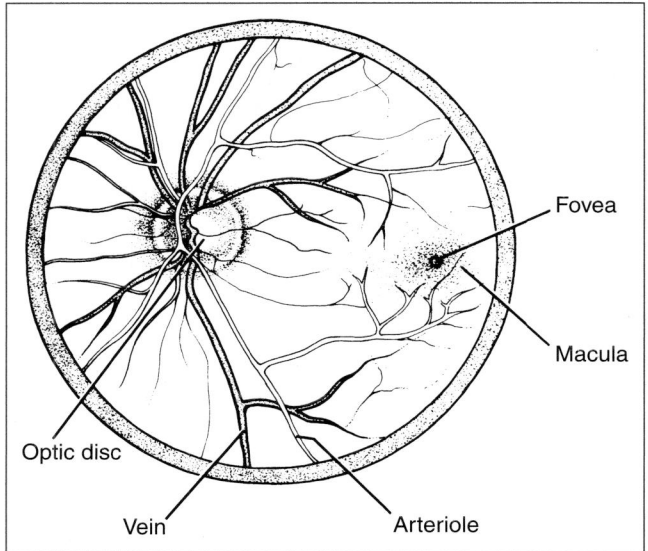

(A)

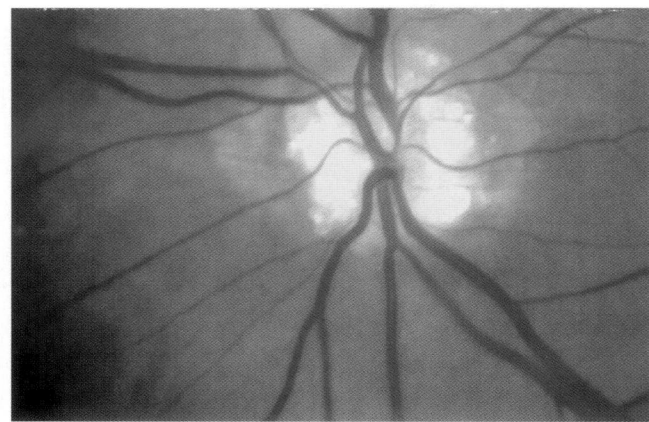

(A)

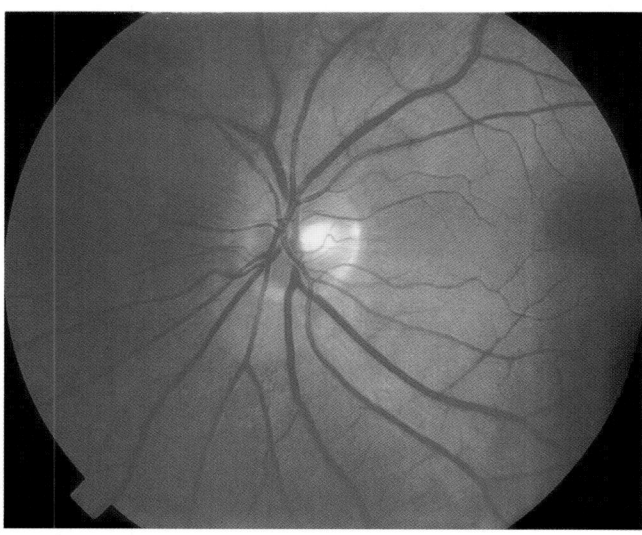

(B)

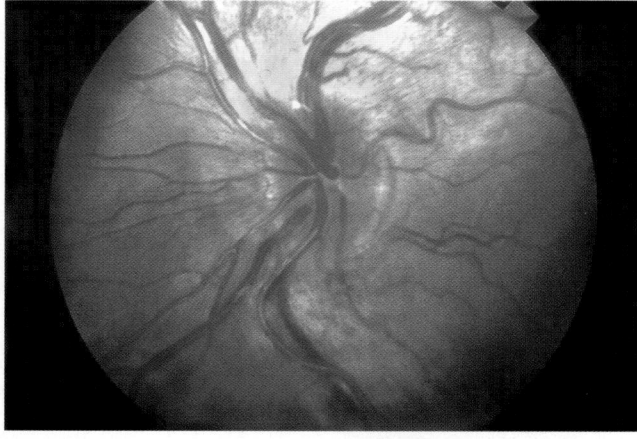

(B)

Figure 161.4 *A*, Color fundus photograph demonstrating optic disk drusen; note that the drusen have an appearance that resembles "rock candy." *B*, Optic disk photograph from a patient with Leber's hereditary optic neuropathy (LHON) demonstrating characteristic circumpapillary telangiectatic vessels and pseudoedema of the nerve fiber layer.

Photograph in part A courtesy of Dr Grant Liu.

Figure 161.1 *A*, Diagram of normal left fundus demonstrating optic disk and macula. *B*, Color fundus photograph of normal left eye.

Part A from Liu GT. Disorders of the eyes and eyelids. *In:* Samuels MA, Feske S, eds. Office Practice of Neurology. 1st ed. New York: Churchill Livingstone, 1996:41, with permission. Parts A and B also from Balcer LJ. Anatomic review and topographic diagnosis. Neurosurg Clin North Am 1999;10:541–561, with permission.

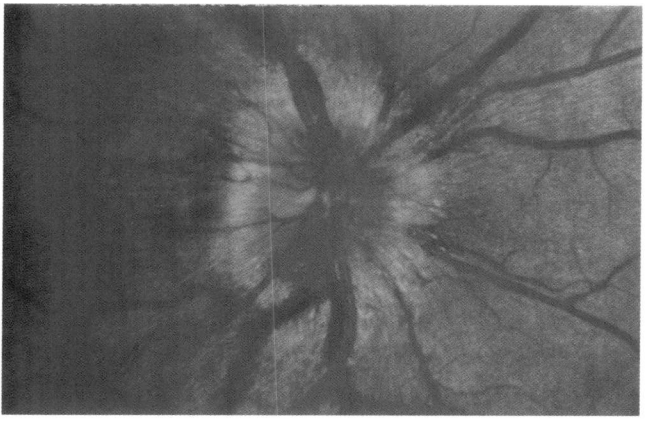

(A)

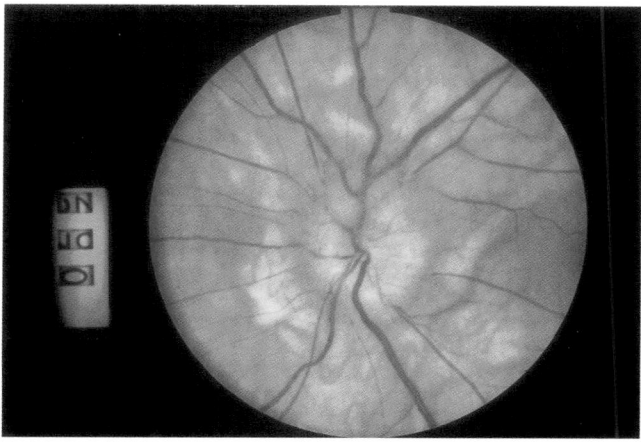

(B)

Figure 161.6 Optic disk swelling in optic neuritis and anterior ischemic optic neuropathy. *A*, Swollen optic disk of patient with acute demyelinating optic neuritis; disk swelling was present in 35% of patients in the Optic Neuritis Treatment Trial. *B*, Swollen optic disk of patient with nonarteritic anterior ischemic optic neuropathy (AION).

Photograph in part A courtesy of Dr Nicholas J Volpe. Part B from Balcer LJ. Anatomic review and topographic diagnosis. Neurosurg Clin North Am 1999;10:541–561, with permission.

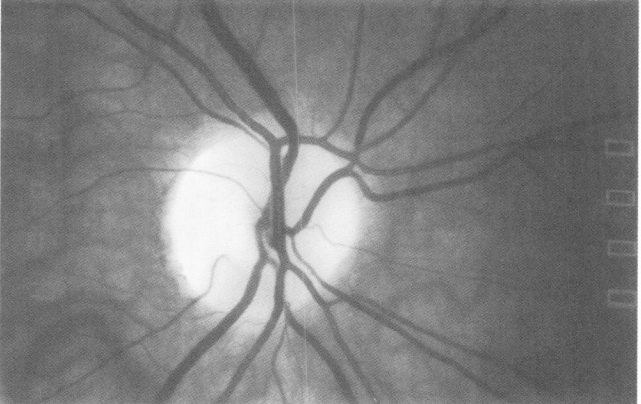

Figure 161.7 Optic disk pallor in a patient with a history of pituitary adenoma and bilateral optic neuropathies; pallor is most pronounced in the temporal region.

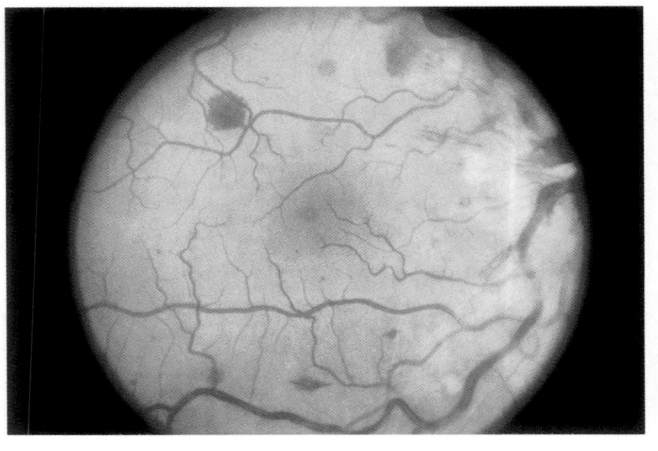

(A)

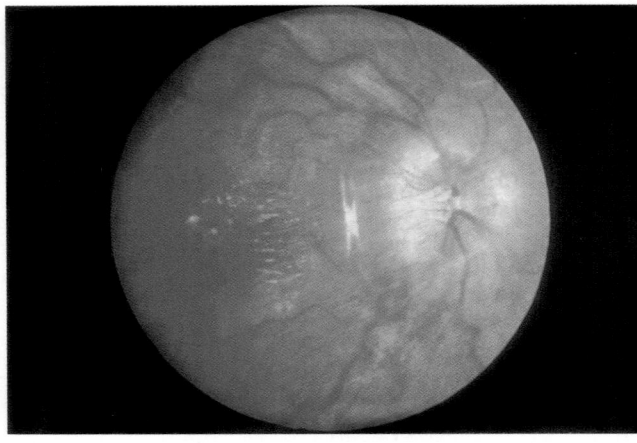

(B)

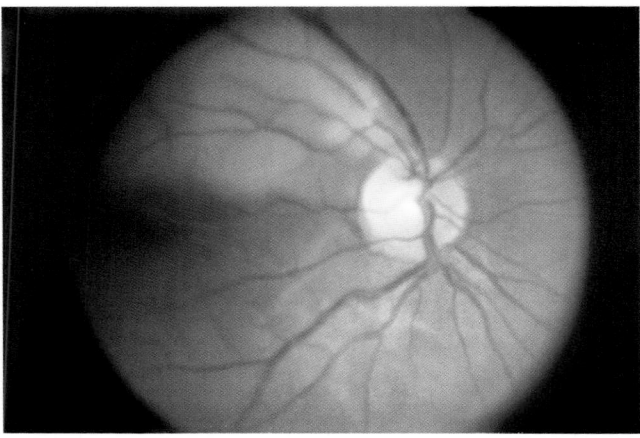

(C)

Figure 161.8 Retinal disorders that may have clinical signs and symptoms similar to optic neuropathy. *A,* Fundus photograph from patient with central retinal vein occlusion; note presence of swollen optic disk and retinal hemorrhages beyond the peripapillary region. *B,* Neuroretinitis with macular lipid exudates. *C,* Photograph from patient with branch retinal artery occlusion demonstrating retinal whitening superiorly, consistent with infarction. Note the presence of preserved reddish coloration in the superior area of the fovea, analogous to the macular "cherry-red spot."

Part C from Balcer LJ. Anatomic review and topographic diagnosis. Neurosurg Clin North Am 1999;10:541–561, with permission.

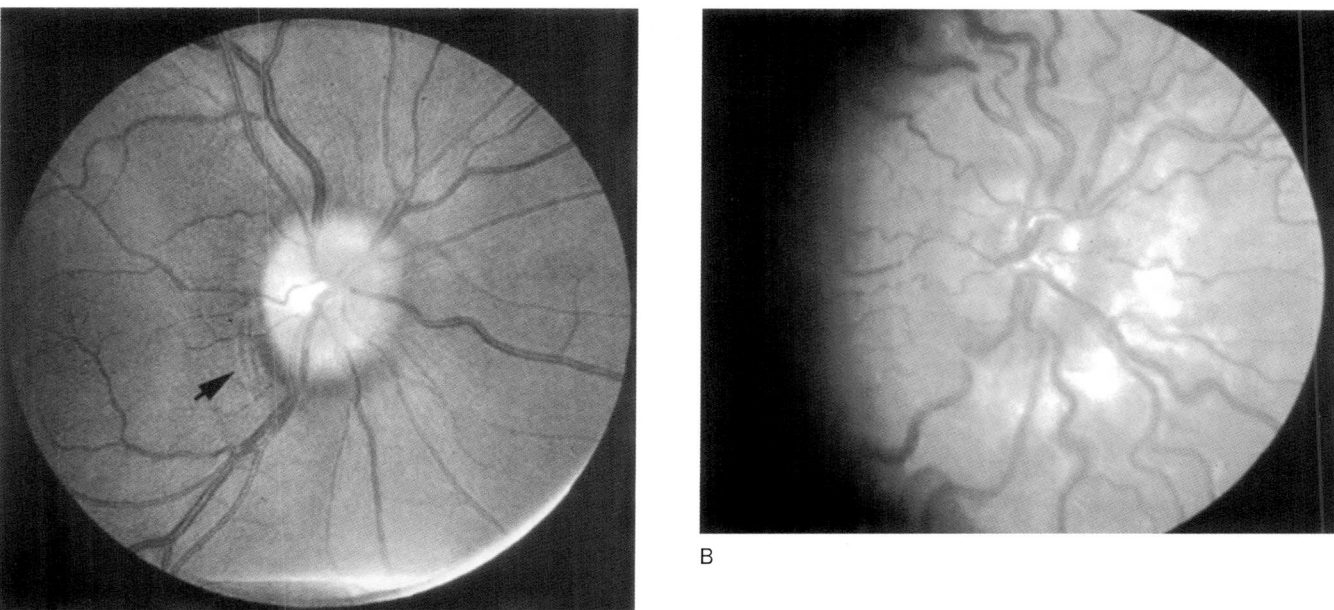

A

B

Figure 162.2 *A,* Optic disk with Frisén grade I papilledema. The disk has a C-shaped halo of nerve fiber layer edema around the disk, with a temporal gap. Choroidal folds are also present (*arrow*). *B,* pseudopapilledema. This is an anomalous disk with considerable anomalies of blood vessel branching.

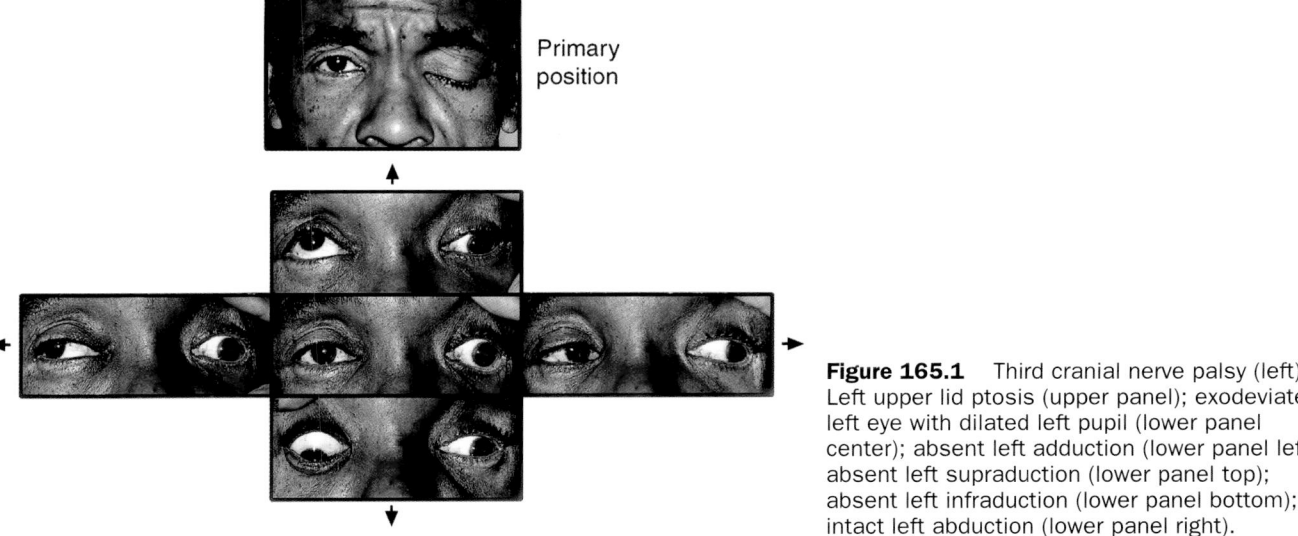

Primary position

Figure 165.1 Third cranial nerve palsy (left). Left upper lid ptosis (upper panel); exodeviated left eye with dilated left pupil (lower panel center); absent left adduction (lower panel left), absent left supraduction (lower panel top); absent left infraduction (lower panel bottom); intact left abduction (lower panel right).

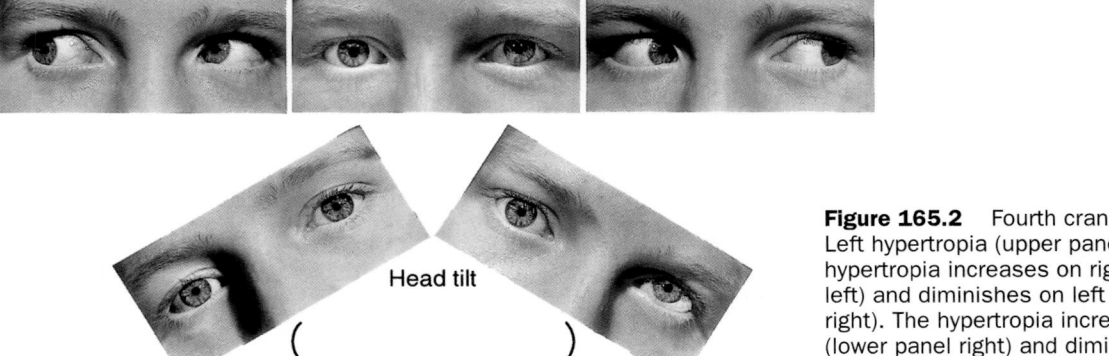

Figure 165.2 Fourth cranial nerve palsy (left). Left hypertropia (upper panel center); the left hypertropia increases on right gaze (upper panel left) and diminishes on left gaze (upper panel right). The hypertropia increases on left head tilt (lower panel right) and diminishes on right head tilt (lower panel left).

Head tilt

Right   Left

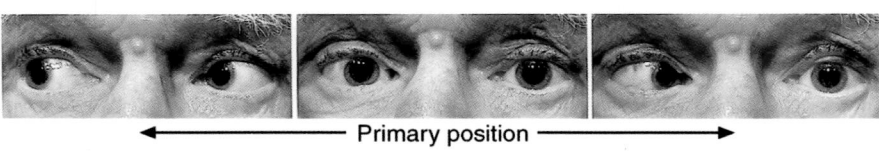

Primary position

Figure 165.3 Sixth cranial nerve palsy (left). Esotropia (center) increases on left gaze as left eye does not abduct (right) and disappears on right gaze (left).

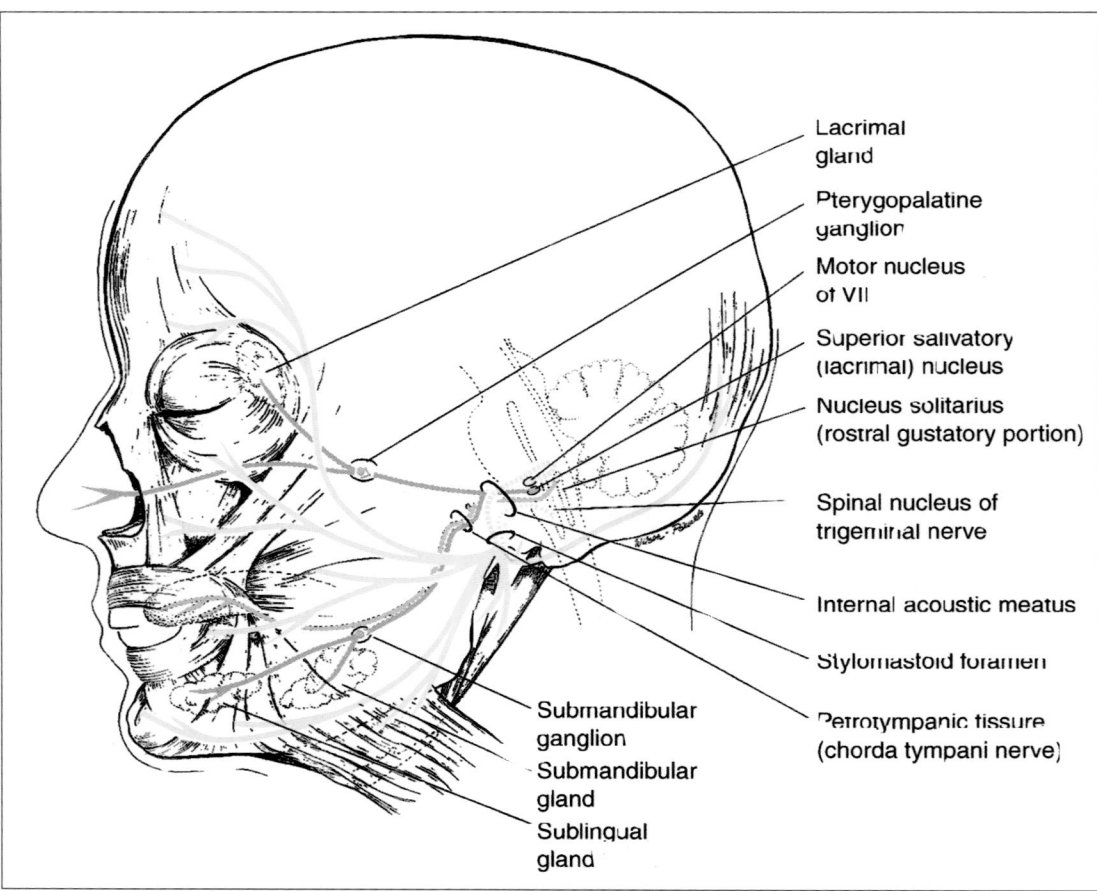

Lacrimal gland

Pterygopalatine ganglion

Motor nucleus of VII

Superior salivatory (lacrimal) nucleus

Nucleus solitarius (rostral gustatory portion)

Spinal nucleus of trigeminal nerve

Internal acoustic meatus

Stylomastoid foramen

Petrotympanic fissure (chorda tympani nerve)

Submandibular ganglion

Submandibular gland

Sublingual gland

Figure 171.1 Schematic of facial nerve anatomy. Color codes: yellow, special visceral efferent fibers; orange, general visceral efferent; blue, general somatic afferent; green, special afferent (taste). Reprinted with permission from: Wilson-Pauwels L, Akesson EJ, Stewart PA. Cranial Nerves: Anatomy and Clinical Comments. Hamilton (Canada): BC Decker, 1988:83.

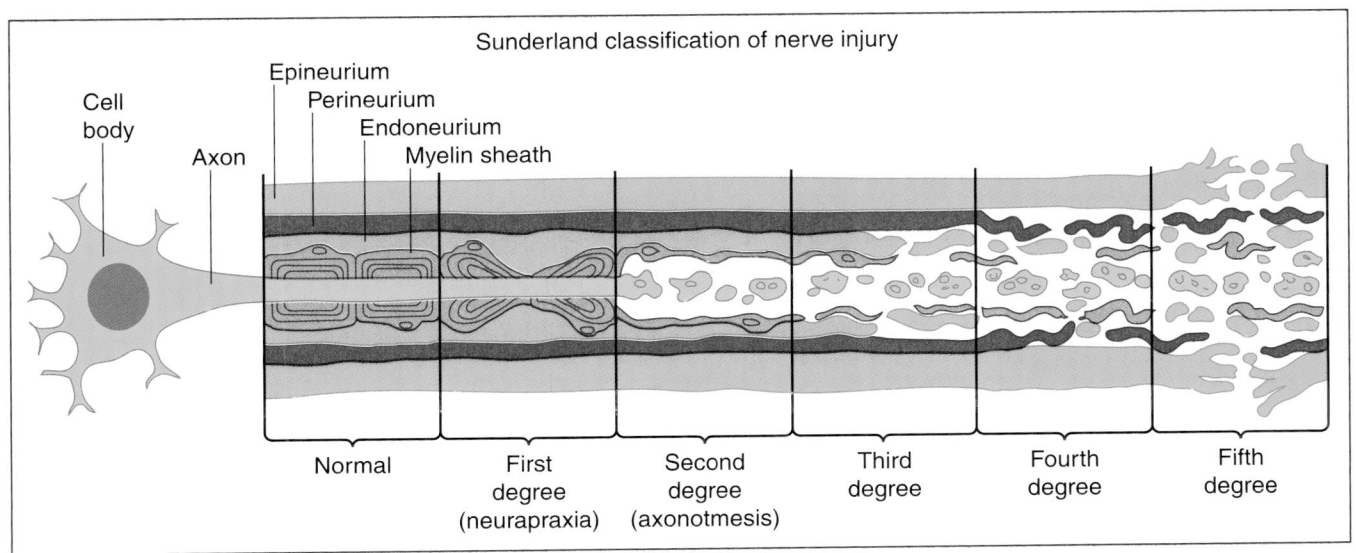

Figure 178.1 Classification of nerve injury by degree of involvement of various neural elements. (From Rayan GM. Compression neuropathies, including carpal tunnel syndrome. Clinical Symposia 1997;49(2):1–32. By permission of *Novartis*.)

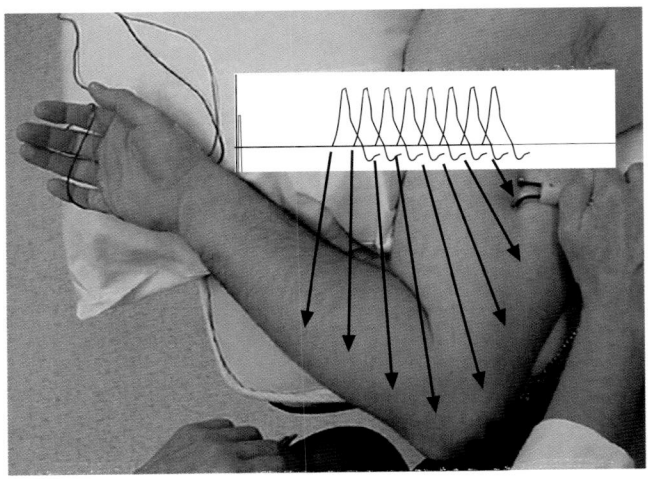

Figure 178.8 Normal ulnar nerve motor conduction study with short segment incremental stimulation ("inching"). Compound muscle action potential (*upper right*) recorded from hypothenar muscles after percutaneous supramaximal stimulation of motor axons along the length of a healthy ulnar nerve beginning at the mid forearm and moving the stimulating site proximally at equally spaced intervals up to the axilla. Note that the amplitude and configuration of the evoked potentials are essentially the same from stimulation at all the levels but the latency from the stimulus becomes progressively longer with more proximal stimulation.

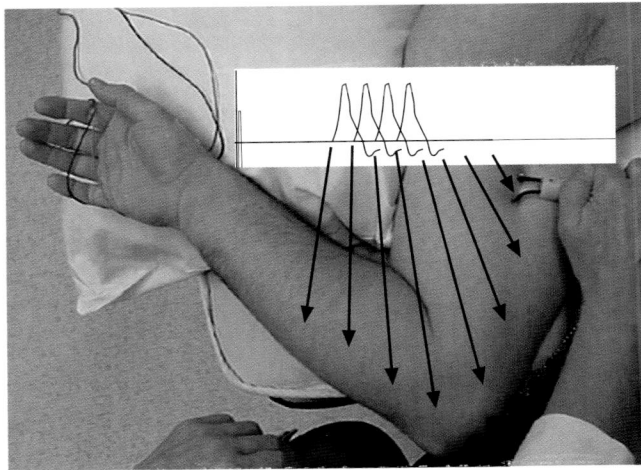

Figure 178.9 Ulnar nerve motor conduction study with short segment incremental stimulation ("inching") in a complete neuFigurapractic lesion at the elbow. The recording of the compound muscle action potential (*upper right*) from hypothenar muscles after percutaneous supramaximal stimulation of motor axons along the length of the ulnar nerve, as described in Figure 178.8. Note that the potentials from stimulation of the four most distal sites (below the elbow) evoke a potential resembling that of a normal subject (Figure 178.8). At and above the elbow, no potential is elicited. These findings would be typical for the first 36 to 48 hours after nerve transection at the elbow or a neurapractic lesion at the elbow.

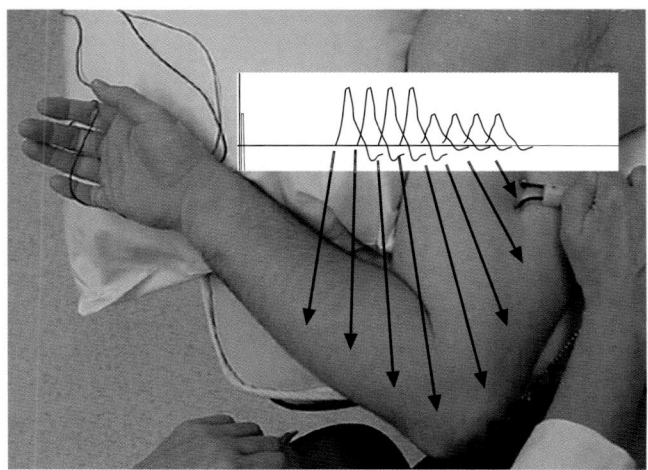

Figure 178.10 Ulnar nerve motor conduction study with short segment incremental stimulation ("inching") in a 50% neurapractic lesion at the elbow. The recording of the compound muscle action potential (*upper right*) from hypothenar muscles after percutaneous supramaximal stimulation of motor axons along the length of the ulnar nerve, as described in Figure 178.8. Note that the potential from stimulation of the four most distal sites (below the elbow) evokes a potential resembling that of a normal subject (Figure 178.8). At and above the elbow, the amplitude of the potential is reduced. These findings are typical of the first 36 to 48 hours after partial nerve transection at the elbow or a partial neurapractic lesion at the elbow.

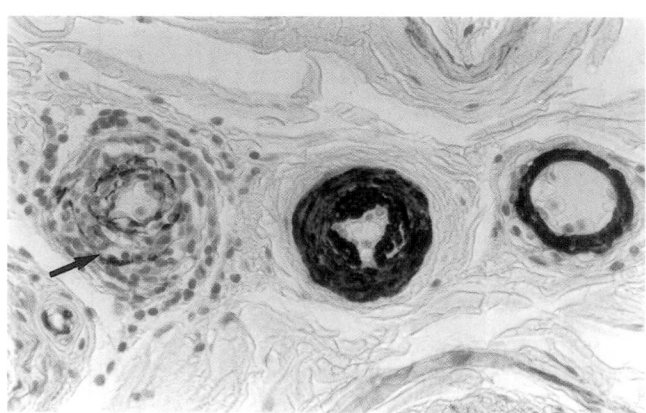

Figure 187.1 Sural nerve from a patient with lumbosacral radiculoplexus neuropathy immunoreacted to smooth muscle actin. The vessel on the left is a thin-walled microvessel with fragmentation of its wall (*arrow*); the fragments are separated by mononuclear cells. The vessels in the middle and on the right are unaffected.

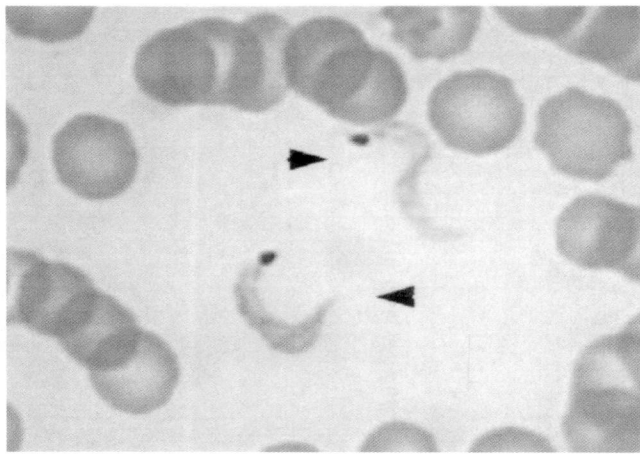

Figure 184.1 Circulating forms of *Trypanosoma cruzi* (trypomastigotes) ×1534.

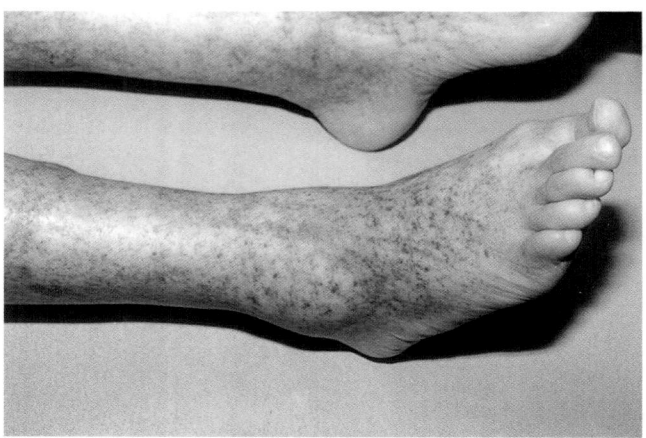

Figure 190.1 Purpura of legs of woman with painful sensorimotor polyneuropathy associated with hepatitis C virus-related mixed cryoglobulinemia.

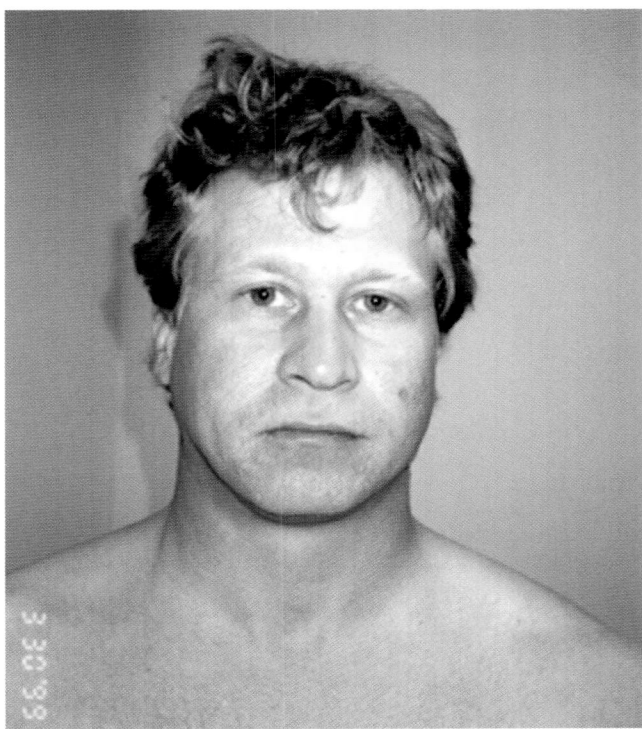

Figure 195.1 A patient with hereditary neuralgic amyotrophy (HMA) showing some dysmorphic features, namely, long narrow face, facial asymmetry, and hypotelorism.

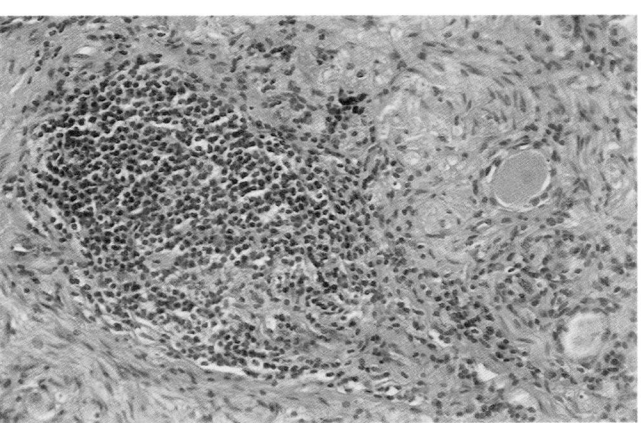

Figure 197.1 Dorsal root ganglion from a patient with sensory ganglionopathy associated with Sjögren syndrome. A mononuclear inflammatory infiltrate is present. Two neuronal cell bodies are seen to right. (Hematoxylin and eosin, ×250.)

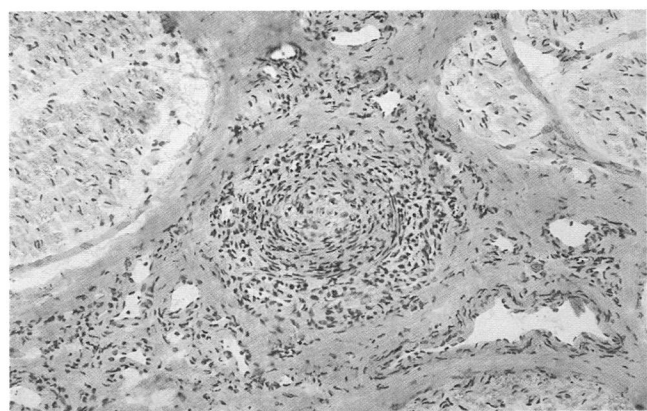

Figure 198.2 This superficial peroneal nerve biopsy specimen shows a necrotic epineurial blood vessel destroyed by a marked perivascular and transmural inflammatory cell infiltration.

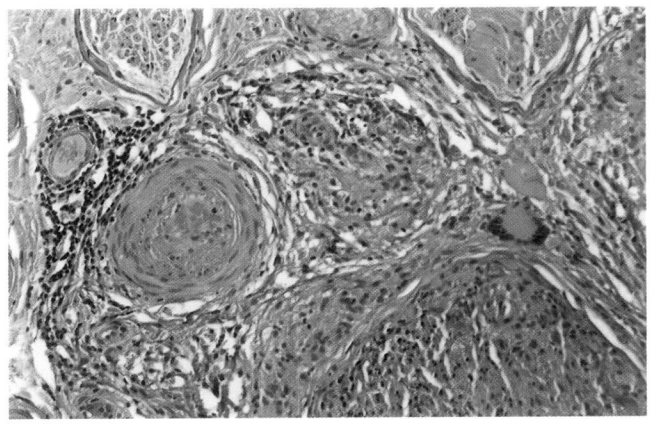

(A)

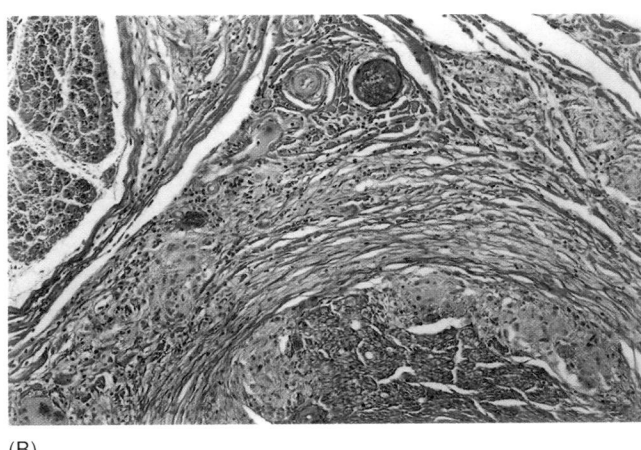

(B)

Figure 200.1 Transverse, paraffin-embedded tissue sections of a sural nerve biopsy from a patient with sarcoidosis. Hematoxylin-eosin stain (*A*) and Masson stain with trichrome (*B*) of tissue sections show multinucleated giant cells, epithelioid granuloma, and mononuclear inflammatory cell infiltrates associated with nerve fascicles. (Courtesy of PJ Dyck and J Englestad, Mayo Clinic, Rochester, Minnesota.)

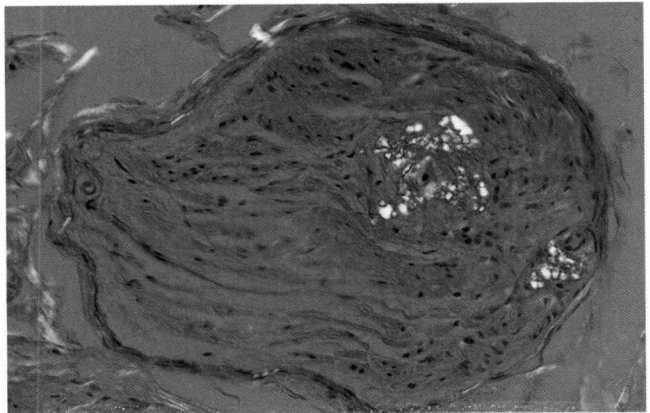

Figure 202.5 Congo red stain of sural nerve viewed under polarizing light showing selective loss of unmyelinated and small myelinated fibers in a patient with familial amyloidosis.

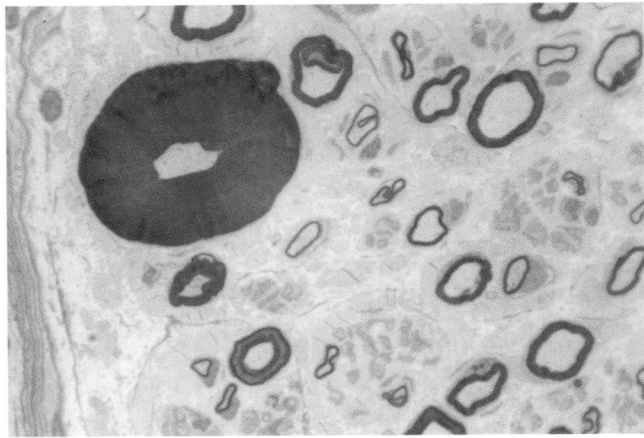

Figure 209.1 Cross-section of a sural nerve biopsy from a patient with HNPP showing a tomaculum. Thinly myelinated axons are also seen. One-micron section prepared from plastic embedded specimen, toluidine blue staining. Original magnification ×400.

Courtesy of Dr. Zarife Sahenk, Dept. of Neurology, Ohio State University, Columbus, Ohio.

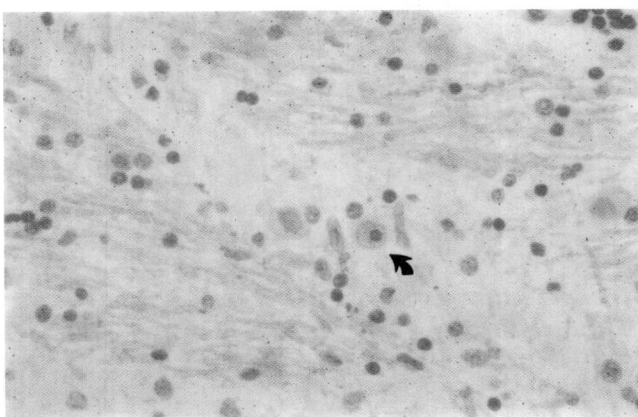

Figure 210.1 Histopathological findings in spinocerebellar ataxia-3. Note neuronal loss, gliosis, and ubiquitin-immunoreactive neuronal intranuclear inclusion body (*arrow*). (Basal pons immunostained with anti-ubiquitin antibody and counterstained with hematoxylin-eosin; ×100.) (Courtesy of Brent Clark, M.D., University of Minnesota.)

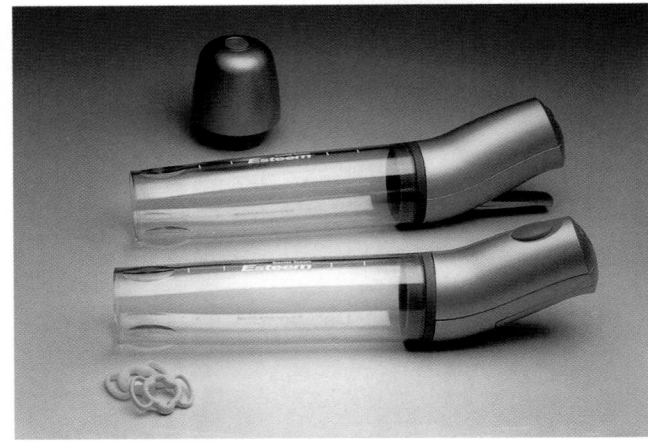

Figure 215.1 Vacuum constriction device. (Photograph courtesy of Timm Medical Technologies, Inc., Eden Prairie, MN)

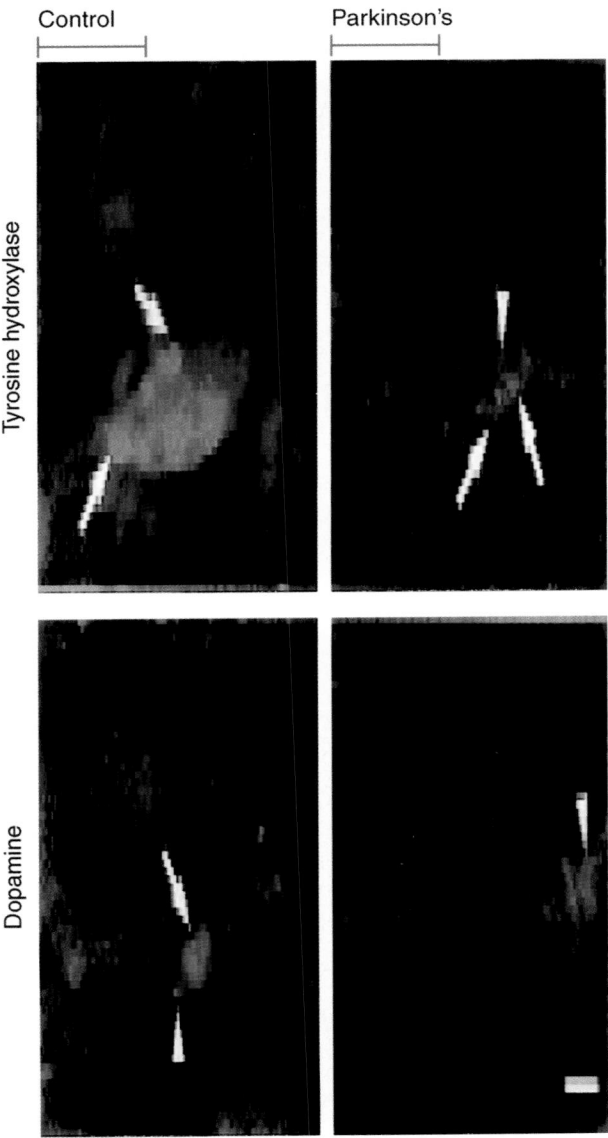

Figure 216.4 Immunohistochemistry of myenteric plexus showing positively stained neurons (*arrows*) in healthy control and patient with Parkinson disease; bar = 1 μm. Note the significantly greater reduction in dopamine (*arrows*) compared to tyrosine hydroxylase neurons. (From Singaram et al.[11] By permission of Lancet Ltd.)

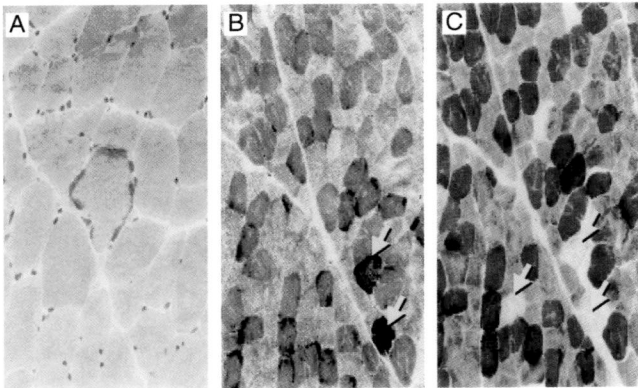

Figure 216.5 Mitochondrial cytopathy in mitochondrial neurogastrointestinal encephalomyopathy. *A*, Note the ragged red fibers on modified Gomori stain reflecting a few muscle fibers with prominent subsarcolemmal mitochondria. *B*, In contrast, ragged blue fibers indicate succinate dehydrogenase positive fibers (*arrow*) are *C*, cytochrome c oxidase-negative, indicating the mitochondrial enzyme deficiency (*arrow*). (From Mueller et al.[29] By permission of American Gastroenterological Association.)

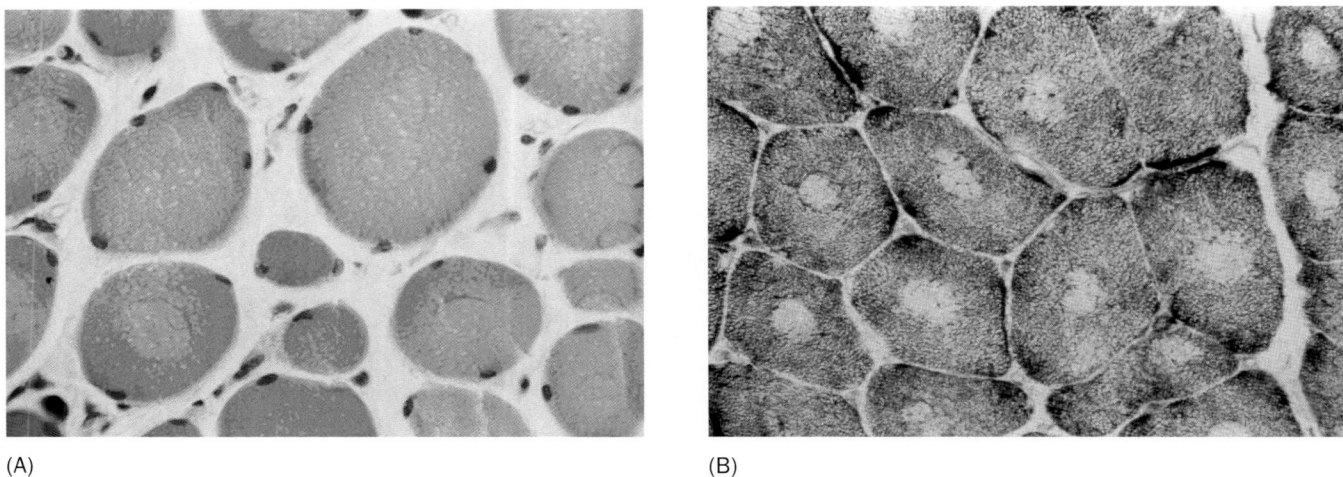

(A)   (B)

Figure 221.2   Central Core Disease A. The cores are not apparent on haematoxylin endcosin staining. B. Transverse sections stained for NADH show absence of enzyme activity in single large central cores.

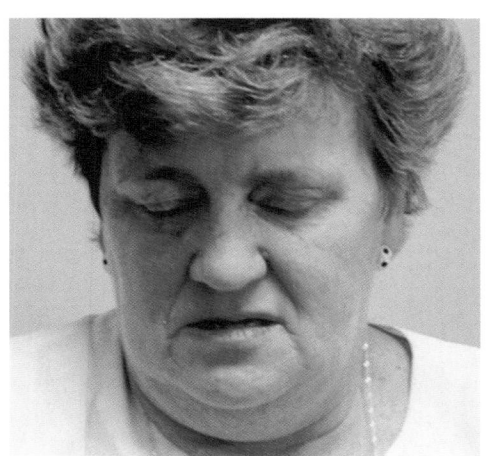 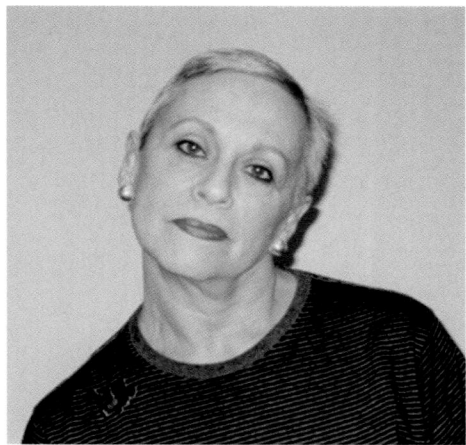

Figure 236.1   *A*, Patient with blepharospasm. *B*, Patient with cervical dystonia, manifested mainly by left laterocollis.

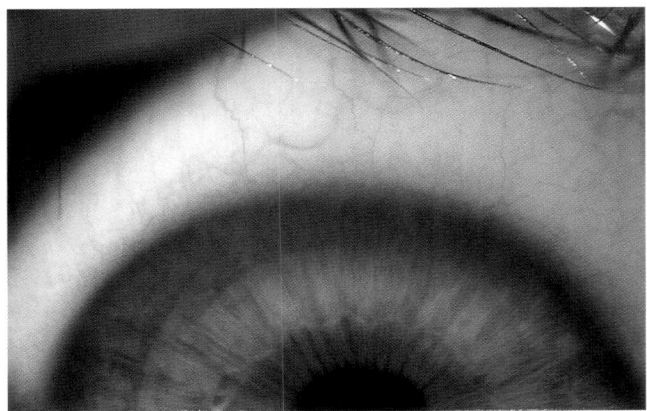

Figure 253.1 Wilson's disease Kayser-Fleischer ring. Courtesy of Dr Brian R Younge.

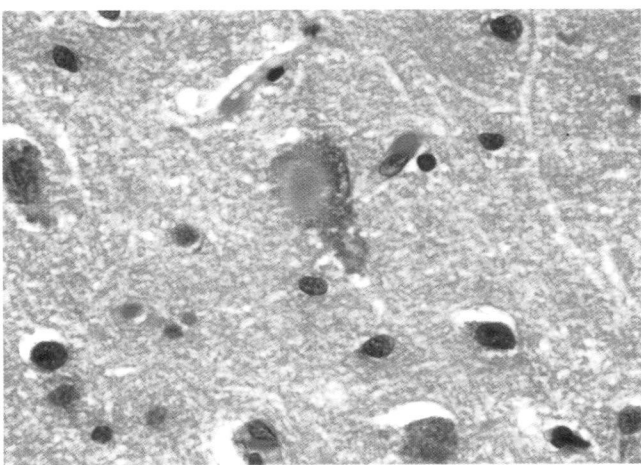

Figure 269.1 Lewy body (cingulate cortex) characteristic of Lewy body disease (H&E ×60). Courtesy Joseph E Parisi, MD.

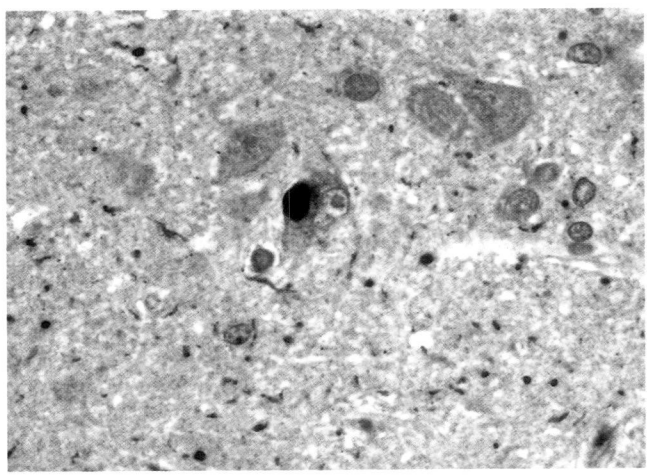

Figure 269.2 α-synuclein-positive Lewy body (cingulate cortex) characteristic of Lewy body disease (α-synuclein ×60). Courtesy Joseph E Parisi, MD.

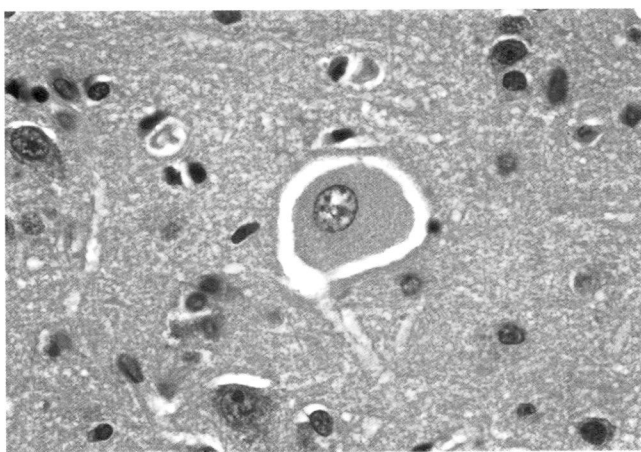

Figure 269.4 Ballooned, achromatic neuron (frontal cortex) typical of corticobasal degeneration (H&E ×60). Courtesy Joseph E Parisi, MD.

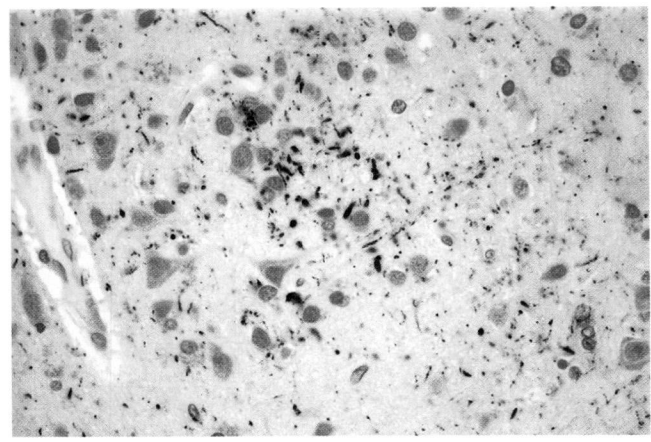

Figure 269.5 Tau-positive astrocytic plaque (parietal cortex) typical of corticobasal degeneration (tau ×40). Courtesy Joseph E Parisi, MD.

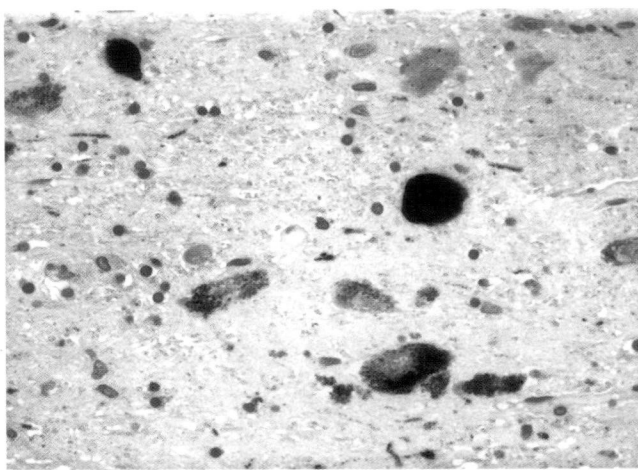

Figure 269.6 Tau-positive globose neurofibrillary tangle (substantia nigra) typical of progressive supranuclear palsy (tau ×40). Courtesy Joseph E Parisi, MD.

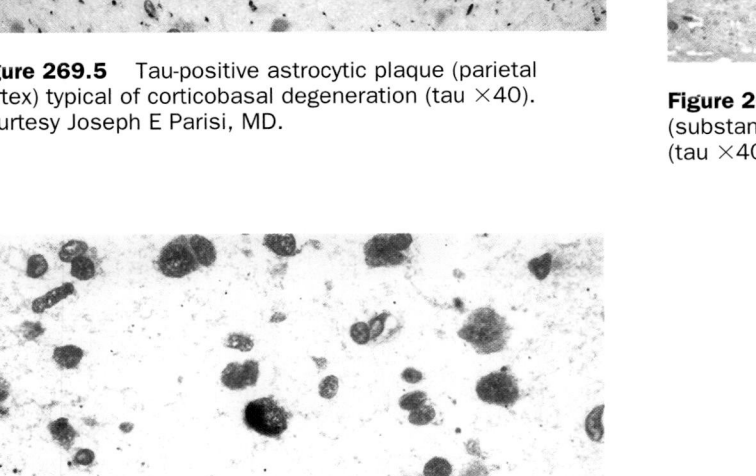

Figure 269.7 Intraneuronal inclusion (frontal cortex) that is positive for ubiquitin but negative for tau and α-synuclein associated with frontotemporal dementia (ubiquitin ×60). Courtesy Joseph E Parisi, MD.

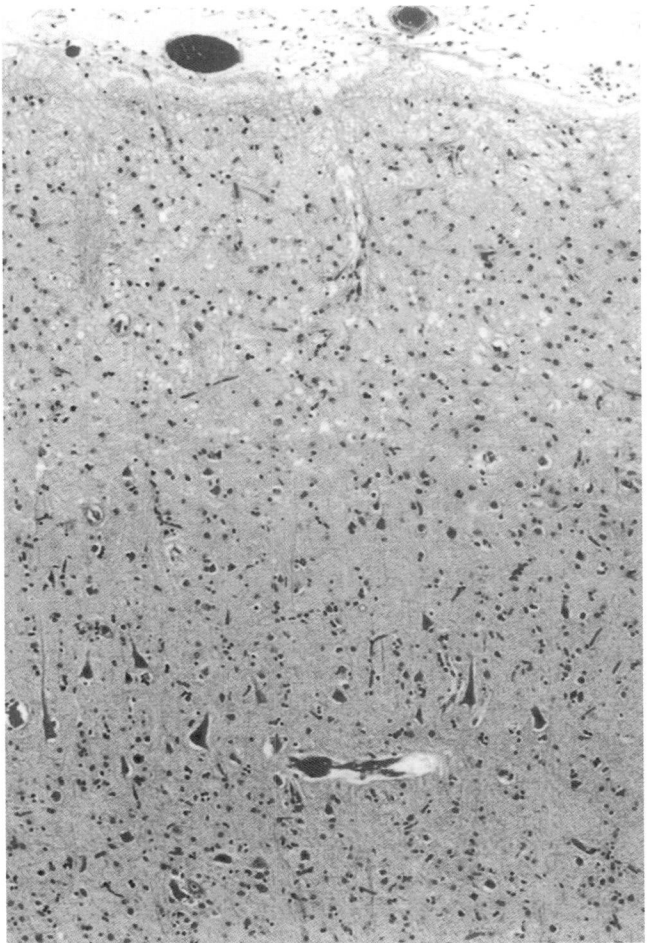

Figure 269.8 Marked neuronal loss, gliosis, and status spongiosis (frontal cortex) with no abnormalities revealed by tau, ubiquitin, α-synuclein, and prion immunocytochemistry, associated with parkinsonism and cognitive impairment—often termed "dementia lacking distinctive histopathology" (H&E ×25). From Boeve BF, Maraganore DM, Parisi JE, et al. Corticobasal degeneration and frontotemporal dementia presentations in a kindred with nonspecific histopathology. Dement Geriatr Cogn Disord 2002;13:80–90. By permission by S Karger AG, Basel.

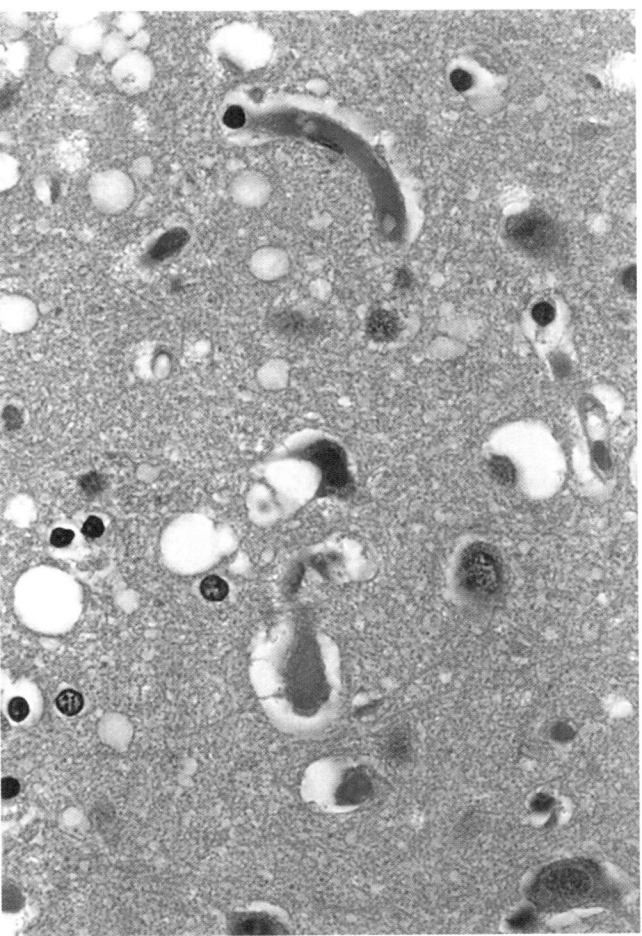

Figure 269.9 Marked spongiform changes characteristic of Creutzfeldt-Jakob disease (H&E ×150). Courtesy Joseph E Parisi, MD.

VIII   Neurological Complications of Systemic Illness

Section editor: Martin A Samuels

110 Neurological Complications of Cardiac Procedures: Catheterization, Interventional Procedures and Surgery

Cathy A Sila

Brief overview

Coronary artery angiography began in the 1940s but modern imaging evolved with selective, high speed cine filming and percutaneous techniques for arterial access.[1] After Rene Favalaro introduced coronary artery bypass graft surgery, coronary angiography became the reference standard for assessing patients with coronary artery disease.[2] The era of endovascular therapy for vascular disease began with the first percutaneous transluminal coronary angioplasty (PTCA) by Gruentzig in 1977.[3] The neurological complications of interventions for cardiac disease are important components of outcomes-based research as adverse neurological events substantially increase procedural mortality, hospital length of stay, and the use of care facilities upon discharge.[4]

Epidemiology

Cardiac angiographic procedures

Ischemic stroke complicates 0.1% to 1% of cardiac catheterization and catheter-based coronary interventions, 1% to 10% of endovascular balloon valvuloplasties, and 1% to 2% of atrial septal closures.[5–9] Transient cortical blindness after catheterization occurs even less frequently at 0.01% to 0.05%.[10] Peripheral nerve complications related to vascular access are uncommon, occurring in fewer than 1% and related to the site of access: brachial artery approaches can injure the median nerve, and femoral access can injure the femoral nerve.[11] The femoral nerve or lumbar plexus is more commonly injured by retroperitoneal hemorrhage, which complicates up to 5% of endovascular interventions employing antithrombotic therapies, particularly after femoral artery puncture.[12] Intra-aortic balloon counter-pulsation support (IABP) is associated with a 15% rate of femoral nerve injury or ischemic monomelic neuropathy and rarely infarction of the thoracic spinal cord.[13]

Intracranial hemorrhage (ICH) has been reduced to 0.14% in contemporary series of coronary angioplasty, stent implantation and atherectomy employing glycoprotein IIb/IIIa inhibitors with weight-adjusted heparin regimens, but ICH after thrombolytic therapy for acute myocardial infarction continues at 0.3% to 1%, with risk related to the aggressiveness of the drug regimen, advanced patient age, and hypertension.[14,15]

Cardiac surgical procedures

Coronary artery bypass graft surgery (CABG) for myocardial revascularization is the most frequently performed cardiac surgery: more than 500 000 procedures in the US, and 800 000 procedures are performed worldwide. The complications of CABG include ischemic stroke (2% to 5%), encephalopathy (3% to 12% clinically evident, 35% to 75% with neurocognitive testing batteries), coma (0.2%), ICH (0.03%), peripheral nerve injuries (2% to 13%), and rarely optic neuropathy and pituitary apoplexy.[4,9,16–18] More complex cardiac surgeries, such as valvular replacement or repair, ventricular aneurysmectomy, and hypothermic circulatory arrest for reconstruction of the aortic arch are associated with higher rates of stroke at 5% to 15%.[19,20] Hypothermic retrograde cerebral perfusion carries a 15% risk of global or focal neurological deficit and a 6% risk of coma or death.[21]

Etiology, pathophysiology and pathogenesis

Cardiac angiographic procedures

Ischemic stroke due to embolism is the most common neurological complication of diagnostic and therapeutic cardiac catheterization. Atherosclerotic plaque or thrombus can be dislodged during guiding catheter manipulation; platelet–fibrin thrombus formed on the catheters or air can embolize during flushing.[22] The vertebrobasilar predominance of cerebral embolism with angiography differs from other cardioembolic sources and probably relates to catheter position within the aorta.

Encephalopathic states after coronary angiography are often attributed to sedative and analgesic medications, systemic hypotension, and large volumes of contrast material, although patients with vertebrobasilar distribution ischemia can also present with confusion and memory defects.[23] Transient cortical blindness after angiography may have a different mechanism as the patchy cortical enhancement on neuroimaging, vascular headache and hypertension are similar to that seen in hypertensive encephalopathy and eclampsia.[24]

Cardiac surgical procedures

After cardiac surgery, the neurological complications may be classified by the clinical manifestation of the injury (e.g. stroke, encephalopathy, coma, etc.) or by the proposed mechanism of the injury (e.g. macro-embolism, microembolism, hypoperfusion, hypoxic-ischemic injury, hemorrhage, etc.) but for many cases the relationship between the clinical picture and the presumed mechanism is either multifactorial or uncertain. The presumed mechanisms of ischemic stroke after cardiac surgery with cardiopulmonary bypass include embolism from the aortic arch in one-third, one-third evenly distributed between cardioembolism, hypoperfusion and concomitant cerebrovascular disease, the remaining one-third being cryptogenic. Risk factors for stroke after CABG include advanced age, aortic arch atheromatous disease, prior stroke or documented cerebrovascular disease, recent myocardial infarction, left ventricular dysfunction, hypertension, diabetes, chronic renal insufficiency, and postoperative atrial fibrillation.[4,25] Patients with stroke were more likely to have longer cross-clamp and total cardiopulmonary bypass (CPB) times and low postoperative cardiac output.[25]

Intracranial hemorrhage within one week of cardiac surgery is rare and results from hemorrhagic transformation of bland infarcts or coagulopathies in the critically ill or after cardiac transplantation (Figure 110.1).[26] Persistent nonmetabolic coma after open heart surgery is often due to multifocal cerebral infarction, infarction with herniation, or a diffuse global hypoxic-ischemic insult, although at least half remain cryptogenic.

Postoperative encephalopathy has been linked to markers of systemic hypotension, such as postoperative pressor or intra-aortic balloon pump support, as well as multifocal microembolization (Figure 110.2). Other risk factors for cognitive decline include advanced age, hypertension, diabetes, excessive alcohol consumption, postoperative atrial fibrillation, a history of peripheral vascular disease or prior CABG, and cerebral atrophy by neuroimaging.[4]

The cardiopulmonary bypass (CPB) can contribute to cerebral injury by cerebral embolization of atheromatous material and other debris, cerebral hypoperfusion, and through the production of a systemic inflammatory response which produces cerebral edema.[27] CABG performed with CPB ("on-pump") involves excluding the heart by constructing an extra-corporeal circuit through cannulation of the proximal ascending aorta and the right atrium. After systemic heparinization, the ascending aorta is occluded and the heart arrested, allowing the CPB circuit to supply the systemic circulation with oxygenated blood adjusted for pump flow, perfusion pressure, temperature, and venous saturation. Truly open heart surgeries, those which require opening of the cardiac chambers, have a significantly increased risk of embolization with the added elements of valvular debris, chamber thrombus and embolism of air and particulates during mechanical de-airing of the heart.[19] "Off-pump" surgery permits revascularization of the beating heart with the use of a cardiac stabilizer and has been proposed to reduce cerebral embolization by avoiding the risks of aortic manipulation and cardiopulmonary bypass.

Transcranial Doppler (TCD) and transesophageal echocardiography (TEE) monitoring have been used to investigate the role of cerebral emboli in the production of cerebral complications.[28] Several prospective studies have correlated the burden of TCD microemboli during CPB with cognitive deficits on neuropsychological testing.[29,30] The majority of high intensity signals occur during aortic manipulation and at the initiation of bypass (Figure 110.3). Aortic arch atheromatous disease, defined by surgical palpation or epiaortic ultrasound, has been identified as a major risk factor for atheroemboli during CABG.[4,31]

During hypothermic CPB, neuronal metabolism is slowed and cerebral autoregulation mechanisms operate to produce a state of luxury perfusion. However, cerebral autoregulation becomes dysfunctional at mean arterial pressures less than 20 or more than 100 mm Hg and temperatures lower than 22°C, particularly in patients with diabetes, which may explain the increased risk of neurological complications seen in diabetics.[32,33]

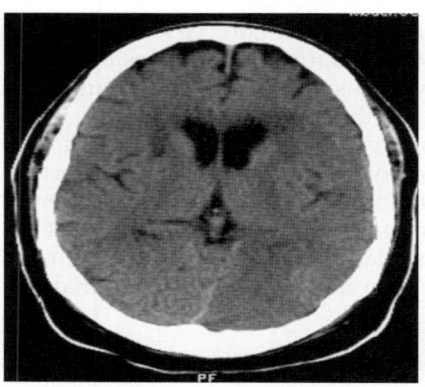
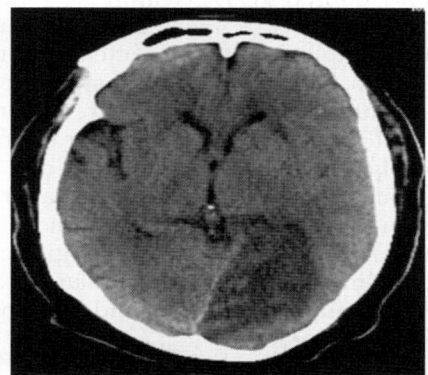
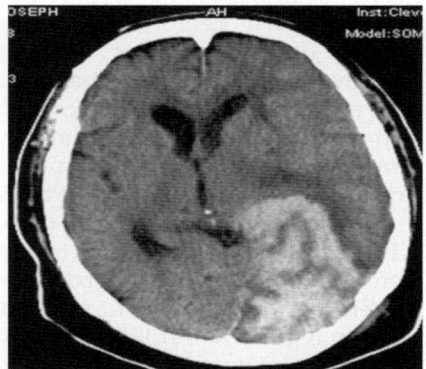

Figure 110.1   A, Acute left posterior cerebral artery infarct. B, Asymptomatic hemorrhagic transformation. C, Symptomatic parenchymal hemorrhage.

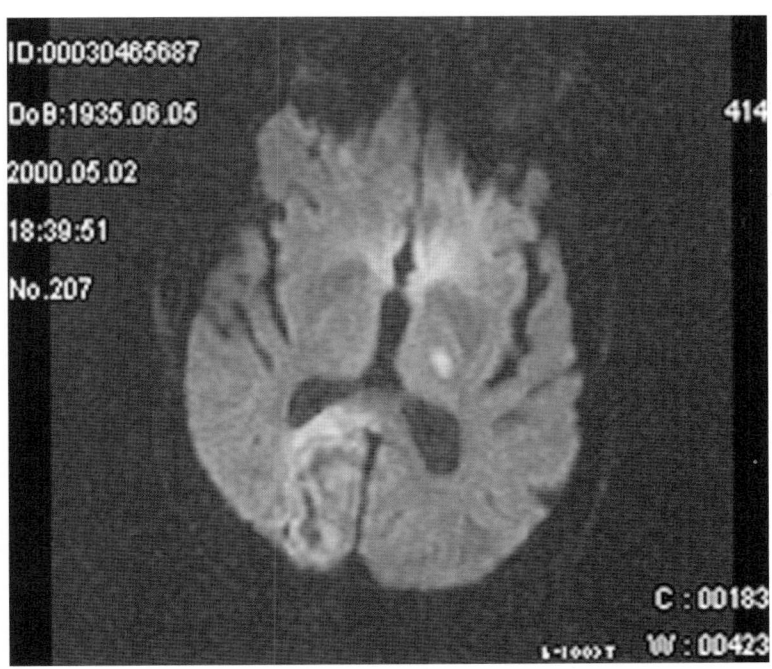

Figure 110.2 Confusion post open heart surgery—multifocal embolization.

Circulatory arrest is required when the aortic arch is too diseased to permit cross-clamping or during aortic reconstruction and repair of congenital malformations. Various studies have demonstrated that cognitive deficits increase with circulatory arrest time and increasing age, so hypothermic retrograde cerebral perfusion is used when circulatory arrest is expected to exceed a safe interval.

Genetics

Autopsy studies from patients with intracranial hemorrhage complicating thrombolytic therapy for acute myocardial infarction often reveal underlying amyloid angiopathy. This has been proposed to explain the increased risk of hemorrhage with advancing age.

Clinical features

Cardiac angiographic procedures

Cerebral embolism complicating coronary angiographic procedures affects the vertebrobasilar distribution in 60% of cases and presents with combinations of cortical blindness, hemianoptic visual field defects, intrinsic brainstem signs, confusion and amnesia. The carotid circulation accounts for 30% to 40% of focal

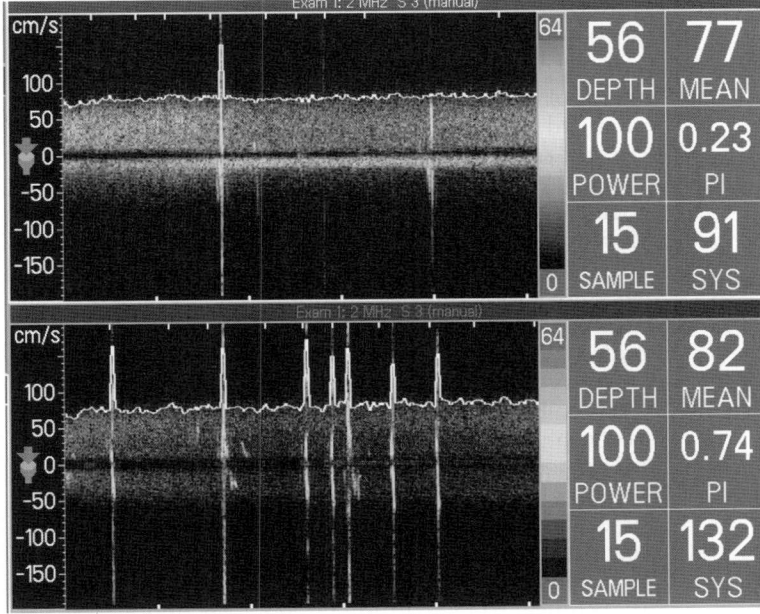

Figure 110.3 Embolus during bypass—transcranial Doppler. (See color plate section.)

deficits, consisting of combinations of hemiparesis, hemisensory deficits, retinal ischemia, and dysphasia. In the setting of coronary angiography, about half of the focal defects resolve within 48 hours but disabling and fatal stroke can also occur.[5]

Most of the hemorrhages complicating thrombolysis for acute myocardial infarction are solitary and lobar in location although multifocal hemorrhage, subdural hemorrhage, and ventricular rupture are common and their appearance tends to be bizarre with mottling and blood–fluid levels. Many are clinically recognized during the infusion of the lytic or shortly afterward; most occur within 24 hours of therapy. Half of those affected die within the first week but one-third achieve at least a good recovery. Predictors of mortality include hemorrhage volume, Glasgow Coma Scale score, and early onset of hemorrhage.[34]

Cardiac surgical procedures

Patients who develop stroke after CABG have a 3 to 5 fold higher in-hospital mortality rate as well as greater intensive care unit and hospital length of stay and discharge to extended care facilities. The prognosis of postoperative nonmetabolic coma is extremely poor, with an 85% mortality and a less than 5% chance of useful neurological recovery.

Clinically recognizable encephalopathy persisting to the fourth postoperative day occurs in 3% to 12% of patients although 80% of these recover to be able to perform normally on a simple mental status test by the time of discharge.[16] Prospective investigations employing extensive neuropsychological test batteries have found that 35% to 75% of patients have impairments in cognitive function, 20% severe, within the first 7 to 10 days, and 10% to 30% have persistent significant deficits, particularly in attention, concentration, memory and the speed of mental and motor responses, at 3 to 6 months. Those who experience early cognitive decline, particularly older patients and those with lower levels of education, are also more likely to develop late cognitive deterioration.[35]

Diagnostic criteria/process

The diagnosis of stroke in the setting of a cardiac intervention is no different than in other situations but some general observations about stroke subtype can be made. In the setting of nontransplant cardiac surgery, stroke is almost exclusively ischemic in nature. After thrombolysis for acute myocardial infarction, intracranial bleeding should be considered the cause of any acute neurological deterioration until proven otherwise.

Differential diagnosis
Treatment

Cardiac angiographic procedures The first opportunity for treatment begins with prevention. The complication rates of angiographic procedures have been reduced through proper patient selection, modifications in catheterization technique and design, acquisi-

tion of experience by the angiographers, and clinical trials designed to titrate various antithrombotic regimens for optimal outcome.

Acute neurological deterioration after thrombolysis for acute myocardial infarction should be presumed to be an intracranial hemorrhage until proven otherwise.[36] All thrombolytic, antithrombotic and antiplatelet therapies should be stopped immediately while the patient is stabilized and blood is drawn for coagulation studies including platelet count, prothrombin time (PT), and activated clotting time (ACT) or activated partial thromboplastin time (aPTT). Reversal of the coagulation disturbance should not be delayed by awaiting confirmation of the clinical suspicion with an emergency CT brain scan as the hemorrhage can expand rapidly within several hours.

Cardiac surgical procedures Concomitant cerebrovascular disease is a risk factor for stroke during CABG, but the role of prophylactic carotid endarterectomy (CE) to reduce stroke risk remains controversial. The patients at highest risk include those with symptomatic and severe stenoses, carotid occlusion, and bilateral, greater than 50% carotid stenosis as well as those with significant intracranial stenoses. Meta-analysis of 16 non-randomized studies concluded that the risk of stroke or death was significantly increased for combined surgery versus staged surgery. The rates of stroke, death, and stroke or death were 6.0%, 4.7%, and 9.5% for combined surgery versus 3.2%, 2.9%, and 5.7% for staged surgery.[37] Until the requisite data are available, a reasonable approach to patients with carotid disease undergoing CABG surgery is to attempt to view the carotid disease independently. Based on clinical trials, CE should be performed for symptomatic, greater than 70% carotid stenosis, prior to CABG if the coronary status is stable, or combined if both diseases are unstable as the long term prognosis of this group is poor with 36% mortality at 3.4 years.[38] Prophylactic endarterectomy prior to or combined with CABG for most patients with asymptomatic carotid stenosis is not supported by the data available but the management of this subgroup is likely to be significantly changed with the completion of clinical trials of carotid angioplasty and stenting in high risk patients.

Limiting embolization during CPB has long been a focus for technological improvements. In-line filtration with 40 micron filters and membrane oxygenators were introduced to filter macroemboli such as air, fat, glove powder, PVC tubing debris, and silicone antifoaming agents. Heparin-bonded and closed circuits have been developed to reduce activation of the inflammatory and coagulation system while on bypass. Eliminating CPB with "off-pump" surgery is accomplished via special stabilizers to minimize movement of the beating heart during vascular anastomoses. Although embolism from an atheromatous or calcific aortic arch may be less, the longer, more technically challenging surgery and increased risk of hypotension with the procedure warrants comparative clinical trials to guide patient selection.

Numerous "neuroprotective" therapies, efficacious in animal models when administered prior to an ischemic insult, have not been beneficial in the treatment of acute ischemic stroke. However, cardiac surgery offers a clinical scenario in which the nature and exact timing of a potential cerebral injury can be predicted and affords a unique opportunity to ameliorate neural injury with treatment prior to and during the operation.

The current options for treating acute ischemic stroke are restricted by the difficulty with timing onset in an anesthetized patient as well as the postoperative state posing an increased risk of bleeding. Recent surgery is an exclusion criterion in all the trials of thrombolytic therapy for acute ischemic stroke, however catastrophic cerebral embolism after a successful cardiac surgery often occurs in a monitored setting with rapid access to interventional therapies. Preliminary experience with intra-arterial thrombolysis within hours of acute ischemic stroke has met with mixed success in recanalization but few major hemorrhagic complications when performed within several days of cardiac surgery.[39] With the advent of mechanical clot disruption and extraction methods as an adjunct to thrombolysis, progress in effective stroke management in the postoperative setting is likely to improve.

References

1. Sones MF, Shirey EK, Proudfit WL, Westcott RN. Cine coronary angiography. Circulation 1959;20:773
2. Favalaro RG. Saphenous vein autograft replacement of severe segmental coronary artery occlusion: operative techniques. Ann Thorac Surg 1968;5:334–339
3. Gruentzig AR, Senning A, Siegenthaler WE. Non-operative dilatation of coronary artery stenosis: Percutaneous transluminal coronary angioplasty. N Engl J Med 1979;301:61–68
4. Roach GW, Kanchuger M, Mangano CM, et al. Adverse cerebral outcomes after coronary bypass surgery. N Engl J Med 1996;335:1857–1863
5. Dawson DM, Fischer EG. Neurologic complications of cardiac catheterization. Neurology 1977;27:496–497
6. Holmes DR, Holubkov R, Vlietstra RE, et al. Comparison of complications during percutaneous transluminal coronary angioplasty from 1977–1981 and 1985–1986. The NHLBI Percutaneous Transluminal Coronary Angioplasty Registry. J Am Coll Cardiol 1988;12: 1149–1155
7. The NHLBI Balloon Valvuloplasty Registry. Complications and mortality of percutaneous balloon mitral commissurotomy. Circulation 1992;85:2014–2024
8. NHLBI Balloon Registry Participants. Percutaneous balloon aortic valvuloplasty. Acute and 30 day followup results in 674 patients from the NHLBI balloon valvuloplasty registry. Circulation 1991;84:2383–2387
9. Sila CA. Neurologic complications of vascular surgery. In: Evans RW, ed. Neurology and Iatrogenic Disorders, Neurologic Clinics of North America. Philadelphia: WB Saunders, 1998:9–20
10. Sticherling C, Berkefeld J, Auch-Schwelk W, Lanfermann H. Transient cortical blindness after coronary angiography. Lancet 1998;351(9102):570
11. Kennedy AM, Grocott M, Schwartz MS, et al. Median nerve injury: an underrecognised complication of brachial artery catheterization? J Neurol Neurosurg Psychiatry 1997;63:54206
12. Schomig A, Neumann FJ, Kastrati A, et al. A randomized comparison of antiplatelet and anticoagulant therapy after the placement of coronary artery stents. N Engl J Med 1996;334:1084–1089
13. Harvey JC, Goldstein JE, McCabe JC, et al. Complications of percutaneous intra-aortic balloon pumping. Circulation 1981;64:1114–1117
14. Sila CA. Cerebrovascular aspects. In: Lincoff AM, ed. Glycoprotein IIb/IIIa Inhibitors in Cardiology. Humana Press, 1999:315–326
15. Vaitkus PT, Berlin JA, Schwartz JS, Barnathan ES. Stroke complicating acute myocardial infarction—a meta-analysis of risk modification by anticoagulation and thrombolytic therapy. Arch Intern Med 1992;152: 2020–2024
16. Breuer AC, Furlan AJ, Hanson MR, et al. Central nervous system complications of coronary artery bypass graft surgery: Prospective analysis of 421 patients. Stroke 1983;14:682–687
17. Murkin JM, Newman SP, Stump DA, Blumenthal JA. Statement of consensus on assessment of neurobehavioral outcomes after cardiac surgery. Ann Thorac Surg 1995;59:1289–1295
18. Lederman RJ, Breuer AC, Hanson MR, et al. Peripheral nervous system complications of coronary artery bypass graft surgery. Ann Neurol 1982;12:297–301
19. Wolman RL, Nussmeier NA, Aggarwal A, et al. Cerebral injury after cardiac surgery: identification of a group at extraordinary risk. Multicenter Study of Perioperative Ischemia Research Group (McSPI) and the Ischemia Research Education Foundation (IREF) Investigators. Stroke 1999;30(3):514–522
20. Svensson LG, Crawford ES, Hess KR, et al. Deep hypothermia with circulatory arrest. Determinants of stroke and early mortality in 656 patients. J Thorac Cardiovasc Surg 1993;106:19–28
21. Stevens GHJ, Brown M, Furlan AJ. Hypothermic retrograde cerebral perfusion: Neurologic complications. Neurology 1996;46:A257
22. Fischer A, Ozbek C, Bay W, Hamann GF. Cerebral microemboli during left heart catheterization. Am Heart J 1999;137:162–168
23. Kosmorsky G, Hanson MR, Tomsak RL. Neuro-ophthalmologic complications of cardiac catheterization. Neurology 1988;38:483–485
24. Hinchey J, Sweeney P. Transient cortical blindness after coronary angiography. Lancet 1998;351(9114): 1513–1514
25. Stamou SC, Hill PC, Dangas G, et al. Stroke after coronary artery bypass: Incidence, predictors, and clinical outcome. Stroke 2001;32:1508–1513
26. Hanna JP, Katzan IL, Sila CA. Intracranial hemorrhage following cardiothoracic surgery. Neurology 1998:A
27. Harris DN, Bailey SM, Smith PL, et al. Brain swelling in the first hour after coronary artery bypass surgery. Lancet 1993;342:586–587
28. Barbut D, Yao FS, Hager DN, et al. Comparison of transcranial Doppler ultrasonography and transesophageal echocardiography to monitor emboli during cardiopulmonary bypass. Stroke 1996;27:87–90
29. Pugsley W, Klinger L, Paschalis C, et al. The impact of microemboli during cardiopulmonary bypass on neuropsychological functioning. Stroke 1994;25:1393–1399
30. Diegler A, Hirsch R, Schneider F, et al. Neuromonitoring and neurocognitive outcome in off-pump versus conventional coronary bypass operation. Ann Thorac Surg 2000;69:1162–1166

31. Blauth CI, Cosgrove DM, Webb BW, et al. Atheroembolism from the ascending aorta. An emerging problem in cardiac surgery. J Thorac Cardiovasc Surg 1992;103: 1104–1112

32. Newman MF, Croughwell ND, White WD, et al. Effect of perfusion pressure on CBF during normothermic CPB. Circulation 1996;94:353–357

33. Croughwell ND, Lyth M, Quill TJ, et al. Diabetic patients have abnormal cerebral autoregulation during CPB. Circulation 1990;82:407–412

34. Gebel J, Sila CA, Sloan MA, et al. Thrombolysis-related intracranial hemorrhage. A radiographic analysis of 244 cases from the GUSTO-I trial. Stroke 1998;29: 563–569

35. Newman MF, Kirchner JL, Phillips-Bute B, et al. Longitudinal assessment of neurocognitive function after coronary artery bypass surgery. N Engl J Med 2001;344: 451–452

36. Sloan MA, Sila CA, Mahaffey KW, et al. Prediction of 30-day mortality among patients with thrombolysis-related intracranial hemorrhage. Circulation 1998;98: 1376–1382

37. Borger MA, Fremes SE, Weisel RD, et al. Coronary bypass and carotid endarterectomy: does a combined approach increase risk? A metaanalysis. Ann Thorac Surg 1999;68:14–20

38. Link MJ, Meyer FB, Orszulak TA, et al. Combined carotid and coronary revascularization. Stroke 1994;25: 272

39. Katzan I, Masaryk TJ, Furlan AJ, et al. Intra-arterial thrombolysis for perioperative stroke after open heart surgery. Neurology 1999;52:1081–1084

111 Cardiac Arrhythmias and Sudden Death

William T Talman

Although cardiac arrhythmias clearly may predispose patients to neurological illness, discussion of the recognition and management of arrhythmias and their pathophysiological contributions is beyond the scope of this chapter. The reader is therefore referred to recent reviews on the topic.[1,2] Suffice it to say that evaluation of the patient with stroke would be incomplete without electrocardiographic evaluation for atrial fibrillation. Similarly, evaluation of sudden unexplained loss of consciousness would not be complete without consideration of possible cardiac tachy- or bradyarrhythmias (ventricular or supraventricular) that could compromise cardiac output and hence cerebral blood flow. Attention to the neurological complications of treatments for the same arrhythmias must also be reserved for another forum.

Instead, this chapter is devoted to a consideration of contributions that the nervous system, particularly the central nervous system (CNS), may make to the development of cardiac arrhythmias. Indeed, the impact that the nervous system may have on autonomic and neurohumoral influences on cardiovascular function in health and disease is profound and may contribute to morbidity and mortality associated with nervous system disease.

Cardiac arrhythmias complicating CNS disease are well recognized,[3,4] as is the need for their aggressive management.[5] The range of central disorders that may lead to arrhythmias is legion,[6] although arrhythmias are best described in patients with subarachnoid hemorrhage. Arrhythmias may contribute to the high incidence (4% to 5%) of sudden death seen in that condition,[7] but fatal outcome from arrhythmia is certainly not restricted to patients with subarachnoid hemorrhage. Some studies report that 5% to 8% of patients with intracerebral hemorrhages also died suddenly.[8,9] Arrhythmias have even occurred briefly during neurosurgical manipulation of the brain and have stopped with cessation of the manipulation.[10] It is worth noting that irritative lesions account for most centrally mediated arrhythmias. Thus, arrhythmias are frequently associated with potentially epileptogenic processes such as intracranial hemorrhage, trauma, surgery and tumors. Of course, not all arrhythmogenic lesions are irritative. Some may lead to arrhythmias by altering the symmetry of sympathetic activity. Such imbalances could be the basis for arrhythmias seen in patients with multiple sclerosis[11] and Alzheimer's disease.[12]

The arrhythmogenic potential of a lesion is dependent not only on the nature of the lesion but also on its location and the age of the patient. The elderly tend to be affected more than the young.[13,14]

Long QT intervals, which may predispose patients to cardiac arrhythmias, occur with particularly high frequency when lesions affect the limbic system,[15] but limbic involvement is not essential. Cortical hemispheric involvement may be arrhythmogenic as well. When it is, there may be a predilection for arrhythmias when the right hemisphere[14] and insular cortex[16,17] are involved. However, whether there is indeed "dominance" of one hemisphere in autonomic control is yet to be proven.

Centrally mediated arrhythmias may occur in the absence of demonstrable cardiac disease. On the other hand, a central mechanism may contribute even when arrhythmias are associated with ischemic cardiac disease. For example, stress such as that induced by an earthquake can lead to a significantly increased incidence of sudden death that seems to affect those at risk.[18] Less prominent stressful events may contribute significantly to episodes of sudden death seen each year in individuals who are at risk.[18,19] The risk of stress-related cardiac events may be further magnified in the presence of cerebral ischemia.[20]

Because of the great danger imposed by some cardiac arrhythmias in patients with cerebral lesions, particularly those with subarachnoid hemorrhages, treatment of arrhythmias should be approached aggressively, as it is in patients who have suffered an acute myocardial infarction.[7] In some situations, such as arrhythmogenic seizures, the best therapy for arrhythmias is direct treatment of the underlying central condition[21] and effective management of ventilatory dysfunction, that may compromise cardiac function.[22]

Much evidence points to altered cardiac autonomic activity as a contributor to cardiac arrhythmias and sudden death associated with central disorders such as subarachnoid hemorrhage, other cerebrovascular events,[7] and epilepsy.[23,24] Although autonomic disturbances may still be suspected, the central cause of sudden death in some conditions remains elusive. Dysfunction in the CNS is certainly a suspected contributor in sudden death in adults,[25] in digitalis-induced arrhythmias,[26,27] and in the idiopathic long QT syndrome.[28] The central events associated with these conditions, even when the accompanying arrhythmia is profound and fatal, may not be related to gross CNS lesions[29] and certainly do not depend on coronary vascular disease.[16,30,31] It appears that the syndrome, which may be triggered by the autonomic nervous system, may occur as a result of an isolated cardiac electrical event. The ECG changes in the long QT syndrome, a well recognized risk factor for sudden death,[28] may clearly result from autonomic stimulation or localized central lesions,[25] and may reflect imbalances between the activity of the left and right sympathetic innervation of the heart.[32] However, although prolongation of the QT interval and even sudden death may result from a central lesion, a specific relationship between the long QT syndrome and a central disorder has not been established. It will be difficult to make an absolute association in that pathological sympathetic activation may be mediated by the CNS without any demonstrable CNS lesion but may instead result from naturally occurring behavioral events.[6] As noted previously, stress itself can lead to arrhythmias through a number of pathophysiological mechanisms. Inescapable, unavoidable stress seems particularly prone to lead to cardiac arrhythmia and sudden death.[33,34] One patient seen at the University of Iowa exemplified how profound the effect of psychological factors can be on cardiac rhythm. This patient, a young woman with clearly documented pseudoseizures, was told that her spells were pseudoseizures and that she did not require continued treatment with antiepileptic medications. She was convinced that her spells were real and that stopping her medication would cause her to die. Nonetheless, her physicians told her they planned to taper her medications. Before the taper had started, she repeatedly manifested her typical pseudoseizures that were consistently accompanied by transient cardiac asystole and apnea. Normal ventilation and correction of her ECG to a normal sinus rhythm occurred without intervention within 30–45 seconds. With the addition of muscarinic antagonists, but no other change in her medical regimen, the patient became symptom free and has remained so for four years.

Clearly, potential central influences on cardiac rhythm may be profound, but those influences may have an even greater impact when there is coexistent disease of the peripheral nervous system. The Guillain–Barré syndrome is a good example. In it, the incidence of arrhythmias and sudden death is increased as an apparent result of increased sympathetic activity.[35] Diabetic polyneuropathy, in which an increased incidence of sudden death also has been described, is yet another example.[36]

This brief review emphasizes how the nervous and cardiovascular systems maintain a balance and how disturbances in one may profoundly affect function in the other. It emphasizes that one must be vigilant in guarding against such imbalances because outcomes from neurologic disorders may be significantly adversely affected by correlative changes in cardiac function.

References

1. Singh BN. Overview of trends in the control of cardiac arrhythmia: past and future. Am J Cardiol 1999;84:3–10
2. Sen S, Oppenheimer SM. Cardiac disorders and stroke. Curr Opin Neurol 1998;11:51–56
3. Danilewsky B. Experimentelle beitrage zur physiologie des gehirns. Pflügers Arch 1875;11:128–138
4. Schiff M. Untersuchungen uber die motorischen functionen des gross-hirns. Naunyn-Schmiedeberg's Arch Pharmacol 1875;3:171–179
5. Parizel G. Life-threatening arrhythmias in subarachnoid hemorrhage. Angiology 1973;24:17–21
6. Talman WT. The central nervous system and cardiovascular control in health and disease. In: Low PA, ed. Clinical Autonomic Disorders: Evaluation and Management, 2nd edn. Boston: Little Brown, 1997:47–59
7. Parizel G. On the mechanism of sudden death with subarachnoid hemorrhage. J Neurol 1979;220:71–76
8. Hamman L. Sudden death. Bull Johns Hopkins Hosp 1934;55:387–415
9. Helpern M, Rabson SM. Sudden and unexpected death—general considerations and statistics. NY State J Med 1945;45:1197–1201
10. Hayashi S, Watanabe J, Miyagawa S, et al. Studies of electrocardiographic patterns in cases with neurosurgical lesions. Jpn Heart J 1961;2:92–111
11. Schroth WS, Tenner SM, Rappaport BA, Mani R. Multiple sclerosis as a cause of atrial fibrillation and electrocardiographic changes. Arch Neurol 1992;49:422–424
12. Aharon-Peretz J, Harel T, Revach M, Ben-Haim SA. Increased sympathetic and decreased parasympathetic cardiac innervation in patients with Alzheimer's disease. Arch Neurol 1992;49:919–922
13. Hachinski VC, Wilson JX, Smith KE, Cechetto DF. Effect of age on autonomic and cardiac responses in a rat stroke model. Arch Neurol 1992;49:690–696
14. Hachinski VC, Oppenheimer SM, Wilson JX, et al. Asymmetry of sympathetic consequences of experimental stroke. Arch Neurol 1992;49:697–702
15. Koepp M, Kern A, Schmidt D. Electrocardiographic changes in patients with brain tumors. Arch Neurol 1995;52:152–155
16. Oppenheimer SM, Wilson JX, Guiraudon C, Cechetto DF. Insular cortex stimulation produces lethal cardiac arrhythmias: a mechanism of sudden death. Brain Res 1991;550:115–121
17. Tokgözoglu SL, Batur MK, Topçuoglu MA, et al. Effects of stroke localization on cardiac autonomic balance and sudden death. Stroke 1999;30:1307–1311
18. Leor J, Poole WK, Kloner RA. Sudden cardiac death triggered by an earthquake. N Engl J Med 1996;334:413–419
19. Muller JE, Verrier RL. Triggering of sudden death-lessons from an earthquake. N Engl J Med 1996;334:460–461
20. Cheung RT, Hachinski VC, Cechetto DF. Cardiovascular response to stress after middle cerebral artery occlusion in rats. Brain Res 1997;747:181–188
21. Liedholm LJ, Gudjonsson O. Cardiac arrest due to partial epileptic seizures. Neurology 1992;42:824–829
22. Johnston SC, Siedenberg R, Min JK, et al. Central apnea and acute cardiac ischemia in a sheep model of epileptic sudden death. Ann Neurol 1997;42:588–594
23. Blumhardt LD, Smith PEM, Owen L. Electrocardiographic accompaniments of temporal lobe epileptic seizures. Lancet 1986;i:1051–1056
24. Van Buren JM, Ajmone-Marsan C. A correlation of autonomic and EEG components in temporal lobe epilepsy. Arch Neurol 1960;3:683–703
25. Oppenheimer SM, Cechetto DF, Hachinski VC. Cerebrogenic cardiac arrhythmias: cerebral electrocardiographic influences and their role in sudden death. Arch Neurol 1990;47:513–519
26. Gillis RA, Quest JA. The role of the nervous system in the cardiovascular effects of digitalis. Pharmacol Rev 1979;31:19–97
27. Natelson BH. Stress, predisposition and the onset of

serious disease: implications about psychosomatic etiology. Neurosci Biobehav Rev 1991;7:511–527

28. Schwartz PJ, Periti M, Malliani A. The long Q-T syndrome. Am Heart J 1975;89:378–390

29. Lown B. Sudden cardiac death: the major challenge confronting contemporary cardiology. Am J Cardiol 1979;43:313–328

30. Lown B, Temte JV, Reich P, et al. Basis for recurring ventricular fibrillation in the absence of coronary heart disease and its management. N Engl J Med 1976; 294:623–629

31. Moss AJ. Prediction and prevention of sudden cardiac death. Ann Rev Med 1980;31:1–14

32. Malliani A, Schwartz PJ, Zanchetti A. Neural mechanisms in life-threatening arrhythmias. Am Heart J 1980; 100:705–715

33. Cannon WB. "Voodoo" death. Am Anthropologist 1942;44:169–181

34. Engel GL. Psychologic factors in instantaneous cardiac death. N Engl J Med 1976;294:664–665

35. Greenland P, Griggs RC. Arrhythmic complications in the Guillain-Barré syndrome. Arch Intern Med 1980; 140:1053–1055

36. Weston PJ, Gill GV. Is undetected autonomic dysfunction responsible for sudden death in type 1 diabetes mellitus? The "dead in bed" syndrome revisited. Diabet Med 1999;16:626–631

112 Endocarditis (Infective and Non-Infective)

Amy Pruitt

Introduction

Well over a century has passed since William Osler highlighted the association of fever, heart murmur, and hemiplegia.[1] Since Osler's detailed description of infective endocarditis (IE), many reports of neurological complications have appeared. Despite markedly changing demographics, there is striking uniformity in the frequency and distribution of neurological problems associated with the condition.[2–7] The author's two series (separated by 17 years), as well as other reports spanning six decades, concur that about 30% of patients with IE will have neurological complications, for about half of whom the neurological event will be the presenting clinical symptom. In most series, patients experiencing neurological complications have mortality rates between 1.5 and 3 times higher than patients without such complications. Table 112.1 summarizes the percentage of neurological complications and mortality in 1097 patients from six series published during the last 24 years.

Epidemiology

The stable incidence and mortality rates mask a changing spectrum of conditions predisposing to IE and an evolving range of causative organisms. The risk of nervous system involvement in endocarditis depends on the predisposing condition. Predisposing conditions include underlying cardiac abnormalities, patient behavior, and medical or surgical therapies of other conditions. In the pre-antibiotic era, rheumatic heart disease accounted for 39% to 76% of cases.[8–10] More recent series report a declining frequency of rheumatic heart disease and a rising percentage of IE cases of which no underlying cardiac condition is apparent. Currently, among identifiable predisposing conditions, mitral valve prolapse and degenerative conditions such as calcific aortic stenosis outweigh congenital heart disease and rheumatic heart disease.[11,12] Ten to twenty percent of cases of IE in patients over age 60 may be hospital-acquired from iatrogenic risk factors, including invasive instrumentation of the gastrointestinal and genitourinary tracks, and indwelling devices such as pacemakers, intra-aortic balloon pumps and central intravenous catheters. Improved treatment of native valve IE has led to an increasing population at risk for prosthetic valve endocarditis; 25% of IE cases occurred on prosthetic valves in a recent series.[7] Intravenous drug abuse accounts for an increasing percentage of community-acquired IE and stroke (with or without IE) among young adults, and several series identify the salient features of drug-abuse-related IE relevant to neurological morbidity.[13–16] Right and left heart valves are affected roughly equally in drug abusers with IE and neurological complications. *Staphylococcus aureus* is the causative organism in two-thirds of these patients.

Etiology

As the population at risk for IE tends to include increasing numbers of very ill patients with systemic neoplasia and multiple organ failure, the distribution of pathogenic micro-organisms increasingly includes virulent, often multiple antibiotic-resistant bacteria and fungi. Non-bacterial thrombotic endocarditis presents with fever, stroke, and sometimes a cardiac murmur in patients with systemic neoplasia and coagulation abnormalities.

Table 112.1 Neurological complications of infective endocarditis

Reference	No. of patients	% Neurological complication	% Stroke[†]	Mortality Neuro+	Neuro−
Pruitt,[2]	216	39	17	58	20
Salgado,[3]	175	36.5	17	20.6	14.6
Gransden,[4]	178*	33	7		
Kaner,[5]	166*	33.5	20	35	19
Pruitt,[6]	144	29	18	32	13
Heiro,[7]	218	25	11	24	10

*Series included only native valve endocarditis; [†] ischemic and hemorrhagic strokes are grouped together.

Table 112.2   Clinical features of _Staphylococcus aureus_ endocarditis[6,7,15–17,45]

Incidence	Up to 40% of endocarditis cases
Risk factors	60% of patients are intravenous drug abusers 50% of intravenous drug abusers have _S. aureus_ as pathogen 50% of prosthetic valve endocarditis cases have _S. aureus_ as pathogen
Mortality	32% _S. aureus_ cases vs 11.2% of cases due to other pathogens Congestive heart failure, conduction disturbances, and neurological complications explain excess mortality
Neurological complications	39% to 50% of _S. aureus_ group vs 25% other pathogens Early cerebral embolism, septic arteritis, purulent meningitis, and mycotic aneurysms are major issues Patients with _S. aureus_ prosthetic valve endocarditis receiving anticoagulants are particularly prone to cerebral hemorrhage 54% to 66% of _S. aureus_ neurological complications occurred at presentation vs 19% for streptococcal cases
S. aureus _bacteremia_	13% to 25% bacteremic patients have definite endocarditis by TTE/TEE* Risk factors for endocarditis are community acquisition, absence of infectious focus, fever/bacteremia more than 3 days after removal of infected intravenous catheter TEE used to determine duration of antibiotic treatment in patients with intravenous catheter-associated bacteremia

*TTE/TEE, transthoracic/transesophageal echocardiography.

The distribution of causative organisms varies somewhat among institutions due to disparate referral patterns and nosocomial issues, but the decline of streptococci as causative organisms from 90% in the pre-antibiotic era to less than 50% is a uniform observation. Of particular neurological relevance because of the frequency of complications in patients affected with them are two streptococci: Group D streptococci, of which _Enterococcus fecalis_ is the most common, is often antibiotic-resistant; and _Streptococcus bovis_, observed in association with digestive tract malignancy, has been associated with late cerebral emboli.

S. aureus now accounts for up to 40% of IE in some institutions. Valves with no apparent underlying cardiac lesions are affected in up to 30% of _S. aureus_ cases.[17,18] Nearly one-half of prosthetic valve endocarditis cases are due to staphylococcal species. Because of its current importance as the causative organism in IE, features of _S. aureus_ endocarditis are summarized in Table 112.2. A wider range of pathogens afflicts elderly patients with multiple system disease and immunocompromised patients, and these organisms include the HACEK bacteria group (_Hemophilus_, _Actinobacillus_, _Cardiobacterium_, _Eikenella_ and _Kingella_) and fungal organisms. In these often heavily pretreated patients, blood cultures may be persistently negative.

In contrast to the statistics from the USA, IE in developing countries has a different patient base and bacteriological spectrum. A review of 110 patients from a southern Indian referral hospital between 1977 and 1994 demonstrated that rheumatic heart disease remains the most frequent underlying cardiac lesion in patients of mean age 24 years. Neurological complications were frequent (52.7%) and mortality higher in the group with nervous system involvement.[19]

Pathophysiology and pathogenesis

Neurological complications of endocarditis can be divided into three general groups: ischemic stroke, hemorrhagic stroke and cerebral infection (abscess, meningitis). The vast majority of neurological complications of IE are due to embolism. It is postulated that the antithrombotic properties of the cardiac endothelial surface are lost during IE. Bacteria adhere to damaged endothelium, with subsequent platelet–fibrin deposition. Both septic and non-septic material may embolize, and either type may cause ischemic stroke, but septic emboli may also produce hemorrhagic stroke through direct vessel wall necrosis (arteritis) or mycotic aneurysm. Initially bland cerebral infarctions may convert to hemorrhagic ones. Emboli may also produce cerebral microabscesses, though macroabscesses are extremely rare, and embolism is also probably the cause of meningitis through seeding of the meninges. The development of infarction, aneurysm and abscess probably represents a continuum of processes whose outcome depends on host defense factors, the timing and appropriateness of antibiotic therapy, and organism virulence. A less common mechanism of neurological involvement in IE is delayed toxic or immune-mediated injury. Circulating immune complexes may play a role in systemic dysfunction such as glomerulonephritis, and in clinical signs such as petechiae, Osler's nodes, and Janeway's lesions, as well as in several infrequent neurological sequelae including late aneurysmal rupture and mononeuropathies.[20]

Clinical features

In most series, about 30% of patients with IE have a neurological complication. Patients with and without neurological complications of IE differ in several important respects. In patients with neurological complications, *S. aureus* is over-represented as the causative organism and intravenous drug abuse is disproportionately represented as a risk factor. Vegetations are more frequently detected by echocardiography in the group with neurological complications, but, in contrast to some earlier studies, the author's recent series at the University of Pennsylvania found no particular cardiac valve or valves to be more consistently affected in patients with neurological complications.[6] The mortality rate in patients with neurological complications is consistently about twice that of patients without such involvement, and about one-half of the mortality can be ascribed directly to the neurological problem.

Table 112.3 summarizes the distribution and timing of neurological complications of IE in the author's 1995 series from the University of Pennsylvania. This institution's experience is quite consistent with that of other large urban hospitals. Cerebral embolism was the most common neurological complication, occurring in 20 patients (14%). Sudden focal neurological episodes were investigated with computed tomography (CT) and in many cases with magnetic resonance imaging (MRI). Cerebral embolism was apparently single in 9 cases and multiple in 11 by

neuroimaging studies. Conversion to hemorrhagic infarction occurred spontaneously (without anticoagulation) in 3 of the 20 patients.

Primary intracranial hemorrhage was a significantly less common stroke mechanism, occurring in only 4.1% of the 144 episodes. Demonstrable mycotic aneurysms were found in only two of these patients, while septic arteritis was believed to account for three others. Subdural hematoma and hemorrhagic conversion of an initially bland infarction complicated one case. CNS infection in the form of brain abscess occurred in only 2% of patients and cerebrospinal fluid (CSF) pleocytosis was present in only 4.1%, a third of whom had culture-positive purulent meningitis (only 18 lumbar punctures were performed to investigate the 144 episodes of IE). Seizures complicated six courses of IE, and paraspinal abscess occurred in two patients.

Diagnostic procedures

The gold standard for definitive clinical diagnosis of IE traditionally has been two positive blood cultures in a patient without another identifiable nidus of infection. However, the current diagnostic criteria for IE, known as the Duke criteria and validated in several prospective studies, have modified the microbiological standard with the addition of echocardiographic demonstration of vegetations as a major criterion in 1994. Major criteria for the diagnosis of IE now include:

1. *Microbiological criteria:* isolation of typical IE-causing organisms from two separate blood cultures, or a single positive blood culture for Coxiella burnetii (Q fever).
2. *Echocardiographic evidence* of endocardial involvement, including new valvular regurgitation or TTE or TEE demonstrated vegetations.

TEE is recommended for patients with prosthetic valves. Minor criteria include predisposition to IE based on certain cardiac conditions and injection drug use, as well as immunological manifestations such as Osler's nodes or Roth spots. Some authors suggest that positive blood cultures for *S. aureus* in the setting of intravenous catheter infections should become a major criterion.

Thus, the diagnosis of IE depends on the presence of clinical risk factors, blood culture confirmation, and echocardiographic criteria, allowing the diagnosis of IE to be made with negative blood cultures if echocardiography and clinical risk factors are consistent. Transesophageal echocardiography (TEE) has proved superior to standard two-dimensional echocardiography for the detection of valvular abscesses, and particularly for definitive diagnosis of prosthetic valve endocarditis (PVE), with as many as 34% of previously "possible" PVE cases reclassified as "definite" by TEE.[21]

This section addresses the major controversies about the association between demonstrable valvular vegetations and risk for subsequent embolism, as well as increased likelihood of requirement for valve

---

Table 112.3 Neurological complications in 144 episodes of infective endocarditis[6]

	n	% of total	% at presentation
Stroke			
Cerebral embolism*	20	14	7
Single	9		
Multiple	11		
Hemorrhagic	3		
Hemorrhagic on warfarin	1		
Intracranial hemorrhage	6	4.1	2.8
Mycotic aneurysm	2		
Septic arteritis	3		
Subdural hematoma	1		
CNS infection			
Brain abscess	3	2	
Meningitis	4	2.6	
Aseptic	2		
Purulent	2		
Miscellaneous			
Seizures	6	4.1	1.3
Paraspinous abscess	2	1.3	1.3
Peroneal palsy	1		
Radial palsy	1		
Postoperative lower brachial plexopathy	1		
Delirium	2		
H. zoster	1		
Opiates	1		

*13 of 20 emboli (65%) occurred within 48 hours of presentation at a time of uncontrolled infection.

replacement for congestive heart failure. Several studies claim that demonstrable vegetations do not correlate with embolism risk and are equally common in patients with and without stroke.[18,22] Two meta-analyses looked at the risk of embolism in patients with and without demonstrable vegetations by transthoracic echocardiography, and found that patients with lesions larger than 10 mm had a higher incidence of emboli than those with smaller lesions (47% versus 19%).[23,24] Patients with left-sided heart valve vegetations greater than 10 mm had an increased risk of requiring valve replacement, with an odds ratio of 2.95.

As further data from TEE become available, more management decisions will be based on the presence and size of cardiac vegetations. DiSalvo and colleagues looked prospectively at both cerebral and systemic embolic events in 178 patients. Positive TEE predictors of embolism included vegetation length and mobility, particularly for patients with right valve endocarditis and *S. aureus* endocarditis.[25] Vila-costa and colleagues documented the ongoing risk of emboli after the institution of antibiotic therapy in 12.9% of their patients, the major risk factors being documented growth in vegetations, mitral valve location, *S. aureus* etiology, and prior embolism.[26] While the advent of TEE has been extremely helpful in diagnosis of IE, echocardiographic demonstration of vegetations in the absence of clinical cerebral embolism does not yet justify prophylactic valve replacement, as healing of such lesions has been clearly demonstrated. An exception to this policy is the identification of large vegetations in fungal endocarditis. Further refinement of TEE technique may lead to firmer guidelines.

Differential diagnosis

Of prime concern to the neurological consultant attempting to make an early diagnosis of IE are those CNS manifestations that precede or coincide with the diagnosis of IE. Early neurological involvement is most characteristic of *S. aureus* endocarditis. Fifty-four percent of neurological events associated with this organism occurred at presentation, whereas only 19% of streptococcal cases presented with a neurological problem. Heiro and colleagues point out in their recent series from Finland that 90% of all neurological complications occurred in the first week, more than half within the first 48 hours after admission.[7]

Because IE has protean initial manifestations, the neurologist must consider the possibility of IE in many different situations. The constellation of fever, elevated erythrocyte sedimentation rate, and cerebral infarction can be seen in many conditions other than IE, including arteritis, intravascular lymphoma, non-bacterial thrombotic endocarditis, and atrial myxoma. Conversely, the classic situation of a febrile patient with focal neurological deficit and changing heart murmur represents the minority of IE case presentations. The diagnosis of IE should be considered and appropriate blood cultures obtained in any febrile patient with a focal neurological deficit or headache,

or with an intracranial hemorrhage in a clinical setting lacking conventional risk factors for cerebral hemorrhage. Patients whose underlying heart condition dictates antimicrobial prophylaxis for various dental or surgical procedures should be questioned about compliance with the regimens outlined by Dajani and Seto.[27,28]

Culture-negative endocarditis (CNE) has become an increasing problem, as many hospitalized patients with nosocomially-acquired infections and possible endocarditis have received antibiotics. However, the major cause of CNE is Q fever, infection caused by *Coxiella burnetii*. Patients with Q fever endocarditis are particularly prone to embolism, and Q fever serology has been added to the Duke criteria for IE.[29,30] Useful diagnostic studies in a patient with suspected CNE include serological studies for Bartonella species, Chlamydia serology, PCR or culture of vegetation for *Tropheryma whipplei*, Brucella serologies, and continued blood culture surveillance for fungal species.

Treatment

Table 112.4 summarizes the major management issues confronting the neurologist who cares for patients with neurological complications of IE. As emphasized above, the majority of neurological complications occur early in the course of IE and the best treatment for ongoing or potential neurological problems is appropriate antibiotic therapy. Table 112.5 summarizes currently recommended antimicrobial strategies for common IE-causing organisms.

Management of cerebral embolism

The advent of CT scanning has revealed that nearly 50% of cerebral emboli in IE are multiple, compared with the reported 18% in the pre-CT era.[31] Computerized tomography to differentiate bland from hemorrhagic infarctions is the diagnostic procedure of choice for emergent investigation of sudden focal neurological deficit in IE. Magnetic resonance imaging (MRI), which demonstrates better the evolution of neuropathological processes from cerebral emboli to cerebritis to microabscess, aneurysm, or macroabscess formation, is useful in follow-up of cerebral emboli.

Anticoagulation for IE-associated cerebral embolism
Cerebral emboli cluster at IE presentation early in the course of the disease, during uncontrolled infection, and are accompanied by systemic emboli in nearly half of all cases. Only 15% of emboli occur more than 2 weeks after initiation of antibiotic therapy.[6] Despite the early morbidity and mortality from cerebral embolism, a case of cured native valve endocarditis (NVE) does not change future stroke risk in patients with valvular heart disease. These data suggest that anticoagulation is not indicated to prevent recurrent embolism in cured NVE.

A more urgent question is the role of anticoagulation during an episode of IE. Experimental evidence suggests that the risk of hemorrhage during anticoag-

Table 112.4   Major issues in the management of patients with infective endocarditis and neurological complications

Anticoagulation
- What are the risks and benefits of anticoagulation during an episode of endocarditis?
- Is there a role for heparin or antiplatelet agents?
- Should anticoagulation be discontinued when patients with prosthetic valves develop endocarditis?
- After an embolic stroke, when can anticoagulation be reinstituted safely in patients receiving antibiotics for endocarditis?
- Is a cured episode of native valve endocarditis a risk factor for future stroke?

Cardiac surgery
- What is the risk of neurological deterioration if a patient with a stroke requires emergent valve replacement?
- Should a single cerebral embolus be an indication for valve replacement?
- Is there an echocardiographically-defined group of patients who will benefit from valve repair surgery and avoiding prosthetic valves?
- Are there echocardiographic criteria for vegetations at great enough risk for cerebral embolism to warrant prophylactic cardiac surgery?

Infectious intracranial (mycotic) aneurysms
- Should a search for mycotic aneurysms be undertaken in every endocarditis patient?
- What is the role of magnetic resonance angiography in the detection and follow-up of mycotic aneurysms?
- What is the proper management of mycotic aneurysms?

Table 112.5   Antimicrobial therapy for common causes of infective endocarditis[45]

Pathogen	Native valve endocarditis	Prosthetic valve endocarditis
Penicillin-sensitive streptococci	Penicillin G for 4 weeks	Penicillin G for 6 weeks and gentamicin for 3 weeks
Methicillin-sensitive staphylococci	Nafcillin for 6–8 weeks and gentamicin for first 5 days	Nafcillin/Oxacillin for 8 weeks and gentamicin for 3 weeks
Methicillin-resistant staphylococci	Vancomycin for 8 weeks and gentamicin for 2 weeks	Vancomycin for 8 weeks and gentamicin for 2 weeks
HACEK organisms*	Ceftriaxone for 8 weeks	Ceftriaxone for 8 weeks

Clinicians should consult the infectious disease specialists in their individual hospitals for local antimicrobial resistance patterns and specific recommendations that may differ from the ones given here.
*See text for organisms in this group.

ulation may be very high when cerebral emboli are septic, and clinical series have produced disturbing statistics, such as the 1978 observation that one-half of cerebral hemorrhages occurred in the 3% of patients anticoagulated at the time of embolism.[2]

The advent of CT and MRI have given a better understanding of the rate of transformation of bland to hemorrhagic infarction and the time course of resolution of blood. In NVE, embolic recurrence rate is low after infection is controlled. Because virtually all emboli occur within the first 48 hours, anticoagulation is of no benefit in prevention of recurrent embolism. Vigorous effort should be made to control infection, including consideration of cardiac surgery for patients with large or growing vegetations. On the other hand, the development of uncomplicated prosthetic valve endocarditis (PVE) does not dictate cessation of otherwise indicated anticoagulation therapy. Insufficient data are available to make a recommendation about low molecular weight heparin therapy in this setting.

Patients with bioprosthetic or mechanical cardiac valves have a 1% to 4% incidence of IE, conventionally divided into "late" (more than 60 days postoperatively) and "early" (less than 50 days postoperatively). Aggregate data from more than 200 PVE patients in the literature suggest that inadequately anticoagulated patients with mechanical valves are at greatest risk for embolism during IE.[32,33] Thus, anticoagulation should be continued at the onset of PVE in a high-risk mechanical valve. However, the occurrence of a hemorrhage after embolization in an anticoagulated patient is associated with a roughly 80% mortality. Some authors believe that heparin may be safer than warfarin in the high-risk population of IE patients with mechanical prosthetic valves. If embolism occurs in an anticoagulated patient, the recommendations given above for NVE apply. For patients developing endocarditis with the highest risk mechanical valves, such as those manufactured by St Jude Medical or Bjork–Shiley, most authorities advise continuous heparinization. Table 112.6 summarizes the anticoagulation recommendations for NVE and PVE.

Table 112.6   Recommendations for anticoagulation in infective endocarditis

Endocarditis without neurological complications
- The development of native or prosthetic valve infective bacterial endocarditis does not mandate automatic cessation of otherwise indicated warfarin therapy
- If fungal prosthetic valve endocarditis is present, consider discontinuation of anticoagulation in all but the highest risk prostheses*
- Routine initiation of anticoagulants to prevent stroke in bioprosthetic valve endocarditis is not justified.

Endocarditis with cerebral embolism
- Anticoagulation should be withheld for 48 hours in patients suffering a cerebral embolism while receiving anticoagulation; CT should be obtained prior to reinstitution of anticoagulation
- Anticoagulation is not indicated for the prevention recurrent embolic stroke in native valve endocarditis

Follow-up after cerebral embolism
- Follow-up MRI, if clinically feasible, should be done in 1 to 2 weeks to allow documentation of resolution of cerebritis and/or microabscesses

*Some experts recommend discontinuation of anticoagulation when *S. aureus* endocarditis develops on prosthetic valves because of the high risk of embolism and subsequent hemorrhage.

Cardiac surgery in patients with neurological complications of IE

The occurrence of cerebral emboli may contribute to the decision about timing of valve replacement. The neurologist is frequently asked to comment about the risk of bleeding into an ischemic stroke during cardiac bypass or about the effect of non-pulsatile blood flow or hypotension on a recent cerebral infarction. Most consultants believe that cardiac valve replacement is not mandatory for patients with an episode of cerebral embolism in the absence of other cardiac indications. If emergent cardiac surgery is required for hemodynamic reasons, several studies suggest that patients operated on within the first week after stroke may suffer further neurological deterioration. The neurological complication rate of cardiac surgery was 30% for patients who required valve replacement within 2 weeks of a stroke.[6,34–36] More recently, Gillinov has documented that patients undergoing valve replacement at 3 weeks after stroke have no excess neurological morbidity when their CT scans show no evidence of hemorrhagic conversion of cerebral infarction.[37]

Absolute indications for cardiac surgery may preempt neurological considerations. These include refractory congestive heart failure, myocardial or perivalvular abscess, repeated relapses of IE despite antibiotic therapy, unstable prostheses, and fungal endocarditis. A relative indication may be multiple cerebral embolic episodes. The relative risk of embolism for patients with vegetations greater than 10 mm has been discussed previously. Future studies with transesophageal echocardiography may help to refine these recommendations.

Mycotic aneurysms

Infectious intracranial aneurysms, still often referred to by the slightly misleading Oslerian term "mycotic aneurysm," are recognized in 1% to 5% of IE cases. The true incidence almost certainly exceeds the reported one, since many aneurysms may heal after antibiotic therapy. Aneurysms in IE tend to be more peripheral than congenital aneurysms, and at least 20% are multiple. Fungal IE is associated with large proximal aneurysms.

Few debates in neurological management have generated as many pages of controversy as have discussions of the detection and therapy of mycotic aneurysms. Adding 28 of their own cases to numerous prior reports, Brust and colleagues have become the major advocates for early aggressive search for mycotic aneurysms in all cases of IE. They emphasize the high morbidity and mortality from aneurysms, and conclude that all patients should undergo CT and lumbar puncture. Those with neurological abnormalities, including isolated CSF pleocytosis, should undergo four-vessel cerebral angiography. Brust further recommends that single accessible mycotic aneurysms in medically stable patients be promptly excised.[38]

Opposing this view are Hart, Kanter, and others, who emphasize the rarity of mycotic aneurysms, their symptomatic clustering in the early stages of infection, and the extremely low incidence of later rupture after bacteriological cure.[39] Corr's recent longitudinal study of mycotic aneurysms on treatment found that no new aneurysms developed during appropriate treatment.[40] Four-vessel angiography remains the gold standard for the detection and follow-up of mycotic aneurysms. This author interprets the above data to suggest that the prevalence of unruptured mycotic aneurysms in patients with IE is really unknown, so that for the 1% to 2% of patients who experience rupture of aneurysms after hospital admission, there is no accurate denominator for the frequency of unruptured mycotic aneurysms to determine real risk. Current management at the author's institution includes emergent CT for patients with neurological symptoms. The presence of blood on CT dictates four-vessel angiography, and decisions about emergent surgery will depend on the patient's medical condition and the location and integrity of the aneurysm or aneurysms. Surgical techniques for mycotic aneurysm have evolved in the past few years, and CT now allows localized stereotactic craniotomy with laser-guided localization and excision of affected distal arterial branches.[41,42]

Although not every patient with IE requires cerebral angiography, several important clinical symptoms should not be ignored even when the neurological examination and the CT are normal. Severe persistent headache or "sentinel" transient embolic symptoms dictate lumbar puncture. Because minimal aneurysmal leakage can result in a focal meningeal reaction, CSF pleocytosis should sway the decision in favor of four-vessel angiography. Optimal treatment of mycotic aneurysms in IE remains unclear. Chun and colleagues reported successful outcomes in 16 of 20 patients (80%) with 27 infectious aneurysms, the majority due to IE. They suggest that unruptured aneurysms be treated medically with antibiotics and followed with serial angiography. Ruptured aneurysms without hematoma in non-eloquent brain areas can be treated with endovascular coiling. Surgical treatment is reserved for patients with ruptured aneurysms and hematomas who are unstable or who have failed endovascular treatment.[43] Since the true incidence of unruptured aneurysms in the IE populations is unknown, these data must be interpreted cautiously. Serial prospective CT and MRI/angiography correlation in high-risk groups such as patients with *S. aureus* endocarditis would allow definitive determination of the true incidence and clinical consequences of these aneurysms. Table 112.7 summarizes management recommendations for mycotic aneurysms.

Summary of management issues

The algorithm in Figure 112.1 summarizes our current approach to the management of a patient with known or suspected IE and a neurological abnormality in accordance with the following clinical series-based conclusions:

1. Anticoagulation is not indicated to prevent recurrent cerebral emboli in NVE. Anticoagulation should not be discontinued because of the development of uncomplicated IE in patients with mechanical valves. Anticoagulation should be withheld 48 hours after a cerebral embolus to minimize the risk of hemorrhage.
2. If emergent valve replacement is necessary in a patient with recent cerebral infarction, if possible, surgery should be delayed for 2 to 3 weeks following the stroke.
3. Routine search for mycotic aneurysm in all IE patients is not justified. Medical treatment may suffice for many aneurysms and for most macroabscesses. Advances in surgical technique may decrease the morbidity of vessel ligation, and each case should be considered on the basis of the aneurysm's location and the patient's medical condition.

Evolving diagnostic and management issues

Major management dilemmas continue to plague the clinician who seeks to provide optimal care for a patient with IE and neurological abnormalities. Diagnostic techniques allowing early identification and appropriate treatment of IE continue to evolve. The use of polymerase chain reaction amplification of specific gene targets and universal loci for bacteria continues to be investigated and may be incorporated into the Duke criteria, allowing specific identification of previously culture-negative cases.[44]

The major challenge in the management of IE is to keep abreast of the evolving spectrum of host factors and organisms and their impact on both neurological and systemic complications of IE. Mylonakis and Calderwood have recently provided an excellent review of IE in adults.[45] The most pressing concern for neurological management is the refinement of criteria to identify the few patients for whom surgical intervention either with valve replacement or aneurysm repair can minimize neurological morbidity. Other issues for which clinicians must look to future clinical investigations for definitive answers include:

1. The role of TEE in defining patients with bacteremia who can receive a shorter course of antibiotics.

Table 112.7   Summary of management recommendations for infectious intracranial (mycotic) aneurysms[6,38-43]

Angiography Routine angiography for all patients with endocarditis and cerebral embolism is not justified. Four-vessel angiography is prompted by:
- CT-documented blood
- CSF pleocytosis with persistent focal headache
- Magnetic resonance angiography is not a substitute for four-vessel arteriography in high-risk situations

Neurosurgery The indications for neurosurgical repair of aneurysm must be individualized by organism, location, number, and size, and by the patient's medical condition:
- Unruptured aneurysms can be treated medically and followed with serial angiography
- Ruptured aneurysms without hematoma in non-eloquent brain areas can be treated with endovascular coiling
- Ruptured aneurysms with hematomas or patients who are unstable or who have failed endovascular treatment are treated with conventional surgical clipping

Cardiac surgery
- Arteriography in all patients to detect asymptomatic aneurysm is not required prior to anticoagulation
- Patients with documented aneurysms should have cardiac surgery delayed, if possible, to allow healing of aneurysms

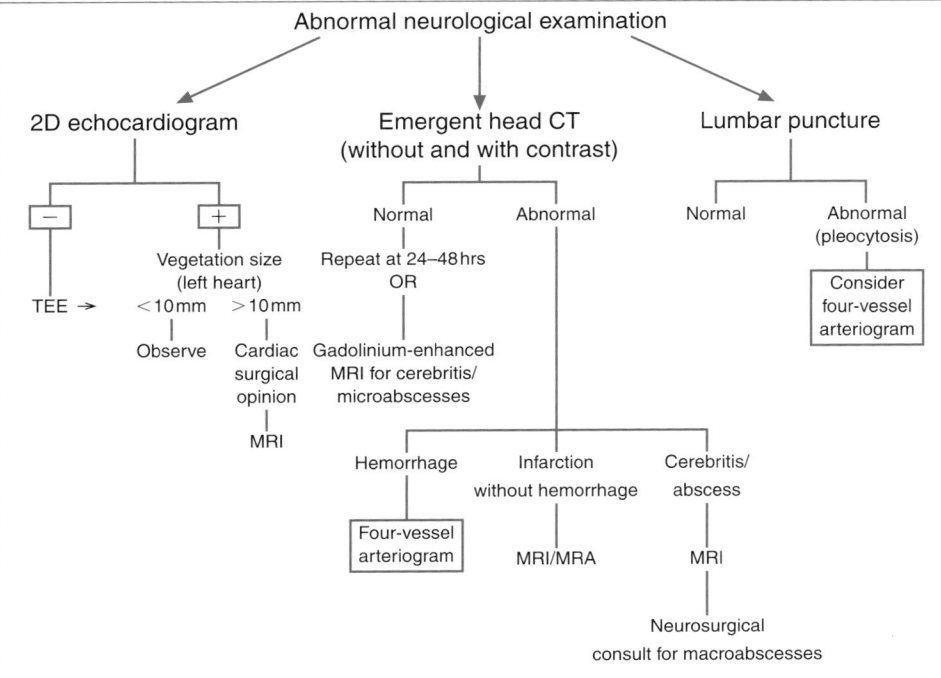

Figure 112.1 Management algorithm: the patient with known or suspected infective endocarditis and neurological abnormalities.

Pathways leading to four-vessel arteriography to diagnose mycotic aneurysms include: 1) CT-demonstrated hemorrhage; 2) Purulent meningitis even with a normal CT. MRI is the preferred neuro-imaging technique to define number of cerebral emboli and to follow resolution of cerebritis and abscesses. Arteriography is not mandatory for all patients with cerebral embolism requiring urgent cardiac valve replacement.

TEE, transesophageal echocardiography; MRI/MRA, magnetic resonance imaging/angiography.

2. The possible role of antiplatelet agents or low molecular weight heparinoids.
3. The sensitivity of MRA for detection of unruptured mycotic aneurysms.
4. The true incidence, consequences, and management of mycotic aneurysms in the group of patients at greatest risk for cerebral embolism (those with *S. aureus* endocarditis). Such patients should be studied prospectively with CT/MRI/MRA, and ateriography.

References

1. Osler W. Gulstonian lectures on malignant endocarditis. Lancet 1885;1:415–508
2. Pruitt AA, Rubin RH, Karchmer AW, et al. Neurologic complications of bacterial endocarditis. Medicine 1978; 57:329–343
3. Salgado SAV, Furlan AJ, Keyes TF, et al. Neurologic complications of endocarditis: a 12-year experience. Neurology 1989;39:173–178
4. Gransden WR, Eykyn SJ, Leach RM. Neurological presentations of native value endocarditis. QJM 1989;73: 1135–1142
5. Kanter MC, Hart RG. Neurologic complications of infective endocarditis. Neurology 1991;41:1015–1020
6. Pruitt AA. Neurologic complications of infective endocarditis: a review of an evolving disease and its management issues in the 1990s. Neurologist 1995;1: 20–34
7. Heiro M, Nikoskelainen J, Engblom E, et al. Neurologic manifestations of infective endocarditis: a 17-year experience in a teaching hospital in Finland. Arch Intern Med 2000;160:2781–2787
8. Rabinovich S, Evans J, Smith IM, et al. A long-term view of bacterial endocarditis. 337 cases 1924–1963. Ann Intern Med 1965;63:185–198
9. Francioli PB. Central nervous system complications of infective endocarditis. *In:* Scheld WM, Whitley RJ, Durack DT, eds. Infections of the Central Nervous System. New York: Raven Press, 1991
10. Cherubin CE, Neu HC. Infective endocarditis at the Presbyterian Hospital in New York City from 1938–1967. Am J Med 1971;51:83–85
11. Terpenning MS, Buggy BP, Kaufmann CA. Infective endocarditis: clinical features in young and elderly patients. Am J Med 1987;83:626–634
12. McKinsey DS, Ratts TE, Bisno A. Underlying cardiac lesions in adults with infective endocarditis. The changing spectrum. Am J Med 1987;82:681–688
13. Bevan H, Sharma K, Bradley W. Stroke in young adults. Stroke 1990;21:382–386
14. Kaku DA, Lowenstein DH. Emergence of recreational drug abuse as a major risk, factor for stroke in young adults. Ann Intern Med 1990;113:821–827
15. Sloan MA, Kittner SJ, Feeser BR, et al. Illicit drug-associated ischemic stroke in the Washington Young Stroke Study. Neurology 1998;19:1688–1693
16. Mathew J, Addai T, Anand A, et al. Clinical features, site of involvement, bacteriologic findings, and outcome of infective endocarditis in intravenous drug users. Arch Intern Med 1995;155:1641–1648
17. Roder BL, Wandall DA, Espersen F, et al. Neurologic manifestations in *Staphylococcus aureus* endocarditis: a review of 260 bacteremic cases in non-drug addicts. Am J Med 1997;102:379–386
18. Strom BL, Abrutyn E, Berlin JA, et al. Dental and cardiac risk factors for infective endocarditis: a popu-

lation-based case-control study. Ann Intern Med 1998; 129:761–769

19. Santoshkumar B, Radhaakrishnan K, Balakrishnan KG, et al. Neurologic complications of infective endocarditis observed in a south Indian referral hospital. J Neurol Sci 1996;137:139–144

20. Venger GH, Aldama AE. Mycotic vasculitis with repeated intracranial aneurysmal hemorrhage. J Neurosurg 1988;69:775–779

21. Roe MT, Abramson MA, Li J, et al. Clinical information determines the impact of transesophageal echocardiography on the diagnosis of infective endocarditis by the Duke criteria. Am Heart J 2000;139:945–951

22. Hart RG, Foster JW, Luther MF, et al. Stroke in infective endocarditis. Stroke 1990;21:695–700

23. Lutas EM, Roberts RB, Devereux RB, et al. Relation between the presence of echocardiographic vegetations and the complication rate in infective endocarditis. Am Heart J 1986;112:107–113

24. Tischler MD, Vaitkus PT. The ability of vegetation size on echocardiography to predict clinical complications: a meta-analysis. J Am Soc Echocardiogr 1997;10:562–568

25. Disalvo G, Habib G, Pergola V, et al. Echocardiography predicts embolic events in infective endocarditis. J Am Coll Cardiol 2001;37:1069–1076

26. Vilacosta I, Graupner C, San Roman JA, et al. Risk of embolization after institution of antibiotic therapy for infective endocarditis. J Am Coll Cardiol 2002;39:1489–1495

27. Dajani AS, Taubert KA, Wilson W, et al. Prevention of bacterial endocarditis: recommendations by the American Heart Association. JAMA 1997;277:1795–1801

28. Seto TB, Kwiat D, Taira DA, et al. Antibacterial prophylaxis to prevent endocarditis. JAMA 2000;284:68–71

29. Salamand AC, Collart F, Caus T, et al. Q fever endocarditis: over 14 years of surgical experience in a referral center for rickettsioses. J Valve Dis 2002;11:84–90

30. Kupferwasser LI, Darius H, Muller AM, et al. Diagnosis of culture negative endocarditis: the role of the Duke criteria and the impact of transesophageal echocardiography. Am Heart J 2001;142:146–152

31. Le Cam B, Guivarch G, Boles JM, et al. Neurological complications in a group of 86 bacterial endocarditis cases. Eur Heart J 1985;5(Suppl C):97–100

32. Davenport J, Hart RG. Prosthetic valve endocarditis 1978–1987: antibiotics, anticoagulation and stroke. Stroke 1990;21:993–999

33. Keyser DL, Biller J, Coffman TT, et al. Neurologic complications of late prosthetic valve endocarditis. Stroke 1990;21:472–475

34. Maruyama M, Kuriyama Y, Sawada T, et al. Brain damage after open heart surgery in patients with acute cardioembolic stroke. Stroke 1989;20:1305–1310

35. Ting W, Silverman N, Levitsky S. Valve replacement in patients with endocarditis and cerebral septic emboli. Ann Thorac Surg 1991;51:18–22

36. Eishi K, Kawazoe K, Kuriyama HY, et al. Surgical management of infective endocarditis associated with cerebral complications: a multi-center retrospective study in Japan. J Thorac Cardiovasc Surg 1995;110:1645–1755

37. Gillinov AM, Shah RV, Curtis WE, et al. Valve replacement in patients with endocarditis and acute neurological deficit. Ann Thorac Surg 1996;61:1125–1130

38. Brust JCM, Dickinson PCT, Hughes JED, et al. The diagnosis and treatment of cerebral mycotic aneurysms. Ann Neurol 1990;27:238–246

39. Kanter MC, Webb RM, Hart RG, et al. Management of acute stroke in infective endocarditis. Neurology 1990;40(Suppl 1):S417

40. Corr P, Wright M, Handler LC. Endocarditis-related cerebral aneurysms. Radiologic changes with treatment. Am J Neuroradiol 1995;16:745–748

41. Elowiz EH, Johnson WD, Milhorat TH. CT-localized stereotactic craniotomy for excision of a bacterial intracranial aneurysm. Surg Neurol 1995;44:265–269

42. Malik LM, Kamiryo T, Goble J, et al. Stereotactic laser-guided approach to distal middle cerebral artery aneurysm. Acta Neurochir Wien 1995;132:138–144

43. Chun JY, Smith W, Halach VV, et al. Current multi-modality management of infectious intracranial aneurysms. Neurosurgery 2001;48:1203–1213

44. Millar B, Moore J, Mallan P, et al. Molecular diagnosis of infective endocarditis: a new Duke's criterion. Scand J Infect Dis 2001;33:673–680

45. Mylonakis E, Calderwood SB. Infective endocarditis in adults. N Engl J Med 2001;345:1318–1330

113 Syncope

Horacio Kaufmann

Overview

Syncope (Greek *synkope*—cessation, pause) is a transient loss of consciousness and postural tone with spontaneous recovery and no neurological sequelae. Syncope is caused by a global reversible reduction of blood flow to the reticular activating system, the neuronal network in the brainstem responsible for supporting consciousness.

Abnormalities in autonomic cardiovascular control result in orthostatic hypotension and syncope in two different disorders: autonomic failure and neurally mediated syncope. In autonomic failure, sympathetic efferent activity is chronically impaired so that vasoconstriction is deficient and, upon standing, blood pressure always falls and syncope or presyncope occurs. Conversely, in patients with neurally mediated syncope, the failure of sympathetic efferent vasoconstrictor traffic (and hypotension) occurs episodically and, frequently, in response to a trigger. Between syncopal episodes, these patients have normal blood pressure.

Neurally mediated syncope, also referred to as vasovagal, vasodepressor or reflex syncope, is the most frequent cause of hypotension and syncope or presyncope in apparently normal subjects.[1] Syncope is a very frequent problem. In the 26-year surveillance period of the Framingham study, syncope occurred in 3% of men and in 3.5% of women.[2] The prevalence of syncope increases with age, occurring in 0.7% of subjects 35 to 44 years old and in 5.6% of those older than 74. Syncope accounts for 3% of emergency room visits and 6% of hospital admissions.[3] In this chapter, the mechanisms responsible for neurally mediated syncope, its diagnosis and management are reviewed.

Neurally mediated syncope

Neurally mediated syncope has been much scrutinized but remains incompletely understood and is still frequently misdiagnosed. During neurally mediated syncope, parasympathetic (vagal) outflow to the sinus node of the heart increases, producing bradycardia.[4] Bradycardia, however, is not the main cause of the fall in blood pressure, because preventing the bradycardia by implantation of a pacemaker or administration of atropine does not prevent the hypotension and syncope.[5,6] Blood pressure falls because of vasodilation, which, interestingly, is heterogeneous—vasodilation occurs in skeletal muscle and probably in the splanchnic vascular bed, but not in the skin. The mechanisms responsible for vasodilation are not well understood. There is a marked reduction in sympathetic vasoconstrictor

outflow to blood vessels in leg skeletal muscles, as has convincingly been shown with direct microneurography recordings,[7] and measurements of plasma norepinephrine, which falls. Vasopressin, endothelin-1, and angiotensin II all increase normally during neurally mediated syncope.[8]

The main unanswered question is whether vasodilation is solely due to a reduction in sympathetic vasoconstrictor traffic (i.e. "passive" vasodilation) or whether there is also activation of a vasodilator system (i.e. "active" vasodilation).[9] Several vasodilator mechanisms have been proposed. Although sympathetic postganglionic outflow to blood vessels decreases, epinephrine release by the adrenal medulla increases during vasovagal syncope. Hence, vasodilation from activation of beta-2 adrenergic receptors, induced by a rise in circulating epinephrine, has been suggested as a possible mechanism.[10] Blockade of beta-2 adrenergic receptors in the forearm, however, does not prevent forearm vasodilation during syncope.[11]

Recently, the discovery of nitric oxide (NO), a powerful vasodilator released by endothelial and other cells, has stimulated new interest in the active vasodilation hypothesis of syncope. The role of NO-mediated vasodilation is still uncertain, however. The finding that subjects with tilt-induced syncope have a doubling in the urinary concentration of cGMP, a marker of NO activity,[12] supports a role for NO-mediated vasodilation. Furthermore, Dietz et al. showed that skeletal muscle vasodilation in response to mental stress, which may induce vasodilation by a mechanism similar to that occurring during fainting, is mediated by nitric oxide.[13] However, recent work from the same group showed no prevention of forearm vasodilation during fainting after administration of the NO synthase inhibitor N^G-monomethy-L-arginine (L-NMMA).[11]

Causes of neurally mediated syncope

Clinical observation shows that a variety of seemingly different causes can trigger neurally mediated syncope. Depending on the trigger mechanism, two distinct syndromes emerge. First, neurally mediated syncope may be of central origin, when vasodilation and bradycardia occur in response to emotions such as intense fear or revulsion. In these cases, the stimulus must act on neocortical and limbic structures first. Neurons in the amygdala relay to hypothalamic and brainstem autonomic nuclei the information based on conscious evaluation and interpretations of stressors. These neurons may play a key role in emotionally induced syncope.

Neuroendocrine and autonomic changes during fainting are similar to those produced by intense fear. Threatening stimuli elicit two types of neuroendocrine-autonomic responses depending on whether the emotional response is anger or fear.[14] When the emotional response is anger, there is sympathetic neuronal activation and increased norepinephrine release (as in the fight-or-flight response); when the emotion is fear, there is mainly adrenomedullary activation with increased epinephrine release but little or no sympathetic postganglionic activation and no increase in norepinephrine release.

Emotionally induced fainting represents a specific autonomic response to situations of extreme fear or particular displeasure. It is tempting to speculate that when individuals perceive the futility of fighting or fleeing, they may choose a response resembling primitive freezing or "playing dead."[15]

The second type of neurally mediated syncope occurs as the result of failure of normal homeostatic reflexes or due to excessive excitation of a depressor reflex. One example of syncope thought to be due to an inappropriate reflex response is so-called "carotid sinus syncope." The suggested mechanism is that the sinus baroreceptors are abnormally stimulated, in the original classic case by pressure from a stiff-winged collar, and this leads to a hypotensive reaction. This condition is now diagnosed by carotid sinus massage, which when positive results in bradycardia, hypotension, or both. Carotid sinus syncope is probably greatly overdiagnosed, as a more physiological distension of sinus baroreceptors by applying controlled negative pressures rarely induces such large responses.

Syncope has also been associated with a number of other reflexes including micturition, defecation, and coughing. Defecating and coughing are essentially Valsalva-like maneuvers involving raised intra-abdominal and intrathoracic pressures that may result in a reduction in the venous return to the extent that cardiac output and blood pressure fall to critical levels. Micturition syncope may involve several mechanisms acting in concert to reduce the blood pressure. Typically, it occurs when a man stands to urinate after leaving a warm bed. The cutaneous blood vessels are dilated, and pooling of blood reduces venous return. In addition, straining will further reduce venous return. An additional factor may arise from relief of bladder distension, which may cause reflex vasodilation as the result of decreasing stimulus to bladder stretch receptors. Most episodes of neurally mediated syncope are associated with a reduction in central blood volume occurring during orthostatic (gravitational) stress, when the volume of the blood increases in dependent vessels. Part of the stress is also due to actual loss of blood volume from capillaries in dependent regions. Orthostatic stress is greatest when standing motionless, but may also occur when sitting still for long periods, particularly on high stools or aircraft seats for lengthy flights.

The normal "appropriate" response to hypo-volemia is vasoconstriction. However, at some stage this is abruptly inhibited, leading to vasodilation, bradycardia, and syncope. The ability to tolerate orthostatic stress before "switching" to a vasovagal reaction varies greatly between subjects. In general, younger women have lower tolerance than other subjects.[16] Orthostatic stress can usually be countered by contraction of muscles in dependent regions to compress veins and enhance return of blood to the heart. Not surprisingly, since syncope occurs when venous return is inadequate, individuals with relatively large blood and plasma volumes tend to have greater tolerance to orthostatic stress. Also, procedures that increase these volumes, such as salt loading[17] or exercise training,[18] also increase orthostatic tolerance and reduce the frequency of syncopal attacks.

The trigger mechanism for converting vasoconstriction and tachycardia to vasodilation and bradycardia remains unknown. The view formerly held was that it was due to abnormal stimulation of afferent nonmyelinated nerves from the ventricle as the nearly empty heart was stimulated to contract powerfully. This led to the term "neurocardiogenic" syncope. The postulated mechanism was based on the findings of Oberg and Thoren[19] that some nonmyelinated vagal afferents were paradoxically stimulated during hemorrhage and that this induced a Bezold–Jarisch type of response. However, the evidence against this mechanism now seems overwhelming. First, even in the original report, relatively few receptors showed this paradoxical response, and most nerves actually decreased their discharge as the ventricular volume decreased. Second, in animals, where the left ventricle was bypassed and sympathetic nerves strongly stimulated, there was no hypotensive response. Third, patients who have had cardiac transplants show similar vasodilation even though there could have been no afferent neural activity from their ventricles.[20]

Neurally mediated syncope thus remains an intriguing physiological problem. It is not an abnormal response as it can be induced in anyone provided the stress is sufficiently great, although some individuals may be abnormally susceptible. The trigger mechanism remains elusive but it does seem often to involve central mechanisms, peripheral reflexes, or possibly both. It is related to decreases in effective blood volume, and volume expansion is often an effective method for the management of patients with recurrent attacks.

Diagnosis

The history and physical examination may determine the cause of syncope in up to 50% of cases. Neurally mediated syncope needs to be differentiated from several other disorders such as chronic autonomic failure, syncope due to cardiac arrhythmias, and seizures. A thorough history of the circumstances preceding syncope and eyewitness accounts are invaluable. Many of the well known neurally mediated syncopal syndromes occur in typical scenarios. Syncope occurring after standing immobile for a prolonged period of time, particularly in hot weather or after prolonged bedrest (physical deconditioning), syncope during micturition or in conjunction with trigeminal or glossopharyngeal neuralgia, and syncope preceded by emotional stress or painful stimuli are likely to be neurally mediated in origin.

Hyperventilation preceding syncope may indicate a panic disorder. The reduction in carbon dioxide in the blood may result in cerebral vasoconstriction sufficient to induce cerebral hypoperfusion and syncope. Syncope during or after exercise suggests fixed or dynamic aortic stenosis, reflecting obstruction to flow, arrhythmias or reflex vasodilation. The latter results from increased ventricular mechanoreceptor discharge, a mechanism similar to that of neurally mediated syncope.

Symptoms of autonomic activation typically precede neurally mediated syncope. Sympathetic activation results in piloerection, sweating and pallor (cutaneous vasoconstriction); a peculiar phenomenon referred to as "cold sweat." Blurred vision is caused by pupillary dilatation. Vagal activation causes abdominal discomfort and nausea. With the onset of cerebral hypoperfusion and acute reversal of sympathetic activation, lightheadedness and darkening of vision precedes loss of consciousness. In marked contrast, patients with chronic autonomic failure never have prodromal symptoms of autonomic activation. Therefore such patients experience only lightheadedness and gradual loss of vision with cerebral hypoperfusion.

Patients with seizure disorders, particularly of temporal lobe origin, experience aura, which may be difficult to distinguish from symptoms of autonomic activation. Symptoms include epigastric discomfort, "deja-vu," gustatory and auditory phenomena.

Patients with neurally mediated syncope typically lose postural tone and fall. The horizontal position improves cerebral blood flow and consciousness is quickly regained. Hypotension and bradycardia can persist for several minutes, so that attempting to stand too early can result in a further episode of loss of consciousness. Patients should be told to lie down for at least 15 to 20 minutes after syncope and then to rise slowly. Individuals witnessing a syncopal event should be advised not to hold the patient up and to leave the victim in the horizontal position, on the ground if necessary.

A few myoclonic jerks, tonic contractions of the limbs or "rolling of the eyes" can occur in syncope. Frank tonic–clonic convulsion, tongue-biting, urinary incontinence and confusion on regaining consciousness are diagnostic of seizures rather than syncope. Patients with neurally mediated syncope may feel dazed momentarily on regaining consciousness but this is very brief and there is never frank confusion.

Drug history A detailed drug history should be obtained to determine the potential for iatrogenic syncope. Both neurally mediated syncope and autonomic failure can manifest for the first time with medications that cause vasodilation. This is a common overlooked cause of syncope, particularly in the elderly in whom baroreflexes may be impaired. Common culprits include antihypertensive agents, alpha-adrenergic blockers used in bladder outflow obstruction, antidepressants, neuroleptics and antiparkinsonian medications, all capable of lowering blood pressure and triggering orthostatic hypotension. Nitrates reduce afterload, and can cause outflow obstruction in patients with aortic stenosis and thus can induce syncope.

Family history A family history of recurrent syncope and sudden death in younger patients points toward a diagnosis of cardiac syncope, for example, secondary to hypertrophic obstructive cardiomyopathy and congenital abnormalities of the Q–T interval.[21]

Physical examination Neurally mediated syncope is the most frequent cause of syncope in otherwise normal individuals; therefore, in the majority of cases there are no abnormalities on systemic, cardiological and neurological examination. The presence of physical abnormalities suggests an alternative diagnosis. Special attention should be given to cardiac signs such as added heart sounds. Bruits over the supraclavicular area may indicate subclavian steal syndrome with induction of symptoms on exercising of the arm. A neurological examination revealing extrapyramidal signs alone or in conjunction with cerebellar and pyramidal signs points toward a diagnosis of Parkinson's disease with autonomic failure or multiple system atrophy.[22] Normal physical examination can also occur in pure autonomic failure, another, much rarer cause of chronic autonomic failure and syncope.[23] Therefore, blood pressure and heart rate should always be taken after supine rest for 20 minutes and after standing upright for at least 3 minutes, checking for orthostatic hypotension with or without a compensatory increase in heart rate.

12 lead electrocardiograph Ventricular hypertrophy, bundle branch block, first-degree atrioventricular (AV) block, and premature ventricular or atrial complexes are extremely frequent (documented in 75% of patients) and are thus generally considered as incidental findings, not necessarily related to the cause of syncope.[24] Electrocardiograph findings that may be helpful in identifying a potential cause of syncope include evidence of a previous myocardial infarction, prolongation of the Q–T interval, a short P–R interval and delta waves indicative of the Wolff–Parkinson–White syndrome, and high-degree AV block.

Ambulatory electrocardiograph and loop monitors Because syncope is often sporadic and infrequent, ambulatory ECG is rarely diagnostic. Only in 1% to 3% of patients has syncope been documented during 24 to 48 hours of ambulatory ECG monitoring.[24,25] Unless syncope or severe presyncope is temporarily associated with an arrhythmia, the arrhythmia should not be considered as the cause of syncope. Abnormalities such as sinus pauses of less than 3 seconds, AV Wenckebach block, or bursts of nonsustained ventricular tachycardia are frequently observed in elderly patients, thus unless they are temporarily associated with syncope they should be interpreted as incidental findings. Loop monitors have recently been introduced for the assessment of patients with recurrent unexplained syncope. These chronic, long-term, patient-activated devices have the ability to record between 1 and 5 minutes of ECG during the syncopal episode. The major limitation is that the device needs to be self-activated; therefore, in patients with short prodromes or no warning symptoms, syncopal episodes may be lost. Nonetheless, the diagnostic yield with loop monitors has been reported at 25% in one series[25] and more recently at 55%. The most common diagnosis was bradycardia and these patients were frequently treated with a pacemaker. Heart rate event monitors, however, cannot distinguish bradycardias resulting from intrinsic cardiac conduction abnormalities or from neurocardiogenic syncope. At least one patient in this series had recurrent syncope after pacemaker implantation, suggesting unrecognized neurally mediated syncope.

Head-up tilt testing   Head-up tilt testing is the best diagnostic tool for the evaluation of recurrent unexplained syncope.[26] Passive head-up tilt, by preventing the pumping effect of skeletal muscle contraction, exaggerates the reduction in venous return of the upright posture and triggers neurally mediated syncope in susceptible individuals. Hemodynamic profiles in response to head-up tilt are diagnostic. In patients with neurally mediated syncope, the initial blood pressure and heart rate response to passive tilt is normal. However, following a variable period of time with appropriately maintained blood pressure and heart rate, sudden hypotension and bradycardia develops. In marked contrast, patients with chronic autonomic failure typically have a progressive fall in blood pressure beginning immediately after tilt onset. If the fall in blood pressure is pronounced syncope occurs but there is never acute bradycardia (Figure 113.1).

In some patients with frequent syncope, particularly the elderly with multiple medical problems, head-up tilt testing shows that blood pressure starts to fall immediately after assuming the upright position, similar to the response of patients with autonomic failure, but the slow steady fall in blood pressure is interrupted by typical neurally mediated syncope (acute vasodilation and bradycardia).

Another characteristic response to tilt is that of the postural tachycardia syndrome (POTS) consisting in an exaggerated heart rate response, of more than 30 beats per minute, without a fall in blood pressure but a propensity to suffer neurally mediated syncope. Patients with the postural tachycardia syndrome are a heterogeneous group but they may share an excessive sympathetic activation in response to physiological stimuli. Symptoms may include dizziness, lightheadedness, giddiness, feeling faint, fatigue, and inability to concentrate, as well as palpitations, diaphoresis, tremulousness, and visual blurring, all suggestive of sympathetic overactivity. The cause of the syndrome is unknown, but recent studies suggest two different

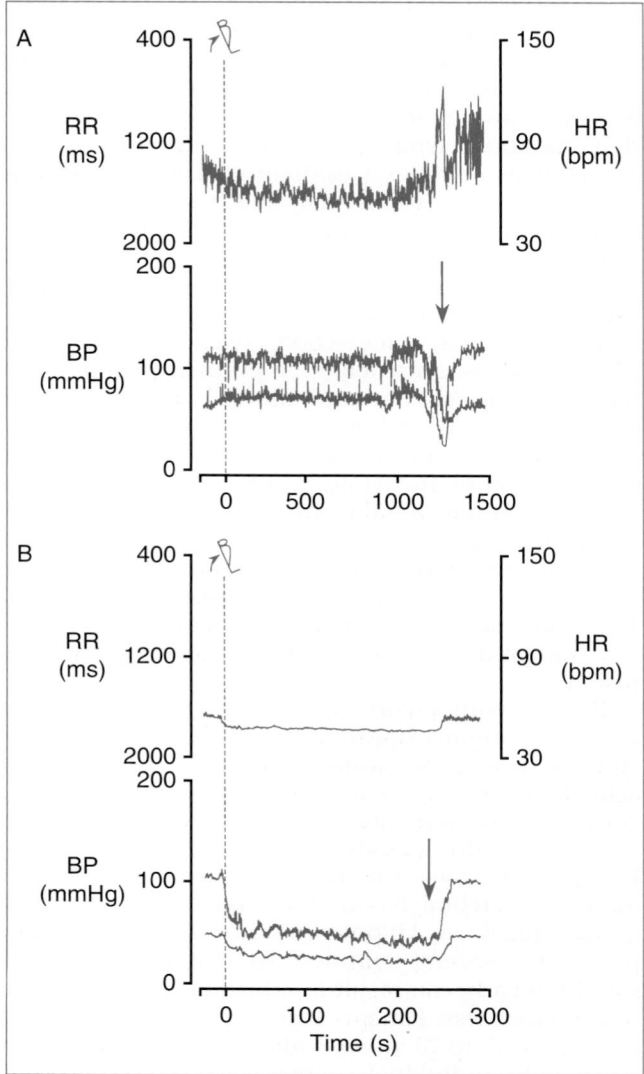

Figure 113.1   *A*, A 33-year-old male with history of recurrent episodes of neurally mediated syncope. Tracings show R–R interval and heart rate (upper panel) and blood pressure (lower panel) before and during 60 degrees passive head-up tilt. Dashed line indicates beginning of head-up tilt. Arrow shows time of syncope, following which the patient was immediately returned to horizontal position. Note increase in heart rate variability after syncope, indicative of increased parasympathetic (vagal) outflow. *B*, A 58-year-old male with chronic autonomic failure due to multiple system atrophy and recurrent episodes of syncope. Tracings show R–R interval and heart rate (upper panel) and blood pressure (lower panel) before and during 60 degrees passive head-up tilt. Dashed line indicates beginning of head-up tilt. Arrow shows time of syncope, following which the patient was immediately returned to horizontal position. Note lack of appropriate increase in heart rate during tilt despite the prominent decrease in blood pressure.

mechanisms of pathogenesis. First, some patients may have a neuropathy affecting sympathetic nerves to blood vessels in the lower part of the body, resulting in vascular denervation and excessive pooling of blood in the legs when standing. Because autonomic innervation to the heart is preserved, these patients have pronounced reflex tachycardia upon standing—a normal, expected response to their decreased central blood volume. This denervation hypothesis is supported by the finding of decreased norepinephrine spillover in the legs in affected patients.[27] Second, a genetic or an acquired impairment of synaptic norepinephrine clearance may explain the disorder. Specifically, a deficiency in the neuronal norepinephrine transporter may occur in some patients, increasing the synaptic concentration of norepinephrine in response to physiological stimuli such as standing. This hypothesis is supported by the recent finding of a patient with postural tachycardia who was heterozygous for a mutation in the norepinephrine-transporter gene that resulted in pronounced (more than 98%) loss of function.[28]

Essentially, two tilt-table test protocols have been proposed—drug-free prolonged tilt, lasting between 40 and 60 minutes, and upright tilt with graded isoproterenol infusions, lasting between 10 and 30 minutes.[26,29–33] The advantages of the drug-free protocol include good sensitivity (ranging between 40% and 75%), excellent specificity (93%) and acceptable short-term reproducibility (80%). One disadvantage, however, is the prolonged duration, which may be a limiting factor in busy electrophysiology laboratories. The infusion of isoproterenol significantly decreases the duration of the protocol and increases sensitivity but decreases specificity, i.e. there is a greater incidence of false positives. Other pharmacological agents that have been used to induce neurally mediated syncope during tilt-table testing include edrophonium, nitroglycerin, and adenosine.[30,34–36] Most laboratories define a positive tilt test as the induction of presyncope or syncope associated with a systolic blood pressure less than or equal to 70 mmHg and/or bradycardia less than or equal to 50 bpm. Most importantly, the reproduction of symptoms that resemble the clinical presentation is necessary to establish correctly the diagnosis of neurally mediated syncope. Head-up tilt is the diagnostic method of choice in subjects with unexplained syncope and no structural heart disease.

Signal-averaged ECG and electrophysiological studies Signal-averaged ECG is a technique that increases several thousand times the amplitude of the QRS, allowing the detection of late potentials from electrically abnormal ventricular myocytes secondary to an old myocardial infarction. The presence of late potentials has a high correlation with inducibility of ventricular tachycardia during electrophysiological assessment.[37,38] On the other hand, a negative signal-averaged ECG (no evidence of late potentials) indicates that ventricular tachycardia is unlikely to be the cause of the syncopal episode. Invasive electrophysio-

logical testing is used in patients with organic heart disease, particularly those with previous myocardial infarction and depressed left ventricular ejection fraction (< 40%).[39–41] Abnormal findings include sinus node dysfunction, abnormal His-bundle conduction and ventricular tachycardia. Multiple abnormalities may be documented in the same patient. Dizziness and syncope are frequently observed in elderly patients with sinus bradycardia. Persistent bradycardia of less than 40 beats per minute is a potential indication for electrophysiological study. Permanent pacing may be indicated if bradycardia persists. If sinus node recovery time is abnormal, permanent pacing is indicated.[42]

Treatment

Patient education and recognition and avoidance of recognized triggers are invaluable in the treatment of neurally mediated syncope. It is important for the patient to identify symptoms, such as nausea, blurred vision, abdominal discomfort and diaphoresis, as premonitory to a syncopal episode. In this way the patient, on experiencing such symptoms, knows to lie down flat, and so restore cerebral perfusion.

Volume expansion Some subjects with neurally mediated syncope may have a true "salt deficit syndrome" because of severe dietary salt restriction or a putative defect in renal sodium conservation, perhaps secondary to impaired renin–aldosterone responses to volume loss. Increasing salt intake should expand intravascular volume and reduce the frequency of neurally mediated syncope. Several recent studies support this. Eight weeks after salt or placebo treatment, 70% of the patients given salt and 30% of the placebo group showed increases in plasma and blood volumes and in orthostatic tolerance. The patients in the placebo group who improved also showed increases in urinary salt excretion, suggesting that they had increased their salt intake. Thus, the first line of treatment in subjects with susceptibility to neurally mediated syncope should be increasing dietary salt intake.

Exercise and orthostatic training Another complementary strategy is resistance training of leg muscles (i.e. isometric exercise) which improves muscle tone and therefore increases venous return to the heart during orthostasis. Resistance training may also increase plasma volume, which further improves orthostatic tolerance.

In subjects with recurrent syncope, irrespective of drug treatment, the incidence of positive head-up tilt tests falls with repeated tilts. Based on these observations, orthostatic training has been tried as a treatment of neurally mediated syncope.[43] In a controlled study of 47 adolescents with recurrent syncope,[44] orthostatic training was started in-hospital and then performed at home by standing against a wall twice a day for up to 40 minutes, depending on the in-hospital orthostatic tolerance. After 1 month, 26% of patients in the control group and 96% of patients in the training group became tilt negative ($P < 0.0001$).

Pharmacological treatment   In some patients non-pharmacological treatment is ineffective. Over the years several pharmacological agents have been proposed to prevent recurrent neurally mediated syncope. Fludrocortisone, beta-blockers, serotonin reuptake inhibitors (SSRIs), disopyramide and alpha-agonists are the most widely used.

Fludrocortisone   is effective mainly because of plasma volume expansion ameliorating the decrease in preload, which is believed to trigger syncope. Long term use of fludrocortisone is associated with hypertension, and the drug should be used with caution in patients with only occasional episodes of neurally mediated syncope.

Beta-blockers   are popular in the treatment of neurally mediated syncope. They could work in various ways. By decreasing the force of ventricular contraction beta-blockade could prevent excessive stimulation of ventricular mechanoreceptors, the hypothetical source of neurally mediated syncope. They may also prevent epinephrine-induced arterial vasodilation through β2-adrenergic receptor blockade.

The study of Mahanonda et al.[45] is frequently quoted as the best study supporting the effectiveness of beta-blockers. The authors randomized 42 patients who had suffered syncope and had it reproduced during tilt-table test with isoproterenol infusion to receive either atenolol or placebo. After a 1-month period, 62% of patients receiving atenolol had a negative tilt test versus 5% of those receiving placebo. Moreover, patients who received atenolol reported feeling better compared with those who received placebo (71% vs. 29%, $P = 0.02$). The strongest conclusion of the study was that atenolol prevented isoproterenol-induced syncope. However, the assumption that isoproterenol-induced syncope is similar to spontaneous syncope is disputed.

A recent prospective, double-blind, randomized and placebo-controlled study,[46] however, showed lack of efficacy of atenolol in preventing neurally mediated syncope. Fifty patients with recurrent syncope (at least two episodes in the previous year) were randomized to receive either atenolol 50 mg/day or a placebo and followed for one year. The primary end-point of the study was the time to first recurrence of syncope. The group treated with atenolol had a similar number of patients with recurrent syncopal episodes as the placebo group. The recurrence of neurocardiogenic syncope in highly symptomatic patients treated with atenolol is similar to that of patients treated with placebo.

Alpha-agonists   Another approach to treatment is the use of alpha-adrenergic agonists, which could prevent neurally mediated syncope in a variety of ways. By stimulating arterial alpha-adrenergic vasoconstrictor receptors, alpha-agonists could diminish the passive vasodilation during reduction of sympathetic outflow, characteristic of neurally mediated syncope, and therefore lessen hypotension. Alpha-agonists could also reduce venous pooling of blood by causing venoconstriction.

A recent multicenter, randomized, placebo-controlled study evaluated the efficacy of the alpha-agonist etilefrine in the long term management of patients with recurrent vasovagal syncope.[47] In 20 participating centers, 126 patients with recurrent vasovagal syncope and a baseline head-up tilt response that reproduced syncope were randomly assigned to placebo or etilefrine (75 mg/day) and were followed up for one year or until syncope recurred. The primary end-point of the study was the first recurrence of syncope. During follow-up, the group treated with etilefrine had a similar incidence of first syncopal recurrence to that of placebo group (26% versus 24%). Moreover, the median time to the first syncopal recurrence was similar in the two study groups (106 days in the etilefrine arm and 112 days in the placebo arm). Thus, oral etilefrine was not superior to placebo in preventing spontaneous episodes of vasovagal syncope.

An alpha-agonist available in the US is midodrine, which has been used successfully to treat patients with chronic autonomic failure.[48–50] Midodrine is an interesting alpha-agonist because it does not cross the blood–brain barrier, so it does not have central nervous system effects such as anxiety, agitation, and insomnia, which are common with other alpha-agonists. It can be taken by mouth and has a predictable 3 to 4 hour blood pressure effect. A few studies suggest that midodrine may be effective in treating neurally mediated syncope. Recently, in a randomized, double-blind, placebo-controlled study Ward et al.[51] assessed the benefit of midodrine on symptom frequency and hemodynamic responses during head-up tilt in 16 patients with frequent hypotensive symptoms and reproducible neurally mediated syncope with glyceryl trinitrate (GTN) during head-up tilt. During one month, patients on midodrine had an average of 7 more symptom free days in comparison to those who received placebo. Fourteen patients who were given placebo had tilt-induced syncope compared with 6 given midodrine ($P = 0.01$). Supine systolic blood pressure was higher and heart rate lower in patients who received midodrine than in those who were given placebo ($P < 0.05$).

Kaufmann et al.[52] recently conducted a double-blind, randomized, crossover, placebo-controlled trial to investigate the efficacy of midodrine in preventing neurally mediated syncope triggered by passive head-up tilt. Twelve patients with a history of recurrent neurally mediated syncope, mean age 42 ± 15, were randomized to receive midodrine 5 mg or placebo on day 1 and the opposite 2 days later. In the supine position, midodrine produced no significant change in blood pressure or heart rate but the responses to head-up tilt were significantly different on the midodrine and the placebo day. During the placebo day 58% (7/12) of the subjects developed neurally mediated syncope. In contrast, during the midodrine day, only 8% (1/12) of the subjects developed neurally mediated syncope ($P < 0.03$, Fisher's exact test) suggesting that midodrine significantly improves orthostatic tolerance during head-up tilt. In patients with frequent symptoms, midodrine should be considered. A clinical trial to determine the chronic effect of midodrine in patients with recurrent neurally mediated syncope is warranted.

Disopyramide The antiarrhythmic disopyramide was tried because of its anticholinergic and negative inotropic effects. Although it appeared effective in small trials, a double-blind crossover study showed this drug to be no better than placebo in preventing syncope.[53]

Serotonin reuptake inhibitors In small uncontrolled trials, serotonin reuptake inhibitors have been reported to be effective in preventing neurally mediated syncope. Recently, the effect of paroxetine hydrochloride, a selective serotonin reuptake inhibitor, was evaluated in patients with vasovagal syncope in a randomized, double-blind, placebo-controlled study.[54] Sixty-eight patients with recurrent syncope and positive head-up tilt randomly received either paroxetine 20 mg a day or placebo. After one month of treatment, 62% of patients receiving paroxetine had a negative tilt test versus 38% of negative tilt tests in patients on placebo ($P < 0.001$).

Pacemakers The utility of cardiac pacing in vasovagal syncope is controversial.[55] Guidelines from several professional societies including the American College of Cardiology, American Heart Association,[56] and British Pacing and Electrophysiology Working Group[57] provide a class 2 indication for pacing in vasovagal syncope. It is well established that bradycardia is not the cause of hypotension in neurally mediated syncope. In 1932, in his classic paper on vasovagal syncope, Sir Thomas Lewis reported that atropine "while raising the pulse rate up ... leaves the blood pressure below normal and the patient not fully conscious".[6] It has been postulated, however, that by preventing bradycardia, cardiac pacing could lessen the severity of the fall in blood pressure or increase the time from premonitory symptoms to syncope.[58] Pacing would be particularly useful in those patients in whom syncope is associated with a few seconds of sinus arrest. In the recently completed North American Vasovagal Pacemaker Study[59] the investigators concluded that dual-chamber pacing with rate-drop response reduces the likelihood of syncope in patients with recurrent vasovagal syncope. However, as Benditt points out in an editorial accompanying the article, the study has several significant limitations.[60]

Fifty-four patients, with at least 6 lifetime episodes of syncope and with a tilt-table test that induced syncope or presyncope, as well as a relative bradycardia, were randomized to receive no pacemaker or a dual chamber pacemaker. The pacemaker provided high-rate pacing if a predetermined drop in heart rate occurred (rate-drop response). The primary outcome was the first recurrence of syncope. Recurrent syncope occurred in 70% of no pacemaker patients and in 22% of pacemaker patients. The mean time from randomization to syncope was 54 days in the nonpacemaker group and 112 days in the pacemaker group. What do these results mean? First, there was no proof that the pacemaker actually aborted or prevented syncope; i.e. there was no information on whether the pacemaker was triggered and prevented loss of consciousness in any of the patients. This is important because El-Bedawi et al. had shown that a functioning pacemaker has no effect on the magnitude of the blood pressure fall during neurally mediated syncope,[5] confirming that hypotension was due to profound vasodilation while bradycardia played little or no role in the fall in blood pressure. One may conclude that, rather than the ability of a functioning pacemaker to abort syncope, the treatment tested in the North American Vasovagal Pacemaker Study was pacemaker implantation itself, a surgical procedure with profound psychological impact, in addition to the additional care and follow-up that a pacemaker requires. Therefore, a potentially powerful placebo effect may have occurred which could account for the apparent positive results of pacemaker implantation. Finally, the study does not permit assessment of the merits of pacing relative to pharmacological approaches; only 32 of the 54 patients had received drug treatment, mainly beta-adrenergic blockers or disopyramide—agents that are not universally accepted as effective.

A recent study[61] compared cardiac pacing in the treatment of cardioinhibitory neurally mediated syncope and pharmacological treatment with atenolol (100 mg/day). No placebo group was included. Patients (n = 93) with more than 3 episodes of neurally mediated syncope in the previous 2 years were enrolled if they had syncope reproduced during tilt-table testing in association with relative bradycardia (heart rate < 60 bpm). The primary outcome was recurrence of syncope. The study was suspended because an interim analysis revealed beneficial effects of pacing. Recurrence of syncope occurred in 2 patients (4%) in the pacing arm after a median of 390 days, versus 12 patients (26%) in the atenolol arm after a median of 135 days. The authors concluded that cardiac pacing was significantly more effective compared to beta-blockers in patients with the cardioinhibitory type of neurally mediated syncope. There are several problems with this study. First, beta-blockers are not an effective treatment for neurally mediated syncope. Despite this, over 60% of patients remained syncope-free in the atenolol group. By its nature, the study could not be blinded. A placebo effect associated with surgical implantation of a pacemaker could only be excluded in a crossover design study where the pacemaker is blindly deactivated.

Conclusion

Once tilt-table testing confirms the diagnosis of neurally mediated syncope, it may suffice to reassure the patient and teach him or her to avoid known triggers and to recognize and act upon early warning symptoms (Figure 113.2). Subjects with susceptibility to

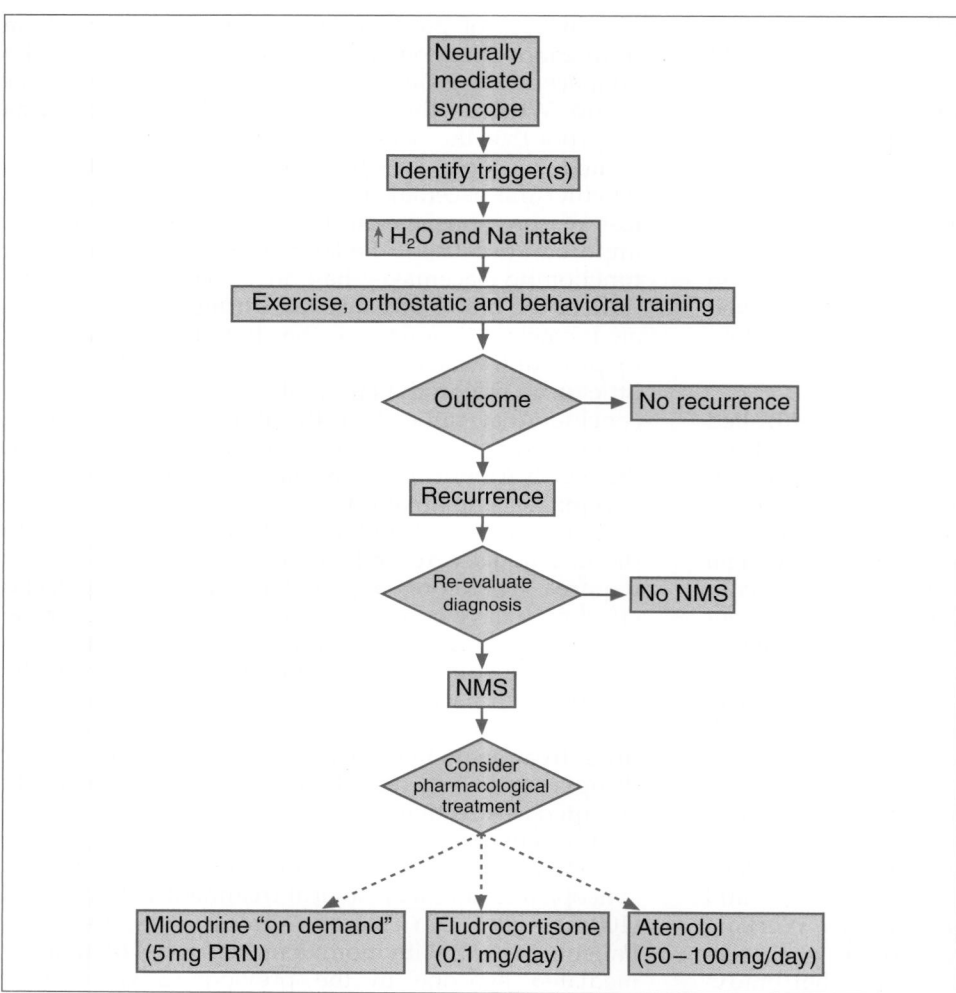

Figure 113.2 Algorithm for the treatment of neurally mediated syncope (NMS). Dashed lines indicate treatments for which there is no conclusive proof of efficacy. See text for details.

neurally mediated syncope may potentially be sodium depleted, and an increase in dietary salt intake should be the first line of treatment. If salt alone is not effective, a low dose of fludrocortisone could be used for a short period of time.

Fludrocortisone and increased salt intake are effective in preventing neurally mediated syncope but whether the benefits outweigh the risk of potential mineralocorticoid induced hypertension during chronic administration is unknown. Further, serum electrolytes have to be checked periodically because of potential hypokalemic metabolic alkalosis. Despite good theoretical reasons for their use, in the author's experience beta-blockers are not useful. Moreover, they should be used with caution because they can prolong asystole in patients with neurally mediated syncope.[62] The alpha-agonist midodrine may be useful in some patients. Pacemakers have not proven to be more effective than pharmacological treatment. There are still no adequately powered large-scale double-blind controlled studies that prove the effectiveness and safety of chronic administration of any drugs; pharmacological treatment of neurally mediated syncope should therefore be approached with caution.

References

1. Kaufmann H. Syncope. A neurologist's viewpoint. Cardiol Clin 1997;15:177–194
2. Savage DD, Corwin L, McGee DL, et al. Epidemiologic features of isolated syncope: The Framingham Study. Stroke 1985;16:62
3. Silverstein MD, Singer DE, Mulley AG, et al. Patients with syncope admitted to medical intensive care units. JAMA 1982;248:1185–1189
4. Kaufmann H. Neurally mediated syncope: pathogenesis, diagnosis, and treatment. Neurology 1995;45:S12–S18
5. el-Bedawi KM, Wahbha MA, Hainsworth R. Cardiac pacing does not improve orthostatic tolerance in patients with vasovagal syncope. Clin Auton Res 1994;4:233–237
6. Lewis T. Lecture on vasovagal syncope and the carotid sinus mechanism. BMJ 1932;1:873–876
7. Wallin B, Sundlof G. Sympathetic outflow to muscles during vasovagal syncope. J Auton Nerv Syst 1982;6:287–291
8. Kaufmann H, Oribe E, Oliver JA. Plasma endothelin during upright tilt: relevance for orthostatic hypotension? Lancet 1991;338:1542–1545
9. Barcroft HEO. On the vasodilatation in human skeletal muscle during post-hemorrhagic fainting. J Physiol 1945;104:161–175

10. Glover W, Greenfield A, Shanks R. The contribution made by adrenaline to the vasodilation in the human forearm during emotional stress. J Physiol 1962;161: 42P–43P

11. Dietz NM, Halliwill JR, Spielmann JM, et al. Sympathetic withdrawal and forearm vasodilation during vasovagal syncope in humans. J Appl Physiol 1997;82: 1785–1793

12. Kaufmann H, Berman J, Oribe E, Oliver J. Possible increase in the synthesis of endothelial derived relaxing factor (EDRF) during vasovagal syncope. Clin Auton Res 1993;3:69 (Abstract)

13. Dietz NM, Engelke KA, Samuel TT, et al. Evidence for nitric oxide-mediated sympathetic forearm vasodilatation in humans. J Physiol 1997;498:531–540

14. Ekman P, Levenson RW, Friesen WV. Autonomic nervous system activity distinguishes among emotions. Science 1983;221:1208–1210

15. Goldstein D. Stress response patterns. Stress, catecholamines, and cardiovascular disease. New York: Oxford University Press, 1995:287–328

16. Hainsworth R, el-Bedawi KM. Orthostatic tolerance in patients with unexplained syncope. Clin Auton Res 1994;4:239–244

17. El-Sayed H, Hainsworth R. Salt supplement increases plasma volume and orthostatic tolerance in patients with unexplained syncope. Heart 1996;75:134–140

18. Mtinangi BL, Hainsworth R. Increased orthostatic tolerance following moderate exercise training in patients with unexplained syncope. Heart 1998;80:596–600

19. Oberg B, Thoren P. Increased activity in left ventricular receptors during hemorrhage or occlusion of caval veins in the cat. A possible cause of the vaso-vagal reaction. Acta Physiol Scand 1972;85:164–173

20. Fitzpatrick AP, Banner N, Cheng A, et al. Vasovagal reactions may occur after orthotopic heart transplantation. J Am Coll Cardiol 1993;21:1132–1137

21. Towbin JA, Vatta M. Molecular biology and the prolonged QT syndromes. Am J Med 2001;110:385–398

22. Kaufmann H. Multiple system atrophy. Curr Opin Neurol 1998;11:351–355

23. Kaufmann H, Hague K, Perl D. Accumulation of alpha-synuclein in autonomic nerves in pure autonomic failure. Neurology 2001;56:980–981

24. Kapoor WN, Karpf M, Wieand S, et al. A prospective evaluation and follow-up of patients with syncope. N Engl J Med 1983;309:197–204

25. Linzer M, Yang EH, Estes NA III, et al. Diagnosing syncope. Part 1: Value of history, physical examination, and electrocardiography. Clinical Efficacy Assessment Project of the American College of Physicians. Ann Intern Med 1997;126:989–996

26. Oribe E, Perera R, Caro S, et al. Syncope: The diagnostic value of head-up tilt testing. Pacing Clin Electrophysiol 1997;20:874–879

27. Jacob G, Costa F, Shannon JR, et al. The neuropathic postural tachycardia syndrome. N Engl J Med 2000;343:1008–1014

28. Shannon JR, Flattem NL, Jordan J, et al. Orthostatic intolerance and tachycardia associated with norepinephrine-transporter deficiency. N Engl J Med 2000; 342:541–549

29. Kenny RA, Ingram A, Bayliss J, Sutton R. Head-up tilt: a useful test for investigating unexplained syncope. Lancet 1986;1:1352–1355

30. Raviele A, Gasparini G, Di Pede F, et al. Usefulness of head-up tilt test in evaluating patients with syncope of unknown origin and negative electrophysiologic study. Am J Cardiol 1990;65:1322–1327

31. Waxman MB, Yao L, Cameron DA, et al. Isoproterenol induction of vasodepressor-type reaction in vasodepressor-prone persons. Am J Cardiol 1989;63:58–65

32. Sheldon R, Killam S. Methodology of isoproterenol-tilt table testing in patients with syncope. J Am Coll Cardiol 1992;19:773–779

33. Morillo CA, Klein GJ, Zandri S, Yee R. Diagnostic accuracy of a low-dose isoproterenol head-up tilt protocol. Am Heart J 1995;129:901–906

34. Lurie KG, Dutton J, Mangat R, et al. Evaluation of edrophonium as a provocative agent for vasovagal syncope during head-up tilt-table testing. Am J Cardiol 1993;72:1286–1290

35. Voice RA, Lurie KG, Sakaguchi S, et al. Comparison of tilt angles and provocative agents (edrophonium and isoproterenol) to improve head-upright tilt-table testing. Am J Cardiol 1998;81:346–351

36. Shen W, Hamill S, Munger T, et al. Adenosine: potential modulator for vasovagal syncope. J Am Coll Cardiol 1996;28:146–154

37. Steinberg JS, Regan A, Sciacca RR, et al. Predicting arrhythmic events after acute myocardial infarction using the signal-averaged electrocardiogram. Am J Cardiol 1992;69:13–21

38. Winters SL, Stewart D, Gomes JA. Signal averaging of the surface QRS complex predicts inducibility of ventricular tachycardia in patients with syncope of unknown origin: a prospective study. J Am Coll Cardiol 1987;10(4):775–781

39. Teichman SL, Felder SD, Matos JA, et al. The value of electrophysiologic studies in syncope of undetermined origin: report of 150 cases. Am Heart J 1985;110: 469–479

40. Krol RB, Morady F, Flaker GC, et al. Electrophysiologic testing in patients with unexplained syncope: clinical and noninvasive predictors of outcome. J Am Coll Cardiol 1987;10:358–363

41. Muller T, Roy D, Talajic M, et al. Electrophysiologic evaluation and outcome of patients with syncope of unknown origin. Eur Heart J 1991;12:139–143

42. Gann D, Tolentino A, Samet P. Electrophysiologic evaluation of elderly patients with sinus bradycardia: a long-term follow-up study. Ann Intern Med 1979;90: 24–29

43. Ector H, Reybrouck T, Heidbuchel H, et al. Tilt training: a new treatment for recurrent neurocardiogenic syncope and severe orthostatic intolerance. Pacing Clin Electrophysiol 1998;21:193–196

44. Di Girolamo E, Di Iorio C, Leonzio L, et al. Usefulness of a tilt training program for the prevention of refractory neurocardiogenic syncope in adolescents: A controlled study. Circulation 1999;100:1798–1801

45. Mahanonda N, Bhuripanyo K, Kangkagate C, et al. Randomized double-blind, placebo-controlled trial of oral atenolol in patients with unexplained syncope and positive upright tilt table test results. Am Heart J 1995;130:1250–1253

46. Madrid AH, Ortega J, Rebollo JG, et al. Lack of efficacy of atenolol for the prevention of neurally mediated syncope in a highly symptomatic population: a prospective, double-blind, randomized and placebo-controlled study. J Am Coll Cardiol 2001;37:554–559

47. Raviele A, Brignole M, Sutton R, et al. Effect of etilefrine in preventing syncopal recurrence in patients with vasovagal syncope: a double-blind, randomized, placebo-controlled trial. Circulation 1999;99:1452–1457

48. Kaufmann H, Brannan T, Krakoff L, et al. Treatment of orthostatic hypotension due to autonomic failure with

a peripheral alpha-adrenergic agonist (midodrine). Neurology 1988;38:951–956

49. Jankovic J, Gilden JL, Hiner BC, et al. Neurogenic orthostatic hypotension: a double-blind, placebo-controlled study with midodrine. Am J Med 1993;95:38–48

50. Wright RA, Kaufmann HC, Perera R, et al. A double-blind, dose-response study of midodrine in neurogenic orthostatic hypotension. Neurology 1998;51:120–124

51. Ward CR, Gray JC, Gilroy JJ, Kenny RA. Midodrine: a role in the management of neurocardiogenic syncope. Heart 1998;79:45–49

52. Kaufmann H, Saadia D, Voustianiouk A. Midodrine in neurally mediated syncope: a double-blind, randomized, crossover study. Ann Neurol 2002;52(3):342–345

53. Morillo C, Leitch J, Yee R, Klein G. A placebo-controlled trial of intravenous and oral disopyramide for prevention of neurally mediated syncope induced by head-up tilt. J Am Coll Cardiol 1993;22:1843–1848

54. Di Girolamo E, Di Iorio C, Sabatini P, et al. Effects of paroxetine hydrochloride, a selective serotonin reuptake inhibitor, on refractory vasovagal syncope: a randomized, double-blind, placebo-controlled study. J Am Coll Cardiol 1999;33:1227–1230

55. Kaufmann H. Head up tilt, lower body negative pressure, pacemakers and vasovagal syncope. Clin Auton Res 1994;4:231–232

56. Gregoratos G, Cheitlin MD, Conill A, et al. ACC/AHA guidelines for implantation of cardiac pacemakers and antiarrhythmia devices: a report of the American College of Cardiology/American Heart Association Task Force on Practice Guidelines (Committee on Pacemaker Implantation). J Am Coll Cardiol 1998;31:1175–1209

57. British Pacing and Electrophysiology Working Group. Recommendations for pacemaker prescription for symptomatic bradycardia. Br Heart J 1991;66:185–191

58. Petersen ME, Chamberlain-Webber R, Fitzpatrick AP, et al. Permanent pacing for cardioinhibitory malignant vasovagal syndrome. Br Heart J 1994;71:274–281

59. Connolly SJ, Sheldon R, Roberts RS, Gent M. The North American Vasovagal Pacemaker Study (VPS). A randomized trial of permanent cardiac pacing for the prevention of vasovagal syncope. J Am Coll Cardiol 1999;33:16–20

60. Benditt DG. Cardiac pacing for prevention of vasovagal syncope. J Am Coll Cardiol 1999;33:21–23

61. Ammirati F, Colivicchi F, Santini M. Permanent cardiac pacing versus medical treatment for the prevention of recurrent vasovagal syncope: a multicenter, randomized, controlled trial. Circulation 2001;104:52–57

62. Dangovian MI, Jarandilla R, Frumin H. Prolonged asystole during head-up tilt table testing after beta blockade. Pacing Clin Electrophysiol 1992;15:14–16

114 Cardiomyopathy

Gilbert H Mudge

The cardiomyopathies are a relatively common abnormality of myocardial contraction that is clinically manifest by producing symptoms of congestive heart failure or eliciting atrial or ventricular dysrhythmias, the latter which predisposes to sudden death. The term "cardiomyopathy" implies an abnormality that replaces, alters, or infiltrates between normal myocytes, and hence designation of cardiomyopathy implies that ischemic, valvular, pericardial, and congenital heart disease have been excluded by conventional clinical criteria as an etiology to a patient's presentation.

The number of possible causes of cardiomyopathy is enormous. Since the condition is considered to be a diagnosis of exclusion with multiple etiologies, the cardiomyopathies are primarily classified based upon physiological presentation (see Table 114.1). The most common one is a dilated cardiomyopathy, evident by systolic dysfunction manifested by ventricular dilatation. Hypertrophic cardiomyopathy is evident by an inappropriate and unexplained increase in left ventricular mass with preservation of ventricular dimensions. Restrictive cardiomyopathy is considered in cases in which the early clinical manifestations reflect diastolic impairment. These operational distinctions are virtually always apparent by conventional echocardiographic assessment of ventricular size, thickness, and function. Epidemiological data suggest that the incidence of cardiomyopathy is increasing, but the relevance of such a conclusion must be tempered by earlier diagnosis, an expanding list of clinical and subclinical causes of cardiomyopathy, and new clinical insights into the genetic importance of both dilated and hypertrophic forms of the disease.

Conventional clinical wisdom lists distinct and separate etiologies for each of the three types of cardiomyopathy. Hypertrophic and restrictive cardiomyopathy may initially be confused with each other and with constrictive pericardial disease, but careful clinical analysis will ultimately define marked differences in pathophysiology. A very small percentage of patients with hypertrophic cardiomyopathy may progress to a dilated cardiomyopathy late in their clinical course; when such occurs, systolic dysfunction and dilatation of the ventricle rarely approach the dimensions that are anticipated with the dilated form of the disease. Hence, the etiologies of cardiomyopathy are most often mutually exclusive.

Dilated cardiomyopathy

The literature will support an encyclopedic listing of potential courses of dilated cardiomyopathy. Each of these would suggest that an inflammatory myocardial process or myocarditis is the initial common pathway to a dilated cardiomyopathy. Be the etiology infectious, immunological, metabolic, toxic, drug-induced, familial, or infiltrative, the final result of myocyte destruction and intracellular fibrosis is systolic dysfunction. Left ventricular dilatation and depression of ejection fraction ensue. Right ventricular dilatation may occur, but usually not until the late stages of the disease; four chamber enlargement is a very advanced finding.

Acute viral myocarditis has often been assumed to be the major infectious etiology in the evolution of dilated cardiomyopathy. Various viruses have been incriminated, most commonly the adenovirus and Coxsackie B virus.[1] Coxsackie A virus, poliovirus, influenza virus, arbovirus, and cytomegalovirus have also been frequently identified.[2] Dilated

Table 114.1 Pathophysiological presentation of cardiomyopathies

	Dilated cardiomyopathy	Hypertrophic cardiomyopathy	Restrictive cardiomyopathy
Etiology	Infectious, immunological, metabolic, toxic, or familial causes	Primarily familial, or sustained hypertension	Amyloid, sarcoid, and hemochromatosis are most common etiologies
Echocardiogram	Four chamber enlargement Systolic dysfunction Thin ventricle	Preserved systolic function Disproportionate diastolic dysfunction Increased wall thickness Asymmetric hypertrophy	Preserved systolic function Disproportionate diastolic dysfunction Increased wall thickness
Symptoms	Left-sided heart failure before right-sided heart failure	Heart failure Angina Syncope	Right-sided heart failure occurs early

cardiomyopathy is common in human immunodeficiency virus (HIV) disease. Recent studies have isolated viral specific RNA within myocardium of patients with clinical myocarditis—additional presumptive evidence of a viral etiology.

However, virus replication may not be the primary insulting event. Rather, the immunological response to new antigens, or to disrupted cell surfaces, may be of greater importance.[3–5] Cytokine activation may be critical in the pathogenic cascade.[6] Moreover, in the rare patient who has biopsy proven acute myocarditis with a diffuse lymphocytic infiltrate, pinpointing a virus etiology by conventional methods has been often exceedingly difficult. There is little evidence that antiviral agents can be used in this patient population.[7] These etiological nuances are of particular relevance, for endomyocardial biopsy has not shown to be of definitive assistance in detecting and monitoring patients with suspected myocarditis, and there is little clinical evidence to suggest that immunosuppressive therapy offers any particular benefit to this patient population.[8] High-dose intravenous gamma globulin is reported to have a clinical impact in the pediatric population.[9]

Other infectious etiologies are better established. Trypanosomiasis notoriously causes a dilated cardiomyopathy, manifested by heart block, high-grade ventricular dysrhythmias, an history of endemic exposure, and positive serology. Release of diphtheria toxin is a time-honored differential to dilated cardiomyopathy of an infectious etiology. Lyme myocarditis is secondary to the spirochete *Borrelia burgdorferi* and is of increasing frequency. Atrioventricular (AV) conduction defects are the usual clinical presentation and symptomatic dilated cardiomyopathy is rare.

The most common toxic etiology of a dilated cardiomyopathy must be excess alcohol consumption.[10] This is presumed to be a direct toxic effect of alcohol on the myocyte as well as the underlying nutritional deficiencies often associated with this patient population. Cocaine-induced cardiomyopathy may also present with typical features of dilated cardiomyopathy, although myocardial infarction and regional wall motion abnormalities are also documented in this patient population.[11,12] Free-base cocaine is associated with greater predisposition to cardiomyopathy or to sudden death. Doxorubicin and daunorubicin are the primary toxic chemotherapeutic agents incriminated in the evolution of dilated cardiomyopathy.[13] Attention has been paid to dose-related toxicity, cardiotoxicity rarely being seen below doses of doxorubicin of 500 mg per square meter. Another anthracenedione, mitoxantrone, closely related to doxorubicin, has recently been approved by the Food and Drug Administration for use in severe, relapsing or progressive multiple sclerosis. Reports suggest that cardiomyopathy is uncommon in otherwise healthy patients who have received less than 140 mg per square meter, although many neurologists currently prefer not to exceed a total dose of 96 mg per square meter (usually administered as 5 to 12 mg per square

meter every 12 weeks). Noninvasive assessment of patients throughout their chemotherapy is required. Monitoring for histological changes with endomyocardial biopsy is accepted in this particular instance but not for mitoxantrone when this is used in multiple sclerosis. Other potential toxic etiologies include cyclophosphamide administration, methysergide, carbon monoxide, and lead exposure. Prolonged exposure to catecholamines can induce profound myocyte destruction and left ventricular dysfunction, be this the result of sustained infusion or underlying pheochromocytoma. Catecholamine cardiomyopathy can often be reversed if properly recognized.[14]

Metabolic etiologies of dilated cardiomyopathy include uremia, hypocalcemia, hypercalcemia, hemochromatosis, hyperthyroidism and hypothyroidism, homocystinuria, a variety of glycogen storage diseases, of which Fabry disease is the most common, and selenium deficiency. Identifying a metabolic cause may be curative, and hence routine assessment of a patient with dilated cardiomyopathy must include customary chemistry panels along with thyroid and iron analysis.

Genetic etiologies of dilated cardiomyopathy have received much recent attention. The current elucidation of their role in the evolution of such a devastating disease is one of the more exciting interfaces between molecular biology and clinical medicine. Inherited genetic defects may account for as much as 30% of dilated cardiomyopathies.[15–17] Moreover, genetic predisposition to the disease may be enhanced when such individuals are exposed to other secondary etiologies. Mutations in the sarcomere protein genes may well account for approximately 10% of all familial dilated cardiomyopathy, and seem to be more prominent in those individuals with early onset of ventricular dilatation and symptomatic congestive heart failure.[18] Moreover, the same gene mutations are now noted to cause either a dilated or hypertrophic cardiomyopathy, suggesting that the effects of mutant proteins on muscle mechanics precipitate two different responses within the myocyte that remodel the heart.

Hypertrophic cardiomyopathy

While the initial clinical description in this form of cardiomyopathy was in those patients with dynamic subaortic obstruction, more recent studies define a larger group of patients who do not have any outflow gradient, but rather profound and unexplained left ventricular hypertrophy. This often results in an increase in biventricular muscle mass, with small ventricular cavities. As a result, clinical presentation reflects abnormalities in diastolic function, and hence often confusion with restrictive cardiomyopathy. The histological examination of hypertrophic cardiomyopathy reveals classic whorling of myocytes with cell to cell fiber disarray in a large percentage of the heart.

While unrecognized or untreated systemic hypertension must always be considered a cause, the primary etiology of hypertrophic cardiomyopathy must now be recognized to be familial.[19,20] Autosomal dominant mendelian-inherited traits are now identified in more than 50% of patients reported. More than 125 different mutations have been reported, many of these spontaneous; many loci may have genetic defects. Prognosis and clinical presentation may depend solely upon the genetic abnormality: mutations on the troponin T gene characterize individuals with less hypertrophy but a poor prognosis and higher risk for sudden death; other mutations may have a more benign prognosis.[21–23] The complexity of the genetic mutations means that genetic testing is not a routine clinical screen at the present time, but special analysis may be important in some predisposed individuals to assist in genetic counseling.

Hypertrophic cardiomyopathy may at times be confused with other infiltrative processes, including Pompe and Fabry disease.

Restrictive cardiomyopathy

Restrictive cardiomyopathy is the least common of the cardiomyopathies. Patients with restrictive cardiomyopathy will have restricted diastolic function, but the echocardiogram that assesses ventricular dimensions and contraction will appear normal.[24] Many of the initial clinical features of restrictive cardiomyopathy may be identical to those of constrictive pericarditis, hence precise distinction between the two is mandatory, given the potential for successful surgical treatment of the latter condition. Infiltrative etiologies of restrictive cardiomyopathy are probably the most common and include amyloid, sarcoidosis, hemochromatosis, and Gaucher disease. Advanced cases of amyloid restrictive cardiomyopathy may be suggested by speckling or visualization of infiltrate on echocardiogram.[25] Other less frequent etiologies include hypereosinophilic syndrome, carcinoid syndrome and endomyocardial fibrosis, the most frequent cause of congestive heart failure in equatorial Africa. Diagnosis of the infiltrative process is often secured by endomyocardial biopsy.

Cardiomyopathies and neurological disorders

A large number of myopathies and the muscular dystrophies may be associated with one of the three forms of cardiomyopathy (Table 114.2). Duchenne and Becker muscular dystrophy are often associated with an X-linked dilated cardiomyopathy, the abnormality being on the dystrophin gene. Cardiac manifestations of the diseases are often obscured by unrelenting progression of skeletal muscle weakness, but approximately 25% of the patients may succumb to progressive heart failure or sudden death. Transplantation has been successfully reported in this patient population. Emery–Dreifuss muscular dystrophy may often present with progressive cardiomyopathy. While atrial and ventricular dysrhythmias and AV block are the most common cardiac manifestations of this muscular dystrophy, patients also may progress to develop symptomatic dilated cardiomyopathy and rarely hypertrophic cardiomyopathy. Myotonic muscular dystrophy is often associated with degeneration and fibrosis of the conduction system and hence dysrhythmias and conduction abnormalities are the anticipated cardiac presentation. In each of the muscular dystrophies, echocardiogram findings usually reveal asymptomatic dilated cardiomyopathy, and sudden death from dysrhythmias is a more common presentation than progressive heart failure.

Friedreich's ataxia is inherited as an autosomal recessive disease. Abnormalities in frataxin, a mitochondrial protein, lead to mitochondrial dysfunction manifest by apoptosis. Cardiac manifestations are frequently associated with a hypertrophic cardiomyopathy rather than a dilated cardiomyopathy, and asymmetric hypertrophy has been reported.

Other less frequent neurological diseases may also be associated with cardiac abnormalities, but progression to overt congestive heart failure is unusual. Kearns–Sayre syndrome often presents with AV block, the spinal muscular atrophies are associated with complex congenital heart disease, dysrhythmias and dilated cardiomyopathy, and myasthenia gravis is reported to be associated with histological evidence of myocarditis which is rarely clinically manifested.

Clinical presentation

There are slight variations to the presentation in cardiomyopathies that may assist in differentiating the etiology at the bedside, and will certainly direct initial therapeutic efforts. Dilated cardiomyopathies usually present with symptoms of left-sided heart failure, manifested by progressive dyspnea, fatigue, and progressive weakness. Later in the clinical course patients develop symptoms of right-sided heart failure, manifested by peripheral edema, hepatomegaly, and venous distension. Weight loss in a setting of symptoms of left-sided heart failure forebodes an adverse prognosis, for weight loss implies inadequate cardiac output to meet metabolic demands. Patients with hypertrophic cardiomyopathy may have a similar degree of exertional dyspnea, but may also have anginal discomfort due to mismatch between enhanced left ventricular muscle mass and increased ventricular pressures. They will have similar symptoms of fatigue, and right-sided heart failure is once again a finding for the late disease process. Restrictive cardiomyopathy, representing a primary diastolic abnormality, will present with symptoms of dyspnea, but right-sided heart failure is more common earlier in the patient's clinical course. This reflects diastolic dysfunction of both right and left ventricles, and the initial clinical presentation may be that of peripheral edema, or hepatomegaly with hepatic dysfunction and cirrhosis.

The physical examination of patients with cardiomyopathy will be of marginal assistance in differentiating etiology. S3 and S4 gallops and severe cardiomegaly will be appreciated in the physical examination of dilated cardiomyopathy, but these findings often are not evident in patients with restrictive and hypertrophic cardiomyopathy.

The chest radiograph is of also of little assistance in

Table 114.2   Myopathies associated with cardiomyopathy

Myopathy	Cardiomyopathy	Clinical clues
Duchenne dystrophy	D, H	X-linked, age of onset 3–5 years, pseudohypertrophy of calves, high CK
Becker dystrophy	D, H	X-linked, onset usually early adulthood, slowly progressive, high CK, cardiomyopathy may be the presenting symptom
Dystrophinopathy manifesting female carrier	D	Slowly progressive weakness, high CK
Emery–Dreifuss muscular dystrophy	A, D, R	X-linked or AD, slowly progressive weakness, prominent contractures
Sarcoglycanopathies	A, D	AR, slowly progressive, usually proximal weakness
Myotonic dystrophy	A, D	AD with anticipation, onset neonatal to late adulthood, facial, and distal > proximal weakness, myotonia
Proximal myotonic myopathy	A	AD, onset usually adulthood, slowly progressive proximal weakness, myalgia
Facioscapulohumeral dystrophy	A (infrequent)	AD, facial and proximal > distal weakness, winging of scapulae
Merosin-negative congenital muscular dystrophy	D	AR, onset infancy or childhood, contractures, demyelinating polyneuropathy, T_2 signal changes of white matter
Myofibrillar myopathy	H, R, A, D	AD, AR, or X-linked, onset infancy, childhood or adult life, distal and proximal weakness, neuropathy

Congenital myopathies
  Nemaline myopathy
  Centronuclear myopathy
  Multicore myopathy
	D, H, A	AR, AD, or X-linked, onset infancy, usually nonprogressive or slowly progressive

Mitochondrial myopathy	A, D, H	Maternal, AR, multisystem involvement
Systemic carnitine deficiency	H, D	AR, proximal weakness, metabolic crises
Infantile acid maltase deficiency	H, D	AR, progressive weakness, hypotonia
Childhood onset branching enzyme deficiency	H	AR, onset after age 1 year, liver involvement
Infantile debrancher enzyme deficiency	H	AR, recurrent hypoglycemia, seizures, hepatomegaly
Danon disease (Lamp-2 deficiency)	A, H	X-linked, usually with mental retardation, mild proximal and distal weakness
Barth syndrome	D, H	X-linked, onset, infancy, hypotonia, mild weakness, cyclic neutropenia
McLeod syndrome	D, R, A	X-linked, onset adulthood, movement disorder, seizures, acanthocytosis
Polymyositis	D	Acute onset, may be associated with anti-SRP antibodies

D, dilated; H, hypertrophic; A, arrhythmogenic; R, restrictive; CK, creatine kinase; AD, autosomal dominant; AR, autosomal recessive; SRP, signal recognition peptide. (The author and the editor [JN] thank Dr. Duygu Selcen, Mayo Clinic, for creating this table.)

differentiating etiologies. Electrocardiograms usually reveal diffuse ST and T wave changes, atrial and ventricular dysrhythmias, and intraventricular conduction defects. While left ventricular hypertrophy (LVH) should be expected on the electrocardiogram in an individual with hypertrophic cardiomyopathy, voltage criteria for LVH may also be met in patients who have dilated cardiomyopathy, the result of an increase in left ventricular size rather than left ventricular muscle mass. Hence, electrocardiographic criteria for left ventricular hypertrophy are not usually of assistance in differentiating etiologies.

The echocardiogram becomes essential to the differential diagnosis, for the echocardiogram of a dilated cardiomyopathy by definition depicts ventricular dilatation and systolic dysfunction. The echocardiogram of hypertrophic cardiomyopathy will document enhanced muscle mass, as reflected in an increase in wall thickness, a small or normal-sized ventricle, and may also define the degree of subvalvu-

lar obstruction to left ventricular outflow. In the case of restrictive cardiomyopathy, left ventricular wall mass may be minimally enhanced, diastolic abnormalities suggested by Doppler flow characteristics, left ventricle normal in size, pericardial effusions excluded, and characteristics of echogenicity within the myocardial tissue may suggest either amyloid or hemochromatosis.

The results of cardiac catheterization will often supplement the echocardiographic findings. In the case of a dilated cardiomyopathy, elevated right and left heart filling pressures, diminished cardiac output, and the degree of mitral and/or tricuspid regurgitation are important diagnostic features that further characterize the stage of the disease. In the patient with either restrictive or hypertrophic cardiomyopathy, diastolic abnormalities of left ventricular noncompliance will be reflected in an elevated end-diastolic pressure and the morphology of the left ventricular diastolic pressure contour. In these two types of cardiomyopathy, diagnostic cardiac catheterization becomes central in differentiating the cardiomyopathies from constrictive pericarditis. In patients with cardiomyopathy, there will usually be elevated right- and left-sided pressures, pulmonary hypertension, and a wide pulse pressure in the right ventricular pressure tracing. This is to be contrasted to constrictive pericarditis, which may have similar elevations of right- and left-sided filling pressures, but rarely pulmonary hypertension, and usually has a very narrow pulse pressure in the right ventricle; right ventricular diastolic pressure may often be 30% to 50% of right ventricular systolic pressure. When this hemodynamic profile is recorded, surgical exploration for constrictive pericarditis is often justified.

Treatment of cardiomyopathies

Unfortunately, there are very few specific treatments for any of the three forms of cardiomyopathy once they are clinically apparent (see summary in Table 114.3). Obviously, metabolic causes of a restrictive process are readily reversed with conventional medical therapy, but such represents a small majority of clinical presentations. Once these metabolic causes are excluded, the therapy of all three forms of cardiomyopathy follows a common pathway for the treatment of congestive heart failure that will include dietary modulation and sodium restriction, physical exercise, and institution of a medical regimen. Sodium restriction to 2 grams intake per 24 hours, and a fluid restriction of 2 liters per day are often overlooked at the bedside in the management of recurrent congestive symptoms. In this regard, proper patient education as to precipitating factors for congestive symptoms is essential.

Major therapeutic approaches in the medical therapy of cardiomyopathy are directed toward abnormalities incurred by activation of the renin–angiotensin and the adrenergic system in patients with congestive heart failure. The degree of medical therapy to address each of the potential abnormalities of neural-hormonal deregulation depends in large part on the symptomatic status of the patient.

In the truly asymptomatic individual who has evidence of cardiomyopathy, it is difficult to make a compelling case for medical therapy beyond the institution of angiotensin converting enzyme inhibitors.[26] There is limited clinical experience to suggest that treating the asymptomatic patient will reduce the probability of overt heart failure and reduce the combined end-points of mortality plus hospitalization. The beta-adrenergic blocking agents and the angiotensin II receptor blocking agents have not been documented to be effective in the asymptomatic patient population.

In those individuals with mild to moderate symptoms of congestive heart failure, medical therapy is directed toward improving symptomatic status as well as preventing further remodeling and dysfunction of the ventricle. The angiotensin converting enzyme inhibitors have a proven record for both end-points, and there is now compelling evidence that angiotensin II blocking agents and beta-adrenergic blocking agents are similarly effective.[27–30] It is more difficult to show a similar beneficial effect for the cardiac glycosides; a single randomized study with digoxin does report reduced hospitalization and improved symptoms, although the impact on mortality is not as convincing as with other neural-hormonal agents. The addition of diuretic therapy in the symptomatic patient continues to be a cornerstone of therapy, with obvious improvement in the patient's overall volume status. Conventional loop diuretics may often be sufficient, and there is now renewed enthusiasm for adding an aldosterone antagonist to the diuretic regimens. A recent randomized study reports improved survival in patients on an aldosterone antagonist,[31] and the clinical benefit is clearly more manifest in patients who present with right heart failure.

As the symptomatic status of the patient deteriorates, the impact of both beta-adrenergic blocking agents and angiotensin converting enzyme inhibitors

Table 114.3   Treatment options for cardiomyopathies

Dilated cardiomyopathy	Hypertrophic cardiomyopathy	Restrictive cardiomyopathy
Sodium restriction	Sodium restriction	Sodium restriction
Fluid restriction	Fluid restriction	Fluid restriction
Afterload reduction therapy	Diuresis	Diuresis
Diuresis	Prophylactic antiarrhythmics	Treatment of any reversible systemic disease
Aldosterone antagonists	Implantable defibrillators	
Beta-adrenergic blocking therapy	Cardiac transplantation	
Cardiac glycosides		
Prophylactic antiarrhythmics		
Implantable defibrillators		
Anticoagulation		
Parenteral infusion of inotropic agents		
Ventricular synchronization		
Cardiac transplantation		
Ventricular assist devices		

becomes more pronounced. Diuretics and an aldosterone antagonist must be maintained. The therapy for advanced heart failure is usually stratified, initiating angiotensin converting enzyme inhibitors and diuretics to stabilize the patient, and once clinically improved, adding beta-adrenergic blocking agents for long-term protection from excess catacholamines;[5] this may well result in further improvement in overall functional status. The angiotensin II receptor blocking agents are developing a promising role in the management of heart failure, especially for those patients who are intolerant of converting enzyme inhibitors. Other vasodilators, in particular the combination of hydralazine and nitrates, are also very effective.

The therapeutic benefit of the medical regimen in those individuals with persistent and refractory decompensation remains poor. The mortality of this population may approach 80% at 2 years. Clinical studies with more potent inotropic agents have been indeed discouraging for the oral inotropic agents are all associated with enhanced mortality.[32,33] While home dopamine or dobutamine infusions are theoretically possible options to return a patient to a home or hospice environment, the impact of these agents on a long-term functional status remains dubious.

The proper role of anticoagulant therapy in the management of cardiomyopathies remains controversial, and has not been the subject of the same outcome research as the angiotensin converting enzyme inhibitors or beta-adrenergic blocking therapy. In patients with advanced left ventricular dysfunction, there remains a risk of arterial thromboembolic events, most often resulting in cerebral ischemia. This may approach a risk of 5% per 100 patient years.[34] Coexistent atrial fibrillation certainly enhances this risk. Since long-term warfarin therapy lowers the overall risk of arterial thromboembolism, it seems reasonable to recommend this to patients who have severe and symptomatic cardiomyopathy.[35] Although such therapy is not without risk, it can now be safely followed by conventional anticoagulation clinics and, with proper patient education, adverse consequences of anticoagulation can be reduced to minimum. Moreover, in an individual with right heart failure, anticoagulation may prevent venostasis, and hence pulmonary emboli complicating the patient's overall clinical presentation. This has not been confirmed in randomized clinical trials.

The role of prophylactic antiarrhythmic therapy remains controversial. Some of the agents have been found to be detrimental in patients with advanced left ventricular dysfunction, particularly those with ischemic heart disease.[36,37] Type 1 antiarrhythmic agents are now generally contraindicated in patients with significant left ventricular dysfunction. Amiodarone, a type 3 antiarrhythmic agent with some adrenergic blocking properties, may have some role in the patient population with asymptomatic ventricular arrhythmias.[38] Despite an extensive list of toxicities that include hyper- and hypothyroidism, hepatic dysfunction, and pulmonary toxicity, studies suggest that it may be safe and effective in patients with advanced left ventricular dysfunction and heart failure. However, any enthusiasm for the use of amiodarone must now be tempered by the unusual strides that have been made in the technology and indications for implantable cardiac defibrillators. These compact devices can now be effectively placed with minimal compromise to a patient's overall lifestyle, and have convincingly been shown to reduce the incidence of cardiac death in patients thought to be at high risk with advanced left ventricular dysfunction and symptomatic congestive heart failure. Given the impact of implantable defibrillators on the incidence of sudden death in select populations, one can now anticipate expansion of their indications for patients with all forms of left ventricular dysfunction.[39]

Future innovative therapies for the management of congestive heart failure will include a number of different strategies. The use of atrial natriuretic peptide is rapidly emerging as a potential option for decompensated patients, and may supplement current strategies directed toward the angiotensin–renin system and the adrenergic system. Biventricular pacing may be of benefit in patients who have significant intraventricular conduction defects and symptomatic congestive heart failure.[40] By synchronizing right and left ventricular contraction, improvements in ejection fraction, cardiac output, and ventricular filling pressures have all been recorded. In limited studies, this is associated with an improvement in the overall symptomatic status. Long-term randomized studies are currently underway.

Cardiac transplantation continues to be the most definitive intervention for end-stage congestive heart failure. Cardiac transplant centers follow relatively rigid recipient selection criteria, for the donor supply continues to be limited. There is a multiplicity of immunosuppressive regimens, with improved long-term survival, reduced infectious complications, and less long-term morbidity. Options include prednisone, azathioprine, mycophenolate mofetil, cyclosporine, sirolimus (rapamycin), tacrolimus, interleukin II blocking agents, and OKT3 monoclonal antibodies, all of which provide clinicians with a broad spectrum of immunosuppressive capabilities.

Left ventricular assist devices, and perhaps artificial hearts will prove to be of long-term benefit to patients with refractory congestive heart failure. A recent randomized study showed that an electric left ventricular assist device was superior to medical therapy in patients who were not candidates for cardiac transplantation.[41] Currently used devices develop pulsatile flow, and discharge to the home setting is now possible. Whether such technology becomes a definitive form of therapy rather than a bridge to cardiac transplantation remains conjecture at the present time, but the evolution of the technology for this particular population is indeed impressive. The major complication of such devices is thromboembolism. Only one device does not require long-term anticoagulation. Infectious complications are also well documented. The long-term clinical impact of this technology will rest not only upon potential medical complications, but many ethical and financial issues that have not even yet been addressed regarding the use of artificial hearts.

Acknowledgments

Dr. Duygu Selcen of the Mayo Clinic Department of Neurology created Table 114.2 for this chapter.

References

1. Hingorani AD. Postinfectious myocarditis. BMJ 1992; 304:1676
2. Partanen J, Nieminen MS, Krogerus L, et al. Cytomegalovirus myocarditis in transplanted heart verified by endomyocardial biopsy. Clin Cardiol 1991; 14:847
3. Nakamura H, Yamamura T, Umemoto S, et al. Autoimmune response in chronic ongoing myocarditis demonstrated by heterotopic cardiac transplantation in mice. Circulation 1996;94:3348
4. Seko Y, Matsuda H, Kato K, et al. Expression of intercellular adhesion molecule-1 in murine hearts with acute myocarditis caused by coxsackievirus B3. J Clin Invest 1993;91:1327
5. Wessely R, Henke A, Zell R, et al. Low-level expression of a mutant coxsackieviral cDNA induces a myocytopathic effect in culture: An approach to the study of enteroviral persistence in cardiac myocytes. Circulation 1998;98:450
6. Knowlton KU, Badorff C. The immune system in viral myocarditis: Maintaining the balance. Circ Res 1999;85:559
7. Yamamoto N, Shibamori M, Ogura M, et al. Effects of intranasal administration of recombinant murine interferon-gamma on murine acute myocarditis caused by encephalomyocarditis virus. Circulation 1998;97:1017
8. Mason JW, O'Connell JB, Herskowitz A, et al. A clinical trial of immunosuppressive therapy for myocarditis: The Myocarditis Treatment Trial Investigators. N Engl J Med 1995;333:269
9. McNamara DM, Rosenblum WD, Janosko KM, et al. Intravenous immune globulin in the therapy of myocarditis and acute cardiomyopathy. Circulation 1997;95:2476
10. Fernandez-Sola J, Estruch R, Grau JM, et al. The relation of alcoholic myopathy to cardiomyopathy. Ann Intern Med 1994;120:529
11. Chakko S, Fernandez A, Mellman TA, et al. Cardiac manifestations of cocaine abuse: A cross-sectional study of asymptomatic men with a history of long-term abuse of "crack" cocaine. J Am Coll Cardiol 1992; 20:1168
12. Kloner RA, Hale S. Unraveling the complex effects of cocaine on the heart. Circulation 1993;87:1046
13. Henderson IC, Frei E III. Adriamycin and the heart. N Engl J Med 1979;300:310
14. Jiang JP, Downing SE. Catecholamine cardiomyopathy: Review and analysis of pathogenetic mechanisms. Yale J Biol Med 1990;63:581
15. Baig MK, Goldman JH, Caforio AL, et al. Familial dilated cardiomyopathy: Cardiac abnormalities are common in asymptomatic relatives and may represent early disease. J Am Coll Cardiol 1998;31:195
16. McKenna CJ, Codd MB, McCann HA, et al. Idiopathic dilated cardiomyopathy: Familial prevalence and HLA distribution. Heart 1997;77:549
17. Leiden JM. The genetics of dilated cardiomyopathy— emerging clues to the puzzle. N Engl J Med 1997; 337:1080
18. Ortiz-Lopez R, Li H, Su J, et al. Evidence for a dystrophin missense mutation as a cause of X-linked dilated cardiomyopathy. Circulation 1997;95:2434
19. McKenna WJ, Coccolo F, Elliott PM. Genes and disease expression in hypertrophic cardiomyopathy. Lancet 1998;352:1162
20. Lewis JF, Maron BJ. Clinical and morphologic expression of hypertrophic cardiomyopathy in patients > or = 65 years of age. Am J Cardiol 1994;73:1105
21. Watkins H, McKenna WJ, Thierfelder L, et al. Mutations in the genes for cardiac troponin T and alpha-tropomyosin in hypertrophic cardiomyopathy. N Engl J Med 1995;332:1058
22. Keating M. The devil's in the details: Progress in familial hypertrophic cardiomyopathy. J Clin Invest 1994; 93:2
23. Fananapazir L. Advances in molecular genetics and management of hypertrophic cardiomyopathy. JAMA 1999;281:1746
24. Kushwaha SS, Fallon JT, Fuster V. Restrictive cardiomyopathy. N Engl J Med 1997;336:267
25. Kyle RA. Amyloidosis. Circulation 1995;91:1269
26. The SOLVD Investigators. Effect of enalapril on mortality and the development of heart failures in asymptomatic patients with reduced left ventricular ejection fractions. N Engl J Med 1992;327:685–691
27. The SOLVD Investigators. Effect of enalapril on survival in patients with reduced left ventricular ejection fractions and congestive heart failure. N Engl J Med 1991;325:293–302
28. Packer M, Poole-Wilson PA, Armstrong PW, et al. Comparative effects of low and high doses of the angiotensin-converting enzyme inhibitor, lisinopril, on morbidity and mortality in chronic heart failure. ATLAS Study Group. Circulation 1999;100:2312–2318
29. Packer M, Bristow MR, Cohn JN, et al. Effect of carvedilol on morbidity and mortality in patients with chronic heart failure. N Engl J Med 1996;334:1349–1355
30. CIBIS-II Investigators and Committees. The Cardiac Insufficiency Bisoprolol Study II: A (CIBIS-II): A randomized trial. Lancet 1999;353:9–13
31. Pitt B, Zannad F, Remme WJ, et al. The effect of spironolactone on morbidity and mortality in patients with severe heart failure. N Engl J Med 1999;341: 709–717
32. Packer M, Carver JR, Rodeheffer RJ, et al. Effect of oral milrinone on mortality in severe chronic heart failure. The prospective randomized milrity in severe chronic heart failure. Study Research Group PROMISE. N Engl J Med 1991;325:1468–1475
33. Cohn JN, Goldstein SO, Greenberg BH, et al. A dose-dependent increase in mortality with vesnarinone among patients with severe heart failure. Vesnarinone Trial Investigators. N Engl J Med 1998;339:1810–1816
34. Dunkman WB, Johnson GR, Carson PE, et al. Incidence of thromboembolic events in congestive heart failure. The V-HeFT VA Cooperative Studies Group. Circulation 1993;87(Suppl 6):94–101
35. Garg RK, Gheorghiade M, Jafri SM. Antiplatelet and anticoagulant therapy in the prevention of thromboemboli in chronic heart failure. Prog Cardiovasc Dis 1998;41:225–236
36. Echt DS, Liebson PR, Mitchell LB, et al. Mortality and morbidity in patients receiving encainide, flecainide, or placebo. The Cardiac Arrhythmia Suppression Trial. N Engl J Med 1991;324:781–788

37. The Cardiac Arrhythmia Suppression Trial Investigators. Effect of the antiarrhythmic agent moricizine on survival after myocardial infarction. N Engl J Med 1992;327:227–233

38. Singh SN, Fletcher RD, Fisher SG, et al. Amiodarone in patients with congestive heart failure and asymptomatic ventricular arrhythmia. Survival Trial of Antiarrhythmic Therapy in Congestive Heart Failure. N Engl J Med 1995;333:77–82

39. Moss AJ, Zareba W, Hall WJ, et al. Prophylactic implantation of a defibrillator in patients with myocardial infarction and reduced ejection fraction. N Engl J Med 2002;346:887–933

40. Kass DA, Chen CH, Curry C, et al. Improved left ventricular mechanics from acute VDD pacing in patients with dilated cardiomyopathy and ventricular conduction delay. Circulation 1999;99:1567–1573

41. Rose EA, Gelijns AC, Moskowitz AJ, et al. Long-term use of a left ventricular assist device for end-stage heart failure. N Engl J Med 2001;345:1435–1443

115 Cardiac Tumors

Patricia H Davis and Harold P Adams

Epidemiology of cardiac tumors

In a review of 22 autopsy series primary cardiac tumors were found in 0.02% of the population, and in approximately three-quarters of instances these tumors were histologically benign.[1,2] About 50% of benign cardiac tumors are comprised of myxomas, 10% are lipomas, 10% are papillary fibroelastomas and 10% are rhabdomyomas. The remaining 20% include fibromas, hemangiomas, teratomas, mesotheliomas, and rarely granular cell tumors, neurofibromas and lymphangiomas.[2] Myxomas most commonly arise from the interatrial septum and are attached by a pedicle.[3] About 75% arise in the left atrium and 20% in the right atrium.[3] The age group most commonly affected is that between the third and sixth decades of life, but these tumors have been found in persons ranging from a stillborn child to a 95-year-old.[3] They are more frequently found in women than in men: in one series the ratio was 3:1.[4] Approximately 7% of cases of atrial myxoma are familial, and these tumors are often bilateral or multicentric. In the autosomal dominant Carney complex, affected individuals have cutaneous lesions (lentigines, blue nevi and ephelides) as well as cutaneous hyperpigmentation on the face and trunk, endocrine overactivity (Cushing's syndrome, acromegaly), testicular tumors and schwannomas, as well as intracardiac myxomas. This syndrome has been associated with two gene defects on chromosomes 17q or 2p.[5] It is important to recognize this syndrome, as a close follow-up for recurrence is needed and family members should be screened for the presence of myxoma before they develop symptoms. In children the most common benign cardiac tumor is a rhabdomyoma, but there are few cases reported in the literature with neurologic symptoms.[6]

Lesions arising from the cardiac valve comprise 10% of all cardiac tumors. The most common histological type is the papillary fibroelastoma, which accounts for 80% of all heart valve tumors.[7] In a series of 53 patients reviewed retrospectively with this pathological diagnosis, 79% were male and their mean age was 52 years.[7]

Primary malignant tumors of the heart are rare and usually affect the right side of the heart, so that neurological symptoms are uncommon, and these lesions are not discussed further in this chapter.

Atrial myxoma

Clinical presentation

There are three main presentations for patients with left atrial myxoma. The most common reflects cardiac dysfunction and is reported in 30% to 70% of cases.[8] Symptoms include dyspnea, syncope, pulmonary edema and myocardial infarction.[9] The latter is due to tumor embolization to the coronary arteries. Sudden death can result from obstruction of a valvular orifice. Patients may have heart murmurs or a loud pulmonic component of the second heart sound. A diastolic rumble which changes with position or a tumor "plop" occurs in only 15% of patients.[9] Electrocardiographic abnormalities are non-specific and include left atrial enlargement or right ventricular hypertrophy. Atrial fibrillation is uncommon.[3] Another frequent presentation involves non-specific constitutional symptoms, including weight loss, fatigue, fever, myalgias, arthralgias, livedo reticularis, splinter hemorrhages and Raynaud's phenomenon. This occurs in 30% to 89% of patients.[8] Laboratory findings include elevated erythrocyte sedimentation rate (ESR), leukocytosis, thrombocytopenia and hypergammaglobulinemia.[9]

The third presentation is with neurological symptoms, which occurs in 25% to 45% of cases,[8] and most frequently manifests as ischemic stroke or transient ischemic attack. Any vascular territory can be involved, including the retina and spinal cord.[8,9] Multiple infarcts may lead to a clinical picture of progressive dementia.[9] Hemorrhagic infarction and subarachnoid hemorrhage[8] are infrequent in patients with myxoma. The latter may be due to rupture of an aneurysm that arises secondary to a tumor embolus. No particular characteristics of these cerebrovascular events identify them as probably being due to myxoma, although some authors have suggested that this diagnosis should be considered in young patients and those without cardiovascular risk factors.[4] Accompanying symptoms and signs suggesting constitutional or cardiac involvement would also prompt consideration of this diagnosis. In approximately 25% of patients with cardiac myxoma the presenting symptoms are neurological.[9] The literature contains numerous reports of patients presenting with neurological findings as the sole manifestation of atrial myxoma,[4,8,10–14] so the neurologist must maintain a high index of suspicion.

Right atrial myxomas are not usually associated with cerebral embolic events unless there is a patent foramen ovale with paradoxical embolism. Clinically evident embolic events affecting the lung are uncommon, although there have been case reports of lethal pulmonary embolism and pulmonary hypertension.[3] Other findings include right-sided heart failure and syncope.[4]

Differential diagnosis

The differential diagnoses in a patient with myxoma include collagen vascular disease, vasculitis including polyarteritis nodosa, and subacute bacterial endocarditis. The latter can be difficult to distinguish because at least 40 cases have been reported in the literature of patients with myxoma who were secondarily infected with microorganisms. It may be difficult to differentiate those with infected from those with uninfected tumors, although constitutional symptoms, including fever and elevated ESR, were more often found in the presence of infection.[15] Blood cultures should be considered in patients with suspected myxoma.

Diagnostic tests

Before 1951, atrial myxoma was a postmortem diagnosis[3] and the first living patient was diagnosed with cardiac angiography. Now, the diagnostic test of choice is echocardiography. Two-dimensional transthoracic echocardiography (TTE) is frequently diagnostic, and in a series of 62 patients with myxomas reviewed retrospectively the sensitivity of TTE was 95.2%[16] (Figure 115.1). With transesophageal echocardiography (TEE), tumors as small as 1–3 mm can be detected and the sensitivity approaches 100%.[16] CT and MRI scans of the heart may be useful in determining the tissue composition of the tumor more accurately, but sensitivity is only about 70%.[16] TEE may also be useful to determine the site of attachment of the tumor to the left atrium.[3] Tumors that are highly mobile tend to be associated with a higher risk of embolization.[16]

Imaging studies

CT or MRI scans of the brain typically demonstrate cerebral infarcts in patients with neurological abnormalities due to myxoma. The lesions are more frequent in the hemispheres than the brainstem, and hemorrhagic infarction or subarachnoid hemorrhage are uncommon.[17] In one report of serial MRI scans in a patient assessed several times prior to surgery, there were multiple small bilateral white matter infarcts which increased in number up to the time of surgery

and then remained stable.[18] Cerebral angiography in some cases of cardiac myxoma has shown that multiple small fusiform peripheral aneurysms form, similar to mycotic aneurysms, and these tend to affect small branches of the middle cerebral arteries.[19–21] These have been reported to develop months after surgical resection of the cardiac tumor, and to enlarge over time.[19,21] In one case report the pathological examination of an excised aneurysm showed myxoma cells invading and destroying the subendothelial space.[21] The other postulated mechanism of aneurysm formation is recanalization of a thrombus, with damage to the vessel wall causing subsequent pseudoaneurysm formation.[21] Although there have been several case reports of myxomatous emboli to the brain that subsequently enlarged after surgical resection of the cardiac tumor,[3] the malignant potential of cardiac myxomas is controversial. Some authors suggest that "malignant" myxomas are in fact cardiac sarcomas, if careful histological examination is performed.[22]

Therapy

The treatment of choice for myxoma is surgical excision as soon as it is feasible (Figure 115.2). There are reports of patients experiencing recurrent cerebral infarction while awaiting surgery, despite anticoagulation.[8] In one case report, no cardiac evaluation was done after an initial cerebral infarction and the patient went on to have showers of emboli from an atrial myxoma, resulting in severe brain necrosis and death within 24 hours.[12] There is a case report of a patient treated with intra-arterial urokinase for a middle cerebral artery thrombus due to an underlying myxoma. The artery partially recanalized with no evidence of intracerebral hemorrhage, but the patient did not improve neurologically and subsequently had a further embolus to the aorta and died. The authors cautioned that a careful search for pseudoaneurysms was necessary prior to instituting this therapy in a patient with myxoma.[11] Operative mortality associated with surgical resection of the cardiac tumor is usually low, at 0% to 3%.[3] Follow-up neuroimaging

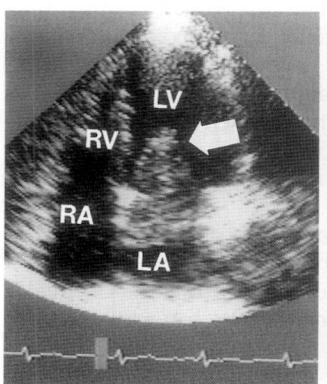
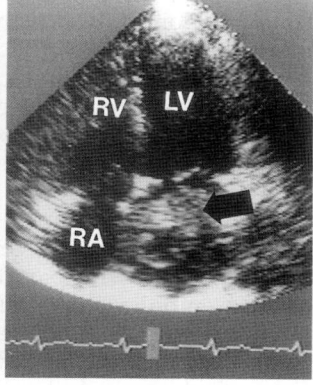

Figure 115.1 Transthoracic echocardiogram demonstrating an atrial myxoma (arrow) in the left atrium.

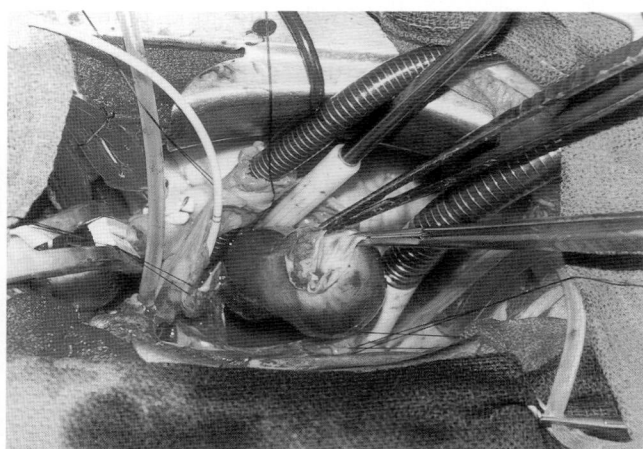

Figure 115.2 Intraoperative photograph demonstrating excision of a large left atrial myxoma. (See color plate section.)

studies most commonly show no new lesions once the cardiac lesion is excised.[8,17,18,23] Routine repeat imaging studies and angiography are probably not indicated following surgery. Recurrence of the cardiac tumor occurs in 1% to 3% of patients,[3] although those with the Carney complex are at higher risk as these lesions are frequently multifocal and require closer observation.[9]

Papillary fibroelastoma

The most common benign cardiac valve tumor is the papillary fibroelastoma.[7] These affect all of the heart valves equally in autopsy series,[7] but in case series involvement of the mitral valve is most frequent.[24] Although initially thought to be harmless, it has become clear that there is a potential for embolism to the brain, retina and coronary arteries. The first reported complication of this tumor was sudden death due to tumor embolism into the coronary arteries.[25] At least 45 cases have now been reported of patients presenting with neurological events thought to be due to embolism from a papillary fibroelastoma.[1,24,26–39] Including all these reports, 26 patients had ischemic strokes, 19 had transient ischemic attacks and four had retinal ischemia. The age range was from 3.5 to 77 years. At least 18 of the cases reported were under the age of 45 years.[24,28,29,34,37–39] Most patients present with neurological symptoms, and cardiac symptoms are less common in patients with fibroelastomas. Howard et al.[34] reviewed 97 cases confirmed pathologically and 8% had myocardial infarction, 5% had angina and 1% had a murmur; 39% had neurological symptoms and 35% were asymptomatic. Many of the patients had recurrent events and did not have other documented risk factors for stroke.[24,26] In all the patients who underwent TEE the tumor was seen, but TTE was a less sensitive test in these case series. Characteristic ultrasound features include small size (<1.5 cm), pedicle attachment to the endocardium of the valve, high mobility, and echolucency within the tumor (Figure 115.3). These features can be used to differentiate papillary fibroelastoma from myxoma (location), Lambl's excrescence (larger size of papillary fibroadenoma) and fibroma (a more highly refractive mass).[1] Lambl's excrescences are filamentous mobile processes attached to the aortic or mitral valve which occur with aging and are not associated with an increased risk of stroke recurrence.[40] Surgical excision with reconstitution or replacement of the valve is the recommended therapy because of the potential for recurrent embolism, but there are no large series of cases.[35] Surgical morbidity is usually less than 5%.[34] In one retrospective review, 17 patients had surgical excision with no recurrent embolic events in 34.2 months of follow-up, whereas there were nine new neurological events in a mean follow-up of 30.7 months in the 37 patients treated medically.[1] Although these data are biased by the unknown selection criteria for surgery, they do confirm the potential for recurrent events in these patients. Other case reports also document recurrent events in patients

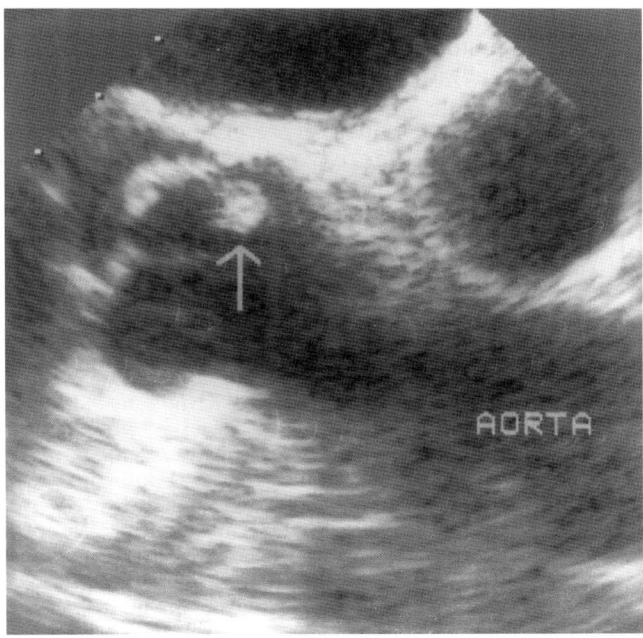

Figure 115.3   Transthoracic echocardiogram of a patient with a papillary fibroelastoma (arrow) on the aortic valve which was subsequently confirmed at autopsy.

who were treated with anticoagulants[24,26] and no recurrences in surgically treated patients.[24,26,31,34] There is controversy about whether the emboli are due to thrombi forming on the tumor, or pieces of tumor itself.[41] The tumor is very friable, and intraoperative TEE may be useful in guiding excision so that aggressive manipulation of the tumor is avoided.[34] Although anticoagulation is commonly used postoperatively, even in the absence of valve replacement or repair, there is no available evidence to support this therapy or which addresses the appropriate duration of anticoagulation.[34] With the increased use of TEE as a diagnostic test following ischemic stroke, it is likely that this disorder will be more commonly detected.

Summary

Cardiac tumors are infrequent causes of ischemic stroke or transient ischemic attack, and there may be few clinical clues to alert the neurologist to look for this underlying disorder. However, if a patient with stroke also has constitutional or cardiac obstructive symptoms, a cardiac myxoma should be strongly considered in the differential diagnosis. Cardiac imaging studies are the key to diagnosis. TEE approaches 100% sensitivity in detecting these tumors and is superior to TTE. Echocardiographic characteristics can be useful in predicting the type of cardiac tumor. In young patients or those with no risk factors for ischemic stroke, transesophageal echocardiography may be useful to exclude these rare but eminently treatable tumors, although there is no consensus on this issue.[26,42] Surgical excision is the treatment of choice if it can be accomplished with reasonable morbidity, and should be performed expeditiously, particularly in patients with myxoma. Anticoagulation would be the second choice of therapy in patients who are not eligible for surgery, but recurrences may occur despite this therapy. Neurologists need to consider this unusual cause of cerebrovascular events because of the importance of early surgical therapy.

References

1. Klarich KW, Enriquez-Saranao M, Gura GM, et al. Papillary fibroelastoma: echocardiographic characteristics for diagnosis and pathologic correlation. J Am Coll Cardiol 1997;30:784–790
2. Reynen K. Frequency of primary tumors of the heart. Am J Cardiol 1996;77:107
3. Reynen K. Medical progress: cardiac myxomas. N Engl J Med 1995;333:1610–1617
4. Sandok BA, von Estorff I, Giuliani ER. CNS embolism due to atrial myxoma. Clinical features and diagnosis. Arch Neurol 1980;37:485–488
5. Casey M, Mah C, Merliss AD, et al. Identification of a novel genetic locus for familial cardiac myxomas and Carney complex. Circulation 1998;98:2560–2566
6. Bayir H, Morelli PJ, Smith TH, Biancaniello TA. A left atrial myxoma presenting as a cerebrovascular accident. Pediatr Neurol 1999;21:569–572
7. Edward FH, Hale D, Cohen A, et al. Primary cardiac valve tumors. Ann Thorac Surg 1991;52:1127–1131
8. Knepper LE, Biller J, Adams HP Jr, Bruno A. Neurologic manifestations of atrial myxoma. Stroke 1988;19:1435–1440
9. Schmidley JW. Neurological presentations of atrial myxoma. Heart Dis Stroke 1993;2:483–486
10. Bloom C, del Carpio-O'Donovan R, Wein T, Begin LR. Cardiovascular radiology. Left atrial myxoma presenting as Gerstmann syndrome. Can Assoc Radiol J 1996;47:16–19
11. Bekavac I, Hanna JP, Wallace RC, et al. Intra-arterial thrombolysis of embolic proximal middle cerebral artery occlusion from presumed atrial myxoma. Neurology 1997;49:618–620
12. Browne WT, Wijdicks EFM, Parisi JE, Viggiano RW. Fulminant brain necrosis from atrial myxoma showers. Stroke 1993;24:1090–1092
13. Lazarevic AM, Neskovic AN, Popovic AD. Hypertensive crisis associated with cerebellar embolization due to left atrial myxoma. Int J Cardiol 1997;61:287–289
14. Robinson DC. An unusual cause of stroke in a young adult. J Fam Pract 1997;44:401–404
15. Revankar SG, Clark RA. Infected cardiac myxoma. Case report and literature review. Medicine 1998;77:337–344
16. Engberding R, Daniel WG, Erbel R, et al. Diagnosis of heart tumors by transesophageal echocardiography: a multicentre study in 154 patients. Eur Heart J 1993;14:1223–1228
17. Hofmann E, Becker T, Romberg-Hahnloser R, et al. Cranial MRI and CT in patients with left atrial myxoma. Neuroradiology 1992;34:57–61
18. Kawamura T, Muratani H, Inamura T, et al. Serial MRI of cerebral infarcts before and after removal of an atrial myxoma. Neuroradiology 1999;41:573–575
19. Suzuki T, Nagai R, Yamazaki T, et al. Rapid growth of intracranial aneurysms secondary to cardiac myxoma. Neurology 1994;44:570–571
20. Damasio H, Seabra-Gomes R, da Silva JP, et al. Multiple cerebral aneurysms and cardiac myxoma. Arch Neurol 1975;32:269–270
21. Furuya K, Sasaki T, Yoshimoto Y, et al. Histologically verified cerebral aneurysm formation secondary to embolism from cardiac myxoma. J Neurosurg 1995;83:170–173
22. Burke AVR. More on cardiac myxomas [Correspondence]. N Engl J Med 1996;335:1462–1464
23. Reichmann H, Romberg-Hahnloser R, Hofmann E, et al. Neurological long-term follow-up in left atrial myxoma. J Neurol 1992;239:170–174
24. Giannesini C, Kubis N, N'Guyen A, et al. Cardiac papillary fibroelastoma. Cerebrovasc Dis 1999;9:45–49
25. Amr SS, Abu AL, Ragheb SY. Sudden unexpected death due to a papillary fibroma of the aortic valve. Report of a case and review of the literature. Am J Forensic Med Pathol 1991;12:143–148
26. Brown RD, Khandheria BK, Edwards WD. Cardiac papillary fibroelastoma: a treatable cause of transient ischemic attack and ischemic stroke detected by transesophageal echocardiography. Mayo Clin Proc 1995;70:863–868
27. Gorton ME, Soltanzadeh H. Mitral valve fibroelastoma. Ann Thorac Surg 1989;47:605–607
28. Bailbe M, Coisne D, Babin P, et al. Fibroelastome papillaire. [French] Rev Med Interne 1998;19:119–122
29. Graca A, Nunes R, Costeira A, et al. Cardiac papillary fibroelastoma of a mitral valve chordae revealed by stroke. [Portuguese] Rev Port Cardiol 1999;18:937–939
30. al-Mohammad A, Pambakian H, Young C. Fibroelastoma: case report and review of the literature. Heart 1998;79:301–304
31. Carmi D, Touati GD, Roux N, et al. Papillary fibroelastoma. Report of 3 cases. [French]. Arch Mal Coeur Vaiss 1999;92:331–335
32. Grinda JM, Couetil JP, Chauvaud S, et al. Cardiac valve papillary fibroelastoma: surgical excision for revealed or potential embolization. J Thoracic Cardiovasc Surg 1999;117:106–110
33. Gunter C, Jenni R. What is your diagnosis? Papillary fibroelastoma of the right coronary aortic sinus—embolism with 2 transient cerebral ischemic attacks. [German]. Schweiz Rund Med Prax 1998;87:1009–1011
34. Howard RA, Aldea GS, Shapira OM, et al. Papillary fibroelastoma: increasing recognition of a surgical disease. Ann Thorac Surg 1999;68:1881–1885
35. Madhu Sankar N, Odayan MK, Morris M, et al. Cardiac valvular papillary fibroelastoma: a report of 2 cases. Texas Heart Inst J 1999;26:298–299
36. McFadden PM, Lacy JR. Intracardiac papillary fibroelastoma: an occult cause of embolic neurologic deficit. Ann Thorac Surg 1987;43:667–669
37. Moraes D, Philippides GJ, Shapira OM. Papillary fibroelastoma of the mitral valve with systemic embolization. Circulation 1998;98:1251–1252
38. Pinelli G, Carteaux JP, Mertes PM, et al. Mitral valve tumor revealed by stroke. J Heart Valve Dis 1995;4:199–201
39. Conte FJ, Katz AS. Fibroelastoma and embolic stroke. Circulation 1998;97:1648
40. Goldman JH, Foster E. Transesophageal echocardiographic (TEE) evaluation of intracardiac and pericardial masses. Cardiol Clin 2000;18:849–860
41. Veinot JP. Fibroelastoma and embolic stroke. Circulation 1999;99:2709
42. Kapral MK, Silver FL. Preventive health care, 1999 update: 2. Echocardiography for the detection of a cardiac source of embolus in patients with stroke. Canadian Task Force on Preventive Health Care. Can Med Assoc J 1999;161:989–996

116 Arterial Hypertension and Hypertensive Encephalopathy

Thomas J Moore

Cardiovascular disease is the leading cause of death in almost all developed countries, accounting for 20% to 50% of total mortality. In the United States, American Heart Association statistics indicate that there were 950 000 deaths from cardiovascular disease (CVD) in 1998,[1] half of which were due to coronary heart disease. Stroke killed 160 000 people (16% of CVD mortality). Williams et al. reported an even higher stroke estimate: in 1995, 750 000 individuals suffered a stroke in the US.[2] Twenty-nine percent of strokes result in death within one year. Although stroke is more common in the elderly, 28% of strokes occur in people under 65 years of age. For many patients, the risk of stroke-induced disability is even more terrifying than the mortality risk: 30% of stroke survivors need help caring for themselves and, three months after the event, 20% require institutionalization. Stroke also carries a staggering economic burden. For 2001, the cost of stroke is expected to be $45.4 billion: about two-thirds for direct medical expenses and one-third for lost productivity.

Hypertension and other stroke risk factors

There are a number of factors that increase the risk of stroke (Table 116.1). Of the modifiable risk factors, hypertension is the most important. In the United States, the National Health and Nutrition Examination Survey III (NHANES III) estimated that 42 million people have hypertension, i.e. one in four American adults. Despite a massive public and physician education campaign in the past three decades, 31% of those with hypertension are unaware they have it. This lack of awareness is especially common in Mexican Americans, males and the elderly.[3] Only 53% of hypertensive Americans are on therapy and only 25% are controlled to recommended goals

($<140/<90$ mmHg). Hypertension is particularly devastating in African Americans. Hypertension affects a higher percentage of blacks than whites, and it appears at an earlier age. On an age-adjusted basis, blacks have more strokes than whites and those strokes are more often fatal. The southeastern United States is particularly stroke prone: both the prevalence of hypertension in the population and the incidence of stroke are higher than in other regions.

Benefits of antihypertensive treatment

Several large placebo-controlled clinical trials have demonstrated conclusively that antihypertensive therapy reduces stroke frequency by about 40% compared to placebo. Recent meta-analyses demonstrated that antihypertensive therapy provides statistically significant improvement in all the major endpoints: stroke, coronary disease, cardiovascular mortality and the development of congestive heart failure.[4]

A comparison of trials performed in younger versus older subjects indicates significant benefit in both age groups. For example, in MacMahon and Rodgers' analysis, stroke incidence was reduced by 34% in trials of elderly patients versus 43% in younger subjects.[5] However, because the absolute number of strokes is greater in the elderly, the absolute reduction in strokes in antihypertensive trials was nearly twice as great in older as in younger subjects (5.1 strokes were prevented per 1000 patient-years of treatment in older subjects, versus 2.6 per 1000 patient-years in younger subjects). A similar pattern was seen for reduction in coronary events. In pooled clinical trials of elderly subjects, coronary events were reduced by 19% in the active treatment versus the placebo groups; in younger subjects the reduction was 14%. The absolute reduction in coronary events was 2.6 events prevented per 1000 patient-years in older subjects, versus 1.0 events per 1000 patient-years in younger subjects.

Another way to quantify the benefit of treatment is to calculate the number of patients one would need to treat to prevent one cardiovascular event or death (compared to placebo-treated patients). The number-needed-to-treat (NNT) is commonly calculated for a five-year treatment period. For patients with mild-to-moderate hypertension, the five-year NNT for preventing one fatal or non-fatal stoke is 135 in younger patients and 45 in the elderly (Table 116.2).[6]

Isolated systolic hypertension (i.e. systolic BP > 140 and diastolic <90 mmHg) (ISH) is a common blood

Table 116.1	Risk factors for stroke
Modifiable	**Non-modifiable**
Hypertension	Increasing age
Smoking	African American
Hyperlipidemia	Family history
Obesity	Prior stroke
Diabetes mellitus	
Atrial fibrillation	
Carotid stenosis	

Table 116.2 Number needed to treat (NNT) for five years to prevent one cardiovascular event or death (from Pearce et al.,[6] with permission)

	Middle-aged patients (7 trials)	Elderly (>60 years) (8 trials)
Fatal/non-fatal stroke	135	45
Fatal/non-fatal CHD	390*	70
Death (all causes)	271*	72

*Event reduction not significantly different from middle-aged control groups.

pressure pattern among people over 60 years of age. It is now clear that treating ISH in patients with systolic pressure >160 mmHg with medical therapy reduces cardiovascular events. Two large randomized placebo-controlled trials including 9000 participants showed that treatment with diuretics in the Systolic Hypertension in the Elderly Project (SHEP)[7] and with a long-acting calcium channel blocker in the Syst-Eur trial[8] reduced stroke frequency by approximately 40%. Neither trial achieved a significant reduction in total or cardiovascular mortality, and no trial has evaluated the benefit of treating ISH in the 140–160 mmHg range.

Measuring the benefit from placebo-controlled trials may underestimate the potential benefit of hypertension treatment. Most such trials use an intention-to-treat assumption: once assigned to the active therapy or placebo group, a subject's results are analyzed as part of that group regardless of what they did with their treatment. Antihypertensive trials typically have an escape blood pressure policy which dictates that active therapy must be started in "placebo" patients whose blood pressure rises above a safe level. In most trials, the number of subjects in the placebo arm who are given active therapy is approximately 15% (so-called "treatment drop-ins"). These treated "placebo" patients probably derive some benefit from antihypertensive therapy and reduce the measured benefit between treatment and placebo groups.

It is important to note that all of the benefits of treatment in clinical trials were achieved with average blood pressure reductions in the active therapy versus placebo groups of 12–15 mmHg systolic and 5–6 mmHg diastolic. Most trials completed to date used diuretics or β-blockers as the therapy tested. Over 30 trials are currently under way, testing the effect of newer antihypertensive agents on cardiovascular events and mortality. However, because of the conclusive evidence that hypertension treatment prevents cardiovascular events, long-term placebo-controlled trials are now considered unethical. Current and future trials will compare newer therapies against diuretics or β-blockers or other new therapies.

The earliest of these "newer-therapy" treatment trials have been completed and published. Three trials deserve individual mention. In the Swedish Trial in Old Patients with Hypertension–2 study (STOP-2), 6614 elderly subjects (two-thirds women) were randomly assigned to three treatments: "conventional" drugs (diuretics or β-blockers), angiotensin-converting enzyme (ACE) inhibitors or calcium channel blockers.[9] The primary combined endpoint of fatal myocardial infarction, fatal stroke and fatal other CVD was similar in the three treatment arms: conventional therapies, 19.8 deaths per 1000 patient-years; ACE inhibitors, 20.5 deaths per 1000 patient-years, calcium channel blockers, 19.2 deaths per 1000 patient-years. The frequency of individual fatal and non-fatal events was also similar in the three treatments, with the exceptions that ACE inhibitors reduced the frequency of myocardial infarction and developing congestive heart failure significantly more than did the calcium channel blockers.

The Captopril Prevention Project (CAPPP) was a prospective randomized trial comparing the ACE inhibitor captopril versus conventional therapies (diuretics and β-blockers) in 10 985 subjects with hypertension.[10] The primary endpoint of the trial was a composite of fatal and non-fatal myocardial infarction, stroke and other cardiovascular deaths. The two treatment groups proved similar: 7.0% of the captopril group and 6.4% of the "conventional therapy" group suffered a primary endpoint event. However, an analysis of secondary endpoints revealed some differences. The combined fatal/non-fatal stroke frequency was significantly greater in the captopril group (P = 0.04). The captopril group had 20 fatal and 173 non-fatal strokes; the conventional therapy group had 22 fatal and 127 non-fatal strokes. In contrast, significantly fewer captopril-treated patients developed diabetes mellitus during the trial (337 vs. 380).

A third recently completed trial (the Heart Outcomes Prevention Evaluation Study, HOPE) evaluated the benefit of adding the ACE inhibitor ramipril or placebo to conventional therapy in subjects at high cardiovascular risk (age at least 55 years; history of coronary disease, stroke or peripheral vascular disease; or diabetes plus at least one other cardiovascular risk factor).[11] Only about 50% of the participants had hypertension, and most were already on therapy (excluding ACE inhibitors). The primary outcome was the same as for the CAPPP trial: fatal and non-fatal myocardial infarction, fatal and non-fatal stroke, and other cardiovascular deaths. Thus, the purpose of the trial was to test whether an ACE inhibitor could reduce risk of cardiovascular events in high-risk patients already on conventional therapies. Overall, 14.1% of the ramipril group suffered a primary endpoint event versus 17.7% in the placebo group (relative risk 0.78: P < 0.001). Ramipril improved several individual endpoints as well: fewer cardiovascular deaths (relative risk 0.75), fewer myocardial infarctions (relative risk 0.80) and fewer strokes (relative risk 0.69). The ramipril group also had significantly fewer coronary revascularizations, complications related to diabetes, developments of new heart failure, worsening angina, and new diagnoses of diabetes. This event reduction is probably not due to ramipril's blood pressure-lowering effect, as the ramipril group displayed a mean reduction in blood pressure of only 3/2 mmHg. Based upon the reduction in events in previous antihypertensive trials, this small reduction would only account for about 40% of the reduction in strokes and 25% of the reduction in myocardial infarction seen in the HOPE trial.

The results of CAPPP and HOPE indicate that ACE inhibitors may offer benefits of antihypertensive therapy comparable to those of diuretics and β-blockers, although differences may exist in certain outcomes (e.g. stroke frequency and development of diabetes). The HOPE trial suggests that ACE inhibition may offer additional cardiovascular risk reduction beyond just blood pressure lowering. It is known that angiotensin II can be synthesized in cardiac and vascular tissues and has a number of tissue effects that could contribute to vascular damage. These include inducing receptor sites for oxidized low-density lipoprotein, increasing monocyte recruitment to sites of vascular injury, and increasing tissue superoxide production. The beneficial effects of ACE inhibition (with only minimal blood pressure lowering) in the HOPE trial could be due to blockade of one or more of these tissue effects of angiotensin II. The results of the many ongoing trials of other ACE inhibitors, angiotensin II receptor antagonists and calcium channel blockers are needed to determine whether there are important differences between the several classes of antihypertensive agent.

Treatment considerations

There are several national and international hypertension guidelines. They agree on general principles but differ in some details. The recommendations below are based on the Sixth Report of the Joint National Committee on Prevention, Detection, Evaluation, and Treatment of High Blood Pressure (JNC VI).[12]

Who should be treated?

JNC VI has stratified blood pressure levels (Table 116.3). Because a considerable number of cardiovascular events occur in people with blood pressure 130–139/85–89 mmHg, surveillance and non-pharmacological treatment are advised for all people in this "high normal" range. Lifestyle and/or medication are recommended for those with systolic higher than 140 or diastolic higher than 90. The intensity of treatment depends on both the level of BP and also on other cardiovascular risk factors. For example, an otherwise healthy person with BP 142/92 should be encouraged to try non-phar-

macological measures (see below). The same BP in a person with a previous stroke, myocardial infarction or diabetes should be treated with medication.

Clinical trials have indicated treatment benefit regardless of gender, age and ethnic background.

Available treatments?

A number of non-pharmacological measures have been shown to lower BP. These have been recommended to prevent the progression from high normal to hypertensive BP levels, as sole treatment for minimally elevated BP, and to enhance the response to antihypertensive medications.

Weight loss (if overweight), reducing dietary sodium intake (to less than 100 mEq/day), regular aerobic physical activity (e.g. brisk walking 30 min/day, 5 days/week), and increasing dietary potassium intake have been shown to reduce BP modestly (2–4 mmHg). A diet rich in fruits, vegetables and dairy foods and reduced in saturated fat, red meat and sugar-sweetened foods and beverages (the so-called DASH diet—Dietary Approaches to Stop Hypertension) has been shown to lower BP by 11/5 mmHg in stage 1 hypertensives. Coupled with sodium reduction (70 mEq/day), the DASH diet is even more effective.[13] It is also effective in stage 1 isolated systolic hypertension.[14] Although all these measures are widely recommended, it is important to note that no non-pharmacological BP treatment has been shown to reduce cardiovascular events in a controlled clinical trial.

Other measures (calcium and magnesium supplements, dietary fat reduction, fish oil, and relaxation/biofeedback) have been recommended, but there is little evidence from controlled clinical trials to support their blood pressure-lowering effectiveness.

More than 80 medications have been approved for BP treatment. Five general classes of drug have achieved broad use based on their antihypertensive effectiveness and side-effect profiles (Table 116.4). These include thiazide diuretics, β-blockers, angiotensin-converting enzyme (ACE) inhibitors, calcium channel blockers (CCB) and angiotensin II receptor antagonists. There are also numerous combination products. JNC VI and the 1999 British Hypertension Society guidelines both recommend diuretics or β-blockers as initial therapy for uncomplicated hypertension, because these agents have produced significant reductions in cardiovascular events in clinical trials. However, both guidelines also acknowledge that some other drug classes may be preferred in selected patient groups, such as those with congestive heart failure (ACE inhibitors, diuretics), diabetes with proteinuria (ACE inhibitors), isolated systolic hypertension in older subjects (diuretics, long-acting dihydropyridine CCB), and post myocardial infarction (β-blockers, ACE inhibitors if myocardial systolic dysfunction). Angiotensin II receptor antagonists are the newest class of antihypertensives. Because they interrupt the renin–angiotensin axis, most experts consider these agents for blood pressure lowering in the same situations where they would consider ACE inhibitors. Recent trials have shown that in type 2 diabetics with

Table 116.3 JNC VI definitions of blood pressure levels (mmHg)

	Systolic		Diastolic
Optimal	<120	and	<80
Normal	<130	and	<85
High normal	130–139	or	85–89
Stage 1	140–159	or	90–99
Stage 2	160–179	or	100–109
Stage 3	>180	or	>110

Table 116.4   The classes of agents most often used for initiating antihypertensive therapy. The usual starting dose for one of the more commonly prescribed drugs in each class is shown

CLASS (example)	Commonly used agent/starting dose	Side effects	Comments*
Thiazide diuretics (hydrochlorothiazide, chlorthalidone)	Hydrochlorothiazide 12.5–25 mg po q.d.	Hypokalemia, hyperuricemia increased glucose level	Thiazides have been proved to reduce CV morbidity and mortality. Contraindicated in patients with sulfa allergy
β-Blockers (propranolol, metoprolol, atenolol nadolol)	Atenolol 50 mg po q.d.	Bronchospasm, bradycardia, cold extremities, depression, fatigue	β-Blockers have been proved to reduce CV morbidity and mortality. Especially recommended post myocardial infarction. β-Blockers are contraindicated in patients with sinus bradycardia or greater than first-degree heart block
Angiotensin-converting enzyme inhibitors (ACE) (captopril, enalapril, lisinopril, benazepril, quinapril, ramipril)	Lisinopril 5–10 mg po q.d.	Cough, headache, rarely angioedema	Especially recommended for patients with heart failure or diabetes (to prevent nephropathy)
Calcium channel blockers (CCB) (dihydropyridine: nifedipine, amlodipine, vicadipine; non-dihydropyridine: diltiazem, verapamil)	Amlodipine 5 mg po q.d.	Headache Flushing peripheral edema; verapamil and diltiazem can slow conduction through AV mode	CCB reduce CV morbity in Isolated systolic hypertension. CCB are also used to reduce anginal symptoms
Antiotensin-receptor blockers (losartan, valsartan, candesartan, irbesartan)	Losartan 50 mg po q.d.	No major side effects	Especially recommended to prevent renal complications in diabetes

*Any of these agents is contraindicated if patients have had previous allergic reaction to the agent.

nephropathy, angiotensin receptor antagonists (losartan and irbesartan) slow the progression to chronic renal failure more effectively than therapies that do not block the renin–angiotensin system.[15,16]

When beginning therapy in subjects with systolic BP 140–160 mmHg and diastolic 90–105 mmHg, the first agent chosen, regardless of which it is, on average normalizes BP in about 40% to 50% of subjects. In the remainder, the options include increasing the dose of the initial agent, changing to a different class of agent, or adding a low dose of another agent. Of these options, the one most likely to be successful is to add a second agent (especially if one agent is a thiazide diuretic). Combination therapy is successful in about 60% to 70% of subjects. The remainder require higher doses or additional agents.

How aggressively should blood pressure be treated?

The goal of therapy for most hypertensive individuals is systolic below 140 mmHg and diastolic below 90 mmHg. The goal for patients with diabetes or renal disease and urinary protein excretion over 1 g/day is systolic under 130 and diastolic less than 85.

There is still uncertainty about whether lowering pressure below these goal levels would provide more benefit or perhaps do harm. Evidence from observational studies suggests that very low blood pressure is associated with an increased mortality rate. Because of this, there has been concern that treating hypertension to levels below 80 mmHg diastolic might cause an increase in mortality rate. The Hypertension Optimal Treatment (HOT) trial addressed this issue by assigning 18 790 hypertensive patients to blood pressure treatment regimens designed to lower diastolic to less than 90 mmHg, less than 85 mmHg and less than 80 mmHg.[17] Patients were treated with a standardized hypertension regimen which began with the long-acting calcium channel blocker felodipine and then added ACE inhibitors, β-blockers and diuretics. From a baseline of 105 mmHg, the three treatment target groups achieved diastolic pressures of 85.2, 83.2 and 81.1 mmHg. There was no significant trend that lower BP was associated with lower event rates for all major cardiovascular events combined, for stroke, or for cardiovascular mortality. However, there was a significant trend for lower rates of myocardial infarction in the lower blood pressure groups, but this significance was lost when silent myocardial infarctions were included in the estimate. It is important to note, however, that there was also no suggestion of increased event rates as long as on-therapy diastolic pressures remained above 75 mmHg. Finally, participants in the HOT trial were also randomly assigned to aspirin or placebo. Overall (i.e. regardless of diastolic pressure target group), the aspirin group showed a 15% reduction in major cardiovascular events ($P = 0.03$). There was no difference in stroke incidence between patients randomized to aspirin or placebo. Fatal bleeds, including cerebral bleeds, were equal in the two groups. The aspirin group did suffer more non-fatal bleeds than the placebo group (relative risk 1.8), but there was no difference in non-fatal cerebral bleeds. Thus, the HOT trial suggests that it is safe to lower diastolic pressure to 80 mmHg in a hypertensive population.

Hypertensive encephalopathy

If the level of arterial pressure rises to exceed the ability of the cerebral vasculature to autoregulate flow, the resulting disruption of the blood–brain barrier and cerebral edema result in hypertensive encephalopathy. The clinical presentation consists of very high blood pressure (typically >240/140 mmHg) and evidence of neurologic dysfunction ranging from confusion to stupor to coma. Papilledema, reflecting increased intracerebral pressure, is a hallmark physical finding.

Hypertensive encephalopathy requires immediate treatment to lower blood pressure. The goal is a reduction of up to 25% within one to two hours. This degree of blood pressure lowering can lead to a dramatic improvement in neurologic function even though the blood pressure level may still be quite elevated. Blood pressure can then be lowered more gradually toward a goal of 160/100 mmHg.

Treatment of hypertensive encephalopathy should be performed under close observation, either with continuous arterial pressure monitoring via an arterial line or with frequent measurements using a standard sphygmomanometer. A number of drugs have been used to treat hypertensive emergencies, but the ideal drug should have a rapid onset and short duration of action to allow careful blood pressure titration. The two most popular agents for this purpose are intravenous sodium nitroprusside or intravenous nitroglycerine. Both require special handling and administration. With prolonged administration, sodium nitroprusside can cause thiocyanate intoxication and methemoglobinemia. Nitroglycerine administration can cause methemoglobinemia, headache and flushing. Patients should be started on oral hypertensive therapy as soon as possible, and the intravenous agent should be gradually withdrawn as tolerated. The use of sublingual nitroglycerine or calcium channel blockers is not recommended for the treatment of hypertensive emergencies. Administered in this way the blood pressure-lowering effect of these drugs is unpredictable, as is their duration of action. The intravenous agents recommended above provide far superior control and can be titrated to maintain blood pressure at the desired level.

References

1. American Heart Association. Heart and Stroke Statistical Update. 2001 Http://www.americanheart.org/statistics/cvd.html
2. Williams GR, Jiang JG, Matchar DB, Samsa GP. Incidence and occurrence of total (first-ever and recurrent) stroke. Stroke 1999;30:2523
3. Hyman DJ, Pavlik VN. Characteristics of patients with uncontrolled hypertension in the United States. N Engl J Med 2001;345:479–486
4. Psaty BM, Smith NL, Siscovick DS, et al. Health outcomes associated with antihypertensive therapies used as first-line agents. JAMA 1997;277:739–745
5. MacMahon S, Rodgers A. The effects of blood pressure reduction in older patients: an overview of five randomized controlled trials in elderly hypertensives. Clin Exp Hypertens 1993;15:967–978
6. Pearce KA, Furberg CD, Psaty BM, Kirk J. Cost-minimization and the number needed to treat in uncomplicated hypertension. Am J Hypertens 1998;11:618–629
7. SHEP Cooperative Group Investigators. Prevention of stroke by antihypertensive drug treatment in older persons with isolated systolic hypertension. JAMA 1991;265:3255–3264
8. Systolic Hypertension in Europe Trial Investigators. Randomised double-blind comparison of placebo and active treatment for older patients with isolated systolic hypertension. Lancet 1997;350:757–764
9. Hansson L, Lindhold LH, Ekbom T, et al. Randomised trial of old and new antihypertensive drugs in elderly patients: cardiovascular mortality and morbidity the Swedish Trial in old patients with hypertension-2 study. Lancet 1999;354:1751–1756
10. Hansson L, Lindholm LH, Niskanen L, et al. Effect of angiotensin-converting-enzyme inhibition compared with conventional therapy on cardiovascular morbidity and mortality in hypertension: the captopril prevention project (CAPP) randomized trial. Lancet 1999;353:611–616
11. Yusuf S, Sleight P, Pogue J, et al. Effects of an angiotensin-converting-enzyme inhibitor, ramipril, on cardiovascular events in high-risk patients. N Engl J Med 2000; 342:145–153
12. Joint National Committee on Prevention, Detection, Evaluation and Treatment of High Blood Pressure. The sixth report of the Joint National Committee on Prevention, Detection, Evaluation and Treatment of High Blood Pressure. Arch Intern Med 1997;157:2413–2446
13. Appel LJ, Moore TJ, Obarzanek E, et al. A clinical trial of the effects of dietary patterns on blood pressure. N Engl J Med 1997;336:1117–1124
14. Moore TJ, Conlin PR, Ard J, Svetkey LP. DASH (dietary approaches to stop hypertension) diet is effective treatment for stage 1 isolated systolic hypertension. Hypertension 2001;38:155–158
15. Lewis EJ, Hunsicker LG, Clarke WR, for the Collaborative Study Group. Renoprotective effect of the angiotensin-receptor antagonist irbesartan in patients with nephropathy due to type 2 diabetes. N Engl J Med 2001;345:851–860
16. Brenner BM, Cooper ME, de Zeeuw D, for the RENAAL study investigators. Effects of losartan on renal and cardiovascular outcomes in patients with type 2 diabetes and nephropathy. N Engl J Med 2001;345:861–869
17. Hansson L, for the HOT Study Group. The hypertension optimal treatment study (the HOT study). Blood Pressure 1993;2:62–68

117 Hepatic Encephalopathy—Diagnosis and Management

Kozhikade V Narayanan Menon and Patrick S Kamath

Introduction

"Hepatic encephalopathy" is a term applied to the wide range of neuropsychiatric manifestations seen in patients with advanced liver dysfunction. Similar neuropsychiatric manifestations may also be seen after the creation of portosystemic shunts or with disorders of the urea cycle. Hepatic encephalopathy may be classified as "acute" or "chronic" according to the duration of the encephalopathy and as "encephalopathy secondary to chronic liver disease" or "encephalopathy secondary to fulminant hepatic failure" on the basis of the underlying liver disease. Rarely, hepatic encephalopathy may be caused by the development of portosystemic venous shunts in the absence of advanced liver disease.

The four grades of severity of hepatic encephalopathy range from subtle behavioral abnormalities (grade I) to deep coma (grade IV) (Table 117.1).[1] In addition, a subset of patients with cirrhosis of the liver exhibit subclinical encephalopathy that is diagnosed primarily with psychometric and electrophysiological testing.[2-6] Hepatic encephalopathy secondary to chronic liver disease and hepatic encephalopathy associated with fulminant liver failure are discussed below.

Hepatic encephalopathy associated with chronic liver disease

Pathogenesis

The exact pathophysiological process for the development of hepatic encephalopathy is unclear and several mechanisms have been implicated, including increased production and absorption of ammonia, production of false neurotransmitters and activation of central γ-aminobutyric acid (GABA)-benzodiazepine receptors by ligands of endogenous origin, altered cerebral metabolism, disturbed activity of Na^+/K^+-ATPase, zinc deficiency, and deposition of manganese in the brain. Ammonia is considered to have an important role in the pathogenesis of hepatic encephalopathy, and most treatment measures of proven value are aimed at decreasing ammonia levels. Central nervous system inhibition at the level of the GABA-benzodiazepine receptor complex by increased levels of endogenous benzodiazepine-receptor ligands has also been proposed as a mechanism for the development of hepatic encephalopathy. Additionally, increased numbers of peripheral-type benzodiazepine receptors have been demonstrated in the brains of patients with cirrhosis, but the

Table 117.1	Grading system for hepatic encephalopathy			
Grade	Level of consciousness	Personality and intellect	Neurological abnormalities	EEG abnormalities
0	Normal	No abnormality	None	None
Subclinical	Normal	No abnormality	None except impaired psychomotor testing	None
I	Inverted sleep pattern, restless	Forgetful, mild confusion, agitation, irritable	Tremor, apraxia, incoordination, impaired handwriting	Slowing 5-cps triphasic waves
II	Lethargic, slow responses	Disorientation for time, amnesia, decreased inhibitions, inappropriate behavior	Asterixis, dysarthria, ataxia, hypoactive reflexes	Slowing triphasic waves
III	Somnolent but arousable, confused	Disorientation for place, aggressive	Asterixis, hyperactive reflexes, Babinski sign, muscle rigidity	Slowing triphasic waves
IV	Coma/unarousable	None	Decerebrate	Slow 2–3-cps delta activity

EEG, electroencephalographic.

Table 117.2   Factors precipitating hepatic encephalopathy in chronic liver disease

Possible mechanism	Precipitant
Increased ammonia production	Excess dietary protein,* constipation,* anorexia, fluid restriction, gastrointestinal tract hemorrhage,* infection (including bacterial peritonitis),* blood transfusion
Increased diffusion of ammonia across blood–brain barrier	Azotemia,* hypokalemia,* systemic alkalosis*
Activation of central GABA-benzodiazepine receptors compounding CNS depressant effect	Use of other psychoactive drugs
Decreased metabolism of toxins because of liver hypoxia	Dehydration, fluid restriction, diuretic effect, excessive paracentesis, diarrhea due to osmotic laxatives, arterial hypotension, gastrointestinal tract hemorrhage, peripheral vascular dilatation, arterial hypoxemia, anemia, use of benzodiazepines
Decreased liver metabolism of toxins because of diversion of portal blood	Portosystemic shunts,* spontaneous, surgical, TIPS
Decreased liver metabolism of toxins because of decreased functional reserve	Progressive hepatic parenchymal damage*
Multiple factors	Development of hepatocellular carcinoma*

GABA, γ-aminobutyric acid; TIPS, transjugular intrahepatic portosystemic shunt. *Common precipitants.

implications of this finding are not clear.[7] Cerebral edema has also been described in patients with hepatic encephalopathy complicating cirrhosis and following placement of transjugular intrahepatic portosystemic shunts (TIPS) for control of variceal bleeding.[8,9]

Hepatic encephalopathy associated with chronic liver disease is often precipitated by various factors (Table 117.2) or develops as a result of spontaneous portosystemic shunting. Thus, management includes various measures to decrease the production and absorption of ammonia and to identify and treat a precipitating cause.

Clinical features

Patients with hepatic encephalopathy related to cirrhosis usually present with an altered sensorium on a background of chronic liver disease. However, because there are no specific manifestations of hepatic encephalopathy, it is important to exclude other causes of an altered sensorium. Asterixis, or flapping tremor, is a characteristic feature of hepatic encephalopathy. Asterixis is a disorder of motor control characterized by myoclonic lapses of posture. These lapses occur as a result of involuntary 50- to 200-ms periods of electrical silence appearing in muscles that are tonically active. Asterixis has also been described in various other conditions (Table 117.3). It may be unilateral or bilateral and is best detected in the hands, although it can be demonstrated in other parts of the body such as the feet. It is elicited by asking the patient to extend the elbows fully and to dorsiflex the wrists with the fingers spread apart, while the arms are off the bed. A rapid flexion-extension movement is characteristically seen at the wrist and metacarpophalangeal joints. Patients with hepatic encephalopathy or metabolic derangements demonstrate bilateral asterixis; unilateral asterixis usually results from structural cerebral lesions. Asterixis is seen characteristically in patients with grade II or grade III encephalopathy. As the encephalopathy progresses, the level of consciousness gradually decreases, ultimately resulting in coma. In addition to alterations in the sensorium, these patients exhibit signs of chronic liver disease, including the loss of secondary sexual characteristics, gynecomastia in men, parotid enlargement, palmar erythema, spider nevi, ascites, and prominent veins on the anterior abdominal wall.

Investigations

Subclinical encephalopathy may be detected with a combination of neurophysiological and neuropsychological testing. Simple bedside tests such as the number connection tests and trail-making tests may be useful. Patients with overt hepatic encephalopathy may have increased arterial levels of ammonia.

Table 117.3   Causes of asterixis[10–15]

Hepatic encephalopathy
Metabolic
    Uremia and dialysis-related encephalopathy
    Hypercapnia
    Nonketotic hyperglycemia
Drugs
    Phenytoin sodium
    Lithium
    Carbamazepine
    Clozapine
Structural cerebral lesions

However, levels of arterial ammonia correlate poorly with the grade of hepatic encephalopathy and cannot be relied upon in making the diagnosis. Several techniques have been used to image the brain in patients with hepatic encephalopathy. These include magnetic resonance imaging (MRI), magnetic resonance spectroscopy (MRS), single photon emission tomography, and positron emission tomography. The primary role of imaging techniques is to exclude structural lesions in patients who have cirrhosis and an altered sensorium. However, investigators have reported increased signal intensity in the globus pallidus on T_1-weighted images of patients with cirrhosis. This change has been described both in the presence and in the absence of hepatic encephalopathy and its significance remains unclear. The intensity of this change has not been found to correlate with the degree of hepatic encephalopathy. In addition, this change has been described in other conditions such as manganese toxicity, fulminant liver failure, parenteral nutrition, neurofibromatosis, and portal vein thrombosis in the absence of cirrhosis.[16] Increased concentrations of manganese have been found in this area, raising the possibility of a role for manganese in the pathogenesis of hepatic encephalopathy and in the production of the increased signal intensity in the globus pallidus seen on MRI. Proton MRS has also been used to determine the role of various molecules in the pathogenesis of hepatic encephalopathy. Decreased myo-inositol:creatine and choline:creatine ratios along with increased glutamate and glutamine:creatine ratios have been described on 1H MRS, with changes occurring after liver transplantation. However, these findings have not been consistent in all studies, and the use of these imaging techniques is confined to research studies.

Management

Management of hepatic encephalopathy in patients with cirrhosis involves 1) identifying and treating the precipitating cause, 2) decreasing the production and absorption of ammonia, 3) administering centrally acting drugs such as flumazenil, levodopa, and bromocriptine, and 4) administering other drugs such as zinc.

Identification and treatment of a precipitating cause In many patients with cirrhosis of the liver, exacerbation of hepatic encephalopathy is usually related to a precipitating cause (Table 117.2). Some of the more common precipitating causes include gastrointestinal tract hemorrhage, infection (e.g., bacterial peritonitis), constipation, benzodiazepine or opiate use, hypokalemia, dehydration, and large-volume paracentesis. Less commonly, the development of hepatocellular carcinoma or portal vein thrombosis may precipitate hepatic encephalopathy. TIPS, which now has largely replaced surgical portosystemic shunting, is associated with a 25% incidence of either new or worsening encephalopathy. An increased risk of encephalopathy after TIPS is associated with a cause of liver disease other than alcohol, female sex, age older than 60

years, or hypoalbuminemia. All patients presenting with an exacerbation of hepatic encephalopathy should have screening tests for infection, including abdominal paracentesis to detect the presence of spontaneous bacterial peritonitis. The presence of an ascitic fluid absolute neutrophil count greater than $250/mm^3$ indicates spontaneous bacterial peritonitis and should prompt the administration of an antibiotic (third-generation cephalosporin, e.g., cefotaxime, 2 g every 8 hours, or a fluroquinolone).[17] Gastrointestinal tract bleeding that is not immediately manifest may also result in hepatic encephalopathy. Associated features such as anemia and hypotension may provide a clue to the diagnosis. In some patients with hepatic encephalopathy, no precipitating factor is identified and the encephalopathy is related to worsening liver function.

Decreasing the production and absorption of ammonia The conventional treatment of hepatic encephalopathy relies largely on decreasing the production and absorption of ammonia. Various strategies include the following:

Dietary measures If hepatic encephalopathy is refractory to lactulose therapy, dietary protein is restricted to 0.8 to 1 g/kg daily. Dietary protein restriction serves to decrease the substrate available in the colon for the production of ammonia. If the patient presents with grade IV encephalopathy, all dietary protein is restricted. With improvement in the level of consciousness, protein intake is increased by 10 g every 3 to 5 days as tolerated. Long-term restriction of dietary protein to less than 0.8 to 1 g/kg daily should be avoided if possible. Supplementation with vegetable protein may be advantageous for patients in whom the total dietary animal and dairy protein tolerance is less than 0.8 to 1 g/kg daily. Most patients will accept a diet supplemented with 30 to 40 g of vegetable protein daily. A pure vegetable protein diet with protein intake up to 120 g/day is usually well tolerated, although sodium restriction may render the diet unpalatable.

The use of oral branched-chain amino acids has been studied in the treatment of chronic hepatic encephalopathy.[18] Although no benefit was found, these agents may have a specific role in improving nitrogen balance without precipitating hepatic encephalopathy in malnourished patients with cirrhosis who are intolerant of protein supplementation.

Nonabsorbable disaccharides Nonabsorbable disaccharides such as lactulose (β-galactosidofructose) or lactitol (β-galactosidosorbitol) help to remove both dietary and endogenous ammoniagenic substrates from the intestinal lumen and have been shown to improve hepatic encephalopathy.[19] Lactulose has become the standard therapy in the United States for the treatment of hepatic encephalopathy. Lactulose is also effective in controlling encephalopathy in the majority of patients with post-TIPS encephalopathy. Although the exact mechanism of action is still unclear, lactulose administration has been associated with a lowering of blood ammonia levels and an increase in fecal nitrogen excretion. After oral administration, lactulose passes relatively unchanged into the large bowel, where it is metabolized by colonic bacteria. Experimental and clinical evidence suggests that lactulose exerts its action by several mechanisms that include 1) acting as an osmotic laxative, 2) facilitating the incorporation of ammonia into bacterial protein that is then excreted, and 3) decreasing ammonia production by intestinal bacteria through a direct action on bacterial metabolism as a result of lowering colonic pH.

The dose of lactulose should be titrated to result in two to four soft acidic (pH < 6) stools daily. To comatose patients, lactulose may be administered through a nasogastric tube at a dose of 30 mL every 4 hours until catharsis occurs. The usual daily maintenance dose of lactulose for patients in whom the encephalopathy has resolved ranges from 30 to 60 g. Doses larger than 90 g/day may produce marked diarrhea and cause dehydration and hypernatremia, resulting in worsening of hepatic encephalopathy. If oral or nasogastric administration is not possible because of ileus or the risk of aspiration, especially in patients with deep coma, lactulose can be administered as an enema (300 mL of lactulose in 700 mL of water administered as a retention enema). This dose can be repeated at 6-hour intervals as needed for a clinical response.

Lactilol, another disaccharide, is not licensed for use in the United States, but it has been shown to be as effective as lactulose in the treatment of hepatic encephalopathy.[20] It is more palatable than lactulose and is associated with less nausea and abdominal distention. The recommended dose is 0.3 to 0.5 g/kg daily, titrated to produce one to two semiformed stools daily. Oral lactose is another alternative for lactase-deficient patients.

Antibiotics Antibiotics with activity against urease-producing bacteria are useful in the management of hepatic encephalopathy. Neomycin (4 to 6 g/day) is similar to lactulose in efficacy and is the most commonly used agent for this purpose.[19] A small percentage (1% to 3%) of the drug may be absorbed and can cause nephrotoxicity and ototoxicity, especially when used for several months. Thus, it should be prescribed with caution for patients with renal failure. Although the data available are limited, they suggest that combination therapy with lactulose and neomycin may be of benefit in patients with hepatic encephalopathy who have an inadequate response to lactulose alone.[20] Because prolonged administration of neomycin can inhibit disaccharidase-metabolizing bacteria, which results in increased stool pH and increased ammonia production, neomycin therapy longer than 3 to 4 continuous weeks is not recommended.

The efficacy of metronidazole (800 mg/day) treatment for 1 week is similar to that of neomycin, although the possibility of gastrointestinal and systemic side effects limits its use for longer periods.

Ornithine aspartate (L-ornithine-L-aspartate) In small clinical trials, oral or parenteral ornithine aspartate, a substrate for the conversion of ammonia to urea and glutamine, has been found to have a benefit similar to that of lactulose but with fewer side effects for patients with grade I or grade II hepatic encephalopathy. Ornithine aspartate stimulates ammonia fixation by increasing glutamine synthetase in the liver. Larger clinical trials are needed to demonstrate that the combination of ornithine aspartate and lactulose may have an additive benefit because both compounds act through different pathways. Until such evidence is available, the routine use of ornithine aspartate in the treatment of hepatic encephalopathy is not recommended.

Zinc Zinc is a cofactor of urea cycle enzymes and also has a role in central nervous system neurotransmission. Clinical trials of zinc supplementation (600 mg of zinc sulphate daily) in hepatic encephalopathy have shown mixed results.[20] Also, the characteristics of patients who may benefit from zinc therapy have not been identified. However, although zinc-deficient patients with cirrhosis should receive supplementation, the benefit of zinc supplementation in the absence of zinc deficiency in hepatic encephalopathy has not been demonstrated.

Centrally acting agents Flumazenil, a benzodiazepine receptor antagonist, has been used in the treatment of hepatic encephalopathy. Although uncontrolled trials initially showed promising results,[21-23] prospective, controlled trials have shown that flumazenil improves neurological scores only in a small proportion of patients with severe (grade III to IVa) encephalopathy.[24-31] However, for patients who had dramatic improvement with flumazenil, the previous administration of benzodiazepines could not be ruled out entirely. Because flumazenil has to be administered intravenously and is short-acting, its use in the treatment of hepatic encephalopathy is limited.

Portosystemic shunt obliteration For refractory encephalopathy secondary to TIPS insertion, the diameter of the shunt may be reduced with interventional radiological techniques. This is often successful in controlling encephalopathy if conventional treatment fails. Similarly, transhepatic embolization or surgical ligation of portosystemic shunts has been beneficial in some patients with refractory encephalopathy secondary to the development of spontaneous portosystemic shunts.

Liver transplantation Liver transplantation offers effective therapy and prolongs the survival of patients with intractable encephalopathy and cirrhosis of the liver. Patients with chronic encephalopathy should be referred for transplantation in accordance with the local criteria for listing for transplantation. The 1- and 5-year overall survival rates after liver transplantation are 87.9% and 74.2%, respectively.[32]

Table 117.4   Some principal causes of fulminant liver failure

Cause	Agent responsible
Viral hepatitis	Hepatitis A, B, D, or E virus Herpes simplex virus
Drug-related liver injury	Acetaminophen Idiosyncratic reactions
Toxins	Carbon tetrachloride *Amanita phalloides* Phosphorus
Vascular events	Ischemic hepatitis Veno-occlusive disease
Miscellaneous	Heatstroke Malignant infiltration Wilson disease Acute fatty liver of pregnancy Reye syndrome

Hepatic encephalopathy associated with fulminant liver failure

Pathogenesis

Fulminant liver failure is defined by the development of hepatic encephalopathy within 8 weeks after the onset of the first symptoms of the disease or the onset of encephalopathy within 2 weeks after the onset of jaundice. Compared with chronic liver disease, fulminant liver failure is characterized by the development of cerebral edema, intracranial hypertension, and subsequent brain herniation. Cerebral edema is the leading cause of death in patients who progress to grade IV encephalopathy and can occur in 75% to 80% of these patients. Two theories have emerged to explain the pathogenesis of cerebral edema in fulminant liver failure. In the glutamine hypothesis, glutamine (the end product of ammonia metabolism in the brain) accumulates in the astrocyte, causing it to swell, thus resulting in cerebral edema. Alternatively, cerebral vasodilatation and increased cerebral blood flow resulting from failure of cerebral autoregulation may also produce cerebral edema. However, recent studies have suggested that both excess glutamine and increased cerebral blood flow may contribute to the development of cerebral edema in fulminant hepatic failure. Cerebral edema leads to increased intracranial pressure in the fixed confines of the cranium, ultimately producing cerebral herniation and death. Intracranial hypertension also leads to a decrease in cerebral perfusion pressure, causing cerebral ischemia, the sequelae of which may progress even during recovery of liver function.

Clinical features

Fulminant liver failure has various causes[33] (Table 117.4). The common causes include viruses, drugs, and toxins. Most patients present with jaundice, followed by the development of hepatic encephalopathy. The onset of hepatic encephalopathy in patients with fulminant liver failure is rapid and characterized

by the development of an altered sensorium, rapidly progressing to coma if untreated. The differential diagnosis for patients presenting with an altered sensorium is broad, and alternative diagnoses should be excluded (Table 117.5). Patients with grade II or III encephalopathy may demonstrate asterixis. Agitation and delusions may occur before the onset of grade III or IV encephalopathy. A few patients may not have characteristic features of liver disease, such as jaundice and ascites, because of the rapidity of progression of liver necrosis. A high degree of clinical suspicion may be necessary to diagnose hepatic encephalopathy in patients who present with an altered sensorium but without overt evidence of liver disease. In these patients, the presence of a prolonged prothrombin time may provide a clue to the diagnosis. Ammonia levels correlate poorly with the severity of hepatic encephalopathy, and their measurement is of little clinical value, both for diagnosis and follow-up of patients with acute hepatic encephalopathy. Other laboratory abnormalities seen in patients with fulminant liver failure include increased transaminase levels, low plasma levels of glucose, and respiratory alkalosis on arterial blood gas analysis.

As cerebral edema develops, patients manifest systemic hypertension, bradycardia, and increased muscle tone, with progression to decerebrate posturing, sluggish pupillary reflexes, papilledema, seizures, and, finally, brainstem respiratory patterns and apnea. Clinical signs of increased intracranial pressure appear late in the course of the disease and do not help guide therapeutic management. Computed tomography, although useful in excluding other causes of increased intracranial pressure, is not helpful in the diagnosis of cerebral edema.

Treatment

Because of the propensity for the rapid progression to deep coma and death from cerebral herniation, patients with fulminant liver failure should be considered for urgent liver transplantation on the basis of the underlying nature of the liver disease. Once fulminant liver failure is diagnosed or suspected, the patient should be transferred to a center capable of performing urgent liver transplantation.

Management of increased intracranial pressure General measures for the management of increased intracranial pressure are shown in Table 117.6. Patients with grade III or IV encephalopathy should be transferred to an intensive care unit, sedated, paralyzed, and electively ventilated. Factors that increase intracranial pressure should be avoided (Table 117.6). The classic neurological findings of increased intracranial pressure and cerebral edema (pupillary changes, abnormal posturing, papilledema) are late changes in hepatic encephalopathy; hence, intracranial pressure catheters are recommended to monitor intracranial pressure in patients with grade III or IV encephalopathy. The major complication arising from the use of these pressure-monitoring devices is intracranial hemorrhage, which in the face of coagu-

Table 117.5   Differential diagnosis of hepatic encephalopathy

Disorder	Diagnostic test

Metabolic encephalopathies
    Hypoglycemia*
    Electrolyte imbalance*
    Hypoxia*
    Carbon dioxide narcosis
    Azotemia*
    Ketoacidosis
	Blood biochemical analysis

Toxic encephalopathies
    Alcohol*
        Acute intoxication
        Withdrawal syndrome
        Wernicke-Korsakoff syndrome
    Psychoactive drugs
    Salicylates
    Heavy metals
	Measurement of blood alcohol level, erythrocyte
	    transketolase activity, therapeutic response to thiamine
	
	Toxicologic screening

Intracranial lesions
    Subarachnoid, subdural, or intracerebral hemorrhage*
    Cerebral infarction
    Cerebral tumor
    Cerebral abscess
    Meningitis
    Encephalitis
    Epilepsy or post-seizure encephalopathy
	Computed tomography, cerebrospinal fluid analysis,
	    arteriography, electroencephalography, virologic testing

Neuropsychiatric disorders	Tests for organic brain syndromes

*This diagnosis is especially pertinent to patients with liver disease.

lopathy can be fatal. Epidural catheters have been shown to have a lower risk of hemorrhage (5%) than subdural bolts or intraparenchymal monitors, for which the risk of hemorrhage can be as high as 20%.[34] Although epidural monitors are less accurate, their lower complication rate and ease of placement make them the optimal choice for intracranial pressure monitoring. Noninvasive techniques such as transcranial Doppler ultrasonography and magnetic resonance angiography may prove useful in selected situations if invasive procedures are contraindicated. An increase in intracranial pressure greater than 20 mmHg or a decrease in cerebral perfusion pressure (Cerebral Perfusion Pressure = Mean Arterial Pressure − Intracranial Pressure) less than 60 mmHg is commonly taken as an indication to commence specific therapy. Mean arterial pressure should be supported with phenylephrine (or norepinephrine) if necessary to maintain cerebral perfusion pressure above 60 mmHg. Mean arterial pressure greater than 150 mmHg or a mean arterial pressure resulting in a cerebral perfusion pressure more than 80 mmHg is reduced with sodium nitroprusside or hydralazine if necessary. To rapidly lower intracranial pressure that is increased to more than 20 mmHg and to improve cerebral perfusion pressure to more than 60 mmHg, hyperventilating the patient to a $PaCO_2$ of 25 mmHg is recommended. For more prolonged reductions of intracranial pressure, the use of mannitol boluses (100 mL of 20% mannitol) at 10-minute intervals is recommended (hold mannitol if serum osmolality is greater than 320 mEq/L or if oliguric renal failure develops). Furosemide can be given intravenously to treat fluid overload or hyperosmolality from mannitol.

Dexamethasone, useful in managing some causes of increased intracranial pressure, is not useful in fulminant liver failure.[35] Extracorporeal liver-assist devices incorporating porcine or human hepatocyte cell lines may be useful in decreasing intracranial pressure in some patients; however, these devices are still considered experimental and have not been approved for use by the United States Food and Drug Administration.[36–38] Mild hypothermia to 32°C to

Table 117.6   Management of intracranial hypertension in fulminant liver failure

Head elevation to 20°
Tracheal intubation at onset of grade 3
Placement of ICP transducer at onset of grade 3
Treat fever and seizures adequately
Avoid
    Valsalva maneuver
    Head turning and moving
    Neck vein compression
    Respiratory suctioning
    Vasodilator agents

ICP, intracranial pressure.

Table 117.7   King's College Hospital criteria for liver transplantation in fulminant liver failure

Acetaminophen
 pH < 7.3
 or
 All 3 of the following
  Prothrombin time > 100 seconds or INR > 6.5
  Creatinine > 2.3 mg/dL
  Grade III or IV encephalopathy

Non-acetaminophen patients
 Prothrombin time > 100 seconds or INR > 6.7
 or
 Any 3 of the following (irrespective of the grade of
   encephalopathy)
  Age < 10 or > 40 years
  Etiology—seronegative hepatitis or drug reaction
  Duration of jaundice before onset of
    encephalopathy > 7 days
  Prothrombin time > 50 seconds or INR > 3.5
  Serum bilirubin > 2.3 mg/dL

INR, international normalized ratio. Modified from O'Grady et al.[43] By permission of the American Gastroenterological Association.

33°C, with the use of cooling blankets, has been shown to decrease intracranial pressure in patients with fulminant liver failure and may be useful as a bridge to liver transplantation for selected patients.[39] Increased intracranial pressure can also be treated with thiopentone (a barbiturate) infusions.[40] This is especially useful in the presence of renal failure, which precludes the use of mannitol. The exact mechanism of action is unclear, but barbiturates are thought to reduce cerebral metabolism, thereby causing a decrease in cerebral blood flow and intracranial pressure. However, the use of barbiturates is considered controversial and may be complicated by the development of arterial hypotension, which offsets the beneficial effect of decreasing intracranial pressure.

Specific therapy   Specific therapy for the underlying liver disease should be commenced as soon as possible. This includes corticosteroid therapy for autoimmune hepatitis, N-acetylcysteine for acetaminophen overdose, and D-penicillamine for Wilson disease. Other therapeutic interventions considered experimental in the management of fulminant liver failure include prophylactic phenytoin to prevent subclinical seizures and N-acetylcysteine for non-acetaminophen poisoning.[41,42] Liver transplantation generally is considered the most definitive therapy for fulminant liver failure. Criteria from King's College Hospital in London (Table 117.7) are useful for identifying the cohort of patients who are most likely to benefit from liver transplantation. However, these criteria may not be wholly applicable to patients with fulminant liver failure that results from rare causes such as Wilson disease or pregnancy-related liver disease.[43] With improvements in surgical techniques, postoperative care, and immunosuppression, 1-year survival after

liver transplantation has been reported to be as high as 76% for patients in the United States with fulminant liver failure.[44] Thus, an urgent effort must be made to perform liver transplantation in these patients before brain herniation and death occur.

References

1. Parsons-Smith BG, Summerskill WH, Dawson AM, Sherlock S. The electroencephalograph in liver disease. Lancet 1957;273:867–871
2. Groeneweg M, Moerland W, Quero JC, et al. Screening of subclinical hepatic encephalopathy. J Hepatol 2000;32:748–753
3. Hartmann IJ, Groeneweg M, Quero JC, et al. The prognostic significance of subclinical hepatic encephalopathy. Am J Gastroenterol 2000;95:2029–2034
4. Groeneweg M, Quero JC, De Bruijn I, et al. Subclinical hepatic encephalopathy impairs daily functioning. Hepatology 1998;28:45–49
5. Amodio P, Quero JC, Del Piccolo F, et al. Diagnostic tools for the detection of subclinical hepatic encephalopathy: comparison of standard and computerized psychometric tests with spectral-EEG. Metab Brain Dis 1996;11:315–327
6. Quero JC, Hartmann KJ, Meulstee J, et al. The diagnosis of subclinical hepatic encephalopathy in patients with cirrhosis using neuropsychological tests and automated electroencephalogram analysis. Hepatology 1996;24:556–560
7. Costa E, Guidotti A. Diazepam binding inhibitor (DBI): a peptide with multiple biological actions. Life Sci 1991;49:325–344
8. Donovan JP, Schafer DF, Shaw BW, Jr, Sorrell MF. Cerebral oedema and increased intracranial pressure in chronic liver disease. Lancet 1998;351:719–721
9. Jalan R, Dabos K, Redhead DN, et al. Elevation of intracranial pressure following transjugular intrahepatic portosystemic stent-shunt for variceal haemorrhage. J Hepatol 1997;27:928–933
10. Kim JS. Asterixis after unilateral stroke: lesion location of 30 patients. Neurology 2001;56:533–536
11. Tatu L, Moulin T, Martin V, et al. Unilateral pure thalamic asterixis: clinical, electromyographic, and topographic patterns. Neurology 2000;54:2339–2342
12. Rittmannsberger H. Asterixis induced by psychotropic drug treatment. Clin Neuropharmacol 1996;19:349–355
13. Rio J, Montalban J, Pujadas F, et al. Asterixis associated with anatomic cerebral lesions: a study of 45 cases. Acta Neurol Scand 1995;91:377–381
14. Morres CA, Dire DJ. Movement disorders as a manifestation of nonketotic hyperglycemia. J Emerg Med 1989;7:359–364
15. Young RR, Shahani BT. Asterixis: one type of negative myoclonus. Adv Neurol 1986;43:137–156
16. Nolte W, Wiltfang J, Schindler CG, et al. Bright basal ganglia in T1-weighted magnetic resonance images are frequent in patients with portal vein thrombosis without liver cirrhosis and not suggestive of hepatic encephalopathy. J Hepatol 1998;29:443–449
17. Rimola A, Garcia-Tsao G, Navasa M, et al. Diagnosis, treatment and prophylaxis of spontaneous bacterial peritonitis: a consensus document. International Ascites Club. J Hepatol 2000;32:142–153
18. Fabbri A, Magrini N, Bianchi G, et al. Overview of randomized clinical trials of oral branched-chain amino acid treatment in chronic hepatic encephalopathy. JPEN J Parenter Enteral Nutr 1996;20:159–164

19. Conn HO, Leevy CM, Vlahcevic ZR, et al. Comparison of lactulose and neomycin in the treatment of chronic portal-systemic encephalopathy: a double blind controlled trial. Gastroenterology 1977;72:573–583

20. Riordan SM, Williams R. Treatment of hepatic encephalopathy. N Engl J Med 1997;337:473–479

21. Ferenci P, Grimm G. Benzodiazepine antagonist in the treatment of human hepatic encephalopathy. Adv Exp Med Biol 1990;272:255–265

22. Gyr K, Meier R. Flumazenil in the treatment of portal systemic encephalopathy: an overview. Intensive Care Med 1991;17(Suppl 1):S39–S42

23. Bansky G, Meier PJ, Riederer E, et al. Effects of the benzodiazepine receptor antagonist flumazenil in hepatic encephalopathy in humans. Gastroenterology 1989;97:744–750

24. Barbaro G, Di Lorenzo G, Soldini M, et al. Flumazenil for hepatic encephalopathy grade III and IVa in patients with cirrhosis: an Italian multicenter double-blind, placebo-controlled, cross-over study. Hepatology 1998;28:374–378

25. Barbaro G, Di Lorenzo G, Soldini M, et al. Flumazenil for hepatic coma in patients with liver cirrhosis: an Italian multicentre double-blind, placebo-controlled, crossover study. Eur J Emerg Med 1998;5:213–218

26. Amodio P, Marchetti P, Del Piccolo F, et al. The effect of flumazenil on subclinical psychometric or neurophysiological alterations in cirrhotic patients: a double-blind placebo-controlled study. Clin Physiol 1997;17:533–539

27. Gyr K, Meier R, Haussler J, et al. Evaluation of the efficacy and safety of flumazenil in the treatment of portal systemic encephalopathy: a double blind, randomised, placebo controlled multicentre study. Gut 1996;39:319–324

28. Groeneweg M, Gyr K, Amrein R, et al. Effect of flumazenil on the electroencephalogram of patients with portosystemic encephalopathy: results of a double blind, randomised, placebo-controlled multicentre trial. Electroencephalogr Clin Neurophysiol 1996;98:29–34

29. Van der Rijt CC, Schalm SW, Meulstee J, Stijnen T. Flumazenil therapy for hepatic encephalopathy: a double-blind cross over study. Gastroenterol Clin Biol 1995;19:572–580

30. Cadranel JF, el Younsi M, Pidoux B, et al. Flumazenil therapy for hepatic encephalopathy in cirrhotic patients: a double-blind pragmatic randomized, placebo study. Eur J Gastroenterol Hepatol 1995;7:325–329

31. Pomier-Layrargues G, Giguere JF, Lavoie J, et al. Flumazenil in cirrhotic patients in hepatic coma: a randomized double-blind placebo-controlled crossover trial. Hepatology 1994;19:32–37

32. Transplant Patient DataSource (2000, September 5). Richmond, VA: United Network for Organ Sharing. Retrieved September 5, 2000 from the World Wide Web: http://www.patients.unos.org/data.htm

33. Lee WM. Acute liver failure. N Engl J Med 1993;329:1862–1872

34. Blei AT, Olafsson S, Webster S, Levy R. Complications of intracranial pressure monitoring in fulminant hepatic failure. Lancet 1993;341:157–158

35. Canalese J, Gimson AE, Davis C, et al. Controlled trial of dexamethasone and mannitol for the cerebral oedema of fulminant hepatic failure. Gut 1982;23:625–629

36. Watanabe FD, Mullon CJ, Hewitt WR, et al. Clinical experience with a bioartificial liver in the treatment of severe liver failure: a phase I clinical trial. Ann Surg 1997;225:484–491

37. Watanabe FD, Shackleton CR, Cohen SM, et al. Treatment of acetaminophen-induced fulminant hepatic failure with a bioartificial liver. Transplant Proc 1997;29:487–488

38. Chen SC, Hewitt WR, Watanabe FD, et al. Clinical experience with a porcine hepatocyte-based liver support system. Int J Artif Organs 1996;19:664–669

39. Jalan R, Damink SW, Deutz NE, et al. Moderate hypothermia for uncontrolled intracranial hypertension in acute liver failure. Lancet 1999;354:1164–1168

40. Forbes A, Alexander GJ, O'Grady JG, et al. Thiopental infusion in the treatment of intracranial hypertension complicating fulminant hepatic failure. Hepatology 1989;10:306–310

41. Ellis AJ, Wendon JA, Williams R. Subclinical seizure activity and prophylactic phenytoin infusion in acute liver failure: a controlled clinical trial. Hepatology 2000;32:536–541

42. Walsh TS, Hopton P, Philips BJ, et al. The effect of N-acetylcysteine on oxygen transport and uptake in patients with fulminant hepatic failure. Hepatology 1998;27:1332–1340

43. O'Grady JG, Alexander GJ, Hayllar KM, Williams R. Early indicators of prognosis in fulminant hepatic failure. Gastroenterology 1989;97:439–445

44. Schiodt FV, Atillasoy E, Shakil AO, et al. Etiology and outcome for 295 patients with acute liver failure in the United States. Liver Transpl Surg 1999;5:29–34

118 Acute Respiratory Failure in Neurological Disease

Galen V Henderson

Acute respiratory failure in neurological critical illness may accelerate rapidly, becoming severe in a matter of minutes. Therefore, assessment and timely management are crucial when one is suddenly faced with a deteriorating patient. When acute respiratory failure is associated with impaired gas exchange, the situation is even more urgent. Catastrophic illness in the neurologically critically ill patient is either the result of a progression of underlying illness, or of respiratory or cardiac dysfunction caused by the neurological illness. Neurological impairment caused by respiratory or circulatory embarrassment reduces oxygen delivery to the effected neurons and increases the neurological injury and cardiorespiratory dysfunction. This ultimately results in increased morbidity and mortality. By supporting the respiration and circulation this prevents increased neurological injury resulting from tissue hypoxia, and may allow for stabilization sufficient to initiate disease-specific therapy.

Management of acute respiratory failure in patients with neurological critical illness is different for several reasons. First, coexistent neck trauma may make airway management more difficult. This may apply to patients with traumatic brain injury, status epilepticus, or falls from acute hemiplegia of any source. Hyperextension of the neck may potentially worsen or introduce spinal cord lesions. Second, many patients struck with acute neurological illness have normal baseline pulmonary function, unlike patients with critical medical illnesses, who often have newly acquired serious pulmonary parenchymal disease.[1] Gas exchange in acute neurological catastrophes more often becomes less efficient owing to impaired mechanisms of breathing involving the respiratory muscles, the musculature of the upper airway and central drive to breathe, rather than to impaired pulmonary function. Third, when pulmonary disorders occur they are most often restricted to aspiration pneumonitis, pneumonia or neurogenic pulmonary edema. Therefore, ventilator dependency is less common, and most acutely ill neurological patients can later be successfully weaned from the ventilator. Finally, the assessment of respiratory drive and indications for mechanical intubation are unique in neurologically injured patients.

Respiratory failure usually is divided into two types. Type I respiratory failure is a primary defect in oxygenation, usually as a consequence of diseases affecting the pulmonary parenchyma, and sometimes the alveoli as well. The patient becomes tachypneic and, if consciousness is not impaired, develops symptomatic air hunger. Cyanosis may be present if the arterial blood is sufficiently desaturated. Measurement of arterial blood gases shows hypoxemia, usually accompanied by a respiratory alkalosis, unless the underlying condition is severe enough to cause a defect in CO_2 clearance. In patients with neurological disease the major causes of de novo type I respiratory failures are pneumonia (often caused by aspiration) and neurogenic pulmonary edema. Patients with underlying lung disorders, such as chronic obstructive lung disease, also may manifest worsening hypoxemia in the course of an acute neurological disorder.

Type II respiratory failure occurs when ventilation is inadequate to maintain normal levels of blood oxygen and CO_2. This may occur as a consequence of failure of the central nervous system to respond adequately to the need to take in oxygen and excrete CO_2, or failure of the neuromuscular system involved in respiration. Conditions affecting the ability of the central nervous system to respond to changes in arterial oxygen and CO_2 tensions include drug intoxication and brainstem damage. Conditions causing failure of the neuromuscular system include amyotrophic lateral sclerosis and other motor neuron diseases, Guillain–Barré syndrome, myasthenia gravis or myopathy.

Conditions causing type II respiratory failure often also impair protection of the upper airway, so the assessment of the patient must consider both airway and ventilation. With type II respiratory failure no specific measurement defines when a patient should be intubated, but the patient's distress is usually evident and is itself a reason for intubation. Patients typically have concordant difficulty with secretions and usually require endotracheal intubation to protect the airway.

Etiology of acute respiratory failure in neurologically ill patients

Disorders can be divided into acute brain injury, acute neuromuscular failure and pulmonary complications.

Acute brain injury

The major clinical etiologies of acute respiratory failure are usually ischemic or hemorrhagic stroke, seizures with a decreased level of consciousness or from its treatment, or brain swelling. Primary insults to the CNS may result in inadequate respiratory drive, abnormal breathing patterns such as severe ataxic or cluster breathing, or ability to protect the airway. Some patients may hyperventilate to compensate for hypoxemia,[2,3] acidosis, or fever. Patients with severe central causes of ventilatory failure may experience an immediate inability to sense or control blood pH, resulting in an increasing partial pressure of carbon dioxide, and fail to respond to declining partial-pressure oxygen. Such conditions rapidly produce a profound respiratory acidosis, accompanied by hypoxemia as hypoventilation persists. As tissue hypoxemia becomes critical, aerobic metabolism fails and the patient develops a metabolic acidosis. If the underlying condition is not quickly managed with mechanical ventilation, permanent cerebral damage or death follows. Patients with acute CNS injury who are intubated may be able to maintain efficient gas exchange and can be monitored at the bedside with pulse oximetry and arterial blood gas results.

When managing patients who may develop dangerous increases in intracranial pressure, there is no rationale for prophylactically instituting hyperventilation in a patient at risk for brain swelling because of the considerable risk of decreasing cerebral perfusion and increasing neuronal damage.[4] Depression of the level of consciousness is not an absolute indication for mechanical ventilation.

Acute neuromuscular failure

The indications for ventilatory support because of neuromuscular failure are complex; therefore, bedside measurements of respiratory mechanics or by pulse oximeter may not be adequate. Laboratory measurements in combination with clinical manifestations are sensitive to detect ventilation failure. The respiratory mechanical values may be low for inadequate mouth closure, particularly in patients with bilateral facial palsy (see Table 118.1 for critical values). Patients with diaphragmatic failure usually have tachycardia and tachypnea.[5,6] Many have interrupted speech and need to pause after a few words. Restlessness is very typical and patients are usually quiet, answering with signals such as nods.

Vital capacity can be estimated at the bedside by asking patients to take a deep breath and count to 20. Inability to perform this simple bedside test is related to vital capacity at 15–18 mL/kg or less.[7] These values may be low because of inadequate mouth closure, particularly in patients with bilateral facial palsy or poor patient participation. Palpation of the sternoclei-

domastoic muscle, rather than visualization, may disclose increased muscle activity during breathing.[8] Contraction of paradoxical breathing is a consequence of profound weakness of the diaphragm. Diaphragmatic failure is manifested by dyspnea at relatively low levels of physical exercise. The work of breathing is increased in the supine position owing to the increased pressure of the abdominal contents against the weak and less resistant diaphragm. Patients with neuromuscular disease often have severe weakness of the diaphragm during acute ventilatory failure, and the degree of failure seems to correlate with diaphragmatic weakness. Sleep reduces the clearance of secretions owing to decreased expiratory muscle function and impaired cough, and because of supine positioning. Weakness of the respiratory muscles is not uniform in acute neuromuscular disease, and peripheral strength may not correlate with respiratory strength.[9] With respiratory failure, diaphragmatic failure seems to correlate with diaphragmatic weakness.[10]

Generally, mechanical ventilation in neuromuscular respiratory failure is indicated when clinical deterioration is associated with a vital capacity of 15 mL/kg or less and maximum inspiratory pressure of less than −25 cmH$_2$O. Other clinical abnormalities should override laboratory values in the final decision to intubate and mechanically ventilate. In patients with Guillain–Barré syndrome mechanical ventilation will be needed if the initial baseline values are decreased by 50% in 36 hours.[11]

In myasthenic patients, worsening dyspnea is less common than in most other neuromuscular patients. In this patient population, respiratory problems may be triggered by a pulmonary infection, resulting in progressive hypercapnia and hypoxia.

Pulmonary complications

In the critically ill neurological patient with acute brain lesions, intubation for pulmonary complications is less common. When there is impaired gas exchange it is usually attributed to aspiration causing a pneumonia or pneumonitis. Having an altered level of consciousness is a major risk for aspiration. Other risk factors for aspiration include emergency intubation, vomiting, obesity, nasogastric feeding, and a diabetes mellitus-associated gastrointestinal motility disorder.

Occasionally neurogenic pulmonary edema (NPE) is seen acutely after acute head injury.[12] In addition to trauma, NPE has been associated with a variety of

Table 118.1 Normal and critical respiratory parameters in the neurological patient

Measurement	Normal value	Critical value
Vital capacity	Male 40–70 mL/kg	15 mL/kg
Maximal inspiratory pressure	Male ⩾ 100 cmH$_2$O	−25 cmH$_2$O
	Female > 70 cmH$_2$O	
Maximal expiratory pressure	Male > 200 cmH$_2$O	40 cmH$_2$O
	Female > 140 cmH$_2$O	

neurological conditions, including subarachnoid hemorrhage, electroconvulsive therapy, seizures and meningitis, and with the diagnosis of brain death.[13–18] Although this is a diagnosis of exclusion, the true frequency seems very low.[19] NPE may be potentially life-threatening because it impairs oxygenation. This syndrome was first recognized in an autopsy series of 100 soldiers who died in combat during the Vietnam war. Regardless of thoracic injury, pulmonary edema and thoracic hemorrhage were present in 89% of these soldiers.[20] Neurogenic pulmonary edema is believed to arise from massive sympathetic overflow, probably mediated by the anterior hypothalamus and triggered by an initial increase in intracranial pressure during the head injury or aneurysmal rupture. This leads to an increased peripheral and pulmonary vascular resistance,[21,22] possibly damaging the endothelial cells of the pulmonary vessels. Initially, increased hydrostatic forces caused by abnormally high pulmonary artery pressures force transudate into the alveolar space. Over time, pulmonary capillary endothelial damage can occur, leading to persistent pulmonary edema with high protein content. This diagnosis is one of exclusion and can only be made in the presence of normal cardiac function and left ventricular filling pressures.

There is increasing evidence that pulmonary edema in subarachnoid hemorrhage may have a cardiogenic origin. Earlier concepts of its pathogenesis postulated a large, abrupt increase in systemic arterial pressure as a consequence of a catecholamine surge at the time of the acute neurological insult. This would increase the afterload seen by the left ventricle, resulting in congestive heart failure. Structural damage to the myocardium, contraction band necrosis and subendocardial ischemia are characteristic histological features that have been documented. Experimental studies of neurogenic pulmonary edema demonstrate, however, that no increase in left atrial or ventricular pressures is required for its development. A 1992 case report has documented a medullary demyelinating lesion as the presumptive etiology of acute pulmonary hypertension, supporting the contention that bilateral injury to the nucleus solitarius may be responsible for this phenomenon.[23] Mayer et al. have suggested that impaired left ventricular hemodynamic performance may contribute to cardiovascular instability and pulmonary edema formation.[24] The clinical entity may be mistaken for other pulmonary conditions, such as a massive aspiration pneumonia or pulmonary confusion. Delayed neurogenic pulmonary edema should be differentiated from multiple pulmonary emboli. The clinical picture is remarkable for excessive sweating; hypertension, tachypnea and the production of frothy sputum are typical. Usually it is extremely rapid in onset.[25] Chest radiography demonstrates diffuse pulmonary infiltrates. The diagnosis of neurogenic pulmonary edema is supported by the combination of marked hypoxemic respiratory failure with a normal wedge pressure, and excluding a cardiogenic cause for pulmonary edema. Management of neurogenic pulmonary edema is focused on the recruitment of collapsed alveoli to correct the marked ventilation–perfusion mismatch. Mechanical ventilation with positive end-expiratory pressure ventilation usually reverses the condition, and definite radiographic improvement is evident within hours.[26]

References

1. Tobin MJ. Respiratory monitoring in the intensive care unit. Am Rev Respir Dis 1988;138:1625–1642
2. Fein IA, Rackow EC. Neurogenic pulmonary edema. Chest 1982;81:318–20
3. Carlson RW, Schaeffer RC Jr, Michaels SG, Weil MH. Pulmonary edema following intracranial hemorrhage. Chest 1979;75:731–734
4. Muizelaar JP, Marmarou A, Ward JD et al. Adverse effects of prolonged hyperventilation in patients with severe head injury: a randomized clinical trial. J Neurosurg 1991;75:731–739
5. Cohen CA, Zagelbaum G, Gross D et al. Clinical manifestations of inspiratory muscle fatigue. Am J Med 1982;73:308–316
6. O'Donohue WJ Jr, Baker JP, Bell GM et al. Respiratory failure in neuromuscular disease. Management in a respiratory intensive care unit. JAMA 1976;235:733–735
7. Ropper AH, ed. Neurological and Neurosurgical Intensive Care, 3rd ed. New York: Raven Press, 1993
8. Roussos C, Macklem PT. The respiratory muscles. N Engl J Med 1982;307:786–797
9. Ferguson IT, Murphy RP, Lascelles RG. Ventilatory failure in myasthenia gravis. J Neurol Neurosurg Psychiatry 1982;45:217–222
10. Borel CO, Tilford C, Nichols DG et al. Diaphragmatic performance during recovery from acute ventilatory failure in Guillain–Barré syndrome and myasthenia gravis. Chest 1991;99:444–451
11. Chevrolet C, Deleamont P. Repeated vital capacity measurements as predictive parameters for mechanical ventilation need and weaning success in the Guillain–Barré syndrome. Am Rev Respir Dis 1991;144: 814–818
12. Rogers FB, Shackford SR, Trevisani GT et al. Neurogenic pulmonary edema in fatal and nonfatal injuries. J Trauma Inj Infect Crit Care 1995;39:860
13. Carlson RW, Schaeffer RC Jr, Michaels SG, Weil MH. Pulmonary edema following intracranial hemorrhage. Chest 1979;75:731–734
14. Hardmann JM, Earle KM. Meningococcal infections: a review of 200 fatal cases. J Neuropathol Exp Neurol 1967;26:119
15. Darnell JC, Jay SJ. Recurrent postictal pulmonary edema: a case report and review of the literature. Epilepsia 1982;23:499
16. Chen HI, Sun SC, Chai CY. Pulmonary edema and hemorrhage resulting from cerebral compression. Am J Physiol 1973;224:223–229
17. Colice GL. Neurogenic pulmonary edema. Clin Chest Med 1982;81:318–320
18. Yabumoto M, Kuriyama T, Iwamoto M et al. Neurogenic pulmonary edema associated with ruptured intracranial aneurysm: case report. Neurosurgery 1986;19:300–304
19. Fein IA, Rackow EC. Neurogenic pulmonary edema. Chest 1982;81:318–320
20. Martin AM, Simmons RL, Heisterkamp CA. Respiratory insufficiency in combat casualties: I. Pathologic changes in the lungs of patients dying of wounds. Ann Surg 1969;170:30

21. Theodore J, Robin ED. Speculations on neurogenic pulmonary edema (NPE). Am Rev Respir Dis 1976;113:405–411
22. Ell SR. Neurogenic pulmonary edema: a review of the literature and a perspective. Invest Radiol 1991;26:499
23. Eberhardt KE. Dose-dependent rate of nosoicomial pulmonary infection in mechanically ventilated patients with brain oedema receiving barbiturates: a prospective case study. Infection 1992;20:12
24. Mayer SA, Fink ME, Homma S, et al. Cardiac injury associated with neurogenic pulmonary edema following subarachnoid hemorrhage. Neurology 1994;44:815–820
25. Fisher A, Aboul-Nasr NT. Delayed nonfatal pulmonary edema following subarachnoid hemorrhage. J Neurosurg 1979;51:856–859
26. Wauchob TD, Brooks RJ, Harrison KM. Neurogenic pulmonary oedema. Anesthesia 1984;39:529–534

119 Disorders of Excessive Sleepiness

Atul Malhotra, Robert B Fogel and David P White

Introduction

The initial approach to a patient with an apparent disorder of excessive sleepiness is to ensure that the complaint is truly sleepiness and not fatigue or lethargy. "Sleepiness" is an increased propensity to fall asleep at inopportune times, for example while driving or during conversations. Conversely, fatigue and lethargy are symptoms of malaise, without increased sleep propensity, and may be caused by several medical or psychological problems, such as anemia, congestive heart failure, malignancy and depression. Because the approach to these two problems is quite different, the distinction is an important one.[1]

Once hypersomnolence has been confirmed historically, the approach is relatively straightforward, with the three categories of disorder of excessive sleepiness outlined in Table 119.1. Patients with insufficient duration of sleep should try to achieve 7.5 to 8 hours of sleep nightly before an extensive evaluation is performed. In most cases, overnight polysomnography is used to diagnose sleep fragmentation, and polysomnography plus multiple sleep latency testing are required to document excessive sleep drive. Multiple sleep latency testing measures the elapsed time to sleep and onset of rapid eye movement (REM) sleep during a repeated series of daytime naps following overnight polysomnography. Shortened sleep latency is a general characteristic of pathological sleepiness, and shortened REM latency is seen most often in narcolepsy, although it can occur in other conditions.

Insufficient nocturnal sleep

Chronic partial sleep deprivation is an exceedingly common problem in modern society and almost certainly is the most frequent cause of waking hypersomnolence. However, data on the actual prevalence or long-term consequences are sparse. Evidence suggests that almost all persons require at least 7 hours of sleep per night to optimize neurocognitive performance.[2,3] Despite claims to the contrary, most of those who sleep fewer than 7 hours per night have measurable declines in cognitive function. Therefore, lifestyle modification (e.g., fixed bedtime and wakeup time, avoidance of stimulants such as caffeine, and treatment of underlying insomnia if present) should be encouraged to obtain adequate sleep duration by patients who complain of sleepiness yet sleep fewer than 7.5 to 8 hours per night.

Sleep fragmentation

"Sleep fragmentation" is the category of disorder of excessive sleepiness most frequently encountered in sleep clinics and laboratories.[4] The most common causes include obstructive sleep apnea, periodic limb movements, and medical conditions (e.g., pain or shortness of breath). Although central sleep apnea can also fragment sleep, it is uncommon outside the setting of congestive heart failure (Cheyne–Stokes respiration).[5–8] Less common causes of central apnea such as idiopathic central sleep apnea, primary alveolar hypoventilation (Ondine's curse), and apneas occurring during sleep transitions are not discussed in this chapter.

Obstructive sleep apnea

"Obstructive sleep apnea" is characterized by repetitive collapse of the pharyngeal airway during sleep.[9,10] It is common in North America, afflicting an estimated 4% of middle-aged men and 2% of women.[4] Repetitive pharyngeal collapse has two potential consequences. First, to reestablish airway patency, the patient must awaken from sleep. The resulting sleep fragmentation can lead to neurocognitive sequelae such as reduced quality of life, daytime somnolence, and increased risk of motor vehicle accidents.[11] Second, during pharyngeal collapse, reduction or cessation of airflow leads to hypoxia, hypercapnia, vagal withdrawal, and surges in catecholamines. Increasing evidence suggests that this is associated with adverse cardiovascular sequelae such as hypertension, myocardial infarction, and stroke.[12–15] The diagnosis of obstructive sleep apnea should be suspected when the patient reports loud snoring, has witnessed (by bed

---

Table 119.1   Differential diagnosis of excessive daytime sleepiness

Insufficient duration of sleep
  Fewer than 7 hours per night (usually behavioral-
    and/or lifestyle-determined)

Fragmentation of sleep
  Obstructive sleep apnea
  Central sleep apnea (e.g., Cheyne–Stokes respiration)
  Periodic limb movements
  Medical conditions (pain, shortness of breath)

Increased sleep drive
  Narcolepsy
  Idiopathic central nervous system hypersomnia
  Sedating medications
  Previous head injury
  Severe depression
  Viral infection of central nervous system

partner) apneas or gasping, and is obese (increased neck circumference [mean >16.5 in, women >15.5 in]).[16–18] The diagnosis is confirmed by polysomnography, which shows repetitive attenuations in airflow despite ongoing respiratory effort.

Options for treatment of obstructive sleep apnea include nasal continuous positive airway pressure (CPAP), oral appliances, and upper airway surgery.[19] A recent randomized sham placebo-controlled trial showed improved outcome among patients with apnea who received nasal CPAP, as compared with controls.[20] On the basis of this and other publications, CPAP is the treatment of choice, although adherence remains a problem.[21–25] Oral appliances are generally fabricated by a dentist, with the goal of advancing the mandible, thereby alleviating retroglossal pharyngeal compromise.[26–28] On balance, these devices are less effective than nasal CPAP, but they are better tolerated and, thus, useful in selected patients intolerant of CPAP.[29] Multiple upper airway surgical procedures (e.g., uvulopalatopharyngoplasty, genioglossal advancement, and radiofrequency ablation of the soft palate [somnoplasty]) are available but should be reserved for cases refractory to other forms of therapy because substantial improvement in sleep-disordered breathing is uncommon with all procedures short of facial reconstruction procedures (i.e., mandibular maxillary advancement).[30–33]

Periodic limb movements

"Periodic limb movements" during sleep are a common phenomenon of uncertain significance. By definition, they are movements of the lower extremities (generally, contraction of the anterior tibialis muscle) that occur during sleep, with a 20- to 90-second periodicity, with occasional electroencephalographic evidence of arousal or autonomic fluctuation (or both). Several diseases have been associated with these movements, including restless leg syndrome, iron deficiency anemia, peripheral neuropathy, renal failure, and certain medications (e.g., tricyclic antidepressants and selective serotonin reuptake inhibitors).[1] When periodic limb movements are frequent (more than 10 to 20 per hour of sleep), they can lead to sleep fragmentation and daytime sleepiness. The usual treatment for this disorder includes correction of reversible factors or medication (hypnotics, dopaminergic agonists, or narcotics or both; dopaminergic agonists are the preferred agent[34–38]). Although the largest clinical experience is with the combination of levodopa and carbidopa (Sinemet CR 50/200), pramipexole ([Mirapex] 0.125 to 0.5 mg orally at bedtime) is emerging as the drug of choice because of the results of recent clinical trials.[39,40] Therefore, periodic limb movements should be considered in the differential diagnosis of sleep fragmentation with waking hypersomnolence.

Underlying illness

Medical patients often experience sleep fragmentation related to underlying illnesses. For example, shortness of breath such as nocturnal asthma, gastro-esophageal reflux disease, and pain can all contribute to sleep disruption. They are easily overlooked causes of poor sleep quality, but they can be readily confirmed with a careful history. Appropriate treatment of the underlying disease can be helpful in promoting improved sleep quality.

Increased sleep drive

"Increased sleep drive" is defined as ongoing sleepiness despite sufficient quantity and quality of sleep. Several causes exist, but the most commonly encountered are narcolepsy, idiopathic central nervous system hypersomnia, and sedating medications. Although many historical details are helpful in the differential diagnosis, firm documentation generally requires polysomnography plus multiple sleep latency testing.

Narcolepsy

"Narcolepsy" is a disorder characterized by the classic tetrad of waking hypersomnolence, cataplexy (abrupt loss of motor tone, often with emotional stimuli [anger, laughter]), hypnogogic hallucinations, and sleep paralysis. The onset of these symptoms typically occurs in the teens or twenties.[41–43] Sleepiness is described as "irresistible," with the resulting sleep episodes being refreshing but yielding only a short-lived improvement in symptoms. The condition is diagnosed on the basis of the findings of polysomnography plus multiple sleep latency testing. Multiple sleep latency testing shows a shortened latency of sleep onset and early onset of REM sleep.[44–47] Very recent studies indicate that narcolepsy, at least in animals, results from a defect in the hypocretin (orexin) receptor, suggesting an important role for hypocretin in sleep modulation.[48,49] In humans, evidence suggests that narcolepsy is caused by a loss of cells that produce hypocretin.

Because the treatment of narcolepsy is only symptomatic, separate approaches are used to address daytime sleepiness and cataplexy. Both planned naps and stimulants are useful in the treatment of hypersomnolence. Although several stimulants are available, methylphenidate ([Ritalin] 20 mg SR orally twice daily and/or 5 to 10 mg orally 3 times daily) is used most commonly and currently is the treatment of choice.[43] Modafinil ([Provigil] 200 to 400 mg orally every morning) is a new stimulant drug that has less potential for abuse, but it likely is a weaker stimulant than methylphenidate or amphetamines.[50] Medications used to treat cataplexy are generally REM-suppressing agents such as selective serotonin reuptake inhibitors (e.g., fluoxetine [Prozac], 20 to 60 mg orally every morning), sertraline ([Zoloft] 50 to 150 mg orally every morning), paroxetine ([Paxil] 25 to 50 mg orally every morning) or tricyclic antidepressants (e.g., protriptyline [Vivactil], 5 to 30 mg orally daily). The individualization of therapy (dosage and timing) is crucial for effective treatment of narcolepsy.

Idiopathic central nervous system hypersomnia

As the name implies, "idiopathic central nervous system hypersomnia" is a diagnosis of exclusion based on excessive sleep drive of unknown etiology. The hypersomnia is similar to narcolepsy, but the patients generally lack early-onset REM sleep and cataplexy and do not describe their sleep as refreshing. The treatment is symptomatic, with amphetamine type medications or modafinil (or both).

Sedating medications

The use of sedating medications may increase sleep drive. However, drugs are frequently overlooked as a cause of excessive sleepiness. Anticonvulsants (e.g., barbiturates and phenytoin), muscle relaxants (e.g., baclofen and benzodiazepines), and psychoactive agents (antidepressants) are the most frequent offenders, although the list is extensive. Adjustments in medication dose or class (or both) can lead to resolution of the symptoms.

Patients with disorders of excessive sleepiness commonly present to physicians for evaluation. A careful history and an organized approach can help lead to prompt diagnosis and treatment. Because the majority of these disorders are readily treatable, patient and physician satisfaction usually is high.

References

1. Malhotra A, Fogel R, Pillar G, Winkelman JW. Non-Respiratory Disorders of Sleep. Pulmonary and Critical Care Update for the American College of Chest Physicians 1999; Volume 14, Lesson 4:1–11
2. Dinges DF. An overview of sleepiness and accidents. J Sleep Res 1995;4:4–14
3. Dinges DF, Pack F, Williams K, Gillen KA, Powell JW, Ott GE, Aptowicz C, Pack AI. Cumulative sleepiness, mood disturbance, and psychomotor vigilance performance decrements during a week of sleep restricted to 4–5 hours per night. Sleep 1997;20:267–270
4. Young T, Palta M, Dempsey J, Skatrud J, Weber S, Badr S. The occurrence of sleep-disordered breathing among middle-aged adults. New England Journal of Medicine 1993;328:1230–1235
5. Bradley TD, Floras JS. Pathophysiologic and therapeutic implications of sleep apnea in congestive heart failure. J Card Fail 1996;2:223–240
6. Bradley TD. Sleep disturbances in respiratory and cardiovascular disease. J Psychosom Res 1993;37(Suppl 1):13–17
7. Javaheri S. Central sleep apnea-hypopnea syndrome in heart failure: prevalence, impact, and treatment. Sleep 1996;19(Suppl):S229–S231
8. Javaheri S, Parker TJ, Liming JD, Corbett WS, Nishiyama H, Wexler L, Roselle GA. Sleep apnea in 81 ambulatory male patients with stable heart failure. Types and their prevalences, consequences, and presentations. Circulation 1998;97:2154–2159
9. White DP. Sleep-related breathing disorder. 2. Pathophysiology of obstructive sleep apnoea. Thorax 1995;50:797–804
10. Malhotra A, White DP. The Pathogenesis of Obstructive Sleep Apnea, for Breathing Disorders in Sleep. McNicholas W, Phillipson E, eds. WB Saunders: 43–63.
11. Teran-Santos J, Jimenez-Gomez A, Cordero-Guevara J. The association between sleep apnea and the risk of traffic accidents. Cooperative Group Burgos-Santander. N Engl J Med 1999;340:847–851
12. Brooks D, Horner RL, Kozar LF, Render-Teixeira CL,

Phillipson EA. Obstructive sleep apnea as a cause of systemic hypertension. Evidence from a canine model. J Clin Invest 1997;99:106–109
13. Lavie P, Herer P, Hoffstein V. Obstructive sleep apnea syndrome as a risk factor for hypertension. BMJ 2000; 320:479–482
14. Shahar E, Whitney CW, Redline S, Lee ET, Newman AB, Javier Nieto F, O'Connor GT, Boland LL, Schwartz JE, Samet JM. Sleep-disordered breathing and cardiovascular disease. Cross-sectional results of the Sleep Heart Health Study. Am J Respir Crit Care Med 2001; 163:19–25
15. Peppard PE, Young T, Palta M, Skatrud J. Prospective study of the association between sleep-disordered breathing and hypertension. N Engl J Med 2000;342: 1378–1384
16. Stradling JR, Crosby JH. Predictors and prevalence of obstructive sleep apnoea and snoring in 1001 middle aged men. Thorax 1991;46:85–90
17. Davies RJ, Stradling JR. The relationship between neck circumference, radiographic pharyngeal anatomy, and the obstructive sleep apnoea syndrome. Eur Respir J 1990;3:509–514
18. Davies RJ, Ali NJ, Stradling JR. Neck circumference and other clinical features in the diagnosis of the obstructive sleep apnoea syndrome. Thorax 1992;47:101–105
19. Ayas N, Malhotra A, Epstein L. Non-surgical treatments of obstructive sleep Apnea. Drugs of Today 1999;35:811–821
20. Jenkinson C, Davies RJ, Mullins R, Stradling JR. Comparison of therapeutic and subtherapeutic nasal continuous positive airway pressure for obstructive sleep apnoea: a randomised prospective parallel trial. Lancet 1999;353:2100–2105
21. Redline S, Adams N, Strauss ME, Roebuck T, Winters M, Rosenberg C. Improvement of mild sleep-disordered breathing with CPAP compared with conservative therapy. Am J Respir Crit Care Med 1998;157: 858–865
22. Engleman HM, Martin SE, Kingshott RN, Mackay TW, Deary IJ, Douglas NJ. Randomised placebo controlled trial of daytime function after continuous positive airway pressure (CPAP) therapy for the sleep apnoea/hypopnoea syndrome. Thorax 1998;53:341–345
23. Engleman HM, Kingshott RN, Wraith PK, Mackay TW, Deary IJ, Douglas NJ. Randomized placebo-controlled crossover trial of continuous positive airway pressure for mild sleep apnea/hypopnea syndrome. Am J Respir Crit Car Med 1999;159:461–467
24. Engleman HM, Martin SE, Deary IJ, Douglas NJ. Effect of continuous positive airway pressure treatment on daytime function in sleep apnoea/hypopnoea syndrome. Lancet 1994;343:572–575
25. Engleman HM, Martin SE, Douglas NJ. Compliance with CPAP therapy in patients with the sleep apnoea/hypopnoea syndrome. Thorax 1994;49:263–266
26. Schmidt-Nowara WW, Meade TE, Hays MB. Treatment of snoring and obstructive sleep apnea with a dental orthosis. Chest 1991;99:1378–1385
27. Schmidt-Nowara W, Lowe A, Wiegand L, Cartwright R, Perez-Guerra F, Menn S. Oral appliances for the treatment of snoring and obstructive sleep apnea: a review. Sleep 1995;18:501–510
28. Lowe AA. Can we predict the success of dental appliance therapy for the treatment of obstructive sleep apnea based on anatomic considerations? Sleep 1993;16(Suppl):S93–S95
29. Ferguson KA, Ono T, Lowe AA, Keenan SP, Fleetham

JA. A randomized crossover study of an oral appliance vs nasal-continuous positive airway pressure in the treatment of mild-moderate obstructive sleep apnea. Chest 1996;109:1269–1275

30. Woodson BT. Retropalatal airway characteristics in uvulopalatopharyngoplasty compared with transpalatal advancement pharyngoplasty. Laryngoscope 1997;107: 735–740

31. Woodson BT, Conley SF. Prediction of uvulopalatopharyngoplasty response using cephalometric radiographs. American Journal of Otolaryngology 1997;18: 179–184

32. Sher AE, Schechtman KB, Piccirillo JF. The efficacy of surgical modifications of the upper airway in adults with obstructive sleep apnea syndrome. Sleep 1996;19: 156–177

33. Powell NB, Riley RW, Robinson A. Surgical management of obstructive sleep apnea syndrome. Clin Chest Med 1998;19:77–86

34. Hening W, Allen R, Earley C, Kushida C, Picchietti D, Silber M. The treatment of restless legs syndrome and periodic limb movement disorder. An American Academy of Sleep Medicine Review. Sleep 1999;22: 970–999

35. Hening WA, Walters AS, Wagner M, Rosen R, Chen V, Kim S, Shah M, Thai O. Circadian rhythm of motor restlessness and sensory symptoms in the idiopathic restless legs syndrome. Sleep 1999;22:901–912

36. Benes H, Kurella B, Kummer J, Kazenwadel J, Selzer R, Kohnen R. Rapid onset of action of levodopa in restless legs syndrome: a double-blind, randomized, multicenter, crossover trial. Sleep 1999;22:1073–1081

37. Winkelmann J, Wetter TC, Stiasny K, Oertel WH, Trenkwalder C. Treatment of restless leg syndrome with pergolide—an open clinical trial. Mov Disord 1998;13:566–569

38. Walters AS, Wagner ML, Hening WA, Grasing K, Mills R, Chokroverty S, Kavey N. Successful treatment of the idiopathic restless legs syndrome in a randomized double-blind trial of oxycodone versus placebo. Sleep 1993;16:327–332

39. Lin SC, Kaplan J, Burger CD, Fredrickson PA. Effect of pramipexole in treatment of resistant restless legs syndrome. Mayo Clin Proc 1998;73:497–500

40. Montplaisir J, Nicolas A, Denesle R, Gomez-Mancilla B. Restless legs syndrome improved by pramipexole: a double-blind randomized trial. Neurology 1999;52: 938–943

41. Mignot E. Genetics of narcolepsy and other sleep disorders. Am j Hum Genet 1997;60:1289–1302

42. Mignot E, Tafti M, Dement WC, Grumet FC. Narcolepsy and immunity. Adv Neuroimmunol 1995;5: 23–37

43. Mignot E. Perspectives in narcolepsy research and therapy. Curr Opin Pulm Med 1996;2:482–487

44. Spielman AJ, Adler JM, Glovinsky PB, Pressman MR, Thorpy MJ, Ellman SJ, Ackerman KD. Dynamics of REM sleep in narcolepsy. Sleep 1986;9:175–182

45. Thorpy MJ, Wagner DR, Spielman AJ, Weitzman ED. Objective assessment of narcolepsy. Arch Neurol 1983; 40:126–127

46. Aldrich MS. The clinical spectrum of narcolepsy and idiopathic hypersomnia. Neurology 1996;46:393–401

47. Aldrich MS, Chervin RD, Malow BA. Value of the multiple sleep latency test (MSLT) for the diagnosis of narcolepsy. Sleep 1997;20:620–629

48. Lin L, Faraco J, Li R, Kadotani H, Rogers W, Lin X, Qiu X, de Jong PJ, Nishino S, Mignot E. The sleep disorder canine narcolepsy is caused by a mutation in the hypocretin (orexin) receptor 2 gene. Cell 1999;98: 365–376

49. Nishino S, Ripley B, Overeem S, Lammers GJ, Mignot E. Hypocretin (orexin) deficiency in human narcolepsy. Lancet 2000;355:39–40

50. Mignot E, Nishino S, Guilleminault C, Dement WC. Modafinil binds to the dopamine uptake carrier site with low affinity. Sleep 1994;17:436–437

120 Parasomnias

Robert B Fogel and John W Winkelman

Introduction

Parasomnias are undesirable motor, verbal or experiential phenomena that occur during sleep. An understanding of the nature of parasomnias requires some discussion of the activity of the central nervous system during sleep. Sleep is composed of two very different states: non-rapid eye movement (NREM) and rapid eye movement (REM). NREM sleep is characterized by a relatively high-voltage, low-frequency synchronous EEG. During REM, on the other hand, one sees a low-voltage high-frequency EEG along with active paralysis of postural muscles. Although these states are described as mutually exclusive, features of one can intrude into the other or into wakefulness.[1] Parasomnias are often classified as NREM- or REM-related, depending on the state in which they originate (Figure 120.1).

Parasomnias associated with NREM sleep

The NREM parasomnias have several unifying features. They each represent disorders of incomplete or partial arousal from sleep, resulting in wakeful motor behavior with sleep-initiated cognition.[2] Other common features include a positive family history,[3] as well as a tendency for these disorders to arise from slow-wave sleep (SWS), typically in the first third of the night.[1] All are associated with body movement, varying degrees of autonomic activation, confusion, automatic behavior, and impaired recall for the event.

Many of these features can be reproduced by arousing normal subjects from SWS.

Confusional arousals

Confusional arousals (also termed sleep drunkenness) are characterized by partial awakenings from slow-wave sleep, with marked confusion, disorientation and inappropriate behavior. The marked autonomic activation seen in sleep terrors and the complex behaviors of sleepwalking are absent. They are extremely common in children, and may be universal before the age of five years.[4] In children they are usually benign and disappear before adolescence. In adults they tend to be more stable. Polysomnography (PSG) usually confirms their origination in SWS, and EEG may show residual slow waves and θ activity during the arousal. Endogenous or exogenous stimuli which produce inappropriate arousals (including prior sleep deprivation,[5] CNS depressants,[6] restless legs syndrome[7] and the obstructive sleep apnea syndrome[8]) can precipitate these events in predisposed individuals.[9] Treatment (other than reassurance) is rarely necessary for the majority of patients. Avoidance of precipitating factors is indicated.

Sleepwalking (somnambulism)

Sleepwalking is characterized by recurrent episodes of motor activity arising from sleep in which patients

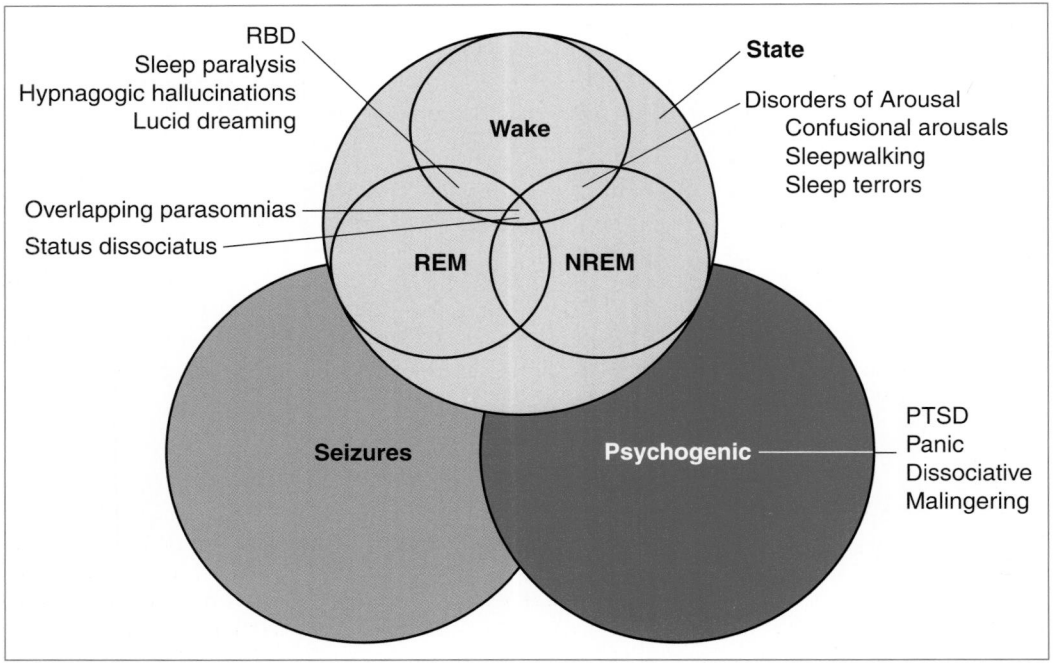

Figure 120.1 The overlapping nature of sleep and wake states along with their relationship to parasomnias. RBD = REM behavior disorder; PTSD = post-traumatic stress disorder. (From Mahowald MW, Schenck CH. Parasomnias including the restless legs syndrome. Clin Chest Med 1998;19: 183, with permission.)

exhibit complex automatic behaviors that may include walking or vocalization. Patients do not achieve full alertness, are relatively unresponsive to external stimuli during the event, and retrograde amnesia is common. Aggressive behavior can occur, and somnambulism has been successfully used as a defense in homicide cases.[10,11] Sleepwalking has been reported to occur in 15% to 30% of children and up to 1% to 2.5% of adults.[12,13] As with confusional arousals, somnambulism may be precipitated by sleep deprivation, fever, stress and certain drugs.[6] Although early studies suggested an increased prevalence of psychopathology in adult sleepwalkers, more recent studies have not confirmed this finding.[14]

The differential diagnosis of somnambulism includes partial-complex seizures, REM behavior disorder (see below), psychogenic fugue, dissociation, and nocturnal paroxysmal dystonia.[15] Diagnostic evaluation is probably not indicated in a subject with a strong family history or in whom sleepwalking has persisted since childhood. Polysomnography may show the event, but more frequently may provide suggestive evidence of a slow-wave sleep arousal disorder. These findings may include hypersynchronous δ waves or abrupt awakenings from SWS.[16,17]

Treatment for somnambulism is indicated if the attacks are associated with injurious or dangerous behaviors, and perhaps if they occur frequently. Treatment or avoidance of precipitating factors (see above) and safety precautions (locking windows, removing hazardous objects etc.) are essential. Pharmacological therapy typically consists of benzodiazepines, although few controlled trials of such therapy exist. Use of short-acting benzodiazepines is recommended (e.g. triazolam or lorazepam) to avoid excessive daytime sedation. In the only study of long-term follow-up of such therapy Schenck et al. reported on the use of chronic (>6 months) nightly use of benzodiazepines in 170 patients with injurious parasomnias and found sustained efficacy in 80%.[18] Other drugs have been less well studied, but there are case reports describing the efficacy of tricyclic antidepressants[19] and trazadone. Behavioral therapy such as hypnosis has also been reported to be successful in up to 50% of patients.[20]

Night terrors

Night terrors occur primarily in children and consist of a sudden arousal from sleep, often punctuated by a piercing scream, motor activity and extreme autonomic discharge (increased heart rate, pupillary dilation, sweating and blood pressure elevation). Crying, inconsolability and amnesia are typical features. The differential diagnosis is similar to that for sleepwalking, but also includes nightmares. Classic nightmares can usually be differentiated from true night terrors by less prominent autonomic features and greater dream recall. Therapy is similar to that for sleepwalking.

Parasomnias associated with REM sleep

REM sleep behavior disorder (RBD)

RBD is characterized by an intermittent absence of the normal atonia associated with REM sleep, leading to dream-enacting behaviors that are potentially injurious to self or bed-partner. Intense dream recall after the event, often of fighting or fleeing, is common.[21] RBD typically occurs in older men (80% to 90%) and is thought to be due to dysfunction of the brainstem mechanisms responsible for suppression of motor tone during REM sleep. Although the majority of cases are idiopathic, a significant minority occur in patients with identifiable underlying neuropathology. Diseases associated with RBD include Parkinson's disease (and may be the initial manifestation),[22] other neurodegenerative disorders such as Lewy body disease and multisystem atrophy,[22] chronic alcohol abuse,[23] dementia, and the use of REM-suppressing medications.[24] PSG recording typically shows elevated tonic and phasic EMG tone during REM sleep. Therapy is usually indicated, given the potential for injury. Clonazepam has been the most extensively used agent and is effective in the majority of cases at a dose of 0.5–2.0 mg.[22] Again, shorter-acting benzodiazepines may be of value if daytime sedation is a problem.

Other parasomnias

Nocturnal enuresis

Nocturnal enuresis or bedwetting is a relatively common problem in children and may occur in as many as 1% of adults. Enuresis is divided into primary (having never been continent) and secondary (develops after at least a six-month period of continence) forms.[25] Patients with primary enuresis are more likely to have a positive family history and structural urological abnormalities.[26] Occasionally enuresis has been described in patients with sleep apnea or with abnormalities of the antidiuretic hormone axis.[27] Diagnostic evaluation should include the history of the disorder, along with an evaluation to rule out structural abnormalities or chronic bacteriuria. Treatment options for enuresis include pharmacological therapy or behavioral conditioning. The tricyclic antidepressants (primarily imipramine) are efficacious in approximately one-third of cases, probably secondary to their anticholinergic properties.[28] Desmopressin, an analog of vasopressin, can provide long-term relief in 60% to 70% of cases.[29] However, enuresis often recurs when the drugs are stopped. Conditioning therapy consists of an alarm system attached to a pad that wakes the individual when the first drops of urine are detected. Although this system takes several weeks to work, it can be highly successful (>70%) and provides the best long-term control of enuresis.[30]

Bruxism

Bruxism is a stereotyped movement disorder characterized by grinding or clenching the teeth during sleep. It often comes to clinical attention[31] because the noise may disturb the bed-partner, but it can also produce dental abnormalities (abnormal tooth wear), jaw pain, masseter muscle hypertrophy or temporomandibular joint symptoms.[32–34] The exact prevalence is hard to determine, but it may occur in up to 6% to 12% of adults on a chronic basis.[35] Although bruxism has been reported to occur in those with a variety of neurological disorders,[36] it usually occurs in normals and may be precipitated by stress.[37] PSG typically shows repeated phasic increases in masseter tone at a frequency of 0.5–1.5 Hz. Treatment should focus on relieving symptoms and preventing permanent sequelae. Evaluation by a dentist is often helpful. Treatments that have been used with varying success rates include behavioral approaches (biofeedback, aversive conditioning, relaxation techniques) and intraoral appliances designed to correct muscle posture and protect the teeth.[31]

References

1. Mahowald MW, Schenck CH. NREM sleep parasomnias. Neurol Clin 1996;14:675–696
2. Broughton RJ. Sleep disorders: disorders of arousal? Enuresis, somnambulism, and nightmares occur in confusional states of arousal, not in "dreaming sleep." Science 1968;159:1070–1078
3. Kales A, Soldatos CR, Bixler EO, et al. Hereditary factors in sleepwalking and night terrors. Br J Psychiatry 1980;137:111–118
4. Ferber R. Sleep disorders in children. In: Kryger M, Roth T, Dement W, eds. Principles and Practice of Sleep Medicine. Philadelphia, PA: 1989:640–642.
5. Kales JD, Kales A, Soldatos CR, et al. Sleepwalking and night terrors related to febrile illness. Am J Psychiatry 1979;136:1214–1215
6. Glassman JN, Darko D, Gillin JC. Medication-induced somnambulism in a patient with schizoaffective disorder. J Clin Psychiatry 1986;47:523–524
7. Lauerma H. Nocturnal wandering caused by restless legs and short-acting benzodiazepines. Acta Psychiatr Scand 1991;83:492–493
8. Pressman MR, Meyer TJ, Kendrick-Mohamed J, et al. Night terrors in an adult precipitated by sleep apnea. Sleep 1995;18:773–775
9. Kushida CA, Clerk AA, Kirsch CM, et al. Prolonged confusion with nocturnal wandering arising from NREM and REM sleep: a case report. Sleep 1995;18:757–764
10. Broughton R, Billings R, Cartwright R, et al. Homicidal somnambulism: a case report. Sleep 1994;17:253–264
11. Broughton RJ, Shimizu T. Sleep-related violence: a medical and forensic challenge. Sleep 1995;18:727–730
12. Bixler EO, Kales A, Soldatos CR, et al. Prevalence of sleep disorders in the Los Angeles metropolitan area. Am J Psychiatry 1979;136:1257–1262
13. Ohayon MM, Guilleminault C, Priest RG. Night terrors, sleepwalking, and confusional arousals in the general population: their frequency and relationship to other sleep and mental disorders. J Clin Psychiatry 1999;60:268–276
14. Llorente MD, Currier MB, Norman SE, Mellman TA. Night terrors in adults: phenomenology and relationship to psychopathology. J Clin Psychiatry 1992;53:392–394
15. Montagna P. Nocturnal paroxysmal dystonia and nocturnal wandering. Neurology 1992;42(7 Suppl 6):61–67
16. Halasz P, Ujszaszi J, Gadoros J. Are microarousals preceded by electroencephalographic slow wave synchronization precursors of confusional awakenings? Sleep 1985;8:231–238
17. Blatt I, Peled R, Gadoth N, Lavie P. The value of sleep recording in evaluating somnambulism in young adults. Electroencephalogr Clin Neurophysiol 1991;78:407–412
18. Schenck CH, Mahowald MW. Long-term, nightly benzodiazepine treatment of injurious parasomnias and other disorders of disrupted nocturnal sleep in 170 adults. Am J Med 1996;100:333–337
19. Cooper AJ. Treatment of coexistent night-terrors and somnambulism in adults with imipramine and diazepam. J Clin Psychiatry 1987;48:209–210
20. Hurwitz TD, Mahowald MW, Schenck CH, et al. A retrospective outcome study and review of hypnosis as treatment of adults with sleepwalking and sleep terror. J Nerv Ment Dis 1991;179:228–233
21. Schenck CH, Bundlie SR, Patterson AL, Mahowald MW. Rapid eye movement sleep behavior disorder. A treatable parasomnia affecting older adults. JAMA 1987;257:1786–1789
22. Schenck CH, Mahowald MW. REM sleep parasomnias. Neurol Clin 1996;14:697–720
23. Barthlen GM, Stacy C. Dyssomnias, parasomnias, and sleep disorders associated with medical and psychiatric diseases. Mt Sinai J Med 1994;61:139–159
24. Louden MB, Morehead MA, Schmidt HS. Activation by selegiline (Eldepryle) of REM sleep behavior disorder in parkinsonism. West Virginia Med J 1995;91:101
25. Tietjen DN, Husmann DA. Nocturnal enuresis: a guide to evaluation and treatment. Mayo Clin Proc 1996;71:857–862
26. Husmann DA. Enuresis. Urology 1996;48:184–193
27. Norgaard JP, Djurhuus JC, Watanabe H, et al. Experience and current status of research into the pathophysiology of nocturnal enuresis. Br J Urol 1997;79:825–835
28. Miller K, Atkin B, Moody ML. Drug therapy for nocturnal enuresis. Current treatment recommendations. Drugs 1992;44:47–56
29. Schmitt BD. Nocturnal enuresis. Pediatr Rev 1997;18:183–190
30. Monda JM, Husmann DA. Primary nocturnal enuresis: a comparison among observation, imipramine, desmopressin acetate and bed-wetting alarm systems. J Urol 1995;154:745–748
31. Thompson BA, Blount BW, Krumholz TS. Treatment approaches to bruxism. Am Fam Phys 1994;49:1617–1622
32. Faulkner KD. Bruxism: a review of the literature. Part I. Aust Dent J 1990;35:266–276
33. Faulkner KD. Bruxism: a review of the literature. Part II. Aust Dent J 1990;35:355–361
34. Kleinberg I. Bruxism: aetiology, clinical signs and symptoms. Aust Prosthodont J 1994;8:9–17
35. Lavigne G, Montplaisir J. Restless legs syndrome and sleep bruxism: prevalence and association among Canadians. Sleep 1994;17:739–743
36. Richmond G. Survey of bruxism in an institutionalized mentally retarded population. Am J Ment Defic 1984;88:418–424
37. Hartman E, Mehta N, Fortgione A. Bruxism: personality traits and other characteristics. Sleep Res 1987;16:350–354

121 Disorders of Water and Sodium Balance

Robert Laureno

Either hyponatremia or hypernatremia can cause encephalopathy, especially when the respective sodium derangement is acute or numerically severe. In addition, correction of either hyponatremia or hypernatremia can induce distinctive neurological disorders: myelinolysis after correction of hyponatremia, and brain swelling following correction of hypernatremia. These iatrogenic conditions are more likely to occur when the sodium correction has been rapid and large and when the precorrection sodium derangement has been prolonged. Accordingly, the following discussion about the treatment of hyponatremia and hypernatremia emphasizes precautions, that lessen the incidence of neurological complications of therapy.[1]

Hyponatremia and myelinolysis following its correction

The more severe and the more acute the hyponatremia, the more likely it is to be symptomatic. Symptoms range from mild confusion to coma and status epilepticus. Patients rarely die from hyponatremia. However, when the hyponatremia is clinically severe (coma, status epilepticus, or agitation with confusion) it may be lethal. In such circumstances saline therapy is indicated. Although 3% saline therapy for severe hyponatremia can be lifesaving, the osmotic insult of aggressive correction of serum Na can induce central pontine and extrapontine myelinolysis, which in itself can be fatal. Typically, the symptoms of myelinolysis appear two to three days after the onset of correction of hyponatremia. Early symptoms include mutism and behavioral problems. Later, spastic quadriparesis and pseudobulbar palsy develop in the typical case; cognitive problems, psychiatric disorders and movement disorders may occur. Severe disability is a common long-term outcome.

Thus the physician must weigh the danger of uncorrected hyponatremia against the risk of myelinolysis with correction. When the hyponatremia is not clinically severe and when brain imaging shows no cerebral edema, there is no need for active therapy. Following hospitalization a spontaneous water diuresis often will correct hyponatremia without the doctor's intervention, especially in thiazide-treated individuals, alcoholics and psychogenic polydipsia patients. When hyponatremia is due to inappropriate secretion of antidiuretic hormone (ADH) or to treatment with vasopressin, fluid restriction (800 mL daily) or withdrawal of medicine may suffice to correct hyponatremia. As a general rule, it is preferable to tolerate the confusion or drowsiness of chronic hyponatremia, even when it is numerically severe, than to suddenly raise the Na level. Caution is the master word.

When the hyponatremia is clinically severe, saline therapy is appropriate. Hypertonic (3%) saline, a dangerous medicine, may be infused in 100 mL aliquots, which treatment should be terminated as soon as the neurological signs show improvement (cessation of convulsions or agitation). The goal is to raise the Na by 4 meq/L over four hours. (When water intoxication is so severe that scans reveal critical brain swelling, more aggressive saline therapy may be appropriate.) Furosemide will facilitate the correction. Even when formal calculations of saline dose are employed, the resulting rate and extent of rise of Na are unpredictable for a specific individual. The physician should urgently check the serum Na level every one to two hours during saline infusion. Only by doing so can the physician know how the Na is in fact rising, and thereby properly adjust therapy. The risk of myelinolysis is minimized when the rise in Na is limited to less than 10 meq/L over the first 24 hours. Whenever possible, rise of Na should be even more slow over subsequent 24-hour periods.

Should the Na rise more than anticipated, relowering it by the use of DDAVP (desmopressin acetate) and hypotonic intravenous fluids should be considered in consultation with a nephrologist. There is convincing animal evidence that such intervention lowers the incidence of myelinolysis. In one human case report, even after corticospinal tract signs had developed with correction of Na, relowering of serum Na was followed by resolution of the postcorrection neurological disorder. When such relowering is attempted, the Na should be lowered to a level no less than 10 meq/L above the level of serum Na that had necessitated the treatment of hyponatremia initially.

When paralysis from myelinolysis is established, physical therapy and good medical care (maintenance of nutrition, support of respiration, treatment of infection, prevention of deep vein thrombosis etc.) may allow some patients to regain upper extremity function and independent ambulation. This recovery may take many months. Conventional symptomatic therapy for parkinsonism or psychiatric sequelae should be used when appropriate.[2]

Hypernatremia

The more severe and the more acute the hypernatremia, the more likely it is to be symptomatic. Manifestations of the encephalopathy range from drowsiness and/or mild confusion to convulsions and/or coma. Neurological manifestations are more severe when the hypernatremia is numerically severe or when it is acute in onset. Hypernatremia as severe as Na = 175 meq/L may cause no symptoms, when it has developed slowly. On the other hand, extreme hypernatremia can cause not only metabolic encephalopathy but also structural changes, namely brain shrinkage and intracranial hemorrhage.

Osmoprotective mechanisms to some extent lessen the metabolic effects of hypernatremia on the brain. Because NaCl is primarily an extracellular salt, hypernatremia causes osmotic movement of intracellular water to the extracellular compartment. In response, even in the initial hours of hypernatremia, uptake of plasma K by brain cells occurs. This electrolyte shift lessens osmotic loss of intracellular water, thereby decreasing brain cell shrinkage. During the initial days of hypernatremia there develops further osmoprotection by the intracellular accumulation of amino acids, polyols and amines. As intracellular osmolality comes to equal that of the hyperosmolar extracellular environment, water shifts back into the brain, which becomes fully compensated to the hypernatremic state.

This osmoprotective adaptation becomes important when one is treating hypernatremia. The intracellular organic osmolytes, which have accumulated for osmoprotection, cannot return to normal levels quickly. Thus, if extracellular osmolality rapidly drops with therapy for hypernatremia, these elevated levels of osmolytes draw water into brain cells and the brain swells. This brain edema during rehydration may cause focal seizures, generalized convulsions and death. To avoid such complications the physician must be gentle in treating hypernatremia.

Although some authors advise rates of correction as high as 2 mEq/L/h, this guideline could bring a 48 mEq/L decrement in 24 hours, when hypernatremia is extreme. It is preferable to limit the correction to 0.5 mEq/L/h. When extracellular volume depletion is a major feature, initiate therapy with normal saline infusion. Otherwise utilize hypotonic 0.45% saline alternating with 5% dextrose in water (D5W) or D5W alone. Frequent monitoring of serum Na is essential because the response to therapy is not predictable for a given individual, despite sophisticated calculations.[3]

Conclusions

Aggressive treatment of hyponatremia is dangerous and usually unnecessary. However, when acute and/or severe hyponatremia causes coma, convulsions, or agitation with confusion, life may be threatened; intravenous 3% saline infusion and furosemide should be given with the aim of increasing the serum Na by 4 meq/L over four hours. As soon as convulsions and/or agitation are controlled, the rate of correction of hyponatremia should be slowed so that the total rise in Na over the first 24 hours is less than 10 meq/L, whenever possible. Over subsequent days it is preferable that the sodium rise even more slowly. Because the response to therapy in a given individual is unpredictable, one should frequently measure the Na to monitor its rise.

Hypernatremia indicates that the patient needs water. Thus, the physician should provide it with dilute intravenous fluid, usually D5W. To avoid overcorrection of hypernatremia, it is important to monitor the Na level frequently during the infusion. The therapeutic decrement in sodium, when possible, should be limited to 12 meq/L/24 h in order to avoid iatrogenic brain swelling.

References

1. Laureno R. Neurologic syndromes accompanying electrolyte disorders. *In:* Goetz CG, Tanner CM, Aminoff MJ, eds. Handbook of Clinical Neurology: Systemic Diseases, Part I, vol. 63. Amsterdam: Elsevier, 1993
2. Laureno R, Karp BI. Myelinolysis after correction of hyponatremia. Ann Intern Med 1997;126:57–62
3. Sterns RH. Hypernatremia in the intensive care unit: instant quality—just add water. Crit Care Med 1999;27:1041–1042

122 Acid–Base Disturbances and the Central Nervous System

Julia H Hayes and Julian L Seifter

Introduction

Neurological dysfunction is a common sequela of both systemic and cerebral acid–base disturbances. An understanding of the interactions of systemic acid–base status with the CNS is important for several reasons. First, the CNS plays a pivotal role in determining the nature and extent of systemic compensation for both respiratory and metabolic disturbances. In addition, although the CNS is well-equipped to defend against systemic acid–base imbalances, neurological symptoms are common in these disorders. And lastly, manipulation of systemic acid–base status has been shown to be therapeutically effective in certain neurological and systemic conditions. Understanding the basis of both systemic and cerebral changes in these disorders permits physicians to assess and treat them appropriately.

Cerebral acid–base disorders are commonly seen in response to primary CNS lesions. In addition to producing profound changes within the CNS, these imbalances have been postulated to affect systemic acid–base status. This chapter will address the effects of systemic acid–base disturbances on the CNS, as well as the effects of primary CNS lesions on both cerebral and systemic acid–base status.

Anatomy

Blood–brain barrier

The CNS is separated from the systemic circulation by the blood–brain barrier, which permits neurons, the brain's interstitial fluid and the CSF to maintain an environment distinct from that of the rest of the body. The blood–brain barrier is a complex of several types of cells located at the brain's capillary interface. The innermost layer is formed by specialized overlapping endothelial cells joined by tight junctions. These cells rest on a thick basal lamina containing smooth muscle cells and pericytes. This layer is surrounded by astrocytic foot processes from glial cells, characterized by a thick cell wall, which cover approximately 85% of the capillary surface.

The brain's endothelial cells differ from peripheral endothelial cells in that they are joined by tight junctions of high electrical resistance, as opposed to the fenestration or low electrical resistance tight junctions of peripheral endothelial cells. In addition, they lack the fluid-phase and receptor-mediated endocytosis characteristic of peripheral endothelial cells, and therefore are capable only of limited transcellular transport of compounds. As a result of these characteristics, passage of molecules from the blood into the brain is determined by lipid solubility, molecular size, configuration and charge, and acid ionization constant, with the diffusion of lipophilic substances and weak acids being favored. Specific carrier systems in the brain's endothelial cells are responsible for controlled exchange between the blood and the central nervous system.

However, not all areas of the brain are separated from the systemic circulation in this manner. Certain regions, which include the posterior pituitary and the circumventricular organs, are characterized by fenestrated capillaries similar to those in the periphery. Endothelial cells in these regions also contain many vesicles in the cytoplasm, believed to function in transcellular transport. These areas are important for the release of neuropeptides into the blood and in sensing chemical changes in the blood to maintain water balance and perform other homeostatic functions.

Brain–CSF interface

There is relatively unrestricted exchange of substances between the CSF and the extracellular space of the brain. The barrier between these compartments is composed primarily of the ependymal cells lining the ventricles and the pia. Both ependymal cells and pial cells are joined by gap junctions, which permit the passage of certain substances, including large protein molecules as well as fluids and ions. Extensions of the subarachnoid space follow blood vessels into the brain in the Virchow–Robinson spaces. The nature of this barrier allows for the movement of molecules between the brain parenchyma and the CSF.

However, in certain regions of the brain the interstitial fluid is separated from the CSF by cells with tight junctions. These areas include the choroid plexus and the circumventricular organs, where the blood–brain barrier is absent. However, it is believed that gap junctions are present in the region of the ventral medullary respiratory center, permitting CSF to enter the interstitial fluid surrounding chemoreceptive cells. This phenomenon proves to be very important in the body's response to acid–base disturbances affecting the CSF.

Choroid plexus and CSF

The choroid plexus in the lateral ventricles secretes most of the CSF. It is composed of villous choroidal epithelium joined by tight junctions surrounding a fenestrated capillary network and interstitial connective tissue. The epithelial cells are structurally similar to the distal and collecting tubules of the kidney and contain transporters which generate the unique environment of CSF. Cerebral capillaries are responsible for the production of the rest of the CSF, primarily by generating an osmotic gradient that pulls fluid into the interstitial space, from which it passes to the CSF.

Transporters in the choroid plexus are responsible for the composition of the CSF, which differs significantly from that of blood (Table 122.1). Some of the transporters that have been identified include an apical Na-K-ATPase pump which exchanges potassium from the CSF for sodium. Carbonic anhydrase within the cell generates bicarbonate, which enters the CSF by what is thought to be an active process; the hydrogen ion is exchanged for sodium on the basolateral membrane. A chloride–bicarbonate exchanger on the basolateral membrane extrudes Cl in exchange for bicarbonate, and systemic hypocarbia has been shown to reduce CSF formation. The composition of the CSF is determined by secretion by the choroid plexus, subsequent adjustment via ion exchange with the interstitial fluid and brain cells, and active and passive transport across the capillary endothelium.

Acid–base status of brain and CSF

Despite being in a steady state, the acid–base components of the CSF and arterial blood differ significantly (Table 122.1). The unique composition of CSF is made possible by the choroid plexus regulated carrier-mediated active transport and the anatomic barriers described above. The pH of cisternal CSF is lower than that of arterial blood, at approximately 7.32 vs 7.40. This relative acidity is in part the result of higher pCO_2 in the CSF (48 mmHg vs 40 mmHg) which, despite diffusing readily across the blood–brain barrier, is maintained at increased partial pressures by continuous metabolic generation and release of pCO_2 by brain cells. Also, the bicarbonate concentration of CSF is slightly less than that of blood. However, bicarbonate forms the primary buffer in CSF, in contrast to the blood, owing to the lower concentrations of protein (40 mg/dL vs 7 g/dL), phosphorus and hemoglobin found in the CSF. In addition, lactic acid is higher in the CSF than in blood and may contribute to the lower pH of CSF.

The acid–base status of CSF has been established by many studies and is technically relatively simple to measure. However, it is important to bear in mind that the intracellular environment of brain cells is distinct from that of the CSF, and therefore is not reflected in these values. The brain's intracellular acid–base status is more difficult to characterize, and many studies have done so indirectly. Therefore, there is less agreement among experts as to the actual composition and responses of these cells to changes in local and systemic conditions.[1]

Effects of respiratory acid–base disturbances on CNS

CNS control of ventilation

Before discussing the effects of respiratory acid–base disturbances on the CNS, it is useful to review briefly the CNS control of ventilation. The CNS is responsible for the total body content of CO_2, achieved as a result of the modulation of both voluntary and involuntary respiration. Voluntary respiration, and the hyperventilation seen in anxiety and certain primary CNS lesions, is determined by higher cortical centers. Involuntary respiration is controlled by areas in the brainstem and is dependent upon input from both central and peripheral sensory receptors that respond to the concentrations of hydrogen, pCO2 and pO2 of the blood and CSF.

The central component in involuntary ventilatory control is the respiratory control center in the medulla oblongata, comprised of several nuclei that both create and modify the respiratory pattern. The best understood of these centers is the family of medullary centers, consisting of the dorsal and ventral respiratory groups of neurons. This area is responsible for the establishment of the basic respiratory pattern and integrates input from multiple sources, including higher brain centers as well as central and peripheral chemoreceptors and baroreceptors.

Input from these peripheral and central sensors allows this center to modify respiration based on the acid–base status of the blood and CSF. Central chemoreceptors are distinct from the respiratory control center but are located adjacent to it at the ventrolateral surface of the medulla. Two areas of chemosensation have been identified in this region, one caudal and one rostral, which sense changes in the pH and pCO2 of the brainstem interstitial fluid. As discussed above, it has been suggested that in this region, gap junctions in the pia may permit mixing of the brain interstitial fluid and CSF, allowing the chemosensitive areas to sense changes in the pH, pCO2 and bicarbonate concentrations of the CSF.

The central chemoreceptors have been shown to be exquisitely sensitive to changes in hydrogen ion concentration. In one experiment in goats, a change of CSF hydrogen ion of only 15 nEq/L led to an increase in ventilation from 5 to 45 L/min.[3] pCO2 is also a

Table 122.1   Constituents of normal CSF and serum (average values)[1]

	CSF	Plasma
Osmolarity (mosnol/L)	295	295
pH	7.33	7.41 (art)
pCO2 (mmHg)	48	38 (art)
Bicarbonate (mEq/L)	23.0	23.0
Chloride (mEq/L)	119.0	101.0
Sodium (mEq/L)	138.0	138.0
Potassium (mEq/L)	2.8	4.1
Calcium (mEq/L)	2.1	4.8
Phosphorus (mg/dL)	1.6	4.0
Total protein	15–50	6.5–8.4
	(mg/dL)	(g/100 dL)
Lactate (mEq/L)	1.6	1.0

potent stimulus for these cells: in normal young men a 2 mmHg increase in pCO2 has been shown to double ventilation. However, the response to pCO2 diminishes with age. The central chemoreceptors are relatively insensitive to changes in pO2 except in cases of severe hypoxia.

Peripheral sensory input is contributed by pulmonary stretch receptors and carotid sinus and aortic arch chemo- and baroreceptors. The most important of these for the maintenance of systemic acid–base balance is the carotid chemoreceptor, though the aortic appears to play a minor role. The carotid bodies, surrounded by a capillary plexus affording close proximity to systemic blood, respond to hypoxia, hypercapnia and hydrogen ion concentrations. Their response to both pCO2 and to hydrogen ion concentration is virtually linear, in the range from a pCO2 of 25–65 mmHg and a hydrogen ion concentration of 25–60 nEq/L. The response to hypoxemia varies among individuals, but the carotid bodies appear to respond when the pO2 decreases below 60 mmHg. The carotid chemoreceptors' sensitivity to combined hypoxia and hypercapnia exceeds the additive effect of the response to each stimulus individually: hypoxia renders the chemoreceptors more sensitive to hypercapnia, and vice versa. It has been suggested that the effect of hydrogen ion concentration is independent of hypercapnia or hypoxemia, increasing the chemoreceptors' sensitivity to hypercapnia at any pCO2 concentration. The sensitivity of these receptors is also dependent upon the degree of change in conditions: a sudden increase in pCO2, for example during recovery from metabolic acidosis, can lead to an overshoot phenomenon resulting in hyperventilation. This response is thought to be the result of the sudden intracellular acidification of the receptors that overwhelms the normal mechanisms for maintaining pH homeostasis. The aortic bodies have been shown to respond to changes in pO2 and pCO2, but not to hydrogen ion concentration.

Respiratory acid–base disturbances

Respiratory acid–base disturbances have a profound effect on the CNS. This phenomenon stems from the fact that the CNS must respond to changes in systemic pCO2, reflected immediately in the CNS as a result of the permeability of the blood–brain barrier to CO_2, as well as to changes in the peripheral concentration of hydrogen ions as reflected in the bicarbonate concentration. However, despite these changes, the CNS is able to maintain a remarkably constant pH in the face of even significant respiratory acid–base disturbances.

Respiratory acidosis

Respiratory acidosis is characterized by a primary elevation in pCO2 reflected in reduced arterial pH with variable elevation in bicarbonate concentration. It is most frequently caused by a decrease in alveolar ventilation.

Causes of respiratory acidosis Respiratory acidosis is most frequently seen clinically in cases of pulmonary insufficiency and can be the result of pulmonary disease, respiratory muscle fatigue, or abnormalities of ventilatory control. Examples of such disorders include central etiologies such as the effects of drugs, stroke and infection; etiologies related to airway obstruction; primary parenchymal processes such as COPD and ARDS; and neuromuscular diseases such as myasthenia gravis or muscular dystrophies.

Clinical findings in respiratory acidosis Clinical findings in respiratory acidosis are related to the degree and duration of the respiratory acidosis and whether or not hypoxemia is present. Neurological symptoms figure prominently in this disorder. A precipitous rise in pCO2 can lead to confusion, anxiety, psychosis, asterixis, seizures and myoclonic jerks, with progressive depression of the sensorium to coma at an arterial pCO2 greater than 60 mmHg (CO_2 narcosis). Hypercapnia has been shown to increase cerebral blood flow and volume and to decrease cerebral compliance. As a result, hypercapnia can lead to symptoms and signs reflecting elevated intracranial pressure, including headaches and papilledema. Other findings in acute respiratory acidosis include signs of catecholamine release, including skin flushing, diaphoresis, and increased cardiac contractility and output.

Symptoms of chronic hypercapnia include fatigue, lethargy and confusion, in addition to the findings seen in acute hypercapnia. However, patients may not show signs of hypercapnia even at pCO2 levels as high as 110 mmHg.

It can be difficult clinically to distinguish the signs of hypercapnia from those of hypoxemia, as the two often present together. However, in many patients the correction of hypoxemia does not improve the clinical picture; as a result, it can be surmised that hypercapnia is responsible for many of the findings seen.

CNS effects of acute respiratory acidosis The effect of acute respiratory acidosis on the CSF pH and the intracellular pH of brain cells is almost instantaneous, reflecting the ability of pCO2 to cross the blood–brain barrier. However, the initial acidosis caused by elevated pCO2 levels is compensated for more quickly in the CNS than in the periphery. In experiments in humans and animals, isolated acute hypercapnia has been shown to result initially in a similar decrease in both arterial and CSF pH. In one experiment in dogs[4] breathing 10% CO_2, both arterial and cisternal CSF pH dropped to 7.1 after one hour of hypercapnia. However, after six hours the CSF pH had risen from 7.1 to almost 7.2, although the arterial pH remained at 7.1. The reason for this increase was an increase in CSF bicarbonate. The concentration of bicarbonate in the CSF began to rise within one hour, before the peripheral bicarbonate had changed significantly. After six hours of sustained hypercapnia the CSF bicarbonate had risen from 19 to 30 mEq/L, compared with an arterial bicarbonate change of only

24–25 mEq/L. It has been shown that within one day of sustained hypercarbia the CSF pH returns to normal, with a bicarbonate level of 35 mmol/L, whereas the arterial pH remains acidotic.[5]

The intracellular pH of brain cells returns to normal even more quickly than the pH of CSF. In similar experiments inducing acute hypercarbia, Arieff et al. have shown that the intracellular pH falls from 7.06 to 6.90 in one hour, contrasted with an arterial pH drop from 7.36 to 7.07 over the same period. However, within three hours the intracellular pH has returned to normal, accompanied by an increase in bicarbonate from 11.3 to 24.4 mmol/kgH$_2$O.[6] These experiments demonstrate that both the CSF and brain cells return to a normal pH significantly before systemic compensation is evident.

The primary mechanism by which the brain and CSF compensate for acute hypercapnia rests in an increase in bicarbonate concentration. It is now commonly believed that two mechanisms are largely responsible for this increase, called the dual contribution theory. The first is an increase in carbonic anhydrase activity in the cells of the choroid plexus, producing bicarbonate which is then transported into the CSF. The mechanism by which these cells are stimulated to increase bicarbonate is not yet established. However, this hypothesis has been supported by the finding that acetazolamide is capable of blocking the increase in bicarbonate seen in the CSF in acute hypercapnia. Second, it is believed that bicarbonate diffuses into the CSF from plasma as a result of the positive electrochemical gradient existing between the CSF and capillary blood. Other mechanisms that may contribute to increased CSF bicarbonate concentration include a decrease in lactic acid production. As stated earlier, lactic acid concentration is higher in the CNS than in the periphery and may contribute to its relative acidosis. However, in hypercapnic states the increase in cerebral blood flow secondary to CO$_2$'s vasodilatory effects would tend to decrease the production of lactic acid. In addition, intracellular bicarbonate could be released into the extracellular environment by a chloride shift into neurons similar to that occurring in red blood cells. And finally, increased ammonia production via the glutamine-α-ketoglutarate pathway during acute respiratory acidosis could buffer hydrogen ions via the creation of ammonium, though this process requires some time to take effect.[7]

The mechanisms of increased intracellular bicarbonate are less well understood but probably overlap with those described for the CSF. The generation of bicarbonate in brain cells does not appear to be carbonic anhydrase dependent, however, as it is not blocked by acetazolamide. Additional possibilities for the intracellular increase in bicarbonate are carboxylation reactions producing CO$_2$, including those involving glucose metabolism and the conversion of glutamic acid to GABA. In addition, certain steps in glucose metabolism are pH-dependent, and CO$_2$-producing steps may be favored in intracellularly acidotic states.[8]

In addition to the mechanisms for increased bicarbonate production and release described above, the brain has been shown to have an as yet unidentified non-bicarbonate buffer equivalent to approximately 33 mmol/kg brain tissue, which would help to return pH to normal values.[8]

Chronic hypercapnia   Chronic hypercapnia is generally seen in patients as the result of chronic disease due to any of the etiologies listed above. These patients show a decreased ventilatory response to increased pCO2, decreased pO2 and increased hydrogen ion concentration. The slow time course of many of these diseases allows the kidney to compensate adequately as the disease progresses, increasing its excretion of hydrogen ion and the generation and reabsorption of bicarbonate to restore systemic pH towards normal values. This compensation allows the normal balance of bicarbonate between CSF and plasma, with CSF bicarbonate slightly lower, to be maintained. The same mechanisms responsible for the CSF's adaptation to acute hypercapnia are probably responsible.

Effects of respiratory acidosis on respiratory drive   In acute respiratory acidosis the peripheral and central chemoreceptors work in concert, both responding to increases in hydrogen ion concentrations to increase ventilation. However, with the rapid restoration of CSF pH to normal values the stimulus for ventilation becomes entirely dependent upon the peripheral chemoreceptors, which will sustain an increase in ventilation until renal compensation is complete. This process has been shown to take three days to take effect, and is not maximal until five days after the onset of respiratory acidosis.

Treatment of respiratory acidosis   Treatment of both chronic and acute respiratory acidosis is aimed primarily at correcting the underlying etiology and ensuring adequate ventilation. Acute respiratory acidosis can be very dangerous, and measures to relieve severe hypoxemia and acidemia should be instituted immediately, including intubation and mechanically assisted ventilation if necessary.

Two complications can be seen in chronic respiratory acidosis patients as a result of renal compensation. In patients breathing spontaneously, oxygen should be carefully titrated: ventilation may be driven by hypoxemia, and correction of the hypoxemia can result in suppression of respiratory drive.

In patients with compensated chronic respiratory acidosis, rapid and complete correction of hypercapnia can also result in posthypercapnic alkalosis (see discussion below). Patients recovering from an acute-on-chronic respiratory acidosis should be monitored carefully for hypokalemia, hypovolemia and chloride levels in order to ensure that adequate renal excretion of bicarbonate can occur.

Bicarbonate therapy should not be considered unless the pH falls below 7.1 and the patient is about to be intubated: in these cases it can be used transiently until the patient is ventilated. There is also a role for bicarbonate therapy in renal failure, in cases in which adequate acid excretion cannot take place.

Permissive hypercapnia

Recently, permissive hypercapnia has been utilized clinically in patients with ARDS to limit pulmonary damage secondary to mechanical ventilation. In order to maintain normal pCO2 levels in ARDS patients, it is necessary to deliver tidal volumes and pressures that can result in overdistension of and damage to alveoli, potentially leading to rupture. By decreasing tidal volume and pressures, pulmonary injury is limited. This technique has been associated with improved survival in ARDS patients and improved outcomes in patients with status epilepticus.

However, clinically significant respiratory acidosis can result from elevations in pCO2 using this approach. Effects are most commonly seen when the pCO2 is allowed to rise precipitously, and include increased intracranial pressure, increased cardiac output and increased organ perfusion in some studies. Cardenas et al.[9] studied the effect of acute hypercapnia in intubated ewes and found that these effects of respiratory acidosis could be lessened by administration of sodium bicarbonate to correct blood pH. The dangers of this technique rest in the fact that many patients will have significant comorbidities that make the complications of respiratory acidosis particularly dangerous. By controlling peripheral pH, many of these potentially lethal effects could be attenuated.

Respiratory alkalosis

Respiratory alkalosis is characterized by a primary decrease in pCO2 reflected in an increased arterial pH and variably decreased plasma bicarbonate concentration. It is commonly the result of alveolar hyperventilation.

Causes of respiratory alkalosis Alveolar hyperventilation leading to respiratory alkalosis can have multiple causes. Etiologies include those secondary to hypoxemia, such as pulmonary disease, CHF, high-altitude living, or anemia. Direct stimulation of the medullary respiratory center can also result in hyperventilation, as seen in cortical hyperventilation resulting from anxiety or pain, as well as systemic conditions including endotoxemia, hepatic cirrhosis, salicylate intoxication, correction of metabolic acidosis, hyperthermia and pregnancy. Mechanical ventilation is also a common cause of respiratory alkalosis.

Primary neurological diseases have also been shown to stimulate alveolar hyperventilation. The causes include CVA, infection, trauma and tumors. Two patterns of respiration are seen: central hyperventilation and Cheyne–Stokes respiration. Central hyperventilation is described as regular but with increased rate and tidal volume, whereas Cheyne–Stokes breathing is characterized by periods of hyperventilation alternating with apnea. Which pattern a patient manifests appears to depend on the location of the lesion, rather than its underlying etiology.

Central hyperventilation is associated with lesions at the pontine–midbrain level, and though its cause is unknown it does not seem to correlate with changes in pCO2 or pO2. Some investigators have described an association between central hyperventilation and increased CSF lactate in hemorrhagic stroke patients, but these results have not been substantiated by others, and many patients without blood in the CSF also exhibit central hyperventilation. Cheyne–Stokes respiration is seen in patients with bilateral cortical and upper pontine lesions and may be related to the increased sensitivity of the respiratory center to pCO2 exhibited in these patients. Both altered respiratory patterns are associated with a poor prognosis.[10]

Clinical findings in respiratory alkalosis The clinical manifestations of respiratory alkalosis depend on the degree and duration of the condition, but are primarily those of the underlying disorder. Symptoms of acute hypocapnia include dizziness, perioral or extremity paresthesias, confusion, asterixis, hypotension, seizures and coma. Most symptoms are manifested only when the pCO2 has fallen below 25–30 mmHg, and can be related to decreased cerebral blood flow or to reduced free calcium (as alkalosis increases calcium's protein-bound fraction). Some symptoms frequently seen in the hyperventilation syndrome secondary to pain or anxiety do not appear to be related to hypocapnia, and include shortness of breath and chest wall pain. Chronic hypocapnia does not appear to be associated with significant clinical symptoms.

Cerebral blood flow is significantly decreased by hypocapnia, which is a potent vasoconstrictor. Cerebral blood flow has been shown to decrease 4% with every 1 mmHg decrease in pCO2 down to 30 mmHg. This phenomenon is used clinically to decrease intracranial pressure by hyperventilating patients with cerebral edema. Patients are hyperventilated to a goal of 25–30 mmHg pCO2. The time course of initial patient response appears to vary based on the severity and cause of the underlying lesion. The effect is relatively short-lived: CSF bicarbonate concentration decreases and CSF pH normalizes rapidly, which probably decreases the effectiveness of hyperventilation, though this fact has not been shown. Renal compensation over 36–72 hours returns systemic pH to normal values and restores cerebral blood flow to normal. Because there is significant variability in patient response throughout the course of this therapy, ICP should be monitored carefully during both hyperventilation and recovery to prevent rebound edema secondary to cerebral acidosis.[11] This technique is commonly used as an adjunct to other forms of treatment, such as osmotic and corticosteroid therapies.

CNS effects of acute respiratory alkalosis As in respiratory acidosis, the CNS is immediately affected by decreases in systemic pCO2 because of the blood–brain barrier's permeability to CO_2. And, as in respiratory acidosis, the CSF and intracellular pH show an initial short-lived response that parallels the systemic increase in pH.

Acute hypocapnia results in an initial increase in the pH of both the CSF and the brain's intracellular environment. However, this increase is quickly offset by a decrease in bicarbonate levels. In acute respiratory alkalosis one of the primary mechanisms of this fall in bicarbonate appears to be the generation of lactate. Experiments in anesthetized dogs have shown that hyperventilation results in an initial increase in CSF pH, followed by a return to normal values after five hours. This change in pH is accompanied by a decrease in bicarbonate levels from approximately 25 to 20 mmol/L and an increase in lactate concentration from 18 to 33 mg/100mL. Systemic pH continued to rise over the entire six hours of the experiment.[12] The increase in lactate seen in similar experiments is not sufficient to account for the decrease in bicarbonate observed in the CSF, however, although measurements of CSF lactate may underestimate the role of lactate production in lowering bicarbonate as a result of lactate transport across the blood–brain barrier.

By contrast, in experiments studying the intracellular pH of brain cells the decrease in intracellular bicarbonate is almost stoichiometric with an increase in lactate, which has been shown to return intracellular pH to normal values with two hours in experimental animals maintained at a pCO2 of 20 mmHg.[6]

The mechanism of this increase in lactate, both in the CSF and intracellularly, is thought to arise from tissue hypoxia secondary to cerebral vasoconstriction and increased hemoglobin affinity for oxygen. Alkalosis produces a transient left shift in the hemoglobin–oxygen dissociation curve via its effects on 2,3-DPG in red blood cells, reducing the delivery of oxygen to brain cells. Increased phosphofructokinase activity in brain cells may also contribute to increased lactate production.

Chronic respiratory alkalosis   Chronic respiratory alkalosis can be seen in patients with chronic conditions caused by any of the etiologies listed above. As previously discussed, CNS compensation for this alkalosis occurs within hours. Chronic respiratory alkalosis does not appear to have a distinct symptomatology.

Renal compensation for sustained hypocapnia is complete in 36–72 hours. The mechanism rests primarily in the kidney's net reduction of hydrogen ion excretion, which it accomplishes largely by decreasing ammonium and titratable acid excretion. The threshold for bicarbonate excretion is also lowered, resulting in bicarbonaturia. As a result, systemic bicarbonate levels decrease and arterial pH returns towards normal values.

Effects of respiratory alkalosis on respiratory drive   Because of the many possible causes of respiratory alkalosis, the effects of this condition on the responses of the central and peripheral chemorecep-

tors are variable. Primary stimulation of the central chemoreceptor is a common cause of respiratory alkalosis, as seen in cortical hyperventilation, endotoxemia and pregnancy. In these cases, the signals from central and peripheral chemoreceptors will be in opposition to each other, with central signals overriding peripheral input until the primary stimulus is removed. However, in cases in which the primary stimulus is the result of systemic conditions, such as hypoxia secondary to pulmonary disease or anemia, the peripheral and central chemoreceptors initially receive similar signals to reduce ventilation from an increase in both peripheral and CSF pH. However, the CSF pH returns quickly to normal values, at which point the stimulus is derived solely from the peripheral chemoreceptors, which will act to reduce hyperventilation until renal compensation is complete.

Treatment of respiratory alkalosis   Treatment of respiratory alkalosis must address the underlying etiology of the disturbance. Hyperventilation syndrome is a diagnosis of exclusion, but patients who exhibit symptoms, such as tetany and syncope, and who have been ruled out for more serious causes of hyperventilation, can be treated with a rebreathing mask. Hypophosphatemia can be seen in these patients, but it usually improves with treatment of the alkalosis.

Adaptation to high altitude

The respiratory response to high altitude is complex. Acute exposure to high altitude results in hypoxia-induced hyperventilation. Compensation requires at least several days to take effect and is characterized by a gradual increase in hyperventilation. The result of this continuing increase in hyperventilation is a steadily decreasing pCO2 and increasing pO2 over this period. It has been shown that after a few days at 3000 m pCO2 decreases from 37 to 30 mmHg, and pO2 increases from 57 to 65 mmHg.[13] It is thought that this phenomenon may be the result of conflicting signals from peripheral and central chemoreceptors. The effect of the hypoxic stimulus to ventilate on the peripheral chemoreceptors is initially modulated by the effects of alkalosis, both peripherally and centrally. However, as bicarbonate in the CSF falls, inhibition of the central stimulus to ventilate decreases. Therefore, the changing balance between hypoxemia, alkalosis and CSF pH in adaptation to high altitude may be responsible for this gradual increase in hyperventilation over time. Once a steady state is achieved, the drive to ventilate is determined by the effects of hypoxemia and alkalemia on the peripheral chemoreceptors.[10]

Effects of metabolic acid–base disturbances on the CNS

In contrast to respiratory acid–base disturbances, in metabolic acidosis and alkalosis the CNS is confronted only with systemic changes in hydrogen ion and bicarbonate concentrations. The CNS is able to protect its unique environment by regulating bicarbonate levels and as a result of the blood–brain barrier. Studies of CSF and brain intracellular pH in animals and of CSF in humans have shown only minimal change in response to sustained metabolic acidosis or alkalosis. However, despite a stable pH, metabolic acid–base disturbances can have profound effects on the CNS which can be the result of either the disturbance itself or respiratory compensation.

Metabolic acidosis

Metabolic acidosis is characterized by a low arterial pH associated with a reduced plasma bicarbonate concentration and a compensatory decrease in pCO2. Causes include a primary renal failure to excrete hydrogen ion, an increase in systemic hydrogen ion load owing to other causes, or the loss of bicarbonate from the GI tract or kidney.

Causes of metabolic acidosis   Metabolic acidosis can be caused by an increase in systemic acid load or loss of bicarbonate. Disorders resulting from the kidney's failure to excrete hydrogen ion include decreased ammonia production, as seen in hypoaldosteronism or renal failure, or decreased hydrogen ion excretion, as seen in type I (distal) RTA. This type of disorder tends to result in a hyperchloremic metabolic acidosis, as the kidney retains chloride in its attempt to conserve extracellular volume. As a result, no anion gap is detected unless renal function is impaired.

Increased systemic hydrogen ion load can be due to endogenous or exogenous sources, as seen in lactic acidosis, ketoacidosis, or the ingestion of salicylates, methanol, ethylene glycol, paraldehyde and other substances. When the acid load overwhelms the kidney's excretory capability, the accumulation of hydrogen ion leads to a fall in bicarbonate. The acid anion concentration then rises, resulting in an increased anion gap. In response, the kidney attempts to excrete as much acid and anion as possible, which can lead to loss of other electrolytes such as sodium and potassium.

Primary bicarbonate loss is a common cause of metabolic acidosis and can be the result of GI or renal disturbances. Diarrhea frequently leads to GI bicarbonate loss, as the body loses fluid disproportionately high in bicarbonate. However, chloride concentration increases with fluid loss, and these cases often present with a hyperchloremic metabolic acidosis. Renal bicarbonate loss produces a similar picture and can result from type 2 (proximal) RTA or carbonic anhydrase inhibitor administration.

Clinical findings in metabolic acidosis   Symptoms and signs of metabolic acidosis are dependent upon the underlying etiology of the disorder, but prominent findings include hyperventilation (Kussmaul respiration); nausea and vomiting; pulmonary edema secondary to pulmonary and systemic vasoconstriction; and decreased cardiac contractility and cardiac arrhythmias. Neurological manifestations of these disorders include headache and progress to depres-

sion of sensorium, seizures and even coma in some patients, as will be discussed below.

CNS effects of metabolic acidosis   The changes in CNS acid–base status that result from metabolic acidosis appear to be primarily in response to respiratory compensation rather than the underlying acid–base disturbance. In order to compensate for metabolic acidosis the body increases alveolar ventilation, leading to a decrease in pCO2 and increase in arterial pH. Once a new respiratory steady state has been achieved, the pH of the CSF and brain cells remains remarkably constant in the face of these changes. This stability is primarily the result of the brain's ability to generate bicarbonate to offset bicarbonate losses to plasma and, to a lesser extent, the blood–brain barrier's relative impermeability to bicarbonate. An increase in cerebral blood flow secondary to vasodilatation in response to local acidosis contributes by increasing CO_2 transport out of brain cells and decreasing lactic acid production, both of which counteract the effects of systemic acidosis. However, before a new respiratory steady state is reached the CSF does exhibit alterations in acid–base status which may affect the initial ventilatory response to acute metabolic acidosis.

Acute metabolic acidosis   The CNS exhibits only transient alterations in CSF pH in response to metabolic acidosis. Studies of intracellular pH in experimental animals during acute metabolic acidosis have shown little or no response. In one experiment in rats, the intracellular pH and bicarbonate concentration remained constant after six hours of NH4Cl injection, despite an arterial pH of 7.31 and plasma bicarbonate concentration decrease of 8 mEq/L.[14]

The CSF does show a response to metabolic acidosis but this is transient and paradoxical, resulting in a period of CSF alkalosis. It is thought that this shift may account for the delay that has been observed in the respiratory response to metabolic acidosis.

Many experiments inducing acute metabolic acidosis in both dogs and humans have demonstrated this initial CSF alkalosis.[15] This shift is the result of an acute decrease in CSF pCO2, which diffuses freely across the blood–brain barrier leaving elevated bicarbonate levels behind. In some studies the alkalinity of CSF has been shown to persist for up to two to five days and is presumed to be the result of the active nature of bicarbonate transport across the blood–brain barrier and into brain cells.[7,15]

Studies in dogs have shown that it can take up to six to eight hours for a new respiratory steady state, as determined by decreased baseline pCO2, to be achieved in response to acute metabolic acidosis.[16] The effect of the initial CSF alkalosis on central chemoreceptors may help to explain this phenomenon. In acute metabolic acidosis, peripheral chemoreceptors are stimulated by the increase in hydrogen ion concentration to increase alveolar ventilation. However, during this period of CSF alkalosis central chemoreceptors may modulate this response, delaying full respiratory compensation until bicarbonate levels in the CSF have decreased.

Sustained metabolic acidosis   In sustained cases of metabolic acidosis the CSF attains a neutral pH which has been shown to be stable even in patients with a systemic pH as low as 6.8. Once a new respiratory steady state is achieved, the bicarbonate concentration of CSF is maintained by the action of intracellular carbonic anhydrase, which is able to offset continuing losses to the periphery due to diffusion across the blood–brain barrier.[17] In uncomplicated cases of metabolic acidosis the drive to increase alveolar ventilation then derives entirely from peripheral chemoreceptors. The ventilatory response to sustained metabolic acidosis is highly predictable, as was shown by Albert et al.[18] in a landmark series of experiments published in 1967.

To determine the relationship between the degree of metabolic acidosis and respiratory compensation, the investigators analyzed the plasma bicarbonate, blood base excess or blood pH, and plasma $pCO2$ of 60 children who had had untreated metabolic acidosis for at least 24 hours. They found that the relationship between the level of either plasma bicarbonate or blood base excess and the change in $pCO2$ measured in these patients was highly predictable. And as a result, by analyzing deviations from projected values they could determine whether a second process was affecting respiration. When the $pCO2$ level was higher than predicted, they projected that a second process preventing adequate respiratory compensation was present. Likewise, if the $pCO2$ was below predicted values they concluded that the patient probably had a stimulus to ventilation in addition to the metabolic acidosis, as seen in salicylate intoxication.[16]

The formula derived from these experiments is commonly used to predict the adequacy of respiratory compensation to metabolic acidosis, and is as follows:

$$pCO2 = 1.54 \times HCO3- + 8.36 \pm 2^{18}$$

Recovery from metabolic acidosis   In addition to affecting the time course of respiratory compensation to acute metabolic acidosis, it has been suggested that the CSF pH may account for the 'respiratory overshoot' observed during the correction of metabolic acidosis. It has been shown that patients whose blood pH has returned to normal may continue to hyperventilate. This continued ventilatory drive may be the result of a transiently acidotic CSF stimulating the central chemoreceptors. The sudden increase in $pCO2$ resulting from decreased peripheral stimulation to ventilate creates an acidic environment that perpetuates hyperventilation. In dogs this respiratory overshoot has been shown to last approximately six hours, but the estimate for humans is between 6 and 12 hours.[16] This observation emphasizes one of the hazards of rapid complete correction of metabolic acidosis with

bicarbonate: severe respiratory alkalosis can develop in some patients.

Neurological complications of metabolic acidosis   Neurological manifestations associated with metabolic acidosis can include severe depression of the sensorium and coma. However, although there appears to be a link between depression of the sensorium and metabolic acidosis, this condition does not appear to cause coma. Experiments in both humans and animals have failed to show a causal relationship between acute metabolic acidemia and coma. In addition, coma is not a feature of many diseases leading to metabolic acidosis, such as uremia or cholera. And despite early studies that indicated to the contrary, CSF acidosis has not been shown to be correlated with depression of the sensorium.[1]

However, neurological outcomes are often dependent upon coexisting morbidities, as well as the underlying cause of metabolic acidosis. Patients with hyperglycemia, hypoglycemia and cerebral ischemia have been shown to have an increase in neuronal damage and adverse outcomes with superimposed metabolic acidosis. Cerebral acidosis will be discussed below.

Treatment of metabolic acidosis   If possible, the treatment of metabolic acidosis should focus on correcting the underlying etiology and permitting the body's homeostatic mechanisms to correct the acid–base disturbance. Studies have shown that the body is capable of restoring acid–base balance without intervention even after the arterial pH has reached 6.9–7.0.

It is generally recommended to treat patients whose pH decline below 7.1 with alkali infusion. Sodium bicarbonate is most frequently used, but other possibilities include Ringer's lactate solution or sodium citrate. However, as discussed above, rapid correction of arterial pH can lead to complications, including a paradoxical CSF acidosis and continued hyperventilation, hypokalemia and hypocalcemia. Formulas have been developed that allow the physician to estimate roughly the base deficit:

$$\text{Amount of } HCO_3 = (25 - [HCO_3]) \times wt\,(kg)/2$$

and to replace the bicarbonate lost. Specific recommendations for various types of metabolic acidosis are listed below.

Specific cases of metabolic acidosis

The causes and neurological manifestations of several specific metabolic acidoses are discussed below.

Diabetic ketoacidosis   Diabetic ketoacidosis (DKA) is defined as hyperglycemia with metabolic acidosis resulting from generation of the ketones β-hydroxybutyrate and acetoacetate in response to insulin deficiency and elevated counter-regulatory hormones such as glucagon. It is most commonly seen in patients with type I diabetes mellitus. Symptoms include nausea and vomiting, anorexia, polydipsia and polyuria, and occasionally abdominal pain. Patients often present with Kussmaul respiration and volume depletion. Neurological symptoms include fatigue and lethargy, with depression of the sensorium progressing to coma in approximately 10% of patients. Seizures are rare in these patients.

The etiology of the neurological changes in DKA remains unclear and is discussed extensively elsewhere. Studies have examined hyperosmolality, cerebral hypoxia, ketonemia and metabolic acidosis, among other features of DKA, as potential contributing factors to the depression of sensorium seen.[5] As in other cases of metabolic acidosis, in DKA the acid–base disturbance per se does not appear to have a significant effect on the acid–base status of the CNS. In human studies of patients with DKA the CSF pH remains unchanged, and experiments using animal models have shown normal intracellular pH and lactate levels in brain cells. However, it is postulated that patients with arterial pH of less than 7.0 may develop intracellular acidosis, which could result in depression of the sensorium by inhibiting the Krebs' cycle.[20]

However, treatment of DKA may precipitate acid–base disturbances in the CNS, with potentially devastating results. The administration of bicarbonate to these patients occasionally results in cerebral edema significant enough to lead to loss of consciousness and even death. Some degree of elevated CSF pressure is believed to be present in most patients during this process, but rarely becomes clinically evident. It is postulated that transient intracellular acidosis may cause some patients to progress to clinically evident edema.[20]

This intracellular acidosis may be related to decreased oxygen delivery to brain tissue resulting from the withdrawal of the compensatory effect of acidemia on hemoglobin's affinity for oxygen. Hemoglobin's affinity for oxygen is generally in the normal range in metabolic acidosis, despite systemic phosphate depletion and the resultant decrease in 2,3-DPG activity, as acidemia counteracts this effect. With the removal of acidemia, oxygen delivery to tissues decreases.

The CSF also exhibits a change in acid–base status with treatment of DKA. Even without bicarbonate administration, the CSF pH falls as a result of the ventilatory response to correction of acidosis and the sudden rise in pCO2. However, as discussed above, no correlation of decreased CSF pH and depression of sensorium has been established in DKA or any other condition.

Treatment of DKA consists of volume repletion, insulin administration with dextrose if necessary to avoid hypoglycemia, and potassium replacement. Bicarbonate administration should be considered only if DKA is accompanied by shock or coma, or if the arterial pH is less than 7.1, and bolus infusion should be avoided.

Lactic acidosis Lactic acidosis results from increased production of lactic acid, the final product in the anaerobic pathway of glucose metabolism. It is most frequently caused by conditions that increase the NADH : NAD ratio and is usually the result of tissue hypoxia, though it can be seen in cases of drug and toxin ingestion, such as phenformin or metformin use and ethanol intoxication, and in predisposing illnesses such as diabetes mellitus and liver failure. Symptoms are those of metabolic acidosis in addition to those of the underlying etiology.

Lactic acidosis can result from seizure activity, when lactate is released from muscle cells that have undergone a period of anaerobic metabolism. The lactate is quickly metabolized to bicarbonate by the liver, kidneys and other as yet unidentified sites, and the acidosis often resolves within 60 minutes. Therefore, administration of bicarbonate is unnecessary and may in fact precipitate metabolic alkalosis, a development of particular concern in a patient with seizures as it lowers the seizure threshold. Seizures have also been associated with cerebral lactic acidosis, discussed below.

Treatment of lactic acidosis is aimed at correcting the underlying cause. Tissue perfusion should be restored if possible. Bicarbonate therapy should be considered only when arterial pH is below 7.1 and should be directed to achieve a pH of 7.2 over 30–40 minutes.

D-Lactic acidosis is a rare cause of anion-gap metabolic acidosis associated with significant neurological symptoms. It is seen in patients with blind loop syndrome, most frequently after jejunoileal bypass, or with other causes of bacterial overgrowth. D-Lactate is produced by anaerobic instestinal flora and under normal conditions is not absorbed. However, in cases of decreased intestinal motility it can achieve high levels in the blood.

D-Lactic acidosis has been associated with an increased anion-gap acidosis and hyperchloremia. Neurological manifestations include ataxia, weakness, lethargy, dysarthria, and mental status changes. The cause of these neurological changes is not known. Treatment consists of oral vancomycin or neomycin, and leads rapidly to resolution of symptoms.[21]

Metabolic acidosis associated with ethanol ingestion Ethanol ingestion has been associated with both ketoacidosis and lactic acidosis. Patients who chronically abuse alcohol can develop moderate to severe ketoacidosis, typically presenting after an episode of binge drinking, starvation or recurrent vomiting. Some studies have suggested that this phenomenon occurs more frequently in women, although this assertion has not been confirmed. Alcoholic ketoacidosis is associated with abdominal pain, vomiting, starvation and volume depletion. In contrast to diabetic ketoacidosis, coma is rare in these patients. Blood glucose levels are generally low or normal, and insulin is frequently low, with elevated glucagon and cortisol levels. Blood alcohol levels may be absent or elevated on presentation.

The pathophysiology of this disorder is thought to be overproduction of β-hydroxybutyrate and, to a lesser extent, acetoacetate secondary to increased free fatty acid circulation in the altered hormonal milieu. This increase in the ratio of β-hydroxybutyrate to aceto-acetate is believed to result from the oxidation of ethanol, which increases the ratio of NAD+ to NADH and favors β-hydroxybutyrate production. Damage to mitochondria by alcohol could further elevate this ratio by preventing reoxidation of NADH.

Chronic alcoholics can also present with lactic acidosis, most frequently seen clinically in association with alcoholic ketoacidosis. Alcohol inhibits the conversion of lactate to glucose in the liver, and plasma lactate levels are elevated in normal individuals after ethanol ingestion. Alcohol-induced lactic acidosis is generally mild unless accompanied by another predisposing condition.

These patients will typically present with a high plasma osmolar gap (defined as the difference between measured and calculated osmolality).

Calculated osmolality = 2(Na) + glucose, mg/dl/18 + BUN, mg/dl/2.8.

This gap should be equal to the ethanol concentration (mg/dL)/4.6; if it is not, ingestion of another alcohol, such as methanol, isopropanol or ethylene glycol, should be suspected. This population is at increased risk for ingestion of these alcohol substitutes.

Treatment of alcoholic metabolic acidosis consists of volume repletion and thiamine and glucose administration, with correction of hypophosphatemia, hypokalemia and hypomagnesemia if present. The acid–base disturbance usually resolves after several hours. Hypophosphatemia generally presents 12–24 hours after the initiation of treatment and is exacerbated by glucose administration.

Occasionally patients in the intensive care unit setting are given high doses of intravenous benzodiazapines, such as lorazepam. They may develop a high osmolar gap owing to the diluent propylene glycol and develop a clinical picture of sedation, failure to wean from the respirator and increased lactate, a metabolite of propylene glycol.

Ethylene glycol intoxication Ethylene glycol is commonly found in antifreeze and used as an industrial solvent. It has a sweet taste and is occasionally seen clinically after ingestion as a substitute for alcohol. Intoxication is characterized by profound CNS toxicity, including seizures and coma, severe metabolic acidosis, and cardiac, pulmonary and renal failure.

Although ethylene glycol itself does not appear to be particularly damaging, its metabolites are highly toxic and include glycolic acid, ketoaldehydes and oxalic acid. Glycolic acid appears to be primarily responsible for the metabolic acidosis observed in this condition. For unclear reasons, metabolic acidosis appears to increase the severity of ethylene glycol's effects: experimental animals whose arterial pH is maintained in the normal range exhibit symptoms at much higher doses. The ketoaldehyde metabolites appear to be responsible for the CNS dysfunction by inhibiting oxidative phosphorylation. Lactic acid pro-

duction is also increased with the inhibition of the Krebs' cycle. Oxalate crystals as well as other metabolites are believed to be responsible for the renal failure.[22]

The increased anion gap seen in ethylene glycol intoxication is attributable to ethylene glycol and its metabolites. As discussed earlier, a high osmolar gap will also be present. Treatment includes immediate institution of a saline or osmotic diuresis, i.v. ethanol or fomepizole, and dialysis. Ethanol competes with ethylene glycol for metabolism by alcohol dehydrogenase and decreases the production of toxic metabolites. It has traditionally been a mainstay of treatment, but its use was characterized by difficulty in controlling plasma levels and monitoring mental status. Fomepizole is an inhibitor of alcohol dehydrogenase and has recently been shown to be a safe and effective antidote to ethylene glycol intoxication.[23]

Renal failure and uremia Renal failure is a major cause of metabolic encephalopathy, and many of the signs and symptoms attributable to uremia are related to CNS dysfunction. Neurological findings in acute renal failure are evident early in the course of the disorder and include fatigue, mental status changes such as disorientation and psychosis, and dysarthria, progressing to depression of sensorium and even coma if untreated. Motor symptoms are also prominent and include myoclonus, restless legs syndrome and asterixis. Abnormalities in deep tendon reflexes are common. Seizures are now infrequently seen as sequelae of ARF as a result of dialysis treatment. Patients with chronic renal failure can exhibit transient hemiplegias and hearing deficits in addition to the above manifestations. In both acute and chronic renal failure the symptoms of uremia tend to wax and wane, even from day to day.

Despite the profound neurological effect of uremia on the CNS, the precise pathogenesis of uremic encephalopathy has not been established. The degree of encephalopathy correlates with BUN levels only at very high concentrations, and no other indicators of renal failure have proved predictive of clinical findings. Currently, the role of parathyroid hormone is being studied.[24]

The systemic acid–base disturbance in renal failure is attributable to the kidney's inability to excrete hydrogen and generate and reabsorb bicarbonate. It is particularly pronounced in oliguric renal failure and is exacerbated by catabolic states such as infection. However, as in other cases of metabolic acidosis, the CNS acid–base status remains relatively unaffected by the decrease in systemic pH.

In both animal and human experiments, uremia with concomitant metabolic acidosis has no effect on the pH of brain cells or the CSF. In models of both acute and chronic renal failure, animals with metabolic acidosis showed no change in intracellular pH in the brain. Both humans and animals maintain normal CSF pH under these conditions as well.[24]

Treatment of metabolic acidosis of renal failure is directed at maintaining plasma bicarbonate concentration and potassium balance. It includes oral bicarbonate administration and furosemide if hyperkalemia is present.

Salicylate intoxication Salicylate intoxication produces a complex acid–base picture. The most common manifestation is a combined metabolic acidosis and respiratory alkalosis (50%), though it can present as either one or the other, or as a combined respiratory and metabolic acidosis. It is most often seen as a result of accidental overdose, therapeutic overdose or suicide attempt. Manifestations of intoxication include nausea and vomiting, hyperventilation, diaphoresis, tinnitus, and occasionally polyuria followed by oliguria. Non-cardiogenic pulmonary edema is seen in up to 30% of adults. An anion-gap metabolic acidosis may develop and in severe cases can lead to seizures, respiratory depression and coma.

The effects of salicylate are age dependent. However, certain characteristics of salicylate intoxication are seen in all age groups. The first of these results is a respiratory alkalosis and is the result of a direct stimulatory effect of salicylate on the medullary respiratory control center. Experiments in which salicylate was injected directly into the cisterna magna of dogs produced almost immediate marked hyperventilation. The respiratory alkalosis is classically described as presenting before other acid–base disturbances, with hyperventilation a common presenting symptom.

The second characteristic of salicylate intoxication affecting patients of all ages is an increase in metabolic rate. Salicylate functions as an uncoupler of oxidative phosphorylation, resulting in increased oxygen consumption and CO_2 production. However, the increase in alveolar ventilation resulting from stimulation of central chemoreceptors overcomes this increase in pCO2.

In children younger than one year an increase in organic acid production, in particular ketones, is frequently seen as well.[16] As a result these children often present with metabolic acidosis, whereas adults often present with respiratory alkalosis. Fever is also seen in young children presenting with salicylate intoxication.

Treatment of salicylate intoxication is aimed at correcting the metabolic acidosis and removing salicylate. Bicarbonate should be administered if metabolic acidosis predominates, and titrated carefully to the patient's response to avoid hypocapnia, which may be exacerbated by respiratory alkalosis in these patients. Salicylates will be removed by this alkaline diuresis. In cases of severe intoxication, other methods include gastric lavage, osmotic diuresis and dialysis. Urinary alkalinization with acetazolamide is controversial because it may impair tissue to blood CO_2 transport and in theory worsen acidosis in the respiratory center.

Metabolic alkalosis

Metabolic alkalosis is characterized by an elevated arterial pH associated with an increased plasma bicarbonate concentration and a compensatory increase in pCO2. This condition can result either from hydrogen ion loss of an increase in bicarbonate.

Causes of metabolic alkalosis Hydrogen ion losses resulting in metabolic alkalosis can be the result of GI, renal or systemic conditions. Causes of hydrogen ion loss from the GI tract include nasogastric suction of gastric secretions, vomiting, or congenital chloridorrhea. Renal losses can result from mineralocorticoid excess, diuretic use, hypoparathyroidism and hypercalcemia, and postchronic hypercapnia. Entry of hydrogen ions into cells can also lead to metabolic alkalosis, as seen in hypokalemia.

An absolute elevation in total body bicarbonate can be the result of exogenous administration or milk-alkali syndrome. Increased bicarbonate concentration is commonly seen in contraction alkalosis secondary to diuretic use, and occurs when NaCl and water are lost but bicarbonate is retained.

Metabolic alkalosis is generally divided into two categories based on its responsiveness to chloride. Chloride-responsive metabolic alkalosis is associated with extracellular fluid and chloride depletion and is seen in gastric fluid loss and diuretic use. Chloride-unresponsive metabolic alkalosis is seen in patients with extracellular fluid expansion in cases such as primary aldosteronism and hypokalemia.

Under normal conditions the kidney is capable of responding promptly to an increased bicarbonate load by retaining acid and increasing bicarbonate excretion. Metabolic alkalosis only persists when some factor prevents this adaptation. Therefore, metabolic alkalosis is described as having a generative stage, in which bicarbonate concentration increases, and a maintenance stage, in which the alkalosis is perpetuated as a result of the kidney's failure to excrete bicarbonate. This failure is usually because of volume depletion, a reduced GFR, hypokalemia, or low chloride levels.

Clinical findings in metabolic alkalosis Metabolic alkalosis has a profound effect on the CNS and is frequently associated with metabolic encephalopathy. Alkalosis leads to significant cerebral tissue hypoxia as a result of cerebral vasoconstriction and increased hemoglobin affinity for oxygen. Symptoms include confusion, obtundation, delirium and coma. The seizure threshold is lowered, and tetany, paresthesias, muscular cramping and other symptoms reflecting low free calcium levels are observed. Neurological manifestations are generally seen when the pH exceeds 7.55, although patients with hypocalcemia may exhibit signs at lower pH values. Other findings include cardiac arrhythmias and hypotension.

Respiratory compensation for metabolic alkalosis The compensatory response to metabolic alkalosis is respiratory. In response to increased systemic pH, alveolar ventilation is decreased in order to increase pCO2 and thereby decrease pH. However, compensation is generally believed to be less effective in metabolic alkalosis than in metabolic acidosis for reasons that have yet to be definitively established, although some studies have shown a linear relationship between increasing pCO_2 and increasing bicarbonate between 25 and 50 mEq/L in humans. Contributing factors may include the fact that hypoventilation also decreases pO_2, a potent stimulus for the peripheral chemoreceptors to increase alveolar ventilation, as discussed above. A second mechanism that may blunt respiratory compensation is intracellular acidosis in the brain in the setting of hypokalemia. Whatever the causes, the result is that the ventilatory response to metabolic alkalosis is highly varied and unpredictable. Many patients with metabolic alkalosis maintain normal pCO_2 levels, and the level rarely rises above 60 mmHg.

CNS effects of metabolic alkalosis   The effects of metabolic alkalosis on the CNS are the result both of the alkalosis itself and of compensatory hypoventilation, and are largely due to changes in blood flow and oxygenation. In addition to producing systemic hypoxia from hypoventilation, metabolic alkalosis itself is a potent cerebral vasoconstrictor which can lead to tissue hypoxia in the brain. This response is amplified by the increased affinity of hemoglobin for oxygen in alkalemia, resulting in less effective delivery of oxygen to tissues than the arterial pO_2 may suggest. However, despite these findings, the CSF and intracellular pH of brain cells remain relatively constant in metabolic alkalosis.

Acute metabolic alkalosis   Although there are fewer data on the effects of metabolic alkalosis on CNS pH than there are for metabolic acidosis, experiments in humans and animals have shown that in acute metabolic alkalosis there is an initial paradoxical acidotic shift in CSF pH secondary to a sudden increase in pCO_2.[15] This phenomenon is similar to the alkaline shift in CSF pH seen in acute metabolic acidosis. It may contribute to the irregular and unpredictable respiratory response to metabolic alkalosis by activating central chemoreceptors and increasing ventilatory drive in the face of peripheral stimulation to decrease alveolar ventilation.

The intracellular pH in brain cells also shows no significant change in acute metabolic alkalosis in experiments conducted on animals. Normocapnic rats given $NaHCO_3$ injections to achieve an arterial pH of 7.52 showed no change in intracellular pH compared to normal values.[14] Some experiments have demonstrated an increase in intracellular lactate concentration under similar conditions. Lactate production in the brain has been shown to increase at pH values above 7.5, and the increase seen in these experiments may reflect increased anaerobic glycolysis secondary to an increased affinity of hemoglobin for oxygen.[4]

Chronic metabolic alkalosis   Although fewer experiments have evaluated the CNS response to chronic metabolic alkalosis, the CSF has been shown to return to normal values and to remain so up to a systemic

pH of 7.6. In one experiment in humans, five patients who had been kept alkalotic for two days by ingesting $NaHCO_3$ (base excess of 9) showed no change in CSF pH from normal values.[15] This neutral pH would result in respiratory drive deriving entirely from the peripheral chemoreceptors. The mechanisms for CNS adaptation to chronic metabolic alkalosis have been less well studied.

Treatment of metabolic alkalosis   In treating metabolic alkalosis it is important to distinguish whether the condition is chloride responsive (urinary Cl less than 10–20) or unresponsive (urinary Cl > 10–20), as discussed above.

In chloride-responsive patients treatment is directed at increasing urinary excretion of bicarbonate. In patients with mild to moderate alkalosis , the administration of NaCl and KCl is effective in suppressing renal acid excretion and increasing renal HCO_3 excretion. In patients with more severe alkalemia with volume expansion, mineral acids (e.g. HCl or arginine monohydrochloride) may also be necessary. In the absence of renal failure acetazolamide may be effective.

Chloride-unresponsive patients include those with mineralocorticoid excess. The hypokalemia and hyperaldosteronism seen lead to increased hydrogen secretion and bicarbonate reabsorption in the kidney. These patients respond to potassium replacement, which reverses the intracellular shift of hydrogen ions and increases bicarbonate excretion, and to agents that reduce aldosterone activity (spironolactone).

In patients presenting with metabolic alkalosis and volume depletion, potassium levels must be returned to normal values in order to restore chloride responsiveness.

If patients cannot tolerate fluid therapy, for example because of significant edema, acetazolamide with KCl replacement will increase bicarbonate excretion as well as help to diurese the patient.

Posthypercapnic metabolic alkalosis

Posthypercapnic alkalosis is a condition in which patients who are chronically hypercapnic experience a sudden decrease in pCO_2, leading to metabolic alkalosis. This is commonly seen in patients with chronic pulmonary disease who acutely require mechanical ventilation because of respiratory failure. The renal adaptation to chronic respiratory acidosis results in high systemic bicarbonate levels, and when pCO_2 is quickly lowered patients can become acutely and severely alkalemic. These patients are also commonly on low-chloride diets or diuretics, and this condition may persist as the kidney continues to reabsorb bicarbonate as a result of low chloride levels. This development can have severe consequences, resulting in arrhythmias, seizures, coma, and even death in some cases. To avoid this condition, pCO_2 should be allowed to rise as slowly as is possible to avoid hypoxemia, and chloride stores should be repleted if necessary.

The effect of primary CNS lesions on systemic acid–base status

Cerebral acidosis

Causes of cerebral acidosis   Cerebral acidosis is seen in many primary CNS lesions. It is most commonly the result of cerebral hypoxia and can be secondary to generalized or focal cerebral ischemia, tumor or head injury. *Grand mal* seizures have been associated with cerebral as well as systemic metabolic acidosis, though the mechanism appears to be secondary to increased cerebral metabolic activity rather than hypoxia.

The acidosis seen in these conditions is primarily the result of increased tissue lactate production and cell catabolism. As discussed earlier, hypoxic conditions favor the conversion of pyruvate to lactate, instead of to acetyl CoA, via anaerobic glycolysis as a result of an increased NADH : NAD ratio. A second mechanism, perhaps responsible for increased lactate production in seizures, is the development of a hypermetabolic state in which all available pathways for the generation of ATP are recruited at once. In addition, increased levels of free fatty acids leading to increased arachidonic acid accumulation has been implicated in cerebral acidosis.

Effects of cerebral acidosis   The effects of increased lactate on brain cells and the extracellular environment is profound. In cerebral ischemia lactate has been shown to rise after only 15 minutes and can reach levels of 20–30 mmol/kg, with a resulting extracellular pH of 6.0. In in vitro experiments with glial cells even modest levels of lactate resulting in an extracellular pH of 6.8 have been shown to be associated with significant cell swelling. It is postulated that the mechanisms underlying this swelling involve the activation of membrane transporters in an attempt to correct the intracellular acidosis, such as the Na/H-antiporter, the Na/HCO3-cotransporter, and the Cl/HCO3 exchanger. Subsequent intracellular accumulation of Na and Cl results in osmotic entry of water into the cells. In addition to these effects secondary to intracellular acidosis, lactate itself has been implicated in abnormalities of neurotransmitter release and calcium homeostasis in brain cells.[25]

Arachidonic acid has also been shown in vitro to result in significant cell edema at levels comparable to those found in pathological states, although the mechanism is believed to be secondary to free radical and lipid peroxidase disruption of the cell membrane and sodium, followed by water entry into cells.[25]

Effects of cerebral acidosis on respiratory drive   The intra- and extracellular acidity resulting from these conditions might be expected to increase ventilatory drive via its effects on the medullary respiratory center. However, many investigators have shown that cerebral hypoxia in fact produces respiratory depression. In a series of experiments on peripherally chemodenervated cats, Neubauer et al.[26] examined the effects of cerebral lactic acidosis on the ventral medullary respiratory center's medulation of ventilatory drive. By inhibiting the formation of lactic acid using sodium dichloroacetate, both topically at the ventral medullary surface and systemically, and by measuring phrenic nerve stimulation, they were able to show that the respiratory depression seen in cerebral hypoxia is in fact slightly ameliorated by the chemosensitive neurons at this location. They postulated that the overall respiratory depression seen in cerebral hypoxia is secondary to other processes, including the fact that acidosis has been shown to have a depressive effect on all neurons, including respiratory neurons. The finding that there is only a slight increase in ventilatory drive with central stimulation by lactic acid may be due to the fact that metabolic acidosis is a less potent stimulator of central chemoreceptors than CO_2. The mechanism of acid's activation of these neurons is unknown, and the primarily intracellular acidosis of hypoxia may not stimulate them significantly. They conclude that despite a demonstrable but slight response of ventral medullary chemoreceptors to local lactic acidosis, the overriding response to cerebral hypoxia is respiratory depression.

Cerebral acidosis and seizures   Cerebral lactic acidosis has also been found in patients presenting with seizures. In contrast to the systemic lactic acidosis seen in seizure patients, the elevated lactate levels in the CNS do not reflect systemic or cerebral hypoxia. The levels of lactate in CSF and brain tissue have been studied in patients with status epilepticus and found to be elevated to levels which appear to be independent of systemic lactate levels, reflecting the inability of lactate to cross the blood–brain barrier readily. It is thought that the production of lactate is secondary to increased metabolic activity, which results in the recruitment and utilization of all available pathways to generate ATP. One study has linked high levels of CSF lactate to a poor prognosis in status epilepticus,[27] possibly resulting from the mechanisms of cellular damage outlined above.

References

1. Adapted from Adams RD, Victor M, Ropper A. Principles of Neurology. 6th edition. New York: McGraw-Hill Information Services Company, Health Professions Division, 1997:16.
2. Arieff A. Acid–base balance in specialized tissues: central nervous system. *In:* Seldin DW, Giebisch G, eds. The Regulation of Acid–Base Balance. New York: Raven Press, 1989:107–121
3. Madias NE, Cohen JJ. Respiratory acidosis. *In:* Cohen JJ, Kassirer JP, eds. Acid–Base. Boston: Little, Brown & Co, 1982:307–348
4. Kazemi H, Shannon DC, Carvallo-Gil E. Brain CO_2 buffering capacity in respiratory acidosis and alkalosis. J Appl Physiol 22: 1967;241
5. Arieff A, Schmidt RW. Fluid and electrolyte disorders and the central nervous system. *In:* Maxwell MH, Kleeman CR, eds. Clinical Disorders of Fluid and Electrolyte Metabolism. New York: McGraw-Hill, 1980: 1409–1480

6. Arieff AI et al. Intracellular pH of brain: alterations in acute respiratory acidosis and alkalosis. Am J Physiol 1976;230:804–812

7. Molony DA, Schiess MC, Dosekun AK. Respiratory acid-base disturbances. In: Kokko JP, Tannen RL, eds. Fluids and Electrolytes. 3rd edition. Philadelphia: WB Saunders, 1996:267–342 (p 284)

8. Arieff A, Schmidt RW. Fluid and electrolyte disorders and the central nervous system. In: Maxwell MH, Kleeman CR, eds. Clinical Disorders of Fluid and Electrolyte Metabolism. New York: McGraw-Hill, 1980: 1409–1480 (p. 1417)

9. Cardenas VJ et al. Correction of blood pH attenuates change in hemodynamics and organ blood flow during permissive hypercapnia. Crit Care Med 1996;24: 827–834

10. Gennari FJ, Kassirer JP. Respiratory alkalosis. In: Cohen JJ, Kassirer JP, eds. Acid–Base. Boston: Little, Brown & Co, 1982:349–376

11. Heffner JE, Sahn SA. Controlled hyperventilation in patients with intracranial hypertension. Arch Intern Med 1983;143:765–769

12. Van Vaerenbergh PJJ, Demeester G, Leusen I. Lactate in cerebrospinal fluid during hyperventilation. Arch Int Physiol Bio 1965;73:738–747

13. Lenfant C, Sullivan K. Adaptation to High Altitude. N Engl J Med 284: 1298, 1971

14. Siesjo BK, Ponten U. Acid–base changes in the brain in non-respiratory acidosis and alkalosis. Exp Brain Res 1966;2:176–190

15. Irsigler GB, Stafford MJ, Severinghaus JW. Relationship of CSF pH, O2, and CO2 responses in metabolic acidosis and alkalosis in humans. J Appl Physiol 1980;48:355–361

16. Winters RW. Physiology of acid–base disorders. In: Winters RW, ed. The Body Fluids in Pediatrics. Boston: Little, Brown and Co, 1973:46–77

17. Herrera L, Kazemi H. CSF bicarbonate regulation in metabolic acidosis: role of HCO3− formation in CNS. J Appl Physiol 1980;49:778–783

18. Albert MS, Dell RB, Winters RW. Quantitative displacement of acid–base equilibrium in metabolic acidosis. Ann Intern Med 1967;66:312–322

19. Arieff A. Acid-base balance in specialized tissues: central nervous system. In: Seldin DW, Giebisch G, eds. The Regulation of Acid-Base Balance. New York: Raven Press, 1989: 107–121 (pp. 117–8)

20. Arieff A. Acid-base balance in specialized tissues: central nervous system. In: Seldin DW, Giebisch G, eds. The Regulation of Acid-Base Balance. New York: Raven Press, 1989: 107–121 (p 118)

21. Charney AN, Goldfarb DS, Dagher PC. Metabolic disorders associated with gastrointestinal disease. In: Arieff AI, DeFronzo RA, eds. Fluid, Electrolyte, and Acid–Base Disorders. New York: Churchill Livingstone, 1995:813–837

22. Harrington JT, Cohen JJ. Metabolic acidosis. In: Cohen JJ, Kassirer JP, eds. Acid–Base. Boston: Little, Brown & Co, 1982:121–226

23. Brent J et al. Fomepizole for the treatment of ethylene glycol poisoning. N Engl J Med 1999;340:832–838

24. Fraser CL, Arieff AI. Metabolic encephalopathy. In: Arieff AI, DeFronzo RA, eds. Fluid, Electrolyte, and Acid–Base Disorders. New York: Churchill Livingstone, 1995:813–837

25. Staub F, Winkler A, Haberstok J, Plesnila N, Peters J, Chang RCC, Kempski O, Baethmann A. Swelling, intracellular acidosis, and damage of glial cells. Acta Neurochir 1996;66Suppl: 56–62

26. Neubauer JA, Simone A, Edelman NH. Role of brain lactic acidosis in hypoxic depression of ventilation. J Appl Physiol 1988; 65:1324–1331

27. Calabrese VP et al. Cerebrospinal fluid lactate levels and prognosis in status epilepticus. Epilepsia 32: 816–821

123 Use of Therapeutic Plasma Exchange and Intravenous Immunoglobulin for the Treatment of Neurological Disease

Bradley E Bernstein and Winthrop H Churchill

Introduction

Evidence supporting the use of plasma exchange and intravenous immunoglobulin for the treatment of neurological disease is rapidly evolving. A decade ago, decisions were based largely on observations, case reports, or a lack of alternative therapy, but now controlled studies have been performed that have shown efficacy for both modalities in various conditions. This chapter summarizes these studies and outlines how plasma exchange and intravenous immunoglobulin therapy are accomplished. Because both therapies occasionally are used for conditions for which their efficacy is uncertain, it is important to consider untoward consequences of the treatments. These are also reviewed and compared in this chapter.

Myasthenia gravis

In myasthenia gravis (MG), IgG antibodies with affinity for the acetylcholine receptor are associated with defective neuromuscular transmission. The titer of these pathological antibodies correlates with disease severity. By the early 1980s, plasma exchange became an accepted treatment on the basis of empirical observations. Despite the lack of well-controlled studies, one volume exchanges on a daily or every-other-day basis for 1 to 2 weeks remain standard therapy for an acute crisis. Occasionally, patients require long-term maintenance, with exchanges every 2 to 4 weeks, typically in conjunction with immunosuppressive therapy. Response rates extrapolated from published series vary between 60% and 100%.[1] A decrease in acetylcholine antibody titer has been documented and has been associated with clinical improvement in observational studies.[2] On the basis of reports of small series, intravenous immunoglobulin has also been used for MG, with a slightly lower response rate.[1,3] A randomized study that compared plasma exchange and intravenous immunoglobulin for the treatment of MG exacerbations similarly found plasma exchange to be slightly better, although the difference was not statistically significant (Table 123.1).[4] Plasma exchange appears to be more effective for the treatment of acute MG (e.g., in preparation for a surgical procedure). However, the relative merits of the two therapies in chronic maintenance are not well defined.

Guillain–Barré syndrome

Guillain–Barré syndrome (GBS) results from an immune-mediated attack on the myelin of peripheral nerves. It is associated with antecedent infection by a viral or bacterial agent or as a complication of immunization. Because GBS is the most common cause of neuromuscular paralysis in developed countries, it has been the subject of several excellent studies that have assessed and compared plasma exchange and intravenous immunoglobulin treatments (Table 123.1). In two large randomized control trials conducted by the Guillain–Barré Study Group and the French Cooperative Group, plasma exchange was shown to shorten disease duration.[5,6,21] Both studies stressed the importance of early treatment. These early trials relied on 3 to 5 exchanges over 1 to 2 weeks. Recently, results of a trial designed to determine the optimal number of exchanges suggested that mild disease could be treated with two exchanges and more severe disease, with four exchanges.[22] This result is unexpected because five exchanges are required to decrease IgG levels to 10% of the starting levels. If confirmed in subsequent studies, these findings could lead to a substantial reduction in the usual treatment course for GBS. Two other randomized trials have found that intravenous immunoglobulin is as effective as plasma exchange in treating GBS.[7,8] The combination of the two modalities was not found to provide additional benefit.[8]

Chronic inflammatory demyelinating polyneuropathy

Chronic inflammatory demyelinating polyneuropathy (CIDP), another presumed autoimmune disorder, presents with proximal and distal weakness. In contrast to GBS, CIDP has a chronic course that is either progressive or relapsing. Two subtypes, one associated with monoclonal gammopathy of undetermined significance (MGUS) and the other idiopathic, differ subtly in presentation and response to treatment. Randomized, blinded, sham-controlled crossover trials, smaller than the GBS studies, have shown that both subtypes of CIDP respond to plasma exchange (Table 123.1).[9,12,23] Response rates were similar for progressive and relapsing courses. Among patients with MGUS, those with IgG or IgA had a response to treatment, particularly if both proximal and distal weakness was present. Patients with IgM monoclonal

Table 123.1   Selected trials assessing the efficacy of therapeutic plasma exchange and intravenous immunoglobulin in the treatment of neurological disease

Condition	Outcome	Studies* (n)	References
Myasthenia gravis	TPE, 100% response	Series (36)	Mahalati et al., 1999[1]
	IVIg, 56% response	Series (14)	Jongen et al., 1998[3]
	TPE vs. IVIg, NSD (both effective)	Random (18)	Gajdos et al., 1997[4]
GBS	TPE beneficial in early disease course	Random (245)	GBS Study Group, 1985[5]
	TPE beneficial in early disease course	Random (220)	French Cooperative Group, 1987[6]
	IVIg as effective as TPE	Random (147)	Van der Meche and Schmitz, 1992[7]
	TPE vs. IVIg, NSD (both effective)	Random (379)	PE/Sandoglobulin, 1997[8]
CIDP			
Idiopathic	TPE, 80% response	Random (18)	Hahn et al., 1996[9]
	IVIg, 63% response	Random (30)	Hahn et al., 1996[10]
	TPE vs. IVIg, NSD (both effective)	Random (20)	Dyck et al., 1994[11]
	Maintenance therapy required		
With MGUS	TPE, effective; IgG & IgA >IgM	Random (39)	Dyck et al., 1991[12]
	TPE, IVIg, or corticosteroids, 66% response	Series (67)	Gorson et al., 1997[13]
IgM, anti-MAG	TPE with cytoxan, modest response	Series (4)	Blume et al., 1995[14]
	IVIg, no response	Random (10)	Mariette et al., 1997[15]
IgM, anti-GM$_1$ (MMN)	TPE with cytoxan, modest response	Series (4)	Pestronk et al., 1994[16]
	IVIg, 86% response	Series (7)	Van den Berg et al., 1998[17]
	IVIg, 67% response	Series (18)	Azulay et al., 1997[18]
	High-titer IgM predicts response to IVIg, maintenance required		
Multiple sclerosis	TPE, 42% response	Random (22)	Weinshenker et al., 1999[19]
	IVIg, 31% improved (vs. 14% placebo)	Random (150)	Fazekas et al., 1997[20]

CIDP, chronic inflammatory demyelinating polyneuropathy; GBS, Guillain–Barré syndrome; IVIg, intravenous immunoglobulin; MAG, myelin-associated glycoprotein; MGUS, monoclonal gammopathy of undetermined significance; MMN, multifocal motor neuropathy; NSD, no significant difference; TPE, therapeutic plasma exchange.
*Random, randomized trial; series, retrospective analysis or uncontrolled trial.

gammopathy and distal sensory motor findings were unlikely to have a response to plasma exchange or intravenous immunoglobulin.[11,24] On the basis of their experience, Hahn et al.[9] stressed the importance of adjuvant immunosuppressive medication and tapering exchanges to minimize rebound effect.

Efficacy for intravenous immunoglobulin in the treatment of CIDP has also been demonstrated. In a blinded, sham-controlled crossover study performed in parallel with a plasma exchange study, Hahn et al.[10] showed that the intravenous administration of immunoglobulin resulted in substantial neurological improvement. Although the plasma exchange trial yielded greater clinical improvement, the discreet study designs did not allow direct comparison of the two modalities. However, that comparison was made in a randomized trial by Dyck et al.,[11] who found that both modalities resulted in clinical improvement, with no statistically significant differences between them. Both groups had a high rate of relapse, necessitating continued treatment at regular intervals. Dyck et al.[11] concluded that, given comparable efficacy, intravenous immunoglobulin may be preferable because of the ease of infusion. However, the recently described acute renal failure that occurs with the use of intravenous immunoglobulin may require that this conclusion be reconsidered.[25]

From their experience with 67 consecutive patients with or without MGUS, Gorson et al.[13] noted similar response rates with plasma exchange, intravenous immunoglobulin, and corticosteroids, but greater functional improvement occurred with plasma exchange. They concluded that most patients will have a response to one of the three therapies and recommended that alternative modalities be tried if initially there is no response.[13]

IgM-associated neuropathies

IgM autoantibodies directed against GM$_1$ are associated with multifocal motor neuropathy, and those directed against myelin-associated glycoprotein (anti-MAG) are associated with a demyelinating peripheral neuropathy. Evidence of the effectiveness of plasma exchange and intravenous immunoglobulin in multifocal motor neuropathy is derived primarily from case series (Table 123.1). In multifocal motor neuropathy, both modalities provide short-term benefit for some patients.[16–18,26] Responses are correlated with high titers of anti-GM$_1$ IgM antibodies.[16,18] In a recent review, Pestronk[27] recommended intravenous immunoglobulin as an initial therapy and discussed strategies for minimizing its use while preventing relapse. The response of anti-MAG-associated neuropathy to treatment remains a matter of controversy.[14,15,24] Neuropathy associated with anti-MAG antibodies may respond to a combination of plasma exchange and cyclophosphamide (Cytoxan).[14] However, in a randomized trial comparing this treatment with interferon alpha, intravenous immunoglobulin was found to be of no benefit in anti-MAG polyneuropathy.[15]

Multiple sclerosis

Studies that have assessed the effect of plasma exchange in multiple sclerosis are few in number and the results conflicting. Vamvakas et al.[28] analyzed six controlled plasma exchange trials, each consisting of 20 to 112 patients with progressive neurological worsening. Treatment regimens varied from three exchanges per week for 2 weeks to weekly exchanges over several months. Meta-analysis showed that plasma exchange "reduced the proportion of patients who experienced neurologic decline" at 12-month follow-up. The authors concluded that further studies are necessary to confirm the results and to identify subgroups likely to benefit from the treatments. A subsequent trial assessed the ability of plasma exchange in combination with azathioprine to alter disease progression in multiple sclerosis by examining gadolinium-enhancing lesions by magnetic resonance imaging (MRI).[29] The authors found some effect on the lesions but concluded that, with the promise of new immunomodulatory drugs, the effect was not substantial enough to justify plasma exchange.[29] A controlled study at the Mayo Clinic assessed the efficacy of plasma exchange in patients with recent and severe deficits from inflammatory demyelinating disease that did not respond to corticosteroid treatment.[19] Of 34 eligible patients, 22 were enrolled, and 6 of 11 patients in each arm had multiple sclerosis; the others had other inflammatory central nervous system demyelinating disease. The study concluded that some proportion of these patients have a response to plasma exchange and those who have a response have improvement early in treatment, but relapse continues to be a problem. This is a promising result that needs to be confirmed in a larger study.

Similarly, the use of intravenous immunoglobulin for the treatment of multiple sclerosis remains controversial. A large randomized trial completed in 1997 concluded that monthly doses of immunoglobulin were effective in patients with relapsing-remitting disease.[20] The authors suggested that the treatment is a feasible option, at least as effective as interferon beta. In another study that used MRI to assess disease progression, monthly intravenous immunoglobulin was also found effective.[30] A randomized trial by Achiron et al.[31] showed that a regimen of intravenous immunoglobulin for 5 consecutive days, followed by treatments every other month, reduced the number of relapses by 39%. Nonetheless, the modest gains associated with intravenous immunoglobulin in these studies and the lack of direct comparisons with other less expensive therapies do not support a major role for this modality in the treatment of multiple sclerosis.[32,33]

Treatments

Plasma exchange can be performed with various instruments based on a rotating membrane system.[34,35] Two peripheral access catheters or, when necessary, a single double-lumen catheter provides venous access. The peripheral access requires an 18-gauge catheter for return and an 18-gauge apheresis needle on the draw side. Double-lumen catheters can be placed percutaneously in either the subclavian or femoral vein. Femoral vein placement is safer in patients who have concurrent pulmonary disease or thrombocytopenia, but it has several disadvantages. A patient with a femoral catheter is restricted to bed rest, and catheters placed at this site are more likely to become infected. For patients requiring long-term central access, it is essential to use a tunneled pheresis catheter placed in the subclavian or internal jugular vein.

Typically, one volume plasma exchange is carried out, with the replacement fluid usually being 5% albumin supplemented with 500 mL of saline. Depending on the volume requirements of the patient, replacement can be less than, equal to, or more than the amount removed. Generally, the volume of the replacement fluid is from 80% to 120% that of the fluid removed. In adults, citrate is the usual anticoagulant, although it is possible to use heparin and citrate if citrate-induced hypocalcemia is a problem. In most patients, hypocalcemia from citrate can be controlled with oral supplements or intravenous infusions of calcium gluconate (or both) before or during the procedure. Pretreatment with ionized calcium is useful in identifying patients likely to require replacement therapy. Most commonly, treatment is given every other day to permit reequilibration between the intravascular and extravascular spaces and regeneration of coagulation components that are removed during exchange. A daily schedule is acceptable for proteins such as IgM antibodies, which are mainly intravascular, or for patients with antibody-mediated disease in whom more rapid removal may influence the evolution of the disease, for example, GBS of recent onset or myasthenia crisis.

The intravenous administration of immunoglobulin requires only a single peripheral access and has a different spectrum of complications from that of plasma exchange (see below). The standard protocol consists of five consecutive daily infusions (0.4 g/kg daily for a total dose of 2.0 g/kg). The alternate schedule of two consecutive daily infusions of 1 g/kg has been used less frequently in the treatment of neurological diseases and there is less clinical evidence supporting the effectiveness of this schedule. A trial bolus of a 5% solution of immunoglobulin is infused at 0.01 to 0.02 mL/kg per minute for 30 minutes. If no reaction occurs, the rate can be increased in increments of 0.02 mL/kg per minute to a maximum of 0.08 mL/kg per minute. Premedication with antihistamines is desirable because of the increased chance of allergic reactions in patients given immunoglobulin intravenously. If allergic symptoms are controlled by antihistamines, there is no need to discontinue the infusion.

Complications of therapy

The use of plasma exchange is limited by the availability of expertise and equipment and the patient's capacity to tolerate associated fluid shifts. The use of

Table 123.2   Complications of therapeutic plasma exchange and intravenous immunoglobulin

Therapeutic plasma exchange (per treatment)*	Intravenous immunoglobulin (per patient)†
Citrate effects in 1.2% of treatments	Headache (23/88), fever (3/88), rash (5/88)
Vasovagal events in 1%–2% of treatments, but 2.7% of treatments for neurological disease	Vasomotor symptoms in 26/88 (chills, nausea, flushing, chest tightness, wheezing)
Reactions to blood product in 0.4% of treatments not using plasma as replacement	Leukopenia in 4/88
Infections related to central access in 0.12% of treatments	One patient (1/88) had each of following: CHF, DVT, severe hypotension, ARF

ARF, acute renal failure; CHF, congestive heart failure; DVT, deep venous thrombosis.
*Data from McLeod et al., 1999.[36]
†Data from Brannagan et al., 1996.[39]

intravenous immunoglobulin is limited by cost and availability; also, good kidney function is required to handle the associated osmotic loads. Complications of plasma exchange include problems associated with citrate toxicity, replacement fluid, volume shifts, and venous access. Adverse events were compiled recently by McLeod et al.[36] (Table 123.2). Citrate effects, including paresthesias and muscle cramps, were minor and generally preventable with calcium taken orally. The risk of serious reaction to blood product was very rare when 5% albumin was used as replacement in the treatment of neurological disease. However, vasovagal events were more common among patients with neurological disease, occurring in 2.7% of treatments. Side effects such as blood pressure change, chills, wheezing, or flushing sometimes can be controlled by rate reduction. The most severe complications were associated with catheter placement and catheter infection, which the authors found in 0.12% of treatments.[36] It has been suggested that by removing immunoglobulins and complement, plasma exchange predisposes patients to infection, although little evidence supports this.[37] In their review of 381 plasma exchanges, Couriel and Weinstein[38] reported four severe complications: hemopneumothorax, pneumothorax, bacteremia, and hematoma. All these complications were associated with catheter placement.

The use of intravenous immunoglobulin has escalated considerably in recent years because of its safety and efficacy in various conditions. Often, it is used to treat conditions for which no data are available from controlled trials. This approach has been criticized because of the shortage of the product and its increasing cost. Also, intravenous administration of immunoglobulin is not without risk. Brannagan et al.[39] reviewed adverse events among 88 patients who received intravenous immunoglobulin for various neurological disorders (Table 123.2) and found that 59% of patients had some complication from treatment, but they usually were minor events, such as vasomotor symptoms, headache, fever, or dyspnea. This series was notable for the absence of aseptic meningitis, a documented side effect of unknown frequency.[40] Four patients in the study of Brannagan et

al.[39] experienced severe complications during the administration of immunoglobulin, including congestive heart failure, hypotensive crisis, deep venous thrombosis, and acute renal failure. These complications occurred in patients with substantial risk factors, for example, congestive heart failure in association with cardiomyopathy and paroxysmal atrial fibrillation or acute renal failure concomitant with diabetic nephropathy. The incidence of acute renal failure following intravenous immunoglobulin is unknown, but increasing recognition of this problem resulted in an advisory being issued by the United States Food and Drug Administration in 1999.[25,41,42] Caution is urged with the use of any immunoglobulin product, particularly in patients with risk factors such as age older than 65 years, diabetes mellitus, or previous renal insufficiency. The mechanism is unclear, but it may be a consequence of stabilizing carbohydrates (usually sucrose) present in the immunoglobulin preparations. Proposals for minimizing risk include decreasing infusion rate, diluting the immunoglobulin preparation, and using caution in the treatment of patients with previous renal dysfunction.[43]

Conclusion

The effects of plasma exchange and intravenous immunoglobulin in managing neurological diseases clearly needs more study. Where comparisons have been made, the responses appeared similar. However, these studies lack the power to distinguish subtle differences. The spectrum of side effects is different for the two treatment modalities, but both treatments have significant consequences. The choice of therapy in a particular instance will depend on the availability of plasma exchange and intravenous immunoglobulin and the clinical circumstances.

References

1. Mahalati K, Dawson RB, Collins JO, Mayer RF. Predictable recovery from myasthenia gravis crisis with plasma exchange: thirty-six cases and review of current management. J Clin Apheresis 1999;14:1–8
2. Tindall RS. Scientific overview of myasthenia gravis and an assessment of the role of plasmapheresis. Prog Clin Biol Res 1982;106:113–142

3. Jongen JL, van Doorn PA, van der Meche FG. High-dose intravenous immunoglobulin therapy for myasthenia gravis. J Neurol 1998;245:26–31

4. Gajdos P, Chevret S, Clair B, et al. Clinical trial of plasma exchange and high-dose intravenous immunoglobulin in myasthenia gravis. Myasthenia Gravis Clinical Study Group. Ann Neurol 1997;41:789–796

5. The Guillain–Barré Syndrome Study Group. Plasmapheresis and acute Guillain–Barré syndrome. Neurology 1985;35:1096–1104

6. French Cooperative Group on Plasma Exchange in Guillain-Barré Syndrome. Efficiency of plasma exchange in Guillain–Barré syndrome: role of replacement fluids. Ann Neurol 1987;22:753–761

7. van der Meche FG, Schmitz PI. A randomized trial comparing intravenous immune globulin and plasma exchange in Guillain–Barré syndrome. Dutch Guillain–Barré Study Group. N Engl J Med 1992;326:1123–1129

8. Plasma Exchange/Sandoglobulin Guillain–Barré Syndrome Trial Group. Randomised trial of plasma exchange, intravenous immunoglobulin, and combined treatments in Guillain–Barré syndrome. Lancet 1997;349:225–230

9. Hahn AF, Bolton CF, Pillay N, et al. Plasma-exchange therapy in chronic inflammatory demyelinating polyneuropathy. A double-blind, sham-controlled, cross-over study. Brain 1996;119:1055–1066

10. Hahn AF, Bolton CF, Zochodne D, Feasby TE. Intravenous immunoglobulin treatment in chronic inflammatory demyelinating polyneuropathy. A double-blind, placebo-controlled, cross-over study. Brain 1996;119:1067–1077

11. Dyck PJ, Litchy WJ, Kratz KM, et al. A plasma exchange versus immune globulin infusion trial in chronic inflammatory demyelinating polyradiculoneuropathy. Ann Neurol 1994;36:838–845

12. Dyck PJ, Low PA, Windebank AJ, et al. Plasma exchange in polyneuropathy associated with monoclonal gammopathy of undetermined significance. N Engl J Med 1991;325:1482–1486

13. Gorson KC, Allam G, Ropper AH. Chronic inflammatory demyelinating polyneuropathy: clinical features and response to treatment in 67 consecutive patients with and without a monoclonal gammopathy. Neurology 1997;48:321–328

14. Blume G, Pestronk A, Goodnough LT. Anti-MAG antibody-associated polyneuropathies: improvement following immunotherapy with monthly plasma exchange and IV cyclophosphamide. Neurology 1995;45:1577–1580

15. Mariette X, Chastang C, Clavelou P, et al. A randomised clinical trial comparing interferon-alpha and intravenous immunoglobulin in polyneuropathy associated with monoclonal IgM. The IgM-associated Polyneuropathy Study Group. N Neurol Neurosurg Psychiatry 1997;63:28–34

16. Pestronk A, Lopate G, Kornberg AJ, et al. Distal lower motor neuron syndrome with high-titer serum IgM anti-GM$_1$ antibodies: improvement following immunotherapy with monthly plasma exchange and intravenous cyclophosphamide. Neurology 1994;44:2027–2031

17. Van den Berg LH, Franssen H, Wokke JH. The long-term effect of intravenous immunoglobulin treatment in multifocal motor neuropathy. Brain 1998;121:421–428

18. Azulay JP, Rihet P, Pouget J, et al. Long term follow up of multifocal motor neuropathy with conduction block under treatment. J Neurol Neurosurg Psychiatry 1997;62:391–394

19. Weinshenker BG, O'Brien PC, Petterson TM, et al. A randomized trial of plasma exchange in acute central nervous system inflammatory demyelinating disease. Ann Neurol 1999;46:878–886

20. Fazekas F, Deisenhammer F, Strasser-Fuchs S, et al. Randomised placebo-controlled trial of monthly intravenous immunoglobulin therapy in relapsing-remitting multiple sclerosis. Austrian Immunoglobulin in Multiple Sclerosis Study Group. Lancet 1997;349:589–593

21. French Cooperative Group on Plasma Exchange in Guillain–Barré syndrome. Plasma exchange in Guillain–Barré syndrome: one-year follow-up. Ann Neurol 1992;32:94–97

22. The French Cooperative Group on Plasma Exchange in Guillain–Barré Syndrome. Appropriate number of plasma exchanges in Guillain–Barré syndrome. Ann Neurol 1997;41:298–306

23. Dyck PJ, Daube J, O'Brien P, et al. Plasma exchange in chronic inflammatory demyelinating polyradiculoneuropathy. N Engl J Med 1986;314:461–465

24. Katz JS, Saperstein DS, Gronseth G, et al. Distal acquired demyelinating symmetric neuropathy. Neurology 2000;54:615–620

25. Anonymous. Renal insufficiency and failure associated with immune globulin intravenous therapy—United States, 1985–1998. MMWR Morb Mortal Wkly Rep 1999;48:518–521

26. Meucci N, Cappellari A, Barbieri S, et al. Long term effect of intravenous immunoglobulins and oral cyclophosphamide in multifocal motor neuropathy. J Neurol Neurosurg Psychiatry 1997;63:765–769

27. Pestronk A. Multifocal motor neuropathy: diagnosis and treatment. Neurology 1998;51 Suppl 5:S22–S24

28. Vamvakas EC, Pineda AA, Weinshenker BG. Meta-analysis of clinical studies of the efficacy of plasma exchange in the treatment of chronic progressive multiple sclerosis. J Clin Apheresis 1995;10:163–170

29. Sorensen PS, Wanscher B, Szpirt W, et al. Plasma exchange combined with azathioprine in multiple sclerosis using serial gadolinium-enhanced MRI to monitor disease activity: a randomized single-masked cross-over pilot study. Neurology 1996;46:1620–1625

30. Sorensen PS, Wanscher B, Jensen CV, et al. Intravenous immunoglobulin G reduces MRI activity in relapsing multiple sclerosis. Neurology 1998;50:1273–1281

31. Achiron A, Gabbay U, Gilad R, et al. Intravenous immunoglobulin treatment in multiple sclerosis. Effect on relapses. Neurology 1998;50:398–402

32. Noseworthy JH, Gold R, Hartung HP. Treatment of multiple sclerosis: recent trials and future perspectives. Curr Opin Neurol 1999;12:279–293

33. Lisak RP. Intravenous immunoglobulins in multiple sclerosis. Neurology 1998;51 Suppl 5:S25–S29

34. Kaplan AA, Halley SE. Evaluation of a rotating filter for use with therapeutic plasma exchange. ASAIO Trans 1988;34:274–276

35. Kaplan AA, Halley SE, Reardon J, Sevigny J. One year's experience using a rotating filter for therapeutic plasma exchange. ASAIO Trans 1989;35:262–264

36. McLeod BC, Sniecinski I, Ciavarella D, et al. Frequency of immediate adverse effects associated with therapeutic apheresis. Transfusion 1999;39:282–288

37. Mokrzycki MH, Kaplan AA. Therapeutic plasma exchange: complications and management. Am J Kidney Dis 1994;23:817–827

38. Couriel D, Weinstein R. Complications of therapeutic

plasma exchange: a recent assessment. J Clin Apheresis 1994;9:1–5

39. Brannagan TH III, Nagle KJ, Lange DJ, Rowland LP. Complications of intravenous immune globulin treatment in neurologic disease. Neurology 1996;47:674–677

40. Mathy I, Gille M, Van Raemdonck F, et al. Neurological complications of intravenous immunoglobulin (IVIg) therapy: an illustrative case of acute encephalopathy following IVIg therapy and a review of the literature. Acta Neurol Belg 1998;98:347–351

41. Pasatiempo AM, Kroser JA, Rudnick M, Hoffman BI. Acute renal failure after intravenous immunoglobulin therapy. J Rheumatol 1994;21:347–349

42. Winward DB, Brophy MT. Acute renal failure after administration of intravenous immunoglobulin: review of the literature and case report. Pharmacotherapy 1995;15:765–772

43. Ahsan N, Wiegand LA, Abendroth CS, Manning EC. Acute renal failure following immunoglobulin therapy. Am J Nephrol 1996;16:532–536

124 Megaloblastic Anemias—Vitamin B$_{12}$, Folate

Laurence J Kinsella

Brief overview

Megaloblastic anemia refers to abnormalities seen on bone marrow examination that reflect disordered DNA synthesis. Macrocytosis—the enlargement of erythrocytes to more than 100 fL on the peripheral smear—may or may not be associated with megaloblastosis. "Oval" macrocytosis and megaloblastosis may be seen in cobalamin (B$_{12}$) deficiency, folate deficiency, cancer chemotherapy and myelodysplastic syndromes.[1] "Round" macrocytosis without megaloblastosis occurs in alcoholism, liver disease and hypothyroidism. Macrocytosis may also be due to abundant reticulocyte formation. Many patients with cobalamin deficiency may have significant neurological symptoms without evidence of either macrocytosis or anemia. Neurological illness is associated with cobalamin and folate deficiency, and therefore this discussion will be limited to cobalamin and folate.

The history of vitamin B$_{12}$ (cobalamin) deficiency begins with JS Combe in 1822 and Thomas Addison in 1855, who published early descriptions of pernicious anemia. Austin Flint, in 1860, speculated that pernicious anemia was due to a defect in gastric juice: this was later confirmed by Fenwick in 1870. The missing substance in the gastric juice of patients with pernicious anemia was identified by William Castle in 1948[2] and named "intrinsic factor." Vitamin B$_{12}$, or "extrinsic factor," was identified later that year. Schilling[3] identified the rate of excretion of radio-labeled cobalamin in the urine of normal and B$_{12}$-deficient patients and developed the test that bears his name in the mid-1950s. Lindenbaum and colleagues[4] recognized that many patients with neurological syndrome of B$_{12}$ deficiency have no hematological abnormalities, and popularized the use of methylmalonic acid and homocysteine assays as more sensitive indicators of biochemical deficiency than the vitamin B$_{12}$ level.

Epidemiology

Vitamin B$_{12}$ deficiency is bimodal.[5] It occurs in young women, usually as a result of autoimmune parietal cell dysfunction, otherwise known as pernicious anemia. It also occurs in elderly men and women, most likely as a result of the high incidence of atrophic gastritis,[6] which leads to food-bound cobalamin malabsorption due to achlorhydria.[7]

In the Framingham Study, 5% of elderly subjects had serum B$_{12}$ levels less than 200 pg/ml (normal for radioassay 200–900 pg/mL), 40.5% had values less than 350 pg/ml (low normal). Fifteen percent had serum methylmalonic acid levels greater than 376 nmol/L. After excluding patients with elevated creatinines, a cause of falsely elevate methylmalonic acid, the prevalence of B12 deficiency was estimated to be greater than 12% in elderly individuals living independently, and 15% had serum methylmalonic acid levels greater than 376 nmol/L.[8] Therefore, 15% of the elderly demonstrate biochemical evidence of B$_{12}$ deficiency. Eighty-seven percent of folate deficiency occurs in alcoholics, whereas only 11% to 13% of B$_{12}$-deficient patients are alcoholics.[9,10] B$_{12}$ deficiency is uncommon in this population for unclear reasons. Anemia and macrocytosis (MCV > 100 fL) occur in respectively 72% and 83% of B$_{12}$-deficient patients, and 100% and 75% respectively of those with folate deficiency.[9]

Etiology

The majority of patients—roughly 50% to 78%—have autoimmune parietal cell dysfunction (pernicious anemia).[4] Another 10% to 40% have food-bound cobalamin malabsorption due to achlorhydria.[11] The rest have a variety of etiologies, mainly due to malabsorption from medical, surgical or pharmacological interruptions of gastric acid secretion or intrinsic factor secretion. These include patients following gastric surgery[12] or bypass procedures for weight reduction,[13] as well as those on long-term H$_2$ blocker therapy, owing to inhibition of acid secretion.[14] Nitrous oxide administration may precipitate acute B$_{12}$ deficiency in patients with asymptomatic low cobalamin levels.[15]

Pathophysiology and pathogenesis

Vitamin B$_{12}$ deficiency probably exerts its effect on the nervous system by the impairment of the two mammalian enzymes systems that require it.[16] The first is the conversion of homocysteine to methionine. In the absence of vitamin B$_{12}$, homocysteine accumulates and prevents the methylation of myelin basic proteins necessary for normal neural function. The second enzyme system is the conversion of methylmalonyl-CoA to succinyl-CoA in the Krebs–citric acid cycle. Inhibition leads to the accumulation of methylmalonyl-CoA, which is shunted to methylmalonic acid. This may lead to the formation of "funny fatty acids," which are incorporated into sphingomyelin, thereby leading to abnormal neural transduction.

It should be noted, however, that the exact pathogenesis of neural dysfunction in vitamin B$_{12}$ deficiency is unknown.

Folate deficiency leads to poor methylation of DNA, which may increase susceptibility to cancer. Folate deficiency also leads to an accumulation of homocysteine, which has been associated with increased cardiovascular and cerebrovascular disease.[17] The conversion of homocysteine to methionine is a cytosolic process both requiring methylcobalamin and accompanied by the conversion of methyltetrahydrofolate to tetrahydrofolate. Homocysteine elevations occur with deficiency of either cofactor.

Genetics

A variety of hereditary enzymatic defects can manifest themselves as vitamin B_{12} deficiency or disorders of cobalamin metabolism.[18] They are found primarily in infancy and early childhood. There is also a hereditary predisposition to autoimmune dysfunction, namely in those patients with polyglandular autoimmune syndromes. Pernicious anemia may be seen in conjunction with other autoimmune disorders, including Hashimoto's thyroiditis, Addison's disease, vitiligo, diabetes, myasthenia gravis and hypopituitarism. There are a number of genetic disturbances of folate metabolism.[19]

Clinical features

Subacute combined degeneration of the spinal cord, peripheral nerve dysfunction and cerebral dysfunction are classic features of the disorder. Healton et al. have provided an excellent and current portrait of the natural history of the disorder. They reviewed 143 patients having 153 episodes of cobalamin deficiency.[20] The majority of patients present with paresthesias and ataxia. Seventy-four percent of the episodes presented with neurological symptoms, including paresthesias, numbness, gait ataxia, fecal incontinence, leg weakness, impaired manual dexterity, impaired memory and impotence. Rarely, patients had orthostatic lightheadedness, anosmia, diminished taste, paranoid psychosis and diminished visual acuity. The remaining 26% presented with nonneurological symptoms classically associated with pernicious anemia, including tiredness, syncope, palpitations, sore tongue, diarrhea and other bowel disturbances.

On examination, 25% of patients demonstrate a neuropathy, 12% isolated myelopathy, and 41% a combined neuropathy and myelopathy. Peripheral neuropathic symptoms and signs were combined with other manifestations, such as myelopathy, cortical dysfunction and autonomic dysfunction in 65% of cases. Only 3% have a neuropathy as the only abnormality. Memory dysfunction and affective and behavioral changes were seen in 8%. Cognitive deficits included psychosis, affective disturbances and memory disturbances, as well as changes in personality. Orthostatic hypotension has been reported and is thought to be due to a disordered release or norepinephrine.[21,22] Fourteen percent had normal examinations.

In the pretreatment era pernicious anemia had a high spontaneous remission rate of 30% to 60%, but the anemia as well as the neurological sequelae often recurred.[23]

Of 529 patients examined, 36% of B_{12}-deficient and 29% of folate-deficient patients developed neuropsychiatric symptoms some time during the course of their illness, including peripheral neuropathy, ataxia or cerebral dysfunction.[9] Because of the high prevalence of alcoholism in patients with folate deficiency it is difficult to separate the effects of alcohol from the folate deficiency itself.

Folate deficiency has been implicated in neural tube defects, increased susceptibility to cancer, accelerated atherosclerosis due to hyperhomocysteinemia, restless legs syndrome and depression.[17,24] The neuropathy or myeloneuropathy may be indistinguishable from cobalamin deficiency.[25–27]

Diagnostic criteria

The diagnostic criteria for vitamin B_{12} deficiency include a consistent clinical syndrome of ataxia, paresthesias, cognitive dysfunction, and evidence of neuropathic or myelopathic dysfunction. A megaloblastic anemia is often missing in patients with neurological symptoms.[4] In fact, a quarter have no anemia or macrocystosis.[20] The most characteristic presentation is gait dysfunction and paresthesias in an elderly individual. The hallmark finding of myeloneuropathy, absent ankle reflexes and extensor plantar responses is present in only 41%.[20]

As mentioned above, patients may have other associated autoimmune conditions, including Hashimoto's thyroiditis, adrenal insufficiency, myasthenia gravis, hypophysitis, and other endocrinopathies related to autoimmune antibody destruction. Low cobalamin levels have also been found in occasional patients with multiple sclerosis and HIV infection, although no pathogenic relationship or treatment response has been established in either disorder.

The serum cobalamin level is the test most commonly used to determine the presence or absence of the disease. However, when using methylmalonic acid levels as a gold standard of biochemical deficiency, the sensitivity and specificity of B_{12} is reduced. Using serum metabolite assays, 90% to 95% of cobalamin-deficient patients have B_{12} levels less than 200 pg/mL, 5% to 10% have levels of 200–300 pg/mL, and 1% may have levels greater than 300 pg/mL.[28] An elevation in either or both of these enzymes in a patient with a borderline or even normal serum B_{12} level has a high sensitivity for the diagnosis. Therefore, patients with B_{12} levels in the lower range of normal but who have a consistent clinical syndrome should have serum methylmalonic acid levels determined.[29]

In addition to sensitivity, the specificity of low cobalamin levels has also been called into question. Falsely low B_{12} levels have been seen in folate deficiency, nitrous oxide exposure, oral contraceptive use, transcobalamin deficiency and multiple myeloma. The cobalamin radioassay may give falsely low readings if performed soon after radionuclide isotope studies, such as bone scans.

Increasingly, chemiluminescence assays are being used instead of the more labor-intensive and expensive radioassays. Many laboratories have switched in recent years for economy, and the lower limit of normal may be up to 50 pg/mL more than the radioassay. Because metabolite assays have only been compared to the radioassay for B$_{12}$, clinicians should be aware of the type of assay used in their laboratory. Patients with B$_{12}$ levels greater than 250 pg/mL by chemiluminescence may have a higher percentage of abnormal metabolite levels than shown by the radioassay.[30]

Other helpful tests include serum gastrin and intrinsic factor and antiparietal cell antibodies. Intrinsic factor-binding antibodies have a sensitivity of 60% and are highly specific for pernicious anemia. Antiparietal cell antibodies are present in 90% of patients with percinious anemia, but may also be present in up to 10% of normal individuals. In patients with renal dynsfunction a urinary methylmalonic acid may be helpful to exclude a falsely elevated serum level due to renal insufficiency. An elevated serum gastrin is a marker for hypo- or achlorhydria, which is present in up to 30% of the elderly.[29] This is a risk factor for food-bound cobalamin malabsorption, which represents approximately 10% to 40% of all patients with B$_{12}$ deficiency. In an individual with serum cobalamin deficiency the finding of an intrinsic factor-binding antibody is diagnostic of pernicious anemia. However, if a low serum B$_{12}$ level and an elevated serum methylmalonic acid is found with a negative intrinsic factor antibody, a Schilling test is appropriate to look for the site of the defect, as this offers a guide to treatment (Figure 124.1).[30]

Elevations in homocysteine levels are more specific for folate deficiency, but both homocysteine and methylmalonic acid may be elevated in cobalamin deficiency. In 96% of patients with B$_{12}$ deficiency both metabolites were elevated, as opposed to 4% with folate deficiency. Eighty-six percent of folate-deficient patients have isolated elevations of homocysteine and normal methylmalonic acid levels.[9]

The pathology of subacute combined degeneration is characterized by demyelination of the posterior and lateral columns of the spinal cord. In the peripheral nerves, nerve conduction studies have demonstrated predominantly an axonal neuropathy, but conduction block and demyelination have also been reported. Teased-nerve fiber studies have shown both axonal degeneration and demyelination. There are a variety of reports of neuroimaging in vitamin B$_{12}$ deficiency, showing classic white matter changes in the posterior and lateral columns of the spinal cord. Resolution of the abnormalities on MRI may occur following replacement therapy.[31,32]

Evaluation

An algorithm for diagnosis and treatment of cobalamin (Figure 124.1) is based on two assumptions: (1) a normal cobalamin assay does not fully exclude cobalamin deficiency; and (2) the normal range may vary depending on the assay type. As mentioned above, many laboratories are switching from radioassay to chemiluminescence assay, which may have a higher normal reference range (230–931 pg/mL in our laboratory).

In a patient with signs and symptoms of cobalamin deficiency, a cobalamin assay should be ordered initially. If the assay is less than the lower limit of normal, intrinsic factor antibodies should be measured. In pernicious anemia, other laboratory evidence of an autoimmune process is frequently present. Serum antibodies are present against parietal cells in 90% and against intrinsic factor antibodies in 60% of patients with pernicious anemia. Unfortunately, false positive results for the parietal cell antibody are common, occurring in 10% of people over age 70. Although the test for intrinsic factor antibodies lacks sensitivity, it is much more specific than antiparietal cell antibodies. If the intrinsic factor antibody is present, a Schilling test is not necessary.

In patients with serum cobalamin levels in the lower normal range (250–350 pg/mL) measurement of metabolite levels is appropriate if cobalamin deficiency is still suspected. If either metabolite is elevated, intrinsic factor antibodies should be measured. If the test for intrinsic factor antibodies is negative, then measurement of the serum gastrin level may be useful to establish the presence of achlorhydria, which is almost invariably associated with percinious anemia as well as food-bound cobalamin malabsorption. The presence of hypersegmentation may be a sensitive marker for cobalamin deficiency, even in the absence of anemia or macrocytosis.

If metabolites or the serum gastrin levels are elevated but the intrinsic factor antibody is absent, a Schilling test may be performed to evaluate cobalamin absorption, which is usually the result of autoimmune parietal cell dysfunction characteristic of pernicious anemia. Technically, patients with classic pernicious anemia have an abnormal test result when radioactive cobalamin alone is given by mouth (Part I). This abnormality is corrected when the test is repeated with intrinsic factor (Part II). Abnormally low secretion of cobalamin in the Part II Schilling test indicates an intestinal cause for the cobalamin malabsorption, such as inflammatory bowel disease. The Part II Schilling test may be repeated after giving antibotics or vermicides to exclude bacterial overgrowth ("blind loop syndrome") or fish tapeworm infestation due to *Diphyllobothrium latum*. A normal Part I test in a patient with cobalamin deficiency may be observed in total vegetarians. It may also occur in patients with food-bound cobalamin malabsorption who show normal absorption of crystalline cobalamin but who are unable to digest and absorb cobalamin present in food due to achlorhydria. This defect can be identified using a modified Schilling test in which radioactive cobalamin is administered with food.

Some authors have advocated treating cobalamin deficiency without performing the Schilling test,

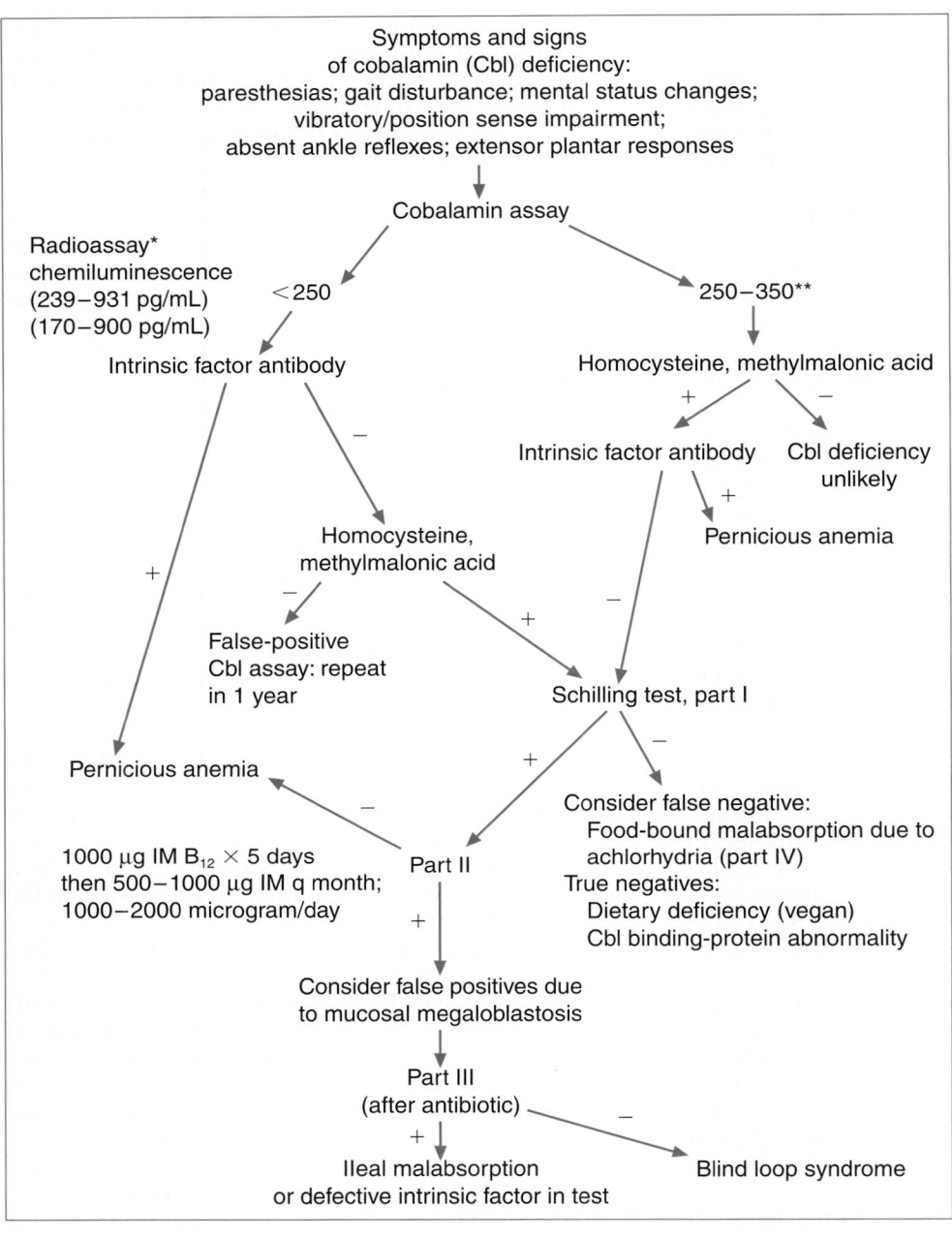

Figure 124.1   Algorithm for cobalamin (Cbl) deficiency diagnosis and treatment. *A higher normal reference range should be applied if chemiluminescence or other nonradioisotopic ligand-binding assays are used. **If the clinical picture is suggestive of possible Cbl deficiency, patients with serum Cbl >350 pg/mL should be investigated similarly. IM = intramuscular.

arguing that it is cumbersome and has problems with sensitivity and specificity. There are times, though, when testing allows for earlier diagnosis of intestinal malabsorption such as Crohn's disease,[15] and can also be used to determine the best form of treatment. Patients with food-bound cobalamin malabsorption due to achlorhydria may be supplemented with 50–100 µg cyanocobalamin orally, whereas those with pernicious anemia require far higher doses orally (1000–2000 µg) or intramuscular replacement on a monthly basis (see below).

Folate levels are subject to diet and may be falsely low in the fasting state. The red cell folate is considered a more reliable assessment of tissue stores of folic acid, but may be falsely elevated if the cells have undergone hemolysis during collection of the sample.

Differential diagnosis

The differential diagnosis is broad, given the variety of clinical manifestations of this disorder. Patients with cognitive dysfunction, ataxia and paresthesias should be considered for possible cobalamin deficiency. Other entities that give extensor plantar responses with absent ankle reflexes (the coexistence of an upper motor neuron and lower motor neuron disorder) include syphilis, Friedreich's ataxia, vitamin E deficiency, metachromatic leukodystrophy, adrenal leukodystrophy and amyotrophic lateral sclerosis. Cervical spondylitic myelopathy with lumbar osteoarthropathy and radiculopathy may also give a similar clinical pattern.

Treatment

The history of the treatment of this disorder begins with Minot and Murphy who, in 1926, documented the efficacy of feeding half a pound of cooked calf's liver daily in 45 consecutive patients.[23] Within a week, reticulocyte counts climbed from 1% to 15%, and at the end of two weeks the sallow icteric appearance of the patients' skin resolved. No mention, however, is made of neurological recovery. In 1949, Ungley documented resolution or arrest of the neurological manifestations in 46% of the patients treated in his series.[33] Of the expected improvement, 95% occurred within the first six months of therapy. Following treatment, improvement was seen earliest and most completely in the following descending order: difficulty using hands, incontinence, proprioception, astereognosis, coordination in the arms, rombergism, paresthesias, plantar response, touch, pinprick, gait abnormality, proprioception of the upper extremities, paresthesias in the lower extremities, coordination of the legs, vibratory sense impairment, and touch pinprick in the lower extremities.

The definitive treatment in the United States since the 1950s has been intramuscular cobalamin in doses ranging from 100 to 1000 µg daily for five days, followed by monthly or quarterly injections. The Anti-Anemia Advisory Board in 1959 established intramuscular B$_{12}$ as the therapeutic standard, despite the successes of Minot and Murphy in curing the disease with oral liver.[34] Concerns regarding the need for higher doses orally rather than intramuscularly, erratic absorption, intrinsic factor impurities, non-standardized oral preparations, delayed reticulocyte response, and reports of relapses on oral B$_{12}$, doomed oral therapy in the United States for the next 40 years.

However, these early clinical studies used subtherapeutic doses of only 25–250 µg of oral B$_{12}$. In Sweden, 1000 µg tablets of B$_{12}$ without intrinsic factor were introduced as standard therapy for pernicious anemia in 1964, with excellent efficacy and restoration of serum cobalamin levels. In 1968, Berlin[35] documented that approximately 1% of oral cobalamin without intrinsic factor could be absorbed regardless of dose or the cause of B$_{12}$ deficiency, presumably by passive diffusion across the gut wall. Others have documented the benefits of oral therapy.[40,42–44] With the introduction of higher doses, serum cobalamin levels rise quickly, rivaling parenteral administration in onset of action and serum levels.[36] Intramuscular B$_{12}$ injections given monthly are painful and more costly than oral treatment because of the need for medical personnel. Given the relapse rate of 25% with i.m. injections,[20] compliance with daily tablets is likely to be better, given the current popularity of dietary supplements.[37]

Sublingual administration of 2000 µg B$_{12}$ has been demonstrated to be as effective as parental cobalamin supplementation.[38] Intranasal B$_{12}$ is also an effective alternative.[39] Recently, Kuzminski demonstrated that 2000 µg B$_{12}$ orally is as or more effective than i.m.

injections given monthly for maintaining normal serum B$_{12}$ levels and correcting elevation in serum methylmalonic acid, with a comparable onset of action.[36] This effect occurred regardless of etiology, and included patients with pernicious anemia, food-cobalamin malabsorption, and those with a history of gastric surgery. A loading dose was not necessary for oral replacement, as serum metabolite elevations normalized as rapidly as did those in patients receiving i.m. loading doses.

Because 15% of 1000 µg B$_{12}$, or approximately 150 µg, will be retained after intramuscular injection, the author's practice has been to administer 1000 µg intramuscular daily for one week in an effort to replace depleted total body stories, followed by 1000 µg orally daily as maintenance therapy. Berlin has demonstrated that all patients respond to 1000 µg, obviating the need for higher doses. This regimen would yield 750 µg delivered by the i.m. route, and 10 µg absorbed orally by passive diffusion, exceeding the minimum daily requirement of 6 µg.

The earlier intervention begins, the more likely the patient is to recover completely.[20,33] Paresthesias often improve within several weeks, whereas spinal cord dysfunction may require several months. About 2% of patients experience an acute worsening of paresthesias immediately following B$_{12}$ supplementation, but this does not impair the long-term response to therapy. Folate supplementation may reverse the hematological abnormalities but will not prevent neurological deterioration. With early recognition, patients may resume a normal lifestyle with limited impairment of gait or cognition. Spasticity due to spinal cord dysfunction, when established, is often difficult to reverse, but may continue to improve over many months to years. Ten percent to 20% of patients may relapse as a result of non-compliance with long-term supplementation. These patients often develop identical symptoms that respond equally well to repeat treatment.[20]

Hyperhomocysteinemia has been directly linked to an increasing incidence of coronary and cerebrovascular disease. It is present in cobalamin, pyridoxine and folate deficiency, hypothyroidism, renal failure and heterozygous homocysteinemia. Therefore, B$_{12}$ deficiency, as well as folate and pyridoxine deficiencies, may be an independent risk factor for the development of carotid and coronary disease. Approximately 40% of patients with biochemical cobalamin deficiency may be asymptomatic. A high index of suspicion for B$_{12}$ deficiency is warranted in view of its high prevalence in the elderly.

The quality of evidence of efficacy dates back to the early studies of Ungley and Minot and Murphy, and is best classified as class 2 evidence or even class 3, based on large case series.

There is always difficulty with compliance, as demonstrated by Healton.[20] A number of patients discontinue intramuscular therapy and will have relapses. Patients used to taking a daily vitamin every day may find compliance with oral therapy easier.

Adverse events are uncommon. One issue

commonly raised is whether or not replacing B_{12} deficiency with folate will not only mask but accelerate the appearance of neurological manifestations. There is no documentation to support this. Nevertheless, any patient with megaloblastic anemia should be evaluated for both folate and B_{12} deficiency and supplemented appropriately.[41]

Trials in progress at the present time include observational studies of patients who are being exposed to nitrous oxide. Pre- and postoperative vitamin B_{12} and serum methylmalonic acid levels are being measured to test the incidence of this potential drug interaction. Nitrous oxide permanently oxidizes the available stores of B_{12} in patients who are deficient. For the average individual a several-hour exposure to nitrous oxide would be of no consequence. However, in those who are borderline B_{12} deficient a short exposure of one to two hours may be enough to precipitate acute deficiency.

Several unanswered questions remain. One is the relationship of serum B_{12} deficiency and folate deficiency to cardiovascular and cerebrovascular disease. Given the fact that both are potent stimuli to elevations in homocysteine, it is reasonable to suppose that these vitamin deficiencies may result in accelerated atherosclerosis and morbidity and mortality.[17]

References

1. Pruthi RK, Tefferi A. Pernicious anema revisited. Mayo Clin Proc 1994;69:144–150
2. Castle WB. Development of knowledge concerning the gastric intrinsic factor and its relation to pernicious anemia. N Engl J Med 1953;249:603–614
3. Woodson RD. Robert F Schilling—a tribute. Am J Hematol 1990;34:81–82
4. Lindenbaum J, Healton EB, Savage DG, et al. Neuropsychiatric disorders caused by cobalamin deficiency in the absence of anemia or macrocytosis. N Engl J Med 1988;318:1720–1728
5. Bolann BJ, Solli JD, Schneede J, et al. Evaluation of indicators of cobalamin deficiency defined as cobalamin-induced reduction in increased serum methylmalonic acid. Clin Chem 2000;46:1744–1750
6. Hurwitz A, Brady DA, Schaal SE, et al. Gastric acidity in older adults. JAMA 1997;278:659–662
7. Carmel R. Subtle and atypical cobalamin deficiency states. Am J Hematol 1990;34:108–114
8. Lindenbaum J, Rosenberg IH, Wilson PW, et al. Prevalence of cobalamin deficiency in the Framingham elderly population. Am J Clin Nutr 1994;60:2–11
9. Savage DG, Lindenbaum J, Stabler, SP, Allen RH. Sensitivity of serum methylmalonic acid and total homocysteine determinations for diagnosing cobalamin and folate deficiencies. Am J Med 1994;96:239–246
10. Fernando OV, Grimsley EW. Prevalence of folate deficiency and macrocytosis in patients with and without alcohol-related illness. South Med J 1999;92:841
11. Carmel R. Cobalamin, the stomach, and aging. Am J Clin Nutr 1997;66:750–759
12. Sumner AE, Chin MM, Abrahm JL, et al. Elevated methylmalonic acid and total homocysteine levels show high prevalence of vitamin B sub 12 deficiency after gastric surgery. Ann Intern Med 1996;124:469–476
13. Halverson JD. Micronutrient deficiencies after gastric bypass for morbid obesity. Am Surg 1986;52:594–598
14. Marcuard SP, Albernaz L, Khazanie PG. Omeprazole therapy causes malabsorption of cyanocobalamin (vitamin B_{12}). Ann Intern Med 1994;120:211–215
15. Kinsella LJ, Green R. "Anesthesia paresthetica": nitrous oxide-induced cobalamin deficiency. Neurology 1995;45:1608–1610
16. Tefferi A, Pruthi RK. The biochemical basis of cobalamin deficiency. Mayo Clin Proc 1994;69:181–186
17. Green R, Miller JW. Folate deficiency beyond megaloblastic anemia: hyperhomocysteinemia and other manifestations of dysfunctional folate status. Semin Hematol 1999;36:47–64
18. Rosenblatt DS, Cooper BA. Inherited disorders of vitamin B12 utilization. Bioessays 1990;12:331–334
19. Rosenblatt DS. Inherited disorders of folate transport and metabolism. In: Scriver CR, Beaudet AL, Sly WS, Valle D, eds. The metabolic basis of inherited disease. Vol II, 6th edn. New York: McGraw Hill, 1989; 2049–2064
20. Healton EB, Savage DG, Brust JCM, et al. Neurologic aspects of cobalamin deficiency. Medicine 1991;70:229–244
21. White WB, Reik L Jr, Cutlip DE. Pernicious anemia seen initially as orthostatic hypotension. Arch Intern Med 1991;141:1543–1544
22. Eisenhofer G, Lambie DG, Johnson RH, et al. Deficient catecholamine release as the basis of orthostatic hypotension in pernicious anemia. J Neurol Neurosurg Psychiatry 1982;45:1053–1055
23. Minot GR, Murphy WP. Treatment of pernicious anemia by a special diet. JAMA 1926;37:470–476
24. Alpert JE, Fava M. Nutrition and depression: the role of folate. Nutr Rev 1997;55:145–149
25. Lever EG, Elwes RD, Williams A, Reynolds EH. Subacute combined degeneration of the cord due to folate deficiency: response to methyl folate treatment. J Neurol Neurosurg Psychiatry 1986;49:1203–1207
26. Manzoor M, Runcie J. Folate-responsive neuropathy: report of 10 cases. Br Med J 1976;1:1176–1178
27. Parry TE. Folate-responsive neuropathy. Presse Med 1994;23:131–137
28. Stabler SP, Allen RH, Savage DG, Lindenbaum J. Clinical spectrum and diagnosis of cobalamin deficiency. Blood 1990;76:871–881
29. Hurwitz A, Brady DA, Schaal SE, et al. Gastric acidity in older adults. JAMA 1997;278:659–662
30. Green R, Kinsella LJ. Current concepts in the diagnosis of cobalamin deficiency. Neurology 1995;45:1435–1440
31. Hemmer B, Glocker FX, Schumacher M, et al. Subacute combined degeneration: clinical, electrophysiological, and magnetic resonance imaging findings. J Neurol Neurosurg Psychiatry 1998;65:822–827
32. Timms SR, Cure JK, Kurrent JE. Subacute combined degeneration of the spinal cord: MR findings. Am J Neuroradiol 1993;14:1224–1227
33. Ungley CC. Subacute combined degeneration of the cord: I. Response to liver extracts. II. Trials with B12. Brain 1949;72:382–427
34. Bethell FH, Castle WB, Conley CL, London IM. Present status of treatment of pernicious anemia: Ninth announcement of USP Anti-Anemia Preparations Advisory Board. JAMA 1959;171:2092–2094
35. Berlin H, Berlin R, Brante G. Oral treatment of pernicious anaemia with high doses of vitamin B12 without intrinsic factor. Acta Med Scand 1968;184:247–258
36. Kuzminski AM, Del Giacco EJ, Allen RH, et al. Effective treatment of cobalamin deficiency with oral cobalamin. Blood 1998;92:1191–1198

37. Koehler KM, Romero LJ, Stauber PM, et al. Vitamin supplementation and other variables affecting serum homocysteine and methylmalonic acid concentrations in elderly men and women. J Am Coll Nutr 1996;15:364–376
38. Delpre G, Stark P, Niv Y. Sublingual therapy for cobalamin deficiency as an alternative to oral and parenteral cobalamin supplementation. Lancet 1999; 354:740–742
39. Slot WB, Merkus FW, Van Deventer SJ, Tytgat GN. Normalization of plasma vitamin B12 concentration by intranasal hydroxocobalamin in vitamin b12-deficient patients. Gastroenterol 1997;113:430–433
40. Adachi SA, Kawamoto T, Otsuka M, et al. Enteral vitamin B12 supplements reverse postgastrectomy B12 deficiency. Ann Surg 2000;232:199–201
41. Snow CF. Laboratory diagnosis of vitamin B12 and folate deficiency: a guide for the primary care physician. Arch Intern Med 1999;159:1289–1298
42. Elia M. Oral or parenteral therapy for B12 deficiency. Lancet 1998;352:1721–1722
43. Verhaeverbeke I, Mulkens K. Normalization of low vitamin B12 serum levels in older people by oral treatment. J Am Geriatr Soc 1997;45:124–125
44. Lederle FA. Commentary: oral cobalamin for pernicious anemia: medicine's best kept secret?. JAMA 1991;265:94–95

125 Hemoglobinopathies and Thalassemias: Treatment of Stroke and Other Neurological Complications

Christiana E Hall and Robert J Adams

Introduction

The hemoglobinopathies result from genetically determined abnormalities in the structure of the hemoglobin (Hb) molecule (as in HbS or HbC) or the rate of synthesis of normal α or β-globin chains (as in thalassemias). Neurological complications are most frequently seen in sickle cell disease (SCD).[1] These include stroke and intracranial hemorrhage, cognitive disability, seizures, meningitis, headache, neuropathy and myopathy. Of these, stroke is the entity of greatest clinical import to neurologists, owing to its frequency, impact and recent advances in prevention. For patients at high risk, the standard of care for treatment and prevention of many of the complications of hemoglobinopathies is transfusion therapy, but with it come the risks of iron overload, possible transmissible disease and alloimmunization.

Since Pauling established SCD as the "first molecular disease" in the 1940s, a long tradition of research in the field has brought to light many aspects of its pathophysiology. Based on what has been learned of the mechanisms of this disease, novel treatment options are appearing. The challenge at present is to further clarify the mechanism(s) of disease so as to identify targets for specific therapies with excellent safety profiles. Until this ideal is fully realized, the critical task is to identify with specificity those patients at highest risk for complications and institute preventive treatment where available.

Focusing on stroke: mechanisms, prevention strategies and treatment issues will be addressed, followed by a discussion of less common neurological complications of hemoglobinopathies.

Epidemiology

Sickle cell anemia (HbS/HbS) is detected in 1 of 600 black newborns in the US, but prevalence is reduced in adults owing to early mortality. Nearly as large a population of compound heterozygotes exists wherein HbS is combined with a second abnormal hemoglobin, leading to a sickling disorder of varying severity. Common examples are HbSC (HbS/HbC) and HbS-thalassemia (HbS/B⁰ and HbS/B⁺). Sickle trait, the heterozygous carrier state (HbS/HbA), exists in 8% of black Americans, although with rare exceptions it is not considered a sickling disorder.[2,3]

Pathophysiology

In SCD the majority of clinical manifestations are caused by a phenomenon known as vaso-occlusion. Sickling of red cells directly and indirectly influences these events. The β-globin gene in SCD codes for the substitution of valine for glutamic acid at position 6 of the protein. This substitution enables an abnormal hydrophobic interaction with other such Hb chains, leading to rigid polymer formation and red cells of abnormal or frankly sickled configurations. At least initially, sickling is reversible upon reoxygenation. The tendency of a particular HbSS erythrocyte to sickle is influenced primarily by deoxygenation, intracellular Hb concentration, and the intracellular concentration of fetal hemoglobin (HbF).[4]

At body temperature the solubility of deoxy-HbS is only about half that of normal HbA or oxy-HbS, but an equal mix of HbS and HbF has twice the solubility of HbS alone, owing to HbF's unique ability to block polymerization.[5] Polymer formation sufficiently extensive to cause sickling requires a certain amount of time to develop, which is designated *delay time* (T_d). Fortunately, circulatory transit times in vivo are shorter than T_d, and so at least 80% of cells escape sickling as they traverse the microcirculation.[6] It has become clear that vaso-occlusive events cannot be explained simply by mechanical clogging of postcapillary venules by sickled cells, and that other mechanisms must be at play. These may include abnormal adhesion, hypercoagulability, inflammation and endothelial activation. Vaso-occlusion explains one of the most common clinical manifestations, which is the "painful crisis," but the role of this well studied sickle cell phenomenon in organ infarction such as stroke is not clear.

Stroke

Epidemiology

Earlier reports of the prevalence of stroke in SCD range from 5% to 17%.[1,7–11] Recently the Cooperative Study of Sickle Cell Disease (CSSCD) has provided prevalence and incidence estimates of stroke from a 10-year natural history study of more than 4000 SCD patients observed in 23 US centers. The highest incidence of stroke in HbSS is seen in children and the elderly. For compound heterozygote groups the incidence is generally lower, and is basically nil for sickle β-thalassemia groups (Figure 125.1). For HbSS patients hemorrhagic events peak in the third decade, when the incidence of infarct is lowest, and hemorrhage may explain increased event rates seen in heterozygotes of this age. The chances of having a first stroke by 20 years of age was 11% in HbSS patients vs. 2% in HbSC patients, and essentially 0% for sickle-thalassemia patients, confirming the higher risk of stroke in HbSS and for those strokes to occur in childhood, with no effect of gender. Risk factors for infarction included prior transient ischemic attack (TIA), low steady-state Hb, rate and recency of episodes of acute chest syndrome, and elevated systolic blood pressure. Risk factors for intracranial hemorrhage included low steady-state hemoglobin and high leukocyte count.[12]

Stroke incidence data have traditionally been based on clinical signs and symptoms. MRI has allowed the estimation of the prevalence and incidence of subclinical ischemic events noted incidentally on neuroimaging. Analysis of this question by the CSSCD group revealed that silent infarcts were present in 18.3% of 230 subjects with HbSS selected on the basis of no prior clinical history of stroke.[13] Another CSSCD report sought to define the spectrum of MRI abnormalities in 312 unselected SCD children. Thirteen percent showed abnormalities in the absence of a clinical stroke history, and overall 22% of the population studied had abnormal findings. Interestingly, in those with a clinical stroke history infarcts involved the cortex and deep white matter, whereas silent infarcts tended to be limited to deep white matter only. Although the prevalence of MRI lesions did not change for those aged 6–14 years, older patients tended to have a greater number of lesions than their juniors, consistent with the notion of progressive brain injury as children with the disease mature.[14]

Common infarction patterns seen by conventional neuroimaging, in order of frequency, are: wedge-shaped lesions of large vessel territories; border-zone infarctions, particularly of the middle anterior cerebral artery watershed region; and small punctate lesions of the deep white matter (Figure 125.2). Fat embolism patterns and venous thromboses are rarely encountered.[15,16]

The majority of hemorrhagic events, intracranial hemorrhages (ICH) and subarachnoid hemorrhage (SAH) occur in adults and in children over 14 years of age.[8,17] Incidence peaks in the 20–29-year age range.[12] Hemorrhage is also more frequent in patients with prior infarction.[18] SAH is less often seen than intracerebral hemorrhage.[8,19] It is particularly uncommon in children, but when it does occur angiograms usually show multiple distal branch occlusions, leptomeningeal collateralization and absence of aneurysm. CT scans reveal blood in the superficial cortical sulci.[20] Adults with SAH typically have aneurysms, often multiple, with blood seen by CT in the basal cisterns.[17,21] Sickle cell disease patients seem to be at higher risk for SAH than the general population, and smaller aneurysms tend to bleed at a younger age.[22] A case report meta-analysis[23] adds credence to earlier observations[24] that there is a heightened incidence of multiple aneurysms, and for these to show an unusual predilection for the posterior circulation in SCD patients compared to the general population. Conditions present in the SCD state that might engender aneurysm development include: large vessel vasculopathy with stenosis increasing local and alternative path hemodynamic stress; increased cerebral blood flow and velocities secondary to low hematocrit; and abnormal HbS erythrocyte interactions with endothelial surfaces inducing vessel wall damage. With the life expectancy of SCD patients in developed countries now extending into the fifth and sixth decades, it is possible that aneurysm and SAH may be seen with increased frequency in this population.[25]

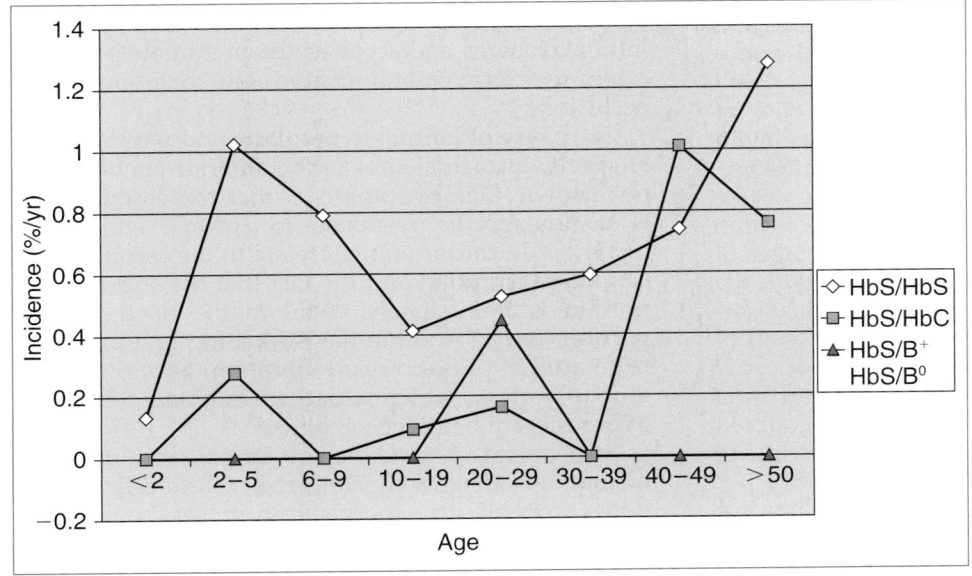

Figure 125.1 Stroke incidence by age in a sickle cell disease population (adapted from Ohene-Frempong[12]).

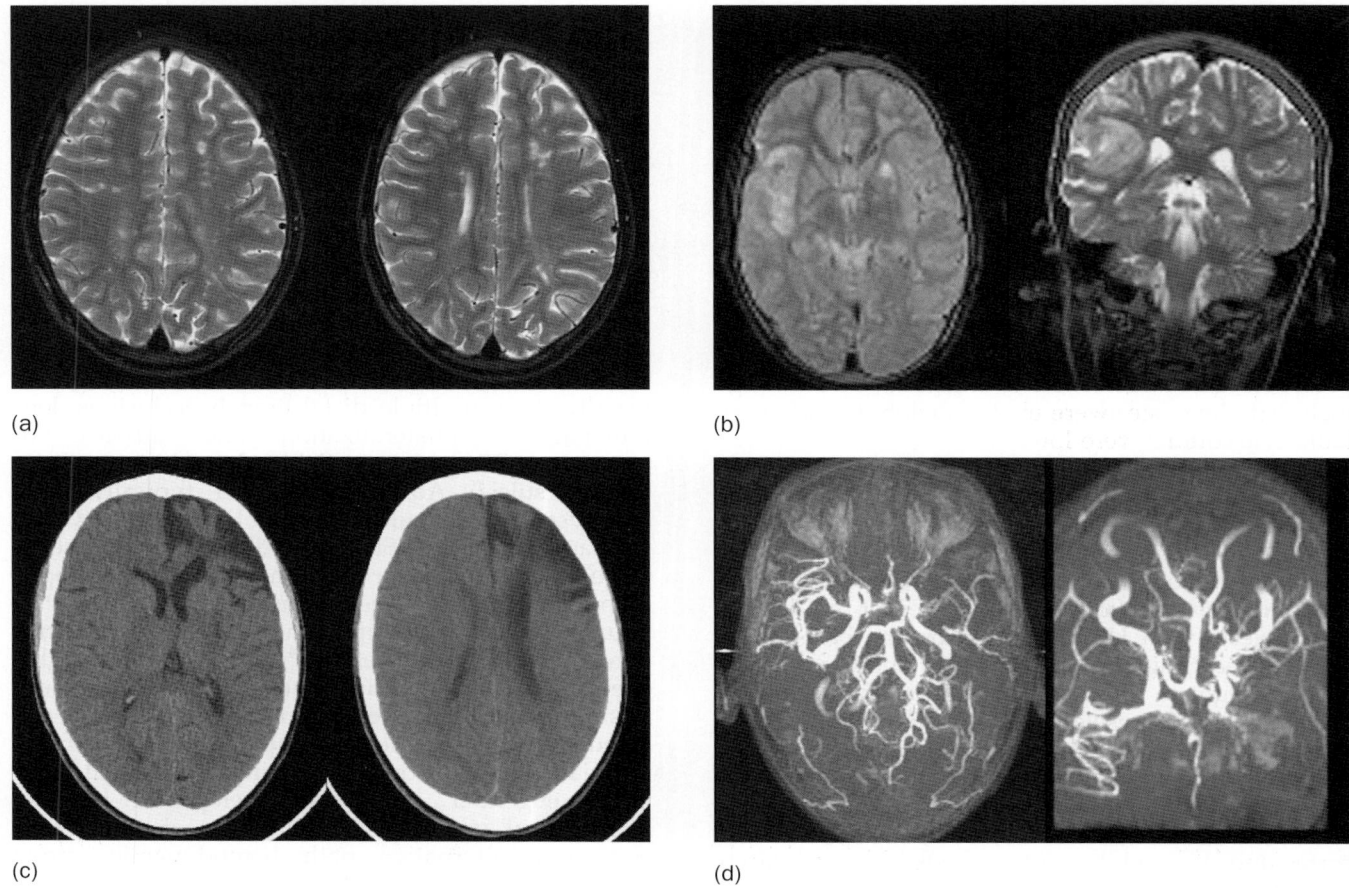

Figure 125.2   Some common infarction patterns and vasculopathy-related occlusions. (a) Border-zone infarct; (b) right MCA infarct; (c) left ACA–MCA infarct; (d) left ICA occlusion.

Pathophysiology of stroke

Counterintuitively, the majority of strokes in SCD do not result from vaso-occlusive phenomena in the microcirculation but are associated with a large vessel vasculopathy primarily localized to the distal supraclinoid internal carotid artery (ICA) (Figure 125.2) and the proximal portions of the middle cerebral artery (MCA) and anterior cerebral artery (ACA). Such lesions have been demonstrated in about 80% of angiograms in sickle cell anemia patients with stroke.[26–30] Also consistent with large vessel etiology, MRI and CT studies of patients with SCD and stroke have shown 80% to have major distal vessel occlusion or distal insufficiency patterns.[15] In the later stages of vasculopathy there may be a striking similarity to the angiographic picture of "moyamoya," with its abnormal network of subcortical vessels giving the "puff of smoke" appearance in as many as 30% of SCD patients with vasculopathy.[26,31] Moyamoya and SCD show parallels in the risk of early infarction coupled with a later risk of hemorrhage, possibly owing to rupture of dilated weakened collateral vessels.[32]

Pathological examination of large vasculopathic segments reveals striking intimal proliferation with discontinuity of the internal elastic lamina. Although endothelial cells may proliferate to resurface denuded areas, they remain a monolayer, whereas components of the hyperplastic intima include fibroblasts, fibrous tissue and scattered smooth muscle cells.[33] Concomitant thrombus formation in areas of endothelial damage may both perpetuate the vicious cycle of intimal changes and serve as the proximate source of artery-to-artery emboli responsible for some distal occlusions.[34,35]

The cause of intimal hyperplasia and why it occurs at specific proximal sites in the anterior circulation is not known. One hypothesis is that the vasculopathy is a non-specific response to chronic endothelial injury.[11,30] Localization may relate to the carotid bifurcation branch point and the fact that the supraclinoid portion is immediately distal to the fixed petrous portion (resistant to intimal thickening and protected from arterial pulsation and vibration) and to the cavernous portion, which is bathed in blood containing byproducts of hemolytic anemia.[33–36]

Mechanical (hemodynamic stress) and chemical mediators, along with abnormal cell-to-cell interactions, probably act synergistically to set the stage for stroke. A detailed discussion of these issues is beyond the scope of this chapter. The interested reader is directed to excellent reviews[33,35–37] and to the work of Hebbel and colleagues, who have been active in areas of abnormal adhesion and endothelial cell activation, with implications for inflammatory processes.[38–41] Another line of investigation that warrants mention has sought to establish the presence of an underlying hypercoagulable state in sickle cell anemia. The patient with stroke and sickle cell disease may have additional factors that place them at risk, such as a hypercoagulable state or antiphospholipid antibodies. A recent study compared 20 HbSS with 17 HbSC patients on measures of coagulation. They found that antiphospholipid antibodies (particularly IgG to phosphatidylserine, which is exposed with red cell membrane damage) were elevated, and that proteins C and S activities were lower in HbSS than in HbSC. These findings were related to each other and with other measures of coagulation activation, which were abnormal in HbSS but not in HbSC subjects. The authors felt the significant differences in coagulation indices were consistent with observed differences in the clinical severity between the two diseases.[42]

Stroke treatment and prevention

Transfusion

Significant evidence has accrued to support the hypothesis that primary and secondary stroke prevention in children with SCD may be accomplished with transfusion therapy. Following the first stroke, as many as two-thirds of untreated children experience a subsequent stroke, with the majority of these occurring within 36 months.[8] Although not tested in a clinical trial, chronic transfusion therapy with a goal of HbS reduction to less than 30% has been associated with a reduced stroke recurrence to as low as 10%.[26,43] A primary prevention strategy using transfusion was tested in a randomized controlled trial. The Stroke Prevention Trial in Sickle Cell Anemia (STOP) recently established that transfusion therapy can reduce the risk of first stroke by 92% in high-risk children aged 2–16 years, selected on the basis of screening with transcranial Doppler ultrasonography (TCD). The children randomized in this study, none of whom had a history of stroke at entry, were identified by two TCDs showing time-averaged mean (as opposed to peak systolic) velocities greater than or equal to 200 cm/s in the ICA or MCA. Children with SCD generally have TCD velocities in the range of 130–140 cm/s, and the 200 cm/s cutoff is about two standard deviations above normal for children of this age and degree of anemia. Children in the untreated arm had a stroke risk of 10% per year. Eleven events occurred in the untreated group vs. only one in the transfused group ($P < 0.001$). These results led to early termination of the trial and the publication of a Clinical Alert by the National Heart Lung and Blood Institute that encouraged TCD screening and consideration of transfusion in cases of high risk based on the STOP study results.[44,45]

A transfusion program should be developed in consultation with the pediatric hematologist.

Exchange transfusion or simple transfusions are options. Exchange may have some advantages. In the acute setting exchange transfusions avoid the potential adverse effect of bringing hemoglobin towards a more normal level, thereby raising viscosity. In the long term iron loading is reduced, but exchange transfusion requires more blood and exposes the patient to more units of blood. To maintain HbS less than 30% transfusion is generally required every three to four weeks. Transfusion is indicated in acute stroke in children immediately following stabilization, as well as for the prevention of stroke in children with abnormal TCD based on the STOP study, and for prevention of recurrent stroke in those who have already developed brain infarction. Wayne et al.[46] provide further detail on transfusion management of sickle cell disease.

Despite being effective in carefully selected cases, transfusion is not a panacea. There are no data supporting its use in adults with infarction. It is unclear whether transfusion is helpful in preventing recurrent brain hemorrhage, although it is frequently given in this setting in preparation for cerebral angiography, which is recommended to rule out treatable vascular lesions. It may also be of some benefit on a continuing basis by reducing hemodynamic stress, which may lower the risk of aneurysm rupture, but this has not been systematically studied.

The risk of alloimmunization with chronic transfusion is 30%,[47] although careful phenotypic matching may reduce this problem.[44,46] In the STOP study transfused children's ferritin levels rose from an average of 164 ± 155 ng/mL at baseline to 1804 ± 773 ng/mL within 12 months. Chelation therapy with the only available agent, desferrioxamine, is usually recommended when serum ferritin reaches 2500 ng/mL. The initial dose is 50 mg/kg administered by subcutaneous infusion over an eight-hour period daily. The treatment is arduous, painful, may cause hearing loss, and has rarely caused adult respiratory distress syndrome (ARDS). Compliance estimates average 50%.[48] Untreated, transfusional siderosis leads to organ damage, most prominently cardiomyopathy[49] or liver problems. Measurement of serum ferritin is less accurate for estimating tissue iron load than are quantitative liver biopsy and magnetic susceptometry,[50] but the availability of latter method is extremely limited.[51] With ever-improving surveillance of the blood supply the threat of transmissible disease has lessened, but remains a risk. In STOP, for instance, there were no cases of HIV or hepatitis C transmission in over 1500 transfusions delivered as part of the study. There is some evidence that a modified transfusion protocol allowing HbS of 50% may also be effective in preventing recurrent stroke.[52,53] This may be reasonable after several years of standard transfusion, but has not been widely embraced.

It has not been established when it is safe to discontinue chronic transfusion following stroke or to prevent first stroke. In practice, many hematologists discontinue this therapy in young adulthood, or patients tire of the program and fail to continue with regular transfusions. The rate of stroke after discontinuation in these cases is unknown. A few small case series have reported event rates following transfusion cessation,[10,27,54–56] but from the available data it is difficult to determine any age cut-off point after which it would appear safe to discontinue transfusion (Table 125.1). Existing guidelines recommending transfusion after infarction to continue for at least five years or until the age of 18 are reasonable in the absence of better data.[57]

Hydroxyurea (Hdu)

This therapy emerged from efforts to identify agents capable of elevating the HbF%, as observations of populations and a study of natural history have shown that increased HbF% correlates negatively with disease severity.[58] Hdu is the only chemotherapeutic agent available for the treatment of SCD. The double-blind placebo-controlled study of Hdu in 299 adults with SCD for the reduction of painful episodes was terminated early when significant reductions in pain episode frequency, acute chest syndrome, need for hospitalization and blood transfusions became evident.[59] There were too few strokes in this study to determine any

effect of the drug on risk of stroke. No study has addressed the issue of whether Hdu is effective in stroke prevention in a controlled fashion. Ware et al.[56] did report the outcomes of treatment with Hdu and phlebotomy in 16 young patients in whom transfusion was no longer an option. Their results of a 19% recurrent event incidence compares favorably with the 50% or higher recurrence that might be expected untreated.[8,55] In this single report the sample size was small and controls and randomization lacking.

On theoretical grounds Hdu offers promise for stroke prevention. In addition to elevating HbF% in the majority of those treated, it reduces many of the events felt to be markers for severe disease. Unexpected benefits include improved red blood cell (RBC) deformability, reduction in cellular dehydration and potassium content, decrement in the irreversibly sickled cell fraction, and improvements in rheology and RBC survival.[60] Abnormal adhesion of blood cells may also be modified.[61–63] Increased granulocytes, reticulocytes and platelets are putative markers of increased risk of cerebral vasculopathy,[48] and Hdu has been shown to reduce these.[64] Pretreatment elevation of these markers also seems to predict a good response to Hdu.[65]

Table 125.1 Stroke, TIA or death after transfusion cessation

Study year	Number of subjects	Average number of years on TX post index stroke (range)	Average post-TX observation period (range)	Number and type of event	*Age of subject with events	*Age of subject without events (number in category)
Williams et al.[27] 1980	10	(1–2)	(5 wks–11 mos)	7 strokes	all < 15 yrs	all < 15 yrs
Moohr et al.[10] 1982	7	2	(9–44 mos)	0	–	–
†Rana et al.[54] 1997	9	6.3 (10.5–16)	9 yrs (3–18.5 yrs)	0 infarcts 1 ICH (resulting in death) 1 death (liver disease)	17.5 yrs	9.5 10 17 (2) 18 (3) 25
Wang et al.[55] 1991	10	9.5 (5–12)	1 yr	3 infarcts 1 infarct plus ICH 1 ICH 1 death unknown cause	10 13 15 16 17 23	7 17 20 21
(*) Ware et al.[56] 1999	16	4.7 (0.58–10.6)	22 months (3–52 months)	3 infarcts	10 13 18	2 6 7 8 (3) 11 12 13 16 (2) 19 (2)

TX: Transfusion   ICH: Intracranial hemorrhage
† Some patients received hydroxyurea after TX cessation
(*) All patients received hydroxyurea after TX cessation
* Age at time TX stopped

Hdu therapy begins at 15 mg/kg/day and escalates by 5 mg/kg/day each 8–12 weeks, with monitoring of platelets, reticulocytes and neutrophils. Reductions of these parameters below a critical level triggers holding of the drug and restarting of a modified dose when suppression recovers.[56,59] Mean corpuscular volume (MCV) increases linearly to normal levels along with increasing HbF%, and so may provide an estimate of HbF response.[63]

In the short term Hdu appears to be safe in both adults and children,[59,64] but questions remain about the long-term risks. Concern for negative effects on growth and development cannot be excluded, and questions regarding the development of malignancy remain to be answered with long-term observation. A large well-designed clinical trial is needed to establish whether Hdu is efficacious in the primary and secondary prevention of stroke in SCD. Such a trial may need to call upon subjects who are ineligible for transfusion, or very young patients displaying markers for severe disease[66] in whom early Hdu treatment might conceivably prevent the development of those indicators of stroke risk as identifiable by TCD screening.

Bone marrow transplant

Bone marrow transplant (BMT) may be curative in SCD. Combining European and US experience, published data are now available on more than 120 patients to show that HLA-identical sibling stem cell allografts can successfully replace sickle cells with normal donor-derived RBCs, and that stable mixed chimerism, even with a relatively low proportion of donor cells, can ameliorate the symptoms and complications of SCD. Survival and event-free survival have been respectively 94% and 84% in the US, 92% and 75% in France, and 93% and 82% in Belgium.[67] The cumulative incidence of graft rejection or return of SCD is 11%. Although most transplanted patients have survived free of SCD approximately 8% have died, and about half of these deaths occurred in the setting of graft-versus-host disease (GVHD).[68] Acute and chronic GVHD and gonadal dysfunction resulting from requisite myeloablative conditioning, and more clinically evident in girls than boys, are realities associated with this therapy. With the early transplants acute neurological complications were unacceptably high, particularly intracerebral hemorrhage (ICH), and patients with a history of prior stroke were noted to be at increased risk.[69–71] The institution of preventative measures has reduced significant peritransplant neurological complications. These include phenytoin prophylaxis, control of hypertension, repletion of hypomagnesemia, maintenance of hemoglobin between 9 and 11 g/dL, and platelet counts higher than 50 000/uL and pretransplant transfusion to achieve HbS less than 30%. There remains about a 20% incidence of peritransplant seizure, which appears more likely to affect patients with evidence of prior cerebral vasculopathy. Most complications are transient and relatively benign.[67,68]

Walters et al.[67] reported the impact of BMT on CNS disease for 22 patients with stable donor engraftment followed for at least two years. Ten patients had a history of stroke, four had silent infarcts by MRI, one had TIA, and one had positive TCD screening prior to BMT. Conclusions based on clinical and MRI follow-up were that no significant CNS events had occurred and that most had shown "stabilization" of the underlying cerebral vasculopathy.[67] Bernaudin[72] reports from France that, with the advent of Hdu, history of stroke has become the main indication for BMT, and he asserts that it should be considered in patients with silent cerebral infarcts associated with cognitive impairment or TCD evidence of stroke risk.[72] Others have been more cautious, suggesting that BMT should occur only in the context of clinical trials, pointing to the fact that in exchange for the possibility of cure BMT entails a sizeable initial risk, versus a more distributed risk of modern supportive care and other treatments available to enable prolonged life and a less severe disease course.[2] The paucity of available HLA-identical sibling donors is a major obstacle to transplantation. Consideration of unrelated donor transplants is premature at this time and would entail long-term immunosuppression, with its attendant risks.[68] BMT, if feasible, is worth considering on a case-by-case basis because of its curative potential. It has usually been reserved for those with severe complications; however, evidence exists that a higher rate of transplant-related adverse events is seen in older symptomatic patients than in those who are younger and asymptomatic.[73] This suggests that BMT may be best used early in life in those at highest risk for significant adverse events, including stroke.

Other treatments

Gene therapy offers hope as a future intervention in SCD but appears years away from clinical application. Obstacles include the expected problems of efficient gene transfer into hematopoietic cells, and regulation of gene expression. Successful gene therapy in SCD must not only increase the production of a normal hemoglobin chain, but also ameliorate the effects of abnormal HbS. Because patients with increased HbF% are known to have a milder course, efforts are currently directed toward gene therapy that would increase the production of HbF. Preliminary findings in mice suggest the possibility of an Hb chain regulatory mechanism such that, as HbF gene product increases, the production of HbS declines.[74,75] Such a switching mechanism, if identified and manipulated through gene therapy, could be of benefit in the treatment of SCD.

Management of the acute stroke patient

There are no data available to guide management in an adult patient with SCD with first-time stroke. Treatment planning therefore relies on the practices of stroke neurologists experienced in the care of the SCD patient with stroke, and informed by existing guidelines and data for the treatment of stroke patients without SCD.[76–79] Acutely, ischemic stroke patients with SCD over the age of 18 may be considered for intravenous recombinant tissue plasminogen activator (r-TPA), if therapy can be delivered within three hours of symptom onset and there are no contraindications according to existing guidelines.[77] There is no clear justification to exclude adult SCD patients from thrombolytic therapy. Adequate hydration, normothermia and euglycemia should be maintained and hypotension avoided in the setting of acute stroke.

Beyond the immediate CT scan, additional neurodiagnostics are indicated to demonstrate parenchymal injury and assess the current status of cerebral vasculature. In adults with stroke, or in children who cannot be transfused long term, warfarin may be an alternative if there is evidence of intracranial arterial stenosis. In the presence of moyamoya anticoagulation is best avoided, and antiplatelet therapy is an option. There is no systematic experience with either anticoagulation or antiplatelet agents in this setting, but, given the support for use of these agents in adults generally, it is reasonable to use them in adults with SCD when no other specific stroke prevention strategy is available. In cases of treatment failure and recurrent strokes despite medical therapy, and in the setting of severe vascular disease, surgical management is an option. There are a few reports of the successful establishment of collateral supply using an elegant surgical strategy called encephaloduroarteriosyangiosis (EDAS), in which a superficial scalp artery with galea is mobilized and passed through the dura to lie on the arachnoid surface of the brain.[80]

The prevalence of SCD-related vasculopathy is high, but other mechanisms and risk factors for stroke should also be considered, especially in adults with SCD and stroke. Drug abuse, anticardiolipin antibodies and other hypercoagulable states, vasculitides, arterial dissection, cardioembolic or paradoxical emboli, and elevated homocysteine should all be considered. A "stroke in the young adult" work-up should be contemplated in adults with SCD. Hypercoagulable states are best treated with anticoagulation. Data are conflicting as to whether elevation of serum homocysteine is a risk factor for stroke in SCD;[81,82] however, it is an established risk factor for stroke in other settings.[83] Because treatment with low-dose folate and B vitamins easily modifies elevated homocysteine levels, screening of plasma homocysteine is reasonable. Other modifiable stroke risks—smoking, diabetes, hypertension, obesity—should all be addressed in SCD patients (Figures 125.3, 125.4).

Other neurological manifestations
Cognitive disability

There is a growing body of literature to suggest that cognitive disability detectable by neuropsychological testing (NST) may exist in a high proportion of SCD patients. The degree of impairment probably follows a continuum worse in those with clinically evident stroke > silent infarct > radiographically normal with SCD vs. siblings without SCD or relevant controls.[84–86] Deficits may be present at a very young age, possibly reflecting a generalized effect of inadequate oxygen delivery relative to the increased demands of the

rapidly developing brain.[85] Work is in progress to establish the interplay of NST and several other neurodiagnostic modalities (conventional and quantitative MRI,[85–87] proton MR spectroscopy[88] and PET scanning[89,90]) in assessing early cognitive impairment and in relating the composite information to stroke or the prediction of stroke.[48] Brief cognitive screening measures have been identified which are sensitive and specific indicators of the presence of overt and silent infarction.[91] NST is appropriate for the early identification of those SCD children with special educational needs.

Seizures

Seizure incidence appears to be higher in SCD than in the general population—12% to 16% vs. 1% to 2%.[1,7,11,92] The risk of seizure as a side effect of meperidine treatment may also be somewhat higher among SCD patients.[92] The combination of neuroimaging and EEG is the typical work-up for SCD patients with seizures and abnormalities supportive of epilepsy, leading to consideration of treatment with anticonvulsant agents. Other analgesics may be preferable to meperidine in SCD patients, particularly those with a history of cortical stroke or renal insufficiency.[92] In the SCD patient presenting with seizure, the possibility should not be overlooked that seizure may be an indicator of acute brain ischemia.

Meningitis

Progressive splenic dysfunction places the youngest children with SCD at risk for sepsis and meningitis.[93,94] Strong data are available to support the following recommendations.[95–97] Prophylactic oral penicillin should be initiated in infants by eight weeks and continued until the fifth year of life. Pneumococcal vaccine is recommended at 24 months, but alone is not sufficient to prevent sepsis. Dosing of oral penicillin is 125 mg b.i.d. until age three, and 250 mg b.i.d. thereafter. The conjugate *Haemophilus influenzae* type b vaccine is recommended in infancy.[98]

Headaches

Recurrent headaches in the absence of serious underlying pathology may be present in over one-quarter of sickle cell patients. Many of these are of the "vascular" type.[99] A recent survey of 102 Jamaicans, half of whom had SCD, compiled reports of headache from 77% of the SCD group vs. 47% of matched controls. The overall findings pointed to an etiology for orofacial and dental pain which related not to dental pathology but presumably to sickling crises in the facial bones, dental pulps, and small foci of necrosis in bone marrow.[100] Similarly, there are a few reports of skull or marrow infarcts leading to headaches with skull or orbital edema, and sometimes with subperiosteal or epidural hematomas. These are managed conservatively unless the hematomas are large or orbital compression syndrome with optic nerve dysfunction arises, in which case surgical decompression is appropriate.[101–103] Pediatric vascular headache is more common in SCD patients than in others, and those on

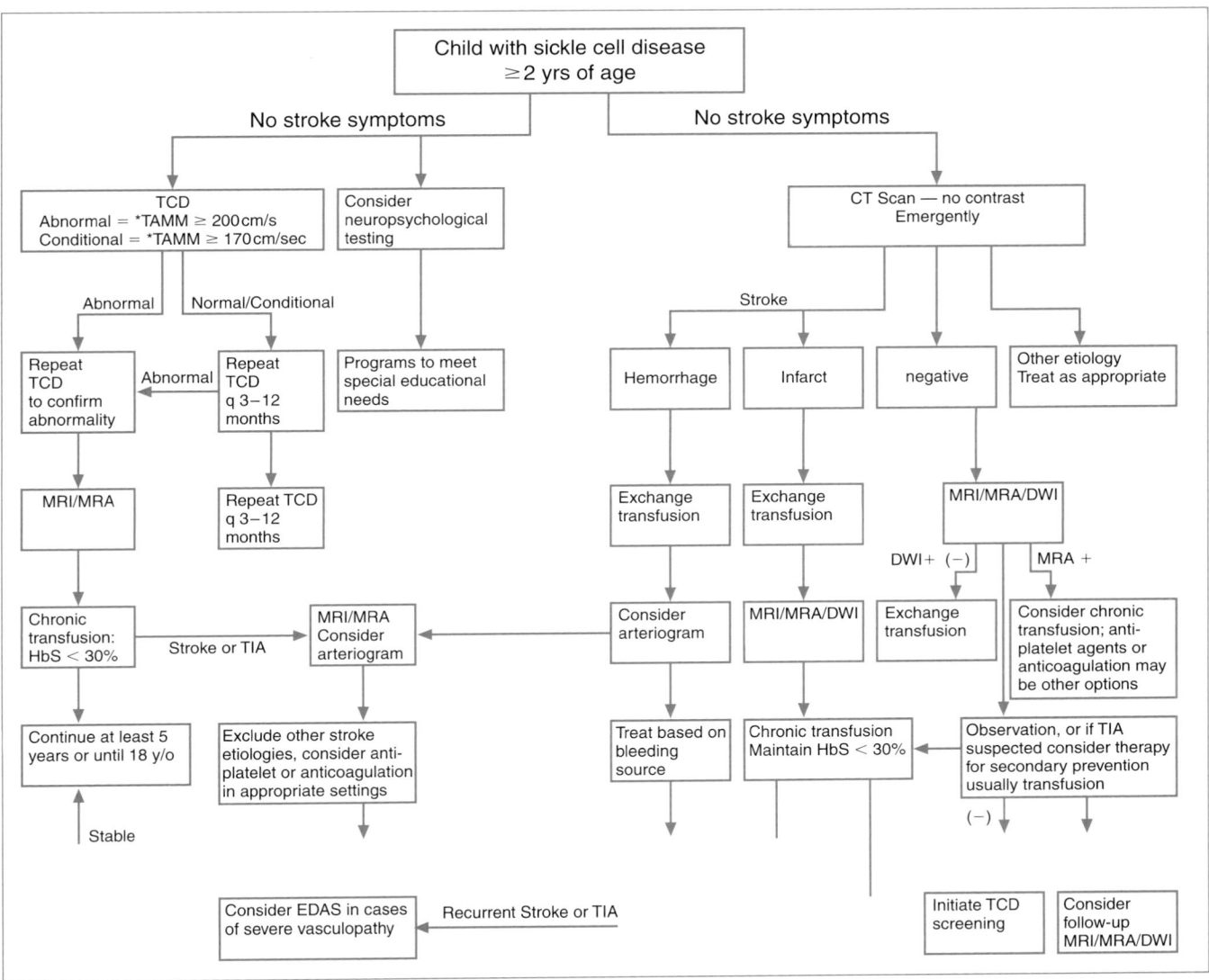

Figure 125.3 Evaluation and treatment algorithm for child sickle cell patient. *TAMM—time-averaged maximum of the mean velocity. The closer this value is to 200 cm/s the more frequently follow-up TCD studies should be done.

transfusion for other indications have reported reduced headache frequency post transfusion, as well as worsening of headaches when chronic transfusion is discontinued. This may suggest a possible relationship between increased cerebral blood flow and vascular headache in SCD.[104] Vascular headache in SCD may be managed with the same acute and prophylactic measures available to patients without SCD; however, some have urged caution in the use of propranolol, tryptans and, presumably, ergots, owing to the prevalence of cerebrovascular disease.[105] Whether a relationship exists between chronic headache and stroke in SCD has not been established. Vigilance for the possibility of acute underlying pathology, such as ICH, is important in compatible presentations.

Neuropathy and myopathy

Peripheral neuropathies are infrequent complications of SCD. Ischemic optic neuropathy[106,107] and mental

and mandibular neuropathies[108–113] are reported. Mononeuropathies involving the limbs are more rare.[114] Children with SCD who suffer lead poisoning may be especially vulnerable to peripheral nerve damage.[115] Recently, three SCD patients with difficulty in walking and nerve conduction study-confirmed sensorimotor neuropathy were described. All had abnormalities of B_{12} coupled with a history of frequent painful crises treated with prolonged nitrous oxide analgesia. The association between nitrous oxide and neuropathy discourages routine use of this modality in the treatment of painful crises.[116]

There is disagreement as to whether a syndrome of myopathy exists in SCD as a consequence of microvascular ischemia in muscle during sickle cell crisis. Four patients suggesting such a syndrome have been presented. These patients had recurrent bouts of proximal muscle pain and swelling with their crises, and chronic muscle induration, atrophy and contrac-

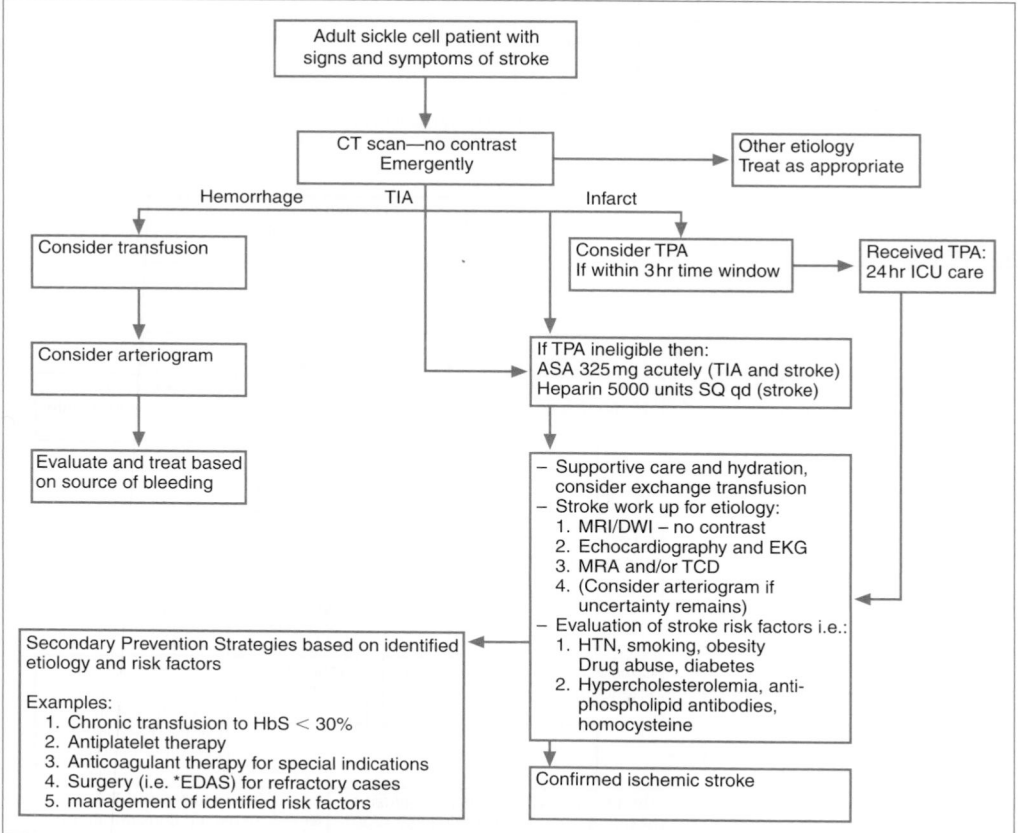

Figure 125.4 Treatment algorithm for adult sickle cell patient with signs and symptoms of stroke. *EDAS = encephaloduro-arteriosynangiosis.

ture resulted. Myonecrosis and fibrosis were seen on muscle biopsy.[117] The exact cause and optimal management of muscle involvement in SCD is unknown. The patients above improved with standard supportive treatment of sickle cell crisis, although the development of compartment syndrome would require fasciotomy.[117,118]

Hearing loss

Two frequent etiologies for hearing loss are seen in SCD. First, ischemia of cranial nerve VIII may cause sensorineural hearing loss in 10% to 15% of patients.[119] Second, largely reversible high-frequency hearing loss is seen in about 30% with long-term desferrioxamine chelation. Because this may be subclinical, baseline and yearly audiometric testing is advisable, with dose reduction in cases of detected abnormality.[120]

References

1. Portnoy BA, Herion JC. Neurologic manifestations in sickle cell disease: with a review of the literature and emphasis in the prevalence of hemiplegia. Ann Intern Med 1972;76:643–652

2. Steinberg MH. Management of sickle cell disease. N Engl J Med 1999;340:1021–1030

3. Steinberg M, Embury S. Natural history: Overview. In: Embury SH, Hebbel RP, Mohandas N, Steinberg M, eds. Sickle Cell Disease: Basic Principles and Practice. New York: Raven Press, 1994:349–352

4. Bunn HF. Pathogenesis and treatment of sickle cell disease. N Engl J Med 1997;337:762–769

5. Schechter AN, Noguchi CT. Sickle hemoglobin polymer: structure–function correlates. In: Embury SH, Hebbel RP, Mohandas N, Steinberg M, eds. Sickle Cell Disease: Basic Principles and Practice. New York: Raven Press, 1994:33–51

6. Mozzarelli A, Holrichter J, Eaton WA. Delay time of HbS polymerization prevents most cells from sickling in vivo. Science 1987;237:500–506

7. Greer M, Schotland D. Abnormal hemoglobin as a cause of neurological disease. Neurology 1962;12: 114–120

8. Powers D, Wilson B, Imbus C, et al. The natural history of stroke in sickle cell disease. Am J Med 1978;65:461–471

9. Sarniak SA, Lusher JM. Neurological complications of sickle cell anemia. Am J Pediatr Hematol Oncol 1982;4:386–394

10. Moohr JW, Wilson H, Pang E. Strokes and their management in sickle cell disease. In: Fried W, ed. Comparative Clinical Aspects of Sickle Cell Disease. New York: Elsevier, 1982:101–111

11. Sergeant G. The nervous system. In: Sergeant G, ed. Sickle Cell Disease. Oxford: Oxford University Press, 1985:233–246

12. Ohene-Frempong K, Weiner SJ, Sleeper LA, et al. Cerebrovascular accidents: rates and risk factors. Blood 1998;91:288–294

13. Kinney TR, Sleeper LA, Wang WC, et al. Silent cerebral infarcts in sickle cell anemia: a risk factor analysis. Pediatrics 1999;103:640–645

14. Moser FG, Miller ST, Bello JA, et al. The spectrum of

brain MR abnormalities in sickle cell disease: a report from the Cooperative Study of Sickle Cell Disease. Am J Neuroradiol 1996;17:965–972

15. Adams RJ, Nichols FT, McKie V, et al. Cerebral infarction in sickle cell anemia: mechanism based on CT and MRI. Neurology 1988;38:1012–1017

16. Adams RJ, Neurologic complications. In: Embury SH, Hebbel RP, Mohandas N, Steinberg M, eds. Sickle Cell Disease: Basic Principles and Practice. New York: Raven Press, 1994:599–621

17. Van Hoff J, Ritchey AK, Shaywitz BA. Intracranial hemorrhage in children with sickle cell disease. Am J Dis Child 1985;139:1120–1122

18. Powers D, Adams RJ, Nichols FT, et al. Delayed intracranial hemorrhage following cerebral infarction in sickle cell anemia. J Assoc Acad Minor Phys 1990;1:79–82

19. Wood DH. Cerebrovascular complications of sickle cell anemia. Stroke 1978;9:73–75

20. Carey J, Numaguchi Y, Nadell J. Subarachnoid hemorrhage in sickle cell disease. Childs Nerv Syst 1990;6:647–650

21. Love LC, Mickle JP, Sypert GW. Ruptured intracranial aneurysms in cases of sickle cell anemia. Neurosurgery 1985;16:808–812

22. Anson JA, Koshy M, Ferguson L, Crowell RM. Subarachnoid hemorrhage in sickle cell disease. Hematology 1991;75:552–558

23. Preul MC, Cendes F, Just N, Mohr G. Intracranial aneurysms and sickle cell anemia: multiplicity and propensity for vertebrobasilar territory. Neurosurgery 1998;42:971–977

24. Oyesiku NM, Barrow DL, Eckman JR, et al. Intracranial aneurysms in sickle cell anemia: clinical features and pathogenesis. J Neurosurg 1991;75:356–363

25. Diggs LW, Brookoff D. Multiple cerebral aneurysms in patients with sickle cell disease. South Med J 1993;86:377–379

26. Russell MO, Goldberg HI, Hodson A, et al. Effect of transfusion therapy on arteriographic abnormalities and on recurrence of stroke in sickle cell disease. Blood 1984;4:162–169

27. Wilimas J, Goff JR, Anderson HR, et al. Efficacy of transfusion for one to two years in patients with sickle cell disease and cerebrovascular accidents. J Pediatr 1980;96:205–208

28. Jeffries BF, Lipper MH, Kishore PRF. Major intracerebral involvement in sickle cell disease. Surg Neurol 1980;14:291–295

29. Gerald B, Sebes JI, Langston JW. Cerebral infarction secondary to sickle cell disease: arteriographic findings. Am J Radiol 1980;134:1209–1212

30. Baird RL, Weiss DL, Ferguson AD, et al. Studies in sickle cell anemia: XII clinico-pathological aspects of neurological manifestations. Pediatrics 1964;34:92–100

31. Seeler RA, Royal JE, Powe L, Goldbarg HR. Moya Moya in children with sickle cell anemia and cerebrovascular occlusion. J Pediatr 1978;93:808–810

32. Suzuki J, Takaku A. Cerebrovascular moya moya disease: disease showing abnormal net-like vessels in the base of the brain. Arch Neurol 1969;20:288–299

33. Hess DC, Adams RJ, Nichols FT. Sickle cell anemia and other hemoglobinopathies. Semin Neurol 1991;11:314–328

34. Merkel KHH, Ginsberg PL, Parker JC, Post MJD. Cerebrovascular disease in sickle cell anemia: a clinical pathological and radiological correlation. Stroke 1978;9:45–52

35. Rothman SM, Fulling KH, Nelson JS. Sickle cell anemia and central nervous system infarction a neuropathological study. Ann Neurol 1986;20:684–690

36. Stehbens WE. Localization of atherosclerotic lesions in relation to hemodynamics. In: Olson AG, ed. Atherosclerosis: Biology and Clinical Science. New York: Churchill Livingstone, 1987:175–182

37. Kaul DK, Fabry ME, Nagel RL. The pathophysiology of vascular obstruction. Blood Rev 1996;10:29–44

38. Solovey A, Gui L, Key NS, Hebbel RP. Tissue factor expression by endothelial cells in sickle sell anemia. J Clin Invest 1998;101:1899–1904

39. Solovey A, Lin Y, Browne P, et al. Circulating activated endothelial cells in sickle cell anemia. N Engl J Med 1997;337:1584–1590

40. Hebbel RP. Adhesive interactions if sickle erythrocytes with endothelium. J Clin Invest 1997;99:2561–2564

41. Barabino GA, Wise RJ, Woodbury VA, et al. Inhibition of sickle erythrocyte adhesion to immobilized thrombospondin by von Willebrand factor under dynamic flow conditions. Blood 1997;89:2560–2567

42. Westerman MP, Green D, Gilman-Sacks A, et al. Antiphospholipid antibodies, proteins C and S and coagulation changes in sickle cell disease. J Clin Invest 1999;134:352–362

43. Pegelow CH, Adams RJ, Mckie V, et al. Risk of recurrent stroke in patients with sickle cell disease treated with erythrocyte transfusions. J Pediatr 1995;126:896–899

44. Adams RJ, Mckie VC, Hsu L, et al. Prevention of first stroke by transfusions in children with sickle sell anemia and abnormal results on transcranial ultrasonography. N Engl J Med 1998;339:5–11

45. National Heart, Lung and Blood Institute, Department of Health and Human Services. Clinical Alert. 18 September 1997

46. Wayne AS, Kevy SV, Nathan DG. Transfusion management of sickle cell disease. Blood 1993;81:1109–1123

47. Rosse WR, Gallagher D, Kinney TR, et al. Transfusion and alloimmunization in sickle cell disease. Blood 1990;76:1431–1437

48. Powers D. Management of cerebral vasculopathy in children with sickle cell anemia. Br J Haematol (in press)

49. Andrews NC. Disorders of iron metabolism. N Engl J Med 1999;341:1986–1995

50. Brittenham GM, Farrell DE, Harris JW, et al. Magnetic-susceptibility measurement of human iron store. N Engl J Med 1982;307:1671–1675

51. Olivieri NF. The β-Thalassemias. N Engl J Med 1999;341:99–109

52. Cohen AR, Martin MB, Silber JH, et al. A modified transfusion program for prevention of stroke in sickle cell disease. Blood 1992;79:1657–1661

53. Miller ST, Jensen D, Rao SP. Less intensive long-term transfusion therapy for sickle cell anemia and cerebrovascular accident. J Pediatr 1992;79:1657–1661

54. Rana S, Houston PE, Surana N, et al. Discontinuation of long term transfusion therapy in patients with sickle cell disease and stroke. J Pediatr 1997;131:757–760

55. Wang WC, Kovnar EH, Tonkin IL, et al. High risk of recurrent stroke after discontinuation of five to twelve years of transfusion therapy in patients with sickle cell disease. J Pediatr 1991;118:377–382

56. Ware WE, Zimmerman SA, Schultz WH. Hydroxyurea as an alternative to blood transfusions for the prevention of recurrent stroke in children with sickle cell disease. Blood 1999;94:3022–3026

57. Charache S, Lubin B, Reid CD. Management and therapy of sickle cell disease. Washington DC: US Dept of Health and Human Services Public Health Service, National Institutes of Health. Publication No. 92–2117, 1992: p.22

58. Platt OS, Thorington BD, Brambilla DJ, et al. Pain in sickle cell disease: rates and risk factors. N Engl J Med 1991:325:11–16

59. Charache S, Terrin ML, Moore RD, et al. Effect of hydroxyurea on the frequency of painful crisis in sickle cell anemia. N Engl J Med 1995;332:1317–1322

60. Ballas SK, Marcolina MJ, Dover GJ, Barton FB. Erythropoietic activity in patients with sickle cell anaemia before and after treatment with hydroxyurea. Br J Haematol 1999;105:491–496

61. Bridges KR, Barabino GD, Brugnara C, et al. A multiparameter analysis of sickle erythrocytes in patients undergoing hydroxyurea therapy. Blood 1996;88: 4701–4710

62. Saleh AW, Hillen HF, Duits AJ. Levels of endothelial, neutrophil and platelet-specific factors in sickle cell anemia patients during hydroxyurea therapy. Acta Haematol 1999;102:31–37

63. Styles LA, Lubin B, Vichinsky E, et al. Decrease of very late activation of antigen-4 and CD-36 on reticulocytes in sickle cell patients treated with hydroxyurea. Blood 1997;89:2554–2559

64. Kinney TR, Helms RW, O'Branski EE, et al. Safety of hydroxyurea in children with sickle cell disease: results of the Hug-Kids Study, a phase I/II trial. Pediatric hydroxyurea group. Blood 1999;94:1550–1554

65. Charache S, Barton FB, Moore RD, et al. Hydroxyurea and sickle cell anemia clinical utility of a myelosuppressive "switching" agent: the multicenter study of hydroxyurea in sickle cell anemia. Medicine (Baltimore) 1996;75:300–326

66. Miller ST, Sleeper LA, Pegelow CH, et al. Prediction of adverse outcomes in children with sickle cell disease. N Engl J Med 2000;342:82–89

67. Walters MC, Storb R, Patience M, et al. Impact of bone marrow transplantation for symptomatic sickle cell disease: an interim report. Blood 2000;95: 1918–1924

68. Walters MC. Bone marrow transplantation for sickle cell disease: where do we go from here? J Pediatr Hematol Oncol 1999;21:467–474

69. Walters MC, Sullivan KM, Bernaudin F, et al. Neurologic complications after allogeneic marrow transplantation for sickle cell anemia. Blood 1995;85:879–884

70. Ferster A, Christophe C, Dan B, et al. Neurologic complications after bone marrow transplantation for sickle cell anemia. Blood 1995;86:408–409

71. Abboud MR, Jackson SM, Barredo J, et al. Neurologic complications following bone marrow transplant for sickle cell disease. Bone Marrow Transplant 1996; 17:405–407

72. Bernaudin F. Results and current indications of bone marrow allograft in sickle cell disease. Pathol Biol (Paris) 1999;47:59–64

73. Vermylen C, Cornu G, Ferster A, et al. Haematopoietic stem cell transplantation for sickle cell anemia: the first 50 patients transplanted in Belgium. Bone Marrow Transplant 1998;22:1–6

74. Karsson S. The first steps on the gene therapy pathway to anti-sickling process. Nature Med 2000;6:139–140

75. Blouin M-J, Beauchemin H, Wright A, et al. Genetic correction of sickle cell disease: insights using transgenic models. Nature Med 2000;6:177–182

76. Albers GW, Easton JD, Sacco RL, Teal P. Antithrombotic and thrombolytic therapy for ischemic stroke. Chest 1998;114(Suppl):683S–698S

77. Adams HP, Brott TG, Furlan AJ, et al. Guidelines for thrombolytic therapy for acute stroke: a supplement to the guidelines for the management of patients with acute ischemic stroke. A statement for healthcare professionals from a special writing group of the stroke council, American Heart Association. Stroke 1996; 27:1711–1718

78. Wolf PA, Clagett GP, Easton JD, et al. Preventing ischemic stroke in patients with prior stroke and transient ischemic attack: a statement for healthcare professionals from the stroke council of the American Heart Association. Stroke 1999;30:1991–1994

79. Adams RJ. Update on sickle cell disease. Neurologist 2000;6:12–17

80. Vernet O, Montes JL, O'Gorman AM, et al. Encephaloduroarteriosynangiosis in a child with sickle cell disease and moyamoya disease. Pediatr Neurol 1996;14:226–230

81. Houston PE, Rana S, Sekhsaria S, et al. Homocysteine in sickle cell disease: relationship to stroke. Am J Med 1997;103:192–196

82. Balasa V, Gruppo R, Gartside PS, Kalinyak KA. Correlation of the C677T MTHFR genotype with homocysteine levels in children with sickle cell disease. J Pediatr Hematol Oncol 1999;21:397–400

83. Perry IJ, Refsum H, Morris RW, et al. Prospective study of serum homocysteine concentration and risk of stroke in middle aged British men. Lancet 1995;346:1395–1398

84. Armstrong F, Thompson R, Wang W, et al. Cognitive functioning and brain magnetic resonance imaging in children with sickle cell disease. Pediatrics 1996;97: 864–870

85. Steen RG, Xiong X, Mulhern JW, et al. Subtle brain abnormalities in children with sickle cell disease: relationship to blood hematocrit. Ann Neurol 1999;45: 279–286

86. Steen RG, Reddick WE, Mulhern RK, et al. Quantitative MRI of the brain in children with SCD reveals abnormalities unseen by conventional MRI. Magn Reson Imag 1998;8:535–543

87. Steen RG, Langston JW, Ogg RJ, et al. Diffuse T1 reduction in gray matter of sickle cell disease patients: evidence of selective vulnerability to damage? Magn Reson Imag 1999;17:503–515

88. Wang Z, Zimmerman R, Sauter R. Proton MR spectroscopy of the brain: clinically useful information obtained in assessing CNS disease in children. Am J Radiol 1996;167:191–199

89. Reed W, Jagust W, Al-Mateen M, Vichinsky E. Positron emission tomography in determining the extent of CNS ischemia in patients with sickle cell disease. Am J Hematol 1999;60:268–272

90. Powers DR, Conti PS, Wong W-Y, et al. Cerebral vasculopathy in sickle cell anemia: diagnostic contribution of positron emission tomography. Blood 1999;93:71–79

91. DeBaun MR, Schatz J, Siegel MJ, et al. Cognitive screening examinations for silent cerebral infarcts in sickle cell disease. Neurology 1998;50:1678–1682

92. Liu JE, Gzesh DJ, Ballas SK. The spectrum of epilepsy in sickle cell anemia. J Neurol Sci 1994;123:6–10

93. Robinson MG, Watson RJ. Pneumococcal meningitis in sickle cell anemia. N Engl J Med 1966;274:1006–1008

94. Overturf GD, Powers D, Baraff LJ. Bacterial meningitis

and septicemia in sickle cell disease. Am J Dis Child 1977;131:784–787

95. Gaston MH, Verter JI, Woods G, et al. Prophylaxis with oral penicillin in children with sickle cell anemia: a randomized trial. N Engl J Med 1986;25:1593–1599

96. Falletta JM, Woods GM, Verter JI. Discontinuing penicillin prophylaxis in patients with sickle cell anemia. J Pediatr 1995;127:685–690

97. Pai VB, Nahata M. Duration of penicillin prophylaxis in sickle cell anemia: issues and controversies. Pharmacotherapy 2000;20:110–117

98. Murphy TV, White KL, Pastor P, et al. Declining incidence of *Haemophilus influenzae* type b disease since introduction of the vaccination. JAMA 1993;269:246–248

99. Pavlakis SG, Prohovnic I, Piomelli S, DeVivo DC. Neurologic complications of sickle cell disease. Adv Pediatr 1989;36:247–276

100. O'Rourke CA, Hawley GM. Sickle cell disorder and orofacial pain in Jamaican patients. Br Dent J 1998;185:90–92

101. Resar LM, Oliva MM, Casella JF. Skull infarction and epidural hematomas in a patient with sickle cell anemia. J Pediatr Hematol Oncol 1996;18:413–415

102. Curran EL, Flemming JC, Rice K, Wang WC. Orbital compression syndrome in sickle cell disease. Ophthalmology 1997;104:1610–1615

103. Pari G, Schipper HM. Headache and scalp edema in sickle cell disease. Can J Neurol Sci 1996;23:224–226

104. Al-Mateen M, DeGraca A, Koblenz L, Vichinsky E. Headaches in children with sickle cell anemia. Neurology 1995;45(Suppl 4):A348 [Abstract]

105. Salman MS. Migraine and sickle cell disorders: is there a cause for concern? Med Hypoth 1996;46:569–571

106. Lana-Peixoto MA, Barbosa A. Anterior ischaemic optic neuropathy in a child with AS haemoglobinopathy and migraine. Br J Ophthalmol 1998;82:199–200

107. Perlman JI, Forman S, Gonzalez ER. Retrobulbar ischemic optic neuropathy associated with sickle cell disease. J Neuroophthalmol 1994;14:45–48

108. Gregory G, Olujohungbe A. Mandibular nerve neuropathy in sickle cell disease. Local factors. Oral Surg Oral Med Oral Pathol 1994;77:66–69

109. Cherry-Peppers G, Davis V, Atkinson JC. Sickle cell anemia: a case report and literature review. Clin Prev Dent 1992;14:5–9

110. Seeler RA, Royal JE. Mental nerve neuropathy in a child with sickle cell anemia. Am J Pediatr Hematol Oncol 1982;4:212–213

111. Friedlander AH, Genser L, Swerdloff M. Mental nerve neuropathy: a complication of sickle-cell crisis. Oral Surg Oral Med Oral Pathol 1980;49:15–17

112. Konotey-Ahulu FI. Mental-nerve neuropathy: a complication of sickle-cell crisis. Lancet 1972;2:338

113. Kirson LE, Tomaro AJ. Mental nerve paresthesia secondary to sickle cell crisis. Oral Surg 1979;48:509–512

114. Shields RW Jr, Harris JW, Clark M. Mononeuropathy in sickle cell anemia: anatomical and pathophysiological basis for its rarity. Muscle Nerve 1991;14:370–374

115. Imbus CE, Warner J, Smith E, et al. Peripheral neuropathy in lead-intoxicated sickle cell patients. Muscle Nerve 1978;1:168–171

116. Ogundipe O, Pearson MW, Slater NG, et al. Sickle cell disease and nitrous oxide-induced neuropathy. Clin Lab Haematol 1999;21:409–412

117. Valeriano-Marcet J, Kerr LD. Myonecrosis and myofibrosis as complications of sickle cell anemia. Ann Intern Med 1991;115:99–101

118. Dorwart BB, Gabuzda TG. Symmetric myositis and fasciitis: a complication of sickle cell anemia during vasoocclusion. J Rheumatol 1985;12:590–595

119. Sergeant GR. The Nervous System in Sickle Cell Disease, 2nd edn. Oxford: Oxford University Press, 1992:292–314

120. Styles LA, Vichinsky EP. Ototoxity in hemoglobinopathy patients chelated with desferrioxamine. J Pediatr Hematol Oncol 1966;18:42–45

126 Therapy of the Neurological Complications of Lymphoma and Leukemia

Fred H Hochberg and Roberto Ciordia

Overview

Approximately 55 000 new cases of non-Hodgkin's systemic lymphoma will be diagnosed in United States in the year 2000.[1] Neurologists are exposed to the complications of these in addition to those of Hodgkin's disease and acute leukemia. On the shoulders of these clinicians falls the burden of the neurological syndromes associated with the direct involvement of the brain, spinal cord and nerve roots; the non-metastatic complications (paraneoplastic illnesses, toxicity) and the effects of ionizing radiation and chemotherapy. By providing descriptions of the clinical syndromes and their treatment we offer the basics for appropriate therapy. No consensus exists as to the therapy of many of the neuraxis complications of lymphoma and leukemia.

Hodgkin's lymphoma (HD) and non-Hodgkin's lymphoma (NHL)

Neurological involvement occurs in advanced-stage disease (IV or IV B) and commonly with disease in recurrence (Table 126.1). Less than 1% of HD patients have intracranial involvement. When this occurs it is usually dural based[2] and involves the calvarium and the dural membrane, but does not enter the subarachnoid space. Approximately 5% of patients develop spinal cord compression,[3] most frequently in the thoracic or lumbar spine. When this occurs, retropleural or retroperitoneal masses erode into a vertebral body or through an intervertebral foramen. In comparison, NHL involvement of the brain occurs in 10% of patients, as many as 50% of Burkitt's lymphoma cases, and 15% of mycosis fungoides cases with or without Sézary's syndrome. Spinal cord involvement appears in 4%. Tumor infiltrates commonly emerge from contiguous vertebrae or lymph nodes. However, NHL, a remarkable neuraxis-seeking disease, can invade the nervous system in unique ways.

Metastatic NHL to the nervous system Although HD is unlikely to involve brain parenchyma or eye or spinal fluid, NHL patients are at risk of all three types of neuraxis invasion. Common as a late effect of primary testicular NHL, brain involvement is usually multifocal, with the CSF likely to be coincidentally involved.

Primary central nervous system lymphoma represents 2% of all primary neuraxis tumors. Patients with prior immunosuppression (AIDS, organ transplantation, prior steroid or chemotherapy use) develop multiple MRI-enhancing masses in close proximity to the ventricular system. The masses produce psychotic thought disorders or abnormalities of fluid balance (SIADH or diabetes insipidus as a result of peri-third ventricular lesions), seizure activity or alterations of memory and mood. These lesions occur in the absence of known systemic lymphoma.

Neurolymphomatosis results from NHL infiltrates within the intradural and extradural nerve roots. These may be in cranial nerves to produce painless involvement of facial movements (Bell's palsy), visual abnormalities (optic nerve), auditory defects or alterations of facial sensation. These infiltrates may appear absent invasion of brain parenchyma or spinal fluid. As common are painful infiltrates of nerve roots in the extradural cervical or lumbar spinal cord. The tumor cells, without contiguous adenopathy, lead to paresis of extremities in the setting of electrical lancinating pain. The afflicted root sleeves are both thick and enhance on gadolinium-injected MRI studies.

Intravascular lymphoma, or angioendotheliomatosis, reflects intraluminal foci of malignant clonal lymphocytes in small arterioles and capillaries of the brain and spinal cord. Also involved are the skin (a violaceous raised papule) and adrenal glands. Fever, "B symptoms" and neutropenia with thrombocytopenia coexist, but scanning procedures to identify chest or abdominal extranodal deposits or bone marrow biopsies are futile. Tumor foci within vessels of the brain produce stroke-like syndromes. The afflicted brain appears abnormal on diffusion-weighted MRI images.

Eye lymphoma involves the orbital cone as an extranodal B-cell mass. The vitreous and retina are afflicted either before or after diagnosis of brain involvement in 15% of patients.

Richter's syndrome is the lymphomatous conversion of chronic lymphocytic leukemia.[4]

Table 126.1   Neurologic complications of lymphoma and leukemia

Disease stage	Neuraxis involvement	Symptoms	Diagnostic procedure	Staging after diagnosis
Non-Hodgkin's lymphoma Hodgkin's lymphoma	Brain mass	Focal deficits, seizures, headaches	MRI with gadolinium-enhancing mass Stereotactic biopsy	Slit lamp examination of eye CSF if possible Systemic restage
	Vitreal or retinal lymphoma	Blurred vision, floaters, eye pain	Slit lamp examination Vitreal aspirate or vitrectomy Fluorescent cell sorting	Brain MRI
Lymphoma or leukemia	Spinal cord compression—epidural mass	Back pain, bladder paresis, leg weakness	MRI—whole spine CT vertebrae for bone stability CT retro—thorax or peritoneum	Brain MRI
Lymphoma or leukemia	Meningeal disease—meningeal lymphoma/ventricular lymphoma	Diplopia, confusion, bladder or radicular symptoms	Brain MRI—to exclude mass CSF—fluorescent cell sorting/cytology	[111]In scan MRI of spine for nodular disease
	Peripheral nerve or root infiltration—neurolymphomatosis	Cranial or peripheral root pain or deficit(s)	MRI—contrast coronal images Nerve root biopsy	CSF studies Brain MRI if not already done
	Nasopharynx lymphoma	**NOTE**	Coronal MRI through sinuses Biopsy	Brain MRI with contrast
	Stroke from intravascular lymphoma	Multifocal brain and/or eye involved	Brain MRI—diffusion weighted Stereotactic biopsy of brain	Skin examination and CT of adrenal glands
	Stroke secondary to L-asparaginase	Multifocal brain and/or eye involved	Brain MRI—diffusion weighted	MRI venogram or CT venogram of large vessels and lung Coagulation studies
	Stroke from circulating anticoagulant or endocarditis	Multifocal brain and/or eye involved	Brain MRI—diffusion weighted	Echocardiogram Coagulation studies
	Paraneoplastic—cerebellar degeneration, Guillain–Barré, myelopathy	Ataxia, weakness in legs or four extremities	Serologies for anti-Hu, Ri, Yo	
	Toxic effects of chemotherapy	Distal sensory deficit with pain	1. EMG	

Direct infiltration of the central nervous system

Leptomeningeal disease

This is the most frequent neurological complication in NHL. Patients develop headache, deficits of the facial, trigeminal or optic cranial nerves, or altered mentation. Cerebrospinal fluid (CSF) cells are abnormal in appearance or monoclonal on immunochemical studies. Immunoglobulin gene rearrangement can be demonstrated using consensus polymerase chain reaction (PCR) primers, or monoclonal populations demonstrated by fluorescent activated cell sorting techniques.

Treatment of free-floating cells provides intrathecal (IT) drug (methotrexate 12 mg in 8 mL Ringer's lactate twice weekly, *or* cytarabine 50 mg in 8 mL Ringer's lactate) administered via lumbar puncture or Ommaya reservoir. A recent development is liposomal cytarabine (50 mg every two weeks with systemic steroids) or high-dose intravenous systemic methotrexate (MTX) 8 g/m². Radiation (40 Gy in fractions of 1.8 Gy) is provided for localized symptomatic or nodular or bulky disease not likely responsive to intrathecal drugs. The authors' own predisposition is towards high-dose intravenous MTX therapy. This reflects the frequent disorders of CSF percolation in the setting of dense clusters of leptomeningeal tumor. Intrathecal drugs may not reach the symptomatic cranial nerve locations if administered through lumbar routes, nor the lumbar root involvement if provided through an Ommaya catheter. Both approaches carry the risk of providing unacceptably high levels of chemotherapy at the injection site. Both leukoencephalopathy and radiculopathy have been reported after MTX or ARA-C administration into the CSF. Lastly, spinal fluid administration does not penetrate into tumor nodules larger than several millimeters, a situation not likely to be the case following high-dose venous administration.

Epidural lymphoma

Epidural lymphoma causes back pain and leg weakness. Fat-saturated gadolinium scans of the entire spine disclose both the level(s) of tumor and the changes in contiguous cord and nerve roots. Emergency therapy mandates the use of **dexamethasone** (100 mg i.v. followed by 24 mg/6 h for three days) to reduce edema of the spinal cord and lyse contiguous tumor.[5] Unmeasured are the benefits of **mannitol** (50–100 g i.v.) and equivocal[6] are the benefits of **surgery**, which is indicated for tissue diagnosis, maintenance of spine stability, or for radiation therapy failure. **Radiation therapy** (Table 126.2) is an emergency therapy: 2 Gy in 20 fractions to 40 Gy[7] will preserve gait in three-quarters of patients treated immediately upon diagnosis. Sporadic responses are reported to systemic chemotherapy (ABVD, or ProMACE-CytaBOM)[8] when irradiation has failed or cannot be provided.

Prophylactic treatment of brain or meninges is provided for lymphoma of testicular, eye, or cranial sinus origin.[9,10] Some experimental therapies for systemic lymphoma require neuraxis prophylaxis. This can be achieved with intrathecal MTX (12 g weekly for five doses) or MTX and cytarabine or methotrexate i.v. (3.5 g/m^2). Patients in whom the lymphoma involves the skull base or cranial sinus, who have an approximately one-quarter chance of brain or cranial nerve involvement, are better protected from central nervous system involvement when the prophylactic treatment is whole-brain radiation therapy (WBXRT) 36 Gy at 1.8 Gy/day in 20 fractions.

Non-infiltrating brain or spinal cord involvement

Paraneoplastic syndromes

Paraneoplastic syndromes can result in **cerebellar degeneration** (Hodgkin's disease) with ataxia. Weakness can reflect **subacute motor neuropathy**, **motor neuron disease**, similar to amyotrophic lateral sclerosis, and **polyradiculopathy**, whose motor difficulties are similar to those of Guillain–Barré syndrome. In general, the proximal leg muscles are afflicted first. Weakness is followed by a syndrome not unlike paraparesis with areflexia. Sensory findings are few. The diagnosis is often made because of the absence of MRI abnormalities suggesting direct tumor infiltration, and the lack of identified tumor cells in CSF. Several serum markers (Yo, Hu, Ma) may serve as surrogates of the paraneoplastic syndrome, but commercial assays detect these in fewer than 20% of patients. Optimal therapy involves treatment of the underlying lymphoma and the exclusion of direct involvement. The inflammatory disorders, polyradiculopathy and cerebellar, sometimes respond to high doses of methylprednisolone (1000 mg i.v. for five days), and anecdotal reports exist of efficacious treatment of the others with immunoglobulin (0.5 g/kg/day i.v. for five days) or plasmapheresis.

The leukemias

The leptomeninges and spinal fluid are sanctuaries for leukemia. For patients with **acute lymphocytic leukemia (ALL)** prophylaxis of these areas with radiation has reduced to 9% the previously reported 75% risk of neuraxis invasion.[11] The radiation approaches result in late toxicities, apparent at two years, and include bone marrow suppression, neuroendocrine difficulties (elevated prolactin level with amenorrhea or impotence *or* Addison's disease) and memory difficulties. For children with ALL, unfavorable prognostic factors include age less than one or more than 10 years, more than five leukoblasts per milliliter of spinal fluid, and peripheral white blood cell count above 50 000. It is likely that the immunophenotype of B- and T-cell stage correlates with risk of neuraxis involvement. A low risk of neuraxis invasion is associated with ALL of B-cell precursors; standard risk is associated with T-cell leukemia, and high-risk with rearrangements of t(9;22), or MLL or BCR-ABL fusion proteins combining with genes. For adults with ALL the unfavorable factors are male gender, non-white race, age under 30 years at diagnosis, white blood cell count more than 50 000, splenomegaly, serum lactate dehydrogenase (LDH) level higher than 600 U/mL, high leukemic cell proliferation index, and short duration of first remission.[12] At special risk are those patients with T-cell immunophenotype, those with mature B-cell (Burkitt type) (usually possessing translocations t(8;14), t(8;22) and t(2;8) or FAB-L3 surface immunoglobulin), and those with Philadelphia chromosome translocation, t(9;22). The nuclear marker TdT, present on cells within CSF, is probably pathognomonic of meningeal infiltration.

Patients with AML (acute myeloid leukemia) classified into eight types (M0 to M7). Those with M4 and M5 types have a 30% incidence of CNS involvement, compared to 5% for those with M1, M2, M6 or M7.

Prophylaxis for patients at high or intermediate risk of CNS involvement has been provided with intrathecal MTX or MTX in combination with cytarabine and steroids. For children with ALL the most logical prophylaxis, providing five-year control in all but 5% of patients, is achieved with the latter (methotrexate 15 mg/m^2 or less than 15 mg, cytarabine 30 mg/m^2 or less than 60 mg and prednisone 60 mg/m^2) twice a week for each of three weeks and every eight weeks for 17 additional doses. Similar rates of control of potential disease, but higher rates of neurotoxicity, are associated with the provision of combinations of intrathecal and intravenous methotrexate *or* intrathecal MTX alone (Pediatric Oncology Group 9005) or parenteral MTX and triple intrathecal prophylaxis.[13] Whole-brain XRT (24 Gy at 2 Gy/day in 12 fractions) also provides appropriate prophylaxis in adults and in the high-risk pediatric population (18 Gy at 1.8 Gy/day in 10 fractions).

Leptomeningeal leukemia

ALL and AML spread to the subarachnoid space through the choroid plexus or veins within the cortical

Table 126.2   Therapy of leukemia or lymphoma involving the neuraxis

Disease stage	Involvement	Primary therapy	Secondary therapy	Experimental therapy
Non-Hodgkin's lymphoma Hodgkin's lymphoma	Brain mass	Methotrexate 8 g/m^2 i.v. q10d until resolution	Cranial radiation (1.8–40 Gy)	1. Topotecan 1.5 mg/m^2 for 5 days every 3 weeks 2. MAB anti-CD20 (rituxamab) 375 or 500 mg/m^2 i.v. q wk for 4–8 doses
	Vitreal or retinal lymphoma	Radiation 18–30 Gy to posterior orbit	Intraocular methotrexate at 400 µg/every 3 days until resolution	High doses i.v. MTX
	Spinal cord compression —epidural mass	**Emergency:** • **Dexamethasone 100 mg i.v. then 24 mg q.i.d.** • Mannitol 25 g every 4 h • **Radiation 1.8 Gy for 20 fractions to 36 Gy**	Surgical decompression for: • Spinal stability • Tissue diagnosis	Systemic chemotherapy— CHOP (NHL) or ABVD (HD)
	Meningeal disease, meningeal lymphoma/ ventricular lymphoma	• Methotrexate 12.5 mg intrathecal (lumbar or Ommaya) every 3 days until resolution of cells • Depocyte (Depo ARA-C) as 50 mg intrathecal every 14 days with dexamethasone 4 mg/day for meningitis prophylaxis	1. Methotrexate 8 g/m^2 every 7–10 days i.v. 2. Radiation (30 Gy) for nodular disease or symptomatic disease	Mafosfamide 4–20 mg once or twice weekly until remission achieved
	Peripheral nerve or root infiltration Neurolymphomatosis Nasopharyngeal lymphoma	Methotrexate 8 g/m^2 i.v. every 7–10 days WBXRT for brain prophylaxis, 36 Gy at 1.8 Gy/day in 20 fractions	1. Topotecan 1.5 mg/m^2/day i.v. for 5 days every 3 weeks	
	Stroke from intravascular lymphoma Stroke secondary to L-asparaginase	Methotrexate 8 g/m^2 i.v. every 7–10 days • Fresh frozen plasma and cryoprecipitate • Stop L-asparaginase		
	Stroke secondary to paraprotein hyperviscosity Stroke from circulating anticoagulant or endocarditis	Plasmapheresis Possible use of anticoagulation (i.v. heparin or S.Q. low weight heparin)		
	Paraneoplastic—cerebellar degeneration, Guillain– Barré, myelopathy	• Therapy for underlying lymphoma • Dexamethasone 6 mg q 8 h • Intravenous immunoglobulin (IVIG) 0.4 g/kg i.v. daily for 3 days or 0.5 g/kg/day from days 1–5	1. Plasmapheresis: 4 L/day inline at 2/week for 3 weeks, then IVIG 2. Cytoxan	1. Staphylococcal protein A absorption
Leukemia	Prophylaxis:	• *Low-risk patient: IT MTX 12.5 mg/m^2 or TIT (MTX 15 mg/m^2, ARA-C 30 mg/m^2, hydrocortisone 15 mg/m^2) • †High-risk patient: Craniospinal radiation 18–24 Gy		
	Meningeal leukemia	• IT methotrexate or TIT • WBXRT 24 Gy in 12 fractions • IT maintenance (MTX or TIT)	1. IT methotrexate or TIT (26 total doses) 2. Craniospinal XRT	Autologous bone marrow transplantation (ABMT)
	Epidural disease—leukemia or chloroma CNS Aspergillosis	Radiation 40 Gy at 2 Gy/ fraction in 20 fractions Liposomal amphotericin B		

*Low risk of neuraxis invasion is associated with ALL of B-cell precursors.
†High risk of neuraxis invasion is associated with age less than 1 year or more than 10 years, more than five leukoblasts per mL of spinal fluid, and peripheral white blood cell count above 50 000. For adults with ALL unfavorable factors are male gender, non-white race, age under 30 years at diagnosis, white blood cell count higher than 50 000, splenomegaly, serum lactate dehydrogenase (LDH) level higher than 600 U/mL, high leukemic cell proliferation index and short duration of first remission.[39] At special risk are those patients with T-cell immunophenotype, those with mature B-cell (Burkitt type) as well as the following rearrangements t(9;22), or MLL or BCR-ABL fusion, translocations t(8;14), t(8;22) and t(2;8) or FAB-L3 surface immunoglobulin).

sulci. Presumably the cells are capable of passing through these thin-walled vessels. The meningeal infiltrates occur in addition to neurological symptoms,[15] which occur in one-quarter of ALL patients. These symptoms, which require symptomatic therapy, include migraine or CSF hyperproduction. When meningeal leukemia occurs the diagnosis is heralded by headache with double vision, facial numbness or radicular complaints. Adults are usually afflicted by AML or CML (chronic myeloid leukemia), whereas children suffer ALL. The CSF from the lumbar or ventricular locations may be sampled three times to achieve diagnosis. The specimens are sent for Cytospin cytological evaluation or immunohistochemical diagnosis[14] or cell sorting[15] for confirmation. Less accurate are diagnoses based on enhanced MRI demonstration of nodular disease. These changes may also reflect infection or the effects of numerous samples of CSF and the resulting "low-pressure syndrome." Following diagnosis, many clinicians perform cisternograms using indium-111 (^{111}In) which is injected into the lumbar CSF. Sequential scans delineate regions of the CSF circulation with localized diminished flow as a result of tumor foci. These areas are not likely to be addressed by intrathecal drugs and must be treated with radiation therapy (if symptomatic) or by the administration of high doses of parenteral methotrexate. As CNS relapse precedes systemic failure, meningeal therapy should be accompanied by intensified systemic treatment. Treatment is provided with neuraxis irradiation or intrathecal chemotherapy, which provide similar event-free survival[16] approaching 90% at two years.[17] For children and most adults an Ommaya reservoir provides uniform drug distribution into the ventricles. Access is easy for the clinician and patient acceptance is excellent. The Ommaya catheters carry a 5% risk of infection or malfunction.[18] For children, therapy based on triple chemotherapy (MTX 15 mg/m² to a maximum of 15 mg, cytarabine 30 mg/m² maximum dose 60 mg, and prednisone 60 mg/m²) as six weekly injections is the mainstay of treatment. To this, for high-risk patients, is added either cranial or craniospinal irradiation at 1400–2400 Gy.[19] Radiation therapy is also the basis for treatment of recurrences after failed prophylaxis.[20] In adults, therapy is commonly based on MTX (12.5 mg every three days) or the liposomal cytarabine, whose half-life is 40 times longer than that of the parent drug.[21] High CSF levels can be achieved following systemic administration of MTX,[22] topotecan and cytarabine.[23] Radiation therapy is provided for localized nodular or symptomatic leukemia refractory to chemotherapy. Experimental therapies include mafosfamide as intrathecal medication,[24] radiolabeled monoclonal antibodies[25] and high-dose chemotherapy with marrow transplant.[26]

Special forms of leukemia

Acute promyelocytic leukemia (APL), characterized by t(15;17), rarely afflicts the brain or meninges. The exception is for recipients of *trans* retinoic acid.[27] Acute myeloid leukemia (AML) afflicts 2.2% of patients and rarely benefits from therapy.[28] Chronic lymphocytic leukemia (CLL) rarely infiltrates the CNS but is associated with neuropathy of peripheral and cranial nerves or epidural spinal cord compression.[29,30] Meningeal disease is responsive to intrathecal MTX or XRT.

Spinal cord compression from epidural acute leukemia afflicts the thoracic spinal cord in one in 200 patients. Pain and sensory deficits are explained by MRI-identified epidural masses. As with lymphoma, emergency treatment is dexamethasone 100 mg i.v. In the setting of rapidly progressive steroid-resistant paresis or plegia, the authors will commonly use mannitol (20 g every four to six hours for serum osmolality below 300 mmol. Radiation therapy (40 Gy at 2 Gy/day in 20 fractions) is provided on an emergency basis irrespective of the time of day. Cloroma, or granulocytic sarcoma, is formed by immature myeloid cells, usually in AML patients with t(8;21) or chromosome 16 rearrangement. The name reflects the greenish color of the mass, which invades brain parenchyma, meninges, or the bones of the skull or orbits. Depending on the areas involved, chemotherapy is successfully provided into the CSF or by systemic routes.

The long-term sequelae of CNS leukemia and its treatment are less apparent in the modern era. Previous combinations of drugs and radiation were associated with damage to white matter,[31] causing intellectual changes[32,33] or neuroendocrine difficulties. These changes reflected a calcific disorder of small blood vessels within the white matter. Myelin loss occurred and patients developed myoclonus and dementia. Stroke and hemorrhage in leukemia can reflect non-bacterial thrombotic endocarditis, disseminated intravascular coagulopathy or functional disorders of platelets. Non-cardial infections can alter vessels. The stroke manifestations are treated with supportive care, leukopheresis, frozen plasma and platelet transfusions. Drug toxicities occur in the setting of leukemia and lymphoma therapy. L-Asparaginase produces thrombosis and hemorrhage, which may improve with the provision of frozen plasma and immediate cessation of the drug. Vincristine administration produces a dose-related disorder of sensory nerves in the face or extremities, in addition to paresis of gastrointestinal motility and visual function. Some improvement is noted with cessation of the medication and the provision of neurontin for painful paresthesias. Cytarabine induces cerebellar and spinal cord toxicity.[34] Methotrexate administered by intrathecal routes can produce a localized disorder of white matter. This reflects the high local concentrations of the drug. Patients may have seizures or confusion, with MRI evidence of demyelination as seen on T_2 or FLAIR images. Underlying these changes is a calcific microangiopathy[35] afflicting white matter. Cyclosporin A, used in allogeneic marrow transplant, induces cortical blindness and seizures. The complications of radiation therapy have been identified but include the induction of second tumor occurrences at a rate which approaches

2% per year. These tumors include meningiomas, anaplastic astrocytoma and paranasal carcinoma, in addition to non-tumor hyalinization changes of intracranial arterioles. Unlike vascular disorders in non-tumor patients, the **cerebrovascular complications of leukemia** are non-atherosclerotic, afflict young patients, and are best treated by prompt treatment of the underlying coagulation disorders. **Intracerebral hemorrhage** occurs in those patients with leukocyte counts above $300\,000/\text{mm}^3$ and those with acute promyelocytic leukemia.[36] **Venous and arterial thrombosis**, identified on MRI venography or arteriography, reflects coagulopathy or the vascular effects of L-asparaginase. **CNS infections in leukemia** are commonly vascular-based fungal diseases. The fungi are visualized on biopsies of brain tissue. *Aspergillus*[37] and mucor are treated with minimal success by liposomal amphotericin.[38]

References

1. Greenlee RT, Murray T, Bolden S, et al. Cancer statistics, 2000. CA Cancer J Clin 2000;50:7–33
2. Sapoznick MD, Kaplan HS. Intracranial Hodgkin's disease. Cancer 1983;52:1301–1307
3. Mullins GM, Flynn JPG, El-Mahdi AH, et al. Malignant lymphoma of the spinal epidural space. Ann Intern Med 1971;74:416–423
4. Mahe B, Moreau P, Bonnemain B, et al. Isolated Richter's syndrome of the brain: two recent cases. Nouv Rev Fr Hematol 1994;36:383–385
5. Vecht CJ, Haaxma-Reiche H, van Putten WLJ, et al. Initial bolus of conventional versus high-dose dexamethasone in metastatic spinal cord compression. Neurology 1989;39:1255–1257
6. Perry JR, Deodhare SS, Bilbao JM, et al. The significance of spinal cord compression as the initial manifestation of lymphoma. Neurosurgery 1993;32:157–162
7. Aabo K, Walbom-Jorgensen S. Central nervous system complications by malignant lymphomas: radiation schedule and treatment results. Int J Radiat Oncol Biol Phys 1986;12:197–202
8. Buch PA, Grossman SA. Treatment of epidural cord compression from Hodgkin's disease with chemotherapy. Am J Med 1988;84:555–558
9. Van Besien K, Ha CS, Murphy S, et al. Risk factors and outcome of central nervous system recurrence in adults with intermediate-grade and immunoblastic lymphoma. Blood 1998;91:1178–1184
10. Liang R, Chiu E, Loke SL. Secondary central nervous system involvement by non-Hodgkin's lymphoma: the risk factors. Hematol Oncol 1990;8:141–145
11. Bleyer AW. Central nervous system leukemia. *In:* Henderson HS, Lister TA, eds. Leukemia, 5th edn. Philadelphia: WB. Saunders, 1990:207–224
12. Kreuger A, Garwicz S, Hertz H, et al. Central nervous system disease in childhood acute lymphoblastic leukemia:prognostic factors and results of treatment. Pediatr Hematol Oncol 1991;8:291–299
13. Mahoney DH Jr, Shuster JJ, Nitschke R, et al. Acute neurotoxicity in children with B-precursor acute lymphoid leukemia: an association with intermediate-dose intravenous methotrexate and intrathecal triple therapy—a Pediatric Oncology Group study. J Clin Oncol 1998;16:1712–1722
14. Kaplan J, DeSousa T, Farkash A, et al. Leptomeningeal metastasis: comparison of clinical features and laboratory data of solid tumors, lymphomas and leukemias. J Neurol Oncol 1990;92:225–229
15. Cibas E, Malkin M, Posner J, Melamed M. Detection of DNA abnormalities by flow cytometry in cells from cerebrospinal fluid. Am J Clin Pathol 1987;88:570–577
16. Winick NJ, Smith SD, Shuster J, et al. Treatment of CNS relapse in children with acute lymphoblastic leukemia: a Pediatric Oncology Group study. J Clin Oncol 1993;11:271–278
17. Gelber R, Sallan S, Cohen HJ, et al. Central nervous system treatment in childhood acute lymphoblastic leukemia: long-term follow up of patients diagnosed between 1973 and 1985. Cancer 1993;72:261–270
18. Chamberlain MC, Kormanick PA, Barbara D. Complications associated with intraventricular chemotherapy in patients with leptomeningeal metastasis. J Neurosurg 1997;87:694–699
19. Land VJ, Thomas PRM, Boyett JM, et al. Comparison of maintenance treatment regimens for first central nervous system relapse in children with acute lymphocytic leukemia. Cancer 1985, 56:81–87
20. Winick NJ, Smith SD, Shuster J, et al. Treatment of CNS relapse in children with acute lymphoblastic leukemia: a pediatric oncology group study. J Clin Oncol 1993;11:271–278
21. Kim S, Chatelut E, Kim J, et al. Extended CSF cytarabine exposure following intrathecal administration of DTC 101. J Clin Oncol 1993;11:2186–2193
22. Balis F, Savitch J, Bleyer B, et al. Remission induction of meningeal leukemia with high-dose intravenous methotrexate. J Clin Oncol 1985;11:74–86
23. Morra E, Lazzarino M, Inverardi D, et al. Systemic high dose ara-C for treatment of meningeal leukemia in adult acute lymphoblastic leukemia and non-Hodgkin's lymphoma. J Clin Oncol 1986;4:1207–1211
24. Slavc I, Schuller E, Czech T, et al. Intrathecal mafosfamide therapy for pediatric brain tumors with meningeal dissemination. J Neurooncol 1998;38:213–218
25. Coakham HB, Kemshead JT. Treatment of neoplastic meningitis by targeted radiation using (131)I-radio-labelled monoclonal antibodies. Result of responses and long term follow-up in 40 patients. J Neurooncol 1998;389:225–232
26. Messina C, Valsecchi MG, Arico M, et al. Autologous bone marrow transplantation for treatment of isolated central nervous system relapse of childhood acute lymphoblastic leukemia. Bone Marrow Transplant 1998; 21:9–14
27. Evans G, Grimwade D, Prentice HG, Simpson N. Central nervous system relapse in acute promyelosytic leukemia in patients treated with all-trans retinoic acid. Br J Hematol 1997;98:437–439
28. Castagnola C, Nozza A, Corso A, Bernasconi C. The value of combination therapy in adult acute myeloid leukemia with central nervous system involvement. Hematologica 1997;82:577–580
29. Cramer SC, Glaspy JA, Efird JT, Louis DN. Chronic lymphocytic leukemia and the central nervous system: A clinical and pathological study. Neurology 1996;46:19–25
30. Miller K, Budke H, Orazi A. Leukemic meningitis complicating early stage chronic lymphocytic leukemia. Arch Pathol Lab Med 1997;121:524–527
31. Butler RW, Hill JM, Steinherz PG, et al. Neuropsychologic effects of cranial irradiation, intrathecal methotrexate, and systemic methotrexate in childhood cancer. J Clin Oncol 1994;12:2621–2629

32. Cousens P, Waters B, Said J, et al. Cognitive effects of cranial irradiation in leukemia: a survey and meta-analysis. J Child Psychol Psychiatry 1988;29:839–852

33. Mulhern RK, Fairclough D, Ochs J. A prospective comparison of neuropsychologic performance of children surviving leukemia who received 18-Gy, 24-Gy or no cranial irradiation. J Clin Oncol 1991;9:1348–1356

34. Damon LE, Mass R, Linker CA. The association between high-dose cytarabine neurotoxicity and renal insufficiency. J Clin Oncol 1989;7:1563–1568

35. Lovblad K, Kelkar P, Ozdoba C, et al. Pure methotrexate encephalopathy presenting with seizures: CT and MRI features. Pediatr Radiol 1998;28:86–91

36. Graus F, Rogers LR, Posner JB. Cerebrovascular complications in patients with cancer. Medicine 1985;64: 16–35

37. Pagano L, Ricci P, Montillo M, et al. Localization of aspergillosis to the central nervous system among patients with acute leukemia: report of 14 cases. Gruppo Italiano Malattie Ematologiche dell'Adulto Infection Program. Clin Infect Dis 1996;23:628–630

38. Khoury H, Adkins D, Miller G, et al. Resolution of invasive central nervous system aspergillosis in a transplant recipient. Bone Marrow Transplant 1997;20: 179–180

39. Kreuger A, Garwicz S, Hertz H, et al. Central nervous system disease in childhood acute lymphoblastic leukemia:prognostic factors and results of treatment. Pediatr Hematol Oncol 1991;8:291–299

127 Neurologic Disorders in Benign and Malignant Plasma Cell Dyscrasias

John J Kelly

Introduction

Plasma cell dyscrasias (PCD), synonymous with monoclonal gammopathies (MG), and their accompanying monoclonal proteins (M-protein, MP) or immunoglobulins, are rare. They are, however, interesting to neurologists as they are frequently associated with neurological diseases.[1] These syndromes may be distinctive, and in some cases appear to be due to the direct effects of the M-proteins on peripheral nerves (paraneoplastic syndromes).[2] This chapter describes the recognition and treatment of these patients.

Historical

The recognition of epidemiological and etiologic associations between plasma cell dyscrasias and neurological diseases, especially paraneoplastic syndromes, is a recent phenomenon.[3] Formerly, M-proteins produced by PCDs were assumed to be immunologically inert for the most part, and except for direct, non-immunological effects, such as deposition in kidneys, were not thought directly to cause neurological disease. In the 1970s and 1980s, however, a number of investigators[4,5] reported an increased frequency of peripheral neuropathies associated with both malignant and non-malignant PCDs. In addition, reports appeared linking M-proteins secreted by the PCDs to direct immunological nerve damage. The binding of M-proteins to specific epitopes was described,[2] implying a pathophysiologic mechanism.

Now, most investigators in this field accept that monoclonal antibodies or other secretory products can cause several distinct neurological syndromes. Indeed, treatment by removal or neutralization of these immunoglobulins can halt disease progression and, in some cases, improve these patients. As a result, the biology of PCDs and their remote effects on neurological and other tissues is now a fruitful area for research for many basic and clinical investigators.

Evaluation of monoclonal gammopathies

A plasma cell dyscrasia (Table 127.1) is defined as a proliferation of a single clone of plasma cells, either neoplastic or non-neoplastic, and is usually associated with a monoclonal serum or urine protein (see Chapter 202 for a detailed discussion).[1,6] M-proteins consist of a single heavy chain (M, G or A) and a single light chain (κ or λ).[1] Polyclonal gammopathies are not considered plasma cell dyscrasias. They consist of immunoglobulins containing both light chains and generally more than one heavy chain. They do not directly cause neuropathy and are considered non-specific immunological reactions to an inflammatory disease or neoplasia. Occasionally, in a monoclonal gammopathy, only the light chain or the heavy chain may be secreted (light- or heavy-chain disease) in either serum or urine (Bence-Jones protein).[6]

The M-protein is detected by screening patients with serum protein (cellulose acetate) electrophoresis

Table 127.1 Classification of plasma cell dyscrasias	
Disorder	**Diagnostic criteria**
Monoclonal gammopathy of undetermined significance	MP in serum < 3 g/dL; no malignancy or amyloid
Osteosclerotic myeloma	Solitary or multiple plasmacytomas with osteosclerotic features—requires tissue confirmation
Multiple myeloma	>10% abnormal plasma cells in bone marrow *or* plasmacytoma and MP in serum or urine *or* osteolytic lesions
Waldenström's macroglobulinemia	IgM-MP > 3 g/dL *and* >10% lymphs or plasma cells in bone marrow
Primary systemic amyloidosis	Presence of light-chain amyloid by histology
γ-Heavy-chain disease	Monoclonal heavy chain in serum or urine

MP, monoclonal protein; IgM, immunoglobulin M.
Data from Kelly JJ Jr, Kyle RA, Latov N. Polyneuropathies associated with plasma cell dyscrasias. Boston: Martinus-Nijhoff, 1987[8]

(SPEP).[1] In cases where a suspicious peak is seen on SPEP, and in all cases where a monoclonal gammopathy is suspected as a possible cause, such as idiopathic polyneuropathy or atypical motor neuron disease, serum immunoelectrophoresis (IEP) or immunofixation electrophoresis (IFE) should be performed, even with a normal SPEP.[6] IEP and IFE are more sensitive than SPEP for the presence of a small M-protein and allow characterization of the single heavy and light chains, thus verifying the monoclonal nature of the immunoglobulin.[6] Of these two, IFE is the more sensitive and will occasionally detect M-proteins when IEP and SPEP are negative. A concentrated urine specimen should also be examined, as monoclonal light chains may appear in urine when serum is normal, suggesting either a malignant PCD or light chain amyloidosis (AL).

After identification and characterization of an M-protein in serum or urine, further hematologic evaluation should be carried out to classify the PCD.[1,4] If a diagnosis of monoclonal gammopathy of undetermined significance (MGUS), the new and more accurate term for "benign monoclonal gammopathy," is established, M-protein levels should be monitored on a yearly basis. A sudden increase can indicate malignant transformation of a benign plasma cell dyscrasia, which can occur in up to 20% of cases, hence the term MGUS.[7]

Epidemiology

There are no accurate prevalence or incidence data for these neuropathies. In general, PCDs with neurological manifestations caused by remote effects, mostly peripheral neuropathy, are rare (Table 127.2). For example, neuropathies due to the remote effects of PCDs account for only a few percent of unselected patients with polyneuropathy (Table 127.3).[4] Roughly half of these are due to IgM-secreting PCDs, either benign or malignant, and most of the other half are due to MGUS secreting IgG or IgA M-proteins. The prevalence of neuropathy is, however, very high in those patients with benign or malignant IgM gammopathy, osteosclerotic myeloma and light-chain amyloidosis (AL).

Pathophysiology and pathogenesis

The mechanism for the remote effects of plasma cell dyscrasias is known in only a few instances. In some, circulating monoclonal antibodies—almost always IgM—are directed against neural antigens, with resultant complement-dependent nerve damage. In others, a direct link between the MP and nerve damage is less clear. MGs of all types are overrepresented in patients with idiopathic polyneuropathy.[4] However, whether the neuropathy in individual patients is due to damage by the immunoglobulin or to a secondary toxic or metabolic effect is often unknown. For example, some IgM gammopathies cause type I cryoglobulinemia, which can damage nerve fibers in addition to direct immunological effects. These factors will be discussed below in more detail.

The pathogenesis of light chain-derived amyloid neuropathy has been debated for years. Most likely, the direct toxic effects of amyloid on neural tissue damage the nerve, either through primary toxicity to neurons or axons, or due to compression, as in carpal tunnel syndrome.

Osteosclerotic myeloma neuropathy and POEMS

Table 127.2 Clinical syndromes of plasma cell dyscrasias

	Toxic/metabolic	Root/cord	Polyneuropathy	Other
MGUS	No	No	Yes	No
MM	Yes	Yes	Yes	Infections
OSM	No	No	Yes	POEMS
Amyloid	No	No	Yes	R, C, GI

MGUS, monoclonal gammopathy of undetermined significance; MM, typical lytic multiple myeloma; OSM, osteosclerotic myeloma; R, renal; C, cardiac; GI, gastrointestinal.

Table 127.3 Hematological diagnosis of 28 patients with PCD and polyneuropathy

Diagnosis	Number
Monoclonal gammopathy of undetermined significance	16
Primary systemic amyloidosis	7
Multiple myeloma (includes osteosclerotic myeloma)	3
Waldenström's macroglobulinemia	1
γ-Heavy-chain disease	1

PCD, plasma cell dyscrasia.
Adapted from Kelly JJ Jr, Kyle RA, O'Brien PC, et al. Prevalence of monoclonal protein in peripheral neuropathy. Neurology 1981;31:1480[4]

syndrome is a fascinating disorder that is probably caused by a circulating factor. Whether this is due to the monoclonal protein or to secretory products of the tumor is unclear at present.

Clinical and laboratory features

MGUS neuropathy

Monoclonal gammopathy of undetermined significance, formerly known as benign monoclonal gammopathy, is the most common condition associated with neurological disorders, most of which are peripheral neuropathies (Table 127.4). These disorders are best approached clinically by classifying them as IgM and non-IgM types (IgG and IgA). By definition, these patients have non-malignant gammopathies with MP levels of less than 3 g/dL, less than 10% plasma cells in the bone marrow and no evidence of anemia, hypercalcemia, hepatosplenomegaly, renal failure or bony plasmacytomas (Table 127.1).

IgM-associated neuropathies

Anti-MAG neuropathy (Latov's syndrome) Roughly 50% of MGUS neuropathies are associated with an IgM gammopathy.[8,9] Studies have shown that sera from about half of these in turn have antinerve antibody activity directed against myelin-associated glycoprotein (anti-MAG),[10] which is a minor glycoprotein in the myelin sheath. Anti-MAG polyneuropathies are the most common of all the PCD-associated polyneuropathies, accounting for about 25% of the total.

1. *Clinical manifestations* Anti-MAG neuropathy has a fairly homogeneous clinical presentation.[11–15] These patients are older (sixth to ninth decades) and present with a slowly progressive and relatively painless sensory neuropathy. Patients complain of numbness and paresthesias of the feet and distal legs, and gradually increasing unsteadiness due to sensory ataxia. Weakness is less prominent, although as the disease progresses it becomes more so. An action tremor of the hands is evident in some patients.[16] Examination reveals striking discriminative sensory loss, including loss of vibration and position sense in the feet. This causes sensory ataxia associated with a markedly positive Romberg's sign. Pain and temperature sensation is less severely affected and clinically evident autonomic dysfunction rarely occurs. Motor strength is usually impaired distally to a much lesser extent. Reflexes are typically absent in the legs and depressed in the arms. Nerves may be thickened and firm to palpation. The symptoms are very chronic and slowly progressive over months to years, with long periods of apparent stability. At their worst, patients are unable to walk, mostly because of sensory ataxia with varying degrees of weakness.

2. *Laboratory tests* In all but the earliest cases, EMG shows the classic findings of a demyelinating polyneuropathy with marked slowing of motor conduction velocities, very prolonged distal latencies, and areas of conduction block and dispersal on proximal stimulation, with secondary axonal degenerative changes.[13,17] Sensory potentials are absent or severely attenuated. Cerebrospinal fluid has a high protein concentration, with non-specific features and a normal glucose and cell count. Nerve biopsy can be pathognomonic, typically showing IgM deposition on the myelin sheath using immunofluorescent techniques, and splitting and separation of the outer layers of compacted myelin on electron microscopy.[9,18–21] General laboratory and hematological tests are negative in these patients, which helps to exclude the more serious gammopathies. The SPEP usually shows a small monoclonal spike in the γ region. However, a negative SPEP may occur and should not obviate further testing for antinerve antibodies in the appropriate setting. IEP or IFE confirms the presence of an IgM gammopathy, usually with κ light chains. Further testing using ELISA and Western blotting shows that the IgM antibody reacts with MAG and other sphingoglycolipid epitopes,[10,14,22,23] thereby establishing the diagnosis.

3. *Pathophysiology* There is now overwhelming evidence that the MP directly causes the neuropathy. There is a close relationship between the clinical and laboratory manifestations of this syndrome and the presence in serum of IgM anti-MAG antibodies. However, small studies comparing IgM-MP patients with and without anti-MAG antibody activity could not demonstrate a difference in the characteristics of neuropathy between the two

Table 127.4	**Features of dysproteinemia polyneuropathy syndromes**				
Class	**Weakness**	**Sensory**	**Autonomic**	**CSF**	**MNCV**
MGUS-IgM	+	+++	−	++	D
MGUS-IgG,A	++	++	−	+	D
Amyloidosis	+/++	+++	+++	+	A or D
OSM	+++	++	−	+++	D
WM	++	++	−	++	D or A

CSF, cerebrospinal fluid protein concentration; MNCV, motor nerve conduction velocity; MGUS, monoclonal gammopathy of undetermined significance; OSM, osteosclerotic myeloma; WM, Waldenström's macroglobulinemia; D, segmental demyelination pattern; A, axonal degeneration pattern.
Adapted from Kelly JJ Jr, Kyle RA, Latov N. Polyneuropathies associated with plasma cell dyscrasias. Boston: Martinus-Nijhoff, 1987[8]

groups.[24–26] Laboratory data are much more convincing. The anti-MAG antibodies are deposited in the layers of the myelin sheath, where complement-mediated damage to the sheath can be demonstrated.[9,18,20] Separation of the outer lamellae of myelin occurs,[9,18] presumably owing to the specificity of these antibodies for the adhesion molecules of the myelin sheath. In addition, although intraneural injections of serum into rats have not demonstrated pathological changes comparable to those in humans, injection systemically (passive transfer) into higher animals has demonstrated changes identical to those of the human disease.[27] Also, although exceptions occur, clinical improvement is generally associated with a reduction of the MP level in serum.[12,28,29] In addition, the presence of anti-MAG antibodies predicts the future development of neuropathy.[30] Variability of the clinical course and time of onset in individual patients may be related to differing binding affinities of the anti-MAG proteins.[31] Thus most investigators now accept anti-MAG neuropathy as an autoimmune disease, although further work needs to be done to elucidate the specific epitopes affected and the exact mechanism of myelin damage.

4. *Treatment* Most treatments are aimed at lowering the concentration of the IgM protein. This is often problematic, as the M-protein is difficult to eliminate. There are no controlled studies and thus as yet no definitive proof of efficacy of any treatment. Plasmapheresis should, theoretically, work simply by physically lowering the concentration of the M-protein,[32] but the marked chronicity of this disorder would necessitate lifelong pheresis, which is not practical. However, pheresis can be used to rapidly lower the concentration of IgM at the onset of treatment.[12] Likewise, intravenous γ-globulin and corticosteroids by themselves are generally not helpful and should not be used.[19,26,33–35] Cytotoxic drugs such as cyclophosphamide and fludarabine in conventional doses have been shown to help some patients,[12,18,29,36] presumably by lowering the M-protein level in serum. However, some patients respond without lowering of the M-protein level.[36] The mechanism of action of these drugs is therefore unclear. The toxicity of cytotoxic drugs is the limiting factor, especially in elderly patients. Generally, monthly intravenous therapy is thought to be less toxic than daily oral therapy. Unless a neurologist is very experienced in using these drugs, I recommend referral to an oncologist to implement the chemotherapy protocol. The neurologist should follow them neurologically on a monthly basis during treatment. Careful consideration in each case must be given to whether or not to treat and, if so, how aggressively to treat. Many patients with mild disease should not be treated aggressively unless their disease accelerates.[8] A recent preliminary study found that interferon-α seemed to help some patients.[37] Other treatments warranting further investigation, based on preliminary studies, include immunoabsorption with selective affinity

columns,[15,38,39] and perhaps immunological reconstitution with bone marrow transplantation. Undoubtedly, better, more selective and less toxic treatments will be developed when the molecular pathology of this disorder is fully understood.

Non-MAG IgM MGUS neuropathy syndromes Non-IgM polyneuropathies are more heterogeneous than the IgM type (Table 127.4).

1. *Demyelinating type* Based on nerve conduction studies and nerve biopsy the majority of non-MAG IgM neuropathies appear to be demyelinating in type. They resemble anti-MAG neuropathy, based on clinical[24–26] and electrophysiologic attributes.[24,26] However, tests for antinerve antibodies are usually negative or reveal antibody relationships of unclear significance, including those against sulfatides,[22,40] myelin basic protein[41] and others. The nerve biopsy does not show the typical myelin deposition of antibodies or the characteristic myelin splitting of anti-MAG neuropathy. With further study, these disorders may also prove to be caused by specific antineural antigens. These neuropathies, like anti-MAG neuropathy, respond poorly to the first-line anti-immune treatments such as steroids, plasmapheresis and IVIG, and respond better to cytotoxic drugs.

2. *Axonal type* The neuropathies with IgM gammopathy, which have mainly axonal changes on pathology and nerve conduction studies, are common,[42] some associated with antisulfatide antibodies.[40,43] In all cases, amyloidosis needs to be excluded by appropriate testing (see below). If this is excluded, most of these patients have mild, painful axonal neuropathies which can be managed symptomatically.

IgG and IgA-MGUS polyneuropathies

Axonal type IgG- and IgA-MGUS-associated neuropathies represent the other 50% of neuropathies in the MGUS group. Most patients in this group will have axonal neuropathies. These are often minor, affect mainly the feet and legs, and cause intractable dysesthesias without much functional deficit. Amyloid must be excluded in this group (see below). Amyloid neuropathy is generally much more severe, has prominent autonomic involvement and commonly affects other organs (Table 127.5). Biopsy is sometimes necessary to make this distinction. If amyloid is excluded on tissue or clinical grounds, these neuropathies are rarely severe. They can usually be managed by controlling pain with medications used in other painful neuropathies. The author generally follows these patients for two to three years. If the symptoms and findings suddenly accelerate, or if the MP spike suddenly increases, a more sinister form of PCD, such as amyloidosis or myeloma,[44] may have developed and should be searched for.

Demyelinating type These patients have a clinical syndrome resembling chronic inflammatory demyelinating polyradiculoneuropathy (CIDP).[45,46] Some

Table 127.5   Medical syndromes in amyloid polyneuropathy

Syndrome	Percentage frequency
Orthostatic hypotension	42
Nephrotic syndrome	23
Cardiac failure	23
Malabsorption	16

Adapted from Kelly JJ Jr, Kyle RA, O'Brien PC, et al. The natural history of peripheral neuropathy in primary systemic amyloidosis. Ann Neurol 1979;5:271[75]

think this disorder, referred to by some as CIDP-MGUS, represents the chance co-occurrence of two rare disorders. However, antineural antibodies of unclear significance have been described in these patients.[45] Treatments usually successful in CIDP, such as plasmapheresis, IVIG and steroids, are more likely to be helpful in these patients than in those with IgM-MGUS.[24,26]

Multiple myeloma (MM)

Multiple myeloma is a malignant PCD with high serum and urinary concentrations of MP, infiltration of bone marrow by malignant plasma cells, and multiple bony plasmacytomas.[6]

Direct effects of myeloma   Most neurological symptoms are due to malignant infiltration of the vertebral column or metabolic and toxic manifestations. Patients with spinal involvement usually present with segmental spinal pain and symptoms of spinal cord or cauda equina disruption. If there is no clinical evidence of root or cord compression, plain X-ray or CT is often adequate for diagnosis, although subsequent MRI may be warranted to judge whether there should be concern for later epidural encroachment and cord compression. Treatment of uncomplicated vertebral involvement consists of adequate pain control, localized radiation therapy and possibly chemotherapy. The patient needs to be followed carefully to watch for cord compression.

Root and spinal cord compression cause local pain plus a radicular or cord syndrome or both, depending on the level and extent of compression. Diagnosis is suspected by the association of local symptoms (spinal pain, radicular pain and findings) and/or a spinal cord pattern of involvement of the lower extremities. Diagnosis is urgent in these cases to prevent further worsening. Emergency MRI is warranted, with imaging of the suspected area. Because incomplete spinal lesions are often difficult to localize with confidence, a lateral screening total spine MRI (MRI "myelogram") is often helpful as an initial step to detect suspicious areas, allowing careful localized imaging. In patients who cannot have MRI, spinal plain films and radionuclide bone scans can be helpful in localizing collapsed vertebrae and eroded pedicles, thereby suggesting the level of compression, with the realization that radionuclide scans may be negative with bony involvement in myeloma.[47–49] This

can be followed by CT of this area to look for an epidural mass. If the findings fit the clinical picture, treatment can commence without myelography. However, as the lesion seen on CT may not be the proximate cause, careful follow-up must be maintained and any worsening should prompt urgent CT myelography.

Treatment generally consists of high-dose corticosteroids, pain control, localized irradiation of the area and chemotherapy. As mentioned above, careful monitoring is necessary to detect deterioration that may necessitate surgical decompression, although usually this is not necessary if treatment is commenced promptly. Surgery is complicated in addition by the frequent involvement of adjacent vertebrae, which may render the postoperative spine unstable. Outcome usually depends on speed of diagnosis, rapidity of treatment and the neurological status before treatment. Severe pretreatment impairment usually predicts a poor result.

Mononeuropathies or plexopathies due to localized deposits in the peripheral nerves are quite rare. Direct involvement of plasma cell disorders in the intracranial compartment is also rare but well documented. Leptomeningeal myelomatosis typically occurs in advanced cases of multiple myeloma and is managed according to the usual guidelines for leptomeningeal leukemia.[50] Myelomatous infiltration of the dura occurs rarely, presumably the result of spread from contiguous bone. This entity has responded favorably to radiation therapy.[51] Solitary extramedullary plasmacytomas also rarely involve the dura and are successfully managed with surgery and radiotherapy.[52] Parenchymal brain plasmacytomas are exceedingly rare.[53]

Metabolic, toxic and infectious effects of myeloma   Metabolic, toxic and infectious disorders can also cause neurological syndromes in myeloma. These patients can develop encephalopathy, sometimes with seizures, from renal insufficiency, dehydration, hypercalcemia and associated metabolic failure. Light-chain deposition can cause a rapidly progressive nephropathy. Anemia, immunosuppression and secondary infections are common. In patients with IgM myeloma a hyperviscosity syndrome with CNS changes (Bing–Neel syndrome) can develop (see below).

In these patients a thorough metabolic screening is indicated, with careful review of medications. If the patient is febrile or no obvious metabolic or toxic cause is found, evaluation for infection should include a CSF examination for bacteria, fungi and tuberculosis. Brain MRI and EEG are indicated in all cases where the cause is not clear. These patients generally do well once the cause is found, with rapid reversal of the underlying problem, but recovery to baseline often takes several days or longer.

Remote effects of myeloma   Remote effects consist mostly of peripheral neuropathies of various types. Other remote effects, such as paraneoplastic cerebellar ataxia, are extremely rare.

Typical lytic multiple myeloma These polyneuropathies occur in only a few percent of MM patients[54–57] and are diverse in nature, similar to the polyneuropathies associated with other malignancies. The exception is osteosclerotic myeloma (OSM), discussed separately below. Neuropathies associated with typical lytic MM include a distal sensorimotor axonopathy, a chronic inflammatory demyelinating polyneuropathy (CIDP-like syndrome), and a sensory neuropathy resembling carcinomatous ataxic sensory neuropathy.[54] In addition, these patients may also develop amyloid polyneuropathy, also known as primary systemic amyloid (PSA) neuropathy or AL neuropathy, owing to deposition of light chain-derived amyloid in nerve and other tissues. In one series, 20% of neuropathies associated with MM were due to AL.[54] In occasional patients, superimposed root involvement may confuse the clinician by mistakenly suggesting a picture of mononeuritis multiplex. The root and cord compressive syndromes should be managed by conventional means, as discussed above. The neuropathies should be separately classified by the usual techniques and treated according to type. Electromyography can be very helpful in properly classifying these disorders. Of the four types mentioned above, only the CIDP-like neuropathy is amenable to treatment using conventional immunosuppression.

Osteosclerotic myeloma (OSM) and polyneuropathy (and related syndromes)[47,54] Osteosclerotic myeloma is a rare and relatively benign variant of MM. Less than 3% of untreated myeloma patients have sclerotic bony lesions. In addition, polyneuropathy (rare with typical MM) occurs in 50% or more of reported cases with OSM. In contrast to typical MM, patients with OSM are usually not systemically ill. They present with symptoms due to neuropathy or other remote effects of the malignancy, instead of to a direct effect of the malignancy. Anemia, hypercalcemia and renal insufficiency are uncommon in OSM, the bone marrow is rarely infiltrated with malignant plasma cells, and the serum M-protein concentration is low. Finally, the course of OSM is indolent and these patients have prolonged survival even without treatment, often for years.

1. *Clinical features* Unlike MM, the polyneuropathy accompanying OSM is distinctive and homogeneous. Deficits are predominantly motor and slowly progressive, without sudden changes in tempo or severity of progression. OSM neuropathy is occasionally mistaken for slowly progressive CIDP even by experienced neuropathy experts. Therefore, any patient with slowly progressive monophasic CIDP should have a bone X-ray survey performed, even if the SPEP and IFE are negative. The deficit is usually very symmetrical and the speed of progression slow, often over months to years.

2. *Laboratory studies* General laboratory studies are usually relatively uninformative. However, a small serum M-protein is present in approximately 75% to 80% of patients. It may be very small and obscured by the normal serum protein components in the electrophoresis, emphasizing the importance of IEP or IFE in all patients with idiopathic polyneuropathy resembling this disorder. The M-protein is characteristically IgG or IgA with a λ light chain (occasionally κ), and is rarely present in the urine, unlike with MM and AL. Neurodiagnostic studies are more helpful but undiagnostic.[47] Nerve histopathology discloses a reduced concentration of myelinated fibers with changes of mixed demyelination and axonal degeneration.[47,58] There may be mild foci of mononuclear cells in the epineurium surrounding blood vessels. These changes are non-specific and characteristic of a number of neuropathies, including CIDP and diabetic polyneuropathy. The EMG reveals a mixed axonal and demyelinating picture, often with disproportionately long distal latencies, which is also non-specific but helpful in categorizing the neuropathy into the limited group with clear-cut demyelinating features.[13,47] Cerebrospinal fluid typically discloses a normal cell count but a very high protein concentration, generally greater than 100 mg/dL. As all these findings are non-specific, the diagnosis often hinges on the discovery of the characteristic bony lesion on radiographs and subsequent bone biopsy. The osteosclerotic lesions may be solitary or multiple,[47] and are best detected on plain radiographs rather than radionuclide bone scans.[47–49] They tend to affect the axial skeleton and very proximal long bones, but spare the distal long bones and skull. They may be purely sclerotic or mixed sclerotic and lytic. Thus, all patients with unexplained polyneuropathies that fit this clinical profile should be screened with a radiographic skeletal survey, even in the absence of a serum or urine MP. In our experience open biopsy is preferable to needle biopsy.

3. *Pathogenesis* The cause of the polyneuropathy is not known, but most theories of pathogenesis have focused on some secretory product of the tumor, perhaps circulating cytokines[59] or vascular endothelial growth factor (VEGF).[60–64] Others have found evidence for infection with human herpesvirus 8 in POEMS syndrome associated with multicentric Castleman's disease.[65] Unlike with anti-MAG neuropathy, there is little evidence that the M-protein itself causes the neuropathy and systemic features.

4. *Treatment* The diagnosis of this disorder is important, as these patients may be helped by tumoricidal treatment.[47,66] Patients with solitary lesions do best. Radiation therapy in tumoricidal doses to the lesion and/or surgical excision results in elimination of the M-protein from the serum and gradual recovery of the neuropathy and other symptoms over the ensuing months in most patients. However, these patients should continue to be followed, as they have a tendency to relapse with the development of new lesions months to years later. This is usually

heralded by the return of the neuropathy and other symptoms and the reappearance of the serum M-protein. Patients with multiple lesions are more difficult to treat. Radiation therapy is generally not an option because of the risk of toxicity. In some cases aggressive chemotherapy, with or without local radiation therapy to large lesions, can help these patients,[6,47,67] but in general the outcome is less favorable than for solitary lesions. Treatment usually requires large doses of steroids and alkylating agents.[68] High-dose corticosteroids, azathioprine, plasmapheresis and IVIG, which are usually effective in autoimmune inflammatory neuropathies, are typically ineffective or impractical in these patients.

5. *Systemic features* This disorder is also of considerable interest as many patients develop a multisystem syndrome (Table 127.6) which goes by a variety of names, including the POEMS syndrome (polyneuropathy, organomegaly, endocrinopathy, M-protein, skin changes)[69] or the Crow–Fukase syndrome.[70] In addition to polyneuropathy these patients have other features (Table 127.6) suggesting the presence of an underlying endocrinopathy or malignancy.[47,69–71] The reason for the endocrinopathy is unclear. Limited data suggest a disturbance of the hypothalamopituitary axis rather than primary end-organ failure.[46] The organomegaly is usually non-specific pathologically. Biopsy of affected lymph nodes generally discloses hyperplastic changes, sometimes resembling the pathological findings in the syndrome of angiofollicular lymph node hyperplasia (Castleman's disease), which is a benign localized or generalized hyperplastic lymph node syndrome of unknown etiology. Interestingly, patients with generalized angiofollicular lymph node hyperplasia without bony lesions may also have the manifestations of Crow–Fukase syndrome associated with serum M-proteins or polyclonal gammopathies. Thus, it is likely that the main pathogenetic determinant of these syndromes is the oversecretion of a serum product such as cytokines[59] or VEGF.[60–64] The term POEMS syndrome is, however, not entirely accurate for these patients, and focuses attention on a small number of them to the exclusion of others.[47,71] For example, most patients with OSM polyneuropathy have features other than neuropathy which are fragments of a multisystemic disorder, but only a few would qualify for the term POEMS (Table 127.6). Also, patients without myeloma may develop all the features of the POEMS syndrome. Thus, the term Crow–Fukase syndrome is preferable when referring to patients with polyneuropathy and multisystemic disorder, as suggested by Nakanishi and colleagues.[70]

Primary systemic amyloidosis (PSA)

PSA can occur in the setting of multiple myeloma[54] or Waldenström's macroglobulinemia,[72] although most commonly it presents in the absence of a malignant

Table 127.6 Non-neurological abnormalities in 16 patients with OSM and polyneuropathy

Abnormality	Patients
Gyneomastia	2
Hepatomegaly	5
Splenomegaly	2
Hyperpigmentation	5
Edema	3
Lymphadenopathy	2
Papilledema	4
Digit clubbing	3
White nails	2
Hypertrichosis	3
Atrophic testes	3
Impotence	4
Polycythemia	5
Leucocytosis	3
Thrombocythemia	12
Hypotestosterone	5
Hyperestrogen	3
Hypothyroid	2
Hyperglycemia	1

OSM, osteosclerotic myeloma.
Adapted from Kelly JJ Jr, Kyle RA, Miles JM, et al. Osteosclerotic myeloma and peripheral neuropathy. Neurology (NY) 1983; 33; 202[47]

plasma cell dyscrasia.[73–76] It should always be considered when a patient develops a neuropathy in the setting of a malignant or apparently benign plasma cell dyscrasia, or in any patient who presents with a predominantly small-fiber neuropathy with attendant autonomic symptoms.

1. *Clinical presentation* This syndrome is perhaps the best characterized of the polyneuropathies associated with M-proteins and accounts for up to one-quarter of cases in some series.[4] It characteristically occurs in older men and is rare prior to the sixth decade. Most cases are unassociated with an underlying illness, but a few are associated with hematological malignancies such as myeloma and Waldenström's macroglobulinemia.[47] PSA generally presents as a multisystem disease owing to the deposition of fragments of the variable portion of a monoclonal light chain, most often λ, in tissue.[74–76] Patients present with a medical disease with associated polyneuropathy (60%), or severe polyneuropathy with minimal organ involvement (40%).[75] A similar illness can occur in a variety of inherited amyloid polyneuropathies owing to an abnormal circulating prealbumin (transthyretin) protein with a single amino acid substitution. Polyneuropathy does not occur in amyloidosis secondary to chronic inflammatory disease or familial CNS amyloidosis.

2. *Medical syndromes* These (see Table 127.5) include the nephrotic syndrome caused by amyloid infiltration of the kidneys, cardiac failure due to amyloid cardiomyopathy, chronic diarrhea with wasting due to amyloid infiltration of the gut wall, and autonomic neuropathy with prominent orthostatic hypoten-

sion.[75] General laboratory studies reflect the medical syndromes, with proteinuria occurring in a high percentage, elevated erythrocyte sedimentation rate in about half, and a mild increase in benign-appearing plasma cells in bone marrow in many. Up to 90% have an M-protein in serum or a monoclonal light chain in urine when thoroughly screened with serum and urine IFE.[75] Those lacking an M-protein may have inherited amyloid neuropathy. However, most have primary systemic amyloidosis and are called non-secretory. Immunocytological studies of their tissue disclose amyloid derived from single (monoclonal) light chains. Presumably the serum concentration is too low to detect light chains in these patients. The light chains are deposited in tissue, where they are digested by macrophages with the production of amyloid fibrils, which are insoluble.

3. *Clinical findings* The polyneuropathy has been well characterized.[75,76] Sensory symptoms are typically most prominent and the earliest to appear. Almost all present with numbness of the hands and legs, with complaints such as burning, aching, stabbing and shooting pains. In more than half of patients cutaneous sensation (light touch, pain, temperature) is more frequently and severely affected than discriminatory sensation (vibration and position sense). Occasional patients (about 20%) present with the typical symptoms of carpal tunnel syndrome due to amyloid infiltration of the flexor retinaculum of the wrist before distal neuropathy symptoms appear. Rare patients present with symptoms of autonomic dysfunction without symptoms of somatic sensory dysfunction. Symptoms and signs of weakness generally follow. These are usually less prominent than the sensory findings, although rare patients may present with predominantly motor findings.[77] Occasional patients with amyloid infiltrative myopathy present with proximal muscle weakness,[78] and patients with malignant plasma cell dyscrasias, such as myeloma, may present with additional compressive radiculopathies which can mimic mononeuropathies or plexopathies. Otherwise the findings tend to be symmetrical and predominantly distal, with gradual proximal spread. Most patients soon complain of autonomic dysfunction, with orthostatic lightheadedness and syncope,

bowel and bladder disturbances, impotence, and sweating disturbances. Hypoactive pupils and orthostatic blood pressure drop with a fixed heart rate are the most easily detected autonomic signs at the bedside.

4. *Laboratory studies* Electrophysiological studies confirm the presence of a distal axonopathy which is maximal in the legs.[75] Motor conduction velocities in the very slow range occur rarely and then only in severely affected nerves, where the evoked compound muscle action potential is very low in amplitude. Sensory nerve action potentials are usually absent. Often there is evidence of carpal tunnel syndrome, which can suggest the diagnosis. Needle EMG shows the changes expected of a distal axonopathy, with abundant signs of distal denervation and reinnervation. Cerebrospinal fluid is usually acellular and there are typically mild elevations of protein levels, in the range 50–70 mg/dL. Diagnosis depends on the discovery of amyloid in tissue. Sural nerve biopsy is very useful in the detection of amyloid in virtually all cases, although occasionally it has to be sought through multiple sections. One study, however, reported that six of 10 patients with PSA neuropathy had negative nerve biopsies,[79] so biopsy of more than one tissue is generally advisable (Table 127.7). Other useful tissues to biopsy include rectum, fat pad aspiration—reported to be 82% sensitive[80]—and other affected organs, such as kidney. Because fat pad biopsy is so simple and innocuous, we now biopsy this organ first and, if negative, proceed with nerve or other tissue biopsy. Amorphous deposits of amyloid on Congo red or cresyl violet stains typically appear in the perivascular regions of the epineurium, or occasionally in the endoneurium. Amyloid is classically defined by its appearance under polarized light, where the Congo red-stained deposits emit an apple-green birefringence. Electron microscopy can also be used to identify the characteristic β-pleated fibrils. Immunofluorescent staining for monoclonal light-chain fragments is helpful but is technically more demanding and should be limited to experienced laboratories. Teased fiber studies show predominant axonal degeneration. The reason for nerve fiber damage, however, is not always readily apparent in all

Table 127.7   Results of biopsy in primary amyloidosis with neuropathy

Site	Number of patients	Percentage positive
Rectum	25	88
Kidney	4	75
Liver	2	100
Small intestine	2	100
Bone marrow	21	33
Sural nerve	10	100
Other (skin, gingiva)	2	100

Adapted from Kelly JJ Jr, Kyle RA, O'Brien PC, et al. The natural history of peripheral neuropathy in primary systemic amyloidosis. Ann Neurol 1979;5:1–7)[75]

cases. In some instances, marked axonal degeneration appears with minimal amyloid infiltration, possibly caused by more proximal amyloid, perhaps at the level of the dorsal root ganglion.

5. *Pathogenesis* These findings have led to many theories about the pathogenesis of the neuropathy, including vascular and pressure changes by the amyloid deposits. However, direct toxic effects of the amyloid fibrils on nerve fibers and dorsal root ganglion cells seem more likely.[1]

6. *Treatment* Treatment is problematic. The amyloid fibrils are insoluble once deposited in tissue. It is therefore unlikely that much improvement would appear even with cessation of amyloid deposition. So far, the neuropathy has resisted all attempts to halt its progression with combinations of anti-inflammatory medications, including steroids, alkylating agents such as melphalan and cyclophosphamide, and even more intensive combination chemotherapy[81] designed to slow production of the light chains. In addition, prolonged plasma-pheresis is aimed at lowering the light-chain concentration in serum.[75,82,83] However, the nephropathy due to light-chain deposition has been shown to be partially responsive to a combination of melphalan and prednisone.[82,83] These patients usually progress inexorably, with increasing numbness and pain, autonomic failure and weakness, with added multiorgan failure in many cases. Death usually occurs in two to four years from the time of diagnosis and is generally due to major organ failure, most commonly cardiac. Diagnosis is delayed most in patients with relatively pure neuropathies without significant organ failure (median 26 months).[78,84] The disease has a dismal prognosis and 85% are dead within 25 months.[75] The role of high-dose chemotherapy and stem cell rescue in this disorder is yet to be determined.

Miscellaneous syndromes

Waldenström's macroglobulinemia (WM) Separating WM from IgM-MGUS is difficult and the latter

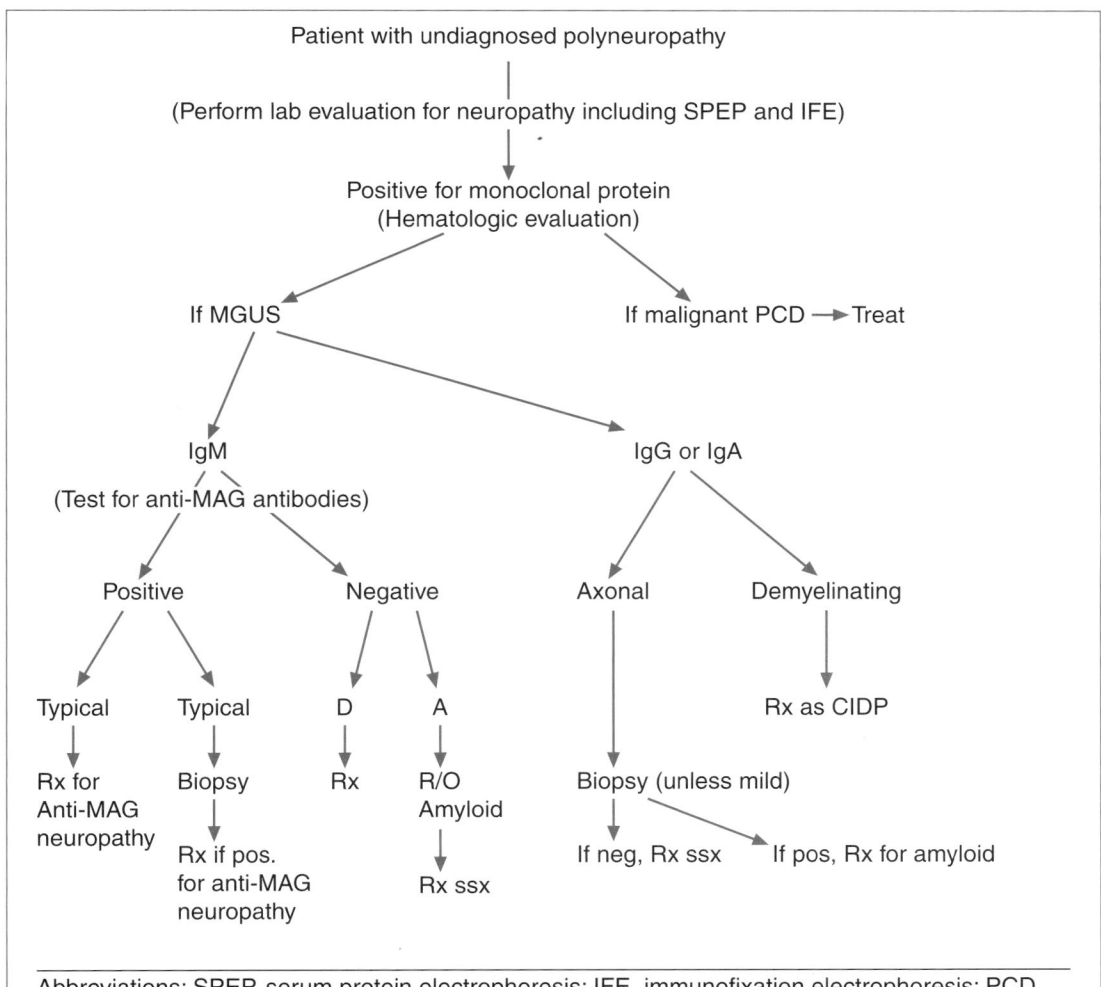

Abbreviations: SPEP, serum protein electrophoresis; IFE, immunofixation electrophoresis; PCD, plasma cell dyscrasia; MGUS, monoclonal protein of undetermined significance; IgM, IgG or IgA, immunoglobulins M, G or A; anti-MAG antibodies, anti-Myelin-Associated-Glycoprotein antibodies; Rx, treat; ssx, symptoms; D, demyelinating neuropathy pattern; A, axonal neuropathy pattern.

Figure 127.1   Treatment algorithm for managing a patient with neuropathy and monoclonal gammopathy.

may evolve into WM over time.[72] Thus, similar polyneuropathy syndromes occur. The most frequent polyneuropathy encountered is probably that associated with anti-MAG antibodies.[14] This syndrome has the same features and clinical course as in IgM-MGUS because, despite the presence of a malignant plasma cell dyscrasia, the anti-MAG antibody probably determines the type of neuropathy. One patient with anti-MAG neuropathy and WM was reported to respond to bone marrow transplantation.[72] Other patients may have a CIDP-like picture, a distal axonal neuropathy, typical amyloid polyneuropathy, or even the sensory neuronopathy syndrome usually seen with small cell cancer of the lung. Rare patients develop central nervous system symptoms due to hyperviscosity, requiring urgent lowering of viscosity via plasmapheresis. These patients present with encephalopathy with or without seizures. Treatment is based on rapid lowering of IgM levels, hydration, and chemotherapy to lower IgM production. The prognosis is often poor unless the patient is treated promptly before there is significant neurological deterioration.

Cryoglobulinemia   This disorder is usually divided into three types.[85,86] In type 1, the M-protein itself is a cryoglobulin in the setting of a plasma cell disorder. In type 2 the cryoglobulin is a mixture of an M-protein of IgM type with rheumatoid factor activity against polyclonal immunoglobulins, usually occurring in the setting of a lymphoproliferative disorder. Type 3 occurs in the setting of a collagen–vascular or other chronic inflammatory disease, and the cryoglobulin consists of polyclonal immunoglobulins. The polyneuropathy in all these syndromes is painful, symmetrical or asymmetrical, sensorimotor and axonal in nature. Purpura occurs in distal limbs in a high percentage of patients, and the neuropathy is generally considered to be due to a vasculopathy or vasculitis of skin and vasa nervorum.

Lymphoma, leukemia, cancer   These disorders can be associated with MP and polyneuropathy.[14] In lymphoma with IgM M-protein the IgM may have anti-MAG activity with the usual clinical and pathological features. Other syndromes without clear antinerve activity in the M-protein fraction may respond to ablation of the malignancy. Still others have an unclear relation to the malignancy and show little response to tumoricidal treatment or to lowering of the M-protein concentration in serum.

Conclusion

The topic of plasma cell dyscrasias and neurological disease has been a fruitful area for active research over the last two decades. These patients frequently develop or present with neurological disease, and an organized approach, as presented here, aids diagnosis (Figure 127.1). Prompt treatment can reverse many of these patients, and prompt recognition and treatment may lead to remission in some cases. Study of these patients may lead to a better understanding of the

pathogenesis of polyneuropathies, and possibly of motor neuron disease. This may in turn lead to effective treatment for conditions which are currently untreatable. Therefore, despite their relative infrequency, increased recognition of these neuropathies will continue to be a high priority for both peripheral nerve specialists and general neurologists.

References

1. Kelly JJ Jr. Peripheral neuropathies associated with monoclonal proteins: a clinical review. Muscle Nerve 1985;8:138–150
2. Latov N, Sherman WH, Nemni R, et al. Plasma cell dyscrasia and peripheral neuropathy with a monoclonal antibody to peripheral nerve myelin. N Engl J Med 1980;303:618–621
3. Osby LE, Noring L, Hast R, et al. Benign monoclonal gammopathy and peripheral neuropathy. Br J Haematol 1982;51:531–539
4. Kelly JJ Jr, Kyle RA, O'Brien PC, et al. Prevalence of monoclonal protein in peripheral neuropathy. Neurology 1981;31:1480–1483
5. Khan SN, Riches PG, Kohn J. Paraproteinemia in neurological disease: incidence, association and classification of monoclonal immunoglobulins. J Clin Pathol 1980;33:617–621
6. Kyle RA. Plasma cell dyscrasias. *In:* Spitell JA Jr, ed. Clinical Medicine. Philadelphia: Harper & Row, 1981: 1–35
7. Kyle RA. "Benign" monoclonal gammopathy: A misnomer? JAMA 1984;251:1849–1854
8. Kelly JJ Jr, Kyle RA, Latov N. Polyneuropathies associated with plasma cell dyscrasias. Boston: Martinus-Nijhoff, 1987
9. Latov NR, Hays AP, Sherman WH. Peripheral neuropathy and anti-MAG antibodies. CRC Crit Rev Neurobiol 1988;3:301–332
10. Latov N, Braun PE, Gross RA, et al. Plasma cell dyscrasia and peripheral neuropathy; identification of the myelin antigens that react with human paraproteins. Proc Natl Acad Sci 1981;78:7139–7142
11. Chassande B, Leger JM, Younes-Chennoufi AB, et al. Peripheral neuropathy associated with IgM monoclonal gammopathy: correlations between M-protein antibody activity and clinical/electrophysiological features in 40 cases. Muscle Nerve 1998;21:55–62
12. Kelly JJ Jr, Adelman LS, Berkman E, et al. Polyneuropathies associated with IgM monoclonal gammopathies. Arch Neurol 1988;45:1355–1359
13. Kelly JJ Jr. The electrodiagnostic findings in polyneuropathies associated with IgM monoclonal gammopathies. Muscle Nerve 1990;13:1113–1117
14. Latov N, Wokke JHJ, Kelly JJ Jr. Immunological and Infectious Diseases of the Peripheral Nerves. Cambridge: Cambridge University Press, 1997
15. Melmed C, Frail DE, Duncan I, et al. Peripheral neuropathy with IgM kappa monoclonal immunoglobulin directed against myelin-associated glycoprotein. Neurology 1983;33:1397–1405
16. Bain PG, Britton TC, Jenkins IH, et al. Tremor associated with benign IgM paraproteinemia. Brain 1996; 119:789–799
17. Kaku DA, England JD, Sumner AJ. Distal accentuation of conduction slowing in polyneuropathy associated with antibodies to myelin-associated glycoprotein and sulphated glucuronyl paragloboside. Brain 1994; 117:941–947

18. Ellie E, Vital A, Steck A, et al. Neuropathy associated with "benign" anti-myelin-associated glycoprotein IgM gammopathy: clinical, immunological, neurophysiological and pathological findings and response to treatment in 33 cases. J Neurol 1996;243:34–43

19. Jacobs JM. Morphological changes at paranodes in IgM paraproteinaemic neuropathy. Microsc Res Tech 1996;34:544–553

20. Nemni R, Galassi G, Latov N, et al. Polyneuropathy in non-malignant IgM plasma cell dyscrasia: a morphological study. Ann Neurol 1983;14:43–54

21. Vallat J-M, Tabaraud F, Sindou P, et al. Myelin widening and MGUS-IgA: An immunoelectron microscopic study. Ann Neurol 2000;47:808–811

22. Ilyas AA, Cook SD, Dalakas MC, Mithen FA. Anti-MAG IgM paraproteins from some patients with polyneuropathy associated with IgM paraproteinemia also react with sulfatide. J Neuroimmunol 1992;37:85–92

23. Yu RK, Ariga T. The role of glycosphingolipids in neurological disorders. Mechanisms of immune action. Ann NY Acad Sci 1998;19:285–306

24. Gosselin S, Kyle R, Dyck P. Neuropathy associated with monoclonal gammopathies of undetermined significance. Ann Neurol 1991;30:54–61

25. Simovic D, Gorson KC, Ropper AH. Comparison of IgM-MGUS and IgG-MGUS polyneuropathy. Acta Neurol Scand 1998;97:194–200

26. Suarez GA, Kelly JJ Jr. Polyneuropathy associated with monoclonal gammopathy of undetermined significance: further evidence that IgM-MGUS neuropathies are different than IgG-MGUS. Neurology 1993;43:1304–1308

27. Tatum AH. Experimental paraprotein neuropathy, demyelination by passive transfer of human IgM anti-myelin-associated glycoprotein. Ann Neurol 1993:33;502–506

28. Gorson KC. Clinical features and treatment of patients with polyneuropathy associated with monoclonal gammopathy of undetermined significance (MGUS). J Clin Aperesis 1991;14:149–153

29. Notermans NC, Lokhorst HM, Franssen H, et al. Intermittent cyclophosphamide and prednisone treatment of polyneuropathy associated with monoclonal gammopathy of undetermined significance. Neurology 1996;47:1227–1233

30. Meucci N, Baldini L, Cappellari A, et al. Anti-myelin-associated antibodies predict the development of neuropathy in asymptomatic patients with IgM monoclonal gammopathy. Ann Neurol 1999;46:119–222

31. Weiss MD, Dalakas MC, Lauter CJ, et al. Variability in the binding of anti-MAG and anti-SGPG antibodies to target antigens in demyelinating neuropathy and IgM paraproteinemias. J Neuroimmunol 1999;95:174–184

32. Dyck PJ, Low PA, Windebank AJ, et al. Plasma exchange in polyneuropathy associated with monoclonal gammopathy of undetermined significance. N Engl J Med 1991;325:1482–1486

33. Dalakas MC, Quarles RH, Farrer RG, et al. A controlled study of intravenous immunoglobulin in demyelinating neuropathy with IgM gammopathy. Ann Neurol 1996;40:792–795

34. Ernerudh JH, Vrethem M, Andersen O, et al. Immunochemical and clinic effects of immunosuppressive treatment in monoclonal IgM neuropathy. J Neurol Neurosurg Psychiatry 1992;55:930–934

35. Nobile-Orazio E, Meucci N, Baldini L, et al. Long-term prognosis of neuropathy associated with anti-MAG IgM M-proteins and its relationship to immune therapies. Brain 2000;123:710–717

36. Wilson HC, Lunn MP, Schey S, Hughes RA. Successful treatment of IgM paraproteinemia with fludarabine. J Neurol Neurosurg Psychiatry 1999;66:575–580

37. Mariette X, Chastang C, Clavelou P, et al. A randomized clinical trial comparing interferon-alpha and intravenous immunoglobulin in polyneuropathy associated with monoclonal IgM. The IgM-associated Polyneuropathy Study Group. J Neurol Neurosurg Psychiatry 1997;63:28–34

38. Toepfer M, Schroeder M, Muller-Felber W, et al. Successful management of polyneuropathy associated with IgM gammopathy of undetermined significance with antibody-based immunoadsorption. Clin Nephrol 2000;53:404–407

39. Niemierko E, Weinstein R. Response of patients with IgM and IgA-associated peripheral polyneuropathies to "off-line" immunoabsorption treatment using the Prosorba protein A columns. Endocr Res 1991; 25:371–380

40. Dabby R, Weimer LH, Hays AP, et al. Antisulfatide antibodies in neuropathy: clinical and electrophysiologic correlates. Neurology 2000;54:1448–1452

41. Noerager BD, Inuzuka T, Kira J, et al. An IgM anti-MBP Ab in a case of Waldenström's macroglobulinemia with polyneuropathy expressing an idiotype reactive with an MBP epitope immunodominant in MS and EAE. J Neuroimmunol 2001;113:163–169

42. Gorson KC, Ropper AH. Axonal neuropathy associated with monoclonal gammopathy of undetermined significance. J Neurol Neurosurg Psychiatry 1997; 63:163–168

43. Steck AJ, Murray N, Dellagi K, et al. Peripheral neuropathy associated with monoclonal IgM autoantibody. Ann Neurol 1987;22:764–767

44. Ponsford S, Willison H, Veitch J, et al. Long-term and neurophysiological follow-up of patients with peripheral neuropathy associated with benign monoclonal gammopathy. Muscle Nerve 2000:23;150–152

45. DiTroia A, Carpo M, Meucci N, et al. Clinical features and anti-neural reactivity in neuropathy associated with IgG monoclonal gammopathy of undetermined significance. J Neurol Sci 1999;15:64–71

46. Simmons Z, Albers JW, Bromberg MB, et al. Presentation and initial clinical course in patients with chronic inflammatory demyelinating polyradiculoneuropathy: comparison of patients without and with monoclonal gammopathy. Neurology 1993;43:2202–2209

47. Kelly JJ Jr, Kyle RA, Miles JM, et al. Osteosclerotic myeloma and peripheral neuropathy. Neurology (NY) 1983;33:202–210

48. Lindstrom E, Lindstrom FD. Skeletal scintigraphy with technetium diphosphonate in multiple myeloma—a comparison with skeletal x-ray. Acta Med Scand 1980;208:289–291

49. Tamir R, Glanz I, Lubin E, et al. Comparison of the sensitivity of ^{99m}Tc-methyl diphosphonate bone scan with the skeletal X-ray survey in multiple myeloma. Acta Haematol 1983;69:236–242

50. Leifer D, Grabowski T, Simonian N, Demirjian ZN. Leptomeningeal myelomatosis presenting with mental status changes and other neurologic findings [Review]. Cancer 1992;70:1899–1904

51. Lebrun C, Chanalet S, Paquis P, et al. Solitary meningeal plasmacytomas. Ann Oncol 1997;8:791–795

52. Roddie P, Collie D, Johnson P. Myelomatous involvement of the dura mater: a rare complication of multiple myeloma. J Clin Pathol 2000;53:398–399

53. Wisniewski T, Sisti M, Inhirami G, et al. Intracerebral solitary plasmacytoma. Neurosurgery 1990;27:826–829; discussion 829

54. Kelly JJ Jr, Kyle RA, Miles JM, et al. The spectrum of peripheral neuropathy in myeloma. Neurology (NY) 1981;31:24–31

55. Kyle RA. Clinical aspects of multiple myeloma and related disorders including amyloidosis. Pathol Biol 1999;47:148–157

56. Scheinker I. Myelom und nervensystem. Deutsch Zeits Nervenheikenstalt 1938;147:247–273

57. Victor M, Banker B, Adams RD. The neuropathy of multiple myeloma. J Neurol Neurosurg Psychiatry 1958;21:73–78

58. Adams D, Said G. Ultrastructural characterisation of the M protein in nerve biopsy of patients with POEMS syndrome. J Neurol Neurosurg Psychiatry 1998;64: 809–812

59. Gherardi RK, Authier FJ, Belec L. Les cytokines pro-inflammatoires: une pathogénique du syndrome POEMS. Rev Neurol 1996;64:809–812

60. Nakano A, Mitsui T, Endo I, et al. Solitary plasmacytoma with VEGF overproduction: report of a patient with polyneuropathy. Neurology 2001;56:818–819

61. Watanabe O, Arimura K, Kitajami I, et al. Greatly increased growth factor (VEGF) in POEMS syndrome. Lancet 1996;347:702

62. Watanabe O, Maruyama I, Arimura K, et al. Overproduction of vascular endothelial growth factor/vascular permeability factor is causative in Crow–Fukase (POEMS) syndrome. Muscle Nerve 1998;21:1390–1397.

63. Watanabe O, Arimura K, Kitajami I, et al. Greatly increased growth factor (VEGF) in POEMS syndrome. Lancet 1996;347:702

64. Nakano A, Mitsui T, Endo I, et al. Solitary plasmacytoma with VEGF overproduction: report of a patient with polyneuropathy. Neurology 2001;56:818–819

65. Belec L, Mohamed AS, Authier FJ, et al. Human herpesvirus 8 infection in patients with POEMS syndrome-associated multicentric Castleman's disease. Blood 1999;93:3643–3653

66. Davison C, Balser BH. Myeloma neuropathy: successful treatment of two patients and review of cases. Arch Surg 1937;35:913–936

67. Donofrio PD, Albers JW, Greenberg HS, et al. Peripheral neuropathy in osteosclerotic myeloma: clinical and electrodiagnostic improvement with chemotherapy. Muscle Nerve 1984;7:137–141

68. Kuwabara S, Hattori T, Shimoe Y, Kamitsukasa I. Long term melphalan-prednisolone chemotherapy for POEMS syndrome. J Neurol Neurosurg Psychiatry 1997;63:385–387

69. Bardwick PZ, Zvaifler NJ, Gill GN, et al. Plasma cell dyscrasia with polyneuropathy, organomegaly, endocrinopathy, M-protein and skin changes: the POEMS syndrome. Medicine 1980;59:311–322

70. Nakanishi T, Sobue I, Toyokura Y, et al. The Crow–Fukase syndrome: a study of 102 cases in Japan. Neurology 1984;34:712–720

71. Miralles GD, O'Fallon J, Talley NJ. Plasma cell dyscrasia with polyneuropathy: the spectrum of POEMS syndrome. N Engl J Med 1992;327:1919–1923

72. Rudnicki SA, Harik SI, Dhodapkar M, et al. Nervous system dysfunction in Waldenström's macroglobulinemia: response to treatment. Neurology 1998;51: 1210–1213

73. DeNavasquez S, Treble HA. A case of primary generalized amyloid disease with involvement of the nerves. Brain 1938;61:116–128

74. Gertz MA, Lacy MQ, Dispenzieri A. Amyloidosis: recognition, confirmation, prognosis and therapy. Mayo Clin Proc 1999;74:490–494

75. Kelly JJ Jr, Kyle RA, O'Brien PC, et al. The natural history of peripheral neuropathy in primary systemic amyloidosis. Ann Neurol 1979;5:1–7

76. Trotter JL, Engel WE, Ignaczak TF. Amyloidosis with plasma cell dyscrasia: an overlooked cause of adult onset sensorimotor polyneuropathy. Arch Neurol 1947;34:209–214

77. Quattrini A, Nemni R, Sferrazza B, et al. Amyloid neuropathy simulating lower moor neuron disease. Neurology 1998;51:600–602

78. Spuler S, Emslie-Smith A, Engel AG. Amyloid myopathy: an underdiagnosed entity. Ann Neurol 1998; 43:719–728

79. Simmons Z, Blaivas M, Aguilera AJ, et al. Low diagnostic yield of sural nerve biopsy in patients with peripheral neuropathy and primary amyloidosis. J Neurol Sci 1993;120:60–63

80. Masouye I. Diagnostic screening of systemic amyloidosis by abdominal fat aspiration: an analysis of 100 cases. Am J Dermatopathol 1997;19:41–45

81. Gertz MA, Lacy MQ, Lust JA, et al. Prospective randomized trial of melphalan and prednisone versus vincristine, carmustine, melphalan, cyclophosphamide, and prednisone in the treatment of primary systemic amyloidosis. J Clin Oncol 1999;17:262–267

82. Gertz MA, Kyle RZ, Greipp PR. Response rates and survival in primary systemic amyloidosis. Blood 1991;77:257–262

83. Gertz MA, Kyle RA. Amyloidosis: prognosis and treatment. Semin Arthritis Rheum 1994;24:124–138

84. Rajkumar SV, Gertz MA, Kyle RZ. Prognosis of patients with primary systemic amyloidosis who present with dominant neuropathy. Am J Med 1998;104:232–237

85. Logothetis J, Kennedy WR, Ellington A, et al. Cryoglobulinemic neuropathy. Arch Neurol 1968;19:389–397

86. McLeod JG, Walsh JC, Pollard JD. Neuropathies associated with paraproteinemias and dysproteinemias. In: Dyck PJ, Thomas PK, Lambert EH, Bunge R, eds. Peripheral Neuropathy, 2nd edn. Philadelphia: WB Saunders, 1984:1857–1860

128 Neurological Manifestations of Systemic Disease: Cryoglobulinemia

Caroline M Klein, Eric Logigian and Guillermo A Suarez

Overview

Cryoglobulins are serum immunoglobulins that precipitate in vitro at temperatures below 37°C.[1,2] Initially, they were thought to be artifacts. However, they have been found to be a marker of systemic vasculitis of small- and medium-sized blood vessels that result in particular clinical manifestations and may either be associated with various systemic diseases or be idiopathic. According to the classification scheme of Brouet et al,[1] there are 3 types (types I, II, and III) of cryoglobulins, according to their composition (Table 128.1). Type I is a monoclonal immunoglobulin and is found typically in association with various lymphoproliferative disorders such as Waldenström macroglobulinemia or multiple myeloma. Types II and III are considered "mixed cryoglobulins" because they contain more than a single component. Type II consists of a monoclonal protein (usually IgM) that has rheumatoid factor activity against a polyclonal IgG, and type III is a polyclonal IgG with rheumatoid factor activity.

Mixed cryoglobulinemias account for the majority of cases of cryoglobulinemia.[3,4] Traditionally, they have been subdivided further into those secondary to other systemic diseases such as infections (viral, parasitic), autoimmune diseases (systemic lupus erythematosus, rheumatoid arthritis), or lymphoproliferative disorders (non-Hodgkin lymphoma) and those without associated systemic disease (i.e., "essential" mixed cryoglobulins.[2,3,5] This latter category has been modified to some extent over the last 10 years with the discovery that up to 80% to 90% of patients classified with essential mixed cryoglobulinemia were actually infected with chronic hepatitis C virus.[2,4–11] This finding has had important implications for treatment approaches to this disease.

Although cryoglobulins may be detected in low titers in otherwise normal persons,[9] their presence usually is associated with a systemic vasculitic syndrome, with multiple possible clinical features that include neurological involvement. Symptomatic cryoglobulinemia commonly includes skin involvement (purpura), polyarthralgias, or fatigue and may also manifest with more severe organ involvement of the kidney (glomerulonephritis), liver (chronic liver disease), or the nervous system (Table 128.2).[1,4,5,12] The typical patient is female, with age at onset in the fifth decade.[3,4,12] The overall clinical course of the systemic disease is that of slow progression with superimposed exacerbations and remissions.[4] The cause of death may be due to renal failure, overwhelming infection, or lymphoproliferative disease.[3]

Although not every patient with cryoglobulinemia has neurological symptoms or findings, these occur frequently[4] and denote a poorer prognosis overall because they are, especially if severe, resistant to currently available therapies.[13,14] The most common manifestation of neurological involvement is peripheral neuropathy, ranging from painful paresthesias to axonal sensorimotor peripheral neuropathy or multiple mononeuropathies with severe neurological impairment. Central nervous system (CNS) symptoms such as stroke, encephalopathy, corticobulbar or corticospinal tract involvement, communicating hydrocephalus, and seizures have been reported but are rare[1,4,9,12,15–22] (Table 128.3). Involvement of the

Table 128.1 Classification of cryoglobulinemia

Type I	Monoclonal immunoglobulin Associated with lymphoproliferative disorders such as Waldenstrom macroglobulinemia, multiple myeloma
Mixed	
Type II	Monoclonal immunoglobulin (usually IgM) with rheumatoid factor activity + polyclonal IgG
Type III	Polyclonal IgG with rheumatoid factor activity Associated with infections (viral, parasitic), autoimmune diseases, lymphoproliferative disorders (non-Hodgkin lymphoma, polyarteritis nodosa)
Essential	Type II or Type III *without* associated underlying disease except Sjögren syndrome (up to 80% to 90% are positive for hepatitis C antibody/viral RNA)

Table 128.2 Systemic clinical features associated with cryoglobulinemia

Purpura
   Ulceration
     Gangrene
Raynaud phenomenon
Polyarthralgias
Nephropathy
   Membranoproliferative glomerulonephritis
Chronic liver disease
Sicca or Sjögren syndrome

Table 128.3   Neurological complications associated with cryoglobulinemia

Peripheral neuropathy (most common)
  Distal, symmetrical, axonal sensory
  Distal, symmetrical, axonal sensorimotor
  Multiple mononeuropathies (mononeuritis multiplex)
  Combination of distal symmetrical sensorimotor
    peripheral neuropathy and superimposed multiple
    mononeuropathies (mixed pattern)
Other neurological complications (rare)
  Encephalopathy
  Coma
  Seizures
  Stroke (ischemic, cerebral hemorrhage)
  Central nervous system vasculitis
  Communicating hydrocephalus
  Myelopathy

nervous system represents severe cryoglobulinemia and treatment is appropriately aggressive and may include various immunosuppressive agents as well as antiviral regimens if hepatitis C infection is documented.

Clinical features

Peripheral neuropathy may be the initial symptom of cryoglobulinemia in some patients,[21,23–25] but the neurological symptoms generally present in association with the typical triad of purpura (typically affecting the lower extremities), polyarthralgias, and fatigue.[9,11,16,23,26–28] Purpura is the most common initial presenting symptom or finding of cryoglobulinemia[1,12] and may[1] or may not be elicited by cold environmental temperatures.[27] The incidence of peripheral neuropathy in patients with cryoglobulinemia ranges from 7%[27,29] to 90%[4,21,30] depending on the series reported. In a comprehensive, retrospective review of patients evaluated at Mayo Clinic between 1975 and 1999,[31,32] we investigated the peripheral neuropathy associated with cryoglobulinemia and found that type II cryoglobulinemia was most often associated with peripheral neuropathy.

Distal lower extremity paresthesias and numbness are the most common neurological symptoms, with weakness subsequently developing as part of a generalized sensorimotor peripheral neuropathy or mononeuritis multiplex.[1,3,4,9,12,17,24,29–31,33] Pure motor neuropathy is rare, reportedly occurring in 5% of patients.[4] The pattern of peripheral nerve involvement may be asymmetrical, as in mononeuritis multiplex, but more commonly is distal and symmetrical.[5,11–13,31,32,34–37] The initial sensory symptoms, which may include pain as well as paresthesias and numbness, may be asymmetrical[14,21,27] before progressing to a more symmetrical pattern.[14,27,31] In the Mayo Clinic retrospective series, purpura was the most common presenting symptom of the disease, occurring before the onset of sensory symptoms of tingling or numbness and burning pain, which were typically symmetrical in distribution, and preceded motor symptoms of weakness.[31] Autonomic dysfunc-

tion has not been described or documented in these patients.[34] Findings on neurological examination may include sensory loss, decreased deep tendon reflexes, and variable degrees of weakness, usually limited to the lower extremities.[14,38]

The clinical course of the more common distal symmetrical sensorimotor peripheral neuropathy is usually insidious,[13] whereas mononeuritis multiplex may present more acutely with severe deficits at onset.[13] In a group of 15 patients with peripheral neuropathy and essential mixed cryoglobulinemia, Apartis et al.[34] found that those with positive anti-hepatitis C viral antibodies were more likely to have a more severe sensorimotor neuropathy, with involvement of both the upper and lower extremities. Crespi et al.[39] followed prospectively a group of nine patients with essential mixed cryoglobulinemia over 3 to 6 years and found that the peripheral neuropathy in one-half of the patients tended to worsen slightly over time, although the degree of peripheral nerve involvement at the onset was mild (symmetrical, axonal sensory).

Gemignani et al.[33] reported on a group of patients who had symmetrical sensory neuropathy associated with mixed cryoglobulinemia and prominent symptoms of restless legs syndrome. They thought that the restless legs symptoms were due to moderate sensory loss from the neuropathy.

On electrophysiological and pathological evaluations, the peripheral nerve involvement in cryoglobulinemia has been characterized as axonal degeneration, with minimal demyelinating features.[7,11–13,24,25,27,30,32,34–37,39–44] In the Mayo Clinic retrospective series, electrodiagnostic testing performed on a total of 56 patients with cryoglobulinemic peripheral neuropathy revealed axonal sensorimotor abnormalities in the majority of patients with multiple mononeuropathies or mixed pattern seen less commonly.[31,32] Sural nerve biopsy specimens have findings diagnostic or suggestive of necrotizing vasculitis,[3,11,13–16,19,24,25,28,31,33,34,36,37,40,41,45,46] focal ischemia,[11] or axonal degeneration and myelinated fiber loss without inflammation.[26,30,35,38,47] Demyelination is rarely seen in biopsy specimens[16,25,30] and may be secondary to axonal degeneration. Alterations in the structure of the wall of endoneurial blood vessels, that is, thickening and luminal occlusion, have also been described in sural nerve biopsy specimens.[24,26,35,45]

On the basis of nerve biopsy data, the peripheral nerve manifestations of cryoglobulinemia are thought to be due to vasculitis. The various CNS features have been investigated less extensively but presumably are due at least partly to vasculopathy or vasculitis in the CNS.[15,20,22] Gorevic et al.[12] reported on a group of 40 patients with essential mixed cryoglobulinemia who were evaluated between 1960 and 1978 (before the association with hepatitis C virus was known), and on postmortem, the authors found systemic vasculitis involving small- and medium-sized blood vessels in the heart, gastrointestinal tract, muscle, skin, lung, peripheral nerve, and CNS of nine subjects.

The pathophysiological mechanism of neurological complications in cryoglobulinemia is not certain. Although the vasculitic changes observed pathologically in nervous tissue biopsy specimens likely account for axonal degeneration and fiber loss in peripheral nerve,[14] the initial triggering factors for the inflammation have not been determined. Despite viral antigens having been localized by immunofluorescent techniques to the walls of blood vessels in areas of purpura as well as healthy skin[9,48,49] in patients with cryoglobulinemia and associated hepatitis C infection, no viral antigens have been found in peripheral nerve or kidney.[9,49] With the reverse transcription-polymerase chain reaction (RT-PCR), Bonetti et al.[36] found hepatitis C RNA in five nerve biopsy specimens and determined that the RNA localized to the nerve was the same genotype as that in the serum. These investigators also demonstrated in situ RT-PCR positivity in macrophages surrounding epineurial blood vessels in three of five nerve biopsy specimens examined, suggesting that hepatitis C viral infection of perivascular cells may lead to lymphocytic infiltration and tissue damage. Immune complexes have been localized to these tissues;[14,15,19,45,50] thus, neurological involvement may be part of a systemic immune-complex disease.[3,16,21,24,29,51–53] This systemic immune involvement appears to be related directly to a certain degree of clonal B lymphocyte expansion.[53] Damage of local blood vessels from immune-complex deposition could lead to local ischemic changes and, eventually, to axonal degeneration in peripheral nerves.[12,19,41]

Because active hepatitis C viral infection (with isolation of hepatitis C viral RNA by PCR) has been found in the majority of patients with essential mixed cryoglobulinemia, its role in the pathogenesis of cryoglobulinemic neuropathy has been aggressively sought. There are several potential mechanisms. Chronic viral infection of circulating lymphocytes could lead to infection of endothelial cells in nerve (and other tissue) with subsequent release of cytokines and an expanding inflammatory response.[6,9,49] Also, hepatitis C viral infection may disrupt the reticuloendothelial system in the liver so that appropriate clearance of immune complexes, formed from the circulating cryoglobulins, is impaired, with deposition of these complexes in susceptible organs or tissues.[3,54] Because hepatitis C has an affinity for lymphocytes and hepatocytes,[51] it may trigger an autoimmune or lymphoproliferative disorder.[53,55–57] In fact, concomitant development of autoimmune hepatitis type I in patients with hepatitis C-associated mixed cryoglobulinemia has led to particular treatment dilemmas.[53] The concentration of hepatitis C viral antibody and RNA in cryoprecipitates[2,10,40,54,58] suggests that the virus may have a crucial role in the formation of circulating immune complexes.[10,47,53,54] Although this has not been proved,[3] the beneficial clinical effects of interferon alfa in treating mixed cryoglobulinemia associated with hepatitis C provides possible evidence of a link between the presence of the virus and cryoglobulins.[6,51,54]

Diagnosis

The diagnostic evaluation of a patient with suspected cryoglobulinemia begins with the demonstration of a cryoprecipitate of measurable quantity from the patient's serum, a procedure that requires scrupulous and standardized laboratory technique (Figure 128.1). This test should be performed when symptoms of polyneuropathy are accompanied by purpura, polyarthralgias, fatigue, Raynaud phenomenon (Table 128.2), hepatitis C viral infection, or any other systemic condition associated with cryoglobulin formation.[1,3,12] Testing for cryoglobulins should also be considered in patients with polyneuropathy of unknown cause. Other general laboratory findings may include low serum levels of total complement or C4, increased rheumatoid factor activity, increased erythrocyte sedimentation rate, increased antinuclear antibody levels, abnormal liver function tests, and possibly increased cerebrospinal fluid protein concentration.[7,13,14,25,27,41–43,55] Serum protein electrophoresis may show a monoclonal protein spike,[43] although it more commonly shows only polyclonal hypergammaglobulinemia. In testing for hepatitis C, viral antibody titers should be confirmed with the RNA PCR of the serum or the cryoprecipitate (if the serum is negative).[10,43]

If a patient with cryoglobulinemia reports symptoms of peripheral neuropathy, including burning pain, paresthesias, focal weakness, then nerve conduction studies and electromyography should be performed to document and characterize the neuropathy. As part of this evaluation, other causes of peripheral neuropathy should be considered and excluded. Cutaneous nerve biopsy may be useful to verify the presence of vasculitis before immunosuppressive therapy is initiated and it may also serve to exclude other causes of neuropathy such as amyloidosis or sarcoidosis.

Patients with suspected involvement of the CNS should have magnetic resonance imaging and possibly cerebral arteriography to help document CNS vasculitis. Leptomeningeal biopsy is rarely necessary, but it may be helpful in certain situations, particularly when other diagnoses such as CNS lymphoma are under consideration.

The differential diagnosis for vasculitic neuropathy includes diabetes mellitus, polyarteritis nodosa, Churg-Strauss vasculitis, Wegener granulomatosis, rheumatoid arthritis and vasculitis, systemic lupus erythematosus, neurosarcoidosis, syphilis, Lyme disease, Sjögren syndrome, and nonsystemic vasculitis affecting peripheral nerve,[43] each of which generally is associated with distinctive clinical and laboratory features. Note that sicca or Sjögren syndrome is commonly associated with mixed cryoglobulinemia.[10,12,29,58] However, the other clinical manifestations of cryoglobulinemia, such as purpura and glomerulonephritis, are not part of Sjögren syndrome.

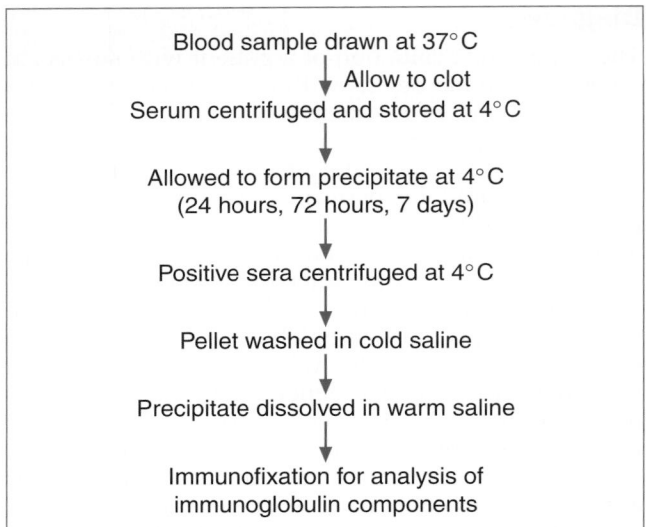

Blood sample drawn at 37°C
↓ Allow to clot
Serum centrifuged and stored at 4°C

↓

Allowed to form precipitate at 4°C
(24 hours, 72 hours, 7 days)

↓

Positive sera centrifuged at 4°C

↓

Pellet washed in cold saline

↓

Precipitate dissolved in warm saline

↓

Immunofixation for analysis of
immunoglobulin components

Figure 128.1   Laboratory method for demonstrating cryoprecipitates for diagnosis of cryoglobulinemia

Treatment

Treatment of neurological manifestations of cryoglobulinemia depends on the presence or absence of underlying or associated disease such as hepatitis C viral infection. Traditionally, neurological disease associated with cryoglobulinemia has been considered a "major" clinical indicator of severe disease and one that warrants aggressive immunosuppressive therapy.[1] Therefore, neurological disease was equated in severity with renal involvement as a requirement for treatment. However, attempts to treat the neurological manifestations with immunomodulating therapy have had limited benefit.[3] With the discovery that a substantial number of patients with "essential" mixed cryoglobulinemia have hepatitis C viral infection, alternative strategies have evolved.

Because CNS manifestations of cryoglobulinemia rarely occur, their treatment has not been studied systematically. Successful outcomes have been reported with high-dose oral prednisone,[20] plasmapheresis,[15,19] or combination therapy with cyclophosphamide and intravenous methylprednisolone,[22] but it is uncertain which of these therapeutic regimens is most effective.

Treatment of peripheral neuropathy has been investigated more thoroughly but with mixed success. Improvement in sensory symptoms and findings (without electrophysiological correlation) has been reported in individual patients or small series of patients given treatment with high-dose prednisone.[14,25] Others also have reported improvement in peripheral neuropathy[12,13,45,47] with individual or combination immunosuppressive therapies, including corticosteroids, interferon, cyclophosphamide, chlorambucil, azathioprine, or plasmapheresis, but treatment failure is not uncommon.[12,24,41]

Data from individual and small case series indicate that patients with mixed cryoglobulinemia and hepatitis C viral infection experience only minimal improvement in neurological symptoms when treated with corticosteroids, cyclophosphamide, or plasmapheresis.[28,34,42,46] Outcome is better with interferon alpha, and clinical improvement is associated with the disappearance of hepatitis C viremia and a reduction in cryocrit.[7,28,34] However, a patient who did not have a response initially to intravenous cyclophosphamide with oral corticosteroids had a reduction in cryocrit and improvement in the peripheral neuropathy after treatment with oral cyclophosphamide, intravenous methylprednisolone, and plasmapheresis.[42] This particular patient could not be given interferon because of advanced age and pre-morbid depression, so the remission was maintained with methotrexate (0.3 mg/kg given intravenously weekly) and 5 mg of oral prednisone daily.[42] In a series of patients who had mononeuritis multiplex due to cryoglobulinemia with hepatitis C, Ghini et al.[59] described a patient who had no clinical improvement after 1 year of treatment with corticosteroids and interferon-alfa but did have symptomatic and electrophysiological improvement with cyclophosphamide. Souayah and Khella[37] recently reported three patients who had hepatitis C infection and cryoglobulinemic neuropathy and who did not have a response initially to interferon alfa therapy but had sustained improvement in the peripheral neuropathy after treatment with cyclophosphamide. Adverse effects of various treatments are listed in Table 128.4.

After interferon was established as a potentially effective treatment for hepatitis C viral infection,[60,61] its use in patients with mixed cryoglobulinemia was investigated. Pellicano et al.[62] treated 62 patients who had hepatitis C (32 patients with and 30 patients without mixed cryoglobulinemia) with interferon alfa at a dose of 3 million units three times weekly for 6 to 12 months and determined there was no difference in rate of response between the two groups. In both groups, approximately 50% of patients had an initial response and a subsequent relapse, 25% had no response, and 25% had a sustained response, with improvement in viremia and cryoglobulin levels. Misiani et al.[63] performed a prospective, randomized controlled trial of interferon alfa in 53 patients with cryoglobulinemia and hepatitis C. One-half of the patients were given recombinant interferon alfa (1.5 million units three times a week for 1 week and then 3 million units three times a week for 23 weeks), and 15 of them had a complete response, with undetectable hepatitis C RNA in the serum. Viremia returned in 13 patients within 6 months after treatment was stopped. This was associated with worsening of the symptoms of cryoglobulinemia, but three of the four patients who had relapse received an additional 6-month course of treatment and had a sustained reduction in RNA levels. Treatment of peripheral neuropathy, with interferon has had mixed results. A beneficial response of peripheral neuropathy to interferon therapy has been reported as complete,[64] partial,[65–67] or absent,[68] but those who had relief from neuropathic symptoms were in the minority.[64]

Table 128.4   Adverse effects of treatment

Drug	Adverse effect	Possible intervention
Interferon	Flu-like symptoms (fever, headache, myalgias)	Predosing treatment with acetaminophen
	Leukopenia, thrombopenia	Monitor CBC monthly
		If pronounced, lower dose
	Depression	Lower dose
	Confusion/encephalopathy	Lower dose
	Peripheral paresthesias	Lower dose or discontinue treatment
	Nausea	Antiemetics
	Alopecia	If pronounced, lower dose
	Anorexia	If pronounced, lower dose
	Insomnia	If pronounced, lower dose
Ribavirin	Hemolytic anemia	Monitor CBC monthly
		If pronounced, lower dose or discontinue treatment
Plasmapheresis	Systemic hypotension	Slow rate of pheresis
	Electrolyte depletion	Monitor posttreatment and replace as needed
	Depletion of clotting factors	Treat every other day or at greater intervals
Corticosteroids	Weight gain	Nutritional counseling
	Glucose intolerance	Monitor blood glucose level
	Hypertension	Monitor blood pressure
	Osteopenia	Supplemental calcium and vitamin D for patients at risk
	Glaucoma/cataracts	Regular eye exam
	Gastritis	Histamine (H_2) blockers
Cyclophosphamide	Hemorrhagic cystitis	Increase oral fluid intake
	Nausea	Give antiemetic with intravenous therapy
	Carcinogenicity	Intermittent intravenous dosing vs. oral dosing
	Hematological	Monitor CBC monthly
	Teratogenicity	Appropriate contraception
Methotrexate	Hepatotoxicity	Liver biopsy after each 1 g cumulative dose
	Mucositis	Give folate 1 mg orally daily
	Teratogenicity	Appropriate contraception
	Hematological	Monitor CBC monthly
	Renal toxicity	Avoid if creatinine > 3
		Instruct patient to limit use of NSAIDs
		Monitor renal function tests
Azathioprine	Hematological	Monitor CBC monthly
	Nausea	Divided dosing
	Teratogenicity	Appropriate contraception
Cyclosporine	Hypertension	Frequent monitoring
	Renal toxicity	Monitor renal function tests
	Hematological malignancies	Monitor CBC during and after treatment

CBC, complete blood count; NSAID, nonsteroidal anti-inflammatory drug.

Patients with mixed cryoglobulinemia but without evidence of hepatitis C infection have also been shown to respond to interferon-alfa therapy. Casato et al.[69] reported two patients who had type II essential mixed cryoglobulinemia, and both had a complete clinical response that was sustained for 2 years. Overall, sustained remission is expected in only 15% to 20% of patients with hepatitis C-associated mixed cryoglobulinemia treated with interferon alfa.[60,70]

Predictors of positive response of hepatitis C, and thus indirectly of hepatitis C-associated cryoglobulinemia, to interferon alfa treatment reportedly include absence of cirrhosis, younger age, female sex, low hepatitis C viral titer before treatment, and viral genotype other than 1b.[3,29,56,67,68,70–72] For patients without these factors, higher and more frequent dosing of interferon with a prolonged course of therapy may be helpful.[3,70] In one randomized trial, African-American patients who had chronic hepatitis C had a reduced response to interferon alfa monotherapy or combination interferon and ribavirin therapy, presumably because they had a higher incidence (96%) of hepatitis C genotype 1 than the white patients (65%) in the study.[73] In that study, race was not determined to be an independent predictor of response to treatment.

Treatment with a combination of interferon-alfa and corticosteroids has been reported. Dammacco et al.[71] compared treatment with 1 year of interferon versus a combination of interferon with 16 mg/day 6-methylprednisolone versus 6-methylprednisolone alone in patients with hepatitis C-associated mixed cryoglobulinemia. Patients receiving combination therapy had a more prompt response and prolonged remission, but the authors refrained from recommending combination therapy over interferon alone because of the increased risk of viremia and greater incidence of nausea in the combination therapy group.[71] Similarly, Lauta and De Sangro[74] reported a higher response rate among patients receiving the combination of interferon and oral prednisone (10 mg daily) than among those receiving prednisone alone. Moreover, the clinical response occurred despite persistent viremia, perhaps because the cryoglobulin levels also decreased.[74]

The combination of interferon alfa and ribavirin, a synthetic nucleoside analogue with antiviral activity, has been shown to have therapeutic benefit.[3,29,75,76] Ribavirin is administered in doses from 800 to 1200 mg daily in two divided doses.[3,75] It appears to have a synergistic effect with interferon alfa,[75] with longer sustained remissions and higher response rates.[75] Ribavirin monotherapy has not been shown to produce sustained absence of hepatitis C viral RNA.[75-77] Its most common side effect is mild hemolytic anemia[3,75-78] (Table 128.4).

Davis et al.[78] recently published the results of a double-blind, placebo-controlled trial that evaluated interferon alfa alone or in combination with ribavirin in 173 patients with chronic hepatitis C who had been treated previously with interferon but had disease relapse within 1 year after discontinuing treatment. Of the patients receiving combination therapy, 82% had undetectable hepatitis C RNA levels after 24 weeks, compared with 47% of the patients receiving interferon alone. Also, 49% of the patients receiving combination therapy maintained a response, compared with only 5% of those receiving interferon only.[78] The presence of cryoglobulins does not appear to affect the response to the combined regimen.[79] Positive predictors of a response to combination therapy include low pretreatment hepatitis C RNA serum level, history of previous virological response to interferon monotherapy, and hepatitis C genotype other than type 1.[78,80] Calleja et al.[81] evaluated the therapeutic response of patients with hepatitis C-associated symptomatic mixed cryoglobulinemia to combination interferon and ribavirin therapy who had disease relapse or did not have a response to an initial course of interferon monotherapy. Of the eight patients who initially did not have a response to interferon, five had a response to combination therapy, three of whom had a sustained virological response. The combination therapy has not been found to have any greater efficacy in treating the neurological complications of mixed cryoglobulinemia.[81]

Side effects of interferon alfa include flu-like symptoms (fever, headache, and myalgias that typically occur during the initial phases of treatment and may be relieved with acetaminophen), neutropenia/thrombocytopenia (up to 20% to 25% decrease in cell counts), depression, anorexia, alopecia, and insomnia[60,61,63-65,67,70,78,81] (Table 128.4). Any of these side effects may become severe enough to warrant decreasing the dose of interferon or discontinuing treatment.[70] Rare adverse effects of interferon therapy have included seizures, acute renal failure, cardiac arrhythmias, autoimmune thyroiditis, and congestive heart failure.[58,61,70,82] Frequent monitoring of serum aminotransferase levels, complete blood counts, and thyroid function tests may help detect such effects.[70] Worsening symptoms of peripheral neuropathy such as paresthesias have occurred in a small number of patients given interferon[64,65,82-84] and pretreatment neuropathy usually required discontinuation of therapy in patients with pretreatment neuropathy.[64,65,82,84] The development of serum neutralizing antibodies against recombinant interferon alfa may also occur and prevent a therapeutic response.[60,64,67,70] Changing formulations to natural human interferon alfa has been shown to be of benefit in patients who have disease relapse from antibody formation.[3,64] Patients with breakthrough symptoms or worsening laboratory findings such as hepatitis viremia or increasing cryocrit may also benefit from a trial of an increased dose of interferon, such as 6 million units three times weekly[85] or the addition of ribavirin to interferon. In summary, in about one-fourth of patients, interferon alfa with or without ribavirin may be beneficial in the treatment of cryoglobulinemia associated with hepatitis C, but the therapeutic yield in terms of neurological complications, including peripheral neuropathy, so far has been poor.

A low antigen content diet has been proposed as a nonpharmacological treatment for mildly symptomatic mixed cryoglobulinemia. The diet provides decreased amounts of certain macromolecular antigens for a specified time, followed by reintroduction of certain food groups over a period of time.[86] A group of 24 patients who followed this dietary regimen had a significant decrease in cryocrit and improvement in purpura but no reported change in peripheral neuropathy.[86] Other reports suggest that this diet may benefit patients with mild sensory neuropathy.[3,87] The theoretical basis of the diet is the "functional rescue" of the body's intrinsic phagocytic system by decreasing the ingested macromolecular burden, thus allowing the body to clear the accumulated circulating immune complexes from the disease.[86]

Intravenous immunoglobulin has not been recommended for treatment of cryoglobulinemia because case reports have documented acute renal failure[88-90] and the development of cutaneous vasculitis.[89,90] Worsening vasculitis developed in these patients, presumably from increased formation of immune complexes from the iatrogenic supply of immunoglobulin provided intravenously.[89,90]

Newer treatments for cryoglobulinemia that may lead to better efficacy in relieving neurological symp-

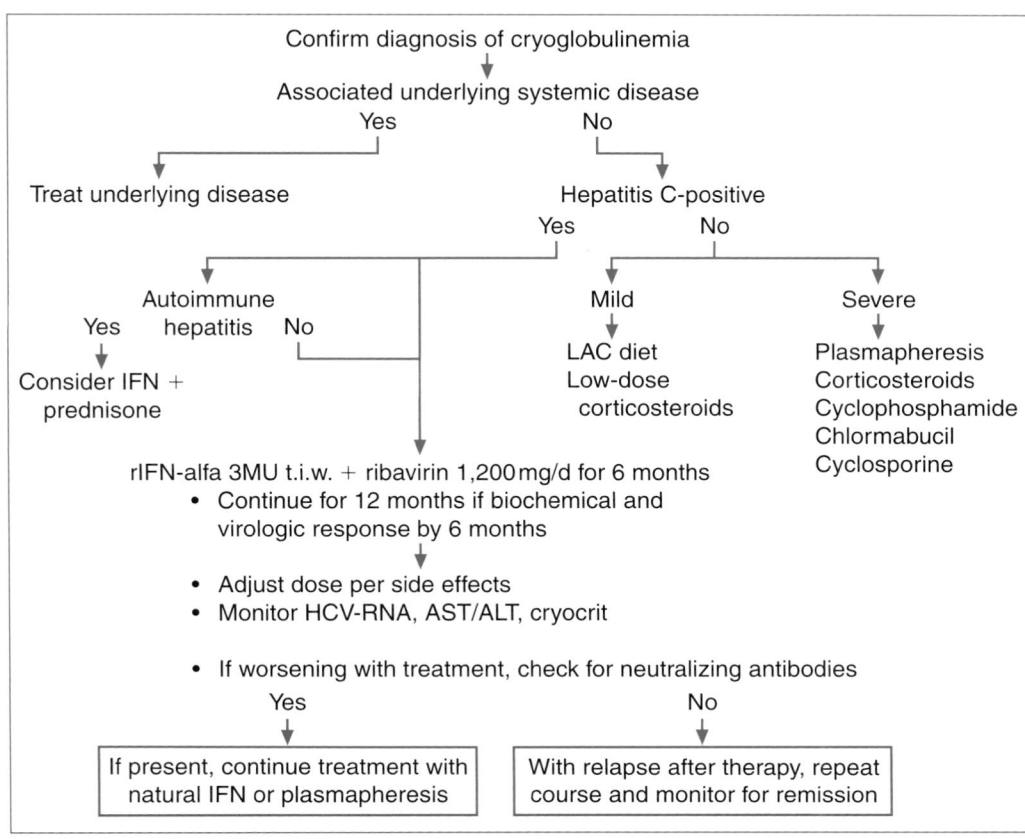

Figure 128.2 Treatment protocol for neurological complications of cryoglobulinemia. ALT, alanine aminotransferase; AST, aspartate aminotransferase; HCV, hepatitis C virus; IFN, interferon; LAC, low antigen content; rIFN, recombinant IFN.

toms include peginterferon, a conjugate of polyethylene glycol and interferon alfa-2a. Compared with interferon alone, the pharmacokinetics of peginterferon are improved in terms of reduced systemic clearance and administration on a once weekly basis (compared with three times a week for interferon).[80,91] Recently, peginterferon, alone or in combination with ribarvirin, was approved in the United States for the treatment of hepatitis C. Currently, treatment trials for its use in treating hepatitis C-associated mixed cryoglobulinemia are pending.[92] Zeuzem et al.[93] recently published data from their phase III, open-label, randomized clinical trial of patients with chronic hepatitis C to receive 180 µg of peginterferon alfa-2a subcutaneously once a week for 48 weeks or 6 million units of interferon alfa-2a subcutaneously three times a week for 12 weeks, followed by 3 million units three times a week for 36 weeks. Treatment with peginterferon resulted in a higher rate of sustained virological response (39% vs. 19%), defined as an undetectable level of hepatitis C virus RNA at week 72. The side effects of peginterferon are similar to those of interferon alfa and included headache, fatigue, fever, depression, and myalgias.[91,93,94] In summary, treatment of hepatitis C with peginterferon alfa-2a appears to be equivalent in efficacy to combination therapy with interferon alfa-2a and ribavirin.[93]

Recent data have indicated that combination therapy with peginterferon alfa-2a and ribavirin may be equally or slightly more effective than treatment with interferon alfa-2b plus ribavirin in eradicating

hepatitis C virus,[80,94] leading to the recommendation that this be considered the preferred therapy for this group of patients.[80,94] In fact, this regimen seems to be particularly effective for patients infected with hepatitis C viral genotype 1.[94] It has been suggested that peginterferon monotherapy (without the addition of ribavirin) should be considered for patients who cannot tolerate the side effects of ribavirin, who require long-term maintenance therapy, who have cirrhosis, who have predominant extrahepatic manifestations of hepatitis C,[80] which may include patients with cryoglobulinemia and its neurological manifestations. No clinical trials have evaluated the effectiveness of peginterferon, with or without ribavirin, in the treatment of hepatitis C-associated cryoglobulinemia, including its neurological complications.

A pilot study that evaluated the effectiveness of cyclosporine in the treatment of two patients with type II mixed cryoglobulinemia, hepatitis C, and peripheral neuropathy who did not have a substantial response to previous treatment with corticosteroids, cyclophosphamide, interferon, and plasmapheresis, showed a good response, that is, reduction in cryocrit, normalization of liver function tests (despite no change in hepatitis C RNA levels), and normalization of electrophysiological test results in one patient (the other had marked improvement in the peripheral neuropathy).[95] Although treatment with interferon, cyclophosphamide, prednisone, and plasmapheresis failed in a patient who had type II mixed cryoglobulinemia and hepatitis C, treatment with rituximab, an

Table 128.5   Recommended drug doses for treatment

Drug	Recommended dose
Interferon alpha	3–6 million units subcutaneously, 3 times a week for 24 weeks (if response, continue for 48 weeks)
Ribavirin	800–1200 mg orally daily in divided doses
Peginterferon	180 μg subcutaneously weekly for 1 year (monotherapy) 1.5 μg/kg body weight weekly (combination therapy with 800 mg ribavirin orally daily)
Cyclophosphamide	2 mg/kg orally daily
Corticosteroids	30–60 mg orally daily; 120 mg orally every other day; 0.5–1.5 mg/kg orally daily

anti-CD20 monoclonal antibody, produced transient improvement in the symptoms of purpura and joint pain.[96] However, after two infusions of rituximab, retinal artery thrombosis developed, and no additional treatment was given except for oral prednisone, which controlled the patient's symptoms.[96] Thymosin α_1, an immunomodulatory peptide, has been given in combination with interferon to treat chronic hepatitis C, and the biochemical and virological responses were better than with interferon monotherapy, although the relapse rate was high.[97]

In summary, the first step in deciding on a course of treatment after neurological involvement has been established in a patient with cryoglobulinemia is to refer to the type of cryoglobulins present and to determine whether any associated systemic illness is present (Figure 128.2). If the cryoglobulinemia is type I or mixed but due to an identified infectious, lymphoproliferative, or autoimmune disease, treatment should be directed at the underlying condition.[3,5] In patients with mixed cryoglobulinemia classified as "essential," the presence of hepatitis C viral infection should be investigated. If present, additional testing for autoimmune hepatitis, including anti-smooth muscle antibody and anti-liver/kidney/microsomal antibody, should be done to determine whether autoimmune hepatitis is present because this information may also affect the type of treatment selected.[56,72] If autoimmune disease due to hepatitis C is present, a trial of corticosteroids before or concomitant with interferon alfa may be benficial[70,72] because interferon alone may exacerbate autoimmunity.[56,98] Patients with true essential mixed cryoglobulinemia who do not have an underlying or associated disorder (except sicca or Sjögren syndrome) should be subdivided further into those with mild neurological involvement (sensory symptoms, mild sensory neuropathy) and those with severe manifestations (motor involvement, mononeuritis multiplex, CNS disease). For patients with milder neurological involvement, treatment with a low antigen content diet on an intermittent basis,

possibly in combination with a low dose of corticosteroids, may control the symptoms. For patients with more severe involvement, a course of plasmapheresis in combination with one or more cytotoxic agents, including high doses of corticosteroids, should be considered (Table 128.5).

References

1. Brouet JC, Clauvel JP, Danon F, et al. Biologic and clinical significance of cryoglobulins: a report of 86 cases. Am J Med 1974;57: 775–788
2. Gorevic PD, Galanakis D, Finn AF Jr. "Cryoglobulins." *In:* Manual of Clinical Laboratory Immunology. Rose. 5th ed., 1997
3. Dispenzieri A, Gorevic PD. Cryoglobulinemia. Hematol Oncol Clin N America 1999;13:1315–1349
4. Della Rossa A, Trevisani G, Bombardieri S. Cryoglobulins and cryoglobulinemia: diagnostic and therapeutic considerations. Clin Rev Allergy Immunol 1998;16:249–264
5. Foerster J. "Cryoglobulins and cryoglobulinemia." *In:* Wintrobe's Clinical Hematology. 10th ed., 1999
6. Agnello V. The etiology and pathophysiology of mixed cryoglobulinemia secondary to hepatitis C virus infection. Springer Semin Immunopathol 1997;19:111–129
7. Agnello V. Mixed cryoglobulinemia and hepatitis C virus. Hosp Pract (Hosp Ed) 1995;30:35–42
8. Ferri C, Greco F, Longombardo G, et al. Association between hepatitis C virus and mixed cryoglobulinemia. Clin Exp Rheumatol 1991;9:621–624
9. Dammacco F, Sansonno D. Mixed cryoglobulinemia as a model of systemic vasculitis. Clin Rev Allergy Immunol 1997;15:97–119
10. Agnello V, Chung RT, Kaplan LM. A role for hepatitis C virus infection in type II cryoglobulinemia. N Engl J Med 1992;327:1490–1495
11. Authier FJ, Pawlotsky JM, Viard JP, et al. High incidence of hepatitis C virus infection in patients with cryoglobulinemic neuropathy. Ann Neurol 1993;34:749–750
12. Gorevic PD, Kassab HJ, Levo Y, et al. Mixed cryoglobulinemia: clinical aspects and long-term follow-up of 40 patients. Am J Med 1980;69:287–308
13. Garcia-Bragado F, Fernandez JM, Navarro C, et al. Peripheral neuropathy in essential mixed cryoglobulinemia. Arch Neurol 1988;45:1210–1214
14. Nemni R, Corbo M, Fazio R, et al. Cryoglobulinaemic neuropathy: a clinical, morphological and immunocytochemical study of 8 cases. Brain 1988;111:541–552
15. Berkman EM, Orlin JB. Use of plasmapheresis and partial plasma exchange in the management of patients with cryoglobulinemia. Transfusion 1980;20:171–178
16. Cream JJ, Hern JEC, Hughes RAC, MacKenzi ICK. Mixed or immune complex cryoglobulinemia and neuropathy. J Neurol Neurosurg Psychiatry 1974;37:82–87
17. Abramsky O, Slavin S. Neurologic manifestations in patients with mixed cryoglobulinemia. Neurology 1974;24:245–249
18. Palazzi C, D'Amico E, Fratelli V, et al. Communicating hydrocephalus in a patient with mixed cryoglobulinemia and chronic hepatitis C. Clin Exp Rheumatol 1996;14:75–77
19. Chad D, Pariser K, Bradley WG, et al. The pathogenesis of cryoglobulinemic neuropathy. Neurology 1982;32:725–729
20. Petty GW, Duffy J, Huston J III. Cerebral ischemia in

patients with hepatitis C virus infection and mixed cryoglobulinemia. Mayo Clin Proc 1996;71:671–678

21. Ferri C, La Civita L, Cirafisi C, et al. Peripheral neuropathy in mixed cryoglobulinemia: clinical and electrophysiologic investigations. J Rheumatol 1992;19: 889–895

22. Origgi L, Vanoli M, Carbone A, et al. Central nervous system involvement in patients with HCV-related cryoglobulinemia. Am J Med Sci 1998;315:208–210

23. Abel G, Zhang Q-X, Agnello V. Hepatitis C virus infection in type II mixed cryoglobulinemia. Arth Rheum 1993;36:1341–1349

24. Gemignani F, Pavesi G, Fiocchi A, et al. Peripheral neuropathy in essential mixed cryoglobulinaemia. J Neurol Neurosurg Psychiatry 1992;55:116–120

25. Lippa CF, Chad DA, Smith TW, et al. Neuropathy associated with cryoglobulinemia. Muscle Nerve 1986;9: 626–631

26. Tredici G, Petruccioli MG, Cavaletti G, et al. Sural nerve bioptic findings in essential cryoglobulinemic patients with and without peripheral neuropathy. Clin Neuropathol 1992;11:121–127

27. Logothetis J, Kennedy WR, Ellington A, Williams RC. Cryoglobulinemic neuropathy: incidence and clinical characteristics. Arch Neurol 1968;19:389–397

28. Khella SL, Frost S, Hermann GA, et al. Hepatitis C infection, cryoglobulinemia, and vasculitic neuropathy. Treatment with interferon alpha: case report and literature review. Neurology 1995;45:407–411

29. Ramos-Casals M, Trejo O, Garcia-Carrasco M, et al. Mixed cryoglobulinemia: new concepts. Lupus 2000;9: 83–91

30. Ciompi ML, Marini D, Siciliano G, et al. Cryoglobulinemic peripheral neuropathy: neurophysiologic evaluation in twenty-two patients. Biomed Pharmacother 1996;50:329–336

31. Klein CM, Suarez GA. The natural history of peripheral neuropathy associated with cryoglobulinemia. Neurology 2000;54(Suppl 3):A385

32. Klein CM, Suarez GA. The electrophysiologic findings of peripheral neuropathy associated with cryoglobulinemia. Clin Neurophysiol 2001;112(Suppl 1):S39

33. Gemignani F, Marbini A, DiGiovanni G, et al. Cryoglobulinaemic neuropathy manifesting with restless legs syndrome. J Neurol Sci 1997;152:218–223

34. Apartis E, Leger JM, Musset L, et al. Peripheral neuropathy associated with essential mixed cryoglobulinaemia: a role for hepatitis C virus infection? J Neurol Neurosurg Psychiatry 1996;60:661–666

35. Cavaletti G, Petruccioli MG, Crespi V, et al. A clinicopathological and follow up study of 10 cases of essential type II cryoglobulinaemic neuropathy. J Neurol Neurosurg Psychiatry 1990;53:886–889

36. Bonetti B, Scardoni M, Monaco S, et al. Hepatitis C virus infection of peripheral nerves in type II cryoglobulinaemia. Virchows Arch 1999;434:533–535

37. Souayah N, Khella SL. Peripheral neuropathy associated with hepatitis C and cryoglobulinemia: treatment with cyclophosphamide. Ann Neurol 1999;46:A492

38. Valli G, De Vecchi A, Gaddi L, et al. Peripheral nervous system involvement in essential cryoglobulinemia and nephropathy. Clin Exp Rheumatol 1989;7:479–483

39. Crespi V, Cavaletti G, Pioltelli P, et al. Cryoglobulinaemic neuropathy: lack of progression in patients with good haematological control. Acta Neurol Scand 1995;92:372–375

40. Marcellin P, Descamps V, Martinot-Peignoux M, et al. Cryoglobulinemia with vasculitis associated with hepatitis C virus infection. Gastroenterology 1993;104: 272–277

41. Konishi T, Saida K, Ohnishi A, Nishitani H. Perineuritis in mononeuritis multiplex with cryoglobulinemia. Muscle Nerve 1982;5:173–177

42. Lamprecht P, Gause A, Gross WL. Cryoglobulinemic vasculitis resistant to intermittent intravenous pulse cyclophosphamide therapy. Scand J Rheumatol 2000; 29:201–202

43. Menkes DL, Palmer-Toy DE, Hedley-Whyte ET. Weekly clinicopathological exercises: case 3—1999: a 41 year old woman with muscle weakness, painful paresthesias and visual problems. N Engl J Med 1999;340: 300–307

44. Munoz-Fernandez S, Barbado FJ, Martin Mola E, et al. Evidence of hepatitis C virus antibodies in the cryoprecipitate of patients with mixed cryoglobulinemia. J Rheumatol 1994;21:229–233

45. Vital C, Deminiere C, Lagueny A, et al. Peripheral neuropathy with essential mixed cryoglobulinemia: biopsies from 5 cases. Acta Neuropathol 1988;75:605–610

46. David WS, Peine C, Schlesinger P, Smith SA. Nonsystemic vasculitic mononeuropathy multiplex, cryoglobulinemia and hepatitis C. Muscle Nerve 1996;19: 1596–1602

47. Murai H, Inaba S, Kira J, et al. Hepatitis C virus associated cryoglobulinemic neuropathy successfully treated with plasma exchange. Artif Organs 1995;19:334–338

48. Sansonno D, Cornacchiulo V, Iacobelli AR, et al. Localization of hepatitis C virus antigens in liver and skin tissues of chronic hepatitis C virus-infected patients with mixed cryoglobulinemia. Hepatology 1995;21: 305–312

49. Agnello V, Abel G. Localization of hepatitis C virus in cutaneous vasculitic lesions in patients with type II cryoglobulinemia. Arthritis Rheum 1997;40:2007–2015

50. Boom BW, Brand A, Bavinck JN, et al. Severe leukocytoclastic vasculitis of the skin in a patient with essential mixed cryoglobulinemia treated with high-dose gamma-globulin intravenously. Arch Dermatol 1988; 124:1550–1553

51. Ferri C, La Civita L, Longombardo G, et al. Hepatitis C virus and mixed cryoglobulinemia. Eur J Clin Invest 1993;23:399–405

52. Lamprecht P, Gause A, Gross WL. Cryoglobulinemic vasculitis. Arthritis Rheum 1999;42:2507–2516

53. Ferri C, Zignego AL. Relation between infection and autoimmunity in mixed cryoglobulinemia. Curr Opin Rheumatol 2000;12:53–60

54. Cacoub P, Hausfater P, Musset L, Piette JC. Mixed cryoglobulinemia in hepatitis C patients. GERMIVIC. Ann Med Interne (Paris) 2000;151:20–29

55. Gordon SC. Extrahepatic manifestations of hepatitis C. Dig Dis 1996;14:157–168

56. McMurray RW, Elbourne K. Hepatitis C virus infection and autoimmunity. Semin Arthritis Rheum 1997;26: 689–701

57. Pawlotsky JM. Hepatitis C: virology, clinical aspects and the relation to cryoglobulinemia. Acta Gastroenterol Belg 2000;63:200–201

58. Cosserat J, Cacoub P, Bletry O. Immunological disorders in C virus chronic hepatitis. Nephrol Dial Transplant 1996;11(Suppl 4):31–35

59. Ghini M, Mascia MT, Gentilini M, Mussini C. Treatment of cryoglobulinemic neuropathy with alpha-interferon. Neurology 1996;46:588–589

60. Davis GL, Balart LA, Schiff ER, et al. Hepatitis Interventional Therapy Group, Treatment of chronic hepati-

tis C with recombinant interferon alfa: a multicenter randomized, controlled trial. N Engl J Med 1989;321: 1501–1506

61. Di Bisceglie AM, Martin P, Kassianides C, et al. Recombinant interferon alfa therapy for chronic hepatitis C: a randomized, double-blind, placebo-controlled trial. New Engl J Med 1989;321:1506–1510

62. Pellicano R, Marietti G, Leone N, et al. Mixed cryoglobulinaemia associated with hepatitis C virus infection: a predictor factor for treatment with interferon? J Gastroenterol Hepatol 1999;14:1108–1111

63. Misiani R, Bellavita P, Fenili D, et al. Interferon alpha-2a therapy in cryoglobulinemia associated with hepatitis C virus. N Engl J Med 1994;330:751–756

64. Casato M, Lagana B, Antonelli G, et al. Long-term results of therapy with interferon-alpha for type II essential mixed cryoglobulinemia. Blood 1991;78: 3142–3147

65. Ferri C, Marzo E, Longombardo G, et al. Interferon alpha in mixed cryoglobulinemia patients: a randomized, crossover-controlled trial. Blood 1993;81: 1132–1136

66. Adinolfi LE, Utili R, Zampino R, et al. Effects of long-term course of alpha-interferon in patients with chronic hepatitis C associated to mixed cryoglobulinemia. Eur J Gastroenterol Hepatol 1997;9:1067–1072

67. Casato M, Agnello V, Pucillo LP, et al. Predictors of long-term response to high-dose interferon therapy in type II cryoglobulinemia associated with hepatitis C virus infection. Blood 1997;90:3865–3873

68. Cresta P, Musset L, Cacoub P, et al. Response to interferon alpha treatment and disappearance of cryoglobulinaemia in patients infected by hepatitis C virus. Gut 1999;45:122–128

69. Casato M, Lagana B, Pucillo LP, Quinti I. Interferon for hepatitis C virus-negative Type II mixed cryoglobulinemia. N Engl J Med 1998;338:1386–1387

70. Fried MW, Hoofnagle JH. Therapy of hepatitis C. Semin Liver Dis 1995;15:82–91

71. Dammacco F, Sansonno D, Han JH, et al. Natural interferon-alfa versus its combination with 6-methyl-prednisolone in the therapy of type II mixed cryoglobulinemia: a long-term, randomized, controlled study. Blood 1994;84:3336–3343

72. Lunel F, Cacoub P. Treatment of autoimmune and extra-hepatic manifestations of HCV infection. Ann Med Interne (Paris) 2000;151:58–64

73. McHutchison JG, Poynard T, Pianko S, et al. The impact of interferon plus ribavirin on response to therapy in black patients with chronic hepatitis C. The International Hepatitis Interventional Therapy Group. Gastroenterology 2000;119:1317–1323

74. Lauta VM, De Sangro MA. Long-term results regarding the use of recombinant interferon alpha-2b in the treatment of II type mixed essential cryoglobulinemia. Med Oncol 1995;12:223–230

75. Trepo C, Bailly F, Bizollon T. Treatment of chronic hepatitis C: another therapeutic option. Nephrol Dial Transplant 1996;11(Suppl 4):62–64

76. DiBisceglie AM, Shindo M, Fong T-L, et al. A pilot study of ribavirin therapy for chronic hepatitis C. Hepatology 1992;16:649–654

77. Camps J, Garcia N, Riezu-Boj JI, et al. Ribavirin in the treatment of chronic hepatitis C unresponsive to alpha interferon. J Hepatol 1993;19:408–412

78. Davis GL, Esteban-Mur R, Rustgi V, et al. Interferon alpha-2b alone or in combination with ribavirin for the treatment of relapse of chronic hepatitis C. International Hepatitis Interventional Therapy Group. N Engl J Med 1998; 339:1493–1499

79. Donada C, Crucitti A, Donadon V, et al. Interferon and ribavirin combination therapy in patients with chronic hepatitis C and mixed cryoglobulinemia. Blood 1998;92:2983–2984

80. Gordon SC. Treatment of viral hepatitis—2001. Ann Med 2001;33:385–390

81. Calleja JL, Albillos A, Moreno-Otero R, et al. Sustained response to interferon-alfa or to interferon-alfa plus ribavirin in hepatitis C virus-associated symptomatic mixed cryoglobulinaemia. Aliment Pharmacol Ther 1999;13:1179–1186

82. Harle JR, Disdier P, Pelletier J, et al. Dramatic worsening of hepatitis C virus-related cryoglobulinemia subsequent to treatment with interferon alpha. JAMA 1995; 274:126

83. Gastineau DA, Habermann TM, Hermann RC. Severe neuropathy associated with low-dose recombinant interferon-alpha. Am J Med 1989;87:116

84. Ferri C, Marzo E, Longombardo G, et al. Alpha interferon in the treatment of mixed cryoglobulinaemia patients. Eur J Cancer 1991;27(Suppl 4):S81–S82

85. Schirren CA, Zachoval R, Schirren CG, et al. A role for chronic hepatitis C virus infection in a patient with cutaneous vasculitis, cryoglobulinemia, and chronic liver disease: effective therapy with interferon-alfa. Dig Dis Sci 1995;40:1221–1225

86. Ferri C, Pietrogrande M, Cecchetti R, et al. Low-antigen-content diet in the treatment of patients with mixed cryoglobulinemia. Am J Med 1989;87:519–524

87. Tavoni A, Mosca M, Ferri C, et al. Guidelines for the management of essential mixed cryoglobulinemia. Clin Exp Rheumatol 1995;13(Suppl 13):S191–S195

88. Barton JC, Herrera GA, Galla JH, et al. Acute cryoglobulinemic renal failure after intravenous infusion of gamma globulin. Am J Med 1987;82:624–629

89. Odum J, D'Costa D, Freeth M, et al. Cryoglobulinemic vasculitis caused by intravenous immunoglobulin treatment. Nephrol Dial Transplant 2001;16:403–406

90. Wooten MD, Jasin HE. Mixed cryoglobulinemia and vasculitis: a novel pathogenic mechanism. J Rheumatol 1996;23:1278–1281

91. Perry CM, Jarvis B. Peginterferon-alfa-2a (40 kD): a review of its use in the management of chronic hepatitis C. Drugs 2001;61:2263–2288

92. Schafer DF, Sorrell MF. Conquering hepatitis C, step by step. N Engl J Med 2000;343:1723–1724

93. Zeuzem S, Feinman SV, Rasenack J, et al. Peginterferon alfa-2a in patients with chronic hepatitis C. N Engl J Med 2000;343:1666–1672

94. Manns MP, McHutchison JG, Gordon SC, et al. Peginterferon alfa-2b plus ribavirin compared with interferon alfa-2b plus ribavirin for the initial treatment of chronic hepatitis C: a randomised trial. Lancet 2001; 358:958–965

95. Ballare M, Bobbio F, Poggi S, et al. A pilot study on the effectiveness of cyclosporine in type II mixed cryoglobulinemia. Clin Exp Rheumatol 1995;13(Suppl 13):S201–S203

96. Zaja F, Russo D, Fuga G, et al. Rituximab for the treatment of type II mixed cryoglobulinemia. Haematologica 1999;84:1157–1158

97. Sherman KE, Sjögren M, Creager RL, et al. Combination therapy with thymosin alpha 1 and interferon for the treatment of chronic hepatitis C infection: a randomized, placebo-controlled double-blind trial. Hepatology 1998;27:1128–1135

98. Papo T, Marcellin P, Bernuau J, et al. Autoimmune chronic hepatitis exacerbated by alpha-interferon. Ann Intern Med 1992;116:51–53

129 Neurological Aspects of Transplantation

Joseph H Antin

Introduction

Although hematopoietic stem cell transplantation and organ transplantation are common and effective therapies for otherwise fatal diseases, the intensity of these treatments is associated with substantial morbidity. Neurological toxicity is common and often multifactorial. A critical challenge is for the clinician to distinguish between the items on a complex differential diagnosis promptly, so effective intervention can be initiated. Often, more than one cause contributes, and features of the underlying disease or intrinsic effects of the transplantation make routine neurological testing difficult. Empirical therapy with continuous reevaluation is often the only feasible approach. A common error is to ascribe neurological symptoms erroneously to metabolic disturbances or psychiatric causes, when they were related to occult infection or drug toxicity. The primary causes of neurological injury are: (1) the intensive immunosuppression and immunoincompetence required to prevent graft rejection and the associated susceptibility to infection, (2) intrinsic drug toxicity from a panoply of medications given to the patients, (3) second malignancies, (4) metabolic encephalopathy, (5) hemorrhage, and (6) in the case of hematopoietic stem cell grafting, neurological toxicity from the high-dose chemoradiotherapy that is used to prepare the patient for transplantation ("transplant conditioning"). These manifestations are summarized in Table 129.1.

The prevalence of neurological toxicity is difficult to determine because many of the studies that addressed these complications were retrospective and

Table 129.1   Neurological complications of transplantation in the early and late post-transplant periods

Complication	Transplant			
	Kidney	Liver	Heart–lung	Bone marrow
Early post-transplant period				
Disease-related	Metabolic encephalopathy	Metabolic encephalopathy	Hypoxia, poor cardiac output	Meningeal or parenchymal involvement with the malignancy Infection
Procedure-related		Central pontine myelinolysis	Embolic disease, anoxic injury	Conditioning-related seizures, SIADH, cerebellar toxicity
Infections	Wide spectrum of opportunistic infections related to the degree of immunosuppression More prevalent in marrow transplantation because of associated myelosuppression			
Calcineurin inhibitors	Seizures, cortical blindness, numerous nonspecific manifestations, drug interactions are important because they may increase blood levels of calcineurin inhibitor HUS/TTP			
Vascular injury		CNS hemorrhage	Atheroemboli, pump complications, antiarrhythmic drugs	Nonbacterial thrombotic endocarditis
Late post-transplant period				
Infections	CMV, other herpesvirus infections, EBV lymphoproliferative disorders, aspergillus and other fungi, toxoplasmosis, progressive multifocal leukoencephalopathy			
Drug-related	Tremor, steroid myopathy, muscle spasms	Tremor, steroid myopathy, muscle spasms	Tremor, steroid myopathy, muscle spasms	Tremor, steroid myopathy, muscle spasms
Inflammatory disorders				Guillain-Barré syndrome, myasthenia gravis, focal demyelinization

CMV, cytomegalovirus; CNS, central nervous system; EBV, Epstein–Barr virus; HUS/TTP, hemolytic-uremic syndrome/thrombotic thrombocytopenic purpura; SIADH, syndrome of inappropriate antidiuretic hormone secretion.

often postmortem analyses. Furthermore, improvements in transplantation technology have resulted in a general reduction in toxicity and opportunistic infections. For example, air embolism was once a common cause of stroke after liver transplantation. However, a review of the literature shows that a broad range of patients (5% to 80% depending on the type of transplantation) have significant neurological injury. A much larger percentage have more non-specific problems of sedation, tremors, confusion, insomnia, delirium, myopathies, and neuropathies that never come to the attention of a neurologist.

It is convenient to consider the risk of neurological injury (1) early after the transplantation and (2) late complications. No arbitrary number divides these periods, and they merge imperceptibly. Susceptibility to toxicity and the type of injury may be quite different depending on the stage of the transplantation achieved by the patient. Early toxicity tends to be related to immediate problems with transplantation surgery or stem cell transplantation conditioning-regimen effects. Preexistent neurological problems related to malignancy or metabolic encephalopathy are likely to increase the risk of immediate post-transplantation neurological symptoms; thus, the early period can be considered to begin days to months before the procedure is performed. Later events in stem cell and organ transplantation are often related to prolonged immunoincompetence and the effects of calcineurin inhibitors.

Early post-transplant period

Early after transplantation is a critical period in which they may be massive fluid shifts, hypoxia, unstable liver or kidney function, severe coagulopathies, and initiation of treatment with multiple medications with overlapping toxicities and opportunities for drug interactions. In kidney transplantation, central nervous system (CNS) toxicity is uncommon, and when it occurs, it most likely is related to vascular disease from an underlying disease such as diabetes mellitus or hypertension. A small number of kidney transplant recipients develop compressive neuropathies of the femoral nerve because of surgical injury. Recipients of liver transplants are often in worse metabolic condition than other transplant recipients and, thus, have a proportionately increased risk of complications. Some degree of hepatic encephalopathy is usually present, but there is a specific risk of central pontine myelinolysis and extrapontine myelinolysis. These problems appear to result from perioperative electrolyte imbalances, although often the expected association with the correction of hyponatremia or hypernatremia is not observed. This appears to be more common after liver transplantation, although it is occasionally seen in stem cell grafting, particularly in association with hepatic veno-occlusive disease. Cardiopulmonary bypass used in heart and lung transplantation may result in atheromatous embolic disease or diffuse anoxic injury. Also, there is a substantial risk of problems with memory after the procedure. Brachial plexus lesions may occur related to chest wall retraction or hematoma formation. In stem cell transplantation, most encephalopathies are related to transplant conditioning toxicity. The use of narcotics, antiemetics, and calcineurin inhibitors, often in combination, is probably the most frequent cause of seizures or altered mental status.

Opportunistic infections

Opportunistic infections in the early transplant period are more of a concern in stem cell transplantation than they are in organ transplantation, because many of the recipients will enter the transplant either intrinsically immunocompromised from the underlying disease or from previous chemotherapy. Furthermore, the conditioning regimen is extremely myelotoxic and immunosuppressive. Nevertheless, although systemic and local infections are common, CNS infections at this stage in the treatment are relatively unusual. Reactivation of herpesviruses such as herpes simplex is usually prevented with acyclovir prophylaxis, but, increasingly, resistant strains are encountered. The most frequent CNS infections are due to reactivation of toxoplasmosis and metastatic fungal infections, most commonly *Aspergillus* species. Disseminated candidiasis is also relatively common. It must be remembered that in stem cell transplantation, the severity of the immunosuppression and myelo-suppression is so extreme that even extremely unusual organisms, such as *Fusarium*, *Trichosporon*, and others can be observed. The presentation of these infections is often dramatic, with seizures, altered consciousness, and focal defects. It is noteworthy that toxoplasmosis can be more insidious, resulting in delayed diagnosis; the characteristic ring enhancement may not be seen on computed tomography because the macrophages and lymphocytes that generate granulomas have not yet recovered.

Calcineurin inhibitors

The immunophilin inhibitors cyclosporine and tacrolimus (FK 506) are probably the most frequent cause of neurological toxicity in these patients. Neurological toxicity occurs in approximately 20% of patients after kidney or liver transplant. Arguably, depending on the sensitivity of the examiner, it occurs in up to 100% of patients after stem cell grafting. Both drugs work by binding to an immunophilin(s) and inhibiting the phosphatase activity of calcineurin. The most common manifestations are tremor and burning palmar and plantar dysesthesias. However, headache, depression, confusion, somnolence, and nystagmus may be observed. Seizures may occur, especially in association with hypomagnesemia, hypertension, hypocholesterolemia, infections, and high blood levels, although the association with hypocholesterolemia has been questioned. It needs to be recognized when treating seizures that cyclosporine and tacrolimus levels may be altered by anticonvulsants. For instance, phenobarbital induces cytochrome P450 to the degree that massive doses of calcineurin inhibitors may be required to maintain adequate levels to prevent graft rejection or graft-versus-host disease. Furthermore, clinicians who perform stem cell transplants are reluctant to use carbamazepine, phenytoin, and other anticonvulsants because of concern about the effect on incipient marrow recovery. Valproate, benzodiazepines, and gabapentin may be more useful because of their limited drug interactions and low risk of marrow toxicity. A particularly unique complication of these drugs is cortical blindness and posterior leukoencephalopathy (Figure 129.1). This complication, or syndrome, may be associated with methylprednisolone treatment, but it is not associated with high blood levels of the drug per se. This syndrome is often observed in association with the new onset of hypertension, suggesting that there is cerebral edema due to abnormalities of pressure regulation in the posterior circulation. Many of the radiological manifestations are similar to those seen in hypertensive encephalopathy. The most common pattern is white matter edema in the area of the posterior circulation. It may or may not persist despite continued treatment with the drug. Despite reports to the contrary, most clinicians believe that cyclosporine and tacrolimus are cross-reactive; therefore, substitution of one for the other may not be useful. Establishing a successful immunosuppressive regimen in this setting can be difficult and may

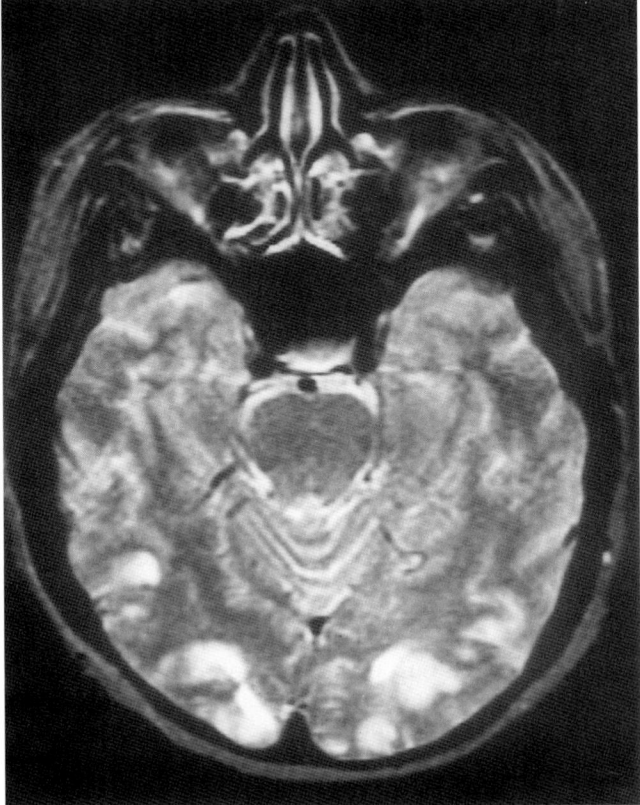

Figure 129.1 Posterior leukoencephalopathy in a patient receiving cyclosporine. The clinical manifestation was cortical blindness. (Courtesy of Dr. Richard Schwartz, Neuroradiology, Brigham and Women's Hospital).

require persistent use of the offending agent, with an effort to maintain excellent blood pressure control. Other less common manifestations of these agents include coma, optic disk edema, aphasia, paralysis, insomnia, somnolence, and rigidity.

Vascular injury

Vascular complications may be related to primary vascular disease, or to surgical complications such as air embolus or microemboli from cardiopulmonary bypass. Nonbacterial thrombotic endocarditis commonly develops in severely ill patients and may embolize to various organs, including the brain. A frequent complication of cyclosporine and tacrolimus therapy is the development of hemolytic uremic syndrome or thrombotic thrombocytopenic purpura. These microangiopathies are associated with evidence of hemolysis; typically, schistocytes are observed in the blood smear and haptoglobin levels are decreased. Because of the involvement of renal vasculature, hypertension and azotemia generally are observed concomitantly. Subarachnoid, subdural, or parenchymal hemorrhages are observed most commonly after liver transplantation. The extremely severe coagulopathy that occurs is related to the lack of an effective source for clotting factors and the massive blood replacement necessary in this procedure. Stem cell transplantation is often associated with severe thrombocytopenia due to the underlying disease or to the intensity of the myelotoxic conditioning regimen that occasionally is refractory to platelet transfusion. Also, veno-occlusive disease of the liver may result in severe liver failure and consequent coagulopathy (in addition to metabolic encephalopathy). Cardiopulmonary bypass may cause a partial platelet release reaction as well as some consumption of platelets. The platelet release reaction occurs when platelets adhere to the membrane oxygenator, partially degranulate, and are released back into the circulation. The dysfunctional platelets that pass through the pump may increase the risk of hemorrhage despite a relatively normal platelet count. This should be treated with platelet transfusions. These coagulopathies generally are responsive to replacement therapy.

Cardiac-specific agents

Heart transplantation requires several antiarrhythmic agents that may have neurological toxicity. Calcium channel blockers, β-blockers, amiodarone, bretylium, lidocaine, procainamide, and others can cause seizures, agitation, tremor, weakness, confusion, psychosis, vertigo, headache, ataxia, tinnitus, neuropathy, diplopia, and myoclonus. Sedatives and hypnotics as well as hypoxic encephalopathy may contribute to or exacerbate these problems.

Stem cell transplantation-specific toxicity

Risks that are limited to stem cell grafting include the development of conditioning regimen-related neurological injury. High-dose cyclophosphamide therapy can cause the syndrome of inappropriate antidiuretic hormone secretion, presumably through a central mechanism. Rarely, if incorrectly treated, this can result in central pontine myelinolysis. High-dose cytosine arabinoside therapy may cause severe and sometimes irreversible cerebellar and cerebral cortical toxicity. Busulfan, in the doses used in stem cell transplantation, produces generalized seizures in approximately 5% of patients unless they receive prophylactic treatment with anticonvulsant agents. Leukemic or lymphomatous meningitis that occurs before transplantation increases the risk of relapse after the transplantation and the risk of nonspecific injury such as leukoencephalopathy. Total body irradiation does not appear to have intrinsic brain toxicity; however, in patients with previous irradiation of the mediastinum, it must be avoided or spinal cord tolerance may be exceeded and cord transection occur.

Late post-transplant period

After the graft is functioning acceptably and the patient has recovered, the causes of neurological injury change. During the late post-transplant period, the major risks are the manifestations of opportunistic infections and the long-term toxicity of strategies used to prevent or control rejection and graft-versus-host disease.

Opportunistic infections

As mentioned above for early complications of transplantation, patients are susceptible to a wide variety of organisms. Viral meningoencephalitis may occur from infection by most of the herpesvirus family, especially cytomegalovirus, varicella-zoster virus, and herpes simplex virus. Early diagnosis and aggressive therapy with appropriate antiviral therapy such as acyclovir, ganciclovir, or foscarnet are often effective, resulting in complete resolution of the infection. Varicella-zoster virus reactivation typically results in the cutaneous manifestation of shingles, but in severely immunocompromised patients, it has a propensity to manifest as severe abdominal pain without dermatomal vesicles. It is critical to suspect this entity early and to treat it aggressively, because it has a propensity to disseminate. High-dose acyclovir therapy can cause a reversible encephalopathy in susceptible patients. Post-herpetic neuralgia is observed occasionally and may be ameliorated with agents such as amitriptyline and gabapentin.

Another serious herpesvirus complication of immunosuppression is the development of Epstein–Barr virus (EBV)-related lymphoproliferative disorders. In contrast to most lymphomas, these disorders tend to occur in extranodal sites, such as the brain and gastrointestinal tract. Depending on the degree of immunosuppression administered, EBV-related lymphoproliferative disorders have been reported in up to 25% of patients with organ transplants and a similar number of those with stem cell grafts. Typically, this complication occurs in recipients of T-cell-depleted marrow grafts and is uncommon in standard transplantation using calcineurin inhibitors and methotrexate. This presumably is related to some degree of passive immunity transmitted with the donor T cells. Often, these tumors can be detected when they represent a polyclonal proliferation of EBV-transformed B cells. A reasonable therapeutic strategy is to decrease the immunosuppression as much as possible, to allow reestablishment of some T-cell-mediated control of the infection. This strategy is most useful in kidney transplantation, in which graft failure can be salvaged with the initiation of dialysis. For other organ and stem cell transplantation, reduction of immunosuppression is not feasible. Local radiotherapy, systemic chemotherapy, and the administration of humanized monoclonal antibodies directed against B cells (rituximab) are sometimes useful. In stem cell transplantation, a useful strategy is intravenous administration of T cells from the donor to reestablish effective immunity. Although this approach can be quite effective, it has the risk of inducing graft-versus-host disease.

Long-term use of adrenal corticosteroids increases the risk of aspergillosis and other fungal infections. Typically, brain involvement follows pulmonary or sinus infection. The infection is extremely difficult to treat, but occasionally it responds to surgery and aggressive therapy with amphotericin B. Toxoplasmosis typically occurs during the 6 months after transplantation, but it also can occur as a later manifestation. Trimethoprim-sulfamethoxazole for pneumocystis prophylaxis often prevents CNS toxoplasmosis. Computed tomography and magnetic resonance imaging usually show the typical ring-enhancing lesions when the infection occurs late, in contrast to the less definitive appearance in the early post-transplant period. Other viral and bacterial infections are common and are related to the degree and duration of immunosuppression, myelosuppression, and the use of indwelling venous catheters. The organisms are varied and often unexpected. Occasionally, progressive multifocal encephalopathy is encountered, but it is rare. Some authors have reported improvement with purine analog therapy, but no consistently beneficial therapy is available for this degenerative disease.

Drug-related toxicity

Calcineurin-related toxicity is less prevalent as a late complication, presumably because susceptible patients have already experienced complications that were managed by either decreasing the dose of the drug or correcting concomitant metabolic problems. The most bothersome long-term toxicity is a coarse tremor that resists all efforts of control. It is often severe enough to interfere with handwriting and can make drinking a cup of hot coffee an extreme sport. Muscular and neuromuscular complications are common. Steroid myopathies are often quite debilitating. Efforts to improve muscle strength involve the use of supplemental immunosuppressants to allow a decrease in corticosteroid dose. In this regard, mycophenolate mofetil appears to be useful. Thalidomide is sometimes used to treat chronic graft-versus-host disease resistant to other therapy, but the major complications of this drug—constipation, peripheral neuropathy, and sedation—may limit its use. Muscle spasms are a particular aggravation for many patients after allogeneic stem cell grafting. Although they can occur in almost any muscle, they are most common in the lower extremities and hands. The spasms may or may not be painful, and they often are triggered by such activity as writing or typing. Calcineurin inhibitors are implicated in the development of this complication; however, many patients continue to have the spasms long after treatment with cyclosporine or tacrolimus has been stopped. Typically, therapeutic trials with quinine, baclofen, diazepam, high-dose vitamin E, magnesium replacement, and potassium replacement are tried. Some manipulations appear to work for some patients, but there is no consistently useful approach.

Inflammatory disorders

Neurological injury that results from inflammatory cell dysregulation can occur after stem cell transplantation, but it is unusual. Both Guillain-Barré syndrome and myasthenia gravis have been reported at increased frequency after allogeneic stem cell transplantation. Myasthenia gravis appears to be a complication primarily of chronic graft-versus-host disease, and it may respond to immunosuppression, plasmapheresis, and anticholinesterase therapy. Guillain-Barré syndrome does not appear to be a direct complication of graft-versus-host disease, and it usually responds to standard treatments. There are rare cases of focal demyelination of the CNS that appear similar to multiple sclerosis. It has been suggested that this is a manifestation of graft-versus-host disease, although there is little objective support for this. Although the nervous system is not immune to T-cell-mediated injury, there are no well-accepted CNS manifestations of graft-versus-host disease.

Summary

Increasingly, organ and stem cell transplantations are being performed for the treatment of life-threatening organ failure or malignancies. It is likely that these procedures will be refined further and become more complex as stem cell grafting is used as a support for organ transplantation and as efforts are made to use xenografts. Typically, transplant toxicity has become better recognized and prevented as more experience is gained with these procedures. However, the trend only encourages transplant teams to take on greater challenges. Neurological toxicity is a frequent complication of all forms of transplantation, and it will continue to be so for the foreseeable future. In approaching neurological symptoms associated with transplantation a broad differential diagnosis is critical so that serious treatable causes are identified early and treated aggressively.

References

1. Lee JM, Raps EC. Neurologic complications of transplantation. Neurol Clin 1998;16:21–33
2. Martinez AJ. The neuropathology of organ transplantation: comparison and contrasts in 500 patients. Pathol Res Pract 1998;194:473–486
3. Patchell RA. Neurological complications of organ transplantation. Ann Neurol 1994;36:688–703
4. Schwartz RB, Bravo SM, Klufas RA, et al. Cyclosporine neurotoxicity and its relationship to hypertensive encephalopathy: CT and MR findings in 16 cases. AJR Am J Roentgenol 1995;165:627–631
5. Ferreiro JA, Robert MA, Townsend J, Vinters HV. Neuropathologic findings after liver transplantation. Acta Neuropathol (Berl) 1992;84:1–14
6. Goldstein LS, Haug MT III, Perl J II, et al. Central nervous system complications after lung transplantation. J Heart Lung Transplant 1998;17:185–191
7. Pratschke J, Neuhaus R, Tullius SG, et al. Treatment of cyclosporine-related adverse effects by conversion to tacrolimus after liver transplantation. Transplantation 1997;64:938–940

130 Immunodeficiency Diseases

Joseph R Berger

Introduction

The immune system is complex and a review is beyond the general scope of this chapter. The immune system may be comprised of a number of genetic disorders, disease processes and therapeutic interventions. In simple terms, these defects may be divided into those resulting from abnormalities of cell-mediated immunity, humoral immunity, neutrophil dysfunction, and defects in integument or mucosal barrier disruption. Not uncommonly, these immunological defects may coexist. The spectrum of neurological disorders occurring as a consequence of immunological impairment is dictated by the specific nature of the immune defect and, to a lesser extent, the degree of immunological impairment. The neurological diseases that are most commonly observed in the setting of a particular form of underlying immunodeficiency are categorized in Table 130.1.

For each category of alteration in a host's defenses, specific classes of infection result. For example, interruptions in the integument result in bacterial and fungal infections, and defects in neutrophil function are associated with recurrent bouts of infections caused by encapsulated organisms. Cell-mediated immunity is of particular importance in relation to viral, protozoal and fungal infections. Given the relative frequency of acquired defects in cell-mediated immunity, a large portion of this chapter will be devoted to discussing the specific infectious complications of infection with the human immunodeficiency virus (HIV) and organ transplantation. Many of the causes of immunosuppression may also have a direct pernicious effect on the nervous system. Perhaps none is capable of causing as wide a spectrum of neurological disorders as HIV.

General classes of immunosuppression

Defects in cell-mediated immunity

Human immunodeficiency virus and AIDS The acquired immunodeficiency syndrome (AIDS) is caused by the lentivirus, human immunodeficiency virus type 1 (HIV). These viruses are retroviruses, a group of enveloped single-stranded RNA viruses dependent on the enzyme reverse transcriptase to copy the viral genome into proviral double-stranded DNA.[1] Like all retroviruses, HIV is rapidly inactivated outside the body and can be transmitted only through direct contact with the infecting source. The mechanism of infection is typically sexual contact, transmission via blood products, or vertically from mother to child. HIV is capable of infecting a large number of cell types, albeit chiefly those involved in

the immune system. Its primary pathogenic effect results from a reduction in both the numbers and the effectiveness of CD4 T lymphocytes,[2] predisposing HIV-infected persons to a wide range of opportunistic infections. In addition to infecting immune cells systemically, HIV can also infect brain glial cells, both astrocytes and fixed tissue macrophages, the microglial cells. Therefore, it can be detected in brain parenchyma as well as isolated from cerebrospinal fluid.

HIV infection commonly involves the nervous system. Clinically evident neurological disease occurs in as many as 60% of patients prior to death, and autopsy series indicate that many neurological complications of HIV infection are unrecognized clinically.[3,4] The latter suggest involvement of the nervous system in 80% or more of patients.[3] Between 10% and 20% of persons with HIV will have neurological disease heralding the infection.[5] The neurological complications of HIV can be divided into two major

Table 130.1 Correlation of the nature of underlying immunosuppression with likely infectious agent

Neutrophil deficits (absolute neutropenia or functional abnormalities)
Bacteria
    Enteric Gram-negative bacteria
    Staphylococcus
Fungi
    Candida
    Aspergillosis
    Mucormycosis

Abnormal T cell or monocytes
Viruses
    Herpes (CMV, HSV 1 and 2, VZV)
    JC virus
Parasites
    Toxoplasmosis
    Strongyloides
Fungi (typically yeast forming)
    Cryptococcus
    Histoplasmosis
    Blastomycosis
Bacteria
    Mycobacteria
    Nocardia
    Listeria

Disorders of humoral immunity
Bacteria
    Streptococcus pneumoniae
    Neisseria meningitidis
    Hemophilus influenzae

categories (Table 130.2). In the first, the virus is believed to be directly responsible for the neurological disorder. However, increasing evidence suggests that HIV-associated myelopathy may be the consequence of a metabolic disturbance in vitamin B_{12} pathways consequent upon HIV infection. The second category is chiefly (although not exclusively) the result of the overwhelming cellular immunodeficiency that attends HIV infection. Opportunistic infections of the nervous system occur on this basis. Opportunistic infection may also contribute to the development of certain neoplasms and some forms of cerebrovascular disease that occur in association with HIV. Other causes of neurological disorders in HIV infection include toxic and metabolic disorders and drug side effects.

It is essential that the clinician realize that several neurological abnormalities may coexist in the HIV-infected patient. Also, these patients are not exempt from other neurological disorders that affect the general population. Every neurological complaint must be systematically evaluated and, when possible, promptly treated.

HIV meningitis Acute infection with HIV often results in a clinical illness resembling infectious mononucleosis. The incubation time from infection to the appearance of this acute illness is three to six weeks. Symptoms include sweating, arthralgia, myalgia, nausea and vomiting, sore throat, abdominal cramps and diarrhea. During this acute illness, meningitis or meningoencephalitis may occur. Headache, meningismus, photophobia, seizures, and alterations in mental status characterize the latter. Less frequently, acute myelopathy or brachial plexopathy may be seen in association with acute HIV infection.[6,7] CSF findings during this acute phase typically reveal mildly increased protein levels (less than 100 mg%), mononuclear pleocytosis (200 cells/mm^3 or less), and normal glucose concentrations.[8] Although HIV can be isolated from the CSF during this acute phase, special virological techniques, e.g. polymerase

chain reaction (PCR), are typically required to document its presence.

Subacute meningitis with symptoms persisting for months or longer is also observed. CSF findings tend to be less striking.[8,9] Sporadic episodes of acute meningitis presumably attributable to HIV as well as chronic meningitis may also complicate established HIV infection.[8] These disorders are generally characterized by chronic headaches with or without meningeal signs.[10,11]

HIV dementia Both alterations in cognitive abilities and a decline in overall level of consciousness may be associated with HIV infection. The spectrum of illnesses that may result in global encephalopathy in the setting of HIV infection is broad. Therefore, its evaluation requires a thorough physical and neurological evaluation, as well as radiographic and laboratory studies. Because of its greater sensitivity, cranial magnetic resonance imaging (MRI) with gadolinium is preferred to computed tomography (CT). In addition to routine hematological and electrolyte studies, it is essential that metabolic screens for renal, liver and thyroid dysfunction and vitamin B_{12} and folate levels be performed. Infections, such as syphilis, cryptococcus and toxoplasmosis, and primary central nervous system lymphoma must always be considered in the differential diagnosis and appropriate studies performed. Unless contraindicated, a lumbar puncture should be performed to measure opening pressure, as well as to obtain CSF for determining the cell count with differential, for determination of protein and glucose concentrations, and for detailed microbiological studies, VDRL and cryptococcal antigen studies. Further evaluations, such as PCR analysis for cytomegalovirus (CMV) or other pathogens, may also be indicated.

Most frequently, the decline in intellectual function is a consequence of HIV dementia. This illness often presents in a rather stereotypical fashion. The affected patient presents with features of advanced AIDS, exhibiting systemic features such as general wasting, alopecia, seborrheic dermatitis and generalized lymphadenopathy. Although typically a disorder that occurs in the setting of advanced AIDS, it may on rare occasions be the presenting or even the sole manifestation of HIV infection.[12,13] Mental processes are slow (bradyphrenia) and patients demonstrate little facial expression and a hypophonic, monotonous voice. A variety of eye movement abnormalities are noted which commonly affect both saccadic and pursuit movements. Fine motor movements are slow and imprecise.[14,15] Postural instability, gait disturbances and altered motor tone occur. Frontal release signs are common. The features of this illness have the hallmarks of a "subcortical" dementia. The annual incidence of HIV dementia has been reported to be 7%[16] or 14%.[17] However, by the time of death approximately one-third of AIDS patients will exhibit this dementia. The widespread use of highly active antiretroviral therapy, beginning in 1996, appears to have altered the frequency of HIV dementia, but this remains controversial.

Table 130.2 The effects of HIV on the nervous system

Direct effects
Acute meningitis
Chronic meningitis
AIDS dementia
HIV-associated vacuolar myelopathy
HIV-associated peripheral neuropathy
HIV myopathy/myositis

Indirect effects
Opportunistic infections
Neoplastic diseases
    Primary central nervous system lymphoma
    Metastatic disease
Neurotoxic effects of therapy
Malnutrition
Cerebrovascular disorders

Neuroimaging studies of the brain are critically important in evaluating the patient with suspected HIV dementia. These studies may on occasion be normal, but more commonly reveal diffuse atrophy with sulcal widening and a proportional ventriculomegaly. MRI (Figure 130.1) is better than CT in revealing the white matter abnormalities often seen in association with HIV infection. These lesions are usually manifest as widespread, relatively symmetrical hyperintensities on T_2-weighted images,[18] but may appear focal, patchy or punctate, and be difficult to differentiate from those commonly seen with progressive multifocal leukoencephalopathy (PML).[19] Hyperintense signal abnormalities of the basal ganglia on T_2-weighted MRI may be observed on occasion.

Laboratory studies are seldom diagnostic. CSF evaluation may reveal a mild pleocytosis with an increased protein concentration, similar to that of HIV-infected patients without encephalopathy. The CSF protein concentration is seldom greater than 200 mg/dL and the cell count is usually less than 50 cells/mm³.[12] Oligoclonal bands and intrathecal synthesis of HIV-specific antibody are frequently present, but are not predictive of the development of CNS disease.[20] The isolation of HIV from the CSF is not a useful marker as it may be found in the absence of HIV dementia. On the other hand, HIV viral copy numbers, as determined by quantitative PCR, do appear to correlate with degree of dementia.

Gross pathological findings of HIV dementia include diffuse brain atrophy with sulcal widening and large ventricles. Often, meningeal fibrosis is observed. The histopathological hallmark of the disease is the presence of multinucleated giant cells (MGC), which are believed to result from direct virus-induced cell fusion.[4,17] Other common features of HIV encephalopathy include white matter pallor, microglial nodules, diffuse astrocytosis and perivascular mononuclear infiltration.[4] Thinning of the neocortex and neuronal loss in specific brain regions, as demonstrated by quantitative assessment, have also been reported.[21,22]

Therapy for patients with HIV dementia generally consists of antiretroviral agents. The first available therapy for HIV dementia was zidovudine, which was demonstrated to be effective in large controlled trials of both children and adults with the disorder.[23,24] Highly active antiretroviral therapy (HAART) has subsequently been demonstrated to be very valuable. However, a salutary response to therapy is not universal. Therapeutic measures other than those directed at the virus per se, but rather at the potential underlying mechanisms of cellular injury in HIV dementia, are currently being studied.

HIV vacuolar myelopathy Autopsy studies show that approximately 30% of persons dying with AIDS exhibit stereotypical abnormalities of their spinal cords, referred to as vacuolar myelopathy.[25] Pathologically, a striking loss of myelin, with spongy degeneration and microvacuolization of the cord, characterizes this myelopathy. The lesions are typically symmetrical and most severe in the lateral and posterior columns of the thoracic spinal cord, although not always confined to anatomical tracts.[4] Initially believed to be unique to HIV infection, a similar myelopathy has been observed very rarely pathologically in other disorders, particularly in the setting of immunosuppression.

Leg weakness and gait disturbances, often developing insidiously, herald the disorder. Paresthesias, vague leg discomfort, and bowel and bladder incontinence are also common.[25–27] Not infrequently, many of the complaints are attributed to the generalized debilitated condition of the patient, and the true nature of the illness remains undiagnosed until a careful neurological examination or at autopsy. Physical examination reveals a spastic paraparesis. Asymmetrical leg weakness, monoparesis and quadriplegia are less common. Gait ataxia and lower limb dysmetria are usually present. Muscle stretch reflexes are generally increased, but may be diminished or absent as the result of a concomitant peripheral neuropathy. In keeping with the preponderance of the lesions in the posterior columns, sensory examination typically reveals a greater loss of vibratory and position sense than perception of pinprick, temperature or light touch. A discrete sensory level is unusual and should suggest other spinal cord pathology. Symptoms correlate with the severity of pathological findings in this condition.[25]

MRI of the spinal cord is critical in excluding other causes of myelopathy. The spectrum of myelopathies that can be seen in association with HIV infection is given in Table 130.3. Other causes of cellular immunosuppression may also predispose individuals to a similar spectrum of myelopathies. Generally, if the results of spinal MRI are negative for mass lesions, myelography is probably not indicated, although the presence of radicular findings, a discrete sensory level or severe back pain dictate a more

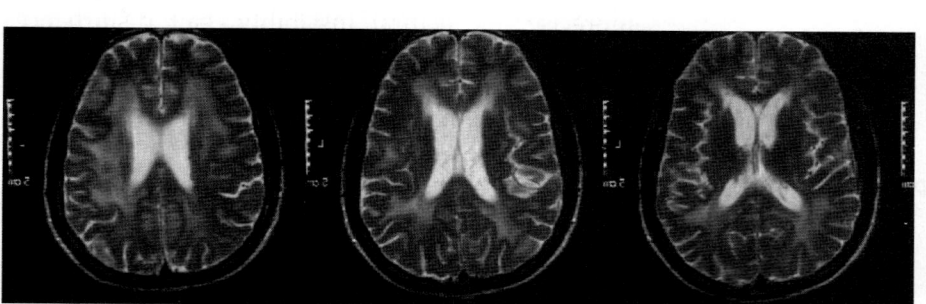

Figure 130.1 MRI of HIV dementia. Axial T_2-weighted MRI scan shows chiefly a symmetrical increased signal within the periventricular white matter. (Reproduced from Berger JR, Levy RM. AIDS and the Nervous System. 2nd ed. Philadelphia: Lippincott Raven, 1996.)

Table 130.3 Spinal cord disorders with HIV infection

Infectious
Viral
  HIV
    Acute transient myelopathy occurring at the time of
      seroconversion
    Chronic progressive myelopathy (vacuolar)
  HTLV-I
  Cytomegalovirus
  Herpes simplex
  Herpes zoster
Bacterial
  Epidural abscess
  Mycobacterium tuberculosis
  Treponema pallidum
Fungal
  Cryptococcus neoformans
  Others
Parasites
  Toxoplasma gondii

Non-infectious etiologies
Multiple sclerosis-like illness
Tumors
  Plasmacytoma
  Spinal cord astrocytomas
  Others
Vascular injury of the cord
  Epidural hemorrhage secondary to thrombocytopenia
  Vasculitis

aggressive diagnostic approach. CSF should be obtained and examined for other viral pathogens, and bacterial, fungal and cryptococcal studies should be performed. There is currently no effective therapy for this condition. Some investigators have postulated that the clinicopathological similarity to subacute combined degeneration suggest a role of the B_{12} pathways in its pathogenesis, and have suggested high-dose methylmethionine.

HIV peripheral neuropathy A diverse group of peripheral neuropathies have been described in association with HIV infection. As many as 50% of patients with advanced HIV infection may suffer from one or more types of peripheral neuropathy.[28] Clearly, many factors play a role in their pathogenesis. Among these are HIV per se, nutritional deficiencies, side effects of antiretroviral and other medications, and opportunistic infections. Four primary types of peripheral neuropathy are associated with HIV infection. The most common form is a distal, symmetrical peripheral neuropathy. Other forms are an inflammatory demyelinating type, mononeuritis multiplex and polyradiculopathy.

Distal symmetrical peripheral neuropathy is the most common form seen with HIV infection and is increasingly common with advanced immunosuppression.[29] Clinically, this condition is characterized by painful debilitating dysesthesias, with numbness of the feet. Sensory deficits are distal and symmetrical and involve a stocking-and-glove loss of response to pain and temperature, with decreased vibratory sense. Strength and proprioception are relatively spared, although reflexes are depressed distally.

Symptomatic treatment of the dysesthesias with carbamazepine or tricyclic antidepressants may be of benefit, and withdrawal of nucleoside analog antiretroviral therapy may be required. Patients may have transient worsening of symptoms for an extended period following withdrawal of an offending drug.[29]

An inflammatory demyelinating polyneuropathy (IDP) and acute Guillain–Barré syndrome (GBS) are also associated with HIV infection. Nerve conduction studies are consistent with a primary demyelinating neuropathy, which may be the presenting symptom of HIV infection. Corticosteroids, plasmapheresis and intravenous immunoglobulin may be beneficial in patients with these conditions, although they have not been tested in controlled clinical trials.

Mononeuritis multiplex and a progressive polyradiculopathy have also been described in HIV-infected patients. Mononeuritis multiplex may occur early in the disease and resolve spontaneously, although more commonly it occurs late and is rapidly progressive. The late-occurring rapidly progressive form of the disease may be associated with cytomegalovirus (CMV) infection, in which case anti-CMV therapy may be of benefit. Progressive polyradiculopathy is also believed to be associated with CMV infection, usually in association with advanced immunosuppression. Lower extremity and sacral paresthesias, followed by a rapidly progressive paraparesis, sensory loss and urinary retention clinically characterize progressive polyradiculopathy. Treatment with anti-CMV agents such as ganciclovir or foscarnet may be effective, but recovery is typically very slow.

HIV-associated myopathy Myopathy has been recognized in association with HIV infection. The chief symptoms are proximal weakness, myalgias, and fatiguability.[30] Serum creatine kinase (CK) is increased and EMG findings are similar to those of polymyositis. A polymyositis-like syndrome consequent upon mitochondrial toxicity due to zidovudine therapy may also be seen.

Neurological complications of immunosuppression for organ and bone marrow transplantation The remarkable success of organ and bone marrow transplantation in recent years has been largely related to the greater sophistication with which the immune system of the recipient can be manipulated by immunosuppressive agents. A wide variety of these agents are currently employed. Many have direct neurological toxicity and also result in opportunistic CNS infection as a consequence of associated systemic immunosuppression. The infectious complications of iatrogenic immunosuppression differ somewhat from those associated with congenital and other acquired forms of immunosuppression.

Infectious neurological complications of organ transplantation are not uncommon, occurring in approximately 5% to 10% of transplant recipients.[31] CNS infection following organ transplantation has a very poor prognosis, with reported mortality rates varying between 44% and 77%.[31] Delayed diagnosis and treatment may in part be responsible for the high morbidity and mortality rates of these disorders. The presentation may be subtle and characteristic diagnostic features are often lacking, rendering diagnosis difficult. As in other immunosuppressive conditions, organ transplant patients often have multiple organ system involvement and, not infrequently, more than one offending infectious agent. As is the case with all immunosuppressed patients with CNS infections, meaningful survival depends largely on rapid diagnosis and the prompt institution of effective medical therapy.

Commonly seen infectious agents that cause neurological disease after organ transplantation are, with a few exceptions, similar to those seen with AIDS and other immunosuppressed states. The transplant patient is particularly at risk for disease resulting from viral, bacterial and fungal pathogens. The herpes group of viruses, hepatitis and papova viruses are all common among transplant patients. Bacterial infections from listeria, nocardia, and mycobacterial infections are common, and fungal infections caused by *Aspergillus*, Mucoraceae, *Candida* and *Cryptococcus* are frequent complications of iatrogenic immunosuppression.

The infectious complications of organ and bone marrow transplantation are closely related not only to the nature and degree of immunosuppression experienced by the host, but also to the underlying disease mechanisms that necessitated the transplant. Intensive medical care with invasive systemic lines and monitoring procedures necessitated by transplantation also predispose the patient to superinfection. Patients are very susceptible to the wide variety of pathogens to which they are routinely exposed.[32] Although many of the agents used for controlling graft rejection in transplant recipients are similar, the infectious complications of transplantation are often specific for the type of underlying pathology necessitating the transplant. Thus, aspergillosis is a relatively common terminal infection in all transplant recipients. On the other hand, viral infections are relatively rare among patients receiving bone marrow transplants, but common among other transplant patients.[33]

Agents commonly in use for immunosuppression are cyclosporine (CsA), corticosteroids, methotrexate, cytarabine, OKT3 monoclonal antibody, antithymocyte antibody and azathioprine. With the exception of azathioprine and antithymocyte antibody, all of these agents have direct neurotoxic effects in addition to their immunosuppressive action.[34] A brief discussion of cyclosporine and corticosteroids, both of which are widely used immunosuppressive agents in organ transplantation and are known to have direct neurological toxicity, follows.

Cyclosporine (CsA)   Since its initial use for renal transplantation in the 1970s, a wide range of transplant recipients have been treated with cyclosporine, a derivative of *Fungi imperfecta*. Cyclosporine has a compound mechanism of action but acts primarily as a selective inhibitor of T-helper cells, with relative sparing of T-suppressor cells.[35] Animal studies of CsA show the relative preservation of T cell-independent B-lymphocyte responses to lipopolysaccharide antigens, accompanied by a modest adverse effect on polymorphonuclear leukocytes, blood monocytes and macrophages.[34,36] Neurological complications occur in 10% to 15% of patients treated with CsA. The drug exhibits a wide variety of neurotoxic effects, including tremor, seizures, ataxia, leukoencephalopathy, cortical blindness, neuropathy, para- and quadriparesis, and mental status changes. In addition to its direct neurotoxic side effects, CsA causes renal wasting of magnesium, which may result in seizures due to hypomagnesemia. The liver extensively metabolizes CsA, and drugs that induce cytochrome P450 activity, such as phenytoin, will lower CsA levels. Conversely, the levels of antiepileptic drugs need to be carefully monitored during therapy with CsA.

Treatment of virtually all the neurotoxic side effects of cyclosporine is achieved by decreasing the dose or discontinuing the drug.[34] Serious infections from listeria, mycobacteria and fungi, which are dependent on their clearance by cell-mediated immunity, is uncommon among patients receiving cyclosporine despite its effect on helper T cells.[37] Furthermore, despite the impairment of T cell-mediated resistance to viral infection associated with CsA,[38] 10% or less of patients receiving CsA and prednisone for allograft renal transplantation develop Herpes virus infections, including CMV.[37] Indeed, with the possible exception of urinary tract infections, immunosuppression by CsA may not result in a significant increase in opportunistic infection during more than 24 months of therapy.[37]

Corticosteroids   Corticosteroids are also used extensively, not only to prevent organ and tissue rejection in transplant patients, but also to suppress the immune system in patients with autoimmune disorders. This class of drugs is known to impair the immune response at virtually all levels, thereby resulting in a greater risk of opportunistic infections than with newer, more specific immunosuppressive agents.[32] Corticosteroids may permit the uncontrolled spread of infection as well as increasing the risk of superinfection.[39] Corticosteroid therapy is known to have both systemic and neurological side effects. Their systemic effects are well described and beyond the scope of this chapter. The direct neurological effects are chiefly altered mental status and myopathy. The mental disturbances associated with corticosteroids include changes in mood and affect, and are seen in as many as 40% of patients.[34] Sleeplessness and irritability are common. Mania and frank psychosis occur more rarely. Mental status changes are most common within the first five days of treatment, but may present at any time during therapy. Corticosteroid-induced myopathy is characterized by symmetrical involvement of proximal muscles with relative preservation of reflexes. This is more common with the fluorinated corticosteroids, and symptoms may respond to the administration of a non-fluorinated corticosteroid such as prednisone or hydrocortisone, or to decreasing the dose of medication. Symptoms typically resolve within two to eight months after discontinuing the drug. Epidural lipomatosis resulting in myelopathy or a cauda equina syndrome has been reported as a complication of corticosteroid therapy and may require decompressive surgery.[34]

Neurological complications associated with immunosuppressive therapy for cancer and autoimmune disorders The spectrum of antineoplastic agents used in the treatment of cancer and autoimmune disorders is very broad. It is of the utmost importance to distinguish those neurological complications arising as a result of these therapies from those associated with the underlying disorder. Corticosteroid therapy is employed in a number of these conditions and is addressed in the preceding section. Drugs such as cytosine arabinoside, methotrexate and azathioprine chiefly affect the cell-mediated arm of immunity. Therefore, the neurological illnesses observed with their use are those seen in association with this dysfunction.

DiGeorge syndrome Among the inherited causes of compromised cell-mediated immunity, DiGeorge syndrome is perhaps the best characterized. It results from a failure of evolution of the thymus and parathyroid glands consequent upon abnormal development of the third and fourth pharyngeal pouches. Associated abnormalities of the heart and kidneys are common. Neonates with DiGeorge syndrome often present initially with hypocalcemia and cardiac abnormalities.

Infants with this disorder have a marked reduction in the number and function of T lymphocytes. B cells and immunoglobulin levels appear normal; however, antibody responses are diminished because of a lack of T-helper cells. Patients with the disease suffer from chronic viral, fungal and protozoal infections caused by defective cell-mediated immunity.

The infectious complications of DiGeorge syndrome are treated by transplantation of fetal thymus tissue. Prolonged survival after transplantation is observed; however, the associated congenital anomalies may complicate treatment and prognosis.[40]

Defects in humoral (antibody-mediated) immunity

X-linked agammaglobulinemia X-linked agammaglobulinemia (XLA), also known as Bruton's agammaglobulinemia, is a genetically transmitted disease that affects boys during the first year of life. The defect results in an abnormality in Bruton's tyrosine kinase gene.[41] Early B-cell lineage is affected. Pre-B cells can be found in the bone marrow, but few (if any) blood lymphocytes bear surface immunoglobu-

lin or react with monoclonal antibodies to B cell-specific antigens. The faulty gene has been isolated and is known to be a member of the *src* family of proto-oncogenes that encode tyrosine kinases. Carriers of the gene can be detected by finding nonrandom X-chromosome inactivation of B cells in restriction fragment length polymorphisms (RFLP) studies. Prenatal diagnosis is also possible by RFLP.[42]

Until age six to nine months the persistence of maternal antibodies protects infants with XLA. Thereafter, the infant suffers recurrent infections with extracellular pyogenic organisms such as pneumococci, streptococci and *Hemophilus*, unless treated with prophylactic antibiotics or γ-globulin therapy.[42] Otitis media, bronchitis, septicemia, pneumonia, arthritis, meningitis and dermatitis occur commonly. Malabsorption caused by bacterial overgrowth of *Giardia lamblia* is commonly observed. Because many of these infections do not respond well to antibiotic therapy, the treatment of choice is periodic injections of large amounts of IgG. Chronic fungal infections are uncommon and resistance to *Pneumocystis* and viral pathogens seems to be preserved, with the notable exception of the hepatitis viruses and enteroviruses.[43] T-cell function is almost always normal.

The central nervous system is commonly affected by recurrent bouts of bacterial meningitis. In addition, fatal and persistent enteroviral meningitis and meningoencephalitis have been reported among these patients.[44]

Current therapy for X-linked agammaglobulinemia, X-linked severe combined immunodeficiency and X-linked hyper-IgM syndrome can be successful, and patients can survive into their mid-20s and 30s. However, their survival is associated with significant morbidity associated with recurrent infection and high medical costs because of the repeated γ-globulin injections and antibiotic therapy. Approximately one-third of all children born with these disorders in the recent past died before reaching 10 years of age, either because of severe infection contracted before the diagnosis of immunodeficiency was made or because of treatment failure.[45] Gene therapy is attractive, as such treatment has proved effective for related disorders such as severe combined immunodeficiency (SCID).[46] However, the genetic defects responsible for many of these defects are complex, and the practical implications of delivery, duration of effect and potential side effects are not yet clear.

Other disorders Selective IgA deficiency is characterized by an isolated absence or near absence of secretory IgA and is the most common primary defect of humoral immunity. It affects approximately 1 in 500 persons.[40,42] Affected individuals, when symptomatic, usually suffer from recurrent sinopulmonary viral or bacterial infections, but, neurological disorders are relatively rare.

X-linked immunodeficiency with hyper-IgM (HIGM1) is a rare X-linked disorder characterized by recurrent infections associated with very low or absent levels of IgG and IgA, and normal to increased levels of IgM. Presentation is usually within the first year of life, with recurrent bacterial infections as maternally acquired antibodies decline. However, the disorder affects the immune system in a complex fashion, resulting in a degree of impairment of cell-mediated immunity as well. Presumably the latter is responsible for the recurrent bouts of *Pneumocystis carinii* pneumonia and cryptosporidial intestinal infections that may be observed. Neutropenia also occurs and may affect the nature of the offending microorganism.

Combined defects in B- and T-cell function

Wiskott–Aldrich syndrome (WAS)   Wiskott–Aldrich syndrome (WAS) is an inherited X-linked recessive immunodeficiency disease characterized by thrombocytopenia, abnormal platelets, eczema and recurrent infections. Wiskott–Aldrich syndrome is rare, with an incidence of 4 in 1 000 000 live male births.[47] The abnormal gene is believed to code for a surface glycoprotein that plays an important role in regulating the normal senescence of blood cells, resulting in the progressive decline in number and function of T cells.[48] In the absence of curative bone marrow transplantation the mean age of survival is 6.5 years. Infection is the leading cause of death (59%), followed by hemorrhage (27%) and lymphoreticular malignancies (12%).[47]

Patients with WAS have complex defects in both humoral and cell-mediated immunity and suffer from bleeding caused by thrombocytopenia, as well as from recurrent meningitis, otitis and pneumonia. In additional to intracranial hemorrhage and bacterial meningitis, brain lymphoma and progressive multifocal leukoencephalopathy have been seen in association with this disorder.[49]

Severe combined immunodeficiency (SCID)   Severe combined immunodeficiency (SCID) includes a group of syndromes that are characterized by the absence of all adaptive immune function from the time of birth. Both B and T cells are affected, and several cellular, molecular and genetic abnormalities have been described. Patients with SCID have the most severe defects in immune function of all patients with primary immunodeficiencies. The diagnosis is usually made within the first few months of life. Patients usually develop recurrent infections caused by a wide variety of pathogens that can involve any organ system, including the nervous system. Untreated, the disease is invariably fatal. Bone marrow transplantation is curative for all forms of SCID.[42]

Defects in phagocytic function

Chronic granulomatous disease   Chronic granulomatous disease (CGD) is a rare disorder that results in an inability of phagocytic cells to produce the oxidative burst required for intracellular lysis of phagocytosed organisms consequent upon a heterogeneous group of defects in NADPH or NADH oxidase. These enzymes normally assist in generating the superoxide radicals necessary for the effectiveness of phagocytic

cells; the intracellular survival of the ingested organisms contributes to the formation of granulomas. CGD occurs with an estimated incidence of between 1 in 250 000 and 1 in 1 000 000 in the general population. The disease is found primarily among boys, and tends to manifest itself in early childhood. It is characterized by recurrent bacterial and fungal infections that commonly involve the subcutaneous tissues, lungs and lymph nodes. *Aspergillus* pneumonia is a serious complication for these patients, even though antibody levels and cell-mediated immunity are believed to be normal.[22] Central nervous system infections from these bacterial and fungal pathogens are a recognized and serious complication for these patients. The prognosis with CGD is poor, although bone marrow transplantation and gene therapy are promising new methods of treating this disease.

Other inherited conditions affecting phagocytic function have been described, such as Chediak–Higashi syndrome. Like CGD, these conditions tend to manifest early in childhood with recurrent infections by organisms of low virulence. Meningitis is not uncommon among these patients. In addition, acquired disorders may affect phagocytic function. Chief among them is diabetes mellitus, which affects neutrophil function at many levels.[50] Fortunately, severe or recurrent neurological infection associated with these conditions is rare.

Opportunistic infectious agents commonly seen in a variety of immunosuppressed states

Pathogenic viruses

Progressive multifocal leukoencephalopathy   Progressive multifocal leukoencephalopathy (PML) is a disease that results from infection of oligodendrocytes by JC virus, a papovavirus.[51] Seroepidemiological studies indicate that, worldwide, approximately 70% to 80% of adults have been infected with JC virus in the absence of recognized symptomatic illness.[52] Before the worldwide AIDS pandemic PML was rare and seen primarily in association with lymphoproliferative disorders, as well as other malignancies, antineoplastic therapy, organ transplantation, and other immunodeficient states.[53] However, following the AIDS pandemic it became increasingly common. Approximately 5% of HIV-infected persons will ultimately develop PML[52,54] (Berger, personal communication). Although chiefly observed in the setting of advanced immunosuppression, the neurological findings of PML may even be the presenting manifestation of AIDS[10] (Berger, personal communication).

Immunocompromised patients with PML may present with clinical symptoms such as decline in mental status, personality change, memory loss, cognitive and speech disturbances, motor and sensory abnormalities, and deterioration of visual capacity. Focal neurological signs are common in the initial presentation. The region of the brain affected dictates the clinical features. PML usually progresses rapidly to death over a period of several weeks to months. Mean survival of PML in AIDS is approximately four months (Berger, personal communication). There is currently no convincingly demonstrated effective therapy for PML. Every attempt should be made to restore immunological function, for instance by removing offending therapeutic agents when possible. In the setting of AIDS, HAART with the associated increase in CD4 helper lymphocytes has shown promise.[55] Curiously, as many as 8% of AIDS patients with PML will survive for more than one year after the diagnosis, and some reports describe patients with partial or complete neurological recovery in the absence of specific therapy.[56]

CSF studies are usually normal, although a mildly increased protein concentration, increased IgG levels, and mild pleocytosis of mononuclear cells have all been reported. Polymerase chain reaction (PCR) has been used to detect the DNA of the JC virus in cerebrospinal fluid, with a sensitivity of approximately 80%.[57] Radiographic studies of the brain are quite helpful. CT and MRI findings will typically reveal non-enhancing or minimally peripherally enhancing hypodense white-matter lesions without mass effect.[58] These lesions are typically found in the subcortical region and often have a "scalloped" appearance resulting from the involvement of subcortical U-fibers (Figure 130.2). Posterior fossa involvement is seen up to 32% of the time, and isolated posterior fossa involvement is found in approximately 10% of cases.[58]

The coupling of typical clinical and radiographic findings with the amplification of JCV DNA from the CSF by PCR is believed to be sufficiently diagnostic to preclude brain biopsy. However, brain biopsy remains the gold standard for diagnosis and will be required in those instances in which CSF PCR is falsely negative. The histopathology of PML is characterized by a triad of focal areas of demyelination, prominent oligodendrocytes containing enlarged basophilic nuclei and intranuclear inclusions, and bizarre giant astrocytes with basophilic nuclei.[4] Immunohistochemical techniques or electron microscopy can demonstrate JC virus.

Cytomegalovirus (CMV) Cytomegalovirus is ubiquitous: the serum of at least 80% of adults contains anti-CMV antibodies. CMV is most frequently acquired during the first five years of life or during young adulthood. The virus has been isolated from most body fluids and is known to be sexually transmissible. Transmission by blood transfusion can be avoided by using blood products from seronegative donors or blood that has been treated to remove potentially infective white cells.[59] Primary infection in the immunocompetent host is usually asymptomatic; however, clinical illness, if it occurs, can result in an infectious mononucleosis-type illness, complete with an atypical lymphocytosis but lacking a heterophil antibody. The virus becomes latent in leukocytes, and although primary infection in the immunocompromised host can be severe, most patients with AIDS are positive for CMV antibody before becoming infected with HIV.[60] Autopsy and clinical studies indicate that 90% of patients with AIDS develop active CMV infec-

tion during their illness, and that 25% will develop life- or sight-threatening illness as a result.[61]

CMV infection in immunocompromised hosts is commonly manifest by progressive retinitis, colitis, encephalitis and pneumonia. The diagnosis of CMV in association with nervous system disease is often challenging. Despite histopathological and virological evidence implicating CMV in the cause of HIV encephalitis, the clinical features of CMV encephalitis among the AIDS population remain poorly characterized, and clinical recognition of the condition is difficult. CMV may localize to the CNS without significant clinical sequelae; however, neurological involvement by CMV has resulted in ventriculitis, encephalitis, polyradiculopathy, myelopathy and multifocal neuropathy.[60,62] Routine CSF or radiographic imaging studies are not always helpful, and are seldom specific enough to allow a confirmatory diagnosis.[10] Polymerase chain reaction (PCR) has been used to identify CMV-specific DNA from patients with neurological disease and HIV infection.[63]

Treatment of CMV infection of the CNS is problematic. Ganciclovir, a synthetic analog of thymidine that is structurally similar to aciclovir, has been used successfully to treat patients with CMV, as has foscarnet.[60] These medications are the current recommended therapy for CNS cytomegalovirus. In severely immunocompromised patients with AIDS, as indicated by a CD4 lymphocyte count below $50\,\mathrm{cells/mm^3}$, prophylactic anti-CMV therapy is warranted. In those patients who have had CMV infection and continue to have significant immunosuppression, secondary prophylaxis with anti-CMV therapy is appropriate. The use of primary and secondary prophylaxis in other conditions associated with persistent and severe immunosuppression is not as well studied.

Varicella zoster virus Varicella zoster virus (VZV), like HSV and CMV, is also a herpes virus. Until the adoption of widespread vaccination programs it was ubiquitous. As a consequence, most people developed chickenpox following childhood exposure. The virus is highly contagious and has an attack rate in susceptible hosts of 75%.[59] The virus is neurotropic and becomes latent in the dorsal root ganglia. Reactivation is closely associated with advancing age, as well as immunosuppression from a variety of causes. It results in a painful, dermatomal vesicular rash known clinically as shingles.

Varicella or herpes zoster is usually readily diagnosed clinically. When there is uncertainty in the clinical diagnosis, a Tzanck smear – a test of scrapings of the lesions for characteristic multinucleated giant cells – may be helpful. A more rapid diagnostic method is the use of immunofluorescent antibody staining of exfoliated cells to demonstrate varicella zoster antigen. Because of the extreme lability of the virus, recovery of infectious virus from clinical specimens is difficult, although PCR for VZV DNA may be applied to clinical specimens.

Shingles is not infrequently the heralding manifes-

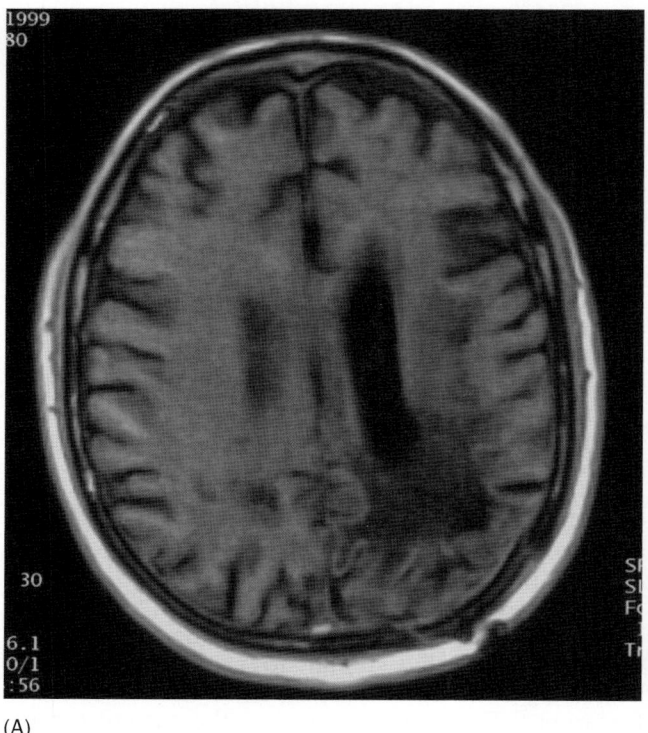
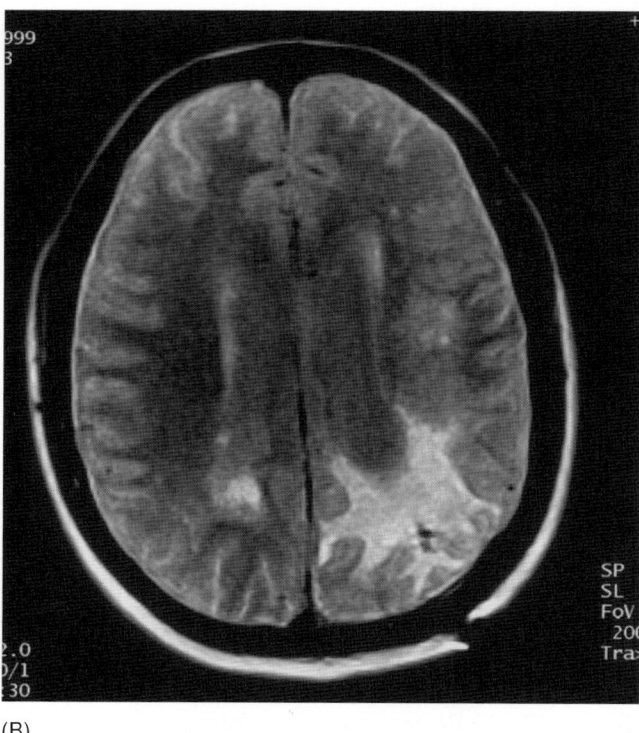

(A)   (B)

Figure 130.2   CT scan of PML. Non-contrast axial CT scan demonstrates focal hypodense lesion in the right parietal region (Reproduced from Berger JR, Levy RM. AIDS and the Nervous System. 2nd ed. Philadelphia: Lippincott Raven, 1996.)

tation of AIDS, and frequent and severe zoster infections are commonly seen in this disorder. Despite the relatively common cutaneous manifestations of zoster among AIDS patients, VZV infection of the CNS is relatively uncommon, accounting for, at the most, 2% of neurological disease.[64] In general, it occurs only in the setting of very advanced immunosuppression with marked depletion of CD4 lymphocytes.[65] VZV involvement of the CNS may present a variety of clinicopathological patterns in AIDS patients. The most characteristic is a multifocal leukoencephalitis with or without a non-inflammatory vasculopathy.[64,66] Ventriculitis and meningomyeloradiculitis have also been described.[66] These patterns are probably dependent on the severity of the infection and on the different routes of spread to the brain from latent viral infections.[65] VZV has been associated with a wide spectrum of neurological diseases, including transverse myelitis, ascending myelitis, encephalitis, leukoencephalopathy, and CNS vasculitis causing focal neurological signs.[65] The clinical signs and symptoms of VZV encephalitis include headache, fever, hallucinations, delirium, mild confusion and meningeal irritation. Focal neurological signs, seizures or coma are rarely associated with VZV encephalitis; if these clinical findings are present, they should prompt further evaluation of the CNS for other disease processes.[11]

The gross pathology of VZV infection of the CNS is characterized by multiple macroscopic well-defined foci of gray-yellow necrosis of the white matter. These lesions may involve the spinal cord as well as the brain. Histologically, the central area of necrosis is surrounded by demyelination, with eosinophilic intranuclear inclusions in oligodendrocytes, astrocytes and neurons. These contain VZV, as demonstrated by immunocytochemical and ultrastructural methods.[65]

The only indicated treatment for VZV infection in the immunosuppressed patient is aciclovir, although valaciclovir, famciclovir and foscarnet have all demonstrated efficacy. Aciclovir-resistant VZV infection should be treated with foscarnet. Unlike CMV in AIDS, the benefit of maintenance antiviral therapy remains uncertain. A live attenuated VZV vaccine was approved in the United States in 1995, and is recommended for all healthy chickenpox-negative persons over 12 months of age. It is not recommended for immunosuppressed individuals.

Herpes simplex virus (HSV)   The herpes simplex virus has two similar but distinct antigenic types, HSV-1 and HSV-2. Like all herpes viruses, they have genomes that consist of linear double-stranded DNA. They are found worldwide, and humans are their only known reservoir. The neurotropism of the human herpes viruses has been well described.[67,68] Autopsy studies using PCR assays to detect HSV-1 in the trigeminal ganglia have found that the virus is age-specific: as humans age, they are more likely to harbor the virus (20% by the age of 20 years to 100% by the age of 60).[69] Detection of HSV-2 antibody in patients who have not yet reached puberty is unusual.[6] HSV-1 can be demonstrated in approximately 15% of human olfactory bulbs at autopsy, without an age-specific prevalence.[69] Although the pathogenesis is not completely understood, the neuronal latency of HSV-1 may play a role in the etiology of HSV encephalitis. Curiously, despite the high frequency of recurrent and severe herpes simplex infections (both HSV-1 and HSV-2) in individuals with impaired cellular immunity, HSV neurological complications are not proportionately increased and remain relatively uncommon. Furthermore, HSV encephalitis in the immunocompromised host often contrasts with infection in the immunocompetent host by a more indolent nature, suggesting the importance of the immune response in the pathogenesis of the classic disorder. Both HSV-1 and HSV-2 have been associated with myelitis in the immunocompromised host.

In the immunocompetent host, CT scans reveal poorly defined areas of low attenuation in the anterior or medial temporal lobes, with relative sparing of the basal ganglia. Contrast enhancement is variable but may show minimal and asymmetrical enhancement in a meningeal pattern. The focal hemorrhages that are invariably found at autopsy may not be evident on CT scans. MRI studies more consistently show bilateral involvement and can better define the acute hemorrhages that are characteristic of HSV encephalitis.[70] In the immunocompromised patient, the typical neuroradiological features may be lacking.

Treatment of herpetic encephalitis with aciclovir has resulted in a striking improvement in morbidity and mortality compared to the natural history of the disease. Newer-generation antiherpetic agents, e.g. famciclovir and valaciclovir, are probably equally effective, but experience with these agents in herpetic CNS infections is limited. Foscarnet is effective in treating aciclovir-resistant HSV seen in immunocompromised patients and is the recommended therapy.[71]

Epstein–Barr virus (EBV) and primary CNS lymphoma Epstein–Barr virus has been implicated as a causal factor in a variety of lymphoid and epithelial malignancies, including Hodgkin's and non-Hodgkin's lymphomas and nasopharyngeal carcinoma. Immunosuppression may be contributory to their development. Epstein–Barr virus is consistently associated with AIDS-related primary CNS lymphoma (PCNSL), and less often with primary CNS lymphoma in non-immunocompromised patients.[72] PCNSL is the second most common cause of brain mass lesions in the AIDS population of the developed world.

Primary CNS lymphoma occurs in as many as 5% of patients with AIDS, and may herald the disorder in a significant percentage. Clinical features include headache, altered mentation, and focal neurological findings in the absence of systemic illness consequent upon the lymphoma. CT and MRI findings are often variable. No features on radiographic imaging reliably differentiate CNS lymphoma from other intracra-

nial mass lesions.[18] The high metabolic rate of primary CNS lymphoma allows FDG-PET scanning or thallium-201 single-photon emission CT to differentiate cerebral infections from malignancy, and this technology may come to play an important role in the clinical diagnosis and subsequent treatment of patients.[73,74] The definitive diagnosis of primary CNS lymphoma currently requires a brain biopsy. This procedure has been shown to be both safe and effective, with low surgical and perioperative morbidity and mortality rates.[75] Primary CNS lymphoma among AIDS patients is treated with whole-brain radiotherapy (RT). The tumor is extremely radiosensitive and clinical and radiographic responses to treatment are rapid. The survival times of patients treated promptly are increased compared with those not treated with whole-brain RT. Treated patients often succumb to systemic opportunistic infections rather than to CNS pathology.[75]

Bacteria

Nocardia *Nocardia* spp., an atypical, filamentous Gram-positive bacterium often confused with fungi, are related to mycobacteria. More than 80% of individuals infected by these bacteria are immunosuppressed from a variety of causes, generally those resulting in impaired cell-mediated immunity.[76,77] Between 0.3% and 1.8% of all infections in AIDS patients have been reported to have CNS nocardial involvement.[77] Primary infection typically involves the lungs, followed by subsequent systemic spread to the brain and elsewhere. Other sites of primary infection include the skin and soft tissue, which may occur after direct inoculation following local trauma. The CNS is the most common site of extrapulmonary involvement, and such involvement is seen in 15% to 44% of patients.[78] The lung lesions may be highly suggestive of malignancy, and their association with contrast-enhancing mass lesions in the CNS due to nocardial abscess (Figure 130.3) may lead to an incorrect diagnosis of metastatic lung cancer. Therefore, tissue diagnosis is required, unless the diagnosis is established by other means. Sulfonamides remain the mainstay of treatment.

Listeria monocytogenes *Listeria monocytogenes*, an aerobic and facultatively Gram-positive non-spore-forming rod, is distributed widely in the environment. Listeriosis has a predilection for the immunocompromised as well as pregnant women and neonates. Sepsis and meningitis are the typical clinical presentations in the former group. Patients with listeria meningitis may display fluctuating levels of consciousness, tremors, seizures and ataxia. Features of meningeal irritation tend to be less commonly observed than with other bacterial meningitides.[79] Other CNS manifestations include meningoencephalitis, cerebritis, brainstem abscess (for unknown reasons, *L. monocytogenes* has a propensity to cause cerebral abscesses in the brainstem) and spinal cord abscess.[79] CNS manifestations may also occur as a result of listeria endocarditis. Despite the name of the

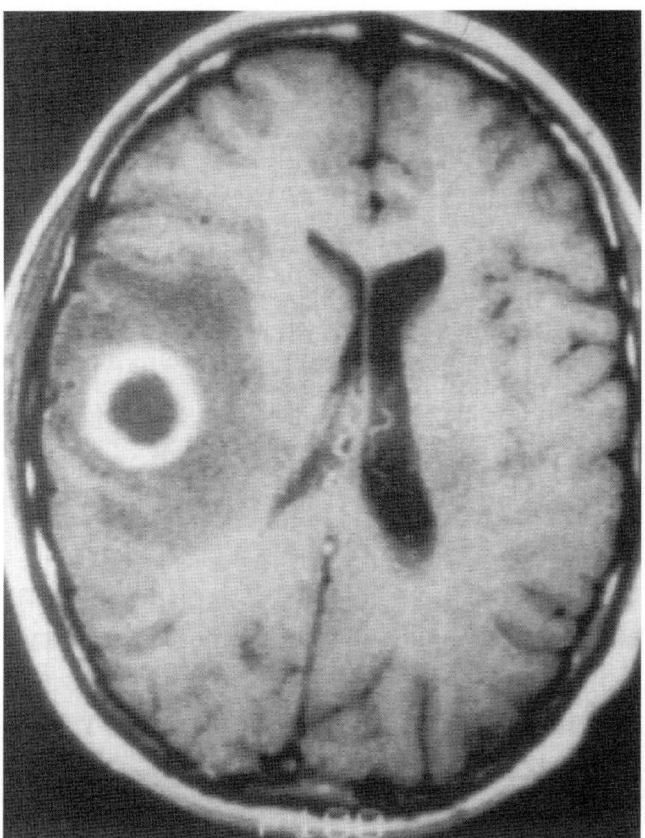

Figure 130.3   MRI of nocardial abscess. Ring-enhancing lesion observed in subcortical white matter, with adjacent edema. (Reproduced from Berger JR, Levy RM. AIDS and the Nervous System. 2nd ed. Philadelphia: Lippincott Raven, 1996.)

organism, monocytosis is not a feature of the illness. CSF parameters in listeria meningitis are abnormal, but specific values for cell count, protein and glucose may vary widely.

The organism grows well in culture, but fluorescent antibody reagents and PCR may also expedite its identification. Ampicillin is generally recommended in the treatment of listeria infections, although penicillin may be equally effective, and synergy with aminoglycosides has been reported. Prolonged antibiotic therapy (five to six weeks) is required for focal CNS listerial infections.[79]

Mycobacterial diseases Tuberculosis is caused by *Mycobacterium tuberculosis*, a slim rod-shaped organism that is resistant to basic aniline dyes, hence the term "acid-fast bacillus". Cell-mediated immunity is critical for the control of *M. tuberculosis* infection. Despite their elicitation of a considerable humoral antibody response, the latter appears to have a limited role in the control of mycobacterial infection. *M. tuberculosis* is capable of surviving for extended periods of time within macrophages and monocytes. Hypersensitivity reaction to the infection is responsible for many of the manifestations of the disease.

Tuberculosis and other mycobacterial infections are relatively common complications of HIV infection. Tuberculosis is also observed in other forms of impaired cell-mediated immunity, particularly in persons previously exposed to tuberculosis placed on long-term corticosteroid therapy in the absence of suppressive antibiotic treatment.

Central nervous system involvement is a common manifestation of mycobacterial infection. In areas with high endemic incidences of tuberculosis, tuberculous meningitis is a frequent complication of AIDS and may exceed all other causes of meningeal infection, including cryptococcus.[80] The most common clinical symptoms of tuberculous meningitis are fever, headache and altered consciousness. On examination, meningeal signs may be absent in one-third of these patients and altered mentation may be present in only half. CNS disease may also present as a mass lesion (tuberculomas or tuberculous abscesses) and with focal neurological symptoms and signs of increased intracranial pressure.[81] Unlike many other opportunistic infections in immunocompromised patients, HIV infection does not appear to change the outcome of tuberculous meningitis.[80]

The optimal treatment regimen remains undefined and largely empirical. Isoniazid, pyrazinamide and ethionamide penetrate readily into cerebrospinal fluid, whereas rifampicin, ethambutol and streptomycin do so poorly, especially in non-inflamed meninges.[82] Various regimens employing isoniazid and rifampicin with or without pyrazinamide, streptomycin, and ethambutol have been proposed. Therapy must continue over a six-month period or longer.

Fungi

Cryptococcus   Cryptococcus is a frequent cause of meningitis in patients with compromised cell-mediated immunity. Although cryptococcal meningitis may be seen in the absence of a disruption to the immune system, prior to the AIDS pandemic it occurred most commonly in patients with neoplastic disease, organ transplants, or on corticosteroid therapy.[83] The estimated incidence of cryptococcus among patients with AIDS varies from 1.9% to 11%[53,84] and may be the initial AIDS-defining event in some.[5,85]

Cryptococcus neoformans is a saprophytic fungus found worldwide in the soil, particularly soil contaminated by bird droppings. It has a characteristic polysaccharide capsule that is the primary determinant of virulence, as unencapsulated organisms are not pathogenic. Human-to-human transmission of the disease does not occur.[86] Yeasts are normally phagocytosed and killed by polymorphonuclear leukocytes in association with complement, despite the antiphagocytic effect of the capsule. Tissue reaction to *C. neoformans* varies from none to purulent or granulomatous.[87] Infection is usually caused by direct inhalation of fungal conidia into the lungs. Generally, the initial infection will be mild and rarely correctly diagnosed. After initial infection the yeast remains localized or disseminates to other organ systems, particularly the CNS. In immunocompetent patients infection with *C. neoformans* is usually restricted to the lungs, whereas an underlying immunodeficiency increases the risk of dissemination.[88]

The clinical symptoms of cryptococcal meningitis are variable. More than 75% of patients will demonstrate features of a subacute meningitis or meningoencephalitis.[89] The disease characteristically has a slow, insidious onset with relatively non-specific findings, including fever, malaise and headache during the two to four weeks before the patient seeks treatment. Only 25% to 33% of patients exhibit overt signs of meningitis, such as neck stiffness and photophobia. Encephalopathy characterized by lethargy, altered mentation, difficulty with complex cerebral function and memory loss may herald the infection.[90] Focal neurological disturbances, such as cranial nerve palsies, hemiparesis, language disturbances, seizures, cerebellar findings and psychosis, occur less frequently and are often seen later in the course of the disease.[10] A more rapid course may be seen in patients with severely compromised cell-mediated immunity, and many of the clinical findings may be absent or non-specific until late in the course of the disease. As a result of the highly variable and relatively non-specific clinical findings associated with cryptococcal meningitis among immunocompromised patients, it must always be considered in the differential diagnosis of patients presenting with these neurological findings and the appropriate laboratory studies obtained.

Lumbar puncture will usually show an elevated opening pressure, and examination of the CSF will often show a mononuclear pleocytosis, elevated protein concentrations, and a depressed glucose level.[91] However, standard CSF values may, surprisingly, be relatively normal.[10] The frequency with which India ink staining of fresh CSF shows the yeast by its characteristic polysaccharide capsule is variable, and may approach 75% in some series.[90] More than 95% of patients with cryptococcal meningitis will have a positive titer of cryptococcal antigen in the serum, and a titer of more than 1:8 should be regarded as presumptive evidence of cryptococcal infection.[90] The appearance of antigen in the CSF is considered diagnostic for cryptococcal meningitis, because the antigen is not believed to cross the blood–brain barrier. CSF cryptococcal antigen is positive in approximately 95% of patients. However, in some patients with early signs of meningitis the antigen will remain detectable only in the serum. Results of serum antigen tests are routinely positive in cases of cryptococcal meningitis, and cultures of the CSF and blood have been reported as 100% sensitive in one study.[92] The value of fungal cultures in diagnosing cryptococcal meningitis is limited by the fact that growth is indolent and a positive culture may require as much as three weeks, even in optimal media. The severity of infection can be inferred from the laboratory studies: it has been suggested that a CSF cryptococcal antigen titer over 1:10 000 or a positive India ink smear is associated with a worse prognosis.[91]

The pathological findings of central nervous system involvement often reveal a basilar, chronic meningitis that is neither thick nor exudative. An inconspicuous chronic inflammation of the leptomeninges is typical, although occasionally the leptomeninges will be studded with small, 2–3 mm lesions.[3] Cystic lesions, referred to as cryptococcomas, contain clusters of budding yeast and may be found throughout the brain, chiefly in superficial layers of the cerebral cortex. They typically exhibit little surrounding inflammation and can attain macroscopic sizes.[83]

Many authorities advocate the institution of antifungal therapy for immunosuppressed patients with serological evidence of cryptococcus, even in the absence of CNS findings.[83] In the absence of treatment, cryptococcal meningitis is fatal in 86% within one year of onset.[93] Despite aggressive therapy, the disease remains associated with a high morbidity and mortality. The acute mortality rate for AIDS-associated cryptococcal meningitis is 10% to 20%, and 12-month survival rates for all patients are 30% to 60%.[89] The latter is partly the consequence of associated underlying illnesses. Current antibiotic regimens for cryptococcal meningitis consist of intravenous amphotericin B, either alone or in combination with flucytosine or one of the triazoles (fluconazole or itraconazole). At the end of two weeks of aggressive therapy, oral fluconazole may be used at high doses (400 mg/day) for the next eight to ten weeks. If at the end of this time the results of CSF culture are negative for *C. neoformans*, the fluconazole dose may be reduced to 200 mg daily and continued indefinitely to prevent relapse.[83] The current standard of care for patients with AIDS and CNS cryptococcosis mandates maintenance therapy. Relapse rates as low as 3% have been reported with daily fluconazole administration;[93] in comparison, a 50% to 60% rate of relapse and shorter life expectancies are reported for patients not receiving chronic suppressive therapy.[88] Even with long-term prophylactic therapy, many patients will continue to have *C. neoformans* in the genitourinary (GU) tract. The prostate is a known nidus of residual infection.[89] The clinical implications of persistent GU cryptococcus are unclear, and even fluconazole, which achieves high levels in the urine, is not always effective in sterilizing the GU tract.[83]

Aspergillosis Aspergillosis is caused by infection with *Aspergillus*, a ubiquitous mold that is found worldwide in soil, water, decaying vegetation or other organic debris. This fungus grows rapidly and exhibits septate hyphae and characteristic asexual conidia. Nosocomial sources have included hospital air and air ducts. The lungs are the most frequent site of primary infection, with intracranial disease most often seen secondary to hematologic spread. Direct CNS contamination during surgery has been reported[94] and sinus infection may lead to intracranial extension.[95] The CNS is involved in 10% to 15% of patients with pulmonary aspergillosis. As is the rule with invasive molds having a hyphal growth pattern, such as *Mucor*, *Aspergillus* tends to invade blood vessels, causing ischemic and hemorrhagic infarcts. The infection usually spreads radially into fresh tissue, circumscribing an enlarging necrotic center.[96]

The clinical presentation of intracranial aspergillosis is variable. The most common symptom is an unremitting fever, despite the administration of broad-spectrum antibiotics, with the subsequent appearance of pulmonary infiltrates on chest radiography. Headache, seizures and meningeal signs are uncommon. The CNS involvement is often heralded by focal neurological deficits consequent upon underlying ischemic and infectious brain lesions.[97,98] CSF studies are believed to be of little benefit, showing a mildly elevated protein concentration and a nonspecific white blood cell count. Cultures are rarely positive, and although *Aspergillus* antigens have been demonstrated in the serum and pleural fluid, they have not been reported in the CSF.[98] Contrast-enhanced MRI and CT scans will often reveal the lesions, which tend to have variable degrees of enhancement and edema. The characteristic ring-enhancing abscess lesion is a late development in the evolution of intracranial aspergillosis. CT scans often underestimates the degree of tissue involvement.[24]

Pathological studies commonly show multiple abscesses. Hematological dissemination of the CNS may uncharacteristically favor the posterior circulation and the cerebellum.[99] The most common pathological feature is that of a stroke syndrome secondary to thrombosis of small and large blood vessels. Isolated granulomata without abscesses, meningitis, meningoencephalitis, arachnoiditis and subarachnoid hemorrhage have also been reported.[99] Light microscopy reveals a combination of coagulative necrosis and various stages of hemorrhage, and vessels may show thrombosis by *Aspergillus* hyphae.[99] Culture for *Aspergillus* may be negative, even when the organism is morphologically identified in pathological specimens.

The prognosis for patients with CNS aspergillosis is extremely poor, although survival is reported.[97] Therapy usually involves combination chemotherapy and surgical excision or biopsy if possible.[97,98] Often surgery is precluded by the patient's underlying clinical condition and the presence of multiple lesions and extensive infarcted tissue. Timely diagnosis, prompt antifungal therapy and the discontinuation of immunosuppressive agents, when possible, may improve survival.

Mucormycoses   Mucormycosis, also referred to as zygomycosis, describes a diverse group of infections caused by the zygomycetes. The most common of these are *Rhizopus* and *Mucor*. Rhinocerebral mucormycosis is acquired by inhalation of conidia and produces a dramatic clinical syndrome of cerebral invasion, after penetration of the mucosa of the nose or paranasal sinuses. Corticosteroid therapy and diabetes mellitus are strongly associated with mucormycosis.

Clinical symptoms often begin with headaches and progress to death, usually within two weeks. Orbital cellulitis, cranial nerve palsies and vascular thrombosis may also complicate rhinocerebral mucormycosis. Diagnosis requires tissue biopsy to reveal the invasive hyphae. Cultures are often negative, even from grossly involved tissue, and should not be allowed to delay the diagnosis.[86] Therapy consists of correcting the underlying disease, surgical debridement and amphotericin B.

Candida   Neutropenic patients are particularly susceptible to infection with *Candida* spp., particularly *C. albicans*. These organisms are small, thin-walled fungi that reproduce by budding. In 50% of persons with proven disseminated candidiasis, CNS involvement has been demonstrated at autopsy.[99] The finding of multiple microabscesses pathologically explains the frequent absence of focal neurological findings and the often normal brain radiographic imaging. Macroabscesses, granulomatous vasculitis, and meningitis may also be observed.[100,101] These illnesses are generally nosocomial. CSF findings include a pleocytosis with either polymorphonuclear cells or mononuclear cells predominating, increased protein, and low to normal glucose values. The organisms are seen on Gram stain in less than 50% of cases. The diagnosis is often missed initially, with delays in the correct diagnosis of two or more months being typical. Single-agent therapy with amphotericin B has a cure rate exceeding 85%.[102]

Parasites

Toxoplasmosis   Humans typically acquire *Toxoplasma gondii*, an obligate intracellular parasite for which the primary host is the cat, either by the fecal–oral route or by eating undercooked meat that contains tissue cysts from infected domestic animals.[103] The parasite may also be acquired by maternofetal transmission and result in severe systemic and neurological disease in the neonate. Except in the latter instance primary infection is usually asymptomatic. Following primary infection, the organism is distributed throughout the body, where it forms cysts and becomes latent. With the possible exception of persons undergoing heart transplantation, these cysts are the source of recrudescent infection in the immunocompromised host.[104–107] Serological evidence of exposure to toxoplasmosis is found in from 20% to 90% of adults, depending upon their geographical location.[108] Despite the high incidence of toxoplasmosis exposure in the general population, disseminated or neurological disease is rare in immunocompetent adults.

Before the AIDS pandemic, cerebral toxoplasmosis was a relatively rare disorder that occurred principally in the setting of disorders accompanied by defects in cell-mediated immunity, such as lymphoreticular malignancies and organ transplantation.[109] In contrast, cerebral toxoplasmosis is the most common cause of a focal neurological deficit in patients with AIDS, affecting 5% to 30%.[108] It is frequently the index illness for AIDS.

Toxoplasmosis of the CNS is multifocal in approximately 80% of cases. The mechanism by which the reactivation of toxoplasmosis takes place is poorly understood, but seems to be linked to specific defects in cell-mediated immunity.[110] Animal models suggest that the tachyzoites are less efficiently cleared from the brain. The clinical presentation of patients with CNS toxoplasmosis is variable, and either focal or non-focal signs of cerebral dysfunction are often present. Onset is often insidious, with a gradual progression of symptoms from disorientation and confusion to frank psychosis and even coma. In 50% or more instances patients present with encephalopathic features of headache, confusion and fever, and subsequently develop focal neurological deficits, such as hemiparesis, hemiplegia, tremor, visual field defects, cranial nerve palsies and focal seizures as the disease progresses. Seizures are the presenting symptom in approximately 30% of patients.[104] Infrequently the presentation may be acute, with the rapid development of a diffuse encephalitic process and death over a period of days to weeks.[107]

CT and MRI scans of the brain typically show single or, more commonly, multiple lesions that display various patterns of enhancement, generally either homogeneous or ring-enhancing (Figure 130.4). The lesions have a predilection for subcortical locations and the basal ganglia. Perilesional edema may be extensive. Standard laboratory tests of serum and cerebrospinal fluid from patients with *Toxoplasma encephalitis* (TE) are seldom diagnostic. Serum antitoxoplasma IgG titers are helpful in that it is seldom negative in the presence of CNS toxoplasma. PCR for *T. gondii* in the CSF is a reliable and sensitive indicator;[111] however, lumbar puncture is often precluded by the presence of brain lesions with significant mass effect. Brain biopsy is usually reserved for patients with diagnostic problems who are suspected to have TE, or who fail to have a timely response to empirical therapy. A protocol for the evaluation of brain mass lesions in AIDS has been proposed.[112] Single-photon emission computed tomography (SPECT) and positron emission tomography may be helpful in distinguishing toxoplasmosis and other non-malignant etiologies from CNS lymphoma.[73,113,114]

Combination chemotherapy for CNS toxoplasmosis is recommended, usually with pyrimethamine and either sulfadiazine or clindamycin. The initial response to treatment is excellent, with 90% of patients showing both radiographic and clinical improvement within two weeks.[104,107] Provided corticosteroid therapy has not been coadministered, the response to antitoxoplasma therapy may be used for diagnostic purposes. Patients treated with the above regimens often experience drug toxicity, and 44% will have side effects severe enough to require a change in medication or dosage.[104] Maintenance therapy is recommended to prevent relapses of TE, in either daily or twice-weekly dosing regimens.[115]

Strongyloides stercoralis *Strongyloides stercoralis* is a small nematode that may parasitize the human small intestine. The invading infective larvae are found in

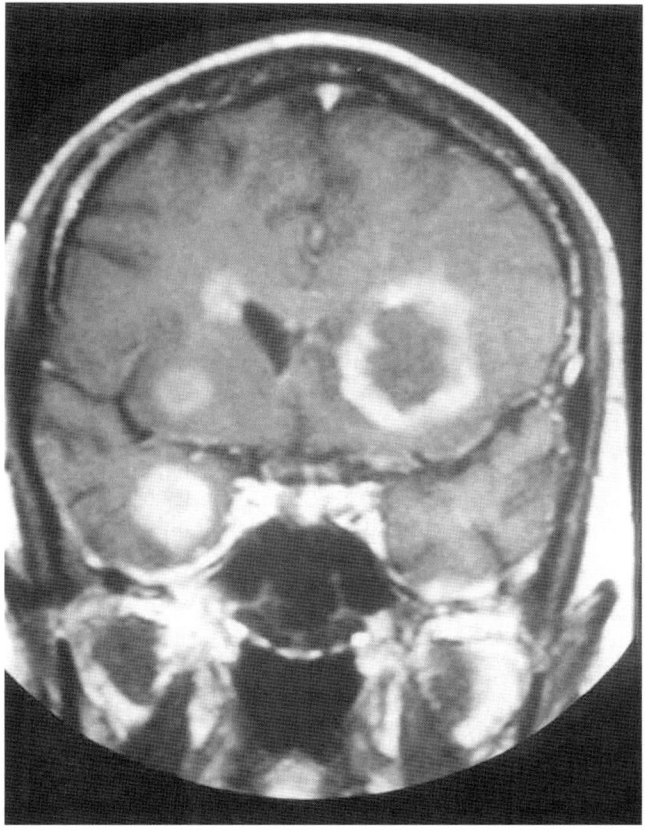

Figure 130.4 CT scan of toxoplasmosis. Contrast-enhanced CT using double-dose enhancement technique shows multiple ring-enhancing lesions with surrounding edema. (Reproduced from Berger JR, Levy RM. AIDS and the Nervous System. 2nd ed. Philadelphia: Lippincott Raven, 1996.)

moist soil and can rapidly penetrate the skin, travel through lymphatics to the pulmonary venous system, and from there migrate through alveoli, glottis and ultimately the esophagus to the small bowel. Autoinfection may also occur and may be quite prominent in the face of impaired immunity, e.g. with cytotoxic chemotherapy or in AIDS, resulting in hyperinfection. In hyperinfection larvae are widely distributed in many tissues, including the intestines, lung, lymph nodes, liver, peritoneal cavity, adrenals, heart and CNS.

CNS manifestations only occur in the setting of hyperinfection. Symptoms include headache with or without features of meningeal irritation, altered mentation, seizures and focal neurological findings. The chief abnormality is meningitis, but brain edema, focal hemorrhages with necrosis and microinfarcts may also be observed. The latter may be the consequence of larval deposition in small blood vessels. Viable larvae may be found in the brain without associated inflammation or necrosis.[116] Survival in this condition is poor; however, occasional patients may be rescued with thiabendazole 25 mg/kg twice daily if therapy is administered promptly.[117]

Summary

The etiologies of neurological complications occurring in the immunosuppressed host are quite diverse. A working knowledge of the most commonly encountered entities and their characteristics is important for developing a systematic approach to diagnosis and treatment. Antimicrobial therapy must often be initiated on a presumptive basis prior to the establishment of a definitive diagnosis. The widespread presence of AIDS, bone marrow and organ transplantation, and the aggressive management of malignancy necessitates a working knowledge of these infectious complications for all treating physicians.

References

1. Gallo RC, Sarin PS, Gelmann EP, et al. Isolation of human T-cell leukemia virus in acquired immune deficiency syndrome (AIDS). Science 1983;220:865–867

2. Wiley CA, Schrier RD, Nelson JA, et al. Cellular localization of human immunodeficiency virus infection within the brains of acquired immune deficiency syndrome patients. Proc Natl Acad Sci USA 1986;83:7089–7093

3. Levy JA, Shimabukuro J, Hollander H, et al. Isolation of AIDS-associated retroviruses from cerebrospinal fluid and brain of patients with neurological symptoms. Lancet 1985;2:586–588

4. Gray F, Belec L, Lescs MC, et al. Varicella-zoster virus infection of the central nervous system in the acquired immune deficiency syndrome. Brain 1994; 117:987–999

5. Berger JR, Kaszovitz B, Post MJ, Dickinson G. Progressive multifocal leukoencephalopathy associated with human immunodeficiency virus infection. A review of the literature with a report of sixteen cases. Ann Intern Med 1987;107:78–87

6. Denning DW, Anderson J, Rudge P, Smith H. Acute myelopathy associated with primary infection with human immunodeficiency virus. Br Med J (Clin Res Ed) 1987;294:143–144

7. Calabrese LH, Proffitt MR, Levin KH, et al. Acute infection with the human immunodeficiency virus (HIV) associated with acute brachial neuritis and exanthematous rash. Ann Intern Med 1987;107:849–851

8. Holtzman DM, Kaku DA, So YT. New-onset seizures associated with human immunodeficiency virus infection: causation and clinical features in 100 cases. Am J Med 1989;87:173–177

9. Gotswami KK, Kaye S, Miller R, et al. Intrathecal IgG synthesis and specificity of oligoclonal IgG in patients infected with HIV-1 do not correlate with CNS disease. J Med Virol 1991;33:106–113

10. Berger JR, Mucke L. Prolonged survival and partial recovery in AIDS-associated progressive multifocal leukoencephalopathy. Neurology 1988;38:1060–1065

11. Berger JR, Levy RM, Dix R. Aids and other immunocompromised states. In: Schlossberg D, ed. Infections of the Nervous System. New York: Springer-Verlag, 1990: 268–303

12. Nguyen N, Rimmer S, Katz B. Slowed saccades in the acquired immunodeficiency syndrome. Am J Ophthalmol 1989;107:356–360

13. Beal MF, O'Carroll P, Kleinman GM, Grossman RI. Apergillosis of the central nervous system. Neurology 1982;32:473–479

14. Norman SE, Chediak AD, Kiel M, Cohn MA. Sleep disturbances in HIV-infected homosexual men. AIDS 1990;4:775–781

15. Moret H, Guichard M, Matheron S, et al. Virological diagnosis of progressive multifocal leukoencephalopathy: detection of JC virus DNA in cerebrospinal fluid and brain tissue of AIDS patients. J Clin Microbiol 1993;31:3310–3313

16. McKendall RR, Klawans HL. Nervous system complications of varicella-zoster virus. In: Vinken PJ, Bruyn GW, eds. Handbook of Clinical Neurology. New York: Elsevier, North Holland, 1978:161–183

17. Day JJ, Grant I, Atkinson JH, et al. Incidence of AIDS dementia in a two-year follow-up of AIDS and ARC patients on an initial phase II AZT placebo-controlled study: San Diego cohort. J Neuropsychiatry Clin Neurosci 1992;4:15–20

18. Liedtke W, Opalka B, Zimmermann CW, Lignitz E. Age distribution of latent herpes simplex virus 1 and varicella-zoster virus genome in human nervous tissue. J Neurol Sci 1993;116:6–11

19. Uttamchandani RB, Daikos GL, Reyes RR, et al. Nocardiosis in 30 patients with advanced human immunodeficiency virus infection: clinical features and outcome. Clin Infect Dis 1994;18:348–353

20. Buffet R, Agut H, Chieze F, et al. Virological markers in the cerebrospinal fluid from HIV-1-infected individuals. AIDS 1991;5:1419–1424

21. Wiley CA, Masliah E, Morey M, et al. Neocortical damage during HIV infection. Ann Neurol 1991; 29:651–657

22. Forrest CB, Forehand JR, Axtell RA, et al. Clinical features and current management of chronic granulomatous disease. Hematol Oncol Clin North Am 1988;2: 253–266

23. Selnes OA, Miller E, McArthur J, et al. HIV-1 infection: no evidence of cognitive decline during the asymptomatic stages. The Multicenter AIDS Cohort Study. Neurology 1990;40:204–208

24. Plorde JJ. An introduction to infectious disease. In: Ryan KJ, ed. Sherris's Medical Microbiology. Norwalk, CT: Appleton and Lange, 1994:651–658

25. Pierce MA, Johnson MD, Maciunas RJ, et al. Evaluating contrast-enhancing brain lesions in patients with AIDS by using positron emission tomography. Ann Intern Med 1995;123:594–598

26. Hooper DC, Pruitt AA, Rubin RH. Central nervous system infection in the chronically immunosuppressed. Medicine (Baltimore) 1982;61:166–188

27. Snider WD, Simpson DM, Nielsen S, et al. Neurologic complications of the acquired immunodeficiency syndrome: analysis of 50 patients. Ann Neurol 1983; 14:403–418

28. Javaly K, Horowitz HW, Wormser GP. Nocardiosis in patients with human immunodeficiency virus infection. Report of 2 cases and review of the literature. Medicine (Baltimore) 1992;71:128–138

29. St. Gerogiev V. Opportunistic/nocosomial infections. Med Res Rev 1993;13:493–506

30. Dalakas MD. Neuromuscular complications of AIDS. Muscle Nerve 1986;9:92

31. Conti DJ, Rubin RH. Infection of the central nervous system in organ transplant recipients. Neurol Clin 1988;6:241–260

32. Perry GS 3rd, Spector BD, Schuman LM, et al. The Wiskott–Aldrich syndrome in the United States and Canada (1892–1979). J Pediatr 1980;97:72–78

33. Patchell RA. Neurological complications of organ transplantation. Ann Neurol 1994;36:688–703

34. Weber T, Turner RW, Frye S, et al. Specific diagnosis of progressive multifocal leukoencephalopathy by polymerase chain reaction. J Infect Dis 1994;169: 1138–1141

35. Kalayjian RC, Cohen ML, Bonomo RA, Flanigan TP. Cytomegalovirus ventriculoencephalitis in AIDS. A syndrome with distinct clinical and pathologic features. Medicine (Baltimore) 1993;72:67–77

36. Borel JF, Feurer C, Gubler HU, Stahelin H. Biological effects of cyclosporin A: a new antilymphocytic agent. Agents Actions 1976;6:468–475

37. Kahan BD, Flechner SM, Lorber MI, et al. Complications of cyclosporine-prednisone immunosuppression in 402 renal allograft recipients exclusively followed at a single center for from one to five years. Transplantation 1987;43:197–204

38. Drath DB, Kahan BD. Phagocytic cell function in response to immunosuppressive therapy. Arch Surg 1984;119:156–160

39. Baumgartner JE, Rachlin JR, Beckstead JH, et al. Primary central nervous system lymphomas: natural history and response to radiation therapy in 55 patients with acquired immunodeficiency syndrome. J Neurosurg 1990;73:206–211

40. Beckett A, Summergrad P, Manschreck T, et al. Symptomatic HIV infection of the CNS in a patient without clinical evidence of immune deficiency. Am J Psychiatry 1987;144:1342–1344

41. Pienaar S, Eley B, Beatty DW, Henderson HE. X-linked agammaglobulinaemia and the underlying genetics in two kindreds. J Paediatr Child Health 2000;36:453–456

42. Buckley RH. Primary immunodeficiency diseases. In: Paul W, ed. Fundamental Immunology. 3rd ed. New York: Raven Press, 1993:1353–1374

43. Wilfert CM, Buckley RH, Mohanakumar T, et al. Persistent and fatal central-nervous-system ECHOvirus infections in patients with agammaglobulinemia. N Engl J Med 1977;296:1485–1489

44. Merrill PT, Paige GD, Abrams RA, et al. Ocular motor abnormalities in human immunodeficiency virus infection. Ann Neurol 1991;30:130–138

45. Conley ME, Parolini O, Rohrer J, Campana D. X-linked agammaglobulinemia: new approaches to old questions based on the identification of the defective gene. Immunol Rev 1994;138:5–21

46. Anderson WF. Gene therapy. Sci Am 1995;273:124–128

47. Petito CK, Navia BA, Cho ES, et al. Vacuolar myelopathy pathologically resembling subacute combined degeneration in patients with the acquired immunodeficiency syndrome. N Engl J Med 1985;312:874–879

48. Ryan KJ. Medical Microbiology. 3rd ed. Norwalk, CT: Appleton and Lange, 1994

49. Klatt EC, Nichols L, Noguchi TT. Evolving trends revealed by autopsies of patients with the acquired immunodeficiency syndrome. 565 autopsies in adults with the acquired immunodeficiency syndrome, Los Angeles, California 1982–1993 [corrected]. Arch Pathol Lab Med 1994;118:884–890

50. Delamaire MEA. Impaired leucocyte functions in diabetic patients. Diabetic Med 1997;14:29–34

51. Patchell RA, White CL 3rd, Clark AW, et al. Neurologic complications of bone marrow transplantation. Neurology 1985;35:300–306

52. Hall WA. Neurosurgical infections in the compromised host. Neurosurg Clin North Am 1992;3:435–442

53. Levy RM, Rosenbloom S, Perrett LV. Neuroradiologic findings in AIDS: a review of 200 cases. AJR Am J Roentgenol 1986;147:977–983

54. Levy RM, Berger JR. Neurosurgical aspects of human immunodeficiency virus infection. Neurosurg Clin North Am 1992;3:443–470

55. Gray CM, Schapiro JM, Winters MA, Merigan TC. Changes in CD4+ and CD8+ T cell subsets in response to highly active antiretroviral therapy in HIV type 1-infected patients with prior protease inhibitor experience. AIDS Res Hum Retrovirus 1998;14:561–569

56. Berger JR, Moskowitz L, Fischl M, Kelley RE. Neurologic disease as the presenting manifestation of acquired immunodeficiency syndrome. South Med J 1987;80: 683–686

57. Whiteman ML, Post MJ, Berger JR, et al. Progressive multifocal leukoencephalopathy in 47 HIV-seropositive patients: neuroimaging with clinical and pathologic correlation. Radiology 1993;187:233–240

58. Hoffman JM, Waskin HA, Schifter T, et al. FDG-PET in differentiating lymphoma from nonmalignant central nervous system lesions in patients with AIDS. J Nucl Med 1993;34:567–575

59. Corey L. Persistent viral infections of the central nervous system. In: Sherries JC, ed. Medical Microbiology. 2nd ed. New York: Elsevier, 1990

60. Drew WL. CMV infection in patients with AIDS. J Infect Dis 1988; 158:449–456

61. Resnick L, Berger JR, Shapshak P, Tourtellotte WW. Early penetration of the blood-brain barrier by HIV. Neurology 1988;38:9–14

62. Katz DA, Berger JR, Hamilton B, et al. Progressive multifocal leukoencephalopathy complicating Wiskott–Aldrich syndrome. Report of a case and review of the literature of progressive multifocal leukoencephalopathy with other inherited immunodeficiency states. Arch Neurol 1994;51:422–426

63. Clifford DB, Buller RS, Mohammed S, et al. Use of PCR to demonstrate CMV DNA in CSF of patients with HIV. Neurology 1993;43:75–79

64. Petito CK, Cho ES, Lemann W, et al. Neuropathology of acquired immunodeficiency syndrome (AIDS): an autopsy review. J Neuropathol Exp Neurol 1986; 45:635–646

65. Gray F, Gherardi R, Scaravilli F. The neuropathology of the acquired immune deficiency syndrome (AIDS). A review. Brain 1988;111:245–266

66. Chretien F, Gray F, Lescs MC, et al. Acute varicella-zoster virus ventriculitis and meningo-myelo-radiculitis in acquired immunodeficiency syndrome. Acta Neuropathol 1993;86:659–665

67. Banjamini E, Coico R, Sunshine G. Immunology: A Short Course. 4th edn. New York: Wiley-Liss, 2000

68. Whitley R, Lakeman AD, Nahmias A, Roizman B. DNA restriction-enzyme analysis of herpes simplex virus isolates obtained from patients with encephalitis. N Engl J Med 1982;307:1060–1062

69. Luft BJ, Remington JS. Toxoplasmic encephalitis in AIDS. Clin Infect Dis 1992;15:211–222

70. Bowen BC, Post JD. Diagnostic imaging of CNS infection and inflammation. In: Scholssberg D, ed. Infections of the Nervous System. New York: Springer-Verlag, 1990

71. Wutzler P. Antiviral therapy of herpes simplex and varicella-zoster virus infections. Intervirology 1997;40: 343–356

72. Matthews WB. Slow viruses on the central nervous system. In: Lambert HP, ed. Infections of the Central Nervous System. Philadelphia: Marcel Decker, 1991

73. Hollander H, Stringari S. Human immunodeficiency

virus-associated meningitis. Clinical course and correlations. Am J Med 1987;83:813–816

74. Pinto AN. AIDS and cerebrovascular disease. Stroke 1996;27:538–543

75. Baringer JR, Swoveland P. Recovery of herpes-simplex virus from human trigeminal ganglions. N Engl J Med 1973;288:648–650

76. Berkey P, Bodey GP. Nocardial infection in patients with neoplastic disease. Rev Infect Dis 1989;11:407–412

77. Kahan BD. Cyclosporine: the agent and its actions. Transplant Proc 1985;17(4 Suppl 1):5–18

78. Villringer K, Jager H, Dichgans M, et al. Differential diagnosis of CNS lesions in AIDS patients by FDG-PET. J Comput Assist Tomogr 1995;19:532–536

79. Mylonakis E, Hohmann EL, Calderwood SB. Central nervous system infection with *Listeria monocytogenes*. 33 years' experience at a general hospital and review of 776 episodes from the literature. Medicine (Baltimore) 1998;77:313–336

80. Berenguer J, Moreno S, Laguna F, et al. Tuberculous meningitis in patients infected with the human immunodeficiency virus. N Engl J Med 1992;326:668–672

81. Bishburg E, Sunderam G, Reichman LB, Kapila R. Central nervous system tuberculosis with the acquired immunodeficiency syndrome and its related complex. Ann Intern Med 1986;105:210–213

82. Ellard GA, Humphries MJ, Allen BW. Cerebrospinal fluid drug concentrations and the treatment of tuberculous meningitis. Am Rev Respir Dis 1993;148:650–655

83. Dismukes WE. Management of cryptococcosis. Clin Infect Dis 1993;17(Suppl 2):S507–S512

84. Steinmetz H, Arendt G, Hefter H, et al. Focal brain lesions in patients with AIDS: aetiologies and corresponding radiological patterns in a prospective study. J Neurol 1995;242:69–74

85. Krick JA, Remington JS. Toxoplasmosis in the adult-an overview. N Engl J Med 1978;298:550–553

86. Schmitt FA, Bigley JW, McKinnis R, et al. Neuropsychological outcome of zidovudine (AZT) treatment of patients with AIDS and AIDS-related complex. N Engl J Med 1988;319:1573–1578

87. Casadevall A. Antibody immunity and invasive fungal infections. Infect Immun 1995;63:4211–4218

88. Clark RA, Greer D, Atkinson W, et al. Spectrum of *Cryptococcus neoformans* infection in 68 patients infected with human immunodeficiency virus. Rev Infect Dis 1990;12:768–777

89. Chuck SL, Sande MA. Infections with *Cryptococcus neoformans* in the acquired immunodeficiency syndrome. N Engl J Med 1989;321:794–799

90. Price RW, Brew B, Sidtis J, et al. The brain in AIDS: central nervous system HIV-1 infection and AIDS dementia complex. Science 1988;239:586–592

91. Zuger A, Louie E, Holzman RS, et al. Cryptococcal disease in patients with the acquired immunodeficiency syndrome. Diagnostic features and outcome of treatment. Ann Intern Med 1986;104:234–240

92. Gal AA, Evans S, Meyer PR. The clinical laboratory evaluation of cryptococcal infections in the acquired immunodeficiency syndrome. Diagn Microbiol Infect Dis 1987;7:249–254

93. Subauste CS, Remington JS. Immunity to *Toxoplasma gondii*. Curr Opin Immunol 1993;5:532–537

94. Baxter JD, Forsham PH. Tissue effects of glucocorticoids. Am J Med 1972;53:573–589

95. Hunter CA, Remington JS. Immunopathogenesis of toxoplasmic encephalitis. J Infect Dis 1994;170:1057–1067

96. Simpson DM. Neuromuscular complications of human immunodeficiency virus infection. Semin Neurol 1992;12:34–42

97. Coleman JM, Hogg GG, Rosenfeld JV, Waters KD. Invasive central nervous system aspergillosis: cure with liposomal amphotericin B, itraconazole, and radical surgery-case report and review of the literature. Neurosurgery 1995;36:858–863

98. Bhupalam L, Bhupalam R, Roy TM, Powers J. Invasive aspergillosis of the central nervous system. J Ky Med Assoc 1993;91:454–459

99. Denning DW, Stevens DA. Antifungal and surgical treatment of invasive aspergillosis: review of 2121 published cases. Rev Infect Dis 1990;12:1147–1201

100. Lipton SA, Hickey WF, Morris JH, Loscalzo J. Candidal infection in the central nervous system. Am J Med 1984;76:101–108

101. Walsh TJ, Hier DB, Caplan LR. Fungal infections of the central nervous system: comparative analysis of risk factors and clinical signs in 57 patients. Neurology 1985;35:1654–1657

102. Smego RA Jr, Perfect JR, Durack DT. Combined therapy with amphotericin B and 5-fluorocytosine for *Candida* meningitis. Rev Infect Dis 1984;6:791–801

103. Podzamczer D, Miro JM, Bolao F, et al. Twice-weekly maintenance therapy with sulfadiazine-pyrimethamine to prevent recurrent toxoplasmic encephalitis in patients with AIDS. Spanish Toxoplasmosis Study Group. Ann Intern Med 1995;123:175–180

104. Powderly WG. Cryptococcal meningitis and AIDS. Clin Infect Dis 1993;17:837–842

105. Kroczek RA, Graf D, Brugnoni D, et al. Defective expression of CD40 ligand on T cells causes "X-linked immunodeficiency with hyper-IgM (HIGM1)". Immunol Rev 1994;138:39–59

106. Nahmias AJ, Whitley RJ, Visintine AN, et al. Herpes simplex virus encephalitis: laboratory evaluations and their diagnostic significance. J Infect Dis 1982;145:829–836

107. MacArthur JC, Cohen BA, Selnes OA, et al. Low prevalence of neurological and neuropsychological abnormalities in otherwise healthy HIV-1 infected individuals: results from the AIDS Cohort Study. Ann Neurol 1989;26:601–611

108. Wistanley P. Drug treatment of toxoplasmosic encephalitis in acquired immunodeficiency syndrome. Postgrad Med J 1995;71:404–408

109. Navia BA, Jordan BD, Price RW. The AIDS dementia complex: I. Clinical features. Ann Neurol 1986;19:517–524

110. van de Schoondermark VE, Galama J, Kraaijeveld C, et al. Value of the polymerase chain reaction for detection of toxoplasma gondii in cerebrospinal fluid from patients with AIDS. Clin Infect Dis 1993;16:661–666

111. Sepkowitz K, Armstrong D. Space occupying fungal lesions of the CNS. *In:* Scheld, Whitley, Durack, eds. Infections of the Central Nervous System. New York: Raven Press, 1991:741–764.

112. Evaluation and management of intracranial mass lesions in AIDS. Report of the Quality Standards Subcommittee of the American Academy of Neurology. Neurology 1998;50:21–26

113. Pizzo PA, Eddy J, Faloon J. Acquired immune deficiency syndrome in children. Current problems and therapeutic considerations. Am J Med 1988;85:195–202

114. Walker RW, Brochstein JA. Neurologic complications

of immunosuppressive agents. Neurol Clin 1988;6: 261–278

115. Portegies P, de Gans J, Lange JM, et al. Declining incidence of AIDS dementia complex after introduction of zidovudine treatment. Br Med J 1989;299:819–821

116. Neefe LI. Pinella D, Gavagusi VF, Bauer H. Disseminated strongyloidiasis with cerebral involvement. A complication of corticosteroid therapy. Am J Med 1973;55:832–838

117. Scowdon EB, Schaffner W, Stone WJ. Overwhelming strongyloidiasis: an unappreciated opportunistic infection. Medicine 1987;57:527–544

131 Vasculitis Involving the Nervous System

Clarence W Legerton III and Jerome E Kurent

Introduction

Vasculitis involving the nervous system represents an important group of disorders. Establishing a diagnosis of CNS vasculitis is challenging for the clinician. The vasculitides are an increasingly treatable group of disorders. This chapter will focus on therapies for vasculitis involving the nervous system. Potent agents may be used individually or in combination. Therapies commonly utilized for the treatment of vasculitis are often not the result of controlled clinical trials but have become accepted approaches, especially in patients with life-threatening or refractory symptoms of vasculitis affecting the nervous system. Devastating clinical consequences may result from vasculitis involving vital neural structures. Early diagnosis and institution of effective therapies are critical in minimizing risk to the patient.

The vasculitides affecting the nervous system represent a group of disorders that share histological features consisting of inflammation and necrosis of blood vessels. Vasculitis may occur as a primary pathological process or may occur secondary to other conditions.[1-3] The classification of vasculitis has been based on a combination of clinical, laboratory and pathological features. Ischemia of vital neural structures represents the final common pathway of tissue injury caused by vasculitis.

As the nervous system exhibits a limited number of ways of manifesting ischemic injury, there are few unique or characteristic features to indicate a specific clinicopathological entity as the underlying cause of vasculitis affecting an individual patient. Laboratory and pathological evaluation is therefore critical in establishing a definitive diagnosis, but may also yield abnormalities not highly specific for any particular clinicopathological entity. The clinical features, in conjunction with supporting data, should be utilized when attempting to institute a diagnosis of vasculitis.

The evolution of neurological injury may be acute or slowly progressive. Signs and symptoms are often non-specific and may include headache, acute and chronic encephalopathy, coma, seizures, stroke, visual symptoms and myelopathies.[4-6] Vasculitis of the peripheral nerve and muscle may also occur.

Pathophysiology and pathogenesis

The specific causes of most vasculitis syndromes affecting the nervous system are unknown. Occasionally a relationship can be identified between a specific antigen and the onset of vasculitis, and may involve a drug or infectious agent.[7-9]

Primary immunopathogenetic mechanisms are responsible for ischemic injury due to vasculitis. These include immune complex formation; direct antibody-mediated damage to the blood vessel, usually involving the endothelial cell; and cell-mediated immunity, usually reflecting T-cell–endothelial cell interactions.[10,11]

Key mechanisms of vasculitic injury may include the release by the vascular endothelium of cytokines and other immune mediators that influence chemotaxis and leukocyte adherence. These may be associated with changes in blood vessel permeability. The perivascular microglial cell has also been demonstrated to be the target of some immunopathogenetic mechanisms in CNS vasculitis. Eosinophils are also implicated in a more limited number of vasculitic conditions, such as the Churg–Strauss syndrome. Extensive descriptions of the cellular immune mechanisms leading to vasculitic injury are described elsewhere in this volume.

Clinical features

Vasculitis-mediated nervous system injury may occur as a sudden unexpected event or may be a manifestation of established systemic vasculitis, such as polyarteritis nodosa. Primary angiitis of the central nervous system may cause ischemic injury to the brain, such as stroke. Vasculitis may also be restricted to the peripheral nervous system, or may be involved in causing multiorgan system disease.

Vasculitis affecting the peripheral nerve may be manifest as mononeuritis multiplex, involving one or more different motor or sensory nerves. A confluent symmetrical neuropathy may develop over time after vasculitic involvement of multiple peripheral nerves. Electrophysiological testing, including nerve conduction studies, followed by nerve biopsy, may provide confirmatory evidence for vasculitis of the peripheral nerve.

The devastating consequences of CNS vasculitis may include ischemic or hemorrhagic stroke syndrome, which may occur as solitary or multiple events. Impaired cognition, seizures and coma are frequent manifestations of CNS vasculitis. The spinal cord may also be the target of vasculitis syndromes, and may lead to paraplegia.

On clinical grounds alone, signs and symptoms occurring in an individual patient with vasculitis are usually difficult to attribute to a specific vasculitis syndrome. Evidence of systemic illness with multiorgan dysfunction often indicates an underlying vasculitis as the basis for the neurological event. The need for laboratory evaluation, including cerebral angiography, as well as histopathological confirmation is emphasized, but the clinician must recognize that these test results may be non-specific.

Classification of vasculitis

Many attempts to classify vasculitis have been discussed and are summarized in an editorial by Lie[12] and elsewhere in this volume. Given the lack of understanding of the etiology and pathogenesis of these syndromes, any classification scheme is imperfect. For the clinician, the essential attributes of a useful scheme are to define primary versus secondary forms, and to differentiate the various syndromes and their predominant clinical manifestations. Classically, this latter feature has been accomplished by focusing on the size of the vessel involved. Although this may be clinically helpful, this approach is limited by the significant overlap between diseases and the inability to relate the syndrome to any unifying pathogenetic construct. One approach is presented in Table 131.1. The major systemic vasculitidies with neurological manifestations are described in this chapter.

Giant cell arteritis

Giant cell arteritis (GCA, also called temporal arteritis) is one of the few true rheumatic and neurological emergencies. Neurological sequelae may include irreversible blindness, stroke and other severe consequences, which are largely preventable by treatment with glucocorticoids. Thus, early recognition and treatment are essential.

Nearly all patients with either polymyalgia rheumatica (PMR) or temporal arteritis are over 50 years of age. Symptoms of PMR usually begin first. Classically, patients will note the acute onset of stiffness, aches, and pain involving the shoulder girdle musculature, perhaps involving the lumbar spine and hip girdle as well. The symptom of stiffness often predominates and is quite severe upon first awaking in the morning. Upon direct questioning, patients often note difficulty arising from the bed and toilet. Constitutional symptoms reflect the systemic inflammatory state and include decreased activity, fatigue, malaise, anorexia and weight loss. True inflammatory arthritis may occur.

Temporal arteritis is a large vessel vasculitis that affects the aorta and its major branches, with a predilection for the large cranial arteries. Thus patients often note headaches, scalp tenderness or jaw claudication. Ominous symptoms of optic nerve arteritis classically include amaurosis fugax, but any transient visual disturbance may be encountered. In one series of 245 patients followed for five years, 14% suffered permanent visual loss, nearly all events occurring prior to the institution of glucocorticoid therapy.[13] Ten percent to 15% of patients will have large artery involvement, manifesting as aortic aneurysm, intermittent claudication of an extremity, or paresthesias.[14] Limb claudication in the absence of typical atherosclerotic disease should raise concern about temporal arteritis, as well as Takayasu's arteritis.

The neurological manifestations of GCA are myriad. In one review of 166 consecutive patients,[15] 51 (31%) developed neurological complications, including neuropathy, central vascular events, tremor, tongue paresthesia, myelopathy, and neuropsychiatric syndromes. Twenty-one percent of these patients experienced neuro-ophthalmological symptoms. The literature is replete with case reports and neurological complications of GCA.

The diagnosis of PMR is based largely on clinical criteria. Most patients will have an elevated erythrocyte sedimentation rate (ESR). In addition to a typical history and an elevated ESR, a brisk response to low-dose corticosteroids is consistent with this diagnosis. The ESR is more consistently elevated in temporal arteritis, averaging approximately 80–100 mmHg, although occasional cases with a normal ESR are reported. When temporal arteritis is considered, the diagnosis is confirmed by typical histological changes in biopsies of involved vessels, usually the temporal arteries. Granulomatous inflammation involves the media of the artery and results in fragmentation of the internal elastic lamina. Multinucleated giant cells are part of the classic picture, but are not required for the diagnosis. If abnormal arterial segments are not clinically evident, then long sections (at least 2.5 cm) of temporal artery should be taken and carefully examined so as not to overlook "skip lesions".[16] One should be attuned to the possibility of healed vasculi-

---

Table 131.1   A classification of vasculitis

Primary vasculitis
Predominantly large vessel
- Takayasu arteritis
- Giant cell (termporal) arteritis

Predominantly medium and small vessels
- Polyarteritis nodosa
- Churg–Strauss syndrome
- ANCA associated vasculitis
  - Wegener's granulomatosis
  - Microscopic polyarteritis nodosa

Predominantly small vessel vasculitis
- Henoch–Schonlein purpura
- Leukocytoclastic vasculitis

Miscellaneous
- Behçet's syndrome
- Cogan syndrome
- Kawasaki disease

Secondary vasculitis
- Infection
- Connective tissue disease
- Drug
- Malignancy
- Other

Adapted from Lie JT. Nomenclature and classification of vasculitis: plus ça change, plus c'est las meme chose. Arthritis & Rheumatism 1994;37:181–186.

tis, represented by intimal and medial fibrosis, if treatment has occurred for a prolonged period of more than a few weeks or if symptoms are remote. Given the age of patients affected by these diseases, one needs to consider the differential of malignancy, cervical spine disease, mechanical shoulder problems such as rotator cuff syndrome, rheumatoid arthritis or other inflammatory diseases, and hypothyroidism and other metabolic and non-inflammatory causes of myalgia.

The dramatic response of PMR to low doses of glucocorticoids is so consistent that the diagnosis should be questioned if the patient fails to improve within a few days to a week. Prednisone is often begun at a dose of approximately 15–20 mg/day, given as a single morning dose. Follow-up can occur at two to three weeks, by which time both the patient's symptoms should have dramatically improved and the ESR should have decreased. Doses may then be tapered gradually, based on the patient's clinical and ESR response.

In contrast to PMR, consideration of GCA warrants the immediate institution of corticosteroids (CS) in high doses to minimize the risks of vascular complications such as blindness, which is most typically unilateral and irreversible. Temporal artery biopsy may occur within a couple of weeks of the institution of steroids without concern about suppressing the histological changes. Unlike most forms of systemic vasculitis, steroids alone are sufficient therapy and other immunosuppressive agents are only rarely employed. Typically, glucocorticoids are instituted at doses approximating 1 mg/kg/day, usually 60 mg of prednisone daily. Divided-dose therapy is more effectively immunosuppressive initially, but more toxic the longer it is continued. The authors often institute prednisone at 20 mg t.i.d. for two weeks, then consolidate to 60 mg each morning for a second two weeks. At this point, or sooner once symptoms are controlled, steroids are tapered. A typical reduction might proceed at 10 mg every two to four weeks to a dose of 20 mg daily, at which point the taper is slowed to 5 mg each two to four weeks to a dose of 10 mg daily. From this point, doses are often reduced in 2.5 mg increments.

In this and other forms of vasculitis the reduction of steroids is as much art as science, and the patient's clinical and ESR response should be considered. The appropriate duration of corticosteroid therapy is debatable and approaches vary widely. Some physicians taper rapidly over six months in the hope that some patients will have minimal exposure to corticosteroids. The obvious risk is that a number of patients will relapse, requiring an increase in dosage and a slower taper. Other physicians advocate a one to two-year course of therapy to minimize the risk that vasculitis will recur. In any event, relapses are not uncommon and may be precipitated by too rapid a taper of steroids. Relapse may present with a recurrence of clinical symptoms and a rise in acute phase reactants, and initial therapy for relapse should consist of an increase in steroids to an effective dose

and a slower taper. One needs to consider malignancy, occult infection or other causes for a persistently elevated ESR. Some elderly patients may continue with an unexplained elevation in ESR. If the disease remains clinically inactive, the ESR itself should not preclude dosage reduction.

In view of the older average age of patients affected by this disorder and the dose of corticosteroids required, most patients will experience adverse effects and need to be appropriately informed. Interventions to ensure the preservation of bone mass should be instituted concomitantly with steroid therapy, and should include at least non-pharmacological measures (e.g. weight-bearing exercise), calcium and vitamin D supplementation, and gonadal hormone replacement in deficient patients. The early use both of more potent pharmacological agents such as bisphosphonates and of bone mineral density assessment is recommended in recent guidelines published by the American College of Rheumatology.[17] Other measures to prevent adverse events due to glucocorticoids should be employed (Table 131.2).

Because of the significant potential toxicity of corticosteroid therapy in temporal arteritis, more recent clinical trials have focused on the use of alternative immunosuppressive therapies in an attempt to reduce

Table 131.2   Therapy for severe or common adverse effects of corticosteroids

Adverse effect	Intervention
Bone loss	• calcium and vitamin D supplementation • hormone replacement therapy in both females and males • early institution of bisphosphonate therapy or other agent proven effective in corticosteroid induced osteoporosis • determination of BMD by DEXA • weight bearing exercise
Weight gain	• dietary counseling • exercise
Hyperglycemia, hypertension	• careful monitoring • adjustment of therapy
Immunosuppression	• early evaluation for febrile illness
Osteonecrosis	• use lowest effective dose
Steroid side effects (depression, euphoria)	• reduce dose if possible; initiate psychotropic medication if symptoms persist

BMD = bone mineral density
DEXA = dual x-ray absorptiometry

the dose and duration of corticosteroids. Methotrexate has been most frequently studied, but the results have been mixed.[18,19] Other reported options include azathioprine,[20] cyclophosphamide[21] and cyclosporin A,[22] although no large randomized trials utilizing these agents exist to demonstrate efficacy across populations. Similarly, only a few small uncontrolled trials have described the treatment of steroid-resistant GCA.[23] Occasionally there is a need to biopsy other arteries if symptoms, physical examination or imaging studies suggest involvement in other distributions.[24]

Polyarteritis nodosa and Churg–Strauss syndrome

Polyarteritis nodosa (PAN) affects predominantly medium-sized and small vessels, especially in the peripheral nerves, kidneys, mesenteric vessels and skin. The majority of patients have neurological involvement,[25] for example mononeuritis multiplex, distal sensorimotor polyneuropathy or peripheral sensory neuropathy. CNS disease is a less common but increasingly recognized complication which can present as diffuse encephalopathy or focal syndromes.[26] Reflecting the widespread vascular disease, various neurological syndromes are reported in the literature. Patients are often systemically ill, with fever, malaise, anorexia, weight loss and abdominal pain. Other symptoms reflect the involvement of various organ systems. Rashes, arthritis and muscle pain are common.

The non-specific variability of presenting symptoms makes the diagnosis difficult. Diagnosis is confirmed with a biopsy demonstrating mural vascular inflammation with fibrinoid necrosis. Multiple microaneurysms on angiography, usually involving the hepatic, mesenteric or renal vasculature, may be diagnostic in a classic case. However, one must be aware of other causes of vascular microaneurysms, such as ischemia, atrial myxoma and other embolic diseases, or other forms of vasculitis. Importantly, tests for antineutrophil antibodies (ANCA) are typically negative.

Therapy should begin with high-dose corticosteroids equivalent to approximately 60 mg of prednisone daily administered in divided doses (see Table 131.6). In contrast to therapy in PMR and GCA, the use of corticosteroids in the systemic necrotizing vasculitis syndromes may be given in various dosing options, depending on the severity of the clinical manifestations (see Table 131.8). Ther has been controversy about whether the immediate institution of other immunosuppressive agents results in improved disease control or survival, but the extensive contributions of the French Vasculitis Study Group have helped to clarify treatment issues.[27] Patients with severe organ-threatening disease should be treated with cyclophosphamide (see Table 131.4) One study has suggested that treatment with daily cyclophosphamide on an intermittent basis was therapeutically equivalent to daily dosing.[28]

As outlined previously, there are many potential complications of prednisone (Table 131.2) and

Table 131.3	Adverse effects of cyclophosphamide

Nausea/vomiting
Leukopenia/neutropenia
Anemia
Thrombocytopenia
Leukemia/lymphoma
Alopecia
Hemorrhagic cystitis
Bladder cancer
Infection
Pulmonary interstitial lung disease
Infertility
Premature ovarian failure
Teratogenesis

Table 131.4	Daily dosing of cyclophosphamide

Begin dosing at 2 mg/kg/day either p.o. or IV. If insufficient response, increase dose 25 mg every 2 weeks until:
  a. a clinical response occurs
  b. a WBC count of approximately 3000 cells/mm^3 is attained

Maximum nadir approximately 8–10 days after dose is administered or increased. Follow CBC 1–2 times weekly. Stop cyclophosphamide if rapid drop in WBC, anticipating maximal drug effect at 8–10 days.

Monitor CBC closely, every 2–4 weeks. Anticipate decreased tolerance of cyclophosphamide over time, required dosage reduction. Follow urinalysis every 3–4 months. Continue therapy for 1 year after remission or switch to agent with less long-term toxicity (e.g. methotrexate) after 3–4 months of cyclophosphamide. After one year in remission, taper dose by 25–50 mg each month.

During and after therapy with cyclophosphamide, life-long observation for other complications (e.g. bladder cancer, leukemia, infertility).

In severe life-threatening disease, may begin cyclophosphamide at 4 mg/kg/day for several days, followed by reduction to 1–2 mg/kg/day and adjusting dose to WBC nadir.

Decrease dose in patients with decreased creatinine clearance.

cyclophosphamide therapy (Table 131.3). Only physicians skilled in the use of these medications should prescribe them. Use and monitoring of cyclophosphamide is outlined in Tables 131.4 and 131.9. Because of the toxicity of these agents, much attention has been focused on the use of other, less toxic agents to maintain the remission once established by cyclophosphamide. Few data exist to support efficacy, but other immunomodulating therapy is occasionally utilized (Table 131.5).

Table 131.5　Alternative immunomodulating therapy in vasculitis

Drug	Typical dose range
Methotrexate	10–25 mg/week
Azathioprine	100–250 mg/day
Cyclosporine A	2–5 mg/kg/day
Chlorambucil	2 mg/day
Mycophenolate mofetil	1–3 grams/day
Gamma globulin	400 mg/kg daily for 4 days
Plasma exchange protocol	

Table 131.6　Corticosteroid therapy in systemic vasculitis: common approaches

Initiate prednisone (or equivalent) at 1 mg/kg/day in single or divided doses, usually 20 mg. p.o. TID, for 2 weeks. Consider pulse therapy if life-threatening disease. Consolidate to 60 mg. p.o. each morning for weeks 2 through 4. Taper over the next few months based on total dose:

- doses >20 mg qd, taper by 10 mg every 2–4 weeks
- doses between 10 and 20 mg qd, taper by 5 mg every 2–4 weeks
- doses ≤10 mg qd, taper by 2.5 mg every 2–4 weeks

Alternatively, taper to an alternate day schedule with a more rapid tapering schedule (perhaps over 2 months). Use of additional immunosuppressive agents may allow faster taper of steroids, depending on the disease being treated. Follow clinical symptoms and signs, laboratory values, or imaging studies and adjust taper accordingly.

Churg–Strauss syndrome (allergic angiitis and granulomatosis) is characterized by an allergic diathesis consisting of asthma, allergic rhinitis and nasal polyposis in the setting of a systemic vasculitis with peripheral eosinophilia. Peripheral nervous system disease is commonly seen, usually mononeuritis or peripheral neuropathy.[29,30] CNS disease is uncommon. Significant renal disease is less common in Churg–Strauss syndrome than in microscopic polyarteritis nodosa or Wegener's granulomatosis. The diagnosis is confirmed by histological evidence of vasculitis in the clinical setting outlined above. Typically, granulomas and extravascular eosinophils are present, though neither is required to establish the diagnosis. Therapy is similar to that of PAN, utilizing prednisone in doses of 40–60 mg/day for pulmonary or milder systemic disease. Cyclophosphamide should be used in the presence of severe manifestations.[27] One study defined five prognostic factors associated with increased mortality, including proteinuria (>1 g/day), renal insufficiency (serum creatinine >1.58 mg/dL), gastrointestinal involvement, cardiomyopathy and CNS signs.[31] Patients are moni-

tored in an effort to demonstrate improved constitutional and organ system function, and for reductions in eosinophilia and ESR.

Wegener's granulomatosis and ANCA-associated diseases

Wegener's granulomatosis (WG) is a granulomatous vasculitis which classically presents as a triad involving both the upper and lower respiratory tract and the kidneys. Hence it is one of the pulmonary–renal syndromes. Patients most commonly present with persistent upper respiratory symptoms involving the sinuses, nose, ears or trachea. Pulmonary symptoms include cough, dyspnea and hemoptysis. Chest radiographs may demonstrate nodules or infiltrates, which may cavitate. Renal disease presents with signs and symptoms of a pauci-immune focal and segmental glomerulonephritis. Ocular involvement is the most common neurological sign, with 15% of patients presenting with eye disease and 52% having ocular involvement at some point in their disease.[32] Neurological involvement is uncommon at presentation. Mononeuritis multiplex developed in 15% of patients. Eight percent eventually developed CNS involvement, including stroke, cranial nerve dysfunction, and one case of diabetes insipidus.[10] Wegener's granulomatosis may range from severe multisystem life-threatening disease to more limited forms involving only one or two organ systems.

Classically, the diagnosis of Wegener's granulomatosis is made by the demonstration of granulomatous vasculitis on tissue biopsy, usually the lung. However, the development of testing for the antineutrophil cytoplasmic antibody (ANCA) has allowed the diagnosis to be made in the appropriate clinical setting in the presence of a cytoplasmic staining pattern positive for serine protease 3.

The therapeutic advances in alkylating agent use have dramatically increased survival from five months without therapy[33] to the point where more than 90% of patients achieve significant improvement in their disease activity.[32] Current therapeutic recommendations include high-dose prednisone and cyclophosphamide, as described for severe systemic necrotizing vasculitis above (Tables 131.4 and 131.6). Because of their significant toxicity, corticosteroids are often tapered to an alternate-day dosing schedule over the initial three to four months. Therapeutic protocols comparing daily cyclophosphamide with intermittent (monthly) dosing schedules have been studied.[34,35] Both are successful at achieving remission, although relapses are more common with intermittent therapy.[34] Daily administration is therefore more often utilized.

Owing to the significant combined toxicity of prednisone and cyclophosphamide, investigations have been conducted to develop an equally efficacious but less toxic regimen. One study treated 42 patients without life-threatening disease in an open fashion with prednisone and methotrexate. Remission was achieved in 30 patients (71%). Eleven of these 30 achieving remission relapsed, most while taking methotrexate alone.[36] Another approach involves the induction of remission by using prednisone and cyclophosphamide for several months and converting cyclophosphamide to an alternative, less toxic immunosuppressive drug for maintenance of remission. Patients who fail to respond may be considered for additional therapies. A recent review summarizes the current experience.[37] An open label trial of the tumor necrosis factor inhibitor etanercept in 20 patients with persistently active disease despite conventional therapy demonstrated promising results,[38] and further studies are under way.

Microscopic polyarteritis nodosa is small vessel vasculitis without granulomas, and was historically classified with classic PAN. However, the facts that the ANCA test is often positive (although in a perinuclear pattern positive for myeloperoxidase) and that clinical symptoms overlap with both PAN and WG has led most experts to favor its inclusion with WG. Microscopic polyarteritis is characterized by a high incidence of renal vasculitis, often presenting clinically as rapidly progressive glomerulonephritis with pulmonary involvement, making it clinically similar to Wegener's granulomatosis. However, pulmonary disease often manifests as diffuse alveolar hemorrhage, which contributes significantly to the high mortality of this syndrome. Ocular and upper respiratory involvement can occur, symptoms also seen in Wegener's granulomatosis. Peripheral neuropathy occurs in up to one-third of patients,[39] which is less frequent than in PAN. Therapy is similar to that of Wegener's granulomatosis, including the initial use of high-dose corticosteroid therapy along with cyclophosphamide.

Takayasu's arteritis

Patients with Takayasu's arteritis often present with non-specific neurological symptoms. These include dizziness, headaches, arthralgias and other constitutional features, and are often associated with delays in establishing a diagnosis. Because it is a disease resulting in occlusion of the aorta and its major branches, patients may experience limb and organ ischemia. Vascular bruits of involved vessels and ischemic symptoms of the carotid and vertebrobasilar systems are the primary neurological signs and symptoms. Funduscopic abnormalities are common. Treatment is initiated with 1 mg/kg of oral prednisone, while monitoring clinical symptoms and ESR. In patients with refractory symptoms or who require prolonged use of corticosteroids, the addition of cyclophosphamide,[40] methotrexate[41] or cyclosporine[42,43] is often advocated. The NIH experience of 60 patients has been described.[44]

Hypersensitivity vasculitis

Hypersensitivity vasculitis is a broad term encompassing several distinct entities (Table 131.7). These share common features of small vessel vasculitis, a predominance of skin involvement and a relatively benign clinical course. Although a discussion of each individual entity is beyond the scope of this chapter,

Table 131.7   Hypersensitivity vasculitis

Henoch–Schonlein purpura
Cryoglobulinemia
Serum sickness
Drug induced*
Hypocomplimentemic vasculitis
Secondary to other connective tissue disease**
Secondary to other inflammatory disease***

*	e.g. penicillin, sulfonamides drugs
**	e.g. rheumatoid arthritis, systemic lupus erythematosis, Sjogren's syndrome
***	chronic active hepatitis, ulcerative colitis, primary biliary cirrhosis, paraneoplastic, infection

several general comments may be made. The most common cutaneous manifestation is leukocytoclastic vasculitis. This term refers to the nuclear debris that remains from the neutrophils which have infiltrated in and around the postcapillary venules. As a result of damage to the vessel wall, erythrocytes extravasate from the small dermal vessels, especially in areas of higher hydrostatic pressure. This results in lesions characterized as palpable purpura. Extradermal involvement is less common and usually less severe. The skin lesions may ulcerate and be quite painful. Neurological involvement is uncommon.

Many of these disorders require no specific therapy as their course is transient. Offending antigens, including drugs, must be eliminated if identified. Systemic disease such as diffuse skin involvement, visceral organ disease or systemic symptoms may be treated with moderate to high doses of corticosteroids, preferably with a rapid taper. Alternatively, therapy with NSAIDs, dapsone[45,46] or colchicine[47,48] may be considered, but results are sporadic. Only rarely does disease severity justify the need for more aggressive immunosuppressive therapy. Before using dapsone, the physician should test the patient for G6PD deficiency, as patients with this enzyme deficiency may experience marked hemolysis with even low doses of dapsone. Dapsone is started at 50–100 mg/day, and the dose titrated upwards to control disease activity. Patients should be monitored for anemia, leukopenia and methemoglobinemia as potential side effects of dapsone therapy. All patients on dapsone will experience dose-dependent hemolysis. Uncommon adverse effects include neuropathy, renal disease, cholestasis and agranulocytosis.

Behçet's disease

Behçet's disease is of unknown cause and is more common in Mediterranean countries and Japan than the United States. Histopathology reflects vasculitis with neutrophilic inflammatory infiltrates. Common manifestations include recurrent oral and genital aphthous ulcers, diffuse mucocutaneous rashes, arthritis and arterial aneurysms. Ocular involvement occurs in approximately two-thirds of patients, classically with anterior uveitis. Posterior uveitis and retinal vasculitis

Table 131.8   Dosing options for corticosteroids

Disease state	Therapy	Dose
Life-threatening or organ-threatening disease	Pulse	1 gram solumedrol (or equivalent) intravenously daily for 3 days, followed by high dose oral prednisone
Life-threatening or organ-threatening disease	High dose	40–60 mg prednisone (oral) daily in divided doses (up to 1–2 mg/kg/day in 3 divided doses)
Severe, but not life or organ threatening disease	Moderate dose	10–40 mg daily, preferably dosed once a day in the morning
Mild disease or as maintenance to control disease while other agents being instituted	Low dose	Less than 10 mg prednisone daily in one morning dose

Table 131.9   Prevention of cyclophosphamide adverse effects

Counsel regarding use of birth control
Consider sperm banking
Consider ovarian suppression with lupron
Antiemetics
Monitor CBC
Monitor urinalysis; cystoscopy for hematuria
Push fluids to maintain urine flow during treatment
Treat any abnormalities of bladder function
Lifelong follow-up for bladder cancer or secondary malignancy, especially hematologic

may also occur. Neurological involvement occurs in Behçet's disease, and can be severe. CNS parenchymal disease predominates, usually as a meningoencephalitis with brainstem involvement.[49] Myriad other neurological syndromes may occur, such as cerebellar ataxia, benign intracranial hypertension, headaches and seizures.[50] Dural sinus thrombosis and intracranial hypertension are reported.[51]

Treatment can be challenging, as ulcers and other severe manifestations can be refractory. Most reported therapeutic trials have involved small numbers of patients and have been uncontrolled. Steroids are often used as first-line therapy. High doses may be required to ameliorate ulcers. Colchicine, interferon-α[52] and dapsone[53,54] have also often been reported. Both ocular and CNS disease are notoriously unresponsive to glucocorticoids, and often require more aggressive therapy. The immunomodulating drug cyclosporin has been used, especially for uveitis.[55,56] Alkylating agents such as cyclophosphamide and chlorambucil have been used for severe disease. Azathioprine may be effective.[57] Recently, thalidomide has been employed for treatment of the mucocutaneous lesions of Behçet's.[58] Physicians must have special registration to prescribe this drug and patients must undergo extensive education and monitoring during its use, primarily to ensure that pregnancy does not occur. Serious poten-

tial adverse effects include birth defects, peripheral neuropathy and neutropenia. Recent case reports have described success with inhibitors of tumor necrosis factor.[59,60]

Vasculitis secondary to other autoimmune diseases

Many of the autoimmune diseases have vasculitis as a component of their systemic manifestations. Most commonly, the features are those of a hypersensitivity vasculitis with involvement of small vessels, but larger vessel vasculitis may occur. Symptoms and signs are usually similar to those of the primary systemic vasculitides described earlier. Rheumatoid arthritis is a good example. Occurring most often in severe seropositive nodular RA, rheumatoid vasculitis most commonly presents with cutaneous manifestations which can range from nailfold infarcts to vasculitic ulcers, to true gangrene. Other organ systems are less commonly involved. Neuropathy can occur in less than half the patients, either as mononeuritis multiplex or as a pure sensory neuropathy.[61] CNS involvement is exceedingly rare.[62] Treatment should be provided relative to the degree of vasculitis present. Nailfold infarcts may require no therapy or a transient increase in steroid dose. Treatment for more severe manifestations, such as mononeuritis multiplex, is similar to that for other severe necrotizing vasculitis.

Similarly, systemic lupus erythematosis (SLE) manifests vasculitis principally as a cutaneous rash. There is periungual involvement, as in RA, but urticaria and leukocytoclastic vasculitis may also occur. Peripheral neuropathy may occur as mononeuritis multiplex or generalized sensory motor neuropathy. Central nervous system involvement is common. Historically, the presence of widespread CNS inflammation ("cerebritis") and vasculitis was assumed. However, it is now clear that most of the cerebral disease is not due to inflammatory or necrotizing vasculitis, although other causes of vasculopathy (e.g. the antiphospholipid syndrome) may play a role. True cerebral vasculitis is rare, and occurred in only 7% of 57 patients with CNS disease verified histopathologically.[63] As a result, the term "cerebritis" has been replaced by the diagnosis of "neuropsychiatric lupus". The absence of vasculitis in the CNS is a clinically important distinction when one is faced with the treatment of the patient with neuropsychiatric manifestations. Although treatment for active lupus is often a part of the therapeutic algorithm, one must be equally aggressive in instituting antipsychotic or other psychiatric therapies. Neuropsychiatric manifestations include cognitive dysfunction, psychosis, organic brain syndrome and vascular headache syndrome. As suggested above, one must be vigilant in the search for coexisting complications that would alter therapy, including the antiphospholipid syndrome, fibromyalgia, cryoglobulinemia and hyperviscosity syndrome, and thrombotic thrombocytopenic purpura and infections due to treatment with systemic immunosuppressive agents occur.

Lastly, any of several other rheumatic diseases may present with small vessel vasculitis consistent with hypersensitivity vasculitis. Chief among these are Sjögren's syndrome and Wegener's granulomatosis.

Isolated angiitis of the CNS

Isolated angiitis of the CNS, or granulomatous angiitis, may result in brain or spinal cord injury restricted to the central nervous system.[64–66] It is a rare syndrome and primarily affects small vessels, although arteries or veins of any size may be involved.

A combination of headache and cognitive impairment with associated CSF pleiocytosis represents the most common manifestation of isolated angiitis of the CNS. Focal brain or spinal cord dysfunction as well as seizures may represent presenting symptoms. Visual symptoms related to choroid and retinal artery vasculitis can also occur. Systemic symptoms often present in more generalized vasculitic syndromes are usually absent in patients with isolated angiitis of the CNS. Malaise, fever, myalgias and arthralgias are associated more with the systemic vasculitides than with isolated CNS angiitis.

The CBC and ESR are usually normal in isolated CNS angiitis. The cerebral spinal fluid usually demonstrates a mild pleiocytosis consisting of 40–500 cells, predominantly lymphocytes. CSF protein elevations with normal glucose levels are typical.[67] The electroencephalogram may reveal diffuse slowing. Cerebral angiography may demonstrate vasculopathic changes.[68] The MRI brain scan may be normal or non-specifically abnormal, unless the patient has experienced a clinical stroke associated with significant brain ischemia. Therapy of isolated CNS angiitis usually consists of corticosteroids and cyclophosphamide,[69,70] although some patients have been managed with corticosteroids alone.

Summary and conclusions

A wide variety of vasculitis syndromes may adversely affect the central and peripheral nervous systems. Although systemic vasculitis syndromes are uncommon, patients are at significant risk for neurological complications which are often severe and permanent.

The definitive diagnosis of vasculitis involving the nervous system usually depends on correlating a combination of clinical signs and symptoms supported by laboratory data. Establishing the diagnosis of a specific clinicopathologic vasculitis entity may be difficult, as overlap between clinical and laboratory features is common. Consultation by a rheumatologist may assist in establishing a diagnosis.

The medical management of vasculitis affecting the nervous system has changed significantly over the last 10–15 years. The cornerstones of pharmacological therapy include corticosteroids and cyclophosphamide. Adjunctive cytotoxic and immunosuppressive agents are often used, but supporting evidence obtained from randomized controlled clinical trials is rare. It has been challenging to identify adequate numbers of patients with vasculitis to enrol in clinical trials, in view of the uncommon incidence of vasculitis syndromes.

Risk–benefit considerations are of paramount importance when treating patients with suspected or confirmed vasculitis involving the nervous system. Because of the significant potential for severe and permanent neurological impairment, there is often a sense of relative urgency to establish the diagnosis of CNS vasculitis and to proceed with appropriate therapies. It is to be expected that more effective therapies will be developed which may have more favorable risk–benefit profiles as our understanding of the underlying causes and immunopathogenetic mechanisms increases.

References

1. Siva A. Vasculitis of the nervous system. J Neurol 2001;248:451–468
2. Ferro JM. Vasculitis of the central nervous system. [Review] J Neurol 1998;245:766–776
3. Calabrese LH, Duna GF. Evaluation and treatment of central nervous system vasculitis. Curr Opin Rheumatol 1995;71:34–44
4. Moore PM. Neurology of vasculitides and connective tissue diseases. J Neurol Neurosurg Psychiatry 1998;65:10–22
5. Guillevin L, Lhote P, Gherardi R. Polyarteritis nodosa, microscopic angiitis, and Churg–Strauss syndrome: clinical aspects, neurologic manifestations, and treatment. Neurol Clin 1997;15:865–886
6. Gross WL. New concepts in treatment protocols for severe systemic vasculitis. Curr Opin Rheumatol 1999;11:41–46
7. Brust JCM. Vasculitis owing to substance abuse. Neurol Clin 1997;15:945–957
8. Glick R, Hoying J, Cerullo L, Perlman S. Phenylpropanolamine: an over the counter drug causing central nervous system vasculitis and intracerebral hemorrhage. Case report and review. Neurosurgery 1987;20:969–974
9. Gilden DH, Kleinschmidt-DeMasters BK, Welish M, Hedley-Whyte ET, et al. Varicella zoster virus, a cause of waxing and waning vasculitis: the New England Journal of Medicine case 5—1995 revisited. Neurology 1996;47:1441–1446

10. Moore PM. Neurological manifestations of vasculitis: update on immunopathogenic mechanisms and clinical features. Ann Neurol 1995;37:S131–S141

11. Cohen Tervaert JW, Popa ER, Bos NA. The role of superantigens in vasculitis. Curr Opin Rheumatol 1999;11:24–33

12. Lie JT. Nomenclature and classification of vasculitis: plus ca change, plus c'est la meme chose. Arthritis Rheum 1994;37:181–186

13. Aiello PD, Trautmann JC, McPhee TJ, et al. Visual prognosis in giant cell arteritis. Ophthalmology 1993; 100:550–555

14. Klein RG, Hunder GG, Stanson AW, Sheps SG. Large artery involvement in giant cell (temporal) arteritis. Ann Intern Med 1975;83:806–812

15. Caselli RJ, Hunder GG, Whisnant JP. Neurologic disease in biopsy-proven giant cell (temporal) arteritis. Neurology 1988;38:352–359

16. Poller DN, Van Wyk Q, Jeffrey MJ. The importance of skip lesions in temporal arteritis. J Clin Pathol 2000;53:137–139

17. Anonymous. Recommendations for the prevention and treatment of glucocorticoid-induced osteoporosis: 2001 update. American College of Rheumatology Ad Hoc Committee on Glucocorticoid-Induced Osteoporosis. [Review]. Arthritis Rheum 2001;44:1496–1503

18. Jover J, Hernandex-Garcia C, Morado I, et al. Combined treatment of giant-cell arteritis with methotrexate and prednisone, a randomized, double-blind, placebo-controlled trial. Ann Intern Med 2001;134:106–114

19. Hoffman GS, Cid M, Hellmann D, et al. A multicenter placebo-controlled study of methotrexate (MTX) in giant cell arteritis (GCA). Arthritis Rheum 2000;43:292

20. DeSilva M, Hazleman B. Azathioprine in giant cell arteritis/polymyalgia rheumatica: a double-blind study. Ann Rheum Dis 1986;45:136–138

21. de Vita S, Tavoni A, Jeracitano G, et al. Treatment of giant cell arteritis with cyclophosphamide. J Intern Med 1992;232:373–375

22. Schaufelberger C, Andersson R, Nordborg E. No addictive effect of cyclosporin A compared with glucocorticoid treatment alone in giant cell arteritis: results of an open, controlled, randomized study. Br J Rheumatol 1998;37:464–465

23. Wilke W, Hoffman G. Treatment of corticosteroid-resistant giant cell arteritis. Rheum Dis Clin North Am 1995;21:59–71

24. Kattah JC, Cupps T, Manz HJ, et al. Occipital artery biopsy: a diagnostic alternative in giant cell arteritis. Neurology 1991;41:949–950

25. Guillevin L, Le Thi Huong D, Godeau P, et al. Clinical findings and prognosis of polyarteritis nodosa and Churg–Strauss angiitis: a study in 165 patients. Br J Rheumatol 1988;27:258–264

26. Reichart MD, Bogousslavsky J, Janzer RC. Early lacunar strokes complicating polyarteritis nodosa: thrombotic microangiopathy. Neurology 2000;54: 883–889

27. Gayraud M, Guillevin L, le Toumelin P, et al. Long-term followup of polyarteritis nodosa, microscopic polyangiitis, and Churg–Strauss syndrome: analysis of four prospective trials including 278 patients. Arthritis Rheum 2001;44:666–675

28. Gayraud M, Guillevin L, Cohen P, et al. Treatment of good-prognosis polyarteritis nodosa and Churg–Strauss syndrome: comparison of steroids and oral or pulse cyclophosphamide in 25 patients. French Cooper-

ative Study Group for Vasculitides. Br J Rheumatol 1997;36:1290–1297

29. Sehgal M, Swanson JW, DeRemee RA, Colby TV. Neurologic manifestations of Churg–Strauss syndrome. Mayo Clin Proc 1995;70:337–341

30. Hattori N, Ichimura M, Nagamatsu M, et al. Clinicopathological features of Churg–Strauss syndrome-associated neuropathy. Brain 1999;122:427–439

31. Guillevin L, Lhote F, Gayraud M, et al. Prognostic factors in polyarteritis nodosa and Churg–Strauss syndrome. A prospective study in 342 patients. Medicine 1996;75:17–28

32. Hoffman GS, Kerr GS, Leavitt RY, et al. Wegener granulomatosis: an analysis of 158 patients. Ann Intern Med 1992;116:488–498

33. Hollander D, Manning RT. The use of alkylating agents in the treatment of Wegener's granulomatosis. Ann Intern Med 1967;67:393–398

34. Guillevin L, Cordier J, Lhote F, et al. A prospective, multicenter randomized trial comparing steroids and pulse cyclophosphamide versus steroids and oral cyclophosphamide in the treatment of generalized Wegener's granulomatosis. Arthritis Rheumat 1997;40:2187–2198

35. Hoffman G, Leavitt R, Fleisher T, et al. Treatment of Wegener's granulomatosis with intermittent high-dose intravenous cyclophosphamide. Am J Med 1990; 89:403–410

36. Sneller MC, Hoffman GS, Talar-Williams C, et al. An analysis of forty-two Wegener's granulomatosis patients treated with methotrexate and prednisone. Arthritis Rheum 1995;38:608–613

37. Langford C, Sneller M. Update on the diagnosis and treatment of Wegener's granulomatosis. Adv Intern Med 2001;46:177–206

38. Stone J, Uhlfelder M, Hellmann D, et al. Etanercept combined with conventional treatment in Wegener's granulomatosis: a six-month open-label trial to evaluate safety. Arthritis Rheum 2001;44:1149–1154

39. Lhote F, Cohen P, Genereau T, et al. Microscopic polyangiitis: clinical aspects and treatment. Ann Med Intern 1996;147:165–177

40. Shelhamer JH, Volkman DJ, Parrillo JE, et al. Takayasu's arteritis and its therapy. Ann Intern Med 1985;103:121–126

41. Hoffman GS, Leavitt RY, Kerr GS, et al. Treatment of glucocorticoid-resistant or relapsing Takayasu arteritis with methotrexate. Arthritis Rheum 1994;37:578–582

42. Anonymous. Case records of the Massachusetts General Hospital. Weekly clinicopathological exercises. Case 4—1995. A 26-year-old woman with recurrent angina after a triple-coronary-artery bypass graft. N Engl J Med 1995;332:380–386

43. Horigome H, Kamoda T, Matsui A. Treatment of glucocorticoid-dependent Takayasu's arteritis with cyclosporine. Med J Aust 1999;170:566

44. Kerr GS, Hallahan CW, Giordano J, et al. Takayasu arteritis. Ann Intern Med 1994;120:919–929

45. Lilic D, Carmichael AJ. Cutaneous vasculitis with partial C4 deficiency responsive to dapsone. Br J Dermatol 1997;137:476

46. Eiser AR, Signgh P, Shanies HM. Sustained dapsone-induced remission of hypocomplementemic urticarial vasculitis—a case report. Angiology 1997;48:1019–1022

47. Sais G, Vidaller A, Jucgla A, et al. Colchicine in the treatment of cutaneous leukocytoclastic vasculitis. Results of a prospective, randomized controlled trial. Arch Dermatol 1995;131:1399–1402

48. Callen JP. Colchicine is effective in controlling chronic cutaneous leukocytoclastic vasculitis. J Am Acad Dermatol 1985;13:193–200

49. Kidd D, Steuer A, Denman AM, Rudge P. Neurological complications in Behçet's syndrome. Brain 1999; 122:2183–2194

50. Chajek T, Fainaru M. Behçet's disease. Report of 41 cases and a review of the literature (Review). Medicine 1975;54:179–196

51. Akman-Demir G, Serdaroglu P, Tasci B. Clinical patterns of neurological involvement in Behçet's disease: evaluation of 200 patients. The Neuro-Behçet Study Group. Brain 1999;122:2171–2182

52. Boyvat A, Sisman-Solak C, Gurler A. Long-term effects of interferon alpha 2A treatment in Behçet's disease. Dermatology 2000;201:40–43

53. Sharquie KE. Suppression of Behçet's disease with dapsone. Br J Dermatol 1984;110:493–494

54. Convit J, Goihman-Yahr M, Rondon-Lugo AJ. Effectiveness of dapsone in Behçet's disease. Br J Dermatol 1984;111:629–630

55. Nussenblatt RB, Palestine AG, Chan CC, et al. Effectiveness of cyclosporin therapy for Behçet's disease. Arthritis Rheum 1985;28:671–679

56. Whitcup SM, Salvo EC, Nussenblatt RB. Combined cyclosporine and corticosteroid therapy for sight-threatening uveitis in Behçet's disease. Am J Ophthalmol 1994;118:39–45

57. Yazici H, Pazarli H, Barnes CG, et al. A controlled trial of azathioprine in Behçet's syndrome. N Engl J Med 1990;322:281–285

58. Hamuryudan V, Mat C, Saip S, et al. Thalidomide in the treatment of the mucocutaneous lesions of the Behçet syndrome. A randomized, double-blind, placebo-controlled trial. Ann Intern Med 1998; 128:443–450

59. Robertson LP, Hickling P. Treatment of recalcitrant orogenital ulceration of Behçet's syndrome with infliximab. Rheumatology (Oxford) 2001;40:473–474

60. Goossens P, Verburg R, Breedveld F. Remission of Behçet's syndrome with tumour necrosis factor alpha blocking therapy. Ann Rheum Dis 2001;60:637

61. Bacon PA, Carruthers DM. Vasculitis associated with connective tissue disorders. Rheum Dis Clin North Am 1995;21:1077–1096

62. Kim RC, Collins GH. The neuropathology of rheumatoid disease. Hum Pathol 1981;12:5–15

63. Ellis SG, Verity MA. Central nervous system involvement in systemic lupus erythematosus: a review of neuropathologic findings in 57 cases, 1955–1977. Semin Arthritis Rheum 1979;8:212–221

64. Vollmer TL, Guarnaccia J, Harrington W, et al. Idiopathic granulomatous angiitis of the central nervous system. Diagnostic challenges. Arch Neurol 1993; 50:925–930

65. Caccamo DV, Garci AJH, Ho KL. Isolated granulomatous angiitis of the spinal cord. Ann Neurol 1992; 32:580–582

66. Fountain NB, Eberhard DA. Primary angiitis of the central nervous system associated with cerebral amyloid angiopathy: report of two cases and review of the literature. Neurology 1996;46:190–197

67. Oliveira V, Pavos P, Costa A, Ducla-Soares J. Cerebrospinal fluid and therapy of isolated angiitis of the central nervous system. Stroke 1994;25:1693–1695

68. Woolfenden AR, Rong DC, Marks MP, et al. Angiographically defined primary angiitis of the CNS: is it really benign? Neurology 1998;51:183–188

69. Riemer G, Lamszus K, Zschaber R, et al. Isolated angiitis of the central nervous system: lack of inflammation after long-term treatment. Neurology 1999;52:196–199

70. McCallum RM, Haynes BF. Vasculitis: systemic necrotizing vasculitis. In: Lichtenstein L, Fauci A, eds. Current Therapy in Allergy, Immunology, and Rheumatology. 5th edn. Mosby: St Louis; 1996:241–260

132 Neurological Manifestations of Rheumatoid Arthritis

Monica L Piecyk and Peter H Schur

Rheumatoid arthritis (RA) is a chronic inflammatory disease characterized by peripheral joint inflammation that is usually symmetrical. Its etiology is unknown. The prevalence of RA is estimated at 0.3% to 1.5%, and women are affected more commonly than men.[1] Extra-articular manifestations occur in 10% to 20% of patients.[1,2] The skin, eyes, lungs, heart, and both the central and peripheral nervous systems may be involved. The pathophysiology of neurological involvement includes synovial inflammation, the formation of invasive rheumatoid synovial tissue or pannus, and vasculitis. Cervical myelopathy, compression neuropathies, sensory and motor neuropathies, and neuromuscular disorders can result.

Central nervous system

Cervical spine involvement

In patients with RA, cervical spine disease may result from bone, cartilage and ligament damage caused by invasive pannus. Thoracic, lumbar and sacral involvement is unusual. Synovial cysts can impinge upon the spinal cord at any level.[3]

Anatomy of the atlantoaxial region The anterior arch of the atlas (C1) is anterior to the odontoid process of the axis (C2). The odontoid is surrounded by two synovium-lined bursae. The transverse ligament of the atlas is posterior to the odontoid process and prevents posterior protrusion of the odontoid process into the spinal cord during neck flexion. The apical and alar ligaments attach the odontoid superiorly and superolaterally to the edge of the foramen magnum.

Pathology Damage to the transverse ligament or erosion or fracture of the odontoid process can lead to atlantoaxial subluxation (AAS). Atlantoaxial subluxation may be anterior, posterior, vertical and/or lateral. Destruction of the atlanto-occipital and lateral atlantoaxial facet joints and their associated ligaments also contributes to upper cervical neurological complications.[2,4,5]

Risk factors for cervical spine RA include male gender, long disease duration, erosive peripheral joint disease, joint instability, the presence of rheumatoid nodules, and a positive rheumatoid factor.[2,6–14] In one radiographic study of 100 consecutive RA patients followed for a mean of 9.5 years, the timing and severity of cervical subluxations coincided with the progression of peripheral erosive disease of the hands

and feet.[14,15] Some authors have suggested that steroid use increases risk,[4,16,17] although it is likely that patients with more severe disease are also those more likely to use steroids.

Symptoms and signs of cervical spine involvement[4,10,12,13,18–26] Radiological subluxation has been reported in 16% to 86% of patients with RA.[4,6,8,9,12,14,15,24,26–30] It is a potentially life-threatening complication when spinal cord compression results. Patients are often asymptomatic, and the severity of radiological subluxation does not correlate well with the severity of neurological abnormalities.[12,13,26,31–33] In one series of 130 patients with radiological cervical subluxations, only 8% had neurological deficits.[26] In another series of 194 patients with radiological evidence for cervical subluxation, 10% had neurological evidence of upper cord compression over a 5.7-year period.[13] Neurological signs and symptoms may not develop even with large subluxations.[32]

In patients with radiological subluxations the earliest and most common symptoms are neck pain and stiffness, reported in 45% to 82% of patients.[32] Neck pain may be due to chronic synovitis and ligamentous inflammation of the cervical spine. Localized neck pain with radiation to the occiput can occur as a result of compression of the second cervical nerve roots.[10,12,25] Patients may have unpleasant sensations of instability, often described as "clunking."[4]

Neurological deficits are due to direct compression of neural tissue by bone or soft tissue, such as pannus.[10] Initial symptoms of cervical myelopathy include numbness and paresthesias in a stocking–glove distribution, which may be confused with peripheral neuropathy.[18,22] Dorsal column and spinothalamic tract involvement results in decreased light touch, vibratory and pain sensation, with decreased tactile discrimination and sparing of proprioception.[10,18,22,23] If the pyramidal tract is affected upper motor neuron symptoms and signs result, and include increased deep tendon reflexes and a Babinski sign.[18,22–25] Spasticity, extremity muscle atrophy and muscle weakness may occur. Late manifestations of cord compression include spastic paraparesis or quadriparesis, and bladder and bowel dysfunction.[25] L'hermitte's sign, which is a sudden electric-like sensation down the spine into the extremities associated with sudden head or neck movement, may also be seen. Previously asymptomatic patients may present acutely quadriplegic.[23]

Vertebrobasilar insufficiency may result when

cervical subluxation leads to torsion of the vertebral artery as it passes through the transverse process foramina of the cervical vertebrae.[18,24–26,31] This complication has been reported in 19% of patients in one series.[25] Symptoms can include dysarthria, diplopia, tinnitus, vertigo, dizziness, nystagmus, ataxia, incoordination and syncope. Compression, stretching or thrombosis of the anterior spinal arteries may affect the anterior horn and result in lower motor neuron signs, including weakness, atrophy and decreased deep tendon reflexes.[18]

Ranawat et al.[34] devised the following grading system for neurological deficits: class 1 = no neurological deficit, class 2 = subjective weakness with hyperreflexia and dysesthesia, and class 3 = objective findings of weakness and long tract signs, a = ambulatory, b = non-ambulatory.

Neuropathology In an autopsy study of nine patients with severe long-standing seropositive RA, clinical myelopathy and craniocervical compression, cranial nerve and brainstem pathology was rare.[35] Findings included craniocervical compression with fragmentation and necrosis of the spinal cord and widespread subaxial changes in the spinal cord, including edema and axonal disruption most severe in the dorsal white matter. There was no evidence for vasculitis or ischemic changes. The authors concluded that myelopathy in RA is probably due to the effects of compression, stretch and movement of the spinal cord, rather than to ischemia.

In another description of two autopsy cases of RA patients with cervical myelopathy, abnormalities were most severe in the central gray matter and adjacent posterior and lateral columns.[25] The authors postulated that direct pressure caused intermittent compression and narrowing of the distal transverse branches of the anterior spinal artery.

Types of subluxation

Anterior atlantoaxial subluxation (AAS) This is the most common type of cervical subluxation in patients with RA.[4,10,28,32] Anterior AAS is reported in 9.5% to 36% of RA patients[6,12,15,17,26,32] and represents 65% of all subluxations.[19] As a result of transverse ligament laxity and/or odontoid process erosion or fracture, the atlas moves anterior to the axis (i.e. the odontoid process migrates posteriorly away from the anterior arch of the atlas). More severe subluxation may occur if the apical and alar ligaments are also involved.[18]

Viewed on lateral flexion films of the neck, anterior AAS is defined as a distance between the posterior–inferior aspect of the anterior arch of the atlas and the most anterior point of the odontoid process greater than 2.5 mm in females and greater than 3.0 mm in males.[4,29,36] The subluxation may be reduced in extension or may be fixed.[10] Anterior subluxation greater than 10–12 mm implies loss of the functional integrity of the transverse, alar and apical ligaments.[4]

Many patients with anterior AAS are asymptomatic. Smith et al.[26] reported that 13% of 150 RA

patients with anterior AAS had signs of brainstem or spinal cord involvement. Severe subluxations without neurological sequelae have been seen.[6,13,14,26,32] According to one study of 194 patients with radiographic evidence for subluxation, the risk for cervical spinal cord compression due to anterior AAS may be increased in males, with anterior subluxation greater than 9 mm, with the coexistence of vertical subluxation, and with the presence of lateral AAS.[13]

Posterior atlantoaxial subluxation In this type of subluxation, the posterior border of the anterior arch of C1 is positioned posterior to the anterior aspect of the body of the axis. This may occur when the odontoid is eroded or fractured.[2,37] Posterior AAS accounts for less than 10% of all cervical subluxations.[13,19] It is rarely associated with symptoms of cervical myelopathy.[10]

Vertical atlantoaxial subluxation This also has been called basilar invagination or impression, atlantoaxial impaction, downward or inferior subluxation, cranial settling, and upward migration or dislocation of the odontoid.[2,13,15,16,23,26] The cranium settles down on the odontoid. Destruction of the cartilage and osseous structures in the region of the atlanto-occipital or lateral atlantoaxial facet joints is required for this to occur.[10,28,38] Lateral mass collapse of the axis can worsen vertical subluxations.[11] The prevalence of vertical subluxation in RA patients is 3% to 8%,[15–17] and it correlates with longer disease duration and severe peripheral joint disease.[16,26] It is seen in 20% to 22% of patients with subluxations, and may occur in patients who also have anterior AAS.[13,19]

The odontoid may be displaced upwards and backwards into the foramen magnum, resulting in compression of the lower brainstem.[28] Cranial nerves V, IX, X and XII may be affected, causing facial numbness, depressed corneal reflexes, dysphagia and dysphonia.[10,16,23,39]

The most recently proposed method for screening and grading vertical AAS is the Sakaguchi–Kauppi[40] method. Cranial settling is determined by the presence of superior migration of the superior aspect of the body of the axis beyond a line drawn between the most inferior point of the anterior and posterior arches of the atlas. Using another method, McGregor's line is drawn from the hard palate to the occiput on a lateral radiograph.[4] Atlantoaxial impaction is present when the tip of the odontoid is 8 mm (men) or 9.7 mm (women) above McGregor's line.[13] Vertical subluxation can incorrectly give the impression of improving anterior AAS on cervical radiographs.[10,13,17,32]

Lateral atlantoaxial subluxation Atlantoaxial facet joint disease leads to lateral displacement of the lateral masses of the atlas.[21] Rotary subluxation of the atlas on the axis may coexist. Lateral AAS may be seen in up to 20% of subluxations[19,41] and may coexist with anterior subluxations.[13] In one study of 650 RA patients,[41] lateral atlantoaxial facet joint involvement was seen in 9%, lateral AAS in 3%, and lateral mass collapse in 4%. Patients with atlantoaxial lateral joint involvement tend to be younger, female and seropositive, and to have a longer disease duration, erosions and nodules.[41]

Radiographic evaluation is done with anteroposterior open-mouthed views and is abnormal if the lateral masses of C1 are 2 mm or more lateral to the lateral masses of C2.[13]

Non-reducible rotational head tilt deformity is another entity caused by changes in the atlantoaxial facet joints.[10,21]

Subaxial cervical spine disease   In the cervical spine, the facet joints help to maintain horizontal stability. The anterior longitudinal ligament stabilizes the spine during extension, and the posterior longitudinal ligament stabilizes the spine during flexion. Longitudinal ligaments, vertebral endplates, facet joints and intervertebral discs may be damaged in patients with RA, resulting in subaxial subluxation, spondylodiscitis and facet joint changes.[2,10] When subluxation occurs below C2, involvement of multiple levels is more common than subluxation at a single level.[2] Cervical nerve roots may be affected.[10] Subaxial subluxations are reported in 7% to 36% of RA patients.[6,8,15,19,30,32,42] Reports on whether there is any correlation with long disease duration are conflicting.[26,42] Vertebral endplate erosions with intervertebral disc narrowing, typically at C2–C3 and C3–C4, are characteristic of cervical spine RA, reported in 14% to 29% of patients,[6,8,18,30] and may occur without subaxial subluxation.

Flexion and extension lateral radiographs are used to visualize horizontal dislocations of vertebral bodies. Displacements between adjacent vertebral bodies of more than 1 mm or more than 15% of the anteroposterior vertebral diameter are consistent with subaxial subluxation. A staircase or stepladder deformity results when subluxations occur at multiple levels.[15,26,28]

Radiographic evaluation

In addition to plain radiographs already described, CT scan, myelography, CT myelography, MRI and somatosensory evoked potentials are also used to evaluate the cervical spine in patients with rheumatoid arthritis. Myelography and CT myelography can determine the presence of medullary and spinal cord compressions.[43,44] On CT scan, transverse ligament attenuation, pannus and bony impingement of the spinal cord may be seen.[45] In one study of patients with anterior AAS, the presence of cord compressions as suggested by loss of posterior subarachnoid space on CT correlated better with neurological signs and symptoms than did abnormalities on plain radiographs.[46] Somatosensory evoked potentials help to identify spinal cord dysfunction and differentiate brachial plexus and cervical root lesions from central nervous system lesions.[47,48]

MRI is the preferred method to examine the cervical spine in patients with RA. In a study by Breedveld et al.,[49] all patients with at least two objective signs of

cervical myelopathy had cord distortion on MRI. No correlation was found between the degree of vertebral dislocation on plain films and the presence of cord distortion on MRI. In another group of RA patients, all those with neurological symptoms had cord or brainstem abnormalities on MRI.[50] In another study, MRI more accurately assessed cord compression than did myelography or CT myelography.[44]

Treatment of cervical spine disease

Conservative management is recommended in the absence of signs of cord compression or progressive neurological deficits. For head and neck pain and limitation of cervical motion, pain medications and physical therapy may be helpful. Gentle neck stretching, range of motion and isometric exercises, heat, and transcutaneous electrical nerve stimulation have been used.[51] There is no evidence that cervical collars prevent neurological progression.[4,26,32,51,52] However, they may give patients a sense of protection, neck stability and warmth. Rigid collars should not be used, as they prevent extension of the neck and may worsen anterior AAS.[52]

Endotracheal intubation, whiplash and minor injuries can be devastating for these patients. It is generally recommended that after a fracture of the odontoid has been ruled out, patients with advanced RA should undergo flexion radiographs of the cervical spine prior to general anesthesia.[31,53]

Indications for surgery include cervical myelopathy or worsening neurological signs.[4,11,20,22,23,25,34,54–57] Possible indications include intractable head and neck pain, asymptomatic cord compression, and prophylaxis for severe subluxations. It is difficult to know which patients should undergo prophylactic surgery, as the correlation between neurological symptoms and the amount of subluxation on plain radiographs is poor. Numerous surgical techniques have been reported.[11,23,25,34,39,54,56] The most common are posterior fusion by internal fixation of C1–C2 for anterior AAS; occiput–C2 fusion, sometimes with transpharyngeal resection of the odontoid process for vertical subluxations; and posterior fusion of the involved cervical vertebrae for subaxial subluxations.[2,34] Cervical cord decompression is sometimes necessary. Postoperative mortality is less than 10%.[2,11,34,57] Following surgery, most patients report decreased pain, and there is neurological stabilization or improvement in the majority.[19,34,54,58] Those who do not improve or worsen tend to have more severe preoperative neurological deficits. Patients may also be at risk for additional subluxation at another location in the cervical spine.[54]

Examples of surgical outcomes include the following:

- Eighteen operatively treated (atlantoaxial fusion or occipitocervical fusion) and 14 non-operatively treated RA patients with various types of cervical subluxation were followed for a mean of 2.2 years.[11] Occipital pain improved in most of the operatively treated patients and did not in most of the non-operative group. In the operative patients neurological function was unchanged or improved, whereas neurological function worsened slightly in the conservatively treated patients.

- Marks et al.[22] followed 31 RA patients with cervical myelopathy; 20 were treated conservatively, and 60% died within 6 months. Eleven patients underwent surgery, and 27% died within 6 months.
- Twenty-eight RA patients who underwent cervical spine stabilization surgery were followed for a mean of 30 months.[58] Of 14 patients with preoperative neurological impairment, nine were unchanged, four improved and one deteriorated; 76% of patients reported an improvement in pain.
- Thirty-one patients with cervical myelopathy were followed for 3 years;[25] 37% of 19 medically treated patients progressed neurologically or died, and 17% of 12 surgically treated patients developed worsening myelopathy.
- Seventy-three patients with RA involvement of the cervical spine were followed for at least two years, with an average follow-up of seven years:[59] 58% developed neurological deficits. The posterior atlanto-odontoid interval and the diameter of the subaxial saggital canal measured on cervical radiography correlated with the presence and severity of paralysis. All patients with a class 3 neurological deficit had a posterior atlanto-odontoid interval of the subaxial canal less than 14 mm. Of the patients with neurological deficits, 83% had operative stabilization, whereas those who refused or were unable to have surgery were treated with a soft cervical collar. All of the non-operative patients developed worsening paralysis, whereas 71% of the surgically treated patients improved. The prognosis for neurological recovery following operation was influenced by the severity of paralysis at the time of operation and not by the duration of paralysis.

These studies suggest that RA patients with signs of cervical myelopathy who do not undergo surgical stabilization have a higher rate of neurological worsening and a higher mortality rate. However, these are not randomized controlled trials but rather case descriptions, which may be influenced by selection bias.

Prognosis of cervical spine disease

- Smith et al.[26] followed 84 patients with anterior AAS without brainstem or cord compression. Over a period of 5–14 years, 25% worsened, 25% improved, and 50% remained unchanged by radiographic criteria; 5% developed cord involvement.
- In a prospective study of 100 patients with early RA followed for 7 years, 36% developed anterior or subaxial subluxations but none developed neurological signs.[15]
- In a six year follow-up study of 171 patients, 32% of 38 patients with baseline anterior AAS had worsening on radiographs.[8] In 41 patients, a new diagnosis of anterior AAS was made. None of the patients had evidence for new or worsening nervous system involvement.

- In one five-year follow-up study of patients with RA, one-third of patients with anteroposterior and half of those with vertical subluxation had long tract signs.[17]
- One hundred and six patients with RA were followed for five years:[32] 43% had radiographic evidence of cervical subluxations at the start of the study. At five years, 70% of patients had radiographic cervical subluxations. Of these patients, there was radiographic progression in 80% and neurological deterioration in 36%; 9% of those with radiographic involvement required surgical stabilization.

These studies suggest that radiographic progression of cervical spine disease in RA is common but does not necessarily correlate with an increased rate of neurological deterioration.

The overall five-year mortality rate of patients with radiographic evidence of cervical subluxation, with or without neurological symptoms, is reported to be 17%.[2,19] This is similar to the rate in patients with severe RA without cervical involvement, but higher than that in the cohort healthy population.[32] Other authors agree that the presence of cervical spine involvement does correlate with increased mortality.[8,17,26] Although deaths due to spinal cord compression have been reported,[13,22,25,59] death is usually due to non-neurological causes.[8,17,26]

Central nervous system vasculitis[24,36,60,61]

CNS vasculitis is rare in patients with RA. The literature consists of case reports of intracranial arteritis.[28,60–66] In one case,[61] the spinal cord also was affected. CNS lesions are infrequent in patients with systemic rheumatoid vasculitis.[61,67,68] Presenting manifestations of CNS vasculitis include seizures, dementia, cranial nerve palsies, strokes, encephalopathy, intracerebral or subarachnoid hemorrhage and myelopathy. Brain biopsy is the gold standard for diagnosis. Cerebral angiography and MRA may also be helpful but are less specific. In an attempt to evaluate RA patients for signs of CNS vasculitis, 33 randomly selected patients underwent cerebral MRI.[69] There was no significant difference in the degree of atrophy or in the number of hyperintense white matter lesions between RA patients and controls. Treatment of CNS vasculitis in RA patients is identical to that of isolated CNS vasculitis, and includes the use of high-dose corticosteroids, cyclophosphamide and other immunosuppressive medications.

Rheumatoid nodules

Rheumatoid nodules have rarely been reported in the central nervous system. Extradural nodules in the spinal canal can cause nerve root compression, spinal cord compression and spinal stenosis.[70,71] Rheumatoid nodules of the cerebral leptomeninges have also been described.[65,72–74] A rheumatoid nodule within the choroid plexus was reported in one patient.[75] Most patients with central nervous system nodules have severe erosive joint disease, extra-articular features and high-titer rheumatoid factors.[70,73,75]

Organic brain syndrome

Organic brain syndrome (OBS), with manifestations including confusion, memory loss and seizures, was described in six RA patients on no or low doses of steroids.[76] It is unknown whether the OBS was due to RA itself. Four of the patients were treated with high-dose steroid therapy. All six patients, including those who were observed without therapy, improved within one week.

Progressive multifocal leukoencephalopathy

This has been reported in at least two patients with RA.[24]

Peripheral nervous system

Compression or entrapment neuropathy

Entrapment neuropathies are diagnosed in more than 45% of patients with severe peripheral disease and subcutaneous nodules at some time in the course of their disease.[77] Inflamed synovia, ligaments or tendon sheaths may compress peripheral nerves that are in close proximity to joints or bursae. Joint deformities also can cause increased pressure on peripheral nerves. In patients with rheumatoid arthritis there is no correlation between compression neuropathies and gender, duration of RA, functional class, the presence of other extra-articular disease, seropositivity, or the level of acute-phase reactants.[78]

Carpal tunnel syndrome (CTS)

This is the most common compression neuropathy associated with RA, occurring in 23% to 69% of patients.[78–81] It is possibly the most common neurological manifestation of RA, and may occur at any time during the disease.[28,31,77,82] In a study by Barnes et al.,[79] 33% of RA patients had both clinical and electrophysiological evidence for CTS, 20% had only clinical evidence, and 16% had electrophysiological abnormalities only. In another study of 72 patients with RA for less than 1 year,[80] 23% had clinical evidence for CTS. Most of these patients also had soft tissue swelling and limitation of movement. Only one of 36 patients who underwent electrodiagnostic testing had characteristic findings of CTS. Another group compared 45 randomly selected patients with seropositive RA against 20 control patients with non-inflammatory arthritic conditions not affecting the neck or upper limbs.[79] In the RA group there was no significant correlation between the duration of RA and the incidence of electrodiagnostic abnormalities. In the RA group, 69% of the patients had clinical or electrodiagnostic evidence for CTS (20% had clinical evidence only, and 15% had electrodiagnostic evidence only). CTS was bilateral in 31%. Twenty percent of controls had clinical and/or electrodiagnostic evidence for CTS.

Anatomy[77]   The transverse carpal ligament forms the anterior border and the carpal bones form the posterior border of the carpal tunnel. Compression of the median nerve within the carpal tunnel results in CTS. The likely cause of CTS in patients with RA is finger flexor tenosynovitis, as these tendons also pass through the carpal tunnel.

Signs and symptoms[77]   Sensory changes occur early, whereas motor involvement occurs late. Nocturnal numbness and paresthesias in the first to the third and half of the ring finger is common. Motor manifestations include atrophy of the radial aspect of the thenar muscles and weak thumb opposition. Bilateral involvement is frequent. A positive Tinel's sign elicits symptoms with percussion of the median nerve over the volar aspect of the wrist. A positive Phalen's sign elicits symptoms with complete flexion of the wrist for at least one minute.

The differential diagnosis for CTS includes C6 or C7 radiculopathy and thoracic outlet syndrome. In addition to RA, the differential diagnosis for etiologies of CTS includes hypothyroidism, amyloidosis, acromegaly, gout, sarcoidosis, pregnancy, and repetitive hand movement.[2]

Sensory nerve conduction studies are the most accurate method of diagnosis[2] and are abnormal in more than 85% of patients with CTS. Because motor fibers are smaller in diameter than sensory fibers compression damage occurs more slowly, and motor nerve conduction studies are less sensitive in mild carpal tunnel syndrome. Electromyography is even less helpful, being abnormal in only 40% to 45% of patients with carpal tunnel syndrome.

Tarsal tunnel syndrome[2,36,77,83–85]

Tarsal tunnel syndrome is less common than CTS in RA patients. Five percent to 25% of RA patients have electrophysiological abnormalities characteristic of tarsal tunnel syndrome, although not all of these patients are symptomatic.[83–85]

Anatomy[84]   The posterior tibial nerve courses through the tarsal tunnel, which is formed by the medial malleolus and the flexor retinaculum of the medial foot and ankle. Compression of the posterior tibial nerve within the tarsal tunnel results in tarsal tunnel syndrome. It may result from tenosynovitis, inflammation of the flexor retinaculum, valgus deformities, adjacent bone fracture or dislocation, or post-traumatic edema and fibrosis.

Signs and symptoms[84]   These include paresthesias, burning, and pain in the soles and first to third toes. These symptoms may initially be intermittent. Symptoms may be worse with tight-fitting shoes, with activity, or at night. Late signs include atrophy and weakness of the intrinsic foot muscles. As in CTS, sensory nerve conduction studies are helpful in the diagnosis.

Other compression neuropathies

These rarely occur in patients with RA.[2,31,36,77,82,86,87]

- The *anterior interosseous nerve* is a motor branch of the median nerve. Compression results in forearm pain and second- and third-finger flexion weakness.

- The *posterior interosseous nerve* is a branch of the radial nerve. Compression at the elbow results in decreased ability to extend the MCP joints.
- *Ulnar nerve* compression at the elbow results in sensory loss at the ulnar surface of the hand and inner half of the fourth fingers, and weak abduction of the wrist, adduction of the thumb, abduction and opposition of the fifth finger, and abduction and adduction of the fingers.
- *Ulnar nerve* compression at the wrist results in the above without sensory loss in the dorsal hand or loss of wrist abduction and fourth and fifth finger flexion.
- The *common peroneal nerve* may be injured by a popliteal cyst or by a cast or brace. This palsy also is described in RA patients following total knee arthroplasty.[88] Compression results in sensory deficits in the lateral leg, dorsal foot, and web interspace of the first and second toes, and weak toe extension, dorsiflexion and eversion of the foot.
- The *tibial nerve* may be injured by a popliteal cyst and results in sensory loss in the soles, heels and posterolateral calf, and decreased toe flexion and foot plantar flexion and inversion.

An entrapment neuropathy and symptomatic cervical spine disease with nerve root compression may present concurrently. This is termed the "double crush" syndrome.[77]

Treatment of compression neuropathies[84,87] Non-surgical management involves treatment of the underlying disease process. Additional modalities include splints, anti-inflammatory medications and local corticosteroid injections. Surgical decompression is indicated if motor deficits or denervation are present, or if sensory symptoms worsen despite adequate non-surgical therapy.

A *distal sensory neuropathy or a sensorimotor neuropathy* occurs in 1% to 18% of RA patients.[81] The former is more common. Vasculopathy and vasculitis have been implicated in the pathogenesis of these neuropathies.[67,82,86,89–91]

Distal sensory neuropathy

Symptoms and signs The development of symptoms is insidious. Symmetrical paresthesias and burning sensations tend to be worse in the feet than in the hands.[82,89,92] These symptoms may be difficult to distinguish from arthritic symptoms.[82,89] Vibratory, pinprick and light touch sensation is decreased, but proprioception is spared. Reflexes may be lost.[89] Both sensory and motor nerve conduction studies may be abnormal.[89,91]

Pathology Sural nerve biopsy demonstrates mild proliferative endarteritis, or normal vasculature with segmental demyelination and remyelination with areas of axonal degeneration.[90,91] There is mild loss of predominantly large myelinated fibers.[31,89] The yield of biopsy may be low, given the mild pathological changes and patchy distribution of lesions.

In one study of 25 patients,[89] neuropathy usually developed after the arthritis, and there was no relation between the time of onset of arthritis and neuropathy. In most patients the severity of neuropathy was not altered with steroid therapy; 75% of patients recovered partially or completely. Overall, distal sensory neuropathy has a good prognosis, and it is uncommon for patients to progress to a more severe neuropathy.[30,86]

Combined sensorimotor neuropathy

This neuropathy is associated with long duration of seropositive nodular RA, male gender, other extra-articular involvement, systemic constitutional symptoms and other signs of vasculitis, including palpable purpura, livedo reticularis, skin ulcerations, nailfold and digital infarcts, and Raynaud's phenomenon.[24,67,82,86,89,91–83] High rheumatoid factor titers, a polyclonal increase in immunoglobulins and low complement levels also are more common in these patients.

Symptoms and signs This neuropathy is more severe and presents more acutely than distal sensory neuropathy. Symptoms include severe asymmetrical pain and paresthesias.[89] Weakness may develop within hours to days of the initial onset of symptoms. Wrist and foot drops are most common.[89] Deep tendon reflexes are decreased or absent.[82,89] Mononeuritis multiplex or a polyneuropathy can be seen.[82,89] Electrophysiological studies demonstrate axonal degeneration or severe demyelination.[89,91]

Pathology Arterial pathology of involved peripheral nerves includes fibrinoid necrosis of the media, with infiltration by polymorphonuclear leukocytes, eosinophils and mononuclear cells. Perivascular infiltration with mononuclear cells, intimal proliferation with minimal cellular infiltrates, and/or fibrosis also can be seen.[91] Vasculitis of the epineural arteries results in vessel ischemia, with resulting axonal degeneration and neuronal demyelination.[2,91] The arteritis may be immune complex mediated. Sural nerve examination has demonstrated IgG, IgM, complement and fibrin depositions in areas of acute necrotizing arteritis, whereas such deposits are usually absent in vessels without acute inflammation.[92]

Treatment There is no standard regimen. Patients are treated as for any type of immune complex-mediated necrotizing vasculitis.[2] Both corticosteroids and cyclophosphamide, in oral doses and intravenous pulses, have been used. There is no convincing evidence that steroids are helpful.[82,89] Antimalarials and gold have not altered the course of disease.[89] Plasmapheresis also has been used in refractory cases, without great success.[93]

This neuropathy has a poor prognosis, with most patients worsening progressively.[24,86,89] Death may result from visceral disease or immunosuppressive therapy-related infections.[82,89] Most individuals who do improve have residual sensory and motor deficits.

Autonomic neuropathy

An increased incidence of autonomic neuropathy was suggested by abnormal cardiovascular reflexes in RA patients in one study.[94]

Neuromuscular disorders

In one series of 220 RA patients,[95] muscle weakness and/or atrophy were seen in one-third of cases. Neuromuscular disorders in patients with RA have been divided into the following categories:

- *Disuse atrophy* due to pain from synovitis. Muscle biopsy reveals type 2 fiber atrophy.[95–97] There is a lack of muscle inflammation, necrosis, regeneration or vasculitis.[90]
- *Denervation atrophy* Motor nerve demyelination and degeneration due to angiopathic neuropathy, such as mononeuritis multiplex, can lead to muscle fiber atrophy, necrosis and regeneration, with minimal muscle inflammation.[90,95]
- Myopathy clinically and pathologically *similar to progressive muscular dystrophy*. There is loss of muscle tissue, replacement by adipose tissue, fiber caliber variations, and fibrosis without inflammatory infiltrates.[90] Motor innervation is not disturbed. This may represent late chronic myositis.
- *Myositis* Myofiber necrosis and regeneration are seen. There is focal or diffuse infiltration of lymphocytes, plasma cells and mononuclear cells into endomysium, perimysium and perivascular areas.[90,95,96,98] It may be impossible to distinguish this from idiopathic polymyositis, and it may represent an overlap syndrome between RA and polymyositis.[28,90,95] One author has suggested that the pathological abnormalities in rheumatoid myositis are less severe and more patchy than those of polymyositis, and that RA patients tend to clinically respond to lower prednisone doses than do polymyositis patients.[96] In this study, rheumatoid myositis also was associated with elevated creatine phosphokinase, reflecting muscle fiber damage, and with disproportionately elevated erythrocyte sedimentation rates for the mild degree of synovitis.
- *Steroid myopathy*[90,97,99] Characterized by proximal muscle weakness without significant muscle enzyme elevations. Muscle biopsy reveals type 2 muscle fiber atrophy.

There is a case report of a patient with RA and a left inferior oblique muscle palsy, or *Brown's syndrome*, presumably secondary to tenosynovitis of this muscle's tendon sheath.[100] This deficit resolved with steroid therapy.

Amyloid

RA may rarely be complicated by secondary amyloidosis, which may result in abnormalities in both the central and peripheral nervous systems.[28,101] Amyloid deposits have been reported in brain arterioles in four patients with RA and CNS vasculitis.[60,63] Peripheral neuropathy also can result from secondary amyloidosis.[28]

Medications

Medications are another major cause of neurological complications in RA patients.[101] Non-steroidal anti-inflammatory drugs (NSAIDs) can cause headaches, drowsiness and aseptic meningitis. Steroids can cause myopathy, depression, psychosis and benign intracranial hypertension. Antimalarials, such as hydroxychloroquine, can cause dizziness, headache, tinnitus, seizures and neuromyopathy. Gold therapy can be complicated by peripheral neuropathy, cranial nerve palsies and Guillain–Barré syndrome.

References

1. Klippel JH, ed. Primer on the Rheumatic Diseases. 11th edn. Atlanta: Arthritis Foundation, 1997
2. Chang DJ, Paget SA. Neurologic complications of rheumatoid arthritis. Rheum Dis Clin North Am 1993;19:955–973
3. Jacob JR, Weisman MH, Mink JH, et al. Reversible cause of back pain and sciatica in rheumatoid arthritis: an apophyseal joint cyst. Arthritis Rheum 1986;29:431
4. Bland JH. Rheumatoid subluxation of the cervical spine. J Rheumatol 1990;17:134–137
5. Martel W. Pathogenesis of cervical discovertebral destruction in rheumatoid arthritis. Arthritis Rheum 1977;20:1217–1225
6. Conlon PW, Isdale IC, Rose BS. Rheumatoid arthritis of the cervical spine: an analysis of 333 cases. Ann Rheum Dis 1966;25:120–126
7. Fujiwara K, Fujimoto M, Owaki H, et al. Cervical lesions related to the systemic progression in rheumatoid arthritis. Spine 1998;23:2052–2056
8. Isdale IC, Conlon PW. Atlanto-axial subluxation: a six-year follow-up report. Ann Rheum Dis 1971;30:387–389
9. Paimela L, Laasonen L, Kankaanpaa E, et al. Progression of cervical spine changes in patients with early rheumatoid arthritis. J Rheumatol 1997;24:1280–1284
10. Santavirta S, Kankaanpaa U, Sandelin J, et al. Evaluation of patients with rheumatoid cervical spine. Scand J Rheumatol 1987;16:9–16
11. Santavirta S, Slatis P, Kankaanpaa U, et al. Treatment of the cervical spine in rheumatoid arthritis. J Bone Joint Surg [Am] 1988;70:658–667
12. Stevens JC, Cartlidge NE, Saunders M, et al. Atlanto-axial subluxation and cervical myelopathy in rheumatoid arthritis. Q J Med 1971;40:391–408
13. Weissman BN, Aliabadi P, Weinfeld MS, et al. Prognostic features of atlantoaxial subluxation in rheumatoid arthritis patients. Radiology 1982;144:745–751
14. Winfield J, Young A, Williams P, et al. Prospective study of the radiological changes in hands, feet, and cervical spine in adult rheumatoid disease. Ann Rheum Dis 1983;42:613–618
15. Winfield J, Cooke D, Brook AS, et al. A prospective study of the radiological changes in the cervical spine in early rheumatoid disease. Ann Rheum Dis 1981;40:109–114
16. Henderson DR. Vertical atlanto-axial subluxation in rheumatoid arthritis. Rheumatol Rehab 1972;14:31–38
17. Mathews JA. Atlanto-axial subluxation in rheumatoid arthritis. A 5-year follow-up study. Ann Rheum Dis 1974;33:526–531
18. Bland JH. Rheumatoid arthritis of the cervical spine. J Rheumatol 1974;1:319–342
19. Boden SD. Rheumatoid arthritis of the cervical spine.

Surgical decision making based on predictors of paralysis and recovery. Spine 1994;19:2275–2280

20. Gurley JP, Bell GR. The surgical management of patients with rheumatoid cervical spine disease. Rheum Dis Clin North Am 1997;23:317–332

21. Halla JT, Fallahi S, Hardin JG. Nonreducible rotational head tilt and lateral mass collapse: A prospective study of frequency, radiographic findings, and clinical features in patients with rheumatoid arthritis. Arthritis Rheum 1982;25:1316–1324

22. Marks JS, Sharp J. Rheumatoid cervical myelopathy. Q J Med 1981;50:307–319

23. Menezes AH, VanGilder JC, Clark CR, et al. Odontoid upward migration in rheumatoid arthritis. J Neurosurg 1985;63:500–509

24. Nakano KK. Neurologic complications of rheumatoid arthritis. Orthop Clin North Am 1975;6:861–880

25. Nakano KK, Schoene WC, Baker RA, et al. The cervical myelopathy associated with rheumatoid arthritis: analysis of 32 patients, with 2 postmortem cases. Ann Neurol 1978;3:144–151

26. Smith PH, Benn RT, Sharp J. Natural history of rheumatoid cervical luxations. Ann Rheum Dis 1972;31:431–439

27. Kauppi M, Hakala M. Prevalence of cervical spine subluxations and dislocations in a community-based rheumatoid arthritis population. Scand J Rheumatol 1994;23:133–136

28. Kim RC, Collins GH. The neuropathology of rheumatoid disease. Hum Pathol 1981;12:5–15

29. Martel W. The occipito-atlanto-axial joints in rheumatoid arthritis and ankylosing spondylitis. AJR Am J Roentgenol 1961;86:223–240

30. Meikle JA, Wilkinson M. Rheumatoid involvement of the cervical spine: Radiological assessment. Ann Rheum Dis 1971;30:154–161

31. Brick JE, Brick JF. Neurologic manifestations of rheumatologic disease. Neurol Clin 1989;7:629–639

32. Pellicci PM, Ranawat CS, Tsairis P, et al. A prospective study of the progression of rheumatoid arthritis in the cervical spine. J Bone Joint Surg [Am] 1981;63:342–350

33. Reijnierse M, Bloem JL, Dijkmans BA, et al. The cervical spine in rheumatoid arthritis: relationship between neurologic signs and morphology of MR imaging and radiographs. Skeletal Radiol 1996;25:113–118

34. Ranawat CS, O'Leary P, Pellicci PM, et al. Cervical spine fusion in rheumatoid arthritis. J Bone Joint Surg [Am] 1979;61:1003–1010

35. Henderson FC, Geddes JF, Crockard HA. Neuropathology of the brainstem and spinal cord in end stage rheumatoid arthritis: implications for treatment. Ann Rheum Dis 1993;52:629–637

36. Hurd ER. Extraarticular manifestations of rheumatoid arthritis. Semin Arthritis Rheum 1979;8:151–176

37. Isdale IC, Corrigan AB. Backward luxation of the atlas: Two cases of an uncommon condition. Ann Rheum Dis 1970;29:6–9

38. Santavirta S, Hopfner-Hallikainen D, Paukku P, et al. Atlantoaxial facet joint arthritis in the rheumatoid cervical spine: a panoramic zonography study. J Rheumatol 1988;15:217–223

39. Davidson RC, Horn JR, Herndon JH, et al. Brain-stem compression in rheumatoid arthritis. JAMA 1977;238:2633–2634

40. Kauppi M, Sakaguchi M, Knottinen YT, et al. A new method of screening for vertical atlantoaxial dislocation. J Rheumatol 1990;17:167–172

41. Halla JT, Hardin JG. The spectrum of atlantoaxial facet joint involvement in rheumatoid arthritis. Arthritis Rheum 1990;33:325–329

42. Wolfe BK, O'Keefe D, Mitchell DM, et al. Rheumatoid arthritis of the cervical spine: early and progressive radiographic features. Radiology 1987;165:145–148

43. Laasonen EM, Kankaanpaa U, Paukku P, et al. Computed tomographic myelography in atlanto-axial rheumatoid arthritis. Neuroradiology 1985;27:119–122

44. Masaryk TJ, Modic MT, Geisinger MA, et al. Cervical myelopathy: a comparison of magnetic resonance and myelography. J Comput Assist Tomogr 1986;10:184–194

45. Braunstein EM, Weissman BN, Seltzer SE, et al. Computed tomography and conventional radiographs of craniocervical region in rheumatoid arthritis: a comparison. Arthritis Rheum 1984;27:26–31

46. Raskin RJ, Schnapf DJ, Wolf CR, et al. Computerized tomography in evaluation of atlantoaxial subluxation in rheumatoid arthritis. J Rheumatol 1983;10:33–41

47. Katz LM, Emsellem HA, Borenstein DG. Evaluation of cervical spine inflammatory arthritis with somatosensory potentials. J Rheumatol 1990;17:508–514

48. Toolanen G, Knibestol M, Larsson SE, et al. Somatosensory evoked potentials (SSEPs) in rheumatoid cervical subluxation. Scand J Rheumatol 1987;16:17–25

49. Breedveld FC, Algra PR, Veilvoye CJ, et al. Magnetic resonance imaging in the evaluation of patients with rheumatoid arthritis and subluxations of the cervical spine. Arthritis Rheum 1987;30:624–629

50. Aisen AM, Martel W, Ellis JH, et al. Cervical spine involvement in rheumatoid arthritis: MR imaging. Radiology 1987;165:159–163

51. Moncur C, Williams HJ. Cervical spine management in patients with rheumatoid arthritis. Phys Ther 1988;68:509–515

52. Althoff B, Goldie IF. Cervical collars in rheumatoid atlanto-axial subluxation: a radiographic comparison. Ann Rheum Dis 1980;39:485–489

53. Kwek TK, Lew TW, Thoo FL. The role of preoperative cervical spine X-rays in rheumatoid arthritis. Anaesth Intens Care 1998;26:636–641

54. Conaty JP, Mongan ES. Surgical fusion in rheumatoid arthritis. J Bone Joint Surg [Am] 1981;63:1218–1227

55. Floyd AS, Learmonth ID, Mody G, et al. Atlantoaxial instability and neurologic indicators in rheumatoid arthritis. Clin Orthop 1989;241:177–182

56. Heywood AW, Learmonth ID, Thomas M. Cervical spine instability in rheumatoid arthritis. J Bone Joint Surg [Br] 1988;70:702–707

57. Zygmunt SC, Christensson D, Saveland H, et al. Occipito-cervical fixation in rheumatoid arthritis—an analysis of surgical risk factors in 163 patients. Acta Neurochir (Wien) 1995;135:25–31

58. McRorie ER, McLoughlin P, Russell T, et al. Cervical spine surgery in patients with rheumatoid arthritis: an appraisal. Ann Rheum Dis 1996;55:99–104

59. Boden SD, Dodge LD, Bohlman HH, et al. Rheumatoid arthritis of the cervical spine. J Bone Joint Surg 1993;75:1282–1297

60. Mandybur TI. Cerebral amyloid angiopathy: possible relationship to rheumatoid vasculitis. Neurology 1979;29:1336–1340

61. Watson P, Fekete J, Deck J. Central nervous system vasculitis in rheumatoid arthritis. Can J Neurol Sci 1977;4:269–272

62. Beck DO, Corbett JJ. Seizures due to central nervous system rheumatoid meningovasculitis. Neurology 1983;33:1058–1061

63. Ramos M, Mandybur TI. Cerebral vasculitis in rheumatoid arthritis. Arch Neurol 1975;32:271–275
64. Singleton JD, West SG, Reddy VV, et al. Cerebral vasculitis complicating rheumatoid arthritis. South Med J 1995;88:470–474
65. Steiner JW, Gelbloom AJ. Intracranial manifestations in two cases of systemic rheumatoid disease. Arthritis Rheum 1959;2:537–545
66. Watson P. Intracranial hemorrhage with vasculitis in rheumatoid arthritis. Arch Neurol 1979;36:58
67. Scott DG, Bacon PA, Tribe CR. Systemic rheumatoid vasculitis: A clinical and laboratory study of 50 cases. Medicine (Baltimore) 1981;60:288–297
68. Sigal LH. The neurologic presentation of vasculitic and rheumatologic syndromes. A review. Medicine (Baltimore) 1987;66:157–180
69. Bekkelund SI, Pierre-Jerome C, Husby G, et al. Quantitative cerebral MR in rheumatoid arthritis. Am J Neuroradiol 1995;16:767–772
70. Friedman H. Intraspinal rheumatoid nodule causing nerve root compression: case report. J Neurosurg 1970;32:689–691
71. Hauge T, Magnaes B, Loken AC, et al. Treatment of rheumatoid pachymeningitis involving the entire thoracic region. Scand J Rheumatol 1978;7:209–211
72. Contin JU, Oka M. Unusual cardiac, pulmonary and meningeal involvement in rheumatoid arthritis. Report of a case. Dis Chest 1966;49:552–556
73. Jackson CG, Chess RL, Ward JR. A case of rheumatoid nodule formation within the central nervous system and review of the literature. J Rheumatol 1984;11:237–240
74. Sunter JP. Rheumatoid disease with involvement of the leptomeninges presenting as symptomatic epilepsy. Beitr Pathol 1977;161:194–202
75. Kim RC, Collins GH, Parisi JE. Rheumatoid nodule formation within the choroid plexus: report of a second case. Arch Pathol Lab Med 1982;106:83–84
76. Gupta VP, Ehrlich GE. Organic brain syndrome in rheumatoid arthritis following corticosteroid withdrawal. Arthritis Rheum 1976;19:1333–1338
77. Nakano KK. The entrapment neuropathies of rheumatoid arthritis. Orthop Clin North Am 1975;6:837–860
78. Herbison GJ, Teng C, Martin JH, et al. Carpal tunnel syndrome in rheumatoid arthritis. Am J Phys Med 1973;52:68–74
79. Barnes CG, Currey HL. Carpal tunnel syndrome in rheumatoid arthritis: a clinical and electrodiagnostic survey. Ann Rheum Dis 1967;26:226–233
80. Chamberlain MA, Corbett M. Carpal tunnel syndrome in early rheumatoid arthritis. Ann Rheum Dis 1970;29:149–152
81. Fleming A, Dodman S, Crown JM, et al. Extra-articular features in early rheumatoid disease. Br Med J 1976;1:1241–1243
82. Pallis CA, Scott JT. Peripheral neuropathy in rheumatoid arthritis. Br Med J 1965;1:1141–1147
83. Baylan SP, Paik SW, Barnert AL, et al. Prevalence of the tarsal tunnel syndrome in rheumatoid arthritis. Rheumatol Rehab 1981;20:148–150
84. Grabois M, Puentes J, Lidsky M. Tarsal tunnel syndrome in rheumatoid arthritis. Arch Phys Med Rehab 1981;62:401–403
85. McGuigan L, Burke D, Fleming A. Tarsal tunnel syndrome and peripheral neuropathy in rheumatoid disease. Ann Rheum Dis 1983;42:128–131
86. Ferguson RH, Slocumb CH. Peripheral neuropathy in rheumatoid arthritis. Bull Rheum Dis 1961;11:251
87. White SH, Goodfellow JW, Mowat A. Posterior interosseous nerve palsy in rheumatoid arthritis. J Bone Joint Surg [Br] 1988;70:468–471
88. Rose HA, Hood RW, Otis JC, et al. Peroneal-nerve palsy following total knee arthroplasty. A review of The Hospital for Special Surgery experience. J Bone Joint Surg [Am] 1982;64:347–351
89. Chamberlain MA, Bruckner FE. Rheumatoid neuropathy: clinical and electrophysiological features. Ann Rheum Dis 1970;29:609–616
90. Haslock DI, Wright V, Harriman DG. Neuromuscular disorders in rheumatoid arthritis: a motor-point muscle biopsy study. Q J Med 1970;39:335–358
91. Weller RO, Bruckner FE, Chamberlain MA. Rheumatoid neuropathy: a histological and electrophysiological study. J Neurol Neurosurg Psychiatry 1970;33:592–604
92. Conn DL, McDuffie FC, Dyck PJ. Immunopathologic study of sural nerves in rheumatoid arthritis. Arthritis Rheum 1972;15:135–143
93. Goldman JA, Casey HL, McIlwain H, et al. Limited plasmapheresis in rheumatoid arthritis with vasculitis. Arthritis Rheum 1979;22:1146–1150
94. Edmonds ME, Jones TC, Saunders WA. Autonomic neuropathy in rheumatoid arthritis. Br Med J 1979;2:173–175
95. Reza MJ, Verity MA. Neuromuscular manifestations of rheumatoid arthritis: a clinical and histomorphological analysis. Clin Rheum Dis 1977;3:565–588
96. Halla JT, Koopman WJ, Fallahi S, et al. Rheumatoid myositis: clinical and histologic features and possible pathogenesis. Arthritis Rheum 1984;27:737–743
97. Haslock DI, Harriman DF, Wright V. Neuromuscular disorders associated with rheumatoid arthritis. Ann Rheum Dis 1970;29:197
98. Wegelius O, Pasternack A, Kuhlback B. Muscular involvement in rheumatoid arthritis. Acta Rheumatol Scand 1969;15:257–261
99. Askari A, Bignos PJ, Moskowitz RW. Steroid myopathy in connective tissue disease. Am J Med 1976;61:485–492
100. Cooper C, Kirwan JR, McGill NW, et al. Brown's syndrome: an unusual ocular complication of rheumatoid arthritis. Ann Rheum Dis 1990;49:188–189
101. Klippel JH, Dieppe PA, eds. Rheumatology. 2nd edn. London: Mosby, 1998

133 Cervical Spondylosis, Ankylosing Spondylitis, and Lumbar Disk Disease

Michael Ronthal

Cervical spondylosis

The term "cervical spondylosis" is used to describe a degenerative disorder of the cervical spine with disk degeneration, secondary osteophyte formation from the vertebral bodies, hypertrophy of the facet joints and ligaments, and, sometimes, segmental instability or subluxation. Nerve roots or the spinal cord may be injured in the process. Cervical spondylosis is common: 50% of persons older than 50 years and 75% of those older than 65 years have radiological changes of spondylosis. Also, 40% of persons older than 50 years have some limitation of neck movement and 60% have neurological signs if examined carefully.[1] In spite of this, no prospective controlled trials of treatment have been published; thus, the treatment offered is based on the clinical experience of "what seems to work."[2]

Treatment is tailored to the symptoms and signs found at examination. The commonest *symptom* is pain due to radiculopathy and neck muscle spasm. The most frequent *signs* are those of nerve root involvement, although the most important signs are related to myelopathy.

Symptoms

Patients frequently complain of pain and stiffness in the neck. The pain radiates from the cervico-occipital region to the vertex, temporal, or bifrontal region. The headache that enures has the typical signature of "muscle contraction headache." The pain is constant and not throbbing and is variously described as squeezing, bursting, or exploding. It frequently is worse in the morning on awakening and may subside during the day. The neck pain, often called a "stiff neck," is aggravated by neck movements. When the nerve roots are involved, radicular pain develops. This typically presents as a diffuse brachalgia, and because cervical spondylosis has its maximal expression at level C5 to C7, the pain usually radiates down the outer aspect of the arm to the thumb or index finger (or both). The pain may be episodic and lancinating or continuous and aching. Brachalgia aggravated by neck movement more or less confirms the diagnosis of radiculopathy. There may be associated numbness, tingling, or other paresthesias.

Depending on the activity of the patient, he or she may complain of clumsiness of the hands or frank weakness, and because of the segmental lesion, elbow flexion or shoulder abduction is likely to be involved. If the spinal cord is involved, the patient may complain of difficulty walking, and there may be a distur-bance of bladder function. Thus, the patient may scuff his or her toes, trip, and have difficulty climbing a staircase. Frequency and urgency of micturition and urgency incontinence of urine are symptoms of dysfunction of bladder upper motor neurons.

Signs

The signs of cervical spondylosis relate to local examination of the neck and a search for neurological deficits. The latter implies careful examination for root signs, either motor or sensory, and a determination of whether spinal cord function is normal.

In cervical spondylosis, neck movement is always restricted and the best test of this is passive or active rotation of the head to the right and the left. Normal subjects can rotate the neck to the point that the chin almost approximates the point of the shoulder. Palpation of the posterior cervical muscles will demonstrate muscle spasm and tenderness.

In cervical spondylosis, the pattern of weakness in the upper limbs is myotomal (Table 133.1). Wasting and weakness of the small muscles of the hands are frequent. This does not necessarily represent lower cervical radiculopathy but may be a "false localizer." Sensory loss, if present, usually is most marked for pinprick and temperature sensations and follows a dermatomal distribution. The absence of a biceps or triceps reflex may help localize the level, but frequently the reflexes are unaffected and may even be increased symmetrically because of a combined upper and lower motor neuron problem.

Of more concern is the possibility of myelopathy. The motor signs may include spasticity and weakness of hip flexion, toe extension, perhaps foot dorsiflexion, and hamstring and thigh abduction. With hypertonia, ankle clonus, hyperreflexia, and extensor plantar responses may occur. Any combination of these can occur, and flexor plantar responses in the presence of hypertonia or weakness do not exclude myelopathy. The commonest sensory deficit is the loss of vibratory sense, and the level may be anywhere from the costal margin distally. At times, an isolated loss of proprioception in the toes is the only sign of myelopathy. If signs of myelopathy are found, the cervical spine should be examined with magnetic resonance imaging (MRI). Lateral radiographs of the cervical spine with flexion and extension show the presence or absence of subluxation; normally, at the extremes of flexion and extension, up to 3 mm of slip between vertebral bodies is acceptable.

Table 133.1   Cervical myotomes*

Segmental level	Muscle(s)	Action
C4	Supra- and infraspinatus	1st 10° of shoulder abduction
		Externally rotate arm
C5	Deltoid	Abducts shoulder
	Biceps/brachialis	Flexes elbow
C6/7	Triceps	Extends elbow
	Brachioradialis	Flexes elbow in half supination
C6	Extensor carpi radialis	Radial wrist extension
C7	Extensor digitorum	Extends fingers
C8	Flexor digitorum	Flexes fingers
T1	Interossei	Abducts fingers
	Abductor digiti V	Abducts little finger

*This table indicates the main radicular motor segmental innervation of the upper limb. Although not entirely anatomically correct, it is a good clinical guide for localization.

Treatment

For pain and stiffness in the neck, the patient should be instructed to sleep on a very firm and bulky feather pillow (Table 133.2). A warming pad applied to the neck relieves spasm and pain. Sleeping in a soft collar achieves the same goal, and the effect can be quite dramatic. Some patients cannot tolerate the collar but can sleep with a hand towel, rolled to the width of a cervical collar, draped around the neck and fastened with a large safety pin. The towel is soft, pliant, and molds itself around the neck in a comforting fashion, protecting the neck from excessive movement during sleep.

Some patients report pain relief from cervical traction,[3] but this may be idiosyncratic; systematic reviews have not demonstrated any benefit.[4] Traction is best applied as "over the door traction." The patient sits on one side of an open door with a head halter attached to a cord that passes over the door to a water bag. The bag is filled to a weight of 5 to 7 lb (never more). The patient can have 20- to 30-minute traction sessions whenever convenient.

Physical therapy provides temporary symptomatic benefit.[5] The therapist is requested to apply gentle massage to tense muscles and to use heat and ultrasound. However, at least one review of physical therapy treatment of patients who had neck pain but no neurological deficit concluded that none of the following physical treatments provided significant benefit: heat or cold, traction, electrotherapy (pulsing electromagnetic field or transcutaneous electrical nerve stimulation), biofeedback, spray and stretch, acupuncture, or laser.[6] Active exercises probably do not help much and are painful in the acute phase, and cervical manipulation has been mentioned only to condemn it. Chiropractic neck manipulation is a dangerous maneuver and occasionally can result in stroke and even death.[7,8]

The failure of the treatments listed above to produce a response suggests that drug therapy should be instituted. Muscle relaxants in combination with antidepressants are the mainstay of treatment. A good combination is diazepam, 2 mg 2 or 3 times daily, with paroxetine, 20 mg at night. Specific muscle relaxants such as metaxalone, 400 mg 3 times daily, are just as effective. The choice of antidepressant is made on the frequency of side effects at low doses. Anti-inflammatory agents are analgesic and provide symptomatic benefit, but whether they treat "inflammation" in the neck is debated.

Table 133.2   Management of neck complaint

No neurological signs, pain and stiffness only
  Sleep with head on hard pillow

If no response

Sleep in a collar
Use local heat, massage
Analgesic agent—acetaminophen, NSAID

If no response in 10–14 days

Add to the above
  Muscle relaxant—diazepam (2 mg 3 times daily)
  Antidepressant, tricyclic agent, or serotonin
    reuptake inhibitor

If still no response

Imaging study of cervical spine
Root signs only
  Same as above but start with collar
Spinal cord signs or bladder symptoms
  Imaging study—MRI (if contraindicated, CT)*
    If spinal cord compression, refer for neurosurgical
      opinion
    If no spinal cord compression, perform lumbar
      puncture

CT, computed tomography; MRI, magnetic resonance imaging; NSAID, nonsteroidal anti-inflammatory drug.
*Myelography is rarely indicated.

Surgery

Myelopathy is an indication for a neuroimaging study and possible decompressive surgery. A contributing cause of myelopathy is a congenitally narrow spinal canal. Patients with cervical spondylosis and a posteroanterior canal diameter greater than 13 to 15 mm almost never have myelopathy. A canal diameter of 8 mm or less is considered "critical."

The benefits of surgical treatment are debated. In a review of the literature published in 1992, Rowland[9] reported that of 261 patients who had posterior cervical laminectomy, 60% improved, 34% had no change, and 6% were worse. Of 385 patients surgically treated with an anterior approach, 52% improved, 24% had no change, and 23% were worse. Of 136 patients treated conservatively without an operation, 44% improved, 33% had no change, and 23% were worse. Perioperative morbidity was 4% to 5%.[9] No prospective controlled trials have been performed, and the condition of some patients continues to deteriorate despite adequate decompression.

Nonetheless, surgical treatment for cervical spondylotic myelopathy is still accepted. It generally is estimated that about 80% of patients with spinal cord compression due to cervical spondylosis have improvement or no change postoperatively.[10]

It is difficult to prove that an anterior approach with or without fusion is better than a posterior approach.[11] It seems reasonable to suggest that the direction of the approach should be the most direct and shortest route to the site of greatest cord compression. If there is considerable instability with subluxation on flexion and extension studies, fusion is the best procedure.

According to the review by Clifton et al.,[12] the causes of poor outcome in 56 patients were wrong diagnosis (14.3%), spinal cord atrophy (26.8%), diffuse spinal stenosis (28.6%), and failure of decompression (57.1%).

Severe brachalgia due to root compression at a single level by acute disk herniation can be cured dramatically by excision of the offending disk via an anterior approach.

Some patients refuse surgery or are not surgical candidates. Many of these patients benefit from using the collar, initially for 24 hours daily and, after about a month, only at night when sleeping. In some instances, the clinical signs of myelopathy are evident but the imaging evidence for severe cord compression is not strong. These patients, too, usually benefit from neck immobilization.

Ankylosing spondylitis

"Ankylosing spondylitis" is a chronic inflammatory disease manifested by back pain and spine stiffness. The combination of radiographic evidence of sacroiliitis, back pain, and decreased movement of the back and chest indicates the diagnosis of this seronegative arthropathy for which there is no cure. The goals of therapy are to prevent deformity (progressive kyphosis) and to suppress inflammation and pain.[13] Prevalence varies from zero to 1.4%, depending on the ethnic group and the prevalence of HLA-B27. Among the white population of Europe and North America, the prevalence is 0.05% to 0.23%, and the risk increases to 1.3% for those who are HLA-B27-positive.[14]

Signs

Decreased movement of the low back can be documented with the Schober test. The patient stands erect, and the position of the spinous process of L5 is marked with a pen and another mark is made 10 cm below it in the midline. Next, the patient bends forward maximally, without bending the knees. Normally, the distance between the two points marked on the skin exceeds 15 cm.

Chest expansion is measured at the level of the fourth intercostal space. The patient is asked to exert a maximal forced expiration, followed by a maximal inspiration. Expansion is usually 5 cm or more, and an expansion less than 2.5 cm is abnormal.

The sacroiliac joint can be stressed to demonstrate a local lesion as evidenced by pain. With the patient supine, the examiner presses on the anterior superior iliac spine, and at the same time, the iliac spine is forced laterally. With the patient lying on the side, the examiner can compress the pelvis from above. Lying supine, the patient is asked to flex a knee and to abduct and externally rotate the ipsilateral hip. Pressure on the flexed knee causes pain in the ipsilateral sacroiliac joint.

Laboratory studies

The results of hematological studies are neither specific nor helpful in establishing the diagnosis of ankylosing spondylitis. Acute phase reactants are frequently abnormal but have poor predictive value for active clinical disease.[15] Although HLA-B27 is frequently present, the usefulness of the test depends on the ethnic group of the patient. In whites of northern European extraction, HLA-B27 is present in approximately 95% of those with ankylosing spondylitis but in only 6% of the general population.[12] The absence of HLA-B27 in a white patient of northern European extraction makes the diagnosis of ankylosing spondylitis unlikely.

The first radiographic changes are in the sacroiliac joints. Subtle changes are open to interpretation, but recent standardizations of scoring systems appear reliable.[16] Sclerosis of the joint and fusion particularly on one side only is often seen best with computed tomography (CT), which is thought to be more specific but less sensitive than MRI.[17] Other imaging techniques include ultrasonography of tendons[18] and bone densitometry, because osteoporosis occurs early in ankylosing spondylitis in association with persistent active disease.[19]

Neurological complications

Spinal cord compression can occur with fractures of the spine, often from relatively mild trauma. Spontaneous subluxation at the atlantoaxial level, as in patients with rheumatoid arthritis, can compromise the spinal cord.[20] Cauda equina dysfunction is a rare complication in patients with chronic ankylosing spondylitis who have marked ankylosis. Arachnoiditis may cause neurological signs or symptoms, and surgical treatment should be avoided.[21]

Treatment

Although the best conservative intervention in acute exacerbations of pain or myelopathy in cervical spondylosis is rest and immobilization, the opposite is true for ankylosing spondylitis. The most important measure probably is exercise.[22] Regular spinal extension exercises and instruction to stand erect in combination with deep breathing exercises should be the rule. To reinforce these recommendations, patient education is important, and support groups are easily contacted through the Internet. Also, the patients should sleep on a hard mattress.

Nonsteroidal anti-inflammatory drugs relieve stiffness and pain but do not alter the course of the disease. Corticosteroid therapy is of no benefit long term, but pulsed therapy is used occasionally for short-term treatment of acute exacerbations of pain. The primary indication is for complicating uveitis or vasculitis. Phenylbutazone, which carries the risk of bone marrow suppression, is not prescribed in the United States, but it is effective symptomatically and may inhibit ossification of the paraspinal ligaments. Neither sulfasalazine nor penicillamine is beneficial in spinal disease. Methotrexate therapy has not been studied in a placebo-controlled trial. Intravenous cyclophosphamide may be useful for some patients with severe disease in whom all other medications have failed. Gold salts and antimalarial agents do not appear to be effective, but appropriate drug trials for ankylosing spondylitis have not been reported.[23]

Atlanto-occipital or atlantoaxial subluxation and spinal stenosis are the most common indications for surgical treatment of ankylosing spondylitis.[24] The ankylosed spine lacks compensatory soft tissue mechanics in trauma and all energy is absorbed by the diseased bone, resulting in fractures of the cervical spine, often from minimal trauma. Neurosurgical intervention may be required to stabilize unstable fractures, but immobilization is the treatment of choice. Complicating epidural hematomas can cause spinal cord decompression. Vertebral osteotomy or hip-joint replacement may compensate for the kyphotic deformity.[25]

Low back pain, lumbar disk disease, and spinal stenosis

Approximately 80% of the general population will have at least one episode of low back pain sometime during life. Low back pain occurs in about 25% of the working population each year and to a disabling degree in 2% to 8%. Back pain that lasts for 2 weeks affects approximately 14% of adults each year, and about 1% to 2% have sciatica.[26] Acute low back pain is usually self-limiting, and 90% of patients recover within 6 weeks, but 2% to 7% develop chronic pain.[27] Low back pain accounts for 33% of all workers' compensation costs (one-third for medical treatment and two-thirds for indemnity). Seventy-five percent of compensation payments go to patients with low back pain, and these patients constitute only 3% of all those who receive compensation.[28]

A good approach to the diagnosis of back pain is to consider the structures in the lumbar spine that are pain-sensitive and to postulate a lesion related to each structure. The diagnosis is based on the combination of the medical history and the physical signs found on neurological examination. If referred pain down the leg is not present, the pain may be considered to have a rheumatological origin in muscle (which is painful, tender, and in spasm), or in a disk, apophyseal joint, or covering membranes. If referred pain down the leg occurs or physical examination demonstrates signs of radiculopathy through segmental weakness, wasting, sensory loss, or an absent reflex, pressure on the exiting nerve roots should be suspected. About 95% of herniated lumbar disks affect the L4–5 and L5–S1 interspace,[29] so that pain is likely to radiate to the big toe (L5 root) or to the little toe or sole (S1 root).

Sciatic pain precipitated by exercise of a fairly specific duration suggests the diagnosis of spinal claudication, which in turn is likely caused by spinal stenosis. Normal pedal pulses exclude peripheral vascular claudication. Neurogenic claudication improves with flexion of the spine, so that patients often stoop forward or sit down to relieve the pain. Conversely, disk pain is often made worse by lumbar flexion.

Findings on neurological examination may be normal at rest, but after exercise, weakness, sensory loss, or an absent reflex may emerge transiently. Rarely, true claudication of the cauda equina is caused by atherosclerotic disease of the aorta, internal iliac arteries, or ileohypogastric vessels that supply the lumbar radicular feeder arteries. In these patients, lumbar spine imaging studies do not demonstrate spinal stenosis or other causes of compression of the cauda equina.

Lasègue sign

The patient is supine, with the uninvolved knee bent 45 degrees and the foot resting on the table. The involved leg is raised straight up, while the ankle is kept at 90 degrees of flexion. Because disk herniation tends to tether the irritated nerve roots, stretching them causes pain to radiate into the lower extremity along the sciatic distribution. The test has a sensitivity of about 80%, but the specificity is about 40%.[30] If the pain is felt in the contralateral symptomatic leg when the asymptomatic leg is raised ("crossed straight leg raising"), a lesion medial to the nerve root, often an extruded disk fragment, should be suspected (specificity, 90%; sensitivity, 25%).

Red flags

Most patients with low back pain or sciatica (or both) have degenerative disk disease with reactive bone spurring. However, occasionally a patient has a more serious lesion. In a study of 1975 patients who presented to a public hospital with back pain, 13 had pain that ultimately was attributed to malignancy.[31] If the patient has unremitting pain (worse at night in bed), bilateral leg signs or symptoms, sphincter disturbance, unexplained weight loss, immunosuppression, and a history of previous cancer or intravenous drug use, an imaging study should be performed. If these indications are not present, a more conservative work-up is indicated.

Laboratory studies

A complete blood count, erythrocyte sedimentation rate, prostate-specific antigen (in appropriate patients) and alkaline phosphatase testing, and protein immunoelectrophoresis are appropriate.

Imaging

Plain radiographs are helpful if malignancy, infection, or fracture is suspected. However, negative findings do not exclude the diagnosis of a serious lesion. Because 90% of patients have spontaneous recovery within 4 weeks,[32] it is reasonable to delay imaging unless major focal signs are present or compression of the cauda equina is a concern. It is wise to image the lumbar spine before initiating epidural corticosteroid treatment to ensure that the lesion is indeed benign. The imaging modality of choice is MRI, which can demonstrate lesions in the disk, apophyseal joints, and exit foramina as well as in the paraspinal tissues. If infection is a consideration, contrast-enhanced studies should be performed.

Treatment

Although virtually no controlled trials have evaluated the treatment of cervical spondylosis, numerous trials have been conducted on the treatment of low back problems.[33] When subjected to scrutiny, many treatments are found wanting, and some practices have been discredited entirely in recent years. For example, for patients with or without radicular complications, prolonged bed rest has been replaced by rest for at most 2 days.[34-36] Bed rest, however, is probably appropriate for patients with the most severe pain or neurological deficit. Chemonucleolysis has fallen into disfavor.[37] Lumbar traction is not effective,[38] and transcutaneous electrical nerve stimulation is no better than placebo or exercise alone.[39,40] There is no evidence for the use of lumbar supports.[41] However, some old and trusted remedies such as local superficial hot or cold packs are helpful in reducing muscle spasm and pain early on.[42]

For acute low back pain, exercise and ordinary activity produce better results than prolonged rest and are cost-effective.[43,44] Recovery is faster and pain and disability are less for patients advised to stay active than for those given no advice.[35] A recent study compared physical therapy, chiropractic treatment, and an educational booklet and found a marginal benefit for the first two modalities over education alone.[45] In some trials, "back school" has not decreased the time to return to work.[46] For acute low back pain, there is no evidence that specific back exercises (flexion, extension, aerobic, or strengthening exercises) are more effective than other conservative treatments; however, for chronic low back pain, back exercises are more effective than other conservative measures.[47]

Spinal manipulation is possibly of short-term benefit for some patients, but it is unproven for chronic low back pain[48] and is not cost-effective compared with conventional supportive care,[49] possibly because of repeated visits to the chiropractor for "adjustments." The complications of spinal manipulation include fractures and cauda equina syndrome.[50]

Epidural corticosteroid injections afford short-term relief of acute sciatica in more than 50% of patients, and although these injections sometimes are useful in the long term, they do not reduce the need for surgical treatment.[51,52] The therapeutic benefit of facet injections is debated; the procedure may be considered if other conservative measures fail.[53,54]

Nonsteroidal anti-inflammatory drugs provide relief from back pain and possibly have an anti-inflammatory effect, but there is no evidence to distinguish one from another and no evidence of an effect for radicular pain.[55] An analgesic response can be obtained with simple analgesics such as acetaminophen in combination with a muscle relaxant, and a short burst of opioid therapy may be necessary. Evidence for the effect of nonsteroidal anti-inflammatory drugs compared with that of acetaminophen, opioids, muscle relaxants, antidepressants, and nondrug treatment is conflicting.[56] For patients with acute disk herniation, some physicians prefer a short course of corticosteroid therapy, but the effectiveness has not been proved.[57] Patients with chronic pain should be given a trial of antidepressant therapy, but the evidence that it offers benefit is debated.[58,59]

Because of the often inconclusive evidence, practitioners who treat acute and chronic low back pain and lumbar radicular pain need a modus vivendi (Table 133.3). Patients with acute severe pain or neurological deficit should have at least 2 or 3 days of bed rest. Patients with milder degrees of pain should continue to be up and around and should be reassured that the condition usually is self-limiting. They should gradually increase their activity so that they are walking and standing by day 3 and walking in 20-minute bursts within about a week. Lifting heavy weights and sitting for long periods should be avoided. Unassisted lifting should be restricted to less than 20 lb and gradually increased to 60 lb for men and 35 lb for women by 3 months. Patients should limit twisting, bending, and reaching when lifting.[60] Analgesics should be given as necessary to control the pain and may be given in combination with muscle relaxants. For patients with persistent pain, antidepressant therapy should be attempted. If disability persists for more than 10 days, an epidural corticosteroid injection should be considered. For patients whose pain is subsiding and for patients with a history of chronic or recurrent low back pain, a program of regular exercise, weight loss, and low stress aerobic activities should be pursued. Regular walking and swimming are recommended, but high-impact activities such as jogging and repetitive bending or twisting activities should be avoided. Flexion and extension exercises to strengthen the abdominal muscles and to reduce lumbar lordosis may be effective.

For patients with severe chronic low back pain, multidisciplinary treatment programs improve pain, functional status, and return to work.[61] This approach includes a workplace visit and intensive physical and

Table 133.3   Management of back complaint

Acute backache, with or without root signs
  Keep active unless pain is extremely severe—if so,
    2–3 days of bed rest
  Analgesic as necessary, NSAIDs
  Hard mattress
  Muscle relaxant
  If no response to conservative management, MRI
  If root signs or symptoms, epidural corticosteroid
    injections
Chronic backache, with or without root signs
  Active exercise program
  Analgesic
  Muscle relaxant
  Antidepressant
  If no response after a few months, MRI
  "Back school" may be of benefit
  Refer for multidisciplinary treatment program
Indications for early/immediate imaging
  Bilateral root signs and/or symptoms
  Sphincter dysfunction
  Unremitting pain, worse at night in bed
  Weight loss
  Immunosuppression
  History of previous cancer
  Intravenous drug abuse
Indications for surgical therapy
  MRI with significant findings and
    Sphincter disturbance
    Severe unremitting pain
    Severe neurological deficit
    Spinal stenosis with disabling neurogenic
      claudication
    Spondylolisthesis

MRI, magnetic resonance imaging; NSAIDs, nonsteroidal anti-inflammatory drugs.

psychosocial training by the team, which includes a physician, physiotherapist, psychologist, social worker, and occupational therapist. Training usually is given in groups and does not involve passive physical therapy.

Surgery

The indications for imaging studies and surgical intervention are cauda equina syndrome with bladder dysfunction, intractable and severe radicular pain, and severe neurological motor deficit. Pressure on the nerve root or cauda equina is relieved by laminectomy. Spondylolisthesis may require surgical fusion. Spinal stenosis with neurogenic claudication may respond to epidural corticosteroid injections, at least in the short term, but decompressive surgery is indicated for disabling symptoms.[62]

References

1. Pallis C, Jones AM, Spillane JD. Cervical spondylosis: incidence and implications. Brain 1954;77:274–289
2. Ronthal M. Neck Complaints. Butterworth Heinemann: Boston, 2000:43–58
3. Harris PR. Cervical traction. Review of literature and treatment guidelines. Phys Ther 1977;57:910–914
4. van der Heijden GJ, Beurskens AJ, Koes BW, et al. The efficacy of traction for back and neck pain: a systematic, blinded review of randomized clinical trial methods. Phys Ther 1995;75:93–104
5. Tan JC, Nordin M. Role of physical therapy in the treatment of cervical disk disease. Orthop Clin North Am 1992;23:435–449
6. Gross AR, Aker PD, Goldsmith CH, Pelosa P. Physical medicine modalities for mechanical neck disorders (Cochrane Review). In: The Cochrane Library, 3, 2001. Oxford: Update Software
7. Lee KP, Carlini WG, McCormick GF, Albers GW. Neurologic complications following chiropractic manipulation: a survey of California neurologists. Neurology 1995;45:1213–1215
8. Powell FC, Hanigan WC, Olivero WC. A risk/benefit analysis of spinal manipulation therapy for relief of lumbar or cervical pain. Neurosurgery 1993;33:73–78
9. Rowland LP. Surgical treatment of cervical spondylotic myelopathy: time for a controlled trial. Neurology 1992;42:5–13
10. Snow RB, Weiner H. Cervical laminectomy and foraminotomy as surgical treatment of cervical spondylosis: a follow-up study with analysis of failures. J Spinal Disord 1993;6:245–250
11. Fairbank J. Trials and tribulations in cervical spondylosis (editorial). Lancet 1998;352:1165–1166
12. Clifton AG, Stevens JM, Whitear P, Kendall BE. Identifiable causes for poor outcome in surgery for cervical spondylosis. Post-operative compute myelography and MR imaging. Neuroradiology 1990;32:450–455
13. Shah BC, Khan MA. Review of ankylosing spondylitis. Compr Ther 1987;13:52–59
14. Khan MA. HLA-B27 and its subtypes in world populations. Curr Opin Rheumatol 1995;7:263–269
15. Spoorenberg A, van der Heijde D, de Klerk E, et al. Relative value of erythrocyte sedimentation rate and C-reactive protein in assessment of disease activity in ankylosing spondylitis. J Rheumatol 1999;26:980–984
16. Calin A, Mackay K, Santos H, Brophy S. A new dimension to outcome: application of the Bath Ankylosing Spondylitis Radiology Index. J Rheumatol 1999;26:988–992
17. Hanly JG, Mitchell MJ, Barnes DC, MacMillan L. Early recognition of sacroiliitis by magnetic resonance imaging and single photon emission computed tomography. J Rheumatol 1994;21:2088–2095
18. Lehtinen A, Taavitsainen M, Leirisalo-Repo M. Sonographic analysis of enthesopathy in the lower extremities of patients with spondylarthropathy. Clin Exp Rheumatol 1994;12:143–148
19. Gratacos J, Collado A, Pons F, et al. Significant loss of bone mass in patients with early, active ankylosing spondylitis: a followup study. Arthritis Rheum 1999; 42:2319–2324
20. Ramos-Remus C, Gomez-Vargas A, Guzman-Guzman JL, et al. Frequency of atlantoaxial subluxation and neurologic involvement in patients with ankylosing spondylitis. J Rheumatol 1995;22:2120–2125
21. Sant SM, O'Connell D. Cauda equina syndrome in ankylosing spondylitis: a case report and review of the literature. Clin Rheumatol 1995;14:224–226
22. Dougados M, Revel M, Khan MA. Spondylarthropathy treatment: progress in medical treatment, physical therapy and rehabilitation. Baillieres Clin Rheumatol 1998;12:717–736
23. Laurent R. Are there any antirheumatic drugs that modify the course of ankylosing spondylitis? Baillieres Clin Rheumatol 1991;4:387–400

24. Fox MW, Onofrio BM, Kilgore JE. Neurological complications of ankylosing spondylitis. J Neurosurg 1993; 78:871–878

25. Simmons EH. Surgery of the spine in ankylosing spondylitis. Part I. Bull Hosp Jt Dis Orthop Inst 1989; 49:111–130

26. Deyo RA, Tsui-Wu YJ. Descriptive epidemiology of low-back pain and its related medical care in the United States. Spine 1987;12:264–268

27. Frymoyer JW. Back pain and sciatica. N Engl J Med 1988;318:291–300

28. Klein BP, Jensen RC, Sanderson LM. Assessment of workers' compensation claims for back strains/sprains. J Occup Med 1984;26:443–448

29. Jonsson B, Stromqvist B. Symptoms and signs in degeneration of the lumbar spine. A prospective, consecutive study of 300 operated patients. J Bone Joint Surg Br 1993;75:381–385

30. Deyo RA, Rainville J, Kent DL. What can the history and physical examination tell us about low back pain? JAMA 1992;268:760–765

31. Deyo RA, Diehl AK. Cancer as a cause of back pain: frequency, clinical presentation, and diagnostic strategies. J Gen Intern Med 1988;3:230–238

32. Papageorgiou AC, Rigby AS. Review of UK data on the rheumatic diseases—7. Low back pain. Br J Rheumatol 1991;30:208–210

33. Seferlis T, Nemeth G, Carlsson AM, Gillstrom P. Conservative treatment in patients sick-listed for acute low-back pain: a prospective randomised study with 12 months' follow-up. Eur Spine J 1998;7:461–470

34. Deyo RA, Diehl AK, Rosenthal M. How many days of bed rest for acute low back pain? A randomized clinical trial. N Engl J Med 1986;315:1064–1070

35. Waddell G, Feder G, Lewis M. Systematic reviews of bed rest and advice to stay active for acute low back pain. Br J Gen Pract 1997;47:647–652

36. Vroomen PC, de Krom MC, Wilmink JT, et al. Lack of effectiveness of bed rest for sciatica. N Engl J Med 1999;340:418–423

37. Brown MD. Update on chemonucleolysis. Spine 1996 Suppl;21:62S-68S

38. Beurskens AJ, de Vet HC, Koke AJ, et al. Efficacy of traction for nonspecific low back pain. 12-week and 6-month results of a randomized clinical trial. Spine 1997;22:2756–2762

39. Deyo RA, Walsh NE, Martin DC, et al. A controlled trial of transcutaneous electrical nerve stimulation (TENS) and exercise for chronic low back pain. N Engl J Med 1990;322:1627–1634

40. Gadsby JG, Flowerdew MW. The effectiveness of transcutaneous electrical nerve stimulation (TENS) and acupuncture-like transcutaneous electrical nerve stimulation (ALTENS) in the treatment of patients with chronic low back pain. In: The Cochrane Library, Issue 3, 2000. Oxford: Update Software

41. Bigos S, Bowyer O, Braen G, et al. Acute low back problems in adults. Clinical Practice Guideline no 14. AHCPR Publication No 95–0642. Rockville MD: Agency for Health Care Policy and Research, Public Health Service, US Department of Health and Human Services. December 1994

42. Lehmann JF, Warren CG, Scham SM. Therapeutic heat and cold. Clin Orthop 1974;99:207–245

43. Malmivaara A, Hakkinen U, Aro T, et al. The treatment of acute low back pain—bed rest, exercises, or ordinary activity? N Engl J Med 1995;332:351–355

44. Moffett JK, Torgerson D, Bell-Syer S, et al. Randomised controlled trial of exercise for low back pain: clinical outcomes, costs, and preferences. Br Med J 1999;319:279–283

45. Cherkin DC, Deyo RA, Battie M, et al. A comparison of physical therapy, chiropractic manipulation, and provision of an educational booklet for the treatment of patients with low back pain. N Engl J Med 1998; 339:1021–1029

46. Leclaire R, Esdaile JM, Suissa S, et al. Back school in a first episode of compensated acute low back pain: a clinical trial to assess efficacy and prevent relapse. Arch Phys Med Rehabil 1996;77:673–679

47. Faas A. Exercises: which ones are worth trying, for which patients, and when? Spine 1996;21:2874–2878

48. Shekelle PG, Adams AH, Chassin MR, et al. Spinal manipulation for low-back pain. Ann Intern Med 1992; 117:590–598

49. Ernst E, Assendelft WJ. Chiropractic for low back pain. We don't know whether it does more good than harm (editorial). Br Med J 1998;317:160

50. Assendelft WJ, Bouter LM, Knipschild PG. Complications of spinal manipulation: a comprehensive review of the literature. J Fam Pract 1996;42:475–480

51. Watts RW, Silagy CA. A meta-analysis on the efficacy of epidural corticosteroids in the treatment of sciatica. Anaesth Intensive Care 1995; 23:564–569

52. Carette S, Leclaire R, Marcoux S, et al. Epidural corticosteroid injections for sciatica due to herniated nucleus pulposus. N Engl J Med 1997;336:1634–1640

53. Carette S, Marcoux S, Truchon R, et al. A controlled trial of corticosteroid injections into facet joints for chronic low back pain. N Engl J Med 1991;325: 1002–1007

54. Malanga GA, Nadler SF. Nonoperative treatment of low back pain. Mayo Clin Proc 1999;74:1135–1148

55. Koes BW, Scholten RJ, Mens JM, Bouter LM. Efficacy of non-steroidal anti-inflammatory drugs for low back pain: a systematic review of randomised clinical trials. Ann Rheum Dis 1997;56:214–223

56. van Tulder MW, Koes BW, Bouter LM. Conservative treatment of acute and chronic nonspecific low back pain. A systematic review of randomized controlled trials of the most common interventions. Spine 1997;22: 2128–2156

57. Haimovic IC, Beresford HR. Dexamethasone is not superior to placebo for treating lumbosacral radicular pain. Neurology 1986;36:1593–1594

58. McQuay HJ, Tramer M, Nye BA, et al. A systematic review of antidepressants in neuropathic pain. Pain 1996;68:217–227

59. Turner JA, Denny MC. Do antidepressant medications relieve chronic low back pain? J Fam Pract 1993;37: 545–553

60. Bigos S, Bowyer O, Braen G, et al. Acute Low Back Problems in Adults. Clinical Practice Guideline, Quick Reference Guide Number 14. Rockville, Maryland: United States Department of Health and Human Services, Public Health Service, Agency for Health Care Policy and Research, AHCPR Publication No. 95–0643, December, 1994

61. Bendix AF, Bendix T, Vaegter K, et al. Multidisciplinary intensive treatment for chronic low back pain: a randomized, prospective study. Cleve Clin J Med 1996; 63:62–69

62. Atlas SJ, Deyo RA, Keller RB, et al. The Maine Lumbar Spine Study, Part III. 1-year outcomes of surgical and nonsurgical management of lumbar spinal stenosis. Spine 1996;21:1787–1794

134 Neurological Complications of Progressive Systemic Sclerosis

Loren A Rolak

Definition

"Progressive Systemic Sclerosis" (PSS) is a worldwide illness that affects all races and generally appears in the third to fifth decades. The female-to-male predilection is 3:1.

PSS encompasses several different disease entities, although each may be a manifestation of a common underlying pathophysiological process.[1] A feature of most of these diseases is scleroderma, a thickening and fibrosis of the skin. The diseases include the following:

1. Diffuse cutaneous scleroderma—This is characterized by symmetric thickening of the skin, primarily in the extremities, proximally and distally, but also involving the face and trunk. The patients also have a high risk for the development of visceral disease, usually within the first 5 years, with the kidney most often affected. The 10-year survival rate is 70% without visceral involvement but only 30% if the kidneys are affected and 50% if the lungs are involved.
2. Limited cutaneous scleroderma—Patients have symmetric skin thickening limited to areas distal to the elbows and knees. Visceral involvement is rare; thus, the prognosis is good. A subgroup of patients with limited cutaneous scleroderma meet criteria for the illness once called CREST syndrome (calcinosis, Raynaud phenomenon, esophageal dysmotility, sclerodactyly, and telangiectasis).
3. Systemic sclerosis without scleroderma—Patients have fibrosis and sclerosis of visceral organs without any involvement of skin.
4. Linear scleroderma—This is characterized by thickening of the skin confined to only one extremity (or to only the face).
5. Morphea—Patients have smaller, well-demarcated localized plaques of skin induration, either a single plaque or several scattered ones. There is no visceral involvement.

Pathogenesis

The key feature of PSS is overproduction and accumulation of collagen and other extracellular matrix proteins in the skin and other organs. The mechanism by which this occurs is unknown.[2]

Another feature is vascular damage to small arterioles and capillaries, with subsequent thickening of the intima and obliteration of the vascular lumen. The microvascular bed becomes insufficient, leading to a chronic ischemic state. The remaining capillaries may become dilated and tortuous as they proliferate, causing visible telangiectases. The mechanism of the vascular damage is unclear.

Endothelial cells may be targeted directly by either humoral or cell-mediated immune mechanisms or they may be damaged secondarily by toxic cytokines released in a bystander immune process. However, a primary immunologic mechanism for PSS has not been proved.[3]

Nonimmunologic abnormalities include aberrant regulation of growth factors in fibroblasts, stimulation of collagen synthesis, and mitogenic changes in smooth muscle cells.

Diagnosis

PSS has no specific biological marker; therefore, the diagnosis rests heavily on clinical criteria. PSS usually is recognized by typical skin changes (scleroderma), accompanied by Raynaud phenomenon in nearly 90% of patients. Laboratory studies are sometimes helpful, but the findings are nonspecific. The creatine kinase concentration may be increased because of muscle involvement. Several autoimmune antibody measurements are also abnormal, including a positive antinuclear antibody (ANA) in 90% of patients. Although none of these are specific to PSS, their presence is reassuring for the diagnosis in patients with appropriate clinical manifestations.

Clinical features

The most prominent clinical features are Raynaud phenomenon and skin changes. Edematous swelling appears in the fingers, hands, forearms, feet, and face. This swelling may last for months, but then the skin becomes firm and thick and tightly bound to the underlying connective tissue. The taut skin may limit full movement over the joints. This results in a characteristic facial appearance: loss of skin wrinkles, blunting of facial expressions, and microstomia (a small, tightly drawn mouth). Calcium deposits may appear in the skin, as may ulcerations. Joint changes resembling rheumatoid arthritis may occur. Interstitial fibrosis of the lungs may lead to shortness of breath. Cardiac changes can include pericarditis, arrhythmias, and congestive heart failure. Renal involvement is the leading cause of death, accounting for at least 50% of all fatalities.

Neurological complications

The nervous system is not involved in PSS nearly as often or as severely as it is in many other connective tissue diseases. Neurological changes are minimal and often nonspecific.[4,5]

Central nervous system

The brain and spinal cord are not affected directly by PSS. Perhaps because blood vessels in the central nervous system lack an external elastic lamina and have very little media, the vascular changes so characteristic in other visceral organs are absent from the brain.[6,7] There are scattered reports of brain ischemia in patients with PSS,[8] but, in most autopsy series, the brain is normal or the blood vessel changes in patients with ischemic disease are due to hypertension (usually from typical renal involvement) rather than from PSS itself. Some patients with PSS also have antiphospholipid antibodies, and these rather than the PSS itself may lead to central nervous system ischemia.

There are a few reports of multiple sclerosis or isolated optic neuritis in patients with PSS, but these are sufficiently infrequent to make direct causation doubtful.

Trigeminal neuralgia

As with many other connective tissue diseases, an increased incidence of trigeminal neuralgia has been reported with PSS, in some series as high as 5%.[5] In a few cases, this has been the initial symptom of PSS. Nevertheless, other series including more than 100 patients with PSS have not found any cases of trigeminal neuralgia, and, thus, the relationship remains uncertain.[4]

Peripheral neuropathy

The relationship of peripheral neuropathy to PSS is unclear.[2,4] Samples and surveys report an incidence of peripheral neuropathy ranging from zero to 34%, with the higher values generally reported in studies that define cases as "neuropathy" even when there is only asymptomatic slowing of nerve conduction velocities. However, clinical diagnoses also can be confusing because numbness and sensory changes in the hands and feet are often due to the skin lesions of PSS rather than an underlying neuropathy. When neuropathy is present, it may be due to the involvement of other internal organs (such as renal failure). There is no conclusive evidence for any unique PSS neuropathy.

A more convincing relationship exists with carpal tunnel syndrome. Fibrotic thickening of tendon sheaths can compress the median nerve and produce carpal tunnel syndrome with greater frequency among patients with PSS than is seen in the general population.

Myopathy

Clinically, muscle weakness generally correlates with the severity of skin disease, but it usually is due to disuse atrophy rather than direct muscle involvement. Because patients are frequently given corticosteroid therapy, steroid myopathy must be considered as a differential diagnosis of weakness

and muscle symptoms. Thyroid disease is another cause of myopathy in patients with PSS.

The most common pattern of weakness is a mild-to-moderate diffuse loss of strength, which often is not progressive and not associated with a significant increase in creatine kinase concentration. Histologically, muscle is dominated by increased connective tissue, which probably represents a complication of widespread fibrosis. No inflammation is present in biopsy specimens. The weakness does not respond to corticosteroid therapy. The best treatment is physical therapy and exercise.

Myositis has been documented in some patients. It is essentially identical to the polymyositis associated with other connective tissue diseases. The serum concentration of creatine kinase is elevated, and the weakness can be severe and progressive.[9] The myositis usually responds to prednisone at initial doses of 1 mg/kg daily. Methotrexate has also been used with anecdotal success.

Dysphagia

Dysphagia is a common symptom. However, it usually does not have a neurological basis but is due to esophageal muscle fibrosis. There are occasional reports of autonomic dysfunction, especially gastrointestinal,[10] in patients with PSS, but it is doubtful that any primary dysautonomia is caused by the disease.

Treatment

Assessment of therapy is difficult because of the highly variable course and severity of the disease and the lack of any large controlled trials. However, no therapy has been shown in blinded controlled studies to improve the overall course of PSS or to prevent neurological complications.[11]

A common treatment is penicillamine, which interferes with the cross-linking of collagen and also has immunosuppressant properties. The dose is usually maintained between 0.5 and 1 g/day (taken without food). Its important toxic effects include renal failure, myasthenia, and anemia, and its therapeutic value is unproven. Other treatments that have been tried, without scientific proof of efficacy, include azathioprine, 5-fluorouracil, colchicine, and chlorambucil.

Corticosteroids are not indicated as chronic therapy, but prednisone may be useful in doses of 40 to 60 mg daily for myositis, pericarditis, or similar acute symptoms.

Studies have not shown any benefit for either aspirin or dipyridamole in preventing vascular complications.

Thus, with few exceptions, neurological problems in patients with PSS are treated as they would be in any other patient. The neurologist should seldom need to intervene in therapy for the PSS itself.

References

1. Pope JE, Seibold JR. International Conference on Systemic Sclerosis. J Rheumatol 1999;26:938–944
2. Rosenbaum RB, Campbell SM, Rosenbaum JT. Clinical Neurology of Rheumatic Diseases. Boston: Butter-

worth-Heinemann, 1996:319–340

3. Rose NR, Leskovesek N. Scleroderma: immunopatho-genesis and treatment. Immunol Today 1998;19:499–501

4. Gordon RM, Silverstein A. Neurologic manifestations in progressive systemic sclerosis. Arch Neurol 1970;22:126–134

5. Cerinic MM, Generini S, Pignone A, Casale R. The nervous system in systemic sclerosis (scleroderma). Clinical features and pathogenetic mechanisms. Rheum Dis Clin North Am 1996;22:879–892

6. Kerin K, Yost JH. Advances in the diagnosis and management of scleroderma-related vascular complications. Compr Ther 1998;24:574–581

7. Heron E, Fornes P, Rance A, et al. Brain involvement in scleroderma: two autopsy cases. Stroke 1998;29:719–721

8. Kanzato N, Matsuzaki T, Komine Y, et al. Localized scleroderma associated with progressing ischemic stroke. J Neurol Sci 1999;163:86–89

9. Jablonska S, Blaszczyk M. Scleromyositis: a scleroderma/polymyositis overlap syndrome. Clin Rheumatol 1998;17:465–467

10. Reynolds JC. Immune-mediated enteric neuron dysfunction in scleroderma. J Lab Clin Med 1999;133:523–524

11. Stone JH, Wigley FM. Management of systemic sclerosis: the art and science. Semin Cutan Med Surg 1998;17:55–64

135 Treatment of Neurosarcoidosis

Thomas F Scott and Barney Stern

Introduction

"Sarcoidosis" is an idiopathic granulomatous disorder that involves multiple organs, primarily the lungs and lymph nodes. Also commonly affected are ocular structures and the skin. Liver and muscle involvement is common and may be asymptomatic. Although involvement of the heart and nervous system is relatively rare (about 5% of patients each), the most severe complications may occur in these patients.[1,2] Renal involvement is rare. Approximately 50% of patients with neurosarcoidosis present with neurological difficulties.

Estimates of the annual incidence of sarcoidosis in the United States and Europe range from 5 to 100/100 000. The wide discrepancy is accounted for partly by an increased prevalence if surveillance chest radiographs are used instead of symptomatic disease. A definite preponderance among blacks is seen in the United States, where an increased incidence among women is also likely.[3] The age at onset tends to be between 30 and 40 years. Although sarcoidosis was once associated with residence in the southeastern United States, it now is recognized to be more widespread and more common than previously estimated.[4]

Sarcoidosis affecting the nervous system presents challenges for both diagnosis and treatment. Multifocal disease, presentation without systemic involvement, and the lack of definitive noninvasive testing contribute to the difficulty of diagnosis. Also, life-threatening neurosarcoidosis is relatively rare and precludes the possibility of controlled treatment trials.

General approach

A definitive diagnosis of sarcoidosis is usually made on the basis of biopsy results. Once sarcoidosis has been demonstrated in a particular organ, involvement of other organs often can be determined with noninvasive testing by demonstrating findings typical of sarcoidosis. Screening for sarcoidosis should include examination of the skin and eyes, complete blood count, thyroid function tests, renal and liver function tests, serum concentration of calcium, and chest radiography. Cerebrospinal fluid (CSF) studies and serum markers of active inflammation (erythrocyte sedimentation rate, angiotensin-converting enzyme, immunoglobulin concentration, oligoclonal bands) are sometimes helpful diagnostically.[5,6]

After sarcoidosis has been "staged" or localized by the interpretation of clinical and paraclinical information, benign chronic lesions, characterized histologically by fibrous scarring, must be differentiated from inflammatory active lesions, which can cause progressive deficits. Granulomas can develop as a microscopic diffuse infiltrating process involving the central nervous system (CNS) parenchyma, meninges, cranial and peripheral nerves, and muscle or coalesce to form large lesions with a mass effect. Inflammatory cytokines likely produce local tissue injury directly as well as mediate the evolution of granuloma formation.[7] Spread of the inflammatory process may occur hematogenously or along CSF spaces.

In neurosarcoidosis, there can be several mechanisms of neuronal injury. For example, in cases of optic nerve involvement, the optic nerve sheath may be compressed extrinsically by a granulomatous mass lesion or the optic nerve may be infiltrated by sarcoidosis, causing a mass effect as well as inflammatory injury.[8] Perivascular inflammation can lead to small infarcts. Also, the optic nerve can be injured by increased intracranial pressure caused by the inflammatory reaction of the meninges and the resulting hydrocephalus. Similarly, multiple sarcoid-associated factors can lead to limb weakness. Weak limbs can result from myopathy, neuropathy, central weakness, or some combination of these. Neuromuscular disease can be complicated by endocrinopathies related to sarcoidosis of the hypothalamic-pituitary axis or to corticosteroid use.

In summary, pretreatment evaluation of patients includes a complete evaluation of all the organ systems that may be involved, precise localization of the neural tissues involved, an estimation of the degree of ongoing inflammation, and a compilation of the various factors contributing to the patient's presentation. Most patients will receive pharmacological treatment, although occasionally surgical intervention is indicated. Management should also take into account the general medical care of the patient. An ideal treatment for neurosarcoidosis would decrease inflammation, inhibit formation of scar tissue, and promote tissue repair processes such as remyelination. Currently, however, pharmacological treatments are limited essentially to anti-inflammatory strategies.

Meningitis and hydrocephalus

Chronic meningitis is fairly common in neurosarcoidosis. An abnormal CSF profile (mild-moderate predominantly mononuclear pleocytosis and increased protein concentration) is common in patients with neurosarcoidosis presenting as peripheral neuropathy, cranial neuropathy, myelopathy, or intracranial disease.[1,9] Normalization of the CSF profile generally is not a goal of treatment, because this usually lags behind a clinical response.

If sarcoidosis is strongly suspected during evaluation of a patient with meningitis and symptoms of increased intracranial pressure are present, a high dose of corticosteroids should be administered immediately rather than waiting for the diagnosis to be verified. This may prevent the rare death due to cerebral herniation.[10–12] Headache, cognitive and visual complaints, nausea, and ataxia suggest the possibility of increased intracranial pressure. In our experience, some patients have headache as the sole clinical manifestation of severe increased intracranial pressure. The risk of severe disability and death due to hydrocephalus requires that physicians advise all patients with neurosarcoidosis to report the onset of headaches. Neuroimaging may or may not demonstrate marked hydrocephalus in these patients, and it does not always distinguish which patients are at risk for severe complications due to increasing intracranial pressure. Also, neuroimaging may show enlarged ventricles in asymptomatic patients with neurosarcoidosis whose condition is stable. Lumbar puncture shows a high opening pressure in patients at risk for cerebral herniation and should be avoided in patients with severe hydrocephalus.

When the condition of patients with increased intracranial pressure appears unstable or does not respond quickly to the intravenous administration of a high dose of corticosteroids, a ventriculostomy should be performed. This will relieve increased intracranial pressure caused by partial or complete obstruction of the cerebral aqueduct or the foramina of the fourth ventricle by granulomatous inflammation. Also, ventricular shunting may relieve pressure in a "trapped" lateral ventricle caused by inflammation or granuloma involving the foramen of Monro.

Increased intracranial pressure appears to occur in some patients with neurosarcoidosis despite patency of the ventricular system, including the outlet foramina of the fourth ventricle.[10–13] The proposed substrate for increased intracranial pressure in these patients is impaired absorption of CSF by the arachnoid villi because of granulomatous disease. Patients may present with symptoms of either increased intracranial pressure (usually headache) or normal-pressure hydrocephalus (cognitive and gait disturbances and incontinence).[13] Neuroimaging may show minimal signs of ventricular enlargement in patients with chronic sarcoid meningitis and dementia that has responded to ventriculoperitoneal shunting. Cisternography may be helpful in documenting the patency of the ventricular system and abnormal CSF dynamics. CSF examination is necessary for all patients with known sarcoidosis who present with cognitive dysfunction.

Intracranial mass lesion

Large or small intra-axial and extra-axial mass lesions of neurosarcoidosis can occur in virtually any location and often seem to evolve as inflammatory lesions that infiltrate the parenchyma from meningeal or ependymal surfaces. Periventricular hypothalamic involvement, ventriculitis, fourth ventricular pseudogliomas,

cerebellopontine angle lesions, and cerebral convexity pseudomeningiomas have all been well described.[1,9,14–18] Periventricular white matter lesions can mimic the magnetic resonance imaging (MRI) appearance of multiple sclerosis.[18,19] Many lesions are asymptomatic.

MRI with gadolinium is best for identifying intracranial neurosarcoidosis and usually has an important role in evaluating the onset of new symptoms, monitoring patients long-term, and evaluating treatment response.[19–22] Lesions generally enhance with a diffuse or irregular pattern when active and show decreasing size and enhancement as the disease responds to treatment.[22,23] Eradication of enhancing lesions is not necessarily a goal of treatment because some chronic inactive meningeal lesions appear to enhance, likely from the formation of a hypervascular scar.[18,22]

Generally, treatment is with moderate doses of corticosteroids, 1 mg/kg daily of prednisone, tapering over 3 to 6 months to 10 to 20 mg daily. This may be followed by tapering the remaining low dose over an additional 6 months or more. Repeating the neuroimaging study 2 to 4 months after therapy has been initiated usually is recommended to determine the response to management, which may be complete, partial, or none. This helps to establish a post-treatment baseline important in subsequent monitoring of disease activity and in making treatment decisions. Response to corticosteroids is often good, but treatment failures occur. Either clinical or neuroimaging evidence of relapse requires resumption of higher doses of corticosteroids. Although serum markers of active sarcoidosis, such as angiotensin-converting enzyme, are useful in the diagnosis of sarcoidosis, they are not reliable for determining the response to therapy.

In refractory disease or in patients unable to tolerate corticosteroids, treatment with immunosuppressive agents is often successful (Table 135.1). Methotrexate is perhaps the best studied immunosuppressant used to treat pulmonary sarcoidosis, but similar studies in neurosarcoidosis have not been feasible because of the small number of patients. Despite this limitation, methotrexate, azathioprine, cyclosporine, cyclophosphamide, and intracranial irradiation have all been reported to be efficacious.[24–35] Cyclophosphamide and intracranial irradiation may have a more rapid onset of effect in patients with life-threatening neurosarcoidosis, such as those with encephalopathy and seizures, but this has not been substantiated.[24,28,34] Azathioprine, methotrexate, and cyclosporine may have a slight advantage compared with cyclophosphamide based on their more common use as reported in small case series[24,25,28,34,35] and overall side-effect profile. Most patients given immunosuppressants also receive a low maintenance dose of corticosteroids. Appropriate monitoring of hematological status, liver function, creatinine, and bone density is required.

It is difficult to determine when an adequate trial of immunosuppression has been completed. We

Table 135.1 Adjunct treatments for neurosarcoidosis

Medication	Dose range	Precautions	Comments
Cyclosporine	Titrate dose to transplantation therapeutic range	Renal toxicity, hypertension	Minimal experience with pulmonary sarcoidosis
Azathioprine	2–3 mg/kg orally daily; titrate dose to leukocyte count of 3000–4000/mm³ or total lymphocyte count of 1000/mm³	Nausea, leukopenia, liver toxicity, neoplasia	Some patients lack enzyme for metabolism
Methotrexate	7.5–15 mg orally weekly; can titrate dose to leukocyte count of 3000–4000/mm³	Leukopenia, liver toxicity, pulmonary fibrosis	Low short-term toxicity, higher long-term toxicity (liver)
Cyclophosphamide	600–800 mg/m² IV pulse monthly 1–2 mg/kg orally daily	Neoplasia, leukopenia, nausea, cystitis	Overall toxicity probably highest of available agents
Intracranial irradiation	1–3000 rads	Radiation toxicity	Few reports, dosage limitations
Chlorambucil	Hematologic end point	Hematologically toxic	
Hydroxychloroquine	200 mg 2 times daily	Ocular toxicity	Limited treatment duration
Pentoxyfulline	25 mg/kg/d in 3 divided doses	Nausea	Well tolerated adjunct therapy

generally are satisfied with 12 to 24 months of disease stability or improvement (by neurological examination and by other monitoring methods such as neuroimaging), and we then begin to taper immunosuppressant therapy. Chronic disabilities can develop in many patients despite several months of intervention.

Myelopathy

There are several reports of sarcoid myelopathy, and in some of these reports, myelopathy was the first clinical manifestation of sarcoidosis.[27,36–42] Biopsy was performed in some patients to establish diagnosis. When evidence of systemic sarcoidosis is lacking, important clues to the diagnosis include concurrent radiculopathy and myelopathy, evidence of inflammation in the CSF, and MRI findings of concurrent meningeal and parenchymal involvement. As in intracranial neurosarcoidosis, treatment is guided primarily by disease severity and response to initial therapy. Initial treatment is with moderate doses of corticosteroids; the disease frequently responds well. A few reports of refractory sarcoid myelopathy indicate that immunosuppressive therapy may sometimes be successful.

Peripheral neuropathy

Virtually all patterns of peripheral neuropathy are found in patients with neurosarcoidosis. These include acute or chronic symmetrical polyneuropathy, mononeuritis multiplex, monoradiculopathy, polyradiculopathy, pure motor neuropathy, and pure sensory neuropathy.[43–51] Nerve conduction studies may demonstrate demyelinating and axonal components of neuropathy, and an electromyographic (EMG) needle examination often shows denervation even in the absence of abnormal findings on nerve conduction studies.[41] Nerve biopsy may be necessary to confirm the diagnosis; it commonly shows epineural and perineural inflammation. Treatment usually is with moderate doses of prednisone,

0.5 mg/kg daily, tapering over 6 to 12 months when the disease is stable or has improved. More aggressive therapies (Table 135.1) may be tried in cases of more severe or refractory disease, but experience with other medications is quite limited. Generally, neuropathy responds well to treatment.

Cranial neuropathy

Bell palsy, the most common cranial neuropathy found in neurosarcoidosis, generally responds well to low-dose corticosteroid treatment, prednisone 0.25 to 0.5 mg/kg daily given over 2 to 6 weeks.[32,33] A peripheral facial nerve palsy, which can be unilateral or bilateral and recurrent, develops in more than 50% of patients with neurosarcoidosis. Optic neuropathy can be acute and clinically indistinguishable from optic neuritis, but it generally evolves slowly and can be refractory to corticosteroid treatment.[7,26] Aggressive treatment with immunosuppressive agents and radiation therapy has been successful. Cerebellopontine angle mass lesions due to sarcoidosis are a rare potential cause of cranial nerve dysfunction, as are intraaxial brainstem lesions. To determine the extent of the illness of patients with cranial neuropathy, cerebral contrast MRI and CSF examination are necessary.

Hypothalamic and pituitary sarcoidosis

Hypothalamic and pituitary involvement occurs in only 0.5% of patients with sarcoidosis; however, this increases to 10% when patients with neurosarcoidosis are considered.[52,53] Inflammatory lesions seem to infiltrate the hypothalamus from the ependymal lining of the third ventricle and infiltrate the pituitary gland and stalk from the basal meninges. A pattern of involvement of basal meninges, pituitary, and hypothalamic structures, seen as enhancing lesions on MRI, is considered classic for sarcoidosis. Less frequently, an intracranial mass lesion mimicking tumor can occur in this region and also produce dysfunction of the pituitary axis.

Diabetes insipidus is the most common endocrine syndrome associated with neurosarcoidosis. Polydipsia and polyuria may be presenting symptoms for neurosarcoidosis. Polyuria and polydipsia also may result from hyperglycemia, hypercalciuria, and nephrogenic diabetes insipidus associated with sarcoidosis.

Symptoms of hypothalamic dysfunction include sleep disorder (especially hypersomnolence), temperature dysregulation, weight gain, and personality changes. Typical symptoms of hypothyroidism, or testosterone secondary amenorrhea, or secondary adrenocortical deficiency have all been reported.

Biopsy of the hypothalamus or pituitary gland and stalk usually can be avoided if the typical pattern of neuroimaging abnormalities is recognized and evidence of sarcoidosis is found in another organ. Assessment of the overall functioning of the pituitary axis through studies of hormone levels and electrolytes is mandatory. In patients with known sarcoidosis, the possibility of endocrine dysfunction should be considered frequently when evaluating other nonspecific complaints such as fatigue, generalized weakness, and weight change.

The treatment of hypothalamic and pituitary sarcoidosis generally is the same as that outlined above for intracranial disease and meningeal disease. Response to treatment with corticosteroids alone has occurred in some cases.

Sarcoid myopathy

Although asymptomatic myopathy seen as granuloma infiltration in skeletal muscle may occur in as many as 50% of patients with sarcoidosis, symptomatic sarcoid myopathy is rare, occurring in 1% or 2% of patients.[54,55] Sarcoid myopathy may present as a slow chronic wasting process, acute myositis, or nodular myositis. The serum level of creatine kinase usually is increased in acute myopathic conditions but may be normal in slow progressive disease. The diagnosis is suggested by abnormalities (myopathic motor unit potentials) on EMG, and it may also be supported by neuroimaging with gallium scanning or MRI findings.

Acute myositis usually responds to high-dose corticosteroid treatment; however, slow progressive sarcoid myopathy appears to be more refractory to this treatment. Treatment with prednisone at 1 mg/kg daily, followed by gradually tapering doses over a 6-month period, has been proposed. Steroid-sparing agents can be given in cases of refractory disease.

Refractory or severe neurosarcoidosis

Treatment of severe, recurrent, or refractory neurosarcoidosis should be individualized. The side-effect profile, ease of use, and therapeutic limitations of the medication should be considered. When optimized corticosteroid therapy has been inadequate in controlling neurosarcoidosis, treatment with an alternative agent can result in improved functional outcome in about 10% to 20% of patients.[24] Each of at least two or three agents in addition to corticosteroids should be given for several months before concluding that the disease is truly refractory. When the condition of patients with known systemic sarcoidosis and neurological disease deteriorates progressively despite optimized therapy, biopsy may be important to establish an alternative diagnosis.[56]

A few particular clinical scenarios of intracranial sarcoidosis seem to be most associated with severe disability and mortality. As mentioned above, aseptic meningitis with hydrocephalus can present acutely as a life-threatening problem and may lead to a chronic or relapsing course despite aggressive intervention. The other clinical scenario we have found most troubling involves seizures and encephalopathy in association with diffuse deep white matter lesions (identified with MRI or other neuroimaging techniques), presumably related to inflammatory vasculopathy.[57] In these scenarios, initial treatment with very high doses of corticosteroids (15 mg/kg daily for 3 to 5 days of intravenous methylprednisolone) and the earlier addition of immunosuppressants may be warranted.

Dosing regimens of medications for patients with refractory neurosarcoidosis remain conjectural. Experience has shown that patients tend to have the best response when they receive maintenance therapy with at least a modest corticosteroid regimen (prednisone 10 to 20 mg daily) when another immunosuppressant is added. The usual doses of immunosuppressants are listed in Table 135.1. We generally seek to lower the total leukocyte count to approximately 3500/mm^3 or the lymphocyte count to 700 to 1000/mm^3.

Other therapeutic agents that have shown promise for the treatment of neurosarcoidosis have been used in a very limited fashion or have been applied only to other forms of sarcoidosis. The latter group includes thalidomide[58,59] and pentoxifylline.[60] Sharma[61] treated a small number of cases of neurosarcoidosis with hydroxychloroquine and reported some success. There also are a few reports on the experience with chlorambucil therapy.[24,26] In fliximab, a monoclonal antibody against tumor necrosis factor alpha may have a role in the treatment of severe disease.

References

1. Stern BJ, Krumholz A, Johns C, et al. Sarcoidosis and its neurological manifestations. Arch Neurol 1985;42: 909–917
2. Delaney P. Neurologic manifestations in sarcoidosis: review of the literature, with a report of 23 cases. Ann Intern Med 1977;87:336–345
3. Rybicki BA, Major M, Popovich J Jr, et al. Racial differences in sarcoidosis incidence: a 5-year study in a health maintenance organization. Am J Epidemiol 1997; 145:234–241
4. Henke CE, Henke G, Elveback LR, et al. The epidemiology of sarcoidosis in Rochester, Minnesota: a population-based study of incidence and survival. Am J Epidemiol 1986;123:840–845
5. Scott TF, Seay AR, Goust JM. Pattern and concentration of IgG in cerebrospinal fluid in neurosarcoidosis. Neurology 1989;39:1637–1639

6. Borucki SJ, Nguyen BV, Ladoulis CT, McKendall RR. Cerebrospinal fluid immunoglobulin abnormalities in neurosarcoidosis. Arch Neurol 1989;46:270–273

7. Moller DR. Cells and cytokines involved in the pathogenesis of sarcoidosis. Sarcoidosis Vasc Diffuse Lung Dis 1999;16:24–31

8. Gudeman SK, Selhorst JB, Susac JO, Waybright EA. Sarcoid optic neuropathy. Neurology 1982;32:597–603

9. Scott TF. Neurosarcoidosis: progress and clinical aspects. Neurology 1993;43:8–12

10. Scott TF. Cerebral herniation after lumbar puncture in sarcoid meningitis. Clin Neurol Neurosurg 2000;102: 26–28

11. Foley KT, Howell JD, Junck L. Progression of hydrocephalus during corticosteroid therapy for neurosarcoidosis. Postgrad Med J 1989;65:481–484

12. Spencer N, Ross G, Helm G, et al. Aqueductal obstruction in sarcoidosis. Clin Neuropathol 1989;8:158–161

13. Scott TF, Brillman J. Shunt-responsive dementia in sarcoid meningitis: role of magnetic resonance imaging and cisternography. J Neuroimaging 2000;10:185–186

14. Cahill DW, Salcman M. Neurosarcoidosis: a review of the rarer manifestations. Surg Neurol 1981;15:204–211

15. Whelan MA, Stern J. Sarcoidosis presenting as a posterior fossa mass. Surg Neurol 1981;15:455–457

16. Clark WC, Acker JD, Dohan FC Jr, Robertson JH. Presentation of central nervous system sarcoidosis as intracranial tumors. J Neurosurg 1985;63:851–856

17. Brooks ML, Wang AM, Black PM, Haikal N. Subdural mass lesion secondary to sarcoid granuloma: MR and CT findings and differential diagnosis. Comput Med Imaging Graph 1989;13:199–205

18. Scott TF, Brillman J, Marquardt M. Slowly progressive en-plaque intracranial sarcoidosis: magnetic resonance imaging and biopsy appearance. J Neuroimaging 1993;3:202–204

19. Miller DH, Kendall BE, Barter S, et al. Magnetic resonance imaging in central nervous system sarcoidosis. Neurology 1988;38:378–383

20. Smith AS, Meisler DM, Weinstein MA, et al. High-signal periventricular lesions in patients with sarcoidosis: neurosarcoidosis or multiple sclerosis? AJR Am J Roentgenol 1989;153:147–152

21. Sherman JL, Stern BJ. Sarcoidosis of the CNS: comparison of unenhanced and enhanced MR images. AJR Am J Roentgenol 1990;155:1293–1301

22. Lexa FJ, Grossman RI. MR of sarcoidosis in the head and spine: spectrum of manifestations and radiographic response to steroid therapy. AJNR Am J Neuroradiol 1994;15:973–982

23. Christoforidis GA, Spickler EM, Recio MV, Mehta BM. MR of CNS sarcoidosis: correlation of imaging features to clinical symptoms and response to treatment. AJNR Am J Neuroradiol 1999;20:655–669

24. Agbogu BN, Stern BJ, Sewell C, Yang G. Therapeutic considerations in patients with refractory neurosarcoidosis. Arch Neurol 1995;52:875–879

25. Stern BJ, Schonfeld SA, Sewell C, et al. The treatment of neurosarcoidosis with cyclosporine. Arch Neurol 1992;49:1065–1072

26. Baughman RP, Lower EE. Steroid-sparing alternative treatments for sarcoidosis. Clin Chest Med 1997; 18:853–864

27. Junger SS, Stern BJ, Levine SR, et al. Intramedullary spinal sarcoidosis: clinical and magnetic resonance imaging characteristics. Neurology 1993;43:333–337

28. Gelwan MJ, Kellen RI, Burde RM, Kupersmith MJ. Sarcoidosis of the anterior visual pathway: successes and failures. J Neurol Neurosurg Psychiatry 1988;51: 1473–1480

29. Garcia-Monco C, Berciano J. Sarcoid meningitis, high adenosine deaminase levels in CSF and results of cranial irradiation (letter). J Neurol Neurosurg Psychiatry 1988;51:1594–1596

30. Feibelman RY, Harman EM. Sarcoid meningoencephalitis treated with high-dosage steroids and radiation (letter). Ann Intern Med 1985;102:136

31. Bejar JM, Kerby GR, Ziegler DK, Festoff BW. Treatment of central nervous system sarcoidosis with radiotherapy. Ann Neurol 1985;18:258–260

32. Grizzanti JM, Knapp AB, Schecter AJ, Williams MH Jr. Treatment of sarcoid meningitis with radiotherapy. Am J Med 1982;73:605–608

33. Rubinstein I, Gray TA, Moldofsky H, Hoffstein V. Neurosarcoidosis associated with hypersomnolence treated with corticosteroids and brain irradiation. Chest 1988;94:205–206

34. Lower EE, Broderick JP, Brott TG, Baughman RP. Diagnosis and management of neurological sarcoidosis. Arch Intern Med 1997;157:1864–1868

35. Chapelon C, Ziza JM, Piette JC, et al. Neurosarcoidosis: signs, course and treatment in 35 confirmed cases. Medicine (Baltimore) 1990;69:261–276

36. Day AL, Sypert GW. Spinal cord sarcoidosis. Ann Neurol 1977;1:79–85

37. Sauter MK, Panitch HS, Kristt DA. Myelopathic neurosarcoidosis: diagnostic value of enhanced MRI. Neurology 1991;41:150–151

38. Terunuma H, Konno H, Iizuka H, et al. Sarcoidosis presenting as progressive myelopathy. Clin Neuropathol 1988;7:77–80

39. Vighetto A, Fischer G, Collet P, et al. Intramedullary sarcoidosis of the cervical spinal cord. J Neurol Neurosurg Psychiatry 1985;48:477–479

40. Clifton AG, Stevens JM, Kapoor R, Rudge P. Spinal cord sarcoidosis with intramedullary cyst formation. Br J Radiol 1990;63:805–808

41. Elkin R, Willcox PA. Neurosarcoidosis. A report of 5 cases. S Afr Med J 1985;67:943–946

42. Kelly RB, Mahoney PD, Cawley KM. MR demonstration of spinal cord sarcoidosis: report of a case. AJNR Am J Neuroradiol 1988;9:197–199

43. Scott TS, Brillman J, Gross JA. Sarcoidosis of the peripheral nervous system. Neurol Res 1993;15:389–390

44. Zuniga G, Ropper AH, Frank J. Sarcoid peripheral neuropathy. Neurology 1991;41:1558–1561

45. Nemni R, Galassi G, Cohen M, et al. Symmetric sarcoid polyneuropathy: analysis of a sural nerve biopsy. Neurology 1981;31:1217–1223

46. Vital C, Aubertin J, Ragnault JM, et al. Sarcoidosis of the peripheral nerve: a histological and ultrastructural study of two cases. Acta Neuropathol (Berl) 1982; 58:111–114

47. Kompf D, Neundorfer B, Kayser-Gatchalian C, et al. Mononeuritis multiplex in Boeck's sarcoidosis [German]. Nervenarzt 1976;47:687–689

48. Baron B, Goldberg AL, Rothfus WE, Sherman RL. CT features of sarcoid infiltration of a lumbosacral nerve root. J Comput Assist Tomogr 1989;13:364–365

49. Oksanen V. Neurosarcoidosis: clinical presentations and course in 50 patients. Acta Neurol Scand 1986; 73:283–290

50. Strickland GT Jr, Moser KM. Sarcoidosis with a Landry-Guillain-Barré syndrome and clinical response to corticosteroids. Am J Med 1967;43:131–135

51. Galassi G, Gibertoni M, Mancini A, et al. Sarcoidosis of the peripheral nerve: clinical, electrophysiological and

histological study of two cases. Eur Neurol 1984;23: 459–465

52. Stuart CA, Neelon FA, Lebovitz HE. Hypothalamic insufficiency: the cause of hypopituitarism in sarcoidosis. Ann Intern Med 1978;88:589–594

53. Raoult D, Guibout M, Jaquet P, et al. Sarcoïdose neuro-endocrinienne: un cas. Ann Méd Interne (Paris) 1984;135:149–152

54. Prayson RA. Granulomatous myositis. Clinicopathologic study of 12 cases. Am J Clin Pathol 1999;112:63–68

55. Ando DG, Lynch JP III, Fantone JC III. Sarcoid myopathy with elevated creatine phosphokinase. Am Rev Respir Dis 1985;131:298–300

56. Peeples DM, Stern BJ, Jiji V, Sahni KS. Germ cell tumors masquerading as central nervous system sarcoidosis. Arch Neurol 1991;48:554–556

57. Krumholz A, Stern BJ, Stern EG. Clinical implications of seizures in neurosarcoidosis. Arch Neurol 1991;48: 842–844

58. Lee JB, Koblenzer PS. Disfiguring cutaneous manifestation of sarcoidosis treated with thalidomide: a case report. J Am Acad Dermatol 1998;39:835–838

59. Rousseau L, Beylot-Barry M, Doutre MS, Beylot C. Cutaneous sarcoidosis successfully treated with low doses of thalidomide (letter). Arch Dermatol 1998; 134:1045–1046

60. Zabel P, Entzian P, Dalhoff K, Schlaak M. Pentoxifylline in treatment of sarcoidosis. Am J Respir Crit Care Med 1997;155:1665–1669

61. Sharma OP. Effectiveness of chloroquine and hydroxychloroquine in treating selected patients with sarcoidosis with neurological involvement. Arch Neurol 1998;55:1248–1254

136 Hypothalamus, Anterior and Posterior Pituitary and Adrenal (Including Disorders of Temperature Regulation)

Paul Cooper

Hypothalamus

Maintaining homeostasis—the constancy of the "internal milieu"—is the primary function of the hypothalamus. From its location above the pituitary, and through its connections with the limbic system, the hypothalamus sends and receives endocrine and neural signals that regulate energy, water and electrolyte balance, body temperature, the response to stress, growth, development and reproduction, immune function and sleep–wake cycles. Although hypothalamic disorders are uncommon, when they do occur, patients present with one (or more commonly two) of the disorders listed in Table 136.1. The causes of hypothalamic dysfunction are listed in Table 136.2. Treatment is very lesion dependent and also must be based on individual patient factors. An overview of the most common forms of therapy is given in Table 136.3.

Disorders of temperature regulation

In an individual at rest, if the hypothalamus did not intervene, metabolic heat would cause the normal body temperature of 37°C (98.6°F) to increase by about 2°C (4°F) per hour. Simple activity, such as walking, would increase that rate of rise by two- to threefold. As body heat increases, the hypothalamus initiates sweating, vasodilation, and increases heart rate to cause heat loss and maintain thermal balance. If body heat falls, the hypothalamus reduces sweating, causes vasoconstriction and may initiate shivering.

Acute hyperthermia In the clinical setting, the most common cause of *acute hyperthermia* will be the response of the hypothalamus to bacterial or other pyrogens. Acute damage to the anterior hypothalamus and preoptic region, as can occur in subarachnoid hemorrhage, stroke, or surgery in the region of the hypothalamus, may lead to temperature elevations up to 41°C (105.8°F). A temperature rise of this magnitude will usually cause depressed level of consciousness. The tachycardia of hypothalamic hyperthermia is said

Table 136.1 Common clinical manifestations of hypothalamic disorders

Disorder	%
Optic nerve or chiasm involvement	78
Corticospinal tract or sensory signs and symptoms	75
Extrapyramidal or cerebellar signs	62
Vomiting	40
Precocious puberty	40
Diabetes Insipidus	35
Hypogonadism	32
Excessive drowsiness	30
Disturbance of temperature regulation	28
Obesity or edema	25
Gelastic seizures	

(From Bronstein et al.,[1] with permission)

Table 136.2 Causes of hypothalamic syndromes

Tumours
  Craniopharyngioma
  Chordoma
  Dermoid
  Epidermoid
  Germ cell tumour
  Hamartoma
  Meningioma
  Glioma
  Pituitary adenoma
  Metastasis

Granulomatous disease
  Tuberculosis
  Sarcoidosis
  Histiocytosis X

Trauma, including surgery

Vascular
  Aneurysm and arteriovenous malformation
  Infarction
  Radiation-induced necrosis

Infection
  Meningitis
  Encephalitis
  Neurosyphilis

Nutritional
  Wernicke's encephalopathy

Other
  Hydrocephalus
  Arachnoid cyst

Table 136.3   Treatment of lesions causing hypothalamic dysfunction

Lesion	Usual treatment	Other treatment	Comments
Craniopharyngioma (2.5% of brain tumours, 5–10% of childhood brain tumors)	Surgery	Partial resection, with postsurgical radiation therapy	Hormonal deficiency is common after surgery and radiation therapy
Germ cell tumors (1% of primary brain tumors in North America but 6% in Japan)	Radiotherapy	Surgery and chemotherapy	Need for pretreatment histological diagnosis is debated
Hamartoma	Management of precocious puberty with long-acting gonadotropin-releasing hormone analogs	Surgery is generally used only for seizure control	90% of patients have precocious puberty May be associated with gelastic seizures
Meningioma	Surgery		Visual loss most common symptom
Glioma (1–3% of brain tumors in children and adolescents)	Controversial—ranges from follow-up only to conventional or stereotactic radiotherapy		Endocrine abnormalities uncommon. 20–23% of optic nerve glioma patients have neurofibromatosis
Chordoma	Surgery		Usually resistant to chemotherapy and radiotherapy
Metastatic tumors (occur in 3.5% of cancer patients) (breast 47%, lung 19%, GI 6%, prostate 6%)	Depends in part on type of tumour—usually radiotherapy	Surgery and chemotherapy	Diabetes insipidus is the first manifestation in 70%
Dermoid and epidermoid tumors	Surgery		Epidermoids are more common
Granulomatous/inflammatory lesions			
Sarcoidosis (5% of cases involve the nervous system, 1.35% the central nervous system, and only 0.53% the hypothalamopituitary	Prednisone 40 mg daily for 2 weeks then reduce to 10–20 mg over 2 weeks, with therapy for 6 months to several years		Diabetes insipidus is seen in 37.5%; 66% have hilar adenopathy
Histiocytosis X—usual type that involves the hypothalamopituitary is Hand–Schüller–Christian disease	Low-dose radiotherapy, corticosteroids and chemotherapy are often tried		Triad of exophthalmos, lytic lesions in bone and diabetes insipidus Diabetes insipidus and hypopituitarism may not resolve with treatment
Tuberculosis	Isoniazid, rifampin and a third drug	Surgical resection of tuberculoma may be necessary	CSF picture is more that of a parameningeal focus of infection rather than tuberculous meningitis
Radiation-induced lesions	Replacement of hormone deficiencies	Radiation-induced gliomas and sarcomas are rare but often fatal	Children and adolescents are more prone to developing hypopituitarism following radiotherapy
Traumatic lesions	Supportive therapy and treatment of hormone deficiencies	Treatment of precocious puberty with long-acting gonadotropin-releasing hormone analogs	

to be less than that seen with hyperthermia secondary to bacterial pyrogens, but patients with suspected hypothalamic hypothermia must be thoroughly investigated for other causes of fever. Treatment of acute hypothalamic hyperthermia is supportive. Patients will usually respond well to cooling blankets to reduce body temperature. By about two weeks after an acute injury the syndrome resolves, although patients who survive may have an ongoing impairment of dissipating body heat in hot environments.

Acute hyperthermia on a hypothalamic basis can usually be readily distinguished from heat-related illness (e.g. heat exhaustion and heat stroke) by virtue of the setting in which it occurs and the clinical picture. Fulminant hyperthermia during anesthesia needs to be thought of in the differential diagnosis of patients with acute anterior hypothalamic injury and temperature rise. The differentiating point in anesthesia-related malignant hyperthermia is the muscular rigidity of rigor mortis-like proportions. Finally, neuroleptic malignant syndrome is the other condition that should be thought of in the differential diagnosis of acute hypothalamic hyperthermia. The clinical settings in which it can occur are:

- Prolonged use or rapid increase in neuroleptic dose
- Use of low-dose neuroleptics in patients with extrapyramidal signs who are on treatment with antiparkinsonian drugs
- Patients with Parkinson's disease who are suddenly withdrawn from antiparkinsonian drugs
- Patients treated with catecholamine-depleting drugs (e.g. tetrabenazine).

In addition to fever, one expects to find impairment of consciousness, autonomic instability (e.g. episodes of pallor, sweating, unstable blood pressure and cardiac arrhythmias) and elevated creatine phosphokinase (CK) levels. Dantrolene, levodopa/carbidopa, bromocriptine and amantadine have all been used in the treatment of the neuroleptic malignant syndrome. There are no controlled trials to guide the clinician. The author's personal preference is to use bromocriptine, as monotherapy, in a dose of 2.5–10 mg orally, three times daily, in addition to general supportive measures.

Chronic hyperthermia Chronic hyperthermia is uncommon when confounding conditions such as malignancy and unrecognized infections have been systematically excluded. It seems to occur either because of ongoing inability to dissipate heat adequately, or because of difficulty in sensing temperature elevations. In general no treatment is necessary, as the elevations are usually mild. Protection from heat stress is indicated. Antipyretics (e.g. salicylates) are ineffective in these individuals because the condition is not due to a prostaglandin-mediated elevation in temperature.

Acute and chronic hypothermia Hypothermia is defined as a core temperature less than 35°C. It may be associated with symptoms of fatigue, decreased alertness, hypoventilation and cardiac arrhythmia. Remember that some devices used clinically for measuring body temperature may not register this low and can miss serious hypothermia. Body temperatures below 32.2°C (90°F) are usually associated with an acute confusional state at the very least, or even frank stupor or coma. *Chronic hypothermia* is uncommon. It has been reported to occur with extensive gliosis of the preoptic anterior hypothalamus, with hypothalamic infarction and following head trauma. Both *acute* and *chronic hypothermia* have been reported in patients with multiple sclerosis.[2,3] Although most cases have been due to demyelination in the hypothalamus, the cause of the hypothermia is not always apparent.[4] Patients with high cervical cord injury may become hypothermic because of their inability to shiver and generate heat, and because of the interruption of the sympathetic connections between the hypothalamus and the thoracic spinal cord. *Acute hypothermia* may occur in a paroxysmal manner. This has led some to postulate that the cause may be epileptic, although only rarely will it respond to

therapy with anticonvulsants.[5] Agenesis of the corpus callosum in association with episodic hyperhidrosis and hypothermia (Shapiro's syndrome) has been found to be caused, in some individuals, by an abnormally low hypothalamic set-point. Symptoms can be controlled with clonidine (an α_2-adrenergic receptor agonist).[6] A similar condition, associated with hyperthermia (so-called "reverse Shapiro's syndrome"), has been found to have a normalization of temperature with low-dose levodopa and hypothermia with higher doses.[7] The differential diagnosis of both acute and chronic hypothermia must include severe hypothyroidism (myxedema coma), Wernicke's disease and drug effects.

Poikilothermia Poikilothermia is a condition in which both heat production and heat dissipation mechanisms are impaired, leading to a tendency for body temperature to fluctuate in parallel with environmental temperature. It is usually seen with damage to the posterior hypothalamus. Patients are seldom aware of this condition, and under most conditions there will be mild hypothermia. Protecting patients from extremes of environmental temperature is the only practical treatment. This is especially important in children who, because of their higher metabolic rates, have a tendency to become hyperthermic more easily than do adults, and who because of their relatively larger surface area can also become hypothermic more easily than adults.

Disorders of food intake

Bilateral destruction of the ventromedial nuclei of the hypothalamus is a well recognized cause of obesity in humans and animals. The most common causes of this are found in Table 136.4. The syndrome of hypothalamic hyperphagia seldom occurs by itself and is often accompanied by evidence of other hypothalamic or parahypothalamic dysfunction (Table 136.5). The obesity in hypothalamic disease is not due to overeating alone: there is evidence that these patients hypersecrete insulin, which contributes to their efficient fat

Table 136.4 Common causes of hypothalamic obesity
Tumor (most commonly craniopharyngioma) Inflammatory or granulomatous lesions Trauma Malignant infiltration (e.g. leukemia)

Table 136.5 Common accompaniments in patients with hypothalamic obesity
Diabetes insipidus Drowsiness Seizures Hypodipsia Anterior pituitary hypofunction Antisocial behavior and aggression

Table 136.6   Syndromes attributed to hypothalamic dysfunction

Syndrome	Clinical features	Pathology	Comments
Diencephalic epilepsy	Episodes of autonomic hyperactivity—flushing, pupillary dilatation, tachycardia, hyperthermia, hypertension and hyperventilation	Described in patients with tumors and other abnormalities in the region of the third ventricle, small thalamic tumors and hypothalamic tumors	Probably not epileptic because EEG does not show seizures and anticonvulsants are usually ineffective. Bromocriptine has been effective in some patients to reduce hyperthermia and diaphoresis. Morphine can terminate episodes in some patients.
Gelastic seizures	Ictal laughter; may go on to multiple seizure types with cognitive decline	Hypothalamic hamartoma	Seizures were previously thought to originate in the temporal lobes; now evidence suggests that the hamartoma itself is the origin of the epileptic discharges
Frölich syndrome	Delayed puberty and obesity	Damage to the ventromedial nucleus of the hypothalamus, with involvement of the median eminence by tumor	The term is really of historical interest only, the syndrome having been described by Frölich in 1901
Kleine–Levin syndrome	Rare, self-limited disorder Seen most commonly in adolescent males but has been described in females Recurring episodes of hypersomnia, excessive food intake and psychic alteration	MRI scans usually normal Neuroendocrinological findings usually normal	May not be a distinct entity but represent a variety of neurophysiological/neuropsychiatric disorders
Diencephalic syndrome of infancy and childhood	Emaciation despite normal or excess food intake and increased appetite High energy, hyperactive children Happy disposition/euphoric Pale skin Horizontal nystagmus (50%) May have tendency to hypoglycemia	Hypothalamic glioma or astrocytoma	Treatment with radiotherapy or chemotherapy has been helpful in individual patients
Laurence–Moon–Bardet–Biedl syndrome	Autosomal dominant Retinal degeneration (rarely retinitis pigmentosa), extra digits (polydactyly), mental retardation, hypogonadism, hypogenitalism, obesity and spastic paraparesis Diabetes insipidus is common	Neuropathologic examination of the pituitary and hypothalamus has been normal, as has hypothalamopituitary testing	Probably actually two syndromes: Laurence–Moon: polydactyly is rare but paraparesis common; Bardet–Biedl syndrome: mental retardation, if present at all, is mild Hypogenitalism occurs in males only
Alström–Hallgren syndrome	Retinal dysplasia, deafness, obesity, non-insulin dependent diabetes mellitus and hypogenitalism	Pathological examination of the pituitary and hypothalamus reveals no abnormality	
Prader–Labhard–Willi syndrome	Obesity, hypotonia, mental retardation, hypogonadism, short stature, small hands and feet	No hypothalamic abnormalities on MRI or pathological examination Genetically there is loss of a paternal gene or genes on chromosome 15, or there is uniparental disomy	
Wolff's periodic syndrome	Periodic hyperthermia, vomiting, weight loss and elevated serum cortisol	Unknown	Single case described in 1964 Of mainly historical interest Cases of periodic hyperthermia have been described with Rathke's cleft cyst and with dysfunction of the central thermoregulatory area

storage. Treatment of hypothalamic obesity is difficult and there are no controlled studies to guide the clinician. Serotonergic substances (i.e. fluoxetine and fenfluramine) failed to alter either food intake or weight in one patient.[8] This may be because the effect of these compounds is blocked by damage to the hypothala-

mus. This seems to be the case for leptin, the peptide that normally inhibits appetite via hypothalamic receptors. Roth et al.[9] found that serum leptin concentrations were elevated in 11 postoperative craniopharyngioma patients. They postulated a disturbed feedback mechanism from the hypothalamic leptin receptors to the adipose tissue. Leptin stimulates the release of α-melanocyte-stimulating hormone (α-MSH) from the hypothalamus. α-MSH binds at the Mc4r melanocortin receptor subtype to decrease food intake and increase energy expenditure, as well as to inhibit the release of agouti-related peptide (AgRP) an antagonist of the Mc4r receptor. Weight loss or starvation reduce leptin levels, resulting in a rise in AgRP and subsequent increased food intake and decreased energy expenditure. Mc4r receptor agonists might be used to bypass the leptin step in individuals with abnormal leptin sensitivity and bring about weight control.[10] Cholecystokinin (CCK), a peptide known to produce satiety, has been studied as a possible treatment for hypothalamic obesity. An 8-amino acid analog of cholecystokinin (CCK-8), when infused into both controls and patients with hypothalamic obesity, produced satiety.[11] Unfortunately, such continuous infusion is not practical for long-term therapy. Octreotide (a long-acting analog of somatostatin) has been shown to be effective at promoting weight loss in patients with hypothalamic obesity.[12] The mechanism of action is thought to be through a reduction in insulin secretion. Because insulin tends to "escape" from the suppressing effect of octreotide after only a few days, long-term therapy may not be feasible.

Syndromes associated with or attributed to hypothalamic dysfunction

There are a number of clinical syndromes in which dysfunction of the hypothalamus has been implicated. The main features of these are summarized in Table 136.6.

Over the years, because of the hypothalamic abnormalities that occur in patients with anorexia nervosa, and to a lesser extent with bulimia nervosa, various authors have postulated a hypothalamic cause for these conditions. In most instances, the so-called hypothalamic abnormalities can be explained on the basis of severe weight loss or accompanying mood disturbance. Whether an underlying hypothalamic abnormality triggers the condition remains unproven. There is growing evidence that there is a substantial genetic contribution to these disorders.[13] Also, persisting elevation of elevated 5-hydroxyindoleacetic acid levels in cerebral spinal fluid following recovery, as well as polymorphisms in 5-HT2a (serotonin) receptors all suggest that a disturbance in serotonin activity may make certain individuals vulnerable to developing this condition.[14]

The pituitary gland

The posterior pituitary gland

The posterior pituitary gland secretes two hormones: oxytocin and vasopressin. The physiological role for oxytocin in humans is unclear. Women who are deficient in oxytocin will go into labor and deliver spontaneously and can even breastfeed, although labor may be prolonged and contractions weak. The role of oxytocin in the human male is unknown.

Vasopressin is the pituitary hormone that is essen-

tial for water balance. To maintain water homeostasis there must be intact thirst and drinking centers in the hypothalamus, there must be ready access to water, renal function must be normal, and vasopressin must be present.

Diabetes insipidus Neurogenic (central) diabetes insipidus is characterized by thirst, polyuria, polydipsia and an inability to maintain water homeostasis in the face of fluid restriction. The clinical features of neurogenic diabetes insipidus are summarized in Table 136.7 and its common causes in Table 136.8.

After metabolic disturbances, drug effects and osmotic diuresis have been ruled out, careful examination of the patient to determine volume status (including a review of weight and intake-and-output charts) is essential. The single best test in the diagnosis of patients with polyuria is the *water deprivation test* (see Box 136.1).

Acute diabetes insipidus, in the alert, oriented patient, can be treated by allowing free access to water. The patient's endogenous fluid balance mechanisms will maintain homeostasis. If the patient is having to drink more than 7 L/day, or is lethargic or unconscious, exogenous vasopressin may be used. In calculating fluid requirements for the unconscious or lethargic patient, remember that in the afebrile adult insensible losses approximate 1 L every 24 hours. Therefore, in any 24-hour period most patients with diabetes insipidus will require 40–60 mmol of potassium chloride (KCl) and 1 L of 0.9% sodium

Table 136.7 Clinical features of diabetes insipidus
Urine specific gravity 1.000–1.005
Urine osmolality always <300 mmol/kg (may be as low as 50 mmol/kg)
Urine excretion >2 mL/kg/h (8–10 L/24 h up to 20 L/24 h)
Plasma osmolality >300 mmol/kg
Serum sodium ≥143 mmol/L

Table 136.8 Common causes of neurogenic (central) diabetes insipidus
Familial or congenital
Dominant or recessive inheritance
Idiopathic
Post-traumatic
Post-neurosurgery
Neoplastic
Granulomatous
Histiocytosis X
Sarcoidosis
Infectious
Tuberculosis
Basal meningitis (e.g. syphilis)
Vascular
Aneurysm (with or without subarachnoid hemorrhage)
Sickle cell disease
Pituitary apoplexy/infarction
Stroke

Box 136.1   Water deprivation test

1. Free access to water overnight.
2. Light breakfast. No coffee, tea or nicotine.
3. Start fluid deprivation at 0800 hours – patient may have dry food if desired
4. Weigh patient every hour. Test is stopped if weight drops by 5% or more.
5. Measure serum and urine osmolality every hour.
6. Ensure that urine osmolality has reached a plateau (i.e. no greater than 30 mmol/kg change in osmolality between successive specimens). If a plateau is not reached, continue the water deprivation. Ensure the patient is not taking water surreptitiously. The patient's serum osmolality should rise above 290 mmol/kg before it is concluded that adequate dehydration has been achieved.
7. When a plateau is reached, give desmopressin (DDAVP) 2 μg i.v.
8. Allow patient free access to food and water.
9. Measure urine osmolality at 1, 2, 4, 8, and 12 hours after DDAVP.

Serum osmolality should rise during the test. If the urine osmolality following the period of dehydration is more than 750 mmol/kg then central diabetes insipidus is excluded. Urine osmolality of less than 300 mmol/kg suggests either neurogenic (central) or nephrogenic diabetes insipidus. In central diabetes insipidus there should be a good response to DDAVP with urine osmolality higher than 750 mmol/kg. Patients with compulsive polydipsia show a slow rise in serum osmolality with water deprivation.

---

chloride. The replacement of urinary losses, on top of this, should be with 5% dextrose and water. Replacement of urinary losses with sodium-containing solutions (even 0.2% NaCl) can lead to salt overload, thereby aggravating the diuresis and causing electrolyte disturbance.

In *chronic diabetes insipidus* treatment with 1-deamino-D-arginine vasopressin (DDAVP) is preferred. It can be given by several routes and the doses are quite variable (see Box 136.2). Avoidance of water intoxication is key.

The anterior pituitary gland

Pituitary adenomas Symptomatic pituitary adenomas account for between 10% and 25% of all intracranial neoplasms.[15] Pituitary tumors that are entirely asymptomatic clinically have been variously reported to occur in 3.7% to 20% of CT scans, 10% of MRI scans and 1.5% to 26.7% of autopsies.[16] The various types of pituitary adenoma and other entities to be considered in the differential diagnosis are listed in Table 136.9.

Prolactin-secreting adenomas Prolactin-secreting pituitary tumors (prolactinomas) account for 60% of all pituitary tumors.[17] Prolactinomas cause the clinical syndrome of amenorrhea/galactorrhea in menstruating women. They may cause little in the way of hormonal symptoms in postmenopausal women, although galactorrhea can occur. In males they are often asymptomatic, producing only decreased libido. Prolactinomas are rare in children but are part of the differential diagnosis of delayed puberty.

Microadenomas (tumors ≤10 mm) in men and in women who do not wish to conceive can be observed. The main concern with observation is that in the long term it will put the patient at risk for developing osteoporosis. In women this risk can be reduced by treatment with the oral contraceptive, without fear of stimulating tumor growth.[18] In patients with macroadenomas (tumors >10 mm) initial treatment is with dopamine agonists to reduce tumor bulk and, if

possible, normalize prolactin levels. The various dopamine agonists used are listed in Table 136.10. In women who wish to conceive, dopamine agonists are discontinued as soon as conception has been confirmed. These women need to be followed carefully during their pregnancy to ensure that adenoma

Table 136.9   Differential diagnosis of pituitary and parapituitary lesions

Pituitary adenomas
Growth-hormone secreting
Prolactin secreting
Thyrotropin secreting
ACTH secreting
Gonadotropin secreting
Plurihormonal secreting
Non-secreting

Congenital anomalies
Empty sella syndrome
Rathke's cleft cyst
Encephalocele
Suprasellar arachnoid cysts

Neoplasms
Craniopharyngioma
Optic chiasm and hypothalamic glioma
Hypothalamic hamartoma
Sellar and parasellar meningioma
Schwannoma and neurofibroma
Germ cell tumors
Dermoid and Epidermoid
Metastasis

Other
Pituitary apoplexy
Aneurysm
Sarcoidosis
Histiocytosis X
Tuberculosis
Lymphocytic hypophysitis

Sphenoid sinus disease – granulomatous, infectious, malignant, inflammatory

Box 136.2   Vasopressin and the treatment of diabetes insipidus

1. Aqueous vasopressin
2. DDAVP:
   Intranasal 10–40 μg qhs (children generally require half that amount) (start with 1–2 μg and titrate upward to avoid water intoxication)
   Subcutaneous or i.v. 1–2 μg every 12 h
   Oral 50–400 μg by mouth every 12 h

Frequent monitoring of electrolytes is necessary to avoid hyponatraemia. In general one tries to slightly underreplace the patient and let them drink to "top up" their requirements.

Table 136.10   Dopamine agonists used in the treatment of hyperprolactinemia

Drug	Pharmacology	Dose	Comments
Bromocriptine	Semisynthetic ergot alkaloid—D_1 and D_2 receptor agonist	Start with 0.625 mg by mouth at bedtime, taken with food Increase as tolerated, every 3–5 days to 2.5 mg twice daily, and then make further increases based on prolactin levels	Drug can be given intravaginally to reduce stomach upset Resistance to the effects of bromocriptine occurs in up to 18% of patients
Long-acting bromocriptine	More prolonged action	50–75 mg by i.m. injection monthly	Side effects similar to oral preparation but tend to occur only the first few days after injection
Cabergoline	Ergoline derivative—higher D_2 receptor affinity than bromocriptine and more prolonged action	0.5 mg once a week or 0.25 mg every Monday and Thursday, to a maximum of 1 mg twice weekly	May be useful in patients who are resistant to bromocriptine or troubled by its side effects
Pergolide	Ergot derivative—long-acting	0.05 mg/day, increased every 3–5 days to 0.3 mg once daily	Similar side-effect profile to bromocriptine
Lisuride	Ergot derivative	0.4–2.0 mg/day given in 3 or more divided doses	Similar side-effect profile to bromocriptine
Quinagolide	Long-acting non-ergot octahydrobenzyl(g)-quinoline—D_2 receptor activity	0.1–0.4 mg once daily	

expansion does not occur. At the first sign of any visual field change or other visual symptoms, MRI or CT should be performed.

Patients who fail to respond to dopamine agonists or who are unable to tolerate the side effects can be treated with surgery. Macroadenomas that continue to grow following surgery can be treated with dopamine agonists or radiotherapy, or both.

Growth hormone-secreting adenomas   Excessive growth hormone levels prior to fusion of the epiphyses leads to the syndrome of pituitary gigantism. After epiphyseal closure, it causes acromegaly. Most patients with acromegaly (over 75%) have macroadenomas at the time of presentation. The primary treatment for acromegaly is surgery. If, after surgery, growth hormone levels fail to suppress to less than 1 μg/L following an oral glucose load, then patients are usually

sent for radiotherapy. Radiotherapy may take up to 15 years to reduce plasma growth hormone levels to the 2 to 5 μg/L range, and full normalization is unusual. While waiting for radiotherapy to have its full effect, treatment with somatostatin analogs (Table 136.11) can be used to normalize growth hormone levels.

Dopamine agonists will decrease growth hormone secretion in patients with acromegaly but seldom normalize the levels. Bromocriptine has been used in doses of 7.5–80 mg/day (in three or four divided doses). Cabergoline has been used in doses of 1–2 mg/week, and quinagolide in doses of 0.3–0.6 mg/day. Most frequently, the dopamine agonists are combined with somatostatin analogs in patients who have completed their surgery and radiotherapy.

Corticotropin-secreting adenomas   Cushing's disease is the result of excessive adrenocorticotrophic hormone

Table 136.11   Somatostatin analogs

Analog	Pharmacology	Dose	Comments
Octreotide	Long-acting synthetic somatostatin analog	100 µg subcutaneously every 8 h, increase as necessary to maximum of 500 µg per dose	40 times more potent than somatostatin at suppressing growth hormone levels Causes some tumor shrinkage 10% of patients do not respond Short-term side effects include diarrhea, fat malabsorption, nausea and flatulence 25% of patients develop asymptomatic gallstones
Long-acting octreotide	Long-acting preparation	20–40 mg every 4–6 weeks by i.m. injection	
Lanreotide	Somatostatin analog	30 mg given every 7–14 days by i.m. injection	Fewer gastrointestinal side effects than octreotide

(ACTH) secretion by a pituitary tumor. Cushing's syndrome is excessive circulating cortisol levels from any cause. Corticotropin-secreting adenomas account for only about 15% of all pituitary tumors, but they are responsible for more than two-thirds of cases of Cushing's syndrome.[17]

Corticotropin-secreting microadenomas can be removed totally in 90% of patients, with complete cure of the condition. In those in whom a surgical cure is not achieved, over 80% will be cured within four years following radiotherapy.[17]

Overall, the medical therapy of Cushing's disease has been quite disappointing. One helpful aspect is the use of inhibitors of glucocorticoid synthesis to lower cortisol levels, in preparation for surgery, while waiting for radiation effect, or in patients with inoperable tumors. The use of these medications is discussed in the section below on the adrenal gland.

Thyrotropin-secreting adenomas   Thyrotropin-secreting adenomas are rare (less than 1% of pituitary tumors) and tend to be large at the time of diagnosis. Patients present with goitre and hyperthyroidism, with inappropriately "normal range" or elevated thyroid-stimulating hormone (TSH) levels. Reliance on TSH alone in these patients may lead to a wrong diagnosis. In a patient who is clinically hyperthyroid, even if the TSH is "normal" or elevated, it is important to measure both free T_3 and free T_4 to determine thyroid status definitively.

Treatment generally relies on a surgical approach to remove as much of the tumor as is safely possible; this is then followed by radiotherapy. Such an approach will restore normal thyroid function in only a third of patients. The next step often involves radioactive ablation of the thyroid gland; however, careful follow-up is needed to ensure that this does not result in accelerated growth of the pituitary adenoma.

Octreotide (50–750 µg subcutaneously every eight hours) can normalize thyroid function and cause adenoma shrinkage and is a useful adjunct in patients who have had surgery and radiotherapy, while awaiting an effect, or in whom surgery and radiotherapy

cannot be used. Lanreotide (30 mg intramuscularly every two weeks) is also effective.

Gonadotropin-secreting adenomas   Most gonadotropin-secreting adenomas present clinically as non-secretory tumors. Although the presence of such a tumor may be suspected when luteinizing hormone (LH) and follicle-stimulating hormone (FSH) levels are high, often the levels are normal because, rather than secreting intact hormone, the tumors secrete only α and β subunits that are not detected in clinical assays of LH and FSH.

Treatment for these tumors is surgery, followed by radiation. Medical treatment has not been overly promising. Octreotide may help shrink tumors in a minority of patients, and is probably worth trying in those who have not responded to standard therapy.

Hypopituitarism   Vasopressin, thyroid hormone and cortisol are essential for life. Patients can survive without sex steroid and growth hormone, although their health will be affected. There seem to be few, if any, health effects from prolactin or oxytocin deficiency.

Prolactin deficiency   In general, hypoprolactinemia is not treated and has been thought to have little effect, if any, on health. There are, however, scattered case reports suggesting that prolactin may have a number of important functions. It has been suggested that one of the causes of male infertility is hypoprolactinemia, and that this can be corrected by treatment with exogenous human prolactin.[19] At present such treatment is only available as part of a research protocol.

Growth hormone deficiency   The treatment of growth hormone deficiency in adults is possible, but to date the risks and benefits remain uncertain. The interested reader is directed to a recently published monograph that deals with this problem in some detail.[20]

In general, the first step is to determine whether a patient is deficient in growth hormone or not. In an adult with known cause for pituitary insufficiency, a rise of growth hormone of less than 3 µg/L in response to insulin-induced hypoglycemia is taken as evidence for growth hormone deficiency. If isolated growth hormone deficiency is suspected, in either a child or an adult, a second provocative test must also be abnormal before the diagnosis is confirmed.

Growth hormone is given in a dose of 0.15–0.30 mg/day (the conversion factor for IU is to multiply by 3). This is given subcutaneously and the dose increased by 0.15 mg/day each month to a maximum of 1.0 mg/day. Patients must be monitored for side effects, such as hypertension and glucose intolerance. If no benefit is achieved after six months, the hormone is discontinued.

Growth hormone secretagogues or growth hormone-releasing peptides can be used to stimulate growth hormone release in individuals with intact pituitary function. Such compounds may prove useful in the treatment of individuals with low-normal growth hormone levels.

Gonadotropin deficiency In males, if fertility is not an issue, LH and FSH deficiency is treated with testosterone. Different formulations are available (Table 136.12). In women, treatment depends on whether the individual is pre- or postmenopausal. In a premenopausal woman an oral contraceptive containing 20–35 µg of ethinylestradiol is indicated.[21] In a postmenopausal woman with an intact uterus, cyclical estrogen and progesterone therapy is given (e.g. conjugated estrogen 0.625–1.25 mg/day for 25 days, with medroxyprogesterone 5–10 mg/day for the last 10–14 days). If the uterus is absent, then the estrogen is administered continuously.

If fertility is desired, therapy with human chorionic gonadotropin (hCG) and human menopausal gonadotropin can be used, or gonadotropins produced by recombinant DNA technology. In males hCG is administered first, to activate testicular testosterone production by the Leydig cells and then, when testosterone levels have been normal for two months, FSH is added to stimulate spermatogenesis. FSH treatment may need to be given for six months to a year. In females, FSH is given to induce follicular maturation and then a single bolus of LH is given to induce ovulation.

Gonadotropin-releasing hormone (GnRH), given in a pulsatile fashion, can treat crypto-orchism and delayed puberty, and be used to initiate spermatogenesis in males with hypogonadotropic hypogonadism and normal pituitary function[22] or to induce normal ovarian function in females with hypogonadotropic hypogonadism and normal pituitary function.[23]

Corticotropin deficiency Patients with adrenocorticotropic hormone (ACTH) deficiency tend to have less severe cortisol deficiency than those with primary adrenal failure. Cortisone acetate (25 mg in the morning and 12.5 mg in the evening) has been the traditional replacement therapy, providing both glucocorticoid and mineralocorticoid effect. Prednisone (5 mg in the morning, with or without 2.5 mg in the evening) is an alternative and is cheaper than cortisone acetate. On this dose, some patients will develop signs of Cushing's syndrome. If this occurs, the first step is to discontinue the evening dose of prednisone. If the problem does not resolve then the dose can be reduced to 3–4 mg of prednisone daily. Most patients with pituitary insufficiency will not require mineralocorticoid supplementation with fludrocortisone. Glucocorticoid deficiency can also be treated with hydrocortisone 15 mg a.m. and 5 mg p.m. A more physiological way of administering steroid supplementation is to give 10 mg of hydrocortisone or equivalent on awakening, followed by 5 mg at noon and 5 mg in the early evening.[24]

Thyrotropin deficiency Pituitary or secondary hypothyroidism is unusual and may be missed if clinicians ignore their suspicions and request only a TSH level. TSH levels are often within the normal range in secondary or tertiary hypothyroidism, and it is only if the free T_3 and free T_4 are ordered that the diagnosis will be confirmed. The treatment of choice for pituitary or hypothalamic hypothyroidism is L-thyroxine. Before thyroxine is started hypocortisolism must be treated if present, otherwise it may precipitate an episode of acute adrenal insufficiency. In healthy young adults, thyroxine can be started in a dose of 100 µg daily. In the elderly, or in patients with a history of cardiac disease, a starting dose of 25 µg daily is more appropriate. Increases are made slowly every three to four weeks. In patients with pituitary hypothyroidism, the TSH level as a measure of adequate hormone replacement is lost. In general, one

---

Table 136.12   Preparations available for testosterone replacement

Preparation	Dose	Comments
Testosterone enanthate or cipionate	200–300 mg i.m. every 2–3 weeks	
Testosterone transdermal – scrotal	4–6 mg/day	May cause pruritus, blistering and redness
Testosterone transdermal – non-scrotal	2.5–5 mg/day	
Testosterone undecanoate	40 mg orally 3 or 4 times daily	Short-acting—gives more erratic levels and compliance is often a problem because of the frequent dosing necessary
Check hemoglobin (or hematocrit) and prostate-specific antigen before and during therapy.		

Table 136.13   Glucocorticoids used clinically

Duration of action	Glucocorticoid potency	Equivalent dose (mg)	Mineralocorticoid activity	$T_{\frac{1}{2}}$ h
Short				
Cortisol (hydrocortisone)	1	20	Yes	1.3–1.9
Cortisone	0.8	25	Yes	0.5
Prednisone	4	5	No	3.4–3.8
Prednisolone	4	5	No	2.1–3.5
Methylprednisolone	5	4	No	1.3–3.1
Intermediate				
Triamcinolone	5	4	No	
Long				
Betamethasone	25	0.60	No	
Dexamethasone	30	0.75	No	1.8–4.7

Modified from Axelrod 1976.[25]

should rely on the free T_4 and free T_3 levels as well as the clinical response. Patients often require free T_4 levels that are at the upper end or just above the normal range in order to be clinically euthyroid. The free T_3 level will usually be in the middle of the therapeutic range.

The adrenal gland

The adrenal cortex

Glucocorticoid therapy Systemic glucocorticoid administration is used in a number of different neurological conditions. The commonly used glucocorticoids can be distinguished on their *half life* $(T_{\frac{1}{2}})$, their *duration of action*, their *potency* and their *mineralocorticoid activity* (Table 136.13). Circulating half-life bears little relationship to glucocorticoid potency. This is because the duration in the circulation does not correlate with the action of the compound, as steroids bind to intracellular receptors to produce their effect. Compounds that induce hepatic enzyme activity may increase the glucocorticoid requirements of patients with glucocorticoid deficiency, or cause breakthrough of disease symptoms in patients treated with glucocorticoids. Glucocorticoids will increase the need for insulin or oral hypoglycemic agents in diabetics. In patients treated with digoxin, glucocorticoid-induced hypokalemia may cause digoxin cardiac toxicity. The use of glucocorticoids can be associated with a number of different side effects (Table 136.14).

Suppression of the hypothalamopituitary–adrenal (HPA) axis in patients treated with glucocorticoids is a valid concern. If a patient has received 20 mg of prednisone or more per day for more than 5 days, HPA axis suppression should be presumed to be present until proved otherwise. If the daily dose is closer to the physiological range (i.e. 7.5–10 mg/day), then suppression should be presumed to be present after one month of therapy.

Alternate-day glucocorticoid therapy can minimize the adverse effects of glucocorticoids while at the same time ensuring appropriate disease control. The use of alternate-day therapy in giant cell arteritis is

Table 136.14   Possible glucocorticoid side effects

Endocrine
Obesity, including lipomatosis
Hyperglycemia
Sodium retention and hypokalemia
Hypothalamopituitary–adrenal axis suppression
Osteoporosis

Cardiovascular
Hypertension
Congestive failure

Gastrointestinal
Peptic ulcer disease
Pancreatitis

Ophthalmological
Cataract
Glaucoma
Exophthalmos

Neurological
Seizures
Personality change, euphoria and psychosis
Myopathy
Benign intracranial hypertension

Orthopedic
Vertebral body collapse
Aseptic necrosis of the femoral head

Dermatological
Acne
Thin skin, easy bruising
Facial erythema
Impaired wound healing

Immunological
Susceptibility to infections
Neutrophilia
Reactivation of tuberculosis

unproven. It can be used in myasthenia gravis, Duchenne muscular dystrophy, dermatomyositis, idiopathic polyneuropathy, Sjögren's syndrome and sarcoidosis. Daily glucocorticoid dosing may be necessary to control breakthrough symptoms on the second day. This is seen most commonly in patients with rheumatoid arthritis, systemic lupus erythematosus, polyarteritis, proctocolitis and giant cell arteritis. In such patients, therapy should be given as a single daily dose in the morning to reduce HPA suppression.

One cannot give hard and fast recommendations with respect to tapering glucocorticoids, as the rate of taper is very dependent on the type of disease being treated. In a patient with multiple sclerosis in whom prednisone is being used to shorten an acute attack, tapering by 5–10 mg every three to five days is reasonable. In myasthenia gravis, tapering by 5 mg per dose may be done as slowly as every two months. A similarly slow taper may be necessary in patients with inflammatory conditions, such as polyarteritis or temporal arteritis.

When switching patients to alternate-day glucocorticoid therapy, one might initially taper the dose by 5 mg/day every three to five days until the dose was reduced to 40 mg/day and then continue to taper by 5 mg/day on the alternate day only, every three to five days, until the patient was taking 40 mg every other day. Thereafter, further tapering could occur. The rate of taper and the ability to go to alternate-day therapy is very dependent on the type of disease being treated and its activity. If there is a disease flare during tapering, or if symptoms of steroid withdrawal develop, then increase the dose to the last asymptomatic level or slightly higher and taper more slowly.

The standard perioperative or "stress" dose of glucocorticoid in patients with suspected HPA suppression or adrenal insufficiency has traditionally been hydrocortisone 100 mg intravenously every eight hours. Salem et al[26] have studied the problem and devised more physiological recommendations (Table 136.15).

Osteoporosis is a concerning and potentially avoidable complication of long-term glucocorticoid therapy. When a patient is going to be treated with glucocorticoids for more than two to three months the author will usually arrange for bone mineral density to be measured so that this can be followed. Patients should be encouraged to stop smoking, as smoking increases the risk of osteoporosis. Screening for hyperthyroidism with TSH is also prudent. Patients with hypogonadism, both male and female, should receive appropriate hormonal supplementation in the absence of contraindications to this type of therapy. Although there is no evidence that vitamin D and calcium will prevent glucocorticoid-induced bone loss, the author usually recommends that patients take 500 mg of calcium carbonate after breakfast and with supper, as well as vitamin D 500 IU daily. A number of recent studies, summarized in a review by Sambrook and Lane,[27] indicate that bisphosphonates are a safe treatment that is effective at preventing the development of osteoporosis and vertebral fractures. One large study by Adachi et al[28] used alendronate in a dose of 5 mg or 10 mg daily.

Prophylactic therapy with trimethoprim-sulfamethoxazole to prevent *Pneumocystis carinii* pneumonia in patients receiving glucocorticoids is controversial. In patients with primary or metastatic central nervous system tumors, only about 1.3% will develop *P. carinii* pneumonia.[29] This attack rate may not be high enough to justify the risk of side effects from prophylactic therapy. In patients receiving chemotherapy, in post-transplant patients and in those with inflammatory disorders, some physicians recommend trimethoprim-sulfamethoxazole (160/800 mg) one tablet daily if prednisone is used in a dose of 20 mg or higher for a month or more.

Therapy for excess glucocorticoid levels A number of compounds with an adrenal site of action have been used to lower glucocorticoid levels both in patients with Cushing's disease, in preparation for surgery or while waiting for the effect of radiotherapy, and in patients with excess adrenal production of glucocorticoid (Table 136.16). Of all of the compounds listed, ketoconazole has proved to be the most useful.

Monitoring drug effects is best done with 24-hour urine assays for urinary free cortisol.

Mineralocorticoid therapy Mineralocorticoids are used most commonly in the treatment of primary

---

Table 136.15 Recommendations for glucocorticoid treatment in patients with suspected or known hypothalamopituitary–adrenal axis suppression

Minor surgical stress (e.g. inguinal hernia repair)
Hydrocortisone (equivalent) 25 mg on morning of surgery
Surgeon and anesthetist aware of potential glucocorticoid deficiency
Restart usual glucocorticoid dose the day after surgery

Moderate surgical stress (e.g. cholecystectomy (non-laparascopic), lower limb revascularization, total joint replacement, segmental colon resection, abdominal hysterectomy)
Give daily glucocorticoid dose in morning on day of surgery and an equivalent dose intraoperatively, and then hydrocortisone (equivalent) 20 mg every 8 hours for 1–2 days

Major surgical stress (e.g. pancreatoduodenectomy, esophagogastrectomy, total proctocolectomy, cardiac surgery involving cardiopulmonary bypass)
Give daily glucocorticoid dose in morning on day of surgery and then hydrocortisone (equivalent) 50 mg every 8 hours thereafter for 2–3 days

Table 136.16   Agents that act at the adrenal gland to decrease glucocorticoid levels

Agent	Mechanism of action	Dose	Comments
Mitotane (o, p' DDD)	Adrenocorticolytic effects Modifications of steroid peripheral metabolism Direct inhibition of steroid biosynthesis Direct inhibition of cholesterol side-chain cleavage and 11β/18-hydroxylase activity	2–4 g/day	Control is not permanent Watch for hypercholesterolemia Gynecomastia may occur Adrenal insufficiency may occur
Metyrapone	Inhibits 11β-hydroxylase	500 mg to 4 g per day	Relatively non-toxic Side effects include acne, hirsutism, hypokalemia and edema
Aminoglutethimide	Inhibits cholesterol side-chain cleavage and 11β/18-hydroxylation	500–750 mg/day	Usually combined with metyrapone to reduce side effects
Ketoconazole	Interferes with cholesterol synthesis by blocking demethylation of lanosterol Blocks C17–20 lyase involved in the formation of sex steroid Inhibits cholesterol side-chain cleavage and 11β/18-hydroxylation	200 mg twice daily, increasing to 300–400 mg twice daily	Does not worsen hirsutism but the antiandrogenic effect may be a problem for male patients Does not elevate cholesterol Patients may eventually escape from pharmacological control Can be combined with aminoglutethimide

adrenal insufficiency. They can also be required in patients with hypoaldosteronism, adrenal hyperplasia with salt-losing state, and in patients with orthostatic hypotension (e.g. idiopathic, diabetic autonomic neuropathy, Shy–Drager syndrome). Fludrocortisone is the drug of choice. The usual starting dose is 0.1 mg daily, but can be as low as 0.1 mg every other day. Some patients will require 0.2 mg daily. Doses should be adjusted to avoid salt retention and edema or supine hypertension.

Adrenal incidentalomas Non-functioning adrenal tumors discovered at the time of imaging for other indications are referred to as "incidentalomas". Conditions that should be thought of are listed in Table 136.17.

The adrenal medulla

The adrenal gland and the sympathetic nervous system work together, as what has been called "the sympathoadrenal system", to maintain homeostasis. The adrenal medulla converts norepinephrine to epinephrine and secretes the latter directly into the circulation. For the neurologist, the most important disease of the adrenal medulla is pheochromocytoma.

Pheochromocytoma Ninety percent of pheochromocytomas occur in the adrenal gland. They are an uncommon tumor, seen in patients with multiple endocrine neoplasia types 2A (Sipple syndrome) (medullary carcinoma of the thyroid and hyperparathyroidism) and 2B (medullary carcinoma of the thyroid, muscosal neuroma, intestinal ganglioneuroma, megacolon and marfanoid habitus); 1% of

patients with neurofibromatosis type 1 (von Recklinghausen disease) have pheochromocytoma.[31] Pheochromocytoma is also seen in patients with cerebelloretinal hemangioblastomatosis type 2 (von Hippel–Lindau syndrome) (retinal angioma, cerebellar and spinal cord hemangioblastoma, renal cell carcinoma, and pancreatic, renal, epididymal and endolymphatic cysts/tumors).

The most common signs and symptoms of pheochromocytoma are listed in Table 136.18.

The treatment of pheochromocytoma is surgical removal of the tumor. Metyrosine, an inhibitor of tyrosine hydroxylation, is a useful adjunct in the

Table 136.17   Adrenal incidentalomas

Adrenal cysts
Hemorrhage
Calcification
Tumors*
    Myelolipoma
    Neuroblastoma
    Adenoma
        Non-functioning
        Glucocorticoid secreting (usually presents with Cushing's syndrome)
        Aldosterone secreting (usually presents with Conn's syndrome)
    Adrenocortical carcinoma
    Metastases

*Adrenocortical tumors may be part of a genetic syndrome, e.g. Beckwith–Wiedemann, Li–Fraumeni, McCune–Albright, Carney, multiple endocrine neoplasia type 1.[30]

Table 136.18   Signs and symptoms of pheochromocytoma

Hypertension (paroxysmal or sustained—equally common)
Severe throbbing headache (when blood pressure
   elevated)*
Profuse sweating over most of the body*
Palpitations (with or without tachycardia)*
Anxiety
Sense of doom
Pallor of the skin
Nausea (with or without vomiting)
Abdominal pain

*Patients with all three symptoms and hypertension can be said
to have a pheochromocytomas with 93.8% specificity and 90.9%
sensitivity. In the absence of hypertension these symptoms
exclude a diagnosis of pheochromocytoma with 99.9%
certainty.[32]

Table 136.19   Causes of orthostatic hypotension

Peripheral (postganglionic) neurons (orthostatic
   hypotension, erectile dysfunction, abnormal sweating
   and sphincter control)
   Diabetes mellitus
   Tabes dorsalis
   Alcoholic polyneuropathy
   Amyloidosis
   Holmes–Adie syndrome

Central (pre-ganglionic) neurons
   Pure autonomic failure without other neurological
      features
   Parkinson's disease with autonomic failure
   Multiple system atrophy
      Striatonigral degeneration (parkinsonian features
         predominate)
      Olivopontocerebellar atrophy (cerebellar features
         predominate)
      Shy–Drager syndrome (autonomic failure
         predominates)

Table 136.20   Treatment of orthostatic hypotension

Practical measures
Increased dietary salt (150–200 mmol/day)
Head-up tilt during sleep: 20°–30°
Avoid rapid postural change and prolonged standing
   (stand with one leg elevated on a stool and change
   frequently)
Support stockings
Avoidance of Valsalva maneuver

Medication
Fludrocortisone (0.1 mg/day up to maximum of
   1 mg/day)
Midodrine (10 mg orally, 3 times daily)
Indomethacin (25–50 mg 3 times daily)
Yohimbine (5.4 mg—$\frac{1}{2}$ to 1 tablet 3 times daily)
Phenylpropanolamine (12.5–25 mg, but no longer readily
   available)

preparation of these patients for surgery. It is given as 250 mg every six hours, increasing the dose by 250 mg/day as necessary to control hypertension, up to a total dose of 1000 mg every six hours.[33] Drowsiness is the most common central nervous system side effect, but it can also cause extrapyramidal symptoms, albeit less commonly.

Orthostatic hypotension   Orthostatic hypotension—a fall in blood pressure on standing of more than 20 mmHg—can be a disabling condition and is part of the differential diagnosis of syncope. The common causes of orthostatic hypotension are listed in Table 136.19. Treatment of this condition is difficult, and some combination of the various modalities listed in Table 136.20 are often used. Serious complications of therapy include hypertension, congestive cardiac failure, edema and hypokalemia. Very often, when patients have an adequate standing blood pressure,

they have supine hypertension. This can sometimes be managed simply by having patients sleep with the head of the bed elevated, but it may be a limiting factor in many of these therapies.

References

1. Bronstein MD, Cunha Neto MBC, de C Musolino NR. Diagnosis and treatment of hypothalamus disease. *In:* Conn PM, Freeman ME, eds. Neuroendocrinology in Physiology and Medicine. Totowa, NJ: Humana Press, 2000:475–497

2. Edwards S, Lennox G, Robson K, Whitley A. Hypothermia due to hypothalamic involvement in multiple sclerosis. J Neurol Neurosurg Psychiatry 1996;61:419–420

3. Sullivan F, Hutchinson M, Bahandeka S, Moore RE. Chronic hypothermia in multiple sclerosis. J Neurol Neurosurg Psychiatry 1987;50:813–815

4. Kurz A, Sessler DI, Tayefeh F, Goldberger R. Poikilothermia syndrome. J Intern Med 1998;244:431–436

5. De Plaen JL, Sepulchre D, Bidingija M. Paroxysmal hypertension and spontaneous periodic hypothermia. Acta Clin Belg 1992;47:401–407

6. Walker BR, Anderson JA, Edwards CR. Clonidine therapy for Shapiro's syndrome. Q J Med 1992;82:235–245

7. Hirayama K, Hoshino Y, Kumashiro H, Yamamoto T. Reverse Shapiro's syndrome. A case of agenesis of corpus callosum associated with periodic hyperthermia. Arch Neurol 1994;51:494–496

8. Jordaan GP, Roberts MC, Emsley RA. Serotonergic agents in the treatment of hypothalamic obesity syndrome: a case report. Int J Eat Disord 1996;20:111–113

9. Roth C, Wilken B, Hanefeld F, et al. Hyperphagia in children with craniopharyngioma is associated with hyperleptinaemia and a failure in the downregulation of appetite. Eur J Endocrinol 1998;138:89–91

10. Wisse BE, Schwartz MW. Role of melanocortins in control of obesity. Lancet 2001;358:857–859

11. Boosalis MG, Gemayel N, Lee A, et al. Cholecystokinin and satiety: effect of hypothalamic obesity and gastric bubble insertion. Am J Physiol 1992;262:R241–R244

12. Lustig RH, Rose SR, Burghen GA, et al. Hypothalamic obesity caused by cranial insult in children: altered glucose and insulin dynamics and reversal by a somatostatin agonist. J Pediatr 1999;135:162–168

13. Kaye WH, Klump KL, Frank GK, Strober M. Anorexia and bulimia nervosa. Annu Rev Med 2000;51:299–313

14. Kaye W, Gendall K, Strober M. Serotonin neuronal function and selective serotonin reuptake inhibitor treatment in anorexia and bulimia nervosa. Biol Psychiatry 1990;44:825–838

15. Kovacs K, Horvath E. Tumors of the pituitary gland. Atlas of Tumor Pathology Second Series, Fascicle 21. Washington, DC: Armed Forces Institute of Pathology, 1986

16. Molitch ME, Russell EJ. The pituitary "incidentaloma". Ann Intern Med 1990;112:925–931

17. Orrego JJ, Barkan AL. Pituitary disorders—drug treatment options. Drugs 2000;59:93–106

18. Corenblum B, Donovan L. The safety of physiological estrogen plus progestin replacement with oral contraceptive therapy in women with pathological hyperprolactinemia. Fertil Steril 1993;59:671–674

19. Ufearo CS, Orisakwe OE. Restoration of normal sperm characteristics in hypoprolactinemic infertile men treated with metoclopramide and exogenous human prolactin. Clin Pharmacol Ther 1995;58:354–359

20. Conceição FL, Bojensen A, Jørgensen JOL, Christiansen JS. Growth hormone therapy in adults. Front Neuroendocrinol 2001;22:213–246

21. Lamberts SWJ, De Herder WW, Van der Lely AJ. Pituitary insufficiency. Lancet 1998;352:127–134

22. Zitzmann M, Nieschlag E. Hormone substitution in male hypogonadism. Mol Cell Endocrinol 2000;161:73–88

23. Young J, Schaison G. Diagnosis and treatment of hypogonadotropism in males and females. Rev Prat 1999;49:1283–1289

24. Howlett TA. An assessment of optimal hydrocortisone replacement therapy. Clin Endocrinol 1997;46:262–268

25. Axelrod L. Glucocorticoid therapy. Medicine 1976;55:39–64

26. Salem M, Tainsh RE Jr, Bromberg J, et al. Perioperative glucocorticoid coverage—a reassessment 42 years after emergency of a problem. Ann Surg 1994;219:416–425

27. Sambrook P, Lane NE. Corticosteroid osteoporosis. Best Pract Res Clin Rheumatol 2001;15:401–413

28. Adachi JD, Saag KG, Delmas PD, et al. Two-year effects of alendronate on bone mineral density and vertebral fracture in patients receiving glucocorticoids: a randomized, double-blind placebo-controlled extension trial. Arthritis Rheum 2001;44:202–211

29. Sepkowitz KA. *Pneumocystis carinii* pneumonia without acquired immunodeficiency syndrome: who should receive prophylaxis? Mayo Clin Proc 1996;71:102–103

30. Gicquel C, Bertherat J, Le Bouc Y, Bertanga X. Pathogenesis of adrenocortical incidentalomas and genetic syndromes associated with adrenocortical neoplasms. Endocrinol Metab Clin North Am 2000;29:1–13

31. Manger WM, Gifford RW Jr. Clinical and experimental pheochromocytoma. 2nd edn. Cambridge, MA: Blackwell Science, 1996

32. Plouin PF, Degoulet P, Tugaye A, et al. Le dépistage du phéochromocytome: chez quel hypertendus?: Étude séminologique chez 2585 hypertendus dont 11 ayant un phéochromocytome. Nouv Press Med 1981;10:869–872

33. Keiser HR. Pheochromocytoma and other diseases of the sympathetic nervous system. In: Becker KL, ed. Principles and Practice of Endocrinology and Metabolism. 3rd edn. Philadelphia: Lippincott Williams & Wilkins, 2001:827–834

137 The Neurological Manifestations of Thyroid Disease

Colin Doherty

Introduction

The neurological disorders associated with thyroid dysfunction span the entire spectrum of neurology. Symptoms range from disorders of emotion and higher cognitive function through movement disorders to neuromuscular diseases and include a range of rare yet significant neurological sequelae. Generally the subject may be divided into the effects on the metabolism and development of neurological structures by intoxication or deprivation of thyroid hormones.

Hyperthyroidism

Thyrotoxicosis is a relatively common illness caused by excessive serum concentrations of thyroid hormones. If untreated, it may result in substantial morbidity and even death.[1] The effects of thyroid hormone excess on the brain and neuromuscular system are complex, and a discussion of the basic biochemical and physiological aspects is often required to understand the myriad clinical effects on the adult neurological system.

General features of hyperthyroidism

In most patients, the most common findings in the hypermetabolic state are heat intolerance, weight loss, palpitations, shortness of breath, dysphagia, hoarseness, and hair loss.[2] The prominent neurological features are manifest in the neuropsychiatric and neuromuscular systems in which the effects of hypermetabolism lead to such diverse systems as myopathy, tremor, movement disorder, seizures, and coma.[1,3,4] Furthermore, local effects from disturbed tissue or tumors of the thyroid can also cause considerable neurological morbidity, with dysthyroid orbitopathy and neuropathies being prominent.[5]

Neuropsychiatric manifestations of hyperthyroidism

Measurement in rat brains of the effects of chronic thyroid hormone excess on neural tissue demonstrates that despite the extremes of thyroxine availability, brain thyroxine and triiodothyronine concentrations and brain triiodothyronine production rates are maintained within narrow limits. This indicates a robust homeostatic mechanism of control.[6] Clearly then, very small changes in brain iodo compounds must produce marked physiological changes. In rats, an increase in β-adrenergic receptor sites over γ-aminobutyric acid (GABA) sites has been shown in response to excessive thyroxine, indicating that these changes probably are manifest at the level of neurotransmission.[6] Similarly, opiate receptors and native pain sensitivity increase.[3] It has been suggested that the above factors may be the basis of psychological and emotional changes accompanying hyperthyroidism.[3]

Thus, hyperactivity, rapid-fire speech, and an inability to sit quietly usually characterize a patient with hyperthyroidism. Often, patients appear jittery, restless, and easily moved to anger, and occasionally, they demonstrate extreme emotional lability.[1] Because of decreased attention, mild cognitive impairment may occur.[7] However, more significant, psychiatric disturbance is not uncommon in hyperthyroidism, and acute psychological distress may sometimes be the first manifestation of the disease.[2] Furthermore, it has been suggested that a predominance of psychological features in thyrotoxicosis may be lead to more formally characterized psychiatric disease such as schizophrenia or depression.[8,9] Despite this, a recent epidemiological study reported that neither a previous history of psychiatric disease nor a positive family history was predictive of the prevalence of major psychiatric illness in hyperthyroidism.[10]

Not all patients with thyrotoxicosis who have neuropsychiatric disease present with florid symptoms. The elderly are a particular example. Hyperthyroidism affects up to 4% of hospitalized geriatric patients.[11] Although nervousness and irritability occur in almost all younger patients with thyrotoxicosis, older patients may present, paradoxically, with apathy and depression, which sometimes is referred to as "apathetic thyrotoxicosis."[2,11,12]

Epilepsy, seizures and coma

Hyperthyroidism may cause seizures or trigger a preexisting seizure disorder.[5] Although it is not entirely clear why the tendency to seizures is increased, experiments have shown that the administration of excess thyroxine to euthyroid nonepileptic animals lowers the seizure threshold.[13] In one clinical series, nearly half of the patients had electroencephalographic (EEG) abnormalities, ranging from generalized slowing to focal abnormalities.[14] It was argued that the degree of abnormality correlated with the amount of excess hormone. However, most would agree that the EEG in nonepileptic patients with thyrotoxicosis tends to be normal, although the alpha-rhythms may be faster than average and the basal metabolic rate tends to correlate with the frequency of the background rhythm.[2,15]

A more profound EEG abnormality occurs in thyrotoxic crisis, which is an exaggerated response of the body to preexisting increases in serum levels of thyroid hormones. It characteristically develops in previously hyperthyroid patients who 1) have had thyroid surgery, 2) are in a postpartum period, 3) have had rapid withdrawal of antithyroid medications, 4) have received radiographic contrast agent, or 5) have a significant infection.[3] Clinical features include severe bradycardia, hyperreflexia, occasionally rhabdomyolysis and renal failure, profound changes in mental status, and seizures.[2,16,17] If untreated, death occurs in up to 20% of patients.[18] A favorable outcome often depends on aggressive management of the metabolic crisis in an intensive care unit setting with the use of β-adrenergic blocking agents, intravenous sodium iodide, antithyroid drugs, glucocorticoids, and temperature regulation.[3,18]

Neuromuscular disease

Thyrotoxic myopathy, thyrotoxic hypokalaemic periodic paralysis, myasthenia gravis, and exophthalmic ophthalmoplegia represent the majority of neuromuscular syndromes that are associated with thyrotoxicosis.[4] A possible common feature of all these disorders is that excess thyroid hormone induces change in skeletal musculature that may be manifested in several ways.[3] For example, although thyrotoxicosis increases cardiac output at rest, it adversely affects muscle bulk and function.[19] Furthermore, excess thyroid hormone has been found to have an overall catabolic effect on muscle.[20]

The changes in skeletal muscle that have been demonstrated with EMG studies of repeated contraction induced by electrical stimuli include an overall slowing and weakness of contraction in thyrotoxicosis.[4] Furthermore, electromyographic (EMG) studies in a population of patients with thyrotoxicosis showed myopathic features in the proximal muscles in 93% of patients and in the distal muscles in 43%.[21] Muscle biopsy specimens have shown decreased proportions of type I (mitochondria-rich) fibers, with lower glycogen content and higher capillary density.[22] Ultrastructural changes include elongated mitochondria and loss of mitochondria, myofibrillar degeneration, focal swelling of tubules, and subsarcolemmal glycogen deposits.[22,23]

Thyrotoxicosis may also produce changes in the metabolic character of skeletal muscle. Thyroid hormone increases the basal metabolic rate, skeletal muscle heat production, mitochondrial oxygen, and pyruvate consumption. It also accelerates gluconeogenesis, protein degradation, and lipid oxidation and enhances β-adrenergic sensitivity.[24,25] Muscle and serum levels of muscle enzymes such as creatine kinase (CK) and aldolase may be mildly increased, but they often are normal because of the slow progression of disease.[2,4] Patients may also have insulin resistance, which in combination with accelerated metabolism results in glycogen depletion and leads to a decrease in ATP, thus inducing easy fatigability and weakness.[24]

Thyrotoxic myopathy   A wide range of effects might be expected from such structural and metabolic changes. It has been suggested that the incidence of weakness in hyperthyroidism may be from 50% to 80%, with the majority being elderly men.[1,24] However, although many patients complain of weakness in a general sense, few have a pattern type weakness such as proximal myopathy.[4] The degree of muscle weakness is roughly correlated with the severity and duration of the thyrotoxic state[1] and the amount of muscle wasting.[4] Fatigue and myalgia are common complaints.[24] Shortness of breath may occur when respiratory muscles are involved, and it usually resolves after treatment.[26] Bulbar weakness resulting in dysarthria and dysphagia has been reported.[27] Tendon reflexes usually are normal, although a small percentage have shortened relaxation times.[24] This has been demonstrated particularly in the Achilles tendon.[28] It is caused by shortening of the twitch duration in slow twitch muscles and is a result of several thyroid hormone-induced effects such as a shift in the expression of myosin heavy and light chains to the characteristics of fast twitch muscle, a shift in calcium sensitivity of contractile protein, and an increase in calcium uptake by sarcoplasmic reticulum.[29] Recently, an inflammatory myopathy with increased CK levels has been described, the enzyme levels decreased with treatment of the hyperthyroidism rather than with corticosteroid therapy.[30]

Thyrotoxic periodic paralysis   The association of periodic paralysis and thyrotoxicosis was made initially in the early 1900s and since then, the clinical characterization, epidemiology, and treatment have evolved slowly.[31] As with all forms of periodic paralysis, the thyrotoxic form is characterized by recurrent attacks of weakness that may last fewer than 30 minutes to several days.[4] Although periodic paralysis is a relatively common complication of thyrotoxicosis in Chinese and Japanese populations, it is rare in the west.[5] Smooth muscle is not affected and cardiac function is seldom disturbed.[3] Exposure to cold or rest after exercising provokes attacks.[4] In severe attacks, of all skeletal muscles, including those controlling respiration, may be completely paralyzed.[3] As in primary periodic paralysis, the serum concentration of potassium in thyrotoxic periodic paralysis (TPP) decreases, but not always below normal values, and high carbohydrate loading may provoke attacks. Unlike primary periodic paralysis, however, thyrotoxic periodic paralysis is common in males of any age and most cases are sporadic and resolve with correction of the hyperthyroid state.[4] Occasionally, the symptoms may subside with treatment with potassium salts.[1] Propranolol therapy reportedly decreases the number of attacks.[32] In 75% of reported cases, the first attack of thyrotoxic periodic paralysis occurred after the onset of hyperthyroid symptoms.[33] However, despite the similarities between these conditions, the exact pathophysiologic mechanism is not known.[1]

Biopsy specimens of muscle fibers are characterized by vacuolar myopathy.[22] Ultrastructural studies have shown various abnormalities, with the most consistent finding being proliferation and focal dilatation of the sarcotubules.[4] The clinical signs and symptoms have been reported in association with Graves disease, toxic nodular goitre, lymphocytic thyroiditis, and thyrotoxicosis resulting from administration of exogenous thyroid hormone.[34]

Myasthenia gravis and thyrotoxicosis The occurrence of clinical thyrotoxicosis occurs in about 6% of cases of myasthenia gravis and about 10% of cases of preclinical hyperthyroidism are unmasked by thyrotropin-releasing hormone stimulation.[35] However, the incidence of myasthenia gravis in the course of thyrotoxicosis is much lower.[36] Nevertheless, the association between these two diseases is not one of chance. They often do not begin simultaneously, and one may precede the other by months or years.[37] The mean age at onset of the combined syndrome is the fourth decade, and women are affected four times more often than men.[4] Autoimmune mechanisms are implicated in the pathogenesis of both Graves disease and myasthenia gravis, and this may account for their coexistence. However, for the pathogenetic connection between the two conditions, the direct effect of thyroid hormone on neuromuscular transmission should be considered.[2,4,36]

The clinical myasthenic syndrome does not differ from that occurring in euthyroid patients. Variable weakness after the use of skeletal muscle, particularly those subserving ocular movement, facial expression, and speech, is the principle feature of the disease.[3] The largest series of patients reported with myasthenia gravis and thyrotoxicosis consisted of 20 women and 5 men.[38] Ophthalmoplegia was documented in 16 patients, bulbar weakness in 12, and limb weakness in 8. No relationship was found between the onset of myasthenia and the stage of thyrotoxicosis, in one-third of patients, thyrotoxicosis developed first and in another one-third myasthenia preceded the clinical thyroid disorder. Patients generally have a response to neostigmine therapy, although the improvement is less than complete because the thyroid hormone defect has not been altered.[3] Thyrotoxic myopathy may contribute to the overall weakness, and this may be reversed only with anti-thyroid treatment.[39]

Other effects

Dysthyroid orbitopathy "Graves disease" usually refers to the combination of hyperthyroidism, exophthalmic ophthalmoplegia or dysthyroid orbitopathy, and goitre. Not all patients with hyperthyroidism have prominent eyes, and exopthalmia is not related merely to excess thyroxine.[2] In a recent cohort study, 90% of patients with the eye disorder had Graves disease, 1% had primary hypothyroidism, 3% had Hashimoto thyroiditis, and the other 6% had these findings but without any disturbance of thyroid hormones.[40] Interestingly, the eye disorder has been shown to have a higher prevalence among patients with Graves disease who have other endocrine disorders such as diabetes mellitus.[41]

Clinically, patients typically describe a gritty sensation in their eyes, blurring of vision, photophobia, increased lacrimation, double vision, or deep orbital pressure. Physical examination findings include exophthalmos, extraocular muscle dysfunction, periorbital and eyelid edema, conjunctival chemosis and injection, lid lag and retraction, and lagophthalmic (exposure) keratitis.[42] Marked asymmetrical involvement of the orbits is not uncommon.[2] Patients who have hyperthyroidism but not Graves disease generally have no eye symptoms but may have lid lag and retraction, which indicates that these signs may be related directly to the effects of either the overactivity of levator palpebrae muscle or sympathetic overdrive causing overactivity of Mueller muscle.[42,43] Eyelid retraction may be manifested in several ways. With downward eye movements, the lids seems to lag, leaving a larger than normal portion of the sclera visible (von Graefe sign). Retraction of the upper and lower lids and the resulting widened palpebral fissure is referred to as "Dalrymple sign." The resultant staring phenomenon brought about by these changes is known as "Stellwag sign," which is added to by the absence of contraction of the frontalis muscle when looking up (Joffroy sign). The exophthalmos may lead initially to decreased ability to converge (Moebius sign) and, rarely, to complete external ophthalmoplegia.[2,5] Pain usually is mild or absent, and the condition may be distinguished readily from other causes of proptosis with computed tomography (CT) or magnetic resonance imaging (MRI) of the orbit, which show muscle enlargement without involvement of the tendons.[5]

The orbitopathy may precede other signs of Graves disease, occur concomitantly with the hyperthyroidism, or develop after treatment of the hyperthyroidism.[44] Once established, the features generally improve with treatment of hyperthyroidism. However, in a few patients, the disease progresses, and in rare instances, optic neuropathy with decreased visual acuity and visual field defects may occur.[2,42] Certain genetic characteristics such as various HLA-DR antigens (especially HLA-DR3) and particular environmental factors such as cigarette smoking may be necessary for the full clinical expression of the disorder.[45,46]

Histological examination shows an accumulation of glycosaminoglycans in the connective tissue components of the orbital fat and muscles, with edema, inflammation and fibrosis in the endomysial connective tissues that invest the extraocular muscle fibres; the muscles cells themselves remain intact.[47] The result is enlargement of the extraocular muscles and surrounding fat. Chemosis is periorbital edema caused by decreased venous drainage from the orbit and by increased intraorbital pressure.[42] There are close histological similarities between these changes and those occurring in pretibial dermopathy. This disorder is found in association with Graves dysthyroid orbitopathy and, although clinically rare, is detected in up to 10% of patients who have skin biopsy, it involves accumulation of glycosaminoglycans in the dermis.[48] Swelling of the extraocular muscles at the apex of the orbit and lack of forward mobility of the orbital contents because of the tight attachment of connective tissue to the orbital walls may lead to ischemic optic neuropathy.[49,50]

Bahn[42] has proposed the following scheme for the pathogenesis of dysthyroid orbitopathy in Graves disease. Circulating T cells directed against an antigen on thyroid follicular cells recognize this antigen on orbital and pretibial fibroblasts. The T cells infiltrate the orbit and skin, resulting in the release of cytokines into the surrounding tissue. This in turn stimulates the expression of immunomodulatory proteins (heat shock proteins and adhesion molecules and HLA-DR) in orbital fibroblasts, thus triggering the autoimmune response on orbital connective issue. The accumulation of glycosaminoglycan is presumed to be due to stimulation of the fibroblasts by particular cytokines such as interferons and growth factors. Thyrotrophin receptor antibodies may have a direct effect on orbital fibroblasts and contribute to the cycle of autoimmune phenomena.

Almost invariably, patients have some relief from their symptoms with treatment of the hyperthyroidism; often, however, additional measures are required to treat dysthyroid orbitopathy. Nevertheless, further therapeutic interventions remains controversial, and the condition usually is treated only when the symptoms become serious or vision is affected.[42] Corticosteroids and radiation therapy are most effective in resolving the acute inflammatory symptoms, and up to 60% of patients have a favorable response.[51] Although the effectiveness of other immunosuppressive regimes such as intravenous immunoglobulins, azathioprine, and plasmapheresis are unproven, a recent report has suggested that they may be useful in combination. In a small cohort of patients, the combination of azathioprine, low-dose prednisolone, and radiotherapy lead to a fourfold reduction in the progression to surgery.[52] Surgical orbital decompression is indicated only for severe eye disease that is unresponsive to the other treatment modalities. In a recent study of a large cohort of 428 patients with so-called severe Graves ophthalmopathy, most patients had a favorable outcome with minimal adverse events over 8 years of follow-up.[53]

Neuropathy   Although neuropathy associated with hyperthyroidism is rare, there is a clinical entity known as "Basedow paraplegia" which is a distal sensorimotor polyneuropathy with slowed conduction velocities indicating a demyelinating disorder.[5] The patients may present with various degrees of symmetrical lower extremity weakness, sensory loss, and absence of reflexes. It must be considered as a possible contributor to weakness in patients who may also have a myopathy.[24] More recently, a chronic peripheral radicular neuropathy has been described in association with hyperthyroidism and has been ascribed to an autoimmune mechanism similar to that in chronic inflammatory demyelinating polyradiculopathy (CIDP).[54] Patients generally have a response

to treatment of the primary cause of hyperthyroidism.[24]

Thyrotoxicosis predisposes to local pressure-type neuropathies because of the goitreous change that occurs. This may be manifested as a postganglionic Horner syndrome from interruption of ascending sympathetic fibers and vocal cord paralysis and hoarseness caused by pressure on the recurrent laryngeal nerve. These conditions may also occur in the setting of thyroid carcinoma, in which the palsies may be indicative of invasion rather than neuropraxia.[2,5] Peripheral neuropathy also may occur in association with propothiouracil treatment of hyperthyroidism.[55]

Movement disorders   Apart from weakness, the most commonly observed motor disorder caused by myopathies is thyrotoxic tremor. The phenomenon is seen best in the outstretched hand or protruding tongue. It is characterized by repeated rapid fine movements.[2] The amplitude of the tremor depends on the speed of muscle contraction, but the frequency is independent of the speed.[28] Thus, thyrotoxic tremor has many characteristics of the action tremor of physiological tremor, and this has led to the theory that thyrotoxic tremor is essentially due to up-regulation of β-adrenergic receptors caused by circulating excess thyroxine.[56] EMG studies show simultaneous bursts of activity in agonist and antagonist muscles. The segmental stretch reflex may have a role in producing the tremor by causing rhythmic motor outflow at a frequency that enhances the mechanical resonant properties of the limb.[57]

Apart from nervousness and an inability to remain still (described above), several reports (some more than a century ago) have mentioned chorea associated with thyrotoxicosis.[58,59] Unlike other choreaform disorders such as Huntington disease, which is caused by a structural lesion in the striatum, the problem in thyrotoxicosis is thought to be due only to increased dopaminergic receptor sensitivity, which has been shown to be affected by thyroxine levels. As in other forms of neuromuscular disease in thyrotoxicosis, the up-regulation of β-adrenergic receptors has also been implicated.[2] These theories of pathogenesis have been borne out by the amelioration of symptoms after treatment with antithyroid drugs, antidopaminergic drugs, or, indeed, β-blockers. However, occasionally, the chorea may persist.[3,59]

Hypothyroidism

The effects of chronic thyroid hormone depletion on the brain are often opposite to the effects described above; however, many neurological effects are unique to deficiency, especially in the developing brain. Hypothyroidism undoubtedly is the most common disorder of thyroid function. It usually is caused by a disorder of the thyroid gland that results in decreased hormone production and secretion of excess thyroid-stimulating hormone (TSH) (primary hypothyroidism). Less often, it is caused by a central disorder of decreased thyroidal stimulation by TSH, "secondary hypothyroidism".[60] The overall prevalence of hypothyroidism is 0.5% to 1% of the general population, but is 2% to 4% among the elderly. Women are three times more likely to have hypothyroidism than men.[60] The general features of hypothyroidism are decreased basal metabolic rate; dry flaky, thickened and cool skin; cold intolerance; weight gain; puffy hands and feet; constipation; bradycardia; hyperlipidemia; and hypertension.[2,60] The clinical effects of hypothyroidism on developing and mature brain are described below.

Effects of hypothyroidism on developing brain

Thyroid hormone is a principle hormonal determinant of normal growth and development of the CNS. Thyroid hormone receptors can be detected in human fetal brain after 9 weeks of gestation. The fetal thyroid begins to accumulate colloid at 12 weeks, and in conditions of iodine deficiency, fetal thyroid hypertrophy has been documented in the fifth fetal month.[61] Treatment of the deficiency must begin before the third trimester to ensure normal development.[62] However, the major effect of thyroid hormone has been suggested to be on later neurological development during the pregnancy, for example, synaptogenesis and myelination.[62]

The effects of thyroid hormone on brain development have been studied most extensively in rat brains. In cretinism, brain is small but has a normal gyral pattern. The microscopic architecture tends to be disrupted, with disordered neurons and dendritic arborization in the pyramidal layer of the cerebral cortex, decreased neuronal size, and decreased number of neurons.[62,63] Furthermore, as predicted, the brain of hypothyroid rats contains less myelin and synaptogenesis is decreased in the cerebellum.[64,65]

In humans, lack of thyroid hormone causes two forms of cretinism. (1) "Sporadic cretinism," caused by defective thyroid gland function in the fetus and infant, is characterized by retardation of mental and physical development that is preventable with early treatment with thyroid hormone in infancy. (2) "Endemic cretinism" is associated with environmental iodine deficiency ("geographical association") and endemic goitre; this form, too, is preventable with correction. Endemic cretinism includes two distinct clinical entities. "Neurological cretinism" is characterized by mental deficiency, deaf mutism, spastic rigid disorder of gait and mobility, and autism (described relatively recently) but not clinical hypothyroidism. "Hypothyroid" or "myxedematous cretinism" is typified neurologically by modestly retarded psychomotor development and slow pyschomotor activity but not deaf mutism or spasticity of the limbs.[2,60,66,67] The patient may have highly specific musculoskeletal abnormalities such as the muscular hypertrophy seen in Kocher-Debré-Sémélaigne syndrome.[68] The most exaggerated form of hypothyroid cretinism is found in Zaire.

The concept of a crucial period for treatment of hypothyroidism has been recognized for many years. The earlier the condition is diagnosed, the better the prognosis.[66] Recently, a cohort of more than 100 children with congenital hypothyroidism detected via newborn screening was followed regularly throughout childhood and into adolescence. Children with congenital hypothyroidism, regardless of treatment, had significantly poorer performance in many cognitive domains.[69] Several authors have described the neurophysiological and radiographic appearance of congenital hypothyroidism. Before treatment the EEG has an excess of slow activity. Sharp waves are seen in a small proportion of patients and may be distributed asymmetrically over the hemisphere. After a few days, the EEG may normalize.[70] On MRI hyperintensity on T1-weighted and hypointensity on T2-weighted images are seen in the globus pallidus and substantia nigra. However, the patients appear to have a normal myelination pattern.[71] Pathological studies of human brains with congenital hypothyroidism are sparse. However, of the brains that have been examined microscopically, the findings seem to confirm predictions based on animal studies, namely, small brains with atrophy, gliosis, and decreased myelination.[72]

Neuropsychiatric manifestations of hypothyroidism

In 1873, Gull first described the neuropsychiatric features of hypothyroidism by "painting a picture" of overall mental and physical slowing. The term "myxedema" was introduced in 1876 by Ord, who postulated that the overall apathy, fatigue, and weariness of the patients was due to a "jelly-like" swelling of connective tissue.[66] About 15 years later, the Clinical Society of London released its classic report on myxedema. In that report, the disease was characterized by acute or chronic mania in more than one-third of patients, and by dementia and melancholia, with a preponderance of suspicion and self-accusation, in the rest.[66] Later, Asher[73] used the term "myxedema madness' to emphasize the prevalence of florid hallucinosis and agitation in patients with untreated hypothyroidism. Although currently frank psychosis is rare as presenting feature of hypothyroidism, significant psychiatric illness in the form of depression can occur, even with subclinical hypothyroidism.[74] Hypothyroidism with circulating antithyroid antibodies from lithium treatment of affective illness has been described.[75] Furthermore, the general behavioral features of hypothyroidism have been recognized as a major differential diagnosis for depression, with slowness, decreased concentration, and poor attention often accompanied by somnolence and lethargy.[5]

The common neuropsychiatric features of hypothyroidism are prevalent particularly among the elderly. Two-thirds of all cases of hypothyroidism in this group present with apathy, psychomotor retardation, and poor attention and memory.[11] In most cases, the disorder improves after treatment with thyroid hormone.[5] The cause of these stereotypical mental changes is unknown, but decreased β-adrenergic receptor sensitivity and decreased central metabolism, which have been implicated as important chemical and metabolic consequences of thyroid deficiency in adult brains, may lead to overall slowness of thought processes.[62] This is supported by neurophysiological data from EEG studies that have demonstrated generalized slowing, with absence of the normal alpha-rhythm.[70] Despite the prevalence of intellectual impairment, few comprehensive neuropsychological investigations have been conducted to identify the specific cognitive domains affected or to document the natural history of the cognitive decline. The lack of these studies also makes it difficult to identify those at risk for psychiatric decompensation.

In the absence of florid psychosis, the most dramatic neuropsychiatric manifestations usually are encountered in combination with gross metabolic or inflammatory dysfunction and may present as a rapidly progressive dementia and progress to coma and death if the disorders are not recognized as manifestations of thyroid disease. These disorders are "myxedematous dementia" and "Hashimoto encephalopathy." Myxedematous dementia is a serious deterioration in cerebral function under conditions of extreme hypothyroidism.[62] All psychic activity is impoverished, and bizarre behavior and abnormal ideation may be present.[62] In the literature, emphasis is placed on excessive somnolence and sleeping.[2,5,60,62] If the condition is untreated, the patient may develop a rapidly accelerated syndrome of myxedematous cachexia, which may progress to seizures and coma.[2,76]

The clinical features include unresponsiveness, hypothermia, hypoventilation, and hypotension. It has a predilection for winter and may be precipitated by stress (infection, anesthesia) or drugs such as chlorpromazine, which may have secondary effects on the hypothalmus (affecting thyrotrophin release) that make it particularly likely to trigger the syndrome.[2,60,62,76] Treatment includes management in an intensive care unit, respiratory and pressor support, correction of electrolyte abnormalities, intravenous administration of thyroid hormone, and concurrent treatment of any precipitating illness.[62]

Of all the syndromes associated with hypothyroidism, the least understood probably is Hashimoto encephalopathy. Since its first description by Brain in 1966 about only 50 cases have been reported.[77] The clinical picture is overwhelmingly one of rapidly progressive dementia, with seizures, extrapyramidal rigidity, myoclonus, and occasional focal stroke-like features.[78-82] The cause is thought to be inflammatory vasculitis on the central nervous system, although only nonspecific evidence from brain biopsy specimens support this.[79,80,83] The clinical features and EEG may mimic those of prion disease, a diagnostic problem not helped by the fact that many patients may be biochemically euthyroid, with the only marker of the disease being an increase in thyroid peroxidase antibodies.[84,85] However, the disease usually responds dramatically to corticosteroid treatment, but relapse may occur.[79,86]

Hypothyroid myopathy

Hypothyroidism affects carbohydrate, protein, and lipid metabolism. It reduces oxygen consumption and the basal metabolic rate by decreasing mitochondrial oxidative capacity, muscle oxidative enzyme activity, and glucose uptake.[24] Muscle glycogenolysis is impaired, resulting in fasting hypoglycemia and glycogen accumulation, and this may contribute to muscle cramping and fatigability. Both protein synthesis and degradation are reduced, with a net catabolic effect.[24] The overall effects of these metabolic changes on skeletal muscle have been observed in a small cohort of patients before and after treatment. Skeletal muscle response was examined in 19 hypothyroid patients by measuring the ankle jerk response time (AJRT), a well known clinical sign of hypothyroidism. Initially, 11 of the patients had delayed AJRT, which returned to normal in all patients after treatment.[87] The sluggish contraction and relaxation of the ankle jerk has been attributed to reduced myosin ATPase activity and impaired calcium uptake by the sarcoplasmic reticulum. Relaxation probably is prolonged because of slowing of calcium sequestration by the sarcoplasmic reticulum.[88]

In patients who actually complain of and manifest muscle weakness in hypothyroidism, disordered muscle function may be the predominant feature of their thyroid dysfunction.[62] Muscle cramps or aching are commonly associated, with or without frank weakness, and reflexes tend to be sluggish. Some cases show ridging of the muscle on percussion (myoedema).[22] In a congenital form of hypothyroidism, originally called "hypertrophia musculorum vera" and subsequently "Kocher-Debré-Sémélaigne syndrome" muscle hypertrophy is a prominent feature.[22,68] Hoffmann syndrome, a myopathic syndrome with mild hypertrophy and prominent myotonia, has been described in adults.[2,22] Typically, a patient presents the firm, large, well-developed muscles and is often described as appearing "muscle bound" or "athletic."[62] In addition to these circumscribed conditions, a large group of hypothyroid patients have a form of proximal muscle weakness similar to that of other endocrine neuromyopathies.[24] In a review of the prevalence of muscle weakness among a group of 20 patients with primary hypothyroidism, 70% had some element of muscular weakness, which was significant in 40%.[89]

Most patients with weakness can be shown to have EMG abnormalities with fibrillations and sharp positive waves as well as low-amplitude, short-duration, polyphasic motor unit action potentials and complex repetitive discharges, which may resolve with treatment.[90] The creatine kinase tends to be increased in hypothyroid myopathy, which may reflect myopathy or delayed turnover of the enzyme in the serum.[87] The histopathological and ultrastructral features of skeletal muscle in hypothyroidism include a predominant type-2 fiber atrophy or enlargement; an increase in internal nuclei, glycogen, and mitochondrial aggregates; dilated sarcoplasmic reticulum; and focal myofibrillar loss.[22,87] Muscle biopsy specimens from two children with congenital hypothyroidism and congenital hypertrophic myopathy showed no abnormality in one child but did show predominant type-1 fiber atrophy, abnormal oxidative enzyme activity, focal accumulations of glycogen, amorphic crescents, and destruction of the sarcoplasmic reticulum in the other child.[68]

Neuropathy

Mononeuropathies are the commonest variety of neuropathy to occur in hypothyroidism. The most frequent complaints are tingling, numbness, and paresthesias of the extremities. Characteristically, the paresthesias occur most often in the hands, in the area of the distribution of the median nerve.[2] The pathophysiological mechanism is thought to be entrapment carpal tunnel syndrome caused by thickening of the connective tissue of the tendon sheaths which allegedly trap the nerve in the retinaculum.[62] It is believed that up to 10% of patients with hypothyroidism have a carpal tunnel-like syndrome, which is more often bilateral than unilateral. As in many thyroid-related syndromes, the condition tends to resolve with supplementation of the deficient hormone.[5] Other entrapment neuropathies resulting in facial weakness, hearing loss, and facial sensory abnormalities have been reported.[2] Rarely, peripheral polyneuropathy may occur in hypothyroidism. In a group of 39 patients with primary hypothyroidism, 25 had clinical evidence of possible neuropathy according to standard electrical conduction criteria. A definitive diagnosis of polyneuropathy was made in 72% of patients, with the commonest abnormality being delayed conduction in sensory nerves.[91] It has been suggested that even patients with subclinical hypothyroidism have electrophysiological features of polyneuropathy. The pattern of abnormalities suggest that both axonal loss and demyelination occur.[92] The droopy eyelid seen so often in myxedema has been attributed to a decrease in sympathetic tone, because it is reversible with phenylephrine.[2]

Other effects

Cerebellar ataxia A subset of patients with hypothyroidism complains of unsteadiness of gait. This has been called "myxedema staggers" and reportedly occurs in up to 10% of patients with hypothyroidism.[93] Although some patients may have only mild awkwardness, others have a definite pattern of ataxia, intention tremor, and dysmetria.[2,62] The pathophysiological mechanism for this is not known, but the pattern of abnormalities suggests a midline lesion and cell loss has been found in the vermis in several cases.[2,5]

Sleep apnea The incidence of sleep apnea in hypothyroidism is relatively high and has been attributed to peripheral obstruction due to edema and myopathy in the laryngeal area.[94] However, in some patients, a syndrome of chronic alveolar hypoventilation has been implicated, possibly related to phrenic nerve involvement or a purely centrally driven disorder.[62] Frequently thyroid substitution therapy is effective, but nasal continuous positive airway pressure can be necessary even after treatment.[94]

Myasthenia gravis Although myasthenia gravis usually is associated with thyrotoxicosis, hypothyroidism has been documented in nearly 2% of patients with myasthenia.[35] However, some of these patients may be in a hypothyroid phase of a primary thyrotoxic disorder.[5] Nevertheless, the association underlines the probable direct and autoantibody effects on neuromuscular transmission.[5]

Conclusion

In many respects the basic cellular pathophysiological mechanism of the peripheral effects of excess or depleted thyroid hormone on muscle and nerve have been comprehensively described. However, the direct and autoimmune effects on higher cognitive function and the natural history of the myriad presentations of mental status changes caused by both hyperthyroidism and hypothyroidism still need to be explained. Also, proper neuropsychological studies and comprehensive functional imaging studies of the brain under these diverse conditions need to be conducted.

References

1. Dabon-Almirante C, Surks M. Thyrotoxicosis. Endocrinology and Metabolism Clinics 1998;27(1):25–35
2. Tyler HR, Samuels MA, Hyman SE. Neurological complications of endocrine and metabolic disorders. *In:* Spittell JA, Jr, ed. Clinical Medicine—Vol 11—Neurology. Philadelphia: Harper & Row, 1986;1–48. vol Chap 21
3. Delong GR. Chapter 43—The neuromuscular system and brain in thyrotoxicosis. *In:* Braverman L, Utiger RD, eds. Werner & Ingbar's The Thyroid: A Fundamental and Clinical Text. 7th ed. Philadelphia, New York: Lippincott-Raven, 1996:645–652
4. Engel A. Neuromuscular manifestations of thyroid disease. Mayo Clin Proc 1971;47:919–925
5. Abend WK, Tyler HR. Thyroid disease and the nervous system. *In:* Aminoff MJ, ed. Neurology and General Medicine. New York: Churchill Livingstone, 1989: 257–271
6. Dratman M, Crutchfield F, Gordon J, Jennings A. Iodothyronine homeostasis in rat brain during hypo- and hyperthyroidism. Am J Physiol 1983;245: E185–E193
7. MacCrimmon D, Wallace J, Goldberg W. Emotional disturbance and cognitive deficits in hyperthyroidism. Psychosom Med 1979;41:331–340
8. Lazarus A, Jaffe R. Resolution of thyroid-induced schizophreniform disorder following subtotal thyroidectomy: Case report. Gen Hosp Psychiatry 1986; 8(1):29–31
9. Bauer M, Whybrow P. The effect of changing thyroid function on cyclic affective illness in a human subject. Am J Psychiatry 1983;143(5):633–636
10. Kathol R, Delahunt J. The relationship of anxiety and depression to symptoms of hyperthyroidism using operational criteria. Gen Hosp Psychiatry 1986;8(1): 23–28
11. Marsh C. Psychiatric presentations of medical illness. Psychiatric Clinics of North America 1997;20(1):181–204
12. Thomas F, Mazzaferri E, Skillman T. Apathetic thyrotoxicosis: a distinctive clinical and laboratory entity. Ann Intern Med 1970;72(5):679–685
13. Seyfried T, Glaser G, Yu R. Thyroid hormone influence on susceptibility of mice to audiogenic seizures. Science 1979;205:598–599

14. Zander Olsen P, Stoier M, Siersbaek-Nielsen K, et al. Electroencephalographic findings in hyperthyroidism. Electroencephalogr Clin Neurophysiol 1972;32(2): 171–177

15. Hermann HT, Quarton GC. Changes in alpha frequency with change in thyroid hormone level. Electroencephalogr Clin Neurophysiol 1964;16:515–518

16. Bennett W, Huston D. Rhabdomyolysis in thyroid storm. Am J Med 1984;77(4):733–735

17. Safe A, Griffiths K, Maxwell R. Thyrotoxic storm presenting as status epilepticus. Post Grad Med 1990;66:150–152

18. Ingbar S. Management of emergencies IX: Thyrotoxic storm. N Engl J Med 1966;274(22):1252–1254

19. Martin W, Spina R, Korte E, et al. Mechanisms of impaired exercise capacity in short duration experimental hyperthyroidism. J Clin Invest 1991;88(6): 2047–2053

20. Gelfland R, Hutchinson-Williams K, Bonde A, et al. Catabolic effects of thyroid hormone excess: the contribution of adrenergic activity to hypermetabolism and protein breakdown. Metabolism 1987;36:562–569

21. Ramsay I. Electromyography in thyrotoxicosis. Q J Med 1965;34(135):255–268

22. Dubowitz V. Chapter 11—metabolic and endocrine myopathies. In: Muscle Biopsy—A practical approach. 2nd ed. London: Baillière Tindall, 1985:465–570

23. Gruener R, Stern L, Payne C, Hannapel L. Hyperthyroid myopathy. Intracellular electrophysiological measurements in biopsied human intercostal muscle. J Neurol Sci 1975;24:339–349

24. Anagous A, Ruff R, Kaminski H. Endocrine neuromyopathies. Neurologic Clinics 1997;15(3):673–696

25. Foss M, Paccola G, Saad M, Pimenta C, et al. Peripheral glucose metabolism in human hyperthyroidism. J Clin Endocrinol Metab 1990;70:1167–1172

26. Siafakas N, Milona I, Salesiotou V, et al. Respiratory muscle strength in hyperthyroidism before and after treatment. Am Rev Resp Disease 1992;146:1025–1029

27. Sweatman M, Chambers L. Disordered oesphageal motility in thyrotoxic myopathy. Postgrad Med J 1985; 61:619–620

28. Marsden C, Medows J, Lange G. Effects of speed of muscle contraction on physiological tremor in normal subjects and in patients with thyrotoxicosis and myxoedema. J Neurol Neurosurg Psychiatry 1970;33(6): 776–782

29. Wiles C, Young A, Jones D, Edwards R. Muscle relaxation rate, fibre type composition and energy turnover in hyper- and hypo-thyroid patients. Clin Sci 1979; 57(4):375–384

30. Hardiman O, Molloy F, Brett F, Farrell M. Inflammatory myopathy in thyrotoxicosis. Neurology 1997;48(2): 339–341

31. Ferreiro J, Arguelles D, Rams H. Thyrotoxic periodic paralysis. Am J Med 1986;80:146–150

32. Yeung R, Tse T. Thyrotoxic periodic paralysis: effect of propranolol. Am J Med 1974;57:584–590

33. Kelley D, Garib H, Duda R, McManis P. Thyrotoxic periodic paralysis: Report of 10 cases and a review of electromyographic findings. Arch Intern Med 1989;149(11):2597–2600

34. Tamai H, Tanaka K, Komaki G, et al. HLA and thyrotoxic periodic paralysis in Japanese patients. J Clin Endocrinol Metab 1987;64:1075–1078

35. Kiessling W, Pflughaupt K, Ricker K, et al. Thyroid function and circulating antithyroid antibodies in myasthenia gravis. Neurology 1981;31:771–774

36. Puvanendran K, Cheah J, Naganthan N, et al. Neuromuscular transmission in thyrotoxicosis. J Neurol Sci 1979;43:47–57

37. Drachman DB. Myasthenia gravis and the thyroid gland. N Engl J Med 1962;266:330–337

38. Millikan CH, Haines SF. The thyroid gland in relation to neuromuscular disease. Arch Intern Med 1953;92: 5–39

39. Teoh R, Chow C, Kay R, et al. Response to control of hyperthyroidism in patients with myasthenia gravis and thyrotoxicosis. Br J Clin Pract 1990;44(12):742–744

40. Bartley G, Fatourechi V, Kadrmas E, et al. Clinical feature of Graves's ophthalmopathy in an incidence cohort. Am J Ophthalmol 1996;121(3):284–290

41. Kalmann R, Mourtis M. Diabetes Mellitus: a risk factor in patients with Graves' orbitopathy. Br J Ophthal 1999;83(4):463–465

42. Bahn R, Heufelder A. Pathogenesis of Graves' Ophthalmopathy. N Engl J Med 1993;329(20):1468–1475

43. Emlen W, Segal D, Mandell A. Thyroid state: effects on pre- and post-synaptic central noradrenergic mechanisms. Science 1972;175(17):79–82

44. Gorman C. Temporal relationship between onset of Graves' ophthalmopathy and diagnosis of thyrotoxicosis. Mayo Clin Proc 1983;58(8):515–519

45. Frecker M, Stenszky V, Balazs C, et al. Genetic factors in Graves' ophthalmopathy. Clin Endocrinol 1986;25: 479–485

46. Bartalena L, Marcocci C, Tanda M, et al. Cigarette smoking and treatment outcomes in Graves' ophthalmopathy. Ann Intern Med 1998;129(8):632–635

47. Campbell RJ. Pathology of Graves' ophthalmopathy. In: Gorman CA, Waller RR, Dyer JA, eds. The eye and orbit in thyroid disease. New York: Raven Press, 1984: 25–31

48. Smith B, Bahn R, Gorman C. Connective tissue, glycosaminoglycans and diseases of the thyroid. Endocr Rev 1989;10:366–391

49. Dosso A, Safran A, Sunaric G, Burger A. Anterior ischaemic optic neuropathy in Graves' disease. Journal of Neuro-ophthalmology 1994;14(3):170–174

50. Koornneef L. Eyelid and orbital fascial attachments and their clinical significance. Eye 1988;2:130–134

51. Bartelena L, Marcocci C, Pinchera A. Treating severe Graves' ophthalmopathy. Baillieres Clin Endo Metabol 1997;11(3):521–536

52. Claridge K, Ghabrial R, Davis G, et al. Combined radiotherapy and medical immunosuppression in the management of thyroid eye disease. Eye 1997;11(5):717–722

53. Garrity J, Fatourechi V, Bergstralh E, et al. Results of transantral orbital decompression in 428 patients with severe Graves' ophthalmopathy. Am J Ophthal 1993;116(5):533–547

54. Konagaya Y, Knoagaya M, Nakamuro T. Recurrent polyradiculopathy with hyperthyroidism. Eur Neurol 1993;33:238–240

55. Van Boekel V, Godoy J, Lamy L, et al. Propylthiouracil and periferal neuropathy. Arquivos de Neuro-Psiquiatria 1992;50(2):239–240

56. Young R, Growdon J, Shahani B. Beta-adrenergic mechanisms in action tremor. N Engl J Med 1975; 293(19):950–953

57. Hagbarth K, Young R. Participation of the stretch reflex in human physiological tremor. Brain 1979;102(3): 509–526

58. Sutherland GA. Chorea and Graves' disease. Brain 1903;26:210–214

59. Javaid A, Hilton D. Persistent chorea as a manifestation

of thyrotoxicosis. Postgrad Med J 1988;64:789–790

60. Braverman LE, Utiger RD. Chapter 54—Introduction to hypothyroidism. *In:* Braverman L, Utiger RD, ed. Werner & Ingbar's The Thyroid. 7th ed. Philadelphia, New York: Lippincott-Raven, 1996:736–737

61. Liu J, Tan Y, Zhuang A, et al. Influence of iodine deficiency on human fetal thyroid gland and brain. *In:* Delong G, Robbins J, Condliffe P, eds. Iodine and the brain. New York: Plenum Press, 1989:249–259

62. Delong GR. Chapter 72—The neuromuscular system and brain in hypothyroidism. *In:* Braverman L, Utiger RD, ed. Werner & Ingbar's The Thyroid. 7th ed. Philadelphia, New York: Lippincott-Raven, 1996: 826–835

63. Ruiz-Marcos A, Salas J, Sanchez-Toscano J, et al. Effect of neonatal and adult-onset hypothyroidism on pyramidal cells of the rat auditory cortex. Dev Brain Res 1983;9:205–213

64. Nicholson J, Altman J. Synaptogenesis in the rat cerebellum: effects of early hypo- and hyperthyroidism. Science 1972;176(34):530–532

65. Rosman N, Malone M, Helfenstein M, Kraft E. The effect of thyroid deficiency on myelination of brain. Neurology 1972;22(1):99–106

66. Greene R. The thyroid gland: its relationship to neurology. *In:* Vinken PJ, Bruyn GW, eds. Handbook of clinical neurology; vol 27; metabolic and deficiency diseases of the nervous system. Part I. New York: American Elsevier Publishing Co., Inc., 1976:255–277

67. Gillberg I, Gillberg C, Kopp S. Hypothyroidism and autism spectrum disorders. J Child Psychol Psychiatry 1992;33(3):531–542

68. Spiro A, Hirano A, Beilin R, Finkelstein J. Cretinism with muscular hypertrophy (Kocher–Debre–Semelaigne syndrome). Arch Neurol 1970;23:340–342

69. Rovet J. Long-term neuropsychological sequelae of early treated congenital hypothyroidism: effects in adolescence. Acta Paediatr Suppl 1999;88(432):88–95

70. Harris R, Della Rovere M, Prior P. Electroencephalographic studies in infants and children with hypothyroidism. Arch Dis Childh 1965;612–617

71. Ma T, Lian Z, Qi S, et al. Magnetic resonance imaging of brain and the neuromotor disorder in endemic cretinism. Ann Neurol 1993;34:91–94

72. Lotmar F. Histopathologische Befunde in Gehirnen von endemischen Kretinismus, Thyreoaplasie, und Kachexia thyreopriva, Ztschr ges. Neurol Psychiat 1933;146:1–53

73. Asher R. Myxedematous madness. Br Med J 1949;2:555–562

74. Haggerty J, Evans D, Prange A. Organic brain syndrome associated with marginal hypothyroidism. AJ Psychiatry 1986;143:785–786

75. Calabrese J, Gulledge A, Hahn K, et al. Autoimmune thyroiditis in manic-depressive patients treated with lithium. Am J Psychiatry 1985;142(11):1318–1321

76. Forester CF. Coma in myxedema: report of a case and review of the world literature. Arch Intern Med 1963:111:734–743

77. Brain L, Jellinek E, Ball K. Hashimoto's disease and encephalopathy. Lancet 1966;2:512–514

78. Seipelt M, Zerr I, Nau R, et al. Hashimoto's encephalitis as a differential diagnosis of Creutzfeldt–Jakob disease. J Neurol Neurosurg Psychiat 1999;66(2):172–176

79. Shaw P, Walls T, Newman P, et al. Hashimoto's encephalopathy: A steroid responsive disorder associated with high anti-thyroid antibody titers—report of five cases. Neurology 1991;41:228–233

80. Shein M, Apter A, Dickerman Z, et al. Encephalopathy in compensated Hashimoto's thyroiditis: A clinical expression of autoimmune cerebral vasculitis. Brain Dev 1986;8:60–64

81. Kothbauer-Margreiter I, Sturzenegger M, Komor J, et al. Encephalopathy associated with Hashimoto Thyroiditis: diagnosis and treatment. J Neurol 1996;243: 585–593

82. Balestri P, Grosso S, Garibaldi G. Letter: Alternating hemiplegia of childhood of Hashimoto's encephalopathy? J Neurol Neurosurg Psychiat 1999;66(4):548–549

83. Nolte K, Unbehaun A, Sieker M, et al. Hashimoto encephalopathy: A brainstem vasculitis. Neurology 2000;54(1):769

84. Seipelt M, Zerr I, Nau R, et al. Hashimoto's encephalitis as a differential diagnosis of Creutzfeldt–Jakob disease. J Neurol Neurosurg Psychiat 1999;66(2):172–176

85. Henhley R, Cibula J, Helveston W. Electroencephalographic findings in Hashimoto's encephalopathy. Neurology 1995;45(5):977–981

86. Cohen L, Mouly S, Tassan P, Pierrot-Deseilligny C. A woman with a relapsing psychosis who got better with prednisone. Lancet 1996;347(9010):1228

87. Khaleeli A, Edwards H. Effect of treatment on skeletal muscle dysfunction in hypothyroidism. Clin Sci 1984; 66:63–68

88. Simonides W, van Hardeveld C. The postnatal development of the sarcoplasmic reticulum Ca2+ transport activity in skeletal muscle of the rat is critically dependent on thyroid hormone. Endocrinology 1989;124:1145

89. del Palacio, Trueba J, Cabello A, et al. Thyroid myopathy: effect of treatment with thyroid hormones. Anales de Medicina Interna 1990;7(3):120–122

90. Torres C, Moxley R. Hypothyroid neuropathy and myopathy: Clinical and electrodiagnostic longitudinal findings. J Neurol 1990;237(4):271–274

91. Beghi E, Delodovici M, Boglium G, et al. Hypothyroidism and polyneuropathy. J Neurol Neurosurg Psychiatry 1989;52(12):1420–1423

92. Misiunas A, Niepomniszcze H, Ravera B, et al. Peripheral neuropathy in subclinical hypothyroidism. Thyroid 1995;5(4):283–286

93. Jellinek EH, Kelly RE. Cerebellar syndrome in myxoedema. Lancet 1960;2:225–227

94. Rosenow F, McCarthy V, Caruso A. Sleep apneoa in endocrine diseases. J Sleep Res 1998;7(1):3–11

138 Reproductive Endocrinology and Gender-Specific Issues in Neurology

Mark N Friedman and Andrew G Herzog

Introduction

Hormones classically act to coordinate mind and body in basic biological processes that are important for the survival of the individual and the species. They coordinate regulatory drive mechanisms in the hypothalamus with primarily cerebral limbic-mediated perceptual, behavioral and emotional functions that are important for the satisfaction of these drives. They help to focus attention and perception on biologically relevant stimuli, influence verbal and spatial learning and memory, promote relevant appetitive and consummatory behaviors, and adjust emotional states to be consistent with motivation. Hormones have a wide assortment of additional, less classic, actions that influence virtually every category of neurological and neuropsychiatric disorder. They promote the synthesis and release of growth factors that affect the development of meningiomas and neurofibromas (relevant to neuro-oncology). They modulate neuronal excitability and seizure occurrence (relevant to epileptology), monoamine synthesis and release (relevant to movement disorders, sleep medicine and neuropsychiatry), and modulate immune mechanisms (relevant to multiple sclerosis and systemic autoimmune disorders). Each neurological disorder can be viewed from an endocrine perspective. This chapter focuses on some of the more common neurological disorders in which a reproductive hormonal contribution may be present.

Epilepsy

Hormones can affect neuronal excitability and seizures; seizures can affect hormonal regulation and secretion. An understanding of the neuroactive properties of specific hormones and how epilepsy may promote the development of reproductive endocrine disorders can lead to a clearer understanding of pathophysiology and the comprehensive treatment of individuals with epilepsy.[1,2]

Estradiol has potent neuroexcitatory and proconvulsant properties. It promotes glutamate, in particular N-methyl-D-aspartate (NMDA)-mediated conductance. Estradiol administration has been shown to potentiate kindling in animal models and to increase seizures in animals as well as clinically. Conversely, some natural progesterone metabolites, such as tetrahydroprogesterone (THP, or allopregnenolone), have potent GABAergic properties that hyperpolarize neurons and can inhibit seizures. Rapid withdrawal of THP, as may occur premenstrually,

results in a change in the subunit composition of the GABA receptor to a form that, in animal models, is insensitive to benzodiazepine, and hence presumably to GABA. In women with partial seizures the intravenous infusion of progesterone, resulting in normal luteal-phase plasma levels, has been shown to suppress interictal epileptiform discharges. Testosterone has more variable effects. This may be related to its ready metabolism by aromatase to estradiol, which has neuroexcitatory effects; by reductase to dihydrotestosterone, which may block NMDA conductance; and by further reduction to androstanediol, a potent GABAergic steroid with antiseizure properties.

Catamenial epilepsy is seizure exacerbation in relation to specific phases of the menstrual cycle. The neuroactive properties of estradiol and progesterone, and the cyclic variations in their concentrations and ratios, may be responsible. An association between seizures and specific phases of the menstrual cycle can be established by analysing charts that record the daily occurrence of seizures and the day of onset of menstrual flow. A midluteal-phase serum progesterone level is also important to establish if ovulation has occurred, as patterns differ between ovulatory and anovulatory or inadequate luteal-phase cycles. The menstrual cycle is divided into four phases: menstrual, days −3 to +3; follicular, days +4 to +9; ovulatory, days +10 to −13; and luteal, days −12 to −4. Day 1 refers to the first day of menstrual bleeding; day −14, i.e. 14 days before the subsequent onset of menses, is the presumed day of ovulation. We define seizure exacerbation as a twofold or greater increase in the average daily seizure frequency during the affected part of the menstrual cycle compared to the midfollicular and midluteal phases. In ovulatory cycles there are type I or perimenstrual (days −3 to 3) and type II or ovulatory (days 10 to −13) patterns of seizure exacerbation.[3] In anovulatory cycles there is a characteristic pattern, type III, that extends from day 10 of one cycle to day 3 of the next.[3] Type I probably relates to rapid premenstrual progesterone withdrawal, as well as to decreased serum antiepileptic drug levels that tend to develop from increased hepatic metabolism following the premenstrual lowering of reproductive steroid levels. Hepatic microsomal enzymes metabolize both gonadal steroids and several anticonvulsants (e.g. phenytoin and carbamazepine), with competition between the two. Type II probably relates to the substantial rise in estradiol levels that occur prior to ovulation. Type III occurs in relation to the rise in serum estradiol that occurs

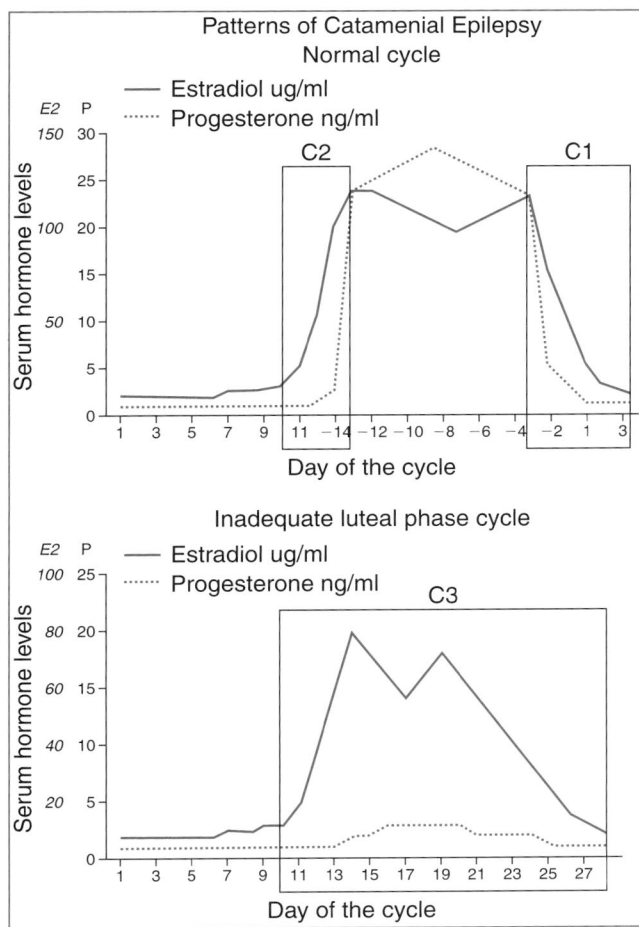

Figure 138.1 Three patterns of catamenial epilepsy: perimenstrual (C1: days −3 to 3) and periovulatory (C2: days 10 to −13) exacerbations during normal cycles and entire second half of the cycle (C3 days 10 to 3) exacerbation during inadequate luteal-phase cycles.

during the second week of the cycle, even in the absence of ovulation, which lasts until menstruation and is unaccompanied during the second half of the cycle by any substantial rise in progesterone (Figure 138.1).

Natural progesterone therapy (100–200 mg lozenges t.i.d. or micronized progesterone capsules 100 mg t.i.d. on days 14–25) may be associated with a substantial reduction in seizure frequency among women with cyclically exacerbated temporal lobe epilepsy (TLE).[4] Such therapy can help to normalize luteal-phase progesterone levels. We typically recommend a gradual withdrawal of the progesterone therapy premenstrually (days 26–28) The induction of ovulation and normalization of the luteal phase using the anti-estrogen clomiphene may be beneficial as well, although undesirable side effects of clinical significance are more common, such as ovarian overstimulation syndrome and unplanned pregnancy. Likewise, GnRH analogs that abolish the cycle may have effi-

cacy, but usually require a stable balanced regimen of estradiol and progesterone replacement to deal with the complications of hypoestrogenism, such as menopausal symptoms (hot flashes, night sweats, vaginal dryness and irritation) and diminished bone density.

Reproductive dysfunction is unusually common among women and men with epilepsy, specifically TLE.[1,2] Such dysfunction may result from the effects of epilepsy itself, the use of antiepileptic drugs, or both. Dysfunction of reproductive function in women typically manifests as menstrual disorders (e.g., amenorrhea (no menses for six or more months), oligomenorrhea (longer than 35-day cycle intervals or fewer than nine menses per year), polymenorrhea (cycles with shorter than 23-day intervals) abnormal variability in cycle intervals (more than four days' variability), and menometrorrhagia (heavy menses and bleeding between periods)) and infertility. There is evidence to suggest that more than one-third of cycles in women with TLE are anovulatory, compared to 8% in the general population, and that anovulatory cycles may be more common in women with localization-related epilepsy than in primary generalized epilepsy. Women with idiopathic epilepsy are only 37% as likely as unaffected female siblings to become pregnant. This finding is not attributable to marital rate, seizure type, age of seizure onset or family history of epilepsy. In men, reproductive dysfunction manifests as diminished potency and abnormal sperm characteristics. Men with idiopathic epilepsy are only 36% as likely as unaffected male siblings to ever father a pregnancy.

Certain reproductive endocrine disorders such as polycystic ovarian syndrome (PCOS) and hypothalamic amenorrhea (HA), are unusually common in women with epilepsy. There is also an overrepresentation of premature menopause and functional hyperprolactinemia. PCOS occurs in 10% to 20% of women with TLE, compared to about 5% in the general population. Both epilepsy and antiepileptic drugs have been implicated. Women with left TLE have been shown to differ from those with right TLE in their patterns of hypothalamic, pituitary and ovarian hormonal secretion. Left TLE is associated with a significantly greater frequency of PCOS, whereas HA is more common with right unilateral TLE. PCOS is also significantly more common in women with epilepsy who take valproic acid, especially if they begin its use before 20 years of age.[5] Although there is an association with weight gain, PCOS is also overrepresented in lean users.

Reproductive endocrine disorders may favor the development of seizures in women with TLE and certain primary generalized forms of epilepsy, such as juvenile myoclonic epilepsy. Reproductive endocrine disorders are characterized by anovulatory cycles. Anovulatory cycles feature elevated serum estrogen to progesterone ratios or unopposed estrogen during the luteal phase. Because estrogen has neuroexcitatory effects and certain progesterone metabolites have potent antiseizure properties in most adult epilepsy, these endocrine alterations appear to be associated with an increased incidence of seizures in women with epilepsy. There is also evidence to suggest that they potentiate kindling in animal models and the occurrence of interictal epileptiform discharges in both animal models and clinically.

Reproductive dysfunction and endocrine disorders are also overrepresented in men with epilepsy.[6] Between one-third and two-thirds may have complaints of diminished sexual interest or potency. The most common hormonal finding is a decreased level of bioactive testosterone. This may be related to the use of enzyme-inducing antiepileptic drugs that increase the hepatic synthesis of sex hormone-binding globulin and thereby reduce the bioactive portion of testosterone. Other drug-related factors, such as direct testicular toxicity, and also an increase in the ratio of estradiol to testosterone, perhaps as a result of aromatase induction, have been implicated. Although estradiol makes up only 1% of the total reproductive steroid concentration in the serum, it exerts almost 50% of the negative feedback on the hypothalamo-pituitary axis. A small incremental increase in estradiol level relative to testosterone may, therefore, have a disproportionately large negative effect on androgen production, and hence sexual interest and function.

Although testosterone replacement has proved only moderately effective in restoring sexual function, one study has reported superior results using combined treatment with testosterone and an aromatase inhibitor that blocked the transformation of testosterone to estradiol.[7]

Migraine

Migraine is three times more common in women (18%) than in men (6%) during adolescence and adulthood, but occurs with similar frequency in boys and girls before puberty. Menstrual exacerbation is reported by 60% of women, and migraine occurs exclusively at that time in about 15%. Migraine without aura (common migraine) usually lessens in frequency and severity during the second and third trimesters of pregnancy, whereas migraine with aura (classic or complicated migraine) commonly worsens. Migraine generally subsides after the menopause, but is frequently exacerbated perimenopausally. Estrogen withdrawal appears to be an important factor.[8] This occurs both premenstrually and after ovulation, as well as at unpredictable times during the perimenopause. Menstrual migraine can be treated or delayed by treatment with estrogen. Women with reproductive endocrine disorders characterized by anovulatory cycles are much more likely to suffer from migraine. Almost 70% of women with PCOS have been reported to have migraine. Apart from its three times greater frequency of occurrence in women with major mood disorders, migraine is also twice as likely to occur in women with premenstrual dysphoric disorder.

Migraine, especially menstrual migraine, is commonly associated with hyperprolactinemia and abnormal prolactin dynamics with increased sensitivity to dopaminergic effects. It is more common in women with prolactin-secreting adenomas, and responds favorably to prolactin reduction with the use of dopaminergic agonists.

Menstrual migraine is often refractory to the usual methods of pharmaceutical prophylaxis, e.g. β-blockers, antidepressants, calcium channel blockers or valproic acid. If these approaches are not efficacious, neuroendocrine intervention or hormonal therapy may be considered.

Migraine is considered to be a contraindication for oral contraceptive use because at least one-quarter of women experience worsening of migraine and some may develop stroke. The risk of stroke in women with migraine who use oral contraceptives is increased by more than 10-fold. Anecdotally, however, some women, especially those with menstrual disorders, may benefit more from oral contraceptive use, especially from continuous active pill use, than from other therapies. Close monitoring and considerable caution must be used, and oral contraceptives should be discontinued if headaches worsen or neurological symptoms develop. Other hormonal therapies include the elimination of the menstrual cycle by reversible abolition of ovarian function using GnRH analogs, usually along with hormonal replacement that includes continuous estrogen and, if the uterus is present, progestin. Estrogen receptor blockade with tamoxifen has also been reported to be effective. Continuous stable estrogen replacement should be carried out with a form of estrogen that has a long half-life, e.g. conjugated estrogen tablets are strongly preferred over estradiol tablets that have a much shorter half-life. Alternatively, and perhaps preferably, estrogen may be replaced in a very stable fashion using a transdermal lotion or patch. Care must be used to maintain a fresh supply of lotion and to overlap the patches by about two hours to prevent estrogen withdrawal following removal of the old patch. Finally, in an open-label trial in 24 women, daily bromocriptine, built up very gradually over the course of a month to a dosage of 2.5 mg t.i.d., has been shown to reduce menstrual migraine episodes by over 25% in 75% of women, and by over 50% in 62.5%.[9] Headache frequency among the 21 women who remained on treatment for over one year declined by 72%. Discontinuation of treatment resulted from nausea and lightheadedness, which are the most common side effects. These are particularly likely to occur if the dosage is not built up very slowly. Cyclic rather than continuous bromocriptine use has benefited premenstrual dysphoric disorder but not menstrual migraine. Unlike bromocriptine, pergolide was poorly tolerated and ineffective. Differences in dopamine receptor and possibly serotoninergic actions may account for the differences between these drugs.

Aging and dementia

Reproductive hormones influence the brain throughout life.[10] As the brain achieves a recognizable form during the third month of human gestation, it elaborates a dense array of reproductive steroid receptors.

By the same time and during the remainder of gestation, the gonads and adrenal secrete reproductive steroids in serum concentrations that are comparable to those attained after puberty and which far surpass the levels achieved during infancy and childhood. Reproductive hormones act as trophic factors for the growth and development of neurons and the neuropil. These hormones are important during critical developmental periods to establish sexual dimorphism and lateralized asymmetry in the structure and function of the brain. Throughout life, the reproductive hormones also have a significant role in those processes that are mediated by the limbic system, such as attention, learning, memory and mood. During adult life, these hormones may have important neuroprotective as well as neurotoxic effects on physiological (e.g. aging, programmed cell death) and pathological (e.g. dementia, stroke, epilepsy) age-related changes in the brain.

Conversely, age-related brain changes are responsible for reproductive and reproductive endocrine changes. For example, in women there is a process of gradual reproductive endocrine decline (i.e. perimenopause) that eventually results in the cessation of ovarian endocrine function and elevated gonadotropin levels (i.e. menopause). With regard to cognitive function, estrogen appears to enhance verbal more than non-verbal skills, and has a minimal effect on visual or spatial memory. Although the magnitude of estrogen effects on verbal function is generally small, it may be very substantial clinically in some women, especially those with heredofamilial or developmental brain anomalies or those with acquired brain lesions, in particular when there is involvement of temporolimbic structures. Physiological occurrence of hormonally related cognitive decline is perhaps most common in relation to the development of perimenopause-menopause. Pathologically or pharmacologically, it is commonly encountered in relation to the suppression of ovarian estrogen production with the use of gonadotropin-releasing hormone (GnRH) analog treatment, as in the management of endometriosis or fibroids, or with tamoxifen use for the adjunctive treatment of female cancers.

Aging in men is associated with a progressive decline in serum concentrations of total and biologically active (i.e. 1.2% per year) testosterone. This may adversely affect muscle mass, hematopoiesis, bone density, insulin sensitivity, energy, mood, sexual interest and potency. The symptom complex has been termed *andropause*. Although the dihydrotestosterone patch has been reported to benefit the symptoms of andropause, well controlled studies are lacking.

With the increase in life expectancy, quality of life issues related to aging and the prevention or slowing of degenerative diseases have assumed increasing importance. In Alzheimer's disease (AD) the cardinal feature is the gradual loss of recent memory and learning ability. It is the most common cause of dementia. A possible role for reproductive hormones is gaining prominence for several reasons, including the gender differences in the occurrence of Alzheimer's disease; basic scientific evidence for the neuroprotective effects of estrogen and its metabolites; and the apparent prophylactic effects of chronic estrogen exposure in epidemiological studies.

Estradiol receptors are most highly concentrated in regions of the brain that bear the brunt of Alzheimer's neurodegenerative changes. These areas are found in the temporolimbic forebrain. Estrogen markedly enhances the activity of choline acetyltransferase in the limbic forebrain. Estrogen may also potentiate the beneficial effects of anticholinesterase drugs on cognitive measures in women with AD.

Estrogen may protect synapses from neurodegenerative changes. It can act directly on synapses and protect critical membrane transport systems from oxidative impairment. Estrogen can reduce plasma levels of apolipoprotein E and modify some of the inflammatory responses (e.g. interleukin-6) that have been implicated in neuritic plaque formation. In addition, estrogen can increase cerebral blood flow and promote the breakdown of the β-amyloid precursor protein to fragments that are less likely to accumulate as β-amyloid.

τ Protein is a major constituent of normal neurofilaments as well as abnormal neurofibrillary tangles. Estrogen stimulates normal τ synthesis for inclusion in the developing cytoskeleton. Abnormally hyperphosphorhylated τ, which is seen in the neurofibrillary tangles of AD, can be prevented by androgen treatment, suggesting a possible neuroprotective role of androgens.

Several epidemiological studies have investigated the relationship between chronic estrogen use and dementia. Some of these suggest that estrogen replacement therapy (ERT) can potentially reduce the risk of developing AD in postmenopausal women, and factors such as a longer duration of estrogen use and recent estrogen exposure may enhance the effectiveness of its risk-reducing properties. Results show that long-term estrogen therapy is associated with a progressive but generally modest improvement in cognition during the course of one year of treatment, and that the progression of AD can be delayed for up to two years. The following is a summary of some of these investigations.

Early clinical studies suggested that long-term estrogen therapy contributes to a progressive but limited improvement in cognition after one year of treatment, and that the progression of Alzheimer's disease can be delayed by up to two years.[11,12] Interestingly, most of the more recent studies that have examined the effects of estrogen on Alzheimer's disease have included much shorter timeframes, making it difficult to ascertain the long-term benefits and risks. For example, Fillit et al.[13] used 2 mg/day of micronized estradiol for six weeks in an open trial consisting of seven female patients with AD. Three patients had a significant improvement in attention, orientation, mood and special interaction, as measured by the MMSE, the Hamilton Depression Rating Scale (HDRS), and the Rand Memory Test. The patients with AD who benefited from estradiol therapy had affective disorders in addition to cognitive dysfunction. Honjo et al.[14] reported that five of seven women with AD who were treated with a dose of 1.25 mg/day of conjugated estrogen for six weeks showed a significant improvement in Hasegawa Dementia Scale scores, and six of seven showed an improvement in the scores of the New Screening Test for Dementia. Statistically significant improvements were noted at both three and six weeks, particularly in memory, orientation and calculation. Ohkura et al.[15,16] studied 15 elderly women with AD who were treated with 0.625 mg of conjugated equine estrogens orally twice a day for six weeks. Psychometric measures showed significant improvements in cognitive performance.

Mortel and Meyer studied 93 postmenopausal women with probable AD, 65 with probable ischemic vascular dementia, and 148 normal controls.[17] The proportion of control subjects on ERT compared to women with either type of dementia who were on ERT was almost 2:1. Their findings suggest that lack of ERT in postmenopausal women is associated with an increased likelihood of cognitive impairments in both the Alzheimer's and vascular forms of dementia. Women with dementia were only 53% as likely to have had ERT as were the control subjects, suggesting that ERT may have neuroprotective properties. Henderson et al.[18] reported on a case–control study of ERT in which subjects were a volunteer sample of consecutively enrolled elderly women who met clinical criteria for probable AD or for non-demented control status. They found that AD case patients were significantly less likely than control subjects to use ERT (7% vs. 18%), and that the mean performance on a cognitive screening examination was significantly better in the demented group who used estrogen. They suggest that postmenopausal ERT may be associated with a decreased risk of AD, and that ERT may improve cognitive performance in women with AD. Paganini-Hill and Henderson also reported in a case–control study that the risk of AD and related dementia was significantly reduced in estrogen users compared to non-users.[19] The risk decreased significantly with both increasing dosages and increasing duration of oral therapy with conjugated equine estrogen. Tang et al.[20] studied 1124 elderly women who were initially free of AD and were taking part in a longitudinal study of aging and health in a New York City community. Overall, 12.5% of the women reported taking estrogen after menopause. The age of AD onset was significantly later in women who had taken estrogen than in those who had not. The relative risk of the disease was significantly reduced in estrogen users (5.8%) compared to non-users (16.3%) even after adjustments in education, ethnic origin, and apo-E genotype. The women who developed AD, however, were significantly older (78.5 ± 7.7 vs. 73.7 ± 6.6). Longer estrogen use was associated with a lower risk of AD. Several recent studies (Mulnard et al.[21]; Seshadri et al.[22]) showed that the use of ERT in postmenopausal women was not associated with a reduced risk of developing AD.

Movement disorders

Reproductive steroids influence the manifestations of movement disorders. Estrogen affects the dopaminergic system and modulates behaviors that are mediated by striatal dopamine. Animal research has shown estrogen to have both pro-and antidopaminergic effects on the mesostriatal dopaminergic system. Estrogen can downregulate monoamine oxidase activity and catechol-O-methyltransferase activity. It can also increase the density of dopamine receptors. There is also evidence to suggest that chronic estrogen treatment in ovariectomized rats can decrease dopamine concentration in the striatum. The effect of progesterone on the dopaminergic system is less clear. It may have an antagonistic or synergistic effect with estrogen.

Parkinson's disease (PD) is a neurodegenerative disorder characterized by a loss of melanin-containing neurons in the substantia nigra pars compacta, the presence of Lewy bodies, and a reduction of striatal dopamine. Estrogen replacement therapy may have several beneficial effects with regard to the manifestations and progression of PD, the severity of motor symptoms, and the cognitive function of women with PD. ERT may also be associated with a delayed age of onset of Parkinson's disease. Postmenopausal ERT has also been associated with a reduced risk of PD and an improvement in parkinsonian symptoms. Conversely, ERT withdrawal can increase motor impairment. An improvement in verbal memory retention and better performance on the Mini-Mental Status Examination has been shown. Cyclic exacerbation of parkinsonian symptoms with loss of medication efficacy has been reported in 25% of menstruating women, particularly during the premenstrual phase. This phenomenon has been associated with and attributed to both estrogen and progesterone withdrawal.

Choreatic disorders involve a state of increased striatal dopaminergic activity. Chorea is a rare complication of oral contraceptives that contain estrogen. The disorder can begin shortly after therapy is started (i.e. an average of nine weeks), follows a subacute pattern of evolution, often resolves with discontinuation of estrogen supplementation, is most frequently hemichorea, and in 41% of the patients there is a history of Sydenham's chorea. ERT may be associated with a variable degree of symptomatic improvement in patients with Huntington's disease or levodopa-induced chorea in patients with PD (30% to 60%).

Cranial and cervical dystonias are more common in women than in men. This is particularly notable for spasmodic torticollis (ST), in which there is a female to male ratio of 1.6:1. Several observations suggest a possible relationship between reproductive function and ST. In one regional epidemiologic study among nine female patients with ST, three had ovarian cysts, two had primary ovarian failure and one had carcinoma of the cervix. ST shows a significantly greater frequency of onset in the fifth decade than at other times. A relationship to perimenopausal hormonal changes has been proposed. Menstrual exacerbation of symptoms, reproductive disorders and hysterectomy are significantly more common than in controls in the general population, as well as in controls with some other chronic neurological disorders. Oral contraceptive use and pregnancy do not have adverse effects.[23] In a case report, treatment of a patient with polycystic ovarian syndrome (PCOS) and ST with progesterone during the second half of each menstrual cycle produced long-lasting reversal of cervical dystonia.[24] The possibility that ST onset and severity may relate to reproductive state and hormonal factors merits further consideration and investigation.

Phenotypic expression of essential tremor may be gender related. One study has found that men were affected more by hand tremor and that women had more severe head or voice tremor.

With regard to tic disorders, the male:female incidence ratio is 4.3:1. Males are also more likely than females to have comorbid disorders. The most common reported comorbidity is attention deficit hyperactivity disorder. Tic disorders and myoclonus may increase in frequency or severity during the premenstrual phase. Symptoms of obsessive-compulsive disorder (OCD) can worsen premenstrually, and relapse during the perimenopause or postpartum. Conversely, there are reports of worsening OCD symptoms with oral contraceptive use, as well as during menarche and pregnancy. Investigations of androgen suppression or androgen receptor blockade therapy in men or boys are currently under way.

Pregnancy in patients with movement disorders is an uncommon occurrence. Pregnancy frequently has a mild exacerbating effect on symptoms of PD and may also unmask an underlying potential for chorea (i.e. chorea gravidarum). However, pregnancy seems to have little effect on other movement disorders.

Mood disorders

The reproductive hormones have variable effects on mood.[25] Estrogen exerts energizing and antidepressant effects. It generally increases serotonin synthesis and levels of 5-hydroxy indole acetic acid (5HIAA). Its antidepressant effect is also the result of increased binding and clinical effects of antidepressant medications. Whereas estrogen decreases monoamine oxidase activity in the amygdala and hypothalamus, progesterone increases it, thereby resulting in lower concentrations of brain serotonin. These neuroactive effects of reproductive hormones may be important in the emotional changes that occur in some women in the following settings: physiological changes in the reproductive state, such as during menarche, menstruation, pregnancy, and menopause; pathological changes, such as reproductive endocrine disorders (e.g. polycystic ovarian syndrome and hypogonadotropic hypogonadism); and pharmacological hormone therapies such as oral contraceptives, estrogen replacement and gonadotropin-releasing hormone analogs.[26,27]

Mood disorders commonly occur or become markedly exacerbated in relation to menopause, especially prior to the cessation of menses. Menopause is a process characterized by gradual menstrual and endocrine changes resulting in amenorrhea, decreased gonadal steroid levels and elevated gonadotropin serum levels. Mood disorder symptoms include depression, anxiety, agitation, restlessness, emotional lability, irritability, fears, insomnia, logorrheic complaints with hypochondriacal content, and weight loss.

Although the majority of women pass through the menopausal stage of life uneventfully, a significant minority develop disabling emotional symptoms. Hormonal factors have been implicated. The pattern of hormonal changes, however, is remarkably common to all menopausal women. The possibility then exists that there may be a special feature of the brain (i.e. an anomalous brain substrate) that predisposes some women to develop hormonally related mood disorders. Brain substrate as well as age-related endocrine changes, therefore, may both be important in the development of perimenopausal depression or anxiety.

Estrogen replacement can enhance mood and subjective wellbeing. In menopausal women receiving estrogen replacement, circulating estrogen levels correlate with positive mood states. The antidepressant effects of estrogen may contribute to the frequently associated improvements in cognitive function. There has been suggestive evidence that depressed mood may also moderately increase the risk of developing dementia, primarily dementia of the Alzheimer's type, and that depression may be a very early manifestation of Alzheimer's disease.

The emotional changes attending the perimenopausal state are quite diverse and may include different forms of depression, including the agitated form, atypical depression with vegetative symptomatology, a combination of the two, and anxiety disorders, including generalized anxiety disorder, panic attacks, phobias, and obsessive-compulsive disorders. This distinction is important, as different emotional changes may be associated with different gonadal hormonal alterations. For example, during the natural perimenopause failure of progesterone secretion can precede the decline in estrogen levels, setting the stage for a relative excess ratio of estrogens to progesterone. This can contribute to the symptoms of depression, with agitated features or anxiety disorders. In contrast, in late menopause or surgical menopause, where there is a loss of production of both hormones, vegetative depressive symptoms may be expected to predominate.

Progesterone therapy can be beneficial in the treatment of women with anxiety disorders and some forms of depression (i.e. those associated with agitation or irritability). Synthetic progestins may affect the brain and behavior differently from natural progesterone, however. Specifically, natural progesterone is converted in the brain to allopregnenolone, whereas synthetic progestins are not. Allopregnenolone has GABAergic neuronal and anxiolytic clinical effects that are much more potent than pentobarbital and comparable to the most potent benzodiazepines. Excessive effects may lead to sedation and depression.

Some intermediaries of cortisol synthesis, especially the sulfated ester of dehydroepiandrosterone (DHEAS), are picrotoxin-like antagonists of the γ-aminobutyric acid A (GABA-A) receptor and exert potent neuroexcitatory and anxiogenic effects. Refractory anxiety disorders have been reported to occur in men and women who have non-classic or so-called late-onset congenital adrenal hyperplasia (CAH).[28] Elevated serum levels of excitatory neurosteroids may act on the brain, especially the anomalous brain, to promote the development of anxiety disorders. These disorders may be unusually resistant to treatment with the usual anxiolytic psychotropic medications and may respond best with adjuvant partial suppression of abnormal steroid secretion (e.g. using low-dose hydrocortisone or, when appropriate, ketoconazole). Combined therapy was found to be more effective in a series of 12 subjects in whom combination therapy resulted in statistically and clinically significantly greater improvement than with optimal baseline psychotherapeutic medicational intervention alone (Jacobs et al. 1999). Hormonal treatment that failed to lower DHEAS was ineffective.

Sleep

Sleep patterns may be affected by the cyclical changes in hormones that characterize the menstrual cycle. Rapid eye movement (REM) latency can be significantly shorter during the postovulatory (luteal) phase than in the preovulatory (follicular) phase, but no significant differences in latency to sleep onset or the percentage of REM sleep has been reported. Although no significant menstrual cycle differences in the percentages of various sleep stages has been found, women with premenstrual affective symptoms can have less δ sleep throughout the menstrual cycle than asymptomatic patients.

Obstructive sleep apnea (OSA) is considerably more common in men than in women. Preliminary data suggest that androgens may play a role in the male predominance of apnea. PCOS is characterized by menstrual disturbances, androgen excess and, frequently, obesity. These features suggest that women with PCOS may be at increased risk for OSA. Women with PCOS have been shown to have a higher apnea–hypopnea index and are more likely to suffer from symptomatic OSA syndrome than are matched reproductively normal women.[29] Sleep-disordered breathing (SDB) and excessive daytime sleepiness (EDS) are also markedly and significantly more frequent in PCOS women than in premenopausal controls.[30] Insulin resistance may be a stronger risk factor for SDB than body mass index or testosterone levels in women with PCOS.

Progesterone has hypnotic effects that can have a beneficial use in the treatment of premenstrual or perimenopause–menopause-related sleep disorders that may be related to rapid progesterone withdrawal or elevated estrogen/progesterone ratios. On the other hand, estrogen is the most important therapy for the treatment of perimenopausal–menopausal symptoms, hot flashes and night sweats, which constitute the commonest cause of sleep disorder in women during midlife. Estrogen and estrogen–progesterone combinations have both been shown to significantly ameliorate OSA. In contrast, treatment of hypogonadal men using testosterone has been shown to exacerbate OSA.

Neoplasms

Throughout life, particularly following the menopause, an increasing percentage of adrenal-secreted androstenedione is converted to estrogen, specifically estrone, by adipose and muscle tissue. There is a high correlation between this conversion rate, body weight, and the frequencies of female malignancies. The most obese women tend to be at a higher risk for female cancers. There is a greater than chance association between breast cancer and meningiomas. Epidemiological evidence suggests a possible role for female reproductive hormones in regulating the growth of meningiomas and neurofibromas.[31]

Intracranial meningiomas have an incidence of 2–7 per 100 000 in women, that is, approximately twice that of men. The possibility that reproductive hormones may have an important influence is supported by the substantially higher incidence in women, the frequent exacerbation of symptoms during pregnancy, and the existence of estrogen and progesterone receptors in the tumors. Estrogen and progesterone receptors are expressed commonly by meningiomas.[32] The frequency is highly variable in reports, perhaps because of pretreatment with corticosteroid hormones and differences between assay techniques. Progesterone receptors have been generally found to be much more common than estradiol receptors.[33] Whereas estradiol and progesterone agonists have been found to have little effect on tumor growth in animal models and in vitro human resected tissue experiments, meningioma growth has been retarded by the competitive progestin inhibitor mifepristone, in three separate investigations.[34] Efficacy has been demonstrated for clinical symptoms and findings, as well as tumor size.

Neurofibromas can grow at remarkably accelerated rates under the influence of female reproductive steroids, including during pregnancy.[35] Conversely, neurofibromatosis is associated with an elevated risk of intrauterine growth retardation, pregnancy-related hypertension (including an exacerbation of pre-existing chronic hypertension), abortion, stillbirth and oligohydramnios.

Stroke

There are sex differences in the pathophysiology and outcome of acute neurological injury that are relevant to stroke. In experimental models and clinically, females show less susceptibility to postischemic injury. This advantage of having greater neuroprotection is probably due to the effects of circulating estrogens and progestins. Both hormones have been shown to improve outcome after cerebral ischemia in experimental models.[36] The beneficial effects of estrogen include its antioxidant effect, the reduction of β-amyloid production and its neurotoxicity, preservation of autoregulatory function, increased expression of the antiapoptotic factor bcl-2, and activation of mitogen-activated protein kinase pathways.[37] Progesterone may provide neuroprotection by suppressing neuronal hyperexcitability. It also has a membrane stabilizing effect that can help reduce the damage caused by lipid peroxidation.

The incidence of ischemic stroke is low in women of reproductive age, and any risk attributable to oral contraceptive (OC) use has been demonstrated to be small.[38] First-generation oral contraceptives that have higher estrogen and progestin content appear to be associated with higher risk than the second- and third-generation pills that are mostly in use today. The risk is lower if users are under 35, do not smoke, do not have hypertension and do not have migraine. The risk of hemorrhagic stroke with OC use is not increased in younger women and only slightly increased in older women.[39]

The findings are similarly divided regarding the risks of postmenopausal hormone replacement, with conclusions ranging from a decrease to almost a twofold increase in stroke risk.[40,41] There is general agreement that the effects of hypertension, diabetes and smoking appear to strongly outweigh the effects of reproductive hormone replacement.

There is evidence that migraine increases stroke risk as follows: migraine without aura is associated with a two- to threefold increase; migraine with aura, a four- to sixfold increase; and migraine in the setting of oral contraceptive use, over a 10-fold increase. Therefore, considerable caution should be exercised in prescribing OC use for women who have migraine. OC use should be discontinued if migraines increase in frequency or severity, or become associated with neurological symptoms or findings.

The role of testosterone therapy as a risk factor for stroke is less clear. On the one hand, androgen therapy in hypogonadal men can increase total cholesterol, low-density lipoprotein and triglycerides, and decrease high-density lipoprotein, independent of the androgen type and the serum androgen levels achieved. On the other hand, total and free testosterone can be inversely associated with stroke severity and six-month mortality in men. Levels of total testosterone in men may be inversely associated with infarct size as well.

Multiple sclerosis

Sex affects the susceptibility to many autoimmune diseases. Compared to men, women have an increased risk of developing autoimmune disorders, including multiple sclerosis (MS), rheumatoid arthritis and systemic lupus erythematosus. The reasons for this may reflect complex interactions between hormonal, immunological, genetic and environmental factors. For example, women tend to have a generally greater humoral immune response than men. There is also an increased representation of HLA-DR2 in women with MS. Women with MS are even more sus-

ceptible to hormonal influences when the onset of symptoms occurs at an early (adolescence) or delayed (midlife) age. Pregnancy is associated with fewer exacerbations of MS, whereas exacerbations are increased during the first three months postpartum. Pregnancy is also associated with a long-term decrease in the risk of exacerbations.

Activated microglia are believed to contribute to the pathogenesis of MS, perhaps in part due to the production of nitric oxide (NO) and tumor necrosis factor (TNF)-α. These molecules can be toxic to oligodendrocytes. Estrogens and progesterone can inhibit NO and TNF-α production by microglial cells. In particular, concentrations of estriol and progesterone that are comparable to those in late pregnancy have been shown to inhibit these molecules, suggesting that hormonal inhibition of microglial cell activation may contribute to the decreased severity of MS that is commonly seen during pregnancy.

MS can show a tendency for worsening during the second half of the menstrual cycle, especially the premenstrual phase, or during the perimenopause. One possible explanation for this could be related to conditions where an elevated ratio of estrogen to progesterone exists, suggesting that progesterone may have protective benefits. Patients with a high estrogen to progesterone ratio can have a greater number of active MRI lesions than those with a low ratio.[42]

Prolactin has been found to be elevated in multiple sclerosis.[43] Although this elevation may represent a non-specific response to stress, prolactin has been found to promote both humoral and cell-mediated immune responses. Suppression of prolactin by bromocriptine, a dopamine agonist, in female rats reduces both the occurrence and severity of neurological signs of acute experimental allergic encephalomyelitis. Bromocriptine shows efficacy not only when used as pretreatment but also when introduced one week after immunization. It inhibits splenic lymphocyte proliferative responses in vitro to both the immunizing antigen and to concanavalin A.

References

1. Herzog AG. Reproductive endocrine considerations and hormonal therapy for women with epilepsy. Epilepsia 1991;32:S27–S33
2. Herzog AG. Reproductive endocrine considerations and hormonal therapy for men with epilepsy. Epilepsia 1991;32:S34–S37
3. Herzog AG, Klein P, Ransil BJ. Three patterns of catamenial epilepsy. Epilepsia 1997;38:1082–1088
4. Herzog AG. Progesterone therapy in women with complex partial and secondary generalized seizures. Neurology 1995;45:1660–1662
5. Herzog AG, Schachter SC. Valproate and the polycystic ovarian syndrome. Epilepsia 2001;42:315–320
6. Friedman MN, Herzog AG. Patient case reports: the evaluation and treatment of sexual dysfunction in men with epilepsy. Epilepsy Q 2000;8:3–16
7. Herzog AG, Klein P, Jacobs AR. Testosterone versus testosterone and testolactone in treating reproductive and sexual dysfunction in men with epilepsy and hypogonadism. Neurology 1998;50:782–784

8. Silberstein S, Merriam GR. Estrogens, progestins and headache. Neurology 1991;786–793

9. Herzog AG. Continuous bromocriptine therapy in menstrual migraine. Neurology 1997;48:101–102

10. Friedman MN, Herzog AG. Reproductive hormones, aging and dementia. J Geriatr Psychiatry 1999;32: 139–182

11. Caldwell BM. Estradiol treatment of Alzheimer's Disease. J Gerontol 1954;9:168–174

12. Kantor HI, Michael CM, Shore H. Estrogen for older women. Am J Obstet Gynecol 1973;116:115–118

13. Fillit H, Weinreb H, Cholst I, et al. Observations in a preliminary open trial of estradiol therapy for senile dementia-Alzheimer's type. Psychoneuroendocrinology 1986; 2:337–345

14. Honjo H, Ogino Y, Naitoh K, et al. In vivo effects by estrone sulfate on the central nervous system–senile dementia (Alzheimer's type). J Steroid Biochem 1989;34: 521–525

15. Ohkura T, Isse K, Akazawa K, et al. Evaluation of estrogen treatment in female patients with dementia of the Alzheimer type. Endocr J 1994;41:361–371

16. Ohkura T, Isse K, Kenji A, et al. Low-dose estrogen replacement therapy for Alzheimer disease in women. Menopause: J North Am Menopause Soc 1994;1: 125–130

17. Mortel KF, Meyer JS. Lack of postmenopausal estrogen replacement therapy and the risk of dementia. J Neuropsychiatr Clin Neurosci 1995;7:334–337

18. Henderson VW, Paganini-Hill A, Emanuel CK, et al. Estrogen replacement therapy in older women. Comparisons between Alzheimer's disease cases and nondemented control subjects. Arch Neurol 1994;51: 896–900

19. Paganini-Hill A, Henderson VW. Estrogen replacement therapy and risk of Alzheimer disease. Arch Intern Med 1996;156:2213–2217

20. Tang MX, Jacobs D, Stern Y, et al. Effect of oestrogen during menopause on risk and age at onset of Alzheimer's disease [see comments]. Lancet 1996;348: 429–432

21. Mulnard RA, Cotman CW, Kawas C, et al. Estrogen replacement therapy for treatment of mild to moderate Alzheimer disease: a randomized controlled trial. Alzheimer's Disease Cooperative Study. JAMA 2000; 283(8):1007–1015.

22. Seshadri S, Zornberg GL, Derby LE, et al. Postmenopausal estrogen replacement therapy and the risk of Alzheimer disease. Arch Neurol 2001;58(3):435–440.

23. Tarsy D, Thulin PC, Herzog AG. Spasmodic torticollis and reproductive function. Parkinsonism Rel Dis 2001;7: 323–327

24. Herzog AG. Hormonal influences on spasmodic torticollis: A case report. Mov Disord 1993;8:118–119

25. Herzog AG. Psychoneuroendocrine aspects of temporolimbic epilepsy: I. Brain, reproductive steroids and emotions. Psychosomatics 1999;40:95–100

26. Herzog AG. Psychoneuroendocrine aspects of temporolimbic epilepsy: II. Epilepsy and reproductive steroids. Psychosomatics 1999;40:102–108

27. Herzog AG. Psychoneuroendocrine aspects of temporolimbic epilepsy: III. Case reports. Psychosomatics 1999;40: 109–116

28. Jacobs AR, Edelheit PB, Coleman AE, Herzog AG. Late onset congenital adrenal hyperplasia: a treatable cause of anxiety. Biol Psychiatry 1999;46:856–859

29. Fogel RB, Malhotra A, Pillar G, et al. Increased prevalence of obstructive sleep apnea syndrome in obese women with polycystic ovary syndrome. J Clin Endocrinol Metab 2001;86:1175–1180

30. Vgontzas AN, Legro RS, Bixler EO, et al. Polycystic ovary syndrome is associated with obstructive sleep apnea and daytime sleepiness: role of insulin resistance. J Clin Endocrinol Metab 2001;86:517–520

31. Longstreth WT, Dennis LK, McGuire VM, et al. Epidemiology of intracranial meningioma. Cancer 1993;72: 639–648

32. Cahill DW, Bashirelahi N, Solomon LW, et al. Estrogen and progesterone receptors in meningiomas. J Neurosurg 1984;60:985–993

33. Smith DA, Cahill DW. The biology of meningiomas. Neurosurg Clin North Am 1994;5:201–215

34. Grunberg SM. Role of antiprogestational therapy for meningiomas. Hum Reprod 1994;9(Suppl 1):202–207

35. Martuza RL, MacLaughlin DT, Ojemann RG. Specific estradiol binding in schwannomas, meningiomas, and neurofibromas. Neurosurgery 1981;9:665–671

36. McCullough LD, Alkayed NJ, Traystman RJ, et al. Postischemic estrogen reduces hypoperfusion and secondary ischemia after experimental stroke. Stroke 2001;32: 796–802

37. Hurn PD, Macrae IM. Estrogen as a neuroprotectant in stroke. J Cerebr Blood Flow Metab 2000;20:631–652

38. Gillum LA, Mamidipudi SK, Johnston SC. Ischemic stroke risk with oral contraceptives: A meta-analysis. JAMA 2000;284:72–78

39. Schwartz SM, Siscovick DS, Longstreth WT, et al. Use of low-dose oral contraceptives and stroke in young women. Ann Intern Med 1997;127:596–603

40. Simon JA, Hsia J, Cauley JA, et al. Postmenopausal hormone therapy and risk of stroke: The Heart and Estrogen-progestin Replacement Study (HERS). Circulation 2001;103:638–642

41. Paganini-Hill A, Perez Barreto M. Stroke risk in older men and women: aspirin, estrogen, exercise, vitamins, and other factors. J Gend Specif Med 2001;4:18–28

42. Bansil S, Lee HJ, Jindal S, et al. Correlation between sex hormones and magnetic resonance imaging lesions in multiple sclerosis. Acta Neurol Scand 1999;99:91–94

43. Riskind PN, Massacesi L, Doolittle TH, Hauser SL. The role of prolactin in autoimmune demyelination: suppression of experimental allergic encephalomyelitis by bromocriptine. Ann Neurol 1991;29:542–547

139 Disorders of Bone and Mineral Metabolism

Ann Sweeney and Robert M Levin

Osteoporosis

Osteoporosis, a common metabolic bone disorder, is a frequent cause of low back pain, for which reason patients are often referred for neurological consultation. This section of the chapter reviews the current evaluation and management of low back pain as a metabolic bone disorder.

Osteoporosis is characterized by low bone mass and microarchitectural deterioration. Therefore, patients are at increased risk for fracture. Fractures may occur after low-intensity trauma, particularly fractures of the spine, hip, and distal radius. Most serious is hip fracture, which is associated with substantial morbidity and mortality.

Multiple compression fractures of the thoracic spine result in a kyphotic deformity called "dowager's hump." The back pain associated with osteoporosis may result from a radiographically apparent compression fracture, an inapparent trabecular microfracture, or a strain on supporting structures that try to maintain a relatively straight spine in the presence of a spinal deformity. Back pain has many causes, ranging from mild muscle sprains to metastatic disease (Table 139.1), but this chapter is concerned primarily with osteoporosis and the role it has in managing a patient with low back pain. Secondary causes of osteoporosis are listed in Table 139.2.

The cause of osteoporosis is unknown. There is an imbalance in bone turnover, with osteoclastic bone resorption exceeding osteoblastic bone formation. Normally, the activity of these two bone cells is linearly correlated. As discussed below, the effective therapeutic agents in osteoporosis are those that inhibit osteoclastic activity. Skeletal radiographs are not helpful in the diagnosis of mild to moderate osteoporosis because osteopenia does not show up on a radiograph until at least one-third of the skeletal mass has been lost. Therefore, a lateral thoracolumbar spine film may be read as "normal" despite the presence of substantial bone loss. As many as 30% to 40% of patients with osteoporosis and spinal compression fractures may be completely asymptomatic. The diagnosis of osteoporosis is often made incidentally during the radiographic evaluation of an unrelated problem.

Risk factors in osteoporosis

A typical presentation of someone at high risk for osteoporosis is a thin postmenopausal white or Asian woman presenting with a recent hip fracture following minor trauma. Other risk factors that may alert the clinician to suspect osteoporosis include cigarette smoking, alcohol excess, history of prolonged immobilization, and a history of hip fracture in either parent. A diet low in calcium and vitamin D is an important cause of bone loss. Other contributing factors include prolonged glucocorticoid therapy, excessive thyroid hormone replacement therapy for hypothyroidism, and a previously incurred fracture.

Evaluation of osteoporosis

The important blood tests recommended to evaluate for osteoporosis are measurements of calcium,

Table 139.1	Causes of back pain

Osteoporosis
Malignancy
Osteoarthritis
Disk herniation
Sciatica
Paget disease
Osteomyelitis
Spinal stenosis
Facet disease
Muscle sprain

Table 139.2	Secondary causes of osteoporosis

Medications	Glucocorticoid excess
	Thyroid hormone excess
	Phenytoin
	Cyclosporine
	Heparin
Endocrinopathies	Hyperparathyroidism
	Hypogonadism
	Postmenopausal
	Anorexia nervosa
	Thyrotoxicosis
	Cushing syndrome
Malignancies	Multiple myeloma
	Lymphoma
	Leukemia
Gastrointestinal tract disorders	Malabsorption
	Primary biliary cirrhosis
Osteogenesis imperfecta	

phosphorus, alkaline phosphatase, and 25-hydroxy-vitamin D. The values for all of these usually are within normal limits in primary osteoporosis. Other tests that may be helpful include serum protein immunoelectrophoresis, serum concentration of testosterone (in men), and 24-hour urinary calcium determination. Primary hyperparathyroidism (PHP) is a common disorder, particularly in the elderly, and is important to consider as a secondary cause of osteoporosis. It is often asymptomatic. Unexpected hypercalcemia is detected incidentally during the evaluation of an unrelated problem. An increased serum level of parathyroid hormone associated with an increased serum concentration of calcium confirms the diagnosis of PHP.

Vitamin D deficiency is important to exclude because it is a common disorder, is easily diagnosed, and is readily corrected with vitamin D replacement therapy.[1] A 25-hydroxyvitamin D level less than 20 ng/mL is considered "vitamin D insufficiency" and a level less than 15 ng/mL is "vitamin D deficiency." Vitamin D is essential for gastrointestinal absorption of calcium and normal bone remodeling. Vitamin D deficiency may lead to a mild decrease in the serum concentration of calcium, which in turn leads to an increased serum level of parathyroid hormone (PTH). The latter stimulates osteoclastic bone resorption.

A bone mineral densitometry study is recommended for all women older than 65 years and for those younger who have other risk factors for osteoporosis. Abnormal results on bone mineral densitometry, best performed by dual-energy X-ray absorptiometry, is helpful in diagnosing osteoporosis and in alerting the clinician and patient of the severity of the bone loss.[2]

Treatment of osteoporosis

The goal of therapy is to prevent osteoporotic bone deformities and fractures. Preventive measures should be instituted before substantial bone loss occurs. The average American diet contains less than 800 mg of calcium daily—less than the recommended daily allowance. Adults should ingest between 1300 and 1500 mg of calcium daily in their diet, and if this cannot be attained, supplements of calcium carbonate or other calcium-containing preparations should be added.[3]

Vitamin D insufficiency is present in 30% to 40% of adults living in the United States. Those who live in the northeast have little to no vitamin D produced in their skin during the winter months because of insufficient ultraviolet light from the sun.[4] Persons younger than 50 years should ingest 400 IU of vitamin D daily, and those older than 70 years should have twice that much. The vitamin D status of a person is easily determined by measuring the serum level of 25-hydroxyvitamin D.

Estrogen replacement therapy Estrogen replacement therapy (ERT) is the reference standard for treatment of postmenopausal osteoporosis. Several well-designed studies have demonstrated the effectiveness of ERT in slowing the rate of bone loss and decreasing the occurrence of fractures in postmenopausal women.[5,6] ERT should be started at the time of menopause because of the exaggerated increase in the rate of bone loss during the first 6 to 8 years of menopause. However, if ERT is discontinued, bone loss accelerates again. The two regimens most frequently recommended for hormonal replacement therapy are "intermittent cyclical therapy" or "continuous hormonal replacement." Intermittent cyclical therapy consists of conjugated equine estrogens (0.625 mg daily) from day 1 to day 25 monthly plus medroxyprogesterone (5 to 10 mg daily) from day 15 to day 25. Progestin is added to convert a proliferative endometrium to a secretory one, to promote endometrial sloughing, and, thereby, to prevent endometrial carcinoma from developing. Continuous therapy consisting of estrogen (0.625 mg daily) plus medroxy progesterone (2.5 mg daily) is also effective in slowing bone loss and, at the same time, in avoiding monthly menstrual bleeding.

Contraindications to ERT include a history of unexplained deep venous thrombosis, pulmonary embolus, active liver disease, history of breast or endometrial cancer, unexplained vaginal bleeding, migraine headaches, or symptomatic uterine fibroids. There is considerable controversy concerning the extraskeletal pros and cons of ERT. On the "plus side," many studies have demonstrated a beneficial effect on the primary prevention of coronary artery disease, but not as effective on secondary prevention.[7,8] ERT has been reported to decrease fatal coronary events by 50% to 60%. On the "negative side" are data that ERT is associated with an increased incidence of breast cancer, particularly in women who have been receiving ERT for more than 10 to 15 years.[9] However, most of these investigations of both coronary artery disease and breast cancer lacked sufficient prospective study. What is needed is a large prospective, placebo-controlled, randomized trial such as the National Institutes of Health-sponsored Women's Health Initiative Study.[10] This study is randomly assigning 27 500 postmenopausal women to hormone replacement therapy or placebo to clarify the risks and benefits of hormonal replacement therapy on coronary artery disease and breast cancer. However, the results of this study will not be available for several years.

Bisphosphonates Currently, these are the most effective agents for increasing bone density and decreasing fractures. They are analogues of endogenous pyrophosphates that become incorporated in the hydroxyapatite crystal of bone. They directly inhibit osteoclast activity and slow bone loss. The two most recent bisphosphonates approved by the Food and Drug Administration (FDA) are alendronate (10 mg daily) and risedronate (5 mg daily). Both have been studied carefully and have been demonstrated to increase bone density of the spine and hip and to decrease hip and vertebral fractures in women and men with osteoporosis.[11,12] These drugs have no effect on coronary arteries or mammary tissue, but they are the most potent agents yet developed to benefit bone. They are particularly valuable in the prevention and treatment of corticosteroid-induced osteoporosis.[13]

Raloxifene This is the drug most recently approved by the FDA for the prevention and treatment of osteoporosis. It is a benzothiophene that acts on estrogen receptors and has an estrogen-like agonist effect on some tissues (bone and lipids) and an antagonist effect on other tissues (breast and uterus).[14] Benzothiophenes, known as "selective estrogen receptor modulators," have specific appeal for postmenopausal women who are at significant risk for the development of breast cancer. In fact, preliminary data suggest that raloxifene may be as effective as tamoxifen in primary breast cancer prevention and, at the same time, act as an antiresorptive agent on bone.

In summary, several agents are now available that can be used alone or in combination for the prevention and treatment of osteoporosis. A tailored approach is now possible for patients who are either at risk for or have well-established osteoporosis.

Paget Disease

"Paget disease" is a common metabolic bone disorder associated with considerable neurological complications. It does not receive the attention that osteoporosis does, probably because 70% to 80% of the patients with Paget disease are asymptomatic.[15] The diagnosis is often made incidentally during the evaluation of an unrelated disorder. A typical scenario is as follows: an elderly person falls, and back pain develops. The person is taken to a nearby emergency department for evaluation. Routine radiographs of the back show a small area of Paget disease in the pelvis, most likely unrelated to the patient's complaint. The radiograph of a pagetic abnormality is readily identified as Paget disease. Neurological complications are uncommon in Paget disease, but when present, they may present with a very dramatic and puzzling clinical picture, and referral to a neurologist is not infrequent.

Definition and pathophysiology

Paget disease is a localized bone disorder that often begins in one and, occasionally, multiple sites. It is characterized histologically by the abrupt onset of accelerated bone resorption (the "osteoclastic" or "destructive" phase), followed by an equally vigorous phase of attempted bone healing, with excessive new bone formation ("osteoblastic" or "sclerotic" phase). The earliest findings are an increased number of large multinucleated osteoclasts and increased vascularity of the bone. Bone normally receives 5% of the cardiac output, compared with 18% by pagetic bone.[16] In response to excessive bone resorption, new bone is formed so rapidly that it is not laid down properly according to lines of stress ("lamellar bone") but rather in a poorly organized pattern ("woven bone"). This results in enlarged distorted bones composed of areas of poorly mineralized bone lying in proximity to areas of sclerotic bone.

Sir James Paget first described this disorder in 1876, and its cause is still uncertain. The histological pattern resembles that of a slow virus infection, with active proliferating cells, fibrosis, and multinucleated osteoclasts.

Up to 15% to 30% of patients with Paget disease have a positive family history for the disorder. An autosomal dominant pattern of inheritance is supported by kindred studies. A first-degree relative of a person with Paget disease has a risk of developing the disorder seven times greater than that of an age-matched unrelated control. The disorder is common in Europe, North America, Australia, and New Zealand, but it is rare in China, Japan, India, and Malaysia.[17] Paget disease affects 3% of persons in North America older than 55 years, and the prevalence increases with age.

Presentation

Paget disease is often discovered incidentally when a routine blood test reveals an unexpected increased level of alkaline phosphatase. After liver disease has been excluded as the cause of the increase in alkaline phosphatase, an evaluation of the skeleton by bone scintigraphy may reveal "hot" spots, which can be confirmed by radiographic study to be Paget disease. Bone pain may be described as a dull ache; it worsens with weight-bearing. Often, the pain is that of osteoarthritis, which is aggravated by the pagetic process abutting the hip or other joints. Pagetic bone is soft and may lead to deformities such as a bowed tibia. Involvement of the skull may cause enlargement of the head, and the patient may complain that the hat size has recently increased.

Neurological complications

Bony overgrowth of vertebrae, a common site of Paget disease, may cause narrowing of the spinal canal, radiculopathies due to compression of a nerve root, spinal stenosis, or cauda equina syndrome. Progressive lower limb weakness may be the patient's only complaint. If evaluation by computed tomography–myelography or magnetic resonance imaging does not show evidence of a mechanical obstruction, consider a vascular steal phenomenon. In such a setting, blood flow is diverted to the highly vascular pagetic bone, resulting in ischemia of the spinal cord.[18] Herzburg and Bayliss[19] described a 76-year-old man with Paget disease of the spine who presented with progressively worsening low back pain and lower extremity weakness and sensory loss. No mechanical obstruction could be identified. A spinal artery steal syndrome was diagnosed. Subcutaneous salmon calcitonin treatment was begun and, within 12 days after he received 100 Medical Reseach Council (MRC) units daily, his neurological findings improved markedly.

Narrowing of bony foramina of the skull can lead to cranial nerve (CN) palsies, especially CNs I, II, III, V, VII, and VIII. Hearing loss may occur as a neurological complication of Paget disease.[20] Compression of CN VIII, diminished hair cell function, a decrease in cochlear capsule bone density, or fixation of the ossicles, leading to a conductive hearing loss, are possible mechanisms. In most cases, after hearing loss has occurred, it is irreversible. Softening of pagetic bone may result in deformities of the base of the skull and produce cerebellar compression, palsies of CNs IX through XII, and, rarely, obstructive hydrocephalus and its sequelae.[21] In addition, new-onset migraine headaches in the elderly, a symptom of a vascular steal syndrome, may alert physicians to consider Paget disease in the differential diagnosis.

What is unique about Paget disease is that the symptoms and signs of the disorder are, for the most part, due to the reparative process, that is, excessive osteoblastic new bone formation resulting in narrowed bony foramina and compressed nerves.

Clinical and laboratory features

The accelerated rate of bone remodeling in Paget disease may lead to increased bone breakdown, hypercalciuria, and kidney stones. If multiple bones are involved, the increased vascularity may lead to arteriovenous shunting and resultant high-output heart failure. Skeletal deformities, bone pain, and fractures also may occur. If multiple bones are involved and the patient is prescribed prolonged bed rest, hypercalcemia due to immobilization may develop. Although osteoclastic bone activity does not slow with bed rest, osteoblastic activity does, resulting in increased bone resorption.

The serum concentrations of calcium and phosphorus are usually normal, but the alkaline phosphatase level is increased. The serum level of alkaline phosphatase correlates well with the rate of bone formation and reflects the osteoblastic activity associated with increased bone turnover. The urinary excretion of hydroxyproline or one of the other currently available bone markers (e.g., N-telopeptide) measures the rate of bone resorption. Because bone resorption and formation rates are closely coupled, the activity of Paget disease can be followed by measuring the serum level of alkaline phosphatase at regular intervals. Within 3 to 12 weeks, this level decreases by more than 50% in two-thirds of the patients given an antiresorptive agent.

The most frequently involved bones in Paget disease are the pelvis, spine, proximal femur, skull, scapula, tibia, and humerus. The clinical phase of the disease usually can be determined by radiological examination. In a long bone, a V-shaped ("blades of grass") advancing edge of osteolysis is characteristic of Paget disease. This phase is followed shortly thereafter by a period of active bone formation, and dense bone begins to replace the radiolucent areas. Small cortical fractures may be noted along the convex side of a bowed tibia or femur. During the late stages of the disease, the bone has a dense, cotton-ball sclerotic appearance, with cortical thickening. Although the radiographic findings of Paget disease may be quite characteristic, a bone scan is the most sensitive way to detect pagetic lesions. A bone scan shows abnormality before a radiograph does.

Treatment

The indications to begin medical treatment of Paget disease are somewhat controversial. For example, there is general agreement to treat patients who have a marked increase in the serum alkaline phosphatase level, bone pain, immobilization hypercalcemia, high-output heart failure, fractures, kidney stones, or any neurological complications. In addition, a focus of pagetic bone abutting any major joint should be treated before undergoing an orthopedic procedure in that vicinity. However, how should a patient who has a small lytic area in a non-weight-bearing bone and who is completely asymptomatic be managed? Will medical treatment of a very early lesion prevent an osteogenic sarcoma from developing many years later? Osteogenic sarcoma, an unusual complication of Paget disease, occurs in fewer than 0.1% of patients.

The earliest effective drugs used to treat Paget disease were calcitonin and etidronate, but newer bisphosphonates have become the treatment of choice. Calcitonin is a potent inhibitor of osteoclastic bone resorption and it reduces bone pain, lessens neurological symptoms, heals osteolytic lesions, and decreases the vascularity of pagetic bone.[22,23] It results in decreasing serum levels of alkaline phosphatase and urinary bone markers. Most of the experience with calcitonin treatment has been with salmon calcitonin, 50 to 100 MRC units daily, and then adjusted to 3 times weekly for 6 to 12 months. Minor adverse effects include nausea and facial flushing. Monitoring the alkaline phosphatase level is helpful in deciding when to stop and restart cycles of therapy. When calcitonin treatment is stopped, the patient's clinical condition often remains improved for many months while the serum level of alkaline phosphatase and the urinary level of hydroxyproline slowly increase, reaching pretreatment levels in about 6 months. Intranasal calcitonin (200 units daily, alternating nasal passages, for 6 months) and human calcitonin have been approved by the FDA, but they are less effective than the new bisphosphonates.

The bisphosphonates that have been studied most recently are etidronate (Didronel), pamidronate (Aredia), alendronate (Fosamax), risedronate (Actonel), and tiludronate (Skelid). Each one effectively slows bone resorption by inhibiting osteoclast activity. They also reduce bone pain, improve neurological complaints, and decrease the serum levels of alkaline phosphatase and urinary bone markers. Etidronate is not the preferred drug because it may cause mineralization defects (focal osteomalacia) in a small percentage of the patients.[24]

Pamidronate, which is available for intravenous use, is highly effective. A single infusion of 60 mg given over 3 hours (in 500 mL of 5% dextrose in water) results in reduced bone turnover and a decrease in the alkaline phosphatase level. Most patients require monthly infusions (often three to six) until the serum alkaline phosphatase level returns to normal. Advantages of pamidronate over etidronate include (1) greater potency in inhibiting bone resorption, (2) longer duration of effectiveness, and (3) absence of focal osteomalacia. The disadvantages are its need to be given intravenously and its cost. Transient mild hypocalcemia may occur. Adverse effects include mild transient (24 hours) fever and myalgias in 20% to 30% of the patients.

Thiebaud et al.[25] reported on the use of pamidronate as a single intravenous infusion in the treatment of Paget disease. Of 11 patients with symptomatic disease, 10 had clinical improvement and normalization of biochemical values (i.e., bone markers returned to normal levels) after a single infusion of 60 mg over 24 hours. Wimalawansa and Gunasekera[26] described 15 patients with extensive Paget disease that had become refractory to calcitonin and etidronate therapy. The disease in all but one of these patients markedly improved clinically and biochemically with pamidronate given intravenously.

Alendronate is an effective treatment. A multicenter trial compared alendronate with etidronate and showed that alendronate was more effective.[27] An oral dose of 40 mg daily for 6 months is recommended. The drug is contraindicated for patients with esophageal dysfunction. The drug must be taken in the fasting state, preferably in the morning, with 6 to 8 ounces of tap water. Breakfast is to be delayed 30 to 45 minutes. The patient should take the drug while standing and remain upright for 30 minutes to expedite the drug's passage through the esophagus.

Risedronate, the most recently FDA-approved bisphosphonate, was recently compared in a randomized double-blinded comparison with etidronate to treat Paget disease.[28] This multicenter trial included 62 patients given risedronate, 30 mg daily for 2 months, and 61 patients given etidronate, 400 mg daily for 6 months. The serum level of alkaline phosphatase normalized by 1 year in 73% of patients given risedronate, compared with 15% of those given etidronate. By the eighteenth month of the study, 53% of the patients receiving risedronate and 14% of those receiving etidronate remained in biochemical remission. There were no reports of esophagitis.

It should be emphasized that pagetic bone may be very vascular, and patients should be given medical treatment with an antiosteoclastic agent for a few months before orthopedic surgery is performed. The goal is to lessen intraoperative bleeding.

Hypocalcemia

This section of the chapter discusses disorders of calcium and magnesium metabolism frequently encountered on a hospital general medical service and often associated with abnormalities of the central and peripheral nervous systems.

The most common causes of hypocalcemia include postoperative hypoparathyroidism, vitamin D deficiency, renal insufficiency, and hypomagnesemia. The differential diagnosis is broad but may be divided into two major categories: parathyroid and nonparathyroid causes of hypocalcemia (Tables 139.3 and 139.4). The inadvertent removal of excess parathyroid

Table 139.3 Parathyroid causes of hypoparathyroidism

Postsurgical
Hypomagnesemia
Polyglandular autoimmune syndrome
Infiltrative diseases
    Metastatic carcinoma
    Wilson disease
    Hemochromatosis
    Thalassemia
Irradiation
Idiopathic
    Branchial dysembryogenesis (DiGeorge syndrome)
    Congenital absence of parathyroids

Modified from Guise TA, Mundy GR. Evaluation of hypocalcemia in children and adults. J Clin Endocrinol Metab 1995;80:1473–1478. By permission of The Endocrine Society.

Table 139.4 Nonparathyroid causes of hypocalcemia

Vitamin D deficiency
    Nutritional
    Renal failure
    Malabsorption
    Anticonvulsant therapy
    Liver disease
1α-Hydroxylase deficiency (vitamin D-dependent rickets type I)
Vitamin D resistance
    Medications
    Plicamycin, calcitonin, bisphosphonates, phosphate
    Phenobarbital, dilantin
    Citrated blood, radiographic contrast dyes
    Fluoride, foscarnet, pentamidine
    Reversible hypoparathyroidism
Malignancy
    Osteoblastic metastases
    Tumor lysis syndrome
PTH resistance
Hypomagnesemia
Acute pancreatitis
Toxic shock syndrome
Acute rhabdomyolysis

PTH, parathyroid hormone.
Modified from Guise TA, Mundy GR. Evaluation of hypocalcemia in children and adults. J Clin Endocrinol Metab 1995;80:1473–1478. By permission of The Endocrine Society.

tissue during surgical exploration for hyperparathyroidism results in a low serum concentration of calcium. Approximately 40% of the total circulating calcium is bound to albumin, 10% is complexed (citrate, sulfate, and phosphate), and 50% remains in the free ionized form. A decrease in the serum concentration of albumin lowers the total blood level of calcium but has no effect on the biologically active ionized fraction. A formula used to correct for a decreased serum concentration of albumin is to add 0.8 mg/dL to the serum calcium concentration for each 1.0 g/dL that the serum albumin concentration is below 4.0 g/dL.

Clinical features

The clinical features associated with hypocalcemia vary widely from an asymptomatic biochemical abnormality to a life-threatening condition. The major signs and symptoms of hypocalcemia are neurological. Low serum concentrations of calcium increase neuromuscular excitability and result in transient paresthesias and muscle cramping and twitching of the distal extremities. Nerves exposed to low levels of calcium experimentally have a decreased threshold of excitation, repetitive responses to a single stimulus, impaired accommodation, and continuous activity.[29,30] These tetanic manifestations are due to spontaneous discharges of sensory and motor fibers in peripheral nerves. Peripheral nerve irritability to mechanical stimuli is the basis of the Chvostek and Trousseau signs.

As the serum concentration of calcium decreases further, overt tetanic signs may occur, such as carpopedal and laryngeal spasms and seizures. The symptoms of hypocalcemia correlate with the absolute calcium concentration but, more importantly, with the rate of decrease in the serum concentration of calcium. Kugelberg[31] described the typical sequence in which tetanic symptoms arise. Initially, tingling occurs around the mouth and at the tips of the fingers and then increases in intensity and spreads over the entire face. Later, a sensation of spasm occurs in the muscles of the mouth, hands, and distal parts of the extremities. This sensation intensifies and becomes a tonic spasm. The spasms usually are not painful, but they are frightening for the patient. Chvostek first described and demonstrated increased irritability of the facial nerve. The Chvostek sign, used to detect latent tetany, is elicited by lightly percussing the facial nerve.[32,33] A response graded +1 may be seen normally in up to 20% of adults. The Trousseau sign is also used to detect latent tetany. The classic main d'accoucheur posture, diagnostic of tetany, is characterized by adduction of the thumb, followed by flexion of the metacarpophalangeal joints, extension of the interphalangeal joints without separation of the fingers, and flexion at the wrist and elbow. Trousseau discovered an artificial production of a tetanic cramp of the hand in a patient with tetany who was bled with the assistance of a bandage applied around the arm.[34] The Trousseau sign is elicited by inflating a blood pressure cuff 30 mm Hg above systolic pressure.[35] Ischemia induced by inflation of the blood pressure cuff results in increased excitability of the nerve. Tactile paresthesias, fasciculations, the sensation of spasm, and the classic main d'accoucheur posture occur in sequential order.

Other features of chronic hypocalcemia include ophthalmologic abnormalities such as posterior lenticular cataracts and dental abnormalities such as absent or delayed tooth eruption and formation as well as enamel malformation. Chronic hypocalcemia may be associated with extrapyramidal signs, including parkinsonism, related to calcification of the basal ganglia.[36] Cardiac manifestations of hypocalcemia include flattening of T waves, U waves, and QTc prolongation.[37] The prolongation of the QTc interval depends not only on the severity of the hypocalcemia but also on the rapidity of the fall in calcium concentration. Ventricular tachycardia with torsades de pointes may also occur.

Treatment

In the setting of acute hypocalcemia, serum levels of PTH, 25-hydroxyvitamin D, calcium, albumin, magnesium, and phosphorus should be determined. In severe cases, it may be necessary for the patient to have cardiac monitoring. Acute symptomatic hypocalcemia should be treated with intravenous calcium gluconate.[38] For frank tetany, 1 or 2 ampules of calcium gluconate (1 ampule contains 1 g of calcium gluconate or 93 mg of elemental calcium) should be infused rapidly over 15 to 20 minutes. This usually results in prompt relief of symptoms, but the infusion may have to be repeated. If prolonged hypocalcemia is anticipated, for example in the hungry bone syndrome following removal of a parathyroid adenoma, continuous intravenous infusion of calcium gluconate (15 mg/kg) may be required. In a 70-kg person, 10 ampules of calcium gluconate should be placed in a liter of 5% dextrose and infused at a rate to be determined according to the patient's symptoms. The serum concentration of calcium needs to be monitored closely.

If the hypocalcemia is complicated by hypomagnesemia (serum level of magnesium <1.5 mg/dL), the serum calcium level may not be corrected until the hypomagnesemia is corrected. Four to 6 g of magnesium sulfate ($MgSO_4$) is administered over 24 hours and repeated for 4 to 6 days. One ampule of $MgSO_4$ contains 1 g of $MgSO_4$ but only 96 mg of elemental magnesium. If renal function is normal, 5 to 6 g of $MgSO_4$ can be administered intravenously daily. If the corrected calcium level remains below 8.5 mg/dL, oral 0.25 μg of calcitriol (1,25-dihydroxyvitamin D) should be given twice daily. If the serum calcium is still less than 8.5 mg/dL after 24 hours, the calcitriol dose should be gradually increased to 0.5 μg twice daily. Also, 2 to 3 g of oral calcium carbonate are recommended daily. The serum calcium level should be monitored closely, particularly early on, to avoid hypercalcemia.

Hypercalcemia
Etiology

The causes of hypercalcemia are listed in Table 139.5. Primary hyperparathyroidism (PHP) and malignancy account for 90% of hypercalcemic cases. These two diagnoses usually are easily distinguished on the basis of the clinical features and laboratory test results. More than 80% of patients with PHP are entirely asymptomatic, and hypercalcemia is detected incidentally during evaluation of an unrelated problem. Review of previous records may show that mild hypercalcemia has been long-standing. In contrast, patients with hypercalcemia of malignancy appear quite ill and are more likely to manifest the clinical features of malignancy. Most patients with PHP have mild hypercalcemia, with serum calcium levels often only 1.0 mg/dL above the upper limit of normal. In contrast, patients with hypercalcemia of malignancy may have serum calcium levels that exceed 14 mg/dL.

Hypercalcemia in the presence of an increased level of PTH is the biochemical hallmark of PHP. Other conditions may produce an identical biochemical profile and should be considered in the differential diagnosis. These include tertiary hyperparathyroidism, medications such as lithium and thiazide diuretics, and the syndrome of familial hypocalciuric hypercalcemia (FHH). Tertiary hyperparathyroidism occurs in the setting of renal failure when hyperplastic chief cells progress to monoclonal proliferation. FHH is an autosomal dominantly inherited trait characterized by mild hypercalcemia and relative hypocalciuria. In FHH, an alteration in the set point for PTH secretion occurs such that the hormone continues to be secreted at higher calcium levels than normal. It is important to exclude this diagnosis because it is a benign condition and surgical treatment is not indicated. Lithium also alters the set point

for PTH secretion, and patients given lithium treatment may become hypercalcemic. Chronic thiazide administration produces mild hypercalcemia associated with a decrease in urinary calcium excretion.

Clinical and laboratory features

The clinical features of hypercalcemia are closely related to the absolute calcium concentration and its rate of increase. Patients with PHP usually have mild hypercalcemia, as noted above, and may not have any symptoms. A neuropsychiatric syndrome described in some patients with PHP is characterized by vague constitutional symptoms such as depression, fatigue, lassitude, sleep disturbances, and memory loss.[39] The patient's family may recognize a personality change. These admittedly are subtle symptoms and difficult to quantitate. At serum concentrations of calcium greater than 13 mg/dL, renal impairment and calcification of the blood vessels, kidneys, skin, lung, and heart may occur. A serum calcium concentration greater than 14 mg/dL is considered a medical emergency and should be treated as such. Patients with calcium levels this high are usually volume-depleted and present with altered mental status. Hypercalcemia may interfere with the action of antidiuretic hormone on the distal nephron and cause nephrogenic diabetes insipidus. Gastrointestinal manifestations include anorexia, nausea, vomiting, and, rarely, pancreatitis. Neurological signs at this degree of hypercalcemia range from apathy, drowsiness, and obtundation to coma. The cardiac manifestations of severe hypercalcemia include enhanced sensitivity to digitalis and electrocardiographic abnormalities such as a shortened QT interval, bradyarrythmia, bundle branch block, complete heart block, and cardiac arrest.

Evaluation

The history should focus on the two most likely causes of hypercalcemia: PHP and malignancy. A history of kidney stones may be elicited in 20% of patients with PHP. The presence of other diseases associated with PHP such as peptic ulcer disease and hypertension as well as other endocrinopathies (that may implicate multiple endocrine neoplasia type 1 or type 2) should be noted. Malignancy occurring with hypercalcemia usually is not occult. The history should be directed at constitutional symptoms, bone pain, weight loss, smoking history, recent mammographic results, and family history of cancer. A careful medication history, specifically regarding hydrochlorothiazide, lithium, calcium supplements, and vitamin D use, should be sought.

The physical examination also should focus on the most likely causes of hypercalcemia. Patients with PHP have few abnormal findings on examination. Band keratopathy, an unusual finding in PHP, is characterized by calcification in the lateral and medial margins of the limbus. Enlarged parathyroid glands usually are not palpable but, if present, are suggestive of parathyroid carcinoma. The patient should be examined carefully for signs of malignancy, with particular attention to the lungs, breast, head, and neck.

Table 139.5 Causes of hypercalcemia

PTH-associated causes
    Primary hyperparathyroidism
    Tertiary hyperparathyroidism
    FHH
    Drugs: lithium, hydrochlorothiazide
Malignancy-related causes
    Solid tumor metastases (breast)
    Humoral hypercalcemia of malignancy (lung and kidney)
    Hematologic malignancies (multiple myeloma, leukemia, lymphoma)
Vitamin D-mediated causes
    Vitamin D intoxication
    $1,25(OH)_2D$ production; sarcoidosis and other granulomatous disorders
    Idiopathic hypercalcemia of infancy
Accelerated bone turnover
    Hyperthyroidism
    Immobilization
    Vitamin A intoxication
Renal failure
    Aluminum intoxication
    Milk-alkali syndrome
Other endocrine diseases
    Addison disease
    Pheochromocytoma

FHH, familial hypocalciuric hypercalcemia; PTH, parathyroid hormone.
Modified from Potts JT Jr. Diseases of the parathyroid gland and other hyper- and hypocalcemic disorders. *In*: Fauci AS, Braunwald E, Isselbacher KJ, et al., eds. Harrison's Principles of Internal Medicine. 14th ed. New York: McGraw-Hill, 1998:2227–2247. By permission of the publisher.

Confirm hypercalcemia with repeated measurement of the serum calcium level. After hypercalcemia has been verified, the intact parathyroid hormone level (iPTH) should be determined, as should the PTH-related peptide level in hospitalized patients. An increased serum calcium level in the presence of an increased level of intact PTH is virtually diagnostic of PHP. A suppressed PTH level in the presence of hypercalcemia is suspicious for malignancy. PTH-related peptide is a 141-amino-acid peptide that has considerable homology with PTH, binds to the PTH receptors on bone, and is produced by squamous cell carcinoma of the lung, renal cell carcinoma, and breast cancer. The following additional tests are also recommended: serum protein electrophoresis, alkaline phosphatase, 25-hydroxyvitamin D, serum creatinine, bone scan, and 24-hour urine collection for calcium and creatinine. Obtaining a 24-hour urine collection for measuring calcium and creatinine to exclude the diagnosis of FHH is essential because it is a benign syndrome. The fractional excretion of calcium in FHH typically is less than 0.01, that is, one-third the usual value of that in classic PHP.

Treatment

Although there is some controversy about the treatment of elderly patients with PHP, most authors agree that PHP is a surgical disease. Mild to moderate hypercalcemia (<12 mg/dL) may be treated conservatively, with the patient's clinical manifestations serving as a guide to therapy. The patient should be kept well hydrated and follow a diet containing only a modest amount of calcium. Surgical treatment is recommended for symptomatic patients with PHP.[40]

Serum calcium levels greater than 13 mg/dL should be treated aggressively.[41] Restoring adequate volume status is the first step in the management of acute hypercalcemia. This may be accomplished by infusing isotonic saline (initially 2.5 to 4 L/day). Hydration allows expansion of the vascular compartment and results in a direct decrease in the serum level of calcium. This expansion of intravascular volume also leads to an increase in renal calcium clearance through a direct link between sodium and calcium excretion. Generally, we do not advocate furosemide as adjunctive therapy in the treatment of acute hypercalcemia unless the patient is susceptible to volume overload. Furosemide facilitates urinary calcium and sodium excretion but should only be administered if the patient is fully rehydrated.

Many pharmacological agents are available to lower the serum calcium level (Table 139.6). The choice of agent depends on the cause of the hypercalcemia. Bisphosphonates, which function as osteoclast

Table 139.6   Therapies for severe hypercalcemia

Treatment	Onset of action	Duration	Advantages	Disadvantages
Most useful				
Hydration with saline	Hours	During infusion		
Forced diuresis; saline + loop diuretic	Hours	During treatment	Rapid onset of action	CHF
Bisphosphonates				
Etidronate	1–2 days	5–7 days	Intermediate onset of action	Hyperphosphatemia
Pamidronate	1–2 days	10–14 days	High potency	Fever in 20%; hypophosphatemia, hypocalcemia, hypomagnesemia
Calcitonin	Hours	2–3 days	Rapid onset of action; useful as an adjunct in severe hypercalcemia	Often limited in calcium lowering; rapid tachyphylaxis
Others				
Gallium nitrate	Day after 5-day infusion	7–10 days	High potency	Length of IV administration
Plicamycin	3–4 days	Days	Potent antiresorptive	Liver, kidney, and marrow toxicity Bleeding
Glucocorticoids	Days	Days, weeks	Oral therapy, antitumor agent	Active in only certain malignancies
Dialysis	Hours	During use and 24–48 hours afterwards	Useful in renal failure; can immediately reverse life-threatening hypercalcemia	Complex procedure; reserved for extreme circumstances

CHF, congestive heart failure; IV, intravenous.
Modified from Potts JT Jr. Diseases of the parathyroid gland and other hyper- and hypocalcemic disorders. In: Fauci AS, Braunwald E, Isselbacher KJ, et al., eds. Harrison's Principles of Internal Medicine. 14th ed. New York: McGraw-Hill, 1998:2227–2247. By permission of the publisher.

inhibitors, are the mainstay of treatment in the management of hypercalcemia associated with malignancy.

Pamidronate This second-generation bisphosphonate is the preferred agent for treating acute hypercalcemia. It is potent and relatively nontoxic. Pamidronate (60 to 90 mg) is infused in 1 L of dextrose in water over 12 to 24 hours. The side effects include transient fever and myalgias on the day of infusion, local infusion site reactions, mild gastrointestinal symptoms, hypophosphatemia, hypokalemia, and hypomagnesemia. The onset of action is usually 24 hours, and the duration of the effect is typically 7 to 10 days.

Calcitonin This is a polypeptide hormone secreted by parafollicular cells of the thyroid. It functions as an osteoclast inhibitor. Calcitonin is only moderately effective when given alone but serves as a useful adjunctive agent to help acutely decrease serum calcium levels. The combination of calcitonin and pamidronate is the preferred therapy for acute hypercalcemic crisis. Calcitonin is available in the form of salmon calcitonin and may be administered intravenously or intramuscularly at a dose of 4 to 8 U/kg every 6 hours. The drug acts rapidly, causing the serum calcium level to decrease within 2 to 6 hours after administration and to reach a nadir within 24 hours. However, the effect is transient and generally lasts only 2 to 3 days. The serum calcium concentration usually decreases by a mean of 2 mg/dL and may begin to increase within 48 hours. Adverse effects associated with calcitonin include mild transient nausea, abdominal cramps, and flushing.

Plicamycin This is a cytotoxic antibiotic that interferes with RNA synthesis in osteoclasts, thereby inhibiting osteoclastic function. The drug typically is given at a dose of 15 to 25 μg/kg of body weight over a period of 4 to 6 hours. The onset of action is 12 hours, and a nadir is usually reached within 48 to 72 hours. The drug is very effective at decreasing serum calcium levels, and often only one dose is needed to achieve normocalcemia. Plicamycin has associated bone marrow, liver, and renal toxic effects and, thus, is used infrequently.

Other approaches These include dialysis, which generally is reserved for patients with severe hypercalcemia associated with acute or chronic renal failure. Gallium has been approved by the FDA for the treatment of acute hypercalcemia, although it is rarely given because of its long infusion time (5 days) and relatively slow decrease in the serum calcium level. Gallium also has considerable toxicity, including nephrotoxicity. Glucocorticoids are useful as therapy in hypercalcemic disorders associated with vitamin D excess (vitamin D intoxication, lymphomas, and granulomatous disease). If possible, treatment of the underlying disease associated with the hypercalcemia should be instituted.

Magnesium deficiency

Magnesium depletion is a commonly overlooked disorder that is prevalent among hospitalized patients, especially those in intensive care units.[42,43] The normal serum concentration of magnesium ranges from 1.5 mEq/L to 1.9 mEq/L (1.8 to 2.5 mg/dL) and levels less than the normal range indicate significant magnesium deficiency. Balance studies performed by Flink[44] measured a total body magnesium deficiency of 1000 mg in patients with a low serum level of magnesium.

Etiology

Magnesium deficiency usually results from excessive gastrointestinal tract or renal magnesium losses. The causes of magnesium deficiency are listed in Table 139.7. However, the history is of major importance in alerting the physician to consider magnesium deficiency because significant magnesium deficiency may occur even if the serum level is normal. Chronic alcoholism is a major cause of magnesium deficiency because alcohol acts as a magnesium diuretic and thus leads to hypermagnesuria. Excess urinary losses may also occur in patients with poorly controlled diabetes mellitus (osmotic diuresis). The chronic use of loop diuretics may also result in large magnesium losses. However, one of the most common ways that

Table 139.7 Common causes of magnesium deficiency

Gastrointestinal disorders
    Prolonged nasogastric suction/vomiting
    Diarrhea
    Intestinal biliary fistulas
    Malabsorption syndromes
    Extensive bowel resection or bypass
    Acute hemorrhagic pancreatitis
Renal losses
    Osmotic diuresis (glucose)
    Hypercalcemia
    Alcohol
    Diuretics
    Aminoglycosides
    Cisplatin
    Cyclosporine
    Amphotericin B
    Pentamidine
    Metabolic acidosis
    Renal disease with Mg wasting
Endocrine and metabolic
    Diabetes mellitus
    Phosphate depletion
    Primary hyperparathyroidism
    Hypoparathyroidism
    Primary aldosteronism
    Hungry-bone syndrome

Modified from Rude RK. Magnesium depletion and hypermagnesemia. *In*: Favus MJ, ed. Primer on the Metabolic Bone Diseases and Disorders of Mineral Metabolism. 4th ed. Philadelphia: Lippincott Williams & Wilkins, 1999:241–245. By permission of the American Society for Bone and Mineral Research.

magnesium deficiency is detected is the presence of unexplained hypocalcemia. Magnesium is an essential cofactor for both the synthesis and secretion of PTH and both processes are impaired in magnesium-deficient patients.

Clinical features

The clinical manifestations of magnesium deficiency are primarily due to associated hypocalcemia. Severe magnesium deficiency (serum magnesium levels <1 mg/dL) results in hypocalcemia. Therefore, many of the clinical features associated with hypomagnesemia are those of hypocalcemia, such as Chvostek and Trousseau signs, fasciculations, frank tetany, and seizures. Other neurological manifestations include tremors, athetoid movements, vertical and lateral nystagmus, and dysphagia (Table 139.8). Cardiac arrhythmias such as atrial tachycardia, atrial fibrillation, ventricular tachycardia, and ventricular fibrillation are also associated with magnesium deficiency.

Management

Therapy to correct hypomagnesemia should be directed at the underlying cause. Patients with hypomagnesemia in whom seizures or an acute arrhythmia develops should be given 8 to 16 mEq of elemental magnesium (8 mEq of magnesium is contained in 1 g MgSO$_4$, which equals 96 mg elemental Mg) intravenously over 5 to 10 minutes, followed by an infusion of 48 mEq of magnesium daily. This is followed with 48 mEq of magnesium given intravenously daily (6 g MgSO$_4$) for 4 or 5 days. Extreme caution should be exercised in treating magnesium deficiency in patients who also have renal insufficiency. In this case, only 1 to 2 g should be given and the serum level of magnesium should be determined again in 24 hours before an additional dose is given.

Hypermagnesemia

Hypermagnesemia is more rare than the other biochemical abnormalities discussed above but deserves attention because of the associated neurological complications. Hypermagnesemia occurs most commonly in persons with renal failure. Generally, magnesium excess occurs when a patient with renal failure receives exogenous magnesium as an enema, antacid, or infusion.

Table 139.8   Neurological manifestations of magnesium deficiency
Neuromuscular irritability
Muscle weakness
Fasciculations
Chvostek and Trousseau signs
Tremors and athetoid movements
Tetany
Seizures
Nystagmus
Dysphagia

Clinical features

Hypermagnesemia decreases transmission across the neuromuscular junction, causing a curare-like effect.[45] One of the earliest clinical signs associated with hypermagnesemia is diminished deep tendon reflexes. This usually occurs when the serum concentration of magnesium is between 4 and 7 mEq/L. More severe hypermagnesemia may result in somnolence, loss of deep tendon reflexes, and muscle paralysis with flaccid quadriplegia. Depressed respiration and apnea follow at magnesium levels in excess of 8 to 10 mEq/L. Hypermagnesemia of this degree may also cause parasympathetic blockade, with fixed and dilated pupils, mimicking a central brainstem herniation syndrome.[46] Cardiac manifestations of magnesium excess include hypotension, complete heart block, and cardiac arrest.

Management

Generally, mild to moderate hypermagnesemia may be treated by withdrawing magnesium therapy. Severe magnesium intoxication may be treated effectively with intravenous calcium (100 to 200 mg elemental calcium).[47,48] Calcium antagonizes the toxic effects of magnesium. Although this treatment is effective, it is transient, lasting only 5 to 10 minutes. A patient in renal failure may be treated with hemodialysis against a low magnesium dialysis bath.

References

1. Chapuy MC, Arlot ME, Duboeuf F, et al. Vitamin D and calcium to prevent hip fractures in the elderly women. N Engl J Med 1992;327:1637–1642
2. Miller PD, Bonnick SL, Rosen CJ. Consensus of an international panel on the clinical utility of bone mass measurements in the detection of low bone mass in the adult population. Calcif Tissue Int 1996;58:207–214
3. Dawson-Hughes B, Harris SS, Krall EA, Dallal GE. Effect of calcium and vitamin D supplementation on bone density in men and women 65 years of age or older. N Engl J Med 1997;337:670–676
4. Holick MF. Vitamin D requirements for the elderly. Clin Nutr 1986;5:121–129
5. Cauley JA, Seeley DG, Ensrud K, et al. Estrogen replacement therapy and fractures in older women. Study of Osteoporotic Fractures Research Group. Ann Intern Med 1995;122:9–16
6. Weiss NS, Ure CL, Ballard JH, et al. Decreased risk of fractures of the hip and lower forearm with postmenopausal use of estrogen. N Engl J Med 1980;303:1195–1198
7. Hulley S, Grady D, Bush T, et al. Randomized trial of estrogen plus progestin for secondary prevention of coronary heart disease in postmentopausal women. Heart and Estrogen/progestin Replacement Study (HERS) Research Group. JAMA 1998;280:605–613
8. Bush TL, Barrett-Connor E, Cowan LD, et al. Cardiovascular mortality and noncontraceptive use of estrogen in women: results from the Lipid Research Clinics Program Follow-up Study. Circulation 1987;75:1102–1109
9. Colditz GA, Hankinson SE, Hunter DJ, et al. The use of estrogens and progestins and the risk of breast cancer in postmenopausal women. N Engl J Med 1995;332:1589–1593

10. The Women's Health Initiative Study Group. Design of the Women's Health Initiative clinical trial and observational study. Control Clin Trials 1998;19:61–109

11. Liberman UA, Weiss SR, Broll J, et al. Effect of oral alendronate on bone mineral density and the incidence of fractures in postmenopausal osteoporosis. The Alendronate Phase III Osteoporosis Treatment Study Group. N Engl J Med 1995;333:1437–1443

12. Harris ST, Watts NB, Genant HK, et al. Effects of risedronate treatment on vertebral and nonvertebral fractures in women with postmenopausal osteoporosis: a randomized controlled trial. Vertebral Efficacy With Risedronate Therapy (VERT) Study Group. JAMA 1999; 282:1344–1352

13. Saag KG, Emkey R, Schnitzer TJ, et al. Alendronate for the prevention and treatment of glucocorticoid-induced osteoporosis. Glucocorticoid-Induced Osteoporosis Intervention Study Group. N Engl J Med 1998;339: 292–299

14. Delmas PD, Bjarnason NH, Mitlak BH, et al. Effects of raloxifene on bone mineral density, serum cholesterol concentrations, and uterine endometrium in postmenopausal women. N Engl J Med 1997;337:1641–1647

15. Delmas PD, Meunier PJ. The management of Paget's disease of bone. N Engl J Med 1997;336:558–566

16. Wootton R, Reeve J, Spellacy E, Tellez-Yudilevich M. Skeletal blood flow in Paget's disease of bone and its response to calcitonin therapy. Clin Sci Mol Med 1978;54:69–74

17. Kanis JA. Pathophysiology and Treatment of Paget's Disease of Bone. 2nd ed. London: Martin Dunitz, 1998

18. Chen JR, Rhee RS, Wallach S, et al. Neurologic disturbances in Paget disease of bone: response to calcitonin. Neurology 1979;29:448–457

19. Herzberg L, Bayliss E. Spinal-cord syndrome due to non-compressive Paget's disease of bone: a spinal-artery steal phenomenon reversible with calcitonin. Lancet 1980;2:13–15

20. Monsell EM, Cody DD, Bone HG, Divine GW. Hearing loss as a complication of Paget's disease of bone. J Bone Miner Res 1999;14 Suppl 2:92–95

21. Poncelet A. The neurologic complications of Paget's disease. J Bone Miner Res 1999;14 Suppl 2:88–91

22. Muff R, Dambacher MA, Perrenoud A, et al. Efficacy of intranasal human calcitonin in patients with Paget's disease refractory to salmon calcitonin. Am J Med 1990;89:181–184

23. Murphy WA, Whyte MP, Haddad JG Jr. Paget bone disease: radiologic documentation of healing with human calcitonin therapy. Radiology 1980;136:1–4

24. Boyce BF, Smith L, Fogelman I, et al. Focal osteomalacia due to low-dose diphosphonate therapy in Paget's disease. Lancet 1984;1:821–824

25. Thiebaud D, Jaeger P, Gobelet C, et al. A single infusion of the bisphosphonate AHPrBP (APD) as treatment of Paget's disease of bone. Am J Med 1988;85:207–212

26. Wimalawansa SJ, Gunasekera RD. Pamidronate is effective for Paget's disease of bone refractory to conventional therapy. Calcif Tissue Int 1993;53:237–241

27. Siris E, Weinstein RS, Altman R, et al. Comparative study of alendronate versus etidronate for the treatment of Paget's disease of bone. J Clin Endocrinol Metab 1996;81:961–967

28. Miller PD, Brown JP, Siris ES, et al. A randomized, double-blind comparison of risedronate and etidronate in the treatment of Paget's disease of bone. Paget's Risedronate/Etidronate Study Group. Am J Med 1999;106:513–520

29. Parfitt AM. Surgical, idiopathic, and other varieties of parathyroid deficient hypoparathyroidism. In: DeGroot L, ed. Metabolic Basis of Endocrinology. New York: Grune and Stratton, 1979;755–768

30. Brink F. The role of calcium ions in neural processes. Pharmacol Rev 1954;6:243–298

31. Kugelberg E. Neurologic mechanism for certain phenomena in tetany. Arch Neurol Psychiatry 1946;56: 507–521

32. Chvostek F. Weitere Beiträge zur Tetanie. Wien med Presse 1878;19, passim, cont in 1879;20:1201, 1233, 1268, 1301

33. Hoffman E. The Chvostek sign; a clinical study. Am J Surg 1958;96:33–37

34. Trousseau A. Clinical Medicine 1868, Volume I, 376. London: New Sydenham Soc.

35. Lewis T. Trousseau's phenomenon in tetany. Clin Sci 1942;4:361–364

36. Uncini A, Tartaro A, Di Stefano E, Gambi D. Parkinsonism, basal ganglia calcification and epilepsy as late complications of postoperative hypoparathyroidism. J Neurol 1985;232:109–111

37. Davis TM, Singh B, Choo KE, et al. Dynamic assessment of parathyroid function in acute malaria. J Intern Med 1998;243:349–354

38. Tohme JF, Bilezikian JP. Hypocalcemic emergencies. Endocrinol Metab Clin North Am 1993;22:363–375

39. Solomon BL, Schaaf M, Smallridge RC. Psychologic symptoms before and after parathyroid surgery. Am J Med 1994;96:101–106

40. Consensus Development Conference Panel. Diagnosis and management of asymptomatic primary hyperparathyroidism: Consensus Development Conference Statement. Ann Intern Med 1991:114;593–597

41. Bilezikian JP. Management of acute hypercalcemia. N Engl J Med 1992;326:1196–1203

42. Wong ET, Rude RK, Singer FR, Shaw ST Jr. A high prevalence of hypomagnesemia and hypermagnesemia in hospitalized patients. Am J Clin Pathol 1983; 79:348–352

43. Desai TK, Carlson RW, Geheb MA. Prevalence and clinical implications of hypocalcemia in acutely ill patients in a medical intensive care setting. Am J Med 1988;84:209–214

44. Flink EB. Magnesium deficiency in human subjects—a personal historical perspective. J Am Coll Nutr 1985; 4:17–31

45. Krendel DA. Hypermagnesemia and neuromuscular transmission. Semin Neurol 1990;10:42–45

46. Rizzo MA, Fisher M, Lock JP. Hypermagnesemic pseudocoma. Arch Intern Med 1993;153:1130–1132

47. Mordes JP, Wacker WE. Excess magnesium. Pharmacol Rev 1977;29:273–300

48. Fishman RA. Neurological aspects of magnesium metabolism. Arch Neurol 1965;12:562–569

140 Lysosomal Storage Diseases

Gregory M Pastores and Edwin H Kolodny

A lysosome is a membrane-bound intracytoplasmic organelle containing various enzymes required for the degradation of lipids, complex carbohydrates, proteins, and nucleotides, that is, the molecules that represent the metabolic by-products of cellular turnover. The existence of lysosomes as subcellular organelles was first recognized by DeDuve in 1957; his observations were based on ultracentrifugation of cellular constituents and their examination with electron microscopy.[1] Disruption of the normal mechanisms involved in the sequential catabolism of several molecules leads to the intracellular accumulation of these molecules (i.e., lysosomal storage) within various tissues, with disease ultimately resulting from organ dysfunction. Collectively, these disorders are referred to as "lysosomal storage diseases" (LSDs). Most individual LSDs have an eponymous designation in recognition of the physicians who have provided the "classic" descriptions of the clinical manifestations of the diseases. In most cases, this occurred before the causal biochemical or molecular defect was identified. The classification of LSDs is provided in Table 140.1.

The LSD concept was first proposed by Hers in 1963,[2] on the basis of the detection of glycogen-filled vesicles of lysosomal origin in cells obtained from a patient with Pompe disease (glycogen storage disease II). Today, it is known that progressive lysosomal storage can occur through various means: 1) a primary deficiency of a specific hydrolase (e.g., Tay-Sachs, Gaucher, and Fabry diseases); 2) deficiency of either a "protective protein" that aids in lysosomal targeting and prevention of premature degradation of enzymes (e.g., galactosialidosis) or an "activator protein" necessary for enzyme-substrate interaction and degradation (e.g., GM$_2$-gangliosidosis, AB variant); 3) abnormal enzyme processing by the required enzymes in the endoplasmic reticulum for functional maturation of the relevant proteins (e.g., multiple sulfatase deficiency); and 4) failure to attach the appropriate targeting signals (mannose-6-phosphate) in the Golgi apparatus (e.g., I-cell disease). Disease mechanisms 3 and 4 represent defects of posttranslational modification.

More recently, it has been shown that LSDs can also result from defects in the removal or transport of the substrate from lysosomes (e.g., Niemann-Pick type C and sialic acid storage diseases) or defects in an integral membrane protein of endosomal-lysosomal membranes leading to abnormalities in endocytosis, in vesicle fusion, or in the internal endosomal or lysosomal environment (e.g., Danon disease).[3] The abnormalities associated with Danon disease refer to defects in processing of autophagic vacuoles. Other disorders of intracellular vesicle formation that result in abnormal lysosome formation and lysosomal storage include Hermansky-Pudlack syndrome and Chédiak-Higashi syndrome.[4]

LSDs are transmitted as autosomal recessive traits except for Fabry disease, Hunter syndrome (mucopolysaccharidosis [MPS] II), and Danon disease, which are inherited in an X-linked recessive manner. Histological demonstration of storage bodies in different tissues (e.g., skin, rectal mucosa, conjunctiva) obtained from patients with certain LSDs may provide diagnostic clues, although the majority of cases can now be diagnosed through a blood test for confirmation of the corresponding biochemical or molecular (DNA) defect. Prenatal diagnosis is possible for almost all LSDs with analysis of enzymatic activity, molecular genetic testing, or ultrastructural examination for inclusion bodies in cells from cultured chorionic villi or amniocytes. In families in which the causal mutation is known, molecular testing enables accurate assignment of carrier status.

The rationale for and potential of treatment of LSDs evolved after the observations of metabolic cross-correction by Fratantoni et al.[5] These studies showed that medium from fibroblasts with nonallelic mutations, in particular MPS I (Hurler syndrome) and MPS II (Hunter syndrome), enabled the clearance of stored material. Subsequently, the "corrective factors" were identified as the functional enzymes secreted from the cells in culture that had been processed normally and bore the proper targeting signals for their incorporation into the deficient cells. Today, cellular correction is achieved in certain clinical subtypes through bone marrow transplantation (BMT) and enzyme replacement therapy (ERT). The characterization of the relevant lectins on the cell surface responsible for the uptake of a lysosomal enzyme enabled targeting of the therapeutic proteins to the pathological sites of storage. Potential therapies being investigated include the use of substrate synthesis inhibitors, chaperone-mediated agents, and gene therapy.

A few animal models of disease have arisen spontaneously, although the field has been dramatically advanced by the ability to create animal models, primarily with mice, of several LSDs. Application of recombinant genetic techniques enabled the generation of knockout or knock-in models, often resulting in complete or partial deficiency of the relevant protein, respectively. These animal models have provided valuable insight into pathophysiological mechanisms and have made possible investigations of various therapeutic options.

Epidemiology

Limited data are available from population-based studies to establish the incidence of LSDs. Factors that help explain this are the general lack of technical knowledge and the great expense associated with the performance of biochemical and molecular assays to establish a clinical diagnosis. Furthermore, the delay in the diagnosis of LSDs can be considerable because the characteristic features may not be recognized until later in childhood or adulthood. Also, the diagnosis can be missed, particularly in patients with an atypical disease course. Epidemiologic data will become increasingly important as new screening programs and novel therapies are introduced. This information will be important in obtaining a reliable estimate of the societal and economic burden associated with LSDs.

Three recent studies—conducted by the central laboratories for the diagnosis of metabolic disease in their respective countries—have provided insight into disease frequencies. All three populations surveyed are represented predominantly by whites. In British Columbia (for the years 1969–1996), the overall minimum incidence of inborn error of metabolism was approximately 40 cases per 100,000 live births.[6] The majority (approximately 60%) of cases involved small molecules, which include diseases of amino acids (including phenylketonuria) and organic acid metabolism, primary lactic acidosis, galactosemia, or a urea cycle defect. Approximately 20% (8 per 100,000 live births) had an LSD (evaluated for years 1972–1996), which together with diseases involving other subcellular organelles (i.e., mitochondria and peroxisomes) accounted for about one-half of the "diagnostic dilemma" group. Among the LSDs, Pompe disease (at 1 in 115,091 live births) was noted as the most common disorder. The incidence of MPSs ($n = 20$ cases) and glycolipid storage diseases ($n = 23$ cases) was estimated at 1 in 51,791 and 1 in 45,035 live births, respectively.

In the Netherlands, the combined birth prevalence for all LSDs was 14 per 100,000 live births (based on all 963 enzymatically confirmed cases diagnosed during the period 1970–1996).[7] Pompe disease (2 per 100,000 live births) was the most frequent LSD, representing 17% of all diagnosed cases. The combined birth prevalence for all lipid storage diseases was 6.2 per 100,000 live births. Within this group, the prevalence for metachromatic leukodystrophy (MLD), involving all subtypes, was most common (1.42 per 100,000 live births), accounting for 24% of the lipidoses. Birth prevalence for Krabbe disease and Gaucher disease were 1.35 and 1.16 per 100,000, respectively. The combined birth prevalence for all the MPSs was 4.5 per 100,000 live births. Within this group, the combined prevalence for MPS III subtypes (47% of cases) was 1.89 per 100,000 live births. MPS I (including all clinical variants) was the most common subtype (25%), with a prevalence of 1.19 per 100,000 live births.

In Australia, retrospective examination of cases from 1980 to 1996 provided data on 27 different LSDs diagnosed in 470 patients.[8] No data were collected on the diagnosis of pyknodysostosis, glycogen storage disease type IIB, or the various forms of neuronal ceroid-lipofuscinosis because during the study period enzyme assays were not performed in Australia for these conditions. As a group, the combined prevalence for the LSDs was 1 per 7,700 births. If prenatally diagnosed cases are excluded, the calculated incidence for the LSDs would be 1 in 9,000. For individual conditions, prevalence ranged from 1 per 57,000 live births for Gaucher disease to 1 per 4.2 million live births for sialidosis.

Certain subtypes of neuronal ceroid-lipofuscinosis represent deficiencies of a specific lysosomal enzyme (e.g., palmitol protein thioesterase in Batten disease and carboxypeptidase in classic late-infantile neuronal ceroid-lipofuscinosis).[9] This group of disorders is among the most common neurodegenerative conditions in children—with an estimated global incidence as high as 1 in 12,500.

The frequency of specific LSDs may be higher in certain ethnic groups, such as the Ashkenazim, when compared with the general population. This most likely is a consequence of founder effects (i.e., descent from a common ancestor). It has been hypothesized that the high carrier frequency for certain lipidoses among the Ashkenazim may be due to selective (heterozygote) advantage, although no satisfactory explanation has been demonstrated to confirm this. Among the Ashkenazim, carrier frequency for three lipidoses (specifically, Gaucher disease, 1 in 15; Tay-Sachs disease, 1 in 30; and Niemann-Pick disease type A, 1 in 80) and mucolipidosis IV (1 in 70 to 100) is relatively high.[10] These observations prompted the development of carrier screening programs, as in the case of screening before marriage introductions within the Orthodox Jewish community and the consideration of prenatal diagnosis in all Ashkenazim carrier couples at risk. Indeed, a few mutations associated with each of the above-mentioned disorders have been identified to account for a substantial proportion of disease alleles among affected patients. This has led to a DNA-based multiplex screening approach, that is, simultaneous screening for several disease mutations on a single blood specimen.

Information on ethnic background may be an important indicator of a probable diagnosis of a particular subtype in a symptomatic patient with a suspected LSD. For example, many of the patients with fucosidosis have Italian ancestry and those with aspartylglycosaminuria are mostly of Scandinavian origin. A variant of Gaucher disease type 3 (the Norrbottnian form) has also been described among patients from Sweden. The incidence of MPS II (Hunter syndrome) among the Jewish population is reportedly increased (estimated prevalence of 1.5 per 100,000 live births), and MPS IV (Morquio A) IVA is reportedly more common in Northern Ireland (1.3 per 100,000 live births) than in other countries.

Increased knowledge about LSDs and the availability of treatment (e.g., BMT and ERT) in some forms

Table 140.1   Classification of lysosomal storage diseases

Stored substrate	Disease	Enzyme deficiency	Gene locus
Sphingolipids			
G_{M2}-gangliosides, glycolipids, globoside oligosaccharides	Tay-Sachs	α-Subunit β-hexosaminidase	15q23-24
	GM_2-gangliosidosis (3 types)* Sandhoff	β-Subunit β-hexosaminidase	5q13
	GM_2-gangliosidosis GM_2-gangliosidosis, AB variant	G_{M2} activator	5q32-33
G_{M1}-gangliosides, oligosaccharides, keratan sulfate, glycolipids	GM_1-gangliosidosis (3 types)*	β-Galactosidase	3p21-3pter
Sulphatides	Metachromatic leukodystrophy (MLD)	Arylsulphatase A (galactose-3-sulphatase)	22q13.31-qter
GM_1-gangliosides, sphingomyelin, glycolipids, sulphatide	MLD variant	Saposin B activator	10q21
Galactosylceramides	Krabbe	Galactocerebrosidase	14q31
α-Galactosyl-sphingolipids, oligosaccharides	Fabry	α-Galactosidase A	Xq22
Glucosylceramide, globosides	Gaucher (3 types)*	β-Glucosidase	1q2l
Glucosylceramide, globosides	Gaucher (variant)	Saposin C	10q2l
Ceramide	Farber (7 types)	Acid ceramidase	8p22-21.2
Sphingomyelin	Niemann-Pick types A and B	Sphingomyelinase	11p15.1-15.4
Mucopolysaccharidoses (glycosaminoglycans)			
Dermatan sulphate and heparan sulfate	MPS I (Hurler Scheie) MPS II (Hunter)	α-L-iduronidase Iduronate-2-sulphatase	4p16.3 Xq27.3-28
Heparan sulfate	MPS IIIA (Sanfilippo A) MPS IIIB (Sanfilippo B) MPS IIIC (Sanfilippo C) MPS IIID (Sanfilippo D)	Sulfamidase α-N-acetylglucosaminidase Acetyl CoA:α-glucosaminide-N-acetyltransferase N-acetylglucosamine-6-sulfatase	17q25.3 17q21.1 – 12q14
Keratan sulphate	MPS IVA (Morquio A) MPS IVB (Morquio B)	Galactosamine-6-sulphatase β-D-galactosidase	16q24.3 3p21.33
Dermatan sulfate	MPS VI (Maroteaux-Lamy)	N-acetylgalactosamine-4-sulfatase	5q13-14
Dermatan sulfate and heparan sulfate	MPS VII (Sly)	β-D-glucuronidase	7q21.1-22
Hyaluronan	MPS IX	Hyaluronidase	3p21.3

Table 140.1 *continued*

Substrate	Disease	Enzyme/Protein	Locus
Glycogen			
Glycogen	Glycogen storage IIA (Pompe)	α-D glucosidase	17q23
Glycogen	Danon	Lysosomal associated membrane protein-2 (LAMP-2)	Xq24-25
Oligosaccharides/glycopeptides			
α-Mannoside	α-Mannosidosis	α-Mannosidase	19p13.2-q12
β-Mannoside	β-Mannosidosis	β-Mannosidase	4q22-25
α-Fucosides, glycolipids	α-Fucosidosis	α-Fucosidase	1p34.1-36.1
α-N-acetylgalactosaminide	Schindler	α-N-acetylgalactosaminidase	22q13.1-13.2
Sialyloligosaccharides	Sialidosis	α-Neuraminidase	6p21.3
Aspartylglucosamine	Aspartylglucosaminuria	Aspartylglucosaminidase	4q34-35
Multiple enzyme deficiencies			
Glycolipids, oligosaccharides	Mucolipidosis II (I-cell disease)	N-acetylglucosamine-1-phosphotransferase	4q21-q23
Sulphatides, glycolipids, glycosaminoglycans	Multiple sulfatases	–	–
Lipids			
Cholesterol esters	Cholesterol ester storage disease (Wolman disease)	Acid lipase	10q23.2-q23.3
Cholesterol, sphingomyelin	Niemann-Pick type C	NPC1; HE1	18q11-12; 14q24.3
Monosaccraides/amino acid/monomers			
Sialic acid, glucuronic acid	Infantile free sialic acid storage (Salla)	Sialin	6q14-15
Cystine	Cystinosis	Cystinosin	17p12
Peptides			
Bone proteins	Pycnodysostosis	Cathepsin K	1q21
S-acylated proteins			
Palmitoylated proteins	Infantile neuronal ceroid-lipofuscinosis	Palmitoyl-protein thioesterase	1p32
Pepstatin-insensitive lysosomal peptidase	Late-infantile neuronal ceroid-lipofusinosis	Pepstatin-insensitive lysosomal peptidase	11p15

MLD, metachromatic leukodystrophy; MPS, mucopolysaccharidosis.
*Three types imply infantile, childhood and adulthood presentations.

has stimulated interest in population-based screening. In the absence of specific and effective therapy for most other clinical types, an advantage to early identification of cases includes the prevention of recurrence in families at risk. Screening blood spots on filter paper (Guthrie card) for by-products of lysosomal metabolism or turnover (lysosomal-associated membrane proteins [LAMPs]-1 and -2) by immunoquantification assays and subsequent analysis of specific substrates in blood or urine using tandem mass spectrometry (the same technique used to screen for metabolites in patients with fatty acid oxidation defects) has been proposed.[11] LAMP-1 is increased in the majority of LSDs, and although LAMP-2 concentrations are also increased, testing for LAMP-2 does not appear to detect additional disorders; thus, LAMP-2 is of limited value as an additional marker. An increase in saposin levels has also been reported, particularly among patients with sphingolipidosis who often do not have increased levels of LAMP-1. This approach may address the limitations of a DNA-based strategy, which can be labor-intensive because of the large number of causal mutations associated with most LSDs and low mutant-allele frequencies (i.e., absence of common mutations). Other approaches being considered include analysis of enzyme activity from blood spots in filter paper for certain disorders resulting from single enzyme deficiencies, which may be appropriate for screening high-risk groups (e.g., screening for Fabry disease in patients with renal failure or receiving dialysis or patients with cardiomyopathy).[12–17] These methods may prove cost-effective, although the absence of specific therapies for most subtypes may create certain dilemmas.

Pathophysiology and clinical manifestations

Lysosomes are involved in the metabolism of various cellular constituents, including glycolipids, glycoproteins, and mucopolysaccharides. The normal pattern and distribution of these compounds and their turnover determine the clinical manifestations associated with each LSD. For example, diseases of ganglioside metabolism such as GM_1-gangliosidosis and Tay-Sachs disease (GM_2-gangliosidosis) primarily affect brain gray matter because the concentration of gangliosides is higher in nerve cells than in extraneural tissue. Similarly, galactolipids are a component of myelin, and diseases that involve its abnormal metabolism, such as Krabbe disease and MLD, predominantly affect brain white matter (leukodystrophy).

The intralysosomal accumulation of incompletely degraded, complex substrates represents the initial and possibly major insult to cells. Substrate storage results in an increase in the number and size of lysosomes, from approximately 1% to as much as 50% of total cellular volume. The mechanical crowding resulting from the infiltration of engorged lysosomes may be a common mechanism of injury. However, it is likely that a host of other factors, including mechanical and vascular changes and immune-mediated events, contribute to the development of various disease-specific complications. For instance, a marked increase and abnormal distribution of endothelin-1 have been noted in neurons and glial cells of a patient with galactosialidosis.[18] Also, evidence of loss of CD31 immunoreactivity and the breakdown of vascular cell adhesion molecules in vacuolated endothelial cells has been reported.[19] These factors are thought to promote development of brain infarction and the other pathological changes seen in galactosialidosis. In Fabry disease, patients have increased serum levels of various endothelial prothrombotic factors and leukocyte adhesion-molecule expression, changes thought to influence the likelihood of stroke.[20] In Krabbe disease (globoid cell leukodystrophy), the death of oligodendrocytes has been attributed to the accumulation of psychosine (galactosylsphingosine). Recently, psychosine has been shown to bind to TDAG8 (a putative G protein-coupled T-cell receptor), leading to a block in cytokinesis. This possibly may represent one of the pathways leading to cell death.[21]

LSDs are a clinically heterogeneous group of disorders that often involve multiple organ systems. A wide spectrum of clinical manifestations can be found within individual diagnostic categories, which to some extent reflects the broad (allelic) heterogeneity in causal mutations. Disease onset may be early or late. In rapidly progressive forms, clinical signs may be evident in the neonatal period or early infancy. With later-onset forms, the condition may not be manifest until adolescence or adulthood. The disease course may be acute, subacute, or chronic. Acute and subacute forms are usually associated with primary central nervous system involvement, developmental delay, and mental retardation. Not all LSDs cause mental deficiency, and intellect is preserved in Fabry disease, Gaucher disease type 1, Niemann-Pick disease type B, MPS I (Scheie syndrome), MPS IV (Morquio syndrome), and mild MPS VI (Maroteaux-Lamy syndrome).

Clinical findings that may serve as clues to the diagnosis of an LSD are listed in Table 140.2. It is important to note that most of the clinical features are nonspecific when viewed in isolation. Thus, when one sign or symptom is recognized, it is important to search for other indications of a multisystem disease. Details about the family history may also be helpful.

Information about the natural history of various LSDs has been derived primarily from case reports. The increase in the number of clinical trials to assess potential therapies for certain subtypes has prompted a more careful examination of the clinical course of these diseases and the creation of disease-specific registries.

LSDs associated with early-onset or acute neurological involvement are often associated with a significantly curtailed life span (i.e., death within the first decade). Early death is a feature noted among patients with neuropathic Gaucher disease types 2 and 3, MPS I (Hurler syndrome), Niemann-Pick disease type A, and Tay-Sachs disease. Long survival can be encountered in several LSDs, including Gaucher disease types 1 and 3, MPS II (Hunter syndrome), MPS III (Sanfilippo syndrome), mucolipidosis III, the juvenile- and adult-onset forms of neuronal ceroid-lipofuscinosis, and the oligosaccharidoses

Table 140.2 Clinical manifestations reported in patients with lysosomal storage disorders

Non-immune hydrops fetalis
- Disseminated lipogranulomatosis (Farber disease)
- Galactosialidosis (neuraminidase deficiency)
- Gaucher disease
- GM_1-gangliosidosis
- ISSD
- Mucolipidosis II (I-cell disease)
- MPS IV and MPS VII
- Niemann-Pick disease type C
- Sialidosis type 1
- Wolman disease

Myoclonic seizures
- Galactosialidosis
- Gaucher disease type 3
- GM_2-gangliosidosis
- Neuronal ceroid lipofuscinosis
- Niemann-Pick disease type C
- Oligosaccharidosis (α-N-acetylgalactosaminidase deficiency, fucosidosis, sialidosis type 1)

Ataxia
- Galactosialidosis
- Gaucher disease type 3
- G_{M1}-gangliosidosis
- Late-onset GM_2-gangliosidosis (cerebellar hypoplasia)
- Krabbe disease
- MLD
- Neuronal ceroid-lipofucinosis
- Niemann-Pick disease type C

Extrapyramidal signs
- Gaucher disease type 3
- GM_1-gangliosidosis (adult form)
- Late-onset GM_2-gangliosidosis
- Krabbe disease
- Niemann-Pick disease type C
- Oligosaccharidosis

Cortical atrophy
- Late stage of GM_1- and GM_2-gangliosidosis
- MLD
- I-cell disease
- Neuronal ceroid-lipofuscinosis

Cytopenia (anemia, thrombocytopenia)
- Gaucher disease
- Niemann-Pick disease
- Wolman disease (acanthocytosis)

Vacuolated lymphocytes
- GM_1-gangliosidosis (Landing disease)
- I-cell disease
- Multiple sulfatase deficiency (Austin disease)
- Neuronal ceroid-lipofuscinosis
- Niemann-Pick disease
- Oligosaccharidosis (aspartylglucosainuria, sialidosis)

Cerebrovascular or stroke-like episodes and other vascular events (e.g., Raynaud's phenomenon)
- Fabry disease

Dementia, psychosis
- Fabry disease
- Gaucher disease type 3
- GM_1-gangliosidosis
- Late-onset GM_2-gangliosidosis
- Krabbe disease
- MLD
- MPS III (Sanfilippo)
- Neuronal ceroid-lipofuscinosis
- Niemann-Pick disease type C

Macrocephaly
- Krabbe disease
- Tay-Sachs disease
- Sandhoff disease

Peripheral neuropathy
- Krabbe disease
- MLD (spastic paraplegia)
- Multiple sulfatase deficiency

Deafness
- Fabry disease
- I-cell disease
- MPS I, II, IV
- Oligosaccharidosis (α- and β-mannosidosis)

Interstitial lung disease
- Gaucher disease
- Niemann-Pick disease

Obstructive airway disease
- Fabry disease
- MPS

Cardiomyopathy
- Fabry disease (arrhythmia, conduction abnormalities)
- MPS (valvular disease)
- Pompe disease (hypotonia)

Cherry-red spot,* optic atrophy
- Galactosialidosis
- GM_1-gangliosidosis
- ISSD
- Mucolipidosis II (I-cell disease)
- MPS IV and MPS VII
- Niemann-Pick disease type A
- Sialidosis type 1
- Sandhoff disease
- Tay-Sachs disease

Retinitis pigmentosa
- Neuronal ceroid-lipofuscinosis

Corneal opacities (clouding)
- Mucolipidosis II (I-cell disease)
- Mucolipidosis IV
- MPS I, IV, VI
- Oligosaccharidosis (late-onset α-mannosidosis)
- Fabry disease

Lenticular opacities (cataracts)
- Oligosaccharidosis (sialidosis, α-mannosidosis)
- Fabry disease

Ophthalmoplegia (abnormal eye movements), nystagmus
- Gaucher disease type 3
- Niemann-Pick disease types C and D

Hepatosplenomegaly
- Gaucher disease
- MPS
- Niemann-Pick disease type A and B
- Niemann-Pick disease type C (cholestatic jaundice)
- Oligosaccharidoses
- Wolman disease and cholesterol ester storage disease

Nephrolithiasis
- Cystinuria

Proteinuria
- Fabry disease

Osteopenia
- Gaucher disease
- I-cell disease

Punctate epiphyseal calcifications
- β-Glucuronidase deficiency

Degenerative arthritis, bone infarcts
- Fabry disease
- Farber disease
- Gaucher disease
- I-cell disease
- Mucolipidosis III
- MPS I

Pain crises
- Gaucher disease types 1 and 3 (bone)
- Krabbe disease
- MLD

Dysostosis multiplex[†]
- MPS (coarse facies)
- Oligosaccharidoses

Angiokeratoma
- Fabry disease
- Oligosaccharidoses (aspartylglucosaminuria, fucosidosis, galactosialidosis, β-mannosidosis, sialidosis)

ISSD, infantile free sialic acid storage disease; MLD, metachromatic leukodystrophy; MPS, mucopolysaccharidosis.

* Describes the presence of the normal red macula surrounded by a pale retina reflecting storage material in the perifoveal ganglion cells.

† Refer to constellation of radiologic findings characterized by several of the following: macrocephaly, thickened calvarium, J-shaped sella turcica, spatulate ribs, bullet-shaped phalanges, rounding and anterior beaking of the vertebral bodies (especially lumbar), and flaring of iliac wings.

(aspartylglycosaminuria, mannosidosis, and fucosidosis). Patients with these particular diseases frequently inhabit residential treatment facilities such as nursing homes and state schools for the mentally retarded. Recent studies that examined the median cumulative survival (50 years) in males with Fabry disease (n = 51) noted a reduction in life span of approximately 20 years.[22] Similar studies examining median cumulative survival (70 years) in symptomatic Fabry disease carrier females noted a reduction in life span of approximately 15 years when compared with women in the general population.[23] Although life span in these females was greater than that noted among affected males, a gradual decline of the survival curve among carrier females was evident from the age of 35. The same investigators also reported several disease-related complications among Fabry disease carrier females, with frequency and severity that are higher than previously appreciated. This observation has prompted some investigators to suggest that Fabry disease may be an X-linked dominant disorder, with variable expression in carrier females that may be explained partly by lyonization (the phenomenon of random X-inactivation wherein the disease phenotype would only be expressed in cells in which the mutant rather than the normal allele is expressed).[24]

Unless the index of suspicion for LSD is high—based on the recognition of tell-tale signs such as angiokeratomas, cherry-red spot, dysostosis multiplex, or a positive family history—diagnosis can be delayed until the phenotype has fully evolved. Early diagnosis may be critical for certain subtypes because intervention (e.g., BMT or ERT) may reduce or eliminate the likelihood of a disease-related complication. In certain subtypes characterized by neurological involvement, BMT at the appropriate time before marked cognitive decline may decrease the risk of neurological sequelae in potentially responsive cases.

Several animal models of LSDs have occurred either naturally or have been generated by recombinant genetic techniques and the introduction of the relevant null allele into mouse embryonic stem cells.[25] These models have proven useful in investigations of pathophysiological mechanisms and therapeutic manipulation. For instance, investigations of the use of substrate synthesis inhibitors in several animal models for sphingolipidoses, including Tay-Sachs disease and Sandhoff disease, provided the rationale for the use of these agents in human clinical trials.

A naturally occurring mouse model of Krabbe disease, twitcher mouse (caused by a mutation of the galactosylceramidase gene), shows pathological changes similar to those of human disease. Classic Krabbe disease in humans is due to galactosylceramidase deficiency, with infantile onset as the most common presentation. A targeted disruption of saposin A (activator of the enzyme galactosylceramidase) also leads to similar findings, except for a later onset and slower rate of disease progression. Although saposin-A deficiency has not been described in humans, the information from the corresponding mouse model has provided some recent interesting insights. During intercrossing of saposin-A null mice, it was observed that affected females that were continually pregnant had greatly improved neurological symptoms compared with affected females that did not experience pregnancy or with affected males.[26] The pathological hallmark of Krabbe disease—demyelination with infiltration of globoid cells—largely disappeared and immune-related gene (monocyte chemotactic protein-1 and tumor necrosis factor-α) expression was significantly downregulated. The findings were attributed to a higher level of estrogen during pregnancy, suggesting that this may be one of the important factors in the protective effect of pregnancy in women with Krabbe disease.[27]

Additional insights have come from the creation of double-knockout animal models (i.e., mice models with mutations in two distinct genes whose expressed product or products involve integrated pathways of metabolism). Although these situations have not been reported in clinical patients with LSD, they provide highly instructive information. G_{M2}-gangliosidosis is characterized by neuronal storage of an anionic glycosphingolipid (G_{M2}-ganglioside) resulting from impaired G_{M2} hydrolysis due to mutant β-hexosaminidase or the absence of its functionally active G_{M2} activator protein (Tay-Sachs disease AB variant). A defect of the β-hexosaminidase α-subunit gene leads to Tay-Sachs disease (variant B), and a defect of the β-subunit gene causes Sandhoff disease (variant O). The mouse model for Tay-Sachs disease, unlike the human form, displays only localized neuropathological features, and the animals have normal balance and motor and behavioral patterns.[28] The milder expression was attributed to the presence of murine sialidase (not active in humans), which is able to convert G_{M2} to G_{A2} for further degradation. In contrast, the mouse model of Sandhoff disease shows progressive neurological deterioration in motor function and gait, with extensive ganglioside storage in nearly all neurons of the nervous system.[29] Double-knockout mice totally deficient in hexosaminidase activity and with a striking accumulation of anionic oligosaccharides have a more severe phenotype than either the Tay-Sachs or Sandhoff mouse model, with physical dysmorphic features and MPS.[30] The latter finding was attributed to secondary activity of hexosaminidase in the degradation of mucopolysaccharides (glycosaminoglycans). These studies have helped to elucidate the pathway of ganglioside metabolism and the role of hexosaminidase.

A second interesting example includes the study performed on double-knockout mice incapable of degrading any sulfolipids (due to arylsulfatase A deficiency) and synthesizing the major sulfolipid S-galactosylceramide (because of deficiency of galactosylceramide synthase). In humans, arylsulfatase A deficiency causes lysosomal accumulation of sulfoglycolipids and MLD. The mice studies suggested that the turnover of sulfolipids in general is highest in the distal nephron and that long thin limbs and distal convoluted tubules are the main sites of turnover of a minor sulfolipid species synthesized in the kidney of galactosylceramide synthase-null mice.[31] Investigations of the role of neuronal and microglial lesions may provide insight into human MLD, which is characterized by widespread demyelination.

In certain cases, however, knockout mice models for certain diseases (e.g., Fabry disease, Pompe disease, MLD, and Tay-Sachs disease) have been shown to reproduce the biochemical defect but not the clinical symptoms characterizing the classic phenotypes of these disorders.[32]

Diagnosis

The diagnosis of an LSD is based on the presence of characteristic clinical features, as noted in Table 140.2. When the specific diagnosis is not immediately apparent, general screening tools may include examination of urine for increased excretion of certain metabolites (e.g., glycosaminoglycans or oligosaccharides) and skin tissue for the presence of storage bodies. When skin biopsy is performed for ultrastructural studies, it usually is advisable to obtain a second sample for culture which then can be used for analysis of the activity of specific enzymes and as a source of DNA for subsequent mutation analysis. In patients with suspected Niemann-Pick disease type C, analysis of cholesterol esterification and staining for filipin may be performed on skin fibroblasts. This method is also the basis of prenatal diagnosis of the disease, using either cultured villi or amniocytes when the causal mutations are not known. Somatic hybridization studies of Niemann-Pick disease type C have demonstrated the existence of two complementation groups (designated "NPC1" and "NPC2") that have overlapping clinical features and biochemical characteristics. Molecular genetic studies in patients with Niemann-Pick disease type C have shown the presence of locus heterogeneity, with a defect of a major locus, NPC1 (approximately 95% of cases) mapped to chromosome 18q11 and a minor locus, the HE1 gene, on 14q24.3.[33,34] Thus, for most families with Niemann-Pick disease type C, biochemical (rather than molecular) studies involving cultured villi or amniocytes is a practical way to monitor future pregnancies at risk (unless a rapid means for mutation detection is established). Biochemical and molecular testing for most LSDs are available through several laboratories (a list of diagnostic referral laboratories can be found at www.genetests.org).

Microscopic examination of tissues (e.g., skin, bone marrow, rectal mucosa, or conjunctiva) from certain patients with suspected LSD may show residual bodies within lysosomes, for example, particulate glycogen in glycogenosis type II (Pompe disease) and Danon disease, lamellar profiles in sphingolipidoses (i.e., membranous cytoplasmic bodies in Tay-Sachs disease and prismatic inclusions in MLD), and zebra bodies in MPS.[35,36] These findings may suggest a diagnosis and help focus testing and avoid random or sequential screening for a battery of lysosomal enzyme activities. The presence of characteristic storage bodies, seen in skin biopsy specimens, is specific for two disorders, neuronal ceroid-lipofuscinosis and mucolipidosis IV. Recently, important progress in identifying the underlying defects in these two LSDs has permitted the characterization of the causal gene defects for these autosomal recessive disorders in clinically suspected cases.[37,38] Molecular genetic (DNA) analysis obviates the need for an invasive diagnostic procedure and the required expertise for accurate interpretation of biopsy findings, which often is not readily available.

The diverse clinical presentations of patients with LSDs can lead to consideration of a wide range of diagnostic possibilities, especially in the early stages of disease. An abbreviated scheme for approaching the diagnosis of an LSD is shown in Figure 140.1. Clinical investigations should be directed by the nature of the problem, the physical examination findings, and family history when contributory. Involvement of the central nervous system may prompt a request for magnetic resonance imaging (MRI) of the brain to look for leukodystrophy (e.g., Krabbe disease and MLD, diseases also associated with increased levels of protein in the cerebrospinal fluid). Testing of brainstem auditory evoked potentials and nerve conduction velocity studies may be informative in disorders associated with primary cranial nerve (e.g., neuropathic Gaucher disease, Krabbe disease, and MLD) and peripheral nerve (e.g., Krabbe disease and MLD) involvement, respectively. Peripheral nerve involvement may also arise from skeletal complications (e.g., nerve root problem as a consequence of vertebral compression in Gaucher disease and MPS) or entrapment within infiltrated soft tissue (e.g., carpal tunnel syndrome in patients with MPS). Electromyography can be used to differentiate anterior horn cell degeneration, as in adult GM_2-gangliosidosis, from other causes of muscle weakness. Assessment of autonomic dysfunction may be revealing in patients with Fabry disease, which is often associated with acroparesthesias, hearing loss, decreased sweating, and intestinal dysmotility. Electroretinography is a sensitive measure of retinal degeneration. The destruction of the outer retinal layer in the infantile form of neuronal ceroid-lipofuscinosis completely abolishes the electroretinographic response. Electroretinographic abnormalities may also be evident in patients with mucolipidosis IV. In patients with hepatosplenomegaly, volumetric organ measurements can be obtained with computed tomography (CT) or MRI. A limited skeletal survey (X-rays of the skull, lateral lumbar spine, and anteroposterior views of the left hand and wrist, pelvis, and femurs) may show signs of dysostosis multiplex in patients with MPS and some of the oligosaccharidoses and sialidosis. The information derived from these studies is useful not only for defining the pattern and severity of disease but also in evaluating disease progression. For certain subtypes in which treatment may be available, clinical studies may provide evidence of disease stabilization or reversal with therapy.

For certain subtypes in which more than one clinical variant may be encountered, age at disease onset

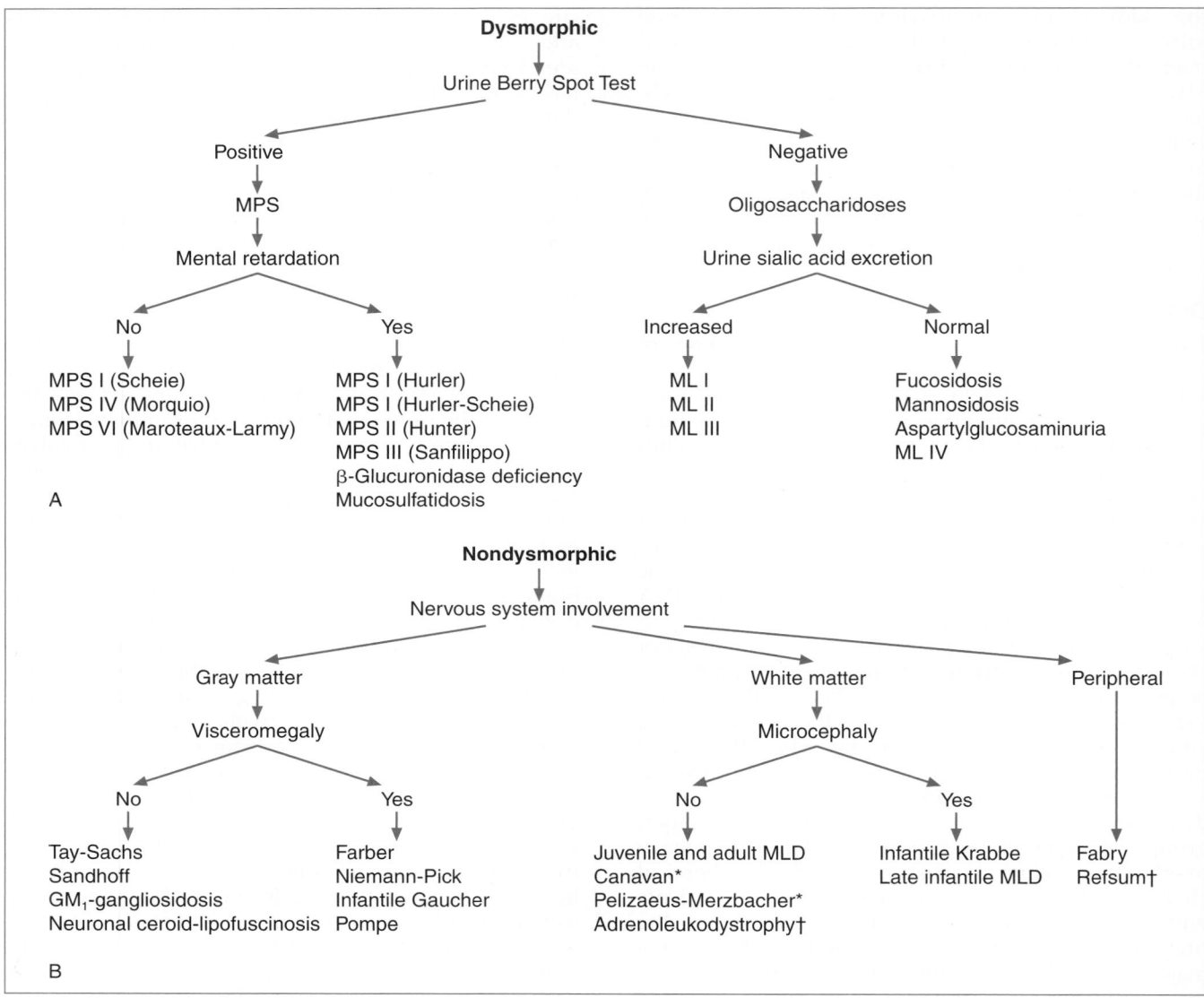

Figure 140.1   *A* and *B*, Algorithm for diagnosing lysosomal storage diseases. ML, mucolipidosis; MLD, metachromatic leukodystrophy; MPS, mucopolysaccharidosis. *Nonlysosomal; †nonlysosomal (defect of peroxisomes).

and clinical course are used for classification. Clinical findings associated with LSDs, based on age at onset, are summarized in Table 140.3. Existing clinical designations were established before the biochemical basis and underlying molecular defects were fully understood. It now is recognized that the clinical classifications are relatively arbitrary because most subtypes do not belong to clear-cut categories but fall somewhere along a broad spectrum of clinical presentations. In certain cases, disease expression can be related to the type of (allelic) mutations, which can be associated with either a mild or severe effect, and in cases characterized by an intermediate course, the expression can be the result of a combination of these two extremes. It is important to note that studies of genotype-phenotype correlation have rarely demonstrated perfect concordance, and the use of genotype information for prognostication in individual cases may not be completely reliable. This underscores the need for regular monitoring of patients in whom LSD has been diagnosed to accurately establish prognosis and to enable appropriate genetic counseling.

Genetic DNA analysis is becoming increasingly available, and it has been used to accurately detect carriers or confirm the clinical diagnosis, complementing the results of biochemical analysis. Carrier testing based on biochemical assays for the majority of LSDs resulting from an enzyme deficiency can be associated with a high rate of misdiagnosis because of considerable overlap in the enzyme activity between those who are obligate (true) carriers and the general population. An exception is Tay-Sachs disease. If the blood specimen is handled and processed properly, an assessment of enzyme activity can be used to reliably identify carriers; this has been the basis for carrier screening among high-risk groups such as the Ashkenazim since the mid-1970s.

Table 140.3 Presenting clinical manifestations associated with lysosomal storage diseases, according to age of onset

Age at onset	Presenting signs and associated clinical features
First year	
Farber disease (ceramide deficiency)	Hoarseness, vomiting, swollen joints, subcutaneous nodules, lymphadenopathy, foamy macrophages
Fucosidosis type 1	Slow development, rapid progression leading to decerebrate rigidity, coarse facies, vacuolated lymphocytes
Gaucher disease type 2	Failure to thrive, hepatosplenomegaly, brainstem signs
GM$_1$-gangliosidosis type 1	Slow development, increased startle reflex, hepatosplenomegaly
GM$_2$-gangliosidosis, Sandhoff variant	Slow development, increased startle reflex, cherry-red macula
Hunter syndrome	Coarse facies, stiff joints
Hurler syndrome	Coarse facies, stiff joints
α-Mannosidosis	Slow development, coarse facies, hepatosplenomegaly, moderate to severe mental retardation
Mucolipidosis II	Wizened face at birth, gingival hyperplasia, stiff joints
Mucolipidosis IV	Slow development, corneal clouding
Mucosulfatidosis	Slow development, coarse facies
Neuronal ceroid-lipofuscinosis, infantile type	Slow development, poor vision
Niemann-Pick disease type A	Slow development, hepatosplenomegaly
Sanfilippo syndrome	Coarse facies, stiff joints, severe mental retardation
Sialic acid storage disease	Slow development, hepatosplenomegaly, coarse facies
Sialidosis type II, late-infantile	Slow development, coarse facies, hepatomegaly
Wolman disease	Vomiting, diarrhea, hepatosplenomegaly, calcified adrenal glands
Second year	
Aspartylglucosaminuria	Slow development, delayed or absent speech, coarse facies, aggressive behavior
Fucosidosis, type 2	Slow neurological deterioration, angiokeratoma
GM$_1$-gangliosidosis type 2	Slow development, increased startle reflex
Maroteaux-Lamy syndrome	Coarse facies, stiff joints, corneal clouding
Morquio syndrome	Dwarfism, skeletal abnormalities, loose joints
Mucolipidosis III	Stiff hands and shoulders
Neuronal ceroid-lipofuscinosis, late infantile type	Seizures, myoclonus, decreased vision, decreased intellect
Niemann-Pick disease type B	Hepatosplenomegaly
Sialidosis type II	Walking difficulties, seizures, myoclonus, mental retardation, macular cherry-red spot
Childhood	
Cholesterol ester storage disease	Hepatomegaly, increased plasma cholesterol and triglycerides
Galactosialidosis	Delayed motor development, mental retardation, seizures, myoclonus, coarse facies
Gaucher disease type 1	Splenomegaly, anemia, thrombocytopenia, osteopenia, osteonecrosis
Maroteaux-Lamy syndrome, mild	Short stature, limitation in joint range of motion, coarse facies, corneal clouding, lumbar lordosis, normal intelligence, cardiac valve disease
Neuronal ceroid-lipofuscinosis, juvenile type	Blindness, seizures, decreased intellect
Niemann-Pick disease, chronic neuropathic form	Tetraparesis, decreased intellect, hepatomegaly
Scheie syndrome	Claw hands, short stature
Adolescence	
Cherry-red spot myoclonus syndrome, sialidosis type I	Unexpected falls, seizures, cherry-red macula, corneal clouding, coarse facies, seizures
Gaucher disease, type 3	Splenomegaly, seizures, myoclonus, osteopenia
GM$_2$-gangliosidosis, late-onset	Dysarthria, walking difficulties from spastic paraparesis, cerebellar ataxia, dystonia
Adulthood	
Gaucher disease type I	Splenomegaly, thrombocytopenia, osteonecrosis
Maroteaux-Lamy syndrome, mild	Short stature, coarse facies, corneal clouding, compressive myelopathy
Neuronal ceroid-lipofuscinosis (Kufs disease)	Dementia, behavioral disturbances, epilepsy, ataxia
Pompe disease, adult type (acid maltase myopathy)	Proximal muscle weakness (limb-girdle myopathy), with intercostal and diaphragm involvement (leading to respiratory insufficiency)

Management

General principles

Improvements in the understanding of the biochemical and molecular basis of LSDs have fostered the development of targeted therapeutic strategies. Promising treatment options include ERT, substrate synthesis inhibition, and gene therapy. Although solid organ (e.g., liver, kidney) transplants have been performed in certain patients (e.g., the liver in Gaucher disease and kidney in Fabry disease) for end-organ failure and have led to functional improvement, enzyme activity within the "healthy" donor organs is not sufficient to achieve effective clearance of systemic substrate storage.[39]

Several technical and practical clinical factors represent potential barriers to the introduction of effective treatments for LSDs. These include the need for safe methods to breach the blood-brain barrier to achieve sufficient drug concentration in the central nervous system for clinical subtypes associated with neuropathic involvement. Because certain abnormalities may develop prenatally, effective delivery of drugs across the blood-brain barrier may still not be adequate to achieve a full response. Moreover, efficient drug delivery to various extraneurological sites of substrate storage is required because most LSDs are multisystem disorders. Cellular processes result in the generation of a steady stream of substrate that needs to be catabolized. Thus, for any treatment to be effective, it is crucial that activity of the enzyme/cofactor or protein involved in transport mechanisms or substrate hydrolysis be sustained or be replenished safely.

The conduct of clinical trials to test the safety and effectiveness of novel agents can be confounded by the 1) small number of eligible patients (because most LSDs are relatively infrequent or rare disorders), 2) heterogeneity of clinical expression, 3) paucity of reliable surrogate markers that correlate with the pattern and severity of disease, and 4) uncertainty a priori of being able to reverse disease (which creates a problem in the selection of the appropriate primary end points).[40] Furthermore, the demonstration of a therapeutic benefit may not be evident when the period of observation is short.

It is likely that clinical responses will be influenced by preexisting lesions. As more specific treatments become available and are shown to be safe in the management of LSDs, earlier intervention may be necessary to achieve the best possible outcomes. Because of the rarity of most LSDs, the estimated cost of treatment is anticipated to be high. This is evident from the high cost of enzyme therapy for Gaucher disease and Fabry disease, which on average amounts to US $150,000 to $300,000 annually. The major morbidity and shortened life span associated with certain clinical types and the poor quality of life experienced by most untreated patients have prompted the development of directed therapies. Health care regulators will need to examine various issues relating to safety, effectiveness, and cost-utility to ensure equitable distribution of resources and to address the concerns of patients and their families.

Because all LSDs are inherited disorders, confirmation of the diagnosis in an individual patient may have implications for other family members. The concerns may not be restricted to reproductive risks, because certain disorders with late-onset may imply that other siblings (particularly younger family members) may be at risk for the development of the condition. It is important that families receive appropriate genetic counseling regarding reproductive risks and other information relating to the specific condition, such as prognosis and treatment if available. Risks are related to the mode of disease inheritance and the proband's familial relationship to the index patient. In cases in which individuals are identified as a carrier, the risk that the spouse may be a carrier is determined by family history or general population risks (based on disease incidence).

Symptomatic treatment

Until recently, the mainstay of treatment for most LSDs has been primarily palliative or supportive care,

with management directed at disease-specific complications. Attention to clinical problems and attempts at providing relief can lead to marked improvement in the patient's quality of life, and it helps families deal with the anxiety and frustration that result from not being able to obtain a cure. General issues include identification of community resources that can be called upon for assistance and attention to the nutritional needs of the patient. Feeding problems, which may arise because of bulbar paralysis, may require attention to ways of reducing the likelihood of choking and aspiration and providing supplemental caloric sources to meet the patient's metabolic needs. It also is important not to overlook dental care and airway maintenance and to manage problems arising from incontinence and constipation.

Often, the presence of a sick family member with a genetic disorder can create tension between parents that leads to separation and threatens the emotional well-being of other healthy siblings. The involvement of a social worker at an early stage is frequently beneficial. A social worker can direct the family to local institutions that can provide assistance, for example, with transportation to the clinic or providing respite care while the rest of the family is on vacation. Special educational programs for handicapped children and programs sponsored by various organizations such as the Cerebral Palsy Association help with promoting skills to facilitate activities of daily living and communication. Communication is an important component of establishing relationships, and attention to the child's needs in this area to foster social interaction may prove to be a rewarding experience for all involved. In counseling of families, it is important that the goals and expectations are realistic. Also, some families may require more time to adjust than others, and the avenue of hope should not be completely shut at the time of diagnosis. Families should be given adequate support, and issues of bereavement should be confronted with the aid of a professional if necessary.

Neurological problems may be primary or secondary. Various medications may be given for effective seizure control and spasticity. Families should be counseled about the difficulty of fully controlling seizures and irritability (e.g., a major issue for infants with Krabbe disease), which helps assuage feelings of helplessness and "not doing enough." Hydrocephalus, which can be a problem in some patients with MPS, may require shunting. Musculoskeletal problems may require tendon release procedures and applications of a splint or brace or enrollment in a regular physical and occupational therapy program. Patients in whom pathological fractures or osteonecrosis and secondary degenerative joint disease (e.g., Gaucher disease) develop may benefit from orthopedic intervention, and patients with osteopenia may show improvement with attention to calcium requirements and treatment with bisphosphonates. End-stage organ damage (e.g., heart or renal failure in patients with Fabry disease) may be corrected by organ transplant. Renal insufficiency, in the absence of a donor kidney, may be adequately managed with peritoneal or hemodialysis and may

Table 140.4   Bone marrow transplantation for lysosomal storage disorders

Disease	Clinical response to transplantation
Aspartylglycosaminuria	Not effective
Farber disease	Reduction in nodule size
Fucosidosis	Effective*
Gaucher disease	
Type 1	Effective* (ERT preferred)
Type 2	Not effective
Type 3	Effective*
Hunter syndrome (MPS II)	Effective for later-onset mild cases only
Hurler syndrome (MPS I)	Effective* (visceral effects improved)
α-Mannosidosis	Probable, if performed early; somatic disease reversed, but lysosomal storage in brain may persist
Maroteaux-Lamy syndrome (MPS VI)	Effective* (but poor skeletal response)
Neuronal ceroid-lipofuscinosis	Not effective
Niemann Pick disease:	
Type A	Not effective
Type B	Effective*
Type C	Liver disease improved, but not CNS involvement
Sanfilippo syndrome (MPS III), all variants	Not effective
Sly syndrome (MPS VII)	Effective*
Wolman disease	Effective*

CNS, central nervous system; ERT, enzyme replacement therapy; MPS, mucopolysaccharidosis.
*If transplant is performed early in clinical course.

result in an increase in physical and functional well-being. Before enzyme therapy was available for Gaucher disease, patients with cardiopulmonary and gastrointestinal tract problems attributed to an enlarged spleen and those with marked hypersplenism obtained relief with a partial or total splenectomy.

Bone marrow transplantation

Cellular replacement, mainly through BMT, has been the method primarily considered in attempting to establish a "cure" for LSDs (Table 140.4). However, the high morbidity and mortality risk associated with BMT has limited its general introduction. BMT has been performed in certain LSDs to prevent or ameliorate the inexorable neurological deterioration.[41,42] The potential benefit of BMT for central nervous system disease may be the ability of marrow-derived elements to penetrate the blood-brain barrier and seed brain parenchyma. Experiments conducted in mice models of some LSDs (e.g., Sandhoff disease) have suggested that BMT may suppress both the explosive expansion of activated microglia and neuronal cell death without detectable decreases in neuronal G_{M2}-ganglioside storage.[43] These results suggest that the mechanism of neurodegeneration includes a vigorous inflammatory response as an important component. They also suggest that BMT may provide added benefit beyond that resulting from correction of the underlying enzyme deficiency. The implications of these observations for human and other sphingolipidoses remain to be determined.

Although patients with certain LSDs (e.g., Gaucher disease type 3 and Hurler syndrome) have evidence of some benefit from BMT, there is no indication of an important change in the clinical course after transplantation in other disorders in which neuronal storage is present (e.g., GM_1-gangliosidosis, Pompe disease, Gaucher disease type 2, and Niemann-Pick disease type A).

Differences in clinical outcome after BMT appear to be influenced by the age at disease onset and the severity of disease at the time the procedure is contemplated. Thus, early identification of patients before the development of marked neurological injury through newborn screening programs may provide a window of opportunity. Also, the naturally suppressed immune system of the neonate may maximize the chances of successful engraftment because the use of immunologically privileged cells may reduce the likelihood of graft-versus-host disease. Because autologous BMT is not a therapeutic option, there is a need to identify an HLA-matched donor for allogeneic transplant. Systematic collection of umbilical cord blood, which has been used increasingly as a source of hematopoietic progenitors, may solve previous problems resulting from a limited donor pool. However, longer-term experience is required to establish the benefit derived from using umbilical cord blood cells, because these precursor cells may not be fully differentiated and able to adequately degrade the excess intracellular storage materials.

It is preferable to obtain cells for transplant from a donor who is not a carrier of the trait for which the procedure is being performed. This is to ensure maximal residual enzyme activity following BMT, even in cases in which full engraftment may not be achieved and there is mixed chimerism.

Several approaches are actively being explored as a means of optimizing the safety and efficacy of BMT, including the use of nonmyeloablative or minimal conditioning to reduce procedural toxicity and mesenchymal stem cells that can undergo multilineage differentiation as an added or alternative cellular resource for the enzyme or protein.[44]

Enzyme replacement therapy

Advances in the application of molecular genetic techniques have enabled the development of directed protein therapies as an alternative to potentially curative procedures such as BMT.[45] Previous attempts based on leukocyte infusions for patients with MPS and subcutaneous injections of amnion epithelial cells in Niemann-Pick disease type B patients have not been shown to be an effective means of endogenous enzyme production.[46,47] Industrial-scale production of recombinant enzyme (using mammalian cell cultures) has enabled clinical trials to be conducted in patients with various LSDs.

In Gaucher disease, the introduction of ERT established "proof of concept" that this approach can induce the clearance of stored lipid and reverse disease manifestations. Slow substrate turnover, restricted sites of abnormality, and targeted macrophage delivery of the recombinant enzyme ensured the success of this approach. The absence of primary central nervous system involvement in

Gaucher disease type 1 (the most common subtype) also obviated the need for breaching the blood-brain barrier to gain access to central nervous system sites of storage. ERT does not appear to ultimately influence the course of the neurological disease in acute Gaucher disease type 2. However, treatment of Gaucher disease type 3 (subacute neuropathic disease) has been reported to stabilize supranuclear palsy and cognitive function, although the condition of some patients has worsened and progressive myoclonic encephalopathy has developed, accompanied by cranial MRI and EEG abnormalities.[48] The assessment of therapeutic response in patients with Gaucher disease type 3 is complicated by wide heterogeneity in clinical expression, and a longer experience in the treatment of these patients is required to determine management guidelines.

The observations of clinical benefit in certain subtypes of Gaucher disease provided the impetus for considering ERT in treating other storage disorders such as Fabry disease and MPS I, II, and VI. In contrast to recombinant glucocerebrosidase for Gaucher disease, which relies on α-mannosyl residues for targeted cellular delivery, the recombinant enzyme for the other LSDs listed uses mannose 6-phosphate and binding to the relevant receptor for their intracellular uptake.[49] Recent clinical trials conducted in patients with Fabry disease showed the effectiveness of ERT in reducing the incidence and severity of neuropathic pain and other changes such as a marked decrease in abnormal cerebral perfusion and vascular reactivity (based on $H_2^{15}O$ positron emission tomography) and the resolution of cerebrovascular hyperdynamicity, that is, abnormally increased blood flow in the absence of arterial stenosis (based on transcranial Doppler study).[50] The latter findings suggest that ERT may potentially lead to reduction of cerebrovascular complications in patients with Fabry disease. Ongoing ERT clinical trials in patients with MPS I also suggest some benefit, including a decrease in hepatosplenomegaly and an increase in joint range of motion.[51]

The limited experience with ERT suggests that it is likely to be effective in eliminating substrate storage in sites to which it can gain access. Thus, most of the therapeutic gains may be derived primarily from extraneurological improvements, unless a method of delivery can be devised to ensure adequate enzyme concentrations within the central nervous system. Clinical responses are likely to be limited by the extent of preexisting lesions because the approach is designed to overcome the block in the catabolism of stored substrate and relies on the intrinsic ability of the cells to regenerate or heal. This concern leads to the suggestion that early intervention may offer the best opportunity for a full response, although the required commitment to regular intravenous infusion and high costs of treatment may limit its consideration as a prophylactic measure.

Future therapeutic prospects

Increasing knowledge from investigations on the various biochemical pathways and mechanisms of disease in the LSDs has raised the prospects for novel treatment strategies. Alternative options under study include the use of substrate synthesis inhibitors, chemical-mediated chaperones, and gene therapy.

The rationale for the use of substrate synthesis inhibitors was based on the hypothesis that a decrease in substrate load to a level that can be handled sufficiently by existing residual enzyme activity may permit adequate substrate turnover to prevent its critical buildup within cells.[52,53] Subsequently, preclinical trials in several animal models of sphingolipidosis demonstrated increased survival and histological improvements. Limited trials using N-butyldeoxynojirimycin, a glucosyltransferase inhibitor, in patients with Gaucher disease type 1 have suggested that it may induce an increase in blood cell counts and a reduction in organomegaly.[54] The drug appears to be relatively well tolerated; most patients initially have gastrointestinal side effects (bloating, flatulence, and diarrhea) and weight loss that appear to diminish with continued treatment. However, certain patients have developed tremors and paresthesias, and although these problems appear to reverse with withdrawal of the drug, they may be of concern because patients with sphingolipidoses who benefit from the use of these drugs will likely require long-term treatment. Subsequent generations of these imino-sugar compounds possibly may have a better toxicity profile. Other agents also being considered include the compound D-threo-1-phenyl-2-decanoylamino-3-morpholino-1-propanol (PDMP), so-called P4 analogues, which simulate the ceramide moiety and reduce substrate synthesis through competitive inhibition.[55] Other disorders for which substrate synthesis inhibitors are under consideration include late-onset GM_2-gangliosidosis, Fabry disease, and Niemann-Pick disease type C.

Certain mutations that involve lysosomal enzymes are found in regions outside the catalytic site and lead to impaired function because of misfolding. Agents that can serve as chemical chaperones that allow for proper refolding of the mutant proteins may lead to resumption of substantial partial or full enzyme activity. This hypothesis received a recent boost from the results of a trial in one patient with Fabry disease in whom intravenous galactose infusions were shown to reverse congestive heart failure due to cardiomyopathy.[56] The effectiveness of this approach for other organs involved, such as the kidneys and central nervous system, remains to be established. The availability of cell lines and animal models for LSDs may permit systematic screening for other similar compounds, with clinical trials using potentially safe and promising agents.

Gene therapy strategies for LSDs have used ex vivo gene transduction of cellular targets with subsequent transplantation of the enzymatically corrected cells or direct in vivo delivery of the viral vectors.[57,58] Oncoretroviral vectors and, more recently, adeno-associated vectors and lentiviral vectors have been tested extensively. Nonviral vectors, in at least one study consisting of lipofectin/integrin-targeting peptide/

DNA complexes, have also been examined because they are potentially safer, simpler, and able to package large DNA molecules.[59] Delivery of therapeutic genes by this method into fibroblasts of patients with fucosidosis or Fabry disease resulted in the production of large amounts of normal enzyme, with secretion into the medium and the potential for uptake by other deficient cells.[59] Clinical gene therapy trials have been conducted in a small number of patients with Gaucher disease. The limited success was characterized by a small but measurable amount of enzyme production that was not sustained. Most of the hydrolytic enzymes within the lysosome are expressed constitutively to keep up with their housekeeping role. Because carriers do not show evidence of disease or substrate storage, a small but persistent expression from corrected cells may be adequate to effect a cure. These observations also suggest that regulation of gene function may not be critical, as also suggested by the wide range of enzyme doses used in treatment of patients with Gaucher disease and Fabry disease. However, transduced cells are not expected to have a proliferative advantage over uncorrected cells because most storage materials are not directly cytotoxic. Thus, a means for the creation of a niche may be essential to ensuring that the gene-corrected cells take hold in the patient. This may involve some measure of ablation in disorders associated with marrow infiltration, a state that possibly may be achieved with pretreatment using enzyme therapy rather than routine measures such as chemotherapy.

A review of recently published reports suggests that novel therapies may become increasingly available for this previously untreatable group of disorders. Obviously, it would be instructive to examine data from trials in animal models of disease, although one should always consider the possibility that species-specific differences exist and may not allow the direct transfer of experience in animals to humans. Ultimately, the cautious introduction into human patients and greater experience with potentially promising treatment may transform the natural history of certain LSDs.

References

1. De Duve C, Wattiaux R. Functions of lysosomes. Annu Rev Physiol 1966;28:435–492
2. Hers HG. The role of lysosomes in the pathogeny of storage diseases. Biochimie 1972;54:753–757
3. Walkley SU. New proteins from old diseases provide novel insights in cell biology. Curr Opin Neurol 2001;14:805–810
4. Huizing M, Anikster Y, Gahl WA. Hermansky-Pudlak syndrome and Chediak-Higashi syndrome: disorders of vesicle formation and trafficking. Thromb Haemost 2001;86:233–245
5. Fratantoni JC, Hall CW, Neufeld EF. Hurler and Hunter syndromes: mutual correction of the defect in cultured fibroblasts. Science 1968;162:570–572
6. Applegarth DA, Toone JR, Lowry RB. Incidence of inborn errors of metabolism in British Columbia, 1969–1996. Pediatrics 2000;105:e10
7. Poorthuis BJ, Wevers RA, Kleijer WJ, et al. The frequency of lysosomal storage diseases in The Netherlands. Hum Genet 1999;105:151–156
8. Meikle PJ, Hopwood JJ, Clague AE, Carey WF. Prevalence of lysosomal storage disorders. JAMA 1999;281:249–254
9. Mitchison HM, Mole SE. Neurodegenerative disease: the neuronal ceroid lipofuscinoses (Batten disease). Curr Opin Neurol 2001;14:795–803
10. Zlotogora J, Bach G, Munnich A. Molecular basis of mendelian disorders among Jews. Mol Genet Metab 2000;69:169–180
11. Meikle PJ, Ranieri E, Ravenscroft EM, et al. Newborn screening for lysosomal storage disorders. Southeast Asian J Trop Med Public Health 1999;30 Suppl 2:104–110
12. Chamoles NA, Blanco M, Gaggioli D, Casentini C. Tay-Sachs and Sandhoff diseases: enzymatic diagnosis in dried blood spots on filter paper: retrospective diagnoses in newborn-screening cards. Clin Chim Acta 2002;318:133–137
13. Chamoles NA, Blanco M, Gaggioli D, Casentini C. Gaucher and Niemann-Pick diseases—enzymatic diagnosis in dried blood spots on filter paper: retrospective diagnoses in newborn-screening cards. Clin Chim Acta 2002;317:191–197
14. Chamoles NA, Blanco MB, Gaggioli D, Casentini C. Hurler-like phenotype: enzymatic diagnosis in dried blood spots on filter paper. Clin Chem 2001;47:2098–2102
15. Chamoles NA, Blanco MB, Iorcansky S, et al. Retrospective diagnosis of GM1 gangliosidosis by use of a newborn-screening card (letter). Clin Chem 2001;47:2068
16. Chamoles NA, Blanco M, Gaggioli D. Fabry disease: enzymatic diagnosis in dried blood spots on filter paper (letter). Clin Chim Acta 2001;308:195–196
17. Chamoles NA, Blanco M, Gaggioli D. Diagnosis of alpha-L-iduronidase deficiency in dried blood spots on filter paper: the possibility of newborn diagnosis. Clin Chem 2001;47:780–781
18. Itoh K, Oyanagi K, Takahashi H, et al. Endothelin-1 in the brain of patients with galactosialidosis: its abnormal increase and distribution pattern. Ann Neurol 2000;47:122–126
19. Arai Y, Edwards V, Takashima S, Becker LE. Vascular pathology in galactosialidosis. Ultrastruct Pathol 1999;23:369–374
20. Altarescu G, Moore DF, Pursley R, et al. Enhanced endothelium-dependent vasodilation in Fabry disease. Stroke 2001;32:1559–1562
21. Im DS, Heise CE, Nguyen T, et al. Identification of a molecular target of psychosine and its role in globoid cell formation. J Cell Biol 2001;153:429–434
22. MacDermot KD, Holmes A, Miners AH. Anderson-Fabry disease: clinical manifestations and impact of disease in a cohort of 98 hemizygous males. J Med Genet 2001;38:750–760
23. MacDermot KD, Holmes A, Miners AH. Anderson-Fabry disease: clinical manifestations and impact of disease in a cohort of 60 obligate carrier females. J Med Genet 2001;38:769–775
24. Whybra C, Wendrich K, Ries M, et al. Clinical manifestation in female Fabry disease patients. Contrib Nephrol 2001;136:245–250
25. Alroy J, Warren CD, Raghavan SS, Kolodny EH. Animal models for lysosomal storage diseases: their past and future contribution. Hum Pathol 1989;20:823–826
26. Matsuda J, Vanier MT, Saito Y, et al. A mutation in the

saposin A domain of the sphingolipid activator protein (prosaposin) gene results in a late-onset, chronic form of globoid cell leukodystrophy in the mouse. Hum Mol Genet 2001;10:1191–1199

27. Matsuda J, Vanier MT, Saito Y, Suzuki K. Dramatic phenotypic improvement during pregnancy in a genetic leukodystrophy: estrogen appears to be a critical factor. Hum Mol Genet 2001;10:2709–2715

28. Yamanaka S, Johnson MD, Grinberg A, et al. Targeted disruption of the Hexa gene results in mice with biochemical and pathologic features of Tay-Sachs disease. Proc Natl Acad Sci U S A 1994;91:9975–9979

29. Sango K, Yamanaka S, Hoffmann A, et al. Mouse models of Tay-Sachs and Sandhoff diseases differ in neurologic phenotype and ganglioside metabolism. Nat Genet 1995;11:170–176

30. Sango K, McDonald MP, Crawley JN, et al. Mice lacking both subunits of lysosomal beta-hexosaminidase display gangliosidosis and mucopolysaccharidosis. Nat Genet 1996;14:348–352

31. Lullmann-Rauch R, Matzner U, Franken S, et al. Lysosomal sulfoglycolipid storage in the kidneys of mice deficient for arylsulfatase A (ASA) and of double-knockout mice deficient for ASA and galactosylceramide synthase. Histochem Cell Biol 2001;116:161–169

32. Elsea SH, Lucas RE. The mousetrap: what we can learn when the mouse model does not mimic the human disease. ILAR J 2002;43:66–79

33. Carstea ED, Morris JA, Coleman KG, et al. Niemann-Pick C1 disease gene: homology to mediators of cholesterol homeostasis. Science 1997;277:228–231

34. Naureckiene S, Sleat DE, Lackland H, et al. Identification of HE1 as the second gene of Niemann-Pick C disease. Science 2000;290:2298–2301

35. Prasad A, Kaye EM, Alroy J. Electron microscopic examination of skin biopsy as a cost-effective tool in the diagnosis of lysosomal storage diseases. J Child Neurol 1996;11:301–308

36. Warren CD, Alroy J. Morphological, biochemical and molecular biology approaches for the diagnosis of lysosomal storage diseases. J Vet Diagn Invest 2000; 12:483–496

37. Weimer JM, Kriscenski-Perry E, Elshatory Y, Pearce DA. The neuronal ceroid lipofuscinoses: mutations in different proteins result in similar disease. Neuromolecular Med 2002;1:111–124

38. Bach G. Mucolipidosis type IV. Mol Genet Metab 2001;73:197–203

39. Groth CG, Ringden O. Transplantation in relation to the treatment of inherited disease. Transplantation 1984;38:319–327

40. Pastores GM, Thadhani R. Advances in the management of Anderson-Fabry disease: enzyme replacement therapy. Expert Opin Biol Ther 2002;2:325–333

41. Krivit W, Peters C, Shapiro EG. Bone marrow transplantation as effective treatment of central nervous system disease in globoid cell leukodystrophy, metachromatic leukodystrophy, adrenoleukodystrophy, mannosidosis, fucosidosis, aspartylglucosaminuria, Hurler, Maroteaux-Lamy, and Sly syndromes, and Gaucher disease type III. Curr Opin Neurol 1999;12:167–176

42. Hoogerbrugge PM, Brouwer OF, Fischer A. Bone marrow transplantation for metabolic diseases with severe neurological symptoms. Bone Marrow Transplant 1991;7 Suppl 2:71

43. Wada R, Tifft CJ, Proia RL. Microglial activation precedes acute neurodegeneration in Sandhoff disease and is suppressed by bone marrow transplantation. Proc Natl Acad Sci U S A 2000;97:10954–10959

44. Tse WT, Egalka MC. Stem cell plasticity and blood and marrow transplantation: a clinical strategy. J Cell Biochem Suppl 2002;38:96–103

45. Schiffmann R, Brady RO. New prospects for the treatment of lysosomal storage diseases. Drugs 2002;62: 733–742

46. Nishioka J, Mizushima T, Ono K. Treatment of mucopolysaccharidosis: clinical and biochemical aspects of leucocyte transfusion as compared with plasma infusion in patients with Hurler's and Scheie's syndromes. Clin Orthop 1979;140:194–203

47. Cerneca F, Andolina M, Simeone R, et al. Treatment of patients with Niemann-Pick type is using repeated amniotic epithelial cells implantation: correction of aggregation and coagulation abnormalities. Clin Pediatr (Phila) 1997;36:141–146

48. Altarescu G, Hill S, Wiggs E, et al. The efficacy of enzyme replacement therapy in patients with chronic neuronopathic Gaucher's disease. J Pediatr 2001;138: 539–547

49. Kaye EM. Therapeutic approaches to lysosomal storage diseases. Curr Opin Pediatr 1995;7:650–654

50. Brady RO, Murray GJ, Moore DF, Schiffmann R. Enzyme replacement therapy in Fabry disease. J Inherit Metab Dis 2001;24 Suppl 2:18–24

51. Wraith JE. Enzyme replacement therapy in mucopolysaccharidosis type I: progress and emerging difficulties. J Inherit Metab Dis 2001;24:245–250

52. Platt FM, Butters TD. New therapeutic prospects for the glycosphingolipid lysosomal storage diseases. Biochem Pharmacol 1998;56:421–430

53. Lachmann RH, Platt FM. Substrate reduction therapy for glycosphingolipid storage disorders. Expert Opin Investig Drugs 2001;10:455–466

54. Cox T, Lachmann R, Hollak C, et al. Novel oral treatment of Gaucher's disease with N-butyldeoxynojirimycin (OGT 918) to decrease substrate biosynthesis. Lancet 2000;355:1481–1485

55. Abe A, Wild SR, Lee WL, Shayman JA. Agents for the treatment of glycosphingolipid storage disorders. Curr Drug Metab 2001;2:331–338

56. Frustaci A, Chimenti C, Ricci R, et al. Improvement in cardiac function in the cardiac variant of Fabry's disease with galactose-infusion therapy. N Engl J Med 2001;345:25–32

57. Barranger JM, Novelli EA. Gene therapy for lysosomal storage disorders. Expert Opin Biol Ther 2001;1: 857–867

58. Yew NS, Cheng SH. Gene therapy for lysosomal storage disorders. Curr Opin Mol Ther 2001;3:399–406

59. Estruch EJ, Hart SL, Kinnon C, Winchester BG. Nonviral, integrin-mediated gene transfer into fibroblasts from patients with lysosomal storage diseases. J Gene Med 2001;3:488–497

141 Whipple Disease of the Nervous System

Jeremy D Schmahmann

Whipple disease (WD) is a chronic multisystem infection caused by a novel actinomycete, the Gram-positive bacillus *Tropheryma whippelii*. It was described in 1907 by George Hoyt Whipple, from the department of pathology of Johns Hopkins University. Whipple subsequently went on to become Professor of Pathology and Dean of the School of Medicine and Dentistry at the University of Rochester. He was the 1934 Nobel Prize winner in Physiology or Medicine, along with Minot and Murphy of Harvard Medical School, for the discovery that oral intake of liver reverses anemia, and pernicious anemia in particular. The original case of the disease that came to bear Whipple's name was a 36-year-old physician–missionary who succumbed after a five-year illness characterized by gradual loss of weight and strength, vague abdominal signs, steatorrhea and polyarthritis. Deposits of fat and fatty acids were observed in the intestinal and mesenteric lymph nodes, and large foamy mononuclear cells, subsequently shown to stain with the periodic acid–Schiff (PAS) reaction, were described by Whipple in the jejunal and ileal mucosa.

Whipple disease presents with systemic symptoms, including chronic diarrhea with malabsorption syndrome, weight loss and abdominal pain; migratory polyarthralgias, polarthritis or polyserositis; lymphadenopathy; and fever of unknown origin. Anemia, chronic cough, and valvular and conduction cardiac defects occur, and gray-brown melanin skin pigmentation is sometimes deposited in exposed areas and old scars. The disorder is rare, with approximately 800 cases reported in the literature to date. It occurs more commonly in males in midlife. A prodromal period lasting a few years may be characterized by fleeting attacks of arthritis, weight loss, diarrhea, fever and malaise. Neurological involvement occurs in 6% to 43% of cases. Whereas only a handful of cases have been reported in which the central nervous system (CNS) is clinically affected in isolation, in many instances the neurological manifestations may be prominent components of the illness, or the most debilitating. Treatment of the intestinal manifestations of WD by antibiotics that have poor CNS penetration may account for the neurological deterioration that occurs late in the course of the illness. It is possible that the incidence of this unusual disorder is underestimated, owing in part to the difficulty of establishing the diagnosis. The differential diagnoses include Wernicke–Korsakoff syndrome, paraneoplastic limbic encephalitis, herpes zoster encephalitis, brainstem and diencephalic infiltrative tumors, infections and granulomatous diseases, and metabolic and degenerative dementias. Failure to recognize and optimally treat CNS WD usually leads to the death of the patient.

The *T. whippelii* bacillus has a predilection for the midbrain and hypothalamus, accounting for many of the principal neurological manifestations. These can be grouped into four main presentations, some more easily identifiable than others.

Oculomasticatory myorhythmia (OMM) is a rare instance of what appears to be a truly pathognomonic sign in clinical neurology, occurring in 25% of patients with CNS WD. The clinical constellation consists of vergence movements of the eyes and co-contractions of the jaw and tongue, occurring at a rate of 0.5–1.2 Hz (Figure 141.1). These may be associated also with semirhythmic blinking, and movements of the proximal upper and lower extremities (oculofacial–skeletal myorhythmia, OFSM). The original report described these movements as persisting during sleep, but this is not always the case.

Supranuclear vertical gaze palsy is a hallmark feature of CNS WD, and although it is not pathognomonic, it should alert the clinician to the diagnosis. Horizontal gaze may be lost, but only when vertical gaze is absent as well. Along with the ophthalmoplegia, there may be dissociation of the pupillary response in the

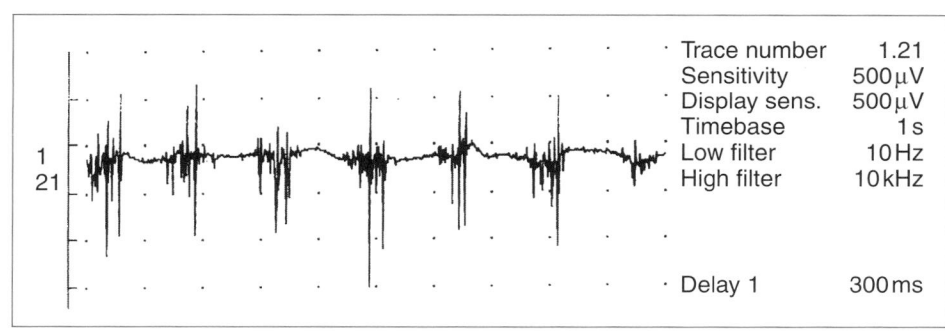

Trace number	1.21
Sensitivity	500 μV
Display sens.	500 μV
Timebase	1 s
Low filter	10 Hz
High filter	10 kHz
Delay 1	300 ms

Figure 141.1 Electromyographic recording from the masseter muscle of a patient with oculomasticatory myorhythmia. This feature is consistent with clinically definite CNS WD, but in this patient the diagnosis could not be established by biopsy or PCR.

direction opposite to that usually seen in Parinaud syndrome, namely, preserved with light and absent with attempted convergence. Paralysis of vertical gaze is almost always present if the patient has OMM.

Cognitive changes may evolve over a period of weeks or months, and present predominantly as an amnestic syndrome including confabulation and delusional thinking. Intellectual function may decline over a period of years, however, and include visual, spatial and executive impairments. Psychiatric manifestations are frequent, and include personality change, irritability, depression, paranoid ideation and hallucinations.

Hypothalamic involvement can present clinically with somnolence, insomnia, polydipsia, hyperphagia, hypothermia, amenorrhea, syndrome of inappropriate antidiuretic hormone secretion, and other disorders of endocrine regulation. A non-specific confusional state that overwhelms isolated neuropsychological deficits may occur in patients with lesions located predominantly in the diencephalon.

Other focal neurological findings, including aphasia, hemiparesis, hemianopia, ataxia, cranial mono- or polyneuropathies and posterior column sensory loss, reflect focal involvement of different brain, brainstem or spinal cord structures, and do not in themselves suggest the nature of the underlying disease.

Magnetic resonance imaging (MRI) reveals lesions in the hypothalamus and rostral brainstem that are hyperintense on T_2-weighted images and fluid-attenuated inversion–recovery (FLAIR) sequences, and they usually enhance with gadolinium (Figure 141.2). Other areas of predilection include the medial temporal region, basal ganglia and pons. The abnormalities may not be demonstrable on computerized tomography.

The diagnosis is confirmed by specific polymerase chain reaction (PCR) primers for the 16S ribosomal RNA gene (16S rDNA) of *T. whippelii*. This has been used successfully in analyses of CSF, peripheral blood, vitreous fluid, pleural fluid and cardiac valve, in addition to its utility on biopsy specimens from duodenum, lymph node and brain. A moderate CSF

pleocytosis may be observed. In some cases CSF cytological analysis reveals the unique morphological feature that characterizes this disorder, namely, foamy mononuclear cells filled with material (mucopeptides of the bacillary cell wall) that stains intensely with the PAS reaction which is diastase resistant. Cerebrospinal fluid PCR is not always definitive despite strong clinical suspicion, and diagnosis may require biopsy in search of the PAS-positive macrophages. These may be present in endoscopically guided biopsies of multiple duodenal sites, even in the absence of overt gastrointestinal symptoms. Other sites that have been biopsied to make the diagnosis include lymph nodes, bone marrow, synovium, lung and vitreous aspirate. Electron microscopy of biopsy specimens reveals remnants of the bacillary cell wall located in membranous inclusions within the macrophages.

If the clinical suspicion remains high and the diagnosis cannot be established by other means, brain biopsy may be necessary. The pathological features include granulomatous inflammation with granular ependymitis, microglial nodules, and neuronal loss. The granulomas are composed of large, foamy PAS-positive macrophages (Figure 141.3). These may be distributed widely throughout the cerebral cortex, white matter and basal ganglia, but they have a predilection for the midbrain and hypothalamus. Rod-shaped bacilli demonstrable with silver stains can be detected within the macrophages and also within glial cells.

The antibiotics used to treat CNS WD must effectively penetrate the blood–brain barrier, and therapy needs to be prolonged. Third-generation cephalosporins are currently the treatment of choice because of their excellent CNS penetration, but given the paucity of clinical cases, recommendations are

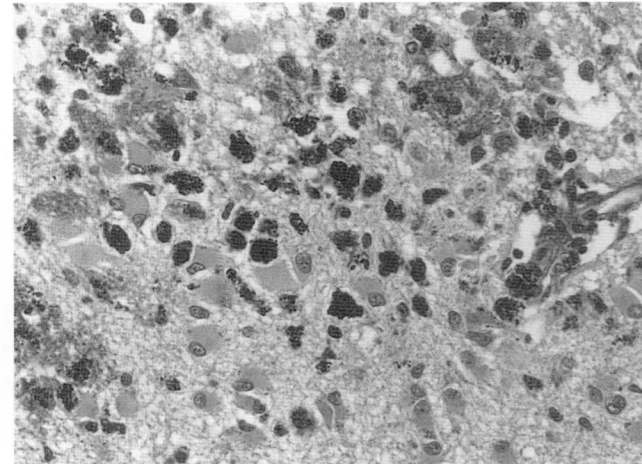

Figure 141.3 Light microscopic features characteristic of infection of the brain with *T. whippelii*, including foamy macrophages filled with PAS-positive and diastase-resistant material. Numerous reactive astrocytes are present. (Stain for periodic acid–Schiff reaction, 40× magnification. Courtesy of Massachusetts General Hospital Department of Neuropathology.) (See color plate section.)

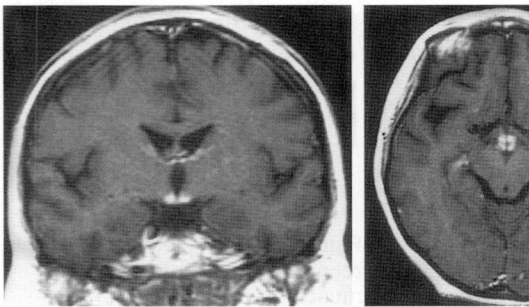

Figure 141.2 Contrast-enhanced T_1-weighted MRI scans of a patient with CNS WD proven by brain biopsy and PCR. Lesions are seen bilaterally in the mammillary bodies and adjacent areas of the hypothalamus in the coronal (left) and axial (right) images.

Table 141.1   Whipple disease. Principal clinical manifestations

Nervous system
Oculomasticatory myorhythmia
Supranuclear vertical gaze palsy
Cognitive decline, with or without psychiatric presentation
Hypothalamic features (SIADH, polydipsia, amenorrhea)

Systemic
Malabsorption syndrome with diarrhea, weight loss and
   abdominal pain
Chronic migratory polyarthralgias and polyserositis
Fever of unknown origin
Lymphadenopathy

Table 141.2   CNS Whipple disease. Stepwise diagnostic evaluation

Brain MRI with gadolinium, FLAIR
Blood, CSF, for *T. whippelii* PCR, and CSF cytology for
   PAS + foamy macrophages
Biopsy—duodenum (endoscopically guided) for light and
   electron microscopy histology; other tissues (lymph
   nodes, marrow) based on presentation
Brain biopsy of clinically and radiographically affected
   region

Table 141.3   CNS Whipple disease. Treatment guidelines

Initial treatment for two weeks
Ceftriaxone 2 g, every 12 hours i.v., and streptomycin 1 g
   daily i.m.

Alternatives:
Penicillin 4 million units, every 4 hours i.v., and
   streptomycin 1 g daily, i.m.
Trimethoprim–sulfamethoxazole 160 mg/800 mg, every
   12 hours i.v.

Long-term oral treatment for a minimum of one year
Cefixime 400 mg twice daily

Alternatives:
Trimethoprim–sulfamethoxazole 160 mg/800 mg twice
   daily
Rifampin 600 mg daily
Doxycycline 100 mg twice daily

Reinstitute long-term therapy (oral or intravenous) if relapse clinically, by MRI or by CSF-PCR.

necessarily based on case reports. Therapy commences with intravenous injection for two weeks of ceftriaxone, 2 g every 12 hours, along with intramuscular streptomycin 1 g daily. Acceptable alternatives are meningeal doses of penicillin, 4 million units i.v. every four hours for two weeks, along with streptomycin 1 g i.m. daily; or trimethoprim–sulfamethoxazole (160 mg/800 mg) every 12 hours intravenously. This is followed by long-term treatment for at least one year with an oral dose of cefixime 400 mg twice daily. In patients unable to tolerate the cephalosporins, alternative choices are rifampin 600 mg daily or doxycycline 100 mg twice daily. Trimethoprim–sulfamethoxazole (160 mg/800 mg twice daily) is a bacteriostatic agent that has been used for the long-term treatment of CNS-WD, but it does not prevent or cure CNS involvement in all patients and it has a mixed record of success. Monitoring response to treatment by repeat PAS staining of duodenal biopsy specimens is not recommended for CNS WD, as disappearance of the intestinal form does not guarantee a CNS cure. Repeat CSF analysis for PCR and for cytology for PAS-laden macrophages is more appropriate, if these were positive at the time of diagnosis. Antibiotics should be reinstituted if clinical relapse occurs following withdrawal after the first year of antibiotic therapy, and may need to be continued indefinitely. Some cases have required long-term intravenous administration of cephalosporins to maintain clinical remission.

References

1. Smith WT, French JM, Gottsman M, et al. Cerebral complications of Whipple's disease. Brain 1965;88:137–150
2. Louis ED, Lynch T, Kaufmann P, et al. Diagnostic guidelines in central nervous system Whipple's disease. Ann Neurol 1996;40:561–568
3. Durand DV, Lecomte C, Cathébras P, et al. Whipple disease. Clinical review of 52 cases. The SNFMI Research Group on Whipple Disease. Société Nationale Française de Médécine Interne. Medicine (Baltimore) 1997;76:170–184
4. Maiwald M, Relman DA. Whipple's disease and *Tropheryma whippelii*: secrets slowly revealed. Clin Infect Dis 2001;32:457–463

142 Alcohol

Michael E Charness

Introduction

Alcoholism is a widespread and serious public health problem in most countries of the world. Alcoholism and alcohol abuse cost the United States approximately $185 billion annually through medical expenses, accidents, injuries, and lost productivity. The nervous system is a major target of alcohol. This chapter focuses on the management of alcohol intoxication, the alcohol withdrawal syndrome, and the chronic neurological complications of alcoholism. More detailed accounts of the pathophysiology and diagnosis of these disorders can be found elsewhere.[1,2]

Ethanol intoxication

Ethanol causes intoxication by interacting specifically with selective neuronal proteins, including the family of ligand-gated ion channels.[1,3] The sedative-hypnotic effects of ethanol arise in part through the potentiation of inhibitory neurotransmission at the $GABA_A$ receptor chloride ion channel complex and the inhibition of excitatory neurotransmission at the NMDA subtype glutamate receptor. These combined actions contribute to ethanol-induced ataxia, incoordination, dysarthria, nystagmus, and sedation. In naïve individuals, blood alcohol concentrations in excess of 100 mM or 461 mg/dL impair medullary control of respiration, leading to respiratory arrest and death. However, higher blood levels are sometimes encountered in sober alcoholics, reflecting their development of tolerance.[4]

Ethanol intoxication is treated with supportive therapy.[5] Ethanol is eliminated at a rate of approximately 15 mg/dL per hour, primarily by metabolism to acetaldehyde and acetate,[6] so blood ethanol concentrations of 150 mg/dL can be eliminated in under 12 hours. The rate of ethanol elimination in children is about twice that of adults.[7,8] Gastric emptying can remove significant amounts of alcohol from the stomach, particularly close to the time of ethanol ingestion; however, this approach is not generally recommended.[9] Hemodialysis is used rarely to treat severe alcohol intoxication with coma, more so in children than in adults. Hypoglycemia is uncommon in intoxicated adults, but occurs with greater frequency in young children and should be managed accordingly.[7] Conservative management in adults should include the administration of glucose-containing fluids with vitamin supplementation.[8] There are no approved medications for reversing ethanol intoxication. Ethanol blocks the reuptake of adenosine,[3] an inhibitory neuromodulator that produces sedation. Caffeine is an adenosine receptor antagonist and is used commonly in social settings to increase arousal after drinking, but its effects are mild.

Alcohol withdrawal syndromes

The central nervous system (CNS) adapts to the molecular and physiological perturbations caused by ethanol to restore normal function in its presence. Tolerance develops even in naïve individuals during the course of a single session of drinking.[10] In alcoholics, adaptation to ethanol may be so successful that almost normal ambulation and arousal are observed in the presence of blood ethanol concentrations several times those that would cause death in non-drinkers.[4] Abrupt ethanol withdrawal unmasks these adaptive changes, leading to CNS excitation, convulsions, hallucinations, and autonomic hyperactivity.

The alcohol withdrawal syndrome unfolds variably.[11] Some individuals manifest only tremulousness, anxiety, and mild agitation. Others experience hallucinations with a clear sensorium, particularly during the first 24 hours after withdrawal. Alcohol withdrawal seizures occur most commonly between 12 and 48 hours after the last drink, sometimes in the absence of antecedent agitation.[12] Delirium tremens begins gradually after a few days of withdrawal, or may be heralded by tremulousness, agitation, hallucinations, or seizures. Treatment of alcohol withdrawal symptoms is summarized in Table 142.1.

Delirium tremens

The full expression of delirium tremens includes marked agitation, an altered sensorium, hallucinations, and delusions. Sympathetic hyperactivity is marked by diaphoresis, tachycardia, hypertension, and hyperreflexia. Diaphoresis, agitation, and hyperventilation may lead to rapid loss of fluids. The clinical course is frequently complicated by concurrent alcohol-related illnesses, included hepatic failure and sepsis. Death occurs in about 5% of individuals, but the death rate rises steeply in the elderly.[13]

Alcohol detoxification is typically undertaken in an outpatient setting, unless patients have a history of withdrawal seizures, delirium tremens, or co-morbid medical and psychiatric illnesses. Mild alcohol withdrawal syndromes can be managed effectively with oral benzodiazepines, which may be titrated against agitation and tremulousness. Symptoms can be scored according to the revised Clinical Institute Withdrawal Assessment for Alcohol scale (CIWA-Ar)[14] http://addiction-medicine.org/ files/15doc.html), which evaluates 10 symptoms and signs of withdrawal. Benzodiazepines are administered for CIWA-Ar score of ≥10. Symptom-triggered administration

Table 142.1   Treatment of alcohol withdrawal syndromes

Outpatient detoxification
- Hourly clinical assessment using the revised Clinical Institute Withdrawal Assessment for Alcohol scale (CIWA-Ar)[14] (http://addiction-medicine.org/files/15doc.html)
- Symptom-triggered administration of benzodiazepines, based on a CIWA-Ar score of ⩾10
- Supportive care: reassurance, reality orientation, and nursing care[15]
- Vitamin supplementation

Single alcohol withdrawal seizure
- If first seizure observed within 6 hours and no other contraindications, consider lorazepam 2 mg iv[16]

Delirium tremens

Agitation:
Benzodiazepines:
- Administer as needed to induce and maintain a calm state
- Efficacy is equivalent for all agents studied
- Choice is based on pharmacokinetic considerations
- Dosing and route of administration is individualized per patient
- Massive doses may be required[17,18]
  Longer half-life: elimination is dependent on hepatic metabolism, more sedation, fewer rebound symptoms, poor im absorption
  Diazepam: e.g. 10 mg iv, then 5 mg iv q 5 minutes until calm[17]
  Chlordiazepoxide: e.g. 50–100 mg iv, repeat as needed
  Shorter half-life: decreased dependence on hepatic metabolism, less sedation
  Lorazepam: e.g. 2–4 mg iv load, then 2 mg iv as needed
  Oxazepam: e.g. 15–30 mg po, repeat as needed

Dehydration
- Aggressive iv fluid and electrolyte replacement
- Monitor electrolytes, renal function, blood pressure, urine output, and urine specific gravity

Hypomagnesemia (begin treatment for low normal or low serum magnesium)
- Assume an average deficit of 2 mEq/kg magnesium and replace as outlined:[19]
- 6 g iv, first 3 hours
- 5 g iv, each of next 12 hours
- 5 g daily, each of next 4 days
- reduce doses and increase monitoring for renal impairment

Malnutrition
- Multivitamins iv
- Thiamine 100 mg iv for 5 days; first dose should be administered before iv glucose

Autonomic hyperactivity (if not controlled by above measures, may add one of the following adjunctive drugs; none is recommended as monotherapy)
- Clonidine
- Beta blockers, e.g. atenolol 50–100 mg per day[20]

Alcoholism
- Treatment for alcoholism should begin after resolution of alcohol withdrawal syndrome.

of benzodiazepines results in shorter durations of treatment and lower total doses than fixed-schedule regimens.[21] Carbamazepine shows efficacy in reducing mild to moderate withdrawal symptoms, and doesn't cause sedation or rebound withdrawal symptoms.[22] Adequate nutrition and correction of vitamin deficiency (see below) are essential. Replacement of most vitamins and minerals can also be accomplished orally, although it is preferable to administer thiamine parenterally, since oral absorption of thiamine is unreliable in alcoholic and malnourished patients.[1] The morbidity of delirium tremens mandates aggressive treatment in an inpatient setting and, when necessary, in an intensive care unit. Intravenous benzodiazepines, hydration, and replacement of magnesium and vitamins are the mainstays of therapy.

Benzodiazepines produce sedation by potentiating the actions of GABA. Animal and human studies suggest that ethanol dependence is associated with compensatory reductions in the expression of GABA receptors and an uncoupling of benzodiazepine enhancement of GABA-mediated chloride flux.[3] This may account for the requirement for high doses of benzodiazepines to sedate alcoholics in withdrawal. Some clinicians administer benzodiazepines every 5 to 10 minutes until sedation is achieved, and then less frequently to maintain sedation.[23] Efficacy does not differ among the benzodiazepines, and the selection of a particular drug is often based on pharmacokinetic considerations. Chlordiazepoxide, diazepam, and lorazepam may be administered orally or parenterally. Oxazepam and lorazepam may be preferable in patients with liver disease because clearance is less dependent on hepatic metabolism. Lorazepam is effectively absorbed after intramuscular injection. Although paraldehyde is also effective in treating alcohol withdrawal, its use is limited by poor availability, instability, adverse effects, and the requirement for oral or rectal administration. Clonidine has been reported to decrease the autonomic hyperactivity of alcohol withdrawal and beta adrenergic receptor antagonists may be useful in suppressing tremulousness as well as autonomic hyperactivity.[24]

Dehydration may develop rapidly during alcohol withdrawal because of agitation and diaphoresis. Vigorous intravenous hydration as well as sedation may be required to prevent hypotension. Venous access provides an opportunity to correct rapidly potential deficiencies of multiple vitamins and electrolytes. Symptomatic hyponatremia should be corrected slowly to prevent central pontine myelinolyis, which occurs more frequently in alcoholics than in nondrinkers.[1] It is important to administer multivitamins as well as additional supplements of thiamine (100 mg per day) because of the high incidence of unrecognized Wernicke's encephalopathy in alcoholics (see below).

Magnesium deficiency is common in alcoholics, and serum magnesium can be normal or low-normal despite tissue depletion.[25] Magnesium replacement has not been shown to reduce alcohol withdrawal severity, seizures, or delirium.[24] However, hypomagnesemia is associated with cardiac arrhythmias and complicates the correction of coexisting hypokalemia and hypocalcemia. Magnesium is also a cofactor for transketolase, one of the thiamine-dependent enzymes implicated in the pathogenesis of Wernicke's encephalopathy. Metabolic balance studies in alcoholics have suggested the need to replace deficits of 2 mEq/kg of magnesium. One suggested regimen is to administer 6 g of magnesium (1 ampoule of magnesium sulfate contains 1 g or 8.13 mEq of magnesium) over 3 hours in intravenous fluids followed by another 10 g of magnesium by continuous intravenous infusion over the next 24 hours and 6 g daily for an additional 3 days.[19] Serum magnesium should be monitored at least twice daily for the development of hypermagnesemia during the first days of treatment. Typically, magnesium levels will rise during the initial period of repletion, only to return to low-normal levels following the first infusion. Magnesium should be replaced cautiously in patients with impaired renal function.

Alcohol withdrawal seizures

Seizures may follow rapid reductions in blood ethanol concentration.[12] Although most ethanol withdrawal seizures occur within 12 to 48 hours after the last drink, patients who abuse ethanol and other sedative hypnotics may have withdrawal seizures after a much longer interval. Ethanol withdrawal typically causes generalized tonic–clonic seizures.[12] Focal seizures in the setting of alcohol withdrawal should suggest a pre-existing seizure disorder or focal brain lesions. In slightly more than half of cases, seizures are multiple, occur within a 6-hour time period, and

are each followed by a rapid return of consciousness. Although ethanol withdrawal seizures do not often progress to status epilepticus, as many as one-third of patients with status epilepticus have a history of ethanol withdrawal.[26] The interictal EEG is normal in uncomplicated ethanol withdrawal seizures, although there may be increased photic driving.[12] The presence of epileptiform activity on an interictal EEG increases the likelihood of recurrent seizures in the absence of ethanol withdrawal.

Benzodiazepines are effective in the primary prevention of ethanol withdrawal seizures during alcohol detoxification.[24] The intravenous administration of 2 mg of lorazepam in patients with a single ethanol withdrawal seizure significantly reduces the incidence of multiple ethanol withdrawal seizures within a 6-hour time period and decreases the likelihood that patients with withdrawal seizures will require hospital admission.[16] In contrast, intravenous phenytoin is not effective in preventing a second ethanol withdrawal seizure.[27] Status epilepticus in the setting of ethanol withdrawal should be treated according to standard protocols, including the use of phenytoin.

Uncomplicated ethanol withdrawal seizures are self-limited and are not likely to recur in the absence of further episodes of ethanol withdrawal. For this reason, patients suspected of having ethanol withdrawal seizures should not be subjected to long-term treatment with anticonvulsants. There is little expectation that anticonvulsants will prevent future episodes of withdrawal seizures, and there is concern that simultaneous withdrawal from ethanol and anticonvulsants will lead to status epilepticus.

Wernicke's encephalopathy

Wernicke's encephalopathy is the neurological manifestation of thiamine deficiency.[28,29] Characteristic lesions occur symmetrically in structures surrounding the third ventricle, aqueduct and fourth ventricle. The mamillary bodies are involved in virtually all cases, and the dorsomedial thalamus, locus ceruleus, periaqueductal gray, ocular motor nuclei, and vestibular nuclei are commonly affected. Atrophy of the mamillary bodies develops in up to 80% of cases after acute Wernicke's encephalopathy, and occurs rarely in other disorders. In the Western world, Wernicke lesions are found most commonly in alcoholics.

In clinically-based series, most patients with Wernicke's encephalopathy present with a classical triad of encephalopathy, oculomotor dysfunction, and gait ataxia.[28] The encephalopathy is characterized by profound disorientation, indifference, and inattentiveness. Some patients exhibit an agitated delirium related to ethanol withdrawal. Ocular motor abnormalities include nystagmus, lateral rectus palsy, and conjugate gaze palsy. Gait ataxia is common, and is likely due to a combination of polyneuropathy, midline cerebellar involvement, and vestibular paresis. In contrast, ataxia of the arms and dysarthria or scanning speech are infrequent.

Neuropathological studies of the past four decades have questioned the reliability of the clinical diagnosis of Wernicke's encephalopathy. Only 1 of 22 patients with lesions of acute Wernicke's encephalopathy was diagnosed clinically, and most of these patients presented with lethargy and coma.[30] From these data, it can be concluded that in many patients with Wernicke's encephalopathy, elements of the clinical triad are absent during hospitalization, not recognized, or not recorded. In an alcoholic population, there is a high probability of finding lesions of Wernicke's encephalopathy in patients who have two of the following four criteria: dietary deficiency, oculomotor abnormalities, cerebellar dysfunction, and either altered mental status or mild memory impairment.[31] MRI may assist in making the diagnosis. Acute lesions appear as areas of increased signal within the diencephalon and periaqueductal gray on T2-weighted images and diffusion-weighted images.[32,33] These signal abnormalities recede following thiamine treatment. In a majority of chronic cases, MRI shows evidence of mamillary body atrophy and enlargement of the third ventricle.[32,34,35]

Although Wernicke's encephalopathy may be difficult to diagnose clinically, it is readily treatable (see Table 142.2). Intravenous administration of thiamine is safe,[36] simple, inexpensive, and effective. Untreated, most patients progress to coma and death. The current author recommends administering 100 mg of thiamine intravenously (at least for the first day) or intramuscularly for 5 consecutive days in all patients with undiagnosed altered mental status, oculomotor disorders, or ataxia. Imaging can confirm the diagnosis in difficult cases, but it is not necessary to initiate treatment. Although dietary requirements for thiamine are 1–2 mg daily, absorption and utilization of thiamine are incomplete, and some patients have genetically determined requirements for much larger doses.[37,38] Gastrointestinal absorption of thiamine is erratic in alcoholic and malnourished patients, making oral administration of thiamine an unreliable treatment for acute Wernicke's encephalopathy.[39] Daily oral administration of 100 mg of thiamine should be continued after the completion of parenteral treatment and after discharge from the hospital.

With prompt administration of thiamine, ocular signs improve within hours to days, and ataxia and confusion within days to weeks.[28] However, a majority of patients are left with horizontal nystagmus, ataxia, and Korsakoff's amnestic syndrome. The prevention of irreversible lesions might be possible through the widespread oral administration of thiamine to outpatients at risk of developing Wernicke's encephalopathy. The autopsy incidence of Wernicke's encephalopathy has declined significantly following the enrichment of flour with thiamine.[40]

Alcoholic cerebellar degeneration

Some alcoholic patients develop a chronic cerebellar syndrome related to the degeneration of Purkinje cells in the cerebellar cortex.[41] Midline cerebellar structures—especially the anterior and superior vermis—are predominantly affected, a pattern identical to that in Wernicke's encephalopathy. Alcoholic cerebellar degeneration typically occurs only after 10 or more years of excessive ethanol use. It usually develops gradually over weeks to months, but may also evolve over years or commence abruptly. Mild and apparently stable cases may become suddenly worse. As in Wernicke's encephalopathy, ataxia affects the gait most severely. Limb ataxia and dysarthria occur more often than in Wernicke's encephalopathy, whereas nystagmus is rare. The diagnosis of alcoholic cerebellar ataxia is based on the clinical history and neurological examination. CT or MRI scans may show cerebellar vermian atrophy.[32] Alcoholic cerebellar degeneration may be caused by a combination of nutritional deficiency and alcohol neurotoxicity.[28,42] Cessation of drinking and nutritional supplementation are the only treatments available, and gait improvement does not occur in most patients.[41] Physical therapy, canes, walkers, and wheelchairs are helpful in maintaining mobility.

Marchiafava–Bignami disease

Marchiafava–Bignami disease is a rare disorder of demyelination or necrosis of the corpus callosum and adjacent subcortical white matter that occurs predominantly in malnourished alcoholics.[43] In some cases there are associated lesions of Wernicke's encephalopathy as well as selective neuronal loss and gliosis in the third cortical layer. A few cases have been described in non-alcoholics, demonstrating that ethanol alone is not responsible for the lesion. The course may be acute, subacute, or chronic, and is marked by dementia, spasticity, dysarthria, and inability to walk. Patients may lapse into coma and die, survive for many years in a demented condition, or occasionally recover. An interhemispheric disconnection syndrome has been reported in survivors.[44] Lesions appear as hypodense areas in portions of the corpus callosum on CT and as discrete or confluent areas of decreased T1 signal and increased T2 signal on MRI.[32] Alcoholics without liver disease, amnesia,

Table 142.2 Treatment of acute Wernicke's encephalopathy

Administer parenteral thiamine to any patient, whether alcoholic or not, suffering one of the following:
- Altered mental status
- Memory loss
- Coma
- Unexplained ataxia
- Unexplained oculomotor dysfunction
- Severe malnutrition

Treatment
- Thiamine 100 mg iv for 5 days; im treatment can replace iv if venous access is problematic
- Thiamine 100 mg po for the rest of the hospitalization and as an outpatient
- Replace magnesium (see Table 142.1)
- Replace fluid and electrolyte losses

or cognitive dysfunction show thinning of the corpus callosum on MRI, particularly in the genu and body, suggesting that alcohol or malnutrition damages the corpus callosum commonly in the absence of the necrotic lesions of Marchiafava–Bignami disease.[45,46] These findings raise the possibility that aggressive nutritional supplementation along with a reduction in drinking can prevent the development of Marchiafava–Bignami disease in alcoholics.

Cognitive dysfunction and dementia in alcoholics

Imaging studies, neuropathological observations, and animal experimentation suggest that ethanol neurotoxicity may contribute to chronic cognitive dysfunction in alcoholics, although a characteristic lesion of ethanol neurotoxicity has not been described.[29] Alcoholics lose a disproportionate amount of subcortical white matter compared with cortical gray matter, and show associated ventricular enlargement.[47] CT and MRI reveal enlargement of the cerebral ventricles and sulci in a majority of alcoholics. The ventricles and sulci become significantly smaller within about 1 month of abstinence,[48] whereas brain water, estimated by MRI or chemical analysis does not change consistently. Therefore, changes in brain parenchyma (but not brain water), may account for the reversible radiographic and cognitive abnormalities of alcoholics.

The partial reversibility of cognitive dysfunction and ventricular enlargement following abstinence suggests that alcohol neurotoxicity plays a role in the neurological complications of alcoholism. It is important to determine whether patients with undiagnosed cognitive decline are alcoholic, because abstinence and nutritional repletion may prevent further worsening. Acetylcholine esterase inhibitors have not been evaluated as treatments for dementia in alcoholics, although such a trial might prove interesting. Like patients with Alzheimer's disease, patients with Korsakoff's amnestic syndrome show reductions in presynaptic cholinergic markers[49] and loss of cholinergic cells in the basal forebrain.[50,51]

Fetal alcohol syndrome

Heavy drinking during pregnancy may cause fetal alcohol syndrome, a disorder of pre- and post-natal growth retardation, microcephaly, neurological abnormalities, facial dysmorphology, and other congenital anomalies.[52] A constellation of less severe "fetal alcohol effects" is more common, but is difficult to diagnose in the absence of a clear history of gestational alcohol exposure. Neuropathological examination in fetal alcohol syndrome reveals microcephaly, cerebellar dysplasia, agenesis of the corpus callosum, and neuronal–glial heterotopias. MRI in children with fetal alcohol syndrome has identified microcephaly, agenesis or hypoplasia of the corpus callosum, and selective reductions in the volume of the cerebrum, cerebellum, and basal ganglia.[53] Overlapping neuropathological abnormalities are observed in children with mutations in the gene for the L1 cell adhesion

molecule, and cellular studies suggest that ethanol decreases L1-mediated cell adhesion.[54] The identification of drugs that block the effects of ethanol on L1 and prevent ethanol teratogenesis in mice raises the possibility of pharmacological interventions to prevent fetal alcohol syndrome and other neurological complications of alcoholism.[55,56] The Surgeon General has recommended that women who are pregnant or trying to conceive should abstain from ethanol, and this remains the most obvious means of prevention.

Neuromuscular complications of alcoholism

Neuropathy

Alcoholic patients have a high incidence of peripheral nerve disorders, including symmetrical polyneuropathy, autonomic neuropathy, and compression mononeuropathies. Alcoholic polyneuropathy is believed to result from inadequate nutrition, and particularly from deficiencies of thiamine and other B vitamins.[28] A direct neurotoxic effect of ethanol may also contribute to this disorder,[57] because ethanol induces a disturbance of fast axonal transport that could promote alcoholic polyneuropathy. Alcoholic polyneuropathy is a gradually progressive disorder of sensory, motor, and autonomic nerves. The clinical abnormalities are usually symmetrical and predominantly distal. Symptoms include numbness, paresthesia, burning dysesthesia, pain, weakness, muscle cramps and gait ataxia. The most common neurological signs are loss of tendon reflexes (beginning with the ankle jerks), defective perception of touch and vibration sensation, and weakness. Cardiac autonomic abnormalities are present in about one quarter of alcoholics with peripheral neuropathy,[57] and are associated with increased mortality. Because malnutrition may contribute to the development of alcoholic polyneuropathy, patients with this disorder should receive parenteral thiamine supplementation. Improved nutrition with cessation of drinking appears to be associated with a good prognosis for improvement. Low doses of tricyclic antidepressants or gabapentin are sometimes effective in controlling the burning dysesthesiae of alcoholic peripheral neuropathy.

Myopathy

Skeletal myopathy is an under-recognized complication of alcohol abuse. Almost half of alcoholic patients visiting an ambulatory clinic and 60% of hospitalized alcoholics had biopsy evidence of myopathy.[58,59] Skeletal muscle can be damaged by the administration of ethanol to well-nourished volunteers, and most patients with alcoholic myopathy are not demonstrably malnourished.[60,61] Alcoholic myopathy may present as either an acute necrotizing disorder or as a more indolent process. The acute form develops predominantly in men, over hours to days, often in relation to an alcoholic binge, and is characterized by weakness, pain, tenderness and swelling of affected muscles. Proximal muscles are often most severely involved, but the distribution of involvement may be asymmetrical or focal. Dysphagia and congestive heart failure may occur. Laboratory findings include moderate to severe elevation of serum creatine kinase (CK), myoglobinuria, fibrillations and myopathic changes in the electromyogram, and selective fiber necrosis of type I muscle fibers. Initial treatment is directed at correcting cardiac arrhythmias, renal failure due to rhabdomyolysis, and electrolyte disturbances such as hypophosphatemia or hypokalemia. Abstinence from ethanol is usually associated with gradual recovery.

Chronic alcoholic myopathy, which evolves over weeks to months, is a more common disorder.[60,61] Pain is less prominent than in acute alcoholic myopathy, but muscle cramps may occur. On examination the major findings are muscle weakness and atrophy, which affect predominantly the hip and shoulder girdles. Although a polyneuropathy coexists in many cases, the clinical and laboratory features of this disorder indicate a primary disturbance of muscle. Muscle biopsies show preferential atrophy of type II fibers. Serum CK is less elevated than in acute alcoholic myopathy, and myoglobinuria does not occur. Cessation of drinking leads to improvement in most cases, while continued heavy ethanol abuse results in clinical deterioration.[62]

Treatment of alcoholism

Abstinence and nutritional repletion are the preferred treatment for most of the neurological complications of alcoholism, and abstinence is the only means for preventing fetal alcohol syndrome. Unfortunately, achieving abstinence remains a formidable challenge. Strong biological, psychological, social, and environmental forces contribute to high rates of relapse to heavy drinking. Psychotherapy and self-help groups, such as Alcoholics Anonymous, are successful in reducing drinking and achieving abstinence in some patients, but relapse rates after 1 year are 40% to 70%.[63] Alcoholism is common among patients with schizophrenia, panic disorder, and depression, and treatment of these primary disorders might reduce drinking; however, treatment with serotonin reuptake inhibitors in unselected populations of alcoholics has not decreased drinking.[63] Ethanol is metabolized to acetaldehyde, whose further metabolism is inhibited by disulfiram, leading to flushing, headache, tachycardia, nausea, and vomiting. Aversive therapy with disulfiram has not been shown to be effective in large double-blind trials, and is not widely utilized.[63] The opiate antagonist naltrexone reduces the craving for alcohol, perhaps by blocking endorphin-mediated release of dopamine in the nucleus accumbens.[64] Naltrexone 50 mg orally per day, in combination with psychotherapy, reduces drinking, relapse to drinking and craving for alcohol better than psychotherapy alone,[65,66] although not all studies show benefit.[67] Naltrexone is tolerated well by most patients; a minority experience nausea, headache, anxiety, and sedation.[63] Acamprosate (calcium acetyl-homotaurine) has shown benefit in European trials, and is under investigation in the United States for use alone and in combination with naltrexone.[68] Early studies with the serotonin-3 receptor antagonist ondansetron also appear promising.[69]

Acknowledgements

The author's work is supported by grants from NIAAA, the Alcoholic Beverage Medical Research Foundation, and the Medical Research Service, Department of Veterans Affairs.

References

1. Charness ME, Simon RP, Greenberg DA. Ethanol and the nervous system. N Engl J Med 1989;321:442–454
2. Charness ME. Neurological complications of alcoholism. In: Samuels MA, Feske S, eds. Office Practice of Neurology. 2nd ed. Philadelphia: Harcourt Health Sciences, 2003: in press
3. Diamond I, Gordon AS. Cellular and molecular neuroscience of alcoholism. Physiol Rev 1997;77:1–20
4. Johnson RA, Noll EC, Rodney WM. Survival after a serum ethanol concentration of 1 1/2% [letter]. Lancet 1982;2:1394
5. Marco CA, Kelen GD. Acute intoxication. Emerg Med Clin North Am 1990;8:731–748
6. Adinoff B, Bone GH, Linnoila M. Acute ethanol poisoning and the ethanol withdrawal syndrome. Med Toxicol 1988;3:172–196
7. Leung AK. Ethyl alcohol ingestion in children. A 15-year review. Clin Ped 1986;25:617–619
8. Lamminpaa A. Acute alcohol intoxication among children and adolescents. Eur J Ped 1994;153:868–872
9. Pollack CV Jr, Jorden RC, Carlton FB, Baker ML. Gastric emptying in the acutely inebriated patient. J Emerg Med 1992;10:1–5
10. Mirsky IR, Piker P, Rosenbaum M, Lederer H. "Adaptation" of the central nervous system to varying concentrations of alcohol in the blood. Q J Stud Alc 1941; 2:35–45
11. Victor M, Adams RD. The effect of alcohol on the nervous system. Res Publ Assn Nerv Ment Dis 1953; 32:526–573
12. Victor M, Brausch C. The role of abstinence in the genesis of alcoholic epilepsy. Epilepsia 1967;8:1–20
13. Feuerlein W, Reiser E. Parameters affecting the course and results of delirium tremens treatment. Acta Psychiatr Scand 1986;73(Suppl 329):120–123
14. Sullivan JT, Sykora K, Schneiderman J, et al. Assessment of alcohol withdrawal: the revised clinical institute withdrawal assessment for alcohol scale (CIWA-Ar). Br J Addiction 1989;84:1353–1357
15. Naranjo CA, Sellers EM, Chater K, et al. Non-pharmacologic intervention in acute alcohol withdrawal. Clin Pharmacol Ther 1983;34:214–219
16. D'Onofrio G, Rathlev NK, Ulrich AS, et al. Lorazepam for the prevention of recurrent seizures related to alcohol. N Engl J Med 1999;340:915–919
17. Thompson WL, Johnson AD, Maddrey WL, Housestaff OM. Diazepam and paraldehyde for treatment of severe delirium tremens: a controlled trial. Ann Intern Med 1975;82:175–180
18. Woo E, Greenblatt DJ. Massive benzodiazepine requirements during acute alcohol withdrawal. Am J Psychiatry 1979;136:821–823
19. Flink EB. Therapy of magnesium deficiency. Ann NY Acad Sci 1969;162:901–905
20. Kraus ML, Gottlieb LD, Horwitz RI, Anscher M. Randomized clinical trial of atenolol in patients with

alcohol withdrawal. N Engl J Med 1985;313:905–909

21. Daeppen JB, Gache P, Landry U, et al. Symptom-triggered vs fixed-schedule doses of benzodiazepine for alcohol withdrawal: a randomized treatment trial. Arch Int Med 2002;162:1117–1121

22. Malcolm R, Myrick H, Roberts J, et al. The effects of carbamazepine and lorazepam on single versus multiple previous alcohol withdrawals in an outpatient randomized trial. J Gen Int Med 2002;17:349–355

23. Thompson WL. Management of alcohol withdrawal syndromes. Arch Int Med 1978;138:278–283

24. Mayo-Smith MF. Pharmacological management of alcohol withdrawal. A meta-analysis and evidence-based practice guideline. American Society of Addiction Medicine Working Group on Pharmacological Management of Alcohol Withdrawal. Jama 1997;278:144–151

25. McLean RM. Magnesium and its therapeutic uses: a review. [Review]. Am J Med 1994;96:63–76

26. Aminoff MJ, Simon RP. Status epilepticus. Causes, clinical features and consequences in 98 patients. Am J Med 1980;69:657–666

27. Alldredge BK, Lowenstein DH, Simon RP. The effectiveness of intravenous phenytoin in the acute treatment of alcohol-withdrawal seizures. Epilepsia 1988;29:496

28. Victor M, Adams RA, Collins GH. The Wernicke–Korsakoff syndrome and related disorders due to alcoholism and malnutrition. Philadelphia: F.A. Davis, 1989

29. Charness ME. Brain lesions in alcoholics. Alcohol Clin Exp Res 1993;17:2–11

30. Torvik A, Lindboe CF, Rodge S. Brain lesions in alcoholics. A neuropathological study with clinical correlation. J Neurol Sci 1982;56:233–248

31. Caine D, Halliday GM, Kril JJ, Harper CG. Operational criteria for the classification of chronic alcoholics: identification of Wernicke's encephalopathy. J Neurol Neurosurg Psychiatry 1997;62:51–60

32. Warach SJ, Charness ME. Imaging the brain lesions of alcoholics. In: Greenberg JO, ed. Neuroimaging: A Companion to Adams and Victor's Principles of Neurology. New York: McGraw-Hill, 1994:503–515

33. Bergui M, Bradac GB, Zhong JJ, et al. Diffusion-weighted MR in reversible Wernicke encephalopathy. Neuroradiology 2001;43:969–972

34. Charness ME, DeLaPaz RL. Mamillary body atrophy in Wernicke's encephalopathy: antemortem identification using magnetic resonance imaging. Ann Neurol 1987;22:595–600

35. Charness ME. Intracranial voyeurism: revealing the mamillary bodies in alcoholism. Alcohol Clin Exp Res 1999;23:1941–1944

36. Wrenn KD, Murphy F, Slovis CM. A toxicity study of parenteral thiamine hydrochloride. Ann Emerg Med 1989;18:867–870

37. Hoyumpa AM. Alcohol and thiamine metabolism. Alcohol Clin Exp Res 1983;7:11–14

38. Mukherjee AB, Svoronos S, Ghazanfari A, et al. Transketolase abnormality in cultured fibroblasts from familial chronic alcoholic men and their male offspring. J Clin Invest 1987;79:1039–1043

39. Thomson AD, Ryle PR, Shaw GK. Ethanol, thiamine, and brain damage. Alcohol Alcoholism 1983;18:27–43

40. Harper CG, Sheedy DL, Lara AI, et al. Prevalence of Wernicke–Korsakoff syndrome in Australia: has thiamine fortification made a difference? [see comments]. Med J Austr 1998;168:542–545

41. Victor M, Adams RD, Mancall EL. A restricted form of cerebellar cortical degeneration occurring in alcoholic patients. Arch Neurol 1959;1:579–688

42. Nicolas JM, Fernandez-Sola J, Robert J, et al. High ethanol intake and malnutrition in alcoholic cerebellar shrinkage. Q J Med 2000;93:449–456

43. Brion S. Marchiafava–Bignami syndrome. In: Vinken PJ, Bruyn GW, eds. Metabolic and Deficiency Diseases of the Nervous System, Part 2. Vol 28. Amsterdam: North-Holland Publishing Company, 1976:317–329

44. Rosa A, Demiati M, Cartz L, Mizon JP. Marchiafava–Bignami disease, syndrome of interhemispheric disconnection, and right-handed agraphia in a left-hander. Arch Neurol 1991;48:986–988

45. Pfefferbaum A, Lim KO, Desmond JE, Sullivan EV. Thinning of the corpus callosum in older alcoholic men: a magnetic resonance imaging study. Alcohol Clin Exp Res 1996;20:752–757

46. Estruch R, Nicolas JM, Salamero M, et al. Atrophy of the corpus callosum in chronic alcoholism. J Neurol Sci 1987;146:145–151

47. Harper CG, Kril JJ, Holloway RL. Brain shrinkage in chronic alcoholics: a pathological study. Br Med J 1985;290:501–504

48. Carlen PL, Wortzman G, Holgate RC, et al. Reversible cerebral atrophy in recently abstinent chronic alcoholics measured by computed tomography scans. Science 1978;200:1076–1078

49. Nordberg A, Adolfsson R, Aquilonius SM, et al. Brain enzymes and Ach receptors in senile dementia of Alzheimer type and chronic alcohol abuse. In: Amaducci L, Davison AN, Antuono P, eds. Aging of the Brain and Dementia. Vol 13. New York: Raven Press, 1980:169–171

50. Arendt T, Bigl V, Arendt A, Tennstedt A. Loss of neurons in the nucleus basalis of Meynert in Alzheimer's disease, paralysis agitans and Korsakoff's disease. Acta Neuropathol (Berl) 1983;61:101–108

51. Cullen KM, Halliday GM, Caine D, Kril JJ. The nucleus basalis (Ch4) in the alcoholic Wernicke–Korsakoff syndrome: reduced cell number in both amnesic and nonamnesic patients. J Neurol Neurosurg Psychiatry 1997;63:315–320

52. Streissguth AP, Landesman-Dwyer S, Martin JC, Smith DW. Teratogenic effects of alcohol in humans and laboratory animals. Science 1980;209:353–361

53. Roebuck TM, Mattson SN, Riley EP. A review of the neuroanatomical findings in children with fetal alcohol syndrome or prenatal exposure to alcohol. Alcohol Clin Exp Res 1998;22:339–344

54. Ramanathan R, Wilkemeyer MF, Mittal B, et al. Ethanol inhibits cell-cell adhesion mediated by human L1. J Cell Biol 1996;133:381–390

55. Chen S-Y, Wilkemeyer MF, Sulik KK, Charness ME. Octanol antagonism of ethanol teratogenesis. FASEB J 2001;15(9):1649–1651

56. Wilkemeyer MF, Menkari C, Spong CY, Charness ME. Peptide antagonists of ethanol inhibition of L1-mediated cell-cell adhesion. J Pharmacol Exp Ther 2002; in press

57. Monforte R, Estruch R, Valls-Sole J, et al. Autonomic and peripheral neuropathies in patients with chronic alcoholism. A dose-related toxic effect of alcohol. Arch Neurol 1995;52:45–51

58. Martin F, Ward K, Slavin G, et al. Alcoholic skeletal myopathy, a clinical and pathologic study. Q J Med 1985;55:233–251

59. Urbano-Marquez A, Estruch R, Navarro-Lopez F, et al. The effects of alcoholism on skeletal and cardiac muscle. N Engl J Med 1989;320:409–415

60. Estruch R, Nicolas JM, Villegas E, et al. Relationship between ethanol-related diseases and nutritional status in chronically alcoholic men. Alcohol Alcoholism 1993;28:543–550

61. Sacanella E, Fernandez-Sola J, Cofan M, et al. Chronic alcoholic myopathy: diagnostic clues and relationship with other ethanol-related diseases. Q J Med 1995;88: 811–817

62. Fernandez-Sola J, Nicolas JM, Sacanella E, et al. Low-dose ethanol consumption allows strength recovery in chronic myopathy. Q J Med 2000;93:35–40

63. Swift RM. Drug therapy for alcohol dependence. N Engl J Med 1999;340:1482–1490

64. Acquas E, Meloni M, Di Chiara G. Blockade of delta-opioid receptors in the nucleus accumbens prevents ethanol-induced stimulation of dopamine release. Eur J Pharmacol 1993;230:239–241

65. O'Malley SS, Jaffe AJ, Chang G, et al. Naltrexone and coping skills therapy for alcohol dependence. A controlled study. Arch Gen Psychiatry 1992;49:881–887

66. Volpicelli JR, Alterman AI, Hayashida M, O'Brien CP. Naltrexone in the treatment of alcohol dependence. Arch Gen Psychiatry 1992;49:876–880

67. Krystal JH, Cramer JA, Krol WF, et al. Veterans Affairs Naltrexone Cooperative Study G. Naltrexone in the treatment of alcohol dependence. N Engl J Med 2001; 345:1734–1739

68. Mason BJ. Treatment of alcohol-dependent outpatients with acamprosate: a clinical review. J Clin Psych 2001; 62:42–48

69. Johnson BA, Roache JD, Javors MA, et al. Ondansetron for reduction of drinking among biologically predisposed alcoholic patients: a randomized controlled trial. JAMA 2000;284:963–971

143 Stimulants, Sedatives, and Opiates

Daniel K Hall-Flavin and Virginia E Hofmann

Introduction

The harmful use of psychoactive drugs, whether licit or illicit, represents a major public health concern of particular relevance to the practice of neurology. Problems associated with the use of these substances exist along a spectrum of severity and often require specialized treatment. Much can be accomplished, however, through timely identification, office-based brief interventions, and referral for further assessment if indicated.

Diagnosis

Both the World Health Organization and the American Psychiatric Association have published diagnostic criteria for substance use disorders. In the most recent revision of the *Diagnostic and Statistical Manual of Mental Disorders* (DSM-IV Text Revision),[1] these disorders are classified as "substance-induced disorders" and "substance-use disorders" (Table 143.1). "Substance-induced disorders" include specific pathophysiological states related directly to the use of a particular drug, whereas the term "substance-use disorders" emphasizes the concepts of abuse and dependence. Physiological dependence may exist alone without other behavioral signs of addiction and not meet the criteria for a substance dependence disorder. This distinction is important in the assessment of patients with certain conditions such as pain disorders who may demonstrate physiological dependence without addiction and, thus, not require formal addiction treatment.

Recently, clarification of the terms "addiction," "tolerance," and "physical dependence" has been approved jointly by the American Academy of Pain Medicine, the American Pain Society, and the American Society of Addiction Medicine.[2] The term "addiction" may be defined as "a primary, chronic neurobiologic disease with genetic, psychosocial, and environmental factors influencing its development and manifestations. It is characterized by behaviors that include one or more of the following: impaired control over drug use, compulsive use, continued use despite harm, and craving." "Physical dependence" is defined as "a state of adaptation that is manifested by a drug class specific withdrawal syndrome that can be produced by abrupt cessation, rapid dose reduction, decreasing blood levels of the drug, and/or administration of an antagonist." The term "tolerance" refers to a state of adaptation in which exposure to a drug induces changes that result in a diminution of one or more of the drug's effects over time.

Although the DSM-IV Text Revision identifies 11 categories of "abusable" substances, many of these substances may be classified alternatively, on the basis of shared properties, into one of three distinct categories: stimulants (caffeine, amphetamines and congeners, cocaine), depressants (alcohol, sedatives and hypnotics, and anxiolytics), and opioids. Other agents (cannabis, hallucinogens, phencyclidine and congeners, inhalants, and nicotine) generally are considered individually.

Identification of substance-use disorders may be particularly challenging even for the most seasoned clinicians; barriers to establishing a diagnosis have been reviewed creatively by Delbanco.[3] Defense mechanisms, including denial, rationalization, and projection, are used in a manner to perpetuate drug use. The most common of these, denial, may be

Table 143.1 Substance use disorders	
Substance-induced disorders	**Substance-use disorders**
Substance-induced intoxication	Substance abuse
Substance-induced withdrawal	A maladaptive pattern of continued substance use leading to
Intoxication delirium	clinically significant impairment or distress
Withdrawal delirium	Substance dependence
Substance-induced persisting dementia	A maladaptive pattern of continued substance use leading to
Substance-induced persisting amnestic disorder	clinically significant impairment or distress, impaired control,
Substance-induced psychotic disorder	preoccupation, tolerance, or withdrawal (or some combination of
With delusions	these)
With hallucinations	
Substance-induced mood disorder	
Substance-induced anxiety disorder	
Substance-induced sexual dysfunction	
Substance-induced sleep disorder	

defined as the range of psychological maneuvers that decrease awareness that drug use is the *cause* of consequences rather than a *solution*. Denial is nearly always a major obstacle to recovery.[4] Thus, identification of these disorders requires diligence, patience, and a straightforward, nonjudgmental, yet thorough, approach to assessment and management. Speaking with persons who know the patient well is critical. Several short self-reporting screening questionnaires are available. The CAGE questionnaire is a four-question screening tool that is easily incorporated into a diagnostic interview setting (Figure 143.1).[5] Signs and symptoms of key substance-induced disorders are summarized in Table 143.2. Laboratory screening is an essential part of the assessment process, and patterns of abnormalities may vary with the substance used. A urine drug screen is an essential part of the assessment.

After key information has been gathered, it is important to review this with the patient and those close to the patient. It is important to recognize that behavioral change proceeds through a series of steps which requires time to effect and that the patient must not only recognize there is a problem but that there is hope for change. General principles of motivational interviewing include 1) expression of empathy, 2) notation of discrepancies between

C	Have you ever felt you ought to **CUT** back on your drinking?
A	Have people **ANNOYED** you by criticizing your drinking?
G	Have you ever felt bad or **GUILTY** about your drinking?
E	Have you ever had a drink first thing in the morning to steady your nerves or to get rid of a hangover? (**EYE-OPENER**)

Note: Index of suspicion for alcohol dependence is directly related to number of positive responses.

Figure 143.1   The CAGE questionnaire.

current and goal behaviors, 3) avoidance of argumentation or direct confrontation of defenses, and 4) support of self-efficacy. Specialty consultation with an addiction medicine specialist should be considered.

Epidemiology

It has been estimated that for every one case of drug dependence that is treated, three are not. According to Epidemiologic Catchment Area Survey data, 3% to 4% of the population of the United States meet the criteria for the diagnosis of dependence on substances other than alcohol.[6] The risk of developing dependence on a drug other than alcohol is greatest for

Table 143.2	Signs and symptoms of key substance-induced disorders

Substance	Signs and symptoms
Opioids	
Intoxication	Behavioral or psychological changes (i.e., initial euphoria followed by apathy, dysphoria, psychomotor agitation or retardation, impaired judgment, or impaired social or occupational functioning) that developed during or shortly after opioid use and *at least 1* of the following: pupillary constriction, drowsiness or coma, slurred speech, impairment in attention or memory
Withdrawal	Cessation or reduction of opioid use that has been heavy or prolonged (several weeks or longer) or administration of an opioid antagonist after opioid use and *at least 3* of the following: dysphoric mood, nausea or vomiting, muscle aches, lacrimation or rhinorrhea, pupillary dilatation, piloerection or sweating, diarrhea, yawning, fever, insomnia
Stimulants	
Intoxication	Behavioral or psychological changes (i.e., euphoria or affective blunting; changes in sociability; hypervigilance; interpersonal sensitivity; anxiety, tension, or anger; stereotyped behaviors; impaired judgment) that developed during or shortly after stimulant use and *at least 2* of the following: tachycardia or bradycardia, pupillary dilatation, increased or decreased blood pressure, perspiration or chills, nausea or vomiting, evidence of weight loss, psychomotor agitation or retardation, muscle weakness, respiratory depression, chest pain or cardiac arrhythmias, confusion, seizures, dyskinesias, dystonias, coma
Withdrawal	Cessation or reduction of sedative-hypnotic use that has been heavy or prolonged, accompanied by dysphoric mood and *at least 2* of the following physiological changes: fatigue, vivid unpleasant dreams, insomnia or hypersomnia, increased appetite, psychomotor agitation or retardation.
Sedative-hypnotics	
Intoxication	Behavioral or psychological changes (inappropriate sexual or aggressive behavior, mood lability, and impaired judgment) that developed during or shortly after sedative-hypnotic use and *at least 1* of the following: slurred speech, incoordination, unsteady gait, nystagmus, impairment in attention or memory, stupor or coma.
Withdrawal	Cessation or reduction of sedative-hypnotic use that has been heavy or prolonged (several weeks or longer), and with *at least 2* of the following developing several hours to a few days after cessation: autonomic hyperactivity; increased hand tremor; insomnia; nausea or vomiting; transient visual, tactile, or auditory hallucinations or illusions; psychomotor agitation; anxiety; generalized tonic-clonic seizures

nicotine (in 33% of nicotine users), followed by cocaine (16.7% of cocaine users), and cannabis (9.1% of cannabis users). Clearly, the risk for developing a major drug-use problem depends on several variables, including biological factors, availability, setting, drug characteristics and route of administration, comorbid conditions, and environmental factors.

Genetics

Most of the work exploring the relationship between genetic factors and the development of substance-use disorders has focused on the risk for developing alcohol-related problems. This has provided a theoretical foundation for the study of other drug-related disorders. Specifically, factors of temperament (which include novelty-seeking, harm avoidance, reward dependence, and persistence) and character traits (notably self-directedness and cooperativeness) are believed to represent causal determinants of drug use, abuse, and dependence. Polysubstance dependence has been most consistently correlated with novelty-seeking.[7] This does not appear to demonstrate important variation by birth cohort or culture. Overall, the heritability of any substance abuse is estimated at 34% (marijuana, stimulants, opioids).

Clinical observations involving candidate gene searches include heritability, age at onset, criminality, severity, number of drugs used, temperament, character, the presence of personality disorder, global assessment of functioning, and evoked potentials (e.g., decreased amplitude of P300 auditory evoked potential in alcohol-naive sons of alcoholic fathers). Specific observations about drugs other than alcohol include associations between 1) polysubstance use in cocaine-dependent persons with the A_2 allele of TaqI on chromosome 11q of the dopamine D_2 receptor polymorphism, 2) novelty-seeking and opioid dependence with the long exon variant of the dopamine D_4 receptor on chromosome 11, and 3) evidence of increased dopamine reuptake and variants of the dopamine transporter.

Etiology/pathophysiology

The etiology and pathophysiology of addictive disorders involve a complex interplay of genetic vulnerability and environmental influences. Brain reward mechanisms that are critical for the pleasurable or euphoric effects of a drug (reinforcing use in the short-term) primarily involve the neurotransmitters dopamine and, to a lesser extent, norepinephrine and serotonin, which may help modulate dopaminergic "hedonistic" tone. Blum et al.[8] have speculated that some substance abusers possess a defect in their ability to experience reward or pleasure naturally. Koob and Le Moal[9] propose that the dysregulation of brain reward systems motivates the development of actual drug-dependent states.

The neuroanatomical substrates of reward have been studied extensively. In the mammalian model (Figure 143.2), moderately fast-conducting neurons in the descending medial forebrain bundle synapse with dopaminergic cell bodies in the ventral tegmental area which function as a synaptic "way station." The axons of these dopaminergic cell bodies (mesolimbic fibers) synapse in the nucleus accumbens, the putative "central processor," to ultimately send reward signals to the frontal cortex and ventral pallidum. Amphetamines, cocaine, opioids, cannabinoids, phencyclidine, and ketamine appear to act preferentially in the nucleus accumbens; opioids, alcohol, barbiturates, benzodiazepines, and nicotine appear to act preferentially in or near the area of the ventral tegmentum.[10]

The chronic, addictive use of a substance, however, reflects additional neuronal changes in intracellular signaling pathways (most notably the cyclic adenosine monophosphate [cAMP] second-messenger pathway) and in neuronal activities (neuroplastic sensitization). Intracellular transcription factors associated with upregulation of cAMP (CREB [cAMP response element binding protein]) or down-regulation of cAMP (delta-FosB) have been the focus of recent research as intracellular predecessors of changes in neuroplasticity that occur in addictive states.[11] "Neuroplasticity" is defined as the ability of the nervous system to modify its response to a stimulus in response to experience. An example of this is found in drug craving or rapid reinstatement of addictive drug use during stress after an extended period of abstinence. Recent research has posited that the neurotransmitter glutamate may have a pivotal role and the neural substrates involved in addictive use may differ in part from those involved in nonaddictive use.

General principles of treatment

"Treatment" may be defined as the broad range of services—identification; brief intervention; assessment; diagnosis; counseling; psychiatric, psychological, and medical services; social services; and follow-up—for persons with addiction. The overall goal of treatment is to eliminate the use of the substance as a contributing factor to physical, psychological, or social dysfunction and to arrest, retard, or reverse the progress of any associated problems.[12] Specific elements of treatment include 1) detoxification, 2) pharmacotherapies designed to treat specific withdrawal symptoms, comorbid conditions, or relapse-specific precipitants, and 3) psychosocial interventions designed to provide peer support, psychological counseling, relapse prevention skills training, and motivational enhancement. Because persons who suffer from addiction are not a homogeneous group, individualized approaches to treatment are necessary. Nonetheless, common goals of psychosocial interventions include enhancing motivation, teaching coping skills, addressing reinforcement contingencies, fostering management of painful affects, improving interpersonal functioning, and enhancing compliance with treatment.

Opioids

Before the development of opioid maintenance strategies in the treatment of opioid addiction, treatment primarily relied on limited detoxification strategies,

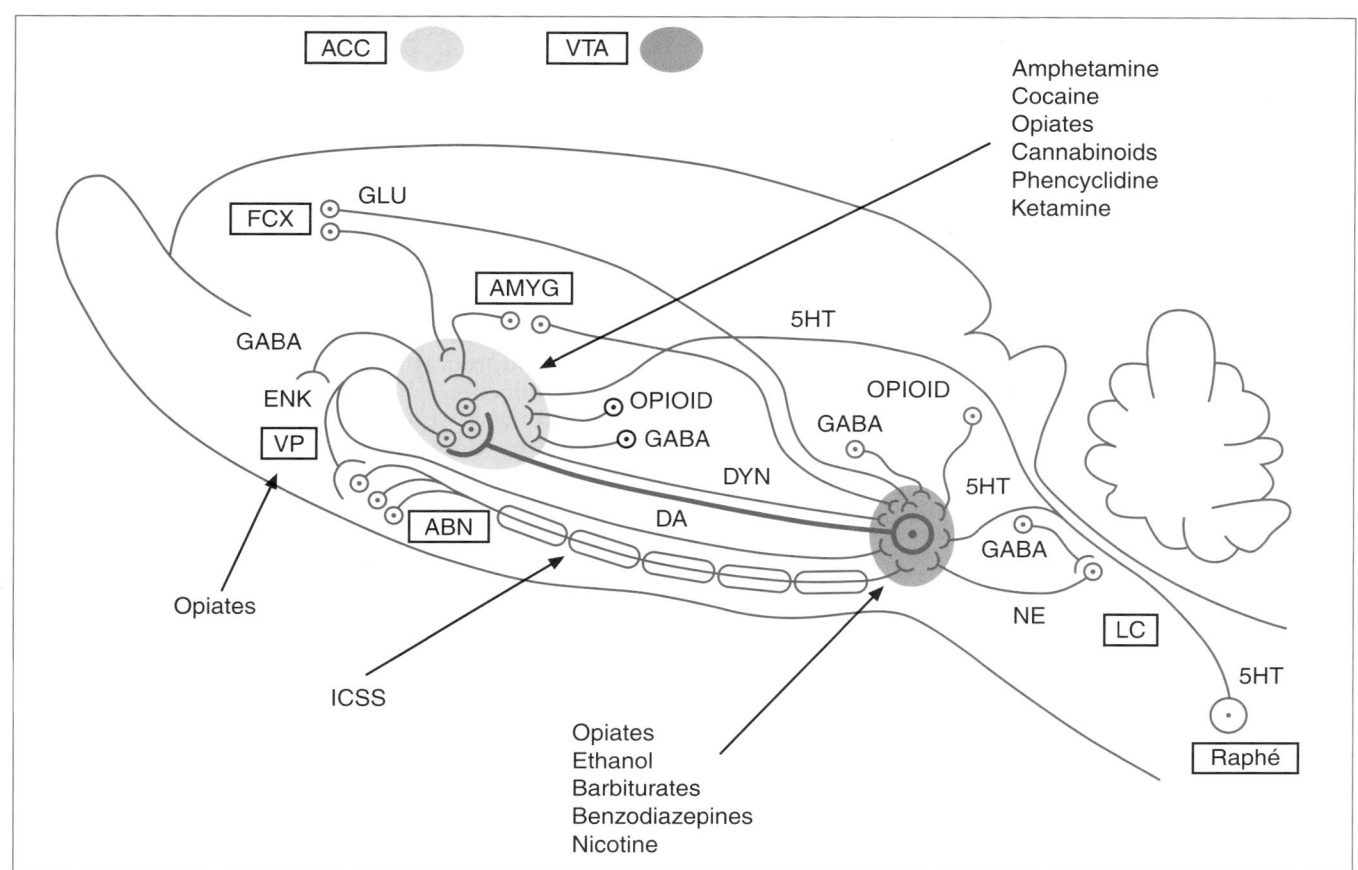

Figure 143.2 Model of mammalian reward pathways in the central nervous system. ABN, anterior bed nuclei of medial forebrain bundle; ACC, nucleus accumbens; AMYG, amygdala; DA, subcomponent of ascending mesolimbic dopaminergic system that appears preferentially activated by abusable substances; DYN, dynorphinergic outflow from ACC; ENK, enkephalinergic outflow from ACC; FCX, frontal cortex; GABA, GABAergic inhibitory fiber systems synapsing in locus ceruleus (noradrenergic cells), VTA, and ACC as well as the GABAergic outflow from ACC; GLU, glutamatergic neural systems originating in FCX and synapsing in VTA and ACC; 5HT, serotonergic fibers originating in anterior raphe nuclei and projecting to VTA and ACC; ICSS, descending, myelinated, and moderately fast conducting component of brain reward system that is preferentially activated by intracranial self-stimulation; LC, locus ceruleus; NE, noradrenergic fibers originating in locus ceruleus and synapsing in vicinity of ventral mesencephalic DA cell fields of VTA; OPIOID, endogenous opioid peptide neural systems synapsing in VTA DA cell fields and ACC dopaminergic terminal projection loci; Raphé, brainstem serotonergic raphe nuclei; VP, ventral pallidum; VTA, ventral tegmental area. (Redrawn from Cooper JR, Bloom FE, Roth RH. The Biochemical Basis of Neuropharmacology. 7th ed. New York: Oxford University Press, 1996:295. By permission of the publisher.)

with long-term abstinence as a goal. This approach was associated with impressive relapse rates and recidivism. Subsequent developments in treatment have improved outcomes substantially. Pharmacotherapies may be classified broadly into "maintenance" and "nonmaintenance" strategies.

Maintenance pharmacological strategies

Maintenance strategies were pioneered nearly 40 years ago when Dole and Nyswander[13] introduced methadone maintenance. Methadone, a μ-opioid agonist with pharmacological properties similar to those of morphine, has a half-life of 15 to 40 hours and does not produce the euphoria seen with short-acting opioids. When given daily in adequate doses, methadone is associated with impressive reductions in illicit, shorter-acting opioid use. Daily monitored doses of 80 to 120 mg of methadone are often needed

to block the euphoria caused by heroin, decrease craving, ensure greater retention in treatment, and decrease the consequences of use. About three-fourths of patients maintained at these levels remain heroin-free for at least 6 months. Federal law requires that for the treatment of opioid dependence, methadone be dispensed at specially licensed and regulated clinics.

An alternative to methadone is levomethadyl acetate hydrochloride (LAAM), a synthetic opioid with a longer half-life than methadone. LAAM is used in specially regulated clinics for the treatment of opioid addiction. It offers the advantage of three times weekly dosing. Studies are under way to compare the efficacy of methadone and LAAM in maintenance treatment.

For the first time in nearly a century, the Drug Addiction Treatment Act of 2000 allows physicians to treat opioid addiction with opioid medications in

Schedules III, IV, and V in the office setting.[14] Specifically, buprenorphine, a partial μ-opioid agonist used either alone (Subutex) or in a sublingual preparation that is a 4:1 combination of buprenorphine and naloxone (Suboxone), is awaiting final approval by the U.S. Food and Drug Administration (FDA) for maintenance-based treatment in this setting. It is expected to expand access to narcotic treatment; physicians who prescribe buprenorphine in this setting must meet certain competency requirements but will not require special licensure. Because of its activity as a partial agonist, the danger of overdose is decreased, but it still produces sufficient tolerance to block the effects of exogenous opioids. Three times weekly dosing will be possible. Buprenorphine initially may produce withdrawal discomfort in persons who have severe opioid addiction. The only fatalities that have been associated with the use of buprenorphine in this setting have involved patients who were also taking benzodiazepines.

Nonmaintenance-based pharmacological strategies

Abstinence-based strategies are appropriate for patients addicted to opioids who are not eligible or who cannot access maintenance treatment in a specialty clinic. Detoxification protocols are generally followed by both pharmacologically and psychosocially based interventions designed to help maintain abstinence. Detoxification is designed to safely minimize the emergence of μ-opioid withdrawal symptoms. Several approaches to detoxification are outlined in Table 143.3.

Selection of an appropriate detoxification strategy must take into account the specific drug or multiple substances used; its duration of action and receptor affinity; the amount, duration, and frequency of use; comorbid medical and psychological factors; and legal issues. Withdrawal signs and symptoms are generally the opposite of those seen with acute activation of μ-opioid receptors. Generally, a cross-tolerant opioid of longer duration than the opioid of use should be prescribed; also, agents of greater dependence risk should not be chosen for detoxification from an agent of lesser dependence risk (Table 143.4). Although methadone is an appropriate choice for withdrawal from many opioids (especially for patients who have a coexisting pain disorder), current federal law prohibits the administration of any opioid for more than 72 hours for the purposes of detoxification only, outside of a methadone maintenance program. Buprenorphine has also been used in withdrawal protocols.

Accordingly, protocols using adjunctive agents designed to decrease the severity of withdrawal symptoms have been developed. The most studied of these agents, the α_2-adrenergic receptor agonist clonidine, has been demonstrated to minimize autonomic

Table 143.4 Opiate analgesics dose equivalents

Drug (brand name)	Dose, mg	Half-life, hr
Codeine	200	2–3
Heroin	5 IM	0.5
Hydromorphone (Dilaudid)	7.5	2–3
Hydrocodone (Lortab and Vicodin [with acetaminophen])	5–10	2–4
Methadone (Dolophine)	10	12–150+
Morphine	60	2–3
Morphine, controlled release (MS Contin, Oramorph SR)	20–60	2–3
Oxycodone with aspirin (Percodan)	5–10	2–3
Propoxyphene (Darvon)	65	6–12

IM, intramuscularly.

Table 143.3 Management of opioid withdrawal

1 Taper the agent of dependence
   a. Using history, collateral information, and evidence of drug use, establish patient's 24-hour dose of the agent
   b. Systematically decrease the daily dose by no more than 5%–10% of baseline dose, and administer in divided doses. Decrease in dose should occur at regular intervals (daily, every 3–4 days, weekly, etc.)
   c. If patient does not comply with taper as an outpatient, consider inpatient taper

2 Substitute methadone and taper it (must be done in inpatient setting)
   a. Establish baseline 24-hour dose
   b. Convert opioid dose to equivalent dose of methadone
   c. If baseline dose is unknown, administer 15–20 mg of methadone as test dose and observe patient's condition (40 mg in 24 hours usually prevents withdrawal in most patients)
   d. Adjust dose empirically by observing the patient's *objective* signs of withdrawal (not subjective complaints)
   e. Systematically decrease daily dose by 10%–20% of baseline dose per day, and administer in divided doses
   f. Monitor patient for withdrawal symptoms and inability to proceed with taper because of withdrawal symptoms. Consider slowing the taper in patients who cannot tolerate a faster rate because of withdrawal symptoms

3 Use of clonidine for autonomic hyperactivity during opioid withdrawal
   a. Administer oral 0.1-mg test dose, monitoring blood pressure carefully (main side effects are hypotension and sedation)
   b. If no significant hypotension after test dose, give patient scheduled doses of clonidine, 0.3–0.4 mg 3 times daily (maximal dose, 1.2 mg/day)
   c. It may still be necessary to administer nonopioid analgesics for pain and antiemetics for nausea

hyperactivity in doses up to 0.3 mg two to four times daily. The persons given this agent were monitored for signs of hypotension. Clonidine does not shorten the period of withdrawal, only the severity of withdrawal symptoms. Kleber and Kosten[15] have developed an approach to detoxification involving pretreatment with clonidine and a benzodiazepine (for agitation), followed by precipitated withdrawal with naltrexone.

Naltrexone is a μ-opioid antagonist that, when taken, can be effective in preventing relapse by blocking the "high" produced by opioids. It is free of agonist properties, it produces no withdrawal symptoms when treatment is stopped, and its side effects are mild. To avoid precipitating withdrawal, patients need to be opioid-free for 5 days or longer depending on the half-life of the drug. Studies have indicated low levels of compliance, with the best success reported among impaired professionals and persons in work-release programs. An implantable form of naltrexone as a maintenance strategy has been in use outside the United States.

At least five peer-reviewed trials have examined the usefulness of lofexidine, an α_2-adrenergic receptor agonist, in managing withdrawal symptoms.[16] Three of these have compared lofexidine with clonidine, and two have examined the time to resolution of withdrawal symptoms in comparison with that of methadone. Lofexidine appeared to offer clear advantages in avoiding the hypotensive effects of the alternative α_2-agent clonidine. A shorter time to the resolution of withdrawal symptoms has been noted with lofexidine, which currently is not available in the United States.

Because of the protracted nature of methadone withdrawal protocols and the sedation and hypotension associated with available α_2-adrenergic receptor agonists, ultrarapid detoxification protocols involving the administration of opioid antagonists to induce withdrawal with concomitant heavy sedation or anesthesia have been developed. A recent evidence-based review of these procedures noted that no comparison studies vis-à-vis other detoxification strategies have been published and the variability in treatment regimes is marked. Complications have been reported, and whether the favorable risk-to-benefit ratio is favorable has not been established.[17]

Nonpharmacological approaches to treatment

Halfway houses and residential programs for opioid-dependent patients use some variation of the therapeutic community approach. Counseling, behavioral treatments, 12-step or other self-help programs, and focused psychotherapy add to a positive outcome. Prevention of relapse, management of craving, dealing with decreased motivation, and decreasing access to drugs are key elements in the counseling and therapy process.

Stimulants

It has been estimated that more than 23 million Americans have tried cocaine or crack, and over 3 million have used it within the past year.[18] A rising trend has been noted in the 18- to 25-year-old age cohort. An earlier version of the National Household Survey noted that 4 to 9 million persons had tried methamphetamine.

Cocaine toxicity is a medical emergency, with the patient presenting with a hyperadrenergic state characterized by hypertension, tachycardia, tonic-clonic seizures, dyspnea, and ventricular arrhythmia. After medical stability has been established, the patient needs a chemical dependence assessment and referral to a treatment program.

Treatment approaches to cocaine abuse and dependence may be classified as "behavioral" and "pharmacological" approaches. The 1999 NIDA Collaborative Cocaine Treatment Study, a multisite randomized control trial, concluded that behavioral treatment approaches improve outcome in cocaine-dependent patients.[19] Other psychosocial therapies include peer support, psychological counseling, relapse prevention skills building, and motivational enhancement.

Pharmacological treatments for cocaine dependence have focused on several areas: 1) treatment of cocaine-induced neurotransmitter derangement, 2) modification of kindling, 3) modification of enzymatic degradation pathways, 4) use of dopamine-selective receptor antagonists, and 5) use of vaccines.[20]

The acute effects of cocaine use include prevention of the reuptake of dopamine, norepinephrine, and serotonin; subsequently, new dopamine synthesis is inhibited by neuronal autoregulation, leading to increased craving and increased use. Theoretically, treatment with amantadine (stimulation of dopamine release) and bromocriptine (a dopamine receptor agonist) held promise, but studies have not demonstrated any efficacy. The results of treatment with antidepressants, including desipramine, fluoxetine, and bupropion, purported to alter receptor supersensitivity, have been mixed. However, these agents may be helpful in treating depression and decreasing cocaine use by cocaine users who have depression. In an open label trial, the antidepressant venlofaxine has demonstrated promise in treating cocaine addiction.

The results of attempts to modify kindling to decrease craving have been inconsistent. Four clinical trials have found that carbamazepine is not particularly helpful. There is some evidence that the calcium channel blockers nifedipine and amlodipine may be helpful. Inconsistencies in the pharmacotherapy trials are due to variations in study design, selection of study populations, and large dropout numbers. Many studies have been conducted in cocaine-dependent patients in methadone maintenance programs.

The alcohol-aversive agent disulfiram may be beneficial in decreasing craving for cocaine and preventing relapse in early recovery. Disulfiram is thought to decrease dopamine β-hydroxylase and plasma esterases involved in the metabolism of cocaine. A 1993 study reported a reduction of alcohol and cocaine use in 16 dually addicted patients.[21] Two studies published in 2000 reported more total days of abstinence from cocaine use and a decrease in total amount used.[22,23]

Other studies have examined the role of D_1 antagonists, central nervous system (CNS) cell membrane repair agents, and agents designed to increase cerebral blood flow. The results of early studies suggested that these agents held promise.

Research continues on the use of vaccines. Normally, cocaine is cleared quickly from the body, preventing the development of an antibody response. Fox[24] has reported on a vaccine designed to prevent entry of cocaine into the CNS via a partially antibody-mediated response. Also, passive immunization with a monoclonal IgG cocaine antagonist may prevent reinstatement of cocaine self-administration.

Research into the treatment of methamphetamine-specific syndromes is in the nascent stage. Neuroimaging studies have shown significant long-lasting damage to dopaminergic terminals and apoptosis in the striatum, hippocampus, and frontal cortex of mouse brains. With positron emission tomography (PET), lower dopamine transporter density has been found in the caudate-putamen, nucleus accumbens, and prefrontal cortex of methamphetamine users who were abstinent for 18 months. The clinical effects in humans include memory dysfunction, alterations in concentration and decision-making capacity, and increased risk for the development of movement disorders or psychosis. Selegiline has been studied for its neuroprotective effects. Cognitive enhancers, glial neurotrophic factors, and other agents are being considered for experimental study.

Sedative-hypnotics

Sedative-hypnotics and anxiolytics include benzodiazepines, barbiturates, and other agents such as buspirone, chloral hydrate, ethchlorvynol, glutethimide, meprobamate, and methyprylon. Benzodiazepines attach to a subunit of the γ-aminobutyric acid (GABA) receptor, the major inhibitory neurotransmitter, and barbiturates attach to an alternate site on the GABA receptor. Long-term use alters the pharmacodynamics of the GABA receptor sites. Acute intoxication with benzodiazepines may be reversed with the benzodiazepine antagonist flumazenil via displacement of benzodiazepine receptor agonists, including benzodiazepines, zolpidem, and zaleplon, at the GABA A receptor complex.[25] Flumazenil may be associated with seizures in patients with seizure disorder, impaired memory retrieval, or emergence of toxic effects of other drugs in the case of mixed drug overdose. It does not reverse the effects of ethanol, barbiturates, or opioids. Barbiturate intoxication or overdose requires hemodynamic and respiratory support and correction of electrolyte imbalance along with the use of diuresis and activated charcoal. Hemodialysis may also be indicated. Flumazenil should be given intravenously at a dose of 0.1 mg at 1-minute intervals until the desired effect occurs or a cumulative dose of 3 mg has been given, with repeat dosing possible. Flumazenil can cause seizures in patients who take stimulants or tricyclic antidepres-

sants and should be avoided in patients with evidence of tricyclic cardiotoxicity.[26]

Both high-dose and low-dose (therapeutic dose) sedative-hypnotic withdrawal syndromes have been reported. Signs and symptoms include anxiety, tremors, nightmares, insomnia, anorexia, nausea, vomiting, postural hypotension, seizures, delirium, and hyperpyrexia. Death may result from precipitous withdrawal. The time to peak symptoms and the length of withdrawal correlate directly with the half-life of the drug. Delirium and seizures are possible. Symptom rebound, an intensification of the symptoms for which the drug was prescribed initially, and protracted withdrawal can occur.[27]

The pharmacological management of benzodiazepine withdrawal may be classified into one of four general approaches: 1) tapering the agent of dependence, 2) substituting phenobarbital or another longer acting barbiturate and tapering it, 3) substituting a longer acting benzodiazepine and tapering it, and 4) using valproate or carbamazepine (or both) (Table 143.5). Tables are available for calculating barbiturate substitution. Tapering occurs after a stabilization phase. Usually, phenobarbital is given for the purpose of detoxifying someone from barbiturates. Equivalency tables also are available for specific benzodiazepine substitution (Table 143.6).

Anticonvulsants have been used supplementally to assist in detoxification. Carbamazepine and valproate have been studied most, and they appear to enhance GABAergic function. According to a recent review by Pages and Ries,[28] most studies have shown positive results, but there has been a lack of randomized studies. Valproate may have the added advantage of treating both benzodiazepine dependence and symptom recurrence.

Other drugs

Currently, no drug-specific treatments are included in routine clinical practice for cannabis, "club" drugs such as MDMA (3,4-methylenedioxymethamphetamine), flunitrazepam (Rohypnol), LSD (lysergic acid diethylamide), phencyclidine, or inhalants. Treatment is aimed toward supportive reassurance, symptomatic relief of subjective distress, treatment of acute psychosis or behavioral inhibition, treatment of associated comorbid states, and psychosocial rehabilitation.

Conclusion

Adequate treatment of substance use disorders requires clinical intuition and appropriate identification as well as innovative approaches to intervention. The first step in successful treatment is detoxification when appropriate. This is followed by care designed to 1) help prevent relapse and craving, 2) treat comorbid states, and 3) offer the resources needed to achieve success. No single therapeutic modality is uniquely effective in this process. It is important to remember that substance abuse disorders represent a chronic disorder with an unpredictable pattern of abstinence and relapse and that the process of change is a complex one that requires dedication, patience, and perseverance on the part of the caregiver.

Table 143.5 Pharmacological management of benzodiazepine withdrawal

1 Taper the agent of dependence
  a. Establish baseline 24-hour dose
  b. Systematically decrease daily dose by no more than 5%–10% of baseline dose, and administer in divided doses. Decrease in dose should occur at regular intervals (daily, every 3–4 days, weekly, etc.)
  c. Monitor patient for withdrawal symptoms and inability to proceed with taper because of withdrawal symptoms
  d. Consider slowing taper in patients who cannot tolerate a faster rate because of withdrawal/anxiety symptoms
  e. Inpatient care/detoxification is indicated if patient is taking doses sufficient to impair functioning or ability to cooperate with an outpatient taper or if taper is not successful in an outpatient setting

2 Substitute phenobarbital or longer acting barbiturate and taper it
  a. Establish baseline 24-hour dose
  b. Convert benzodiazepine dose to equivalent phenobarbital dose for withdrawal (Table 143.6)
  c. Systematically decrease total daily phenobarbital dose by percentage of baseline dose (10% every day for a 10-day taper, 5% daily for a 20-day taper)
  d. This procedure is best done in an inpatient setting to titrate phenobarbital dose under close control and medical supervision

3 Substitute longer acting benzodiazepine (usually chlordiazepoxide or clonazepam) and taper it as in #1 above

4 Use valproate or carbamazepine at therapeutic levels as an adjunct to taper
  a. Useful for patients who must undergo more rapid detoxification or those who cannot tolerate taper because of withdrawal symptoms
  b. Therapeutic levels should be attained before starting the taper

Table 143.6 Benzodiazepines and phenobarbital dose equivalents for withdrawal

Drug (brand name)	Usual daily dose range, mg	Half-life, hr	Equivalent dose to 30 mg phenobarbital, mg
Alprazolam (Xanax)	0.5–4	12	1
Chlordiazepoxide (Librium)	15–100	10	25
Clonazepam (Klonopin)	0.5–4	23	2
Clorazepate (Tranxene)	15–60	65	7.5
Diazepam (Valium)	5–40	43	10
Flurazepam (Dalmane)	15–30	15	15
Lorazepam (Ativan)	1–6	14	2
Oxazepam (Serax)	45–120	8	10
Quazepam (Doral)	7.5–15	39	15
Temazepam (Restoril)	7.5–30	11	15
Triazolam (Halcion)	0.125–0.50	3	0.25

References

1. American Psychiatric Association. Diagnostic and Statistical Manual of Mental Disorders. 4th ed, text revision. Washington, DC: American Psychiatric Association, 2000
2. Definitions related to the use of opioids for the treatment of pain. A consensus document from the American Academy of Pain Medicine, the American Pain Society, and the American Society of Addiction Medicine, February, 2001. Retrieved March 19, 2002, from the World Wide Web: http://www.asam.org/pain/definitions2.pdf
3. Delbanco TL. Patients who drink too much. Where are their doctors? JAMA 1992;267:702–703
4. Morse RM, Flavin DK. The definition of alcoholism. The Joint Committee of the National Council on Alcoholism and Drug Dependence and the American Society of Addiction Medicine to Study the Definition and Criteria for the Diagnosis of Alcoholism. JAMA 1992;268:1012–1014
5. Mayfield D, McLeod G, Hall P. The CAGE questionnaire: validation of a new alcoholism screening instrument. Am J Psychiatry 1974;131:1121–1123
6. Anthony JC. Epidemiology of drug dependence. In: Galanter M, Kleber HD, eds. The American Psychiatric Press Textbook of Substance Abuse Treatment. 2nd ed. Washington, DC: American Psychiatric Press, 1999: 47–58
7. Cloninger CR. Genetics of substance abuse. In: Galanter M, Kleber HD, eds. The American Psychiatric Press Textbook of Substance Abuse Treatment. 2nd ed. Washington, DC: American Psychiatric Press, 1999: 59–66
8. Blum K, Braverman ER, Holden JM, et al. Reward deficiency syndrome: a biogenetic model for the diagnosis and treatment of impulsive, addictive, and compulsive behaviors. J Psychoactive Drugs. 2000;32(Suppl i–iv): 1–112
9. Koob GF, Le Moal M. Drug addiction, dysregulation of reward, and allostasis. Neuropsychopharmacology 2001;24:97–129
10. Gardner EL. Brain reward mechanisms. In: Lowinson JH, Ruiz P, Millman RB, Langrod JG, eds. Substance

Abuse: A Comprehensive Textbook. 3rd ed. Baltimore: Williams & Wilkins, 1997:51–85

11. Wolf ME. The neuroplasticity of addiction. *In:* Shaw CA, McEachern JC. Toward a Theory of Neuroplasticity. Philadelphia: Psychology Press, 2001:359–372

12. Institute of Medicine. Broadening the Base of Treatment for Alcohol Problems. Washington DC, National Academy of Sciences, 1990

13. Dole VP, Nyswander ME. A medical treatment of diacetylmorphine (heroin) addiction. JAMA 1965;193: 646–650

14. Johnson RE, McCagh JC. Buprenorphine and naloxone for heroin dependence. Curr Psychiatry Rep 2000;2: 519–526

15. Kleber HD, Kosten TR. Naltrexone induction: psychologic and pharmacologic strategies. J Clin Psychiatry 1984;95:29–38

16. Strang J, Bearn J, Gossop M. Lofexidine for opiate detoxification: review of recent randomised and open controlled trials. Am J Addict 1999;8:337–348

17. Gowing L, Ali R, White J. Opioid antagonists under heavy sedation or anesthesia for opioid withdrawal. Cochrane Database Syst Rev 2002;(2):CD002022

18. Department of Health and Human Services, Substance Abuse and Mental Health Services Administration. Summary of findings from the 1998 National Household Survey on Drug Abuse. August, 1999. Retrieved March 19, 2002, from the World Wide Web: http://www.samhsa.gov/oas/NHSDA/98SummHtm/ NHSDA98Summ.htm

19. Crits-Christoph P, Siqueland L, Blaine J, et al. Psychosocial treatments for cocaine dependence. Result of the NIDA Collaborative Cocaine Treatment Study. Arch Gen Psychiatry 1999;56:493–502

20. O'Leary G, Weiss RD. Pharmacotherapies for cocaine dependence. Curr Psychiatry Rep 2000;2:508–513

21. Higgins ST, Budney AJ, Bickel WK, et al. Disulfiram therapy in patients abusing alcohol and cocaine. Am J Psychiatry 1993;150:675–676

22. George TP, Chawarski MC, Pakes I, et al. Disulfiram v. placebo for cocaine dependence in buprenorphine-maintained patients: a preliminary trial. Biol Psychiatry 2000;47:1080–1086

23. Petrakis IL, Carroll KM, Nich C, et al. Disulfiram treatment for cocaine dependence in methadone maintained opioid addicts. Addiction 2000;95:215–228

24. Fox BS. Development of a therapeutic vaccine for the treatment of cocaine addiction. Drug Alcohol Depend 1997;48:153–158

25. Hardman JG, Limbird LE, eds. Goodman & Gilman's The Pharmacological Basis of Therapeutics. 9th ed. New York: McGraw-Hill, 1996

26. Schatzberg AF, Cole JO, DeBattista C. Manual of Clinical Psychopharmacology. 3rd ed. Washington, DC: American Psychiatric Press, 1997

27. Smith DE, Wesson DR. Benzodiazepine and other sedative-hypnotic dependence. *In:* Galanter M, Kleber HD, eds. The American Psychiatric Press Textbook of Substance Abuse Treatment. 2nd ed. Washington, DC: American Psychiatric Press, 1999:239–251

28. Pages KP, Ries RK. Use of anticonvulsants in benzodiazepine withdrawal. Am J Addict 1998;7:198–204

144 Treatment of the Neurotoxic Effects of Organic Solvents

Robert G Feldman

Neurotoxicants

A "neurotoxicant" is any synthetic chemical substance that can adversely affect the function of neural tissue and the nervous system. The ability to disrupt normal neurological function is related to the physical properties of a particular chemical and to the biological makeup of the exposed organism and its unique susceptibilities to the neurotoxic effects of exposure to certain chemicals. Many organic chemicals used as solvents are neurotoxicants (Table 144.1).

Organic solvents are nonpolar compounds and are highly soluble in nonpolar solutions (e.g., other organic solvents, fat, and oils). The lipophilic characteristics of organic solvents make them suitable for removing grease and cutting the viscosity of oils. Conversely, organic solvents are not readily miscible with polar compounds such as water. It is this specific property—that is, polarity—of the organic solvents that also accounts for their ability to readily cross the pulmonary alveoli, skin, gastrointestinal tract mucosa, blood–brain barrier, and cell membranes and to accumulate in tissues with a high lipid content, such as adipose tissue and the brain. These biochemical properties of organic solvents are related directly to their ability to disrupt nervous system function.

The neurotoxic effects associated with exposure to

Table 144.1 Sources and neurotoxic effects associated with exposure to selected organic solvents

Solvent	Source of exposure	Associated clinical diagnosis
Trichloroethylene	Degreasers Painting industry Varnishes Spot removers Process of decaffeination Dry cleaning industry Rubber solvents	Acute—narcosis Chronic—encephalopathy, cranial neuropathy
Perchloroethylene	Paint removers Degreasers Extraction agents Dry cleaning industry Textile industry	Acute—narcosis Chronic—peripheral neuropathy, encephalopathy
Toluene	Rubber solvents Cleaning agents Glues Manufacturers of benzene Gasoline and aviation fuels Paints, paint thinners, and lacquers Screen printing industry	Acute—narcosis Chronic—tremor, ataxia, encephalopathy
n-Hexane, methyl n-butyl ketone	Paints, laquers, varnishes Paint removers Metal-cleaning compounds Quick-drying inks Glues and adhesives	Acute—narcosis Chronic—peripheral neuropathy
Carbon disulfide	Manufacture of viscose rayon Preservatives Textiles Rubber cement Varnishes Electroplating industry	Acute—encephalopathy Chronic—peripheral neuropathy, parkinsonism

Modified from Feldman.[32] By permission of Lippincott-Raven Publishers.

an organic solvent depend on the amount of chemical absorbed. Organic solvents are volatile and evaporate readily in the ambient atmosphere, from which they are inhaled and taken up through the lungs. Uptake via the pulmonary route is influenced by respiration rate, heart rate, the blood–air partition coefficient of the solvent, and current blood concentrations of the solvent (faster at the onset of exposure, when blood levels of the solvent have not reached equilibrium or saturation).[1] Physical activity can increase cardiac and respiratory rates and, thus, increase uptake.[2,3] Total dermal absorption is influenced by the condition of the skin, the duration of exposure, and the surface area of the skin exposed.[4] Typically, gastrointestinal tract absorption is slower but more complete than pulmonary absorption.[2]

Organic solvents readily cross the blood–brain barrier and gain access to the central nervous system (CNS). After passing through the lipid-rich cell membrane, organic molecules can react with enzymes of the microsomal oxidizing system inside the cell (i.e., cytochrome P-450). Reaction with cytochrome P-450 enzymes, particularly those in the liver, rapidly converts many organic solvents to alcohols that produce the acute narcotic effects which make these chemicals cheap alternatives to other recreational drugs (e.g., cocaine).[5] Many organic solvents that have entered cells, including neurons in the CNS and peripheral nervous system, as a nontoxic parent molecule are subsequently activated by cytochrome P-450 enzymes to become reactive intermediates (e.g., epoxides) that can react with cellular macromolecules such as neurofilaments and DNA.[6–11] These reactive metabolites are largely responsible for the effects of chronic exposures to organic solvents such as n-hexane, methyl n-butyl ketone (MnBK), and carbon disulfide.[11]

Immediate detection of the hazards associated with exposure to a specific organic solvent and the institution of measures to prevent exposure to toxic levels of these chemicals are optimal when the chemicals are used safely. However, when the amount of a neurotoxicant absorbed exceeds the body's ability to detoxify or excrete it (or both), cellular damage, often irreversible, occurs. Emergency efforts should be used to prevent further neurotoxicant uptake, including removal of the person affected from further exposure. Gastric lavage can be used to remove the solvent from the stomach; pulmonary hyperventilation and replacement of toxic vapors with fresh air or oxygen prevents further metabolism of the neurotoxicant. Additional interventions should include methods to prevent further metabolism of the parent molecules to toxic metabolites (e.g., administration of a competitive inhibitor of the chemical's metabolism) and to enhance their excretion (e.g., hemodialysis).[12–14] Antidotes that prevent or reduce the adverse effects of severe acute exposures have been developed for some organic solvents shown to induce persistent effects after a single incident of exposure. For example, fomepizole and ethanol can be administered to patients exposed to ethylene glycol or methanol (or both) to competitively inhibit the activity of alcohol dehydrogenase, which catalyzes the initial steps in the

metabolism of ethylene glycol to glycolate and oxalate as well as methanol to formate.[14,15] Because there are no specific interventions or therapies as yet for the effects of many organic solvents, this chapter focuses primarily on preventive measures and supportive therapies for selected organic solvents.

Prevention and therapeutic methods for selected organic solvents

Trichloroethylene

Acute exposure The first step in treating acute trichloroethylene (TCE) intoxication is to recognize the condition and to remove the exposed person from risk of further danger. Acute symptoms of TCE exposure are related to the formation of its metabolite, trichloroethanol, and include nausea, vomiting, dizziness, confusion, headache, and stupor and loss of consciousness.[5,16–18] To reduce the risk of a person developing symptoms of exposure, the ambient air levels of TCE should not exceed 100 ppm.[19] An ambient air level of 1000 ppm of TCE is considered to be immediately dangerous to life and health.[20] The urine concentration of the TCE metabolite trichloroacetic acid should not exceed 100 mg/g creatinine at the end of the work shift.[21] Acute inhalation exposure to vapors of TCE, which are degraded to dichloroacetylene after being heated or mixed with an alkali, can cause immediate and irreversible damage to peripheral and cranial nerves.[16,22–24] This potential hazard must be anticipated and prevented by persons responsible for monitoring workers exposed to TCE and by clinicians treating patients who have been exposed to it.

Displacing the TCE-contaminated air in the lungs with fresh air or oxygen sources, while encouraging energetic deep breathing, is essential in emergency care.[17,25] After liquid TCE has been swallowed, gastric lavage should be performed. Syrup of ipecac can be given to initiate vomiting in cases of poison ingestion, but the risk of further inhalation of TCE vapors from the oropharynx or by aspiration of vomitus containing TCE makes controlled stomach lavage a safer method of eliminating residual ingested TCE. Cardiac monitoring can detect arrhythmias induced by TCE. Pulmonary edema and vasomotor instability must be watched for and treated symptomatically in susceptible persons.[26–28] Hemodialysis for acute renal failure may be necessary.[12,13]

The acute narcotic effects of TCE and its metabolites generally subside within hours to days after cessation of exposure.[16,22,24,29] Impairment in neuropsychological performance and emotional disturbances may persist after a single severe toxic exposure.[30,31] Although no specific antidote or treatment has been developed to enhance recovery from TCE or dichloroacetylene injury to the trigeminal nerve, the empirical administration of vitamin E and B-complex vitamins has been recommended. Spontaneous and often incomplete recovery follow cessation of further exposure to TCE.[30,32]

Chronic exposures Symptoms appear gradually after chronic exposure to TCE. Prolonged exposures at low to moderate ambient air levels of TCE vapor or repeated peak level exposure to TCE vapor results in accumulated neurotoxic effects. The toxic effects of chronic low-level exposure to TCE, such as dizziness, incoordination, and confusion, are exacerbated by alcohol.[33] Cardiac dysrhythmias, somnolence, confusion, dizziness, and imbalance may occur in persons who have also taken adrenergic agonists such as epinephrine, amphetamine, or cocaine.[24,26] Normal metabolism of TCE can be impaired with liver failure.[26] Thus, if TCE exposure is suspected, effective management of the effects of chronic exposure requires that the person be removed from further exposure to TCE, refrain from alcohol intake, and avoid exposure to various volatile organic solvents.

Once established, many of the effects of TCE exposure on the CNS are irreversible.[30,32,33] The long-term affective disorders following toxic encephalopathies are particularly difficult to treat, and they adversely affect recovery and prognosis.[34] To compensate for permanent impairments of behavior and cognitive function, treatment must include individualized recommendations for maintaining the patient's vocational and financial security. For example, a patient with a previously highly demanding, well-compensated job will require a vocational change and retraining to accommodate postexposure intellectual capabilities.[31]

Tetrachloroethylene

Acute exposure Acute exposure to tetrachloroethylene or perchloroethylene (PCE), a common solvent used in the dry cleaning industry, induces encephalopathy characterized by a sense of inebriation, dizziness, headache, drowsiness, nausea, and vomiting, and, at high concentrations, coma and death may occur.[35–39] The acute effects of PCE are related to formation of a metabolite, trichloroethanol.[5,18] Dry cleaning and degreasing shops should be properly ventilated, and ambient air levels of PCE should be determined regularly to reduce the risks of hazardous exposure. Handling of wet garments, which emit vapors of TCE, should be kept to a minimum and, then, only in well-ventilated areas. Persons using coin-operated dry cleaning machines should dry any damp items on a line that is in an open and well-ventilated area.[38,39] The 8-hour time-weighted-average ambient air concentration of PCE should not exceed 100 ppm.[19] Urinary excretion of the PCE metabolite trichloroacetic acid is used as an indicator of PCE absorption. The concentration of this metabolite in a urine sample taken before the last work shift of the week should not exceed 3.5 mg/L.[21]

Because inhalation of vapors is the main route of acute intake, displacing the PCE-contaminated air in the lungs with oxygen or fresh air (or both) is essential in the immediate care of an exposed person. Gastric lavage is the preferred method of eliminating residual quantities of the ingested solvent and should be performed as soon as possible after the solvent has been swallowed. Induced emesis (e.g., ipecac) may cause more vapor inhalation from the oropharynx or by aspiration of vomitus containing PCE. Because the elimination kinetics following oral and inhalation exposure are similar, hyperventilation of the patient can increase pulmonary excretion of PCE and any exhaled metabolites after PCE has been absorbed through the gastrointestinal tract.[36] Appropriate general supportive measures as well as specific interventions may be needed for cardiac arrhythmia, pulmonary edema, and vasomotor instability in susceptible persons. Hemodialysis may be necessary.[12,13]

Recovery from acute PCE intoxication depends on the intensity and duration of the exposure. Brief isolated acute exposures typically are not associated with residual neurological effects.[35–37]

Chronic exposure Chronic exposure to PCE may produce many of the symptoms of episodes of acute exposure because the body-burden of PCE and its metabolites accumulates over time. Symptoms may arise at times of peak exposures and at lower levels of exposure when there has been a background of ongoing or repeated contact (or both) with PCE.[40] Long-term low-level PCE exposures may result in mood and memory problems, suggesting a dementing illness.[41] It is important for clinicians to recognize the chronology of exposure events associated with the onset and progression of clinical signs and symptoms. A formal neuropsychological assessment with a comprehensive and standardized test battery usually is necessary to differentiate chronic toxic encephalopathy from a possible neurodegenerative process such as Alzheimer disease, which may produce similar neurological impairments. Estimates of recovery of patients with chronic PCE encephalopathy can vary according to time of follow-up between when exposure ended and the neurological tests were performed.[41,42] Long-term affective disorders following toxic encephalopathies are particularly difficult to treat, and they adversely affect the prognosis for recovery.[34] The persistent and often slowly resolving cognitive disabilities in PCE-exposed persons requires therapeutic approaches similar to those for patients with closed head injury. Anxiolytics and antidepressants are often necessary in conjunction with cognitive rehabilitation programs. Psychotherapy and family counseling to address adaptation and coping mechanisms and to minimize the patient's communication difficulties with family, friends, and coworkers are helpful. Vocational retraining may also be necessary. In some instances, permanent disability results from a severe memory disorder which persists after plateauing following whatever recovery has taken place during the 2 to 4 years following the cessation of exposure.[32,42,43]

Toluene

Acute exposure Toluene is a common organic solvent used in paints and thinners. The acute symptoms of toluene exposure include headache, dizziness, feeling of drunkenness, confusion, incoordination, nausea, vomiting, and unconsciousness and are attributable to the formation of benzyl alcohol.[44,45] The acute euphoria experienced when the vapors of toluene are inhaled make it a popular choice among paint and glue sniffers ("Huffers").[46] Occasional brief episodes of inhalation of toluene vapor produce transient, reversible symptoms and leave no neurological sequelae. However, repeated exposure, causes more permanent disturbances in cognition, memory, mood, and coordination.[47–49] Proper ventilation of work areas, monitoring of ambient air concentrations, and biological monitoring of employees at risk for increased exposure are necessary to prevent toluene intoxication. The urinary metabolite hippuric acid is used to detect exposure to toluene. Urinary levels of hippuric acid should not exceed 1.6 g/g creatinine at the end of the work shift.[21]

If toluene intoxication is detected, the person affected should be removed from further exposure and appropriate measures should be instituted to displace the toluene vapors from the lungs with noncontaminated sources of air or oxygen (or both). Acute neurological symptoms usually disappear after withdrawal from exposure, but cognitive impairments and emotional instabilities persist with repeated acute or chronic exposure.

Chronic exposure Recurrent episodes of acute toxic exposure, such as that related to inhaling the vapors of glues containing toluene ("Huffing") and the chronic low-level exposure experienced on the job, may cause cerebellar symptoms (e.g., nystagmus, intention tremor, head titubation, and truncal ataxia) and a cognitive syndrome characterized by irritability, apathy, and attention and memory deficits. These signs and symptoms of exposure develop insidiously and persist indefinitely after cessation of exposure to toluene.[27,32,50] Clonazepam can be used to treat intention tremor caused by toluene exposure.[51,52] Stereotactic coagulation of the left nucleus ventromedius of the thalamus abolished a persistent tremor in the right hand of a 22-year-old man with a 5-year history of toluene abuse. In this patient, magnetic resonance imaging showed lesions in the red nucleus, basal ganglia, and thalamus which were attributed to the toxic effects of toluene.[52] Although the treatment was successful in this patient, it is an invasive and aggressive procedure that should be considered only for patients who have a severe tremor that (1) interferes with activities of daily living, (2) has persisted at least for several years since documented cessation of exposure, (3) does not respond to pharmaceutical therapy, and (4) has been differentiated from a tremor of nontoxic cause. If formal neuropsychological assessment reveals deficits in specific cognitive functional domains, the remaining functional strengths can be exploited to compensate for deficits. This often requires treatment with antidepressants and anxiolytics as well as specialized psychological rehabilitative therapies and vocation retraining.[31]

n-Hexane and methyl n-butyl ketone

Acute exposure n-Hexane and MnBK are both metabolized to 2-hexanol in vivo. The percentage of 2-hexanol formed is substantially higher after intake of n-hexane than after intake of MnBK, which explains the greater ability of n-hexane to induce narcosis.[53,54] Emergency room personnel should be aware that the peripheral nervous system is affected by n-hexane and MnBK and, with recurrent exposure, unsuspecting glue sniffers are at risk for the development of peripheral neuropathy and central nervous system effects.

Employees and employers must be aware of the potential hazards associated with acute exposure to n-hexane or MnBK (or both). Workers who may have dermal contact with either compound should wear protective clothing and gloves to prevent dermal absorption.[55] Work areas where products containing n-hexane or MnBK are used should be well ventilated to prevent inhalation of vapors.[56] Respirators should be provided for workers who are at risk for acute exposure to high concentrations of either compound.

Acutely exposed persons complain of transient and reversible lightheadedness, dizziness, mucous membrane irritation, drowsiness, and fatigue. Hyperventilation with air or supplemental oxygen should be encouraged to displace the contaminated air from the lungs and to enhance respiratory elimination of the unmetabolized solvent. If the person is unconscious, intubation and the administration of oxygen are necessary. If liquid n-hexane or MnBK has been swallowed, stomach lavage should be performed immediately to empty the stomach of the solvent-containing contents, thus preventing further absorption. Hemodialysis and blood transfusion for acute renal or liver failure also may be necessary after acute oral intake. Hypotension must be treated with appropriate fluid and vasopressor medications. In cases of acute toxicity, clinicians must be alert to cardiac complications from changes in autonomic nervous system function.[57]

The acute narcotic effects of both n-hexane and MnBK disappear rapidly, with no residual sequelae. Recovery from an acute and subacute exposure to n-hexane or MnBK depends on the intensity and duration of the exposure.[58–62] Overlooking clinical symptoms and not removing the worker from further exposure until more overt manifestations of peripheral neuropathy appear, such as neurogenic muscle weakness and atrophy, may lead to greater permanent disability.

Chronic exposure To prevent the effects of chronic exposure, the ambient air concentration of n-hexane or MnBK should be monitored in the workplace and kept below 50 and 100 ppm, respectively.[19,20] Urine samples should be obtained from persons exposed to either compound regularly to analyze for the common metabolite 2,5-hexanedione. Although the American Conference of Governmental Industrial Hygienists has not established a biological exposure index for MnBK, the index for n-hexane can be used to monitor indirectly workers exposed to MnBK and to prevent the effects of chronic exposure because both solvents are metabolized to 2,5-hexanedione. Urinary levels of 2,5-hexanedione should not exceed 5 mg/g creatinine at the end of the work shift.[21]

Chronic exposure to *n*-hexane or MnBK is associated with the insidious paranodal accumulation of neurofilaments, myelin retraction, and a combination of axonal and demyelinating neuropathy.[11,60,63,64] Effective case management of persons exposed chronically to *n*-hexane or MnBK requires immediate removal from further exposure when clinical signs are first manifested, because early removal from exposure may prevent permanent damage to nerve fibers and result in better clinical recovery.[11,56] There is no known therapy to reverse the acute linking of neurofilaments, which causes the paranodal swelling and secondary demyelination, and, thus, to hasten recovery. Administration of vitamins B_{12} and B_6 does not promote recovery from 2,5-hexanedione exposure-induced neuropathy.[65] Residual gait disturbances and other signs of peripheral neuropathy may persist indefinitely.[61,62,66] Even after several years of absence from further exposure, return of function may be incomplete and activities of daily living may be difficult to perform.[56,58–61] The results of long-term exposure may interfere with a worker's ability to concentrate and to perform the job properly. Patients with permanent neurological impairment may require vocational retraining. Significant economic losses are associated with subsequent disability, loss of work, and the very long time needed for rehabilitation.

Carbon disulfide

Acute exposure Acute exposure to carbon disulfide results in transient symptoms of eye and mucous membrane irritation, nausea, irritability, headache, dizziness, hallucinations, and loss of consciousness.[32,67] Gloves, protective goggles, filtered facemask, and protective clothing should be worn to prevent eye contact, pulmonary irritation, and dermal absorption of the compound. Full self-contained respirators should be provided to workers who are at risk for exposure to high concentrations of carbon disulfide. Ambient air concentrations of carbon disulfide should be measured periodically, and workers should be monitored regularly for individual exposure dose. Ambient air levels should not exceed 20 ppm.[19] Urine concentrations of the carbon disulfide metabolite 2-thio-thiazolidine-4-carboxylic acid should not exceed 0.05 mg/g creatinine at the end of the work shift.[21]

Workers who excrete more than 150 μg of diethyldithiocarbamate per milligram creatinine in their urine after intake of a 0.5-g oral dose of disulfiram can be expected to have considerably fewer symptoms of carbon disulfide exposure than persons who excreted lower quantities of the compound.[68] This provocative test has been used to evaluate a person's ability to metabolize sulfur compounds,[68,69] but proper safety practices should make such screening unnecessary.

If acute exposure to a high concentration of carbon disulfide is suspected, the person should be moved immediately to a well-ventilated area. Contaminated exposed skin must be bathed thoroughly. Hyperventilation with fresh air or an oxygen supply increases displacement and elimination of carbon disulfide vapors. Controlled stomach lavage should be used to remove the stomach contents if liquid carbon disulfide has been ingested. Hemodialysis and blood transfusion for acute renal failure and liver dysfunction may be necessary after the compound has been ingested.

Chronic exposure Encephalopathy and overt symptoms of neuropathy, including denervation atrophy, have been reported in workers exposed to carbon disulfide.[70,71] Chronic exposure to carbon disulfide is associated with the accumulation of neurofilaments, paranodal swelling, and secondary demyelination.[11] Careful periodic monitoring of ambient air levels can prevent damage to the nervous system of workers chronically exposed to carbon disulfide.[71,72] The use of hemoglobin adducts to document the biochemical events occurring within an exposed person has been proposed as a novel biological marker not only for carbon disulfide exposure but also for its probable effects on the nervous system.[73]

Symptomatic pharmacological treatment may be needed for central nervous effects, including anxiety, sleeplessness, and even acute psychosis. The central nervous effects of carbon disulfide are related, in part, to its ability to alter levels of catecholamines.[74,75] The behavioral manifestations of carbon disulfide resemble the CNS effects of vitamin B_6 deficiency and have been attributed to the ability of carbon disulfide to deplete levels of vitamin B_6 (pyridoxine, pyridoxamine, and pyridoxal) and nicotinic acid.[76] Carbon disulfide has been shown to react with pyridoxamine, one of the two biologically active forms of vitamin B_6 (pyridoxal being the other), and to deplete the activity of pyridoxamine-dependent enzymes.[77] The association between these reactions and peripheral nervous system dysfunction in patients exposed to carbon disulfide has not been established; nevertheless, the empirical treatment with B-complex vitamins to correct carbon disulfide exposure-induced deficiencies is recommended for symptomatic patients with a history of carbon disulfide exposure.[78] Similarly, the prophylactic administration of B-complex vitamins to chronically exposed workers has possible pragmatic value. Workers in whom persistent symptoms, behavioral manifestations, or peripheral neuropathy develops after recurrent or chronic exposure to carbon disulfide need to be transferred to another job task to prevent further exposure.[31]

Acknowledgment

The author thanks Marcia H Ratner for her assistance with the preparation of this manuscript.

References

1. Astrand I. Uptake of solvents in the blood and tissues of man. A review. Scand J Work Environ Health 1975;1:199–218
2. Cohr KH, Stokholm J. Toluene. A toxicologic review. Scand J Work Environ Health 1979;5:71–90
3. Carlsson A. Exposure to toluene: uptake, distribution and elimination in man. Scand J Work Environ Health 1982;8:43–55

4. Brown HS, Bishop DR, Rowan CA. The role of skin absorption as a route of exposure for volatile organic compounds (VOCs) in drinking water. Am J Public Health 1984;74:479–484

5. Peoples RW, Weight FF. Trichloroethanol potentiation of gamma-aminobutyric acid-activated chloride current in mouse hippocampal neurones. Br J Pharmacol 1994;113:555–563

6. Parkki MG. The role of glutathione in the toxicity of styrene. Scand J Work Environ Health 1978;4 Suppl 2:53–59

7. Dixit R, Das M, Mushtaq M, et al. Depletion of glutathione content and inhibition of glutathione-S-transferase and aryl hydrocarbon hydroxylase activity of rat brain following exposure to styrene. Neurotoxicology 1982;3 no. 1:142–145

8. Srivastava SP, Das M, Seth PK. Enhancement of lipid peroxidation in rat liver on acute exposure to styrene and acrylamide a consequence of glutathione depletion. Chem Biol Interact 1983;45:373–380

9. Parke DV. Activation mechanisms to chemical toxicity. Arch Toxicol 1987;60:5–15

10. Trenga CA, Kunkel DD, Eaton DL, Costa LG. Effect of styrene oxide on rat brain glutathione. Neurotoxicology 1991;12:165–178

11. Graham DG, Amarnath V, Valentine WM, et al. Pathogenetic studies of hexane and carbon disulfide neurotoxicity. Crit Rev Toxicol 1995;25:91–112

12. Olivares Esquer J, Saldana Arevalo M, Garcia Torres R, Trevino Becerra A. Treatment using hemodialysis and exsanguination transfusion of acute renal failure, myopathy and toxic hepatitis, caused by trichloroacethylene. Report of a case and review of the literature [Spanish]. Prensa Med Mex 1974;39:461–467

13. Sasdelli M, Vagnoli E, Duranti E, et al. Treatment of acute "triline" poisoning by plasmapheresis and hemoperfusion. Int J Artif Organs 1986;9:195–196

14. Brent J, McMartin K, Phillips S, et al. Fomepizole for the treatment of ethylene glycol poisoning. Methylpyrazole for Toxic Alcohols Study Group. N Engl J Med 1999;340:832–838

15. Goldfrank LR, Flomenbaum NE. Toxic alcohols. In: Goldfrank LR, Flomenbaum NE, Lewin NA, et al., eds. Goldfrank's Toxicologic Emergencies. 6th ed. Stamford, Connecticut: Appleton & Lange, 1998:1049–1069

16. Feldman RG, Mayer RM, Taub A. Evidence for peripheral neurotoxic effect of trichloroethylene. Neurology 1970;20:599–606

17. Perbellini L, Olivato D, Zedde A, Miglioranzi R. Acute trichloroethylene poisoning by ingestion: clinical and pharmacokinetic aspects. Intensive Care Med 1991;17: 234–235

18. Peoples RW, Lovinger DM, Weight FF. Inhibition of excitatory amino acid currents by general anesthetic agents (abstract). Abstr Soc Neurosci 1990;16:1017

19. United States. National Archives and Records Administration. Code of Federal Regulations. Title 29—Labor, Vol 6, Part 1910.1000/.1047—Occupational Safety and Health Administration, Department of Labor, Washington, DC, revised July 1, 1995:411–431

20. United States. National Institute for Occupational Safety and Health. NIOSH Pocket Guide to Chemical Hazards (DHHS [NIOSH] publication no. 97–140). United States Department of Health and Human Services, Centers for Disease Control and Prevention, Washington, DC, 1997

21. American Conference of Governmental Industrial Hygienists. TLVs and BEIs: Threshold Limit Values for Chemical Substances and Physical Agents; Biological Exposure Indices. Cincinnati, Ohio: ACGIH Worldwide, 2001.

22. Buxton PH, Hayward M. Polyneuritis cranialis associated with industrial trichloroethylene poisoning. J Neurol Neurosurg Psychiatry 1967;30:511–518

23. Reichert D, Liebaldt G, Henschler D. Neurotoxic effects of dichloroacetylene. Arch Toxicol 1976;37:23–38

24. Szlatenyi CS, Wang RY. Encephalopathy and cranial nerve palsies caused by intentional trichloroethylene inhalation. Am J Emerg Med 1996;14:464–466

25. Köppel C, Lanz HJ, Ibe K. Acute trichloroethylene poisoning with additional ingestion of ethanol—concentrations of trichloroethylene and its metabolites during hyperventilation therapy. Intensive Care Med 1988;14: 74–76

26. White JF, Carlson GP. Epinephrine-induced cardiac arrhythmias in rabbits exposed to trichloroethylene: role of trichloroethylene metabolites. Toxicol Appl Pharmacol 1981;60:458–465

27. King MD, Day RE, Oliver JS, et al. Solvent encephalopathy. Br Med J 1981;283:663–665

28. Musclow CE, Wen CF. Glue sniffing: report of a fatal case. Can Med Assoc J 1971;104:315–319

29. Martinelli P, Gulli MR, Gabellini AS. Acute intoxication of trichloroethylene with complete recovery: a case report. Ital J Neurol Sci 1984;5:469

30. Feldman RG, White RF, Currie JN, et al. Long-term follow-up after single toxic exposure to trichloroethylene. Am J Ind Med 1985;8:119–126

31. White RF, Feldman RG, Proctor SP. Neurobehavioral effects of toxic exposure. In: White RF, ed. Clinical Syndromes in Adult Neuropsychology: The Practitioner's Handbook. Amsterdam: Elsevier, 1992:1–51

32. Feldman RG. Occupational and Environmental Neurotoxicology. Philadelphia: Lippincott-Raven Publishers, 1999

33. Kjellstrand P, Lanke J, Bjerkemo M, et al. Irreversible effects of trichloroethylene exposure on the central nervous system. Scand J Work Environ Health 1980; 6:40–47

34. Gregersen P, Angelso B, Nielsen TE, et al. Neurotoxic effects of organic solvents in exposed workers: an occupational, neuropsychological, and neurological investigation. Am J Ind Med 1984;5:201–225

35. Foot EB, Bishop K, Apgar V. Tetrachlorethylene as anesthesic agent. Anesthesiology 1943;4:283–292

36. Köppel C, Arndt I, Arendt U, Koeppe P. Acute tetrachloroethylene poisoning—blood elimination kinetics during hyperventilation therapy. J Toxicol Clin Toxicol 1985;23:103–115

37. Seiji K, Inoue O, Jin C, et al. Dose-excretion relationship in tetrachloroethylene-exposed workers and the effect of tetrachloroethylene co-exposure on trichloroethylene metabolism. Am J Ind Med 1989;16:675–684

38. Garnier R, Bédouin J, Pépin G, Gaillard Y. Coin-operated dry cleaning machines may be responsible for acute tetrachloroethylene poisoning: report of 26 cases including one death. J Toxicol Clin Toxicol 1996;34:191–197

39. Gaillard Y, Billault F, Pépin G. Tetrachloroethylene fatality: case report and simple gas chromatographic determination in blood and tissues. Forensic Sci Int 1995;76:161–168

40. Rozman KK, Klaassen CD. Absorption, distribution, and excretion of toxicants. In: Klaassen CD, ed. Casarett and Doull's Toxicology: The Basic Science of Poisons. 5th ed. New York: McGraw-Hill, 1996:91–112

41. Freed DM, Kandel E. Long-term occupational exposure and the diagnosis of dementia. Neurotoxicology 1988;9 no. 3:391–400

42. Echeverria D, White RF, Sampaio C. A behavioral evaluation of PCE exposure in patients and dry cleaners: a possible relationship between clinical and preclinical effects. J Occup Environ Med 1995;37:667–680

43. Gold JH. Chronic perchlorethylene poisoning. Can Psychiatr Assoc J 1969;14:627–630

44. Lee BK, Lee SH, Lee KM, et al. Dose-dependent increase in subjective symptom prevalence among toluene-exposed workers. Ind Health 1988;26:11–23

45. Williams JM, Howe NR. Benzyl alcohol attenuates the pain of lidocaine injections and prolongs anesthesia. J Dermatol Surg Oncol 1994;20:730–733

46. Hunnewell J, Miller NR. Bilateral internuclear ophthalmoplegia related to chronic toluene abuse. J Neuroophthalmol 1998;18:277–280

47. Metrick SA, Brenner RP. Abnormal brainstem auditory evoked potentials in chronic paint sniffers. Ann Neurol 1982;12:553–556

48. Gupta BN, Kumar P, Srivastava AK. An investigation of the neurobehavioural effects on workers exposed to organic solvents. J Soc Occup Med 1990;40:94–96

49. Foo SC, Jeyaratnam J, Ong CN, et al. Biological monitoring for occupational exposure to toluene. Am Ind Hyg Assoc J 1991;52:212–217

50. Knox JW, Nelson JR. Permanent encephalopathy from toluene inhalation. N Engl J Med 1966;275:1494–1496

51. Sodeyama N, Orimo S, Okiyama R, et al. A case of chronic thinner intoxication developing hyperkinesie volitionnelle three years after stopping thinner abuse. Rinsho Shinkeigaku 1993;33(2):213–215

52. Miyagi Y, Shima F, Ishido K, et al. Tremor induced by toluene misuse successfully treated by a Vim thalamotomy. J Neurol Neurosurg Psychiatry 1999;66:794–796

53. Haydon DA, Hendry BM, Levinson SR, Requena J. The molecular mechanisms of anaesthesia. Nature 1977; 268:356–358

54. Haydon DA, Hendry BM, Levinson SR, Requena J. Anaesthesia by the n-alkanes. A comparative study of nerve impulse blockage and the properties of black lipid bilayer membranes. Biochim Biophys Acta 1977; 470:17–34

55. Cardona A, Marhuenda D, Martí J, et al. Biological monitoring of occupational exposure to n-hexane by measurement of urinary 2,5-hexanedione. Int Arch Occup Environ Health 1993;65:71–74

56. Wang JD, Chang YC, Kao KP, et al. An outbreak of N-hexane induced polyneuropathy among press proofing workers in Taipei. Am J Ind Med 1986;10:111–118

57. Murata K, Araki S, Yokoyama K, et al. Changes in autonomic function as determined by ECG R-R interval variability in sandal, shoe and leather workers exposed to n-hexane, xylene and toluene. Neurotoxicology 1994;15 no. 4:867–875

58. Herskowitz A, Ishii N, Schaumburg H. N-hexane neuropathy. A syndrome occurring as a result of industrial exposure. N Engl J Med 1971;285:82–85

59. Shirabe T, Tsuda T, Terao A, Araki S. Toxic polyneuropathy due to glue-sniffing. Report of two cases with a light and electron-microscopic study of the peripheral nerves and muscles. J Neurol Sci 1974;21:101–113

60. Yokoyama K, Feldman RG, Sax DS, et al. Relation of distribution of conduction velocities to nerve biopsy findings in n-hexane poisoning. Muscle Nerve 1990; 13:314–320

61. Chang YC. Patients with n-hexane induced polyneuropathy: a clinical follow up. Br J Ind Med 1990;47: 485–489

62. Chang YC. An electrophysiological follow up of patients with n-hexane polyneuropathy. Br J Ind Med 1991;48:12–17

63. Ruff RL, Petito CK, Acheson LS. Neuropathy associated with chronic low level exposure to n-hexane. Clin Toxicol 1981;18:515–519

64. Barregård L, Sällsten G, Nordborg C, Gieth W. Polyneuropathy possibly caused by 30 years of low exposure to n-hexane. Scand J Work Environ Health 1991;17:205–207

65. Misumi J, Nagano M, Kaisaku J, Hitoshi T. Effects of vitamin B_{12} and B_6 on 2,5-hexanedione-induced neuropathy. Arch Toxicol 1985;56:204–206

66. Oryshkevich RS, Wilcox R, Jhee WH. Polyneuropathy due to glue exposure: case report and 16-year follow-up. Arch Phys Med Rehabil 1986;67:827–828

67. Lieben J, Williams RA. Five years of experience with CS_2. In: Xintaras C, Johnson BL, de Groot I, eds. Behavioral toxicology; early detection of occupational hazards (HEW publication no. [NIOSH] 74-126). United States Department of Health, Education & Welfare, Public Health Service, Center for Disease Control, National Institute for Occupational Safety and Health, Washington, DC, 1974:60–63

68. Besarabic M. Antabuse test and absenteeism in workers exposed to carbon disulfide. Arhiv za Higijenu Rada I Toksikologiju 1978;29:321–326

69. Djuric D, Postic-Grujin A, Graovac-Leposavic L, Delic V. Disulfiram as an indicator of human susceptibility to carbon disulfide. Excretion of diethyldithiocarbamate sodium in the urine of workers exposed to CS_2 after oral administration of disulfiram. Arch Environ Health 1973;26:287–289

70. Vigliani EC. Carbon disulphide poisoning in viscose rayon factories. Br J Ind Med 1954;11:235–244

71. De Fruyt P, Thiery E, De Bacquer D, Vanhoorne M. Neuropsychological effects of occupational exposures to carbon disulfide and hydrogen sulfide. Int J Occup Environ Health 1998;4:139–146

72. Reinhardt F, Drexler H, Bickel A, et al. Electrophysiological investigation of central, peripheral and autonomic nerve function in workers with long-term low-level exposure to carbon disulphide in the viscose industry. Int Arch Occup Environ Health 1997;70: 249–256

73. Harry GJ, Graham DG, Valentine WM, et al. Carbon disulfide neurotoxicity in rats: VIII. Summary. Neurotoxicology 1998;19:159–161

74. Bus JS. The relationship of carbon disulfide metabolism to development of toxicity. Neurotoxicology 1985;6 no. 4:73–80

75. Stanosz S, Kuligowski D, Pieleszek A, et al. Concentration of dopamine in plasma, activity of dopamine beta-hydroxylase in serum and urinary excretion of free catecholamines and vanillylmandelic acid in women chronically exposed to carbon disulphide. Int J Occup Med Environ Health 1994;7:257–261

76. Calabrese EJ. Nutrition and Environmental Health: The Influence of Nutritional Status on Pollutant Toxicity and Carcinogenicity. Vol 1. New York: Wiley, 1980: 164–171

77. Teisinger J. New advances in the toxicology of carbon disulfide. Am Ind Hyg Assoc J 1974;35:55–61

78. Maroni M, Colombi A, Gilioli R, et al. Effects of ganglioside therapy on experimental CS2 neuropathy. Clin Toxicol 1981;18:1475–1484

145 Treatment of the Neurotoxic Effects of Gases: Carbon Monoxide, Hydrogen Sulfide and the Nitrogen Oxides

Robert G Feldman and Marcia H Ratner

In a gaseous state, the cohesion forces between molecules are relatively small. Thus, in a gas, individual chemical molecules within the space they occupy are free to move about. The unique physical properties of gases explain the various effects these chemicals exhibit in environmental settings and in their medical applications. All gases, including neurotoxic ones, obey the physical laws for gases and thus are dependent upon pressure, volume and temperature. The ability of a gas to diffuse across biological membranes is dependent upon the partial pressure of the gas, temperature, and the size of the molecule. These variables affect the rate and amount of uptake of a gas by an exposed person.

Certain gases (e.g. argon, carbon dioxide, helium, methane) displace oxygen from the lungs and act as simple asphyxiants. The diminution of the normal supply of oxygen results in injury to the brain, which has a high oxygen demand and thus is particularly sensitive to the effects of asphyxiant-induced hypoxia.

Oxygen and carbon dioxide are two gases that are essential to the normal biological functions of all aerobic organisms, including humans. The respiratory process permits the exchange of these gases and others through the lungs in response to metabolic demands. Changes in respiratory rate may therefore reflect a person's metabolic status. For example, a patient with a metabolic acidosis may have acidemia (a blood pH less than 7.40), a decrease in their P_{CO_2}, and an increased respiratory rate (hyperventilation). The increased respiratory rate seen in this patient reflects the body's natural compensatory process designed to alleviate the acidosis and maintain a normal blood pH and P_{CO_2}.

Determination of a patient's blood concentrations of oxygen and carbon dioxide (i.e. P_{O_2} and P_{CO_2}), as well as their blood pH, bicarbonate, electrolytes, glucose, creatinine and blood urea nitrogen (BUN) levels and anion gap, is necessary in order to evaluate acid–base disorders and respiratory dysfunction. A metabolic acidosis is a change in a person's metabolic status characterized by a serum bicarbonate of less than 24 mEq/L with a P_{CO_2} less than 40 mmHg and a pH less than 7.40. By contrast, a respiratory acidosis is characterized by a serum bicarbonate greater than 24 mEq/L with a P_{CO_2} greater than 40 mmHg and a pH less than 7.40. A metabolic alkalosis is character-

ized by a pH greater than 7.40 and can be differentiated from a respiratory alkalosis by the serum bicarbonate and P_{CO_2} levels, which are greater than 24 mEq/L and 40 mmHg, respectively; in a respiratory alkalosis the serum bicarbonate is less than 24 mEq/L and the P_{CO_2} is less than 40 mmHg. A combination of acidosis and alkalosis may be seen in the same patient, and therefore assessment will require a complete history and consideration of the clinical complaints associated with the laboratory abnormalities. Treatment of the metabolic derangement (acidosis and/or alkalosis) must be initiated immediately regardless of the etiology (i.e. gas or solvent exposure, salicylate poisoning or renal dysfunction).

Inhaled gases within the respiratory tract may also induce damage to pulmonary tissues. Gases that penetrate deeply into the lungs produce toxic effects on lung tissues, including chemical pneumonitis and/or pulmonary edema, which often emerge after cessation of exposure and may decrease the arterial oxygen content and subsequently induce lactic acidosis due to the hypoxemia. Hydrogen sulfide is an example of a gas which, because of its chemical structure, produces respiratory and central nervous system symptoms. Pulmonary edema is a common manifestation of exposure to hydrogen sulfide due to the irritant effects of this gas. Edema interferes with the uptake of oxygen and thereby induces tissue hypoxemia, which may contribute to and/or exacerbate the neurological effects mediated by inhibition of cytochrome oxidase which is also associated with exposure to this neurotoxic gas. Relatively insoluble hydrophobic gases such as nitrogen dioxide produce pulmonary edema and symptoms of hypoxia at high concentrations, including headache, nausea and dizziness. These symptoms typically resolve after cessation of exposure.[1]

Therapeutic measures for selected gases

Specific therapeutic interventions are recommended in this chapter for three commonly encountered gases with neurotoxic effects. All patients with suspected exposures to gases should immediately be removed from the source of potentially toxic substances into an area with fresh air and, if possible, immediately provided with a source of 100% oxygen (O_2). Supportive measures, including endotracheal intubation and mechanical ventilation, should be administered to ensure adequate oxygenation of the blood. Arterial blood gas analysis should be performed. Measures to correct acidosis should be administered as necessary, based on the patient's blood gas analysis, serum pH, bicarbonate and electrolyte levels, and the anion gap. The presence of carboxyhemoglobin (COHb) or methemoglobin should be suspected if the measured O_2 saturation is lower than predicted by calculating the O_2 saturation from the partial pressure of O_2 (PO_2), and measures to increase oxygenation of the blood should be employed as necessary.

Carbon monoxide

Acute exposures Carbon monoxide (CO) displaces oxygen from the heme moiety of hemoglobin to form COHb. Impairment of the delivery of oxygen to tissues results in oxygen deprivation. The brain and heart are the first to be affected by acute CO exposure. Symptoms of low-level exposure may include headache, dizziness, difficulty in thinking and concentrating, drowsiness, weakness, fatigue, nausea, vomiting, irritability, hyperventilation and increased heart rate. The symptoms of lower-level acute exposure are mild and reversible upon removal from the source. With continued exposure, blood COHb levels increase further and the severity of these early symptoms increases, and others, including chest pain, loss of consciousness and even death, emerge. Exposure to high levels of CO can cause severe central nervous system edema and necrosis. Permanent neurological effects result from cerebral edema and necrosis[2] (Figure 145..1).

When CO contamination of an area is suspected all persons at risk of exposure should immediately be removed from the source of the gas and placed in a well-ventilated area. Oxygen should be administered by mask as soon as possible. Hypotension is a common clinical manifestation of carbon monoxide poisoning, which should be treated with intravenous fluids.[3] Unconscious patients require endotracheal intubation and mechanical ventilation with an oxygen supply. Cardiac monitoring is recommended for all patients exposed to CO. Patients with severe exposure or pre-existing coronary artery disease should receive (along with cardiac monitoring) a 12-lead electrocardiogram (ECG), as this is essential in documenting ischemia or dysrrhythmias.

A blood sample must be obtained as soon as possible to measure the COHb level. A COHb level greater than 5% indicates exposure to carbon monoxide. The timing of blood sampling and determining COHb level in relation to oxygen administration should be taken into consideration when interpreting the laboratory results. Administration of oxygen before a blood COHb level is obtained will normalize the level. Blood gases (PO_2 and PCO_2), pH, and serum electrolyte and bicarbonate levels and anion gap should also be determined. Blood pH and PCO_2 are typically decreased in those patients presenting with carbon monoxide poisoning, indicating a metabolic acidosis. Any patient who is not responding to 100% oxygen and/or who has a COHb level of greater than 20% may respond to hyperbaric oxygen therapy. Hyperbaric oxygen can be used in pregnant women without consequence and

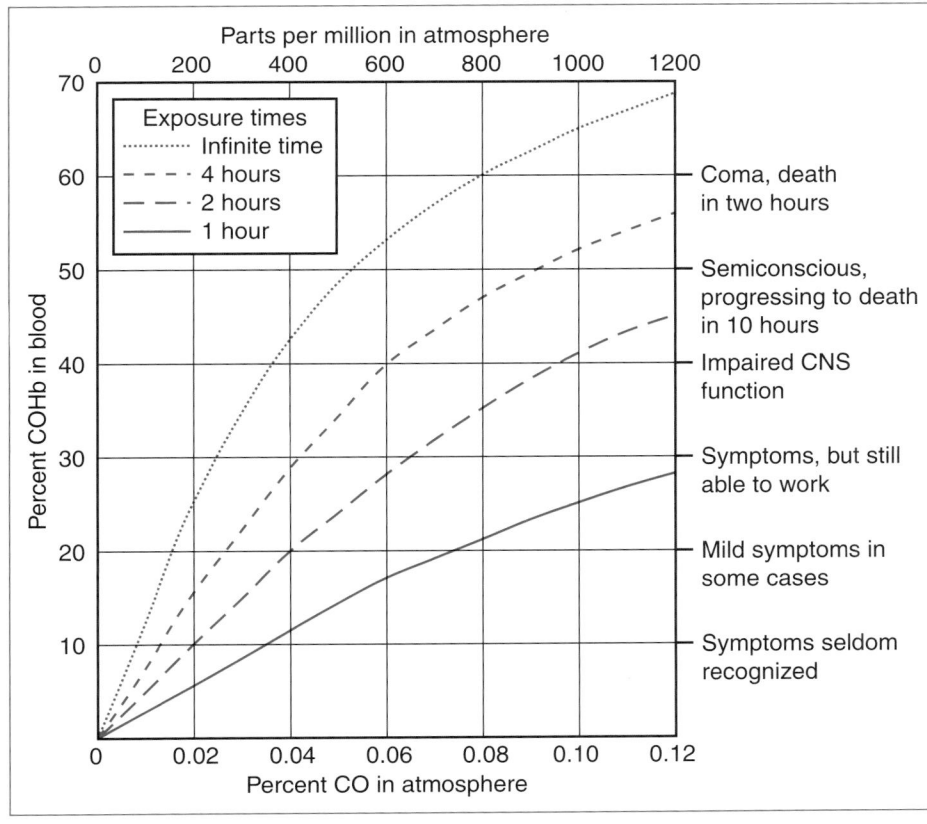

Figure 145..1 Relationships between clinical manifestations, percent carboxyhemoglobin in blood, and atmospheric carbon monoxide levels after 1, 2 and 4 hours, and an infinite duration of exposure to carbon monoxide. (Modified from Forbes, 1970 with permission)

thus should be administered to all pregnant women exposed to CO to reduce the risk of injury to the fetus.

In addition to hemoglobin, CO binds to the heme moieties in other enzymes, including those in myoglobin and cytochrome oxidase. CO inactivates cytochrome oxidase and disrupts cellular respiration. Patients exposed to other inhibitors of cytochrome oxidase, such as hydrogen sulfide, may benefit from administration of sodium nitrite as well as hyperbaric oxygen but this should be used with caution. Sodium nitrite generates methemoglobin, which acts as a scavenger of hydrogen sulfide to reduce its toxicity by removing it from the heme moiety of cytochrome oxidase, permitting aerobic respiration to resume.[4] However, the therapeutic use of sodium nitrite in the management of patients exposed to CO only will not improve the clinical outcome because it does not have any significant impact on the CO bound to the heme moiety of cytochrome oxidase. Furthermore, the methemoglobin generated by administration of sodium nitrite to those patients exposed to CO only may contribute to the adverse neurological effects by reducing the ability of hemoglobin to carry oxygen to tissues where it is needed. The clinical utility of sodium nitrite in the management of persons suffering from the inhalation of smoke, which may include cyanide as well as carbon monoxide, has not been fully elucidated.[5]

Caution must be used in estimating prognosis after acute treatment for CO poisoning. Some patients exposed to CO will develop neurological symptoms after a period of "pseudo" recovery. Symptoms re-emerge as soon as 2 but as many as 20 days after cessation of exposure and include paralysis, dementia, peripheral neuropathy, psychosis, chorea, parkinsonism and incontinence. One explanation for this delayed effect has been the binding of glutamate to N-methyl-D-aspartate (NMDA) receptors, which promotes an increase in intracellular calcium that subsequently induces cell death via apoptosis. The efficacy of the therapeutic administration of NMDA receptor blockers to patients with elevated blood COHb levels in preventing the occurrence of delayed neurological effects of carbon monoxide poisoning has not been fully elucidated in humans. However, studies in animals indicate that pretreatment with non-competitive NMDA receptor antagonists (e.g. MK-801) prevents delayed neurological sequelae.[6,7] Those CO-exposed patients who lose consciousness typically have the poorest prognosis.

The parkinsonian symptoms associated with exposure to CO are often refractory to treatment, but may also remain relatively stable after cessation of exposure. Neuroimaging studies often reveal areas of demyelination and neuronal loss in the globus pallidus. Therefore, response to dopaminergic therapy (e.g. levodopa) is equivocal at best, because cellular structures downstream from the dopamine-producing cells of the substantia nigra, such as the neurons of the globus pallidus, are affected.[2]

Chronic exposures Symptoms of chronic exposure to CO are similar to those seen in acute low-level expo-

sure and may include memory disturbances, emotional liability, aphasia, personality disturbances, seizures, cardiac arrhythmia and angina, and parkinsonism. These symptoms emerge insidiously with chronic or repeated intermittent exposures. This may at first be attenuated or ameliorated during periods away from the source of exposure, but eventually they become more severe until they persist even during extended periods away from the source. Patients with parkinsonism due to chronic CO exposure typically do not exhibit a good response to levodopa.[2]

Hydrogen sulfide

Acute exposure Hydrogen sulfide poisoning should be suspected in those found unconscious in any area where there is the smell of rotten eggs, and particularly if the patient works in an industry where exposure to hydrogen sulfide is likely to occur, such as a petroleum refinery, tannery or paper mill, or where there is escaping sewer gas.

Acute exposures to hydrogen sulfide (e.g. sewer gas) are associated with knockdowns: these sudden collapses and drop attacks are characterized by an abrupt loss of consciousness due to central nervous system depression and loss of muscle tone. Death frequently results from disruption of the functioning of cells located in the brainstem respiratory center and heart. Pulmonary edema due to the irritant effects of the hydrogen sulfide occurs and contributes to the overall clinical picture of respiratory dysfunction, and may contribute to tissue hypoxia.

All persons involved in the rescue of an individual exposed to hydrogen sulfide should wear a respirator with a self-contained breathing apparatus. Entering an area with increased ambient air levels of hydrogen sulfide without an oxygen source is extremely dangerous and may result in severe injury or death to the rescue personnel before they can help the original victim.

Management of hydrogen sulfide poisoning includes the immediate removal of the patient from the source of exposure. Oxygen should be administered immediately. Begin monitoring cardiac function as soon as possible after the patient is removed from the source of exposure, as tachycardia and arrhythmias may need treatment. Advanced life support measures should be administered as necessary. Patients presenting with severe acidosis, respiratory arrest and seizures, severe agitation or coma should be intubated to secure an adequate airway. Acidosis and hypotension should be corrected. Convulsions may occur in association with hypoxia due to acute exposure to hydrogen sulfide. These may resolve spontaneously with the administration of oxygen, or may require intravenous diazepam (10 mg).

Hydrogen sulfide inhibits the activity of cytochrome oxidase, an enzyme essential for cellular aerobic respiration, and thereby induces tissue hypoxia. Inhibition of cytochrome oxidase activity disrupts oxidative phosphorylation and hence the generation of the ATP essential for all cellular processes. The disruption of cellular respiration induces an influx of calcium that triggers programmed cell death via apoptosis, which accounts in part for the delayed effects seen after cessation of exposure among those who survive the acute effects.

Emergency pharmacological interventions include sodium nitrite (3% $NaNO_2$) to induce the formation of methemoglobin, which acts as a scavenger of hydrogen sulfide and thus acts as an antidote by preventing its binding with cytochrome oxidase.[8] Sodium nitrite should be administered intravenously over a 15-minute period. Normal adult dose is 10 mL (300 mg). Blood pressure should be monitored constantly during treatment, and a methemoglobin level should be obtained 30 minutes after dosing. Hyperbaric oxygen has been used in cases of hydrogen sulfide poisoning and is recommended if available, as it may improve prognosis in some patients.[4]

Survivors of a hydrogen sulfide knockdown may have abnormal findings on pulmonary function tests and persistent symptoms of central nervous system dysfunction, including parkinsonism and encephalopathy. Brain CT scans and MRI studies may reveal areas of demyelination and neuronal loss in the globus pallidus and putamen. The parkinsonian symptoms should be treated supportively. The clinical efficacy of dopaminergic therapy (e.g. levodopa) in treating patients exposed to hydrogen sulfide is limited owing to the involvement of structures that are neurochemically located downstream from the dopamine-producing cells of the substantia nigra. Patients with parkinsonism or memory deficits and other behavioral problems due to encephalopathy may require vocational retraining.[9,10]

Chronic exposures Low-level chronic exposures to hydrogen sulfide are associated with non-specific symptoms of irritation of the eyes and mucous membranes, shortness of breath, dizziness, headache, chest tightness and pain, nausea and vomiting. These symptoms often improve when the subject is away from the source of exposure; the temporal pattern of symptom severity may reveal clues as to the location of the source. Low-level exposures do not produce the overt knockdown that characterizes higher-level exposures, but can lead to cell loss in those areas of the central nervous system with high oxygen demands. Encephalopathy and parkinsonism are rare complications of chronic low-level hydrogen sulfide poisoning, but may occur as a result of the disruption of aerobic metabolism in neurons with high oxygen demand. Olfactory dysfunction has also been reported among workers with chronic exposure to hydrogen sulfide.[11]

Patients with encephalopathy may require vocational retraining and psychological counseling. The clinical efficacy of levodopa in treating patients with parkinsonism due to hydrogen sulfide is limited, and the effect of dopamine receptor agonists is undetermined.

Nitrogen oxides

Acute exposures The nitrogen oxides include nitric oxide (NO), nitrogen dioxide (NO_2) and nitrous oxide (N_2O). All of the nitrogen oxides cause tissue hypoxia by displacing atmosphere and ambient sources of air containing oxygen. Once absorbed through the lungs and into the bloodstream, nitric oxide or nitrogen dioxide induce the formation of methemoglobin by transforming the iron in heme from ferrous (Fe^{2+}) to ferric (Fe^{3+}). Methemoglobin is incapable of binding and releasing oxygen molecules; elevated methemoglobin levels lead to tissue hypoxia. Nitric oxide and nitrogen dioxide also damage lung tissue and impair the transport of oxygen across the pulmonary alveoli, thus resulting in hypoxemia. Acute exposure to nitric oxide and nitrogen dioxide is associated with eye irritation, headache, dizziness, dyspnea, chest pain, confusion, incoordination, weakness, nausea and vomiting. High-level exposures are associated with cyanosis, seizures, coma and death.

Treatment of poisoning by nitrogen oxide gases includes immediate removal of the exposed individual from the source of the gas. Oxygen should be administered and the patient treated supportively. Comatose patients should be intubated, and bronchodilators should be administered as necessary to reduce bronchoconstriction and enhance the delivery of oxygen. Methylene blue should be administered i.v. over three to five minutes at an initial dose of 2 mg/kg to those patients presenting with methemoglobinemia (NB: methylene blue should not be given to patients with a deficiency in glucose-6-phosphate dehydrogenase or methemoglobin reductase). If the patient remains symptomatic this initial dose can be followed with a dose of 1 mg/kg. The total dose administered during the first three to four hours should not exceed 7 mg/kg.[12] Hyperbaric oxygen followed by blood transfusions may be a life-saving measure in these patients. Metabolic acidosis may occur and should be treated as necessary.

Mild cases of *nitric oxide* and *nitrogen dioxide* poisoning show good clinical recovery within hours of cessation of exposure. Corticosteroids should be administered to reduce the delayed and subacute respiratory effects of exposure to nitric oxide that often appear after successive periods of pseudo recovery, and which include pulmonary edema and bronchiolitis. The course of corticosteroids should be approximately eight weeks, including a gradual tapering-off period.

Nitrous oxide is a naturally occurring gas with a sweet odor that is commonly used as an anesthetic agent ("laughing gas"). The possibility of exposure to nitrous oxide is greatest among individuals who work in the dental profession, where it is used as an anesthetic agent. Nitrous oxide produces acute narcosis by activation of mesocortical dopaminergic projections.[13] Persistent neurological problems after acute exposure may include encephalopathy and a combination of myelopathy with distal axonopathy (myeloneuropathy). The clinical features of nitrous oxide-induced myeloneuropathy closely resemble those of combined systems disease due to vitamin B_{12} deficiency; the peripheral neuropathy is, however, more pronounced in the nitrous oxide syndrome than it is when due to B_{12} deficiency.

The explanation for the neurotoxic effects of nitrous oxide is its interference with vitamin B_{12} (cobalamin) metabolism. Vitamin B_{12} is essential to DNA synthesis and to the maintenance of the myelin sheath by the methylation of myelin basic protein. Active vitamin B_{12} contains cobalt in its reduced form (Co^+). Nitrous oxide forms complexes with the cobalt in methylcobalamin (the cofactor for methionine synthase), resulting in irreversible oxidation of this cofactor and inactivation of the enzyme.[14]

Parenteral (intramuscular) vitamin B_{12} should be administered to patients suspected of having nitrous oxide poisoning. A baseline blood level of B_{12} should be obtained before initiating B_{12} therapy. Normal plasma values of vitamin B_{12} range from 200 to 750 pg/mL. Patients with low or marginal B_{12} depots (<250 pg/mL) prior to exposure may be at greater risk for neurological sequelae, including myeloneuropathy, following nitrous oxide anesthesia. Prophylactic administration of vitamin B_{12} (3.0–6.0 μg/day) beginning several weeks before surgery is recommended for higher-risk groups such as the elderly, to reduce the risk of neurotoxic effects.[15] The Shilling test, which measures the absorption of radioactive vitamin B_{12} with and without intrinsic factor, can be used to confirm the diagnosis of B_{12} deficiency, an intrinsic factor problem, or poor gastrointestinal absorption of the vitamin.

Symptoms of poisoning emerge within two weeks to two months after exposure. Vitamin B_{12} (500–1000 μg i.m.) should be given two to four times per week until hematological abnormalities are corrected. The hematological symptoms typically improve within six weeks, but the neurological deficits may persist indefinitely. Nerve conduction studies can be used to objectively document the patient's clinical recovery.

Chronic exposures Chronic exposure to the nitrogen oxides occurs among silo workers, dental professionals, anesthesiologists, and those who use nitrous oxide recreationally to achieve euphoric states of mind.

Treatment for the effects of chronic exposure begins with the immediate cessation of exposure. Patients presenting with posterior column myeloneuropathy after chronic exposure to nitrous oxide should be administered vitamin B_{12} and treated supportively.[16] Methionine treatment may be beneficial in some cases of chronic nitrogen oxide poisoning. Vitamin B_{12} is essential for converting L-methylmalonyl coenzyme A into succinyl coenzyme A, and for the formation of methionine by methylation of homocysteine ethionine, and therefore supplemental administration of methionine (13 mg/kg/day) is recommended for patients who develop myeloneuropathy after exposure to nitrous oxide.

Acknowledgements

The authors would like to thank Ms Paulette Allen, Program in Biomedical Laboratory and Clinical Sciences, Boston University School of Medicine and Metropolitan College, for her assistance with the preparation of this manuscript.

References

1. Lipsett MJ, Shusterman DJ, Beard RR. Inorganic compounds of carbon, nitrogen and oxygen. In: Clayton GD, Clayton FE, eds. Patty's Industrial Hygiene and Toxicology, 4th edn. New York: John Wiley & Sons, 1994:4523–4643
2. Feldman RG. Carbon monoxide. In: Occupational and Environmental Neurotoxicology. Philadelphia: Lippincott-Raven, 1999:378–399
3. Tomaszewski C. Carbon monoxide. In: Goldfrank LR, Flomenbaum NE, Lewin NA, Weisman RS, Howland MA, Hoffman RS, eds. Goldfrank's Toxicologic Emergencies, 6th edn. Stanford, Appleton & Lange, 1998: 1551–1568
4. Vicas IMO. Hydrogen sulfide. In: Haddad LM, Shannon MW, Winchester JF, eds. Clinical Management of Poisoning and Drug Overdose, 3rd edn. Philadelphia: WB Saunders, 1998:906–912
5. Moore SJ, Norris JC, Walsh DA, Hume AS. Antidotal use of methemoglobin forming cyanide antagonists in concurrent carbon monoxide/cyanide intoxication. J Pharmacol Exp Ther 1987;242:70–73
6. Ishimaru H, Nabeshima T, Katoh A, Suzuki H, Fukuta T, Kameyama T. Effects of successive carbon monoxide exposures on delayed neuronal death in mice under the maintenance of normal body temperature. Biochem Biophys Res Commun 1991;179:836–840
7. Liu Y, Fechter LD. MK-801 protects against carbon monoxide-induced hearing loss. Toxicol Appl Pharmacol 1995;132:196–202
8. Hall AH, Rumack BH. Hydrogen sulfide poisoning: an antidotal role for sodium nitrite? Vet Hum Toxicol 1997;39:152–154
9. White RF, Feldman RG, Proctor SP. Neurobehavioral effects of toxic exposures. In: White RF, ed. Clinical Syndrome in Adult Neuropsychology. New York: Elsevier 1992;1–51.
10. Kerns WP, Kirk MA. Cyanide and hydrogen sulfide. In: Goldfrank LR, Flomenbaum NE, Lewis NA, Weisman RS, Howland MA, Hoffman RS, eds. Goldfrank's Toxicologic Emergencies, 6th edn. Stanford: Appleton and Lange, 1998:1569–1582
11. Hirsch AR, Zavala G. Long-term effects on the olfactory system of exposure to hydrogen sulphide. Occup Environ Med 1999;56:284–287
12. Dotsch J, Demirakca S, Kratz M, Repp R, Knerr I, Rascher W. Comparison of methylene blue, riboflavin, and N-acetylcysteine for the reduction of nitric oxide-induced methemoglobinemia. Crit Care Med 2000;28:958–961
13. Scelsa SN. Nitrous oxide. In: Spencer PS, Schaumburg HH, Ludolph AC, eds. Experimental and Clinical Neurotoxicology, 2nd ed. New York: Oxford University Press, 2000:882–889
14. Flippo TS, Holder WD. Neurologic degeneration associated with nitrous oxide anesthesia in patients with vitamin B12 deficiency. Arch Surg 1993;128: 1391–1395
15. Lindstedt G. Nitrous oxide can cause cobalamin deficiency. Vitamin B12 is a simple and cheap remedy. Lakartidningen 1999;96:4801–4805
16. Butzkueven H, King JO. Nitrous oxide myelopathy in an abuser of whipped cream bulbs. J Clin Neurosci 2000;7:73–75

146 Pesticides

Christopher G Goetz and Steven L Lewis

Introduction

Pesticides are agents used deliberately to kill organisms. They include agents that kill insects (*insecticides*), plants (*herbicides*) and rodents (*rodenticides*). The utility of the insecticides that are currently marketed is based on the greater relative toxicity of these chemicals towards pests than to humans and most other animals. However, significant neurological toxic effects from some of these agents can occur, particularly among workers involved in their manufacture and use, as well as among individuals who intentionally or unintentionally expose themselves to these compounds. Toxicity from bipyridyl herbicide exposure is primarily pulmonary,[1] with only rare reports of toxicity from chlorophenoxy herbicides causing neurological symptoms in the setting of severe systemic toxicity.[2,3] The rodenticides with significant primary neurological toxicity are strychnine and crimidine, powerful convulsants,[4] but these are now rarely used and are no longer marketed in the United States. This chapter will therefore focus on the insecticides.

The major classes of insecticides are the organophosphates and carbamates, the organochlorine insecticides and the botanical insecticides. The organophosphate and carbamate insecticides are the most commonly used insecticides in the world.[5,6] These agents are a very important cause of neurological toxicity, due primarily to their ability to inhibit acetylcholinesterase. The organochlorine insecticides, of which dichlorodiphenyltrichloroethane (DDT) is a prototype, have been largely banned in the United States.[7] Because of their persistence in the environment and the food chain, their use is strictly controlled in most countries.[8] However, lindane, an organochlorine derivative, continues to be used as an insecticide and as a topical treatment and shampoo for the treatment of scabies and head lice. The botanical insecticides, which are produced from natural sources, are very common household and garden insecticides. They include the pyrethroids, which are prepared from chrysanthemum flowers, and rotenone, which is prepared from the roots of certain plant species.[8]

Epidemiology of insecticide toxicity

The American Association of Poison Control Centers reported approximately 59 000 cases of insecticide exposure in 1999, of which approximately 17 500 were to organophosphate or carbamate insecticides.[9]

Exposure to pesticides can occur occupationally or otherwise, or because of accidental or intentional ingestion. Those at greatest risk from occupational exposure include individuals involved in the manufacture and transport of these compounds, and those involved in their use, including farm workers and farm families, veterinary workers, gardeners, and pest-control workers.[10] Children can also be exposed when pets are treated for pests.[5] Accidental ingestion can occur as a result of storage of compounds in poorly labeled containers, or by intentional poisoning by another individual. Intentional ingestion of pesticides as a suicide attempt is an important and common cause of poisoning in some countries. For example, the frequency of suicide attempts due to organophosphate ingestion in India, Germany, England and Wales allowed investigators in those countries to extensively study the neurophysiological effects of these compounds.[11-14]

Mass human exposure to organophosphates in particular has occurred in various parts of the world owing to contamination of food or beverages, or to exposure in the form of organophosphate nerve gases. In 1995, mass exposure to the organophosphate nerve gas sarin, from a terrorist attack on the Tokyo subway, killed 12 and injured 5000 others.[15] Exposure to organophosphate compounds in the form of triarylphosphates, currently used as plasticizers and lubricants, can occur. The epidemic known as Jamaica ginger paralysis occurred in the United States in 1930 as a result of contamination of an illicit alcoholic beverage with triorthocresyl phosphate, a triaryl phosphate lubricant.[16] In that epidemic an estimated 20 000 people were affected.[17]

Etiology of insecticide-related neurotoxicity

Not all classes of pesticide have clinically significant neurological toxicity. Even among the organophosphates, compounds can vary in their potential for neurological or systemic toxicity. The organophosphates are the most important pesticides causing clinical neurotoxicity, owing to the common use of these compounds, their specific effects as acetylcholinesterase inhibitors, their late sequelae, and the treatment used to counteract their toxicity. Organophosphate insecticides are rapidly absorbed through dermal, respiratory, gastrointestinal and conjunctival routes.[5] The most important route of occupational exposure is via skin contamination and dermal absorption.[10]

Lindane, the most commonly available pesticide of the organochlorine class, can cause neurotoxicity after ingestion, prolonged or excessive dermal exposure, and increased absorption through abraded skin.[5,18]

The botanical insecticides are generally very safe.[5,19] Only a few reports document significant neurological or systemic toxicity from pyrethrins. Local transient paresthesias from dermal exposure to pyrethrins are, however, common.[20,21] The botanical insecticide rotenone has also been considered to be without significant acute neurological toxicity; however, rotenone infusion in rats produced a syndrome resembling Parkinson's disease, both behaviorally and neuropathologically.[22,23]

Pathophysiology of neurotoxicity form insecticides

Organophosphate and carbamate insecticides

The organophosphate insecticides inhibit acetylcholinesterase, leading to excess acetylcholine at cholinergic synapses throughout the peripheral and central nervous system. This causes excess cholinergic stimulation and often depolarization blockade, both responsible for much of the clinical symptomatology of toxicity from these compounds.[24] In the peripheral nervous system acetylcholine is the neurotransmitter at the parasympathetic and sympathetic ganglia (primarily nicotinic), at postganglionic parasympathetic nerve endings (muscarinic), at a few postganglionic (muscarinic) sympathetic nerve endings such as sweat glands, and at the neuromuscular junction (nicotinic).[25]

Organophosphates are considered "irreversible" acetylcholinesterase inhibitors. Their action occurs via phosphorylation of the enzyme, and the stability and irreversibility of the phosphorylated enzyme is further enhanced through a process known as "aging", which occurs as a result of loss of an alkyl group from the phosphorylated enzyme.[24] Aging takes 24–48 hours.[5] Before aging has occurred the process is still reversible by treatment with the acetylcholinesterase reactivator pralidoxime, which regenerates active enzyme.[5,24] After aging has occurred, active enzyme can only be produced through new protein synthesis.

In the acute syndrome of organophosphate intoxication, muscarinic effects usually dominate the clinical symptomatology, although nicotinic effects at the neuromuscular junction (such as fasciculations, cramps and weakness) are also seen. Sometimes, days after the onset of acute organophosphate poisoning, as the muscarinic effects are resolving, predominant nicotinic effects at the neuromuscular junction cause more severe weakness; this has sometimes been referred to as the intermediate syndrome.[12,26]

In addition to their effect on acetylcholinesterase at nerve endings and ganglia, organophosphate insecticides also inhibit an enzyme called neuropathy target esterase (NTE), an integral membrane protein found in all neurons.[27] Inhibition of NTE occurs by a process analogous to the inhibition of acetylcholinesterase, by phosphorylation and rapid "aging" of the phosphorylated enzyme by loss of an alkyl group. This is felt to be the cause of the delayed central and peripheral axonopathy, called organophosphate-induced delayed neurotoxicity (OPIDN), that has been seen after intoxication by some organophosphates.[27,28] The pathological lesion of OPIDN is a distal axonopathy that preferentially affects large-diameter long fibers of the peripheral and central nervous systems.[17,28] Degeneration of the anterior columns of the thoracic and lumbar spinal cord has been described.[28] Fortunately, not all organophosphates produce significant inhibition of NTE or clinical OPIDN. The potential for NTE inhibition and OPIDN is screened for in animal models,[17,28] and most pesticides with known clinical neuropathic potential in man have been screened out of the market.[27]

Carbamate insecticides also inhibit acetylcholinesterase. However, carbamates act via transient, reversible carbamoylation of acetylcholinesterase, resulting in a shorter duration and a more benign clinical syndrome than with organophosphates.[10] In addition, unlike organophosphates, carbamates penetrate the central nervous system poorly.[5]

Organochlorine insecticides

The organochlorine insecticides produce toxic effects primarily via a generalized increase in neuronal excitability, inducing repetitive axonal discharges to single stimuli in experimental models.[29] There is evidence that a major action of these compounds is antagonism of γ-aminobutyric acid (GABA) receptor-mediated inhibition.[29,30]

Botanical insecticides

Although significant neurotoxicity is rare, the pyrethroid insecticides are sodium channel toxins. The major site of action is the voltage-dependent sodium channel, slowing the activation and inactivation properties of the channel and leading to hyperexcitability.[19–21] The other major botanical insecticide, rotenone, although without significant known human toxicity at normal concentrations in normal use,[5] was chosen for a study of toxin-induced parkinsonism in rats because it is an inhibitor of complex I, an enzyme involved in oxidative phosphorylation.[22]

Clinical features of insecticide toxicity

Organophosphate and carbamate insecticides

The timing of onset and the severity of symptoms of organophosphate toxicity depend upon the toxicity of the specific agent, the amount of exposure and the route of exposure. The onset of symptoms generally occurs within 12 hours of exposure.[5,31] Table 146.1 lists some commonly available organophosphate insecticides.

The acute clinical features of toxicity from organophosphate insecticides relate to their effect on inhibition of acetylcholinesterase, and the symptoms and signs can reflect both muscarinic and nicotinic dysfunction due to involvement of the various levels of the nervous system in which acetylcholine is the neurotransmitter (Table 146.2). The mnemonic SLUDGE has been suggested to remember the prominent parasympathetic muscarinic effects that may dominate the acute clinical picture: salivation, lacrimation, urination, diarrhea, gastrointestinal

Table 146.1 Some common organophosphate insecticides

Acephate
Azinphos-methyl
Bromophos
Carbophenothion
Chlorpyrifos
Coumaphos
Crotoxyphos
Demeton
Diazinon
Dichlorofenthion
Dichlorvos
Dicrotophos
Dimethoate
Dioxathion
Disulfoton
EPN
Ethion
Fenamiphos
Fensulfothion
Fonofos
Fosamine ammonium
Malathion
Methamidophos
Methomyl
Methyl parathion
Mevinphos
Monocrotophos
Naled
Parathion
Phorate
Phosalone
Phosphamidon
Phosmet
Schradan
Temephos
Terbufos
Trichlorfon
Zinofos

Table 146.2 Signs and symptoms of organophosphate toxicity

*Muscarinic effects**
Bradycardia, hypotension†
Excessive sweating, salivation and tearing
Miosis, blurred vision
Nausea, vomiting, abdominal cramps, diarrhea
Urinary incontinence
Wheezing, bronchial constriction

Nicotinic effects
Neuromuscular junction: fasciculations, cramps, weakness
Sympathetic ganglia: tachycardia, hypertension†

Central nervous system effects
Anxiety, confusion
Ataxia
Coma
Convulsions
Depression
Headaches
Insomnia
Respiratory and circulatory depression
Slurred speech
Tremor

* The mnemonic SLUDGE is helpful to remember the muscarinic effects of organophosphate toxicity: salivation, lacrimation, urination, diarrhea, gastrointestinal distress and emesis.
†The blood pressure and pulse of the patient will depend on the relative balance of parasympathetic effects and sympathetic ganglia effects.

distress and emesis.[32] Other acute muscarinic effects include miosis, bronchial hypersecretion and bronchoconstriction, urinary and fecal incontinence, and cardiac dysfunction, especially bradycardia. Although the predominant autonomic signs are usually related to muscarinic stimulation, sympathetic signs such as mydriasis or tachycardia can be present as well, owing to dysfunction at the sympathetic autonomic ganglia.[31,32] Acute nicotinic effects at the neuromuscular junction cause muscle cramping, fasciculations and weakness, including weakness of respiration. The combination of weakness with increased bronchial secretions and bronchoconstriction is an important cause of respiratory failure.[10]

Central nervous system symptoms can vary. In mild intoxication patients may be alert. More severe intoxication can lead to more severe symptoms, including anxiety, restlessness, tremor, ataxia, seizures or coma.[5,31]

Profound weakness may be seen in some patients during the illness and may relate to depolarization blockade at the neuromuscular junction. This weakness usually develops after a delay of 24–96 hours after the onset of poisoning, during or after resolution of the acute cholinergic crisis, despite apparently adequate treatment of the intoxication.[26,33] This clinical picture is called the intermediate syndrome and is characterized by weakness that may involve the neck flexors, proximal limb muscles, respiratory muscles and cranial nerves.[12,26,32,33] The risk of developing the intermediate syndrome appears to be greatest with severe and prolonged acetylcholinesterase inhibition.[34] Recovery from this weakness may take several weeks.[12,26,32]

In some patients, after organophosphate intoxication a delayed peripheral and central axonopathy (organophosphate-induced delayed neurotoxicity, OPIDN) develops.[17] Jamaica ginger paralysis due to triorthocresyl phosphate intoxication was an example of OPIDN.[16] The symptoms of OPIDN begin one to three weeks after the acute exposure. Symptoms usually start with cramping muscle pain, followed by distal numbness and paresthesias, and progressive leg weakness. The upper extremities may then become involved. Examination shows severe weakness and wasting of distal limb muscles. Motor signs usually dominate the clinical picture, with only minimal if any sensory findings. Pyramidal and other signs of central nervous system dysfunction may be present. There may be some functional recovery over time, especially in mild to moderate cases.[17,28]

Table 146.3   Some common carbamate insecticides

Aldicarb
Aminocarb
Bendiocarb
Bufencarb
Carbaryl
Carbofuran
Cloethocarb
Dimetan
Dioxacarb
Fenoxycarb
Formetanate hydrochloride
Isolan
Isoprocarb
Methiocarb
Methomyl
Mexacarbate
Oxamyl
Pirimicarb
Promecarb
Propoxur
Thiodicarb
Trimethacarb

The signs and symptoms of carbamate insecticide exposure are generally milder and of shorter duration than with organophosphate toxicity. Also, because carbamates do not penetrate the central nervous system well, CNS effects are less prominent and convulsions are rare.[5] Table 146.3 lists some commonly available carbamate insecticides.

Organochlorine insecticides

Toxic effects from lindane, the most common currently available insecticide of the organochlorine class, usually occur as a result of prolonged dermal exposure and can include signs and symptoms of central nervous system hyperexcitability, such as confusion, muscle twitching, tremors, paresthesias, seizures or coma.[5]

Pyrethroid insecticides

The most common clinical syndrome related to pyrethroids occurs from dermal exposure. Affected patients describe a sensation of burning, itching, numbness or paresthesias that begins within one to two hours of exposure and may last up to 24 hours before resolving spontaneously.[21] The rare reports of systemic toxicity from massive exposure describe clinical effects of CNS stimulation, including tremors and seizures.[5,19,20]

Diagnosis

Organophosphate and carbamate insecticides

The diagnosis of poisoning by these compounds is straightforward when a patient presents with the prototypical clinical signs, symptoms and exposure history. In the absence of known exposure, one should be alert to the possibility of cholinesterase-inhibiting insecticide exposure by recognizing the characteristic symptoms and signs. In addition to the usually prominent muscarinic and nicotinic signs and symptoms, clinical diagnosis may be aided by the finding of a characteristic garlic-like odor in organophosphate poisoning.[5]

Laboratory tests are important adjuncts in the diagnosis of toxicity from the organophosphates. Organophosphates cause a decrease in circulating levels of acetylcholinesterase, measured in the form of red blood cell (RBC) cholinesterase or plasma cholinesterase. Plasma cholinesterase is also called pseudocholinesterase, a liver acute-phase protein. Although RBC cholinesterase is generally considered to be more representative of the cholinesterase found in the nervous system, and a more specific indicator of poisoning, plasma cholinesterase is sensitive, easier to assay, and more widely and quickly available.[10,32] From a laboratory standpoint, mild poisoning has been defined as a depression in cholinesterase activity of 20% to 50% of normal, moderate poisoning 10% to 20% of normal, and severe poisoning being less than 10% of normal.[32] Cholinesterase values vary, however, in normal individuals: workers at significant occupational risk for cholinesterase-inhibiting insecticide exposure can benefit from baseline pre-exposure cholinesterase levels.[35] In the absence of a known baseline, the finding of a progressive increase in cholinesterase levels after acute presentation and treatment is also a strong indicator of cholinesterase-inhibiting insecticide toxicity, even if the initial cholinesterase level at presentation is within the "normal" range.[32] In addition to cholinesterase levels, pesticide screens (of urine, blood or gastric contents) are available for some of the common organophosphate compounds.[36] Brain imaging is not helpful in the diagnosis of organophosphate, carbamate or other insecticide exposure, except to exclude other processes if necessary.

Cholinesterase levels are not reliable in the diagnosis of carbamate toxicity because of the short duration of inhibition by the carbamates; the diagnosis of carbamate toxicity is primarily clinical.[5]

Although not often necessary from a diagnostic standpoint, electrophysiological studies, if performed, may show some characteristic features when patients are weak from acute organophosphorus intoxication. The earliest electrophysiological finding in these patients is a spontaneous repetitive compound muscle action potential (CMAP) after a single stimulus. Abnormalities after repetitive stimulation can also be seen, including a decremental response of the compound muscle action potential (CMAP) at high rates of stimulation in severely weak patients. In milder, or earlier, cases, repetitive stimulation has shown a CMAP decrement on the second stimulus followed by some recovery of amplitude on repetitive stimulation ("decrement–increment response").[12]

The diagnosis of carbamate insecticide toxicity is primarily clinical, by recognition of the signs and symptoms of cholinergic stimulation, especially in the setting of known or possible exposure. Because of the shorter duration of action of cholinesterase inhibition by carbamates, cholinesterase levels may not be abnormal at the time of clinical presentation. For this reason cholinesterase levels are generally not as reliable for diagnosis as they are for the organophosphates.[5,37]

Organochlorine insecticides

The diagnosis of organochlorine insecticide toxicity is clinical, based on the finding of signs of central nervous system stimulation after dermal, oral or inhalational exposure to one of these agents,[18] such as lindane. No specific laboratory test can be used to diagnose organochlorine intoxication.

Pyrethroid insecticides

There are no specific tests for exposure to pyrethroid insecticides. A history of exposure is the primary method of diagnosis.[5]

Differential diagnosis

Organophosphate and carbamate insecticides

Even if no history is available, the finding of peripheral muscarinic cholinergic dysfunction superimposed on peripheral nicotinic dysfunction in the form of muscle fasciculations should lead the clinician to consider cholinesterase-inhibiting insecticide toxicity. However, the differential diagnosis of intoxication by the cholinesterase-inhibiting insecticides can be vast, and includes systemic illnesses, viral illnesses and meningoencephalitides, metabolic disorders and other intoxications. The finding of coma or seizures would also suggest the possibility of a further vast neurological differential diagnosis, including focal or diffuse central nervous system processes. Standard emergency management and diagnostic testing, as indicated, should help exclude other urgent and treatable diagnoses.

Organochlorine insecticides

The differential diagnosis of poisoning by these compounds includes any other processes that may present with symptoms such as encephalopathy, seizures or coma, including metabolic processes, meningoencephalitis, and focal or diffuse central nervous system disorders. Standard emergency diagnostic testing should be employed, as appropriate, to exclude other important and treatable causes of the clinical syndrome.

Pyrethroid insecticides

The differential diagnosis for the dermal symptoms of pyrethroid exposure would include other dermatological exposures or sensitivities. Focal or other neuropathies might be considered, except for the time course and resolution. The rare cases of central nervous system dysfunction after massive pyrethroid exposure would have the same differential diagnosis as described for the organochlorines.

Treatment

General principles

The general principles of emergency treatment of pesticide intoxication include attention to, and maintenance of, the patient's airway, respiration and oxygenation. Endotracheal intubation and mechanical ventilation may be necessary. Respiratory distress is particularly common in organophosphate intoxication because of excessive bronchial secretions or bronchospasm, superimposed on possible respiratory muscle weakness.[5,31] Severe hypotension or life-threatening cardiac arrhythmias should be treated as appropriate, to maintain adequate circulation. Even patients whose initial signs and symptoms suggest mild poisoning should be observed closely, preferably in an intensive care setting, for they may progress rapidly as the absorption of the poison or its physiological effects progresses.[31]

When ingestion is the route of intoxication, another important aspect of emergency care is to attempt to empty the stomach contents. In the awake and alert patient this can be accomplished by inducing emesis by administering syrup of ipecac. The usual dose is 15 mL followed by 200–300 mL of water; this can be repeated in 20 minutes if the first dose is not effective.[38] In the stuporous or unconscious patient with a risk of aspiration during emesis, gastric lavage is appropriate, performed after intubation and protection of the airway with a cuffed endotracheal tube.[31,38] Activated charcoal should be administered in an attempt to adsorb the compound within the gastrointestinal tract, and cathartics should be given to increase the rate of evacuation of poison through the intestines.[38]

After external exposure the affected areas should be decontaminated as soon as possible to avoid continued absorption of the material. If the eyes have been exposed they should be washed with generous amounts of water. After skin exposure, all contaminated clothing, including shoes, should be removed and the skin washed with detergent and water. Vigorous rubbing of the skin should be avoided, however, as this may promote absorption.[38] Healthcare personnel should wear protective clothing and gloves during these procedures, so as to avoid being exposed to the toxin.[5] With organophosphates in particular, contaminated clothing has been reported as an important source of continued exposure to the patient and others,[39] and contamination of clothing has even been used as a surreptitious source of poisoning.[40]

Organophosphate and carbamate insecticides

Treatment of toxicity from organophosphate compounds (Table 146.4) is centered on two goals: the relief of acute muscarinic toxicity at cholinergic synapses, and the regeneration of acetylcholinesterase. Evidence for the efficacy of modern treatment of organophosphate exposures is based on class 3 evidence, but is supported by knowledge of the pathophysiology of the toxins and the physiology of the antidotes, animal and in vitro models[38,41] and clinical experience.

Table 146.4   Treatment of acute organophosphate toxicity

1. General emergency measures: attention to airway, breathing and circulation; intubation and mechanical ventilation may be necessary

2. Atropine administration to treat muscarinic symptoms

    Adults: Initially 1.0–2.0 mg intravenously, repeat 2 mg intravenously every 15 minutes until signs of atropinization, including drying of airway secretions, flushing, mydriasis and tachycardia (if miosis and bradycardia present prior to atropine)

    Children: Initially 0.05 mg/kg intravenously, repeat 0.02–0.05 mg/kg every 15 minutes until signs of atropinization

3. Pralidoxime administration to regenerate active acetylcholinesterase

    Adults: 1.0–2.0 g by slow intravenous infusion (mixed in 100 mL normal saline, infused no faster than 0.2 g/min); may be repeated in 1–2 hours, then every 10–12 hours as needed

    Children: 20–50 mg/kg (depending upon severity of syndrome) intravenously, infused slowly, and may be repeated as above

4. Remove all contaminated clothing and dispose of carefully; wash contaminated skin and hair; flush eyes with water if exposed (healthcare personnel should wear protective clothing and rubber gloves to avoid self-exposure)

5. If ingestion has occurred:

    If patient is awake and alert, induce vomiting with ipecac, 15 mL orally, followed by 200–300 mL of water. If the patient is stuporous or unconscious, and at risk of aspiration, perform gastric lavage after intubation and airway protection

    Administer activated charcoal and cathartics

6. Symptomatic treatment of additional symptoms (such as persistent seizures: intravenous diazepam or lorazepam; intravenous phenobarbitol if necessary)

7. Continued close observation: observe for weakness that may occur up to 96 hours after initial presentation (intermediate syndrome)

Atropine is used to relieve the acute toxicity at peripheral cholinergic synapses and in the central nervous system by competitively blocking the effect of acetylcholine at muscarinic receptors. Atropine is particularly effective in drying excessive secretions, including bronchial secretions. It has no effect at the neuromuscular junction. The recommended initial dose of atropine for adults is 1–2 mg given intravenously (0.05 mg/kg for children), although it may be given intramuscularly if there is no intravenous access. Continued treatment with atropine is based on the patient's symptoms and response to treatment. It is generally recommended that doses be repeated, as necessary, by giving an additional 2 mg intravenously for adults (0.02–0.05 mg/kg for children) every 15 minutes until signs of "atropinization" appear. These include flushing, xerostomia, dilated pupils if they were small before treatment, and tachycardia or normal heart rate if there was bradycardia before treatment. The total dosage of atropine will vary depending upon the severity of poisoning, but is generally required for 24 hours and should then be tapered before discontinuing. Cases of severe organophosphate poisoning have been described requiring large total doses of atropine, and some authors have used continuous intravenous administration in some of these cases.[5,31,32]

Pralidoxime (pyridine-2-aldoxime, also called 2-PAM) is a specific antidote for organophosphate poisoning; this compound reactivates acetyl-cholinesterase that has been inhibited by the organophosphate. Pralidoxime is used concomitantly with atropine. Whereas atropine treats the acute muscarinic symptoms of the illness, pralidoxime has its primary effect throughout the body on the underlying mechanism of the enzymatic dysfunction. Pralidoxime, the only cholinesterase-reactivating agent available in the United States,[42] is one of a class of drugs called oximes. Oximes have the ability to restore acetylcholine after it has been phosphorylated by the organophosphate; this is because the oxime has a greater affinity for the phosphorus than the cholinesterase enzyme has.[38] The development of oximes came as a result of a direct and successful effort in the 1950s, based on pharmacological and biochemical theory, to find compounds that would correct the enzymatic dysfunction created by organophosphates.[43] Although pralidoxime has also been shown in experimental studies to have some anticholinergic effects, its primary clinically relevant therapeutic role is as a reactivator of inhibited acetyl-cholinesterase.[38] Pralidoxime has no effect on "aged" phosphorylated acetylcholinesterase, thereby emphasizing the need to begin pralidoxime therapy as early as possible after organophosphate intoxication.

Pralidoxime should be given intravenously by slow infusion, but can be given intramuscularly if intravenous infusion is not possible. The usual adult dose is 1–2 g (20–50 mg/kg in children, depending upon the severity of the poisoning) given as a slow intravenous infusion dissolved in saline and infused over 30 minutes. The rate of infusion should not exceed 0.2 g/min. The dosage may be repeated in one to two hours and every 10–12 hours as needed, and may be necessary for several days depending on the severity of the clinical syndrome.[5,6,31,38] The effects of pralidoxime may be seen clinically quite quickly, with improvement of muscle weakness and fasciculations within 10–40 minutes of administration.[31] Pralidoxime is considered to be a very safe drug, but is best tolerated with slow infusions: dizziness, blurred vision, hypotension, and respiratory and cardiac arrest have been attributed to rapid infusions,[36] although it is difficult to determine whether such occurrences were actually due to the poisoning itself.[38] Hypertensive crisis have also been described during pralidoxime administration, and patients should be monitored closely.[6]

Continued close observation of the organophosphate-intoxicated individual is indicated, despite apparently adequate control of symptoms, especially because maximal muscle weakness that can be severe enough to impair respiration (the intermediate syndrome) can occur after a delay of several days.[26,33,34] Continued supportive treatment, including mechanical respiration if necessary, is important during the duration of this syndrome.[6]

Prevention of organophosphate insecticide toxicity is primarily through good occupational practice, including protective clothing and gloves for workers involved in the manufacture, use and transport of these compounds. Workers who have been affected by organophosphate poisoning should not return to work involving potential further exposure to these compounds until their RBC cholinesterase has fully regenerated, because a low level would make them particularly vulnerable to repeat clinical toxicity.[35] Workers at risk of occupational exposure should not be given prophylactic antidotes, because these drugs could mask the early signs and symptoms of organophosphate poisoning and thereby allow continued exposure to the toxin.[6] In the setting of a credible threat of organophosphate nerve gas attack (such as from sarin or tabun) during the Gulf War, however, prophylactic pyridostigmine (30 mg orally t.i.d. during the threat) was given in order to provide some protective effect.[44] This strategy was based on animal studies showing that pretreatment with pyridostigmine, a reversible carbamate-type acetylcholinesterase inhibitor, by binding to acetylcholinesterase, may induce some protection from binding by the organophosphate.[24,32]

Patients with carbamate insecticide toxicity should be treated with atropine, similar to the treatment of organophosphate toxicity above. However, carbamate toxicity is generally a more benign syndrome, and atropine may be necessary for only 6–12 hours, followed by observation. Because the mechanism of carbamate toxicity is via reversible cholinesterase inhibition, pralidoxime is not indicated when it is known that the only compound producing toxicity is a carbamate insecticide. However, pralidoxime is indicated in a mixed carbamate–organophosphate intoxication, or when the agent is not known but the clinical symptoms and signs suggest the agent could be either an organophosphate or a carbamate.[5]

Organochlorine toxicity

In addition to the general principles of emergency treatment described at the beginning of this section, the treatment of organochlorine toxicity is symptomatic. It has generally been recommended that seizures should be managed with a benzodiazepine (e.g. lorazepam or diazepam) followed by phenobarbitol infusion (see chapter on status epilepticus). The use of phenobarbitol as the agent of choice, after benzodiazepines, for seizures secondary to organochlorine-induced excitation, is based on anecdote and theoretical considerations.[18]

Pyrethroid toxicity

Pyrethroid-induced paresthesias from dermal exposure resolve spontaneously within 24 hours,[21] and management consists simply of an attempt at local skin decontamination.[20,45] Treatment of the very rare cases of systemic and neurological symptoms from pyrethroids has been symptomatic.[5,20,45]

References

1. Winchester JF. Paraquat and the bipyridyl herbicides. *In:* Haddad LM, Shannon MW, Winchester JF, eds. Clinical Management of Poisoning and Drug Overdose, 3rd edn. Philadelphia: WB Saunders, 1998:845–855
2. Bradberry SM, Watt BE, Proudfoot AT, Vale JA. Mechanisms of toxicity, clinical features, and management of acute chlorophenoxy herbicide poisoning: a review. Clin Toxicol 2000;38:111–122
3. Kulig K. Chlorophenoxy herbicides and dioxin contaminants; other herbicides and fungicides. *In:* Haddad LM, Shannon MW, Winchester JF, eds. Clinical Management of Poisoning and Drug Overdose, 3rd edn. Philadelphia: WB Saunders, 1998:856–863
4. Reigart JR, Roberts JR. Rodenticides. *In:* Recognition and Management of Pesticide Poisonings, 5th edn. Washington DC: US Environmental Protection Agency, 1999:169–182
5. Carlton FB, Simpson WM, Haddad LM. The organophosphates and other insecticides. *In:* Haddad LM, Shannon MW, Winchester JF, eds. Clinical Management of Poisoning and Drug Overdose, 3rd edn. Philadelphia: WB Saunders, 1998:836–845
6. Reigart JR, Roberts JR. Organophosphate insecticides. *In:* Recognition and Management of Pesticide Poisonings, 5th edn. Washington DC: US Environment Protection Agency, 1999:34–47 (www.epa.gov/pesticides/safety/healthcare/handbook/handbook.htm)
7. Reigart JR, Roberts JR. Solid organochlorine insecticides. *In:* Recognition and Management of Pesticide Poisonings, 5th edn. Washington DC: US Environment Protection Agency, 1999:55–73
8. Ecobichon DJ. Introduction. *In:* Ecobichon DJ, Joy RM, eds. Pesticides and Neurological Diseases, 2nd edn. Boca Raton: CRC Press, 1994:1–23
9. Litovitz TL, Klein-Schwartz W, White S et al. 1999 annual report of the American Association of Poison Control Centers toxic exposure surveillance system. Am J Emerg Med 2000;18:517–574

10. Fuortes LJ, Ayebo AD, Kross BC. Cholinesterase-inhibiting insecticide toxicity. Am Fam Phys 1993;47: 1613–1620

11. Wadia RS, Chitra S, Amin RB, Kiwalkar RS, Sardesai HV. Electrophysiological studies in acute organophosphate poisoning. J Neurol Neurosurg Psychiatry 1987;50:1442–1448

12. Besser R, Gutmann L, Dillman U, Weilemann LS, Hopf HC. End-plate dysfunction in organophosphate intoxication. Neurology 1989;39:561–567

13. Gutmann L, Besser R. Organophosphate intoxication: pharmacologic, neurophysiologic, clinical, and therapeutic considerations. Semin Neurol 1990;10:46–51

14. Thompson JP, Casey PB, Vale JA. Deaths from pesticide poisoning in England and Wales 1990–1991. Hum Exp Toxicol 1995;13:437–445

15. Satoh T, Hosokawa M. Organophosphates and their impact on the global environment. Neurotoxicology 2000;21:223–227

16. Morgan JP, Penovich P. Jamaica ginger paralysis. Forty-seven-year follow-up. Arch Neurol 1978;35:530–532

17. Weiner ML, Jortner BS. Organophosphate-induced delayed neurotoxicity of triarylphosphates. Neurotoxicology 1999;20:653–674

18. Howland MA. Insecticides: chlorinated hydrocarbons, pyrethrins, and DEET. In: Goldfrank LR, Flomenbaum NE, Lewis NA, Weisman RS, Howland MA, Hoffman RS, eds. Goldfrank's Toxicologic Emergencies, 6th edn. Stamford: Appleton and Lange, 1998:1451–1458

19. Joy RM. Pyrethrins and pyrethroid insecticides. In: Ecobichon DJ, Joy RM, eds. Pesticides and Neurological Diseases, 2nd edn. Boca Raton: CRC Press; 1994:291–312

20. Ray DE, Forshaw PJ. Pyrethroid insecticides: poisoning syndromes, synergism and therapy. Clin Toxicol 2000;38:95–101

21. Wilks MF. Pyrethroid-induced paresthesia—a central or local toxic effect? Clin Toxicol 2000;38:103–105

22. Betarbet R, Sherer TB, MacKenzie G, Garcia-Osuna M, Panov AV, Greenamyre JT. Chronic systemic pesticide exposure reproduces features of Parkinson's disease. Nature Neurosci 2000;3:1301–1306

23. Giasson BI, Lee VMY. A new link between pesticides and Parkinson's disease. Nature Neurosci 2000;3: 1227–1228

24. Taylor P. Anticholinesterase agents. In: Hardman JG, Limberd LE, Molinoff PB, Ruddon RW, Gilman AG, eds. Goodman & Gilman's The Pharmacological Basis of Therapeutics, 9th edn. New York: McGraw-Hill, 1996:161–176

25. Lefkowitz RJ, Hoffman BB, Taylor P. Neurotransmission. The autonomic and somatic motor nervous systems. In: Hardman JG, Limberd LE, Molinoff PB, Ruddon RW, Gilman AG, eds. Goodman & Gilman's The Pharmacological Basis of Therapeutics, 9th edn. New York: McGraw-Hill, 1996:105–140

26. Senanayake N, Karalliedde LK. Neurotoxic effects of organophosphorus insecticides. An intermediate syndrome. N Engl J Med 1987;316:761–763

27. Glynn P. Neuropathy target esterase. Biochem J 1999; 344:625–631

28. Lotti M, Becker CE, Aminoff MJ. Organophosphate polyneuropathy: pathogenesis and prevention. Neurology 1984;34:658–662

29. Joy RM. Chlorinated hydrocarbon insecticides. In: Pesticides and Neurological Diseases, 2nd edn. Boca Raton: CRC Press, 1994:81–170

30. Albertson TE, Walby WF, Stark LG, Joy RM. The effects of lindane and long-term potentiation (LTP) on pyramidal cell excitability in the rat hippocampal slice. Neurotoxicology 1997;18:469–478

31. Tafuri J, Roberts J. Organophosphate poisoning. Ann Emerg Med 1987;16:193–202

32. Aaron CK, Howland MA. Insecticides: organophosphates and carbamates. In: Goldfrank LR, Flomenbaum NE, Lewis NA, Weisman RS, Howland MA, Hoffman RS, eds. Goldfrank's Toxicologic Emergencies, 6th edn. Stamford: Appleton and Lange, 1998:1429–1449

33. Sudakin DL, Mullins ME, Horowitz BZ, Abshier V, Letzig L. Intermediate syndrome after malathion ingestion despite continuous infusion of pralidoxime. Clin Toxicol 2000;38:47–50

34. De Bleeker J, Van Den Neucker K, Colardyn F. Intermediate syndrome in organophosphorus poisoning: a prospective study. Crit Care Med 1993;21:1706–1711

35. Midtling JE, Barnett PG, Coye MJ, et al. Clinical management of field worker organophosphate poisoning. West J Med 1985;142:514–518

36. Leikin JB, Paloucek FP. Poisoning & Toxicology Compendium. Cleveland: Lexi-Comp, 1998

37. Reigart JR, Roberts JR. N-methyl carbamate insecticides. In: Recognition and Management of Pesticide Poisonings, 5th edn. Washington DC: US Environmental Protection Agency, 1999:48–54

38. Laws ER. Diagnosis and treatment of poisoning. In: Hayes WJ, Laws ER, eds. Handbook of Pesticide Toxicology. San Diego: Academic Press, 1991:361–403

39. Clifford NJ, Nies AS. Organophosphate poisoning from wearing a laundered uniform previously contaminated with parathion. JAMA 1989;262:2035–2036

40. Bjornsdottir US, Smith D. Case report: South African religious leader with hyperventilation, hypophosphataemia, and respiratory arrest. Lancet 1999;354:2130

41. Worek F, Backer M, Thiermann H, et al. Reappraisal of indications and limitations of oxime therapy in organophosphate poisoning. Hum Exp Toxicol 1997; 16:466–472

42. Howland MA, Aaron CK. Pralidoxime. In: Goldfrank LR, Flomenbaum NE, Lewis NA, Weisman RS, Howland MA, Hoffman RS, eds. Goldfrank's Toxicologic Emergencies, 6th edn. Stamford: Appleton and Lange, 1998:1445–1449

43. Wilson IB, Ginsburg S. A powerful reactivator of alkylphosphate-inhibited acetylcholinesterase. Biochim Biophys Acta 1955;18:168–170

44. Keeler JR, Hurst CG, Dunn MA. Pyridostigmine used as a nerve agent pretreatment under wartime conditions. JAMA 1991;266:693–695

45. Bateman DN. Management of pyrethroid exposure. Clin Toxicol 2000;38:107–109

147 Toxemia of Pregnancy

Steven K Feske

Historical overview

Pre-eclampsia is a multisystem disorder of mid to late pregnancy, occurring generally after 20 weeks' gestation and traditionally characterized by hypertension, edema and proteinuria. In its most severe form, encephalopathy and seizures ensue. The onset of seizures has traditionally defined the progression from pre-eclampsia to eclampsia. The term HELLP syndrome was coined by Weinstein in 1982 to describe patients with hemolytic anemia, elevated liver enzymes, and low platelets occurring in late pregnancy.[1] This syndrome is now considered to be a severe form of pre-eclampsia–eclampsia. Although the syndrome of pre-eclampsia–eclampsia has been recognized since antiquity, an adequate understanding of its cause and pathogenesis remains elusive.

Epidemiology

Pre-eclampsia affects 3% to 5% of pregnant women.[2] Worldwide, approximately 50 000 women die each year from eclampsia.[3] Risk factors for pre-eclampsia include nulliparity, poor nourishment, obesity, multiple gestations, age greater than 35 years, extrauterine pregnancy and molar pregnancy. Pre-existing maternal hypertension, diabetes mellitus and thrombophilic disorders also increase risk. These last conditions all cause microvascular disease, and they may contribute to risk by promoting compromise of placental perfusion.[2] In recent years multiple change of partner has also been correlated with risk.[4,5] This finding has more recently been called into question by the finding that the risk lowering conferred by parity is only transient, and that risk increases with increasing interbirth interval. In one recent study, correction for the interbirth interval effect eliminated the effect of a change of partner.[6]

Etiology, pathophysiology and pathogenesis

The cause and pathophysiology of pre-eclampsia–eclampsia are still poorly understood, and many different directions of investigation continue to pursue the many hypotheses. However, several features appear to be fundamental. Abnormal placentation leads to placental hypoperfusion. Normal remodeling of the spiral arteries, which creates the low-resistance system perfusing the intervillous space, does not occur in pre-eclampsia. Mothers with pre-eclampsia exhibit increased vascular tone and reactivity causing vasospasm and widespread decreased organ perfusion. They also exhibit evidence of endothelial cell dysfunction. This underlies the abnormal vasomotor responses and hypertension, as well as the increased vascular permeability, that characterize the syndrome. The link between the placental insufficiency and the endothelial and vasomotor dysfunction has not been established, but various mechanisms have been suggested. These include immune mediation of both the placental abnormality and the endothelial dysfunction, genetic factors, and the transfer of oxidative stress from the hypoperfused placenta to the systemic circulation by activated neutrophils and monocytes, by cytokines, or by other mediators.[2]

Hypertension, or relative hypertension, is present in almost all patients with other features of pre-eclampsia–eclampsia and contributes to its clinical definition. The nature and distribution of the brain lesions in eclampsia are identical to those of hypertensive encephalopathy (HTE) as demonstrated by MRI and SPECT imaging.[7] That the changes of HTE occur at relatively low absolute blood pressure values in pre-eclampsia–eclampsia suggests that (1) the endothelial cell dysfunction is not merely secondary to hypertension, and (2) that these two pathogenetic features, endothelial cell dysfunction and hypertension, interact to produce the clinical syndrome.

The primary result of hypertension and endothelial cell dysfunction in the brain is vasogenic edema. The changes of edema are most prominent in the subcortical white matter of the occipital lobes and other posterior fossa structures, although lesions also occur in the cortex and in other regions of the brain.[8,9] This cerebral edema is reversible. Intraparenchymal hemorrhage may occur. Less commonly, infarctions due to vasospasm or thrombosis will cause irreversible focal brain injury. As in other forms of hypertensive encephalopathy, cortical and subcortical edema may lead to seizures.

Genetics

Population studies have focused on the questions whether pre-eclampsia–eclampsia is due to maternal or fetal factors, and whether single or multiple genetic influences are involved. Although most data argue for maternal susceptibility, several findings suggest a fetal influence as well. The lack of concordance between monozygotic twins, the risk of changed paternity (if this finding is sustained), and the recent finding that risk is increased in partners of fathers whose mothers had pre-eclampsia, all argue for a fetal contribution to susceptibility.[10–12] HLA genes and genes associated with many features associated with pre-eclampsia have been investigated, with no firm correlations. It appears likely that multiple genetic factors contribute. Although modern linkage techniques might further the

Table 147.1   Standard criteria for the diagnosis of pre-eclampsia and eclampsia
Pre-eclampsia Hypertension: diastolic BP ⩾90 mmHg or systolic BP ⩾140 mmHg, or rise of diastolic BP by 15 mmHg or systolic BP by 30 mmHg on at least two readings 6 h apart, *and* Proteinuria: ⩾300 mg protein/24 h or ⩾1 g/L protein in at least two random specimens ⩾6 h apart, *or* Edema: >1+ pitting edema after 12 h bedrest or weight gain of ⩾5 lb in one week *Eclampsia* Seizures: convulsions not caused by any coincidental neurological disease, such as epilepsy, in a woman who meets the criteria for pre-eclampsia
(Reprinted with permission from 13.)

search, the lack of a clear definition of the boundaries of the clinical syndrome hamper this effort.[2]

Clinical features

The most common neurological manifestations of the cerebral edema of eclampsia are headache, cortical visual phenomena consistent with the occipital lobe localization, and ultimately seizures. Seizures can be partial or generalized, although generalized seizures are probably secondarily generalized after an inapparent focal onset. Patients may present without seizures but with other features of encephalopathy, such as headache, confusion, aphasia and other cognitive deficits, and depressed level of consciousness.

Although commonly occurring in women who fulfill the standard criteria for pre-eclampsia, not uncommonly patients present in late pregnancy or in the early postpartum period with new, and often mild, hypertension and with seizures or encephalopathy as the first and only manifestations of toxemia.

Classification and diagnostic criteria

Traditional classifications define pre-eclampsia as hypertension (diastolic BP higher than 90 or systolic BP higher than 140, or rise in diastolic BP of 15 mmHg or of systolic BP of 30 mmHg on repeated readings) and either proteinuria (>300 mg/24 h or >1 g/L on repeated tests) or edema (Table 147.1).[13] Updated classifications, though perhaps less precise, recognize the varied multisystemic nature of this syndrome. These eliminate edema as a defining symptom, as it is such a common feature of normal pregnancy, although sudden severe widespread edema without another cause should add weight to the diagnosis. They also recognize that women with hypertension without proteinuria but with other features of pre-eclampsia–eclampsia, such as fetal compromise, headache, seizures, encephalopathy, hyperuricemia, and features of the HELLP syndrome without another explanation, should be considered to have toxemia. Such an inclusive definition is meant to capture patients broadly for clinical purposes. A more exclusive definition will often be appropriate for research purposes.[14]

Differential diagnosis

Hypertension, proteinuria and edema have many causes, which must be considered in patients with pregnancy as in others. Table 147.2 lists many of the disorders that may resemble severe pre-eclampsia–eclampsia. Disseminated intravascular coagulation may complicate pregnancy. Laboratory features that demonstrate consumption of fibrinogen and clotting factors should distinguish this disorder. The five major clinical features of thrombocytopenic purpura (TTP) (fever, thrombocytopenia, microangioplastic hemolytic anemia, renal insufficiency, and focal or diffuse brain involvement) may all occur in the HELLP syndrome. However, in TTP the encephalopathy rarely occurs with platelet counts greater than 20 000/cm³. Patients who present with features of the HELLP syndrome can usually be distinguished from those with TTP by (1) relative hypertension, (2) lack of fever, (3) lack of renal failure, (4) characteristic CT/MRI changes of HTE, and (5) response to therapy for pre-eclampsia–eclampsia (antihypertensive agents, $MgSO_4$, and delivery). In hemolytic uremic syndrome (HUS) the renal failure is typically more severe. Table 147.3 compares and contrasts HELLP, DIC and TTP/HUS. When the clinical context suggests possible sepsis, systemic lupus and antiphospholipid antibody syndrome, evidence of these diagnoses should be sought with appropriate laboratory studies. Patients with "postpartum angiitis" have been reported, based on encehalopathies and angiograms with segmental vascular narrowings. Such an angiogram is non-specific and consistent with eclampsia, and this was probably the correct diagnosis in many reported patients.

Diagnosis

Diagnosis of toxemia of pregnancy remains clinical, based on the traditional criteria: late pregnancy, hypertension and proteinuria, without or without

Table 147.2   Differential diagnosis of toxemia of pregnancy
Pre-eclampsia–eclampsia/HELLP syndrome Disseminated intravascular coagulation Thrombotic thrombocytopenic purpura Hemolytic uremic syndrome Sepsis Systemic vasculitis Systemic lupus erythematosus Antiphospholipid antibody syndrome

Table 147.3   Differentiation of HELLP syndrome from DIC and TTP/HUS

Parameter	HELLP	DIC	TTP/HUS
BP	Elevated	Any	Any
Edema	Variable	Variable	Variable
Proteinuria	Usually present	Variable	Variable
LFTs	Elevated	Often elevated	Often elevated
LDH	Elevated	Elevated	Elevated
BUN/Creat	Variable	Variable	Highest in HUS
CT/MRI	HTE changes	Normal/var	Normal/var
Anemia	MAHA[¶]	MAHA	MAHA
Platelets	Low, usually mildly	Low	Very low if neurological
Coagulation tests	Normal	DIC	Normal
ANA	Normal	Normal	20% positive
Biopsy	Not done	None rec	[†]Gingival biopsy positive
vWF-CP*	Normal	Normal	Antibodies/low level activity
AT III[†]	Low	Normal	Normal

*von Willebrand factor-cleaving protein studies are not currently available for routine clinical use.
[†]Hyaline platelet clots in microvessels.
[‡]Antithrombin III.
[¶]MAHA = microangiopathic hemolytic anemia.

seizures or encephalopathy. With our current understanding of this disorder and available diagnostic neuroimaging, it seems clear that many patients will have encephalopathy on this basis without satisfying the traditional clinical definitions, and this fact has been recognized in some newer classifications.[14] It is also clear that seizures, which have traditionally defined eclampsia, are merely a severe manifestation of encephalopathy caused by reversible brain edema, and major encephalopathy can occur without seizures.[15]

Patients who present with confusion, depressed conscious level, cortical visual loss, brainstem signs, focal hemispheric deficits, or seizures in late pregnancy or the puerperium should undergo neuroimaging to look for evidence of alternative diagnoses and evidence of characteristic brain edema. These findings of edema are best seen on MRI. Diffusion-weighted imaging can distinguish acute ischemic stroke (high intensity, decreased apparent diffusion coefficient (ADC)) from reversible edema secondary to increased blood flow (normal or low intensity, increased ADC).[16] Perfusion-weighted imaging can show evidence of increased cerebral blood flow, as can SPECT, although this is rarely needed to establish the diagnosis. Transcranial Doppler ultrasound will often show increased velocities due to vasocontriction and possibly to increased blood flow. Angiography is rarely necessary; however, it may show multifocal vascular narrowings.

Possible preventive therapies

Placental perfusion defects, release of placental factors, promoters of vasoconstriction and vascular permeability and inhibitors of vasodilation (decreased prostaglandin E_2 and prostacyclin; increased thromboxane A_2, serotonin, and endothelin; inhibited nitric oxide (endothelial-derived relaxing factor) and nitric oxide synthase), platelet and neutrophil activation, oxidative stress and autoimmunity are just some of the proposed mechanisms of dysfunction. Such abnormalities suggest possible therapies, including vasodilators, aspirin, selective serotonin-2 receptor antagonists, corticosteroids, plasmapheresis and antioxidants. Although little is known about the clinical importance of most of these identified abnormalities and potential therapies directed at them, aspirin and the antioxidants vitamins C and E have undergone controlled clinical study.

Several studies in the late 1980s suggested that by inhibiting the formation of thromboxane A_2, low-dose aspirin (60–100 mg/day) and other platelet inhibitors might prevent pre-eclampsia in patients at increased risk.[17–24] Although two large studies in the 1990s failed to find such a benefit of low-dose aspirin, one of these (CLASP) did find a decrease in the rate of preterm delivery in treated women and a trend in favor of therapy to prevent pre-eclampsia.[25,26] Although controversy remains, many authors recommend low-dose aspirin for certain groups of women at high risk for pre-eclampsia.

Based on evidence that oxidative stress contributes to the pathogenesis of pre-eclampsia, Chappell and colleagues[27] identified women at risk and compared treatment with vitamin C 1000 mg/day and vitamin E 400 IU/day ($n = 141$) with placebo ($n = 142$) beginning at 16–22 weeks of gestation. Pre-eclampsia occurred in 17% of those in the placebo group and in 8% in the treatment group ($P = 0.02$). The authors concluded that vitamin C and E supplementation may be beneficial in women at high risk.

Aspirin, antioxidants and other potential therapies that address the underlying pathogenesis will require further study that, it is hoped, will lead to effective preventive therapies. Such early therapeutic decisions will in most cases be made by obstetricians providing prenatal care.

Blood pressure control and invasive monitoring

When prophylactic therapies are unsuccessful and patients are deemed to have poor control of pregnancy-induced hypertension or pre-eclampsia, they will typically be admitted for bedrest and obstetric monitoring and care, including observation for symptoms such as headache, visual changes, epigastric pain, and serial measurement of body weight, blood pressure, urine protein and volume output, and plasma creatinine, hemoglobin, hematocrit, platelets and liver enzymes, and fetal monitoring.[28]

It is usually when neurological symptoms emerge during this phase of the illness that neurologists are consulted in these obstetric patients. Headache and hypertension raise the possibility of hypertensive encephalopathy (HTE). Because occipital lobe edema is common in this disorder, visual changes are often a clue to the diagnosis. However, because cerebral venous sinus thrombosis, ischemia and hemorrhage cannot be reliably distinguished from pre-eclampsia with HTE, MRI with diffusion-weighted sequences and arterial and venous flow studies are often indicated to rule out these disorders and to establish a positive diagnosis of HTE based on the characteristic MRI findings.[8] In pre-eclampsia–eclampsia HTE may occur at blood pressure levels that are usually well tolerated in non-pregnant patients.[7] This is presumed to occur because of the increased vascular permeability that results from the endothelial dysfunction which is fundamental to pre-eclampsia–eclampsia.

Prompt control of blood pressure is crucial to prevent the progression of encephalopathy – worsening cerebral edema and the risk of seizures and intracranial hemorrhage. Antihypertensive therapy will often have been started as part of the high-risk obstetric care. However, occasionally patients will present with new hypertension and encephalopathy postpartum.

To achieve rapid blood pressure control, favored therapeutics agents include labetalol and hydralazine. Other β-blocking agents and calcium channel blocking agents, such as nifedipine, may also be used. Nitroprusside and nitroglycerin raise the issue of possible fetal cyanide toxicity and are best avoided during pregnancy; however, they may be used when pre-eclampsia–eclampsia occurs after delivery. Angiotensin-converting enzyme inhibitors are contraindicated during pregnancy, because they have been shown to cause fetal morbidity and death (category D).[29]

Blood pressure should be lowered to a diastolic of about 90–105. In most cases this will translate into a decrease of 15% to 20% in the mean arterial pressure (MAP). For example, a blood pressure of 160/110 (MAP = 127) might be lowered to 140/94, (MAP = 107), a 16% reduction. Excessive blood pressure lowering can cause a decrease in placental perfusion, and during aggressive antihypertensive therapy the obstetrician should monitor the fetus for signs of distress. Most patients respond to medical therapy of

hypertension and careful fluid management with non-invasive monitoring.[30] However, because the hemodynamic profiles of women with pre-eclampsia–eclampsia are heterogeneous, invasive hemodynamic monitoring with a pulmonary artery catheter may be indicated in some patients with refractory hypertension, oliguria or pulmonary edema. In this way, individualized use of vasodilators, β-blockers or diuretics can be guided by a clear definition of the cardiac output and systemic vascular resistance.[31,32]

Magnesium sulfate and traditional anticonvulsant agents

In North America and much of the world, magnesium sulfate has been the mainstay of therapy for severe pre-eclampsia and eclampsia for many years. Although magnesium has been reported to have many salutary effects in women with toxemia (decreased systemic vascular resistance and blood pressure, increased cardiac output, increased uterine blood flow, enhanced prostacyclin activity in endothelial cells), there has been some controversy in the neurological literature concerning the benefit of this therapy for eclamptic seizures.[33–35] Recent clinical trials have brought controlled clinical data to bear on this debate, supporting the use of magnesium sulfate for both treatment and prevention of seizures. The Eclampsia Trial Collaborative Group study compared magnesium sulfate with diazepam and with phenytoin in women who had had an eclamptic seizure.[36] The intravenous magnesium maintenance regimen in this study was a conservative 1 mg/h. Magnesium sulfate was superior to both diazepam and phenytoin when both seizure recurrence and maternal mortality were compared (Table 147.4). In the phenytoin versus magnesium sulfate comparison, neonates also fared better in the magnesium sulfate group. Although it is not clear that the phenytoin dosing was adequate, as it was not checked against serum levels, the doses used were those that are commonly given.

Magnesium sulfate has also been shown to prevent seizures in women with pre-eclampsia. Lucas and colleagues[37] compared patients with pregnancy-induced hypertension who received magnesium sulfate by intravenous loading and intramuscular maintenance dosing with patients treated with a phenytoin 1000 mg loading dose and a second dose of 500 mg after 10 hours. Fewer patients in the magnesium sulfate group developed seizures ($MgSO_4$ 0/1049 vs phenytoin 10/1089, $P = 0.004$).[37] In this study, phenytoin levels were measured at 2 and 10 hours and at the time of the seizure in the 10 patients who developed eclamptic seizures. In 9 of the 10, the serum level exceeded 10 μg/mL and in 8 of the 10 it exceeded 15 μg/mL.

The empirical evidence of benefit offered by these trials has been paralleled by speculation about potential mechanisms of action, such as blockage of calcium flux through N-methyl-D-aspartate receptors that mediate glutamate neurotoxicity causing seizures and cerebral vasospasm causing ischemia.[38–42]

A regimen for magnesium sulfate therapy used in

Table 147.4   Outcome of Eclampsia Trial Collaborative Group Study[22]

	MgSO$_4$ (%)	Diazepam (%)	2p	MgSO$_4$ (%)	Phenytoin (%)	2p
Recurrent seizures	13.2	27.9	<0.00001	5.7	17.1	<0.00001
Maternal mortality	3.8	5.1	NS	2.6	5.2	NS

NS = not significant.

Table 147.5   Protocol for magnesium sulfate therapy for pre-eclampsia–eclampsia

1. MgSO$_4$ 4–6 g in 50 mL normal saline, infused over 20–30 min*
2. MgSO$_4$ 20 g/500 mL H$_2$0, begin at 2 g/h by infusion pump
3. May give additional MgSO$_4$ 2 g i.v. over 3–5 min, if further seizures occur
4. Discontinue MgSO$_4$ if:
    (a) the patellar reflexes are lost (test in upper extremities if epidural anesthesia is used)
    (b) respirations are depressed, or
    (c) urine output <100 mL in previous 4 h
5. If serious toxicity occurs, give calcium gluconate 1 g slow i.v. push and repeat until signs begin to abate

*If a more rapid effect is desired, give an MgSO$_4$ 4 g loading dose over 5 min, and if seizures persist an additional 2 g over 3–5 min.
With permission from and thanks to the Center for Labor and Birth, Brigham and Women's Hospital, Boston, Massachusetts.

the Center for Labor and Birth at Brigham and Women's Hospital is presented in Table 147.5. Such high intravenous doses should always be given with an infusion pump to avoid overdosing. Although the expected response to different serum levels has been defined, it is not clear that serum levels guide therapy reliably. Serum magnesium levels of 4–7 mEq/L are considered desirable. At 8–10 mEq/L reflex depression is typically apparent, and above 10–12 mEq/L respiratory depression is likely. Respiratory depression should be treated by discontinuing magnesium sulfate and administering calcium gluconate intravenously. In patients with renal insufficiency, it is advised that a low-side loading dose (4 g) be used, that the maintenance dose be halved (to 1 g/h), and that serum magnesium levels be closely monitored.

When patients with severe pre-eclampsia progress to convulsions, the term eclampsia is applied. Sometimes this term is also applied to women with severe pre-eclampsia and coma without seizures. These distinctions are largely arbitrary, and convulsions and coma occur as manifestations on the most severe end of the spectrum of the pre-eclampsia–eclampsia syndrome. Seizures may occur in late pregnancy, during labor and delivery, or postpartum. Although, most postpartum eclamptic seizures occur within 48 hours of delivery they may occur much farther out, and standard definitions probably understate the duration.[43] Still, especially when seizures occur beyond 48 hours after delivery, careful consideration should be given to other possible causes. Pre-eclampsia is said to precede seizures in almost all cases; however, cases have been reported when typical preceding symptoms and signs are lacking.

Should traditional anticonvulsants be given as well as magnesium sulfate? This issue has not been ade-quately addressed by clinical trials. Available clinical trials have compared magnesium sulfate to more traditional anticonvulsants but not assessed their combined use. The Eclampsia Trial Collaborative Group study suggests that magnesium is the drug of choice for seizures in pre-eclampsia, and in most cases no additional anticonvulsant will be needed. However, when given properly and carefully monitored, it is unlikely that phenytoin will cause serious side effects to either mother or child. Certainly, when seizures recur despite appropriate therapy with magnesium sulfate, and when lesions are identified by MRI, and therapy prolonged beyond 24–48 hours postpartum is anticipated, then traditional AEDs should be given, usually lorazepam and phenytoin, for prompt control. Refractory seizures should be treated aggressively as status epilepticus. When recurrent seizures or status epilepticus occur, causes other than eclampsia should also be sought.

References

1. Weinstein L. Syndrome of hemolysis, elevated liver enzymes, and low platelet count: a severe consequence of hypertension in pregnancy. Am J Obstet Gynecol 1982;142:159–167
2. Roberts JM, Cooper DW. Pathogenesis and genetics of pre-eclampsia. Lancet 2001;357:53–56
3. Duley L. Maternal mortality associated with hypertensive disorders of pregnancy in Africa, Asia, Latin America and the Caribbean. Br J Obstet Gynaecol 1992;99:547
4. Trupin LS, Simon LP, Eskenazi B. Change in paternity: a risk factor for preeclampsia in multiparas. Epidemiology 1996;7:240–244
5. Tubbergen P, Lachmeijer AM, Althuisius SM, et al. Change in paternity: a risk factor for preeclampsia in multiparous women? J Reprod Immunol 1999;45:81–88

6. Skjærven R, Wilcox AJ, Lie RT. The interval between pregnancies and the risk of preeclampsia. N Engl J Med 2002;346:33–38

7. Schwartz RB, Feske SK, Polak JF, et al. Clinical and neuroradiographic correlates in pre-eclampsia–eclampsia: insights into the pathogenesis of hypertensive encephalopathy. Radiology, 2000;217:371–376

8. Mantello MT, Schwartz RB. Jones KM, et al. Imaging of neurologic complications associated with pregnancy. Am J Roentgenol 1993;160:843–847

9. Hinchey J, Chaves C, Appignani B, et al. A reversible posterior leukoencephalopathy syndrome. N Engl J Med 1996;334:494–500

10. Thornton JG, Macdonald AM. Twin mothers, pregnancy, hypertension and pre-eclampsia. Br J Obstet Gynaecol 1999;106:570–575

11. Lachmeijer AM, Aarnoudse JG, ten Kate LP, et al. Concordance for pre-eclampsia in monozygous twins. Br J Obstet Gynaecol 1998;105:1315–1317

12. Esplin MS, Fausett MB, Fraser A, et al. Paternal and maternal components of the predisposition to preeclampsia. N Engl J Med 2001;344:867–872

13. Kaplan PW, Repke JT. Eclampsia. Neurol Clin 1994; 12:566

14. Higgins JR, de Swiet M. Blood-pressure measurement and classification in pregnancy. Lancet 2001;357: 131–135

15. Feske SK, Sperling RA, Schwartz RB. Extensive reversible brain magnetic resonance lesions in a patient with HELLP syndrome. J Neuroimag 1997;7:247–250

16. Schaefer PW, Buonanno FS, Gonzalez RG, et al. Diffusion-weighted imaging discriminates between cytotoxic and vasogenic edema in a patient with eclampsia. Stroke 1997;28:1082–1085

17. Wallenburg HCS, Dekker GA, Makovitz JW, Rotmans P. Low-dose aspirin prevents pregnancy-induced hypertension and pre-eclampsia in angiotensin-sensitive primigravidae. Lancet 1986;1:1–3

18. Beaufils M, Uzan M, Donsimoni R. Colau JC. Prevention of pre-eclampsia by early antiplatelet therapy. Lancet 1985;1:840–842

19. Benigni A, Gregorini G, Frusca T, et al. Effect of low-dose aspirin on fetal and maternal generation of thromboxane by platelets in women at risk for pregnancy-induced hypertension. N Engl J Med 1989; 321:357–362

20. Schiff E, Peleg E, Goldenberg M, et al. The use of aspirin to prevent pregnancy-induced hypertension and lower the ratio of thromboxane A_2 to prostacyclin in relatively high risk pregnancies. N Engl J Med 1989;321:351–356

21. Spitz B, Magness RR, Cox SM, et al. Low-dose aspirin, 1. Effect on angiotensin II pressor responses and blood prostaglandin concentrations in pregnant women sensitive to angiotensin II. Am J Obstet Gynecol 1988;159: 1035–1043

22. Brown CEL, Gant NF, Cox K, et al. Low-dose aspirin, II. Relationship of angiotensin II pressor responses, circulating eicosanoids, and pregnancy outcome. Am J Obstet Gynecol 1990;163:1853–1861

23. Hault JC, Goldenberg RL, Parker CR Jr, et al. Low-dose aspirin therapy to prevent preeclampsia. Am J Obstet Gynecol 1993;168:1083–1093

24. Sibai BM, Caritis SN, Thom E, et al. National Institute of Child Health and Human Development Network of Maternal–Fetal Medicine Units, Prevention of preeclampsia with low-dose aspirin in healthy, nulliparous pregnant women. N Engl J Med 1993;329: 1213–1218

25. CLASP (Collaborative Low-dose Aspirin Study in Pregnancy) Collaborative Group, CLASP: A randomized trial of low-dose aspirin for the prevention and treatment of pre-eclampsia among 9364 pregnant women. Lancet 1994;343:619–629

26. ECPPA (Estudo Colaborativo para Prevençao da Pré-eclampsia com Aspirina) Collaborative Group: ECPPA: Randomized trial of low dose aspirin for the prevention of maternal and fetal complications in high risk pregnant women. Br J Obstet Gynaecol 1996;103:39–47

27. Chappell LC, Seed PT, Briley AL, et al. Effect of antioxidants on the occurrence of pre-eclampsia in women at increased risk: a randomized trial. Lancet 1999;354: 810–816

28. Cunningham FG, MacDonald PC, Grant NF, et al. Hypertensive disorders of pregnancy. In: Williams Obstetrics. 20th edn. Stamford, Conn: Appleton and Lange, 1997:715

29. Cunningham FG, MacDonald PC, Grant NF, et al. Hypertensive disorders of pregnancy. In: Williams Obstetrics. 20th edn. Stamford, Conn: Appleton and Lange, 1997:716

30. Easterling TR, Benedetti TJ, Schmucker BC, Carlson KL. Antihypertensive therapy in pregnancy directed by noninvasive hemodynamic monitoring. Am J Perinatol 1989;6:86–89

31. Clark SL, Cotton DB. Clinical indications for pulmonary artery catheterization in the patient with severe preeclampsia. Am J Obstet Gynecol 1988;158: 453–458

32. Cotton DB, Lee W, Huhta JC, Dorman KF. Hemodynamic profile of severe pregnancy-induced hypertension. Am J Obstet Gynecol 1988;158:523–529

33. Dinsdale HB. Does magnesium sulfate treat eclamptic seizures? Yes. Arch Neurol 1988;45:1360–1361

34. Kaplan PW, Lesser RP, Fisher RS, et al. No, magnesium sulfate should not be used in treating eclamptic seizures. Arch Neurol 1988;45:1361–1364

35. Chua S, Redman CWG. Are prophylactic anticonvulsants required in severe pre-eclampsia? Lancet 1991; 337:250–251

36. Eclampsia Trial Collaborative Group. Which anticonvulsant for women with eclampsia? Evidence from the collaborative eclampsia trial. Lancet 1995;345:1455–1463

37. Lucas MJ, Leveno KJ, Cunningham FG. A comparison of magnesium sulfate and phenytoin for the prevention of eclampsia. N Engl J Med 1995;333:201–205

38. Goldman RS, Finkbeiner SM. Therapeutic use of magnesium sulfate in selected cases of cerebral ischemia and seizures. N Engl J Med 1988;319:1224–1225

39. Cotton DB, Janusz CA, Berman BF. Anticonvulsant effects of magnesium sulfate on hippocampal seizures. Therapeutic implications in pre-eclampsia–eclampsia. Am J Obstet Gynecol 1992;166:1127–1136

40. Belfort MA, Moise KJ. Effect of magnesium sulfate on maternal brain blood flow in preeclampsia: a randomized, placebo-controlled study. Am J Obstet Gynecol 1992;167:661–666

41. Belfort MA, Saade GR, Moise KJ. The effect of magnesium sulfate on maternal retinal blood flow in preeclampsia: a randomized placebo-controlled study. Am J Obstet Gynecol 1992;167:1548–1553

42. Lipton SA, Rosenberg PA. Excitatory amino acids as a final common pathway for neurologic disorders. N Engl J Med 1994;330:613–622

43. Raps EC, Galetta SL, Broderick M, Atlas SW. Delayed peripartum vasculopathy: Cerebral eclampsia revisited. Ann Neurol 1993;33:222–225

Therapy of Neurological Disorders: Neuropathies and Neuromuscular Junction Disorders of Pregnancy

David C Preston

Introduction

Pregnancy is associated with various disorders of the peripheral nerves and neuromuscular junction. The physical changes that occur during pregnancy may result in various entrapment neuropathies, most of which resolve spontaneously in the postpartum period. Alteration in the immune system during pregnancy may place the mother at greater risk for various infectious, postinfectious, and autoimmune neuropathies. The process of birth places substantial strain on the birth canal and adjacent structures, including the lumbosacral plexus and nearby major nerves of the lower extremity. Some neurological disorders are more common in women of child-bearing age (e.g., myasthenia gravis). This chapter reviews the major neuropathies and neuromuscular junction disorders that occur during pregnancy and post partum and their treatment.

Neuropathies

Mononeuropathies

Carpal tunnel syndrome Entrapment of the median nerve as it goes through the carpal tunnel at the wrist is the most common mononeuropathy of the upper extremity. Carpal tunnel syndrome (CTS) is associated with various conditions, including pregnancy, especially in the third trimester.[1] Pregnant women with CTS present with wrist and arm pain that is associated with paresthesias of the hands. The pain may be localized to the wrist or may radiate to the forearm, arm, or, rarely, the shoulder. Some patients describe a diffuse, poorly localized ache involving the entire arm. Paresthesias frequently are bilateral and present in a median nerve distribution (i.e., medial thumb and index, middle, and lateral ring fingers), although it is not uncommon for a patient to describe the whole hand as "falling asleep."

Symptoms are often provoked when either a flexed or extended wrist posture is assumed. Most commonly, this occurs during ordinary activities such as driving or holding a telephone receiver, book, or newspaper. Nocturnal paresthesias are particularly common. During sleep, persistent wrist flexion or extension leads to increased carpal tunnel pressure, nerve ischemia, and subsequent paresthesias. Patients frequently awaken from sleep and shake or ring out their hands or hold them under warm running water.

Pain and paresthesias usually bring patients to medical attention. If motor fibers are involved, weakness of thumb abduction and opposition may develop, followed by atrophy of the thenar eminence. Some patients describe difficulty buttoning shirts, opening a jar, or turning a doorknob.

Although the cause of CTS was long considered to be tenosynovitis of the transverse carpal ligament, pathological examination typically shows little evidence of inflammation. In most cases, edema, vascular sclerosis, and fibrosis are seen, findings consistent with repeated stress of connective tissue. Occupations or activities that involve repetitive hand use clearly increase the risk of CTS. Also, any condition that results in increased fluid volume is associated with an increased incidence of CTS. Accordingly, the CTS in pregnancy likely is related to the increase of whole body fluid volume.

Hand symptoms, including mild pain and paresthesias, are common in pregnancy, occurring in 35% of women.[2] However, CTS that is severe enough to warrant treatment is far less common, in the range of 0.34% to 2.3%.[3,4] In pregnant women with clinically definite CTS, symptoms most often develop in the third trimester, are more common in primiparas, and are associated with excessive weight gain or edema (or both).[4] If questioned closely, some women report mild symptoms before pregnancy, likely indicating an exacerbation of preexistent CTS by pregnancy.

Evaluation and treatment are generally conservative because the symptoms resolve within a few weeks after delivery in nearly all patients. In mild cases, no specific treatment is needed. In cases with pain and nocturnal paresthesias (which may lead to a sleep disturbance), splinting the wrist in the neutral position is indicated. Splinting is associated with excellent results in 80% of patients.[5] If symptoms persist, local injection of corticosteroids (20 to 40 mg of methylprednisolone acetate [Depo-Medrol]) adjacent to the carpal tunnel may be of use.[6] Surgical treatment is required for a small proportion of patients. Generally, women who require an operation (1) had symptoms before pregnancy, (2) have symptoms that developed early in pregnancy, (3) have fixed or advancing neurological deficits with sensory loss or muscle wasting (or both), (4) have symptoms that do not respond to splinting and corticosteroid injections, and (5) have symptoms that continued after delivery.[7] Before proceeding to surgery, all patients should have nerve conduction studies and electromyography (EMG) to confirm that the median neuropathy localizes to the carpal tunnel at the wrist.

Femoral neuropathy   Isolated femoral neuropathies are uncommon in pregnancy, but they may occur, especially during labor and delivery. With modern obstetrical care, the incidence of postpartum femoral neuropathy has decreased and now is 2.8/100 000.[8] Most cases result from prolonged placement in the lithotomy position or from compression during cesarean section. The femoral nerve normally runs anteriorly in the thigh under the inguinal ligament. In the lithotomy position, with the thigh flexed and externally rotated, the nerve can be compressed against the inguinal ligament. During cesarean section, abdominal retractors against the abdominal wall may compress the femoral nerve against the pelvis.

The femoral nerve is derived from the lumbar plexus and receives innervation from the L2, L3, and L4 nerve roots. It supplies muscular innervation primarily to the hip flexors and knee extensors and sensory innervation to the medial calf and the anterior and medial thigh. Accordingly, during the postpartum period, women with femoral neuropathy often note that the knee buckles (from quadriceps weakness) and sensation over the anterior thigh and medial calf is altered. Weakness of hip flexion is an important sign because it indicates involvement of the iliopsoas muscle, localizing the lesion proximal to the inguinal ligament. Femoral neuropathies due to the lithotomy position typically spare the iliopsoas, but intra-abdominal lesions may be associated with weakness of this muscle. In femoral neuropathy, the quadriceps reflex is depressed or absent. Other reflexes should be normal.

Postpartum femoral neuropathy usually has an excellent prognosis because the mechanism of the injury is usually compression.[9] However, if the neuropathy occurs after cesarean section, pelvic imaging with either computed tomography (CT) or magnetic resonance imaging (MRI) should be performed to exclude a hematoma. EMG and nerve conduction studies can be used to assess the degree of demyelination versus axonal loss to help predict the length of time to recovery. Demyelination is associated with relatively rapid improvement, often over a few weeks. However, axonal loss requires more time and, in the case of femoral neuropathy, may require at least several months for recovery. In the interim, simple observation is indicated for mild cases. Physical therapy is indicated for more advanced cases. For patients with severe weakness, bracing, crutches, or canes may be needed to assist with ambulation and to reduce the risk of falling.

Obturator neuropathy   The obturator nerve is the other major nerve derived from the lumbar plexus, being derived from the L2, L3, and L4 nerve roots. The obturator nerve supplies muscular innervation to the thigh adductors and sensory innervation to a small area of skin in the upper medial thigh. Rare isolated cases of obturator neuropathy have been associated with labor and delivery.[6,10] The cause of this neuropathy is not well defined; possibilities include (1) compression of the nerve by the fetal head during delivery, (2) compression by forceps or retractors during surgery, and (3) secondary pelvic hematoma formation. In most cases of postpartum obturator neuropathy, the femoral and other nerves are also involved, representing part of a widespread lumbosacral plexopathy. Obturator neuropathies primarily produce weakness of hip adduction, leading to a disturbed, wide-based gait. As with other nerve injuries, pain and paresthesias may occur in the distribution of the nerve.

Similar to femoral neuropathies, obturator neuropathy usually is treated conservatively with observation or physical therapy (or both). Pelvic imaging is indicated, especially after cesarean section or complicated delivery. Because the cause of these rare neuropathies is likely compression, recovery is expected to be complete, but it may be delayed depending on the amount of demyelination versus axonal loss. Nerve conduction studies and EMG can be useful in assessing the contributions of each of these factors. Also, electrophysiologic studies can be helpful in excluding a more widespread lumbosacral plexopathy.

Lateral femoral cutaneous neuropathy   The lateral femoral cutaneous nerve is a pure sensory nerve derived from the L2 and L3 nerve roots (Figure 148.1). It runs under the inguinal ligament near the superior iliac spine, where it may be injured or entrapped. The lateral femoral cutaneous nerve supplies sensory innervation to a large oval area of skin over the lateral and anterior thigh. Entrapment may occur as the nerve passes under the inguinal ligament. This entrapment occurs more commonly in patients who have gained weight or who wear tight clothing, both of which occur during pregnancy. The clinical syndrome, known as "meralgia paresthetica," results in a painful, burning, numb patch of skin over the anterior and lateral thigh. Because the nerve does not have any muscular innervation from this nerve, there is no associated muscle atrophy, weakness or loss of reflexes.

Because the syndrome of lateral femoral cutaneous neuropathy usually is easily recognized clinically, no further evaluation is needed. In cases in which there is a question of sensory loss beyond the typical territory of the lateral femoral cutaneous nerve or the possibility of weakness, nerve conduction studies and EMG are useful for excluding lumbar plexopathy or radiculopathy. In pregnant women, the syndrome typically resolves spontaneously within a few months after delivery, as weight and abdominal girth return to normal.[1] In cases with marked burning and pain, neuropathic pain medications, such as amitriptyline or gabapentin can be used to treat the symptoms.

Peroneal neuropathy   The common peroneal nerve is derived from the L4, L5, and S1 nerve roots, which

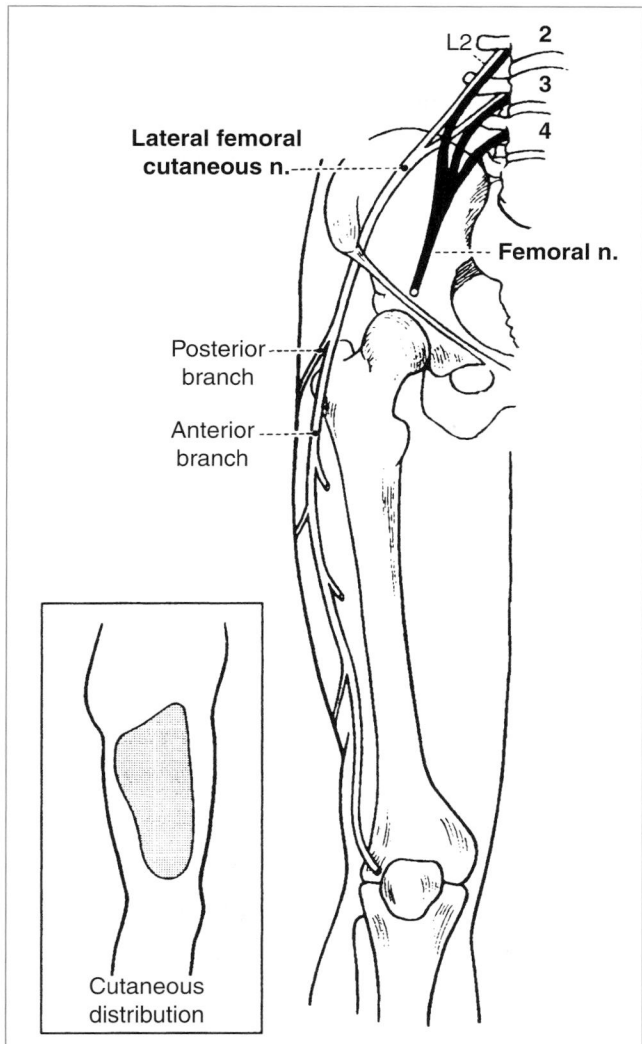

Figure 148.1 Anatomy of the lateral femoral cutaneous nerve. The lateral femoral cutaneous nerve is a pure sensory nerve derived from the L2–L3 roots which supplies sensation to a large oval area of skin over the lateral and anterior thigh. In pregnancy, the nerve may become entrapped as it passes under the inguinal ligament. Adapted from Haymaker W, Woodhal, B. Peripheral Nerve Injuries, Philadelphia: WB Sander, 1953.

travel through the lumbosacral plexus and join the sciatic nerve. Above the popliteal fossa, the sciatic nerve bifurcates into the common peroneal and tibial nerves. The common peroneal nerve winds around the neck of the fibula and passes through the "fibular tunnel" between the peroneus longus muscle and the fibula. The common peroneal nerve then divides into superficial and deep branches. The deep peroneal nerve supplies motor innervation to ankle and toe dorsiflexors and sensory innervation to the webspace between the first and second toes. The superficial peroneal nerve innervates the ankle evertors and supplies sensory innervation to the lateral calf and dorsum of the foot.

Patients with common peroneal neuropathy present with the characteristic neurological picture of footdrop and loss of sensation on the lateral calf and dorsum of the foot. Acute common peroneal neuropathy across the fibular neck often occurs after trauma, forcible stretch injury, or compression. Also, repetitive stretch from squatting has been associated with peroneal neuropathy. Common peroneal neuropathy can occur in association with pushing in a squatting position during childbirth.[11]

Women with postpartum footdrop should have nerve conduction studies and EMG to localize the neuropathy to the fibular neck to exclude postpartum lumbosacral plexopathy (see below). Recovery from peroneal neuropathies at the fibular neck is usually complete. A plastic molded brace (AFO) often helps with ambulation and prevents tripping and falling during the recovery period.

Facial neuropathy The most common cranial mononeuropathy is unilateral facial nerve palsy ("Bell's palsy"). Although associated with various causes, many cases result from an infectious event. There is increasing evidence that herpes simplex virus 1 is an important etiologic agent. In the third trimester of pregnancy and the immediate postpartum period, the incidence of idiopathic facial palsy increases significantly.[1,12–15] One study reported that the incidence of facial palsy was 45.1/100 000 for pregnant women, compared with 17.4/100 000 for age-matched controls. No clear relationship has been established with toxemia, hypertension, or the primigravida state. Except for the higher incidence, there is no important clinical difference in the neuropathy between pregnant and nonpregnant patients.

Bell's palsy results in muscle weakness or paralysis of both the upper and lower facial musculature. Thus, patients are not able to wrinkle the forehead, to close the eye, or to smile. Also, there may be decreased production of tears and saliva, hyperacusis, and absence of taste sensation over the anterior tongue, reflecting involvement of the sensory and autonomic branches of the facial nerve. In patients with Bell palsy, facial weakness/paralysis generally occurs within 24 hours of onset and is often accompanied by pain behind the ipsilateral ear.

No diagnostic testing is required when the typical clinical syndrome is recognized. For most patients, the prognosis is excellent, with full recovery of function occurring over several weeks to months. However, in severe cases, usually those associated with marked axonal loss, some degree of permanent facial weakness remains or aberrant reinnervation may occur as the nerve regenerates and produce synkinesis of facial movements (e.g., closing the eye may be accompanied by movement of the lips or tears may flow rather than saliva when eating). Facial nerve conduction studies that compare the symptomatic and asymptomatic sides can be helpful in assessing the amount of axonal loss and prognosis.

The most important treatment in Bell's palsy is local care of the eye to prevent drying and corneal abrasion in cases in which eye closure is incomplete, especially at night, because of weakness of the obicularis oculi muscle. The use of artificial tears during the day and the application of ophthalamic lubricating cream and taping of the eye at night are often needed. The value of directed therapy at the onset of Bell's palsy has not been settled. Prednisone has been given to nonpregnant women at a dose of 1 mg/kg for 5 days, followed by taper over several days, along with acyclovir, 400 mg 5 times daily for 10 days.[16] The use of this treatment in pregnant women has not been established.

Plexopathies

Postpartum lumbosacral plexopathy Compression injury to the lumbosacral plexus during labor and delivery, known as "postpartum lumbosacral plexopathy," is underappreciated and often misdiagnosed.[17,18] It has been described in the literature under various names, including maternal peroneal palsy, maternal birth palsy, neuritis puerperalis, and maternal obstetric paralysis. Although most large series place the incidence of this disorder at 1:2600 births, many milder cases likely never reach medical attention.

The mechanism of injury involves compression of the fetal head against the underlying pelvis and lumbosacral plexus. Postpartum lumbosacral plexopathy results primarily from compression of the lumbosacral trunk (Figure 148.2). Fibers from the L4 and L5 nerve roots join and descend into the pelvis to reach the sacral plexus. When the lumbosacral trunk crosses the pelvic outlet, the fibers are exposed (i.e., no longer protected by the psoas muscle) as they rest against the sacral ala near the sacroiliac joint. At this point, the fibers are most exposed and susceptible to compression. The fibers that eventually form the peroneal division of the sciatic nerve lie posteriorly, closest to the bone, and are more vulnerable than the fibers of the tibial division. Accordingly, peroneal fibers are affected often most, and some women present with postpartum footdrop, not infrequently misdiagnosed as peroneal palsy at the fibular neck.

Weakness may be noticed immediately or within the first few days after delivery. In addition to peroneal weakness, examination often shows mild weakness of knee flexion, hip abduction, and extension and internal rotation, demonstrating that the lesion clearly is outside the territory of the peroneal nerve. Sensory disturbance is most marked over the dorsum of the foot and lateral calf, but it may be patchy and involve the sole of the foot and the posterior calf and thigh.

Several factors predispose to this injury, including a first pregnancy, a large fetal head with a small pelvis ("cephalopelvic disproportion"), a small mother (<5 feet tall), and a prolonged or difficult labor. Women who have had a previous episode are predisposed to this complication with additional pregnancies.

Nerve conduction studies and EMG are helpful in localizing the lesion to the lumbosacral plexus and in excluding peroneal neuropathy across the fibular neck and L5 radiculopathy, both of which may mimic

postpartum lumbosacral plexopathy. In atypical cases, MRI of the pelvis and lumbosacral spine may be indicated. Rarely, patients may be left with permanent weakness, but in most cases the prognosis is excellent, with recovery occurring over the ensuing weeks to months, depending on the amount of axonal loss versus demyelination. For marked weakness, treatment involves physical therapy, appropriate bracing, and walking aids to prevent falls.

Polyneuropathies

Vitamin deficiency Severe malnutrition may result in distal symmetrical polyneuropathy from vitamin deficiency, especially thiamine (or vitamin B_1).[1,19,20] Pregnant women with hyperemesis gravidarium are potentially at risk for this complication. Symptoms and signs of polyneuropathy from thiamine deficiency usually present with more serious central nervous system dysfunction in the form of Wernicke's

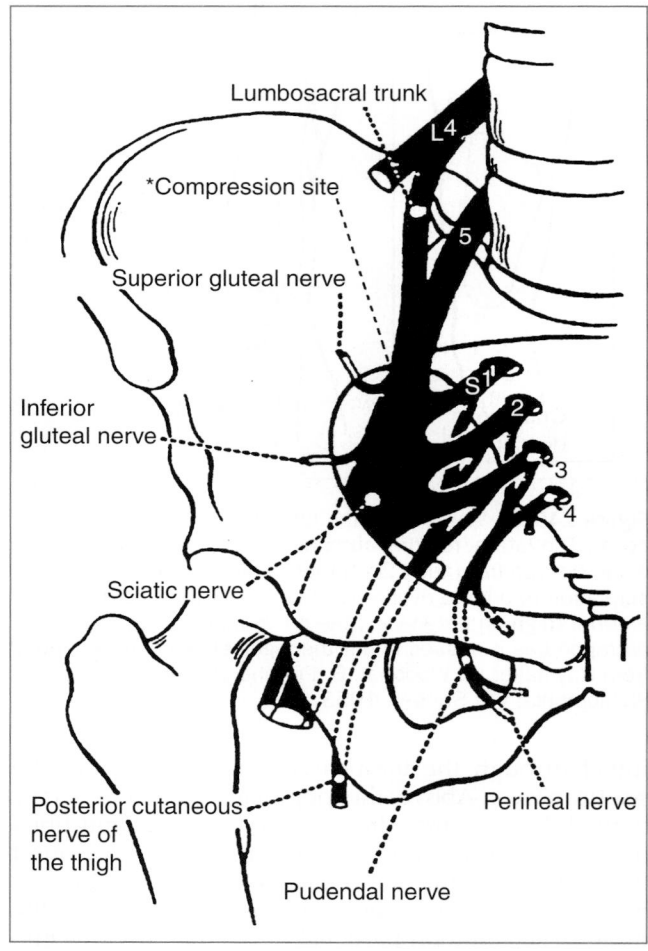

Figure 148.2   Postpartum lumbosacral plexopathy. Postpartum lumbosacral plexopathy results primarily from compression of the lumbosacral trunk which is formed from the L5 and part of the L4 nerve roots. When the lumbosacral trunk crosses the pelvic outlet, the fibers lie exposed as they rest against the sacral ala near the sacroiliac joints (*Compression site). Adapted from Haymaker W, Woodhal, B. Peripheral Nerve Injuries, Philadelphia: WB Sander, 1953.

encephalopathy. If not recognized early, permanent memory loss and other neurological sequelae may occur (i.e., Korsakoff psychosis). Prompt recognition and treatment with parenteral thiamine often produces marked improvement. Parenteral supplementation needs to be continued until normal oral intake resumes; thereafter, continued supplementation of oral thiamine is advisable.

Guillain-Barré syndrome Guillain-Barré syndrome (GBS), also known as "acute inflammatory demyelinating polyneuropathy," is an immune-mediated, rapidly progressive, predominantly motor polyneuropathy that often leads to bulbar and respiratory compromise. Although the prognosis is favorable for more than 80% of patients, the hospital course is frequently long, followed by prolonged recuperation. All ages can be affected, but it is most common in young adults, including pregnant women. An antecedent event is identified in approximately 60% of cases. This is often an upper respiratory tract infection or gastroenteritis. *Campylobacter*, cytomegalovirus, Epstein-Barr virus, human immunodeficiency virus, vaccination, surgery, trauma, and malignancy have all been associated with GBS. The risk of GBS increases after labor and delivery, especially during the first 2 weeks post partum.[21]

The classic presentation of GBS is a rapidly ascending paralysis. Early in the course, patients may complain of imbalance or poor coordination when walking. Sensory symptoms with little objective sensory loss are common. Often, distal paresthesias occur in the fingers and toes at the same time, an unusual finding in other polyneuropathies. Hyporeflexia or areflexia develops early. Bifacial weakness occurs in 50% of patients. Although bulbar weakness with dysarthria and dysphagia are also frequent, other cranial neuropathies are uncommon. Back and radicular pain occur in up to 25% of patients and often requires treatment with narcotics. Autonomic dysfunction can also occur. A fixed resting tachycardia is most common. Ileus, transient bladder dysfunction, arrhythmia, labile blood pressure, syndrome of inappropriate secretion of antidiuretic hormone, and impaired thermoregulation can also be seen.

In most patients, the disease continues to progress for days to weeks, followed by a plateau, before recovery commences. The plateau usually is reached by 3 weeks. Intubation is required in one-third of patients, usually between days 6 and 18. Progression beyond 4 weeks is rare for any patient with GBS.

Pregnancy and the postpartum period do not change the natural history of GBS. After the diagnosis has been established, the disease needs to be managed, whether the woman is pregnant or post partum, as it is in other patients with GBS. Close attention to pulmonary function and avoidance of medical complications are key elements. Treatment with either plasma exchange or intravenous immunoglobulin is indicated for nonambulatory patients. The number of reported pregnant women given either of these treatments is small, but both appear to be safe and appropriate.[22,23]

Chronic inflammatory demyelinating polyneuropathy Chronic inflammatory demyelinating polyneuropathy (CIDP) is an acquired, demyelinating, motor and sensory neuropathy that is presumed to be immune-mediated. It may be idiopathic or occur in association with human immunodeficiency virus (HIV) infection, monoclonal gammopathies, osteosclerotic myeloma, or lymphoma. Similar to other immune-related conditions (i.e., GBS and Bell's palsy), the risk is increased during pregnancy, especially the third trimester, and the postpartum period.[24] Both proximal and distal muscles are affected. The time course in CIDP is longer than that in GBS (>6 weeks), and the disease may have a monophasic progression, a stepwise progression, or a relapsing/remitting course. Early in the illness, it may not be possible to differentiate the initial presentation of CIDP from GBS. CIDP generally progresses slowly (over weeks to months), with the major disability usually being a gait disturbance. Areflexia or hyporeflexia is the rule. Large-fiber sensory loss (touch, vibration, and position sense) is more common than small-fiber loss (pain and temperature). A Romberg sign is commonly present. However, marked bulbar or respiratory weakness is unusual.

Because of the increased risk in this age group, pregnant women with CIDP should have testing to exclude associated HIV. CIDP often improves with plasma exchange, intravenous gamma globulin, or immunosuppressive therapy (prednisone, azathioprine, cyclophosphamide, cyclosporine). Plasma exchange and intravenous gamma globulin are the treatments of choice for pregnant women. Corticosteroids can be used if necessary; immunosuppressives are contraindicated during pregnancy.

Charcot-Marie-Tooth polyneuropathy Charcot-Marie-Tooth polyneuropathy type 1 (CMT1) is the most common of the inherited polyneuropathies. It is a distal, motor greater than sensory demyelinating neuropathy associated with pes cavus, hammer toes, and hypertrophic nerves. Sensory symptoms are uncommon, although mild sensory signs are usually discovered on careful examination. The onset commonly occurs in early childhood and typically presents as a foot deformity or delay in motor milestones. However, many patients are affected so minimally that they do not come to medical attention until middle age or later. CMT1 is most often associated with a duplication error of a 1.5-megabase DNA region on chromosome 17, a region containing the peripheral myelin gene *PMP22*.

There is no evidence that CMT affects pregnancy and labor. However, pregnancy may result in worsening of the neuropathy in some women.[25] Worsening is more common in women with childhood-onset disease (50%) than in those with adult-onset disease. Of the women whose CMT worsens during pregnancy, the increased symptoms and deficits are temporary in 35%; the others have persistent neurological deficits.

Neuromuscular junction disorders

Myasthenia gravis

Myasthenia gravis (MG) is caused by an autoimmune IgG-directed attack on the neuromuscular junction, aimed specifically at nicotinic acetylcholine receptors. Patients with MG present with muscle fatigue and weakness. Myasthenic weakness characteristically affects the extraocular muscles, bulbar muscles, or proximal limb muscles (or a combination of these). Eye findings are the most common, with ptosis and extraocular muscle weakness occurring in more than 50% of patients at the time of presentation and developing in more than 90% sometime during illness. The next most common is bulbar muscle weakness, which results in difficulty swallowing, chewing, and speaking. When limb weakness develops, it usually is symmetrical and proximal. The distinguishing clinical feature of MG is "pathological fatiguability" (i.e., muscle weakness that develops with continued use). This improves after rest. Muscle weakness is less pronounced upon arising in the morning and worsens as the day proceeds.

Most patients with MG have generalized disease; however, as many as 15% have the restricted ocular form of the disease. In these patients, myasthenic symptoms are restricted to the extraocular and eyelid muscles. If the symptoms are restricted to the ocular muscles for 1 to 2 years, there is a high probability that the disease will not generalize and will remain limited to the extraocular and eyelid muscles.

Autoimmune MG can affect all ages, but it is most common in younger women of childbearing age. The effect of pregnancy on MG is highly variable and unpredictable.[26] There is no correlation between the underlying severity of the disease and the risk of exacerbation with pregnancy. The first trimester and postpartum periods are times of greatest risk. If the disease is asymptomatic, the risk of an exacerbation during pregnancy is 17%.[26] In patients with symptomatic MG, 39% had improvement, 42% had no change, and 6% had deterioration of their condition during pregnancy.[26] However, 28% of women experienced exacerbations in the postpartum period.[26]

Because MG has no effect on smooth muscle, it does not affect uterine contractibility and, thus, has no effect on labor and delivery.[1] However, during labor and delivery, magnesium supplementation is contraindicated for the treatment of toxemia because it can provoke a myasthenic crisis. Also, if cesarean section is required, spinal anesthesia is preferable to general anesthesia; curare and other neuromuscular junction blocking agents are contraindicated.

For pregnant women, treatment with acetylcholinesterase inhibitors, corticosteroids, plasma exchange, and intravenous gamma globulin can be administered as they are in nonpregnant patients with MG. Immunosuppressive agents, including azathioprine and cyclosporine, are given with caution and best avoided if possible. Azathioprine crosses the placenta, and animal experiments suggest it has a teratogenic effect.[27] On the basis of reports of azathioprine and cyclosporine treatment administered to pregnant women with other conditions, the risk in humans appears low; however, the risk of using these drugs needs to be balanced for each patient, weighing the risk of relapse of a potentially life-threatening condition if a drug treatment is withdrawn during pregnancy.[26]

Transient neonatal MG may occur in babies of mothers with MG. This occurs when maternal autoantibodies pass through the placenta and produce the same clinical syndrome in newborn infants. The illness is usually mild and self-limited and disappears after the first few months of life as the maternal antibodies are degraded.

Iatrogenic hypermagnesemia

Hypermagnesemia is often used in the treatment of toxemia of pregnancy. Increased magnesium levels results in decreased release of acetylcholine quanta and presynapic blockade of the neuromuscular junction. As magnesium levels increase, paralysis of smooth muscle and autonomic nerves occur, resulting in dry mouth, hypotension, cutaneous flush, nausea, and vomiting.[28] As magnesium levels continue to increase, muscle stretch reflexes become depressed, followed by frank muscle weakness.

Hypermagnesemia has been used safely as a therapeutic agent in toxemia of pregnancy by following clinical examination findings (especially muscle stretch reflexes) and serum levels of magnesium. However, this therapy is contraindicated for patients with an underlying neuromuscular junction disorder (i.e., myasthenia gravis or Lambert-Eaton myasthenic syndrome). Increased magnesium levels in these patients can provoke a crisis with severe bulbar or respiratory weakness (or both).

References

1. Shaner DM. Neurological problems of pregnancy. In: Bradley WG, Daroff RB, Fenichel GM, Marsden CD, eds. Neurology in Clinical Practice, 3rd ed. Boston: Butterworth-Heinemann, 2000:2257–2268
2. McLennan HG, Oats JN, Walstab JE. Survey of hand symptoms in pregnancy. Med J Aust 1987;147:542–544
3. Stolp-Smith KA, Pascoe MK, Ogburn PL Jr. Carpal tunnel syndrome in pregnancy: frequency, severity and prognosis. Arch Phys Med Rehabil 1998;79:1285–1287
4. Ekman-Ordeberg G, Salgeback S, Ordeberg G. Carpal tunnel syndrome in pregnancy. A prospective study. Acta Obstet Gynecol Scand 1987;66:233–235
5. Courts RB. Splinting for symptoms of carpal tunnel syndrome during pregnancy. J Hand Ther 1995;8:31–34
6. Dawson DM, Hallett M, Millender LH. Entrapment Neuropathies. Boston: Little, Brown & Co., 1983
7. Stahl S, Blumenfeld Z, Yarnitsky D. Carpal tunnel syndrome in pregnancy: indications for early surgery. J Neurol Sci 1996;136:182–184
8. Vargo MM, Robinson LR, Nicholas JJ, Rulin MC. Postpartum femoral neuropathy: relic of an earlier era? Arch Phys Med Rehab 1990;71:591–596
9. Montag TW, Mead PB. Post partum femoral neuropathy. J Reprod Med 1981;26:563–566
10. Lindner A, Schulte-Mattler W, Zierz S. Postpartum obturator nerve syndrome: case report and review of

the nerve compression syndrome during pregnancy and delivery. (German) Zentralbl Gynäkol 1997;119: 93–99

11. Babayev M, Bodack MP, Creatura C. Common peroneal neuropathy secondary to squatting during childbirth. Obstet Gynecol 1998;91:830–832

12. Walling D. Bell's palsy in pregnancy and the puerperium. J Fam Pract 1993;36:559–563

13. Falco NA, Eriksson E. Idiopathic facial palsy in pregnancy and the puerperium. Surg Gynecol Obstet 1989;169:337–340

14. McGregor JA, Guberman A, Amer J, Goodlin R. Idiopathic facial nerve paralysis (Bell's palsy) in late pregnancy and the early puerperium. Obstet Gynecol 1987;69:435–438

15. Hilsinger RL Jr, Adour KK, Doty HE. Idiopathic facial paralysis, pregnancy, and the menstrual cycle. Ann Otol Rhinol Laryngol 1975;84:433–442

16. Adour KK, Ruboyianes JM, Von Doersten PG, et al. Bell's palsy treatment with acyclovir and prednisone compared with prednisone alone: a double-blind, randomized, controlled trial. Ann Otol Rhinol Laryngol 1996;105:371–378

17. Feasby TE, Burton SR, Hahn AF. Obstetrical lumbosacral plexus injury. Muscle Nerve 1992;15:937–940

18. Preston DC, Shapiro BE. Electromyography and Neuromuscular Disorders. Boston: Butterworth-Heinemann, 1997

19. Ohkoshi N, Ishii A, Shoji S. Wernicke's encephalopathy induced by hyperemesis gravidarum, associated with bilateral caudate lesions on computed tomography and magnetic resonance imaging. Eur Neurol 1994;34: 177–180

20. Gardian G, Voros E, Jardanhazy T, et al. Wernicke's encephalopathy induced by hyperemesis gravidarum. Acta Neurol Scand 1999;99:196–198

21. Cheng Q. Jiang GX, Fredrikson S, et al. Increased incidence of Guillain-Barré syndrome postpartum. Epidemiology 1998;9:601–604

22. Hurley TJ, Brunson AD, Archer RL, et al. Landry Guillain-Barré Strohl syndrome in pregnancy: report of three cases treated with plasmapheresis. Obstet Gynecol 1991;78:482–485

23. Clark AL. Clinical uses of intravenous immunoglobulin in pregnancy. Clin Obstet Gynecol 1999;42:368–380

24. McCombe PA, McManis PG, Frith JA, et al. Chronic inflammatory demyelinating polyradiculoneuropathy associated with pregnancy. Ann Neurol 1987;21: 102–104

25. Rudnik-Schoneborn S, Rohrig D, Nicholson G, Zerres K. Pregnancy and delivery in Charcot-Marie-Tooth disease type 1. Neurology 1993;43:2011–2016

26. Batocchi AP, Majolini L, Evoli A, et al. Course and treatment of myasthenia gravis during pregnancy. Neurology 1999;52:447–452

27. Tuchmann-Duplessis H, Mercier-Parot L. Production in rabbits of malformations of the limbs by azathioprine and 6-mercaptopurine (French) CR Soc Biol (Paris) 1966;160:501–506

28. Layzer RB. Neuromuscular Manifestations of Systemic Disease. Philadelphia: FA Davis, 1985:62–63

149 Pregnancy and Multiple Sclerosis: Therapeutic Aspects

Karim Makhlouf and Samia J Khoury

Multiple sclerosis (MS) is one of the most common chronic neurological diseases affecting young adults in the western countries. The female-to-male ratio is at least 2:1, and women are often affected during their reproductive age.

For many years, pregnancy was believed to worsen the course of MS and even to trigger its onset. Both MS and pregnancy induce dramatic changes in the immune system. Recent progress in immunology has allowed us to understand better some of the mechanisms of the disease and the physiological events occurring during pregnancy. Counseling a patient with MS about pregnancy must be based largely on her specific needs.

Interactions between MS and pregnancy

Effects of MS on pregnancy

MS has no substantial effect on fertility, conception, fetal viability, prematurity, incidence of toxemia, infant mortality, or delivery.[1,2] Studies have shown no increase in abortion rate or frequency of congenital malformations in children of MS patients of both sexes.[3,4] However, these results may be biased because women with severe disease and frequent relapses are more likely to avoid pregnancy.[5] The significantly greater frequency of childlessness[5] among the MS population most likely is attributable to the influence of MS on sexuality and general behavior concerning conception (of both the woman and her partner).

Effects of pregnancy on MS

Most studies report a trend toward a lower rate of disease relapse during pregnancy and a higher rate during the first 6 months postpartum.[2,3,5–16] However, most studies were retrospective, and the few prospective studies are based on a small number of cases with short-term follow-up. The rate of disease relapse, widely accepted as an indicator of disease activity, is not the only concern when studying pregnancy and MS.

Effect on disease activity The largest prospective study of the natural history of relapsing-remitting MS in pregnant women (PRIMS study) included 256 women (269 pregnancies) who were followed from 1 year before pregnancy until 1 year after delivery.[4] In spite of some drawbacks in the design of the study,[17] the results confirmed the previously observed trend: a decreased rate of relapse during pregnancy, especially in the third trimester, and an increased rate

during the first trimester postpartum. It also showed a return of the relapse rate to the prepregnancy level within the first year postpartum. The total frequency of relapses during the pregnancy-year (defined as the 9 months of pregnancy and the first 3 months postpartum) was very similar to the frequency before pregnancy. van Walderveen et al.[18] showed a clear decrease in the number of active lesions (defined as new or enlarging lesions) on sequential brain magnetic resonance imaging (MRI) during the second half of pregnancy in two patients with MS, followed by an increase in disease activity, as seen on MRI, in the first month postpartum.

Pregnancy and risk of MS onset The onset of MS occurs during pregnancy in less than 10% of the women with the disease.[19] A population-based Swedish study found that pregnancy is associated with a significantly lower risk of MS onset; also, the risk of entering a progressive course is less for women who become pregnant after the onset of MS.[5] Furthermore, no association has been found between oral contraceptive use and the risk of developing MS.[20]

Effect on long-term disability Long-term disability is usually measured by functional scales such as the Expanded Disability Status Scale (EDSS) of Kurtzke or the time to wheelchair dependence. Of the eight studies that considered this issue, none has demonstrated any adverse effect of pregnancy on long-term disability from MS (Table 149.1). Similarly, neither breast-feeding[4,11] nor epidural analgesia has been reported to have an adverse effect on the rate of relapse or the progression of disability in MS.[4]

Immunologic changes in pregnancy and MS

A successful pregnancy is dependent on maternal tolerance to paternal antigens expressed in the fetus. This maternal tolerance is based on, among other mechanisms, a strong shift in cytokine balance toward a type 2 or Th2 anti-inflammatory cytokine (interleukin [IL]-4, IL-5, IL-10) dominance, whereas the proinflammatory cytokines of the Th1 type (IL-2, IL-12, interferon-γ) are suppressed.[25,26] This pattern is reversed during the postpartum period. Because MS is believed to be Th1-mediated,[27] the temporary suppression of Th1 cytokine expression may explain the observed decrease in disease relapse during pregnancy and the increase during the postpartum period. Moreover, progesterone and corticosteroids, which

Table 149.1   Summary of studies that considered the long-term effects of pregnancy on disability in multiple sclerosis

Reference	Type of study	Patient base	Pregnancy after onset, no. of women	Duration of follow-up, years	Outcome measure	Method	Overall effect
Poser and Poser[3]	R	Clinic	91	...	EDSS/yr	Cross-sectional	None
Thompson et al.[21]	R	Clinic	23	13.9	EDSS	Cross-sectional	None
Weinshenker et al.[22]	R	Population	40	13–17	EDSS	Cross-sectional, longitudinal	None
Roullet et al.[14]	P	Clinic	33	0.5–22	EDSS	Cross-sectional	None
Verdru et al.[23]	R	Clinic	40	18.6 (mean)	Time to wheelchair	Longitudinal	Decreased disability
Worthington et al.[15]	P	Clinic	15	3	EDSS or FSS	Cross-sectional	None
Runmarker and Andersen[5]	P	Population	28	25	Time to EDSS 6 or progression	Longitudinal	Decreased disability
Stenager et al.[24]	P	Clinic	12	5	EDSS	Cross-sectional	None

EDSS, Expanded Disability Status Scale of Kurtzke; FSS, Functional Status Score; P, prospective; R, retrospective.
From Damek and Shuster.[2] By permission of Mayo Foundation.

Table 149.2   Immunologically active substances that are increased in the serum of pregnant women

Cytokine
    Transforming growth factor-β
    Interferon-β
Steroid hormones
    Androgens
    Cortisol
    Estrogens
    Progesterone
Peptide hormones
    Human chorionic gonadotropin
    Human placental lactogens
Pregnancy-associated proteins
    Early pregnancy factors
    Pregnancy-associated plasma proteins
    Pregnancy-associated α_2-glycoprotein
    Placental proteins
    Progesterone-induced blocking factor
    α-Fetoprotein
Immunologically specific factors
    Immune complexes
    Anti-major histocompatibility complex autoantibodies
    Autoantibodies specific for maternal T cells

From Damek and Shuster.[2] By permission of Mayo Foundation.

are produced in increased amounts during pregnancy, have the ability to induce a cytokine shift toward Th2 dominance.[25,28] Many other substances with immunomodulating capabilities are also present at higher concentrations in the maternal serum during pregnancy (Table 149.2).

Drugs, MS, and pregnancy

Many of the drugs currently used to manage MS are known to be either teratogenic or to have uncertain effects on the fetus. Few data have been published specifically on MS therapy during pregnancy.[2] The U.S. Food and Drug Administration (FDA) has classified the drugs used to treat MS into 4 categories (Table 149.3).

Although no well-controlled studies have been conducted on the effects of interferon beta-1a or interferon beta-1b in pregnant women, both drugs are associated with an increased abortion rate in monkeys (manufacturers' product information). Thus, they are not recommended for treating MS in pregnant women (FDA pregnancy category C). Similarly, breast-feeding is to be avoided if one of these drugs is used prophylactically during the postpartum period. In rat and rabbit studies, glatiramer acetate at very high doses did not have any teratogenic effect (FDA pregnancy category B), but it was not studied in monkeys. However, extrapolating from animal studies to human results is always difficult, and the pharmaceutical companies that manufacture these drugs are gathering data from patient records throughout the world, usually in cases in which treatment was ongoing when pregnancy occurred.

The recently discovered ovine interferon tau is a unique type 1 interferon, which has an important role in the animal reproductive cycle. It differs from other type 1 interferons (e.g., interferon β) in that it is remarkably less toxic even at high concentrations, is able to cross species barriers, and is not inducible by viral infection.[29,30] Ovine interferon tau has been shown to be effective in the treatment of animal models of MS.[31] Human clinical trials of ovine recombinant interferon tau are in progress. If these trials show that it is effective and safe, it may become an alternative treatment for MS during pregnancy, because it is an interferon of pregnancy in animals.

Orvieto et al.[32] recently reported that immunoglob-

Table 149.3 FDA pregnancy classification for drugs used to treat multiple sclerosis

Category	Drug
A—Controlled studies in pregnant women showing no risk for the fetus in any trimester	None listed
B—Animal data showing no harm to the fetus, but no human data available	Glatiramer (copolymer 1) Pemoline Oxybutynin Immunoglobulin
C—To be used during pregnancy only if no safer drugs are available or the benefit justifies the known risk	Corticosteroids Interferon beta-1a Interferon beta-1b Baclofen Amantadine Tizanidine Carbamazepine
D—Known teratogenic when given to pregnant women; must only be given after cautiously weighing risks and benefits	Azathioprine Cladribine
X—Contraindicated	Methotrexate Cyclophosphamide

FDA, U.S. Food and Drug Administration.
Modified from Damek and Shuster.[2] By permission of Mayo Foundation.

ulin given intravenously 1 to 3 days after delivery to 15 women with relapsing-remitting MS was beneficial in preventing acute postpartum-associated attacks.

The symptomatic treatment of relapses during pregnancy is also controversial because no controlled studies of the safety of short-term immunosuppression (usually with high doses of corticosteroids) during pregnancy have been performed. In studies of women with other autoimmune diseases, neonatal adrenal suppression has been shown after maternal use of corticosteroids. Most neurologists do not treat mild relapses that occur during pregnancy. The more severe exacerbations usually are treated with methylprednisolone (e.g., 1 g/day for 3 to 5 days given intravenously) after the treatment plan has been discussed with the patient and her obstetrician. Long-term treatment (longer than 2 weeks) with oral corticosteroids was common a few years ago, but it is not recommended for pregnant women with MS, because of possible side effects both in the mother and fetus. Studies in pregnant women with chronic asthma have shown that although a short course of corticosteroids (less than 2 weeks) is not associated with any adverse outcome, women with severe asthma requiring constant corticosteroid treatment have an increased incidence of premature delivery and low birth-weight infants.[33]

Treatment with nonessential symptomatic drugs should be discontinued before conception or as soon as pregnancy is recognized, especially if the drugs are potentially teratogenic.

The role of the neurologist is to provide as much information as possible for the patient and her partner to make the most appropriate decision. There is no reason to counsel women with MS against pregnancy, especially if they have only mild disability. It should be made clear that pregnancy does not worsen the long-term course of the disease, but that exacerbations may be expected after delivery.

References

1. Weinreb HJ. Demyelinating and neoplastic diseases in pregnancy. Neurol Clin 1994;12:509–526
2. Damek DM, Shuster EA. Pregnancy and multiple sclerosis. Mayo Clin Proc 1997;72:977–989
3. Poser S, Poser W. Multiple sclerosis and gestation. Neurology 1983;33:1422–1427
4. Confavreux C, Hutchinson M, Hours MM, et al. Rate of pregnancy-related relapse in multiple sclerosis. Pregnancy in Multiple Sclerosis Group. N Engl J Med 1998;339:285–291
5. Runmarker B, Andersen O. Pregnancy is associated with a lower risk of onset and a better prognosis in multiple sclerosis. Brain 1995;118:253–261
6. Millar JHD, Allison RS, Cheeseman EA, Merrett JD. Pregnancy as a factor influencing relapse in disseminated sclerosis. Brain 1959;82:417–426
7. Schapira K, Poskanzer DC, Newell DJ, Miller H. Marriage, pregnancy and multiple sclerosis. Brain 1966;89:419–428
8. Ghezzi A, Caputo D. Pregnancy: a factor influencing the course of multiple sclerosis? Eur Neurol 1981;20:115–117
9. Korn-Lubetzki I, Kahana E, Cooper G, Abramsky O. Activity of multiple sclerosis during pregnancy and puerperium. Ann Neurol 1984;16:229–231
10. Frith JA, McLeod JG. Pregnancy and multiple sclerosis. J Neurol Neurosurg Psychiatry 1988;51:495–498
11. Nelson LM, Franklin GM, Jones MC. Risk of multiple sclerosis exacerbation during pregnancy and breastfeeding. JAMA 1988;259:3441–3443
12. Birk K, Ford C, Smeltzer S, et al. The clinical course of multiple sclerosis during pregnancy and the puerperium. Arch Neurol 1990;47:738–742

13. Bernardi S, Grasso MG, Bertollini R, et al. The influence of pregnancy on relapses in multiple sclerosis: a cohort study. Acta Neurol Scand 1991;84:403–406

14. Roullet E, Verdier-Taillefer MH, Amarenco P, et al. Pregnancy and multiple sclerosis: a longitudinal study of 125 remittent patients. J Neurol Neurosurg Psychiatry 1993;56:1062–1065

15. Worthington J, Jones R, Crawford M, Forti A. Pregnancy and multiple sclerosis—a 3-year prospective study. J Neurol 1994;241:228–233

16. Sadovnick AD, Eisen K, Hashimoto SA, et al. Pregnancy and multiple sclerosis. A prospective study. Arch Neurol 1994;51:1120–1124

17. Whitaker JN. Effects of pregnancy and delivery on disease activity in multiple sclerosis. N Engl J Med 1998;339:339–340

18. van Walderveen MAA, Tas MW, Barkhof F, et al. Magnetic resonance evaluation of disease activity during pregnancy in multiple sclerosis. Neurology 1994;44: 327–329

19. Davis RK, Maslow AS. Multiple sclerosis in pregnancy: a review. Obstet Gynecol Surv 1992;47:290–296

20. Villard-Mackintosh L, Vessey MP. Oral contraceptives and reproductive factors in multiple sclerosis incidence. Contraception 1993;47:161–168

21. Thompson DS, Nelson LM, Burns A, et al. The effects of pregnancy in multiple sclerosis: a retrospective study. Neurology 1986;36:1097–1099

22. Weinshenker BG, Hader W, Carriere W, et al. The influence of pregnancy on disability from multiple sclerosis: a population-based study in Middlesex County, Ontario. Neurology 1989;39:1438–1440

23. Verdru P, Theys P, D'Hooghe MB, Carton H. Pregnancy and multiple sclerosis: the influence on long term disability. Clin Neurol Neurosurg 1994;96:38–41

24. Stenager E, Stenager EN, Jensen K. Effect of pregnancy on the prognosis for multiple sclerosis. A 5-year follow up investigation. Acta Neurol Scand 1994;90:305–308

25. Wilder RL. Hormones, pregnancy, and autoimmune diseases. Ann N Y Acad Sci 1998;840:45–50

26. Wegmann TG, Lin H, Guilbert L, Mosmann TR. Bidirectional cytokine interactions in the maternal-fetal relationship: is successful pregnancy a Th2 phenomenon? Immunol Today 1993;14:353–356

27. Khoury SJ, Weiner HL, Hafler DA. Immunological mechanisms in multiple sclerosis. In: Cook SD, ed. Handbook of Multiple Sclerosis. 2nd ed. New York: Marcel Dekker, 1996:145–155

28. Szekeres-Bartho J, Wegmann TG. A progesterone-dependent immunomodulatory protein alters the Th1/Th2 balance. J Reprod Immunol 1996;31:81–95

29. Soos JM, Subramaniam PS, Hobeika AC, et al. The IFN pregnancy recognition hormone IFN-tau blocks both development and superantigen reactivation of experimental allergic encephalomyelitis without associated toxicity. J Immunol 1995;155:2747–2753

30. Khan OA, Jiang H, Subramaniam PS, et al. Immunomodulating functions of recombinant ovine interferon tau: potential for therapy in multiple sclerosis and autoimmune disorders. Mult Scler 1998;4: 63–69

31. Soos JM, Mujtaba MG, Subramaniam PS, et al. Oral feeding of interferon tau can prevent the acute and chronic relapsing forms of experimental allergic encephalomyelitis. J Neuroimmunol 1997;75:43–50

32. Orvieto R, Achiron R, Rotstein Z, et al. Pregnancy and multiple sclerosis: a 2-year experience. Eur J Obstet Gynecol Reprod Biol 1999;82:191–194

33. Fitzsimons R, Greenberger PA, Patterson R. Outcome of pregnancy in women requiring corticosteroids for severe asthma. J Allergy Clin Immunol 1986;78:349–353

150 Movement Disorders During Pregnancy

Nutan Sharma and Michael Schwarzschild

The majority of movement disorders rarely occur during the reproductive years. The effect of pregnancy on the prognosis of various movement disorders is not well understood. In addition, the safety of movement disorder medications during pregnancy has not been systematically studied. This chapter briefly summarizes what is known about pregnancy and movement disorders, and focuses on the effects of relevant drugs on maternal and fetal health.

Chorea

Chorea is defined as abnormal, involuntary movements that are brief, usually in the distal portion of the extremities, and without purpose. Chorea gravidarum (CG) is used to describe any chorea, due to any cause, with onset during pregnancy. The most common causes of chorea during the reproductive years are systemic lupus erythematosus (SLE), Sydenham's chorea and neuroleptic-induced chorea. Less common but treatable causes include hyperthyroidism and Wilson's disease.

The evaluation of CG is similar to that of chorea occurring at any period of life. SLE can be evaluated by examining the titer of antinuclear antibodies (ANA), anticardiolipin antibodies and lupus anticoagulant assay. Wilson's disease can be diagnosed by evaluating serum copper and ceruloplasmin, measuring 24-hour urine copper excretion and by slit-lamp examination. Thyroid function studies can rule out the possibility of hyperthyroidism. CNS imaging by MRI (without contrast) should be considered in all pregnant women who develop chorea. MRI is particularly important in those who develop chorea, particularly if unilateral, to rule out caudate atrophy, basal ganglia tumor or hemorrhage and focal infarction.

CG is typically a benign complication of pregnancy and can be managed without pharmacological treatment. Drugs are reserved for those in whom the chorea is so disabling that their health or that of the fetus is endangered by risks such as malnutrition, dehydration or injury. Medications used to treat nonpregnant individuals include dopamine-depleting agents, dopamine receptor blockers (i.e. neuroleptics) and benzodiazepines. Dopamine-depleting agents, such as reserpine, are potentially toxic to the fetus and are relatively contraindicated during pregnancy. Neuroleptics should also be avoided, particularly during the limb genesis period of the first trimester. Low-dose benzodiazepines, which are known to cause fetal CNS and respiratory depression, may be considered in the second or third trimester when the risk from uncontrolled chorea outweighs the risk that treatment may harm the fetus.

Essential tremor

Essential tremor (ET) is rarely disabling during the childbearing years and typically does not interfere with pregnancy or delivery. Accordingly, women with ET should be reassured and encouraged to taper off tremor medication during pregnancy. The medications commonly used for symptomatic treatment of ET include β-blockers, primidone and benzodiazepines. Although all of these medications do carry teratogenic risk, propranolol may be the safest choice for treatment of disabling ET in pregnancy.

Parkinson's disease (PD)

Only a small minority of PD cases are diagnosed during the childbearing years. Information regarding pregnancy and PD is therefore limited to retrospective studies and case reports. There is some anecdotal evidence that pregnancy increases the risk of either worsening pre-existing symptoms or developing new symptoms.

Information regarding the teratogenic effects of PD therapy is also limited. Although well-designed human studies are lacking, most studies in rodents and rabbits have not shown any teratogenic effects of levodopa (L-dopa). However the peripheral dopa decarboxylase inhibitors carbidopa and benserazide, which are administered with L-dopa, have been shown to cause visceral and skeletal fetal abnormalities in rabbits. In addition, levodopa inhibits lactation and should be avoided by women who are planning to breastfeed. Treatment with the D_2 and D_1 receptor agonist pergolide has not shown significant evidence of harm to fetuses in mice or rabbits. The relatively new D_2 receptor agonist ropinirole causes decreased fetal survival and digital malformations in rats. Both amantadine and the monoaminoxidase-B inhibitor selegiline are embryotoxic in rodents.

In summary, no antiparkinsonian medication has been conclusively shown to be safe in pregnancy. The prudent management of PD in pregnant women should include efforts to minimize pharmacotherapy. Nevertheless, drug therapy for PD is often warranted to ensure maternal health and safety. At present, treatment with levodopa/carbidopa and/or bromocriptine may offer the greatest overall efficacy and safety for both mother and fetus.

Dystonia

One of the most common causes of acute generalized dystonia during pregnancy is the acute dystonic reaction to dopamine-blocking agents. The most frequent indication for giving such a drug during pregnancy is

Table 150.1 The potential risks during pregnancy of medications used for various movement disorders

Drug	Potential risks during pregnancy	Other side effects
Carbidopa	Visceral and skeletal abnormalities in animals	None when used alone in the recommended dose range
Benserazide	Visceral and skeletal abnormalities in animals	
Levodopa	Inhibits lactation	Nausea, diarrhea, confusion, hallucinations, hypotension
Pergolide	No evidence of fetal abnormalities in animals	Leg edema, nausea, confusion, hallucinations, hypotension
Ropinirole	Decreased fetal survival and digit malformation in animals	Leg edema, sleep attacks, nausea, confusion, hallucinations, hypotension
Pramipexole	Increased frequency of early embryonic loss in rodents	Nausea, hallucinations, hypotension
Lorazepam, diazepam	Increased risk of congenital malformations in rabbits	Sedation, dizziness
Amantadine	Embryotoxic in rodents	Leg edema, livedo reticularis, confusion, hallucinations
Selegiline	Embryotoxic in rodents	Nausea, confusion, hallucinations
Bromocriptine	Inhibits lactation Fetal abnormalities in animals	Nausea, abdominal pain, confusion, hallucinations
Trihexyphenidyl	Effect on pregnancy has not been studied in animals	Dry mouth, blurred vision, dizziness, nausea
Botulinum toxin	Effect on pregnancy has not been studied in animals	Diffuse skin rash
Penicillamine	Visceral abnormalities in animals	Abdominal pain, bone marrow depression, glomerulonephritis
Trientine	Visceral abnormalities in animals	Iron deficiency, systemic lupus erythematosus
Zinc	No evidence that it is teratogenic in animals	

nausea. Avoiding the use of dopamine-blocking antiemetics is the best method of preventing this complication of pregnancy.

The focal dystonias of early adulthood are commonly treated with oral anticholinergic agents such as trihexyphenidyl, or locally injected botulinum toxin A. The safety of anticholinergic agents during pregnancy has not been established. The safety of locally injected botulinum toxin A during pregnancy has not been established either, although its use as a local rather than a systemic agent makes the risk of fetal toxicity less likely.

Wilson's disease

Wilson's disease (WD), caused by an autosomal recessive defect in copper metabolism, can produce multiple signs of basal ganglia dysfunction, including rigidity, bradykinesia, dystonia, chorea and tremor. It is generally agreed that treatment for WD should continue during pregnancy, as cessation of treatment can lead to marked worsening of the disease and death. Treatments for WD include penicillamine, trientine and zinc. Penicillamine is teratogenic in animals and humans. Trientine is teratogenic in animals but has not been shown to cause birth defects in humans. Zinc has been studied for its teratogenic potential but there is no evidence that it is a teratogen in humans. Recent data indicate that zinc is a reasonable choice for pregnant women with WD, as it protects both maternal health and fetal outcome.

Restless legs syndrome

Perhaps most common among movement disorders appearing in pregnancy is restless legs syndrome (RLS), a poorly localized lower extremity discomfort that compels the patient to seek relief by moving her legs. This typically deep-seated bilateral sensation of the calves or legs is variably described as crawling, aching, itching, burning or pulling. It is most prominent at rest later in the day, particularly in bed at night. Neurological examination shows no associated central or neuropathic deficits. Although generally benign, this condition is particularly common during the latter half of gestation, with estimates of its occurrence during pregnancy ranging from 10% to 30%. When RLS develops during pregnancy the symptoms generally resolve upon delivery. In patients with pre-existing RLS, particularly those with a family history, symptoms may be exacerbated during the later trimesters.

The etiology of RLS in pregnancy and otherwise is not well understood, although contributing factors such as folate deficiency have been implicated in some cases. Beyond treatment for any folate deficiency, anemia, uremia or diabetes that may be identified, management of RLS in pregnancy is symptomatic. Explanation, reassurance and suggestions for local massage (by hand or with a vibrator applied to the calves) typically suffice. If symptoms persist and are severe enough to warrant drug therapy, consideration should be given to the lowest effective doses of levodopa with carbidopa (or with benserazide), or a dopaminergic agonist. Among the numerous agents found to be of benefit in RLS (including benzodiazepines and opioids), these may be most likely to be of benefit while offering the lowest risk of side effects to the patient and her fetus. Should the phenomenon of intolerable daytime augmentation of RLS symptoms develop during pregnancy after initiating levodopa therapy, switching to a dopaminergic agonist should be considered, as in the management of RLS in general. And although efficacy for RLS may be greater with other dopaminergic agonists, such as pramipexole, at present bromocriptine is a prudent first choice in this class of drugs, given our considerably greater experience with it in pregnancy.

We thank Drs Juliane Winkelmann and John Winkelman for their helpful discussions.

Selected reading

Brewer GJ, Johnson VD, Dick RD, et al. Treatment of Wilson's disease with zinc. XVII: treatment during pregnancy. Hepatology 2000;31:364–370

Golbe LI. Pregnancy and movement disorders. Neurol Clin 1994;12:497–508

Shulman LM, Minagar A, Weinder WJ. The effect of pregnancy in Parkinson's disease. Mov Disord 2000; 15:132–135

Trenkwalder C, Walters AS, Hening W. Periodic limb movements and restless legs syndrome. Neurol Clin 1996;14:629–650

151 Mitochondrial Disease

Dominic Thyagarajan

In 1962, Luft et al.,[1] showed "loose coupling" between respiration and phosphorylation of adenosine diphosphate (ADP) in isolated skeletal muscle mitochondria from a 35-year-old woman with: life-long non-thyroidal hypermetabolism; muscle hypotonia, wasting and weakness; and absent deep tendon reflexes. By EM (electron microscopy), the mitochondria varied in size, contained very densely packed cristae, and lacked opaque bodies. This was the first well documented defect in mitochondrial enzyme organization. Identical patients have not frequently been reported since, but in the following decades many patients with mitochondrial morphological changes, biochemical evidence of electron transport chain (ETC) defects and various clinical features have been described. Shy et al.,[2] investigated ultrastructural morphological changes in muscle mitochondria and divided certain childhood myopathies into a group with proliferated mitochondria and normal appearance (*pleoclonial myopathy*) and another group with enlarged, abnormal mitochondria with disoriented cristae (*megaconial myopathy*). Drachman[3] and Kearns and Sayre[4] described chronic progressive external ophthalmoplegia (CPEO) with other features. In 1972, Olson et al.,[5] reported seven patients with CPEO who had a distinctive subsarcolemmar clustering of skeletal muscle mitochondria on the Gomori modified trichrome stain (introduced in 1963 by Engel and Cunningham),[6] which they termed "ragged-red" fibers. Ultrastructurally, the mitochondria were enlarged, had abnormal cristae and sometimes contained paracrystalline inclusions. It emerged that these "mitochondrial encephalomyopathies"[7] or "mitochondrial cytopathies"[8] were clinically diverse, not necessarily associated with CPEO and included disorders of vision (retinal degeneration, optic atrophy, cataract and glaucoma), deafness, proximal myopathy or CPEO, neuropathy, encephalopathy, short stature, renal tubular disorders, endocrinopathies and lactic acidosis. In some of these cases, specific ETC defects were identified biochemically, including in cytochrome *b*, ATPase, reduced nicotinamide adenine dinucleotide coenzyme Q (NADH-CoQ) reductase, and cytochrome *c* oxidoreductase (COX). Through the 1970s a number of mitochondrial enzyme deficiencies other than ETC defects were characterized, including pyruvate dehydrogenase complex deficiency,[9] carnitine palmitoyltransferase deficiency,[10] and carnitine deficiency.[11] A systematic biochemical classification of mitochondrial disorders was devised[12] and included: (1) substrate transport defects into the mitochondrial matrix, (2) substrate utilization defects in the mitochondrial matrix (3) Kreb's cycle defects, (4) ETC defects and (5) defects of oxidation/phosphoryla-

tion coupling. Although classifications (1)–(3) are mitochondrial disorders in the strict sense, the term is often taken to mean defects of the ETC or oxidative phosphorylation coupling, and this is the focus of this chapter.

The turning point came in the 1980s with an understanding of the genetics of mitochondrial disorders. Egger and Wilson[13] noted the excess of maternal inheritance in pedigrees with mitochondrial cytopathy, and maternal inheritance in Leber's Hereditary Optic Atrophy (LHON). They postulated mitochondrial genetic inheritance, since mammalian mitochondrial DNA (mtDNA) (discovered in 1963[14] and sequenced in the human in 1981),[15] was known to be maternally inherited.[16] In 1988, a specific point mutation of mtDNA in LHON, and large-scale deletions in muscle mtDNA from patients with mitochondrial encephalomyopathies were found. An explosion in genotype-phenotype correlation followed and now there are over 50 point mutations and hundreds of deletions of mtDNA known in various mitochondrial encephalomyopathies.[17] In most, but not all instances (LHON is a notable example), the mutant mtDNA coexists with the normal "wild-type" (heteroplasmy). In general, mtDNA mutations impairing mitochondrial protein synthesis (tRNA mutations and deletions) are associated with the "ragged red" fibers on muscle biopsy, whilst a morphological clue is absent in mutations of the mitochondrial structural genes.

Only 10% of mitochondrial protein is encoded by mtDNA and it is possible that most mitochondrial disease originates in the nuclear DNA (nDNA). Zeviani et al.,[18] showed dominant inheritance of multiple mtDNA deletions in 1989, clearly implicating a nuclear factor. In 1995, Bourgeron et al.,[19] identified a mutation in the flavoprotein subunit of Complex II (nucleus-encoded) in two siblings with recessively inherited Leigh syndrome (LS) and Suomalainen et al.,[20] showed linkage to chromosome 10q in autosomal dominant CPEO pedigrees with multiple mtDNA deletions. In the last two years, mutations in three different genes have been found in this genetically heterogeneous group of disorders: in a gene encoding a phage T7 gene 4-like protein, probably with a helicase function in the chromosome 10-linked form;[21] in the gene for polymerase gamma on chromosome 15;[22] and in the gene encoding the heart and skeletal muscle-specific isoform of the adenine nucleotide transporter (ANT1) in the chromosome 4-linked form.[23] Mutations have been found in the thymidine phosphorylase gene in a recessive form of progressive external ophthalmoplegia (PEO), myo-neuro-gastrointestinal encephalomyopathy (MNGIE).[24] Nuclear mutations have been found in Complex I deficiency, affecting different nuclear subunits.[25-30] In isolated COX deficiency, mutations have been found in different COX assembly genes[31-34] and similar findings have emerged in Complex III deficiency with the finding of mutations in a gene involved in assembly of Complex III.[35] As the nucleus-encoded defects affecting subunits of the respiratory chain and intergenomic signalling have been identified, there has been increasing interest in the role of mitochondrial abnormalities in the pathogenesis of common neurodegenerative diseases such as Parkinson's disease (PD), Alzheimer's disease (AD), Huntington's disease (HD) and ageing.[36,37]

Epidemiology

There are no good population-based estimates of the prevalence of mtDNA disorders in the community. Data from a diagnostic referral center in England are that 12.48 per 100 000 individuals in the adult and child population either had mtDNA disease or were at risk of developing mtDNA disease.[38] A high index of suspicion will invariably lead to greater detection but diagnostic methods lack both sensitivity and specificity.

Aetiology

Mitochondrial disorders are largely genetic in origin, due to a genetic defect of nuclear or mtDNA, an intergenomic signalling defect or in some other process affecting the mitochondrial respiratory chain. Drugs and toxins of interest to the movement disorder specialist may affect mitochondrial function, but it is not always certain these directly cause or exacerbate human disease. Chronic L-dopa administration at high doses was found by one group to cause reversible Complex I deficiency in rats, but not by another, and, in L-dopa treated patients with multiple system atrophy (MSA), there is no reduction in Complex I activity in post-mortem substantia nigra or platelets. 3-Nitroproprionic acid (3-NPA), an irreversible inhibitor of succinate dehydrogenase (SDH, Complex II) causes age dependent striatal excitotoxic damage in rats and non-human primates and when accidentally ingested by humans causes delayed putaminal necrosis and dystonia. MPP$^+$, the active metabolite of the neurotoxin MPTP (1-methyl-4-phenyl-1,2,3,6-tetrahydropyridine), that produces an irreversible clinical, biochemical and neuropathological condition similar to idiopathic PD, inhibits Complex I of the respiratory chain. MPTP also shares structural similarity with haloperidol, chlorpromazine, thiothixene and clozapine, neuroleptics which cause a dose-dependent reduction of Complex I activity in disrupted rat brain mitochondria and in platelets from five psychiatric patients chronically exposed to one or more of these agents. Rats chronically challenged with rotenone, a Complex I inhibitor, develop behavioral and pathological features of PD.[39] This finding is particularly relevant to the movement disorder specialist interested in the pathogenesis of idiopathic PD as rotenone is a plant-derived compound used as a household pesticide and in the control of fish populations.

Pathophysiology and pathogenesis

Mitochondria are cellular organelles with a central role in energy metabolism. They have the key function of generating adenosine triphosphate (ATP) through the electron transport chain (ETC). Pyruvate and fatty acids are transported into the mitochondrial matrix where oxidative pathways convert them to acetyl coenzyme A (acetyl-CoA). Acetyl-CoA is oxidized to the CO_2 and H_2O by the Kreb's cycle, generating NADH and FMNH (a reduced form of flavin mononucleotide), which donate electrons to the ETC. The ETC comprises five multisubunit enzymes and two mobile electron carriers (coenzyme Q and cytochrome c), embedded in the mitochondrial membrane. A series of redox reactions in the ETC results in the reduction of O_2 to water and generates a pH gradient across the inner mitochondrial membrane. The H$^+$ gradient generates proton flow through the fifth enzyme complex which catalyses the synthesis of ATP from ADP and inorganic phosphate (Pi).

Unlike other organelles, mitochondria contain their own genetic material: in humans, 2–10 copies of a double-stranded 16 569 kb circular DNA.[15] At fertilization, the sperm, containing 50–75 mitochondria, each with one copy of mtDNA, enters the oocyte, containing 10^5–10^8 mitochondria (and 10^5 copies of mtDNA in human oocytes), complete with mitochondria in the mid-piece. In embryogenesis, the paternal contribution to the individual's mtDNA is eliminated by unknown mechanisms. In mice, Kaneda et al.,[40] showed that the specific elimination of paternal mtDNA occurred early in embryogenesis in intraspecific crosses but not interspecific crosses, where paternal mtDNA could be detected by polymerase chain reaction (PCR) even in the neonates. Mitochondrial DNA only encodes 13 subunits of the ETC, 22 tRNAs, and two rRNAs. The remaining 70 or so proteins of the ETC and the proteins required for replication, transcription, and translation of mtDNA are encoded by nuclear DNA (nDNA). Nucleus-encoded subunits of the ETC are synthesized in the cytoplasm, usually as larger precursor polypeptides with N-terminal presequences that direct them to mitochondria in an energy-dependent process. Nuclear and mitochondrial-encoded subunits assemble in the inner mitochondrial membrane after cleavage of the pre-sequence by a Ca^{++}/Mg^{++} dependent protease.

In such a complex mechanism, hundreds of molecular lesions could ultimately disrupt ETC function. We presently recognize only comparatively few of these lesions. How ETC dysfunction results in disease is not fully understood. There may be several pathogenetic mechanisms operating:

1. Necrotic and apoptotic cell death appear to be downstream events of ETC dysfunction due to mtDNA mutations.[41,42] A variety of mechanisms may be important, including the opening of the mitochondrial transition pore (MTP). The MTP,

present at contact sites between the inner and outer membrane, is formed from a complex of the voltage-dependent anion channel (VDAC), the adenine nucleotide translocase and cyclophilin-D (CyP-D) and interacts with pro- and anti-apoptotic members of the Bcl-2 family. Many signals, including in vitro conditions of oxidative stress, relatively high Ca^{2+} and low ATP, cause pore opening, an increase in the inner membrane permeability to small solutes, mitochondrial swelling, and release into the cytosol of proteins crucial in the induction of apoptosis such as apoptosis inhibitory factor and cytochrome c.[43-45]

2. Inhibition of the ETC causes accumulation of electrons in the early steps, particularly Complex I. Single electron transfer produces superoxide radicals. Through the action of manganese-superoxide dismutase (MnSOD) in the mitochondrial matrix, these generate H_2O_2 that can lead to the production of highly reactive oxygen radical species in the redox environment of the inner mitochondrial membrane. Damage to lipids, proteins and DNA by these free radicals is postulated to lead to cell death.[36,46]

3. Beal[47] proposed a role for ETC dysfunction in excitotoxic cell damage in neurodegenerative diseases. The energy-dependent Na^+/K^+ ATPase pump is impaired, inhibiting the repolarization of neuronal synaptic membranes after depolarizing glutamatergic stimuli. Voltage-dependent Ca^{2+} channels remain inappropriately open and the block of voltage-dependent Mg^{2+} NMDA channels is reduced, leading to their activation with endogenous glutamate. The Na^+ and Ca^{2+} enter the cell through the high-conductance Ca^{2+} permeable NMDA channels. Inside the cell, the ATP-dependent sequestration of the Ca^{2+} into the endoplasmic reticulum is reduced and the high Na^+ levels will reduce the removal of Ca^{2+} from the cell through the Na^+–Ca^{2+} antiport system. The elevated intracellular Ca^{2+} level activates proteases, lipases and endonucleases, leading to auto-destructive processes and excitotoxic cell injury. Defects of Ca^{2+} homeostasis have been observed in cell lines with mtDNA mutations.[48] The hypothesis explains the selective vulnerability of certain neuronal cell groups, observed in some mitochondrial encephalomyopathies[49,50] and neurodegenerations, by the anatomic distribution of excitatory pathways. Evidence for the hypothesis comes from the effect 3-NPA (see above). Neurotoxicity of 3-NPA can be blocked in vivo in rats by removal of excitatory inputs or in vitro with antagonists of excitatory amino acids.

Genetics

The ETC is a complex assembly of multisubunit enzymes encoded by two genetic systems, one with Mendelian and one with non-Mendelian (maternal) transmission.[36] Mitochondrial diseases may thus be autosomal dominant or autosomal recessive, when some nucleus-encoded subunit of the ETC[19,25-27] or other protein important in biogenesis of the ETC is affected, or maternally inherited when mtDNA is mutated. For reasons still unexplained, single large-scale rearrangements of mtDNA are usually, though not invariably, sporadic. Single large-scale rearrangements coexist with the wild-type mtDNA, a phenomenon called heteroplasmy. In general, they are not found in significant amounts in all tissues, tending to be present in highest amount in post-mitotic tissues like muscle and brain.[51] Mitochondrial DNA point mutations are generally maternally-inherited. Heteroplasmy is a common feature of mtDNA point mutations, except those causing LHON which are usually homoplasmic. Like mtDNA deletions, the mutant load varies from tissue to tissue and can change with time in a particular tissue of an individual. It is generally believed that the mutant load in a tissue and the metabolic demands of the tissue determine the detrimental effects of the mutation. Commonly, a certain mutant load has to be reached before the tissue suffers—the concept of the "threshold effect."[51] There are now well over 50 described.[17]

Multiple mtDNA deletions follow Mendelian inheritance. Autosomal dominant forms are caused by dysfunction of a protein important in the maintenance of stability or replication of mtDNA. In the last couple of years, mutations in genes for three of these forms, a gene encoding a phage T7 gene 4-like protein, probably with a helicase function on chromosome 10,[21] the gene for polymerase gamma on chromosome 15,[22] and the gene encoding the heart and skeletal muscle-specific isoform of the adenine nucleotide transporter (ANT1)[23] have been found. Mutations in the thymidine phosphorylase gene cause an autosomal recessive form, MNGIE.[24] Another, probably autosomal recessive defect of intergenomic signalling causes grossly reduced mtDNA copy number: mtDNA depletion.[51] In other examples, generally recessive, the mutation is in a gene encoding a component of the mitochondrial import machinery for carrier proteins, for example, the deafness/dystonia peptide 1 (DDP1) gene in the X-linked Mohr-Trajenberg syndrome,[52] or an assembly protein, e.g., a COX assembly protein, in isolated recessive COX deficiency (e.g., SCO2,[33] SURF1,[31,32] or COX10 mutations[34]), or the Complex III assembly gene BCS1L in neonatal proximal tubulopathy, hepatic involvement and encephalopathy associated with Complex III deficiency.[35] In one recessive form of hereditary spastic paraplegia linked to chromosome 16q, "ragged fibres" are present in muscle and there are mutations in a gene called paraplegin. The paraplegin product is highly homologous to the yeast mitochondrial ATPases, AFG3, RCA1, and YME1, which have both proteolytic and chaperone-like activities at the inner mitochondrial membrane.[53] Freidreich's ataxia, the most common cause of recessive ataxia, is associated with loss of function of frataxin, usually due to a homozygous intronic expansion. Frataxin is mitochondrial protein conserved through evolution. In yeast, knockout of the frataxin homologue causes mitochondrial iron accumulation. Thus, defective

Table 151.1   Clinical manifestations of mitochondrial disease

System	Manifestations
CNS	Seizures, stroke-like episodes, dementia, sensorineural deafness, movement disorders including ataxia, myoclonus, dystonia, chorea, migraine, psychomotor regression/retardation, parkinsonism
Skeletal muscle	Hypotonia, myopathy, ptosis, CPEO, recurrent myoglobinuria
Peripheral nerves	Neuropathy
Bone marrow	Pancytopenia, sideroblastic anemia
Kidney	De-Toni-Fanconi renal tubular acidosis
Endocrine	Type II diabetes mellitus, hypoparathyroidism, growth hormone deficiency
Heart	Cardiomyopathy, conduction defect
Gastrointestinal system	Pancreatic failure, pseudoobstruction, hepatopathy
Eye	Retinal pigmentary degeneration, optic atrophy, cataract
Systemic	Systemic lactic acidosis

mitochondrial iron transport with free radical damage and oxidative stress with deficiency of aconitase and iron-sulphur proteins may be the pathogenic mechanism of disease.[54]

Mitochondrial genetic factors are implicated in neurodegenerations like AD and PD.[37] Evidence for involvement of mitochondrial genetic factors is greatest in PD. Complex I activity is reduced in post-mortem substantia nigra (but not other brain regions), platelets and muscle. This Complex I deficiency has been transferred from platelets of PD patients to rho zero cells (cells lacking mtDNA) by cybrid fusion,[55,56] implying that the origin of the ETC defects in PD is mtDNA. However, this does not necessarily establish a cause and effect relationship between mtDNA mutations and PD. Damage to mtDNA might be a bystander phenomenon secondary to some other factor such as direct oxidative damage. Several mtDNA mutations have been recognized in association with Parkinsonism[57–60] but these are only in a handful of pedigrees and work in the last few years has indicated a more important role for other molecular pathways in PD such as ubiquitin-mediated proteolysis. It is not clear how oxidative stress interacts with defects in some of the proteins involved, such as parkin and alpha-synuclein, whose genes are mutated in some instances, although some work suggests that the presence of abnormal alpha-synucleins in substantia nigra in PD may increase neuronal vulnerability to a range of toxic agents producing oxidative stress.[61]

Clinical features

The clinical features of mitochondrial disease are protean and range from mild disease affecting one organ or system to severe multisystem disease. Table 151.1 shows some of the more common manifestations. Typical syndromes have been defined including mitochondrial encephalomyopathy with lactic acidosis and stroke (MELAS), myoclonus epilepsy with ragged red fibers (MERRF), neurogenic weakness, ataxia and retinitis pigmentosa (NARP), Pearson's marrow pancreas syndrome (PS), Leigh syndrome/ Familial bilateral striatal necrosis(LS/FBSN), and LHON.

Classification

A molecular classification of mitochondrial disorders is presented in Table 151.2. Biochemical[51] and clinical[62] classifications have been very useful but a genetically based classification reflects the rapid recent advances in our understanding of these disorders at a fundamental level.

Diagnostic criteria

Diagnostic criteria have been proposed[62] but the genetic complexity and protean clinical and biochemical manifestations of these disorders, pose difficulties for diagnostic aids of this type. Applied knowledge of the patterns of clinical presentation, transmission genetics, laboratory findings, neuroradiological patterns, standardized exercise testing results, muscle morphology, muscle biochemistry, and molecular genetic screening is necessary for effective diagnosis.[63]

Differential diagnosis

Because of the protean clinical manifestations, these disorders share similarities with virtually all disorders in Neurology and many in General Medicine. Clues to the possibility of a mitochondrial disease may be clinical (i.e., a clinically recognizable syndrome e.g., MELAS, adPEO), genetic (e.g., maternal inheritance) or come from laboratory investigations (e.g., "ragged-red" fibers on a muscle biopsy or lactic acidemia). Confirmation of the clinical suspicion may involve one or more special investigations (e.g., standardized exercise test, muscle biopsy for morphology and biochemical ETC analysis, or genetic screening for mtDNA point mutations and rearrangements).[63]

Treatment

Therapies for mitochondrial disease are pharmacological and non-pharmacological (Table 151.3). Because mitochondrial diseases are comparatively uncommon, genetically and clinically heterogeneous, vary so greatly in severity and course and we lack validated clinical outcome measures, there are no good randomized, double-blind controlled treatment trials. Thus, pharmacological therapy is very difficult to

Table 151.2   Classification of mitochondrial disease

Molecular defect	Inheritance	Some phenotypic examples
mtDNA		
Single large scale rearrangement	Nearly all	CPEO
	Sporadic	PS
Point mutation		
In structural genes	Maternal	NARP, LS, LHON, FBSN
In mitochondrial RNA genes	Maternal	MELAS, MERRF, SNHL, cardiomyopathy, myopathy, multisystem disorders
nDNA coded subunits of the ETC		
Mutation in SDH flavoprotein subunit	Recessive	LS[19]
Mutations in NDUFS4, NDUFV1, NDUFS8, NDUFS7, NDUFS2, NDUFS1 subunits of Complex I	Recessive	Fatal multisystem disorder[25,29] Leucodystrophy/myoclonic epilepsy,[27] LS,[26,189] Cardiomyopathy and encephalopathy,[190] Hypotonia, ataxia, psychomotor retardation[30]
Defects of intergenomic signalling		
Mitochondrial depletion	Recessive	Infantile encephalopathy,[191] hepatopathy[191]
Multiple deletions of mtDNA		
Twinkle (phage T7 gene 4-like protein on chromosome 10)	Dominant	CPEO[21]
ANT1 (chromosome 4)	Dominant	CPEO[23]
Polymerase gamma (chromosome 15)	Dominant	CPEO[22]
Mutation in thymidine phosphorylase	Recessive	MNGIE[24]
Other recessive forms	Recessive	Sensory neuropathy,[192] cardiomyopathy,[193] Wolfram syndrome[194]
Nuclear mutations affecting mitochondrial biogenesis		
Mutations in the DDP1 gene	X-linked	Mohr-Trajenberg syndrome[52]
Mutations in SURF1	Recessive	LS[31,32]
Mutations in SCO2	Recessive	Infantile cardioencephalomyopathy[33]
Mutation in COX10	Recessive	COX deficiency[34]
Mutation in BCS1L	Recessive	Complex III deficiency with neonatal proximal tubulopathy, hepatic involvement and encephalopathy[35]
Mutations in Paraplegin	Recessive	Hereditary spastic paraplegia[53]
Other		
Mutations in frataxin	Recessive	Freidreich's ataxia
? mutations in mtDNA	?	Parkinson's disease and other neurodegenerative disorders[37]

CPEO = chronic progressive external ophthalmoplegia; PS = Pearson's marrow pancreas syndrome; NARP = Neurogenic weakness, ataxia and retinitis pigmentosa; LS = Leigh syndrome; LHON = Leber's hereditary optic atrophy; FBSN = Familial bilateral striatal necrosis; MELAS = mitochondrial encephalomyopathy with lactic acidosis and stroke; MERRF = Myoclonus epilepsy with ragged red fibres; SNHL = Sensorineural hearing loss; MNGIE = myo-neuro-gastrointestinal encephalomyopathy; COX = cytochrome c oxidoreductase

evaluate. Most reports of success are based on single or few patients. Where randomized trials have been done, the treated group has been mixed. ^{31}P magnetic resonance spectroscopy of brain or muscle[64,65] or non-invasive tissue oximetry during exercise[66] may be useful *in vivo* biochemical endpoints, but do not necessarily inform us on clinical effects.

Physical and supportive therapies

General principles of neurological care apply to patients with mitochondrial disease. A discussion around special features of mitochondrial disease follows.

Exercise Short-term aerobic training, consisting of eight weeks of treadmill exercise at 70–85% of estimated maximum heart rate reserve showed improvements in estimated aerobic capacity, heart rate, and blood lactate, and ^{31}P NMR spectroscopy showed increased oxidative capacity of muscle in patients with mitochondrial myopathies compared with normals and non-metabolic myopathy disease controls.[67,68] A recent study of lactate and catecholamines in a 10 week aerobic exercise program in 12 patients with mitochondrial myopathies showed lactate accumulation during exercise was decreased and that the effect was partially dissociated from the catecholaminergic response, suggesting improved muscle oxidative metabolism during the training program.[69] Concentric exercise training may also result in "gene shifting" from satellite cells to mature myofibers (see below).[70]

Drugs including anesthetic agents Anticonvulsant therapy in patients with seizures should be modified because the deleterious effects of valproic acid (VPA) on mitochondrial energy metabolism. Valproic acid decreases plasma carnitine levels, which may inhibit

Table 151.3   Treatment of mitochondrial disease

Intervention	Type	Examples
Non-pharmacological	Aerobic exercise	
	Biomedical devices	*Pacemaker, cochlear implant*
	Organ transplantation	*Orthotopic liver/heart transplant (single-organ disease)*
Pharmacological	Quinones	*Ubiquinone (CoQ$_{10}$)*
		Idebenone
	Vitamins	*Menadione (Vitamin K$_3$)*
		Phylloquinone/phytonadione (Vitamin K$_1$)
		Thiamine
		Riboflavin
	Corticosteroids	
	Miscellaneous	*Dichloroacetate*
		Carnitine
		Succinate
		Creatine
		Chloramphenicol
	Genetic complementation	*Protein-DNA chimera*
Gene therapy	Protein complementation	*Recoded mitochondrial genes*
	Sequence specific inhibition	*Peptide nucleic acids*
	Other	*Induced muscle regeneration*
		Pre-implantation selection
		Forced paternal inheritance

beta-oxidation of fatty acids,[71] impairs pyruvate uptake by brain mitochondria,[72] pyruvate oxidation in hepatocytes,[73] and the ETC.[74] The rare coma that may result from VPA intoxication may be treated by direct hemoperfusion.[75] Infections should be vigorously treated, but certain antibiotics (e.g., aminoglycosides) may impair mitochondrial protein synthesis, particularly those acting on the mitochondrial ribosomal RNA (rRNA), which is similar to the prokaryotic rRNA. The A1555G mutation in the mitochondrial 12SrRNA is thought to confer a maternally inherited susceptibility to gentamicin-induced deafness by a structural change in the drug binding site that increases binding to the small subunit of the mitochondrial ribosome.[76] Thus, this drug is contraindicated in those with this mutation. Other mutations,[77] including one in the 12SrRNA gene, T1095C, found in a patient with parkinsonism, neuropathy and maternally inherited sensorineural deafness may confer a similar susceptibility.[58] Most antiviral agents inhibit mitochondrial DNA γ polymerase. Azidothymidine (AZT) may cause a mitochondrial myopathy associated with carnitine deficiency[78] and mtDNA depletion, and fialuridine can cause a fatal hepatocerebral syndrome.[79] In HepG2 cells, there are differential effects of the various antiretroviral nucleoside analogues, with AZT showing the most profound inhibition of oxidative phosphorylation.[80] Acylovir has no reported mitochondrial toxicity. Patients with Kearns-Sayre syndrome (KSS) may suffer anaesthesiological complications because of sensitivity to muscle relaxants, etomidate and thiopentone. Sudden third degree AV (atrioventricular) conduction block may occur in the absence of an artificial pacemaker and lead to death, particularly with halothane anesthesia; isoflurane is

preferable.[81] Sensitivity to vercuronium,[82] rocuronium and atracuronium[83] have been reported. Depressed ventilatory drive and impaired responses to hypercapnia and hypoxemia may complicate the course in a ventilated patient.[84] In a patient with MELAS, hypoxic ventilatory depression observed in the isocapnic progressive hypoxic response test was partially blocked by pretreatment with aminophylline.[85]

Biomedical devices In KSS, pacemaker insertion should be considered early to prevent fatality from cardiac conduction block that is ultimately almost invariable.[86] Cochlear implantation is a valuable treatment for deafness associated with mitochondrial disease.[87,88]

Organ transplantation Successful cardiac transplantation has been reported in KSS.[89] Multi-organ involvement is usually regarded as a contraindication for heart transplantation in metabolic disorders. However, in mitochondrial cardiomyopathies, since the clinical defect may be limited to the myocardium, transplantation may be considered. Results of orthotopic cardiac transplantation in six children with diverse severe dilated mitochondrial cardiomyopathies with sole or predominant cardiac involvement have recently been published.[90] Two have died from acute or subacute rejection, one died seven years after successful transplantation from endocarditis and the remaining three patients are doing well after a mean follow up of 55.6 months (range 2.6–6.5 years). Clinically important extracardiac manifestations in two patients with other organ involvement only on laboratory investigation have not become apparent. Similarly, orthotopic liver transplantation may be considered if extrahepatic involvement is excluded preoperatively because, as recent reports show, neurological or muscle involvement predicts a poor outcome.[91,92]

Counselling Prenatal diagnosis and genetic counselling is problematic in mitochondrial genetic disorders. It is generally acknowledged that single mtDNA deletions are sporadic although exceptions are recorded.[93] Although mtDNA point mutations are maternally inherited, disease expression depends on mutant load and tissue distribution. Furthermore, the mutant load in a particular tissue can change with time. In the NARP 8993 mutation, there is some relationship between the mutant load in the mother and the risk of an affected offspring.[94] A similar relationship exists in the MERRF 8344 mutation. Although there is only limited information on the predictive capability of chorionic villous sampling (CVS), it may be used in asymptomatic women with relatively low mutant load of these mutations since the available data is that embryonic and extra-embryonic tissues bear similar mutant loads.[95] Of course, these women should be prepared to consider termination of pregnancy. Women with high mutant loads may wish to consider oocyte donation. Pre-implantation diagnosis is yet to be reported although it is used routinely in other nuclear genetic disorders.[96] Detection of MELAS is more problematic since there may not be a close relationship between mutant load and disease burden.[97]

Metabolic therapies

CoQ_{10} and other quinones Reports of metabolic therapies, aiming to increase mitochondrial ATP production are most consistent with ubiquinone, discovered by Crane in 1957.[98] Quinones are reversibly reduced to hydroxyquinones. They function as mobile electron acceptors in ETCs of plants, microorganisms and animals, hence the name ubiquinones. The length of the isoprenoid side chain alters properties like lipid solubility. CoQ_{10}, with 10 isoprenyl subunits in the side chain, is a physiological, lipid soluble inner mitochondrial membrane electron acceptor in animals, receiving electrons from Complex I (deriving electrons from NADH), Complex II (deriving electrons from the TCA cycle) and ETF dehydrogenase (deriving electrons from the b-oxidation of fatty acids). In rats, exogenous CoQ_{10} accumulates in the inner mitochondrial membrane and promotes mitochondrial enzyme activity.[99] However in two humans with mitochondrial myopathies, it failed to accumulate in muscle though serum levels increased.[100] It diffuses in the mitochondrial membrane bilayer independently of other redox components, and if administered orally, is readily absorbed with a plasma half life of 33.9 hours. Normal serum levels are $637 \pm 84\,ng/ml$, but may be influenced by gender, alcohol, serum triglycerides and exercise ingestion of statins. There are no important adverse effects even when used in doses of $100\,mg/day$ for up to six years.[101–105] There are several theories regarding the mechanism of action of quinones in mitochondrial disease.

(a) The quinone redox pair may provide a path for electrons to bypass defective ETC complexes and sustain the H^+ gradient.

(b) Ubiquinones may function as antioxidants.[106] Mitochondrial membranes contain high concentrations of unsaturated lipid, making them susceptible to oxidative stress. High levels of heme and non-heme Fe, the availability of molecular O_2 and the production of free radicals by the ETC increase this oxidative damage considerably. Protection against free radical attack was suggested when ubiquinone-6 derived from exogenous ubiquinone-6 was found to inhibit lipid peroxidation of the inner mitochondrial membrane.[107]

(c) CoQ_{10} appears to stabilize components of the respiratory chain. In several case reports, CoQ_{10} has been extremely beneficial for muscle and brain symptoms in familial, probably autosomal recessive deficiency of CoQ_{10}. This is a triad of seizures, proximal myopathy sparing the extraocular muscles and recurrent myopathy. Investigations show lactic acidosis, elevated CK (creatinekinase), marked CoQ_{10} deficiency in muscle (but not serum or fibroblasts). In muscle there is lipid stasis and mitochondrial accumulation in Type I muscle fibers and polarographic evidence of decreased respiration of NADH-dependent substrates and succinate, but normal levels of cytochromes with spectral analysis.[108–110] Here, CoQ_{10} appears correct a biosynthetic deficiency in brain and muscle. Oral CoQ_{10} supplementation failed to provide benefit in one reported case of neonatal CoQ_{10} deficiency.[111]

In collected reports of patients with mitochondrial encephalomyopathies, a beneficial effect of CoQ_{10} has been reported.[66,101,102,108–110,112–120] In KSS, doses of $3\,mg/kg/day$ and $60–150\,mg/day$ lowered serum lactate,[101,112,121] and improved eye movements,[101,112] and cardiac parameters.[101] In doses of $30–90\,mg/day$ and $300\,mg/day$, CoQ_{10} monotherapy was reported to improve some parameters in MELAS, including pancreatic beta cell dysfunction,[120] tissue oximetry,[66] serum lactate[66,122] and others.[114] Single patients with COX deficiency improved in strength[118,122] and ^{31}P NMR spectroscopic findings.[102] Of interest to the movement disorder neurologist, CoQ_{10} was found to protect the nigrostriatal tract in MPTP treated rats[123] and has some anti-apoptotic effects *in vivo*.[124] However, benefits were not confirmed in other reports of KSS,[89,100] and in 44 patients with various mitochondrial encephalomyopathies,[103] a multicenter trial with a double-blind phase in apparent responders. In another open trial, using CoQ_{10} and a vitamin cocktail, there were no objective, reproducible clinical benefits or changes in oxidative metabolism in 16 patients with various mitochondrial encephalomyopathies despite a substantial increase in serum CoQ_{10}.[125] In an open trial in eight patients with various mitochondrial encephalomyopathies,

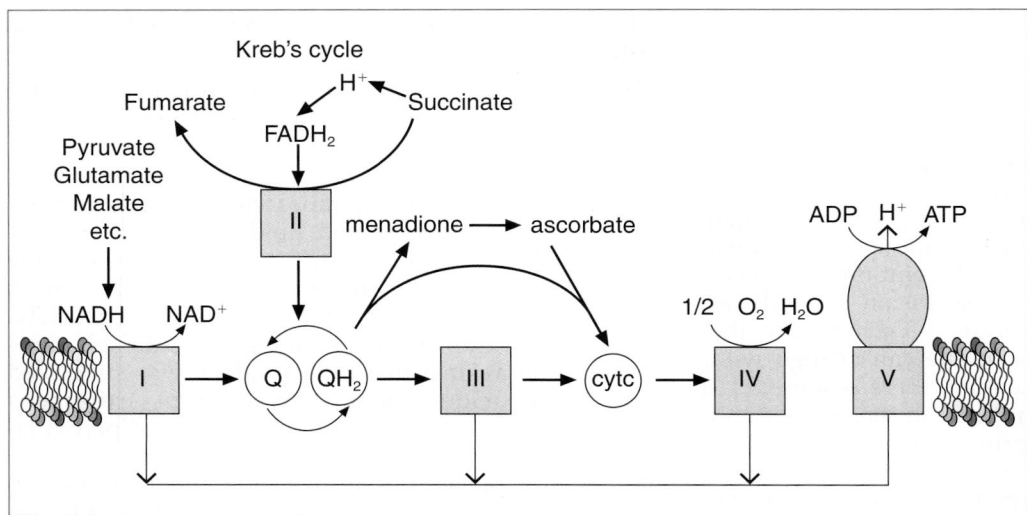

Figure 151.1 The mitochondrial respiratory chain. Bypass of block with menadione and ascorbate

^{31}P-NMR showed improved mean post-exercise ratio of phosphocreatine (PCr) to inorganic phosphate, but this was the effect of a single responder.[126] Idebenone is a benzoquinone derivative which stimulates oxidative metabolism in the myocardium, rat brain mitochondria, has a neuroprotective effect in brain ischemia and inhibits lipid peroxidation.[127-129] In two patients with MELAS, combination treatment with CoQ$_{10}$ improved the EEG and CSF protein, lactate and pyruvate.[114] In another single case of MELAS, high oral doses markedly increased cerebral metabolic ratio of oxygen and oxygen extraction fraction without increased cerebral blood flow shown by PET.[130] Dramatic resolution of heart failure has been reported after idebenone treatment in a patient with ubiquinone dependent combined respiratory deficiency,[131] suggesting CoQ$_{10}$ deficiency.

Menadione (vitamin K$_3$), phylloquinone (vitamin K$_1$) and ascorbate   In a patient with Complex III deficiency, later found to have a heteroplasmic cytochrome b stop codon mutation[132] (see Figure 151.1), Eleff et al.,[133] reasoned they could bypass the ETC block by using menadione (40–80 mg/day) and ascorbate (4 g/day) as electron acceptors and reducers of cytochrome c oxidase. They based the reasoning on the redox midpotential of these compounds and experiments in antimycin treated yeast (a model for Complex III deficiency) showing reactivation of respiration and increase of ATP production with menadione and ascorbate.[134] ^{31}P NMR showed an increase in the PCr/P$_i$ ratio at rest and an increase in its rate of recovery after exercise.[133,135] Withdrawal of vitamin K resulted in increased fatigue and weakness, which improved within 24 hours of recommencing therapy.[135] Cooper et al.,[136] used menadione to treat experimental NADH ubiquinone reductase deficiency in rats treated with diphenylene iodonium. Treated rats gained weight, lived longer and had improved muscle function shown by isometric twitch tension, but there was no difference between controls and treated animals in the decline in PCr and delay during

stimulation and recovery in PCr after stimulation. Shoffner et al.,[137] used phylloquinone (25 mg/day) and ascorbate (4 g/day) to produce a 62% improvement in retinal cone function in a single patient with CPEO. Addition of CoQ$_{10}$ produced and additional 46% improvement. Phylloquinone may be preferred to menadione: it is lipophilic, whilst menadione must first alkylate to menadione-4 to be lipophilic and biologically active; it is concentrated more in mitochondria; and there are no reported side effects, whilst menadione has been reported to produce hemolytic anemia and hyperbilirubinemia and kernicterus in newborns. However, electron carriers like menadione and ascorbate may also generate superoxide anion.[138] A larger trial of 16 patients in which ascorbate and menadione were used in combination with CoQ$_{10}$ and other vitamins in patients with assorted mitochondrial disorders showed no benefit.[125]

Thiamine (Vitamin B$_1$) and Riboflavin (Vitamin B$_2$)
Thiamine pyrophosphate is a coenzyme for pyruvate decarboxylase. The rationale for its use is that it may lower pyruvate and lactate levels and stimulate NADH production making more reducing equivalents available for the ETC via Complex I. In large doses of 300 mg/day, thiamine reduced lactate and pyruvate levels in three patients with Kearns-Sayre syndrome, but failed to produce important clinical benefit.[139] One patient with myopathy, lactic acidosis, cardiomyopathy and cardiac failure, responded to thiamine and prednisone.[140] Thiamine was part of cocktail containing flavin mononucleotide and intravenous cytochrome c, which produced clinical improvement in muscle fatigability, and severity of stroke-like episodes in eight of nine patients with mitochondrial encephalomyopathies, four of whom had MELAS.[141] However, a larger study, in which thiamine (100 mg/day for two months) was part of a vitamin and CoQ$_{10}$ cocktail, showed no benefit in 16 patients with different mitochondrial encephalomyopathies.[125] High doses are well tolerated except in occasional cases of hypersensitivity. Riboflavin is a

precursor of the electron transport cofactors flavin monophosphate (Complex I) and flavin adenine dinucleotide (Complex II). At a dose of 100 mg/day, it improved exercise capacity in a patient with Complex I deficiency.[142] Penn et al.,[143] noted that in a patient with Complex I deficiency and a known tRNA[Leu] mutation, encephalopathy ceased with nicotinamide and riboflavin treatment. PCr/ATP recovery rates fell in parallel with sural nerve sensory amplitudes, and a drop in muscle bioenergetic efficiency (relationship of Pi/PCr to the accelerating force of contracting muscle) coincided with development of encephalopathy before treatment was instituted. A sustained clinical response was noted in an infant with Complex I deficiency and a myopathy.[144] In a larger trial of riboflavin in six patients with Complex I deficiency with encephalomyopathy and pure myopathy, the two patients with pure myopathy improved clinically, but only one of the patients with an encephalomyopathy improved and there was no good correlation between clinical response and normalization of Complex I activity.[145] Sato et al.,[146] reported two siblings with the MELAS mutation from a pedigree with familial thiamine deficiency. Thiamine supplementation improved myopathy and reduced lactate levels in one sibling, but not the other.

Steroids Low doses of glucocorticoids have improved muscle strength, lowered lactate levels and improved other clinical features in case reports of mitochondrial encephalomyopathies.[140,147–149] However steroids should be used with caution. Methylprednisolone inhibits the oxidation of NAD-linked substrates between the primary NADH dehydrogenase flavoprotein and coenzyme Q, and inhibits succinate oxidation *in vitro*, suggesting that any therapeutic effect in mitochondrial disease result from indirect rather than direct effects on the mitochondrial membrane. Also, estradiol and related steroids in therapeutic doses inhibit Complex V *in vitro*.[150] Furthermore, there is one report of fatal ketoacidosis and hyperglycemia in two patients with KSS who received a brief course of corticosteroids.[151]

Miscellaneous
Dichloroacetate (DCA). In mitochondrial encephalomyopathies, high intracerebral lactate levels, evident on magnetic resonance spectroscopy (MRS), may contribute to neuronal death. Dichloroacetate, which stimulates conversion of lactate to CO_2 and acetyl-coenzyme A, has been used to lower lactic acidemia in adult and congenital lactic acidosis,[152] although a controlled trial has shown the effect is clinically insignificant and does not lengthen survival.[153] In a patient with MELAS and a stroke-like episode, who clinically improved with DCA treatment, an elevated lactate-creatine ratio in the "stroke" region decreased on MRS studies with improvement. During a second episode, the lactate-creatine ratio rose from baseline in a region of the brain that was normal on MRI scans.[154] In other anecdotal reports of MELAS treated with DCA alone,[155,156] or in combination with

thiamine[157] there have been clinical improvements in addition to reduction of lactic acidemia. Similar observations have been made in Pearson's marrow-pancreas syndrome,[158] muscle COX deficiency,[159] and other disorders of the ETC.[160,161] The only randomized, double-blind study of DCA in mitochondrial encephalomyopathies was a small, short term, placebo-controlled, crossover trial in 11 patients with various mitochondrial disorders in whom blood lactate and several indices of brain oxidative metabolism on proton MRS improved after one week, but ^{31}P-NMR spectroscopy, clinical symptoms, the neurological examination and quantitative muscle strength testing did not change.[162] Peripheral neuropathy, not always symptomatic, appears to be a common side effect in chronic DCA treatment, even with co-administration of oral thiamine and nerve conduction should be monitored.[163]

Carnitine Carnitine deficiency may be found in the muscle of a third and in the plasma of half of patients with mitochondrial myopathies.[164,165] Evidence suggests that an increased $NADH/NAD^+$ ratio generated by reduced flux through the respiratory chain inhibits beta-oxidation, producing secondary carnitine deficiency.[166] In an open trial of L-carnitine (50–200 mg/kg per day in four daily doses) in patients with "mitochondrial myopathy" and plasma carnitine deficiency, muscle weakness improved in 19 of 20 patients, failure to thrive in four of eight, encephalopathy in one of nine, and cardiomyopathy in eight of eight patients.[165] There are similar anecdotal reports in the literature, but there are no placebo-controlled, randomized trials.

Succinate Succinate is a Kreb's cycle intermediate that donates electrons directly to the ETC (Figure 151.1). Treatment of a single patient with Complex I deficiency with 6 g/day resulted in disappearance of stroke-like episodes[167] and respiratory failure resolved in a patient with combined deficiency of Complex I, IV and V on a regimen of 300 mg/day of CoQ_{10} and 6 g/day of succinate.[115]

Creatine Another treatment strategy is increasing flux through non-mitochondrial energy pathways. Increasing flux through glycogenolysis/glycolysis may be expected to increase lactic acidemia, but ATP may be regenerated from PCr using creatine without increasing lactic acid production. This has been exploited in short-term, randomized, double-blind, crossover trial in seven patients, six with MELAS[168] of 5 g, reducing to 2 g bd creatine monophosphate. A variety of strength measurements were used as end points and the trial indicated an improvement in strength in high-intensity anaerobic, and aerobic activities, but no effect in low intensity aerobic activities. The treatment may be useful in weaning the fatigued patient from a ventilator.

Chloramphenicol In Luft's disease, the hypermetabolism has been reduced by Lugol's iodine and methylthiouracil[1] and by inhibition of mitochondrial protein synthesis by chloramphenicol.[169]

Gene therapy

Gene therapy for mitochondrial disorders is in its infancy. A major obstacle to all the somatic gene therapy approaches is the delivery of a therapeutic gene into the mitochondrial matrix in cells throughout the body, including the brain. Some potential strategies have been recently reviewed.[170]

Prospects for somatic gene therapy

Genetic complementation by delivered genes expressed in the mitochondrion   Heteroplasmic mtDNA mutations are functionally recessive. There is a "threshold effect" in which a proportion of mutant mtDNA is required before the mutation has biochemical and clinical consequences. By intramitochondrial genetic complementation, even a small reduction in mutant DNA may correct the ETC defect. No-one has yet succeeded in transforming mammalian mitochondria with a full length, functioning, replicating mtDNA. DNA can be transferred into the mitochondria of yeast by biolistic techniques,[171] the plastome (analogous organelle in plants) of Chlamydomonas,[172] and the tobacco plastome[173] with polyethylene glycol. Seibel et al., (1996)[174] recently reported that a small double-stranded linear segment of mtDNA linked covalently to the amino terminal leader peptide of the rat ornithine transcarbamylase (a mitochondrial matrix protein) was imported into isolated rat liver mitochondria. This holds promise for the transformation of cells with exogenous mitochondrial genes but the isolated mitochondria must then either be returned undamaged to the cells, or it must be shown that the cells can be successfully transfected with the DNA-protein chimera, that it is not degraded in the cytoplasm by exonucleases etc., and mitochondrial import of the chimera also occurs within cells. Furthermore, the DNA molecule must either be processed to a mitochondrial replicon, or recombined with an existing replicon. At each step, there are difficult technical obstacles to overcome. Mitochondria may be returned to cells by microinjection,[175] but this is laborious and inefficient. Although Clarke and Shay[176] reported the efficient transfer of chloramphenicol resistance (CAPr)—a cytoplasmically inherited phenotype in mammalian cells—by simple mixing of mitochondria isolated from CAPr cells and CAPs cells, numerous attempts to replicate these experiments using mouse or human cells lacking their own mtDNA (rho zero cells) as recipients, including those of the author, have failed. Novel delivery vectors such as bola-amphiphiles with delocalized charge centers may solve some of the technical problems involved.[177] Conceptually, transport of other small nucleic acid species across both mitochondrial membranes known in some species, for example, tRNAs in yeast[178] and 5SrRNA in mammalian cells[179] may be exploited for gene delivery to the mitochondrial matrix, but this has yet to be shown in mammalian cells.

Protein complementation by recoded mitochondrial genes expressed in the cytoplasm   Another approach, pioneered by Nagley et al.,[180] in yeast, has been to insert a recoded, corrected copy of the defective mitochondrial gene coupled to a leader sequence in the nucleus, and express it in the cytosol (the mitochondrial genetic code differs from the code employed by nuclear DNA). The recoded gene product is targeted to mitochondria by the attached protein import sequence. The cytosolically-synthesized protein was correctly imported into mitochondria, functionally assembled into the ATPase complex and phenotypic rescue occurred. A similar approach designed to correct the homologous human ATPase 6 gene mutation has been tried using mouse mtDNA and the N-terminal leader sequence for the Fp subunit of succinate dehydrogenase.[181,182] However, when the recoded gene—targeting sequence was expressed in NIH3T3 fibroblasts, the construct was found to be toxic to the host cells.

Sequence-specific inhibition of mutant mtDNA replication   Yet another approach has been taken by Taylor et al.,[183,184] to selectively inhibit replication of the mutant mtDNA using sequence specific peptide nucleic acid (PNAs) complementary to the mutant sequence of a mtDNA base change or deletion breakpoint. The antigenomic PNAs specifically inhibited replication of mutant but not wild-type mtDNA templates in an in vitro replication runoff assay and the PNAs were taken up into cultured human myoblasts.

Other genetically based therapies

Induced muscle regeneration   In injured muscle, satellite cells, the myogenic precursor cells are activated and proliferate to form new muscle fibers. Because there is varied mutant load in different tissues due to segregation of mutant mtDNA molecules during embryogenesis and the mitotic activity of the cells, the normally quiescent satellite cells may contain much lower mutant mtDNA loads that myofibers. Clark et al.,[185] used bupivacaine to cause necrosis of muscle fibers leaving satellite cells intact in a patient with a tRNALeu(CUN) mutation which was absent in satellite cells, and showed reversal of the genetic defect in the injected muscle. A similar effect has been reported in concentric exercise training, presumably because the signals for muscle growth and repair stimulate satellite cell fusion with mature myofibers.[70] However an attempt to correct ptosis by the same approach has been unsuccessful in five patients.[186]

In vitro fertilization with pre-implantation selection   One group has shown skewed segregation of the NARP mutation in oocytes from women, with mutant load of the mutation ranging from none to more than 95%.[187] This has not been confirmed, but if it occurs generally for point mutations of mtDNA, then it is technically possible to harvest eggs from an affected woman, fertilize them in vitro, determine if the embryos contain the mutation by single cell PCR, and implanting only those free of mutation. Sampling error makes this approach fraught with danger and there are no published reports of its application.

Forced paternal inheritance Maternal inheritance of the mtDNA is almost universal in the animal kingdom but the mechanisms are unknown. It appears that at conception, the sperm's mitochondria enter the egg. Paternally derived sperm may be recognized and actively destroyed. Manipulation of this mechanism may allow interference with the vertical transmission of mtDNA mutations from mother to child. The threshold effect of mtDNA mutations means a small reduction in mutant load may be sufficient to convert from a devastating to mild phenotype. In somatic cells, the elimination of paternally derived mitochondria occurs in 48 hours.[188] If this also occurs in the egg and it is possible to promote admixture of mtDNA between the sperm and oocyte soon after conception, the zygote may be genetically "rescued." However the mechanisms of maternal transmission of mtDNA are still obscure. In summary, this and other forms of genetic therapy are mostly conceptual and in the earliest stages of development. However, they may be the future of treatment in this group of devastating disorders. Compared with knowledge of the molecular genetics of mitochondrial disorders, our understanding of disease mechanisms is still rudimentary. It is only recently that the mode of cellular death and damage in mitochondrial disease has been the subject of detailed study. It is clear that mitochondrial energy metabolism has a central role not just in the living, but also in the dying cell. Greater insight into the processes involved may lead to new and effective pharmacological treatments.

Acknowledgements

The author is supported by Grant# 980729 from the National Health and Medical Research Council of Australia.

References

1. Luft R, Ikkos D, Palmieri G, et al. A case of severe hypermetabolism of nonthyroid origin with a defect in the maintenance of mitochondrial respiratory control: a correlated clinical, biochemical, and morphological study. J Clin Invest 1962;41:1776–1804
2. Shy G, Gonatas N, Perez M. Two childhood myopathies with abnormal mitochondria. I. Megaconial myopathy. II. Pleoclonial myopathy. Brain 1966; 89:133–158
3. Drachman D. Ophthalmoplegia plus: the neurodegenerative disorders associated with progressive external ophthalmoplegia. Arch Neurol 1968;18:654–674
4. Kearns T, Sayre G. Retinitis pigmentosa, external ophthalmoplegia, and complete heart block. Unusual syndrome with histologic study in one of two cases. Arch Ophthal 1958;60:280–289
5. Olson W, King Engel W, Walsh G, Einaugler R. Oculocraniosomatic neuromuscular disease with "ragged-red" fibres. Arch Neurol 1972;26:193–211
6. Engel W, Cunningham C. Rapid examination of muscle tissue: an improved trichrome stain method for fresh-frozen biopsy sections. Neurology 1963;13:919–923
7. Shapira Y, Harel S, Russel A. Mitochondrial encepha-

lomyopathies: a group of neuromuscular disorders with defects in oxidative metabolism. Is J Med 1977; 13:161–164
8. Egger J, Lake B, Wilson J. Mitochondrial cytopathy. A multisystem disorder with ragged red fibres on muscle biopsy. Arch Dis Child 1981;56:741–752
9. Blass J, Avigan J, Uhlendorf B. A defect of pyruvate decarboxylase in a child with an intermittent movement disorder. J Clin Invest 1970;49:423–432
10. DiMauro S, Melis-DiMauro P. Muscle carnitine palmiryl-transferase deficiency and myoglobinuria. Science 1973;182:929–931
11. Engel A, Angelini C. Carnitine deficiency of human skeletal muscle with associated lipid storage myopathy: a new syndrome. Science 1973;179:899–902
12. DiMauro S, Bonilla E, Zeviani M, et al. Mitochondrial myopathies. J Inherit Metab Dis 1987;10:113–128
13. Egger J, Wilson J. Mitochondrial inheritance in a mitochondrially mediated disease. New Engl J Med 1983; 309:142–146
14. Nass S, Nass M. Intramitochondrial fibres with DNA characteristics. I. Fixation and electron staining reactions. J Cell Biol 1963;19:593–612
15. Anderson S, Bankier A, Barrell B, et al. Sequence and organization of the human mitochondrial genome. Nature 1981;290:457–465
16. Hutchison C, Newbold J, Potter S, Edgell M. Maternal inheritance of mammalian mitochondrial DNA. Nature 1974;251:536–538
17. Anonymous. Mitochondrial encephalomyopathies: gene mutation. Neuromuscul Disord 2000;10:X–XV
18. Zeviani M, Servidei S, Gellera C, et al. An autosomal dominant disorder with multiple deletions of mitochondrial DNA starting at the D-loop region. Nature 1989;339:309–11
19. Bourgeron T, Rustin P, Chretien D, et al. Mutation of a nuclear succinate dehydrogenase gene results in mitochondrial respiratory chain deficiency. Nat Genet 1995; 11:144–149
20. Suomalainen A, Kaukonen J, Amati P, et al. An autosomal locus predisposing to deletions of mitochondrial DNA. Nat Genet 1995;9:146–151
21. Spelbrink JN, Li FY, Tiranti V, et al. Human mitochondrial DNA deletions associated with mutations in the gene encoding Twinkle, a phage T7 gene 4-like protein localized in mitochondria. Nat Genet 2001;28:223–231
22. Van Goethem G, Dermaut B, Lofgren A, et al. Mutation of POLG is associated with progressive external ophthalmoplegia characterized by mtDNA deletions. Nat Genet 2001;28:211–212
23. Kaukonen J, Juselius JK, Tiranti V, et al. Role of adenine nucleotide translocator 1 in mtDNA maintenance. Science 2000;289:782–785
24. Nishino I, Spinazzola A, Hirano M. Thymidine phosphorylase gene mutations in MNGIE: a human mitochondrial disorder. Science 1999;283:689–692
25. van den Heuvel L, Ruitenbeek W, Smeets R, et al. Demonstration of a new pathogenic mutation in human complex I deficiency: a 5-bp duplication in the nuclear gene encoding the 18-kD (AQDQ) subunit. Am J Hum Genet 1998;62:262–268
26. Loeffen J, Smeitink J, Triepels R, et al. The first nuclear-encoded complex I mutation in a patient with Leigh syndrome. Am J Hum Genet 1998;63:1598–1608
27. Schuelke M, Smeitink J, Mariman E, et al. Mutant NDUFV1 subunit of mitochondrial complex I causes leukodystrophy and myoclonic epilepsy [letter]. Nat Genet 1999;21:260–261

28. Triepels RH, van dHLP, Loeffen JL, et al. Leigh syndrome associated with a mutation in the NDUFS7 (PSST) nuclear encoded subunit of complex I. Ann Neurol 1999;45:787–790

29. Petruzzella V, Vergari R, Puzziferri I, et al. A nonsense mutation in the NDUFS4 gene encoding the 18 kDa (AQDQ) subunit of complex I abolishes assembly and activity of the complex in a patient with Leigh-like syndrome. Hum Mol Genet 2001;10: 529–535

30. Benit P, Chretien D, Kadhom N, et al. Large-scale deletion and point mutations of the nuclear NDUFV1 and NDUFS1 genes in mitochondrial complex I deficiency. Am J Hum Genet 2001;68:1344–1352

31. Tiranti V, Hoertnagel K, Carrozzo R, et al. Mutations of SURF-1 in Leigh disease associated with cytochrome c oxidase deficiency. Am J Hum Genet 1998;63:1609–1621

32. Zhu Z, Yao J, Johns T, et al. SURF1, encoding a factor involved in the biogenesis of cytochrome c oxidase, is mutated in Leigh syndrome [see comments]. Nat Genet 1998;20:337–343

33. Papadopoulou LC, Sue CM, Davidson MM, et al. Fatal infantile cardioencephalomyopathy with COX deficiency and mutations in SCO2, a COX assembly gene. Nat Genet 1999;23:333–337

34. Valnot I, von Kleist-Retzow J, Barrientos A, et al. A mutation in the human heme A: farnesyltransferase gene (COX10) causes cytochrome c oxidase deficiency. Hum Mol Genet 2000;9:1245–1249

35. de Lonlay P, Valnot I, Barrientos A, et al. A mutant mitochondrial respiratory chain assembly protein causes complex III deficiency in patients with tubulopathy, encephalopathy and liver failure. Nat Genet 2001;29:57–60

36. Wallace D. Mitochondrial DNA mutations and bioenergetic defects in aging and degenerative diseases. In: Rosenberg R, Pruisner S, DiMauro S, Barchi R, eds. The molecular and genetic basis of neurologic disease. 2 ed. Boston: Butterworth-Heinemann, 1997:189

37. Leonard JV, Schapira AH. Mitochondrial respiratory chain disorders II: neurodegenerative disorders and nuclear gene defects. Lancet 2000;355:389–394

38. Chinnery PF, Johnson MA, Wardell TM, et al. The epidemiology of pathogenic mitochondrial DNA mutations. Ann Neurol 2000;48:188–193

39. Betarbet R, Sherer TB, Mackenzie G, et al. Chronic systemic pesticide exposure reproduces features of Parkinson's disease. Nat Neurosci 2000;3:1301–1306

40. Kaneda H, Hayashi J, Takahama S, et al. Elimination of paternal mitochondrial DNA in intraspecific crosses during early mouse embryogenesis. Proc Natl Acad Sci USA 1995;92:4542–4546

41. Mirabella M, Di GS, Silvestri G, et al. Apoptosis in mitochondrial encephalomyopathies with mitochondrial DNA mutations: a potential pathogenic mechanism. Brain 2000;123:93–104

42. Monici MC, Toscano A, Girlanda P, et al. Apoptosis in metabolic myopathies. NeuroReport 1998;9:2431–2435

43. Bernardi P, Scorrano L, Colonna R, et al. Mitochondria and cell death. Mechanistic aspects and methodological issues. Eur J Biochem 1999;264:687–701

44. Jacotot E, Costantini P, Laboureau E, et al. Mitochondrial membrane permeabilization during the apoptotic process. Ann NY Acad Sci 1999;887:18–30

45. Loeffler M, Kroemer G. The mitochondrion in cell death control: certainties and incognita. Exp Cell Res 2000;256:19–26

46. Bandy B, Davison A. Mitochondrial mutations may increase oxidative stress: implications for carcinogenesis and aging? Free Radic Biol Med 1990;8:523–539

47. Beal F. Does impairment of energy metabolism result in excitoxic neuronal death in neurodegenerative illnesses? Ann Neurol 1992;31:119–130

48. Brini M, Pinton P, King MP, et al. A calcium signaling defect in the pathogenesis of a mitochondrial DNA inherited oxidative phosphorylation deficiency. Nat Med 1999;5:951–954

49. Tatuch Y, Christodoulou J, Feigenbaum A, et al. Heteroplasmic mtDNA mutation (T→G) at 8993 can cause Leigh disease when the percentage of abnormal mtDNA is high. Am J Hum Genet 1992;50:852–858

50. Thyagarajan D, Shanske S, Vazquez-Memije M, et al. A novel mitochondrial ATPase 6 point mutation in familial bilateral striatal necrosis. Ann Neurol 1995;38: 468–472

51. DiMauro S, Bonilla E. Mitochondrial encephalomyopathies. In: Rosenberg R, Pruisner S, DiMauro S, Barchi R, eds. The molecular and genetic basis of neurologic disease. 2 ed. Boston: Butterworth-Heinemann, 1997:189

52. Jin H, May M, Tranebjaerg L, et al. A novel X-linked gene, DDP, shows mutations in families with deafness (DFN-1), dystonia, mental deficiency and blindness. Nat Genet 1996;14:177–180

53. Casari G, De FM, Ciarmatori S, et al. Spastic paraplegia and OXPHOS impairment caused by mutations in paraplegin, a nuclear-encoded mitochondrial metalloprotease. Cell 1998;93:973–983

54. Puccio H, Koenig M. Recent advances in the molecular pathogenesis of Friedreich ataxia. Hum Mol Genet 2000;9:887–892

55. Gu M, Cooper JM, Taanman JW, Schapira AH. Mitochondrial DNA transmission of the mitochondrial defect in Parkinson's disease. Ann Neurol 1998;44: 177–186

56. Swerdlow RH, Parks JK, Miller SW, et al. Origin and functional consequences of the complex I defect in Parkinson's disease. Ann Neurol 1996;40:663–671

57. Chalmers RM, Brockington M, Howard RS, et al. Mitochondrial encephalopathy with multiple mitochondrial DNA deletions: a report of two families and two sporadic cases with unusual clinical and neuropathological features. J Neurol Sci 1996;143:41–45

58. Thyagarajan D, Bressman S, Bruno C, et al. A novel mitochondrial 12SrRNA point mutation in parkinsonism, deafness and neuropathy. Ann Neurol 2000;48: 730–736

59. De Coo IF, Renier WO, Ruitenbeek W, et al. A 4-base pair deletion in the mitochondrial cytochrome b gene associated with parkinsonism/MELAS overlap syndrome. Ann Neurol 1999;45:130–133

60. Simon DK, Pulst SM, Sutton JP, et al. Familial multisystem degeneration with parkinsonism associated with the 11778 mitochondrial DNA mutation. Neurology 1999;53:1787–1793

61. Lee M, Hyun D, Halliwell B, Jenner P. Effect of the overexpression of wild-type or mutant alpha-synuclein on cell susceptibility to insult. J Neurochem 2001; 76:998–1009

62. Walker U, Collins S, Byrne E. Respiratory chain encephalomyopathies: a diagnostic classification. Eur Neurol 1996;36:260–267

63. DiMauro S, Bonilla E, De VDC. Does the patient have a mitochondrial encephalomyopathy? J Child Neurol 1999;14(Suppl 1):S23–S35

64. Barbiroli B, Iotti S, Lodi R. In vivo assessment of

human skeletal muscle mitochondria respiration in health and disease. Mol Cell Biochem 1997;174:11–15

65. Barbiroli B, Iotti S, Lodi R. Improved brain and muscle mitochondrial respiration with CoQ. An in vivo study by ^{31}P-MR spectroscopy in patients with mitochondrial cytopathies. Biofactors 1999;9:253–260

66. Abe K, Matsuo Y, Kadekawa J, et al. Effect of coenzyme Q_{10} in patients with mitochondrial myopathy, encephalopathy, lactic acidosis, and stroke-like episodes (MELAS): evaluation by noninvasive tissue oximetry. J Neurol Sci 1999;162:65–68

67. Taivassalo T, De SN, Argov Z, et al. Effects of aerobic training in patients with mitochondrial myopathies, Neurology 1998;50:1055–1060

68. Taivassalo T, De SN, Chen J, et al. Short-term aerobic training response in chronic myopathies. Muscle Nerve 1999;22:1239–1243

69. Siciliano G, Manca ML, Renna M, et al. Effects of aerobic training on lactate and catecholaminergic exercise responses in mitochondrial myopathies. Neuromuscul Disord 2000;10:40–45

70. Taivassalo T, Fu K, Johns T, et al. Gene shifting: a novel therapy for mitochondrial myopathy. Hum Mol Genet 1999;8:1047–1052

71. Ohtani Y, Endo F, Matsuda I. Carnitine deficiency and hyperammonemia associated with valproate acid therapy. J Pediatr 1982;101:782–785

72. Benavides J, Martin A, Ugarte M, Valdivieso F. Inhibition by valproic acid of pyruvate uptake by brain mitochondria. Biochem Pharmacol 1982;31:1633–1636

73. Turnbull D, Bone A, Bartlett K, et al. The effects of valproate on intermediary metabolism in isolated rat hepatocytes and intact rats. Biochem Pharmacol 1983;32:1887–1892

74. Haas R, Stumpf D, Parks J, Eguren L. Inhibitory effects of sodium valproate on oxidative phosphorylation. Neurology 1981;31:1473–1476

75. Matsumoto J, Ogawa H, Maeyama R, et al. Successful treatment by direct hemoperfusion of coma possibly resulting from mitochondrial dysfunction in acute valproate intoxication. Epilepsia 1997;38:950–953

76. Prezant TR, Agapian JV, Bohlman MC, et al. Mitochondrial ribosomal RNA mutation associated with both antibiotic-induced and non-syndromic deafness. Nat Genet 1993;4:289–294

77. Bacino C, Prezant TR, Bu X, et al. Susceptibility mutations in the mitochondrial small ribosomal RNA gene in aminoglycoside induced deafness. Pharmacogenetics 1995;5:165–172

78. Dalakas MC, Leon-Monzon ME, Bernardini I, et al. Zidovudine-induced mitochondrial myopathy is associated with muscle carnitine deficiency and lipid storage [see comments]. Ann Neurol 1994;35:482–487

79. Lewis W, Dalakas M. Mitochondrial toxicity of antiviral drugs. Nat Med 1995;1:417–422

80. Pan-Zhou XR, Cui L, Zhou XJ, et al. Differential effects of antiretroviral nucleoside analogs on mitochondrial function in HepG2 cells. Antimicrobial Agents and Chemotherapy 2000;44:496–503

81. Lauwers M, Van Lersberghe C, Camu F. Inhalation anaesthesia and the Kearns-Sayre syndrome. Anaesthesia 1994;49:876–878

82. Wisely NA, Cook PR. General anaesthesia in a man with mitochondrial myopathy undergoing eye surgery. Eur J Anaesthesiol 2001;18:333–335

83. Finsterer J, Stratil U, Bittner R, Sporn P. Increased sensitivity to rocuronium and atracurium in mitochondrial myopathy. Can J Anaesth 1998;45:781–784

84. Barohn R, Clanton T, Sahenk Z, Mendell J. Recurrent respiratory insufficiency and depressed ventilatory drive complicating mitochondrial myopathies. Neurology 1990;40:103–106

85. Osanai S, Takahashi T, Enomoto H, et al. Hypoxic ventilatory depression in a patient with mitochondrial myopathy, encephalopathy, lactic acidosis and stroke-like episodes. Respirology 2001;6:163–166

86. Polak PE, Zijlstra F, Roelandt JR. Indications for pacemaker implantation in the Kearns-Sayre syndrome. Eur Heart J 1989;10:281–282

87. Tono T, Ushisako Y, Kiyomizu K, et al. Cochlear implantation in a patient with profound hearing loss with the A1555G mitochondrial mutation. Am J Otol 1998;19:754–757

88. Rosenthal EL, Kileny PR, Boerst A, Telian SA. Successful cochlear implantation in a patient with MELAS syndrome. Am J Otol 1999;20:187–190

89. Tranchant C, Mousson B, Mohr M, et al. Cardiac transplantation in an incomplete Kearns-Sayre syndrome with mitochondrial DNA deletion. Neuromuscul Disord 1993;3:561–566

90. Bonnet D, Rustin P, Rotig A, et al. Heart transplantation in children with mitochondrial cardiomyopathy. Heart 2001;86:570–573

91. Sokal EM, Sokol R, Cormier V, et al. Liver transplantation in mitochondrial respiratory chain disorders. Eur J Pediatr 1999;158(Suppl 2):S81–S84

92. Dubern B, Broue P, Dubuisson C, et al. Orthotopic liver transplantation for mitochondrial respiratory chain disorders: a study of 5 children. Transplantation 2001;71:633–637

93. Ballinger SW, Shoffner JM, Hedaya EV, et al. Maternally transmitted diabetes and deafness associated with a 10.4 kb mitochondrial DNA deletion. Nat Genet 1992;1:11–15

94. White SL, Collins VR, Wolfe R, et al. Genetic counseling and prenatal diagnosis for the mitochondrial DNA mutations at nucleotide 8993. Am J Hum Genet 1999;65:474–482

95. White SL, Shanske S, Biros I, et al. Two cases of prenatal analysis for the pathogenic T to G substitution at nucleotide 8993 in mitochondrial DNA. Prenat Diagn 1999;19:1165–1168

96. Harper JC, Wells D. Recent advances and future developments in PGD. Prenat Diagn 1999;19:1193–1199

97. Chinnery PF, Taylor DJ, Brown DT, et al. Very low levels of the mtDNA A3243G mutation associated with mitochondrial dysfunction in vivo. Ann Neurol 2000;47:381–384

98. Crane F, Hatefi Y, Lester R, Widmer C. Isolation of a quinone from beef heart mitochondria. Biochemica et Biophys Acta 1957;25:2201

99. Nakamura T, Sanma H, Himeno M, Kato K. Transfer of exogenous coenzyme Q_{10} into the inner membrane of heart mitochondria in rats. Amsterdam: Elsevier, 1980

100. Zierz S, von Wersebe O, Bleistein J, Jerusalem F. Exogenous coenzyme Q (CoQ) fails to increase CoQ in skeletal muscle of two patients with mitochondrial myopathies. J Neurol Sci 1990;95:283–290

101. Ogasahara S, Nishikawa Y, Yorifuji S, et al. Treatment of Kearns-Sayre syndrome with coenzyme Q_{10}. Neurology 1986;36:45–53

102. Nishikawa Y, Takahashi M, Yorifuji S, et al. Long-term coenzyme Q_{10} therapy for a mitochondrial encephalomyopathy with cytochrome c oxidase deficiency: a ^{31}P NMR study. Neurology 1989;39:399–403

103. Bresolin N, Doriguzzi C, Ponzetto C, et al. Ubide-carenone in the treatment of mitochondrial myopathies: a multi-center. J Neurol Sci 1990;100:70–78

104. Kaikkonen J, Nyyssonen K, Tuomainen T, et al. Determinants of plasma coenzyme Q_{10} in humans. FEBS Lett 1999;443:163–166

105. Overvad K, Diamant B, Holm L, et al. Coenzyme Q_{10} in health and disease. Eur J Clin Nutr 1999;53:764–770

106. Beyer R, Ernester L. The antioxidant role of coenzyme Q. London: Taylor and Francis, 1990

107. Mellors A, Tappel A. The inhibition of mitochondrial peroxidation by ubiquinone and ubiquinol. J Biol Chem 1966;241:4353–4356

108. Ogasahara S, Engel AG, Frens D, Mack D. Muscle coenzyme Q deficiency in familial mitochondrial encephalomyopathy. Proc Natl Acad Sci USA 1989;86:2379–2382

109. Servidei S, Spinazzola A, Crociani P. Coenzyme Q_{10} therapy is effective in familial mitochondrial encephalomyopathy with muscle CoQ_{10} deficiency. Neurology 1996;46:A420

110. Hirano M, Sobreira C, Shanske S. Coenzyme Q_{10} deficiency in a woman with myopathy, recurrent myoglobinuria, and seizures. Neurology 1996;46:A231

111. Rahman S, Hargreaves I, Clayton P, Heales S. Neonatal presentation of coenzyme Q_{10} deficiency. J Pediatr 2001;139:456–458

112. Ogasahara S, Yorifuji S, Nishikawa Y, et al. Improvement of abnormal pyruvate metabolism and cardiac conduction defect with coenzyme Q_{10} in Kearns-Sayre syndrome. Neurology 1985;35:372–377

113. Goda S, Hamada T, Ishimoto S, et al. Clinical improvement after administration of coenzyme Q_{10} in a patient. J Neurol 1987;234:62–63

114. Ihara Y, Namba R, Kuroda S, et al. Mitochondrial encephalomyopathy (MELAS): pathological study and successful therapy with coenzyme Q_{10} and idebenone. J Neurol Sci 1989;90:263–271

115. Shoffner JM, Lott MT, Voljavec AS, et al. Spontaneous Kearns-Sayre/chronic external ophthalmoplegia plus syndrome. Proc Natl Acad Sci USA 1989;86:7952–7956

116. Zierz S, Jahns G, Jerusalem F. Coenzyme Q in serum and muscle of 5 patients with Kearns-Sayre syndrome. J Neurol 1989;236:97–101

117. Bendahan D, Desnuelle C, Vanuxem D, et al. ^{31}P NMR spectroscopy and ergometer exercise test as evidence for muscle oxidative performance improvement with coenzyme Q in mitochondrial myopathies. Neurology 1992;42:1203–1208

118. Arpa J, Campos Y, Gutierrez-Molina M, et al. Benign mitochondrial myopathy with decreased succinate cytochrome C reductase activity. Acta Neurol Scand 1994;90:281–284

119. Barbiroli B, Frassineti C, Martinelli P, et al. Coenzyme Q_{10} improves mitochondrial respiration in patients with mitochondrial cytopathies. An in vivo study on brain and skeletal muscle by phosphorous magnetic resonance spectroscopy. Cell Mol Biol 1997;43:741–749

120. Liou CW, Huang CC, Lin TK, et al. Correction of pancreatic beta-cell dysfunction with coenzyme Q(10) in a patient with mitochondrial encephalomyopathy, lactic acidosis and stroke-like episodes syndrome and diabetes mellitus. Eur Neurol 2000;43:54–55

121. Bresolin N, Bet L, Binda A, et al. Clinical and biochemical correlations in mitochondrial myopathies treated with coenzyme Q_{10}. Neurology 1988;38:892–899

122. Yamamoto M, Sato T, Anno M, et al. Mitochondrial myopathy, encephalopathy, lactic acidosis, and stroke-like episodes with recurrent abdominal symptoms and coenzyme Q_{10} administration. J Neurol Neurosurg Psychiatr 1987;50:1475–1481

123. Shults CW, Haas RH, Beal MF. A possible role of coenzyme Q_{10} in the etiology and treatment of Parkinson's disease. Biofactors 1999;9:267–272

124. Kagan T, Davis C, Lin L, Zakeri Z. Coenzyme Q_{10} can in some circumstances block apoptosis, and this effect is mediated through mitochondria. Ann NY Acad Sci 1999;887:31–47

125. Matthews PM, Ford B, Dandurand RJ, et al. Coenzyme Q_{10} with multiple vitamins is generally ineffective in treatment of mitochondrial disease. Neurology 1993;43:884–890

126. Gold R, Seibel P, Reinelt G, et al. Phosphorus magnetic resonance spectroscopy in the evaluation of mitochondrial myopathies: results of a 6-month therapy study with coenzyme Q. Eur Neurol 1996;36:191–196

127. Suno M, Nagaoka A. Inhibition of lipid peroxidation by a novel compound (CV-2619) in brain mitochondria and mode of action of the inhibition. Biochem Biophys Res Commun 1984;125:1046–1052

128. Sugiyama Y, Fujita T. Stimulation of the respiratory and phosphorylating activities in rat brain mitochondria by idebenone (CV-2619), a new agent improving cerebral metabolism. FEBS Lett 1985;184:48–51

129. Barkworth MF, Dyde CJ, Johnson KI, Schnelle K. An early phase I study to determine the tolerance, safety and pharmacokinetics of idebenone following multiple oral doses. Arzneimittelforschung 1985;35:1704–1707

130. Ikejiri Y, Mori E, Ishii K, et al. Idebenone improves cerebral mitochondrial oxidative metabolism in a patient with MELAS. Neurology 1996;47:583–585

131. Lerman-Sagie T, Rustin P, Lev D, et al. Dramatic improvement in mitochondrial cardiomyopathy following treatment with idebenone. J Inherit Metab Dis 2001;24:28–34

132. Keightley JA, Anitori R, Burton MD, et al. Mitochondrial encephalomyopathy and complex III deficiency associated with a stop-codon mutation in the cytochrome b gene. Am J Hum Genet 2000;67:1400–1410

133. Eleff S, Kennaway N, Buist N, et al. ^{31}P NMR study of improvement in oxidative phosphorylation by vitamins K3 and C in a patient with a defect in electron transport at complex III in skeletal muscle. Proc Natl Acad Sci USA 1984;81:3529–3533

134. Nosoh Y, Kajioka J, Itoh M. Effect of menadione on the electron transport pathway of yeast. Arch Biochem Biophys 1968;127:1–6

135. Argov Z, Bank W, Maris J, et al. Treatment of mitochondrial myopathy due to Complex III deficiency with vitamins K_3 and C: a ^{31}P-NMR follow-up study. Ann Neurol 1986;19:598–602

136. Cooper JM, Hayes DJ, Challis RA et al. Treatment of experimental NADH ubiquinone reductase deficiency with menadione. Brain 1992;115:991–1000

137. Shoffner J, Voljavec A, Costigan D, et al. Chronic external ophthalmoplegia and ptosis (CEOP): improved retinal cone function with ascorbate, phylloquinone, and coenzyme Q_{10}. Neurology 1989;39(Suppl 1):404

138. McCord J, Fridovich I. The utility of superoxide dismutase in studying free radical reactions. II. The mechanism of the mediation of cytochrome c reduction by a variety of electron carriers. J Biol Chem 1970;245:1374–1377

139. Lou H. Correction of increased plasma pyruvate and

plasma lactate levels using large doses of thiamine in patients with Kearns-Sayre syndrome. Arch Neurol 1981;38:469

140. Mastaglia FL, Thompson PL, Papadimitriou JM. Mitochondrial myopathy with cardiomyopathy, lactic acidosis and responseto prednisone and thiamine. Aust NZ J Med 1980;10(6):660–664

141. Tanaka J, Nagai T, Arai H, et al. Treatment of mitochondrial encephalomyopathy with a combination of cytochrome C and vitamins B_1 and B_2. Brain Dev 1997; 19:262–267

142. Arts W, Scholte H, Bogaars J, et al. NADH-CoQ reductase deficiency: successful treatment with riboflavin. Lancet 1983;2:581–582

143. Penn AM, Lee JW, Thuillier P, et al. MELAS syndrome with mitochondrial tRNA(Leu)(UUR) mutation: correlation of clinical state, nerve conduction, and muscle ^{31}P magnetic resonance spectroscopy during treatment with nicotinamide and riboflavin. Neurology 1992;42: 2147–2152

144. Ogle RF, Christodoulou J, Fagan E, et al. Mitochondrial myopathy with tRNA(Leu(UUR)) mutation and complex I deficiency responsive to riboflavin. J Pediatr 1997;130:138–145

145. Bernsen PL, Gabreels FJ, Ruitenbeek W, Hamburger HL. Treatment of complex I deficiency with riboflavin. J Neurol Sci 1993;118:181–187

146. Sato Y, Nakagawa M, Higuchi I, et al. Mitochondrial myopathy and familial thiamine deficiency. Muscle Nerve 2000;23:1069–1075

147. Shapira Y, Cederbaum SD, Cancilla PA, et al. Familial poliodystrophy, mitochondrial myopathy, and lactate acidemia. Neurology 1975;25:614–621

148. Montagna P, Gallassi R, Medori R, et al. MELAS syndrome: characteristic migrainous and epileptic features and maternal transmission. Neurology 1988; 38(5):751–754

149. Gubbay SS, Hankey GJ, Tan NT, Fry JM. Mitochondrial encephalomyopathy with corticosteroid dependence. Med J Aust 1989;151(2):100–108

150. Zheng J, Ramirez VD. Rapid inhibition of rat brain mitochondrial proton F0F1-ATPase activity by estrogens: comparison with Na+, K+-ATPase of porcine cortex. Eur J Pharmacol 1999;368:95–102

151. Curless RG, Flynn J, Bachynski B, et al. Fatal metabolic acidosis, hyperglycemia, and coma after steroid therapy for Kearns-Sayre syndrome. Neurology 1986; 36(6):872–873

152. Stacpoole PW, Lorenz AC, Thomas RG, Harman EM. Dichloroacetate in the treatment of lactic acidosis. Ann Intern Med 1988;108:58–63

153. Stacpoole PW, Wright EC, Baumgartner TG, et al. A controlled clinical trial of dichloroacetate for treatment of lactic acidosis in adults. The Dichloroacetate-Lactic Acidosis Study Group. N Engl J Med 1992;327: 1564–1569

154. Pavlakis SG, Kingsley PB, Kaplan GP, et al. Magnetic resonance spectroscopy: use in monitoring MELAS treatment. Arch Neurol 1998;55:849–852

155. Saitoh S, Momoi MY, Yamagata T, et al. Effects of dichloroacetate in three patients with MELAS. Neurology 1998;50:531–534

156. Saijo T, Naito E, Ito M, et al. Therapeutic effect of sodium dichloroacetate on visual and auditory hallucinations in a patient with MELAS. Neuropediatrics 1991;22:166–167

157. Kuroda Y, Ito M, Naito E, et al. Concomitant administration of sodium dichloroacetate and vitamin B_1 for

lactic acidemia in children with MELAS syndrome. J Pediatr 1997;131:450–452

158. Seneca S, De ML, De SJ, et al. Pearson marrow pancreas syndrome: a molecular study and clinical management. Clin Genet 1997;51:338–342

159. Burlina AB, Milanesi O, Biban P, et al. Beneficial effect of sodium dichloroacetate in muscle cytochrome c oxidase deficiency [letter]. Eur J Pediatr 1993;152:537

160. Tulinius MH, Eriksson BO, Hjalmarson O, et al. Mitochondrial myopathy and cardiomyopathy in siblings. Pediatr Neurol 1989;5:182–188

161. North K, Korson MS, Krawiecki N, et al. Oxidative phosphorylation defect associated with primary adrenal insufficiency. J Pediatr 1996;128:688–692

162. De Stefano N, Matthews P, Ford B, et al. Short-term dichloroacetate treatment improves indices of cerebral metabolism in patients with mitochondrial disorders. Neurology 1995;45:1193–1198

163. Spruijt L, Naviaux RK, McGowan KA, et al. Nerve conduction changes in patients with mitochondrial diseases treated with dichloroacetate. Muscle Nerve 2001;24:916–924

164. Campos Y, Huertas R, Bautista J, et al. Muscle carnitine deficiency and lipid storage myopathy in patients with mitochondrial myopathy. Muscle Nerve 1993;16: 778–781

165. Campos Y, Huertas R, Lorenzo G, et al. Plasma carnitine insufficiency and effectiveness of L-carnitine therapy in patients with mitochondrial myopathy. Muscle Nerve 1993;16:150–153

166. Infante JP, Huszagh VA. Secondary carnitine deficiency and impaired docosahexaenoic (22:6n-3) acid synthesis: a common denominator in the pathophysiology of diseases of oxidative phosphorylation and beta-oxidation. FEBS Lett 2000;468:1–5

167. Kobayashi M, Morishita H, Sugiyama N, Wada Y. Successful treatment with succinate supplement in a patient with a deficiency of Complex I (NADH-CoQ reductase). The Fourth International Congress of Inborn errors of metabolism, Sendai, Japan, 1987

168. Tarnopolsky MA, Roy BD, MacDonald JR. A randomized, controlled trial of creatine monohydrate in patients with mitochondrial cytopathies. Muscle Nerve 1997;20:1502–1509

169. DiMauro S, Bonilla E, Lee C, et al. Luft's disease. Further biochemical and ultrastructural studies of skeletal muscle in the second case. J Neurol Sci 1976; 27:217–232

170. Taylor RW, Chinnery P, Clark K, et al. Treatment of mitochondrial disease. J Bioenerg Biomembr 1997;29: 195–205

171. Johnston S, Anziano P, Shark K, et al. Mitochondrial transformation in yeast by bombardment with microprojectiles. Science 1988;240:1538–1541

172. Boynton J, Gillham N, Harris E, et al. Chloroplast transformation in Chlamydomonas with high velocity microprojectiles. Science 1987;240:1534–1538

173. Koop H, Steinmüller K, Wagner H, et al. Integration of foreign sequences into the tobocco plastome via polyethylene glycol-mediated protoplast transformation. Planta 1996;199:193–201

174. Seibel P, Trappe J, Villani G, et al. Transfection of mitochondria: strategy towards a gene therapy of mitochondrial diseases. Nuc Acid Res 1996;23:10–17

175. King M, Attardi G. Injection of mitochondria into human cells leads to a rapid replacement of the endogenous mitochondrial DNA. Cell 1988;52:811–819

176. Clarke M, Shay J. Mitochondrial transformation of mammalian cells. Science 1982;295:605–607

177. Weissig V, Torchilin VP. Cationic bolasomes with delocalized charge centers as mitochondria-specific DNA delivery systems. Adv Drug Deliv Rev 2001;49: 127–149

178. Entelis N, Kieffer S, Kolesnikova O, et al. Structural requirements of tRNALys for its import into yeast mitochondria. Proc Natl Acad Sci, USA 1998;95: 2838–2843

179. Magalhaes PJ, Sjo O, Norby S. Ocular myopathy and mitochondrial DNA deletion. A presentation of seven identified Danish patients. Acta Ophthalmologica Scandinavica Supplement 1996;29–32

180. Nagley P, Farrell L, Gearing D, et al. Assembly of functional proton-translocating ATPase complex in yeast mitochondria with cytoplasmically synthesized subunit 8, a polypeptide normally encoded within the organelle. Proc Natl Acad Sci USA 1988;85:2091–2095

181. Sutherland L, Davidson J, Jacobs H. Nuclear expression of mitochondrial genes implicated in human encephalomyopathies. Biochem Soc Trans 1994;22:413S

182. Sutherland L, Davidson J, Glass LL, Jacobs HT. Multisite oligonucleotide-mediated mutagenesis: application to the conversion of a mitochondrial gene to universal genetic code. Biotechniques 1995;18:458–464

183. Taylor R, Chinnery P, Turnbull D, Lightowlers R. Selective inhibition of mutant human mitochondrial DNA replication in vitro by peptide nucleic acids. Nat Genet 1997;15:212–215

184. Chinnery PF, Taylor RW, Diekert K, et al. Peptide nucleic acid delivery to human mitochondria. Gene Ther 1999;6:1919–1928

185. Clark KM, Bindoff LA, Lightowlers RN, et al. Reversal of a mitochondrial DNA defect in human skeletal muscle [letter]. Nat Genet 1997;16:222–224

186. Andrews RM, Griffiths PG, Chinnery PF, Turnbull DM. Evaluation of bupivacaine-induced muscle regeneration in the treatment of ptosis in patients with chronic progressive external ophthalmoplegia and Kearns-Sayre syndrome. Eye 1999;13:769–772

187. Blok R, Gook D, Thorburn D, Dahl H. Skewed segregation of the mtDNA nt 8993 (T→G) mutation in human oocytes. Am J Hum Genet 1997;60:1495–1501

188. Manfredi G, Thyagarajan D, Papadopoulou LC, et al. The fate of human sperm-derived mtDNA in somatic cells. Am J Hum Genet 1997;61:953–960

189. Triepels RH, van den Heuvel LP, Loeffen JL, et al. Leigh syndrome associated with a mutation in the NDUFS7 (PSST) nuclear encoded subunit of complex I. Ann Neurol 1999;45:787–790

190. Loeffen J, Elpeleg O, Smeitink J, et al. Mutations in the complex I NDUFS2 gene of patients with cardiomyopathy and encephalomyopathy. Ann Neurol 2001;49: 195–201

191. Moraes CT, Shanske S, Tritschler HJ, et al. mtDNA depletion with variable tissue expression: a novel genetic abnormality in mitochondrial diseases. Am J Hum Genet 1991;48:492–501

192. Fadic R, Russell JA, Vedanarayanan VV, et al. Sensory ataxic neuropathy as the presenting feature of a novel mitochondrial disease. Neurology 1997;49:239–245

193. Bohlega S, Tanji K, Santorelli F, et al. Multiple mitochondrial DNA deletions associated with autosomal recessive ophthalmoplegia and severe cardiomyopathy. Neurology 1996;46:1329–1334

194. Barrientos A, Casademont J, Saiz A, et al. Autosomal recessive Wolfram syndrome associated with an 8.5-kb mtDNA single deletion. Am J Hum Genet 1996;58: 963–970

IX   Pediatric and Adolescent Neurology

Section editor: Russell D Snyder

152 The Neurological Examination of the Infant and Child

Neil R Friedman and Bruce H Cohen

Despite the proliferation of diagnostic and investigational tools available to medical practitioners, a thorough, precise history and a detailed clinical examination remain the cornerstone for establishing a diagnostic differential analysis and for directing further evaluation. The examination of a child or infant—as for an adult—is directed toward establishing 1) whether the problem is neurological, 2) the nature of the problem, and 3) where the problem lies within the neuraxis. A child, however, is not merely a "little adult," and it is necessary to be aware that one is dealing with a rapidly developing and maturing brain, both structurally (e.g., maturation of myelin) and physiologically (e.g., the formation of neural networks). Compare a neonate who is nonambulant and wholly dependent on others for its care with an infant at the end of the first year of life, who is now ambulant, developing language, and starting to manipulate the environment. Head growth, one reflection of the development and maturation of the brain, on average is 12 cm during the first 2 years of life, compared with approximately 5 cm during the subsequent 16 years. Progressive myelination occurs from early in the second trimester of pregnancy until well into childhood. It is myelination of the corticospinal tracts in the first year of life that ultimately allows the infant to sit and subsequently to walk independently. Thus, although the fundamentals of the neurological examination are the same for an infant/child and adult, the milieu of the developmental aspects is very different. Other differences include the inability of an infant or younger child to recount the history; the age-dependent acquisition of gross motor, fine motor, and social skills; and the diverse group of neurological conditions that can affect children. Furthermore, obtaining a diagnosis may provide crucial genetic information and information important for counseling parents who wish to have more children.

History: "Listen to the parent"

The art of history taking requires good listening and interpersonal communication skills and good powers of deduction. Although typically a history is obtained from a parent or other third party, some young children are able to describe their symptoms and should be encouraged and given the opportunity to do so. When possible, the history should include the child's or parent's words rather than the physician's medical interpretation of them. It is important to distinguish between the subjective interpretations of symptoms by third parties and objective observations. Symptoms should be described in plain language rather than in medical jargon. As the history taking progresses, the physician should begin to develop a differential diagnosis, and further questioning should be directed at trying to confirm or exclude these possibilities. When doing this, it is useful to have in mind a framework of major pathophysiological causes of disease (Table 152.1).

Presenting symptom or symptoms

The history typically begins with elucidating the nature of the presenting complaint. A chronological approach is often helpful. The temporal pattern of the problem should be determined: static, progressive, or regressive. Is the problem limited to one area of the neuraxis or is a combination of systems involved? With respect to development, it is critical to determine if the delay is global or limited to one of the four main areas of development, that is, gross motor, fine motor, social, or speech/language skills. The severity of the problem and its changes over time should be assessed. In addition, any associated features and previous interventions should be documented.

Past history

It should be established whether the patient has had any previous hospitalizations or surgical treatment (or both). Any chronic underlying illness that may affect the presenting symptoms or may be a factor in considering treatment options (e.g., avoiding β-blockers for patients with migraine headache who have asthma, diabetes mellitus, or depression) should be noted.

Birth history

This is an essential part of the history of the infant and child and may provide a clue to the cause of the

Table 152.1 Major pathophysiological causes of disease
Congenital
Traumatic
Inflammatory
Infectious
Ischemic/vascular
Toxic/drug
Metabolic
Neoplastic

current problem. Trauma, hypoxic-ischemic events, infection, drug use or abuse, and malnutrition all affect the developing brain. The history should examine the three main areas of interest:

- The antenatal course
  1. Gestation: It is important to establish the duration of the pregnancy and the reliability of that assessment. A term pregnancy is 37 to 42 weeks of gestation. Preterm infants have a unique set of complications affecting the brain, for example, approximately a 20% incidence of intraventricular hemorrhage in neonates weighing less than 1500 grams, and hypoxic-ischemic injury leading to periventricular leukomalacia and the classic resultant spastic diplegia that may affect these children. Chorioamnionitis is a frequent cause of preterm labor, and sepsis may result in shock and hypoxic-ischemic injury or even meningitis. Multiple births also carry the risk of premature delivery.
  2. Infection: Inquiry should be made about any problems during the labor with regard to fever, rash, or infection, especially TORCHS (toxoplasmosis, rubella, cytomegalovirus, herpes simplex, and syphilis) and HIV infections. These infections may be relatively silent in the mother. Defects of cortical migration, microcephaly, mental retardation, spasticity, and quadriplegia are potential complications.
  3. Drug or toxin exposure: A history of both illicit and prescription drug use should be documented. Many drugs are teratogenic and associated with well-established syndromes and phenotypes (e.g., phenytoin and fetal hydantoin syndrome). Illicit drugs such as cocaine or "crack" may be associated with neonatal stroke or intracranial hemorrhage. Smoking and alcohol both affect fetal development. Cigarette smoking may result in intrauterine growth retardation and a stressed baby at delivery. Alcohol abuse may result in fetal alcohol syndrome or fetal alcohol effects, which have neurological complications, especially impaired cognitive development and behavioral disturbances.
  4. Prenatal care and ultrasonography: Brain malformations, choroid plexus cysts, spinal dysraphism, and hydrocephalus can all be detected antenatally. The results of prenatal ultrasonography, if performed, should be recorded. The amount of amniotic fluid is important, particularly with regard to suspected neuromuscular disease. Impaired swallowing may result in polyhydramnios. Oligohydramnios may result in diminished fetal movement and subsequent joint contractures (arthrogryposis). Fetal movements specifically should be addressed. Diminished fetal movement is often found in neuromuscular disorders, especially spinal muscular atrophy type 1 (Werdnig–Hoffmann disease). An abrupt cessation of movement for a prolonged period may be indicative of fetal dis-

tress and possible hypoxemia. Prenatal seizure activity has been described in utero. More than one-half the cases of cerebral palsy have an antenatal cause.

- Labor and delivery
  Important factors to consider include birth weight, gestation, Apgar score, need for resuscitation, type of resuscitation, and the presence or absence of meconium (indicating possible fetal distress). The mode of delivery is also important. If a cesarean section was performed, why was it necessary? Forceps delivery has been implicated in facial nerve palsy at birth and shoulder dystocia *may* result in a brachial plexopathy. However, these types of injuries are not always caused by events during labor and delivery and may be of prenatal onset. With suspected perinatal hypoxia, it is important to try to determine whether the stress of labor exacerbated a preexisting condition or was the primary cause. In the latter case, no further neurological work-up is necessary for the cause, but in the former case, it may be necessary to consider and evaluate for a primary metabolic or neuromuscular disorder.
- Postnatal course
  Inquiry should be made about complications such as sepsis and the need for mechanical ventilation and extracorporeal membrane oxygenation. It is particularly important to document hypoglycemia and neonatal seizures. The most common cause of neonatal seizures is hypoxic-ischemic encephalopathy, typically occurring within the first 24 hours after birth, and frequently within 12 hours. Other causes include hypoglycemia, hypocalcemia, drug withdrawal, intracranial hemorrhage, meningitis, metabolic disorder (such as nonketotic hyperglycinemia and neonatal adrenoleukodystrophy), and defect of cortical migration. Results of neuroimaging studies and neurophysiological studies are also important. Ultrasonography of the head is performed routinely in premature infants and is useful for detecting both intraventricular and parenchymal hemorrhages and for assessing ventricular size. The grade of intraventricular hemorrhage and the size of periventricular echodensity are important prognostically for neurological outcome. A burst suppression electroencephalogram at birth invariably is associated with poor neurological outcome.

Developmental history

An appreciation of normal developmental milestones is crucial when evaluating an infant or child. It is best to use standardized screening tests (e.g., the Denver developmental screening test, Gesell developmental test, and the Binet test). Particularly in the first year of life, deviation from the mean needs to be interpreted in relation to gestational age. It is important to determine what aspect of development is delayed and by how many months. Equally important is to determine whether there is any evidence of regression that could suggest a neurodegenerative process such as leukodystrophy. Because this may not be evident the first time a child is evaluated, subsequent follow-up and observation are crucial. A strong hand preference in an infant younger than 12 to 18 months suggests weakness or apraxia of the opposite hand and side of the body. For a school-aged child, information about cognitive functioning is often available from school proficiency tests or multifactorial evaluations that include psychometric and achievement tests. Stereotypes, poor socialization, lack of understanding of interpersonal interactions and social cues, and developmental language delay raise concern of a possible pervasive developmental disorder or autistic spectrum disorder. A history of true language regression should be sought because of the possibility of acquired epileptic aphasia or Landau–Kleffner syndrome.

Family history

With the ever-increasing application of molecular genetic techniques to the investigation of neurological disorders, a genetic basis is possible for many disorders. Thus, a thorough and careful family history is important in establishing a possible autosomal, X-linked, or mitochondrial genetic link for the problem under review. Even in the absence of an established genetic basis, many problems are clearly familial, for example, migraine headache, learning disability, epilepsy, and Tourette syndrome. Social circumstances and environment also affect the expression of certain disorders.

Review of systems

A systematic review of all major organ systems should complete the medical history, especially how they may affect or modify the neurological problem. For example, complex congenital heart disease may be associated with learning disability, stroke, or, rarely, choreathetosis as a complication of cardiopulmonary bypass. When a metabolic disorder is suspected, parents should be asked whether the child's breath or urine has a strange odor, especially at times of illness. Marked decompensation at the time of illness, with vomiting, pallor, and delayed recovery, suggests a disorder of intermediary energy metabolism or urea cycle defect.

Examination: "Observe the patient"

The examination of a neonate, infant, and child relies heavily on the power of observation. Unlike the adult neurological examination, which is performed in a coherent, systematic manner, the examination of a child should be flexible and nonthreatening. For example, this may require the examiner to delay ophthalmoscopy until the end of the examination. In older children and adolescents, the approach to the neurological examination is the same as that for adults. Watching the child at play, at rest, and interacting with caregivers is often very revealing. Behavioral problems, interactions with their environment, asymmetries in posture or movement, abnormal

movements (dystonia, posturing, tremor, infantile spasms, etc.), weakness, and gait abnormalities may all be apparent.

General examination

Dysmorphology   In contradistinction to adult neurological disease, genetic syndromes and dysmorphology are important in pediatric neurological disease. Common genetic syndromes that may have neurological involvement include trisomy 21 syndrome (Down syndrome), Turner syndrome, fragile X syndrome, Angelman syndrome, Prader–Willi syndrome, Cornelia de Lange syndrome, and velocardiofacial syndrome. The phenotypic appearance usually is obvious from direct observation. Midline defects such as cleft lip and palate, central incisors, and congenital heart disease may be associated with abnormalities of cortical migration.

Neurocutaneous stigmata   The skin should be examined carefully for evidence of neurocutaneous lesions, because several disorders are associated with a combination of skin and central or peripheral nervous system problems (Table 152.2). Examination with a Wood lamp is usually more sensitive than visual inspection alone for detecting these lesions.

Head size and shape   Head circumference should be measured and percentiles for all growth variables (weight, height, and head circumference) should be plotted for all children. Head size directly reflects intracranial contents. Macrocephaly is most commonly familial, and if found, the head circumference of the parents should be documented. Benign external hydrocephalus is another common cause of macrocephaly and has a distinctive radiographic appearance (increased extra-axial cerebrospinal fluid spaces predominantly over the frontal convexities) and mild motor delay. This needs to be distinguished from communicating or obstructive hydrocephalus, which may produce signs of increased intracranial pressure (lethargy, vomiting, and "sunsetting" sign). Unlike benign external hydrocephalus, in which the head circumference follows its own appropriate percentile, there is crossing of percentiles of head circumference in hydrocephalus proper. Macrocephaly may also occur with several neurocutaneous disorders, especially neurofibromatosis. Other rare causes of macrocephaly include Alexander disease, Canavan disease, glutaricaciduria type I, and thickening of the skull (as in myelodysplasias or sickle cell disease). Microcephaly may also be familial or result from defects of cortical migration (e.g., schizencephaly, lissencephaly, and polymicrogyria), hypoxic-ischemic brain injury, congenital infections (e.g., toxoplasmosis, rubella, and cytomegalovirus), or premature fusion of the sutures (craniosynostosis).

It is also important to assess skull shape. The anterior fontanelle remains open until approximately 18 months of age. Premature closure may be associated with microcephaly or craniosynostosis. A large anterior fontanelle raises the suspicion of hypothyroidism

Table 152.2   Neurocutaneous lesions and associated conditions

Lesion	Associated condition
Café-au-lait macule	Neurofibromatosis
	Tuberous sclerosis
	Hypomelanosis of Ito
Hypopigmented macule	Tuberous sclerosis
	Hypomelanosis of Ito
Shagren patch	Tuberous sclerosis
Adenoma sebaceum	Tuberous sclerosis
Nevus flammeus	Sturge–Weber syndrome
Gottron papules	Dermatomyositis
Unilateral linear nevus (usually face)	Linear sebaceous nevus syndrome
Telangiectasia	Ataxia-telangiectasia

or increased intracranial pressure. The posterior fontanelle typically closes between 3 and 6 months of age. Plagiocephaly, especially occipital, suggests decreased mobility due to hypotonia or weakness (or both), with resultant flattening of the bone. Dolichocephaly (a long narrow head) is commonly seen in premature infants. Several craniofacial syndromes, including Pfeiffer syndrome (brachycephaly), Crouzon disease (acrocephaly), and Saethre–Chotzen syndrome (brachycephaly), are associated with abnormally shaped heads.

Neurological examination

Mental status   A brief reference to a child's alertness, appropriateness, and interactiveness with the examiner should be noted. Age-based language ability, expressive and receptive language ability, fluency, and articulation should be assessed. A comment on mood may be important, particularly for patients with chronic headache or pain syndrome. Attention, impulsiveness, and motor activity are particularly important if academic difficulties or disorders of behavior are of concern. However, this should always be interpreted in the context of the age of the child and reasonable expectations. A more detailed examination is rarely necessary and should be dictated by the presenting symptoms and history. With older children and adolescents, a formal mini-mental assessment can be performed if necessary.

Cranial nerves   The cranial nerve examination for children is similar to that for adults, with some notable exceptions. Cranial nerve I (olfactory nerve) is rarely tested except when anosmia is an important consideration (e.g., Kallman syndrome). In the newborn, the absence of a red reflex on direct ophthalmoscopic examination raises the concern of retinoblastoma. Confrontational visual field testing (cranial nerve II or optic nerve) is not possible in a very young child, but a blink response to a threat provides a crude assessment of visual field integrity. Although a very young infant will fix on and follow a face, "doll's head" movements (oculocephalics) are usually necessary for assessing extraocular move-

ments during the neonatal period. Exotropia and esotropia are frequently encountered in the infant and young child, and latent strabismus can be unmasked by the cover–uncover test. When these are detected, the child should be referred to an ophthalmologist for further evaluation and possible patching to allow for fusion and the development of binocular vision. Head tilt or torticollis in a child may be the only clue to cranial nerve IV (trochlear nerve) palsy, because the child may not complain of diplopia. In the first month of life, a neonate will quieten to a bell presented at it's ear and, by 5 or 6 months, should localize the sound. This provides a useful assessment of cranial nerve VIII (vestibulocochlear nerve) function.

Motor examination   The motor examination involves testing the integrity of the pyramidal, extrapyramidal, and cerebellar systems. It principally involves seven aspects of motor function (Table 152.3).

1. Muscle bulk: examination begins with inspection of the muscles and assessment of muscle bulk. This involves looking for evidence of generalized (arthrogryposis) or focal contractures or abnormal fasciculations of muscle. Pseudohypertrophy, particularly of calf muscles but other muscle groups as well, occurs in several muscular dystrophies, including Duchenne, Becker, and limb-girdle muscular dystrophy. Generalized muscular hypertrophy is seen in myotonia congenita (so-called little Hercules appearance). Atrophy of muscle occurs with disuse or cachexia or can be due to neurogenic or anterior horn cell disease (e.g., Charcot–Marie–Tooth disease or spinal muscular atrophy). Scapular winging due to weakness and wasting of the supraspinatus and infraspinatus muscles is apparent in some forms of limb-girdle muscular dystrophy as well as in facioscapulohumeral muscular dystrophy. Arthrogryposis in children generally is associated with arthrogryposis multiplex congenita or with certain neuromuscular conditions such as congenital myotonic dystrophy or congenital muscular dystrophy.

Table 152.3   Motor examination

Muscle bulk
Muscle tone
Strength
Reflexes
Coordination of movement
Gait
Involuntary movements

Percussion of the muscle is important if the history indicates a possible myotonic muscle disorder. Percussion over the thenar eminence, tongue, or deltoid muscle may elicit a sustained muscle contraction (myotonia). Sustained grip or eye closure may result in difficulty opening the hand or eyes, respectively, confirming myotonia, and may be the only clue to the diagnosis in a young child. Palpation of the muscle may reveal tenderness, as in myositis (viral or dermatomyositis), or a "doughy" feel, as in muscular dystrophy.

2. Muscle tone: tone reflects the state of tension or contraction in muscle and may be normal, increased (hypertonic), or decreased (hypotonic). Hypertonia resulting from upper motor neuron damage to the corticospinal tracts gives rise to spasticity with the characteristic pattern of flexion of the upper extremity and extension and plantar flexion of the lower extremity. A "soft" neurological sign in the infant, suggesting possible injury to these tracts, is plantar flexion of the feet when the infant is suspended vertically. With more severe involvement, scissoring of the legs may occur. Severe spasticity may result ultimately in hip flexor, hip adductor, and tendo Achilles contractures. During the first year of life, it is important to note that following an injury to the corticospinal tract an infant often presents with hypotonia before hypertonia develops. A useful sign, when present, is the obligatory fisting (so-called cortical thumb) that may be seen despite hypotonia. An infant up to about 3 months old may hold the hand in a fist, with the thumbs adducted most of the time, but after 4 months, the hand should be held mostly open, and if it is not, suggests possible injury to the central nervous system. Injury to the basal ganglia results in a different form of hypertonia called "extrapyramidal rigidity" (sometimes referred to as "cogwheeling rigidity"). In this form, the hypertonia tends to be more uniform than the "clasp-knife" hypertonia of spasticity.

Hypotonia is felt as decreased resistance or the absence of resistance to passive movement of the limbs. Hyperextensibility of joints may be associated with hypotonia. Posture at rest may give an indication of tone, for example, the "frog leg" position and internal rotation of the shoulders seen in spinal muscular atrophy. A premature infant is hypotonic because flexor tone develops at about 32 weeks of gestation and is strongly established by term. Head lag on pull-to-sit and poor head and trunk posture with vertical suspension help establish that an infant has axial hypotonia. By 3 months of age, an infant should be able to maintain the head horizontally while suspended ventrally, and, after 4 months, should be able to elevate and maintain the head above the midline. Although classically hypotonia is due to a lesion of lower motor neurons, it also may result from cerebral dysfunction, especially if the cerebellum or cerebellar pathways are involved. With "cerebral hypotonia," other upper motor neuron features (hyperreflexia, pathological reflexes, and extensor plantar responses) should be present. In some situations, a combination of central and peripheral nervous system involvement (peripheral neuropathy) may occur, for example, Krabbe disease, metachromatic leukodystrophy, or mitochondrial cytopathy.

3. Muscle strength: direct observation of a child playing or a neonate/infant moving spontaneously gives invaluable information about strength. Watching the child walk into the room, climbing onto and off a chair, reaching for toys, and jumping and hopping will readily identify marked weakness. Even in a newborn or infant, antigravity strength can be assessed by watching the child move spontaneously or offering him or her a toy to grab. Strength can be tested reliably in children as young as 3 or 4 years. Many different scales exist for testing manual strength, but the most common is the Medical Research Council 5-point grade scale, with grade 0 representing complete paralysis of movement and grade 5 representing normal strength. The key level is the presence of antigravity strength (grade 3). With marked weakness of the proximal lower extremity, Gower sign can be elicited. In this maneuver, the child is told to lie flat on the back on the floor and then attempt to stand as quickly as possible without the assistance of furniture. A child who has marked weakness will roll over onto the stomach and adduct and "lock" the legs before using the arms to push off the floor and "walk" or climb up the legs. With infants, counter traction on pull-to-sit can provide useful information about strength and symmetry. The same applies to eliciting the Moro reflex in infants younger than 6 months. Patterns of weakness should be documented because they provide useful clues about cause, for example, monoplegia or hemiplegia in focal cerebral injury or neonatal stroke, diplegia in injury to the premature brain, or quadriplegia in diffuse cortical or cerebral injury. A proximal-to-distal distribution of weakness or vice-versa may be helpful in differentiating myopathy from neuropathy or distinguishing among various myopathies.

4. Reflexes: the major reflexes tested in infants and children are the same as those tested in adults (Table 152.4). Additional specific reflexes are evaluated as appropriate. Reflexes may be increased (hyperreflexia), normal, or decreased (hyporeflexia) and are often graded on a scale of 0 to 4,

Table 152.4 Common reflexes and levels

Reflex	Level
Corneal	CN V and VII
Pharyngeal	CN IX and X
Biceps	C5–6
Triceps	C7–8
Brachioradialis	C5–6
Knee (quadriceps)	L3–4
Ankle	S1–2
Superficial abdominal	
Epigastric	T6–9
Midabdominal	T9–11
Hypogastric	T11–L1
Cremasteric	L1–2
Anal	S2–4

with 0 indicating absence of the reflex and 4 indicating clonus.

An important difference between adults and children is the appearance and disappearance of certain primitive reflexes that serve as important indicators of the maturation of the nervous system (Table 152.5). Asymmetries or persistence of these reflexes in certain instances is pathological. Many of these reflexes (e.g., the grasp, snout, and sucking reflexes) occur because of the lack of inhibition in degenerative conditions in adults. It is debated when an extensor toe reflex (Babinski sign) should be considered abnormal during the first year of life. Certainly, a Babinski sign is abnormal after a child starts walking, and an asymmetry, even in children younger than 1 year, should be regarded as pathological. An obligate tonic reflex ("fencing posture") is always abnormal. The crossed adductor reflex (that is, contraction of both hip adductors on eliciting the knee jerk) is normally present for the first few months of life, but its presence after 6 to 8 months of age should be regarded as pathological and indicative of an upper motor neuron lesion. This is true also of ankle clonus. A few beats may be elicited in the first 1 or 2 months of life, but after this time, more than 1 or 2 beats of clonus is abnormal.

5. Coordination of movement: formal testing of the coordination of movement in a young child can be difficult. Disorders of the cerebellum or its afferent or efferent pathways inhibit smooth, integrated, coordinated movement of the limb, resulting in a jerky, nonrhythmic movement or ataxia. This is best elicited by having the patient perform rapid alternating movements or reaching for a small target. To be certain that the ataxia is of cerebellar origin, proprioceptive loss has to be excluded; proprioception is difficult to test reliably in a child younger than 5 or 6 years. Proximal muscle weakness may also resemble ataxia, but its presence is usually obvious. Observation of the child playing, undressing, and doing zippers or buttons provides useful information about dexterity, steadiness of reach, and accuracy. Finger–nose testing provides a sense of distance judgment. By 18 months, a child should know many body parts and, with the use of a toy, can be encouraged to go back and forward between a doll's nose and his or her own nose. Rapid alternating movement can be more difficult, but with patience, it is possible to get even a young child to mimic the action. Tandem gait is not performed reliably until about age 8 years.

6. Gait: assessment of gait should start when the child enters the room. The normal toddler gait is somewhat wide-based and unsteady. Typically, walking is achieved between 12 and 18 months and running, by 18 months. Characteristic gait patterns include hemiplegic, spastic, ataxic, high steppage (footdrop or proprioceptive loss), waddling, and antalgic patterns. Rarely, astasia-abasia or hysterical gait patterns may be found, with elaborate attempts to maintain balance. Toe walking is particularly important to identify because it may suggest early tightness or contractures of the tendo Achillis or imbalance of the gastrocnemius muscle. When toe walking is unilateral, hemiplegia should be suspected, and when bilateral, muscle disease, such as muscular dystrophy. Intermittent toe walking is often seen in autistic-spectrum disorders and also is occasionally volitional. Therefore, it needs to be evaluated in the context of the entire examination. Even before a child can walk, dragging of a leg or arm when crawling may indicate hemiplegia. The appearance of asymmetric pat-

Table 152.5 Primitive reflexes and the time of normal appearance and disappearance

Reflex	Appearance	Disappearance
Moro	Birth	6 mo
Palmar and plantar grasp	32 wk	2 mo
Rooting and sucking	32 wk	4 mo
Stepping and placing	37 wk	Persists as voluntary standing
Tonic neck reflex	1 mo	6 mo
Neck righting reflex	4 mo	Persists voluntarily
Parachute	6–9 mo	Persists

terns of shoe wear may be seen in even mild hemiparesis.

7. Involuntary movements: it is beyond the scope of this chapter to discuss all the involuntary movements that may occur in childhood. Most involuntary movements in children are the same types as in adults and include tics, tremors, chorea, athetosis, dystonia, ballismus, dyskinesia, myoclonus, and myokymia. However, some special situations need to be mentioned. Abnormal movements in an infant raise the question of possible seizure activity, and this often needs to be excluded. Dystonia is frequently a consequence of gastroesophageal reflux (Sandifer syndrome). Chorea in childhood most commonly is due to rheumatic fever (Sydenham chorea) or drugs (phenothiazines). Juvenile Huntington disease usually presents as stiffness rather than chorea in childhood. Choreoathetosis or dystonia may be a late sequela of cerebral palsy, occurring many years after the insult. Choreoathetosis also may occur with metabolic disorders or inborn errors of metabolism of childhood or with brain tumors affecting the basal ganglia or, rarely, as a complication of bypass surgery for congenital heart disease. Tics frequently are seen in children and adolescents as part of Tourette syndrome (chronic vocal and motor tic disorder).

Sensory examination The sensory examination involves testing primary and secondary (cortical sensory) modalities. The former involves testing pain and temperature (spinothalamic tracts) and proprioception and vibration (dorsal columns). Light touch probably involves both tracts. Cortical sensory modalities include graphesthesia, two-point discrimination, and stereognosis. Usually, only a rudimentary sensory examination is performed in children unless the history suggests a spinal cord lesion or peripheral nerve problem. Discrimination and withdrawal to light touch and pain can be assessed readily even in a newborn, by watching the facial response and grimacing. In older children, sensory examination findings frequently are inconsistent, requiring repetition of the examination on multiple occasions.

Selected readings

1. Aids to the Examination of the Peripheral Nervous System. Rev. ed. London: Baillière Tindall, 1986
2. Frankenburg WK, Dodds J, Archer P, et al. The Denver II: a major revision and restandardization of the Denver Developmental Screening Test. Pediatrics 1992;89:91–97
3. Members of the Department of Neurology, Mayo Clinic. Clinical Examinations in Neurology. 6th ed. St. Louis: Mosby Year Book, 1991
4. Swash M, ed. Hutchison's Clinical Methods. 20th ed. London: WB Saunders, 1995
5. Volpe JJ: Neurology of the Newborn. 3rd ed. Philadelphia: WB Saunders, 1995

153 Perinatal Neurology

Alan Hill

Introduction

Improved survival of premature and critically ill term newborns is shifting the focus of perinatology from the management of cardiorespiratory disorders to the prevention of long-term neurological sequelae in survivors. Neurological problems in the newborn require separate discussion because of the major differences in the vulnerability and expression of dysfunction of the immature nervous system. Furthermore, the principles of diagnosis and management that have been established for the evaluation of dysfunction of the mature nervous system cannot necessarily be extrapolated directly to the neonatal infant. It may be anticipated that the most dramatic advances in neonatal critical care will center around the development of techniques for fetal diagnosis and intervention, which in turn may prevent or minimize neurological morbidity in the newborn.

Symptoms and signs of neonatal neurological problems

A detailed history, including a review of complications of pregnancy, labor and delivery and a careful clinical examination, forms the basis for diagnosis of neurological problems in the newborn. However, neurological examination is often hampered by associated systemic illness and the use of complex life support systems, which may necessitate reliance on adjunctive diagnostic techniques, e.g. neuroimaging, electroencephalography, for the assessment of neurological injury. Although the general framework of the neurological examination used in older children is applicable to the newborn, observations must be interpreted in the light of normal maturational changes which occur at different gestational ages.

Clearly, the hallmark of cerebral abnormality in the newborn is the presence of encephalopathy, which may be manifest as an altered level of consciousness, cranial nerve dysfunction, abnormalities of tone and movement, or seizures. However, the more premature the infant, the less reliable are these signs. Thus, prior to 28 weeks of gestation it is difficult to identify specific periods of wakefulness. Even in normal term newborns, alertness may be influenced considerably by the timing of the last feed and recent environmental stimuli. Seizures are an important and treatable feature of encephalopathy that will be discussed in more detail in a later section.

The most common motor abnormality which may be indicative of neurological dysfunction is hypotonia, which must always be evaluated in relation to gestational age. It is important to distinguish between hypotonia and weakness, although both often occur together in the newborn. Specific patterns of focal weakness may indicate focal cerebral injury, e.g. focal cerebral infarction may be associated with contralateral hemiparesis, and periventricular white matter injury may result in bilateral weakness of lower extremities. Weakness of both upper and lower limbs with preservation of facial movement may indicate cervical spinal cord injury or anterior horn cell disease. Limb weakness, which may be assessed on the basis of diminished recoil movement in response to painful stimuli, usually indicates disease of the motor unit, e.g. anterior horn cell disease (spinal muscular atrophy), peripheral neuropathy or muscle disease.

Because hypotonia and weakness often occur together, abnormalities of tendon reflexes may assist in the differentiation between upper and lower motor neuron disease. In the latter, tendon reflexes are characteristically absent or diminished. In contrast, in newborns with disease of the upper motor neuron, tendon reflexes may be normal initially and become hyperactive weeks or months later.

Neonatal seizures

As discussed previously, neonatal seizures are a common manifestation of significant neurological disease.

Clinical features

Generalized tonic–clonic seizures or the orderly progression of partial seizures are uncommon in the newborn because of the immature organization of the cerebral cortex and incomplete myelination. In contrast, oral–buccal–lingual movements, oculomotor abnormalities and autonomic dysfunction are common and reflect the relatively more advanced stage of development of the brainstem and diencephalon in this age group.[1,2] Cardiorespiratory disturbances, which frequently accompany seizure activity, may increase the likelihood of hemorrhagic or ischemic brain injury because of the ineffective cerebrovascular autoregulation and the consequent direct relationship between cerebral blood flow and systemic hemodynamics that occurs in the newborn. Neonatal seizures must be distinguished from non-epileptic movements, e.g. jitteriness, benign sleep myoclonus, stimulus-evoked myoclonus and hyperekplexia, in order to avoid inappropriate intervention with anticonvulsant medications and to permit a more accurate prediction of outcome.

Diagnosis

Neonatal seizures are identified principally on the basis of observation of unusual repetitive and stereotypical behavior, as described above. In addition, it is important to recognize that seizures in this age group may manifest as isolated autonomic dysfunction, e.g. bradycardia, change in blood pressure or oxygenation. There is an inconsistent relationship between clinical manifestations and epileptiform activity on surface-recorded electroencephalography (EEG) which has raised the notion that some abnormal movements may be brainstem-release phenomena rather than seizures. Furthermore, EEG abnormalities are usually not useful for establishing the specific etiology of seizures. Nevertheless, the confirmation of neonatal seizures may depend on the use of EEG, especially in infants who are paralyzed pharmacologically for the purpose of ventilation. Modifications of EEG technique, e.g. serial or prolonged continuous EEG monitoring, synchronized video/EEG recordings, have been developed in an attempt to improve diagnostic accuracy. In addition, background abnormalities on the interictal EEG may have important prognostic value.

In contrast to seizures in older children, neonatal seizures are rarely idiopathic. This necessitates immediate investigation for the underlying etiology, which may permit specific treatment as well as more accurate prediction of outcome. Although there are many possible causes for neonatal seizures, a relatively small number of etiologies account for the majority of cases (Table 153.1). The time of onset and characteristics of the seizures may suggest the most probable cause. Initial screening investigations should address common metabolic derangements, such as hypoglycemia, hypocalcemia, hyponatremia and acidosis. Neuroimaging may identify hypoxic–ischemic cerebral injury, intracranial hemorrhage or cerebral dysgenesis. Lumbar puncture should be considered if there is concern about intracranial infection or hemorrhage. More specific investigations may be required for diagnosis of inborn errors of metabolism, congenital viral infections, chromosomal and genetic abnormalities, and drug withdrawal or intoxication.

Management

Initial treatment must include maintenance of cardiorespiratory stability, control of ongoing or recurrent seizures by correction of specific underlying metabolic derangements (when present), and use of anticonvulsant medications. A scheme for routine management of neonatal seizures is outlined in Table 153.2. Serial blood levels of anticonvulsants may be required because of variable pharmacokinetics. Recent studies on the efficacy of anticonvulsants for the treatment of neonatal seizures suggest that phenobarbital and phenytoin are equally effective, but seizures are controlled in less than 50% of cases when either of these drugs is administered alone. When combined therapy is used, seizure control is achieved in approximately 60% of cases.[3] For treatment of refractory seizures the addition of intermittent doses of lorazepam should be considered. There is only anecdotal experience reported about the use of other anticonvulsants for treatment of neonatal seizures, e.g. primidone, lamotrigine, thiopentone, carbamazepine. The duration of anticonvulsant therapy must be guided by the risk of seizure recurrence, which is determined principally by awareness of the specific underlying etiology.[1,4] Unnecessary prolongation of therapy for transient disorders should be avoided because of unresolved concerns regarding possible adverse effects of anticonvulsants on the developing nervous system.[5,6]

Periventricular–intraventricular hemorrhage
Incidence

Periventricular–intraventricular hemorrhage (PIVH) occurs principally in premature newborns, with a reported incidence of more than 20% in infants of birthweight less than 1500 g compared to a less than 3% occurrence in healthy term newborns.[1,7] Approximately 50% of PIVH occurs on the first day of life, and 90% before four days of age. Approximately 15% of

Table 153.1 Neonatal seizures–common etiologies

Etiology	Outcome
Hypoxic–ischemic encephalopathy	Variable (50% normal development)
Intracranial hemorrhage	Intraventricular hemorrhage: poor outcome; subarachnoid hemorrhage: good outcome
Cerebral infarction	Variable
Intracranial infection	Variable
Hypoglycemia	Variable
Hypocalcemia, hypomagnesemia	Good
Rapidly changing serum sodium	Good
Cerebral dysgenesis	Poor
Inborn errors of metabolism	Poor; possibly better with early correction of metabolic derangement
Maternal drug withdrawal	Variable
Benign familial neonatal seizures	Good
Pyridoxine-dependent seizures	Variable

Table 153.2   Acute management of neonatal seizures

Treatment	Usual dosage
Ensure cardiorespiratory stability	
Specific treatments (as indicated):	
Glucose	10% solution; 2 mL/kg intravenously (i.v.)
Calcium gluconate	5% solution: 4 mL/kg i.v.
Magnesium sulfate	50% solution: 0.2 mL/kg i.m.
Phenobarbital	20 mg/kg i.v. followed by additional doses 5 mg/kg (every 10–15 min) as needed to max 20 mg/kg
Phenytoin	20 mg/kg (rate: 1 mg/kg/min) i.v.
Lorazepam	0.05–0.1 mg/kg i.v.
Pyridoxine	50–100 mg orally (duration 14 days)

infants with severe PIVH have associated intra-parenchymal hemorrhage.

Pathogenesis

In the vast majority of instances in the premature newborn, PIVH originates from the rupture of small, fragile endothelium-lined vessels located in the subependymal germinal matrix. In approximately 80% of cases, hemorrhage extends into the adjacent lateral ventricles. PIVH may occur spontaneously or as a result of a variety of stresses (which may be relatively minor), for example hypoxic–ischemic insult, venous congestion, and fluctuations in cerebral perfusion owing to the immaturity of cerebrovascular autoregulation in the premature brain. Effective management of PIVH must focus primarily on the prevention of pathogenetic mechanisms and subsequent management of complications.[1,7,8]

The principal sites of origin of IVH in the term newborn differ from those in the premature infant. Neuropathological studies indicate that the majority of cases originate from bleeding in the choroid plexus. However, ultrasound studies of live term newborns suggest that the subependymal germinal matrix is at least as common as the choroid plexus as the site of PIVH in the term newborn.

Diagnosis

Clinical abnormalities may be recognized in less than 50% of cases. When present, they may include a stepwise deterioration over several days, or rapid catastrophic deterioration with coma, apnea, seizures and brainstem dysfunction. Associated systemic derangements may include metabolic acidosis, hypotension, bradycardia and hyponatremia. Bloody or xanthochromic cerebrospinal fluid (CSF) at lumbar puncture may suggest PIVH. The limited clinical manifestations have led to the routine use of cranial ultrasonography (US) at around four days of age for all newborns less than 32 weeks of gestation, which may be performed repeatedly at the bedside without concern about ionizing radiation. Serial head circumference measurements and serial US scanning are required to monitor the development of complications, e.g. posthemorrhagic hydrocephalus. Com-

puted tomography (CT) remains the technique of choice for diagnosis of epidural, subdural and subarachnoid hemorrhage, as well as most intracerebral and posterior fossa hemorrhage.

Management

Optimal management strategies must focus on the prevention of PIVH which, under ideal circumstances, implies the prevention of premature delivery. Unfortunately, in most instances premature delivery is unavoidable, and alternative strategies have been proposed which address the multifactorial pathogenesis of PIVH and its complications.[1,7–9] The rationale for the principal prenatal and postnatal interventions that show promise for reducing either the occurrence or the severity (extent) of PIVH is summarized in Table 153.3.

Because the outcome following PIVH is determined largely by the occurrence of complications of PIVH, e.g. posthemorrhagic hydrocephalus and periventricular hemorrhagic infarction and associated hypoxic–ischemic brain injury, for example periventricular leukomalacia (PVL), these aspects deserve close attention. For example, severe PIVH may decrease circulating blood volume enough to result in systemic hypotension, which in turn may cause hypoxic–ischemic cerebral injury unless correction with volume expansion is undertaken.

With posthemorrhagic hydrocephalus it is important to appreciate that significant progressive ventriculomegaly may precede measurable increases in head circumference.[1,8] Thus, serial cranial ultrasonography often provides the earliest indications of developing hydrocephalus. Clearly, rapid ventricular enlargement associated with clinical features of raised intracranial pressure requires early intervention. More typically, ventriculomegaly that progresses slowly may be observed for several weeks without intervention, or with the use of temporizing measures only, such as serial lumbar punctures, ventricular catheter with subcutaneous reservoir for removal of CSF, or drugs that decrease CSF production. In fact, in more than 50% of cases the ventriculomegaly will arrest, and in some instances resolve spontaneously. In the remainder with progressive ventriculomegaly,

Table 153.3   Interventions for periventricular-intraventricular hemorrhage

Prenatal interventions	Common mechanisms
Delay of premature delivery (tocolytic therapy: indomethacin, magnesium sulfate)	Indomethacin: inhibits prostaglandin synthesis and platelet aggregation
	Magnesium sulfate: glutamate receptor antagonist
Antenatal corticosteroids	Induce maturation of fetal lungs and other organs
	Stabilize germinal matrix vessels
?Antenatal phenobarbital	?Neuroprotective effect
	?Dampens fluctuations of blood pressure/cerebral blood flow
Postnatal interventions	
Muscle paralysis (pancuronium bromide)	Correction of hemodynamic perturbations and fluctuations in cerebral perfusion
?Fresh-frozen plasma	Correction of coagulation disturbance
?Indomethacin	Reduces baseline cerebral blood flow
	Inhibits prostaglandins, free radicals
	Accelerates maturation of germinal matrix vessels
?Vitamin E	Minimizes oxidative damage to capillaries

definitive treatment with placement of a ventriculoperitoneal shunt is usually indicated, despite the morbidity associated with repeated shunt obstructions and infections.[8,10] Shunted posthemorrhagic hydrocephalus has a notoriously poor outcome, which may be a result of hemorrhagic or ischemic injury to the cerebral parenchyma that may occur at the time of the PIVH.[8,10,11] Thus, in a multicenter randomized controlled study of 157 cases of posthemorrhagic hydrocephalus, 20% died and 76% had major motor impairment. Early drainage of CSF did not appear to improve outcome significantly compared with controls.[11]

In addition to posthemorrhagic hydrocephalus, the other major complication which occurs in approximately 15% of infants with PIVH and which carries major prognostic significance is periventricular hemorrhagic infarction. This unilateral or grossly asymmetrical lesion of white matter is characteristically fan-shaped in appearance and closely follows the distribution of the medullary veins in the periventricular white matter. Neuropathological studies demonstrate that this lesion, which often occurs in association with ipsilateral large PIVH, results from venous congestion and infarction rather than from simple extension of intraventricular blood into the cerebral white matter. Clearly, prevention of this complication involves the avoidance of hypoxia–ischemia and consequent increases in cerebral venous pressure, which occur most frequently in association with labor and delivery, asphyxia and respiratory complications. Although the long-term neurological outcome of infants with small frontal hemorrhagic infarction may be benign, the majority of those with extensive parieto-occipital infarcts develop significant motor impairment, usually contralateral hemiparesis with more marked involvement of the lower limbs, often combined with major cognitive problems owing to interference with the developmental process of organization within the cerebral cortex.

Other intracranial hemorrhage

Other types of hemorrhage, for example subdural, epidural, subarachnoid and intracerebral, may occur in the context of birth trauma, hypoxic–ischemic insult or coagulation disturbances. However, minor degrees of such hemorrhage, which may be suspected on the basis of bloody CSF or visualization on CT, may be asymptomatic and occur following routine delivery. Severe hemorrhage may require surgical evacuation.

Hypoxic–ischemic cerebral injury

Incidence

Epidemiological studies of large populations of children with cerebral palsy suggest that approximately 12% to 20% of cases of cerebral palsy[12–15] and 10% of mental retardation[16] may be related to intrapartum hypoxic–ischemic insult. Clearly, these epidemiological data have drawn attention to the significance of prenatal factors in the genesis of chronic neurological handicap in children, which may have been underestimated previously. This emphasizes the importance of thorough investigation before a definitive diagnosis of hypoxic–ischemic brain injury is made.[17]

Pathogenesis

Hypoxic–ischemic cerebral injury is often associated with impaired cerebrovascular autoregulation, diminished cerebral glucose substrates, lactic acidosis, accumulation of free radicals and toxic excitatory amino acids, e.g. glutamate, and other metabolic derangements.[1] The topographical distribution of injury is determined principally by the maturity of the brain at the time of insult, and the severity and duration of the insult.[1,17] For example, periventricular leukomalacia, which is the principal hypoxic–ischemic lesion in the premature infant, is determined principally by the location of border zones of cerebral perfusion, together with the specific vulnerability of developing oligodendroglial cells in the periventricular white matter of the premature brain. Data from experimental animal studies suggest that the immature brain appears to have greater resistance generally to the development of hypoxic–ischemic injury. However, specific populations of neurons in the neonatal brain may have relatively increased vulnerability, related perhaps to regional activation of excitatory amino acids.

Focal or multifocal ischemic brain lesions (cerebral infarction) implies localized areas of necrosis corresponding to the distribution of specific major vessels. Although this discussion is limited to ischemic lesions, it must be recognized that a variety of fetal and neonatal insults, e.g. hemorrhagic, infections, trauma, may cause focal necrosis and cavitation if they occur during the period from approximately the second trimester of gestation to early postnatal life. The topography of perinatal arterial cerebral infarction is distinctive: nearly 90% of lesions are unilateral and involve the middle cerebral artery. Of all unilateral middle cerebral artery infarcts, approximately 75% are left-sided. Venous thrombosis is less common, and approximately 85% affect the superior sagittal sinus; the remainder involve the lateral sinus or deep venous system.

Although it is speculated that intravascular occlusion (e.g. embolus or thrombus) or a vascular maldevelopment may be the underlying etiology, documentation of such structural abnormalities is usually lacking and the etiology remains unknown in more than 50% of cases. Nevertheless, it is presumed that emboli, including placental fragments or clots, or thrombi from involuting fetal vessels, could enter the arterial circulation by passage from the venous system across the foramen ovale, and the transient right-to-left shunting through the patent ductus arteriosus would favor a predilection for left hemisphere involvement. Cardiac sources of emboli are considered rare in the newborn. Hypercoagulable states and abnormalities of blood volume, e.g. hypernatremia–dehydration, account for a small percentage of cases. The most common conditions are polycythemia and disseminated intravascular coagulation in association with sepsis, or a twin pregnancy with a dead co-twin. Inherited deficiences of protein C, protein S, antithrombin III, antiphospholipid antibodies and Factor V Leiden mutation are rare in the absence of associated systemic thrombosis. Vasculitis from bacterial meningitis and vascular injury from cranial trauma or extreme neck movement may be relevant.

The observation that a considerable percentage (i.e. approximately 35%) of focal infarcts occur in the context of generalized circulatory insufficiency or hypoxic–ischemic insult is puzzling. It is possible that asphyxia may induce vasoconstriction affecting primarily the anterior circulation, which has particularly dense sympathetic innervation. Vasospasm is also postulated to be the mechanism causing focal cerebral infarction with intrauterine exposure to cocaine.

The clinical features of neonatal cerebral infarction may be subtle. Acute unilateral weakness is uncommon. More commonly, lesions are asymptomatic or present with focal seizures. Diagnosis is confirmed by neuroimaging. Late sequelae include hemiparesis, seizures and cognitive dysfunction, although the long-term outcome is often better than might have been anticipated from the extent of cerebral necrosis demonstrated by neuroimaging.

Diagnosis

Diagnosis must begin with a detailed history of maternal factors and complications of pregnancy, labor and delivery. Several clinical indicators have been suggested as markers of perinatal hypoxic–ischemic insult, e.g. prolonged bradycardia or repetitive late decelerations of fetal heart rate, low Apgar scores, low fetal scalp or cord pH, and a requirement for prolonged resuscitation. It is important to emphasize that these clinical indicators may suggest that acute hypoxic insult has probably occurred, but they are not diagnostic of hypoxic–ischemic brain injury or predictive of long-term outcome. The actual diagnosis requires the occurrence of an acute hypoxic–ischemic insult followed by an encephalopathy during the first days of life. The neurological outcome may be predicted on the basis of the severity of the encephalopathy, together with additional data from adjunctive investigations, especially neuroimaging.[1,17]

Infants who sustain hypoxic–ischemic brain injury earlier in gestation may exhibit no clinical abnormalities in the neonatal period. In addition, features of encephalopathy may be difficult to recognize in premature newborns, and in term infants who require complex life support apparatus which precludes accurate examination. However, term newborns who sustain an acute insult of sufficient severity to result in long-term neurological sequelae invariably have an encephalopathy during the first days of life. Although there is a spectrum of severity of hypoxic–ischemic encephalopathy in the term newborn, a classification scheme of severity is useful for prognostic purposes (Table 153.4).[18–20] Seizures, which occur in approximately 50% of asphyxiated infants, are an important clinical sign in that they are indicative of moderate or severe encephalopathy. In this context, seizures usually begin during the first 24 hours of life and may be difficult to control with anticonvulsant medication.

Specific motor abnormalities on examination may suggest specific neuropathological patterns of involvement. Thus, infants with focal infarction may have focal seizures and unilateral limb weakness (hemiparesis); premature newborns with periventricular white matter injury may have bilateral mild leg weakness; term newborns with parasagittal watershed injury may have hypotonia involving the shoulder girdle musculature. However, the lack of demonstrable motor abnormality on neurological examination at this time does not preclude the presence of neuropathological injury.[1]

In addition to neurological dysfunction, there may be evidence of hypoxic–ischemic injury to organs other than the brain, e.g. kidneys, liver or myocardium. Involvement of other organs is often transient and reversible, even in the context of severe

Table 153.4   Classification of severity of hypoxic–ischemic encephalopathy

Severity	Clinical features	Outcome
Mild	Increased irritability, jitteriness Seizures: absent Primitive reflexes: exaggerated Brainstem function: intact Intracranial pressure: normal Duration: <24 h	Excellent
Moderate	Lethargy Seizures: variable Primitive reflexes: suppressed Brainstem function: intact Intracranial pressure: normal Duration: variable	Variable
Severe	Stupor, coma Seizures: present Primitive reflexes: absent Brainstem function: abnormal Intracranial pressure: may be elevated Duration: >5 days	Poor

Modified from[18].

encephalopathy.[21,22] Furthermore, hypoxic–ischemic brain injury may occur without evidence of injury to other organs on routine investigations.

Clinical observations may be corroborated by neuroimaging. Cranial ultrasonography (US) is of limited value in the term newborn because of the relatively poor visualization of cortical and posterior fossa structures, and difficulty distinguishing between hemorrhagic and hypoxic–ischemic abnormalities using this modality. However, following hypoxic–ischemic insult, serial US scans performed with identical technique on successive occasions may demonstrate increased echogenicity in affected areas around 24–48 hours of age. Computed tomography (CT) performed between three and five days following the insult, may demonstrate areas of decreased tissue attenuation that correspond to known neuropathological patterns.[23,24] The CT abnormalities and neuropathological patterns that have been correlated with abnormal neurological outcome include diffuse or patchy decrease of attenuation of the cerebral hemispheres, bilateral parasagittal watershed regions, unilateral focal areas or central injury, involving predominently thalami/basal ganglia/brainstem with relative preservation of cortex and subcortical white matter.[25,26] This latter pattern corresponds to the neuropathological abnormalities documented in experimental animals following an "acute total" hypoxic–ischemic insult.[27] In human term newborns a similar pattern has been observed following acute insult, e.g. umbilical cord prolapse, uterine rupture, massive placental abruption, or prolonged and severe fetal bradycardia. There is mounting evidence that magnetic resonance imaging (MRI) may demonstrate additional patterns of injury. For example, in newborns with cerebral infarction the extent of the lesion on MRI

appears to be more predictive of outcome than the neonatal clinical examination. Thus, in a recent study concomitant involvement of cerebral hemispheres, internal capsule and basal ganglia was associated with the subsequent development of hemiplegia, whereas involvement of only one or two of these three locations tended to be associated with a normal outcome.[28] Diffusion-weighted MRI may be more sensitive than standard MRI during the first hours following hypoxic–ischemic injury.[23] However, technical difficulties related to prolonged scanning time and difficulties with monitoring the sick newborn within the scanner limit the clinical application of MRI during the early neonatal period.

In contrast to its major role in the term newborn, CT is of limited value for the assessment of acute hypoxic–ischemic brain injury in the premature neonate. This is because of the normally high water content of brain tissue in this age group, which results in normally low tissue attenuation. Serial US scanning may demonstrate increased echogenicity of periventricular white matter during the first days of life, followed by the development of periventricular cysts in these regions after several weeks in severe cases. Serial US scanning has the practical advantages of lack of ionizing radiation and that it can be performed at the bedside. However, in older infants and children, features of end-stage periventricular leukomalacia (PVL) on CT or MRI include decreased volume of periventricular white matter, ventriculomegaly with irregular ventricular walls and deep sulci that abut directly onto the ventricles.[29] In addition, MRI may show more extensive signal changes diffusely throughout the white matter.[30]

In addition to neuroimaging, electrodiagnostic techniques have a role in the evaluation of hypoxic–

ischemic brain injury. Thus, electroencephalography may assist with the diagnosis of seizures. This is of particular importance in infants who are sedated or paralyzed pharmacologically. In addition, EEG recordings that are isoelectric, have suppressed background activity or a burst-suppression pattern are generally indicative of poor outcome. Although evoked responses have been shown to have prognostic value, their clinical application has been limited by technical difficulties in many instances.

Management

Under ideal circumstances, the optimal approach to hypoxic–ischemic cerebral injury is prevention by close monitoring of the high-risk fetus and urgent delivery if there is persistent fetal distress. Newborns with hypoxic–ischemic encephalopathy require immediate intervention to prevent additional postnatal injury via the provision of adequate ventilation and perfusion, maintenance of normal blood pressure, normoglycemia and control of seizures. With regard to maintenance of adequate ventilation, hypoxemia and hypercapnia should be avoided because they may worsen intracellular acidosis and impair cerebrovascular autoregulation. The effects of hypocapnia on cerebral perfusion have not been fully established. Experimental animal and human data do not support the use of hyperventilation, except perhaps in the context of persistent fetal circulation. Seizures associated with hypoxic–ischemic encelphalopathy may be notoriously difficult to control: their management has been outlined previously (see section on Neonatal seizures). Inappropriate antidiuretic hormone secretion may occur, resulting in hyponatremia and decreased osmolality, with a consequent risk of cerebral edema. Fluid overload should therefore be avoided. Elevated intracranial pressure, which may occur in the context of severe encephalopathy, reflects extensive cerebral necrosis and is predictive of a poor outcome.[24] Thus, although it is possible to reduce elevated intracranial pressure with the use of antiedema agents such as mannitol, such intervention has not been shown to improve outcome.[31]

In addition to the management of neurological dysfunction, there is a high incidence of dysfunction of other organ systems, e.g. heart, kidneys, gastrointestinal tract, which requires careful monitoring. Myocardial dysfunction, which may contribute to systemic hypotension in asphyxiated newborns, may require aggressive use of inotropic agents, e.g. dopamine, to avoid additional decrease in cerebral perfusion postnatally, especially in the context of impaired cerebrovascular autoregulation.

Neonatal meningitis

Bacterial meningitis in the newborn may be acquired from the mother, either transplacentally at the time of delivery, or postnatally. Alternatively, the other major source of infection is the nursery environment. Group B β-hemolytic streptococcus and *Escherichia coli* account for approximately 75% of all cases; less common organisms include *Listeria monocytogenes*, other streptococci and staphylococci, other Gram-negative enterics (i.e. *Pseudomonas aeruginosa*, *Klebsiella*, *Enterobacter* species, *Proteus* species, *Citrobacter*, *Serratia marcescens*, *Hemophilus influenzae* and *Salmonella* species.[32] Ventriculitis and hydrocephalus are common complications in this age group, whereas subdural effusions occur rarely.

Diagnosis

The clinical manifestations of meningitis are non-specific and are often indistinguishable from neonatal septicemia, e.g. lethargy, feeding problems, temperature instability, respiratory distress, vomiting and diarrhea. Seizures are common. Signs of meningeal irritation, e.g. neck retraction, opisthotonus, and signs of raised intracranial pressure, e.g. bulging fontanelle, are uncommon in the early stages. Thus, the absence of these signs should not be used to guide diagnosis and treatment. Lumbar puncture should be performed in all suspected cases, which should include a Gram stain and culture of the CSF. Other CSF findings, such as pleocytosis (if mild), elevation of protein and decreased glucose levels, may be difficult to interpret because of the wide range of normal values in this age group.[33,34] Latex agglutination in the CSF may identify group B streptococcal infection.

Management

Initial treatment of a newborn with bacterial meningitis of unknown cause should include a combination of ampicillin, an aminoglycoside such as gentamicin, and possibly cefotaxime administered intravenously.[35] The selection of antibiotics may be refined subsequently based on the resistance of the infecting organism. Parenteral antimicrobial therapy should be continued for at least 21 days.

In addition to antimicrobial therapy, supportive measures are essential, e.g. maintenance of normal fluid and electrolyte balance, blood pressure and blood gases. Fluid restriction should be considered because of the risk of inappropriate antidiuretic hormone secretion. Seizures may necessitate treatment with anticonvulsants. Serial measurements of head circumference and cranial US permit surveillance for the possible development of complications of ventriculitis and hydrocephalus. Ventriculitis commonly causes hydrocephalus, either during the acute phase of the illness or subsequently. Infants with meningitic hydrocephalus may be treated initially with external ventricular drainage, followed by the insertion of a permanent ventriculoperitoneal shunt after the infection has been eradicated.

Cerebral abscess is a rare complication of neonatal meningitis which should be considered in infants who do not appear to respond to appropriate treatment. It occurs most commonly with *Citrobacter* infection.[36] Treatment is controversial and involves prolonged antibiotic therapy, and possibly surgical exploration and drainage. In the case of *Citrobacter* infection, the addition of trimethoprim-sulfamethoxazole to the antibiotic regimen is particularly important.

Maternal substance abuse

The two major consequences of maternal substance abuse on the newborn are teratogenic effects and passive addiction. In addition, maternal cocaine abuse carries a significant risk of intracranial hemorrhage and focal cerebral infarction related to cerebral vasoconstriction in the fetus.[37]

The teratogenic effects of maternal substance abuse may be difficult to diagnose with certainty in the context of common confounding influences, e.g. genetic factors, poor nutrition, infection. Nevertheless, maternal alcohol abuse is a known cause of growth retardation, microcephaly and intellectual deficits.[38] Microcephaly has been reported in approximately 40% of infants who are passively addicted to heroin.[39] It is estimated that passive addiction occurs in 60% to 90% of newborns whose mothers used drugs that affect the central nervous system during pregnancy.

The prognosis of passive addiction to heroin involves consideration of the acute neonatal withdrawal syndrome, subacute symptoms of withdrawal, and long-term outcome. With modern neonatal intensive care the mortality from acute neonatal withdrawal syndrome is negligible. However, approximately 80% of affected infants experience a recurrence or exacerbation of symptoms, including restlessness, agitation, stimulus-sensitive tremors, colic, vomiting and disturbed sleep patterns, which may persist for three to six months. In addition, passively addicted infants are at significantly higher risk for sudden infant death syndrome (SIDS), presumably related to impaired regulation of respiration and arousal. The long-term outcome of prenatal exposure to opiates is variable, although there appears to be an increased incidence of cognitive and behavioral dysfunction. However, it is difficult to exclude the effect of confounding variables such as poor prenatal care, poor maternal nutrition, prenatal infection and a defective home environment.[1]

In addition to the acute neonatal encephalopathy and increased risk for SIDS, fetuses exposed to cocaine are at risk for serious ischemic and hemorrhagic destructive cerebral lesions, especially cerebral infarction in the distribution of major cerebral arteries.

Diagnosis

Passive addiction may be anticipated when there is known maternal addiction or drug abuse. However, such background information is notoriously unreliable and difficult to obtain. Screening for the presence of toxins in mother and newborn, e.g. urine, meconium, hair, may confirm clinical suspicions of recent drug exposure and withdrawal. The time of onset of withdrawal varies according to the elimination half-life of the specific drug. Thus, withdrawal symptoms often begin on the first day with heroin, alcohol, diazepam, short-acting barbiturates, propoxyphene and pentazocine; at two to three days of age with methadone and cocaine; and as late as seven days for longer-acting barbiturates and 21 days for chlordiazepoxide.

The clinical features of withdrawal are similar for most drugs. Initial abnormalities reflect central nervous system overactivity, e.g. jitteriness, irritability, disturbed sleep–wake cycles, shrill cry and frantic sucking. There may also be gastrointestinal disturbances, such as poor feeding, vomiting, diarrhea, as well as excessive sneezing, sweating and tachypnea. Fever and seizures are not common and their occurrence requires investigation for other potential problems, such as sepsis or meningitis. Symptoms of withdrawal may persist for several weeks following exposure to long-acting barbiturates, and heroin withdrawal may last as long as six months.[40]

Management

Early diagnosis requires a high index of suspicion. Respiratory abnormalities, dehydration and metabolic derangements must be corrected. In cases of severe irritability, vomiting and diarrhea, additional treatment with paregoric, laudanum, phenobarbital, chlorpromazine or diazepam may be required.[40] Paregoric, laudanum and chlorpromazine control both the neurological and the gastrointestinal symptoms. Paregoric or laudanum (0.4%) are the preferred treatments, because chlorpromazine may cause extrapyramidal abnormalities and a lowered seizure threshold. Either paregoric or laudanum (0.4%) is administered at a dose of three to six drops every four to six hours orally for several days or weeks, and tapered gradually to avoid the recurrence of symptoms. Alternatively, the recommended dose for chlorpromazine is 2–3 mg/kg/day given in four divided doses. Phenobarbital (loading dose of 20 mg/kg followed by a maintenance dose of 5 mg/kg/day) or diazepam (0.5–1.0 mg every 8 h) control only neurological abnormalities, and their sedative properties may worsen feeding problems. The recommended protocol for management involves the initial use of paregoric or laudanum alone, with the addition of phenobarbital if neurological abnormalities are not controlled.

References

1. Volpe JJ. Neurology of the Newborn. 4th ed. Philadelphia: WB Saunders, 2001
2. Roland EH, Hill A. Neonatal seizures. In: Maria B, ed. Current Management in Child Neurology. London: Marcel Decker, 1999:285–289
3. Painter MJ, Sher MS, Stein AD, et al. Phenobarbital compared with phenytoin for the treatment of neonatal seizures. N Engl J Med 1999;341:485–489
4. Sher MS, Seizures in the newborn infant. Clin Perinatol 1997;24:735–772
5. Holmes GL. Epilepsy in the developing brain: lessons from the laboratory and clinic. Epilepsia 1997;38:2–30
6. Farwell JR, Lee YJ, Hirtz DG, et al. Phenobarbital for febrile seizures—effects on intelligence and on seizure recurrence. N Engl J Med 1992;326:144–149
7. Hill A. Intraventricular hemorrhage: emphasis on prevention. Semin Pediatr Neurol 1998;5:152–161
8. Roland EH, Hill A. Intraventricular hemorrhage and posthemorrhagic hydrocephalus—current and potential future interventions. Clin Perinatol 1997;24:589–605

9. Horbar JD. Prevention of periventricular-intraventricular hemorrhage. *In:* Sinclair JC, Bracken MC, eds. Effective Care of the Newborn Infant. New York: Oxford University Press, 1992:562–589

10. du Plessis AJ. Posthemorrhagic hydrocephalus and brain injury in the preterm infant: dilemmas in diagnosis and management. Semin Pediatr Neurol 1998;5: 161–179

11. Ventriculomegaly Trial Group. Randomized trial of early tapping in neonatal posthemorrhagic ventricular dilatation: results at 30 months. Arch Dis Child 1990; 65:3–10

12. Stanley FJ, Watson L. Trends in perinatal mortality and cerebral palsy in Western Australia, 1967 to 1985. Br Med J 1992;304:1658–1663

13. Blair E, Stanley FJ. Intrapartum asphyxia: a rare cause of cerebral palsy. J Pediatr 1988;112:515–519

14. Freeman JM, Nelson KB. Intrapartum asphyxia and cerebral palsy. Pediatrics 1988;82:240–249

15. Nelson KB, Ellenberg JH. Antecedents of cerebral palsy: multivariate analysis of risk. N Engl J Med 1986;315:81–86

16. Paneth N, Stark RI. Cerebral palsy and mental retardation in relation to indicators of perinatal asphyxia: an epidemiologic overview. Am J Obstet Gynecol 1983; 147:960–966

17. Roland EH, Hill A. How important is perinatal asphyxia in the causation of brain injury? MRDD Res Rev 1997;3:22–27

18. Sarnat HB, Sarnat MS. Neonatal encephalopathy following fetal distress. Arch Dis Child 1976;33:696–699

19. Robertson CMT, Finer NN. Term infants with hypoxic-ischemic encephalopathy: outcome at 3.5 years. Dev Med Child Neurol 1985;27:473–485

20. Robertson CMT, Finer NN. Longterm follow-up of term neonates with perinatal asphyxia. Clin Perinatol 1993;20:483–496

21. Martin-Ancel A, Garcia-Alix A, Gaya F, et al. Multiple organ involvement in perinatal asphyxia. J Pediatr 1995;127:786–793

22. Perlman JM, Tack ED, Martin T, et al. Acute systemic organ injury in the term infant after asphyxia. Am J Dis Child 1989;143:617–620

23. Barkovitch AJ, Hallam D. Neuroimaging in perinatal hypoxic–ischemic injury. MRDD Res Rev 1997;3:28–41

24. Lupton BA, Hill A, Roland EH, et al. Brain swelling in the asphyxiated term newborn: pathogenesis and outcome. Pediatrics 1988;82:139–146

25. Roland EH, Poskitt K, Rodriguez E, et al. Perinatal hypoxic–ischemic thalamic injury: clinical features and neuroimaging. Ann Neurol 1998;44:161–166

26. Pasternak JF, Gorey MT. The syndrome of near total intrauterine asphyxia in the term infant. Pediatr Neurol 1998;18:391–398

27. Myers RE. Few patterns of perinatal brain damage and their conditions of occurrence in primates. Adv Neurol 1975;10:223–234

28. Mercuri E, Rutherford M, Gwan F, et al. Early prognostic indicators of outcome in infants with neonatal cerebral infarction: a clinical, electroencephalogram and magnetic resonance imaging study. Pediatrics 1999;103: 39–46

29. Flodmark O, Roland EH, Hill A, Whitfield M. Periventricular leukomalacia: radiologic diagnosis. Radiology 1987;162:119–124

30. Flodmark O, Lupton BA, Li D, et al. Magnetic resonance imaging of periventricular leukomalacia (PVL) in childhood. Am J Neuroradiol 1988;10:111–118

31. Levene MI, Evans DH. Medical management of raised intracranial pressure after severe birth asphyxia. Arch Dis Child 1985;60:12–16

32. Smith AL. Neonatal bacterial meningitis. *In:* Scheld WM, Wintley RJ, Durack DT, eds. Infections of the Central Nervous System. 2nd ed. Philadelphia: Lippincott-Raven, 1997:313

33. Ahmed A, Hickey SM, Ehrett S, et al. Cerebrospinal fluid values in the term neonate. Pediatr Infect Dis J 1996;15:298–302

34. Sarff LD, Platt LH, McCracken GH Jr. Cerebrospinal fluid evaluation in neonates: comparison of high risk infants with and without meningitis. J Pediatr 1976; 88:473–476

35. Kaplan SL, Patrick CC. Cefotaxime and aminoglycoside treatment of meningitis caused by Gram-negative enteric organisms. Pediatr Infect Dis J 1990;9:810–817

36. Foreman SD, Smith EE, Ryan NJ, Hogan GR. Neonatal *Citrobacter* meningitis: pathogenesis of cerebral abscess formation. Ann Neurol 1984;16:655–659

37. Roland EH, Volpe JJ. The effect of maternal cocaine use on the fetus and newborn: review of the literature. Pediatr Neurosci 1989;15:88–94

38. Committee on Substance Abuse. Fetal alcohol syndrome and fetal alcohol effects. Pediatrics 1993;91: 1004–1006

39. Vargas GC, Piles RS, Vidyasagar D, et al. Effect of maternal heroin addiction on 67 liveborn neonates. Clin Pediatr 1975;14:751–758

40. Ostrea EM Jr, Posecion EC, Villanueva ME. The infant of the drug-dependent mother. *In:* Avery GB, Fletcher MA, MacDonald MG, eds. Neonatology: Pathophysiology and Management of the Newborn. 5th ed. Philadelphia: Lippincott William & Wilkins, 1999:1407–1445

154 Developmental Problems of the Brain, Skull, and Spine

John B Bodensteiner

Overview

Because the formation of the central nervous system (CNS) encompasses the entire gestational period, disruptive factors occurring at any time during pregnancy may disturb the process.[1] The first trimester is particularly vulnerable, but the second and third trimesters are not exempt from risk. Disruptive factors may be intrinsic (genetic) or extrinsic (teratogens or injuries).[2] Alcohol, maternal rubella, vitamin excess (vitamin A) or deficiency (folate in spina bifida), maternal fever, and antiepileptic drugs are among the recognized causes of disturbed development of the CNS.[3-5]

Any discussion of the developmental structural abnormalities of the CNS and its housing (brain, spinal cord, spine, and skull) begins with an overview of the embryology of the neural tube and its derivatives. Tremendous advances have been made in developmental neurobiology in the last decade. Only recently have some of the molecular mechanisms that control the timing of the expression of the myriad of genes whose proper function is necessary for the normal development of the nervous system come to light. Thus, emphasis is shifting from the traditional developmental epochs, including induction, proliferation, migration, organization, synaptogenesis, and myelination, to an understanding of preprogrammed mechanisms that allow these overlapping processes to proceed in concert, resulting in the development of the normal nervous system.

We are beginning to understand, for example, that induction, both dorsal and ventral, is the result of the activation or expression of genes causing the differential growth of cells from notochord, mesoderm, and ectoderm. The process of induction was first demonstrated by showing that cells—the equivalent of Hensen node in the human embryo—induce the formation of a second ectopic nervous system when transplanted to another site in another embryo.[6] It is now clear that the same induction process can be produced by the application of the protein product of a homeodomain gene without the presence of the tissue itself.[7]

The genes involved in the orchestration of the development of the embryonic nervous system are being identified, and their products and functions are being delineated. The known genes can be divided into two groups: organizer genes and regulator genes.[8] "Organizer genes" control cell proliferation, identify organ or tissue specificity of precursor cells, and determine the axes of polarity for growth of tissues (e.g., ventrodorsal or rostrocaudal), segmentation, and right–left symmetry. "Regulator genes" control differentiation of structures within organs and specialization of individual cells and inhibit other genetic programs to change the course of cell differentiation. The molecular genetics of the development of the nervous system have been reviewed recently.[8,9] Not only is a detailed discussion of gene control of embryogenesis of the nervous system beyond the scope of this chapter, but the information would be obsolete by the time the book is published.

Epidemiology

Approximately 3% of newborn infants have life-threatening congenital anomalies, including ones of the CNS. A significantly higher percentage of fetuses have CNS malformations that are incompatible with extrauterine life and end in spontaneous abortion. Twenty percent of neonatal mortality is a result of birth defects.[10] Major defects of the CNS occur at a rate of 1 or 2 per 1000 live births in the general population, with a 2% to 5% recurrence rate.[11] Minor malformations, less life threatening but important as a cause of physical and mental handicap, are probably more common than the more severe malformations. Their frequent occurrence was not appreciated until the development of magnetic resonance imaging (MRI) allowed noninvasive ante-mortem identification of some of these anomalies.[1] Minor malformations may not have clinically apparent effects on the function of the nervous system but may cause focal epilepsy, static motor deficiencies, dyslexia, or apraxia.[12-15] Neural tube defects, the most common and complex neurological malformation compatible with meaningful existence, occurred with an incidence of 1.3 per 1000 births in the United States in 1970.[16] The incidence decreased to 0.6 per 1000 births in 1989.[17]

Defects of neural tube closure

Recent information on the genetic control of the closure of the neural tube has altered the way the genesis of the dysraphic conditions has been viewed and has provided an explanation for the striking decrease in the incidence of this malformation in recent years. Normal closure of the developing neural tube is under the control of five distinct genes, each responsible for the closure of a portion of the primitive tube.[18] The portion of the neural tube for which each gene is responsible (its domain) is as follows: gene 1, from the lumbosacral junction to the cervical region; gene 2, from the hairline to the occipital region; gene 3, the face from the nose to the forehead, roughly at the hairline; gene 4, from the occipital region to the cervical region; and gene 5, from the lumbar region to the end of the sacrum (Fig. 154.1). Complete failure of one of the five genes results in a major anomaly such as merocranium, holocranium, faciocraniorachischisis, or craniorachischisis (Table 154.1). All these are incompatible with life. The milder defects, which usually are compatible with survival, occur at the junctions between the domains of two of the five genes. A defect between the caudal end of the domain of gene 2 and the rostral end of gene 4, for example, results in the development of an occipital encephalocele. The most common location for the development of a meningomyelocele is at the junction of the domains of gene 1 and gene 5, or the lumbosacral region. The concept that multiple genes are involved in neural tube closure explains several unusual cases, including the occasional case of multiple closure defects that result in sinus tracts and meningeal defects at the junction zones between the domains of three or more genes. The dramatic

decrease in the incidence of neural tube defects coincident with folic acid supplementation can be better understood now because it is known that three of the five genes are dependent on folate as a cofactor for normal function.

Neural tube defects, collectively referred to as "spinal dysraphisms," are classified according to the location and the tissues involved in the lesion. A lesion on the lower back with a sack containing meninges and neural elements is a "lumbosacral meningomyelocele." If the lesion consists of a cutaneous sack with meningeal elements only (no neural elements), it is a "meningocele." However, close examination of these lesions shows that neural elements nearly always occur within the lesion. Furthermore, the spinal cord underneath is dysplastic to some degree. Meningoceles, as the term is generally used, are not usually associated with identifiable neurological deficits. Protrusion of the meninges and neural tissue through a defect in the skull is referred to as an "encephalocele" and usually is accompanied by variable degrees of dysplasia of the brain, resulting in varying degrees of dysfunction of the nervous system.

Occult spinal dysraphism

Some degree of dysraphism occurs in up to 5% of the population. Most of these lesions are asymptomatic and designated as "spina bifida occulta," and most of them probably remain unidentified. The diagnosis is made by the identification of a defect in closure of the vertebral arch on radiographs of the lumbosacral spine or computed tomographic (CT) scans of the same area. A few patients have symptoms related to myelodysplasia, tethered cord, or expansion of congenital tissue remnants consisting of dermal or lipomatous tissue (Fig. 154.2). These patients usually are said to have "occult spinal dysraphism." Cutaneous features associated with occult spina bifida, which suggest a more prominent or extensive lesion (i.e., occult spinal dysraphism), are listed in Table 154.2.

Symptoms of occult spinal dysraphism may vary considerably from minor nonprogressive motor or sensory deficits, foot deformities, or gait abnormalities to progressive weakness and bowel and bladder dysfunction. The findings commonly include decreased tendon reflexes, tendon contractures, and skeletal deformities (foot and leg shortening) in the affected extremity. Upper extremity involvement or a Babinski sign, when present, suggests a more extensive abnormality of the nervous system, with involvement of the brainstem, craniovertebral junction, or higher levels of the spinal cord.

Therapy

There is little argument that for symptomatic patients, particularly with evidence of progression of symptoms, surgical intervention is appropriate. The goal of the operation is to remove any tissue remnants (lipoma, dermoid), to release adhesions binding the nerve roots, and to release the tether of the filum terminalis and conus medularis.[19] Generally, it is

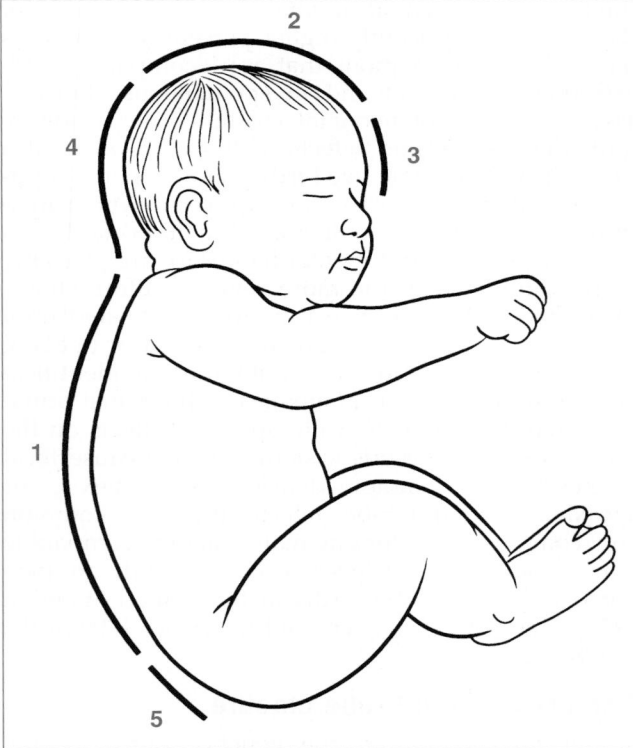

Figure 154.1   Multisite closure of the neural tube. Closure of the neural tube depends on normal function of at least five genes (1–5), each of which has an area of effect or domain, as shown. Sporadic defects of neural tube closure are most likely to occur at the junction between two domains, and failure of one gene will more likely produce a lesion involving much of the domain of that gene.[18] (For examples, see Figs. 154.3 and 154.4.)

Table 154.1 Definitions of selected terms

Term	Definition
Holocraniam	Defect in formation of cranium, including brain and skull, extending to foramen magnum
Merocraniam	Partial defect of formation of skull and brain not extending as far as foramen magnum
Rachischisis	Congenital fissure of spinal column resulting from failure of neural tube closure, involving neural and cutaneous elements
Occult spinal dysraphism	Congenital failure of complete formation of spinal column without obvious continuity with overlying cutaneous structures
Diplomyelia/diastematomyelia	More or less complete duplication of spinal cord, often with a fibrous or bony spur separating the halves
Basilar invagination	Congenital anomaly of base of the skull occurring when tip of odontoid process extends above Wackenheim clivus canal line
Basilar impression	Anomaly of base of skull defined in same fashion as basilar invagination but representing an acquired abnormality
Platybasia	Flattening of base of skull; the angle formed by a line along base of anterior fossa to tuberculum sella and another line drawn along clivus from tuberculum sella (Welcker basal angle normally 125°–143°) exceeds 143°
Colpocephaly	Persistence of "fetal configuration" of lateral ventricles, with posterior horns proportionately larger than in normal term infants
Macrocephaly/megalocephaly	Large head
Macrencephaly/megalencephaly	Large head due to large brain
Plagiocephaly	Abnormal shape of skull; deformational plagiocephaly is abnormal head shape due to external forces applied to pliable infant skull (position)

unlikely that such treatment will restore function that was not present at the time of the operation. Although natural history data are scant and controlled studies have not been performed, it is widely believed that surgical intervention can prevent future deterioration of neurological function.[19–21] Another clear indication for surgical intervention is the occurrence of meningitis from contamination of the cerebrospinal fluid (CSF) via a dermal sinus tract communicating with the subarachnoid space.[22] Sinus tracts can exist also in midline lesions in the occipital region, the base of the skull, and the nasofrontal region. These lesions are potentially present at the junction between any two of the five genes controlling neural tube closure. Frequently, lipomatous lesions within the spinal canal cannot be removed completely even with modern surgical techniques. Of interest, the long-term outcome of patients in whom lesion removal was incomplete is indistinguishable from that of patients in whom resection was complete.[23]

Improved neuroimaging technology with ultrasonography and MRI has greatly facilitated the non-invasive diagnosis and follow-up of these lesions.[24,25] According to some authors, prophylactic surgical intervention in asymptomatic patients to prevent future deterioration of neurological function is now the standard of care.[19,24] However, little information is available about the natural history of these asymptomatic lesions; thus, many physicians still require

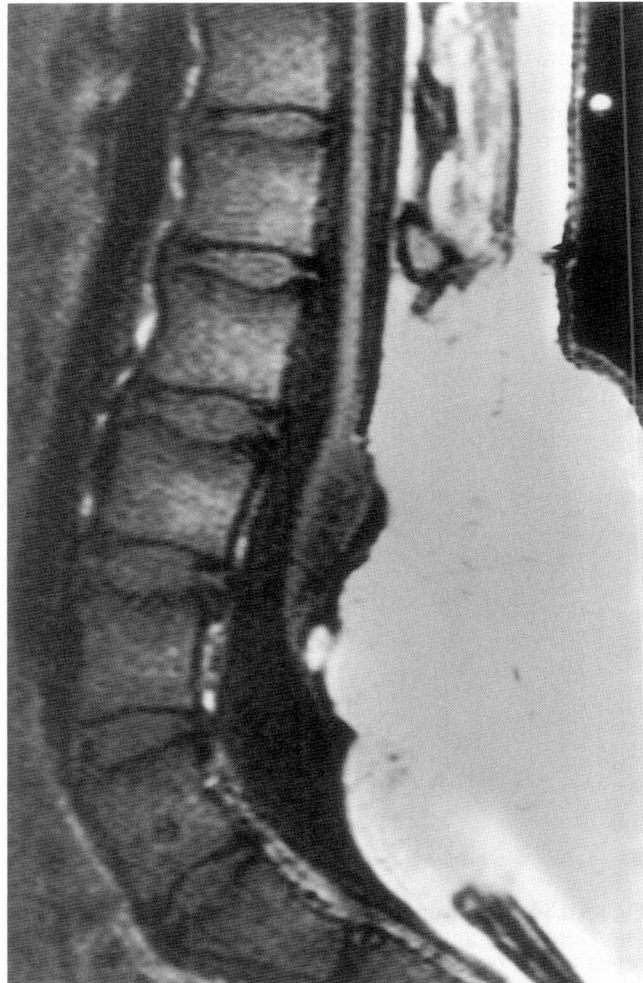

Figure 154.2 Lipomeningocele. Sagittal MRI showing neural placode at caudal end of low-lying, dysplastic spinal cord. The placode is "tethered" to a large lipomatous lesion (lipomeningocele) posteriorly at L5 spinal level. Lipomatous tissue is seen in caudal end of spinal canal.

Table 154.2   Cutaneous features of occult spinal dysraphism suggesting intraspinal involvement

Pigmented dermal patch or port-wine stain
Patch of hair in midline, particularly coarse and/or hair that is darker than rest of patient's hair
Lump in midline of lower sacral region
Dermal sinus tract, the bottom of which cannot be identified

clinical evidence of neurological dysfunction before surgical intervention is justified.[26]

Meningocele

"Meningocele" is defined as a protrusion of meninges through a defect in the spine or skull without inclusion of any underlying neural tissue. However, if these lesions are examined carefully from a histopathological standpoint, neural elements almost always are identifiable in the lesion, and the underlying cord (with spinal lesions) or brain (with cranial lesions) is nearly always somewhat dysplastic. Nevertheless, the term "meningocele" is used to identify patients with no grossly identifiable neural tissue in the lesion and no clinically identifiable neurological manifestations (Fig. 154.3).

Therapy

Surgical removal of the meningocele and repair of the defect in the dura mater eliminates the risk of injury or infection. Depending on the size of the lesion, the procedure is low risk and, most often, cosmetically satisfactory. However, the occurrence of this lesion in one child increases the risk that other children of the

same parents will have the lesion, and it may indicate disordered function of one of the neural tube closure genes. In the future, molecular examination of these genes will be possible. Currently, folic acid supplementation is the only treatment available. Future pregnancies should be considered high risk and followed closely for the possibility of neural tube defects.

Myelomeningocele

By definition, a defect of neural tube closure that includes all the layers from the skin to the spinal cord is a "myelomeningocele." If the lesion, is not covered with skin, it usually is referred to as "myeloschisis." The most common location of myelomeningoceles is the lumbosacral region, but they may occur at any level of the spine. The level of the lesion largely determines the degree of neurological dysfunction. The usual clinical features include more or less complete loss of voluntary function below the level of the lesion. Neurogenic bladder and bowel, clubfoot (talipes equinovarus deformity), dislocated hips, and joint contractures all result from the absence of innervation in the lower segment in utero (Fig. 154.4). More

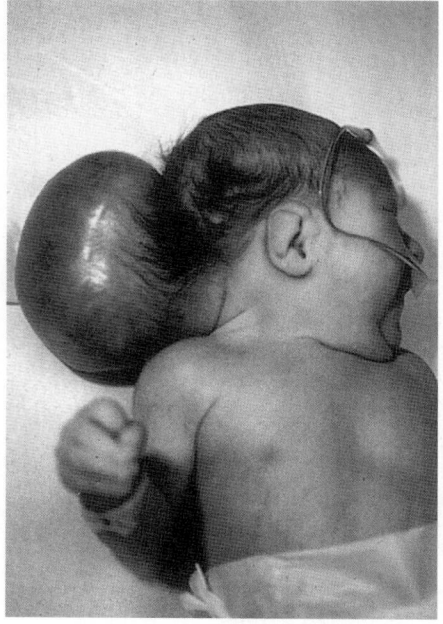
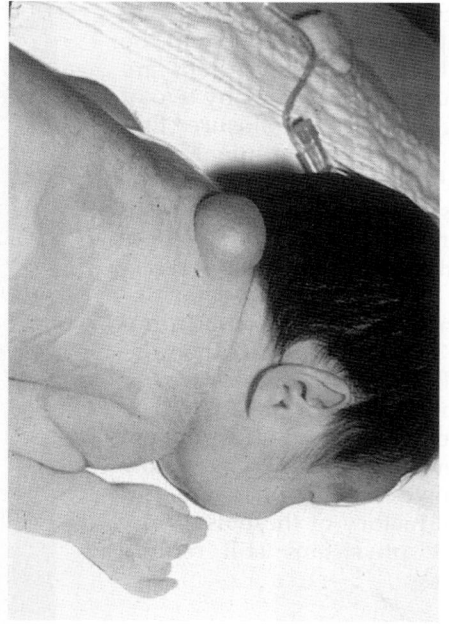

A   B

Figure 154.3   Encephalocele and meningocele. *A,* Large encephalocele containing a considerable volume of brain tissue. The brain remaining in the skull was insufficient to sustain life after the encephalocele was surgically removed. This lesion would result from a defect of function of neural tube closure gene 4 (see Fig. 154.1). *B,* This meningocele was not associated with any identifiable neurological deficit. The lesion occurs approximately at the junction between neural tube closure genes 1 and 4.

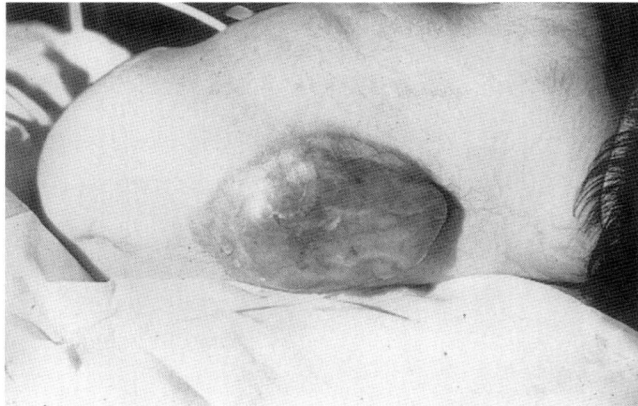

A

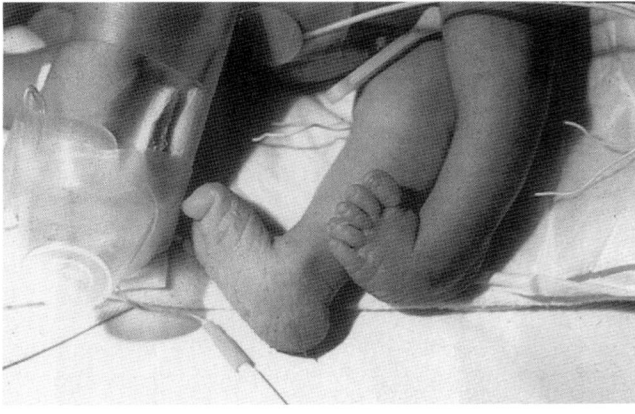

B

Figure 154.4 Myelomeningocele. *A,* Myelomeningocele resulting from defect of failure of neural tube closure gene 1 (a folate-dependent gene). The large lesion extends from mid-lumbar to mid-thoracic spine levels and is covered by a membrane of dura mater and fibrous tissue but not by skin. *B,* Deformity of lower extremities caused by lack of neural innervation in utero. Note position-dependent deformities of feet, ankles, and knees. Deformities of the hips would also likely be present but cannot be seen in this photograph.

than 80% of the patients have hydrocephalus, which nearly always is associated with a complex malformation of the craniovertebral junction, brain, and brainstem called "Chiari II malformation." Grossly, this malformation consists of (1) a beak-like deformity of the quadrigeminal plate of the midbrain, (2) distorted formation of the medulla, with elongation of the structure into the cervical spinal canal, (3) dysplastic formation and herniation of the cerebellar tonsils into the cervical canal, and (4) malformed cerebral aqueduct, with resulting hydrocephalus.

Commonly, neural tube defects are identified antenatally by an increased concentration of alpha-fetoprotein (AFP) in the maternal serum or amniotic fluid or ultrasonic examination of the fetus. After an increased concentration of AFP has been identified, an acetylcholine esterase (AChE) test usually is per-

formed to confirm the diagnosis, because positive results have a specificity approaching 100%. Because the AFP concentration is also increased in the maternal serum when a neural tube defect exists in the fetus, general screening is possible by determining AFP levels in pregnant females; the sensitivity is approximately 80%.[27] The current recommendations for screening include determining the AFP or AChE value, ultrasonically confirming the defect, and, if the fetus is aborted (spontaneously or otherwise), checking the tissue for chromosomal aberrations. The risk of recurrence after the birth of one affected child, in the absence of an identifiable chromosome abnormality, is 4% to 8% and 10% after the birth of two affected children.[28] With the identification of an affected fetus with hydrocephalus which will be carried to delivery, delivery by Caesarian section should be considered because of evidence that the level of spinal cord function and cognitive ability is affected adversely when the infant is delivered vaginally.[29]

Therapy

The diagnosis usually is obvious on casual observation, but delineation of the extent and nature of the associated malformations may require extensive evaluation. Because of the variety of associated defects, including spinal deformities, neurogenic bowel and bladder, and hydrocephalus, initial therapy is most efficient with the coordinated efforts of a multidisciplinary team of physicians from neurosurgery, orthopedics, urology, and, frequently, general and plastic surgery.[30–32]

To some extent, the potential for meaningful survival can be determined by the features identifiable at birth.[33] If the lesion is at the mid-thoracic level or higher or if the patient has severe hydrocephalus with less than 1 cm of cerebral mantle, severe hydronephrosis, severe vertebral anomalies, or birth defects in other systems, the long-term outlook is bleak, with or without therapy.[33] The choice to treat or not to treat involves complex ethical issues, and currently in the U.S., withholding therapy is not usually an option.

Early management of myelomeningocele is directed toward closure of the lesion, with repair of the CSF leak and provision for covering the spinal cord with an intact epithelial barrier.[20] Closure within the first 24 hours has been advocated to maximize neurological outcome.[20,30] However, if the neural placode or dural sack can be kept clean and infection avoided, there is no requirement to close the defect within the first 24 hours; furthermore, extra time frequently is required to ascertain the status of the urinary bladder, Chiari II malformation, and other malformations.[20,30] Best results are obtained if the infant is given broad-spectrum antibiotics from birth until 2 days after the defect has been closed. A CSF diversionary procedure may be necessary at the time of initial closure if hydrocephalus is well developed at birth. More often, however, one can wait several days or longer to determine whether the procedure is necessary and to allow time for a more thorough study of the situation. Frequently, plastic surgery is part of the initial procedure, but orthopedic and uro-logic procedures usually are performed later unless hydronephrosis is present at birth.

After the newborn period, the children should be monitored for signs of deteriorating spinal cord func-tion, increased intracranial pressure, orthopedic abnormalities, development, growth, and bladder and bowel function.[30] These issues may be pertinent for the rest of the patient's life, and it is not uncommon for patients with myelomeningocele to have progres-sive decline in upper cervical cord and lower brain-stem function beginning well into their second decade and beyond. Late-onset deterioration of function may be the result of several problems unique to this group of children. The presence of Chiari II malformation may result in compression of the upper cervical cord at the level of the foramen magnum because of herni-ation of the cerebellar tonsils into the foramen (Fig. 154.5). In fact, medullary dysfunction is the leading cause of death in older patients with myelomeningo-cele.[34] Also, syringomyelia may develop either at the end of the dysplastic spinal cord or in the cervical region. Tethering of the caudal end of the spinal cord is almost universal, and frequently procedures are performed on multiple occasions to release the tether.[19,20,34] As the patients with myelomeningocele grow, a progressive deformity of the odontoid process tends to develop in the midline in a posterior direction. This deformity of the dens produces basilar invagination, compressing the lower medulla and upper cervical cord at the craniovertebral junction (Fig. 154.5). This can produce the symptoms of pro-gressive dysfunction of the upper spinal cord and brainstem, which will not respond to "untethering" or posterior decompression of the foramen magnum. Sometimes, these patients can be helped by anterior decompression, if stability can be maintained with such an approach, or by preventing flexion of the head, which stretches the brainstem and upper spinal cord over the invaginating odontoid process.[35] Fur-thermore, there are well-documented cases of patients who have progressive deterioration of spinal cord function without tethering or compression at the craniovertebral junction (Ketonen R, personal com-munication, April 1995).[36]

The goal of orthopedic management is to maximize mobility and maintain normal spine alignment and normal hip–knee–ankle alignment. Accomplishing these goals frequently requires multiple operations as well as advice from orthotists, physical therapists, and others. The level of motor function that can be expected depends largely on the level of the lesion and, thus, the joints at which the patient can exert some voluntary control, at least to the point of being able to stabilize the joint. Functional outcome based on the level of the lesion is given in Table 154.3.

An area that is controversial in the management of patients with myelomeningocele is the use of a wheel-chair for community ambulation. Although children with high lesions necessarily use wheelchairs, some experts advocate the use of wheelchairs at an early age, even for some children who might be able to

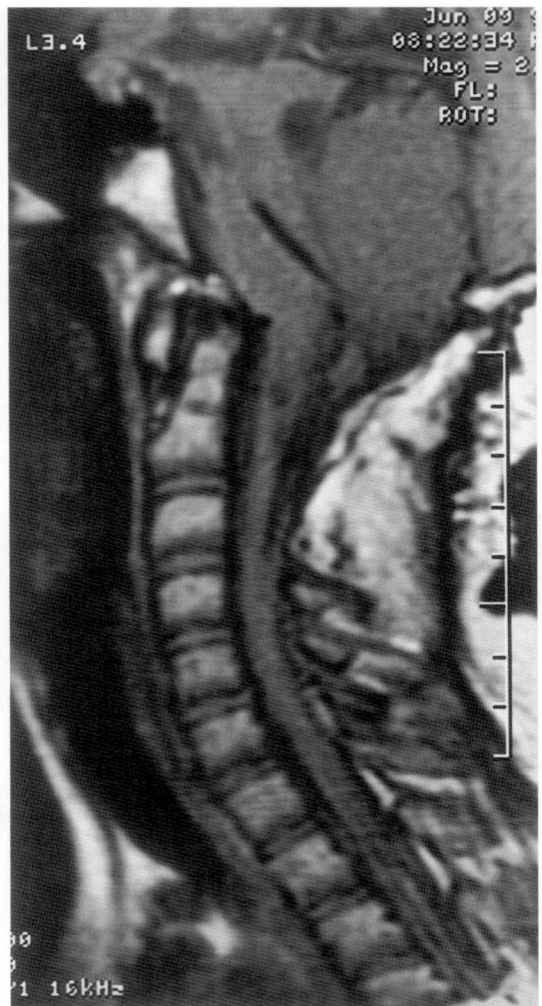

Figure 154.5   Chiari II malformation. MRI of craniovertebral junction of 16-year-old girl with myelomeningocele. The posterior lip of foramen magnum has been removed surgically to decompress neural tissue. Note distorted fourth ventricle, beaked tectum of midbrain, extension of cerebellar tissue several centimeters into the cervical canal, and posterior angulation of odontoid process of C2. The patient had progressive neurological dysfunction of lower brainstem and upper spinal cord, which was relieved temporarily by extension of the neck and head. More permanent relief of compression of the craniovertebral junction in this setting requires an anterior approach to offending bony structures.[35]

ambulate with long leg braces and a parapodium. These experts believe that a wheelchair gives the patient greater ability to interact with others and more social opportunities and results in less need for surgical treatment and a better psychological outcome. Others think that an upright posture improves the health of the bones, promotes growth, improves urinary function, and enhances cardiovas-cular fitness.[30]

The urologic management of myelomeningocele is directed toward prevention of reflux and subsequent hydronephrosis, prevention of infection, improve-

Table 154.3 Outcome of patients with myelomeningocele based on level of lesion

Level of lesion	Joint control	Ambulation prognosis	Deformity	Hydrocephalus, %	Survival, %	% with NL IQ
Thoracic	Trunk	Wheelchair only		96	51	34
L1	Pelvis	Exercise	Hip only	86	50+	34+
L2–3	Hip	Household	Hip and knee	80+	50+	50
L4–5	Knee	Community	Hip, knee, and ankle	80+	50	50
S1–2	Ankle	Functional	Ankle	60	72	77

Adapted from Lorber[33] (with addition of personal experience).

ment of urinary continence, and early detection of signs of renal dysfunction (uremia and hypertension).[30] Vesicoureteral reflux commonly begins during the second or third year of life and threatens long-term function of the kidneys. Ureteral reimplantation or external drainage of the ureters directly or through an ileal conduit helps prevent progressive reflux damage to the kidneys. In addition to urinary problems, chronic constipation is an ever-present problem because of sphincter dysfunction. Management includes dietary manipulation, periodic treatment with laxatives, stool softeners, enemas, and manual evacuation.

Psychological counseling is essential to ensure that first the parents and then the patients understand the nature and severity of the deficits as well as the long-term outlook. Few of the patients, even those with normal cognitive ability, become employed adults living independently. Many require special attention in an educational setting for both their academic and physical problems. Generalizations are difficult in this setting, but there is evidence that children with myelomeningocele do better psychologically when they are schooled in a class with physically normal children regardless of the appropriateness of the learning environment.[37]

Other defects of neural tube closure

Sacral agenesis

More or less complete failure of the development of the sacral portion of the spinal column and accompanying genitourinary and anorectal anomalies is referred to as "caudal regression syndrome of sacral agenesis."[38,39] The neurological abnormalities are similar to those of myelodysplasia and range from a minimal detectable deficit of innervation of the lower extremities to complete lack of sensory and motor function in the lower extremities, with neurogenic bladder and bowel. The motor deficit corresponds to the level of the skeletal anomaly, but sensory function is less often involved.[40] Often, the spinal cord is dysplastic, truncated, and tethered. Although the majority of these lesions are sporadic, maternal diabetes mellitus increases the risk of sacral agenesis several-fold.[41] Also, an inheritable deletion on chromosome 7 can result in sacral agenesis and may be allelic or contiguous with a holoprosencephaly gene.[42]

Therapy issues for patients with sacral agenesis are similar to those for patients with myelomeningocele, except that patients with sacral agenesis generally do not have associated Chiari II malformations with hydrocephalus, and the likelihood of having significant problems with bowel and bladder innervation is considerably greater. Also, patients are at risk for the development of progressive cord dysfunction that may require release of a tethered cord. Follow-up is necessary to prevent kidney damage from reflux from the urinary bladder; obstipation or constipation is a constant problem. Counseling of the patient and family is especially important to establish expectations and to anticipate ego and self-image problems. Schooling is less of a problem than for patients with myelomeningocele, because children with sacral agenesis are not as likely to have cognitive problems.

Split cord malformations (diplomyelia and diastematomyelia)

Duplication of the spinal cord, usually side by side, may result in two individual spinal cords with distinct dural coverings and intervening mesenchymal tissue (either a bony or cartilaginous spur) or two partial cords that share one set of meningeal structures and, thus, have no mesenchymal tissue between them. These possibilities have been labeled "SCM (split cord malformation) I" and "SCM II."[43]

The clinical features encountered are those of myelodysplasia. They vary in severity and spinal level, although the deficits generally are mild. Scoliosis, kyphosis, deformities of the feet, and leg length discrepancy are frequent features. These patients commonly have the cutaneous features of occult spinal dysraphism (Table 154.2).[44] Although this lesion has been detected prenatally, the definitive neuroimaging study is MRI.[45] Patients with the cutaneous features of occult spinal dysraphism or the clinical features of myelodysplasia or diastematomyelia should be considered candidates for diagnostic neuroimaging. Most of the lesions are found in the lumbosacral region but may occur at other spinal cord levels (Fig. 154.6).

Patients whose symptoms are limited to leg length discrepancy or minor foot asymmetries may not require intervention. In some patients, the neurological deficits or the kyphosis or scoliosis appears to be

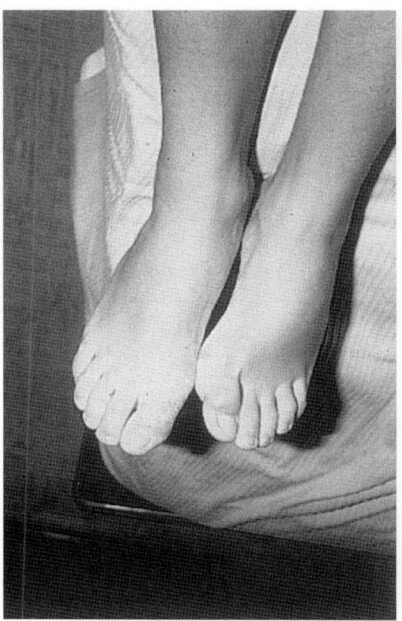
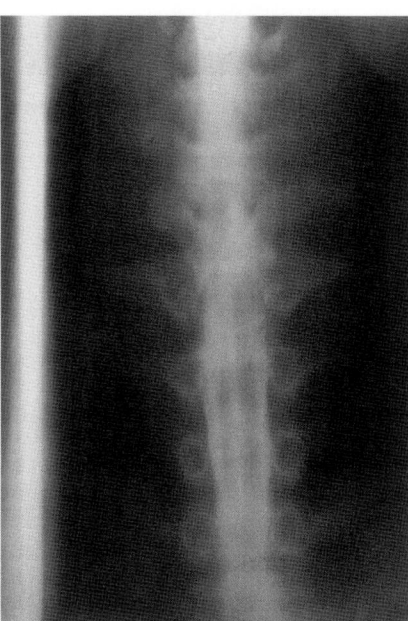
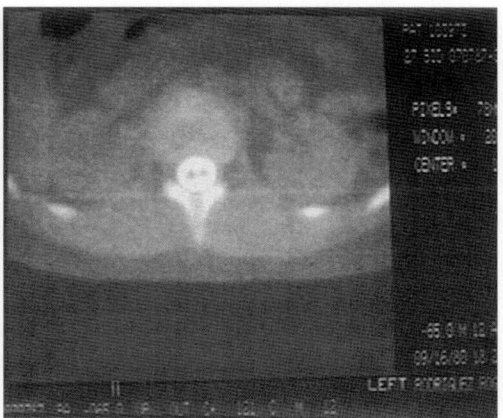

C

A   B

Figure 154.6   Diastematomyelia/diplomyelia. *A*, Feet of a 14-year-old boy who had subtle features of occult spinal dysraphism on the skin of the lower back and foot length discrepancy, with hammer toes of the left foot. Reflexes were decreased, and there was no plantar response on the left. *B*, Myelography of the lower thoracic, upper lumbar spine showing duplication of the shadow of the spinal cord. The cartilaginous spur between the halves of spinal cord could not be visualized on this study. *C*, Computed tomogram of the back, following the myelogram in *B*, in axial plane at level of vertebra L1. Note two apparently separate and nearly equal-sized spinal cord shadows.

progressive. The presumption is that the progression of the neurological symptoms is due to tethering of the spinal cord by the peg of mesenchymal tissue. Most often, the approach is to surgically remove the peg and release the tethering of the spinal cord.[46] In my experience, this does not always halt the progression of the neurological deficit, which occasionally proceeds in the absence of tethering in patients with myelodysplasia. These patients should be followed for impaired urinary bladder function, because urodynamics are abnormal in the majority of patients.[44]

Encephalocele

Traditionally, a lesion consisting of a defect in closure of the skin, skull, and meninges without the inclusion of neural tissue is designated "cephalocele."[47] If the sac contains portions of the ventricle, it is sometimes referred to as "ventriculocele." These distinctions are more apparent than real because nearly all meningoceles contain some neural elements and the only difference between encephalocele and ventriculocele is the extent to which brain tissue herniates into the meningeal sac (thus, the difference is quantitative, not qualitative). Most often encephaloceles are located between the domains of neural tube closure genes. The most common site is occipital (75% of cases, between the domains of gene 2 and gene 4), followed by frontal (most common in Asian populations, between the domains of gene 3 and gene 2). Fundamentally identical lesions occur between the

domains of neural tube closure genes 4 and 1 at the junction between the occipital bone and the cervical spine and may contain portions of the cervical spinal cord or brain tissue from the posterior fossa.[18] Encephaloceles also occur in the midline between the sphenoid and ethmoid sinuses and may present as an intranasal mass.[48] The latter lesions likely are related to defects in the formation of the skull base and may not be related to malfunction of the neural tube closure gene.[49]

Encephaloceles usually present as an obvious mass protruding from the skull or between the eyes (Fig. 154.3). They usually are soft and fluctuant and covered by tissue, often by a full thickness of skin. Typically, the degree of neurological involvement is related to the amount of brain tissue within the mass and the degree of dysplasia of the underlying brain.[50] Other malformations may also be present, including Klippel–Feil, Dandy–Walker, Chiari II, agenesis of the corpus callosum, optic nerve hypoplasia, cleft palate, and myelodysplasia.[51] Several disorders have been associated with encephaloceles, including chromosomal deletions and trisomies, Meckel–Gruber syndrome, Joubert syndrome, and Walker–Warburg syndrome.[28]

Encephalocele can be diagnosed prenatally on the basis of increased concentrations of AFP in the serum and amniotic fluid or fetal ultrasonographic findings. A large sac may require cesarean section to prevent rupture. Surgical closure of the lesion with repair of the defect in the dura mater and restoration of a full skin barrier are the only therapeutic interventions available. Children who have had repair need to be observed for possible development of hydrocephalus. The outcome is correlated with the quantity of cerebral tissue in the encephalocele and the degree of associated cerebral dysgenesis. The quantity of cerebral tissue in the encephalocele is correlated with the size of the infant's head after repair. If head size is normal, hydrocephalus does not occur, and the underlying brain is not grossly dysplastic, prognosis is good.[52] For those patients with a substantial amount of cerebral tissue in the encephalocele, the outlook for normal function is not good.

Other anomalies of the spine

Fusion-segmentation anomalies

"Segmentation" of the vertebral column is the process of separation of each vertebral segment from its neighbors to form individual vertebral bodies. Failure of segmentation leads to anomalies, with fusion of two or more vertebral segments into a single block of bone. Other vertebral anomalies in which the vertebral body is malformed, such as hemivertebrae or wedge vertebrae, also result in clinically significant deformities of the back. Fusion and segmentation anomalies may produce kyphosis or scoliosis with an acute angle curve. In more subtle malformations, called "short-segment" scoliosis or kyphosis, the majority of the curve occurs over one to three vertebral segments. Congenital scoliosis or kyphosis involving the thoracic or lumbar spine results from wedge vertebrae, hemivertebrae, or block vertebrae, in order of descending frequency.[53] The most common of these anomalies, the Klippel–Feil syndrome, occurs in the cervical region and consists of two or more cervical vertebrae fusing into a single block.

Congenital scoliosis and congenital kyphosis are coronal and sagittal plane curvature deformities resulting from segmentation anomalies. Processes such as partial unilateral failure of vertebral body formation ("wedge vertebrae"), complete unilateral failure of vertebral body formation ("hemivertebrae"), unilateral segmentation failure ("fusion of pedicles"), or bilateral segmentation failure ("block hemivertebrae") are responsible for congenital deformities of the spinal column. Underlying myelodysplasia is found in 20% of cases of fusion segmentation anomalies with genitourinary and cardiac anomalies occurring in 20% also.[53] Although congenital scoliosis and kyphosis are the result of developmental anomalies, about 50% of scoliotic lesions and nearly all kyphotic lesions in fact progress over time,[54] particularly unilateral fusion bars of the pedicles of the vertebral bodies.

Because of the likelihood of underlying spinal cord anomalies, neuroimaging of the spinal cord should be performed before surgical repair of congenital curves of the spine. Also, the patient should have a neurological examination preoperatively to investigate the possibility of a defect in innervation of the lower extremities, bladder, or bowel. Syringomyelia, tethered cord, and less easily identifiable myelodysplasia are spinal cord anomalies commonly associated with congenital curves of the spine. If an underlying anomaly of the spinal cord (syrinx or tethered cord) is identified, it should be repaired before the orthopedic correction to obviate approaching the lesion after the spine has been corrected. Urodynamics are often abnormal in these patients and should be documented before definitive surgical correction. Intraoperative monitoring of spinal cord function during correction of a major spinal curve should be considered.[55]

Congenital kyphosis is the most common noninfectious cause of spinal deformity related to paraplegia in childhood. Congenital kyphosis is generally divided into two types: type I and type II. Type I results from failure of vertebral body formation, with complete or nearly complete absence of one or more vertebral segments. The risk of spinal cord damage and the angle of the kyphosis depend on the shape of the vertebral body, the alignment of the spinal canal, and the status of the posterior arch. Partial vertebral absence with a dislocated spinal canal (congenitally dislocated spine) usually occurs at the thoracolumbar junction and is associated with a step-off in canal alignment and deficiency of the posterior arch.[53] In patients with total failure of vertebral body formation, no posterior arch is present, the deformity is unstable, and the underlying spinal cord is thin or flattened. Type II kyphosis results from failure of segmentation, most commonly in the thoracolumbar region, is associated with a smooth contour of the curve, and has a low risk of damage to the underlying spinal cord.

The prognosis for patients with congenital kyphosis depends on several factors. The presence or absence of underlying anomalies or injury to the spinal cord is critical to the outlook for neurological function. The stability of the spine with movement (flexion and extension), the amount of room in the spinal canal, and the alignment of the canal are important with respect to the likelihood of injury to the spinal cord. These factors and the degree of posterior arch abnormality also affect the likelihood of compromise of spinal cord function in the future with growth of the spine.[54]

Klippel–Feil anomaly

Klippel–Feil anomaly consists of the triad of short neck, low posterior hairline, and limitation of neck movement.[56] It results from a failure of segmentation in the cervical spine, with fusion of two or more vertebrae. It is associated with a wide spectrum of potential abnormalities,[35] including assimilation of the atlas (segmentation anomaly resulting in more or less complete fusion of the atlas with one or more of the lower cervical vertebrae) associated with atlantoaxial instability and basilar invagination. The incidence of syringomyelia or Chiari I malformation (or both) in these patients is about 20%. Developmental anomalies of the skull, Sprengel deformity of the scapula, cardiovascular system anomalies, pulmonary abnormalities, and genitourinary anomalies may all occur in association with Klippel–Feil anomaly. Klippel–Feil anomaly usually is sporadic, but it has been reported as a dominantly inherited disorder associated with a pericentric inversion of chromosome 8 (q22.2–q23.3) and a balanced translocation between 5q11.2 and 17q23.[57,58] The gene has been called *segmental-1*, or *SGM1*, and malfunction of the gene causes vertebral fusion and failure of segmentation.[59]

Clinical characteristics in patients with Klippel–Feil anomaly include a short neck with limited motion and a low hairline. The head appears to be sitting on the shoulders, and frequently one scapula is higher than the other and malpositioned (Sprengel deformity). Facial asymmetry with torticollis may be observed. The most common presenting complaint is the appearance of the neck, followed by torticollis and symptoms of spinal cord compression, either slowly progressive, or, more commonly in childhood, induced suddenly by hyperextension of flexion of the neck. Two interesting associations with Klippel–Feil anomaly are the striking tendency for patients to have mirror movements of the upper extremities and syringomyelia. Mirror movements are thought to be due to incomplete decussation of the pyramidal tracts, which is the mild end of the spectrum of myelodysplasia frequently present in patients with Klippel–Feil anomaly.

Therapy is directed at ensuring stability of the spine. With excessive movement at the junction between the block vertebrae and the more normal vertebral bodies or at the atlantoaxial junction, there may be chronic repeated compression of the cervical cord resulting in progressive neurological deficits that localize to the lower brainstem, cervical-medullary junction, or upper cervical spine. Although fusion of the vertebral column at the site of excessive mobility is necessary to protect the spinal cord, the procedure often further limits the mobility of the neck. Unstabilized Klippel–Feil anomalies represent a hazard to the patient, because if the neck undergoes uncontrolled flexion-extension (as might occur during anesthesia) the spinal cord is at risk for being damaged.[60,61] This is also a problem for other groups of patients, notably those with Down syndrome who have atlantoaxial instability due to ligamentous laxity rather than a developmental anomaly of the cervical spine.[62,63]

Syringomyelia

"Syringomyelia" is a formation of a fluid-filled cavity within the spinal cord. If the cavity is lined with ependymal cells, the lesion is called "hydromyelia" and if the cavity occurs in the brainstem, the lesion is called "syringobulbia." Although syringomyelia may occur as an isolated anomaly of the spinal cord, it occurs more often in association with Chiari I (Fig. 154.7) and II malformations, Klippel–Feil fusion segmentation anomaly, and anomalies of the base of the skull such as platybasia and basilar invagination. The lesion also occurs after spinal cord injury or a tether release in children with spinal dysraphism. The mechanism of the formation of the syrinx has not

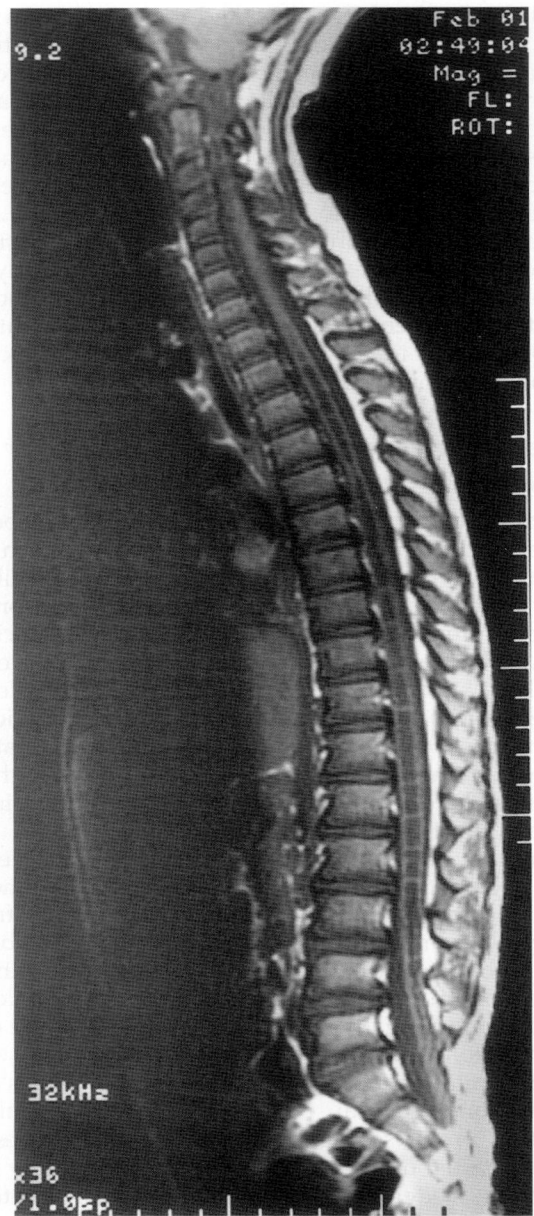

Figure 154.7   Syringomyelia. Midsagittal MRI of the entire spinal cord showing an associated Chiari I malformation, low-lying tethered caudal end, and an apparently septated syrinx cavity extending the entire length of the spinal cord. When the lower end of the syrinx cavity was opened with the release of the spinal cord, the entire cavity collapsed, indicating free communication between the various levels of the cavity.

been clearly established, but in congenital forms, the lesion probably represents incomplete closure of the neural tube. Other purported mechanisms include hydrostatic pressure acting at the obex, traumatic delivery, and arachnoiditis.[64] Syringomyelia, particularly when not present as a congenital anomaly, may also be associated with intramedullary glial tumors in which the canal of the syrinx is filled with proteinaceous fluid (the equivalent of a tumor cyst).[65] In theory, it should be possible with modern neuroimaging techniques to differentiate syringomyelia associated with tumor from congenital syringomyelia. In practice, however, this distinction is not easy to make. The clinical features of congenital syringomyelia are variable and may include a combination of upper and lower motor neuron symptoms, with weakness in the arms or legs (due to anterior horn cell dysfunction), lower cranial nerve dysfunction, or long tract signs, with spasticity in the legs.

Therapy for syringomyelia is primarily surgical. Drainage of the syrinx cavity usually results in stabilization of the neurological deficits and eliminates the pressure on the functional cord surrounding the cavity. In patients who have a syrinx cavity that extends the entire length of the spinal cord, drainage at the caudal end of the lesion may decompress the entire cord even though the cavity may appear to be septated on MRI.[34] In other patients, the various segments of the cavity do not communicate freely, and adequate drainage of the lesion may require extensive surgical "splitting" of the cord, sometimes with the insertion of a drainage device to maintain decompression. If syringomyelia is associated with an intramedullary glial tumor, treatment is directed at the neoplasm and may include tumor removal, with intraoperative drainage of the syrinx. Treatment of the intramedullary neoplasm may also include irradiation and chemotherapy.

Anomalies of the skull base and craniovertebral junction

Craniovertebral junction anomalies

Atlantoaxial instability Craniovertebral junction anomalies may also be classified as fusion segmentation abnormalities and would include Klippel–Feil anomaly. The craniovertebral junction is the most complex portion of the axial skeleton. Congenital or acquired abnormalities of this region may cause neurological deficits by compression or distortion of neural structures, compromise of the vertebrobasilar arterial system, or occlusion of CSF flow channels. A wide spectrum of congenital anomalies arise at this level because of the complexity of the developmental anatomy, the mobility of the craniovertebral junction, and the complexity of the transition between brainstem and spinal cord.[66,67] Advances in neuroimaging have made it easier to identify these lesions and, noninvasively, to delineate the osseous, soft tissue, and neural components (Ketonen R, personal communication, 1995).[60]

The occipito-atlantoaxial complex functions as a single unit, with the atlas serving as the site of greatest rotational movement between the skull and cervical spine (Ketonen R, personal communication, 1995). Flexion and extension of the head and cervical spine occurs largely at the occipitoatloid and atlantoaxial articulations. In children, the anteroposterior movement that occurs between the dens of the axis and the anterior ring of the atlas is greater than in adults and can be up to 5 mm, because of the relative laxity of the cruciate

ligament.[68] In children older than 8 years and in adults, the predental space (between the dens and the ring of the atlas) should be less than 3 mm. The problem of spinal cord injury due to increased movement of the atlas on the odontoid process as a result of laxity of the cruciate ligament has received considerable attention because some patients with Down syndrome have developed severe neurological deficits during participation in the Special Olympics.[69] Atlantoaxial instability may be present in 14% to 25% of patients with Down syndrome, although the incidence of symptomatic instability is much less. The Committee on Sports Medicine of the American Academy of Pediatrics has determined that stabilization of the cervical spine should be considered when the predental space is greater than 4.5 mm.[63] Although the recommendation is somewhat controversial, some authors have recommended that atlantoaxial fusion be considered for patients in whom the instability is limited to the C1–C2 interspace and if cranial settling, reducible basilar invagination, or dislocation of the spine (either anteroposteriorly or laterally) is documented.[70]

A common anomaly of the craniovertebral junction is "assimilation of the atlas," in which the bone of the first vertebral body is incorporated into the base of the skull as part of the occipital bone. This lesion is commonly associated with Klippel–Feil anomaly and other fusion segmentation abnormalities of variable severity. Normally, rotation of the head of about more than 35 degrees compresses the contralateral vertebral artery. Normal functioning of the cervical musculature serves to stabilize the vertebral column so that rotation is limited and the lower vertebral segments are forced to do some of the rotating. In patients with assimilation of the atlas, rotation of the head through an angle of 40 degrees or greater occludes the contralateral vertebral artery. In situations that produce sudden rotation of the head (wrestling or football) or in persons who are unconscious (during anesthesia, sleep, or trauma), the vertebral artery may be damaged or occluded without evident injury to the ligamentous or bony portions of the spine (Ketonen R, personal communication, 1995).[71] Various neurological abnormalities may result from such maneuvers, but the mechanism is occlusive cerebrovascular disease resulting in dysfunction or infarction of tissue in the distribution of the vertebrobasilar arterial system.[71]

Basilar invagination The terms "basilar invagination" and "basilar impression" are often used interchangeably, although some reserve the latter term to describe an acquired anatomical abnormality of the craniovertebral junction, most often due to softening of the skull as a result of metabolic bone disease. Among the recognized causes of softening of the base of the skull that allow basilar impression to occur are hypoparathyroidism, Paget disease, achondroplasia, rickets, and osteogenesis imperfecta. A line drawn down the clivus into the cervical canal should pass above or tangential to the tip of the odontoid process. This is known as the "Wackenheim clivus canal line." Basilar invagination is present if the tip of the odontoid process extends above the line (Fig. 154.8). The cause of basilar invagination may be deformity of the dens, as occurs in older patients with myelomeningocele or from dislocation of C1–C2 and anterior movement of the skull in relationship to the odontoid process (Fig. 154.5) (Ketonen R, personal communication, 1995).

Abnormality of the odontoid process and compromise of the size of the foramen magnum may be made worse by a deformity of the clivus called "platybasia," which causes the anterior lip of the foramen to be higher than normal. With basilar impression, the vertebral column is pushed up into the base of the skull and the lateral dimension of the foramen magnum is narrowed. When the sagittal diameter of the foramen magnum is less than 19 mm, neurological function at the craniovertebral junction is usually compromised. Basilar impression is identified when the tip of the odontoid process is above the Wackenheim clivus canal line or above the Chamberlain palato-occipital line. Basilar invagination can be suspected when the atlantoaxial articulation cannot be visualized in the open-mouth view of a cervical spine radiographic series (Ketonen R, personal communication, 1995).[68]

Thus, radiographic evaluation of craniovertebral anomalies should include lateral skull and cervical spine radiographs, anteroposterior or open-mouth views, and oblique views of the cervical spine; usually a Towne view of the foramen magnum is necessary. MRI of the region is very useful for identifying the neural elements and their relative positions within the skeletal components, but it does not provide sufficient visualization of the bony structures to be used without standard radiographs (Ketonen R, personal communication, 1995). CT, particularly with the spiral technique and three-dimensional reconstruction, may provide additional information but usually is not necessary for identifying the problem. Flexion and extension views with any imaging modality (MRI, CT, plain radiographs) frequently add information about the stability of the craniovertebral junction, which may alter the approach to repair and stabilization of the spine.

Basilar invagination frequently is seen in conjunction with Chiari malformations. Furthermore, instability of the craniovertebral junction may be seen in any of the conditions that soften the skull base enough to allow basilar impression to develop. The clinical features arising from these conditions may range from sleep apnea to progressive quadriparesis. These patients also may have obstruction of CSF flow, particularly those with associated Chiari II malformations. Other symptoms may include dysfunction of lower cranial nerves such as voice quality and speech articulation problems, swallowing difficulties, eye movement abnormalities, and decreased gag response.[60]

The therapeutic approach to symptomatic patients with craniovertebral junction anomalies is determined partly by the nature of the compression. Traumatic lesions and many acquired lesions are managed by skull traction for a minimum of 2 months and up to 6 months to reduce the lesion and to allow healing of

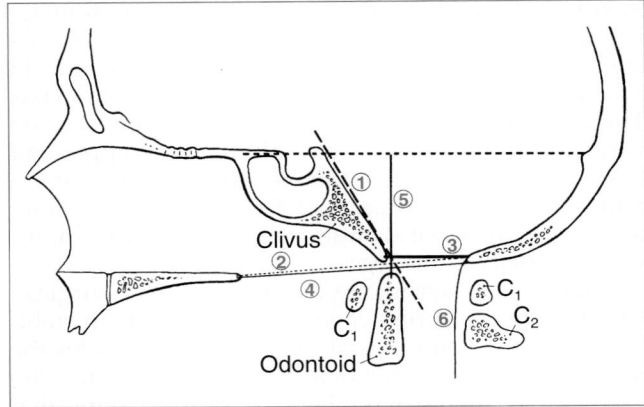

Figure 154.8   Radiographic reference lines at the craniocervical junction. (1) Wackenheim clivus line—Line drawn along the plane of the clivus and extended into the cervical canal. The odontoid process should be at or below this line. The odontoid process is above this line in basilar invagination, anterior occipitocervical dislocation, and C1–2 dislocation. (2) Chamberlain line—Line drawn from the hard palate to the posterior edge of the foramen magnum. The tip of the odontoid process should be less than 6 mm (usually <3 mm) above this line. The odontoid process is above this level in basilar invagination. (3) McRae line—Line from the anterior lip of the foramen magnum to the posterior edge of the foramen magnum. The tip of the dens is above this line in basilar invagination. This line should be at least 20 mm long. (4) McGregor line—Line drawn from the posterior margin of the hard palate to the inferior margin of the occipital squama. Normally very close to the Chamberlain line, the McGregor line may be significantly lower in conditions causing basilar impression. (5) Height index of Klaus—The distance between the tip of the dens and the tuberculum-cruciate line. The index normally is greater than 40 mm. An index less than 30 mm suggests distortion of the base of the skull to a significant degree. (6) Spinous interlaminar line—Line drawn from the posterior margin of the foramen magnum along the inner aspect of the spinous processes of the cervical vertebrae. Transgression of this line may be present in posterior spinal cord compression.

the ligamentous elements. In congenital lesions in which the likelihood of mechanical reduction of the lesion is slim, surgical fixation of the bony elements usually is required. For best results, immobilization of the neck after bony fixation is crucial. Usually a minimum of 3 months of immobilization postoperatively is required (Ketonen R, personal communication, 1995).[67] These fixation procedures are difficult to perform in young infants, and immobilization of children 2 to 3 years old is almost impossible. Furthermore, surgical fixation of the spine in a growing child has implications with respect to the length of the spine at maturity. Therapy is also determined by whether the compression of the brainstem and cervical cord is dorsal or ventral. In ventral compressive lesions, the operative approach is to perform fusion via an anterior or lateral approach. In dorsal compressive lesions, decompression can be accomplished by unroofing the foramen magnum by removing the posterior lip of the foramen.[67] If instability is present after posterior decompression, posterior fixation is mandatory (Ketonen R, personal communication, 1995).

Chiari malformations The malformations of the brain, brainstem, and spine called "Chiari I" and "Chiari II" are the most common of the several malformations described by Professor Hans Chiari in Prague in the 1890s (Table 154.4).[34,47] The malformations represent various degrees of herniation of the brainstem and cerebellum (hindbrain) through the foramen magnum, with resultant compression of the neural tissue at the foramen, and they are associated with different degrees of dysplasia of the nervous system (Fig. 154.5 and 154.7).

Chiari I malformation, usually an incidental finding, is defined radiographically as the herniation of the cerebellar tonsils into the cervical canal more than 3 mm below the lower edge of the foramen magnum.[72] Symptoms, when present, are usually milder than with other Chiari malformations and include hydrocephalus (25% of patients), headache (15% to 75% of patients), neck pain, nystagmus, and apnea.[34,73] The headache usually is identifiable by its clinical characteristics: typically protracted, suboccipital in location, not throbbing, and exacerbated by cough, exertion, or the Valsalva maneuver.[34] Chiari I malformation probably is most important because of its association with fusion-segmentation anomalies of the cervical spine (Klippel–Feil syndrome), syringomyelia, occult spinal dysraphism, hydrocephalus, and abnormalities of the skull base and craniovertebral junction. Herniation of the cerebellar tonsils through the foramen magnum may exacerbate the structural abnormality produced by bony malformations of the skull or craniovertebral junction, making surgical intervention more likely with this combination of findings. Patients with Chiari I malformations may suffer sudden death because of acute compression of the spinal cord; more commonly, however, they have slowly progressive dysfunction of the lower cranial nerves, with symptoms ranging from stridor and swallowing difficulties to esotropia, nystagmus, vertigo, and ataxia. Downbeating nystagmus on downward gaze is typical and may be a localizing feature of disorders of the craniovertebral junction.[74,75]

Often, treatment of Chiari I malformations is directed at the associated vertebral or skull anomalies or syringomyelia. The goal is to relieve compression of the nervous system and, thus, prevent progression of symptoms, which are thought to result from vascular compromise. The most commonly performed operation for Chiari I malformation is removal of the posterior lip of the foramen magnum and enlargement of the dural sac to some degree. If there is an associated anomaly of the craniovertebral junction or the skull base, a Chiari I malformation may be a complicating factor in the treatment of the primary anomaly.[34,60]

Chiari II malformation, associated with myelomeningocele in more than 90% of cases, involves extensive dysplastic changes in the brain, brainstem, and spinal cord. Hydrocephalus occurs in up to 80% of patients with Chiari II malformation. The malformation includes dysplasia of the medulla, with elongation of its structure and herniation into the cervical spinal canal. The cerebellar tonsils are dysplastic and also displaced into the cervical spinal canal. Other features include dysplastic changes in the pons; beaking of the midbrain tectum, sometimes with aqueductal stenosis; dysplasia of the cerebral hemispheres, with colpocephaly; frequently agenesis of the corpus callosum; and neuronal heterotopias. Many of the children (40% to 60%) have dysfunction of the lower cranial nerves, with high morbidity and mortality among those who present early in childhood with progressive neurological dysfunction.[76] The majority of these patients have feeding and swallowing dysfunction.[77]

Therapeutic issues in this complex malformation are discussed above with myelomeningocele.

Hydrocephalus

CSF is formed mostly (70%) by an energy-requiring secretory process in the choroid plexuses of the lateral, third, and fourth ventricles.[78] Another 20% to 50% of CSF is extracellular fluid that is a by-product of cerebral metabolism.[78] In normal adults, the volume of CSF within the cerebral ventricles and cerebral and spinal subarachnoid spaces is about 150 mL.[79] Term infants have about 50 mL of CSF and

Table 154.4 Hindbrain malformations described by Chiari

Type	Anatomical abnormality	Neurological features
I	Cerebellum and tonsils displaced downward, 4th ventricle and brainstem elongated	Relatively mild features, including headache, lower brainstem dysfunction, syrinx, hydrocephalus, apnea
II (Arnold–Chiari)	Displacement of cerebellum and tonsils, elongated dysplastic medulla, beaked midbrain, displaced 4th ventricle	Myelomeningocele, hydrocephalus, syrinx, brainstem dysfunction, apnea
III	Encephalocele in occipital-upper cervical region, cerebellar tissue involved	Functionally similar to type II without associated myelomeningocele
IV	Hypoplasia of cerebellum	Cerebellar dysfunction of variable severity

Data from Cai and Oakes[34] and Norman et al.[47]

very premature infants may have as little as 15 to 20 mL. CSF is formed at a rate of about 0.35 mL/min, which remains constant regardless of intracranial pressure and age, beginning at about 5 years. CSF flows from the lateral cerebral ventricles through the foramina of Monro into the third ventricle and thence through the aqueduct of Sylvius into the fourth ventricle. It exits from the fourth ventricle and enters the subarachnoid space through the foramina of Luschka and the foramen of Magendie in the posterior caudal portion of the fourth ventricle. From the subarachoid space in the posterior fossa (the cisterna magna), some of the CSF circulates into the spinal subarachnoid space and some circulates up over the surface of the cerebellum, through the tentorial notch, and over the surface of the cerebral hemispheres to the vertex, where it is absorbed through the arachnoid villi into the superior sagittal sinus of the venous system.[80] Although some CSF is also absorbed by the choroid plexus, leptomeninges, ependymal surface, and lymphatics, these mechanisms combined generally are not sufficient to compensate for serious impairment of the absorptive function of the arachnoid villi.

Hydrocephalus develops when there is an imbalance in the dynamics of the CSF with obstruction to flow of the fluid or obstruction of or insufficient capacity for absorption of the fluid into the arachnoid villi. Whether the ventricles enlarge and to what extent depends on the degree of obstruction in relation to the reabsorptive capacity, the tissue turgor of the brain, and the compliance (stiffness) of the cerebral tissue.[78]

Obstruction to the flow of CSF within the ventricular system is generally referred to as "obstructive" or "noncommunicating hydrocephalus." The most common site of obstruction in noncommunicating hydrocephalus is the cerebral aqueduct, which may be congenitally malformed or atretic because of inflammatory or mechanical factors. The second most common site of obstruction is the outlet foramina of the fourth ventricle. These patients often have malformation of the cerebellum, particularly the cerebellar vermis as in Dandy–Walker syndrome or Joubert syndrome.

Obstruction of CSF flow outside the ventricular system generally is referred to as "communicating hydrocephalus." The most common site of obstruction is increased resistance to absorption of the CSF into the venous system at the arachnoid villi, usually the result of "clogging the drain" by proteinaceous debris after hemorrhage into the subarachnoid space or after an inflammatory process such as meningitis. Increased resistance to absorption of the CSF may also occur from increased venous pressure within the vascular system (probably the mechanism in many cases of pseudotumor cerebri). Increased resistance may be due to decreased venous return to the heart, arterialization of the venous blood from an arteriovenous shunt within the head, or venous obstruction due to the placement of central catheters.[82]

Aqueductal stenosis may be a developmental anomaly with a genetic origin. The best known example is X-linked hydrocephalus, which has been shown to be caused by a defect in the function of neural cell adhesion molecule (L1CAM).[82] Localization of genes for other genetic forms of hydrocephalus with aqueductal stenosis and other anomalies have been reported.[78,83] At least as common as the genetic forms is hydrocephalus associated with developmental syndromes that include Chiari II malformation and Dandy–Walker syndrome. Although the hydrocephalus associated with Chiari II malformation may be due to aqueductal malformations, it most commonly is due to obstruction of CSF flow over the cerebellar surface and through the tentorial notch. A similar mechanism may explain hydrocephalus in patients with large cysts in the cisterna magna or other hindbrain malformations. Communicating hydrocephalus, more frequent than noncommunicating hydrocephalus, is usually the end result of meningitis, intraventricular or subarachnoid hemorrhage, intrauterine viral infection, or an increased concentration of CSF protein.

Increased production of CSF is a rare cause of hydrocephalus and may result from the production of fluid by a choroid plexus papilloma or papillocarcinoma such that the demand for absorption of CSF exceeds the capacity of the arachnoid villi. In patients with increased venous pressure, pressure-dependent absorption of CSF at the arachnoid villi may not permit adequate quantities of fluid to be absorbed (Table 154.5).

Clinical features of hydrocephalus in very young infants may include rapid head enlargement, vomiting, decreased feeding, irritability, and lethargy. The infant may have a bulging anterior fontanelle and separation of cranial sutures, with dilated veins visible in the scalp and orbits. Eye movements are characteristically abnormal, with downward or down and inward deviation of the eyes or limitation of up gaze. Older patients with hydrocephalus may not have head enlargement (at least, not early on); more often, they complain of headache, lethargy, and vomiting. Chronic increased CSF pressure may be associated with a gradual decrease in cognitive function and a slow change in personality, which may not be identified until someone notices that the head is larger than normal. When CSF pressure increases sufficiently to cause enhanced absorption, equilibrium may be reached in which the ventricles are large and the pressure is increased but the process is stable. This is called "arrested" or "compensated hydrocephalus," and the patients may be asymptomatic; however, with intercurrent illness or minor head trauma, they are at risk for rapid decompensation, with acutely increased pressure.

Examination often shows an enlarged head with spread sutures and dilated veins on the scalp. There may be limitation of up gaze or preferential down gaze. Papilledema is not usually found in young patients unless the pressure changes are extreme and acute. Commonly after hydrocephalus severe enough to warrant a diversionary procedure, the optic nerves are pale, demonstrating a form of optic atrophy. The development of this feature precludes papilledema

Table 154.5 Causes of hydrocephalus

Type	Cause
Noncommunicating (obstructive)	Aqueductal stenosis
	Genetic
	Developmental
	Intrauterine viral infection
	Acquired
	Neoplastic
	Inflammatory
	Posterior fossa
	Dandy–Walker malformation
	Chiari II and other malformation syndromes
	Acquired
	Neoplastic
	Inflammatory
Communicating	Post-hemorrhagic
	Inflammatory (meningitis)
	Metabolic (mucopolysaccharidosis, achondroplasia)
	Increased venous pressure
	Arterialization of venous circulation (arteriovenous malformation)
	Cerebral venous thrombosis
	Extracerebral venous thrombosis (superior vena cava syndrome)
	Left-to-right shunts with cardiac malformations
	Increased cerebrospinal fluid production
Hydrocephalis ex-vacuo	

being a sign of increased intracranial pressure, and the examiner cannot rely on the appearance of the optic disk to indicate the degree of intracranial pressure. Examination of the optic fundus is still useful, particularly in the initial evaluation when the finding of chorioretinitis, colobomas, or retinal hamartoma—indicative of conditions such as intrauterine infections or genetic malformation syndromes—provides a clue to the cause of the hydrocephalus. Tendon reflexes usually are increased, with up-going plantar responses and increased tone in the lower extremities. In the early stages of subacute hydrocephalus, progressive enlargement of the head may be the only clue to the condition. Head circumference should be measured by the pediatrician at each visit and plotted on the appropriate graph for the patient's age and sex.[84,85] The head circumference of a full-term male infant is about 35 cm and for a term female infant, about 34 cm. At 1 year of age, the average head circumference has grown 12 cm, half in the first 3 months, half of the remainder in the next 3 months, and the rest during the third 3-month period. If the head grows faster than the normal rate at this age, the cause should be determined, whether or not the patient is symptomatic at the time. Head shape is often abnormal, with occipital prominence and frontal bossing—the two most notable abnormalities in infants with hydrocephalus.

The differential diagnosis of hydrocephalus includes chronic subdural effusions, metabolic abnormalities of bone or brain, mass lesions within the head (e.g., abscess or neoplasm), and developmental syndromes that include large heads and familial macrencephaly.[84,85] The most common cause of macrocephaly in infants between the ages of 4 months and 1 year is "benign extracerebral fluid collections" (BECFC), also called "external hydrocephalus" and "benign enlargement of the subarachnoid spaces" (Fig. 154.9).[86] These patients have large heads, usually over the 98th percentile, but are otherwise free of symptoms; usually one or both parents also have a large head.[87–89] The confusion about the proper name reflects that the location of the fluid collection has been studied carefully in only a few patients, and in these patients, the fluid spaces do not appear to be in communication with the subarachnoid space.[90,91] BECFC represents a subset of the group of patients with benign familial macrencephaly. If these infants are followed for several months, the fluid spaces disappear but the head remains large an the patient remains asymptomatic.[92]

A radiographic evaluation of hydrocephalus might include skull films, which show such evidence of chronic increased intracranial pressure as thinning of the dorsum sellae and a "beaten silver" appearance of the flat bones of the calvarium; however, CT and MRI have largely replaced plain films in the evaluation of hydrocephalus. The goals of neuroimaging studies are to identify the cause of the hydrocephalus, to determine the degree of enlargement of the ventricular system, and to identify which ventricles are involved. The use of contrast agents (metrizamide) in the CSF may help delineate the complex anatomy of some malformations associated with hydrocephalus. Potentially, magnetic resonance spectroscopy, positron emission tomography, and single photon emission CT can add information about the metabolism of the brain parenchyma but usually are not

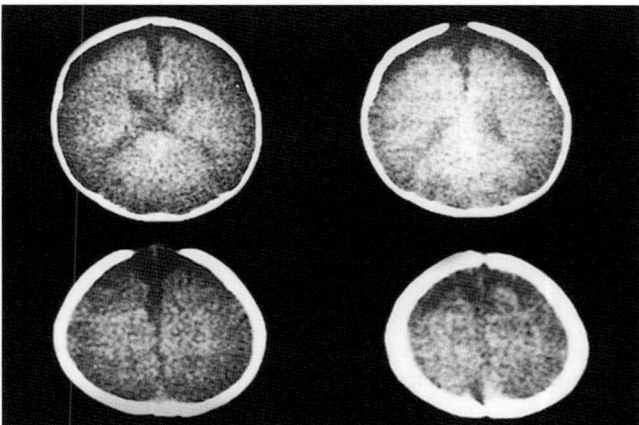

Figure 154.9   Benign extracerebral fluid collections. CT scan of 6-month-old infant with macrocephaly. Both parents were macrencephalic. Subsequent CT scan at 16 months showed resolution of fluid collections but persistence of macrocephaly/macrencephaly.

necessary in the diagnostic evaluation. In most cases, CT provides enough information to plan and initiate therapy. MRI is more useful in some of the complex cases, primarily because of its multiplanar capability and better resolution.

Treatment of hydrocephalus

Most discussions of treatment for hydrocephalus include nonsurgical options. However, for nearly all forms of hydrocephalus, effective long-term therapy requires surgery, usually the implantation of a device to divert CSF from the ventricular system to another site, such as the abdomen. Still, medical or nonsurgical therapy can be useful if no site of obstruction has been demonstrated, as in communicating hydrocephalus. This is particularly true in the early phases of hydrocephalus when a medical approach may provide time, for example, for collateral venous pathways to develop in a patient with venous outflow obstruction and, consequently, increased intravenous pressure with decreased CSF absorption.[93] Nonsurgical approaches include pharmacological therapy with acetazolamide or isosorbide to decrease the formation of CSF, osmotic diuretics, including glycerol, or repeated lumbar puncture to decrease the volume of CSF, and wrapping the head to encourage the development of alternative drainage pathways. Most often, a nonsurgical approach is used to provide time to prepare the patient for surgery. This includes the treatment of sepsis or other intercurrent problem and, in the case of increased venous pressure, to give collateral flow pathways an opportunity to develop, obviating placement of a more permanent diversionary device.

Surgical options for hydrocephalus   The surgical options available depend on the site of obstruction and the experience of the neurosurgeon. Historically, three approaches have been tried to relieve obstruc-

tive hydrocephalus: (1) removal of the cause of the obstruction, (2) bypass of the obstruction, and (3) prevention of the formation of CSF. For communicating hydrocephalus, the surgical options include (1) reduction of CSF production, (2) improvement of CSF absorption, and (3) disposal of excess fluid (shunt).[94] Generally, operations to decrease CSF formation (choroid plexectomy) have not been successful and, currently, are rarely performed except to resect tumors of the choroid plexus (papilloma or papillocarcinoma).

Noncommunicating hydrocephalus

For noncommunicating hydrocephalus, removal of the obstruction is appropriate for acquired lesions such as neoplasm but generally is not appropriate for congenital developmental lesions. The obstruction is bypassed in two ways. (1) One way is to create an artificial communication between the ventricular system and the subarachnoid space. Third ventriculostomy was among the first operations attempted for developmental hydrocephalus and has been revived recently because neuroendoscopy has made it possible to perform the procedure successfully in older patients.[78,95] Success has not been common in younger children and infants.[96] Failure of the procedure in infants may be related to underdevelopment of the arachnoid granulations, which requires that CSF be diverted to another site where it can be absorbed more readily. (2) Another way to bypass an obstruction is to place a relatively permanent diversionary device (shunt). Early shunts were simple tubes without valves; they were not successful because they were position-dependent and overdrained the lateral ventricles. The distal end was often placed in the superior vena cava, leading to considerable difficulty with infection, clotting, and embolization from the tip of the catheter.[97,98] With modern shunt devices, the distal end is implanted into the peritoneal space, and valve technology has improved greatly. Shunt devices now are designed to avoid overshunting and have variable pressure valves that, in some cases, can be adjusted externally.[78] Currently, surgical implantation of a shunt device appropriate for the clinical situation is the most common therapeutic intervention for hydrocephalus.

It now is possible to identify congenital hydrocephalus in utero. Techniques have been developed that allow in utero decompression of the lateral ventricles with a ventriculoamniotic shunt.[99,100] The procedure is performed with the intention of preventing injury to the cerebral cortex from compromise of cortical perfusion. The early results of antenatal therapy of hydrocephalus have been mixed, and the outcome is dependent largely on the associated anomalies that these patients often have but which cannot be evaluated carefully until after the infant has been delivered.

Intraoperative complications are uncommon with shunt placement operations. Once the shunt is in place, it is subject to various complications, including overdrainage, subdural hematoma, mechanical failure, abdominal pseudocysts, and infection. Infection, early and delayed, is a major problem, and 8% of shunts implanted for the first time become infected regardless of the patient's age (but the risk is higher in infants younger than 6 months).[101] The first-year failure rate for all shunts is 38%, and the threat to the development of cognitive function of the patient is significant, particularly a young patient if the shunt device becomes infected or develops other complications.[102,103] Shunt infection may result in nephritis, meningitis, ventriculitis, peritonitis, abdominal pseudocysts, or shunt failure with uncontrolled increased intracranial pressure.

Little progress has been made in the prevention of complications of shunt placement, compared with the technological advances in device manufacture.[78] The common practice is to give antibiotics prophylactically during shunt insertion and for the following 24 hours. This may decrease the infection rate, although the data are not entirely convincing.[94] Most shunt failures, whether because of mechanical reasons or infection, occur during the first 2 years after insertion. Because the shunt represents a foreign body in the system, prophylactic antibiotic treatment should be considered for these patients anytime they undergo a surgical or dental procedure.

The outcome of a patient with hydrocephalus, intellectual and otherwise, depends partly on the presence of associated anomalies of the brain, spine, and other organs. Of a recent series of patients with hydrocephalus followed more than 2 decades, 13.7% died, 49% had normal results on intellectual testing, 30% had mild impairment, and 7.4% had severe impairment.[104] Children with congenital hydrocephalus have less risk of intellectual impairment than those in whom hydrocephalus develops as a complication of meningitis.[105] Behavior problems and psychological problems are considerably more common in children with hydrocephalus than in the general population.[37,106]

Although hydrocephalus is no longer a lethal disease, it still represents an important threat to the life and well-being of patients.[78] The complication rate leading to death or serious neurological deterioration in patients with hydrocephalus during the transition from childhood to adulthood is high and suggests the need for increased awareness of these patients and their problems among adult neurological specialists.[107] In a poll of adults with hydrocephalus, 25% had had shunt failure that resulted in coma. Patients who lived alone either ignored the early signs of impending shunt failure or could not convince their physicians of the significance of the symptoms. Such patients were at substantial risk for being found dead or in coma. It is clear that a patient with hydrocephalus must maintain access to a medical practitioner who is knowledgeable about the signs and symptoms of shunt malfunction and about the appropriate steps to investigate and remedy the situation.[78] The average patient requires 2.7 shunt revisions during the first 3 decades; this poses a substantial financial burden.[78,104] These patients also are at risk because frequent changes in the insurance or health care delivery system may impair access to the specialists necessary for proper care.

Posterior fossa and cerebellar anomalies

Several conditions involve the posterior fossa and cerebellum. Chiari malformations, neural tube closure defects such as encephalocele and syringomyelia, and fusion segmentation abnormalities all have associated anomalies of the brainstem or posterior fossa CSF spaces. These conditions are discussed above. Only conditions for which treatment is available are included in this section.

Errors in the development of the cerebellum may result from several adverse events: (1) damage to the embryonic tissue, as in early exposure to isotretinoin, may cause incomplete development of the cerebellar vermis, (2) in utero infection with various viruses may result in hypoplasia of the entire cerebellum, vermis, or hemispheres, (3) various genetic conditions, including chromosomal, metabolic, single-gene, and contiguous gene syndromes, may be associated with cerebellar abnormalities. The most important in the context of potential therapeutic interventions is Dandy–Walker syndrome.

"Dandy–Walker syndrome" consists of cystic transformation of the fourth ventricle, with dysplasia of the cerebellar vermis; although the outlet foramina of the fourth ventricle may be patent, they frequently are not. Aqueductal stenosis is also a frequent feature of this anomaly; thus, obstruction of the outlet foramina of the fourth ventricle and aqueductal stenosis may occur in the same patient, producing an encysted fourth ventricle. Dandy–Walker syndrome is relatively frequent (1 in 30 000), with a high risk of recurrence when associated with a genetic syndrome such as Walker–Warburg, Meckel–Gruber, or Fryns syndrome, but only a 1% to 5% risk of recurrence when it occurs in isolation. Even when Dandy–Walker malformation occurs without the presence of an identifiable genetic multiple malformation syndrome, it usually is accompanied by brain anomalies, including agenesis of the corpus callosum, heterotopias, and hemimegalencephaly.[47]

The clinical features of patients with Dandy–Walker syndrome include delayed motor development, usually with prominent hypotonia, titubation, nystagmus, and hydrocephalus. When the patient is old enough to be tested, most demonstrate ataxia, and increased intracranial pressure (if untreated). Intellectual function depends on the presence of associated anomalies of the brain.[108] In patients with hydrocephalus, the condition of the fourth ventricle should be evaluated after a shunt has been placed in the lateral ventricles, because if the fourth ventricle does not decompress after the shunt has been placed, a second diversionary procedure will be needed to decompress the fourth ventricle.[109]

A relatively uncommon finding in patients undergoing a neuroimaging study for any reason is a large cisterna magna or "macro cisterna magna" (Fig. 154.10).[110] This condition presents as a large CSF space posterior to the cerebellum. It is different from

Dandy–Walker syndrome, in which the cerebellar vermis is absent or dysplastic and the fourth ventricle is incorporated into the cyst. Some believe that macro cisterna magna represents an arachnoid cyst of the posterior fossa, and clearly, this sometimes occurs but more commonly large spaces posterior to this cerebellum represents an enlarged CSF space without any obstruction to CSF flow. It has been shown that patients with macro cisterna magna have a vague clinical syndrome consisting of hypotonia, apraxia of lateral gaze, decreased facility of complex movements, and a tendency to nonspecific clumsiness.[1] No treatment is required for macro cisterna magna; however, failure to recognize the anomaly may result in diagnostic confusion and unnecessary diagnostic studies.

Another condition that must be distinguished from Dandy–Walker syndrome is Joubert syndrome. In Joubert syndrome, aplasia of the cerebellar vermis and distortion of the fourth ventricle occur in conjunction with a deformity of the midbrain and aqueduct, producing what has been called the "molar" sign seen on MRI scans of the lower midbrain and upper cerebellum.[111] The characteristic clinical features of Joubert syndrome include retinal dystrophy, episodic hyperpnea and apnea as an infant, developmental delay, hypotonia, and ataxia. Joubert syndrome is an autosomal recessive condition that only rarely requires diversionary shunts but has a serious risk (25%) of recurring in families.[112]

Craniosynostoses

The growth of the skull occurs at the cranial sutures and in a plane perpendicular to a suture. Several sutures are important to the growth and shape of the skull. The "sagittal suture" is an unpaired suture that extends from the junction of the lambdoid sutures at the rostral end of the occipital bone to the forehead. The portion of the suture anterior to the intersection with the coronal sutures is called the "etopic suture." The "coronal sutures" are paired and extend from the squamosal sutures in the temporal region to the sagittal suture at the anterior fontanelle. The "lambdoid sutures" separate the occipital bone from the parietal bones and meet at the posterior fontanelle with the posterior end of the sagittal suture. Growth of the skull occurs in response to pressure exerted from within by the growing brain. When the brain stops growing and, thus, stops exerting pressure on the skull, the sutures close. If one suture closes but growth continues at other cranial sutures, the head becomes increasingly "out of round," or "plagiocephalic," and the deformity increases as growth occurs.

"Deformational plagiocephaly" is a distorted head shape caused by forces applied to the outside of the skull, such as in utero positioning or consistently placing the infant in an awkward position before the infant is able to effectively object. For example, there has been a rash of "flat heads" as a result of the American Academy of Pediatrics "Back to sleep" campaign that was important in decreasing the incidence of

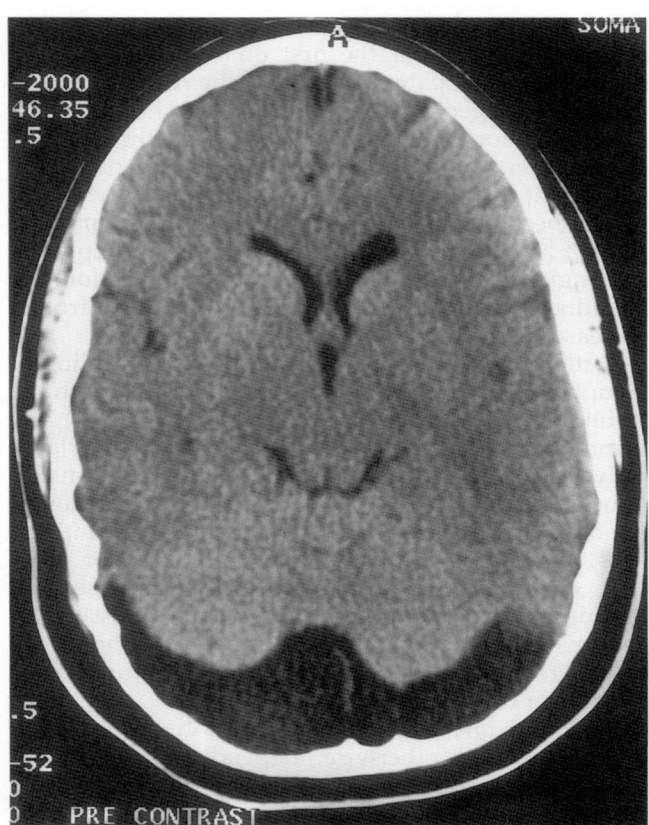

Figure 154.10   Macro cisterna magna. CT scan of 16-year-old boy who was clumsy and hypotonic and had apraxia of lateral gaze. Acquisition of motor skills was mildly delayed.

sudden infant death syndrome (SIDS) in the mid 1990s. Deformational plagiocephaly can be distinguished from plagiocephaly due to suture synostosis because infants with the former have improvement as growth occurs, have no identifiable ridging of the suture, demonstrate some movement at the suture line with pressure, and usually have no finding of synostosis on radiographic study (plain skull films or CT). Currently, it is popular to recommend the application of a helmet to redirect the external forces applied to the skull in infants with more severe deformational plagiocephaly. No controlled studies have investigated the effectiveness of this procedure, and because all these infants have improvement as they grow, with or without the helmet, the criteria for the initiation of the helmet therapy are not clear.

If brain growth is not sufficient, the sutures fuse. Fused sutures usually are not present at the time patients with brain growth failure are evaluated, even if they are microcephalic, because considerable time is required for fusion to occur. In infants with small but normally shaped heads, head size is not the result of suture closure but the failure of brain growth. If the head is not shaped normally, the examiner should determine which suture or sutures are closed. The head shapes that result from common suture closures can be identified visually (Table 154.6). In patients in whom several sutures may not be functional, CT with three-dimensional reconstruction is often useful for delineating the extent of involvement and planning the appropriate intervention (Fig. 154.11).

In addition to the mechanical forces exerted by the growing brain, several genetic factors are related to normal suture growth and function. Many syndromes are characterized by premature closure of one or more cranial sutures (Tables 154.6 and 154.7). More commonly, however, only one suture is involved and failure is sporadic. Recent studies have shown that many of the genetic craniosynostosis syndromes result from inherited mutations of the gene for fibroblast growth factor receptors (FGFR) or genes that regulate the transcription of FGFR genes (TWIST).[113,114] Most cases of isolated single-suture synostosis probably represent somatic mutations of FGFR genes.

The clinical features of craniosynostosis depend on the sutures involved and whether synostosis is part of a larger syndrome, which may include developmental anomalies of the underlying brain (Table 154.7). Progressive skull deformity is the most obvious feature. The shape depends on which sutures are involved and to what extent. A fused suture usually is palpable as a bony ridge, and the skull on either side of the suture cannot be moved by manual pressure applied to the scalp. Increased intracranial pressure is an often-expressed concern and frequently considered a threat to the normal growth and function of the brain; thus, it is cited as an indication for surgical repair of the fused suture. In fact, isolated suture closure rarely produces increased intracranial pressure; moreover, any brain dysfunction is more likely the result of anomalies of brain development (associated or not) than of impaired function due to pressure or perfusion changes.[115] Only about one-half of patients with multiple suture synostosis have unequivocally increased intracranial pressure.[115] In the complex, multiple-suture synostosis syndromes, the brain frequently is abnormal and mental retardation is a frequent accompaniment regardless of intracranial pressure. Patients with increased intracranial pressure

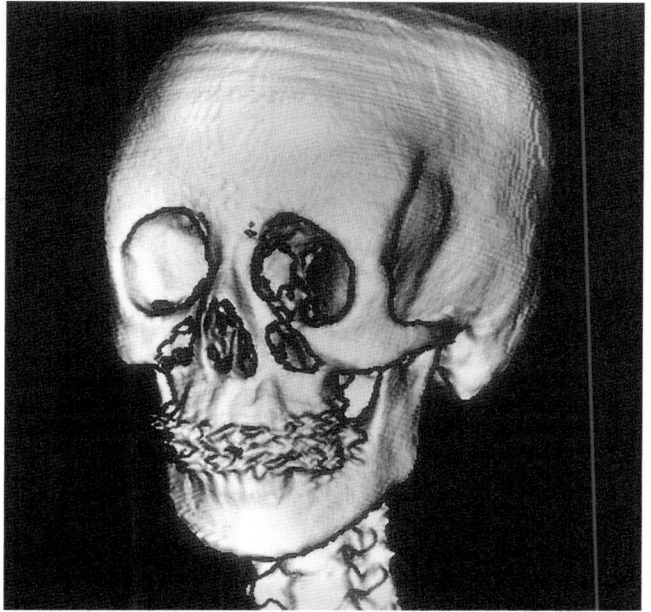

Figure 154.11   CT three-dimensional computer reconstruction. CT data were obtained via thin slices, with no gap between slices. Patient had fibrous dysplasia of skull, with thickening of zygomatic process on the left. This technique is also helpful in evaluation of head shape and suture closure.

may have abnormalities of the skull, with increased digital markings on the internal surface of the calvaria (Fig. 154.12). In addition, sleep apnea and hydrocephalus may result from craniosynostosis.[116]

Treatment

When craniosynostosis affects only one suture and the associated cranial deformity is not severe, intervention may not be required. In this clinical setting, the chief reason for intervention is cosmetic.[117] Operative intervention is indicated if the deformity is severe, increased intracranial pressure is present, or increased intracranial pressure is likely to develop.

Table 154.6   Skull deformities associated with premature closure of cranial sutures

Deformity	Suture affected	Frequency Isolated, %	Part of complex syndrome (%)
Scaphocephaly	Sagittal	45–50	Crouzon (30–40)
Trigonocephaly	Metopic	5	Carpenter (?)
Frontal plagiocephaly	Unilateral coronal and sphenofrontal	20–25	Saethre–Chotzen
Occipital plagiocephaly	Unilateral lambdoid	?10	Rare
Turricephaly	Bilateral coronal and sphenoid	5–10	Apert (100) Crouzon (50–60)
Pachycephaly	Bilateral lambdoid	Rare	Rare
Oxycephaly/triphyllocephaly (kleeblattschädel)	Multiple	Rare	Crouzon + hydrocephalus

Modified from Simpson and David.[117] By permission of Blackwell Scientific Publications.

Table 154.7   Genetic craniosynostosis syndromes

Syndrome	Gene basis/locus	Clinical features
Major		
Apert (ACS I)	AD, 10q26, *FGFR2*	Multiple synostosis, coronal most prominent, severe fusion syndactyly, hypertelorism, antimongoloid slant, MR
Carpenter (ACS II)	AR	Turricephaly, brachydactyly, polydactyly, MR, obesity
Crouzon (CFD I)	AD, *FGFR2*	Coronal synostosis, maxillary hypoplasia, shallow orbits, beaked nose
Pfeiffer (ACS V)	AD, *FGFR1, FGFR2*	Coronal synostosis, broad thumbs and toes, polysyndactyly (3 subgroups)
Saethre–Chotzen (ACS III)	AD, TWIST* gene, *FGFR3, FGFR2*	Asymmetrical coronal synostosis, plagiocephaly, hearing loss, craniovertebral junction anomalies, seizures, low frontal hairline
Minor		
Baller–Gerold	AR	Radial aplasia, multiple sutures, short stature, imperforate anus, MR
Hunter–McAlpine	AD, deletion 17q23–24	Allelic with Ruvalcaba syndrome?, MR, down-turned small mouth, short stature
Jackson–Weiss	AD, *FGFR2*	Coronal and basal skull sutures, broad large toes, syndactyly, tarsal fusion
Shprintzen–Goldberg	AD, *fibrillin-1* gene	Multiple suture synostosis, mandibular and maxillary hypoplasia, exophthalmos, MR

*A transcription factor.
ACS, acrocephalosyndactyly; AD, autosomal dominant; AR, autosomal recessive; CFD, craniofacial dysostosis; FGFR, fibroblast growth factor receptor; MR, mental retardation.

Surgical intervention for craniosynostosis can be described in three different age periods. In the early period, the first year of life, the skull and brain are growing rapidly and the chief goal of the operation is to allow the brain to assume a normal configuration. The suture is opened and an artificial suture is created by the placement of a substance such as Silastic between the ends of the skull bones, thus preventing re-fusion of the bones before the completion of brain growth. To accomplish this effectively and to prevent further operations, the artificial suture needs to be extensive.[117]

In the second period, ages 1 to 10 years, the velocity of brain growth and skull enlargement slows and sutural growth is less marked. Failure of multiple sutures to grow may still cause increased pressure, however, and if sutures at the base of the skull are involved, bony encroachment of the cranial nerve foramen such as the foramen for the optic nerve may occur, leading to progressive neurological disability (Fig. 154.12). In children with complex craniofacial anomalies, major complex cranial and facial reconstruction may be necessary to compensate for the lack of growth at the cranial sutures at the base of the skull.

In the late period, after age 10 years, there is little effect on the brain except that hydrocephalus may develop, presumably from alteration of CSF or venous flow dynamics due to the skull deformity. The chief reason for a surgical procedure in this age group is cosmetic, relief of cranial nerve impingement, or relief of hydrocephalus.

Abnormalities of ossification of the skull— hyperostotic bone diseases

Several diseases of bone result in thickening of the skull and subsequent neurological problems. Osteopetrosis, several types of craniometaphyseal and craniodiaphyseal dysplasia, and other diseases characterized by thickening of the skull are all included in the category of "hyperostotic bone diseases." These conditions share several clinical features neurologically, including the tendency to develop increased venous pressure, hydrocephalus, and multiple cranial nerve compression syndromes (Fig. 154.13). These neurological symptoms are believed to occur from increased resistance to CSF and venous outflow due to thickening of the skull and narrowing of the vascular and cranial nerve foramina.[118] Similar neurological symptoms may also result from extensive involvement of the skull by "fibrous dysplasia" (i.e., thickening and replacement of bone with fibrous tissue) or from McCune–Albright syndrome with fibrous dysplasia of the skull.

Effective therapy for osteopetrosis is bone marrow transplantation.[119] The defect, a mutation in the gene for macrophage colony-stimulating factor 1 (Mcsf-1), cannot be corrected effectively by any other means, and, to date, the results of metabolic interventions have been disappointing. I have followed children who were symptom-free for a decade after bone marrow transplantation before headaches, hydrocephalus, optic nerve compression, or other cranial nerve dysfunction developed as the skull began to thicken. Retransplantation is the only effective therapeutic option, because over time the transplanted cells are expunged from the patient and the Mcsf-1

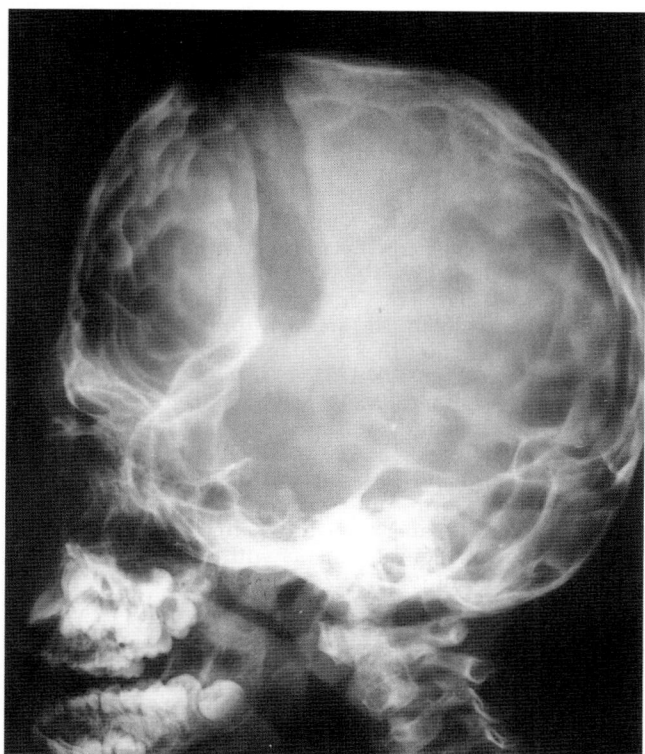

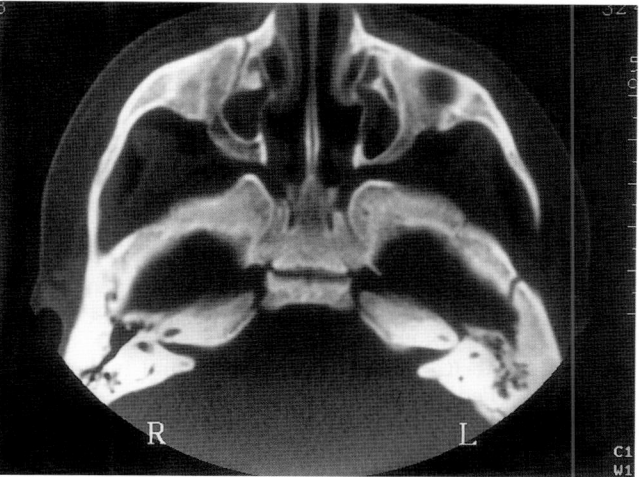

Figure 154.13 Osteopetrosis. CT scan through nasal and facial structures of the skull of 12-year-old patient with osteopetrosis who had undergone bone marrow transplantation as an infant. Recently, thickening of the skull had begun to impinge on the optic, auditory, and facial cranial nerves. Note the lack of trabecular structure in the bones of the skull.

Figure 154.12 Coronal synostosis. Lateral skull radiograph of a 13-year-old patient with Apert syndrome. There is evidence of long-standing increased intracranial pressure, with thinning of posterior and anterior clinoid processes and extensively increased digital markings of inner table of calvaria. Note that surgical opening of the coronal sutures has been attempted.

deficient state recurs. It has not been established whether the results of retransplantation match those of the initial transplantation.

To date, no effective therapy for craniometaphyseal dysplasias has been devised. The thickening of the skull impinges on the vascular and neural foramina. Also, the thickening may cause communicating hydrocephalus, but ordinary decompression fails quickly. Attempts to remove portions of the calvaria to provide decompression of the brain have been unsuccessful, perhaps because an important venous egress from the skull is through the emissary veins, and patients do not tolerate the removal of significant areas of the calvaria.[120] Surgical intervention to remove the fibrous thickened bone and to enlarge the foramina of the cranial nerves is indicated in patients with extensive fibrous dysplasia of the skull.[121]

References

1. Schaefer GB, Sheth RD, Bodensteiner JB. Cerebral dysgenesis: an overview. Neurol Clin 1994;12:773–788
2. Volpe JJ. Neuronal proliferation, migration, organization, and myelination. Major Probl Clin Pediatr 1987;22:33–68
3. Autti-Ramo I, Gaily E, Granstrom ML. Dysmorphic features in offspring of alcoholic mothers. Arch Dis Child 1992;67:712–716
4. Lindhout D, Omtzigt JG, Cornel MC. Spectrum of neural-tube defects in 34 infants prenatally exposed to antiepileptic drugs. Neurology 1992;42:111–118
5. Schardein JL. Chemically Induced Birth Defects. Drug and Chemical Toxicology Series. Vol 2. New York: Marcel Dekker, 1985
6. Spemann H, Mangold H. Über Induktion von Embryonalanlagen durch Implantation Aftfremder organisatoren. Wilhelm Roux Arch Entwick 1924;100:599–638
7. De Robertis EM, Kim S, Leyns L, et al. Patterning by genes expressed in Spemann's organizer. Cold Spring Harb Symp Quant Biol 1997;62:169–175
8. Sarnat HB, Menkes JH. How to construct a neural tube. J Child Neurol 2000;15:110–124
9. Ashwal S. Congenital structural defects. In: Swaiman KF, Ashwal S, eds. Pediatric Neurology. Vol 1, 3rd ed. St. Louis: Mosby, 1999:234–300
10. D'Alton ME, DeCherney AH. Prenatal diagnosis. N Engl J Med 1993;328:114–120
11. Contribution of birth defects to infant mortality—United States, 1986. MMWR Morb Mortal Wkly Rep 1986;38:633–635
12. Brodtkorb E, Nilsen G, Smevik O, Rinck PA. Epilepsy and anomalies of neuronal migration: MRI and clinical aspects. Acta Neurol Scand 1992;86:24–32
13. Cohen M, Campbell R, Yaghmai F. Neuropathological abnormalities in developmental dysphasia. Ann Neurol 1989;25:567–570
14. Sarnat HB. Disturbances of late neuronal migrations in the perinatal period. Am J Dis Child 1987;141:969–980
15. Stoll C, Alembik Y, Dott B, Roth MP. An epidemiologic study of environmental and genetic factors in congenital hydrocephalus. Eur J Epidemiol 1992;8:797–803

16. Shurtleff D, Lemire R, Warkany J. Embryology, etiology, and epidemiology. *In*: Shurtleff DB, ed. Myelodysplasias and Exstrophies: Significance, Prevention, and Treatment. New York: Grune & Stratton, 1986:39–64

17. Yen IH, Khoury MJ, Erickson JD, et al. The changing epidemiology of neural tube defects: United States 1968–1989. Am J Dis Child 1992;146:857–861

18. Van Allen MI, Kalousek DK, Chernoff GF, et al. Evidence of multi-site closure of the neural tube in humans. Am J Med Genet 1993;47:723–743

19. McLone DG, La Marca F. The tethered spinal cord: diagnosis, significance, and management. Semin Pediatr Neurol 1997;4:192–208

20. McComb JG. Spinal and cranial neural tube defects. Semin Pediatr Neurol 1997;4:156–166

21. Hemphill M, Freeman JM, Martinez CR, et al. A new, treatable source of recurrent meningitis: basiooccipital meningocele. Pediatrics 1982;70:941–943

22. Thomas JE, Miller RH. Lipomatous tumors of the spinal canal: a study of their clinical range. Mayo Clin Proc 1973;48:393–400

23. Gundry CR, Heithoff KB. Neuroimaging evaluation of patients with spinal deformity. Orthop Clin North Am 1994;25:247–264

24. Kriss BM, Kriss TC, Desai NS, Warf BC. Occult spinal dysraphism in the infant: clinical and sonographic review. Clin Pediatr 1995;34:650–654

25. Herman JM, McLone DG, Storrs BB, et al. Analysis of 153 patients with myelomeningocele or spinal lipoma reoperated upon for tethered cord. Presentation, management and outcome. Pediatr Neurosurg 1993; 19:243–249

26. Bodensteiner JB. Standard of care: the blind leading the blind? (Editorial.) Clin Pediatr 1995;34:655–656

27. Brennand DM, Jehanli AM, Wood PJ, et al. Raised levels of maternal serum secretory acetylcholinesterase may be indicative of fetal neural tube defects in early pregnancy. Acta Obstet Gynecol Scand 1998;77:8–13

28. McKusick VA. Mendelian Inheritance in Man: A Catalog of Human Genes and Genetic Disorders. 11th ed. Baltimore: Johns Hopkins University Press, 1994

29. McLone DG, Naidich TP. Myelomeningocele: outcome and late complications. *In*: McLaurin RL, Schut L, Benes JL, et al., eds. Pediatric Neurosurgery: Surgery of the Developing Nervous System. 2nd ed. Philadelphia: WB Saunders, 1989, pp. 53–71

30. Liptak GS, Bloss JW, Briskin H, et al. The management of children with spinal dysraphism. J Child Neurol 1988;3:3–20

31. Park TS. Spinal Dysraphism. Boston: Blackwell Scientific Publications, 1992

32. Chambers GK, Cochrane DD, Irwin B, et al. Assessment of the appropriateness of services provided by a multidisciplinary meningomyelocele clinic. Pediatr Neurosurg 1996;24:92–97

33. Lorber J. Spina bifida cystica: results of treatment of 270 consecutive cases with criteria for selection for the future. Arch Dis Child 1972;47:854–873

34. Cai C, Oakes WJ. Hindbrain herniation syndromes: the Chiari malformations (I and II). Semin Pediatr Neurol 1997;4:179–192

35. Menezes AH. Craniovertebral junction anomalies: diagnosis and management. Semin Pediatr Neurol 1997;4:209–223

36. reference inserted in text

37. Zurmöhle UM, Homann T, Schroeter C, et al. Psycho-

social adjustment of children with spina bifida. J Child Neurol 1998;13:64–70

38. Towfighi J, Housman C. Spinal cord abnormalities in caudal regression syndrome. Acta Neuropathol Berl 1991;81:458–466

39. Davidoff AM, Thompson CV, Grimm JM, et al. Occult spinal dysraphism in patients with anal agenesis. J Pediatr Surg 1991;26:1001–1005

40. Estin D, Cohen AR. Caudal agenesis and associated caudal spinal cord malformations. Neurosurg Clin North Am 1995;6:377–391

41. Miller E, Hare JW, Cloherty JP, et al. Elevated maternal hemoglobin Alc in early pregnancy and major congenital anomalies in infants of diabetic mothers. N Engl J Med 1981;304:1331–1334

42. Lynch SA, Bond PM, Copp AJ, et al. A gene for autosomal dominant sacral agenesis maps to the holoprosencephaly region at 7q36. Nat Genet 1995;11:93–95

43. Dias MS, Pang D. Split cord malformations. Neurosurg Clin North Am 1995;6:339–358

44. Kothari MJ, Bauer SB. Urodynamic and neurophysiologic evaluation of patients with diastematomyelia. J Child Neurol 1997;12:97–100

45. Anderson NG, Jordan S, MacFarlane MR, Lovell-Smith M. Diastematomyelia: diagnosis by prenatal sonography. AJR Am J Roentgenol 1994;163:911–914

46. Miller A, Guille JT, Bowen JR. Evaluation and treatment of diastematomyelia. J Bone Joint Surg Am 1993;75:1308–1317

47. Norman MG, McGillivray BC, Kalousek DK, et al. Congenital Malformations of the Brain: Pathologic, Embryologic, Clinical, Radiologic and Genetic Aspects. New York: Oxford University Press, 1995

48. Harley EH. Pediatric congenital nasal masses. Ear Nose Throat J 1991;70:28–32

49. Marin-Padilla M. Cephalic axial skeletal-neural dysraphic disorders: embryology and pathology. Can J Neurol Sci 1991;18:153–169

50. Mealey J Jr, Dzentis AJ, Hockey AA. The prognosis of encephaloceles. J Neurosurg 1970;32:209–218

51. Cohen MM, Lemire RJ. Syndromes with cephaloceles. Teratology 1982;25:161–172

52. Martinez-Lage JF, Poza M, Sola J, et al. The child with a cephalocele: etiology, neuroimaging and outcome. Childs Nerv Syst 1996;12:540–550

53. Barnes PD. Developmental abnormalities of the spine and spinal neuroaxis. *In*: Wolpert SM, Barnes PD, eds. MRI in Pediatric Neuroradiology. St. Louis: Mosby, 1992:331–411

54. McMaster M, Ohtsuka K. The natural history of congenital scoliosis: a study of two hundred and fifty-one patients. J Bone Joint Surg Am 1982;64:1128–1147

55. Ben-David B. Spinal cord monitoring. Orthop Clin North Am 1988;19:427–448

56. Klippel M, Feil A. Un cas d'absence des vertèbres cervicales avec cage thoracique remontant jusqu' à base du crâne. Nouv Icon Salpêtrière Paris 1912;25:223–250

57. Clarke RA, Singh S, McKenzie H, et al. Familial Klippel-Feil syndrome and paracentric inv (8)(q22.2–q23.3). Am J Hum Genet 1995;57:1364–1370

58. Fukushima Y, Ohashi H, Wakui K, et al. De novo apparently balanced reciprocal translocation between 5q.2 and 17q23 associated with Klippel–Feil anomaly and type A1 brachydactyly. Am J Med Genet 1995; 57:447–449.

59. Clarke RA, Kearsley JH, Walsh DA. Patterned expression in familial Klippel–Feil syndrome. Teratology 1996;53:152–157

60. Menezes AH. Primary craniovertebral anomalies and the hindbrain herniation syndrome (Chiari I): data base analysis. Pediatr Neurosurg 1995;23:260–269

61. Piper JG, Menezes AH. Chiari malformation in the adult. In: Menezes AH, Sonntag VKH, eds. Principles of Spinal Surgery. Vol 1. New York: McGraw-Hill, 1996:379–394

62. Burke SW, French HG, Roberts JM, et al. Chronic atlantoaxial instability in Down syndrome. J Bone Joint Surg Am 1985;67:1356–1360

63. Pueschel SM, Scola FH. Atlantoaxial instability in individuals with Down syndrome: epidemiologic, radiographic and clinical studies. Pediatrics 1987; 80:555–560

64. Williams B. Pathogenesis of syringomyelia. In: Batzdorf U, ed. Syringomyelia: Current Concepts in Diagnosis and Treatment. Baltimore: Williams & Wilkins, 1991:59–90

65. Williams B, Timperley WR. Three cases of communication syringomyelia secondary to midbrain gliomas. J Neurol Neurosurg Psychiatry 1977;40:80–88

66. McRae DL. Bony abnormalities in the region of the foramen magnum: correlation of the anatomic and neurologic findings. Acta Radiol 1953;40:335–355

67. Menezes AH, VanGilder JC, Graf CJ, McDonnell DE. Craniocervical abnormalities. A comprehensive surgical approach. J Neurosurg 1980;53:444–455

68. VanGilder JC, Menezes AH, Dolan KD. The Craniovertebral Junction and Its Abnormalities. Mount Kisco, New York: Futura, 1987:109–158

69. Menezes AH. Congenital and acquired anomalies of the craniovertebral junction. In: Youmans JR, ed. Neurological Surgery. Philadelphia: WB Saunders, 1996: 1035–1089

70. Menezes AH, Ryken TC. Craniovertebral abnormalities in Down's syndrome. Pediatr Neurosurg 1992;18: 24–33

71. Hope EE, Bodensteiner JB, Barnes PD. Cerebral infarction related to neck position in an adolescent. Pediatrics 1983;72:335–337

72. DeLaPaz RL, Brady TJ, Buonanno FS, et al. Nuclear magnetic resonance (NMR) imaging of Arnold–Chiari type I malformation with hydromyelia. J Comput Assist Tomogr 1983;7:126–129

73. Keefover R, Sam M, Nicholson A, et al. Hypersomnolence and pure central sleep apnea associated with the Chiari-I malformation. J Child Neurol 1995;10:65–67

74. Cogan DG. Down-beat nystagmus. Arch Ophthalmol 1968;80:757–768

75. Lewis AR, Kline LB, Sharpe JA. Acquired esotropia due to Arnold-Chiari malformation. J Neuro-ophthalmol 1996;16:49–54

76. Dyste GN, Menezes AH, Van Gilder JC. Symptomatic Chiari malformations. An analysis of presentation, management, and long-term outcome. J Neurosurg 1989;71:159–168

77. Pollack IF, Pang D, Albright AL, Krieger D. Outcome following hindbrain decompression of symptomatic Chiari malformations in children previously treated with meningomyelocele closure and shunts. J Neurosurg 1992;77:881–888

78. Rekate HL. Recent advances in the understanding and treatment of hydrocephalus. Semin Pediatr Neurol 1997;4:167–178

79. Fishman RA. Cerebrospinal Fluid in Diseases of the Nervous System. Philadelphia: WB Saunders, 1980

80. Leech RW. Normal physiology of cerebrospinal fluid. In: Leech RW, Brumback RA, eds. Hydrocephalus: Current Clinical Concepts. St. Louis: Mosby Year Book, 1991:30–38

81. Rosman NP, Shands KN. Hydrocephalus caused by increased intracranial venous pressure: a clinicopathological study. Ann Neurol 1978;3:445–450

82. Rosenthal A, Jouet M, Kenwrick S. Aberrant splicing of neural cell adhesion molecule L1mRNA in a family with X-linked hydrocephalus. Nat Genet 1992;2: 107–112

83. Vincent C, Kalatzis V, Compain S, et al. A proposed new contiguous gene syndrome on 8q consists of branchio-oto-renal (BOR) syndrome, Duane syndrome, a dominant form of hydrocephalus and trapeze aplasia; implications for the mapping of the BOR gene. Hum Molec Genet 1994;3:1859–1866

84. DeMyer W. Megalencephaly: types, clinical syndromes, and management. Pediatr Neurol 1986;2: 321–328

85. Bodensteiner JB, Chung EO. Macrocrania and megalencephaly in the neonate. Semin Neurol 1993;13: 84–91

86. Hamza M, Bodensteiner JB, Noorani PA, Barnes PD. Benign extracerebral fluid collections: a cause of macrocrania in infancy. Pediatr Neurol 1987;3:218–221

87. Schreier H, Rapin I, Davis J. Familial megalencephaly or hydrocephalus? Neurology 1974;24:232–236

88. Alvarez AL, Maytal J, Shinnar S. Idiopathic external hydrocephalus: natural history and relationship to benign familial macrocephaly. Pediatrics 1986;77: 901–907

89. Briner S, Bodensteiner JB. Benign subdural collections of infancy. Pediatrics 1981;67:802–804

90. Bodensteiner JB. Benign macrocephaly: a common cause of big heads in the first year. J Child Neurol 2000;15:630–631

91. Sunder TR. Benign subdural collections: a metrizamide study (abstract). Neurology 1988;38 Suppl 1: S293

92. Alper G, Ekinci G, Yilmaz Y, et al. Magnetic resonance imaging characteristics of benign macrocephaly in children. J Child Neurol 1999;14:678–682

93. Gascon GG. Medical management. In: Leech RW, Brumback RA, eds. Hydrocephalus: Current Clinical Concepts. St. Louis: Mosby Year Book, 1991:161–165

94. Christoferson LA. Surgical treatment. In: Leech RW, Brumback RA, eds. Hydrocephalus: Current Clinical Concepts. St. Louis: Mosby Year Book, 1991:166–180

95. Jones RF, Stening WA, Kwok BC, Sands TM. Third ventriculostomy for shunt infections in children. Neurosurgery 1993;32:855–859

96. Walker ML, McDonald J, Wright LC. The history of ventriculoscopy: where do we go from here? Pediatr Neurosurg 1992;18:218–223

97. Meirovitch J, Kitai-Cohen Y, Keren G, et al. Cerebrospinal fluid shunt infections in children. Pediatr Infect Dis J 1987;6:921–924

98. Goldblum RM, Pelley RP, O'Donell AA, et al. Antibodies to silicone elastomers and reactions to ventriculoperitoneal shunts. Lancet 1992;340:510–513

99. Birnholz JC, Frigoletto FD. Antenatal treatment of hydrocephalus. N Engl J Med 1981;304:1021–1022

100. Frigoletto FD Jr, Birnholz JC, Greene MF. Antenatal treatment of hydrocephalus by ventriculoamniotic shunting. JAMA 1982;248:2496–2497

101. Pople IK, Bayston R, Hayward RD. Infection of cerebrospinal fluid shunts in infants: a study of etiological factors. J Neurosurg 1992;77:29–36

102. McLone DG. Effects of complications on intellectual

function in 173 children with myelomeningocele. Child's Brain 1979;5:61–70

103. Mapstone TB, Rekate HL, Nulsen FE, et al. Relationship of CSF shunting and IQ in children with myelomeningocele: a retrospective analysis. Child's Brain 1984;11:112–118

104. Lumenta CB, Skotarczak U. Long-term follow-up in 233 patients with congenital hydrocephalus. Childs Nerv Syst 1995;11:173–175

105. Casey AT, Kimmings EJ, Kleinlugtebeld AD, et al. The long-term outlook for hydrocephalus in childhood: a ten-year cohort study of 155 patients. Pediatr Neurosurg 1997;27:63–70

106. Fletcher JM, Brookshire BL, Landry SH, et al. Behavioral adjustment of children with hydrocephalus: relationships with etiology, neurological, and family status. J Pediatr Psychol 1995;20:109–125

107. Sgouros S, Malluci C, Walsh AR, Hockley AD. Long-term complications of hydrocephalus. Pediatr Neurosurg 1995;23:127–132

108. Gerszten PC, Albright AL. Relationship between cerebellar appearance and function in children with Dandy–Walker syndrome. Pediatr Neurosurg 1995;23: 86–92

109. Elterman RD, Bodensteiner JB, Barnard JJ. Sudden unexpected death in patients with Dandy–Walker malformation. J Child Neurol 1995;10:382–384

110. Bodensteiner JB, Gay CT, Marks WA, et al. The macro cisterna magna: a marker for maldevelopment of the brain? Pediatr Neurol 1988;4:284–286

111. Maria BL, Hoang KBN, Tusa RJ, et al. "Joubert syndrome" revisited: key ocular motor signs with magnetic resonance imaging correlation. J Child Neurol 1997;12:423–430

112. Bodensteiner JB, Sheth RD. Mental retardation plus macrocephaly in a 16-year-old boy. Semin Pediatr Neurol 1996;3:177–181

113. Muller U, Steinberger D, Kunze S. Molecular genetics of craniosynostotic syndromes. Graefes Arch Clin Exp Ophthalmol 1997;235:545–550

114. Steinberger D, Reinhartz T, Unsold R, Muller U. FGFR2 mutation in clinically nonclassifiable autosomal dominant craniosynostosis with pronounced phenotypic variation. Am J Med Genet 1996;66:81–86

115. Renier D, Sainte-Rose C, Marchac D, Hirsch JF. Intracranial pressure in craniostenosis. J Neurosurg 1982;57:370–377

116. Noetzel MJ, Marsh JL, Palkes H, et al. Hydrocephalus and mental retardation in craniosynostosis. J Pediatr 1985;107:885–892

117. Simpson DA, David DJ. Craniosynostosis. *In*: Hoffman HJ, Epstein F, eds. Disorders of the Developing Nervous System: Diagnosis and Treatment. Boston: Blackwell Scientific Publications, 1986: 323–345

118. Kirkpatrick DB, Rimoin DL, Kaitila I, Goodman SJ. The craniotubular bone modeling disorders: a neurosurgical introduction to rare skeletal dysplasias with cranial nerve compression. Surg Neurol 1977;7: 221–232

119. Solh H, Da Cunha AM, Giri N, et al. Bone marrow transplantation for infantile malignant osteopetrosis. J Pediatr Hematol Oncol 1995;17:350–355

120. Schaefer B, Stein S, Oshman D, et al. Dominantly inherited craniodiaphyseal dysplasia: a new craniotubular dysplasia. Clin Genet 1986;30:381–391

121. Papay FA, Morales L Jr, Flaharty P, et al. Optic nerve decompression in cranial base fibrous dysplasia. J Craniofac Surg 1995;6:5–14

155 Mental Retardation and Cerebral Palsy

Ann H Tilton and Grant Butterbaugh

Introduction

The clinical management of mental retardation (MR) and cerebral palsy (CP) requires a knowledge of diagnostic definitions, the heterogeneity of associated functional impairments, and an appreciation of medical, allied health, educational and family services. In addition, both MR and CP often occur with other treatable medical or psychiatric disorders, necessitating clinical knowledge and use of multidisciplinary services for the affected individual and their families.

Mental retardation

Theories of MR differ according to whether or not affected children are assumed to develop similar (but eventually lower) multiskill profiles via normal (but slower) sequential developmental stages, regardless of etiology.[1] Recent research has shown, however, that distinct patterns of skills may be associated with different causes of MR. For example, whereas in Down's syndrome language deficits are greater than spatial–perceptual deficits, in Williams Syndrome the inverse is observed.[2] Such heterogeneous skill profiles illustrate the need for individualized multidisciplinary evaluations and treatment approaches.

Diagnostic criteria and classification of mental retardation

The diagnosis of MR requires IQ and adaptive behavioral test scores of less than 70 (i.e. with standard score mean = 100; standard deviation ± 15) and the onset of impairments occurring before 18 years of age.[3] With the limitations of traditional tests of infant cognition in predicting future IQ in childhood, the diagnosis of MR usually follows repeated evaluations and intensive early interventions to observe the child's cognitive and behavioral growth[4] (Table 155.1).

As many IQ tests assume some requisite communication skills, children for whom English is a second language or for whom oral speech or language is significantly impaired may have their true IQ unfairly underestimated. Likewise, the motor demands of many common IQ tests may unfairly underestimate the IQ of children with motor impairments. Children with severe acute psychiatric disorders often demonstrate a higher IQ with lower current adaptive behavior. Children for whom educational opportunities are poor demonstrate lower IQ with higher adaptive behavior. These examples illustrate the importance of considering both verbal and non-verbal based IQ scores, as well as the importance of considering various adaptive behavioral scores in fairly diagnosing MR.

The American Association of Mental Retardation (AAMR) recently redefined MR as a score of 75 which increases diagnostic labeling and the prevalence rate of MR.[5] Although some parental desire to have children with borderline IQs better served is understandable, the risk of overdiagnosing MR in educationally disadvantaged or minority children results in this controversial definition not being recommended.[5,6]

Epidemiology

Epidemiological estimates of MR depend on which IQ and adaptive behavioral test cutoff scores are used. The estimates in Table 155.3 are based on an IQ less than 70.[7]

Table 155.1 Definition and severity of MR	
Criterion A. Sub-average intellectual functioning: IQ of approximately 70 or below	
Borderline intellectual functioning	71–84
Mild mental retardation	50–55 to 70
Moderate mental retardation	35–40 to 50–55
Severe mental retardation	20–25 to 35–40
Profound mental retardation	below 20–25
Criterion B. Concurrent impairment in adaptive functioning in two or more of these areas	
Communication	Self-direction
Self-care	Functional academic skills
Home living	Work
Social/interpersonal skills	Health
Use of community resources	Safety
Criterion C. Onset before 18 years of age	

Modified from DSM-IV.[3]

Table 155.2   Mental retardation: IQ and adaptive behavior matrix

		Adaptive behavior	
		<70	>70
IQ	<70	MR	Educationally disadvantaged
	>70	Psychiatric disorder	WNL*

*Within normal limits

Neurological disorders associated with MR include autism (5%), CP (7% to 18%), epilepsy (12% to 35%), as well as visual (10% to 14%) and hearing (2% to 11%) impairments.[7,8]

Etiology and pathophysiology

Hundreds of conditions occurring during prenatal, perinatal or postnatal development are associated with MR.[5] McLaren and Bryson,[7] however, noted that in 30% of cases with severe MR, and in 50% of cases with mild MR, no cause could be identified. MR attributable to known neurological causes is found disproportionately in children with lower functioning MR (i.e. IQ < 50).[7] By contrast, familial MR accounts for a disproportionately greater number of cases with mild MR in the 50–70 IQ range.[9] Genetic causes of MR are often commonly associated with identified X-linked syndromes, e.g. Fragile X.[10] Fetal alcohol, Fragile X and Down's syndromes are common causes of MR that may account for as many as 30% of all cases.[11]

Cerebral palsy

In 1843, Little[12] described three forms of paralysis or cerebral palsy (CP): congenital hemiplegic, dyskinetic and spastic diplegic (i.e. Little's disease), which he attributed to "difficult deliveries." In the late 1800s Freud[13] recognized the role of prenatal complications leading to CP. His hypothesis has been supported by research in premature and full-term births.[14]

Diagnostic criteria and classification

In clinical practice, cerebral palsy is often a term of convenience, defining a clinical condition and implying nothing about pathology, etiology or prognosis.[15] Nelson[16] defined CP as "... an aberrant control of motor posture ... appearing early in life secondary to a central nervous system lesion, damage, or dysfunction, and not the result of recognized progressive or degenerative brain disease."[16]

The diagnosis of CP is based on combinations of several findings, including documented motor milestone delays, persistence of primitive reflexes, failure to develop protective reflexes, and the presence of pathological reflexes, rather than on any individual abnormal sign.[17] Although brain MRI is reported to detect abnormalities in 93% of patients, there is no definitive diagnostic test for cerebral palsy.[18]

The initial evaluation that leads to the diagnosis of CP (Table 155.5) is often based on early parental or physician concerns. The timeframe may be variable, spasticity may not be appreciated before the age of six months, and dyskinetic CP may not be manifest until 18 months of age. However, it is prudent to wait and perform subsequent examinations, particularly with

Table 155.3   Epidemiological estimates of mental retardation[7]

	Mild	Moderate	Severe	Profound
Prevalence (n per 100)	3.7–5.9	2	1.3	0.4
Percentage of all MR (%)	50–61	21–27	14–18	4–5

Table 155.4   Estimated rates of "mild" and "severe" by etiology (%)[7]

Etiological factor	Mild MR (IQ 50–70)	"Severe" MR (IQ < 50)
Idiopathic	45–62	14–40
Prenatal		
Chromosomal	4–7	13–38
Single gene	1–8	3–21
Multifactorial	11–23	1–24
Environmental	8	0.7–11
Perinatal		
Infections or other	1	0–5
Hypoxia	5–18	0.7–25
Prematurity/low birthweight	0.6–4	0.6–5
Postnatal		
Trauma or deprivation	2–14	0.6–4
Disease or other	2–3	1–11

Table 155.5   Considerations for diagnosis of CP[17]

Complete history and physical and neurological examination
Correlation of clinical history with physical findings
Investigation of delayed milestones (ensure not a progressive disorder)
Evaluation of vision and hearing
Integrate the information from therapists and other healthcare providers
If cognition spared despite significant spasticity:
   Ensure cervical spine status
   Ensure not DOPA-responsive dystonia
In unknown etiologies: other genetic and metabolic evaluations

Table 155.6   Classification of cerebral palsies[23]

Spastic CP 86%	Dyskinetic CP 14%
Diplegia 33%	Mainly dystonic
	Mainly athetoid
Hemiplegia 29%	Ataxic
Quadriplegia 24%	Atonic

premature infants. Some patients who had suspicious early examinations later proved to normalize.[19,20] Notably, some children who appear to have "outgrown" initial motor problems may subsequently demonstrate language or attention deficits.[21,22]

The classification of CP (Table 155.6) is primarily based on motor abnormalities and includes spastic and dyskinetic groups. The more common spastic group includes diplegic, quadriplegic and hemiplegic subgroups. Within the dyskinetic group are patients with dystonic, athetoid, ataxic, atonic, and often mixed motor movements.

Physiologically pure motor syndromes are rare; other types of tone and movement abnormalities, alone or in conjunction with spasticity, occur in at least 25% of cases.[24]

Epidemiology

Cerebral palsy, like mental retardation, is a major neurological disorder of childhood. In spite of advances in medical care, CP appears to be increasing in prevalence since the mid-1970s because of advances in neonatal care for premature infants.[25,26] Current prevalence estimates range from 1.5 to 2.5 per 1000 live births. The risk of CP is 90 per 1000 if the birthweight is less than 1500 g.[17] Overall, this represents more than 100 000 Americans with neurological symptoms of CP under the age of 18 years.[27] In addition, the 30-year survival rate is approximately 87%.[28] The economic impact of CP on society is significant. Reports in 1992 estimated the cost per new case as $503 000.[29]

Etiology and pathophysiology

Neuroimaging supports the current thought that antepartum causes of CP are far more common than birth asphyxia.[18,30] Brain malformations, intrauterine vascular malformations and infection are well recognized. Fifty percent of CP cases occur in infants with a birthweight of less than 1000 g.[31] Intrapartum asphyxia accounts for 10% to 20% of cases.[32,33] Postnatal causes typically result in spastic CP and represent only about 10% to 18% of cases.[34]

Associated issues and treatment

The evaluation is best accomplished by a multidisciplinary approach to address the multilevel service needs of these patients. CP is associated with other disorders, including autism and MR (65%), and visual (10%) and hearing impairment (4%).[26,35] Seizures occur in 25% of patients and typically begin in the first two years of life (Table 155.7). The risk is higher if the pathological process involves the cortical gray matter, and highest in patients with spastic quadriparesis.[36]

Orthopedic problems often evolve over time because muscles require to be stretched for growth and elasticity. CP often precludes adequate stretching, resulting in muscles that become overcontracted and, as bone grows, relatively shorter. Contractures may progress rapidly.[37] In addition, osteoporosis resulting from inadequate nutrition or immobility may occur, leading to fractures.[38]

Failure to thrive is a major issue, especially in patients with spastic quadriparesis and dyskinetic syndromes. A complex combination of factors may contribute, including poor feeding, dental problems, gastroesophageal reflux, recurrent aspiration and increased energy demands.[17]

Communication is often reduced because oral motor skills are affected, similar to other motor skills. Educational and recreational opportunities are often limited because of the motor speed and dexterity required. Augmentative communication and computer technology should always be considered.

Although there is often an overlap of symptoms, cerebral palsy is defined mainly by the associated motor disabilities. Within the past 10 years more therapeutic options have become available for these disabilities, which will be discussed. Family, psychiatric and educational issues common to CP and MR will be discussed after the treatment of CP.

Treatment approach to motor impairment   All of the treatment modalities attempt to establish appropriate

Table 155.7   Probability of epilepsy in cerebral palsy

Spastic diplegia	16–27%
Spastic hemiplegia	34–60%
Spastic quadriplegia	50–90%
Dyskinetic	23–26%

muscle balance, improve musculoskeletal alignment and improve the quality of movement and functional abilities. Spasticity is the most frequent motor abnormality, characterized by a velocity-dependent increase in tonic stretch reflexes (muscle tone). The current theory of the pathophysiology of spasticity involves a chronic reduction of inhibitory input and hyperexcitability of the α motor neurons, resulting in abnormal processing at the spinal cord level of peripheral afferent input.[39] The model in the other movement disorders is less clear.

The clinical characteristics that define spasticity are fairly uniform and are best described as "positive and negative" (Table 155.8). The positive symptoms are those associated with the *release* of the intact motor system from control, and are the most amenable to medical interventions. The negative are linked with the *loss* of a specific skill of central nervous system origin, and are often the most disabling symptoms.[39] If spasticity goes untreated, the health consequences may include contractures, pain, spasms and sleep disturbances.

Effective intervention for motor impairments combines traditional and new treatment therapies while encouraging family compliance (Table 155.9).

The "ladder" theory helps prioritize interventions for patients with CP. The current treatment perspective does not, however, imply "rung by rung" implementation: rather, it advocates using the least invasive and then more invasive techniques, with different modalities applied in varying combinations and orders (Figure 155.1).

Physical and occupational therapy

Physical and occupational therapies have been the cornerstone of treatment for the CP patient. The different theories of motor therapies, including motor retraining, sensory reintegration and neurodevelopmental treatments, all seek to minimize impairment, maximize function and emphasize independence.[40] In addition, therapists integrate orthotics, casting, tran-

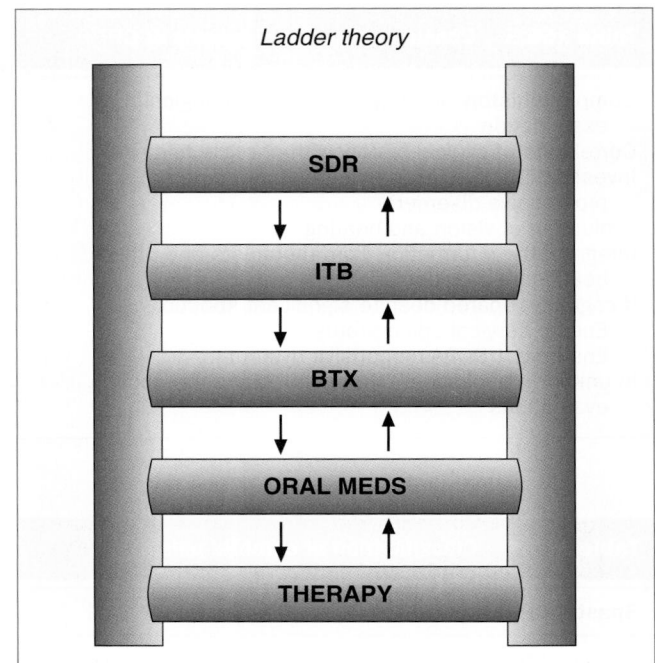

Figure 155.1 "Ladder" theory for CP treatment. SDR, selective dorsal rhizotomy; ITB, intrathecal baclofen; BTX, botulinum toxin.

scutaneous electrical stimulation and dynamic bracing to address difficulties such as motor weakness and contractures.[41] The determination of appropriate seating devices (manual or power) to promote mobility is another major goal.

Efficacy Debate is ongoing about both the clinical efficacy and the theoretical basis for these therapies.[42,43] No adequately randomized controlled studies exist to support their long-term efficacy.[44] Only cohort, case or retrospective studies have reported treatment benefits.[45]

Pharmacological management Pharmacological management targets either generalized or regional spasticity needs. Modalities include oral medications, botulinum toxin, phenol and alcohol.

Generalized spasticity
Oral medications (Table 155.10).

There are several physiological mechanisms for the action of oral medications. Their systemic effects preclude "targeting" a focal or regional area of spasticity.

- *Benzodiazepines* Diazepam facilitates the postsynaptic effects of GABA-A. Diazepam binds to the brainstem reticular formation and spinal synaptic pathways. Diazepam's clinical efficacy in athetosis, as well as spasticity, in cerebral palsy indicates that generalized relaxation is a major component of its action.[46] Side effects, including excessive somnolence, dizziness, mild weakness and withdrawal syndrome, may limit its potential use.[47]

Table 155.8   Positive and negative symptoms in CP

Positive	Negative
Increased reflexes	Lack of agility
Clonus	Fatiguability
Increased tone	Weakness

Table 155.9   Traditional and new therapies

Traditional	New
Allied health therapy	Selective dorsal rhizotomy
Orthotics and casting	New oral medications
Oral medications	Botulinum toxin
Nerve and motor point blocks	Intrathecal baclofen
Orthopedic interventions	

Table 155.10   Oral antispasticity medications

	Mechanism	Dosage	Side effect	Monitor	Studies
Diazepam	Facilitates GABA-A Inhibits at the spinal cord and brain stem	0.1–0.8 mg/kg per day Divided q 6–8 h Increase weekly	3+ Sedation 2+ Weakness Dizziness	Avoid abrupt withdrawal	DBPC (child/adult)
Clonazepam	Facilitates GABA-A Inhibits at the spinal cord and brainstem	0.01–0.2 mg/kg per day Divided q 8 h Begin slowly Increase weekly Max dose 20 mg	3++ Sedation 2+ weakness	Avoid abrupt withdrawal	Open trial only
Clorazepate	Facilitates GABA-A Inhibits at the spinal cord and brainstem	>9–12 yr. max 60 mg/day >12 yr. max 90 mg Divided q 8–12 h Begin slowly Increase weekly	1–2+ Sedation 2+ Weakness	Avoid abrupt withdrawal	DBPC (adult)
Baclofen	GABA-B agonist Inhibits at the spinal cord level	2–8 yr. max 40 mg/day >8 yr. max 80 mg/day Divided q 6–8 h Begin slowly Increase q 3 days	2+ Sedation Confusion 2+ Weakness ± Seizure control	Avoid abrupt withdrawal Monitor LFT	DBPC (child/adult)
Dantrolene	Interferes with skeletal muscle contraction by interruption of calcium release from sarcoplasmic reticulum	0.5–3 mg/kg per dose Divided q 6–12 h Increase 4–7 days Adult max 400 mg/day	1+ Sedation 3+ Weakness Hepatotoxicity GI complaints	Not for use in hepatic disease Monitor LFT Caution in cardiac and pulmonary impairment Avoid excessive sunlight	DBPC (child/adult)
Tizanidine	α_2 Adrenergic agonist with presynaptic inhibition	0.2–0.5 mg/kg per day Divided q 4–6 h Increase weekly Adult max 36 mg/day	2++ Sedation 1+ Weakness Hypotension	Avoid abrupt withdrawal Monitor LFT	DBPC (adult)

DBPC, Double-blind placebo-controlled clinical trials; LFT, liver function test.

Efficacy: Although diazepam has been observed to provide greater improvement in behavior and general relaxation than in spasticity, double-blind placebo-controlled studies in CP have shown significant improvement in spasticity, especially in younger children and those with athetosis.[48–51] In addition, diazepam in combination with dantrolene was superior to either medication alone.[52]

Clorazepate and clonazepam also have demonstrated antispasticity action in adult studies, with sedation being a limiting factor with clonazepam.[47] Chlorazepate is less sedating, but no studies of this medication in childhood spasticity have been conducted.[47]

• *Baclofen* Baclofen, a presynaptic inhibitor of GABA-B, is frequently prescribed. The medication is most effective in spinal cord lesions and less so in spasticity of cerebral origin. The side-effect profile includes central depression, confusion and weakness. Baclofen also has fewer potential liver and weakness problems than dantrolene.[53,54]

Efficacy: In adult studies baclofen compares favorably to diazepam, with equal efficacy but less sedation.[53,54] A placebo-controlled double-blind crossover study of oral baclofen in childhood cerebral palsy has reported significant reductions in spasticity and improved movement of the extremities.[51,55]

• *Dantrolene* Dantrolene is a unique medication that acts directly on the muscle contractility mechanism. Side effects include excessive weakness and functional impairment, with mild sedation and gastrointestinal complaints. Hepatotoxicity is reported in 1% of patients, with fatal hepatitis occurring in 0.1% to 0.2% of those taking it for longer than 60 days.[53,56]

Efficacy: Dantrolene would be a logical choice for spasticity of cerebral origin. However, its side-effect profile has limited its use in children despite proven benefits in placebo-controlled studies of children with CP.[57,58]

• α_2 *Agonists* Tizanidine has a novel mechanism of action as an α_2 agonist inhibiting the release of excitatory amino acids and facilitating the action of glycine at spinal and supraspinal levels. Because of its mechanism of action, tizanidine may be used in conjunction with other antispasticity medications.[59]

Side effects of tizanidine include dry mouth and notable sedation. Although it does not have the significant blood pressure effect seen with clonidine, it may be associated with symptomatic hypotension. Caution should be exercised in using

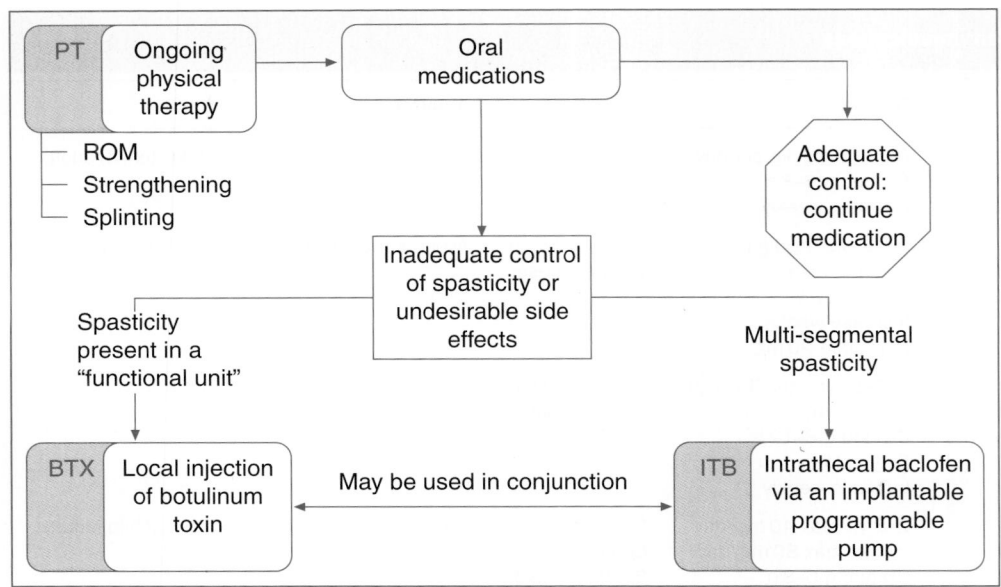

Figure 155.2 Therapy for spasticity "Decision tree." PT = physical therapy, ROM = range of motion, BTX = botulinum toxin, ITB = intrathecal baclofen. (Reprinted with permission from WE MOVE. Spasticity: Etiology, Evaluaton, Management and the Role of Botulinum Toxin. Mayer NH, Simpson DM, editors. New York: WE MOVE, 2002.)

it with other antihypertensives. Dose-related effects on liver function and even hallucinations, have been reported in 3% to 5% of subjects.[47] It does have a short half-life, with food accelerating absorption and untoward effects. Frequent dosing with a very slow upward titration is beneficial.[59]

Efficacy: In a review of several adult studies, tizanidine was compared to baclofen. Tizanidine demonstrated better effects on clonus and resulted in less compromise of strength. Compared to diazepam, tizanidine was less sedating. Overall, the data supported a 30% reduction in tone.[60] Studies in children are currently in progress.

Regional management
• *Nerve and motor blocks* Although less frequently used, nerve and motor point blocks are useful in the management of regional or focal spasticity. Diagnostic nerve blocks use anesthetic agents to

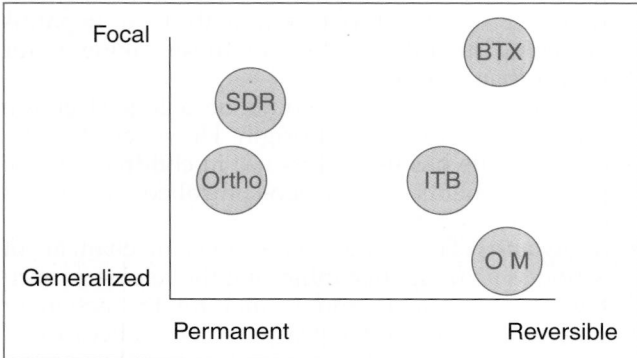

Figure 155.3 Treatment options in spasticity. SDR = selective dorsal rhizotomy, Ortho = orthopedic intervention, BTX = botulinum toxin, ITB = intrathecal baclofen, O M = oral medications. (Reprinted with permission from Gait and Posture 11;2000: 67–79. Elsevier Science.)

relax the muscle and to identify the presence and extent of contracture. Neurolytic blocks with phenol and ethanol decrease spasticity by directly damaging the nerve and causing tissue necrosis.[61] Nerve blocks are variably effective and may last from one to more than 12 months. Motor point blocks are more graded, but may be less effective because of difficulty in identifying and treating the multiple motor points within the muscle.

There are concerns regarding these techniques because about 10% of patients experience dysesthesia and causalgia following the injection of mixed motor nerves. Vascular complications, sensory loss and excessive weakness may also occur. The procedure is time-consuming and requires an understanding of the multiple technical requirements for its effective use.[61]

Efficacy: Studies from the 1960s detailed the beneficial effects of injecting children with CP with 45% alcohol into muscle motor points. Spasticity was reduced without associated muscle weakness.[61] In addition, studies have shown the benefit of phenol use in children with CP.[61,62] Well controlled studies are needed to compare the effects of alcohol, phenol and botulinum toxin.

• *Botulinum toxin* Botulinum toxin is derived from *Clostridium botulinum*. There are seven serologically separable potent neuroparalytic toxins. The FDA has approved the use of botulinum toxin A (BTX A) for strabismus and blepharospasm associated with dystonia. Both botulinum toxin A (BTX A) and botulinum toxin B (BTX B) are approved for use in cervical dystonia (Tables 155.11, 155.12).

The mechanism of action is the inhibition of acetylcholine release at the neuromuscular junction by bonding of the toxin to peripheral presynaptic cholinergic nerves. As a result, chemical denervation is provided on a temporary basis in the injected muscles. Once the muscle stops experienc-

Table 155.11　Dosing guideline based on BTX-A (Botox)

Dose	Total dose	Dose per single injection site	Dilution	Sites	LD50
Small muscles (upper ext) 1–3 U/kg Large muscles (hamstrings) 3–6 U/kg	Up to 12 U/kg Typical max dose; 300 U (child) 400 U (adult)	50 U	100 U/mL or 100 U/2mL 0.9% Preservative-free saline	4–5 cm apart if possible 1–2 sites/muscle	39 U/kg

Table 155.12　Delivery guidelines – botulinum toxin

Anxiolytics	Anesthesia	Local anesthetic	Localization	Action
Nasal, rectal or oral versed	Rarely needed	EMLA cream 1–2 h prior to procedure Ethyl chloride at the time of injection	Anatomic landmark EMG improves localization in difficult to identify muscles	Initial response 1–2 h Peak effect 4–6 wks Useful 10–16+ wks

ing excitatory stimulation, decreased tone and weakness result. Although dosage limitations preclude simultaneous injections in multiple muscle groups, the treatment is effective for focal or local spasticity.[63]

The main action is localized to an area 4–5 cm^2, with clinical effects apparent within 24–72 hours and peak action at approximately four weeks. Duration of effect is estimated to be three to four months. There are benefits that clearly exceed the projected chemical effects, possibly related to improved balance of the previously overstretched antagonists in conjunction with actual muscle lengthening at the injected site in the agonist muscles.[64]

Electromyography is frequently used to administer the medication to difficult-to-locate muscles such as the posterior tibialis and the small muscles of the forearm and hand. Using superficial landmarks to localize targeted muscles was not predictive of appropriate localization in 25% of instances.[65]

Appropriate patients are those for whom weakening a limited number of specific muscles could potentially provide increased function. Fixed contractures and bony deformities do not benefit from BTX and are only amenable to orthopedic intervention, such as inhibition casting or surgery.

Botulinum toxin A has a relatively small (6%) reported rate of minor self-limiting side effects[66,67] (Table 155.13).

Efficacy: Well controlled studies of botulinum toxin A have observed significantly decreased tone and functional improvements in the upper and lower extremities.[63,66–70] Improvement in gait has been demonstrated by 3D analysis, electromyography and subjective reports, as well as by functional outcome measures. The studies also support that botulinum toxin effects are more sustained than casting and may delay lower extremity surgery in selected patients.[71,72] Studies supporting botulinum toxin treatment have been criticized because of heterogeneous etiologies, ages and types of spasticity, precluding comparison of findings across studies.[73]

Multisegmental therapy
Intrathecal baclofen therapy Continuous intrathecal baclofen infusion (ITB) has FDA approval for the treatment of spasticity of cerebral or spinal cord origin. It is also recognized as an effective medical treatment for patients with dystonia.[74,75]

Baclofen is a GABA analog affecting GABA-B receptors that provides presynaptic inhibition at the spinal cord level. Although oral baclofen does not easily cross the blood-brain barrier and has systemic side effects that limit its clinical use, the intrathecal dose requirement is substantially less, at 0.5% to 1%, than that of the oral route, and is better tolerated.[47] With the four-hour half-life, continuous intrathecal infusion is necessary to maintain an adequate intrathecal level.

Table 155.13　BTX-A side-effect profile

Bruising/discomfort at injection site
Antibody formation
Excessive weakness in target and neighboring muscles
Fever
Flu-like feeling
Dysphagia in patients with pseudobulbar symptoms
Incontinence
Constipation – both worse and improved

Baclofen is delivered by a SynchroMed infusion system via a catheter in the intrathecal space, a pump in the abdomen, and telemetry programming. With the current catheter tip placement at the T11–12 level, the lumbar to cervical medication concentration gradient is 4:1. Catheter placement at T6–7 or higher has been successfully recommended in patients with significant upper extremity involvement and dystonia.[24,76,77] The rate, mode and pattern of infusion may be modified non-invasively to meet specific patient requirements.

Appropriate candidates for this treatment typically have a score of 3 or higher on the Ashworth scale (Box 155.1) in the lower extremities, involvement of four or more muscle groups, a body mass that can support the system, and a family commitment to refill the pump every six to 12 weeks. Patients who generally benefit from ITB include those with poor underlying strength whose lower extremity movements are impeded by spasticity; non-ambulatory spastic quadriparetics whose spasticity interferes with daily living skills; non-functional patients for whom the goal is to enhance quality of caregiving; and patients with dystonia or other movement disorders.[24,78] Although initially its use was recommended for 4-year-olds who weighed at least 40 pounds, subfascial pump placements are currently used in smaller patients or those with less than optimum subcutaneous tissue.

- *Screening and infusion* A screening trial is accomplished using a spinal tap or external catheter with infusion of the medications. An adequate response in spasticity of cerebral origin is a one-point score decline on the Ashworth scale. Patients with dystonia may benefit from ITB, but higher dosing is required delivered over several days via the external catheter.[24] A catheter trial also may be needed for access if the patient has had posterior spinal fusion or if there are other limitations to direct spinal infusion. Following a successful trial, the pump is implanted.
- *Complications and side effects* In both oral baclofen use and indwelling technology there is the poten-

tial for side effects. The drug-related complications include hypotonia, weakness, nausea and vomiting, and changes in urinary or bowel function. The frequency of seizures in patients who were previously diagnosed with epilepsy does not seem to be influenced by ITB. The most common device- and surgical-related events were seroma, infection and catheter-related problems.[79] One of the more serious issues is the potential for overdose. Over-infusion of ITB, primarily related to programming errors, can lead to flaccidity, respiratory suppression and reversible coma.[80] Rapid withdrawal is also a major concern and may be life-threatening.[81]

Efficacy: Numerous studies strongly support the use of intrathecal baclofen in children with cerebral palsy.[75–77,79,82–93] Four studies were double-blind randomized trials of treatment effects in children with CP.[77,79,82,88] Although the majority of these studies measured the improvement in spasticity using technical measures such as the Ashworth scale, rather than functional improvements, a recent prospective placebo-controlled double-blind dose reduction study demonstrated the efficacy of intrathecal baclofen on functional abilities and pain relief.[77] Other beneficial effects include, improvements in swallowing and speech.[77] Recent literature supports the use of ITB in hemiplegic cerebral palsy, with benefits reported on the paretic side but without side effects on the non-paretic side.[77,94]

- *Additional issues* Cost is a consideration. However, ITB may well affect the patient's number of hospitalizations, orthopedic surgery, and other health care related to the known complications of CP.[87] Gerszten[91] reported that ITB for the treatment of spastic cerebral palsy reduces the need for subsequent orthopedic surgery.

Surgical management

Selective dorsal rhizotomy (SDR) In 1987 Dr Warwick Peacock repopularized the surgical technique of dorsal rhizotomy when a selective approach to severing the posterior spinal rootlets was improved.[95] The original non-selective procedure had fallen out of favor when complications, including sensory deficits, weakness, and bowel and bladder problems, were observed.

The surgical goal is to reduce spasticity by limiting stimulatory inputs from the muscle spindle that arrive via afferent fibers in the dorsal roots. The procedure consists of a lumbar laminectomy. Limiting the procedure to severing 40% to 60% of the rootlets in L4–S1 or L5–S1 distribution results in less risk of sensory loss and hypotonia, with a similar improvement in reduced muscle tone and functional improvement.[96]

The best candidates are typically children 3–7 years old with spastic diplegia, good trunk control, good lower extremity strength and isolated leg movements.[97] Predictors of the ability to walk after SDR include the type of CP (hemiplegic and diplegic > quadriplegic) and the preoperative gait

Box 155.1	Ashworth scale

Muscle tone

Score	Criteria
1	No increase in tone
2	Slight increase in tone
3	Marked increase in tone, but affected part(s) easily flexed
4	Considerable increase in tone; passive movement difficult
5	Affected part(s) rigid in flexion or extension

Table 155.14   Treatment options

	Oral medicine	Botulinum toxin	Nerve/motor block	Intrathecal baclofen	Selective dorsal rhizotomy	Orthopedic
Appropriate spasticity candidate	Generalized	Focal	Focal	Generalized	Focal	Focal or generalized
Appropriate candidate	Spasms Sleep disturbance Need Anxiolytics	Not fixed contracture Strong antagonists	Not fixed contracture Pure motor nerve	Significant spasticity Underlying weakness Older children Dystonia	Diplegia Individual leg movement Good trunk control and L ext strength	Sjeketally mature Fixed contracture Bone/joint deformity
Age	All	1–5+ yr for lower ext 3–4+ yr for upper ext	> 6 yr	> 3–4 yr	> 3 yr < 7 yr	Skelatally mature if possible
Advantages	Delivery Cost Sedation Reversible	Minimal side effects Effective Reversible Selective	1–12 mo effect Reversible Low cost	Adjustable Reversible	Permanent L>>U EXT	Permanent
Disadvantages	Sedation Potential liver issue Cognition Non-selective	Reversible Cost	May require anesthesia Dysesthesia Pain Lack of selectivity	Surgery Cost Refills Foreign body Battery replacement	Surgery Cost Orthopedic problems Permanent	Surgery Cost Recurrent problems Permanent
Efficacy	Older studies DBPC	DBPC Cohort studies	Case reports Cohort studies in children	DBPC Dose reduction studies Cohort studies	DBPC Cohort studies Technical and function studies	Observational studies
Cost estimate ($)	15–300/mo	500–2500/ treatment	300–1000/ treatment + anesthesia	15–30 000 initial 300–1000/refill	30 000+ initial 6 mo PT/OT 10–15 000	8000–100 000/ procedure

score.[98] In the past, patients with severe spastic quadriparesis were candidates for SDR: their suitability is now controversial, with ITB being the recommended modality.

Postrhizotomy management requires aggressive physical therapy four to five times a week and occupational therapy once or twice a week for six months to return motor function to preoperative levels.

Efficacy: Randomized clinical trials have demonstrated that SDR results in a decrease in tone and improved motor function. It may be most effective for marginal ambulators.[99–101]

Orthopedic surgery   Orthopedic surgery has been a major treatment for CP. Fixed contractures and bone and joint deformities are substantial issues and most amenable to surgical intervention. Soft tissue lengthening and transfers also have a role in the care of these patients. Orthopedic surgery is advocated when patients are more skeletally mature, thereby providing one balanced multilevel procedure, as opposed to multiple procedures with each growth spurt.[102]

Efficacy: The published reports are primarily observational and based on studies of specific procedures.[103]

Table 155.14 lists the various treatment options.

Psychiatric and school services for MR and CP

It is essential to understand the normal heterogeneity of parent perspectives regarding their child's developmental disability. It has been compared to the "grief" reaction owing to "loss of the ideal child" and the recurrent "sorrow" reaction.[104,105] Professionals may view a child's needs from a time-limited intervention perspective; parents are looking at their needs from a lifelong functional, social and daily living perspective.[106]

Episodic or chronic psychiatric comorbidities are associated with MR and CP.[8,107,108] Diagnosis of psychiatric disorders in children with MR or CP can be difficult, with underdiagnosis or misdiagnosis affecting both the child's quality of life and the appropriateness of pharmacotherapy or other mental health interventions.[109,110] Despite advances in pharmacotherapy, child, parenting and classroom behavioral psychological therapies are necessary to teach new

Table 155.15 Consensus regarding psychotropic medications in MR/DD	
Diagnosis/symptom	**Medications**
Adjustment disorder	Anxiolytics
Aggression (chronic and neurological)	β-Blockers Buspirone Anticonvulsants
Akathesia (neuroleptic induced)	β-Blockers (propranolol)
Attention deficit/ hyperactivity disorder	Stimulants Tricyclic antidepressants
Autism	Neuroleptics Serotonin reuptake inhibitors
Depressive disorders	Antidepressants
Enuresis	Tricyclic antidepressants
Generalized anxiety disorder	Anxiolytics Antidepressants
Hyperactivity	Clonidine
Mania	Lithium Valproate, carbamazepine Benzodiazepine
Obsessive–compulsive disorder	Clonimpramine, fluoxetine, paroxetine
Panic disorder	Antidepressants Benzodiazepine
Pica (zinc deficiency)	Zinc supplement
Schizophrenia	Neuroleptics
Self-injurious behaviour	Naltrexone Neuroleptics Antidepressants β-Blockers
Sleep problems (primary)	Melatonin Benzodiazepines Clonidine
Tourette syndrome (or tics)	Neuroleptics Anxiolytics Clonidine

Table 155.16 Timelines and procedures for individualized school plans	
Early intervention (<3 years old)	**Special education (≥3 years old)**
Referral for early evaluation	Referral for pupil appraisal
Evaluation of eligibility and needs	Evaluation of eligibility and needs
Individualized health care (IHCP) and family service plans (IFSP)	Individualized health care (IHCP) and education (IEP) or transition plan (ITP)
Annual review of IFSP	Annual review of IEP or ITP
Transition planning re IEP	Transition planning for adult services

coping, educational and daily living skills.[111] Although psychotropic medications are often used, few well controlled clinical trials have been conducted to provide evidence-based pharmacotherapy guidelines in children. However, practice guidelines for multimodal pharmacotherapy and behavioral interventions for psychiatric comorbidities are available[112,113] (Table 155.15)

Community, school and adult transition services

Community or school-based resources can be critical for children with CP and MR. Physicians and other professionals must be aware of services and any documentation required.

Federal and state laws, including the Disabilities Education Act (IDEA 1997), mandate that eligible children be provided with free, appropriate appraisal and educational intervention services in the least restrictive educational setting. Classifications include isolated or multiple disabilities, including MR, orthopedic impairment (e.g. motor impairments of CP), speech (e.g. speech impairments of CP), traumatic brain injury, autism, learning disabilities, and other health impairments (e.g. attention deficit/hyperactivity disorder). Multidisciplinary evaluations are followed by parental conferences to design an individualized program. Special education is mandated until high school graduation or the patient's 22nd birthday. For the purposes of the individualized health care plan (IHCP), professionals are the only authorities who can document the child's diagnosis, their healthcare needs and physical education and other medical restrictions (Table 155.16).

IFSP is designed for disabled or at-risk infants or toddlers (birth to age 3) who have, or who will have, substantial developmental delays if early intervention services are not provided. Funding limitations may constrain the availability of IFSP-recommended services at school or in the community.

IEP conferences involve parents, the affected child if appropriate, school professionals and community-based professionals. The goal is to design an individualized education plan for eligible children from 3 to 21 years of age. The IEP specifies annual instructional goals, classroom placement and school-based therapy.

The ITP conferences begin after 14 years of age, the goal being to ease patients into functional adulthood. The ITP helps patients and their families develop a plan for achieving adult lifestyle goals, including physical and mental health, and a residential, vocational, financial and social services plan.[114]

Summary

The clinical management of MR and CP requires a knowledge of their developmental course, the heterogeneity of functional impairments, as well as children's long-term multidisciplinary health care, educational and adult transition service needs. MR and CP often are complicated by numerous medical or psychiatric disorders requiring the physician's participation and leadership in recommending, implementing and revising the individualized school, family and community services necessary to achieve greater functional independence.

Family resources

The Arc (formerly Association of Retarded Citizens of
the United States)
500 East Border Street
Arlington, TX 76010
817-261-6003
www.thearc.org

American Association of Mental Retardation (AAMR)
1719 Kalorama Rd., NW
Washington, DC 20009-2683
800-424-3688; 202-387-1968
www.aamr.org

United Cerebral Palsy Association, Inc.
1660 L St., NW
Washington, DC 20036-5602
800-USA-5-UCP
202-776-0406
www.ucpa.org

References

1. Zigler E. Developmental versus differences: theories of retardation and the problem of motivation. Am J Ment Defic 1969;73:536–556
2. Bellugi U, Wang P, Jernigan T. Williams syndrome: an unusual neuropsychological profile. In: Broman SH, Grafman J, eds. Atypical Cognitive Deficits in Developmental Disorders. Hillsdale: Lawrence Erlbaum Associates, 1994:23–56
3. American Psychiatric Association. Diagnostic and Statistical Manual of Mental Disorders. 4th edn. Washington, DC: ADA Press, 1994
4. Butterbaugh G. Selected psychometric and clinical review of neurodevelopmental infant tests. Clin Neuropsychol 1988;2:350–364
5. Luckasson R. Mental Retardation: Definition, Classification, and Systems of Support. Washington DC: American Association on Mental Retardation, 1992
6. MacMillan D, Gresham F, Siperstein G. Conceptual and psychometric concerns about the 1992 AAMR definition of mental retardation. Am J Ment Retard 1995;98:325–335
7. McLaren J, Bryson S. Review of recent epidemiological studies of mental retardation: prevalence, associated disorders, and etiology. Am J Ment Retard 1987;96:243–254
8. Gillberg C, Persson E, Grufman M, et al. Psychiatric disorders in mildly and severely mentally retarded urban children and adolescents: epidemiological aspects. Br J Psychiatry 1986;149:68–74
9. Zigler E, Hodapp R. Understanding mental retardation. Cambridge: Cambridge University Press, 1986
10. Feldman EJ. The recognition and investigation of X-linked learning disability syndromes. J Intellect Disabil Res 1996;40:400–411
11. Batshaw M. Mental retardation. Pediatric Clinics of North America, 1993;40:507–521
12. Little WJ. Course of lectures on the deformities of the human frame. Lancet 1843;1:318–322
13. Freud S. Infantile Cerebral Paralysis. Coral Gables: University of Miami Press, 1968
14. Naeyi R, Peters E, Bartholmew M, et al. Origins of cerebral palsy. Am J Dis Child 1989;143:1154–1161
15. Badawi N, Watson L, Petterson B, et al. What constitutes cerebral palsy? Dev Med Child Neurol 1998;40:520–527
16. Nelson KB, Ellenberg JH. Epidemiology of cerebral palsy. Adv Neurol 1978;19:421–435
17. Miller G. Cerebral palsies: an overview. In: Miller G, Clark GD, eds. The Cerebral Palsies: Causes, Consequences, and Management. Boston: Butterworth-Heinemann, 1998:1–35
18. Truwit CL, Barkovich AJ, Kock TK, et al. Cerebral palsy: MR findings in 40 patients. Am J Neuroradiol 1992;13:67–78
19. Allen MC, Alexander GR. Using motor milestones as a multistep process to screen preterm infants for cerebral palsy. Dev Med Child Neurol 1997;39:12–16
20. Burns YR, O'Callaghan M, Tudehope DI. Early identification of cerebral palsy in high risk infants. Aust Paediatr J 1989;25:215–219
21. Nelson K, Ellenberg J. Children who "outgrow" cerebral palsy. Pediatrics 1982;59:529–536
22. Dargassies SS. Neurodevelopmental symptoms during the first year of life: I. Essential landmarks for each key-age. Dev Med Child Neurol 1972;14:235–246
23. Miller G, Clark G. The Cerebral Palsies Causes, Consequences, and Management. Boston: Butterworth-Heineman, 1998
24. Albright AL. Intrathecal baclofen in cerebral palsy movement disorders. J Child Neurol 1996;11:S29–S35
25. Bhushan V, Paneth N, Kiely J. Impact of improved survival of very low birth weight infants on recent secular trends in the prevalence of cerebral palsy. Pediatrics 1993;91:1094–1100
26. Murphy C, Yeargin-Allsopp M, Decoufler P, et al. Prevalence of cerebral palsy among 10-year-old children in metropolitan Atlanta 1985–1987. J Pediatr 1993;123:S13–S19
27. Newacheck P, Taylor W. Childhood chronic illness: prevalence, severity and impact. Am J Public Health 1992;82:364–371
28. Crichton J, Mackinnon M, White C. The life expectancy of persons with cerebral palsy. Dev Med Child Neurol 1995;37:364–371
29. Kuben K, Leviton A. Cerebral palsy. N Engl J Med 1994;330:188–195
30. Bax M, Nelson K. Birth asphyxia: a statement. Dev Med Child Neurol 1993;71:235–238
31. Pharoah P, Platt M, Cooke T. The changing epidemiology of cerebral palsy. Arch Dis Child 1996;75:169–173
32. Nelson KB, Ellenberg JH. Antecedents of cerebral palsy-multivariate analysis. N Engl J Med 1986;315:81–86
33. Perlman JM. Intrapartum hypoxic-ischemic cerebral injury and subsequent cerebral palsy: medicolegal issues. Pediatrics 1997;99:851–857
34. Pharoah P, Cooke T, Rosenbloom L. Acquired cerebral palsy. Arch Dis Child 1989;64:1013–1016
35. Fernell E, Gillberg C, von Wendt L. Autistic symptoms in children with severe hydrocephalus. Acta Paediatr Scand 1991;80:451–457
36. Tharp BR. The electroencephalogram, seizures, and epileptic syndromes in the cerebral palsies. In: Miller G, Clark GD, eds. The Cerebral Palsies: Causes, Consequences, and Management. Boston: Butterworth-Heinemann, 1998:273–297
37. Reimers J. Clinically based decision making for surgery. In: Sussman MD, ed. The Diplegic Child: Evaluation and Management. Rosemont: American Academy of Orthopedic Surgeons, 1991:151–161
38. Shaw N, White C, Fraser W, et al. Osteopenia in cerebral palsy. Arch Dis Child 1994;71:235–238

39. Young RR. Spasticity: a review. Neurology 1994; 44(Suppl 9):S12– S20

40. Barry MJ. Physical therapy interventions for patients with movement disorders due to cerebral palsy. J Child Neurol 1996;11:S51–S60

41. Carmick J. Clinical use of neuromuscular electrical stimulation for children with cerebral palsy. Phys Ther 1993;73:505–527

42. Russman BS, Romness M. Neurorehabilitation for the child with cerebral palsy. In: Miller G, Clark GD, eds. The Cerebral Palsies: Causes, Consequences, and Management. Boston: Butterworth-Heinemann, 1998: 321–332

43. Bobath B. The very early treatment of cerebral palsy. Dev Med Child Neurol 1996;9:373–393

44. Palmer FB, Shapiro BK, Wachtel RC. The effects of physical therapy on cerebral palsy. A controlled trial in infants with spastic diplegia. N Engl J Med 1988;318: 803–808

45. Scherzer AL, Mike V, Jolson J. Physical therapy as a determinant of change in the cerebral palsied infant. Pediatrics 1976;58:47–52

46. Marsh HO. Diazepam in incapacitating cerebral palsied children. JAMA 1965;191:797–800

47. Gracies JM, Nance P, Elovic E, et al. Traditional pharmacological treatments for spasticity Part II: General and regional treatments. Muscle Nerve 1997;20(Suppl 6):S92–S120

48. Engle HA. The effects of diazepam (valium) in children with cerebral palsy: a double blind study. Dev Med Child Neurol 1966;8:661–667

49. Denhoff E. Cerebral palsy-a pharmacologic approach. Clin Pharmacol Ther 1964;5:947–954

50. Holt KS. The use of diazepam in childhood cerebral palsy. Report of a small study including electromyographic observations. Ann Phys Med 1964(Suppl): 16–24

51. Pranzatelli MR. Oral pharmacotherapy for the movement disorders of cerebral palsy. J Child Neurol 1996;11(Suppl 1):S13–S22

52. Nogen AG. Effect of dantrolene sodium of the incidence of seizures in children with spasticity. Childs Brain 1979;5:420–425

53. Young RR, Delwaide PJ. Drug therapy spasticity (first of two parts). N Engl J Med 1981 Jan 1;304(1):28–33

54. Young RR, Delwaide PJ. Drug therapy: spasticity (second of two parts). N Engl J Med 1981 Jan 8;304(2):96–99

55. Milla PJ, Jackson ADM. A controlled trial of baclofen in children with cerebral palsy. J Int Med Res 1977;5:398–404

56. Katz RT. Management of spasticity. Am J Phys Med Rehab 1988 Jun;67(3):108–116

57. Haslam RH, Walcher JR, Leitman PS. Dantrolene sodium in children with spasticity. Arch Phys Med Rehab 1974;55:384–388

58. Joynt RL, Leonard JA. Dantrolene sodium suspension in treatment of spastic cerebral palsy. Dev Med Child Neurol 1980;22:755–767

59. Coward DM. Neuropharmacology and mechanism of action of tizanidine. Neurology 1994;44(Suppl 9): 6–11

60. Lataste X, Emre M, Davis C, et al. Comparative profile of tizanidine in the management of spasticity. Neurosurgery 1994;44(Suppl 9):s53–s59

61. Gracies JM, Elovic E, McGuire J, et al. Traditional pharmacological treatments for spasticity Part I: Local treatments. Muscle Nerve 1997;20(Suppl 6):S61–S91

62. Yadav SL, Singh U, Dureja GP. Phenol block in the management of spastic cerebral palsy. Ind J Pediatr 1994;61:249–255

63. Koman LA, Mooney JF III, Smith BP, et al. Management of cerebral palsy with botulinum-A toxin: preliminary investigation. J Pediatr Orthop 1993;13: 489–495

64. Koman LA, Mooney JF III, Smith BP. The use of botulinum toxin in the management of cerebral palsy in pediatric patients. In: DasGupta BR, ed. Botulinum and Tetanus Neurotoxins. New York: Plenum Press, 1993:581–587

65. Ajax T, Ross MA, Rodnitzky RL. The role of electromyography in guiding botulinum toxin injections for focal dystonia and spasticity. J Neuro Rehab 1998;12:1–4

66. Delgado MR. The use of botulinum toxin type A in children with cerebral palsy: a retrospective study. Eur J Neurol 1999;6(Suppl 4):S11–S18

67. Boyd RN, Graham JE, Nattrass GR, et al. Medium-term response characterization and risk factor analysis of botulinum toxin type A in the management of spasticity in children with cerebral palsy. Eur J Neurol 1999;6:S37–S45

68. Cosgrove AP, Corry IS, Graham HK. Botulinum toxin in the management of the lower limb in cerebral palsy. Dev Med Child Neurol 1994;36:386–396

69. Calderon-Gonzalez R, Calderon-Sepulveda R, Rincon-Reyes M, et al. Botulinum toxin A in management of cerebral palsy. Pediatr Neurosurg 1994;10:284–288

70. Corry IS, Cosgrove AP, Walsh EG, et al. Botulinum toxin A in the hemiplegic upper limb: a double-blind trial. Dev Med Child Neurol 1997;39:185–193

71. Corry IS, Cosgrove AP, Duffy CM, et al. Botulinum toxin A compared with stretching casts in the treatment of spastic equinus: a randomised prospective trial. J Pediatr Orthop 1998;18:304–311

72. Koman LA, Smith BP, Tingey CT, et al. The effect of botulinum toxin type A injections on the natural history of equinus foot deformity in paediatric cerebral palsy patients. Eur J Neurol 1999;6(Suppl 4):S19–S22

73. Forssberg H, Tedroff KB. Botulinum toxin treatment in cerebral palsy: intervention with poor evaluation? Dev Med Child Neurol 1997;39:635–640

74. Albright AL, Barry MJ, Fasick P, et al. Continuous intrathecal baclofen infusion for symptomatic generalized dystonia. Neurosurgery 1996;181:934–939

75. Albright AL. Baclofen in the treatment of cerebral palsy. J Child Neurol 1996;11:77–83

76. Grabb PA, Guin-Renfroe S, Meythaler JM. Midthoracic catheter tip placement for intrathecal baclofen administration in children with quadriparetic spasticity. Neurosurgery 1999;45:833–837

77. Van Schaeybroeck P, Nuttin B, Lagae L, et al. Intrathecal baclofen for intractable cerebral spasticity: a prospective placebo-controlled, double-blind study. Neurosurgery 2000;46:603–612

78. Damiano DL, Kelly LE, Vaughan CL. Effects of quadriceps strengthening in crouched gait in children with spastic diplegia. Phys Ther 1995;75:658–667

79. Gilmartin R, Bruce D, Abbott R, et al. Intrathecal baclofen for the management of spastic cerebral palsy: multicenter trial. J Child Neurol 2000;15:71–77

80. Medtronic. Intrathecal Baclofen Therapy: Clinical Reference Guide for Spasticity Management. Minneapolis: Medtronic, 1996

81. Green LB, Nelson VS. Death after withdrawal of intrathecal baclofen: case report and literature review. Arch Phys Med Rehab 1999;80:1600–1604

82. Albright AL, Cervi A, Singletary J. Intrathecal baclofen

for spasticity in cerebral palsy. JAMA 1991;265: 1418–1422

83. Albright AL, Barron WB, Fasick MP, et al. Continuous baclofen infusion for spasticity of cerebral origin. JAMA 1993;270:2475–2477

84. Albright AL, Barry MJ, Fasick MP, et al. Effects of continuous intrathecal baclofen infusion and selective posterior rhizotomy on upper extremity spasticity. Neurosurgery 1995;23:82–85

85. Penn RD, Gianino JM, York MM. Intrathecal baclofen for motor disorders. Movement Dis 1995;10:675–677

86. Latash ML, Penn RD. Changes in voluntary motor control induced by intrathecal baclofen in patients with spasticity of different etiology. Physiother Res Int 1996;1:229–246

87. Steinbok P, Daveshvar H, Evans D, et al. Cost analysis of continuous intrathecal baclofen versus selective functional posterior rhizotomy in the treatment of spastic quadriplegia associated with cerebral palsy. Pediatr Neurosurg 1995;22:255–264

88. Alemeida GL, Campbell SK, Girolami GL, et al. Multidimensional assessment of motor function in a child with cerebal palsy following intrathecal administration of baclofen. Phys Ther 1997;77:751–764

89. Armstrong RW, Steinbok P, Cochrane DD, et al. Intrathecally administered baclofen infusion for treatment of children with spasticity of cerebral origin. J Neurosurg 1997;87:409–414

90. Gerszten PC, Albright AL, Barry MJ. Effect on ambulation of continuous intrathecal baclofen infusion. Pediatr Neurosurg 1997;27:40–44

91. Gerszten PC, Albright AL, Johnstone G. Intrathecal baclofen infusion and subsequent orthopedic surgery in patients with spastic cerebal palsy. J Neurosurg 1998;88:1009–1013

92. Meythaler JM, Guin-Renfroe S, Hadley MN. Continuously infused intrathecal baclofen for spastic/dystonic hemiplegia. Am J Phys Med Rehab 1999;78:247–254

93. Rawicki B. Treatment of cerebal origin spasticity with continuous intrathecal baclofen delivered via an implantable pump: long-term follow-up review of 18 patients. J Neurosurg 1999;91:733–736

94. Meythaler JM, Guin-Renfroe S, Grabb PA, et al. Long-term continuously infused baclofen for spastic-dystonic hypertonia in traumatic brain injury: 1-year experience. Arch Phys Med Rehab 1999;80:13–19

95. Peacock WJ, Staudt L. Selective posterior rhizotomy: history and results. Neurosurg: State of the Art Rev 1989;4:403–408

96. Lazareff JA, Garcia-Mendez MA, De Rosa R, et al. Limited (L4–S1, L5–S1) Selective dorsal rhizotomy for reducing spasticity in cerebral palsy. Acta Neurochir 1999;141:743–751

97. Engsberg JR, Ross SA, Park TS. Changes in ankle spasticity and strength following selective dorsal rhizotomy and physical therapy for spastic cerebral palsy. J Neurosurg 1999;91:727–732

98. Chicoine MR, Park TS, Voger GP, et al. Predictors of ability to walk after selective dorsal rhizotomy in children with cerebral palsy. Neurosurgery 1996;38:711–714

99. McLaughlin JF, Bjornson KF, Astley SJ, et al. Selective dorsal rhizotomy: efficacy and safety in an investigator-masked randomized clinical trial. Dev Med Child Neurol 1998;40:220–232

100. Wright F, Sheil EM, Drake JM, et al. Evaluation of selective dorsal rhizotomy for the reduction of spasticity in cerebral palsy: a randomized control study. Dev Med Child Neurol 1998;40:239–247

101. Lin JP. Dorsal rhizotomy and physical therapy. Dev Med Child Neurol 1998 Apr;40(4):219

102. Renshaw TS, Green NE, Griffin PP, et al. Cerebral palsy: orthopedic management. J Bone Joint Surg 1995;77-A:1590–1606

103. Rang M, Wright J. What have 30 years of medical progress done for cerebral palsy? Clin Orthop Rel Res 1989;247:55–60

104. Solnit A, Stark M. Mourning and the birth of a defective child. Psychoanalytic Study of the Child 1961:523–537

105. Olshansky S. Chronic sorrow: a response to having a defective child. Social Casework 1962:190–193

106. Leff P, Walizer E. Building the Healing Partnership: Parents, Professionals, and Children with Chronic Illnesses and Disabilities. Cambridge: Brookline Books, 1992

107. Graham P, Rutter M. Organic brain dysfunction and child psychiatric disorder. Br Med J 1968;iii:695–700

108. Breslau N, Marshall I. Psychological disturbance in children with physical disabilities: continuity and change in a 5-year follow-up. J Abnormal Child Psychol 1985;13:199–216

109. Sundheim M, Ryan R, Voeller K. Mental retardation. In: Coffey E, Brumbach R, eds. Textbook of Pediatric Neuropsychiatry. Washington DC: American Psychiatric Association Press, 1998:649–690

110. Reiss S, Levitan G, Syszko J. Emotional disturbance and mental retardation's diagnostic overshadowing. Am J Ment Defic 1982;86:567–574

111. Kalachnik J, Leventhal B, James D, et al. Guidelines for the use of psychotropic medication. In: Reiss S, Aman M, eds. Psychotropic Medications and Developmental Disabilities. Columbus: Ohio State Press, 1998:45–72

112. Syzmanski L. Diagnosis of mental disorder in people with mental retardation. In: Reiss S, Aman M, eds. Psychotropic Medications and Developmental Disabilities. Columbus: Ohio State Press, 1998:3–17

113. Reiss S, Aman M. Psychotropic Medications and Developmental Disabilities. Columbus: Ohio State Press, 1998

114. Everson J. Youth with Disabilities. Boston: Andover Medical Publishers, 1998

156 Disorders of Learning and Behavior in Children

Peter B Rosenberger

Introduction

Cognition and social engagement are arguably the two most important agendas of the human organism during its developing years. Because both depend heavily upon the brain, it is no surprise that they occupy so much of the practice effort of the child neurologist. At the same time, both are addressed in detail by many other therapeutic disciplines with which neurology must share the patient's attention. It is thus important that the practitioner be aware of the *neurological perspective* on these questions.

To begin with, neurological nosologies of learning disability have traditionally focused on the functional deficit, borrowing from syndromes of altered cortical function in adults. This approach has occasionally been misleading, as in the case of developmental dyslexia, the most common mechanism of which—phonemic unawareness—is seldom found in cases of acquired dyslexia. Nevertheless, it provides valuable clues to diagnosis and recognition which are often unavailable to the psychologist or educator. Thus a left-handed male child with a history of spoken language delay who is having difficulty learning to read, and who has a father and brother with the same problem, is dyslectic until proven otherwise, regardless of the level of reading skills on standard tests.

The neurological perspective also has implications for dealing with allied medical specialities. Thus although behavior is obviously to a significant extent a product of brain function, this chapter will not deal in detail with disorders of conduct or emotional stability. Whenever possible, such matters are better left to specialists in child psychiatry.

Disorders of learning in early life

Disorders of language

Of the specific learning disorders recognized during the preschool years, the most readily identifiable and thoroughly studied are those of language function. The usual presenting symptom is that the child is not talking as well as expected for age, and thus the clinician needs first to establish (a) that hearing is normal, and (b) that the primary speech mechanism is functioning. The latter can be difficult. An anatomical lesion, such as a submucous cleft palate, or bilateral corticospinal tract malfunction due to cerebral palsy, can severely incapacitate speech in a child with normal language function.

The nosology of the developmental language disorders is complex and has undergone considerable evolution in recent years. Rapin[1] suggests that the clinician needs to be aware of three main categories involving (1) phonology, (2) verbal expression, and (3) language processing. The subtypes under these main categories are of theoretical interest as questions for further research. However, only a few have known therapeutic relevance at present.

1. For a child who is not acquiring spoken language at the expected rate, the prognosis for spontaneous resolution is directly related to the degree to which general intelligence, and in particular receptive language, is preserved. Thus when phonologic encoding and/or verbal dyspraxia are identified as the principal deficits, parents can be reassured that there is a high probability that the child will be speaking intelligibly by school age. Formal measurement of receptive language function by a speech–language pathologist is the most useful laboratory assessment in such cases. Based on the studies of Tallal and coworkers,[2] a technique has been devised for training of phonemic awareness[3] which may prove useful as a rational therapy for developmental expressive language delay.

2. When phonologic *de*coding is the primary deficit, the result is a verbal auditory agnosia, or pure word deafness. In this case an acquired epileptic aphasia, or Landau–Kleffner syndrome,[4] should be suspected, even when the problem is of such early onset that no clear deterioration of language function can be documented. The electroencephalographic finding of temporal lobe epileptic discharges, or of continuous spike–wave activity during sleep (ESES), can be helpful, although the absence of such findings does not rule out the diagnosis when the clinical picture is characteristic. Anticonvulsant medications are helpful for seizures in this syndrome, but usually have no effect on the language deficit. Recently treatment with high-dose corticosteroids[5] or with intravenous immunoglobulin[6] has been shown to be helpful in small numbers of cases.

3. Deficits involving higher-order language processing may be more difficult to recognize, as sentence structure may be relatively intact. When the deficit is one of semantics, the child will exhibit problems with word-finding and may actually circumlocute. When pragmatics are primarily affected, verbal output may resemble that of the adult with very mild Wernicke's aphasia ("Casey Stengel speech"). Echolalia, either immediate or delayed (nursery

rhymes, radio commercials etc.) may be a feature. In either case therapy is basically educational, and there is unfortunately a dearth of information from controlled studies to support the claims of any specific method.

Disorders of speech fluency

Fluency is a relative attribute of speech, occurring along a spectrum in the normal population. Dysfluency of some degree is practically universal among young children, but nearly always resolves as language skills are acquired. The most common dysfluency, stuttering, can either be acquired as result of a specific brain lesion, or can be spontaneous in onset during early to middle childhood, constituting a significant handicap in about 4% of children. As a general rule, the longer a child speaks fluently before beginning to stutter ("fluent interval"), the worse the prognosis. Thus, the child who does not begin to stutter until early adolescence is usually in for a prolonged struggle. However, nearly 80% of all stutterers eventually show some improvement, with virtual disappearance by middle adulthood in about 50%. Stuttering is more common in males, and has long been recognized to have a strong genetic component.

There has been a long-standing controversy as to whether stuttering is primarily a disorder of language or of motor planning. Evidence from imaging studies supports both hypotheses. Although neurophysiological and pharmacological studies strongly confirm deficits in motor integration and planning,[7] there is much evidence for association with language disorders. Stutterers whose fluency is improved by reading aloud perform better on tests of reading comprehension and spelling than their counterparts who remain dysfluent while reading. Stuttering is associated with non-right handedness and dyslexia, both in individuals and in families.

The mainstay of treatment for stuttering is speech therapy. Traditional therapies have focused on slowing the rate of speech, entraining it or giving it rhythm; associated motor behaviors such as pencil strokes; or declaiming as if from the stage or pulpit. Intensive programs based on operant conditioning principles, some employing delayed auditory feedback, have a sound rationale and have been dramatically effective in severe cases, although carryover outside the laboratory is variable. A wide variety of medications have been shown to be effective in selected cases, but none has proved beneficial for stutterers in general. Those of greatest theoretical interest include antidopaminergic agents, especially haloperidol,[8] and anticompulsive medications such as fluoxetine and clomipramine. Stuttering is currently under investigation as a candidate PANDAS disorder (see below).

Disorders of social awareness and engagement

Autism Autism, once thought to represent a psychodynamic reaction to traumatic events in early childhood, is now practically universally recognized as a disorder of brain function. Although the core features

of the syndrome (social isolation, atypical language development and a restricted behavioral repertoire) are seen in the context of a wide variety of developmental disorders, there remains a cohort of children for whom these are essentially the only deficits. Onset before age 30 months is usually required as a criterion for the diagnosis, and signs are frequently seen in early infancy. The language disorder may be one of several of those mentioned above, but prominent receptive language deficit is practically universal. The prognosis is highly variable; as a rule, social isolation resolves somewhat as receptive language improves.

Every autistic child should have an electroencephalogram some time before age five; depending upon selection criteria, as many as 50% will have seizures at some point. If there is clinical reason to suspect focal encephalopathy, an MRI scan should be obtained, with careful attention to medial temporal, hippocampal and amygdalar areas. Many studies over the years have attempted to define a specific cognitive deficit in autism. Those of Frith and colleagues[9] concerning "theory of mind" have most successfully explained the disorder of social awareness. Simple tests are now available for assessment of this ability in young children; most involve talking about pictures, but some are ingeniously constructed so as not to require verbal interchange.

Of behavioral interventions to cope with autistic deficits, those currently believed most effective combine intensive language stimulation with systematic behavioral management.[10] The most convincing demonstration of the long-term effects of intensive intervention comes from the studies of Lovaas and co-workers.[11] Pharmacotherapy is for the most part symptomatic for associated symptoms. The attention deficits sometimes (but by no means always) respond to the stimulant medications in small doses. Clonidine and guanficine can be useful for reducing impulsiveness. Major neuroleptics should be used with care, as the disorder is lifelong. The one class of medication that appears helpful in improving social engagement and awareness are the selective serotonin reuptake inhibitors, especially fluvoxamine.[12] This finding is of especial interest in view of recent demonstrations of abnormal brain serotonin synthesis capacity in autistic children.[13]

As is frequently the case with serious disorders of unknown etiology, autism has been the target of many unconventional therapies. Mega-doses of common vitamins were popular for many years. More recently, a report of a small number of children with both autism and gastrointestinal malabsorption spurred interest in the use of the gastric enzyme secretin, and enthusiastic testimonials about improvement have generated a cottage industry in this treatment. None of these therapies has withstood the test of properly controlled trials.

Asperger syndrome Clinical reviews have traditionally lumped this syndrome together with others of the "autistic spectrum"; however, the distinctions are beginning to be of therapeutic relevance. The feature that most importantly distinguished Asperger children from other autistic children is the relative preservation of receptive language. Asperger children are typically introverted, rigid and obsessive in thinking, and resistant to change or novelty. They are particularly inept at reading social messages or cues – "can't take a hint". Their cognitive disorder tends to be of the non-verbal variety, with spatial awareness deficits, dyscalculia and "overfocused" attention (see below), all suggestive of right hemisphere dysfunction. The clinical spectrum has been reviewed by Frith.[14] Management is chiefly by accommodation, and here the clinician can be of great assistance to the child, family and friends, and teachers. Pharmacological intervention, if any, is again symptomatic for attention deficits, anxiety, and obsessive–compulsive tendencies. Again, "overfocused" attention does not respond particularly well to the stimulant medications typically used for attention deficit. It is too early to say whether the serotoninergic medications will be beneficial for the social difficulties of Asperger children.

Disorders with autistic features   Recognition of autistic features in children with other identifiable brain disorders has been primarily responsible for the recent shift toward viewing autism as a functional deficit rather than a specific disease process. Many children with profound mental retardation show some autistic features, but they are particularly striking in Rett syndrome, the fragile-x genetic deficit, and in untreated phenylketonuria (fortunately a rarity in modern times). They are seen in perhaps half of children with the Landau–Kleffner syndrome, a fact which has led to much misplaced parental enthusiasm for steroid treatment of autistic children. We have also seen autistic features in children recovering from encephalitis involving the medial temporal lobes. Management is the same as for the core autistic syndrome, except that identification of an underlying disease process is frequently helpful for genetic or other counseling.

Disorders of academic function
General principles

In the management of disorders of learning in the school-age child the clinician will be dealing even more frequently with non-medical professionals, chiefly psychologists and educational specialists. It thus becomes especially important to recognize that the biological perspective on these disorders is only one of several. It will frequently be heard that a particular educational professional "doesn't believe in" a particular learning disorder. It must then be borne in mind that one would no more ask the teacher to diagnose dyslexia in a poor reader than one would expect the track coach to recognize muscular dystrophy in a poor runner. This does not mean that the teacher's or the psychologist's perspective is less valid—it is merely different.

Principles axiomatic to the biological perspective include the following, which are reviewed in greater detail elsewhere:[15]

- The term "ability" is often applied interchangeably to aptitude and skill. Learning *disabilities are aptitude* deficits, which in turn are *reflected* in skill deficits. This becomes important when one is asked to exclude a particular child from a diagnosis of learning disability, because skills do not fall below the norm by a criterion amount.
- Learning disabilities are relatively specific aptitude deficits, but the aptitudes they involve do not differ in kind from the other aptitudes that go together to make up learning ability in general (intelligence). There is thus no logical justification for the assumption that a child with a specific learning disability would not in some sense be smarter without it.

Diagnosis   The basic diagnosis of learning disabilities, as with other neurological conditions, is by history and physical examination. However, formal psychometry is essential in most cases. Testing is best obtained from an experienced educational psychologist; although a neuropsychological approach is helpful, formal neuropsychological evaluation is usually not required. Information is needed regarding general scholastic aptitude (intelligence), specific aptitudes (language, perceptual), and achievement in basic academic skills. A detailed discussion of the available tests has been prepared for the medical clinician.[16]

Management   The management of specific learning disabilities has three basic goals: to help the child acquire the skill in question despite the lack of aptitude; to help the child cope with academic challenges despite the lack of skill; and to preserve self-esteem and motivation in the process. The first of these is accomplished by *remedial instruction*, the recommendation for which can be more or less specific depending upon our understanding of the mechanism involved, as noted below. The second is achieved by *curriculum support*, which is what is usually provided by resource rooms and learning centers in the state schools. It is important for all involved to understand that these two missions differ, and that educational plans, especially beyond the third grade, must provide for both. The third is less well defined, but none the less important. Children need to be involved with activities in which they can excel publicly, and it is a rare child for whom some such activity cannot be found. It is not difficult for a child to be the best archer on the block: there usually aren't any others.

Dyslexia

Dyslexia, or specific reading disability, is the longest-recognized and most thoroughly studied of the learning disabilities. It favors males by a ratio of at least three to one, and is strongly familial. Although a single gene locus has not been established with certainty, a genetic tendency is supported by studies of concordance in monozygotic and dizygotic twins.

Problems with spoken language during the preschool years place a child at high risk for dyslexia.

The great majority, perhaps 90%, of all children with developmental specific reading disability can be shown to have a deficit in phonemic awareness, which multiple studies have correlated with dysfunction in the major temporal lobe. This finding unfortunately does not explain the difficulty many dyslectic children have with recognition of letters of the alphabet, but it does provide a valuable clue to treatment. Dyslectic children need to be taught the principles of phonetic analysis: they cannot be relied on to pick up this skill for themselves. This is best accomplished by tutorials (individual, or in groups of three or fewer), outside the regular classroom, at the hands of an experienced tutor of the dyslectic reader, according to a highly systematic rule-based method that directly addresses the phonetic structure of the spoken language. The Orton–Gillingham technique is the prototype of such methods, although somewhat tedious in intensive application. Derivative techniques such as the Stevenson method, the Wilson method or Project READ can be effective as well. A specific program for training of phonemic awareness, known as "Fast ForWord", has a sound rationale, but its efficacy over the long term in large-scale studies remains to be proven.

To whatever extent functional illiteracy persists

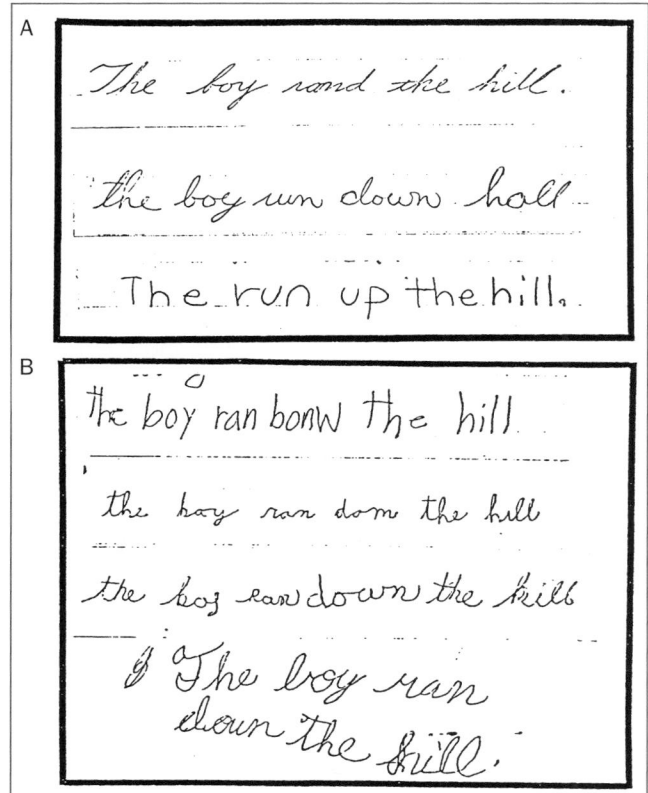

Figure 156.1 Written response of several learning-disabled boys to a dictated sentence. "Linguistic" dysgraphia (group A) is distinguished from "mechanical" dysgraphia (group B). (From[15] with permission.)

beyond the third grade, dyslectic students will need curriculum support as well, to help them learn what they need to learn despite being unable to extract information from the printed page. Group study, audiovisual aids and books on tape all serve this purpose. Accommodations that can be helpful in the upper grades and beyond include additional time for examinations that require reading, proofreading of written compositions for errors of spelling and punctuation, and waivers of foreign language requirements for school admission or graduation.

Dysgraphia

The consensus of research on developmental dysgraphia is that two main types can be distinguished: linguistic, and mechanical (Figure 156.1). The majority of children of either type are also dyslectic, but especially the mechanical or "dysorthographic" type can be found in the absence of reading disability. The key to management is accommodation. Children with either type need to be given sufficient time to get their thoughts down on paper at a rate that produces a coherent and legible output. Homework assignments need to be proofread before being handed in. The wordprocessor is a godsend for the dysgraphic student, especially of the dysorthographic type: it allows the production of a legible letter with a simple keystroke, and eliminates the need for complete rewriting after proofreading. Parents providing such prosthetic devices on a doctor's prescription can usually deduct the purchase price from their taxable income as a medical expense. Improvement of handwriting legibility is often one of the most dramatic effects of stimulant medications on attention deficit.

Dyscalculia

The mechanisms of developmental dyscalculia are less well understood than those of dyslexia or dysgraphia. The conventional wisdom, supported by considerable research, is that deficits of spatial awareness and visuomotor coordination are characteristic of these children; however, this mechanism probably accounts for only one of several subtypes of dyscalculia. Analysis of the types of errors made by dyscalculic children (Figure 156.2) has thus far been of only limited help in clarifying these subtypes.

The majority of children having specific difficulties with maths also have attention deficits, and in a substantial portion of that group the "dyscalculia" is actually secondary to the attention problem. When the child has problems with factual recall, makes careless errors or cannot finish enough examples within the required time, attention deficit should be suspected as the chief culprit.

Management, apart from treatment of the attention deficit in appropriate cases, will consist largely of remedial instruction. A competent special education teacher will discern at what stage the obstruction has been encountered, whether with basic concepts of addition and subtraction, place value, regrouping or beyond. Counseling for realistic choices of future maths courses can also be helpful.

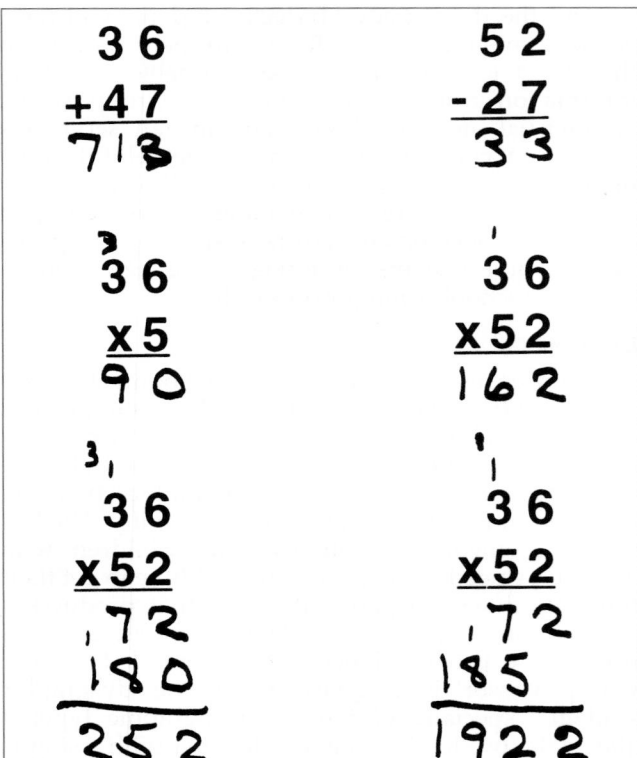

Figure 156.2 Some of the types of errors most commonly made by dyscalculic children.

Attention deficit

Attention deficit is an important cognitive handicap, recognized by neurologists for over a century to be the sequela of a large variety of diffuse insults to the brain. This history is reviewed in detail elsewhere.[17] Attention deficit as a disease entity is thus in very much the same category as epilepsy. The neurologist is well advised to leave the diagnosis of "attention deficit disorder" to colleagues in psychiatry, and side-step the controversy over whether such a syndrome exists. We do disagree with educational administrators who maintain that attention deficit is not a learning disorder.

Attention deficit is measured in a variety of ways. In addition to direct measures, including physiological, psychophysical and psychometric instruments, a number of useful indirect (questionnaire) assessments are available (see[17] for a list).

Attention deficit is not only comorbid to a significant degree with most other specific learning disorders, it also interacts with them; and the aggravation is mutual. This is most obvious in the case of dyscalculia, but is also clearly seen with the others (see above).

Management of attention deficit is a combination of direct treatment and counseling to improve coping strategies by the patient, and accommodations by school, home and workplace. The only direct therapeutic intervention of proven benefit to attention itself is stimulant medications in small doses. The two

classes of drug most widely used are amphetamine preparations and methylphenidate; pemoline is equally effective, but has fallen into disfavor because of liver toxicity. A new combination of amphetamine salts including the racemic form (Adderall) has been shown to have a longer duration of action than methylphenidate sustained release (Ritalin SR), but newer extended-action methylphenidate preparations currently being tested may prove equally effective. For school-age children, a four-week trial is usually sufficient for a reliable judgment about effectiveness. For those in the lower grades the class teacher should be asked to fill out a brief standard checklist, preferably one using items directly from the DSM criteria. The medication, e.g. Adderall 5 mg in the morning for children under 30 kg, 10 mg for those above, is given on schooldays for four weeks, after which the teacher is asked to fill out the checklist once again, and the child returns to see the physician. If either Ritalin or Adderall is ineffective or poorly tolerated, the other should be tried. When the effect is reported in later months to have "worn off", increasing the dose may be helpful, but this is a "slippery slope" and should be avoided whenever possible.

Coping strategies are extremely important, especially for students in the higher grades. The teacher needs to understand that the classroom may not be a setting in which the child performs most effectively. Classroom exercises that cannot be completed during class time should be sent home for completion there. Important examinations may require additional time and, when possible, administration in a separate quiet setting. At home, it is essential that the child has a place for study that is for his/her exclusive use, as well as only for study. A rigid schedule for activities on schooldays can also be helpful.

Attention deficit-related syndromes

Tourette syndrome A high prevalence of attention deficit has long been recognized among children with the syndrome of Gilles de la Tourette (*tic convulsif*). As many as half of such children will show evidence of attention deficit prior to the onset of tics. The problem is that the medications most helpful for attention deficit are highly likely to precipitate or aggravate tics in such patients.

The consensus of experts in this disorder is that careful administration of small doses of stimulant medications, with frequent monitoring, is appropriate in cases in which the attention deficit is sufficiently handicapping. Denckla and co-workers,[18] who have studied the cognitive deficit in Tourette syndrome extensively, believe that the primary problem is one of speed and celerity of motor response, and that "pure Tourette's" patients actually show less difficulty with executive function than those with comorbid attention deficit disorder.

The "overfocused" child Kinsbourne[19] described an atypical form of attention deficit in which the child obsessively chooses a single focus of attention, sometimes to the detriment of effective function. Such children are usually introverted and socially inept, and may show evidence of right hemisphere dysfunction, with low performance IQ scores and visuomotor coordination deficit. There may be no essential difference between this disorder and mild forms of the Asperger syndrome (see above). Clinical consensus (not well supported by formal studies) is that this type of attention deficit does not react well to stimulant medications. Treatment of allied symptoms (anxiety, obsessive–compulsive tendencies) may be more profitable.

PANDAS Swedo and co-workers[20] have found evidence of an autoimmune response to previous streptococcal infection in some patients with tic disorders and obsessive–compulsive symptoms, and have coined the term "PANDAS" (*p*ediatric *a*utoimmune *n*europsychiatric *d*isorders *a*ssociated with *s*treptococcal infection) to describe this syndrome. These findings are of interest to the clinician treating attention deficits, in view of the comorbidity of these disorders with attention deficit disorder, the high prevalence of attention deficits in patients with Sydenham's chorea, and numerous demonstrations of basal ganglia abnormality in patients with attention deficit. Intravenous immunoglobulin has been tried in a small number of especially severe cases, with some apparent success.

References

1. Rapin I. Developmental language disorders: a clinical update. J Child Psychiatry Psychol 1996;37:643–655
2. Tallal P, Stark R. Speech discrimination abilities of normally developing and language-impaired children. J Acoust Soc Am 1981;69:568
3. Merzenich M, Jenkins W, Johnston P, Schreiner C, Miller S, Tallal P. Temporal processing deficits of language-learning impaired children ameliorated by training. Science 1996;271:77–80
4. Landau W, Kleffner F. Syndrome of acquired aphasia and convulsive disorders in children. Neurology 1957;7:523–530
5. Lerman P, Lerman-Sagie T, Kively S. Effect of early corticosteroid therapy for Landau–Kleffner syndrome. Dev Med Child Neurol 1991;33:257–260
6. Lagae L, Silberstein J, Gillis P, Caesar P. Successful use of intravenous immunoglobulin in Landau–Kleffner syndrome. Pediatr Neurol 1998;18:165–168
7. Nudelman H, Herbrich K, Hoyt B, Rosenfield D. A neuroscience model of stuttering. J Fluency Dis 1989; 14:399–427
8. Rosenberger P. Dopaminergic systems and speech fluency. J Fluency Dis 1980;5:255–267
9. Frith U, Morton J, Leslie A. The cognitive basis of a biological disorder: autism. Trends Neurosci 1991;14: 433–438
10. Rogers S, Lewis H. An effective day treatment model for young children with pervasive developmental disorders. J Am Acad Child Adolesc Psychiatry 1989;28: 207–214
11. McEachin J, Smith T, Lovaas O. Long-term outcome for children with autism who received early intensive behavioral treatment. Am J Ment Retard 1993;97: 359–372
12. McDougle C, Naylor S, Cohen D, Volkmar F, Heninger G, Price L. A double-blind, placebo controlled study of fluvozamine in adults with autistic disorder. Arch Gen Psychiatry 1996;53:1001–1008
13. Chugani D, Muzik O, Behen M, et al. Developmental changes in brain serotonin synthesis capacity in autistic and nonautistic children. Ann Neurol 1999;45:287–295
14. Frith U. Asperger and his syndrome. In: Frith U, ed. Autism and Asperger Syndrome. Cambridge: Cambridge University Press, 1991:16–21
15. Rosenberger P. Learning disorders. In: Berg B, ed. Principles of Child Neurology. New York: McGraw-Hill, 1996:355–369
16. Rosenberger P. The pediatrician and psychometric testing. Pediatr Rev 1981;2:301–310
17. Rosenberger P. Attention deficit. Pediatr Neurol 1991; 7:397–405
18. Harris E, Schuerholz L, Singer H, et al. Executive function in children with Tourette syndrome and/or attention deficit hyperactivity disorder. J Int Neuropsychol Soc 1995;1:511–516
19. Kinsbourne M. Overfocusing: an apparent subtype of attention deficit hyperactivity disorder. In: Amir N, Rapin I, Branski D, eds. Pediatric Neurology: Behavior and Cognition of the Child with Brain Dysfunction. Basel: Karger, 1991:18–35
20. Swedo S, Leonard H, Garver M, et al. Pediatric autoimmune neuropsychiatric disorders associated with streptococcal infections: clinical description of the first 50 cases. Am J Psychiatry 1998;155:264–271

Glossary of terms

Dyscalculia – disorder of calculation or number manipulation
Dysgraphia – disorder of writing
Dyslexia – disorder of reading
Entraining – regulation of behavior through an exteroceptive signal
Operant conditioning – regulation of behavior through manipulation of consequences
Orthography – the mechanical process of construction of written letters and words
Phonic – pertaining to sounds
Phonemic – pertaining to *combination* of sounds to form the speech code
Phonetic – pertaining to *written representation* of the speech code
Phonologic – pertaining to the *study* of any or all of the above
Pragmatic – the employment of language to achieve a goal or purpose
Semantic – the employment of language to convey meaning

157 Chromosomal Disorders, Inborn Errors of Metabolism and Degenerative Diseases

Michael I Shevell

Introduction

An extraordinarily diverse and numerous group of entities are contained within the rubric of this chapter. Individually they are rare, collectively these disorders constitute a considerable burden of morbidity, and indeed mortality, in the practice of pediatric neurology. This individual rarity challenges the practitioner, who may see but a handful of cases of a specific disorder over a career lifetime. The challenge is not only with respect to the accurate and timely recognition of a specific diagnosis, but also with regard to providing appropriate therapeutic interventions that may lessen, or more rarely reverse, disease progression. The rarity of these entities, together with the frequent lack of therapeutic alternatives, also provides an often insurmountable barrier to undertaking therapeutic trials that meet the burdens of proof imposed by randomized prospective double-blind controlled clinical trials. Reports in the literature of the effects of specific treatments are often anecdotal case reports or small series which compare outcomes in a few individuals against the known natural history of a disorder.

In addition to their rarity, these disorders challenge the clinician by their frequent heterogeneity. A single disorder may have protean clinical manifestations, depending on the age of onset (e.g. metachromatic leukodystrophy). Furthermore, clinical presentation may resemble that noted for far more common conditions (e.g. organic aciduria and infantile sepsis). Accurate diagnosis of these rare disorders is the necessary precondition for meaningful therapeutic intervention. As a result of an accurate early diagnosis, specific therapy may be available to alleviate symptoms or lessen disease progression. Such interventions are almost inevitably more effective if instituted at an early stage.

Accurate diagnosis also provides an insight into the genetic and biochemical mechanisms of disease occurrence. Recent advances in molecular genetics frequently permit gene identification, raising the possibility of prenatal diagnosis, presymptomatic diagnosis and/or carrier detection in other family members. Diagnosis also provides a means of access to a clearer understanding of prognosis and, via a diverse array of support groups, to others who are struggling with the challenge of coping with a child with a rare and frequently devastating, illness. A specific diagnostic label may also provide the key to accessing special-ized services (both rehabilitation and nursing). All of these serve to empower the child's family and lessen the overall effects of illness on the child and family.

General treatment issues

Certain issues and symptoms cut across the necessity for a specific diagnosis, and their proper management can be applied in toto to the entire spectrum of disorders considered in this chapter. These issues and symptoms will be presented and considered initially, as together they form a background template for an effective comprehensive clinical management and therapeutic approach.

Seizures occur frequently within the context of these disorders. For some (e.g. neuronal ceroid lipofuscinosis and epileptic myoclonus), the seizures experienced are a prominent part of the disorder's presentation and evolution. For others (e.g. Down syndrome and infantile spasms), the seizures occur at an increased frequency compared to the general pediatric population. Seizures may occur as a result of metabolic disturbances (e.g. non-ketotic hyperglycinemia) or cortical dysgenesis (e.g. Zellweger syndrome). Seizures are frequently mixed in type and may be intractable. Complete seizure control may at times be elusive, but should be strived for so as to lessen intermittent additional encephalopathy and the familial burden of care. General principles of anticonvulsant management apply. Specifically, drug selection should be determined by the seizure type experienced by the individual, and polypharmacy avoided if at all possible. Seizures (e.g. complex partial, atypical absences) may be subtle in character and masked by an already existing cognitive disability or behavioral disturbance. The clinician should be particularly sensitive to the sedating effect of excessive anticonvulsant usage (i.e. phenobarbital, benzodiazepines), given the often limited cognitive reserve of this patient population. Some authors recommend the avoidance of valproic acid derivatives in the setting of a known mitochondrial cytopathy. Disorders of carbohydrate or fatty acid metabolism should effectively preclude consideration of the ketogenic diet as a therapeutic alternative.

Spasticity, especially that which is progressive and quadriparetic in distribution, may also be a prominent feature of these disorders. It may initially limit acquired mobility and, if unchecked, may lead to progressive scoliosis, compromised respiratory function and an enhanced burden of care. For some of these disorders (e.g. leukodystrophies) spasticity is an early and salient feature of illness. Regular physiotherapy and stretching exercises are the initial step in preventing contracture formation, together with the use of appliances. For some individuals with prominent spasticity that is painful or which limits the provision of daily care (e.g. dressing, bathing, transferring), alternatives include antispasticity medications (i.e. baclofen, an analog of γ-aminobutyric acid—a GABA-B agonist) given either orally or continuously into the subarachnoid space by a subcutaneously implanted pump. Selective dorsal rhizotomy, popular in the comprehensive management of the spastic diplegic variant of cerebral palsy, has not yet been systematically studied in this group of disorders.

Several of the degenerative diseases and inborn errors of metabolism have a prominent effect on basal ganglia structures and may thus display extrapyramidal symptoms such as dystonia, choreoathetosis or tics, which may be disabling to the affected individual either by limiting functional skills or enhancing the burden of care. Examples of such disorders include dopa-responsive dystonia, dystonia musculorum deformans, Hallervorden–Spatz disease, Lesch–Nyhan syndrome, Wilson disease, glutaric aciduria type I and cobalamin C disease. Specific pharmacological treatment depends on the predominant targeted movement disorder: (a) dystonia–dopa agonists or anticholinergics, (b) choreoathetosis–dopamine antagonists, (c) tic-selective dopamine blockers or α_1-adrenergic blockers.

Inappropriate behaviors may also be prominent in these disorders to an extent requiring therapeutic, including pharmacological, intervention. Inattention, with or without associated hyperactivity and impulsivity, may occur. It has been noted with particular frequency in children with the fragile X syndrome. Existing significant cognitive disability may prevent caregivers, educators and clinicians from appreciating inattention as a significant issue limiting learning and participation. Non-pharmacological and pharmacological strategies can be utilized to improve attention and lessen distractability along the same lines as in non-cognitively disabled children with ADHD. The response to stimulant medication (i.e. methylphenidate) in this population tends not to be as frequently positive, with a higher frequency of observed side effects, thus necessitating a slower introduction of medication and stepwise increments. Agitation, disinhibition and aggression, towards self and others, also occur with increased frequency in this population. Indeed, self-mutilation is frequently a diagnostic hallmark of Lesch–Nyhan syndrome or hereditary tyrosinemia. Psychological intervention utilizing behavior management and positive reinforcement principles is the initial approach. Pharmacological management of these symptoms has been largely "hit or miss", with a wide variety of agents being used on speculation, with recent enthusiasm for the use of risperidone evident.

Regular restful sleep which is time-locked to the diurnal cycle of caregivers may also be elusive at times. Frequently there may be difficulty in initiating and maintaining sleep, with frequent nocturnal awakenings and excessive daytime somnolence. Nocturnal awakenings may be particularly disruptive to the household unit, especially if accompanied by agitation. Sleep deprivation can be a prominent disruptive stress to the family unit that may effectively limit the ability to provide continuous ongoing quality care, despite the very best of intentions. Pharmacological options exist for this symptom and include bedtime use of chloral hydrate, benzodiazepines (e.g. ativan) or melatonin.

The medical clinician providing either ongoing or specialty care to children with these disorders needs to be explicitly cognisant of the multiplicity of care needs that demands an interdisciplinary approach, utilizing skills from a variety of healthcare and allied professionals. Occupational therapists provide expertise and input to maximize function in relation to activities of daily living and lessen the burden of care. Physiotherapists strive to maximize mobility and limit contracture formation. Speech–language pathologists assist in realizing communication potential that may require the use of augmentative or assistive technologies and, in some instances, non-verbal means of communication (i.e. American Sign Language, Bliss boards). Behavioral issues often require the intervention of psychologists who can also ably assist in determining cognitive ability, which may be a major factor in determining proper school placement and the need for supplemental educational resources. Special educators sensitive to the different learning skills and styles possessed by cognitively disabled children often provide such supplemental education. Frequently these disorders have a known genetic mechanism, which requires the expertise of geneticists and genetic counselors to assist in management. In addition, they assist in explaining and interpreting within the family context such issues as future prenatal diagnosis, carrier detection and screening of asymptomatic family members.

The best caregiver possible for these children is their own loving, supportive and nurturing family. This is evident by the widespread trend away from institutionalization. However, the burdens placed upon such a family to take care of a child with a handicapping and rare illness that is often progressive should not be underestimated, nor taken for granted. Tangible supports provided by nursing contacts and services concerning basic issues such as daily care, feeding and medicating, need to be put into place, as well as options for respite care if the burden become too great. Frequently there are emotional issues regarding acceptance, anger, guilt or loneliness that may become paramount and which need to be addressed through resources provided by social workers, family counselors and psychologists. The value of contact with other individuals and families struggling with the same rare disorder should also not be overlooked. Families welcome the knowledge that a support group exists and find comfort among those who truly understand what they are going through. Information technology such as the Internet has created many "virtual" communities among those in need. Finally, towards the end of life for these children, palliative care provided by an established team with pediatric expertise may be necessary.

Chromosomal disorders

Chromosomal disorders may be considered diagnostically within the context of several discrete clinical situations. These include the dysmorphic child, whose pattern of dysmorphic features may suggest a specific syndromic diagnosis (e.g. Down syndrome, fragile X), the child with multiple congenital anomalies, and the child with a global developmental delay or mental retardation, especially if associated with microcephaly. Indeed, global delay or cognitive disability may be the predominant symptom of an underlying chromosomal disorder in the absence of any obvious dysmorphology.

Laboratory investigations that may diagnose chromosomal disorders include standard high-resolution G-banding (i.e. karyotype); fluorescent in situ hybridization (FISH) employing fluorescent tagged segments of molecular DNA to reveal microdeletion syndromes; and chromosome painting employing a diverse array of tagged molecular probes against particular chromosomes, which is effective in detecting subtelomeric deletions. Actual chromosomal abnormalities of diagnostic relevance include (a) alterations in the actual number of chromosomes (aneuploidy), (b) expansions, deletions, duplications, inversions or translocations of a segment of chromosomal DNA, and (c) alterations in imprinting expression.

For practical purposes, discussion in this section will be limited to the following entities: Down syndrome, fragile X syndrome, Williams syndrome, Miller–Dieker syndrome, Di George syndrome, Prader–Willi syndrome and Angelman syndrome.

Down syndrome

First described in the mid-1800s in a group of institutionalized patients, this syndrome was well delineated long before the discovery of the actual underlying chromosomal defect in 1959. All individuals with Down syndrome have a full or partial trisomy of chromosome 21. For the vast majority this is the result of a non-dysjunction event occurring during the first phase of maternal meiosis. This is a phenomenon that increases with advancing maternal age. For a small minority (typically less than 5%) an unbalanced translocation of a portion of chromosome 21, usually with chromosome 14, is found. Down syndrome is the most common of the aneuplodies and is a relatively frequent cause of cognitive disability.

The child with Down syndrome does not usually present a diagnostic challenge except for those who are mosaic for the disorder, in whom facial dysmorphic features may be quite subtle. The dysmorphic features of the child with Down syndrome, which

often prompt the diagnosis shortly after birth, are well described and easily recognized and will not be repeated here. Non-neurological medical issues that occur with increased prevalence in individuals with Down syndrome include congenital cardiac defects (particularly involving the atrial septum and endocardial cushion), hypothyroidism, gastrointestinal abnormalities including celiac disease, and hematologic malignancies (typically non-lymphocytic leukemias). The American Academy of Pediatrics has established guidelines for the ongoing management of children with Down syndrome.

From a neurological perspective a number of issues arise, including hypotonia, atlantoaxial instability which may impair spinal cord integrity, cognitive disability (which may be quite variable), seizures, behavioral disorders, and a later-onset dementing process. It is pronounced ligamentous laxity that underlies both the observed hypotonia and atlantoaxial instability. Clinicians need to be sensitive to the early signs and symptoms of evolving spinal cord compression (i.e. neck pain, gait changes, bowel or bladder dysfunction, new pyramidal tract signs) in this population that should prompt radiological investigation. Universal screening for this entity is no longer considered necessary. The cognitive disability is related to underlying reduced neuronal density, altered synaptic density and impaired myelination. This probably also relates to an increased observed seizure frequency, particularly of infantile spasms, that warrants specific directed anticonvulsant management. Behavioral disorders include inattention, hyperactivity and agitation that may require pharmacological intervention (see above). Finally, individuals with Down syndrome may undergo Alzheimer-like changes in their brains, featuring the formation of neurofibrillary plaques and neuritic tangles pathologically at an early age which manifests clinically as a cognitive decline from baseline. This is thought to be related to the chromosome 21 location of the amyloid precursor protein (APP) gene that has been linked to familial Alzheimer disease. Treatment for this process, when it occurs, includes the elimination of treatable conditions such as hypothyroidism or depression as a cause for the observed dementia. Treatment with acetylcholinesterase inhibitors has not yet been systematically attempted in this subgroup.

Fragile X syndrome

Over 50 X-linked disorders account for the predominance of cognitive disability among males compared to females. All of these disorders are relatively rare, with the exception of the fragile X syndrome, which is one of the more common causes of mental retardation. First described clinically in an extended family in the 1940s, it was only in 1969 that its chromosomal basis became apparent. Cytogenetically, a fragile site prone to breakage at the distal end of the X chromosome was noted in cells from affected individuals grown in thymidine-deficient media (typically one in which folic acid was omitted). The gene (FMR-1) underlying fragile X syndrome was cloned in the early 1990s and the molecular mechanism responsible for the disorder elucidated. Specifically, a triplet repeat (CGG) expansion beyond a critical number (more than 200 repeats) near the promoter region of this gene results in hypermethylation of the promoter region, lack of *FMR-1* gene expression, chromosomal fragility and the associated syndromic clinical features.

The fragile X syndrome demonstrates X-linked inheritance; however, females can be affected (reflecting uneven Lyonization in critical tissues) and unaffected males can have unaffected daughters, who can then have affected children (Sherman paradox). This is related to the phenomenon of an unstable premutation (between 50 and 200 repeats) that may undergo expansion to a full mutation during oogenesis but not spermatogenesis. Molecular diagnosis of the *FMR-1* premutation and full mutation is possible using a standardized Southern blot analysis employing DNA probes and restriction enzyme digestion. This analysis is far more sensitive than the previously relied-upon cytogenetic means of diagnosis.

Individuals with fragile X syndrome, especially males, have a characteristic dysmorphology that is usually more apparent with puberty. This includes long facies, prominent ears, jaws and forehead and, among the males, macroorchidism. These dysmorphic features may be less apparent in the younger child at the time of initial presentation for evaluation of a developmental or cognitive disability. Cognitive disability is the major neurological issue for individuals with fragile X, mandating access to appropriate developmental and educational resources. Behavioral issues such as inattention, impulsivity and hyperactivity may also be prominent, interfering with the ability of the individual to derive benefit from supplemental resources and preventing social and educational participation. Psychological intervention and pharmacological agents (i.e. methylphenidate) may be useful adjuncts in this setting. The genetic complexity of the mode of fragile X inheritance has enormous implications for the affected family and maternal relatives, thus mandating referral to genetic resources for full counseling regarding screening of family members and the risk of affected offspring.

Microdeletion syndromes

These disorders feature a submicroscopic deletion of a segment of DNA corresponding to a contiguous gene sequence. Diagnosis is by FISH study utilizing specific molecular DNA probes undertaken in the setting of clinical diagnostic suspicion. Each has an attached characteristic dysmorphology and clinical features. Williams syndrome is the result of a deletion on the long arm of chromosome 7 involving the elastin gene locus. It is characterized by an elfin facies, outgoing voluble personality, supravalvular aortic stenosis and cognitive disability. Despite the cognitive disability, these individuals are frequently musically gifted. Di George syndrome involves a deletion on the long arm of chromosome 22, conotruncal cardiac abnormalities, absent thymus and parathyroids, and frequently

developmental delay. Miller–Dieker syndrome features a deletion on the short arm of chromosome 17 involving the *LIS1* gene locus. These children have type 1 lissencephaly, microcephaly with temporal pinching, severe global developmental delay and frequent seizures. For these disorders, access to developmental services represent the major mode of neurological intervention. Children with Miller–Dieker frequently require seizure-specific anticonvulsant therapy and additional support and nursing services appropriate to the level of their significant delay.

Both Prader–Willi syndrome and Angelman syndrome are also microdeletion syndromes frequently diagnosed by FISH study of an identical region on the long arm of chromosome 15. Phenotypically quite distinct, they are examples of imprinting in which phenotypic expression is determined by whether the deletion is maternal or paternal in origin. In Prader–Willi syndrome the deletion is on the paternally derived chromosome, or there is maternal isodisomy (i.e. two maternal copies) for the critical region of chromosome 15. In Angelman syndrome the deletion is on the maternally derived chromosome 15, or there is paternal isodisomy (i.e. two paternal copies) for the critical region. In children with suspected Prader–Willi or Angelman in whom FISH study is negative, DNA methylation patterns can be analyzed by molecular means to ascertain differential imprinting effects. Prader–Willi syndrome is characterized by early hypotonia, facial dysmorphism, small puffy hands and feet, developmental delay/cognitive disability, later hyperphagia leading to morbid obesity, and disproportionately small genitalia. Angelman syndrome features microcephaly, triangular facies, widely spaced teeth, ataxic gait, an inappropriately happy affect and frequent seizures. Both of these microdeletion syndromes require access to appropriate developmental services. In addition, Prader–Willi individuals require nutrition, psychology and endocrine intervention to deal with the hyperphagia-driven obesity and the frequently resulting type 2 diabetes. The seizures of Angelman syndrome may challenge the best efforts at seizure control.

Inborn errors of metabolism/degenerative diseases

The distinction between degenerative disorders and inborn errors of metabolism can be an arbitrary one that varies from reference to reference. Many inborn errors of metabolism are indeed degenerative, and many degenerative disorders are metabolic in pathogenesis.

Traditionally, inborn errors of metabolism affect the synthesis, metabolism, transport or storage of biochemical compounds. Typically, this refers to amino acid, organic acid, glucose, purine/pyrimidine or mitochondrial metabolism. Disturbances in the biosynthesis of complex macromolecules such as sphingolipids or mucopolysaccharides may or may not be included under this heading. Abnormalities in the metabolism of such macromolecules typically

Table 157.1   Mitochondrial disorders

Pyruvate dehydrogenase complex deficiency
  X-linked (lethal in males)
  Lactic acidosis
  Microcephaly, developmental delay, dysmorphic,
    callosal agenesis
  Leigh disease phenotype
Complex I deficiency
  AR
  Lactic acidosis
  Fatal infantile multisystem disorder
  Myopathy with exercise intolerance
Complex III deficiency
  AR
  Lactic acidosis
  Myopathy/cardiomyopathy
Complex IV (COX) deficiency
  AR
  Lactic acidosis
  Myopathy/encephalomyopathy
  Leigh disease phenotype
Kearns–Sayre–Shy
  Maternal inheritance
  Lactic acidosis
  Progressive external ophthalmoplegia
  Pigmentary retinopathy
MERRF
  Maternal inheritance
  Lactic acidosis/ragged red fibers (muscle biopsy)
  Progressive myoclonic epilepsy
  Myopathy/ataxia
MELAS
  Maternal inheritance
  Lactic acidosis
  Seizures/strokes/headaches
NARP
  Maternal inheritance
  Lactic acidosis
  Developmental delay/neuropathy/ataxia
  Retinitis pigmentosa
Mitochondrial β-oxidation defects
  Non-ketotic hypoglycemia
  Hepatic insufficiency
  Hypotonia/weakness/exercise intolerance
  Cardiomyopathy
Carnitine deficiency
  Non-ketotic hypoglycemia
  Decrease serum carnitine
  Myopathy
  Lipid storage (muscle biopsy)
Carnitine palmityl transferase deficiency
  Non-ketotic hypoglycemia
  Fasting induced lethargy, coma, seizures
  Developmental delay

Rx: coenzyme Q10 (ubiquinone)
  Thiamine (vitamin B_1)
  Riboflavin (vitamin B_2)
  Ascorbic acid (vitamin C)
  Carnitine/creatine supplementation
  Dichloroacetate (?)

AR = Autosomal recessive.

Table 157.2   Peroxisomal disorders

Zellweger
  AR
  Elevated VLCFA/phytanic acid, decreased plasmalogen
  Absent peroxisomal biogenesis
  Dysmorphic facies, hypotonia, renal cysts
  Severe developmental delay
Adrenoleukodystrophy
  X-linked
  Elevated VLCFA
  Behavioral changes, regression, spasticity, visual
    impairment
  Addisonian features
  Adrenomyeloneuropathy
  Rx: bone marrow transplant
Refsum disease
  AR
  Elevated phytanic acid
  Peripheral neuropathy, retinitis pigmentosa, ataxia
  Deafness
  Rx: dietary restriction, plasmapharesis

VLCFA = Very long chained fatty acids.

results in evidence of storage (i.e. lysosome–sphingolipidosis, mucopolysaccharidosis, mucolipidosis, neuronal ceroid lipofuscinosis), white matter disease (i.e. leukodystrophies–Pelizaeus–Merzbacher, adrenoleukodystrophy, metachromatic leukodystrophy, Krabbe, Alexander, Canavan) or disturbances in peroxisomal biogenesis (e.g. Zellweger syndrome). Abnormalities in vitamin (e.g. biotin, Hallervorden–Spatz), metal (e.g. Wilson, Menkes) and cholesterol (e.g. Niemann–Pick type C, Smith–Lemli–Opitz) metabolism have also been described. A comprehensive and inclusive approach will be taken in this chapter.

To further assist readers through what can be a bewildering thicket of eponyms and diseases, tables have been formulated that classify and group these disorders in a simplified manner. Salient mode of inheritance, major clinical features, physical findings, laboratory clues to diagnosis, metabolic defect and specific therapeutic options (where applicable) are listed in these tables.

These disorders present in myriad ways and their accurate diagnosis can challenge the diagnostic vigilance of even the most astute clinician. A single disorder may display clinical heterogeneity in terms of mode of presentation and age of onset even within the same family. Frequently the age of onset predicts the rate of disease progression, with an earlier onset heralding a more rapid rate of progression. Some may present with the non-specific profile of an acute neonatal metabolic distress following a variable postnatal symptom-free interval. Others may present with recurrent symptoms of acute distress occurring later in infancy, childhood, adolescence, or even adulthood. These episodes may be precipitated by minor illness, immunizations, excessive protein intake, or catabolism brought on by fasting. Recurrent symptoms of acute

Table 157.3　Leukodystrophies

Canavan
    AR
    Increased NAA (urine, brain (proton-MRS))
    Spongiform changes on MRI
    Aspartoacylase
    Macrocephaly, developmental delay,
        hypotonia → spasticity
    Seizures
Alexander
    AR
    Cystic white matters changes on CT/MRI
    Astrocytic Rosenthal fibers
    Macrocephaly
    Psychomotor regression
Pelizaeus–Merzbacher
    X-linked
    Hypomyelination/abnormal white matter signal (MRI)
    Proteolipid protein
    Nystagmus, spasticity, psychomotor regression
Adrenoleukodystrophy
    X-linked
    Elevated very long chained fatty acids
    White matter changes (posterior)—MRI
    Behavioral changes, regression, spasticity, visual
        impairment
    Addisonian features
    Adrenomyeloneuropathy
    Rx: BMT
Krabbe
    AR
    Galactocerebrosidase
    Central and peripheral white matter (myelin) changes
    Early onset
    Psychomotor delay → regression
    Spasticity
    Rx: BMT
Metachromatic leukodystrophy
    AR
    Arylsulfatase
    Central and peripheral white matter (myelin) changes
    Motor impairment, regression
    Intellectual deterioration/spasticity
    Rx: BMT

NAA = N-acetylaspartate.

Table 157.4　Progressive myoclonic epilepsies

Lafora body disease
    AR
    PAS + inclusion bodies (muscle or skin biopsy)
    Myoclonic seizures (mid-teens)
    Dementia/psychosis
Baltic myoclonus (Unverricht–Lundborg)
    AR
    Myoclonus
    Dementia
Neuronal ceroid lipofuscinosis
    AR
    Lipofuscins + (rectal biopsy)
    Early infantile/infantile/juvenile/adult forms
    Myoclonus
    Dementia/visual loss

See MERRF/sialidosis.
PAS = Periodic-acid Schiff.

Table 157.5　Neuropathies

Hereditary tyrosinemia
    AR
    Hepatic/renal insufficiency
    Episodic painful neuropathy
    Self-mutilation
    Rx: liver transplant
Giant axonal neuropathy
    AR
    Neurofilament accumulation (nerve biopsy)
    Developmental delay/psychomotor regression
    Ataxia/dysarthria/loss of ambulation
Friedreich's ataxia
    AR
    Frataxin (mitochondrial) deficiency
    Areflexia/ataxia/cardiomyopathy/pes cavus/scoliosis
    Loss of ambulation

Table 157.6　Purines and metals

Lesch–Nyhan
    X-linked
    Elevated uric acid
    Developmental delay/dystonia/choreoathetosis
    Self-injurious behaviors
    Rx: allopurinol
Wilson
    AR
    Decreased serum copper, increased urinary copper
    Hepatic insufficiency/Keyser–Fleischer rings (eye)
    Tremor/dystonia/rigidity
    Psychosis
    Rx: D-penicillamine, liver transplant
Menkes
    X-linked
    Decreased serum copper and ceruloplasmin
    Dysmorphic/friable colorless hair
    Hypotonia/psychomotor regression
    Seizures
    Rx: parenteral copper

distress may include obtundation, stupor or coma, vomiting with lethargy, ataxia, and exercise intolerance featuring myalgia and painful cramps. Others may present with a relentless, either insidious or inexorable, decline in acquired capabilities, highlighted by the loss of either intellectual or motor skills. Disorders evolving in this manner often feature an earlier, more subtle maturational delay in the acquisition of developmental skills. In the older child, alterations in school performance or behavior coupled with incoordination or evidence for a movement disorder may be the presenting clinical picture.

Clinical clues that should prompt the search for one of these disorders include a low threshold for the recognition of the above modes of presentation. Additional clues can include documentation of parental

Table 157.7   Vitamins

Pyridoxine dependency
   AR
   Intractable neonatal seizures
   Rx: pyridoxine (pharmacological)
Biotinidase deficiency
   AR
   Organic aciduria
   Seizures/hypotonia/developmental delay
   Skin rash/alopecia
   Rx: biotin supplementation
Cobalamin metabolism
   AR
   Methylmalonic acidemia and/or homocysteinemia
   Megaloblastic anemia
   Developmental delay/seizures/myelopathy
   Rx: cobalamin (pharmacological), protein restriction,
     carnitine supplementation
     betaine, metronidazole
Biopterin deficiency
   AR
   Elevated phenylalanine, decreased
     serotonin/noradrenaline
   Developmental delay, seizures
   Hypotonia evolving into spasticity and dystonia
   Rx: tetrahydrobiopterin supplementation,
     L-dopa/carbidopa, 5-OH tryptophan

Table 157.8   Basal ganglia disorders

Juvenile Huntington
   AD (paternal)
   Caudate atrophy
   Rigidity/choreoathetosis/behavioral changes/
     dementia
   Rx: dopamine blockers (neuroleptics)
Dystonia musculorum deformans
   AD (Ashkenazi Jews—variable penetrance)
   Progressive dystonia
   Rx: dopamine blockers (neuroleptics)
Dopa-responsive dystonia (Sagawa)
   AD (variable penetrance)
   Parkinsonian features/dystonia
   Rx: L-dopa + carbidopa
Hallervorden–Spatz PKAN-Pantotherate Kinase-
   Associated
   AR
   Neuroaxonal swellings (spheroids)
   Rigidity/dystonia/dementia
   Basal ganglia iron accumulation
   Rx: iron chelators (ineffective)

See also glutaric acidemia type 1.

Table 157.9   Urea cycle

Ornithine transcarbamylase
   X-linked
   Elevated ammonia
   Feeding difficulties/vomiting/seizures/ataxia/
     obtundation
Carbamyl phosphate synthetase/arginosuccinic acid
   synthetase/arginosuccinase/arginase deficiency
   AR
   Elevated ammonia
   Hepatomegaly
   FTT/feeding difficulty/lethargy/obtundation
Rx: dialysis for acute crises
   Arginine, sodium benzoate, sodium phenylacetate
   Dietary restriction of nitrogen intake

Table 157.10   Aminoacidopathies

Hartnup disease
   AR
   Aminoaciduria (neutral aminoacids)
   Intermittent ataxia
   Behavioral changes/ataxia
   Rx: tryptophan supplementation
Maple syrup urine disease
   AR
   Elevated branched-chain amino acids (leucine,
     isoleucine, valine)
   Neonatal metabolic decompensation
   Vomiting/spasticity
   Rx: dietary restriction, dialysis, thiamine
     supplementation
Phenylketonuria
   AR
   Elevated phenylalanine
   Developmental delay/spastic paresis/extrapyramidal
     signs
   Rx: dietary restriction of phenylalanine
Non-ketotic hyperglycinemia
   AR
   Elevated serum and CSF glycine
   Neonatal seizures (intractable)/obtundation and coma
   Severe delay
   Microcephaly
   Rx: sodium benzoate
Homocystinuria
   AR
   Elevated homocysteine
   Lens subluxation
   Developmental delay/seizures/strokes
   Rx: methionine restriction, betaine, pyridoxine
     supplementation

consanguinity (most of these disorders are recessive) and a prior affected child or unexplained loss of a child. Documentation of early seizures suggest the possibility of biotin deficiency, pyridoxine dependency or glucose transporter protein defect. Later myoclonic seizures (i.e. progressive myoclonic epilepsy) are a hallmark of the neuronal ceroid lipofuscinosis, sialidosis, and certain of the mitochondrial disorders (e.g. MELAS, MERRF).

Findings on examination may also provide insight into etiology. Macrocephaly suggests the possibility of Canavan, Alexander, Tay–Sachs or glutaric

Table 157.11   Organic acidemias

Symptom-free interval followed by vomiting, anorexia,
    lethargy (resembles sepsis)
Dehydration/obtundation/coma
Ketosis and acidosis
Abnormal organic acid screen
Multiple carboxylase deficiency
    AR
    Biotin requiring carboxylases affected
    Alopecia/rash
    Rx: biotin supplementation
Methylmalonic aciduria
    AR
    Methylmalonyl CoA mutase
    FTT/RTA
    Stroke (basal ganglia)
    Rx: protein restriction, cobalamin supplementation,
        carnitine
Propionic acidemia
    AR
    Propionyl CoA carboxylase
    Hypotonia/seizures
    Rx: protein restriction, carnitine
Isovaleric acidemia
    AR
    Isovaleryl CoA dehydrogenase
    Rx: protein restriction, glycine supplementation,
        carnitine
Glutaric acidemia type I
    AR
    Glutaryl CoA dehydrogenase
    Macrocephaly
    Developmental delay/spasticity/dystonia/
        choreoathetosis
    Rx: decreased dietary lysine and tryptophan, carnitine,
        riboflavin

Table 157.12   Glucose/carbohydrate disorders

Glucose transporter defect
    AR
    Markedly decreased CSF glucose
    Neonatal–infantile seizures/developmental
        delay/ataxia/microcephaly
    Rx: carbohydrate loading, thioatic acid
Acid maltase deficiency
    Infantile (Pompe)
        Elevated CK/myopathic EMG
        Severe hypotonia/weakness
        Cardiomyopathy
    Childhood
        Elevated CK/myopathic EMG
        Proximal myopathy
        Weakness/motor delay
Muscle phosphorylase deficiency (McArdle)
    AR
    Myoglobinuria
    Exercise intolerance/myalgia/cramps
    Relief by rest
Phosphorylase b kinase deficiency
    AR
    Exercise intolerance
    Myopathy
    Hepatomegaly
Muscle phosphofructokinase deficiency (Tarui)
    Exercise intolerance/myalgia/cramps
    Weakness

Table 157.13   Cholesterol metabolism

Smith–Lemli–Opitz
    AR
    Elevated 7-dehydrocholesterol
    Dysmorphic/microcephaly/FTT
    Developmental delay
    Rx: dietary cholesterol supplementation
Nieman–Pick type C
    AR
    Decreased cholesterol esterification
    Hepatomegaly/hepatic dysfunction
    Developmental delay/ataxia/spasticity
    Vertical gaze paresis
    Rx: cholestyramine, lovostatin

aciduria type 1; microcephaly the possibility of
Smith–Lemli–Opitz. Observed dysmorphic features
may suggest more specifically such entities as Zellweger, mucopolysaccharidosis, mucolipidosis, or
Smith–Lemli–Opitz. Ophthalmological abnormalities
are very common among this group of disorders,
including the classic cherry-red spot (actually a
normal macula surrounded by retinal ganglion
cells swollen with storage material) associated
with Tay–Sachs, GM1 gangliosidosis, sialidosis,
Niemann–Pick type A and Gaucher. Corneal clouding
is a feature of mucopolysaccharidosis and mucolipidosis disorders. Hepatosplenomegaly is a hallmark
of the storage disorders (i.e. sphingolipidosis,
mucopolysaccharidosis, Niemann–Pick, Gaucher). The
white matter tract involvement of the leukodystrophies
leads to an evolving spasticity. Sometimes, owing to
peripheral nerve involvement (i.e. Krabbe, metachromatic leukodystrophy), a mixed spastic and flaccid
paresis of the limbs may be apparent. Hypotonia and
areflexia characterizes the neuroaxonal dystrophies.
Extrapyramidal movement disturbances provide evidence for the basal ganglia involvement that is a prominent feature of juvenile Huntington, Hallervorden–
Spatz, Lesch–Nyhan and Wilson diseases.

The laboratory evaluation of a child with a suspected inborn error of metabolism or degenerative
disease is potentially extensive. Essential investigations
include determination of acid–base balance, glucose,
ammonia, liver function (ALT, AST, γ-GT), lactate,
very long-chain fatty acids, serum amino acid profile,
and a urine screen for organic acids and ketones. Neuroimaging studies are inevitable and a useful adjunct
to document white matter or basal ganglia involvement. Additional investigations should be selectively
undertaken. Specific diagnostic suspicions may prompt
the measurement of serum carnitine (fatty acid oxidation disorders), ceruloplasmin and serum and urine
copper (Wilson, Menkes), 7-dehydrocholesterol

Table 157.14   Lysosomal mucopolysaccharidosis (MPS)

MPS I (Hurler)
    AR
    α-L-Iduronidase
    Coarse features, organomegaly
    Dysostosis multiplex, corneal clouding
    Developmental regression
    Rx: BMT
MPS II (Hunter)
    X-linked
    Iduronosulfate sulfatase
    Coarse features, organomegaly
    Dysostosis multiplex
    Developmental regression
    Rx: BMT(?)
MPS III (Sanfilippo A–D)
    AR
    Accumulation of heparan sulfate
    Coarse features, organomegaly
    Dysostosis multiplex
    Developmental delay → regression
MPS IV (Morquio A/B)
    AR
    Skeletal dysplasia (atlantoaxial
        dislocation/kyphoscoliosis)
    Corneal clouding
    Normal development
MPS VI (Maroteaux–Lamy)
    AR
    Coarse features, organomegaly
    Dysostosis multiplex
    Corneal clouding
    Rx: BMT

Table 157.15   Lysosomal mucolipoidosis and glycoprotein degradation

Mucolipidosis I (sialidosis)
    AR
    Neuraminidase
    PME
    Dysostosis multiplex, organomegaly, coarse facies
    Cherry-red spot
    Developmental regression
Mucolipidosis II (I-cell disease)
    AR
    UDP-N-acetylglucosamine
    Coarse features
    Dysostosis multiplex
    Mental retardation
Sialidosis
    AR
    N-acetylneuraminidase
    Action myoclonus
    Ataxia, spasticity
    Cherry-red spot
Fucosidosis
    AR
    Fucosidase
    Coarse features
    Dystosis multiplex, short stature
    Psychomotor regression
    Rx: BMT (single case report)
Mannosidosis
    AR
    α-mannosidase
    Coarse features, organomegaly
    Developmental delay, mental retardation
    Rx: BMT (single case report)

(Smith–Lemli–Opitz), urinary N-acetylaspartic acid (Canavan), CSF glucose (glucose transporter defect), CSF lactate (pyruvate dehydrogenase deficiency), electrophysiological studies of nerve (neuroaxonal dystrophy, metachromatic leukodystrophy, Krabbe) or muscle (mitochondrial disorders, fatty acid oxidation disorders), and a skeletal survey (mucopolysaccharidosis, mucolipidosis). Definitive diagnosis may ultimately depend on tissue biopsy (skin, liver, smooth muscle, skeletal muscle/nerve), which may yield a diagnosis on either microscopic analysis or enzymatic study. In some of these disorders peripheral leukocytes (e.g. Krabbe) may be an adequate source for enzymatic diagnosis.

For these disorders, apart from medical interventions focusing on observed symptoms (see General principles, above), specific broad therapeutic strategies exist that can be implemented. These include substrate restriction to prevent accumulation to toxic levels (e.g. dietary alteration in PKU), promotion of alternative metabolic elimination pathways (e.g. penicillamine in Wilson), pharmacological metabolic inhibitors (e.g. allopurinol in Lesch–Nyhan), replacement of deficient product (e.g. pyridoxine in pyridoxine dependency), cofactor activation (cobalamin in methylmalonic aciduria) and protein replacement (e.g. bone marrow transplantation in metachromatic leukodystrophy).

Recent advances in molecular genetics have led to raised hopes regarding eventual gene therapy for many of these disorders. This is currently an area of intense research interest at both public funding and private corporate levels. The objective is to introduce a normal copy of the defective gene leading to expression of the responsible deficient protein, and the restoration of metabolic homeostasis. The literature is replete with reports of attempts to correct enzymatic defects in either cell culture or animal models of a variety of inborn errors of metabolism/degenerative diseases. Barriers to the success of gene therapy include the development of reliable delivery systems (either viral or non-viral) that reach the target tissue of interest at a time in the disease course to still be clinically effective in either preventing disease progression or fostering amelioration. At the present time successful gene therapy for any of these diseases remains elusive (possible with the exception of metachromatic leukodystrophy), but is a source of much family hope. Breakthroughs in this area can be reasonably expected within the coming decade.

Table 157.16	Lysosomal sphingolipidosis

Niemann–Pick type A
 AR
 Sphingomyelinase
 Hepatic dysfunction, organomegaly
 Progressive neurological deterioration
 Cherry-red spot
Gaucher
 AR
 Glucocerebrosidase
 Organomegaly
 Psychomotor regression, pyramidal tract signs
 Rx: splenectomy, i.v. glucocerebrosidase
GM₁ gangliosidosis
 AR
 β-galactosidase
 Primary sensory impairments (vision, hearing)
 Psychomotor delay → regression
 Cherry-red spot
GM₂ gangliosidosis (Tay–Sachs)
 AR
 Hexosaminidase A
 Macrocephaly
 Spasticity
 Psychomotor delay → regression
 Cherry-red spot
Sandhoff
 AR
 Hexosaminidase A/B
 Gait disturbance, clumsiness
 Tremors, dystonia

References

Texts

Jones KL. Smith's Recognizable Patterns of Human Malformation. 5th ed. Philadelphia: WB Saunders, 1997

Lyon G, Adams RD, Kolodny EH. Neurology of Hereditary Metabolic Diseases of Children. New York: McGraw-Hill, 1996

Maria BL. Current Management in Child Neurology. 2nd ed. Hamilton, Ontario: BC Decker, 2002

Rosenberg RN, Prusiner SB, DiMauro S, Barchi RL. The Molecular and Genetic Basis of Neurological Disease. 2nd ed. Boston: Butterworth-Heinemann, 1997

Scriver CR, Beaudet AL, Sly WS, Valle D. The Metabolic and Molecular Basis of Inherited Disease. 8th ed. New York: McGraw-Hill, 2001

Swaiman KF, Ashwal S. Pediatric Neurology: Principles and Practice. 3rd ed. St. Louis: Mosby, 1999

Articles

Anon. Health supervision for children with fragile X syndrome. American Academy of Pediatrics Committee on Genetics. Pediatrics 1996;98:297–300

Balicki D, Beutler E. Gene therapy of human disease. Medicine 2002;81:69–86

Berardelli A, Curra A, Manfredi M. Torsion dystonia. Curr Opin Neurol 1996;9:317–320

Berger J, Moser HW, Forst-Pettr S. Leukodystrophies: recent developments in genetics, molecular biology, pathogenesis and treatment. Curr Opin Neurol 2001;14: 305–312

Berkovic SF, Andermann F, Carpenter S, Wolf LS. Progressive myoclonus epilepsy: specific causes and diagnosis. N Engl J Med 1986;315:296–305

Blau V, Thony B, Renneberg A, et al. Dihydropteridine reduc-

tase deficiency localized to the central nervous system. J Inherit Metab Dis 1998;21:433–434

Brady RO. Therapy for the sphingolipidoses. Arch Neurol 1998;55:1055–1056

Brusilow SW, Maestri NE. Urea cycle disorders: diagnosis, pathophysiology and therapy. Adv Pediatr 1996;43: 127–170

Chinnery PF, Turnbull DM. Epidemiology and treatment of mitochondrial disorders. Am J Med Genet 2001;106: 94–101

Cohen WI. Health care guidelines for individuals with Down syndrome—1999 revision. Down Syndrome Q 1999;4:1–15

Fowler B. Genetic defects of folate and cobalamin metabolism. Eur J Pediatr 1998;157(Suppl 2):S60–S66

Furukawa Y, Kish SJ. Dopa responsive dystonia: recent advances and remaining issues to be addressed. Movement Dis 1999;14:709–715

Gillis L, Kaye E. Diagnosis and management of mitochondrial diseases. Pediatr Clin North Am 2002;49:203–219

Gordon N. Pyridoxine dependency: an update. Dev Med Child Neurol 1997;39:63–65

Hynes J, Wolf B. Biotinidase and its role in brain metabolism. Clin Chim Acta 1996;255:1–11

Kelley RI. Inborn errors of cholesterol biosynthesis. Adv Pediatr 2000;47:1–53

Krivan G, Timar L, Goda V, et al. Bone marrow transplantation in non-malignant disorders. Bone Marrow Transplant 1998;22(Suppl 4):S80–S83

Leonard JV, Morris AA. Inborn errors of metabolism around the time of birth. Lancet 2000;356:583–587

Leonard JV, Walter JH, McKiernan PJ. The management of organic acidemias. J Inherit Metab Dis 2001;24:309–311

Menkes JH. Menkes disease and Wilson disease: two sides of the same copper coin. Part I and Part II. Eur J Pediatr Neurol 1999;3:147–158; 245–253

Miano M, Poeta F, Locatelli F, et al. Unrelated donor marrow transplantation for inborn errors. Bone Marrow Transplant 1998;21(Suppl 2):S37–S41

Mitchell GA, Wang SP, Ashmarina L, et al. Inborn errors of ketogenesis. Biochem Soc Trans 1998;20:136–140

Moser HW. Neurometabolic disease. Curr Opin Neurol 1998;11:91–95

Nyhan WL, Wong DF. New approaches to understanding Lesch–Nyhan disease. N Engl J Med 1996;334: 1602–1604

Patel PI, Isaya G. Friedreich ataxia: from GAA triplet repeat expansion to frataxin deficiency. Am J Hum Genet 2001;69:15–24

Raymond GV. Peroxisomal disorders. Curr Opin Pediatr 1999;11:572–576

Scriver CR, Treacy EP. Is there treatment for "genetic" disease? Mol Genet Metab 1999;68:93–102

Shapira SK. An update on chromosome deletion and microdeletion syndromes. Curr Opin Pediatr 1998;10: 622–627

Stone JE. Urine analysis in the diagnosis of mucopolysaccharide disorders. Ann Clin Biochem 1998;315 (Pt 2): 207–225

Swaiman KF. Hallervorden–Spatz syndrome. Pediatr Neurol 2001;25:102–108

Selected online resources

1. Health professional
   www.ncbi.nlm.nih.gov/omim
   www.geneclinics.org
2. Patient/family oriented
   www.rarediseases.org
   www.umdf.org
   www.ndss.org
   www.geneticalliance.org

158 Neurocutaneous Disorders

Robert S Rust

In 1933 van der Hoeve classified five hereditary neurocutaneous conditions as phakomatoses, because four of them were associated with hamartoma formation.[1] Subsequently, more than 140 additional conditions have been termed "neurocutaneous," conditions wherein cutaneous findings disclose the presence of or risk for neurological abnormalities. Tumor formation is not a required feature and cutaneous findings may be less diagnostic than characteristic changes of hair, eyes, or noncutaneous blood vessels. Most neurocutaneous conditions are hereditary, although some do not as yet have a clearly identified mechanism of inheritance and many individual cases arise as the result of new mutations, although the participation of germline mutation or mosaic inheritance is not always easy to discern. A fairly inclusive working list of neurocutaneous conditions is found in Table 158.1, grouped by mode of inheritance. The list of these conditions would be much longer if patients with cutaneous markers whose sole neurological manifestation is mental retardation were included.

Within the space assigned for this review, only a small selection of the most important neurocutaneous conditions can be included and with these conditions emphasis will be placed on management rather than the burgeoning subject of the genetics and mechanisms of neurocutaneous diseases. Suffice it to say that many of these conditions are pleomorphic and many are evolutive in manifestations, and that there are considerable areas of semiological overlap between various entities. The rate of evolution and degree of expression of many conditions may be influenced by environmental exposures, trauma, infection, age and state of tissue development, hormonal milieu, or other influences. Clinical expression may be gradual, saltatory, fulminant, or may arrest in a very partial state. A great deal of effort has been expended in the past two decades to identify the genetic substrate and mechanisms that govern variability in these conditions and to establish consensus diagnostic criteria.

Most neurocutaneous conditions are dysembryoblastic developmental disturbances of embryonic plates, differing in the type and degree of germ layer (exoblastic, mesoblastic, or endoblastic) involvement.[2] The particular conjunction of abnormalities of skin, hair, nails, and nervous system, eyes, and ears in many neurocutaneous conditions reflects these variable effects on these specialized tissues of ectodermal origin. But many neurocutaneous conditions affect mesodermal tissues (blood vessels, bone, connective tissues) and somewhat fewer involve entodermal tissue derivatives. Only conditions that are associated with the development of hamartomas or other tumors should be termed "phakomatoses." These include neurofibromatosis, tuberous sclerosis, von Hippel–Lindau disease, and nevoid basal cell carcinoma syndrome.

Major autosomal dominant neurocutaneous disorders

Neurofibromatosis (von Recklinghausen's disease, neuroectodermosis, congenital neuroectodermal dysplasia)

Some of the distinctive features of the neurofibromatosis (NF) spectrum were recognized long before von Recklinghausen's classic 1882 account.[3–5] NF2 was thought to be a variant of NF1 prior to its designation as a clinically and genetically distinct disease. Both of these conditions exhibit marked variability of clinical expression.[6] The fundamental disturbances in these conditions involve migration, localization, and maturation of cells derived from the neural crest and entail risk for excessive growth of various tissues. They are prototypic hereditary tumor syndromes, most tumors arising from the Schwann cell sheaths of cranial, spinal, sympathetic, or peripheral nerves. However, many abnormal processes may occur in additional systems, involving endocrine, gastrointestinal, and both peripheral and central nervous tissues. Diagnostic manifestations are often present at birth, although in many instances they are overlooked or difficult to detect. The age at which manifestations become evident or at diagnosis does not predict severity of disease.[7]

NF1 is the most commonly encountered phakomatosis and neurocutaneous syndrome and is one of the most common human autosomal dominant conditions. NF1 is found in approximately 1/3000–3500 live births, as compared to an incidence of 1/50 000–100 000 live births for NF2. Thus, NF1 accounts for at least 85% of all examples of NF.[8] The gene for NF1, encoding neurofibromin, is in the pericentric region of chromosome 17 (band 11.2).[9] Penetrance of NF1 is very nearly 100% in adults and the molecular mechanisms of this disease are increasingly well understood.[10] Between 30% and 50% of all NF1 cases are new mutations, of which more than 240 have been catalogued.[8] The reproductive capacity of affected individuals with an NF1 engendering mutation is reduced, on average, and for unclear reasons, by about 50%.[11] NF2 has been associated with defects of a tumor suppressor gene located on chromosome 22 (22q11.2) that is responsible for the expression of a protein termed merlin or schwannomin.[12] Penetrance

Table 158.1 Neurocutaneous disorders

Autosomal dominant conditions
  Neurofibromatosis-1
    Variant and related conditions
      Isolated familial intestinal neurofibromatosis
      Isolated neurofibromatosis with multiple endocrine
        neoplasia
      Neurofibromatosis–Noonan syndrome
      Isolated hereditary spinal neurofibromatosis
      Watson syndrome
      Syndrome of complete absence of NF1 gene
      Familial multiple neurofibromas, schwannomas, and
        uterine leiomyomas
  Neurofibromatosis-2
    Variant and related conditions
      Multiple schwannomatosis
      Familial multiple plexiform schwannomas
      Sporadic meningioangiomatosis
  Tuberous sclerosis complex
    von Hippel–Lindau Disease
    Hereditary hemorrhagic telangiectasis (Rendu–Osler–
      Weber Disease)
    HID syndrome
    IFAP syndrome
    KID syndrome
    LEOPARD syndrome (multiple lentigines syndrome)
    Nevoid basal cell carcinoma syndrome (Gorlin syndrome)
    Noonan syndrome (cardiofaciocutaneous syndrome)
    Piebald trait with neurological deficits
    Preaxial anonychia with neurological defects
    Tangier Island disease
    Variegate porphyria
    Verbov–Sharland syndrome
    Waardenburg syndrome

X-linked, male-lethal syndromes
  CHILD syndrome
  Focal dermal hypoplasia syndrome
  Incontinentia pigmenti (Bloch–Sulzberger syndrome)
  MIDAS syndrome
  OFD I syndrome

X-linked nonlethal inheritance
  Adrenoleukodystrophy
  Albinism–deafness syndrome
  Bullous dystrophy of the Mendes da Costa type
  Dyskeratosis congenita
  Fabry disease
  Hoyeraal–Hreidarsson syndrome
  Lesch–Nyhan syndrome
  Menkes disease

Possible mosaicism of autosomal lethal mutations
  Sturge–Weber syndrome
  Variant and related conditions
    Klippel–Trenaunay syndrome
    Epilepsy with bilateral occipital calcification
    Syndrome of bilateral facial nevi, mosaicism, anomalous
      venous return
    Syndrome of facial angioma, posterior fossa cyst, partial
      ACC
    Leptomeningeal angiomatosis
  Delleman syndrome (oculocerebrocutaneous syndrome)
  Encephalocraniocutaneous lipomatosis
  Neurocutaneous melanosis
  Pallister–Killian syndrome
  Phakomatosis pigmentokeratitis
  Phakomatosis pigmentovascularis
  Pigmentary mosaicism of the Ito type
  Proteus syndrome
  Schimmelpenning syndrome
  Van Lohuizen syndrome

Autosomal recessive conditions
  Acrodermatitis acidemica
  Amish brittle hair syndrome (BIDS, Tay syndrome)
  Aspartylglucosaminoaciduria
  Ataxia–telangiectasia
  Björnstad syndrome
  CHIME syndrome
  Cockayne syndrome
  Cross syndrome
  De Basry syndrome
  Divry–Van Bogaert syndrome
  Dubowitz syndrome
  Elejalde syndrome
  Hartnup's syndrome
  Meckel–Gruber syndrome
  Multiple sulfatase deficiency
  Neutral lipoid storage disease
  Oculocutaneous albinism
  Refsum disease
  Shapira syndrome
  Sjögren–Larson syndrome
  Steijlman syndrome
  Urbach–Weithe disease (lipoid proteinosis)
  Xeroderma pigmentosum

Sex chromosome aneuploidy
  Ullrich–Turner syndrome

Sporadic conditions of known mechanism of inheritance
  Angelman syndrome

*Sporadic, known mechanism of inheritance (could include those
listed as due to mosaicism of autosomal lethal mutations)*
  Brachman–De Lange syndrome
  Blue rubber nevus syndrome
  Chediak–Higashi syndrome
  Cobb syndrome (cutaneomeningioangiomatosis)
  Johnston syndrome
  Maffucci syndrome (multiple enchondromatosis)
  Nevus unius lateris
  Nevus sebaceus of Jadassohn
  Nicolaides–Baraitser syndrome
  Ollier syndrome
  Parry–Romberg syndrome
  Rothmund–Thomson syndrome
  Rud syndrome
  Satoyoshi syndrome

*Heritable mental retardation syndromes with manifestations of
skin, bone, or hair*
  Biotinidase deficiency
  Cobalamin C deficiency
  Fucosidosis II
  Fucosidosis III
  GM_1 gangliosidosis type II
  Homocystinuria
  Isovaleric acidemia
  Lowe disease
  α-mannosidosis
  β-mannosidosis
  Methylmalonic acidemia
  Mucolipidosis II (I-cell)
  Mucolipidosis III
  Mucopolysaccharidosis I
  Mucopolysaccharidosis II
  Mucopolysaccharidosis III
  Propionic acidemia
  Sialidosis II

Table 158.2   Diagnostic criteria for neurofibromatosis–1[15]

Two or more of the following:
  At least six *café au lait* macules: greatest diameter
    >5 mm if prepubertal, >15 mm if postpubertal
  Axillary freckling
  Two or more iris hamartomas (Lisch nodules)
  Optic glioma
  At least two neurofibromas of any type
  One or more plexiform neuroma
  Typical bone lesion (sphenoid dysplasia, cortex
    thinning, tibial pseudarthrosis)
  At least one first degree relative with NF1 by these
    criteria

Table 158.3   Conditions that may manifest multiple *café au lait* macules[22]

Neurofibromatosis-1
Neurofibromatosis-2
Bannayan–Riley–Ruvalcaba syndrome
Familial multiple *café au lait* macules
Maffucci syndrome
McCune–Albright syndrome
Multiple lentigines syndrome
Multiple neuroma syndrome (multiple endocrine
neoplasia syndrome type IIb)
Tuberous sclerosis
Watson's syndrome

by adulthood is greater than 95%. Between 50% and 75% of cases arise as new mutations.[13] Understanding of the molecular aspects of NF2 has also advanced greatly in recent years.[14] There is no known ethnic predilection for either form of NF.[11] The diagnostic criteria for each type of neurofibromatosis are listed in Tables 158.2 and 158.4 respectively.

Neurofibromatosis-1 NF1's former designation as "peripheral" NF was applied because of the prominent cutaneous manifestations, which may be the only findings. However, the term "peripheral" does not adequately convey the appreciable risk for central nervous system and visceral complications. *Café au lait* macules, the hallmark of NF1, are often the first recognizable sign. At least one is found in almost every case, and in most instances six spots greater than 0.5 cm in one dimension are seen by one year of age. Lesions darken, enlarge, and increase in number with age. In prepubertal individuals finding six of that size is considered unique and diagnostic of NF1. Six such *café au lait* macules of at least 1.5 cm indicate NF1 in postpubertal individuals, and are found in approximately 80% of cases.[16] They may occur anywhere on the body, but are more common on the trunk than the limbs. Palms, soles, eyebrow regions, and scalp are typically spared. Most are ovoid, with smooth margins. As a rule, pigmentation is uniform and of a darker hue than that of the surrounding skin. Few entirely new *café au lait* macules arise in NF patients after 1 to 2 years of age. Excepting the fact that some fading of these macules may occur late in life,[17] the subsequent cutaneous pigmentary evolution of NF1 is typically limited to the possible appearance of freckling. Histological examination of pigmented lesions can confirm the diagnosis of NF1 due to characteristic melanosome abnormalities, but is seldom necessary.[18]

Some patients with six or more *café au lait* macules remain free of other known NF1 manifestations.[19] Thus, caution must be maintained in assigning a diagnosis to very young children with six or more *café au lait* spots but no family history or other manifestations of NF1. Nonetheless, most such individuals will be found, in time, to have NF1. The confinement of numerous *café au lait* macules to a single unilateral

body segment has been termed "segmental NF."[20] Approximately 5% to 10% of normal and 15% of all neurologically handicapped individuals as well as 26% of those with tuberous sclerosis have at least one or two but rarely three *café au lait* spots.[21] Various other conditions that manifest multiple *café au lait* macules are listed in Table 158.3.

Freckling (multiple 1–4 mm *café au lait* macules) in the axillary and inguinal intertriginous regions is another finding that strongly supports the diagnosis of NF1. Freckles are found in approximately 80% of patients[23] and usually develop before 6 years of age. They may also be found on areas of "skin–skin" contact in the axillary and inguinal regions. Patches of freckles may be found just below the breasts of some older women with NF1.[7] Early childhood total body "freckling" suggests NF even in individuals with somewhat less than the requisite number and size of typical *café au lait* macules.[24] Nonfamilial hyperpigmentation involving most or all of the skin should also prompt consideration of the diagnosis of NF1.[20] Hypopigmented macules resembling those of tuberous sclerosis and "white freckles" are also reasonably common in NF1. These lesions may be pseudoatrophic or hypoplastic macular neurofibromas.[25]

Fibromata molluscum are flat, sessile, or pedunculated tumors that arise from the dermis in some patients with NF1 at some point after infancy. Soft or firm, they are readily compressible into the underlying dermal tissues. They are the same hue as skin or slightly darker and range in size from millimeters to several centimeters. Benign skin angiomas may occur. Juvenile xanthogranulomas are found in less than 10% of young NF1 patients. They involute after a few years, but signify enhanced risk for juvenile chronic myelogenous leukemia.[26] Other dermal features of NF1 include glabrous, velvety skin texture and laxity of skin, subcutaneous tissues, and joints. In the face this renders the appearance of premature aging. Joints may be hyperextensible and secondary creases of palms, interphalangeal joints, and finger pads may be found.[27]

Peripheral nervous system in NF1 Peripheral neurofibromas are, with *café au lait* macules, one of the two most characteristic and conspicuous features of NF1, although they occasionally arise in individuals that do not have NF1. They arise from nerve sheath Schwann cells and almost always involve the skin.[28] They may be found in any portion of a peripheral nerve or in sympathetic ganglia and range in size from a few millimeters up to two centimeters in diameter. Three types of neurofibromas are highly specific for NF1: multiple cutaneous neurofibromas, subcutaneous plexiform neuromas, and massive soft tissue neurofibromas. A fourth type, the localized intraneural neurofibroma of the spine, occurs in NF1 and in individuals not known to have neurofibromas. Plexiform neuromas and localized intraneural neurofibromas are subject to sarcomatous transformation.

Neurofibromas occur rarely in children with NF1 that are as young as 4 to 5 years of age. They arise more typically at 8 to 12 years of age; growth may be stimulated by puberty, trauma, or pregnancy.[7] Eyelid neurofibromas are important exceptions, typically congenital and detectable very early in life. Detection of these by eyelid palpation indicates an enhanced risk for congenital glaucoma. Areolar neurofibromas are found in about 80% of postpubertal women with NF1.[23] Although neurofibromas of NF1 provoke self-consciousness, they do not alter the appearance of affected individuals to the degree represented by John Merrick, the "elephant man," who had Proteus syndrome rather than NF1. The venerable misattribution of his deformities to NF has been the source of immeasurable psychosocial stress in individuals with NF1.[29]

Cutaneous neurofibromas are the color of surrounding skin or may have a slightly violaceous hue. They are pedunculated or broad based and move with surrounding skin. A moderate amount of digital pressure may induce invagination of some lesions through an underlying dermal defect ("buttonholing") that is "almost specific" for NF1.[21] Some appear to be little more than skin tags. Some patients may have few and some have countless neurofibromas.

Palpable subcutaneous neurofibromas develop along the course of peripheral nerves. One fifth of NF1 patients have at least one. Some patients have many, some arranged along a given nerve like a "string of large beads."[30] They are firmer than cutaneous neurofibromas, but their nontender rubbery roundness and mobility distinguish them from invasive or aggressive tumors. Newly developing and enlarging cutaneous or subcutaneous neurofibromas may itch, probably due to the presence of mast cells.[31] Perhaps 5% of NF1 patients experience pain from one of more of their subcutaneous neurofibromas.

Subcutaneous neurofibromas only occasionally interfere with the function of nerves from which they arise.[32] Growth of these lesions within a bony canal such as vertebral foramina may result in severe pain and neuropathy due to compression, scoliosis, or vertebral collapse. Paraspinous neurofibromas may compress anterior spinal roots or the spinal cord. Sarcomatous transformation of neurofibromas may result in neuropathy. In 2% to 8% of individuals with NF1, a plexiform neuroma will undergo transformation into a highly malignant neurofibrosarcoma,

a tumor for which the prognosis is poor. This process must be considered in any individual with NF1 who has rapid enlargement of a subcutaneous neurofibroma or who manifests neuropathic changes or worsening pain.[16]

Plexiform neuromas develop in some NF1 patients; one third are quite large.[33] They combine the features of cutaneous and subcutaneous neurofibromas and may result in significant morbidity due to disfigurement, functional disturbances, or transformation into life-threatening malignant peripheral nerve sheath tumors (MPNSTs)[34] including the "Triton tumor."[35] Plexiform neuromas may be nodular or diffuse. The nodular variety consist of an intertwined network of large subcutaneous neurofibromas; firm and often tender nodules are arrayed along the cords of nerve plexuses or dorsal spinal roots. The diffuse variety arise congenitally in about 5% of NF1 patients, although the lesion may not become palpable until later in childhood. The nexus of limb and trunk and the orbit are favored locations. A relatively modest degree of cutaneous hyperpigmentation and hypertrichosis may overlie an extensive lesion involving subjacent fascia, muscle and bone. They include highly vascular masses of neurofibromas, and the regional bone and connective tissues may hypertrophy resulting in disfigurement.[36]

Orbital/periorbital plexiform neuromas occur in about 5% of NF1 patients. Diffuse growth may produce hemimegalencephaly,[37] a condition to which the unfortunate term "cranial elephantiasis" is sometimes applied. Proptosis, visual dysfunction, or buphthalmos may also develop.[38] A plexiform neuroma behind the ear may overlie a defect in the occipital bone.[39] Various intracranial tumors, such as optic nerve and temporal lobe gliomas, occur in contiguity with head plexiform neuromas.[32] Lesions overlying the spine may mark an underlying lesion that may compress the spine and spinal roots, including intraspinal tumors. Trunk lesions may extensively involve the mediastinum, gut, or retroperitoneum; bowel obstruction or hemorrhage may occur. Lesions at the junction of limb and trunk may be associated with limb hypertrophy and diffuse regional limb–trunk hyperpigmentation (often the earliest manifestation of the plexiform neuroma, darker than that of the café au lait macules found elsewhere on the skin of the same individual). The skin of the region may manifest marked laxity or "droopiness" and true lymphostasis of the limb may occur, producing further enlargement.[40]

Although they are not precursors of MPNSTs, plexiform neuromas conceal such tumors (arising from contiguous intraneural neurofibromas) within their bulk in about 2% of NF1 patients.[35] MPNSTs are usually solitary, deep, firm, globoid, or fusiform. Although they are locally invasive, diagnosis is often delayed. Between 85% and 90% are highly malignant, with a high rate of distant metastases. The remaining 10% to 15% of MPNSTs are low-grade tumors. The five-year survival rate after detection and resection of an MPNST ranges from 34% to 52%.[35]

Visual and central nervous systems in NF1   Most of the wide variety of visual and CNS abnormalities of NF1 are due to tumors.[32] Three diagnostic manifestations of NF1 involve the visual system: Lisch nodules, optic glioma, and sphenoid hyperplasia. Lisch nodules, benign yellow–brown melanocytic hamartomas of the iris, are found in one third of NF1 patients under 6 years of age, 50% to 90% of those 30 years old, and 94% of 60-year-old NF1 patients.[7] The combination of these and *café au lait* macules of appropriate size and number is pathognomonic of NF1. Congenital eyelid neurofibromas signify a risk for congenital glaucoma (buphthalmos).[41] Evaluation for glaucoma is also important in NF1 patients with ocular plexiform neuromas or findings that indicate risk for plexiform neuromas, such as facial hemihypertrophy, orbital enlargement or downward displacement, exophthalmos, enophthalmos, or asymmetrical bulging of a temple. Exophthalmos in NF1 may be unilateral and pulsatile; an associated bruit may be audible. Pulsatile exophthalmos may result from defective formation of the posterior orbital wall with herniation of the temporal tip, from a neurofibroma behind the eye but within the orbit, or from erosion of a middle fossa cyst through the superior wall of the orbit.[30] The posterior wall defect of the orbit is caused by congenital sphenoid dysplasia. Optic pathway gliomas occur in 10% to 20% of all patients with NF1 and are the most frequently encountered intracranial complication of NF1 in childhood. Among the important sites of such tumors are the optic nerves, optic chiasm, hypothalamus, and optic radiations. Hypothalamic involvement may result in the diencephalic syndrome or precocious puberty.[42] Many unilateral and almost all bilateral optic nerve gliomas are found in patients with NF1.[43] NF1 optic gliomas are indolent tumors that resemble congenital hamartomas or pilocytic astrocytomas. They seldom show malignant progression and two thirds remain asymptomatic. Acquired optic disk atrophy in individuals with NF1, especially those under 10 years of age, strongly implies optic glioma. Most such lesions are now first diagnosed radiographically as part of the systematic evaluation of NF1 by computed tomography (CT) or better by magnetic resonance imaging (MRI).[43]

MRI scans disclose extensive contiguous and noncontiguous signal abnormality in the majority of patients with optic gliomas. These abnormalities may disappear on follow-up, as new areas of transient abnormality may develop, rendering the process of evaluating tumor extent and growth particularly difficult.[44] Symptomatic optic nerve or tract gliomas are not biopsied, excised, or otherwise treated unless clinical progression prompts action. Contiguous or noncontiguous T_2 bright lesions are usually insignificant if there is no corresponding T_1-weighted or CT-apparent lesion. They are found in the globus pallidus, periventricular white matter, cerebral peduncles, deep gray nuclei, brainstem, and cerebellum. Although sometimes termed "hamartomas," the pathological character of these lesions is unknown and their relationship to neuropsychological or behavioral aspects of NF1 is controversial.[45] They are found much less frequently in older than younger NF1 patients.[46] Bilateral acoustic neuromas are rarely, if ever, found in NF1.[47] Hamartomas occasionally arise along the peripheral course of almost any of the remaining cranial nerves. Aside from hamartomas, astrocytomas are the most common intracranial tumors found in patients with NF1. However, medulloblastomas or ependymomas may develop.

Other features of NF1   Although a wide variety of cognitive and behavioral disorders have been discerned in 30% to 74% of cases of NF1, it remains unclear to what extent these abnormalities are intrinsic features of the disease itself. Some studies suggest lowering of full-scale IQ as compared to siblings (mean 94 vs. 105)[48] or impairment of language, nonverbal, and executive functions, but no clear pattern of deficits has as yet been discerned.[49] Careful evaluation for learning problems should be undertaken where indicated: such problems may be due to impaired expression of specific populations of neurons.[50] Seizures occur in approximately 10% of NF1 cases, and mental retardation, with or without seizures, in about 8%.[49]

Although one population-based study found mental retardation, usually mild, in 45% of NF1 patients,[51] other authorities have found mental retardation to be uncommon.

Electroencephalographic abnormalities are found in about 15% of patients.[7] Rare migrational disturbances, heterotopias, or hemimegalencephaly [52] do not appear to account for most of the intellectual problems or seizures that are found in patients with NF1.

Presymptomatic brain images disclosing lesions likely to be slow-growing CNS tumors represent a difficult management problem, often arousing considerable anxiety in patient and family without indicating any well-established program of management other than clinical and radiographic follow-up of such indolent lesions. Frequency of imaging is initially guided by the principle that 96% of optic pathway tumors arising anterior to the chiasm are likely to be more indolent and less invasive than those in chiasmatic and retrochiasmatic locations.[32] Enlarging lesions involving the optic chiasm have been treated with chemotherapy in children under 5 years, and with irradiation in doses of as much as 5200 rad in older children. Unfortunately, effective radiation doses have been associated with serious intellectual and endocrinological consequences in as many as one third of treated children. Surgical intervention is sometimes required.[43] Single or multiple astrocytomas may occur in other CNS locations, including cerebral hemispheres, deep gray nuclei, brainstem, or cerebellum.[53] These lesions must be distinguished from the insignificant and evanescent bright signal abnormalities on T_2-weighted MR images ("UBOs"). Calcification in the periventricular region or deep gray nuclei without other changes is not usually indicative of tumor.[54]

Although megalencephalic macrocephaly is found

in 16% to 45% of patients with NF1,[7] obstructive hydrocephalus due to slowly evolving aqueductal stenosis due to membranous gliosis is only occasionally found. Ventriculomegaly may also result from obstruction due to posterior fossa tumors or Chiari I malformation.[55] Various forms of craniofacial or skull osseous dysplasia may be found in patients with NF1. Dysplasia of all or part of the greater sphenoid wing, sometimes associated with pulsating exophthalmos, has already been discussed.[56] Dysplasia of the lesser wing, disturbed contour of the sella turcica (enlarged, "box"- or J-shaped), and ballooning of the middle fossa may be found, changes that may indicate the presence of a plexiform neuroma. These developmental abnormalities must be distinguished from acquired defects due to an enlarging optic glioma. Bilateral enlargement of the auditory canal may be found. Although similar in appearance to changes that occur due to acoustic schwannomas in NF2, this enlargement in NF1 patients is due to dural ectasia.[44]

Calvarial defects, especially in the occipital bones adjacent to the lambdoid suture, may also be found in NF1 patients. Scalp tumors may occasionally be indicated by the presence of a patch of hypertrichosis or of alopecia. Migraine and tension-type headaches or both may afflict patients with NF1. Severe, recurrent or chronic headaches may also prove symptomatic of tumor or hydrocephalus, an etiological distinction that is not always easily ascertained.

Spine and spinal cord Uncommonly, tumors may develop in the intradural or extradural compartments of the spinal cord, arising from spinal nerve roots. Pathological designation is controversial. These tumors are usually designated neurofibromas, but they may arise in individuals or families without other evidence for neurofibromatosis.[57] Most of these tumors grow slowly and present more commonly in adults. Second decade of life presentations occur in about 9%, first decade in less than 1%. A thoracic is slightly more common than a cervical or lumbar location and in a small number of cases these tumors arise in the cauda equina.[57] Pain is the most frequent presenting symptom of spinal neurofibroma, developing in approximately 50% of cervical, 68% of thoracic, and 91% of lumbosacral cases. Pain may be local spine pain, root pain, or remotely referred to various sites distal to the lesion along the spine or in the legs (especially in cases of cervical or thoracic tumor).

Motor or sensory cord deficits typical of extrinsic cord lesions are found in a majority of thoracic and in just under half of cervical tumors. These signs are uncommon in lumbosacral tumors, which may on the other hand give rise to root-localized motor and sensory dysfunction. Cervical spinal neurofibromas tend to present at an earlier age than thoracic or lumbosacral and are those most likely to present suddenly as compressive lesions. Some of these acutely manifesting lesions are found to be "dumbbell" tumors, extending through the intervertebral foramina and occupying both intra- and extradural compartments, occasionally in association with vertebral

dysplasia or an overlying cutaneous plexiform neuroma or hair whorl.[57] Sarcomatous transformation occurs in 2% to 7% of spinal tumors in patients with NF1, usually after the second decade.[58]

Endocrine, gastrointestinal, renal and hematological manifestations Hypothalamic hamartomas with diencephalic syndrome, neurofibromas of the adrenal medulla, or multiple endocrine neoplasia syndrome (MENS) may complicate NF1. MENS-related tumors include medullary thyroid carcinoma and pheochromocytoma. Patients with NF1 are also at increased risk for either neuroblastoma. Between 4% and 23% of all pheochromocytomas arise in NF1 patients.[59]

Short stature is common; short macrocephalic individuals deserve careful assessment for NF1. Approximately 10% to 15% of NF patients develop neurofibromas or ganglioneuromas of the intestinal wall, splanchnic nerves, or pelvic plexuses; megacolon, giant appendix, papillary adenomatosis of the intestinal mucosa, or intestinal obstruction may develop.[60] These intestinal manifestations may occur as a constituent of MENS.[61] Neurofibromas of the tongue, multiple subungual glomus tumors, or mediastinal neurofibromas may arise.[62] Routine ascertainment of blood pressure is important in NF1 since vascular intimal proliferation and fibromuscular changes of the media of small renal arteries may result in hypertension and elevation of risk for vascular accidents.[63] Risk for either Wilms tumor or chronic myelogenous leukemia is elevated in NF1.[26]

Orthopedic manifestations The spine is the skeletal region most frequently affected by NF1.[64] Abnormalities include enlargement of intervertebral foramina, dural ectasia with lateral or anterior meningocele, and vertebral scalloping. Scoliosis is detectable at some point after mid-childhood in 10% to 40% of patients; kyphosis is common and may become severe with cervical spondyloptosis.[7] Prevention of the progressive severe pain and neurological deficits that may result from these spinal changes may require timely stabilization of the spine with anterior and posterior spinal fusion.[64] Other potential orthopedic manifestations of NF1 include cortical rarefaction of long bones that may be especially prominent subjacent to subperiosteal neurofibromas. Rarely, cortical thinning results in early-onset tibulofibular bowing or pathological fractures at the junction of the middle and distal thirds of tibia or fibula with pseudarthrosis. Similar changes may occur in other long bones.[65] Bone overgrowth may occur in hypertrophic limbs in association with a plexiform neuroma.

Possible variant forms of NF1 Segmental neurofibromatosis is a condition wherein typical café au lait macules and neurofibromas occur unilaterally, often restricted to just one or a few dermatomes; four subtypes have been designated. Most, but not all cases are the sporadic result of early embryonic somatic mutation or mosaicism. Individuals with segmental NF1 may have a child with classic NF1 due to germinal mosaicism. Entire loss of the NF1 gene results in the syndrome of facial dysmorphia, dull intelligence, and early onset of a large number of neurofibromas. Large deletions in the NF1 gene may result in Watson syndrome, consisting of multiple *café au lait* macules, short stature, pulmonary valve stenosis, dull intelligence, and a small number of neurofibromas.[66] The combination of NF1 features with short stature, low intelligence, ptosis, facial dysmorphia, pectus carinatum, and cardiac defects is termed the neurofibromatosis–Noonan syndrome, a condition that is genetically distinct from true Noonan syndrome.[67] Other possible NF1 variants, some of which were noted in various sections of the preceding text are: 1) dominantly inherited isolated *café au lait* macules; 2) isolated familial intestinal neurofibromatosis; 3) intestinal neurofibromatosis with multiple endocrine neoplasia; 4) isolated hereditary spinal neurofibromatosis; and 5) syndrome of multiple nevi, multiple schwannomas, and multiple vaginal leiomyomas. Current understanding of the clinical and molecular aspects of these rare variant phenotypes has been the subject of a recent review.[11]

Neurofibromatosis-2 (Central neurofibromatosis, syndrome of bilateral acoustic neuroma)   As noted, NF2 is genetically distinct from NF1. Only one instance of simultaneous inheritance of both NF1 and NF2 has been documented,[68] although other possible cases have been reported.[69] The risk for clinical manifestations of this autosomal dominant condition in offspring of an affected parent is about 50%.[70] Diagnostic criteria for NF2 are shown in Table 158.4. Clinically silent acoustic schwannomas may be present from very early stages of development. At earliest, signs and symptoms of NF2 become apparent at 10 years of age, but usually considerably later in life. There is considerable mutation-specific variation in distribution of findings, and severity ranges from mild forms ("Gardner variant") to intermittent and severe forms ("Whishart variant"). Intellect is not impaired in NF2.[71]

Few if any cutaneous manifestations are found in the majority of patients. The few *café au lait* macules that may be found tend to have a less distinct appearance. Cutaneous neurofibromas are uncommon and, if present, are typically limited to the nasal alae and the palms. Plexiform neurofibromas are quite

Table 158.4   Diagnostic criteria for neurofibromatosis 2[15]

Either of the following:
1) Bilateral VIIIth cranial nerve neurofibromas
   or
2) First degree relative with NF2 by these criteria and either:
   a) Unilateral VIIIth cranial nerve neurofibroma
      or
   b) Any two of the following: meningioma, non-VIIIth cranial nerve neurofibroma, schwannoma, juvenile posterior subcapsular cataracts

unusual, although not unknown, in NF2. Schwannomas are the most common dermatological manifestations of NF2. The cutaneous variety appear as discrete, slightly raised, rough papules, pigmented and covered by an excess of hair. Subcutaneous schwannomas are palpable spherical tumors found along the course of peripheral nerves, often with palpable nerve thickening at either end of the schwannoma.[72] The characteristic NF2 lesions are specific non-neoplastic ocular abnormalities and multiple slow-growing CNS tumors, especially vestibular schwannomas and meningiomas.

Highly specific ocular findings that may be found are clinically unapparent pre-senile posterior cortical cataracts, optic disk gliomas or meningiomas, and retinal hamartomas. Eyelid ptosis may develop.[73] Lisch nodules are not found, or are exceedingly rare.

Bilateral acoustic schwannomas, the most common characteristic feature of NF2, are found in at least 90% of cases. The compressive effects of the enlargement of these tumors result in hearing loss, noted first in one ear. An identical process almost always becomes manifest in the other ear within months to years. Onset at earliest is in the second or third decades (especially in familial "Gardner variant" cases), at latest in the seventh decade, and may be accompanied by tinnitus. Vestibular reactions are lost early, producing unsteadiness, but typically without the episodes of paroxysmal vertigo seen in Ménière's disease. The process is relentlessly progressive to total deafness. Mass effects at the cerebellopontine angle may result in homolateral facial numbness or paresis, unilateral extinction of spontaneous blink, loss of corneal reflex, lateral diplopia due to abducens dysfunction, nystagmus, gait or appendicular ataxia. Papilledema may be found.[74]

Seizures may occur in NF2 patients, especially those that develop the rare complication of meningioangiomatosis. This process of malformative meningovascular proliferation results in the development of calcified hamartomas either at the periphery of one cerebellar hemisphere, or as a linear collection elsewhere in the subependymal region. These lesions are occasionally confused with invasive meningioma on radiographs or even histopathology. This may prompt excessively aggressive therapy, especially in young patients, in whom meningiomas often follow an unusually malignant course. Meningioangiomatosis may occur sporadically without other NF2 manifestations.[75]

NF2 patients are at risk for the development of single or multiple meningiomas, as well as other intracranial or intraspinal tumors. One particular NF2 gene mutation results in bilateral vestibular schwannomas, foramen magnum and supratentorial meningiomas, and multiple subcutaneous tumors.[71] Other NF2 mutations may result in single or multiple schwannomas in any of the cranial nerves except olfactory and optic; lower (V–XII) cranial nerves are those most commonly involved. Optic nerve gliomas are not features of NF2; astrocytomas are exceptional.[44] Spinal cord tumors arising in NF2 patients differ from those found in NF1 and include meningiomas, schwannomas (sometimes multiple and difficult to manage), astrocytomas, and ependymomas.[76] Spinal cord meningiomas occur at a younger age than the sporadic variety and tend to be bilateral. Dorsal nerve root paraspinal schwannomas are quite common in NF2. They are sometimes multiple and difficult to manage; their growth results in considerable morbidity in NF2, due to compression of the involved nerve or of the spinal cord.

NF2 variants or closely related conditions Patients with significant numbers of schwannomas arising in skin or spinal cord who have neither vestibular schwannomas nor stigmata characteristic of NF1 are set apart by some authorities as examples of *multiple schwannomatosis*.[75] A subset of these patients have multiple cutaneous plexiform schwannomas that do not manifest progression to MPNSTs. Some patients from these groups have been shown, by molecular methods, to have NF2, while others have had pigmentary changes of the skin suggesting that they were cases of NF1.[74] The appropriate categorization of the residue from each group remains uncertain. *Familial meningiomatosis* arises from a gene locus on the long arm of chromosome 22 that is not distant from the NF2 gene locus but is genetically distinct and has no other features characteristic of NF2.[78] *Sporadic meningioangiomatosis* is not associated with the development of vestibuloacoustic schwannomas.

Management of neurofibromatosis Although NF1 is a protean illness entering into the differential diagnosis of a wide variety of illnesses and NF2 may have few or no visible findings, either illness is usually easy to diagnose, based on the characteristics and diagnostic criteria already reviewed. Current molecular diagnostic strategies are only useful in families with known mutations. One major NF1 manifestation in the child of a parent with that condition renders a diagnosis of NF1 highly probable without molecular confirmation. The absence of any manifestation in the child of a parent with NF1 by age 5 renders the ultimate diagnosis of NF1 in that child highly unlikely since penetrance by that age approaches 100%. For that same reason, there is usually no mystery as to which parent is carrying the dominant NF1 mutation.

Genetic testing for NF2 has considerably greater potential value since manifestations may not be apparent for a very long time. Typical auditory and visual manifestations of NF2 are often not detectable until long after the achievement of fertility.[79] If it is not possible to assay for a specific NF2 mutation, imaging for an as yet asymptomatic vestibuloauditory schwannoma should enable diagnosis of NF2 in sexually mature, consenting individuals, after careful genetic counseling. Newer techniques (e.g. protein truncation assays) for diagnosis of presymptomatic individuals raise ethical and social questions about diagnostic ascertainment in presymptomatic and especially prepubertal individuals. Individuals with

equivocal manifestations in families with known mutations may elect for testing since a negative result may alleviate considerable degrees of anxiety.

In all cases, counseling should be provided by individuals thoroughly familiar with the limitations of the assays, pleiotropic variation of neurofibromatoses, and lack of clear genotype–phenotype correlations in most instances of positive results.[80] Prenatal linkage analysis of the presence of a known familial mutation may be possible, although counseling and parental decisions relevant to the unborn child are made quite difficult by the phenotypic variability of these conditions.[8] It is not as yet known whether this variation is mediated by modifying genes or environmental contributions.[81]

Once the diagnosis of NF1 or NF2 is made, frank discussion of the potential consequences should be undertaken. This requires accurate knowledge and understanding of the risk for various manifestations, upon the basis of which a plan for follow-up evaluation must be formulated. Unjustified anxiety about risk for severe deformities of the "elephant man" variety should be dispelled. Current extent of disease should be determined, imaging studies supplementing thorough examination. A program of retesting to monitor disease progression should be designed, including yearly imaging of known intracranial or intraspinal lesions. Visual fields and acuity should be followed at least yearly in NF1 patients in order to detect and monitor optic pathway gliomas. Careful documentation of fundoscopic appearance with routine follow-up examination is important in both NF1 and NF2 for detection of changes produced by intracranial tumors.[7] Headache, changes in vision or hearing, precocious puberty, diencephalic syndrome or complaints referable to the spinal cord should also prompt investigation for tumor.

Surgical removal of neurofibromas for cosmetic reasons has been considered, by many, to be inappropriate unless they are considerably disfiguring or painful.[20] Some large, deep neurofibromas require biopsy to exclude malignancy. In addition to likely or proven malignant lesions, lesions quite likely to engender malignant tumors (e.g. giant hairy bathing suit nevi) should be excised. The mast-cell stabilizer ketotifen may decrease the rate of growth of neurofibromas and reduce the pain, pruritus, or tenderness that they may impart.[31] Current research is designed to develop ras-signaling cascade component suppressors that blockade NF1 tumor formation.[82]

Management of tumors of optic, vestibular, and other cranial nerves is challenging, since the only available treatments, surgery or radiation, carry significant potential morbidity. Early detection may reduce the magnitude of surgical intervention. Other brain and spinal tumors are often managed with quite gratifying results. Surgical management may be indicated for visceral tumors or for orthopedic problems. The care of neurofibromatosis may require a team composed of neurologists, pediatricians, internists, neuro-otologists, neurosurgeons, ophthalmologists, geneticists, renal specialists, gastroenterologists, endocrinologists, psychologists, counselors, psychiatrists, and various rehabilitative specialists.[83]

Tuberous sclerosis complex (Bourneville disease, Pringle's disease; epiloia)

Tuberous sclerosis (TS) is another autosomal dominant hamartomatosis that is readily diagnosed upon the basis of a distinctive collection of cutaneous, visceral, and cerebral manifestations. Although some characteristic lesions were noted more than 160 years ago, it was not until 1862 that von Recklinghausen provided the first clinical description of a patient with TS.[84] Between 1880 and 1900 a fairly comprehensive view of the constituents of this disorder was formulated by Bourneville and others.[85] Additional hamartomatous lesions (benign tumors composed of various cell types derived from all of the primary germ cell lines) have subsequently been demonstrated in brain, lungs, kidneys, heart, and bones,[86,87] and the rare occurrence of malignant tumors, chiefly in kidneys, has been appreciated. Given the sometimes indistinct diagnostic margins of TS, particularly in patients with limited or localized manifestations, the establishment of diagnostic criteria has been important. Of great importance was promulgation of the Gomez criteria for probability of diagnosis in 1988[88] and their recent modification into simplified consensus criteria by Roach et al.,[89] shown in Table 158.5.

Genetics and pathophysiology The actual prevalence of TS is difficult to estimate since the condition is so variable in its manifestations; many paucisymp-

tomatic patients are likely to remain undiagnosed. Estimates range between 1/10000 and 1/100000 live births. Approximately two thirds of cases arise as new mutations and it is uncommon for TS to develop in siblings of affected children when neither parent is found to have clinical manifestations. However, 2% to 10% of TS cases occur in siblings of such parents, presumably on the basis of *de novo* gonadal or somatic germline mosaicism of one of those parents.[90] Extrinsic and "second hit" factors may play a role in clinical expression, accounting for the remarkable discordance of expression of TS that has been observed in some monozygotic twins with TS, one of whom may have many or quite serious features of TS while the other has few, trivial, or no TS manifestations.[91]

Approximately half of familial TS cases have been linked to abnormality of the *TSC-2* tumor suppressor gene located at 16p13, half to the *TSC-1* tumor suppressor gene located at 9q31. New mutations are more likely to be due to *TSC-2* than *TSC-1* mutations,[92,93] but in a considerable number of sporadic cases neither mutation is found.[94] The gene product of *TSC-2* is tuberin, while that of *TSC-1* is hamartin. The rapidly emerging cellular understanding of TS, which has contributed enormously to investigation of brain development and tumor biology, is the subject of several excellent reviews.[95,96]

Cutaneous manifestations At least one cutaneous feature of TS is found in 96% of TS patients.[97] No single feature is universal and there is considerable age-related variation in likelihood of cutaneous expression. White macules and fibromatous plaques of the forehead are early, facial angiofibromas and shagreen patches intermediate, and peri and subungual fibromas late manifestations. Four cutaneous findings are especially strongly supportive of a TS diagnosis: facial angiofibromas, periungual/subungual angiofibromas, forehead fibrous plaques, and shagreen patches.

Facial angiofibromas are papules that range in hue from flesh-colored to red–brown. At first they are small erythematous papules that then slowly enlarge while new examples appear. In time, fine vascular telangiectases may be found on the surface of larger papules.[21] They are concentrated on the nose and symmetrically across the adjacent nasolabial folds and cheeks but may be found on the chin. Only 7% to 13% of patients manifest them in the first year of life, 27–50% by 3 years of age. Most of the remaining 50% to 83% of TS patients who develop these lesions will do so by 6 years of age.[98] Vogt's term "adenoma sebaceum" has been used for nearly a century to incorrectly designate the facial angiofibromas of TS. Vogt noted that the combination of these fibrous facial hamartomas with mental retardation and seizures ("Vogt's triad") was highly suggestive of TS.[99] This triad is found is less than half of all TS patients.

Periungual or subungual angiofibromas ("Könen tumors") are found more commonly on the toes than the fingers and tend to be less vascular and more

Table 158.5 Consensus diagnostic criteria for tuberous sclerosis

Major features
- Cortical tubers
- Subependymal glial nodules
- Three or more typical hypomelanotic macules
- Retinal phakomas (= peripapillary retinal hamartomas or "pseudo-drusen")
- Midfacial ("adenoma sebaceum") or ungual/periungual angiofibromas/fibromas
- Multiple renal angiomyolipomas
- Cardiac rhabdomyomas
- Pulmonary lymphangiomyomatosis
- Shagreen patch

Minor features
- Fibrous forehead or scalp plaques
- Gingival fibromas
- Wedge-shaped cortical or subcortical brain calcification
- Multiple subcortical changes: hypodense by CT, high signal T_2-weighted MRI
- Renal cysts
- Dental enamel pits
- Bone cysts
- Hamartomatous rectal polyps
- First degree relative with TS

Diagnosis by consensus criteria: one major and first degree relative with tuberous sclerosis or one major and two minor. One major and one minor = probable. One major or two or more minor = possible.[89]

fibrous than facial angiofibromas. They are found in only 15% to 16% of cases, are never present before 2 years of age, and may develop as late as the fifth decade of life.[98] In some cases they are the only cutaneous manifestation of TS.[21] Similar fibrous patches may be found on the forehead, scalp, and gums. Forehead fibrous plaques (FFP) and similar lesions on the scalp exceeding several centimeters in diameter are pathognomonic of TS. The FFP are found in 6% of 2-year-olds and in as many as 20% of all children and adolescents with TS.[98] Gingival fibromas, which develop at some stage in approximately one third of TS patients, are supportive of the diagnosis. They tend to occur on the anterior portions of the gums. Rarely, fibrous hamartomas are found on the occiput or forearm.[97]

White macules (achromic nevi), a form of hypomelanotic leukoderma, develop in 66% to 97% of patients with TS. They are more common than most other cutaneous manifestations and are often the earliest cutaneous indication of diagnosis.[100] It is important to note, however, that they are considered supportive of TS diagnosis rather than pathognomonic. With careful assessment these lesions may be found in nearly two thirds of neonates, 80% of infants, and 90% of 2-year-olds with TS.[98] Most are found on the abdomen, back, and anterior and lateral surfaces of the legs. They increase in number and visibility with age and probably persist throughout life. Only a minority are lanceolate "ash leaf" macules with serrated margins. Most are oval "thumbprint" macules with quite irregular margins. The longest diameter of the macules is usually 1 to 3 cm (range 0.4 to 7 cm). At least three are found on most TS patients, but some have none and some have as many as 32.[21,98,100]

White macules may tan slightly on sun exposure, although tanning usually sets the lesions into greater relief from surrounding normally tanning areas. Wood's lamp illumination also renders the lesions easier to discern in fair-skinned individuals, especially in body regions that receive little or no sun exposure. Slight perifollicular pigmentation within TS white macules sets these lesions apart from the uniformly milk-white appearance of vitiligo.[101] As many as 3% to 13% of TS patients exhibit hundreds of 2 to 3 mm white freckles (guttate macular leukoderma) on their legs. These "confetti-like" macules support the diagnosis of TS.[102] One or two and rarely three *café au lait* spots are found in 23% to 28% of TS patients, apparent by 2 years of age. Ash leaf-shaped examples found alongside a white macule of similar size and configuration are highly suggestive of TS.[21,98]

Shagreen patches are found in 21% to 48% of patients with TS, and are strongly suggestive of TS diagnosis. They are flesh-colored lesions that have a palpable pebbly consistency of the feel and appearance of soft pigskin with prominent follicular openings. They are usually found in the dorsal lumbosacral region, although examples have been found anywhere on the trunk. If they do develop, they are likely to do so before puberty and are found in as many as 6% of 2-year-olds with TS.[21,98] The lesion

may be the only cutaneous manifestation of TS and should be sought where infants or young children manifest seizures with developmental delay or mental retardation.[103] Shagreen patches must be distinguished from two fairly obscure lesions: 1) dermatofibrosis lenticularis disseminata, and 2) disseminated connective tissue nevi.[104] Molluscum fibrosum pendulum is a cutaneous finding in 23% of individuals with TS, but these lesions do not develop until after early childhood.[98]

Kidney manifestations Renal angiomyolipomas, if multiple (bilateral or in just one kidney), are the only visceral tumor sufficiently characteristic of TS as to be considered pathognomonic; in some cases they are the only discernible TS manifestation.[105] Although they are found in 50% to 67% of TS patients (more commonly adults than children), evaluation for such lesions by ultrasonography, CT, MRI, or angiography is too often neglected.[106] Since multiple renal tumors rarely occur in children, this tumor type and TS must be suspected in young patients exhibiting such multiplicity. Since these tumors are subject, especially if large or multiple, to hemorrhage, these diagnoses must also be excluded in young patients whose renal tumors present in that way. Occasionally the tumors become malignant.[107] Conservative surgical resection is the usual treatment, given the fact that tumors are commonly bilateral. However, interventional radiological treatment with super-selective tumor embolization can be considered.[108] Multicystic renal tumors are less common in adults but more common in children with TS than angiomyolipomas, lesions that support the diagnosis of TS. The cysts are typically small, numerous and widely scattered, but vary in size and may enlarge. The appearance may resemble polycystic kidney disease. Renal insufficiency and hypertension may develop in TS patients; involvement of both kidneys often makes management difficult.[109]

Heart manifestations Cardiac rhabdomyomas occur in nearly half of patients with TS and suggest TS diagnosis. The most common cardiac tumor of neonates and infants, rhabdomyomas occur in some who do not have TS. Single or multiple multinodular lesions may be found in TS patients and many remain asymptomatic. Symptoms include arrhythmias (e.g. paroxysmal atrial tachycardia), cyanosis with right to left shunt, and hemodynamic obstruction that may produce profound intractable pre- or post-natal cardiac failure. Murmurs are not usually present. Rhabdomyoma is the most likely cause of heart disease in infants with TS and should be considered in every case of prenatal-onset arrhythmia or anasarca. In infants, heart failure may come on with great suddenness with rapid deterioration and demise. Rhabdomyomas may be prenatally symptomatic; the diagnosis should be considered in every case of prenatal-onset arrhythmia or anasarca. Suspected diagnosis is readily confirmed with ultrasonography, even prenatally.[110]

Since severe heart failure is uniformly lethal with medical therapy, alleviation of the obstruction produced by rhabdomyoma in such cases is the only therapeutic option. Neither very young age nor diagnosis of TS are contraindications to such an approach. With symptomatic relief from partial resection, involution of residual tumor will subsequently occur.[111] Management of some infants with TS and cardiac rhabdomyoma is further and seriously complicated by diffuse myocardial dysfunction. Nonsymptomatic rhabdomyomas are left to their natural course of involution and loss of significance as infants grow.[112] Children who have had cardiac rhabdomyomas may be found to have persistent calcification of the ventricular wall and papillary muscles that appear hyperechoic on cardiac ultrasound.[110]

Lungs manifestations Lymphangioleiomyomatosis (LAM) of the lungs is a very rare hamartomatous proliferation of lymphatic vessel smooth muscle that is supportive of the diagnosis of TS. It occurs in less than 0.1% of individuals with TS, almost exclusively females. Female sex hormones likely play a role in the proliferation of these noncancerous lesions.[113] Intelligence is normal and the TS is often otherwise mild, additional manifestations being limited to skin hamartomas. The dyspnea and spontaneous pneumothorax that announce the condition rarely appear before early adulthood. Serial chest radiographs in mild cases of TS in females may permit early diagnosis, especially in patients who must undergo surgery with anesthesia and assisted ventilation. As many as half of all patients with pulmonary LAM and TS die unnecessary deaths due to spontaneous, unanticipated pneumothorax.[114] Extrapulmonary forms such as retroperitoneal or uterine lymphangioleiomyomatous cysts or kidney angiomyolipomas may also complicate TS.[21,113]

Other non-neurological problems that afflict some individuals with TS include cyst development and patchy sclerosis of the bones of hands or feet, pitting of dental enamel (deciduous or permanent teeth), bone cysts, hamartomatous rectal polyps, and a variety of endocrine disturbances. Some of these features have assumed importance in the consensus diagnostic criteria.[89]

Eye manifestations Retinal phakomas are glial hamartomas that may calcify but do not typically produce visual disturbances. Found in approximately 53% of patients with TS, they are pathognomonic. They appear as multiple elevated nodules near the optic disk or in the midperipheral retinal field. Their appearance prompted the term "mulberry lesions." Peripapillary retinal hamartomas are another retinal finding supportive of the diagnosis of TS. One or more of these flat or slightly elevated grayish lesions with indistinct margins may be present. Some may overlie retinal vessels and some are indistinguishable from drusen.[115] Detection of papilledema is important in TS, but must be distinguished from findings due to optic disk drusen, retinal angiomas, phakomas, or peripapillary hamartomas. The causes of papilledema in TS include hydrocephalus secondary to obstruction of the foramina of Monro by subependymal giant cell astrocytomas or the presence of bilateral fusiform carotid aneurysms.[116]

Central nervous system manifestations Three types of brain hamartomas may occur in TS, each so distinctive as to be pathognomonic: cortical tubers, subependymal nodules (SEN), and subependymal giant cell astrocytomas (SEGA). The cortical tubers which prompted the name tuberous sclerosis are hard dysplastic nodules of variable size that are found in more than 80% of cases. They arise very early in corticogenesis and are in essence isolated areas of disturbed brain architecture with abnormal cellular and laminar development which may in some instances span several gyri. They contain several types of abnormal or unusual cells. Between the tubers and the subependymal germinal zones abnormal-appearing heterotopic neurons are frequently found in an apparent state of migrational arrest.[95,117] They have been identified in some fetal and neonatal brain images.[118] Tubers are often calcified. Patches of focal cortical dysplasia or of gliosis, distinct from tubers, may also be found in the brains of TS patients.[95] Tubers and the developmental and migrational disturbances they represent are likely to play a major role in the neurological morbidity of TS, including mental retardation, learning difficulties, seizures, and possibly autism. Tubers are not subject to malignant transformation.

Subependymal nodules are found in approximately 80% of TS patients and have been detected in scans of some fetuses or neonates with TS.[119] They are found in subependymal white matter up to the surface of deep gray nuclei. They enlarge and then protrude into the lateral ventricles as linear excrescences termed "candle gutterings." Rarely, they develop in the cerebral aqueduct or in the fourth ventricle.[118] They are also composed of various unusual cells, more densely packed than cortical tubers, imparting the appearance of malignancy although they do not become malignant.[32] They appear to remain clinically silent, unless with enlargement they become SEGA, whose histological appearance even more strongly resembles a malignant lesion—indeed, they do rarely become malignant. SEGAs are the least common TS brain hamartomas. They have a strong predilection to arise in the ventricular wall near the foramina of Monro. They usually become apparent during the first two decades of life, occasionally as early as infancy, provoking headache, mental status changes, hemiparesis, or other abnormalities due to obstruction of third ventricular CSF outflow.[95]

Abnormalities of CT and MR images of brain that support the diagnosis are found in most patients with TS. Normal CT and MR scans of brain are very reassuring concerning cerebral involvement of TS.[88] Cortical tubers, SEN and SEGA appear hypodense on CT. Calcification of these lesions is characteristic, usually appearing after the second year of life, most apparent in SEN and SEGA near the foramina of Monro. Hamartomas are larger and more numerous on T_2-weighted MRI than on CT images, often showing wedge-shaped extension into subcortical or subependymal brain parenchyma. SEGA near the foramen of Monro may appear heterogeneous on T_2-weighted images and are the lesions most likely to enhance brightly after gadolinium administration. MRI demonstration of ventricular "candle gutterings" is diagnostic of TS. Imaging shows atrophy of cerebellar folia or cerebellar tubers in approximately 30% of cases. Curiously, the spinal cord is typically spared in TS.[120]

Although epilepsy and mental retardation do not always develop in patients with numerous tubers,[32] patients with 10 or more CNS tubers are at considerable risk for intractable epilepsy.[120] Epilepsy is the most common neurological feature of TS, found in 93% to 98% of patients. One of the earliest of TS manifestations, found in 75% of patients during the first year of life, it is epilepsy that brings affected infants and children to medical attention for the first time.[121] Infants usually present with infantile spasms. As many as 25% of children with infantile spasms (IS) may be found to have TS.[88] Although this form of epilepsy is no longer a supportive diagnostic feature, the diagnosis of TS should be excluded in every child with IS. White macules are the only cutaneous marker likely to be present in the first year of life. The combination of IS, hypomelanotic macules, and developmental delay is highly suspicious of the diagnosis of TS. Atypical hypsarrhythmia is found in one third of infants with TS, often emphasized in one hemisphere. Early diagnosis and effective treatment of infantile spasms may lead to normal outcome by 4 years of age in some TS patients.[122]

With increasing age a wide variety of partial or generalized motor seizures (tonic, clonic, akinetic, myoclonic) may manifest themselves in patients with TS. Indeed, epilepsy may develop at almost any age. More than half of children who have TS with epilepsy will develop complex partial seizures, regardless of what other types of seizures occur.[123] Older children with TS, mixed seizures, and significant neurological handicaps often have generalized spike and slow wave activity admixed with independent multifocal spike discharges.[124] Focality is found in fully 40% of EEGs obtained in patients with TS.[123]

Mental retardation is found in 47% to 82% of TS patients.[115,125] It is found only in cases with epilepsy, and the likelihood and degree of retardation is greater the earlier in life that seizures, especially infantile spasms, become apparent.[88,126] Some series have found normal intelligence in as many as 44% of TS cases.[88] Patients with sporadic *TSC-2* mutations have a greater tendency to intellectual disabilities than patients with sporadic *TSC-1* mutations.[127] Some children with TS-related infantile spasms may manifest withdrawal, isolation, "strangeness," agitation, hyperkinesia, autism, or pervasive developmental disturbance.[128] Seizures are not always found in such patients. Thus, careful examination of the skin for

signs of TS is an important element of the assessment of every child with early infantile autism.[128] A small number of TS patients manifest intellectual deterioration at some point during the interval of 2 to 20 years of age. In some instances this is due to hydrocephalus, which occurs in about 3% of TS cases, typically after 5 years of age. A number of patients with TS and mental retardation show behavioral deterioration after puberty.

The variability of expression of TS necessitates consideration of this diagnosis in individuals with epilepsy, mental retardation, autism, and other diagnoses, in addition to those who exhibit a more classical combination of these conditions. Skin signs of TS, usually present before 1 year of age, are often overlooked. On the other hand, it may be difficult or inappropriate to assign the TS diagnosis to young individuals with one or two white patches and epilepsy. It is as yet impractical to use genetic probes to confirm TS except in families with known mutations. The Wood's lamp (unnecessary in individuals with darker-hued skin) and brain imaging are usually the most helpful diagnostic adjuvants. At times the characteristic lesions of heart, kidney, or lung indicate the diagnosis.

Treatment Ameliorative treatments for TS include laser techniques that flatten and diminish the erythema of stigmatizing facial angiofibroma. Shagreen patches may be rendered less evident by shaving elevated portions with a Reese dermatome.[129] Where any surgery is undertaken, especially in mildly affected women with TS, the risk of positive pressure ventilation and the possibility that pulmonary lymphangioleiomyomatosis is present must be considered. Prompt and effective treatment of epilepsy is of obvious importance. Despite the risk for retinal injury, vigabatrin has appeared to have particular efficacy in the treatment of the infantile myoclonic seizures associated with TS in some patients. Large cortical or subcortical tubers may be removed surgically, especially when they are the source of epileptic fits or of ventricular obstruction. Epilepsy surgery is more likely to prove beneficial where video-EEG monitoring has demonstrated that the electrographic discharge related to most or all seizures is confined to a particular resectable region of cortex. Intraoperative monitoring may define appropriate surgical margins better than relying on visual determination of cortical tuber margins since zones of subcortical migrational arrest may prove epileptogenic. Radiotherapy for brain tumors is not advisable in TS. Symptomatic renal angiomyofibromas can be treated with selective embolization. Management of renal insufficiency due to cysts and angiomyolipomas entails a range of therapeutic options that includes medical management, dialysis, and transplantation.[130] Management of the intellectual, behavioral, and psychiatric aspects of TS is a challenging but often rewarding endeavor. Recognition and treatment of disturbances of sleep or mood may have a particularly gratifying impact. Psychiatry and involvement of increasingly prevalent support groups and other resources for pervasive developmental disturbances may provide particular benefit.[128] Genetic counseling requires careful examination of both parents, a full family history, and where necessary, parental renal ultrasonography, brain imaging by CT or MRI, and neuroophthalmological examination.[131]

Von Hippel–Lindau disease (angiomatosis retinae et cerebelli, Von Hippel–Lindau complex)

The retinal and many of the other lesions of von Hippel–Lindau disease (VHLD) were characterized between 1879 and 1933, when it was designated as the third of the autosomal dominant phakomatoses by van der Hoeve.[1,132,133] Lindau's detailed observations of 1926 drew attention to the occurrence of cerebellar hemangioblastomas with the similar retinal lesions of von Hippel's disease.[134] VHLD occurs in approximately 1/36 000 individuals.[135] In addition to the occurrence of hemangioblastomas in the retina and cerebellum (more commonly than brainstem or spinal cord), cystic tumors may develop in kidney, liver, pancreas, or epididymis. The risk for various malignant tumors renders VHLD a pleiomorphic familial multisystem tumor/cancer syndrome.[136] Cutaneous lesions are quite exceptional; cases exhibiting such changes are more likely to have been examples of Sturge–Weber or related conditions.

VHLD results from any of more than 140 different germline or other mutations of a tumor suppressor gene located at chromosome 3p25-26.[135] There is insufficient genotype–phenotype correlation to permit mutation-specific counseling except as regards the risk for development of pheochromocytoma.[137] Heritable VHLD-related hemangioblastomas are associated with germline, while sporadic VHLD hemangioblastomas are due to new somatic mutations of the *VHL* gene.[138] The mechanisms whereby abnormalities of vascular endothelium and the various tumors may develop, details of the encoded cytoplasmic protein, and explanations for pleomorphism are the subject of recent reviews.[136,139]

Retinal hemangioblastomas of VHLD can be detected in children known to harbor a *VHL* gene mutation, although they do not usually become clinically apparent until after the second decade of life.[140] Early lesions may be mistaken for dilated retinal vessel aneurysms.[141] With maturation, lesions assume the classical round, elevated, whitish-pink "mulberry tumor" appearance.[139] They are subserved by a single artery and vein.[142] They may be bilateral and multicentric and are more likely to be located in the periphery of the retina, although they may also be found near the optic disk. Very peripheral lesions may be missed without careful dilated fundoscopy. Peripheral and early lesions are more easily detected with fluorescein angiography.[139] Retinal hemangioblastomas predispose to development of subretinal edema and retinal detachment. Detachment with sudden progressive visual loss is often the incident that leads to diagnosis of VHLD, usually during or after the second decade. Between 38% and 58% of all individuals found to have retinal angiomas express a VHLD mutation.[143]

Approximately 20% of patients with VHLD retinal hemangioblastoma develop symptomatic manifestations of an associated cerebellar hemangioblastoma.[144] These otherwise benign tumors are subject to hemorrhage that produces local compressive effects, with significant risk for increased intracranial pressure and herniation. Cerebellar hemangioblastomas are rare tumors. At least 25% to 40% are found in patients with VHLD.[145] Cerebellar hemangioblastomas, usually found in the paramedian cerebellar cortex, are the most characteristic lesions of VHLD. They are the lesions most likely to bring patients to medical attention and the chief source of morbidity and mortality. They exhibit a characteristic pathology.[138] There is a strong tendency to multiple occurrence. Rarely, hemangioblastomas are found in extracerebellar subtentorial sites such as pons, medulla, or cervical spinal cord. Very rarely, they occur in such supratentorial locations as the optic nerve, temporal lobe, basal ganglia, or ventricle.[146,147]

Repeated radiographic surveillance initiated as early as the second decade of life in individuals known to have VHLD and at-risk relatives permits asymptomatic tumors to be detected. This surveillance is especially important for women of childbearing age, since peripartum or postpartum intracranial or spinal hemorrhages may occur with devastating impact.[148] The tumors typically have a single mural nodule, apparent on angiography, and a cyst that is apparent on CT or MR images. A ring of increased signal surrounding the cyst is characteristic on MR scans, whether or not contrast has been administered.[149] Occasionally, cerebellar hemangioblastomas are solid masses that resemble meningiomas radiographically.[150] Spinal cord hemangioblastomas may provoke cystic degeneration of the central cord with development of syrinx that may extend over many cord levels. The tumors tend to be located in the mediodorsal portion of the cord, but may be central or lateral. MR scans are helpful in distinguishing hemangioblastomatous cavitation from non-tumor induced syrinx.[146] Fairly large lesions cause little if any neurological dysfunction unless hemorrhage occurs. Even sensory function, which should be carefully assessed, is often spared.

After retinal and cerebellar hemangioblastomas, malignant hypernephroma is the third most common tumor of VHLD and an important cause of morbidity and mortality. Indeed, in some series hypernephroma is found in 70% of VHLD patients.[151] Multiple renal clear cell carcinomas may be found in patients with VHLD, in one or both kidneys, and single or multiple tumors within involved kidneys. They are the leading cause of death in VHLD.[152] Familial clusters of renal clear cell carcinoma without other VHLD features do *not* appear to be caused by VHLD-related mutations.[153] Nephron-sparing surgery has been developed to manage VHLD-related renal cell carcinoma and can be employed in selected cases without compromising duration of survival.[154] Rarely, renal cell

Table 158.6 Diagnostic criteria for von Hippel–Lindau disease[151]

If positive family history, one of the following:
Single retinal or cerebellar hemangioblastoma
Renal cell carcinoma
Pheochromocytoma
Multiple pancreatic cysts

If no family history, one of the following:
Two or more retinal or cerebellar hemangioblastomas
One hemangioblastoma and one visceral tumor (renal clear cell or pheochromocytoma)

carcinoma may metastasize to the cerebellar hemangioblastoma.[155]

Patients with VHLD may also develop renal hemangiomas or adenomas. Benign renal cysts of varied size occur in VHLD, usually multiple and bilateral, in some instances resembling polycystic kidney disease.[156] Pancreatic cysts may also be found. It is estimated that either renal or pancreatic cysts or both are detectable in at least 75% of VLD cases.[157] Cystic or cystadenomatous lesions may also be found in adrenal glands or epididymis, and less commonly in the lung, liver, or spleen.[158,159] Papillary adenomas may develop in the skull and other bones.[160]

Pheochromocytoma is found in 3% to 20% of VHLD patients, occasionally bilateral,[161] accounting for a substantial percentage of familial pheochromocytoma.[152,153] Mutations analysis assists in deciding which VHLD patients require surveillance for this tumor.[153] A positive family history of pheochromocytoma with VHLD provides the same information.[135] Screening clues include elevation of serum and urine catecholamines, particularly norepinephrine, and of fasting serum glucose.[161] Pancreatic islet cell tumors and endolymphatic sac tumors also occur in VHLD.[137,162] The unusual combination of pancreatic islet cell tumor with pheochromocytoma occurs in either VHLD or multiple endocrine neoplasia syndrome.[136] Abnormal somatostatin receptors in VHLD-related islet cell tumors can be targeted for imaging and for provision of β-emitting radionuclide chemotherapy. Somatostatin analogs can be employed to control the flushing, diarrhea, hypoglycemia, and electrolyte abnormalities that occur in the neuroendocrine tumors associated with VHLD.[163] VHLD should be excluded in all patients with endolymphatic sac tumors, the manifestations of which include tinnitus and progressive deafness.[151]

Clinical diagnostic criteria for VHLD are shown in Table 158.6. Genetic diagnosis by mutations analysis is also possible and may be helpful in assessing risk for some VHLD tumors. The lesions of VHLD are detected by fundoscopy, retinal fluorescein angiography, ultrasonography, CT, or MRI.[162] Annual physical, neurological, and ophthalmological examination should begin at diagnosis or, in individuals with a positive family history, at 5 years of age. Biennial cranial and abdominal CT should also be commenced at diagnosis. If renal cysts are found, abdominal CT

scans should be performed every 6 months to follow these lesions. Undiagnosed individuals at risk for VHLD because of a positive family history should have cranial and abdominal CT at 10, 15, and 20 years of age. Biennial cranial and abdominal CT should be obtained in individuals with isolated cerebellar or retinal hemangioblastoma.[32,144] Yearly screening of urine for catecholamine elevations should be undertaken in individuals with a positive family history of pheochromocytoma, those with pheochromocytoma-associated VHL gene mutations, and in cases with unknown family history or without mutation analysis.[151] A negative thorough initial evaluation and mutation analysis in members of a kindred known to harbor a given mutation alleviates the need for further follow-up for such individuals.[151]

Elevation of hematocrit or red blood cell mass in patients with VHLD may indicate the presence of cerebellar hemangioblastoma or malignant hypernephroma due to erythropoietin stimulation by the cyst fluid of either tumor, although either tumor may be present without producing such an effect. Hemangioblastomas of brain, brainstem, or spinal cord may elevate CSF protein concentration. As noted, screening of urine for elevation of catecholamines (epinephrine, norepinephrine, and vanillymandelic acid) is a valuable initial and periodic screening test in patients with VHLD.[164]

Retinal hemangioblastomas, once detected, should be followed carefully. If lesions are large or if visual loss or retinal detachment are noted, treatment is undertaken with photo- or cryo-coagulation. Surgical management of cerebellar hemangioblastomas entails removal of mural nodule and cyst. An 8% to 15% rate of post-surgical recurrence has been estimated.[143] Radiation should be avoided unless surgery is contraindicated or is not feasible. Surveillance for renal carcinomas and pheochromocytomas is important, since early detection improves outlook and permits more limited therapeutic interventions such as nephron-sparing surgery.[152] Patients who develop end-stage renal disease due to bilateral extensive clear cell carcinoma have achieved excellent results from kidney transplantation and have shown limited risk of recurrence.[154]

Life expectancy for VHLD discerned in older studies was typically less than 50 years. Death was chiefly due to hemorrhagic complications of hemangioblastoma or to renal cell carcinoma. It is likely that modern surveillance and intervention strategies have prolonged life expectancy as well as quality of life in VHLD.[151] Innovations such as the use of angiogenesis inhibitors may have a considerable further impact on improving the outcome of VHLD.[165]

Other autosomal dominant neurocutaneous syndromes

Additional autosomal dominant neurocutaneous syndromes are listed in Table 158.7.

Table 158.7   Autosomal dominant neurocutaneous syndromes

Name	Cutaneous features	Neurological features	Other organs
Blue rubber-bleb nevus syndrome[166]	Blue, compressible angiomatous blebs (pedunculated or sessile)	Rare: Cavernous angiomas of the eye, brain, or spinal cord Seizures, paresis, pain Medulloblastoma?	Angiomatous malformations of heart, mouth, parotid glands, lung, liver, spleen, genitourinary tract, or muscles may bleed Coagulopathy
Hereditary hemorrhagic telangiectasia (Osler–Rendu–Weber syndrome)[167]	Telangiectases (skin, mucous membranes, face, ears, fingers, conjunctivas, and nasopharynx)	Vascular malformations of brain, brainstem, spinal cord Hypoxemia, stroke due to pulmonary A-V fistulae Rare: portal-systemic encephalopathy	Recurrent epistaxis GI, hepatic, bladder telangiectases may bleed Pulmonary, liver, GI, bladder A-V fistulae Polycythemia may occur
HID syndrome 1989[168] usually sporadic?	Ichthyosis hystrix	Bilateral sensorineural deafness	
IFAP syndrome overlaps KID syndrome[169]	*I*chthyosis *f*ollicularis, *a*lopecia atricha, follicular hyperkeratosis, keratitis	*P*hotophobia, seizures, mental retardation	Chronic candidiasis Inguinal hernia
KID syndrome[170]	*K*eratitis, *i*chthyosis erythroderma, follicular keratosis, pachydermatoglyphy, hypertrichosis, atricha, alopecia	Sensorineural *d*eafness, corneal keratitis Rare Dandy–Walker	Mucocutaneous candidiasis
LEOPARD (multiple lentigines) syndrome[171,172]	*L*entiginosis	Sensorineural *d*eafness Rare ventriculomegaly, Gerstmann syndrome, mental retardation	*E*KG abnormalities, pulmonic stenosis, ventricular hypertrophy, *o*cular hypertelorism, *p*ulmonic stenosis, *a*bnormal genitalia, growth *r*etardation, orthopedic *d*abnormalities
Gorlin (nevoid basal cell carcinoma) syndrome[173]	Basal cell carcinoma, x- and gamma-irradiation sensitivity, palmar and plantar dermal pits	Medulloblastoma and other posterior fossa tumors, agenesis corpus callosum, brain calcification, mild mental retardation	Rhabdomyosarcoma, jaw cysts, vertebral abnormalities
Cardiofaciocutaneous/ Noonan syndrome	Melanocytic nevi, keratosis pilaris	Occasional mild mental difficulties	Dysmorphia, growth retardation, cardiac defects (PS, ASD), lymphedema
Piebald trait with neurological deficits[174]	White forelock and largely unpigmented skin macule	Poor coordination, cerebellar ataxia, variable mental retardation, hearing impairment	Short stature, bone or tooth growth delay, dysmorphia
Lynch syndrome[175]	Absence of thumb and toe nails	Developmental delay, epilepsy, kinesiogenic choreoathetosis	Preaxial anonychia
Variegate porphyria[176]	Waxy/withered prematurely aged skin, other dermatoses	Intermittent sensory/motor dysfunction, abdominal pain Confusion, seizures, psychosis	
Verbov–Sharland syndrome[177]	Palmoplantar keratoderma	Sensorineural hearing loss	
Waardenburg syndrome[178]	White forelock, heterochromia irides, leukoderma	Cochlear deafness	

Table 158.8	Neurocutaneous diseases with X-linked male-lethal inheritance		
Name	**Cutaneous features**	**Neurological features**	**Other features**
CHILD syndrome[179]	Lateralized *ich*thyosiform nevus, streaky lesions, claw nails	*H*emi-*h*ypoplasia of cerebral hemispheric, cranial nerves or spinal cord Occasional intellectual or hemisensory abnormalities	Congenital *h*emidysplasia with and *li*mb *d*efects Occasional cardiac, lung, or kidney abnormalities
Focal dermal hypoplasia (Xp22.3: Goltz syndrome)[180]	Linear or patchy dermal hypoplasia, poikiloderma, multiple periorificial papillomas, Blashko pigmentary streaks	Mild mental retardation, hearing loss, hydrocephalus, meningomyelocele Optic nerve abnormalities	Long bone dysplasia/aplasia, hypodontia, cleft lip and palate, diaphragmatic hernia
MIDAS syndrome[181]	Linear *d*ermal *a*plasia (head, neck)	Cortical hypoplasia, (focal), agenesis septum pellucidum or corpus callosum, microcephaly Occasional Aicardi syndrome	Unilateral or bilateral *mi*crophthalmia, and *s*clerocornea Occasional cardiac defects
Oral–facial–digital syndrome I (Xp22.3-p22.2)[182]	Cheek/ear milia (infantile), linear mucobuccal bands, alopecia	Mental retardation, hydrocephalus, porencephaly, partial agenesis corpus callosum	Dysmorphia, finger abnormalities, polycystic kidney disease

Neurocutaneous syndromes with X-linked male-lethal inheritance

Syndromes with X-linked male-lethal inheritance, which occur almost exclusively in girls, are listed in Table 158.8.

Neurocutaneous syndromes with X-linked, non male-lethal inheritance

Fabry disease (angiokeratoma corporis diffusum)

Fabry disease (FD) is an X-linked recessive disease, caused by deficiency of α-galactosidase A, a lysosomal hydrolase. More than 50 different mutations and polymorphisms have been identified at the site of the defective gene, Xq22.1.[183] It is largely a disease of hemizygous males, but milder forms of illness may express themselves in heterozygous females. Disease manifestations are chiefly due to lysosomally predominant accumulation of neutral α-galactosyl substituted glycosphingolipids (ceramides), especially trihexosylceramide (globotriaosylceramide or GL3) within blood vessels. This in turn leads to proliferative small vessel endarteritis with microaneurysm formation, especially in the skin, kidneys, heart, and nervous system. Direct accumulation of ceramides occurs in cardiac smooth muscle (especially left ventricular myocardium), endocardium, mitral valve leaflets, renal glomerular and tubular cells, corneal epithelial cells, and lymph nodes, prompting dysfunction of these tissues. Sites of neuronal accumulation and ensuing dysfunction include hypothalamus, substantia nigra, nuclei gracilis and cuneatus, dorsal vagal and salivary nuclei, nucleus ambiguus, the dorsal root ganglia, and the myenteric plexus. Aging may exacerbate the metabolic defect.[184]

Boys manifest disease in late childhood or early adolescence. The pathognomonic cutaneous finding is angiokeratoma corporis diffusum: punctate, telangiectatic, horny vascular and slightly elevated papules of the epidermis that increase in number with age. Flat macules and variable amounts of scaling may also be found. The papules are no larger than 4 to 5 mm in diameter, ranging in color from reddish-black to blue. They are symmetrically distributed between the umbilicus and the knees, concentrated in the "bathing suit" region (especially the hips and genitalia). Occasionally they are found on the face and oral mucosa.[21] Frequent stretching or distortion of skin rather than sun exposure is thought to provoke papule development.

Vasculopathy of conjunctiva and retina may impart a tortuous vascular contour to both retinal and conjunctival blood vessels. Corneal opacities termed "verticillata" are diagnostically important as they are virtually pathognomonic and appear quite early, detectable with slit lamp in some instances by 6 months of age. Initially diffuse, hazy, and subtle, the opacities may become a web of lines converging upon the center of the cornea. Linear "feathery" cataracts may also develop.[185] Thus the eye examination may permit presymptomatic members of a Fabry kindred to be diagnosed and may confirm the diagnosis in individuals not known to be at risk who manifest an appropriate clinical history.

Neuropathy of small unmyelinated fibers results in severe acroparesthesiae with reddening that has been termed erythromelalgia or acromelalgia of Weir Mitchell. The process is likely in part ischemic, due to autonomic dysregulation of vasa nervosa subserving central or peripheral nerves. The regulatory dysfunction may result from abnormalities of hypothalamus or other central or peripheral autonomic regulatory tissues. Burning, shooting, or lancinating pains and paresthesiae are common early symptoms of FD in boys, problems that often bring undiagnosed patients to medical attention. The severity and distal predilection (fingers or toes) resembles gout. Physical activity and fever are provocative. Boys may also experience arthritic limb and joint pains, especially of the distal interphalangeal joints. Hip pain and necrosis of the femoral head may occur.[186] Acromelalgia is a disturbingly persistent intermittent problem in FD, with painful epochs lasting days to weeks, often associated with other manifestations of autonomic instability, such as fevers (persistent or undulating) or bouts of diarrhea. Hands and feet may become edematous. Hypohidrosis may contribute to fever.[187]

Cardiac, renal, or cerebral vasculopathic dysfunction tend to become overt in the third or fourth decades of life. Any of these may lead to death by the fifth decade. Renal tubular dysfunction leads to impaired urine concentration, polyuria and nocturia. This gradually progressive process may be detectable by laboratory testing in childhood, but overt renal failure and hypertension are uncommon except in adults with FD. Cerebrovascular manifestations often lead to considerable cumulative neurological morbidity, including recurrent thrombotic or embolic infarction. Renal, cardiac, or cerebrovascular abnormalities may each contribute to the stroke risk. The tendency to enhanced platelet aggregation, another FD manifestation, increases the risk for stroke as well as for renal, cardiac, and cerebrovascular abnormality. Adult men with FD are at risk for seizures and epilepsy, and vascular dementia of adults has been ascribed to FD.[188]

Cardiac ceramide accumulation may lead to sick sinus syndrome, angina pectoris, and hypertrophic nonobstructive cardiomyopathy.[189] Preferential accumulation predisposes especially to left ventricular myocardial dysfunction.[190] Valvular disease may result from coronary artery disease or from deposition of lipids on mitral valve leaflets. The cardiomegaly caused by these various processes may be enormous.[191] Cardiac disease may in turn result in embolic cerebral, renal, pulmonary, or other organ system disease. Possible gastrointestinal disturbances in FD include episodic abdominal pain, nausea, vomiting, diarrhea and intestinal diverticuli.[192]

Chronic pulmonary insufficiency is a potential late complication of Fabry disease.[193]

Mild or restricted forms of Fabry disease
It is possible that some boys develop congenital cyanotic cardiac abnormalities due to FD, and some mutations result in severe heart problems in otherwise mild FD.[194] Some individuals with relatively modest α-galactosidase A deficiency remain asymptomatic or manifest mild symptoms such as proteinuria or recurrent acroparesthesiae in adulthood. A progeroid syndrome with pathological changes in heart, great vessels, and kidneys that resemble those of FD has been reported.[195]

Females
Heterozygous females are among those who remain asymptomatic or whose manifestations have a late onset, remaining relatively minor. Some women with FD manifest heart disease, while other FD manifestations are absent or minor. Another isolated FD manifestation found in heterozygous women is the appearance of the corneal verticilla. Other women exhibit only the angiokeratomatous rash, pain, proteinuria, or elevated urinary trihexosylceramide.[196] Diagnosis in such limited disease forms may be challenging, since ceramide and enzyme studies may not distinguish affected patients from the broad range of normal values. Therefore biopsies of affected tissue may be required to confirm diagnosis, disclosing the typical lamellar inclusions.[197] Limited expression is likely the result of lionization. Occasionally, very unfavorable X-inactivation will permit full expression of FD in a woman.[196] Enzymatic activity in heterozygous females may range from normal to, in those rare instances of fully-affected females, undetectable.[198]

Diagnosis
Complete absence of enzyme from plasma, leukocytes, tears, or fibroblasts is characteristic of affected or presymptomatic hemizygous males. Enzymatic deficiency also permits diagnosis of some heterozygous female carriers, depending upon their type of X-chromosome inactivation. Fluorescence-based molecular techniques permit reliable diagnosis of hemizygous or heterozygous individuals, including prenatal diagnosis by analysis of amniocytes or chorionic villi.[183,198] However, these techniques require identification of the precise mutation that has caused FD in a given family.[199,200] Electron microscopic demonstration of characteristic inclusions of skin, conjunctival, or kidney tissues may also establish the diagnosis of FD in homozygous males and some heterozygous females.[197] Small, unmyelinated cutaneous nerves are particularly likely to disclose ceramide storage, while Schwann cells are characteristically spared.[201] Significant (greater than 12-fold) elevations of trihexosylceramide in plasma and urine sediment are usually found in homozygous males and may be of use in monitoring therapeutic efficacy; the technique is far less helpful in diagnosing heterozygous females.[202] Foam cells in bone marrow and lipid-laden cells in the urinary sediment support the diagnosis of FD. Sedimentation rate may be elevated during pain crises.

Treatment
Bouts of pain and acroparesthesiae may respond to treatment with anticonvulsant drugs such as phenytoin, carbamazepine, or gabapentin. Hydration, antipyretic analgesics, and avoidance of heat and sunshine may have prophylactic and therapeutic effects on pain. Prophylactic use of antiplatelet-aggregation agents such as aspirin or ticlopidine has been advocated. Kidney or heart transplantation has been performed successfully in patients with FD. In addition to replacing dysfunctional organs, transplantation provides the patients with tissues that produce α-galactosidase. Liver and bone marrow transplantation for enzyme replacement and gene transfer are currently under investigation.[203] Genetic counseling and screening are of considerable importance.

Table 158.9   X-linked neurocutaneous diseases that are not lethal for males

Name	Cutaneous features	Neurological features	Other features
Incontinentia pigmenti (Xq28)[204]	Hyperpigmented whorls, splatters, and linear lesions	Visual disturbances, CNS vasculopathy, ataxia, weakness, mental retardation	Dental, orthopedic deformities
Albinism–deafness syndrome (Xq26.3-q27.1)[205]	Piebald pigmentary disturbance	Profound deafness in males, with mutism; lesser deafness in girls	
Bullous dystrophy of Mendes da Costa (Xq27.3qter)[206]	Macular hyper-depigmentation, alopecia totalis	Microcephaly, mental retardation	
Dyskeratosis congenita (Zinnser–Cole–Engman syndrome; DKC1 gene Xq28)[207]	Reticular facial hyperpigmentation, telangiectases, alopecia, mucosal premalignant leukoplakia, palmar hyperkeratosis	Mental deficiency, dentate/ basal ganglia calcification, deafness, cerebellar hypoplasia	Conjunctivitis, blepharitis, ectropion, excessive lacrimation Osteoporosis, carious teeth, testicular hypoplasia, cancer, pancytopenia Immunodeficiency
Hoyeraal–Hreidarsson syndrome	Similar to Zinnser–Cole–Engman	Ditto	Ditto
Kallmann syndrome (Xp2.3t)[208]	Occasional ichthyosis, chondrodysplasia punctata	Agenesis of olfactory lobes with anosmia	Hypogonadotropic hypogonadism
Partington syndrome (Xp22-p21)[209]	Generalized reticulate hyperpigmentation	Hemiparesis, epilepsy	Failure to thrive, recurrent pneumonia

Approximately half the sons of a heterozygous female carrier will have FD, half the daughters will be carriers. All daughters of affected males will be carriers; sons will not inherit the disease.

Other X-linked neurocutaneous diseases that are not lethal for males are listed in Table 158.9.

Mosaicism of autosomal lethal mutations

Sturge–Weber syndrome (encephalofacial angiomatosis; encephalotrigeminal angiomatosis)

The clinical description of Sturge–Weber syndrome (SWS) was refined between 1860 and 1929.[210–212] It is a highly variable but recognizable entity of uncertain inheritance, although clinically variable familial clusters have been reported.[213] Mosaic inheritance of spontaneous autosomal lethal mutations with occasional paradominant passage has been proposed as a genetic mechanism, although this intriguing hypothesis is as yet incompletely proven. SWS is not actually a phakomatosis since it is a vascular rather than a cancer syndrome. The complete form of SWS is defined by the presence of three forms of ipsilateral angioma: upper facial, leptomeningeal, and choroidal.[214] The vascular anlage of these affected tissues share embryological origin in the same region of the neural crest and primitive facial cleft from which the optic cup originates.[215] This explains the occasional development of macrophthalmia, glaucoma, or exudative retinal detachment ipsilateral to the portwine stain.[216] Developmental abnormalities,

epilepsy, headache, and stroke-like episodes are the consequences of the leptomeningeal abnormality. Visual disturbances are common and are chiefly due to choroidal angiomatosis.[217] Although classically SWS is a lateralized illness, bilateral manifestations, usually quite asymmetrical, are not uncommonly detected in carefully examined adults.[218]

The nevus flammeus is the most important diagnostic clue, present in almost all SWS cases. It is a mature capillary hemangioma that occurs most commonly in regions of the upper face that receive sensory innervation from the first division of the trigeminal nerve, especially the forehead, upper eyelid, and periorbital inner canthus. It may extend into regions innervated by the second and, even less commonly, by the third trigeminal sensory divisions, but some portion of the lesion is almost always found cephalad to the palpebral fissure in patients with SWS.[219] The flat angiomatous nevus has often been termed, on the basis of its typical tawny to bluish-red color, a "portwine stain." It is present from birth, grows only in proportion to the growth of the affected part, and does not involute. These features and the hue distinguish it from the bright red strawberry hemangioma, which may enlarge for the first 6 to 8 months of life, then involute.[21] The appearance is more subtle but appreciable in moderately pigmented skin, but difficult to ascertain in darkly pigmented skin.

In some instances the nevus is found on nasopharyngeal surfaces, mucous membranes (lips, gingiva, palate, floor of mouth, tongue, uvula, pharynx, larynx), ipsilateral jaw, or skull. Rarely the angioma is cavernous.[220] Gingival tumor or intraoral vascular hyperplasia of lip, tongue, cheek and gingiva may also be found, occasionally requiring repeated periodontal intervention. These changes may be prevented by careful control of plaque.[220] The SWS portwine stain may also be found to extend to the neck, trunk, or extremities. Trunk and extremity nevi may be ipsilateral or contralateral to the facial nevus or even bilateral and may contain hypertrophic vascular nodules.[21,221] Other cutaneous nevi may rarely be seen in SWS, including cavernous hemangiomas, phacomatosis pigmentovascularis type II, pyogenic granulomas, or nevus of Ota.[222]

Not every patient with a facial portwine stain will have pial angiomatosis, and not all patients with pial angiomatosis will have portwine stains. It is estimated that the risk for pial angiomatosis is at least 6% in patients with a unilateral portwine stain in the upper to midface. If found, angiomatosis is ipsilateral to the stain in about 90% of cases, although an additional lesser degree of angiomatosis of the contralateral leptomeninges is found in about 10%. Bilateral portwine stains indicate at least a 24% risk for associated pial angiomatosis, which may be bilateral or unilateral.[223] If present, the likelihood of anteriorly located pial angiomatosis is roughly proportional to the degree to which the portwine stain approaches the midface. Extent of laterofrontal involvement is roughly proportional to likelihood of occipitoparietal pial angiomatosis.[32,224] Unusually, a portwine stain may bilaterally straddle the midface, with limited lateral extension. Occasional instances of cavernous leptomeningeal venous angiomas have been described in patients with SWS.[216]

Magnetic resonance images with gadolinium often quite clearly demonstrate gyral enhancement proportional to the extent of pial angiomatosis, even in patients without clinical manifestations.[225] T_2-weighted MRI also reliably demonstrates the cortical thickening, diminished convolutional complexity, and subcortical white matter abnormality consistent with pial angiomatosis. Increase in size of the ipsilateral choroid plexus, proportional to the degree of pial angiomatosis, is an early and reliable sign of pial angiomatosis.[226] Classical angiography, single-photon emission CT (SPECT), and positron emission tomography (PET) techniques also disclose characteristic changes of pial angiomatosis.[217,227,228] SPECT studies have shown bilateral abnormalities of perfusion and glucose metabolism during and after the second decade in as many as 60% of SWS patients.[217] Approximately one third of SWS patients are found to have arteriovenous malformations, dural sinus abnormalities, and vascular thromboses by MRI and other angiographic techniques.[229]

Calcification in areas of pial angiomatosis is best demonstrated by CT scans.[230] Calcification increases over time and is initially subcortical with subsequent extension toward the cortical surface. It is often greatest in the occipital region. CT is the most sensitive

technique and may prove abnormal in some neonates, many infants, and probably as many as 90% of adolescents or adults with SWS.[231] Calcification within the walls of small cerebral blood vessels results in the characteristic radiographic "tram-track sign," usually most evident in the parieto-occipital region. Convolutional undulating calcification may also be found in the parieto-occipital region.[109] Bilateral calcification may be found in as many as 10% of older patients, including those who appear to have only unilateral pial angiomatosis.[32,217] CT scans of older patients often also disclose unilateral hemispheric atrophy (especially frontal, parietal, and temporal), enlargement of the choroid plexus, and abnormal contrast drainage along the ventricular angle into the vein of Galen system. Transient cortical enhancement may appear after prolonged seizures.[225]

The progressive nature of the neurological dysfunction seen in SWS is probably due to oligemia, tissue hypoxemia, and venous stagnation with retention of potentially toxic byproducts of metabolism in the region of pial angiomatosis.[217] Tenuous circulation may be intermittently compromised by impaired hemodynamic response, thrombotic events, or the enhanced energy cost exacted by seizures.[232] Oligemia and vascular dysregulation may affect areas of brain not known to have pial angiomatosis, including an apparently uninvolved hemisphere.[233] Epilepsy may be provoked by these cumulative tissue injuries, in addition to possible abnormalities of cortical development. Earlier onset and greater severity of seizures, associated with greater initial severity of SWS-associated dysfunction, enhance likelihood and severity of subsequent neurological regression.[234] Neurological deficits, such as hemianopsia, hemiparesis, or aphasia, at times observed in SWS, may be ascribed to transient mismatches of blood flow and energy demand from these various mechanisms. Deficits may be transient, resolving over days to months, but saltatory or steadily progressive hemiparesis, hemiatrophy, progressive, worsening epilepsy, and loss of intellectual capacity are quite common in SWS, especially where repeated episodes of status epilepticus occur.[232,234] A better outlook is found in individuals with relatively mild epilepsy of comparatively late onset.

Among the ocular complications of SWS is glaucoma, which develops in approximately 25% to 35% of cases. Most or possibly all of these patients are among the 40% of SWS patients that have ocular choroidal membrane angiomas, the third characteristic vascular lesion of SWS. Glaucoma may be unilateral or bilateral, even if the portwine stain is strictly unilateral. One half of those with glaucoma have buphthalmos ipsilateral to the facial angioma. Other possible ocular findings of SWS include heterochromia irides, choroidal atrophy, megalocornea, exophthalmos, macrophthalmia, optic atrophy, optic neuropathy, dilated retinal veins, and strabismus. SWS should be considered in all infants with congenital glaucoma or megalocornea.[235] Hemianopsia of variable degree is found in 25% to 50% of patients with SWS, with or without associated ipsilateral hemiparesis.[21,109]

Epilepsy develops in 75% to 90% of SWS patients, often as early as a few months of age, as one of the first manifestations.[217,224,236] The risk for epilepsy is greater than 70% if pial angiomatosis is confined to one hemisphere, with mean age of onset of 24 months. Bihemispheric pial angiomatosis increases that risk to 93%, with a mean age of onset of 6 months of age.[224] Patients with SWS-associated epilepsy can be usefully segregated into two groups: early (mean 6 to 7 months) and later (mean 3.7 years) onset. The earlier onset group has more severe neurological abnormality, and a greater tendency to experience stroke-like episodes.[217]

Partial motor events originating in the hemisphere with pial angiomatosis, ranging from quite focal to hemiconvulsive, occur in 80% of patients with SWS and epilepsy. In half of afflicted patients these remain focal; in half there is a combination of focal and primary or secondary generalized motor seizures. The remaining 20% of patients with SWS and epilepsy manifest primary or secondarily generalized tonic–clonic seizures, which may also progressively worsen.[224] Myoclonic, atonic, mixed seizures, and infantile spasms may occur in SWS patients with unilateral angiomatosis.[237] There is a significant risk for status epilepticus or for postictal (Todd's) paralysis, and for steadily worsening severity of epilepsy and saltatory progression of associated postictal deficits, such as the progressive hemiparesis observed in 25% to 35% of cases. However, some individuals with SWS have only mild or occasional seizures, and some have none at all.

Bilateral epileptic manifestations suggest bilateral pial abnormalities, especially where the facial nevus is bilateral, and carry greater risk for cumulative bilateral motor deficits and intellectual deterioration. However, bilateral epileptic manifestations are occasionally found in patients whose facial nevus is strictly unilateral.[109] Interictal EEG recording of an affected hemisphere typically discloses slowing and diminished amplitude, in association with multiple, widespread, independent spike foci.[124] Bisynchronous generalized EEG discharges may be found in patients with unilateral pial angiomatosis.[237]

Migrainous headaches afflict approximately 30% of patients with SWS and may have onset in the first decade of life. Transient hemiplegia may follow some headaches. Similar transient non-postconvulsive episodes may occur without associated headache. These episodes do not appear to have the same ominous significance as do episodes of postconvulsive hemiparesis. It is possible that some patients with bilateral occipital calcification and migraine have a limited form of SWS.[238,239]

Nearly half of all SWS and fully 75% of those with epilepsy exhibit mental subnormality, especially if evaluated in adolescence or adulthood. Mental retardation is found in nearly 20%. Intellectual deficit is likely proportional to extent of leptomeningeal involvement (especially if bilateral), degree of hemi-

paresis/hemiatrophy, and especially severity of epilepsy.[236] Although it is possible that severity of epilepsy merely reflects severity of underlying structural disease, it is quite likely that seizures worsen structural abnormality. Early severe neurological manifestations including epilepsy imply a considerable risk for ultimate IQ scores ranging only from 40 to 68.[240] Where leptomeningeal angiomatosis is confined to one hemisphere and there are no seizures, average intelligence is the rule. Some patients with bihemispheric pial abnormality but no seizures also have normal intelligence.[224]

Elevation of spinal fluid protein is a common finding in SWS. Hydrocephalus is an occasional feature.[241] Macrocephaly without hydrocephalus has occasionally been noted.[221] Extrafacial portwine stains may be associated with hypertrophy of soft tissues and bones, usually due to enhancement of regional blood flow by an associated cavernous hemangioma.[21] This feature represents an important clinical overlap between SWS and Klippel–Trenaunay syndrome (see below).

Management Sturge–Weber syndrome is a disease of variable severity. It is possible that the percentage of patients who experience a favorable outcome may be increased by early very aggressive treatment of epilepsy with anticonvulsants or epilepsy surgery in order to prevent the cascade of epilepsy-related deterioration of function.[225,242] Provision of rectal valium for home use and aggressive management of status epilepticus are especially important. Delays in treatment entailed by scans and clinical obscuration by neuromuscular paralysis should scrupulously be avoided. The early prophylactic use of aspirin and other agents to prevent vasospasm, platelet activation, and blood constituent clumping may also improve outlook, possibly reducing the risk for stroke-like episodes by as much as two thirds.[217]

There is evidence that functional reorganization preserves motor, language, and other capacities that might otherwise be lost due to the degenerative potential of pial angiomatosis. Some of these functions may be assumed by the hemisphere contralateral to pial angiomatosis. These preserved functions may be compromised or lost by uncontrolled seizure activity.[243] These facts may explain the recovery of function observed after epilepsy surgery achieves control of seizures. Improvement has even been observed in SWS patients with mutism or very low levels of language function if surgery is undertaken before 8.5 years of age.[240] Even without evidence for early improvement after surgery, patients may experience better long-term psychomotor outlook due to surgical control of intractable seizures,[244] although further efficacy studies are needed. Amelioration of seizures in SWS has been achieved with lesionectomy, selective lobar corticectomy, lobectomy (occipital or parietal), modified (functional) or anatomical hemispherectomy, or callosotomy.[225,233,242] Postsurgical complications may include hemiparesis and hemianesthesia, but even these deficits may exhibit varying degrees of recovery.[225] Particular anesthetic risks may be encountered in patients with SWS.[245]

The migrainous headaches of SWS patients should be recognized and adequately treated, distinguishing the post-headache hemiparetic episodes from the much more ominous non-headache related onset of hemiparesis. The usual armamentarium of abortive and prophylactic approaches to migraine may be employed, although it may be prudent to avoid such vasoactive medications as ergotamines and triptans. The stigmatizing portwine stain of SWS can be ameliorated with various forms of laser therapy.[246] Careful ophthalmological evaluation and follow-up is an essential aspect of the management of SWS, given the risk for glaucoma and other ophthalmological complications.

Possible Sturge–Weber variants and other possible examples of mosaic inheritance of autosomal lethal neurocutaneous conditions

These conditions are listed in Table 158.10.

Autosomal recessive neurocutaneous diseases

Ataxia–telangiectasia (Louis–Bar syndrome)

Described in 1941,[263] the incidence of ataxia–telangiectasia (AT) disease is approximately 1/40 000.[264] Immunological and neurological dysfunction, the earliest findings, become apparent in the first few years of life. Cutaneous and conjunctival changes develop in mid-childhood, while lymphomatous malignancies develop and further neurological deterioration occurs during adolescence. The mutant gene, on chromosome 11q22.3, encodes ATM protein, which is involved in check-point regulation of the cell cycle. Five complementation groups and more than 100 different mutations have been described, accounting for the clinical heterogeneity of AT.[265] Immunodeficiency and malignancies result from sensitivity to induction of DNA injury and chromosomal instability by X-irradiation and radiomimetic chemicals as well as from defective cell cycle regulation. Dysfunctional DNA synthetic and repair enzymes result in chromosomal rearrangements and incorporation of abnormal segments that become breakpoints,[266,267] which tend to occur on chromosomes 7 (bands 7p14 and 7p35), 14 (14q2, 14q32, and 14qter),[268] and 2 (2p12 and 2q11).[269]

Immunoglobulin superfamily gene defects on chromosome 11 may increase susceptibility to certain kinds of infection due to failure of maturation of T-cell receptors and of immunoglobulin synthetic shift from IgM to IgA, IgG, or IgE heavy chain production.[270] Chromosomal instability may predispose to the development of hematological malignancies because of deficient immunosurveillance or other causes. The 14–14 translocation at breakpoint 14q32, found in about 10% of AT cases, is particularly associated with lymphoreticular malignancies, especially leukemia.[271] Translocation at the 11q22.3 site has been found in some AT-associated nonlymphoid leukemias.[232] Synapsis and recombination of meiotic chromosomes may account for gonadal atrophy in some AT cases.[273]

The causes of oculocutaneous telangiectases, thymic aplasia or hypoplasia, diminished spleen size, poor growth, impaired organ maturation, and progressive cerebellar and extrapyramidal neurological dysfunction in AT are not well understood.[274] Light exposure promotes the progress oculocutaneous changes, either because of enhanced vascular sensitivity or defective repair. Progressive ataxia and hypotonia are associated with degeneration of cerebellar cortex (with Purkinje and granule cell loss), as well as the loss of posterior column myelinated fibers. Degeneration of other spinal tracts and loss of anterior spinal horn and sympathetic ganglia cells may also occur in AT.[275] Basal ganglia lesions, found in a large minority of AT patients, may account for choreoathetosis.[274] Other poorly understood pathological findings of AT include late degenerative gliovascular nodules within cerebral white matter, peripheral nerve abnormalities with or without slowed nerve conduction velocities, and the curious finding of nucleocytomegaly in diverse cell types of various body tissues.[276]

Clinical features Approximately 70% of children with AT are small, manifesting "failure to thrive" in the first few years of life. Infections and endocrine dysfunction may contribute to this tendency. Recurrent bouts of sinusitis, otitis media, and bronchopulmonary infections, caused by common bacterial pathogens or viruses, provide a diagnostic clue in 65% to 80% of AT patients. Recurrent bouts of severe impetigo are common, as are blepharitis and seborrheic dermatitis. In half of the AT patients that manifest recurrent infections, progressive pulmonary difficulties including bronchiectasis or clubbing of fingers are especially distinctive. The predilection to sinopulmonary infections is due to both humoral and cellular deficiencies and may be proportional to their severity,[277] although other investigators have failed to confirm such a relationship.[228] Humoral defects include low or absent IgA, IgG_2 and IgG_4, and IgE, and B cells have been shown to have intrinsic defects. Production of antibodies specific for viral or bacterial antigens is often inadequate. Defective immunoregulation occurs with inadequate T-lymphocyte proliferative responses and excessive T-suppressor activity.[277] Pulmonary diseases are the most frequent causes of early death in individuals with AT. On the other hand, one third of children with AT do not have an infectious history that is distinguishable from that of other children.[279]

The cardinal neurological manifestations of AT, found in almost all cases, are progressive ataxia and abnormal eye movements. Ataxia, associated with hypotonia, typically becomes apparent at the time children with AT start to walk, long before the oculocutaneous telangiectases appear. The ataxia involves head, trunk, and limbs, imparting an unsteady axio-proximal "loose jointedness" for patterned movement, together with awkward compensatory swaying postures, titubation, and intention tremor.[32] True

Table 158.10 Neurocutaneous conditions or Sturge–Weber related conditions with possible mosaic inheritance of autosomal lethal traits

Name	Cutaneous features	Neurological features	Other features
Epilepsy with occipital calcifications[247]	None	Epilepsy, occipital calcifications	
Leptomeningeal angiomatosis[236]	None	Pial and ocular choroidal angiomatosis	
Klippel–Trenaunay syndrome[248]	Resemble SWS	Intracranial AVMs, hemimegalencephaly, mental retardation, abnormal neck or skull bones	Lymphangiomas, varicosities, A-V fistulas, body segment hypertrophy
Syndrome of bilateral facial nevi, macrocrania, and anomalous venous return[249]	Resemble SWS	Cerebral venous drainage through superficial veins, macrocrania, some SWS features	
Syndrome of facial angiomas, posterior fossa cyst and partial corpus callosum agenesis[250]	Cutaneous features resemble SWS	Dandy–Walker, cerebellar hypoplasia, callosal agenesis, cerebral arterial occlusion/aneurysm as in Wyburn-Mason	
Syndrome of facial angiomatosis, ocular changes, and hypotonia[216]	Resemble SWS, but facial AVMs	Hypotonia	Uveal tract AVMs, microphthalmos, heterochromia irides
Oculocerebrocutaneous (Delleman) syndrome[251]	Goldenhar-like unilateral periorbital skin tags, focal aplastic skin lesions, focal scalp alopecia	Hydrocephalus, macrocephaly, porencephaly or other malformations, cerebral hemiatrophy, neuroendocrine, seizures	Unilateral eyelid/iris colobomas, orbital cysts, microtia, microphthalmia or anophthalmia, facial microsomia, midline facial clefts
Encephalocranio-cutaneous lipomatosis (Haberland syndrome)[252]	Unilateral hairless fatty scalp hamartoma with dermal hypoplasia (nevus psiloliparus)	Mental retardation, epilepsy, unilateral intracranial lipomas, vascular dysplasia, porencephaly	Limbal conjunctival lipodermoids, ectopia pupillae, aberrant iris tissue
Neurocutaneous melanosis[253]	Pigmented nevi, including the giant hairy melanocytic nevus	Leptomeningeal melanoma of brain or spinal cord	
Nevus comedonicus syndrome[254]	Lateralized nevus comedonicus	EEG abnormalities	Ipsilateral cataract and skeletal deformities
Oculoauriculo-vertebral syndrome[255]	Resemble Delleman syndrome	Resemble Delleman syndrome	Resemble Delleman syndrome
Pallister–Killian (isochromosome 12p) syndrome[256]	Hypopigmented patches, sparse hair	Severe mental retardation, seizures, hearing loss, ptosis	Growth deficiency, characteristic facies, sparse hair
Phakomatosis pigmentokeratotica[257]	Twin organoid sebaceous and speckled lentiginous nevi	Mental retardation, seizures, ptosis, strabismus, deafness, weakness, segmental dysesthesia or hyperhidrosis	
Phakomatosis pigmentovascularis[258]	Nevus flammeus, spilus, or anemicus, linear telangiectatic nevi, extensive aberrant Mongolian spots	Seizures, moyamoya, hemiparesis	Ocular melanosis, discrepant limb length, scoliosis, pelvic obliquity, renal agenesis or angiomatous lesions
Pigmentary mosaicism of the Ito type[259]	Whorls or streaks of reduced pigmentation in "Christmas tree" pattern	Mental retardation, weakness, seizures, hemimegalencephaly	Orthopedic problems of legs, abnormalities of nails

Table 158.10 *continued*

Name	Cutaneous features	Neurological features	Other features
Proteus syndrome[260]	Nonepidermolytic, nonorganoid epidermal nevus, dermal hypoplasia or lipohypoplasia	Macrocephaly, mental retardation, hydrocephalus, seizures	Asymmetrical partial gigantism or hemihypertrophy, hamartomas, neoplasms; renal or pulmonary anomalies
Schimmelpenning (Feuerstein–Mims) syndrome[261]	Systematized sebaceous nevus	Mental retardation and seizures	Conjunctival lipodermoid, colobomas, and orbital bone or skull defects
Van Lohuizen syndrome[262]	Cutis marmorata, nevus flammeus	Developmental delay, seizures, macrocephaly	Limb anomalies, syndactyly

AVM, arteriovenous malformation; SWS, Sturge–Weber syndrome.

appendicular dysmetria, dyssynergia, and intention tremor may be less prominent than these axial ataxic findings. Head thrusting and forced blinking due to impairments of gaze are also common at this stage of illness, and although facial movement and animation are present, facies are often dull or inexpressive at rest. Aicardi noted that this combination of findings brings to mind the movements of "little clowns" and that one particularly characteristic feature is the peculiar "slow-spreading smile."[32] Drooling and slow, cerebellar dysarthric speech are often noted.

The movements of AT are due to failure of cerebellar and extrapyramidal regulation of movement and loss of joint position sense. Atrophy of cerebellum, basal ganglia, posterior columns, and posterior sensory nerve roots is often detectable by 2 to 3 years of age.[280] In some patients extrapyramidal signs predominate. Choreoathetosis develops in approximately 25% of patients.[274] Dystonia, myoclonus,[281] posterior column signs, diminution or absence of muscle stretch reflexes, and spinal muscular atrophy are found in some older AT patients. The progression of this combination of features may suggest spinocerebellar degeneration.[277] Rarely, AT evolves as a predominantly pyramidal disease with spasticity and mental retardation.[282] In other patients, peripheral neuropathy is the most prominent neurological abnormality.[283] Although motor and sensory abnormalities are relentlessly progressive, the rate of neurological progression is quite variable even among siblings. Since deterioration is often slow, many toddlers initially receive the label "ataxic CP."

The correct diagnosis is often suggested at about age 7, with the appearance of telangiectases. However, oculomotor apraxia and abnormal saccadic eye movements, which appear before the telangiectases, distinguish AT from ataxic CP. Saccades are slow and hypometric, and may be preceded by forced blinking or head thrusting to interrupt gaze fixation in order to initiate movement, especially from the primary position of gaze. In instances of severe gaze apraxia, refixation is obtained almost entirely by head movement.[284]

Optokinetic nystagmus is absent. Approximately one third of AT patients become mentally retarded, usually in the mild range, after slow deterioration of mental function in association with disease progression.

Conjunctival telangiectases usually appear at 5 to 6 years of age, occasionally as early as 3 years of age, and sometimes not until adolescence or adulthood. The bilateral changes are first detectable at the lateral ocular canthi and subsequently spread across the equatorial bulbar conjunctival plane. The lower tarsal conjunctivae tend also to become involved. Because recurrent blepharitis, impetigo, and dermatitis often precede the development of ocular telangiectases, the telangiectases are often mistakenly viewed as representing allergic or infectious blepharoconjunctivitis. Telangiectases may be found on the eyelids, cheek eminences, ears, and to a lesser extent on the anterior chest, antecubital and popliteal fossae, and dorsal surfaces of hands and feet. In regions of skin flexures, the telangiectases may be subtle, resembling fine petechiae.[285] Sun exposure may provoke the development of telangiectases, which are less common in individuals with darkly pigmented skin.[286]

Cutaneous pigmentary and progeric manifestations, including xerosis and diffuse premature graying of hair, develop in late childhood or early adolescence in 90% of AT patients. Mottled hyperpigmented macules, some resembling *café au lait* patches, and areas of hypopigmentation resembling vitiligo have been noted in many older AT patients.[286] Persistent noninfectious cutaneous granulomas that are prone to ulceration are common in AT. They improve with intralesional administration of triamcinolone, although they do not then resolve.[287] Progressive sclerodermatous atrophy and loss of subcutaneous fat may render the face of older AT patients gaunt and mask-like; similar changes may occasionally be noted in the ears, arms, and hands. The combination of cutaneous pigmentary changes, atrophy, and sclerosis may result in an appearance that resembles the poikiloderma found in scleroderma, actinic, or radiodermatoses. Other abnormalities of skin or hair found in patients with AT include alopecia areata, limb hirsutism, atopic dermatitis, keratitis pilaris, nummular eczema, acanthosis nigricans, warts, and ephelides.[286]

Patients with AT may not achieve normal puberty. Girls with AT may not have normal differentiation of ovarian tissues; boys may have testicular hypoplasia. Insulin-dependent diabetes mellitus may develop in older patients.[279] Elevation of hepatic transaminases is found in 40% to 50% of AT patients.[288]

The risk for malignancy in AT is 60 to 300 fold greater than for other children and adolescents. Malignancy is the second most common cause of early death in AT. Lymphoreticular tumors are noted in 10% to 15% of AT patients by adolescence, although the actual prevalence of such tumors is probably much higher. Almost half of AT patients in one autopsy series were found to harbor malignant tumors, although many had died of pulmonary failure before malignancy was clinically apparent.[289] Hodgkin's and nonHodgkin lymphomas and lymphocytic leukemias (especially B-cell lymphomas and chronic T-cell leukemias) are the most commonly encountered malignancies of the first 15 years of life of those with AT. After 15 years of age epithelial tumors predominate.[290] Even AT heterozygotes (approximately 1% of the population of North America) are at increased risk for malignancy, albeit to a much lesser degree than homozygotes.[291] Heterozygotic female carriers of AT are at a 3 to 5 fold increased risk for the development of breast cancer.[291] Surveillance for breast tumors is complicated by the fact that these heterozygotic women are also subject to X-irradiation-induced chromosomal breaks, and therefore routine mammography is contraindicated.

Diagnosis Ataxia with oculomotor apraxia strongly suggests the diagnosis of AT prior to the appearance of the pathognomonic telangiectases. AT must be considered in all children thought to have ataxic cerebral palsy[292] and in those who suggest the variant presentations noted above. Supportive laboratory tests include the almost universal elevation of α-fetoprotein (AFP) and carcinoembryonic antigen (CEA). Inversions and translocations of chromosomes 7 and 14 are found in most,[293] but not all[294] AT patients. Rarely, individuals manifest AFP elevation and typical cytogenetic abnormalities without neurological abnormalities.[32] Most individuals with AT are found to have the characteristic dysgammaglobulinemia, with little or no detectable serum IgA or IgE, low total IgG, selective deficiency of IgG_2 and IgG_4 subclasses, but normal IgM.[278] Circulating anti-IgA antibodies are commonly found in AT patients who have IgA deficiency.[295]

Two thirds of AT patients are anergic to skin testing to common antigens and show diminished mitogen-induced T-cell proliferation.[277] T-cell marker studies show an increase in those bearing γ/δ receptors.[296] Induction of characteristic chromosomal breakage in the presence of ionizing radiation has been employed in pre- and postnatal diagnosis of AT.[297] Prenatal diagnosis can also be ascertained with measurement of amniotic AFP or clastogenic factor, or by molecular methods.[297] A gene that accounts for as many as two thirds of cases of AT in Scandinavians has been identified.[298] As with all genetic testing of degenerative conditions, the availability of that diagnostic test has posed ethical and psychological dilemmas.[299] Hepatic transaminases and glucose tolerance should be studied in all individuals known to have AT. Although cerebellar atrophy is found in some AT patients, CT and MRI are of greater value in excluding other illnesses than in the establishment of the diagnosis of AT. Electromyography and nerve conduction testing may demonstrate denervation due to anterior horn cell loss or slowing of nerve conduction in older patients.[300]

Much of the differential diagnosis, including static and progressive/degenerative cerebellar, spinocerebellar, extrapyramidal and other diseases relevant to the oculocutaneous findings, has been mentioned in passing. Patients with a combination of motor findings suggesting AT who lack expected telangiectases or laboratory abnormalities may have the syndrome of ataxia–oculomotor apraxia. The combination of spastic diplegia, ataxia, and immunodeficiency, with normal immunoglobulin studies may indicate dysequilibrium–diplegia syndrome.[301] Other diseases associated with DNA repair disturbances that may be considered include Bloom or Cockayne syndromes, and xeroderma pigmentosum. The rare Nijmegen chromosomal breakage syndrome may be either a separate disease or a variant form of AT.[302]

There are no specific treatments for AT. Ionizing radiation (X-rays, radiomimetic drugs) and sources of infection should be avoided. Full doses of conventional radiation and most chemotherapeutic agents are contraindicated for the treatment of AT-associated malignancy since they may provoke extreme tissue necrosis, chromosomal disturbances, and development of secondary malignancies. These modalities are sometimes employed at reduced and highly fractionated dosage, but complete avoidance of actinomycin D, cyclophosphamide, and especially bleomycin is of great importance. Avoidance of sunlight may prevent actinic and progeric changes. Antibiotics have clearly prolonged the survival of patients subject to severe sinopulmonary disease. Physiotherapy is important for the prevention and amelioration of bronchiectasis. Administration of gamma globulins may be beneficial. Various types of stimulation of the immune system and provision of fetal thymus implants have not been shown to be of clear benefit.

Rehabilitation may aid in compensating for motor deficits. Propranolol or tiapride may alleviate some forms of tremor. Much remains to be learned about the pharmacological management of the extrapyramidal dysfunction of AT and there is no effective therapy for ataxia. Most AT patients become wheelchair bound early in the second decade of life. Death typically occurs between late childhood and early adulthood, although at least one patient has survived until age 50.[303] In 50% to 60% of AT patients, death is caused by respiratory failure due to progressive

Table 158.11   Other autosomal recessive neurocutaneous conditions

Name	Cutaneous features	Neurological features	Other features
Acrodermatitis acidemica[304]	Periorificial, acral erythema/ desquamation; hypopigmented, sparse, brittle hair	Episodic lethargy, hypotonia, weakness, coma	Failure to thrive; episodic acidemia, vomiting, acidemia, dehydration, dyspnea
Amish brittle hair (BIDS) syndrome[305]	Brittle hair	Mental retardation, ataxia, intention tremor, EEG abnormalities	Low birthweight, short stature, hypogenitalism, diminished fertility
Aspartylglucosaminuria[306]	Large nevi, angiokeratoma, crystal-like lens opacities	Psychomotor and language retardation, photosensitivity, abnormal behavior, seizures	Characteristic facial dysmorphia, short stature, joint laxity, hepatomegaly, hernias, heart abnormalities, arthritis
Beraidinelli lipodystrophy syndrome	Hyperpigmented skin, especially axillary; variable acanthosis nigricans; hirsutism not including pubic and axillary areas; curly scalp hair	Mental deficiency is variable	Corneal opacities
Bjørnstad's syndrome[307]	Pili torti	Sensorineural hearing loss	
CHIME (neuroectodermal) syndrome[308]	Ichthyosis, hyperkeratosis of palms and soles, sparse fine hair	Mental retardation, hearing loss, seizures	Colobomas of the eye, heart and ear defects
Cockayne syndrome[309]	Photosensitivity dermatitis, abnormal pigment, blistering, scarring	Intellectual and motor degeneration, ataxia, peripheral neuritis	Progeric appearance, growth retardation, renal failure, DNA repair deficits Growth retardation
Cross (oculocerebral hypopigmentation) syndrome[310]	Silvery hair, cutaneous and retinal hypopigmentation, abnormal electroretinogram	Psychomotor retardation, spasticity, ataxia, cerebellar hypoplasia, posterior fossa cyst, EEG abnormalities	
Divry–van Bogaert syndrome[311]	Generalized cutis marmorata, capillary angiomatosis	Cortico-meningeal angiomatosis, diffuse sclerosis, stroke, dementia, seizures, leukodystrophy, paraparesis, visual loss	
Dubowitz syndrome[312]	Infantile eczema, sparse hair and lateral eyebrows	Mental retardation, muscular hypotonia, ocular albinism, retinal degeneration, colobomas	Microcephaly with characteristic facies, growth failure, malignancies, aplastic anemia
Elejalde (neuroectodermal melanolysosomal) disease[313]	Characteristic hair shafts, bronzed skin	Retinopathy, blindness, nystagmus, retardation, paresis, ataxia, seizures	Early death
Hartnup disease[314]	Pellagraform dermatitis	Progressive cerebellar ataxia	
Meckel–Gruber syndrome[315]	Ichthyosis	Encephalomeningocele, anencephaly, hydrocephaly, Dandy–Walker, eye deficits	Facial clefts; kidney, liver, or pancreas cysts; genital, cardiac abnormalities
Multiple sulfatase deficiency (Austin disease)[316]	Mild ichthyosis	Leukodystrophy, neuropathy, loss of speech, blindness	Coarse features, hepatosplenomegaly, skeletal abnormalities
Neutral lipid storage (Dorfman–Chanarin) disease[317]	Congenital ichthyotic erythroderma	Mental retardation, deafness, weakness, ataxia	Fatty degeneration of liver, cataracts, vacuolar neutrophils

continued

Table 158.11 *continued*

Name	Cutaneous features	Neurological features	Other features
Oculocutaneous albinism[318]	Albinism of skin, hair, iris; melanoma	Photophobia, reduced vision, strabismus, nystagmus	
Refsum disease[319]	Mild ichthyosis, yellow melanocytic nevi	Pigmentary retinopathy night blindness, anosmia, hearing loss, ataxia, tremor, neuropathy, areflexia	Cardiac conduction defects
Shapira syndrome[320]	Brittle, sparse, light hair, pili torti	Psychomotor delay, neurological findings	Short stature
Sjögren–Larsson syndrome[321]	Ichthyosis with lichenification	Macular dystrophy, mental retardation, weakness, spasticity	
Tangier disease[322]	Xanthomatous papulosis	Recurrent peripheral neuropathy	Absence of high-density lipoproteins, yellow tonsils, splenomegaly
Tay (IBIDS) syndrome[323]	Ichthyosis, brittle hair, trichothiodystrophy, nail dysplasia	Intellectual deficit, microcephaly, hoarse voice, hearing loss, incoordination, brain calcification, ataxia, weakness, spasticity	Short stature, progeroid facies, cataracts
Urbach–Weithe disease[324]	Cutaneomucous hyalinosis, facial and oropharyngeal nodules	Hoarse voice, brain calcification, seizures	Dwarfism
Xeroderma pigmentosum (De Sanctis–Cacchione syndrome)[325]	Photosensitivity dermatitis, ulcers, telangiectases, melanoma	Mental or motor degeneration, ataxia, weakness, deafness, brain atrophy, peripheral neuritis	Iritis, keratitis, ocular melanoma, dwarfism, gonadal hypoplasia

Table 158.12 **Hereditary neurometabolic syndromes with abnormalities of skin, hair, and bone**

Disease	Skin	Hair	Dysmorphia	Bone
Adrenomyeloneuropathy (XL)	AddM			
Aspartylglucosaminuria	Acne/AK		yes	PDM*
Biotinidase deficiency	SSR	Alop		
Cobalamin C deficiency	EryR			
Fucosidosis II	ES/KD	C-H	yes	PDM**/RLD
Fucosidosis III	AK/KD	C-H	yes	PDM**/RLD
GM$_1$ gangliosidosis type II				PDM**/RLD
Homocystinuria	LR/MalF			
Isovaleric acidemia		Alop		
Lowe disease				RLD
α-mannosidosis			yes	PDM**
β-mannosidosis	AK		yes	
Methylmalonic acidemia	EryR			
Mucolipidosis II (I-cell)	KD	C-H	yes	PDM***/RLD
Mucolipidosis III			yes	PDM***
Mucopolysaccharidosis I	KD	C-H		PDM***/RLD
Mucopolysaccharidosis II	KD	C-H		PDM***/RLD
Mucopolysaccharidosis III	KD	C-H		PDM**/RLD
Propionic acidemia	EryR			
Sialidosis II	Tel/AK			PDM***

* = mild; ** = moderate; *** = severe.
AddM, Addisonian melanoderma; AK, angiokeratoma; Alop, alopecia; C-H, coarse hair and eyebrows, hirsute; EryR, erythematous rash; ES, excessive sweating; KD, keratoderma, thickened skin; LR, livedo reticularis; MalF, malar flush; PDM, progressive dysostosis multiplex; RLD, rickets-like changes; SSR, seborrheic skin rash (resembling atopic dermatitis); Tel, telangiectatic skin rash; XL, X-linked.

Table 158.13   Rare neurocutaneous conditions with other or unknown mechanisms of inheritance

Sex chromosome aneuploidy
  Ullrich–Turner syndrome[326]

Sporadic, but known genetic mechanism
  Angelman syndrome[327]

Neurocutaneous syndromes with incompletely understood inheritance
  Blue rubber bleb nevus syndrome
  Bonnet–Dechaume–Blanc syndrome[328]
  Brachman–De Lange syndrome[329]
  Chediak–Higashi[330]
  Cobb metameric angiomatosis[331]
  Costello syndrome[332]
  Johnston syndrome[333]
  Maffucci syndrome (multiple enchondromatosis)[334]
  Muir–Torre syndrome[335]
  Nevus comedonicus (follicularis keratosis)[336]
  Nevus sebaceus of Jadassohn[337]
  Nevus unius lateris[338]
  Nicolaides–Baraitser syndrome
  Ollier syndrome[339]
  Parry–Romberg syndrome[340]
  Rothmund–Thomson syndrome (poikiloderma congenitale)[341]
  Rud syndrome[342]
  Satoyoshi syndrome (generalized Komuragaeri disease)[343]
  Sneddon syndrome[344]
  Van Lohuizen's cutis marmorata telangiectatica congenita[345]
  Wyburn-Mason syndrome[346]

bronchiectasis. Between 15% to 40% of patients die from lymphoreticular malignancies.

Other autosomal recessive neurocutaneous conditions and hereditary neurometabolic syndromes with abnormalities of skin, hair, and bone are listed in Tables 158.11 and 158.12, respectively.

Neurocutaneous syndromes with other or unknown modes of inheritance

These conditions are listed in Table 158.13, together with references for interested readers.

References

1. Van der Hoeve J. Les phacomatoses de Bourneville, de Recklinghausen, et de von Hippel–Lindau. J Neurol Psychiatry 1933;33:752
2. Andre JM, Picard L, Jacquier A. [Phacomatoses. Pathogenesis—Classification—Vascular aspects]. Phlebologie 1980;33:7–20
3. Tilesius WG. Historia pathologica singularis cutis turpitudinis. Leipzig, Germany, 1793
4. Wishart J. Cases of tumors of the skull, dura mater, and brain. Edinburgh Med J 1822;18:393
5. von Recklinghausen F. Ueber die multiplen fibrome der Haut und ihre Bezeihung zu den multiplen Neuromen. Berlin: A. Hirschwald, 1882
6. Carey JC, Viskochil DH. Neurofibromatosis type 1: A model condition for the study of the molecular basis of variable expressivity in human disorders. Am J Med Genet 1999;89:7–13
7. Riccardi V. Neurofibromatosis—Phenotype, Natural History, and Pathogenesis. Baltimore: Johns Hopkins University Press, 1986
8. Ars E, Kruyer H, Gaona A, et al. Prenatal diagnosis of sporadic neurofibromatosis type 1 (NF1) by RNA and DNA analysis of a splicing mutation. Prenat Diagn 1999;19:739–742
9. Barker D, Wright E, Nguyen K, et al. A genomic search for linkage of neurofibromatosis to RFLPs. J Med Genet 1987;24:536–538
10. Buske A, Gewies A, Lehmann R, et al. Recurrent NF1 gene mutation in a patient with oligosymptomatic neurofibromatosis type 1 (NF1). Am J Med Genet 1999; 86:328–330
11. Friedman JM. Epidemiology of neurofibromatosis type 1. Am J Med Genet 1999;89:1–6
12. Wolff RK, Frazer KA, Jackler RK, et al. Analysis of chromosome 22 deletions in neurofibromatosis type 2-related tumors. Am J Hum Genet 1992;51:478–485
13. Evans DG, Huson SM, Donnai D, et al. A genetic study of type 2 neurofibromatosis in the United Kingdom. II. Guidelines for genetic counselling. J Med Genet 1992;29:847–852
14. Sanson M. [A new tumor suppressor gene responsible for type 2 neurofibromatosis is inactivated in neurinoma and meningioma]. Rev Neurol (Paris) 1996;152: 1–10
15. Stumpf P. National Institutes of Health Consensus Development Conference: Neurofibromatosis. Statement 6, 1987;12:1
16. Crowe S, Schull W, Neil J. A Clinical, Pathological Study of Neurofibromatosis. Springfield, Ill: Charles C. Thompson, 1956
17. Huson SM. Recent developments in the diagnosis and management of neurofibromatosis. Arch Dis Child 1989;64:745–749
18. Martuza RL, Philippe I, Fitzpatrick TB, et al. Melanin macroglobules as a cellular marker of neurofibromatosis: a quantitative study. J Invest Dermatol 1985;85: 347–350
19. Riccardi VM. Neurofibromatosis: clinical heterogeneity. Curr Probl Cancer 1982;7:1–34
20. Riccardi VM. Type 1 neurofibromatosis and the pediatric patient. Curr Probl Pediatr 1992;22:66–106; discussion 107
21. Braverman I. Skin Signs of Systemic Disease. Philadelphia: WB Saunders, 1970
22. Korf BR. Diagnostic outcome of children with multiple cute au lait spots. Pediatr 1992;90(Suppl 6):924–927
23. Obringer AC, Meadows AT, Zackai EH. The diagnosis of neurofibromatosis-1 in the child under the age of 6 years. Am J Dis Child 1989;143:717–719
24. Riccardi VM. Cutaneous manifestation of neurofibromatosis: cellular interaction, pigmentation, and mast cells. Birth Defects Orig Artic Ser 1981;17:129–145
25. Pique E, Olivares M, Farina MC, et al. Pseudoatrophic macules: a variant of neurofibroma. Cutis 1996;57: 100–102
26. Shannon KM, O'Connell P, Martin GA, et al. Loss of the normal NF1 allele from the bone marrow of children with type 1 neurofibromatosis and malignant myeloid disorders. N Engl J Med 1994;330:597–601
27. Pallotta R, Carlone G, Petrucci A, Chiarelli F. Dermatoglyphics in von Recklinghausen neurofibromatosis. Am J Med Genet 1989;34:233–236
28. Harkin JC. Pathology of nerve sheath tumors. Ann N Y Acad Sci 1986;486:147–154
29. Cohen MM Jr. Understanding Proteus syndrome,

unmasking the elephant man, and stemming elephant fever. Neurofibromatosis 1988;1:260–280

30. Ford F. Diseases of the Nervous System In Infancy, Childhood, and Adolescence. Springfield, Ill: Charles C. Thomas, 1960

31. Nurnberger M, Moll I. Semiquantitative aspects of mast cells in normal skin and in neurofibromas of neurofibromatosis types 1 and 5. Dermatology 1994;188:296–299

32. Aicardi J. Diseases of the Nervous System in Childhood. London: MacKeith Press, 1992

33. Huson SM, Harper PS, Compston DA. Von Recklinghausen neurofibromatosis. A clinical and population study in south-east Wales. Brain 1988;111:1355–1381

34. Korf BR. Plexiform neurofibromas. Am J Med Genet 1999;89:31–37

35. Woodruff JM. Pathology of tumors of the peripheral nerve sheath in type 1 neurofibromatosis. Am J Med Genet 1999;89:23–30

36. Riccardi VM. Von Recklinghausen neurofibromatosis. N Engl J Med 1981;305:1617–1627

37. Ross GW, Miller JQ, Persing JA, Urich H. Hemimegalencephaly, hemifacial hypertrophy and intracranial lipoma: a variant of neurofibromatosis. Neurofibromatosis 1989;2:69–77

38. Boltshauser E, Stocker H, Sailer H, Valavanis A. Intracranial abnormalities associated with facial plexiform neurofibromas in neurofibromatosis type 1. Neurofibromatosis 1989;2:274–277

39. Rosendal T. Some cranial changes in Recklinghausen's neurofibromatosis. Acta Radiol Scand 1938;19:373

40. Riccardi VM. Pathophysiology of neurofibromatosis. IV. Dermatologic insights into heterogeneity and pathogenesis. J Am Acad Dermatol 1980;3:157–166

41. Grant WM, Walton DS. Distinctive gonioscopic findings in glaucoma due to neurofibromatosis. Arch Ophthalmol 1968;79:127–134

42. Holt JF. 1977 Edward BD. Neuhauser lecture: neurofibromatosis in children. AJR Am J Roentgenol 1978;130:615–639

43. Packer RJ, Sutton LN, Bilaniuk LT, et al. Treatment of chiasmatic/hypothalamic gliomas of childhood with chemotherapy: an update. Ann Neurol 1988;23:79–85

44. Aoki S, Barkovich AJ, Nishimura K, et al. Neurofibromatosis types 1 and 2: cranial MR findings. Radiology 1989;172:527–534

45. North K, Joy P, Yuille D, et al. Specific learning disability in children with neurofibromatosis type 1: significance of MRI abnormalities. Neurology 1994;44:878–883

46. DiPaolo DP, Zimmerman RA, Rorke LB, et al. Neurofibromatosis type 1: pathologic substrate of high-signal-intensity foci in the brain. Radiology 1995;195:721–724

47. Michels VV, Whisnant JP, Garrity JA, Miller GM. Neurofibromatosis type 1 with bilateral acoustic neuromas. Neurofibromatosis 1989;2:213–217

48. Eldridge R, Denckla MB, Bien E, et al. Neurofibromatosis type 1 (Recklinghausen's disease). Neurologic and cognitive assessment with sibling controls. Am J Dis Child 1989;143:833–837

49. Ozonoff S. Cognitive impairment in neurofibromatosis type 1. Am J Med Genet 1999;89:45–52

50. Gutmann DH, Zhang Y, Hirbe A. Developmental regulation of a neuron-specific neurofibromatosis 1 isoform. Ann Neurol 1999;46:777–782

51. Samuelsson B, Riccardi VM. Neurofibromatosis in Gothenburg, Sweden. II. Intellectual compromise. Neurofibromatosis 1989;2:78–83

52. Cusmai R, Curatolo P, Mangano S, et al. Hemimega-

lencephaly and neurofibromatosis. Neuropediatrics 1990;21:179–182

53. Hochstrasser H, Boltshauser E, Valavanis A. Brain tumors in children with von Recklinghausen neurofibromatosis. Neurofibromatosis 1988;1:233–239

54. Arts WF, Van Dongen KJ. Intracranial calcified deposits in neurofibromatosis. J Neurol Neurosurg Psychiatry 1986;49:1317–1320

55. Riviello JJ Jr, Marks HG, Lee MS, Mandell GA. Aqueductal stenosis in neurofibromatosis. Neurofibromatosis 1988;1:312–317

56. Binet EF, Kieffer SA, Martin SH, Peterson HO. Orbital dysplasia in neurofibromatosis. Radiology 1969;93:829–833

57. Gautier-Smith PC. Clinical aspects of spinal neurofibromas. Brain 1967;90:359–394

58. Halliday AL, Sobel RA, Martuza RL. Benign spinal nerve sheath tumors: their occurrence sporadically and in neurofibromatosis types 1 and 2. J Neurosurg 1991;74:248–253

59. Lamovec J, Frkovic-Grazio S, Bracko M. Nonsporadic cases and unusual morphological features in pheochromocytoma and paraganglioma. Arch Pathol Lab Med 1998;122:63–68

60. Hegstrom JL, Kircher T. Alimentary tract ganglioneuromatosis-lipomatosis, adrenal myelolipomas, pancreatic telangiectasias, and multinodular thyroid goiter. A possible neuroendocrine syndrome. Am J Clin Pathol 1985;83:744–747

61. Heimann R, Verhest A, Verschraegen J, et al. Hereditary intestinal neurofibromatosis. I. A distinctive genetic disease. Neurofibromatosis 1988;1:26–32

62. Okada O, Demitsu T, Manabe M, Yoneda K. A case of multiple subungual glomus tumors associated with neurofibromatosis type 1. J Dermatol 1999;26:535–537

63. Pellock JM, Kleinman PK, McDonald BM, Wixson D. Childhood hypertensive stroke with neurofibromatosis. Neurology 1980;30:656–659

64. Goffin J, Grob D. Spondyloptosis of the cervical spine in neurofibromatosis. A case report. Spine 1999;24:587–590

65. Andersen KS. Congenital pseudarthrosis of the leg. Late results. J Bone Joint Surg Am 1976;58:657–662

66. Allanson JE, Upadhyaya M, Watson GH, et al. Watson syndrome: is it a subtype of type 1 neurofibromatosis? J Med Genet 1991;28:752–756

67. Colley A, Donnai D, Evans DG. Neurofibromatosis/Noonan phenotype: a variable feature of type 1 neurofibromatosis. Clin Genet 1996;49:59–64

68. Sadeh M, Martinovits G, Goldhammer Y. Occurrence of both neurofibromatoses 1 and 2 in the same individual with a rapidly progressive course. Neurology 1989;39:282–283

69. Stachura Z, Zralek C, Siemianowicz S, et al. [Selected problems of neurofibromatosis with presentation of a case of multiple intracranial and intramedullary tumors]. Neurol Neurochir Pol 1998;32:1563–1569

70. Eldridge R. Central neurofibromatosis with bilateral acoustic neuroma. Adv Neurol 1981;29:57–65

71. Harada H, Kumon Y, Hatta N, et al. Neurofibromatosis type 2 with multiple primary brain tumors in monozygotic twins. Surg Neurol 1999;51:528–535

72. Evans DG, Huson SM, Donnai D, et al. A clinical study of type 2 neurofibromatosis. QJM 1992;84:603–618

73. Rettele GA, Brodsky MC, Merin LM, et al. Blindness, deafness, quadriparesis, and a retinal malformation: the ravages of neurofibromatosis 2. Surv Ophthalmol 1996;41:135–141

74. Martuza RL, Eldridge R. Neurofibromatosis 2 (bilateral acoustic neurofibromatosis). N Engl J Med 1988; 318:684–688

75. Giangaspero F, Guiducci A, Lenz FA, et al. Meningioma with meningioangiomatosis: a condition mimicking invasive meningiomas in children and young adults: report of two cases and review of the literature. Am J Surg Pathol 1999;23:872–875

76. Rubinstein LJ. The malformative central nervous system lesions in the central and peripheral forms of neurofibromatosis. A neuropathological study of 22 cases. Ann N Y Acad Sci 1986;486:14–29

77. Pou Serradell A. [Central lesions in neurofibromatosis: clinical, MRI and histopathologic correlations. An attempted classification]. Rev Neurol 1991;147:17–27

78. Pulst SM, Rouleau GA, Marineau C, et al. Familial meningioma is not allelic to neurofibromatosis 2. Neurology 1993;43:2096–2098

79. Mautner VF, Tatagiba M, Guthoff R, et al. Neurofibromatosis 2 in the pediatric age group. Neurosurgery 1993;33:92–96

80. Heim RA, Kam-Morgan LN, Binnie CG, et al. Distribution of 13 truncating mutations in the neurofibromatosis 1 gene. Hum Mol Genet 1995;4:975–981

81. Easton DF, Ponder MA, Huson SM, Ponder BA. An analysis of variation in expression of neurofibromatosis (NF) type 1 (NF1): evidence for modifying genes. Am J Hum Genet 1993;53:305–313

82. Weiss B, Bollag G, Shannon K. Hyperactive Ras as a therapeutic target in neurofibromatosis type 1. Am J Med Genet 1999;89:14–22

83. Bance M, Ramsden RT. Management of neurofibromatosis type 2. Ear Nose Throat J 1999;78:91–94, 96

84. von Recklinghausen F. Ein Herz von einen Neugeborene welches mehrere theils nach aussen, theils nach den Höhlen prominirende Tumoren (Myomen) trug. Monatsschr Geburtsk 1862;20:1

85. Bourneville D, Brissaud E. Idiotie et épilepsie symptomatique de sclérose tubéreuse ou hypertrophique. Arch Neurol (Paris) 1900;10:29

86. Gomez MR. History of the tuberous sclerosis complex. Brain Dev 1995;17:55–57

87. O'Callaghan FJ, Clarke AC, Joffe H, et al. Tuberous sclerosis complex and Wolff-Parkinson-White syndrome. Arch Dis Child 1998;78:159–162

88. Gomez M. Tuberous Sclerosis. New York: Raven Press, 1988

89. Roach ES, Gomez MR, Northrup H. Tuberous sclerosis complex consensus conference: revised clinical diagnostic criteria. J Child Neurol 1998;13:624–628

90. Verhoef S, Bakker L, Tempelaars AM, et al. High rate of mosaicism in tuberous sclerosis complex. Am J Hum Genet 1999;64:1632–1637

91. Kondo S, Yamashina U, Sato N, Aso K. Discordant expression of tuberous sclerosis in monozygotic twins. J Dermatol 1991;18:178–180

92. The European Chromosome 16 Tuberous Sclerosis Consortium. Identification and characterization of the tuberous sclerosis gene on chromosome 16. Cell 1993;75:1305–1315

93. Au KS, Rodriguez JA, Finch JL, et al. Germ-line mutational analysis of the TSC2 gene in 90 tuberous-sclerosis patients. Am J Hum Genet 1998;62:286–294

94. Jones AC, Daniells CE, Snell RG, et al. Molecular genetic and phenotypic analysis reveals differences between TSC1 and TSC2 associated familial and sporadic tuberous sclerosis. Hum Mol Genet 1997;6: 2155–2161

95. Crino PB, Henske EP. New developments in the neurobiology of the tuberous sclerosis complex. Neurology 1999;53:1384–1390

96. van Slegtenhorst M, Nellist M, Nagelkerken B, et al. Interaction between hamartin and tuberin, the TSC1 and TSC2 gene products. Hum Mol Genet 1998;7: 1053–1057

97. Webb DW, Clarke A, Fryer A, Osborne JP. The cutaneous features of tuberous sclerosis: a population study. Br J Dermatol 1996;135:1–5

98. Jozwiak S, Schwartz RA, Janniger CK, et al. Skin lesions in children with tuberous sclerosis complex: their prevalence, natural course, and diagnostic significance. Int J Dermatol 1998;37:911–917

99. Vogt H. Zur Diagnostik der tuberosen Sklerose. Zeit Erforsch Behandl Schwachsinns 1908;2:1

100. Gold A, Freeman J. Depigmented nevi: The earliest sign of tuberous sclerosis. Pediatrics 1965;335:1003

101. Fitzpatrick TB, Szabo G, Hori Y, et al. White leaf-shaped macules. Earliest visible sign of tuberous sclerosis. Arch Dermatol 1968;98:1–6

102. Hurwitz S, Braverman IM. White spots in tuberous sclerosis. J Pediatr 1970;77:587–594

103. Yoshida T, Nakagawa SI, Tabata K, Yanagisawa N. [A case of "forme fruste" of tuberous sclerosis having been treated as genuine epilepsy]. Rinsho Shinkeigaku 1994;34:925–927

104. Danielsen L, Kobayasi T, Jacobsen GK. Ultrastructural changes in disseminated connective tissue nevi. Acta Derm Venereol 1977;57:93–101

105. Gomez M. Tuberous Sclerosis. New York: Raven Press, 1979

106. Hunt A. Tuberous sclerosis: a survey of 97 cases. II: Physical findings. Dev Med Child Neurol 1983;25: 350–352

107. Jardin A, Richard F, Le Duc A, et al. Diagnosis and treatment of renal angiomyolipoma (based on 15 cases). Arguments in favor of conservative surgery (based on 8 cases). Eur Urol 1980;6:69–82

108. Chatterjee T, Heindel W, Vorreuther R, et al. Recurrent bleeding of angiomyolipomas in tuberous sclerosis. Urol Int 1996;56:44–47

109. Berg B. Developmental disorders of the nervous system. In: Berg B, ed. Principles of Child Neurology. San Francisco: McGraw-Hill, 1996

110. Di Liang C, Fat Ko S, Chei Huang S. Echocardiographic evaluation of cardiac rhabdomyoma in infants and children. J Clin Ultrasound 2000;28:381–386

111. Gutierrez de Loma J, Villagra F, Perez de Leon J, et al. Rhabdomyoma of the heart: surgical treatment. J Cardiovasc Surg (Torino) 1982;23:149–154

112. Crawford DC, Garrett C, Tynan M, et al. Cardiac rhabdomyomata as a marker for the antenatal detection of tuberous sclerosis. J Med Genet 1983;20:303–304

113. Torres VE, Bjornsson J, King BF, et al. Extrapulmonary lymphangioleiomyomatosis and lymphangiomatous cysts in tuberous sclerosis complex. Mayo Clin Proc 1995;70:641–648

114. Wendt JR, Watson LR. Cosmetic treatment of shagreen patches in selected patients with tuberous sclerosis. Plast Reconstr Surg 1991;87:780–782

115. Lagos JC, Gomez MR. Tuberous sclerosis: reappraisal of a clinical entity. Mayo Clin Proc 1967;42:26–49

116. Schwartz PL, Beards JA, Maris PJ. Tuberous sclerosis associated with a retinal angioma. Am J Ophthalmol 1980;90:485–488

117. Huttenlocher PR, Wollmann RL. Cellular neuropathology of tuberous sclerosis. Ann NY Acad Sci 1991;615: 140–148

118. Hirose T, Scheithauer BW, Lopes MB, et al. Tuber and subependymal giant cell astrocytoma associated with tuberous sclerosis: an immunohistochemical, ultrastructural, and immunoelectron and microscopic study. Acta Neuropathol 1995;90:387–399
119. Sonigo P, Elmaleh A, Fermont L, et al. Prenatal MRI diagnosis of fetal cerebral tuberous sclerosis. Pediatr Radiol 1996;26:1–4
120. Roach ES, Williams DP, Laster DW. Magnetic resonance imaging in tuberous sclerosis. Arch Neurol 1987;44:301–303
121. Jozwiak S, Goodman M, Lamm SH. Poor mental development in patients with tuberous sclerosis complex: clinical risk factors. Arch Neurol 1998;55:379–384
122. Lane VW, Samples JM. Tuberous sclerosis: case study of early seizure control and subsequent normal development. J Autism Dev Disord 1984;14:423–427
123. Yamamoto N, Watanabe K, Negoro T, et al. Long-term prognosis of tuberous sclerosis with epilepsy in children. Brain Dev 1987;9:292–295
124. Aminoff M. Electrodiagnosis in Clinical Neurology. New York: Churchill Livingstone, 1992
125. Monaghan HP, Krafchik BR, MacGregor DL, Fitz CR. Tuberous sclerosis complex in children. Am J Dis Child 1981;135:912–917
126. Lagos J, Gomez M. Tuberous sclerosis: Reappraisal of a clinical entity. Mayo Clin Proc 1967;46:26
127. Jones AC, Shyamsundar MM, Thomas MW, et al. Comprehensive mutation analysis of TSC1 and TSC2 and phenotypic correlations in 150 families with tuberous sclerosis. Am J Hum Genet 1999;64:1305–1315
128. Reich M, Lenoir P, Malvy J, et al. [Bourneville's tuberous sclerosis and autism]. Arch Pediatr 1997;4:170–175
129. Boixeda P, Sanchez-Miralles E, Azana JM, et al. CO2, argon, and pulsed dye laser treatment of angiofibromas. J Dermatol Surg Oncol 1994;20:808–812
130. Fleury P. [Tuberous sclerosis, changes in the diagnostic and therapeutic approach]. Tijdschr Kindergeneeskd 1989;57:158–164
131. Fleury P, de Groot WP, Delleman JW, et al. Tuberous sclerosis: the incidence of sporadic cases versus familial cases. Brain Dev 1980;2:107–117
132. Panas F, Remy D. Anatomie Pathologique de l'oeil. Paris: Delahaye, 1879
133. von Hippel E. Die anatomische Grundlage der von mir beschreibenen "sehr seltenen Erkrankung der Netzhaut." Albrecht Graefe's Arch Ophthalmol 1911;79:350
134. Lindau A. Studien ueber kleinhirncysten: bau, pathogenese, und bezeihungen zur angiomatosis retinae. Arch Pathol Microbiol Scand 1926;1:1
135. Richard S, Giraud S, Beroud C, et al. [Von Hippel–Lindau disease: recent genetic progress and patient management. Francophone Study Group of von Hippel–Lindau Disease (GEFVH)]. Ann Endocrinol 1998;59:452–458
136. Richard S, Giraud S, Hammel P, et al. [Von Hippel–Lindau disease: a hereditary disease that impacts multiple tissues]. Presse Med 1998;27:1112–1120
137. Richards FM, Webster AR, McMahon R, et al. Molecular genetic analysis of von Hippel–Lindau disease. J Intern Med 1998;243:527–533
138. Richard S, Martin S, David P, Decq P. [Von Hippel–Lindau disease and central nervous system hemangioblastoma. Progress in genetics and clinical management]. Neurochirurgie 1998;44:258–266
139. Webster AR, Maher ER, Moore AT. Clinical characteristics of ocular angiomatosis in von Hippel–Lindau disease and correlation with germline mutation. Arch Ophthalmol 1999;117:371–378
140. Ridley M, Green J, Johnson G. Retinal angiomatosis: the ocular manifestations of von Hippel–Lindau disease. Can J Ophthalmol 1986;21:276–283
141. Fuchs E. Aneurysma arteri-venosum retinae. Arch Augenheilkd 1882;11:440
142. Macmichael IM. Von Hippel Lindau's disease of the optic disc. Trans Ophthalmol Soc UK 1970;90:877–885
143. Niemela M, Lemeta S, Sainio M, et al. Hemangioblastomas of the retina: impact of von Hippel–Lindau disease. Invest Ophthalmol Vis Sci 2000;41:1909–1915
144. Huson SM, Harper PS, Hourihan MD, et al. Cerebellar haemangioblastoma and von Hippel–Lindau disease. Brain 1986;109:1297–1310
145. Neumann HP, Eggert HR, Weigel K, et al. Hemangioblastomas of the central nervous system. A 10-year study with special reference to von Hippel–Lindau syndrome. J Neurosurg 1989;70:24–30
146. Roessler K, Dietrich W, Haberler C, et al. Multiple spinal "miliary" hemangioblastomas in von Hippel–Lindau (vHL) disease without cerebellar involvement. A case report and review of the literature. Neurosurg Rev 1999;22:130–134
147. Kouri JG, Chen MY, Watson JC, Oldfield EH. Resection of suprasellar tumors by using a modified transsphenoidal approach. Report of four cases. J Neurosurg 2000;92:1028–1035
148. Othmane IS, Shields C, Singh A, et al. Postpartum cerebellar herniation in von Hippel–Lindau syndrome. Am J Ophthalmol 1999;128:387–389
149. Spetzger U, Bertalanffy H, Huffmann B, et al. Hemangioblastomas of the spinal cord and the brainstem: diagnostic and therapeutic features. Neurosurg Rev 1996;19:147–151
150. Young S, Richardson AE. Solid haemangioblastomas of the posterior fossa: radiological features and results of surgery. J Neurol Neurosurg Psychiatry 1987;50:155–158
151. Friedrich CA. Von Hippel–Lindau syndrome. A pleomorphic condition. Cancer 1999;86:2478–2482
152. Atuk NO, McDonald T, Wood T, et al. Familial pheochromocytoma, hypercalcemia, and von Hippel–Lindau disease. A ten year study of a large family. Medicine (Baltimore) 1979;58:209–218
153. Richard S, Beroud C, Joly D, et al. [Von Hippel–Lindau disease and renal cancer: 10 years of genetic progress. GEFVHL (French-Speaking Study Group on von Hippel–Lindau disease)]. Prog Urol 1998;8:330–339
154. Goldfarb DA. Nephron-sparing surgery and renal transplantation in patients with renal cell carcinoma and von Hippel–Lindau disease. J Intern Med 1998;243:563–567
155. Bret P, Streichenberger N, Guyotat J. Metastasis of renal carcinoma to a cerebellar hemangioblastoma in a patient with von Hippel Lindau disease: a case report. Br J Neurosurg 1999;13:413–416
156. Renal mass in a man with von-Hippel Lindau disease [clinical conference]. Am J Med 1981;71:287–297
157. Paraf F, Chauveau D, Chretien Y, et al. Renal lesions in von Hippel–Lindau disease: immunohistochemical expression of nephron differentiation molecules, adhesion molecules and apoptosis proteins. Histopathology 2000;36:457–465
158. Choyke PL, Glenn GM, Walther MM, et al. von Hippel–Lindau disease: genetic, clinical, and imaging

features [published erratum appears in Radiology 1995 Aug;196(2):582]. Radiology 1995;194:629–642

159. Raimoldi A, Berti GL, Canclini L, et al. [Papillary cystadenoma of the epididymis. 2 case reports]. Arch Ital Urol Androl 1997;69:309–311

160. Palmer JM, Coker NJ, Harper RL. Papillary adenoma of the temporal bone in von Hippel–Lindau disease. Otolaryngol Head Neck Surg 1989;100:64–68

161. Kubota Y, Furuya Y, Ueda T, et al. [Bilateral pheochromocytomas with von Hippel–Lindau's disease: a case report]. Nippon Hinyokika Gakkai Zasshi 1998;89:726–729

162. Hes FJ, Feldberg MA. Von Hippel–Lindau disease: strategies in early detection (renal-, adrenal-, pancreatic masses). Eur Radiol 1999;9:598–610

163. Lamberts SW, Hofland LJ, Lely AJ, de Herder WW. Somatostatin receptor expression in multiple endocrine neoplasia and in von Hippel–Lindau disease. J Intern Med 1998;243:569–571

164. Scully RE, Galdabini JJ, McNeely BU. Case records of the Massachusetts General Hospital. Weekly clinicopathological exercises. Case 17-1978. N Engl J Med 1978;298:1014–1021

165. Harris AL. von Hippel–Lindau syndrome: target for anti-vascular endothelial growth factor (VEGF) receptor therapy. Oncologist 2000;5:32–36

166. Kim SJ. Blue rubber bleb nevus syndrome with central nervous system involvement. Pediatr Neurol 2000;22:410–412

167. Savin JA. Osler and the skin. Br J Dermatol 2000;143:1–8

168. Koenig A, Kuester W, Berger R, Happle R. European J Dermatol 1997;7(Suppl 8):554–555

169. Boente MC, Bibas-Bonet H, Coronel AM, Asial RA. Atrichia, ichthyosis, follicular hyperkeratosis, chronic candidiasis, keratitis, seizures, mental retardation and inguinal hernia: a severe manifestation of IFAP syndrome? Eur J Dermatol 2000;10:98–102

170. Andre N, Kone-Paut I, Koeppel MC, Berbis P. [KID syndrome (keratitis, ichthyosis and deafness)]. Arch Pediatr 1999;6:302–306

171. Gorlin RJ, Anderson RC, Blaw M. Multiple lentigenes syndrome. Am J Dis Child 1969;117:652–662

172. Garty BZ, Waisman Y, Weitz R. Gerstmann tetrad in leopard syndrome. Pediatr Neurol 1989;5:391–392

173. Kimonis VE, Goldstein AM, Pastakia B, et al. Clinical manifestations in 105 persons with nevoid basal cell carcinoma syndrome. Am J Med Genet 1997;69:299–308

174. Fujimoto A, Reddy KS, Spinks R. Interstitial deletion of chromosome 4, del(4)(q12q21.1), in a mentally retarded boy with a piebald trait, due to maternal insertion, ins(8;4). Am J Med Genet 1998;75:78–81

175. Lynch SA, Gardner-Medwin D, Burn J, Bushby KM. Absent nails, kinesogenic choreoathetosis, epilepsy and developmental delay—a new autosomal dominant disorder? Clin Dysmorphol 1997;6:133–138

176. Meyer UA, Schuurmans MM, Lindberg RL. Acute porphyrias: pathogenesis of neurological manifestations. Semin Liver Dis 1998;18:43–52

177. Sharland M, Bleach NR, Goberdhan PD, Patton MA. Autosomal dominant palmoplantar hyperkeratosis and sensorineural deafness in three generations. J Med Genet 1992;29:50–52

178. Asher JH Jr, Harrison RW, Morell R, et al. Effects of Pax3 modifier genes on craniofacial morphology, pigmentation, and viability: a murine model of Waardenburg syndrome variation. Genomics 1996;34:285–298

179. Happle R, Mittag H, Kuster W. The CHILD nevus: a distinct skin disorder. Dermatology 1995;191:210–216

180. Barre V, Drouin-Garraud V, Marret S, et al. [Focal dermal hypoplasia: description of three cases]. Arch Pediatr 1998;5:513–516

181. Happle R, Daniels O, Koopman RJ. MIDAS syndrome (microphthalmia, dermal aplasia, and sclerocornea): an X-linked phenotype distinct from Goltz syndrome. Am J Med Genet 1993;47:710–713

182. Feather SA, Winyard PJ, Dodd S, Woolf AS. Oral-facial-digital syndrome type 1 is another dominant polycystic kidney disease: clinical, radiological and histopathological features of a new kindred. Nephrol Dial Transplant 1997;12:1354–1361

183. Germain DP, Poenaru L. Fabry disease: identification of novel alpha-galactosidase A mutations and molecular carrier detection by use of fluorescent chemical cleavage of mismatches. Biochem Biophys Res Commun 1999;257:708–713

184. Ohshima T, Schiffmann R, Murray GJ, et al. Aging accentuates and bone marrow transplantation ameliorates metabolic defects in Fabry disease mice. Proc Natl Acad Sci USA 1999;96:6423–6427

185. Sher NA, Letson RD, Desnick RJ. The ocular manifestations in Fabry's disease. Arch Ophthalmol 1979;97:671–676

186. Cailleux N, Levesque H, Joly P, et al. [Childhood acromelalgia a propos of a case revealing Fabry's disease]. J Mal Vasc 1995;20:142–145

187. Sakakihara Y. [Autonomic dysfunction in metabolic diseases]. Nippon Rinsho 1992;50:811–817

188. Mendez MF, Stanley TM, Medel NM, et al. The vascular dementia of Fabry's disease. Dement Geriatr Cogn Disord 1997;8:252–257

189. Nakayama Y, Tsumura K, Yoshimaru K. Images in cardiology. Echocardiographic features of cardiac involvement in Fabry's disease. Heart 2000;83:695

190. Desnick RJ, Blieden LC, Sharp HL, et al. Cardiac valvular anomalies in Fabry disease. Clinical, morphologic, and biochemical studies. Circulation 1976;54:818–825

191. Elleder M, Ledvinova J, Vosmik F, et al. An atypical ultrastructural pattern in Fabry's disease: a study on its nature and incidence in 7 cases. Ultrastruct Pathol 1990;14:467–474

192. Argoff CE, Barton NW, Brady RO, Ziessman HA. Gastrointestinal symptoms and delayed gastric emptying in Fabry's disease: response to metoclopramide. Nucl Med Commun 1998;19:887–891

193. Shirai T, Ohtake T, Kimura M, et al. Atypical Fabry's disease presenting with cholesterol crystal embolization. Intern Med 2000;39:646–649

194. Lewin MB, Belmont J, McNamara DG, et al. Further associations of congenital heart disease and genetic syndromes: report of a case of tetralogy of Fallot and Fabry's disease [letter]. Pediatr Cardiol 1999;20:236–237

195. Moynahan EJ. Progeria in childhood with description of a new progeroid syndrome displaying gross Fabry-like changes in heart, great vessels and kidneys. Mod Probl Paediatr 1976;20:14–17

196. Broadbent JC, Edwards WD, Gordon H, et al. Fabry cardiomyopathy in the female confirmed by endomyocardial biopsy. Mayo Clin Proc 1981;56:623–628

197. Roth J, Roth H. [Electron microscopic observations in internal organs in morbus Fabry (author's transl)]. Virchows Arch A Pathol Pathol Anat 1978;378:75–90

198. Ashton-Prolla P, Ashley GA, Giugliani R, et al. Fabry disease: comparison of enzymatic, linkage, and mutation analysis for carrier detection in a family with a novel mutation (30delG). Am J Med Genet 1999;84: 420–424

199. Eng CM, Desnick RJ. Molecular basis of Fabry disease: mutations and polymorphisms in the human alpha-galactosidase A gene. Hum Mutat 1994;3:103–111

200. Eng CM, Niehaus DJ, Enriquez AL, et al. Fabry disease: twenty-three mutations including sense and antisense CpG alterations and identification of a deletional hot-spot in the alpha-galactosidase A gene. Hum Mol Genet 1994;3:1795–1799

201. Cable WJ, Dvorak AM, Osage JE, Kolodny EH. Fabry disease: significance of ultrastructural localization of lipid inclusions in dermal nerves. Neurology 1982;32: 347–353

202. Zeidner KM, Desnick RJ, Ioannou YA. Quantitative determination of globotriaosylceramide by immuno-detection of glycolipid-bound recombinant verotoxin B subunit. Anal Biochem 1999;267:104–113

203. Takenaka T, Murray GJ, Qin G, et al. Long-term enzyme correction and lipid reduction in multiple organs of primary and secondary transplanted Fabry mice receiving transduced bone marrow cells. Proc Natl Acad Sci USA 2000;97:7515–7520

204. Kasmann-Kelluer B, Jurin-Bunte B, Ruprecht KW. Incontinentia pigmenti (Block-Sulzberger Syndrome): Case report and differential diagnosis related to dermato-ocular syndrome. Ophthalmologia 1999; 213(Supp 1):63–69

205. Zlotogora J. X-linked albinism-deafness syndrome and Waardenburg syndrome type II: a hypothesis [letter]. Am J Med Genet 1995;59:386–387

206. Wijker M, Ligtenberg MJ, Schoute F, et al. The gene for hereditary bullous dystrophy, X-linked macular type, maps to the Xq27.3-qter region. Am J Hum Genet 1995;56:1096–1100

207. Heiss NS, Knight SW, Vulliamy TJ, et al. X-linked dyskeratosis congenita is caused by mutations in a highly conserved gene with putative nucleolar functions. Nat Genet 1998;19:32–38

208. Quinton R, Duke VM, de Zoysa PA, et al. The neuroradiology of Kallmann's syndrome: a genotypic and phenotypic analysis [published erratum appears in J Clin Endocrinol Metab 1996;81:3614]. J Clin Endocrinol Metab 1996;81:3010–3017

209. Gedeon AK, Mulley JC, Kozman H, et al. Localisation of the gene for X-linked reticulate pigmentary disorder with systemic manifestations (PDR), previously known as X-linked cutaneous amyloidosis. Am J Med Genet 1994;52:75–78

210. Schirmer R. Ein Fall von Telangiekrasie. Graefe's Arch Ophthalmol 1860;7:119

211. Sturge WA. Case of rare vaso-motor disturbance in the leg. Trans Clin Soc Lond 1879;12:156

212. Weber F. A note on the association of extensive haemangiomatous naevus of the skin with cerebral meningeal haemangioma, especially cases of facial vascular naevus with contralateral hemiplegia. Proc R Soc Med 1929;22:431

213. Debicka A, Adamczak P. [A case of hereditary Sturge–Weber syndrome (author's transl)]. Klin Oczna 1979;81:541–542

214. Weber FP. Encephalotrigeminal angiomatosis. BMJ 1955;I:726

215. Norman MG, Schoene WC. The ultrastructure of Sturge–Weber disease. Acta Neuropathol (Berl) 1977; 37:199–205

216. Gass JD. Ipsilateral facial and uveal arteriovenous and capillary angioma, microphthalmos, heterochromia of the iris, and hypotony: an oculocutaneous syndrome simulating Sturge–Weber syndrome. Trans Am Ophthalmol Soc 1996;94:227–237

217. Maria BL, Neufeld JA, Rosainz LC, et al. Central nervous system structure and function in Sturge–Weber syndrome: evidence of neurologic and radiologic progression. J Child Neurol 1998;13:606–618

218. Sujansky E, Conradi S. Outcome of Sturge–Weber syndrome in 52 adults. Am J Med Genet 1995;57:35–45

219. Enjolras O. [Systematized complex vascular malformations]. Rev Prat 1992;42:2048–2052

220. Huang JS, Chen CC, Wu YM, et al. Periodontal manifestations and treatment of Sturge–Weber syndrome—report of two cases. Kao Hsiung I Hsueh Ko Hsueh Tsa Chih 1997;13:127–135

221. Meyer E. Neurocutaneous syndrome with excessive macrohydrocephalus. (Sturge–Weber/Klippel–Trenaunay syndrome). Neuropadiatrie 1979;10:67–75

222. Hagiwara K, Uezato H, Nonaka S. Phacomatosis pigmentovascularis type IIb associated with Sturge–Weber syndrome and pyogenic granuloma. J Dermatol 1998;25:721–729

223. Tallman B, Tan OT, Morelli JG, et al. Location of port-wine stains and the likelihood of ophthalmic and/or central nervous system complications. Pediatrics 1991; 87:323–327

224. Bebin EM, Gomez MR. Prognosis in Sturge–Weber disease: comparison of unihemispheric and bihemispheric involvement. J Child Neurol 1988;3: 181–184

225. Hata D, Isu T, Nakanishi M, Tanaka T. Intraoperative electrocorticography and successful focus resection in a case of Sturge–Weber syndrome. Seizure 1998;7: 505–508

226. Griffiths PD, Blaser S, Boodram MB, et al. Choroid plexus size in young children with Sturge–Weber syndrome. AJNR Am J Neuroradiol 1996;17:175–180

227. Chugani HT, Mazziotta JC, Phelps ME. Sturge–Weber syndrome: a study of cerebral glucose utilization with positron emission tomography. J Pediatr 1989;114: 244–253

228. Aylett SE, Neville BG, Cross JH, et al. Sturge–Weber syndrome: cerebral haemodynamics during seizure activity. Dev Med Child Neurol 1999;41:480–485

229. Bentson J, Wilson G, Newton T. The cerebral venous drainage pattern in Sturge Weber syndrome. Radiology 1957;68:327

230. Elster AD, Chen MY. MR imaging of Sturge–Weber syndrome: role of gadopentetate dimeglumine and gradient-echo techniques. AJNR Am J Neuroradiol 1990;11:685–689

231. Nellhaus G, Haberland C, Hill BJ. Sturge–Weber disease with bilateral intracranial calcifications at birth and unusual pathologic findings. Acta Neurol Scand 1967;43:314–347

232. Coley SC, Britton J, Clarke A. Status epilepticus and venous infarction in Sturge–Weber syndrome. Childs Nerv Syst 1998;14:693–696

233. Okudaira Y, Arai H, Sato K. Hemodynamic compromise as a factor in clinical progression of Sturge–Weber syndrome. Childs Nerv Syst 1997;13:214–219

234. Salman MS. Is the prophylactic use of antiepileptic drugs in Sturge–Weber syndrome justified? Med Hypotheses 1998;51:293–296

235. Sadda SR, Miller NR, Tamargo R, Wityk R. Bilateral optic neuropathy associated with diffuse cerebral

angiomatosis in Sturge–Weber syndrome. J Neuroophthalmol 2000;20:28–31

236. Gomez MR, Bebin EM. Sturge–Weber syndrome. *In:* Gomez MR, ed. Neurocutaneous Diseases: A Practical Approach. London: Butterworth, 1987:356–367

237. Chevrie JJ, Specola N, Aicardi J. Secondary bilateral synchrony in unilateral pial angiomatosis: successful surgical treatment. J Neurol Neurosurg Psychiatry 1988;51:663–670

238. Terdjman P, Aicardi J, Sainte-Rose C, Brunelle F. Neuroradiological findings in Sturge–Weber syndrome (SWS) and isolated pial angiomatosis. Neuropediatrics 1991;22:115–120

239. Narbone MC, D'Amico D, Bramanti P, et al. Bilateral cortical calcifications with benign clinical course: an unusual case of Sturge–Weber syndrome? Acta Neurol (Napoli) 1989;11:423–427

240. Vargha-Khadem F, Carr LJ, Isaacs E, et al. Onset of speech after left hemispherectomy in a nine-year-old boy. Brain 1997;120:159–182

241. Fishman MA, Baram TZ. Megalencephaly due to impaired cerebral venous return in a Sturge–Weber variant syndrome. J Child Neurol 1986;1:115–118

242. Carson BS, Javedan SP, Freeman JM, et al. Hemispherectomy: a hemidecortication approach and review of 52 cases. J Neurosurg 1996;84:903–911

243. Chugani HT, Muller RA, Chugani DC. Functional brain reorganization in children. Brain Dev 1996;18:347–356

244. Hoffman HJ, Hendrick EB, Dennis M, Armstrong D. Hemispherectomy for Sturge–Weber syndrome. Childs Brain 1979;5:233–248

245. Ceyhan A, Cakan T, Basar H, et al. Anaesthesia for Sturge–Weber syndrome. Eur J Anaesthesiol 1999;16:339–341

246. Enjolras O, Herbreteau D, Lemarchand F, et al. [Hemangiomas and superficial vascular malformations: classification]. J Mal Vasc 1992;17:2–19

247. Gobbi G, Sorrenti G, Santucci M, et al. Epilepsy with bilateral occipital calcifications: a benign onset with progressive severity. Neurology 1988;38:913–920

248. Hamm H. Cutaneous mosaicism of lethal mutations. Am J Med Genet 1999;85:342–345

249. Shapiro K, Shulman K. Facial nevi associated with anomalous venous return and hydrocephalus. J Neurosurg 1976;45:20–25

250. Bordarier C, Aicardi J. Dandy-Walker syndrome and agenesis of the cerebellar vermis: diagnostic problems and genetic counselling. Dev Med Child Neurol 1990;32:285–294

251. McCandless SE, Robin NH. Severe oculocerebrocutaneous (Delleman) syndrome: overlap with Goldenhar anomaly. Am J Med Genet 1998;78:282–285

252. Happle R, Kuster W. Nevus psiloliparus: a distinct fatty tissue nevus. Dermatology 1998;197:6–10

253. Demirci A, Kawamura Y, Sze G, Duncan C. MR of parenchymal neurocutaneous melanosis. AJNR Am J Neuroradiol 1995;16:603–606

254. Happle R. Lethal genes surviving by mosaicism: a possible explanation for sporadic birth defects involving the skin. J Am Acad Dermatol 1987;16:899–906

255. Ming JE, Katowitz J, McDonald-McGinn DM, et al. Hemifacial microsomia in a newborn with hypoplastic skin lesions, an eyelid skin tag, and microphthalmia: an unusual presentation of Delleman syndrome. Clin Dysmorphol 1998;7:279–283

256. Schubert R, Viersbach R, Eggermann T, et al. Report of two new cases of Pallister-Killian syndrome confirmed by FISH: tissue-specific mosaicism and loss of i(12p) by in vitro selection. Am J Med Genet 1997;72:106–110

257. Boente MC, Pizzi de Parra N, Larralde de Luna M, et al. Phacomatosis pigmentokeratotica: another epidermal nevus syndrome and a distinctive type of twin spotting. Eur J Dermatol 2000;10:190–194

258. Di Landro A, Tadini GL, Marchesi L, Cainelli T. Phakomatosis pigmentovascularis: A new case with renal angiomas and some considerations about the classification. Pediatr Dermatol 1999;16:25–30

259. Fritz B, Kuster W, Orstavik KH, et al. Pigmentary mosaicism in hypomelanosis of Ito. Further evidence for functional disomy of Xp. Hum Genet 1998;103:441–449

260. Sayama K, Hato N, Matsuda O, et al. Proteus syndrome. Dermatology 1994;189:392–395

261. Happle R. Mosaicism in human skin. Understanding the patterns and mechanisms. Arch Dermatol 1993;129:1460–1470

262. Clayton-Smith J, Kerr B, Brunner H, et al. Macrocephaly with cutis marmorata, haemangioma and syndactyly—a distinctive overgrowth syndrome. Clin Dysmorphol 1997;6:291–302

263. Louis-Bar D. Sur un syndrome progressif comprenant des téléngiectasies capillaires cutanées et conjunctivales symétriques à disposition naevoïde et des troubles cérébelleux. Confin Neurol 1941;4:32–42

264. Boder E, Sedgwick RP. Ataxia-telangiectasia. A familial syndrome of progressive cerebellar ataxia, oculocutaneous telangiectasia, and frequent pulmonary infection. Pediatrics 1958;4:526–554

265. Lavin MF. ATM: the product of the gene mutated in ataxia-telangiectasia. Int J Biochem Cell Biol 1999;31:735–740

266. Li S, Ting NSY, Zheng L, et al. Functional link of BRCA-1 and ataxia telangiectasia gene product in DNA damage response. Nature 2000;406:210–215

267. Takao N, Li Y, Yamamoto K. Protective roles for ATM in cellular response to oxidative stress. FEBS Lett 2000;472:133–136

268. Aurias A, Dutrillaux B. Acquired inversions in human leucocytes. Ann Genet 1986;29:203–206

269. Gatti RA, Boehnke M, Crist M, Sparkes RS. Genetic linkage studies in ataxia-telangiectasia: Gm markers. Kroc Found Ser 1985;19:163–172

270. Carbonari M, Cherchi M, Paganelli R, et al. Relative increase of T cells expressing the gamma/delta rather than the alpha/beta receptor in ataxia-telangiectasia. N Engl J Med 1990;322:73–76

271. Stern MH. Ataxia telangiectasia: a model for T-cell leukemogenesis. Nouv Rev Fr Hematol 1993;35:29–31

272. Lange E, Borresen AL, Chen X, et al. Localization of an ataxia-telangiectasia gene to an approximately 500-kb interval on chromosome 11q23.1: linkage analysis of 176 families by an international consortium. Am J Hum Genet 1995;57:112–119

273. Plug AW, Peters AH, Xu Y, et al. ATM and RPA in meiotic chromosome synapsis and recombination. Nat Genet 1997;17:457–461

274. Boder E. Ataxia-telangiectasia: an overview. Kroc Found Ser 1985;19:1–63

275. Paula-Barbosa MM, Ruela C, Tavares MA, et al. Cerebellar cortex ultrastructure in ataxia-telangiectasia. Ann Neurol 1983;13:297–302

276. De Leon GA, Grover WD, Huff DS. Neuropathologic changes in ataxia-telangiectasia. Neurology 1976;26:947–951

277. Waldmann TA, Misiti J, Nelson DL, Kraemer KH.

Ataxia-telangiectasis: a multisystem hereditary disease with immunodeficiency, impaired organ maturation, x-ray hypersensitivity, and a high incidence of neoplasia [clinical conference]. Ann Intern Med 1983;99: 367–379

278. Roifman CM, Gelfand EW. Heterogeneity of the immunological deficiency in ataxia-telangiectasia: absence of a clinical-pathological correlation. Kroc Found Ser 1985;19:273–285

279. McFarlin DE, Strober W, Waldmann TA. Ataxia-telangiectasia. Medicine (Baltimore) 1972;51:281–314

280. Aguilar MJ, Kamoshita S, Landing BH, et al. Pathological observations in ataxia-telangiectasia. A report of five cases. J Neuropathol Exp Neurol 1968;27:659–676

281. Bodensteiner JB, Goldblum RM, Goldman AS. Progressive dystonia masking ataxia in ataxia-telangiectasia. Arch Neurol 1980;37:464–465

282. Meshram CM, Sawhney IM, Prabhakar S, Chopra JS. Ataxia telangiectasia in identical twins: unusual features. J Neurol 1986;233:304–305

283. Terenty TR, Robson P, Walton JN. Presumed ataxia-telangiectasia in a man. BMJ 1978;2:802

284. Baloh RW, Yee RD, Boder E. Eye movements in ataxia-telangiectasia. Neurology 1978;28:1099–1104

285. Paller AS. Ataxia-telangiectasia. Neurol Clin 1987;5: 447–449

286. Cohen LE, Tanner DJ, Schaefer HG, Levis WR. Common and uncommon cutaneous findings in patients with ataxia-telangiectasia. J Am Acad Dermatol 1984;10:431–438

287. Paller AS, Massey RB, Curtis MA, et al. Cutaneous granulomatous lesions in patients with ataxia-telangiectasia. J Pediatr 1991;119:917–922

288. Beaudry PH, Bergsteinsson H, Dupont C, et al. alpha-Fetoprotein and cystic fibrosis. Clin Invest Med 1982;5: 45–47

289. Gatti RA, Good RA. Occurrence of malignancy in immunodeficiency diseases. A literature review. Cancer 1971;28:89–98

290. Hecht F, Hecht BK. Cancer in ataxia-telangiectasia patients. Cancer Genet Cytogenet 1990;46:9–19

291. Swift M, Chase CL, Morrell D. Cancer predisposition of ataxia-telangiectasia heterozygotes. Cancer Genet Cytogenet 1990;46:21–27

292. Byrne E, Hallpike JF, Manson JI, et al. Ataxia-without-telangiectasia. Progressive multisystem degeneration with IgE deficiency and chromosomal instability. J Neurol Sci 1984;66:307–317

293. Hecht F, Hecht BK. Ataxia-telangiectasia breakpoints in chromosome rearrangements reflect genes important to T and B lymphocytes. Kroc Found Ser 1985;19: 189–195

294. Richkind KE, Boder E, Teplitz RL. Fetal proteins in ataxia-telangiectasia. JAMA 1982;248:1346–1347

295. Homburger HA, Smith JR, Jacob GL, et al. Measurement of anti-IgA antibodies by a two-site immunoradiometric assay. Transfusion 1981;21:38–44

296. Carbonari M, Cherchi M, Paganelli R, et al. Relative increase of T cells expressing the gamma/delta rather than the alpha/beta receptor in ataxia-telangiectasia. N Engl J Med 1990;322:73–76

297. Schwartz S, Flannery DB, Cohen MM. Tests appropriate for the prenatal diagnosis of ataxia telangiectasia. Prenat Diagn 1985;5:9–14

298. Telatar M, Teraoka S, Wang Z, et al. Ataxia-telangiectasia: identification and detection of founder-effect mutations in the ATM gene in ethnic populations. Am J Hum Genet 1998;62:86–97

299. Fanos JH, Mackintosh MA. Never again joy without sorrow: the effect on parents of a child with ataxia-telangiectasia. Am J Med Genet 1999;87:413–419

300. Dunn HG. Nerve conduction studies in children with Friedreich's ataxia and ataxia-telangiectasia. Dev Med Child Neurol 1973;15:324–337

301. Hagberg B, Hansson O, Liden S, Nilsson K. Familial ataxic diplegia with deficient cellular immunity. A new clinical entity. Acta Paediatr Scand 1970;59: 545–550

302. Girard PM, Foray N, Stumm M, et al. Radiosensitivity in Nijmegen Breakage Syndrome cells is attributable to a repair defect and not cell cycle checkpoint defects. Cancer Res 2000;60:4881–4888

303. Broeks A, Urbanus JH, Floore AN, et al. ATM-heterozygous germline mutations contribute to breast cancer-susceptibility. Am J Hum Genet 2000;66: 494–500

304. Ledley FD, Rosenblatt DS. Mutations in mut methylmalonic acidemia: clinical and enzymatic correlations. Hum Mutat 1997;9:1–6

305. Hora RK, Murthy VS. Mental retardation, short stature and brittle hair (BIDS syndrome; hair brain syndrome). Indian J Pediatr 1996;63:117–120

306. Autti T, Rapola J, Santavuori P, et al. Bone marrow transplantation in aspartylglucosaminuria—histopathological and MRI study. Neuropediatrics 1999;30: 283–288

307. Cremers CW, Geerts SJ. Sensorineural hearing loss and pili torti. Ann Otol Rhinol Laryngol 1979;88:100–104

308. Shashi V, Zunich J, Kelly TE, Fryburg JS. Neuroectodermal (CHIME) syndrome: an additional case with long term follow up of all reported cases. J Med Genet 1995;32:465–469

309. Conforti G, Nardo T, D'Incalci M, Stefanini M. Proneness to UV-induced apoptosis in human fibroblasts defective in transcription coupled repair is associated with the lack of Mdm2 transactivation. Oncogene 2000;19:2714–2720

310. Tezcan I, Demir E, Asan E, et al. A new case of oculocerebral hypopigmentation syndrome (Cross syndrome) with additional findings. Clin Genet 1997;51: 118–121

311. de Felipe I, Quintanilla E. [Neurocutaneous syndromes with vascular alterations]. Rev Neurol 1997;25 Suppl 3:S250–S258

312. Wallerstein R, Kacmar J, Anderson CE, Jackson L. Dubowitz syndrome in a boy without developmental delay: further evidence for phenotypic variability. Am J Med Genet 1997;68:216–218

313. Elejalde BR, Holguin J, Valencia A, et al. Mutations affecting pigmentation in man: I. Neuroectodermal melanolysosomal disease. Am J Med Genet 1979;3: 65–80

314. Symula DJ, Shedlovsky A, Dove WF. Genetic mapping of hph2, a mutation affecting amino acid transport in the mouse. Mamm Genome 1997;8:98–101

315. Bartels I, Caesar J, Sancken U. Prenatal detection of X-linked ichthyosis by maternal serum screening for Down syndrome. Prenat Diagn 1994;14:227–229

316. Schmidt B, Selmer T, Ingendoh A, von Figura K. A novel amino acid modification in sulfatases that is defective in multiple sulfatase deficiency. Cell 1995;82: 271–278

317. Srebrnik A, Brenner S, Ilie B, Messer G. Dorfman-Chanarin syndrome: morphologic studies and presentation of new cases. Am J Dermatopathol 1998;20:79–85

318. Spritz RA. Hermansky-Pudlak syndrome and pale ear:

melanosome-making for the millennium. Pigment Cell Res 2000;13:15–20

319. Ramsay BC, Meeran K, Woodrow D, et al. Cutaneous aspects of Refsum's disease. J R Soc Med 1991;84: 559–560

320. Shapira SK, Neish AS, Pober BR. Unknown syndrome in sibs: pili torti, growth delay, developmental delay, and mild neurological abnormalities. J Med Genet 1992;29:509–510

321. Vasiliou V, Pappa A. Polymorphisms of human aldehyde dehydrogenases. consequences for drug metabolism and disease. Pharmacology 2000;61:192–198

322. Rust S, Rosier M, Funke H, et al. Tangier disease is caused by mutations in the gene encoding ATP-binding cassette transporter 1. Nat Genet 1999;22: 352–355

323. Blomquist HK, Back O, Fagerlund M, et al. Tay or IBIDS syndrome. A case with growth and mental retardation, congenital ichthyosis and brittle hair. Acta Paediatr Scand 1991;80:1241–1245

324. Costagliola C, Verolino M, Landolfo P, et al. Lipoid proteinosis (Urbach-Wiethe disease). Ophthalmologica 1999;213:392–396

325. Lefkowitz A, Schwartz RA, Janniger CK. Melanoma precursors in children. Cutis 1999;63:321–324

326. Ross JL, Roeltgen D, Feuillan P, et al. Use of estrogen in young girls with Turner syndrome: effects on memory. Neurology 2000;54:164–170

327. Glenn CC, Deng G, Michaelis RC, et al. DNA methylation analysis with respect to prenatal diagnosis of the Angelman and Prader-Willi syndromes and imprinting. Prenat Diagn 2000;20:300–306

328. Brodsky MC, Hoyt WF, Higashida RT, et al. Bonnet-Dechaume-Blanc syndrome with large facial angioma. Arch Ophthalmol 1987;105:854–855

329. Hyman P, Oliver C, Hall S. Self-injurious behavior, self-restraint, and compulsive behaviors in Cornelia de Lange syndrome. Am J Ment Retard 2002;107:146–154

330. Barak Y, Nir E. Chediak-Higashi syndrome. Am J Pediatr Hematol Oncol 1987;9:42–55

331. Gray F, Gherardi R, Benhaiem-Sigaux N. [Vertebral hemangioma. Definition, limitations, anatomopathologic aspects]. Neurochirurgie 1989;35:267–269

332. Pratesi R, Santos M, Ferrari I. Costello syndrome in two Brazilian children. J Med Genet 1998;35:54–57

333. Johnston K, Aarons R, Schelley S, Horoupian D. Joint contractures, hyperkeratosis, and severe hypoplasia of the posterior columns: a new recessive syndrome. Am J Med Genet 1993;47:246–249

334. Hofman S, Heeg M, Klein JP, Krikke AP. Simultaneous occurrence of a supra- and an infratentorial glioma in a patient with Ollier's disease: more evidence for nonmesodermal tumor predisposition in multiple enchondromatosis. Skeletal Radiol 1998;27:688–691

335. Schwartz RA, Torre DP. The Muir-Torre syndrome: a 25-year retrospect. J Am Acad Dermatol 1995;33: 90–104

336. Filosa G, Bugatti L, Ciattaglia G, et al. Naevus comedonicus as dermatologic hallmark of occult spinal dysraphism [letter]. Acta Derm Venereol 1997;77:243

337. Van der Warrenburg BP, van Gulik S, Renier WO, et al. The linear naevus sebaceous syndromes. Clin Neurol Neurosurg 1998;100(Suppl 2):126–132

338. Larroque G, Cantaloube D, Ndiaye B, et al. [Verrucous epidermal nevus of the face]. Ann Chir Plast Esthet 1991;36:169–172

339. Mainzer F, Minagi H, Steinbach HL. The variable manifestations of multiple enchondromatosis. Radiology 1971;99:377–388

340. Cory RC, Clayman DA, Faillace WJ, et al. Clinical and radiologic findings in progressive facial hemiatrophy (Parry-Romberg syndrome). AJNR Am J Neuroradiol 1997;18:751–757

341. Baro PR, Bastart FM, Bartrina JR, et al. Case report 529: Osteosarcoma of calcaneus with Rothmund-Thompson syndrome (RTS). Skeletal Radiol 1989;18:136–139

342. Maldonado RR, Tamayo L, Carnevale A. Neuroichthyosis with hypogonadism (Rud's syndrome). Int J Dermatol 1975;14:347–352

343. Satoyoshi E. [Establishment of a syndrome of progressive muscle spasm, alopecia and diarrhea (author's transl)]. Rinsho Shinkeigaku 1978;18:731–739

344. Zipper SG, Lambert S, Seemann WR, et al. [Sneddon syndrome: vasculitis or thrombotic disorder?]. Med Klin 2000;95:158–162

345. Rupprecht R, Hundeiker M. [Cutis marmorata telangiectatica congenita. Important aspects for dermatologic practice]. Hautarzt 1997;48:21–25

346. Wyburn-Mason R. Arteriovenous aneurysm of midbrain and retina, facial naevi and mental changes. Brain 1943;66:163–203

159 Pediatric Brain and Spinal Cord Injury

John P Phillips

Epidemiology

Brain injury is common in children and has devastating consequences for them and their families. Injuries are the leading cause of death of children in the United States, and those who die of injury usually do so because of brain damage.[1] Traumatic brain injury (TBI) occurs in approximately 1/500 children annually,[2] resulting in 100000 children younger than 15 years being admitted to hospitals.[3] Of all TBIs among children, 82% are classified as mild, 14% as moderate to severe, and 5% as fatal.[4] Therefore, the estimated fatality rate among children in the United States from TBI is 1/10000, which far exceeds that of leukemia, the second leading cause of childhood mortality, with a death rate of approximately 1/50000.[5] Many survivors of TBI experience life-long consequences of the injury, and 20% have marked disability.[4]

Spinal cord injury (SCI) also has dire consequences in childhood, but it is less common than TBI. Each year between 230 and 500 children younger than 15 years sustain SCI.[6] It is more common among adolescents and young adults: the prevalence of SCI in the United States among persons younger than 25 years is approximately 1/10000, or 26000 people.[7-9] Appropriate care of patients with SCI requires lifelong support to achieve optimal health and integration into society. Although the life expectancy for children and adolescents with SCI is from 10 to 25 years less than that for the general population,[10] patients with SCI still require decades of care. The care for all persons with SCI in the United States in 1990 was estimated to cost $4 billion.[11] Clearly, pediatric brain and spinal cord injury are issues of tremendous public health importance.

TBI is defined as "physical damage to, or functional impairment of, the cranial contents from acute mechanical energy exchange (exclusive of birth trauma)."[12] TBI in children is different from that in adults. The types of injuries that occur, the acute response to injury, and the long-term consequences vary in large part according to age. As pointed out by Symonds[13] more than 50 years ago, it is not only the kind of head injury that is important but the kind of head that is injured.

Closed head injury accounts for 95% of all pediatric TBIs.[14] Mobility of the head at the moment of impact is critical in the genesis of closed head injury. Most TBIs are the result of a dynamic injury: the head is freely mobile and force is rapidly applied (within 1/5 second), causing the head to accelerate or decelerate rapidly.[15] Experiments with animals have established the importance of rotational head movement in producing TBI and coma.[16,17]

Brain injury is less severe when the head is stationary. In children, crush injuries (impact occurring over more than 1/5 second) happen when a heavy object is pulled onto a child who then falls over with the object on his or her head or when the child is run over by a motor vehicle. This usually causes basilar skull fractures and cranial nerve palsies in addition to brain injury. With appropriate care, the prognosis is excellent for these types of injuries; prolonged unconsciousness is rare, and full cognitive recovery is frequent.[18]

More common in the pediatric population are brain injuries due to falls,[19,20] all-terrain vehicles,[21] child abuse,[22] lawn darts,[23] skateboarding,[24] and walkers.[25] As shown in Table 159.1, the cause of brain injury changes with age. Child abuse and falls are common for infants and young children, but by late childhood to adolescence, motor vehicle accidents, assaults, and sporting injuries account for the majority of TBIs. Children as well as adults share the disturbing increased incidence of firearm injuries, which carry a high mortality rate.[26,27] For adults in the United States, firearms are the second leading cause of death by injury. Firearm death rate in the United States is 90 times higher than in any other country in the world; this includes homicides (39%), suicides (56%), and unintentional deaths (5%).[28] At highest risk for unintentional firearm injury are children 10 to 14 years old.[29] Firearm injury to children results in considerable morbidity even when low-velocity firearms are involved.[30]

Table 159.1	Etiology of TBI in children[4,191,314]
Age (years)	**Etiology**
< 1	Falls Child abuse Motor vehicle accidents
1–4	Falls Motor vehicle accidents Child abuse
5–9	Motor vehicle accidents Falls Sporting injuries
10–14	Motor vehicle accidents Falls Sporting injuries
15–19	Motor vehicle accidents Assaults Sporting injuries

Child abuse is a particularly troubling cause of TBI. It occurs in young children who are often subjected to repeated brain injuries, unlike a TBI from a fall or motor vehicle accident in which the brain is injured by a single impact (Figure 159.1). Severe brain damage can occur, often with retinal hemorrhages, despite little external injury. The term "shaken baby syndrome" aptly describes the repeated trauma often associated with child abuse.[31] Without intervention, child abuse often recurs with increasing severity. Alexander et al.[32] found a 71% incidence of previous abuse among children with "shaken baby syndrome." Jenny et al.[33] reported a series of 173 children with head injuries caused by abuse and found that for approximately 1/3 of the children the diagnosis was not correct at initial presentation. Of the cases of missed child abuse, 1/3 were reinjured, and 4 of 5 deaths could have been prevented by early recognition of child abuse as the cause of the head injuries.

Social and sex factors influence TBI in children. Boys are twice as likely to sustain a TBI as girls[34] except for children younger than 1 year, for whom the incidence is closer to equal.[35] Poverty and marital instability are associated with an increased risk of TBI.[36] Head injury occurs more often in the afternoons or on weekends and during the spring or summer months.[4]

As with adults, the most common cause of SCI in children and adolescents is motor vehicle accidents, with violence and athletics being the second or third most common depending on age.[37] Causes of SCI unique to children include C1-C2 subluxation due to tonsillitis or pharyngitis,[38] birth injury,[39] and child abuse.[40] Lap-belt injuries are also a pediatric cause of SCI. They generally occur in children who weigh less than 60 pounds and for whom the seat belt rests above the pelvic brim. In this position, the seat belt can act as a fulcrum during a motor vehicle accident, causing severe flexion/extension injury.[41,42]

Among several pediatric syndromes at increased risk for SCI is Down syndrome, which is associated with ligamentous laxity of the cervical spine.[43] Approximately 15% of patients with Down syndrome have an atlantodens interval greater than 4.5 mm, which is abnormal, and this increases the risk of cervical subluxation. Asymptomatic persons often are counseled against high-risk activities, and those with symptoms are offered C1-C2 fusion.[37] Juvenile rheumatoid arthritis[44] and achondroplasia[45] also place children at risk for SCI.

A fairly common spine injury unique to the pediatric population is "spinal cord injury without radiographic abnormality" (SCIWORA). This occurs primarily in children younger than about 8 years.[46] It is due to ligamentous laxity of the pediatric spine in combination with a relatively large head and weak neck muscles, which predispose young children to hyperflexion and hyperextension injury. Before about the age of 8 years, the pediatric spine is capable of stretching up to 5 cm before fracturing; however, the pediatric cord remains firmly anchored and ruptures with only 5 to 6 mm of traction.[47] In addition to spinal cord rupture, ischemic injury can follow SCIWORA, either from direct vessel compression or avulsion (Figure 159.2).[48,49]

Prevention is the best treatment. Seat belts and car safety seats clearly help prevent childhood deaths from motor vehicle accidents[50,51] and are particularly important for children younger than 4 years.[52] Seat belts for children of all ages have decreased severe brain injury by 45% to 55%.[53] Air bags offer additional protection for adolescents and adults but are dangerous for children. For a right front seat passenger in a car with dual air bags, the risk of death from a frontal crash is 14% lower for adults wearing seat belts and 23% lower for those not wearing seat belts. However, children younger than 10 years have a higher risk of dying if sitting in the front seat of a car with dual air bags, even if they are wearing a seat belt.[54] The worst injuries are to children placed in rear-facing car seats; they have an extremely high fatality rate because of intracranial injuries. Fatal cervical spine injuries often occur in children who are unrestrained or improperly restrained and who slump forward as the vehicle is braking; a severe hyperextension neck injury occurs as the airbag explodes at 200 to 300 miles per hour into the child's head. Children should be at least 12 years old and capable of reliably wearing a lap and shoulder belt before they sit in the front seat of a car equipped with a passenger-side frontal air bag (personal communication, Bull MJ, 2000).

Bicycle helmets are also effective and decrease the incidence of brain injury by 88%.[55] However, riding a motorcycle is a high-risk activity, particularly if a safety helmet is not worn. The death rate per mile for motorcycles is 20 times that for cars.[56] Riders who do not wear helmets are six times more likely to have a

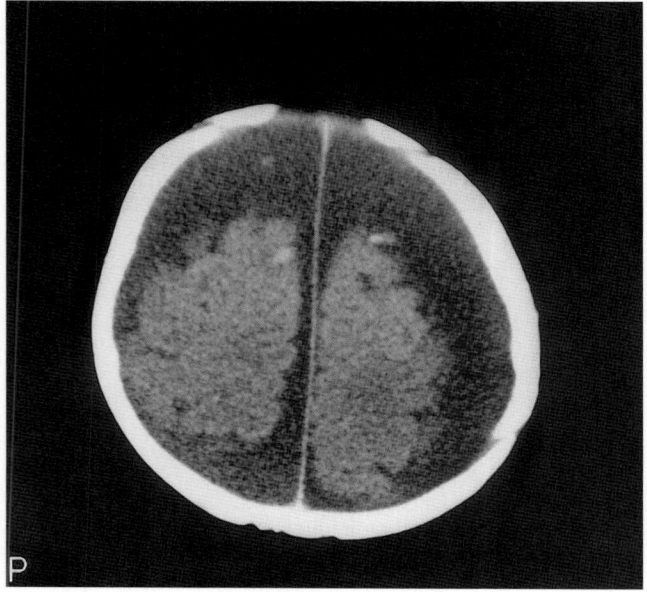

Figure 159.1   Computed tomography of head demonstrating bilateral chronic subdural fluid collections, small acute hemorrhages near anterior convexities, and left parietal skull fracture (right side of figure) in 5-month-old victim of child abuse (Photo courtesy of Blaine L Hart, MD).

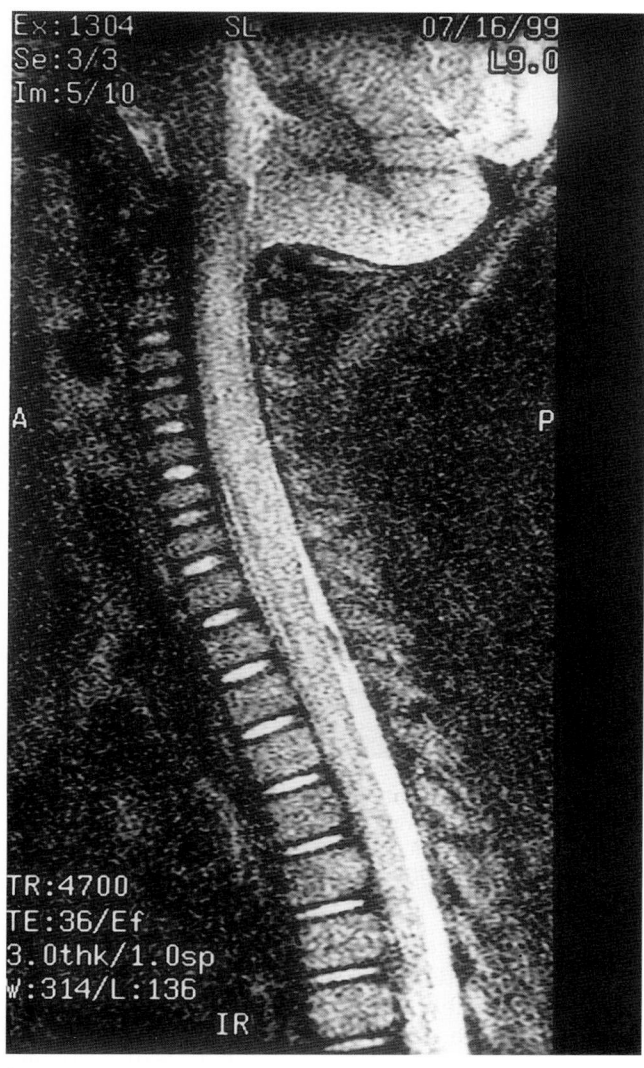

A

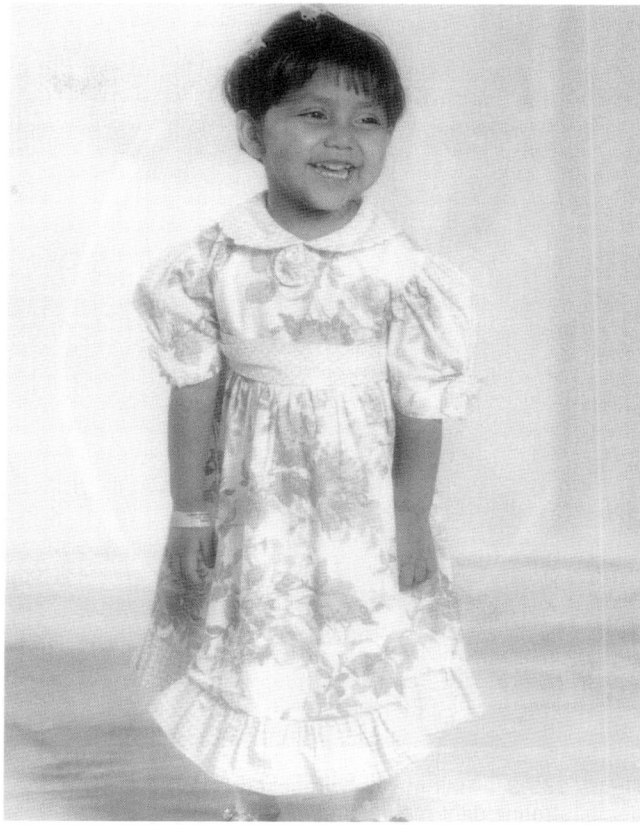

B

Figure 159.2 *A,* Sagittal magnetic resonance image, fast spin echo inversion recovery sequence, showing edema of cervical spinal cord in a 2.5-year-old child, *B,* with spinal cord injury without radiographic abnormality (SCIWORA). A central cord syndrome developed after a trampoline accident, and the child had loss of pain sensation and strength in the upper extremities.

severe brain injury[57] and 3.4 times more likely to die than riders who wear helmets.[58] Wearing a helmet makes no difference in preventing or causing neck injury.[58]

Pathophysiology

Trauma to the central nervous system initiates a cascade of events that leads to neuronal death. Understanding this cascade offers potential opportunities for treatment because it is now clear that much of the pathological reaction of traumatic brain and spinal cord injury develops after the initial impact occurs. There are primary and secondary effects of mechanical injury to the central nervous system. The primary injury occurs at impact and results in mechanical disruption of brain tissue and neuronal circuitry, often associated with hemorrhage, infarction, and contusion. The normal response of the brain to this injury includes breakdown of the blood–brain barrier, vasospasm, loss of cerebral autoregulation, and edema.[60]

Secondary injury develops over hours to days after an impact, and causes diffuse axonal injury (for review, see Gennarelli 1998).[61–63] In the first days after injury, histological examination of brain tissue from humans and animals shows multiple swollen and detached axons, which have been termed "retraction balls."[64,65] Axonal disruption may occur even in mild traumatic head injury.[66] Several recent animal experiments have demonstrated how traumatic injury leads to formation of retraction balls.[67–69] Two major components of the axon cytoskeleton are neurofilaments and microtubules. Neurofilaments provide structure and stability to the axon, and microtubules are involved in intracellular transport.[70] Within 5 minutes after moderate TBI, focal alterations occur in axonal permeability.[71] Adjacent to these sites of permeability change, neurofilaments become compact and microtubular density decreases.[71,72] Thus, axoplasmic flow is disrupted, followed by secondary axotomy.[68] The initial trigger for this cascade appears to be a change in membrane permeability. It is not clear whether this allows the influx of calcium that triggers proteolytic cleavage of neurofilaments and neurofilament sidearms or if some other mechanism alters but does not degrade the neurofilament sidearms.[72,73] What is

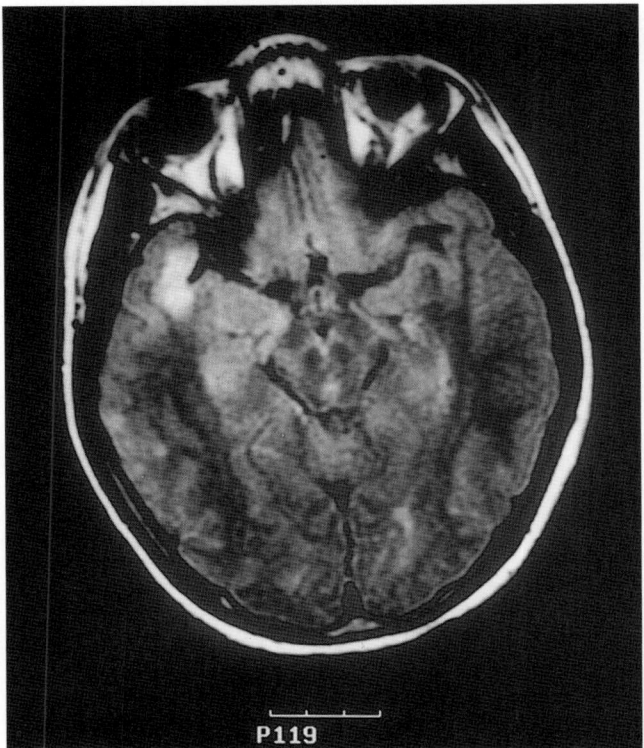

Figure 159.3 Flair magnetic resonance image demonstrating right medial and lateral temporal lobe contusions in 16-year-old after traumatic brain injury.

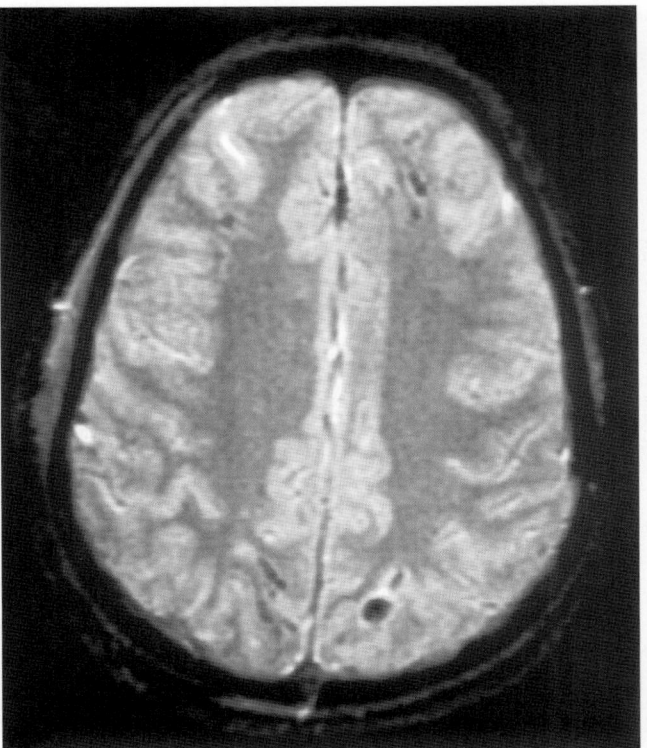

Figure 159.4 T$_2$-weighted gradient recall magnetic resonance image showing multiple small foci of low signal intensity in subcortical locations, representing small areas of hemorrhagic subcortical shear injury in child with traumatic brain injury (Photo courtesy of Blaine L Hart, MD).

clear is that focal membrane permeability occurs at sites of neurofilament compaction, microtubules are lost, and axoplasmic flow is disrupted, leading to secondary axotomy. Diffuse axonal injury affects scattered areas of the cerebral cortex, subcortex, hippocampus, thalamus, and brainstem (Figures 159.3 and 159.4).[70]

In addition to causing cytoskeletal disruption, TBI initiates several other neurochemical processes that lead to neuronal dysfunction and death. These include production of intracellular free radicals, excessive release of glutamate and other excitatory amino acids, initiation of the inflammatory response, generation of widely fluctuating levels of acetylcholine, and change from aerobic to anaerobic glycolysis.

Acetylcholine may have an important role in the development of the cognitive deficits seen after brain injury. Damage to the cholinergic basal forebrain septohippocampal pathways has been demonstrated in animal models of TBI.[75–78] Lesions of cholinergic basal forebrain cell bodies cause cognitive deficits, including problems with learning and memory.[79,80] Initial work indicated that acetylcholine levels were increased after brain trauma,[81] but a more recent investigation has suggested a "swing theory" of cholinergic hyperfunction immediately after brain injury, followed by a longer period of cholinergic hypofunction.[82] In animals, functional outcome after

TBI is improved if anticholinergic medications are given immediately after the injury[83] or if cholinergic medications are given later.[84] Drugs that affect the cholinergic system are not yet used clinically. Clearly, timing will be critical for successful treatment of brain injury with anticholinergic or cholinergic agents.

Glutamate is the major excitatory neurotransmitter of the central nervous system and has a critical role in learning and memory. The hippocampus has a particularly high concentration of glutamate receptors.[85] However, excessive glutamate is neurotoxic, and direct applications to neurons in vitro or injected into brain cause cell swelling and death.[86,87] Glutamate concentration increases for up to several days after brain injury,[88–90] and the degree of increase may reach neurotoxic levels.[91] Several animal studies have evaluated the use of glutamate receptor antagonists in the treatment of brain injury, and most have shown improved outcome (for review, see Myseros JS and Bullock R, 1995).[92,93] However, the results of large-scale clinical trials of glutamate receptor antagonists have been disappointing.[94,95]

Free radicals are molecules or atoms with an unpaired electron in the outer orbit. This unpaired electron makes the free radical highly reactive.[96] Within a neuron, oxygen free radicals such as hydroxy radical or superoxide are formed in response to TBI[97] and SCI.[98] Free radical-induced central

Table 159.2 Glasgow Coma Scale

Best motor response	Score	Best verbal response	Score	Eye opening	Score
Obeys	6	Oriented	5	Spontaneous	4
Localizes	5	Confused conversation	4	Reaction to speech	3
Withdraws	4	Inappropriate words	3	Reaction to pain	2
Abnormal flexion	3	Incomprehensible sounds	2	No response	1
Extension response	2	No response	1		
No response	1				

Source: Teasdale G, Jennett B. Assessment of coma and impaired consciousness. A practical scale. Lancet 2:81–84, 1974

nervous system injury has been implicated in the pathophysiology of TBI (for review, see Shohami 1997).[99,100] Antioxidants have been shown to be beneficial in animal models of traumatic injury to the central nervous systems,[101–103] however, a phase III multicenter clinical trial involving 463 patients with TBI treated with the free radical scavenger superoxide dismutase failed to show any benefit.[104]

Excessive intracellular calcium also contributes to neuronal destruction in TBI.[105,106] Total calcium is higher in areas of the brain subjected to traumatic injury.[107–109] Intracellular calcium concentration increases directly because of membrane permeability changes after physical stress and as a result of excessive glutamate release in a response to brain trauma.[110] By binding to mitochondrial membranes and interrupting oxidative phosphorylation and ATP production, excessive calcium is cytotoxic to neurons.[111] Excessive intracellular calcium also stimulates the additional release of excitatory amino acids and activates several degradative enzymes, including lipases and proteases, that lead to membrane breakdown. In animal models of moderate TBI, there is an immediate decrease in ATP, and marked lipid peroxidation begins within 30 minutes after surgery.[112] Calpains, a type of calcium-activated protease that degrades neurofilaments and microtubules, have been implicated in key processes of cytoskeletal disruption induced by TBI. In animal models of TBI, cognitive outcome improved after the administration of calpain inhibitors and calcium channel blockers.[113,114] However, double-blind, placebo-controlled human studies of calcium antagonists in TBI have not demonstrated any clinical benefit.[115,116]

Neurotrophic factors are peptides that, in the normal brain, function to maintain neurons and to support neurite outgrowth, including guiding neurons to their target sites.[117,118] Common neurotrophic factors are nerve growth factor, basic fibroblast growth factor, brain-derived neurotrophic factor, and insulin-like growth factor. Neurotrophic factors increase in response to traumatic central nervous system injury,[119–121] suggesting a role in the recovery process. In experimental models of TBI, neurotrophic factors improve cognitive outcome and decrease cell loss.[122–124] Clinical trials of treatment with neurotrophic factors for TBI have not been reported.

Acute treatment

The initial treatment of a child with TBI is similar to that for any seriously injured child—airway, breathing, circulation. Nothing takes precedence over these fundamental ABCs of emergency care. During initial stabilization, the cervical spine is immobilized until SCI or vertebral fracture can be ruled out. The expedient general trauma examination evaluates for other injuries. A rapid neurological examination is performed, including assessment of the level of consciousness, cranial nerve function, motor and sensory systems, and reflexes. Palpation of the skull may reveal bogginess, suggesting a depressed skull fracture. Battle sign or "racoon eyes" may indicate a basilar skull fracture. The patient's score on the Glasgow Coma Scale is determined (Table 159.2). In preverbal children or those with a developmental disability, a modified Glasgow Coma Scale such as the Children's Coma Scale (Table 159.3) may be more appropriate. The injured brain of a child is particularly sensitive to hypoxia and ischemia;[125] therefore, maintenance of adequate blood pressure and oxygenation is essential. Rapid assessment and treatment of increased intracranial pressure, decreased cerebral perfusion pressure, electrolyte disturbance, neurosurgical lesions, and seizures are also important. Expedient transport to a pediatric trauma center improves outcome.[126]

Children with TBI have diffuse injury with edema and increased intracranial pressure more often than adults with TBI.[127,128] Diffuse cerebral edema develops in up to 44% of children after severe TBI.[129] Increased intracranial pressure may compromise cerebral perfusion pressure, with devastating results. Poor clinical outcome is correlated with high intracranial pressure in patients with severe brain injury.[130–134] Thus, the appropriate management of increased intracranial pressure is an essential part of caring for children or adults with acute TBI.

Intracranial pressure is important because of its effect on cerebral perfusion pressure:

Cerebral Perfusion Pressure = Mean Arterial Blood Pressure − Intracranial Pressure

Adequate cerebral perfusion pressure can be maintained in spite of increased intracranial pressure if moderate systemic hypertension exists; conversely, if

Table 159.3 Children's Coma Scale (modified Glasgow Coma Scale)[35]

Best motor response	Score	Best verbal response	Score	Eye opening	Score
Spontaneous (obeys verbal command	6	Oriented; or smiles, oriented to sound, follows objects, interacts	5	Spontaneous	4
Localizes pain	5	Confused/disordered; or crying but consolable, inappropriate interaction	4	Reaction to speech	3
Withdraws in response to pain	4	Inappropriate words; or inconsistently consolable, moaning	3	Reaction to pain	2
Abnormal flexion in response to pain (decorticate posture)	3	Incomprehensible sounds; or inconsolable, irritable and restless	2	No response	1
Abnormal extension in response to pain (decerebrate posture)	2	No response	1		
No response	1				

a patient is hypotensive, any increase in intracranial pressure can markedly decrease cerebral perfusion pressure. For this reason, avoiding systemic hypotension is extremely important, and indeed, hypotension is correlated with a poorer outcome after TBI.[135] Cerebral blood flow needs to meet metabolic demands to prevent ischemia.

Cerebral perfusion pressure determines cerebral blood flow. Normally, the cerebral circulation maintains a constant cerebral blood flow despite changes in cerebral perfusion pressure because of autoregulation. Autoregulation is mediated by changes in cerebral vascular resistance[136] and can be disturbed after brain injury.[60,137,138] In children, the exact relationship among cerebral perfusion pressure, cerebral blood flow, autoregulation, and TBI is unclear.

Normal cerebral blood flow is 50 mL/100 g of tissue per minute.[135] Under normal metabolic conditions, ischemic injury occurs when cerebral blood flow is less than 15 to 18 mL/100 g per minute.[139,140] Cerebral blood flow is lowest immediately after injury, decreasing to potentially ischemic levels in one-third of children with severe TBI.[136,141,142] However, after traumatic injury, total brain metabolism is typically depressed, and this may be neuroprotective because a lower cerebral blood flow is necessary to avoid ischemia.[143] Thus, the precise cerebral blood flow required to avoid ischemic injury after TBI is not known.

Brain edema peaks from 24 to 72 hours after TBI.[59] The cause is likely multifactorial; cytotoxicity and delayed tissue damage occur through many mechanisms, including excitotoxicity, release of free radicals, calcium influx, inflammation, and energy failure with dysfunction of cellular ion pumps. Treatment of increased intracranial pressure includes judicious use of hyperventilation, osmotic agents, sedation, and cerebrospinal fluid drainage. Barbiturate-induced

coma may help by decreasing cerebral metabolism (Table 159.4).

Hyperventilation decreases intracranial pressure by causing vasoconstriction and, thus, decreasing cerebral blood flow.[144] Vasoconstriction occurs because cerebral arteries are sensitive to changes in the pH of cerebrospinal fluid in addition to changes in cerebral vascular resistance.[145] Acute hyperventilation causes a decrease in arterial carbon dioxide and a concomitant increase in pH, in response to which cerebral arteries constrict. If hyperventilation continues, the cerebrospinal fluid pH is corrected over several hours by carbonic anhydrase in the choroid plexus.[146,147] The clinical consequence is that as the pH is corrected, cerebral blood flow returns to baseline levels and intracranial pressure increases. In a study of three healthy adults, a decrease in PCO_2 to 15 to 20 mm Hg by hyperventilation caused a 40% decrease in cerebral blood flow within 30 minutes. After 4 hours, cerebral blood flow returned almost to baseline, and when the original PCO_2 was restored at 5 hours, there was a 31% rebound in cerebral blood flow over the baseline level.[148] A clinical trial of prophylactic hyperventilation in adults with TBI demonstrated a poorer outcome for patients who were treated with 5 days of hyperventilation to a $PaCO_2$ of 25 ± 2 mm Hg.[149] Therefore, prophylactic hyperventilation is not recommended for adults, although hyperventilation can be effective in acutely decreasing intracranial pressure for brief periods.[150] Moderate hyperventilation to a PCO_2 of 30 to 35 mg Hg helps control intracranial pressure without inducing ischemia.[151] Aggressive hyperventilation should be avoided, particularly during the first 24 hours after TBI when cerebral blood flow is lowest and brain ischemia can be aggravated.[143] It is not clear whether the clinical response of children with TBI to hyperventilation is substantially different from that of adults.

Table 159.4   Increased intracranial pressure treatment

	Onset of action	Mechanism of action	Dose/endpoint	Comments
Hyperventilation	Minutes	Cerebral artery vasoconstriction	P CO_2 = 30–35 mm Hg	Acutely decreases ICP; chronic use contraindicated, watch for rebound increased ICP
Mannitol	Bimodal: 1) several minutes 2) 15 to 30 minutes	1) immediate decreased blood viscosity causes increased O_2 delivery and reflex vasoconstriction 2) Delayed effect due to osmotic gradient across blood–brain barrier	0.5–1.0 g/kg loading dose, 0.25–0.5 g/kg/ 4 hours Keep serum osmolarity less than 320 mOsm	Bolus dosing more effective than constant infusion
Barbiturates	Minutes	Decreases cerebral metabolism	Pentobarbital loading dose: 3–5 mg/kg Maintenance 1–1.5 mg/kg/hour Goal is burst-suppression EEG pattern, or ICP control	Use after other methods fail, monitor for cardiac depression
Head position	Minutes	Encourages venous drainage	Head midline and raised 30 degrees decreases ICP but no effect on cerebral blood flow or perfusion pressure	Unclear efficacy Raising head more than 30 degrees may decrease cerebral blood flow

Mannitol is commonly used to treat increased intracranial pressure after TBI. Several studies have suggested its effectiveness both in animals[152] and humans,[153–155] although no placebo-controlled clinical trials have been conducted of its use for increased intracranial pressure associated with brain injury.[156] Several mechanisms of action occur when mannitol is used. First, there is an immediate decrease in blood viscosity and hematocrit, which increases cerebral blood flow and cerebral oxygen delivery.[152,157,158] This may result in reflex cerebral vasoconstriction, decreasing intracranial pressure.[159] Second, a delayed effect occurs with the osmotic action of mannitol. Mannitol does not cross the intact blood–brain barrier. Osmotic gradients between plasma and cells develop 15 to 30 minutes after a bolus of mannitol, and this decreases brain edema.[60,157] Bolus administration is more effective than slow or continuous infusion, and the effect on intracranial pressure can persist for up to 6 to 8 hours or longer.[153,160] Mannitol may be more effective in treating increased intracranial pressure when cerebral perfusion pressure is less than 70 mm Hg,[159] although it is effective in lowering even normal intracranial pressure. In a study of adults with normal intracranial pressure, mannitol decreased the mean pressure from 11 to 4 mm Hg.[161] Caution must be used with prolonged treatment with mannitol because it causes breakdown of the blood–brain barrier, result-

ing in the accumulation of mannitol in the brain. This creates a reverse osmotic gradient that may exacerbate intracranial pressure.[162,163] At all times, the fluid status of the patient must be assessed carefully to avoid hypovolemia. Serum osmolarity should be kept below 320 mOsm to avoid renal complications.[164] A commonly used starting dose of mannitol is 0.5 to 1.0 g/kg, then 0.25 to 0.5 g/kg every 4 hours.

Barbiturates also have been used to treat increased intracranial pressure associated with TBI. The cerebral metabolic rate is decreased, and this is believed to decrease oxygen demand and cerebral blood flow.[165–167] In primates, pretreatment with barbiturates has been shown to protect against ischemic injury.[168] Commonly, to control intracranial pressure, a loading dose of pentobarbital, 3 to 5 mg/kg, is given, followed by a continuous infusion at 1 to 1.5 mg/kg per hour. Continuous EEG monitoring is performed. The end point is either adequately controlled intracranial pressure or a burst-suppression pattern on EEG.[169] Because of possible side effects, including cardiac depression, barbiturates are given only after other methods have failed to control intracranial pressure. In a prospective comparison study of adults with TBI, mannitol was better than barbiturates for control of intracranial pressure; mortality was higher in the barbiturate group.[170]

Raising the patient's head and maintaining it in the

neutral position is commonly done to decrease intracranial pressure. However, the efficacy of this maneuver is not clear. In an adult study, raising the head to 30 degrees decreased intracranial pressure, although there was no effect on cerebral perfusion pressure or cerebral blood flow. Raising the head to 60 degrees decreased cerebral blood flow.[171] A similar study has not been conducted for children. Increased intracranial pressure often is decreased by sedation and paralysis, particularly if the patient is agitated or the intracranial pressure increases in response to medical care, for example suctioning or drawing blood. However, prophylactic neuromuscular blockade is not warranted without a specific indication, because it increases the risk of pneumonia and sepsis and prolongs the stay in an intensive care unit without clearly improving outcome.[172]

Early administration of a high dose of corticosteroid in some cases may be helpful for adult SCI.[173] However, despite numerous studies of corticosteroid treatment for brain injury, no clear benefit has been demonstrated (for review, see Alderson 1997).[174] The Brain Trauma Foundation does not recommend corticosteroids for management of severe brain injury.[175]

The recognition of increased intracranial pressure is essential for treating it. Unless herniation has occurred, clinical signs are not a reliable method for determining that intracranial pressure is increased.[176,177] If an adult is in a coma after TBI and the findings on CT of the head are abnormal, the risk of increased intracranial pressure is significant but even if the CT findings are normal, intracranial pressure can be increased and cerebral perfusion pressure decreased.[178] An intracranial monitor allows accurate, continuous assessment of intracranial pressure. This helps to guide treatment and to avoid unnecessary therapy and permits early diagnosis of mass lesions (such as an expanding hemorrhage) and provides information about prognosis. Several types of monitors are available. An external ventriculer drainage system monitors intracranial pressure and has the added advantage of allowing drainage of cerebrospinal fluid when necessary. A common practice is to adjust the ventriculostomy so that it drains when cerebrospinal fluid pressure exceeds a specified level, usually from 15 to 20 mm Hg. Because edematous brains are stiff and poorly compliant, draining just a few milliliters of cerebrospinal fluid through a ventriculostomy can markedly reduce intracranial pressure.[179] Complications are rare with intraventricular monitoring of intracranial pressure and include risks of infection, hemorrhage, malfunction, or obstruction. In adults, intracranial pressure monitoring is recommended if the patient is comatose and has abnormal CT findings. If a comatose patient has normal CT findings, monitoring is recommended if the patient is older than 40 years, has unilateral or bilateral motor posturing, or has systolic blood pressure less than 90 mm Hg.[180] Formal guidelines for monitoring intracranial pressure in children are still under development (Storrs BB, personal communication, 2000).

Appropriate fluid management is essential for children with acute TBI. Cerebral blood flow is lowest during the first 24 hours after injury, which makes this a critical time to avoid hypotension.[125] Children younger than 4 years have a higher incidence of hypotension after TBI.[181] In a study of severe head injuries in children, an episode of hypotension decreased survival fourfold.[125] Older reports have advocated fluid restriction for patients with increased intracranial pressure,[182] but this is no longer the standard of care, because fluid restriction is of questionable value and, indeed, may be harmful. In dogs denied access to water for 72 hours, body weight decreased by 8%, plasma osmolality increased from 307 to 349 mOsm/kg, and brain water decreased by only 1%.[183]

Volume resuscitation is achieved best with isotonic or hypertonic fluids; hypo-osmolar solutions can have a deleterious effect by increasing brain water and intracranial pressure.[184] Hypertonic solutions have been advocated specifically for fluid resuscitation in patients with TBI. Animal experiments using hypertonic solutions to treat shock in the presence of brain injury have shown that intracranial pressure and cerebral blood flow are either improved[185–187] or unaffected.[188] Randomized, double-blind clinical trials of a hypertonic saline and dextran solution for adults (mean age, 30 years) with TBI and hypotension have shown improved outcome.[189] A reasonable approach is to aggressively maintain adequate blood volume in all children with TBI by using either isotonic or hypertonic solutions.

The optimal treatment of neurosurgical lesions requires rapid identification of the lesion. An expanding hemorrhage can be life-threatening and requires immediate surgical intervention.[179] The incidence of surgical lesions varies with severity of TBI; in some reports, up to 23% of children with severe TBI required neurosurgical intervention.[190] The incidence is much lower if the brain injury is less severe.[191] Clinical predictors of intracranial injury include altered mental status, focal neurological signs, loss of consciousness for more than 5 minutes, signs of basilar skull fracture, or presence of any skull fracture. Even children without neurological findings can have a neurosurgical lesion, although this is rare. Quayle et al.[191] reported a series of 322 children with nontrivial TBI who had head CT studies. Of the 27 children who had intracranial injury, 10 required surgery. One of the 10 had normal mental status and no focal neurological findings. This stresses the importance of continued follow-up of all children who have nontrivial TBI, even those without an identifiable intracranial injury. When deciding whether to perform CT, a reasonable approach, based on published case series, is to obtain a CT study of the head for any head-injured child who has focal neurological findings, altered mental status, seizures, signs of basilar skull fracture, or a palpable skull depression. Also, a CT study of the head should be considered for any child who has normal findings on examination but has a history of loss of consciousness, vomiting, headache, amnesia, or sleepiness.[191]

A CT study of the head should be considered for any child with mild traumatic brain injury, particularly one who is being dismissed from the emergency department. Epidural hematomas are rare in children younger than 2 years, because at this age the middle meningeal artery has not become embedded in the bony surface of the temporal bone.[192] Still, epidural hemorrhages may occur after childhood TBI and have been reported even in a child with normal mental status and no focal abnormalities on examination.[191,193] Rare cases of significant intracranial injury have been reported in children after mild TBI, including basal ganglia infarction,[194] transient global amnesia,[195] transient blindness,[196–198] and epidural hematoma requiring late surgical evacuation.[199]

Falls are a common cause of minor head injury in infants. Falls from heights less than 3 ft or after rolling off furniture rarely cause injury of significance,[200,201] although skull fractures can be caused by such falls in infants and are difficult to identify by clinical features alone.[202] Even with an isolated skull fracture, children younger than 2 years often can be dismissed to home if caretakers are reliable, nonaccidental trauma has been ruled out, and there is no other reason for hospitalization.[203]

Plain radiographs are used primarily to assess the cervical spine from C1 to T1. Three views are standard: anteroposterior, lateral, and open mouth. Questions of abnormality may prompt CT or magnetic resonance imaging (MRI). Plain radiographs of the skull are rarely indicated because of the availability of CT: CT provides better resolution of bone and permits assessment of underlying brain parenchyma.[191] Occasionally, fractures can be missed on CT because of the plane of orientation of the image; this is true particularly in children.

Skull fractures are common in TBI and, by themselves, usually are not of clinical importance. However, the presence of a skull fracture makes intracranial injury more likely, and in these cases, CT is indicated.[204] In a study of more than 4000 children with TBI, 27% had a skull fracture: 62% of the fractures were of a single bone and 7% were depressed fractures.[205] Fractures that depress more than the thickness of the skull are surgically elevated.[179] A "growing fracture" is an injury unique to children usually younger than 3 years. It results from a linear skull fracture that tears the dura mater. Dura mater, arachnoid, and cerebrospinal fluid evaginate into the fracture site and, over time, grow, causing the fracture to enlarge. Growing fractures often require surgical intervention.[192]

Young children can be particularly difficult to evaluate because of limited verbal skills, and a careful evaluation is needed to rule out important intracranial lesions. Even with no history of loss of consciousness or neurological abnormalities on examination, intracranial abnormalities may occur in very young children.[201] Thus, in these youngest of children, a CT study of the head is a good way to examine for intracranial injury. With normal CT and neurological examination findings, most children can be safely dismissed from the emergency department with careful dismissal instructions.[206,207]

It is important that flexion and extension films be obtained to rule out subluxation in any child with suspected SCIWORA. MRI should be performed to examine for an underlying spinal cord lesion such as a rare tumor or epidural hematoma. Any neurological signs or symptoms in a child, such as transient paresthesias, weakness, or numbness, associated with cervical trauma raises the question of SCIWORA with incipient spinal instability.[208] Devastating SCI can be avoided by careful evaluation of these children and by the use of immobilization if necessary and counseling against activities that put the child at risk for repeated neck injury.[47]

Initial management of any child suspected of having SCI involves careful spine stabilization until appropriate imaging and neurosurgical consultation are available. SCI is managed best by an experienced multidisciplinary team. This not only improves outcome but also reduces costs.[209] As with TBI, it is important to limit secondary ischemic damage by ensuring adequate oxygenation and perfusion. Although young children have not been studied, corticosteroids may improve outcome in adults. Several double-blind, randomized clinical trials involving adults and adolescents older than 13 years have demonstrated possible improved outcome if high-dose methylprednisolone, 30 mg/kg, is given within 8 hours after injury, followed by methylprednisolone infusion, 5.4 mg/kg per hour, for 24 hours.[173,210] However, recent evidence suggests there may not be a significant benefit to using corticosteroids to treat SCI, and using corticosteroids is therefore not standard of care but rather can be used at the treating physician's discretion.[211]

Athletic-related head injuries are common and often require treatment decisions on the field. Generally, the head injuries are mild, but occasionally, severe TBI can result from an athletic-related injury and several deaths occur each year. In the United States, approximately 10 to 15 deaths annually are associated with football.[212] Statistics are not as well kept for boxing, but from 1945 to 1979, 335 deaths were recorded among amateur and professional boxers; that is, each boxer had approximately a 0.1% chance of being killed.[213] Concussion and minor TBI due to athletics are far more common, occurring at an estimated rate of 250000 annually in the United States.[214] For high school football players, the chance of minor head injury for each year of play is approximately 20%, and after the first concussion, the rate increases fourfold.[215] Proper equipment can help reduce the chance of brain injury. For football players, the type of helmet affects the chance of injury.[216] Guidelines for the evaluation and management of potential head injury in a sports setting recommend that any player with a potential head injury be removed from play for observation (Table 159.5).[217] A second head injury can be lethal if the athlete still has symptoms from the first injury.[217]

Table 159.5   Management of concussion[217]

Grade	Signs and symptoms	Management
1	Transient confusion No loss of consciousness Symptoms resolve within 15 minutes	Remove from play Examine every 15 minutes May return to play if symptoms resolve within 15 minutes Second grade 1 concussion eliminates player from competition that day; may return to play after one asymptomatic week
2	Transient confusion No loss of consciousness Symptoms last more than 15 minutes	Remove from play Frequent examinations on day of injury to rule out evolving intracranial pathology; reexamine following day May return to play after one asymptomatic week and normal neurologic examination Neuroimaging for persistent signs or symptoms after one week Second grade 2 concussion eliminates player from competition for at least 2 asymptomatic weeks
3	Any loss of consciousness	Transport to emergenty room if still unconscious, with cervical spine precautions as indicated Neurologic evaluation and treatment as indicated, including neurosurgical evaluation or transport to trauma center Daily neurologic assessment until symptoms resolve or stabilize After brief (seconds) concussion, may return to play after 1 asymptomatic week After prolonged (minutes) concussion, may return to play after 2 asymptomatic weeks After second grade 3 concussion, may return to play only after at least one asymptomatic month and physician's clearance Symptoms lasting longer than 1 week, consider neuroimaging

Subacute treatment

Rehabilitation after TBI or SCI ideally begins in the intensive care unit. Early efforts are directed toward preventing secondary complications. Physical and occupational therapists help maintain extremity range of motion, preventing contractures and checking for skin breakdown. Special mattresses may help prevent decubitus ulcers, particularly over bony prominences.

In the case of brain injury, speech therapists begin work with oral motor function, evaluate safety of swallowing, and help guide a structured stimulation program. Families should be introduced to the social worker, who will have an important role in providing support and education about recovery from brain injury. Families also may require help in developing strategies to solve the daunting financial problems that can arise when raising a child who has brain injury. Almost 80% of families report financial problems 6 months after a child has had a severe TBI, and in 29% of families, one parent stopped working to care for the injured child.[218] Even before a patient emerges from coma, a psychologist can help identify issues surrounding changing family dynamics. Individual or family therapy may be of benefit. At all stages of recovery, a well-coordinated team approach is necessary to identify and achieve appropriate goals.

Agitation is a common problem after brain injury. From 33% to 50% of adults emerging from coma after TBI exhibit agitated behavior.[219] The incidence in children is not clear, but agitation certainly exists and can

persist for weeks. Agitation creates problems with nursing care, and patents are at risk for hurting themselves, particularly when ambulatory. The common practice is to begin treatment by controlling the patient's environment and avoiding excessive sensory stimulation. One-on-one "technicians" or "sitters" can provide a helpful non pharmacological method of ensuring safety. Medications are available to treat post-traumatic agitation, but few data are available about their use in treating children with TBI. In addition to side effects such as sedation, it is unclear what long-term effects these medications might have on an injured brain. For this reason, drugs should be given sparingly and only when necessary to control post-traumatic agitation.[220] Medications that have been used after TBI in adults include carbamazepine,[221] amitriptyline,[222] trazodone,[223] buspirone,[224] haloperidol,[225] amantadine,[226] lithium,[227] and propranolol.[228]

Several neurotransmitter systems are affected in brain injury, and this may be relevant to agitation. Catecholamines (dopamine, epinephrine, and norepinephrine) have important roles in memory, learning, arousal, and motivation. Catecholamine metabolites increase acutely in the cerebrospinal fluid after diffuse TBI,[229,230] although catecholamine levels in the cerebrospinal fluid may be suppressed in agitated patients with frontotemporal lobe contusions.[231] Serotonin levels of the cerebrospinal fluid are also affected by TBI,[229,232] and among the large number of studies that have linked mood and behavior disorders to serotonin are ones that have suggested a role for serotonin in aggressive behavior.[233] Indeed, lower cerebrospinal fluid levels of serotonin usually are associated with violent behavior, and patients who are agitated after TBI may have lower levels of serotonin than patients who are not agitated.[231] Acetylcholine is also involved in cognition and behavior and may have a key role in memory. Acetylcholine levels fluctuate after TBI and are likely related to the memory deficits seen after injury to cholinergic basal forebrain septohippocampal pathways.[82] It is unclear whether acetylcholine has a role in agitation that occurs after TBI.

Seizures are a known complication of TBI. In children, the incidence of seizures occurring within a week after brain injury is as high as 30% and decreases to about 6% after 1 week.[234] The severity of the injury determines the risk of seizures, as does the presence of focal signs on examination, depressed fracture, or intracerebral hemorrhage.[235,236] The risk of epilepsy is as high as 50% after penetrating trauma.[237] In the acute period after TBI, seizures may interfere with diagnostic studies or medical care, and anticonvulsants such as phenytoin are often given prophylactically. However, data do not support the prophylactic use of anticonvulsants to prevent posttraumatic epilepsy. Therefore, long-term anticonvulsant therapy is not recommended unless a diagnosis of epilepsy (i.e., two or more seizures) is made on clinical grounds.[238] Indeed, anticonvulsant medication may impede recovery from brain injury.[239]

Attention to bladder function begins immediately in a child with SCI. Most children can begin a program of intermittent self-catheterization after about 5 years of age (clean technique is probably as safe as sterile catheterization), usually in combination with an anticholinergic medication such as oxybutynin, up to 0.4 mg/kg orally.[240] Periodic urodynamic testing, including an annual renal ultrasonographic study, should be performed to ensure that management is successful in preserving renal function. In the past, renal failure was a leading cause of death of patients with SCI.[241] Asymptomatic bacteriuria is not an indication for antibiotic therapy; therefore, routine urine cultures are not done.[242]

A daily bowel program should be started in any child with TBI or SCI. Fiber, stool softeners, suppositories, or enemas can help prevent fecal impaction and keep bowel movements soft and regular. For recalcitrant constipation, milk and molasses enemas are successful either for disimpaction or as part of a daily program.[243]

Autonomic dysreflexia occurs in patients with spinal cord lesions at T6 or higher. Noxious stimuli below the level of the lesion reflexively increase sympathetic activity below the lesion, causing vasoconstriction and hypertension. Above the lesion, the response is increased vagal tone and bradycardia. Patients clinically present with abrupt headache, hypertension, warm and blotchy skin above the lesion, and cool skin below the lesion.[244] Bradycardia is not always present. Treatment is aimed at correcting the underlying inciting event. Possible causes

include bladder distention, constipation, infection, or pain from any cause. If symptoms persist, the bladder should be catheterized; for persistent hypertension, sublingual nifedipine or hydralazine can be prescribed.[244]

Approximately 50% of children with SCI develop spasticity,[245] which is also common after TBI.[246] Spasticity should be treated if it interferes with function or comfort or if there is risk of contractures forming. Treatment begins with range of motion exercises.[247] This often is augmented with oral medications, injections of botulinum toxin, implantation of a baclofen pump or selective dorsal rhizotomy (Table 159.6). Splinting or serial casting is often a helpful adjuvant.

Other medical issues also should be addressed during rehabilitation. Patients with SCI should be cared for in a latex-free environment because they are at high risk for the development of latex allergy.[248] Spinal deformities commonly result from SCI. Up to 98% of children injured before puberty develop scoliosis, with 67% of them requiring surgery.[249] Only 20% of those injured after skeletal maturity develop scoliosis, with 5% needing surgery. Sexuality is an issue that often is overlooked in the management of SCI and should be dealt with in a developmentally sensitive manner. Female fertility is not affected, although the spectrum of female sexuality after SCI has not been well studied.[250] In males, fertility and function depend on the level of the injury and how complete it is. Erection is primarily under parasympathetic control (S2-S4) and ejaculation is under sympathetic control (T12-L2). Even for high lesions, treatment is often possible with penile implants, vibratory stimulation, or medications such as sildenafil.[251]

Cognitive sequelae of TBI can be debilitating. Emanuelson et al. followed a series of 25 children after severe TBI for several years and found that most were ambulatory and two-thirds had a normal IQ; however, none were able to function normally in society because of overwhelming behavioral problems.[252] Other studies have confirmed the importance of behavioral and social dysfunction after childhood TBI.[253] Indeed specific diagnoses such as attention deficit hyperactivity disorder place children at higher risk for TBI, but the injury itself may cause new behavioral problems or exacerbate previously existing ones. Children with severe head injury have three times the incidence of behavioral problems than those with mild brain injury or orthopedic injury.[254] Adaptive function is worse in children after severe TBI than in those with mild or moderate TBI.[255]

Children with closed head injury are particularly vulnerable to persistent deficits in memory, attention, planning, response inhibition, and performance-based intelligence tasks.[256–259] Younger children are more vulnerable to attention problems after TBI than adolescents with similar injuries.[260] Focused attention may not be affected as much by TBI in childhood as is divided, sustained, or alternating attention.[259] A proposed explanation of this is that "emerging" skills are more vulnerable to injury than fully developed

Table 159.6	Spasticity treatment after CNS injury			
Modality	**Mechanism**	**Indications**	**Frequency/dose**	**Advantages/ disadvantages**
Range of motion exercises	Muscle stretching encourages new sarcomere growth	All spasticity	Daily	Taught by PT/OT, requires periodic reassessment, may not suffice with significant spasticity
Oral medications Baclofen	GABA B receptor agonist primarily at spinal level	Generalized spasticity	5 mg/day to 60 + mg/day divided TID	Sedation, may increase weakness, rare liver dysfunction
Diazepam	GABA A receptor agonist at brain and spinal level	Generalized spasticity	5 mg/day to 20 + mg/day divided BID–QID	Sedation, risk respiratory depression at high doses
Dantrolene	Inhibits release of calcium from sarcoplasmic reticulum	Generalized spasticity	0.5 mg/kg/dose to 3 mg/kg/dose TID to QID (adult maximum is 100 mg QID)	Weakness, stomach upset, risk of liver dysfunction (check liver function tests periodically)
Clonidine	Alpha 2 adrenergic agonist		0.05 mg to 0.4 mg/day divided BID to QID	Sedation, hypotension, rare cardiac rhythm abnormality (consider EKG)
Tizanidine	Alpha 2 adrenergic agonist	Generalized spasticity	2.0 mg/day to 8.0 + mg/day divided BID to TID	Sedation, hypotension, stomach upset
Botulinum toxin injections	Inhibits presynaptic release of acetylcholine from neuromuscular junction	Focal spasticity	8 units to 12 units/kg depending on muscles injected— reinject no more often than every 3 months	Requires skilled injector, effect lasts 3 to 6 months, often good in combination with range of motion exercises, serial casting, bracing
Intrathecal baclofen pump	Direct constant infusion of baclofen onto spinal cord	Spastic diplegia	Refill pump every 2 to 3 months; reimplant pump every 4 to 5 years	10% perioperative complication rate, programmable pump allows various infusion rates
Selective dorsal rhizotomy	Surgically lesion hyperactive sensory rootlets	Spastic diplegia	Single operation	Active participation required in aggressive post-operative physical therapy program; permanent results (therefore select patient carefully)
Orthopedic surgery	Lengthens tendons, corrects bony abnormalities	Contractures	Operation as indicated	Addresses results of spasticity, not the spasticity itself; tendon lengthening procedures may weaken muscles, growing patients may "outgrow" surgery and require repeat operations

skills.[261] Attention matures throughout childhood and into adolescence, making it particularly vulnerable to injury during this period. It has been proposed that focused attention develops first and reaches adult levels by mid-childhood and other types of attention develop later.[262]

Psychopharmacology and behavioral intervention are used to treat attention problems in children regardless of the cause. Strategies such as alerting teachers to the importance of presenting information in short segments, using frequent reminders and cues to stay on task, decreasing distracting stimuli, and preferential classroom placement, can be helpful. Stimulant medication is also beneficial. Dextroamphetamine and methylphenidate affect several different neurotransmitter systems, and part of their effect in treating attention deficits may be the enhancement of function of dopaminergic circuits in the frontal neocortex,[263] an area often affected in TBI. Stimulant treatment reportedly is helpful for attention deficits of adults[264–271] and children[272–274] after TBI. Attention retraining programs for adults with brain injury have been developed.[275,276]

Memory in children is commonly affected after severe TBI. This impairment is related to severity, as based on the Glasgow Coma Scale score, and persists for at least 1 year after the injury.[277] In a detailed memory study of children and adolescents with TBI, Levin et al.[278] demonstrated that verbal memory is relatively spared in childhood compared with verbal memory in adolescence or visual memory in all age groups. Because visual memory reaches adult performance levels earlier (at age 10 years) than verbal memory, it has been hypothesized that deficits in verbal learning and memory become more apparent during adolescence when these skills normally develop. Thus, deficits do not become evident until the developmental stage at which they usually emerge. The practical implication is that children with severe TBI need to be followed closely for several years because deficits may emerge over time that need to be identified and treated. Various memory strategies and devices can be used if necessary.[279]

Mild traumatic brain injury

Mild TBI is common and has provoked debate about its long-term consequences. Mild TBI has been defined by the Head Injury Interdisciplinary Special Interest Group of the American Congress of Rehabilitation Medicine as a traumatically induced physiological disruption of brain function, as manifested by one of the following: (1) any period of loss of consciousness, (2) any loss of memory for events occurring immediately after the accident or before it, (3) any alteration in mental state at the time of the accident, and (4) focal neurological deficits, which may or may not be transient.[280] Other investigators have defined mild head injury as anyone with a Glasgow Coma Scale score of 13 or higher with a history of the loss of consciousness or amnesia related to the injury.[281] Concern has been raised about sequelae from mild TBI in children,[277,282,283] although several studies have

not found differences between control groups and children with mild TBI.[284–287] There has been concern that even "heading" a soccer ball may cause brain injury in adults.[288] Confirmation of this is awaiting further study, and it is not known whether this has any relevance for a child playing soccer (for review, see Baroff 1998).[289] Indeed, the outcome of mild TBI in childhood may be multifactorial, involving such factors as genetics (presence of *APOE-ε4*, psychosocial environment, presence of previous subclinical head injuries, and developmental age at the time of the injury. Until a clear marker of prognosis is available, it may be prudent to follow children after even mild TBI to provide early identification and treatment for any problems that develop with behavior or cognition.

Prognosis

The prognosis of TBI in childhood varies depending on several factors. In a large prospective study, Luerssen et al.[181] found significantly decreased mortality among children younger than 14 years compared with adults, although specific neuropsychometric functions such as memory and attention may be more vulnerable in children.[290,291] The Glasgow Coma Scale score, duration of coma, and duration of post-traumatic amnesia correlated to some extent with outcome in children.[292–294] Among children younger than 3 years, poor outcome was associated with fixed dilated pupils, absence of the oculovestibular reflex, a Glasgow Coma Scale or Children's Coma Scale score of 3 or 4, or intracranial pressure greater than 40 mm Hg.[35] Overall, children may have a better prognosis than adults after TBI, but young children do worse than older children and adolescents.[60,295] Children with isolated head injuries have a much better neurological prognosis than those with multiple trauma, likely because of the effects of hypotension, hypoxemia, or sepsis that are more frequent with multiple injuries.[296] Child abuse carries a poorer prognosis than accidental trauma to children.[297]

The impact of carrying *APOE-ε4* has not been studied in children; however, in adults this allele is associated with a poorer outcome.[298] It may be prudent to test for the presence of the *APOE-ε4* allele in children and adolescents who wish to participate in activities that place them at risk for head injury (e.g., boxing or hockey), but this raises ethical issues about consent between parents and children, some of whom may have different wishes.[299] The results of proton magnetic resonance spectroscopy correlate with outcome of TBI in adults, and studies of children are in progress.[300]

Patients with SCI often ask about prognosis for ambulation. Generally, functional walking is possible for children with SCI who have *complete* lesions at or below L3, if incomplete lesions above L3 spare motor function, and if there are no lower extremity contractures.[301] Experiments have indicated that ambulation may be possible even with high, complete lesions. In cats with spinal cord transection, locomotion is possible after treadmill training.[302] Locomotor training programs also may help humans who have SCI.[303]

Also, specific medications may have a role; for example, gait pattern may improve in animals and humans after treatment with dextroamphetamine and is worse after treatment with clonidine.[304,305]

Persistent vegetative state carries a poor prognosis in childhood, whether from anoxic or traumatic brain injury. If this state persists for longer than 3 months, minimal improvement is expected,[306] although one group reported that a cohort of children who were in a persistent vegetative state for at least 1 month after TBI continued to have improvement over 12 months.[307]

Conclusion

After severe injury to the brain or spinal cord, many children face a lifetime of special challenges. Helping children and families meet these challenges is the goal of rehabilitation. The goal of acute and long-term rehabilitation is to help improve functional recovery and to develop compensatory strategies in areas in which full recovery is not possible. The Americans With Disabilities Act, passed in 1990, recognizes the need to integrate persons with disabilities into society.[308] Terminology developed by the World Health Organization helps view disabilities along a continuum from biology to a person's social environment. "Pathology" is the change in structure or function of a specific tissue or organ; "impairment" is the loss or abnormality of psychological, physiological, or anatomical structure or function; "disability" is the effect of the impairment on a person's ability to perform an activity; and "handicap" refers to the net effect of the disabilities on the person's general ability to function in society.[309]

A child with SCI, for example, has spinal cord ischemia (pathology) and hemiparesis (impairment) as a result of the lesion and is not able to ambulate (disability) and, thus, cannot play on the high school basketball team (handicap). A wheelchair sports program does not affect "pathology," "impairment," or "disability" but does potentially remove one of the child's handicaps. These are important issues: the long-term outcome of pediatric SCI has been shown to reflect satisfaction with education, employment, and social opportunities. Life satisfaction has less to do with the level of injury, age at the time of injury, or duration of injury.[310] Thus, rehabilitation includes the essential component of community reintegration.

Research on the effectiveness of rehabilitation is inherently difficult. In today's environment, a randomized, double-blind clinical study of rehabilitation is nearly impossible because of the many social, financial, and ethical problems involved.[311] Still, considerable data support the idea that a formal rehabilitation program improves outcome for patients with TBI. Although most studies have involved only adults, rehabilitation for children may produce even greater long-term benefits. Brain-injured patients referred early to an inpatient rehabilitation program had a total decrease in number of inpatient days compared with a matched group that was referred later.[312] Other studies have documented long-term functional improvement

after rehabilitation,[313] particularly when compared with similar populations that did not receive formal rehabilitation (for review, see Cope 1995).[311,314,315]

Brain and spinal cord injury in children rightly commands attention. It is common, often deadly, and, in many cases, preventable. For those who survive—and for their families—the consequences can be devastating. However, progress is being made in several areas. Safety belts and helmets are effective in preventing morbidity and mortality. Greater awareness of child abuse helps protect children from worsening violence. Recognizing firearm injury as a public health problem has pushed gun control issues to national attention. As more is known about the secondary physiological effects of traumatic injury to the central nervous system, effective therapy may become available to help in the first hours or days after injury to protect against toxic biochemical cascades activated by the trauma. A better understanding is emerging about the effect of trauma on the developing nervous system. Also, the science of rehabilitation is defining ways to improve recovery long after the initial injury has occurred. Children are different from adults and potentially have the most to gain from continued work on brain and spinal cord injury.

Acknowledgment

The author would like to thank Bruce B Storrs, MD, for critical review of this manuscript, and Janice K Phillips and Michael J Phillips for thoughtful comments and editing.

References

1. Conroy C, Kraus JF. Survival after brain injury. Cause of death, length of survival, and prognostic variables in a cohort of brain-injured people. Neuroepidemiology 1988;7:13–22
2. Division of Injury Control, Center for Environmental Health and Injury Control, Centers for Disease Control. Childhood injuries in the United States. Am J Dis Child, 1990;144:627–646
3. Kraus JF, Fife D, Conroy C. Pediatric brain injuries: The nature, clinical course, and early outcomes in a defined United States' population. Pediatrics 1987;79: 501–507
4. Kraus JF, Rock A, Hemyari P. Brain injuries among infants, children, adolescents, and young adults. Am J Dis Child, 1990;144:684–691
5. McLaurin RL, Towbin R. Diagnosis and treatment of head injury in infants and children. In: Youmans JR, ed. Neurological Surgery, 3rd ed. Philadelphia: WB Saunders, 1990:2149–2193
6. Kewalramani LS, Kraus JF, Sterling HM. Acute spinal-cord lesions in a pediatric population: epidemiological and clinical features. Paraplegia 1980;18:206–219
7. Berkowitz M, Harvey C, Greene CG, Wilson SE. The economic consequences of traumatic spinal cord injury. New York: Demos Publications, 1992
8. DeVivo MJ, Fine PR, Maetz HM, Stover SL. Prevalence of spinal cord injury. A reestimation employing life table techniques. Arch Neurol 1980;37:707–708
9. harvey C, Rothschild BB, Asmann AJ, Stripling T. New estimates of traumatic SCI prevalence: a survey-based approach. Paraplegia 1990;28:537–544

10. Vogel LC, DeVivo MJ. Etiology and demographics. *In:* Betz RR, Mulcahey MJ, eds. The Child with a Spinal Cord Injury. Rosemont, IL: American Academy of Orthopaedic Surgeons, 1996:3–12

11. Stripling TE. The cost of economic consequences of traumatic spinal cord injury. Paraplegia News 1990; August:50–54

12. Michaud LJ, Duhaime A, Batshaw ML. Traumatic Brain Injury in Children. Pediatr Clin North Am 1993; 40:553–565

13. Rosenthal M, Bond MR. Behavioral and psychiatric sequelae. *In:* Rosenthal M, Griffith ER, Bond MR, Miller JD, eds. Rehabilitation of the Adult and Child with Traumatic Brain Injury. Philadelphia: FA Davis Co, 1990:179–192

14. Levin HS, Aldrich EF, Saydjari C, et al. Severe head injury in children: experience of the Traumatic Coma Bank. Neurosurgery 1992;31:435–444

15. Gennarelli TA, Thibault LE. Biomechanics of head injury. *In:* Wilkins RH, Rengachary SS, eds. Neurosurgery, vol. 2. New York: McGraw-Hill, 1985: 1531–1536

16. Denny-Brown D, Russell WR. Experimental cerebral concussion. Brain 1941;64:93–164

17. Pudenz RH, Shelden CH, Lucite calvarium—a method for direct observation of the brain. II. Cranial trauma and brain movement. J Neurosurg 1946;3:487–505

18. Duhaime AC, Eppley M, Margulies S, et al. Crush injuries to the head in children. Neurosurgery 1995;37: 401–407

19. Jaffe M, Ludwig S. Stairway injuries in children. Pediatrics 1988;82:457–461

20. Musemeche CA, Barthel M, Cosentino C, Reynolds M. Pediatric falls from heights. J Trauma, 1991;31: 1347–1349

21. Kriel RL, Sheehan M, Krach LE, et al. Pediatric head injury resulting from all-terrain vehicle accidents. Pediatrics 1986;78:933–935

22. Christoffel KK. Violent death and injury in US children and adolescents. Am J Dis Child 1990;144:697–708

23. Sotiropoulos SV, Jackson MA, Tremblay GF, et al. Childhood lawn dart injuries. Summary of 75 patients and patient report. Am J Dis Child 1990;144:980–982

24. Retsky J, Jaffe D, Christoffel K. Skateboarding injuries in children. A second wave. Am J Dis Child 1991;145:188–192

25. Rieder MJ, Schwartz C, Newman J. Patterns of walker use and walker injury. Pediatrics 1986;78:488–493

26. Beaver BL, Moore VL, Peclet M, et al. Characteristics of pediatric firearm fatalities. J Pediatr Surg 1990;25:97–99

27. Miner ME, Ewing-Cobbs L, Kopaniky DR, et al. The results of treatment of gunshot wounds to the brain in children. Neurosurgery 1990;26:20–24

28. Runge JW. The cost of injury. Emerg Med Clin North Am 1993;11:241–253

29. Wintemute JG, Teret SP, Kraus JF, et al. When children shoot children: 88 unintended deaths in California. JAMA 1987;257:3107–3109

30. Kountakis SE, Rafie JJ, Ghorayeb B, Stiernberg CM. Pediatric gunshot wounds to the head and neck. Otolaryngol Head Neck Surg 1996;114:756–760

31. Caffey J. On the theory and practice of shaking infants. Its potential residual effects of permanent brain damage and mental retardation. Am J Dis Child 1972;124:161–169

32. Alexander R, Crabbe L, Sato Y, et al. Serial abuse in children who are shaken. Am J Dis Child 1990;144: 58–60

33. Jenny C, Hymel KP, Ritzen A, et al. Analysis of missed cases of abusive head trauma. JAMA 1999;281:621–626

34. Division of Injury Control, Center for Environmental Health and Injury Control, Centers for Disease Control. Childhood injuries in the United States. Am J Dis Child 1990;144:627–646

35. Hahn YS, Chyung C, Barthel MJ, et al. Head injuries in children under 36 months of age. Childs Nerv Syst 1988;4:34–40

36. Klonoff H. Head injuries in children: Predisposing factors, accident conditions, accident proneness and sequelae. Am J Public Health 1971;61:2405–2417

37. Vogel LC. Unique management needs of pediatric spinal cord injury patients: etiology and pathophysiology. J Spinal Cord Med 1997;20:10–13

38. Wilberger JE. Clinical aspects of specific spinal injuries. *In:* Wilberger JE Jr, ed. Spinal Cord Injuries in Children. Mount Kisco, NY: Futura Publishing Company, 1986:69–95

39. MacKinnon JA, Perlman M, Kirpalani H, et al. Spinal cord injury at birth: diagnostic and prognostic data in twenty-two patients. J Pediatr 1993;122:431–437

40. Swischuk LE. Spine and spinal cord trauma in the battered child syndrome. Radiology 1969;92:733–738

41. Garrett JW, Braunstein PW. The seat belt syndrome. J Trauma 1962;2:220–238

42. Apple DF, Murray HH. Lap belt injuries in children. *In:* Betz RR, Mulcahey MJ, eds. The Child with a Spinal Cord Injury. Rosemont, IL: American Academy of Orthopaedic Surgeons, 1996:169–177

43. Committee on Sports Medicine, American Academy of Pediatrics. Atlantoaxial instability in Down syndrome. Pediatrics 1984;74:152–154

44. Nathan FF, Bickel WH. Spontaneous axial subluxation in a child as the first sign of juvenile rheumatoid arthritis. J Bone Joint Surg Am 1968;50:1675–1678

45. Yang SS, Corbett DP, Brough AJ, et al. Upper cervical myelopathy in achondroplasia. Am J Clin Pathol 1977;68:68–72

46. Pang D, Wilberger JE Jr. Spinal cord injury without radiographic abnormalities in children. J Neurosurg 1982;57:114–129

47. Kriss VM, Kriss TC. SCIWORA (spinal cord injury without radiographic abnormality) in infants and children. Clin Pediatr (Phila) 1996;35:119–124

48. Scher AT. Trauma of the spinal cord in children. S Afr Med J 1976;50:2023–2025

49. Ahmann PA, Smith SA, Schwartz JF, Clark DB. Spinal cord infarction due to minor trauma in children. Neurology 1975;25:301–307

50. Scherz RG. Fatal motor vehicle accidents of child passengers from birth through 4 years of age in Washington State, Pediatrics 1981;68:572–575

51. Williams AF. Children killed in falls from motor vehicles. Pediatrics 1981;68:576–578

52. Decker MD, Dewey MJ, Hutcheson RH, Schaffner W. The use and efficacy of child restraint devices. The Tennessee experience. JAMA 1984;252:2571–2575

53. Hartlage LC, Rattan G. Brain injury from motor vehicle accidents. *In:* Templer DL, Hartlage LC, Cannon WG, eds. Preventable Brain Damage: Brain Vulnerability and Brain Health. New York, NY: Springer Publishing Co, 1992:3–14

54. Braver ER, Ferguson SA, Greene MA, Lund AK. Reductions in deaths in frontal crashes among right front passengers in vehicles equipped with passenger air bags. JAMA 1997;278(17):1437–1439

55. Thompson RS, Rivara FP, Thompson DC. Case-control

study of the effectiveness of bicycle safety helmets. N Eng J Med 1989;320:1361–1367

56. US Department of Transportation, National Highway Traffic Safety Administration: Fatal Accident Reporting System. Washington, DC, Department of Transportation, 1990

57. Bachulis BL, Sangster W, Gorrell GW, Long WB. - Patterns of injury in helmeted and nonhelmeted motorcyclists. Am J Surg 1988;155:708–711

58. Braddock M, Schwartz R, Lapidus G, et al. A population-based study of motorcycle injury and costs. Ann Emerg Med 1992;21:273–278

59. Kelly P, Sanson T, Strange G, Orsay E. A prospective study of helmet usage on motorcycle trauma. Ann Emerg Med 1991;20:852–856

60. Adelson PD, Kochanek PM. Head injury in children. J Child Neurol 1998;13:2–15

61. Gennarelli TA, Thibault LE, Graham DI. Diffuse Axonal Injury: An important form of traumatic brain damage. Neuroscientist 1998;4:202–215

62. Adams JH, Doyle D, Ford I, et al. Diffuse axonal injury in head injury: Definition, diagnosis and grading. Histopathology 1989;15:49–59

63. Gennarelli TA, Thibault LE, Adams JH, et al. Diffuse axonal injury and traumatic coma in the primate. Ann Neurol 1982;12:564–574

64. Adams JH. Head injury. In: Adams JH, Duchen LW, eds. Greenfield's Neuropathology, 5th ed. New York: Oxford University Press, 1992:106–152

65. Christman CW, Grady MS, Walker SA, et al. Ultrastructural studies of diffuse axonal injury in humans. J Neurotrauma 1994;11:173–186

66. Povlishock JT, Becker DP, Cheng CLY, Vaughan GW. Axonal change in minor head injury. J Neuropathol Exp Neurol 1983;42:225–242

67. Maxwell WL, Watt C, Graham DI, Gennarelli TA. Ultrastructural evidence of axonal shearing as a result of lateral acceleration of the head in non-human primates. Acta Neuropathol 1993;86:136–144

68. Povlishock JT, Pettus EH. Traumatically induced axonal damage: evidence for enduring changes in axolemmal permeability with associated cytoskeletal change. Acta Neurochir Suppl 1996;66:81–86

69. Povlishock JT, Christman CW. The pathobiology of traumatically induced axonal injury in animals and humans: A review of current thoughts. J Neurotrauma 1995;12:555–564

70. Saatman KE, Graham DI, McIntosh TK. The neuronal cytoskeleton is at risk after mild and moderate brain injury. J Neurotrauma 1998;15:1047–1058

71. Pettus PH, Povlishock JT. Characterization of a distinct set of intra-axonal ultrastructural changes associated with traumatically induced alteration in axolemmal permeability. Brain Res 1996;722:1–11

72. Jafari SS, Maxwell WL, Neilson M, Graham DI. Axonal cytoskeletal changes after non-disruptive axonal injury. J Neurocytol 1997;26:207–221

73. Maxwell WL, Povlishock JT, Graham DL. A mechanistic analysis of nondisruptive axonal injury: a review. J Neurotrauma 1997;14:419–440

74. Okonkwo DO, Pettus EH, Moroi J, Povlishock JT. Alteration of the neurofilament sidearm and its relation to neurofilament compaction occurring with traumatic axonal injury. Brain Res 1998;784:1–6

75. Schmidt RH, Grady MS. Loss of forebrain cholinergic neurons following fluid-percussion injury: implications for cognitive impairment in closed head injury. J Neurosurg 1995;83:496–502

76. Gorman LK, Fu K, Hovda DA, et al. Effects of traumatic brain injury on the cholinergic system in the rat. J Neurotrauma 1996;13:457–463

77. Leonard JR, Maris DO, Grady MS. Fluid percussion injury causes loss of forebrain choline acetyltransferase and nerve growth factor receptor immunoreactive cells in the rat. J Neurotrauma 1994;11:379–392

78. Leonard JR, Grady MS, Lee ME, et al. Fluid percussion injury causes disruption of the septohippocampal pathway in the rat. Exp Neurol 1997;143:177–187

79. Hepler DJ, Olton DS, Wenk GL, Coyle JT. Lesions in nucleus basilis magnocellularis and medial septal area of rats produce qualitatively similar memory impairments. J Neurosci 1985;5:866–873

80. Miyamoto M, Kato J, Narumi S, Nagaoka A. Characteristics of memory impairment following lesioning of the basal forebrain and medial septal nucleus in rats. Brain Res 1987;419:19–31

81. Tower D, McEachern D. Acetylcholine and neuronal activity: cholinesterase patterns and acetylcholine in cerebrospinal fluids of patients with craniocerebral trauma. Can J Res, Sect. E, 1949;27:105–119

82. McIntosh TK, Juhler M, Wieloch T. Novel pharmacologic strategies in the treatment of experimental traumatic brain injury: 1998. J Neurotrauma 1998;15:731–769

83. Lyeth BG, Ray M, Mann RJ, et al. Postinjury scopolamine administration in experimental traumatic brain injury. Brain Res 1992;569:281–286

84. Dixon CE, Ma X, Marion DW. Effects of CDP-choline treatment on behavioral deficits after TBI and on hippocampal and neocortical acetycholine release. J Neurotrauma 1997;14:161–169

85. Monaghan DT, Cotman CW. Identification and properties of N-methyl-D-aspartate receptors in rat brain plasma membranes. Proc Natl Acad Sci USA 1986;83:7532–7536

86. Choi DW. Ionic dependence of glutamate neurotoxicity. J Neurosci 1987;7:369–379

87. Coyle JT, Schwarcz R. Lesion of striatal neurones with kainic acid provides a model for Huntington's chorea. Nature 1976;263:244–246

88. Baker AJ, Moulton RJ, MacMillan VH, Shedden PM. Excitatory amino acids in cerebrospinal fluid following traumatic brain injury in humans. J Neurosurg 1993;79:369–372

89. Palmer AM, Marion DW, Botscheller ML, et al. Increased transmitter amino acid concentration in human ventricular CSF after brain trauma. Neuroreport 1994;6:153–156

90. Zauner A, Bullock R. The role of excitatory amino acids in severe brain trauma. Opportunities for therapy: a review. J Neurotrauma 1995;12:547–554

91. Palmer AM, Marion DW, Botscheller LM, et al. Traumatic brain injury-induced excitotoxicity as assessed in a controlled cortical impact model. J Neurochem 1993;61:2015–2024

92. Myseros JS and Bullock R. The rationale for glutamate antagonists in the treatment of traumatic brain injury. Ann NY Acad Sci 1995;765:262–271

93. Katoh H, Sima K, Nawashiro H, et al. The effect of MK-801 on extracellular neuroactive amino acids in hippocampus after closed head injury followed by hypoxia in rats. Brain Res 1997;758:153–162

94. Morris GF, Bullock R, Marshall SB, et al. Failure of the competitive N-methyl-D-aspartate antagonist Selfotel (CGS 19755) in the treatment of severe head injury: results of two phase III clinical trials. The Selfotel

Investigators. J Neurosurg 1999;91:737–743

95. Doppenberg EMR, Bullock R. Clinical neuro-protection trials in severe traumatic brain injury: lessons from previous studies. J Neurotrauma 1997;14:71–80

96. Kerr ME, Bender CM, Monti EJ. An introduction to oxygen free radicals. Heart Lung 1996;25:200–209

97. Hall ED, Andrus PK, Yonkers PA. Brain hydroxyl radical generation in acute experimental head injury. J Neurochem 1993;60:588–594

98. Xu J, Beckman JS, Hogan EL, Hsu CY. Xanthine oxidase in experimental spinal cord injury. J Neurotrauma 1991;8:11–18

99. Shohami E, Beit-Yannai E, Horowitz M, Kohen R. Oxidative stress in closed-head injury: brain antioxidant capacity as an indicator of functional outcome. J Cereb Blood Flow Metab 1997;17:1007–1019

100. Braughler JM, Hall ED. Involvement of lipid peroxidation in CNS injury. J Neurotrauma 1992;9(Suppl 1):S1–S7

101. Anderson DK, Saunders RD, Demediuk P, et al. Lipid hydrolysis and peroxidation in injured spinal cord: partial protection with methylprednisolone or vitamin E and selenium. J Neurotrauma 1985;2:257–267

102. Wei EP, Kontos HA, Dietrich WD, et al. Inhibition by free radical scavengers and by cyclooxygenase inhibitors of pial arteriolar abnormalities from concussive brain injury in cats. Circ Res 1981;48:95–103

103. Xiong Y, Peterson PL, Muizelaar JP, Lee CP. Amelioration of mitochondrial function by a novel antioxidant U-101033E following traumatic brain injury in rats. J Neurotrauma 1997;14:907–917

104. Young B, Runge JW, Waxman KS, et al. Effects of pegorgotein on neurologic outcome of patients with severe head injury. A multicenter, randomized controlled trial. JAMA 1996;276:538–543

105. McIntosh ST, Saatman KE, Raghupathi R. Calcium and the pathogenesis of traumatic CNS injury: cellular and molecular mechanism. The Neuroscientist 1997;3:169–175

106. Tymianski M, Tator CH. Normal and abnormal calcium homeostasis in neurons: a basis for the pathophysiology of traumatic and ischemic central nervous system injury. Neurosurgery 1996;38:1176–1195

107. Thomas WJ, Breault D, Nolan B, Smith DH, McIntosh TK. Effects of experimental brain injury on regional cation homeostasis. Neuroscientist 1990;Abstract 16:777

108. Nilsson P, Hillered L, Olsson Y, et al. Regional changes in interstition K^+ and Ca^{2+} levels following cortical compression contusion trauma in rats. J Cereb Blood Flow Metab 1993;13:183–192

109. Fineman I, Hovda DA, Smith M, et al. Concussive brain injury is associated with a prolonged accumulation of calcium: a ^{45}Ca autoradiographic study. Brain Res 1993;624:94–102

110. Luer MS, Rhoney DH, Hughes M, Hatton J. New pharmacologic strategies for acute neuronal injury. Pharmacotherapy 1996;16:830–848

111. Okonkwo DO, Buki A, Siman R, Povlishock JT. Cyclosporin A limits calcium-induced axonal damage following traumatic brain injury. Neuroreport 1999;10:353–358

112. Sullivan PG, Keller JN, Mattson MP, Scheff SW. Traumatic brain injury alters synaptic homeostasis: implications for impaired mitochondrial and transport function. J Neurotrauma 1998;15:789–798

113. Saatman KE, Murai H, Bartus RT, et al. Calpain inhibitor AK295 attenuates motor and cognitive deficits following experimental brain injury in the rat.

Proc Natl Acad Sci USA 1996;93:3428–3433

114. Badie H, Fu K, Samii A, Hovda DA. A selective N-channel calcium blocker attenuates the injury-induced accumulation of calcium following experimental traumatic brain injury (abstract). J Neurotrauma 1993;10(Suppl 1):S161

115. Compton JS, Lee T, Jones NR, et al. A double blind placebo controlled trial of the calcium entry blocking drug, nicardipine, in the treatment of vasospasm following severe head injury. Br J Neurosurg 1990;4:9–15

116. Teasdale G, Bailey I, Bell A, et al. A randomized trial of nimodipine in severe head injury: HIT 1. British/Finnish Co-operative Head Injury Trial Group. J Neurotrauma 1992;9(Suppl 2):S545–S550

117. McIntosh TK, Smith DH, Garde E. Therapeutic approaches for the prevention of secondary brain injury. Eur J Anaesthesiol 1996;13:291–309

118. Mocchetti I, Wrathall JR. Neurotrophic factors in central nervous trauma. J Neurotrauma 1995;12:853–870

119. DeKosky ST, Goss JR, Miller PD, et al. Upregulation of nerve growth factor following cortical trauma. Exp Neurol 1994;130:173–177

120. Patterson SL, Grady SM, Bothwell M. Nerve growth factor and a fibroblast growth factor-like neurotrophic activity in cerebrospinal fluid of brain injured human patients. Brain Res 1993;605:43–49

121. Mattson MP, Scheff SW. Endogenous neuroprotection factors and traumatic brain injury mechanisms of action and implications for therapy. J Neurotrauma 1994;11:3–33

122. Sinson G, Perri BR, Trojanowski JQ, et al. Improvement of cognitive deficits and decreased cholinergic neuronal cell loss and apoptotic cell death following neurotrophin infusion after experimental traumatic brain injury. J Neurosurg 1997;86:511–518

123. Dietrich WD, Alonso O, Busto R, Finklestein SP. Posttreatment with intravenous basic fibroblast growth factor reduces histopathological damage following fluid-percussion brain injury in rats. J Neurotrauma 1996;13:309–316

124. Kromer LF. Nerve growth factor treatment after brain injury prevents neuronal death. Science 1987;235:214–216

125. Pigula FA, Wald SL, Shackford SR, Vane DW. The effect of hypotension and hypoxia on children with severe head injuries. J Pediatr Surg 1993;28:310–314

126. Johnson DL, Krishnamurthy S. Send severely head-injured children to a pediatric trauma center. Pediatr Neurosurg 1996;25:309–314

127. Aldrich EF, Eisenberg HM, Saydjari C, et al. Diffuse brain swelling in severely head-injured children. A report from the NIH Traumatic Coma Data Bank. J Neurosurg 1992;76:450–454

128. Zimmerman RA, Bilaniuk LT, Bruce D, et al. Computed tomography of pediatric head trauma: acute general cerebral swelling. Radiology 1978;126:403–408

129. Berger MS, Pitts LH, Lovely M, et al. Outcome from severe head injury in children and adolescents. J Neurosurg 1985;62:194–199

130. Becker DP, Miller JD, Ward JD, et al. The outcome from severe head injury with early diagnosis and intensive management. J Neurosurg 1977;47:491–502

131. Johnston IH, Johnston JA, Jennett WB. Intracranial-pressure changes following head injury. Lancet 1970;2:433–436

132. Miller JD, Butterworth JF, Gudeman SK, et al. Further

experience in the management of severe head injury. J Neurosurg 1981;54:289–299

133. Narayan RK, Greenberg RP, Miller JD, et al. Improved confidence of outcome prediction in severe head injury: A comparative analysis of the clinical examination, multimodality evoked potentials, CT scanning, and intracranial pressure. J Neurosurg 1981;54:751–762

134. Troupp J. Intraventricular pressure in patients with severe brain injuries. J Trauma 1965;5:373–378

135. Chesnut RM, Marshall LF, Klauber MR, et al. The role of secondary brain injury in determining outcome from severe head injury. J Trauma 1993;34:216–222

136. Yundt KD, Diringer MN. The use of hyperventilation and its impact on cerebral ischemia in the treatment of traumatic brain injury. Crit Care Clin 1997;13:163–184

137. Sharples PM, Stuart AG, Matthews DSF, et al. Cerebral blood flow and metabolism in children with severe head injury. Part 1. Relation to age, Glasgow coma score, outcome, intracranial pressure, and time after injury. J Neurol Neurosurg Psychiatry 1995;58:145–152

138. Muizelaar JP, Ward JD, Marmarou A, et al. Cerebral blood flow and metabolism in severely head-injured children. Part 2. Autoregulation. J Neurosurg 1989;71:72–76

139. Astrup J, Siesjo BK, Symon L. Thresholds in cerebral ischemia: The ischemic penumbra. Stroke 1981;12:723–725

140. Powers WJ, Grubb RL Jr, Darriet D, Raichle ME. Cerebral blood flow and cerebral metabolic rate of oxygen requirements for cerebral function and viability in humans. J Cereb Blood Flow Metab 1985;5:600–608

141. Muizelaar JP, Marmarou A, DeSalles AAF, et al. Cerebral blood flow and metabolism in severely head-injured children. Part 1. Relationship with GCS score, outcome, ICP, and PVI. J Neurosurg 1989;71:63–71

142. Robertson CS, Contant CF, Narayan RK, Grossman RG. Cerebral blood flow, AVDO$_2$, and neurologic outcome in head-injured patients. J Neurotrauma 1992;9(Suppl 1):S349–S358

143. Obrist WD, Langfitt TW, Jaggi JL, et al. Cerebral blood flow and metabolism in comatose patients with acute head injury. Relationship to intracranial hypertension. J Neurosurg 1984;61:241–253

144. Raichle ME, Plum F. Hyperventilation and cerebral blood flow. Stroke 1972;3:566–575

145. Kontos HA, Raper AH, Patterson JL. Analysis of vasoactivity of local pH, Pco$_2$ and bicarbonate on pial vessels. Stroke 1977;8:358–360

146. Albrecht RF, Miletich DJ, Ruttle M. Cerebral effects of extended hyperventilation in unanesthetized goats. Stroke 1987;18:649–655

147. Plum F, Posner JB. Blood and cerebrospinal fluid lactate during hyperventilation. Am J Physiol 1967;212:864–870

148. Raichle ME, Posner JB, Plum F. Cerebral blood flow during and after hyperventilation. Arch Neurol 1970;23:394–403

149. Muizelaar JP, Marmarou A, Ward JD, et al. Adverse effects of prolonged hyperventilation in patients with severe head injury: A randomized clinical trial J Neurosurg 1991;75(5):731–739

150. Brain Trauma Foundation. The use of hyperventilation in the acute management of severe traumatic brain injury. J Neurotrauma. 1996;13:699–703

151. Narayan RK, Kishore PRS, Becker DP, et al. Intracranial pressure: to monitor or not to monitor? A review of our experience with severe head injury. J Neurosurg 1991;56:650–659

152. Israel RS, Marks JA, Moore EE, Lowenstein SR. Hemodynamic effect of mannitol in a canine model of concomitant increased intracranial pressure and hemorrhagic shock. Ann Emerg Med 1988;17:560–566

153. Marshall LF, Smith RW, Rauscher LA, Shapiro HM. Mannitol dose requirements in brain-injured patients. J Neurosurg 1978;48:169–172

154. Mendelow AD, Teasdale GM, Russell T, et al. Effect of mannitol on cerebral blood flow and cerebral perfusion pressure in human head injury. J Neurosurg 1985;63:43–48

155. Miller JD, Piper IR, Dearden NM. Management of intracranial hypertension in head injury: Matching treatment with cause. Acta Neurochir Suppl 57. 1993:152–159

156. Brain Trauma Foundation. The use of mannitol in severe head injury. J Neurotrauma 1996;13:705–709

157. Barry KG, Berman AR. Mannitol infusion. III. The acute effect of the intravenous infusion of mannitol on blood and plasma volumes. N Engl J Med 1961;264:1085–1088

158. Brown FD, Johns L, Jafar JJ, et al. Detailed monitoring of the effects of mannitol following experimental head injury. J Neurosurg 1979;50:423–432

159. Rosner MJ, Coley I. Cerebral perfusion pressure: A hemodynamic mechanism of mannitol and the post-mannitol hemogram. Neurosurgery 1987;21:147–156

160. Jafar JJ, Johns LM, Mullan SF. The effect of mannitol on cerebral blood flow. J Neurosurg 1986;64:754–759

161. Rudehill A, Gordon E, Ohman G, et al. Pharmacokinetics and effects of mannitol on hemodynamics, blood and cerebrospinal fluid electrolytes, and osmolality during intracranial surgery. J Neurosurg Anesthesiol 1993;5:4–12

162. Kaufmann AM, Cardoso ER. Aggravation of vasogenic cerebral edema by multiple-dose mannitol. J Neurosurg 1992;77:584–589

163. Cold GE. Cerebral blood flow in acute head injury. Acta Neurochir 1990;49(Suppl):18–21

164. Becker DP, Vries JK. The alleviation of increased intracranial pressure by the chronic administration of osmotic agents. In: Brock M, Dietz H, eds. Intracranial Pressure: Experimental and Clinical Aspects. New York: Springer-Verlag, 1972:309–315

165. Marshall LF, Smith RW, Shapiro HM. The outcome with aggressive treatment in severe head injuries. Part II. Acute and chronic barbiturate administration in the management of head injury. J Neurosurg 1979;50:26–30

166. Rockoff MA, Marshall LF, Shapiro HM. High-dose barbiturate therapy in humans: A clinical review of 60 patients. Ann Neurol 1979;6:194–199

167. Nordstrom CH, Messeter K, Sundbarg G, et al. Cerebral blood flow, vasoreactivity, and oxygen consumption during barbiturate therapy in severe traumatic brain lesions. J Neurosurg 1988;68:424–431

168. Hoff JT, Smith AL, Hankinson HL, Nielsen SL. Barbiturate protection from cerebral infarction in primates. Stroke 1975;6:28–33

169. Marion DW. Head and spinal cord injury. Neurol Clin 1998;16:485–502

170. Schwartz ML, Tator CH, Rowed DW, et al. The University of Toronto Head Injury Treatment Study: A prospective randomized comparison of pentobarbital and mannitol. Can J Neurol Sci 1984;11:434–440

171. Feldman Z, Kanter MJ, Robertson CS, et al. Effect of head elevation on intracranial pressure, cerebral perfusion pressure, and cerebral blood flow in head-injured patients. J Neurosurg 1992;76:207–211

172. Hsiang JK, Chesnut RM, Crisp CB et al. Early, routine paralysis for intracranial pressure control in severe head injury: Is it necessary? Crit Care Med 1994;22: 1471–1476

173. Bracken MB, Shepard MJ, Holford TR, et al. Administration of methylprednisolone for 24 to 48 hours or tirilazad mesylate for 48 hours in the treatment of acute spinal cord injury. JAMA 1997;277:1597–1604

174. Alderson P, Roberts I. Corticosteroids in acute traumatic brain injury: systematic review of randomised controlled trials. BMJ 1997;314:1855–1859

175. Task Force of the American Association of Neurological Surgeons and Joint Section in Neurotrauma and Critical Care, Guidelines for the management of severe head injury. Brain Trauma Foundation Website, 1995

176. Browder J, Meyers R. Observations on behavior of the systemic blood pressure, pulse, and spinal fluid pressure following craniocerebral injury. Am J Surg 1936;31:403–426

177. Lundberg N. Continuous recording and control of ventricular fluid pressure in neurosurgical practice. Acta Psychiatr Neurol Scand 1960;36(Suppl 149):1–193

178. O'Sullivan MG, Statham PF, Jones PA, et al. role of intracranial pressure monitoring in severely head-injured patients without signs of intracranial hypertension on initial computerized tomography. J Neurosurg 1994;80:46–50

179. Greenwald BM, Ghajar J, Notterman DA. Critical care of children with acute brain injury. Adv Pediatr 1995; 42:47–89

180. Brain Trauma Foundation. Indications for intracranial pressure monitoring. J Neurotrauma 1996;13:667–679

181. Luerssen TG, Klauber MR, Marshall LF. Outcome from head injury related to patient's age. A longitudinal prospective study of adult and pediatric head injury. J Neurosurg 1988;68:409–416

182. Shenkin HA, Bezier HS, Bouzarth WF. Restricted fluid intake. Rational management of the neurosurgical patient. J Neurosurg 1976;45:432–436

183. Jelsma LF, McQueen JD. Effect of experimental water restriction on brain water. J Neurosurg 1967;26:35–40

184. Zornow MH, Prough DS. Fluid management in patients with traumatic brain injury. New Horiz 1995; 3:488–498

185. Gunnar W, Jonasson O, Merlotti G, et al. Head injury and hemorrhagic shock: studies of the blood brain barrier and intracranial pressure after resuscitation with normal saline solution, 3% saline solution, and dextran-40. Surgery 1988;103:398–407

186. Prough DS, Whitley JM, Taylor CL, et al. Regional cerebral blood flow following resuscitation from hemorrhagic shock with hypertonic saline: Influence of a subdural mass. Anesthesiology 1991;75:319–327

187. Ducey JP, Mozingo DW, Lamiell JM, et al. A comparison of the cerebral and cardiovascular effects of complete resuscitation with isotonic and hypertonic saline, hetastarch, and whole blood following hemorrhage. J Trauma 1989;29:1510–1518

188. Prough DS, DeWitt DS, Taylor CL, et al. Hypertonic saline does not reduce intracranial pressure or improve cerebral blood flow after experimental head injury and hemorrhage in cats (abstract). Anesthesiology 1991;75(Suppl):A544

189. Wade CE, Grady JJ, Kramer GC, et al. Individual patient cohort analysis of the efficacy of hypertonic saline/dextran in patients with traumatic brain injury and hypotension. J Trauma 1997;42(Suppl):S61–S65

190. Alberico AM, Ward JD, Choi SC, et al. Outcome after severe head injury. Relationship to mass lesions, diffuse injury, and ICP course in pediatric and adult patients. J Neurosurg 1987;67:648–656

191. Quayle KS, Jaffe DM, Kuppermann N, et al. Diagnostic testing for acute head injury in children: when are head computed tomography and skull radiographs indicated? (abstract) Pediatrics 1997;99(5):726. Full text article at www.pediatrics.org

192. Zuckerman GB, Conway EE Jr. Accidental head injury. Pediatr Ann 1997;26:621–632

193. Bor-Seng-Shu E, Aguiar PH, Matushita H, et al. Actual asymptomatic epidural hematomas in childhood. Report of three cases. Childs Nerv Syst 1997;13: 605–607

194. Maki Y, Akimoto H, Enomoto T. Injuries of basal ganglia following head trauma in children. Childs Brain 1980;7:113–123

195. Vohanka S, Zouhar A. Transient global amnesia after mild head injury in childhood. Activitas Nervosa Superior (Praha) 1988;30:68–74

196. Yamamoto LG, Bart RD Jr. Transient blindness following mild head trauma. Criteria for a benign outcome. Clin Pediatr (Phila) 1988;27:479–483

197. Hochstetler K, Beals RD. Transient cortical blindness in a child. Ann Emerg Med 1987;16:218–219

198. Kaye EM, Herskowitz J. Transient post-traumatic cortical blindness: brief v prolonged syndromes in childhood. J Child Neurol 1986;1:206–210

199. Geller E, Yoon MS, Loiselle J, et al. Head injuries in children from plastic hairbeads. Pediatr Radiol 1997; 27:790–793

200. Tarantino CA, Dowd MD, Murdock TC. Short vertical falls in infants. Pediatr Emerg Care 1999;15:5–8

201. Gruskin KD, Schutzman SA. Head trauma in children younger than 2 years: are there predictors for complications? Arch Pediatr Adolesc Med 1999;153:15–20

202. Ros SP, Cetta F. Are skull radiographs useful in the evaluation of asymptomatic infants following minor head injury? Pediatr Emerg Care 1992;8:328–330

203. Greenes DS, Schutzman SA. Infants with isolated skull fracture: what are their clinical characteristics, and do they require hospitalization? Ann Emerg Med 1997;30: 253–259

204. Ward JD. Pediatric issues in head trauma. New Horiz 1995;3:539–545

205. Harwood-Nash CE, Hendrick EB, Hudson AR. The significance of skull fractures in children. A study of 1,187 patients. Radiology 1971;101:151–156

206. Roddy SP, Cohn SM, Moller BA, et al. Minimal head trauma in children revisited. Is routine hospitalization required? Pediatrics 1998;101:575–577

207. Davis RL, Hughes M, Gubler KD, et al. The use of cranial CT scans in the triage of pediatric patients with mild head injury. Pediatrics 1995;95:345–349

208. Pang D, Pollack IF. Spinal cord injury without radiographic abnormality in children: the SCIWORA syndrome. J Trauma 1989;29:654–664

209. Tator CH, Duncan EG, Edmonds VE, et al. Neurological recovery, mortality and length of stay after acute spinal cord injury associated with changes in management. Paraplegia 1995;33:254–262

210. Bracken MB, Shepard MJ, Collins WF, et al. A randomized, controlled trial of methylprednisolone or naloxone in the treatment of acute spinal-cord injury. Results of the Second National Acute Spinal Cord Injury Study. N Eng J Med 1990;322:1405–1411

211. Hurlbert R John. The role of steroids in acute spinal cord injury: an evidence-based analysis. Spine 2001;26(Suppl 24):S39–S46

212. Wilberger JE Jr, Maroon JC. Head injuries in athletes. Clin Sports Med 1989;8:1–9

213. Council on Scientific Affairs. Brain injury in boxing. JAMA 1983;249:254–257

214. Cantu C. When to return to contact sports after a cerebral concussion. Sports Med Digest 1988;10:1–2

215. Gerberich SG, Priest JD, Boen JR, et al. Concussion incidences and severity in secondary school varsity football players. Am J Public Health 1983;73:1370–1375

216. Zemper ED. Analysis of cerebral concussion frequency with the most commonly used models of football helmets. J Athletic Train 1994;29(1):44–49

217. Practice parameter: The management of concussion in sports (summary statement). Report of the Quality Standards Subcommittee. Neurology 1997;48:581–585

218. Osberg JS, Brooke MM, Baryza MJ, et al. Impact of childhood brain injury on work and family finances. Brain Inj 1997;11:11–24

219. Sandel ME, Mysiw WJ. The agitated brain injured patient, Part 1. Definitions, differential diagnosis, and assessment. Arch Phys Med Rehabil 1996;77:617–623

220. Krach LE, Kriel RL. Traumatic Brain Injury. In: Molnar GE, Alexander MA, eds. Pediatric Rehabilitation, 3rd edn. Philadelphia: Hanley and Belfus, 1999:245–268

221. Pourcher E, Filteau MJ, Bouchard RH, Baruch P. Efficacy of the combination of buspirone and carbamazepine in early posttraumatic delirium. Am J Psychiatry 1994;151:150–151

222. Mysiw WJ, Jackson RD, Corrigan JD. Amitriptyline for post-traumatic agitation. Am J Phys Med Rehabil 1988;67:29–33

223. Rowland TR, Mysiw WJ, Bogner JA, Corrigan JD. Trazodone for post-traumatic agitation (abstract). Arch Phys Med Rehabil 1992;73:963

224. Ratey JJ, Leveroni CL, Miller AC, et al. Low-dose buspirone to treat agitation and maladaptive behavior in brain-injured patients: two case reports. J Clin Psychopharmacol 1992;12:362–364

225. Rao N, Jellinek HM, Woolston DC. Agitation in closed head injury: haloperidol effects on rehabilitation outcome. Arch Phys Med Rehabil 1985;66:30–34

226. Chandler MC, Barnhill JL, Gualtieri CT. Amantadine for the agitated head-injury patient. Brain Inj 1988;2:309–311

227. Glenn WB, Wroblewski B, Parziale J, Levine L, Whyte J, Rosenthal M. Lithium carbonate for aggressive behavior or affective instability in ten brain-injured patients. Am J Phys Med Rehabil 1989;68:221–226

228. Brooke MM, Patterson DR, Questad KA, Cardenas D, Farrel-Roberts L. The treatment of agitation during initial hospitalization after traumatic brain injury. Arch Phys Med Rehabil 1992;73(10):917–921

229. Markianos M, Seretis A, Kotsou A, Christopoulos M. CSF neurotransmitter metabolites in comatose head injury patients during changes in their clinical state. Acta Neurochir (Wien) 1996;138(1):57–59

230. Markianos M, Seretis A, Kotsou S, Baltas I, Sacharogiannis H. CSF neurotransmitter metabolites and short-term outcome of patients in coma after head injury. Acta Neuro Scand 1992;86:190–193

231. van Woerkom TCA-M, Teelken AW, Minderhoud JM. Difference in neurotransmitter metabolism in frontotemporal-lobe contusion and diffuse cerebral contusion. Lancet 1977;1:812–813

232. Vecht CJ, van Woerkom TC, Teelken AW, Minderhoud JM. On the nature of brain stem disorders in severe head injured patients. Acta Neurochir (Wien) 1976;34(1–4):11–21

233. Burrowes KL, Hales RE, Arrington E. Research on the biologic aspects of violence. Psychiatr Clin North Am 1988;11:499–509

234. Annegers JF, Grabow JD, Groover RV, Laws ER Jr, Elveback LR, Kurland LT. Seizures after head trauma: a population study. Neurology 1980;30:683–689

235. Pohlmann-Eden B, Bruckmeir J. Predictors and dynamics of posttraumatic epilepsy. Acta Neurologica Scandinavica 1997;95:257–262

236. Asikainen I, Kaste M, Sarna S. Early and late posttraumatic seizures in traumatic brain injury rehabilitation patients: brain injury factors causing late seizures and influence of seizures on long-term outcome. Epilepsia 1999;40(5):584–589

237. Salazar AM, Jabbari B, Vance SC, Grafman J, Amin D, Dillon JD. Epilepsy after penetrating head injury. I. Clinical correlates: a report of the Vietnam Head Injury Study. Neurology 1985;35:1406–1414

238. Hernandez TD, Naritoku DK. Seizures, epilepsy, and functional recovery after traumatic brain injury: A reappraisal. Neurology 1997;48:803–806

239. Dikmen SS, Temkin NR, Miller B, Machamer J, Winn R. Neurobehavioral effects of phenytoin prophylaxis of posttraumatic seizures. JAMA 1991;265:1271–1277

240. Pannek J, Diederichs W, Botel U. Urodynamically controlled management of spinal cord injury in children. Neurourol Urodyn 1997;16:285–292

241. Nyquist RH, Bors E. Mortality and survival in traumatic myelopathy during nineteen years, from 1946 to 1965. Paraplegia 1967;5:22–48

242. National Institute on Disability and Rehabilitation Research consensus statement. The prevention and management of urinary tract infections among people with spinal cord injuries. J Am Paraplegia Soc 1992;15:194–204

243. Armstrong M, Robbins A, Rose E, Phillips JP. Treatment of Intractable Constipation with Milk and Molasses Enemas. Poster presentation. Am Acad Cereb Palsy Dev Med Annual Meeting, Washington DC, September 1998

244. Vogel L, Mulcahy MJ, Betz RR. The child with a spinal cord injury. Dev Med Child Neurol 1997;39:202–207

245. Vogel LC. Spasticity: diagnostic workup and medical management. In: Betz RR, Mulcahey MJ, eds. The Child with a Spinal Cord Injury. Rosemont, IL: American Academy of Orthopaedic Surgeons, 1996:261–268

246. Brink JD, Imbus C, Woo-Sam J. Physical recovery after severe closed head trauma in children and adolescents. J Pediatr 1980;97:721–727

247. Katz RT. Management of spasticity. Am J Phys Med Rehabil 1988;67:108–116

248. Vogel LC, Schrader T, Lubicky JP. Latex allergy in children and adolescents with spinal cord injuries. J Pediatr Orthop 1995;15:517–520

249. Dearolf WW III, Betz RR, Vogel LC, Levin J, Clancy M, Steel HH. Scoliosis in pediatric spinal cord-injured patients. J Pediatr Orthop 1990;10:214–218

250. Sipski ML, Alexander CJ. Female sexuality after spinal cord injury: current knowledge and future direction. Topics in Spinal Cord Inj Rehabil 1995;1:1–10

251. Brindley GS. Neurophysiology of ejaculation and treatment of infertility in men with spinal cord injuries. In: Hargreave TB, ed. Male Infertility, 2nd edn. New York: Springer-Verlag, 1994:307–317

252. Emanuelson I, von Wendt L, Lundalv E, Larsson J. Rehabilitation and follow-up of children with severe traumatic brain injury. Childs Nerv Syst 1996;12: 460–465

253. Cattelani R, Lombardi F, Brianti R, Mazzucchi A. Trau-

matic brain injury in childhood: intellectual, behavioural and social outcome into adulthood. Brain Inj 1998;12(4):283–296

254. Brown G, Chadwick O, Shaffer D, Rutter M, Traub M. A prospective study of children with head injuries: III. Psychiatric sequelae. Psychol Med 1981;11:63–78

255. Fletcher JM, Ewing-Cobbs L, Miner ME, Levin HS, Eisenberg HM. Behavioral changes after closed head injury in children. J Consult Clin Psychol 1990;58(1): 93–98

256. Fletcher JM, Levine HS. Neurobehavioral effects of brain injury in children. In: Rough D, ed. Handbook of Pediatric Psychology. New York: Guilford Press, 1988:258–298

257. Gutentag SS, Naglieri JA, Yeates KO. Performance of children with traumatic brain injury on the Cognitive Assessment System. Assessment 1998;5(3):263–272

258. Catroppa C, Anderson V, Stargatt R. A prospective analysis of the recovery of attention following pediatric head injury. J Int Neuropsychol Soc 1999;5(1): 48–57

259. Anderson V, Fenwick T, Manly T, Robertson I. Attentional skills following traumatic brain injury in childhood: a componential analysis. Brain Inj 1998;12(11): 937–949

260. Kaufmann PM, Fletcher JM, Levin HS, Miner ME, Ewing-Cobbs L. Attentional disturbance after pediatric closed head injury. J Child Neurol 1993;8(4):348–353

261. Dennis M. Language and the young damaged brain. In: Dennis M, Boll T, Bryant BK, eds. Clinical Neuropsychology and Brain Function: Research, Measurement and Practice. Washington, DC: American Psychological Association, 1988:89–123

262. Cooley EL, Morris RD. Attention in children: A neuropsychologically-based model for assessment. Dev Neuropsychol 1990;6:239–274

263. Gualtieri CT, Hicks RE. The neuropharmacology of methylphenidate and a neural substrate for childhood hyperactivity. Psychiatr Clin North Am 1985;8:875–892

264. Gualtieri CT, Evans RW. Stimulant treatment for the neurobehavioural sequelae of traumatic brain injury. Brain Inj 1988;2:273–290

265. Evans RW, Gualtieri CT, Patterson DR. Treatment of chronic closed injury with psychostimulant drugs: a controlled case study and an appropriate evaluation procedure. J Nerv Ment Dis 1987;175:106–110

266. Lipper S, Tuchman MM. Treatment of chronic post-traumatic organic brain syndrome with dextroamphetamine: first reported case. J Nerv Ment Dis 1976;162:366–371

267. Mooney GF, Haas LJ. Effect of methylphenidate on brain injury-related anger. Arch Phys Med Rehabil 1993;74:153–160

268. Kaelin DL, Cifu DX, Matthies B. Methylphenidate effect on attention deficit in the acutely brain-injured adult. Arch Phys Med Rehabil 1996;77:6–9

269. Plenger PM, Dixon CE, Castillo RM, Frankowski RF, Yablon SA, Levin HS. Subacute methylphenidate treatment for moderate to moderately severe traumatic brain injury: a preliminary double-blind placebo-controlled study. Arch Phys Med Rehabil 1996;77:536–540

270. Speech TJ, Rao SM, Osmon DC, Sperry LT. A double-blind controlled study of methylphenidate treatment in closed head injury. Brain Inj 1993;7:333–338

271. Whyte J, Hart T, Schuster K, Fleming M, Polansky M, Coslett HB. Effects of methylphenidate on attentional function after traumatic brain injury. A randomized placebo-controlled trial. Am J Phys Med Rehabil 1997;76:440–450

272. Mahalick DM, Carmel PW, Greenberg JP, et al. Psychopharmacologic treatment of acquired attention disorders in children with brain injury. Pediatr Neurosurg 1998; 29(3):121–126

273. Williams SE, Ris MD, Ayyangar R, Schefft BK, Berch D. Recovery in pediatric brain injury: is psychostimulant medication beneficial? J Head Trauma Rehab 1998; 13(3):73–81

274. Hornyak JE, Nelson VS, Hurvitz EA. The use of methylphenidate in pediatric traumatic brain injury. Pediatric Rehabil 1997;1:15–17

275. Niemann H, Ruff RM, Baser CA. Computer-assisted attention retraining in head-injured individuals: a controlled efficacy study of an outpatient program. J Consult Clin Psychol 1990;58:811–817

276. Sohlberg MM, Mateer CA. Effectiveness of an attention-training program. J Clin Exp Neuropsychol 1987; 9:117–130

277. Levin HS, Eisenberg HM. Neuropsychological outcome of closed head injury in children and adolescents. Childs Brain 1979;5:281–292

278. Levin HS, Eisenberg HM, Wigg NR, Kobayashi K. Memory and intellectual ability after head injury in children and adolescents. Neurosurgery 1982;11: 668–673

279. Wilson BA, Evans JJ, Emslie H, Malinek V. Evaluation of NeuroPage: a new memory aid. J Neurol Neurosurg Psychiatry 1997;63:113–115

280. Kay T, Harrington DE. Definition of mild traumatic brain injury. J Head Trauma Rehab 1993;8:86–87

281. Stein SC, Ross SE. The value of computed tomographic scans in patients with low-risk head injuries. Neurosurgery 1990;26:638–640

282. Rimel RW, Giordani B, Barth JT, et al. Disability caused by minor head injury. Neurosurgery 1981;9: 221–228

283. Ewing-Cobbs L, Fletcher JM, Levin HS, et al. Longitudinal neuropsychological outcome in infants and preschoolers with traumatic brain injury. J Int Neuropsychol Soc 1997;3:581–591

284. Bijur PE, Haslum M, Golding J. Cognitive and behavioral sequelae of mild head injury in children. Pediatrics 1990;86:337–344

285. Max JE, Robin DA, Lindgren SD, et al. Traumatic brain injury in children and adolescents: psychiatric disorders at two years. J Am Acad Child Adolesc Psychiatry 1997;36:1278–1285

286. McLean A Jr, Temkin NR, Dikmen S, Wyler AR. The behavioral sequelae of head injury. J Clin Neuropsychol 1983;5:361–376

287. Fay GC, Jaffe KM, Polissar NL, et al. Outcome of pediatric traumatic brain injury at three years: cohort study. Arch Phys Med Rehabil 1994;75:733–741

288. Matser EJ, Kessels AG, Lezak MD, et al. Neuropsychological impairment in amateur soccer players. JAMA 1999;282:971–973

289. Baroff GS. Is heading a soccer ball injurious to brain function? J Head Trauma Rehab 1998;13:45–52

290. Levin HS, Eisenberg HM, Wigg NR, Kobayashi K. Memory and intellectual ability after head injury in children and adolescents. Neurosurgery 1982;11: 668–673

291. Taylor HG, Alden J. Age-related differences in outcomes following childhood brain insults: an introduction and overview. J Int Neuropsychol Soc 1997; 3: 555–567

292. McDonald CM, Jaffe KM, Fay GC, et al. Comparison of indices of traumatic brain injury severity as predictors of neurobehavioral outcome in children. Arch Phys Med Rehabil 1994;75(3):328–337

293. Bruce DA, Raphaely RC, Goldberg AI, et al. Pathophysiology, treatment and outcome following severe head injury in children. Childs Brain 1979;5:174–191

294. Filley CM, Cranberg LD, Alexander MP, Hart EJ. Neurobehavioral outcome after closed head injury in childhood and adolescence. Arch Neurol 1987;44: 194–198

295. Thakker JC, Splaingard M, Zhu J, et al. Survival and functional outcome of children requiring endotracheal intubation during therapy for severe traumatic brain injury. Crit Care Med 1997;25:1396–1401

296. Mayer T, Walker ML, Shasha I, et al. Effect of multiple trauma on outcome of pediatric patients with neurologic injuries. Childs Brain 1981;8:189–197

297. Ewing-Cobbs L, Kramer L, Prasad M, et al. Neuroimaging, physical, and developmental findings after inflicted and noninflicted traumatic brain injury in young children. Pediatrics 1998;102:300–307

298. Friedman G, Froom P, Sazbon L, et al. Apolipoprotein E-epsilon-4 genotype predicts a poor outcome in survivors of traumatic brain injury. Neurology 1999;52: 244–248

299. Caulfield TA. The law, adolescents, and the APOE epsilon-4 genotype: a view from Canada. Genet Test 1999;3:107–113

300. Friedman SD, Brooks WM, Jung RE, et al. Quantitative proton MRS predicts outcome after traumatic brain injury. Neurology 1999;52(7):1384–1391

301. Vogel LC, Lubicky JP. Ambulation in children and adolescents with spinal cord injuries. J Pediatr Orthop 1995;15:510–516

302. Barbeau H, Rossignol S. Recovery of locomotion after chronic spinalization in the adult cat. Brain Res 1987;412:84–95

303. Dietz V, Wirz M, Jensen L. Locomotion in patients with spinal cord injuries. Phys Ther 1997;77:508–516

304. Feeney DM, Sutton RL. Pharmacotherapy for recovery of function after brain injury. Crit Rev Neurobiol 1987;3:135–197

305. Dietz V, Colombo G, Jensen L, Baumgartner L. Locomotor capacity of spinal cord in paraplegic patients. Ann Neurol 1995;37:574–582

306. Ashwal S. The persistent vegetative state in children. Adv Pediatr 1994;41:195–222

307. Heindl UT, Laub MC. Outcome of persistent vegetative state following hypoxic or traumatic brain injury in children and adolescents. Neuropediatrics 1996;27:94–100

308. Gordon CG, Kaplan ??. Physical Medicine and Rehabilitation: State of the Art Reviews. 1992;6:341–358

309. International Classification of Impairments, Disabilities, and Handicaps: A Manual of Classification Relating to the Consequences of Disease. Geneva: World Health Organization, 1980

310. Vogel LC, Klaas SJ, Lubicky JP, Anderson CJ. Long-term outcomes and life satisfaction of adults who had pediatric spinal cord injuries. Arch Phys Med Rehabil 1998;79:1496–1503

311. Cope DN. The effectiveness of traumatic brain injury rehabilitation: a review. Brain Inj 1995;9:649–670

312. Cope DN, Hall K. Head injury rehabilitation: benefit of early intervention. Arch Phys Med Rehabil 1982;63: 433–437

313. Cope DN, Cole JR, Hall KM, Barkan H. Brain injury: analysis of outcome in a post-acute rehabilitation system. Part 2: Subanalyses. Brain Inj 1991;5:127–139

314. Aronow HU. Rehabilitation effectiveness with severe brain injury: translating research into policy. J Head Trauma Rehab 1987;2(3):24–36

315. Mackay LE, Bernstein BA, Chapman PE, et al. Early intervention in severe head injury: long-term benefits of a formalized program. Arch Phys Med Rehabil 1992;73:635–641

316. Goldstein FC, Levin HS. Epidemiology of pediatric closed head injury: Incidence, clinical characteristics, and risk factors. J Learn Disabil 1987;20:518–525

X Cranial Nerve Disorders, Neuro-otology and Neuro-ophthalmology

Section editor: James A Sharpe

160 Disturbances of Smell and Taste

Richard L Doty*

Overview

The senses of taste and smell determine the flavors of foods and beverages, purvey esthetic pleasures, and provide warning of such dangers as spoiled food, leaking natural gas, and fire or smoke. Disorders of these senses have been reported in the medical literature for many years. Indeed, anosmia due to head injury and nasal blockage was recognized as early as the third century BC.[1] Johns Hughlings Jackson, the great nineteenth century British neurologist, was among the first to bring attention to the fact that olfactory and gustatory aberrations are associated with neurological disturbances of the temporal and frontal lobes, and that chemosensory auras can precede paroxysms associated with epilepsy.[2,3]

Etiology

The most common cause of *permanent* olfactory loss in patients appears to be a severe upper respiratory infection, usually viral in origin, in which the olfactory neuroepithelium is damaged.[4] Such loss most typically occurs after the age of 45 years. The second most common cause of olfactory dysfunction is head trauma. It is estimated that between 7% and 15% of patients suffering from severe head trauma have demonstrable olfactory loss, usually anosmia or severe microsmia.[5,6] In most such cases, the loss reflects a shearing of the olfactory filaments at the level of the cribriform plate, although contusions of the frontal and temporal poles can also be present.[6,7] Resolution of function over time is noted in some cases when brain swelling subsides or hematomas resolve; such resolution occurs within a few months of the trauma. The third most common cause of smell loss is nasal and sinus disease. While some patients with loss due to this cause are benefited by steroidal therapy or surgical intervention, such treatments typically do not completely return function to normal levels.[8] Thus, factors other than gross airway access to the receptor sheet appear responsible for the dysfunction (e.g. damage to the receptors as a result of chronic inflammation).

We now know, largely as the result of the proliferation of easy-to-use commercially available tests of olfactory function,[9] that decreased smell function is the first sign, or at least among the first signs, of a number of common neurological disorders, including Alzheimer's disease, idiopathic Parkinson's disease, and schizophrenia.[10,11] In the case of schizophrenia, a strong and inverse correlation has been noted between disease duration and odor identification test scores, suggesting that there may be a progressive, perhaps degenerative, component of this disorder that heretofore has gone unrecognized.[12] The prevalence of olfactory loss in Parkinson's disease (90%) is higher than the prevalence of several cardinal signs of Parkinson's disease (e.g. tremor).[13] Unfortunately, the olfactory loss in Parkinson's disease does not respond to medical therapy; it also does not correlate with disease severity and, unlike the motor symptoms, does not progress over time.[14,15] Interestingly, olfactory testing differentiates well between idiopathic Parkinson's disease and both progressive supranuclear palsy (PSP) and MPTP-induced parkinsonism, since olfactory loss is uncommon in the latter two disorders.[16,17]

Recently it has been shown that scores on a simple three-item microencapsulated odor test differentiate better between Alzheimer's disease and depression than scores on the Mini-Mental State Examination, although both of these tests usually make this distinction.[18,19] Moreover, there is now strong evidence that smell testing may be of considerable prognostic value in early detection of Alzheimer's disease. Graves et al.[20] administered a 12-item commercially available smell identification test and several cognitive tests to 1985 Japanese-American people around the age of 60, and then readministered these tests to 1604 of these people 2 years later. Sixty-nine percent of the follow-up participants were genotyped for apolipoprotein E (apoE). Low odor identification test scores in the presence of one or more APOE-e4 alleles were associated with a very high risk of subsequent cognitive decline, and the smell test identified persons who came to exhibit later cognitive decline better than did a global cognitive test (grade B efficacy—level II). In another longitudinal study, Devanand et al.[21] administered the 40-item University of Pennsylvania Smell Identification Test (UPSIT) to 90 outpatients with mild cognitive impairment and to matched healthy controls at 6-month intervals over a 5-year time period. Patients with mild cognitive impairment had lower UPSIT scores than did controls. Most importantly, patients with low UPSIT scores (<34) were more likely to develop Alzheimer's disease than the other patients. Low UPSIT scores, combined with lack of awareness of olfactory deficits on the part of the patients, predicted the time to development of Alzheimer's disease. UPSIT scores from 30 to 35 showed moderate

*Supported, in part, by Grants PO1 DC 00161, RO1 DC 04278, RO1 DC 02974, and RO1 AG 27496 from the National Institutes of Health, Bethesda, MD, USA (R.L. Doty, Principal Investigator).

to strong sensitivity and specificity for diagnosis of Alzheimer's disease at follow-up (grade B efficacy—level II).

The cause of the olfactory loss of most neurological diseases is generally unknown. An exception to this rule is multiple sclerosis (MS), where the olfactory loss is inversely and strongly correlated with the number of MS-related plaques within the subtemporal and subfrontal lobes—regions containing neurons involved in central olfactory processing (Figure 160.1A).[22,23] An analogous association is not present between the olfactory loss and plaque numbers in brain regions outside of these two areas (Figure 160.1B). Longitudinal studies have shown that olfactory function waxes and wanes over time in direct association with the number of active plaques in these target regions.[24]

Olfaction seems to be particularly influenced by aging or factors correlated with aging, with greater and earlier loss occurring in men than in women. Such decrements explain, at least in part, why a disproportionate number of elderly persons die from accidental gas poisoning,[25] and why many older persons report that their food lacks flavor.[26] While less than 2% of the American population under the age of 65 years is estimated to have meaningful olfactory loss,[26–28] approximately half of the population between the ages of 65 and 80 years has such loss; over the age of 80 years, three quarters of the population exhibits this problem.[26] The mechanisms responsible for age-related decrements are likely varied. In some cases, the smell loss may reflect impending neurological disease, such as Alzheimer's

disease, as noted earlier in this chapter. In other cases, such loss may simply be a reflection of cumulative damage to the olfactory epithelium from insults from viruses, bacteria, and exposure to airborne toxins.[29] Another cause of age-related olfactory loss appears to be sclerotic or ossification-related occlusion of the cribriform plate foramina through which the olfactory fila project.[30]

Although decreased "taste" perception during chewing and swallowing usually reflects attenuation of food flavor via retronasal olfactory stimulation (such sensations as chocolate, coffee, vanilla, steak sauce, pizza, cheese, etc., are mediated via cranial nerve I),[31] decrements in the taste-bud mediated sensations of sweet, sour, bitter and salty are also present in many elderly persons. Such losses are particularly evident when small regions of the tongue are evaluated.[32] Additionally, distortions of taste perception (dysgeusias) often occur in older persons and can be very debilitating and difficult to manage.[33] Such distortions, along with persistent and unpleasant phantom tastes, can arise from the use of various medications (e.g. antihypertensive and antibacterial agents),[34,35] poor oral hygiene, radiation therapy, and the presence of dissimilar metals in dental fillings and appliances, as well as from small infarcts in the brainstem and thalamus.

Aside from the major etiologies noted above, chemosensory dysfunction can arise from other sources, including congenital causes, intranasal and intracranial neoplasms (e.g. olfactory groove meningiomas, frontal lobe gliomas, paraoptic chiasma tumors, temporal lobe tumors), nutritional and meta-

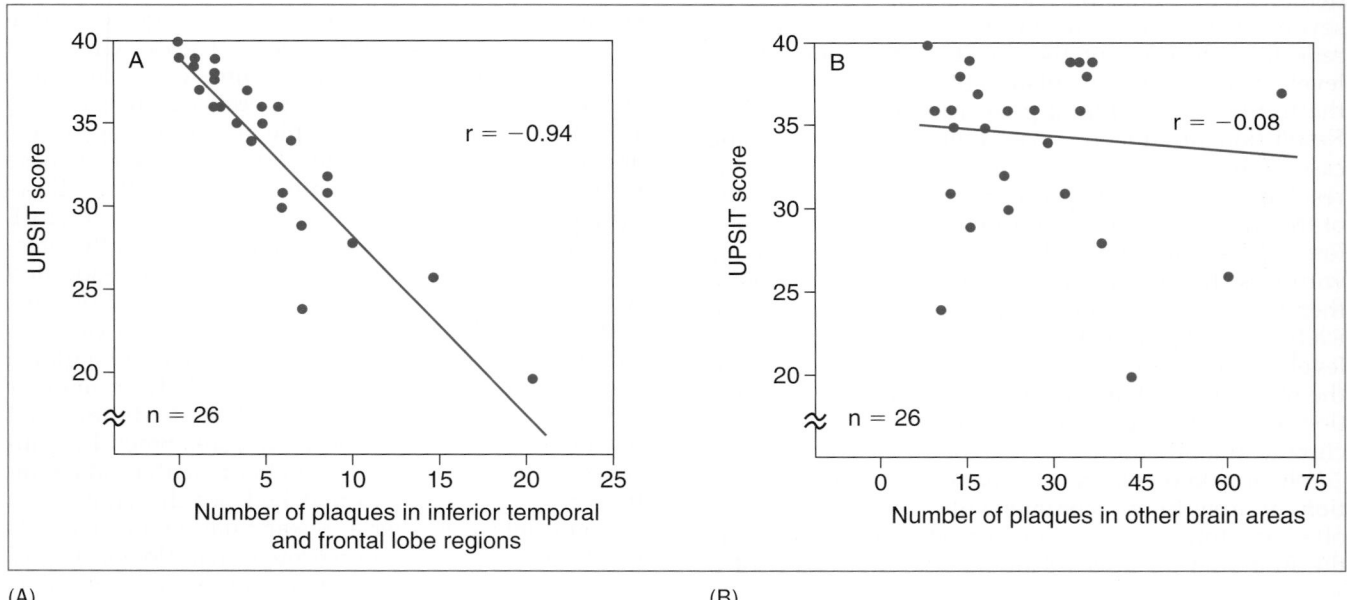

(A)   (B)

Figure 160.1   Relationship between the number of MS-related plaques found in olfactory (A) and non-olfactory (B) brain regions and scores on the University of Pennsylvania Smell Identification Test (UPSIT), a widely-used standardized test of olfactory function. r-value reflects the Spearman correlation coefficient.

From Doty et al.[19] Reprinted by permission from the New England Journal of Medicine. Copyright © 1997, The Massachusetts Medical Society.

bolic deficiencies (e.g. cirrhosis of the liver, thiamine deficiency), lesions or blockages of the nose and oral cavity (e.g. polyposis, hypertrophied adenoids), endocrine problems (e.g. Addison's disease, diabetes, Kallmann's syndrome, pseudohypoparathyroidism, hypothyroidism), iatrogenesis (e.g. damage to cranial nerve IX during tonsillectomy), radiation therapy, epilepsy, and hemodialysis, among others.

Diagnosis

Although many smell and taste problems reflect irreversible neurological damage, therapeutic intervention is possible in some cases. Before initiating therapeutic maneuvers, however, an accurate assessment of the problem is desirable using quantitative taste and smell tests, which are now commercially available.[36,37] Such testing allows the physician: (a) to verify or more definitively clarify the nature and degree of the condition (most taste problems are really smell problems; some patients exaggerate their dysfunction or are unaware of return of function); (b) to detect malingering; (c) to provide an objective basis for establishing insurance compensation; and (d) to help some patients, particularly older ones, to put into perspective their dysfunction relative to peers (e.g. as a result of the determination of a percentile score). The physician should be aware that many patients suffering from taste and smell disorders experience considerable depression which, in some cases, reflects not only the loss of a major sensory system, but a sense of alienation from peers and, in some cases, from members of the medical establishment, who often lack empathy and an understanding of the consequences of the condition.

Treatment

A reversal of a number of chemosensory problems is possible by treating medically or surgically (grade C, levels IV or V evidence of efficacy) an underlying medical condition (e.g. allergies, central tumors, oral disease or growths, rhinosinusitis, renal dysfunction, nutritional deficiencies, liver disease, hypothyroidism, or diabetes). In some patients, a brief course of systemic steroid therapy can be useful in distinguishing between conductive and sensorineural olfactory loss, as patients with the former will often respond positively to the treatment. Longer term systemic steroid therapy, however, is not advised. Topical nasal steroids may be ineffectual in altering smell dysfunction because the medication fails to penetrate the higher recesses of the nose. Administering nasal drops or sprays in the head-down Moffett's position can sometimes increase efficacy.

The majority of patients with dysosmia (parosmia) do not exhibit, upon careful testing, marked smell loss, implying a requirement for at least some degree of olfactory system function for the sensory expression. Although, as noted above, central nervous system lesions or tumors can produce dysosmic sensations, such cases are rare. More typically, dysosmias reflect dynamic changes within the olfactory epithelium proper and spontaneously remit over time.[4,38]

However, many dysgeusias are caused by medications (e.g. antibiotics and antihypertensive, antilipid and antifungal agents) and disappear or are greatly mitigated after drug discontinuance, dosage adjustment, or substitution. Such reversal can, however, take many weeks or months. In rare instances dysosmias can last for years and can be extremely debilitating. Surgical intervention is appropriate in some such cases, particularly those where daily function is markedly impaired, weight loss has occurred, and the quality of life has diminished to the point that suicide may be contemplated. Of the surgical approaches, intranasal ablation or stripping of tissue from the olfactory epithelium on the affected side is more conservative and less invasive than removal of the olfactory bulb and/or tract via a craniotomy.[39] Should the dysosmia reappear after intranasal intervention, additional or repeat ablations can be performed.

References

1. Doty RL. Introduction and historical perspective. In: Doty RL, ed. Handbook of Olfaction and Gustation. 1st edn. New York: Marcel Dekker, 1995:1–32
2. Jackson JH, Beevor CE. Case of tumour of the right temporo-sphenoidal lobe, bearing on the localization of the sense of smell and on the interpretation of a particular variety of epilepsy. Brain 1890;12:346
3. Jackson JH, Stewart P. Epileptic attacks with a warning of a crude sensation of smell and the intellectual aura (dreamy state) in a patient who had symptoms pointing to gross organic disease of the right temporo-sphenoidal lobe. Brain 1899;22:534–550
4. Deems DA, Doty RL, Settle RG, et al. Smell and taste disorders, a study of 750 patients from the University of Pennsylvania Smell and Taste Center. Arch Otolaryngol Head Neck Surg 1991;117:519–528
5. Costanzo RM, DiNardo LJ, Zasler ND. Head injury and olfaction. In: Doty RL, ed. Handbook of Olfaction and Gustation. New York: Marcel Dekker, 1995:493–502
6. Doty RL, Yousem DM, Pham LT, et al. Olfactory dysfunction in patients with head trauma. Arch Neurol 1997;54:1131–1140
7. Yousem DM, Geckle RJ, Bilker WB, et al. Posttraumatic smell loss: relationship of psychophysical tests and volumes of the olfactory bulbs and tracts and the temporal lobes. Acad Radiol 1999;6:264–272
8. Doty RL, Mishra A. Olfaction and its alteration by nasal obstruction, rhinitis, and rhinosinusitis. Laryngoscope 2001;111:409–423
9. Doty RL, Kobal G. Current trends in the measurement of olfactory function. In: Doty RL, ed. Handbook of Olfaction and Gustation. 1st edn. New York: Marcel Dekker, 1995:191–225
10. Mesholam RI, Moberg PJ, Mahr RN, Doty RL. Olfaction in neurodegenerative disease: a meta-analysis of olfactory functioning in Alzheimer's and Parkinson's diseases. Arch Neurol 1998;55:84–90
11. Doty RL. Olfactory dysfunction in neurogenerative disorders. In: Getchell TV, Doty RL, Bartoshuk LM, Snow JB Jr, eds. Smell and Taste in Health and Disease. New York: Raven Press, 1991:735–751
12. Moberg PJ, Doty RL, Turetsky BI, et al. Olfactory identification deficits in schizophrenia: correlation with duration of illness. Am J Psychiatry 1997;154:1016–1018
13. Doty RL, Bromley SM, Stern MB. Olfactory testing as an aid in the diagnosis of Parkinson's disease: development

of optimal discrimination criteria. Neurodegeneration 1995;4:93–97

14. Doty RL, Deems DA, Stellar S. Olfactory dysfunction in parkinsonism: a general deficit unrelated to neurologic signs, disease stage, or disease duration. Neurology 1988;38:1237–1244

15. Doty RL, Stern MB, Pfeiffer C, et al. Bilateral olfactory dysfunction in early stage treated and untreated idiopathic Parkinson's disease. J Neurol Neurosurg Psychiatry 1992;55:138–142

16. Doty RL, Golbe LI, McKeown DA, et al. Olfactory testing differentiates between progressive supranuclear palsy and idiopathic Parkinson's disease. Neurology 1993;43:962–965

17. Doty RL, Singh A, Tetrude J, Langston JW. Lack of olfactory dysfunction in MPTP-induced parkinsonism. Ann Neurol 1992;32:97–100

18. McCaffrey RJ, Duff K, Solomon GS. Olfactory dysfunction discriminates probable Alzheimer's dementia from major depression: A cross validation and extension. J Neuropsychiatry Clin Neurosci 2000;12:29–33

19. Solomon GS, Petrie WM, Hart JR, Brackin HB Jr. Olfactory dysfunction discriminates Alzheimer's dementia from major depression. J Neuropsychiatry Clin Neurosci 1998;10:64–67

20. Graves AB, Bowen JD, Rajaram L, et al. Impaired olfaction as a marker for cognitive decline: interaction with apolipoprotein E epsilon4 status. Neurology 1999;53:1480–1487

21. Devanand DP, Michaels-Marston KS, Liu X, et al. Olfactory deficits in patients with mild cognitive impairment predict Alzheimer's disease at follow-up. Am J Psychiatry 2000;157:1399–1405

22. Doty RL, Li C, Mannon LJ, Yousem DM. Olfactory dysfunction in multiple sclerosis: Relation to plaque load in inferior frontal and temporal lobes. Ann NY Acad Sci 1998;855:781–786

23. Doty RL, Li C, Mannon LJ, Yousem DM. Olfactory dysfunction in multiple sclerosis. N Engl J Med 1997;336:1918–1919

24. Doty RL, Li C, Mannon LJ, Yousem DM. Olfactory dysfunction in multiple sclerosis: relation to longitudinal changes in plaque numbers in central olfactory structures. Neurology 1999;53:880–882

25. Chalke HD, Dewhurst JR, Ward CW. Loss of smell in old people. Public Health 1958;72:223–230

26. Doty RL, Shaman P, Applebaum SL, et al. Smell identification ability: changes with age. Science 1984;226:1441–1443

27. Hoffman HJ, Ishii EK, Macturk RH. Age-related changes in the prevalence of smell/taste problems among the United States adult population. Results of the 1994 disability supplement to the National Health Interview Survey (NHIS). Ann NY Acad Sci 1998;855:716–722

28. Doty RL, Gregor T, Monroe C. Quantitative assessment of olfactory function in an industrial setting. J Occup Med 1986;28:457–460

29. Nakashima T, Kimmelman CP, Snow JB Jr. Structure of human fetal and adult olfactory neuroepithelium. Arch Otolaryngol 1984;110:641–646

30. Kalmey JK, Thewissen JG, Dluzen DE. Age-related size reduction of foramina in the cribriform plate. Anat Rec 1998;251:326–329

31. Burdach KJ, Doty RL. The effects of mouth movements, swallowing, and spitting on retronasal odor perception. Physiol Behav 1987;41:353–356

32. Matsuda T, Doty RL. Regional taste sensitivity to NaCl: relationship to subject age, tongue locus and area of stimulation. Chem Senses 1995;20:283–290

33. Cohen T, Gitman L. Oral complaints and taste perception in the elderly. J Gerontol 1959;14:294–298

34. Ackerman BH, Kasbekar N. Disturbances of taste and smell induced by drugs. Pharmacotherapy 1997;17:482–496

35. Frank ME, Hettinger TP, Mott AE. The sense of taste: neurobiology, aging, and medication effects. Crit Rev Oral Biol Med 1992;3:371–393

36. Doty RL. Olfaction. Annu Rev Psychol 2001;52:423–452

37. Frank ME, Smith DV. Electrogustometry: a simple way to test taste. In: Getchell TV, Doty RL, Bartoshuk LM, Snow JB Jr, eds. Smell and Taste in Health and Disease. New York: Raven Press, 1991:503–514

38. Deems DA, Yen DM, Kreshak A, Doty RL. Spontaneous resolution of dysgeusia. Arch Otolaryngol Head Neck Surg 1996;122:961–963

39. Leopold DA, Schwob JE, Youngentob SL, et al. Successful treatment of phantosmia with preservation of olfaction. Arch Otolaryngol Head Neck Surg 1991;117:1402–1406

161 Optic Neuropathies

Laura J Balcer and Steven L Galetta

Overview

Nonglaucomatous disorders of the optic nerve comprise many of the most frequently encountered clinical problems in neuro-ophthalmology. The diagnosis of optic neuropathy should generally be considered under the following circumstances: (1) visual loss in association with a swollen, pale, or anomalous optic disk; or (2) a normal disk appearance in the setting of vision loss (visual acuity, color vision, or visual field) combined with an afferent pupillary defect (APD).[1] This chapter will present a broad overview of the potential etiologies, pathophysiological mechanisms, clinical features, and appropriate diagnostic testing for patients with optic neuropathies. An approach to the patient based on optic disk appearance at presentation (swollen, pale, normal, or anomalous) will also be presented.[1] Particular emphasis will be placed on the clinical features and current treatment recommendations for several of the most common optic neuropathies encountered in neurological practice. The evaluation and treatment of papilledema (optic disk swelling caused by increased intracranial pressure) is discussed in Chapter 162.

Epidemiology of common optic neuropathies

Optic nerve dysfunction is frequently encountered in neurological and neuro-ophthalmological practice. The prevalence of various forms of optic neuropathy varies among patient populations with respect to age group and other demographic factors. For example, acute demyelinating optic neuritis affects primarily young patients (peak incidence in the 20s and 30s), and is more common among women.[1–3] The incidence of optic neuritis is highest among Caucasian populations of northern European ancestry, particularly those residing in areas away from the equator. Studies in the U.S. (Rochester, MN) have estimated the annual incidence rate for optic neuritis to be 6.4/100 000/year.[4] Optic neuritis may also occur in children, and the clinical profile of pediatric optic neuritis often differs from that seen in adults (including an increased likelihood of disk swelling and bilateral involvement).[5–7]

In contrast, among adults over the age of 50 years, nonarteritic anterior ischemic optic neuropathy (nonarteritic AION) represents the most common cause of unilateral optic neuropathy and disk swelling.[1,8] The annual incidence of nonarteritic AION has been estimated to be 2.3/100 000/year; NAION, like optic neuritis, is also more common among Caucasians.[1,8] Arteritic AION, which occurs in the setting of giant cell (temporal) arteritis, demonstrates an

increasing prevalence with age (1/1000 patients over the age of 80 years), and affects women more frequently than men (3:1).[1,9–12]

Leber's hereditary optic neuropathy (LHON) affects men predominantly (80% to 90% of patients are male).[13–16] This disorder is caused by mutations in mitochondrial DNA (mt DNA), and demonstrates a maternal inheritance pattern.[17,18] In one series[13] the mean age of onset of visual loss was 27.6 years, with most patients presenting between the ages of 26 and 37 years. The reason for the male predominance in this disorder is, however, unknown, and it remains of interest that women who develop LHON generally do so at an older age.[1]

The demographics of other forms of optic neuropathy are less well defined, although, as will be discussed in the next section on etiology, there are several etiological categories that must be considered for all patients with signs and symptoms of optic neuropathy, regardless of age or other demographic factors.

Etiologies for optic neuropathy

Potential etiologies for optic neuropathy are numerous, and fall into several broad categories:

- Inflammatory (e.g. idiopathic/demyelinating optic neuritis, sarcoidosis)
- Infectious (e.g. syphilis, Lyme disease)
- Ischemic (e.g. anterior/posterior ischemic optic neuropathy, giant cell arteritis)
- Infiltrative (e.g. optic nerve glioma, lymphoma, leukemia, metastatic tumor)
- Compressive (e.g. meningioma, pituitary adenoma, orbital tumors, thyroid eye disease)
- Toxic/nutritional (e.g. amiodarone toxicity, B$_{12}$ deficiency)
- Traumatic
- Hereditary (e.g. Leber's hereditary optic neuropathy, dominant optic atrophy)
- Congenital (e.g. optic disk anomalies—hypoplasia, drusen, coloboma, myopic tilting).

In addition to historical and demographic data, the diagnosis and determination of etiology for optic neuropathies may be aided by the presence or absence of other neuro-ophthalmological and systemic signs and symptoms. As discussed below in the section on classification, the optic disk appearance at presentation (swollen, pale, normal, or anomalous) is often an important factor in narrowing the list of potential etiologies and in determining initial treatment and evaluation.

Pathophysiology and pathogenesis: Optic nerve structure and function

A thorough knowledge of optic nerve anatomy and blood supply is necessary in order to understand the pathophysiology of optic neuropathies (Figures 161.1–161.3).[19–23] The optic nerve itself is composed of 1.2 million retinal ganglion cell axons.[1,24–26] These

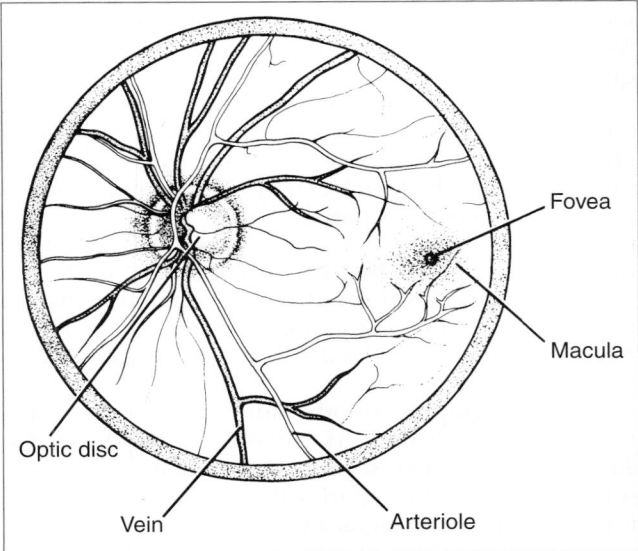

(A)

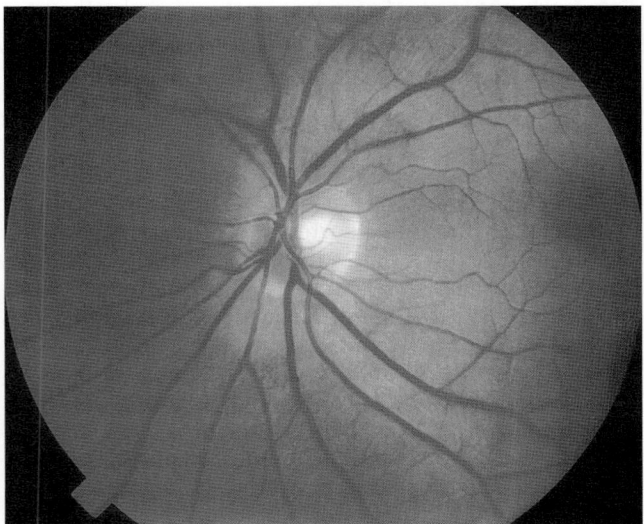

(B)

Figure 161.1   *A*, Diagram of normal left fundus demonstrating optic disk and macula. *B*, Color fundus photograph of normal left eye.
Part A from Liu GT. Disorders of the eyes and eyelids. *In*: Samuels MA, Feske S, eds. Office Practice of Neurology. 1st ed. New York: Churchill Livingstone, 1996:41, with permission. Parts A and B also from Balcer LJ. Anatomic review and topographic diagnosis. Neurosurg Clin North Am 1999;10:541–561, with permission. (See color plate section.)

axons travel through the optic nerves, chiasm, and optic tracts, eventually synapsing in the lateral geniculate body of the thalamus, the pretectum of the midbrain, the superior colliculus, the accessory optic nuclei, and the suprachiasmatic nuclei of the hypothalamus.[1] The optic nerve represents, therefore, a brain white matter tract. Unlike other cranial and peripheral nerves, the optic nerve is myelinated by oligodendrocytes beyond the lamina cribrosa, and does not regenerate.[1]

Within the optic canal, the optic nerve and its adjacent dura are fixed to the periosteum; this short segment of the optic nerve (10 mm in length) is thus vulnerable to traumatic injury and mass lesions within this tight space.[1] Intracranially, the optic nerves join to form the optic chiasm. The length of the intracranial optic nerve proximal to its junction with the chiasm is variable (4–15 mm), and is dependent upon the position of the optic chiasm with respect to the sella turcica (prefixed, postfixed, or directly above the sella).[1] The intracranial optic nerve courses upward toward the optic chiasm at a 45 degree angle. The internal carotid arteries lie just lateral to the intracranial optic nerves; the ophthalmic artery–internal carotid artery junction is located immediately below each optic nerve.

The blood supply to the retina and optic nerve originates primarily from the ophthalmic artery, the first major intracranial branch of the internal carotid artery. The inner two thirds of the retina is supplied by the central retinal artery (Figure 161.3).[19,21] This artery travels within the optic nerve for a short distance behind the disk, supplying intraorbital portions of the optic nerve, and then branches out to supply the four main quadrants of the retina (Figure 161.1).[19,23] The short and long posterior ciliary arteries are also branches of the ophthalmic artery. The long posterior ciliaries supply the ciliary body (responsible for lens accommodation), while the short posterior ciliary arteries provide the main blood supply to the optic nerve head and the outer one third of the retina. While the optic disk itself is supplied by a network fed mostly by the posterior ciliary arteries (anastomotic circle of Zinn–Haller), the portion of the optic nerve directly behind the lamina cribrosa (intraorbital optic nerve) is supplied by perforating branches of the ophthalmic artery. Capillaries feeding the intraorbital optic nerve are also supplied by branches from the central retinal artery (Figure 161.3).[1,19,21] Within the optic canal and intracranially, the pial plexus supplying the optic nerve is fed by branches of the internal carotid artery. The intracranial optic nerve may also receive circulation from branches of the anterior cerebral or anterior communicating arteries.[1]

The retinal ganglion cells, whose axons comprise the optic nerves, are maintained by the process of axonal transport. Disruption of axonal transport has been implicated as a mechanism for optic nerve damage in papilledema (optic disk swelling due to increased intracranial pressure),[26] optic nerve ischemia, compressive lesions, and inflammatory and toxic optic neuropathies.[27] Axonal transport within

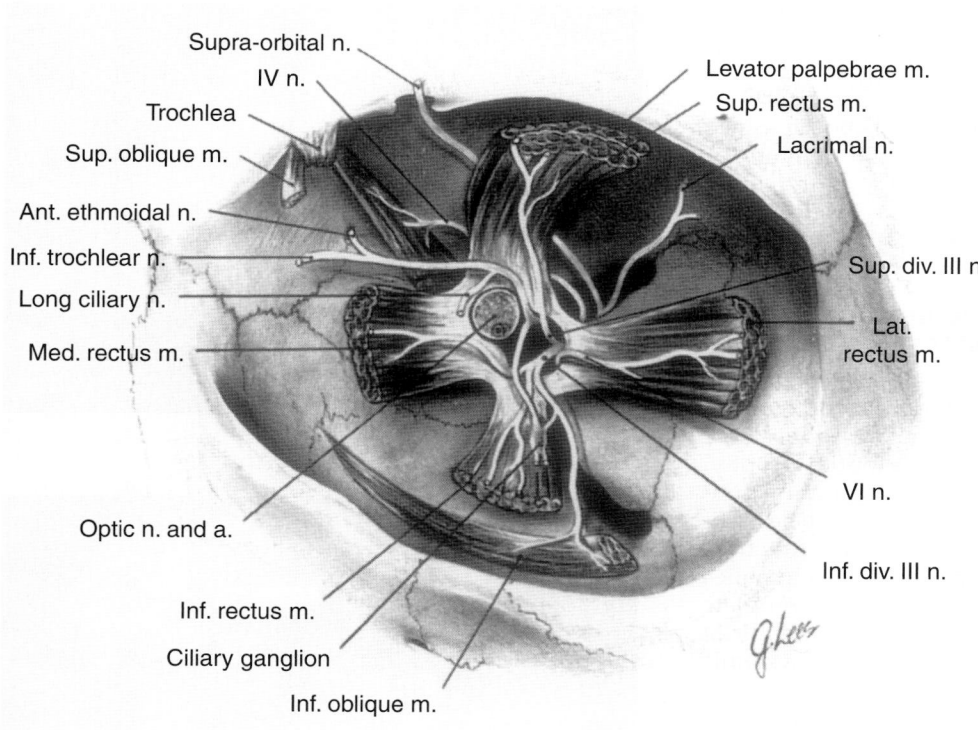

Supra-orbital n.
IV n.
Trochlea
Sup. oblique m.
Ant. ethmoidal n.
Inf. trochlear n.
Long ciliary n.
Med. rectus m.

Optic n. and a.
Inf. rectus m.
Ciliary ganglion
Inf. oblique m.

Levator palpebrae m.
Sup. rectus m.
Lacrimal n.

Sup. div. III n.
Lat. rectus m.

VI n.

Inf. div. III n.

Figure 161.2 View of the posterior orbit and orbital apex demonstrating relationships of the optic nerve, extraocular muscles, cranial nerves, and blood vessels. The tendon origins of the lateral, superior, inferior, and medial rectus muscles form a sheath, the annulus of Zinn, through which the optic nerve, third nerve, and sixth nerve pass at the orbital apex.

From Balcer LJ. Anatomic review and topographic diagnosis. Neurosurg Clin North Am 1999;10:541–561, and from Porter JD, Baker RS. Anatomy and embryology of the ocular motor system. *In:* Miller NR, Newman NJ, eds. Walsh and Hoyt's Clinical Neuro-Ophthalmology. 5th ed. Baltimore: Williams & Wilkins, 1998:1044, with permission. Adapted from Warwick R. Eugene Wolff's Anatomy of the Eye and Orbit. Philadelphia: WB Saunders, 1976, with permission.

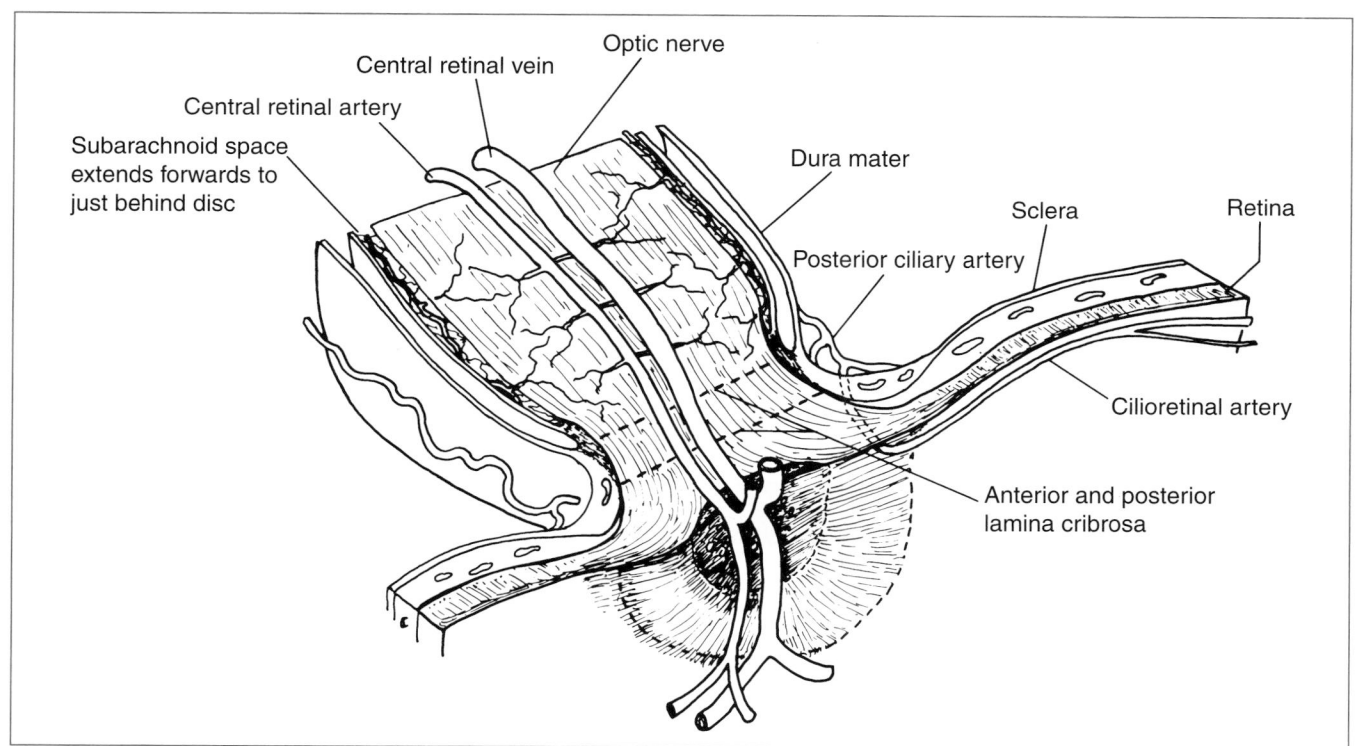

Central retinal vein
Central retinal artery
Subarachnoid space extends forwards to just behind disc

Optic nerve

Dura mater

Posterior ciliary artery

Sclera
Retina

Ciliary artery

Anterior and posterior lamina cribrosa

Figure 161.3 Diagram of the optic nerve demonstrating circulation to the optic nerve head (posterior ciliary arteries) and retina (central retinal artery).

From Patten J. Vision, the visual fields, and the olfactory nerve. *In:* Patten J. Neurological Differential Diagnosis. 2nd ed. Berlin: Springer-Verlag, 1996:23, with permission, and from Balcer LJ. Anatomic review and topographic diagnosis. Neurosurg Clin North Am 1999;10:541–561, with permission.

optic nerve axons occurs in two directions: (1) orthograde axonal transport, or movement away from the ganglion cell body and toward the lateral geniculate body; and (2) retrograde axonal transport, or movement toward the ganglion cell body. Since axonal transport is dependent upon the delivery of adequate energy and oxygen supply to the optic nerve, optic nerve dysfunction may be produced by any process that disrupts axonal transport, including ischemia, anoxia, or compression.

Genetics of hereditary optic neuropathies and congenital disc anomalies

The genetics of optic neuropathies are particularly relevant to discussions of mitochondrial optic neuropathies, certain forms of congenital optic disk anomalies, and hereditary forms of optic atrophy. Table 161.1 provides a list of the most common congenital optic disk anomalies, all of which may be associated with variable degrees of visual dysfunction. Visual loss in the setting of congenital disk anomalies may range from mild visual field loss to complete blindness. These anomalies are present from birth, and occasionally may be associated with systemic conditions, such as endocrine dysfunction or septo-optic dysplasia in the setting of optic nerve hypoplasia, or moyamoya disease in the setting of morning glory disk anomaly.[28-36] Congenital anomalies of the optic disk may be most important to recognize in children, who may develop strabismus or nystagmus as a first sign of visual dysfunction.

Optic disk drusen (Figure 161.4) are a form of pseudopapilledema, and the appearance of the optic nerve heads may be difficult to distinguish from true papilledema. The identification of pseudopapilledema due to optic nerve head drusen may be aided by the examination of first-degree relatives, who may have similar disk abnormalities. An autosomal dominant pattern of inheritance has been implicated. Antcliff and Spalton[37] recently conducted an analysis of the families of several patients with optic disk drusen to examine the prevalence of disk drusen and related optic disk anomalies. Among the relatives of patients with optic disk drusen examined in this study, only one (3.7%) had evidence of disk drusen. Other optic

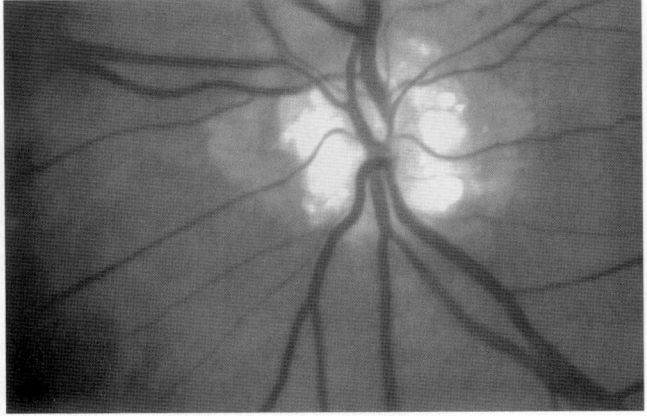

(A)

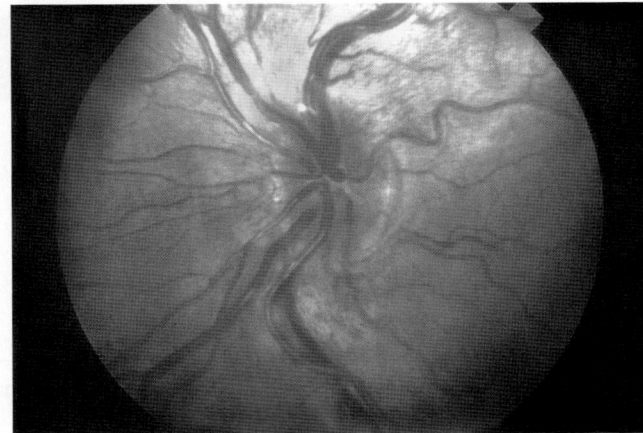

(B)

Figure 161.4 *A,* Color fundus photograph demonstrating optic disk drusen; note that the drusen have an appearance that resembles "rock candy." *B,* Optic disk photograph from a patient with Leber's hereditary optic neuropathy (LHON) demonstrating characteristic circumpapillary telangiectatic vessels and pseudoedema of the nerve fiber layer. (See color plate section.)
Photograph in part A courtesy of Dr Grant Liu.

disk anomalies, however, were common among family members, with 30/53 eyes (57%) demonstrating anomalous vessels, and 26/53 eyes (49%) containing no optic cup. While the low prevalence of optic disk drusen among relatives of affected patients is somewhat surprising, the authors[37] suggested that such patients may inherit a dysplasia of the optic disk and its blood supply. This abnormality may, in turn, predispose to the formation of optic disk drusen in some patients.

Despite the fact that many patients with optic disk drusen are asymptomatic, visual field defects may be found in up to 70% of patients.[38,39] Such visual loss is usually insidious, and often manifests as nerve fiber bundle defects on visual field testing. Rarely, acute visual loss involving central vision may occur secondary to superimposed ischemic optic neuropathy.

Table 161.1 Congenital optic disk anomalies
Optic nerve hypoplasia Myopic tilting Staphyloma Optic disk drusen Pseudopapilledema Optic disk colobomas Optic pits Morning glory disk anomaly
Adapted with permission from: Liu GT. Visual loss: optic neuropathies. *In:* Liu GT, Volpe NJ, Galetta SL, eds. Neuro-Ophthalmology: Diagnosis and Management. Philadelphia: WB Saunders, 2000.

Table 161.2   Common hereditary optic neuropathies

Ataxias
    Spinocerebellar degenerations (SCAs)
    Friedreich's ataxia
    Olivopontocerebellar atrophy
Leber's hereditary optic neuropathy (LHON)
Dominant optic atrophy
Recessive optic atrophy
Wolfram (DIDMOAD) syndrome

DIDMOAD; Diabetes Insipidus, Diabetes Mellitus, Optic Atrophy and Deafness.
Adapted with permission from: Liu GT. Visual loss: optic neuropathies. *In:* Liu GT, Volpe NJ, Galetta SL, eds. Neuro-Ophthalmology: Diagnosis and Management. Philadelphia: WB Saunders, 2000.

There is no established treatment for visual loss associated with optic disk drusen.[1]

Other forms of hereditary optic neuropathy produce optic disk pallor at initial presentation, or may be associated with pseudoedema of the nerve fiber layer (Figure 161.4B), as in Leber's hereditary optic neuropathy (LHON). These disorders are often accompanied by other neurological manifestations, particularly ataxia. Inheritance patterns for hereditary optic neuropathies may be spontaneous, dominant, recessive, or mitochondrial.[1] The diagnosis depends upon family history, clinical signs and symptoms, and, in some cases, specific genetic testing. Table 161.2 lists the most common hereditary forms of optic neuropathy. A detailed discussion of the clinical presentation, mitochondrial genetics, and potential treatment of LHON is provided in the section on treatment.

Clinical features of optic neuropathy

The history and neuro-ophthalmological examination are in many cases the most important elements used to identify potential etiologies for optic neuropathy. The clinical history is particularly important, and information should be sought from the patient and/or family regarding each of the following: (1) temporal profile of visual loss (sudden vs. insidious onset, episodic vs. constant presence of symptoms, time course of progression to maximal visual loss); (2) associated ocular and nonocular neurological symptoms (pain on eye movement, proptosis, redness, photophobia, headache, diplopia, anosmia, numbness, weakness, hearing loss); (3) symptoms of underlying systemic illness (infection, giant cell arteritis and other rheumatological disorders, vascular disease); and (4) family history of visual loss or degenerative neurological illness.[1]

Patients with optic neuropathy have a characteristic combination of visual acuity loss, color vision loss (dyschromatopsia), visual field defects, afferent pupillary defect (APD), and abnormal optic disk appearance (swollen, pale, or anomalous). Several of these features are often present on neuro-ophthalmological examination. Visual acuity loss in the setting of optic

neuropathies is highly variable, and likely represents the least sensitive indicator of optic nerve dysfunction. In fact, severe optic nerve dysfunction, manifested by dyschromatopsia, visual field loss, and an APD, may be present despite excellent (20/20 or better) visual acuity. Conversely, any level of visual acuity loss (ranging from none to severe) may be associated with virtually any cause of optic neuropathy.

Color vision loss is one of the most important and sensitive features of optic nerve dysfunction. Patients may have color vision defects measurable by color plate testing, or may have only subtle color desaturation when asked to compare a red object between the two eyes. Contrast sensitivity, or the threshold for detection of objects (such as letters) of varying shades of gray against a white background, is also often abnormal in patients with optic neuropathy. One of the most sensitive indicators of visual impairment in patients with optic neuritis and multiple sclerosis, contrast sensitivity is frequently abnormal in patients with visual acuities of 20/20 or better.[40–42]

Perhaps the most important localizing feature for optic nerve-related visual loss is the afferent pupillary defect (APD). Optic nerve dysfunction is the most common underlying cause for the APD; the APD is the hallmark of asymmetric disease of the pregeniculate afferent visual pathways.[1] A related clinical manifestation of optic neuropathy that may produce symptoms for the patient both during formal testing and daily activities is the Pulfrich phenomenon.[43] The Pulfrich phenomenon is a stereo illusion in which the to-and-fro motion of an object (pen or ball on string) in the plane perpendicular to the visual axis is perceived as an elliptical movement by the patient with unilateral optic neuropathy.[44,45] The elliptical movement of the object is perceived as counterclockwise if the right eye has optic nerve dysfunction, and clockwise if the left eye is affected. Patients may also report symptoms of the Pulfrich phenomenon when performing activities in which the motion of objects must be judged using stereopsis, such as driving or walking.[43] Since the Pulfrich phenomenon is only infrequently encountered in the setting of retinal disease or ocular media opacities, this sign is highly specific for unilateral or asymmetric optic nerve dysfunction.

Visual field testing frequently reveals abnormalities in patients with optic neuropathy. Such testing may be performed using computerized perimetry (static perimetry, in which stimuli are presented in single locations within the visual field) or Goldmann kinetic perimetry. Visual field defects indicative of optic nerve disease are variable, and most often include generalized constriction, enlargement of the blind spot, central and cecocentral scotomas, arcuate defects, and altitudinal defects (Figure 161.5).[1,19] Generalized constriction and blind spot enlargement are seen most often in patients with papilledema (discussed in Chapter 162), but are non-specific and may be present in patients with other causes of optic neuropathy, retinal disease, or media opacities.

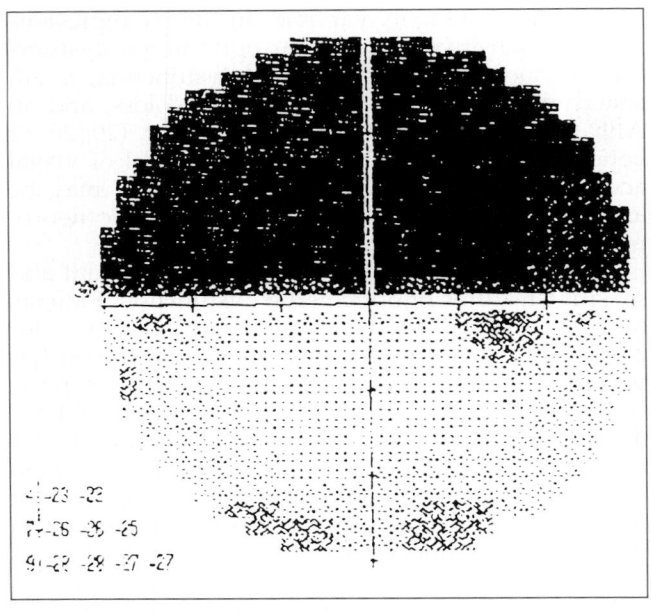

(A)

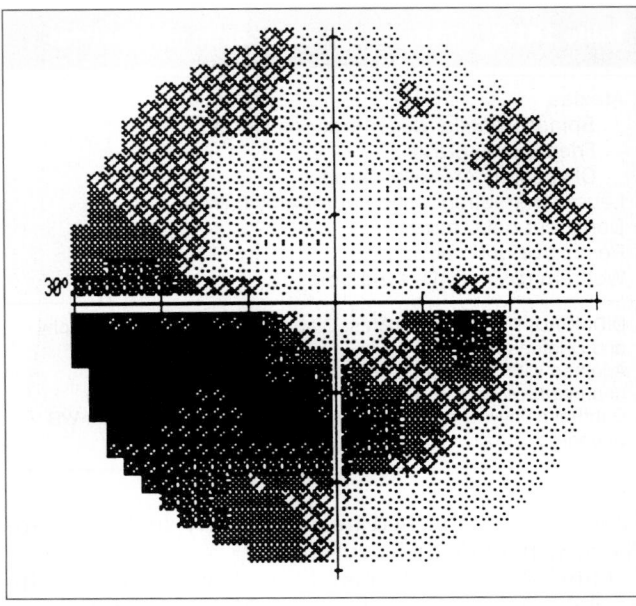

(B)

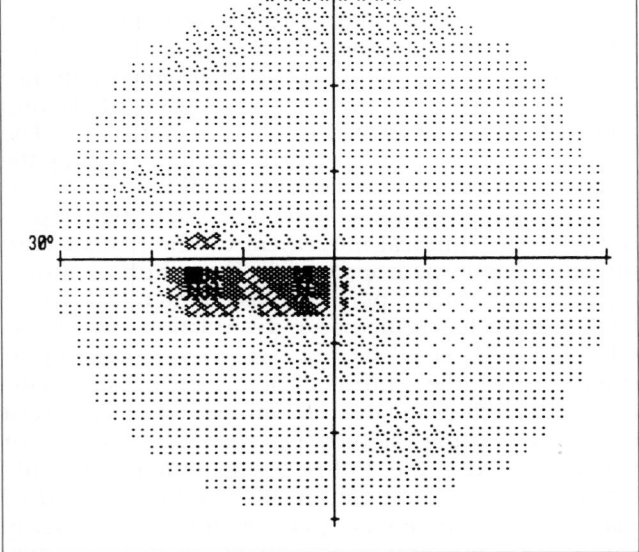

(C)

Figure 161.5   Common visual field defects for patients with optic neuropathy. *A,* Superior altitudinal visual field defect from patient with nonarteritic anterior ischemic optic neuropathy; note that this defect respects the horizontal meridian, a characteristic of optic nerve-related field defects. *B,* Arcuate defect with extension from the physiological blind spot. *C,* Cecocentral scotoma with involvement of both central vision and the physiological blind spot.

Part A from Balcer LJ. Anatomic review and topographic diagnosis. Neurosurg Clin North Am 1999;10:541–561, with permission. Parts B, C from Liu, GT. Visual loss: optic neuropathies. *In:* Liu GT, Galetta SL, Volpe NJ, eds. Neuro-Ophthalmology: Diagnosis and Management. Philadelphia: WB Saunders, 2000, with permission.

Ischemic, compressive, or inflammatory optic neuropathies, however, are often associated with altitudinal defects (Figure 161.5A), or arcuate defects (radiating from the blind spot but not involving an entire half of the visual field—Figure 161.5B). Central scotomas and cecocentral scotomas (Figure 161.5C) also occur in the setting of optic nerve dysfunction. Although certain patterns of visual field loss are commonly associated with particular causes of optic neuropathy (i.e. altitudinal defects in ischemic optic neuropathy, or central and cecocentral scotomas in toxic/nutritional optic neu-

ropathies), there is considerable overlap of field loss amongst the various optic neuropathies.

The funduscopic features and optic nerve appearance in patients with optic neuropathy are often useful for classifying optic neuropathies with regard to potential etiology (see below, classification). The optic nerve head in patients with unilateral or bilateral optic neuropathy may be swollen, or edematous (Figure 161.6). The funduscopic features of optic disk swelling include elevation of the optic nerve head, disk hyperemia, blurring of the disk margins, and edema of the nerve fiber layer. Other features may be

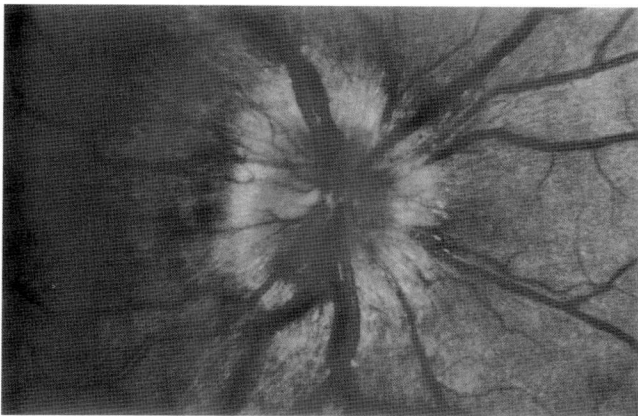

(A)

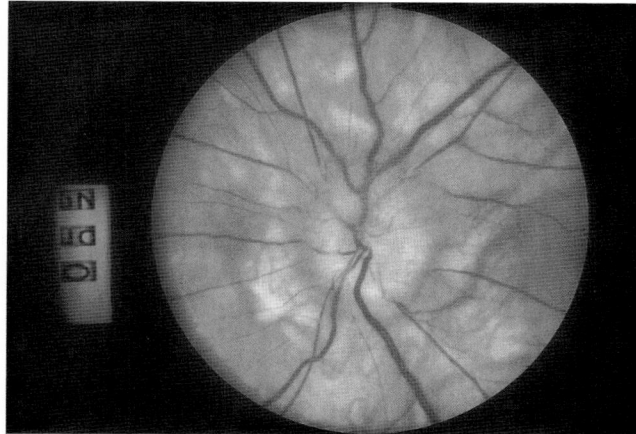

(B)

Figure 161.6   Optic disk swelling in optic neuritis and anterior ischemic optic neuropathy. *A*, Swollen optic disk of patient with acute demyelinating optic neuritis; disk swelling was present in 35% of patients in the Optic Neuritis Treatment Trial. *B*, Swollen optic disk of patient with nonarteritic anterior ischemic optic neuropathy (AION). (See color plate section.)
   Photograph in part A courtesy of Dr Nicholas J Volpe. Part B from Balcer LJ. Anatomic review and topographic diagnosis. Neurosurg Clin North Am 1999;10:541–561, with permission.

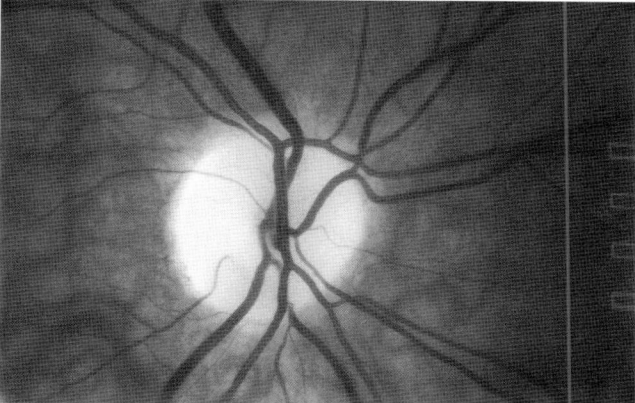

Figure 161.7   Optic disk pallor in a patient with a history of pituitary adenoma and bilateral optic neuropathies; pallor is most pronounced in the temporal region. (See color plate section.)

present, including venous distension, obliteration of the optic cup, peripapillary hemorrhages, exudates, and cotton wool spots. The presence or absence of certain features of disk swelling may be helpful in judging its chronicity (i.e. presence of hemorrhages in the setting of acute disk swelling), but are not diagnostic. Optic disk pallor, or optic atrophy, often accompanies optic neuropathies of a more chronic nature (Figure 161.7). Disk pallor is a sign of permanent optic nerve damage, and is characterized by a loss of the usual pink color of the optic nerve head. Both optic disk swelling and optic disk pallor may be diffuse (involving the entire disk) or segmental

(involving only part of the disk). For instance, segmental atrophy of one disk may be a clue to a prior ischemic optic neuropathy in the appropriate clinical situation. Optic atrophy may follow optic disk swelling (secondary optic atrophy), or may occur in the absence of significant swelling or gliosis (primary optic atrophy).

While optic disk swelling and optic disk pallor are common funduscopic features of optic neuropathy, patients with optic nerve dysfunction may have a normal disk appearance (most often in the setting of acute retrobulbar optic neuritis), or may have one of several congenital optic disk anomalies (Table 161.1).[1] Optic disk anomalies may be associated with visual loss and visual field defects.

Classification of optic neuropathies: Optic disk appearance at presentation

Optic disk appearance at presentation is one of the most important features that may be used to classify optic neuropathies, and to focus the list of most likely etiologies. Liu et al.[1] have suggested the following classification scheme based on optic disk appearance at presentation: (1) swollen optic disk(s); (2) pale optic disk(s); (3) normal optic disk(s); (4) anomalous optic disk(s). Table 161.3 presents a listing of various types of optic neuropathies that may manifest with a swollen, pale, or normal disk. A list of congenital anomalies, for which the disk appearance is characteristic, is included in Table 161.1.

In the setting of bilateral optic disk swelling, papilledema (disk swelling due to increased intracranial pressure) must be considered, and an intracranial mass lesion, venous sinus thrombosis, meningitis, hydrocephalus, or idiopathic intracranial hypertension must be excluded. Unlike optic neuropathies due to inflammatory, ischemic, compressive, or infiltrative causes, the visual loss that occurs in the setting of early papilledema is generally mild despite the degree of disk swelling (mismatch of degree of disk swelling and visual function). Preserved visual acuity

Table 161.3   **Classification of optic neuropathies based on optic disk appearance at presentation**

Swollen optic disk(s)	Pale optic disk(s)	Normal optic disk(s)
Idiopathic optic neuritis	Compressive	Idiopathic optic neuritis
AION	Toxic/nutritional (B_{12})	PION
Papilledema	Hereditary (dominant optic atrophy)	Compressive (early)
Diabetic papillopathy		Radiation-induced
Compressive (meningioma)		Traumatic
Inflammatory (sarcoid)		
Infectious (syphilis, Lyme)		
Infiltrative (glioma, lymphoma)		
Radiation-induced		
Toxic (amiodarone, methanol)		
Uveitis-associated optic neuropathy		
LHON (pseudoswollen appearance)		

AION, anterior ischemic optic neuropathy; PION, posterior ischemic optic neuropathy; LHON, Leber's hereditary optic neuropathy.
Adapted with permission from: Liu GT, Visual loss: optic neuropathies. *In:* Liu GT, Volpe NJ, Galetta SL, eds. Neuro-Ophthalmology: Diagnosis and Management. Philadelphia: WB Saunders, 2000.

in the setting of marked bilateral optic disk swelling is a hallmark of early papilledema. Enlarged blind spots and constriction on visual field testing are important characteristics that may help distinguish papilledema from other causes of optic neuropathy.

Among optic neuropathies that may manifest with unilateral disk swelling, the most common diagnoses to consider are optic neuritis (in younger patients) and anterior ischemic optic neuropathy (AION) (in older patients). The clinical features, evaluation, and treatment for optic neuritis and AION are discussed in detail in the section on treatment, below. Acute demyelinating optic neuritis, in fact, most often presents with a normal optic disk appearance (retrobulbar optic neuritis).[3] Other entities that may manifest acutely with a normal appearing optic disk, implying involvement of the retrobulbar portion of the optic nerve, are listed in Table 161.3. Optic disk pallor frequently also develops during the period following initial presentation, and thus may follow optic disk swelling or a previously normal optic disk appearance. Entities that commonly present with optic disk pallor are presented in Table 161.3. Such disorders are most frequently associated with a chronic, progressive course of visual loss, which may be insidious or attributed initially to other causes (such as need for new glasses).

Diagnostic criteria: Role for neuroimaging and laboratory testing

In addition to history and neuro-ophthalmological examination findings, the etiology of optic nerve dysfunction is often assisted by neuroimaging and laboratory testing. Table 161.4 presents a list of the diagnostic entities to consider in patients with clinical profiles that are atypical for acute demyelinating optic neuritis or anterior ischemic optic neuropathy. MR imaging has a critical role in the diagnosis of most optic neuropathies (especially those of compressive, inflammatory, or infiltrative origin), and is also

important in determining prognosis and appropriate treatment for acute demyelinating optic neuritis, see below.

Differential diagnosis: Other potential causes of visual loss

Visual dysfunction caused by optic neuropathy must be distinguished from retinal disease or other disorders of the eye or brain. In patients with bilateral visual loss, processes affecting the optic chiasm or other regions of the afferent visual pathways must be considered. Clinical features are often helpful in making these distinctions, including the presence or absence of visual acuity loss, color vision loss, or an afferent pupillary defect (APD). The fundus examination may be particularly important, not only in demonstrating evidence of optic nerve disease, but also in excluding the presence of visible retinal pathology. Dilated fundus examination should be performed, since particular funduscopic findings in the setting of optic disk swelling may raise suspicion for retinal processes. The combination of dilated, tortuous retinal veins and retinal hemorrhages away from the peripapillary region suggests a retinal vein occlusion (Figure 161.8A). Neuroretinitis, such as that caused by cat-scratch disease (*Bartonella henselae*), is suggested by the presence of macular lipid deposition (macular star) (Figure 161.8B). In the absence of optic disk swelling or pallor, visual loss due to a macular lesion, which may mimic optic neuropathy, must be excluded. Retinal infarction may have a clinical profile similar to optic neuropathy. However, characteristic retinal whitening on funduscopic examination (Figure 161.8C)[19] should readily distinguish these entities.

Visual field testing is especially helpful in localizing visual loss within the afferent visual pathways. Neuroimaging may also reveal structural lesions at the optic chiasm and elsewhere. In patients with otherwise unexplained visual loss, electroretinography

Table 161.4   Diagnostic considerations, laboratory evaluation, and distinguishing features for patients with clinical profiles that are atypical for acute demyelinating optic neuritis or anterior ischemic optic neuropathy

Diagnostic entity	Laboratory evaluation	Distinguishing features
Optic nerve compression	MRI brain and orbits w/gadolinium	Progressive loss of vision beyond 1–2 weeks
Carcinomatous meningitis	CSF cytology	Systemic tumor usually present
Syphilis	MHATP	Papillitis with hemorrhage
		Optic perineuritis, uveitis
Lyme disease	Serum Lyme titer	Residence in endemic area
		Erythema migrans rash
		Optic perineuritis
Sarcoidosis	Serum ACE level	Optic nerve granuloma
	Chest radiograph	Uveitis, retinal periphlebitis
Lupus	Serum ANA	Arthritis
	Double-stranded DNA antibodies	Antiphospholipid antibodies
Nutritional	Serum B$_{12}$ level	Progressive optic atrophy
		Pernicious anemia
		Ileum dysfunction
LHON	Mitochondrial DNA analysis	More common in males
		Pseudoedematous disk
		Telangiectasias

MRI, magnetic resonance imaging; CSF, cerebrospinal fluid; MHATP, microhemagglutinin treponema pallidum; ACE, angiotensin converting enzyme; ANA, antinuclear antibody; LHON, Leber's hereditary optic neuropathy.
Adapted with permission from: Liu GT, Visual loss: optic neuropathies. *In:* Liu GT, Volpe NJ, Galetta SL, eds. Neuro-Ophthalmology: Diagnosis and Management. Philadelphia: WB Saunders, 2000.

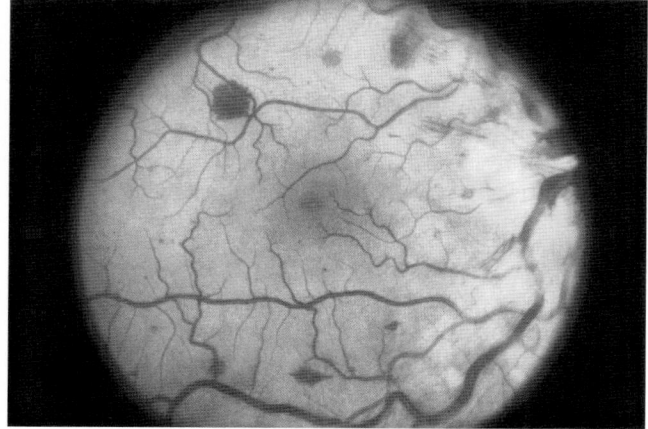

(A)

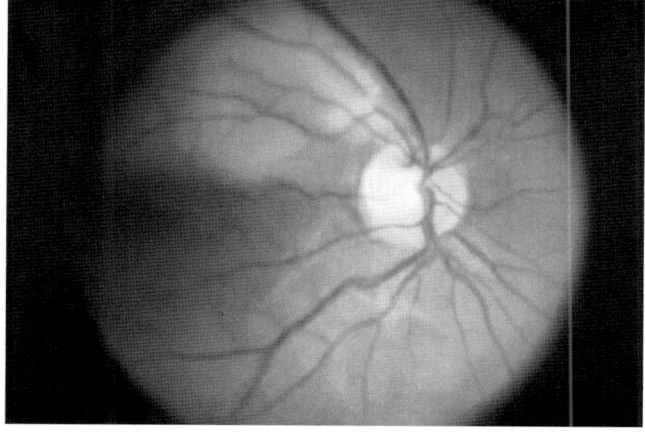

(C)

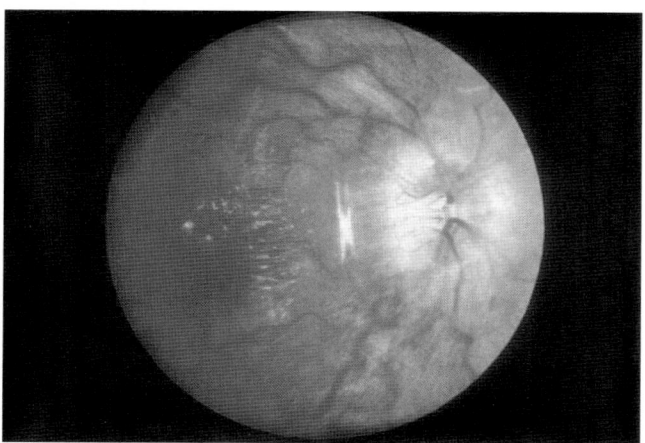

(B)

Figure 161.8 Retinal disorders that may have clinical signs and symptoms similar to optic neuropathy. *A,* Fundus photograph from patient with central retinal vein occlusion; note presence of swollen optic disk and retinal hemorrhages beyond the peripapillary region. *B,* Neuroretinitis with macular lipid exudates. *C,* Photograph from patient with branch retinal artery occlusion demonstrating retinal whitening superiorly, consistent with infarction. Note the presence of preserved reddish coloration in the superior area of the fovea, analogous to the macular "cherry-red spot." (See color plate section.)

Part C from Balcer LJ. Anatomic review and topographic diagnosis. Neurosurg Clin North Am 1999;10:541–561, with permission.

(ERG) may be useful in diagnosing paraneoplastic retinopathies, many of which are associated with optic disk pallor and retinal arteriolar attenuation. Slit lamp examination is important to exclude ocular causes of visual loss, including corneal opacities, keratoconus, cataract, uveitis, vitritis, and other processes. Refractive error as a cause of visual dysfunction may be suspected if blurring is present exclusively at near or distance, and if corrected by a pinhole device.

Treatment and clinical presentation of common optic neuropathies in neurological practice

The treatment of many inflammatory, infectious, and neoplastic or cancer-associated optic nerve disorders is often dictated by recommendations for treatment of the underlying systemic disease (i.e. sarcoidosis or syphilis). Such treatments are frequently undertaken by neurologists in conjunction with experts in other specialties. In contrast, patients with acute demyelinating optic neuritis, ischemic optic neuropathy, and hereditary optic neuropathies, including those of mitochondrial origin, often present to the neurologist primarily. In addition, because of their association with other neurological disorders (such as multiple sclerosis in the case of optic neuritis), these forms of optic neuropathy are also most frequently managed and treated by neurologists.

Optic neuritis

The term optic neuritis refers to inflammation of the optic nerve. Conditions that may be associated with acute or chronic optic neuritis are numerous, and include sarcoidosis and other inflammatory or autoimmune disorders (see etiologies, above). The treatment of optic neuritis in the setting of such systemic disorders is dictated by guidelines for appropriate treatment of the underlying inflammatory or autoimmune disorder itself.

The most common form of optic neuritis, and the type most familiar to neurologists, is acute demyelinating optic neuritis.[46] This form of optic neuritis most often occurs in the setting of multiple sclerosis (MS), either as a first symptom or in patients in whom the diagnosis of clinically definite or laboratory-supported definite MS[46] has been established. In the absence of signs or symptoms of MS or other systemic disease, optic neuritis may be referred to as idiopathic or monosymptomatic.[46] With the advent of new immunomodulatory therapies for MS, the recommendations for treatment of monosymptomatic optic neuritis in patients who are at high risk for the development of CDMS (more than two white matter lesions by brain MRI) continues to evolve.

Symptoms of optic neuritis   Patients with optic neuritis are typically young (aged 20–50 years), and are most commonly female[46] (see also epidemiologies, above). The most common symptoms of acute demyelinating optic neuritis are loss of central vision and ocular/periorbital pain.[1,46]

Although some of the most common signs and symptoms of acute optic neuritis, such as an afferent pupillary defect and visual field loss, were included as entry criteria for the Optic Neuritis Treatment Trial (ONTT),[3,41,46–61] the ONTT has provided important information about the clinical features of optic neuritis, including their relative frequencies. For example, loss of central visual acuity was reported by more than 90% of patients in the ONTT.[3] Such loss of vision is usually subacute, progressing over hours to days. In general, progression or worsening of visual loss or symptoms beyond a one-week period is considered atypical for acute demyelinating optic neuritis, and should prompt suspicion for an alternative cause for visual loss. Other forms of optic neuropathy should also be suspected if visual recovery does not occur within 2 to 4 weeks following the onset of symptoms.

Pain in or around the eye is also present in more than 90% of patients with acute demyelinating optic neuritis.[46] This pain may precede or occur concomitantly with visual loss, and is usually exacerbated by eye movement.[3] In typical cases of optic neuritis, the pain generally lasts no longer than a few days.[46] Among participants in the ONTT, ocular or periorbital pain was reported by 92%; 87% of these patients noted worsening of the pain by eye movement.[3,48]

Many patients with acute demyelinating optic neuritis note loss of peripheral vision or describe field defects. Such defects may be described as inferior, superior, temporal, or nasal, and may be reported by patients whose visual acuity is 20/20 or better.[40] Patients with optic neuritis may also describe color desaturation in the affected eye. During and even beyond the recovery of vision following acute optic neuritis, patients often experience a temporary worsening of symptoms with exposure to heat (hot shower or exercise). This is referred to as Uhthoff's symptom.[62,63] Patients with optic neuritis may also experience positive visual phenomena, consisting of flashing bright lights or photopsias in the affected eye.[3,48] These symptoms may be precipitated by eye movement or by sounds, and were reported by 30% of ONTT participants.[3,48]

Neuro-ophthalmological signs and clinical features of optic neuritis   Clinical signs and neuro-ophthalmological examination findings in acute demyelinating optic neuritis are those typical of optic nerve dysfunction. The visual profile of optic neuritis, like its clinical symptoms and natural history, has been established most definitively by the ONTT.[3] The ONTT enrolled 455 patients with acute unilateral optic neuritis. Patients were randomized to one of three treatment groups: (1) oral prednisone (1 mg/kg/day) for 14 days (oral prednisone group); (2) intravenous methylprednisolone sodium succinate (250 mg 4 times/day) for 3 days, followed by oral prednisone (1 mg/kg/day) for 11 days (IV methylprednisolone group); or (3) oral placebo for 14 days (placebo group).[48] Each steroid regimen was followed by an oral taper.

Visual function outcome measures were administered at baseline, at seven follow-up visits during the first 6 months, after 1 year, and then at yearly intervals. The primary measure of outcome was visual function at 6 months. The following measures were used to assess visual function: (1) visual acuity (retro-illuminated Bailey–Lovie chart at 4 meters); (2) color vision (Farnsworth–Munsell 100-hue test); (3) contrast sensitivity (Pelli–Robson chart); (4) visual field testing/perimetry (Humphrey Field Analyzer program 30-2, Goldmann perimeter). Detailed standard neurological examinations were also performed at baseline, 6 months, 1 year, and then on a yearly basis or when patients developed new symptoms. The purpose of these examinations was to assess for the development of clinically definite MS (CDMS—defined as new neurological symptoms attributable to demyelination in one or more regions of the CNS, other than new optic neuritis, confirmed by neurological exam, occurring at least 4 weeks after the initial episode of optic neuritis, and lasting at least 24 hours). The development of CDMS was a secondary end point for the ONTT.[53]

The ONTT confirmed that visual acuity is reduced, at least mildly, in most patients with acute demyelinating optic neuritis.[3,48] Baseline visual acuities in affected eyes ranged from 20/20 (11%) to no light perception (3%); most had visual acuities in the 20/25 to 20/190 range (54%).[3] Color vision is also almost always abnormal in patients with acute demyelinating optic neuritis, and is often more severely affected than visual acuity. In the ONTT, color vision using the Ishihara plates was abnormal in 88% of affected eyes. The Farnsworth–Munsell 100-hue test, a more sensitive test of color vision, was abnormal in 94% of affected eyes.[3] Visual field loss, which may be diffuse (48% of 415 ONTT patients tested) or focal (52%—nerve fiber bundle defects, central/cecocentral scotomas, hemianopic defects), is also common in acute optic neuritis.[64] Recent analyses of visual fields from the ONTT cohort[58–61] have indicated that, even among patients with apparently focal defects on Humphrey perimetry, there was also a superimposed generalized depression of the visual field, at least within the central 30 degrees. Reductions in contrast sensitivity were also present among both affected and fellow eyes of patients in the ONTT.[3] Much evidence indicates that contrast sensitivity is one of the most sensitive measures of afferent visual dysfunction in patients with optic neuritis and MS, and often demonstrates abnormalities even among patients with visual acuities of 20/20 or better.[40–42] In fact, contrast sensitivity (along with visual acuity) served as the primary visual outcome measure in the ONTT.[41,48] An afferent pupillary defect (APD) is usually always present in patients with acute unilateral optic neuritis; one notable exception may be patients with a history of optic neuritis in the fellow eye, or simultaneous fellow eye involvement.[46] Finally, the funduscopic appearance in patients with acute optic neuritis is characterized by disk swelling in 20% to 40% of cases (Figure 161.6A).[46] In the ONTT, 35% of patients were noted to have disk swelling.[3] Importantly, peripapil-

lary or disk hemorrhages were uncommon (6% of ONTT participants), and their presence should suggest an alternative diagnosis, such as AION.[46] In most patients with acute demyelinating optic neuritis, the optic disk appears normal (retrobulbar optic neuritis).

Diagnostic and prognostic studies for optic neuritis Diagnostic testing, including MRI, cerebrospinal fluid (CSF) studies, and serologic studies, is usually performed for the following reasons:[46] (1) to determine if the cause of the acute optic neuropathy is non-inflammatory (such as a compressive lesion); (2) to determine if the etiology for an inflammatory optic neuritis is one other than demyelination (such as sarcoidosis or other autoimmune disorder); (3) to determine the visual and neurological prognosis, particularly with respect to development of CDMS.

In patients with suspected optic neuritis, MRI scanning of the brain and orbits with fat suppression and gadolinium should be performed, even in typical cases, to confirm the diagnosis and to assess for the presence of other white matter lesions.[46] Gadolinium enhancement of the retrobulbar optic nerve is often present, as demonstrated in Figure 161.9. The ONTT demonstrated that the number of white matter lesions is highly predictive of the development of CDMS (Figure 161.10).[46,53] Follow-up of the ONTT cohort to 5 years and beyond has indicated that the presence of more than two white matter lesions was associated with a 51% risk of CDMS (at 5 years), while the risk was 37% for those with one or two white matter lesions, and only 16% if the MRI was normal (excluding optic nerve enhancement).[56] Continued follow-up of the ONTT cohort will determine the long-term value of MRI in predicting MS risk in patients with

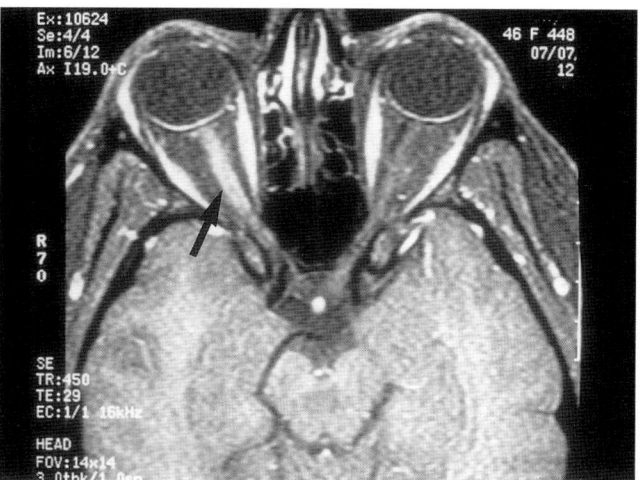

Figure 161.9 Axial T_1-weighted magnetic resonance (MR) image of the brain and orbits demonstrating gadolinium enhancement of the optic nerve (arrow) in a patient with acute demyelinating optic neuritis. This finding is also common in patients with other causes of inflammatory optic neuropathy, such as sarcoidosis.
Photograph courtesy of Dr Nicholas J Volpe.

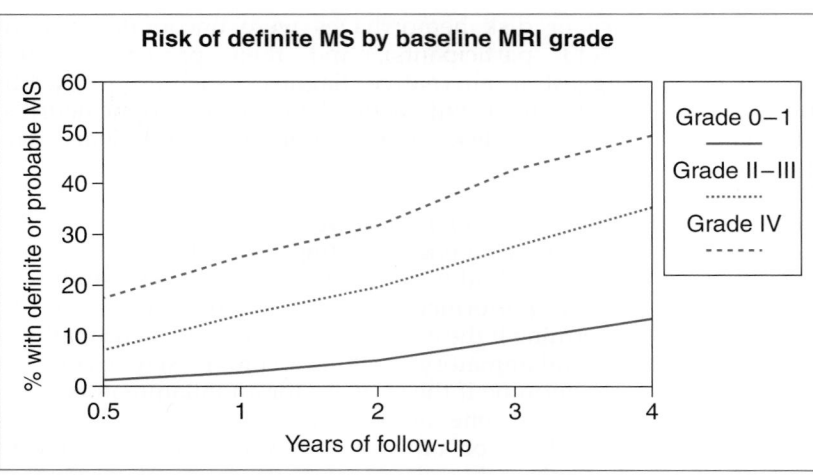

Figure 161.10   Graph showing cumulative incidence of development of multiple sclerosis (MS) correlated with magnetic resonance (MR) imaging of the brain in patients with acute isolated optic neuritis enrolled in the Optic Neuritis Treatment Trial and Longitudinal Optic Neuritis Study. Note that the risk of developing MS increases with increasingly abnormal MR imaging at the time of the episode of optic neuritis. Grade 0–I = 0–1 white matter lesions in brain; Grade II–III = 2–3 white matter lesions; Grade IV = >3 white matter lesions.

   From Beck RW. Optic neuritis. *In:* Miller NR, Newman NJ, eds. Walsh and Hoyt's Clinical Neuro-Ophthalmology. 5th ed. Baltimore: Williams & Wilkins, 1998:599–647, with permission.

acute optic neuritis. In patients with a clinical course that is atypical for demyelinating optic neuritis, MRI is important for identifying or excluding other potential etiologies for optic neuropathy, including compressive and other inflammatory lesions which may have characteristic MRI findings (such as meningeal enhancement in patients with sarcoid).

Cerebrospinal fluid (CSF) testing is again important most often in patients with an atypical clinical course for optic neuritis. The same is true for most serological studies, including antinuclear antibodies (ANA), Lyme titers, rapid plasma reagin (RPR), and microhemagglutinin treponema pallidum (MHATP) testing. One notable exception might be human leukocyte antigen (HLA) testing. Certain HLA antigens, such as HLA-DR2, have been associated with an increased likelihood of the development of clinically definite multiple sclerosis (CDMS) following acute demyelinating optic neuritis.[65,66] Such studies are generally unrevealing in patients with typical acute demyelinating optic neuritis. The CSF in patients with acute demyelinating optic neuritis often reveals a mild pleocytosis (>6 WBC/mm³—present in 36% of 131 ONTT participants who underwent lumbar puncture), mild protein elevation, elevated levels of myelin basic protein (18% of ONTT participants), and increased CSF/serum IgG ratio (22% of ONTT participants).[46] Recent studies have revealed CSF abnormalities in up to 79% of patients with acute optic neuritis, with oligoclonal bands present in approximately 69% of patients.[67] Söderström et al.[65] also found the presence of oligoclonal banding at presentation to be significantly associated with the development of CDMS in patients with acute optic neuritis ($P < 0.001$, Fisher's exact test). Life table analysis demonstrated that the probability of developing MS at 5 years was approximately 85% for those with three or more MRI lesions vs. 20% for those with none to two lesions. For patients with CSF oligoclonal bands, the 5-year probability of MS by life table analysis was 65% (vs. <10% for those without bands). Twenty-five percent of patients with either a positive MRI (three or more lesions) or CSF oligoclonal banding had been

diagnosed with MS by 6 months following the optic neuritis episode. Furthermore, the combination of a normal brain MRI and absent CSF oligoclonal bands had a negative predictive value of 100%; that is, none of these patients were diagnosed with MS within the 5-year follow-up period.

Treatment of optic neuritis   The ONTT is the most definitive study to date on the treatment of acute demyelinating optic neuritis.[3,41,46–61,68] Patients in the ONTT were randomized to one of three treatment groups as follows: (1) oral prednisone (1 mg/kg/day) for 14 days (oral prednisone group); (2) intravenous methylprednisolone sodium succinate (250 mg 4 times/day) for 3 days, followed by oral prednisone (1 mg/kg/day) for 11 days (IV methylprednisolone group); or (3) oral placebo for 14 days (placebo group).[48] Each steroid regimen was followed by an oral taper.[47,48]

The major findings, which dictate treatment of acute demyelinating optic neuritis to the present time, and have influenced clinical practice,[57] may be summarized as follows: (1) intravenous methylprednisolone hastened the recovery of visual function in acute optic neuritis, but did not affect visual outcome at 6 months or beyond compared to oral prednisone or placebo—this benefit for intravenous corticosteroids was greatest within the first 15 days of follow-up; (2) unexpectedly, patients treated with oral prednisone alone demonstrated an increased rate of recurrent attacks of optic neuritis in both the affected and fellow eyes compared with the IV methylprednisolone and placebo groups (Figure 161.11);[46,48] (3) patients in the IV methylprednisolone group had a reduced rate of development of CDMS during the first 2 years follow-up[53,56]—this benefit did not persist, however, at 3 years and beyond, and was only seen in patients who had significantly abnormal brain MRI (more than two lesions) at the time of acute optic neuritis. Patients in all three treatment groups had good visual recovery;[48] the median visual acuity in affected eyes at 6 months was 20/16. Fewer than 10% of patients in each group had a visual acuity of 20/50 or

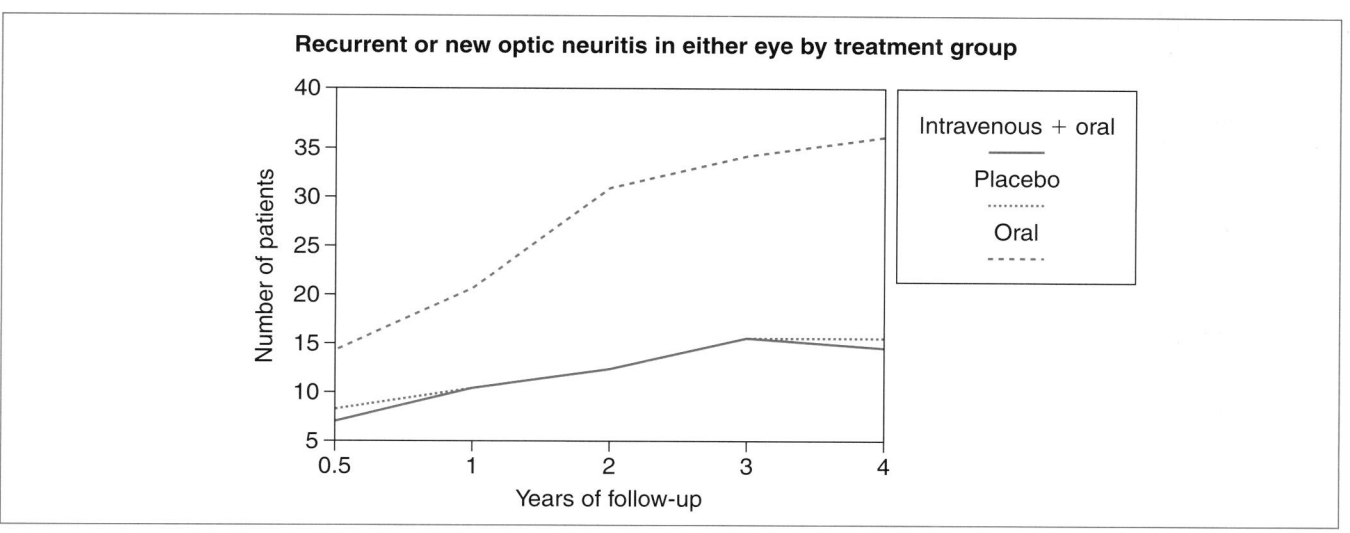

Figure 161.11   Graph showing incidence of recurrent attacks of optic neuritis in the previously affected eye and new attacks of optic neuritis in the fellow eye of patients enrolled in the Optic Neuritis Treatment Trial and Longitudinal Optic Neuritis Study by treatment groups. Note that patients who were treated with oral prednisone alone, at a dose of 1 mg/kg/day for 14 days, have had a much higher incidence of such attacks than have patients who were given oral placebo or patients who were treated with intravenous methylprednisolone at a dose of 250 mg every 6 hours for 3 days, followed by 11 day course of oral prednisone at a dose of 1 mg/kg/day.

From Beck RW. Optic neuritis. *In:* Miller NR, Newman NJ, eds. Walsh and Hoyt's Clinical Neuro-Ophthalmology. 5th ed. Baltimore: Williams & Wilkins, 1998:599–647, with permission.

worse. There were no significant differences between treatment groups at 1 year with respect to mean visual acuity, color vision, contrast sensitivity, or visual field (mean deviation).[54]

On the basis of these data, as emphasized by Beck,[46] there is no treatment for acute demyelinating optic neuritis that changes the long-term visual outcome or visual prognosis compared with placebo (natural history).[49,50,68] Intravenous methylprednisolone, followed by oral prednisone at doses given in the ONTT, may hasten the speed of visual recovery by 2 to 3 weeks when started within 1 to 2 weeks of the onset of symptoms.[48] Intravenous corticosteroids may also lessen the risk of CDMS within the first 2 years of follow-up in monosymptomatic patients, especially in those determined to be at high risk by MRI (more than two white matter lesions).[52] The decision to treat with IV methylprednisolone patients with acute monosymptomatic demyelinating optic neuritis is thus based upon the need or preference for hastening visual recovery (perhaps as dictated by the patient's occupation or circumstances), and the potential delay in MS development during the first 2 years. These potential benefits should be discussed with the patient, and weighed against the potential side effects of high-dose steroid therapy. Based on the increased incidence of recurrent optic neuritis observed in the affected and fellow eyes of ONTT participants who received oral prednisone, it is inappropriate to treat any patient with typical acute demyelinating optic neuritis with oral steroids alone at a 1 mg/kg/day dose.[53,56,68] It is possible that higher doses of oral steroids may be effective, but further studies are

needed.[69] A recent study[38] showed that treatment practices for acute optic neuritis have indeed been influenced by the results of the ONTT.

A small pilot study in 1992 suggested that intravenous immunoglobulin may have some benefit in patients with resolved optic neuritis who have significant visual deficits. However, use of this therapy awaits the publication of larger clinical trials.[70] In animal models, intravenous immunoglobulin has been demonstrated to promote remyelination of the CNS in experimental allergic encephalomyelitis and in Theiler's virus model of MS.[71,72]

Occasionally, the pain associated with acute demyelinating optic neuritis may be disabling. In this situation, a short course of nonsteroidal anti-inflammatory agents may be helpful. Likewise, intravenous corticosteroid treatment may rapidly ameliorate this symptom. During and even beyond the recovery of vision following acute optic neuritis, patients often experience a temporary worsening of symptoms with exposure to heat (hot shower or exercise). This is referred to as Uhthoff's phenomenon.[62,63] This symptom may be very difficult to treat, though limited success may be achieved by keeping the patient cool with an ice vest or by having them take a cold drink. We have had some success using gabapentin in one patient with very frequent episodes of Uhthoff's phenomenon. Sustained-release 4-aminopyridine improves motor conduction and performance of motor tasks in patients with MS, and may thus improve symptoms of temporary weakness or visual loss. Routine use of this medication, however, has been limited by toxicity.[73,74]

The most recent development in the treatment of acute monosymptomatic optic neuritis has been the results of the Controlled High-Risk Avonex Multiple Sclerosis Prevention Study (CHAMPS).[75] Given the high risk of the development of CDMS among patients with more than two MRI white matter lesions in the ONTT and other studies, a randomized, placebo-controlled trial was undertaken to test the effect of interferon beta-1a (IFN β-1a, 30 μg once per week) on the development of CDMS in patients with (1) monosymptomatic acute demyelinating optic neuritis, or (2) a first attack of demyelination in the brainstem, or (3) a first attack of demyelination in the spinal cord (incomplete myelopathy). To be eligible, patients also were required to have brain MRI findings consistent with a high risk for development of CDMS—two or more white matter lesions, 3 mm in diameter or larger, at least one lesion periventricular). This trial enrolled 383 patients between the ages of 18 and 50 years. All patients were initially given a short course of IV methylprednisolone, and were then randomized to receive IFN β-1a or placebo. The results of this study demonstrated that the 3-year probability of CDMS was significantly reduced for the IFN β-1a group vs. placebo (rate ratio 0.56, $P = 0.002$, Kaplan–Meier analysis/Mantel log-rank test).[75] Even more dramatic was the effect of IFN β-1a on the MRI scans of these patients. Those patients on active treatment had reduced number and volume of gadolinium enhancing lesions ($P < 0.0001$ at 18 months), reduced accumulation of new lesions on T_2-weighted images ($P < 0.0001$ at 18 months), and reduced T_2 lesion volume ($P = 0.0001$ at 18 months). The results of this important trial thus indicate that patients with acute monosymptomatic optic neuritis and other white matter lesions on MRI (more than two lesions) should be considered for treatment with IFN β-1a. Although the potential for long-term benefit is not yet known, results from the CHAMPS Study provide a rationale for early therapy in patients with a first demyelinating event and MRI findings suggesting a high risk for CDMS.

Anterior ischemic optic neuropathy

While optic neuritis typically occurs in younger patients (<50 years of age), and is characterized by pain on eye movement, anterior ischemic optic neuropathy (AION) is the most common cause of acute unilateral optic neuropathy in older patients. Although there is some overlap in the age distribution, symptom profile, and clinical characteristics of AION and optic neuritis, and both produce an optic neuropathy that is usually unilateral, there are some features that are suggestive of AION.

Symptoms of anterior ischemic optic neuropathy
Patients with AION have sudden visual loss due to optic nerve head ischemia. Microvascular occlusive disease of the posterior ciliary artery branches (Figure 161.3) has been implicated as a mechanism of AION, but this has not been confirmed pathologically.[1] AION may be nonarteritic, or may occur in the setting

of giant cell (temporal) arteritis (arteritic AION). In the patient with AION, the distinction between the arteritic and nonarteritic forms is often first made on the basis of clinical history and symptoms. This distinction has important implications for the treatment of AION, and is key to the prevention of second eye involvement and neurological complications from giant cell arteritis.

Patients with nonarteritic AION often experience painless, sudden loss of vision in one eye; these symptoms are frequently first noted upon awakening.[76] There are usually no premonitory symptoms, such as amaurosis fugax, in patients with nonarteritic AION; the presence of such symptoms should suggest giant cell arteritis. Other symptoms that should prompt suspicion for arteritic AION include headache (especially new headache in an elderly patient), scalp tenderness, jaw claudication, weight loss, myalgias, and arthralgias. Simultaneous or sequential involvement of both eyes is rare in the setting of nonarteritic AION, but is common in the arteritic form.

Neuro-ophthalmological signs of anterior ischemic optic neuropathy As the ONTT provided important data on the clinical features, visual profile, and natural history of optic neuritis, the Ischemic Optic Neuropathy Decompression Trial (IONDT) has provided similar information for nonarteritic AION.[76] This trial was designed to assess the efficacy and safety of optic nerve sheath decompression surgery (ONSD) vs. careful medical follow-up for nonarteritic AION. Performance of this study was inspired by observations that patients (12/14 in one study)[77] demonstrated improvement of visual function following ONSD, a surgical treatment that is often used for severe visual loss in the setting of idiopathic intracranial hypertension with severe visual loss. As discussed below (treatment of AION), the IONDT also provided invaluable information on the natural history of nonarteritic AION, particularly with respect to visual recovery. Baseline clinical features of patients enrolled in the IONDT (244 patients) are shown in Table 161.5.[76] Entry criteria included age over 50 years, and visual acuity of 20/64 or worse (retroilluminated Bailey–Lovie chart) in the affected eye.

As illustrated in Table 161.5, examination findings in nonarteritic AION include visual acuity loss (as severe as no light perception), dyschromatopsia, afferent pupillary defect (APD), and visual field loss (most commonly inferior altitudinal defects as shown in Figure 161.5).[1,76,78] Patients have optic disk swelling that is characterized by a pallid appearance, splinter hemorrhages, and sectoral disk involvement (Figure 161.6B). The fellow eye optic disk is often crowded and cupless, an anatomical feature which has been demonstrated to be a risk factor for nonarteritic AION (Figure 161.6C).[79]

Clinical features which would suggest arteritic AION include temporal artery tenderness, bilateral ocular involvement, and evidence of central or branch retinal artery occlusion (macular cherry-red spot or

Table 161.5   Ischemic Optic Neuropathy Decompression Trial (IONDT)—Patient characteristics at randomization

Patient characteristics	Careful follow-up group Number (%), N = 122	Surgery group Number (%), N = 115
Age (years)		
50–59	19 (15.6)	17 (14.8)
60–69	49 (40.2)	53 (56.1)
70–79	42 (34.4)	34 (29.6)
80–89	12 (9.8)	11 (9.6)
≥90	0	0
Sex—female	52 (42.6)	50 (43.5)
Hypertension	63 (52.1)	54 (47.0)
Diabetes	39 (32.2)	21 (18.3)
Visual acuity (Snellen equivalent)		
20/64 → 20/100	23 (19.3)	28 (24.6)
20/100 → 20/200	16 (13.5)	26 (22.8)
20/200 → 20/800	42 (35.3)	27 (23.7)
20/800 → count fingers (CF)	13 (10.9)	10 (8.8)
CF—no light perception	25 (21.0)	23 (20.2)

Adapted with permission from: The Ischemic Optic Neuropathy Decompression Trial Research Group. Optic nerve decompression surgery for nonarteritic anterior ischemic optic neuropathy (NAION) is not effective and may be harmful. JAMA 1995;273:625–632.

retinal whitening; Figure 161.8). Elderly patients who have sudden visual loss and a normal optic disk appearance may also have posterior ischemic optic neuropathy. This is most often caused by giant cell arteritis, and such patients should undergo appropriate treatment (corticosteroids) and evaluation. While AION is the most common etiology of visual loss in patients with giant cell arteritis (88% of 63 patients in one series),[80] posterior ischemic optic neuropathy, central/branch retinal artery occlusion, and choroidal ischemia are also features of giant cell arteritis that are not present in patients with nonarteritic AION.

Diagnostic studies for anterior ischemic optic neuropathy   In patients with suspected AION, the most important roles for diagnostic testing include the following: (1) exclusion of other causes of optic disk swelling, such as compressive, inflammatory, or infiltrative lesions (see etiology, above, and Table 161.4), which may mimic typical AION; and (2) evaluation for possible giant cell (temporal) arteritis. Thus, while MRI is not particularly useful in the diagnosis of AION, it may be important in some cases to exclude an alternative etiology for optic neuropathy.[1] MRI may also demonstrate evidence for small-vessel ischemic disease in the white matter, a feature that is likely reflective of the presence of vasculopathic risk factors in patients with NAION.[81] Patients with arteritic AION may also demonstrate optic nerve enhancement on MR imaging.[82] Fluorescein angiography, which when carefully timed may demonstrate delayed optic nerve head filling, may be helpful in distinguishing AION disk swelling from other causes.[1] Choroidal filling defects on fluorescein angiography suggest giant cell arteritis.

The identification of giant cell arteritis in patients with AION is perhaps the most important aspect of

diagnostic testing. As emphasized by Liu,[1] patients with giant cell arteritis can be identified by any combination of the following factors: (1) age over 50 years; (2) typical fundus appearance—"chalky white" disk edema and/or retinal infarctions and cotton wool spots; (3) systemic symptoms—headache, jaw claudication, scalp tenderness, myalgias, arthralgias, weight loss; (4) elevated ESR (erythrocyte sedimentation rate); (5) positive temporal artery biopsy; (6) elevated C-reactive protein; (7) abnormal fluorescein angiography. In the absence of systemic symptoms (occult giant cell arteritis), the ESR is usually elevated.[80] Conversely, in patients with a normal ESR and AION or other ophthalmic manifestations, systemic symptoms are almost always present in the setting of giant cell arteritis. Therefore, visual loss due to giant cell arteritis rarely occurs in the absence of both systemic symptoms and elevated ESR and/or C-reactive protein.[1]

Treatment of anterior ischemic optic neuropathy

Nonarteritic AION   There is no known effective treatment for nonarteritic AION. Unlike acute optic neuritis, for which corticosteroids may hasten visual recovery, no such benefit has been demonstrated for nonarteritic AION.[1,48] Although optic nerve sheath decompression surgery (ONSD) initially appeared to improve vision in some patients with progressive visual loss and nonarteritic AION, these findings were not supported by other series.[77,83,84]

The IONDT ultimately demonstrated, however, that ONSD does not improve visual outcome in the setting of nonarteritic AION, and may be potentially harmful.[76] Patients in the IONDT who received ONSD actually had a lower rate of visual recovery, and a higher rate of visual loss (loss of three or more lines of visual acuity on the ETDRS chart).[76] Patients assigned to the surgical group in the IONDT thus did no better

Table 161.6   Ischemic Optic Neuropathy Decompression Trial (IONDT)—Association between follow-up visual acuity and treatment group, all participants

	No. pts.	Follow-up Visual Acuity			Relative Risk (95% CI)	
		≥3 Lines Better (%)	Little Change (%)	≥3 Lines Worse (%)	≥3 Lines Better	≥3 Lines Worse
3 months						
Follow-up	109	39.5	53.2	7.3	0.69 (0.47–1.02)	2.51 (1.19–5.30)
Surgery	103	27.2	54.4	18.5	$P = 0.06$	$P = 0.02$
6 months						
Follow-up	89	42.7	44.9	12.4	0.76 (0.52–1.12)	1.94 (1.02–3.69)
Surgery	92	32.6	43.5	23.9	$P = 0.16$	$P = 0.04$
12 months						
Follow-up	51	41.2	51.0	7.8	0.71 (0.42–1.22)	3.25 (1.23–8.58)
Surgery	51	29.4	45.1	25.5	$P = 0.22$	$P = 0.02$

Adapted with permission from: The Ischemic Optic Neuropathy Decompression Trial Research Group. Optic nerve decompression surgery for nonarteritic anterior ischemic optic neuropathy (NAION) is not effective and may be harmful. JAMA 1995;273:625–632.

than patients who received careful follow-up alone.[76] At 6 months following enrolment, 32.6% of patients in the surgical group demonstrated three or more lines improvement in visual acuity, compared with 42.7% in the follow-up group (Table 161.6).[76] Furthermore, at 3, 6, and 12 months following enrolment, the risk of visual loss (three or more lines worsening of visual acuity) was significantly greater for patients who received ONSD. Such visual loss was observed in 12.4% of the follow-up group vs. 3.9% of the surgical group (relative risk 1.94, $P = 0.04$).

Despite the observation that ONSD is ineffective and potentially harmful in the setting of nonarteritic AION, one of the most important findings of the IONDT was the demonstration that the natural history of nonarteritic AION is often marked by improvement of vision. At 3, 6, and 12 months, 40% of patients in the careful follow-up group demonstrated improvement of visual acuity by three or more lines over their acuity at enrolment. The IONDT, therefore, demonstrated that patients with nonarteritic AION may, in fact, show improvement of vision; this is in contrast to the fixed deficit and static course that have long been thought to represent the natural history for most patients with nonarteritic AION.

While the recurrence of nonarteritic AION in affected eyes is extremely rare, the lifetime risk of second eye involvement is 30% to 40%.[85] Studies of the use of aspirin for prophylaxis of second eye involvement in nonarteritic AION have not demonstrated definitive evidence for efficacy.[86,87] However, the use of 325 mg of aspirin per day, if tolerated, is often suggested since patients with nonarteritic AION frequently have other vasculopathic risk factors.[88]

Arteritic AION When AION is accompanied by systemic signs or symptoms of giant cell arteritis, elevated ESR and/or C-reactive protein, or suggestive ocular signs, immediate therapy with high-dose corticosteroids is recommended. The primary goal in such patients is the prevention of second eye involvement and neurological complications. As emphasized by Liu,[1] evidence from retrospective studies and case series have suggested the following: (1) corticosteroids may retard the progression of visual loss; (2) corticosteroids may diminish the risk of fellow eye involvement; (3) on occasion (15% to 34% of patients) steroids may restore some vision; (4) intravenous steroids may be more effective than oral steroids in protecting the fellow eye and in enhancing visual prognosis, both due to higher dosing and greater bioavailability.[1,80,89–91]

Therefore, for patients with AION or other visual loss in whom giant cell arteritis is suspected, we recommend the following: (1) immediate initiation of intravenous corticosteroid therapy (methylprednisolone 250 mg 4 times/day); (2) temporal artery biopsy to confirm the diagnosis.[1] Corticosteroid therapy should not be delayed while awaiting temporal artery biopsy. Histopathological evidence of arteritis may be seen beyond one week following the start of steroid treatment.[92] In fact, positive temporal artery biopsies, with chronic changes consistent with arteritis, may be obtained for months and even years beyond the initiation of corticosteroids.[80,93–96] Since dramatic recovery of vision is rare once vision is lost in patients with ischemic optic neuropathy or central retinal artery occlusion and giant cell arteritis, the importance of immediate corticosteroid treatment in protecting the fellow eye cannot be overemphasized.[80,97,98]

Despite prompt treatment with high-dose intravenous corticosteroids, however, some patients with giant cell arteritis may demonstrate continued progression or new onset of visual loss or neurological manifestations, including spinal cord infarction.[80,89,96–102] Symptoms and signs in such patients may be related to a decrease in blood flow to the ocular or vertebral artery circulations.[96,102–104] Galetta et al.[96,102] recently reported two patients with giant cell arteritis who presented with unusual flow-related ophthalmic and brainstem signs. One patient stabilized with the combination of intravenous heparin and hydration. Although the optimal treatment for patients with giant cell arteritis and flow-related symptoms remains uncertain, intravenous hydration and anticoagulation may be considered for selected patients.

Giant cell arteritis has a self-limited course that may last for several months, but more commonly lasts 1 to 2 years or longer.[105] Treatment with corticosteroids for this duration, however, may result in significant side effects.[106] The search for effective alternatives to steroids for giant cell arteritis has thus far been of limited success.[97] Nonsteroidal anti-inflammatory drugs and cytotoxic agents have not been demonstrated to be effective when used alone or in combination with corticosteroids.[107,108] A controlled trial of methotrexate in conjunction with systemic corticosteroids, however, is in progress.[97]

Leber's hereditary optic neuropathy

Leber's hereditary optic neuropathy (LHON) is a genetic optic neuropathy which usually causes subacute, sequential visual loss.[1,13–16,18,109] Although LHON most commonly affects young men, the age of onset may vary substantially even within families. Women are thought to be affected less commonly than men, although this has recently been questioned. LHON is caused by point mutations at specific locations in the mitochondrial genome, giving rise to a maternal inheritance pattern. However, the relatively high penetrance in males is best explained by genetic modifying factors on the X chromosome.[1,109,110] Alternatively, this variable penetrance may be related to sex linked environmental factors.

Symptoms of LHON Patients with LHON experience loss of central vision. This may vary in severity, although visual acuities worse than 5/200 are not typical for LHON. Although headache occasionally occurs, visual loss in LHON is usually painless.[1,109] Uhthoff's symptom (worsening of vision in the setting of heat exposure) has also been reported.[13] Visual dysfunction most commonly occurs over weeks to months in patients with LHON. Visual loss is often unilateral initially, but second eye involvement may occur simultaneously (55% of cases) or within weeks to months.[13]

Neuro-ophthalmological signs of LHON Signs of acute optic neuropathy, with loss of central vision and dyschromatopsia, are the most common presenting features of LHON.[1] Visual acuities typically range between 20/200 and 5/200, but are rarely reduced to hand motions or worse.[1,109] Visual field testing reveals dense central or cecocentral defects. Recent studies have demonstrated that, as in patients with other forms of optic neuropathy, afferent pupillary defects are noted in patients with asymmetric visual loss and LHON.[111,112] On fundus examination, circumpapillary telangiectatic vessels are present (Figure 161.4B), and create an appearance of pseudoedema in the nerve

fiber layer. Fluorescein angiography may reveal an absence of staining of the optic disk.[113] Later in the course of LHON (and in some patients at presentation), the vascular features may not be present and the fundus may display only optic atrophy.

In some patients, partial visual recovery has been well documented clinically, but the mechanism of this remains unclear.[114] When more sensitive measures of visual function are used, visual recovery (at a subclinical level) may be noted in higher proportions of patients (up to one third).[115] The association of LHON with mitochondrial dysfunction has suggested that other features of mitochondrial illness may be present in affected patients. These include cardiac conduction abnormalities, peripheral neuropathy, skeletal deformities, and CNS manifestations, such as dystonia.[13,113–119] White matter abnormalities have been demonstrated by MR imaging in association with LHON and a multiple sclerosis-like syndrome.[13,116,120] In one patient with the 11778 mutation, LHON has been associated with basal ganglia degeneration.[121] Mutations of guanine to adenine at base 13513 appear to cause a syndrome of optic neuropathy followed by a MELAS-like syndrome.[122]

Diagnostic studies and genetic testing for LHON Genetic testing for specific mitochondrial mutations is crucial to the diagnosis of LHON, and may also be used to identify individuals at risk for this disorder.[1] There are three primary mutations for LHON (11778, 14484, and 3460), and many secondary mutations. In addition, distinct mitochondrial mutations appear to be associated with slightly different clinical courses. The highest rate of visual recovery has been noted in patients harboring the 14484 mutation, while this recovery rate is lowest for those with mutations at 11778.[1] Although MRI scanning may reveal white matter abnormalities,[116] cerebrospinal fluid analysis, electroretinography, and visual evoked potential testing are not particularly helpful in the diagnosis of LHON.[1,16]

Treatment of LHON and other mitochondrial disorders At present, no therapy has been shown to prevent the onset of LHON or to enhance recovery. However, the presence of mitochondrial mutations in this disorder has created an interest in the use of agents that enhance mitochondrial function. Coenzyme Q and its synthetic analog, idebenone, are capable of reversing the abnormal muscle spectroscopy findings seen in mitochondrial disorders.[123–126] However, a clear effect on visual function has yet to be demonstrated. In two patients with mitochondrial disease, neurological manifestations, and optic neuropathy, administration of coenzyme Q reversed the CNS symptoms and MRI findings, but had no effect on visual outcome.[127,128] One of these two patients carried the 11178 mutation, the most common mutation seen in LHON. Therefore the treatment of symptomatic patients with coenzyme Q and its analogs has an anecdotal basis for use in LHON. Since coenzyme Q is available on a nonprescription basis and has no known side effects, it is frequently self-administered by patents with LHON and other mitochondrial disorders. This factor may complicate the design of potential clinical trials of these agents in LHON.

Another important aspect of therapy in LHON is the prevention of symptom onset in patients at risk. Many individuals who carry LHON mutations never develop clinically evident visual dysfunction. This suggests a potential role for environmental factors in the development of visual loss in LHON. For example, Dotti et al.[129] reported a patient who harbored the 11778 mutation and developed an optic neuropathy following ethambutol exposure. This suggests that toxic exposure may increase the likelihood of developing optic neuropathy in individuals with LHON mutations. Similarly, in one large series,[130] patients harboring the 11178 mutation were more likely to develop visual dysfunction if they were also cigarette smokers, again suggesting that risk factor modification may be one mechanism of preventing visual loss in at-risk patients.

References

1. Liu GT. Visual loss: optic neuropathies. *In:* Liu GT, Volpe NJ, Galetta SL, eds. Neuro-Ophthalmology: Diagnosis and Management. Philadelphia: WB Saunders, 2001
2. Wray SH. Optic neuritis. *In:* Albert DM, Jakobiec FA, eds. Principles and Practice of Ophthalmology. Philadelphia: WB Saunders, 1994:2539–2568
3. Optic Neuritis Study Group. The clinical profile of optic neuritis: experience of the Optic Neuritis Treatment Trial. Arch Ophthalmol 1991;109:1673–1678
4. Percy AK, Nobrega FT, Kurland LT. Optic neuritis and multiple sclerosis: an epidemiologic study. Arch Ophthalmol 1972;87:135–139
5. Kriss A, Francis DA, Cuendet B. Recovery of optic neuritis in childhood. J Neurol Neurosurg Psychiatry 1988;51:1253–1258
6. Kennedy C, Carroll FD. Optic neuritis in children. Arch Ophthalmol 1960;63:747–755
7. Riikonen R, Donner M, Erkkila H. Optic neuritis in children and its relationship to multiple sclerosis: a clinical study of 21 children. Dev Med Child Neurol 1988;30:349–359
8. Johnson LN, Arnold AC. Incidence of nonarteritic and arteritic anterior ischemic optic neuropathy: population-based study in the state of Missouri and Los Angeles County, California. J Neuroophthalmol 1994;14:38–44
9. Biller J, Asconape J, Weinblatt ME, et al. Temporal arteritis associated with a normal sedimentation rate. JAMA 1982;247:486–487
10. Bengtsson B-A, Malmvall B-E. The epidemiology of giant cell arteritis including temporal arteritis and polymyalgia rheumatica: incidences of different clinical presentations and eye complications. Arthritis Rheum 1981;24:899–904
11. Hauser WA, Ferguson RH, Holley KE, et al. Temporal arteritis in Rochester, Minnesota, 1951 to 1967. Mayo Clin Proc 1971;46:597–602
12. Huston KA, Hunder GG, Lie JT, et al. Temporal arteritis: a 25-year epidemiologic, clinical, and pathologic study. Ann Intern Med 1978;88:162–167
13. Newman NJ, Lott MT, Wallace DC. The clinical characteristics of pedigrees of Leber's hereditary optic neuropathy with the 11778 mutation. Am J Ophthalmol 1991;111:750–762
14. Nikoskelainen E, Hoyt WF, Nummelin K. Ophthalmoscopic findings in Leber's hereditary optic neuropathy: I. Fundus findings in asymptomatic family members. Arch Ophthalmol 1982;100:1597–1602
15. Nikoskelainen EK, Savontaus ML, Wanne OP. Leber's hereditary optic neuroretinopathy, a maternally inherited disease: a genealogical study in four pedigrees. Arch Ophthalmol 1987;105:665–671
16. Carroll WM, Mastaglia FL. Leber's optic neuropathy: a clinical and visual evoked potential study of affected and asymptomatic members of a six generation family. Brain 1979;102:559–580
17. Singh G, Lott MT, Wallace DC. A mitochondrial DNA mutation as a cause of Leber's hereditary optic neuropathy. N Engl J Med 1989;320:1300–1305
18. Wallace DC, Singh G, Lott MT, et al. Mitochondrial DNA mutation associated with Leber's hereditary optic neuropathy. Science 1988;242:1427–1430
19. Balcer LJ. Anatomic review and topographic diagnosis. Neurosurg Clin North Am 1999;10:541–561
20. Porter JD, Baker RS. Anatomy and embryology of the ocular motor system. *In:* Miller NR, Newman NJ, eds. Walsh and Hoyt's Clinical Neuro-Ophthalmology. 5th ed. Baltimore: Williams & Wilkins, 1998:1044
21. Patten J. Neurological Differential Diagnosis. 2nd ed. Berlin: Springer-Verlag, 1996:23
22. Warwick R. Eugene Wolff's Anatomy of the Eye and Orbit. Philadelphia: WB Saunders, 1976
23. Liu GT. Disorders of the eyes and eyelids. *In:* Samuels MA, Feske S, eds. Office Practice of Neurology. 1st ed. New York: Churchill Livingstone, 1996
24. Kupfer C, Chumbley L, Downer JC. Quantitative histology of optic nerve, optic tract, and lateral geniculate nucleus of man. J Anat 1967;101:393–401
25. Potts AM, Hodges D, Sherman CB, et al. Morphology of the primate optic nerve: I–III. Invest Ophthalmol Vis Sci 1972;11:980–1016
26. Minckler DS, Tso MO. Experimental papilledema produced by cyclocryotherapy. Am J Ophthalmol 1976;82:577–589
27. Morrison JC. Anatomy and physiology of the optic nerve. *In:* Kline LB, ed. Optic Nerve Disorders. San Francisco: American Academy of Ophthalmology and Palace Press, 1996:1–20
28. Hoyt CS, Good WV. Do we really understand the difference between optic nerve hypoplasia and optic atrophy? Eye 1992;6:201–204
29. Hoyt WF, Kaplan SK, Grumbach MM, et al. Septooptic dysplasia and pituitary dwarfism. Lancet 1970;1:893–894
30. Margalith D, Tze WJ, Jan JE. Congenital optic nerve hypoplasia with hypothalamic-pituitary dysplasia. Am J Dis Child 1985;139:361–366
31. Costin G, Murphee AL. Hypothalamic-pituitary function in children with optic nerve hypoplasia. Am J Dis Child 1985;139:249–254
32. Siatkowski RM, Sanchez JC, Andrade R, et al. The clinical, neuroradiologic, and endocrinologic profile of patients with bilateral optic nerve hypoplasia. Ophthalmology 1997;104:493–496
33. Hanson RR, Price RL, Rothner AD, et al. Developmental anomalies of the optic disc and carotid circulation: a new association. J Clin Neuroophthalmol 1985;5:3–8

34. Massaro M, Thorarensen O, Liu GT, et al. Morning glory disc anomaly and moyamoya vessels. Arch Ophthalmol 1998;116:253–254

35. Bakri SJ, Siker D, Masaryk T, et al. Ocular malformations, moyamoya disease, and midline cranial defects: a distinct syndrome. Am J Ophthalmol 1999;127:356–357

36. Goldhammer Y, Smith JL. Optic nerve anomalies in basal encephalocele. Arch Ophthalmol 1975;93:115–118

37. Antcliff RJ, Spalton DJ. Are optic disc drusen inherited? Ophthalmology 1999;106:1278–1281

38. Lorentzen SE. Drusen of the optic disc: a clinical and genetic study. Acta Ophthalmol 1966(Suppl 90):1–180

39. Savino PJ, Glaser JS, Rosenberg MA. A clinical analysis of pseudopapilledema. II: visual field defects. Arch Ophthalmol 1979;97:71–75

40. Kupersmith MJ, Nelson JI, Seiple WH, et al. The 20/20 eye in multiple sclerosis. Neurology 1983;33:1015–1020

41. Trobe JD, Beck RW, Moke PS, Cleary PA. Contrast sensitivity and other vision tests in the Optic Neuritis Treatment Trial. Am J Ophthalmol 1996;121:547–553

42. Balcer LJ, Baier ML, Pelak VS, et al. New low-contrast vision charts: reliability and test characteristics in patients with multiple sclerosis. Multiple Sclerosis 2000;6:163–171

43. Diaper CJM, Dutton GN, Heron G. The Pulfrich phenomenon: its symptoms and their management. J Neuroophthalmol 1999;12:12

44. Diaper CJM. Pulfrich revisited. Surv Ophthalmol 1997;41:493–499

45. Mojon DS, Rosler KM, Oetliker H. A bedside test to determine motion stereopsis using the Pulfrich phenomenon. Ophthalmology 1998;105:1337–1344

46. Beck RW. Optic neuritis. In: Miller NR, Newman NJ, eds. Walsh and Hoyt's Clinical Neuro-Ophthalmology. 5th ed. Baltimore: Williams & Wilkins, 1998:599–647

47. Beck RW. Optic Neuritis Study Group, The Optic Neuritis Treatment Trial. Arch Ophthalmol 1988;106:1051–1053

48. Beck RW, Cleary PA, Anderson MM Jr, et al. A randomized, controlled trial of corticosteroids in the treatment of acute optic neuritis. N Engl J Med 1992;326:581–588

49. Beck RW. Optic Neuritis Study Group, The Optic Neuritis Treatment Trial: implications for clinical practice. Arch Ophthalmol 1992;110:331–332

50. Beck RW. Optic Neuritis Study Group, Corticosteroid treatment of optic neuritis: a need to change treatment practices. Neurology 1992;42:1133–1135

51. Beck RW, Kupersmith MJ, Cleary PA, et al. Fellow eye abnormalities in acute unilateral optic neuritis: experience of the Optic Neuritis Treatment Trial. Ophthalmology 1993;100:691–698

52. Beck RW, Arrington J, Murtagh FR, et al. Brain MRI in acute optic neuritis: experience of the Optic Neuritis Study Group. Arch Neurol 1993;8:841–846

53. Beck RW, Cleary PA, Trobe JD, et al. The effect of corticosteroids for acute optic neuritis on the subsequent development of multiple sclerosis. N Engl J Med 1993;329:1764–1769

54. Beck RW, Cleary PA. Optic Neuritis Study Group, Optic Neuritis Treatment Trial: one-year follow-up results. Arch Ophthalmol 1993;111:773–775

55. Beck RW, Cleary PA, Backlund J, et al. The course of visual recovery after optic neuritis: experience of the Optic Neuritis Treatment Trial. Ophthalmology 1994;101:1771–1778

56. Optic Neuritis Study Group. The 5-year risk of MS after optic neuritis: experience of the Optic Neuritis Treatment Trial. Neurology 1997;47:1404–1413

57. Trobe JD, Sieving PC, Guire KE, Fendrick AM. The impact of the Optic Neuritis Treatment Trial on the practices of ophthalmologists and neurologists. Ophthalmology 1999;106:2047–2053

58. Keltner JL, Johnson CA, Spurr JO, Beck RW, for the Optic Neuritis Study Group. Comparison of central and peripheral visual field properties in the Optic Neuritis Treatment Trial. Am J Ophthalmol 1999;128:543–553

59. Fang JP, Donahue SP, Lin RH. Global visual field involvement in acute unilateral optic neuritis. Am J Ophthalmol 1999;128:554–565

60. Fang JP, Lin RH, Donahue SP. Recovery of visual field function in the Optic Neuritis Treatment Trial. Am J Ophthalmol 1999;128:566–572

61. Arnold AC. Visual field defects in the Optic Neuritis Treatment Trial: central vs. peripheral, focal vs. global. Am J Ophthalmol 1999;128:632–634

62. Parkin PJ, Hierons R, McDonald WI. Bilateral optic neuritis: a long term follow-up. Brain 1984;107:951–964

63. Scholl GB, Song HS, Wray SH. Uhthoff's symptom in optic neuritis: relationship to magnetic resonance imaging and development of multiple sclerosis. Ann Neurol 1991;30:180–184

64. Keltner JL, Johnson CA, Spurr JO, et al. Baseline visual field profile of optic neuritis: the experience of the Optic Neuritis Treatment Trial. Arch Ophthalmol 1993;111:231–234

65. Söderström M, Ya-Ping J, Hillert J, Link H. Optic neuritis: prognosis for multiple sclerosis from MRI, CSF, and HLA findings. Neurology 1998;50:708–714

66. Frederiksen JL, Madsen HO, Ryder LP, et al. HLA typing in acute optic neuritis: relation to multiple sclerosis and magnetic resonance imaging findings. Arch Neurol 1996;54:76–80

67. Frederiksen JL, Larsson HBW, Oleon J. Correlation of magnetic resonance imaging and CSF findings in patients with acute monosymptomatic optic neuritis. Acta Neurol Scand 1992;86:317–322

68. The Optic Neuritis Study Group. Visual function 5 years after optic neuritis: experience of the Optic Neuritis Treatment Trial. Arch Ophthalmol 1997;115:1545–1552

69. Sellebjerg F, Nielsen HS, Frederiksen JL, et al. A randomized, controlled trial of oral high-dose methylprednisolone in acute optic neuritis. Neurology 1999;52:1479–1484

70. van Engelen BGM, Hommes OR, Pinkers A, et al. Improved vision after intravenous immunoglobulin in stable demyelinating optic neuritis (letter). Ann Neurol 1992;32:834–835

71. Raine CS, Hintzen R, Traugott U, et al. Oligodendrocyte proliferation and enhanced CNS remyelination after therapeutic manipulation of chronic relapsing EAE. Ann NY Acad Sci 1988;540:712–714

72. van Engelen BGM, Miller DJ, Pavelko KD, et al. Promotion of remyelination by polyclonal immunoglobulin and IVIg in Theiler's virus induced demyelination and in MS. J Neurol Neurosurg Psychiatry 1994;57(Suppl):65–68

73. Schwid SR, Petrie MD, McDermott MP, et al. Quantitative assessment of sustained-release 4-aminopyridine for symptomatic treatment of multiple sclerosis. Neurology 1997;48:817–821

74. Fujihara K, Miyoshi T. The effects of 4-aminopyridine

on motor evoked potentials in multiple sclerosis. J Neurol Sci 1998;159:102–106

75. Jacobs LD, Beck RW, Simon JH, et al. Intramuscular interferon beta-1a therapy initiated during a first demyelinating event in multiple sclerosis. N Engl J Med 2000;343:898–904

76. Ischemic Optic Neuropathy Decompression Trial Research Group. Optic nerve decompression surgery for nonarteritic anterior ischemic optic neuropathy (NAION) is not effective and may be harmful. JAMA 1995;273:625–632

77. Sergott RC, Cohen MS, Bosley TM, Savino PJ. Optic nerve decompression may improve the progressive form of nonarteritic ischemic optic neuropathy. Arch Ophthalmol 1989;107:1743–1754

78. Rizzo JF, Lessell S. Optic neuritis and ischemic optic neuropathy: overlapping clinical profiles. Arch Ophthalmol 1991;100:1668–1672

79. Beck RW, Servais GE, Hayreh SS. Anterior ischemic optic neuropathy. IX. Cup-to-disc ratio and its role in pathogenesis. Ophthalmology 1987;94:1502–1508

80. Liu GT, Glaser JS, Schatz NJ, et al. Visual morbidity in giant cell arteritis: clinical characteristics and prognosis for vision. Ophthalmology 1994;101:1779–1785

81. Arnold AC, Hepler RS, Hamilton DR, et al. Magnetic resonance imaging of the brain in nonarteritic ischemic optic neuropathy. J Neuroophthalmol 1995;15:158–160

82. Lee AG, Eggenberger ER, Kaufman DI, Manrique C. Optic nerve enhancement on magnetic resonance imaging in arteritic ischemic optic neuropathy. J Neuroophthalmol 1999;19:235–237

83. Glaser JS, Temory M, Schatz NJ. Optic nerve sheath fenestration for progressive ischemic optic neuropathy: results in a second series consisting of 21 eyes. Arch Ophthalmol 1994;112:1047–1050

84. Yee RD, Selky AK, Purvin VA. Outcomes of optic nerve sheath decompression for nonartertic ischemic optic neuropathy. J Neuroophthalmol 1994;14:70–76

85. Beri M, Klugman MR, Kohler JA, et al. Anterior ischemic optic neuropathy. VII. Incidence of bilaterality and various influencing factors. Ophthalmology 1987;94:1020–1028

86. Beck RW, Hayreh SS, Podhajsky P, et al. Aspirin therapy in nonarteritic anterior ischemic optic neuropathy. Am J Ophthalmol 1997;123:212–217

87. Kupersmith MJ, Frohman L, Sanderson M, et al. Aspirin reduces the incidence of second eye NAION: a retrospective study. J Neuroophthalmol 1997;17:250–253

88. Salomon O, Huna-Baron R, Jurtz S, et al. Analysis of prothrombotic and vascular risk factors in patients with nonarteritic anterior ischemic optic neuropathy. Ophthalmology 1999;106:739–742

89. Aiello PD, Trautmann JC, McPhee TJ, et al. Visual prognosis in giant cell arteritis. Ophthalmology 1993;100:550–555

90. Model DG. Reversal of blindness in temporal arteritis with methylprednisolone (letter), Lancet 1978;1:340

91. Diamond JP, IV steroid treatment in giant cell arteritis (letter). Ophthalmology 1993;100:291–292

92. Allison MC, Gallagher PJ. Temporal artery biopsy and corticosteroid treatment. Ann Rheum Dis 1984;43:416–417

93. Achkar AA, Lie JT, Hunder GG, et al. How does previous corticosteroid therapy affect the biopsy findings in giant cell (temporal) arteritis? Ann Intern Med 1994;120:987–992

94. To KW, Enzer YR, Tsiaras WG. Temporal artery biopsy after one month of corticosteroid therapy. Am J Ophthalmol 1994;117:265–267

95. Guevara RA, Newman NJ, Grossniklaus HE. Positive temporal artery biopsy 6 months after prednisone treatment. Arch Ophthalmol 1998;116:1252–1253

96. Galetta SL, Balcer LJ, Lieberman AP, et al. Refractory giant cell arteritis with spinal cord infarction. Neurology 1997;49:1720–1723

97. Galetta SL. Vasculitis. In: Miller NR, Newman NJ, eds. Walsh and Hoyt's Clinical Neuro-Ophthalmology. 5th ed. Baltimore: Williams & Wilkins, 1998:3725–3885

98. Myles AB, Perera T, Ridley MG. Prevention of blindness in giant cell arteritis by corticosteroid treatment. Br J Rheumatol 1992;31:103–105

99. Slavin ML, Margolis AJ. Progressive anterior ischemic optic neuropathy due to giant cell arteritis despite high-dose intravenous corticosteroids (letter). Arch Ophthalmol 1988;106:1167

100. Rauser M, Rismondo V. Ischemic optic neuropathy during corticosteroid therapy for giant cell arteritis. Arch Ophthalmol 1995;113:707–708

101. Cornblath WT, Eggenberger ER. Progressive visual loss from giant cell arteritis despite high-dose intravenous methylprednisolone. Ophthalmology 1997;104:854–858

102. Galetta SL, Balcer LJ, Liu GT. Giant cell arteritis with unusual flow-related neuro-ophthalmologic manifestations. Neurology 1997;49:1463–1465

103. Hwang JM, Girkin CA, Perry JD, et al. Bilateral ocular ischemic syndrome secondary to giant cell arteritis progressing despite corticosteroid treatment. Am J Ophthalmol 1999;127:102–104

104. Diego M, Margo CE. Postural vision loss in giant cell arteritis. J Neuroophthalmol 1998;18:124–126

105. Kyle V, Hazelman BL. Stopping steroids in polymyalgia rheumatica and giant cell arteritis: treatment usually lasts for two to five years. Br J Med 1990;300:244–245

106. Kyle V, Hazelman BL. Treatment of polymyalgia rheumatica and giant cell arteritis. II. Relation between steroid dose and steroid associated side effects. Ann Rheum Dis 1989;48:662–666

107. De Silva M, Hazelman BL. Azathioprine in giant cell arteritis/polymyalgia rheumatica: a double blind study. Ann Rheum Dis 1986;45:136–138

108. Wilke WS, Hoffman GS. Treatment of corticosteroid resistant giant cell arteritis. Rheum Dis Clin North Am 1995;21:59–71

109. Newman NJ. Hereditary optic neuropathies. In: Miller NR, Newman NJ, eds. Walsh and Hoyt's Clinical Neuro-Ophthalmology. 5th ed. Baltimore: Williams & Wilkins, 1998:741–773

110. Mashima Y, Hiida Y, Oguchi Y. Lack of differences among mitochondrial DNA in family members with Leber's hereditary optic neuropathy and differing visual outcomes. J Neuroophthalmol 1995;15:15–19

111. Jacobson DM, Stone EM, Miller NR, et al. Relative afferent pupillary defects in patients with Leber hereditary optic neuropathy and unilateral visual loss. Am J Ophthalmol 1998;126:291–295

112. Ludtke H, Kriegbaum C, Leo-Kottler B, et al. Pupillary light reflexes in patients with Leber's hereditary optic neuropathy. Graefe's Arch Clin Exp Ophthalmol 1999;237:207–211

113. Smith JL, Hoyt WF, Susac JO. Ocular fundus in acute Leber optic neuropathy. Arch Ophthalmol 1973;90:349–354

114. Lessell S, Gise RL, Krohel GB. Bilateral optic neuropa-

thy with remission in young men: variation on a theme by Leber? Arch Neurol 1983;40:2–6

115. Nakamura M, Yamamoto M. Variable pattern of visual recovery of Leber's hereditary optic neuropathy. Br J Ophthalmol 2000;84:534–535

116. Kermode AG, Moseley IF, Kendall BE, et al. Magnetic resonance imaging in Leber's optic neuropathy. J Neurol Neurosurg Psychiatry 1989;52:671–674

117. Rose FC, Bowden AN, Bowden P. The heart in Leber's optic atrophy. Br J Ophthalmol 1970;54:388–393

118. Nikoskelainen E, Wanne O, Dahl M. Pre-excitation syndrome in Leber's hereditary optic neuropathy. Lancet 1985;1:696

119. Funalot B, Ranoux D, Mas JL, et al. Brainstem involvement in Leber's hereditary optic neuropathy: association with the 14484 mitochondrial DNA mutation. J Neurol Neurosurg Psychiatry 1996;61:533–534

120. Bhatti MT, Newman NJ. A multiple sclerosis-like illness in a man harboring the mtDNA 14484 mutation. J Neuroophthalmol 1999;19:28–33

121. Simon DK, Pulst SM, Sutton JP, et al. Familial multisystem degeneration with parkinsonism associated with the 11778 mitochondrial DNA mutation. Neurology 1999;53:1787–1793

122. Pulkes T, Eunson L, Patterson V, et al. The mitochondrial DNA G13513A transition in ND5 is associated with a LHON/MELAS overlap syndrome and may be a frequent cause of MELAS. Ann Neurol 1999;46:916–919

123. Bresolin N, Bet L, Binda A, et al. Clinical and biochemical correlations in mitochondrial myopathies treated with coenzyme Q10. Neurology 1988;38:892–899

124. Shoffner JM, Lott MT, Voljavec AS, et al. Spontaneous Kearns-Sayre/chronic external ophthalmoplegia plus syndrome associated with a mitochondrial DNA deletion: a slip-replication model and metabolic therapy. Proc Natl Acad Sci USA 1989;86:7952–7956

125. Wallace DC. Mitochondrial DNA mutations and neuromuscular disease. Trends Genet 1989;5:9–13

126. Lodi R, Taylor DJ, Tabrizi SJ, et al. In vivo skeletal muscle mitochondrial function in Leber's hereditary optic neuropathy assessed by 31P magnetic resonance spectroscopy. Ann Neurol 1997;42:573–579

127. Chariot P, Brugieres P, Eliezer-Vanerot MC, et al. Choreic movements and MRI abnormalities in the subthalamic nuclei reversible after administration of coenzyme Q10 and multiple vitamins in a patient with bilateral optic neuropathy. Mov Disord 1999;14:855–859

128. Cortelli P, Montagna P, Pierangeli G, et al. Clinical and brain bioenergetics improvement with idebenone in a patient with Leber's hereditary optic neuropathy: a clinical and 31P-MRS study. J Neurol Sci 1997;148:25–31

129. Dotti MT, Plewnia K, Cardaioli E, et al. A case of ethambutol-induced optic neuropathy harbouring the primary mitochondrial LHON mutation at nt 11778. J Neurol 1998;245:302–303

130. Tsao K, Aitken PA, Johns DR. Smoking as an aetiological factor in a pedigree with Leber's hereditary optic neuropathy. Br J Ophthalmol 1999;83:577–581

Papilledema and Idiopathic Intracranial Hypertension (Pseudotumor Cerebri)

Michael Wall

Introduction

Idiopathic intracranial hypertension (IIH), also called "pseudotumor cerebri", is a disorder of increased intracranial pressure that occurs in women of the childbearing years. Its cause is not known. It is a syndrome characterized by increased intracranial pressure and its associated signs and symptoms in an alert and oriented patient, but without localizing neurological findings. There is no evidence of deformity or obstruction of the ventricular system, and neurodiagnostic studies are otherwise normal except for increased cerebrospinal fluid (CSF) pressure. Furthermore, no secondary cause of intracranial hypertension is apparent. IIH can have a self-limited or a life-long chronic course.

Although obesity and weight gain have been established as related factors, as has female sex, the cause of the disorder has eluded investigators. The major morbidity of the disease is loss of vision related to papilledema, with blindness as a potential outcome of treatment failure.

Epidemiology

The annual incidence if IIH is 0.9/100 000 persons and 3.5/100 000 in females 15 to 44 years old.[1,2] Among obese women 20 to 44 years who are 20% or more over ideal weight, the incidence is 19/100 000.[1] More than 90% of IIH patients are obese and more than 90% are women of childbearing age. Female preponderance and the association of obesity is true only for postpubertal patients.[3] This mean age at diagnosis is about 30 years.[1]

Etiology

Most studies of conditions associated with IIH have been uncontrolled and retrospective. This has led to erroneous conclusions because investigators have reported chance and spurious associations with common medical conditions and medications. Also, many of the case reports of associations with intracranial hypertension do not meet the modified Dandy criteria for IIH. For example, pregnancy, irregular menses, and oral contraceptive use have been reported to be associated with IIH, but these associations have been shown to be due to chance alone.[4–6] In case-control studies, no significant association has been found between IIH and multivitamin, oral contraceptive, or antibiotic use.[5,6] A case-control study has found strong associations between IIH and obesity and weight gain during the 12 months before diagnosis.[6]

Pathophysiology and pathogenesis

Any hypothesis of pathogenesis of IIH should explain the following observations of patients with the disorder: (1) high rate of occurrence in women of childbearing years, (2) association of obesity, (3) decreased conductance to CSF outflow, and (4) normal ventricular size and no hydrocephalus.

Changes in cerebral hemodynamics, that is, increased cerebral blood volume and decreased cerebral blood flow, have been reported. However, others have found no significant changes in these factors. The most popular hypothesis is that IIH is a syndrome of reduced CSF absorption. Decreased conductance to CSF outflow may be due to dysfunction of the absorptive mechanism of the arachnoid granulations. Intracranial pressure, then, must increase for CSF to be absorbed. Although interstitial and intracellular edema have been reported in brain biopsy specimens,[7] study with current methods of analysis has concluded that the histological features of the brain parenchyma are normal.[8]

Genetics

There are case reports of familial occurrence of the disease, and a specific phenotype for the disease exists, that is, an obese woman of childbearing years. However, the genetics of IIH are unknown.

Clinical features

Symptoms

The symptoms of IIH are headache in 94% of patients, transient visual obscurations in 68%, pulse synchronous tinnitus in 58%, photopsia in 54%, and retrobulbar pain in 44%. Diplopia (38% of patients) and loss of vision (30% of patients) are less common. Some of these symptoms are common in controls (Figure 162.1).

The presence of headache is nearly ubiquitous among patients with IIH and is the usual presenting symptom. The headache profile is that of severe daily headaches described as pulsatile.[9] They are different from previous headaches, may awaken the patient, and usually last hours. Nausea is common, and vomiting is uncommon. The headache usually is reported as the worst head pain the person has experienced.

Transient visual obscurations Visual obscurations are episodes of transient blurred vision that usually last less than 30 seconds and are followed by restoration of vision. Visual obscurations occur in about three-fourths of patients with IIH.[6] The attacks may

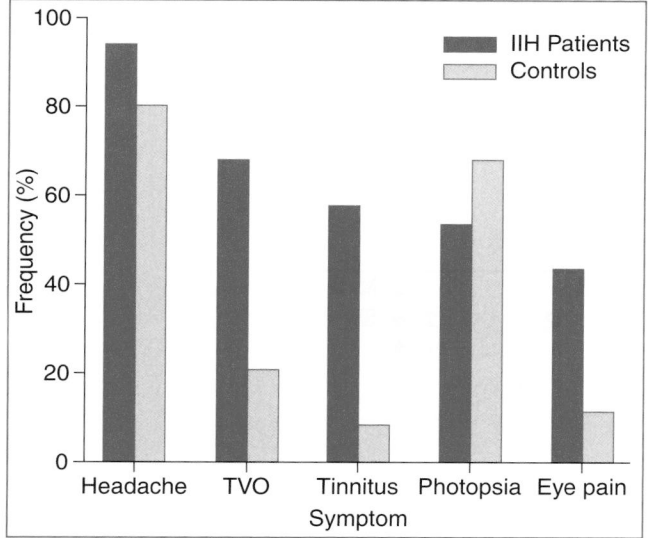

Figure 162.1 Frequency of symptoms among patients with idiopathic intracranial hypertension (IIH) patient and control subjects. TVO, transient visual obscurations.

be monocular or binocular. The cause of these episodes is thought to be transient ischemia of the optic nerve head caused by increased tissue pressure.[10] Visual obscurations do not appear to be associated with an outcome of poor vision.[11–13]

Pulse-synchronous tinnitus Pulsatile intracranial noise or pulse synchronous tinnitus is common in IIH (60% of patients).[6] The sound is often unilateral, with neither side predominating. In patients with intracranial hypertension, jugular compression ipsilateral to the sound abolishes it.[14] The sound is thought to be due to transmission of intensified vascular pulsations by means of CSF under high pressure to the walls of the venous sinuses.[15]

Signs

The major signs of IIH are papilledema and paresis of cranial nerve (CN) VI.

Ophthalmoscopic examination Papilledema is the cardinal sign of IIH (Figure 162.2A); care must be taken to differentiate true papilledema from pseudopapilledema (Figure 162.2B). Optic disk edema, either directly or indirectly, is the cause of the loss of vision in IIH. The higher the grade of papilledema, the worse the visual loss.[16] However, in a patient, the severity of visual loss cannot easily be predicted from the severity of the papilledema. A partial explanation for this is that with axonal death from compression of the optic nerve, the amount of papilledema decreases.

Ocular motility disturbances Horizontal diplopia occurs in about 33% of patients with IIH and CNVI palsies in 10% to 20%.[17] Motility disturbances other than CNVI palsies have been reported. Some of these reflect erroneous conclusions from the small vertical ocular motor imbalance that is known to accompany CNVI palsies. The diagnosis of IIH should be viewed with suspicion in patients with ocular motility disturbances other than CNVI palsies.

Sensory visual function Visual acuity usually is normal in patients with papilledema except when the condition is long-standing and severe. Snellen acuity

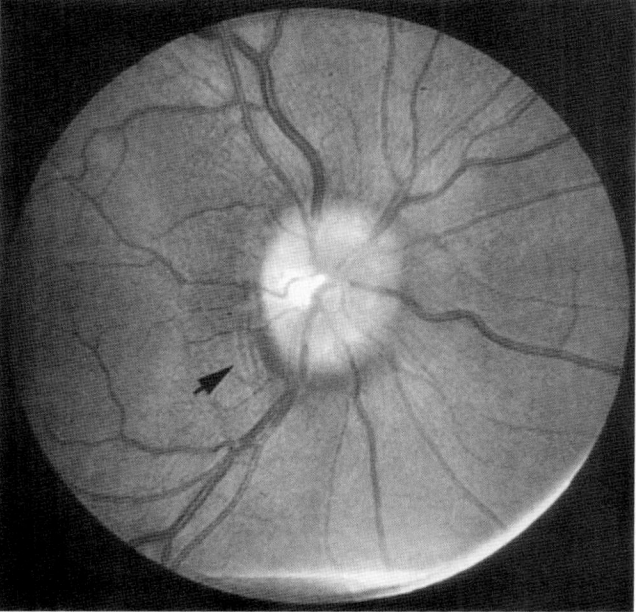

A

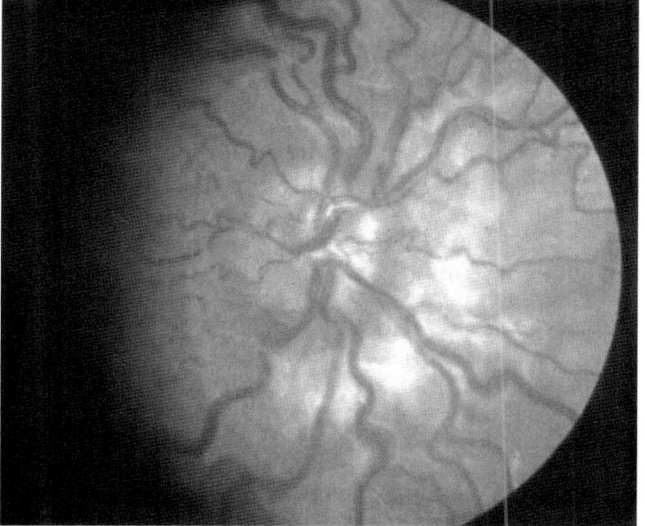

B

Figure 162.2 *A*, Optic disk with Frisén grade I papilledema. The disk has a C-shaped halo of nerve fiber layer edema around the disk, with a temporal gap. Choroidal folds are also present (*arrow*). *B*, pseudopapilledema. This is an anomalous disk with considerable anomalies of blood vessel branching. (See color plate section.)

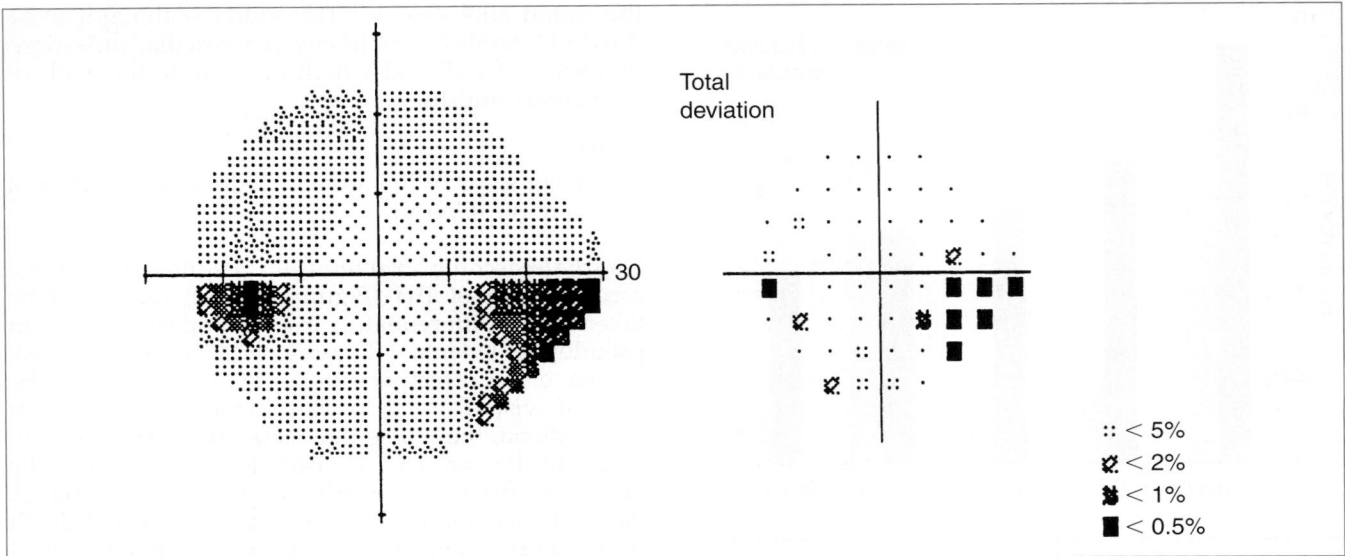

Figure 162.3   Conventional automated perimetry results from patients with idiopathic intracranial hypertension, showing the prototypically enlarged blind spot coupled with inferonasal loss.

testing is insensitive to the amount visual loss found with perimetry and to worsening of the grade of papilledema.[17] Contrast sensitivity testing is more sensitive.

Perimetry   Visual field loss is ubiquitous in IIH. In a prospective study, the loss of vision in at least one eye (other than enlargement of the physiological blind spot) was found with Goldmann perimetry, using a disease-specific strategy, in 96% of patients and with automated perimetry in 92%. About one-fourth of this loss of vision is mild and unlikely to be noticed by the patient.[17]

The visual field defects found in IIH are the same types that occur in papilledema due to other causes. These "disk-related defects" are the same as those found in glaucoma. The most common defects are enlargement of the physiological blind spot and loss of inferonasal portions of the visual field (Figure 162.3) along with constriction of isopters. Central defects are distinctly uncommon and warrant a search for another diagnosis unless there is a large serous retinal detachment from high-grade optic disk edema. The loss of visual field may be progressive and severe and lead to blindness (Figure 162.4). The temporal profile of visual loss is usually gradual; however, acute severe loss of vision of the type found in ischemic optic neuropathy can occur.

Enlargement of the blind spot is ubiquitous in IIH. Because refraction often eliminates this defect, it should not be considered significant visual loss unless it encroaches on fixation. Also, because the size of the blind spot is so dependent on refraction, it should not be used to follow the course of therapy.

With treatment, about 50% of patients have marked improvement in the visual field.[17] Although the vision of most patients improves, a study that evaluated a subgroup of patients with worsening of

vision showed recent weight gain was the only factor significantly associated with deteriorating vision.[17] Other groups at risk for severe loss of vision are black males, patients with glaucoma, and patients whose corticosteroid therapy is being tapered rapidly. The course of IIH is often chronic, with recurrence especially during periods of weight gain.

Classification

"Pseudotumor cerebri" is classified as either primary (idiopathic intracranial hypertension) or secondary (pseudotumor cerebri syndrome). Causes of pseudotumor cerebri syndrome that meet criteria for the

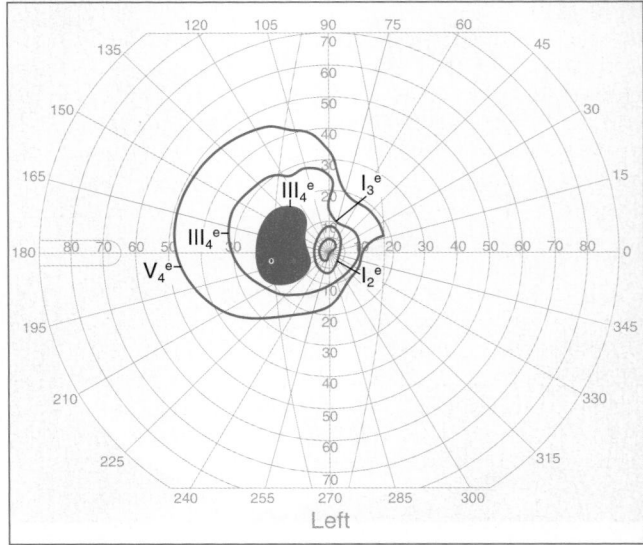

Figure 162.4   Visual field of left eye of patient with idiopathic intracranial hypertension. Note severe constriction of the visual field, with markedly enlarged blind spot.

idiopathic form, except that a secondary cause is found, are listed in Table 162.1.[18]

Diagnostic criteria

The accepted criteria initially proposed by Dandy have been modified.[19] For patients who fulfill these criteria, the diagnosis is the idiopathic form of the disease. These criteria are given in Table 162.2. Alternative criteria have been proposed by the International Headache Society and are also listed in Table 162.2.

Whatever criteria are used, if the examination findings are other than papilledema and CNVI paresis a diagnosis other than IIH should be strongly suspected. Laboratory test results are normal except for increased intracranial pressure on CSF manometry. Abnormal neuroimaging results (except for empty sella and optic nerve enlargement) should lead to another diagnosis.

Differential diagnosis

The differential diagnosis of papilledema is broad. Brain tumors, venous sinus thromboses, and other space-occupying lesions severe enough to cause increased intracranial pressure and papilledema are usually obvious on neuroimaging. More challenging are cases in which neuroimaging findings and CSF constituents are normal. There is reasonable evidence that the following disease associations exist and cause increased intracranial pressure: nalidixic acid,[20] nitrofurantoin,[21] indomethacin[22] or ketoprofen in Bartter syndrome,[23] vitamin A intoxication,[24] isotretinoin,[25] thyroid replacement therapy in hypothyroid children,[26] lithium,[27] and anabolic steroids.[28] Although tetracycline or minocycline therapy might be a related cause,[29,30] the common use of these medications in the age group in conjunction with incomplete proof of the association suggests further study is needed. Cryptic arteriovenous malformations or dural fistulae with high flow may overload venous return and increase intracranial pressure. Although corticosteroid withdrawal and Addison disease clearly are associated with IIH,[31–33] as is hypoparathyroidism, links to other endocrine abnormalities are unproved. For example, corticosteroid use has been associated with many suspected cases of IIH; however, non have fulfilled the modified Dandy criteria of IIH. A more in-depth discussion of differential diagnosis is found elsewhere.[18]

Treatment

Once intracranial hypertension has been discovered, first eliminate presumed causal factors (e.g., discontinue excessive vitamin A, begin weight reduction, discontinue nalidixic acid treatment, or restart corticosteroid therapy and taper more slowly). Next, begin therapy aimed at reversing and preventing loss of vision. Finally, direct treatment at the headache if it persists despite use of intracranial pressure-lowering agents and procedures. Many treatments have been attempted for IIH with varying success. To date, all reports have been anecdotal; that is, they meet grade C, level 4 quality of evidence efficacy. The loss of vision is the only serious complication, and it may

Table 162.1 Causes and disease associations of intracranial hypertension*

Highly likely†
  Decreased flow through arachnoid granulations
    Scarring from previous inflammation,
      e.g., meningitis, sequelae to subarachnoid
      hemorrhage
  Obstruction of venous drainage
    Venous sinus thromboses
      Hypercoaguable states
      Contiguous infection (e.g., middle ear or
        mastoid–otitic hydrocephalus)
    Bilateral radical neck dissection
    Glomus tumor
    Superior vena cava syndrome
    Increased pressure on right side of heart
  Endocrine disorders
    Addison disease
    Corticosteroid withdrawal
    Hypoparathyroidism
    Obesity
  Nuritional disorders
    Hypervitaminosis A (vitamin, liver, or isotretinoin
      intake)
    Hyperalimentation in deprivation dwarfism
  Arteriovenous malformations and dural shunts

Probable causes‡
  Anabolic steroids (may cause venous sinus
    thrombosis)
  Chlordecone (kepone)
  Ketoprofen or indomethacin in Bartter syndrome
  Systemic lupus erythematosus
  Thyroid replacement therapy in hypothyroid children
  Uremia

Possible causes§
  Amiodarone
  Phenytoin
  Iron deficiency anemia
  Lithium carbonate
  Nalidixic acid
  Sarcoidosis
  Sulfa antibiotics
  Tetracycline

Frequently cited causes that are unproved‖
  Corticosteroids
  Hyperthryoidism
  Hypovitaminosis A
  Menarche
  Menstrual irregularities
  Multivitamin intake
  Oral contraceptives
  Pregnancy

*The Table lists the causes of intracranial hypertension that meet the modified Dandy criteria except a cause is associated.
†The "highly likely" category is a list of cases with many reports of the association with multiple lines of evidence.
‡"Probable causes"—reports that provide some convincing evidence.
§Possible causes—suggestive evidence or common conditions or medications with intracranial hypertension as a rare association.
‖Frequently cited but poorly documented or unlikely causes; three case control studies suggest this group of associations is not valid.

Table 162.2   Criteria for idiopathic intracranial hypertension

Modified Dandy Criteria
1. Signs and symptoms of increased intracranial pressure[19]
2. Absence of localizing findings on neurological examination
3. Absence of deformity, displacement, or obstruction of the ventricular system and otherwise normal neurodiagnostic studies, except for increased cerebrospinal fluid pressure (> 250 mm of water in obese patients)[96]
4. Awake and alert patient
5. No other causes of increased intracranial pressure present

International Headache Society diagnostic criteria[97]
A. Patient has benign intracranial hypertension fulfilling the following criteria:
   1. Increased intracranial pressure (> 200 mm of water) measured by epidural or intraventricular pressure monitoring
   2. Normal neurological examination findings except for papilledema and possible CNVI palsy
   3. No mass lesion and no ventricular enlargement on neuroimaging
   4. Normal or low protein concentration and normal leukocyte count in CSF
   5. No clinical or neuroimaging suspicion of venous sinus thrombosis
B. Headache intensity and frequency related to variations of intracranial pressure with a time lag of less than 24 hours.

CN, cranial nerve; CSF, cerebrospinal fluid.

occur at any time from the first appearance of the disease to many years later. Therefore, the author recommends the treatment be tailored mainly to the presence and progression of the loss of vision.

Medical therapy

Treatment of increased intracranial pressure can be both medical and surgical. It is aimed at decreasing intracranial pressure and treating symptoms directly (e.g., headache). However, no controlled clinical treatment trials have been conducted for IIH.

Weight loss

Weight loss has been used to treat IIH for many years. In 1974, Newborn[34] reported remission of papilledema in all nine patients placed on a strict diet. She used a low calorie adaptation of Kempner's rice diet. The patient's intake was 400 to 1000 calories daily by fruits, rice, vegetables, and, occasionally, 1 to 2 oz of meat. Fluids were limited to 750 to 1250 mL/day and sodium to less than 100 mg/day. All patients had reversal of their papilledema. However, visual testing was not mentioned.

The beneficial effects of weight loss have also been reinforced more recently. Kupersmith et al.[35] retrospectively reviewed the records of 56 medically treated IIH patients from two centers who had at least 6 months of follow-up. The mean time to improve one grade of papilledema was about 4 months in patients with weight loss, compared with about 1 year in patients without weight loss. Papilledema resolved in 28 or 38 patients with weight loss, compared with 8 of 20 without weight loss.

Johnson et al.[36] retrospectively studied 15 patients with IIH treated with acetazolamide and weight loss for 24 weeks and reported a 3.3% weight loss in patients having one grade of improvement. Of 10 patients who had improvement, 9 had received acetazolamide, as did 4 patients who did not lose weight and had no improvement in papilledema grade. The author's experience from a pilot study with 29

patients has also been that improvement often occurs with only modest degrees of weight loss. However, Greer[37] reported a group of six obese patients who became asymptomatic without weight loss.

Resolution of IIH in a patient after surgically induced weight loss (gastric exclusion procedure) was first reported by Amaral.[38] Sugarman et al.[39] performed gastric weight reduction procedures in 24 morbidly obese women with IIH. Five patients were lost to follow-up. Symptoms resolved in all but one patient within 4 months after the procedure. Two patients regained weight, and this was associated with the return of their symptoms. There were many serious but treatable complications related to the surgical procedures.

Recent marked weight gain is a predictor of the deterioration of vision.[17] Because the author has observed that papilledema resolves with weight loss as the only treatment, his patients are strongly encouraged to pursue a supervised weight loss program. As Friedman et al.[40] have shown, a subset of patients with IIH has orthostatic edema.[40] Institution of a low salt diet and mild fluid restriction appear to be beneficial for many patients. This may be true especially for patients who lose only a small percentage of their total body mass yet have resolution of optic disk edema. It is not clear whether improvement occurs because of weight loss per se or other changes in diet such as fluid or sodium restriction or decrease in the intake of a molecule, for example, vitamin A.

Lumbar puncture

Repeated lumbar puncture, although still used by some neurologists, leaves much to be desired as a treatment. Lumbar puncture has only a short-lived effect on CSF pressure; Johnston and Paterson[41] found a return of pressure to pre puncture level after only 82 minutes. Weisberg,[42] however, reported that 6 of 28 patients treated with serial lumbar punctures had symptomatic improvement.

Repeated lumbar puncture also increase the risk of

the development of intraspinal epidermoid tumors, presumably caused by implantation of epidermal cells.[43] Manno et al.[44] reported that 41% of intraspinal epidermoid tumors in their series could be traced to previous lumbar punctures. Also, repeated lumbar puncture measures CSF pressure at only one point in time. Because CSF pressure fluctuates widely, this information has limited clinical use for modifying treatment plans.

Corticosteroids

Paterson[45] first reported the efficacy of corticosteroids for treating IIH in five of six consecutive patients. In Weisberg's[42] series of 15 patients treated with corticosteroids, 13 who did not have a response to repeated lumbar punctures had resolution of their symptoms within 3 days after corticosteroid therapy and had no recurrence after this therapy was stopped 7 to 14 days later. Another subgroup of 35 patients initially received corticosteroid therapy and 32 had a prompt response. Of those who had a favorable response to corticosteroid therapy, all showed improvement of symptoms or signs within 4 days.

In a study of 38 children given various regimens for treating IIH, 4 received corticosteroid therapy after repeated lumbar punctures failed.[46] In all four, the symptoms and signs resolved. Twelve other children had clinical improvement with a combination of repeated lumbar puncture and corticosteroids. The study concluded that corticosteroid dosage and intracranial pressure are inversely related. However, there was recurrence with rapid tapering of the dose.

Corticosteroids are still used occasionally to treat IIH, but their mechanism of action is not clear. The side effects of weight gain, striae, and acne are especially unfortunate for these obese patients. Although patients given corticosteroid treatment often have a good response, papilledema may recur with rapid tapering of the dose. This may be accompanied by marked deterioration of visual function. Prolonged tapering may prevent the return of symptoms and signs in some patients. Corticosteroid treatment of IIH has been abandoned by most neuro-ophthalmologists.

Thiazide diuretics

Jefferson and Clark[47] treated 30 patients with IIH with various types of oral dehydrating agents (chlorthalidone, hydroflumethiazide, glycerol, and urea). All patients were also placed on a weight reduction diet. The size of the blind spot size was the main outcome measure. This measure can be problematic for several reasons, including changes in refractive error[48,49] and changes in perimetric stimulus speed and reaction times during and between examinations. Of the 30 patients, 14 had decreased visual acuity and, with therapy, all had improved vision. Friedman[50] treated 30 women with IIH with chlorthalidone and spironolactone (dextroamphetamine or phentermine was added to the regimen of 15 women and acetazolamide to that of 18). This treatment did not consistently reduce headache and papilledema improved in only 4 of the 30 patients.

Acetazolamide

In 1974, McCarthy and Reed[51] showed that acetazolamide decreases CSF flow but not until more than 99.5% of the carbonic anhydrase in the choroid plexus is inhibited. Lubow and Kuhr,[52] in 1976, reported that with acetazolamide (Diamox) and weight reduction were successful in treating IIH in many of their patients. Gücer and Viernstein[53] used intracranial pressure monitoring of IIH in four patients before and after treatment. Two patients received acetazolamide treatment and had a gradual decrease in CSF pressure (the dose of acetazolamide, 4 g daily, was reported for only one of the patients. Ten years later, Tomsak et al.,[54] documented the resolution of papilledema with photographs of the optic disks of four patients given 1 g acetazolamide daily. Acetazolamide treatment appeared to be effective, with results occurring over several months. The most effective dose has not yet been determined. Most neuro-ophthalmologists start with 0.5 to 1 g daily in divided doses and gradually increase the dose until symptoms and signs regress, side effects become intolerable, or a dose of 3 to 4 g daily is reached.

The mechanism of action of acetazolamide is likely multifactorial. It decreases CSF production in humans by 6% to 50%.[55] It has been thought to work by inhibiting carbonic anhydrase which causes a reduction in transport of sodium ions across the choroid plexus epithelium. Also, acetazolamide changes the taste of food and sometimes causes anorexia, which may be desirable. Also, it causes carbonated beverages to taste metallic. These side effects may help the patient lose weight.

Patients who take acetazolamide nearly always experience tingling in the fingers, toes, and perioral region and, less commonly, have malaise. Renal stones, although painful, are treatable and occur in a small percentage of patients. Metabolic acidosis, evidenced by decreased serum bicarbonate, is a good measure of compliance. Younger patients tolerate acetazolamide better than older ones, and azetazolamide (Diamox) 500 mg sustained-release sequels appear to be better tolerated.[56,57] A rare but serious side effect of acetazolamide is aplastic anemia, which occurs in 1/15000 patient-years of treatment and usually occurs in the first 6 months of therapy. Aplastic anemia from acetazolamide has been reported most often in the elderly and is probably less common in younger patients with IIH. Because this side effect is so rare and finding the case and stopping the medication does not necessarily produce a cure, repeated blood testing is not usually performed.[58] Also, testing is not cost-effective; in 1987, Zimran and Beutler[58] estimated that the cost of finding one case was $1.5 million (US).

Furosemide

Furosemide (Lasix) has also been used to treat IIH.[12] It can decrease intracranial pressure.[59–61] Furosemide usually is given in combination with mannitol in neurosurgical emergencies such as herniation syndromes, and its effects appear to be additive to those of mannitol.[59,60,62] Furosemide appears to work both by producing diuresis and reducing sodium transport into the brain.[63]

On the basis of the assumption of McCarthy and Reed[51] that the effects of acetazolamide and furosemide may be additive, Schoeman[64] treated IIH in pediatric patients with this combination therapy. In a controlled trial of children with tuberculous meningitis, 57 with communicating hydrocephalus were randomly assigned to three treatment groups: antituberculous drugs only, additional intrathecal hyaluronidase, or oral acetazolamide and furosemide in addition to antituberculous treatment. Acetazolamide and furosemide in combination were significantly more effective in achieving normal intracranial pressure than antituberculous drugs alone.[65]

Schoeman[64] then treated IIH in eight pediatric patients with oral acetazolamide (37 to 100 mg/kg) and furosemide (1 mg/kg) until the papilledema cleared. He used continuous 1-hour lumbar cerebrospinal fluid pressure monitoring at admission and at weekly intervals until the baseline pressure became normal. Six children had increased CSF pressure at baseline, and increased intracranial pressure was diagnosed in three children on the basis of abnormal pulse wave or pressure wave. The mean baseline pressure normalizedrin all patients within 6 weeks after the start of therapy.

The author initiates furosemide treatment at a dose of 20 mg orally twice daily and gradually increases the dose, if needed, to a maximum of 40 mg orally 3 times daily. Potassium supplementation is often necessary. This appears to be effective treatment for IIH.

Glycerol

Oral glycerol is a form of cerebral dehydration first recommended in 1963 to decrease intracranial pressure. A single dose of 1 g/kg of glycerol increases serum osmolality from 295 to 320 mOsm/L in 90 minutes and decreases CSF pressure for 3 to 5 hours. Doses every 4 hours can cause a reversed osmotic gradient and a rebound increase in intracranial pressure,[48,49] whereas a 6-hour interval is too long and allows the raised intracranial pressure to recur. Together, the additional calories, the large volume of glycerol needed, and the nauseating side effects make this a cumbersome medication for IIH. Currently, glycerol is seldom used to manage increased intracranial pressure.

Surgery

The surgical forms of therapy currently used are various shunting and decompression procedures, including lumbar subarachnoid-peritoneal shunt and optic nerve sheath fenestration.

Subtemporal or suboccipital decompression

Subtemporal or suboccipital decompression was used from the 1940s to the 1960s for patients with loss of vision due to IIH. Although some patients had improvement, others did not and some became blind.[66-68] These procedures have been abandoned because of their many complications, including seizures, otorrhea, subdural hematoma, and postoperative deterioration of vision.[42,69-71] However, long-term success has been reported.[72]

Optic nerve sheath fenestration

De Wecker[73] pioneered treatment for papilledema in 1856 when he performed the first optic nerve sheath fenestration. The procedure fell into disfavor until the 1960s when Hayreh,[74] using a primate model, demonstrated bilateral relief of papilledema with a unilateral optic nerve sheath fenestration; he also demonstrated communication between the lumbar subarachnoid space and the orbital subarachnoid space. Smith et al.[75] reported successful relief of papilledema in a human in 1969. Optic nerve sheath fenestration consists of either creating a window or making a series of slits in the optic nerve sheath just behind the globe. This treatment is preferred for patients who have progressive loss of vision and mild or easily controlled headaches, although more than 50% of the patients who have the procedure achieve adequate headache control. Because papilledema in the unoperated eye may improve and because fistula formation[76] has been demonstrated, Keltner et al.[77] proposed that the mechanism of action is local decompression of the subarachnoid space. Occasional failure of the other eye to improve and the asymmetry of papilledema may be explained by the resistance to CSF flow produced by the trabeculations of the subarachnoid space or tightness of the optic canal. Others have proposed that the long-term mechanism of action of optic nerve sheath fenestration may be closure of the subarachnoid space in the retrolaminar optic nerve by scarring.[78] It is likely that both mechanisms contribute to protect the optic nerve head from high CSF pressure.

Many large case series attest to the efficacy of the technique.[79-82,83-85] In these series, postoperative visual acuity or fields were as good or better than those of preoperative studies in 88.6% of patients (Table 162.3). However, occasional patients lose vision in the perioperative period.[83] The loss of vision can be due to traumatic optic neuropathy, anterior ischemic optic neuropathy, orbital hemorrhage, retinal artery occlusions, outer retinal ischemia or choroidal infarcts.[84,86] Other complications are ocular motility disorders and tonic pupils.

Spoor and McHenry[87] have raised the issue that patients undergoing optic nerve sheath fenestration may have substantial long-term failure rates. They reported results in 75 eyes of 54 patients undergoing optic nerve sheath fenestration who had stable visual acuity and four or more visual field examinations during 6 to 60 months of follow-up.[87] They defined "stability" as a mean deviation within 2 dB of the preoperative visual field and "worsening" as more than a 2-dB mean deviation deterioration. With these definitions, 51 eyes (68%) showed improvement (36%) or stabilization and 24 (32%) showed worsening. The

Table 162.3   Results of optic nerve sheath fenestration

Investigators	No. of patients	Vision, no. of patients		Worse vision, % of patients
		Worse	Better	
Sergott[82] (1988)	23	0	23	0.0
Brourman[85] (1988)	10	0	10	0.0
Kelman[81] (1992)	22	1	21	4.5
Goh[79] (1997)	29	3	26	10.3
Plotnik[84] (1993)	31	4	27	12.9
Acheson[80] (1994)	20	3	17	15.0
Corbett[83] (1988)	40	9	31	22.5
Total	**175**	**20**	**155**	**11.4**

problem with this analysis is that 2 dB or greater mean deviation is well within observed retest variability with moderate visual field damage.[88] Therefore, the clinical course of optic nerve sheath fenestration awaits further study. The author's experience, with considerable long-term follow-up using predominantly Goldmann perimetry, is that late deterioration requiring refenestration is uncommon.

CSF shunting procedures

Various shunting procedures have been used to treat IIH, including lumbar subarachnoid-peritoneal shunts; ventriculoatrial, ventriculojugular, and ventriculoperitoneal shunts; and cisternoatrial shunts.[89–92] The case series are difficult to compare because the types of shunts were different, the shunts that were used had different complications, and the indications and techniques used were different. Generally, the indication for a CSF diversion procedure in these series was failed medical therapy or intractable headache.

Eggenberger et al.[91] retrospectively studied lumboperitoneal shunt in 27 patients with IIH that had been treated with at least one shunt. The average duration of follow-up was 77 months (median, 47 months). The shunting procedure was initially successful in all patients; however, 56% required shunt revision. No major complications from lumboperitoneal shunting were found.

Rosenberg et al.[92] reviewed the efficacy of CSF shunting for IIH in patients from six institutions. Thirty-seven patients had 73 lumboperitoneal shunts and 9 ventricular shunts. The procedure had modest success, with the treatment being successful in 38% of patients after one shunting procedure. The mean time between shunt insertion and replacement was 9 months, with 64% of shunts lasting less than 6 months. The most common causes for reoperation were shunt failure (55% of patients) and low-pressure headache (21% of patients). In most patients, vision improved or stabilized after the procedure, but three patients who initially had improved vision later lost vision and six others had a decrease in vision postoperatively. Four patients lost vision despite apparently

adequate shunt function. Serious complications occurred in 3.6% of patients. Rosenberg et al. concluded that CSF shunting procedures have a high failure rate.

Burgett et al.[90] retrospectively examined the clinical data from 30 patients who had a shunt procedure for IIH. Symptoms of increased intracranial pressure improved in 82% of patients. Among the 28 eyes with abnormal findings on Goldmann perimetry, 18 (64%) improved and none became worse. Johnston et al.[89] analyzed data from 36 patients from a consecutive series of 41 patients with IIH treated with CSF shunting. In 12 patients, shunting was used as the primary treatment becasuse of severe deterioration of vision, and all 12 had rapid and complete resolution of the disease. In 24 patients, a shunt was inserted after other forms of treatment failed; all these patients also had rapid resolution of the disease. Johnston et al. concluded that shunting is effective in the treatment of IIH, but it has a substantial complication rate.

In summary, shunting procedures are successful in selected patients. The common complications are shunt occlusion and intracranial hypotension. shunt occlusion can be accompanied by severe loss of vision, limiting the effectiveness of this procedure. Less common complications are back pain, abdominal pain, infection of the disk space, meningitis, disconnection of tubing, and descent of the cerebellar tonsils. Because a single shunt procedure is successful in about half of the patients, it is a viable treatment for IIH, especially if the patient's main problem is severe headache.

Gastric exclusion surgery

As discussed above, gastric exclusion procedures have been successful for morbidly obese patients.[39] This procedure may be useful especially in treating other conditions that coexist with obesity, such as arterial hypertension, diabetes mellitus, and sleep apnea. Complications include major wound infection and stenosis at the gastrojejunal anastomosis.

Treatment strategies

First, the patient is educated about IIH, and the risk to vision is explained. This usually motivates the patient to follow through on the course of therapy. Next, individualized therapy is designed. Medical and surgical treatment is often challenging, requiring integration of the history, examination findings, and clinical course. Many factors are involved and each is weighed in creating individualized therapy. The most important factor usually is the amount and progression of visual loss. Next in importance is the severity of the patient's symptoms with regard to how much they interfere with the patient's activities of daily living. Headache is the most difficult symptom to treat, but pulse synchronous tinnitus, diplopia, transient visual obscurations, and neck pain can be a challenge, too. Also factored into the design of the treatment is the degree and progression of optic disk edema.

When loss of vision is the major factor driving treatment decisions, the algorithm in Figure 162.5 is

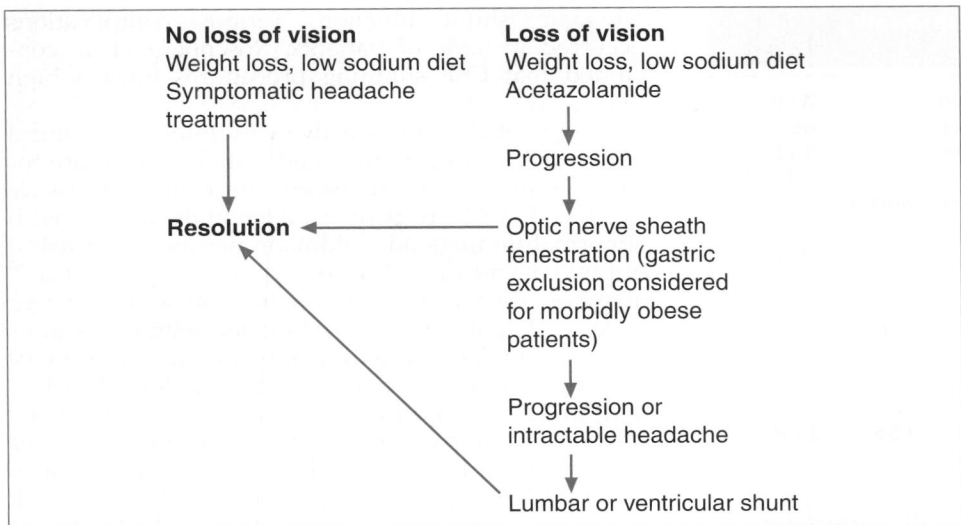

No loss of vision
Weight loss, low sodium diet
Symptomatic headache
treatment

Loss of vision
Weight loss, low sodium diet
Acetazolamide

↓

Progression

↓

Resolution ← Optic nerve sheath
fenestration (gastric
exclusion considered
for morbidly obese
patients)

↓

Progression or
intractable headache

↓

Lumbar or ventricular shunt

Figure 162.5 Algorithm for treating idiopathic intracranial hypertension. Visual loss does not include blind spot enlargement unless it is symptomatic.

useful.[93] Treatment options are summarized in Table 162.4. For a patient with a headache that is easily controlled with analgesics, and without demonstrable loss of vision, the author recommends modest weight loss, a low salt diet, and mild fluid restriction.

It is recommended that patients lose 1 or 2 pounds a week for 2 months, or about 5% of their total body weight, and maintain the weight loss. Not only is this usually sufficient to decrease papilledema, it is a more realistic goal than that of many other dietary plans. More ambitious regimens have a dismal 5-year success rate. In the author's experience, modest weight loss is often successful when the patient understands that his or her vision is "at stake." In addition, patients are asked to consume a diet rich in vegetables and low in processed foods, that is, to follow a low salt diet. Many patients consume large quantities of plain water because they have been told, "it is healthy." This may be true, but excessive water

intake may contribute to increased intracranial pressure. The suggestion is made to patients, especially those taking acetazolamide, that they drink adequate amounts of water but drink when they are thirsty instead of forcing water intake.

At initial presentation, most patients are symptomatic, have mild loss of vision, and have a moderate degree of papilledema. For these patients, the author recommends pharmacological therapy in addition to a change in diet. Patients with a mild loss of vision or symptoms that interfere with the activities of daily living should have medical therapy. The regimen the author prescribes is initiate treatment with acetazolamide, 250 mg orally 3 times daily with meals. If the symptoms do not improve, add 250 mg every 4 days until reaching a dose of 500 mg orally 3 times daily. If necessary, the dose can be increased gradually to 4 g of acetazolamide daily until the symptoms and signs regress or intolerable side effects intervene. Patients

Table 162.4   Treatments for idiopathic intracranial hypertension and the major side effects

Treatment	Indication	Major side effects
Weight loss, salt and fluid restriction	Presence of disease	None
Acetazolamide (250 mg to 4 g daily)	Significant symptoms not responding to weight loss Presence or progression of loss of vision	Nausea, renal stones
Furosemide (20–120 mg daily)	Failure of acetazolamide	Electrolyte disturbance, especially potassium loss
Prednisone (high dose)	Failure of diuretics, and surgery contraindicated or unavailable	Well known
Optic nerve sheath fenestration	Failure of medical treatment (see text)	Loss of vision, diplopia
Shunting procedures	Intractable headache, failure of medical treatment	Shunt failure with loss of vision, low-pressure headaches
Gastric exclusion procedure	Selected patients with morbid obesity	Major wound infection, gastrojejunal anastomosis stenosis

are warned about the small risk of renal stones and the remote risk of aplastic anemia. These and other side effects are discussed above. If patients are unable to tolerate the 250-mg preparation of acetazolamide, the 500-mg sequels are tried (this preparation is substantially more expensive). Alternatively, treatment can be switched to furosemide, 20 mg orally twice daily. The dose can be increased gradually until the desired effect is obtained or 40 mg orally 3 times daily is reached. Close monitoring of the serum level of potassium is recommended. The evidence for using the combination of acetazolamide and furosemide is discussed above, and this treatment can be given in cases of refractory disease. The author does not use corticosteroids to treat IIH. If medical therapy fails or the patient has severe loss of vision at the onset, the surgical options (usually optic nerve sheath fenestration) discussed below are instituted.

It is well accepted that if patients lose vision in spite of full medical therapy, surgical treatment is indicated. What constitutes "worsening disease" can be difficult to define. For example, patients may say they are worse because the headache is worse. However, if this is found to be an analgesic or caffeine rebound headache, surgical treatment would be ill advised. What criteria should be used to define worsening of the visual field? Spoor et al.[87] have suggested that worsening of 2 dB in the mean deviation of automated perimetry. However, this much change can occur with retesting the patient the same day with automated perimetry. The problem with conventional automated perimetry is that variability increases with increasing damage of the visual field. Therefore, the amount of worsening due to fluctuation of the test alone worsens with progressive visual field loss. Consequently, conventional automated perimetry has serious limitations in following patients who have moderate to severe visual field loss. Once patients have between 3 and 5 dB mean deviation, the author follows them with manual (Goldmann bowl) perimetry. This form of kinetic perimetry, in which the perimetrist performs many retests during the examination to verify any change, is less prone to large fluctuations on retesting. Also, it is important to use the trend of a group of perimetric examinations.

If the loss of vision progresses in spite of full medical therapy or if the loss is initially moderate or severe, optic nerve sheath fenestration is recommended. It appears that the earlier this is performed in the course of the disease, the more likely it will be successful. The indications for surgical intervention are 1) serious loss of vision in one or both eyes at the initial examination, 2) loss of vision in spite of full medical therapy, 3) presence of papilledema or increased intracranial pressure in the presence of a risk of hypotension (e.g., renal dialysis or treatment for systemic arterial hypertension), 4) inability to perform visual tests or unlikely to return for follow-up examinations, 5) intractable headache (optic nerve sheath fenestration for headache appears to work best when the patient has fronto-orbital pain, with eye movements. Since this pain may be due to distended

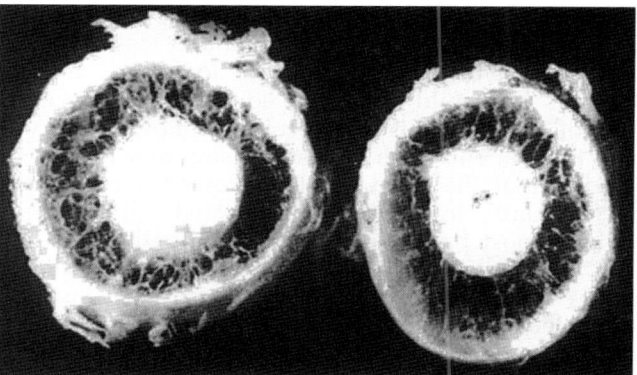

Figure 162.6 Gross pathological specimen of optic nerve (central core), optic nerve sheath, and arachnoid trabeculations. Note the well-developed series of arachnoid trabeculations and the full distended optic nerve sheaths (from [82]).

optic nerve sheaths [Figure 162.6], fenestration may be effective), and 6) moderate visual loss with severe papilledema that is not improving. The relationship between papilledema and loss of vision is complex. With the loss of axons, papilledema can regress while vision worsens. More often, however, the more severe the papilledema, the worse the loss of vision. This is true for case series,[16] but occasionally patients have marked papilledema and little loss of vision. Generally, because the worse the papilledema, the worse the visual loss, this factor has to be used in treatment decisions, especially if the grade of papilledema is increasing.

Optic nerve sheath fenestration usually produces immediate results, with improvement in vision occurring over several months. The procedure usually is performed on the eye with the worse vision, and often vision recovers and papilledema is decreased in the unoperated eye, and this can persist for months or even years. However, patients should expect eventually to have fenestration performed on both eyes. Although headache relief can occur after optic nerve sheath fenestration, the definitive procedure for intractable headache in IIH is a shunting procedure.

Who should treat patients who have IIH? If a neuro-ophthalmologist is not available, a neurologist should collaborate with an ophthalmologist. The ophthalmologist should provide quantitative assessment of visual function (perimetry testing) and should monitor the degree of papilledema. The latter should be done with serial fundus photographs. The neurologist should not use visual evoked potential to follow patients with IIH. This test is insensitive for monitoring the loss of vision associated with IIH,[94] because the loss occurs predominantly outside the central 10° until late in the disease and is not adequately monitored with visual evoked potentials. Also, visual acuity measurements are insensitive until late in the disease.

Follow-up

There is no "fixed" formula for the time needed to monitor patients with IIH. The frequency of re-evaluation after beginning therapy depends mainly on the severity of the papilledema and loss of vision and the rate of progression of the loss. For example, patients with mild optic disk edema who have mild loss of vision that is stable can be followed every 6 months. Patients with a loss of vision that is mild to moderate at the onset can be followed every 2 to 4 weeks until improvement is noted. The author follows most patients every 1 to 3 months until the loss of vision is stable. However, patients with a severe loss of vision should have emergency surgery (optic nerve sheath fenestration or a shunting procedure) or be followed daily to weekly until their condition improves.

When the patient's condition becomes stable or improves, the examination intervals are gradually extended. The follow-up examination should include quantitative visual field examination, stereophotographs of the optic disks if there has been any change in their appearance, and screening for a relative afferent pupillary defect with the alternating light test.

The success of a therapy is judged by the stability or recovery of vision, headache relief, elimination of transient visual obscurations and diplopia, and decreased papilledema. Repeated fundus photographs are more helpful in accurately assessing papilledema than descriptions of the optic disk. However, Frisén's papilledema grading scheme of Frisén should be used if fundus photographs are not available.[95]

Treatment failure is defined as the persistence of headache, diplopia, transient obscurations of vision, or loss of vision. Although papilledema usually disappears within months after treatment is initiated, it may remain for a year or more, with varying effects on vision.

Treatment of headache

The headaches occasionally improve after a single lumbar puncture, but more often, they remain as a major management problem even after medications have been given to reduce edema and CSF production. The author has had reasonably good success with standard prophylactic vascular headache remedies. However, try to avoid medications that cause hypotension, such as β-blockers or calcium channel blockers, because they may decrease perfusion of the optic nerve head. Tricyclic antidepressants can cause a problem because weight gain is one of the side effects. The author prescribes tricyclics at low dose (e.g., amitriptyline, 25 mg orally at bedtime) and nonsteroidal anti-inflammatory agents but only 2 days per week. Topiramate may be useful both for its migraine prophylaxis and carbonic anhydrase inhibition.

It is rare that repeated lumbar puncture is useful or necessary as treatment for headache. Uncommonly, lumboperitoneal shunting or another CSF diversion procedure is needed for persistent headache, but it can produce the "hindbrain herniation" headache. Patients with IIH also have other headache syndromes. Especially in patients with a history of migraine, analgesic rebound or caffeine rebound headaches may coexist. These patients may require dihydroergotamine administered intravenously to treat this troublesome headache syndrome.

Treatment of pregnant women

Digre et al.[4] have reviewed the relationship of IIH and pregnancy and reported that pregnancy occurs among women with IIH at the same rate as among women in the general population and IIH occur in any trimester. Pregnant women with IIH do not have an increased rate of spontaneous abortion. Digre et al. concluded that therapeutic abortion to limit progressive disease is not indicated. The author agrees that a pregnant woman with IIH should be given the same treatment as any other patient with IIH.[4] Also, the pregnancy should be managed as any other. The only exception is caloric restriction, because of its adverse effect of ketosis on the fetus. Weight gain can be limited to 20 lb, which is usually sufficient to help control the disease.

Summary

IIH is a disease of young overweight women that can result in blindness if not treated adequately. Effective treatment strategies appear to be available. Headaches usually become manageable, papilledema regresses, and vision improves in most patients. Treatment is as much art as a science because there are no controlled clinical trials. A properly constructed and controlled treatment trial surely would teach us much about managing IIH.

References

1. Durcan FJ, Corbett JJ, Wall M. The incidence of pseudotumor cerebri. Population studies in Iowa and Louisiana. Arch Neurol 1988;45:875–877
2. Radhakrishnan K, Ahlskog JE, Cross SA, et al. Idiopathic intracranial hypertension (pseudotumor cerebri). Descriptive epidemiology in Rochester, Minn, 1976 to 1990. Arch Neurol 1993;50:78–80
3. Balcer LJ, Liu GT, Forman S, Pun K, et al. Idiopathic intracranial hypertension: relation of age and obesity in children. Neurology 1999;52:870–872
4. Digre KB, Corbett JJ. Pseudotumor cerebri in men. Arch Neurol 1988;45:866–872
5. Ireland B, Corbett J, Wallace RB. The search for causes of idiopathic intracranial hypertension. A preliminary case-control study. Arch Neurol 1990;47:315–320
6. Giuseffi V, Wall M, Siegel PZ, Rojas PB. Symptoms and disease associations in idiopathic intracranial hypertension (pseudotumor cerebri): a case-control study. Neurology 1991;41:239–244
7. Sahs AL, Joynt RJ. Brain swelling of unknown cause. Neurology 1956;6:791–803
8. Wall M, Dollar JD, Sadun AA, Kardon R. Idiopathic intracranial hypertension: Lack of histologic evidence for cerebral edema. Arch Neurol 1995;52:141–145
9. Wall M. The headache profile of idiopathic intracranial hypertension. Cephalalgia 1990;10:331–335
10. Sadun AA, Currie JN, Lessell S. Transient visual obscurations with elevated optic discs. Ann Neurol 1984;16:489–494

11. Bulens C, Meerwaldt JD, Koudstaal PJ, van der Wildt GJ. Spatial contrast sensitivity in benign intracranial hypertension. J Neurol Neurosurg Psychiatry 1988;51: 1323–1329

12. Corbett JJ. The 1982 Silversides lecture. Problems in the diagnosis and treatment of pseudotumor cerebri. Can J Neurol Sci 1983;10:221–229

13. Rush JA. Pseudotumor cerebri: clinical profile and visual outcome in 63 patients. Mayo Clin Proc 1980;55: 541–546

14. Meador KJ, Swift TR. Tinnitus from intracranial hypertension. Neurology 1984;34:1258–1261

15. Sismanis A. Otologic manifestations of benign intracranial hypertension syndrome: diagnosis and management. Laryngoscope 1987;97(Suppl 42):1–17

16. Wall M, White WN II. Asymmetric papilledema in idiopathic intracranial hypertension: prospective interocular comparison of sensory visual function. Invest Ophthalmol Vis Sci 1998;39:134–142

17. Wall M, George D. Idiopathic intracranial hypertension. A prospective study of 50 patients. Brain 1991; 114:155–180

18. Wall M. Idiopathic intracranial hypertension. Neurol Clin 1991;9:73–95

19. Smith JL. Whence pseudotumor cerebri? J Clin Neuroophthalmol 1985;5:55–56

20. Deonna T, Guignard JP. Acute intracranial hypertension after nalidixic acid administration. Arch Dis Child 1974;49:743

21. Mushet GR. Pseudotumor and nitrofurantoin therapy (letter). Arch Neurol 1977;34:257

22. Konomi H, Imai M, Nihei K, et al. Indomethacin causing pseudotumor cerebri in Bartter's syndrome (letter). N Engl J Med 1978;298:855

23. Larizza D, Colombo A, Lorini R, Severi F. Ketoprofen causing pseudotumor cerebri in Bartter's syndrome (letter). N Engl J Med 1979;300:796

24. Feldman MH, Schlezinger NS. Benign intracranial hypertension associated with hypervitaminosis A. Arch Neurol 1970;22:1–7

25. Spector RH, Carlisle J. Pseudotumor cerebri caused by a synthetic vitamin A preparation. Neurology 1984;34: 1509–1511

26. Van Dop C, Conte FA, Koch TK, et al. Pseudotumor cerebri associated with initiation of levothyroxine therapy for juvenile hypothyroidism. N Engl J Med 1983;308:1076–1080

27. Saul RF, Hamburger HA, Selhorst JB. Pseudotumor cerebri secondary to lithium carbonate. JAMA 1985;253: 2869–2870

28. Shah A, Roberts T, McQueen IN, et al. Danazol and benign intracranial hypertension. Br Med J 1987;294: 1323

29. Chiu AM, Chuenkongkaew WL, Cornblath WT, et al. Minocycline treatment and pseudotumor cerebri syndrome. Am J Ophthalmol 1998;126:116–121

30. Gardner K, Cox T, Digre KB. Idiopathic intracranial hypertension associated with tetracycline use in fraternal twins: case reports and review. Neurology 1995;45: 6–10

31. Greer M. Benign intracranial hypertension. II. Following corticosteroid therapy. Neurology 1963;13:439–441

32. Neville BG, Wilson J. Benign intracranial hypertension following corticosteroid withdrawal in childhood. Br Med J 1970;3:554–556

33. Walsh FB. Papilledema associated with increased intracranial pressure in Addison's disease. Arch Ophthalmol 1952;47:86

34. Newborg B. Pseudotumor cerebri treated by rice reduction diet. Arch Intern Med 1974;133:802–807

35. Kupersmith MJ, Gamell L, Turbin R, et al. Effects of weight loss on the course of idiopathic intracranial hypertension in women. Neurology 1998;50:1094–1098

36. Johnson LN, Krohel GB, Madsen RW, March GA Jr. The role of weight loss and acetazolamide in the treatment of idiopathic intracranial hypertension (pseudotumor cerebri). Ophthalmology 1998;105: 2313–2317

37. Greer M. Benign intracranial hypertension. VI. Obesity. Neurology 1965;15:382–388

38. Amaral JF, Tsiaris W, Morgan T, Thompson WR. Reversal of benign intracranial hypertension by surgically induced weight loss. Arch Surg 1987;122:946–949

39. Sugerman HJ, Felton WL III, Sismanis A, et al. Gastric surgery for pseudotumor cerebri associated with severe obesity. Ann Surg 1999;229:634–640

40. Friedman DI, Streeten DH. Idiopathic intracranial hypertension and orthostatic edema may share a common pathogenesis. Neurology 1998;50:1099–1104

41. Johnston I, Paterson A. Benign intracranial hypertension. II. CSF pressure and circulation. Brain 1974;97: 301–312

42. Weisberg LA. Benign intracranial hypertension. Medicine (Baltimore) 1975;54:197–207

43. Batnitzky S, Keucher TR, Mealey T Jr, Campbell RL. Iatrogenic intraspinal epidermoid tumors. JAMA 1977; 237:148–150

44. Manno NJ, Uihlein A, Kernohan JW. Intraspinal epidermoids. J Neurosurg 1962;19:754–765

45. Paterson R, DePasquale N, Mann S. Pseudotumor cerebri. Medicine (Baltimore) 1961;40:85–99

46. Weisberg LA, Chutorian AM. Pseudotumor cerebri of childhood. Am J Dis Child 1977;131:1243–1248

47. Jefferson A, Clark J. Treatment of benign intracranial hypertension by dehydrating agents with particular reference to the measurement of the blind spot area as a means of recording improvement. J Neurol Neurosurg Psychiatry 1976;39:627–639

48. Guisado R, Tourtellotte WW, Arieff AI, et al. Rebound phenomenon complicating cerebral dehydration with glycerol. Case report. J Neurosurg 1975;42:226–228

49. Rottenberg DA, Hurwitz BJ, Posner JB. The effect of oral glycerol on intraventricular pressure in man. Neurology 1977;27:600–608

50. Ahmad S. Amiodarone and reversible benign intracranial hypertension (letter). Cardiology 87:90

51. McCarthy KD, Reed DJ. The effect of acetazolamide and furosemide on cerebrospinal fluid production and choroid plexus carbonic anhydrase activity. J Pharmacol Exp Ther 1974;189:194–201

52. Lubow M, Kuhr L. Pseudotumor cerebri: comments on practical management. In: Glaser JS, Smith JL, eds. Neuro-ophthalmology, Vol. IX. St Louis: CV Mosby 1976:199–206

53. Gucer G, Viernstein L. Long-term intracranial pressure recording in management of pseudotumor cerebri. J Neurosurg 1978;49:256–263

54. Tomsak RL, Niffenegger AS, Remler BF. Treatment of pseudotumor cerebri with Diamox (acetazolamide). J Clin Neuroophthalmol 1988;8:93–98

55. Rubin RC Henderson ES, Ommaya AK, et al. The production of cerebrospinal fluid in man and its modification by acetazolamide. J Neurosurg 1966;25:430–436

56. Lichter PR. Reducing side effects of carbonic anhydrase inhibitors. Ophthalmology 1981;88(3):266–269

57. Garner LL, Carl EF, Ferwerda JR. Advantages of sus-

tained-release therapy with acetazolamide in glaucoma. Am J Ophthalmol 1963;55:323–327

58. Zimran A, Beutler E. Can the risk of acetazolamide-
induced aplastic anemia be decreased by periodic monitoring of blood cell counts? Am J Ophthalmol 1987;104:
654–658

59. Pollay M, Fullenwider C, Roberts PA, Stevens FA.
Effect of mannitol and furosemide on blood–brain
osmotic gradient and intracranial pressure. J Neurosurg 1983;59:945–950

60. Roberts PA, Pollay M, Engles C, et al. Effect on
intracranial pressure of furosemide combined with
varying doses and administration rates of mannitol. J
Neurosurg 1987;66:440–446

61. Vogh BP, Langham MR Jr. The effect of furosemide and
bumetanide on cerebrospinal fluid formation. Brain
1981;221:171–183

62. Cottrell JE, Robustelli A, Post K, Turndorf H.
Furosemide- and mannitol-induced changes in
intracranial pressure and serum osmolality and electrolytes. Anesthesiology 1977;47:28–30

63. Buhrley LE, Reed DJ. The effect of furosemide on
sodium-22 uptake into cerebrospinal fluid and brain.
Exp Brain Res 1972;14:503–510

64. Schoeman JF. Childhood pseudotumor cerebri: clinical
and intracranial pressure response to acetazolamide
and furosemide treatment in a case series. J Child
Neurol 1994;9:130–134

65. Schoeman J, Donald P, van Zyl L, et al. Tuberculous
hydrocephalus: comparison of different treatments
with regard to ICP, ventricular size and clinical
outcome. Med Child Neurol 1991;33:396–405

66. Dandy WE. Intracranial pressure without brain tumor:
diagnosis and treatment. Ann Surg 1937;106:492–513

67. Bradshaw P. Benign intracranial hypertension. J Neurol
Neurosurg Psychiatry 1956;19:28–41

68. Bulens C, De Vries WA, van Crevel H. Benign intracranial hypertension. A retrospective and follow-up study.
J Neurol Sci 1979;40:147–157

69. Wilson DH, Gardner WJ. Benign intracranial hypertension with particular reference to its occurrence in fat
young women. Can Med Assoc J 1966;95:102–105

70. Greer M. Benign intracranial hypertension. Pseudotumor cerebri. In: Vinken PJ, Bruyn GW, eds. Handbook
of Clinical Neurology. New York: Elsevier, 1974:
150–166

71. Davidoff LM. Pseudotumor cerebri. Benign intracranial
hypertension. Neurology 1956;6:605–615

72. Kessler LA, Novelli PM, Reigel DH. Surgical treatment
of benign intracranial hypertension-subtemporal
decompression revisited. Surg Neurol 1998;50:73–76

73. DeWecker L. On incision of the optic nerve in cases of
neuroretinitis. Int Ophthalmol Congr Rep 1872;4:11–14

74. Hayreh SS. Pathogenesis of oedema of the optic disc
(papilloedema): a preliminary report. Br J Ophthalmol
1964;48:522–543

75. Smith JL, Hoyt WF, Newton TH. Optic nerve sheath
decompression for relief of chronic monocular choked
disc. Am J Ophthalmol 1969;68:633–639

76. Hamed LM, Tse DT, Glaser JS, et al. Neuroimaging of
the optic nerve after fenestration for management of
pseudotumor cerebri. Arch Ophthalmol 1992;110:
636–639

77. Keltner JL, Albert DA, Lubow M, et al. Optic nerve
decompression. A clinical pathologic study. Arch Ophthalmol 1977;95:97–104

78. Smith CH, Orcutt JC. Surgical treatment of pseudotumor cerebri. Int Ophthalmol Clin 1986;26:265–275

79. Goh KY, Schatz NJ, Glaser JS. Optic nerve sheath fenestration for pseudotumor cerebri. J Neuroophthalmol
1997;17:86–91

80. Acheson JF, Green WT, Sanders MD. Optic nerve
sheath decompression for the treatment of visual
failure in chronic raised intracranial pressure. J Neurol
Neurosurg Psychiatry 1994;57:1426–1429

81. Kelman SE, Heaps R, Wolf A, Elman MJ. Optic nerve
decompression surgery improves visual function in
patients with pseudotumor cerebri. Neurosurgery
1992;30:391–395

82. Sergott RC, Savino PJ, Bosley TM. Modified optic nerve
sheath decompression provides long-term visual
improvement for pseudotumor cerebri. Arch Ophthalmol 1988;106:1384–1390

83. Corbett JJ, Nerad JA, Tse DT, Anderson RL. Results of
optic nerve sheath fenestration for pseudotumor
cerebri: the lateral orbitotomy approach. Arch Ophthalmol 1988;106:1391–1397

84. Plotnik JL, Kosmorsky GS. Operative complications of
optic nerve sheath decompression. Ophthalmology
1993;100:683–690

85. Brourman ND, Spoor TC, Ramocki JM. Optic nerve
sheath decompression for pseudotumor cerebri. Arch
Ophthalmol 1988;106:1378–1383

86. Rizzo JF III, Lessell S. Choroidal infarction after optic
nerve sheath fenestration. Ophthalmology 1994;101:
1622–1626

87. Spoor TC, McHenry JG. Long-term effectiveness of
optic nerve sheath decompression for pseudotumor
cerebri. Arch Ophthalmol 1993;111:632–635

88. Wall M, Johnson CA, Kutzko KE, et al. Long- and
short-term variability of automated perimetry results in
patients with optic neuritis and healthy subjects. Arch
Ophthalmol 1998;116:53–61

89. Johnston I, Besser M, Morgan MK. Cerebrospinal fluid
diversion in the treatment of benign intracranial hypertension. J Neurosurg 1988;69:195–202

90. Burgett RA, Purvin VA, Kawasaki A. Lumboperitoneal
shunting for pseudotumor cerebri. Neurology 1997;49:
734–739

91. Eggenberger ER, Miller NR, Vitale S. Lumboperitoneal
shunt for the treatment of pseudotumor cerebri. Neurology 1996;46:1524–1530

92. Rosenberg M, Smith C, Beck R, et al. The efficacy of
shunting procedures in pseudotumor cerebri (abstract).
Neurology 1989;39:209

93. Wall M, Weisberg LA. Treatment of pseudotumor
cerebri. In: Johnson RT, ed. Current Therapy in Neurologic Disease. Philadelphia: BC Decker, 1984:226–230

94. Verplanck M, Kaufman DI, Parsons T, et al. Electrophysiology versus psychophysics in the detection of
visual loss in pseudotumor cerebri. Neurology
1988;38:1789–1792

95. Frisén L. Swelling of the optic nerve head: a staging
scheme. J Neurol Neurosurg Psychiatry 1982;45:13–18

96. Corbett JJ, Mehta MP. Cerebrospinal fluid pressure in
normal obese subjects and patients with pseudotumor
cerebri. Neurology 1983;33:1386–1388

97. Headache Classification Committee of the International
Headache Society. Classification and diagnostic criteria
for headache disorders, cranial neuralgias and facial
pain. Cephalalgia 1988;8(Suppl 7):1–96

163 Chiasm and Retrochiasmal Disorders

Andrew G Lee and Paul W Brazis

Overview

The optic chiasm, from the Greek letter *chi* (χ), is formed by the convergence of the optic nerves anteriorly and the divergence of the optic tracts posteriorly.[1] Chiasmal syndromes may be divided into those that affect the anterior chiasm (junction of the optic nerve and chiasm), the body of the optic chiasm, or the posterior chiasm. Thorough knowledge of the topographical anatomy allows the clinician to differentiate these syndromes.

Optic chiasm

Anterior chiasm: anatomy of the junction of the optic nerve and chiasm

The nerve fibers originate in the retina and follow a specific topographical path in the optic nerve and chiasm. The intracranial optic nerves extend posteriorly from the optic foramen and join at the optic chiasm. Within the chiasm, fibers from the nasal retina of each eye cross into the contralateral optic tract, and fibers from the temporal retina pass uncrossed into the ipsilateral optic tract. Within the intracranial optic nerve, the crossed (nasal retinal) and uncrossed (temporal retinal) fibers are separated anatomically at the junction of the optic nerve and chiasm. In addition, inferior nasal crossing fibers had previously been postulated to loop anteriorly for a short distance into the contralateral optic nerve. These fibers were traditionally referred to as the "anterior knee" or "Wilbrand knee."

Recently, the existence of Wilbrand knee has been questioned. Wilbrand was restricted to examining human subjects who had undergone enucleation. In the enucleated eye, the nerve fibers atrophied and became distinct from the nerve fibers of the normal eye and could be distinguished with myelin staining. With the use of axon-labelling techniques in nonenucleated monkeys, Horton[2] was not able to demonstrate crossing fibers looping into the contralateral optic nerve (Wilbrand knee). However, in a monkey that had undergone enucleation 4 years earlier, the nerve fiber topography was similar to that described by Wilbrand. Horton[2] hypothesized that Wilbrand knee may be an artifact of enucleation caused by atrophy of the optic nerve and not a normal anatomical finding. Nevertheless, whether Wilbrand knee exists anatomically, the localizing value of junctional visual field loss to the junction of the optic nerve and chiasm is not diminished because chiasmal compression alone may result in a contralateral superotemporal visual field defect (junctional scotoma).

Clinical features

Junctional lesions Because of the unique topographical anatomy of the junction, compressive lesions at the junction of the intracranial optic nerve and optic chiasm produce characteristic visual field defects. Involvement of the optic nerve at its junction with the optic chiasm may result in unilateral visual field loss (ipsilateral optic neuropathy with loss of acuity, color vision, etc.), and if fibers from the inferonasal retina of the contralateral eye (chiasm or presumed Wilbrand knee) are involved, there is also a superotemporal visual field defect in the contralateral eye (junctional scotoma) (Figure 163.1).[3]

In addition, selective compression of the crossed or uncrossed visual fibers at the junction may result in a unilateral temporal or nasal hemianopic field defect, respectively (Figure 163.2).

Traquair[4] used the term "junction scotoma" to refer to a unilateral temporal hemicentral field defect due to compression of the nasal fibers in the intracranial optic nerve at the junction of the optic nerve and chiasm. Miller[5] emphasized that the junctional

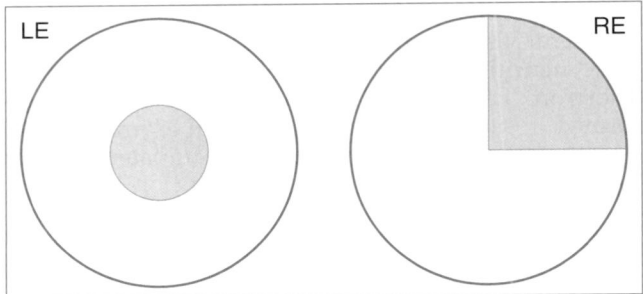

Figure 163.1 Junctional scotoma. Left eye (*LE*) has a dense central scotoma, and the right eye (*RE*) has a superotemporal visual field defect.

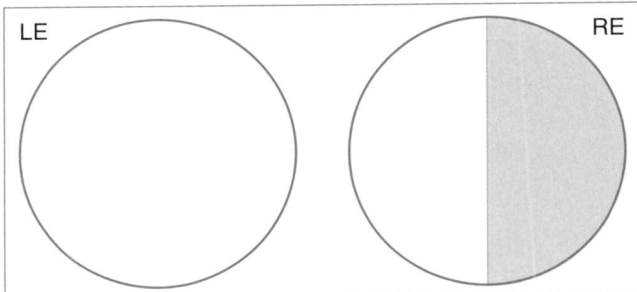

Figure 163.2 Junctional scotoma of Traquair. Left eye (*LE*) is normal, and right eye (*RE*) has a dense monocular temporal hemianopic visual field defect.

scotoma described by Traquair refers to a strictly unilateral temporal scotoma that is assumed to arise from
a lesion at the junction of the optic nerve and chiasm.
However, confusion has arisen regarding the use of
the term "junctional scotoma." In contrast to the
defect described by Traquair, some authors have used
junctional scotoma to refer to ipsilateral optic neuropathy with a contralateral superotemporal visual
field defect. This superotemporal defect is due to
compression of the inferonasal fibers from the contralateral eye travelling in the presumed Wilbrand
knee or the optic chiasm itself.

To clarify this, Smith recommended that the unilateral temporal visual field defect described by
Traquair should be referred to as the "junctional
scotoma of Traquair" to differentiate it from the contralateral superotemporal defect more commonly
referred to as "junctional scotoma."[5]

Trobe and Glaser[6] thought that junctional visual
field loss would be due to a mass lesion in 98 out of
100 cases. The differential diagnosis for junctional
syndrome includes pituitary tumors, suprasellar
meningiomas, supraclinoid aneurysms, craniopharyngiomas, and gliomas.[7–10] Chiasmal neuritis, pachymeningitis, and trauma are rare causes of the
junctional syndrome.[11,12]

Thus, patients with the junctional scotoma of
Traquair or junctional scotoma should be considered
to have a compressive lesion at the junction of
the optic nerve and chiasm until proven otherwise.
Neuroimaging (preferably magnetic resonance
imaging [MRI]) should be directed to this location.
Patients with junctional scotoma may be unaware of a
small superotemporal visual field defect, and strictly
unilateral visual complaints may be misdiagnosed as
optic neuritis or other unilateral optic neuropathy.
Therefore, careful visual field testing should be performed in the contralateral (and often asymptomatic)
eye of any patient with presumed unilateral visual
loss.

Body of the chiasm lesions Lesions of the body of
the chiasm typically produce bitemporal hemianopic
field loss (Figure 163.3). The bitemporal hemianopia
may be peripheral, paracentral, or central, and it may
"split" or "spare" the macular central 5-degree field
(Figure 163.4). The defect usually is the result of a

compressive mass lesion at the level of the optic
chiasm (Figure 163.5).[5,13] Neuroimaging (preferably
MRI) should be directed at the optic chiasm.

Posterior chiasm lesions Posterior chiasm lesions
may produce paracentral bitemporal hemianopic field
defects that may be mistaken for cecocentral field loss
(Figure 163.6). However, color vision and visual
acuity are usually spared (unlike true cecocentral scotomas caused by bilateral optic neuropathies such as
toxic-nutritional disease). Further posterior extension
of a posterior chiasmal lesion may result in homonymous hemianopia because of involvement of the optic
tract or a combination of visual field defects involving
both the chiasm and tract.

Treatment of suprasellar or chiasmal lesions

Treatment of a suprasellar or chiasmal lesion depends
on the cause (Tables 163.1 and 163.2). Exposure to
toxins should be discontinued. Vitamin deficiency
(e.g., vitamin B_{12}) may improve after replacement
therapy. Demyelinating lesions often improve spontaneously or after a short course of corticosteroid
treatment (e.g., intravenous methylprednisolone).

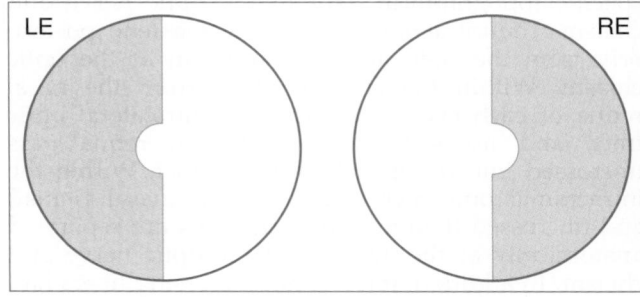

Figure 163.4 Bitemporal hemianopia with macular
sparing. *LE*, left eye; *RE*, right eye.

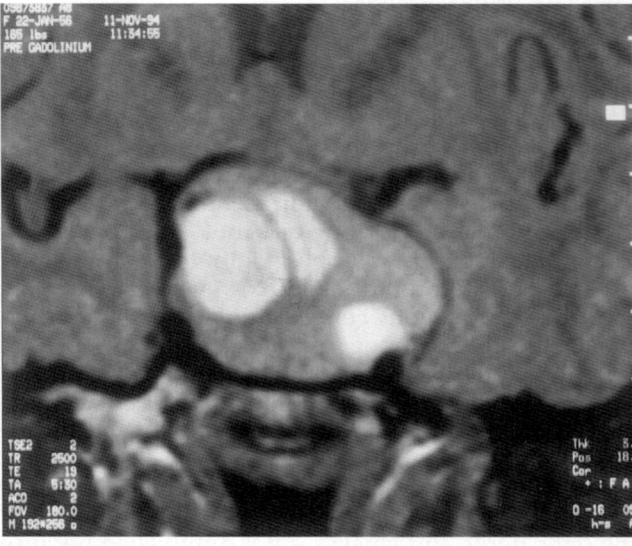

Figure 163.5 Coronal magnetic resonance image showing
large intracellular mass with suprasellar extension. (By
permission of Andrew G Lee MD.)

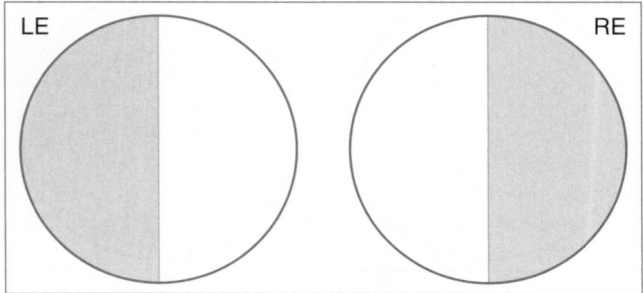

Figure 163.3 Bitemporal hemianopia. *LE*, left eye; *RE*,
right eye.

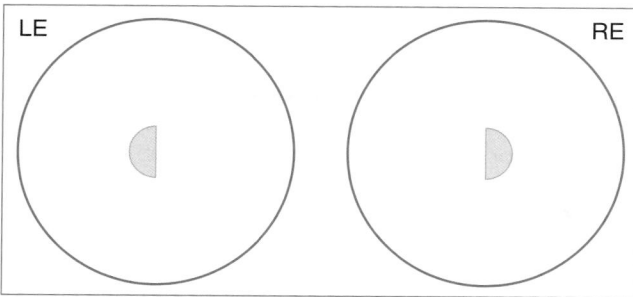

Figure 163.6 Bitemporal paracentral defects. *LE*, left eye; *RE*, right eye.

Infectious causes (e.g., syphilis, tuberculosis) should be treated with specific antibiotic agents. Inflammatory causes (e.g., sarcoidosis, vasculitis) may respond to immunosuppressive treatment (e.g., corticosteroids). Traumatic lesions are usually observed. The options for treatment of a suprasellar or chiasmal mass lesion include no treatment, medical therapy, surgery, or radiotherapy.

Observation An asymptomatic suprasellar mass may not require surgery. Visual loss due to external compression on the optic nerve, chiasm, or tract is usually an indication for treatment. Nevertheless, some patients with a suprasellar mass have systemic medical problems that place them at an unacceptably high risk for perioperative morbidity or mortality. These patients are often observed. In addition, intrinsic parenchymal chiasmal lesions such as chiasmal glioma cannot be surgically resected without unacceptable morbidity and are often observed clinically and radiographically for progression. Other lesions such as giant internal carotid artery aneurysms are too large for a safe surgical approach or have too wide a neck for endovascular treatment.

Medical treatment Medical therapy has been a mainstay of treatment for prolactinoma. Dopamine from the hypothalamus is a physiological regulator (tonic inhibitor) of normal prolactin secretion. Bromocriptine is an effective dopamine agonist that has been used in the treatment of prolactin-secreting pituitary adenomas. Other dopamine agonists include lisuride, pergolide, and cabergoline.[168–175] The alleviation of symptoms and signs (e.g., galactorrhea, amenorrhea, libido, and fertility restoration), normalization of prolactin level, and tumor shrinkage have been well documented during dopaminergic treatment.[168–170] The benefits of medical therapy have to be weighed against the relatively high success rate for selective transsphenoidal surgery (as high as 80%) for small adenomas. Nevertheless, medical therapy should be considered for patients with prolactinoma. In cases of pituitary apoplexy, systemic corticosteroid replacement therapy should be initiated.

Surgical treatment Surgical decompression or excision of suprasellar lesions may be considered if

Table 163.1	Compressive chiasmal syndromes

Most common
    Pituitary apoplexy[14,15]
    Pituitary tumor (especially pituitary adenoma)[10,16–26]
    Meningioma[27–30]
    Craniopharyngioma[31–33]
    Dysgerminoma[34–36]
    Suprasellar aneurysm[7,8,37–41]
    Chiasmal glioma[42–45]
Less common
    Abscess[46,47]
    Arachnoid cyst[48–51]
    Aspergillosis[52,53]
    Cavernous hemangioma[54–59]
    Chiasmal hematoma[60–62]
    Chordoma[63,64]
    Choristoma
    Colloid cyst of the third ventricle
    Dermoid
    Dolichoectatic sclerotic internal carotid arteries[65–67]
    Ependymoma[68]
    Epidermoid
    Fibrous dysplasia
    Granular cell myoblastoma[69]
    Ganglioglioma[70]
    Hemangioblastoma[71]
    Histiocytosis X[72,73]
    Hydrocephalus and distention of the third ventricle
    Leukemia and lymphoma[74–76]
    Lymphocytic hypophysitis[77–87]
    Lymphohistiocytosis[88]
    Melanoma[89]
    Meningeal carcinomatosis
    Metastatic disease[90] to brain or pituitary gland[63,91–95]
    Mucocele or mucopyocele[96]
    Sphenoid sinus disease[97]
    Multiple myeloma[98]
    Nasopharyngeal cancer
    Non-neoplastic pituitary gland enlargement[99,100]
    Plasmacytoma[101]
    Rathke cleft cyst[102–106]
    Sarcoid granuloma[107–109]
    Septum pellucidum cyst[110]
    Sinus tumors
    Syphilitic granuloma
    Teratoma[34]
    Vascular malformation[111–113]
    Venous angioma[114]

From Lee AG, Brazis PW. Clinical Pathways in Neuro-Ophthalmology: An Evidence-Based Approach. New York: Thieme, 1998:151–170. By permission of the publisher.

medical therapy fails or if the patient is intolerant of, not a candidate for, or declines medical therapy. Visual symptoms (e.g., loss of vision or diplopia) may improve after decompression. The advantages of surgery are that smaller tumors may be resected completely, a pathological diagnosis can be made, and compressive effects (e.g., visual loss) are relieved immediately.

The results of transsphenoidal surgery in pituitary adenoma have been studied extensively. Giovanelli et al.[176] reviewed the surgical results in 36 series of

Table 163.2   **Less common causes of chiasmal syndrome**
Cobalamin deficiency[115]
Demyelinating disease[11,115–121]
Empty sella syndrome (primary or secondary)[44,110,122–126]
Chiasmal ischemia[127–129]
Optochiasmatic arachnoiditis[130–132]
Foreign body-induced granuloma (e.g., muslin)
Idiopathic
Infection[133]
Chronic fungal infection
Cryptococcus[134]
Encephalitis
Meningitis
Mucormycosis[135]
Nasopharyngeal and sinus infections
Syphilis[136]
Tuberculosis[137,138]
Inflammatory[133]
Collagen vascular disease[139]
Rheumatoid pachymeningitis[12]
Sarcoidosis[140,141]
Multiple sclerosis[142]
Posthemorrhagic
Posttraumatic[143]
Radiation necrosis[144–147]
Shunt catheter[148–150]
Fat packing after transsphenoidal hypophysectomy[151,152]
Toxic
Ethchlorvynol (Placidyl)
Pheniprazine (Catron)
Trauma, including postsurgical[153–165]
Vascular occlusion[65,128,166]
Vasculitis[115]
Venous aneurysm arising from carotid-cavernous sinus fistula[167]

From Lee AG, Brazis PW. Clinical Pathways in Neuro-Ophthalmology: An Evidence-Based Approach. New York: Thieme, 1998:151–170. By permission of the publisher.

acromegaly and reported a mean rate of 79.3% (range, 56% to 100%) for the control of growth hormone levels. Luedecke et al[177] reviewed 7 series on transsphenoidal surgery for Cushing syndrome and reported total remission rates between 70% and 85%, and Reilly[178] reviewed 16 series of prolactinomas, and the improvement rate ranged from 60% to 90%. Visual function improved postoperatively in most patients (70% to 75%) who had visual loss preoperatively.

Radiotherapy   Radiotherapy may be administered to selected suprasellar tumors. Patients with radiosensitive tumors who are poor candidates for surgical treatment or in whom this treatment fails may benefit from radiotherapy. Invasive tumors (e.g., cavernous sinus or internal carotid artery involvement) often cannot be totally resected and may be candidates for radiotherapy.

Retrochiasmal disorders

The retrochiasmal pathway is composed of the optic tracts, lateral geniculate body, optic radiations (in the temporal and parietal lobes), and the occipital cortex. Homonymous visual field loss is the rule with lesions of retrochiasmal pathways. Lesions of the anterior retrochiasmal pathway, including the optic tract and lateral geniculate body, tend to produce incongruous visual field defects (less similar in density and shape), but more posteriorly located lesions in the optic radiations and occipital cortex produce more congruous visual field defects. Generally, tumors produce sloping visual field defects, whereas vascular lesions produce sharply defined visual field defects. The localization of homonymous visual field defects depends on the nature of the visual field defect and associated neuro-ophthalmological and neurological findings. Complete homonymous hemianopias generally are only lateralizing and not localizing.

Clinical features of lesions of the optic tract

A complete unilateral lesion of the optic tract usually causes a complete macular-splitting homonymous hemianopia without impaired visual acuity unless the lesion involves the optic chiasm or nerve.[179] Partial optic tract lesions are more common than complete ones and result in incongruous visual field defects that may be relative scotomatas (Figure 163.7).[179–181] Optic tract lesions often are associated with a relative afferent pupillary defect (RAPD) in the eye with the temporal field loss (contralateral to the side of the lesion).[180,182,183] The presence of relative afferent pupillary defect, normal visual acuity, and a complete homonymous hemianopia usually localizes the lesion to the optic tract.[1] In addition, patients with optic tract lesions may develop a characteristic "wedge," "band," or "bow-tie" pallor in the contralateral optic nerve and more generalized pallor in the ipsilateral optic nerve (hemianopic optic atrophy).[1,179–183] Hemianopic optic atrophy indicates postchiasmal, preoptic radiation involvement (i.e., optic tract or lateral geniculate body damage); it also has been described rarely in congenital retrogeniculate lesions.[1,184,185]

Causes of optic tract lesions include space-occupying lesions (e.g., glioma, meningioma, craniopharyngioma, metastasis, pituitary adenoma, ectopic pinealoma, abscess), vascular lesions (e.g., aneurysms, arteriovenous malformations), demyelinating disease, and trauma (e.g., temporal lobectomy).[1,48,179,181,185–189] Iatrogenic causes include the tip of a catheter shunt impaling the tract[190,191] and after pallididotomy for Parkinson disease. A complete neurological examina-

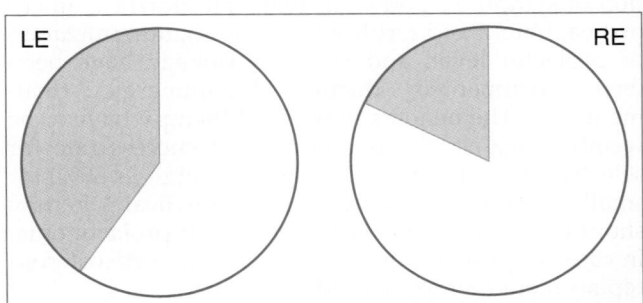

Figure 163.7   Left homonymous hemianopia, incongruous, denser superiorly. *LE*, left eye; *RE*, right eye.

tion and MRI study, with specific attention to the optic tract, are warranted. If MRI does not demonstrate the lesion, then angiography (magnetic resonance or cerebral) should be considered in nontraumatic cases to investigate for the presence of vascular lesions (e.g., aneurysm).[192]

Clinical features of lesions of the lateral geniculate body

Lesions of the lateral geniculate body may also cause a complete macular-splitting homonymous hemianopia.[1,193–195] Partial lesions result in an incongruous homonymous field defect. Hemianopic optic atrophy may develop, but no RAPD is present.

Although lesions of the optic tract or lateral geniculate body often cause incongruous field defects, two relatively specific patterns of congruous homonymous field defects with abruptly sloping borders, associated with sectorial optic atrophy, have been attributed to focal lesions of the lateral geniculate body caused by infarction in the territory of specific arteries. Occlusion of the anterior choroidal artery may cause a homonymous defect in the upper and lower quadrants with sparing of a horizontal sector (Figure 163.8).[196–198] This defect occurs because the lateral geniculate body is organized in projection columns oriented vertically that represent sectors of the field parallel to the horizontal meridians, and the anterior choroidal artery supplies the hilum and anterolateral part of the nucleus. Thus, bilateral lateral geniculate lesions may cause bilateral hourglass-shaped visual field defects[199,200] or bilateral blindness. In three reported cases of isolated bilateral involvement of the lateral geniculate bodies, the pathogenesis included anterior choroidal syphilitic arteritis, methanol toxicity producing coagulative necrosis of the nuclei, and geniculate myelinolysis associated with the rapid correction of hyponatremia.[199,201,202] Interruption of the posterior lateral choroidal artery, which perfuses the central portion of the lateral geniculate body, causes a horizontal (wedge-shaped) homonymous sector defect (Figure 163.9).[198,203–206] With infarction in the posterior lateral choroidal territory, the homonymous quadrantanopia may be associated with hemisensory loss, neuropsychological dysfunction (transcortical aphasia, memory disturbances), and delayed contralateral abnormal movements.[205] This visual field defect is not diagnostic of a lesion of the lateral geniculate body lesion because a similar defect may occur with a lesion affecting the optic radiations,[207] occipital cortex,[208] occipitotemporal junction, or parietotemporal region.[209]

Causes of lateral geniculate damage include infarction, arteriovenous malformation, trauma, tumor, inflammatory disorders, demyelinating disease, and toxic exposure (e.g., methanol).[193,194,196–206] MRI, with attention to the lateral geniculate body, is indicated in all cases.[203,205,210]

Clinical features of lesions of the optic radiations

Temporal lobe optic radiations   Lesions of the proximal portion of the optic radiations may result in com-

plete homonymous hemianopia with macular splitting.[211,212] Superior homonymous quadrantic defects ("pie-in-the-sky") may result from a lesion in the temporal lobe (Meyer loop) optic radiations (Figure 163.10).[213] The visual field defect is usually incongruous,[1] the inferior margins of the defects may have sloping borders and may cross the horizontal midline,[212] and the ipsilateral nasal field defect is often denser and comes closer to fixation than the defect in the contralateral eye. Macular vision may or may not be split.[1,214,215]

With involvement of the dominant temporal lobe, aphasic syndromes may occur. Lesions of the nondominant hemisphere may be associated with impaired recognition of facial expression of emotion, sensory amusia (inability to appreciate various

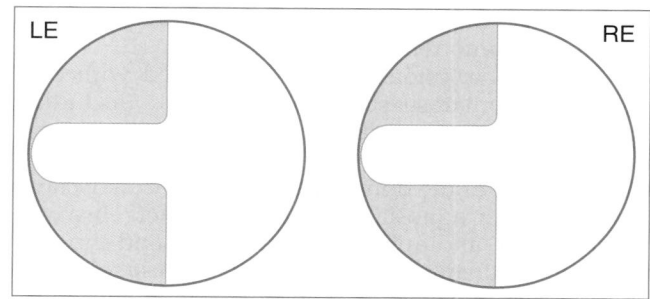

Figure 163.8   Left homonymous hemianopia with sparing of a wedge of central visual field extending to fixation. *LE*, left eye; *RE*, right eye.

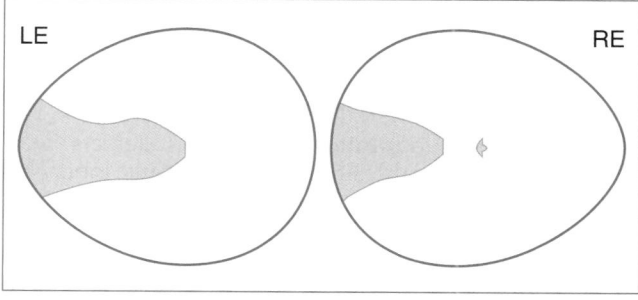

Figure 163.9   Left homonymous incongruous sectoranopia.

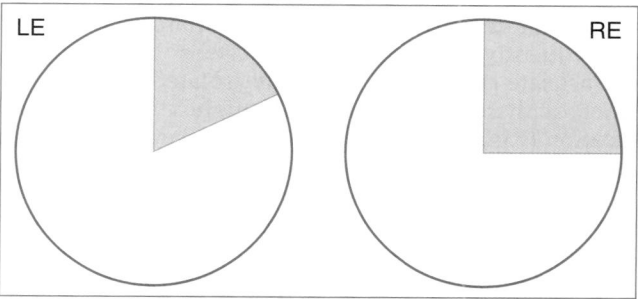

Figure 163.10   Right homonymous superior quadrantanopia, incongruous. *RE*, right eye; *LE*, left eye.

characteristics of heard music), and aprosodias (impaired appreciation of emotional overtones of spoken language). Other abnormalities that occur with temporal lobe dysfunction include memory impairment and seizures. The causes of temporal lobe dysfunction include space-occupying lesions (e.g., tumors, abscesses, hemorrhage), vascular lesions (arteriovenous malformations or infarction), infections, congenital lesions, demyelinating lesions, and trauma (e.g., temporal lobectomy).[189,211,214–216] MRI is required for all patients.

Parietal lobe optic radiations   Involvement of the optic radiations in the parietal lobe causes a congruous homonymous hemianopia, denser inferiorly (Figure 163.11). This defect usually is more congruous than the defect produced by a lesion of the temporal lobe, and because the entire optic radiation passes through the parietal lobe, a large lesion may produce a complete homonymous hemianopia.[1]

Parietal lobe lesions may be associated with contralateral somatosensory impairment (including impaired object recognition, impaired position sense, impaired touch and pain sensation, and tactile extinction). Lesions of the dominant parietal lobe may cause apraxia, finger agnosia, acalculia, right–left disorientation, alexia, and aphasic disturbances, and those of the nondominant lobe may be associated with anosognosia (denial of neurological impairment), autotopagnosia (failure to recognize hemiplegic limbs as belonging to self), spatial disorientation, hemispatial neglect, constructional apraxia (abnormal drawing and copying), and dressing apraxia. Pathological processes associated with parietal dysfunction are essentially the same as those associated with temporal lobe dysfunction and are best evaluated with MRI.[217]

Clinical features of lesions of the occipital lobe

Homonymous quadrantic visual field defects may occur with unilateral lesions of the occipital lobe.[213,218] Superior quadrantic defects may be seen with lesions of the inferior calcarine cortex and inferior quadrantic defects may occur with lesions of the superior calcarine cortex (Figure 163.12). Horton and Hoyt[218] have suggested that a lesion of the extrastriate cortex (areas V2 and V3) would be more likely to explain the sharp horizontal edge of the defect (Figure 163.13) because these areas are divided along the horizontal meridian into separate halves flanking the striate (V1) cortex; consequently, the upper and lower quadrants in extrastriate cortex are physically isolated on opposite sides of the striate cortex. Although a lesion in this location (e.g., tumor) may have irregular margins, if it crosses the representation of the horizontal meridian in extrastriate cortex, it will produce a quadrantic visual field defect with a sharp horizontal border because of the split arrangement of the upper and lower quadrants of V2 and V3. However, a congruous inferior quadrantanopia with borders aligned on both the vertical and horizontal meridians has also been described with a lesion of the superior fibers of the

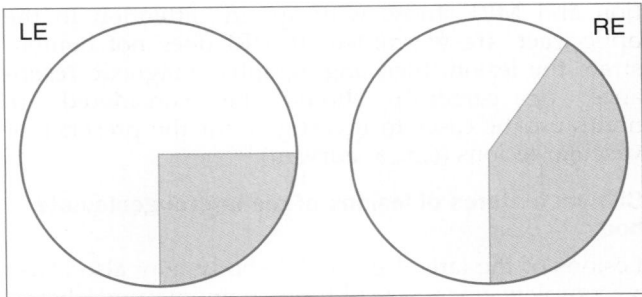

Figure 163.11   Right congruous inferior homonymous hemianopia. *LE*, left eye; *RE*, right eye.

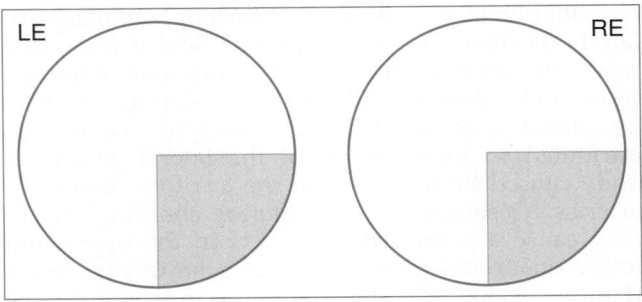

Figure 163.12   Right inferior congruous homonymous quadrantanopia. *LE*, left eye; *RE*, right eye.

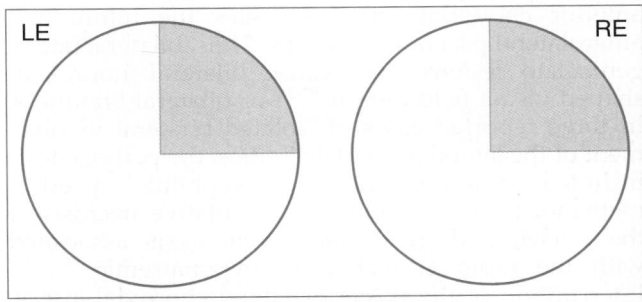

Figure 163.13   Right superior congruous homonymous quadrantanopia. *LE*, left eye; *RE*, right eye.

optic radiations near the contralateral trigone, where the fascicles of the axons in the radiation become compact as they approach calcarine cortex.[219]

Medial occipital lesions cause highly congruous homonymous field defects.[220,221] When both the upper and lower calcarine cortices are affected, a complete homonymous hemianopia, often with macular sparing, develops (Figure 163.14). Sparing of the central 5 degrees of vision (macular sparing) is common with occipital lesions, probably because of the combination of a large macular representation and dual blood supply.[1] The representation of the central 10 to 15 degrees of vision occupies as much as 50% to 60% of the total surface area of the occipital cortex.[220,222] Patients with purely occipital lesions are often aware of the hemianopia, as compared with patients who have larger or more anterior lesions affecting the parietal region or associative pathways to the primary or secondary visual association cortex who may be unaware of their deficit.[223]

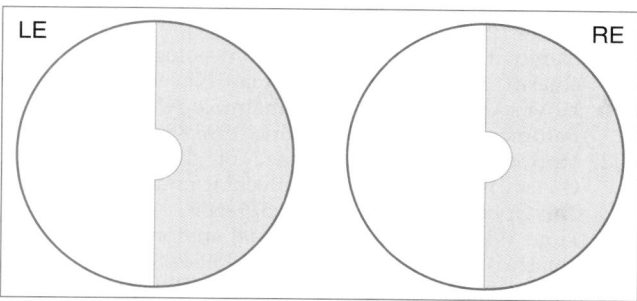

Figure 163.14 Right homonymous, macular-sparing hemianopia. *LE*, left eye; *RE*, right eye.

Lesions of the striate cortex may be classified into anterior, intermediate, and posterior lesions.[1,220,222,224–227] Anterior lesions lie adjacent to the parieto-occipital fissure and may result in a monocular contralateral temporal crescent field loss (temporal crescent or half-moon syndrome).[228] This area constitutes less than 10% of the total surface area of the striate cortex and the defect begins approximately 60 degrees from fixation. Both upper and lower temporal crescents may be scotomatous in the field of one eye or only the upper or lower temporal crescent may be involved. Conversely, the temporal crescent may be spared with lesions that destroy the entire calcarine cortex except for the anterior tip (Figure 163.15).[225]

Lesions in the posterior 50% to 60% of the striate cortex, including the occipital pole and operculum, often affect macular vision (i.e., the central 10 degrees in the contralateral hemifield) and, thus, cause scotomatous defects.

Intermediate lesions lie between the anterior and posterior confines and affect from 10 to 60 degrees in the contralateral hemifield.

The most common cause of unilateral occipital disease is infarction in the distribution of the posterior cerebral artery.[191,216,221,224,226,229–234] Other causes include venous infarction, hemorrhage, arteriovenous malformation, tumor, abscess, and trauma.[235–239] Thus, MRI is warranted for all patients.

Bilateral occipital lobe lesions may cause bilateral homonymous scotomas, usually with some macular sparing ("ring" scotomas), that respect the vertical midline.[1,240] In some cases of macular sparing, there

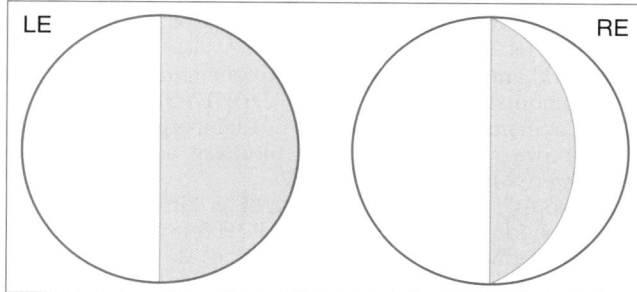

Figure 163.15 Right homonymous hemianopia with sparing of the monocular temporal crescent, RE. *LE*, left eye; *RE*, right eye.

may be "tunnel" or "keyhole" fields with bilateral complete homonymous hemianopias. Bilateral lesions affecting the superior or inferior calcarine cortices may produce bilateral altitudinal defects that may mimic the visual field abnormalities associated with bilateral optic nerve or retinal disease.[241–243] Bilateral lesions of the upper calcarine bank may have associated neurological findings, including Balint syndrome (apraxia of gaze, optic ataxia, decreased visual attention, and simultanagnosia), abnormal depth perception, defective spatial relations, topographic disorientation, and disorientation to place.[244,245] Bilateral lesions of the inferior bank of the calcarine fissure may be associated with prosopagnosia (inability to identify faces visually), cerebral dyschromatopsia, amnesia, and difficulty revisualizing the morphology and appearance of people and objects.[244,245] Bilateral lesions of the visual cortex, often due to large bilateral infarcts of the posterior cerebral artery involving both banks of the calcarine fissure and both temporal lobes, may cause cortical blindness that often is associated with agitated delerium and amnesia.[244,245]

The causes of cortical blindness include hypoxia, infarction, hemorrhage, eclampsia, hypertensive encephalopathy, tentorial herniation, tumor, arteriovenous malformation, infection (e.g., progressive multifocal leukoencephalopathy, Creutzfeldt-Jakob disease, subacute sclerosing panencephalitis, human immunodeficiency virus encephalitis, syphilis, encephalitis, abscess), inflammation (e.g., sarcoidosis), demyelinating disease, trauma, metabolic disorders (e.g., adrenoleukodystrophy, hypoglycemia, porphyria, mitochondrial encephalopathies), toxins (e.g., lead, mercury, ethanol, carbon monoxide), medications (e.g., cyclosporine, tacrolimus, interleukin-2), radiation therapy, Alzheimer disease, postictal after seizures, and complications of cerebral angiography.[1,229,231,232,237,246–267] Occasionally, patients with cortical blindness deny having a visual defect (Anton syndrome).

Evaluation of retrochiasmal defects

MRI is indicated for all patients who have a homonymous visual field defect, except for acute traumatic cases (for which computed tomography [CT] is usually adequate), cases of suspected hemorrhage (CT is better for acute blood), or for those in whom MRI is contraindicated (e.g., ferromagnetic aneurysmal clip, metallic fragments, pacemakers). There are several clinical situations in which MRI findings may be normal in a patient who has a homonymous hemianopia:

1. Homonymous hemianopia or cortical blindness may occur with the Heidenhain variant of Creutzfeldt-Jakob disease.[268–273] Electroencephalography may show characteristic periodic complexes, the cerebrospinal fluid may be abnormal (14-3-3 protein), and patients usually have impaired mentation, myoclonus, and other signs of Creutzfeldt-Jakob disease.

2. Patients with Alzheimer disease or diffuse Lewy

body disease may develop a homonymous field defect.[274,275] MRI findings may be normal or show only diffuse atrophy, and electroencephalograms are normal or show only mild diffuse slowing.

3. Most patients with field defects from cerebral infarction or hypoxia have MRI changes compatible with ischemia. However, Moster et al.[276] described two patients, one with bilateral homonymous congruous hemianopic central scotomata after carbon monoxide poisoning and the other with bilateral congruous inferior visual scotomata after global hypoxia, for whom the initial diagnosis was "functional" visual loss. Neither CT nor MRI adequately demonstrated the source of the visual dysfunction, but single photon emission computed tomography (SPECT) and positron emission tomography (PET) imaging confirmed the organic substrate of the visual impairment. Thus, functional imaging techniques such as SPECT or PET should be considered for patients with suspected cortical visual loss and normal CT or MRI findings.

4. Nonorganic hemianopias may be detected[277] with saccadic eye movement testing into the supposedly absent field (the patient usually assumes that eye movements and not the visual fields are being tested).[278] Another method is to place a 30-prism-diopter Fresnel prism into the upper quadrants of a trial frame.[279] After visual fields have been mapped without the prism, the prism is placed first base-out and then base-in, and with each change, the fields are mapped again. Patients with pathological hemianopsias shift their superior field 15 degrees to the right or to the left of the central vertical meridian with the prism base-in or base-out, respectively, but not patients who have a nonorganic hemifield defect.

Treatment of retrochiasmal lesions

As for a suprasellar lesion, treatment of a retrochiasmal lesion depends on the cause. Exposure to toxic agents (lead, mercury, methanol, alcohol) should be discontinued. Vitamin deficiency (e.g., vitamin B_{12}) may improve after replacement therapy. Demyelinating lesions may improve spontaneously or after a short course of corticosteroid treatment (e.g., intravenous methylprednisolone). Infectious causes (e.g., syphilis, tuberculosis, viral meningitis, encephalitis) should be treated with specific and sensitive antibiotics. Inflammatory causes (e.g., sarcoid, primary and secondary vasculitis of the central nervous system) may respond to immunosuppressive treatment (e.g., corticosteroids). Traumatic lesions are usually observed. The options for treatment of retrochiasmal mass lesions include no treatment, medical therapy (e.g., corticosteroids, chemotherapy), surgery, or radiotherapy, depending on the location, type, and symptoms of the lesion.

References

1. Slamovits TL. Anatomy and physiology of the optic chiasm. In: Miller NR, Newman NJ, eds. Walsh and Hoyt's Clinical Neuro-Ophthalmology. Vol 1, 5th ed. Baltimore: Williams & Wilkins, 1998;88–100
2. Horton JC. Wilbrand's knee of the primate optic chiasm is an artefact of monocular enucleation. Trans Am Ophthalmol Soc 1997;95:579–609
3. Hoyt WF. Correlative functional anatomy of the optic chiasm. Clin Neurosurg 1970;17:189–208
4. Traquair HM. An Introduction to Clinical Perimetry. 6th ed. St. Louis, Mosby, 1949.
5. Miller NR. Walsh and Hoyt's Clinical Neuro-Ophthalmology. Vol 1, 4th ed. Baltimore: Williams & Wilkins, 1982:108–152
6. Trobe JD, Glaser JS. The Visual Fields Manual: A Practical Guide to Testing and Interpretation. Gainesville, Florida: Triad Publishing Company, 1983:176
7. Cullen JF, Haining WM, Crombie AL. Cerebral aneurysms presenting with visual field defects. Br J Ophthalmol 1966;50:251–256
8. Farris BK, Smith JL, David NJ. The nasal junction scotoma in giant aneurysms. Ophthalmology 1986;93:895–905
9. Hershenfeld SA, Sharpe JA. Monocular temporal hemianopia. Br J Ophthalmol 1993;77:424–427
10. Trobe JD, Tao AH, Schuster JJ. Perichiasmal tumors: diagnostic and prognostic features. Neurosurgery 1984;15:391–399
11. Reynolds WD, Smith JL, McCrary JA III. Chiasmal optic neuritis. J Clin Neuroophthalmol 1982;2:93–101
12. Weinstein GW, Powell SR, Thrush WP. Chiasmal neuropathy secondary to rheumatoid pachymeningitis. Am J Ophthalmol 1987;104:439–440
13. Wybar K. Chiasmal compression: presenting ocular features. Proc R Soc Med 1977;70:307–317
14. Bills DC, Meyer FB, Laws ER Jr, et al. A retrospective analysis of pituitary apoplexy. Neurosurgery 1993;33:602–608
15. Embil JM, Kramer M, Kinnear S, Light RB. A blinding headache. Lancet 1997;350:182
16. Abe T, Matsumoto K, Kuwazawa J, et al. Headache associated with pituitary adenomas. Headache 1998;38:782–786
17. Elkington SG. Pituitary adenoma: preoperative symptomatology in a series of 260 patients. Br J Ophthalmol 1968;52:322–328
18. Falconer MA, Stafford-Bell MA. Visual failure from pituitary and parasellar tumours occurring with favourable outcome in pregnant women. J Neurol Neurosurg Psychiatry 1975;38:919–930
19. Ikeda H, Yoshimoto T. Visual disturbances in patients with pituitary adenoma. Acta Neurol Scand 1995;92:157–160
20. Kirkham TH. The ocular symptomatology of pituitary tumours. Proc R Soc Med 1972;65:517–518
21. Kupersmith MJ, Rosenberg C, Kleinberg D. Visual loss in pregnant women with pituitary adenomas. Ann Intern Med 1994;121:473–477
22. Lee AG, Sforza PD, Fard AK, et al. Pituitary adenoma in children. J Neuroophthalmol 1998;18:102–105
23. Moster ML, Savino PJ, Schatz NJ, et al. Visual function in prolactinoma patients treated with bromocriptine. Ophthalmology 1985;92:1332–1341
24. Peter M, De Tribolet N. Visual outcome after transsphenoidal surgery for pituitary adenomas. Br J Neurosurg 1995;9:151–157

25. Petruson B, Jakobsson KE, Elfverson J, Bengtsson BA. Five-year follow-up of nonsecreting pituitary adenomas. Arch Otolaryngol Head Neck Surg 1995;121:317–322

26. Wilson P, Falconer MA. Patterns of visual failure with pituitary tumours: clinical and radiological correlations. Br J Ophthalmol 1968;52:94–110

27. Ehlers N, Malmros R. The suprasellar meningioma: a review of the literature and presentation of a series of 31 cases. Acta Ophthalmol Suppl 1973;1–74

28. Gregorius FK, Hepler RS, Stern WE. Loss and recovery of vision with suprasellar meningiomas. J Neurosurg 1975;42:69–75

29. Kinjo T, al-Mefty O, Ciric I. Diaphragma sellae meningiomas. Neurosurgery 1995;36:1082–1092

30. Rosenberg LF, Miller NR. Visual results after microsurgical removal of meningiomas involving the anterior visual system. Arch Ophthalmol 1984;102:1019–1023

31. Bartlett JR. Craniopharyngiomas—a summary of 85 cases. J Neurol Neurosurg Psychiatry 1971;34:37–41

32. Crane TB, Yee RD, Hepler RS, Hallinan JM. Clinical manifestations and radiologic findings in craniopharyngiomas in adults. Am J Ophthalmol 1982;94: 220–228

33. Mikelberg FS, Yidegiligne HM. Axonal loss in band atrophy of the optic nerve in craniopharyngioma: a quantitative analysis. Can J Ophthalmol 1993;28:69–71

34. Camins MB, Mount LA. Primary suprasellar atypical teratoma. Brain 1974;97:447–456

35. Isayama Y, Takahashi T, Inoue M. Ocular findings of suprasellar germinoma: long term follow-up after radiotherapy. Neuro-Ophthalmology 1980;1:53–61

36. Kageyama N. Ectopic pinealoma in the region of the optic chiasm: report of five cases. J Neurosurg 1971;35: 755–759

37. Berson EL, Freeman MI, Gay AJ. Visual field defects in giant suprasellar aneurysms of internal carotid: report of three cases. Arch Ophthalmol 1966;76:52–58

38. Bird AC, Nolan B, Gargano FP, David NJ. Unruptured aneurysm of the supraclinoid carotid artery: a treatable cause of blindness. Neurology 1970;20:445–454

39. Krauss HR, Slamovits TL, Sibony PA, et al. Carotid artery aneurysm simulating pituitary adenoma. J Clin Neuroophthalmol 1982;2:169–174

40. Norwood EG, Kline LB, Chandra-Sekar B, Harsh GR III. Aneurysmal compression of the anterior visual pathways. Neurology 1986;36:1035–1041

41. Rush JA, Balis GA, Drake CG. Bitemporal hemianopsia in basilar artery aneurysm. J Clin Neuroophthalmol 1981;1:129–133

42. Glaser JS, Hoyt WF, Corbett J. Visual morbidity with chiasmal glioma: long-term studies of visual fields in untreated and irradiated cases. Arch Ophthalmol 1971; 85:3–12

43. Horwich A, Bloom HJ. Optic gliomas: radiation therapy and prognosis. Int J Radiat Oncol Biol Phys 1985;11:1067–1079

44. McFadzean RM, Brewin TB, Doyle D, Grossart K. Glioma of the optic chiasm and its management. Trans Ophthalmol Soc U K 1983;103:199–207

45. Rossi LN, Pastorino G, Scotti G, et al. Early diagnosis of optic glioma in children with neurofibromatosis type 1. Childs Nerv Syst 1994;10:426–429

46. Domingue JN, Wilson CB. Pituitary abscesses: report of seven cases and review of the literature. J Neurosurg 1977;46:601–608

47. Nelson PB, Haverkos H, Martinez AJ, Robinson AG. Abscess formation within pituitary tumors. Neurosurgery 1983;12:331–333

48. Chun BB, Lee AG, Coughlin WF, et al. Unusual presentations of sellar arachnoid cyst. J Neuroophthalmol 1998;18:246–249

49. Meyer FB, Carpenter SM, Laws ER Jr. Intrasellar arachnoid cysts. Surg Neurol 1987;28:105–110

50. Murali R, Epstein F. Diagnosis and treatment of suprasellar arachnoid cyst: report of three cases. J Neurosurg 1979;50:515–518

51. Segall HD, Hassan G, Ling SM, Carton C. Suprasellar cysts associated with isosexual precocious puberty. Radiology 1974;111:607–616

52. Fuchs HA, Evans RM, Gregg CR. Invasive aspergillosis of the sphenoid sinus manifested as a pituitary tumor. South Med J 1985;78:1365–1367

53. Larranaga J, Fandino J, Gomez-Bueno J, et al. Aspergillosis of the sphenoid sinus simulating a pituitary tumor. Neuroradiology 1989;31:362–363

54. Castel JP, Delorge-Kerdiles C, Rivel J. Cavernous angioma of the optic chiasm [French]. Neurochirurgie 1989;35:252–256

55. Corboy JR, Galetta SL. Familial cavernous angiomas manifesting with an acute chiasmal syndrome. Am J Ophthalmol 1989;108:245–250

56. Hwang JF, Yau CW, Huang JK, Tsai CY. Apoplectic optochiasmal syndrome due to intrinsic cavernous hemangioma: case report. J Clin Neuroophthalmol 1993;13:232–236

57. Klein LH, Fermaglich J, Kattah J, Luessenhop AJ. Cavernous hemangioma of optic chiasm, optic nerves and right optic tract: case report and review of literature. Virchows Arch A Pathol Anat Histol 1979;383:225–231

58. Mohr G, Hardy J, Gauvin P. Chiasmal apoplexy due to ruptured cavernous hemangioma of the optic chiasm. Surg Neurol 1985;24:636–640

59. Regli L, de Tribolet N, Regli F, Bogousslavsky J. Chiasmal apoplexy: haemorrhage from a cavernous malformation in the optic chiasm. J Neurol Neurosurg Psychiatry 1989;52:1095–1099

60. Maitland CG, Abiko S, Hoyt WF, et al. Chiasmal apoplexy: report of four cases. J Neurosurg 1982;56: 118–122

61. Riishede J, Seedorff HH. Spontaneous hematoma of the optic chiasma: report of a case. Acta Ophthalmol (Copenh) 1974;52:317–322

62. Crowe NW, Nickles TP, Troost BT, Elster AD. Intrachiasmal hemorrhage: a cause of delayed post-traumatic blindness. Neurology 1989;39:863–865

63. Neetens A, Bultinck J, Martin JJ, et al. Intrasellar adenoma and chordoma. Neuro-Ophthalmology 1980; 2:225–265

64. Takahashi T, Asai T, Isayama Y, et al. Chordoma. J Clin Neuroophthalmol 1983;3:251–257

65. Hilton GF, Hoyt WF. An arteriosclerotic chiasmal syndrome: bitemporal hemianopia associated with fusiform dilatation of the anterior cerebral arteries. JAMA 1966;196:1018–1020

66. Matsuo K, Kobayashi S, Sugita K. Bitemporal hemianopsia associated with sclerosis of the intracranial internal carotid arteries: case report. J Neurosurg 1980; 53:566–569

67. Slavin ML. Bitemporal hemianopia associated with dolichoectasia of the intracranial carotid arteries. J Clin Neuroophthalmol 1990;10:80–81

68. O'Connor PS, Smith JL. Chiasmal ependymoma. Ann Ophthalmol 1979;11:1424–1428

69. Waller RR, Riley FC, Sundt TM Jr. A rare cause of the chiasmal syndrome. Arch Ophthalmol 1972;88: 269–272

70. Liu GT, Galetta SL, Rorke LB, et al. Gangliogliomas involving the optic chiasm. Neurology 1996;46: 1669–1673

71. Sawin PD, Follett KA, Wen BC, Laws ER Jr. Symptomatic intrasellar hemangioblastoma in a child treated with subtotal resection and adjuvant radiosurgery: case report. J Neurosurg 1996;84:1046–1050

72. Goodman RH, Post KD, Molitch ME, et al. Eosinophilic granuloma mimicking a pituitary tumor. Neurosurgery 1979;5:723–725

73. Smolik EA, Devecerski M, Nelson JS, Smith KR Jr. Histiocytosis X in the optic chiasm of an adult with hypopituitarism: case report. J Neurosurg 1968;29: 290–295

74. Cantore GP, Raco A, Artico M, et al. Primary chiasmatic lymphoma. Clin Neurol Neurosurg 1989;91: 71–74

75. Howard RS, Duncombe AS, Owens C, Graham E. Compression of the optic chiasm due to a lymphoreticular malignancy. Postgrad Med J 1987;63:1091–1093

76. McFadzean RM, McIlwaine GG, McLellan D. Hodgkin's disease at the optic chiasm. J Clin Neuroophthalmol 1990;10:248–254

77. Abe T, Matsumoto K, Sanno N, Osamura Y. Lymphocytic hypophysitis: case report. Neurosurgery 1995;36: 1016–1019

78. Beressi N, Cohen R, Beressi JP, et al. Pseudotumoral lymphocytic hypophysitis successfully treated by corticosteroid alone: first case report. Neurosurgery 1994; 35:505–508

79. Honegger J, Fahlbusch R, Bornemann A, et al. Lymphocytic and granulomatous hypophysitis: experience with nine cases. Neurosurgery 1997;40:713–722

80. Hungerford GD, Biggs PJ, Levine JH, et al. Lymphoid adenohypophysitis with radiologic and clinical findings resembling a pituitary tumor. AJNR Am J Neuroradiol 1982;3:444–446

81. Jabre A, Rosales R, Reed JE, Spatz EL. Lymphocytic hypophysitis. J Neurol Neurosurg Psychiatry 1997;63: 672–673

82. Kerrison JB, Lee AG, Weinstein JM. Acute loss of vision during pregnancy due to a suprasellar mass. Surv Ophthalmol 1997;41:402–408

83. Lee JH, Laws ER Jr, Guthrie BL, et al. Lymphocytic hypophysitis: occurrence in two men. Neurosurgery 1994;34:159–162

84. Naik RG, Ammini A, Shah P, et al. Lymphocytic hypophysitis: case report. J Neurosurg 1994;80:925–927

85. Nishioka H, Ito H, Fukushima C. Recurrent lymphocytic hypophysitis: case report. Neurosurgery 1997;41: 684–686

86. Stelmach M, O'Day J. Rapid change in visual fields associated with suprasellar lymphocytic hypophysitis. J Clin Neuroopthalmol 1991;11:19–24

87. Thodou E, Asa SL, Kontogeorgos G, et al. Clinical case seminar: lymphocytic hypophysitis: clinicopathological findings. J Clin Endocrinol Metab 1995;80:2302–2311

88. Galetta SL, Stadtmauer EA, Hicks DG, et al. Reactive lymphohistiocytosis with recurrence in the optic chiasm. J Clin Neuroophthalmol 1991;11:25–30

89. Aubin MJ, Hardy J, Comtois R. Primary sellar haemorrhagic melanoma: case report and review of the literature. Br J Neurosurg 1997;11:80–83

90. Cohen MM, Lessell S. Chiasmal syndrome due to metastasis. Arch Neurol 1979;36:565–567

91. Buonaguidi R, Ferdeghini M, Faggionato F, Tusini G. Intrasellar metastasis mimicking a pituitary adenoma. Surg Neurol 1983;20:373–378

92. Duvall J, Cullen JF. Metastatic disease in the pituitary: clinical features. Trans Ophthalmol Soc UK 1982;102: 481–486

93. Leramo OB, Booth JD, Zinman B, et al. Hyperprolactinemia, hypopituitarism, and chiasmal compression due to carcinoma metastatic to the pituitary. Neurosurgery 1981;8:477–480

94. Max MB, Deck MD, Rottenberg DA. Pituitary metastasis: incidence in cancer patients and clinical differentiation from pituitary adenoma. Neurology 1981;31: 998–1002

95. Morita A, Meyer FB, Laws ER Jr. Symptomatic pituitary metastases. J Neurosurg 1998;89:69–73

96. Abla AA, Maroon JC, Wilberger JE Jr, et al. Intrasellar mucocele simulating pituitary adenoma: case report. Neurosurgery 1986;18:197–199

97. Goodwin JA, Glaser JS. Chiasmal syndrome in sphenoid sinus mucocele. Ann Neurol 1978;4:440–444

98. Poon MC, Prchal JT, Murad TM, Galbraith JG. Multiple myeloma masquerading as chromophobe adenoma. Cancer 1979;43:1513–1515

99. Elias Z, Powers SK, Grimson BS, Bouldin TW. Chiasmal syndrome caused by pituitary-sellar disproportion. Surg Neurol 1987;28:395–400

100. Yamamoto K, Saito K, Takai T, et al. Visual field defects and pituitary enlargement in primary hypothyroidism. J Clin Endocrinol Metab 1983;57:283–287

101. Poon A, McNeill P, Harper A, O'Day J. Patterns of visual loss associated with pituitary macroadenomas. Aust N Z J Ophthalmol 1995;23:107–115

102. Fischer EG, DeGirolami U, Suojanen JN. Reversible visual deficit following debulking of a Rathke's cleft cyst: a tethered chiasm? J Neurosurg 1994;81:459–462

103. Iraci G, Giordano R, Gerosa M, et al. Ocular involvement in recurrent cyst of Rathke's cleft: case report. Ann Ophthalmol 1979;11:94–98

104. Rao GP, Blyth CP, Jeffreys RV. Ophthalmic manifestations of Rathke's cleft cysts. Am J Ophthalmol 1995; 119:86–91

105. Voelker JL, Campbell RL, Muller J. Clinical, radiographic, and pathological features of symptomatic Rathke's cleft cysts. J Neurosurg 1991;74:535–544

106. Yamamoto M, Jimbo M, Ide M, et al. Recurrence of symptomatic Rathke's cleft cyst: a case report. Surg Neurol 1993;39:263–268

107. Godlewski J, Charlin JF, Brasseur G, Freger P. Hypothalamic sarcoidosis with chiasmatic involvement [French]. Rev Otoneuroophtalmol 1984;56:347–355

108. Tang RA, Grotta JC, Lee KF, Lee YE. Chiasmal syndrome in sarcoidosis. Arch Ophthalmol 1983;101: 1069–1073

109. Walsh TJ, Smith JL. Sarcoidosis and suprasellar mass. Smith JL, ed. In: Neuro-Ophthalmology Symposium of the University of Miami and the Bascom Palmer Eye Institute. Vol 4. St. Louis: CV Mosby, 1968:167–177

110. Kansu T, Bertan V. Fifth ventricle with bitemporal hemianopsia: case report. J Neurosurg 1980;52:276–278

111. Carter JE, Wymore J, Ansbacher L, Reid WS. Sudden visual loss and a chiasmal syndrome due to an intrachiasmatic vascular malformation. J Clin Neuroophthalmol 1982;2:163–167

112. Hankey GJ, Khangure MS. Chiasmal apoplexy due to intrachiasmatic vascular malformation rupture. Aust N Z J Med 1987;17:444–446

113. Lavin PJ, McCrary JA III, Roessmann U, Ellenberger C Jr. Chiasmal apoplexy: hemorrhage from a cryptic vascular malformation in the optic chiasm. Neurology 1984;34:1007–1011

114. Fermaglich J, Kattah J, Manz H. Venous angioma of the optic chiasm. Ann Neurol 1978;4:470–471

115. Wilhelm H, Grodd W, Schiefer U, Zrenner E. Uncommon chiasmal lesions: demyelinating disease, vasculitis, and cobalamin deficiency. Ger J Ophthalmol 1993; 2:234–240

116. Edwards MK, Gilmor RL, Franco JM. Computed tomography of chiasmal optic neuritis. AJNR Am J Neuroradiol 1983;4:816–818

117. Newman NJ, Lessell S, Winterkorn JM. Optic chiasmal neuritis. Neurology 1991;41:1203–1210

118. Sacks JG, Melen O. Bitemporal visual field defects in presumed multiple sclerosis. JAMA 1975;234:69–72

119. Spector RH, Glaser JH, Schatz NJ. Demyelinative chiasmal lesions. Arch Neurol 1980;37:757–762

120. Spector RH, Glaser JS, Schatz NJ. Demyelinative chiasmal lesions. Arch Neurol 1980;37:757–762

121. Waespe W, Haenny P. Bitemporal hemianopia due to chiasmal optic neuritis. Neuro-Ophthalmology 1987;7: 69–74

122. Berke JP, Buxton LF, Kokmen E. The "empty" sella. Neurology 1975;25:1137–1143

123. Kaufman B. The "empty" sella turcica—a manifestation of the intrasellar subarachnoid space. Radiology 1968;90:931–941

124. Kosmorsky GS, Straga JM. A descent thing to do for the chiasm. J Neuroophthalmol 1997;17:53–56

125. Neelon FA, Goree JA, Lebovitz HE. The primary empty sella: clinical and radiographic characteristics and endocrine function. Medicine (Baltimore) 1973;52: 73–92

126. Randall RV. Empty sella syndrome. Compr Ther 1984; 10:57–65

127. Ahmadi J, Keane JR, McCormick GS, et al. Ischemic chiasmal syndrome and hypopituitarism associated with progressive cerebrovascular occlusive disease. AJNR Am J Neuroradiol 1984;5:367–372

128. Lee KF, Schatz NJ. Ischemic chiasmal syndrome. Acta Radiol Suppl 1976;347:131–148

129. Lee KF. Ischemic chiasma syndrome. AJNR Am J Neuroradiol 1983;4:777–780

130. Coyle JT. Chiasmatic arachnoiditis: a case report and review. Am J Ophthalmol 1969;68:345–349

131. Iraci G, Pellone M, Scuccimarra A. Optochiasmatic arachnoiditis: remarks on a case of the cystic form of the disease. Ann Ophthalmol 1977;9:147–154

132. Iraci G, Giordano R, Gerosa M, et al. Cystic suprasellar and retrosellar arachnoiditis: a clinical and pathologic follow-up case report. Ann Ophthalmol 1979;11: 1175–1179

133. Krohel GB, Charles H, Smith RS. Granulomatous optic neuropathy. Arch Ophthalmol 1981;99:1053–1055

134. Takahashi T, Isayama Y. Chiasmal meningitis. Neuro-Ophthalmology 1980;1:19–25

135. Lee BL, Holland GN, Glasgow BJ. Chiasmal infarction and sudden blindness caused by mucormycosis in AIDS and diabetes mellitus. Am J Ophthalmol 1996; 122:895–896

136. Oliver M, Beller AJ, Behar A. Chiasmal arachnoiditis as a manifestation of generalized arachnoiditis in systemic vascular disease: clinico-pathological report of two cases. Br J Ophthalmol 1968;52:227–235

137. Navarro IM, Peralta VH, Leon JA, et al. Tuberculous optochiasmatic arachnoiditis. Neurosurgery 1981;9: 654–660

138. Scott RM, Sonntag VK, Wilcox LM, et al. Visual loss from optochiasmatic arachnoiditis after tuberculous meningitis: case report. J Neurosurg 1977;46:524–526

139. Lessell S. The neuro-ophthalmology of systemic lupus erythematosus. Doc Ophthalmol 1979;47:13–42

140. Ingestad R, Stigmar G. Sarcoidosis with ocular and hypothalamic-pituitary manifestations. Acta Ophthalmol (Copenh) 1971;49:1–10

141. Kirkham TH. Neuro-ophthalmic presentations of sarcoidosis. Proc R Soc Med 1973;66:167–169

142. Bell RA, Robertson DM, Rosen DA, Kerr AW. Optochiasmatic arachnoiditis in multiple sclerosis. Arch Ophthalmol 1975;93:191–193

143. Iraci G, Pellone M, Scuccimarra A, Fiore D. Posttraumatic optochiasmatic arachnoiditis. Ann Ophthalmol 1976;8:1313–1328

144. Hammer HM. Optic chiasmal radionecrosis. Trans Ophthalmol Soc U K 1983;103:208–211

145. Harris JR, Levene MB. Visual complications following irradiation for pituitary adenomas and craniopharyngiomas. Radiology 1976;120:167–171

146. Pasquier F, Leys D, Dubois F, et al. Chiasm and optic nerve necrosis following radiation therapy: report of two cases. Neuro-Ophthalmology 1989;9:331–337

147. Schatz NJ, Lichtenstein S, Corbett JJ. Delayed radiation necrosis of the optic nerves and chiasm. In: Glaser JS, Smith JL, eds. Neuro-Ophthalmology. St. Louis: CV Mosby, 1975:131–139

148. Coppeto JR, Gahm NH. Bitemporal hemianoptic scotoma: a complication of intraventricular catheter. Surg Neurol 1977;8:361–362

149. Coppeto JR, Monteiro MLR. Bitemporal hemianopic scotomas from intraventricular catheter: the pinched chiasm syndrome? Neuro-Ophthalmology 1989;9: 343–346

150. Slavin ML, Rosenthal AD. Chiasmal compression caused by a catheter in the suprasellar cistern. Am J Ophthalmol 1988;105:560–561

151. McHenry JG, Spoor TC. Chiasmal compression from fat packing after transsphenoidal resection of intrasellar tumor in two patients (letter). Am J Ophthalmol 1993;116:253

152. Slavin ML, Lam BL, Decker RE, et al. Chiasmal compression from fat packing after transsphenoidal resection of intrasellar tumor in two patients. Am J Ophthalmol 1993;115:368–371

153. Domingo Z, de Villiers JC. Post-traumatic chiasmatic disruption. Br J Neurosurg 1993;7:141–147

154. Fisher NF, Jampolsky A, Scott AB. Traumatic bitemporal hemianopsia. I. Diagnosis of macular splitting. Am J Ophthalmol 1968;65:237–242

155. Gilad E, Dickerman Z, Laron Z, et al. Traumatic chiasmal syndrome with panhypopituitarism. Neuro-Ophthalmol 1986;6:79–83

156. Heinz GW, Nunery WR, Grossman CB. Traumatic chiasmal syndrome associated with midline basilar skull fractures. Am J Ophthalmol 1994;117:90–96

157. Laursen AB. Traumatic bitemporal hemianopsia. Survey of the literature and report of a case. Acta Ophthalmol (Copenh) 1971;49:134–142

158. Logan WC, Gordon DS. Traumatic lesions of the optic chiasm. Br J Ophthalmol 1967;51:258–260

159. Noble MJ, McFadzean R. Indirect injury to the optic nerves and optic chiasm. Neuro-Ophthalmology 1987; 7:341–348

160. Obenchain TG, Killeffer FA, Stern WE. Indirect injury of the optic nerves and chiasm with closed head injury: report of three cases. Bull Los Angeles Neurol Soc 1973;38:13–20

161. Prosperi L, Bernasconi S, Cantarelli A, Voccia E. Traumatic hypopituitarism associated with bitemporal hemianopia in a prepuberal child. J Pediatr Ophthalmol Strabismus 1978;15:376–382

162. Resneck JD, Lederman IR. Traumatic chiasmal syndrome associated with pneumocephalus and sellar fracture. Am J Ophthalmol 1981;92:233–237

163. Savino PJ, Glaser JS, Schatz NJ. Traumatic chiasmal syndrome. Neurology 1980;30:963–970

164. Tibbs PA, Brooks WH. Traumatic bitemporal hemianopsia: case report. J Trauma 1979;19:129–131

165. Walsh FB. Pathological-clinical correlations. I. Indirect trauma to the optic nerves and chiasm. II. Certain cerebral involvements associated with defective blood supply. Invest Ophthalmol 1966;5:433–449

166. Schneider RC, Kriss FC, Falls HF. Prechiasmal infarction associated with intrachiasmal and suprasellar tumors. J Neurosurg 1970;32:197–208

167. Wolansky LJ, Shaderowfsky PD, Sander R, et al. Optic chiasmal compression by venous aneurysm: magnetic resonance imaging diagnosis. J Neuroimaging 1997;7:46–47

168. Bevan JS, Webster J, Burke CW, Scanlon MF. Dopamine agonists and pituitary tumor shrinkage. Endocr Rev 1992;13:220–240

169. Molitch ME. Pregnancy and the hyperprolactinemic woman. N Engl J Med 1985;312:1364–1370

170. Prescott RW, Johnston DG, Kendall-Taylor P, et al. Hyperprolactinaemia in men: response to bromocriptine therapy. Lancet 1982;1:245–248

171. Wass JA, Williams J, Charlesworth M, et al. Bromocriptine in management of large pituitary tumours. Br Med J (Clin Res Ed) 1982;284:1908–1911

172. Verhelst J, Abs R, Maiter D, et al. Cabergolin in the treatment of hyperprolactinemia: a study in 455 patients. J Clin Endocrinol Metab 1999;84:2518–2522

173. Cannavo S, Curto L, Squadrito S, et al. Cabergoline: a first-choice treatment in patients with previously untreated prolactin-secreting pituitary adenoma. J Endocrinol Invest 1999;22:354–359

174. Abs R, Verhelst J, Maiter D, et al. Cabergoline in the treatment of acromegaly: a study in 64 patients. J Clin Endocrinol Metab 1998;83:374–378

175. Ferrari CI, Abs R, Bevan JS, et al. Treatment of macroprolactinoma with cabergoline: a study of 85 patients. Clin Endocrinol (Oxf) 1997;46:409–413

176. Giovanelli M, Losa M, Mortini P. Acromegaly: surgical results and prognosis. In: Landolt AM, Vance ML, Reilly PL, eds. Pituitary Adenomas. New York: Churchill Livingstone, 1996:333–351

177. Luedecke DK, Knappe UJ, Glagla G. Cushing's disease: surgical results and prognosis. In: Landolt AM, Vance ML, Reilly PL, eds. Pituitary Adenomas. New York: Churchill Livingstone, 1996:353–361

178. Reilly PL. Prolactinomas: surgical results and prognosis. In: Landolt AM, Vance ML, Reilly PL, eds. Pituitary Adenomas. New York: Churchill Livingstone, 1996:363–376

179. Savino PJ, Paris M, Schatz NJ, et al. Optic tract syndrome: a review of 21 patients. Arch Ophthalmol 1978;96:656–663

180. Bell RA, Thompson HS. Relative afferent pupillary defect in optic tract hemianopias. Am J Ophthalmol 1978;85:538–540

181. Bender MB, Bodis-Wollner I. Visual dysfunctions in optic tract lesions. Ann Neurol 1978;3:187–193

182. Burde RM. The pupil. Int Ophthalmol Clin 1967;7:839–855

183. O'Connor PS, Kasdon D, Tredici TJ, Ivan DJ. The Marcus Gunn pupil in experimental tract lesions. Ophthalmology 1982;89:160–164

184. Bajandas FJ, McBeath JB, Smith JL. Congenital homonymous hemianopia. Am J Ophthalmol 1976;82:498–500

185. Hoyt WF, Rios-Montenegro EN, Behrens MM, Eckelhoff RJ. Homonymous hemioptic hypoplasia: fundoscopic features in standard and red-free illumination in three patients with congenital hemiplegia. Br J Ophthalmol 1972;56:537–545

186. Anderson DR, Trobe JD, Hood TW, Gebarski SS. Optic tract injury after anterior temporal lobectomy. Ophthalmology 1989;96:1065–1070

187. Groom M, Kay MD, Vicinanza-Adami C, Santini R. Optic tract syndrome secondary to metastatic breast cancer. Am J Ophthalmol 1998;125:115–118

188. Liu GT, Galetta SL. Homonymous hemifield loss in childhood. Neurology 1997;49:1748–1749

189. Slavin ML. Acute homonymous field loss: really a diagnostic dilemma. Surv Ophthalmol 1990;34:399–407

190. Shults WT, Hamby S, Corbett JJ, et al. Neuro-ophthalmic complications of intracranial catheters. Neurosurgery 1993;33:135–138

191. Molia L, Winterkorn JM, Schneider SJ. Hemianopic visual field defects in children with intracranial shunts: report of two cases. Neurosurgery 1996;39:599–603

192. Biousse V, Newman NJ, Carroll C, et al. Visual fields in patients with posterior GPi pallidotomy. Neurology 1998;50:258–265

193. Gunderson CH, Hoyt WF. Geniculate hemianopia: incongruous homonymous field defects in two patients with partial lesions of the lateral geniculate nucleus. J Neurol Neurosurg Psychiatry 1971;34:1–6

194. Hoyt WF. Geniculate hemianopias: incongruous visual defects from partial involvement of the lateral geniculate nucleus. Proc Aust Assoc Neurol 1975;12:7–16

195. Kosmorsky G, Lancione RR Jr. When fighting makes you see black holes instead of stars. J Neuroophthalmol 1998;18:255–257

196. Fisen L. Quadruple sectoranopia and sectorial optic atrophy: a syndrome of the distal anterior choroidal artery. J Neurol Neurosurg Psychiatry 1979;42:590–594

197. Helgason C, Caplan LR, Goodwin J, Hedges T III. Anterior choroidal artery-territory infarction: report of cases and review. Arch Neurol 1986;43:681–686

198. Luco C, Hoppe A, Schweitzer M, et al. Visual field defects in vascular lesions of the lateral geniculate body. J Neurol Neurosurg Psychiatry 1992;55:12–15

199. Donahue SP, Kardon RH, Thompson HS. Hourglass-shaped visual fields as a sign of bilateral lateral geniculate myelinolysis. Am J Ophthalmol 1995;119:378–380

200. Greenfield DS, Siatkowski RM, Schatz NJ, Glaser JS. Bilateral lateral geniculitis associated with severe diarrhea. Am J Ophthalmol 1996;122:280–281

201. Mackenzie I, Meighan S, Pollock EN. On the projection of the retinal quadrants on the lateral geniculate bodies, and the relationship of the quadrants to the optic radiations. Trans Ophthalmol Soc U K 1933;53:142–169

202. Merren MD. Bilateral lateral geniculate body necrosis as a cause of amblyopia. Neurology 1972;22:263–268

203. Borruat FX, Maeder P. Sectoranopia after head trauma: evidence of lateral geniculate body lesion on MRI. Neurology 1995;45:590–592

204. Frisen L, Holmegaard L, Rosencrantz M. Sectorial optic atrophy and homonymous, horizontal sectoranopia: a lateral choroidal artery syndrome? J Neurol Neurosurg Psychiatry 1978;41:374–380

205. Neau JP, Bogousslavsky J. The syndrome of posterior choroidal artery territory infarction. Ann Neurol 1996;39:779–788

206. Shacklett DE, O'Connor PS, Dorwart RH, et al. Congruous and incongruous sectoral visual field defects with lesions of the lateral geniculate nucleus. Am J Ophthalmol 1984;98:283–290

207. Carter JE, O'Connor P, Shacklett D, Rosenberg M. Lesions of the optic radiations mimicking lateral geniculate nucleus visual field defects. J Neurol Neurosurg Psychiatry 1985;48:982–988

208. Grossman M, Galetta SL, Nichols CW, Grossman RI. Horizontal homonymous sectoral field defect after ischemic infarction of the occipital cortex. Am J Ophthalmol 1990;109:234–236

209. Grochowicki M, Vighetto A. Homonymous horizontal sectoranopia: report of four cases. Br J Ophthalmol 1991;75:624–628

210. Horton JC, Landau K, Maeder P, Hoyt WF. Magnetic resonance imaging of the human lateral geniculate body. Arch Neurol 1990;47:1201–1206

211. Falconer MA, Wilson JL. Visual field changes following anterior temporal lobectomy: their significance in relation to Meyer's loop of the optic radiation. Brain (London) 1958;81:1–14

212. Van Buren JM, Baldwin M. The architecture of the optic radiation in the temporal lobe of man. Brain (London) 1958;81:15–40

213. Jacobson DM. The localizing value of a quadrantanopia. Arch Neurol 1997;54:401–404

214. Jensen I, Seedorff HH. Temporal lobe epilepsy and neuro-ophthalmology: ophthalmological findings in 74 temporal lobe resected patients. Acta Ophthalmol (Copenh) 1976;54:827–841

215. Marino R Jr, Rasmussen T. Visual field changes after temporal lobectomy in man. Neurology 1968;18: 825–835

216. Trobe JD, Lorber ML, Schlezinger NS. Isolated homonymous hemianopia: a review of 104 cases. Arch Ophthalmol 1973;89:377–381

217. Beck RW, Savino PJ, Schatz NJ, et al. Plaque causing homonymous hemianopsia in multiple sclerosis identified by computed tomography. Am J Ophthalmol 1982;94:229–234

218. Horton JC, Hoyt WF. Quadrantic visual field defects: a hallmark of lesions in extrastriate (V2/V3) cortex. Brain 1991;114:1703–1718

219. Borruat FX, Siatkowski RM, Schatz NJ, Glaser JS. Congruous quadrantanopia and optic radiation lesion. Neurology 1993;43:1430–1432

220. Horton JC, Hoyt WF. The representation of the visual field in human striate cortex: a revision of the classic Holmes map. Arch Ophthalmol 1991;109:816–824

221. Pessin MS, Lathi ES, Cohen MB, et al. Clinical features and mechanism of occipital infarction. Ann Neurol 1987;21:290–299

222. McFadzean R, Brosnahan D, Hadley D, Mutlukan E. Representation of the visual field in the occipital striate cortex. Br J Ophthalmol 1994;78:185–190

223. Koehler PJ, Endtz LJ, Te Velde J, Hekster RE. Aware or non-aware: on the significance of awareness for the localization of the lesion responsible for homonymous hemianopia. J Neurol Sci 1986;75:255–262

224. Benton S, Levy I, Swash M. Vision in the temporal crescent in occipital infarction. Brain 1980;103:83–97

225. Landau K, Wichmann W, Valavanis A. The missing temporal crescent. Am J Ophthalmol 1995;119:345–349

226. McAuley DL, Russell RW. Correlation of CAT scan and visual field defects in vascular lesions of the posterior visual pathways. J Neurol Neurosurg Psychiatry 1979;42:298–311

227. Walsh TJ. Temporal crescent or half-moon syndrome. Ann Ophthalmol 1974;6:501–505

228. Chavis PS, al-Hazmi A, Clunie D, Hoyt WF. Temporal crescent syndrome with magnetic resonance correlation. J Neuroophthalmol 1997;17:151–155

229. Beal MF, Chapman PH. Cortical blindness and homonymous hemianopia in the postpartum period. JAMA 1980;244:2085–2087

230. Fugino T, Kigazawa K, Yamada R. Homonymous hemianopia: a retrospective study of 140 cases. Neuro-Ophthalmology 1986;6:17–21

231. Gittinger JW Jr. Occipital infarction following chiropractic cervical manipulation. J Clin Neuroophthalmol 1986;6:11–13

232. Hoyt WF. Vascular lesions of the visual cortex with brain herniation through the tentorial incisura: neuro-ophthalmologic considerations. Arch Ophthalmol 1960;64:44–57

233. Pessin MS, Kwan ES, DeWitt LD, et al. Posterior cerebral artery stenosis. Ann Neurol 1987;21:85–89

234. Sato M, Tanaka S, Kohama A, Fujii C. Occipital lobe infarction caused by tentorial herniation. Neurosurgery 1986;18:300–305

235. Bartolomei J, Wecht DA, Chaloupka J, et al. Occipital lobe vascular malformations: prevalence of visual field deficits and prognosis after therapeutic intervention. Neurosurgery 1998;43:415–421

236. Kupersmith MJ, Vargas ME, Yashar A, et al. Occipital arteriovenous malformations: visual disturbances and presentation. Neurology 1996;46:953–957

237. Monteiro ML, Hoyt WF, Imes RK. Puerperal cerebral blindness: transient bilateral occipital involvement from presumed cerebral venous thrombosis. Arch Neurol 1984;41:1300–1301

238. Parkinson D, Craig WM. Tumours of the brain, occipital lobe; their signs and symptoms. Can Med Assoc J 1951;64:111–113

239. Troost BT, Newton TH. Occipital lobe arteriovenous malformations: clinical and radiologic features in 26 cases with comments on differentiation from migraine. Arch Ophthalmol 1975;93:250–256

240. Halpern JI, Sedler RR. Traumatic bilateral homonymous hemianopic scotomas. Ann Ophthalmol 1980;12: 1022–1026

241. Hansen HV. Bilateral inferior altitudinal hemianopia. Neuro-Ophthalmol 1993;13:81–84

242. Lakhanpal A, Selhorst JB. Bilateral altitudinal visual fields. Ann Ophthalmol 1990;22:112–117

243. Newman RP, Kinkel WR, Jacobs L. Altitudinal hemianopia caused by occipital infarctions: clinical and computerized tomographic correlations. Arch Neurol 1984;41:413–418

244. Brazis PW, Masdeu JC, Biller J. Localization in Clinical Neurology. 3rd ed. Boston: Little, Brown and Company 1996:449–534

245. Caplan LR. Visual perception abnormalities, read at the 42nd annual meeting of the American Academy of Neurology, Miami, Florida, 1990

246. Aldrich MS, Alessi AG, Beck RW, Gilman S. Cortical blindness: etiology, diagnosis, and prognosis. Ann Neurol 1987;21:149–158

247. Coughlin WF, McMurdo SK, Reeves T. MR imaging of postpartum cortical blindness. J Comput Assist Tomogr 1989;13:572–576

248. Eldridge PR, Punt JA. Transient traumatic cortical blindness in children. Lancet 1988;1:815–816

249. Gibson JM, Cullen JF. Blindness and visual field defects following cerebral poisoning. Neuro-Ophthalmology 1982;2:297–303

250. Greenblatt SH. Posttraumatic transient cerebral blindness: association with migraine and seizure diatheses. JAMA 1973;225:1073–1076
251. Hinchey J, Chaves C, Appignani B, et al. A reversible posterior leukoencephalopathy syndrome. N Engl J Med 1996;334:494–500
252. Horwitz NH, Wener L. Temporary cortical blindness following angiography. J Neurosurg 1974;40:583–586
253. Jaffe SJ, Roach ES. Transient cortical blindness with occipital lobe epilepsy. J Clin Neuroophthalmol 1988; 8:221–224
254. Karp BI, Yang GC, Khorsand M, et al. Multiple cerebral lesions complicating therapy with interleukin-2. Neurology 1996;47:417–424
255. Katafuchi Y, Nishimi T, Yamaguchi Y, et al. Cortical blindness in acute carbon monoxide poisoning. Brain Dev 1985;7:516–519
256. Keane JR. Blindness following tentorial herniation. Ann Neurol 1980;8:186–190
257. Kupferschmidt H, Bont A, Schnorf H, et al. Transient cortical blindness and biocciptal brain lesions in two patients with acute intermittent porphyria. Ann Intern Med 1995;123:598–600
258. Lantos G. Cortical blindness due to osmotic disruption of the blood–brain barrier by angiographic contrast material: CT and MRI studies. Neurology 1989;39: 567–571
259. Mehler MF. The neuro-ophthalmologic spectrum of the rostral basilar artery syndrome. Arch Neurol 1988; 45:966–971
260. Nepple EW, Appen RE, Sackett JF. Bilateral homonymous hemianopia. Am J Ophthalmol 1978;86:536–543
261. Ormerod LD, Rhodes RH, Gross SA, et al. Ophthalmologic manifestations of acquired immune deficiency syndrome-associated progressive multifocal leukoencephalopathy. Ophthalmology 1996;103:899–906
262. Pomeranz HD, Henson JW, Lessell S. Radiation-associated cerebral blindness. Am J Ophthalmol 1998;126: 609–611
263. Powers JM. Sarcoidosis of the tentorium with cortical blindness. J Clin Neuroophthalmol 1985;5:112–115
264. Salmon JH. Transient postictal hemianopsia. Arch Ophthalmol 1968;79:523–525
265. Studdard WE, Davis DO, Young SW. Cortical blindness after cerebral angiography: case report. J Neurosurg 1981;54:240–244
266. Wilson SE, de Groen PC, Aksamit AJ, et al. Cyclosporin A-induced reversible cortical blindness. J Clin Neuroophthalmol 1988;8:215–220
267. Zihl J, von Cramon D. Restitution of visual function in patients with cerebral blindness. J Neurol Neurosurg Psychiatry 1979;42:312–322
268. Aguglia U, Gambarelli D, Farnarier G, Quattrone A. Different susceptibilities of the geniculate and extrageniculate visual pathways to human Creutzfeldt-Jakob disease (a combined neurophysiological-neuropathological study). Electroencephalogr Clin Neurophysiol 1991;78:413–423
269. Felton WL, read at the 28th annual meeting of the Frank B. Walsh Meeting, Salt Lake City, Utah, February 10 to 11, 1996
270. Kovanen J, Erkinjuntti T, Iivanainen M, et al. Cerebral MR and CT imaging in Creutzfeldt-Jakob disease. J Comput Assist Tomogr 1985;9:125–128
271. Purvin V, Bonnin J, Goodman J. Palinopsia as a presenting manifestation of Creutzfeldt-Jakob disease. J Clin Neuroophthalmol 1989;9:242–246
272. Vargas ME, Kupersmith MJ, Savino PJ, et al. Homonymous field defect as the first manifestation of Creutzfeldt-Jakob disease. Am J Ophthalmol 1995;119: 497–504
273. Warren FE, Vargas ME, Seidman I, Kupersmith MJ. Homonymous field defect in a HIV negative at risk individual, read at the 24th annual Frank B. Walsh Society Meeting, Los Angeles, California, February 28 to 29, 1992
274. Bashir K, Elble RJ, Ghobrial M, Struble RG. Hemianopsia in dementia with Lewy bodies. Arch Neurol 1998;55:1132–1135
275. Trick GL, Trick LR, Morris P, Wolf M. Visual field loss in senile dementia of the Alzheimer's type. Neurology 1995;45:68–74
276. Moster ML, Galetta SL, Schatz NJ. Physiologic functional imaging in "functional" visual loss. Surv Ophthalmol 1996;40:395–399
277. Thompson JC, Kosmorsky GS, Ellis BD. Field of dreamers and dreamed-up fields: functional and fake perimetry. Ophthalmology 1996;103:117–125
278. Weller M, Wiedemann P. Hysterical symptoms in ophthalmology. Doc Ophthalmol 1989;73:1–33
279. Carlow TJ. Functional hemianopsia: identified with Fresnel prisms and quantitative perimetry, read at the North American Neuro-Ophthalmology Society Meeting, Tucson, Arizona, February 1995

164 Disturbances of the Pupil

Randy Kardon

Clinical aspects of pupil function (Figure 164.1) consist of the following features: (1) pupil movement as an objective indicator of afferent input; (2) pupil size as an indicator of wakefulness; (3) pupil inequality (anisocoria) as a reflection of autonomic nerve output to each iris, integrity of the iris sphincter, or external pharmacological influence; (4) the effect of a large pupil size on the optical properties of the eye and (5) the pupil response to drugs as a means of monitoring pharmacological effects.

The pupil light reflex consists of three major divisions of neurons (Figure 164.2) that integrate a light stimulus to produce a pupil contraction: (1) an afferent division; (2) an interneuron division, and (3) an efferent division.

The afferent division of the light reflex consists of retinal input from photoreceptors, bipolar neurons, and ganglion cells. Axons of retinal ganglion cells from each eye provide light input information that is conveyed via synapses to interneurons located in the pretectal olivary nucleus of the midbrain. These interneurons, in turn, distribute pupil light input to neurons in the right and left Edinger-Westphal nuclei through crossed (decussating) and uncrossed (non-

decussating) connections. From here, the neurons of the Edinger-Westphal nucleus send their preganglionic parasympathetic axons along the oculomotor nerve to synapse at the ciliary ganglion in each orbit. The neurons in the ciliary ganglion give rise to post-ganglionic parasympathetic axons that travel in the short ciliary nerves to the globe where they synapse with the iris sphincter muscle.

The pupil constriction to a near stimulus involves activation of neurons in the rostral brainstem that relay their signal to the same Edinger-Westphal neurons that are activated in the light reflex. Therefore, the efferent pathway for the near pupil constric-

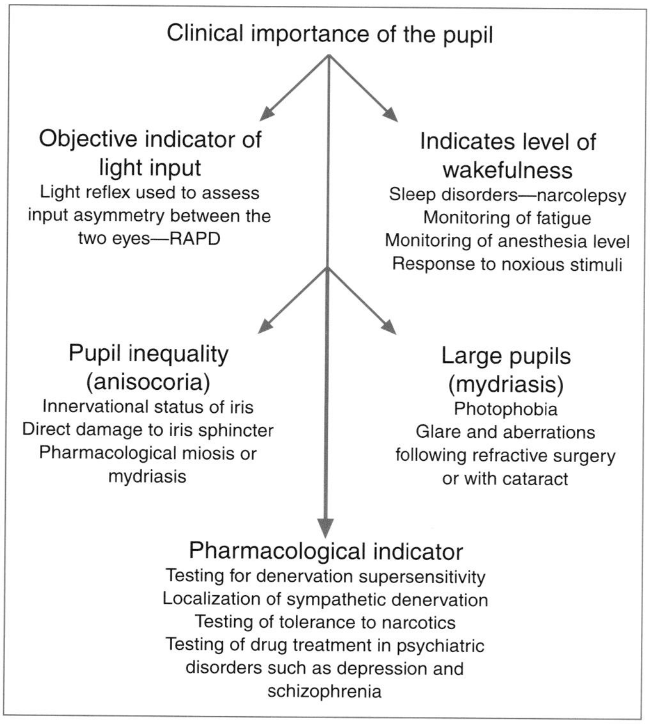

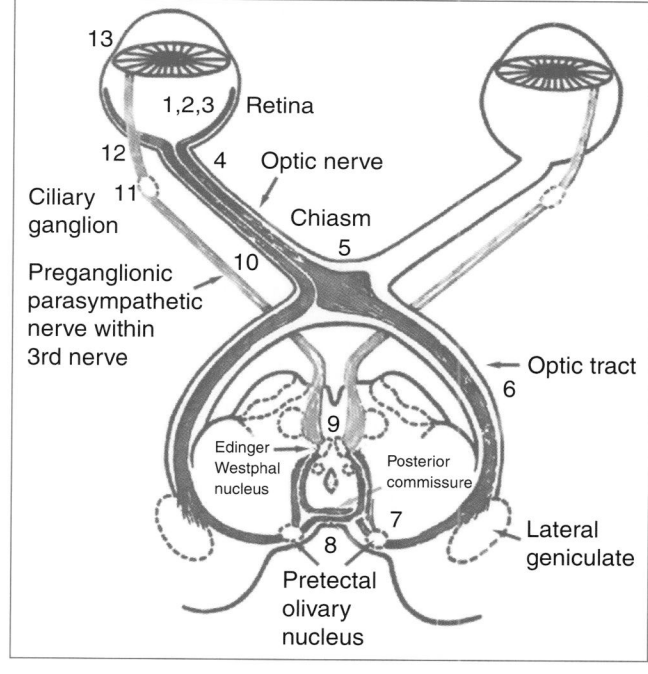

Figure 164.2 Diagram of the nerve pathways involved in the pupil light reflex. The numbers refer to locations where damage can occur (see Table 164.1). Afferent input from the nasal retina crosses to the contralateral side and the pupil input from retinal ganglion cell axons exits the optic tract in the brachium of the superior colliculus to synapse at the pretectal olivary nucleus. The temporal retinal input from the same eye follows a similar course on the ipsilateral side. The neurons in the pretectal olivary nucleus send crossed and uncrossed fibers via the posterior commissure to the Edinger-Westphal nucleus on each side. From here, the preganglionic parasympathetic fibers travel with the oculomotor nerve and then synapse at the ciliary ganglion. The postganglionic parasympathetic neurons pass from the ciliary ganglion via the short ciliary nerves to the iris sphincter muscle.

Figure 164.1 Clinical importance of the pupil.

tion is the same as for the light reflex, but the input pathway to the Edinger-Westphal nucleus differs.

The integration of the pupil light reflex and pupil near response, including the anatomy of the involved neurons, their receptive field properties, and their response to various attributes of light stimuli has been recently reviewed.[1,2]

Almost all disorders of the pupil can be divided into the following disturbances at the following specific locations in the pupil pathway: (1) disorders affecting the afferent pupil pathway (damage to the retina, optic nerve, chiasm, or optic tract); (2) disorders affecting the efferent pupil pathway (damage to the midbrain interneuron, oculomotor nucleus or nerve, ciliary ganglion, ciliary nerves or direct damage to the iris sphincter muscle) and (3) disorders of supranuclear pathways, which may affect pupil size and extent of movement bilaterally to light stimuli or near effort through changes in supranuclear inhibitory influence on the neurons in the Edinger-Westphal nucleus in the midbrain (the preganglionic, efferent neurons of the pupil pathway).

To better understand how various disorders affect the pupil, the neuronal pathways influencing pupil movement and size are shown in Figure 164.2 and the location of lesions (numbered 1–13) are indicated. The most important aspects of Figure 164.1 as they relate to clinical disorders of the pupil are summarized in Table 164.1.

Disorders affecting the afferent pupil pathway

In general, the most important clinical use of the pupil has to do with assessing afferent input from the retina, optic nerve, and anterior visual pathways (chiasm, optic tract, and midbrain pathways). This is because the pupil light reflex is one of the few objective indicators of afferent input that can be assessed. Unlike visual evoked potentials (VEPs) that are weighted toward the central five degrees of visual field, the pupillary input reflects the input of the entire visual field (with some central weighting) to a diffuse full-field light stimulus. Peripheral visual field defects caused by glaucoma or anterior ischemic optic neuropathy would yield a normal visual evoked potential or false negative result, but the pupillary light reflex would be reduced.[3]

The pupil light reflex is not only affected by light input to the retina and optic nerve, but also is modulated by supranuclear input from the reticular activating formation to the midbrain. This accounts for much of the variation in the degree of pupil contraction observed between normal subjects. This intersubject variation in pupil light reflex places constraints on the clinical usefulness of the pupil light reflex in diagnosing symmetric damage to either retinas or optic nerves. However, the input to the pupil light reflex is very symmetric when comparing the two eyes of normal subjects. Therefore, any asymmetric or unilateral damage to the pregeniculate visual system can be sensitively detected and quantified by comparing the pupil light reflex of the two

eyes by alternating the light from one eye to the other while observing for any asymmetry in pupil contraction. The detection of asymmetry of afferent input has been termed the relative afferent pupil defect (Figures 164.3 and 164.4).

The relative afferent pupil defect (RAPD) or Marcus Gunn pupil

Since the pupillary light reflex sums up the entire neuronal input (photoreceptors, bipolar cells, ganglion cells, and axons of ganglion cells), damage anywhere along this portion of the visual pathway will reduce the amplitude of pupillary movement in response to a light stimulus.[1,2] This allows the clinician to pick up any asymmetric damage between the two eyes by simply comparing how well the pupil contracts to a standard light shined into one eye compared to swinging the light over to the other eye.[3,4] Observation of the pupil movement in response to alternating the light back and forth between the two eyes is the basis for the alternating light test or "swinging flashlight" test for assessing the relative afferent pupillary defect.[5,6]

A common impression among clinicians has been that retinal damage causes less of an afferent pupil defect than optic nerve damage for a similar degree of visual field defect. This impression may be partly due to the non-linear relationship between number of optic nerve axons damaged and the resulting amount of visual field defect. Newer instruments used to

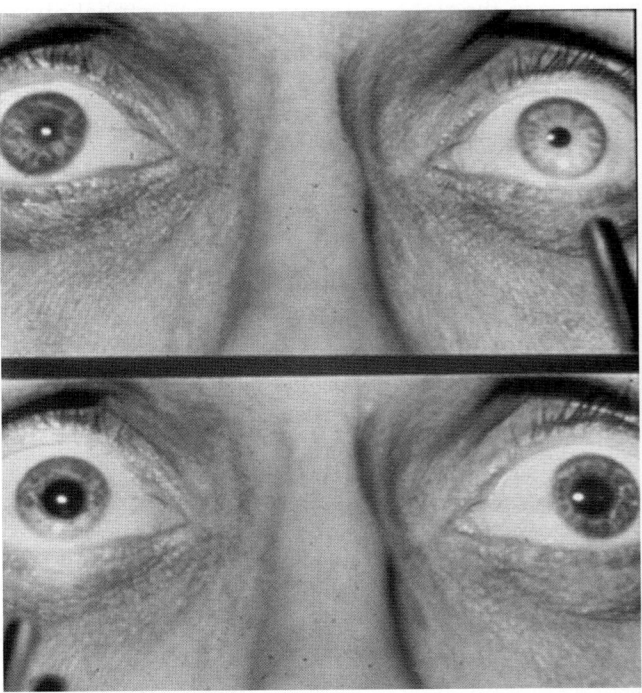

Figure 164.3   A patient is shown with a large relative afferent pupil defect of the right eye. In the top photograph a light is shined in the normal left eye and both pupils constrict to a small size. When the light is alternated to stimulate the right eye (bottom photograph), the pupils do not or hardly constrict at all.

Table 164.1 Localization of lesions in the pupil light reflex pathway

Neuron in pupil pathway	Location in Figure 164.2	Neuron features	Common disorders	Pupil consequences
Afferent Neuron Retinal Photoreceptors	1	Same cells used for visual and pupil input	Retinitis pigmentosa and other retinal dystrophies, posterior uveitis, rarely cancer associated autoimmune	Loss of pupil sensitivity to light parallels visual system
Bipolar cells	2	Same cells used for visual and pupil input	Branch or central retinal artery or vein occlusion, rarely melanoma associated autoimmune damage	Loss of pupil sensitivity to light parallels visual system
Ganglion cells	3	Only about 10^3 out of 10^6 project to midbrain pretectal nucleus	Intraretinal disease (branch or central retinal artery occlusion, diabetic retinopathy)	Relative Afferent Pupil Defect (RAPD) proportional to extent of visual field loss
Ganglion axons (optic nerve)	4	Follow distribution of visual axons up until lateral geniculate	All optic neuropathies (glaucoma, ischemic optic neuropathy, trauma, compression, demyelination)	(RAPD) depending on degree of asymmetry of visual field loss between the two eyes
Optic chiasm	5	Pupil input fibers begin to segregate from visual input fibers	Compression due to pituitary adenoma or meningioma	Usually only small or no RAPD due to symmetry of input damage between two eyes
Optic tract	6	Pupil input fibers of contralateral temporal hemifield join ipsilateral nasal hemifield pupil input	Demyelination, stroke, compression	Usually a small RAPD (0.3–0.6 log units) in the eye contralateral to the tract lesion due to loss of temporal field input which is greater than ipsilateral nasal field
Inter-Neuron Pretectal Olivary Nucleus	7	Pretectal Olivary Nucleus (midbrain)	Midbrain stroke or gliomas	"Tectal" RAPD (for reasons similar to optic tract RAPD) but without visual field loss; small anisocoria in light may be present with unilateral damage
Decussating and non-decussating fibers to Edinger-Westphal Nucleus	8	In primates the decussations are approximately 50–60% of total and travel within the posterior commissure	Dorsal Midbrain Syndrome (pinealomas, stroke). CNS Infections (Argyl-Robertson Pupils due to tertiary syphilis)	Loss of light reflex in both pupils with preservation of near pupil contraction (light near dissociation)
Efferent Neurons (Parasympathetic) Edinger-Westphal Nucleus	9	Same preganglionic neurons are utilized for light reflex and near pupil contraction	Midbrain strokes or tumors with accompanying ocular motility disorders	Anisocoria in light, depending on the degree of asymmetric damage and loss of near pupil reflex
Oculomotor Nerve	10	Pupil fibers are peripheral to oculomotor nerve and lie on medial aspect in subarachnoid portion	Posterior communicating artery aneurysm, pituitary apoplexy, trauma, tumor compression (generally, ischemia will have little effect on pupil)	Unilateral deficit in light and near pupil reflex to light shined in either eye or to near effort; accompanied by degrees of ocular motility deficits and ptosis

continued

Table 164.1   *continued*

Neuron in pupil pathway	Location in Figure 164.2	Neuron features	Common disorders	Pupil consequences
Ciliary ganglion	11	Postganglionic parasympathetic neurons for accommodation (innervating the ciliary body) outnumber those for pupil light and near constriction 30:1	Adie's pupil Orbital surgery	Unilateral deficit in light and near pupil reflex acutely (usually segmental); after months there is aberrant regeneration and return of near reflex but not light reflex
Short ciliary nerves	12	Travel from orbit through sclera and pass to iris sphincter via iris root	Surgery or trauma to globe	Unilateral deficit in light and near pupil reflex acutely (usually segmental)
Iris sphincter muscle	13	20–30 separately innervated segments circumferentially oriented	May be directly damaged by ischemia from very high intraocular pressure, anterior segment ischemia, trauma, or by herpes zoster iritis	Usually segmental areas of damage that do not respond to direct acting topical cholinergic drops (pilocarpine)
Efferent Neurons (Sympathetic) Central neuron (1st order preganglionic)		Travels from hypothalmus, down brainstem, and synapses in lateral cord at lower cervical-upper thoracic levels	Lateral medullary infarct (Wallenberg's syndrome) Spinal cord pathology (trauma, stroke, tumor, arthritis)	Central Horner's Syndrome (miosis, pupil "dilation lag," mild ptosis, anhidrosis) accompanied by other neurological deficits depending on extent and location of lesion
2nd order neuron (preganglionic)		Passes from lateral cord over apex of lung and synapses at superior cervical ganglion at carotid bifurcation	Often damaged by surgical trauma, chest tubes, metastatic lung or breast carcinoma	Horner's syndrome, indistinguishable from central Horner's on pupil exam
3rd order neuron (postganglionic)		Postganglionic axons of superior cervical ganglion follow the internal carotid artery and into the orbital apex and travel in the long ciliary nerves to supply the iris dilator	May be associated with carotid artery dissections, intracranial masses or trauma (surgery or basilar skull fractures), and also with cluster headaches	Horner's syndrome that may be distinguished from preganglionic 1st or 2nd order lesions by failure of pupil dilatation to topical hydroxyamphetamine, compared to contralateral eye

assess the thickness of the retinal nerve fiber layer (which is proportional to the number of axons) as well as autopsy and animal studies seem to indicated that a large percentage of axon loss is required (30–50%) before visual field defects are picked up. However, the pupil response may be more linearly proportional to axon damage. This could explain why it might seem like in some cases, optic nerve damage seems to cause more pupil deficit than retinal damage.

The pupillary light reflex is one of the few objective reflexes that can be used as a clinical test for detecting and quantifying abnormalities of the retina, optic nerve, optic chiasm or optic tract. Because the amount of the relative afferent pupillary defect is correlated to a large extent with the amount of asymmetry of visual field deficit between the two eyes, it can also be used to help substantiate abnormal results of visual field testing.[7–10] This can often help the clinician to determine whether a patient's visual field defects are believable and trustworthy. This correlation between the visual field asymmetry and the relative afferent pupillary defect is also useful in following the course of disease to determine if there is a worsening or improvement in function over time. To this extent, it is important to emphasize that the relative afferent pupillary defect is indeed, relative to the input of one

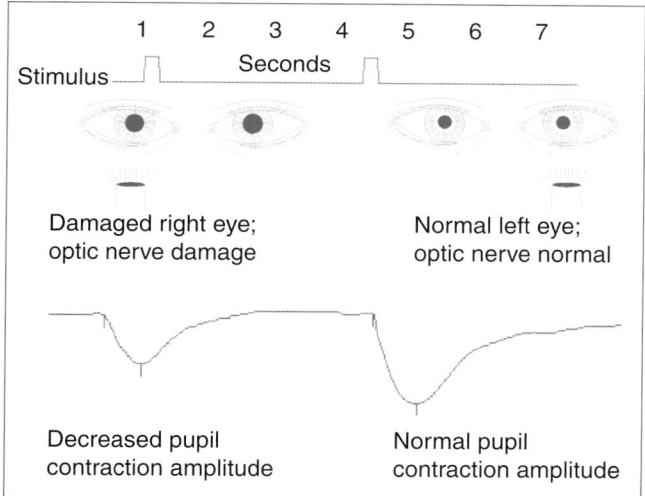

Figure 164.4 Pupillographic demonstration of a right relative afferent pupil defect. With short light pulses the pupil light reflex (bottom tracings) are of lesser amplitude when the stimulus was given to the right eye compared to stimulus to the left eye.

eye compared to the other. Bilateral symmetric damage will produce no relative afferent pupillary defect. Similarly, a patient with a definite relative afferent pupillary defect in one eye on the first visit, when returning for follow-up may show no relative afferent pupillary defect. This may represent improvement in the previously damaged eye. However, it may also indicate that there is now damage in what was previously the better eye, matching the damage to the other eye, so that there are now symmetric visual field defects and no relative afferent pupillary defect. Therefore, it is always important to remember that the relative afferent defect is indeed, relative to the other eye.

Lesions distal to the optic nerve (chiasm and optic tract) may also produce an RAPD, depending on the asymmetry of visual field defect between the two eyes. For example, a complete chiasmal lesion with a bitemporal field defect would not produce an RAPD, but in most cases, the field loss is asymmetric and often involves the intracranial portion of one optic nerve; this is why an RAPD may be common in a chiasmal lesion. An optic tract lesion also commonly produces an RAPD in the eye with the temporal field loss. This is because the temporal visual field provides more input to the pupil light reflex compared to the nasal field in most individuals. During the alternating light test of a patient with an optic tract lesion, the input of the working nasal hemifield of the eye contralateral to the optic tract lesion is compared to the intact temporal field of the eye ipsilateral to the optic tract lesion, and this produces an RAPD. Therefore, a patient with homonymous field loss can usually be localized to a pregeniculate (optic tract lesion) versus a postgeniculate lesion based on whether an RAPD is present.

Recent studies using computerized pupillography

to more precisely quantify the log unit relative afferent pupillary defect has also revealed that some normal subjects with normal visual fields and exam can have a small 0.3 log unit relative afferent pupillary defect.[11,12] Therefore, small relative afferent pupillary defects discovered incidentally in a patient without ocular complaints and a normal exam can probably be dismissed.

Estimating the amount of the pupillomotor input asymmetry (the "relative afferent pupillary defect") can of course be done roughly using the alternating light test—without any neutral density filters by subjectively grading the asymmetry of pupil response as +1, +2, +3 or +4. This subjective grading can also be classified according to the amount of "pupil escape" or dilation of the pupils as the light is alternated to the opposite eye.[13] Subjective grading of the relative afferent pupillary defect has serious limitations; it is subject to some wild errors due to age variations in pupil size and pupil mobility. For example, a patient with small pupils and small pupil contractions to light may have a large relative afferent pupillary defect that may appear deceptively small based on the small differences in pupil excursion observed as the light is alternated between the two eyes. However, the amount of neutral density filter needed to dim the better eye until the small contractions are equal could easily approach 0.9 to 1.2 log units, representing substantial input damage. For clinical purposes, more accurate quantification of the relative afferent pupillary defect is accomplished by determining the log unit difference needed to "balance" the pupil reaction between the two eyes.[5,6] This is done using photographic neutral density filters, that can be purchased through local photo supply stores in increments of 0.3 log, 0.6 log, and 0.9 log units.

Measuring the relative afferent pupillary defect

Measuring the relative afferent pupillary defect (RAPD) is the most important part of the pupil examination—it is the most frequently used part of the exam, and it gives the most valuable clinical information. The alternating light test for an afferent defect is usually based on the assumption that you are working with a matched pair of irises—each of them with structurally normal sphincter and dilator muscles and properly innervated, so that the light reactions can be compared. As the light is alternated back and forth between the two eyes in dim room lighting, the contraction amplitude of the pupil of the eye being illuminated is compared to that of the other pupil when the light is switched over to the contralateral eye (Figure 164.3 and 164.4). Therefore, the direct pupil movement to light is most often used, but it is imperative that the direct and consensual pupil movement is equal under this paradigm and no efferent pupil defect exists. This is best checked by brightly illuminating both eyes with the room light turned up or a bright spot light; if the efferent movement of both pupils is matched, then there should be no anisocoria in bright light. If there is, then the next best thing is to observe only one pupil's movement using an accessory dim sidelight, so that pupil's movement can be observed even when the stimulating light is abruptly moved to the other eye.

To check for a relative afferent pupillary defect, start alternating the light from one eye to the other. It is best to hold the light in front of the eye for approximately three seconds, to induce a pupil constriction, and to allow the pupils to dilate or escape (due to adaptation) toward the end of the three seconds. The escape component is important because it ensures that there will still be some initial contraction when the light is alternated to the other eye. If the light is too bright the pupils will not re-dilate or escape promptly and you will see very little pupillary movement as the light is alternated to the other eye. If this is the case, either reduce the stimulus intensity, or reduce the distance between the light and the eye to three or four inches and then continue to alternate the light. Alternately, one can increase the darkness interval by deliberately passing the light under the patient's nose on the way from one eye to the other. This allows for an extended dark interval between the alternation of the light, allowing the pupils to dilate and sets the starting pupil diameter of the about-to-be-illuminated eye at a higher level. This gives a more visible light reaction but it reduces that slight amplification of the difference between the two responses that comes with prompt alternation of the light. If the pupils react relatively weakly when one eye is stimulated and better when the other is stimulated, then an afferent defect has been identified relative to the better eye and is termed a "relative afferent pupil defect" (RAPD).

Balancing the pupil responses with filters to obtain the log unit RAPD is done by holding a neutral density filter up over the better responding eye and repeating the alternating light test. If the input asymmetry is still visible, increase the density of the filter over the good eye until the amplitude of the direct light reactions of the two eyes is balanced. Deliberately overshoot the balance point and then return to it, to be certain of your measurement. When a dense filter is used it may be necessary to angle the filter so that you can still peek behind the filter just to see the pupil, but at the same time the stimulus light to the eye is dimmed. Sometimes a very small asymmetry is found (e.g., a defect of less than 0.3 log in the left eye) and the examiner is not sure whether he is just seeing noise in the system (i.e., "hippus" or variability in response) or an actual RAPD. In such cases, an effort can be made to confirm a real asymmetry by "tilting" the RAPD to the right and to the left with a 0.3 log filter. The 0.3 log unit filter is held over one eye to see how much asymmetry is induced (in a normal subject, a small RAPD is induced in the eye behind the filter). The filter is then placed over the other eye to see if the same amount of asymmetry is induced in the other eye. In a patient with no RAPD an asymmetry should be induced by the same amount in either eye. In a patient with a small RAPD, the 0.3 log unit filter will amplify the RAPD when held over that eye and will minimize it (or neutralize it) when held over the other eye.

The pupillary response to a repeated light stimulus is far from constant; it changes from moment to moment.[11,12] A common mistake is to make a judgment about apparent asymmetry of the light reflex too quickly. It is important to alternate the light back and forth at least three times to get a mental average of any asymmetry. By doing this, moment to moment fluctuations in the pupil response can be "averaged out."

Infants and children (and even some anxious adults) may appear to have weak pupillary responses to light. This is due to excitement and apprehension, which act to inhibit the pupillary light reflex at the supranuclear level in the midbrain. Usually, when the light stimulus is repeated several times the light reaction begins to improve and "loosen up," especially as the child becomes less anxious. A baby's pupils can be checked from about a meter away with a direct ophthalmoscope. In a dark room, use the brightest light and the smallest spot, focus on the red reflex and alternate the light from eye to eye. The baby is usually fascinated, and a filter can sometimes be placed in the beam to one eye.

Instrumentation is also available in some centers for more precise evaluation of the pupillary light reflex. This includes infrared video recording equipment and in some cases, a computerized interface for presenting controlled light stimuli and quantifying the dynamics of pupil movement in response to each light stimulus:

Infrared videography   Sometimes it is important to see the magnified movement of both pupils at once, and infrared videography enables the examiner to see both pupils clearly in the dark. This is especially helpful for checking difficult afferent pupil defects, such as when one pupil is fixed, or both irises are very darkly pigmented. Since melanin reflects infrared light, dark irises appear light and allow the black pupils to stand out in contrast for easy viewing. Videography is also useful when looking for dilation lag of a Horner's pupil, for catching the brief paradoxical constriction when the lights are turned out in patients with some retinal abnormalities, and for trans-illuminating the iris in pigment dispersion syndrome and in Adie's syndrome.[14]

Computerized pupillometry   Various computerized, infrared-sensitive pupillometers are commercially available. Most of these elegant instruments can precisely record the dynamics of pupillary movement in the light or in the dark. Once recorded, the pupillary information can be analyzed by sophisticated software. This allows very quantitative information about the pupillary light reflex to be assessed which, in the future may help to automate the clinical determination of pupillary input deficits caused by retinal and optic nerve diseases.[11,12,15-17] In addition, new information has been obtained using computerized pupillography that provides evidence that a number of different types of visual stimuli can produce changes in the pupillary light reflex related to color, form, movement, and acuity.[18-24]

Pupil perimetry An automated perimeter can be modified to record pupillary responses to small focal light stimuli. A video camera is pointed at the pupil and the amplitude of each light reaction is measured and stored in the computer. This has turned out to be helpful as an objective form of perimetry and for localizing lesions in the pupillary pathways.[25,26] Pupil perimetry is useful in cases of non-organic, functional visual loss to show objectively that messages are indeed going normally into the brain from parts of the visual field in which the patient claims to see nothing. Of interest is that many of these studies with small, focal stimuli or stimuli having attributes of spatial frequency have shown that lesions of the postgeniculate pathway *do* cause deficits of the pupil light reflex in areas of homonymous field loss, but do not show an

RAPD when the full field is stimulated by diffuse light. Therefore, evidence is accumulating to indicate that visual cortex may indeed play a role in modulating some aspects of the pupil light reflex (Table 164.2).

Disorders affecting the efferent pupil pathway

Lesions that interrupt the pupillary pathway starting from the intercalated neuron (arising from the olivary pretectal nucleus in the midbrain), and including the preganglionic or postganglionic parasympathetic pathway and direct damage to the iris sphincter muscle may produce various degrees of deficit in the pupil light reflex. Lesions along this pathway and also lesions along the sympathetic pathway usually produce pupil inequality (anisocoria). Often, the

Table 164.2   Common diseases producing relative afferent pupillary defects (RAPD) and expected magnitude of defect

Condition	Site	Log unit RAPD	Influencing factors
Intraocular hemorrhage	Anterior chamber or vitreous (dense)	0.6–1.2 log units	Density of hemorrhage
Intraocular hemorrhage	Anterior chamber (diffuse)	0.0–0.3 log units	Density of hemorrhage
Intraocular hemorrhage	Preretinal (central vein occlusion or diabetic)	0.0 log units	Preretinal location does not significantly reduce light
Diffusing media opacity	Cataract corneal scar	0.0–0.3 log units in opposite eye	Dispersion of light producing increase in light input
Unilateral functional visual field loss	None	0.0 log units	
Central serous retinopathy (CSR) or cystoid macular edema (CME)	Retina (fovea)	0.3 log units	Area of retina involved
Central or branch retinal vein occlusion (CRVO, BRVO)	Inner retina	0.3–0.6 log units (non-ischemic) ≥ 0.9 log units (ischemic)	Area of visual field defect and degree of ischemia
Central or branch retinal artery occlusion (CRAO, BRAO)	Inner retina	0.3–3.0 log units	Area and location of retina involved
Retinal detachment	Outer retina	0.3–2.1 log units	Area and location of detached retina (e.g., 0.6 log units for macula +0.3 log units for each quadrant)
Anterior ischemic optic neuropathy	Optic nerve head	0.6–2.7 log units	Extent and location of visual field defect
Optic neuritis (acute)	Optic nerve	0.6–3.0 log units	Extent and location of visual field defect
Optic neuritis (recovered)	Optic nerve	0.0–0.6 log units	No visual field defect, residual RAPD
Compressive optic neuropathy	Optic nerve	0.3–3.0 log units	Extent and location of visual field defect
Chiasmal compression	Optic chiasm	0.0–1.2 log units	Asymmetry of visual field loss, unilateral central field involvement
Optic tract lesion	Optic tract	0.3–1.2 log units in the eye with temporal field loss	Incongruity of homonymous field defect, hemifield pupillomotor input asymmetry
Postgeniculate damage	Visual radiations Visual cortex	0.0 log unit RAPD	Stimulus light area (no RAPD but definite pupil perimetry defects)
Midbrain tectal damage	Olivary pretectal area of pupil light input region of midbrain	0.3–1.0 log units	Similar to optic tract lesions, but no visual field defect

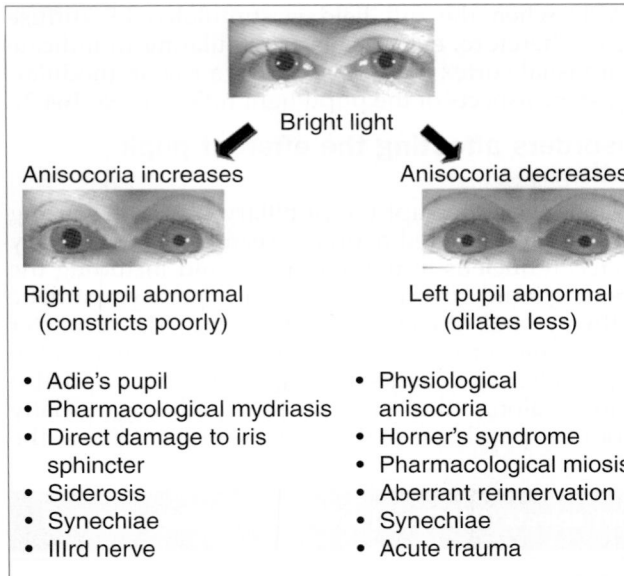

Figure 164.5 The cause of anisocoria in room light is determined by first adding bright light to determine if the anisocoria increases (left) or decreases (right). The two eyes were brought closer together using base out prisms while recording with an infrared video camera.

clinical dilemma is to identify the cause of anisocoria (Figure 164.5), some of which may be benign, while others may be life threatening.

Anisocoria

When a pupillary inequality is seen, it usually means that one of the four iris muscles, or its innervation, is damaged in the efferent pupil pathway. In order to sort out which muscle is not working right, it helps to know how the anisocoria is influenced by light. It is worth noting that an anisocoria always increases in the direction of action of the paretic iris muscle. Therefore, a weak iris sphincter muscle will be most apparent in bright light and under these lighting conditions the resulting anisocoria will be maximal. Conversely, a weak dilator muscle will be most evident in dim light, where the anisocoria will be most apparent (Figure 164.5).

Pupil inequality that is greatest in dim light (lesions of the sympathetic pathway) In such patients, the problem is distinguishing a Horner's syndrome (oculosympathetic deficit causing a weak dilator muscle) from a "simple anisocoria" (or "physiological anisocoria"). In both conditions, the inequality is greater in dim light. A simple anisocoria may vary from day to day, or even from hour to hour and is visible in about a fifth of the normal population and is not related to refractive error. In physiological anisocoria, both pupils dilate promptly to a decrement in light or with excitatory stimuli. In contrast, Horner's syndrome is recognized by looking for an impaired reflex dilation of the smaller pupil compared to the contralateral pupil. In addition, other associated signs, such as

ptosis, "upside down ptosis" of the lower lid, anhidrosis, and in a fresh case, conjunctival injection and lowered intraocular pressure are present.

Physiological anisocoria "Simple Anisocoria" is common, (about 10% of normal subjects, examined in room light, will have an anisocoria of 0.4 mm or more), it is not associated with disease, and it may change from day to day. Simple anisocoria also, like Horner's syndrome, decreases slightly in light, but it does not show a dilation lag of the smaller pupil. Current thinking indicates that simple anisocoria is most likely due to asymmetric inhibition at the Edinger-Westphal nucleus in the midbrain. Normally, during wakefulness there is some inhibition from the reticular activating formation to keep the pupils midsize or larger. During sleep, this inhibition fades and allows the neurons in the Edinger-Westphal nucleus to discharge resulting in miotic pupils. If during wakefulness, the inhibition is greater to the right Edinger-Westphal nucleus compared to the left, then the right pupil will be larger, especially in dim light. When light is added, or a near reflex is generated, this inhibition is overcome and the pupils become smaller and any asymmetric inhibition becomes less. This results in a reduction of the anisocoria as the pupils become smaller.

Oculosympathetic defects (Horner's syndrome) The characteristic "dilation lag" of the Horner's pupil can be easily seen in the office with a hand light shining from below. The room lights should be switched off and the smaller pupil examined to see if it appears reluctant to dilate. Pupillary dilation is normally a combination of sphincter relaxation and dilator contraction. This combination produces a prompt dilation. The patient with Horner's syndrome has a weak dilator muscle in one iris and, as a result, that pupil dilates more slowly than the normal pupil. If the sympathetic lesion is complete, the affected pupil will dilate only by sphincter relaxation. This asymmetry of pupillary dilation produces an anisocoria, which is largest four to five seconds, after the lights are turned out. This is a much slower process than most people imagine. Ten to twenty seconds after the lights are out, the anisocoria lessens as the sympathectomized pupil gradually catches up, a process referred to as "dilation lag" (Figure 164.6). This test is a quick and simple way of distinguishing Horner's syndrome from simple anisocoria, and it is a test that does not require pupillary drug testing. It works well most of the time, especially in young people with mobile pupils, but if the dilation lag is inconclusive, cocaine eye drops may be used to confirm the diagnosis of Horner's syndrome. Cocaine's action is to block the re-uptake of the norepinephrine that is normally released from the nerve endings. If, because of an interruption in the sympathetic pathway, norepinephrine is not being released, cocaine has no adrenergic effect. A Horner's pupil will dilate less to cocaine than the normal pupil, regardless of the location of the lesion. Forty-five minutes after putting cocaine drops

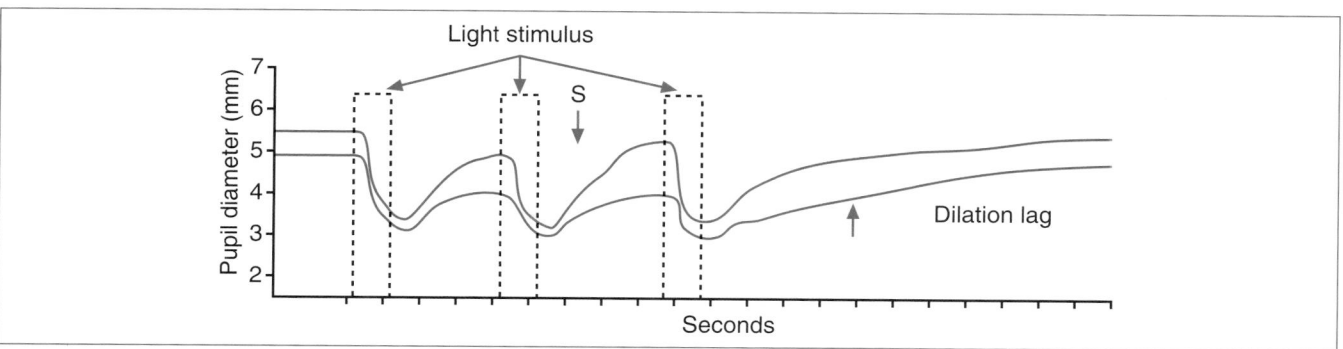

Figure 164.6 Example of a pupillographic demonstration of dilation lag of the pupil in the eye with Horner's syndrome. The smaller pupil is slow to dilate, causing an increase in anisocoria during the early phase of dilation and accentuated by a loud sound (S). In the last part of the tracing, no further stimulus was given to allow the dilation lag to be observed in the tracing. The dilation lag is a delayed dilation of the smaller pupil; after five seconds in darkness (arrow), the smaller pupil slowly dilates due to inhibition of the sphincter muscle, in spite of loss of sympathetic nerve contribution to pupil dilation.

in both eyes the anisocoria should have clearly increased because the normal pupil has dilated more than the Horner's pupil. It is recommended that 10% cocaine HCl be topically placed in both eyes (never more than two drops) to be sure that even the darkest iris gets a full mydriatic dose. It should be said that 2%, 4%, and 5% cocaine have also been used as a diagnostic test for Horner's syndrome and also work well. Forty to sixty minutes should be allowed to elapse before the anisocoria is measured. If there is very little dilation of the eye with a suspected oculosympathetic defect, and this pupil never dilated well in darkness even after 30 seconds, then a false positive cocaine test also needs to be considered. This can occur if the iris is in some way held in a miotic state by either scarring or aberrant reinnervation of the iris sphincter. In such cases, adding a direct acting sympathomimetic agent to both eyes (i.e., 2.5% neosynephrine) at the conclusion of a positive cocaine test should easily dilate the suspected eye and the cocaine-induced anisocoria is almost eliminated. A pseudo-Horner's syndrome due to the reason's stated above would result in inadequate dilation to direct acting sympathetic agents. The likelihood of a diagnosis of Horner's syndrome increases steadily with increasing degrees of pupillary inequality (measured after the instillation of cocaine). If there is at least 0.8 mm of pupillary inequality after cocaine, the presence of a Horner's syndrome is highly likely.[27] Localization of the damage to the sympathetic pathway to either the preganglionic or postganglionic neuron is of considerable clinical importance. Many postganglionic defects are caused by benign vascular headache syndromes or carotid dissections. A preganglionic lesion is sometimes due to the spread of a malignant neoplasm to the second order neuron, a spinal cord problem or damage to the first order neuron (central Horner's) secondary to a stroke such as a lateral medullary infarct. Hydroxyamphetamine eyedrops help in localizing the lesion to either the preganglionic (first or second order preganglionic lesions cannot be differentiated with the test) or postganglionic in Horner's syndrome. The clinician would

like to know where the lesion is because that knowledge directs the radiographic work-up, for example, to the internal carotid artery rather than to the pulmonary apex. Horner's syndrome sometimes presents itself in such a characteristic setting that further efforts at localizing the lesion are not needed. This is true of patients with "cluster headaches." Hydroxyamphetamine acts by releasing norepinephrine from storage in the sympathetic nerve endings. When the lesion is postganglionic, the nerve is dead and no norepinephrine stores are available for release. When the lesion is complete, a pupil like this will not dilate at all. However a time period of almost a week from the onset of damage may be needed before the dying neurons and their stores of norepinephrine are gone. Therefore, a hydroxyamphetamine test given within a week of a postganglionic lesion, such as a carotid dissection, may give a false preganglionic localization if the norepinephrine stores had not yet disappeared. Horner's pupils due to preganglionic or central lesions will dilate at least normally, because the postganglionic neuron with its stores of norepinephrine, although disconnected, is still intact. In fact, when the lesion is in the preganglionic neuron, the Horner's pupil often becomes larger than the normal pupil—due apparently to "decentralization supersensitivity." In the hydroxyamphetamine test, the pupils are measured before and 40–60 minutes after hydroxyamphetamine drops have been put in both eyes, and the change in anisocoria in room light is noted. If the Horner's pupil (the smaller one) dilates less than the normal pupil, and the anisocoria increases, the lesion is in the postganglionic neuron. If the smaller pupil dilates well so that the anisocoria becomes less (or it becomes the larger pupil), then the lesion is preganglionic and the postganglionic neuron is intact. The examiner should wait at least three days after using cocaine before using hydroxyamphetamine, as cocaine seems to block its effectiveness by competing for its uptake into the presynaptic terminal. Postganglionic lesions (along the carotid artery) can be separated from the non-postganglionic lesions (in the brainstem, spinal cord, upper lung and lower neck) with a degree of certainty that varies with the amount of anisocoria induced when the drops are put in both eyes.[28] In infants, hydroxyamphetamine drops are not helpful in localizing the lesion because orthograde transynaptic dysgenesis takes place at the superior cervical ganglion after an early interruption of the preganglionic oculosympathetic neuron. This results in fewer postganglionic neurons, even though there was no postganglionic injury, and this, in turn, produces weak mydriasis and ambiguous answers from the hydroxyamphetamine test in children.[29] A Horner's syndrome that has been clearly acquired in infancy should be evaluated for neuroblastoma—a treatable tumor.

Pupillary inequality that is greatest in bright light Pupil inequality that increases with greater illumination may be due to direct damage to the iris sphincter muscle, pharmacological blockade, or to interruption of the pre- or postganglionic parasympathetic innervation. In order to differentiate these sites, it is advantageous to evaluate the iris directly under high magnification (usually done with the aid of a slit lamp in the emergency room or in an eye examination room).

Direct damage to the iris sphincter muscle or pharmacological mydriasis Trauma to the globe will usually result in a torn sphincter and an iris that trans-illuminates at the slit lamp. The pupil is often not round and there may be other evidence of ocular injury. Naturally, such a pupil will not constrict well to light. The residual reaction is often segmental in a traumatic iridoplegia. An atrophic sphincter due to previous herpes zoster iritis may also reveal trans-illumination defects seen with the slit lamp from previous ischemic insults to the iris. If, however, the iris looks normal, and there is no residual pupil light reflex (or very little) and no evidence of sectors of the iris sphincter behaving asymmetrically, then the possibility of atropinic mydriasis should be considered.[30] However, a completely blocked light reaction can sometimes be seen when the sphincter is denervated by either a preganglionic lesion (third nerve palsy) or a postganglionic lesion (fresh tonic pupil) or in acute angle closure (iris ischemia) or in the presence of an intraocular iron foreign body (iron mydriasis). If the dilated pupil still has some response to light, the dilation could be due to partial denervation of the sphincter or to incomplete atropinization or to adrenergic mydriasis. When the light reaction is poor because the dilator muscle is in spasm (due to adrenergic mydriatics like phenylephrine or sympathetic activation), then the pupil will be very large. However, it may still contract some to bright light due to a working iris sphincter muscle, which can overpower the dilator spasm. In cases of mydriasis due to over-activation of the dilator muscle, other associated signs may help to make the diagnosis. These include conjunctival blanching from sympathomimetic influences on the conjunctival blood vessels, and eyelid retraction due to activation of Mueller's smooth muscle. In such a

case of sympathetic activation induced mydriasis, the amplitude of accommodation will hardly be affected and any decrease in focus will be due to spherical aberration and to a shallow depth of field, both purely optical results of the dilated pupil. When there is some residual light reaction, the next step is to look with the slit lamp under high magnification for sector palsy of the iris sphincter when the illuminating light is turned off and on. When the dilator is in a drug-induced adrenergic spasm or when an atropine-like drug blocks the cholinergic receptors in the iris sphincter, then the entire sphincter muscle (all 360 degrees of it) is symmetrically affected. This is not the case when postganglionic parasympathetic nerve fibers have been interrupted. For example, all Adie's pupils with a residual light reaction (about 90% of them) have segmental contractions of some sections of normally innervated iris sphincter. Many patients with an associated diabetic autonomic neuropathy show a similar picture. This means that when you see a pupil with a weak light reaction and no segmental palsy is seen, the examiner should think about a drug-induced mydriasis and then perhaps look again for lid and motility signs of a third nerve paresis with preganglionic parasympathetic denervation of the iris sphincter. In some cases where it is still unclear if the weakness of the iris sphincter is due to denervation, then cholinergic supersensitivity testing may help. Weak pilocarpine (0.0625%, 0.1%, 0.125%), or weak methacholine (2.5%) is applied to both eyes. In testing for cholinergic supersensitivity, it is important to ensure equal penetration of the drug to both eyes, since the miotic response will be compared. Corneas should be healthy and untouched, tear function should be normal, and the eyelids should be working properly in both eyes. Otherwise unequal penetration of the dilute cholinergic drops may give false positive results. Typically, the relative response of the two pupils is observed in dim light after 30 minutes. If the affected (more dilated) pupil constricts more than the normal pupil after the test, so that it actually becomes the smaller pupil, then the iris sphincter has probably lost some of its innervation and is showing signs of receptor supersensitivity. It seems likely that with a postganglionic denervation (ciliary ganglion to the eye) the sphincter will show a bit more supersensitivity than in the preganglionic case (third nerve palsy). It appears, however, that the differences are not great. Ptosis or diplopia in extreme gazes should be looked for once more to ensure that the oculomotor nerve is intact. It is very rare for an ambulatory patient to have isolated iris sphincter palsy as a result of damage to the third nerve without some other signs of involvement of the eyelid or extraocular muscles. If the normal pupil constricts a little in response to dilute topical cholinergics and the dilated pupil not at all, then the dilation of the pupil may be due to a local dose of an anticholinergic drug like atropine. A stronger concentration of 1% pilocarpine is then instilled in both eyes and if the affected pupil still does not constrict as well as the contralateral normal pupil, then either there is pharmacological cholinergic blockade or direct damage to the iris sphincter muscle. The following are non-neuronal causes of mydriasis that fails to constrict properly to direct acting, non-dilute cholinergic agents: (a) anti-cholinergic mydriasis (e.g., scopolamine, cyclopentolate, atropine, hyoscine); (b) traumatic iridoplegia (look for other signs of trauma, such as sphincter rupture, pigment dispersion in the anterior chamber, or angle recession on gonioscopy performed by an ophthalmologist); (c) angle closure glaucoma in the past, causing infarct of all or parts of the iris sphincter muscle and (d) fixed pupil following anterior segment surgery (may also be due to post-operative spike in intraocular pressure).

Iris sphincter denervation   A common cause of an efferent pupil defect due to postganglionic denervation is Adie's tonic pupil. Adie's pupil is an efferent pupil defect in which the light reaction of one or more iris sphincter segments is lost due to injury of the postganglionic parasympathetic nerves originating in the ciliary ganglion.[31] The exact cause of the injury is usually not known, but in most cases it is benign. The pathological process begins with an acute denervation of smooth muscle segments in both the iris sphincter and ciliary body, followed by re-innervation of the muscles by accommodative neurons over time. Acutely, there is loss of part or all of the pupil light reflex and decrease in accommodative function at near. Chronically, with re-growth of axons of accommodative neurons, focusing improves somewhat, but contraction of the pupil to light does not (Figures 164.7, 164.8 and 164.9). Young adults (more women than men) may suddenly find that one pupil is large or that they cannot focus one eye up close. Slit lamp exam usually shows segmental denervation of the iris sphincter. Within the first week, supersensitivity to cholinergic substances can be demonstrated. After about two months, nerve regrowth has been active and fibers originally bound for the ciliary muscle (they outnumber the sphincter fibers by 30:1) start arriving (aberrantly) to re-innervate the iris sphincter. This produces the characteristic "light-near dissociation" of Adie's syndrome. Eventually the affected pupil becomes the smaller of the two pupils, especially in dim light. It turns out that the segmental palsy of the iris sphincter can be seen especially well by infrared video recording of trans-illumination of the iris (Figure 164.9).[14] As the ciliary body becomes re-innervated, accommodation may also improve over time. However, the dynamics of focusing are not normal and commonly cause symptoms when a patient with chronic Adie's syndrome changes focus from near targets to objects in the distance. A number of terms have been used to describe the condition of postganglionic parasympathetic denervation of the iris sphincter. Some of these terms refer to the authors of early publications of case series on this condition and some terms describe associated dysfunction. The following are terms often encountered with their description:

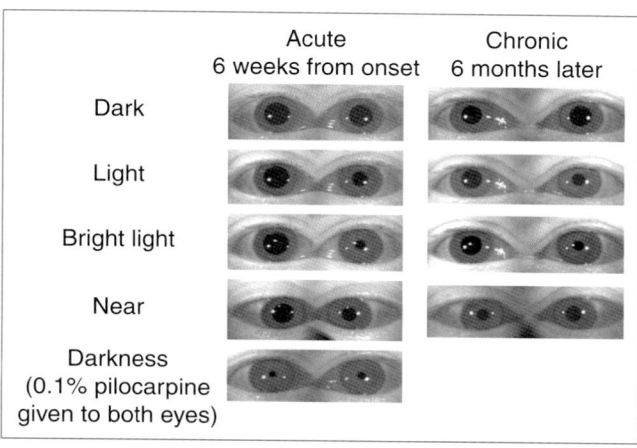

Figure 164.7   Example of a relatively new onset (six weeks old) Adie's pupil (left panel) showing only a small anisocoria in darkness (upper left), and an increasing anisocoria in room light (sequence on left below top picture). With a near effort, there is only a small pupil contraction with resulting decrease in pupil size in the affected right eye, indicating the beginning of re-innervation of the iris sphincter by accommodative fibers. When dilute 0.1% pilocarpine is added to both pupils, miosis occurs in both eyes, but more in the right eye, indicating cholinergic supersensitivity. Six months later the same patient was re-examined (right panel). The right pupil was now smaller than the left pupil in darkness due to re-innervation by accommodative nerve fibers. The light reflex remains damaged, as indicated by an increasing anisocoria with light and bright light. A light-near dissociation with a greater contraction of the left pupil to a near stimulus compared to light (lower right) indicates a chronic state due to re-innervation of the iris sphincter by accommodative neurons.

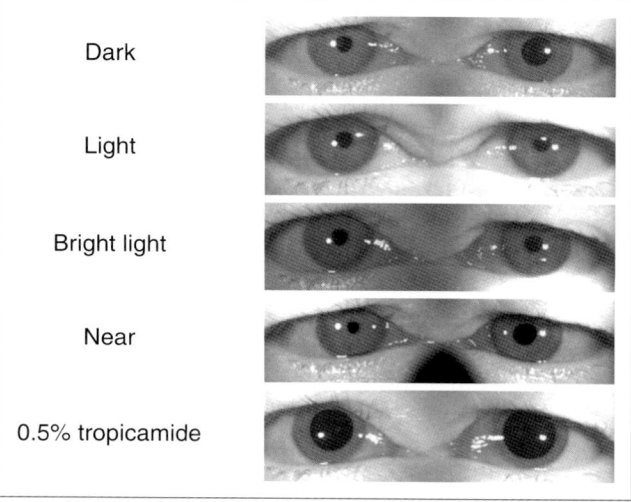

Figure 164.8   Infrared video frames of a patient with a chronic right Adie's pupil, demonstrating a small pupil that does not dilate well in darkness and does not constrict in light, but does constrict more to near effort. Although the pupil does not dilate well in darkness, it does dilate well to topical anticholinergic drops (tropicamide 0.5%).

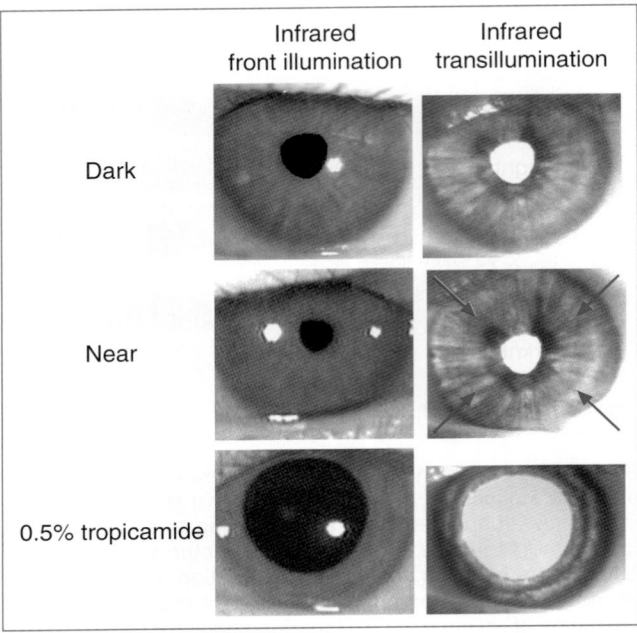

Figure 164.9   Infrared iris trans-illumination in Adie's pupil. Front infrared illumination of a chronic Adie's pupil that is irregular in shape is shown in the left panel of photos and the corresponding infrared trans-illumination of the iris is shown in the right panel. The normal iris sphincter appears as a dark ring at the pupillary border when it contracts, as observed with infrared iris trans-illumination. In the patient shown, the iris sphincter was denervated at the 12 o'clock, 4 o'clock, and 8 o'clock meridians and appears lighter on trans-illumination at these locations. The intervening sphincter areas (arrows) appear darker due to a state of chronic constriction caused by iris re-innervation by accommodative nerves. After cholinergic blockade with topical tropicamide, the sphincter relaxes in all segments and appears light in color over 360 degrees.

- *Adie's pupil or Holmes-Adie's pupil* Most people refer to the postganglionic parasympathetic denervation of the pupil as an Adie's pupil (the student of Holmes) since he described a large case series of patients, however, he was not the first to describe this condition.[32] Although Adie's description included patients with loss of deep tendon reflexes, this association is not required for a patient to have an "Adie's pupil." Although it may be historically unjustifiable, the term "Adie's pupil" now seems to be used to refer to any peripheral parasympathetic internal ophthalmoplegia that is any interruption of the postganglionic parasympathetic nerves to the intraocular muscles. The list of causes is, therefore, long and includes trauma, tumor, infection, and ischemia in addition to the idiopathic and apparently non-syphilitic form that caught the attention of doctors early in the twentieth century. Whether this last, and commonest form is due to "organ specific autoimmune response" is something that is yet to be proven.
- *"Adie's like" pupil* Iatrogenic causes of postganglionic parasympathetic denervation may result from orbital surgery, cryotherapy to the sclera and

underlying short ciliary nerves, laser treatment to the trabecular meshwork, or heavy photocoagulation treatment of the retina. Presumably, these procedures inadvertently damage the short ciliary nerves, and produce a condition that resembles the idiopathic form of Adie's pupil.
- *Adie's syndrome* This term is used when a patient with an Adie's pupil also exhibits other associated dysfunction, such as decrease in deep tendon reflexes or loss of vibratory sensation. The loss of deep tendon reflex may be common (i.e., 75% of patients with Adie's pupil), but is still thought to be benign. It may well be a manifestation of a similar process of denervation occurring at other neuronal locations.
- *Adie's tonic pupil, tonic pupil, and "little old Adie's pupil"* Following acute postganglionic parasympathetic denervation, aberrant re-innervation of the iris sphincter commonly occurs over time (at least 8–12 weeks following acute injury). Dense re-innervation of multiple segments of the iris sphincter by accommodative neurons results in a tonic state of contraction of the re-innervated sphincter segments (Figure 164.8). This causes the pupil to become small, even in dim light, giving rise to the "tonic pupil." Therefore, strictly speaking, the term "tonic pupil" should be reserved for the chronic form of Adie's pupil, when aberrant re-innervation of the iris sphincter has taken place, and not during the acute phase.
- *Ross syndrome* This syndrome refers to patients with Adie's syndrome but in addition, there is segmental loss of sweating on certain areas of the body, implying coexisting sympathetic denervation of the sweat glands. This may also be part of a widespread autonomic neuropathy.

Third nerve palsy   There is an old clinical rule of thumb that says that if the pupillary light reaction is spared, then the third nerve palsy is probably not due to compression or injury, but more likely due to small vessel disease, such as might be seen in diabetes. It is still a fairly good rule, provided one bears in mind that a small but definite number of pupil-sparing third nerve palsies are due to midbrain infarcts and should have neuroimaging studies. Because the pupillary and accommodative fibers are located at the peripheral circumference of the third nerve, they are very sensitive to external compression. In the subarachnoid space, these fibers are located on the medial side of the oculomotor nerve and hence are particularly susceptible to compression by aneurysms of the posterior communicating artery. The third cranial nerve carries instructions to several different muscles, so when the nerve is injured and the fibers re-grow, they often end up in the wrong place. For example, the eye may inappropriately turn in when the patient is trying to look down, or the pupil may inappropriately constrict with depression, adduction, or supraduction of the globe (Figure 164.10).

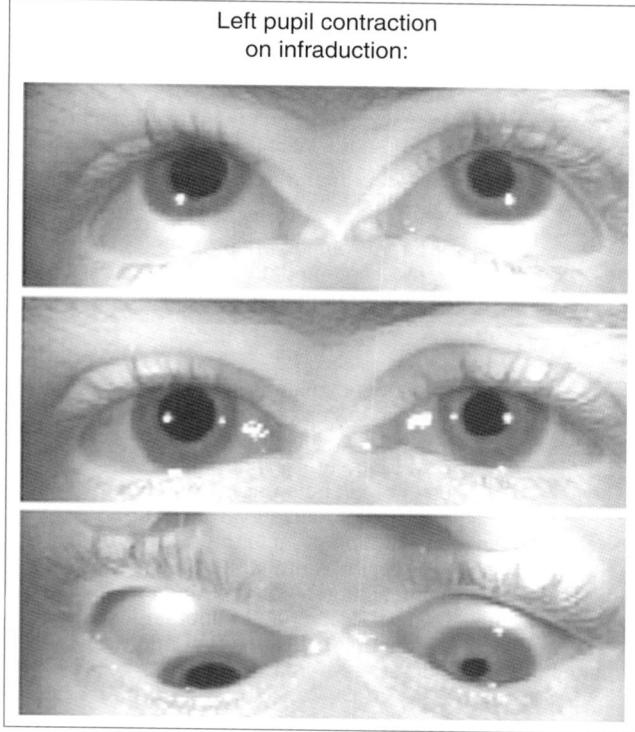

Left pupil contraction
on infraduction:

Figure 164.10 Primary aberrant regeneration of the left third nerve following chronic compression of the oculomotor nerve by a meningioma. In darkness (top and center panels) the left pupil is the smaller of the two pupils due to innervation by motor nerves. Nerves that normally would have supplied the inferior rectus muscle now are innervating the iris sphincter muscle, causing left pupil contraction on down-gaze (lower panel).

Disorders of supranuclear pathways

The preganglionic neurons in the Edinger-Westphal nucleus are unusual in that their baseline state is to continuously discharge. Inhibitory supranuclear neuronal input modulates the discharge rate of these neurons, and hence controls pupil size and reactivity to light and near stimuli. These inhibitory pathways originate from the reticular activating formation and project to the Edinger-Westphal nuclear region via the periaqueductal gray area. Reduction of input from this supranuclear inhibitory source during sleep, anesthesia, with centrally acting narcotic drugs, or from lesions in the periaqueductal gray tissue may cause the pupils to become small. Conversely, activation of the reticular activating formation during excitation may cause the pupils to become large and poorly reactive to light. Disorders of sleep, such as narcolepsy and seizure disorders commonly cause fluctuations in pupil size and reactivity depending on the status of the reticular activating formation providing the inhibitory input to the midbrain.

Other supranuclear inputs, such as for the near pupil response, originate from parietal-occipital cortical areas and project directly to the Edinger-Westphal nucleus. Modulating input for the near pupil response may also arise from the cerebellum.

Light-near dissociation: evaluation of the near response

The pupillary response to a near effort should be observed as a standard part of the pupillary evaluation. Any time the light reaction seems a little weak, the examiner should look to see if the pupils constrict better to near than they do to light. If they do, this is called a "light-near dissociation." Causes of light near dissociation are summarized in Table 164.3. These are categorized by three major mechanisms: (1) loss of light input due to severe damage to the afferent visual system (retina or optic nerve pathways); (2) interruption of the light input pathways from the intercalated neuron in the pretectum to the Edinger-Westphal nucleus (Argyl-Robertson pupils, dorsal midbrain syndrome) and (3) aberrant regeneration of the pupillary sphincter either from postganglionic parasympathetic accommodative fibers (Adie's syndrome) or from preganglionic neurons of the oculomotor nerve (i.e., medial rectus fibers from third nerve aberrant regeneration).

How to test for a pupillary near response

The pupillary near reaction is usually weak when tested in dim light or in the dark. The patient needs to see what he is looking at before trying to get it into focus. Do not try to induce a near response at the slit

Table 164.3 Causes of light-near dissociation of the pupil

Cause	Location	Mechanism
Severe loss of afferent light input to both eyes	Anterior visual pathway (retina, optic nerves, chiasm)	Damage to the retina or optic nerve pathways
Loss of pretectal light input to Edinger-Westphal nucleus	Tectum of the midbrain, lesions of the posterior commissure, dorsal midbrain	Infectious (Argyl Robertson pupils) or compression (pinealoma) or ischemia (stroke), often associated with dorsal midbrain syndrome
Adie's syndrome	Postganglionic parasympathetic innervation to the iris sphincter	Aberrant reinnervation of sphincter by accommodative neurons
Third nerve aberrant reinnervation	Postganglionic innervation to the iris sphincter	Aberrant reinnervation of sphincter by accommodative neurons or medial rectus neurons

Table 164.4   Causes of poor pupil dilation in darkness

Cause	Location	Mechanism
Past inflammation or surgical trauma	Posterior iris surface or sphincter	Scarring or synechiae of the iris due to past iritis
Acute trauma	Sphincter	Prostaglandin release causing sphincter spasm
Adie's tonic pupil	Sphincter	Aberrant reinnervation of iris sphincter by accommodative or extraocular motor neurons that are not inhibited in darkness
Third nerve aberrant reinnervation		
Pharmacological miosis	Iris sphincter	Cholinergic influence
Unilateral episodic spasm of miosis	Postganglionic parasympathetic neuron	Uninhibited episodic activation of postganglionic neurons
Congenital miosis (bilateral)	Sphincter	Developmental abnormality
Fatigue, sleepiness	Edinger-Westphal nucleus	Loss of inhibition at midbrain from reticular activating formation
Lymphoma, inflammation, infection	Periaqueductal gray matter	Interruption of inhibitory fibers to the Edinger-Westphal nucleus
Central acting drugs	Reticular activating formation, midbrain	Narcotics, general anesthetics
Old age (bilateral miosis)	Reticular activating formation, midbrain	Loss of inhibition at midbrain from reticular activating formation
Oculosympathetic defect	Sympathetic neuron interruption	Horner's syndrome

lamp unless you need the magnification to see segmental contractions of the iris sphincter; the room is usually dark and there is too much equipment in the patient's face.

The near response should be looked for in moderate room light so that the patient's pupils are mid-sized, and the near object is clearly visible. Give the patient an accommodative target to look at something of interest or with fine detail on it. Sometimes a better response is obtained if some other sensory input is added to the stimulus—something auditory, for example, such as a ticking watch or clicking fingernails or something proprioceptive. For example, the patient's own thumbnail can be held up in front of him; perhaps, in the case of a child, with a little face drawn on it.

Watch for convergence to help you judge how hard the patient is trying. Remember that the near response, although it may be triggered by blurred or disparate imagery, has a large volitional component, and the patient may need encouragement. If, for some reason, the patient has not been making a near effort recently (for example, because stereopsis is not achieved at near), then the patient may need a few practice runs ("There, you're getting the hang of it; try it one more time"). Often on the third or fourth try he will do a good one. When you do not get a near response, it is usually because the patient (or the doctor) has not been trying hard enough.

A patient who is completely blind and has no pupillary reaction to light will still sometimes do a good near response if you ask him to "cross your eyes like you did when you were a child." If you cannot get a patient to do a near response, try the "lid closure reflex": ask the patient to look at you and squeeze his eyes shut while you try, with both hands, to hold one of them open. This will often produce a surprisingly strong near response. This is called the "eye-closure pupil reaction."

Sometimes, in a doubtful case, it is hard to know where to draw the line. When is the near response clearly greater than the light reaction? When you face the patient, with pocket light in hand, there are usually three levels of light available to the examiner: (1) darkness, with a light shining tangential on the pupils from below; (2) room light and (3) room light with an additional bright light in the eyes. With the patient looking in the distance, shine the bright light in the eye three or four times, each time for only one or two seconds. This tells you how small the pupils will go with just a light stimulus. Never judge the near response by adding a near stimulus to a bright light stimulus; this almost always produces an apparent light-near dissociation because the near stimulus inevitably adds something to the light stimulus. A real light-near dissociation is present only if the near response (tested in moderate light) exceeds the best constriction that bright light can produce.

The pupil that dilates poorly in dim light

When one or both pupils stay small and miotic, even in darkness, a number of reasons may be responsible (Table 164.4). To better understand the different possible mechanisms it is important to understand what normally happens in darkness to allow the pupil to dilate. When a light stimulus is terminated, two mechanisms cause the pupil to dilate. The majority of pupil dilation comes about from inhibition to the Edinger-Westphal nucleus in the midbrain. This reduces the firing of the preganglionic parasympathetic neurons in the Edinger-Westphal nucleus, causing relaxation of the iris sphincter. Within a few seconds, sympathetic nerve firing increases, serving to augment the pupil dilation by active contraction of the dilator muscle. The combined inhibition of the iris sphincter and stimulation of the iris dilator is a carefully integrated neuronal reflex. Therefore, inability of the pupil to dilate in darkness may be due to mechanical limitations of the pupil (senechiae or scarring of the iris tissue), pharmacological miosis, aberrant reinnervation of cholinergic neurons to the iris sphincter that are not normally inhibited in darkness (accommodative or extraocular motor neurons), or lack of inhibitory input signal getting to the Edinger-Westphal nucleus.

References

1. Lowenstein O, Kawabata H, Loewenfeld I. The pupil as indicator of retinal activity. Am J Ophthalmol 1964;57:569–596

2. Loewenfeld IE. The pupil: anatomy, physiology, and clinical applications. Vol 1. Boston, Mass: Butterworth Heinemann, 1999:1080–1130

3. Cox TA, Thompson HS, Hayreh SS, Snyder JE. Visual evoked potential and pupillary signs. A comparison in optic nerve disease. Arch Ophthalmol 1982;100:1603–1607

4. Levatin P. Pupillary escape in disease of the retina or optic nerve. Arch Ophthalmol 1959;62:768–779

5. Thompson HS, Corbett JJ, Cox TA. How to measure the relative afferent pupillary defect. Surv Ophthalmol 1981;26:39–42

6. Thompson HS, Corbett JJ. Asymmetry of pupillomotor input. Eye 1991;5:36–39

7. Thompson HS, Montague P, Cox TA, Corbett JJ. The Relationship between visual acuity, pupillary defect, and visual field loss. Am J Ophthalmol 1982;93:681–688

8. Brown RH, Zillis JD, Lynch MG, Sanborn GE. The afferent pupillary defect in asymmetric glaucoma. Arch Ophthalmol 1987;105:1540–1543

9. Johnson LN, Hill RA, Bartholomew MJ. Correlation of afferent pupillary defect with visual field loss on automated perimetry. Ophthalmol 1988;95:1649–1655

10. Kardon RH, Haupert C, Thompson HS. The relationship between static perimetry and the relative afferent pupillary defect. Am J Ophthalmol 1993;115:351–356

11. Kawasaki A, Moore P, Kardon RH. Variability of the relative afferent pupillary defect. Am J Ophthalmol 1995;120:622–633

12. Kawasaki A, Moore P, Kardon RH. Long-term fluctuation of relative afferent pupillary defect in subjects with normal visual function. Am J Ophthalmol 1996;122:875–882

13. Bell RA, Waggoner PM, Boyd WM, et al. Clinical grading of relative afferent pupillary defects. Arch Ophthalmol 1993;111:938–942

14. Kardon RH, Corbett JJ, Thompson HS. Segmental denervation and reinnervation of the iris sphincter as shown by infrared videographic transillumination. Ophthalmology 1998;105:313–321

15. Fison PN, Garlick DJ, Smith SE. Assessment of unilateral afferent pupillary defects by pupillography. Br J Ophthalmol 1979;63:195–199

16. Cox TA. Pupillography of a relative afferent pupillary defect. Am J Ophthalmol 1986;101:320–324

17. Cox TA. Pupillographic characteristics of simulated relative afferent pupillary defects. Invest Ophthalmol Vis Sci 1989;30:1127–1131

18. Young RSL, Han B, Wu P. Transient and sustained components of the pupillary responses evoked by luminance and color. Vision Res 1993;33(4):437–446

19. Young RSL, Kennish J. Transient and sustained components of the pupil response evoked by achromatic spatial patterns. Vision Res 1993;33(16):2239–2252

20. Barbur JL, Harlow AJ, Sahraie A. Pupillary responses to stimulus structure, color, and movement. Ophthal Physiol Opt 1992;12:137–141

21. Slooter, JH, van Noren D. Visual acuity measured with pupil responses to checkerboard stimuli. Invest Ophthalmol Visual Sci 1980;19:105–108

22. Ukai K. Spatial pattern as a stimulus to the pupillary system. J Opt Soc Am 1985;1094–1100

23. Barbur JL, Thomson WD. Pupil response as an objective measure of visual acuity. Ophthal Physiol Opt 1987;7:425–429

24. Cocker KD, Moseley MJ. Visual acuity and the pupil grating response. Clin Vision Sci 1992;7(2):143–146

25. Kardon RH, Kirkali PA, Thompson HS. Automated pupil perimetry. Pupil field mapping in patients and normal subjects. Ophthalmol 1991;98:485–496

26. Kardon RH. Pupil perimetry. In: Current Opinion in Ophthalmology. Philadelphia: Current Science, 1992;3:565–570

27. Kardon RH, Denison CE, Brown CK, Thompson HS. Critical evaluation of the cocaine test in the diagnosis of Horner's syndrome. Arch Ophthalmol 1990;108:384–387

28. Cremer SA, Thompson HS, Digre KB, Kardon RH. Hydroxyamphetamine mydriasis in Horner's syndrome. Am J Ophthalmol 1990;110:71–76

29. Weinstein JM, Zweifel TJ, Thompson HS. Congenital Horner's syndrome. Arch Ophthalmol 1980;98:1074–1078

30. Thompson HS, Newsome DA, Loewenfeld IE. The fixed dilated pupil: sudden iridoplegia or mydriatic drops? A simple diagnostic test. Arch Ophthalmol 1971;86:21

31. Loewenfeld IE, Thompson HS. Mechanism of tonic pupil. Ann Neurol 1981;10:275–276

32. Loewenfeld IE. Lesions in the ciliary ganglion and short ciliary nerves: the tonic pupil ("Adie's" syndrome). In: The pupil: anatomy, physiology and clinical applications. Vol 1. Boston, Mass: Butterworth Heinemann, 1999:1080–1130

165 Ocular Motor Nerve Palsies

Jonathan D Trobe

The three ocular motor nerve palsies—oculomotor (cranial nerve III), trochlear (cranial nerve IV), and abducens (cranial nerve VI)—produce a characteristic misalignment of the eyes. In most cases, this ocular misalignment evokes the symptom of diplopia, or seeing the same object in two different places. However, those with visual, attentional or other cognitive deficits may not appreciate diplopia. If the palsy develops within the first decade of life, the second image may be quickly suppressed. Finally, if the two images are narrowly separated, patients may interpret the disturbance as blurred rather than double vision.

The major impediment to proper management of ocular motor palsies is making the correct diagnosis.[1,2] There are two hurdles. First, minimal palsies may preserve eye movements, forcing the examiner to rely on alignment measurements—a task that requires skill and proper technique.[1] Second, ocular motor palsies are not the only cause of impaired eye movements; other considerations are convergence spasm, internuclear ophthalmoplegia, and disorders of the neuromuscular junction and extraocular muscles.[2]

Third cranial nerve palsy

Overview

In its complete form, cranial nerve (CN) III palsy produces ipsilateral complete ptosis, a fixed, dilated pupil, and paralysis of adduction, supraduction, and infraduction. Incomplete CN III palsies produce incomplete involvement of each of these components, or sparing of one or more of them (Figure 165.1). The clinician's challenge is to recognize the CN III palsy, determine the appropriate diagnostic studies, and institute proper therapy based on the results.

Epidemiology

The incidence and prevalence of CN III in the general population has never been properly studied. It is rare before age 40, except after severe head trauma. In individuals aged over 40 years, it occurs most commonly among those who have a propensity to microvascular occlusive disease, as in diabetes mellitus, hypertension, and arteriosclerosis.

Etiology

The etiology of a CN III palsy[3–10] (Tables 165.1 and 165.2) depends on five principal factors: 1) whether the palsy is isolated or a component of multiple neurological findings; 2) the patient's age at onset of the CN III palsy; 3) whether the patient has ample risk factors for ischemic microvascular disease; 4) whether the pupil is spared; and 5) whether there are signs of aberrant regeneration of CN III.

Nonisolated palsies Nonisolated CN III palsies—those embedded among other neuro-ophthalmic findings—are often caused by trauma, mass lesions, or meningeal inflammations and neoplasms. For example, CN III palsy may be a sign of a cerebral hemispheric mass lesion that has induced herniation of the temporal lobe uncus over the tentorium, compressing CN III against the rigid posterior clinoid process ("tentorial herniation syndrome").[11] Injury to

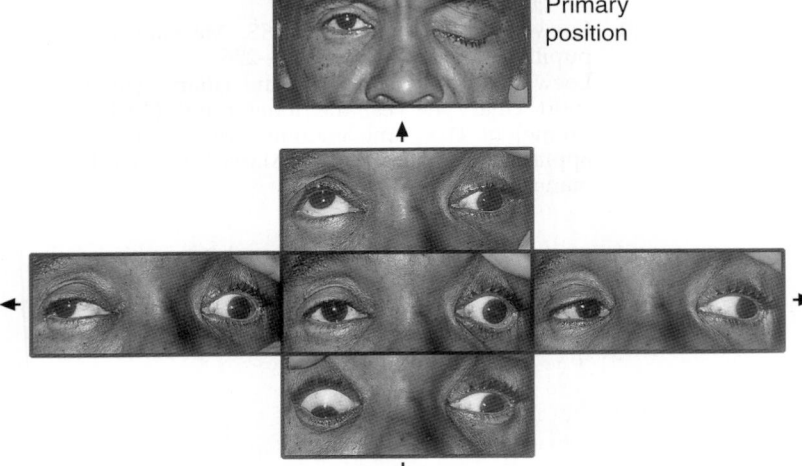

Primary
position

Figure 165.1 Third cranial nerve palsy (left). Left upper lid ptosis (upper panel); exodeviated left eye with dilated left pupil (lower panel center); absent left adduction (lower panel left), absent left supraduction (lower panel top); absent left infraduction (lower panel bottom); intact left abduction (lower panel right). (See color plate section.)

Table 165.1   Nontraumatic causes of isolated ocular motor palsies in adults*

CN III palsy	CN IV palsy	CN VI palsy
Ischemia Berry aneurysm Meningeal or cavernous sinus inflammation, neoplasm Miscellaneous[†]	Breakdown of compensated congenital lesion Ischemia Meningeal, collicular, or tentorial inflammation, neoplasm Dorsal midbrain lesion Miscellaneous[†]	Ischemia Increased intracranial pressure Cranial base inflammation, neoplasm Miscellaneous[†]

*In order of estimated frequency.
[†]Brainstem demyelination; radiation injury, nerve sheath tumor, carotid-cavernous fistula, cavernous sinus aneurysm, orbital lesion, dental anesthesia, migraine, postlumbar puncture (CN IV and VI only), Wernicke's disease (CN VI only).

Table 165.2   Nontraumatic causes of isolated ocular motor palsies in children*

CN III palsy	CN IV palsy	CN VI palsy
Congenital Meningeal or cavernous inflammation, neoplasm Miscellaneous[†]	Congenital Meningeal, collicular, tentorial inflammation, neoplasm Miscellaneous[†]	Congenital Cranial base inflammation, neoplasm Pontine glioma Increased intracranial pressure Miscellaneous[†]

*In order of estimated frequency.
[†]Brainstem demyelination; radiation injury, nerve sheath tumor, migraine, postlumbar puncture (CN IV and VI only), berry aneurysm (CN III only).

the peripherally-situated pupillomotor fibers comes first, so that a fixed, dilated pupil may be the initial sign of CN III dysfunction. Hemiparesis and reduced consciousness are invariably present as well. CN III palsy may also result from infarcts, masses, and demyelination within the midbrain.[2]

Isolated palsies Isolated congenital CN III palsies[10,12–15] are often attributed to cephalic trauma during birth, but in many cases there is no history or external evidence of such trauma. Dysplasia may be the explanation in these cases. Aberrant regeneration is common, but recovery is limited. Amblyopia is a major concern in such patients. The rare acquired CN III palsies of childhood are attributable to head trauma and infectious, inflammatory, and neoplastic conditions. Recovery is variable.

Among isolated CN III palsies acquired in adulthood, ischemia of the peripheral segment of CN III accounts for over 75% of cases.[3,8,16] Most patients have a family history, personal history, or current evidence of conditions associated with small caliber vasculopathy, including diabetes, hypertension, cigarette smoking, and hyperlipidemia.[17] The ischemia typically damages only the core of the nerve, leaving the peripherally-situated iris sphincter fibers relatively or completely intact.[18–21] As a result, anisocoria rarely exceeds 1 mm.[22] Progression of the deficit occurs in two thirds of cases within the first 14 days of onset,[23] but full recovery eventually occurs in nearly 100% of

patients within three months.[24] Recurrences develop in CN III or other cranial nerves in 15% of patients.[25] Occlusion of paramedian midbrain perforating vessels may rarely produce an isolated CN III palsy.[26–28] In most midbrain infarcts, however, other neurological manifestations are present.[29]

A critical cause of isolated CN III palsy is cerebral berry aneurysm.[30–32] It is usually located at the junction of the carotid and posterior communicating arteries, but may also lie at the apex of the basilar artery. Such an aneurysm becomes clinically evident during middle age, and is extraordinarily rare before the second decade. CN III palsy results from expansion, not necessarily rupture, of the aneurysmal wall. CN III is therefore a "sentinel sign" of impending rupture, which may be imminent and fatal in 50% of cases. Treatment at the sentinel stage is much more successful than after the aneurysm has ruptured. Not all patients present acutely with severe headache. The CN III palsy may be incomplete. More than 95% of cases will have anisocoria and a weakly reactive pupil, but the pupil may be normal if the extraocular muscle palsy is incomplete.[33,34]

Isolated CN III palsies may rarely be caused by cranial base (meningeal or cavernous sinus) inflammation or neoplasm, radiation, head trauma, carotid cavernous fistulas, intracavernous aneurysms, and nerve sheath tumors.[2] These lesions may produce sufficient disruption of the nerve that its axons sprout to the wrong destinations. This phenomenon, known as

Table 165.3	Imitators of ocular motor palsies	
CN III palsy	**CN IV palsy**	**CN VI palsy**
CN IV palsy	Partial CN III palsy	Spasm of the near reflex
Extraocular myopathy	Extraocular myopathy	Extraocular myopathy
Myasthenia gravis	Myasthenia gravis	Myasthenia gravis
Skew deviation	Skew deviation	
Internuclear ophthalmoplegia		

"aberrant regeneration," causes the upper lid to elevate on adduction and sometimes on depression of the affected eye.[35,36] Aberrant regeneration never follows microvascular ischemia; it is always a sign of a more disruptive process.

Pathophysiology and pathogenesis

CN III palsy arises from trauma, ischemia, compression by mass lesions, and infiltration by inflammation or neoplasm. Severe head trauma, generally associated with loss of consciousness and other neurological deficits, causes shearing and contusion of the nerve in its subarachnoid segment.[37] Recovery is variable, depending on the severity of the injury.

In patients with microvascular occlusive disease, watershed ischemia of the peripheral segment occurs in precavernous and cavernous portions of the nerve that lie midway between branches of the internal and external carotid arteries.[18–21] Ischemia of the brainstem segment occurs from occlusion of paramedian midbrain perforators, branches of the basilar artery.[26,28] The ischemic event may be prompted by an episode of hypotension in a setting of feeder vessels narrowed by arteriosclerosis. Ischemia of the peripheral nerve is typically mild and centered in the core of the nerve. The pupilloconstrictor fibers are located on the nerve's dorsomedial surface,[38] thus the pupil is often totally or relatively spared. The levator palpebrae and extraocular muscles recover their function fully within three months. Brainstem ischemia to CN III is often more enduring, with recovery less assured.

Compression of CN III may exert its damaging effects by impairing axoplasmic flow or by interfering with the blood supply. The pupilloconstrictor fibers are relatively affected because the periphery of the nerve is most damaged.

Infiltration of CN III produces dysfunction by metabolic and ultimately structural damage. Damage may affect either the nerve core or its periphery, thus pupil-sparing is variable.

Genetics

CN III palsy is a sporadic event without genetic implications.

Clinical features

CN III palsy causes complete or incomplete ipsilateral weakness of adduction, supraduction, and infraduction, sometimes combined with upper lid ptosis, and a dilated, poorly reactive pupil (Figure 165.1).

Classification

A practical classification of CN III palsies is based on the five factors listed under Etiology.

Diagnostic criteria

The diagnosis of CN III palsy is suggested by clinical features. Imitators may be excluded with such tests as intravenous edrophonium chloride administration, repetitive stimulation and single fiber electromyography, and acetylcholine receptor antibody levels (myasthenia gravis); forced ductions (orbitopathy); and brain imaging (orbitopathy, internuclear ophthalmoplegia, skew deviation). The diagnosis of the cause of a CN III palsy is based on clinical presumption and supported by these ancillary studies, including, in some cases, lumbar puncture and cerebral angiography. In many cases, the full battery of ancillary studies is negative, and the cause of the CN III remains presumptive. In such cases, observation of the patient's clinical course is often helpful in fortifying or altering the presumptive diagnosis.

Differential diagnosis

CN III palsies may be mimicked by five conditions[39] (Table 165.3): 1) extraocular myopathy; 2) myasthenia gravis; 3) fourth nerve (CN IV) palsy; 4) internuclear ophthalmoplegia; and 5) skew deviation.

Extraocular myopathy results most commonly from orbital trauma or inflammation (Graves disease, idiopathic orbital inflammation, connective tissue diseases). Signs of orbital congestion (proptosis, soft tissue swelling, conjunctival hyperemia) will usually suggest an orbital process, but they may not be present if the condition is long-standing or indolent.

Myasthenia gravis may fortuitously affect only those muscles innervated by CN III. CN IV palsy produces a vertical misalignment that can be mistaken for a partial CN III palsy.

Internuclear ophthalmoplegia produces an adduction deficit which can be differentiated from CN III palsy by the fact that the eyes are usually aligned in straight-ahead gaze, and there is abducting nystagmus of the contralateral eye.

Skew deviation, caused by a lesion that interrupts vestibular-ocular brainstem pathways, produces a vertical misalignment that, like CN IV palsy, may be confused with a partial CN III palsy. Other manifestations of a brainstem lesion (nystagmus, ataxia) are usually present.[40]

Table 165.4   Work-up of nontraumatic isolated* third cranial nerve palsy

Clinical characteristics	Studies
Onset before age 40	MRI; if negative, angio, LP
Onset after age 40 with aberrant regeneration features present	MRI; if negative, angio, LP
Onset after age 40 with anisocoria >1 mm	MRI; if negative, angio, LP
Onset after age 40 with anisocoria <1 mm and incomplete ductional deficits	MRI, MRA; if negative, LP. (Angio only if no vascular risk factors)
Onset after age 40 with anisocoria <1 mm and complete ductional deficits	Tests directed at detecting arteriosclerotic risk factors; if none present, perform MRI, LP

*No contributory systemic or neurological features to suggest a nonischemic cause.

Treatment

Evaluation of CN III palsies (Table 165.4) depends heavily on the five factors previously cited in Etiology: 1) the patient's age; 2) whether the patient has ample risk factors for ischemic microvascular disease; 3) whether the palsy is isolated; 4) whether the pupil is spared; and 5) whether aberrant regeneration features are present.

All patients whose nontraumatic CN III palsy cannot be reliably attributed to microvascular ischemia should undergo magnetic resonance imaging (MRI). If MRI fails to suggest a nonvascular diagnosis, the clinician must determine whether the possibility of a berry aneurysm is high enough to warrant conventional cerebral angiography, or whether magnetic resonance angiography (MRA) is a sufficient screening study. MRA is sensitive to 95% of aneurysms that would cause an isolated CN III palsy, and is therefore an adequate screening tool for cerebral aneurysm if the index of suspicion is low or the risk of conventional angiography is high.[41,42] Otherwise, conventional cerebral angiography is the study of choice and must be performed promptly. Lumbar puncture is indicated when a meningeal process is suspected.

Some patients who have a nonresolving CN III palsy may be candidates for surgical realignment of the eyes. Surgery involves weakening the lateral rectus muscle, strengthening the other rectus muscles, and transposing the superior oblique to the insertion of the medial rectus muscle. Unfortunately, these pro-cedures rarely restore a useful field of single binocular vision (level 5 evidence).[43–46] For those who cannot be helped with eye muscle surgery, diplopia can often be eliminated by means of occluding the vision in one eye, either with a spectacle occluder, an eye patch, or an opaque contact lens.

Fourth cranial nerve palsy

Overview

Fourth cranial nerve (CN IV) palsy is less common than CN III or CN VI palsy, but can be very difficult to diagnose. In its complete form, it produces a vertical misalignment of the eyes that is accentuated in the field of gaze in which the superior oblique is active (contralaterally downward) (Figure 165.2). Incomplete forms typically preserve eye movements. Because the superior oblique is a powerful intorter, damage to this muscle causes excyclotorsion of the affected eye, and the patient may appreciate that the vertically-separated images are also tilted with respect to one another. The patient often affects a head tilt.

The major causes of CN IV palsy are breakdown of a compensated congenital CN IV lesion and head trauma. Peripheral nerve ischemia and dorsal midbrain lesions are less common causes. Berry aneurysm is not a consideration (Tables 165.1 and 165.2).

Epidemiology

The incidence and prevalence of CN IV have not been formally studied.

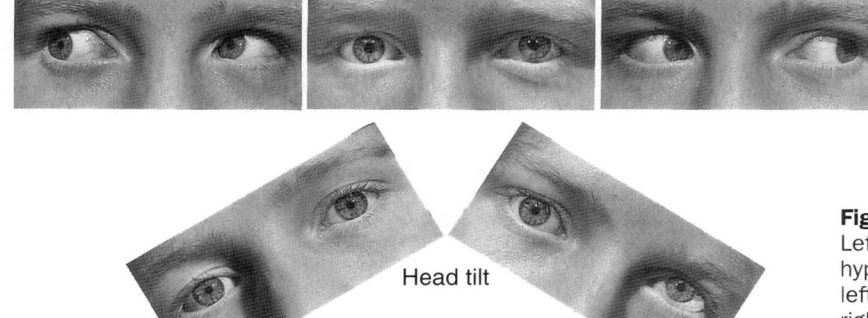

Head tilt

Right   Left

Figure 165.2   Fourth cranial nerve palsy (left). Left hypertropia (upper panel center); the left hypertropia increases on right gaze (upper panel left) and diminishes on left gaze (upper panel right). The hypertropia increases on left head tilt (lower panel right) and diminishes on right head tilt (lower panel left). (See color plate section.)

Etiology

As with CN III and VI palsies, the etiology of CN IV palsy[4–6,9,47–51] (Tables 165.1 and 165.2) depends heavily on the following factors: 1) whether the palsy is isolated or a component of multiple neurological findings; 2) the patient's age at onset of the CN IV palsy; and 3) whether the patient has ample risk factors for ischemic microvascular disease.

Nonisolated palsies   Nonisolated CN IV palsies are usually caused by traumatic, neoplastic, or inflammatory lesions of the brainstem or cranial base.

Isolated palsies   Among isolated CN IV palsies, trauma is a very common cause.[52] The dorsal exit of CN IV in the anterior medullary velum makes it particularly vulnerable to closed head injury, in which both CN IVs are often damaged.[53] Neurosurgical manipulation in the tentorial region is another frequent traumatic cause.[54,55]

Breakdown of a congenital CN IV lesion typically occurs in adulthood, but it may begin earlier.[9,49] The patient reports episodic diplopia that can be eliminated by "focusing," changing gaze position, or tilting the head. Eventually even these maneuvers do not prevent diplopia, and the patient seeks relief. Examination shows features of a long-standing but compensated CN IV palsy (see Clinical features below).

As with CNs III and VI, ischemia of the peripheral nerve segment is another common cause of adult CN IV palsy. Patients have ample arteriosclerotic risk factors. The palsy disappears within three months.

A less common cause of isolated CN IV palsies is dysfunction in the region of the dorsal midbrain (pineal tumors, hydrocephalus, midbrain demyelination, tumor, infarction). Damage to this region usually produces other neuro-ophthalmic signs, but CN IV palsy may be the first manifestation.[56,57]

Infiltration of the peripheral segment of the nerve by inflammation or meningeal neoplasm is a rare but important cause of CN IV palsy.[2]

Pathophysiology and pathogenesis[58]

Of the three ocular motor nerves, CN IV seems to be most vulnerable to closed head injury, in that it occurs with fewer other neurological consequences than does traumatic CN III or VI palsy. The anterior medullary velum is the common site of injury.

Breakdown of a congenital CN IV lesion is attributed to loss of fusion with advancing age. (Fusion is the ability to maintain ocular alignment under binocular viewing conditions against forces that would drive the eyes out of alignment.)

CN IV ischemia is believed to represent a watershed perfusion problem in patients with underlying microvascular stenosis.

Genetics

As with CN III, affections of CN IV are sporadic. There are no genetic considerations.

Clinical features

Patients with CN IV lesions typically report vertical diplopia, often with one tilted image. The patient often tilts the head away from the side of the CN IV palsy. (When CN IV palsy has its onset within the first decade, patients suppress the second image and do not report diplopia; some tilt their heads out of long-standing habit.)

Examination discloses vertical misalignment of the eyes ("hypertropia"), the higher eye being on the lesioned side (Figure 165.2). The extent of the misalignment increases with gaze directed away from the lesioned side and with the head tilted toward the lesioned side. These phenomena are noted in the "three-step test."[59–61] Step one measures the hypertropia in straight-ahead gaze. Step two compares the hypertropia in right and left gaze. Step three compares the hypertropia in right and left head tilt. A right CN IV palsy produces a "right-left-right" pattern of misalignment: right hypertropia in straight-ahead gaze; greater hypertropia on left than right gaze; and greater hypertropia on right than left head tilt. A left CN IV palsy produces a "left-right-left" pattern.

In measuring the vertical misalignment, the examiner notes whether the patient has pathologically high vertical fusional reserves (4 prism-diopters or greater), an indication of a long-standing and probably decompensated congenital CN IV lesion.

A final diagnostic measure is the double Maddox Rod test for torsional misalignment. Maddox Rod lenses are placed in the trial spectacle frames of both eyes with their axes aligned vertically. As the patient views a light with both eyes, he will see two horizontal lines. He is asked if the lines appear tilted with respect to each other. If so, he is instructed to adjust the knob that controls the orientation of the Maddox Rod lens in the right spectacle frame so as to make the two lines parallel. If the eyes are extorted with respect to each other, he will move the Maddox Rod lens to a counterclockwise position. The torsional deviation is then read in degrees from the trial frame. Excyclotorsional misalignment of more than 3 degrees is common in CN IV palsies and is not found in other causes of vertical misalignment except extraocular muscle scarring.[62]

Classification

In order to guide diagnosis and management, nontraumatic CN IV palsies are divided into those that are isolated and those that are not isolated (see Etiology, above). Isolated palsies are subdivided into those that represent breakdown of a congenital CN IV lesion and those that are acquired.

Diagnostic criteria

CN IV palsy is diagnosed on the basis of the ocular misalignment pattern (see the three-step test under Clinical features above), and supported by ancillary studies such as those used in the evaluation of suspected CN III and CN VI palsies.[63]

Table 165.5	Work-up of nontraumatic isolated* fourth cranial nerve palsy	
Clinical characteristics	**Studies**
Pathological vertical fusional amplitudes	None
Adults with ample arteriosclerotic risk factors	None initially; MRI, LP if no recovery within three months
Children and adults without ample arteriosclerotic risk factors	MRI; if negative, LP

*No contributory systemic or neurological features to suggest a nonischemic cause.

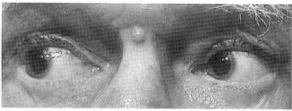 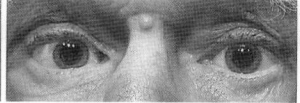 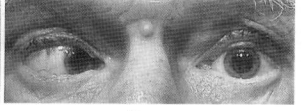

◄――――― Primary position ―――――►

Figure 165.3 Sixth cranial nerve palsy (left). Esotropia (center) increases on left gaze as left eye does not abduct (right) and disappears on right gaze (left). (See color plate section.)

Differential diagnosis

CN IV palsy may be mimicked by four conditions[39,64] (Table 165.3): 1) partial CN III palsy; 2) extraocular muscle disorder; 3) myasthenia gravis; and 4) skew deviation (see Differential diagnosis of CN III palsy, above). Each of these conditions can produce a vertical misalignment that has features of a CN IV palsy. The firmest evidence in favor of a CN IV palsy is a strongly positive three-step test and a double Maddox Rod test showing at least 3 degrees of excyclotorsion. Where evidence is equivocal, appropriate ancillary studies are indicated (see CN III palsy).

Treatment

Traumatic CN IV palsies require no brain imaging or other diagnostic studies unless the trauma is considered too trivial or remote to have been etiological. The management of nontraumatic CN IV palsies (Table 165.5) depends heavily on the following three factors: 1) whether the palsy is isolated or a component of multiple neurological findings; 2) the patient's age at onset of the CN IV palsy; and 3) whether the patient has ample risk factors for ischemic microvascular disease.

Nonisolated palsies These cases should undergo brain imaging guided by the constellation of neurological findings.

Isolated nontraumatic palsies Patients who have pathological vertical fusional amplitudes, suggesting a breakdown of a congenital CN IV lesion, require no diagnostic studies. Neither do acquired isolated CN IV palsies in adults with ample arteriosclerotic risk factors. They can be presumptively attributed to microvascular ischemia and observed for recovery, which should occur within three months. All other acquired isolated CN IV palsies, as well as nonrecovering presumptively ischemic CN IV palsies, should undergo MRI, and if negative, lumbar puncture. Cerebral angiography is not necessary because cerebral aneurysm is not a diagnostic consideration.

Among patients who have troublesome diplopia from persistent CN IV palsies where the cause is known, eye muscle surgery is often successful in restoring single binocular vision over a wide gaze range (level 5 evidence).[65–67] Surgery consists either of strengthening the superior oblique muscle or weakening its yoke muscle, the contralateral inferior rectus muscle.

Sixth cranial nerve palsy
Overview

Sixth cranial nerve (CN VI) palsy produces a simple pattern of ocular misalignment—an esodeviation greatest on the affected side, with or without an abduction deficit (Figure 165.3). Underdiagnosis occurs when there is no obvious abduction deficit. Overdiagnosis occurs when the examiner fails to consider that an obvious abduction deficit may also be caused by extraocular muscle contracture, spasm of convergence, and myasthenia gravis.

CN VI palsy in adults is most commonly a self-limited condition caused by microvascular ischemia to the peripheral segment of the nerve, but in children, and in adults who lack arteriosclerotic risk factors, it may be a manifestation of cranial base tumors or inflammation, and of increased intracranial pressure.

Epidemiology

As with CN III and IV palsies, no study has addressed the incidence and prevalence of CN VI palsy.

Etiology

As with CN III and IV palsies, the etiology of CN VI palsy[4,6,9,68,69] (Tables 165.1 and 165.2) depends on: 1) whether the palsy is isolated or a component of multiple neurological findings; 2) the patient's age at onset of the CN VI palsy; 3) whether the patient has ample risk factors for ischemic microvascular disease.

Nonisolated palsies Congenital CN VI palsies are rare. They are often part of dysplastic syndromes which may have other neurological and systemic manifestations. The most common is Duane's syndrome, in which the abducens neurons in the CN VI nucleus fail to develop.[70] The result is reduced or absent ipsilateral abduction, often accompanied by palpebral fissure narrowing on attempted adduction.

The fissure narrowing is a consequence of retraction of the globe produced by co-firing of the medial and lateral rectus muscles, the latter supplied by aberrant axons from CN III. The lack of diplopia and narrowing of the lid fissure are clues to the diagnosis. Mobius syndrome consists of esotropia with bilateral horizontal gaze paresis, together with atrophic weakness of facial or tongue muscles and other malformations. Multiple cranial nerve nuclear aplasias are found pathologically.[71]

Acquired CN VI palsies may also be caused by brainstem lesions which damage its nucleus or fascicles.[2] The CN VI nucleus contains abducens neurons that mediate abduction of the ipsilateral eye and interneurons that mediate adduction of the contralateral eye, thus nuclear lesions typically cause an ipsilateral gaze palsy. These lesions may be congenital dysplasias (see above) or acquired—usually infarcts. Infarcts of the nucleus usually affect the adjacent medial longitudinal fasciculus to produce a "one-and-one-half syndrome," consisting of an ipsilateral gaze palsy and an ipsilateral adduction deficit.[72,73] Infarcts, tumors, or inflammation affecting the CN VI fascicles may cause an isolated abduction deficit,[74,75] but are often combined with other neurological manifestations such as ataxia, nystagmus, facial palsy, or contralateral hemiparesis.[76]

Isolated palsies In children, isolated nontraumatic CN VI palsies are extraordinarily rare. One must consider meningeal and cranial base inflammation and tumor, and increased or decreased intracranial pressure. In adults, most isolated CN VI palsies are caused by extra-axial microvascular ischemia, but the nonischemic conditions that affect children are also important causes.[2]

Pathophysiology and pathogenesis

Trauma to CN VI produces direct mechanical injury. Ischemic damage probably represents a watershed perfusion problem in patients with underlying microvascular stenosis. Infectious, inflammatory, and neoplastic infiltrative lesions probably gain access to the nerve via the meninges.

CN VI has some predispositions to disease that are not shared by CN III and IV. They derive from the nerve's long course along the cranial base, with two sharp-angled turns at the basal pons and at the junction of the clivus and cavernous sinus. Caudally, CN VI is vulnerable to cerebellopontine angle masses; along the clivus to clival tumors; and at the clivo-cavernous junction to temporal bone (middle ear) lesions, trigeminal ganglion and nasopharyngeal masses. As the only cranial nerve that travels within the cavernous sinus (the others travel in its lateral wall), it is vulnerable to intracavernous carotid lesions—aneurysms and fistulas. It is tethered at the clivo-cavernous junction, and is therefore readily injured by downward shifts in the brainstem, as occur with increased intracranial pressure,[77] spontaneous intracranial hypotension,[78] acutely decreased intracranial pressure following lumbar puncture,[79] spinal anesthesia,[80] or shunting[81] ("false-localizing CN VI palsy").

Genetics

As with CN III and IV, CN VI damage is sporadic. There are no genetic considerations.

Clinical features

Patients with CN VI lesions report horizontal diplopia that may be present in one or more positions of gaze, but the image separation is greatest in the field of action of the affected nerve. An abduction deficit may be apparent on the affected side (Figure 165.4).

Classification

As with CN III and IV palsies, nontraumatic CN VI palsies are divided into those that are isolated and those that are not (see Etiology, above).

Diagnostic criteria

CN VI palsy is diagnosed on the basis of the ocular misalignment pattern (see the three-step test on page 1776), and supported by ancillary studies such as are used in the evaluation of suspected CN III and CN IV palsies. The nonisolated CN VI palsies are easier to diagnose, and localization depends on the accompanying manifestations. Isolated CN VI palsies are more difficult to diagnose, and may be confused with mimickers (see Differential diagnosis, below).

Differential diagnosis

CN VI palsy may be mimicked by three conditions[39] (Table 165.3): 1) myasthenia gravis; 2) extraocular muscle disorder; and 3) spasm of the near reflex.

Although myasthenia gravis often produces concomitant ptosis and reduced eye movements in several directions, it may present with an isolated abduction deficit in one eye.

Inflammation, contusion, entrapment, or scarring of the medial rectus muscle may also cause an isolated abduction deficit. Diagnosis depends on clinical or imaging evidence of soft tissue abnormalities in the orbit.

Spasm of the near reflex is a psychogenic disturbance that consists of excessive convergence, pupil constriction, and overaccommodation.[82] Although both eyes are adducted, one eye will be fixating the target, the other turned inward. On lateral gaze, one or both eyes will have reduced abduction. Pupil constriction is always difficult to recognize because pupil size is so variable between individuals. Excess accommodation normally produces artificial myopia, except in older individuals whose lenses are too stiff to respond to ciliary muscle contraction. In younger individuals, the myopia will not be apparent unless the examiner tests visual acuity at distance and finds it subnormal.

Spasm of the near reflex usually gives itself away because the convergent misalignment is variable within a single clinical encounter. Moreover, abduction usually becomes full when tested with the other eye occluded. This maneuver interrupts the visual cues that allow the

Table 165.6 Work-up of nontraumatic isolated* sixth cranial nerve palsy	
Clinical characteristics	**Studies**
Adults with ample arteriosclerotic risk factors	None initially; MRI, LP if no recovery within three months
Children and adults without ample arteriosclerotic risk factors	MRI; if negative, LP

*No contributory systemic or neurological features to suggest a nonischemic cause.

patient to maintain an artificial state of hyperconvergence. Patients who have spasm of the near reflex have a somatoform disorder or are malingering.

Treatment

Traumatic CN VI palsies require no brain imaging or other diagnostic studies unless the trauma is considered too trivial or remote to have been etiological. The management of nontraumatic CN VI palsies (Table 165.6) depends on the following factors: 1) whether the palsy is isolated or a component of multiple neurological findings; 2) the patient's age at onset of the CN VI palsy; 3) whether the patient has ample risk factors for ischemic microvascular disease.

Nonisolated palsies These palsies should undergo brain imaging that is guided by the constellation of neurological findings.

Isolated palsies If the CN VI palsy can be attributed to an ischemic microvascular event, no diagnostic studies are necessary unless the condition evolves or fails to resolve within three months. Otherwise, MRI with enhancement and attention to the cranial base is the appropriate study, followed by lumbar puncture in accordance with the MRI results. As with CN IV palsy, vascular studies are not important because berry aneurysm does not cause CN VI palsy. If the diagnosis of an unremitting CN VI palsy remains elusive, however, conventional cerebral angiography would be indicated to rule out a posterior-draining cavernous sinus fistula.[83] (These lesions are not visible on MRI or MRA.)

Among patients who have troublesome diplopia from persistent CN VI palsies where the cause is known, eye muscle surgery is often successful in restoring single binocular vision in straight-ahead gaze. However, surgery provides a wide range of single binocular vision only when some lateral rectus function is present preoperatively (level 5 evidence).[84,85] The operations consist either of weakening the medial rectus and strengthening the lateral rectus muscles ("recess-resect procedure") or transposing the vertical rectus muscles to the insertion of the lateral rectus muscle ("tranposition procedure"), often combined with chemodenervation of the medial rectus muscle with intramuscular injection of botulinum toxin. Level 5 evidence suggests that the addition of chemodenervation to the transposition procedure improves postoperative ocular alignment.[86] The recess-resect procedure is typically used when at least 50% of abduction is present.

Botulinum toxin denervation of the medial rectus has also been successfully used without surgery to restore normal alignment in patients with acute sixth cranial nerve palsy (level 5 evidence).[87,88] An additional rationale for its use in this setting is to prevent contracture of the medial rectus, which might worsen the chances of natural recovery of normal alignment. However, a randomized study of 47 patients showed that early botulinum toxin treatment did not affect ultimate ocular alignment (level 2 evidence).[89]

References

1. Borchert MS. Principles and techniques of the examination of ocular motility and alignment. *In:* Miller NR, Newman NJ, eds. Walsh & Hoyt's Clinical Neuro-Ophthalmology. Vol 1, 5th ed. Baltimore: Williams & Wilkins, 1998:1169–1188
2. Smith CH. Nuclear and infranuclear ocular motility disorders. *In:* Miller NR, Newman NJ, eds. Walsh & Hoyt's Clinical Neuro-Ophthalmology. Vol 1, 5th ed. Baltimore: Williams & Wilkins, 1998:1189–1281
3. Richards BW, Jones FR, Younge BR. Causes and prognosis in 4278 cases of paralysis of the oculomotor, trochlear, and abducens cranial nerves. Am J Ophthalmol 1992;113:489–496
4. Rucker CW. Paralysis of the third, fourth, and sixth cranial nerves. Am J Ophthalmol 1958;46:787–794
5. Rucker CW. The causes of paralysis of the third, fourth and sixth cranial nerves. Am J Ophthalmol 1966;61:1293–1298
6. Rush JA, Younge BR. Paralysis of cranial nerves III, IV, and VI: Cause and prognosis in 1000 cases. Arch Ophthalmol 1981;99:76–79
7. Berlit P. Isolated and combined pareses of cranial nerves III, IV and VI: A retrospective study of 412 patients. J Neurol Sci 1991;103:10–15
8. Green WR, Hackett ER, Schlezinger NS. Neuro-ophthalmologic evaluation of oculomotor nerve paralysis. Arch Ophthalmol 1964;72:154–167
9. Harley RD. Paralytic strabismus in children: Etiologic incidence and management of the third, fourth, and sixth nerve palsies. Ophthalmology 1980;86:24–43
10. Miller NR. Solitary oculomotor palsy in childhood. Am J Ophthalmol 1977;83:106–111
11. Kerr FWL, Hollowell OW. Location of pupillomotor and accommodation fibers in the oculomotor nerve: Experimental observations on paralytic mydriasis. J Neurol Neurosurg Psychiatry 1964;27:473–481
12. Ing EB, Sullivan TJ, Clarke MP, et al. Oculomotor nerve palsies in children. J Pediatr Ophthalmol Strabismus 1992;29:331–336
13. Victor DI. The diagnosis of congenital unilateral third-nerve palsy. Brain 1976;99:711–718
14. Balkan R, Hoyt CS. Associated neurologic abnormalities in congenital third nerve palsies. Am J Ophthalmol 1984;97:315–319

15. Hamed LM. Associated neurologic and ophthalmologic findings in congenital oculomotor nerve palsy. Ophthalmology 1991;98:708–714

16. Goldstein JE, Cogan DG. Diabetic ophthalmoplegia with special reference to the pupil. Arch Ophthalmol 1960;64:592–600

17. Jacobson DM, McCanna TD, Layde PM. Risk factors for ischemic ocular motor nerve palsies. Arch Ophthalmol 1994;112:961–965

18. Dreyfus P, Hakim S, Adams R. Diabetic ophthalmoplegia. Arch Neurol Psychiatry 1957;77:337–349

19. Asbury AK, Aldredge H, Hershberg R, et al. Oculomotor palsy in diabetes mellitus: A clinical-pathological study. Brain 1970;93:555–566

20. Weber RB, Daroff RB, Mackey EA. Pathology of oculomotor nerve palsy in diabetics. Neurology 1970;20:835–838

21. Nadeau SE, Trobe JD. Pupil sparing in oculomotor palsy: A brief review. Ann Neurol 1983;13:143–148

22. Jacobson DM. Pupil involvement in patients with diabetes-associated oculomotor nerve palsy. Arch Ophthalmol 1998;116:723–727

23. Jacobson DM, Broste SK. Early progression of ophthalmoplegia in patients with ischemic oculomotor nerve palsies. Arch Ophthalmol 1995;113:1535–1538

24. Capo H, Warren F, Kupersmith MJ. Evolution of oculomotor nerve palsies. J Clin Neuroophthalmol 1992;12:21–25

25. Jacobson DM, Broste SK. Early progression of ophthalmoplegia in patients ischemic oculomotor nerve palsies. Arch Ophthalmol 1995;113:1535–1538

26. Breen LA, Hopf HC, Farris BK, Gutman L. Pupil-sparing oculomotor palsy due to midbrain infarction. Arch Neurol 1991;48:105–106

27. Hopf HC, Gutmann L. Diabetic 3rd nerve palsy: Evidence for a mesencephalic lesion. Neurology 1990;40:1041–1045

28. Tomke F, Tettenborn B, Hopf HC. Third nerve palsy as the sole manifestation of midbrain ischemia. Neuroophthalmology 1995;15:327–335

29. Liu GT, Crenner CW, Logigian EL, et al. Midbrain syndromes of Benedikt, Claude, and Nothnagel: Setting the record straight. Neurology 1992;42:1820–1822

30. Keane JR. Aneurysms and third nerve palsies. Ann Neurol 1983;14:696–697

31. Kissel JT, Burde RM, Klingele TG, et al. Pupil-sparing oculomotor palsies with internal carotid-posterior communicating artery aneurysms. Ann Neurol 1983;13:149–154

32. Soni SR. Aneurysms of the posterior communicating artery and oculomotor paresis. J Neurol Neurosurg Psychiatry 1974;37:475–484

33. Trobe JD. Isolated pupil-sparing third nerve palsy. Ophthalmology 1985;92:58–61

34. Trobe JD. Third nerve palsy and the pupil: Footnotes to the rule. Arch Ophthalmol 1988;106:601–602

35. Forster RK, Schatz NJ, Smith JL. A subtle eyelid sign in aberrant regeneration of the third nerve. Am J Ophthalmol 1969;67:696–698

36. Lepore FE, Glaser JS. Misdirection revisited: A critical appraisal of acquired oculomotor nerve synkinesis. Arch Ophthalmol 1980;98:2206–2209

37. Memon MY, Paine KWE. Direct injury of the oculomotor nerve in craniocerebral trauma. J Neurosurg 1971;35:461–464

38. Sunderland S, Hughes ESR. The pupillo-constrictor pathway and the nerves to the ocular muscles in man. Brain 1946;69:301–309

39. Burde RM, Savino PJ, Trobe JD. Clinical Decisions in Neuro-ophthalmology. 2nd ed. St. Louis: Mosby, 1993

40. Keane JR. Ocular skew deviation: Analysis of 100 cases. Arch Neurol 1975;32:185–190

41. Jacobson DM, Trobe JD. The emerging role of magnetic resonance angiography in the management of patients with third cranial nerve palsy. Am J Ophthalmol 1999;128:94–96

42. Cullom ME, Savino PJ, Sergott RC, et al. Relative papillary sparing third nerve palsies: To arteriogram or not? J Clin Neuroophthalmol 1995;15:136–141

43. Noonan CP, O'Connor M. Surgical management of third nerve palsy. Br J Ophthalmol 1995;79:431–434

44. Gottlob L, Catalano RA, Reinecke RD. Surgical management of oculomotor nerve palsy. Am J Ophthalmol 1991;111:71–76

45. Reinecke RD. Surgical management of third and sixth cranial nerve palsies. Int Ophthalmol Clin 1985;25:139–148

46. Saunders RA, Rogers GL. Superior oblique transposition for third nerve palsy. Ophthalmology 1982;89:310–316

47. Khawam E, Scott AB, Jampolsky A. Acquired superior oblique palsy: Diagnosis and management. Arch Ophthalmol 1967;77:761–768

48. Rougier J, Girod M, Bongrand M. Etiology of and recovery from trochlear nerve paralysis: Apropos of 40 cases. Bull Soc Ophthalmol Fr 1973;73:739–744

49. Younge BR, Sutula F. Analysis of trochlear nerve palsies: Diagnosis, etiology, and treatment. Mayo Clin Proc 1977;52:11–18

50. Keane JR. Fourth nerve palsy: Historical review and study of 215 inpatients. Neurology 1993;43:2439–2443

51. Burger LJ, Kalvin NH, Smith JL. Acquired lesions of the fourth cranial nerve. Brain 1970;93:567–574

52. Sydnor CF, Seaber JH, Buckley EG. Traumatic superior oblique palsies. Ophthalmology 1982;89:134–138

53. Lavin PJM, Troost BT. Traumatic fourth nerve palsy: Clinicoanatomic correlations with computed tomographic scan. Arch Neurol 1984;41:679–680

54. Jacobson DM, Warner JJ, Ruggles KH. Transient trochlear nerve palsy following anterior temporal lobectomy for epilepsy. Neurology 1995;45:1465–1468

55. Grimson BS, Ross MJ, Tyson G. Return of function after intracranial suture of the trochlear nerve. J Neurosurg 1984;61:191–192

56. Cobbs WH, Schatz NJ, Savino PJ. Nontraumatic bilateral fourth nerve palsies: A dorsal midbrain sign. Ann Neurol 1980;8:107–108

57. Keane JR. Trochlear nerve pareses with brainstem lesions. J Clin Neuroophthalmol 1986;6:242–246

58. Brazis PW. Palsies of the trochlear nerve: Diagnosis and location—recent concepts. Mayo Clin Proc 1993;68:501–509

59. Haagedorn A. A new diagnostic motility scheme. Am J Ophthalmol 1942;25:726

60. Parks MM. Isolated cyclovertical muscle palsy. Arch Ophthalmol 1958;60:1027–1035

61. Hardesty HH. Diagnosis of paretic vertical rotators. Am J Ophthalmol 1963;56:811–816

62. Trobe JD. Cyclodeviation in acquired vertical strabismus. Arch Ophthalmol 1984;102:717–720

63. Ellis FD, Helveston EM. Superior oblique palsy: Diagnosis and classification. Int Ophthalmol Clin 1976;16:127–135

64. Spector RH. Vertical diplopia. Surv Ophthalmol 1993;38:31–62

65. Knapp P. Treatment of unilateral fourth nerve paralysis. Trans Ophthalmol Soc UK 1981;101:273–275

66. Maruo T, Iwashige H, Akatsu S, et al. Superior oblique palsy: Results of surgery in 443 cases. Binoc Vis Q 1991; 6:143–149

67. Klainguti G, Lang J. Diagnostique et traitement chirurgical de la paresie du grand oblique. Klin Monatsbl Augenheilkd 1994;204:353–359

68. Shrader EC, Schlezinger NS. Neuro-ophthalmologic evaluation of abducens nerve paralysis. Arch Ophthalmol 1960;63:84–91

69. Robertson DM, Hines JD, Rucker CW. Acquired sixth-nerve paresis in children. Arch Ophthalmol 1970;83:574–579

70. Miller NR, Kiel SM, Green WR, et al. Unilateral Duane's retraction syndrome (Type 1). Arch Ophthalmol 1982;100:1468–1472

71. Towfighi J, Marks K, Palmer E, et al. Möbius syndrome: Neuropathologic observations. Acta Neuropathol 1979; 48:11–17

72. Fisher CM. Some neuro-ophthalmological observations. J Neurol Neurosurg Psychiatry 1967;30:383–392

73. Sharpe JA, Rosenberg MA, Hoyt WF, et al. Paralytic pontine exotropia: A sign of acute unilateral pontine gaze palsy and internuclear ophthalmoplegia. Neurology 1974;24:1076–1081

74. Donaldson D, Rosenberg NL. Infarction of abducens nerve fascicle as cause of isolated sixth nerve palsy related to hypertension. Neurology 1988;38:1654–1657

75. Johnson LN, Hepler RS. Isolated abducens nerve paresis from intrapontine, fascicular abducens nerve injury. Am J Ophthalmol 1989;108:459–461

76. Silverman IE, Liu GT, Volpe NJ, et al. The crossed paralysis: The original brainstem syndromes of Millard-Gubler, Foville, Weber, and Raymond-Cestan. Arch Neurol 1995;52:635–638

77. Van Allen MW. Transient recurring paralysis of ocular abduction: A syndrome of intracranial hypertension. Arch Neurol 1967;17:81–88

78. Horton JC, Fishman RA. Neurovisual findings in the syndrome of spontaneous intracranial hypotension from dural cerebrospinal fluid leak. Ophthalmology 1994;101:244–251

79. Insel TR, Kalin NH, Risch SC, et al. Abducens palsy after lumbar puncture. N Engl J Med 1980;303:703–704

80. De Veuster I, Smet H, Vercauteren M, et al. The time course of a sixth nerve paresis following epidural anesthesia. Bull Soc Belge Ophthalmol 1994;252:45–47

81. Espinosa JA, Girous M, Johnston K, et al. Abducens palsy following shunting for hydrocephalus. Can J Neurol Sci 1993;20:123–125

82. Sarkies NJC, Sanders MD. Convergence spasm. Trans Ophthalmic Soc UK 1985;104;782–786

83. Kurata A, Takano M, Tokiwa K, et al. Spontaneous carotid-cavernous fistula presenting only with cranial nerve palsies. Am J Neuroradiol 1993;14:1097–1101

84. Lee DA, Dyer JA, O'Brien PC, Taylor JZ. Surgical treatment of lateral rectus muscle paralysis. Am J Ophthalmol 1984;97:511–518

85. Reinecke RD. Surgical management of third and sixth cranial nerve palsies. Int Ophthalmol Clin 1985;25:139–148

86. Repka MX, Lam GC, Morrison NA. The efficacy of botulinum neurotoxin A for the treatment of complete and partially recovered chronic sixth nerve palsy. J Pediatr Ophthalmol Strabismus 1994;31:79–83

87. Metz HS, Dickey CF. Treatment of unilateral acute sixth nerve palsy with botulinum toxin. Am J Ophthalmol 1991;112:381–384

88. Murray AD. Early botulinum toxin treatment of acute sixth nerve palsy. Eye 1991;5:45–47

89. Lee J, Harris S, Cohen J, et al. Results of a prospective randomized trial of botulinum toxin therapy in acute unilateral sixth nerve palsy. J Pediatr Ophthalmol Strabismus 1994;31:283–286

166 Nystagmus and Saccadic Oscillations

James A Sharpe

Overview

Nystagmus consists of oscillations of the eyes that are initiated by smooth eye movements. If one phase is a saccade, it is called jerk nystagmus. Although the fundamental defect is a smooth eye movement imbalance that drives the eyes slowly off their target, the direction of nystagmus is conventionally named in the direction of the saccadic phases that return the eyes toward their target. The smooth eye movement imbalance may arise in the vestibulo-ocular, smooth pursuit, optokinetic, or gaze holding systems, or rarely in the vergence system. If both phases are smooth eye movements, nystagmus is pendular.

Involuntary fast eye movements that intermittently take the fovea off a viewed object are saccadic intrusions. Saccadic oscillations are sustained and are also initiated by fast eye movements. Saccades are fast eye movements that normally drive the eyes to a target. They include voluntary refixations to targets, reflex movements toward a visual stimulus appearing suddenly off the fovea, and the fast phases of nystagmus. The goal of saccades is to move the target image to the fovea. In contrast to normal saccades, saccadic intrusions and saccadic oscillations disrupt visual fixation.

Epidemiology

Ocular oscillations have the population distribution and environmental and genetic determinants of the many neurological diseases that cause them.

Etiology

Nystagmus

Diseases involving the brainstem and its connections with the vestibulocerebellum (flocculus, paraflocculus and nodulus) give rise to vestibular imbalance or defective eye position holding, that is evident as gaze evoked nystagmus.[1] Infarction, hemorrhage, demyelination and neoplasms are common causes. Spinocerebellar degenerations that involve the flocculus and paraflocculus cause symmetrical gaze evoked nystagmus to both sides and upward, as well as rebound nystagmus, and sometimes primary position downbeat nystagmus.[2] Developmental disorders include the Chiari malformation, which is often accompanied by primary position downbeat nystagmus and by gaze evoked nystagmus. Peripheral vestibular causes of jerk nystagmus are considered in the chapter on inner ear disorders.

Pendular nystagmus is a sinusoidal or quasi-sinusoidal smooth eye movement oscillation (Figure 166.1). Acquired pendular nystagmus in adulthood is typically a manifestation of multiple sclerosis.[3] It also accompanies palatal tremor in the syndrome of oculopalatal tremor.[4,5] In childhood, acquired pendular nystagmus is a feature of two rare leukodystrophies, Pelizaeus-Merzbacher[6] disease, and Cockayne's syndrome.[7] Pendular vergence nystagmus with synchronous jaw contractions, called oculomasticatory myorhythmia, is characteristic of Whipple's disease.[8] Monocular blindness can cause vertical pendular nystagmus in that eye.[9,10] It has low amplitude. If vision is restored, it may subside, or it may persist leading to oscillopsia. In children an optic nerve tumor should be sought by imaging. Spasmus nutans is a syndrome of early childhood consisting of a triad of signs: head nodding, uniocular or asymmetrical binocular pendular nystagmus, and anomalous head position.[11] Ophthalmological, neurological, and imaging findings are otherwise normal. Spasmus nutans is benign and resolves spontaneously.

Congenital nystagmus is present from infancy, and usually in the absence of any structural brain disease. It can be accompanied by ocular albinism, foveal hypoplasia and congenital achromatopsia, but most often it is an isolated disturbance.[12,13] Congenital nystagmus can be both jerk and pendular in waveform (Figure 166.1), and is characteristically purely horizontal and conjugate, even during vertical gaze. Latent nystagmus is a special type of congenital horizontal jerk nystagmus that occurs when only one eye is used for fixation. By semantic convention latent nystagmus and congenital nystagmus retain distinct names, and latent nystagmus is not termed congenital. Quick phases of latent nystagmus are directed conjugately in the direction of the nonfixating eye. In patients with impaired vision from strabismic amblyopia, latent nystagmus persists while both eyes are viewing and beats toward the side of the eye with defective acuity; this persisting form of latent nystagmus is given the paradoxical name, manifest latent nystagmus.[14] Latent nystagmus typically has no recognized neurological dysgenesis, but can be a feature of trisomy 21 (Down syndrome).[15]

Saccadic intrusions

Square wave jerks (SWJ) (Table 166.1) are the most common ocular dyskinesia[16–18] (Figure 166.2). Square wave jerks that exceed normal 15 per minute frequencies and amplitudes over 0.5 degrees are a feature of cerebellar system disease.[17] They are prominent in cerebellar degenerations[2] and in multiple sclerosis

Supported by Canadian Institutes of Health Research (CIHR) Grants MT 15362 and ME 5504

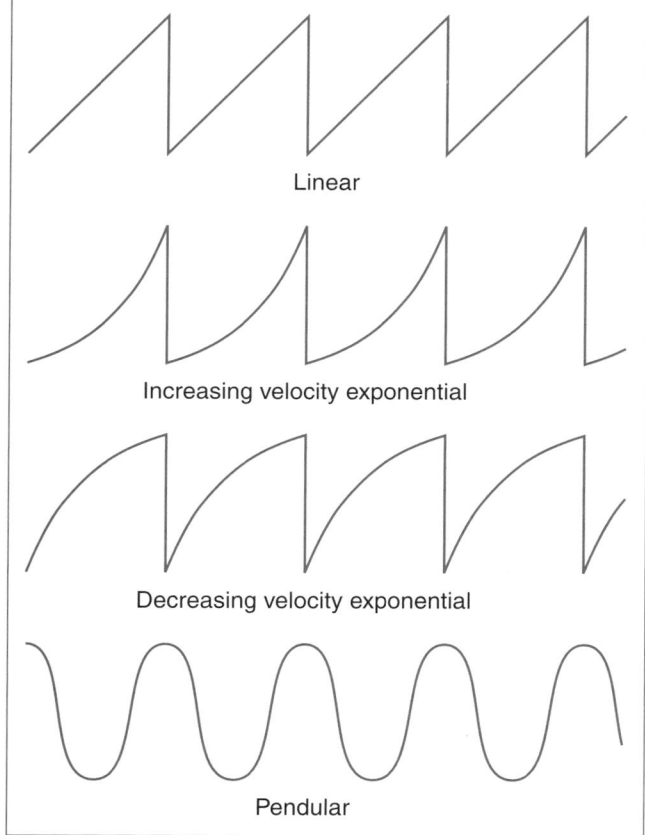

Figure 166.1 Jerk nystagmus has three waveforms: Slow phases are linear, increasing velocity, or decreasing velocity. Vestibular nystagmus has constant velocity (linear) slow phases. Decreasing velocity slow phases signify defective eye position holding by the velocity-to-position integrator, and are typical of gaze paretic nystagmus. Increasing velocity slow phases usually indicate congenital nystagmus. Bidirectional slow phases create pendular or sinusoidal nystagmus. Pendular nystagmus is characteristic of congenital nystagmus when the eyes are in the neutral range, and of acquired nystagmus in multiple sclerosis and oculopalatal tremor.

with cerebellar involvement. They also occur in parkinsonism. SWJ are more frequent in progressive supranuclear palsy and multiple system atrophy than in idiopathic Parkinson's disease,[18] probably reflecting the cerebellar degeneration of the former conditions, rather than basal ganglia dysfunction alone. SWJ also occur in patients with focal cerebral lesions.[17] Comparison of the metrics of SWJ in patients with cerebellar system disease reveal that cerebral SWJ are significantly lower in amplitude than cerebellar SWJ; the frequencies do not differ.[17] Square wave pulses are conjugate larger amplitude (10 to 40 degrees) horizontal saccades to one side of fixation and back, each separated by a brief interval, about 100 milliseconds (Figure 166.2). Square wave pulses often consist of a sustained salvo of oscillation. They have been observed in multiple sclerosis. Both conjugate sac-

cadic pulses and monocular saccadic pulses (Figure 166.3) occur in patients with multiple sclerosis.[19] Double saccadic pulses (Figure 166.3) have been reported in multiple sclerosis and metabolic encephalopathy.[20,21]

Anticipatory saccades are a feature of Alzheimer's disease. Clinically, the intrusions appear as furtive glances away from the examiner.[22] Saccadic anticipation becomes quite prominent during attempted fixation of targets which shift position and during smooth pursuit. Anticipatory saccades occur in the direction of expected target motion. These anticipatory saccadic intrusions are involuntary in the sense that patients cannot wilfully prevent their occurrence. Similar jerks occur sporadically in Huntington's chorea.

Saccadic oscillations

Square wave oscillations (Table 166.1) occur in progressive supranuclear palsy,[23] a condition characterized pathologically by degeneration of nigrostriatal pathways, the brainstem tegmentum, and the deep cerebellar nuclei. We have also encountered them in Parkinson's disease combined with alcoholic cerebellar degeneration (Figure 166.2).

Macro saccadic oscillations (Figure 166.2) are a sign of relatively acute structural damage in the dorsal cerebellum,[24] likely affecting the fastigial nucleus. Metastatic tumor, hematoma, and demyelination at this site are usual causes. Rarely they occur in cerebellar degenerations.[5] Micro saccadic oscillations occur in cerebellar degeneration.[25] They are detected by high resolution oculography but may be seen during funduscopy. The pathological oscillations are distinguished from normal micro saccadic oscillations only by their higher frequency. In cerebellar degeneration the frequency of spindles is about eight per minute, as opposed to normal micro saccadic oscillations which occur about twice per minute.[25]

Opsoclonus (Figure 166.4) accompanies cerebellar ataxia, myoclonic jerks of the limbs, and postural tremor in a benign rhomboencephalitis of early childhood. A variety of posterior fossa lesions can cause opsoclonus.[21,26] Coxsackie B virus, Epstein–Barr virus and *Haemophilus influenzae* meningitis have been incriminated in the myoclonic encephalopathy of childhood.[27–29] Remote, nonmetastatic carcinoma of the lung, breast, or uterus should be sought in adults, and in children an occult neuroblastoma is often responsible.[26,30] Intoxication with lithium, thallium, amitriptyline, or chlordecone also causes this dyskinesia.[21,26] Opsoclonus is occasionally a transient phenomenon in otherwise healthy infants. One normal person has been reported to produce opsoclonus voluntarily.[31]

Pathological ocular flutter (Figure 166.4) can occur as an isolated oscillation in multiple sclerosis, or a continuum of opsoclonus that is observed as it or the underlying disease begins or resolves; ocular flutter that heralds or follows opsoclonus has all of the causes mentioned above for opsoclonus.[21,26,32] Flutter is typically horizontal but it occurs occasionally in the vertical plane. The ability to voluntarily flutter the

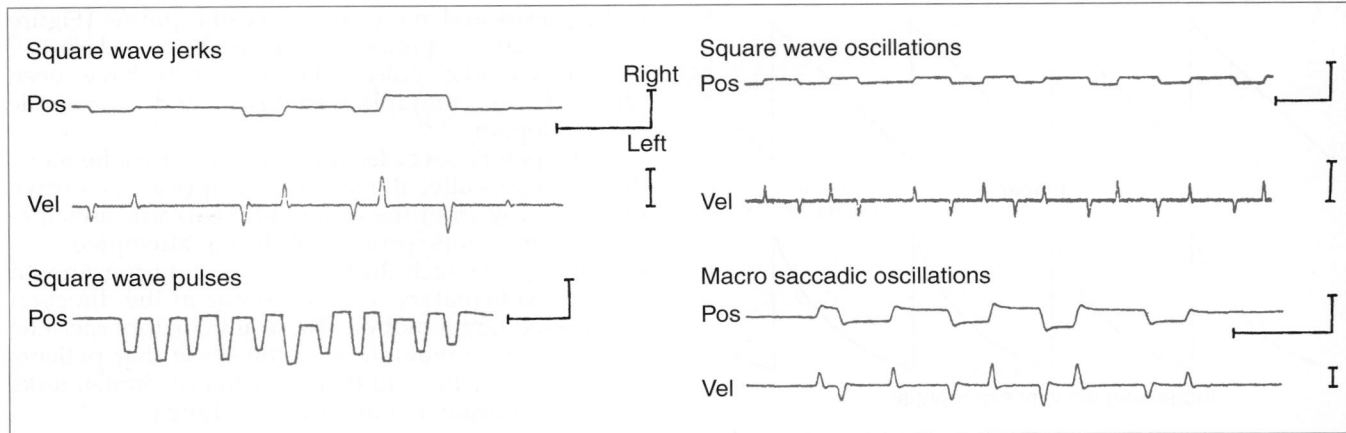

Figure 166.2   Saccadic intrusions and oscillations with intersaccadic intervals. Square wave jerks occur sporadically, and macro saccadic oscillations occur in bursts. Square wave pulses occur horizontally to one side of the fixation position, but macro saccadic oscillations straddle the intended fixation position. Square wave oscillations occur in prolonged trains or nearly continuously. Ordinate calibration bars are 10 degrees for position (Pos), and 200 degrees/s for velocity (Vel). Abscissa calibration bars are time base of 500 ms.

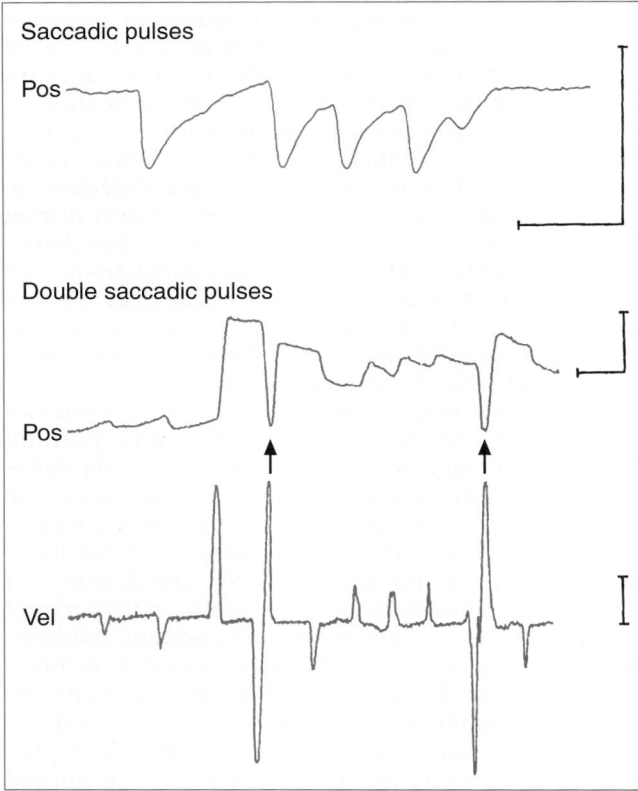

Figure 166.3   Saccadic pulses and double pulses. Saccadic pulses occur sporadically as saccadic intrusions that take the eyes off target, each being followed by a decelerating drift back to the fixation position. They are stepless saccades. Saccadic double pulses consist of two back-to-back saccades. The first drives the eyes off their position and the second returns them. Ordinate calibration bars are 10 degrees for position (Pos), and 200 degrees/s for velocity (Vel). Abscissa calibration bars are time base of 500 ms.

eyes is possessed by fewer than 10% of normal persons.[33]

Convergent-retraction saccades are associated with paresis of upward saccades caused by pretectal or periaqueductal midbrain damage.[34] Severe obstructive hydrocephalus can distend the rostral aqueduct of Sylvius and stretch the posterior commissure. More often pretectal neoplasms (dysgerminoma, pinealoma) or hemorrhage are responsible, and any destructive process in the pretectum can cause these bursts of oscillation.

Ocular bobbing is called typical when it is associated with paralysis of horizontal eye movements. Pontine hemorrhage or infarction is usually responsible.[35] Atypical bobbing refers to bobbing with intact horizontal eye movements. Metabolic encephalopathy, obstructive hydrocephalus, or cerebellar hematoma cause atypical bobbing. Reverse bobbing is a saccadic oscillation in which the eyes move rapidly up from the midposition and show delayed slow return. Metabolic encephalopathy is the usual cause.[36] These upward and downward saccadic oscillations should be distinguished from ocular dipping (also named inverse bobbing).[37,38] Ocular dipping is not a saccadic oscillation since it is initiated by slow downward eye movements and followed by rapid return to the midposition. Dipping is a sign of anoxic coma;[36,38] it has no known localizing significance, in contrast to ocular bobbing.

Superior oblique myokymia is the name for intermittent uniocular microtremor that occurs in bursts causing monocular oscillopsia and vertical diplopia. This dyskinesia is not a saccadic oscillation but is presented here because it resembles bursts of saccadic pulses; it arises from spontaneous discharges of trochlear nerve motor units. The dyskinesia usually lasts seconds, and occurs in clusters at varying intervals. Superior oblique myokymia is typically not

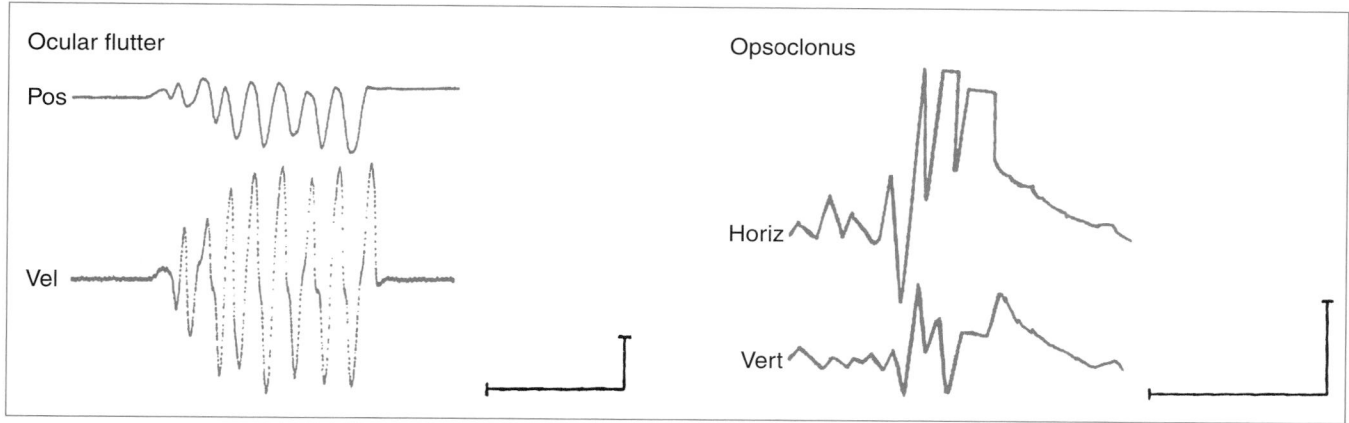

Figure 166.4 Flutter and opsoclonus. Ocular flutter consists of bursts of back-to-back saccades, typically in the horizontal plane. Opsoclonus also consists of bursts of saccades without intervals between them, but the saccades occur in vertical, horizontal and torsional directions. Ordinate calibration bars are 10 degrees for position (Pos), and 200 degrees/s for velocity (Vel). Abscissa calibration bars are time base of 500 ms.

associated with any other neurological or orbital disease.[39] Nonetheless, CT or MRI of the course of the fourth nerve may be warranted since structural lesions in the ambient cistern are rarely responsible[40] and angiography may be required if a dural arteriovenous malformation is suspected, as identified in one report.[41]

Pathophysiology and pathogenesis

Nystagmus

Nystagmus can arise from imbalance in vestibulo-ocular pathways, defective gaze holding by the neural integrator (discussed below), or high gain instability in the neural integrator. Rarely, imbalance in smooth pursuit or optokinetic tracking circuits, or instability in the vergence system is responsible.[42]

Neurotransmitters in the vestibulo-ocular reflex (VOR) Knowledge of neurotransmitter actions in vestibulo-ocular reflex and other smooth eye movement pathways may lead to logical and effective treatments. Excitatory transmission between first and second order vestibular neurons is probably effected by glutamine and by substance P. Both NMDA (N-methyl-D-aspartate) and AMPA (α-amino-3-hydroxy-5 methyl-4-isoxalone propionate) glutamate receptors are involved. Acetylcholine receptors, both nicotinic and muscarinic, are found in the medial vestibular nucleus, and acetylcholine facilitates transmission between first and second order neurons. Cholinergic second order vestibular neurons transmit movement related information to the flocculus, uvula and inferior olivary nucleus.[43]

Glutamate acts as a neurotransmitter in excitatory VOR pathways and its AMPA receptors are likely responsible for transmission to abducens nucleus motoneurons, but glutamate NMDA receptors are also found on abducens motoneurons. Aspartate and glutamate are the excitatory neurotransmitters uti-

lized by abducens internuclear synaptic endings, whose burst-tonic activity conveys vestibular information related to eye position to medial rectus motoneurons. For activity related to head velocity in the ascending tract of Deiters, glutamate is the excitatory neurotransmitter to medial rectus motoneurons.[44]

Glycine and GABA (γ-aminobutyric acid) are inhibitory transmitters in the vestibular nuclei. Glycine is the inhibitory transmitter for the horizontal VOR, acting at the abducens nucleus. On the other hand, GABA mediates inhibition for the vertical VOR on $GABA_A$ receptors of neurons of the trochlear and oculomotor nuclei.[43]

Vestibular nystagmus Peripheral disease of the labyrinth or vestibular nerve, or central imbalance of vestibular projections in the brainstem causes jerk nystagmus with slow phases directed toward the side of damage. The slow phases are typically linear, i.e. of constant velocity (Figure 166.1). Nystagmus is suppressed by visual fixation or smooth pursuit, and may appear only in darkness, although acute lesions typically cause nystagmus of such intensity that it is present during attempted fixation. The intensity of vestibular nystagmus increases during gaze in the direction of the quick phase, a phenomenon known as Alexander's law. Indeed, vestibular nystagmus may be only gaze evoked, appearing when gaze is directed away from the side of the vestibular lesion.[45]

Downbeat nystagmus This type of central vestibular nystagmus occurs in the primary position.[46] It is often encountered in cerebellar system degenerations and in the Chiari malformation, but a variety of structural lesions, or anticonvulsant drugs (phenytoin and carbamazepine), lithium intoxication or magnesium depletion can be responsible. In about 20% of cases, the cause remains undiagnosed.[47,48] Downbeating is maximal in lateral gaze.

Upward vestibular bias caused by disruption of

posterior semicircular canal projections to the brain tegmentum gives rise to downbeat nystagmus. The posterior canals activate the downward VOR and the anterior canals excite the upward VOR.[46,49] Disruption of the posterior canal projections in the brainstem causes the eyes to glide up in downbeat nystagmus; the fast phases correct orbital position.[46,49] Midsagittal section at the pontomedullary junction causes downbeat nystagmus in monkeys.[50] Downbeating is also produced experimentally by flocculectomy in the monkey.[1] Floccular Purkinje cells inhibit vestibular nucleus neurons that carry excitatory signals from the anterior semicircular canals. A few patients demonstrate downbeat nystagmus only with convergence, or in the dark with positioning of the head upside down or supine.[51,52] The slow phase velocity is often dependent on head position; some cases have an imbalance in otolith–ocular reflexes.[52] Many patients also have gaze evoked and rebound nystagmus.[42,48]

Upbeat nystagmus Primary position upbeat nystagmus likely results from disruption of anterior semicircular canal projections, which mediate the upward VOR, thereby causing the eyes to glide down.[49,53,54] Upbeat nystagmus occurs with lesions in the tegmentum at the ponto-medullary junction, and has also been attributed to lesions of the brachium conjunctivum and superior cerebellar vermis. Disruption of projections from both anterior semicircular canals could result from either cerebellar outflow lesions in the brachium conjunctivum or from damage to a ventral tegmental pathway of the upward VOR in the pontomedullary tegmentum,[53,54] where all but one of the pathologically verified lesions have occurred.[54–56]

Multiple sclerosis, tumor, infarcts and cerebellar degeneration are the most common causes. Drugs are seldom responsible. Nicotine from tobacco smoking can induce upbeat nystagmus in darkness;[57] nicotinic acetylcholinergic stimulation seems to be responsible. Like other forms of jerk nystagmus, upbeat usually increases in intensity during gaze in the direction of fast phase, in accord with Alexander's law.

Torsional nystagmus Rotation around the anteroposterior visual axis is called torsional. Torsional nystagmus accompanies horizontal vectors in peripheral vestibular disease. Pure torsional nystagmus indicates brainstem damage. Torsional jerk nystagmus occurs in medullary disease; torsional nystagmus with upward beating is occasionally seen. Pure torsional nystagmus signifies central disruption of input from the anterior and posterior semicircular canals on one side; the upper poles of the eyes beat away from the side of medullary damage.[58,59] Large amplitude pendular torsion is a component of see-saw nystagmus in patients with diencephalic-midbrain lesions who often have bitemporal hemianopia. In see-saw nystagmus the rising eye intorts as the falling eye extorts.[60,61] See-saw nystagmus with jerk half-cycles can result from unilateral midbrain or lateral medullary lesions.[58,62,63]

Periodic alternating nystagmus Periodic alternating nystagmus (PAN) is a form of central vestibular nystagmus that sifts direction every 90 seconds or so. Between right beating cycles (about 90 seconds) and left beating cycles (about 90 seconds) there is a null period of 0 to 10 seconds. It occurs with Chiari malformation, multiple sclerosis, fourth ventricle tumors, spinocerebellar degenerations, and anticonvulsant drug (phenytoin) intoxication. This nystagmus has been modeled by depriving the vestibulo-ocular reflex (VOR) of visual signals and by increasing the gain of a central velocity storage mechanism of the VOR.[64] PAN is produced experimentally in monkeys by removing the cerebellar nodulus and uvula, and depriving them of vision.[65]

Gaze paretic nystagmus Gaze evoked nystagmus with decelerating slow phases is called gaze paretic (Figure 166.1). It signifies cerebellar parenchymal disease, particularly of the flocculus or its projections in the brainstem, involving the eye velocity-to-position neural integrator.[1] Gaze paretic nystagmus in both horizontal directions and during up gaze is usually a sign of intoxication by alcohol or sedative or anticonvulsant drugs.[42] The nystagmus is variable in frequency and amplitude. Gaze paretic nystagmus occurs during deviation of the eyes toward the side of lesions of the cerebellum or its connections to the brainstem tegmentum. The decelerating slow phases are attributed to leakiness of the neural integrator, which sustains eccentric eye position.[1] The slow phase waveform is verified by quantitative oculography. However, slow phase waveform cannot always be relied upon to distinguish the causes of nystagmus, since vestibular nystagmus may occasionally have decelerating or accelerating slow phases.[66]

Brun's nystagmus Gaze paretic nystagmus toward the side of cerebellar pontine angle tumors, combined with vestibular nystagmus that is evoked by gaze to the contralateral side, is called Brun's nystagmus. The contraversive vestibular nystagmus is explained by vestibular nerve damage and ipsiversive gaze paretic nystagmus by compression of the brainstem or cerebellar flocculus.[45,67]

Rebound nystagmus is a variant of gaze evoked nystagmus which fatigues or changes direction with sustained lateral gaze. Upon refixation to the midposition, it transiently rebounds to beat in the direction of gaze shift.[68,69] It persists in the primary position for less than 30 seconds. This oscillation is a sign of cerebellar parenchymal disease and is produced experimentally by flocculectomy.[1] Rebound nystagmus is commonly seen in cerebellar degenerations, multiple sclerosis, and anticonvulsant (phenytoin) intoxication.

Acquired pendular nystagmus The pathogenesis of acquired pendular nystagmus is uncertain. In multiple sclerosis, delay in visual feedback secondary to demyelination in the optic nerves might contribute to it, and electronic manipulation of delay does elicit oscillations of lower frequency in normal subjects and patients; however, delay does not change the characteristics of acquired pendular nystagmus.[70] Neither delayed visual feedback nor a disorder of central vestibular mechanisms is primarily responsible for acquired pendular nystagmus.[70] This nystagmus is likely produced by abnormalities of internal feedback circuits, such as the reciprocal connections between brainstem nuclei and cerebellum. Instability in feedback control of the eye velocity-to-position integrator has been invoked as a mechanism of acquired pendular nystagmus.[71]

The nucleus prepositus hypoglossi, the medial vestibular nucleus, and the cerebellar flocculus are elements of the velocity-to-position integrator, which converts eye velocity signals to position signals, and thereby serves maintenance of steady gaze.[72,73] The interstitial nucleus of Cajal and the vestibular nucleus are elements of the velocity-to-position integrator for vertical eye motion.[74]

Acquired pendular nystagmus often appears a year or more after the first symptom of disease. MRI lesions are found in areas containing the red nucleus, the central tegmental tract, the medial vestibular nucleus and the inferior olivary nucleus.[75] Patients with horizontal pendular nystagmus show predominantly pontine lesions whereas patients with torsional pendular nystagmus show predominantly medullary involvement. Patients with conjugate pendular nystagmus have a higher incidence of symmetrical, "mirror image" lesions on MRI than patients with disconjugate nystagmus. Large or multiple structural lesions, predominantly in the pons but also in the midbrain and medulla, may be required to elicit pendular nystagmus.[75] Involvement of structures projecting to the inferior olive supports the hypothesis that oscillatory properties of neurons in the inferior olivary nuclei cause the rhythm of pendular nystagmus.[5,76]

Oculopalatal tremor Acquired pendular nystagmus is often associated with tremor of the palate. Vertical eye motion predominates in this combined dyskinesia. A misnomer, ocular myoclonus, was used for the nystagmus but can be abandoned. Oculopalatal tremor is sometimes associated with synchronous rhythmic movement of the pharynx, face, tensor tympani, vocal cords, shoulders or respiratory muscles. The palatal tremor and the nystagmus indicate damage to the dentate to superior cerebellar peduncle to central tegmental tract to inferior olivary nucleus to cerebellum circuit, called the triangle of Guillain and Mollaret. Appearance of the tremor and nystagmus is delayed for many months after the insult. The delay supports a mechanism dependent on neural deafferentation. Infarcts, hemorrhages, and rarely demyelination cause this oscillation. Hypertrophic degeneration of the inferior olivary nucleus is necessary, but not sufficient, for the genesis of ocular oscillations. Rostral cerebellar or brainstem damage that denervates the dorsal cap of the inferior olive is a possible foundation for the development of the pendular nystagmus associated with palatal tremor.[5]

Saccadic intrusions and oscillations

Saccadic intrusions are sporadic biphasic disruptions of fixation. Although one phase can be smooth eye movement, the phase that takes the eyes off the target is always a saccade (Figures 166.2 and 166.3). They include square wave jerks, saccadic pulses, double saccadic pulses, and sporadic ocular bobbing (Table 166.1). Sequences of these elements form saccadic oscillations.[21]

Saccades are initiated by supranuclear trigger signals from the frontal eye field, the parietal eye field, and the superior colliculus that inhibit omnipause (pause) neurons located in the midline pontine tegmentum.[77] Inhibition of pause cells releases the discharge of excitatory burst neurons (BN). The frequency of BN firing determines the speed of saccades, and the duration of their firing determines the amplitude of saccades. A command signal of desired eye position (for example, retinal target error), which is independent of the trigger signal, determines how long the burst cells fire (Figure 166.5). Collaterals of BN excite inhibitory burst neurons, which inhibit the pause cells during the saccade. The burst output is also mathematically integrated in the velocity-to-position neural integrator (NI); the output of this integrator is a new eye position command, called a step of innervation. The BN pulse is also believed to be integrated by another re-settable integrator to provide a feedback signal of eye position which inhibits the BN. Once the actual eye position matches the desired eye position, the burst cells cease firing, the pause cells resume activity, and the saccade ends.[21,77,78]

Intrusions and oscillations having an interval between sequential saccades (square wave jerks, square wave pulses, macro saccadic oscillations) (Table 166.1) signify integrity of both pause cells that stop saccades and the neural integrator that sustains eye position between saccades (Figure 166.2).

Neurotransmitters for saccadic premotor neurons Immunocytochemical techniques applying antibodies against putative transmitter molecules or their synthetic enzymes are revealing the chemical messengers of transmission in ocular motor synapses. Omnipause neurons utilize glycine to inhibit excitatory burst neurons. Omnipause neurons are inhibited by serotonin, and probably by γ-aminobutyric acid (GABA) and glycine.[79,80] Glycine is the transmitter of inhibitory burst neurons. Vertical excitatory medium-lead burst neurons likely secrete glutamate and aspartate as their synaptic transmitters. The transmitters of long-lead burst neurons and horizontal medium-lead burst neurons remain unknown. GABA is the inhibitory neurotransmitter, and glutamate and aspartate are the excitatory neurotransmitters utilized by premotor neurons in the rostral interstitial nucleus of the medial longitudinal fasciculus that project to the oculomotor and trochlear nuclei and generate vertical saccades.[81]

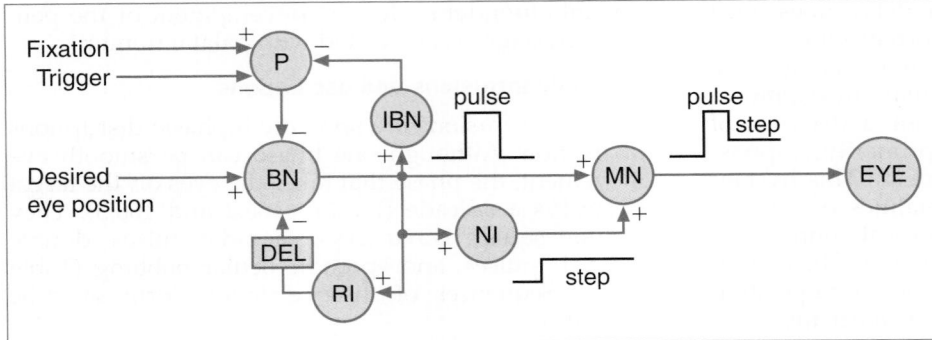

Figure 166.5   Model for generation of saccades. Fixation maintains activity of omnipause pause neurons (P) until a trigger signal inhibits them, releasing excitatory medium lead burst neurons (BN). BN excite inhibitory burst neurons (IBN) which stop pause cell activity and also inhibit motor neurons of antagonist muscles. The burst neurons send a velocity command (the pulse) to motoneurons (MN) and to the neural integrator (NI) which creates a position command (the step) for the eye. Another integrator, resettable after each saccade (RI), creates a negative feedback signal of eye position, delivered after a delay (DEL), to BN. When actual eye position equals desired eye position, BN cease firing, pause cells are disinhibited and the saccade stops.

Adapted from Sharpe JA. Neural control of ocular motor systems. *In:* Miller NR, Newman NJ, eds. Walsh and Hoyt's Clinical Neuro-ophthalmology. Vol 1. Baltimore: Lippincott, Williams and Wilkins, 1998:1101–1167

Square wave jerks   Sporadic horizontal conjugate saccades away from the intended position of fixation are followed after an interval by saccadic return to the fixation position. They vary in amplitude from 0.5 to about 10 degrees. Many normal subjects have low amplitude, low frequency SWJ.[16,17,82,83] The mean amplitude of normal square wave jerks is 1.2 degrees (SD 0.3) and their frequency is less than 15 per minute.[16] Some elderly normal subjects have more frequent SWJ. About 200 ms after the primary saccade which takes the eyes off target, visual feedback triggers the return saccade of each SWJ couplet. Some SWJ have much shorter intervals and their return saccades are not triggered by vision.[17] Injection of the GABA analog muscimol into the substantia nigra pars reticulata (SNpr) of monkeys disinhibits fixation cells in the rostral part of the superior colliculus, causing irrepressible square wave jerks.[84] In humans, the drug α-methyl paratyrosine (which depletes dopamine and norepinephrine) causes frequent square wave jerks.[85]

Saccadic pulses   These intrusions are composed of pulses of motor neuron innervation, without steps.[19–21,23] They are stepless saccades (Figure 166.3). During steady fixation saccades are held in abeyance by the pause neurons in the midline (Figure 166.5) of the caudal pontine tegmentum. Saccadic pulses probably signify damage to the pause cells or their supranuclear inputs combined with disruption of burst cell input to the integrator.

Double saccadic pulses   These saccadic intrusions are composed of isolated pairs of back-to-back saccades (Figure 166.3). They are sporadic conjugate movements. Brief disruption of the tonic input to pause cell activity may cause the intermittent back-to-back saccadic couplets.[20,21]

Opsoclonus and ocular flutter   Computer simulation studies of a feedback model of the saccade system predict that BN on each side of the pontine tegmentum will break into oscillations of back-to-back saccades under any of three conditions: (1) the delay in the feedback loop from the NI to the BN is prolonged; (2) input to the pause neurons is inadequate to keep them active; or (3) if the pause cells are sick.[86] The lower amplitude, higher frequency horizontal oscillations of voluntary flutter and micro flutter might be explained by lower tonic input to the pause neurons.[78] Poisoning with strychnine, a glycine antagonist, is reported to cause opsoclonus;[87] glycine is the neurotransmitter of pause cells.[79] However, patients with opsoclonus associated with lung cancer have been shown to have normal pause cells,[88,89] and experimental chemical lesions of pause cells in monkeys cause slow saccades, not back-to-back saccadic oscillation.[90] The back-to-back saccades of double saccadic pulses, opsoclonus and flutter might be explained by a delay in the feedback loop to the BN, even when pause cell activity is normal (Figure 166.5).

The fastigial nucleus has shown inflammation and degeneration in paraneoplastic opsoclonus.[91] Glycine is the inhibitory transmitter of Purkinje cells. Computer modeling indicates that disinhibition of the caudal part of the fastigial nucleus, resulting from Purkinje cell dysfunction, is a mechanism that can generate opsoclonus.[91]

Genetics

A familial incidence of voluntary flutter, albeit low, suggests either a genetic mechanism or learned behavior.[33] Hereditary spinocerebellar ataxias are associated with gaze evoked, rebound and downbeat nystagmus and square wave jerks.[92–94] Oculopalatal tremor can be a manifestation of brain degeneration in the syndrome of progressive ataxia and palatal tremor (PAPT).[76] Congenital nystagmus may be accompanied by ocular anomalies of autosomal dominant inheritance,[95] or with night blindness in an X linked calcium channel gene mutation,[96] or with albinism, or achromatopsia, but usually no genetic influence is identified and it appears sporadically. Latent and congenital nystagmus are encountered in Down syndrome of trisomy 21.[15]

Clinical features

The clinical features of nystagmus and saccadic oscillations are presented below, with their diagnostic criteria.

Classification

Saccadic dyskinesias are divided into intrusions and oscillations.[21,97] Each in turn is divided into those with and without intervals between sequential saccades (compare Figure 166.2 with Figures 166.3 and 166.4).[21] In the case of saccadic pulses, retraction saccades and bobbing there is no interval between the initiating fast eye movement and the return slower movement (Table 166.1).

Nystagmus can be classified as jerk or pendular and according to the waveform of its smooth eye movement phases (Table 166.2) or according to its specific etiology or its pathogenesis.

Diagnostic criteria and clinical features
Nystagmus

As with saccadic intrusions, nystagmus may be most apparent during funduscopy, which magnifies the eye movements. The examiner must bear in mind that the direction of movement of fundus landmarks is opposite to the direction of the nystagmus since the axis of rotation is through the middle of the eyeball. Thus in upbeat nystagmus, for example, the fundus beats downward. During funduscopy one may mistake torsional nystagmus for vertical nystagmus; since the axis of torsional rotation is through the anterior–posterior axis of the globe which passes near the fovea, the optic disk of one eye beats up and the optic disk of the other eye beats down.[42,58] Frenzel goggles, consisting of illuminated plus 20 or plus 30 diopter lenses, should be used to blur fixation, simulating examination in darkness. They also magnify the examiner's view of the nystagmus.[42]

Congenital nystagmus is almost invariably conjugate and horizontal in all positions of fixation. It remains horizontal during upward and downward gaze, in contrast to acquired nystagmus of central origin (Table 166.3). Fixation effort enhances congenital nystagmus. It subsides in darkness. Head oscillation may accompany the nystagmus.

Most congenital nystagmus is jerk in waveform.

Table 166.1 Classification of saccadic intrusions and oscillations

Saccadic intrusions	Saccadic oscillations
Interval between phases	
Square wave jerks	Square wave oscillation
	Square wave pulses
Anticipatory saccades	Macro saccadic oscillation
	Micro saccadic oscillation
No interval between phases	
Saccadic pulses	Convergence-retraction saccades*
	Ocular bobbing
	Opsoclonus
Double saccadic pulses	Flutter
	Micro flutter
	Voluntary flutter*

*Although usually referred to as nystagmus, convergence-retraction saccadic pulses and voluntary flutter are not genuine nystagmus. They are initiated by saccades rather than by the slow (smooth) eye movements that initiate nystagmus.

Table 166.2 Nystagmus waveforms

	Jerk nystagmus	Pendular nystagmus
Nystagmus slow phase waveform		
Decreasing velocity exponential, decelerating	Gaze paretic	
Linear, constant velocity	Vestibular	
Increasing velocity exponential, accelerating	Congenital, rarely acquired	
Sinusoidal		Acquired, sometimes congenital

Table 166.3   Pendular nystagmus: acquired versus congenital

	Acquired pendular nystagmus	Congenital pendular nystagmus
Form	Purely sinusoidal	Variable waveforms
Dissociation between eyes	Frequent	Rare
Direction	Omnidirectional (vertical, circular, elliptical)	Horizontal, uniplanar (rarely vertical or torsional)
Optokinetic nystagmus reversal	No	Frequent
Oscillopsia	Frequent	Rare and brief

Congenital jerk nystagmus typically has slow phases with velocities that accelerate before the next quick phase (Figure 166.1).[98] However, accelerating slow phases may also occur in acquired nystagmus.[58,66,99] When it is pendular, congenital nystagmus becomes jerk while gaze is directed to either side of a neutral region. Within this neutral region is a null region of minimum nystagmus intensity and optimal visual acuity. Reversed optokinetic nystagmus (OKN), beating in the direction of target motion, occurs in many patients with congenital nystagmus.[100] Reversal is attributed to shift of the neutral point in the direction opposite to optokinetic (or pursuit) target motion. If the null region is eccentric, a head turn permits straight-ahead vision with the eyes in the null region.

Oculography with direct current amplifiers can be used to establish the waveform of nystagmus (Table 166.2). With experience, examiners can detect accelerating (increasing velocity exponential) slow phases and decelerating (decreasing velocity exponential) slow phases and distinguish them with some confidence from linear slow phases (Figure 166.1).

Convergence usually dampens nystagmus. However, convergence may elicit a nystagmus that is absent during distant fixation or amplify it when present during distant fixation.[101,102] In convergence-evoked nystagmus, pendular vergence oscillations of each eye are 180 degrees out of phase. Multiple sclerosis is the usual cause. Neurological involvement in Whipple's disease can cause distinctive pendular vergence nystagmus combined with synchronous jaw contractions, called oculomasticatory myorhythmia.[103] Pendular convergence nystagmus is a genuine vergence oscillation which should be distinguished from convergent-retraction oscillations caused by pretectal midbrain damage.[104] Convergent-retraction oscillation is not nystagmus, since it begins with a fast (saccadic) co-contraction of extraocular muscles. It is elicited by upward saccades. Convergence may also amplify or induce upbeat or downbeat nystagmus or even cause it to reverse direction.

Saccadic intrusions and oscillations

Couplets of to-and-fro horizontal small saccades, each being separated by an interval, signify SWJ (Figure 166.2). Low amplitude SWJ are often undetected during inspection of the eyes. During ophthalmoscopy, saccades as small as 10 minutes of arc can be detected as flicks of fundus landmarks. Blood vessels near the optic disk margin provide convenient landmarks to estimate the amplitudes of saccadic intrusions. Arteries adjacent to the poles of the disk, just distal to the second bifurcation of the central retinal artery, subtend an angle of about 0.5 degrees. While the patient fixates a small distant object with one eye, low amplitude saccadic intrusions can be detected during funduscopy of the other eye.[17] Horizontal flicks that equal or exceed the diameters of peripapillary arteries signify fixation instability. Their frequency can be timed for 1 minute. To-and-fro flicks of 0.5 degrees or more, each separated by an interval, are SWJ. Observation of 15 or more to-and-fro flicks implicates abnormal SWJ.[17] Although not of specific localizing value, they are a sensitive index of brain dysfunction, and may be regarded as the "ocular motor sed rate."

Saccadic pulses appear as intermittent abrupt small flicks of the eyes (Figure 166.3). Flutter appears as intermittent bursts of trains of back-to-back saccades, typically in the horizontal plane (Figure 166.4). Double saccadic pulses take the form of a sporadic single biphasic flutter movement (Figure 166.3). Opsoclonus appears like flutter (Figure 166.4), but occurs in horizontal, vertical, diagonal and torsional directions.[91] Macro saccadic oscillations are recognized as bursts of horizontal to-and-fro saccades that straddle the primary gaze position and have delay between each saccade.[21,24,25] These spindles of oscillation usually occur during forward fixation, but sometimes they are precipitated only by refixation saccades, or during smooth pursuit.

The nature of these dyskinesias can be confirmed by high resolution eye movement recordings. Micro flutter and micro saccadic oscillations may be detected during funduscopy[21,78,105] and are verified by oculography.

Differential diagnosis

Unidirectionality and increase of its slow phase velocity when fixation is impaired by Frenzel goggles or eliminated by darkness are features of peripheral vestibular nystagmus that distinguish it from central nystagmus (Table 166.4). It beats opposite to the side of labyrinthine or vestibular nerve damage. Vestibular end-organ dysfunction usually has a torsional component mixed with a major horizontal vector.[42] Distinctions between benign paroxysmal vertigo and nystagmus and central paroxysmal nystagmus

Table 166.4	Central versus peripheral vestibular nystagmus	
Feature	**Peripheral vestibular nystagmus**	**Central vestibular nystagmus**
Form	Mixed horizontal-torsional	Purely vertical, purely horizontal, purely torsional, or mixed
Direction	Unidirectional	Reverses direction with gaze, or unidirectional
Effect of vision	Suppression	No suppression
Adaptation	Subsides in days	Often persists
Vertigo	Prominent	Mild
Hearing	May be decreased	Usually normal
	Tinnitus may occur	
Other neurological signs	None	Brainstem or cerebellar

brought out be head hanging maneuvers are considered in another chapter. Central vestibular nystagmus is typically not inhibited by fixation. The slow phase velocity remains the same in darkness or behind Frenzel goggles. Failure of vision to inhibit central nystagmus may be explained by impairment of smooth pursuit. Indeed, pursuit and vestibular signals share pathways from the vestibular nuclei to ocular motor nuclei. Vestibular imbalance in one direction, together with failure of fixation suppression by smooth pursuit, may explain the endurance of upbeat and downbeat primary position nystagmus.[41,54]

Gaze evoked nystagmus and its subtype, gaze paretic nystagmus, must be differentiated from physiological end-point nystagmus, a normal phenomenon during extreme gaze in any direction. End-point nystagmus is often unsustained, occurring for only a few beats. Sustained end point nystagmus is normal if it is present in both horizontal directions, and low in amplitude (under 4 degrees); it may be unequal in the two eyes[69,106,107] and has decelerating slow phases.[69,106] Fatigue-induced end-point nystagmus occurs after eccentric fixation for 30 seconds or so in many normal subjects. Pathological nystagmus that is evoked by eccentric gaze (gaze evoked nystagmus) is considered pathological when it is high in amplitude (over 4 degrees), or asymmetrical in two directions, but the most decisive distinguishing feature is the effect of darkness. End-point nystagmus increases its slow phase velocity by over 300% on average in darkness (at least by 36%), whereas the velocity of gaze evoked nystagmus changes little, under 15% on average.[106,108]

Acquired pendular nystagmus is readily distinguished from congenital nystagmus by multidirectional vectors and by the illusionary appearance of oscillation of the environment (oscillopsia) in the former (Table 166.3). In acquired pendular nystagmus vertical and horizontal oscillations are usually present in the same eye, and the two eyes are often disconjugate in direction or amplitude. Diagonal nystagmus occurs if the vertical and horizontal components of acquired pendular nystagmus are in phase or 180 degrees out of phase. If the vertical and horizontal oscillations are of equal amplitude and 90 degrees out of phase, circular nystagmus occurs. Elliptical nystagmus results from different amplitudes between the

vertical and horizontal movements when they are 90 degrees out of phase, or from any phase difference other than 90 or 180 degrees. In contrast, the oscillations characteristic of congenital nystagmus are horizontal and conjugate, and they remain horizontal during upward and downward gaze.

Distinctions among the saccadic oscillations are important in localizing neurological diseases. Macro saccadic oscillations might be confused with opsoclonus, but the former is predominantly horizontal and oculography can be used show intervals of about 200 ms between sequential saccades. Oculopalatal tremor is readily distinguished from ocular bobbing by observing the palate for oscillation and recognition that the upward and downward phases are symmetrical in the former. Voluntary flutter is evoked at will in some 8% of the population.[33] Although the oscillations have been habitually referred to as voluntary nystagmus, they are not truly nystagmus, since smooth (slow) eye movements are absent. Some individuals exhibit a forced facial expression or converge their eyes when making them flutter, which often lasts only a few seconds at a time. In the absence of other neurological signs, pathological ocular flutter, which has the same saccadic composition, must be excluded by prolonged observation and lack of other eye movement signs such as saccadic pursuit, and brain imagining may be warranted.

Treatment

Drug therapy of acquired nystagmus

Pharmacological intervention is effective in some patients. Trial and error is often the treatment strategy (Table 166.5).

Baclofen is an effective treatment for periodic alternating nystagmus[109] (Grade C, level 4 evidence). Baclofen is a GABA analog. It disengages velocity storage in the VOR. It is postulated to work by substituting for damaged Purkinje cells of the nodulus, thereby dumping the activity of the velocity storage mechanism in the vestibular nuclei that is responsible for reflex eye movements at very low frequencies of head motion.[110] A congenital type of PAN does not respond.

A double-blind crossover trial compared gabapentin (up to 900 mg/day) to baclofen (up to

Table 166.5　Treatments for oscillopsia due to acquired nystagmus

Drugs
　Downbeat/upbeat nystagmus
　　Baclofen (Lioresal)*
　　Carbamazepine (Tegretol)
　　Scopolamine dermal patch
　　Clonazepam (Clonopin)*
　　Gabapentin (Neurontin)*
　　Isoniazid
　　Memantine (Akatinol)*
　　Trihexyphenidyl or other anticholinergics*
　　Valproic acid
　Acquired pendular nystagmus
　　Gabapentin (Neurontin)*
　　Memantine*
　　Trihexyphenidyl
　　Valproic acid
　Periodic alternating nystagmus
　　Baclofen*

Optical management
　Base-out prism spectacles, occasionally base-in
　　prisms
　Rotational magnificent device

Invasive techniques
　Suboccipital craniotomy for Arnold–Chiari malformation
　Muscle reattachment (Anderson–Kestenbaum
　　operation)
　Botulinum toxin

*Drugs considered to warrant trial of treatment in individual patients.

30 mg/day) as therapy for acquired nystagmus[111] (Grade B evidence). In patients with acquired pendular nystagmus, visual acuity improved significantly with gabapentin, but not with baclofen. Gabapentin (Neurontin) significantly reduced median pendular eye speed in all planes, but baclofen did so only in the vertical plane. The reduction of nystagmus with gabapentin is substantial in some patients, and they choose to continue taking the drug.

In downbeat nystagmus, changes in median slow phase eye speed are less consistent with either gabapentin or baclofen, either increasing or decreasing it, and being dependent on viewing conditions. Few patients show consistent reduction of median eye speed with either drug. Gabapentin may be an effective treatment for many patients with pendular nystagmus, and occasional patients with downbeat nystagmus respond to gabapentin or baclofen[111] (Grade B evidence).

Memantine is a noncompetitive glutamate antagonist that acts at NMDA receptors. It has therapeutic potential in dementia. spasticity and Parkinson's disease, but is not available for prescription in Canada or the United States. Acquired pendular nystagmus caused by multiple sclerosis may benefit. In one unmasked study, 11 patients with fixational pendular nystagmus who were given memantine experienced complete cessation of the nystagmus. In contrast, scopolamine caused no or only minor (10% to 50%) reduction of the nystagmus.[112] It was concluded that memantine is a safe treatment option for acquired pendular nystagmus (Grade C, level 4 evidence).

Treatment of disabling oscillopsia with other drugs is worth a trial in individual patients (Table 166.5). Trihexyphenidyl in large doses (15 to 20 mg daily) may decrease acquired pendular nystagmus and oscillopsia (Grade C, level 5 evidence)[113] but the side effects are sometimes intolerable, and one randomized double-blind crossover trial showed no benefit (Grade B evidence).[114] Tridihexethyl chloride, a peripherally acting anticholinergic, reduces, but does not abolish, oscillopsia.[114] However, a double-blind randomized crossover study[115] showed that intravenous benztropine or scopolamine (both centrally acting drugs, like trihexyphenidyl) dramatically reduce acquired pendular and downbeat nystagmus (Grade B evidence). While tridihexethyl is a selective M1 muscarinic receptor antagonist, scopolamine has antagonist effects on M2 and M3 muscarinic receptors in cerebellar cortex and M2 receptors in the tegmentum, perhaps accounting for its effectiveness.[115] An acetylcholinesterase inhibitor, physostigmine, given by intravenous injection, transiently increases downbeat nystagmus (Grade C, level 4 evidence).[116] These results provide some rationale for further treatment trials with centrally acting anticholinergic drugs.[115]

The GABAergic drug baclofen (5 mg PO t.i.d.) reduces nystagmus slow phase velocity and distressing oscillopsia by 25% to 75% in some patients with upbeat nystagmus or downbeat nystagmus (Grade C, level 4 evidence).[116] The response to baclofen appears to be a GABA-B-ergic effect with augmentation of the physiological inhibitory influence of the vestibulo-cerebellum on the vestibular nuclei. Baclofen also has an inhibitory effect on the velocity storage mechanism.[110]

Clonazepam, valproic acid, or carbamazepine may also improve central vestibular or acquired pendular nystagmus[58,117–121] (Grade C, level 5 evidence). but controlled trials are not available to exclude placebo effects or spontaneous changes in the oscillations. Moreover, carbamazepine can induce nystagmus.[120] 5-hydroxytryptophan with carbidopa is reported beneficial in acquired pendular nystagmus (Grade C, level 5 evidence),[122] but in our experience, effective doses cause intolerable side effects, including visual hallucinations.

Acetazolamide is useful in preventing attacks in familial periodic ataxia type 2 with interictal nystagmus but prospective studies are not available to indicate whether it can prevent progressive ataxia or improve chronic cerebellar deficits (Grade C, level 5 evidence).[93,123]

Superior oblique myokymia often responds to carbamazepine (Grade C, level 4 evidence)[39–41,124] or propranolol (anecdotal evidence). Spontaneous remissions occur. If medication fails and symptoms are very obtrusive, tenectomy of the superior oblique muscle and myectomy of the inferior oblique muscle may be effective.[124] A Harada–Ito procedure transposes the anterior portion of the superior oblique tendon nasally to create an effective weakening of the anterior portion of the tendon (instead of the temporal displacement utilized for superior oblique muscle paresis).[125] One patient had immediate cessation of myokymia following microvascular decompression of the fourth nerve at the root exit zone (Grade C, level 5 evidence).[126] Temporary double vision at downgaze resolved 5 months after surgery, and no recurrence of oscillopsia occurred during a follow-up of 22 months.[126] This may have been a spontaneous resolution, but vascular compression of the trochlear nerve could be a pathophysiological factor contributing to the myokymia.

Ocular neuromyotonia is a related phenomenon of phasic and tonic contraction of muscles innervated by the sixth or third cranial nerves; it follows radiation therapy to pituitary or other juxtasellar tumors, or rarely nerve compression without radiation. Carbamazepine relieves the episodes in many patients (Grade C, level 5 evidence).[127,128]

Optical treatments for nystagmus

Since convergence sometimes dampens acquired nystagmus, treatment of downbeat, upbeat, or acquired pendular nystagmus with base-out prisms in spectacle lenses can induce convergence and dampen nystagmus and oscillopsia (Grade C, level 5 evidence).[51,119] Images are displaced in the direction of the prism apex, making the eyes converge to achieve binocular single vision. However, in some cases the nystagmus is increased by convergence, and base-in prisms that reduce the need to converge would then be appropriate treatment.[51,101,102,129]

Treatment of congenital nystagmus with base-out prisms also dampens the nystagmus, and may improve visual acuity (Grade C, level 5 evidence).[130,131] Prisms can also be used to shift the viewing position into the null region of minimum nystagmus intensity. Vibration or electrical stimulation to the neck or forehead may also improve visual acuity (Grade C, level 5 evidence).[132] Soft contact lenses provide trigeminal nerve stimulation that dampens nystagmus in some patients (Grade C, level V evidence).[133] Auditory biofeedback is reported to transiently improve vision (Grade C, level 5 evidence).[134] Benefits outside the laboratory have not been demonstrated, and controlled trials are required to confirm results and exclude placebo effects of these therapies.[135] Baclofen has been claimed to be effective (Grade C, level 5 evidence),[136] but any benefits in acuity from drug therapy of congenital nystagmus may not be sufficient to compensate for their side effects.

Rotational magnification lenses can be used to stabilize retinal images in the treatment of oscillopsia from acquired pendular nystagmus or central vestibular nystagmus (Grade C, level 5 evidence).[137,138] Image stabilization is achieved by two lenses for each eye. A powerful plus spectacle lens is worn in front of a powerful minus contact lens. The plus lens focuses

the image on the center of rotation of the eye, and the minus contact lens (which moves with the eye) then focuses the image on the retina. In that way, the image remains stable on the retina and oscillopsia is reduced. Unfortunately, the head must be stationary, since the vestibulo-ocular reflex is negated. The field of view is restricted to about 30 degrees.[138] One device senses eye movements and, by the use of motor-driven prisms, oscillates images in lockstep with the nystagmus, to negate its visual effects while leaving voluntary and reflex eye movements unaffected. It decreases oscillopsia in pendular nystagmus (Grade C, level 5 evidence),[139] but a practical wearable version is not available.

Botulinum toxin for nystagmus

Attempts to stop the eye motion by detaching muscles or paralyzing them with injection of botulinum toxin into extraocular muscles or the retrobulbar space are occasional measures (Grade C, level 5 evidence). Botulinum toxin can stop the horizontal oscillations but is not well accepted by patients and it does not prevent vertical motion without injections that cause blinding ptosis.[140,141] Although nystagmus can be reduced, diplopia, keratitis, ptosis and transience of effectiveness limit patient acceptance. Moreover, if movement of only one eye is paralyzed, the nystagmus may increase in the other eye.[140] Botulinum injections can be tried in patients who are prepared to trade off side effects for improved vision and reduced oscillopsia.[142,143] Botulinum injections have also been used to treat latent and congenital nystagmus (Grade C, level 5 evidence).[144,145]

Surgery for nystagmus

The Kestenbaum operation for congenital nystagmus moves the attachment of extraocular muscles or resects and recesses them so that the null or quiet zone of nystagmus corresponds to the primary position of the eyes (Grade C, level 5 evidence).[146,147] Prisms that shift the gaze angle to the null angle are used to fine tune the surgery. In patients whose nystagmus is much reduced by convergence, base-out prisms can be tried first and if they are unsatisfactory, artificial divergence surgery is available (Grade C, level 5 evidence).[148] Combinations with the Anderson–Kestenbaum procedure may yield better results (Grade C, level 5 evidence).[147,148]

Recession of the four horizontal rectus muscles is a third procedure that can improve acuity and reduce head turn without reducing the range of gaze (Grade C, level 5 evidence).[149,150] Tenotomy of the four horizontal recti muscles with immediate reattachment at their original insertions is reported effective for improving vision in adults with congenital nystagmus, provided they do not have an associated sensory defect, such as from albinism, that sometimes accompanies congenital nystagmus (Grade C, level 5 evidence).[151]

Suboccipital decompression in the Chiari type 1 malformation resolves downbeat nystagmus in some patients and improves it in others (Grade C, level 5 evidence).[152,153] The improvement in oscillopsia and nystagmus may be gradual over about six months.

Treatments of saccadic intrusions and oscillations

Square wave jerks and macro saccadic oscillations were abolished after diazepam, clonazepam, and barbiturates administration to one patient (Grade C, level 5 evidence).[154] The first patient reported with microflutter had cerebellar atrophy, and carbamazepine reduced the frequency of episodes of oscillopsia.[105] In other individual patients, microflutter has been reduced after treatment with propranolol or verapamil (Grade C, level 5 evidence).[78]

Opsoclonus associated with neural crest tumors responds to ACTH treatment, but it has no established benefit over corticosteroids, and therapy to the underlying neoplasm is paramount.[26,155] In a retrospective study of treatment of 29 children with neuroblastoma and opsoclonus–myoclonus,[156] 19 received surgery and 10 received surgery plus chemotherapy. No patient received radiotherapy. Treatment for opsoclonus–myoclonus varied (Grade C, level 3 evidence). Six other children received no treatment for opsoclonus–myoclonus. The following agents were used: ACTH (n = 14), prednisone (n = 12), IV IgG (n = 6), azathioprine (Imuran) (n = 2), divalproex sodium (Depakote) (n = 1), and propranolol (n = 1). Eighteen of 29 children (62%) had resolution of opsoclonus–myoclonus symptoms. The range of time for recovery was a few days to 3 years; the majority recovered over several months. Twenty of 29 children (69%) had persistent neurological deficits including speech delay, cognitive deficits, motor delay, and behavioral problems. Nine children had complete recovery of opsoclonus–myoclonus without neurological sequelae. Their age at diagnosis and duration of symptoms did not differ from the entire group. Six of the nine children with complete recovery received chemotherapy as part of their treatment. Persistent neurological deficits are characteristic of children with neuroblastoma and opsoclonus–myoclonus.[156]

Children with parainfectious or idiopathic opsoclonus–myoclonus syndrome may also respond to corticosteroids or adrenocorticotrophic hormone (ACTH). Eight children in one series[157] were all ACTH responsive with 50% to 70% improvement in multiple clinical features of opsoclonus–myoclonus (Grade C, level 5 evidence). Treatment with ACTH was associated with significant correlations between dopaminergic markers such as homovanillic acid (HVA), dihydroxyphenylacetic acid (DOPAC), and dopa in the CSF. Beneficial effects of ACTH in opsoclonus–myoclonus are not associated with normalization of lowered HVA or 5-HIAA levels. The pattern of decreased HVA and unchanged DOPAC levels could reflect decreased extraneuronal uptake of catecholamines (which steroids inhibit) or decreased O-methylation of catecholamines in nonneuronal cells.[157]

Opsoclonus in adults associated with malignant tumors tends to vary in frequency and intensity and may stop even without removal of the primary neoplasm; this makes assessment of treatment of the opsoclonus and ataxia or other paraneoplastic complications difficult to assess. Immunoadsorption of immune complexes and the Fc portion of IgG protein using a protein A column during plasma exchange is reported to improve opsoclonus and other paraneoplastic complications. In a series of 12 patients treated with immunoadsorption,[158] three had a complete response of the primary clinical symptom/sign while six had a partial response, for a total response rate of nine (75%) (Grade C, level 5 evidence). Complete and durable responses to this treatment were reported in three patients with opsoclonus–myoclonus (Grade C, level 5 evidence).[159] Intravenous human immunoglobulin has been reported effective in occasional patients having opsoclonus with or without neuroblastoma (Grade C, level 5 evidence).[160,161]

References

1. Zee DS, Yamazaki A, Butler PH, Gucer G. Effects of ablation of flocculus and paraflocculus on eye movements in primate. J Neurophysiol 1981;46:878–899
2. Zee DS, Yee RD, Cogan DG, et al. Ocular motor abnormalities in hereditary cerebellar ataxia. Brain 1976;99(2):207–234
3. Gresty MA, Ell JJ, Findley LJ. Acquired pendular nystagmus: its characteristics, localising value and pathophysiology. J Neurol Neurosurg Psychiatry 1982;45(5):431–439
4. Nakada T, Kwee IL. Oculopalatal myoclonus. Brain 1986;109:431–441
5. Sharpe JA, Kim JS. Ocular oscillations and intrusions with palatal tremor. Neurology 2000;54(7)(Suppl 3):A250–A251
6. Trobe JD, Sharpe JA, Hirsh DK, Gebarski SS. The nystagmus of Pelizaeus–Merzbacher disease. Arch Neurol 1991;48:87–91
7. Coker S, Susac JO, Sharpe JA, Smallridge B. Cochayne's syndrome: neuro-ophthalmic, C.A.T. scan and endocrine observations. In: Smith JL, ed. Neuro-ophthalmology-focus 1980. New York: Masson, 1979:379–385
8. Schwartz MA, Selhorst JB, Ochs AL, et al. Oculomasticatory myorhythmia: a unique movement disorder occurring in Whipple's Disease. Ann Neurol 1986;20:677–683
9. Yee RD, Jelks GW, Baloh RW, Honrubia V. Uniocular nystagmus in monocular visual loss. Ophthalmology 1979;86:511–518
10. Farmer J, Hoyt CS. Monocular nystagmus in infancy and early childhood. Am J Ophthalmol 1984;98:504–509
11. Weissman BM, Dell'Osso LF, Abel LA, Leigh RJ. Spasmus nutans. A quantitative prospective study. Arch Ophthalmol 1987;105(4):525–528
12. Dell'Osso LF. Congenital and other types of infantile nystagmus: recording, diagnosis, and treatment. In: Sharpe JA, Barber HO, eds. The Vestibulo-ocular Reflex and Vertigo. New York: Raven Press, 1993:229–247
13. Gresty M, Page N, Barratt H. The differential diagnosis of congenital nystagmus. J Neurol Neurosurg Psychiatry 1984;47:936–942
14. Gresty MA, Metcalfe T, Timms C, et al. Neurology of latent nystagmus. Brain 1992;115:1303–1321
15. Averbuch-Heller L, Dell'Osso LF, Jacobs JB, Remler

BF. Latent and congenital nystagmus in Down syndrome. J Neuroophthalmol 1999;19(3):166–172

16. Herishanu YO, Sharpe JA. Normal square wave jerks. Invest Ophthalmol Vis Sci 1981;20:269–272

17. Sharpe JA, Herishanu YO, White OB. Cerebral square wave jerks. Neurology 1982;32:57–62

18. Rascol O, Sabatini U, Simonetta-Moreau M, et al. Square wave jerks in Parkinsonian syndromes. J Neurol Neurosurg Psychiatry 1991;54:599–602

19. Herishanu YO, Sharpe JA. Saccadic intrusions in internuclear ophthalmoplegia. Ann Neurol 1983;14:67–72

20. Dolsac MJ, Dell'Osso LF, Daroff RB. Multiple double saccadic pulses occurring with other saccadic intrusions and oscillations. Neuroophthalmology (Amsterdam) 1983;3:109–116

21. Sharpe JA, Fletcher WA. Saccadic intrusions and oscillations. Can J Neurol Sci 1984;11:426–433

22. Fletcher WA, Sharpe JA. Saccadic eye movement dysfunction in Alzheimer's disease. Ann Neurol 1986;20:464–471

23. Abel LA, Traccis S, Dell'Osso LF, et al. Square wave oscillation: the relationship of saccadic intrusions and oscillations. Neuroophthalmology 1984;4:21–25

24. Selhorst JB, Stark L, Ochs AL, Hoyt WF. Disorders in cerebellar ocular motor control. II. Macrosaccadic oscillation. An oculographic control system and clinico-anatomical analysis. Brain 1976;99:509–522

25. Hotson JR. Cerebellar control of fixation eye movements. Neurology 1982;32:31–36

26. Digre K. Opsoclonus in adults: report of three cases with review of the literature. Arch Neurol 1986;43:1165–1175

27. Kuban KC, Ephos MA, Freeman RL, et al. Syndrome of opsoclonus-myoclonus caused by Coxsackie B3 infection. Ann Neurol 1983;13:69–71

28. Rivner MH, Jay WM, Green JB, Dyken PR. Opsoclonus in hemophilus influenzae meningitis. Neurology 1982;32:661–663

29. Sheth RD, Horwitz SJ, Aronoff S, et al. Opsoclonus myoclonus syndrome secondary to Epstein–Barr virus infection. J Child Neurol 1995;10(4):297–299

30. Mitchell WG, Snodgrass SR. Opsoclonus-ataxia due to childhood neural crest tumors. A chronic neurologic syndrome. J Child Neurol 1990;5:153–158

31. Yee RD, Spiegel PH, Yamada T, et al. Voluntary saccadic oscillations, resembling ocular flutter and opsoclonus. J Neuroophthalmol 1994;14(2):95–101

32. Ellenberger C, Keltner JL, Stroud MH. Ocular dyskinesia in cerebellar disease: evidence for the similarity of opsoclonus, ocular dysmetria and flutter like oscillations. Brain 1972;95:685–692

33. Zahn JR. Incidence and characteristics of voluntary nystagmus. J Neurol Neurosurg Psychiatry 1978;41:617–623

34. Gay A, Brodkey J, Miller JE. Convergence retraction nystagmus. Arch Ophthalmol 1963;70:456–461

35. Susac JO, Hoyt WF, Daroff RB, Lawrence W. Clinical spectrum of ocular bobbing. J Neurol Neurosurg Psychiatry 1970;33:771–775

36. Rosenberg ML. Spontaneous vertical eye movements in coma. Ann Neurol 1986;20(5):635–637

37. Knobler RL, Somasundaram M, Schutta HS. Inverse ocular bobbing. Ann Neurol 1981;9:194–197

38. Roper AH. Ocular dipping in anoxic coma. Arch Neurol 1981;138:297–299

39. Rosenberg ML, Glaser JS. Superior oblique myokymia. Ann Neurol 1983;13:667–679

40. Morrow MJ, Sharpe JA, Ranalli PJ. Superior oblique myokymia associated with a posterior fossa tumour. Oculographic correlation with an idiopathic case. Neurology 1990;40:367–370

41. Geis TC, Newman NJ, Dawson RC. Superior oblique myokymia associated with a dural arteriovenous fistula. J Neuroophthalmol 1996;16(1):41–43

42. Fletcher WA. Nystagmus: an overview. In: Sharpe JA, Barber HO, eds. The Vestibulo-ocular Reflex and Vertigo. New York: Raven Press, 1993:195–215

43. de Waele C, Muhlethaler M, Vidal PP. Neurochemistry of the central vestibular pathways. Brain Res Brain Res Rev 1995;20(1):24–46

44. Nguyen LT, Spencer RF. Abducens internuclear and ascending tract of Deiters inputs to medial rectus motoneurons in the cat oculomotor nucleus: neurotransmitters. J Comp Neurol 1999;411(1):73–86

45. Robinson DA, Zee DS, Hain TC, et al. Alexander's law: its behavior and origin in the human vestibulo-ocular reflex. Ann Neurol 1984;16(6):714–722

46. Baloh RW, Spooner JW. Downbeat nystagmus: a type of central vestibular nystagmus. Neurology 1981;31(3):304–310

47. Halmagyi GM, Rudge P, Gresty MA, Sanders MD. Downbeating nystagmus. A review of sixty-two cases. Arch Neurol 1983;40:777–784

48. Yee RD. Downbeat nystagmus: characteristics and localization of lesions. Trans Am Ophthalmol Soc 1989;87:984–1032

49. Sharpe JA, Johnston JL. The vestibulo-ocular reflex: clinical anatomic and physiologic correlates. In: Sharpe JA, Barber HO, eds. The Vestibulo-ocular Reflex and Vertigo. New York: Raven Press, 1993:15–39

50. de Jong JM, Cohen B, Matsuo V, Uemura T. Midsagittal pontomedullary brain stem section: effects on ocular adduction and nystagmus. Exp Neurol 1980;68(3):420–442

51. Lavin P, Traccis S, Dell'Osso LF, et al. Downbeat nystagmus with a pseudocycloid waveform: improvement with base-out prism. Ann Neurol 1983;13:621–624

52. Chambers BR, Ell JJ, Gresty MA. Case of downbeat nystagmus influenced by otolith stimulation. Ann Neurol 1983;13(2):204–247

53. Ranalli PJ, Sharpe JA. Upbeat nystagmus and the ventral tegmental pathway of the upward vestibulo-ocular reflex. Neurology 1988;38:1329–1330

54. Hirose G, Kawada J, Tsukada K, et al. Primary position upbeat nystagmus. J Neurol Sci 1991;105:159–167

55. Fisher A, Gresty M, Chambers B, Rudge P. Primary position upbeating nystagmus. Brain 1983;106:949–964

56. Nakada T, Remler MP. Primary position upbeat nystagmus. Another central vestibular nystagmus? J Clin Neuroophthalmol 1981;1:185–189

57. Sibony PA, Evinger C, Manning KA. Tobacco induced primary-position upbeat nystagmus. Ann Neurol 1987;21:53–58

58. Morrow MJ, Sharpe JA. Torsional nystagmus in the lateral medullary syndrome. Ann Neurol 1988;24:390–398

59. Lopez L, Bronstein AM, Gresty MA, et al. Torsional nystagmus. Brain 1992;115:1107–1124

60. Daroff RB. See-saw nystagmus. Neurology 1965;15:874–877

61. Rambold H, Helmchen C, Straube A, Buttner U. Seesaw nystagmus associated with involuntary torsional head oscillations. Neurology 1998;51(3):831–837

62. Ranalli PJ, Sharpe JA, Fletcher WA. Palsy of upward and downward saccadic, pursuit, and vestibular movements with a unilateral midbrain lesion: patho-

physiologic correlations. Neurology 1988;38(1):114–122

63. Halmagyi GM, Aw ST, Dehaene I, et al. Jerk-waveform see-saw nystagmus due to unilateral meso-dien-cephalic lesion. Brain 1994;117:789–803

64. Leigh RJ, Robinson DA, Zee DS. A hypothetical explanation for periodic alternating nysatagmus: instability in the optokinetic-vestibular system. Ann N Y Acad Sci 1981;374:619–635

65. deWaele C, Waespe W, Cohen B, Raphan T. Dynamic modification of the vestibulo-ocular reflex by the nodulus and uvula. Science 1985;228:199–202

66. Fetter M, Zee DS. Recovery from unilateral labyrinthectomy in rhesus monkey. J Neurophysiol 1988;59(2):370–393

67. Baloh RW, Konrad HR, Dirks D, Honrubia V. Cerebellar-pontine angle tumors. Results of quantitative vestibulo-ocular testing. Arch Neurol 1976;33(7): 507–512

68. Bondar RL, Sharpe JA, Lewis AJ. Rebound nystagmus in olivocerebellar atrophy: a clinicopathological correlation. Ann Neurol 1984;15:474–477

69. Eizenman M, Sharpe JA. End point, gaze-evoked, and rebound nystagmus. In: Sharpe JA, Barber HO, eds. The Vestibulo-ocular Reflex and Vertigo. New York: Raven Press, 1993:257–267

70. Averbuch-Heller L, Zivotofsky AZ, Das VE, et al. Investigations of the pathogenesis of acquired pendular nystagmus. Brain 1995;118:369–378

71. Das VE, Oruganti P, Kramer PD, Leigh RJ. Experimental tests of a neural-network model for ocular oscillations. Soc Neurosci Abstr 1999;25:1922

72. Cannon SC, Robinson DA. Loss of the neural integrator of the oculomotor system from brainstem lesions in the monkey. J Neurophysiol 1987;57:1383–1409

73. Arnold DB, Robinson DA. The oculomotor integrator: testing of a neural network model. Exp Brain Res 1997;113:57–74

74. Fukushima K, Kaneko CR. Vestibular integrators in the oculomotor system. Neurosci Res 1995;22(3): 249–258

75. Lopez LI, Bronstein AM, Gresty MA, et al. Clinical and MRI correlates in 27 patients with acquired pendular nystagmus. Brain 1996;119:465–472

76. Sperking MR, Herrmann C. Syndrome of palatal myoclonus and progressive ataxia: two cases with magnetic resonance imaging. Neurology 1985;35: 1212–1214

77. Sharpe JA. Neural control of ocular motor systems. In: Miller NR, Newman NJ, eds. Walsh and Hoyt's Clinical Neuro-ophthalmology. Vol 1. Baltimore: Lippincott, Williams and Wilkins, 1998:1101–1167

78. Ashe J, Hain TC, Zee DC, Schatz NJ Microsaccadic flutter. Brain 1991;114:461–472

79. Horn AKE, Büttner-Ennever JA, Wahle P, Reichenberger I. Neurotransmitter profile of saccadic omnipause neurons in nucleus raphe interpositus. J Neurosci 1994;14:2032–2046

80. Horn AKE, Büttner-Ennever JA, Suzuki Y, Henn V. Histological identification of premotor neurons for horizontal saccades in monkey and man by parvalbumin immunostaining. J Comp Neurol 1995;359:350–363

81. Spencer RF, Wang SF. Immunohistochemical localization of neurotransmitters utilized by neurons in the rostral interstitial nucleus of the medial longitudinal fasciculus (riMLF) that project to the oculomotor and trochlear nuclei in the cat. J Comp Neurol 1996;366(1): 134–148

82. Shallo-Hoffmann J, Petersen J, Muhlendyck H. How

normal are "normal" square wave jerks? Invest Ophthalmol Vis Sci 1989;30(5):1009–1011

83. Shallo-Hoffmann J, Sendler B, Muhlendyck H. Normal square wave jerks in different age groups. Invest Ophthalmol Vis Sci 1990;31:1649–1652

84. Hikosaka O, Wurtz RH. Modification of saccadic eye movements by GABA related substances. I. Effect of muscimol in monkey substantia nigra pars reticulata. J Neurophysiol 1985;53:292–308

85. Tychsen L, Sitaram N. Catecholamine depletion produces irrepressible saccadic eye movements in normal humans. Ann Neurol 1989;25:444–449

86. Zee DS, Robinson DA. A hypothetical explanation of saccadic oscillations. Ann Neurol 1979;5:405–414

87. Blaine PG, Nightingale S, Stoddart JC. Strychnine poisoning: abnormal eye movements. J Toxicol Clin Toxicol 1982;19:215–217

88. Ridley A, Kennard C, Scholtz CL, et al. Omnipause neurons in two cases of opsoclonus associated with oat cell carcinoma of the lung. Brain 1987;110:1699–1709

89. Wong AMF, Shannon P, Sharpe JA. Opsoclonus in three dimensions: an oculographic and neuropathological correlation. Neuroophthalmology 2000;23:196

90. Kaneko CRS. Effect of ibotenic acid lesions of the omnipause neurons on saccadic eye movements in Rhesus Macaques. J Neurophysiol 1996;75:2229–2242

91. Wong AMF, Musallam S, Tomlinson RD, et al. Opsoclonus in three dimensions: an oculographic and neuropathologic correlation. In: Sharpe JA, ed. Neuro-ophthalmology at the Beginning of the New Millennium. Englewood, New Jersey: Medimond Publishing, 2000:87–92

92. Shizuka M, Watanabe M, Ikeda Y, et al. Spinocerebellar ataxia type 6: CAG trinucleotide expansion, clinical characteristics and sperm analysis. Eur J Neurol 1998;5(4):381–387

93. Baloh RW, Yue Q, Furman JM, Nelson SF. Familial episodic ataxia: clinical heterogeneity in four families linked to chromosome 19p. Ann Neurol 1997;41:8–16

94. Burk K, Fetter M, Abele M, et al. Autosomal dominant cerebellar ataxia type I: oculomotor abnormalities in families with SCA1, SCA2, and SCA3. J Neurol 1999;246:789–797

95. Sonoda S, Isashiki Y, Tabata Y, et al. A novel PAX6 gene mutation (P118R) in a family with congenital nystagmus associated with a variant form of aniridia. Graefes Arch Clin Exp Ophthalmol 2000;238(7): 552–558

96. Boycott KM, Pearce WG, Bech-Hansen NT. Clinical variability among patients with incomplete X-linked congenital stationary night blindness and a founder mutation in CACNA1F. Can J Ophthalmol 2000;35(4): 204–213

97. Daroff RB. Ocular oscillations. Ann Otol Rhinol Laryngol 1977;86:102–107

98. Dell'Osso LF. Congenital and other types of infantile nystagmus: recording, diagnosis, and treatment. In: Sharpe JA, Barber HO, eds. The Vestibulo-ocular Reflex and Vertigo. New York: Raven Press, 1993: 229–247

99. Barton JS, Sharpe JA. Oscillopsia and horizontal nystagmus with accelerating slow phases following lumbar puncture in the Arnold-Chiari malformation. Ann Neurol 1993;33:418–421

100. Halmagyi GM, Gresty MA, Leech J. Reversed optokinetic nystagmus (OKN): mechanism and clinical significance. Ann Neurol 1980;7:429–435

101. Sharpe JA, Hoyt WF, Rosenberg MA. Convergence

evoked nystagmus. Congenital and acquired forms. Arch Neurol 1975;32:191–194

102. Averbuch-Heller L, Zivotofsky AZ, Remler BF, et al. Convergent-divergent pendular nystagmus: possible role of the vergence system. Neurology 1995;45: 509–515

103. Schwartz MA, Selhorst JB, Ochs AL, et al. Oculomasticatory myorhythmia: a unique movement disorder occurring in Whipple's Disease. Ann Neurol 1986; 20:677–683

104. Ochs AL, Stark L, Hoyt WF, D'Amicio D. Opposed adducting saccades in convergence-retraction nystagmus. A patient with sylvian acqueduct syndrome. Brian 1979;102:497–508

105. Sharpe JA, Fletcher WA. Disorders of visual fixation. In: Smith JL, ed. Neuro-ophthalmology Now. New York: Field, Rich and Associates, 1986:267–284

106. Eizenman M, Cheng P, Sharpe JA, Frecker RC. End point nystagmus and ocular drift: an experimental and theoretical study. Vision Res 1990;30:863–877

107. Abel LA, Parker L, Daroff RB, Dell'Osso LF. End-point nystagmus. Invest Ophthalmol Vis Sci 1978;17:539–544

108. Sharpe JA, Cheng P, Eizenman M. End-point nystagmus in the vertical plane. In: Fuchs AF, Brandt T, Buettner U, Zee D, eds. Contemporary Ocular Motor and Vestibular Research: A Tribute to David A. Robinson. New York: Thieme Medical Publishers, 1994:348–350

109. Halmagyi GM, Rudge P, Gresty MA, et al. Treatment of periodic alternating nystagmus. Ann Neurol 1980;18:609–611

110. Cohen B, Helwig D, Raphan T. Baclofen and velocity storage: a model of the effects of the drug on the vestibulo-ocular reflex in the rhesus monkey. J Neurophysiol 1987;393:703–725

111. Averbuch-Heller L, Tusa RJ, Fuhry L, et al. A double-blind controlled study of gabapentin and baclofen as treatment for acquired nystagmus. Ann Neurol 1997;41(6):818–825

112. Starck M, Albrecht H, Pollmann W, et al. Drug therapy for acquired pendular nystagmus in multiple sclerosis. J Neurol 1997;244(1):9–16

113. Herishanu Y, Louzoun Z. Trihexyphenidyl treatment of vertical pendular nystagmus. Neurology 1986;36: 82–84

114. Leigh RJ, Burnstine TH, Ruff RL, Kasmer RJ. Effect of anticholinergic agents upon acquired nystagmus: a double-blind study of trihexyphenidyl and tridihexethyl chloride. Neurology 1991;41:1737–1741

115. Barton JJS, Huaman AG, Sharpe JA. Muscarinic antagonists in the treatment of acquired pendular and downbeat nystagmus. Ann Neurol 1994;35:319–325

116. Dieterich M, Staube A, Brandt T, et al. The effects of baclofen and cholinergic drugs on upbeat and downbeat nystagmus. J Neurol Neurosurg Psychiatry 1991; 54:627–632

117. Lefkowitz D, Harpold G. Treatment of ocular myoclonus with valproic acid. Ann Neurol 1985;17: 103–104

118. Currie JN, Matuso V. The use of clonazepam in the treatment of nystagmus-induced oscillopsia. Ophthalmology 1986;93:924–932

119. Traccis S, Rosati G, Monaco MF, et al. Successful treatment of acquired pendular elliptical nystagmus in multiple sclerosis with isoniazid and base-out prisms. Neurology 1990;40:492–494

120. Chrousos GA, Cowdry R, Schuelein M, et al. Two cases of downbeat nystagmus and oscillopsia associated with carbamazepine. Am J Ophthalmol 1987; 103(2):221–224

121. Leigh RJ, Averbuch-Heller L, Tomsak RL, et al. Treatment of abnormal eye movements that impair vision: strategies based on current concepts of physiology and pharmacology. Ann Neurol 1994;36(2):129–141

122. Williams A, Goodenberger D, Calne D, Calne DB. Palatal myoclonus following herpes zoster ameliorated by 5-hydroxytryptophan and carbidopa. Neurology 1978;28:358–359

123. Brandt T, Strupp M. Episodic ataxia type 1 and 2 (familial periodic ataxia/vertigo). Audiol Neurootol 1997;2(6):373–383

124. Brazis PW, Miller NR, Henderer JD, Lee AG. The natural history and results of treatment of superior oblique myokymia. Arch Ophthalmol 1994;112(8): 1063–1067

125. Kosmorsky GS, Ellis BD, Fogt N, Leigh RJ. The treatment of superior oblique myokymia utilizing the Harada–Ito procedure. J Neuroophthalmol 1995;15(3): 142–146

126. Samii M, Rosahl SK, Carvalho GA, Krzizok T. Microvascular decompression for superior oblique myokymia: first experience. Case report. J Neurosurg 1998;89(6):1020–1024

127. Ezra E, Spalton D, Sanders MD, et al. Ocular neuromyotonia. Br J Ophthalmol 1996;80(4):350–355

128. Yee RD, Purvin VA. Ocular neuromyotonia: three case reports with eye movement recordings. J Neuroophthalmol 1998;18(1):1–8

129. Barton JJ, Cox TA, Digre KB. Acquired convergence-evoked pendular nystagmus in multiple sclerosis. J Neuroophthalmol 1999;19(1):34–38

130. Dickinson CM. The elucidation and use of the effect of near fixation in congenital nystagmus. Ophthalmic Physiol Opt 1986;6(3):303–311

131. Dell'Osso LF, van der Steen J, Steinman RM, Collewijn H. Foveation dynamics in congenital nystagmus. I: Fixation. Doc Ophthalmol 1992;79(1):1–23

132. Sheth NV, Dell'Osso LF, Leigh RJ, et al. The effects of afferent stimulation on congenital nystagmus foveation periods. Vision Res 1995;35(16):2371–2382

133. Dell'Osso LF, Traccis S, Erzurum SI. Contact lenses and congenital nystagmus. Clin Vision Sci 1988;3: 229–232

134. Mezawa M, Ishikawa S, Ukai K. Changes in waveform of congenital nystagmus associated with biofeedback treatment. Br J Ophthalmol 1990;74(8):472–476

135. Evans BJ, Evans BV, Jordahl-Moroz J, Nabee M. Randomised double-masked placebo-controlled trial of a treatment for congenital nystagmus. Vision Res 1998;38(14):2193–2202

136. Yee RD, Baloh RW, Honrubia V. Effect of baclofen on congenital nystagmus. In: Lennerstrand G, Zee DS, Keller EL, eds. Functional Basis of Ocular Motility Disorders. Oxford: Pergamon Press, 1982:151–157

137. Rushton D, Cox N. A new optical treatment for oscillopsia. J Neurol Neurosurg Psychiatry 1987;50:411–415

138. Leigh RJ, Rushton DN, Thurston SE, et al. Effects of retinal image stabilization in acquired nystagmus due to neurologic disease. Neurology 1988;38:122–127

139. Stahl JS, Lehmkuhle M, Wu K, et al. Prospects for treating acquired pendular nystagmus with servo-controlled optics. Invest Ophthalmol Vis Sci 2000; 41(5):1084–1090

140. Leigh RJ, Tomsac RL, Grant MP, et al. Effectiveness of botulinum toxin administered to abolish acquired nystagmus. Ann Neurol 1992;32:633–642

141. Tomsak RL, Remler BF, Averbuch-Heller L, et al. Unsatisfactory treatment of acquired nystagmus with

retrobulbar injection of botulinum toxin. Am J Ophthalmol 1995;119:489–496

142. Repka MX, Savino PJ, Reinecke RD. Treatment of acquired nystagmus with botulinum neurotoxin A. Arch Ophthalmol 1994;112(10):1320–1324

143. Ruben ST, Lee JP, O'Neil D, et al. The use of botulinum toxin for treatment of acquired nystagmus and oscillopsia. Ophthalmology 1994;101(4):783–787

144. Carruthers J. The treatment of congenital nystagmus with Botox. J Pediatr Ophthalmol Strabismus 1995;32(5):306–308

145. Liu C, Gresty M, Lee J. Management of symptomatic latent nystagmus. Eye 1993;7(4):550–553

146. Flynn JT, Dell'Osso LF. The effects of congenital nystagmus surgery. Ophthalmology 1979;86(8):1414–1427

147. Lee IS, Lee JB, Kim HS, et al. Modified Kestenbaum surgery for correction of abnormal head posture in infantile nystagmus: outcome in 63 patients with graded augmentation. Binocul Vis Strabismus Q 2000; 15(1):53–58

148. Sendler S, Shallo-Hoffmann J, Muhlendyck H. Die Artifizielle-Divergenz-Operation beim kongenitalen Nystagmus. [Artificial divergence surgery in congenital nystagmus]. Fortschr Ophthalmol 1990;87(1):85–89

149. Helveston EM, Ellis FD, Plager DA. Large recession of the horizontal recti for treatment of nystagmus. Ophthalmology 1991;98(8):1302–1305

150. von Noorden GK, Sprunger DT. Large rectus muscle recessions for the treatment of congenital nystagmus. Arch Ophthalmol 1991;109(2):221–224

151. Del'Osso LF, Hertle RW, FitzGibbon JE, et al. Preliminary results of performing the tenectomy procedure on adults with congenital nystagmus (CN)—"a gift from man's best friend." In: Sharpe JA, ed. Neuro-ophthalmology at the Beginning of the New Millennium, Englewood, New Jersey: Medimond Publishing, 2000: 101–105

152. Spooner JW, Baloh RW. Arnold–Chiari malformation. Improvement in eye movements after surgical treatment. Brain 1981;104:51–60

153. Pedersen RA, Troost BT, Abel LA, Zorub D. Intermittent downbeat nystagmus and oscillopsia reversed by suboccipital craniectomy. Neurology 1980;30(11): 1239–1242

154. Fukazawa T, Tashiro K, Hamada T, Kase M. Multisystem degeneration: drugs and square wave jerks. Neurology 1986;36(9):1230–1233

155. Shawkat FS, Harris CM, Wilson J, Taylor DS. Eye movements in children with opsoclonus-polymyoclonus. Neuropediatrics 1993;24(4):218–223

156. Russo C, Cohn SL, Petruzzi MJ, de Alarcon PA. Long-term neurologic outcome in children with opsoclonus-myoclonus associated with neuroblastoma: a report from the Pediatric Oncology Group. Med Pediatr Oncol 1997;28(4):284–288

157. Pranzatelli MR, Huang YY, Tate E, et al. Monoaminergic effects of high-dose corticotropin in corticotropin-responsive pediatric opsoclonus-myoclonus. Mov Disord 1998;13(3):522–528

158. Batchelor TT, Platten M, Hochberg FH. Immunoadsorption therapy for paraneoplastic syndromes. J Neurooncol 1998;40(2):131–136

159. Cher LM, Hochberg FH, Teruya J, et al. Therapy for paraneoplastic neurologic syndromes in six patients with protein A column immunoadsorption. Cancer 1995;75(7):1678–1683

160. Sugie H, Sugie Y, Akimoto H, et al. High-dose I.V. human immunoglobulin in a case with infantile opsoclonus polymyoclonia syndrome. Acta Paediatr 1992; 81(4):371–372

161. Veneselli E, Conte M, Biancheri R, et al. Effect of steroid and high-dose immunoglobulin therapy on opsoclonus-myoclonus syndrome occurring in neuroblastoma. Med Pediatr Oncol 1998;30(1):15–17

167 Gaze Disorders

James A Sharpe

Overview

Gaze serves vision by placing the image of an object on the fovea of each retina, and by preventing slippage of images on the retina. Foveal vision achieves optimal acuity. Stability of retinal images is also necessary, since slippage of images on the retina over two to three degrees per second blurs visual acuity.

The brain employs two modes of ocular motor control: fast eye movements (saccades) and smooth slow eye movements. Fast eye movements bring the fovea to a target, and smooth eye movements prevent retinal image slip. Six distinct ocular motor systems are utilized to achieve clear vision: (1) saccadic system; (2) smooth pursuit system; (3) optokinetic system; (4) vestibulo-ocular system; (5) vergence system; and (6) fixation system.[1,2] The first four of these systems generate conjugate movements, called version, but the fifth system generates disjunctive horizontal movements, called vergence. The vergence system achieves binocular vision by generating disjunctive eye movements that align the two foveas on an object as it approaches the head; the vergence system is also responsible for maintaining stereo-acuity.

Gaze refers here to conjugate eye movements and combined eye-head movements, the eye movements being achieved by saccades, smooth pursuit or optokinetic tracking, and the vestibulo-ocular reflex (VOR).[1,2] Central and peripheral disorders of the VOR are presented in other chapters of the Section. This chapter considers saccadic and smooth pursuit disorders of gaze.

Epidemiology

The epidemiology is that of the many diseases that cause gaze disorders.

Etiology

Most diseases of the brain can affect gaze. Infarction, hemorrhage, demyelination, neoplasia, and neurodegenerative diseases are most common.

Pathophysiology and pathogenesis

Brainstem control of horizontal gaze

Recordings from ocular motor neurons in alert monkeys demonstrate that the innervational change during all types of eye movements consists of an eye velocity command (a phasic discharge) and an eye position command (a tonic discharge). During saccades, the phasic discharge consists of a high frequency pulse of innervation that moves the eyes rapidly against orbital viscous forces. When a new eye position is attained, the position command, called a step change in innervation, is required to sustain eye position against elastic restoring forces of the eye muscles. This is the pulse-step change of innervation for saccades.[3] The pulse and step must be appropriately matched to prevent slow drift of the eyes after saccades.

Saccades are generated by excitatory burst neurons in the paramedian pontine reticular formation (PPRF) that project to the ipsilateral abducens nucleus. Lesions of the PPRF burst neurons cause conjugate paralysis of ipsilateral saccades, but leave smooth eye movement intact.[4–6] Between saccades, the burst neurons are kept silent by pause neurons located in the midline of the caudal pons (Figure 167.1).[7] Inhibitory burst neurons, located laterally in the rostral medulla, serve to turn antagonist moto-neurons off, while the excitatory burst neurons drive the agonist moto-neurons.[8] Trigger signals from the cerebral cortex and superior colliculus inhibit the pause neurons, thereby releasing the burst neurons to create the pulse. The step discharge (a position command) is generated from the pulse (a velocity command) by a neural integrator that "integrates" (in the mathematical sense) the pulse. This velocity-to-position neural integrator for horizontal gaze is located in the medial vestibular nucleus (MVN) and the nucleus prepositus hypoglossi, which lies just medial to the vestibular nuclei.[9,10]

Similarly, eye velocity commands for smooth pursuit, vestibular, and optokinetic smooth eye movements are transmitted directly to ocular motor neurons and also integrated by the neural integrator to yield appropriate position commands. The position commands are transmitted to ocular motor neurons from cells of the neural integrator. All eye movement systems utilize the same integrator.[1,9]

The abducens nucleus contains both motor neurons to the lateral rectus muscle, and internuclear neurons that project in the contralateral medial longitudinal fasciculus (MLF) to medial rectus motor neurons (Figure 167.1). These internuclear neurons transmit the saccadic and pursuit signals to the medial rectus, and they may be the most important horizontal VOR pathway to the medial rectus.[11,12] Thus a lesion of the abducens nucleus causes ipsilateral conjugate palsy of saccades, pursuit, and vestibular movements, not isolated sixth nerve (lateral rectus) palsy.

Routes through which pursuit motor commands are transmitted to motor neurons in the brainstem are being identified. The dorsolateral pontine nucleus

Supported by Canadian Institutes of Health Research (CIHR) Grants MT 15362 and ME 5504.

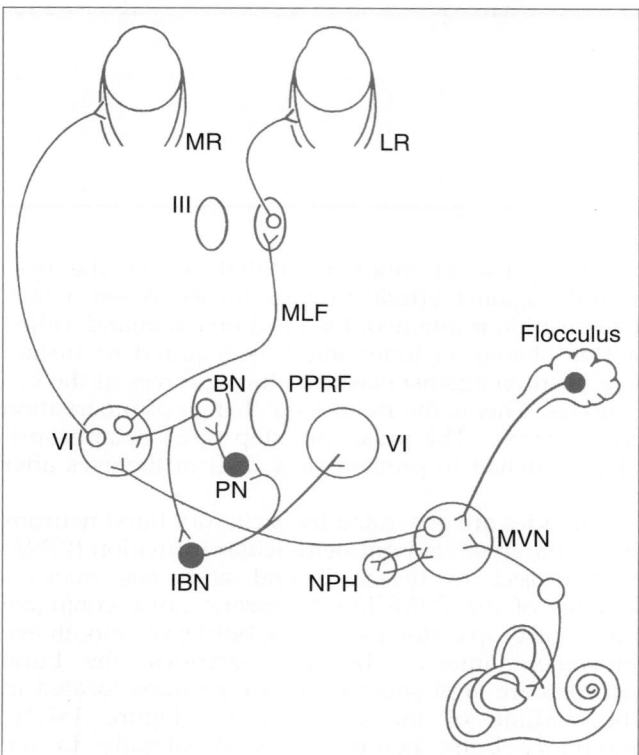

Figure 167.1   Schema of some brainstem projections for horizontal gaze. Saccades are dispatched when a trigger signal turns off pause neurons, which inhibit burst neurons. Reciprocal inhibition of antagonist muscles is achieved by excitation of inhibitory burst neurons. MR, medial rectus; LR, lateral rectus; III, oculomotor nucleus; MLF, medial longitudinal fasciculus; PPRF, paramedian pontine reticular formation; PN, pause neurons; BN, excitatory burst neurons; IBN, inhibitory burst neurons; NPH, nucleus prepositus hypoglossi; MVN, medial vestibular nucleus; VI, abducens nucleus.

From Sharpe JA, Morrow MJ, Newman NJ, Trobe JD, Wall M. Neuro-ophthalmology. Continuum: American Academy of Neurology. Baltimore: Williams and Wilkins, 1995. Reference 106.

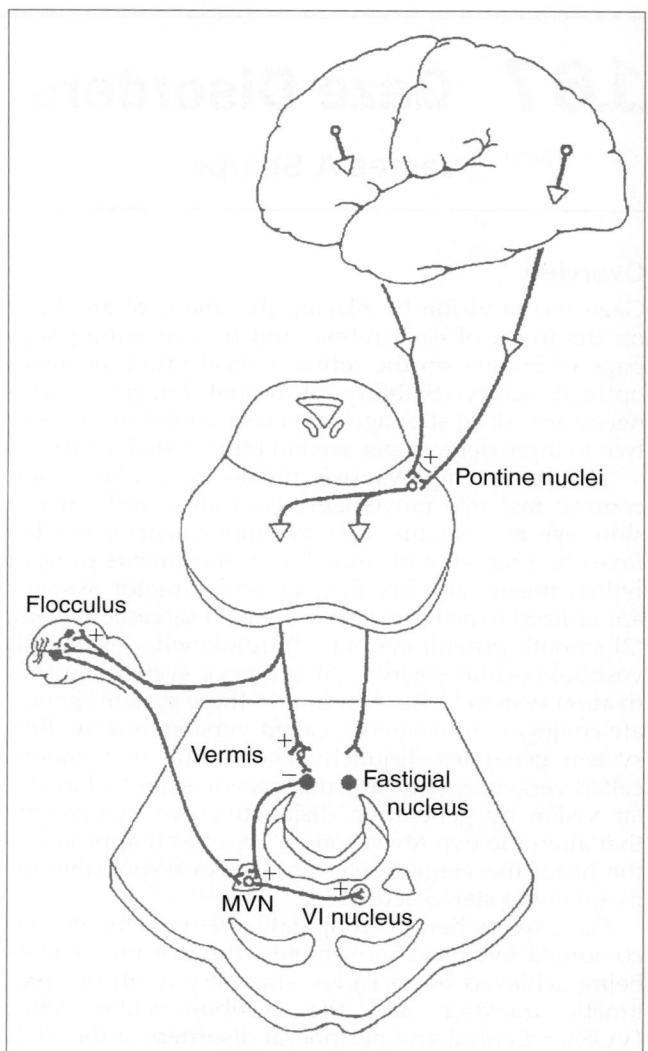

Figure 167.2   Putative brainstem pursuit pathway showing double decussation. The first decussation is from pontine nuclei (mainly the dorsolateral pontine nucleus) to the cerebellar flocculus. Mossy fibers excite basket and stellate cells which inhibit Purkinje cells. Purkinje cells, in turn, inhibit neurons in the medial vestibular nucleus (MVN). Excitatory projections from the MVN to the contralateral abducens nucleus (VI) constitute a second decussation.

Adapted from Johnston JL, Sharpe JA, Morrow MJ. Paresis of contralateral smooth pursuit and normal vestibular smooth eye movements after unilateral brainstem lesions. Ann Neurol 1992;31:495–502. Reference 18.

(DLPN) relays excitatory mossy fiber efferents to the cerebellum.[13] The DLPN projects to the contralateral cerebellar flocculus, paraflocculus, uvula, and the posterior vermis. The fastigial nucleus receives projections from the vermis, and chemical lesions to its caudal part impair contraversive smooth pursuit, requiring catch-up saccades to attain the target.[14–16] Hemicerebellectomy in monkeys causes lower ipsilateral pursuit eye velocities.[17] It is unclear how smooth pursuit neurons in the caudal fastigial nucleus gain access to the smooth pursuit machinery in the brainstem, and whether floccular and fastigial signals merge at common brainstem structures.[14] Direct connections from the vestibular nuclei to ocular motor nuclei complete the principal pursuit circuit in the brainstem (Figure 167.2).

The excitatory circuit from the cerebral cortex to the ipsilateral pontine nuclei, then to the contralateral cerebellar vermis and flocculus, next to the vestibular nucleus, and finally from the vestibular nucleus to activate lateral rectus motor neurons and medial rectus interneurons in the contralateral abducens nucleus (and inhibit them in the ipsilateral abducens nucleus) constitutes a functional-anatomical double decussation of the pathway mediating horizontal smooth pursuit.[2,18] The pontocerebellar projections, through the contralateral middle cerebellar peduncle, form the first decussation, and the effect of MVN neurons on the contralateral abducens nucleus is the second decussation (Figure 167.2).

Vertical gaze

As a general principle, vertical gaze is mediated by bilateral circuits, and vertical gaze palsies signify bilateral or paramedian lesions.

Saccadic commands descending from the cerebral hemispheres and ascending from the caudal PPRF are carried in the brainstem tegmentum to the rostral interstitial nucleus of the MLF (riMLF), located rostral to the third nerve nucleus and within the MLF. Excitatory burst neurons for vertical saccades reside in the riMLF.[19,20] Excitatory burst neurons in the riMLF that generate upward saccades project across the posterior commissure and then to motor neurons in the third nerve nucleus. Excitatory riMLF burst neurons that generate downward saccades project, predominantly ipsilaterally, to the third and fourth nerve nuclei. The riMLF projects to the interstitial nucleus of Cajal, that serves as an element of the velocity-to-position integrator for vertical eye motion.[21] The interstitial nucleus of Cajal is located within the medial longitudinal fasciculus (MLF) just caudal to the riMLF in the rostral midbrain. The cerebellar flocculus also regulates the step of discharge via its connections with the neural integrator. Lesions of the integrator or its cerebellar connections cause gaze paretic nystagmus.[22]

Vertical smooth pursuit channels in the brainstem are distinct from those that control horizontal pursuit. The y group of the vestibular nucleus, which is located at the junction of the brainstem and cerebellum, and the adjacent dentate nucleus have neurons that fire for upward pursuit, and stimulation in this area produces smooth upward eye movements.[23] The MLF and the superior cerebellar peduncle in monkeys carry signals used for vertical pursuit.[24,25] Patients with MLF damage have only mildly impaired vertical smooth pursuit,[26] suggesting that pathways outside of the MLF carry much of the vertical smooth pursuit command signal in humans. Vertical smooth pursuit is selectively impaired by damage in the midbrain. Lesions in the dorsal pretectum that affect the posterior commissure degrade upward pursuit.[27,28] Both upward and downward smooth pursuit are limited by damage in the ventral tegmentum of the midbrain, involving the interstitial nucleus of Cajal and probably commissural projections ventral as well as dorsal to the aqueduct of Sylvius.[29] Neurons of the interstitial nucleus of Cajal modulate their firing during vertical pursuit.[30]

Cerebellar control of gaze

The cerebellum mediates control of gaze through connections to the vestibular nuclei and the reticular formation by way of the deep cerebellar nuclei. The cerebellum participates in major ocular motor functions including: (1) stabilization of images upon the retina during smooth pursuit; (2) regulation of the duration of vestibulo-ocular responses; (3) regulation

of saccadic amplitude and repair of saccadic dysmetria.

The cerebellar flocculus is critical for stabilizing retinal images. Lesions of the flocculus reduce the velocity of ipsiversive smooth pursuit, impair cancellation of the VOR, and make the neural integrator leaky, so that eye position commands are not sustained and the eyes drift centripetally, causing gaze paretic nystagmus.[22] The flocculus is also required for matching the size of the saccade step to the pulse; if the step is too small for the pulse or vice versa, the eyes drift away from their target after each saccade.

The cerebellar vermis and fastigial nucleus and its outflow pathways control saccade accuracy. Saccadic dysmetria indicates a lesion of the vermis or deep nuclei.[31-33] Overshoot dysmetria is apparent when the patient makes refixation saccades between two targets. Multiple-step hypometric saccades consisting of three or more saccadic steps,[34] occur toward the side of lesions involving the cerebellar hemisphere.[27]

Cerebral cortical regions controlling saccades

The cerebral hemispheres generate contraversive saccades. The frontal eye field (FEF) of monkeys is reciprocally connected with posterior cerebral regions that include the posterior parietal cortex and the superior temporal sulcus (Figure 167.3). The FEF projects directly to the ipsilateral superior colliculus and the midbrain tegmentum and the contralateral pontine

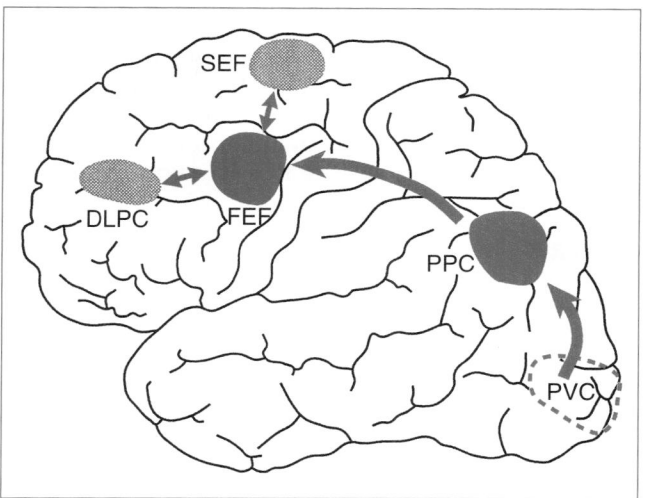

Figure 167.3 Cortical areas involved in generating voluntary and reflexive saccades to visual targets. The parietal eye field in posterior parietal cortex (PPC) governs the accuracy and latency of visually guided saccades. The frontal eye field (FEF), supplementary eye field (SEF) in the mesial cortex, and dorsolateral prefrontal cortex (DLPC) regulate voluntary sequences of saccades, memory guided saccades and suppress unwanted saccades (see text for description). PVC, primary visual cortex (area V1).

From Sharpe JA, Morrow MJ, Newman NJ, Trobe JD, Wall M. Neuro-ophthalmology. Continuum: American Academy of Neurology. Baltimore: Williams and Wilkins, 1995. Reference 106.

tegmentum.[35,36] In monkeys, FEF neurons discharge before saccades to targets but not before spontaneous saccades.[37] Neurons in the supplementary eye field of the supplementary motor area discharge before both visually triggered and spontaneous saccades. Homologs of the simian FEF, supplementary motor area, and parietal eye field areas that participate in generating saccades have been demonstrated in the human brain by functional imaging studies of cerebral blood flow during saccades.[38–40]

The FEF, supplementary eye field, and superior colliculus probably dispatch contraversive saccades by delivering trigger signals to the brainstem circuits that generate the immediate premotor commands for saccades. In monkeys, ablation of either the superior colliculus or the FEF produces only transient ipsilateral deviation of the eyes and reduced frequency of contralateral saccades. Bilateral ablation of the FEF and the superior colliculus produces enduring paralysis of saccades,[41,42] indicating that redundant, parallel pathways subserve the generation of voluntary and visually guided saccades.

The supplementary eye field probably plays a predominant role in directing voluntary sequences of saccades to specific positions in the orbit. The dorsolateral prefrontal cortex may contribute mainly to the advanced planning of environmental scanning using memory of target location. Regional cerebral blood flow in the human FEF increases progressively from tasks requiring fixation, to paradigms that elicit reflexive saccades to visual targets, to paradigms for volitional saccades guided by memory or away from targets. This suggests a hierarchy of FEF functions. The parietal eye field (PEF) in the posterior parietal cortex initiates visually guided reflexive saccades, and it may participate in disengaging fixation.[2] Whereas the FEF is involved mainly in intentional saccade generation to visual targets, the PEF is involved more in reflexive visual exploration.[43,44]

Basal ganglia

The basal ganglia participate in saccadic eye movements. The pars reticulata of the substantia nigra (SNr) and globus pallidus are major outflow pathways of the basal ganglia. In monkeys, neurons of the SNr decrease their tonic discharge rate before saccades to visual, auditory or remembered targets. The FEF projects to the caudate nucleus which in turn projects to the SNr. The SNr projects to the superior colliculus and inhibits it. Saccades are triggered when SNr inhibition of the superior colliculus is removed by suppression of the tonic activity of SNr neurons.[45–50]

Cerebral control of smooth pursuit

The afferent limb of the smooth pursuit system comprises the pathway from retina to lateral geniculate nucleus, to striate cortex and then to extrastriate visual areas. Striate visual cortex relays signals to the ipsilateral parietal and temporal lobe. Discrete cortical areas have retinotopic maps of the visual fields. These are organized into two parallel pathways, one concerned with analyzing motion, the other with processing form and color. In the monkey, the magnocellular motion detection pathway includes the middle temporal visual area (MT) of the superior temporal sulcus. From MT, signals are related to adjacent areas of the superior temporal sulcus and parietal cortex, including the middle superior temporal visual area (MST) and inferior parietal lobe (IPL) or area 7a. Both MST and IPL project to the FEFs. MT, MST, and IPL contain neurons that respond to image motion and are direction selective.[51–53]

Lesions of the simian striate visual cortex or area MT cause retinotopic pursuit defects that are related to target position on the retina. Pursuit eye movements achieve normal speed and accuracy unless the target falls upon the "blind" region of the visual field represented by the damaged area. In contrast, lesions of area MST cause directional pursuit defects. Ipsiversive pursuit speed is reduced, regardless of target location on the retina.[53] Unilateral lesions of the FEF cause ipsiversive pursuit defects whereas bilateral lesions cause symmetric disturbances.[54,55] Combined lesions of the FEF and MT (area V5) cause greater impairment than either alone, implying redundancy of their function.

Lesions of MT also impair the accuracy of saccades toward moving targets in areas of the contralateral visual field that correspond to receptive fields of MT neurons. MT contributes to the analysis of visual motion.[53,56] Unidirectional lowering of smooth pursuit speed occurs toward the side of lesions at the junction of areas 19 and 39, the homolog of simian areas MT/MST, and designated as area V5 in monkeys and humans.[57]

Genetics

Familial paralysis of horizontal gaze is an autosomal recessive disorder, with nonprogressive paralysis of saccadic, smooth pursuit and vestibular movements in both directions.[58,59] Scoliosis is an associated feature. Aplasia or degeneration of the abducens nuclei may explain the gaze palsy. Familial paralysis of vertical gaze is a rare autosomal dominant disorder associated with progressive spasticity and dystonia of gait.[60] Congenital ocular motor apraxia can be inherited as an autosomal dominant trait.[61]

Autosomal dominant cerebellar ataxia type I (ADCAI), having the mutations of spinocerebellar ataxia types 1 or 2 (SCA1, SCA2), is associated with slow saccades.[62]

Gaze palsy may be a sign of lipid storage diseases. Vertical gaze paresis, mental deterioration, and presence of foam cells or sea-blue histiocytes in the bone marrow is described as neurovisceral storage disease with vertical supranuclear ophthalmoplegia and as dystonic lipidosis. The clinical manifestations and profiles of lipid analysis are similar to those in patients with Niemann–Pick disease, type C (NPC). Sphingomyelinase activities in leukocytes and skin fibroblasts are normal.[63] Cholesterol accumulates in lysosomes. The recent identification of the NPC gene, *NPC1*, provides a definitive diagnosis and a means of

studying this key component of intracellular cholesterol transport and homeostasis.[64] Paresis of horizontal saccades is a feature of Gaucher's disease (GD).[65]
Saccade initiation failure (ocular motor apraxia, a
supranuclear gaze palsy) is often the earliest neurological sign in GD3. This sign may be difficult to
detect clinically, but is readily revealed as missed
quick-phases during induced optokinetic and vestibular nystagmus.

Progressive supranuclear palsy (PSP) with characteristic defective vertical gaze and extrapyramidal
signs is associated with mutations in the tau gene on
chromosome 17, namely a mutation (S305S) that
results in an increase in the splicing of exon 10, and
the presence of tau containing 4 microtubule-binding
repeats. This is molecular evidence for a functional
mutation that may cause the disease.[66] Several tau
gene sequence variations from normal have been
identified in PSP.[67] Autosomal dominant frontotemporal dementia and parkinsonism linked to chromosome 17, and its subset of families with
pallido-ponto-nigral degeneration, are a group of 4
repeat tauopathies that often have vertical gaze palsy
identical to that in PSP.[68,69]

Clinical features

Brainstem paralysis of horizontal gaze

Unilateral lesions of the caudal pontine tegmentum
cause contraversive deviation of the eyes. Ipsiversive
saccades are paralyzed because the PPRF is
damaged.[6,18,27] Disruption of projections from the
vestibular nuclei to the abducens nucleus, or of the
abducens nucleus itself, also paralyzes ipsiversive
pursuit and the VOR. The eyes cannot be brought
beyond the midline toward the side of damage. Contraversive jerk nystagmus is sometimes evident.[18,70]

Internuclear ophthalmoplegia (INO) consists of
impaired adduction on the side of the lesion in the
medial longitudinal fasciculus (MLF) and abducting
jerk nystagmus of the opposite eye.[71] In total INO,
adduction is paralyzed to saccadic, pursuit and
vestibular stimulation. Slow adducting saccades are

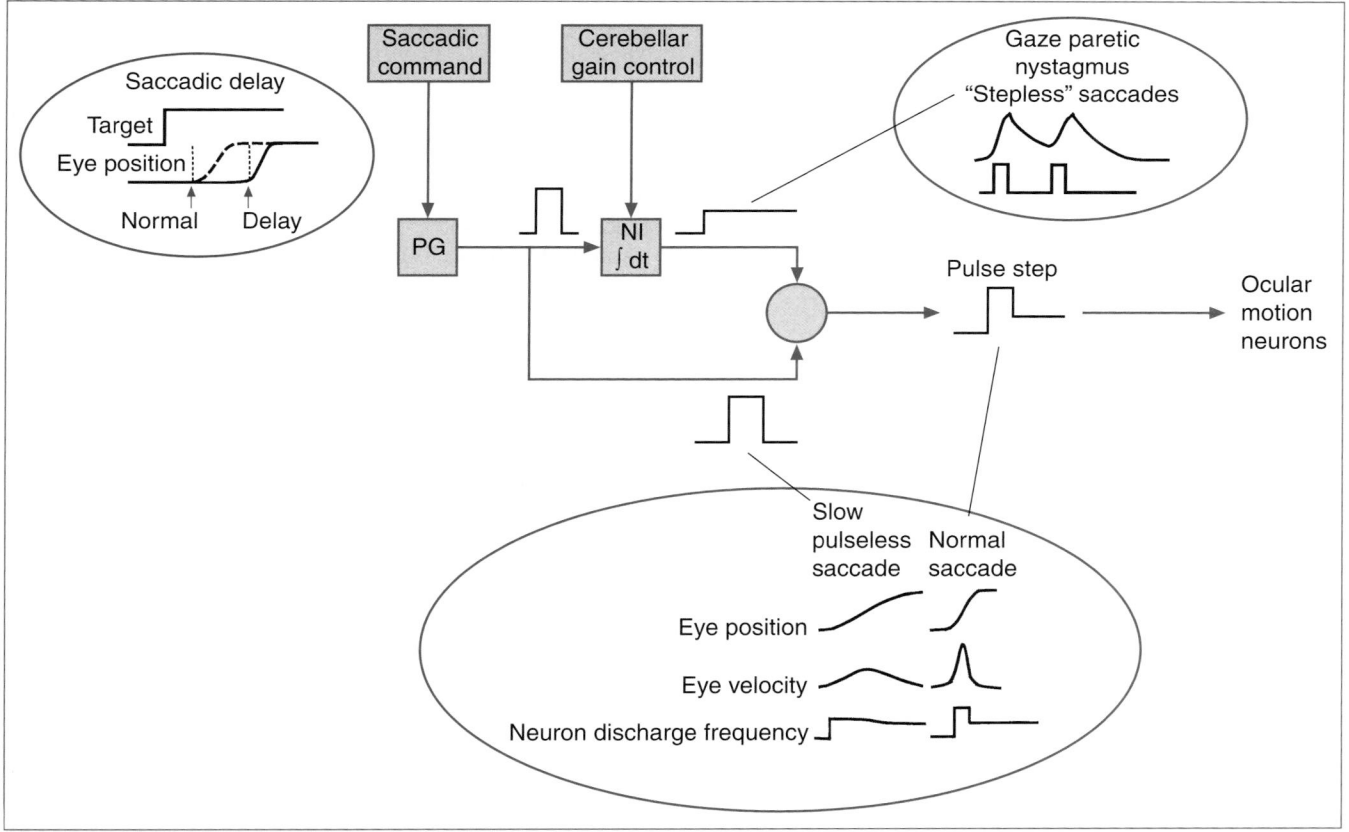

Figure 167.4   Saccadic command from the cerebral hemisphere is delivered to the pulse generator (PG), consisting of burst
neurons in the PPRF for horizontal saccades, and the riMLF for vertical saccades. Saccadic command consists of both a trigger
signal and a retinal error signal. The pulse (an eye velocity command) is transformed to a step (eye position command) by the
neural integrator (NI). The pulse and step are added and delivered to motor neurons. Different parts of the cerebellum
separately control the output of the saccadic command, and the step. Insets depict saccadic delay, gaze evoked nystagmus,
and slow versus normal saccades.
    From Sharpe JA, Morrow MJ, Newman NJ, Trobe JD, Wall M. Neuro-ophthalmology. Continuum: American Academy of
Neurology. Baltimore: Williams and Wilkins, 1995. Reference 106.

the only manifestation of incomplete or chronic lesions. Subtle INO is made obvious by dissociated optokinetic nystagmus (OKN), when targets move in the direction of the paretic eye, that is, toward the side of MLF damage. The intensity of nystagmus is reduced on the side of the INO, when contrasted with active OKN in the fellow eye. Convergence may be lost or spared. Lesions of the MLF disrupt vertical vestibular and pursuit commands that ascend from the vestibular nuclei through the MLF (Figure 167.1). In INO, vertical pursuit and vertical VOR movements are slowed.[26] Vertical saccades are normal. Gaze evoked nystagmus (Figure 167.4) occurs during upward, and sometimes downward, fixation.[26]

The combination of unilateral pontine gaze palsy and INO causes the one and a half syndrome.[72] Damage to the PPRF or abducens nucleus and the MLF on one side is manifested by paralysis of horizontal movements of the ipsilateral eye in both directions and paralysis of adduction in the opposite eye. In the acute phase the opposite eye is exotropic. This "paralytic pontine exotropia" is distinguished from other types of exotropia by slowed adducting saccades in the laterally deviated eye and the horizontal immobility of the eye on the side of pontine damage.[73]

Unilateral lesions of the midbrain reticular formation cause paresis of contraversive saccades and paresis of ipsiversive or bidirectional smooth pursuit. Such lesions are usually associated with involvement of the ipsilateral oculomotor nucleus, or vertical gaze palsy.[74]

Vertical gaze palsy

Upgaze palsy and the pretectal syndrome The pretectal syndrome consists of:

Paralysis of upward saccades
Paralysis of upward saccades and pursuit
Paralysis of upward gaze, VOR and Bell's phenomenon
Retraction and convergent oscillations
Eyelid retraction
Light-near dissociated enlarged pupils.

Paralysis of upward saccades, with variable sparing, or loss, of upward smooth pursuit or the VOR or both, is associated with bursts of binocular adduction and retraction and with light-near dissociation of the pupils.[28,75] Destruction of the posterior commissure is sufficient to cause the pretectal syndrome, but bilateral or unilateral extracommissural pretectal lesions that interrupt its fibers have the same effect. Limitation of upward gaze is also an effect of normal senescence.[76] In the pretectal syndrome, upward saccades are most vulnerable, with the range of vertical pursuit and vestibular smooth eye movements being preserved in many cases.[77] This pretectal syndrome is associated with a variety of ocular signs that encompass the eponyms, sylvian aqueduct and dorsal midbrain syndromes.[78]

Bell's phenomenon refers to the normal upward, often oblique, ocular deviation during forced eyelid closure against manual restraint. When upward sac-

cadic and smooth pursuit eye movements are paralyzed, preservation of Bell's phenomenon indicates a supranuclear cause of ophthalmoplegia. Preservation of Bell's phenomenon often correlates with preservation of upward doll's eye reflexes during oculocephalic stimulation of the VOR, but these two reflex stimuli for ocular elevation may be dissociated by supranuclear brainstem disease. The upward VOR may be absent with preservation of Bell's phenomenon and vice versa.[79]

Retraction and convergent oscillations are evoked by attempted upward saccades. Anomalous co-innervation of extraocular muscles causes the retraction. Nearly synchronous pulses of innervation in horizontally and vertically acting ocular muscles cause saccade-like bursts of retraction.[80] Such lack of reciprocal inhibition of antagonist motor neurons is also a feature of horizontal gaze palsies. Although convergent movements are often prominent in retraction saccades and the phenomenon is sometimes called nystagmus, it is not an oscillation of the smooth eye movements and thus not genuine nystagmus. Downward moving optokinetic targets provide a convenient means of demonstrating the disorder; each upward fast phase of OKN elicits a burst of retraction and often convergence.[27]

Downgaze palsy and ventral lesions Lesions in the midbrain tegmentum, rostral to the third nerve nucleus and ventral to the aqueduct of Sylvius, cause selective paralysis of downward saccades by disrupting projections from the riMLF to the oculomotor and trochlear nuclei.[81,82] The responsible lesions are usually bilateral, but unilateral paramedian lesions can also paralyze downward gaze or both upward and downward gaze;[29,81] the pupils are usually of medium size and poorly reactive to both light and accommodation. We term these distinct ocular motor defects the ventral midbrain syndrome.[79]

In both the dorsal and ventral syndromes, the vertical VOR and smooth pursuit may appear to be spared. However, reduced gain, limited amplitude and abnormal phase lead of the vertical VOR are reported with a unilateral ventral infarct involving the interstitial nucleus of Cajal and rostral interstitial nucleus of the medial longitudinal fasciculus, but sparing the ocular motor nuclei.[29] This indicates that supranuclear lesions of the rostral midbrain can impair the vertical VOR[29,77] and contradicts the prevailing concept that supranuclear lesions spare the vertical VOR. This misconception results from the usual method of testing the vertical VOR at the bedside—the oculocephalic maneuver, in which the patient's head is passively flexed and extended while fixating on a target in a well-lit room. As noted above, the eye movements that result are generated not only by the vertical VOR, but also by visual enhancement of this reflex by smooth pursuit and optokinetic smooth eye movements. The visually enhanced VOR (VVOR) can operate when the VOR is severely reduced or even absent. Thus, although the examiner may judge the amplitude of oculocephalic eye movements to be normal, the gain and phase of the vertical VOR may be abnormal but not detected at the bedside.[77]

Tonic vertical deviation   Sustained downward deviation of the eyes can be a manifestation of caudal thalamic hemorrhage, presumably with compression of the rostral midbrain. Metabolic encephalopathy, usually hepatic, can cause downward deviation and upgaze palsy. Aqueductal distension in patients with hydrocephalus has the same effect.[27,75] Otherwise healthy infants may have unexplained downward deviation during the first few weeks of life.

Sustained upward deviation of the eyes is an infrequent feature of severe hypoxic encephalopathy. The pretectum and midbrain are structurally intact and the deviation has been attributed to damage to cerebellar pathways.[83] Paroxysms of upward deviation are a feature of epileptic seizures and oculogyric crises.[84] Postencephalitic parkinsonism, phenothiazine drugs and carbamazepine intoxication cause oculogyric crises.

Cerebral gaze paralysis   Massive acute cerebral lesions of the frontal, or parieto-occipital regions cause transient ipsiversive deviation of the eyes and inability to trigger contraversive voluntary or visually guided saccades. Quick phases of caloric nystagmus and spontaneous random saccades can be initiated up to the midline of craniotopic space, but not beyond.[85,86] Within hours or days, full bidirectional saccades are evident. Sparing of horizontal VOR motion to oculocephalic stimulation distinguishes this acute hemispheric gaze palsy from that caused by unilateral damage to caudal pontine tegmentum.[6,27] When ipsiversive deviation persists for many days, previous damage to the opposite frontal lobe may be responsible.[87] Rehabilitation of contraversive saccades is nearly complete, but after chronic hemidecortication in man, saccades are delayed and slightly slowed in both horizontal directions and contraversive saccades are hypometric.[85,88]

Ipsilateral gaze deviation is reported to be more prevalent after lesions of the nondominant hemisphere, but conflicting evidence indicates that dominant frontal lobe lesions cause ipsiversive deviation as often as nondominant ones. Occasionally, hemorrhage in one cerebral hemisphere causes transient contralateral deviation of the eyes.[89,90] Caudal thalamic hemorrhage is usually responsible, but frontal or frontoparietal hemorrhage can also cause this wrong side gaze deviation.[91] The mechanism is unknown. The hemorrhage is above the midbrain decussation of pathways that mediate horizontal saccades.

Classification

An operational classification of the direction of horizontal gaze paresis caused by lesions at different levels of the neuraxis is provided in Table 167.1. Some exceptions are noted in the text.

Diagnostic criteria

The gaze deviations outlined above are manifestations of acute and often massive brain damage. Less severe disorders of gaze are apparent with subacute or chronic lesions and often signify quite discrete involvement of eye movement pathways. Their diagnosis requires systematic examination of saccades and smooth eye movements.

Saccadic paresis

Paresis of saccades may be evident as delay in dispatching them, undershooting the target (hypometria), or slowness of their trajectories.

Saccadic delay   Saccades are dispatched about 200 ms after a visual stimulus. Saccadic delay in all directions can be an enduring sign of cerebral cortical and basal ganglia involvement, as in Alzheimer's disease and Parkinson's disease.[92–94] Reflexive saccades to visual targets are delayed mainly contralateral to parietal lobe lesions.[95] Prolonged saccadic latency is an obvious and fundamental defect in congenital ocular motor apraxia.[96] Patients use head motion to dispatch coincident saccades. Combined motor programs for triggering eye and head movement serve to trigger saccades in ocular motor apraxia. This congenital disorder improves with maturation into adulthood. CT scanning is mandatory in ocular motor apraxia, since structural lesions of the posterior fossa or cerebral hemispheres may mimic congenital ocular motor apraxia. Acquired ocular motor apraxia consists of delayed and hypometric voluntary saccades with relative preservation of reflexive saccades to visual targets and intact nystagmus quick phases.[97,98]

Patients with very delayed onset or very slow saccades also use head motion to shift gaze. Head thrusts

Table 167.1 Horizontal gaze paresis					
System involved	**Frontal lobe**	**Parieto-temporal lobes**	**Rostral midbrain**	**Pons**	**Cerebellum**
Saccades	Contraversive	Contraversive	Contraversive	Ipsiversive	Contraversive, acute
Smooth pursuit	Ipsiversive or bidirectional*	Ipsiversive*	Ipsiversive or bidirectional	Ipsiversive	Ipsiversive
Vestibulo-ocular reflex	Spared	Spared	Usually spared	Ipsiversive	Spared
*See Table 167.2 for additional types of pursuit paresis.					

are used to initiate saccades. If saccades are extremely slow, head movements are used to activate vestibular eye movements away from the intended gaze direction. Nystagmus fast phases in the direction of head motion aid refixation.[96] If no fast phase occurs, the head thrusts overshoot the target until the eyes achieve fixation; the head then rotates back with fixation maintained until the eyes reach mid-position in the orbit.

Hypometric saccades Saccadic refixations usually consist of one or two steps. Refixations of three or more dysmetric saccadic steps are called multiple step hypometric saccades.[34] They occur in some normal subjects after fatigue or in advanced age.[76,99] They are conclusively abnormal if they predominate in one direction. Hypometric saccades occur contralateral to cerebral hemispheric damage and ipsilateral to cerebellar cortical lesions.[27,31,100,101] Omnidirectional hypometric saccades accompany bilateral cerebral, basal ganglia or cerebellar disease.[92,93]

   Lateropulsion of saccades is a form of dysmetria that occurs after lateral medullary infarcts, a phenomenon we call ipsipulsion in order to specify the direction of saccadic dysmetria relative to the side of the lesion.[101] It consists of a triad of: (1) overshoot of ipsiversive saccades, (2) undershoot of contraversive saccades, and (3) ipsiversive deviation of vertical saccades.[101–106] Lesions of the superior cerebellar peduncle and uncinate fasciculus (Figure 167.5) cause contrapulsion, which is the triad of overshoot of contraversive saccades, undershoot of ipsiversive saccades, and contraversive deviation of vertical saccades.[101] Ipsipulsion may arise from damage to projections from the inferior olivary nucleus through the inferior cerebellar peduncle to the dorsal vermis (Figure 167.5); this in turn inhibits the ipsilateral fastigial nucleus, which modulates the accuracy of saccades. Damage to the fastigial nucleus itself might cause ipsipulsion,[107] but the typical cause is lateral medullary infarction.[102,106,108] Contrapulsion of saccades can be explained by disruption of the uncinate fasciculus as it passes around the superior cerebellar peduncle, conveying projections from the contralateral fastigial nucleus to the PPRF.[2,101]

Slow saccades Damage to excitatory burst neurons or their projections to the ocular motor nuclei, to inhibitory burst neurons, or to pause neurons (Figure 167.1) causes slow saccades. Lesions of the PPRF severely reduce the peak velocities of ipsiversive saccades.[4,5,18,73,109] Slow saccades are a feature of focal

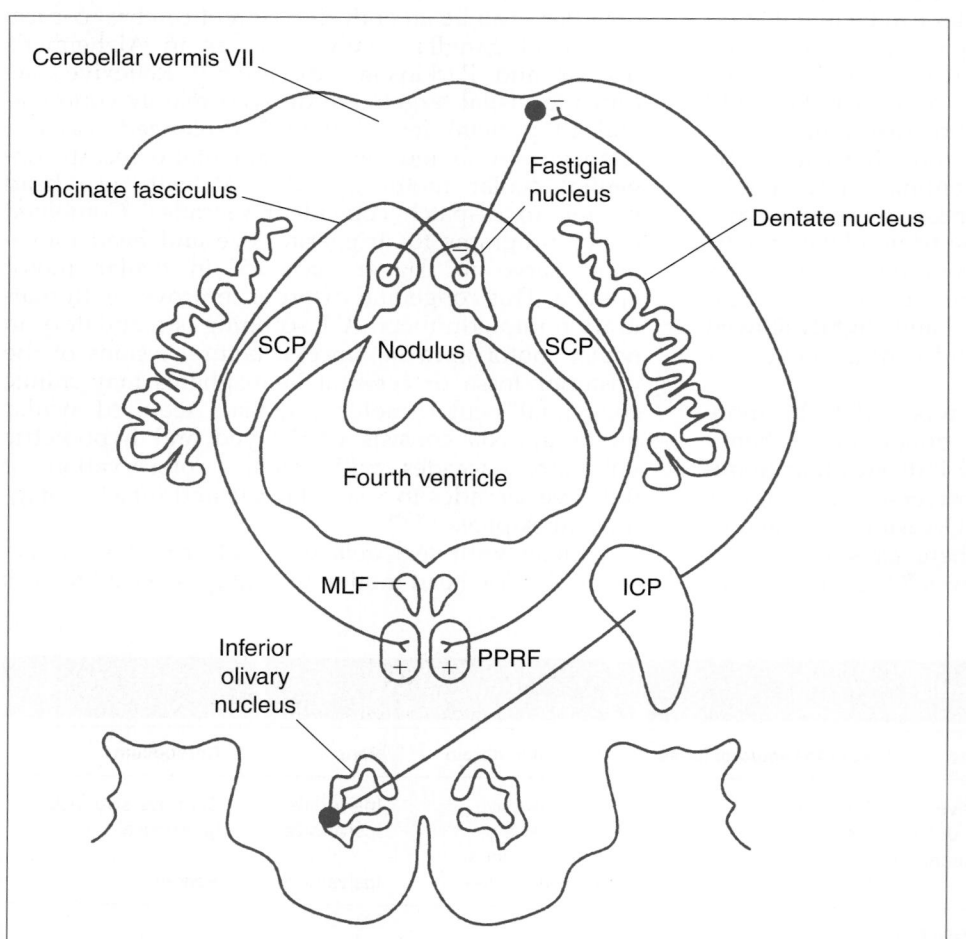

Figure 167.5 Schema of projections from the inferior olivary nucleus through the inferior cerebellar peduncle (ICP) to lobule VII of cerebellar cortex where Purkinje cells inhibit the fastigial nucleus (FN). The FN excites the contralateral paramedian pontine reticular formation (PPRF). A lesion in the left ICP disinhibits Purkinje cells leading to decreased firing of the ipsilateral FN and decreased activation of the contralateral (right) PPRF, leading to ipsipulsion of saccades. A lesion of the left uncinate fasciculus (from the right FN) decreases activity in the ipsilateral (left) PPRF, causing contrapulsion of saccades SCP, superior cerebellar pedurile. MLF, medial longitudinal fasciculus.

   From Sharpe JA, Morrow MJ, Newman NJ, Trobe JD, Wall M. Neuro-ophthalmology. Continuum: American Academy of Neurology. Baltimore: Williams and Wilkins, 1995. Reference 106.

lesions in the pontine tegmentum (Figure 167.4) such as infarcts and tumors and of degenerations such as PSP,[110] Huntington's disease,[111,112] and variants of spinocerebellar degenerations.[62] Multiple sclerosis, lipid storage diseases, or infections (e.g. AIDS, Whipple's disease) involving the tegmentum also cause slow saccades. The fast phases of vestibular and optokinetic nystagmus are also saccadic eye movements; when voluntary and reflex saccades to targets are slowed, they too are slowed.

Slow saccades are also caused by peripheral neuromuscular disease (ocular myopathy and nerve palsies).[113,114] Involvement of cerebral projections to the brainstem by strokes and degenerations in the cerebral hemispheres such as Parkinson's disease and Alzheimer's disease causes mild, but clinically imperceptible slowing.[88,92,93] Mental fatigue, reduced vigilance, and ingestion of sedative drugs cause slight slowing of saccades.

Smooth pursuit paresis

When smooth eye movements fail to match the speed of a slowly moving target, catch-up saccades compensate for the low velocity of smooth tracking. Saccadic pursuit is the sign of paresis in the smooth pursuit system.[2]

Unidirectional pursuit paresis Saccadic pursuit occurs toward the side of posterior parietal and parieto-temporal lesions lobe lesions, particularly involving the angular gyrus and prestriate cortical Brodmann areas 19, 37 and 39 at the temporal-occipital-parietal junction.[57,115] They are the homologs of areas MT and MST (area V5) in the monkey brain. Ipsiversive saccadic pursuit is usually associated with contralateral hemianopia but the smooth eye movement disorder is independent of the visual field defect. It does not accompany hemianopia from pregeniculate, optic radiation, or striate cortical damage.[116] Asymmetric pursuit velocities in patients with hemianopia signify prestriate cortical damage or disruption of commissural connections that transmit retinal information from the normal cerebral hemisphere toward the visually deprived (hemianopic) hemisphere.[88,116]

Optokinetic nystagmus asymmetry Small hand-held striped tapes or drums that are used in the clinic to test optokinetic nystagmus (OKN) activate both smooth pursuit and optokinetic smooth eye movements, but the slow phases of nystagmus stimulated by small targets are generated largely by the pursuit system. The pursuit system is concerned with foveal tracking of small objects, while the optokinetic system is responsible for panretinal tracking of large objects. Genuine optokinetic nystagmus is accompanied by illusionary self-rotation (circularvection) and followed in darkness by OKN-after nystagmus.[2] Nonetheless, small OKN stimuli are useful in the clinical setting since paretic pursuit typically accompanies impaired OKN, and asymmetry of OKN is more readily observed than is asymmetry of pursuit. Like smooth pursuit, OKN evoked by hand-held targets is defective when stimuli move toward the side of cerebral lesions.[117–119] The amplitude and frequency of the nystagmus response is reduced, but the primary deficit is reduction in the slow phase velocity. By convention, nystagmus direction is named by the quick phase direction; therefore, defective slow phases of OKN (and smooth pursuit) toward the side of a posterior parieto-temporal lobe lesion is identified at the bedside as defective OKN beating away from the side of the lesion.

Cerebral hemispheric control of smooth pursuit is not entirely ipsilateral, since unilateral lesions can cause some bidirectional impairment of pursuit.[57,115,120] Cerebral hemidecortication in humans lowers ipsilateral gain, but does not abolish ipsilateral smooth pursuit.[88] Partial sparing of ipsilateral pursuit may be attributed to pathways in the opposite cerebral hemisphere that contribute to contralateral smooth pursuit. The gain (ratio of eye velocity to target velocity) of contralateral low velocity targets may exceed 1.0.[88,115] When smooth eye movement velocity exceeds target velocity, back-up saccades opposite to the direction of smooth eye motion are utilized to refoveate the target. Above normal pursuit gains in patients with large hemispheric lesions can be associated with ipsilaterally beating nystagmus; the slow phase velocities of this pursuit-paretic nystagmus are low (1 to 3 degrees per second). This nystagmus may be explained by imbalanced drive of smooth eye movement tracking systems, either pursuit or optokinetic.

Retinotopic pursuit defects after parieto-temporo-occipital junction lesions can be identified in the laboratory, but not by bedside or clinic examination.[57,121] A target that jumps away from the fovea into one hemifield and then moves at constant speed either toward or away from the fovea is called a step-ramp target. It enables one to examine the initiation of smooth tracking toward a pursuit stimulus from any desired location on the retina close to, or remote from, the fovea. In contrast, pursuit of a continuous to-and-fro target elicits steady-state pursuit (pursuit maintenance) with the fovea at or near the target.

Visual inattention to contralateral space with reference to head position (craniotopic space) does not cause unidirectional pursuit defects. However, unilateral frontal lobe damage space does cause a bidirectional pursuit defect to the contralateral hemirange of eye motion in the orbits.[86] Some patients with acute unilateral parietal or frontal lobe damage do not track targets past the orbital midline into the contralateral craniotopic field of gaze.

Cerebral hemispheric pursuit defects can be grouped into four categories[2,120] (Table 167.2).

Frontal lobe lesions may also cause ipsiversive pursuit paresis,[122] but pursuit paresis after unilateral frontal damage often appears to be symmetrical on clinical examination. Reduced ipsiversive smooth pursuit speed from frontal lobe lesions may result from involvement of the human FEF.[54,123] The ipsiversive pursuit defects caused by damage to either of two distinct cerebral regions, angular gyrus and

Table 167.2   Four classes of cerebral hemispheric pursuit paresis

1. Unidirectional	Saccadic pursuit toward the side of lesions to the posterior parietal and temporal lobe junction, involving V5 or ventral parietal cortex
	Contraversive smooth pursuit velocities may be normal, high, or low (but above the speed of ipsiversive smooth eye movement)
2. Bidirectional	Saccadic pursuit without asymmetry, with bilateral or diffuse cerebral disease
3. Retinotopic	Saccadic pursuit in both horizontal directions in the contralateral visual hemifield, with unilateral lesions of striate cortex, optic radiation or area V5
4. Craniotopic	Loss of pursuit contralateral to the craniotopic midline after acute hemisphere lesions

dorsolateral frontal lobe, imply two parallel routes through which cortical pursuit commands are conveyed to the brainstem. Lesions within the posterior limb of the internal capsule also lower the speed of ipsiversive smooth pursuit.[115,124] Impairment of ipsiversive pursuit accompanies posterior thalamic hemorrhage and may be explained by involvement of the posterior limb of the internal capsule.

Ipsiversive saccadic pursuit also occurs toward the side of lesions that involve the cerebellar flocculus (Figure 167.2). In contrast to unilateral lesions in the cerebral hemisphere, vestibulocerebellum or rostral pons, unilateral tegmental damage in the caudal pons and rostral medulla impairs contraversive smooth pursuit.[18,103,125] Greater paresis of contraversive pursuit after pontomedullary damage may signify disruption of excitatory projections from the vestibular nucleus to the contralateral abducens nucleus, or damage to projections to the cerebellar vermis. The caudal part of the fastigial nucleus drives contraversive pursuit.[14,16] Purkinje cells of the posterior vermis are thought to participate in ipsiversive pursuit by inhibiting the fastigial nucleus.

Omnidirectional pursuit paresis   Saccadic pursuit in all directions results from diffuse cerebral, cerebellar or brainstem disease. For example, multiple sclerosis,[126] Parkinson's disease,[93] Alzheimer's disease,[127] and cerebellar degenerations[128] cause lower smooth pursuit speed, resulting in saccadic tracking of slowly moving targets. Advanced age, sedative drugs, fatigue and inattention also lower smooth pursuit velocities in all directions and thereby cause saccadic tracking.[129–132] When qualified by these influences, horizontal and vertical saccadic pursuit is the most sensitive ocular motor sign of brain dysfunction.

Differential diagnosis

Gaze palsies carry the differential diagnosis of the myriad of disease processes that cause them. Table 167.1 outlines directional defects of gaze that aid localization, which is the first step in neurological diagnosis. Brain imaging is often adequate to determine the cause.

Treatment

Therapy of gaze disorders is aimed at the causative diseases: relevant treatments are presented in other chapters. Below are treatment considerations that apply to selected disorders that disrupt supranuclear control of eye motion.

Gaze deviation and neglect

Long lasting gaze palsies following severe cerebral hemisphere lesions are rare. A report described a patient with a large infarct of the right hemisphere who had a fixed deviated gaze to the right 3 months after onset. Cold caloric vestibular stimulation was used in an attempt to evaluate brainstem integrity. Following three successive injections of cold water into the external auditory canal, the patient regained full voluntary eye movements. The improvement continued for more than 12 months after the last treatment (Grade C, level 5 evidence). A proposed explanation for the improvement was that vestibular input inhibits the tonic phase of antagonistic extraocular muscles while facilitating agonistic extraocular muscles.[133] Natural recovery was more likely responsible.

Ipsiversive gaze deviation keeps the straight-ahead scene on the non-neglected hemifield of vision. Caloric vestibular stimulation may improve hemispatial neglect. Performance on tests of visual neglect and leftward lateral gaze after caloric stimulation in 17 patients with left-sided visual neglect after right hemispheric strokes improved during caloric stimulation—on the left by cold, or on the right by warm water.[134] Improvement seemed to depend on the facilitation of left lateral gaze and on past-pointing to the left. During cold and warm caloric stimulation, patients worked from left to right instead of their usual right to left. Caloric stimulation may be of use in training patients with hemispatial neglect to orient toward the affected field (Grade C, level 5 evidence).[134] Other case studies have supported these results after lesions in either hemisphere,[135,136] but the improvement in neglect is very transient.

Hemianopia

Compensatory ocular motor strategies   Patients with homonymous hemianopia adopt searching staircase patterns of saccades into their blind hemifields. Another strategy is to make large saccades contraversive to their lesions, that overshoot their visual target, while ipsiversive saccades undershoot it.[137,138] This adaptation keeps the target in the seeing hemifield, and then small corrective saccades or drifting smooth eye movements (glissades) bring the fovea to the target. In patients with unidirectional pursuit paresis, the low velocity ipsiversive pursuit also keeps the target on the seeing hemiretina while catch-up saccades attain foveation.[88] This pursuit behavior is not an adaptation to hemianopia, but a consequence of the paresis, since patients with hemianopia from mesial occipital lesions do not develop this pursuit asymmetry.[116,139]

Despite reports of "blindsight" from hemianopic fields, evidence for behaviorally significant saccades toward or pursuit of objects in the blind hemifield is lacking or debated. Patients typically show no evidence of motion perception or saccade or smooth eye movement tracking of targets presented in the hemianopic field.[139] Since it has been shown that monkeys improve their ability to detect and localize light targets in their hemianopic field with practice,[140,141] advocates of the existence of blindsight reasoned that humans might also benefit from specific retraining. Using a forced choice technique, patients practiced discriminating, without looking at, the position of targets flashed in their blind field. Target localization was at first poor, but was restored with practice.[142,143] Feedback on their performance was said to promote the improvement[144] (Grade C, level 5 evidence). Patients who improved felt more confident and less disabled, adding weight to the view that blindsight training may be of therapeutic value. This reasoning is incorrect, since the specific practice technique actually trains patients to make large saccades toward the hemianopic side. Therefore, as a byproduct, the field of search becomes larger, and there is little evidence that the training of blindsight is useful therapy.[145]

Cognitive rehabilitation Compensatory ocular motor training strategies may improve the patients' ability to explore their blind hemifield.[145] Since hemianopic patients use both small amplitude and unsystematic saccades to scan, most training techniques employ two consecutive steps. Patients first practice making large saccades (of amplitude 30 to 40 degrees) into their blind field, to enhance the overshoot, rather than the staircase strategy described above. They are then taught to scan for targets among distracters on projected slides (of eccentricity 30 to 40 degrees) in a systematic way, using a visual search paradigm to improve the spatial organization of their eye movements. The extent of normalization of the eye movements and restoration of the visual search field determines the success of this systematic training. The search field is defined as the perimetrically measured area that a patient can actively scan via eye movements, but without head movements, when searching for a stimulus. The acquisition of compensatory ocular motor strategies appears to depend on systematic stimulation and practice, since the general stimulation from daily activities and even occupational therapy does not achieve the same effect.[145–147]

Hemianopic patients have been trained by instructing them to practice making large saccadic eye move-

ments. Within four to eight sessions their affected visual search field had apparently increased from 10 to 30 degrees[146] (Grade C, level 5 evidence). These results were supported by a study of training hemianopic patients, with and without additional hemineglect, who practiced making large saccades to targets in their blind hemifield, which were presented for a variable duration. They were encouraged to adopt a systematic scanning strategy, involving either horizontal or vertical scanning. Then they practiced searching for targets on projected slides. After about 30 sessions over 6 weeks, the mean search field size increased from 15 to 35 degrees in the hemianopic group without neglect.[147] Those with additional neglect required 25% more training over 2 to 3 months to achieve a similar result. These improvements only occurred during the treatment phase of the study, and at mean follow-up 22 months later there were no further significant changes. Internal controls showed that the magnitude of gain was independent of variables such as etiology, time since lesion, type of field defect, field sparing, and patient age. Patients with the severest defects benefited most from training[147] (Grade C, level 5 evidence).

Head movements during training dramatically increased the number of required treatment sessions.[147] This contradicts the assumption that head movements are helpful to the compensatory mechanisms for hemianopes as has been claimed[148] and supports the view that they are deleterious.[149] A further study[150] quantified the functional benefit of restoring ocular motor functions. After about 25 treatment sessions patients showed a 50% reduction in the time taken to find objects on a table (table test), complementing the subjective improvement in a questionnaire rating their own disability. Following treatment, 91% of this group resumed part-time work[150] (Grade C, level 5 evidence). Similar training, making large saccades and practicing searching for targets, was reported to improve patients' performance to within the normal range after about 26 sessions[151] (Grade C, level 5 evidence). After training, shorter search times were due mainly to fewer fixations and less repetition of scanpaths and of fixations.[151]

Reading has been a focus of rehabilitation attempts since the beginning of this century when First World War veterans with brain damage were trained to overcome reading difficulties.[145,152] Patients with hemianopia have impaired reading proportional to the extent of their field loss. Whereas the fovea possesses the acuity required to discriminate letters and words with sufficient clarity to read, the parafoveal visual field processes forthcoming text in advance of the fovea, in order to guide eye movements while reading. Loss of the parafoveal field retards this perceptual scan and results in a characteristic reading disorder termed "hemianopic dyslexia." Left sided field loss handicaps the return eye movements required to find the beginning of a new line. Right sided hemianopia, however, is more disturbing, since we read from left to right, and is characteristically associated with prolonged fixations, inappropriately small amplitude saccades to the right, and many regressive saccades.[137,153,154]

With training, patients might improve reading eye movements. Left sided hemianopes are encouraged to shift their gaze first to the beginning of the line and the first letter of every word in that line, whereas right sided hemianopes are discouraged to read a word before they have shifted their gaze to the end of it. An electronic computer based reading system was used to train a group of patients[145,155] who were then able to read faster with fewer errors (Grade C, level 5 evidence). Eye movement recordings showed that the improvement was attributable to the emergence of strategies using fewer fixations, larger saccadic jumps, and shorter fixation periods. Right sided hemianopes were more disabled than left, requiring more training sessions, and never reaching the same standard of improvement.[156] An identical protocol had similar success with hemianopic patients after about 3 weeks (mean 13 sessions) of training.[147] At follow-up of 6 months to 2 years the improved reading performance remained stable[147,156] (Grade C, level 5 evidence). Hemianopic patients with additional neglect do not develop adaptive ocular motor reading strategies[157] (Grade C, level 5 evidence).

Visual recovery   The potential for recovery in the defective hemifield corresponding to death of neurons is controversial. Early therapists trained hemianopic patients to read and noticed an enlargement in their visual field.[158] Evidence accumulated that it was possible to shrink the scotoma of monkeys by systematically training them to detect and localize light stimuli.[140,159] In hemianopic humans, light thresholds were repeatedly determined at the visual field border, using a psychophysical method.[160] This was reported to increase the size of the visual field that was confined to the trained area and showed intraocular transfer, indicating its central nature (Grade C, level 5 evidence). A forced choice saccadic technique for training "blindsight" was reported to enlarge the visual field of some patients[161,162] (Grade C, level 5 evidence). In most the field enlargement did not exceed 5 degrees but individual cases showed remarkable recovery. The recovered field included form and color perception and remained stable after the treatment sessions had ended. This result was not attributed to spontaneous recovery because no change occurred during periods without training. Many patients were symptomatically improved[161,162] (Grade C, level 5 evidence). A mechanism was postulated whereby training induces selective attention of the defective field, thereby increasing neuronal activity in areas of the striate cortex surrounding the damaged area.

These results were duplicated in some analogous experiments[147,150] (Grade C, level 5 evidence), but refuted by others[163–165] (Grade C, level 5 evidence). Positive results[162] may have been artifactual.[164] The role of training is disputed. The answer probably lies in patient selection. Visual field enlargement was only found in those cases with partly reversible damage to the striate cortex, as evidenced by the sloping gradient of the border of the field defect and the extent of brain damage on imaging.[162] There has been renewed interest in this challenge, with the publication of encouraging preliminary results[166] (Grade C, level 5 evidence). However, since sharply demarcated field defects are the commonest type it seems unlikely that restoration of vision is a prospect for most patients. Moreover, sloping field margins probably signify partial damage with some viable tissue at the margins, where spontaneous recovery may occur without "training."

Optical management   Hemianopic mirror spectacles consist of a small mirror mounted on the frame of a pair of glasses, at an angle that permits the patient to learn to look into the mirror and see the reflection of objects in the hemianopic field. It is placed beside the left eye in a left hemianope and vice versa, and is suspended so that the patient can adjust it[167] (Grade C, level 5 evidence).

Hemianopic prism spectacles may be used, based on the principle that a prism displaces the images of objects toward its apex. In the case of a left hemianopia, the prism would be placed on the temporal side of the left lens of a pair of spectacles with its base to the left. The prism then displaces the images of objects in the left (hemianopic) field toward its apex and into the seeing nasal field of that eye. Only one lens is fitted with a prism because prisms reduce the acuity of the eye involved. Fifteen to 30 diopter prisms are usually used, increasing the useful field of vision by up to 15 degrees. This is useful for spotting objects. They require careful fitting and a small central area needs to be trimmed to avoid diplopia at fixation.[168] A controlled trial of stick-on Fresnel prisms showed that although the prism treated group performed significantly better on visuospatial tests, no functional improvement in their activities of daily living could be demonstrated[169] (Grade C, level 3 evidence). Furthermore they confuse patients while walking, and require specialized opticians and patients who are highly motivated to practice. Ground-in prisms on a segment of the spectacle may be employed with good patient satisfaction[170,171] (Grade C, level 5 evidence). Opinion is divided as to their efficacy and they have not received general use.[145]

Wernicke's encephalopathy

Wernicke's encephalopathy is an uncommon but treatable cause of vertical or horizontal gaze palsy or INO that must not be overlooked. Early treatment with thiamine results quickly in normal ocular motor function. Evidence based treatment is lacking in the modern epidemiological sense, but is not required. For example, a patient with severe and long-time alcoholism, poor nutrition, and acute Wernicke's disease was reported in whom complete gaze palsy was associated with cerebellar symptoms, disorientation and anterograde amnesia. Lateral gaze palsy disappeared in 3 weeks, but vertical gaze palsy was unchanged after 8 months (Grade C, level 5 evidence).[172] Eye movement disorders rarely persist for more than 1 week in well treated patients. Treatment with thiamine resulted in the disappearance of diplopia in 1 week (pyridoxine and folic acid were also given). It is customary to give parenteral thiamine 50 to 100 mg IV and IM and then 50 mg IM or PO for 3 days, followed by oral daily thiamine supplementation to the diet. Intravenous glucose may precipitate Wernkicke's encephalopathy in patients with low thiamine intake, and thiamine should be administered with glucose in susceptible individuals (Grade C, level 4 evidence).[173]

Multiple sclerosis

Demyelinating events that cause gaze palsy, INO or other ocular motor signs of definite brainstem or cerebellar origin, and are accompanied by two or more clinically silent lesions on MRI, warrant long term treatment with interferon beta-1a, 30 μg IM weekly. This reduces the risk of developing clinically definite multiple sclerosis within 3 years, and the number of new active brain plaques seen on MRI at 18 months (Grade A evidence).[174] Other modes of treatment are discussed in the chapter on multiple sclerosis.

Hydrocephalus and the pretectal syndrome

Obstructive hydrocephalus may be heraded by palsy of upward gaze and other features of the pretectal syndrome. All of these ocular abnormalities often disappear after shunting (Grade C, level 4 evidence).[175] Pretectal dysfunction on the basis of distention of the aqueduct of Sylvius, and perhaps distortion of the posterior commissure from raised intracranial pressure is the probable mechanism. Upward gaze palsy and diplopia from skew deviation may also signify shunt blockage. Resolution of symptoms after shunt revision is usually slow. Transient paradoxical aggravation may occur at the time of shunt revision (Grade C, level 4 evidence).[176]

Ventriculocisternostomy allows resolution of the symptoms and withdrawal of the shunt. Simultaneous supratentorial and infratentorial intracranial pressure recordings show a pressure gradient between the supratentorial and infratentorial compartments, with a higher supratentorial pressure before shunt revision. Inversion of this pressure gradient is observed after shunt revision. Focal midbrain hyperintensity may be evident on T_2-weighted magnetic resonance imaging sequences at the time of shunt malfunction. Third ventriculostomy may be required to equalize cerebrospinal fluid pressure across the tentorium by restoring free communication between the infratentorial and supratentorial compartments, resulting in resolution of the patient's symptoms (Grade C, level 4 evidence).[176]

Parkinson's disease

Diplopia during reading or other near viewing tasks is a frequent complaint of patients with advanced parkinsonism resulting from idiopathic Parkinson's disease[177] or other system degenerations. The diplopia is a consequence of convergence palsy or convergence insufficiency. Treatment with base-out prism glasses may relieve it, but occlusion of one eye with a patch or a frosted spectacle lens is sometimes the only remedy. Dopaminergic drugs are typically not effective, but one case report described diplopia secondary to convergence insufficiency during motor "off" periods, that resolved with onset of motor benefit from levodopa[178] (Grade C, level 4 evidence).

Treatment with dopaminergic drugs can improve saccadic performance in Parkinson's disease. L-dopa therapy is reported to increase the accuracy of hypometric saccades in this disease (Grade C, level 4 evidence).[179,180] However, pergolide does not improve the ability of patients to make saccades away from a target (antisaccades) (Grade C, level 4 evidence).[181] Deep brain stimulation of both subthalamic nuclei is reported to improve the accuracy of memory guided saccades, but has no effect on other voluntary saccades or on visually guided saccades (Grade C, level 4 evidence).[182] Unilateral, stereotactic posteroventral pallidotomy has no beneficial effect on saccades.[183] In contrast, chronic bilateral electrical stimulation of the posteroventral internal pallidum, a recently developed treatment option in advanced Parkinson's disease, shortened the latency of anti-saccades and increased the accuracy of memory-guided saccades in one patient (Grade C, level 5 evidence).[184]

Smooth pursuit speed is reduced in Parkinson's disease, and it is reported to increase after L-dopa treatment (Grade C, level 5 evidence).[185] However, during predictable L-dopa dose-related "off" periods of morning akinesia and wearing off and during "on" periods, smooth pursuit speed remains the same during both on and off phases[186] (Grade C, level 3 evidence). Despite marked fluctuations between parkinsonism and periods of near normal skeletal motion, there are no changes in smooth pursuit gain.[186] Unvarying paresis of smooth pursuit in Parkinson's disease signifies involvement of neural circuits that are distinct from the dopaminergic mechanisms that mediate the on-off phenomenon of skeletal motor control.

Whipple's disease

Whipple's disease is a rare systemic infectious disease that is important to recognize because it is treatable. Central nervous system Whipple's disease may be the cause of gaze palsy, particularly vertical.[187] It has neither been possible to culture the bacillus *Tropheryma whippelii*, nor to infect other individuals with this pathogen. Intestinal biopsy or brain biopsy of lesions seen on imaging can establish the diagnosis and it may also be confirmed by polymerase chain reaction (PCR) technology. Typically, the material for the PCR analysis comes from the duodenum. The diagnosis can also be established in this way on the basis of other tissue, or the cerebrospinal fluid. Treatment should only be carried out with antibiotics which cross into the cerebrospinal fluid (Grade C, level 4 evidence).[188] One favored method of treatment is daily parenteral administration of 1.2 million units of benzylpenicillin (penicillin G) and streptomycin 1 g for a period of 2 weeks. This is followed by treatment with cotrimoxazole (trimethoprim 160 mg and sulfamethoxazole 800 mg) twice daily for 1 to 2 years. The treatment may begin and end with a PCR analysis of cerebrospinal fluid, in order to definitively diagnose infection of the CNS with Whipple's disease and to document the disappearance of the bacillus from the CNS.[189] CNS involvement requires vigorous treatment because there is a high rate of recurrence after apparently successful treatment (Grade C, level 4 evidence).[188]

Gaucher's disease

Gaucher's disease (GD) without primary neurological involvement (GD1) is now treatable with exogenous enzyme replacement therapy, but such treatment does not halt the fatal neurological progression of type 2 (infantile) disease (GD2). However, enzyme replacement therapy in some cases of type 3 disease (GD3) may slow or possibly halt neurological progression (Grade C, level 4 evidence). Distinction between GD1 and GD3 disease is crucial for appropriate treatment. DC electro-oculography or video analysis of optokinetic and vestibular nystagmus can reveal paucity of quick-phases making the eyes "lock up" at the limit of gaze, thus indicating saccadic palsy and confirming GD3 that may not be detected by clinical examination alone.[65]

References

1. Robinson D. The control of eye movements. *In:* Brooks VB, ed. Handbook of Physiology. Bethesda, Md: American Physiology Society, 1981:1275–1320
2. Sharpe J. Neural control of ocular motor systems. *In:* Miller N, Newman NJ, eds. Walsh and Hoyt's Clinical Neuro-ophthalmology. 5th ed. Baltimore: Williams and Wilkins, 1998:1101–1167
3. Robinson DA. The mechanics of human saccadic eye movement. J Physiol (Lond) 1964;174:245–264
4. Henn V, Lang W, Hepp K, Reisine H. Experimental gaze palsies in monkeys and their relation to human pathology. Brain 1984;107:619–636
5. Baloh R, Furman J, Yee RD. Eye movements in patients with absent voluntary horizontal gaze. Ann Neurol 1985;17:283–286
6. Johnston J, Sharpe JA. Sparing of the horizontal vestibulo-ocular reflex with lesions of the paramedian pontine reticular formation. Neurology 1989;39:876
7. Buttner-Ennever JA, Cohen B, Pause M, Fries W. Raphe nucleus of the pons containing omnipause neurons of the oculomotor system in the monkey and its homologue in man. J. Comp. Neurol 1988;267:307–321
8. Scudder C, Fuchs AF, Langer TP. Characteristics and functional identification of saccadic inhibitory burst neurons in the alert monkey. J Neurophysiol 1988;59(5):1430–1454
9. Cannon SC, Robinson DA. Loss of the neural integrator of the oculomotor system from brainstem lesions in monkey. J Neurophysiol 1987;57:1383–1409
10. Anastasio T, Robinson DA. Failure of the oculomotor neurointegrator from a discrete midline lesion between the abducens nuclei in the monkey. Neurosci Lett 1991;127:82–86

11. Skavenski AA, Robinson DA. The role of abducens neurons in the vestibulo-ocular reflex. J Neurophysiol 1973;36:724–738
12. Büttner-Ennever J, Akert K. Medial rectus subgroups of the oculomotor nucleus and their abducens internuclear input in the monkey. J Comp Neurol 1981;197:17–27
13. Suzuki D, May JG, Keller EL, Yee RD. Visual motion response properties of neurons in dorsolateral pontine nucleus of alert monkey. J Neurophysiol 1990;63:37–59
14. Fuchs A, Robinson FR, Straube A. Preliminary observations on the role of the caudal fastigial nucleus in the generation of smooth-pursuit eye movements. *In:* Fuchs AF, Büttner U, Zee D, eds. Contemporary Ocular Motor and Vestibular Research: A Tribute to David A. Robinson. New York: Thieme Medical Publishers, 1994:165–170
15. Straube A, Helmchen C, Robinson F, et al. Saccadic dysmetria is similar in patients with a lateral medullary lesion and in monkeys with a lesion of the deep cerebellar nucleus. J Vestib Res 1994;4:327–333
16. Kurzan R, Straube A, Helmchen C, Buttner U. Muscimol microinjections into the oculomotor part of the fatigial nuclei in alert monkeys. Eur J Neurosci (Suppl) 1991;4:308
17. Westheimer G, Blair SM. Functional organization of primate oculomotor system revealed by cerebellectomy. Exp Brain Res 1974;21:463–472
18. Johnston J, Sharpe JA, Morrow MJ. Paresis of contralateral smooth pursuit and normal vestibular smooth eye movements after unilateral brainstem lesions. Ann Neurol 1992;31:495–502
19. Büttner-Ennever JA, Buttner U, Cohen B, Baumgartner G. Vertical gaze paralysis and the rostral interstitial nucleus of the medial longitudinal fasciculus. Brain 1982;105:125–149
20. Wang S, Spencer RF. Spatial organization of premotor neurons related to vertical upward and downward saccadic eye movements in the rostral interstitial nucleus of the medial longitudinal fasciculus (riMLF) in the cat. J Comp Neurol 1996;366:163–180
21. Fukushima K. The interstitial nucleus of Cajal in the midbrain reticular formation and vertical eye movements. Neurosci Res 1991;10:151–187
22. Zee DS, Yamazaki A, Butler PH, Gucer G. Effects of ablation of flocculus and paraflocculus on eye movements in primates. J Neurophysiol 1981;46:878–899
23. Chubb M, Fuchs AF. Contribution of y-group of vestibular nuclei and dentate nucleus of cerebellum to generation of vertical smooth eye movements. J Neurophysiol 1982;48:75–99
24. Pola J, Robinson DA. Oculomotor signals in medial longitudinal fasciculus of the monkey. J Neurophysiol 1978;41:245–259
25. King WM, Lisberger SG, Fuchs AF. Response of fibers in medial longitudinal fasciculus (MLF) of alert monkeys during horizontal and vertical conjugate eye movements evoked by vestibular or visual stimuli. J Neurophysiol 1976;39:1135–1149
26. Ranalli PJ, Sharpe JA. Vertical vestibulo-ocular reflex, smooth pursuit and eye-head tracking dysfunction in internuclear ophthalmoplegia. Brain 1988;111:1277–1295
27. Daroff R, Hoyt WF. Supranuclear disorders of ocular control systems in man. *In:* Bach-y-Rita P, Collins CC, Hyde J, eds. The Control of Eye Movements. New York: Academic Press, 1971:117–235
28. Baloh R, Furman JM, Yee RD. Dorsal midbrain syn-

drome: clinical and oculographic findings. Neurology 1985;35:54–60

29. Ranalli PJ, Sharpe JA, Fletcher WA. Palsy of upward and downward saccadic, pursuit and vestibular movements with a unilateral midbrain lesion: pathophysiological correlations. Neurology 1988;38:114–122

30. King W, Fuchs AF, Magnin M. Vertical eye movement-related responses of neurons in midbrain near interstitial nucleus of Cajal. J Neurophysiol 1981;46:549–562

31. Ritchie L. Effects of cerebellar lesions on saccadic eye movements. J Neurophysiol 1976;39:1246–1256

32. Fuchs A, Robinson FR, Straube A. Role of the caudal fastigial nucleus in saccade generation. I. Neuronal discharge patterns. J Neurophysiol 1993;70:1723–1740

33. Robinson F, Straube A, Fuchs AF. Role of the caudal fastigial nucleus in saccade generation. II. Effects of Muscimol inactivation. J Neurophysiol 1993;70: 1741–1758

34. Troost B, Weber RB, Daroff RB. Hypometric saccades. Am J Ophthalmol 1974;78:1002–1005

35. Stanton G, Goldberg ME, Bruce CJ. Frontal eye field efferents in the macaque monkey: II Topography of terminal fields in midbrain and pons. J Comp Neurol 1988;27:493–506

36. Seagraves MA. Activity of monkey frontal eye field neurons projecting to oculomotor regions of the pons. J Neurophysiol 1992;68:1967–1985

37. Goldberg ME, Bushnell MC. Behavioral enhancement of visual responses in monkey cerebral cortex: II. Modulation in frontal eye fields specifically related to saccades. J Neurophysiol 1981;46:773–787

38. Anderson T, Jenkins IH, Brooks DJ, et al. Cortical control of saccades and fixation in man. A PET study. Brain 1994;117:1073–1084

39. Sweeney J, Mintun MA, Kwee S, et al. Positron emission tomography study of voluntary saccadic eye movements and spatial working memory. J Neurophysiol 1996;75:454–468

40. Petit L, Orssaud C, Tsourio N, et al. Functional anatomy of a prelearned sequence of horizontal saccades in humans. J Neurosci 1996;16:3714–3716

41. Schiller PH, True SD, Conway JL. Deficits in eye movements following frontal eye field and superior colliculus ablations. J Neurophysiol 1980;44:1175–1189

42. Keating E, Gooley SG. Saccadic disorders caused by cooling the superior colliculus or frontal eye field, or from combined lesions of both structures. Brain Res 1988;438:247–255

43. Li C, Mazzoni P, Andersen RA. Effect of reversible inactivation of macaque lateral intraparietal area on visual and memory saccades. J Neurophysiol 1999; 81(4):1827–1838

44. Heide W, Kompf D. Combined deficits of saccades and visuo-spatial orientation after cortical lesions. Exp Brain Res 1998;123(1–2):164–171

45. Hikosaka O, Wurtz RH. Visual and oculomotor functions of monkey substantia nigra pars reticulata: I. Relation of visual and auditory responses to saccades. J Neurophysiol 1983;49:1230–1253

46. Hikosaka O, Wurtz RH. Visual and oculomotor functions of monkey substantia nigra pars reticulata: II. Visual responses related to fixation of gaze. J Neurophysiol 1983;49:1254–1267

47. Hikosaka O, Wurtz RH. Visual and oculomotor functions of monkey substantia nigra pars reticulata: III. Memory contingent visual and saccade responses. J Neurophysiol 1983;49:1268–1284

48. Hikosaka O, Wurtz RH. Visual and oculomotor functions of monkey substantia nigra pars reticulata: IV. Relation of substantia nigra to superior colliculus. J Neurophysiol 1983;49:1285–1301

49. Hikosaka OWR. Modification of saccadic eye movements by GABA related substances. I. Effect of muscimol in monkey substantia nigra pars reticulata. J Neurophysiol 1985;53:292–308

50. Hikosaka O, Sakamoto M, Miyashita N. Effects of caudate nucleus stimulation on substantia nigra cell activity in monkey. Exp Brain Res 1993;95:457–472

51. Komatsu H, Wurtz RH. Modulation of pursuit eye movements by stimulation of cortical areas MT and MST. J Neurophysiol 1989;62:31–47

52. Komatsu H, Wurtz RH. Relation of cortical areas MT and MST to pursuit eye movements. III. Interaction with full-field stimulation. J Neurophysiol 1988;60: 621–644

53. Dürsteler M, Wurtz RH. Pursuit and optokinetic deficits following chemical lesions of cortical areas MT and MST. J Neurophysiol 1988;60:940–965

54. Keating E. Frontal eye field lesions in predictive and visually-guided pursuit eye movements. Exp Brain Res 1991;86:311–323

55. Keating E. Lesions of the frontal eye field impaired pursuit eye movements but preserved the prediction driving them. Behav Brain Res 1993;53:91–104

56. Dursteler M, Wurtz RH, Newsome WT. Directional pursuit deficits following lesions of the foveal representation within the superior temporal sulcus in the macaque monkey. J Neurophysiol 1987;57: 1262–1287

57. Morrow M, Sharpe JA. Retinotopic and directional deficits of smooth pursuit initiation after posterior cerebral hemispheric lesions. Neurology 1993;43: 595–603

58. Sharpe JA, Silversides JL, Blair RDG. Familial paralysis of horizontal gaze associated with pendular nystagmus, progressive scoliosis and facial contraction with myokymia. Neurology 1975;25:1035–1040

59. Steffen H, Rauterberg-Ruland I, Breitbach N, et al. Familial congenital horizontal gaze paralysis and kyphoscoliosis. Neuropediatrics 1998;29(4):220–222

60. Sharpe JA, Ranalli PJ, Morrow MJ. Familial paralysis of vertical gaze. Neurology 1987;37(3 Suppl 1):140

61. Phillips PBMHP. Congenital ocular motor apraxia with autosomal dominant inheritance. Am J Ophthalmol 2000;129(6):820–822

62. Burk K, Fetter M, Abele M, et al. Autosomal dominant cerebellar ataxia type I: oculomotor abnormalities in families with SCA1, SCA2, and SCA3. J Neurol 1999;246(9):789–797

63. Yan-Go F, Yanagihara T, Pierre RV, Goldstein NPA. A progressive neurologic disorder with supranuclear vertical gaze paresis and distinctive bone marrow cells. Mayo Clin Proc 1984;59(6):404–410

64. Morris JCE. Niemann-Pick C disease: cholesterol handling gone awry. Mol Med Today 1998;4(12):525–531

65. Harris C, Taylor DS, Vellodi A. Ocular motor abnormalities in Gaucher disease. Neuropediatrics 1999; 30(6):289–293

66. Stanford P, Halliday GM, Brooks WS, et al. Progressive supranuclear palsy pathology caused by a novel silent mutation in exon 10 of the tau gene: expansion of the disease phenotype caused by tau gene mutations. Brain 2000;123(pt 5(2)):880–893

67. Higgins J, Adler RL, Loveless JM. Mutational analysis of the tau gene in progressive supranuclear palsy. Neurology 1999;53(7):1421–1424

68. Wszolek Z, Pfeiffer RF, Bhatt MH, et al. Rapidly progressive autosomal dominant parkinsonism and dementia with pallido-ponto-nigral degeneration. Ann Neurol 1992;32(3):312–320

69. Clark L, Poorkaj P, Wszolek Z, et al. Pathogenic implications of mutations in the tau gene in pallido-ponto-nigral degeneration and related neurodegenerative disorders linked to chromosome 17. Proc Natl Acad Sci USA 1998;95(22):13103–13107

70. Goebel H, Komatsuzaki A, Bender MB, Cohen B. Lesions of the pontine tegmentum and conjugate gaze paralysis. Arch Neurol 1971;24(5):431–440

71. Baloh RW, Yee RD, Honrubia V. Internuclear ophthalmoplegia. Arch Neurol 1978;35:484–493

72. Wall MWS. The one-and-a-half syndrome—a unilateral disorder of the pontine tegmentum: a study of 20 cases and review of the literature. Neurology 1983;33(8):971–980

73. Sharpe JA, Rosenberg ME, Hoyt WF, Daroff RB. Paralytic pontine exotropia: a sign of acute unilateral pontine gaze palsy and internuclear ophthalmoplegia. Neurology 1974;24:1076–1081

74. Zackon D, Sharpe JA. Midbrain paresis of horizontal gaze. Ann Neurol 1984;16:495–504

75. Keane JR. Pretectal syndrome: 206 patients. Neurology 1990;40:684–690

76. Huaman A, Sharpe JA. Vertical saccades in senescence. Invest Ophthalmol Vis Sci 1993;34:2588–2595

77. Sharpe J, Ranalli PJ. Vertical vestibulo-ocular reflex control after supranuclear midbrain damage. Acta Otolaryngol 1991;481:194–198

78. Sharpe J. Neuro-ophthalmic implications of vestibular disorders. In: Tusa RJNS, ed. Neuro-ophthalmological Disorders: Diagnostic Work-up and Management. New York: Marcel Dekker, 1994:253–264

79. Sharpe J, Johnston JL. The vestibulo-ocular reflex: clinical anatomic and physiologic correlates. In: Sharpe J, Barber, HO, eds. The Vestibulo-ocular Reflex and Vertigo. New York: Raven Press, 1993:15–39

80. Gay A, Brodkey J, Miller JE. Convergence retraction nystagmus: an electromyographic study. Arch Ophthalmol 1963;70:456–461

81. Buttner-Ennever JA, Buttner U, Cohen B, et al. Vertical gaze paralysis and the rostral interstitial nucleus of the medial longitudinal fasciculus. Brain 1982;105:125–149

82. Kompf D, Pasik T, Pasik P, Bender MB. Downward gaze in monkeys. Brain 1979;102:527–558

83. Keane JR. Sustained up gaze in coma. Ann Neurol 1981;9:409–412

84. Leigh R, Foley JM, Remler BF, Civil RH. Oculogyric crisis: a syndrome of thought disorder and ocular deviation. Ann Neurol 1987;22:13–17

85. Sharpe J. Adaptation to frontal lobe lesions. In: Keller E, Zee DS, eds. Adaptive Processes in Visual and Oculomotor Systems. Oxford: Pergamon Press, 1986:239–246

86. Morrow M. Craniotopic defects of smooth pursuit and saccadic eye movement. Neurology 1996;46(2):514–521

87. Steiner I, Melamed E. Conjugate eye deviation after acute hemispheric stroke: delayed recovery after previous contralateral frontal lobe damage. Ann Neurol 1984;16:509–511

88. Sharpe J, Lo AW, Rabinovitch HE. Control of the saccadic and smooth pursuit systems after cerebral hemidecortication. Brain 1979;102:387–403

89. Fisher C. Some neuro-ophthalmological observations. J Neurol Neurosurg Psychiatry 1967;30(5):383–392

90. Keane J. Contralateral gaze deviation with supratentorial hemorrhage. Arch Neurol 1975;32(2):119–122

91. Sharpe J, Bondar RL, Fletcher WA. Contralateral gaze deviation after frontal lobe hemorrhage. J Neurol Neurosurg Psychiatry 1985;48:86–88

92. Fletcher W, Sharpe JA. Saccadic eye movement dysfunction in Alzheimer's disease. Ann Neurol 1986;20:464–471

93. White OB, Saint-Cyr JA, Tomlinson RD, Sharpe JA. Ocular motor deficits in Parkinson's disease. II. Control of the saccadic and smooth pursuit systems. Brain 1983;106:571–587

94. O'Sullivan E, Shaunak S, Henderson L, et al. Abnormalities of predictive saccades in Parkinson's disease. Neuroreport 1997;8(5):1209–1213

95. Pierrot-Deseilligny C, Rivaus S, Gaymard B, Agid Y. Cortical control of reflexive visually guided saccades in man. Brain 1991;114:1473–1485

96. Zee DS, Yee RD, Singer HS. Congenital ocular motor apraxia. Brain 1977;100:581–599

97. Sharpe JA, Johnston JL. Ocular motor apraxia versus paresis. Ann Neurol 1989;25:209

98. Dehaene I, Lammen M. Paralysis of saccades and pursuit: clinicopathological study. Neurology 1991;41:414–415

99. Sharpe J, Zackon DH. Senescent saccades: effects of aging on their accuracy, latency and velocity. Acta Otolaryngol 1987;104:422–428

100. Sharpe J. Cerebral ocular motor deficits. In: Lenerstrand G, Zee DS, Keller EL, eds. Functional basis of ocular motility disorders. Oxford: Pergamon Press, 1982:479–488

101. Ranalli P, Sharpe JA. Contrapulsion of saccades and ipsilateral ataxia: a unilateral disorder of the rostral cerebellum. Ann Neurol 1986;20:311–316

102. Kommerell G, Hoyt WF. Lateropulsion of saccadic eye movements. Electroculographic studies in a patient with Wallenberg's syndrome. Arch Neurol 1973;28:313–318

103. Waespe W, Wichmann W. Oculomotor disturbances during visual-vestibular interaction in Wallenberg's lateral medullary syndrome. Brain 1990;113:821–846

104. Waespe W, Baumgartner R. Enduring dysmetria and impaired gain adaptivity of saccadic eye movements in Wallenberg's lateral medullary syndrome. Brain 1992;115:1125–1146

105. Solomon D, Galetta SL, Liu GT. Possible mechanisms for horizontal gaze deviation and lateropulsion in the lateral medullary syndrome. J Neuroophthalmol 1995;51:26–30

106. Sharpe J, Morrow MJ, Newman NJ, et al. Neuro-ophthalmology: Continuum, American Academy of Neurology. Baltimore: Williams and Wilkins, 1995

107. Helmchen C, Straube A, Buttner U. Saccadic lateropulsion in Wallenberg's syndrome may be caused by a functional lesion of the fastigial nucleus. J Neurol 1994;241:421–426

108. Morrow M, Sharpe JA. Torsional nystagmus in the lateral medullary syndrome. Ann Neurol 1988;24:390–398

109. Pierrot-Deseilligny C, Goasguen J, Chain F, Lapresle J. Pontine metastasis with dissociated bilateral horizontal gaze paralysis. J Neurol Neurosurg Psychiatry 1984;47:159–164

110. Troost B, Daroff RB. The ocular motor defects in progressive supranuclear palsy. Ann Neurol 1977;2:397–403

111. Leigh R, Newman SA, Folstein SE, et al. Abnormal

ocular motor control in Huntington's disease. Neurology 1983;33:1268–1275

112. Lasker A, Zee DS, Hain TC, et al. Saccades in Huntington's disease: initiation defects and distractibility. Neurology 1987;37:364–370

113. Barton J, Jama A, Sharpe JA. Saccadic duration and intra-saccadic fatigue in myasthenic and non-myasthenic ocular palsies. Neurology 1995;45:2065–2072

114. Sharpe J, Wong AMF, Tweed D. Three dimensional analysis of saccadic abnormalities in unilateral sixth nerve palsy. Invest Ophthalmol Vis Sci 2001; 42(4):S624

115. Morrow M, Sharpe JA. Cerebral hemispheric localization of smooth pursuit asymmetry. Neurology 1990;40:284–292

116. Sharpe J, Deck JHN. Destruction of the internal sagittal stratum and normal smooth pursuit. Ann Neurol 1978;4:473–476

117. Baloh R, Yee RD, Honrubia V. Optokinetic nystagmus and parietal lobe lesions. Ann Neurol 1980;7:269–276

118. Kjallman L, Frisén L. The cerebral ocular pursuit pathways. A clinicoradiological study of small-field optokinetic nystagmus. J Clin Neuroophthalmol 1986;6: 209–214

119. Kömpf D. The significance of optokinetic nystagmus asymmetry in hemispheric lesions. Neuroophthalmology 1986;6:61–64

120. Sharpe J, Morrow MJ. Cerebral hemispheric smooth pursuit disorders. Neuroophthalmology 1991;11:87–98

121. Thurston S, Leigh RJ, Crawford T, et al. Two distinct deficits of visual tracking caused by unilateral lesions of cerebral cortex in humans. Ann Neurol 1988;23: 266–273

122. Morrow M, Sharpe JA. Deficits of smooth pursuit eye movement after unilateral frontal lobe lesions. Ann Neurol 1995;37:443–451

123. Lynch J. Frontal eye field lesions in monkeys disrupt visual pursuit. Exp Brain Res 1987;68:437–441

124. Barton J, Sharpe JA, Raymond JE. Directional defects in pursuit and motion perception in humans with unilateral cerebral lesions. Brain 1996;119:1535–1550

125. Baloh R, Yee RD, Honrubia V. Eye movements in patients with Wallenberg's syndrome. Ann New York Acad Sci 1981;374:600–613

126. Sharpe J, Goldberg HJ, Lo AW, Herishanu YO. Visual-vestibular interaction in multiple sclerosis. Neurology 1981;31:427–433

127. Fletcher W, Sharpe JA. Smooth pursuit dysfunction in Alzheimer's Disease. Neurology 1988;38:272–277

128. Zee D, Yee RD, Cogan DG, et al. Ocular motor abnormalities in hereditary cerebellar ataxia. Brain 1976;99(2):207–234

129. Sharpe J, Sylvester TO. Effect of aging on horizontal smooth pursuit. Invest Ophthalmol Vis Sci 1978;17: 465–468

130. Zackon D, Sharpe JA. Smooth pursuit in senescence: effects of target velocity and acceleration. Acta Otolaryngol 1987;104:290–297

131. Morrow M, Sharpe JA. Smooth pursuit eye movements. In: Sharpe J, Barber HO, eds. The Vestibulo-ocular Reflex and Vertigo. New York: Raven Press, 1993:141–162

132. Kim J, Sharpe JA. The vertical vestibulo-ocular reflex, and its interaction with vision during active head motion: effects of aging. J Vestib Res 2001;11:3–12

133. Marshall CMF. Vestibular stimulation for supranuclear gaze palsy: case report. Arch Phys Med Rehabil 1983;64(3):134–136

134. Rubens A. Caloric stimulation and unilateral visual neglect. Neurology 1985;35:1019–1024

135. Schiff N, Pulver M. Does vestibular stimulation activate thalamocortical mechanisms that reintegrate impaired cortical regions? Proc R Soc Lond B Biol Sci 1999;266:421–433

136. Storrie-Baker H, Segalowitz SJ, Black SE, et al. Improvement of hemispatial neglect with cold-water calorics: an electrophysiological test of the arousal hypothesis of neglect. J Int Neuropsychol Soc 1997; 3(4):394–402

137. Meienberg O, Zangemeister WH, Rosenberg M, et al. Saccadic eye movement strategies in patients with homonymous hemianopia. Ann Neurol 1981;9(6): 537–544

138. Ishiai S, Furukawa T, Tsukagoshi H. Eye-fixation patterns in homonymous hemianopia and unilateral spatial neglect. Neuropsychologia 1987;25:675–679

139. Barton J, Sharpe JA. Smooth pursuit and saccades to moving targets in blind hemifields. A comparison of medial occipital, lateral occipital and optic radiation lesions. Brain 1997;120(4):681–699

140. Mohler C, Wurtz RH. The role of the striate cortex and superior colliculus in visual guidance of saccadic eye movements in monkeys. J Neurophysiol 1977;40:74–94

141. Weiskrantz L, Cowey A, Passingham C. Spatial responses to brief stimuli by monkeys with striate cortex ablations. Brain 1977;100:655–670

142. Zihl J. "Blindsight": improvement of visually guided eye movements by systematic practice in patients with cerebral blindness. Neuropsychologia 1980;18:287–298

143. Zihl J, Von Cramon D. Registration of light stimuli in the cortically blind hemifield and its effect on localisation. Behav Brain Res 1980;1:287–298

144. Zihl J, Werth R. Contributions to the study of "blindsight" II. The role of specific practice for saccadic localisation in patients with postgeniculate visual field defects. Neuropsychologia 1984;22:13–22

145. Pambakian A, Kennard C. Can visual function be restored in patients with homonymous hemianopia? Br J Ophthalmol 1997;81(4):324–328

146. Zihl J. Neuropsychologische rehabilitation. In: Von Cramon DZJ, ed. Neuropsychologische Rehabilitation. Berlin: Springer-Verlag, 1988

147. Kerkhoff G, Müninger U, Haaf E, et al. Rehabilitation of homonymous scotomata in patients with postgeniculate damage of the visual system: saccadic compensation training. Restor Neurol Neurosci 1992;4:245–254

148. Savir H, Michelson I, David C, et al. Homonymous hemianopia and rehabilitation in fifteen cases of CCI. Scand J Rehab Med 1977;9:151–153

149. Zangemeister W, Meienberg O, Stark L, Hoyt WF. Eye-head co-ordination in homonymous hemianopia. J Neurol 1982;226:243–254

150. Kerkhoff G, Müninger U, Meier EK. Neurovisual rehabilitation in cerebral blindness. Arch Neurol 1994; 51:474–481

151. Zihl J. Visual scanning behaviour in patients with homonymous hemianopia. Neuropsychologia 1995; 33:287–303

152. Poppelreuter W. Die Störungen der Niederen und Höreren Sehleistungen durch Verletzungen des Okzipitalhirns. In: Die psychischen Schädigungen durch Kopfschu im Kriege 1914/16. Leipzig: Leopold Voss, 1917

153. Gassel M, Williams D. Visual function in patients with homonymous hemianopia. Part II Oculomotor mechanisms. Brain 1963;86:1–36

154. Zihl J. Eye movement patterns in hemianopic dyslexia. Brain 1995;118:891–912

155. Zihl J, Kennard C. Disorders of higher visual function. *In:* Zihl J, Kennard C, eds. Neurological Disorders: Course and Treatment. London: Academic Press, 1996:201–202

156. Zihl J. Treatment of patients with homonymous visual field disorders (in German). Z Neuropsychol 1990;2: 95–101

157. Schoepf D, Zangemeister WH. Correlation of ocular motor reading strategies to the status of adaptation in patients with hemianopic visual field defects. Ann N Y Acad Sci 1993;682:404–408

158. Luria A. Restoration of Brain Function after Injury. Oxford: Pergamon Press, 1963

159. Cowey A. Perimetric study of field defects in monkeys after cortical and retinal ablations. Q J Exp Psychol 1967;19:232–245

160. Zihl J, Von Cramon D. Restitution of visual function in patients with cerebral blindness. J Neurol Neurosurg Psychiatry 1979;42:312–322

161. Zihl J. Recovery of visual functions in patients with cerebral blindness. Effect of specific practice with saccadic localisation. Exp Brain Res 1981;44:159–169

162. Zihl J, Von Cramon D. Visual field recovery from scotoma in patients with postgeniculate damage. A review of 55 cases. Brain 1985;108:335–365

163. Bach-Y-Rita PBBS. Controlling variables eliminates hemianopia rehabilitation results. Behav Brain Sci 1983;6:448

164. Balliet R, Blood KMT, Bach-Y-Rita P. Visual field rehabilitation in the cortically blind? J Neurol Neurosurg Psychiatry 1985;48:1113–1124

165. Pommerenke K, Markowitsch HJ. Rehabilitation training of homonymous visual field defects in patients with postgeniculate damage of the visual system. Restor Neurol Neurosci 1989;1:47–63

166. Kasten E, Sabel BA. Visual-field enlargement after computer-training in brain-damaged patients with homonymous deficits: an open pilot trial. Restor Neurol Neurosci 1995;8:113–127

167. Walsh T, Lawton Smith J. Hemianopic spectacles. Am J Ophthalmol 1966;61:914–915

168. Smith J, Weiner IG, Lucero AJ. Hemianopic fresnel prisms. J Clin Neuroophthalmol 1982;2:19–22

169. Rossi P, Kheyfets S, Reding MJ. Fresnel prisms improve visual perception in stroke patients with homonymous hemianopia or unilateral visual neglect. Neurology 1990;40:1597–1599

170. Lee A, Perez AM. Improving awareness of peripheral visual field using sectorial prism. J Am Optom Assoc 1999;70(10):624–628

171. Peli E. Field expansion for homonymous hemianopia by optically induced peripheral exotropia. Optom Vis Sci 2000;77(9):453–464

172. Morel-Maroger A. Paralysis of vertical gaze as a sequela of Wernicke's encephalopathy. Rev Neurol (Paris) 1983;139(10):593–594

173. Zubaran C, Fernandes JG, Rodnight R. Wernicke-Korsakoff syndrome. Postgrad Med J 1997;73:27–31

174. Jacobs L, Beck RW, Simon JH, et al. Intramuscular interferon beta-1a therapy initiated during a first demyelinating event in multiple sclerosis. CHAMPS Study Group. N Engl J Med 2000;343(13):898–904

175. Chattha ADG. Sylvian aqueduct syndrome as a sign of acute obstructive hydrocephalus in children. J Neurol Neurosurg Psychiatry 1975;38(3):288–296

176. Cinalli GS, Sainte-Rose C, Simon I, et al. Sylvian aqueduct syndrome and global rostral midbrain dysfunction associated with shunt malfunction. J Neurosurg 1999;90(2):237

177. Repka M, Claro MC, Loupe DN, Reich SG. Ocular motility in Parkinson's disease. J Pediatr Ophthalmol Strabismus 1996;33(3):144–147

178. Racette B, Gokden MS, Tychsen LS, Perlmutter JS. Convergence insufficiency in idiopathic Parkinson's disease responsive to levodopa. Strabismus 1999;7(3): 169–174

179. Gibson J, Pimlott R, Kennard C. Ocular motor and manual tracking in Parkinson's disease and the effect of treatment. J Neurol Neurosurg Psychiatry 1987;50(7):853–860

180. Rascol O, Clanet M, Montastruc JL, et al. Abnormal ocular movements in Parkinson's disease. Evidence for involvement of dopaminergic systems. Brain 1989; 112(5):1193–1214

181. Crevits L, Versijpt J, Hanse M, De Ridder K. Antisaccadic effects of a dopamine agonist as add-on therapy in advanced Parkinson's patients. Neuropsychobiology 2000;42(4):202–206

182. Rivaud-Pechoux S, Vermersch AI, Gaymard B, et al. Improvement of memory guided saccades in parkinsonian patients by high frequency subthalamic nucleus stimulation. J Neurol Neurosurg Psychiatry 2000; 68(3):381–384

183. Blekher T, Siemers E, Abel LA, Yee RD. Eye movements in Parkinson's disease: before and after pallidotomy. Invest Ophthalmol Vis Science 2000;41(8): 2177–2183

184. Straube A, Ditterich J, Oertel W, Kupsch A. Electrical stimulation of the posteroventral pallidum influences internally guided saccades in Parkinson's disease. J Neurol 1998;245(2):101–105

185. Gibson J, Kennard C. Quantitative study of "on-off" fluctuations in the ocular motor system in Parkinson's disease. Adv Neurol 1987;45:329–333

186. Sharpe J, Fletcher WA, Lang AE, Zackon DH. Smooth pursuit during dose-related on-off fluctuations in Parkinson's disease. Neurology 1987;37(8):1389–1392

187. Louis E, Lynch T, Kaufmann P, et al. Diagnostic guidelines in central nervous system Whipple's disease. Ann Neurol 1996;40:561–568

188. Ratnaike R. Whipple's disease. Postgrad Med J 2000; 76:760–766

189. Singer R. Diagnosis and treatment of Whipple's disease. Drugs 1998;55:699–704

168 Ocular Myasthenia Gravis

Mark Moster

Brief overview

Myasthenia gravis ("myasthenia") was first described in 1672 by Willis[1] as a chronic disease with fluctuating weakness, aggravated by exertion and improved by rest. In 1895, Jolly[2] introduced the term "myasthenia gravis pseudoparalytica" and demonstrated muscle fatigue following repeated electrical stimulation.

Walker[3] used physostigmine as a therapy in 1934, and Blalock et al.[4] introduced thymectomy in the late 1930s. In the early days, there were many fatalities from myasthenia. With the advent of the above treatments and, in the 1950s, the application of ventilator support, the mortality rate declined drastically.[5] The autoimmune cause was recognized,[6,7] and medical treatment of the immune response began with corticosteroids in the 1960s.[8] Treatment with immunosuppressant agents such as azathioprine and plasmapheresis began in the 1970s[9] and intravenous immunoglobulin-treatment began in the 1980s. The postsynaptic nature of the defect[10] and the relevant acetylcholine receptor antibodies were appreciated in the 1970s.[11–14]

Although ocular myasthenia is part of a systemic disease, it is useful to consider it a distinct entity because it presents to ophthalmologists and optometrists and has a unique differential diagnosis. Also, the approach to treatment differs from that of generalized myasthenia.

Epidemiology

Estimates of the annual incidence of myasthenia range from 1 per 20 000 annually to 0.4 per million annually. Prevalence estimates have ranged from 1 in 8000 to 1 in 300 000.[15] It may occur at any age but is least common among children younger than 10 years and adults older than 70.

The female-to-male ratio of myasthenia is 3:2,[15] but it tends to present earlier in women than in men. For the population younger than 40 years, the female-to-male ratio is 7:3, the occurrence is equal between 40 and 50 years, and after age 50, the ratio decreases to 4:6.[16] Generalized myasthenia has no racial or geographic predilection, but ocular myasthenia has been reported to be 3 times more common among Chinese than white patients.[17]

In ocular myasthenia, men are affected more frequently than women, especially after age 40.[18,19] The average age at onset of ocular myasthenia is 38 years, compared with 33 years for generalized myasthenia.

Etiology

The cause of myasthenia is an autoimmune response that involves both B and T cells and the thymus. The actual damage to the acetylcholine receptor is caused mainly by acetylcholine receptor antibodies.

Pathophysiology and pathogenesis

The anti-acetylcholine receptor antibodies cause damage by several possible mechanisms, including complement-mediated destruction of the junctional folds and acceleration of the internalization and degradation of acetylcholine receptors. Complement attack causes acetycholine receptors to be shed into the synaptic space, and it destroys segments of the junctional folds, restricting the membrane surface available for the insertion of new acetylcholine receptors.[20] Patients with myasthenia have only 11% to 30% of the acetylcholine receptors present in normal subjects.[10] The decrease in receptors and, thus, the decrease in probability of interaction between acetylcholine and an acetylcholine receptor decreases the "safety margin" normally available in neuromuscular transmission, causing weakness and fatigability.[15]

Genetics

Myasthenia is usually sporadic. There is a slight increased risk in immediate relatives, and there is often a history of other autoimmune diseases, most commonly immune thyroid disease. There have been reports of various HLA types in different populations.

Clinical features

The most common symptom in ocular myasthenia is ptosis, followed by diplopia. These also are the most common findings in generalized myasthenia. Involvement of the levator or extraocular muscles (or both) occurs initially in 70% to 75% of patients and eventually in more than 90%.[21–23] To characterize these symptoms further, 10% of 48 patients with ocular myasthenia had only ptosis, 90% had ptosis and diplopia, and 25% had weakness of the orbicularis oculi.[24] The hallmarks of these deficits are variability and fatigability, so that at different times there are different degress of dysfunction. Thus, as the patient uses the eyes, the muscles fatigue, and the deficit progresses. A characteristic presentation is ptosis that appears on one side, improves, and then develops on the other side.

On examination, ptosis is seen most often. The fatigability can be demonstrated by prolonged upgaze for 90 seconds, with progressive ptosis developing. Enhanced ptosis is demonstrated by elevating one lid, which causes a worsening of ptosis contralaterally.[25] Although frequently seen in myasthenia, enhanced ptosis may occur in other diseases. A Cogan lid twitch sign is often present; this refers to an overshoot and twitching of the eyelid when the patient looks up from a downward position to primary position.[26]

Lid retraction is seen occasionally. It has two mechanisms. One is due to an attempt to overcome contralateral ptosis. According to Hering's law, when the brain provides excess innervation to the ptotic eyelid, the contralateral lid retracts. This pseudoretraction resolves when the ptotic eye is closed or the eyelid is elevated. The other mechanism for eyelid retraction is coexisting thyroid eye disease.

Weakness of extraocular motility has numerous varieties and can mimic any motility defect. The medial rectus muscle is involved most often, with what appears to be a unilateral or bilateral internuclear ophthalmoplegia as a common pattern, and may include abducting nystagmus.[27–29] Eye movement deficits may mimic an individual isolated CNVI, CNIV, or even CNIII palsy with pupil sparing. Although pupillary function may not be entirely normal in myasthenia,[30] anisocoria is present in only rare, isolated cases.

Nystagmus occasionally occurs. In contrast to other types of nystagmus, the nystagmus may become progressively worse with maintained eccentric position.

Saccadic abnormalities result from a combination of peripheral weakness and central adaptation. Saccades may be hypometric, and small saccades may be normal or hypermetric.[31–36]

From 50% to 80% of patients who present with ocular myasthenia subsequently have clinical generalized myasthenia, which usually develops within 2 to 3 years. However, the exceptions are too many to adequately reassure patients. From 10% to 20% of patients have spontaneous remission of ocular myasthenia.[18,19,23,37–46]

In a series of 1487 patients, 40% initially had purely ocular findings for the first month. Subsequently, 66% had generalized myasthenia: 78% within 1 year and 84% within 3 years.[19] In a series of 269 patients, 142 (53%) had only ocular manifestations.[18] Of the 108 patients with adequate follow-up, 40% still had only ocular findings, 49% had generalized myasthenia (in 83%, it developed within 2 years), and 11% had complete remission. Patients older than 50 years were at higher risk for generalized disease.

Classification and diagnostic criteria

Ocular myasthenia gravis is the mildest form of myasthenia gravis. It fits into the classification as grade 1.

Ptosis and diplopia are the most common symptoms. On examination, there is fatigable ptosis and abnormality of ocular motility. Clinical involvement of the pupil should suggest an alternative diagnosis. Involvement of one cranial nerve or multiple cranial nerves on one side suggests a structural lesion. Posterior fossa tumors have presented with fatigable ptosis and diplopia.[47]

Office testing for myasthenia gravis include the edrophonium (Tensilon) test, sleep test, and ice pack test. All three have similar sensitivities and specificities.[48–51] The most specific diagnostic test is the acetyl-choline receptor antibody, but it may be positive in only about 50% of patients with ocular myasthenia.[52–57] Repetitive nerve stimulation shows a decrement greater than 10% in more than 60% of patients.[45] Single fiber electromyography, although not specific, is the most sensitive test for ocular myasthenia and is positive in approximately 70% to 100% of patients.[15,58,59]

Pathologically, the postsynaptic membrane is destroyed and the receptors degraded.[45] The thymus shows hyperplasia, with a typical pattern of lymphofollicular hyperplasia with lymph node-like follicles, so-called germinal centers, in thymic medulla surrounded by areas of T cells.[60,61] Of the patients with myasthenia, 10% have thymoma.

Differential diagnosis

The differential diagnosis of ocular myasthenia includes other entities that produce ptosis or diplopia. Structural lesions in the brainstem or cavernous sinus may mimic myasthenia. Thyroid ophthalmopathy is a consideration and may coexist in approximately 10% of cases. The Miller Fisher variant of Guillain-Barré syndrome presents with ophthalmoplegia, ataxia, and areflexia. Chronic progressive external ophthalmoplegia has symmetric bilateral ptosis and ophthalmoplegia. Botulism may mimic ocular myasthenia, but it is preceded by a gastrointestinal tract syndrome and has pupillary involvement. Myotonic dystrophy presents with ptosis and has the accompanying features of myotonia, cataract, temporalis wasting, and other systemic manifestations.

Treatment

The treatment of myasthenia with anticholinesterase agents was introduced in the 1930s, followed by the introduction of corticosteroids in the 1960s and immunosuppressant agents thereafter. Thymectomy was introduced in the 1930s, too. Although the treatment of myasthenia has been studied, few data are available about isolated ocular myasthenia.

Treatment of ocular myasthenia has to be individualized. The benefit of an excellent response to prednisone or other immunosuppressive agents must be weighed against the potential side effects. The side effects are particularly important because the ocular manifestations of myasthenia most often are a nuisance rather than a medical problem. An individual decision must be made by the patient and physician about how much risk to take for the benefit.

The first-line medical treatment is an anticholinesterase agent. These medications raise the safety factor for neuromuscular transmission by preventing the degradation of acetylcholine and prolonging its action. Pyridostigmine (Mestinon) treatment is initiated at doses of 30 to 60 mg 2 or 3 times daily. The onset of response is within 30 minutes, and the duration of action is 2 to 8 hours. The doses are increased gradually as tolerated and as benefit is seen. The maximal dose is approximately 120 mg every 3 hours. The side effects include abdominal cramps, diarrhea, nausea, sweating, salivation, increased bronchial secretions, muscle cramps, and muscle twitching.

Some of the autonomic effects may be counteracted by giving antimuscarinic agents such as atropine, glycopyrrolate, or loperamide. Ephedrine, 25 mg 2 or 3 times daily, is sometimes helpful as an adjunct to pyridostigmine and is thought to enhance acetylcholine secretion.

A small proportion of patients with ocular myasthenia have an adequate response to pyridostigmine. Most likely to benefit are those troubled by ptosis but not diplopia. Pyridostigmine may improve ocular muscle strength, but unless the strength improves to normal, diplopia persists.

If pyridostigmine does not provide adequate relief, it must be decided whether to use potentially toxic immunosuppressant agents or to rely on the symptomatic treatments mentioned below.

The main immunosuppressant agent for ocular myasthenia is prednisone (grade C evidence in uncontrolled trials). Treatment may be started as low-dose alternate-day therapy, such as 5 to 10 mg every other day, and gradually increased by 5 to 10 mg each week or it may be started at 60 to 100 mg daily. Patients with generalized myasthenia who start receiving high-dose prednisone treatment must be hospitalized because a significant fraction will have worsening of their condition within the first 2 weeks. Although this may not be a problem for patients with ocular myasthenia, the author prefers to begin outpatient treatment with low-dose alternate-day prednisone.[19,24,62,63]

The dose is increased or high-dose treatment is continued until a response occurs or, if no response occurs, for approximately 3 months until the dose is 50 to 60 mg daily. At that time, the move is toward alternate-day treatment, which is less toxic and permits normal adrenal function. One day's dose is decreased by 5 mg and the alternate day's dose is increased by 5 mg, and further, similar changes are made monthly. A benefit usually is seen within a few weeks and becomes maximal within a few months. Eventually, most patients require 20 to 40 mg every other day to maintain clinical remission. Approximately 85% of patients with ocular myasthenia respond well to corticosteroid treatment. Corticosteroids may decrease the rate of progression to generalized myasthenia, but this has not been proved in a controlled study.

The side effects of prednisone include increased glucose level, weight gain, cushingoid appearance, cataracts, osteoporosis with fractures, increased intraocular pressure, steroid myopathy, increased blood pressure, predisposition to infection, and aseptic necrosis of various joints. Blood glucose and electrolyte levels, blood pressure, and intraocular pressure should be monitored. Bone density studies are indicated, and patients should take calcium, vitamin D, and possibly alendronate. Patients should be monitored for gastric irritation, and some should be given antacids and histamine H_2 blockers. Patients receiving corticosteroid or other immunosuppressant therapy should have a tuberculin skin test (PPD) before commencing treatment. If the result is positive,

an alternative treatment should be considered or antituberculous therapy should be initiated along with corticosteroid therapy.

Azathioprine has been shown to be of benefit in myasthenia (grade B evidence).[64] It may be used to treat ocular myasthenia. Also, it is associated with a decreased rate of progression to generalized myasthenia. However, whether this is an effect of ongoing treatment or is actually a change in the course of the disease has not been established. Azathioprine is most useful when corticosteroids are contraindicated, the response to corticosteroids is poor, or dose reduction of prednisone is desired. Azathioprine treatment is begun at low doses of 25 to 50 mg, and the dose is increased gradually to 2 to 3 mg/kg daily. The leukocyte count and mean corpuscular volume (MCV) may be monitored for therapeutic and toxic effects. Liver function tests and serum amylase levels also are monitored. From 3 to 12 months are needed for the effect to occur, and the maximal benefits are seen between 1 and 3 years. Potential side effects include a flu-like syndrome, liver toxicity, gastrointestinal tract symptoms, leukopenia, thrombocytopenia, and a small long-term risk of lymphoproliferative disorder. In a study of ocular myasthenia treated with azathioprine or prednisone (or both), the risk of disease generalization was 12%, compared with 64% without treatment.[46]

Cyclosporine, originally reserved for treating generalized myasthenia, is now frequently used for treating ocular myasthenia. There is grade B evidence for benefit in generalized myasthenia.[65] Dosages are lower than for patients with transplant disorders. The dose begins at 4 to 5 mg/kg daily, divided every 12 hours, and is adjusted to attain trough levels between 100 and 200 mg/mL. After an adequate clinical response has been achieved, the dose may be tapered.

The main toxic effects of cyclosporine are hypertension and nephrotoxicity.[65,66] Because of this, blood pressure, blood urea nitrogen, and creatinine levels are monitored. Less severe side effects include facial hirsutism, gastrointestinal tract disturbance, headache, tremor, seizures, or hepatotoxicity. The onset of benefit is between 2 and 6 weeks, with maximum improvement by about 4 months.

Other medical treatments, described only in case reports, include cyclophosphamide[67] and mycophenolate mofetil.[68]

Plasma exchange or intravenous immunoglobulin is rarely indicated in ocular myasthenia. These treatments are reserved for patients with generalized disease who need rapid improvement (e.g., at the initial diagnosis), who are beginning immunosuppression, or who are preparing for surgery (e.g., thymectomy).

Thymectomy is recommended for patients with ocular myasthenia who have thymoma. Although most practitioners would not use thymectomy to treat ocular myasthenia without thymoma,[69] there is evidence for more frequent remissions and improvement in patients who have thymectomy. Also, it may prevent progression to generalized myasthenia.[70]

Therefore, as the procedure becomes safer, it may be considered for patients with ocular myasthenia. The procedure likely works best when performed early in the course of the disease.

Symptomatic treatments include ones that elevate the eyelids and eliminate diplopia. For ptosis, patients may use specialized lid tapes or lid crutches. For diplopia, occlusion with a patch or frosting the lens of eyeglasses is helpful.

For patients with long-standing fixed ptosis, blepharoplasty may be considered. For patients who have ocular motility defects that are stable with a fixed strabismus, prism therapy or strabismus surgery may be considered.

References

1. Willis T, De Anima Brutorum, Oxford, Theatro Sheldiano, 1672
2. Jolly F. Ueber Myasthenia gravis pseudoparalytica. Berl Klin Wchnschr 1895;32:33
3. Walker MB. Treatment of myasthenia gravis with physostigmine. Lancet 1934;1:1200–1201
4. Blalock A, Mason MF, Morgan HF, Riven SS. Myasthenia gravis and tumors of the thymic region: Report of a case in which the tumor was removed. Ann Surg 1939;110:544–561
5. Grob D, Brunner NG, Namba T. The natural course of myasthenia gravis and effect of therapeutic measures. Ann NY Acad Sci 1981;377:652–669
6. Nastuk WL, Plescia OJ, Osserman KE. Changes in serum complement activity in patients with myasthenia gravis. Proc Soc Exp Biol Med 1960;105:177–184
7. Simpson JA. Myasthenia gravis: A new hypothesis. Scot Med J 1960;5:419–436
8. Grob D, Namba T. Corticotropin in generalized myasthenia gravis. Effect of short intensive courses. JAMA 1966;198:703–707
9. Dau PC, Lindstrom JM, Cassel CK, Denys EH, Shev EE, Spitler LE. Plasmapheresis and immunosuppressive drug therapy in myasthenia gravis. N Eng J Med 1977;297:1134–1140.
10. Fambrough DM, Drachman DB, Satyamurti S, Neuromuscular junction in myasthenia gravis: decreased acetylcholine receptors. Science 1973;182:293–295
11. Almon RR, Andrew CG, Appel SH. Serum globulin in myasthenia gravis: inhibition of alpha-bugarotoxin binding to acetylcholine receptors. Science 1974;186:55–57
12. Appel SH, Almon RR, Levy N. Acetylcholine receptor antibodies in myasthenia gravis. New Engl J Med 1975;293:760–761
13. Bender AN, Ringel SP, Engel WK, et al. Myasthenia gravis: a serum factor blocking acetylcholine receptors of the human neuromuscular junction. Lancet 1975;i:607–609
14. Lindstrom JM, Seybold ME, Lennon VA, et al. Antibody to acetylcholine receptor in myasthenia gravis: prevalence, clinical correlates, and diagnostic value. Neurology (Minneap) 1976;26:1054–1059
15. Weinberg DA, Lesser RL, Vollmer TL. Ocular myasthenia: A protean disorder. Survey of Ophthalmology 1994;39:169–210
16. Grob D. Natural History of Myasthenia. In: Engel AG, ed. Myasthenia Gravis and Myasthenic Disorders. New York: Oxford University Press, 1999:131–145
17. Chiu HC, Vincent A, Newsom-Davis J, et al. Myasthenia gravis: population differences in disease expression and acetylcholine receptor antibody titres between Chinese and Caucasians. Neurology 1987;37:1854–1857
18. Bever CT Jr, Aquino AV, Penn AS, et al. Prognosis of ocular myasthenia. Ann Neurol 1983;14:516–519
19. Grob D, Arsura E, Brunner N, Namba T. The course of myasthenia gravis and therapies affecting outcome. Ann NY Acad Sci 1987;505:472–499
20. Hohlfeld R, Wekerle H. The Immunopathogenesis of Myasthenia Gravis. New York: Oxford University Press, 1999
21. Mattis RD. Ocular manifestations of myasthenia gravis. Arch Ophthalmol 1941;26:969–982
22. Osserman KE. Ocular myasthenia gravis. Invest Ophthalmol 1967;6:277–287
23. Oosterhuis HJGH. The ocular signs and symptoms of myasthenia gravis. Doc Ophthalmol 1982;52:363–378
24. Evoli A, Tonali P, Bartoccioni E, Lo Monaco M. Ocular myasthenia: diagnostic and therapeutic problems. Acta Neurol Scand 1988;77:31–35
25. Gorelick PB, Rosenberg M, Pagano RJ. Enhanced ptosis in myasthenia gravis. Arch Neurol 1981;38:531
26. Cogan DG. Myasthenia gravis: A review of the disease and a description of lid twitch as a characteristic sign. Arch Ophthalmol 1965;74:217–221
27. Glaser JS. Myasthenic pseudo-internuclear ophthalmoplegia. Arch Ophthalmol 1966;75:363–366
28. Finalli PF, Hoyt WF. Myasthenic abduction nystagmus in a patient with hyperthyroidism. Neurology 1976;26:589–590
29. Davis TL, Lavin PJ. Pseudo one-and-a-half syndrome with ocular myasthenia. Neurology 1989;39:1553
30. Lepore FE, Sanborn GE, Slevin JT. Pupillary dysfunction in myasthenia gravis. Ann Neurol 1979;6:29–33
31. Yee RD, Cogan DG, Zee DS, Baloh RW, Honrubia V. Rapid eye movements in myasthenia gravis. Arch Ophthalmol 1976;94:1465–1472
32. Schmidt D, Dell'Osso LF, Abel LA, Daroff RB. Saccadic eye movement waveforms. Exp Neurol 1980;68:346–364
33. Sollberger CE, Meienberg O, Ludin HP. The contribution of oculography to early diagnosis of myasthenia gravis: A study of saccadic eye movements using the infrared reflection method in 22 cases. Eur Arch Psychiatry Neurol Sci 1986;236:102–108
34. Kaminsky HJ, Maas E, Spiegel P, Ruff RL. Why are eye muscles frequently involved in myasthenia gravis? Neurology 1990;40:1663–1669
35. Barton JJS, Sharpe JA. 'Saccadic Jitter' is a quantitative ocular sign in myasthenia gravis. Investigative Ophthalmology & Visual Science 1995;36:1566–1572
36. Barton JJS. Quantitative ocular tests for myasthenia gravis: a comparative review with detection theory analysis. Journal of Neurological Sciences 1998;155:104–114
37. Ferguson FR, Hutchinson EC, Liversedge LA. Myasthenia gravis: Results of medical management. Lancet 1955;2:636–639
38. Garland H, Clark ANG. Myasthenia gravis. A personal study of 60 cases. Br Med J 1956;1:1259–1262
39. Osserman KE. Myasthenia Gravis. New York: Grune & Stratton, 1958
40. Schlezinger NS, Fairfax WA. Evaluation of ocular signs and symptoms in myasthenia gravis. Arch Ophthalmol 1959;62:985–990
41. Perlo VP, Poskanzer DC, Schwab RS, et al. Myasthenia gravis: Evaluation of treatment in 1,355 patients. Neurology 1966;16:431–439
42. Simpson JA, Westerberg MR, Magee KR. Myasthenia

gravis: An analysis of 295 cases. Acta Neurol Scand 1966;42(Suppl):1–27

43. Oosterhuis HJGH. Long term effects of treatment in 374 patients with myasthenia gravis. Monogr Allergy 1988; 25:75–85

44. Sanders DB, Howard JF Jr, Massey JM. Demographic observations on 860 patients with acquired myasthenia gravis (Abstract). Annals of 1992 International Symposium on Myasthenia Gravis and Related Disorders. NY Acad Sci

45. Sommer N, Melms A, Weller M, Dichgans J. Ocular myasthenia gravis. Documenta Ophthalmologica 1993;84:309–333

46. Sommer N, Sigg B, Melms A, Weller M, Schepelmann K, Herzau V. Ocular myasthenia gravis: response to long-term immunosuppressive treatment. J Neurol Neurosurg Psychiatry 1997;62:156–162

47. Ragge NK, Hoyt WF. Midbrain myasthenia: Fatigable ptosis, "lid twitch" sign, and ophthalmoparesis from a dorsal midbrain glioma. Neurology 1992;42:917–919

48. Sethi KD, Riner MH, Swift TR. Ice pack test for myasthenia gravis. Neurology 1987;37:1383–1385

49. Odel JG, Winterkorn JM, Behrens MM. The sleep test for myasthenia gravis. A safe alternative to tensilon. J Clin Neuroophthalmol 1991;11:288–292

50. Golnik KC, Pena R, Lee AG, Eggenberger ER. An ice test for the diagnosis of myasthenia gravis. Ophthalmology 1999;106:1282–1286

51. Kelly JJ, Daube JR, Lennon VA, Howard FM, Younge BR. The laboratory diagnosis of mild myasthenia gravis. Ann Neurol 1982;12:238–242

52. Lefvert AK, Bergstrom K, Matell G, Osterman PO, Pirskanen R. Determination of acetylcholine receptor antibody in myasthenia gravis: Clinical usefulness and pathogenic implications. J Neurol Neurosurg Psychiatry 1978;41:394–403

53. Oda K, Goto I, Kuriowa Y, Onoue K, Ito Y. Myasthenia gravis: Antibodies to acetylcholine receptor with human and rat antigens. Neurology 1980;30:543–546

54. Tindall RSA. Humoral immunity in myasthenia gravis: Biochemical characterization of acquired antireceptor antibodies and clinical correlations. Ann Neurol 1981;10:437–447

55. Limburg PC, The TH, Hummel-Tappel E, Oosterhuis HUGH. Anti-acetylcholine receptor antibodies in myasthenia gravis, Part 1: Relation to clinical parameters in 250 patients. J Neurol Sci 1983;58:357–370

56. Vincent A, Newsom-Davis J. Acetylcholine receptor antibody as a diagnostic test for myasthenia gravis: Results in 153 validated cases and 2967 diagnostic assays. J Neurol Neurosurg Psychiatry 1985;48: 1246–1252

57. Toyka KV, Heininger K. Acetylcholine-receptor antibodies in the diagnosis of myasthenia gravis. Dtsh Med Wochenschr 1986;111:1435–1439

58. Ukachoke C, Ashby P, Basinski A, Sharpe JA. Usefulness of single fiber EMG for distinguishing neuromuscular from other causes of ocular muscle weakness. Can J Neurol Sci 1994;21:125–128

59. Rivero A, Crovetto L, Lopez L, Maselli R, Nogues M. Single fiber electromyography of extraocular muscles: a sensitive method of diagnosis of ocular myasthenia gravis. Muscle Nerve 1995;18:943–947

60. Compston DAS, Vincent A, Newsom-Davis J, Batchelor JR. Clinical, pathological HLA antigen and immunological evidence for disease heterogeneity in myasthenia gravis. Brain 1980;103:579–601

61. Willcox N, Schluep M, Sommer N, Campana D, Janossy G, Brown AN, Newsom-Davis J. Variable corticosteroid sensitivity of thymic cortex and medullary peripheral-type lymphoid tissue in myasthenia gravis patients: Structural and functional effects. Q J Med 1989;73(271): 1071–1087

62. Fischer KC, Schwartzmann RJ. Oral corticosteroids in the treatment of ocular myasthenia gravis. Ann NY Acad Sci 1976;274:652–658

63. Kupersmith MJ, Moster M, Bhuiyan S, et al. Beneficial effects of corticosteroids on ocular myasthenia gravis. Arch Neurol 1996;53:802–804

64. Palace J. A randomized double-blind trial of prednisolone alone or with azathioprine in myasthenia gravis. Myasthenia Gravis Study Group. Neurology 1998;50:1778–1783

65. Tindall RSA, Rollins JA, Phillips JT, Greenlee RG, Wells L, Belendiuk G. Preliminary results of a double-blind, randomized, placebo-controlled trial of cyclosporine in myasthenia gravis. N Eng J Med 1987;316:719–724

66. Schalke B, Kappos L, Dommasch D, Rohrbach E, Merters HG. Cyclosporin A treatment of myasthenia gravis: Initial results of a double-blind trial of cyclosporin A versus azathioprine. Ann NY Acad Sci 1987;505:872–875

67. Perez MC, et al. Stable remissions in myasthenia gravis. Neurology 1981;31:32–37

68. Hauser RA, et al. Successful treatment of a patient with severe refractory myasthenia gravis using mycophenolate mofetil. Neurology 1998;(51)3:912–913

69. Lanska DJ. Indications for thymectomy in myasthenia gravis. Neurology 1990;40:1828–1829

70. Schumm F, Wietholter H, Fateh-Moghadam A, et al. Thymectomy in myasthenia with pure ocular symptoms. J Neuro Neurosurg Psych 1985;48:332–337

169 Cavernous Sinus Disorders

Mark J Kupersmith and Daniel R Lefton

Anatomical, clinical, and radiological features of cavernous sinus disorders

Anatomy of the cavernous sinus region

In order to diagnose, understand, and treat the various clinical syndromes caused by lesions in the cavernous sinus, the complex relationship of the neural, arterial and venous structures must be appreciated. The cavernous sinus is an extradural area comprised of venous channels and dura which contains the third and fourth nerves, the first two divisions of the fifth nerve, the sixth nerve, arachnoid along the cranial nerves (possibly where meningiomas arise), small amounts of fat, the internal carotid artery (ICA), and collateral arteries from the internal maxillary artery. The cavernous sinus is bordered medially by the dura of the sella and the sphenoid sinus, anteriorly by the dura reflected from the sphenoid wing and superior orbital fissure, laterally by the dural leaves which contain the third nerve, posteriorly by the dura of the petrous portion of the temporal bone, superiorly by dura, and inferiorly by dura of the skull base. The parasellar venous anatomy is variable among individuals and between each side. A plexus of venous structures, not a single channel, is formed by trabeculae. The superior and inferior petrosal sinuses provide a venous outlet posteriorly. Small emissary veins provide an outlet inferiorly through the foramen ovale. Venous inflow is through the ophthalmic vein anteriorly, and through the sphenoparietal sinus and the middle cerebral vein superiorly. The cavernous sinus is connected anteriorly and posteriorly to the opposite cavernous sinus via the coronary sinuses, and posteriorly via the basilar venous plexus.

The cavernous sinus is the only region in the body in which an artery is enveloped by a venous structure. The ICA enters the cavernous sinus via the carotid canal. This segment (C5) contains a posterior branch (meningohypophyseal trunk or C5 branch) that divides into posterior inferior hypophyseal, medial clival (anastomoses with ascending pharyngeal artery), and lateral and medial marginal tentorial arteries. A branch off the horizontal segment (inferior lateral trunk or C4 branch) anastomoses with the artery to the foramen rotundum, middle meningeal artery, and accessory meningeal artery (dural branches).[1-3] The ascending portion (C3) of the ICA passes superiorly, passing intradurally (below the anterior clinoid) through a hole in the dura which is separated into two thin rings of dura that have a space between them (area where "ring" aneurysms arise). The arterial supply to the cranial nerves arises predominantly from the branches of the ICA or the external carotid artery collaterals (dural branches) depending on the balance between the two systems.[3-5] The cavernous ICA branches supply many tumors in the cavernous sinus. The dural branches also supply the dural-based tumors such as meningiomas.

The third, fourth, and first division of the fifth nerves course between leaves of lateral dura while the sixth nerve passes in the space of the venous channels below the cavernous ICA. The sympathetics to the pupillary dilator muscle and Müller's muscle of the upper and lower lids run on the surface of the ICA, join the fascicles of the sixth nerve, and enter the orbit with the first division of the fifth nerve. Thus, a single ischemic defect in the cavernous sinus could cause a third order Horner's syndrome as well as a sixth nerve palsy (however, this remains a diagnosis of exclusion). The third (medial to the fourth) and fourth nerves enter the dura of the posterior cavernous sinus through a groove between the tentorial attachments to the posterior clinoid. The third nerve divides into a superior division, which innervates the levator palpebrae and superior rectus muscles, and an inferior division which innervates the pupillary sphincter and ciliary muscle via a synapse in the ciliary ganglion and the medial, inferior oblique and inferior recti muscles. The third and fourth nerves pass through the leaves of dura in the lateral cavernous sinus.

The fifth (first and second divisions) and sixth nerves enter the cavernous sinus posteriorly and inferiorly to the third and fourth nerves, the sixth via a reflection of dura, Dorello's canal, while the fifth nerve enters through the dura nearby. The sixth nerve passes through the cavernous sinus in the lower venous channels. The first division of the fifth nerve passes through the cavernous sinus in the inferior lateral wall dura. The third, fourth, first division fifth, and sixth nerve enter the orbit via the superior orbital fissure. The second division fifth nerve exits through the foramen rotundum and the third division exits via the foramen ovale. The optic nerve is intradural, outside the cavernous sinus, and enters the orbit via the optic canal with the ophthalmic artery. Simultaneous or consecutive dysfunction of ipsilateral cranial nerves three to five localizes the lesion to the cavernous sinus. Rarely, this results from ischemic disease,[4] but this etiology is a diagnosis of exclusion.

Symptoms and clinical findings

Pain, paresthesias and numbness are common with most disorders of the cavernous sinus and are usually located in the distribution of the first division of the trigeminal nerve. The pain can be lancinating, deep and boring, or dull (with the associated fifth nerve or other cranial nerve findings readily distinguished from trigeminal neuralgia). When sensory symptoms involve the second division as well, this suggests that the lesion extends to the posterior cavernous sinus. If the third division is affected, the lesion extends posteriorly outside the cavernous sinus. Motor fifth nerve dysfunction is less common but the associated jaw misalignment can cause pain with chewing. A sixth nerve paresis can be the first clinical manifestation of any cavernous sinus lesion, but dysfunction of the other cranial nerves typically occurs either concomitantly or at a later date. Due to the location of the sixth nerve in the inferior aspect of the cavernous sinus, abducens dysfunction is common with lesions that invade the cavernous sinus from an extracranial locale, such as nasopharyngeal tumors. Patients with meningioma, neurinoma, dural arteriovenous malformation (AVM), and cavernous aneurysm may only have lateral rectus weakness for months to years. In older patients (vasculopathic group) who do not improve over two months, gadolinium magnetic resonance imaging (MRI) with detailed views of the base of the skull and cavernous sinus should be performed (if negative, an edrophonium test should be considered to exclude myasthenia gravis).

A third nerve paresis can be the first and only sign of a cavernous aneurysm, pituitary adenoma, meningioma, dural AVM or neurinoma. Most patients, however, have dysfunction of other cranial nerves at presentation or a later date. When present, the ptosis can be partial or complete. The pupil may appear normal even when the levator and all the third nerve muscles are affected. When patients do not have pupillary dysfunction and lack pain, even though the signs remain strictly unilateral, the third nerve dysfunction has been misdiagnosed as myasthenia gravis, and false positive edrophonium testing has been described.[6,7] When these patients failed to significantly improve with medical therapy, however, the diagnoses were established. When abnormal, the pupil may be larger and fixed to light and accommodation, or the dilation may be as little as 1 mm and slightly less reactive to light. A superior division (monocular paresis of upward movement and upper lid ptosis) or inferior division (weakness of medial rectus, inferior rectus, and pupillary dilation and poor reactivity) third nerve paresis is strongly suggestive of a lesion in the cavernous sinus. Chronic compression of the third nerve can lead to misdirection phenomena due to regrowth of axons into the wrong fascicles. Examples include failure of the lid to completely descend or the lid retracts on attempted downgaze, lid elevation on attempted adduction, pupillary contraction on attempted downgaze or adduction. A misdirection syndrome typically occurs with meningioma and cavernous aneurysms, suggesting that the lesion has been compressing the third nerve for months or years.[8,9] Pupillary dilation without lid or ocular muscle disturbance should not be considered a sign of third nerve compression or infiltration in the cavernous sinus.

The fourth nerve is commonly affected by cavernous sinus lesions, but it is almost always associated with other cranial nerve dysfunction. A fourth nerve paresis is rarely the only sign, and the neuro-ophthalmology axiom—the patient with an isolated fourth nerve palsy (which means there are no other symptoms or neurological findings) does not need extensive testing and neuroimaging—remains an important clinical pearl.

The incidence of third order sympathetic dysfunction is difficult to assess. In the individual with third nerve dysfunction that affects the lid and pupil, the clinical determination of mild sympathetic ptosis and small pupil, particularly in the dark, is difficult. The hydroxyamphetamine drop test may also be difficult to assess. However, the presence of denervation supersensitivity to phenylephrine or upward ptosis of the lower lid suggests sympathetic dysfunction. Few reports have explored this issue.

If a patient develops proptosis, the lesion usually extends into the orbit, via the superior orbital fissure or optic canal, or through bone destruction. Hyperostosis of the sphenoid wing with meningioma or bone metastases (prostate or breast carcinoma) can also cause proptosis with resistance to manual retropulsion. Proptosis can also be caused by orbital congestion from blockage of venous outflow from the orbit. Mild exophthalmos, approximately 2 mm, can occur with total ophthalmoplegia and relaxation of the orbit.

Visual loss is not typical when the lesion is restricted to the cavernous sinus. Compression of the optic nerve in the orbital apex (with proptosis, extraocular muscle limitation), in the optic canal, or intracranially develops with lesion extension. If an anterior visual pathway compromise occurs early in the course or with little or no ocular muscle or lid dysfunction, it suggests that the lesion probably arose outside the cavernous sinus and secondarily invaded the cavernous sinus. Visual loss can also result from corneal lesions due to exposure or a loss of corneal sensation. An anesthetic cornea implies that the lesion extends to involve the posterior cavernous sinus.

Radiological investigations and diagnostic features

MRI is superior to computed tomography (CT) in the investigation of most lesions of the cavernous sinus.[10] However, CT shows bone erosion, remodeling, and hyperostosis.[10] Artifact from dental work can limit the coronal views needed to view the cavernous sinus. The CT can be used to guide aspiration biopsy through the foramen ovale to the parasellar area[11] or into the orbit when the lesion extends anteriorly.[12]

MRI demonstrates the cavernous sinus anatomy, vascular structures, and soft tissue of the cavernous sinus in multiple planes. After intravenous gadolinium, lesions can be seen to extend along the dura and along the cranial nerves when there is perineural spread of a malignancy.

Angiography is no longer a "first-line" diagnostic procedure performed in the evaluation of cavernous sinus lesions. MRI and magnetic resonance angiography (MRA) have replaced angiography for diagnosis even when a cavernous carotid aneurysm, dural AVM, or carotid cavernous fistula is the etiology. However, angiography is still performed in the treatment planning of these lesions. Angiography may also be helpful in evaluation of a lesion with similar CT and MRI appearances. For example, a meningioma in the cavernous sinus that invades the sella can be differentiated from a nonsecretory pituitary adenoma that infiltrates the cavernous sinus if the former lesion has its dural blood supply demonstrated (Figure 169.1).

Angiography may also be used to demonstrate prominent vascularity and the need for presurgical embolization.[13,14] The venous phase of the angiogram shows thrombosis within the cavernous sinus or ophthalmic venous drainage.[15,16]

Venography via the ophthalmic venous system or inferior petrosal sinus is rarely used except in the treatment of arteriovenous shunts that affect the cavernous sinus.[17,18]

Clinical etiologies

Reports on the distribution of the etiologies of clinical cavernous sinus syndromes vary widely depending on whether high resolution contrast imaging was available and on the interests of the reporting service. Refer, for example, to the tables from neuro-ophthalmology series (Table 169.1), neuro-ophthalmology/

neurovascular service series (Table 169.2), and surgical treatment series (Table 169.3).

Other causes of cavernous sinus dysfunction not discussed in this chapter include cavernous sinus thrombosis, invasion or infarct or hemorrhage of pituitary adenoma (Figure 169.2) or carcinoma, chondroma, sarcoma, angiofibroma,[20] Wegener's granulomatosis,[22,23] hemangiopericytoma,[24] epidermoid,[25,26] and sarcoidosis.[27,28] Infectious cavernous sinus thrombosis most commonly arises in immunocompromised or diabetic individuals and is due to adjacent infectious sinus disease (most commonly fungal) which is not always readily apparent.[29] Thrombosis can also develop in patients with hypercoagulable disorders. Minor orbital congestion and conjunctival injection, in

Table 169.1   Distribution of parasellar syndromes[19]

Etiology	Number of patients
Metastatic distant spread	23
Nasopharyngeal tumor	19
Arterial aneurysm	19
Chondroma or chordoma	8
Pituitary adenoma	6
Multiple myeloma, lymphoma	4
Meningioma	3
Herpes zoster	3
Tolosa–Hunt syndrome	3
Arachnoiditis	3
Temporal arteritis	2
Craniopharyngioma	2
Sarcoma	2
Neurofibroma	1
Giant cell tumor	1
Wegener's granulomatosis	1
Lues	1
Cylindroma	1

Table 169.2   Neuro-ophthalmology/neurovascular service distribution of cavernous sinus lesions (Kupersmith)

Etiology	Number of patients
Aneurysm	168
Dural arterial venous malformation	150
Carotid cavernous fistula	100
Pituitary adenoma	75
Meningioma	30
Lymphoma	10
Neurinoma	10
Nasopharyngeal tumor	15
Metastatic carcinoma	10
Chordoma	4
Tolosa–Hunt syndrome	4
Diabetes mellitus	2
Hemangioma	1
Fungal invasion	3
Juvenile angiofibroma[20]	1

Patient with temporal arteritis and herpes zoster not included because localization was in orbit or superior orbital fissure.

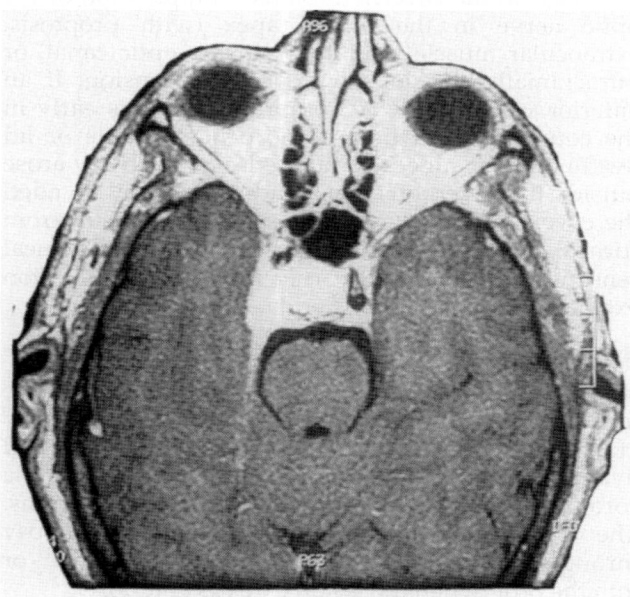

Figure 169.1 A 42-year-old man developed a painless, progressive third nerve palsy over one month. He had diplopia first and later developed a ptosis. On examination, his only finding was a partial pupillary sparing third nerve palsy that affected all of the third nerve innervated eye muscles, and partial ptosis. The MRI with gadolinium demonstrated a mass in the cavernous sinus and in the sella with a suggestion of a "dural tail." The differential included meningioma and pituitary adenoma.

Table 169.3   Tumors involving cavernous sinus from a skull base neurosurgery service[21]

Etiology	Number of patients
Chondrosarcoma	46
Squamous cell carcinoma	30
Adenoid cystic carcinoma	26
Meningioma	21
Chordoma	18
Juvenile angiofibroma	18
Hypernephroma (metastatic)	16
Neurinoma (trigeminal)	13
Chondroblastoma	13
Pituitary adenoma	9
Plasmacytoma	6
Hemangioma	5

addition to visual loss and ophthalmoplegia, are common.

Unilateral ophthalmoparesis with or without ptosis can occur from disorders that do not affect the cranial nerves in the cavernous sinus. Multiple cranial nerves can be affected from carcinomatosis, sarcoid, and infectious meningeal infiltration. Myasthenia gravis can present with unilateral dysfunction but the pupil and sensory fifth nerve dysfunction do not occur. Dysthyroid orbitopathy (usually bilateral) can be unilateral, but lid retraction rather than ptosis, absence of pupil and sensory fifth nerve dysfunction, proptosis, periorbital infiltration, injection over recti muscle insertions, a positive forced duction test, and preferential limitation in abduction or elevation or both are characteristic to this disorder. The Miller Fisher variant of Guillain–Barré syndrome can be markedly asymmetrical and cause pupillary dysfunction, but there is no fifth nerve dysfunction, and cerebellar signs and areflexia are typically present. Ischemia of the muscles in the orbit, rather than the cranial nerves, prior to visual loss occurs with giant cell arteritis, a disorder of elderly individuals. Ophthalmoplegic migraine is a rare disorder that begins in childhood and most commonly affects solely the third nerve.

There have been major diagnostic advances with high resolution contrast enhanced CT and MRI. Reports prior to these developments included a much higher incidence of patients suspected of having Tolosa–Hunt syndrome (inflammatory disorder), many of whom probably had other disorders (Table 169.4). The diagnosis of patients with a parasellar syndrome (either painful or painless ophthalmoparesis with more than one cranial nerve dysfunction) based solely on the clinical presentation is inaccurate because the pattern of dysfunction and evolution of signs and symptoms are nonspecific. This was well recognized by Thomas and Yoss in their review of 102 such patients, found in a database of 1000 patients with ocular motor nerve dysfunction before the introduction of high resolution CT.[19] They also found that the presence of pain (found in 80%) or remission of the symptoms and signs, either spontaneously or in

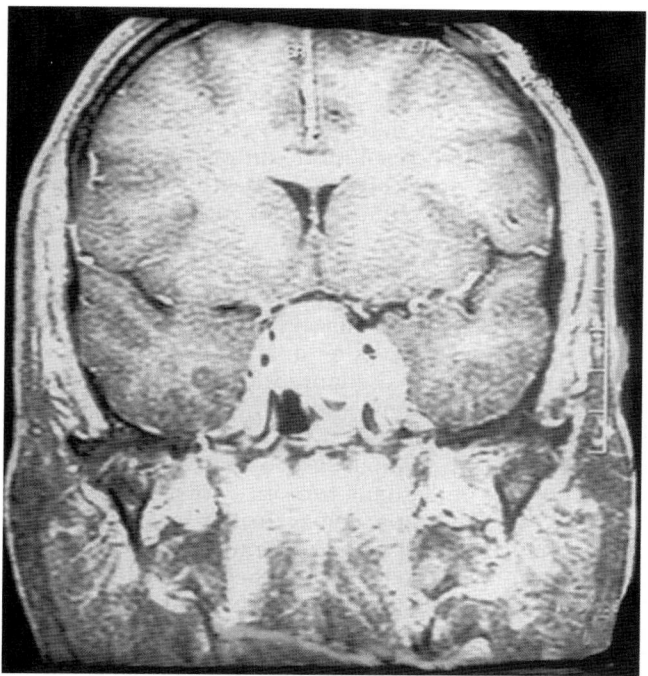

Figure 169.2   A 44-year-old woman had one week of symptoms of a scotoma in the right eye and pain over this eye. The visual acuity was 20/100 OD and 20/25 OS with bitemporal visual field depression, and the remaining cranial nerves were normal. The contrast enhanced coronal MRI showed a uniformly enhancing pituitary tumor confirmed at surgery to be a pituitary adenoma that invaded both cavernous sinuses. Although this was not a meningioma, each cavernous ICA appeared encased by the tumor.

association with steroid therapy, was not an accurate mode of securing a diagnosis. For example, one patient with a chordoma and one with a giant cell tumor had "prompt clearing of symptoms and signs" with steroid therapy and the benefit remained for 4 years. We have seen patients with a "white-eyed" shunt due to a dural AVM or a cavernous carotid aneurysm have spontaneous normalization or

Table 169.4   Differential for painful unilateral ophthalmoplegia not limited to a single cranial neuropathy

Location	Etiology
Cavernous sinus	Aneurysm
	Neoplasm[†]
	Inflammation (idiopathic)[*]
	Infection (from adjacent sinus)
Superior orbital fissure	Neoplasm[†]
	Inflammation (idiopathic)[*]
Orbit	Dysthyroid[†]
	Infection
	Inflammation (idiopathic)
	Neoplasm[†]

[*]Rare; [†]with or without pain.

improvement of the cranial nerve dysfunction and pain.

Therapies

Therapeutic options have increased with better localization using high resolution contrast enhanced MRI and improved surgical approaches to the cavernous sinus,[21,30,31] endovascular embolization methods, and better targeting of radiotherapy. Some success has been gained in developing procedures that are designed to spare cranial nerve function.[32] Cranial nerves injured during surgery can be repaired with end to end anastomosis or intervening nerve graft.[33] Both benign[34] and malignant lesions which have been treated with gamma knife radiotherapy have demonstrated reduction in the size of the lesion and improvement in cranial nerve function. However, recurrence of malignant tumors, worse cranial neuropathy, and radiation injury to the brain and optic nerves have been reported. We must not lose sight of the natural history of many of these disorders, which has revealed that many cause little or no deterioration over long time periods. In many patients, despite available therapies, the best approach is careful follow-up with clinical and MRI evaluations.

Meningioma

Demographics

Meningiomas are currently considered the most common tumor affecting the cavernous sinus. In the older literature, however, meningiomas constitute only 3% of lesions causing cavernous sinus syndromes.[19] Meningiomas in all locations account for up to 18% of all intracranial tumors with women affected twice as often as men. In some reports the gender ratio is 2.3:1 women:men for the cavernous sinus location.[35] In contrast, in our series of 31 cases of meningiomas located in the cavernous sinus, women were affected six times more commonly than men. All intracranial meningiomas, including those that arise in or invade the cavernous sinus, affect individuals in the third to eighth decades and are rare during the first decade of life. Children rarely develop a cavernous sinus meningioma.[36]

Clinical symptoms and findings

Patients commonly report binocular diplopia that is due to sixth[37] or third nerve or multiple nerve compression. The diplopia may be reported as intermittent or might be observed intermittently by the patient if it only affects an eccentric position of gaze.[6] The onset of third nerve dysfunction can be insidious, and, at the first examination, signs of oculomotor nerve aberrant regeneration can be present.[38] Ptosis of varying degrees accompanies the third nerve dysfunction, but as in other cavernous mass lesions, pupillary function may be normal. Numbness or paresthesias in the distribution of the first division of the trigeminal nerve occurs but is less frequent, and severe pain or neuralgia is atypical. However, approximately 50% of patients have some degree of

ipsilateral frontal headache. It is difficult to document third order sympathetic dysfunction, particularly in the setting of third lesion-associated pupillary dilation and ptosis.[6] Patients rarely present with isolated sympathetic dysfunction even when cluster-like symptoms occur.[39] Tumor obstruction in the cavernous sinus can block ophthalmic venous return and cause congestion of the extraocular muscles and orbital soft tissue as well as dilation of the ophthalmic vein. The onset of symptoms can be insidious so that it may take years before patients seek medical evaluation.

A cavernous sinus syndrome can develop from invasion of the cavernous sinus by a meningioma that originates from the dura of the petroclinoid region and cerebellar pontine angle. These patients frequently have dysfunction of the seventh and eighth nerves as well as of all three divisions of the trigeminal nerve.

Neuroimaging

The noncontrast CT shows some degree of hyperostosis in bone (clinoid process and sphenoid wing) adjacent to the mass in approximately 80% of patients. The meningioma can demonstrate a signal of similar attenuation to the brain. Calcification, possibly located in the carotid artery wall or from bone erosion, may be seen in the mass. After contrast, most meningiomas enhance significantly and many demonstrate extension along the tentorium. Bone displacement and thinning, but not destruction, are seen.

On MRI[40] the meningiomas appear isodense with normal brain on T_1-weighted images and bright on T_2-weighted images. Following gadolinium, meningiomas demonstrate considerable enhancement (Figure 169.3). Tumor extension to the petroclinoid ligament or along the tentorium causes a "tail" of enhancement. High resolution contrast enhanced MRI may determine the point of origination for small size tumors, particularly when the meningioma arises from the lateral wall of the cavernous sinus. Outward bulging of the lateral wall is typically demonstrated. Encasement of the ICA is seen in approximately 50% of cases.

On angiography,[41] a tumor stain is seen in the late arterial or early capillary phase due to supply from cavernous ICA arterial feeders. External carotid artery branches, usually via the middle meningeal artery, provide arterial supply to the tumor in less than a third of cases. Prior to the advent of high resolution CT or MRI, mild to severe encasement of the petrous, cavernous or intradural ICA was reported in more than 70% of patients.

Natural history

Meningiomas are rarely malignant but invasion into the brain seems to occur more often when multiple mitoses or anaplasia are found in the tumor.[42] During a follow-up period of 10 years, we have found that many of these tumors do not grow or worsen the presenting cranial nerve dysfunction. This includes tumors that are restricted to the cavernous sinus as

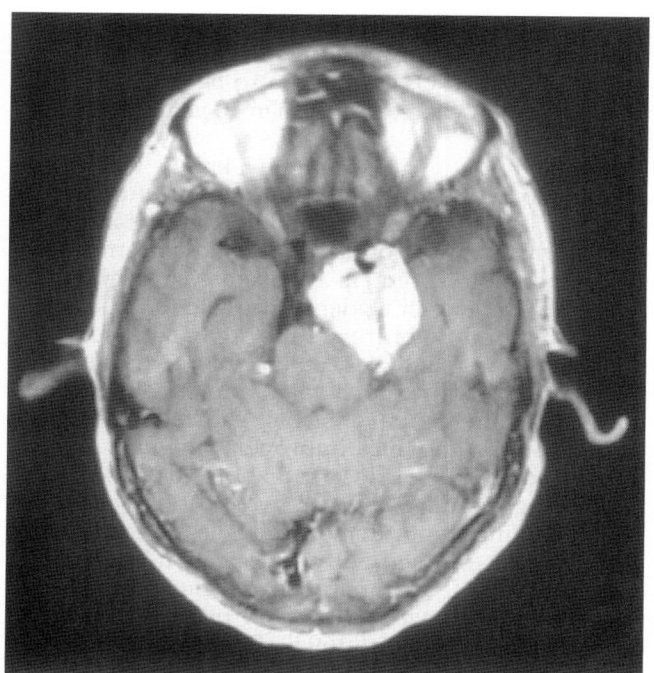

Figure 169.3 A 70-year-old woman had symptoms of painless vertical binocular diplopia for 2 years. The neurological and ophthalmological examinations were normal except for ocular motor function. The versions were full but in primary gaze there was a right hypertropia of 9 prism diopters that was worse on left gaze and estropia of 2 prism diopters that was worse on right gaze. The hypertropia was worse on tilting the head to the right and better tilting to the left. This suggested right fourth and sixth nerve pareses. The T_1-weighted image after gadolinium administration showed a uniformly enhancing mass (meningioma) arising from the cavernous sinus. The examination and MRI were unchanged 4 years later.

well as those that extend into the prepontine cistern to compress the brainstem, into the sella to compress the pituitary gland and stalk, and into the inferior and super orbital fissures. Progressive or new neuropathy of the third, fourth, fifth, and sixth nerves does occur in some cases. Continued growth of the meningioma over years can cause symptomatic compression of the brain, brainstem, and anterior visual pathway. Extension into the orbit can cause proptosis and optic neuropathy from tumor in the orbital apex. The rare meningioma arising in the cavernous sinus in children may affect boys more often and have sarcomatous degeneration.[36]

Most studies report the immediate or moderate duration follow-up, but there is no large series documenting the long term follow-up of patients with these slow growing tumors. Analysis of our 18 patients with primary cavernous sinus meningioma revealed that in the seven untreated patients followed for an average of 3.5 years, one had tumor growth on MRI, and none had a major worsening of the presenting cranial neuropathy. In another small series, one of six patients followed for an average of 4.3 years had minor clinical and MRI progression.[43] And in a third

report, during a briefer follow-up of 2 years, five of six patients had minor or no symptoms.[44] Meningiomas that become symptomatic during pregnancy often remit after delivery, but virtually all of these women become symptomatic again over the ensuing years.

Whether patients are followed expectantly, treated with surgery, surgery and radiotherapy, or radiotherapy alone, yearly clinical follow-up evaluations and gadolinium MRI every 2–3 years seem warranted.

Treatment[45]

Currently, there are three options for the treatment of meningiomas in the cavernous sinus. The first is expectant follow-up with clinical examinations and MRI and the management of the cranial neuropathy and pain. The second is surgical excision of the tumor. The third is radiotherapy. All three approaches must be evaluated in the context of the natural history of this lesion, which is often slowly progressive over the course of 20 years. Most therapeutic approaches are reported with a short duration (1 to 5 years) follow-up. Stabilization or improvement in symptoms and findings that allow individuals to function independently can not be underestimated, particularly for elderly patients where survival for decades may not be a relevant issue.

Surgical removal of meningioma from the cavernous sinus has improved with new methods. However, infiltration of ocular motor nerves can prevent a good result.[35] Incompletely excised tumors are reported to regrow in approximately 15% of patients during a period of less than three years.[46,47] Surgical excision is infrequently curative and can cause worse or new neuropathy or a hemiparesis.[45,46,48,49] Infiltration of the adventitia and muscular media of the cavernous ICA can also limit complete excision. However, if patients have adequate collateral arterial flow (determined preoperatively), the ICA can be sacrificed and removed with the tumor.[50,51] In patients with aggressive tumors and progressive neurological compromise, radical surgery may be indicated and bypass surgery to the distal ICA or middle cerebral artery can be considered. Clearly, this procedure increases the treatment risk and proper case selection is warranted. Some authors report that when radical surgery is accomplished in individuals with less extensive cranial base meningiomas, the 5-year recurrence rate is 4% in contrast to a rate as high as 45% in those with larger tumors and without major excision.[52] However, by 15 years, 25% of the patients with small radically excised tumors experience recurrence. In contrast, others report a 50% recurrence within four years in lesions considered to be completely resected.[53] When the tumor has invaded the pituitary fossa and causes visual loss, the optic apparatus may be decompressed without a craniotomy, using a transphenoidal approach.[54] Surgical excision carries the least risk in the infrequent case when the tumor arises from the lateral dural wall and does not appear to infiltrate the cranial nerves (Figure 169.4).

Radiotherapy is recommended for patients with

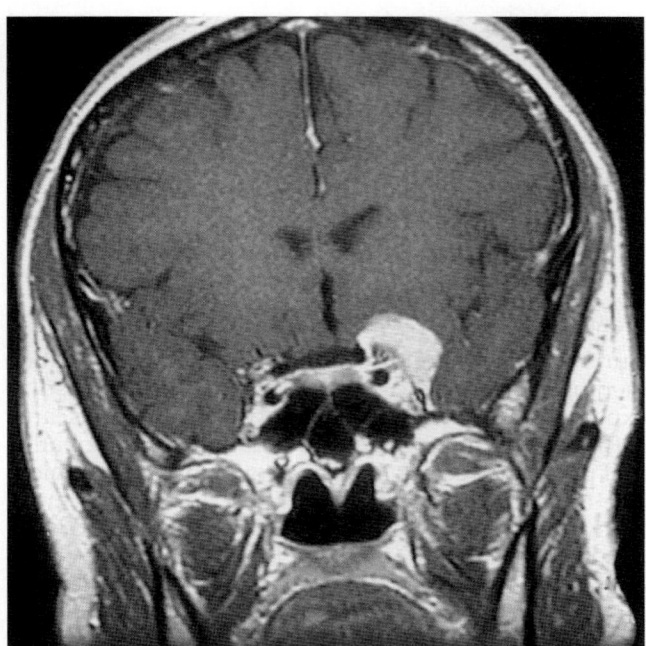

Figure 169.4 A 40-year-old woman had MRI in the evaluation for galactorrhea and elevated prolactin that had been present for many years. She had no neuro-ophthalmological symptoms or findings. The coronal MRI with gadolinium showed a uniformly enhancing mass, presumed meningioma, which seemed to be separated from the cavernous sinus by the dural lateral wall. Surgical excision was recommended and rejected. She has remained clinically normal despite slight tumor growth over a 3-year follow-up.

progressive symptoms and meningiomas that can not be excised without causing a significant new or worse deficit. Conventional dose conformal multiday radiation can be considered in cases where the tumor is abutting the intracranial optic nerve or chiasm or brainstem.[55] Conventional dose radiation, 1.8 to 2 Gy daily delivered via opposed lateral or three-field techniques to the localized field of the tumor and 2 cm margins for a total dose of 45 to 60 Gy, has been demonstrated to prevent tumor growth or clinical deterioration for 5 years in 81% to 88% of patients with parasellar meningiomas.[56,57] Even though the cranial neuropathy frequently improves or resolves, the mass infrequently appears smaller on follow-up MRI. Tumors smaller than 5 cm seem to have better rates of control than larger tumors. Tumor recurrence with invasion through the superior orbital fissure to the orbital apex can cause vision loss.[48] Although at 10 years conventional radiotherapy reduces the mortality rate, by 20 years the difference for radiated and nonradiated patients was not significant.[52] The failures or recurrence frequently seem to occur at tumor margins outside the prescribed isodose. In other reports, the cranial neuropathy and pain improved or resolved but the tumor mass was infrequently reduced.[58,59] Computer-assisted or conformal radiotherapy appears to reduce exposure to surrounding neural structures and radiation-induced neurotoxic-

ity. This type of radiation is most often applied when the risk of complication seems likely with radiosurgery (see below). It should also be considered for use in patients where greater than 10 years' follow-up is not critical.

Radiosurgery with gamma knife technology appears to be useful when the average tumor diameter is less than 3.5 cm and the tumor is at least 4 mm away from the optic nerves and chiasm.[60] Multiple irradiation isocenters are used to cover the mass by the 50% or greater isodense lines (16 to 20 Gy) with the minimum dose of from 10 to 20 Gy applied to the tumor margins and less than 9 Gy to the optic pathway. For two to four years after treatment, two thirds of patients have stable clinical evaluations while less than one third improve.[61] However, in contrast to conventional dose radiation, 37% to 68% of tumors regress on MRI over two to four years.[34,61,62] The remaining tumor demonstrates less enhancement in 24% of cases. Even with the selection criteria discussed above, 7% of patients develop visual loss, which may improve with steroid treatment, and 7% develop seizures (Figure 169.5). Brainstem symptoms, usually steroid responsive, occur in almost 18% of cases and worse cranial neuropathy may develop in 20% or more of patients.[34,63] Some authors have concluded that attempting to limit the dose of treatment to the optic apparatus to less than 8 Gy is unnecessary and could result in 68% of patients receiving suboptimal radiation.[34] Radiation alone (dose and methodology not stated) has prevented tumor progression in six of six patients during an average of 4.3 years.[64] Perhaps targeting the tumor to exclude the portions that abut important central nervous system structures could be considered. In young or middle-aged adults, partial surgical resection to decompress the brainstem and visual pathway in order to create a margin free of tumor might allow the use of radiosurgery in a meningioma otherwise considered unacceptable for this therapy.[55] It is hoped that radiosurgery will have a longer duration of tumor control than conventional radiotherapy. Currently, the follow-up period in most studies is not long enough to draw a clear conclusion.

Medical therapies that block progesterone or estrogen receptors have been ineffective. Hydroxyurea, daily oral dose 1000 to 1500 mg, has been reported to reduce the tumor size in three patients with tumor involvement in the cavernous sinus, two of whom failed radiation therapy. The associated trigeminal pain also improved in two of these cases.[65] Newer therapies such as timazolamide are being evaluated to determine if meningioma growth can be controlled without high risk of complications.

Cavernous hemangioma (cavernoma)
Demographics

Cavernous hemangiomas are much less common than meningiomas, schwannomas, arteriovenous shunts, or aneurysms of the cavernous sinus, but the incidence has been stated to be as high as 2% of all benign intracranial mass lesions and 3% of benign cavernous

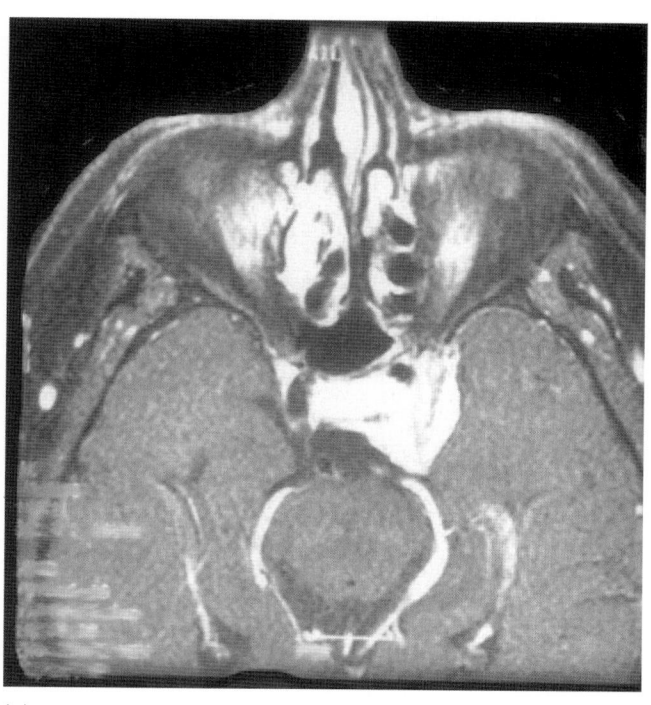
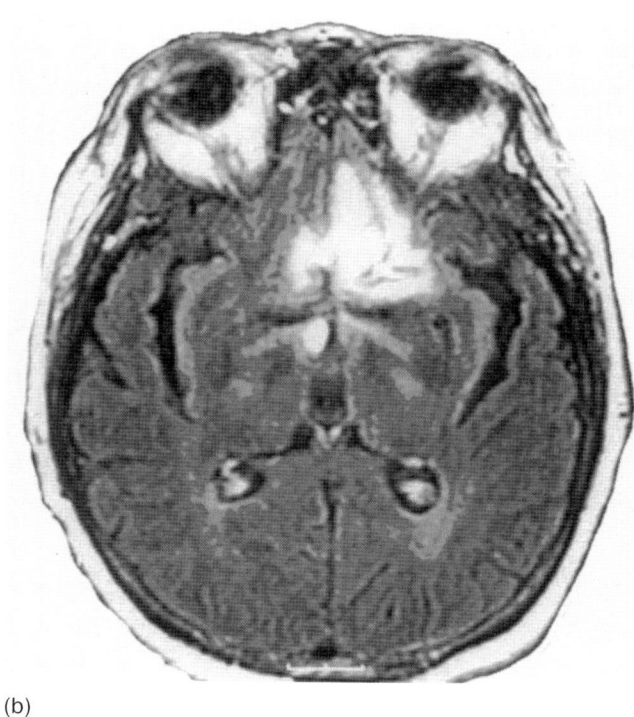

(a)   (b)

Figure 169.5 A 63-year-old man without a history of hypertension or diabetes developed sudden painless loss of vision in the left eye. He had been treated with gamma knife radiosurgery one year previously for a meningioma that invaded the cavernous sinus and was found in the evaluation of tinnitus without diplopia. The examination revealed 20/20 OD and finger counting vision at 2 feet OS, mild disk pallor (not shown), and the remainder of the exam was normal except for the relative afferent pupillary defect OS. MRI performed two weeks after the visual loss demonstrated a uniformly enhancing mass (meningioma) in the cavernous sinus on the T_1-weighted images after gadolinium administration (a). On the fluid attenuated inversion recovery images, there was signal abnormality in the frontal lobes and hypothalamus suggestive of vasogenic edema due to radiation injury (b).

sinus tumors.[66] Women are affected three times more often than men. Symptoms develop during the third to eighth decades of life. Because symptoms have first appeared during pregnancy, some authors have suggested that these lesions are affected by hormonal changes.[67] However, since these lesions appear to contain no hormonal receptors, and most of the affected individuals are women, the presentation during pregnancy most likely is due to blood volume and systemic coagulation alterations.

Clinical symptoms and findings

Patients present with symptoms typical of a mass in the cavernous sinus. The symptoms can develop abruptly, possibly due to thrombus or hemorrhage within the lesion, can occur intermittently, or can progress over years. Diplopia, ptosis, paresthesias in the first or second trigeminal distribution, anesthetic cornea, and headache are common. Patients can present with an isolated sixth nerve paresis.[68] Loss of vision can result from secondary corneal dysfunction but, if the mass expands progressively, visual loss can occur from compression of the optic pathway. In rare instances, painful optic neuropathy occurs early.[69]

Neuroimaging

Prior to contrast administration, the mass can be iso-dense with brain on CT. After contrast, cavernous

hemangioma in this location frequently demonstrates homogeneous marked enhancement. The adjacent sphenoid wing and anterior clinoid bone may show erosion or remodeling, but no hyperostosis or frank destruction.

On MRI the lesion may be isointense on T_1-weighted and bright white on T_2-weighted images. On occasion, the lesion is only mildly bright or there is a heterogeneous reticulated pattern on the T_2-weighted sequence. After gadolinium, the mass enhances brightly, unlike cavernous hemangioma in the brain or orbit, on the T_1-weighted image (Figure 169.6a–c). If there are no bone abnormalities, the appearance on CT and MRI may be indistinguishable from a hemangiopericytoma or a meningioma, particularly the angioblastic type of meningioma.

Angiography may only show the mass effect on the petrous and cavernous portions of the internal carotid artery. The ICA is not narrowed by the tumor. The external carotid artery infrequently supplies the lesion via the middle meningeal and accessory meningeal arteries. Irregular areas of blush may be seen in the late arterial phase due to arterial feeders from the C4 and C5 branches from the cavernous ICA. Contrast dye may pool in areas of the tumor. The angiographic appearance of a tumor blush from the cavernous ICA may appear similar to a meningioma without supply from the middle meningeal artery.

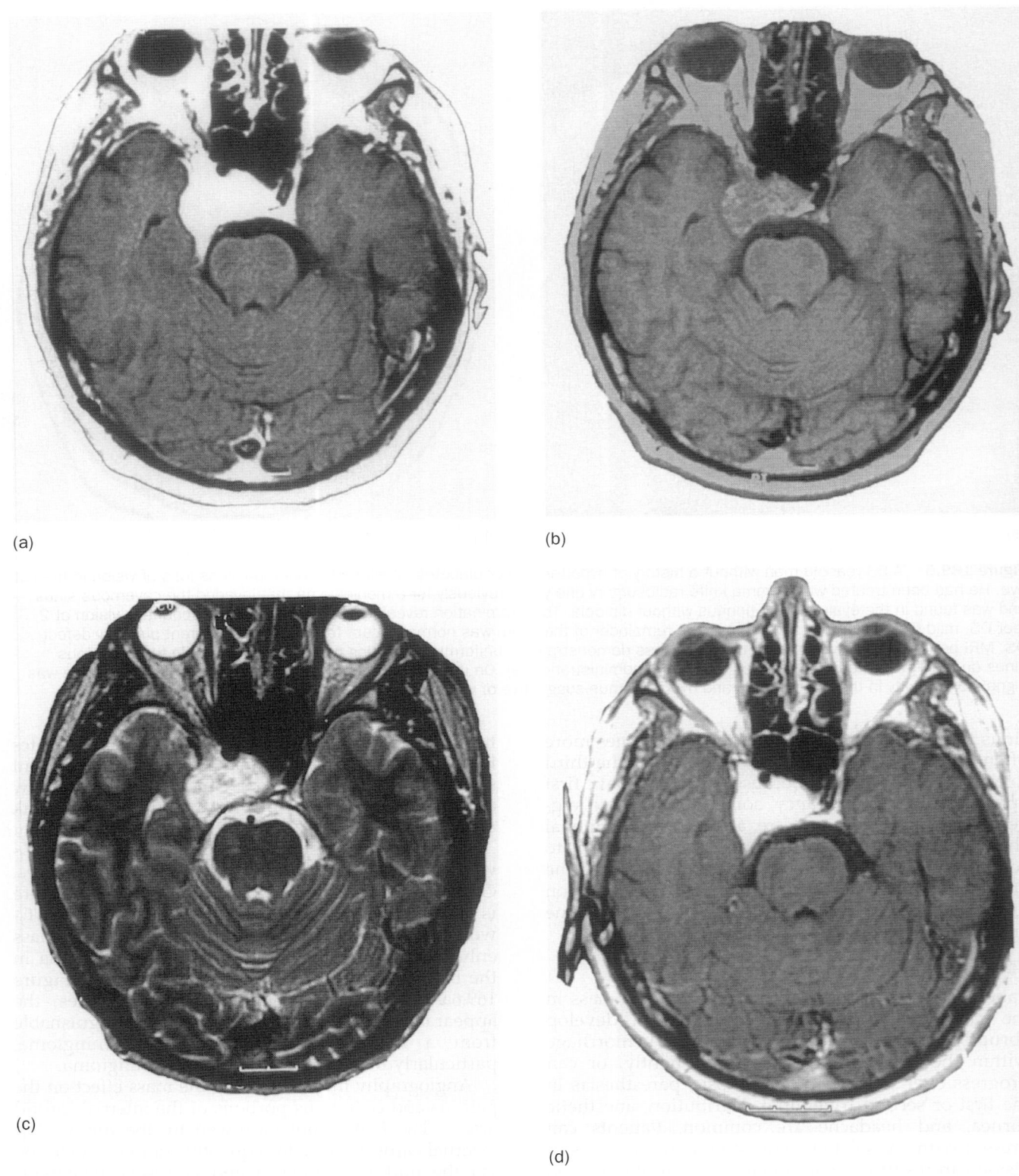

(a)

(b)

(c)

(d)

Figure 169.6   A 50-year-old man developed sudden onset of pain over the right eye and a right upper lid ptosis of one-day duration. On examination, he had 6 mm of right upper lid ptosis and marked underaction of upgaze with right eye suspicious of a superior branch third nerve paresis. The T1-weighted images demonstrated a mass with a reticulated appearance that enhanced uniformly after gadolinium administration (a, b). The lesion had a heterogeneous appearance on the T2-weighted images (c). He was suspected of having a cavernous hemangioma. He received prednisone 60 mg and the pain resolved. Within three months and off the prednisone, his examination was normal. Three years later his examination is entirely normal and MRI demonstrates that the mass is smaller (d).

Natural history

Most of the literature suggests that cavernous hemangiomas in the cavernous sinus commonly increase in size and stretch and compress the cranial nerves resulting in worsening or new cranial nerve dysfunction.[66,67,69–82] Cavernous hemangiomas increase in size due to several mechanisms that include thrombosis and hemorrhage in the vascular channels, capillary growth at the margin of the lesion, and dilation of the vascular spaces. If the lesion grows through the posterior cavernous sinus to involve Meckel's cave, fifth nerve motor dysfunction can develop.[83] The lesion can grow and invade the middle fossa to cause hemispheric dysfunction or into the suprasellar cistern or erode into the orbital apex to cause optic neuropathy or chiasm dysfunction. The mass rarely extends to become life threatening. These lesions may also remain static for years. We have seen the neuropathy and lesion spontaneously regress with no relationship to pregnancy or hormone use (Figure 169.6d). Most of these articles are from neurosurgical or radiation oncology services that were frequently often referred these cases due to a progressive process. Postpartum women can have spontaneous resolution of the cranial neuropathy.[67]

Treatment

Surgical excision has been successfully performed,[70] usually by teams that commonly perform skull base and cavernous sinus surgery, but excessive bleeding from the lesion may prevent complete removal.[68,77] Less than 50% of surgical cases have had complete excision of the hemangioma. The tumor has been reported to peel off the ICA and cranial nerves much more easily than a meningioma. However, new or worse cranial neuropathy and cerebral dysfunction have resulted from surgery. Bleeding can be reduced by preoperative embolization through the C5 and C4 feeders, closure of the ipsilateral cavernous ICA in patients with adequate collaterals, and induced systemic hypotension.[84]

In contrast to cavernomas in the brain, cavernous hemangioma in the cavernous sinus may be radiosensitive. The mass size has been slightly to moderately reduced following 40 Gy of radiation via the Linac method.[85] Conventional multiport radiation from 45 to 50 Gy over 5 weeks has given similar results.[86–88]

Schwannoma (neurinoma)

Demographics

Except for the olfactory and optic nerve, all of the other cranial nerves have schwann cell nerve sheaths that can develop a neurinoma. Most of these tumors arise from sensory branches. Almost 20% of patients with neurinomas have neurofibromatosis. Neurinomas in the cavernous sinus can occur in almost any age group and there is no apparent gender preference.

Clinical symptoms and findings

Neurinomas that arise within the cavernous sinus are rare, and most cavernous sinus dysfunction is due to invasion from trigeminal neurinomas originating in Meckel's cave from the gasserian ganglion or the posterior fossa from a trigeminal branch nerve. In most of the latter cases, fifth nerve sensory symptoms, such as paresthesias, numbness, or pain, develop first. These symptoms can affect the first or second divisions or both. Cluster-like headache without other cranial nerve dysfunction is uncommon.[89] Rarely, neurinomas arise from the first division of the fifth nerve.[90] Diplopia and varying degrees of ophthalmoparesis can develop in patients with abnormal facial sensation.[91] However, even with MRI-demonstrated cavernous sinus invasion, patients may not have other cranial neuropathy. Rarely, a sixth nerve palsy may be the only problem caused by a trigeminal neurinoma.[92,93] Schwannomas arising from a trigeminal branch in the sphenoid sinus are even more rare.[94]

Schwannomas of the cranial nerves that innervate the extraocular muscles are also rare. These cranial nerves are more commonly involved in children with neurofibromatosis type 2 (NF2), although involvement of the eighth nerve is much more common in these patients.[95] Although retinal astrocytic hamartoma, optic nerve sheath meningioma, and lens opacities can occur in NF2, Lisch nodules are rare. Neurinomas of the oculomotor and abducens nerves are even more rare in patients without NF.[96–99] The diplopia associated with tumor of the ocular motor nerves can be painless or associated with a unilateral headache ipsilateral to the tumor. Symptoms of first or second division trigeminal nerve compression can also occur.

Neuroimaging

On CT the bone adjacent to the mass can be seen to be eroded. The medial wall of the cavernous sinus, anterior clinoid, or dorsum sella can be thinned, bowed and remodeled. Prior to contrast, the mass is usually low density or isodense with brain. Following contrast administration, neurinomas typically do not enhance significantly and have a heterogeneous appearance.[98] Rarely, the mass markedly enhances.

Neurinomas are often hypo- or isointense to white matter on T_1-weighted MR images, and bright with a heterogeneous pattern on T_2-weighted MR images[100] (Figure 169.7). These tumors may not enhance or may enhance only mildly after gadolinium administration. Less commonly, a neurinoma will enhance brightly after gadolinium, suggesting a vascular tumor that may correlate with a tumor blush on angiography. Typically, the wall of the cavernous sinus will enhance around the mass. On occasion, the lesion will have an area of cystic degeneration or intratumoral cyst. Most of these lesions are larger than 1.5 cm in symptomatic patients.

Neurinomas tend not to be very vascular but a tumor stain via C4 or C5 blood supply can be demonstrated by angiography. The cavernous ICA can be displaced medially or inferiorly. If the mass has grown into the cavernous sinus from posteriorly, the ICA can be displaced anteriorly. The ICA should not be encased but, if there is marked displacement, the siphon can be narrowed.

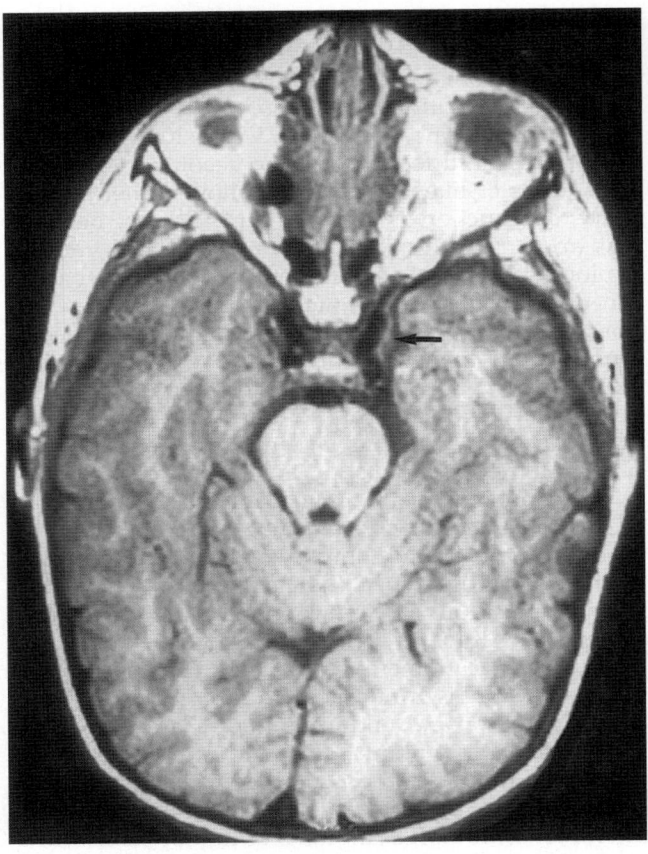

(a)

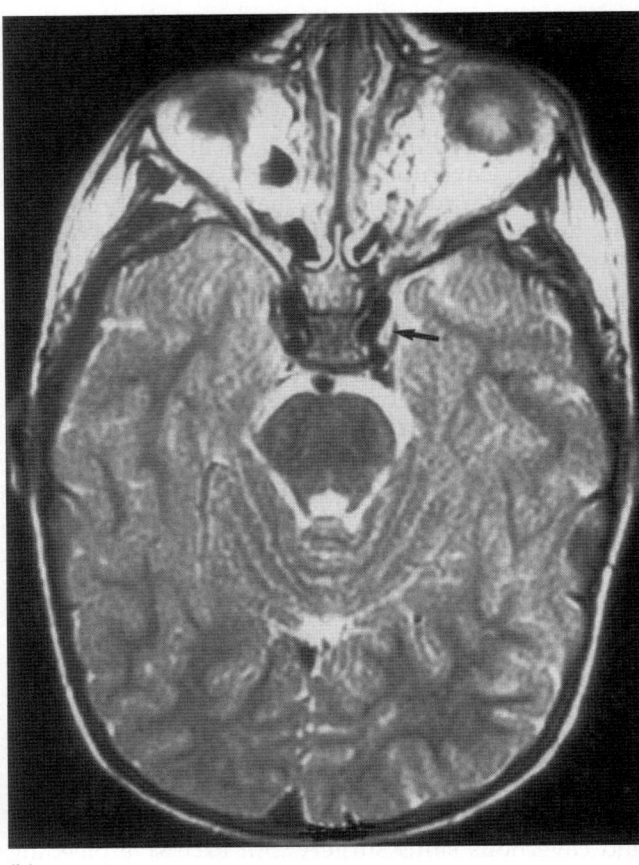

(b)

Figure 169.7 A 4-year-old boy with NF1 developed left upper lid ptosis over two years. His neuro-ophthalmological examination was normal except for 4 mm of left upper lid ptosis. The MRI revealed a subtle left intracavernous abnormal soft tissue mass that was isointense (arrow) with brain gray matter on T_1 (a), and bright (arrow) on T_2 (b), weighted images, suggestive of a schwannoma.

Natural history

The trigeminal sensory dysfunction or pain can progress and the ophthalmoparesis can deteriorate to complete ophthalmoplegia. However, the deficits can remain stable for years or even remit. In children, there are cases that appear to exacerbate with upper respiratory illness and remit afterwards. If the mass increases in size, symptoms and findings develop in relation to the direction of growth. Dysfunction of the brainstem, chiasm, optic tract, pituitary, and orbital apex have all been described.[96]

Treatment

Corticosteroid therapy has not been demonstrated to benefit the neuropathy. The associated pains can be controlled with medications typically used for trigeminal neuralgia or cluster headache.[89]

In patients with progressive unremitting neuropathy, symptomatic compression of the brainstem or secondary hydrocephalus, surgical excision has been performed.[91–93,96,97,99–105] Complete excision is more likely to be accomplished with lesions in the lateral wall of the cavernous sinus.[90,99] Patients tend to have worse cranial neuropathy after surgery, and although improvement can occur, the cranial nerve function

rarely returns to normal.[92] This would appear to be particularly true with neurinoma arising from the ocular motor nerve.[101] Some degree of diplopia often persists with trigeminal neurinomas. Since the cranial nerve is typically removed with an ocular motor nerve tumor, if a complete excision is effected, diplopia in primary gaze is permanent. Cranial nerve function may be partially restored if the proximal and distal portions of the nerve can be sutured together or if an intervening nerve is grafted.[105] Additionally, tumors thought to have been completely removed have recurred. Partial excision or cyst aspiration can preserve cranial nerve function and decompress the optic pathway and the brain.

Radiosurgery with proton beam and gamma knife techniques has been successfully used to treat schwannoma of the vestibular and trigeminal nerves. In a study of 16 patients with a mean follow-up of 44 months, trigeminal origin tumor reduction (56%) and stabilization (44%) was demonstrated after gamma knife treatment with a mean tumor margin dose of 15.3 Gy.[106] In a series with 96 patients primarily treated with gamma knife, vestibular schwannomas decreased in size in 81% or were stable in 13% during a mean follow-up of 4.27 years.[107]

Lymphoma

Demographics

Although previously thought to be rare, lymphoma that arises primarily within the cavernous sinus or presents with features suggestive of cavernous sinus invasion is increasingly reported as the incidence of intracranial lymphomas in all locations appears to be increasing. By 1996, 16 cases had been reported, but many more cases have probably occurred and have not been reported, since our neuro-ophthalmology service has evaluated 10 such cases. All types of non-Hodgkin lymphoma in all locations occur with increased frequency in immunocompromised individuals, from the first to the eighth decade of life. Burkitt's lymphoma is more common in immunocompromised individuals and children.[108] Hodgkin's lymphoma rarely causes a cavernous sinus syndrome.[109,110] Lymphoma in the cavernous sinus has no gender preference.

Clinical symptoms and findings

Varying degrees of ptosis and ocular motor limitation, retrobulbar pain, numbness in the first or second trigeminal divisions, and an anesthetic cornea can be seen at presentation.[111] The sixth nerve seems to be the most frequently affected.[112] A cavernous sinus syndrome can occur in patients with a diagnosed lymphoma, even if the cancer appears to be in remission. The right cavernous sinus appears to be more commonly involved. When the syndrome is due to metastatic lymphoma, other cranial nerves can be affected simultaneously.[113] Bilateral cavernous sinus syndromes can occur.[114]

Neuroimaging

There is no diagnostic feature on CT. Contrast enhanced CT shows diffuse enhancement and infiltration of the cavernous sinus. The mass can arise from tumor in the adjacent paranasal sinuses,[115] particularly in HIV positive[116] or elderly[117] patients. Both cavernous sinuses can become infiltrated with lymphoma.[110,114] Slight or no bone destruction occurs.

MRI may show partial thrombosis of the cavernous sinus and expansion by a soft tissue mass. The lesion appears isointense or slightly brighter to gray matter on T_1-weighted images and slightly bright on T_2-weighted images. The enhancement of the cavernous sinus, normally present after gadolinium, can be heterogeneous with an irregular appearance or uniformly enhancing (Figure 169.8). If the abnormal enhancement involves the meninges and tentorium, lymphoma or an inflammatory disorder due to infection, Wegener's granulomatosis, or vasculitis are in the differential.

Angiography is usually normal but displacement of the cavernous ICA has been seen.[112]

Natural history

Although the pain, ptosis, and ocular motor limitation may improve with a daily dose of 40 to 60 mg of prednisone, there is little or no response to this treatment in many patients and most signs recur as soon as the dose is reduced. Extension to the orbital apex or optic canal causes optic neuropathy.[118] The lymphoma may be confined to the central nervous system but, in most cases, the lymphoma is systemic. Extension into the subarachnoid space leads to carcinomatous meningitis, dysfunction of additional cranial nerves and parenchymal infiltration; death can occur within months of presentation.[111,119]

Treatment

Once a diagnosis is established via a biopsy of the intracranial lesion, extracranial lesion, or via cytology of the cerebrospinal fluid, systemic chemotherapy is initiated.[113] Local radiation therapy is given if a clinical response is not accomplished. Radiosurgery with gamma knife has been used primarily when the mass was presumed to be a meningioma, with resolution of the clinical findings and mass reduction. However, the mass recurred with new cranial neuropathy due to tumor growth outside the irradiation field.[119]

Chordoma

Demographics

Chordomas rarely originate in the cavernous sinus, however, most intracranial chordomas invade the

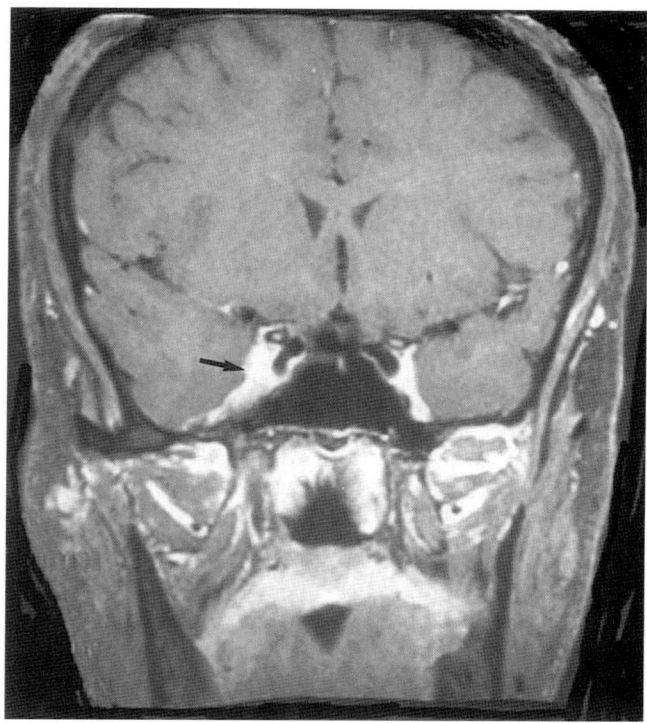

Figure 169.8 A 34-year-old man had symptoms of pain in the right eye for two weeks and then a right sided headache. He developed binocular diplopia one week before his evaluation which revealed 20/30 OD compared to 20/20 OS with a relative afferent pupillary defect and a mild sixth nerve paresis. After gadolinium administration, the T_1-weighted MRI showed a uniformly enhancing lesion (arrow) in the cavernous sinus. The systemic workup revealed a large cell lymphoma.

cavernous sinus and arise from the skull base, principally the clivus. These tumors present from the second to eighth decades of life, but are most common in patients in the 30 to 65 age range. Men and women seem to be equally affected. Chordomas make up approximately 0.2% of all intracranial tumors.

Clinical symptoms and findings

Multiple cranial nerve dysfunction, including bilateral abducens palsies,[120] commonly develops from tumor invasion along the clivus, Dorello's canal, and the base of the skull. With cavernous sinus involvement, most patients present with or soon develop dysfunction of third, fourth, and sixth cranial nerves. Since the clivus is typically involved, bilateral sixth nerve pareses can be present at presentation.[120] Dysfunction of either the first or second division of the trigeminal nerve or both is common. Facial pain is an infrequent major component of the symptoms.

Neuroimaging

Bone destruction of the clivus and base of skull and calcification in the lesion help to distinguish chordoma from other types of tumors on CT[10] (Figure 169.9a). The mass is isodense with the brain before contrast and enhances after contrast administration.

The mass typically has an isointense signal to gray matter on the T_1-weighted MRI images and bright or high signal with small isointense areas on the T_2-weighted MRI images[121] (Figure 169.9b, c). The mass enhances with a heterogeneous pattern (Figure 169.9d). ICA encasement and displacement can be demonstrated.

Angiography reveals minimal tumor blush due to supply from the ICA branches or from the ophthalmic artery if the orbit or ethmoid sinus is invaded. With cavernous sinus invasion, the cavernous ICA can be encased and dislocated by the tumor.[15,122–124]

Natural history

Although chordomas infrequently metastasize, except by local spread, and have a histologically benign appearance, these tumors grow over years and, because of the associated progressive dysfunction, are considered malignant. Progressive ophthalmoplegia, ptosis, and corneal anesthesia occur with lesions that invade the cavernous sinus or the superior orbital fissure. If the lesion crosses to the contralateral cavernous sinus, bilateral cranial nerve dysfunction will occur. Facial numbness and weakness, reduced tearing in the ipsilateral eye, and jaw misalignment due to mandibular branch involvement are common. Extension of the lesion inferiorly causes dysarthria, dysphagia, vocal cord paralysis, and tongue weakness. Brainstem, hypothalamic and pituitary compression are common, and papilledema develops if the lesion reaches a critical size.

Treatment

Radical surgery is the preferred treatment but invasion of the cavernous sinus frequently limits the resection.[125] After complete removal chordomas tend not to recur (over approximately 2-year follow-up),[126] but with partial resection tumor regrowth is typical.[127] In some cases staged operations using more than one approach can be useful.[128] On occasion, a transphenoidal approach may lead to an effective resection of a clival mass.[120] Improvement in ocular motor function can occur in cases with compression but not cavernous sinus invasion. Preoperative determination of whether a patient can tolerate ICA occlusion can facilitate more radical excision. Preoperative endovascular ICA occlusion and embolization of the arterial supply to the tumor can reduce intraoperative blood loss. Patients with total ophthalmoplegia or severe visual loss from optic neuropathy or corneal breakdown due to corneal anesthesia may also be considered for removal of the mass from the cavernous sinus. Despite these considerations, complete surgical removal is accomplished in less than 40% of patients. Surgical complications include cerebral ischemia due to carotid or other arterial injury, worse or new cranial neuropathy, hydrocephalus, hypothalamic/pituitary dysfunction (inappropriate antidiuretic hormone secretion, diabetes insipidus, hypothyroidism, Addison's disorder), and cerebrospinal fluid leak.

Conventional multiport external beam radiation therapy of 55 Gy is not effective.[125,127] Proton beam (heavy-charged particle) fractionated irradiation appears to be effective in preventing or reducing growth of the mass after surgery.[129] This therapy is limited by potential radionecrosis of adjacent neural structures, particularly the chiasm, hypothalamus, and brainstem. Single dose gamma knife radiosurgery also appears to be effective in slowing or reducing tumor growth after surgery but the length of follow-up time has been limited.

Tolosa–Hunt syndrome or idiopathic inflammation of the cavernous sinus
(see Kline[130] for complete overview)

Demographics

Males and females from the second to eighth decades of life can be affected. Idiopathic inflammation that primarily involves the cavernous sinus is rare. In contrast, nongranulomatous chronic inflammation of the orbital structures from the sclera to the orbital apex and superior orbital fissure is not rare. Most patients diagnosed as having Tolosa–Hunt syndrome actually have inflammation in the superior orbital fissure or in the orbit (Figure 169.10). Prior to high resolution contrast enhanced CT the diagnosis was based on clinical criteria of painful ophthalmoplegia that was steroid responsive. If not performed with fat suppression, even gadolinium enhanced MRI can miss a lesion in the superior orbital fissure. The clinical criteria are nonspecific and are clearly not diagnostic.[19] Even though the inflammation can spread from granuloma in the adjacent sinus,[131] in these cases an infectious etiology must be strongly considered and ruled out with the appropriate biopsy.

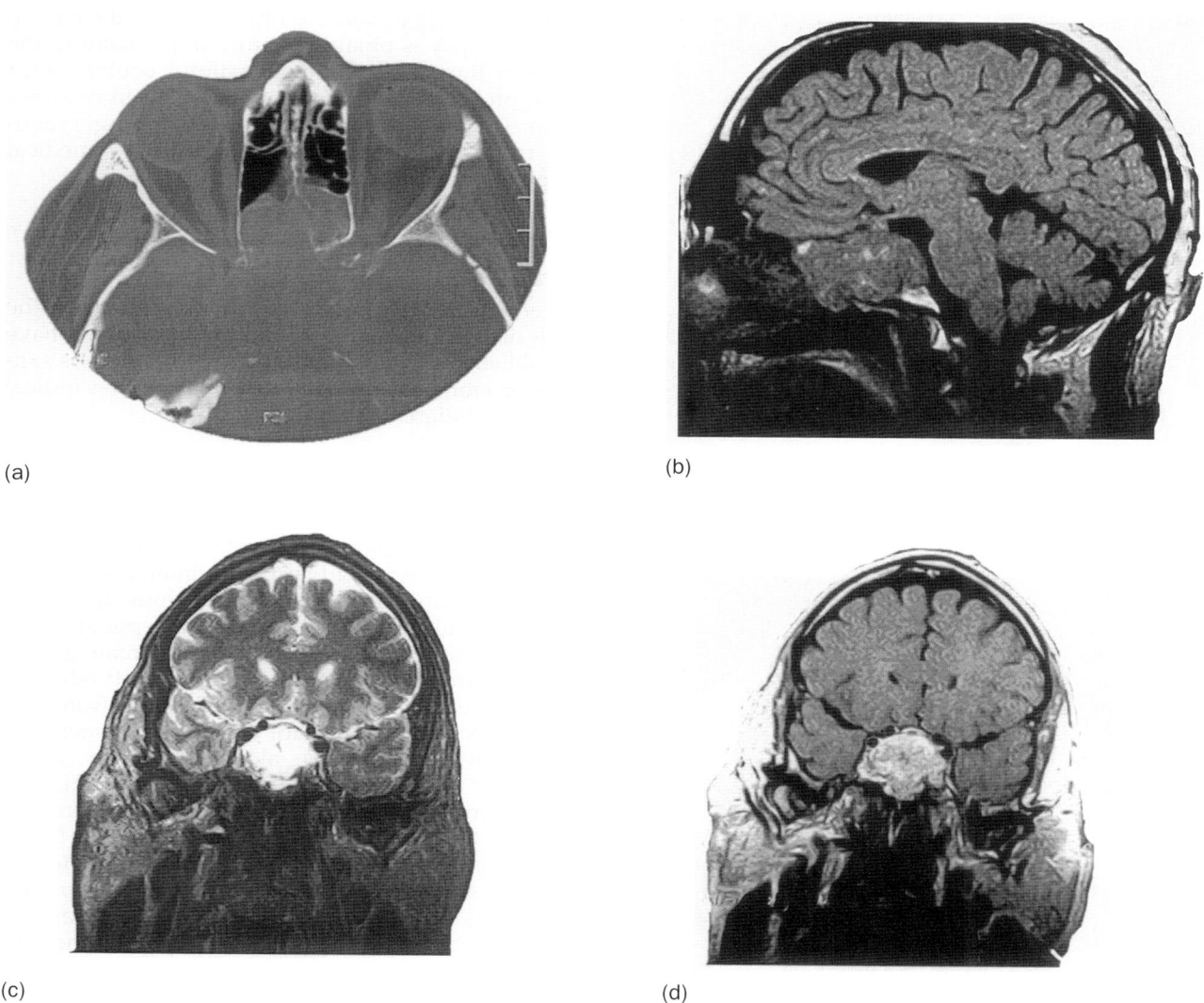

(a)

(b)

(c)

(d)

Figure 169.9 A 54-year-old hypertensive man complained of headache for three months and diplopia for one month. On examination, his only finding was 2–3 mm bilateral upper lid ptosis, and partial left inferior and medial recti restriction. (a) The CT scan showed extensive bone destruction of the sphenoid bone and anterior clivus associated with a mass (typical of chordoma) invading both cavernous sinuses and the suprasellar cistern. (b) MRI showed the mass to be heterogeneous on T_1-weighted images with tumor extension from the clivus to the sphenoid and ethmoid sinuses. (c) The mass was bright on the T_2-weighted images. (d) After gadolinium administration, the mass enhanced intensely and uniformly.

Clinical symptoms and findings

The hallmark of this disorder is pain, which can be severe or a deep ache associated with varying degrees of ophthalmoplegia and ptosis and diplopia.[132,133] The symptoms and signs depend on the location of the inflammation. If the orbit is involved, conjunctival injection and chemosis, orbital congestion and proptosis, lacrimal gland injection and swelling can be observed.

Neuroimaging

Contrast CT may demonstrate increased enhancement in the cavernous sinus without significant mass effect. Chronic inflammation can cause some bone erosion but frank destruction should not be present.[134]

Since the normal cavernous sinus markedly enhances after gadolinium, the MRI findings are not diagnostic.[135]

Angiography may reveal irregularities or narrowing in the cavernous ICA but it is usually normal.[136]

Natural history

Unilateral painful ophthalmoplegia can be acute, chronic, relapsing and remitting (spontaneously or in association with steroid withdrawal and treatment), or progressive. Extension of the inflammation into the orbital apex can cause unilateral optic neuropathy. The symptoms and signs vary with the tissues in the orbit that are inflamed.

Treatment

Corticosteroids, usually starting with the equivalent of 40 to 80 mg of prednisone daily, remain the mainstay of therapy. The dose used is often higher when a significant optic neuropathy is present. The dose is

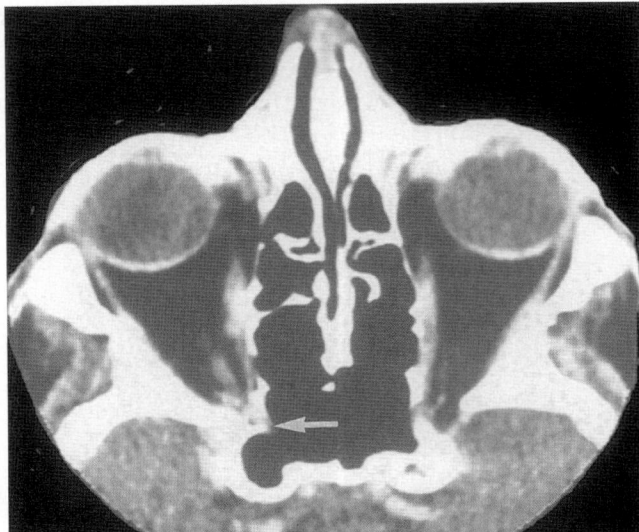

(a)

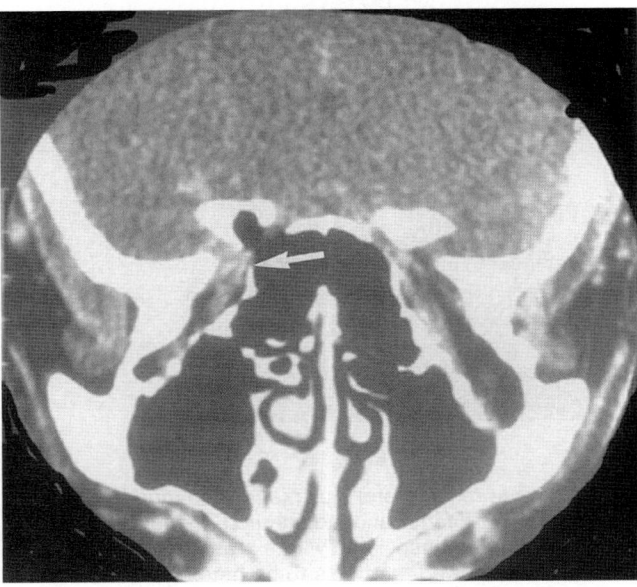

(b)

Figure 169.10   A 50-year-old man had painful diplopia and ptosis over two weeks. On examination he had 3 mm of right upper lid ptosis and moderate to severe limitation of all the right orbital extraocular movements without proptosis and normal pupils. His contrast CT (axial (a) and incompletely coronal (b), views) demonstrated a soft tissue mass (arrow) in the right superior orbital fissure without change in the adjacent bone, suggestive of inflammation. Treatment with oral prednisone improved the diplopia and the pain over several months but, following withdrawal of the medication, he had intermittent pain and no diplopia and no change in the CT for eight years.

gradually lowered and titrated to the amount needed to control the major clinical features. Depending on patient tolerance, clinical course, and development of steroid complications, either low dose radiation or immunosuppressive therapy is added or substituted.

In most cases, if possible without significant risk to vision, a biopsy is obtained before implementing the latter two therapies. Although painful ocular motor palsies, ptosis and recurrent pain have been reported to improve with removal of a noncaseating granuloma from the superior orbital fissure,[137] medical therapy is generally preferred.

Nonlymphomatous metastatic disease

Demographics

The gender and age predilection is dependent on the nature of the underlying tumor. Most patients have an established diagnosis, but the cavernous sinus syndrome or cranial neuropathy may be the first indication that a malignancy is present.[8,138,139]

Clinical symptoms and findings

Painful ophthalmoplegia is a rare complication of renal cell carcinoma,[138] ovarian cancer,[140] breast carcinoma,[141] colon adenocarcinoma,[142] melanoma,[19] and uterine cancer.[19] Adenoid cystic carcinoma of the salivary glands can cause a cavernous sinus syndrome via perineural spread.[143] Perineural spread from adenoid cystic carcinoma of lid meibomian glands can pass intracranially via the foramen rotundum.[144] Squamous cell carcinoma or melanoma from the parotid region, mouth or face can spread epineurally to the cavernous sinus along the fifth nerve branches.[8,145] Anastomoses between the fifth and seventh nerve within the face can lead to perineural spread to the seventh nerve (Figure 169.11). Metastatic carcinoma of prostate, lung and breast to the cavernous sinus, although rare, have been reported more often, probably because these cancers are so common.[19] Patients can present with pain alone, but findings of fifth nerve sensory loss distinguish the problem from trigeminal neuralgia.[8]

Neuroimaging

CT may demonstrate adjacent sinus disease with perineural spread but the cavernous sinus may appear normal until the lesion increases in size.[143] Bone destruction of the parasellar and clival areas occurs with breast metastases.[141,146] Prostate cancer can cause an osteoblastic reaction in affected bone.

Metastases appear as decreased signal of the affected bone marrow on T_1-weighted images and hyperintense relative to bone marrow on T_2-weighted MRI images.[147] Most metastatic lesions enhance after gadolinium on MRI. Perineural invasion causes the nerve to appear enlarged and to enhance after gadolinium.

There are no specific angiographic signs for metastatic disease to the cavernous sinus.

Natural history

Progressive cranial neuropathy, dysesthesia of the forehead, periorbital region or cheek, and trigeminal distribution pain develop over weeks to months without treatment. Patients frequently succumb to the underlying cancer.

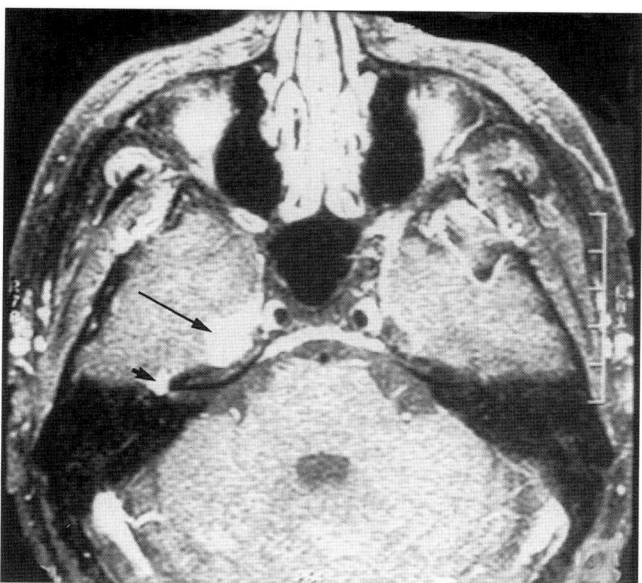

Figure 169.11 A 38-year-old man had symptoms of pain and paresthesias in the right lower jaw for six months and was told that his right pupil was smaller by an oral surgeon one month before neuro-ophthalmological evaluation. His examination revealed 1 mm of upward ptosis of the right lower lid, reduction in the right V_3 sensation, and a 3 mm right pupil compared to a 7 mm left pupil in the dark. MRI after gadolinium administration showed an enhancing mass at the level of the right foramen ovale (arrow) as well as at the level of the ipsilateral seventh nerve near the geniculate ganglion (arrowhead) (indicative of perineural spread). At surgery an adenoid cystic carcinoma was found. Further evaluation revealed that the tumor had spread intracranially from a primary tumor in the nasopharynx.

Treatment

Treatment of the underlying carcinoma is essential. However, most patients with a cavernous sinus syndrome are also treated with radiotherapy. The parasellar area is targeted but if other intracranial lesions are present or if the spinal fluid cytology is abnormal, the entire intracranial contents are treated and possibly the spinal axis. Conventional therapy can be palliative for renal carcinoma (4600 cGy),[148] and colon adenocarcinoma (2000 cGy).[142] Pain and headache may be reduced but ocular motor function may not improve even with 6000 cGy.[138] After conventional radiation therapy, recurrence can occur within 24 months.[8] Corticosteroid therapy may temporarily reduce the pain and improve cranial nerve function but there is no long term benefit.

Nasopharyngeal/sinus tumors

Demographics

Various types of carcinoma of the paranasal sinuses and nasopharynx are not infrequent. Nasopharyngeal carcinoma is uncommon in Caucasian populations with an incidence of approximately 0.4 per year[149] or 0.8 per 100 000.[150] Nasopharyngeal carcinoma is most common in males of North African, Arctic region, or Southeast Asian origin. It is the third leading cause of cancer in men in Southeast Asia. Most patients are adult, typically in the third to eighth decades, but children can be affected. Other risk factors include cigarette smoking and Epstein–Barr virus.[151]

Clinical symptoms and findings

Sinus, pharyngeal and nasal congestion, discharge and hemorrhage are due to the local infiltrative mass.

Trigeminal distribution pain and diplopia can be the first symptoms if the tumor invades the base of the skull. Tumor invasion into the cavernous sinus is not rare. Due to the position of the fifth and sixth nerves in the cavernous sinus, direction of extension of the carcinoma causes dysfunction in these two nerves first. Pain in the face and orbital region is common.

Neuroimaging

Computed tomography demonstrates destruction of the bone at the base of the skull, particularly in the region of the orbital apex and cavernous sinus. The tumor enhances following intravenous contrast administration.

MRI after gadolinium administration is superior to CT in demonstrating tumor invasion into the cavernous sinus, along the cranial nerves, in the superior orbital fissure.[152,153]

Angiography is routinely used in the management of this disorder. Percutaneous embolization can be used to devascularize lesions preoperatively or to stop uncontrolled epistaxis.[154]

Natural history

Progressive cranial neuropathy, extension into the orbit and along the skull base, pituitary dysfunction, and local sinus invasion of the carcinoma develop within months if untreated. Perineural spread along the inferior alveolar nerve to the facial nerve is frequently unrecognized.[8] Compressive optic neuropathy occurs if the orbital apex is invaded.

Undifferentiated carcinoma has a poor prognosis, with 50% of patients dying within 13 months of the diagnosis.[155] Metastatic spread is common;[156] once distant metastases occur, the 5-year overall survival rate is poor.[157] The overall 5- and 10-year survival rates are 19% and 14%, respectively.[158]

Treatment

Surgical resection of the sinus and pharyngeal portion of the tumor is often incomplete. Radiotherapy of the residual lesion and the portion in the parasellar region can prevent local tumor growth[159,160] but does not appear to prevent metastasis to the lymph nodes.[161] Radical surgery of extracranial recurrence despite radiation therapy has a reasonable morbidity and is often recommended.[162,163] Even with fractionated radiation, with the doses of radiation typically used (60 Gy or more), temporal lobe necrosis and optic neuropathy are not uncommon.[164] The superior targeting of conformal radiotherapy should spare central nervous system structures when the tumor is localized and does not infiltrate a wide area.[165] Additional radiation with brachytherapy can enhance the results[166] and can be used for reirradiation of specific areas.[167] Salvage therapy, however, is successful in less than one third of patients.[158] Adjuvant systemic chemotherapy may slow or stop tumor invasion and metastases in some but not all patients; when chemotherapy is combined with radiotherapy, the results appear superior to either alone.[168,169] Chemotherapy is used for remote metastases.[170]

Arteriovenous shunts of the cavernous sinus region—carotid cavernous fistula and dural arteriovenous malformation

Demographics

Carotid cavernous fistula (CCF) is an acquired pathological direct shunt from the cavernous portion of the ICA to the enveloping cavernous sinus. These arteriovenous (AV) shunts can develop spontaneously, usually from pre-existing asymptomatic cavernous carotid aneurysms, but the majority (80%) are the result of a traumatic injury to the ICA or a branch artery.[171] The use of seat belts and air bags have reduced the occurrence of the latter. In most cases, clinical diagnosis is not difficult, but the variable nature of the signs and symptoms can mislead the examining physician. Traumatic CCF more commonly affects males while spontaneous CCF is more common in women. Damage to the ICA sustained during endarterectomy,[172] endovascular procedures for thromboendarterectomy or aneurysm treatment, or angioplasty of the ICA (increasingly performed with stents) can be the inciting injury.[173–175] A CCF can also develop from injury to the ICA during transphenoidal surgery to remove a pituitary tumor. Laceration of the cavernous carotid artery or one of the cavernous branch arteries is likely to occur if the ICA is located medially on the floor of the sella;[176] or if the surgeon unknowingly courses eccentric to the midline. Preoperative MRI which demonstrates an intrasellar location of the cavernous ICA suggests that transphenoidal surgery could be complicated. Specific disorders that cause a defect in the arterial wall media and a CCF can be identified in approximately 60% of spontaneous cases.[177] These include Ehler–Danlos syndrome,[178,179] pseudoxanthoma elasticum,[180] and fibromuscular dysplasia.[181]

Dural arteriovenous malformations (AVM), which are composed of a network of slow flow AV shunts supplied by dural branches of the external carotid artery and cavernous ICA branches, are more common in women, most often postmenopausal, and are rare in children.

Symptoms and clinical findings

Similar orbital and cavernous sinus signs occur with the different types of AV shunts that drain into the cavernous sinus. Although the clinical signs and symptoms can fluctuate, the abnormalities often worsen progressively with the evolution of various hemodynamic processes. Except for the additional direct traumatic injuries, the findings are similar for cases with traumatic or spontaneous CCF or dural AVM. The patients complain of visual blur, diplopia, headache, ocular or orbital pain and subjective bruit.

Neuroimaging

An enlarged superior ophthalmic vein and swelling of the extraocular muscles can be seen on CT or MRI in most of these diseases. Diffuse swelling of the extraocular muscles occurs with a dural AVM or a CCF. Different types of swelling also occur with myositis (affects tendons and causes other orbital soft tissue abnormalities), dysthyroid ophthalmopathy (spares tendons and preferentially affects inferior and medial recti), and metastatic or infiltrative neoplasia (focal masses).

Enlargement of the superior ophthalmic vein can result from any entity that compromises the venous outflow from the posterior orbit. These include: (1) venous congestion due to neoplasm, infection or inflammation related thrombosis in the cavernous sinus; (2) an AV shunt that directs arterial blood flow into the normally low pressure cavernous sinus that already is compromised by some degree of thrombosis; (3) an orbital arteriovenous malformation that mechanically compresses the superior ophthalmic vein or shunts a high volume of blood into the ophthalmic venous system causing venous hypertension; (4) a varix of the ophthalmic vein associated with thrombosis in the superior ophthalmic vein obstructing the blood flow or mechanically compressing the ophthalmic venous outflow; 5) an inflammatory or neoplastic process in the orbit, particularly when located in the apex or in the superior orbital fissure, mechanically compressing the superior ophthalmic vein; 6) dysthyroid orbitopathy enlarging the extraocular muscles, which can compress the superior ophthalmic vein in the orbital apex. High resolution CT or fat suppressed contrast enhanced MRI will differentiate most of the above causes of an enlarged superior ophthalmic vein from a CCF or dural AVM.

A high flow AV shunt will often aneurysmally dilate the involved cavernous sinus. Convex bulging of the cavernous sinus develops as a result of significant congestion or a mass in the cavernous sinus. If this change is subtle, it may be apparent only with coronal views of the contrast enhanced CT. Exophthalmos can be seen on CT, but the clinical measurement of proptosis is superior to the CT evaluation. CT may be less accurate because the eyes are often not in the primary position when the scan is performed or the CT image slices may visualize the two eyes at different levels, so comparison is not exact. If cortical venous drainage from the cavernous sinus is prominent, dilatation of one or more cerebral veins may be demonstrated.

In patients with traumatic CCF, the CT often reveals other sequelae of the head injury. Fractures through the base of the skull along the sphenoid sinus in this location or the petrous bone are best demonstrated with bone windows that eliminate the adjacent soft tissues. Paranasal opacification and/or sinus fluid levels are seen, particularly in the sphenoid sinus. CT will also reveal additional intracranial lesions such as epidural or subdural hematomas, an intracerebral hematoma, or a focal contusion of the brain. One exception is the CCF associated with a pseudoaneurysm of the ICA that extends into the sphenoid sinus and can cause a life-threatening catastrophic epistaxis.

Except for revealing fractures, MRI is superior to CT in evaluating a CCF in demonstrating the above findings. In addition, MRI with gadolinium can demonstrate the presence of dilated cortical veins due to flow reversal and venous hypertension that can cause a venous infarct or intracerebral hemorrhage. MRI and MRA are useful in cases with a spontaneous CCF caused by an aneurysm. MRI frequently demonstrates the abnormal flow voids in the cavernous sinus in cases of dural AVM (Figure 169.12).

Selective cerebral angiography remains the modality used for treatment planning. Potential collaterals between the external and internal carotid artery systems in the orbit and the cavernous sinus area as well as the exact location of the hole in the ICA or branch of the ICA are revealed. The direction of the abnormal venous drainage correlates with the clinical features of these AV shunts.

Natural history

Signs of orbital congestion may develop immediately after trauma, but local orbital injury may mask the signs of a CCF. Trauma may also initially cause a small pseudoaneurysm in a branch artery of the cavernous ICA that ruptures into the venous channels of the cavernous sinus after a latent period of days to weeks. The clinical picture for patients with dural AVM is similar to those with a CCF.

Congestion of the orbital contents from arterialization of the ophthalmic venous system causes elevation of the intraocular pressure (IOP) or secondary glaucoma, venous retinopathy, weakness and mechanical limitation of the eye muscles, arterialization and dilatation of the conjunctival vessels, chemosis, dilation of the veins and edema in the lids. Proptosis results because of congestion and dilatation of the ophthalmic vein. Pulsations that can actually be seen or palpated occur less frequently.[175,182] An objective bruit heard over the orbit or over the direction of the abnormal venous drainage is considerably more common with a CCF than with a dural AVM.

Cranial and sympathetic neuropathies can also occur secondary to the effects of venous hypertension or thrombosis on the nerves within the cavernous sinus or the direct effects of trauma. Isolated third or sixth nerve or combinations of third, fourth, and sixth nerve dysfunction are common. Trigeminal nerve sensory deficits in the first and second divisions are seen in less than 20% of cases. Fifth nerve defects of motor function or of the third division sensation are almost never a complication of these AV shunts and are generally a result of a traumatic neuropathy. Partial ptosis may arise from a partial third nerve or sympathetic paresis, local lid edema or a combination of all three factors.

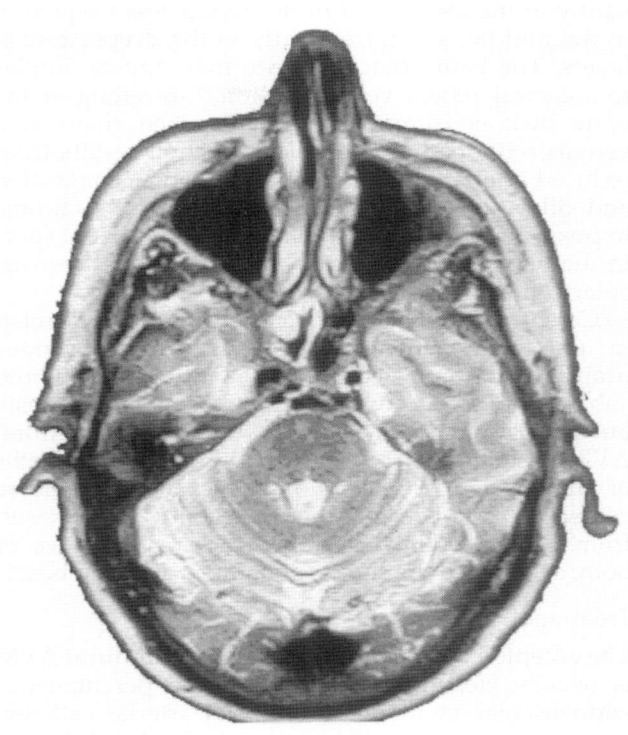

Figure 169.12 A 72-year-old woman had unilateral signs of orbital congestion and a subjective bruit in the opposite ear typical of an AV shunt in the region of the cavernous sinus. MRI showed abnormal flow voids in both cavernous sinuses and in the basilar venous plexus. Abnormally dilated cortical veins (not shown) were confirmed on angiography that was performed in the treatment of a dural AVM.

The ocular motor dysfunction can affect all the eye movements or it can be limited. However, the superior oblique muscle is never affected alone. If the abnormal venous drainage is directed posteriorly to the petrosal sinuses, there will be little or no orbital congestion, and cranial neuropathy with or without a posterior auricular bruit will be found.[182]

The pupil can function normally (even with severe ocular motor dysfunction), or it can be larger or smaller than the unaffected eye. The combination of poor light reactivity and poor dilation in the dark of the pupil suggests the presence of both parasympathetic and sympathetic dysfunction. The pupil may be difficult to evaluate if the trauma has damaged the iris sphincter dysfunction or if a traumatic uveitis is present. An afferent pupillary defect develops in those eyes with a unilateral optic neuropathy.

Venous ischemic-hypoxic retinopathy rarely occurs without concomitant elevation of the intraocular pressure and congestion in the ipsilateral orbit. In fact, the opposite is often found; severe orbital congestion occurs with little or no retinopathy or only mild retinal vein engorement or disk edema. All of the retinal veins can be slightly or severely dilated and engorged. The retinal hemorrhages of venous retinopathy, from any etiology, are located predominantly in the inner layer of the retina, less frequently in the middle, and infrequently in the deeper retinal layers. The hemorrhagic picture may appear similar to a central retinal vein occlusion.[183] Swelling of the optic disk is commonly present when there is a venous retinopathy. Retinal dysfunction results from reduced arterial blood flow into the retina, congestion and dilatation of the retinal veins, and the chronic hypoxia and ischemia of the retina. Cotton wool spots in the nerve fiber layer can occur but retinal neovascularization is rare.[184]

Cerebral hemorrhage or venous infarct can develop in untreated patients who have cortical venous drainage of arterialized blood flowing superiorly into subarachnoid veins. CCF do not close spontaneously but approximately 40% to 50% of cases with dural AVM spontaneous recover, usually within six months of diagnosis, or have a stable nonprogressive course.[185,186] However, visual disability may result from ocular motility dysfunction or visual loss, or both, even when the shunt spontaneously thromboses.

Treatment

The accepted treatment for most CCF and dural AVM is usually closure of the shunt via a percutaneous endovascular method. Through an arterial catheter, one or more detachable balloons or Gugliemi detachable coils are placed into the venous side of the CCF, usually with preservation of the ICA.[175,187–190] Balloons and coils may also be placed into the venous side of the CCF or dural AVM via the inferior petrosal sinus or, in a chronic shunt, through the ophthalmic vein to accomplish closure of the shunt with preservation of the ICA.[191–193] Transarterial embolization of the supplying dural arteries can be accomplished with liquid acrylic and particulate material.[194–197]

Carotid cavernous aneurysm

Demographics

Aneurysms of the cavernous segment of the ICA are extradural and comprise only 3% of all intracranial aneurysms.[198] However, 15% of all symptomatic unruptured aneurysms are found in this location.[199] They are a common cause, along with meningioma, nasopharyngeal cancer, and metastatic cancer, of a cavernous sinus syndrome.[200,201] Most patients with these aneurysms are more than 50 years old (range 30 to 75 years). The authors have seen only one patient who developed this aneurysm during the first decade of life. Women are affected 10 times more often than men. Systemic hypertension does not appear to be a causative factor for developing symptoms, nor is there a greater incidence of high blood pressure in these patients than in the normal population.

Symptoms and clinical findings

The clinical symptomatology and neuro-ophthalmological deficits are similar to the dysfunction caused by any mass located in the cavernous sinus. Typically, a progressive or recurrent unilateral disturbance of the local cranial nerves causes diplopia, ptosis and blurred vision from accommodative paresis; orbital, eye or face pain occur. Less frequently, anesthesia of the forehead and cornea develops.[202] The third, fourth, and sixth nerves are most frequently involved.[203] If the onset of ophthalmoplegia is sudden and painful, it results either from compromise of the blood supply to the cranial nerves because of acute compression, or thrombosis in a branch artery from the cavernous carotid artery.[204,205]

Although a loss of fifth nerve sensation is less common, trigeminal pain is usually an early symptom. Few patients never experience pain. When the pain develops it occurs predominantly in first trigeminal division, ipsilateral to the aneurysm. Some patients present with a combination of ptosis, diplopia, and chronic pain, which develops gradually or abruptly (obviously diplopia is always sudden). The pain can be explosive, possibly because of sudden expansion or hemorrhage into the arterial wall or thrombosis in the lumen of the aneurysm. The pain can be intractable despite the use of narcotics and corticosteroids. Pain along the second trigeminal division, in the maxillary area or upper teeth or jaw, occurs less frequently and never as the sole manifestation of the aneurysm. The pain can remit while other signs of cranial neuropathy remain.

An isolated sixth nerve paresis is common because of the proximity of the nerve to the ICA. An isolated partial third nerve paresis can also develop, but an isolated fourth paresis is extremely rare.[206] In our series of 184 cavernous ICA aneurysms, none had superior oblique weakness without signs of dysfunction in the sixth or third nerves or both. Early on, a partial third nerve paresis, including either an inferior or superior division dysfunction, is possible. Although a total sixth nerve palsy and a moderate paresis of the third nerve can occur alone, a complete absence of third nerve function, without other cranial nerve involvement, is uncommon. Some combination of a partial or complete paresis of the third, fourth, and sixth nerves is common. Longstanding compression of the third nerve may lead to one of the various manifestations of a misdirection syndrome.

On occasion, the pupil is relatively spared in the face of severe paresis of the superior rectus and the levator palpebrae, because the pupillary fibers, which course in the inferior division of the third nerve, are not compromised when the superior division is affected. More commonly, because of both parasympathetic and sympathetic dysfunction, the ipsilateral pupil is the same size or slightly larger than the unaffected pupil. Close inspection reveals reduced dilation in the dark and less reactivity to light and near-accommodative stimuli in the affected pupil. A miotic, poorly reactive pupil with a third nerve paresis usually arises when there is aberrant regeneration.[207] A complete external third nerve ophthalmoplegia with a normal pupil does not occur. Sympathetic dysfunction can occur with a lateral rectus paresis without other cranial nerve dysfunction.

A loss of fifth nerve sensation is found only in longstanding cases. The first and second divisions of the trigeminal nerve are located inferiorly to the aneurysm sac, which usually bulges laterally.[203] The aneurysm must extend posteriorly and inferiorly in order to compress the fifth nerve. The corneal reflex is diminished or absent in approximately 20% and a decrease in sensation in the first division of the trigeminal nerve occurs in approximately 25% of patients, respectively. Corneal anesthesia and a secondary neurotropic keratopathy occur only when the aneurysm is large and compromises the fifth nerve close to the trigeminal ganglion.[208] Less than 10% of the aneurysms expand far enough posteriorly in the cavernous sinus to cause a loss of sensation in the second division of the trigeminal nerve. Aneurysm expansion towards the petrous bone that causes a loss of third division sensation and fifth nerve motor dysfunction is extremely rare.

If the aneurysm is very large and extends anteriorly toward the optic foramen or anterosuperiorly through the dura, the patient can develop an optic neuropathy. The signs of a cavernous sinus dysfunction always precede visual loss and most patients have a complete oculomotor and pupillary paresis. In fact, all of our cases with an optic neuropathy had significant ophthalmoplegia in the affected eye. Once an optic neuropathy begins, the visual loss almost always progresses over months to years, and monocular blindness is inevitable if the aneurysm is untreated. Although chiasm dysfunction can cause a field defect in the eye contralateral to the aneurysm, blindness rarely develops in this eye. In our series, blindness never developed in the second eye of affected patients.

Significant proptosis is also rarely an early finding. The aneurysm must be a massive size and present for years in order to erode through the superior orbital fissure into the orbit. Mild proptosis results from relaxation of the extraocular muscles with complete ophthalmoplegia. The extremely low incidence of proptosis in our patients contrasts with the 60% incidence reported in the older literature.[209] This difference probably reflects earlier diagnosis because of improved neuroimaging.

An orbital or cephalic bruit is ordinarily not found in this disorder because the lesion is not high flow and does not have an arteriovenous shunt like a carotid cavernous fistula. However, if the aneurysm erodes anteriorly an orbital bruit can be auscultated because of turbulent blood flow within the aneurysm.

Other rare presentations result from erosion of the aneurysm into the sella to cause pituitary dysfunction. Pituitary disturbances are always accompanied by symptoms and findings of cavernous sinus dysfunction. Cerebral ischemic episodes due to emboli from thrombus within the aneurysm are rare[210] and are more likely to occur when there is an underlying coagulation disorder.[211]

Neuroimaging

A target sign may be seen on the contrast CT due to enhancement of the wall and part of the lumen with an intervening area of nonenhancing thrombus. The aneurysm may enhance uniformly if no thrombosis is present. Thinning of the adjacent bones or erosion of the aneurysm into the sphenoid sinus or superior orbital fissure can be seen in longstanding cases.

MRI is the best noninvasive method to visualize a cavernous carotid aneurysm and its relationship to the ICA (Figure 169.13). MRI readily differentiates an aneurysm from a neoplastic mass in the cavernous sinus. MRI may also reveal whether the aneurysm has eroded through the dura into the intradural space. MRA will effectively screen for most aneurysms in these cases since most second aneurysms are mirror image cavernous ICA aneurysms.

Cerebral angiography is performed to determine whether treatment can be performed with an acceptable risk. The angiogram may demonstrate a neck of the aneurysm, but more often a definable neck is not seen because the wall of the cavernous ICA is actually part of the aneurysm wall. The mass of the aneurysm exceeds the lumen in most cases and frequently displaces the ICA. Careful study of the angiogram will reveal whether the aneurysm arises within the cavernous sinus or if it is actually an intradural lesion that projects into the cavernous sinus[212] to cause the cranial neuropathy. The angiogram may distinguish whether a cavernous ICA aneurysm extends into the subarachnoid space. Angiography will also reveal if the origin of the ophthalmic artery is subarachnoid or from the cavernous ICA and whether there are adequate collaterals to the affected ICA. In approximately 20% of patients, angiography demonstrates additional aneurysms, 50% of which are mirror aneurysms in the opposite cavernous ICA.

Natural history

Some patients have progression of a combination of third, fourth, and sixth nerve pareses, but the pain may be episodic or continuous. An exacerbating and remitting course occurs in others. In 25% of patients, the clinical course is stable for years. As discussed previously, patients with an anesthetic cornea have reduced vision because of a tropic keratopathy. Permanent visual loss from corneal scarring is rare and we have seen only one such case.

Spontaneous thrombosis within the aneurysm is marked by episodes of severe pain and worsening cranial neuropathy. A reduction or a complete resolution of the pain often follows these periods, within several days to weeks, and there is gradual improvement of the cranial nerve pareses over weeks to months. In these cases, the pain typically resolves completely within approximately six weeks of the ictus. In other patients, stability or spontaneous improvement of the cranial neuropathy gradually occurs without an acute event or severe pain. Once the symptoms have resolved, the patient can remain asymptomatic for months to years.

Many asymptomatic aneurysms, found at the time of the evaluation for symptomatic aneurysms in other locations, are typically small and remain unchanged over years. Approximately 4% of carotid cavernous aneurysms rupture into a venous compartment of the

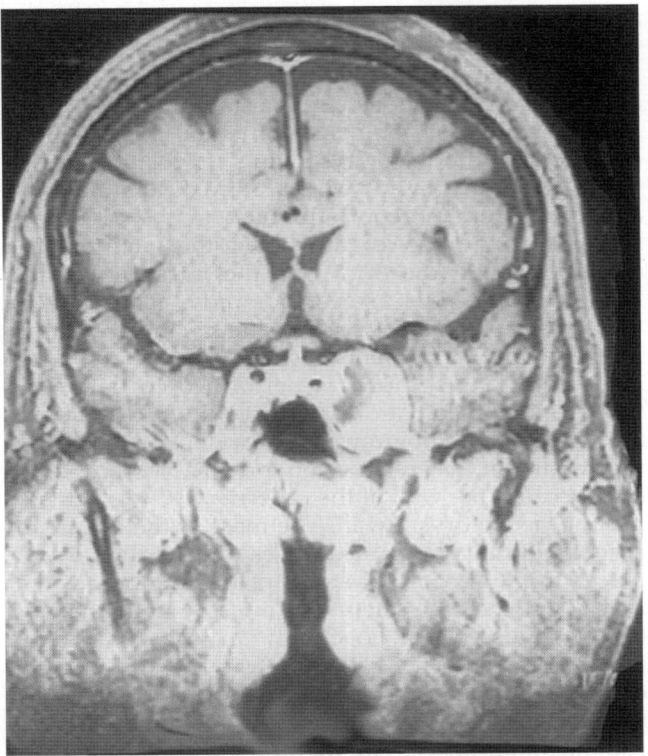

(a)

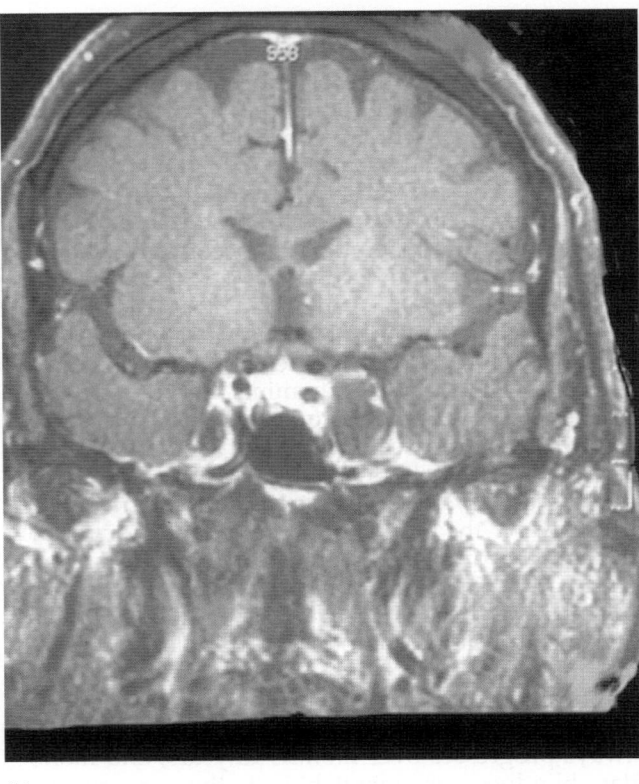

(b)

Figure 169.13   A 70-year-old woman complained of pain over the left eye and diplopia over one month. Her examination only revealed 2 mm of left upper lid ptosis, a 2 mm left pupil compared to a 5 mm pupil in the dark, no left lateral or medial rectus function, and mild limitation in downgaze with the left eye. (a) MRI demonstrated a mass with a central flow void and gadolinium enhancement of thrombus within the aneurysm lumen that arose from the cavernous ICA. The headache and the eye movements spontaneously improved over several months. (b) Contrast enhanced MRI 5 years later showed that the aneurysm is smaller. The patient remains clinically stable.

cavernous sinus, resulting in a carotid cavernous fistula. Prior to rupture, these cases are undiagnosed and typically have small, asymptomatic aneurysms. Similar to other carotid cavernous fistulas, the symptoms depend on the venous drainage, possible thrombosis in the cavernous sinus, and the rate of blood flow through the shunt.

Symptomatic aneurysms can progressively enlarge and attenuate the adjacent dura and bone compartment of the cavernous sinus. Rarely, erosion of the lateral wall of the sphenoid sinus results in the aneurysm bulging into the sphenoid sinus. A rupture of this aneurysm could cause severe epistaxis.[213] However, except for rare cases, this complication has been reported in patients with traumatic pseudo-aneurysms.[214–216]

Cavernous carotid aneurysms rarely cause subarachnoid hemorrhage, even when the lesions are large enough to cause optic neuropathy.[202] One of these cases has been reported more than once.[203] Each of two pathologically studied cases with a subarachnoid space directed rupture had an aneurysm that was definitively shown to have ruptured laterally, in the direction where there is no bone to support the cavernous sinus.[217] We have seen one case with a cavernous

aneurysm that had a projection of a small nipple of the aneurysm into the subarachnoid space that ruptured.[218] Additional cases of subarachnoid hemorrhage have been described with parasellar aneurysms, but clear documentation that the ruptured aneurysm originated from the cavernous ICA was often lacking.[219] The clinical course of a true carotid cavernous aneurysm differs from the aneurysm with an intradural origin and neck that has its sac project extradurally into the cavernous sinus,[212] because the latter aneurysm can cause a subarachnoid hemorrhage.

Treatment

Treatment is indicated if visual loss or cranial neuropathy is debilitating or progressive. Patients who have persistent severe pain that is difficult to control also warrant intervention. Patients with a carotid cavernous fistula are treated as outlined previously. As with other aneurysms, the ideal therapy excludes the aneurysm from the cavernous ICA and preserves the blood flow through the affected ICA. However, in most cases, the ipsilateral ICA is occluded during treatment.[220,221] The cerebral circulation is preserved via the anterior communicating artery from the contralateral ICA, through the posterior communicating artery from the posterior circulation, or via a prophylactic bypass.

If treatment is being considered, a functional tolerance test of ICA occlusion is performed while the patient is awake and under systemic heparinization. A double lumen balloon catheter, placed into the cervical ICA via a percutaneous route, is temporarily inflated for 15 to 20 minutes to occlude the ICA while the patient's neurological status is monitored.[222] If the patient develops a neurological deficit during the tolerance test, a prophylactic extracranial to intracranial arterial bypass procedure is performed before closing the ICA at the level of the aneurysm.[220,223,224]

Until recently, successful direct clipping of an aneurysm in the cavernous sinus had been attempted infrequently and was rarely accomplished without significant complications including ischemia in the ipsilateral cerebral hemisphere.[225,226] Direct surgery of the cavernous aneurysm carries a mortality rate of approximately 20%.[225] Surgical reconstruction of the ICA has been performed with a surgical clip in patients with supraclinoid aneurysms, but it is virtually impossible in the cavernous sinus. Adequate surgical exposure can not be obtained without severely compromising the venous channels and cranial nerves in the cavernous sinus. We have also seen patients develop an optic neuropathy as a complication of this surgery. A surgical procedure that traps the aneurysm by ligating the ICA at supraclinoid and cervical segments accomplishes no more than percutaneous embolization. No matter which method is applied, the same precautions must be taken in a case where occlusion of the ICA is required to treat the aneurysm.

Following embolization or surgical carotid occlusion, sudden thrombosis with expansion of the aneurysm mass can cause temporary worsening of the cranial neuropathy and pain. In most cases, even without obvious thrombosis, there is a temporary increase in the first division trigeminal pain. Over several weeks to months, the pain and the cranial neuropathy improve in all of these cases. However, if the patient has a complete ophthalmoplegia before treatment, recovery of oculomotor function is limited. Patients with partial ophthalmoplegia frequently resolve the diplopia in primary gaze, but rarely become orthophoric in all the cardinal fields of gaze. Following embolization, the pre-embolization optic neuropathy stabilizes in most patients, but significant improvement in the vision occurs in few cases. The pupillary function rarely normalizes and the pupil often remains permanently dilated and poorly reactive to both near and light stimuli.

References

1. Parkinson D. A surgical approach to the cavernous portion of the carotid artery: anatomical studies and case report. J Neurosurg 1965;23:474–483
2. Willinsky R, Lasjaunias P, Berenstein A. Intracavernous branches of the internal carotid artery (ICA): comprehensive review of their variations. Surg Radiol Anat 1987;9:201–215
3. Kupersmith MJ. Neurovascular Neuro-Ophthalmology. Heidelberg: Springer-Verlag, 1993
4. Lapresle J, Lasjaunias LP. Cranial nerve ischaemic arterial syndromes: a review. Brain 1986;109:207–215
5. Capo H, Kupersmith M, Berenstein A, et al. The clinical importance of the inferolateral trunk of the internal carotid artery. Neurosurgery 1991;28:733–738
6. Trobe JD, Glaser JS, Post JD. Meningiomas and aneurysms of the cavernous sinus. Neuro-ophthalmologic features. Arch Ophthalmol 1978;96:457–467
7. Moorthy G, Behrens MM, Drachman DB, et al. Ocular pseudomyasthenia or ocular myasthenia "plus": a warning to clinicians. Neurology 1989;39:1150–1154
8. Trobe JD, Hood CI, Parsons JT, Quisling R. Intracranial spread of squamous carcinoma along the trigeminal nerve. Arch Ophthalmol 1982;100:608–611
9. Lepore FE, Glaser JS. Misdirection revisited. A critical appraisal of acquired oculomotor nerve synkinesis. Arch Ophthalmol 1980;98:2206–2209
10. Moore T, Ganti SR, Mawad ME, Hilal SK. CT and angiography of primary extradural juxtasellar tumors. Am J Roentgenol 1985;145:491–496
11. Sindou M, Chavez JM, Saint Pierre G, Jouvet A. Percutaneous biopsy of cavernous sinus tumors through the foramen ovale. Neurosurgery 1997;40:106–110, discussion 110–111
12. Slamovits TL, Cahill V, Sibony PA, et al. Orbital fine-needle aspiration biopsy in patients with cavernous sinus syndrome. J Neurosurg 1983;59:1037–1042
13. Baker HL Jr. The angiographic delineation of sellar and parasellar masses. Radiology 1972;104:67–78
14. Dilenge D, Metzger J, Ramee A, Simon J. [Angiography of tumors of the cavernous sinus region]. J Radiol Electrol Med Nucl 1966;47:615–628
15. Cophignon J, Doyon D, Djindjian R, Vignaud J. [Tumors of the cavernous sinus and its region: arterial and venous opacification]. Neurochirurgie 1973;19:7–27
16. Theron J, Djindjian R. Comparison of the venous phase of carotid arteriography with direct intracranial venography in the evaluation of lesions at the base of the skull. Neuroradiology 1973;5:43–48
17. Waga S, Kikuchi H, Handa J, Handa H. Cavernous sinus venography. Am J Roentgenol Rad Ther Nucl Med 1970;109:130–137
18. Simon J, Doron Y. Orbital phlebography and cavernography in intra-cranial lesions. Acta Radiol Suppl 1976;347:277–283
19. Thomas J, Yoss RE. The parasellar syndrome: problems in determining etiology. Mayo Clin Proc 1970;45:617–623
20. Close LG, Schaefer SD, Mickey BE, Manning SC. Surgical management of nasopharyngeal angiofibroma involving the cavernous sinus. Arch Otolaryngol Head Neck Surg 1989;115:1091–1095
21. Sekhar LN, Sen CN, Jho HD, Janecka IP. Surgical treatment of intracavernous neoplasms: a four-year experience. Neurosurgery 1989;24:18–30
22. Goldberg AL, Tievsky AL, Jamshidi S. Wegener granulomatosis invading the cavernous sinus: a CT demonstration. J Comput Assist Tomogr 1983;7:701–703
23. Hermann MB, Bobek-Billewicz B, Bullo B, Hermann A, Rutkowski B. Wegener's granulomatosis with unusual cavernous sinus and sella turcica extension. Eur Radiol 1999;9:1859–1861
24. Coffey RJ, Cascino TL, Shaw EG. Radiosurgical treatment of recurrent hemangiopericytomas of meninges: preliminary results. J Neurosurg 1993;78:903–908

25. Kline LB, Galbraith JG. Parasellar epidermoid tumor presenting as painful ophthalmoplegia. J Neurosurg 1981;54:113–117

26. Ikezaki K, Toda K, Abe M, Tabuchi K. Intracavernous epidermoid tumor presenting with abducens nerve paresis—case report. Neurol Med Chir (Tokyo) 1992;32:360–364

27. Nataf F, Devaux B, Lamy C, Fallet-Bianco C, Roux FX. [Sphenocavernous localization of meningeal neurosarcoidosis. Apropos of a case and review of the literature]. Neurochirurgie 1993;39:128–131

28. Keuter EJ. Posterior cavernous syndrome caused by pachymeningitis due to Besnier-Boeck-Schaumann's disease (sarcoidosis). Psychiatr Neurol Neurochir 1970;73:135–144

29. Sekhar LN, Dujovny M, Rao GR. Carotid-cavernous sinus thrombosis caused by Aspergillus fumigatus. Case report. J Neurosurg 1980;52:120–125

30. Cusimano MD, Sekhar LN, Sen CN, et al. The results of surgery for benign tumors of the cavernous sinus. Neurosurgery 1995;37:1–9, discussion 9–10

31. Eisenberg MB, Al-Mefty O, DeMonte F, Burson GT. Benign nonmeningeal tumors of the cavernous sinus. Neurosurgery 1999;44:949–954, discussion 954–955

32. Sekiya T, Hatayama T, Iwabuchi T, Maeda S. A ring electrode to record extraocular muscle activities during skull base surgery. Acta Neurochir 1992;117:66–69

33. Sekhar LN, Lanzino G, Sen CN, Pomonis S. Reconstruction of the third through sixth cranial nerves during cavernous sinus surgery. J Neurosurg 1992;76:935–943

34. Morita A, Coffey RJ, Foote RL, et al. Risk of injury to cranial nerves after gamma knife radiosurgery for skull base meningiomas: experience in 88 patients. J Neurosurg 1999;90:42–49

35. Larson J, van Loveren HR, Balko M, Tew J. Evidence of meningioma infiltration into cranial nerves: clinical implications for cavernous sinus meningioma. J Neurosurg 1995;83:596–599

36. Kuratsu J, Okamura A, Kamiryo T, Ushio Y. A paediatric patient with meningioma arising from the cavernous sinus wall. Acta Neurochir 1997;139:259–260

37. Sakalas R, Harbison JW, Vines FS, Becker DP. Chronic sixth nerve palsy. An initial sign of basisphenoid tumors. Arch Ophthalmol 1975;93:186–190

38. Schatz NJ, Savino PJ, Corbett JJ. Primary aberrant oculomotor regeneration. A sign of intracavernous meningioma. Arch Neurol 1977;34:29–32

39. Hannerz J. A case of parasellar meningioma mimicking cluster headache. Cephalalgia 1989;9:265–269

40. Bradac GB, Riva A, Schorner W, Stura G. Cavernous sinus meningiomas: an MRI study. Neuroradiology 1987;29:578–581

41. Post MJ, Glaser JS, Trobe JD. The radiographic recognition of two clinically elusive mass lesions of the cavernous sinus: meningiomas and aneurysms. Neuroradiology 1978;16:499–503

42. Perry A, Scheithauer BW, Stafford SL, et al. "Malignancy" in mengiomas: a clinicopathologic study of 116 patients, with grading implications. Cancer 1999;85:2046–2056

43. Ojemann RG, Thornton AF, Harsh GR IV. Management of anterior cranial base and cavernous sinus neoplasms with conservative surgery alone or in combination with fractionated photon or stereotactic proton radiosurgery. Clin Neurosurg 1994;42:71–98

44. Sekhar LN, Moller AR. Operative management of tumors involving the cavernous sinus. J Neurosurg 1986;64:879–889

45. O'Sullivan M, van Loveren HR, Tew J. The surgical resectability of meningiomas of the cavernous sinus. Neurosurgery 1997;40:238–247

46. De Jesus O, Sekhar LN, Parikh HK, et al. Long-term follow-up of patients with meningiomas involving the cavernous sinus: recurrence, progression, and quality of life. Neurosurgery 1996;39:915–919, discussion 919–920

47. Bonnal J, Brotchi J, Born J. Meningiomas of the lateral portion of the sella turcica. Acta Neurochir Suppl 1979;28:385–386

48. Cophignon J, Lucena J, Clay C, Marchac D. Limits to radical treatment of spheno-orbital meningiomas. Acta Neurochir Suppl 1979;28:375–380

49. Cioffi FA, Bernini FP, Punzo A, et al. Cavernous sinus meningiomas. Neurochirurgia 1987;30:40–47

50. Shaffrey ME, Dolenc VV, Lanzino G, et al. Invasion of the internal carotid artery by cavernous sinus meningiomas. Surg Neurol 1999;52:167–171

51. Kotapka MJ, Kalia KK, Martinez AJ, Sekhar LN. Infiltration of the carotid artery by cavernous sinus meningioma. J Neurosurg 1994;81:252–255

52. Mathiesen T, Lindquist C, Kihlsrom L, Karlsson B. Recurrence of cranial base meningiomas. Neurosurgery 1996;39:2–9

53. Kim DK, Grieve J, Archer DJ, Uttley D. Meningiomas in the region of the cavernous sinus: a review of 21 patients. Br J Neurosurg 1996;10:439–444

54. Honegger J, Fahlbusch R, Buchfelder M, et al. The role of transsphenoidal microsurgery in the management of sellar and parasellar meningioma. Surg Neurol 1993;39:18–24

55. Sibtain A, Plowman PN. Stereotactic radiosurgery. VII. Radiosurgery versus conventionally-fractionated radiotherapy in the treatment of cavernous sinus meningiomas. Br J Neurosurg 1999;13:158–166

56. Maguire PD, Clough R, Friedman AH, Halperin EC. Fractionated external-beam radiation therapy for meningiomas of the cavernous sinus. Int J Radiat Oncol Biol Phys 1999;44:75–79

57. Connell PP, Macdonald RL, Mansur DB, et al. Tumor size predicts controls of benign meningiomas treated with radiotherapy. Neurosurgery 1999;44:1194–1200

58. van Effenterre R, Bataini JP, Cabanis EA, Iba-Zizen MT. High energy radiotherapy in the treatment of meningiomas of the cavernous sinus. Acta Neurochir Suppl 1979;28:464–467

59. Carella RJ, Ransohoff J, Newall J. Role of radiation therapy in the management of meningiomas. Neurosurgery 1982;10:332–339

60. Duma CM, Lunsford LD, Kondziolka D, et al. Stereotactic radiosurgery of cavernous sinus meningiomas as an addition or alternative to microsurgery. Neurosurgery 1993;32:699–704, discussion 704–705

61. Liscak R, Simonova G, Vymazal J, et al. Gamma knife radiosurgery of meningiomas in the cavernous sinus region. Acta Neurochir 1999;141:473–480

62. Chang SD, Adler JR Jr, Martin DP. LINAC radiosurgery for cavernous sinus meningiomas. Stereotact Funct Neurosurg 1998;71:43–50

63. Kurita H, Sasaki T, Kawamoto S, et al. Role of radiosurgery in the management of cavernous sinus meningiomas. Acta Neurol Scand 1997;96:297–304

64. Friedlander RM, Ojemann RG, Thornton AF. Management of meningiomas of the cavernous sinus: conservative surgery and adjuvant therapy. Clin Neurosurg 1999;45:279–282

65. Schrell UM, Rittig M, Anders M, et al. Hydroxyurea for treatment of unresectable and recurrent meningiomas. II. Decrease in the size of meningiomas in patients treated with hydroxyurea. J Neurosurg 1997;86:840–844

66. Linskey ME, Sekhar LN. Cavernous sinus hemangiomas: a series, a review, and an hypothesis. Neurosurgery 1992;30:101–108

67. Shi J, Hang C, Pan Y, et al. Cavernous hemangiomas in the cavernous sinus. Neurosurgery 1999;45:1308–1313, discussion 1313–1314

68. Lee AG, Miller NR, Brazis PW, Benson ML. Cavernous sinus hemangioma. Clinical and neuroimaging features. J Neuroophthalmol 1995;15:225–229

69. Goto Y, Yamabe K, Aiko Y, et al. Cavernous hemangioma in the cavernous sinus. Neurochirurgia 1993;36:93–95

70. Bristot R, Santoro A, Fantozzi L, Delfini R. Cavernoma of the cavernous sinus: case report. Surg Neurol 1997;48:160–163

71. Lupret V, Negovetic L, Smiljanic D, et al. Cavernous angioma in cavernous sinus: case report of a rare location. Neurol Croat 1992;41:235–240

72. Sepehrnia A, Tatagiba M, Brandis A, et al. Cavernous angioma of the cavernous sinus: case report. Neurosurgery 1990;27:151–154, discussion 154–155

73. Zotta D, Nina P, Martino V, et al. Cavernous angioma of the diencephalon. J Neurosurg Sci 1995;39:159–163

74. Nakasu Y, Handa J, Matsuda M, Koyama T. Cavernous angioma of the middle cranial fossa. Report of two cases and a review. Nippon Geka Hokan 1985;54:364–371

75. Ueki K, Matsutani M, Nakamura O, et al. Cavernous angioma of the middle fossa: a case report and characteristic MRI findings. Radiat Med 1993;11:31–35

76. van Heesewijk JP, Witkamp TD, van Overbeeke JJ. Cavernous haemangioma in the cavernous sinus. CT and MR imaging. Rofo Fortschr Geb Rontgenstr Neuen Bildgeb Verfahr 1992;156:396–397

77. Baskaya MK. Cavernous haemangiomas in the cavernous sinus. Br J Neurosurg 1996;10:422–423

78. Sawamura Y, de Tribolet TN. Cavernous hemangioma in the cavernous sinus: case report. Neurosurgery 1990;26:126–128

79. Shi J, Wang H, Hang C, et al. Cavernous hemangiomas in the cavernous sinus. Case reports. Surg Neurol 1999;52:473–478, discussion 478–479

80. Mawn LA, Jordan DR, Gilberg SM. Cavernous hemangiomas of the orbital apex with intracranial extension. Ophthalmic Surg Lasers 1998;29:680–684

81. Rosenblum B, Rothman AS, Lanzieri C, Song S. A cavernous sinus cavernous hemangioma. Case report. J Neurosurg 1986;65:716–718

82. Bricolo A, De Micheli E, Gambin R, et al. Cavernous malformation of the internal auditory canal. A case report. J Neurosurg Sci 1995;39:153–158

83. Goel A, Nadkarni TD. Cavernous haemangioma in the cavernous sinus. Br J Neurosurg 1995;9:77–80

84. Ohata K, El-Naggar A, Takami T, et al. Efficacy of induced hypotension in the surgical treatment of large cavernous sinus cavernomas. J Neurosurg 1999;90:702–708

85. Maruishi M, Shima T, Okada Y, et al. Cavernous sinus cavernoma treated with radiation therapy—case report. Neurol Med Chir (Tokyo) 1994;34:773–777

86. Miserocchi G, Vaiani S, Migliore MM, Villani RM. Cavernous hemangioma of the cavernous sinus. Complete disappearance of the neoplasma after subtotal excision and radiation therapy. Case report. J Neurosurg Sci 1997;41:203–207

87. Iwai Y, Yamanaka K, Nakajima H, Yasui T. Stereotactic radiosurgery for cavernous sinus cavernous hemangioma—case report. Neurol Med Chir (Tokyo) 1999;39:288–290

88. Jamjoom AB. Response of cavernous sinus hemangioma to radiotherapy: a case report. Neurosurg Rev 1996;19:261–264

89. Masson C, Lehericy S, Guillaume B, Masson M. Cluster-like headache in a patient with a trigeminal neurinoma. Headache 1995;35:48–49

90. el-Kalliny M, van Loveren H, Keller JT, Tew JM Jr. Tumors of the lateral wall of the cavernous sinus. J Neurosurg 1992;77:508–514

91. Cerillo A, Bianco M, Narciso N, et al. Trigeminal cystic neurinoma in the cavernous sinus. Case report. J Neurosurg Sci 1995;39:165–170

92. Inoue T, Fukui M, Matsushima T, et al. Neurinoma in the cavernous sinus: report of two cases. Neurosurgery 1990;27:986–990

93. Yamashita J, Asato R, Handa H, et al. Abducens nerve palsy as initial symptom of trigeminal schwannoma. J Neurol Neurosurg Psychiatry 1977;40:1190–1197

94. De Jesus O, Colon LE. Extradural intrasphenoidal cavernous sinus schwannoma. Case illustration. J Neurosurg 1996;85:359

95. Yu CB, Lyons CJ, Dorrell ED, Taylor D. Congenital cavernous sinus syndrome in a child with neurofibromatosis type 2. Can J Ophthalmol 1999;34:101–103

96. Kachhara R, Nair S, Radhakrishnan VV. Oculomotor nerve neurinoma: report of two cases. Acta Neurochir (Wien) 1998;140:1147–1151

97. Tung H, Chen T, Weiss MH. Sixth nerve schwannomas. Report of two cases. J Neurosurg 1991;75:638–641

98. Hansman ML, Hoover ED, Peyster RG. Sixth nerve neuroma in the cavernous sinus: CT features. J Comput Assist Tomogr 1986;10:1030–1032

99. Kurokawa Y, Uede T, Honda O, Honmou O. Successful removal of intracavernous neurinoma originating from the oculomotor nerve—case report. Neurol Med Chir (Tokyo) 1992;32:225–228

100. Oyoshi T, Hirahara K, Niino M, et al. [Trigeminal neurinoma in the cavernous sinus revealed by intratumoral hemorrhage: a case report]. No Shinkei Geka 1994;22:175–178

101. Lanotte M, Giordana MT, Forni C, Pagni CA. Schwannoma of the cavernous sinus. Case report and review of the literature. J Neurosurg Sci 1992;36:233–238

102. Moscow NP, Newton TH. Angiographic features of hypervascular neurinomas of the head and neck. Radiology 1975;114:635–640

103. Okudera T, Mihara K, Takahashi M, et al. [Neuroradiologic diagnosis of trigeminal neurinoma originating from the gasserian ganglion (author's transl)]. No Shinkei Geka 1975;3:835–848

104. Colin P, Scavarda D, Delemer B, et al. [Fractionated stereotactic radiotherapy: results in hypophyseal adenomas, acoustic neurinomas, and meningiomas of the cavernous sinus]. Cancer Radiother 1998;2:207–214

105. Mariniello G, Horvat A, Dolenc VV. En bloc resection of an intracavernous oculomotor nerve schwannoma and grafting of the oculomotor nerve with sural nerve. Case report and review of the literature. J Neurosurg 1999;91:1045–1049

106. Huang CF, Kondziolka D, Fickinger JC, Lunsford LD. Stereotactic radiosurgery for trigeminal schwannomas. Neurosurgery 1999;45:11–16

107. Prasad D, Steiner M, Steiner L. Gamma surgery for vestibular schwannoma. J Neurosurg 2000;92:745–759

108. Kalina P, Black K, Woldenberg R. Burkitt's lymphoma of the skull base presenting as cavernous sinus syndrome in early childhood. Pediatr Radiol 1996;26:416–417

109. Kasner SE, Galetta SL, Vaughn DJ. Cavernous sinus syndrome in Hodgkin's disease. J Neuroophthalmol 1996;16:204–207

110. Ceyhan M, Erdem G, Kanra G, et al. Lymphoma with bilateral cavernous sinus involvement in early childhood. Pediatr Neurol 1994;10:67–69

111. Julien J, Ferrer X, Drouillard J, et al. Cavernous sinus syndrome due to lymphoma. J Neurol Neurosurg Psychiatry 1984;47:558–560

112. Delpassand ES, Kirkpatrick JB. Cavernous sinus syndrome as the presentation of malignant lymphoma: case report and review of the literature. Neurosurgery 1988;23:501–504

113. Paysse EA, Coats DK, Ellis FD, et al. Simultaneous cavernous sinus syndrome and facial lesion as presenting signs of Ki-1 positive anaplastic large cell lymphoma in a child. J Pediatr Ophthalmol Strabismus 1997;34:313–315

114. Delerue O, Rogelet P, Dupard T, et al. [Bilateral cavernous sinus syndrome: Burkitt's lymphoma]. Rev Neurol (Paris) 1991;147:311–314

115. Koh CS, Tan CT, Alhady SF. Cavernous sinus syndrome. A manifestation of non-Hodgkin's lymphoma of the ethmoid sinus. Med J Aust 1983;2:451–452

116. Rubin MM, Sanfilippo RJ. Lymphoma of the paranasal sinuses presenting as cavernous sinus syndrome. J Oral Maxillofac Surg 1992;50:749–751

117. Williams Z, Norbash A, Goode RL. Cavernous sinus syndrome caused by a primary paranasal sinus non-Hodgkin's lymphoma. J Laryngol Otol 1998;112:777–778

118. Brazis PW, Menke DM, McLeish WM, et al. Angiocentric T-cell lymphoma presenting with multiple cranial nerve palsies and retrobulbar optic neuropathy. J Neuroophthalmol 1995;15:152–157

119. Nakatomi H, Sasaki T, Kawamoto S, et al. Primary cavernous sinus malignant lymphoma treated by gamma knife radiosurgery: case report and review of the literature. Surg Neurol 1996;46:272–278, discussion 278–279

120. Harada T, Ohashi T, Ohki K, et al. Clival chordoma presenting as acute esotropia due to bilateral abducens palsy. Ophthalmologica 1997;211:109–111

121. Oot RF, Melville G, New PF, et al. The role of MR and CT in evaluating clival chordomas and chondrosarcomas. Am J Neuroradiol 1988;9:715–723

122. Launay M, Fredy D, Merland JJ, Bories J. Narrowing and occlusion of arteries by intracranial tumors. Review of the literature and report of 25 cases. Neuroradiology 1977;14:117–126

123. Schechter MM, Liebeskind AL, Azar-Kia B. Intracranial chordomas. Neuroradiology 1974;8:67–82

124. Legre J, Dufour M, Debaene A, et al. [Angiographic signs of tumors of the cavernous sinus region]. Neurochirurgie 1973;19:29–48

125. Arnold H, Hermann HD. Skull base chordoma with cavernous sinus involvement. Partial or radical tumour-removal? Acta Neurochir 1986;83:31–37

126. Lanzino G, Hirsch W, Pomonis S, et al. Cavernous sinus tumors: neuroradiologic and neurosurgical considerations on 150 operated cases. J Neurosurg Sci 1992;36:183–196

127. Krayenbuhl H, Yasargel MG. Cranial chordomas. Prog Neurol Surg 1975;6:380–434

128. Kawase T. [Skull base approaches for clival tumors]. No Shinkei Geka 1990;18:121–128

129. Raffel C, Wright D, Gutin PH, Wilson CB. Cranial chordomas: clinical presentation and results of operative and radiation therapy in twenty-six patients. J Neurosurg 1985;17:703–710

130. Kline LB. The Tolosa–Hunt syndrome. Surv Ophthalmol 1982;27:79–95

131. Iwai Y, Hakuba A, Katsuyama J, et al. [Inflammatory granulomas extending from the sphenoid sinus to the cavernous sinus: report of three cases]. No Shinkei Geka 1991;19:465–470

132. Tolosa E. Periarteritic lesions of the carotid siphon with the clinical features of a carotid infraclinoid aneurysm. J Neurol Neurosurg Psychiatry 1954;17:300–302

133. Hunt WE, Meagher JN, LeFever HE, Zeman W. Painful ophthalmoplegia: its relation to indolent inflammation of the cavernous sinus. Neurology 1961;11:56–62

134. Frohman LP, Kupersmith M, Lang J, et al. Intracranial extension and bone destruction in orbital pseudotumor. Archiv Ophthalmol 1986;104:380–384

135. Goto Y, Hosokawa S, Goto I, et al. Abnormality in the cavernous sinus in three patients with Tolosa–Hunt syndrome: MRI and CT findings. J Neurol Neurosurg Psychiatry 1990;53:231–234

136. Dornan TL, Espir ML, Gale EA, et al. Remittent painful ophthalmoplegia: the Tolosa–Hunt syndrome? A report of seven cases and review of the literature. J Neurol Neurosurg Psychiatry 1979;42:270–275

137. Goadsby PJ, Lance JW. Clinicopathological correlation in a case of painful ophthalmoplegia: Tolosa–Hunt syndrome. J Neurol Neurosurg Psychiatry 1989;52:1290–1293

138. Mehelas TJ, Kosmorsky GS. Painful ophthalmoplegia syndrome secondary to metastatic renal cell carcinoma. J Neuroophthalmol 1996;16:289–290

139. Unsold R, Safran AB, Safran E, Hoyt WF. Metastatic infiltration of nerves in the cavernous sinus. Arch Neurol 1980;37:59–61

140. Merimsky O, Inbar M, Grosswasser-Reider I, et al. Sphenoid and cavernous sinuses involvement as first site of metastasis from a fallopian tube carcinoma. Case report. Tumori 1993;79:444–446

141. Ryan MW, Rassekh CH, Chaljub G. Metastatic breast carcinoma presenting as cavernous sinus syndrome. Ann Otol Rhinol Laryngol 1996;105:666–668

142. Supler ML, Friedman WA. Acute bilateral ophthalmoplegia secondary to cavernous sinus metastasis: a case report. Neurosurgery 1992;31:783–786, discussion 786

143. Yamamoto T, Imai T. [Adenoid cystic carcinoma presenting as cavernous sinus syndrome: a clinico-pathological study of two cases]. No To Shinkei 1989;41:519–525

144. Arcas A, Bescos S, Raspall G, Caspellades J. Perineural spread of epidermoid carcinoma in the infraorbital nerve: case report. J Oral Maxillofac Surg 1996;54:520–522

145. Woodruff WW Jr, Yeates AE, McLendon RE. Perineural tumor extension to the cavernous sinus from superficial facial carcinoma: CT manifestations. Radiology 1986;161:395–399

146. Post MJ, Mendez D, Kline LB, et al. Metastatic disease to the cavernous sinus: clinical syndrome and CT diagnosis. J Comput Assist Tomogr 1985;9:115–120

147. Merimsky O, Reider I, Inbar M, et al. Metastatic

disease of the cavernous sinus: contribution of computed tomography and magnetic resonance imaging to diagnosis. Tumori 1990;76:548–551

148. Spell DW, Gervais DS Jr, Ellis JK, Vial RH. Cavernous sinus syndrome due to metastatic renal cell carcinoma. South Med J 1998;91:576–579

149. Ganzer U. [Carcinoma of the nasopharynx: remarks on its etiology, diagnosis and prognosis]. Strahlenther Onkol 1987;163:519–524

150. Morales-Angulo C, Megia Lopez R, Rubio Suarez A, et al. [Carcinoma of the nasopharynx in Cantabria]. Acta Otorrinolaringol Esp 1999;50:381–386

151. Vasef MA, Ferlito A, Weiss LM. Nasopharyngeal carcinoma, with emphasis on its relationship to Epstein–Barr virus. Ann Otol Rhinol Laryngol 1997; 106:348–356

152. Ng SH, Chong VF, Ko SF, Mukherji SK. Magnetic resonance imaging of nasopharyngeal carcinoma. Top Magn Reson Imaging 1999;10:290–303

153. Koch BL. Imaging extracranial masses of the pediatric head and neck. Neuroimaging Clin N Am 2000; 10:193–214, ix

154. Valavanis A, Christoforidis G. Applications of interventional neuroradiology in the head and neck. Semin Roentgenol 2000;35:72–83

155. Levine PA, Frierson HF Jr, Stewart FM, et al. Sinonasal undifferentiated carcinoma: a distinctive and highly aggressive neoplasm. Laryngoscope 1987;97:905–908

156. Cvitkovic E, Bachouchi M, Armand JP. Nasopharyngeal carcinoma. Biology, natural history, and therapeutic implications. Hematol Oncol Clin North Am 1991;5:821–838

157. Chan AT, Teo PM, Leung TW, Johnson PJ. The role of chemotherapy in the management of nasopharyngeal carcinoma. Cancer 1998;82:1003–1012

158. Lee AW, Law SC, Foo W, et al. Retrospective analysis of patients with nasopharyngeal carcinoma treated during 1976–1985: survival after local recurrence. Int J Radiat Oncol Biol Phys 1993;26:773–782

159. Fujino K, Nonomura M, Fukushima H, et al. Remote afterloading system radiotherapy through sphenoid sinus for T4 nasopharyngeal cancer. Am J Otolaryngol 1994;15:297–300

160. Teo PM, Kwan WH, Chan AT, et al. How successful is high-dose (> or = 60 Gy) reirradiation using mainly external beams in salvaging local failures of nasopharyngeal carcinoma? Int J Radiat Oncol Biol Phys 1998;40:897–913

161. Taguchi J, Sato M, Sasaki M, et al. [A case with nasopharyngeal carcinoma extending into the cavernous sinus]. No Shinkei Geka 1997;25:939–942

162. Wei WI. Salvage surgery for recurrent primary nasopharyngeal carcinoma. Crit Rev Oncology Hematol 2000;33:91–98

163. Eisbruch A, Dawson L. Re-irradiation of head and neck tumors. Benefits and toxicities. Hematol Oncol Clin North Am 1999;13:825–836

164. Lee AW, Sze WM, Fowler JF, et al. Caution on the use of altered fractionation for nasopharyngeal carcinoma. Radiother Oncol 1999;52:207–211

165. Pommier P, Lapeyre M, Ginestet C, et al. [Conformal radiotherapy in cancer of the upper aerodigestive tract]. Cancer Radiother 1999;3:414–424

166. Sanguineti G, Corvo R. Treatment of nasopharyngeal carcinoma: state of the art and new perspectives (review). Oncology Reports 1999;6:377–391

167. Harrison LB. Applications of brachytherapy in head and neck cancer. Semin Surg Oncol 1997;13:177–184

168. Agarwala SS. Adjuvant chemotherapy in head and neck cancer. Hematol Oncol Clin North Am 1999;13: 743–752, vii

169. Chan AT, Teo PM, Johnson PJ. Controversies in the management of locoregionally advanced nasopharyngeal carcinoma. Curr Opin Oncol 1998;10:219–225

170. Ali H, al-Sarraf M. Nasopharyngeal cancer. Hematol Oncol Clin North Am 1999;13:837–847

171. McCormick WF, Boutter TR. Vascular malformations ("angiomas") of the dura mater. Report of two cases. J Neurosurg 1966;25:309–311

172. Barker WF, Stern WE, Krayenbuhl H, et al. Carotid endarterectomy complicated by carotid cavernous fistula. Ann Surg 1968;167:572

173. Eggers F, Lukin R, Chambers AA, et al. Iatrogenic carotid-cavernous fistula following fogarty catheter thromboendarterectomy. Case report. J Neurosurg 1979;51:543–545

174. Kakkasseril JS, Tomsick TA, Arbaugh JA, Cranley JJ. Carotid cavernous fistula following fogarty catheter thrombectomy. Arch Surg 1984;119:1095–1096

175. Kupersmith MJ, Berenstein A, Flamm E, Ransohoff J. Neuroophthalmologic abnormalities and intravascular therapy of traumatic carotid cavernous fistulas. Ophthalmology 1986;93:903–912

176. Takahashi M, Killeffer F, Wilson G. Iatrogenic carotid cavernous fistulas: case report. J Neurosurg 1969; 30:498–500

177. Kupersmith MJ, Berenstein A, Choi IS, et al. Management of nontraumatic vascular shunts involving the cavernous sinus. Ophthalmology 1988;95:121–130

178. Graf CJ. Spontaneous carotid-cavernous fistula: Ehlers-Danlos syndrome and related conditions. Arch Neurol 1965;13:662–672

179. Farley MK, Clark RD, Fallor MK, et al. Spontaneous carotid-cavernous fistula and the Ehlers-Danlos syndromes. Ophthalmology 1983;90:1337–1342

180. Koo AH, Newton TH. Pseudoxanthoma elasticum associated with carotid rate mirable. Am J Roentgenol Radium Ther Nucl Med 1972;116:16–22

181. Kaufman HH, Lind TA, Mullan S. Spontaneous carotid-cavernous fistula with fibromuscular dysplasia. Acta Neurochir 1978;40:123–129

182. Henderson JW, Schneider RC. The ocular findings in carotid cavernous fistula in a series of 17 cases. Am J Ophthalmol 1959;48:585–597

183. Sanders MD, Hoyt WF. Hypoxic ocular sequelae of carotid-cavernous fistulae. Study of the causes and failure before and after neuro-surgical treatment in a series of 25 cases. Br J Ophthalmol 1969;53:82–97

184. Harris MJ, Fine SL, Miller NR. Photocoagulation treatment of proliferative retinopathy secondary to carotid-cavernous fistula. Am J Ophthalmol 1980;90:515–518

185. Grove AS. The dural shunt syndrome. Pathophysiology and clinical course. Ophthalmology 1983;90:31–44

186. Kobayashi H, Hayashi M, Noguchi Y, et al. Dural arteriovenous malformations in the anterior cranial fossa. Surg Neurol 1988;30:396–401

187. Hosobuchi Y. Electrothrombosis of carotid-cavernous fistula. J Neurosurg 1975;42:76–85

188. Brooks B. Discussion, Noland L, Taylor AS. J S Surg 1931;43:176–177

189. Serbinenko FA. Balloon catheterization and occlusion of major cerebral vessels. J Neurosurg 1974;41:125–145

190. Debrun G, Lacour P, Vinuela F. Treatment of 54 traumatic carotid-cavernous fistulas. J Neurosurg 1981; 55:678–692

191. Tsai FY, Hieshima GB, Mehringer CM, et al. Delayed

effects of treatment of carotid-cavernous fistulas. Am J Neuroradiol 1983;4:357–361

192. Berenstein A, Kricheff II. Catheter and material selection for transarterial embolization. Technical considerations I. Catheters. Radiology 1979;132:619–630

193. Berenstein A, Kricheff II. Catheter and material selection for transarterial embolization: Technical considerations II. Materials. Radiology 1979;132:631–663

194. Slusher MM, Lennington BR, Weaver RG, Davis CH. Ophthalmic findings in dural arteriovenous shunts. Ophthalmol AAO 1979;86:720–731

195. Niimi Y, Berenstein A, Kupersmith MJ. Endovascular techniques in the treatment of cavernous sinus aneurysms. In: Eisenberg M and Al-Mefty O. The Cavernous Sinus. A Comprehensive Text. Lippincott William and Wilkins, Philadelphia, 2000:155–176.

196. Berenstein A. Selective and superselective catheterization of the brachiocephalic vessels with a new catheter. Radiology 1983;180:437–441

197. Kikuchi T, Strother CM, Boyar M. New catheter therapy for arteriovenous malformations. Radiology 1987;165:870–871

198. Krayenbuhl H. Klassifikation und Klinische Symptomatologie der zerbralen Aneurysmen. Ophthalmologica 1973;167:122–164

199. Henderson JW. Intracranial arterial aneurysms: A study of 119 cases with special reference to the ocular findings. Trans Am Ophthalmol Soc 1955;53:349–462

200. Jefferson G. Concerning injuries, aneurysms and tumors involving the cavernous sinus. Trans Ophthalmol Soc UK 1953;73:117–152

201. Thomas JE, Yoss RE. The parasellar syndrome: Problems in determining etiology. Mayo Clin Proc 1970;45:617–623

202. Cogan D, Mount HT. Intracranial aneurysms causing ophthalmoplegia. Arch Ophthalmol 1963;70:757–771

203. Barr HWK, Blackwood W, Meadows SP. Intracavernous carotid aneurysms. A clinical-pathological report. Brain 1971;94:607–622

204. Rapport R, Murtagh FR. Ophthalmoplegia due to spontaneous thrombosis in a patient with bilateral cavernous carotid aneurysms. J Clin Opthalmol 1981;1:225–229

205. Markwalder TM, Meienberg O. Acute painful cavernous sinus syndrome in unruptured intracavernous aneurysms of the internal carotid artery. J Clin Neuroophthalmol 1983;3:31–35

206. Rush JA, Younge BR. Paralysis of cranial nerves III, IV and IV: Cause and prognosis in 1000 cases. Arch Ophthalmol 1981;99:76–79

207. Boghen D, Chartrand J, Laflamme P, et al. Primary aberrant third nerve regeneration. Ann Neurol 1979;6:415–418

208. Alper MG. The anesthetic eye: an investigation of changes in the anterior ocular segment of the monkey caused by interrupting the trigeminal nerve at various levels along its course. Trans Am Ophth Soc 1975;LXXIII:323–363

209. Meadows SP. Intracavernous aneurysms of the internal carotid artery. Their clinical features and natural history. Arch Ophthalmol 1959;62:566–579

210. Gauthier G, Rohr J, Wildi E, Megret M. L'hematome dissequant spontane de l'artere carotide interne: revue generale de 205 cas publies dont 10 personnels. Arch Suisse Neurol Psychiatr Neurol Psychiatr 1986;136:53–74

211. Kupersmith MJ, Kalish H, Niimi Y, et al. Cavernous carotid aneurysms should not be included in the analysis of intracranial aneurysms (abstract). Ann Neurol 2000;48:454–455

212. Nutik S. Carotid paraclinoid aneurysms with intradural origin and intracavernous location. J Neurosurg 1978;48:526–533

213. van Beusekom GT, Luyendijk W, Huizing EH. Severe episaxis caused by rupture of non-traumatic infraclinoid aneurysm of the internal carotid artery. Acta Neurochir 1966;15:269–284

214. Linskey ME, Sekhar LN, Hirsch W, et al. Aneurysms of the intracavernous carotid artery: clinical presentation, radiographic features and pathogenesis. Neurosurgery 1990;26:71–79

215. Ding MX. Traumatic aneurysm of the intracavernous part of the internal carotid artery presenting with epistaxis. Case report. Surg Neurol 1988;30:65–67

216. McCormick WF, Beals JD. Severe epistaxis caused by ruptured aneurysm of the internal carotid artery. J Neurosurg 1964;21:678–686

217. Hodes JE, Fletcher WA, Goodman DF, Hoyt W. Rupture of cavernous carotid artery aneurysm causing subdural hematoma and death. J Neurosurg 1988;69:617–619

218. Kupersmith MJ, Hurst R, Choi IS, et al. Carotid cavernous aneurysms—a benign prognosis. Neurology 1991;41(Suppl 1):367

219. Nishioka T, Kondo A, Aoyama I, et al. Subarachnoid hemorrhage possibly caused by a saccular carotid artery aneurysm within the cavernous sinus. J Neurosurg 1990;73:301–304

220. Kupersmith MJ, Berenstein A, Choi I, et al. Percutaneous transvascular treatment of giant carotid aneurysms: neuro-ophthalmologic findings. Neurology 1984;34:328–335

221. Higashida RT, Halbach VV, Dowd C, et al. Endovascular detachable balloon embolization therapy of cavernous carotid artery aneurysms: results in 87 cases. J Neurosurg 1990;72:857–863

222. Kupersmith M, Berenstein A, Flamm ES, et al. Endovascular treatment of giant carotid aneurysms: neuro-ophthalmologic findings. Neurology 1984;34:328–335

223. Fein JN, Flamm E. Planned intracranial revascularizaton before proximal ligation for traumatic aneurysms. Neurosurgery 1979;5:54–57

224. Spetzler RF, Rhodes RS, Roski RA, et al. Subclavian to middle cerebral artery saphenous vein bypass graft. J Neurosurg 1980;53:465–469

225. Dolenc VV, Čerk M, Šušteršič J, et al. Treatment of intracavernous aneurysms of the ICA and CCF's by direct approach. In: Dolenc VV, ed. The Cavernous Sinus: A Multidisciplinary Approach to Vascular and Tumorous Lesions. Wien: Springer–Verlag, 1987:297–310

226. Diaz FG, Ohaegbulam S, Dujovny M, Ausman JI. Surgical alternatives in the treatment of cavernous sinus aneurysms. J Neurosurg 1966;71:215–218

170 Trigeminal Neuropathy and Neuralgia

C Peter N Watson

Overview

Since this book focuses on therapeutics in neurological disorders, the main emphasis in this chapter will be on painful neuropathic disorders of the trigeminal system, particularly the "neuralgias" and their treatment. By "neuralgia" the author means neuropathic pain, usually with a component of a paroxysmal, brief, shock-like pain which is often triggered by non-painful stimulation and is, thus, a form of allodynia (pain from a normally nonpainful stimulus).[1] Sometimes a condition may still be termed neuralgia and not always have this timing and quality, e.g. postherpetic neuralgia (PHN). In this case, the appellation stands because of tradition and its meaning is more "neuropathic" (nerve) pain. Symptomatic trigeminal diseases that may involve nerves such as tumors, cysts, and aneurysms will not be covered in detail except to point out some important anatomical information which can aid in localization. The focus of the chapter will be on trigeminal neuralgia (TN) and PHN, two of the most common and treatable causes of neuropathic pain in the face, with a specific discussion comparing these disorders and emphasizing the differences between them, particularly with regard to treatment. This information can, in the author's view, be extrapolated to other less common or atypical neuropathic facial pain for which there is no good science available. In the author's view, much of so-called "atypical" facial pain is neuropathic when a careful history and physical examination are performed.

Comparing PHN and TN raises more questions than answers, but the questions are intriguing. TN has been recognized for centuries: it is a stereotypical facial pain with a well worked out therapy. It is of particular interest because it appears (along with other, rarer cranial neuralgias such as glossopharyngeal neuralgia) to be unique to the face and head area as are, for example, migraine and cluster headache. PHN is much more like nerve injury pain elsewhere in the body, both clinically and in its pharmacological responsivity. Although PHN has its own idiosyncrasies, it provides a good clinical model for the investigation of neuropathic pain generally, in the search for better therapies, such as for painful diabetic neuropathy, causalgia, and some cases of the failed back syndrome. For more comprehensive information on TN and PHN, the reader is referred to recent books devoted to these conditions.[2,3]

The differences between TN and PHN are striking, particularly from a neuropharmacological point of view. These two disorders are the most easily recognizable and treatable of the facial neuropathic pain problems but by different means (medical and surgical for TN and medical for PHN). If we can find the reasons for these differences, we will come to a greater understanding of the trigeminal system, its disorders, and their treatment.

Some trigeminal neuropathic pain syndromes include:

Trigeminal neuralgia
Postherpetic neuralgia
Post-traumatic neuralgia
Anesthesia dolorosa
Atypical facial pain
Tumor, aneurysm.

The really difficult problems are post-traumatic neuralgia, anesthesia dolorosa, and neuropathic forms of atypical facial pain. Although brain tumor and aneurysm can result in facial pain they are uncommon; however, they should be considered and investigated if appropriate and may be relieved by surgical decompression.

Anatomical considerations

Anatomical considerations are important in localizing the sites of potential lesions in the trigeminal system.[2] There is a somatotopic organization of the three peripheral nerve divisions in the gasserian ganglion in the mediolateral plane. The cell bodies of the ophthalmic (V1) division are located in the anteromedial portion of the ganglion. A somatotopic organization is maintained within the central root and trigeminal tract. This arrangement is laminar with an inverted homuncular representation of the face within the tract. The ophthalmic fibers are most ventral. Termination within the nuclei of the three trigeminal divisions is also an inverted dorsoventral order. All three divisions terminate at all rostrocaudal levels of the nuclear complex, but it is well established that the nucleus caudalis is the main site within the trigeminal brainstem nuclear complex where facial nociceptive information is processed. Within the nucleus there is also a mediolateral somatotopic arrangement of the three divisions of the trigeminal nerve in conjunction with rostrocaudal somatotopy related to the rostrocaudal axis of the orofacial region ("onion peel") with a caudal representation of the forehead. There is also some evidence, especially for intraoral structures, of involvement of more rostral regions of the trigeminal nuclear complex in nociception. The mesencephalic nucleus cells are chiefly bipolar (pseudo-unipolar) and, therefore, resemble the cells in the gasserian ganglion. These cells probably mediate proprioception in masticatory muscles and are analogous to the cells of the gasserian ganglion.

Trigeminal neuralgia (tic douloureux)

Overview

Although earlier authors may have described TN, the term "tic douloureux" was used by Nicholaus Andre (1756) who gave the first accurate clinical description of the disorder.[2] This appellation highlights the tic-like movement of facial muscles resulting from the severe shock-like pain. John Fothergill independently and quite soon after (1769) also described all the clinical aspects of TN.[2] Chapman (1834) described the characteristic spontaneous remissions.[2]

Epidemiology

TN is the most frequent of all the neuralgias, and its overall incidence has been stated to be 155 per million per year.[4] The mean age of onset is in the mid-fifties for the idiopathic form,[5] increasing with age. Patients with the symptomatic disorder are often younger. It has been said that TN is more common in females (1.6:1)[4,6] and more often right-sided (2:1),[5,6] but more recent studies have questioned this. It does affect more commonly the face innervated by the second and third divisions of the trigeminal nerve. There are reports of a familial occurrence[5] and TN is more common in multiple sclerosis (MS) with 2.4% of all patients with TN having MS,[7] and 1.5% of patients with MS having TN.[8]

Etiology

In most cases of TN, no underlying disorder is found with brain imaging and other tests. However, vascular loops compressing the root entry zone are found frequently at surgery,[9] and it is therefore believed that this cause of irritation is a frequent one. The association of TN and MS has previously been mentioned[7,8] and presumably MS plaques in the area are related to the pain. Symptomatic pain similar to TN can be seen in patients with a variety of tumors, vascular malformations and aneurysms, peripheral nerve trauma, and inflammation of the sinuses, teeth, and temporomandibular joint.

Pathophysiology and pathogenesis

Since a variety of peripheral disorders appear to be associated with TN, and pharmacological agents that relieve this pain act centrally, Gerhard Fromm has suggested that there is a peripheral etiology with TN which leads to a central pathogenesis.[10] Specifically, chronic irritation or damage of afferent fibers can produce an afferent bombardment leading to the degeneration of pre- and post-synaptic inhibitory interneurons in the trigeminal nuclear complex and a state of central hyperexcitability involving low threshold mechanoreceptive (LTM) neurons in subnucleus oralis and wide dynamic range (WDR) neurons in subnucleus caudalis. This hypothesis explains clinical features such as tactile triggers, summation, refractory periods and distant radiation. Although some of the details of this concept have been criticized,[11] it remains an attractive explanation of the disorder.

Genetics

Some cases of familial idiopathic TN have been reported.[5]

Clinical features

TN has very characteristic clinical features and is usually readily diagnosed. The temporal profile of the pain is that the attacks are very brief (as of a second or less) but may cluster together. Although spontaneous bursts appear, the attacks are often associated with non-noxious activities which trigger the pain such as brushing the teeth, washing the face, eating, speaking or even cold air blowing on the face. Pain-free intervals thus occur with behavioral quiescence during a flare-up and for weeks or months because of spontaneous remission. The pain is usually unilateral and in the lower face in the trigeminal distribution of V2 and V3. The pain is triggered by non-nociceptive stimuli such as light touch over a small area, often in the nasolabial fold region. The pain itself is like an electric shock. There is minimal or no sensory loss present to ordinary office testing.

Atypical forms can occur such as the concomitant or antecedent presence of a steady background, sometimes burning, pain[12] which can precede the shock-like pain (pre-TN),[13] and sometimes there is an association with cluster headache, the so-called "cluster-tic syndrome." About 3% of patients have bilateral pain, usually not simultaneously but rather at different times in their lives. Symptomatic TN should be suspected in a young patient with V1 involvement, a progressive course, and/or with neurological physical findings.

Classification

TN may be usefully and roughly classified into idiopathic and symptomatic due to multiple sclerosis, tumors, aneurysms, dental disorders, and other conditions.

Diagnostic criteria

Idiopathic TN is usually characterized by: (1) unilateral, brief, electric shock-like pain, usually in the lower face; (2) triggering of these attacks by various nonpainful tactile stimuli to cutaneous and deeper structures of the face innervated by the trigeminal nerve; (3) at least partial responsivity to carbamazepine; (4) spontaneous remissions; and (5) no sensory loss to ordinary sensory testing procedures.

When a progressive course occurs, sometimes with a steady, worsening background pain, when location is atypical, such as V1, and particularly when there is sensory loss and other neurological findings, symptomatic TN should be suspected and appropriate investigations initiated.

Differential diagnosis

The clinical assessment of patients with TN usually leaves no doubt as to the diagnosis. Atypical features may lead to a diagnosis of multiple sclerosis, tumors of various sorts, aneurysms and vascular malformation, cysts, dental problems such as may injure the alveolar nerves, and other disorders. These various lesions are in proximity at some point to the peripheral trigeminal system. There should be no difficulty clinically in discriminating other facial pain syndromes such as PHN, temporal arteritis, cluster headaches, ice pick-like migraine pain, muscular pain, temporomandibular joint pain, atypical odontalgia, or atypical facial pain.

Treatment (historical overview)

Trousseau (1853) thought that the painful attacks of TN resembled epilepsy.[14] Based on this idea, Bergouignan[15] in 1942 described the successful use of phenytoin in this condition very soon after the drug was first approved for use in epilepsy. In the early 1960s, Blom reported that carbamazepine was more effective than phenytoin in preventing the attacks.[16,17]

Grade A evidence A number of randomized, controlled, double-blind trials (RCTs) of carbamazepine followed the reports of Blom.[18–24]

A recent systematic review[25] selected the following three trials of carbamazepine as being eligible for inclusion.[18,19,21] One crossover study reported at least a very good response in 19 of 27 patients (70%) with up to 1000 mg per day (versus no response with placebo).[19] A second crossover design found 15 of 20 (75%) with at least a good response (versus 6 with placebo).[21] A third trial reported a mean fall in pain of 58% with carbamazepine (versus 26% placebo).[18] According to the systematic review of McQuay et al, the number needed to treat (NNT) with carbamazepine for effectiveness versus placebo was 2.6, for minor side effects 3.4, and for drug-related withdrawal 24.

McQuay et al[25] went on to evaluate three RCTs using other agents with carbamazepine as the control. Carbamazepine was found more effective than tizanidine[26] (antispasticity) and no different in comparison with tocainide[27] (antiarrhythmic). Pimozide (antipsychotic) was found to be superior.[28] Unfortunately, tocainide has been found to have serious hematological side effects, including death, and pimozide has frequent adverse reactions.

Baclofen potentiates gamma-amino butyric acid (GABA) and is frequently used for spinal spasticity. It acts to facilitate segmental inhibition and depresses excitatory transmission in the trigeminal nucleus oralis in cats. Successful open label trials and a RCT,[29] using placebo, have demonstrated efficacy. Baclofen has a synergistic action with carbamazepine.[29] Baclofen is a racemic mixture and although the L isomer is five times as potent in TN,[30] the latter is not commercially available.

Grade C evidence Phenytoin was the first drug to be reported effective in TN.[25] A simple blind[31] and three open label trials[32–34] suggest the utility of the benzodiazepine clonazepam. An open label trial suggested that valproate[35] was effective. Other uncontrolled trials report the utility of mephenesin[29,36] and chlorphenesin.[37]

Treatment (definitive treatment)

The following recommendations are based on the scientific evidence as well as the author's clinical experience as a neurologist treating chronic pain patients for 27 years.

First-line approach The most successful treatment of TN occurs with carbamazepine, which relieves the majority of sufferers when used appropriately. The dose of this drug is variable and the range can be from as little as 200 mg to 2000 mg per day in divided doses, 2 to 4 times a day. A start low and go slow approach is best. The author usually begins with a controlled release preparation every 8 to 12 hours using 100 to 200 mg b.i.d. PO with prn doses of the shorter acting preparation of 100 to 200 mg every 4 hours.

Rescue medication may be timed to anticipate attacks that occur with eating, washing the face, or brushing the teeth. Dose escalation with the longer acting preparation may then occur as needed. Blood levels can be used as a guide to compliance and the possibility of further escalation if symptoms are uncontrolled and there are no side effects. The author does not use an arbitrary ceiling for dosing but increases until satisfactory relief occurs or unacceptable side effects, such as drowsiness, ataxia or nausea, supervene.

The most serious potential side effects of carbamazepine are aplastic anemia and hepatitis. Monitoring of hematological and hepatic parameters rarely results in withdrawal of the drug but is prudent every 2 weeks for the first 2 months, when beginning therapy and then quarterly thereafter. Dermatological reactions may be serious, such as Stevens–Johnson syndrome and lupus, and require that therapy be stopped. Most patients will have good control of their pain with carbamazepine and after an appropriate period it may be reduced or withdrawn as remissions are the rule. A further attack may be more readily treated with the knowledge about dosage that is gained from the first therapeutic experience.

Second-line approach Some patients are only partially relieved by carbamazepine, and about 40% of patients experience side effects which often subside with time, but about 10% require discontinuation of the drug. Long-term studies also indicate that only about 50% are helped by carbamazepine after 5 to 16 years of treatment, presumably because of the progression of the disorder. It is the author's practice to next add baclofen if the response to carbamazepine is incomplete or to use it as monotherapy if carbamazepine has to be discontinued.

The dose of baclofen can be slowly increased from 5 mg to 60 mg per day depending on the response and side effects. Often the drug needs to be taken every 4 hours because of its short half life. Baclofen does not have carbamazepine's potential for life threatening side effects, but most commonly causes drowsiness, dizziness, and gastrointestinal reactions. About 10% of patients must cease treatment on monotherapy because of this. One should never stop baclofen suddenly since hallucinations or seizures may occur.

Phenytoin may also be used as monotherapy, but it is much less effective than carbamazepine and the author finds it most useful as an add-on to carbamazepine or to a combination of carbamazepine and baclofen. With add-on therapy it is reasonable to use 100 mg q.h.s. to start and increase slowly every 7 to 10 days, keeping to evening single dosing and using blood levels as a guide to compliance and dose incrementation with the knowledge that there is no proven therapeutic range, the end points being pain relief or intolerable side effects. Phenytoin has the advantage of being available intravenously for very severe pain that makes oral intake difficult. A loading dose may be used as for epilepsy—1000 mg depending on body weight (15 mg/kg) and given at a rate of 25 mg/min or less. The most common side effects of phenytoin are drowsiness, dizziness, diplopia, and ataxia. These are dose related, but may occur at low doses with combined therapy. Other potential difficulties are gingival hyperplasia, low folic acid levels, and idiosyncratic reactions such as hepatitis, lupus, bone marrow depression, Stevens–Johnson syndrome, and lymphadenopathy.

Third-line approaches   Other drugs of potential use in refractory cases are the anticonvulsants clonazepam (3 to 8 mg/day), valproate (250 to 500 mg q.i.d.), and gabapentin (300 mg/day to 1200 mg t.i.d.). The author has seldom had good success with these agents, and refractory patients may have to be referred for surgery. Conventional analgesics, including the opioids, do not satisfactorily relieve this pain. Interestingly, amitriptyline, a drug which relieves the shock-like pains of PHN, is not effective for TN.

Surgical approaches

This article will not extensively review the large literature on the surgical treatment of TN. This approach should only be recommended after the failure of medical therapy or might be offered to a young individual faced with lifelong pharmacotherapy. In this latter instance, a surgical treatment that could be suggested would be the decompression operation, which would aim to cure the disorder.

Surgical treatment may be divided into two categories. The first comprises simple procedures of gangliolysis which have a high chance of relief and a low morbidity and mortality and are hence of particular use in the elderly. The more extensive operation is suboccipital craniectomy with decompression of the trigeminal nerve.

Gangliolysis   The most common procedure has been radiofrequency gangliolysis: there are some large series of 10 000 cases.[38] The main virtue of this procedure is that it has a low risk of complications (less than 0.5%) and is thus suitable for older patients with intractable pain. The goal is deafferentation of the painful region by inserting an insulated needle through the skin lateral to the mouth and guiding this under fluoroscopy to the foramen ovale and trigeminal ganglion. Stimulation aims to produce paresthesia in the area of the pain or trigger zone. When this occurs, a radiofrequency lesion is made. The major complications include anesthesia dolorosa and neuroparalytic keratitis, and are related to the extent of sensory deficit produced. About 80% of patients will have at least a year of relief and 50% will have 5 years, according to one series[39] with complications of less than 0.5% and no mortality. The procedure can be repeated if pain recurs.

Hakansson[40] introduced glycerol gangliolysis. With this procedure, a small amount of glycerol is instilled via a smaller needle introduced via the foramen ovale into the arachnoid cistern of the gasserian ganglion. Patient cooperation is not a requirement, as it is for the radiofrequency procedure, and corneal anesthesia is reported to be less but anesthesia dolorosa remains a low risk. Initial reports suggested a high success rate with low morbidity, but there remains disagreement about this and the complication rate.

A third method is the inflation of a balloon catheter in Meckel's cave. The results are claimed to be similar to other methods of gangliolysis.[41]

Suboccipital craniectomy and microvascular decompression   This operation was popularized by Jannetta[42] and has proven to be very useful for selected patients. It requires general anesthesia, a craniotomy or craniectomy, and the operating microscope. It is stated that more than 90% of patients will have compression of the trigeminal nerve by an artery or vein, but most commonly the superior cerebellar artery. Muscle tissue or synthetic fiber is used to decompress the nerve. The 1-year success rate has been claimed to be around 85%. Early reports claimed no late failures; however, 5-year follow-up has suggested that 80% remain good results, with a 2% to 3% failure rate per annum.[38] In experienced hands, the mortality rate is approximately 0.5%, with permanent cranial nerve problems in the 5% to 10% range.[38] One of the most feared problems is that of anesthesia dolorosa, which may occur in 4% or less.

Other, more rarely used surgical procedures for difficult cases of failure of the above procedures are peripheral nerve avulsion and posterior fossa trigeminal rhizotomy.

Postherpetic neuralgia
Overview

Trigeminal involvement with herpes zoster has been recognized at least since the turn of the century.[43,44] This disorder, usually in the first division, frequently results in PHN.

Epidemiology

The incidence of PHN (defined as pain persisting for more than one month) has been variously estimated from 9% to 14%.[45] Of an original 100 patients with herpes zoster, at three months as few as five, and at one year only three patients will persist with severe pain.[46] These data emphasize that, in order to minimize the sample in any study of the treatment of this disorder, only patients with significant pain at three or six months should be included. Despite this overall low incidence and marked early tendency for PHN to improve with time, the incidence and the severity (as measured by duration) are directly related to age. About 50% of patients at age 60 years and nearly 75% at age 70 years with herpes zoster have PHN one month or more following the rash.[45] This, combined with the knowledge that herpes zoster itself is common and also directly increases with age, means that PHN is a major problem and will increase as age demographics shift upward.

Most studies have found no gender predilection for PHN when normal demographic change with age is considered.[45] The dermatomal distribution of PHN has been found to reflect that of herpes zoster in that a predilection occurs for thoracic dermatomes, especially T5, and for the ophthalmic division of the fifth cranial nerve.[45] Trigeminal pain may be particularly intractable.

Etiology

PHN results from herpes zoster, which is itself a result of varicella infection in childhood. With declining cell mediated immune surveillance resulting from age or disease, the virus re-emerges in a solitary sensory ganglion, spreading both centrally and peripherally and causing segmental central and peripheral neurological injury which may result in persistent pain.

Pathophysiology and pathogenesis

There is pathological evidence of central and peripheral damage in PHN. Spinal cases show atrophy of the dorsal horn, and peripherally there is fibrosis in the ganglion and a loss of large (pain-inhibiting) fibers with a preponderance of the small (excitatory) myelinated and unmyelinated population.[46] The peripheral changes have been corroborated in a single autopsied trigeminal case which, however, showed no central change.[47] It is thought that both peripheral and central mechanisms are important in causing the pain of PHN. This may involve peripheral ectopic generators in a predominantly small fiber population combined with a state of central sensitization.

Genetics

There is no known genetic predisposition for herpes zoster or PHN.

Clinical features, disease course, natural history

When the acute rash has healed, the affected skin often exhibits a reddish, purple, or brownish hue. As this subsides, pale scarring often remains. Occasionally, severe pain with no residual scar may occur or the scars in cases of very long duration are barely perceptible. The scarred areas are usually at least hypoesthetic and often anesthetic, and yet the skin often exhibits marked skin pain on tactile stimulation (allodynia), or increased pain to noxious stimulation

(hyperalgesia), or an increased sensitivity to touch (hyperesthesia) (Figure 170.1). Two types of pain may be found: one a steady burning or aching, the other a paroxysmal, lancinating pain. Both may occur spontaneously and are often aggravated by any contact with the involved skin such as friction from even the lightest clothing. In the same individual, firm pressure on the skin may, curiously, be protective but lighter brushing unbearable. Some patients describe unbearable itch, formication, or dysesthesia. As well as clothing contact, these symptoms may be exacerbated by physical activity, temperature change, and emotional upset.

The examination of the affected, scarred skin often reveals a loss of sensation to pinprick, temperature, and touch over a wider area than the scars, and an even wider area of sensitive or painful skin. This sensitive skin may paradoxically include the anesthetic areas, where pain is elicited by skin stroking or skin traction between the thumb and forefinger, an effect

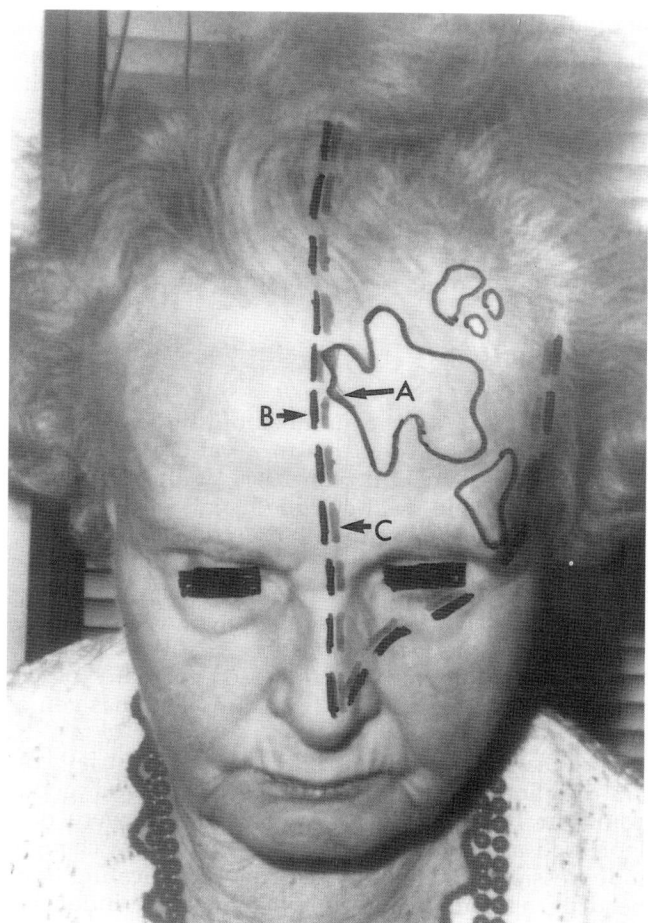

Figure 170.1 Ophthalmic zoster with postherpetic neuralgia and loss of left eye. Solid line outlines scarring; dashed lines outline area of sensory loss and sensitive skin (allodynia).
Trigeminal postherpetic neuralgia; A, scarred area (solid line); B, area of sensory loss (dark interrupted line); C, areas of allodynia (light interrupted line).

which may be caused by summation in hypersensitive, deafferented central neurons with expanded receptive fields.

The natural course of PHN, even of long duration, is of satisfactory pain resolution in 50%; the rest continue to suffer for many years, sometimes until death.[48]

Classification

There is evidence that PHN may have a predominantly central form with little peripheral input contributing to the pain (no allodynia) as well as a peripheral form with prominent allodynia, hyperesthesia, or hyperalgesia.[49] The latter form could result in predominantly peripheral pain mechanisms or a combination of central and peripheral disturbances in the nervous system.

Diagnostic criteria

Trigeminal PHN is diagnosed according to the clinical history and physical examination.

Differential diagnosis

The differential diagnosis is not usually a problem. When rash and scarring have not been prominent, it may be necessary to order brain imaging to rule out a structural cause of neuropathic ophthalmic division pain, sensory loss, and allodynia. There is no need for an investigation for underlying malignancy causing immunosuppression. However, in a young person with herpes zoster or PHN, HIV testing is reasonable since these disorders are uncommon in those below the age of 50.

Treatment

Grade A evidence

Antidepressants A large number of studies support the utility of antidepressants in a variety of chronic pain problems. An important part of this literature concerns favorable, well-designed trials of the use of these agents in neuropathic pain, particularly PHN. PHN is a good model of neuropathic pain for drug trials because, if patients are chosen carefully, the pain is fairly stable over time and sufficient numbers of cases for trials can be readily obtained. Antidepressant therapy, as opposed to many other putative therapies of this difficult problem, has come to have a sound, scientific basis.

The earliest randomized controlled trial of amitriptyline using a placebo control found good results in 16 of 24 (67%).[50] Most patients were not depressed and pain relief occurred without a change in depression ratings in most patients, indicating that the drug appeared to result in pain relief independently of its antidepressant effect. This analgesia occurred at lower doses than those usually used to treat depression (median 75 mg). Follow-up was a median 12 months, with good results maintained in 12 (55%) of 22. A subsequent trial has corroborated these results.[51] Amitriptyline has severe limitations in the long-term because of side effects and the fact that relief is rarely complete and occurs in only about two

thirds of patients. One of the effects of this drug is to potentiate both serotonin and noradrenaline in the central nervous system. Subsequent research has explored whether selective serotonergic or noradrenergic antidepressants might be more effective and have fewer untoward effects.

Experience with serotonergic agents (clomipramine, trazodone, nefazodone, fluoxetine and zimelidine) in PHN has been disappointing.[52] The evidence supporting the use of noradrenergic agents is more compelling. Desipramine, a selective norepinephrine re-uptake inhibitor, has been shown to be more effective than placebo in PHN, and pain relief with this drug as well was found not to be mediated by mood elevation.[53] A randomized, double-blind trial comparing maprotiline (noradrenergic) with amitriptyline found that although both were effective, amitriptyline was more so.[54] Nine patients responded equally well to both drugs, seven responded only to maprotiline whereas eight other responders required amitriptyline for good relief. All three aspects to the pain of PHN responded to treatment in this study, that is, steady pain, brief jabbing pain, and pain on tactile skin contact. Side effects were troublesome with both agents, limiting their effectiveness. Most patients were not depressed and pain relief occurred in most without a change in depression-rating scales. A comparison of nortriptyline (more noradrenergic) with amitriptyline showed about equal efficacy for both drugs, with less side effects with nortriptyline.[55]

Anticonvulsants A randomized controlled trial supports the use of gabapentin in PHN.[56] This study found a 30% advantage over placebo for this drug with few serious side effects. Many patients achieved the target dose of 3500 mg per day.

Opioids For a long time there has been a bias against opioids for nonmalignant pain. There is now increasing support for the view that these drugs are helpful and justifiable in these conditions. Some of these reports have been of neuropathic pain.

Survey data in PHN have indicated that opioids are useful for some patients.[52] Twenty-five of 90 patients with otherwise intractable pain achieved good to excellent results and 50 others had 25% to 50% relief. A placebo-controlled trial of 50 patients treated with sustained release oxycodone has shown that 58% of patients had at least moderate improvement with this drug versus 18% with placebo.[57]

Topical agents A variety of topical agents (capsaicin, aspirin and local anesthetics) have been studied in PHN. Capsaicin, the active ingredient in red peppers and other plants, acts by depleting the neurotransmitter substance P in small primary afferent fibers. Capsaicin has a modest effect according to randomized controlled trials and may best be used as an adjunct to other treatments.[58] The burning sensation induced by capsaicin is often unpleasant or unbearable and limits therapy. A recent randomized controlled trial of lidocaine patch (Lidoderm®) has indicated efficacy in

PHN.[59] The patch itself has been found to offer protection but a significant drug effect was also present with this simple topical approach.

Grade C evidence Russell et al[60] advocated repeated nerve blocks or skin infiltration with procaine hydrochloride for relief of hyperesthesia and spontaneous pain in PHN. They also discussed the use of a hand vibrator over the injured skin. Of 100 patients, they provided details for only five. No duration of antecedent pain was stated. Taverner reported 16 cases treated with ethyl chloride spray to the scarred area.[61] Symptoms for 12 of these (pain duration 10 months to 13 years) were relieved for 3 to 21 months. The spray was applied daily to twice a week. The author commented on the failure of vibration in his experience, cautioning about the risk of skin injury. Todd et al reported on 86 patients with PHN of at least 3 months: 58 (67%) obtained relief with a combination of ethyl chloride spray followed by the application of a hand vibrator; follow-up was 6 months to 6 years.[62] Colding concluded that sympathetic blocks for established PHN were of no value.[63,64]

Nathan and Wall used prolonged transcutaneous electrical nerve stimulation (TENS) and found good results in 11 of 30 patients with established PHN.[65] Voltage, pulse width, frequency, site of application, and duration were all controlled by the patient. Generally, the subjective sensation of the input was nonpainful and tingling. Pain relief often outlasted stimulation by hours. Follow-up duration was not clearly stated in all. Gerson et al found the intermittent use of TENS unsuccessful in 17 patients with chronic PHN.[66] Haas concluded that TENS was helpful in nine of 11 patients, with follow-up over 1 to 18 months.[67] Lewith et al concluded that acupuncture was of little value in PHN when compared with placebo (mock TENS) in 62 patients.[68] Claims have been made for a variety of other therapies, but these studies suffer from small numbers of patients, lack of controls, inadequate data about the patient population, and/or lack of adequate follow-up.

Surgical approaches

No proven surgical cure for PHN has been found. Sugar and Bucy reviewed the surgery for this disease in 1951 and concluded that almost every operation was said to work occasionally, but none consistently.[69] White and Sweet came to similar conclusions.[70] Their list included retrogasserian rhizotomy, avulsion of the supraorbital nerve or gasserian ganglion, greater superficial petrosal neurectomy, trigeminal tractotomy, stereotaxic thalamotomy or mesencephalotomy, sympathectomy, and sensory corticectomy. Resection or undermining of the skin in the involved areas also rarely seemed to provide long-term pain relief, in spite of initial reports of good results. Hitchcock and Schvarcz reported that stereotaxic trigeminal tractotomy was successful in three patients with PHN, all with less than one year of follow-up.[71] No reports of this procedure by other neurosurgeons have been published.

Dorsal root entry zone lesions have been reported useful in 50% of refractory patients but have potential serious side effects and have been largely abandoned.[72-74]

Stimulation of the lateral thalamus (VPL-VPM) has been reported to provide pain relief for some patients with PHN.[75] Approximately one in three patients can be expected to obtain good long-term results. Stereotaxically implanted electrodes can also be directed at other nuclear structures, but the VPM appears to be the best target area. A more comprehensive discussion of surgery for PHN may be found elsewhere.[76]

Conclusions regarding postherpetic neuralgia

None of the putative preventive approaches to PHN can be regarded as conclusively established to be effective at significantly preventing this disorder. Pending final proof, it is reasonable to treat patients early and aggressively to relieve the pain of herpes zoster and to try to prevent PHN if the therapy is safe and well tolerated. It is important to recognize that the population at highest risk for PHN is the age group 60 years and over who may have a risk of 50% or more of developing this complication. Valacyclovir or famciclovir appear safe and modestly reduce the occurrence of PHN. Although no controlled trial has ever been done of nerve blocks to treat herpes zoster pain or prevent PHN, they are reasonable and safe in experienced hands and may be repeated if effective as symptoms dictate. The use of nonsteroidal anti-inflammatory drugs, acetaminophen, and opioids, is justified to relieve severe pain with the acute illness on an as needed or round the clock basis. The initiation of low-dose amitriptyline may be considered at this stage.

For established PHN (neuropathic pain persisting for more than one month after herpes zoster) the most consistently effective agents appear to be antidepressants. Controlled trials support this approach. These data indicate that pain may be reduced from moderate or severe to mild in about two thirds of patients. It is reasonable to commence amitriptyline or nortriptyline at a dose of 10 mg q.h.s. in those over 65 years, and 25 mg in those aged 65 or less. The dose is increased by similar increments in a single h.s. dose every 7 to 20 days until relief is obtained or intolerable side effects supervene. If these agents fail, one can try desipramine or maprotiline in similar doses. Occasional patients failing these may benefit from a serotonergic drug such as trazodone, clomipramine or fluoxetine, but no controlled trial has been done and these do not appear useful for the majority of patients. It is also possible that the addition of a neuroleptic such as fluphenazine, 1 mg up to t.i.d., may give added benefit in some. Gabapentin has a modest effect with few severe side effects and may also be considered a first-line therapy; doses up to 3500 mg may be required. A trial and error approach in refractory patients may also include the anticonvulsants carbamazepine, phenytoin, clonazepam, and valproate. For resistant cases opioids may be safely prescribed on an as needed or round the clock basis.

Long-acting oral forms of oxycodone, morphine and hydromorphone, and the fentanyl skin patch may be of advantage. Trials of different opioids may reveal one that is preferred. The use of topical agents, such as capsaicin, acetylsalicylic acid and local anesthetic agents, is attractive as it is simple and free of systemic effects. For most patients these do not appear useful as sole therapy, but they may be a useful adjunct to other therapies in some individuals. Transcutaneous electrical nerve stimulation (TENS) may be worth trying. Electrode placement, frequency, intensity, and duration of stimulation are a matter of trial and error. Some patients may benefit from nerve blocks which, if efficacious, may be repeated at appropriate intervals. In at least 40% of our patients pain remains totally refractory or unsatisfactorily relieved and our approach with these patients is to see them regularly, try different narcotics for the limited relief they give, and attempt any new or older approach that seems reasonable and safe hoping that improvement will occur with time. Approximately 50% of patients, even those with pain of long duration, will improve over the years, half of these on no treatment.[48]

Differences and similarities between trigeminal and postherpetic neuralgia

There are far more differences than there are similarities between trigeminal and postherpetic neuralgia. Certainly the pain is shock-like in trigeminal neuralgia, and electric shock-like pain is often a component of postherpetic neuralgia, but these pains are really not similar, as will be discussed below. The only similarity is that both disorders occur with increasing frequency with increasing age, which may be due to the decline in inhibitory axo-axonic synapses that occurs with increasing age.[2]

The differences between trigeminal and postherpetic neuralgia are much more striking (Table 170.1).

Postherpetic neuralgia occurs with major injury to ganglion, nerve, nerve root, and spinal cord. Trigeminal neuralgia occurs with presumed irritation or minor injury to the nerve root. Postherpetic neuralgia affects the first division of the trigeminal nerve while trigeminal neuralgia affects the lower face. The difference in the allodynia of the two conditions has already been discussed. In postherpetic neuralgia non-noxious stimulation certainly produces the pain, but the stimulation has to be over a wider area and it usually produces a steady burning pain. Very localized areas in trigeminal neuralgia trigger pain with very light tactile stimulation producing a shock-like pain. Sensory loss is present in postherpetic neuralgia but is usually absent in trigeminal neuralgia, probably reflecting the more minor nature of the injury. There are no painfree intervals in postherpetic neuralgia whereas they do occur in trigeminal neuralgia. The pathology may consist of just demyelination at the nerve root in trigeminal neuralgia but is much more extensive in postherpetic neuralgia.

Surgery has generally been abandoned for postherpetic neuralgia whereas it plays a major role in refractory cases of trigeminal neuralgia. The pharmacological treatment of each disorder is very different (Figure 170.2) with amitriptyline being the standard therapy for postherpetic neuralgia and carbamazepine for trigeminal neuralgia. Overall, about 80% or more of trigeminal neuralgia patients find relief with carbamazepine whereas there is no effect from opioids or amitriptyline. About 60% of postherpetic neuralgia patients respond to amitriptyline and there is a modest opioid effect.

These pharmacological differences led Gerhard Fromm to study the effect of these drugs. Having found amitriptyline-inhibited wide dynamic range neurons in the nucleus caudalis of the trigeminal system, he postulated that postherpetic neuralgia was

Table 170.1   Differences between postherpetic neuralgia and trigeminal neuralgia

	Postherpetic neuralgia	Trigeminal neuralgia
Clinical	Major injury V1 Non-noxious (tactile) trigger in painful area Shock-like pain, steady pain, skin sensitivity Hyperesthesia, dysesthesia, allodynia Allodynia is steady pain Sensory loss No painfree intervals	Minor injury V2, V3 Localized tactile trigger areas in or out of pain area Shock-like pain Allodynia is shock-like pain No or little sensory loss Painfree intervals
Pathology	Damage to dorsal horn, nerve root, nerve and spinal cord	Demyelination at nerve root
Surgery	Some relief in up to 50% of patients with DREZ lesions	(1) Decompression of vessel loops (2) Radiofrequency/glycerol
Drugs	Amitriptyline	Carbamazepine

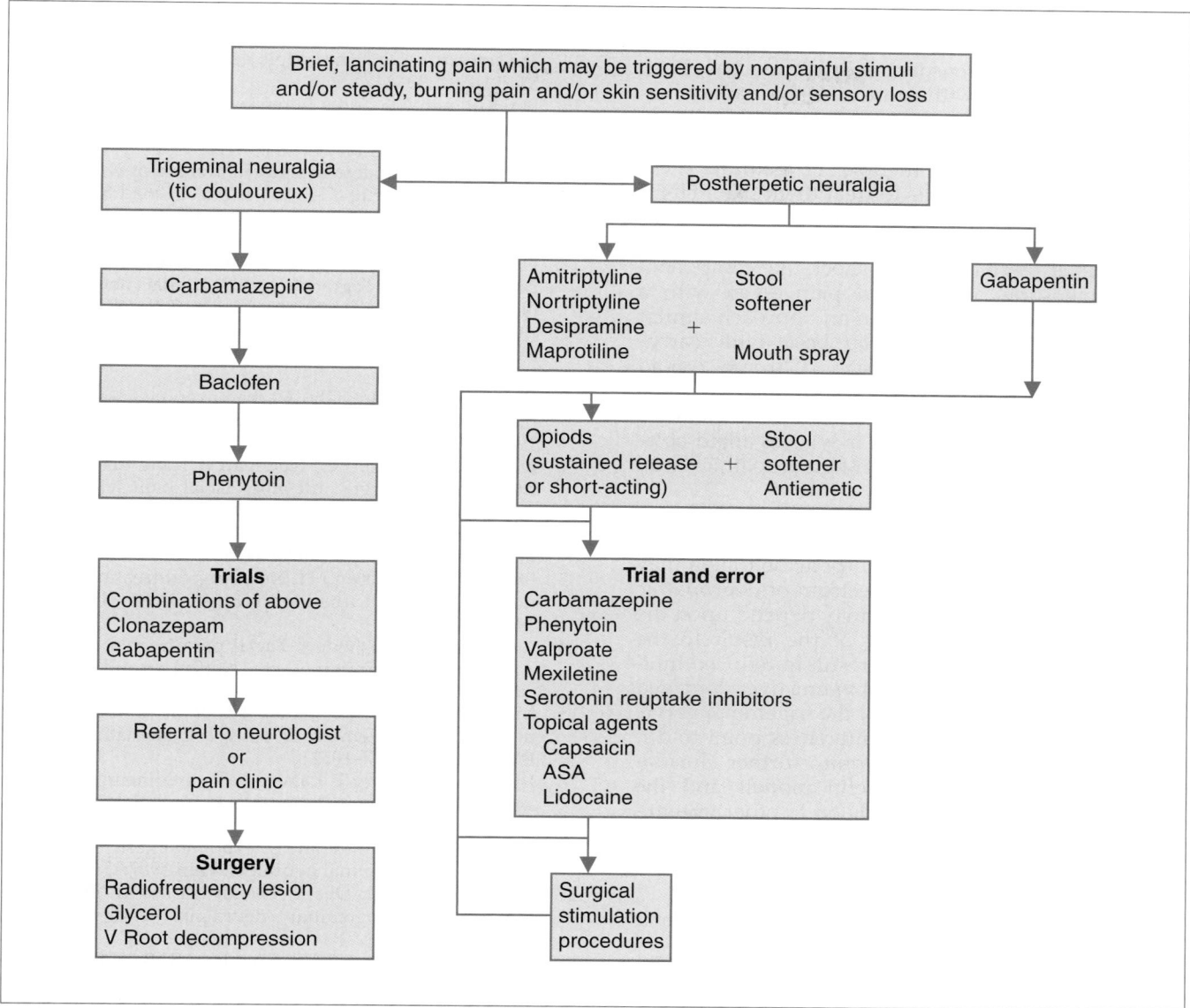

Figure 170.2 Pharmacological management of trigeminal neuropathic pain

a disorder affecting excessive excitation of these neurones.[10] He also found that carbamazepine reduced the excitation of low threshold mechanoreceptive neurons in the nucleus oralis of the trigeminal system and enhanced its segmental inhibition. He therefore postulated that trigeminal neuralgia was a disorder of low threshold mechanoreceptive neurons in this area, which led secondarily to excessive excitation of the wide dynamic range neurons.

Other trigeminal neuropathies

Many other conditions may cause trigeminal neuropathy, with and without pain in the nerve and nerve root. A large group of conditions are difficult to categorize as to cause and have been grouped together as atypical facial pain. In the author's view, a substantial proportion of these are neuropathic

because they occur after situations which can cause nerve injury such as root canals and dental extractions. Trauma to facial structures and the skull may damage branches of the fifth nerve such as the supraorbital and infraorbital nerves. Tumors of various kinds, primary and secondary, may cause progressive trigeminal nerve sensory loss and pain. Mental nerve neuropathy may be the first sign of cancer.[77] Neurotoxins such as trichloroethylene and stilbamidine are known causes of involvement of the fifth nerve. Inflammatory conditions of the middle ear and petrous apex may spread to the nerve root and/or ganglion and also involve the sixth nerve. Trigeminal neuropathy may be caused by collagen diseases such as lupus and scleroderma. Intracranial tumors, including cholesteatomas, acoustic neuromas, and meningiomas, may also affect the fifth root. A benign sensory neuropathy may occur acutely and then resolve slowly.[78] A slowly progressive unilateral or bilateral trigeminal sensory neuropathy has been described associated with numbness and sometimes pain. Some of these cases are associated with collagen diseases.[79]

One approach to the therapy of pain in these usually difficult problems is to treat them like PHN if the pain is steady and burning. One randomized controlled trial supports the efficacy of amitriptyline in this group.[80] If there is a major shock-like component with a suggestion of triggered pain, even with a steady burning component, then an approach similar to the therapy of TN may be best, with carbamazepine as the first approach. Chronic opioid therapy may be necessary to provide at least some relief if the pain is constant, severe, and intractable to all other measures. Generally it is wise to avoid ablative neurosurgical procedures for neuropathic facial pain that is not clearly TN.

Conclusions

Trigeminal neuralgia and postherpetic neuralgia may occupy opposite ends of the spectrum of neuropathic facial pain, and these disorders may depend upon the different location and severity of the insult to the nerve. Probably both disorders result in reduced inhibition and excess excitation of hyperactive, damaged central neurons in the nucleus of the trigeminal nerve. Clinical and pharmacological differences point to different pain mechanisms and require further elucidation. These conditions are useful models and the therapy of each may be extrapolated to other trigeminal neuropathic pain conditions.

References

1. Merskey H, Bogduk N, eds. Classification of Chronic Pain. 2nd ed. Seattle: IASP Press, 1994
2. Fromm GH, Sessle BJ, eds. Trigeminal Neuralgia. Stoneham: Butterworth-Heinemann, 1991
3. Watson CPN, ed. Herpes Zoster and Postherpetic Neuralgia. New York: Elsevier, 1994
4. Penman J. Trigeminal neuralgia. In: Vinken PJ, Bruyn GW, eds. Handbook of Clinical Neurology. Vol 5. Amsterdam: North Holland, 1968:296–322
5. Harris W. An analysis of 1,433 cases of trigeminal neuralgia. Brain 1940;63:209–224
6. Stookey B, Ransohoff J. Trigeminal neuralgia: its history and treatment. Springfield: CC Thomas, 1959
7. Jensen TS, Rasmussen P, Reske-Nielsen E. Association of trigeminal neuralgia with multiple sclerosis. Acta Neurol Scand 1982;65:182–189
8. Huhn A, Daniels L. Die syntropie von encephalomyelitis disseminata und trigeminal neuralgie. Fortschr Neurol Psychiatr 1973;44:477–496
9. Jannetta PJ. Arterial compression of the trigeminal nerve at the pons in patients with trigeminal neuralgia. J Neurosur 1967;26:159–162
10. Fromm GH. Physiological rationale for the treatment of neuropathic pain. APS Journal 1993;2:1–5
11. Sessle BJ. Physiological rationale for the treatment of neuropathic pain. APS Journal 1993;2:17–20
12. Symonds Sir C. Facial pain. Ann R Coll Surg Engl 1949;4:206–212
13. Mitchell RG. Pretrigeminal neuralgia. Br Dent J 1980;140:167–170
14. Trousseau A. De la neuralgie epileptiforme. Arch Gen Med 1853;1:33–44
15. Bergouignan M. Cures hereuses de nevralgies faciales essentielles par le diphenylhydantoin de soude. Rev Laryngol Otol Rhinol 1942;63:34–41
16. Blom S. Trigeminal neuralgia: its treatment with a new anticonvulsant drug (G-32883). Lancet 1962;1:839–840
17. Blom S. Tic douloureux treated with new anticonvulsant. Arch Neurol 1963;9:285–290
18. Campbell FG, Graham JG, Zikha KJ. Clinical trial of carbamazepine (Tegretol) in trigeminal neuralgia. J Neurol Neurosurg Psychiatry 1966;29:265–267
19. Rockliff BW, Davis EH. Controlled sequential trials of carbamazepine in trigeminal neuralgia. Arch Neurol 1966;15:129–136
20. Killian JM, Fromm GH. Carbamazepine in the treatment of neuralgia: use and side effects. Arch Neurol 1968;19:129–136
21. Kiluk KI, Knighton RS, Newman JD. The treatment of trigeminal neuralgia and other facial pain with carbamazepine. Mich Med 1968;67:1066–1069
22. Nicol CF. A four year double-blind study of Tegretol in facial pain. Headache 1969;9:54–57
23. Sturman RH, O'Brien FH. Non-surgical treatment of tic douloureux with carbamazepine (#G32883). Headache 1969;9:88–91
24. Rasmussen P, Riishede J. Facial pain treated with carbamazepine (Tegretol). Acta Neurol Scand 1970;46:385–408
25. McQuay H, Carroll D, Jadad AR, et al. Anticonvulsant drugs for management of pain: a systematic review. BMJ 1995;311:1047–1052
26. Vilming ST, Lyberg T, Lataste X. Tizanidine in the management of trigeminal neuralgia. Cephalalgia 1986;6:181–182
27. Lindstrom P, Lindblom U. The analgesic effect of tocainide in trigeminal neuralgia. Pain 1987;28:45–50
28. Lechin F, van der Dijs B, Lechin ME, et al. Pimozide therapy for trigeminal neuralgia. Arch Neurol 1989;44:960–963
29. Fromm GH, Terrence CF, Chattha AS. Baclofen in the treatment of trigeminal neuralgia: double-blind study and long-term follow-up. Ann Neurol 1984;15:240–244
30. Fromm GH, Terrence CF. Comparison of L-baclofen and racemic baclofen in trigeminal neuralgia. Neurology 1987;37:1725–1728
31. Caccia MR. Clonazepam in facial neuralgia and cluster headache: Clinical and electrophysiological study. Eur Neurol 1975;13:560–563
32. Chandra B. The use of clonazepam in the treatment of tic douloureux (a preliminary report). Proc Aust Assoc Neurol 1976;13:119–122
33. Court JE, Kase CS. Treatment of tic douloureux with a new anticonvulsant (clonazepam). J Neurol Neurosurg Psychiatry 1976;39:297–299
34. Smirne S, Scarlato G. Clonazepam in cranial neuralgia. Med J Aust 1977;1:93–94
35. Peiris JB, Perera GLS, Devendra SV, Lionel NDW. Sodium valproate in trigeminal neuralgia. Med J Aust 1980;2:278
36. King RB. The value of mephenesin carbamate in the control of pain in patients with tic douloureux. J Neurosurg 1966;25:153–158
37. Dalessio DJ. The major neuralgias, postinfectious neuritis, intractable pain, and atypical facial pain. In: Dalessio DJ, ed. Wolff's Headache and Other Head

Pain. New York: Oxford University Press, 1980:233–255

38. Sweet WH. Percutaneous methods for the treatment of trigeminal neuralgia and other faciocephalic pain; comparison with microvascular decompression. Semin Neurol 1988;8:272–279

39. Loeser JD. Tic douloureux and atypical facial pain. *In:* Wall PD, Melzack R, eds. The Textbook of Pain, London: Churchill Livingstone, 1994

40. Hakansson S. Trigeminal neuralgia treated by injection of glycerol into the trigeminal cistern. Neurosurgery 1981;9:638–646

41. Mullan S, Lichtor T. Percutaneous microcompression of the trigeminal ganglion for trigeminal neuralgia. J Neurosurg 1983;59:1007–1012

42. Jannetta PJ. Arterial compression of the trigeminal nerve at the pons in patients with trigeminal neuralgia. J Neurosurg 1967;26:159–162

43. Head H, Campbell AW. The pathology of herpes zoster and its bearing on sensory location. Brain 1900;22:353

44. Head H. Herpes zoster. *In:* Allbutt C, Rolleston HD, eds. A System of Medicine. 2nd ed. London: MacMillan, 1910;7:470–492

45. Watson CPN, Evans RJ. Postherpetic neuralgia: a review. Arch Neurol 1986;43:836–840

46. Watson CPN, Deck JH, Morshead D, et al. Postherpetic neuralgia: Further postmortem studies of cases with and without pain. Pain 1991;44:105–117

47. Watson CPN, Midha R, Devor M, et al. Trigeminal postherpetic neuralgia postmortem: Clinically unilateral, pathologically bilateral. Proc World Congress on Pain, Vienna, Austria, 1999. Seattle: IASP Press, 2000

48. Watson CPN, Watt VR, Chipman M, et al. The prognosis with postherpetic neuralgia. Pain 1991;46:195–199

49. Rowbotham MC, Petersen KL, Fields HL. Is postherpetic neuralgia more than one disorder? Pain Forum 1998;7:231–237

50. Watson CPN, Evans RJ, Reed K, et al. Amitriptyline versus placebo in postherpetic neuralgia. Neurology 1982;32:671–673

51. Max MB, Schafer SC, Culnane M et al. Amitriptyline but not lorazepam relieves postherpetic neuralgia. Neurology 1988;38:1427–1432

52. Watson CPN, Evans RJ, Watt VR, Birkett N. Postherpetic neuralgia: 208 cases. Pain 1988;35:289–298

53. Kishore-Kumar R, Max MB, Shafer SC. Desipramine relieves postherpetic neuralgia. Clin Pharmacol Ther 1990;47:305–312

54. Watson CPN, Chipman M, Reed K, et al. Maprotiline versus amitriptyline in postherpetic neuralgia. Pain 1992;48:29–36

55. Watson CPN, Vernich L, Chipman M, Reed K. Amitriptyline versus nortriptyline in postherpetic neuralgia. Neurology 1998;51:1166–1171

56. Rowbotham M, Harden N, Stacey B. Gabapentin for the treatment of postherpetic neuralgia: a randomized controlled trial. JAMA 1998;280:1837–1842

57. Watson CPN, Babul N. Oxycodone relieves neuropathic pain: a randomized controlled trial in postherpetic neuralgia. Neurology 1998;50:1837–1841

58. Watson CPN. Topical capsaicin as an adjuvant analgesic. J Pain Symptom Manage 1994;9:425–433

59. Rowbotham MD, Davies PS, Verkenpinck C, Galer BS. Lidocaine patch: a double blind controlled trial. Pain 1996;65:39–44

60. Russell WR, Espri MLE, Morganstern FS. Treatment of postherpetic neuralgia. Lancet 1957;1:242–245

61. Taverner D. Alleviation of postherpetic neuralgia. Lancet 1960;2:671–672

62. Todd EM, Crue BL Jr, Vergadamo M. Conservative treatment of postherpetic neuralgia. Bull LA Neurol Soc 1965;30:148–152

63. Colding A. The effect of sympathetic blocks on herpes zoster. Acta Anaesthesiol Scand 1969;13:113–141

64. Colding A. Treatment of pain: Organization of a pain clinic, treatment of herpes zoster. Proc R Soc Med 1973;66:541–542

65. Nathan PW, Wall PD. Treatment of postherpetic neuralgia by prolonged electrical stimulation. BMJ 1974;3:645–647

66. Gerson GR, Jones RB, Luscombe DK. Studies on the concomitant use of carbamazepine and clomipramine for the relief of postherpetic neuralgia. Postgrad Med J 1977;54Suppl4:104–109

67. Haas LF. Postherpetic neuralgia. Trans Ophthalmol Soc NZ 1977;29:133–136

68. Lewith GT, Field F, Machin D. Acupuncture versus placebo in postherpetic pain. Pain 1983;17:361–368

69. Sugar O, Bucy PC. Postherpetic trigeminal neuralgia. Arch Neurol Psychiatr 1951;65:131–145

70. White JC, Sweet WH. Pain and the Neurosurgeon: A 40 Year Experience. Springfield, Ill: C C Thomas Publishers, 1989

71. Hitchcock ER, Schvarcz JR. Stereotaxic trigeminal tractotomy for postherpetic facial pain. J Neurosurg 1972;37:412–417

72. Nashold BS Jr, Ostadhl RH, Bullitt F, et al. Dorsal root entry zone lesions: A new neurosurgical therapy for deafferentation pain. *In:* Bonica JJ, Alhefessard D, eds. Advances in Pain Research and Therapy. New York: Raven Press, 1983:738–750

73. Friedman AH, Nashold BS, Overimann-Levitt J. DREZ lesions for postherpetic neuralgia. J Neurosurg 1984;60: 1258–1262

74. Friedman AH, Nashold BS. DREZ lesions for postherpetic neuralgia. Neurosurgery 1984;15:969–970

75. Mazars GJ. Intermittent stimulation of the nucleus ventralis posterolateralis for pain. Surg Neurol 1975;4: 93–95

76. Loeser J. Surgery for postherpetic neuralgia. *In:* Watson CPN, ed. Herpes Zoster and Postherpetic Neuralgia. Amsterdam: Elsevier, 1993

77. Massey EW, Moore J, Schold SC Jr. Mental neuropathy from systemic cancer. Neurology 191;32:127

78. Blau JN, Harris M, Kennet S. Trigeminal sensory neuropathy. N Engl J Med 1969;281:873

79. Lecky BRF, Hughes RAC, Murray NMF. Trigeminal sensory neuropathy. Brain 1987;110:1453

80. Sharav Y, Singer E, Schmidt E, et al. The analgesic effect of amitriptyline in chronic facial pain. Pain 1987; 31:199–209

171 Disorders of the Facial Nerve

Mark J Morrow

General overview of facial nerve disorders

The facial nerve provides the motor innervation to the face, as well as playing less obvious roles in dampening excessive motion of the tympanic membrane, driving salivary and lacrimal secretions, and transmitting taste information. Abnormalities of facial nerve function may have devastating functional and psychological impact. Facial nerve disorders may be divided into those that reduce function (palsies) and those that produce excessive activation of facial nerve-innervated muscles (e.g. hemifacial spasm). Infectious, inflammatory and neoplastic processes may cause facial neuropathy. This chapter will address treatment of the most common type of facial neuropathy, viral, while conditions that may incidentally affect the facial nerve will be discussed elsewhere. One section will handle treatment and rehabilitation of facial nerve palsy, independent of its cause, and another will address hemifacial spasm.

Facial nerve anatomy

The facial nerve has four distinct components, with efferent fibers that originate in the facial and superior salivatory nuclei and afferent fibers that project to the nucleus solitarius and spinal trigeminal nucleus (see Figure 171.1). The largest portion of the nerve projects from the facial nucleus and provides motor drive to the muscles of facial expression, as well as the stapedius, stylohyoid, digastric and occipitalis muscles. The remaining three components of the nerve are bound together in a separate fascial sheath, forming the nervus intermedius. Visceral motor fibers from the superior salivatory nucleus supply the lacrimal, submandibular and sublingual glands. General sensory fibers carry responses from small areas around the ear to the spinal trigeminal nucleus. Special sensory fibers bring taste information from the anterior two thirds of the tongue into the nucleus solitarius. All components of the facial nerve run together from the brainstem and enter the internal acoustic meatus near the vestibulocochlear (eighth) nerve. They soon divide within the facial canal. First, fibers to the lacrimal and nasal glands exit by the greater petrosal foramen. Then, taste fibers and the motor supply to the submandibular and sublingual glands form the chorda tympani nerve and run through the petrotympanic fissure. The remaining facial motor and general sensory fibers exit the stylomastoid foramen, after giving off the stapedius nerve. Most motor fibers pass through the parotid gland, within which the nerve subdivides into branches for individual facial muscles.

Bell's palsy and herpes zoster oticus

Brief overview

Two viral conditions, Bell's palsy and herpes zoster oticus (Ramsay Hunt syndrome), account for most cases of acute facial neuropathy. Spontaneous improvement is characteristic, but significant residual dysfunction is common. There is moderate evidence supporting the use of steroids and antiviral agents to reduce the risk of these deficits. A variety of supportive measures can be undertaken when facial weakness, spasm or synkinesis persist.

Epidemiology

Bell's palsy is relatively common, with an annual incidence of about 25 cases per 100 000.[1,2] Incidence increases with age, and diabetes and pregnancy are established risk factors. There is a slight female predilection. Herpes zoster oticus is about one fifth as common as Bell's palsy; risk factors include advanced age and immune deficiency.[3]

Etiology

Reactivation of latent varicella zoster virus causes Ramsay Hunt syndrome. Herpes simplex virus type I probably causes most cases of Bell's palsy; it is not certain whether reactivation or exogenous infection with the virus is the prevalent mechanism.

Pathophysiology

In both Bell's palsy and herpes zoster oticus, there is lymphocytic infiltration, demyelination and edema of the affected facial nerve. Axonal compression is a less well-established mechanism of damage. Swelling of an infected nerve against the walls of its narrow conduit in the temporal bone may cause axonal ischemia, adding to other types of injury. Axonal compression has been used as the rationale for surgical treatment of viral facial neuropathy.

Genetics

While the great majority of cases are spontaneous, there is occasionally a genetic predisposition toward Bell's palsy. This is especially true of recurrent cases, sometimes seen with facial edema and lingual plications in the Melkersson–Rosenthal syndrome.

Clinical features

Many patients with Bell's palsy have experienced a prodromal illness of probable viral origin, most commonly upper respiratory infection. Facial weakness is of the lower motor neuron (peripheral) variety, with drooping of the eyebrow and corner of the mouth and

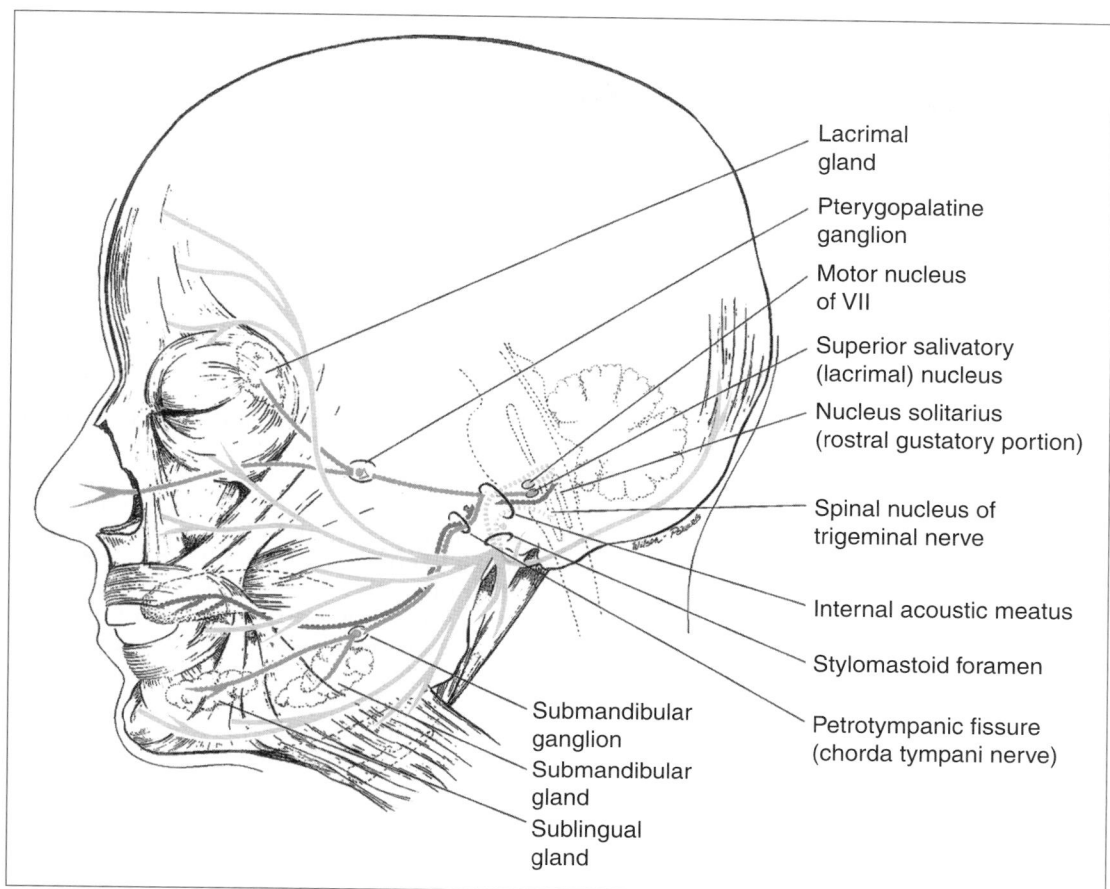

Figure 171.1 Schematic of facial nerve anatomy. Color codes: yellow, special visceral efferent fibers; orange, general visceral efferent; blue, general somatic afferent; green, special afferent (taste). Reprinted with permission from: Wilson-Pauwels L, Akesson EJ, Stewart PA. Cranial Nerves: Anatomy and Clinical Comments. Hamilton (Canada): BC Decker, 1988:83. (See color plate section.)

widening of the palpebral fissure. Ocular irritation from drying and foreign body accumulation may result from inadequate eye closure. Difficulties with mouth closure can cause dysarthria, drooling and chewing difficulty. Facial weakness is unilateral in almost all (about 99%) cases of Bell's palsy and usually reaches peak involvement within five days. Spontaneous improvement usually begins within four to six weeks, and may continue for up to six months in severe cases. Frequent accompanying symptoms include ipsilateral hyperacusis, retroauricular pain and dysgeusia. Some patients demonstrate signs or symptoms of ipsilateral fifth, ninth or tenth nerve involvement, but this is generally mild. Herpes zoster oticus presents in a very similar fashion, but facial weakness is more often severe and evidence of eighth nerve dysfunction, including deafness and vestibular loss, is more common. Zoster vesicles may be found over the auricle, external ear canal, preauricular skin, or pharynx, but may not form until up to two weeks after onset of palsy.

Classification

The distinction between Ramsay Hunt syndrome and Bell's palsy may be difficult, since vesicles may

develop after facial weakness. Moreover, serology has shown evidence of zoster virus reactivation in many patients who never develop vesicles (zoster sine herpete). It is worth trying to identify cases of zoster, since higher levels of antiviral treatment may be indicated. Another important classification is that of partial versus complete facial palsy. The prognosis is considerably better in the former, and a less aggressive approach to treatment may be warranted. Subclassification of complete facial palsy has been done with electroneurography (ENoG) and transcranial magnetic stimulation.

Patients with complete palsy and severe deficits of axonal function on these neurophysiological studies usually have significant residual weakness. ENoG has been used to select patients for more aggressive forms of therapy, such as facial nerve decompression.[4]

Diagnostic criteria

Viral neuropathy can generally be diagnosed with confidence in an otherwise healthy individual with rapid onset of isolated, unilateral peripheral facial weakness. The distinction between Bell's palsy and herpes zoster oticus is based on the presence of vesicles, although this is not infallible (see section above).

Differential diagnosis

A nonviral cause of facial palsy should be suspected when there are bilateral findings, significant involvement of other cranial nerves, progression over more than a week, lack of improvement within three months of onset, or associated systemic symptoms (Table 171.1). Evaluation for other causes should consider *trauma, sarcoidosis, Lyme disease, tuberculosis, otitis media*, and *posterior fossa or parotid gland tumors*. Cranial magnetic resonance imaging (MRI) and lumbar puncture can be very helpful in the search for alternatives to a viral source. MRI may show facial nerve enhancement in both Bell's palsy and herpes zoster oticus, while cerebrospinal fluid can demonstrate mild lymphocytic pleocytosis, elevated protein, and evidence of peripheral demyelination. These findings are nonspecific, however, and of no prognostic value. Ancillary evaluation should be reserved for patients in whom there is reasonable diagnostic uncertainty. Demonstration of the anatomical extent of the facial nerve lesion, for example with taste or stapedius reflex evaluation, has not been shown to provide prognostic or diagnostic information.

Treatment

Without treatment, about 70% of patients with Bell's palsy and 35% of patients with herpes zoster oticus eventually recover normal facial motor function.[1,2,5] Half of the remaining patients are left with moderate to severe deficits, including aberrant regeneration phenomena such as facial synkinesis, crocodile tears, tonic facial contraction, and hemifacial spasm. The severity of facial weakness at peak is the best predictor of outcome. The chief goals of treatment are limiting residual impairment and preventing ocular complications. Rehabilitative techniques are aimed at restoring facial movement, especially eyelid closure.

Oral prednisone has been used extensively in patients with Bell's palsy and herpes zoster oticus.[6–9]

Proof of efficacy is, however, not definitive. At least ten series have compared the use of oral steroids to no treatment or placebo in Bell's palsy; some have suggested benefit in reducing residual weakness or aberrant regeneration, while others have not. Meta-analyses have pointed out flaws in the available steroid treatment studies, including insufficient power. In one meta-analysis, pooled data from better-designed investigations yielded complete recovery rates of 64% in untreated Bell's palsy, compared to 77% with oral steroids.[9] A recent review published by the American Academy of Neurology concluded that steroids were "probably effective" in Bell's palsy.[8] Some authors have suggested that steroids should be used only in patients with complete Bell's palsy, since the prognosis for spontaneous recovery is so good with partial deficits. Citing the low risk and cost, however, others have concluded that prednisone should be started at the initial visit in all patients. Steroids are most likely to be of benefit when initiated early. The duration of the effective therapeutic window for Bell's palsy is not known; most studies have begun prednisone within two weeks of symptom onset. A few limited, uncontrolled series have suggested a benefit of *intravenous steroids* compared with oral steroids in Bell's palsy.[10] The role of steroids in Ramsay Hunt syndrome has not been thoroughly defined. Studies that have employed steroids in this disorder have almost always included antiviral agents.[11] One retrospective review suggested a benefit for oral steroids alone in herpes zoster oticus.[12] Most authors treating viral facial neuropathy have used prednisone 60 to 80 mg/day (1 mg/kg/day) for 5 to 7 days, with a brief (3 to 5 day) taper (Table 171.2).

Acyclovir An antiviral agent that works by inhibiting DNA polymerase. It is most active against viruses of the herpes family, especially herpes simplex type I. In one randomized study, a higher recovery rate and

---

Table 171.1   Differential diagnosis of facial palsy

Atypical features of viral facial neuropathy
Bilateral facial paresis
Significant involvement of cranial nerves V, VIII*, IX, X, XII
Progression over more than a week
Failure to improve after three months
Associated systemic illness

Common alternative diagnoses
Trauma
Sarcoidosis
Lyme disease
Tuberculosis
Otitis media
Posterior fossa tumors (e.g. meningioma, schwannoma)
Parotid gland tumors

*Herpes zoster oticus involves hearing and vestibular function more commonly than Bell's palsy.

Table 171.2   Medical therapy of viral facial neuropathy

Drug treatment
Prednisone 60–80 mg/day × 5–7 days, with 3–5 day taper
plus
Acyclovir* 2000–4000 mg/day (in 5 divided doses) × 7–10 days
or
Famciclovir† 500 mg t.i.d. × 7 days
or
Valacyclovir† 1000 mg t.i.d. × 7 days

General treatment
Artificial tears and eye ointment
Protective eye shades
Lid taping

*Lower doses of acyclovir are usually used for Bell's palsy, higher doses for zoster.
†Famciclovir and valacyclovir have not been studied specifically in viral facial neuropathy, but have proven effective in zoster.

lower frequency of aberrant regeneration was found in Bell's palsy patients given oral acyclovir plus prednisone compared to oral prednisone alone.[6] Other investigations have identified no benefit of acyclovir in Bell's palsy, however. Based on the available evidence, a recent review classified acyclovir as "possibly effective" in Bell's palsy.[8] Oral and intravenous acyclovir has been used in herpes zoster oticus.[7] Reports have been small or uncontrolled and have generally included steroid therapy. A few have shown benefit on recovery rates. Studies of postherpetic neuralgia in various forms of zoster suggest that the combination of acyclovir and prednisone may work better than either drug alone. No advantage has been demonstrated for intravenous versus oral delivery of acyclovir in immunocompetent patients with Ramsay Hunt syndrome. Oral acyclovir has generally been administered for 7 to 10 days in five divided doses, with a total daily dose of 2000 mg for Bell's palsy and 4000 mg for herpes zoster oticus. Because of the relatively poor oral absorption of acyclovir and the requirement for frequent dosing, newer drugs in its class, including valacyclovir and famciclovir, have been employed in various studies of varicella zoster infection. These drugs are more expensive than acyclovir and have not yet been investigated in Bell's palsy or Ramsay Hunt syndrome.

Facial nerve decompression surgery has been used for viral facial neuropathy for almost 70 years. Although a great many articles have been devoted to this subject, very few have presented prospective studies and none has been randomized or blinded. Facial nerve decompression is based upon the premise that permanent damage is induced by axonal ischemia as the inflamed nerve expands within the bony facial canal. It is not clear that this is a major source of pathology, however. Surgery has generally been restricted to patients most likely to suffer residual deficits: those with complete palsies and severely deficient axonal function on electrophysiological testing. Series suggesting benefit have utilized surgery within two weeks after onset of facial palsy, exposing a wide area of the nerve through middle fossa craniotomy.[4] Among the most serious and common complications of this procedure is permanent ipsilateral hearing loss. Given the major cost, hazards and lack of rigorous proof of efficacy, facial nerve decompression must be considered experimental.

General therapy of facial palsy

Weak eyelid closure and decreased tear production associated with facial neuropathy leave the cornea subject to drying and foreign body irritation. For moderate to severe deficits, artificial tears during the daytime and lubricating ointment at night are usually needed.[13] Moisture barriers can be added at night to retain tear film and protect from incidental trauma. The eyelid fissure may be narrowed by elevating the lower lid with tape during the daytime, or by approximating the lids with tape at night. Protective eyewear

should be worn outdoors to avoid irritation from foreign bodies and wind. In severe facial palsy, partial-width eyelid suturing (tarsorrhaphy) may be necessary, at least initially. Physical therapy can be helpful in rehabilitating the paretic face. Feedback techniques, in which electromyographic or visual stimuli are used, may assist in the recovery of symmetric facial tone and expression.[14] Electrical stimulation of affected facial muscles can also be used.[15] Specialized surgical techniques can re-establish function in patients with persistent, severe facial motor loss. These include nerve grafting and anastomosis with the contralateral facial or ipsilateral hypoglossal nerve, often combined with facial muscle grafting.[16] Aberrant regeneration and neural irritability are common features of partially recovered facial nerve deficits. Examples include hemifacial spasm, tonic facial contraction, and various forms of synkinesis. These can usually be treated successfully with botulinum toxin injections (see below).

Hemifacial spasm
Brief overview

Hemifacial spasm causes irregular unilateral activation of the facial musculature. In most cases, it appears to result from compression of the facial nerve by the vertebrobasilar arterial system. Less commonly, it arises from neoplastic, traumatic, or viral facial nerve injury. Microvascular decompression through craniotomy generally offers the best chance of cure. Botulinum toxin injections and oral medications can be effective in alleviating symptoms.

Epidemiology

Hemifacial spasm is a relatively rare condition, with an average annual incidence of just under 1 case per 100 000 and a prevalence of about 10 per 100 000.[17] Women are somewhat more commonly affected, with peak age of onset in the fifth and sixth decades. Hypertension may be a risk factor.

Etiology

It has been postulated that most cases of hemifacial spasm result from compression of the intracranial, extra-axial facial nerve by the vertebral or basilar artery or one of their branches. This idea has been supported by surgical observations and can be demonstrated in many patients by detailed neurovascular imaging.[18,19] The anterior and posterior inferior cerebellar arteries (AICA and PICA) are the most common offending vessels. In about 10% of cases, hemifacial spasm develops as a delayed response to facial nerve injuries from Bell's palsy, herpes zoster oticus, trauma, and other disorders.

Pathophysiology

Two major mechanisms of aberrant facial activation have been proposed for hemifacial spasm. First, ectopic excitation might occur in a demyelinated segment of peripheral facial nerve, possibly with ephaptic crosstalk between fibers. Alternatively, peripheral nerve damage could eventually result in increased spontaneous and stimulus-induced firing upstream in the facial nucleus. With both mechanisms having some experimental support, the pathogenesis of the disorder may really be a mix of the two.

Genetics

There is no genetic basis for most patients with hemifacial spasm. A few familial cases have been reported, in which transmission was autosomal dominant.

Clinical features

Involvement of the periocular muscles is almost always the first and most obvious sign to clinician and patient. Spasm may vary from nearly imperceptible twitching of the orbicularis oculi to sustained, forceful contraction of the entire side of the face, including the platysma. When they appear spasmodic, contractions are irregular in force and rhythm. Hemifacial spasm is typically quite variable in a given patient, with quiescent intervals of minutes to hours interrupted by periods of increased activity. Stress, visual effort and vigorous facial movement are common triggers, while relaxation tends to ameliorate the problem. Unlike tics, the spontaneous movements of hemifacial spasm cannot be voluntarily suppressed. Hemifacial spasm is almost always unilateral. Patients with involuntary movements on both sides of the face generally have a disorder in the blepharospasm–Meige's syndrome spectrum. Onset of hemifacial spasm is subacute to chronic, typically progressing over months to years before reaching plateau. Prolonged spontaneous remission is uncommon. Mild ipsilateral facial weakness can be present, but most patients have little or no motor asymmetry when spasm is absent. Ipsilateral synkinesis between different branches of the facial musculature, for example, activation of the angularis oris or mentalis with blinking, is common. Symptoms of ipsilateral cranial nerve dysfunction, such as vertigo and hearing loss, are reported in 5% to 10% of cases.

Classification

Hemifacial spasm can be separated into more common idiopathic cases, thought to arise from microvascular compression, and symptomatic cases with previous facial nerve injury from tumor, trauma, viral infection, or other cause. This distinction is important, since symptomatic cases might not be expected to improve from surgery at the same rate as idiopathic cases. Some authors have separated a group of "atypical" idiopathic hemifacial spasm patients with initial onset of spasm in the lower face rather than the much more common periocular onset; these patients may have a different pattern of neurovascular compression.[20]

Diagnostic criteria

Hemifacial spasm may be used to describe a unilateral facial movement disorder characterized by spontaneous, involuntary, irregular muscle contraction. Bilateral involvement suggesting a dystonic movement disorder, or evidence of focal seizure activity usually excludes the diagnosis.

Differential diagnosis

Hemifacial spasm is distinguished from *essential blepharospasm* and related disorders that involve both sides of the face, generally symmetrically and synchronously (Table 171.3). *Facial tics* are less complex, forceful and sustained than the movements of hemifacial spasm. Tics usually recur in a stereotypical pattern and are at least temporarily suppressible by force of will. *Facial myokymia* is a generally unilateral disorder characterized by slow, sequential activation and relaxation of adjacent bands of muscle, giving the movement a distinctive wavelike or rippling appearance. It is most common by far in the lower eyelid, where it is usually transient and benign. Rarely, it is more extensive and persistent and is caused by multiple sclerosis or intrinsic brainstem tumors in the region of the facial nucleus. In these cases, it may be associated with *spastic-paretic facial contracture*, in which the affected side of the face is weak, yet tonically contracted. Spastic-paretic facial contracture can resemble the residual from a peripheral nerve injury such as viral neuropathy, but it develops gradually without a history of initial palsy. *Focal motor seizures* can occasionally mimic hemifacial spasm, but begin suddenly, are more rhythmic and not as persistent, and almost always spread below the neck eventually. *Psychogenic facial spasm* lacks the fine, irregular twitching characteristic of hemifacial spasm and is more likely to resemble tic. Evaluation of hemifacial spasm should include MRI with special attention to the posterior fossa and skull base. Mass lesions affecting the facial nerve can thus be excluded and, in many cases, a vessel can be seen to contact the affected nerve, confirming the usual source of the disorder. Electroencephalography can be employed when focal seizures are a serious consideration.

Treatment

Hemifacial spasm is a chronic condition in which spontaneous resolution is rare. Treatment can include:

Table 171.3   Differential diagnosis of hemifacial spasm
Atypical features of hemifacial spasm
Bilateral involvement
Voluntary suppressibility
Significant ipsilateral facial weakness
Involvement below platysma muscle
Predominant or initial spasm in lower face
Regular rhythm of contractions
Common alternative diagnoses
Blepharospasm
Facial tics
Facial myokymia
Focal motor seizures
Psychogenic spasm

Oral medications
    Amitriptyline
    Baclofen
    Carbamazepine
    Clonazepam
    Gabapentin
    Phenytoin
Chemodenervation/myectomy
    Botulinum toxin
    Doxorubicin
Surgery
    Microvascular decompression

Success with oral medications is typically limited, and has only been documented in small, uncontrolled series or case reports. *Carbamazepine, baclofen, clonazepam, amitriptyline, gabapentin* and *phenytoin* are among the drugs that have shown occasional benefit. They may be useful in cases of minimal spasm, or when the patient does not wish to undergo more invasive therapy. A low dose of one of these medications is usually started, with gradual increase until symptoms are satisfactorily controlled or unacceptable side effects ensue.

The generally disappointing experience with oral medication has led to botulinum toxin injections being used as first-line therapy in many patients.[21,22] Botulinum toxin works by irreversible inhibition of acetylcholine release from presynaptic vesicles. Axonal sprouting and regeneration of synaptic boutons makes the induced weakness transient, with a characteristic duration of three to five months. Treatment thus has to be repeated two to four times a year indefinitely. The drug is injected near facial muscle endplates by the subcutaneous/intramuscular route. Between four and 12 sites are usually selected for injection in hemifacial spasm, with doses adjusted for severity and previous experience with a given patient. It is very seldom possible to eliminate all traces of hemifacial spasm with botulinum toxin. The goal of treatment is to reduce functionally and cosmetically limiting spasm, especially around the eye. Excessive weakness of injected muscles or leakage of the drug into areas that are not targeted, such as the levator palpebrae or extraocular muscles, can complicate therapy. Side effects include dry eye, facial droop, ptosis and diplopia, and may occur in up to 30% of patients. Like the therapeutic effect itself, these paretic side effects are transient. Antibodies to botulinum toxin may be demonstrated in the serum of up to a third of long-term recipients of the drug. These might be responsible for occasional patients becoming resistant to therapy. With two serotypes of botulinum toxin (A and B) now available in the US, it may be possible to circumvent problems with drug resistance by switching serotype. Doxorubicin chemomyectomy is an emerging alternative to botulinum toxin chemodenervation.[23] After repeated local injections of doxorubicin over one to two years, permanent destruction of muscle fibers is effected. Complications include persistent disfigurement from loss of subcutaneous fat and scarring.

Although oral medications or botulinum toxin injections may control symptoms, the treatment most likely to abolish the disorder is surgery. Microvascular decompression surgery has been used extensively for over 20 years in hemifacial spasm.[18,20] A retromastoid posterior fossa craniotomy is performed, and any vessels in contact with the facial nerve are separated from it, generally by interposing a pad of synthetic material. Intraoperative neurophysiological monitoring may reduce complications. It is not clear whether benefit arises from the decompression itself, or from manipulation of the nerve. Case series have documented excellent postoperative results, with complete cure or significant improvement in over 90% of cases of idiopathic hemifacial spasm. Delayed recurrence of symptoms occurs in about 10% of patients.[24] The most common serious complications of surgery are permanent ipsilateral facial weakness and hearing loss, each occurring in 3% to 4% of patients in one large series.[20] Meningitis and brainstem stroke occur less frequently, and surgical mortality is rare. Older facial nerve procedures used to treat hemifacial spasm have included partial chemical and surgical ablation and decompression within the temporal bone. These have largely been abandoned in favor of microvascular decompression and botulinum toxin chemodenervation.

References

1. Adour KK, Byl FM, Hilsinger RL Jr, et al. The true nature of Bell's palsy: Analysis of 1000 consecutive patients. Laryngoscope 1978;88:787–801
2. Devriese PP, Schumacher T, Scheide A, et al. Incidence, prognosis and recovery of Bell's palsy. A survey of about 1000 patients (1974–1983). Clin Otolaryngol 1990; 15:15–27
3. Sweeney CJ, Gilden DH. Ramsay Hunt syndrome. J Neurol Neurosurg Psychiatry 2001;71:149–154
4. Gantz BJ, Rubinstein JT, Gidley P, Woodworth GG. Surgical management of Bell's palsy. Laryngoscope 1999;109:1177–1188
5. Devriese PP, Moesker WH. The natural history of facial paralysis in herpes zoster. Clin Otolaryngol 1988;13: 289–298
6. Adour KK, Ruboyianes JM, von Doersten PG, et al. Bell's palsy treatment with acyclovir and prednisone compared with prednisone alone: A double-blind, randomized, controlled trial. Ann Otol Rhinol Laryngol 1996;105:371–378
7. Morrow MJ. Bell's palsy and herpes zoster oticus. Curr Treatment Options Neurol 2000;2:407–416
8. Grogan PM, Gronseth GS. Practice parameter: Steroids, acyclovir, and surgery for Bell's palsy (an evidence-based review): Report of the Quality Standards Subcommittee of the American Academy of Neurology. Neurology 2001;56:830–836
9. Williamson IG, Whelan TR. The clinical problem of Bell's palsy: is treatment with steroids effective? Br J Gen Pract 1996;46:743–747
10. Tani M, Kinishi M, Takahara T, et al. Medical treatment of Bell's palsy. Oral vs. intravenous administration. Acta Otolaryngol Suppl 1988;446:114–118
11. Murikami S, Hato N, Horiuchi J, et al. Treatment of Ramsay Hunt syndrome with acyclovir-prednisone:

Significance of early diagnosis and treatment. Ann Neurol 1997;41:353–357

12. Robillard RB, Hilsiger RL Jr, Adour KK. Ramsay Hunt facial paralysis: Clinical analysis of 185 patients. Otolaryngol Head Neck Surg 1986;95:292–297

13. Seff SR, Chang J. Management of ophthalmic complications of facial nerve palsy. Otolaryngol Clin North Am 1992;25:669–690

14. Ross B, Nedzelski JM, McLean JA. Efficacy of feedback training in long-standing facial nerve paresis. Laryngoscope 1991;101:744–750

15. Targan RS, Alon G, Kay SL. Effect of long-term electrical stimulation on motor recovery and improvement of clinical residuals in patients with unresolved facial nerve palsy. Otolaryngol Head Neck Surg 2000;122: 246–252

16. Hoffman WY. Reanimation of the paralyzed face. Otolaryngol Clin North Am 1992;25:649–666

17. Auger RG, Whisnant JP. Hemifacial spasm in Rochester and Olmsted County, Minnesota, 1960 to 1984. Arch Neurol 1990;47:1233–1234

18. Jannetta PJ, Abbasy M, Maroon JC, et al. Etiology and definitive microsurgical treatment of hemifacial spasm. J Neurosurg 1977;47:321–328

19. Ho SL, Cheng PW, Wong WC, et al. A case-controlled MRI/MRA study of neurovascular contact in hemifacial spasm. Neurology 1999;53:2132–2139

20. Barker FG, Jannetta PJ, Bissonette DJ, et al. Microvascular decompression for hemifacial spasm. J Neurosurg 1995;82:201–210

21. Elston JS. The management of blepharospasm and hemifacial spasm. J Neurol 1992;239:5–8

22. Jost WH, Kohl A. Botulinum toxin: evidence-based medicine criteria in blepharospasm and hemifacial spasm. J Neurol 2001;248(Suppl 1):21–24

23. Wirtschafter JD, McLoon LK. Long-term efficacy of local doxorubicin chemomyectomy in patients with blepharospasm and hemifacial spasm. Ophthalmology 1998;105:342–346

24. Payner TD, Tew JM. Recurrence of hemifacial spasm after vascular decompression. Neurosurgery 1996;38: 686–691

172 Vertigo, Vestibular Nerve, and Central Vestibular Disorders

Ronald J Tusa

Vertigo is defined as sense of motion including rotation, tilt or translation. These symptoms are caused by an imbalance of tonic neural activity to vestibular cerebral cortex from central pathways originating from the semicircular canals and otoliths of the inner ear. Figure 172.1 illustrates the central projections from the vertical semicircular canals of the inner ear. Nystagmus arising from these disorders will be discussed in Chapter 166. Dizziness caused by a variety of other disorders will be discussed in the following chapters; peripheral vestibular (173), hypotension (217, 218), imbalance, and episodic ataxia (210, 255).

Cerebrovascular disorders

Brief overview

Vertigo occurs in up to 50% of all cases of vertebral-basilar ischemia (VBI).[1-3] When vertigo presents as an isolated symptom, however, it is usually due to a peripheral labyrinthine disorder, although it can occasionally occur with VBI.[1,2,4,5] De Kleyn and Nieuwenhuyse first suggested that vertigo and nystagmus might be induced by occlusion of the vertebral artery when the head was held in certain positions.[6] Since then, there have been numerous articles on rotational vertebral artery occlusion. This section will discuss this problem along with other syndromes of vascular-induced vertigo.

Classification

Infarcts Vertigo, pathological ocular tilt reflex (OTR) and central vestibular nystagmus may occur after infarcts in the thalamus and brainstem (Table 172.1). The pathological ocular tilt reflex consists of head tilt, constant ocular torsion of both eyes, and a skew eye deviation. It occurs whenever there is an infarct involving the pathway from the utricle in the inner ear to the interstitial nucleus of Cajal (Figure 172.2).

Thalamus The posteriolateral artery perfuses the vestibular thalamus (ventro-oralis intermedius, ventrocaudalis extrenus and dorsocaudalis) in 65% of cases.[7] In these cases, a stroke in the distribution of this vessel will cause partial OTR (ocular tilt). The paramedian artery perfuses the interstitial nucleus of Cajal (INC) in 50% of cases. In these cases, a stroke in the distribution of this vessel will cause a complete OTR on the contralateral side, falls to the contralateral side, and vertigo with a normal vestibular-ocular reflex (VOR).

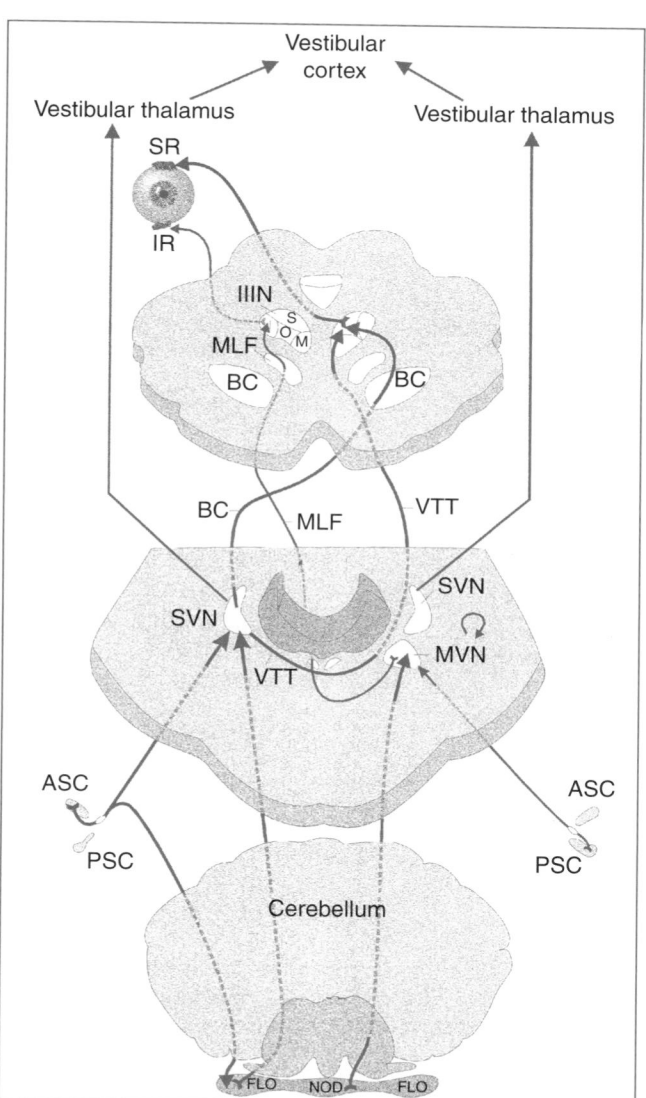

Figure 172.1 Central vestibular pathways that mediate vertical and torsional eye movements. The anterior semicircular canals (ASC) have an excitatory projection directly to the superior vestibular nucleus (SVN) and an inhibitory projection to SVN via the cerebellar flocculus (Flo). The posterior semicircular canals (PSC) project directly to the medial vestibular nucleus (MVN). The MVN projects to the ocular motor nucleus (IIIN) via the medial longitudinal fasciculus (MLF). The SVN projects to the IIIN via the ventral tegmental tract (VTT) and the brachium conjunctivum (BC). The IIIN in turn projects to the superior rectus (SR) and inferior rectus (IR) muscles. The vestibular nuclei project to the vestibular cortex via vestibular thalamus.

Table 172.1   Signs and symptoms from ischemia of central vestibular pathways

Region	Vessel and structures	Symptoms/signs
Thalamus	**Posterolateral artery** 65% Vestibular thalamus (Vim, Vce, Dc) 35% Vestibular thalamus not involved	Ipsilateral or contralateral partial OTR and falls No effect
Thalamus	**Paramedian artery** 50% interstitial nucleus of Cajal (INC) 50% INC not involved	Contralateral OTR, contralateral falls, vertigo (normal VOR) No effect

Dorsolateral pons	**Anterior inferior cerebellar artery**
	• *Cerebellar branch* (lateral cerebellum)
	• *Pontine branch* V, VII
	
	Sympathetic, middle cerebellar peduncle, PPRF
	Spinothalamic tract
	• *Labyrinthine artery* (cochlea and labyrinth)
	   – *Anterior vestibular artery* (HSCC,
	      ASCC, utricle)
	   – *Posterior vestibular artery* (PSCC,
	      saccule, cochlea)
		Ipsilateral (dysmetria)
		Ipsilateral loss pain and temp (face), peripheral
		   VII, dysarthria
		Ipsilateral Horner's, dysmetria, saccade palsy
		Contralateral loss pain and temp (body)
		
		Vertigo (absent ipsilateral VOR), nausea, vomiting,
		   imbalance
		Vertigo (normal VOR), ipsilateral sensorineural
		   hearing loss, tinnitus

Dorsolateral medulla
(Wallenberg
syndrome)
	Posterior inferior cerebellar artery (PICA)
	• *Cerebellar branch* (posterior inferior
	   cerebellum)
	• *Medullary branch* (V nucleus/tract, IX
	   nucleus/tract, X nucleus/tract,
	   sympathetic tract
	Inferior cerebellar peduncle, vestibular
	   nucleus (otolith)
	Lateral spinothalamic tract
	Vestibular nucleus
		Imbalance; ipsilateral (ataxia)
		
		Ipsilateral loss pain and temp (face), decreased
		   gag, vocal cord paresis, ipsilateral Horner's
		   syndrome
		Ipsilateral ataxia, lateropulsion, OTR
		
		Contralateral loss pain and temp (body)
		Vertigo, nausea, vomiting, nystagmus (pure
		   torsional or vestibular with reversal on gaze
		   toward lesion side)

Medial medulla
(lower medulla)
	Penetrator from anterior spinal artery
	XII nucleus
	Pyramidal tract, medial meniscus
	
	Nucleus intercalatus
		Ipsilateral weakness tongue
		Contralateral weakness (body), decreased
		   vibration and proprioception (body)
		Upbeat nystagmus, vertigo, nausea, vomiting,
		   truncal ataxia

ASCC, anterior semicircular canal; Dc, dorsocaudalis nucleus; HSCC, horizontal semicircular canal; OTR, ocular tilt response; PPRF, paramedian pontine reticular formation; PSCC, posterior semicircular canal; Vce, ventrocaudalis extrenus nucleus; Vim, ventro-oralis intermedius nucleus; vestibulo-ocular reflex.

Dorsolateral pontine infarct   The anterior inferior cerebellar artery (AICA) perfuses the lateral cerebellum (cerebellar branch), the dorsolateral pons (pontine branch), and the labyrinth (labyrinth artery). The labyrinthine artery (also called internal auditory artery) in humans is an end artery with very few collateral vessels.[8] Vertigo and hearing loss can occur from infarcts in either the pontine branch or labyrinth artery.[9] The AICA syndrome may present with just peripheral signs if the labyrinth artery is solely involved (vertigo, nausea, vomiting, hearing loss and tinnitus) or may include more central signs if the dorsolateral pons is involved (dysarthria, peripheral facial palsy, trigeminal sensory loss, Horner's syndrome, dysmetria, contralateral temperature and pain sensory loss).[10,11]

Dorsolateral medulla infarct   The posterior inferior

cerebellar artery (PICA) perfuses the posterior inferior cerebellum (cerebellar branch) and the dorsolateral medulla. Vertigo can occur from infarcts in the lateral medulla (Wallenberg syndrome) due to involvement of the vestibular nucleus. Characteristic signs include crossed sensory signs, ipsilateral lateropulsion, ataxia and Horner's sign. Nystagmus may be pure torsion or mixed torsion and horizontal. When the nystagmus contains a horizontal component, it reverses direction on gaze toward the side of infarction, unlike nystagmus from peripheral vestibular lesions.

Medial medulla infarct   A penetrating vessel from the vertebral artery usually perfuses the upper medial medulla, and a branch from the anterior spinal artery perfuses the lower medial medulla. Infarcts in the anterior spinal artery can cause vertigo from involvement of the intercalatus nucleus.[12] The physiological

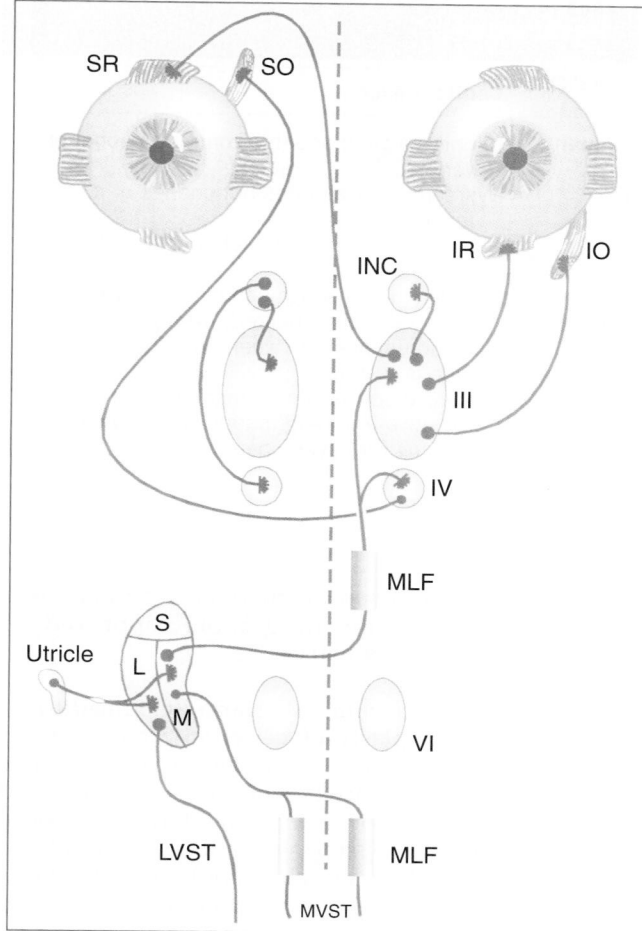

Figure 172.2 Central connections of the utricle mediating the ocular tilt reflex. This figure illustrates the projections for the right utricle. Primary afferents of the utricle project to the lateral (L) and medial (M) vestibular nuclei. Neurons in L cross the midline and travel up the medial longitudinal fasciculus (MLF) to project to the fourth and third nerve nuclei, which innervate eye muscles involved with vertical and torsional eye movements. The third nerve nucleus also innervates the interstitial nucleus of Cajal (INC). The INC in turn projects back to the third and fourth nerve nuclei. Neurons in the L and M vestibular nuclei also project to the spinal cord through the lateral and medial vestibular spinal tracts (LVST and MVST).

role of the intercalatus nucleus is poorly understood, but it is thought to be involved with the vertical neural integrator. Characteristic signs include ipsilateral tongue weakness, contralateral body weakness and sensory loss, and upbeat nystagmus.

Transient ischemic attacks (TIAs)
Vertebrobasilar ischemia (VBI)   TIAs from VBI provoke episodes of dizziness that are abrupt and usually only last for a few minutes. TIAs frequently are associated with other VBI symptoms, most commonly visual disturbance, drop attacks, unsteadiness and weakness.[3] Vertigo is among the initial symptoms in 48% of

patients with VBI. A small percentage of patients with VBI may present with isolated spells of vertigo, presumably due to ischemia in the distribution of the anterior vestibular artery (Table 172.1).

Rotational vertebral artery occlusion   Recurrent attacks of vertigo, nystagmus and ataxia induced by horizontal head rotation can occur from mechanical compression of the vertebral artery by severe cervical spondylosis, anterior scalene muscle or tendinous constriction.[13,14] Patients may be predisposed to rotational occlusion if they have an additional stenosis or vessel malformation beneath the compression, or the opposite vertebral artery is entirely occluded.[14–16]

Vertebrobasilar dolichoectasia   Pathological enlargement of the vertebral or basilar artery is frequently asymptomatic, but may cause vertigo from cranial nerve deficits and brainstem symptoms. The cerebellopontine angle is one of the more common sites for this entity.[17] Cranial nerve defects are due to mechanical pressure (similar to hemifacial spasm or trigeminal neuralgia) and ischemia from thrombosis.[18,19] Dolichoectasia may also present with isolated, sequential sensorineural hearing loss and vestibular hypofunction.[20]

Vascular loops   It has been proposed that compression of the auditory and vestibular nerves by vascular loops of the anterior inferior cerebellar artery (AICA) in the internal auditory canal can cause hearing loss, tinnitus, or vertigo.[21,22] The existence of this disorder is controversial. In a study of 1327 human temporal bone specimens, AICA loops were found within the internal auditory canal 12.3% of the time, yet there was no correlation of this finding with auditory or vestibular complaints.[23]

Vertebral artery dissection   Vertigo and oscillopsia from spontaneous nystagmus may occur acutely up to 20% of patients with vertebral artery dissection.[24] Isolated vertigo, vomiting, horizontal and torsional nystagmus with unsteadiness similar to acute vestibular neuritis due to vertebral artery dissection is rare, but has been reported.[25]

Microangiopathy and Susac's syndrome   The triad of microangiopathy of the brain, retina and inner ear referred to as Susac's syndrome is frequently misdiagnosed as multiple sclerosis.[26] It consists of sudden visual field defects due to branch retinal artery occlusions; a Ménière's-type labyrinth defect with low frequency sensorineural hearing loss (SNHL), tinnitus and vertigo; and encephalopathy. It is caused by arteriolar occlusions of unknown etiology.

Diagnostic criteria

Vertebrobasilar ischemia   Patients with transient vertigo from VBI usually have known cerebrovascular disease or risk factors for this disease.[3] Isolated episodes of vertigo due to VBI do not last longer usually than 6 weeks without the appearance of other

Table 172.2	Features that distinguish peripheral from central causes of vertigo	
Findings	**Peripheral cause**	**Central cause**
Direction of nystagmus	Usually mixed plane (horizontal and torsional)	Usually single plane (horizontal, torsional or vertical)
Effect of gaze	Nystagmus increases with gaze toward direction of quick phase	Nystagmus either does not change or it reverses direction
Effect of fixation	Nystagmus decreases	Nystagmus either does not change or it increases
Ice-water caloric test	Spontaneous nystagmus does not change when affected ear is irrigated; nystagmus decreases or reverses direction when nonaffected side is irrigated	Spontaneous nystagmus increases when affected ear is irrigated; nystagmus reverses direction when nonaffected side is irrigated
Balance	If patient is younger than age 50 years, balance is normal except sharpened Romberg test (tandem stance) may be positive. If patient is older than age 50 years, Romberg's test may be positive	May have severe defect regardless of age (positive Romberg, patient veers when walking with eyes open)

VBI symptoms or stroke.[1] Magnetic resonance arteriography (MRA) usually demonstrates the cause of isolated vertigo in patients with VBI-induced symptoms.[5] The duration of the vertigo in VBI is very helpful in the diagnosis. Most patients report vertigo that lasts minutes, rarely seconds or hours.[1,4,5] Segmental arterial insufficiency in the vertebrobasilar artery documented on magnetic resonance angiography may explain the cause of vertigo in this syndrome.[27]

Rotational vertebral artery occlusion syndrome   The site of vertebral artery occlusion in this disorder can be diagnosed by dynamic angiography during progressive head rotation.[13,14] The entire vertebral artery needs to be visualized in these positions.

Differential diagnosis

Stroke   Ménière's disease, migraine, vestibular neuritis and labyrinthitis need to be considered before a diagnosis of vertebral-basilar artery stroke is made. Clinical features that are helpful in distinguishing peripheral causes of vertigo from central causes are listed in Table 172.2.

Transient ischemic attacks   Benign paroxysmal postural vertigo (BPPV) and orthostatic hypotension need to be considered before diagnosis of VBI or rotational vertebral artery occlusion syndrome. BPPV usually occurs when the patient lies down or turns over in bed and a positive Dix–Hallpike test is present. There may be a 20 mm Hg decrease in systolic blood pressure when patients stand from a supine position.

Treatment

There are only anecdotal comments about the effectiveness of treatment of vertigo from cerebrovascular disorders.

Stroke   Ondansetron (Zofran) may be appropriate for patients with severe vertigo and nausea from stroke, but currently this drug is only approved for chemotherapy-induced nausea.[28]

Vertebrobasilar ischemia   Warfarin (Coumadin) or transluminal angioplasty of vertebral artery stenosis has been found effective in stopping TIAs when there is significant vertebral artery stenosis.[5,29] Warfarin and occasionally aspirin or ticlopidine have also been found to be effective in stopping VBI-induced isolated vertigo.[4] Treatment for VBI also should include reduction of risk factors for cerebrovascular disease.

Rotational vertebral artery occlusion syndrome   In case reports, surgical dilatation of vertebral artery constriction or untethering a mechanical constriction of this vessel has corrected rotational vertebral artery occlusion syndrome.[14,15,30]

Vascular loops   Microsurgical decompression of the eighth cranial nerve from a vascular loop has been advocated for treatment, but no trials have been done.[21,31]

Microangiopathy and Susac's syndrome   This disorder takes an unpredictable course and appears to be unresponsive to anticoagulation and immunosuppressive treatment.[32,33]

Infections: acute vestibular neuritis (or neuronitis) and Ramsay Hunt syndrome

Brief overview

Vestibular neuritis (or neuronitis) and Ramsay Hunt syndrome (herpes zoster oticus) present with intense vertigo and nystagmus for several days and are due to a sudden loss of vestibular function on one side. Hearing loss and facial weakness accompanies vestibular loss in Ramsay Hunt syndrome. The first case of vestibular neuritis was reported in 1909, but the term vestibular neuritis was first used by Hallpike

(1949).[34] Vestibular neuritis has also been referred to as epidemic vertigo and neural labyrinthitis epidemica during the past 40 years.[35]

Epidemiology

Vestibular neuritis is preceded by a common cold 50% of the time. The prevalence of vestibular neuritis peaks at 40 to 50 years of age.[36,37]

The incidence of Ramsay Hunt syndrome is 20/1 000 000/yr. The incidence of Ramsay Hunt syndrome in children is thought to be much lower than in adults but, when all patients with facial palsy are examined, 16.7% (52/311) of the cases were due to Ramsay Hunt syndrome in children (2 to 15 years of age) compared to 18.1% (319/1765) in adults (16 years or older).[38]

Etiology

Postmortem studies indicate that vestibular neuritis is likely due to a virus.[39,40] Herpes simplex type 1 (HSV-1) is the leading candidate, based on finding this virus in human vestibular ganglia and induction of a similar pathology in mice through the ear.[41–43] Vestibular neuritis is thought to frequently represent a reactivated dormant HSV-1 in Scarpa's ganglia.[42] Herpes simplex virus enters the thin mucous membranes of the respiratory tract and travels up the neuronal axons to the ganglion.[44] HSV-1 DNA during necropsy has also been found in the vestibular nuclei ipsilateral and contralateral to infected vestibular ganglia.[45] Based on these studies, Arbusow et al. have suggested that HSV-1 may migrate over the vestibular commissure to potentially cause bilateral infection.[45] Borrelia and post-infectious immune disorder have also been suggested as possible etiologies for vestibular neuritis.[46,47] In a study of 46 cases of Ramsay Hunt syndrome, herpes zoster virus was confirmed 100% of the time by acute and convalescent serum titers.[48]

Pathophysiology and pathogenesis

Vestibular neuritis behaves in a very similar way to Bell's palsy. During the latent period, the virus resides in Scarpa's ganglionic nuclei in a noninfective, nonreplicating form. When the virus is activated, edema of myelin sheath, followed by infiltration of peripheral nerve fiber by lymphocytes and plasma cells, and finally demyelination occurs.[49] The virus primarily affects the superior division of the vestibular nerve, which innervates the anterior and lateral semicircular canals.[50] Axonal degeneration of superior vestibular nerve occurs from focal ganglion cell loss.[51] The infection occasionally can extend from one ganglion to another by axon transport to involve the trigeminal, glossopharyngeal and vagus nerves.[52] With resolution of edema and inflammation, remyelination occurs.[49] Ramsay Hunt syndrome is a variant of vestibular neuritis in which multiple cranial nerves are involved.

Clinical features and natural history

Vestibular neuritis and Ramsay Hunt syndrome

present with intense vertigo, nausea, vomiting, dysequilibrium, horizontal-torsional nystagmus toward the affected side, decreased VOR and normal hearing that persists for days. Usually, only one side is affected. The vertigo is quite severe and patients prefer to lie quietly. Within a few days these symptoms begin to resolve and the patient is left with a dynamic deficit (vertigo and dysequilibrium induced by rapid head movements) which can last for weeks to months until central compensation occurs. Vestibular hypofunction is found, usually on one side. There may be intermittent episodes of vertigo decreasing in severity over the ensuing week.

Ramsay Hunt syndrome also causes facial paresis, tinnitus, and hearing loss.[53] It may also involve cranial nerves V, IX and X. Patients may exhibit vesicular lesions on the ear canal, tympanic membrane, or palate.

Diagnosis criteria

Vestibular neuritis is diagnosed based on the presence of an acute, unilateral peripheral vestibular loss documented on caloric testing with spared hearing.[36] If vestibular loss is associated with significant hearing loss (frequently with tinnitus), it is labeled labyrinthitis. Ramsay Hunt syndrome is usually defined as unilateral loss of vestibular function, hearing, and facial power. There are several case reports of gadolinium enhancement of the seventh and eighth cranial nerves in Ramsay Hunt syndrome on magnetic resonance imaging.[54]

Differential diagnosis

The differential diagnosis of vestibular neuritis and Ramsay Hunt syndrome includes: cerebellar infarcts, hemorrhage or tumors; infarcts in the brainstem distribution of the posterior inferior cerebellar artery and anterior inferior cerebellar artery; otic syphilis; vasculitis; vestibular schwannoma, perilymphatic fistula, migraine, and multiple sclerosis.[55] Certain features on the clinical exam can be used to distinguish peripheral from central causes of vertigo (Table 172.2).

In our clinic, the most common entities in the differential diagnosis are the following:

1. A vestibular schwannoma that bleeds into itself or infarcts. This can be diagnosed with a gadolinium MRI scan that includes eighth nerve levels.
2. A demyelinating plaque on the eighth nerve root entry zone from early multiple sclerosis. This can be diagnosed with a gadolinium MRI scan that includes eighth nerve levels.
3. The first attack of Ménière's disease without hearing loss. In these cases, the vestibular loss usually resolves completely in 10 to 20 days.
4. An infarct in the distribution of the labyrinth artery. This can present with isolated, unilateral vestibular loss. MRI of the head is normal. Patients with these infarcts usually have risk factors for ischemic disease and may have had TIAs preceding the event. It is sometimes impossible to differentiate a labyrinthine artery infarct from vestibular neuritis in elderly patients.

Treatment

Vestibular neuritis   Ariyasu et al.[52] and Ohbayashi et al.[56] found that prednisone during the first 10 days of the attack of vestibular neuritis shortened the course of the illness (Table 172.3). Strupp et al.[57] found that specific vestibular exercises improved balance in 20 patients at 30 days after symptom onset compared to 19 patients without vestibular exercises. This study did not control for the general effect of exercise on the recovery on posture, nor did it examine the effects of vestibular exercises on the dynamic VOR deficits.

Ramsay Hunt syndrome   Murakami et al.[58] found that early treatment with prednisone and acyclovir in Ramsay Hunt syndrome improves recovery (Table 172.4). Reduced facial nerve degeneration and hearing loss occurs if treatment is initiated within 3 days compared to more than 7 days after onset. Some authors have speculate that vaccination against chicken pox (varicella zoster) during childhood may prevent Ramsay Hunt syndrome from developing, but further studies are needed.[38]

Bottom line

The diagnosis of acute vestibular neuritis is based on finding decreased vestibular function on one side on clinical exam in a patient with an otherwise normal neurological exam. MRI scan of the head with gadolinium will help rule out stroke, multiple sclerosis and vestibular schwannoma. Blood work, including a FTA-ABS and ESR, should be obtained to rule out otic syphilis and vasculitis. An audiogram should be obtained if the patient complains of hearing loss. A bedside caloric can be done immediately to help distinguish a peripheral from a central defect.

Management of acute vertigo from vestibular neuritis or Ramsay Hunt syndrome varies depending on how many days have elapsed since the onset of symptoms (Table 172.5). Only admit the patient to the hospital if extreme dehydration is present from vomiting. A quantified caloric study (ENG) should be obtained several days after onset to document the extent of vestibular defect. By this time, the spontaneous nystagmus should be significantly decreased. A variety of medications can be employed for symptomatic treatment (Table 172.6). Vestibular suppressants (phenothiazines, benzodiazepams and anticholinergic drugs) should be used for one week or less, as the acute phase is a self-limited disorder. I use intramuscular Phenergan (promethazine) (25 to 50 mg) in the office at the onset of severe vertigo, and then send the patient home for three days of bed rest with Phenergan suppositories to be taken as needed. This medication causes sedation and reduces nausea. Ondansetron (Zofran) may also be appropriate for patients with severe vertigo and nausea, but currently this is only approved for chemotherapy-induced nausea.[28] I see the patient back in a few days to make certain the symptoms are resolving. It is then important to stop the medication and refer the patient promptly for vestibular rehabilitation.

Currently, prednisone is considered beneficial in patient with vestibular neuritis due to herpes simplex infections, but I believe we may soon start to treat these patients with both prednisone and antiviral agents. A prospective, randomized double-blind controlled study found a favorable effect in adding acyclovir to prednisone alone in recovery of volitional muscle motion and reduction of synkinesia in patients with herpes simplex-induced facial weakness.[60] In this study, 46 patients were treated with prednisone alone (0.5 mg/kg b.i.d. PO for 5 days then tapered to 0 over the next 5 days), and 53 patients were treated with prednisone and acyclovir (400 mg 5 times daily for 10 days). Outcome included an electrical stimulation test and volitional muscle motion. Treatment started within 3 days of facial weakness. Patients with complete Bell's palsy treated empirically with prednisone alone had lower facial function scores and were three times as likely to have unsatisfactory outcome compared with prednisone–acyclovir group.

Based on studies in patients with Bell's palsy, it is unlikely that treatment of vestibular neuritis with antiviral agents alone will be sufficient. In a prospective, randomized study of idiopathic facial palsy, 47 patients treated with PO prednisone (1 mg/kg q.d.) for 10 days and tapered to 0 over the next 6 days did significantly better for 3 months or longer than 54 patients treated with acyclovir (800 mg t.i.d.) for 10 days.[61] Outcome measures included facial power and neural degeneration (electrical stimulation studies). The sequelae were the same in both groups.

There is moderate morbidity with acyclovir including hepatic and renal toxic effects. Patients must be well hydrated during therapy, and hepatic function should be closely monitored. The use of an ester of acyclovir, valacyclovir hydrochloride, is recommended at 1 g, orally, three times a day for 7 days as the absorption rate is higher. Medication needs to be administered within two weeks, as the efficacy is significantly reduced after the inflammatory process has passed.

Migraine

Brief overview

Neurological disorders associated with headache have been described since AD 100, but Bickerstaff in 1961 may have been one of the earliest individuals to clearly describe vertigo as a consequence of migraine (basilar artery migraine.[62] Fenichel may have been the first to relate paroxysms of vertigo in children (benign paroxysmal vertigo of childhood).[63] Slater suggested a similar syndrome in adults (benign recurrent vertigo).[64] Migraine is now recognized as a common cause of episodic vertigo, motion sickness and dysequilibrium in children and adults.

Epidemiology

Migraine is an extremely prevalent disorder. An epidemiological study that involved over 20 000 individuals between 12 and 80 years of age found that 17.6% of all adult females, 5.7% of all adult males and

Table 172.3 Drug treatment for vestibular neuritis

Level of study	Type	Measures	No. of experimental cases	Therapy	Findings	No. of controls	Therapy	Findings	Follow-up	Reference
B	Double-blind, prospective placebo-controlled, crossover study	ENG, subjective	10	PO Methylprednisolone 32 mg, taper to 4 mg by 8th day. If no relief from vertigo or nausea then Methylprednisolone switched to placebo. Drugs started within 72 hr of symptoms	Vertigo improved 9/10. ENG normal in 1 month 16/16. HSV titer >1.8 10/10	10	Placebo. If no relief then switched to Methylprednisolone	Vertigo improved 3/10 ENG normal 1 month 2/4 HSV titer >1.8 8/10	1 month	52
B	Pros	Forced platform	20	Specific vestibular exercises	Improved sway path on forced platform (3.2 ± 1.9 m/min)	19	None	Sway path (16.9 ± 6.1 m/min)	30 days after symptom onset	57
C	Not mentioned. Suspect outcome study	ENG, subjective	34	IV hydrocortisone 500 mg decreased by 100 mg q. 2 days for 10 days or oral prednisolone 30–40 mg tapered for 10 days	Dizzy resolve: 45% 1 month, 60% 3 months, 75% 6 months, 90% 1 year Spontaneous nystagmus resolved: 25% 1 month, 70% at 3 months, 80% at 6 months, 90% 1 year. Caloric (n = 28) 71% recovery; 48% complete recovery	77	None	Dizzy resolve: 45% 1 month, 60% 3 months, 75% 6 months, 90% 1 year Spontaneous nystagmus resolved: 25% 1 month, 45% at 3 months, 60% at 6 months, 90% 1 year Caloric (n = 40) 40% recovery; 20% complete recovery	1, 3, 6, 12 months	56

ENG, electronystagmography; IV, intravenous; PO, by mouth; q., each.

Table 172.4   Drug trial for Ramsay Hunt syndrome

Level of study	Type	Measures	No. of cases	Therapy	Findings	Follow-up	Reference
B	Retrospective	House and Brackmann facial criteria;[59] Nerve conduction time (NCT), audiograms	28 experimental	Within 3 days of facial paralysis initiate acyclovir 800 mg 5×/day × 7 days + prednisone 1 mg/kg × 5 days, then taper next 10 days	Complete facial recovery 75%; normal NCT (18/28); better nerve excitability; near complete or better hearing (5/5)	6–12 months	58
			23 controls	Within 7–10 days of facial paralysis initiate same drugs	Complete facial recovery in 30%; normal NCT (5/23); improved hearing (2/3)		

Table 172.5   Management of vestibular neuritis or Ramsay Hunt

Days one to three	After day three
Perform laboratory tests: If central defect is suspected obtain magnetic resonance imaging of head	Perform laboratory tests: Audiogram (obtain immediately if Ménière's disease is suspected) Caloric test Blood work (rheumatoid factor, sedimentation factor, antinuclear antibody, fluorescent treponemal antibody absorption)
Administer vestibular suppressants and therapeutic drugs Prescribe bed rest (hospitalize if patient is dehydrated)	Stop vestibular suppressants Prescribe vestibular adaptation exercises

Table 172.6   Medications for vestibular neuritis and Ramsay Hunt

Major action	Drug	Indications	Dosage
Anti-inflammatory	Prednisone	Acute vestibular neuritis, labyrinthitis, Ramsay Hunt	60 mg q.d., then taper over 10 days
Antiviral	Acyclovir (Zovirax)	Ramsay Hunt	400 mg 5×/day × 10 days
Phenothiazine	Promethazine (Phenergan), prochlorperazine (Compazine)	Acute vestibular neuritis, labyrinthitis, Ramsay Hunt, severe nausea from central vertigo	25 mg PO, IM or Supp q. 12 hr
Serotonin agonist	Ondansetron (Zofran)	Severe nausea from central vertigo	4 mg q. 8 hr for 3 days

IM, intramuscular; PO, by mouth; q., each; q.d., each day; Supp, suppository.

4% of all children had one or more migraine headaches per year.[65] This study used the diagnostic criteria recommended by the International Headache Society.[66] Of those individuals with migraine, around 18% experienced one or more headaches per month. In both males and females, the prevalence of migraine was highest between the ages of 35 and 45 years. The type and severity of migraine often varies within the same individual.

In practices treating adult patients with headaches, 27% to 33% patients out of a population of 700 patients with migraine report episodic vertigo.[67,68] Thirty-six percent of these patients experience vertigo during their headache-free period, the others experience vertigo either just before or during a headache. The occurrence of vertigo during the headache period is much higher in patients with migraine headaches with aura as opposed to migraine without aura.[69] Episodic motion sickness may occur in up to 67% of patients with migraine. In neurological practices treating adult dizzy patients, migraine was found to be the etiology in 6%.[70]

In a population-based study of 2156 children (5 to 15 years of age), there was a prevalence rate of 2.6% of children with paroxysmal vertigo (at least three episodes of vertigo in the past year).[71] There was a twofold increase in the prevalence of migraine (24%) in this population compared to the general age-matched childhood population (10.6%).

Pathophysiology and pathogenesis

There may be several mechanisms for migraine-induced dizziness. First, direct damage to the peripheral vestibular system may occur. In some individuals, BPPV may occur, possibly due to vasospasm and damage to the inner ear.[72] Migraine is three times more common in patients with BPPV of unknown cause than BPPV secondary to trauma or surgery. An incidence of vestibular hypofunction in up to 29% of individuals has been reported,[68] although the incidence might be much less.[70] Second, migraine may release neuropeptides from efferent neurons to hair cells of the inner ear, which could increase the baseline firing rate of vestibular afferents.[73] Third, migraine may cause dysfunction of vestibular pathways in the brainstem.[62,70] Fourth, migraine may cause spreading cortical depression, possible of vestibular cortex origin. According to the neurogenic hypothesis, the aura of migraine is caused by an area of neuronal dysfunction similar to a wave of spreading depression.[74] This neuronal dysfunction may be mediated by neurons containing serotonin (5-HT) within the trigeminal nucleus.[75] Serotonin is an intracranial vasoconstrictor; its level rises during the migraine aura and falls during the headache. Platelet 5-HT level drops rapidly during the onset of migraine. Through autoregulation, blood flow is reduced to this area of neuronal dysfunction. There are a number of serotonin receptors, but $5-HT1_1$ is the most involved. Agonists of these receptors block neuropeptide release and alter neurotransmission in trigeminovascular neurons.[76] These agonists are the most effective drugs in aborting migraine. Dopamine receptors may also play a role in certain symptoms of migraine including yawning, drowsiness, irritability, nausea, vomiting, gastric paresis and hypotension.[77]

Genetics

The discovery of the genetic cause of certain types of migraine is one of the most promising breakthroughs in understanding and potentially treating this disorder. Familial hemiplegic migraine is an autosomal dominant disorder. In 50% of all families, this disorder is mapped to chromosome 19p13 in the gene called CACNA1A.[78] This gene codes for a subunit of the P/Q voltage-gated neuronal calcium channel.[79]

This same chromosome locus may be involved also in other forms of migraine aura.[80] Defects involving this gene are involved with other autosomal dominant disorders that have neuro-otological symptoms including episodic ataxia-2 (episodic ataxia and vertigo) and SCA 6 (progressive ataxia, decreased VOR cancellation, downbeat nystagmus). The symptoms of these disorders overlap extensively.[81] Only 50% of families with familial hemiplegic migraine map to chromosome 19p13. Other chromosome defects are likely to be found in the future. Mutations in CACNA1A were not found in families with migraine-induced vertigo, but other ion-channel genes in the brain or inner ear may still be a possible cause.[82]

Clinical features and natural history

Spells of dizziness usually last 4 to 60 minutes and may or may not be associated with a headache. The International Headache Society criteria can be helpful for the diagnosis of migraine-induced vertigo,[66] but a recent study suggested that these criteria might only be satisfied in 8% of patients.[70] Since this is a diagnosis of exclusion, the diagnosis is secured with a positive response to treatment.

Classification

Several neuro-otological disorders are caused by or associated with migraine (Table 172.7).

Basilar artery migraine Basilar artery migraine presents with symptoms in the distribution of the basilar artery including vertigo, tinnitus, decreased hearing, and ataxia.[62,83] The initial symptoms are usually visual, followed by vertigo, ataxic gait, dysarthria and hemiparesis. These symptoms usually precede migraine. Impairment of consciousness or stupor can occur in a number of patients. The strict IHS criteria are two or more neurological problems (vertigo, tinnitus, decreased hearing, ataxia, dysarthria, visual symptoms in both hemifields of both eyes, diplopia, bilateral paresthesia or paresis, decreased level of consciousness) followed by a throbbing headache. Vertigo typically lasts between five minutes and one hour. In the majority of cases, audiograms are normal, but many have abnormal ENG studies.[84,85] There is frequently a positive family history for migraine.

Benign recurrent vertigo of adults Benign recurrent vertigo of adults presents with recurrent attacks of vertigo not triggered by movement in young to middle-aged adults.[64] The vertigo can last hours to days and is followed by dysequilibrium. There are no auditory or other neurological symptoms and the caloric test is normal. Triggers of these attacks overlap with those of migraine including alcohol, lack of sleep, emotional stress, female preponderance and a positive family history of migraine.

Benign paroxysmal vertigo of childhood Benign paroxysmal vertigo of childhood presents with sudden attacks associated with ataxia that causes the

Table 172.7   Neuro-otological disorders due to or associated with migraine

Neuro-otological disorders due to migraine	Neuro-otological disorders associated with migraine
Basilar artery migraine Benign recurrent vertigo of adults Benign paroxysmal vertigo of childhood	Benign paroxysmal positional vertigo and central positional vertigo Motion sickness Ménière's disease

child to fall or refuse to walk.[86] Horizontal nystagmus may be evident during the duration of the attack. The child appears frightened and pale. Nausea and vomiting and sweating may be prominent. Consciousness and the ability to verbalize are not disturbed. Vertigo is verbalized in older children. There is no lethargy or drowsiness. Headache is usually not a major feature of these spells initially, and there is no tinnitus or hearing loss. The duration varies from seconds to minutes, and attacks occur daily to monthly. Children with this disorder are more susceptible to motion sickness. There is often a positive family history for migraine. In the majority of cases, the physical exam, audiogram, electronystagmography (ENG) and EEG are normal between spells, although the caloric is occasionally reduced on one side (8/42 cases in the series of Cass et al.[87]). Many of these patients eventually develop more typical migraine headaches and there is frequently a positive family history for migraine. The incidence of migraine, however, is similar to that in the general population.[88] This is still a poorly understood entity even though the IHS lists it as a type of migraine. Since this entity is a diagnosis of exclusion, the diagnosis is aided by a positive response to treatment, which is discussed below. There is one long term follow-up study of 19 children.[89] Age at onset was 5 months to 8 years (mean 3.4 years). Symptoms disappeared after 3 months to 8 years (mean 2 years). At follow-up 13 to 20 years after diagnosis, none had vertigo or balance disorder, but 21% developed migraine.

Diagnostic criteria

In order to help standardize terminology and diagnostic criteria, the International Headache Society (IHS) criteria should be used. Migraine induced dizziness remains a diagnosis of exclusion. Sometimes, the only way to determine if migraine is a significant cause of dizziness is by the response to treatment.

Differential diagnosis

Differentiating vertigo due to migraine from vertigo due to Ménière's disease may be difficult. The classical presentation of Ménière's disease is roaring tinnitus, ear fullness and hearing loss followed by vertigo lasting for hours to days.[70,90] Unfortunately, some patients with Ménière's disease may not have hearing loss until they have had several attacks of vertigo (sometimes referred to as vestibular Ménière's), or may have stable hearing loss that does not seem to fluctuate with their attacks of vertigo. Similarly, some

patients with migraine complain of tinnitus (usually high frequency), hearing disturbance (usually phonophobia), and fullness on the side of the head including the ear. In these situations, both Ménière's disease and migraine should be treated with change in lifestyle including diet, and patients asked to come into the clinic during or immediately after a severe spell of vertigo. Usually, a firm diagnosis can be made after following the patient through several attacks.

Migraine-induced positional vertigo is sometimes confused with central positional vertigo or BPPV. Migraine may even cause some cases of BPPV.[72] Generally, BPPV should be treated if there is doubt and the patient seen back in clinic in a few days. If the symptoms resolve, no further study is necessary. If the symptoms and signs do not resolve, then a thorough neurological exam and possibly MRI of the head should be done to determine if there is a posterior fossa lesion.

Finally, basilar artery migraine may be confused with posterior-vertebral TIA. In general, patients with vertigo from basilar artery migraine have a history of migraine and are younger than patients with posterior-vertebral TIAs, and patients with TIAs have significant risk factors for vascular disease.

Treatment

De Bock et al. have published the only prospective study on the effects of two drugs on migraine-induced dizziness (Table 172.8).[91] They found betahistine to be more effective than flunarizine for reducing severe dizziness due to migraine. Flunarizine is a difluorinated derivate of cinnarizine, which is a piperazine derivative with antihistamine (H1) properties and calcium blocking activity. The limitations of this study are the open design and the use of general practitioners to assess clinical outcomes without diagnostic criteria or an explicit interview format. In addition, no baseline was taken and no standardized dose given.

There are several small, retrospective studies by Johnson,[92] Baloh et al.,[93] and Bikhazi et al.,[94] which were not controlled or randomized (Table 172.8). In addition, there is an observational study that collected questionnaires from 498 general practitioners in Europe on 3186 patients on the effect of flunarizine, propranolol and betahistine on controlling either episodic vertigo (1585 patients) or migraine (1601 patients) for one year.[95] They found that propranolol (80 to 160 mg q.d.) was somewhat better than flunarizine (5 to 10 mg q.d) in the migraine study ($P = 0.02$), and there was no clear difference between flunarizine and betahistine (24 to 48 mg q.d.) in the vertigo study.

Finally, several articles give anecdotal comments about the beneficial effects of an antimigraine regimen (diet, lifestyle, medications) on vertigo and nonvertigo dizziness.[87,92,96]

Bottom line

Spells of vertigo due to migraine respond to the same types of treatment as are used for headaches. Treatment is based on the pathophysiology of this disorder and includes elimination of tyramine from the diet, and the use of drugs that change vascular tone or block serotonin and prostaglandin.[97] In addition, migraine is triggered by a number of factors including stress, anxiety, hypoglycemia, estrogen and nicotine, which should be removed if possible.[98,99] After establishing the diagnosis and reassuring the patient, we give the patient a handout listing the risk factors that may precipitate an aura (Table 172.9). We encourage them to avoid hypoglycemia by eating every 6 to 8 hours, avoid nicotine, avoid or reduce exogenous estrogen and try to maintain a regular sleep schedule. We also give them a diet to follow (Table 172.10). If strict avoidance of these risk factors does not significantly reduce their spells, based on a diary they keep, then a daily anti-serotonergic medication is used. The selective serotonin release-uptake inhibitors (SSRIs) are not approved for treatment of migraine aura. Beta-blockers are among the most effective prophylactic drugs for migraine. Valproic acid can also be used as a prophylactic treatment of migraine.

Multiple sclerosis

Brief overview

Multiple sclerosis can present as acute vestibular loss or positional vertigo and needs to be considered as one of the central causes for these symptoms. See Chapter 97 for a more complete description of multiple sclerosis and treatment. This section will focus only on the literature pertaining to vertigo.

Epidemiology

Vertigo is the initial symptom in 5% to 10% of patients with multiple sclerosis[100,101] and may ultimately occur in 50%.[102] Most patients with multiple sclerosis report imbalance at some time during the course of their disease. It can also be an early presenting finding.[103] In a study of 224 patients with multiple sclerosis, dizziness was self-rated as a severe symptom by 5% of the patients.[104] Although dizziness may be a common symptom among patients with multiple sclerosis, multiple sclerosis is a rare cause of vertigo compared to other etiologies. In a prospective, multidisciplinary study of 812 consecutive patients presenting to a "dizzy" clinic, multiple sclerosis was a rare cause of isolated dizziness in the 8.1% of patients with central causes.[105]

Pathophysiology and pathogenesis

The vestibular pathways are not large, myelinated tracts (unlike the optic nerve, medial longitudinal fasciculus, and spinal tracts), although vestibular structures do lie near the floor of the fourth ventricle, a fairly common site for plaques.[106] Plaques can either simulate a subacute vestibular loss by disrupting transmission at the eighth nerve root entry zone, or cause paroxysmal vertigo lasting seconds to minutes due to ephaptic transmission of adjacent axons within a demyelinated lesion within an area of demyelination in the brainstem.[107,108]

Classification

Several different symptom complexes have been described in patients with multiple sclerosis.

Eighth nerve, root entry zone   Multiple sclerosis may present similar to vestibular neuritis if there are root entry zone or pontine plaques.[109] When a plaque occurs in the lateral pons at the level of the eighth nerve's entry into the brainstem or at the proximal portion of the nerve (Obersteiner–Redlich zone), mixed horizontal-torsional nystagmus and unilateral caloric weakness can occur.[110–113] Plaques can also occur within the pons simulating vestibular neuritis.[114,115] Of 232 consecutive patients with acute peripheral vestibular loss based on caloric tests, 8 patients had multiple sclerosis with a pontine lesion.[107] In most of these cases of root entry zone or pontine plaque-induced dizziness, vertigo resolved with or without treatment within two weeks.

Dorsolateral medulla (Wallenberg's syndrome)   A plaque in the dorsolateral medulla can simulate Wallenberg's syndrome.[116] In these cases a caloric test would not show any decreased response, as the vestibular root entry zone is intact.

Positional vertigo   A variety of different types of positional nystagmus with or without vertigo have been described with multiple sclerosis.[109,117]

Paroxysmal central vertigo   Paroxysms of vertigo, ataxia and dysarthria lasting seconds to minutes, sometimes exacerbated by position change or hyperventilation, can also occur.[118]

Diagnostic criteria

A diagnosis of vertigo induced by multiple sclerosis depends on identifying a plaque as the cause of the symptoms. Routine vestibular tests cannot be relied on to make this diagnosis, although certain vestibular defects may be found in patients with multiple sclerosis. In a study of 20 patients with multiple sclerosis, visual suppression of the VOR was decreased in as many as 75%.[119] A significantly short VOR time constant has been reported in 19% of 130 patients with multiple sclerosis.[120]

Differential diagnosis

Vertigo induced by multiple sclerosis can simulate vestibular neuritis, stroke, or benign paroxysmal positional vertigo.[109,113,115,116] All patients with acute

Table 172.8   Drug treatment of dizziness in patients with migraine

Level of study	Type	No. of experimental cases	Active therapy	Findings	No. of controls	Therapy of control group	Follow-up	Measures	References
B	Prospective open multicenter in the Netherlands	63	Flunarizine for vestibular migraine by IHS criteria	Betahistine more effective on severity of disease (MANOVA $P = 0.03$), but no difference on number of attacks MANOVA ($P = 0.18$). Both drugs effective on number of attacks over time (MANOVA $P = 0.05$). Based on forms sent to general practitioners. No control over dose.	109	Betahistine	4.1 months (SD 1.4) flunarizine and 3.7 months (SD 0.7) betahistine	Severity of disease 1–5 (5 most severe). Number of attacks and over time (first follow-up to second follow-up). No controls	91
D	Retrospective	89	Individualized according to symptoms: benzodiazepines, beta-blockers, SSRIs, tricyclics, diet, physical therapy, lifestyle changes and acupuncture	Complete or substantial control of vestibular symptoms in: 68 (92%) cases of episodic vertigo, 56 (89%) of positional vertigo, and 56 (86%) with nonvertiginous dizziness					92
D	Prospective observation	5	Dominant family (not 19p) with migraine, vertigo and chronic essential tremor. Acetazolamide 250–750 mg/day	Patients reported marked decrease in frequency of headache and vertigo spells.			3–30 months		93
D	Retrospective, survey, patient questionnaire	53	Individualized according to symptoms: headache abortants (NSAIDs, ergots, opiates, sumatriptan) prophylactic (beta-blockers, calcium channel blockers, tricyclics, methysergide, valproic acid, cyproheptadine)	1–4 least–most effective. 3 = sumatriptan (all patients; vertigo); All the rest were 1 or 2				Spearman rank coefficient	94

Table 172.9	Schedule to treat migraine disorders

1) Reduction of stress
   a) Aerobic exercise at end of day (3–4 times/week). Get heart rate above 100 and sustain it for at least 20 minutes
   b) Eat something at least every 8 hours to avoid hypoglycemia. Eat breakfast at same time each morning (breakfast on weekends should be at the same time as on weekdays)
   c) Maintain a regular sleep schedule
2) Do not smoke or chew any products that contain nicotine
3) Avoid exogenous estrogen (oral contraceptives, estrogen replacement)
4) Follow diet
5) Keep a diary
   a) Time and date of all headaches and/or spells that interfere with daily routine
   b) Write down any foods that you had that are listed on the other side of this sheet during the 24 hours prior to the headache and/or spell
   c) Bring diary in with you on your next visit!
6) Medications

Table 172.10	Diet for migraine patients	
	Foods allowed	**Foods to avoid**
Beverages	Decaffeinated coffee, fruit juice, club soda, noncola soda. Limit caffeine sources to 2 cups per day (coffee, tea, cola)	Chocolate, cocoa, certain alcoholic beverages (red wine, port, sherry scotch, bourbon, gin). Excessive Nutrasweet (no more than 24 oz/day of diet drink)
Meats, fish, poultry	Fresh or frozen turkey, chicken, fish, beef, lamb, veal, pork Limit eggs to 3 per week Tuna or tuna salad	Aged, canned, cured, or processed meats including ham or game, pickled herring, salad and dried fish; chicken liver, bologna; fermented sausage; any food prepared with meat tenderizer, soy sauce, or brewer's yeast; any food containing nitrates or tyramine (smoked meats including bacon, sausage, ham, salami, pepperoni, hot dogs)
Dairy products	Milk: homogenized, 2% or skim Cheese: American, cottage, farmer, ricotta, cream, Canadian, processed cheese slice Yogurt (limit 1/2 cup per day)	Buttermilk, sour cream, chocolate milk Cheese: stilton, bleu, cheddar, mozzarella, cheese spread, roquefort, provolone, gruyere, muenster, feta, parmesan, emmenthal, brie, brick, camembert types, cheddar, gouda, romano
Breads, cereals	Commercial bread, English muffins, melba toast, crackers, bagels. All hot and dry cereals	Hot fresh homemade yeast bread, bread or crackers containing cheese. Fresh yeast coffee cake, doughnuts, sourdough bread. Any product containing chocolate or nuts
Potato or substitute	White potato, sweet potato, rice, macaroni, spaghetti, noodles	None
Vegetables	Any except those to avoid	Beans such as pole, broad, lima, Italian, fava, navy, pinto, garbanzo. Snow peas, pea pods, sauerkraut, onions (except for flavoring), olives, pickles
Fruit	Any except those to avoid; limit citrus fruits to 1/2 cup per day (1 orange); limit banana to 1/2 per day	Avocados, figs, raisins, papaya, passion fruit, red plums
Soups	Cream soups made from foods allowed in diet, homemade broth	Canned soup, soup or bouillon cubes, soup base with yeast or MSG (read labels)
Desserts	Any cake, cookies without chocolate, nuts or yeast. Any pudding or ice cream without chocolate or nuts. Flavored gelatin	Any product containing chocolate including ice cream, pudding, cookies, cake or pies. Mincemeat pie
Sweets	Sugar, jelly, jam, honey, hard candy	Chocolate candy or syrup, carob
Miscellaneous	Salt in moderation, lemon juice, butter or margarine, cooking oil, whipped cream, white vinegar, commercial salad dressings	Pizza, cheese sauce, MSG in excessive amounts (including Chinese food and Accent), meat tenderizer, seasoned salt, yeast, yeast extract. Mixed dishes (including macaroni and cheese, beef stroganoff, cheese blintzes, lasagna, frozen TV dinners). Chocolate, nuts (including peanut butter). All nonwhite vinegars. Anything fermented, pickled or marinated.

vestibular loss, or BPPV that does not respond to treatment, should have a gadolinium MRI scan of the head.

Treatment and bottom line

See Chapter 97 for the treatment of multiple sclerosis. There is only one controlled, double-blind study of multiple sclerosis and vertigo. When cinnarizine 75 mg b.i.d. was compared to placebo in 40 patients with vertigo, there was significant improvement ($P < 0.05$) in vertigo from peripheral lesions but no significant difference in patients with central disorders (multiple sclerosis or cerebellar atrophy).[121]

There are several anecdotal reports on the treatment and outcome of vertigo from multiple sclerosis.

Multiple sclerosis causing acute vestibular loss resembling vestibular neuritis or labyrinthitis Based on case reports, vertigo resolves and decreased calorics may or may not resolve for plaques involving the eighth nerve root entry zone within one to two weeks with standard treatment for acute vertigo and intravenous methylprednisolone.[111,112,114] Vertigo may also resolve spontaneously within two weeks in these cases.[111–113,115] Perhaps patients with vertigo from multiple sclerosis should be treated similarly to patients with optic nerve demyelination, where randomized controlled trials have demonstrated a shortened course, better outcome and reduced chance for increased attacks at least during the next three years.[122] Plaques involving more central vestibular pathways frequently cause more prolonged and intractable vertigo, vestibular nystagmus and nausea. In these cases, ondansetron may be helpful.[28]

Paroxysmal central vertigo Paroxysmal central vertigo due to multiple sclerosis may respond to carbamazeine, although it is unclear if this recovery would have occurred spontaneously.[108,123] Double-blind, placebo controlled studies are needed.

Trauma

Brief overview

Head trauma can produce vertigo from injury to structures in the inner ear and the CNS.[124] BPPV is the most common cause of vertigo in patients with head trauma. BPPV can occur as a result of a blow to the head (either directly or associated with a fall), and can also occur after a flexion-extension injury to the neck (whiplash) (see Chapter 108). Other causes of vertigo due to head trauma include perilymphatic fistula from barotrauma (scuba diving or pressure force to the ear), injury to the labyrinth or vestibular nerve from petrous bone fracture, and axon swelling within the brainstem.

Epidemiology

Dizziness (vertigo, dysequilibrium, lightheadedness) following head trauma occurs in 40% to 60% of patients.[125,126] True vertigo is less frequent with an incidence of 2% to 30%. The incidence of vertigo does not appear to be related to the severity of the head trauma.[127]

Etiology

Dizziness may occur from inner ear injury (benign paroxysmal positional vertigo, endolymphatic hydrops, perilymphatic fistula, labyrinth concussion); eighth cranial nerve injury; brain injury (cerebellum, vestibular nuclei, temporal lobe); neck injury (vestibulo-spinal tract, cervical plexus, soft tissue), and from psychological problems (Table 172.11). See Chapter 173 for description and treatment of trauma-induced inner ear disorders.

Pathophysiology and clinical features

Labyrinth concussion and eighth nerve injury from temporal bone fractures Temporal bone fractures are divided into longitudinal (orthogonal to long axis of petrous pyramid) and transverse fractures; longitudinal fractures are four times more common.[128] Meningitis is a late complication of both types of fractures.[129] Longitudinal fractures result from temporal and parietal blows. They cause conductive hearing loss and CSF and hemorrhagic otorrhea.[130] Damage to the vestibular and cochlear nerve is infrequent. The facial nerve is involved in 10% to 20% of cases, usually in the labyrinthine segment or geniculate ganglion.[131]

Transverse fractures usually result from frontal or occipital blows. Eighty to ninety percent of the time the fracture transects the inner ear and lacerates the membranous labyrinth, vestibular nerve and cochlear nerve. This causes severe sensorineural hearing loss and loss of vestibular function. Fifty to 65% of the time the facial nerve is injured, usually in the labyrinthine segment. CSF often fills the middle ear and drains into the eustachian tube. The tympanic membrane usually remains intact, but a hemotympanum is frequently seen. Figure 172.3 is an axial CT scan of a 16-year-old girl who had a transverse fracture through the petrous bone.

Fifty percent of patients with temporal bone fractures will complain of dizziness, and positional nystagmus is the most common vestibular sign.[132] A review of 90 temporal bone fractures of both types revealed hemotympanum as the most common physical finding (46 ears), followed by bleeding from external ear canal (27 ears) and CSF otorrhea (13 patients).[133] Ossicular dislocation or fracture was found in 13 patients and facial paralysis occurred in 14. Battle's sign from extravasation of blood along the path of the posterior auricular artery occurred in 8 patients.

Concussive injury sufficient to cause occipital fracture may also cause complete bilateral loss of cochlear and vestibular function, hypothesized to be due to axonal injury to the eighth nerve and possibly the labyrinth.[134]

Central vestibular nystagmus from brainstem and vestibulocerebellar contusions Severe head trauma may produce axonal swelling and wallerian degeneration in structures throughout the posterior fossa

Table 172.11   Sites and mechanisms of trauma-induced dizziness

Site	Syndrome	Pathophysiology
Inner ear	Benign paroxysmal positional vertigo (BPPV)	Cupula or canal lithiasis
	Post-traumatic endolymphatic hydrops	Decreased endolymphatic absorption
	Perilymphatic fistula	Rupture in round or oval window, or in membranous labyrinth
	Labyrinth concussion	Temporal bone fracture: Disrupts bony or membranous labyrinth
Vestibular nerve	Eighth nerve contusion or section	Temporal bone fracture: disrupts eighth nerve
Brainstem or vestibulocerebellum	Downbeat, upbeat, and torsional nystagmus, central positional vertigo, ocular tilt response	Contusion or hemorrhage
	Postconcussive syndrome	Minor head trauma
	Drug-induced dizziness	Drug-induced dizziness
	Post-traumatic migraine	Post-traumatic migraine
Cerebral cortex	Tornado epilepsy	Post-traumatic seizures
Neck	Whiplash and cervical vertigo	Flexion-extension injury
Psychological	Panic disorder, chronic anxiety, depression, somatization, compensation neurosis	Psychogenic dizziness

based on autopsy review.[135–138] To what extent focal vestibular damage to the brainstem can occur following head trauma is unclear. In animal models, petechial hemorrhages and degenerative changes may occur in vestibular nuclei and vestibular cerebellum with minor head trauma.[139,140] These studies are difficult to extrapolate to human studies since the animals were anesthetized during the head trauma. Careful serial sections of human brainstem in fatal blunt head injury, however, indicate that brainstem damage without damage to the rest of the brain is not found, i.e. brainstem injury is believed to occur as part of diffuse brain damage and not in isolation.[141,142]

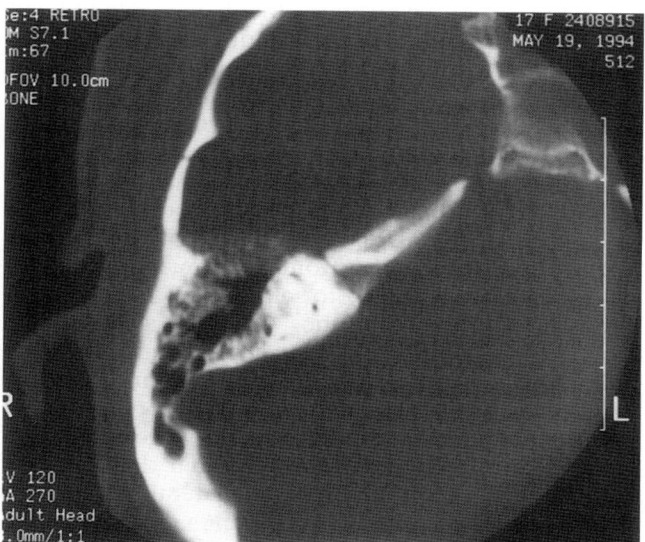

Figure 172.3 CT scan of the skull base (axial view) of a 16-year-old girl who was involved in a car accident and suffered head injury. Her Glasgow Coma Scale was 3 at the scene and 6 in the trauma center. Scan shows a transverse fracture through the left petrous bone.

Following head trauma, a variety of different types of central vestibular nystagmus may occur which are usually not associated with vertigo, including downbeat nystagmus, upbeat nystagmus, and gaze-position nystagmus (see Chapter 166). Positional-induced nystagmus from a central cause is rarely associated with vertigo, and when it occurs is attributed to hemorrhage dorsolateral to the fourth ventricle.[143]

The ocular tilt reaction consists of head tilt, skew eye deviation and cyclodeviation of the eyes (excyclotropia of the hypotropic eye and incyclotropia of the hypertropic eye).[144,145] The patient primarily complains of vertical diplopia. This disorder occurs because there is a unilateral defect in the otolith pathway. Lesions of the labyrinth, eighth nerve, and vestibular nuclei all cause an ipsilateral ocular tilt reaction (head tilt and hypotropic eye ipsilateral to the side of lesion), whereas lesions of the medial longitudinal fasciculus and interstitial nucleus of Cajal cause a contralateral ocular tilt reaction. Variations of the ocular tilt reaction include alternating skew deviation and see-saw nystagmus.[146,147]

Postconcussive syndrome from minor head trauma
Following minor head trauma with concussion and a brief period of amnesia, patients frequently complain of persistent headache (25%), anxiety (19%), insomnia (15%), and dizziness (14%).[148] Depression is also frequently present in patients with head trauma.[149] To what extent these symptoms occur as a result of head trauma is unclear since these same symptoms are reported by patients without head trauma who are involved in litigation.[150] The dizziness described by patients with postconcussive syndrome is usually nonspecific and often consists of a sense of swimming, light-headedness, floating, rocking, and disorientation. Unfortunately, patients with psychogenic dizziness also use these terms. Treatment of dizziness in this syndrome involves reassurance that there is no

structural damage and that the symptoms are not unusual and usually resolve. Medication and psychological intervention is useful when there is underlying anxiety and depression.

There have been two large neuro-otological studies in patients with minor head injury. Tuohimaa[151] studied 82 patients who were unconscious for two hours or less without evidence of skull fractures or intracerebral hemorrhage. Vestibular paresis from presumed labyrinth concussion was found in 17% within four days of the injury and persisted in 5% of patients up to six months. Their exam was not described beyond six months. Griffiths studied 84 patients within a few days of minor head trauma (post-traumatic amnesia of less than 24 hours).[152] Fifty-six percent had hearing loss based on audiogram, the majority of which were sensorineural loss; 24% had vertigo of unknown etiology, 70% of which were associated with deafness. Vestibular studies were not done. Neither of these two studies described the initial neurological exam during the first 24 hours, so the Glasgow Coma Scale could not be determined.

Post-traumatic migraine   Head trauma or whiplash injury may predispose patients to spells of vertigo from migraine.[153,154] These patients may also complain of episodic dysequilibrium.

Drug-induced dizziness   Several hundred drugs may cause dizziness.[155,156] Table 172.12 lists the more common drugs that may be used in patients with head trauma. Certain drugs cause vague complaints of dizziness including dysequilibrium and lightheadedness. These include anticonvulsants, antidepressants, anti-inflammatory agents, hypnotics, muscle relaxants, and tranquilizers. Drugs used to treat dizziness and nausea (vestibular suppressants) also are the cause of dysequilibrium when used chronically. Sensitization may occur to meclizine and scopolamine after a few days of continuous use, and withdrawal symptoms will occur when the medication is stopped. This may be misinterpreted as recurrence of the problem, and physicians should be cautious about restarting these medications. Certain drugs may cause vestibular ototoxicity and dysequilibrium, but spare hearing. These include certain aminoglycosides and loop diuretics.

Tornado epilepsy from post-traumatic seizures   The incidence of seizures following head trauma is 7% to 10%, of which 20% to 36% are partial.[157–159] Ninety-four percent of all seizures occur within 24 hours of the injury. The incidence increases as the GCS decreases ranging from 6% for a GCS greater than 13% to 35% for a GCS of less than 8.[158] Ictal vertigo (tornado epilepsy) is uncommon, and primarily occurs in simple partial seizures that usually evolve into complex partial seizures or generalize with loss of consciousness. In a series of 222 patients with partial seizures from traumatic and nontraumatic causes, nine had ictal vertigo.[160] Vertigo in some patients with partial seizures resembles endolymphatic hydrops without hearing loss.[161] This is most likely due to stimulation of a vestibular cortical area in the superior temporal gyrus.[162] Seizures may also cause other neuro-otological symptoms.

Whiplash syndrome and cervical vertigo from flexion-extension injury of the neck
Whiplash syndrome   Acute flexion-extension injuries of the neck often lead to symptoms referred to as the whiplash syndrome. Neck pain, headache and limited range of motion of the neck are the most common symptoms, but dizziness may follow, usually described as lightheadedness, floating and being off balance. The acute injury is postulated to be mechanical strain with or without contusion or tears of the ligaments and muscles supporting the cervical spine.[163] Following significant neck trauma, dysequilibrium may occur due to central cord syndrome. Vertigo can occur if there is associated vertebral artery thrombosis leading to a posterior inferior cerebellar artery syndrome. Often the physical exam is negative, leading the physician to be skeptical about these subjective complaints. There may be eye movement disorders in patients with whiplash documented on ENG,[164,165] but this is most likely the result of coincidental head trauma. Mallinson and Longridge compared 19 patients with whiplash alone to 17 patients with whiplash and mild head injury.[166] Dizziness persisted for two years in both groups. There were no ENG abnormalities in whiplash but, of mild head injury cases, five had caloric abnormality and three had central ENG findings.

Cervical vertigo   There is cervical input to the vestibular system that can enhance the VOR and contribute to self motion. The cervico-ocular reflex functions synergistically with the vestibular-ocular reflex to generate slow phase eye movements opposite to head movements to stabilize gaze during head movements. The cervico-ocular reflex can be demonstrated by measuring eye movements while moving the trunk with the head fixed. In normal subjects the response is extremely low, but it increases significantly in patients with bilateral vestibular deficits. A multisynaptic pathway from the neck proprioceptors to the vestibular nuclei possibly mediates this reflex. Somatosensory receptors from neck muscles, tendons and joints also contribute to self-motion during active locomotion. "Arthrokinetic nystagmus" can be evoked in the dark by human subjects and primates walking in place on a circular treadmill, and also can be enhanced after bilateral labyrinth defects.[167,168] Despite these findings, there is no evidence that injury to the neck causes significant vestibular deficits. Unilateral anesthesia of the posterior-lateral neck tissue rarely causes spontaneous nystagmus, but can cause transient ipsilateral past pointing, ataxia, and the sensation of numbness or floating.[169] These are the typical features of "cervical vertigo," which is a controversial condition that has been proposed to explain somatic complaints of nonvertiginous dizziness in the absence of true peripheral or central vestibular dysfunction

Table 172.12   Potential dizziness from drugs used in head trauma

Drug	Drugs that can cause dizziness	Drugs that interfere with vestibular compensation	Ototoxic (vestibular) drugs
Anticonvulsants	Barbiturates, carbamazepine, phenytoin, Ethosuximide		
Antidepressants	Amitriptyline, imipramine		
Anti-inflammatory drugs	Ibuprofen, indomethacin		Acetylsalicylic acid (reversible)
Antibiotics			Gentamicin, streptomycin Tobramycin
Hypnotics	Flurazepam, triazolam		
Muscle relaxants	Cyclobenzaprine, orphenadrine Methocarbamol		
Tranquilizers	Chlordiazepoxide, meprobamate		
Vestibular suppressants	Meclizine, scopolamine, chlordiazepoxide Diazepam Lorazepam	Meclizine, scopolamine, chlordiazepoxide Diazepam Lorazepam	

following whiplash injury. Numerous mechanisms had been proposed for cervical vertigo including vertebrobasilar insufficiency, cervical sympathetic irritation causing decreased blood flow to the labyrinth, and altered spinal proprioceptive fiber input.[170,171]

Diagnostic criteria

Electronystagmography   This consists of eye movement recordings during visual tracking and during vestibular testing (rotary chair or caloric). It is difficult to interpret the findings of papers recording ENG in patients complaining of post-traumatic vertigo, since slow phase eye velocity of the spontaneous nystagmus and nystagmus during the caloric is not documented.[172] Despite that, these tests are objective and should be done in patients complaining of dizziness.

Audiogram   An audiogram should be performed on all patients with head trauma-induced tinnitus and hearing loss. Table 172.13 lists trauma-induced disorders in which hearing is impaired or normal. The audiogram should include pure-tone and speech audiometry, acoustic reflexes and middle ear function. Nonpulsatile and constant tinnitus without documented hearing loss is extremely rare. A nonorganic loss of hearing can be determined by the inconsistency of the audiogram (more than a 10 dB change in threshold on successive trials), which may occur in up to 10% of head-injured patients. The Stenger test is helpful in determining a nonorganic or exaggerated loss to hearing. In this test tones are presented simultaneously to both ears and the patient is asked to keep their hand up as long as the tone is on. As long as the tone is above the threshold in the good ear, the patient should respond regardless of the intensity in the suspect ear. A functional disorder is suspected when tones are presented simultaneously, but the tone in the good ear is set below threshold and the tone in the suspect ear is set above true

Table 172.13   Hearing in head trauma-induced acute vertigo

Hearing usually impaired	Hearing usually preserved
Endolymphatic hydrops	BPPV
Labyrinth concussion	Brainstem and vestibulocerebellar injury
Perilymphatic fistula	Postconcussive syndrome
Temporal bone fracture	Post-traumatic seizures
Blast and explosive injury	Cervical trauma
	Post-traumatic migraine
	Psychogenic

threshold. In this case the patient's response is either inconsistent or they fail to respond.

Auditory brainstem evoked responses   The auditory brainstem evoked response (ABR) is the averaged surface-recorded activity of the auditory neural generators of the auditory periphery and lower central auditory pathway. The ABR is an excellent screening test for abnormalities involving eighth nerve and central auditory brainstem pathways. The ABR has been reported to be abnormal in patients with postconcussive syndrome even when all other studies are normal.[173] The sensitivity of finding an abnormality in this test in patients with head trauma may increase when higher repetitive rates are used as the stimulus.[174]

Radiology   High resolution CT imaging of the temporal bone is best for evaluating petrous bone abnormalities including labyrinthine defects, hearing loss, facial nerve paralysis, petrous bone fractures and other pathologies that are likely to entail bone erosion.[175] The location of CSF leaks is also best done with high resolution CT scan of the temporal bone following intrathecal injection of water-soluble contrast material. MRI with gadolinium enhancement with both coronal and horizontal sections through the eighth nerve is the most sensitive test for evaluation of the internal auditory canal, cerebellopontine angle and brainstem.[176]

Treatment and take-home message

General   There are no controlled trials for vertigo induced by head trauma. Vestibular neurectomy has been advocated for treatment of patients with post-traumatic unsteadiness with associated hearing loss, although there have been no controlled trials comparing this form of treatment to vestibular rehabilitation.[177,178] Furthermore, there is no physiological basis for neurectomy except for treatment of intractable spells of vertigo due to post-traumatic endolymphatic hydrops. In the author's opinion, there is no conclusive evidence that neurectomy facilitates vestibular compensation. Meclizine and other vestibular suppressant drugs are used excessively and inappropriately, usually without a good understanding of the cause of dizziness. The use of these medications should be limited to a few days only during acute vestibular hypofunction such as labyrinth concussion or acute eighth nerve transection. Then the drugs should be stopped, otherwise they can interfere with central compensation and frequently cause dizziness in their own right. Peripheral vestibular defects respond much more readily than central causes of dizziness. Patients with brainstem medullary lesions may have nausea lasting for weeks and may require medication for a longer period of time. The most challenging problem in the management of dizziness is the frequently associated psychogenic component. This can be managed with thoughtful discussion by the clinical provider, patient education, behavioral modification, and if necessary supportive psychotherapy and medication including selective serotonin release uptake inhibitors (SSRIs).

Temporal bone fracture   Initial care of temporal bone fractures follows the "a, b, c" preservation of airway, breathing and circulation. The physical exam should include sterile exam of external auditory canal and tympanic membrane to evaluate for blood, CSF and tympanic membrane tear. Cranial nerves VII and VIII should be examined carefully. Patients unable to respond can be electrically stimulated to evoke facial movement. If temporal bone injury is suspected, then high resolution computed tomography is the preferred method with 1.5 mm cuts in coronal and axial planes.[179–182] When CT scan is not available, lateral radiographic projections may reveal longitudinal fractures, and Stenver projections may reveal transverse fractures. Vestibular symptoms from labyrinthine concussion or eighth nerve transection almost always fade by one year due to central compensation, which can be facilitated by vestibular rehabilitation.[132]

Postconcussive syndrome from minor head trauma
Treatment of dizziness in this syndrome involves reassurance that there is no structural damage and that the symptoms are not unusual and usually resolve. Med-ication and psychological intervention are useful when there is underlying anxiety and depression.

Tumors: vestibular schwannoma (or vestibular schwannoma) and neurofibroma

Brief overview

Cushing first described vestibular schwannomas in patients presenting at an advanced stage with multiple cranial nerve defects and central nervous system dysfunction.[183] The most common presentations of vestibular schwannomas are sensorineural hearing loss, dizziness and tinnitus.[184] Up to 12.5% of patients with vestibular schwannoma may present with normal hearing on audiology.[185] These patients were usually younger (39 vs. 49) and complained of tinnitus, dysequilibrium and subjective hearing loss or distortion. The combination of otological and neurotological symptoms in a young patient should prompt the clinician to investigate further even if hearing is normal.

Epidemiology

Vestibular schwannomas are relatively common, constituting approximately 5% to 10% of all intracranial tumors.[186] They are the third largest group of intracranial tumors after gliomas and meningiomas. It is estimated that between 2000 and 3000 vestibular schwannomas are diagnosed in the US each year. The majority of tumors present in the fourth to sixth decades of life. Based on unselected autopsy series, the incidence may be slightly less than 1%, but the incidence of clinical symptoms from acoustic tumors may be only 8 per million per year.[187,188] Based on a population study of 600 000 individuals in a county in Denmark, however, the incidence was 16.8 per million per year.[189] This higher value is thought to be due to the widespread availability of MRI scans of the head.

Etiology

Vestibular schwannomas are thought to arise where the central nerve sheath (glial) meets the peripheral sheath (schwann cell), a transition that is usually located within the internal auditory canal. Vestibular schwannomas originate from both the superior and inferior divisions of the vestibular nerve.

Genetics

Approximately 5% of vestibular schwannomas arise as a manifestation of one of two hereditary syndromes, neurofibromatosis (NF) type 1 (von Recklinghausen's disease, peripheral NF) or NF type 2 (central NF). NF-1 is relatively common, with an incidence of 1 per 4000 births, but unilateral vestibular schwannoma is unusual in NF-1, with a frequency of only about 2%, and virtually no cases of bilateral tumors.[191] The incidence of NF-2 is much less but the actual number is unknown. Bilateral vestibular schwannomas are the rule and are present in over 90% of individuals with NF-2.

Table 172.14 Presenting symptoms in patients with vestibular schwannoma

No. of patients	Hearing loss	Tinnitus	Vertigo/dizziness	Headache	Facial neuropathy	Other	References
68	85%	34%	38% (vertigo)		3%	4%	192
119	95%	65%	46% (dizziness)	2%			193

Table 172.15 Natural history of vestibular schwannoma without treatment

Type	Number of patients	Age	Follow-up	No growth	Growth > 2 mm	References
Retrospective	68	Mean 67.1	0.5–12 years (mean 3.4 years)	48 (71%) (0.36 mm/yr)	20 (29%). 10 no therapy; 10 therapy mean 4 years (3.0 mm/yr)	192
Retrospective	119	Mean = 65 (37–84)	Mean = 2.5 years (5 months to 8 years)		30% at 3.8 mm/yr (maximum 25 mm/yr). 71% tumors > 20 mm onset grew vs. 26% <20 mm	193
Retrospective	52		Image interval 6–24 months depending on growth	21% no growth and 15% remitted	64% 1.6 mm/yr	194
	27	Unilateral tumors = 15 at 59.5 years. Bilateral tumors = 10 at 26.1 years	6.3–14.7 months		63% (including 10 of 12 neurofibroma II)	195
Prospective	64	23–75 (mean 55; SD 13.8 years)	5 months to 15 years	22% regressed 55% no growth	23% grew (>1 mm/yr)	189

Clinical features and natural history

Sensorineural hearing loss, tinnitus, and vertigo or dizziness are the most common presenting symptoms in patients with vestibular schwannoma (Table 172.14).

Several studies have shown that vestibular schwannomas may not grow for several years (Table 172.15). Mirz et al. found that the size of the tumor in the no-growth or regression group was statistically significantly larger than in the growth group ($P = 0.001$).[189] Tumors 12 mm or larger on average showed no growth or regressed to a smaller size. The imaging interval was 6 months to 2 years depending on the growth rate.

Classification

It has been recommended that all tumors arising from the eighth cranial nerve complex be termed vestibular schwannoma instead of acoustic neuroma.[196] This makes sense because the tumors arise from schwann cells surrounding the vestibular portion of the eighth nerve.

Diagnostic criteria

A gadolinium-enhanced T_1-weighted MRI scan with eighth nerve cuts is the gold standard for detecting these tumors. This test reaches 100% sensitivity no matter what the size of the tumor, but the test is also the most expensive of the diagnostic studies. In a study published in 1996, fast spin echo T_2 MRI of one ear correctly diagnosed 98% of surgically confirmed vestibular schwannomas, compared with 100% using conventional enhanced MRI.[197] Since 1996, the resolution of fast spin echo has increased such that it is thought not to miss any of 1070 consecutive cases of unilateral sensorineural hearing loss.[198] Fast spin echo MRI may eventually become the best test to screen patients for vestibular schwannomas.

An auditory brainstem response test (ABR) should be considered as the best current screening test, and should be considered in those patients who cannot have an MRI scan (overweight patients, patients with metal implants and those who cannot afford the cost). ABR has a positive sensitivity of 100% for tumors large than 3 cm, but will miss 9% to 17% if the tumor is smaller than 3 cm.[199] In a retrospective review of 75 patients with surgically confirmed vestibular schwannomas, the cost-effectiveness of screening with ABR followed by MRI in high risk patients was compared to obtaining MRI in all patients.[200] In a "low risk" group (one of the following: isolated vertigo, unilateral tinnitus, explained unilateral hearing loss), a

Table 172.16   Outcomes of the translabyrinthine approach

No. of patients	% CSF leaks	% Bacterial meningitis	References
251	20	15	201
300	11	4	202
215	10	0	203
723	6.8	2.9	204
146	21	3	205
129	6.2	0	206
102	6.9	0.9	207
83	13	1.2	208
258	7.8	1.6	209
331	6.9% first 131 patients; 0% in last 200 after modification of technique	0 at least in last 200 patients	210

Table 172.17   Stereotactically delivered radiation treatments for vestibular schwannomas

Radiation delivery system	No. of patients	Radiation dose	Tumor control	CN palsy V	CN palsy VII	Preservation of useful hearing	Follow-up	References
Gamma Knife	71	8–20 Gy	93%	8%	14%	60%	0.8–5.6 years	212
Gamma Knife	83	16 Gy	94%	8%	11%	N/A	Mean 36 months	213
Gamma Knife	36	16–20 Gy (mean = 15.5)	100%	67%	59%	42%	3 months to 2 years	214
Gamma Knife	452	22–40 Gy (median = 32)	13 (2.9%) needed microsurgery 7–72 months later (27 months median): 10 due to growth and 3 due to increased symptoms (no growth)				12 months to 116 months (mean 41 months)	215
LINAC	56	10–22.5 Gy (70% = 12.5–15)	98%	Combined 21%		N/A	1–5 years	216
LINAC	24	12–45 Gy (median = 30 Gy)	85%	4%	7%	100%	2–8 years	217
Fractionated radiotherapy (LINAC)	27	24–51 Gy (5–27 fractions)	100%	0%	13%	71%	3–27 months	218
Fractionated radiotherapy (LINAC)	12	>53 Gy (over 27–30 fractions)	100%	Combined 8%		100%	16–44 months	219

LINAC, linear accelerator; N/A not available.

Table 172.18   Comparison of treatments for vestibular schwannomas

Level of study	Type	No. of experimental cases	Therapy	Findings	No. of controls	Therapy	Follow-up	Reference
D	Retrospective	50	Fractionated radiotherapy 36–44 Gy (20–22 fractions)	Mean growth rate was 3.87 mm/yr in observation and −0.75 in SRT ($P < 0.0001$)	27	Observation	35 months experimental 30 observations	220

		Table 172.19	Physical therapy after surgery					

Level of study	Type	No. of cases	Therapy	Measures	Findings	Follow-up	Reference
D	Prospective	11 experimental	PT gave VOR enhancement exercises plus ambulation 20 min/day. Started POD 3	1) Visual analog scale for subjective dizziness from POD 1–6 (or post-op day 1–6) 2) Posturography peak-to-peak AP sway test. 3) Gait observation	Subjective: no difference in vertigo, decreased dysequilibrium ($P < 0.05$). Posturography: by POD 6 returned to preoperative state but control still significantly different ($P < 0.023$). Gait: all control and 40% experimental still had abnormal gait	POD 6	221
		8 control	PT directed smooth pursuit eye movements without head movements plus ambulation 20 min/day. Started POD 3				

POD, postoperative day; PT, physical therapy; VOR, vestibulo-ocular reflex.

tumor would have been missed in one out of 16 patients with ABR screening (sensitivity 93%). What must be considered is the number of patients that must be examined in this low risk group to yield one patient with a tumor. Assuming a 1% prevalence rate in this low risk group, the added cost of an MRI as the initial screening for all patients in this group would be $1 612 500. In the "intermediate risk" group (one of the following: sudden SNHL or unexplained persistent tinnitus), four tumors out of 45 were missed (91% sensitivity). Assuming a 5% prevalence rate in this group, the added cost of getting MRI in all patients is $858 000. In the "high-risk" group (all of the following: asymmetric unexplained hearing loss, tinnitus and a less than 30% decreased word recognition), one out of 14 tumors were missed (sensitivity 92%). Assuming a 30% prevalence rate in this group, the added cost of getting MRI in all patients in this group to find 14 tumors is $30 900. In conclusion, it is currently cost-effective to screen with ABR in all patients and get MRI in those who fail screening.[200]

Treatment and take-home message

There are no grade A studies on the treatment of vestibular schwannoma. There are several grade C, level V outcome studies on the effect of surgery or radiation in patients with vestibular schwannoma.

Translabyrinthine surgical removal Table 172.16 lists outcomes of the translabyrinthine approach. Since this approach was introduced in 1960, it has gained widespread acceptance due to its low complication rate (especially facial nerve), total tumor removal, safety and effectiveness even with the largest tumors.[211] It is considered the treatment of choice for patients with nonserviceable hearing.

Radiation therapy Table 172.17 lists the outcomes of stereotactically delivered radiation treatments for acoustic schwannomas. There is only one study that has compared radiotherapy with observation alone (Table 172.18).

Physical therapy after removal of vestibular schwannoma In a grade B, randomized controlled trial (Table 172.19), vestibular adaptation exercises were shown to improve postural stability and diminished perception of dysequilibrium following vestibular schwannoma resection.[221]

Take home message Vestibular schwannomas (a better descriptive name than acoustic neuroma) constitute the third largest group of intracranial tumors. These tumors present usually with SHNL or tinnitus, but can present with acute vertigo. Gadolinium MRI with eighth nerve cuts is the test of choice, but ABR can be done as a screen in patients at low risk for tumor. The author always obtains MRI scans in patients with unilateral loss of vestibular function documented on vestibular testing if this test has not been previously done. Several studies have shown that these tumors may not grow for several years. Therefore, if the patient is not bothered by symptoms and potential tumor growth can be monitored by MRI scans, the patient could be followed. Once tumor growth is documented, the patient has several options for treatment. Translabyrinthine surgical removal is relatively safe and preferred in patients with severe hearing loss. Intracranial resection of the tumor or radiation therapy are options in patients who still have useable hearing. Unfortunately, there are no controlled studies comparing surgery to radiation therapy. Both therapies potentially can cause hearing loss and facial weakness. There are very few studies of long term outcomes (more than 5 years) following radiation therapy.

References

1. Fisher CM. Vertigo in cerebrovascular disease. Arch Otolaryngol 1967;85:529–534
2. Troost BT. Dizziness and vertigo in vertebrobasilar disease. Stroke 1980;11:413–415
3. Grad A, Baloh RW. Vertigo of vascular origin. Clinical and electronystagmographic features in 18 patients. Arch Neurol 1989;46:281–284
4. Fife TD, Baloh RW, Duckwiler GR. Isolated dizziness in vertebrobasilar insufficiency: clinical features, angiography and follow-up. J Stroke Cerebrovasc Dis 1994;4:4–12
5. Gomez CR, Cruz-Flores S, Malkoff S, et al. Isolated vertigo as a manifestation of vertebrobasilar ischemia. Neurology 1996;47:94–97
6. De Kleyn A, Nieuwenhuyse P. Schwindelanfälle und nystagmus bei einer bestimmten stellung des kopfes. Acta Otolaryngol (Stockh) 1927;11:155–157
7. Dieterich M, Brandt T. Thalamic infarctions: differential effects on vestibular function in the roll plane (35 patients). Neurology 1993;43:1732–1740
8. Mazzone A. The vascular anatomy of the vestibular labyrinth in man. Acta Otolaryngol Suppl (Stockh) 1990;472:1–83
9. Kim JS, Lopez I, DiPatre PL, et al. Internal auditory artery infarction: clinicopathologic correlation. Neurology 1999;52:40–44
10. Oas JG, Baloh JG. Vertigo and the anterior inferior cerebellar artery syndrome. Neurology 1992;42: 2274–2279
11. Hinojosa R, Kohut RI. Clinical diagnosis of anterior inferior cerebellar artery thrombosis. Autopsy and temporal bone histopathologic study. Ann Otol Rhinol Laryngol 1990;99:261–267
12. Munro NAR, Gaymard B, Rivaud S, et al. Upbeat nystagmus in a patient with a small medullary infarct. J Neurol Neurosurg Psychiatry 1993;56:1126–1128
13. Kuether TA, Nesbit GM, Clark WM, Barnwell SL. Rotational vertebral artery occlusion: a mechanism of vertebrobasilar insufficiency. Neurosurgery 1997; 41:427–432
14. Strupp M, Planck JH, Arbusow V, et al. Rotational vertebral artery occlusion syndrome with vertigo due to "labyrinthine excitation". Neurology 2000;54: 1376–1379
15. Fox MW, Piepgras DG, Bartleson JD. Anterolateral decompression of the atlantoaxial vertebral artery for symptomatic positional occlusion of the vertebral artery. Case report. J Neurosurg 1995;83:737–740
16. Morimoto T, Kaido T, Uchiyama Y, et al. Rotational obstruction of nondominant vertebral artery and ischemia. Case report. J Neurosurg 1996;85:507–509
17. Passero S, Nuti D. Auditory and vestibular system findings in patients with vertebrobasilar dolichoectasia. Acta Neurol Scand 1996;93:50–55
18. Deeb ZL, Jannetta PJ, Rosenbaum AE, et al. Tortuous vertebrobasilar arteries causing cranial nerve syndrome: screening by computed tomography. J Comput Assist Tomogr 1979;3:774–778
19. Smoker WRK, Corbett JJ, Gentry LR, et al. High resolution computed tomography of the basilar artery. 2. Vertebrobasilar dolichoectasia: clinical pathologic correlation and review. AJNR Am J Neuroradiol 1986; 7:61–72
20. Büttner U, Ott M, Helmchen C, et al. Bilateral loss of eighth nerve function as the only clinical sign of vertebrobasilar dolichoectasia. J Vestib Res 1995;5:47–51
21. Jannetta PJ. Observations on the etiology of trigeminal neuralgia, hemifacial spasm, acoustic nerve dysfunction and glossopharyngeal neuralgia. Definite microsurgical treatment and results in 117 patients. Neurochirurgia (Stuttg) 1977;20:145–154
22. Jannetta PJ, Møller MB, Møller MR. Disabling positional vertigo. N Engl J Med 1984;310:1700–1705
23. Reisser C, Schuknecht HF. The anterior inferior cerebellar artery in the internal auditory canal. Laryngoscope 1991;101:761–766
24. Mokri B, Houser OW, Sandok BA, Piepgras DG. Spontaneous dissections of the vertebral arteries. Neurology 1988;38:880–885
25. Braverman I, River Y, Eliashar R, et al. Spontaneous vertebral artery dissection mimicking acute vertigo. Ann Otol Rhinol Laryngol 1999;108:1170–1173
26. Susac JO, Hardimann JM, Selhorst JB. Microangiopathy of the brain and retina. Neurology 1979;29:313–316
27. Welsh LW, Welsh JJ, Lewin B. Basilar artery and vertigo. Ann Otol Rhinol Laryngol 2000;109:615–622
28. Rice GPA, Ebers GC. Ondansetron for intractable vertigo complicating acute brainstem disorders. Lancet 1995;345:1182–1183
29. Crawley F, Clifton A, Brown MM. Treatable lesions demonstrated on vertebral angiography for posterior circulation ischaemic events. Br J Radiol 1998;852: 1266–1270
30. Nakamura K, Saku Y, Torigoe R, et al. Sonographic detection of haemodynamic changes in a case of vertebrobasilar insufficiency. Neuroradiology 1998;40: 164–166
31. Bergsneider M, Becker DP. Vascular compression syndrome of the vestibular nerve: a critical analysis. Otolaryngol Head Neck Surg 1995;112:118–124
32. Notis CM, Kitei RA, Cafferty MS, et al. Microangiopathy of brain, retina and inner ear. J Neuroophthalmol 1995;15:1–8
33. Susac JO. Susac's syndrome. Neurology 1994;44: 591–593
34. Hallpike C. The pathology and differential diagnosis of aural vertigo. London: Proceedings of the 4th International Congress on Otolaryngology 1949;2:514
35. Aschan G, Stahle J. Vestibular neuritis. J Laryngol Otol 1956;70:497–511
36. Coats AC. Vestibular neuronitis: Acta Otolaryngol Suppl (Stockh) 1969;251:5–32
37. Sekitani T, Imate Y, Noguchi T, et al. Vestibular neuronitis: Epidemiological survey by questionnaire in Japan. Acta Otolaryngol Suppl (Stockh) 1993;503:9–12
38. Hato N, Kisaki H, Honda N, et al. Ramsay Hunt syndrome in children. Ann Neurol 2000;48:254–256
39. Baloh RW, Ishyama A, Wackym PA, Honrubia V. Vestibular neuritis; clinical-pathologic correlation. Otolaryngol Head Neck Surg 1996;114:586–592
40. Schuknecht HF, Kitamura K. Vestibular neuritis. Ann Otol Rhinol Laryngol 1981;90(Suppl 78):1–19
41. Arbusow V, Schulz P, Strupp M, et al. Distribution of herpes simplex virus type 1 in human geniculate and vestibular ganglia: implications of vestibular neuritis. Ann Neurol 1999;46:416–419
42. Furuta Y, Takasu T, Fukuda S, et al. Latent herpes simplex virus type 1 in human vestibular ganglia. Acta Otolaryngol Suppl (Stockh) 1993;503:85–89
43. Hirata Y, Gyo K, Yanagihara N. Herpetic vestibular neuritis: an animal study. Acta Otolaryngol Suppl (Stockh) 1995;519:93–96
44. Nahmias AJ, Roizman B. Infection with herpes-simplex viruses 1 and 2. N Engl J Med 1973;289: 719–725

45. Arbusow V, Strupp M, Wasicky R, et al. Detection of herpes simplex virus type 1 in human vestibular nuclei. Neurology 2000;55:880–882

46. Davis LE, Johnsson LS. Viral infections of the inner ear: clinical, virologic, and pathologic studies in humans and animals. Am J Otolaryngol 1983;4: 347–362

47. Ishizaki H, Pyykko I, Nozue M. Neuroborreliosis in the etiology of vestibular neuronitis. Acta Otolaryngol (Stockh) 1993;503:67–69

48. Robillard RB, Hilsinger RL, Adour KK. Ramsay Hunt facial paralysis: clinical analyses of 185 patients. Otolaryngol Head Neck Surg 1986;95:292–297

49. Adour KK. Cranial polyneuritis and Bell's palsy. Arch Otolaryngol 1976;102:262–264

50. Fetter M, Dichgans J. Vestibular neuritis spares the inferior division of the vestibular nerve. Brain 1996; 119:755–763

51. Gacek RR. The pathology of facial and vestibular neuronitis. Am J Otolaryngol 1999;20:202–210

52. Ariyasu L, Byl FM, Sprague MS, Adour KK. The beneficial effect of methylprednisolone in acute vestibular vertigo. Arch Otolaryngol Head Neck Surg 1990;116: 700–703

53. Adour KK. Otological complications of herpes zoster. Ann Neurol 1994;35:S62–S64

54. Kuo MJ, Drago PC, Proops DW, et al. Early diagnosis and treatment of Ramsay Hunt syndrome: the role of magnetic resonance imaging. J Laryngol Otol 1995; 109:777–780

55. Nadol JB. Vestibular neuritis. Otolaryngol Head Neck Surg 1995;112:162–172

56. Ohbayashi S, Oda M, Yamamoto M, et al. Recovery of vestibular function after vestibular neuronitis. Acta Otolaryngol Suppl (Stockh) 1993;503:31–34

57. Strupp M, Arbusow V, Magg KP, et al. Vestibular exercises improve central vestibulospinal compensation after vestibular neuritis. Neurology 1998;51:838–844

58. Murakami S, Hato N, Horiuchi J, et al. Treatment of Ramsay Hunt syndrome with acyclovir-prednisone: significance of early diagnosis and treatment. Ann Neurol 1997;41:353–357

59. House JW, Brackmann DE. Facial nerve grading system. Otolaryngol Head Neck Surg 1985;93:146–147

60. Adour KK, Ruboyianes JM, Von Doersten PG. Bell's palsy treatment with acyclovir and prednisone compared with prednisone alone: a double-blinded, randomized, controlled trial. Ann Otol Rhinol Laryngol 1996;105:371–378

61. De Diego JI, Prim MP, De Sarria MJ. Idiopathic facial paralysis: A randomized, prospective, and controlled study using single-dose prednisone versus acyclovir three times daily. Laryngoscope 1998;108:573–575

62. Bickerstaff ER. Basilar artery migraine. Lancet 1961; 1:15–19

63. Fenichel GM. Migraine as a cause of benign paroxysmal vertigo of childhood. J Pediatr 1967;71:114–115

64. Slater R. Benign recurrent vertigo. J Neurol Neurosurg Psychiatry 1979;42:363–367

65. Stewart WF, Lipton RB, Celentano DD, Reed ML. Migraine headache: Prevalence in the United States by age, income, race and other sociodemographic factors. JAMA 1992;267:64–69

66. IHS Headache Classification Committee of the International Headache Society. Classification and diagnostic criteria for headache disorders, cranial neuralgias and facial pain. Cephalalgia 1988(Suppl 7):1–96

67. Selby G, Lance JW. Observations on 500 cases of migraine and allied vascular headaches. J Neurol Neurosurg Psychiatry 1960;23:23–32

68. Kayan A, Hood JD. Neuro-otological manifestations of migraine. Brain 1984;107:1123–1142

69. Kuritzky A, Ziegler DK, Hassanein R. Vertigo, motion sickness and migraine. Headache 1981;21:227–231

70. Dieterich M, Brandt T. Episodic vertigo related to migraine (90 cases): vestibular migraine? J Neurol 1999;246:883–892

71. Abu-Arafeh I, Russell G. Paroxysmal vertigo as a migraine equivalent in children: a population-based study. Cephalalgia 1995;15:22–25

72. Ishiyama A, Jacobson KM, Baloh RW. Migraine and benign positional vertigo. Ann Otol Rhinol Laryngol 2000;109:377–380

73. Cutrer FM, Baloh RW. Migraine-associated dizziness. Headache 1992;32:300–304

74. Olesen J, Larsen B, Lauritzen M. Focal hyperemia followed by spreading oligemia and impaired activation of rCBF in classic migraine. Ann Neurol 1981;9: 344–352

75. Moskowitz MA, Nozaki K, Kraig RP. Neocortical spreading depression provokes the expression of c-fos protein-like immunoreactivity within trigeminal nucleus caudalis via trigeminovascular mechanisms. J Neurosci 1993;13:1167–1177

76. Goadsby PJ, Hoskin KL. Serotonin inhibits trigeminal nucleus activity evoked by craniovascular stimulation through a 5-HT receptor: A central action in migraine? Ann Neurol 1998;43:711–718

77. Peroutka SJ. Dopamine and migraine. Neurology 1997;49:650–656

78. Joutel A, Bousser M-G, Biousse V, et al. A gene for familial hemiplegic migraine maps to chromosome 19. Nat Genet 1993;5:40–45

79. Ophoff RA, Terwindt GM, Vergouwe MN, et al. Familial hemiplegic migraine and episodic ataxia type-2 are caused by mutations in the Ca2+ channel gene CACNL1A4. Cell 1996;87:543–552

80. May A, Ophoff RA, Terwindt GM, et al. Familial hemiplegic migraine locus on 19p13 is involved in the common forms of migraine with and without aura. Hum Genet 1995;96:604–608

81. Elliot MA, Peroutka SJ, Welch S, May EF. Familial hemiplegic migraine, nystagmus and cerebellar atrophy. Ann Neurol 1996;39:100–106

82. Kim JS, Yue Q, Jen JC, et al. Familial migraine with vertigo: no mutations found in CACNA1A. Am J Med Genet 1998;79:148–151

83. Harker LA, Rassekh CH. Episodic vertigo in basilar artery migraine. Otolaryngol Head Neck Surg 1987;96: 239–250

84. Eviatar L. Vestibular testing in basilar artery migraine. Ann Neurol 1981;9:126–130

85. Olsson JE. Neurotologic findings in basilar migraine. Laryngoscope 1991;101(Suppl)52:1–41

86. Basser L. Benign paroxysmal vertigo of childhood. Brain 1964;87:141–152

87. Cass SP, Furman JM, Ankerstjerne K, et al. Migraine-related vestibulopathy. Ann Otol Rhinol Laryngol 1997;106:182–189

88. Parker W. Migraine and the vestibular system in childhood and adolescence. Am J Ontol 1989;10:364–371

89. Lindskog U, Ödkvist, Noaksson L, Wallquist J. Benign paroxysmal vertigo in childhood: A long-term follow-up. Headache 1999;39:33–37

90. Kentala E, Pyykkö I. Benign recurrent vertigo—True or artificial diagnosis. Acta Otolaryngol Suppl (Stockh) 1997;529:101–103

91. de Bock GH, Eelhart J, van Marwijk HW, et al. A post-marketing study of flunarizine in migraine and vertigo. Pharm World Sci 1997;19:269–274

92. Johnson G. Medical management of migraine-related dizziness and vertigo. Laryngoscope 1998;108:1–28

93. Baloh RW, Foster CA, Yue Q, Nelson SF. Familial migraine with vertigo and essential tremor. Neurology 1996;46:458–460

94. Bikhazi P, Jackson C, Ruckenstein MJ. Efficacy of antimigrainous therapy in the treatment of migraine-associated dizziness. Am J Otol 1997;18:350–354

95. Verspeelt J, De Locht P, Amery WK. Postmarketing study of the use of flunarizine in vestibular vertigo and in migraine. Eur J Clin Pharmacol 1996;51:15–22

96. Szirmai A. Vestibular disorders in patients with migraine. Eur Arch Otorhinolaryngol 1997;254(Suppl 1):S55–S57

97. Peroutka SJ. The pharmacology of current anti-migraine drugs. Headache 1990;30(Suppl):5–11

98. Diamond S. Strategies for migraine management. Cleve Clin J Med 1991;58:257–261

99. Silberstein SD, Merriam GR. Estrogens, progestins, and headache. Neurology 1991;41:786–793

100. Satoyoshi E, Saku A, Sunohara N, Kinoshita M. Clinical manifestations and the diagnostic problems of multiple sclerosis in Japan. Neurology 1976;26:23–25

101. Mathews WB, ed. McAlpine's Multiple Sclerosis. 2nd ed. New York: Churchill Livingstone, 1991

102. Grenman R. Involvement of the audiovestibular system in multiple sclerosis. An otoneurologic and audiologic study. Acta Otolaryngol Suppl 1985; 420:1–95

103. Williams NP, Roland PS, Yellin W. Vestibular evaluation in patients with early multiple sclerosis. Am J Otol 1997;18:93–100

104. Rae-Grant AD, Eckert NJ, Bartz S, Reed JF. Sensory symptoms of multiple sclerosis: a hidden reservoir of morbidity. Mult Scler 1999;5:179–183

105. Bath AP, Walsh RM, Ranalli P, et al. Experience from a multidisciplinary "dizzy" clinic. Am J Otol 2000;21:92–97

106. Ormerod IEC, Bronstein AM, Rudge P, et al. Magnetic resonance imaging in clinically isolated lesions of the brain stem. J Neurol Neurosurg Psychiatry 1986;49:737–743

107. Thomke F, Hopf HC. Pontine lesions mimicking acute peripheral vestibulopathy. J Neurol Neurosurg Psychiatry 1999;66:340–349

108. Osterman PO, Westerberg CE. Paroxysmal attacks in multiple sclerosis. Brain 1975;98:189–202

109. Rosenhall U. Positional nystagmus. Acta Otolaryngol Suppl (Stockh) 1988;455:17–20

110. Furman JM, Durrant JD, Hirsch WL. Eighth nerve signs in a case of multiple sclerosis. Am J Otolaryngol 1989;10:376–381

111. Gstoettner W, Swoboda H, Müller C, Burian M. Preclinical detection of initial vestibulocochlear abnormalities in a patient with multiple sclerosis. Eur Arch Otorhinolaryngol 1993;250:40–43

112. Commins DJ, Chen JM. Multiple sclerosis: A consideration in acute cranial nerve palsies. Am J Otol 1997;18:590–595

113. Thomke F, Lensch E, Ringel K, Hopf HC. Isolated cranial nerve palsies in multiple sclerosis. J Neurol Neurosurg Psychiatry 1997;63:682–685

114. Sasaki O, Ootsuka K, Taguchi K, Kikukawa M. Multiple sclerosis presented acute hearing loss and vertigo. ORL J Otorhinolaryngol Relat Spec 1994;56:55–59

115. Tsunoda A, Komatsuzaki T, Muraoka H, Gou-Tsu K. A case with symptoms of vestibular neuronitis caused by an intramedullary lesion. J Laryngol Otol 1995;109:545–548

116. Ireland DJ, Jell RM. Symmetrical optokinetic after-nystagmus loss in Wallenberg's syndrome and multiple sclerosis. Acta Otolaryngol Suppl 1984;406:235–238

117. Johnsen NJ, Dam M, Thomsen J, et al. Multiple sclerosis. The value of clinical vestibular examination. Clin Otolaryngol 1976;1:225–232

118. Andermann F, Cosgrove JBR, Lloyd-Smith D, Walters AM. Paroxysmal dysarthria and ataxia in multiple sclerosis. Neurology 1959;9:211–215

119. Sharpe JA, Goldberg JH, Lo AW, Herishanu YO. Visual-vestibular interaction in multiple sclerosis. Neurology 1981;31:427–433

120. Huygen PLM, Verhagen WIM, Hommes OR, Nicolasen MGM. Short vestibulo-ocular reflex time constants associated with oculomotor pathology in multiple sclerosis. Acta Otolaryngol (Stockh) 1990;109: 25–33

121. Hausler R, Sabani E, Rohr M. Effect of cinnarizine on various types of vertigo. Clinical and electronystagmographic results of a double-blind study [in French]. Acta Otorhinolaryngol Belg 1989;43:177–185

122. Beck RW, Cleary PA, Anderson MM Jr, et al. A randomized, controlled trial of corticosteroids in the treatment of acute optic neuritis. The Optic Neuritis Study Group. N Engl J Med 1992;27:326, 581–588

123. Espir MLE, Millac P. Treatment of paroxysmal disorders in multiple sclerosis with carbamazepine (Tegretol). J Neurol Neurosurg Psychiatry 1970;33: 528–531

124. Tusa RJ, Brown SB. Neuro-otological trauma and dizziness. In: Rizzo M, Tranzel D, eds. Head Injury and Post-Concussive Syndrome. New York: Churchill Livingstone, 1996:177–200

125. Friedman AP, Brenner C, Denny-Brown D. Post-traumatic vertigo and dizziness. J Neurosurg 1945;21: 36–46

126. Gannon P, Wilson GN, Roberts ME, Pearse JH. Auditory and vestibular damage in head injuries at work. Arch Otolaryngol 1978;104:404–408

127. Barber HO. Positional nystagmus, especially after head injury. Laryngoscope 1964;74:891–944

128. Goodwin WJ. Temporal bone fractures. Otolaryngol Clin North Am 1983;16:651–659

129. Applebaum E. Meningitis following trauma to the head and face. JAMA 1960;173:1818–1822

130. Tos M. Prognosis of hearing loss in temporal bone fractures. J Laryngol Otol 1971;85:1147–1159

131. Schuknecht HF, Davison RC. Deafness and vertigo from head injury. Arch Otolaryngol 1956;63:513–518

132. Wennmo C, Svensson C. Temporal bone fractures. Vestibular and other related ear sequele. Acta Otolaryngol Suppl (Stockh) 1989;468:379–383

133. Cannon CR, Jahrsdoerfer RA. Temporal bone fractures. Review of 90 cases. Arch Otolaryngol 1983;109: 285–288

134. Feneley MR, Murthy P. Acute bilateral vestibulocochlear dysfunction following occipital fracture. J Laryngol Otol 1994;108:54–56

135. Peerless S, Rewcastle N. Shear injuries of the brain. Can Medical Assoc J 1967;96:577–582

136. Oppenheimer DR. Microscopic lesion in the brain following head injury. J Neurol Neurosurg Psychiatry 1968;31:299–306

137. Pilz P. Axonal injury in head injury. Acta Neurochir Suppl 1983;32:119–123

138. Povlishock JT, Becker DP, Cheng CLY, Vaughan GW. Axonal changes in minor head injury. J Neuropathol Exp Neurol 1983;42:225–242

139. Denny-Brown D, Russell WR. Experimental cerebral concussion. Brain 1941;64:93–164

140. Windle WF, Groat RA, Fox CA. Experimental structural alterations in the brain during and after concussion. Surg Gynecol Obstet 1944;79:561–572

141. Mitchell DE, Adams JH. Primary focal impact damage to the brain stem in blunt head injuries. Does it exist? Lancet 1973;2:215–218

142. Makishima K, Sobel SF, Snow JB. Histopathological correlates of otoneurological manifestations following head trauma. Laryngoscope 1976;86:1303–1314

143. Brandt T. Positional and positioning vertigo and nystagmus. J Neurol Sci 1990;95:3–25

144. Halmagyi GM, Gresty MA, Gibson WP. Ocular tilt reaction with peripheral vestibular lesion. Ann Neurol 1979;6:80–83

145. Brandt T, Dieterich M. Pathological eye–head coordination in roll: tonic ocular tilt reaction in mesencephalic and medullary lesions. Brain 1987;110:649–666

146. Daroff RB. See-saw nystagmus. Neurology 1965;15: 874–877

147. Keane JR. Alternating skew deviation: Analysis of 100 cases. Arch Neurol 1985;32:185–190

148. Rutherford WH, Merrett JD, McDonald JR. Sequelae of concussion caused by minor head injuries. Lancet 1977;1:1–4

149. Szymanski HV, Linn R. A review of the postconcussion syndrome. Int J Psychiatry Med 1992;22(4): 357–375

150. Lees-Haley PR, Brown RS. Neuropsychological complaint base rates of 170 personal injury claimants. Arch Clin Neuropsychol 1993;88:203–209

151. Tuohimaa P. Vestibular disturbances after acute mild head injury. Acta Otolaryngol Suppl 1978;359:1–67

152. Griffiths MV. The incidence of auditory and vestibular concussion following minor head injury. J Laryngol Otol 1979;9:253–265

153. Jacome DF. Basilar artery migraine after uncomplicated whiplash injuries. Headaches 1986;26:515–516

154. Winston KR. Whiplash and its relationship to migraine. Headache 1987;27:452–457

155. Ballantyne J, Ajodhia J. Iatrogenic dizziness. In: Dix MR, Hood JD, eds. Vertigo. Chichester: John Wiley and Sons, 1984:217–247

156. Wennmo K, Wennmo C. Drug-related dizziness. Acta Otolaryngologica Suppl (Stockh) 1988;455:11–13

157. Annegers JF, Grabow JD, Groover RV, et al. Seizures after head trauma: A population study. Neurology 1980;30:683–689

158. Hahn YS, Fuchs S, Flannery AM, et al. Factors influencing posttraumatic seizures in children. Neurosurgery 1988;22:864–867

159. Lee ST, Lui TN. Early seizures after mild closed head injury. J Neurosurg 1992;76:435–439

160. Penfield WG, Kristiansen K. Epileptic Seizure Patterns. Springfield, Ill: Charles C Thomas, 1951

161. Nielsen JM. Tornado epilepsy simulating Ménière's syndrome. Neurology 1959;9:794–796

162. Friberg L, Olsen TS, Roland PE, et al. Focal increase of blood flow in the cerebral cortex of man during vestibular stimulation. Brain 1985;198:609–623

163. Macnab J. The "whiplash syndrome". Orthop Clin North Am 1971;2:389–403

164. Compere WE. Electronystagmographic findings in patients with "whiplash" injuries. Laryngoscope 1968;78:1226–1233

165. Toglia JU. Acute flexion-extension injury of the neck. Electronystagmographic study of 309 patients. Neurology 1976;26:808–814

166. Mallinson AI, Longridge NS. Dizziness from whiplash and head injury. Am J Otol 1998;19:814–818

167. Brandt T, Büchele W, Arnold F. Arthrokinetic nystagmus and ego-motion sensation. Exp Brain Res 1977;30: 331–338

168. Bles W, Klören T, Büchele W, Brandt T. Somatosensory nystagmus: physiological and clinical aspects. Adv Otorhinolaryngol 1983;30:30–33

169. De Jong PTVM, de Jong JMBV, Dohen B, Jongkees LBW. Ataxia and nystagmus induced by injection of local anesthetics in the neck. Ann Neurol 1977;1: 240–246

170. Sandstrom J. Cervical syndrome with vestibular symptoms. Acta Otolaryngol (Stockh) 1962;54:207–226

171. Hinoki M. Vertigo due to whiplash injury: a neurological approach. Acta Otolaryngol Suppl 1985;419:9–29

172. Kirtane MV, Medikeri SB, Karnik PP. ENG after head injury. J Laryngol Otol 1982;96:521–528

173. Noseworthy JH, Miller J, Murray TJ, Regan D. Auditory brainstem responses in post concussive syndrome. Arch Neurol 1981;38:275–278

174. Abd al-Hady MR, Shehata O, el-Mously M, Sallam FS. Audiological findings following head trauma. J Laryngol Otol 1990;104:927–936

175. Hasso AN, Ledington JA. Traumatic injuries of the temporal bone. Otolaryngol Clin North Am 1988;21: 295–316

176. Swartz JD, Harnsberger HR. The temporal bone: magnetic resonance imaging. Top Magn Reson Imaging 1990;2:1–16

177. Ylikoski J, Palva T, Sanna M. Dizziness after head trauma: clinical and morphologic findings. Am J Otol 1982;3:343–352

178. Sanna M, Ylikosky J. Vestibular neurectomy for dizziness after head trauma. A review of 28 patients. ORL J Otorhinolaryngol Relat Spec 1983;45:216–225

179. Schubinger O, Valavanis A, Stuckman G, Antonucci F. Temporal bone fractures and their complications. Examination with high-resolution CT. Neuroradiology 1986;28:93–99

180. Avrahami S, Epstein AD. Ocular motor abnormalities from head trauma. Surv Ophthalmol 1991;35:245–267

181. Liu-Shindo M, Hawkins DB. Traumatic injuries of the temporal bone. Otolaryngol Clin North Am 1988;21:295–316

182. Goligher JE, Lloyd DM. View from within: radiology in focus. Fractures of the petrous temporal bone. J Laryngol Otol 1990;104:438–439

183. Cushing H. Tumors of the nervus acusticus and the syndrome of the cerebellopontine angle. Philadelphia: WB Saunders, 1917

184. Moffat DA, Baguley DM, von Blumenthal H, et al. Sudden deafness in vestibular schwannoma. J Laryngol Otol 1994;108:116–119

185. Saleh EA, Aristegui M, Naguib MB, et al. Normal hearing in acoustic neuroma patients: A critical evaluation. Am J Otol 1996;17:127–132

186. Shiffman F, Dancer J, Rothballer AB. The diagnosis and evaluation of acoustic neuromas. Otolaryngol Clin North Am 1973;6:189–228

187. Leonard JR, Talbot ML. Asymptomatic acoustic neurilemmoma. Arch Otolaryngol 1970;91:117–124

188. Tos M, Thomsen J. Epidemiology of acoustic neuromas. J Laryngol Otol 1984;98:685–692

189. Mirz F, Pedersen CB, Fiirgaard B, Lundorf E. Incidence

and grown pattern of vestibular schwannomas in a Danish county, 1977–1998. Acta Otolaryngol Suppl (Stockh) 2000;543:30–33

190. Clemis JD, Ballad WJ, Baggot PJ, et al. Relative frequency of inferior vestibular schwannoma. Arch Otolaryngol Head Neck Surg 1986;112:190–194

191. Rubenstein AE. Neurofibromatosis: A review of the clinical problem. Ann NY Acad Sci 1986;486:1–13

192. Deen HG, Ebersold MJ, Harner SG, et al. Conservative management of acoustic neuroma: An outcome study. Neurosurgery 1996;39:260–264

193. Fucci MJ, Buchman CA, Brackman DE, et al. Acoustic tumor growth: implications for treatment choices. Am J Otol 1999;20:495–499

194. Mirz F, Jorgensen B, Fiirgaard B, et al. Investigations into the natural history of vestibular schwannomas. Clin Otolaryngol 1999;24:13–18

195. Niemczyk K, Vaneecloo FM, Lemaitre L, et al. The growth of acoustic neuromas in volumetric radiological assessment. Am J Otol 1999;20:244–248

196. NIH Consensus Statement on Acoustic Neuroma, Washington, DC, 1992

197. Allen RW, Harnsberger HR, Shelton C, et al. Low cost high-resolution fast spin-echo MR of acoustic schwannoma: an alternative to enhanced conventional spin-echo MR? Am J Neuroradiol 1996;17:1205–1210

198. Daniels RL, Swallow C, Shelton C, et al. Causes of unilateral sensorineural hearing loss screened by high-resolution fast spin echo magnetic resonance imaging: Review of 1070 consecutive cases. Am J Otol 2000;21:173–180

199. Wilson DF, Talbot JM, Mills L. A critical appraisal of the role of auditory brain stem response and magnetic resonance imaging in acoustic neuroma diagnosis. Am J Otol 1997;5:673–685

200. Robinette MS, Bauch CD, Olsen WO, Cevette M. Auditory brainstem response and magnetic resonance imaging for acoustic neuromas. Costs by prevalence. Arch Otolaryngol Head Neck Surg 2000;126:963–966

201. House WE. Translabyrinthine approach. In: House WF, Luetje CM, eds. Acoustic Tumors. Vol 2: Management. Baltimore: University Park Press, 1979:43–87

202. Tos M, Thomsen J, Harmsen A. Results of translabyrinthine removal of 300 acoustic neuromas related to tumor size. Acta Otolaryngol Suppl (Stockh) 1988;452:38–51

203. Ekvall L. Prevention of cerebrospinal fluid rhinorrhea in translabyrinthine surgery. In: Tos M, Thomsen J, eds. Acoustic neuroma: Proceedings of the First International Conference on Acoustic Neuroma. Amsterdam/New York: Kugler Publications, 1992: 733–734

204. Rodgers GK, Luxford WM. Factors affecting the development of cerebrospinal fluid leak and meningitis after translabyrinthine acoustic tumor surgery. Laryngoscope 1993;103:959–962

205. Hoffman RA. Cerebrospinal fluid leak following acoustic neuroma removal. Laryngoscope 1994;104: 40–58

206. Celikkanat SM, Saleh E, Khashaba A, et al. Cerebrospinal fluid leak after translabyrinthine acoustic neuroma surgery. Otolaryngol Head Neck Surg 1995; 112:654–658

207. Lacombe H, Keravel Y, Nigri F. Prevention of cerebrospinal fluid rhinorrhea in translabyrinthine surgery for vestibular schwannoma. In: Sterkers JM, Charachon R, Sterkers O, eds. Acoustic Neuroma and Skull Base Surgery: Proceedings of the Second International Conference on Vestibular Schwannoma Surgery and Second European Skull Base Society Congress. Amsterdam/New York: Kugler Publications, 1996: 429–433

208. Fishman AJ, Hoffman RA, Roland JT Jr, et al. Cerebrospinal fluid drainage in the management of CSF leak following acoustic neuroma surgery. Laryngoscope 1996;106:1002–1004

209. Mass SC, Wiet RJ, Dinces E. Complications of the translabyrinthine approach for the removal of acoustic neuroma. Arch Otolaryngol Head Neck Surg 1999;125:801–804

210. Falcioni M, Mulder JJS, Taibah A, et al. No cerebrospinal fluid leaks in translabyrinthine vestibular schwannoma removal. Am J Otol 1999;20:660–666

211. House WF, Monograph I. Transtemporal bone microsurgical removal of acoustic neuromas. Arch Otolaryngol 1964;80:598–756

212. Noren G. Long-term complications following gamma knife radiosurgery of vestibular schwannomas. Stereotact Funct Neurosurg 1998;70(Suppl)1:65–73

213. Kondziolka D, Lunsford LD, McLaughlin MR, Flickinger JC. Long-term outcomes after radiosurgery for acoustic neuromas. N Engl J Med 1998;339: 1426–1433

214. Foote RL, Coffey RJ, Swanson JW, et al. Stereotactic radiosurgery using the gamma knife for acoustic neuromas. Int J Radiat Oncol Biol Phys 1995;32:1153–1160

215. Pollock BE, Lunsford LD, Kondziolka D, et al. Vestibular schwannoma management. Part II Failed radiosurgery and role of delayed microsurgery. J Neurosurg 1998;89:949–955

216. Mendenhall WM, Friedman WA, Buatti JM, et al. Preliminary results of linear accelerator radiosurgery for acoustic schwannomas. J Neurosurg 1996;85:1013–1019

217. Valentino V, Raimondi AJ. Tumor response and morphological changes of acoustic neuromas after radiosurgery. Acta Neurochir (Wien) 1995;133:157–163

218. Andrews DW, Silverman CL, Glass J, et al. Preservation of cranial nerve function after treatment of acoustic neuronomas with fractionated stereotactic radiotherapy. Preliminary observations in 26 patients. Stereotact Funct Neurosurg 1995;64:165–182

219. Varolotto JM, Shrieve DC, Alexander E. Fractionated stereotactic radiotherapy for the treatment of acoustic neuromas; preliminary results. Int J Radiat Oncol Biol Phys 1996;36:141–145

220. Shirato H, Sakamoto T, Sawamura Y, et al. Comparison between observation policy and fractionated stereotactic radiotherapy (SRT) as an initial management for vestibular schwannoma. Int J Radiat Oncol Biol Phys 1999;44:545–550

221. Herdman SJ, Clendaniel RA, Mattox DE, et al. Vestibular adaptation exercises and recovery: acute stage after acoustic neuroma resection. Otolaryngol Head Neck Surg 1995;113:77–87

173 Disorders of the Inner Ear

Robert W Baloh

Benign paroxysmal positional vertigo

Overview

Benign paroxysmal positional vertigo (BPPV) is by far the most common cause of vertigo and there is now a simple bedside cure for the vast majority of patients. In 1921, Robert Barany was the first to identify the characteristic paroxysmal positional nystagmus associated with BPPV but it was not until 1952 that Dix and Hallpike described the provocative positioning test and clearly defined the clinical syndrome. Harold Schuknecht was the first to emphasize that the positional vertigo and nystagmus likely originated from the posterior semicircular canal and his cupulolithiasis theory ultimately led to our current understanding of the mechanism of BPPV and the simple bedside cure.

Epidemiology

BPPV is not a disease but rather a syndrome that can be the sequela of several inner ear diseases; in more than half of the cases, no cause can be found.[1] Females outnumber males by a ratio of about 2:1 in the idiopathic group. BPPV can occur at any age, particularly when it is secondary to some other inner ear disease, but the idiopathic variety is much more common in older people, particularly after the age of 60.

Etiology

When BPPV is associated with an inner ear disorder, the two most common diagnostic categories are post-traumatic and postviral.[1] Typically BPPV will begin within a few days of head trauma but it can be delayed for weeks to months after a viral infection of the inner ear.

Pathophysiology

The best current explanation for BPPV is canalithiasis involving the posterior semicircular canal.[2,3] With the patient sitting upright, a clot of calcium carbonate crystals (loosened from the utricular macule) settles at the most dependent portion of the posterior semicircular canal (Figure 173.1). Movement of the head back and to the side in the plane of that posterior semicircular canal (such as with the standard diagnostic test) causes the clot to move in an ampullofugal direction, producing ampullofugal displacement of the cupula due to the plunger effect of the clot moving within the narrow canal. Fatigability with repeated positioning is explained by dispersion of the particles from the clot making the plunger less effective. Reactivation of positional vertigo after prolonged bedrest is explained as the particles re-form into a clot. Finally, the latency before onset of nystagmus is explained by the delay in setting the clot into motion after the position change.

Genetics

Not applicable.

Clinical features

Patients report brief episodes of vertigo (usually lasting less than 30 seconds), typically when turning over in bed, getting in and out of bed, bending over and straightening up, or extending the neck back to look up. Often, after the episodes of positional vertigo, patients will complain of a more prolonged nonspecific motion sick sensation that can persist for hours and may even persist throughout the day. As the name implies, BPPV is a benign disorder that will eventually remit spontaneously even if untreated. About half of patients with BPPV will have at least one recurrence after a remission. In some, bouts of BPPV are intermixed with variable periods of remission over many years.

Classification

Although the vast majority of cases result from debris moving within the posterior semicircular canal, there are also horizontal and anterior canal variants of BPPV.[4] Occasionally, patients with the horizontal canal variant of BPPV will experience episodes of vertigo when turning the head to the side while sitting or even walking. Remissions and exacerbations commonly occur with all types of BPPV but exacerbations are typically shorter in duration with the horizontal canal variant.

Diagnostic criteria

The diagnosis of BPPV rests on finding that characteristic positional nystagmus in a patient with the typical history. The positional nystagmus is induced either by rapidly moving the patient from the sitting to head-hanging position (for the posterior and anterior canal variants) or by turning the patient's head to the side while he is lying supine (for the horizontal canal variant).[4] It is important to prepare the patient in advance by explaining that the goal is to induce positional vertigo and that the patient must keep the eyes open and avoid blinking as much as possible. With the common posterior canal variant, the nystagmus is torsional vertical with the upper pole of the eye beating toward the ground. With the horizontal canal variant, the nystagmus is torsional horizontal with the horizontal component beating toward the ground with the head to either side.

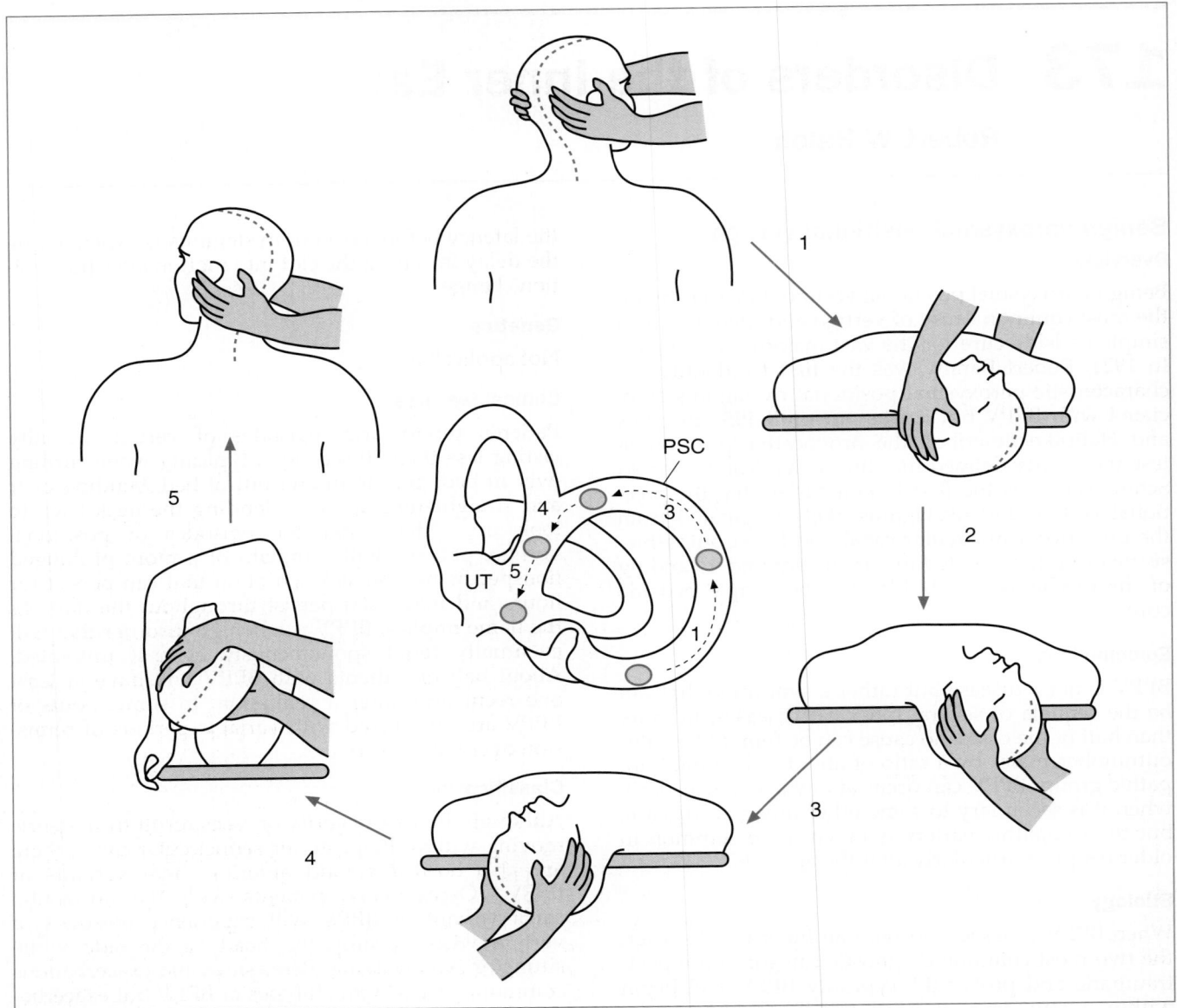

Figure 173.1   Treatment maneuver for benign positional vertigo affecting the right ear (modified Epley maneuver). The procedure can be reversed for treating the left ear. (1) The patient is seated upright, with the head facing the examiner, who is standing on the right. The patient should grasp the forearm of the examiner with both hands for stability. The patient is then moved into the supine position, allowing the head to extend just beyond the end of the examining table, with the right ear downward. This position is maintained until the nystagmus ceases. (2) The examiner moves to the head of the table, repositioning the hands as shown. (3) The head is rotated toward the left, stopping with the right ear upward. This position is maintained for 30 seconds. (4) The patient rolls onto the left side, while the examiner rotates the head leftward until the nose is directed toward the floor. This position is then held for 30 seconds. (5) The patient is lifted into the sitting position, now facing left. The entire sequence should be repeated until no nystagmus can be elicited. Labyrinth in the center shows the position of the debris before and after each position change as it moves around and out of the posterior semicircular canal (PSC) and into the utricle (UT).

Adapted from Foster CA, Baloh RW. Episodic vertigo. *In:* Rakel RE, ed. Conn's Current Therapy. Philadelphia: WB Saunders, 1995:837–841.

Differential diagnosis

The appearance and plane of the induced positional nystagmus defines which semicircular canal it originates from. Although positional vertigo is nearly always a benign condition, in rare cases it can be a

symptom of a central nervous system lesion, particularly one near the fourth ventricle. If the patient exhibits the characteristic fatigable, torsional positioning nystagmus that lasts less than 30 seconds, the diagnosis of benign paroxysmal positional vertigo is made. Central positional nystagmus typically is non-fatiguing and purely vertical (either up- or down-beating). Most cases of central positional vertigo and nystagmus have other associated neurological findings.

Treatment

Once the diagnosis of BPPV is made, a simple explanation of the nature of the disorder and its favorable prognosis can relieve the patient's anxiety. The dramatic nature of the episodes of vertigo leads many patients to believe they have a life-threatening disorder such as a tumor or stroke, and reassurance is important when it can be given. Most patients can be cured at the bedside by a simple particle repositioning maneuver (class 3).[2,4] The basic idea of these maneuvers is to move the patient around the plane of the affected semicircular canal to allow the clot of debris to rotate around the canal and out into the utricle (Figure 173.1). For the posterior and anterior canal variants of BPPV, one can proceed with the particle repositioning maneuver after the diagnosis is confirmed with the Dix–Hallpike positioning test. For the horizontal canal variant of BPPV, the patient is rolled in the plane of the horizontal semicircular canal while lying supine.[4] The patient starts in the supine position and is rolled 90 degrees toward the normal side (the side with the lesser horizontal nystagmus), then in 90 degrees steps to prone, to the abnormal side, and back to the supine. Lying on the side with the normal ear down for a few hours is also effective.[5] Although the majority of patients are cured after a single particle repositioning maneuver, the cure rate is improved by repeating the procedure until no vertigo or nystagmus occurs in any position. Occasionally, a patient will develop severe nausea and have to be rescheduled and premedicated with a vestibular suppressant drug. Also occasionally, vibration applied to the mastoid region is useful, particularly if, rather than a burst of nystagmus with position change, the patient develops a slow persistent nystagmus suggesting that the debris is stuck in the wall of the semicircular canal or is attached to the cupula and not freely moving.

With the posterior canal variant, a reliable sign that the particle repositioning maneuver is going to be successful is the production of a second typical burst of positional nystagmus when the patient is moved from the initial head-hanging position across to the opposite head-hanging position (see Figure 173.1). This indicates that the particles are moving along in the canal in the correct direction toward the utricle. If, on the other hand, a burst of nystagmus in the reverse direction occurs when moving from one head-hanging position to the other, the particles are most likely moving in the wrong direction back toward the cupula, a sign that the particle repositioning maneuver will be unsuccessful. When this occurs, the patient most likely elevated the head during the movement from one head-hanging position to the other so the particles moved back in the opposite direction due to gravity. It is critical that the head stays down during this phase of the positioning maneuver. When returning to the sitting position at the end of the particle repositioning maneuver, patients may have a brief but violent burst of vertigo as late as one to two minutes after assuming the position. This delayed vertigo occurs as the bolus of otolith debris drops out of the canal into the utricle. It is important to keep in mind that there are two factors that must occur before a patient will develop BPPV: first, the otolithic debris must be free floating within the endolymph, but second, the patient must get the head into a critical position that allows the particles to enter the semicircular canal (for example, extended way back for the most common posterior canal variant). For this reason, patients are typically instructed to avoid lying flat for at least 2 days after the particle repositioning maneuver is performed to prevent the clot from reentering the posterior semicircular canal orifice. In patients who have multiple recurrences, we recommend that they avoid all extreme head-back positions such as when visiting the hair dresser or dentist.

Antivertiginous drugs have relatively little use in the management of patients with BPPV since the acute attacks are not suppressed by these drugs. Moreover, the particle repositioning maneuver is much more effective for controlling the condition. Patients who have multiple recurrences of BPPV can be taught to perform the particle repositioning maneuver on their own. They can presedate themselves and often they feel more comfortable performing the maneuver in the controlled environment of their bedroom. Vibration is rarely required, but a simple neck massage vibrator can be used if one is available.

Herdman et al. compared the Epley and Seymont maneuvers for treating the posterior canal variant of BPPV and found a comparable cure rate of 70% to 90% with both.[6] Between 10% and 20% of patients have an exacerbation within a week or two of performing the maneuver; this typically is relieved by repeating the maneuver.

It is still unclear what happens to the otolithic debris once it enters the utricle. It may dissolve in the endolymph fluid or it may be taken up into the membrane by the process of phagocytosis. Calcium concentration of the endolymph seems to be critical for determining whether the otolith debris will dissolve.[7] The otolithic debris apparently cannot be cleared in some patients who have recurrent attacks of BPPV. Hormonal effects on calcium metabolism in women and older people might possibly explain the increased incidence of BPPV in this subpopulation.

In rare cases that do not respond to the particle repositioning maneuver, one might consider surgical procedures to cut the nerve from, or to block, the posterior semicircular canal.[8,9]

Labyrinthitis (acute unilateral peripheral vestibulopathy)

Overview

Labyrinthitis refers to an inflammation of the inner ear although the term is often used to describe an acute vertigo syndrome originating from the inner ear but of unknown cause. Similar terms such as neuro-labyrinthitis, vestibular neuronitis, or vestibular neuritis have also been used to describe the same syndrome. Although the majority of these disorders are probably viral, it is often impossible in any single case to make a definitive diagnosis, so that a less specific term such as acute unilateral peripheral vestibulopathy may be desirable.

Epidemiology

A large percentage of patients with an acute peripheral vestibulopathy report an upper respiratory tract illness within a few weeks prior to the onset of symptoms.[10] The syndrome often occurs in epidemics, may affect several members of the same family, and erupts more commonly in spring and early summer.

Etiology

A long list of viruses has been clinically associated with cases of acute prolonged vertigo. A clear example of a viral syndrome involving the eighth nerve is herpes zoster oticus.[11] Presumably the zoster virus remains dormant in the ganglia associated with the seventh and eighth nerves and is reactivated during a period of lowered immunity. Herpes simplex virus has also been shown to be dormant in the ganglia of the seventh and eighth nerves and there is now convincing evidence that it is the predominant cause of idiopathic Bell's palsy.[12,13] Reactivation of herpes simplex virus from the vestibular ganglia (Scarpa's ganglia) may be a common cause of acute unilateral peripheral vestibulopathy.

Pathophysiology

Studies of temporal bone specimens from patients with isolated auditory and vestibular syndromes indicate a likely viral cause.[14,15] The atrophy of the nerve and endorgans is identical to that associated with well-documented viral syndromes (such as mumps or measles). Furthermore, these pathological studies are supported by experimental studies in animals where it has been shown that several viruses will selectively infect the labyrinth and/or eighth nerve.

Genetics

Not applicable.

Clinical features

Viral neurolabyrinthitis can present with sudden deafness, acute vertigo or some combination of auditory and vestibular symptoms.[14] Although the term "sudden deafness" is commonly used, the hearing loss due to viral infection usually comes on over several hours and may even extend over several days. Vestibular neurolabyrinthitis (vestibular neuronitis, vestibular neuritis) is typically manifested by the gradual onset of vertigo, nausea, and vomiting over several hours. The symptoms usually reach a peak within 24 hours and then gradually resolve over several weeks. Most patients have a benign course with complete recovery within a few months. There

are important exceptions, however, particularly older patients who may have an intractable dizziness that persists for years. Between 20% and 30% of patients will have a recurrent bout of vertigo at some time in the future, possibly representing reactivation of a latent virus since it is often associated with systemic viral illness.

Classification

As noted above, a wide range of terms have been used to describe the viral syndromes affecting the inner ear. Schuknecht preferred the term viral neuro-labyrinthitis since in most cases both the nerve and endorgan are at least partially involved.[14] The terms vestibular neuritis or neuronitis have been used for restricted vestibular syndromes.

Diagnosis

The diagnosis of viral neurolabyrinthitis rests on finding the characteristic clinical profile along with laboratory evidence of peripheral auditory and/or vestibular dysfunction in the absence of neurological symptoms and signs.

Differential diagnosis

Viral neurolabyrinthitis must be differentiated from other forms of labyrinthitis (particularly bacterial) and from labyrinthine infarction and perilymph fistula (Table 173.1). Bacterial labyrinthitis is typically associated with acute or chronic otomastoiditis, which should easily be identified on examination of the ear and with imaging of the temporal bone. Unlike the gradual onset of symptoms over hours with viral neurolabyrinthitis, infarction of the labyrinth results in a sudden profound loss of auditory and vestibular function, often in a setting of prior episodes of transient ischemia within the vertebrobasilar system. Without major risk factors and without a prior history of occlusive vascular disease, there is little reason to suspect a vascular cause for isolated auditory or vestibular symptoms, particularly in young patients. Like viral neurolabyrinthitis, perilymph fistulae can present with hearing loss, vertigo or a combination of auditory and vestibular symptoms. With the latter, however, the onset is usually abrupt and there is nearly always a precipitating event such as head trauma, barotrauma or a sudden strain during heavy lifting, coughing or sneezing. Perilymph fistulae also commonly occur in patients who have undergone stapedectomy surgery for otosclerosis. Fluctuating symptoms, particularly if induced by coughing or sneezing, suggest the likelihood of a perilymph fistula.

Treatment

Treatment of patients who present with isolated episodes of auditory and/or vestibular symptoms due to inner ear damage can be difficult because the pathophysiology in any given case is often uncertain. As suggested above, unless there is convincing evidence to suspect a vascular or nonviral infectious cause the patient should be managed as a presumed viral

Table 173.1   Diagnosis and treatment of acute unilateral peripheral vestibulopathy

	Presentation	Diagnosis	Specific treatments
Viral neurolabyrinthitis	Develops over hours resolves over days, prior viral illness	Unilateral caloric hypoexcitability, hearing may be normal	Brief course of high dose steroids Acyclovir (1 g/day × 10 days) for herpes zoster oticus—no data regarding other viral syndromes
Bacterial labyrinthitis	Abrupt onset, associated hearing loss, prior ear infections	Unilateral absent caloric response and profound sensorineural hearing loss	Antibiotics based on culture and sensitivity tests Surgical eradication of middle ear or mastoid infection may be required
Labyrinthine infarction	Abrupt onset, usually associated neurological symptoms, prior vascular disease	Unilateral absent caloric responses and profound sensorineural hearing loss Neuroimaging may show brain infraction	Control risk factors, antiplatelet drugs (aspirin 75–330 mg/day, ticlopidine 250 mg b.i.d.)
Perilymph fistula	Abrupt onset associated with head trauma, barotrauma, or sudden strain during heavy lifting, coughing or sneezing; chronic infection with cholesteatoma	Unilateral caloric hypoexcitability and hearing loss Imaging may show bony erosion from cholesteatoma	Initially: bedrest, elevated head, avoid straining If symptoms persist, explore ear

neurolabyrinthitis. One small placebo-controlled study suggested that high dose steroids given for their anti-inflammatory effect can significantly shorten the course and severity of symptoms in patients presenting with an acute unilateral peripheral vestibulopathy syndrome (class 2).[16] Since there was no way to be certain of the diagnosis in these patients, it is unclear how many of them had a viral inner ear syndrome. Acyclovir (1 g/day for 10 days) was shown to be effective in treating herpes zoster oticus (class 3),[17] but there have been no studies using antiviral agents in patient with other unilateral peripheral vestibular syndromes. Acyclovir with high dose steroids was no better than high dose steroids alone in managing patients with sudden deafness of presumed viral origin (class 1).[18] Treatment of the other common causes of an acute unilateral peripheral vestibulopathy is summarized in Table 173.1.

Symptomatic treatment   Obviously the best therapy for acute vertigo is to eliminate the underlying cause whenever possible. However, when the illness is not readily treatable and when the symptoms persist, symptomatic therapy is indicated. Two general categories of drugs are used in the symptomatic treatment of vertigo: vestibular suppressants and antiemetics (class 3).

The major classes of vestibular suppressants include antihistamines, benzodiazepines, and anticholinergics, although a variety of other drugs have also been used (Table 173.2).[19] Although the exact mechanism of action of these drugs is unclear, most appear to act at the level of the neurotransmitters involved in propagation of impulses from primary to secondary vestibular neurons and in maintenance of tone in the vestibular nuclei. Drugs used in symptomatic treatment of vertigo can be used either acutely to treat a discrete attack or chronically as prophylaxis against future attacks. It typically takes at least 30 minutes for these drugs to have an effect and it is usually two hours or more before they have their peak effect.[20]

Antiemetic drugs are directed specifically against the areas in the brain controlling vomiting.[21] This system of neurons contains both central components (often called the emetic center) and peripheral components in the gastrointestinal tract. Dopamine, histamine, acetylcholine and serotonin are transmitters thought to act on these sites to produce vomiting. Most of the vestibular suppressants have anticholinergic or antihistaminic qualities, giving them antiemetic properties in addition to their effect on vertigo. When nausea and vomiting are prominent, a mild vestibular suppressant can be combined with an antiemetic to control symptoms (Table 173.2). These medications typically have central dopamine antagonist properties and are believed to prevent emesis by inhibition at the chemoreceptor trigger zone. Occasionally they give rise to serious side effects in patients, particularly in young patients. Although the incidence is less than 1% to 2% in older adults, in young adults and children the incidence can be as high as 25%.[22,23] The major reactions can be categorized symptomatically as parkinsonism, akathisia, dystonia, and dyskinesia. The latter can be acute and reversible or subacute (tardive) and prolonged or permanent.

Overall strategy   Sudden permanent vestibular damage requires careful management. Because the injury is often permanent, central compensation must occur before recovery will be complete. The vestibular suppressants and antiemetics may impair the process of compensation. These medications are most useful over the first few days when nausea and vomiting are

Table 173.2   Vestibular suppressant and antiemetic drugs

Chemical name	Brand name	Form and dosage	Sedative	Antiemetic	Precautions
Anticholinergics					
Scopolamine	Transderm-Scop	Patch: 1 q 3 days	±	+	Asthma, prostate enlargement, liver or kidney disease
Antihistamines					
Diphenhydramine	Benadryl (OTC)	PO: 25–50 mg q 4–6 h IM/IV: 10–50 mg q.i.d.	+	+	Asthma, glaucoma, prostate enlargement
Dimenhydrinate	Dramamine (OTC)	PO: 50 mg q 4–6 h	+	+	Same
Cyclizine	Marezine (OTC)	PO: 50 mg q 4–6 h	+	+	Same
Meclizine	Antivert Bonine (OTC)	PO: 25–50 mg q.d.–q.i.d.	±	+	Same
Promethazine	Phenergan	PO: 25 mg q 6 h Supp: 50 mg q 12 h IM: 25 mg q 4–6 h	++	++	Same; history of seizures
Benzodiazepines					
Diazepam	Valium	PO: 2/5/10 mg b.i.d.–q.i.d. Slow IV: 5–10 mg q 4 h	+++	+	Untreated glaucoma, history of drug addiction, pregnancy
Lorazepam	Ativan	PO: 1–2 mg t.i.d. IM/slow IV: 2 mg	+++	+	Same
Clonazepam	Klonopin	PO: 0.5 mg t.i.d.	+++	+	Same
Phenothiazine					
Prochlorperazine	Compazine	PO: 5–10 mg q 6 h Supp: 25 mg q 12 h IM: 5–10 mg q 6 h IV: 2.5–10 mg slow	+	+++	Liver disease; additive with other CNS suppressants, do not use with benzamides
Benzamide					
Metoclopramide	Reglan, Otamide, Maxolon	PO: 5–10 mg q.i.d. IM: 10 mg q 4–6 h IV: 10 mg q 4–6 h	+	+++	Liver or kidney disease, seizures, bowel obstruction, phenochromocytoma; do not use with phenothiazines or in children
Butyrophenone					
Droperidol	Inapsine	IM/slow IV: 2.5–5 mg q 12 h	+++	++	Liver or kidney disease

OTC, available over the counter

severe. As soon as vomiting ceases, medication should be gradually withdrawn in order to stimulate normal compensation. A course of vestibular rehabilitation (see below) is the appropriate therapy in these cases.

Vestibular rehabilitation   Clinicians have long been aware that vestibular compensation occurs more rapidly and is more complete if the patient begins exercising as soon as possible after a vestibular lesion (class 3). Controlled studies in animals have convincingly shown that an exercise program can accelerate compensation after acute peripheral vestibular lesions.[24,25] During the acute stage when nystagmus is present, the patient should attempt to focus the eyes and hold them in the direction that provokes dizziness.[26] Once the nystagmus diminishes to the point that a target can be held visually in all directions (usually within a few days), the patient should begin eye and head coordination exercises. A useful exercise

involves staring at a visual target while oscillating the head from side to side or up and down. The speed of the movements can be gradually increased, as long as the target can be kept in good focus. Target changes using combined eye and head movements to jump quickly back and forth between two widely separated visual targets are also useful. Blinking during these fast head turns can help reduce symptoms of dizziness or visual blurring.

The patient should try to stand and walk while nystagmus is still present. It may be necessary to walk in contact with a wall or to use an assistant in the early stages. Slow, supported turns should be made initially. As improvement occurs, head movements should be added while standing and walking—at first slow side to side or up and down movements, then fast head turns in all directions. The compensation process occurs at a variable rate, dependent on multiple variables including age, but should be nearly complete within 2 to 6 months after the acute peripheral vestibular injury. Dizziness that persists beyond this time indicates either the presence of ongoing recurrent vestibular damage or poor central compensation.

Meniere's syndrome

Overview

When Prosper Meniere first described the clinical features of his patients with episodic vertigo, hearing loss and tinnitus, he was not aware of a specific clinical syndrome but rather emphasized for the first time that vertigo could originate from the inner ear. Up until that time, vertigo was thought to be symptom of cerebral congestion and was treated with leeches and bloodletting. Meniere convincingly argued that episodic vertigo occurred in isolation from other neurological symptoms and was commonly associated with diseases that damaged the inner ear. More recently, strict diagnostic criteria have been established for Meniere's syndrome and a characteristic pathology has been identified.

Epidemiology

Meniere's syndrome can occur at any age although it is more common between the ages of 30 and 50. In the United States, there is a prevalence of about 200 individuals per 100 000 population or a total of 500 000 afflicted individuals.[27] Approximately a third of patients with Meniere's syndrome are completely disabled because of their symptoms.

Etiology

Meniere's syndrome can be caused by several different diseases but, in the majority of cases, the cause is unknown. Bacterial, viral and syphilitic labyrinthitis can all lead to endolymphatic hydrops and typical symptoms and signs of Meniere's syndrome. Multiple etiologies have been proposed for idiopathic Meniere's syndrome including allergy, metabolic disturbances, prior infection, sympathetic vasomotor disturbances and even psychosomatic factors. A relationship between migraine and Meniere's syndrome dates back to the original description by Meniere himself.[28] Some have suggested that Meniere's syndrome is migraine of the ear. A subclinical viral infection could damage the resorptive mechanism of the inner ear, leading to an eventual decompensation in the balance between secretion and resorption of endolymph. Endolymphatic hydrops can be reliably produced in animals by blocking the endolymphatic duct or destroying the endolymphatic sac.[29]

Pathophysiology

The principal pathological finding in patients with Meniere's syndrome is an increase in the volume of endolymph associated with distension of the entire endolymphatic system.[30] Although the pathological changes in Meniere's syndrome are well described, the mechanism for its fluctuating symptoms and signs is less clear. The leading theory is that episodes of

hearing loss and vertigo are caused by ruptures in the membrane separating endolymph from perilymph, producing a sudden increase in potassium concentration in the perilymph. The dramatic sudden falling spells initially described by Tumarkin probably result from a sudden deformation or displacement of one of the vestibular endorgans.[31,32]

Genetics

Most cases of Meniere's syndrome are sporadic although families have been described with multiple members affected with the disorder. Nearly all of these families also have migraine and most likely it is migraine that is inherited with a subset of the patients with migraine developing Meniere's syndrome.

Clinical features

Meniere's syndrome is characterized by fluctuating hearing loss and tinnitus, episodic vertigo and a sensation of fullness or pressure in the ear. Typically the person first notices the fullness and pressure along with decreased hearing and tinnitus, rapidly followed by vertigo that reaches its intensity within a few minutes and then slowly subsides over several hours. The patient may then be left with a sense of unsteadiness and nonspecific dizziness for days. In the early stages, the hearing loss is completely reversible but in later stages a residual hearing loss remains. So-called "delayed endolymphatic hydrops" develops in an ear that has been damaged years before, usually by a viral or bacterial infection.[33] With this disorder, the patient reports a long history of hearing loss followed years later by typical symptoms and signs of Meniere's syndrome. If the hearing loss is profound, as it often is, the episodic vertigo will not be accompanied by fluctuating hearing loss and tinnitus.

Classification

Rigid diagnostic criteria that require fluctuating hearing loss have been developed for the diagnosis of Meniere's syndrome.[34] Although so-called "vestibular Meniere's" has been proposed as a variation on the classical theme, clinical–pathological correlation of an isolated vestibular disorder with selective endolymphatic hydrops of the vestibular labyrinth is lacking. Current diagnostic criteria do not recognize a vestibular Meniere's syndrome with isolated vestibular symptoms.

Diagnosis

The key to the diagnosis of Meniere's syndrome is to document fluctuating hearing levels in a patient with the characteristic clinical history. A characteristic low frequency trough is identified on audiometric testing, particularly in the early stages of the disease.

Differential diagnosis

The differential diagnosis of the common causes of chronic recurrent vertigo is summarized in Table 173.3. Autoimmune inner ear disease can mimic all of the features of Meniere's syndrome, and early in the course it can be impossible to differentiate from idiopathic Meniere's syndrome. However, autoimmune inner ear disease typically rapidly progresses to bilateral involvement and other systemic symptoms may be present. When in doubt, a trial of high dose steroids should lead to a dramatic response in patients with autoimmune inner ear disease.[35] So-called "vestibular Meniere's" (recurrent episodic vertigo without hearing loss) nearly always turns out be due to migraine.[36] However, fluctuating low frequency hearing loss also occurs with migraine and it is possible that in a subset of patients Meniere's syndrome is caused by migraine. Recurrent vertigo attacks due to transient ischemia typically come on abruptly and last only minutes compared to the several hours' duration of a typical Meniere's attack. Also, associated neurological symptoms are nearly always present.

Treatment

Medical management of Meniere's syndrome consists of a salt restriction diet in the range of 1 to 2 grams of sodium per day with a minimum therapeutic trial of 2 to 3 months (class 3).[37] If a good response is obtained, then the level of salt intake can be gradually increased while symptoms and signs are carefully monitored. Fluid and food intake should be regularly distributed throughout the day and binges (particularly food with high sugar and/or salt content) should be avoided. Occasionally patients will notice that certain foods (for example alcohol, coffee, chocolate) may precipitate attacks. Diuretics (for example hydrochlorothiazide, 50 mg once or twice a day) may provide additional benefit in some patients although they cannot replace a salt restriction diet (class 3). Acetazolamide has been shown to decrease the osmotic pressure of the inner ear in experimental endolymphatic hydrops in guinea pigs,[29] but there have been no controlled studies to see how acetazolamide compares with hydrochlorothiazide or other diuretics in the treatment of Meniere's syndrome. Treatment of other causes of chronic recurrent peripheral vestibulopathy is summarized in Table 173.3.

Two general categories of surgery have been used for treating Meniere's syndrome: 1) shunting procedures, and 2) destructive procedures (class 3).[38] Although shunting the endolymphatic duct and sac is logical based on the presumed pathophysiology of Meniere's syndrome, in practice these procedures have not been very effective, probably because it is technically difficult to maintain an open shunt of the endolymph system. The total endolymph volume is less than 1 cubic centimeter. The rationale for ablative surgery in treating Meniere's syndrome is that the nervous system is better able to compensate for a complete loss of vestibular function than for a partial loss that is fluctuating in degree. Chemical ablation with gentamicin can be performed as an outpatient with minimal risk of hearing loss. Complete ablation of vestibular function is often not necessary to achieve symptomatic relief. The two main types of destructive surgery are labyrinthectomy and vestibular nerve section. Vestibular neurectomy has the advantage of preserving hearing in patients with salvageable residual cochlear function. It is important to conserve hearing whenever possible since about a third of patients with Meniere's syndrome will eventually develop bilateral involvement.

Symptomatic treatment Vestibular suppressants such as meclizine or promethazine (orally or via suppository) are usually effective in suppressing the acute vertigo, nausea and vomiting of an acute attack

Table 173.3   Diagnosis and treatment of common causes of chronic recurrent peripheral vestibulopathy

Cause	Presentation	Diagnosis	Specific treatments
Meniere's disease	Vertigo, fluctuating hearing, ear fullness and tinnitus, usually lasting hours	Low frequency sensorineural hearing loss increases during attack	Salt restriction (1 g Na$^+$/day) Diuretic (hydrochlorothiazide 50 mg or acetazolamide 250 mg/day) Surgery for intractable cases
Autoimmune inner ear disease	Vertigo, fluctuating and sometimes progressive hearing loss; may be systemic symptoms, rapid progression to both ears	Dramatic response to steroids Anticochlear antibodies in about 2/3 of patients	High dose steroids (60–100 mg prednisone, 12–16 mg dexamethasone) for 10 days, then taper Long term immunosuppression may be needed
Migraine	Episodes of vertigo often separate from headaches. May mimic Meniere's disease but not progressive hearing loss	Headaches meet IHS criteria, other causes ruled out	Prophylactic drugs: beta blockers, calcium channel blockers, tricyclic amines, SSRIs
Recurrent ischemia (TIAs)	Abrupt episodes of vertigo usually lasting minutes, other associated neurological symptoms	Exam usually normal but may be signs of prior infarct (exam or imaging)	Control risk factors, antiplatelet drugs. If symptoms continue, anticoagulation

IHS, International Headache Society; TIAs, transient ischemic attacks

(class 3). The drug should be taken as soon as possible, preferably during the prodrome if there are reliable warning symptoms. Additional antiemetics such as prochlorperazine can be useful if the nausea and vomiting are severe. Chronic prophylactic treatment with vestibular suppressants may be used when moderate to severe attacks recur on a frequent basis. During long term therapy, one must balance the need to control vertigo against the need for the patient to maintain full mobility and function. One of the milder suppressants can be used on a daily basis "to take the edge off" the attacks, adding acute antiemetic treatment if spells are very prolonged or are associated with vomiting. In general, the stronger suppressants are more sedating and should be reserved for acute treatment (Table 173.2).

Vestibular rehabilitation As a general rule, vestibular rehabilitation has a minimal role in managing patients with Meniere's syndrome or other causes of recurrent peripheral vestibulopathy. These disorders are typically caused by a transient reversible abnormality, often with return to baseline in between the attacks. Although there may be a gradual progressive loss of unilateral vestibular function, this occurs slowly, typically over several years along with the central compensation process.

Ototoxicity (bilateral vestibulopathy)
Overview

Prior to the 1940s, drugs that damaged the vestibular part of the inner ear were relatively unknown. That all changed with the introduction of streptomycin treatment of tuberculosis. Streptomycin is highly vestibulotoxic and can produce a remarkably selective bilateral vestibulopathy. Subsequently introduced aminoglycosides all have the potential for both auditory and vestibular ototoxicity, although the more recently introduced drugs are less ototoxic.

Epidemiology

The single most important factor in determining potential ototoxicity is the total dose exposure to the drug. However, there is marked variability in individual susceptibility. Patients with renal failure are highly susceptible to ototoxicity from aminoglycosides since these drugs are primarily excreted via the kidney.

Etiology

The relative ototoxicity of the common aminoglycosides to the auditory and vestibular system is summarized in Table 173.4. Other common ototoxins include quinine and salicylates, loop diuretics such as furosemide and ethacrynic acid, and chemotherapeutic agents such as cisplatin.

Pathophysiology

The ototoxicity of the aminoglycosides has been convincingly shown to be due to damage to the hair cells in the inner ear.[39] Aminoglycosides are concentrated

Table 173.4   Relative vestibular and auditory ototoxicities of commonly used aminoglycosides

	Vestibular	Auditory
Streptomycin	+++	+
Gentamicin	+++	+
Tobramycin	++	++
Kanamycin	+	+++
Amikacin	+	+++
Dibekacin	+	+++
Netilmicin	+	+

in the perilymph and endolymph. The earliest effect of the two primary vestibulotoxic aminoglycosides, streptomycin and gentamicin, is a selective destruction of type I hair cells in the crista. With the primary cochleotoxic agents kanamycin and amikacin, there is initially a destruction of the outer hair cells in the basal turn of the cochlea followed by total hair cell loss throughout the cochlea as the dose and duration of treatment are increased.

Genetics

Genetic predisposition may explain the variable sensitivity to the ototoxic effects of aminoglycosides in humans.[40] A mutation in a mitochondrial gene (maternal inheritance) has been shown to predispose to the development of aminoglycoside-induced deafness.

Clinical features

Patients who receive ototoxic drugs are often bedridden and suffer from multiple symptoms of systemic illness so the additional symptoms of auditory and vestibular dysfunction may be easily overlooked. Vestibular symptoms are particularly difficult to identify in this setting. The main symptoms are imbalance and unsteadiness when standing or walking, particularly in the dark, and visual distortion or oscillopsia when the head is moving due to loss of the vestibulospinal and vestibulo-ocular reflexes, respectively. If the vestibular loss is symmetrical, the patient will not experience vertigo.

Classification

There are many causes of progressive bilateral vestibular failure although aminoglycoside ototoxicity is by far most common. In about a third of patients with bilateral vestibular loss, no specific cause can be identified.[41]

Diagnostic criteria

One must be alert to the early symptoms of ototoxic drugs, particularly in patients who are seriously ill and confined to bed. Patients in renal failure are also at high risk. Bedside auditory and vestibular testing, if performed carefully, should identify early cases. Bedside audiometric examinations are available in most hospitals. Bedside vestibular testing is less satisfactory but gait imbalance and unsteadiness are usually apparent early in the course. The head-thrust test, whereby the patient's head is quickly moved a few degrees from side to side to assess the vestibulo-ocular reflex will show corrective saccades if the smooth vestibulo-ocular reflex, is impaired.[42]

Differential diagnosis

Bilateral vestibular loss should be considered in any patient complaining of oscillopsia, unsteadiness of gait, or both. There may or may not be a prior history of vertigo. Common diagnoses in patients with bilateral vestibular loss include ototoxicity, congenital and acquired infections, congenital malformations of the inner ear, autoimmune inner ear disease, and bilateral Meniere's disease. Most of these patients, however, exhibit combined auditory and vestibular loss so that the finding of an isolated bilateral vestibular loss should suggest the possibility of a vestibular ototoxin.

Treatment

Prevention   Prevention is the key to the management of ototoxicity. Kidney function should be monitored when using any potentially ototoxic drugs and patients in high risk groups such as those with kidney failure should probably not be given ototoxic drugs that are excreted via the kidney. All patients should be questioned on a regular basis to identify early symptoms of auditory or vestibular loss. When the earliest effects of ototoxicity are recognized, adjustments in the dosage schedule often can reduce the likelihood of developing permanent symptoms. Often other drugs can be substituted that are less ototoxic. Very often the ototoxic effects will be reversible if the drug is stopped early enough.

Vestibular rehabilitation   The strategy in helping a patient rehabilitate for a bilateral vestibular loss is different from that used for a patient with unilateral vestibular loss. Persons with bilateral vestibular loss demonstrate a series of permanent deficits that require compensation (class 3). Some compensation involves strengthening existing reflexes, such as the cervico-ocular reflex and smooth pursuit, while the remainder requires trained behaviors and a realistic understanding of one's limitations.

If the vestibulospinal reflexes are absent, there is an increased dependence on ankle proprioception and cutaneous sensation from the feet and ankles to provide balance. Such persons are also visually dependent, but there are limitations to their compensation because of oscillopsia. Deficits become apparent when they are exposed to poor support surfaces (soft or shifting surfaces, narrow support base), particularly if visual inputs are misleading. Treatment involves maintaining or improving ankle strength and mobility, increasing cutaneous input through the use of supportive "high-top" shoes, and stressing the importance of solid footing and good lighting at all times.

Due to the absence of the vestibulo-ocular reflex, head movements that are of sufficient velocity to exceed that of smooth pursuit result in visual slip (oscillopsia). Treatment involves maintaining full neck mobility to allow the cervico-ocular reflex to provide compensatory eye movements. Slow head oscillations to strengthen pursuit abilities during head movement are also of value.

References

1. Baloh RW, Honrubia V, Jacobson K. Benign positional vertigo. Clinical and oculographic features in 240 cases. Neurology 1987;37:371–378
2. Epley JM. The canalith repositioning procedure: For treatment of benign paroxysmal positional vertigo. Otolaryngol Head Neck Surg 1992;107:399–403
3. Brandt T, Steddin S. Current view of the mechanism of paroxysmal positional vertigo: Cupulolithiasis or canalithiasis? J Vestib Res 1993;3:373–382
4. Baloh RW. Benign positional vertigo. *In:* Baloh RW, Halmagyi GM, eds. Disorders of the Vestibular System. New York: Oxford University Press, 1996:328–339
5. Vannuchi P, Giannoni B, Pagnini P. Treatment of horizontal semicircular canal benign paroxysmal positional vertigo. J Vestib Res 1997;7:1–6
6. Herdman SJ, Tusa RJ, Zee DS, et al. Single treatment approaches to benign paroxysmal positional vertigo, Arch Otolaryngol Head Neck Surg 1992;119:450–454
7. Zucca G, Valli S, Valli P, et al. Why do benign paroxysmal positional vertigo episodes recover spontaneously? J Vestib Res 1998;8:325–329
8. Gacek RR. Singular neurectomy update II. Review of 102 cases. Laryngoscope 1991;101:855–862
9. Parnes LS, McClure JA. Free floating endolymphatic particles: A new operative finding during posterior semicircular canal occlusion. Laryngoscope 1992;102:988–992
10. Schuknecht HF. Neurolabyrinthitis. Viral infections of the peripheral auditory and vestibular systems. *In:* Nomura Y, ed. Hearing Loss and Dizziness. Tokyo: Igaku-Shoin, 1985
11. Robillard RB, Hilsinger RL Jr, Adour KK. Ramsay Hunt facial paralysis: Clinical analysis of 185 patients. Otolaryngol Head Neck Surg 1986;95:292–297
12. Fukukada S, Furuta Y, Takasu T, et al. The significance of herpes viral latency in the spiral ganglia. Acta Otolaryngol (Stockh) 1994;Suppl 514:108–110
13. Murakami S, Mizobuchi M, Nakashiro Y, et al. Bell palsy and herpes simplex virus: identification of viral DNA in endoneurial fluid and muscle. Ann Intern Med 1996;124:27–30
14. Schuknecht HF. Pathology of the Ear. 2nd ed. Philadelphia: Lea & Febiger, 1993
15. Baloh RW, Lopez I, Ishiyama A, et al. Vestibular neuritis: Clinical-pathologic correlation. Otolaryngol Head Neck Surg 1996;114:586–592
16. Ariyasu L, Byl FM, Sprague MS, Adour KK. The beneficial effect of methlyprednisone in acute vestibular vertigo. Arch Otolaryngol Head Neck Surg 1990;116: 700–703
17. Dickens JRE, Smith JT, Grotlam SS. Herpes zoster oticus: Treatment with intravenous acyclovir. Laryngoscope 1988;98:776–779
18. Stokroos RJ, Albers FWJ, Tenvergert EM. Antiviral treatment of idiopathic sudden sensorineural hearing loss: A prospective, randomized, double-blind clinical trial. Acta Otolaryngol (Stockh) 1998;118:488–495
19. Foster CA, Baloh RW. Drug therapy for vertigo. *In:* Baloh RW, Halmagyi GM, eds. Disorders of the Vestibular System. New York: Oxford University Press, 1996:541–550

20. Davis JR, Jennings RT, Beck BG, Bagian JP. Treatment efficacy of intramuscular promethazine for space motion sickness. Aviat Space Environ Med 1993; 64: 230–233

21. Mitchelson F. Pharmacologic agents affecting emesis: A review. Part I. Drugs 1992;43:295–315

22. Ferrando SJ, Eisendrath SJ. Adverse neuropsychiatric effects of dopamine antagonist medications. Psychosomatics 1992;32:426–432

23. Isah AO, Rawlins MD, Bateman DN. Clinical pharmacology of prochlorperazine in healthy young males. Br J Clin Pharmacol 1991;32:677–684

24. Lacour M, Roll JP, Appaix M. Modifications and development of spinal reflexes in the alert baboon (papio papio) following a unilateral vestibular neurotomy. Brain Res 1976;113:255–269

25. Igarashi M, Levy JK, O-Uchi T, et al. Further study of physical exercise and locomotor balance compensation after a unilateral labyrinthectomy in squirrel monkeys. Acta Otolaryngol (Stockh) 1981;92:101–105

26. Herdman SJ. Vestibular rehabilitation. In: Baloh RW, Halmagyi GM, eds. Disorders of the Vestibular System. New York: Oxford University Press, 1996:255–269

27. National Institute on Deafness and Other Communicative Disorders. Science Panel to Update Strategic National Plan. Bethesda, Maryland, 1991

28. Baloh RW. Neurotology of migraine. Headache 1997;37:615–621

29. Kimura RS. Surgical and drug intervention in experimentally induced endolymphatic hydrops. In: Nomura Y, ed. Hearing Loss and Dizziness. Tokyo: Igaku-Shoin, 1985:16

30. Paparella MM. Pathology of Meniere's disease. Ann Otol Rhinol Laryngol 1984;Suppl 112:31–35

31. Tumarkin I. Otolithic catastrophe: a new syndrome. BMJ 1936;2:175–177

32. Baloh RW, Jacobson K, Winder T. Drop attacks with Meniere's disease. Ann Neurol 1990;28:384–387

33. Schuknecht HF, Delayed endolymphatic hydrops, Ann Otol Rhinol Laryngol 1978;87:743–748

34. Pearson BW, Brackmann DE. Committee on Hearing and Equilibrium guidelines for reporting treatment results in Meniere's disease. Otolaryngol Head Neck Surg 1985;93:579–581

35. Harris JP, O'Driscoll K. Autoimmune inner ear disease. In: Baloh RW, Halmagyi GM, eds. Disorders of the Vestibular System. New York: Oxford University Press, 1996:374–380

36. Harker LA, Rassekh HC. Episodic vertigo in basilar migraine. Otolaryngol Head Neck Surg 1987;96:239–249

37. Santos PM, Hall RA, Snyder JM, et al. Diuretic and diet effect on Meniere's disease evaluated by the 1989 Committee on Hearing and Equilibrium guidelines. Otolaryngol Head Neck Surg 1993;109:680–689

38. Brackmann DE. Surgical procedures: Endolymphatic shunt, vestibular nerve section, and labyrinthectomy. In: Baloh RW, Halmagyi GM, eds. Disorders of the Vestibular System. New York: Oxford University Press, 1996:551–562

39. Hutchin T, Cortopassi G. Proposed molecular and cellular mechanism for aminoglycoside ototoxicity. Antimicrob Agents Chemother 1994;38:2517–2520

40. Casano RA, Johnson DF, Bykhovskaya Y, et al. Inherited susceptibility to aminoglycoside ototoxicity: genetic heterogeneity and clinical implications. Am J Otolaryngol 1999;20:151–156

41. Baloh RW, Jacobson K, Honrubia V. Idiopathic bilateral vestibulopathy. Neurology 1989;39:272–275

42. Halmagyi GM, Curthoys IS. A clinical sign of canal paresis. Arch Neurol 1988;45:737–739

174 Tinnitus and Deafness

Linda M Luxon and Ewa Raglan

Hearing loss is the most common sensory impairment worldwide, and the World Health Organization has estimated that 170 million people have a significant impairment.[1] Tinnitus affects approximately 10% of developed populations,[2] but is virtually unreported in the developing third world.[3] Tinnitus and hearing loss are cardinal symptoms of disordered cochlear function but may also be consequent upon central auditory pathology with normal cochlear function. For the neurologist, hearing loss and/or tinnitus, together with any associated vestibular dysfunction, arising from coincidental otological pathology, must be distinguished from cochlear, eighth nerve or central auditory dysfunction as part of the clinical presentation of the neurological problem. The aim of this chapter is to demonstrate that, armed with some basic knowledge, a diagnostic strategy and some clear principles of management, much can be accomplished for the patient with tinnitus and hearing loss in the context of neurological disease.

Definitions

Tinnitus

Tinnitus may be defined as the perception of sound that originates from within the head rather than the external world. Occasionally, there may be a physical source for this sound such as palatal myoclonus or an arteriovenous fistula or turbulent blood flow through a stenotic artery. The sound may then be audible externally and is known as "objective" tinnitus, as opposed to the much more common "subjective" tinnitus, which is perceived only by the patient himself. The nature of the sound may vary both in quality and intensity, but tinnitus is a universal experience similar to headache and pain. However, a distinction must be drawn between tinnitus experience and tinnitus complaint. It is generally accepted that sufferers complaining of tinnitus demonstrate no direct correlation between psychoacoustic changes and the intrusiveness of tinnitus, whereas there is a strong correlation between psychological factors and the intrusive nature of tinnitus.[4]

Hearing loss

For clinical purposes, the ear may be divided into three sections, the external ear, the middle ear and the internal ear (Figure 174.1). Abnormalities in each of these three subdivisions may give rise to hearing impairment.

Conductive hearing loss The external ear is important in the localization of sound and funnels sound waves to the tympanic membrane, while the middle ear, by means of tympanic membrane and ossicular movement, transfers airborne changes in sound pressure to the fluid-filled compartment of the membranous labyrinth, by way of the oval window. Within the internal ear the mechanical activity at the oval window is transduced into neural responses within the organ of Corti (Figure 174.2).

Pathology affecting the external and middle ear may give rise to abnormalities of the mechanical transmission of sound waves from the environment to the inner ear, leading to a conductive hearing loss. In this condition, bone-conducted sounds applied to the mastoid bone are perceived normally by the cochlea, whereas air-conducted sounds, which are normally perceived more acutely by the cochlea, as a result of the amplifying characteristics of the external and middle ear, are heard less well. Common examples of pathologies giving rise to a conductive hearing loss included impacted wax, chronic middle ear disease, ossicular chain dysfunction secondary to trauma or otosclerosis, and serous otitis media in children.

Sensorineural hearing loss Pathology of the internal ear and eighth cranial nerve characteristically gives rise to a sensorineural hearing loss, in which there is an inability to perceive both bone- and air-conducted sound normally. Both the appreciation of the intensity of sound and the frequency resolution of complex sounds are impaired. Pathologies involving the middle and internal ear, for example chronic middle ear disease, otosclerosis and physical trauma, may give rise to a *mixed hearing loss*, in which there is both a conductive and a sensorineural component (Figure 174.3).

Sensorineural hearing loss may be further divided into that of cochlear origin and that of neural origin, on the basis of two pathological phenomena:

1. *Loudness recruitment* is defined as an abnormally rapid increase in loudness, with an increase of intensity of stimulus, and is characteristic of disorders affecting the hair cells of the organ of Corti, but is absent in pathology of the eighth nerve and brainstem.
2. *Abnormal auditory adaptation* is a decline in discharge frequency with time, observed following an initial burst of neural activity in response to an adequate continuing stimulus applied to the organ of Corti. This phenomenon is characteristic of neural auditory dysfunction arising in both the eighth nerve and brainstem.

Central auditory dysfunction, at the level of the cortex, is rare because of the bilateral representation of both

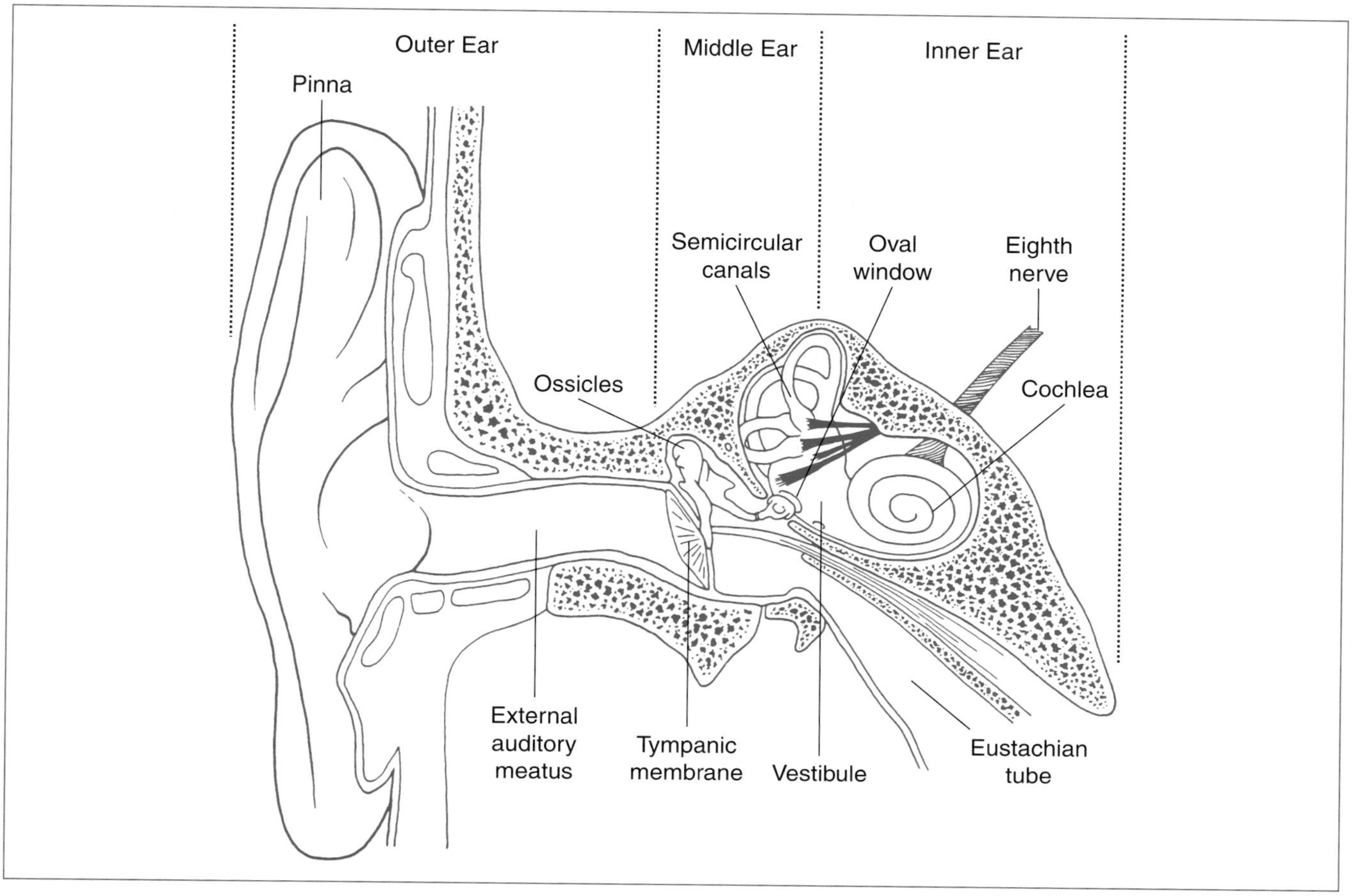

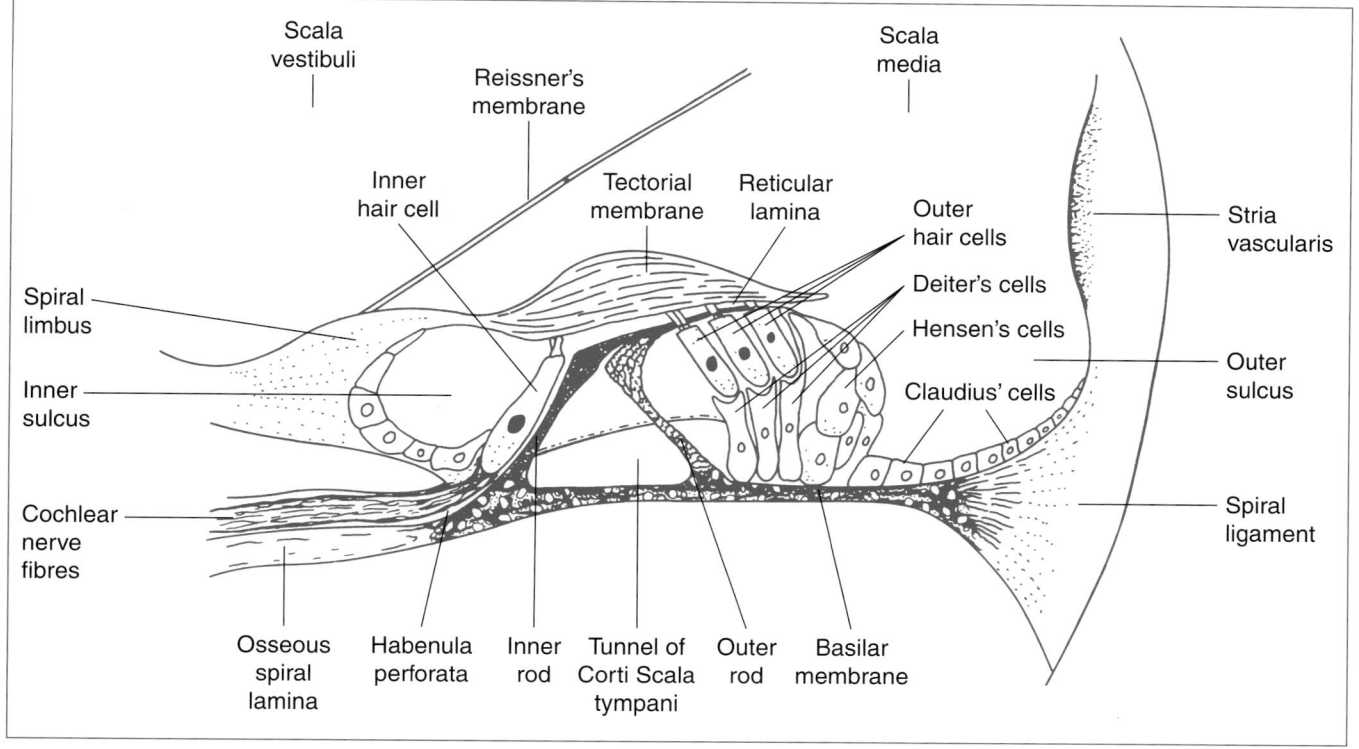

Figure 174.1 Diagram to illustrate anatomy of the ear.

Figure 174.2 Diagram of the structure of the organ of Corti.

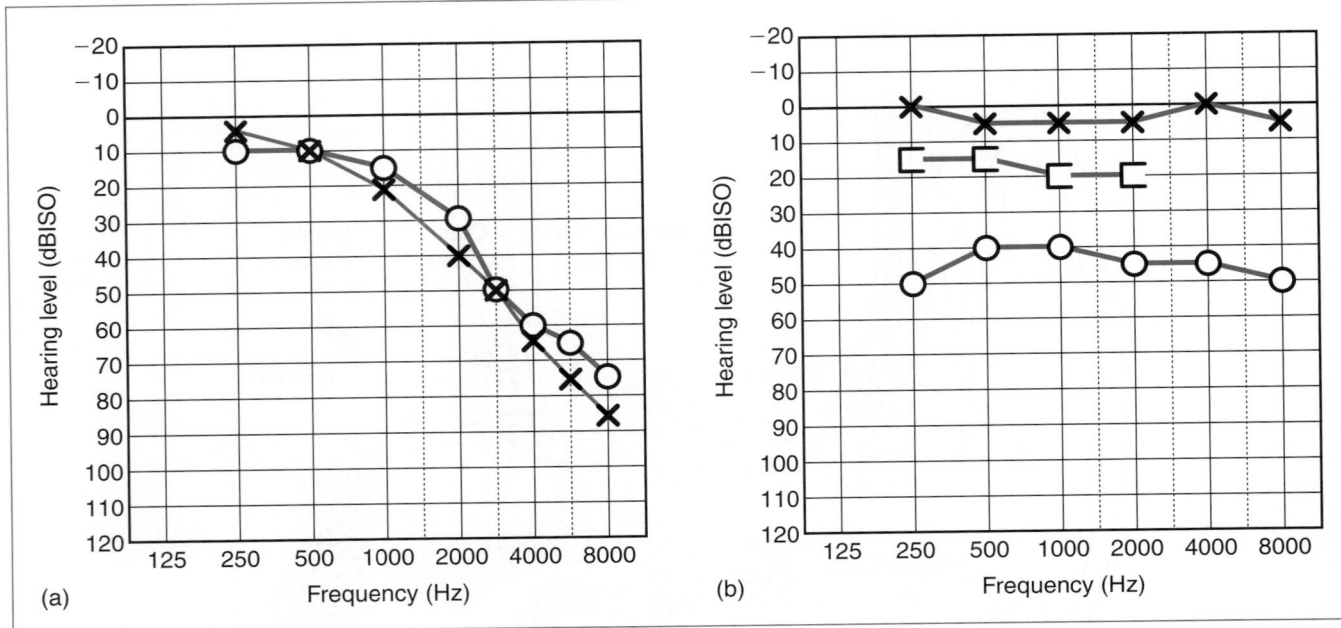

Figure 174.3   Audiometric characteristics of: (a) bilateral high tone sensorineural hearing loss; (b) right conductive hearing loss. *Key:* ◯, right air conduction threshold; ✕, left air conduction threshold; [, right bone duction threshold.

cochleae at this level and the redundancy within the auditory system (Figure 174.4). Thus, both auditory cortices must be involved. Such pathology may or may not show evidence of peripheral hearing loss as judged by standard audiometric tests, although there may be a profound inability to discriminate complex sounds such as speech and music.[5] Hearing impairments are variously defined by severity of loss across the frequency range[6,7] and by configuration/pattern of audiometric findings,[8] for example, high frequency loss, low frequency loss, domed, "cookie-bite," and notched. The time course of the hearing impairment may also be of diagnostic and pathological relevance, for example: the sudden hearing loss of vascular origin; the progressive hearing loss of ototoxicity or noise exposure; the stepwise hearing loss of genetic disorders, such as dilated vestibular aqueduct syndrome; and the fluctuating hearing loss of Ménière's disease and serous otitis media. Equally, the symmetry of hearing loss may be of relevance, for example unilateral hearing loss in certain genetic disorders and cerebellopontine angle tumors, such as acoustic neurinoma, and the bilateral symmetrical characteristic configuration of occupational noise-induced hearing loss.

Etiology

Conductive hearing loss is considerably less common than causes of sensorineural hearing loss in the adult population. In children, the most common cause of conductive hearing loss is otitis media with effusion, while in the elderly population wax and ear canal collapse are frequently encountered causes of conductive hearing loss. In the adult, conductive hearing loss may be seen in head injury following hemotympanum, ossicular discontinuity or middle ear adhesions.

Unilateral or asymmetric conductive hearing loss in an adult with normal middle ear pressure and tympanic membrane compliance should raise the suspicion of otosclerosis, which may be associated with a typical family history or present as a sporadic case. Conductive hearing loss in an adult with negative middle ear pressures or serous otitis media should raise the index of suspicion for a nasopharyngeal carcinoma. A vascular malformation such as a glomus tumor or, more rarely, primary or secondary malignant tumors may also present with a conductive hearing loss.

The causes of sensorineural hearing loss are shown in Table 174.1.

Table 174.1   Causes of sensorineural hearing loss

Genetic	Nonsyndromal
	Syndromal
Trauma	Physical
	Barotrauma
	Acoustic trauma
Vascular	Malformation
	Cardiovascular
	Cerebrovascular
Autoimmune	Isolated inner ear
	Systemic, e.g. SLE, PAN
Infection	Bacterial
	Viral
	Fungal
Iatrogenic	Drugs
	Surgical
	Organic chemicals
Degenerative	Cochlear
	Neuropathy
	Neurological

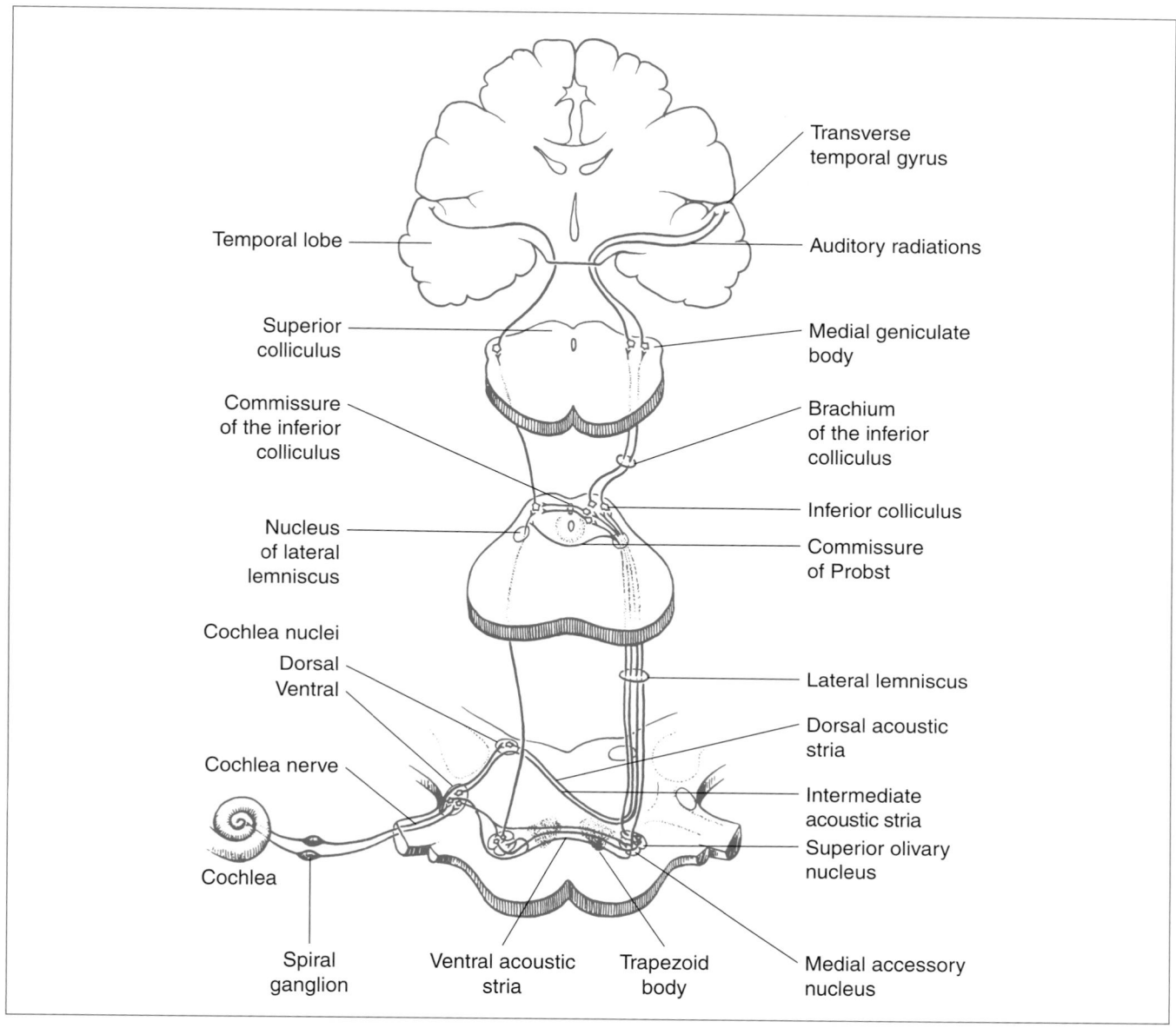

Figure 174.4 Diagram of central auditory pathways.

In the last decade the importance of genetic mutations and deletions in both syndromal and nonsyndromal hearing impairment in children and adults has begun to be clarified. Currently, 27 loci for autosomal recessive inheritance have been defined while 29 loci for autosomal dominant mutations/deletions leading to hearing loss have been identified. A recent paper has reported that 40% of the Spanish population carry a mitochondrial mutation, associated with hearing impairment.[9] Moreover, there is evidence to suggest that much of what was previously known as presbyacusis in fact represents inherited late-onset progressive hearing loss[10] and that specific genetic abnormalities may predispose to environmental triggers giving rise to hearing loss, for example the development of aminoglycoside deafness.[11] Not infrequently, the specific etiology underlying hearing loss defies diagnosis and, thus, identification of the pos-

sible mechanism giving rise to the hearing impairment may be more important than a specific diagnostic label in therapeutic terms. Equally, the recognition of classical clinical presentations such as Ménière's disease[12] is of value in symptomatic treatment, although the underlying pathophysiological mechanism remains elusive and, therefore, rational therapeutic intervention remains ill defined.

Tinnitus is frequently but not always associated with hearing loss, both conductive and sensorineural. The proposed pathophysiological mechanisms giving rise to tinnitus have included the decoupling of the stereocilia of the hair cells,[13] misinterpretation of auditory neural activity in higher auditory centers[14] and self-sustaining oscillation of the basilar membrane.[15] Following Kemp's 1978[16] discovery of acoustic emissions from within the human auditory system, it was thought that spontaneous otoacoustic emissions might provide an explanation for many cases of tinnitus. However, despite the demonstration of such a link, the association has proved to be uncommon.[17]

Other theories of tinnitus generation depend upon abnormalities of neural function. It has been proposed that an abnormality of the spontaneous resting activity of primary auditory nerve fibers, either secondary to hypo- or hyper-excitability of damaged hair cells or as a direct consequence of derangement of the primary neurons themselves, may give rise to the symptom. Møller, in 1984[18] has proposed that damage to the myelin sheath between auditory nerve fibers may allow ephaptic transmission ("cross-talk") between adjacent nerve fibers, while an alternative proposal is that derangement of efferent fibers of the vestibular cochlear nerve produces aberrant auditory behavior. It is also important to note that the majority of people who perceive tinnitus do not complain about it. Psychological factors are highly significant in tinnitus complaint in comparison with psychoacoustical features of the tinnitus. Moreover, the onset of tinnitus complaint has been related to associated negative life events such as retirement, redundancy, bereavement and divorce.

Clinical presentations

In childhood, hearing impairment may be divided into two broad categories: prelingual and postlingual. *Prelingual hearing loss* may be prenatal, perinatal or postnatal in origin and has previously been diagnosed primarily as a result of parental observation that the child is not responding to sound or beginning to develop speech in the normal way. More rarely, it has been identified following at-risk screening programs for children who have a family history of hearing impairment or are at risk of developing hearing loss as a result of infection in utero, postnatal hyperbilirubinemia, or risk factors requiring admission to a special care baby unit. In developed countries, however, there is now a strong movement to establish a universal neonatal screening test for hearing using otoacoustic emissions.[19]

Congenital hearing impairment has genetic and environmental causes. Congenital conductive hearing impairment is uncommon and is associated with congenital defects of the outer and middle ear, for example in such conditions as oto-branchio-renal syndrome or otogenesis imperfecta.

Congenital sensorineural hearing impairment is present in 1 to 1.5 per 1000 children although precise rates vary according to the community: for example, in populations in which consanguineous marriages are common, a prevalence of 12 per 1000 children has been reported. Genetic hearing impairment accounts for at least 50% of congenital hearing loss and may be syndromal (30%) or nonsyndromal (70%), autosomal recessive, autosomal dominant, X-linked or mitochondrially inherited. In children identified as having a hearing impairment, a detailed general medical, neurological and vestibular examination is mandatory to define as accurately as possible the primary condition. For example, Usher's syndrome type 1 is character-

ized by retinitis pigmentosa alone, whereas Usher's syndrome type 2 is associated with a vestibular loss. Craniofacial abnormalities, even such minor defects as ear pits or tags, are particularly associated with hearing impairment, both conductive and sensorineural, and syndromes such as the oto-branchio-renal syndrome. Some syndromes do not present until the third or fourth decade, such as Usher and Refsum (with neuropathy and retinitis pigmentosa), Alport (with renal failure), neurofibromatosis type 2, and Pendred with hypothyroidism and goiter. Other syndromes may present early, but progress during the first two decades of life, for example Waardenburg, Marshall Stickler and Down. It is important to recognize that approximately 30% of congenitally hearing impaired children will have nonsyndromal recessive cochlear hearing impairment and many of these may progress during the first two decades of life.

In adults, hearing loss may be of sudden or progressive type. Sudden hearing loss is almost always of sensorineural type and most commonly of traumatic, infective, vascular or autoimmune etiology. There is no consistent definition of sudden sensorineural hearing loss in the literature and, thus, it is difficult to compare studies as there is no homogeneous group of patients.[20] Nonetheless, the majority of cases fall into an idiopathic group in whom the precise underlying diagnosis cannot be made. About 60% recover spontaneously, the majority of that recovery occurring in the first few weeks after onset.[21]

Progressive hearing loss is frightening for the patient and frustrating for the doctor. It is now recognized that a significant proportion of progressive hearing loss may be of genetic origin, including a number of syndromes associated with neurological disease and hearing loss including Friedreich's ataxia, Charcot–Marie–Tooth disease, dystrophia myotonica and the inherited spinocerebellar degenerations. Specific risk factors include hazardous noise exposure, barotrauma, head injury, ototoxic drugs, and infections such as syphilis. The most prevalent cause of chronic hearing loss is termed presbyacusis, and Schuknecht's seminal work on the subject defined four categories.[22] However, recent work has led to the view that presbyacusis merely represents the cumulative effect of multiple otological insults, as summarized eloquently by Hinchcliffe "...is the deterioration of hearing due to some unavoidable intrinsic degenerative process, or is it merely the result of the individual being exposed to so many surdogens (agents that damage hearing) over the life span?"[23]

Investigation

The investigation of both tinnitus and hearing loss requires a full battery of audiological tests to define the site of auditory pathology, but also a broad knowledge of the plethora of general medical, neurological and otological disorders associated with hearing loss and tinnitus.

Pure tone audiometry is the most widely available quantitative test of auditory thresholds and allows

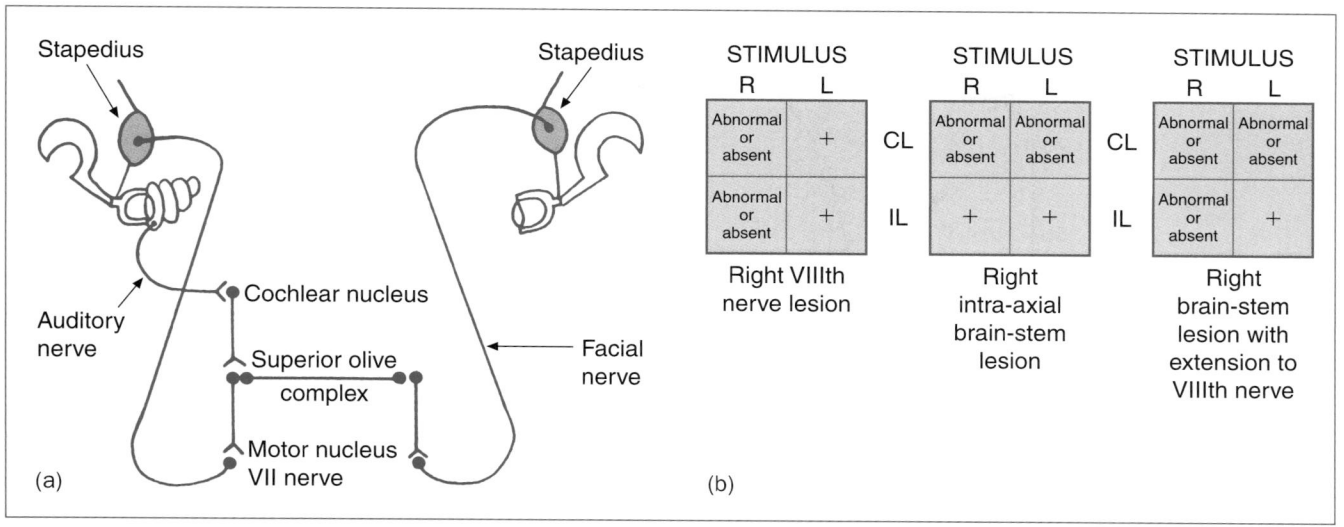

Figure 174.5 Diagrams of: (a) the acoustic reflex arc; (b) characteristic patterns of abnormality.

auditory stimuli to be delivered by both air conduction (through headphones) and bone conduction (using a bone vibrator on the mastoid bone). This technique, performed according to standardized protocols in a soundproofed room, allows the severity, symmetry and configuration of hearing loss to be defined and enables the separation into sensorineural, conductive or mixed disorders.

Acoustic impedance measurements provide information about the middle and internal ear, and the eighth nerve and brainstem function. Passive measurements are made of change in acoustic impedance or admittance, as a function of the pressure in the sealed external acoustic meatus and dynamic changes resulting from the contraction of the stapedius muscles (Figure 174.5).

The development of measurement of *otoacoustic emissions (OAE)* has added a further dimension to audiological testing as OAE represent outer hair cell activity in the cochlea, which can be recorded in the external auditory meatus, either spontaneously, or in response to acoustic stimuli (Figure 174.6). Efferent auditory function can be assessed by the suppression

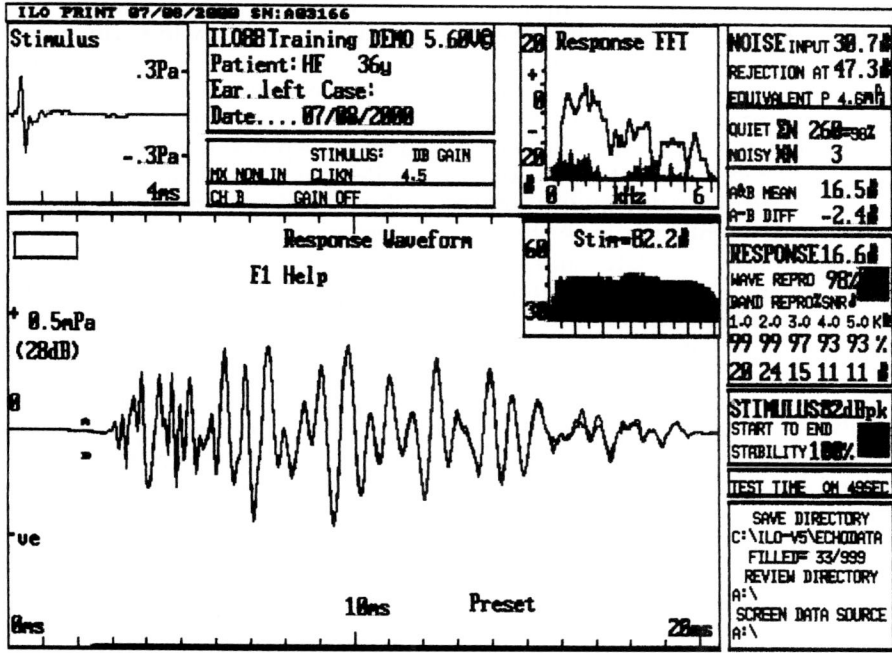

Figure 174.6 Transient evoked otoacoustic emissions recorded with nonlinear click stimuli of 80.4 dB SPL (measurement of sound pressure level) from a normal subject, showing in the response window two alternate (A and B) recorded time waveforms and the FFT (fast fourier transformation) with the frequency spectrum of the response.
With kind permission of Dr. Borka Ceranic.

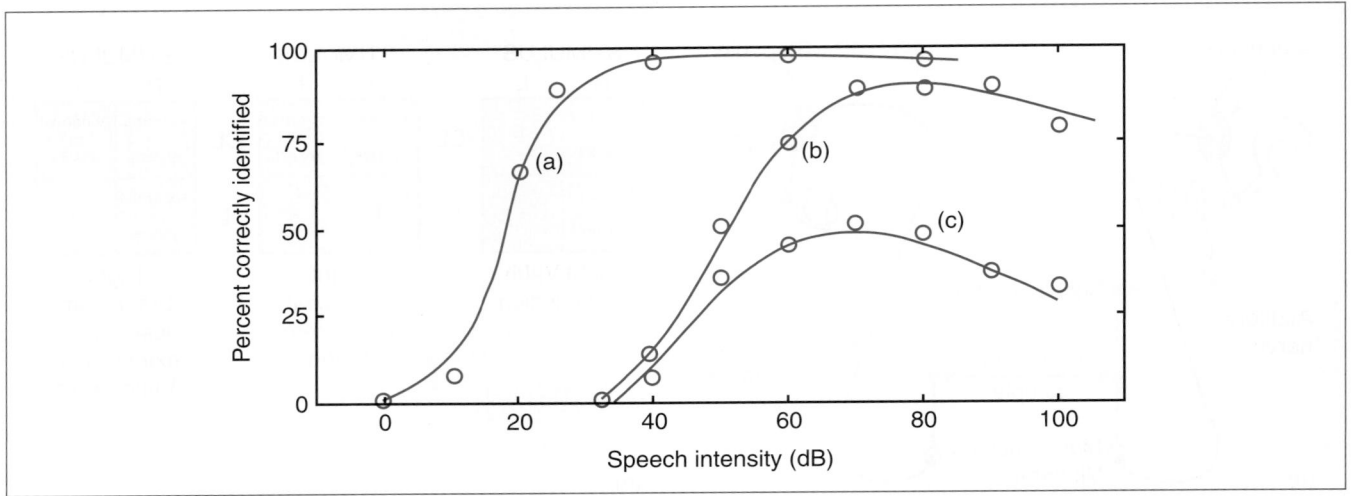

Figure 174.7   Diagram to illustrate: (a) normal speech audiogram; (b) characteristic pattern observed in a moderate cochlear hearing loss; and (c) characteristic "roll-over" phenomenon observed in neural hearing loss.

that noise in the contralateral ear produces on ipsilateral otoacoustic emissions.

Speech audiometry is concerned with the assessment of auditory discriminative ability, as opposed to the assessment of auditory acuity. In combination with other tests, speech material is sensitive in distinguishing sensorineural from conductive loss and in providing information to point toward a sensory or neural impairment (Figure 174.7).

Auditory-evoked potentials may be recorded from many sites in the auditory pathway by varying the stimulus and recording parameters. Electrocochleography is the measurement of the electrical output of the cochlea and eighth cranial nerve, in response to an auditory stimulus, while brainstem-evoked responses are a series of neurogenic potentials that can be recorded using surface electrodes in response to click stimuli in the 10 ms immediately after the stimulus (Figure 174.8). As a diagnostic tool, brainstem-evoked auditory responses are of particular value in discriminating between cochlear and eighth nerve dysfunction. Cortical-evoked responses or late auditory responses are the most effective method of defining auditory thresholds at each frequency in an uncooperative patient and are essential in legal cases in which nonorganic loss should be considered (Figure 174.9).

Central auditory dysfunction

The central auditory nervous system is anatomically and physiologically complex. Thirty thousand neural fibers in the auditory division of the eighth cranial nerve increase to 250,000 in the auditory radiation. In addition, the complexity of auditory processing increases from the cochlea to the auditory cortex, with a greater number of facets of auditory function subserved at higher auditory levels and multiple representations of each ear on each side of the brain at each level of the ascending auditory pathways. Thus, there is intrinsic redundancy within the central auditory system, which renders it resistant to standard

auditory testing. A variety of tests have been designed to challenge the complexity of central auditory processing in the frequency, intensity and temporal domains, although no standard central auditory test battery has been defined. Correlation and interpretation of published results are, therefore, hampered by variability of test procedures, the variety and diffuse nature of central auditory pathologies, the difficulty in extrapolating animal work to man, the complexity of the central auditory nervous system, and the unpredictable manifestations of factors such as age, sex, linguistic ability, intelligence and peripheral labyrinthine pathology.[24]

Central auditory tests can be divided into *behavioral* tests, which require patient cooperation in responding to a given stimulus, and *objective* tests, which do not require patient involvement and provide recordable data in response to acoustical stimulation.

Behavioral tests may be grouped together into tests which share a common parameter such as mode of presentation (e.g. monaural or binaural signals) or type of stimulus employed (e.g. tones or speech). The brainstem auditory nuclei contribute to central auditory processing in two main areas: the extraction of signals from a background of noise, which has led to the development of auditory separation tasks; and binaural integration of auditory information, which has led to the development of binaural interaction tests. Thus, behavioral tests of particular value in the assessment of brainstem disorders include the Masked Speech test, the Synthetic Sentence Identification with Ipsilateral Competing Message test (SSI-ICM), the Masking Level Difference test (MLD) and the Binaural Fusion test (see Figure 174.10).

Behavioral tests are used to assess cortical function and employ speech or speech-like stimuli. In the dichotic paradigm, different stimuli are presented simultaneously to the two ears and the listener is required to respond to one or both stimuli, for example the Dichotic Digit test and the Threshold of

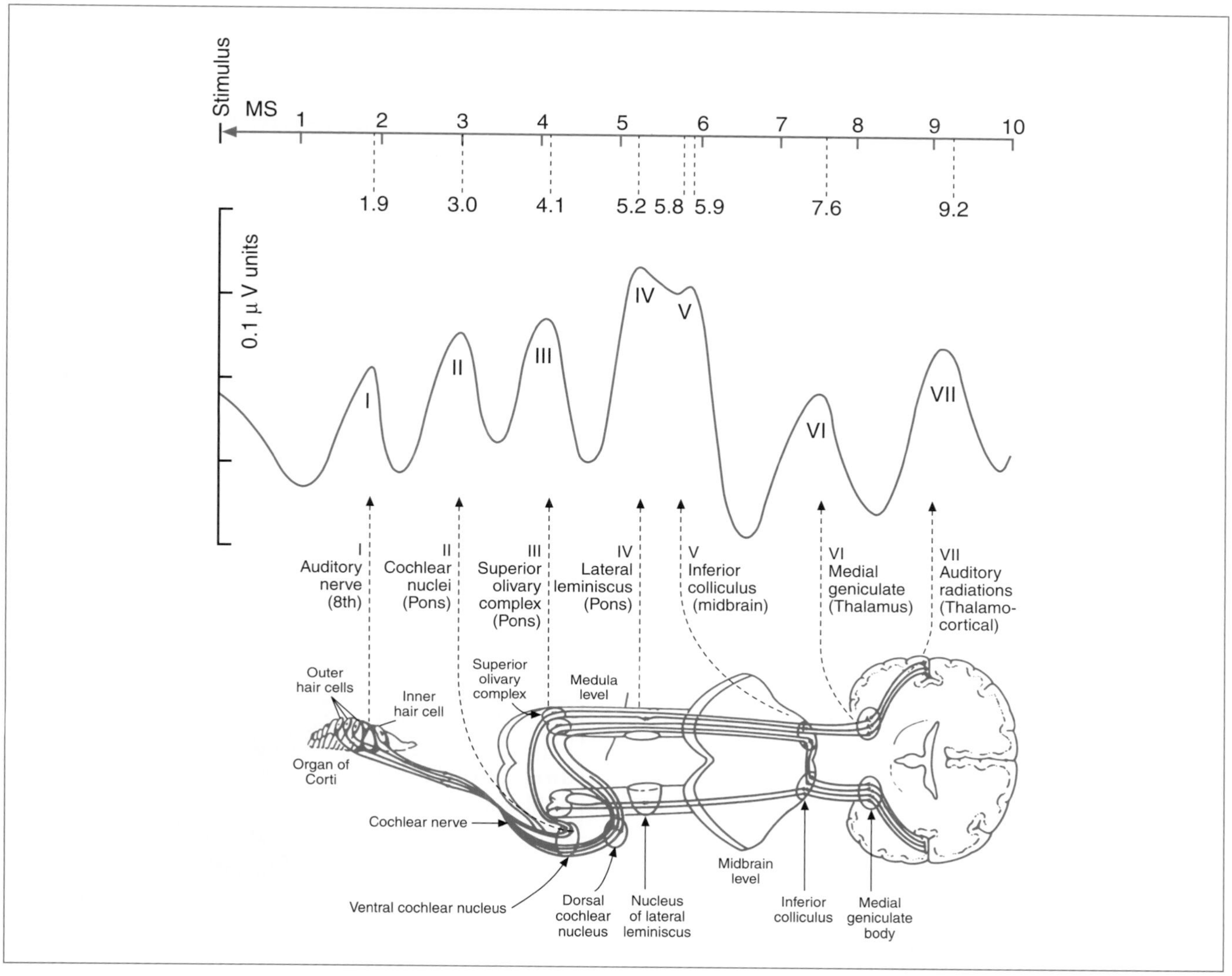

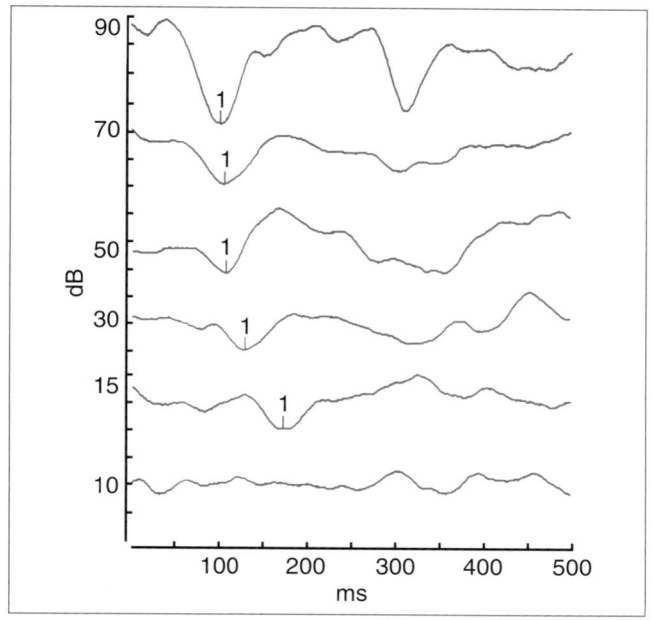

Figure 174.8   Diagram to illustrate generation of waves observed in brainstem evoked response audiometry.

Interference test (Figure 174.10). Sequencing or temporal ordering tasks, in which a sequence of successive stimuli separated by time intervals need to be identified, have also proven of value, for example the Pitch Pattern test and the Psychoacoustic Pattern Discrimination test.

Objective tests of value in brainstem assessment include stapedial reflex threshold measurements, brainstem auditory-evoked potentials and assessment of otoacoustic emissions in the presence and absence of contralateral noise, while for cortical testing, middle latency responses and slow vertex auditory-evoked responses provide valuable information.[25]

Figure 174.9   Figure to illustrate cortical evoked response audiometry in threshold assessment of hearing.

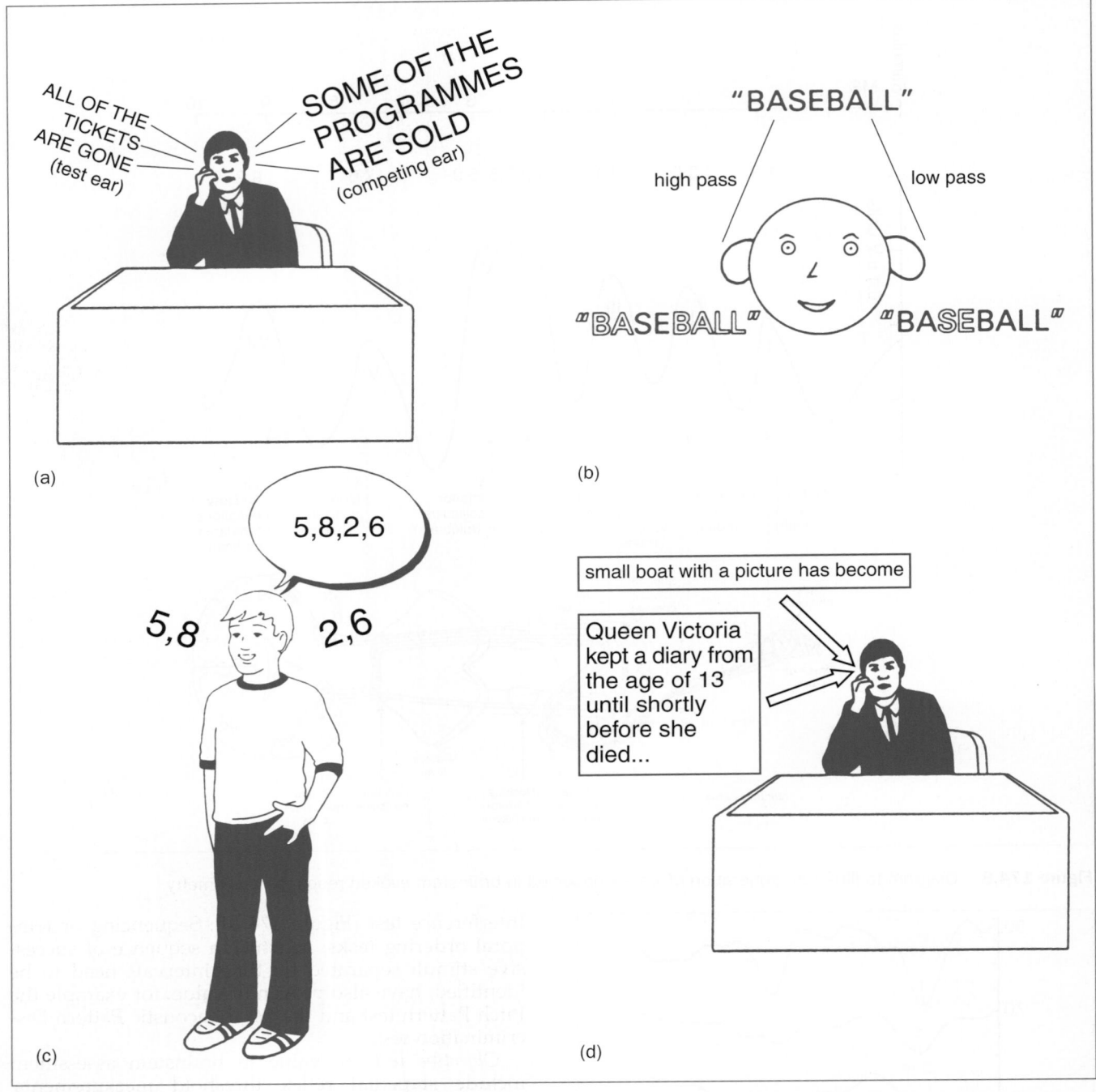

Figure 174.10 Behavioral tests of central auditory function: (a) SSI–ICM (synthetic sentence identification); (b) Filtered Word test; (c) Dichotic Digit test; (d) Threshold of Interference test.

Management of hearing impairment
Conductive hearing loss
Conductive hearing loss is caused by conditions which affect the transmission of sound through the external and middle ears.

Disorders of the external ear The external auditory canal can be blocked by a foreign body, wax, a polyp, carcinoma, or infection.

Acute otitis externa should be treated by the removal of discharge and debris, preferably by suction clearance under microscope.[26] Culture and sensitivity of the organism will enable the indication of the appropriate medication: antifungal or antibacterial, alone or in combination with steroids, to decrease the inflammation and edema of the external auditory canal.[27] Topical ear drops may be applied locally,[28] but in more severe cases systemic antibiotics may be required.[29]

Chronic, nonspecific external otitis, characterized by persistent itching with scaling and erythema but no obvious discharge, is best treated by irrigation of the canal with boric acid or aluminum acetate solution, followed by topical antibiotic and steroid preparations. The treatment may be prolonged for several weeks, often with only limited success.[26,30,31]

Middle ear disorders

Middle ear disorders causing conductive hearing impairment may be treated medically, including amplification, or surgically.

The treatment of *acute otitis media* in children and adults consists of relief of pain, re-establishment of eustachian tube function using nasal drops, inhalations, oral decongestants and mucolytics, and the prescription of systemic antibiotics. The choice of chemotherapy will depend upon the penetration of the drug into middle ear space and the suspected organism causing the infection. Usually, the drug of first choice is amoxicillin; its spectrum of activity can be extended by combining it with clavulanic acid. In patients with sensitivity to penicillin, erythromycin may be used. Increasing antibiotic resistance poses a threat to effective treatment and therefore new drugs are under investigation, such as ketolides, oxazolidinones and quinolones.[32] Myringotomy (incision through the drum) is indicated if the drum is bulging and the pain is severe.

In *recurrent acute otitis media,* especially in children, an underlying immunodeficiency should be excluded and any focus of infection within the upper respiratory tract should be removed. Long term low dose prophylactic antibiotic, e.g. a 3 month course of trimethoprim/amoxicillin, has been shown to be effective in its treatment,[33] but is associated with the emergence of resistant pneumococcus in infants and young children.[33] Therefore, the preferred method of prevention of middle ear infection is surgery such as myringotomy and/or adenoidectomy, with or without insertion of grommets.[34,35] To counter the emergence of antibiotic resistant bacteria, microbial vaccines have been introduced preventatively.[32] Epidemiological data have shown that middle ear infection provides protection against the same organism.[36,37] New vaccines are directed against *S. pneumoniae, M. catarrhalis,* respiratory syncytial virus, adenovirus and influenza A and parainfluenza viruses.[38] Clinical trials are in progress with pneumococcal and attenuated viral vaccines.[39,40]

Chronic otitis media with effusion, "glue ear," is often initially treated with decongestant therapy, mucolytics and antihistamines, although this type of treatment has not proved to be effective in randomized, placebo-controlled, double-blind study.[41] Low dose, long term antibiotics have been shown to be beneficial.[42] Frequently, a period of observation is recommended[43] and allows assessment of whether the condition is chronic and symptomatic. It may become recurrent, with subsequent fluctuation of hearing, may resolve, or the patient may require surgical intervention with myringotomy and grommet insertion, with or without the removal of adenoids. The following criteria are indications for grommet insertion:

- Persistent effusion for more than 12 weeks, not responsive to antimicrobial therapy
- Severe, conductive hearing loss
- Associated behavioral, balance problems
- Cleft palate
- Adhesive otitis media, with severe atelectasis or a retraction pocket of the tympanic membrane.[44,45]

Potential complications of grommet insertion are persistent otorrhea (5% to 15%), residual tympanic membrane perforation, and tympanosclerosis.

Persistent glue ear can be also treated with myringotomy alone or in combination with adenoidectomy. Recent controlled, randomized studies have demonstrated the efficacy of adenoidectomy in reducing OME in children above 4 years of age[46,47] by the elimination of nasopharyngeal pathogens and improved eustachian tube function. Children who suffer with longer periods of glue ear, with subsequent periods of conductive hearing loss resulting in speech delay, should be offered amplification.[48]

The aim of treatment of *chronic suppurative otitis media* is to eliminate infection using antibiotics to control the discharge and, when the ear is free from infection, repair aural damage, e.g. a perforated tympanic membrane, or damage to the ossicles. Coexistent disease in the nose, sinuses or pharynx should be treated. If, in spite of these measures, there is a continual purulent discharge, the possibility of continuing disease in the mastoid area should be considered, and diseased mucosa, granulation tissue, polyps or cholesteatoma surgically removed.[49]

Chronic ear disease, as well as trauma, can cause damage to the structures of the middle ear, such as dislocation, fracture or erosion of the ossicles and perforation of the tympanic membrane. Myringoplasty and ossicular repair (performed when the ear is free of infection, safe and dry for several months[35]), can rectify these deficits, prevent reinfection[50] and allow improvement of sound transmission.[51]

Conductive hearing loss can also be caused by stapes ankylosis such as occurs in *otosclerosis and the hereditary osseous dysplasias* of the petrous temporal bone. The management may be conservative, by use of air conduction aids, or surgical by *stapedectomy.* The head, neck and crura of the stapes are removed, a small opening is made in the middle of the central part of the footplate, and a piston-like prosthesis is inserted, with the tip protruding through the opening in the footplate and a hook clamped on to the incus. This procedure carries a small risk of complications in the hands of an inexperienced surgeon, particularly late, sudden SNHL,[52] and, for this reason, stapedectomy should not be undertaken on both ears.

Congenital malformations of the auditory canal and the middle ear can be treated conservatively with bone conduction or bone anchored hearing aids (BAHA),[53] or surgically. The results of surgery are mixed, with a risk of facial nerve palsy, ear canal restenosis and chronic ear discharge.

Sensorineural hearing loss

Sensorineural hearing loss (SNHL) may be sudden in onset, progressive or chronic. The management is determined on the basis of this classification.

Sudden hearing loss is a medical emergency, requiring admission bed rest and the investigation of possible audiological causes. The management may include not only medication, but also psychological and auditory rehabilitation, especially vital in cases of bilateral hearing loss. There is no universally accepted treatment that demonstrates a response rate beyond that expected for spontaneous recovery (65% of patients).[54]

In most cases (90%), the etiology is difficult to establish,[55] but it is important to exclude treatable systemic vascular disease and tumors. The prevalence of idiopathic cases has led to many hypotheses regarding the pathogenesis of this condition, which in turn have led to a plethora of management regimes, aimed at improving blood flow and oxygenation to the inner ear, treating possible viral infection and reducing inflammation or an autoimmune response. Singly or in combination, the following agents have been used:

- Inhalation of carbogen (95% oxygen and 5% carbon dioxide)[56,57]
- Hyperbaric oxygen[58–60]
- Antiviral treatment: acyclovir, interferon[61,62]
- Immunosuppression[63]
- Calcium channel blockers[64]
- Steroids[65,66]
- Combination of steroids and carbogen[67]
- Blood volume expanders[68,69]
- "Shotgun regimen" including dextran, histamine, diuretic, steroids, vasodilators, and carbogen inhalations.[64,70]

Studies of these various modalities of treatment are small, lack appropriate control groups or blinding, and evaluate different populations, using different outcomes. Thus, the results are not comparable and there is a need for a large, controlled multicenter study. There is one double-blind, randomized, controlled study, which shows a statistically significant benefit of steroids.[66] It is, therefore, recommended to use 60 mg prednisone taken orally for 4 to 7 days with a gradual reduction over the next 6 to 8 days.[71] Contraindications to steroid use are bacterial infection, recent surgery, peptic ulcer, a history of tuberculosis, poorly controlled hypertension or diabetes.[72]

Progressive hearing impairment may be caused by many pathologies, which may be treatable medically or surgically, followed by rehabilitation to reduce disability. Specific conditions are treated appropriately, e.g. *syphilitic labyrinthitis* with steroids and benzylpenicillin, and *acoustic neuroma* by surgical intervention or laser therapy, to secure the preservation of hearing and facial nerve function. Larger tumors have poorer surgical results.[73]

Immune mediated SNHL is usually a rapidly progressive, bilateral or unilateral condition. Once recog-

nized, it should be treated with immunosuppressive medication, in the first instance with steroids (prednisone 60 mg daily) but in more severe cases with the addition of cyclophosphamide, azathioprine or methotrexate.[74]

There is an array of treatments for *Ménière's disease*, but no proven therapy has been defined. Trials of therapy in this condition are particularly difficult because of the lack of diagnostic certainty, the variable frequency and severity of symptoms between and among patients, and the capricious natural history of the condition. Broadly, therapies can be divided into medical and surgical. Medical therapy has classically included dietary modifications, pharmacological intervention, psychological support, physiotherapy and auditory rehabilitation.[75,76] Conventionally, surgical treatment is considered when medical management has failed to control vertigo or progression of hearing impairment, but the possibility of bilateral involvement must be carefully weighed in the consideration of any destructive procedure.

In the early stage, the condition can be treated medically using vestibular sedatives, diuretics or vasodilators, or indeed surgically, using, for example, a saccus decompression procedure. In later stages of the disease, severe hearing loss and incapacitating vertigo may lead to destructive surgical procedures such as labyrinthectomy (surgically or drug induced) or vestibular nerve section, if the aim is to preserve residual hearing.

In an acute attack the patient should be treated with bed rest, vestibular sedatives such as cinnarizine, and antiemetics, e.g. prochlorperazine orally, or, if the patient is vomiting, transbuccally, intramuscularly, intravenously or as a suppository. The aim of long term treatment is to reduce the frequency of attacks, preserve hearing and control tinnitus. A number of therapies have been advocated, such as the restriction of salt, water, alcohol, nicotine and caffeine, and stellate ganglion blocks, diuretics, tranquilizers[77] and the use of subatmospheric pressure chambers,[78] with the aim of reducing endolymphatic hydrops by changes in the inner ear blood flow, osmotic diuresis or central sedation. Review of the literature[79] shows that only diuretics and betahistine have a proven effect in double-blind studies on the long term control of vertigo, but no effect on hearing or the course of disease. The use of diuretic is based on the observation that this may alter fluid balance in the inner ear, leading to depletion of endolymph and correction of hydrops.[80] Similarly, James and Burton,[81] in a systematic review on the effects of betahistine in treatment of Ménière's disease found only one trial of 35 patients of the highest methodological validity and suggested that high dose betahistine had no effect on tinnitus or hearing loss, and unfortunately the effect on vertigo was not assessed.[82] Betahistine is a histamine derivative that improves the microcirculation of the stria vascularis[83] and has an inhibitory effect on polysynaptic vestibular nucleus neurons.[84]

Patients who do not respond to medical therapy may be considered for surgical or chemical ablation of vestibular function.[85] Labyrinthectomy unselectively destroys hearing and vestibular function, while vestibular nerve section is recommended in the patient with vertigo but good hearing, although the morbidity is significant.[86] Chemical labyrinthectomy, achieved by the introduction of aminoglycosides (streptomycin or gentamicin) into the middle ear,[87,88] provides good control of vertigo, but may be complicated by hearing loss. Optimal doses and treatment schedules have not yet been established.[86]

Chronic symptoms of dizziness/imbalance in a patient with Ménière's disease may benefit from a program of vestibular rehabilitation,[89] Those with a hearing impairment may benefit from a suitably chosen hearing aid, followed by a program of auditory rehabilitation.[90]

Chronic sensorineural hearing impairment may be managed along two complementary lines: specific etiological treatment to rectify or halt the progression of the causative condition, and audiological rehabilitation of residual hearing.

The aim of rehabilitation is to minimize disability, prevent handicap, and facilitate as full a recovery as possible, realizing the patient's optimum physical, mental and social potential, and enabling integration into his or her environment.[91] In the process of rehabilitation the patient's motivation, attitude, and expectations of rehabilitation need to be assessed, including factors such as employment, education, and willingness to wear a hearing aid.

Goldstein and Stephens[90] comprehensively described the components of a rehabilitation program: *evaluation* of the patient, including degree of hearing impairment and presence of auditory discomfort, disability, handicap, communication status, mobility, degree of manual dexterity and related aural pathology; and *remediation*, which encompasses personal instrumentation, such as a hearing aid, tactile aid or cochlear implant, as well as general instrumentation (assistive listening devices) such as telephone/TV attachment and alerting warning systems (alarms). The patient is taught how to optimize communication (hearing tactics) and receives further help within the social, psychological, educational and occupational domains.

Hearing tactics include such simple measures as advice on how to position oneself to see as many people as possible while in a group, how to attract an observer's attention before starting to talk, how to take clues from words and body language of a speaker, and how to lip-read and obtain the clues from the shapes/sounds that are missed. The process of aural rehabilitation is concluded by the *assessment of outcome* in terms of patient satisfaction, his or her quality of life and effectiveness of the offered instrumentation.

Selection and fitting of hearing aids

Hearing aids are specific for different types and degrees of hearing loss. The patient's needs are paramount in the choice of the best hearing aid, e.g. a busy person will profit optimally from binaural amplification, while an elderly patient with impaired manual dexterity may prefer monaural fitting.

Air conduction aids are widely used for both conductive and sensorineural hearing loss. They are smaller, have a wider frequency response, are easier to modify and are cosmetically acceptable. They include behind the ear, in the ear, in the canal, body worn and spectacle aids.[92] They may be fitted monaurally or binaurally: the latter improving localization of sound, speech discrimination in noise and speech intelligibility, as well as sense of localization and distance from the sound source.[93] Sounds heard bilaterally are perceived as louder by 3 to 5 dBHL than monaurally, due to binaural summation.[94] Moreover, binaural fitting avoids the attenuation of sound especially at high frequencies, as a result of the "head shadow effect," which blocks the passage of sound waves of shorter wavelength than the width of the head. This leads to an average attenuation of 10 dB at 4 kHz.[95]

Bone conduction aids are retained on the head by a headband, with the receiver placed on the mastoid bone. They are used for conductive hearing losses, with active ear discharge and physical deformity of the pinna or of the ear canal. Additionally, there are implantable hearing aids such as the bone anchored hearing aid (BAHA), middle ear implants, and inner ear implants (cochlear implants). In the past five years, the progress in hearing aid technology has led to consumer programmable and, more recently, digital hearing aids.[96]

How does a hearing aid work? A hearing aid is an amplifier, the function of which is to increase the intensity of the sound energy delivered to the ear, with as little distortion as possible.[97]

In a traditional (*analog*) *hearing aid*, the acoustic energy of sound is converted by the microphone into weak electrical potentials, which are amplified and then converted back into acoustic energy by the receiver[98] (Figure 174.11).

The maximum achievable output is determined by the amplifier and battery and volume control, but can be limited by "peak clipping" or "compression limiting" circuitry, which reduces the output of the aid, with respect to the input, above a predetermined intensity threshold. This prevents amplification of uncomfortably loud sounds. Compression limiting provides undistorted limitation of sound, while peak clipping limits the intensity by cutting off the intensity peaks, which distorts the waveform and, thus, affects the sound quality (Figure 174.12). Peak clipping is less expensive, however, and does provide maximum audibility for profound hearing losses. In addition, the hearing aid frequency response may be adjusted by the "tone control," which allows fine-tuning by the varying degree of high and low pass filtering. Not infrequently, the phenomenon of recruitment is associated with a restricted dynamic range and complicates the assessment of gain required in a particular individual case.

In linear hearing aids, the magnitude of gain is

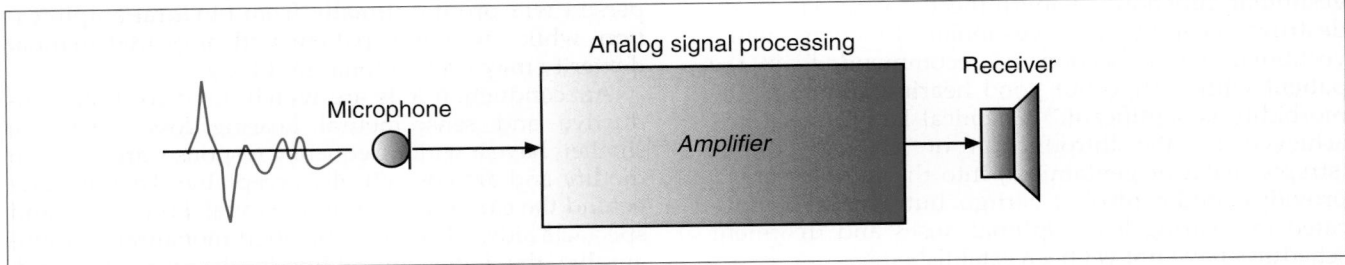

Figure 174.11   Diagram of circuit of an analog hearing aid.

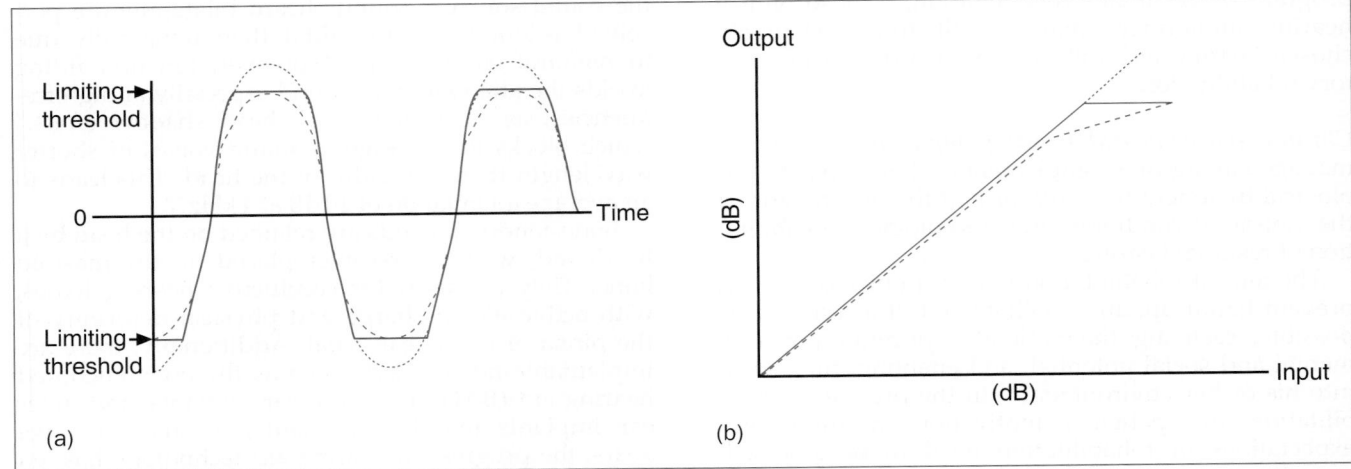

Figure 174.12   Schematic drawings representing the concept of compression and peak clipping of hearing aid circuitry. *A* represents the sound wave and *B* the relationship between input and output of the sound: unlimited, (............), peak clipped (———), and limited by compression (– – – –).

constant for all input levels until saturation occurs, distorting sound quality. These aids provide considerable gain for patients with severe to profound hearing loss, but less for those with mild to moderate losses.

In nonlinear hearing aids (with compression), the gain is gradually reduced as the input intensity increases.[99] It enhances the audibility for soft sounds, while providing comfort for loud sounds, without the need for adjustment of the volume control.[100] However, it may alter the intensity relationship between different segments of the speech signal and lead to poor speech intelligibility for some hearing impaired listeners.[101] "Compression limiting" controls the saturation distortion better than peak clipping and is desirable in all degrees of hearing impairment, except for the very profound. "Wide" dynamic range

compression compresses a wide range of sounds into the residual dynamic range of the hearing impaired ear. Therefore, it produces higher audibility for low input signals and more comfort for high input signals. This is suitable for mild to moderate hearing losses, when frequency resolution remains reasonably good.

Over the last decade, the development of digital technology[102–104] together with progress in understanding the function of the impaired cochlea[105,106] has led to the introduction of *digital hearing aids*. In a digital hearing aid, the analog sound signals are transformed into electrical signals, which are then converted into numerically coded representations of sound. The converter samples the analog signal and creates a binary number, which represents the level of the signal at that instant (Figure 174.13). Such a signal

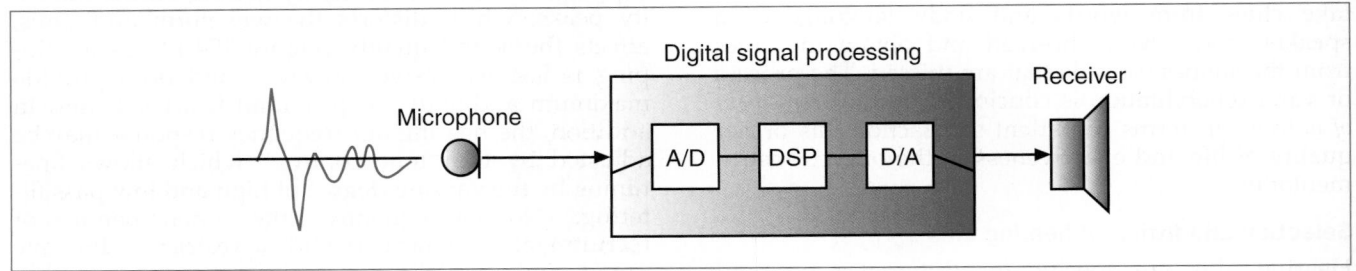

Figure 174.13   Diagram of circuit of a digital hearing aid. DSP, digital processing system; D/A, conversion from digital to analog signal; A/D, conversion from analog to digital signal.

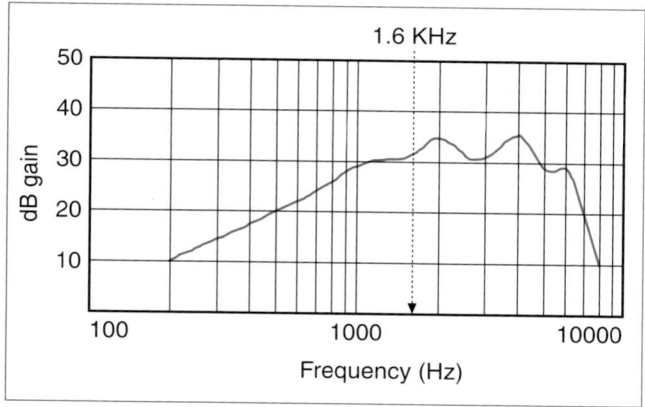

Figure 174.14 Diagram of characteristics of gain of an analog hearing aid.

may be manipulated by any number of mathematical algorithms to control gain and compression characteristics of the aid. The gain at a particular frequency is described by the amplification of the input sound by the hearing aid system, at that frequency. It is usually presented graphically as a system of coordinates[107] (Figure 174.14). The signal is then converted back into the analog mode and fed into the receiver, where it can be converted back into acoustic energy.[108] However, the quality of the digital processing in the hearing aid system is limited by the quality of the analog microphone and receiver.[109]

In analog processing, the electrical signal may become easily distorted or lost, while in digital processing mathematical formulae are used to code the signal, resulting in less distortion, automatic control of signal level, greater precision in adjustment of electroacoustic parameters and control of acoustic feedback, and better programmability.[110] This type of aid brings a significant degree of freedom to the clinician in interfacing the electroacoustic response of the hearing aid to the magnitude and type of hearing loss. Moreover, the acoustic response may easily be altered to meet the changing amplification needs of the patient. Thus, hard of hearing patients are able to distinguish different tones, recognize different voices, perceive the colour and timbre of the individual sound, and recognize specific sounds, e.g. speech in background noise,[111] although it is important to note that these hearing aids do not eliminate background noise.[112]

The question has arisen of the possible advantage of digital over analog aids. Some studies[113] have reported equivocal results in terms of speech recognition in quiet or in noise, while others[114–117] have reported a preference for digital aids. However, there are no randomized controlled trials comparing the two, although there are a few small studies of poor methodological design comparing the effectiveness of more advanced analog aids with digital ones.[118]

Provision of hearing aid relative to auditory deficit In a *moderate cochlear hearing loss* of up to 50 dBHL (consistent with loss of outer hair cell func-

tion and normal inner hair cell function),[119] with normal uncomfortable loudness levels, the differences between thresholds and discomfort levels to sound are small. In such a situation, if a linear hearing aid has enough gain to amplify the quietest sounds, it will have too much gain for louder sound. Thus, a nonlinear hearing aid is required, which will not make loud sounds any louder, but will provide gain to amplify quiet sounds to make them audible and clear.[120]

In *a moderately severe cochlear loss*, in which there is loss of some outer and inner hair cells, there is a loss of both sensitivity for quiet sounds and speech intelligibility. In such a case, more gain will be required for low level sounds and less gain is needed to restore loud sounds to normal loudness.

In a *severe cochlear impairment* in which there is marked outer and inner hair cell loss of function, degradation of speech intelligibility occurs, especially in background noise due to loss of redundant speech cues.[121] In such a situation, there is a need for significant gain for all sounds and for listening near uncomfortable levels in difficult noise situations.[120] The maximum output level of an aid should be related to the loudness discomfort levels to prevent loud sounds causing unacceptable loudness discomfort. However, to achieve good quality of speech discrimination, the aid should use the dynamic range maximally. In such a case, speech sounds should be brought to the level of maximum intelligibility, below the level of discomfort, and the hearing aid gain should be limited by compression. Compensation for recruitment by compression may be treated as an electronic substitute for the physiological dampening of the outer hair cells.[123]

A hearing loss in a specific frequency region can be fitted with a multichannel aid, which allows certain frequency bands to have different gain and compression, thus providing a better match for the patient's needs.[99]

In cases of *asymmetric loss*, the aid should be fitted to the better hearing ear to provide maximal benefit, although the patient's preference may be to use the aid in the poorer hearing ear.[124] Speech discrimination measures may help to decide which ear to aid in cases of asymmetric or severe hearing loss.[125]

In a case of *unilateral severe or profound hearing impairment*, with good or near normal hearing in the other ear and in whom little or no benefit is obtained from a conventional aid, a CROS fitting is used (contralateral routing of signals). The microphone is placed in the "poor" ear, the receiver in the "good" ear, and an open earmold allows the entry of sound to the good ear, in addition to sound received from the impaired ear. The CROS system provides some advantages of binaural fitting. It can also be used in other situations such as in the presence of high frequency loss in the good ear, which prevents overamplification at low frequencies. A Bi-CROS fitting is used when the better ear also has some impairment and requires amplification.[125]

Additionally, any hearing aid may include a special telecoil circuit, which allows the use of the telephone, without interference from sounds in the environment and can also be used with an induction loop for the television, or in the theater, cinema or church.

The aim of optimal amplification is to respond to an individual's needs to provide maximum speech intelligibility in various acoustic conditions and reduce the discomfort of sudden loud sounds. This can be achieved by fitting an aid of particular characteristics, in terms of gain, frequency response and type of signal processing, using specific prescription formulae.[126] Other factors considered in hearing aid fitting are shown in Table 174.2.

Earmolds The electroacoustic specification of a hearing aid may be altered by extrinsic factors such as the way in which the aid is connected to the ear (modifications to the hook, tubing and/or earmold) and intrinsic factors, such as ear canal resonance. The hook may be of various sizes and it retains the aid behind the pinna. It also conducts sound to the tubing, and the hook and/or the tube may house damping material to smooth out the resonance peaks in the frequency response. This allows the user to increase the volume of the control setting and achieve a greater gain with less likelihood of feedback. Unfortunately, such material may easily be contaminated by moisture and debris. High frequency gain may be improved if the tubing is gradually expanded into a horn shape (Libby horn). The earmolds are manufactured from impressions and have a number of functions: to seal the ear canal; to modify an acoustic signal produced by the hearing aid; and to be comfortable, easily handled by the patient and cosmetically appealing. They are made from different materials and are of different styles to fulfil certain requirements of the aid's performance (Figure 174.15):[127]

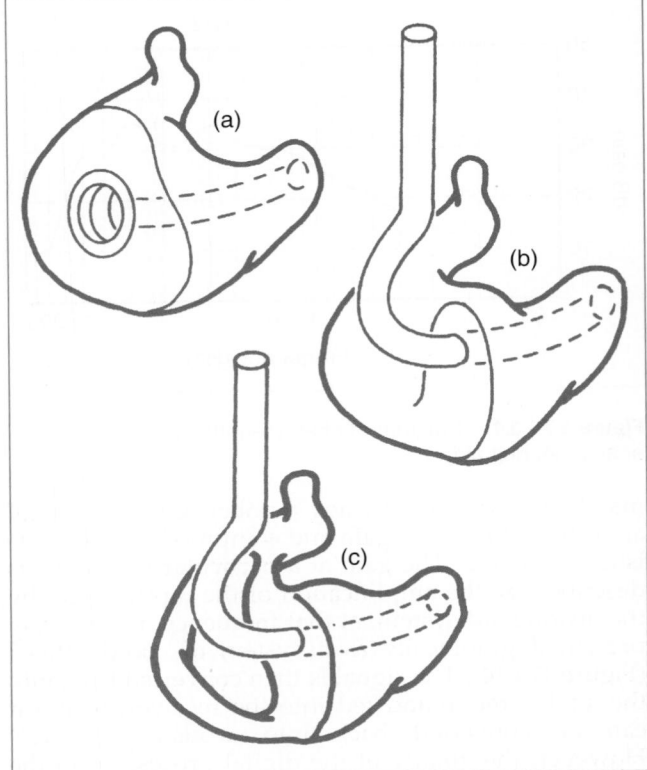

Figure 174.15 Diagrams (*A* and *B*) of types of earmolds: (a) solid; (b) shell; (c) skeleton.
    Reproduced with permission from Hearing Aid Audiology Group, British Society of Audiology. Making the earmould. *In:* Haltby M, ed. The Earmould, Current Practice and Technology. Reading: British Society of Audiology, 1984:19–21[127]

Table 174.2 Factors considered in hearing aid fitting	
1. Characteristics of an aid	
Gain	Adjusted by volume control
Frequency response	Adjusted by tone control
Output control	Adjusted by peak clipping, compression
Type of signal processing	Analog, multiprogrammable, digital
Type of microphone	Directional, omnidirectional
2. Style	
Body worn	
Behind the ear	
In the ear	
3. Type of earmold	
Shape: e.g. solid, shell, skeleton	
Material: e.g. acrylic, silicone, hypoallergenic	
Adjustments: e.g. different sized vents, Libby Horn, soft meatal tip	
Color	
4. Tubing/hooks	
Regular	
Thick walled	
Stay-dry	
Different sizes, with or without filters	
5. Compatibility with assistive listening devices	
6. Binaural/monaural fitting	

- *Solid molds* are made of soft material, not vented, to provide a tight fit to allow a body worn aid to achieve high gain without the risk of a feedback.
- *Shell molds* are rarely vented, often with a long meatal projection providing a good seal, and are used with high power BTE aids.
- *Skeleton molds* are usually vented, with shorter meatal projections, and are used with low/medium powered aids.

A vent is a small hole drilled through the mold to reduce the low frequency gain of the aid. A larger vent is used in patients who have better hearing at low frequencies. The vent additionally reduces the canal occlusion effect, which makes the mold more comfortable but encourages feedback.[122,128] Occlusion of the auditory canal leads to unpleasant louder bone-conducted sounds, including own sounds made by the hearing aid wearer. Feedback occurs when the amplified signal is partially reintroduced to the hearing aid system and reamplified.

Types of hearing aid systems

There are various types of hearing aid systems (Figure 174.16) that may be used depending upon the patient's audiometric or cosmetic need.[129]

Air conduction systems

Body worn aids are used for those with profound deafness and those with manual dexterity problems. They provide a high gain and output and a good low frequency response but a relatively poor high frequency response. The controls are large and easily accessible and the aid is carried in a pocket attached to clothing. The receiver is attached to the earmold and is connected by a lead to the aid. The separation between the microphone and the receiver allows for greater gain and output because of the reduced propensity for feedback.

Behind the ear aid The components of the aid are placed in a small case that sits behind the pinna. Usually the microphone is forward facing. Sound, amplified by the aid, is transmitted through the tube, held in the ear by an earmold, into the external auditory meatus. Such instruments are available for mild

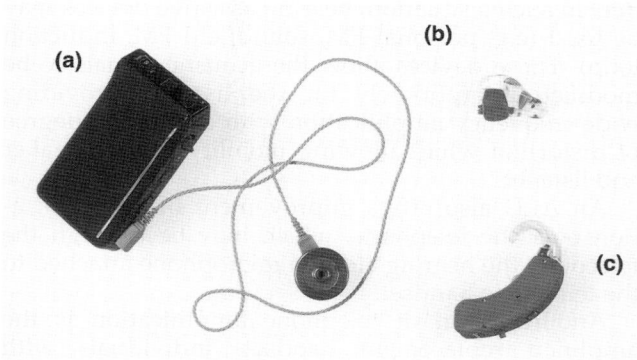

Figure 174.16 Models of analog hearing aids: (a) body worn; (b) in the ear; (c) behind the ear.

to profound hearing losses and offer the greatest possibilities for hearing aid adjustment.

In the ear aid There are three types of in the ear aid; their name indicates their placement position in the ear canal.

1. In the ear (ITE) hearing aids. These fill the bowl of the ear. They are most successful for use with losses having pure tone averages between 35 and 70 dBHL.
2. In the canal (ITC) aid. These may be used for less severe losses than ITE aids. They are more deeply inserted than an ITE, less visible, and provide less gain and output as compared with ITE aids.
3. Completely in the canal (CIC) and peritympanic hearing aids. These are the smallest aids and fit completely in the canal, close to the tympanic membrane. The deep canal fitting provides a number of advantages such as reduction of occlusion effect, reduction of feedback, and the opportunity to fit more severe losses with less gain. The position of an aid near the tympanic membrane leads to an improvement of the gain of an aid between 5 and 13 dBHL, especially in the high frequency region.[130]

Bone conduction hearing aids Bone conduction aids have a large, rigid vibrator, which lies tightly against the mastoid bone, sending vibrations rather than acoustic signals. They have a poor high frequency response and are used for conductive hearing losses where an earmold cannot be placed in the ear canal, e.g. because of gross stenosis of the canal, lack of pinna, or active ear discharge.

Implantable hearing aids

Cochlear implants are used in patients with severe to profound hearing loss who are unable to derive benefit from conventional hearing aids; thus, the possible destruction of residual hearing by the electrode insertion is justified. The cochlea may be nonfunctioning, but the auditory neural pathways from the cochlea to the auditory cortex must be intact. Adults with postlingual deafness due to conditions such as meningitis or ototoxic drug effects and children who suffer with prelingual or profound acquired deafness, as for example due to meningitis, may receive an implant.[131] A detailed selection procedure evaluating surgical, medical, psychological, radiological, social, educational and audiological factors is required.[132,133] The aim of the audiological assessment is to establish that a patient will profit more from cochlear implantation than from conventional hearing aids and to ensure compliance with the intensive rehabilitation program. Potential candidates are required to have a trial of high-powered analog hearing aids with 50–70 dBHL gain and maximum power output of 120–140 dBSPL.[134] Contraindications to implantation include absence of a cochlea (Michel deformity)[135] or absence of the eighth nerve.[136]

Cochlear implantation includes both single and multichannel implant, with intra- and extra-cochlear electrodes, and with a single electrode or an electrode array.[137,138] The system has a microphone, situated above and behind the pinna, which converts an incoming acoustic signal into an electrical impulse. This is sent to the signal processor (worn externally over or under clothes). A modified signal returns to the external transmitter, from where it is transmitted across the skin to an internal receiver. The information is frequency analysed and delivered to the electrodes in a manner specific to the speech processing strategy of the device (interleaved pulses, multipeak, continuous interleaved sampling, compressed analog).[139] Damaged hair cells are bypassed and the electric current stimulates the auditory nerve, producing the sensation of sound[140] (Figure 174.17).

As with all hearing aid provision, the patient has to receive long term auditory training, including listening to speech material, repeating it, and receiving training in the use of the implant. The cochlear implant allows hearing-impaired patients to hear speech information and environmental sounds, it improves the speech quality in an adult and allows the learning of speech in prelingual children. Most adults with postlingual deafness show improvement in speech recognition abilities during the first few months after implantation, but the progress is inversely related to duration of deafness and age.[141,142] Implanted children show improvement over a longer period of time. The most obvious improvement occurs in vocalization followed by spontaneous alerting to sound. There is also a significant improvement in receptive and expressive language development.[143,144] Moreover, implanted children are more likely to attend mainstream schools than schools for the deaf, thus reducing educational costs, improving educational attainments and enhancing integration into normal society.[145]

The benefits of cochlear implantation are measured using both auditory and linguistic tests. Standardized speech discrimination tests are used to measure the ability to hear words and sentences, both pre- and post-implantation, when listening and lip-reading and when lip-reading alone. The majority of implantees report an improved quality of life, with confidence to return to work or education.[146]

Auditory brainstem implants provide electrical stimulation of the auditory system by delivering an electrical signal directly to the complex of the cochlear nucleus, in the case of an absent or nonfunctioning auditory nerve.[147]

Bone anchored hearing aids (BAHA)[148–153] are considered for patients with congenital atresia of the ear canal,[154,155] chronic middle/outer ear infection with a discharging ear,[156,157] bilateral conductive loss due to incorrectable ossicular disease,[158] or mixed losses unaidable by conventional air conduction aids. A BAHA allows the patient to hear by transmitting sound directly through the skull and bypassing the middle ear. A small titanium screw is implanted behind the ear where it osseointegrates with the temporal bone. After a healing period, a percutaneous abutment is attached to the screw and a detachable sound processor can then be connected to the abutment. The process requires two-stage surgery.[159] In comparison with traditional bone conductor aids, a BAHA gives a better sound quality, with improved speech recognition in noisy surroundings[160–162] and the problems associated with acoustic feedback are minimized. Moreover, it is more comfortable and cosmetically acceptable for the user.

Middle ear implants The last 20 years has brought the development of implantable vibrators on one of the auditory ossicles or on the tympanic membrane. These devices are powered by an external source. The degree and type of hearing loss for which these fittings are most suitable has not yet been well established,[163,164] although they can be used with all types of loss.

Assistive listening devices Most types of hearing aid technology offer only minimal benefit to listeners with hearing impairment in adverse listening conditions, e.g. noise. The aim of an assistive listening device (ALD) is to improve communication in noisy or reverberant situations, especially where modifications of the acoustics of the environment are impossible. In such a situation, hearing assistive devices may be used (e.g. personal FM, soundfield FM, induction loop). These devices allow the acoustic signals to be modified appropriately for the listener, providing wide frequency amplification with a minimal degree of distortion while allowing mobility of the speaker and listener.

An ALD also offers improvement in communication over the telephone, which may be through the telecoil of the hearing aid or a microphone attached to the telephone handset.

Another form of telephone amplification is the amplified replacement handset. Individuals with severe to profound hearing losses and poor speech recognition may benefit from telecommunication devices for the deaf (TDD) teletypewriters which

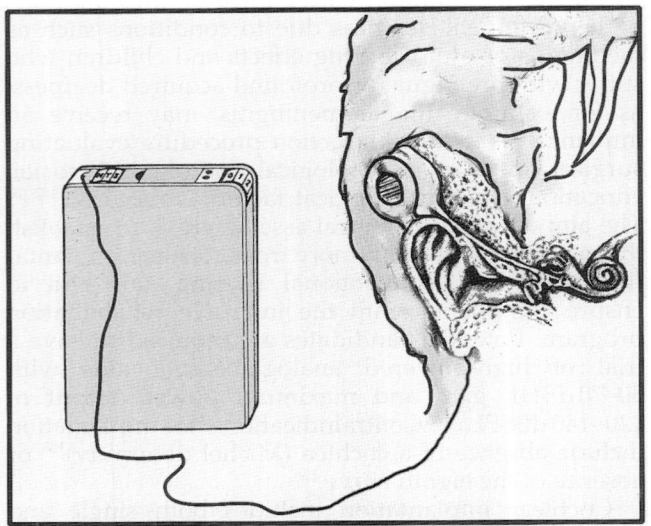

Figure 174.17 Schematic diagram of a cochlear implant.

transmit a typed visual message over a standard telephone line. The typed message may appear on a light emitting diode display or can be printed out. If a TDD user wants to communicate with non-TDD user he needs to do this through a telephone relay service.

Alerting systems are of particular value to profoundly deaf individuals as they alert the user by other senses, such as vision (turning on and off lamp/strobe light), olfaction (pungent scents), or vibration (pocket pagers, bed shakers).[165]

Prescription of hearing aid characteristics

The factors required for successful linear amplification, which ensure optimal utilization of the patient's residual hearing are:

1. Appropriate amplification and gain
2. A maximum output within the level of sound tolerance (LDL)
3. A frequency response shaping, which "mirrors" the configuration of the audiogram with no overt amplification of low frequencies.

Nonlinear amplification requires the appropriate compression ratio.

A variety of prescriptive formulae[126,166] are based on pure tone thresholds and are frequently incorporated into real ear measurement systems and manufacturers' fitting software.

In linear amplification, the *one half gain rule* is widely used.[167] The rule states that the desired gain should be equal to half the value of the hearing impairment averaged over 0.5, 1 and 2 kHz, plus a reserved gain of 15 dBHL. In this formula, no account is taken of the need for different gains at different frequencies, but it does take into account binaural advantages and the need for increased gain with conductive losses.

Many of the *other formulae* are variations of the one half gain rule, but take into consideration varying gains at individual frequencies:

- NAL-R (National Acoustics Laboratory)[168,169]
- Berger procedure[170]
- POGO[171,172]
- Figure 174.6[173]
- DSL.[174]

The *NOAH software system*[175] was introduced in 1994 and is an industry wide software standard for fitting hearing aids. It allows an office computer to link information from hearing aid fitting programs of different manufacturers to patient audiometric data, which may be entered manually or transferred directly from an audiometer connected to the computer. The dispenser may choose one of the manufacturer's hearing aid selection modules for computer assisted fitting of conventional hearing aids. It also allows the dispenser to transfer real ear measurement data and use them in the hearing aid selection, fitting or verification process. To date, there are insufficient data to determine that any one of the prescriptive methods is better than the others.[176]

Evaluation of hearing aid performance

Following the provision of a hearing aid system, a number of aspects need to be evaluated:

- Does the aid meet prescribed characteristics?
- What is the functional benefit of the hearing aid system?
- Does the aid meets the individual's expectations and needs?
- What is the patient's subjective opinion regarding obtained sound quality and clarity?

The insertion gain technique allows the objective assessment of the correlation between the characteristics of the selected aid and the prescribed gain and output, and thus enables monitoring of the effects of modifications to the hearing aid and to the earmold.[177,178] The comparison of aided and unaided thresholds, in freefield, will provide a measure of gain provided by a particular hearing aid and, as this is based on the subjective response from the patient, measures the function of the whole auditory system.

Alternative methods of assessment of the value of a particular aid or aids include measurement of loudness discomfort levels[179] or speech discrimination tests such as the Northwestern University Auditory Test[180] or the Synthetic Sentence Identification Test.[181]

The provision of an appropriate hearing aid forms only a part of the process of the auditory rehabilitation, and reduction of disability and handicap should also be included as part of the rehabilitation process. A number of questionnaires aimed at assessing hearing, e.g. the Abbreviated Profile of Hearing Aid Benefit,[182] provide a measure of disability, while the Client Orientated Scale of Improvement (COSI)[183] provides an individualized assessment of particular situations causing communication difficulties before and after amplification. The Glasgow Hearing Aid Benefit Profile[184,185] is a particularly useful and well-validated tool. A variety of listening circumstances are assessed and the data are pooled to provide a number of different scales encompassing initial disability, handicap, hearing aid use, hearing aid benefit, residual disability and satisfaction.[186]

Management of tinnitus

In the majority of cases, the treatment of tinnitus is symptomatic rather than curative as the underlying cause frequently cannot be established. As the mechanism of tinnitus is not fully understood, the treatment is often empirical and not based on scientific evidence. Moreover, the assessment of treatment is difficult as there are no established objective tinnitus measures, and the course of tinnitus is capricious, with fluctuations in loudness, pitch and duration.

Many therapies have been advocated and reported to be of benefit to some patients, but there is no single established treatment. In a small minority of tinnitus sufferers, in whom the causation can be established, specific treatment may result in a reduction of tinnitus. Surgical management of middle ear disorders, vascular disorders (such as an arterial loop within the internal auditory canal causing auditory nerve compression syndrome) glomus tumor, vascular aneurysms or arteriovenous malformations may alleviate the symptom.[187] Medical management of migraine, hyper- or hypo-thyroid dysfunction, diabetes or hypertension may also bring some improvement in the symptom.

Pharmacological interventions

The first drug to be tested in controlled clinical trials was lidocaine, but this could only be given intravenously and relieved tinnitus for 15 to 30 minutes. Taken orally, it is metabolized by the liver and has no effect on tinnitus.[188] An oral analog, tocainide, has been tried, but only one of 20 patients benefited, and most patients suffered unpleasant side effects.[189] Benzodiazepines such as alprazolam have been shown in a double-blind controlled trial to reduce tinnitus loudness,[190] but the adverse effects, particularly addiction, were noted. Dobie and Sullivan[191] studied the effect of the antidepressant nortriptyline and found that it effectively reduces depressive symptoms in patients with tinnitus and depression but has a questionable effect on the sensation of tinnitus. Fluoxetine has also been used in tinnitus management, but it has significant side effects, and therefore is not recommended.[192] Other drugs such as carbamazepine,[193] furosemide, antihistamines[194] and calcium channel blockers[195] have been used with very limited success.

In pursuit of effective tinnitus treatment, laser therapy has been used on the assumption that the heat produced will promote cochlear healing. In combination with *Ginkgo biloba* extract,[196] a 60% improvement was reported in the elimination of chronic tinnitus, but in a larger, better designed study,[197] no significant difference in the relief of tinnitus was observed.

Physical intervention

Electrical stimulation to suppress tinnitus in deaf patients has been used for more than 200 years. However, it has been established that DC currents cause tissue damage and therefore cannot be used on hearing patients, while AC stimulation is less effective.[198] With the development and increase in application of cochlear implants, the reduction of tinnitus in many profoundly deaf implanted patients has been observed.

Psychological intervention

The aim of psychological techniques is to develop strategies to cope with tinnitus and with the factors that tend to exacerbate it. Psychological treatment of tinnitus focuses on lowering the intrusiveness of the symptom by reducing tension through relaxation therapies[199] and changing the sufferer's attitude toward the tinnitus by cognitive therapy. This latter technique helps the patient to alter negative thoughts about tinnitus and shift his focus of attention away from the symptom.[200] The effectiveness of these forms of therapy has been positively assessed in clinical trials.[199,201]

Psychoacoustic interventions

Feldmann and Vernon[202,203] defined a formalized approach to tinnitus masking, basing the treatment on the rationale that it is easier psychologically to deal with an external sound than to cope with sound generated internally in the head. For the patient with normal hearing thresholds, a simple masker device generates white noise, the intensity of which can be controlled by the patient. For the patient with hearing loss, a combination device of hearing aid and masker may be used, or often a hearing aid alone may be beneficial. The amplification of soft environmental sounds, provided by a hearing aid, is sufficient to produce the masking effect. Controlled studies have shown that patients with tinnitus benefit from the use of maskers or hearing aids.[204,205]

In the late 1980s, Jastreboff developed a neurophysiological model of tinnitus,[206] which postulates the importance of activity within the brain in the perception of tinnitus and proposes that the signal generated in the cochlea is enhanced by the cerebral activity. A sound considered to be "nonthreatening" is only detected subcortically, but if it is considered to be "threatening" it is perceived and evaluated by auditory and other cortical areas. In the latter case, the limbic system becomes activated, producing strong emotional reactions that greatly interfere with the patient's quality of life. These reactions may stimulate the autonomic nervous system with its own systemic reactions, creating a "vicious circle" in which the lack of a rational explanation of tinnitus leads to a sustained negative reaction (Figure 174.18).

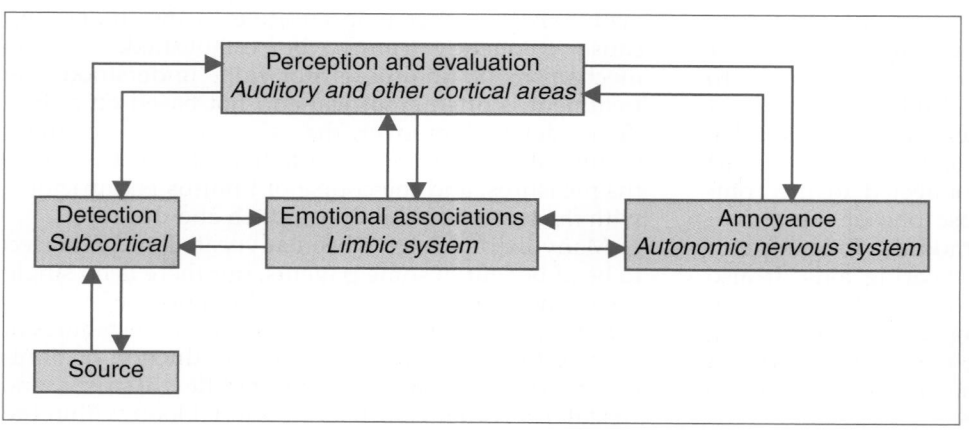

Figure 174.18   Diagram of neurophysiological model of tinnitus generation.
After Jastreboff[208]

The rationale of tinnitus retraining therapy (TRT) is based on this model.[192] Following an explanation of the hearing mechanism of generation of tinnitus, as well as the identification of the patient's reaction to tinnitus, an outline of the tinnitus retraining program is provided. Such therapy includes directive counseling and the use of a white noise generator or hearing aid if appropriate. This is proposed to lead to a reduction of autonomic arousal, and reduction of coexisting or resultant emotional disturbance. This approach is reported to allow the majority of tinnitus sufferers to benefit by removing tinnitus perception from awareness in a consistent and systematic manner. TRT is reported to benefit around 80% of tinnitus sufferers,[192,207] but there is no well-designed independent study to confirm these findings.

In conclusion, as in all branches of science and medicine, there have been major advances in understanding pathophysiology and developments of diagnostic tools and technological approaches to management of hearing disorders over the last two decades. This short chapter highlights the causes and management strategies available to limit disability. This is particularly important in the neurological patient with other sensory and/or motor disability/handicap.

References

1. World Health Organization. Report by the Director General. Prevention of Deafness and Hearing Impairment. A39/14. Geneva: World Health Organization, 1986

2. Coles RRA. Epidemiology of tinnitus: (1) Prevalence and (2) Demographic and clinical features. J Laryngol Otol Suppl 1984;9:(1) 7–15, (2) 195–202

3. Gill BS, Sharma DN. Level of hearing above 50 years of age. Indian J Otolaryngol 1967;19:112–118

4. Hinchcliffe R, King PF. Medicolegal aspects of tinnitus. I: Medicolegal position and current state of knowledge. J Aud Med 1992;i:38–58

5. Benjamin EE, Troost BT. Central auditory disorders. In: English GM, ed. Otolaryngology. Philadelphia: JB Lippincott, 1988:1–33

6. Parving A, Newton V. Editorial: Guidelines for description of inherited hearing loss. J Aud Med 1995;4:ii–v

7. World Health Organization. Report of the Interim Working Group on the Prevention of Deafness and Hearing Impairment Programme Planning. Geneva: World Health Organization, 1991

8. Sorri M, Mäki-Torkko E, Huttunen K, Muhli A. Unambiguous systems for describing audiogram configurations. J Aud Med (In press)

9. Estevill X, Govea N, Barcelo A, et al. Familial progressive sensorineural deafness is mainly due to the mtDNA A1555G mutation and is enhanced by treatment with aminoglycosides. Am J Hum Genet 1998; 62:27–35

10. Sill AM, Stick MJ, Prenger VL, et al. Genetic epidemiology study of hearing impairment. Am J Hum Genet 1994;54:149–153

11. Prezant TR, Agapian JV, Bohlman MC, et al. Mitochondrial ribosomal RNA mutation associated with both antibiotic-induced and non-syndromic deafness. Nat Genet 1993;4:289–294

12. Committee on Hearing and Equilibrium, the American Academy of Ophthalmology and Otolaryngology. Committee on Hearing and Equilibrium guidelines for diagnosis and evaluation of therapy in Ménière's disease. Otolaryngol Head Neck Surg 1995;113:181–185

13. Holgers K-M, Barrenäs M-L. The pathophysiology and assessment of tinnitus. In: Luxon LM, Furman JM, Martini A, Stephens SDG, eds. Textbook of Audiological Medicine.

14. Jastrehoff PJ. An animal model of tinitus: A decade of development. Am J Otol 1994;15:19–27

15. Ceranic B, Luxon LM. Disorders of the auditory system. In: Asbury A, McKhann G, McDonald WI, et al., eds. Diseases of the Nervous System. 3rd ed. Cambridge UK: Cambridge University Press. (In press)

16. Kemp DT. Stimulated acoustic emissions from within the human auditory system. J Acoust Soc Am 1978; 64:1386–1391

17. Penner MJ. An estimate of the prevalence of tinnitus caused by spontaneous otoacoustic emissions. Arch Otolaryngol Head and Neck Surg 1990;116:418–423

18. Møller AR. Pathophysiology of tinnitus. Ann Otol Rhinol Laryngol 1984;93:39–44

19. Bamford J, Davis A. Neonatal hearing screening: a step towards better services for children and families. Br J Audiol 1998;32:1–6

20. Hughes GB, Freedman MA, Haberkamp TJ, Guay ME. Sudden sensorineural hearing loss. Otolaryngol Clin North Am 1996;29:393–405

21. Mattox DE, Simmons FB. Natural history of sudden sensorineural hearing loss. Ann Otol Rhinol Laryngol 1977;86:463–480

22. Schuknecht HF. Pathology of the Ear. 1st ed. Cambridge MA: Harvard University Press, 1974

23. Hinchcliffe R. The age function of hearing—aspects of epidemiology. Acta Otolaryngol Suppl (Stockholm) 1991;476:7–11

24. Luxon LM, Cohen M. In: Kerr AG, ed. Scott Brown's Otolaryngology. 6th ed. Vol 2. Stephens SDG, ed. Adult Audiology. Oxford: Butterworth Heinemann, 1997

25. Musiek FE, Lee WW. Auditory middle and late potentials. In: Musiek FE, Rintelmann WF, eds. Contemporary Perspectives in Hearing Assessment. Boston: Allyn & Bacon, 1999

26. Jahn A. Infection and inflammation of the external ear. In: Ludman H, Wright T, eds. Diseases of the Ear. 6th ed. London: Arnold, 1998:306–318

27. Bojrab D, Bruderly T, Abdulrazzak Y. Otitis externa. Otolaryngol Clin North Am 1996;29(5):761–782

28. Hannley MT, Denneny JC, Holzer SS. Use of ototopical antibiotics in treating 3 common ear diseases. Otolaryngol Head Neck Surg 2000;122(6):934–940

29. Halpern MT, Palmer CS, Seidlin M. Treatment patterns for otitis externa. J Am Board Fam Pract 1999; 12(1):1–7

30. Brook I. Treatment of otitis externa in children. Paediatr Drugs 1999;1(4):283–289

31. Hawke M, Binghaur B, Stammberger H, Benjamin B, eds. Diagnostic Handbook of Otorhinolaryngology. London: Martin Dunitz, 1997:42

32. Klein JO. Management of otitis media: 2000 and beyond. Pediatr Infect Dis J 2000;19(4):383–387

33. Rosenfeld R. What to expect from medical therapy. In: Rosenfeld R, Bluestone C, eds. Evidence-based Otitis Media. Hamilton: BC Decker, 1999:207–222

34. Bluestone C, Dennis L. What to expect from surgical

therapy. *In:* Rosenfeld R, Bluestone C, eds. Evidence-based Otitis Media. Hamilton: BC Decker, 1999: 207–222

35. Burton M, Leighton S, Robson A, Russell JH. *In:* Colman's Diseases of the Ear, Nose and Throat. 15th ed. London: Churchill Livingstone, 2000:29–48

36. Austrian R, Howie VM, Ploussard JH. The bacteriology of pneumoccoccal otitis media. Johns Hopkins Med J 1977;141:104–111

37. Barenkamp SJ, Shurin PA, Marchant CD, et al. Do children with recurrent Haemophilus influenzae otitis media become infected with a new organism or reacquire the original strain? J Pediat 1984;105:533–537

38. Giebink S. Prevention. *In:* Rosenfeld R, Bluestone C, eds. Evidence-based Otitis Media. Hamilton: BC Decker, 1999:223–234

39. Dagan R, Muallem M, Melamed R, et al. Reduction of pneumococcal nasopharyngeal carriage in early infancy after immunisation with tetravalent pneumococcal vaccines conjugated to either tetanus toxoid or diphtheria toxoid. Pediatr Infect Dis J 1997;16: 1060–1064

40. Pitkaranta A, Virolainen A, Jero J, et al. Detection of rhinovirus, respiratory syncytial virus and coronavirus in acute otitis media by reverse transcriptase polymerase chain reaction. Pediatrics 1998;102:291–295

41. Cantekin EI, Mandel EM, Bluestone CD, et al. Lack of efficacy of a decongestant-antihistamine combination for otitis media with effusion in children. Results of a double blind, randomised trial. N Engl J Med 1983; 308:297–301

42. Rosenfeld RM, Post JC. Metanalysis of antibiotics for the treatment of otitis media with effusion. Otolaryngol Head Neck Surg 1992;106:378–386

43. The treatment of persistent glue ear in children. Effective Health Care Bulletin, School of Public Health, University of Leeds, Centre of Health Economics, University of York, Research Unit Royal College of Physicians, funded by Department of Health. November 1992, No. 4.

44. Graham MD, Goldsmith III MM. Infections of the ear. *In:* Lee KJ, ed. Essential Otolaryngology Head & Neck Surgery. 7th ed. Stamford, Connecticut: Appleton & Lange, 1999:673–710

45. Gebhart DE. Tympanostomy tube in the otitis media prone child. Laryngoscope 1981;91:849

46. Gates GAM, Muntz HR, Gaylis B. Adenoidectomy in otitis media. Ann Otol Rhinol Laryngol 1992;101:24–32

47. Paradise JL, Bluestone CD, Rogers KD, et al. Efficacy of adenoidectomy for recurrent otitis media in children treated previously with tympanostomy tube placement: Results of parallel randomised and nonrandomised trials. JAMA 1990;263:2066–2073

48. Downs MP, Jafek B, Wood RP II. Comprehensive treatment of children with recurrent serous otitis media. Otolaryngol Head Neck Surg 1981;89:658–665

49. Youngs RP. Epithelial migration in open mastoidectomy cavities. J Laryngol Otol 1995;109:286–290

50. Frootko N. Reconstruction of the middle ear. *In:* Booth Y, ed. Otology. Scott-Brown's Otolaryngology. 6th ed. Oxford: Butterworth-Heinemann, 1997:3/11/1–3/11/30

51. Robinson J. Reconstruction of the middle ear. *In:* Ludman H, Wright A, eds. Diseases of the Ear. 6th ed. London: Arnold, 1998:429–438

52. Graham MD, Lee KJ, Goldsmith III MM. Noninfectious disorders of the ear. *In:* Lee KJ, ed. Essential Otolaryngology Head & Neck Surgery. 7th ed. Stamford, Connecticut: Appleton & Lange, 1999:711–746

53. Burton MJ, Niparko J, Johansson C, Tjellstrom A. Titanium-anchored prostheses in otology. Otolaryngol Clin North Am 1996;29:301–310

54. Haberkamp TJ, Tanyeri M. Management of idiopathic sensorineural hearing loss. Am J Otol 1999;20(5): 587–593

55. Fetterman BL, Sanders JE, Luxford WM. Prognosis and treatment of sudden sensorineural hearing loss. Am J Otol 1996;17:529–536

56. Kallinen J, Kuttila K, Aitasalo K, Grenman R. Effect of carbogen inhalation on peripheral tissue perfusion and oxygenation in patients suffering from sudden hearing loss. Ann Otol Rhinol Laryngol 1999;108(10):944–947

57. Rahko T, Kotti V. Comparison of carbogen inhalation and intravenous heparin infusion therapies in idiopathic sudden sensorineural hearing loss. Acta Otolaryngol Suppl (Stockholm)1997;529:86–87

58. Tan J, Tange RA, Dreschler WA, et al. Long-term effect of hyperbaric oxygenation treatment on chronic distressing tinnitus. Scan Audiol 1999;28(2):91–96

59. Wattel F, Mathieu D, Neviere R. Indications for hyperbaric oxygen therapy. Organisation of the treatment unit. Training of personnel. Bull Acad Natl Med 1996;180(5):949–963

60. Lamm H. The influence of hyperbaric oxygen therapy on tinnitus and hearing loss in acute and chronic inner ear damage. Oto Rhinol Laryngol Nova 1995; 5/3–4:161–165

61. Kanemaru S, Fukushima H, Nakamura H, et al. Alfainterferon for the treatment of idiopathic sudden sensorineural hearing loss. Eur Arch Otolaryngol 1997;254(30):156–162

62. Hughes GB, Freedman MA, Haberkamp TJ, Guay ME. Sudden sensorineural hearing loss. Otolaryngol Clin North Am 1996;29:393–405

63. Veldman JE. Immune mediated sensorineural hearing loss with or without endolymphatic hydrops, a clinical and experimental approach. Ann NY Acad Sci 1997; 830:179–186

64. Stokroos RJ, Albers FW, Schirm J. Therapy of sudden sensorineural hearing loss. Antiviral treatment of experimental herpes simplex virus infection of the inner ear. Ann Otol Rhinol Laryngol 1999;108(5):423–428

65. Ochi K, Mitsui M, Watanabe S, et al. The effects of high dose of steroid therapy on sudden deafness. Nippon Jibiinkoka Gakkai Kaiho 1998;101(11):1311–1315

66. Wilson WR, Byl FM, Laird N. The efficacy of steroids in the treatment of idiopathic sudden hearing loss. Arch Otolaryngol 1980;106:772–776

67. Russolo M, Bianchi M. Treatment of sudden hearing loss. Acta Otolaryngol Ital 1997;17(5):319–324

68. Redleaf MI, Bauer CA, Gantz BJ, et al. Diatrizoate and dextran treatment of sudden sensorineural hearing loss. Am J Otol 1995;16(3):295–303

69. Probst R, Tschhopp K, Ludin E, et al. A randomised, double-blind placebo controlled study of dextran-pentoxifylline medication in acute acoustic trauma and sudden hearing loss. Acta Otolaryngol 1992;112(3): 435–443

70. Wilkins SA, Mattox DE, Lyles E. Evaluation of a "shotgun" regimen for sudden hearing loss. Otolaryngol Head Neck Surg 1987;97:474–480

71. Shikowitz MJ. Sudden sensorineural hearing loss. Med Clin North Am 1991;75:1239–1250

72. Schwiefurth JM, Parnes SM, Very M. Current concepts in the diagnosis and treatment of sudden sensorineural hearing loss. Eur Arch Otorhinolaryngol 1996;253:117–121

73. O'Connor AF, Otosclerosis. *In:* Ludman H, Wright T, eds. Diseases of the Ear. 6th ed. London: Arnold, 1998:453–462

74. Brookes GB. Inner ear disorders. *In:* Scadding GK. ed. Immunology of ENT Disorders. Dordrecht: Kluwer Academic Publishers, 1994:169–198

75. Brandt T. Ménière's disease. *In:* Brandt T, ed. Vertigo Its Multisensory Syndromes. 2nd ed. London: Springer, 1999:90–93

76. Ruckenstein MJ, Rutka JA, Hawke M. The treatment of Ménière's disease: Torok revisited. Laryngoscope 1991;101:211

77. Slattery W, Fayad J. Medical treatment of Ménière's disease. Otolaryngol Clin North Am 1997;30(6):1027–1038

78. Ödkvist LM, Arlinger S, Billermark E, et al. Effects of therapeutics middle ear pressure changes in patients with Ménière's disease. *In:* Ménière's Disease 1999 Update Proceedings of the 4th International Symposium on Ménière's disease. Paris, April 1999:597–603

79. Claes J, Van de Heyning PH. Medical treatment of Ménière's disease; a review of literature. Acta Otolaryngol Suppl (Stockholm) 1997;526:37–42

80. Klockhoff I, Lindblom U. Ménière's disease and hydrochlorothiazide (Dichlotride). A critical analysis of symptoms and therapeutic effects. Acta Otolaryngol (Stockholm)1967;63:347–350

81. James A, Burton M. Betahistine for Ménière's Disease: a systematic review. *In:* Ménière's Disease 1999 Update Proceedings of the 4th International Symposium on Ménière's Disease. Paris, April 1999:719–726

82. Schmidt JTH, Huizing EH. The clinical drug trial in Ménière's disease. Acta Otolaryngol Suppl (Stockholm) 1992;497:1–189

83. Bertrand RA. Modification of the vestibular function with Betahistine HCL. Laryngoscope 1971;81:889–898

84. Unemoto H, Sasa M, Takaori S, et al. Inhibitory effect of betahistine on polysynaptic neurons in the lateral vestibular nucleus. Arch Otolaryngol 1982;236:229–236

85. Mollfat D, Ballagh R. Ménière's disease. *In:* Booth Y, ed. Scott-Brown's Otolaryngology. 6th ed. Oxford: Butterworth-Heinemann, 1997:3/19/1–3/19/50

86. Hirsch B, Kamerer DL. Role of chemical labyrinthectomy in the treatment of Ménière's disease. Otolaryngol Clin North Am 1997;30(6):1039–1050

87. Bergenius J, Odquist LM. Transtympanic aminoglycosides treatment of Ménière's Disease. *In:* Baloh RW, Halmagyi GM, eds. Disorders of the Vestibular System. New York: Oxford University Press, 1996:575–582

88. Monsell EM, Balkany TA, Gates GA, et al. Guidelines of the Committee on Hearing and Equilibrium. Committee on Hearing and Equilibrium guidelines for the diagnosis and evaluation of therapy in Ménière's Disease. Otolaryngol Head Neck Surg 1995;113:181–185

89. Herdman S, Whitney S. Treatment of vestibular hypofunction. *In:* Herdman S, ed. Vestibular Rehabilitation. 2nd ed. Philadelphia: Davis Co., 2000:387–394

90. Goldstein D, Stephens SDG. Audiological rehabilitation: management model. Audiology 1981;20:432–452

91. World Health Organization. International Classification of Impairments. Disabilities and Handicaps. Geneva: WHO, 1980

92. Volanthen A. Basic components of a hearing instrument. *In:* Volanthen A, ed. Hearing Instrument Technology for the Hearing Healthcare Professional. San Diego: Singular Publishing Group, 1995:7–9

93. De Jonge R. Selecting and verifying hearing aid fittings for symmetrical hearing loss. *In:* Valente M, ed. Strategies for Selecting and Verifying Hearing Aid Fittings. New York: Thieme Medical Publishers, 1994:180–206

94. Dermody P, Byrne D. Loudness summation with binaural hearing aids. Hearing Instruments 1975;26:22–23

95. Tate M. Selection and fitting. *In:* Tate M, ed. Principles of Hearing Aid Technology. London: Chapman and Hall, 1994:155–172

96. Sweetow R. Selection and fitting of programmable and digital hearing aids. *In:* Valente M, Horford-Dunn H, Roeser R, eds. Audiology Treatment. New York: Thieme Medical Publishers, 2000:433–458

97. Volanthen A. Hearing instrument types. *In:* Volanthen A, ed. Hearing Instrument Technology for the Hearing Healthcare Professional, San Diego: Singular Publishing Group, 1995:10–20

98. Pollack MC. Operational overview. *In:* Pollack MC, ed. Amplification for the Hearing-Impaired. 3rd ed. Orlando: Grune & Stratton, 1988:24–37

99. Venema T. The many faces of compression. *In:* Venema T, ed. Compression for Clinicians. San Diego: Singular Publishing Group, 1998:59–83

100. Dillon H. Compression? Yes, but for low or high frequencies, for low or high intensities and for what response time? Ear Hear 1996;17:287–307

101. Verschuure J, Maas AJ, Stikvoort E, et al. Compression and its effects on speech signal. Ear Hear 1996;17:62–175

102. Engebretson AM, Morley FF, Popelka GR. Development of an ear-level digital hearing aid and computer-assisted fitting procedure. An interim report. J Rehabil Res Dev 1987;24(4):55–64

103. Sammeth CA. Current availability of digital and hybrid hearing aids. Sem Hear 1990;11(1):91–100

104. Sammeth CA. Hearing instruments from vacuum tubes to digital microchips. Hearing instruments. J Rehabil Res Dev 1989;40(10):9–12

105. Moore B. Physiological aspects of cochlear hearing loss. *In:* Moore B, ed. Cochlear Hearing Loss. London: Whurr Publishers, 1998:1–39

106. Moore B. Perceptual consequences of cochlear hearing loss and their implications for the design of hearing aids. Ear Hear 1996;17:133–161

107. Gatehouse S. Hearing aids. *In:* Booth Y, ed. Scott-Brown's Otolaryngology. 6th ed. Oxford: Butterworth Heinemann, 1997:2/14/1–2/14/27

108. Schweitzer C. It's about numbers. A primer on the digitization of hearing aids. The Hearing Journal 1998;51(11):15–25

109. Preves D. Current and future applications of digital hearing aid technology. *In:* Sandlin R, ed. Understanding Digitally Programmable Hearing Aids. London: Allyn Bacon, 1994:275–308

110. Cudahy E, Levitt H. Digital hearing aids: A historical perspective. *In:* Sandlin R, ed. Understanding Digitally Programmable Hearing Aids. London: Allyn Bacon, 1994:1–14

111. Holube J, Velde TH. DSP Hearing instruments. *In:* Sandlin R, ed. Textbook of Hearing Aid Amplification. 2nd ed. San Diego: Singular Publishing Group, 2000:285–322

112. Sweetow R. Selection considerations for digital signal processing hearing aids. The Hearing Journal 1998;51:11

113. Fabry D. Do we really need digital hearing aids? The Hearing Journal 1998;151:11

114. Arlinger S, Billemark E, Oberg M, et al. Clinical trial of

a digital hearing aid. Scand Audiol 1998;27:51–61

115. Valente M, Fabry DA, Potts LG, Sandlin RE. Comparing the performance of the Widex sensor digital hearing aid with analog hearing aids. J Am Acad Audiol 1998;9:342–360

116. Boymans M, Dreschler WA, Schoneveld P, Verschuure H. Clinical evaluation of a full digital in-the-ear hearing aid. Audiology 1999;38:99–108

117. Ringdhal A, Magnusson L, Edberg P, Thelin L. Clinical evaluation of a digital power instrument. The Hearing Review 2000;3:59–64

118. National Institute for Clinical Excellence. Guidance on Hearing Aid Technology. Technology Appraisal Guidance No. 8. London: NICE, 2000

119. Venema T. The cochlea, hair cells and compression. In: Venema T, ed. Compression for Clinicians. San Diego: Singular Publishing Group, 1998:1–16

120. Killion M. Talking hair cells. What they have to say about hearing aids. In: Berlin CJ, ed. Hair Cells and Hearing Aids. San Diego: Singular Publishing Group, 1996:125–172

121. Villchur E. A different approach to the noise problem of the hearing impaired. In: Berlin J, Jensen GR, eds. Recent Developments in Hearing Aid Technology. Proceedings of the 15th Danavox Symposium. Danavox Jubilee Foundation Taastrup, Denmark, 1993:69–80

122. British Society of Audiology Recommended Procedures for Uncomfortable Loudness Level. Br J Audiol 1987;21–231

123. Villchur E. Multichannel compression in hearing aids. In: Berlin CJ, ed. Hair Cells and Hearing Aids. San Diego: Singular Publishing Group, 1996:113–124

124. Swan JRC, Gatehouse S. Optimum side for fitting a monaural hearing aid. Measured benefit. Br J Audiol 1987;21:67–71

125. Sandlin R. Fitting binaural amplification to asymmetric hearing loss. In: Valente M, ed. Strategies for Selecting and Verifying Hearing Aid Fittings. New York: Thieme Medical Publishers, 1994:207–222

126. Humes L, Halling D. Overview, rationale and comparison of suprathreshold based gain prescription methods. In: Valente M, ed. Strategies for Selecting and Verifying Hearing Aid Fittings. New York: Thieme Medical Publishers, 1994:19–37

127. Hearing Aid Audiology Group, British Society of Audiology. Making the earmould. In: Haltby M, ed. The Earmould, Current Practice and Technology. Reading: British Society of Audiology, 1984:19–21

128. Kuk F, Hosford-Dunn H, Ross JR, eds. Audiology Treatment. New York: Thieme Medical Publishers, 2000:261–290

129. Staab WJ. Hearing aid selection—an overview. In: Sandlin R, ed. Textbook of Hearing Aid Amplification. 2nd ed. San Diego: Singular Publishing Group, 2000: 55–136

130. Sullivan R. Customs canal and conche hearing instruments, a real ear comparison. Hearing Instrument, 1989;40(4):29–32, 60

131. Chute P, Nevins M. Cochlear implants in children. In: Valente M, Hosford-Dunn H, Roeser R, eds. Audiology Treatment. New York: Thieme Medical, 2000; 511–535

132. Clark G. Cochlear implants. In: Ludman H, Wright T, eds. Diseases of the Ear. 6th ed. London: Arnold, 1998: 149–163

133. Cooper H. Selection of candidates for cochlear implantation—an overview. In: Cooper H, ed. Cochlear

Implants, A Practical Guide. London: Whurr Publishers, 1991:92–100

134. Holden LK, Binzer SM, Skinner MW, Juelich MF. Benefit provided by multi-electrode intracochlear implant to a prelinguistically deaf adult. Missouri Med 1991;88(3):143–148

135. Miyamoto RT, Robbins AM, Osberger MJ. Cochlear implants. In: Harker LA, ed. Otolaryngology, Head and Neck Surgery 2nd ed. St. Louis Mo: Mosby-Year Book, 1993;4:3142–3151

136. Shelton W, Luxford WM, Tonokawa L, et al. The narrow internal auditory canal in children, A contraindication to cochlear implant. Otolaryngol Head Neck Surg 1989;100:227–231

137. Shannon RV. Cochlear implants: What have we learned and where are going? Semin Hear 1996; 17:403–415

138. Beiter AL, Shallop JK. Cochlear implants, past, present and future. In: Estabrooks W, ed. Cochlear Implants in Kids. Washington DC: Alexander Graham Bell Association, 1998;3–29

139. Wilson B. Strategies for representing speech information with cochlear implants. In: Nipaiko J, Kirk K, Mellon N, et al., eds. Cochlear Implants. Principles and Practice. Philadelphia: Lippincott Williams & Wilkins, 2000;129–172

140. Osberger MJ, Koch DB. Cochlear implants. In: Sandlin RE, ed. Textbook of Hearing Aid Amplification. 2nd ed. San Diego: Singular Publishing Group, 1994: 673–698

141. Geier L, Barker M, Fisher L, Opie J. The effect of long term deafness on speech recognition in postlingually deafened adults Clarion cochlear implant users. Ann Otol Rhinol Laryngol 1999;108(177):80–83

142. Tyler RS, Summerfield AQ. Cochlear implantation: Relationship with research on auditory deprivation and acclimatization. Ear Hear 1996;17(3):38–50

143. Bollard PM, Chute PM, Popp A, Parisier SC. Specific language growth in young children using the Clarion cochlear implants. Ann Otol Rhinol Laryngol 1999;108(177):119–123

144. Robbins AM, Bollard PM, Green J. Language development in children implanted with the Clarion Cochlear Implant. Ann Otol Rhinol Laryngol 1999; 108(177):113–118

145. Francis HW, Koch MW, Wyatt R, Niparko JK. Trends in educational placement and cost-benefit considerations in children with cochlear implants. Arch Otolaryngol Head Neck Surg 1999;125:499–505

146. Niparko J, Cheng A, Francis H. Outcomes of cochlear implantation: Assessment of quality of life impact and economic evaluation of the benefits of the cochlear implant in relation to costs. In: Niparko J, Kirk K, Mellon N, et al., eds. Cochlear Implants Principles and Practices. Philadelphia: Lippincott Williams and Wilkins, 2000;269–290

147. Miyamoto R, Wong D, Pisoni D, et al. Positron emission tomography in cochlear implant and auditory brain stem implant recipients. Am Otol 1999; 20: 596–601

148. Tjellstrom A, Granstrom G. One stage procedure to establish osseointegration: a zero to five years follow-up report. J Laryngol Otol 1995;109(7):593–598

149. Powell RH, Burrell SP, Cooper HR, Proops DW. The Birmingham bone anchored hearing aid programme: paediatric experience and results. J Laryngol Otol Suppl 1996;21:21–29

150. Federspil P, Kurt P, Koch A. [Bone-anchored epitheses

and audioprostheses: 4 years' experience with the Branemark system in Germany]. Rev Laryngol Otol Rhinol (Bord) 1992;113(5):431–437

151. Hakansson B, Liden G, Tjellstrom A, et al. Ten years of experience with the Swedish bone-anchored hearing system. Ann Otol Rhinol Laryngol Suppl 1990;151: 1–16

152. Portmann D, Bourdin M. Bone anchored hearing aid: The Bordeaux experience. Rev Laryngol Otol Rhinol (Bord) 1995;116(4):299–300

153. Wazen JJ, Caruso M, Tjellsatrom A. Long term results with the titanium bone-anchored hearing aid: the US experience. Am J Otol 1998;19(6):737–741

154. Van der Pouw KT, Snik AF, Cremers CW. Audiometric results of bilateral bone-anchored hearing aid application in patients with bilateral congenital aural atresia. Laryngoscope 1998;108(4 Pt 1):548–553

155. Granstrom G, Tjellstrom A. The bone-anchored hearing aid (BAHA) in children with auricular malformations. Ear Nose Throat J 1997;76(4):238–247

156. Snik AF, Mylanus EA, Cremers CW. Bone anchored hearing aids in patients with sensorineural hearing loss and persistent otitis externa. Clin Otolaryngol 1995;20(1):31–35

157. Macnamara M, Phillips D, Proops DW. The bone anchored hearing aid (BAHA) in chronic suppurative otitis media (CSOM). J Laryngol Otol Suppl 1996;21: 38–40

158. Burrell SP, Cooper HC, Proops DW. The bone anchored hearing aid—the third option for otosclerosis. J Laryngol Otol Suppl 1996;21:31–37

159. Van der Pouw CT, Mylanus EA, Cremers CW. Percutaneous implants in the temporal bone for securing a bone conductor: surgical methods and results. Ann Otol Rhinol Laryngol 1999;108(6):532–536

160. Ringdahl A, Israelsson B, Caprin L. Paired comparisons between the Classic 300 bone-anchored and conventional bone-conduction hearing aids in terms of sound quality and speech intelligibility. Br J Audiol 1995;29(6):299–307

161. Carlsson P, Hakansson B, Rosenhall U, Tjellstrom A. A speech-to-noise ratio test with the bone-anchored hearing aid: a comparative study. Otolaryngol Head Neck Surg 1986;94(4):421–426

162. Mylanus EA, Snik AF, Cremers CW. Patients' opinions of bone-anchored vs conventional hearing aids. Arch Otolaryngol Head Neck Surg 1995;121(4):421–425

163. Tono T, Inaba J, Takenaka M, et al. Clinical experiences and post operative results with partially implantable middle ear implant. Nippon Jibiinkoka Gakkai Kaiho 1999;102(6):835–845

164. Gyo K, Goode RL. Measurement of stapes vibration driven by the ceramic vibrator of a middle ear implant—human temporal bone experiments. In: Suzuki J, ed. Middle Ear Implant: Implantable Hearing Aids: Advances in Audiology. Basel: Karger AG, 1988;4:107–116

165. Crandell C, Smaldino J. Assistive technologies for the hearing impaired. In: Sandlin R, ed. Textbook of Hearing Aid Amplification. 2nd ed. San Diego: Singular Publishing Group, 1999:643–672

166. McCandless G. Overview and rationale of threshold based hearing aid selection procedures. In: Valente M, ed. Strategies for Selecting and Verifying Hearing Aid fittings. New York: Thieme Medical Publishers, 1994:1–8

167. Lybarger S. Simplified Fitting System for Hearing Aids. Canonsburg PA: Radioear Corporation, 1963

168. Byrne D, Dillon H. The National Acoustic Laboratories (NAL) new procedure for selecting the gain and frequency response of a hearing aid. Ear Hear 1986; 7:257–265

169. Byrne D, Parkinson A, Newall P. Modified hearing selection procedures for severe/profound hearing losses. In: Studebaker GA, Bess FH, Beck NL, eds. Vanderbilt Hearing Aid Report. 11 Parkton MD: York Press, 1991:295–300

170. Berger K, Hagberg E, Rane R. Prescription of Hearing Aids: Rationale Procedures and Results. 5th ed. Kent: Herald Publishing House, 1989

171. McCandless GA, Lyregaard PE. Prescription of Gain/Output (PoGO) for hearing aids. Hearing Instruments 1983;35:16–21

172. Schwartz DM, Lyregaard PE, Lundh P. Hearing aid selection for severe-to-profound hearing loss. Hearing Journal 1988;41:13–17

173. Gitles TC, Niquette PP. FIG 6 in ten. Hearing Review 1995;2:28–30

174. Seewald RC, Cornelisse LE, Ramji KV, et al. DSL 4.1 for windows. A software implementation of the desired sensation level method for fitting linear gain and wide dynamic range compression-hearing instruments. London, Ont: Hearing Healthcare Research Unit, Department of Communicative Disorders, University of Western Ontario, 1997

175. Sandlin R. Observations and future considerations. In: Sandlin R, ed. Textbook of Hearing Aid Amplification. 2nd ed. San Diego: Singular Publishing Group, 1999: 727–733

176. Humes LE. Evolution of prescriptive fitting approaches. Am Audiol 1996;5(2):19–23

177. Revit L. Using coupler tests in the fitting of hearing aids. In: Valente M, ed. Strategies for Selecting and Verifying Hearing Aid Fittings. New York: Thieme Medical Publishers, 1994;6:4–87

178. Tecca J. Use of real ear measurements to verify hearing aid fittings. In: Valente M, ed. Strategies for Selecting and Verifying Hearing Aid Fittings. New York: Thieme Medical Publishers, 1994:88–107

179. Fabry D, Schum D. The role of subjective measurement techniques in hearing aid fittings. In: Valente M, ed. Strategies for Selecting and Verifying Hearing Aid Fittings. New York: Thieme Medical Publishers, 1994: 136–155

180. Beattie RC, Edgerton BJ. Reliability of monosyllabic discrimination tests in white noise for differentiating among hearing aids. J Speech Hear Disord 1976;41: 464–476

181. Jerger J, Hayes D. Hearing aid evaluation. Arch Otolaryngol 1976;102:214–225

182. Cox RM, Alexander GC. The abbreviated profile of hearing aid benefit. Ear Hear 1995;16:176–183

183. Dillon H, James AM, Ginis J. Client Orientated Scale of Improvement (COSI) and its relationship to several other measures of benefits and satisfaction provided by the hearing aids. J Am Acad Audiol 1997;8:27–43

184. Gatehouse S. Glasgow Hearing Aid Benefit Profile and derivation and validation of client centred outcome measure for hearing aid services. J Am Acad Audiol 1999;10:80–103

185. Gatehouse S. A self-report outcome measure for the evaluation of hearing aid fittings and services. Health Bull (Edinb) 1999;57(6):424–436

186. Gatehouse S. The Glasgow Hearing Aid Benefit Profile and what it measures and how to use it. The Hearing Journal 2000;53(3):10–18

187. Storper J, Glasscock M. Tumours of the middle ear and skull base. *In:* Ludman H, Wright T, eds. Diseases of the Ear. 6th ed. London: Arnold, 1998:463–480

188. Den Hartigh J, Hilders CG, Schoemaker RC, et al. Tinnitus suppression by intravenous lidocaine in relation to its plasma concentration. Clin Pharmacol Ther 1993;54:415–420

189. Brummett R. Are there any safe and effective drugs available to treat my tinnitus? Vernon J, ed. Tinnitus, Treatment and Relief. Boston: Allyn & Bacon, 1998:34–41

190. Johnson RM, Brummett R, Schleuning A. Use of Alprazolam for relief of tinnitus. A double-blind study. Arch Otolaryngol Head Neck Surg 1993;119:842–845

191. Dobie R, Sullivan M. Antidepressant drugs and tinnitus. *In:* Vernon J, ed. Tinnitus Treatment and Relief. Boston: Allyn & Bacon, 1998:43–51

192. Hazell J. Management of tinnitus. *In:* Ludman H, Wright T, eds. Diseases of the Ear. 6th ed. London: Arnold, Hodder Headline Group, 1998:203–215

193. Murai K, Tyler RS, Harker LD, Stouffer JC. Review of pharmacologic treatment of tinnitus. Am J Otol 1992;13:454–464

194. Guth PS, Risey J, Amedee R. Drug treatment for tinnitus at Tuhane University School of Medicine. *In:* Vernon J, ed. Tinnitus, Treatment and Relief. Boston: Allyn & Bacon, 1998:52–57

195. Denk DM, Felix D, Brix R, Ehrenberger K. Tinnitus treatment with transmitter antagonists. *In:* Vernon J, ed. Tinnitus Treatment and Relief. Boston: Allyn & Bacon, 1998:60–67

196. Witt U, Felix C. Selektive photobiochemotherapie in der kombination laser und gingko pflanzenextrakt nach der methode Witt. Neve alternativre moglichkeit bei innenohrsstorungen. Informations material der Firma Felas Lasers GmbH Steinredder 1; 2409. Scharbentz Germany, 1989

197. Walger M, Von Wedel H, Calero L, Hoenen S. Effectiveness of low-power-laser and gingko therapy in patients with chronic tinnitus. *In:* Reich G, Vernon J, eds. Proceedings of the Fifth International Tinnitus Seminar (Portland), 1995:99–100

198. Staller S. Suppression of tinnitus with electrical stimulation. *In:* Vernon J, ed. Tinnitus: Treatment and Relief. Boston: Allyn & Bacon, 1998:77–90

199. McKenna L. Psychological treatment for tinnitus. *In:* Vernon J, ed. Tinnitus: Treatment and Relief. Boston: Allyn & Bacon, 1998:140–155

200. Henry J, Wilson P. Psychological treatments for tinnitus. *In:* Vernon J, ed. Tinnitus: Treatment and Relief. Boston: Allyn & Bacon, 1998:99–115

201. Kitajima K, Yamana T, Uchida K, Kitahara M. Biofeedback training for tinnitus control. *In:* Vernon J, ed. Tinnitus: Treatment and Relief. Boston: Allyn & Bacon, 1998:131–139

202. Schleunling AJ, Johnson RM, Vernon JA. Evaluation of a tinnitus masking programme, a follow-up study of 598 patients. Ear Hear 1980;1:71–74

203. Vernon J. Attempts to relieve tinnitus. J Am Acad Audiol 1977;2:124–131

204. Johnson R. The masking of tinnitus. *In:* Vernon J, ed. Tinnitus: Treatment and Relief. Boston: Allyn & Bacon, 1998:164–174

205. Von Wedel S. Tinnitus masking with tinnitus maskers and hearing aids: A longitudinal study of efficacy from 1987 to 1993. *In:* Vernon J, ed. Tinnitus: Treatment and Relief. Boston: Allyn & Bacon, 1998:187–192

206. Jastreboff PJ. Phantom auditory perception (tinnitus), mechanism of generation and perception. Neurosci Res 1990;8:221–254

207. Jastreboff P, Hazell J. Treatment of tinnitus based on neurophysiological model. *In:* Vernon J, ed. Tinnitus: Treatment and Relief. Boston: Allyn & Bacon, 1998:201–216

208. Hazell J. Incidence classification and models of tinnitus. *In:* Ludman H, Wright T, eds. Diseases of the Ear. 6th edn. London: Arnold, Hodder Headline Group, 1998:203–215

175 Disorders of the Glossopharyngeal, Vagus, Accessory, and Hypoglossal Nerves

Colin Chalk

Overview

The ninth, tenth, and twelfth cranial nerves form a natural subset of the cranial nerves, as they share several basic characteristics: origin in the medulla, exit from the base of the skull via common pathways, and integration of function in activities such as swallowing and speech. The eleventh nerve is functionally distinct, but it is frequently involved by lesions affecting the other three lower cranial nerves, as the four nerves are closely related anatomically. Although the discussion following considers the nerves and their disorders individually, clinical reality is often not so tidy. Owing to their anatomical proximity, lesions involving the lower cranial nerves affect multiple nerves at least as often as the individual nerves. A related point is that involvement of more than one of the lower cranial nerves is usually necessary to produce some of the clinical deficits characteristic of these nerves. Some of these clinical syndromes also have a host of other neurological and non-neurological causes. This especially true of dysphagia, which is discussed as a separate section at the end of this chapter.

Glossopharyngeal nerve

Anatomy

The ninth cranial nerve is primarily sensory, carrying somatic sensation from the pharynx, tonsils and posterior tongue, taste information from the posterior third of the tongue, and information from baroreceptors involved in cardiovascular reflexes. Cell bodies of axons carrying somatic sensation and taste are in the superior and inferior glossopharyngeal ganglia, seen as two small swellings on the portion of the nerve traversing the jugular foramen. The central processes of these cells synapse in the nucleus of the solitary tract (taste) and in the spinal trigeminal nucleus (somatic sensation). There is also an efferent component of the ninth nerve, consisting of fibers from parasympathetic neurons in the inferior salivatory nucleus, destined ultimately for the parotid gland, and fibers from motor neurons in the nucleus ambiguous which innervate stylopharyngeus. The ninth nerve leaves the ventrolateral surface of the medulla as a group of rootlets in the groove between the olive and inferior cerebellar peduncle, then runs forward and laterally to the jugular foramen, through which it exits the

skull. In the neck, the nerve descends anterior to the internal carotid artery, curves forward as it innervates stylopharyngeus, pierces the superior and middle constrictors of the pharynx, and is distributed to tonsils, tongue, and pharynx.

Pathophysiology

The glossopharyngeal nerve may be affected by mass lesions (e.g. schwannoma) in the cerebellopontine angle, by lesions of the jugular foramen, or along its course in the neck. Jugular foramen lesions (which include glomus tumors, metastases, chordomas, basal skull fractures, and schwannomas) will also involve the vagus and accessory nerves (Vernet syndrome; a summary of the several eponymous syndromes involving the lower cranial nerves is given in Table 175.1). In the retropharynx and neck the ninth nerve may be injured by nasopharyngeal and other head and neck cancers, abscesses, trauma, or surgery. Such pathologies often involve all four lower cranial nerves (Collet–Sicard syndrome), and may include the adjacent sympathetic chain (Villaret syndrome).

Clinical features

A unilateral ninth nerve palsy produces ipsilateral loss of pharyngeal sensation, and may cause some mild dysphagia. More significant swallowing difficulties generally imply concomitant vagus nerve involvement, or bilateral lesions. It is usually possible to demonstrate impaired pharyngeal sensation on examination, or at least observe that no gag reflex occurs with stimulation of the ipsilateral pharyngeal tonsil. Patients are usually unaware of unilateral loss of pharyngeal taste sensation or impaired parotid gland secretion. Blood pressure abnormalities due to impaired baroreflexes generally occur only with bilateral ninth nerve lesions, although sustained hypertension after unilateral glossopharyngeal section has been described.[1] Lesions affecting the ninth nerve usually involve the vagus nerve also, because of the close proximity of the two nerves.

Glossopharyngeal neuralgia

Glossopharyngeal neuralgia (GPN) is characterized by paroxysmal throat and ear pain, frequently triggered by swallowing. GPN bears many similarities to trigeminal neuralgia.

Table 175.1   Summary of the eponymous syndromes involving the lower cranial nerves

Eponym	Cranial nerves involved	Site of lesion
Vernet	9, 10, 11	Jugular foramen
Schmidt	10, 11	Intracranial or inferior margin of jugular foramen
Hughlings Jackson	10, 11, 12	Intracranial
Collet–Sicard	9, 10, 11, 12	Retroparotid or retropharyngeal space (extracranial)
Villaret	9, 10, 11, 12 + Horner's syndrome	Retroparotid or retropharyngeal space (extracranial)
Tapia	10, 12 (sometimes includes 11 and Horner's syndrome)	High in the neck
Garcin (hemibase syndrome)	All cranial nerves on one side	Base of skull (extensive)

Epidemiology

GPN is a rare condition. Its annual incidence has been estimated to be 0.7 per 100 000, which is 6 to 100 times less than that of trigeminal neuralgia. GPN may also be a milder disease than trigeminal neuralgia. Prolonged or permanent remission of symptoms in GPN appears to be common (experienced by two thirds of patients in the one population-based study), and many patients seem able to tolerate the pain of GPN without any intervention other than explanation.[2]

Pathophysiology

In most patients with GPN no macroscopic lesion can be found, though there are case reports of various unusual causes (e.g. nerve rootlet neuroma,[3] posterior fossa arteriovenous malformation,[4] multiple sclerosis[5]).

Etiology

A popular hypothesis to explain GPN, analogous to trigeminal neuralgia, is chronic mechanical injury of the nerve by ectatic arteriolar loops, usually of the posterior inferior cerebellar artery. The high success rate of microvascular decompression surgical procedures argues in favor of the vascular loop hypothesis, although Adams has argued that surgical trauma to the nerve, rather than removal of vascular loops, is the basis of the procedure's success.[6]

Clinical features

The distribution of pain in GPN corresponds to the sensory territory of the ninth nerve. Pain is usually unilateral, but may be bilateral in up to one quarter of patients. The pain is brief and intense, and, like trigeminal neuralgia, often has an electric shock-like quality. Rarely, the paroxysms of pain are accompanied by paroxysmal hyperactivity in parasympathetic cardioinhibitory fibers. This results in bradycardia or hypotension, and recurrent syncope may be the patient's presenting symptom (exceptionally, there is little or no pain, and diagnosis is difficult).[7]

Treatment

As GPN is rare, it has been difficult to evaluate treatments rigorously. Most treatments have developed from those useful for trigeminal neuralgia, which bears many clinical similarities to GPN. Carbamazepine is the mainstay of medical treatment for trigeminal neuralgia, and its efficacy in GPN has been appreciated since the 1960s.[8] Although the quality of evidence of efficacy is almost entirely grade C, there is little dispute that carbamazepine is efficacious. Good data on the long term response of GPN to carbamazepine are scarce. Among 217 cases seen at Mayo Clinic from 1922 to 1977, 20 were treated with carbamazepine alone. Sustained relief resulted in 7 (4 complete, 3 partial), good but short-lived relief in 6, and no response in 7.[9] As many patients in this series were referred for surgery, the cohort likely overrepresents the failure rate of medical therapy.

Several alternatives to carbamazepine exist. Retrospective data (grade C) suggest that phenytoin is less effective than carbamazepine, and no benefit was found when the two were combined.[9] Baclofen was shown to be efficacious in a double-blind crossover trial in trigeminal neuralgia (grade A evidence),[10] and pain relief in a case of GPN was reported shortly afterward.[11] Ketamine was found to be effective in one patient using a double-blind n-of-1 crossover study.[12] Topical application of cocaine to the tonsillar mucosa provides reliable but short-lived relief, and can be an option for patients with mild or infrequent paroxysms. Gabapentin, which is generally well tolerated, appears to be effective in GPN, although the published experience is small and uncontrolled (grade C).[13]

The main surgical options for GPN are section of glossopharyngeal nerve rootlets (often including the upper two or three vagal rootlets) and microvascular decompression. The relative merit of these two procedures is difficult to assess, as the literature consists largely of retrospective reviews of personal experiences with one procedure or the other (grade C evidence). The reported rates of complete, sustained pain relief in GPN are 80% or higher with either operation,[9,14,15] and operative complications seem to be infrequent. Extracranial procedures, such as the ganglion thermocoagulation or glycerol neurolysis techniques commonly used in trigeminal neuralgia, are either technically difficult or seem to be less effective in GPN.[16] One group has advocated percutaneous trigeminal tractotomy–nucleotomy, which has the advantage of avoiding craniotomy.[17] Syncope due to parasympathetic hyperactivity with GPN paroxysms appears to be abolished effectively by nerve section. If craniotomy is not an option, carbamazepine plus a permanent cardiac pacemaker is an alternative.[18]

In summary, carbamazepine is probably the first-line medical treatment for GPN, although in some patients the symptoms may not be sufficiently severe or sustained to require anything other than reassurance. Baclofen or gabapentin may be tried if carbamazepine fails or is poorly tolerated. Patients in whom medical therapy fails and who are willing to submit to the risks (albeit small) of craniotomy can reasonably be referred to a neurosurgeon. Whether intracranial nerve section or microvascular decompression is performed probably depends more on the experience of the individual surgeon than any intrinsic advantage of either procedure.

Vagus nerve

Anatomy

The tenth cranial nerve is primarily efferent, bearing motor fibers which innervate muscles of the larynx and pharynx, and parasympathetic preganglionic fibers to thoracic and abdominal viscera. There is also a small sensory component, consisting of somatic sensory fibers (from parts of the external auditory meatus and auricle, and from the mucosa of the larynx), and taste fibers from the epiglottis. Vagal motor neurons reside in the nucleus ambiguus, and parasympathetic neurons in the dorsal motor nucleus of the vagus. As with the ninth cranial nerve, vagal fibers leave the ventrolateral surface of the medulla as a group of rootlets in the sulcus between the olive and inferior cerebellar peduncle; determining the precise boundary between vagal and glossopharyngeal rootlets is usually impossible. In the subarachnoid space the vagus runs forward and laterally and exits from the skull via the jugular foramen, in the company of the ninth and eleventh cranial nerves.

In the neck the vagi descend vertically, lying between the internal jugular vein and carotid artery. The *right* vagus nerve crosses the subclavian artery anteriorly, passes behind the right main stem bronchus, and then lies on the esophagus, where it unites with the left vagus to form a common trunk which passes through the diaphragm via the esophageal hiatus. The *left* vagus crosses the lateral side of the aortic arch, passes behind the left main stem bronchus, and then joins the common trunk. Parasympathetic fibers run to cardiac and pulmonary plexuses in the thorax, and the common trunk bears parasympathetic innervation to the abdominal viscera.

Vagal motor fibers are distributed by three branches:

1. The pharyngeal branch, arising just distal to the jugular foramen, is the main motor nerve of the pharynx, supplying the pharyngeal constrictors and muscles of the soft palate (except tensor veli palatini).
2. The superior laryngeal nerve, which arises distal to the pharyngeal branch, supplies cricothyroid, but mostly carries sensory fibers from the laryngeal mucosa.
3. The recurrent laryngeal nerves supply all laryngeal muscles except cricothyroid. On the *right*, the recurrent laryngeal nerve arises in the neck, at the level of the subclavian artery, while the *left* recurrent laryngeal nerve arises in the thorax, below the aortic arch. Both recurrent laryngeal nerves loop under their arterial neighbors and ascend in the groove between trachea and esophagus to reach the larynx.

Pathophysiology

During its course intracranially and through the jugular foramen, the vagus nerve is subject to a range of lesions similar to those that affect the glossopharyngeal nerve (see above). In addition, the proximity of the recurrent laryngeal nerves to the thyroid gland puts them at risk during thyroid surgery or from invasive thyroid carcinoma. The risk of recurrent laryngeal nerve injury during thyroidectomy is about 2% per nerve with experienced surgeons; identification of the nerve by intraoperative stimulation appears to lower the risk.[19] The left recurrent laryngeal nerve may also be compromised by intrathoracic processes such as enlarged hilar lymph nodes or aortic arch aneurysms. Isolated vagus or recurrent laryngeal neuropathy without clear cause is well recognized.[20] Some of these cases may represent inflammatory neuropathies analogous to Bell's palsy.

Clinical features

Vagal lesions proximal to the pharyngeal branch produce ipsilateral paralysis of the soft palate, pharynx, and larynx, manifest as dysphagia and dysphonia. The main signs are unilateral weakness of soft palate elevation during phonation and hoarseness of the voice. Failure of the soft palate to seal off the nasopharynx during swallowing results in nasal regurgitation of fluids; with unilateral vagus lesions, the nasopharynx may be adequately sealed by the actions of the contralateral soft palate. As noted above, lesions of the proximal vagus nerve usually affect the ninth cranial nerve as well, so that pharyngeal weakness may be compounded by impaired pharyngeal sensation.

Lesions of the vagus distal to the pharyngeal branch cause ipsilateral laryngeal weakness but spare swallowing. The weakness of vocal cord abduction and adduction produces a hoarse, breathy voice, a weak cough, and impaired airway protection. Sometimes the vocal cord apparatus on the intact side can compensate quite effectively for the paralyzed side. If the lesion spares the superior laryngeal nerve, cricothyroid acting alone may allow fair preservation of ipsilateral laryngeal function.

While the degree of dysphonia and dysphagia is variable with unilateral vagus palsy, bilateral vagus lesions reliably cause major impairment. Bilateral lesions of the vagus also cause thoracoabdominal parasympathetic failure, which is discussed in the sections of this book dealing with autonomic failure.

Dysphonia

Dysphonia may be a manifestation of vagal palsy, but of course it can be produced by abnormalities in various parts of the phonation apparatus, which includes the larynx, lungs, and upper airway. Potential treatments for laryngeal dysfunction due to vagal palsy (and other causes) are briefly discussed here.

Etiology

During normal phonation, both vocal cords are pulled to the midline of the lumen of the larynx and held in taut opposition. When vagus or recurrent laryngeal palsy causes paresis of the laryngeal musculature, the vocal cord is not stretched appropriately, and it fails to move medially to oppose the contralateral cord. The resulting glottic insufficiency produces a hoarse, breathy voice, often with unwanted multiphonics (due to the two vocal cords vibrating at different frequencies). Glottic insufficiency also impairs airway protection (see below).

Treatment

Several surgical techniques have been developed to treat vocal cord paralysis.[21] At present, these procedures are mainly offered to patients with unilateral vocal cord paralysis, usually after a period of waiting to see whether spontaneous recovery will occur. The basic aims of all techniques are to improve or compensate for the impaired adduction (medialization) of the cord, and to optimize the stiffness of the cord. A simple approach is to augment the size and stiffness of the vocal fold itself by injecting it with Teflon or some other inert substance. More complex procedures such as thyroplasty or arytenoid adduction aim to alter laryngeal anatomy so that the entire vocal fold and supporting tissues are displaced medially, to promote proper opposition of the cords.

There are no prospective, controlled trials of any of these techniques, and most of the literature consists of uncontrolled, retrospective series (grade C evidence). However, some retrospective series describe rigorous, blinded preoperative versus postoperative voice evaluations which provide more convincing evidence of efficacy (grade B).[22] Procedures designed to reinnervate the larynx have also been developed, usually by anastomosing a branch of ansa cervicalis to the distal stump of the recurrent laryngeal nerve. Evidence that functionally useful laryngeal reinnervation can be achieved surgically in humans is lacking.

Dysphagia is discussed at the end of this chapter.

Accessory nerve

Anatomy

The eleventh cranial nerve is purely or predominantly motor. Its spinal root (which most now regard as the accessory nerve proper) is formed by rootlets from motor neurons in the C2–4 segments of the spinal cord. The spinal root proceeds rostrally in the subarachnoid space, enters the cranial cavity via the foramen magnum, then turns laterally toward the jugular foramen. Prior to entering the jugular foramen, it receives some motor axons from the vagus nerve (the "cranial accessory root"), which travel briefly with the accessory nerve but then leave it to rejoin the vagus (these fibers innervate the muscles of the pharynx and soft palate). Once through the jugular foramen, the accessory nerve descends beside the internal jugular vein and innervates sternocleidomastoid. Just above the midpoint of the posterior border of sternomastoid, the nerve turns posteriorly and runs along the floor of the posterior triangle of the neck (formed by levator scapulae), and terminates by innervating trapezius.

Pathophysiology

The most common site of accessory nerve lesions is in the posterior triangle, where the nerve may be injured as a consequence of neck trauma or lymph node or radical neck dissection. There are several descriptions of isolated spontaneous accessory neuropathy, which is presumed to be inflammatory and which may be recurrent.[23] Various other causes of isolated accessory neuropathy have been reported (e.g. schwannoma, stretch injury, love bite, internal jugular vein catheterization), and the nerve may also be involved in the Vernet and Collet–Sicard syndromes (see Table 175.1).

Accessory palsy

Clinical features

The main symptom of accessory palsy is weakness of shoulder elevation and impaired shoulder stability due to trapezius weakness. Patients often have shoulder pain as well, presumably due to altered shoulder mechanics. There is limited information about the time course and extent of recovery in traumatic accessory neuropathy, although in one series spontaneous improvement occurred in 34 of 39 patients who had electromyographic evidence of residual innervation of trapezius.[24]

Treatment

There is a small literature on surgical treatment of accessory palsy, consisting of retrospective reviews of the experience of different surgeons (grade C evidence). A period of observation to await spontaneous recovery is generally advised, but opinions about the optimum interval range from 3[25] to 12[26] months. Several surgical procedures have been used, including neurolysis, nerve suture, or nerve grafting, and good outcomes appear to be surprisingly frequent (e.g. 16 of 28 patients improving from MRC grade 0 to grade 4 following surgery[24]).

If salvage of the accessory nerve is judged to be impossible, other procedures to improve shoulder function have been described, including attempts to reinnervate trapezius with the long thoracic nerve,[27] or by muscle transfer operations. One series reported "excellent" long term results in 13 of 22 patients treated with transfer of levator scapulae and rhomboids (grade C evidence).[28]

In view of the gaps in the available clinical data, it is difficult to formulate clear recommendations for the management of the patient with an accessory neuropathy. Surgery is presumably the only option when the nerve is known to be completely transected. With partial injuries, or when the state of nerve continuity is unknown, the relative merits of conservative versus surgical treatment are unclear. Although there are potential difficulties in trial design, a controlled study of conservative versus surgical treatment, particularly for partial accessory neuropathies, seems ethically justifiable.

Hypoglossal nerve
Anatomy

The twelfth cranial nerve supplies the motor innervation of the tongue. Its nucleus is in the dorsomedial medulla, and the nerve emerges as a series of rootlets between the pyramid and olive on the ventral surface of the medulla. The rootlets coalesce to form the hypoglossal nerve on each side, which passes through the subarachnoid space and exits from the cranial cavity via the hypoglossal canal (anterior condylar canal of the occipital bone). In the neck the nerve initially lies deep to the internal jugular vein and the internal carotid artery. At the level of the angle of the jaw the nerve crosses anterior to the carotid and then runs anteriorly, where it fans out into terminal branches within the tongue. Afferent fibers concerned with proprioception are also carried in the distal hypoglossal nerve; these leave the nerve in the neck and enter the central nervous system via the C2 dorsal root.

Pathophysiology

The hypoglossal nerve may be compromised by skull base lesions (metastasis, chordoma, meningioma, dural arteriovenous fistula[29]) or injured by basal skull fracture. Various intrinsic pathologies (schwannoma, arachnoid cyst) of the nerve have been described. In the neck, the hypoglossal nerve can be affected by carcinoma of the nasopharynx or tongue, cervical lymphadenopathy, and abscesses. As with the tenth and eleventh nerves, isolated hypoglossal palsy with spontaneous recovery may occur and is presumed to be inflammatory.[30]

The hypoglossal nerve is sometimes injured during carotid endarterectomy. A recent prospective study found that cranial nerve injuries occurred in 12.5% of endarterectomies, with the hypoglossal (5.5%) and recurrent laryngeal (4%) nerves chiefly affected, never permanently.[31] Spontaneous carotid dissection produces hypoglossal palsy in about 10% of patients,

often combined with dysfunction of other lower cranial nerves.[32]

Clinical features

Lesions of the hypoglossal nerve cause ipsilateral weakness and wasting of half the tongue. (Supranuclear lesions may also produce contralateral tongue weakness, but the weakness is mild, as each hypoglossal nucleus receives input from both ipsilateral and contralateral corticobulbar tracts; the tongue weakness is usually accompanied by hemiparesis, but *not*, of course, by wasting or fasciculation of the tongue.) Patients with twelfth nerve lesions may observe deviation of the protruded tongue to the side of the lesion, but the main functional difficulties are dysarthria and dysphagia. With unilateral lesions, patients will often compensate effectively with the normal half of the tongue, whereas bilateral lesions produce significant impairment, especially of swallowing (as described below, the tongue is critical to the oral stages of swallowing).

Dysphagia

Inability to swallow adequately and safely can be a major problem for patients with lower cranial neuropathies.

Pathophysiology

Dysphagia has numerous neurological and non-neurological causes. Isolated unilateral lesions of the ninth, tenth, or twelfth cranial nerves may interfere with swallowing, but significant impairment usually requires multiple or bilateral lesions.[33] The most common neurological cause of dysphagia is stroke and, not surprisingly, most of the literature on management of neurological dysphagia is based on patients with stroke. However, all patients with dysphagia, whether due to stroke, lower cranial neuropathies, or other causes, face the same basic problems: ensuring adequate caloric and fluid intake, and protecting the airway from aspiration.

Mechanism of normal swallowing

Swallowing is a complex process which can be divided into four stages (see Figure 175.1). First is the oral preparatory stage, during which food is chewed and shaped into a ball. Second is the oral stage, where the tongue lifts and squeezes the bolus against the hard palate, propelling it toward the pharynx. The first and second stages are critically dependent upon twelfth nerve and tongue function. The third or pharyngeal stage is triggered, usually via the ninth cranial nerve, once the bolus reaches the most posterior level of the tongue. The pharyngeal stage consists of several overlapping activities, including closure of the nasopharynx by the soft palate (to prevent nasal regurgitation), elevation and closure of the larynx (for airway protection), retraction of the tongue base and contraction of the pharyngeal constrictor muscles (to propel the bolus), and relaxation of the cricopharyngeus (upper esophageal sphincter, UES). When the bolus passes the UES, the fourth or

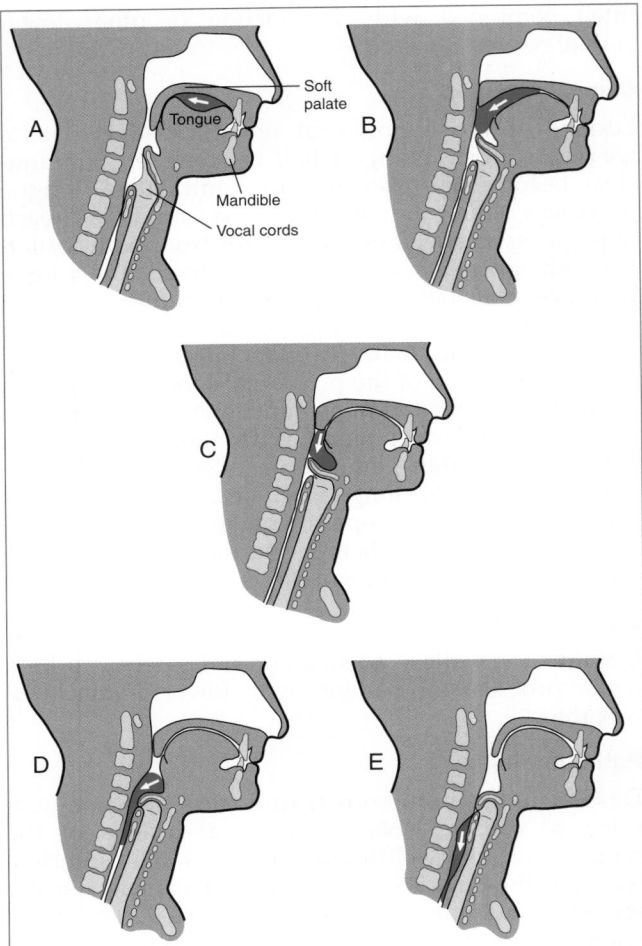

Figure 175.1 The main stages in swallowing. In the oral stage A, the bolus is moved posteriorly by being squeezed against the palate by the tongue. The soft palate serves to seal off the nasopharynx B, and the bolus is forced toward the epiglottis by the base of the tongue. Protection of the airway is accomplished by closure of the vocal cords and by pulling the larynx upward against the epiglottal "lid" (compare the relationship between the vocal cords and the mandible in A and C). Relaxation of the cricopharyngeus/upper esophageal sphincter, D, allows the bolus to pass into the esophagus, E.
From Cummings CW, Frederickson JM, Harker LA, et al. Otolaryngology Head and Neck Surgery. 3rd ed. St. Louis: Mosby-Year Book, 1998:1848

esophageal phase begins, and the bolus is propelled to the stomach. The pharyngeal phase of swallowing is in some sense the most important, as this is when airway protection occurs.

Diagnosis

Complete evaluation of a patient with dysphagia may require several complementary techniques, including videoendoscopy, videofluoroscopy, and manometry of the pharynx and esophagus. A swallowing evaluation has several objectives. The first is to identify, if

possible, exactly how the swallowing process is disturbed, and, in particular, to identify causes for which specific treatment exists (e.g. esophageal stricture, nasopharyngeal carcinoma). A second objective is to determine the patient's risk of aspiration.

Treatment

There is an expanding literature on the treatment of dysphagia (comprehensively reviewed by Cook and Kahrilas[34]). For dysphagia due to lower cranial neuropathies, like most neurological causes of dysphagia, cure of the neurological condition is not available, and treatments are nonspecific. Nonspecific treatments for dysphagia fall into three main classes: swallowing therapies, surgical modification of the oropharynx, and nonoral feeding techniques.

Swallowing therapies include dietary modification (e.g. adding thickeners to liquids), alteration of swallowing techniques (e.g. tilting the head away from the side of a unilateral pharyngeal palsy), and pharyngeal stimulation. One might anticipate that patients with lower cranial neuropathies would be excellent candidates for swallowing therapies, as language and consciousness are not impaired. Though the biological rationale for these therapies is sound, most of the published evidence is grade C.

There are two randomized controlled trials of swallowing therapies in stroke patients, which provide grade A evidence but which reached opposite conclusions. DePippo et al. randomized patients to one of three groups receiving different levels of swallowing therapy, ranging from a single teaching session to daily supervised swallowing exercises plus a precisely modified diet.[35] They could demonstrate no advantage to the more intensive treatments. However, only 15% of patients in any of the groups had an adverse outcome, so that a type II error is possible. In the second trial, patients were randomized to a standard pureed diet with unaltered liquids or to a soft mechanical diet with thickened fluids; at 6 months the rate of pneumonia was decreased by 80% in the group with thickened fluids.[36]

Surgical modification of the oropharynx has an obvious rationale when dysphagia is caused by structural anomalies such as Zenker's diverticulum. Cricopharyngeal myotomy, which is widely used for structural dysphagia, is also advocated for neurogenic dysphagia. The rationale is that if the pharyngeal contractions are weak or poorly coordinated, passage of the bolus into the esophagus will be easier if the resting tone of cricopharyngeus (UES) is decreased. There are no controlled trials of cricopharyngeal myotomy in neurogenic dysphagia. Published retrospective series (i.e. grade C evidence), involving patients with a range of neurological disorders, report that cricopharyngeal myotomy improves swallowing in about 60% of patients, although the subjective outcome measures generally used raise some concern about reporting bias.[34] Unfortunately there seems to be no reliable way preoperatively to distinguish responders from nonresponders. It is not possible to draw definite conclusions about the role of cricopharyngeal myotomy in neurogenic dysphagia, but the technique may have a role in some patients, especially those with concomitant mechanical obstruction in the oropharynx.

A variety of surgical techniques have been developed to limit or prevent passage of oropharyngeal contents into the airway (e.g. tracheostomy with cuffed tube, vocal cord medialization, subperichondrial cricoidectomy, laryngotracheal separation).[37] In the face of gross aspiration, there seems little question that these procedures work, despite the absence of controlled data. There are no data on the relative merits of the various procedures, nor are there good long term outcome studies.

Dysphagic patients who consistently aspirate despite swallowing therapies or surgical modification of the oropharynx generally need to be fed nonorally. Nasogastric intubation with a soft feeding tube is easy and reliable, but unesthetic. Percutaneous gastrostomy, which can be performed endoscopically in most patients, is usually the best alternative for long term feeding. Tube feeding effectively delivers calories and fluids to the patient, but how effectively it protects the patient from aspiration pneumonia is unclear, as the patient's own oral secretions are not diverted by tube feeding. No controlled trials of oral versus tube feeding have been carried out; four retrospective studies found, in fact, that the rates of aspiration pneumonia were higher in tube fed than in orally fed patients (grade C evidence).[38] The additional possibility of aspiration of refluxed gastric contents might be minimized by jejunostosmy or by using feeding tubes with the distal end in the jejunum, but studies comparing outcomes of gastrostomy versus jejunostomy are lacking.

References

1. Alonso T, Pujol J, Ayuso A, Pujol J. Sustained hypertension after section of the glossopharyngeal nerve. J Neurol Neurosurg Psychiatry 1981;44:369
2. Katusic S, Williams DB, Beard CM, et al. Incidence and clinical features of glossopharyngeal neuralgia, Rochester, Minnesota, 1945–1984. Neuroepidemiology 1991;10:266–275
3. Ferroli P, Franzini A, Pluderi M, Broggi G. Vagoglossopharyngeal neuralgia caused by a neuroma of vagal rootlets. Acta Neurochirur (Wien) 1999;141:897–898
4. Galetta SL, Raps EC, Hurst RW, Flamm ES. Glossopharyngeal neuralgia from a posterior fossa arteriovenous malformation: resolution following embolization. Neurology 1993;43:1854–1855
5. Minagar A, Sheremata WA. Glossopharyngeal neuralgia and MS. Neurology 2000;54:1368–1370
6. Adams CB. Microvascular compression: an alternative view and hypothesis. J Neurosurg 1989;1:1–12
7. Reddy K, Hobson DE, Gomori A, Sutherland GR. Painless glossopharyngeal "neuralgia" with syncope: a case report and literature review. Neurosurgery 1987;21:916–919
8. Ekbom KA, Westerberg CE. Carbamazepine in glossopharyngeal neuralgia. Arch Neurol 1966;14:595–596
9. Rushton JG, Stevens JC, Miller RH. Glossopharyngeal (vagoglossopharyngeal) neuralgia: a study of 217 cases. Arch Neurol 1981;38:201–205
10. Fromm GH, Terrence CF, Chattha AS. Baclofen in the treatment of trigeminal neuralgia: Double-blind study and long-term follow-up. Ann Neurol 1984;15:240–244
11. Ringel RA, Roy EP III. Glossopharyngeal neuralgia: successful treatment with baclofen (letter). Ann Neurol 1987;21:514–515
12. Eide PK, Stubhaug A. Relief of glossopharyngeal neuralgia by ketamine-induced N-methyl-aspartate receptor blockade. Neurosurg 1997;41:505–508
13. Garcia Callejo FJ, Velert-Villa MM, Talamantes Escriba F, Blay-Galaud L. Clinical response of gabapentin for glossopharyngeal neuralgia (in Spanish). Rev Neurol 1999;28:380–384
14. Jannetta PJ. Outcome after microvascular decompression for typical trigeminal neuralgia, hemifacial spasm, tinnitus, disabling positional vertigo, and glossopharyngeal neuralgia. Clin Neurosurg 1997;44:331–383
15. Kondo A. Follow-up results of using microvascular decompression for treatment of glossopharyngeal neuralgia. J Neurosurg 1998;88:221–225
16. Taha JM, Tew JM Jr. Long-term results of surgical treatment of idiopathic neuralgias of the glossopharyngeal and vagal nerves. Neurosurgery 1995;36:926–931
17. Kanpolat Y, Savas A, Batay F, Sinav A. Computed tomography-guided trigeminal tractotomy-nucleotomy in the management of vagoglossopharyngeal and geniculate neuralgias. Neurosurgery 1998;43:484–490
18. Johnston RT, Redding VJ. Glossopharyngeal neuralgia associated with cardiac syncope: long term treatment with permanent pacing and carbamazepine. Br Heart J 1990;64:403–405
19. Echeverri A, Flexon PB. Electrophysiologic nerve stimulation for identifying the recurrent laryngeal nerve in thyroid surgery: review of 70 consecutive thyroid surgeries. Am Surg 1998;64:328–333
20. Berry H, Blair RL. Isolated vagus nerve palsy and vagal mononeuritis. Arch Otolaryngol 1980;106:333–338
21. Ford CN. Advances and refinements in phonosurgery. Laryngoscope 1999;109:1891–1900
22. Chhetri DK, Gerratt BR, Kreiman J, Berke GS. Combined arytenoid adduction and laryngeal reinnervation in the treatment of vocal fold paralysis. Laryngoscope 1999;109:1928–1936
23. Chalk C, Isaacs H. Recurrent spontaneous accessory neuropathy. J Neurol Neurosurg Psychiatry 1990;53:621
24. Donner TR, Kline DG. Extracranial spinal accessory nerve injury. Neurosurg 1993;32:907–910
25. Matz PG, Barbaro NM. Diagnosis and treatment of iatrogenic spinal accessory nerve injury. Am Surg 1996;62:682–685
26. Ogino T, Sugawara M, Minami A, et al. Accessory nerve injury: conservative or surgical treatment? J Hand Surg [Br] 1991;16:531–536
27. Schultes G, Gaggl A, Karcher H. Reconstruction of accessory nerve defects with vascularized long thoracic versus non-vascularized thoracodorsal nerve. J Reconstr Microsurg 1999;15:265–270
28. Bigliani LU, Compito CA, Duralde XA, Wolfe IN. Transfer of the levator scapulae, rhomboid major, and rhomboid minor for paralysis of the trapezius. J Bone Joint Surg [Am] 1996;78:1534–1540
29. Blomquist MH, Barr JD, Hurst RW. Isolated unilateral hypoglossal neuropathy caused by dural arteriovenous fistula. AJNR Am J Neuroradiol 1998;19:951–953
30. Combarros O, Alvarez de Arcaya A, Berciano J. Isolated hypoglossal nerve palsy: nine cases. J Neurol 1998;245:98–100
31. Ballotta E, Da Giau G, Renon L, et al. Cranial and cervical

nerve injuries after carotid endartertectomy: a prospective study. Surgery 1999;125:85–91

32. Mokri B, Silbert PL, Schievink WI, Piepgras DG. Cranial nerve palsy in spontaneous dissection of the extracranial internal carotid artery. Neurology 1996; 46:356–359

33. Perie S, Coiffier L, Laccourreye L, et al. Swallowing disorders in paralysis of the lower cranial nerves: a functional analysis. Ann Otol Rhinol Laryngol 1999; 108:606–611

34. Cook IJ, Kahrilas PJ. AGA technical review on management of oropharyngeal dysphagia. Gastroenterology 1999;116:455–478

35. DePippo KL, Holas MA, Mandel FS, Lesser ML. Dysphagia therapy following stroke: A controlled trial. Neurology 1994;44:1655–1660

36. Groher ME. Bolus management and aspiration pneumonia in patients with pseudobulbar dysphagia. Dysphagia 1987;1:215–216

37. Eisele DW. Chronic aspiration. *In:* Cummings CW, Frederickson JM, Harker LA, et al., eds. Otolaryngology Head and Neck Surgery. St Louis: Mosby, 1998: 1989–2000

38. Finucane TE, Bynum JPW. Use of tube feeding to prevent aspiration. Lancet 1996;348:1421–1424

Multiple Cranial Nerve Palsies

James R Perry

Overview

The myriad of disorders causing multiple cranial nerve palsies challenges even the seasoned neurologist. This chapter will focus upon a diagnostic approach to the patient with deficits involving two or more cranial nerves. Intrinsic brainstem lesions may cause multiple cranial nerve palsies; however, these are usually associated with other signs such as long tract findings, are readily detected with computed tomography (CT) or magnetic resonance imaging (MRI) of the brain, and do not present the diagnostic challenge of the other entities considered here. Appropriate therapies for many of the underlying neurological and systemic conditions are located in other portions of the text.

Etiology

An approach to disorders affecting multiple cranial nerves may be found in Tables 176.1 and 176.2. In order to generate a list of diagnostic considerations, the author finds it helpful to categorize cranial neuropathies as localized or nonlocalized. Localized syndromes cause characteristic combinations of cranial neuropathy; for example, involvement of cranial nerves III, IV, VI, and possibly the first and second portions of V suggests localization to the ipsilateral cavernous sinus. A localized syndrome directs attention to specific areas of the nervous system. Consultation with a neuroradiologist may be helpful in these cases since special imaging protocols such as high-resolution CT of the skull base or MRI with orbital views using a fat suppression sequence may be required.

Nonlocalized cranial neuropathy syndromes, in contrast, are not attributable to particular combinations of anatomical structures. For example, while leptomeningeal carcinomatosis affects some cranial nerves more frequently than others, there is no specific pattern of involvement suggesting a precise anatomical location. When a localized syndrome is not present, a process affecting multiple cranial nerves in common areas such as the subarachnoid space, or a process that is diffuse, such as vasculitis, is suggested. As given in Table 176.2, one approach to categorizing the nonlocalized cranial neuropathies is to consider associated systemic conditions. The history and examination of such a patient should include a search for evidence of malignancy, infection, systemic diseases such as sarcoidosis and vasculitis, bone disease such as Paget's, vascular disorders, trauma, toxic exposures, and neurological diseases such as myasthenia gravis.

Pathophysiology and pathogenesis

The pathogenesis of cranial nerve dysfunction is varied. Direct invasion of the cranial nerves may be seen with neurotropic malignancies such as squamous and basal cell carcinoma of the head and neck.[1,2] Entrapment with mechanical compression of cranial nerves is postulated to occur in disorders such as Paget's disease of bone.[3] Vascular involvement of perineural vessels is likely an important factor in sickle cell disease[4] and perhaps in diabetes mellitus.[5] Lastly, compression of the neurovascular bundle is part of the final common pathway leading to cranial nerve dysfunction in the setting of inflammatory disorders such as sarcoidosis[6] and in leptomeningeal carcinomatosis.[7]

Clinical features: localized versus nonlocalized cranial neuropathy syndromes

Localized cranial neuropathy syndromes (Table 176.1)

Cavernous sinus syndromes   In 1976, Hunt proposed criteria for an inflammatory syndrome affecting the cavernous sinus, then widely known as the Tolosa–Hunt syndrome.[8] These criteria included

Table 176.1   Localized syndromes causing multiple cranial nerve palsies (these affect characteristic combinations of cranial nerves)

Cavernous sinus syndrome (all or some of cranial nerves III, IV, VI, V1, and V2)
- Infectious (i.e. mucormycosis)
- Neoplastic (i.e. intracavernous meningioma, dural metastases)
- Inflammatory (i.e. Tolosa–Hunt syndrome)
- Vascular (i.e. carotid-cavernous fistulae, cavernous aneurysm)

Superior orbital fissure syndrome (all or some of cranial nerves III, IV, VI, V1)
Cerebellopontine angle syndrome
Skull base disorders including trauma (primary tumors—chordoma, and metastases to bone, dura)
Gradenigo syndrome (cranial nerves V1 and VI)
Raeder's paratrigeminal syndrome (unilateral oculosympathetic paresis plus V)
Jugular foramen syndrome (Vernet's syndrome—cranial nerves IX, X, XI)

Table 176.2   Nonlocalized syndromes causing multiple cranial nerve palsies (may affect any combination of cranial nerves)

Associated with known or occult cancer
- Primary tumors:
  - skull base tumor (i.e. chordoma)
  - direct invasion by head and neck cancer (i.e. squamous cell carcinoma, nasopharyngeal cancer)
  - primary leptomeningeal neoplasms (i.e. lymphoma, gliomatosis, melanosis)
- Secondary tumors:
  - leptomeningeal carcinomatosis, lymphomatosis

Associated with infection
- Bacterial meningitis
- Fungal disease (mucormycosis, aspergillosis, cryptococcosis)
- Tuberculosis
- Viral (i.e. VZV, EBV)
- Meningovascular syphilis
- Lyme disease

Associated with systemic disease
- Diabetic cranial neuropathies
- Granulomatous disease (i.e. sarcoidosis)
- Vasculitis (i.e. Wegener's granulomatosis)
- Primary amyloidosis[40]
- Sjögren's syndrome[41]

Associated with bone disease
- Paget's disease of bone
- Familial bony disorders (hyperostosis cranialis interna)
- Craniotubular remodeling disorders (i.e. Camurati–Engelmann disease)
- Thalassemia and other disorders associated with extramedullary hematopoiesis

Associated with vascular disease
- Intravascular coagulation
- Sickle cell crisis
- Associated with sepsis and venous or internal jugular thrombosis[42]

Associated with trauma
- Basal skull fracture
- Arterial dissection[43]
- Direct injury to cranial nerves

Associated with toxic exposures
- Ethylene glycol poisoning[44]
- Scorpion sting[45]
- Delayed effect of therapeutic external beam radiation[46]

Associated with neurological disorders
- Myasthenia gravis
- Variant of acute inflammatory demyelinating polyradiculopathy
- Idiopathic intracranial hypertension[47]

Idiopathic cranial polyneuropathy

Familial recurrent multiple cranial neuropathy[48]

steady boring retro-orbital pain, cranial nerve dysfunction affecting the third, fourth, sixth and first division of fifth cranial nerves including the oculosympathetic fibers, symptoms lasting days to weeks, spontaneous remissions and recurrence, and the absence of involvement of structures outside the cavernous sinus. Responsiveness to steroids was later identified.[9,10] In 1988, the International Headache Society (IHS) defined the criteria for Tolosa–Hunt syndrome to include episodes of unilateral orbital pain for an average of eight weeks if untreated, with associated paresis of one or more of the third, fourth, and sixth cranial nerves. Cranial nerve palsies may coincide with the onset of pain or follow it within a period of up to two weeks, and the pain must be relieved within 72 hours after the initiation of corticosteroid therapy. Lastly, other causes are excluded by neuroimaging studies. Several pitfalls exist in the clinical diagnosis of Tolosa–Hunt syndrome according to these criteria.[11–14] Occasionally cranial nerves outside of the boundaries of the cavernous sinus may be involved. For example, facial palsies have been reported in association with otherwise typical presentations of Tolosa–Hunt syndrome.[15] These cases suggest an overlap with the less specific syndrome of idiopathic granulomatous pachymeningitis or idiopathic cranial polyneuropathy.[9,16,17] Imaging investigation of all patients with Tolosa–Hunt syndrome is mandatory as this remains a diagnosis of exclusion. Conventional CT is normal in up to two thirds of patients.[9] Magnetic resonance imaging is often, but not always abnormal, and may demonstrate convex enlargement of the affected cavernous sinus.[14,18,19] Abnormal tissue may be noted in the cavernous sinus and this often enhances markedly following the administration of paramagnetic contrast material. In most cases the abnormal enhancement within the cavernous sinus is noted to decrease over the course of many months while patients are on treatment with corticosteroids.[19]

The differential diagnosis of a cavernous sinus syndrome is diverse. Table 176.1 lists several such entities. Particularly problematic are cavernous sinus syndromes where conventional imaging, including MRI, is normal. Neurotropic spread of cutaneous malignancies,[11] endoneurial invasion of lymphoma and metastatic solid cancers,[13] localized forms of vasculitis,[20] and infectious causes have all been reported to mimic Tolosa–Hunt syndrome both clinically and radiologically. Furthermore, response to the administration of corticosteroids is nonspecific as steroid therapy may improve pain and cranial nerve function in cases of malignant invasion and vasculitis. There have been no controlled trials of corticosteroid use in this setting; however, a short course of oral steroids is often used to relieve pain and in the hope of minimizing neurological morbidity (grade C evidence from case reports and case series without controls).

Orbital pseudotumor   Orbital pseudotumor refers to an idiopathic disorder characterized by ophthalmoplegia due to invasion of orbital and periorbital tissues by an inflammatory lymphoid lesion.[21,22] It affects children and adults, with an equal gender ratio. The acute phase of orbital pseudotumor is often heralded by proptosis, painful ophthalmoplegia, conjunctival injection and edema, eyelid swelling, occasionally associated with decreased corneal sensation, increased intraocular pressure, optic neuropathy, or uveitis.[21,22] Intracranial extension may cause multiple cranial nerve palsies,[23] and if painful is identical to the Tolosa–Hunt syndrome. In adults, orbital pseudotumor is usually unilateral. Unlike children, in whom bilateral involvement may be seen in up to one third of cases, bilateral findings in adults should prompt consideration of an underlying vasculitic or neoplastic syndrome.[21,22] Wegener's granulomatosis and Churg–Strauss vasculitis are both described.[24,25]

The diagnosis of orbital pseudotumor is suggested by the clinical findings. The differential diagnosis includes vasculitis, invasive lymphoma, metastatic carcinoma, infectious processes, orbital cellulites, dural and direct carotid-cavernous fistulae, and thyroid orbitopathy.[21] Imaging is mandatory. CT often reveals thickening of orbital tissues including the extraocular muscles and their affected tendons.[22] Orbital pseudotumor may be thallium avid and therefore mimic neoplastic processes such as lymphoma.[26] Fine-needle aspirates are often diagnostic if the diagnosis is in doubt.[27]

The mainstay of treatment for orbital pseudotumor is systemic corticosteroid therapy, especially if vision is threatened.[27] A high proportion of nonresponders to corticosteroids and a high relapse rate despite treatment led some authors to question the true efficacy of steroid treatment.[28] For patients with corticosteroid intolerance or failure, external beam radiotherapy, cyclophosphamide, and orbital decompression are used.[22,27] None of these strategies has been evaluated in controlled trials (grade C evidence).

Skull base syndromes   A variety of localized cranial neuropathy syndromes depend upon their relationship to the structures of the skull base. Topographic diagnosis of these syndromes requires knowledge of cranial nerve and skull base anatomy. For example, involvement of V2 directs attention to the area of foramen rotundum, V1 to the superior orbital fissure, V1 and V2 together to the cavernous sinus, and V3 to foramen ovale. Cerebellopontine angle, jugular foramen, and paratrigeminal syndromes (Table 176.1) are well known and their presentation should lead to detailed imaging of the skull base. Vestibular schwannoma, glomus tumors, dural metastases, and trauma are amongst the common causes of these syndromes. Basal skull fractures may be associated with involvement of cranial nerves IX through XII.[29] Familial hyperostosis syndromes,[30] craniotubular remodeling disorders,[31] and extramedullary hematopoiesis[32] are rare causes of bony compression of cranial nerves. In addition, Paget's disease of bone causes progressive cranial nerve dysfunction due to foraminal narrowing and, although any cranial nerve may be affected, optic neuropathy, ophthalmoparesis, and the superior orbital fissure syndrome are best described.[3] Dissection of the internal carotid artery may also cause lower cranial neuropathies, often unilaterally, and occasionally in the absence of other signs of ischemic stroke. Directed investigation to detect arterial dissection, with invasive or noninvasive angiography, is appropriate for patients presenting with neck pain and multiple lower cranial neuropathies, especially if conventional imaging is uninformative.

Gradenigo's syndrome refers to the triad of otitis, abducens paresis, and deep pain.[33] Historically this syndrome was used in reference to chronic suppurative petrous apicitis complicating otitis media;[34] however, since the antibiotic era, this is a rare cause of Gradenigo's syndrome. Any lesion near the region of the petrous apex, such as primary or metastatic involvement of temporal bone, may present as Gradenigo's syndrome, and detailed imaging of the skull base is required in these cases.[35]

Paratrigeminal syndrome is a term suggested by Raeder in 1918 to describe the complex of unilateral periorbital pain, meiosis, ptosis, and sensory involvement of the trigeminal nerve.[36] Virtually always, these symptoms are due to a symptomatic structural lesion including neoplasms[37] and chronic infection such as aspergillosis.[38] Carotid dissection may be the cause in cases where skull base imaging is negative.[39]

Nonlocalized cranial neuropathy syndromes

If multiple cranial nerve palsies are identified but do not fit a localized cranial neuropathy syndrome, a useful approach to the differential diagnosis may be to consider the patient's associated systemic conditions (Table 176.2). Many of the entities listed are obscure and presented only for completeness. The following discussion focuses upon the most clinically relevant disease processes.

Cancer causes multiple cranial nerve palsies through several mechanisms including direct involvement of the skull base, extension from the head and neck, and by primary or secondary involvement of the subarachnoid space. Leptomeningeal involvement usually develops in patients with known, rather than occult, cancer and often occurs in the presence of advanced disease affecting other organ systems. The incidence of leptomeningeal disease is increasing due to a combination of better imaging, increased survival from systemic cancer treatment, and the role of the CNS as a sanctuary from drugs with poor blood–brain barrier penetration.[7] Cranial nerve involvement is more commonly seen with the leptomeningeal spread of hematological, rather than solid, malignancies.[49,50] In most series a predilection for cranial nerves II, III, VI, and VII is noted, perhaps because of the relative ease of recognition of deficits in these structures; however, any cranial nerve may be involved.[7,49,50] Furthermore, the pattern of cranial nerve involvement may mimic other syndromes, such as Tolosa–Hunt. Therefore, the clinician must maintain a very high index of suspicion for leptomeningeal disease in any patient with a prior history of cancer, even if the history is remote.

The diagnosis of leptomeningeal involvement by cancer relies upon imaging and cerebrospinal fluid (CSF) examination. Enhancement after administration of contrast material may be detected in the leptomeninges, dural structures and along nerve roots; however, enhancement of these structures is not specific and, in part, the sensitivity of this test depends upon the dose of contrast agent used.[51] CSF examination is usually required to confirm the diagnosis. False-negative results from CSF analysis are found when small volumes of CSF (less than 10 ml) are submitted for analysis, when there is a delay in cytological processing, if the site sampled is remote from the site of clinical involvement, and if repeated sampling is not performed.[52] Several authors have found that a CSF sample taken as near as possible to the site of clinical involvement improves diagnostic yield. For example, if a patient harbors multiple lower cranial nerve palsies and a routine lumbar CSF sample is nondiagnostic, the best strategy may be to perform either an Ommaya tap if available, or a cisternal puncture for cytological analysis.[52–54]

Primary leptomeningeal tumors rarely occur; however, glial tumors,[55] melanoma,[56] and lymphoma[57] may present only with involvement of the leptomeninges and result in multiple cranial nerve palsies. The interpretation of cytological abnormalities in the CSF is difficult, even amongst experienced cytopathologists. In particular, because many diseases cause an atypical lymphocytic pleocytosis with or without elevated CSF protein, caution is appropriate in the interpretation of atypical lymphocytes in a CSF sample. Furthermore, the finding of nonspecific atypical lymphocytosis with abnormal enhancement of peripheral nerve roots occurs in a variety of nonmalignant disorders such as Guillain–Barré syndrome and infectious polyradiculopathies.[58] For these reasons, a biopsy of the dura and leptomeninges may be required to confirm the diagnosis. Special CSF markers, immunomarkers, and molecular analysis may also be helpful. Parotid, oral, and squamous cancers of the head and neck may invade the perineurium of branches of the trigeminal and facial nerves in a retrograde fashion and thereby gain access to the intracranial compartment, causing local compression of adjacent nerves and structures.[1,2]

Infectious processes, especially meningitis, may involve multiple cranial nerves. Bacterial and viral meningitides rarely involve multiple cranial nerves; however, fungal involvement of the subarachnoid space may present with a combination of headache, hydrocephalus and cranial neuropathies. Lyme disease typically involves the facial nerve; however, as with meningovascular syphilis, other cranial nerves can be involved.[59] A cranial polyneuritis occurring with or without rash due to varicella zoster virus has also been described,[60] as have multiple cranial neuropathies in association with infectious mononucleosis.[61–63]

Systemic disorders such as sarcoidosis and vasculitis can present in isolation within the CNS. Sarcoidosis most frequently affects the facial nerve, often bilaterally, and may occasionally present with multiple cranial neuropathies. In these cases, basal meningeal infiltration with granulomatous material often involves adjacent structures causing hydrocephalus, pituitary insufficiency, especially diabetes insipidus, and headache.[64] Cranial CT and MRI studies may demonstrate abnormal leptomeningeal enhancement concentrated in the basal meninges (Figure 176.1). Systemic work-up for pulmonary and cutaneous involvement of sarcoidosis is standard, and the diagnosis may require biopsy of affected tissues. As the finding of diffuse leptomeningeal enhancement is nonspecific, an open biopsy of meningeal tissue is occasionally required to confirm the presence of neurosarcoidosis.

The most common vasculitic syndrome to affect the cranial nerves is Wegener's granulomatosis. Polyarteritis nodosa and giant cell arteritis rarely affect multiple cranial nerves. Wegener's granulomatosis may involve cranial nerves either by direct spread of granulomatous lesions from the paranasal region, or by a focal necrotizing vasculitis.[65] The nervous system is involved in as many as 20% of patients with Wegener's; however, this is usually manifest as a peripheral polyneuropathy. Cranial nerves are less frequently affected. The eighth nerve is the most often

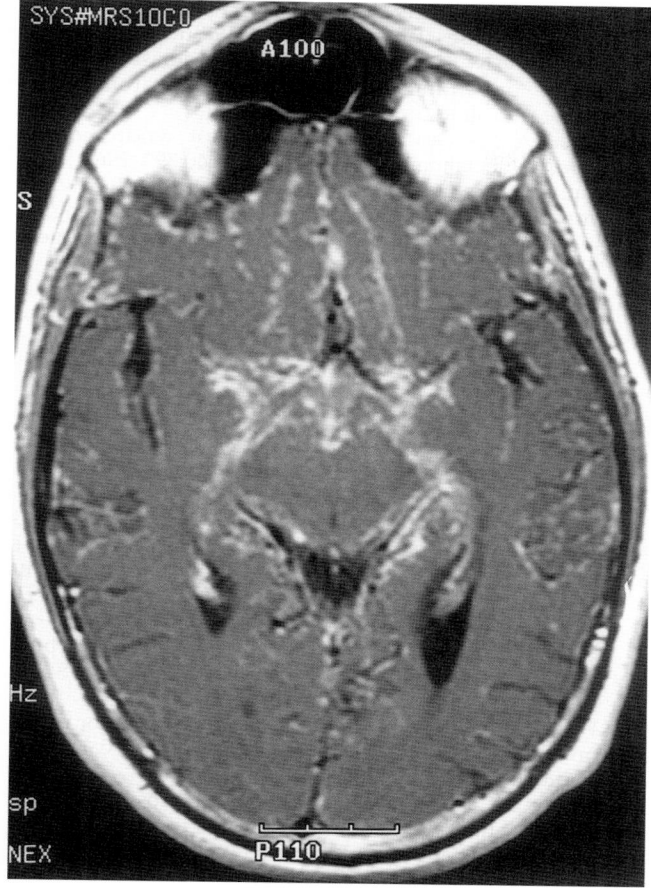

(a)

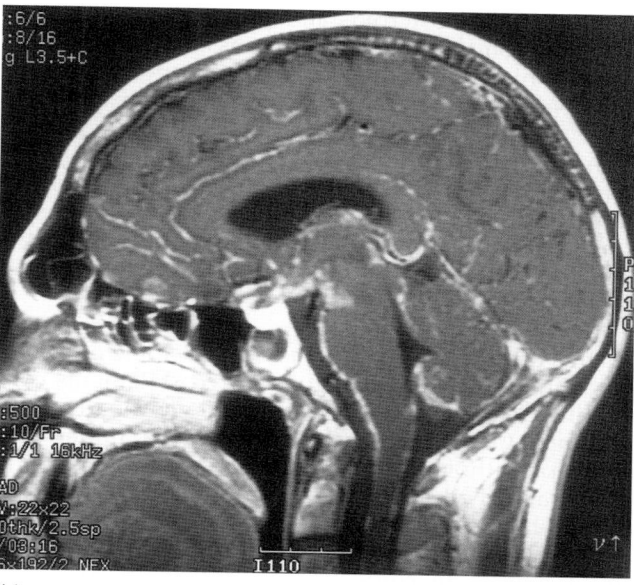

(b)

Figure 176.1   Axial (a) and sagittal (b) T$_1$-weighted magnetic resonance images obtained following intravenous administration of gadolinium. This 27-year-old man presented with bilateral abducens and a unilateral facial palsy in association with headache, polyuria and polydipsia, and optic disk edema. The MRI demonstrates diffuse abnormal leptomeningeal enhancement concentrated in the basal cisterns, but seen throughout the subarachnoid space over the convexities, sylvian fissures, the pituitary fossa, and the brainstem. Neurosarcoidosis was confirmed after mediastinoscopy revealed typical granulomatous involvement of perihilar lymph nodes. The symptoms resolved and the MRI returned to normal after 3 months of oral corticosteroid treatment.

involved and otitis and chronic sinusitis are usually present. A localized form of Wegener's granulomatosis, affecting just cranial nerves, has also been described.[20,66] One reported patient with recurrent Tolosa–Hunt and Raeder's syndromes with enhancing lesions in the cavernous sinus was found to have a cytoplasmic pattern of antineutrophil cytoplasmic autoantibody (c-ANCA), a finding characteristic of Wegener's.[66] This patient received corticosteroids and cyclophosphamide and the authors documented resolution of the syndrome. These reports underscore the difficult overlap between cavernous sinus syndromes, localized forms of diffuse pachymeningitis, and vasculitic syndromes.

Multiple cranial neuropathies occur also as a variant of demyelinating polyradiculopathy (Guillain–Barré) syndromes. Shuaib and Becker described several cases of facial paresis with ophthalmoplegia and lower cranial neuropathies associated with a viral prodrome.[67] In these cases elevated CSF protein and abnormal nerve conduction studies often point in the direction of a demyelinating illness. A description of the unique molecular pathogenesis of the Miller Fisher syndrome is elsewhere in this text.

Intracranial plasma cell granuloma represents another overlap syndrome. The most common site of

plasma cell granuloma is the lung but it may develop in both localized and diffuse intracranial locations.[68] Multiple cranial neuropathies, cavernous, and petrous apex syndromes presenting both with and without pain have been described.[68,69] The radiological appearance may also mimic other dural-based processes such as meningioma and plasmacytoma. In some cases a tissue biopsy is required for diagnosis and reveals an atypical polyclonal plasma cell infiltrate with lymphoid cells.[68,69]

Idiopathic cranial polyneuropathy is a term used to describe a self-limited syndrome recognized since the time of Gowers in his classical textbook of 1888. A comprehensive overview of this syndrome in 1987 emphasized the overlap between this and other clinicopathological entities.[9] Patients present with aching pain, often unilateral and retro-orbital, followed by the sudden development of cranial neuropathies.[9,70] The oculomotor nerves, trigeminal, facial and other lower cranial nerves are most frequently affected. When tested, the CSF reveals a mild inflammatory pleocytosis with elevated protein in some patients. Many patients received corticosteroids and their pain likely improved although no controlled data exist.[9] Idiopathic hypertrophic cranial pachymeningitis overlaps with this syndrome.[16] Most authors report the use of corticosteroids and the resolving nature of the symptoms in these conditions, leaving the true natural history of this syndrome undetermined.[9,16] The syndrome of idiopathic cranial neuropathy is therefore a diagnosis of exclusion.

Appropriate selection of CT and MR imaging with directed studies according to anatomical localization, if any, followed by examination of the CSF and specialized serological tests are required to exclude the spectrum of causes of multiple cranial neuropathies.

Treatment

As this chapter does not focus upon a single or even a few clinical entities, only generalized statements concerning treatment of multiple cranial neuropathies are possible. Of course, the nature of the underlying lesion or pathological process will dictate the first line of therapy. For some conditions, such as Wegener's granulomatosis, disease-specific therapy is available. These conditions are discussed in other portions of this textbook. In contrast, many of the cranial neuropathy syndromes are treated with corticosteroids based upon a proposed inflammatory pathogenesis. Tolosa–Hunt syndrome, for example, responds to the initiation of corticosteroids; however, the level of evidence supporting such treatment is grade C. The rarity of these diseases precludes controlled trials.

References

1. McCord MW, Mendenhall WM, Parsons JT, et al. Skin cancer of the head and neck with clinical perineural invasion. Int J Radiat Oncol Biol Phys 2000;47:89–93
2. Williams LS, Mancuso AA, Mendenhall WM. Perineural spread of cutaneous squamous and basal cell carcinoma: CT and MR detection and its impact on patient management and prognosis. Int J Radiat Oncol Biol Phys 2001;15:1061–1069
3. Chen J-R, Rhee RSC, Wallach S, et al. Neurologic disturbances in Paget disease of bone: response to calcitonin. Neurology 1979;29:448–457
4. Asher SW. Multiple cranial neuropathies, trigeminal neuralgia and vascular headaches in sickle cell disease, a possible common mechanism. Neurology 1980;30:210–211
5. Eshbaugh CG, Siatkowski M, Smith JL, Kline LB. Simultaneous multiple cranial neuropathies in diabetes mellitus. J Neuroophthalmol 1995;15:219–224
6. Boucher RM, Grace J, Java DJ. Sarcoidosis presenting as multiple cranial neuropathies and a parotid mass. Otolaryngol Head Neck Surg 1994;111:652–655
7. Grossman SA, Krabak MJ. Leptomeningeal carcinomatosis. Cancer Treat Rev 1999;25:103–199
8. Hunt WE. Tolosa–Hunt syndrome: one cause of painful ophthalmoplegia. J Neurosurg 1976;44:544–549
9. Juncos JL, Beal MF. Idiopathic cranial polyneuropathy, A fifteen-year experience. Brain 1987;110:197–211
10. Smith JL, Taxdal DSR. Painful ophthalmoplegia: the Tolosa–Hunt syndrome. Am J Ophthalmol 1966;61:1466–1472
11. Esmaeli B, Ginsberg L, Goepfert H, Deavers M. Squamous cell carcinoma with perineural invasion presenting as a Tolosa–Hunt syndrome: a potential pitfall in diagnosis. Ophthal Plast Reconstr Surg 2000;16:450–452
12. Forderreuther S, Straube A. The criteria of the International Headache Society for Tolosa–Hunt syndrome need to be revised. J Neurol 1999;246:371–377
13. Hannerz J. Recurrent Tolosa–Hunt syndrome: a report of ten new cases. Cephalalgia 1999;19(Suppl 25):33–35
14. Harnett AN, Kemp EG, Fraser G. Metastatic breast cancer presenting as Tolosa–Hunt syndrome. Clin Oncol (R Coll Radiol) 1999;11:407–409
15. Tessitore E, Tessitore A. Tolosa–Hunt syndrome preceded by facial palsy. Headache 2000;40:393–396
16. Hatano N, Behari S, Nagatani T, et al. Idiopathic hypertrophic cranial pachymeningitis: clinicopathological spectrum and therapeutic options. Neurosurgery 1999;45:1336–1342
17. Iwasaki Y, Kinoshita M. Idiopathic multiple cranial neuropathy. A twenty year experience. Jpn J Med 1998;28:323–327
18. de Arcaya AA, Cerezal L, Canga A, et al. Neuroimaging diagnosis of Tolosa–Hunt syndrome: MRI contribution. Headache 1999;39:321–325
19. Pascual J, Cerezal L, Canga A, et al. Tolosa–Hunt syndrome: focus on MRI diagnosis. Cephalalgia 1999;19(Suppl 25):36–38
20. Montecucco C, Caporali R, Pacchetti C, Turla M. Is Tolosa–Hunt syndrome a limited form of Wegener's granulomatosis? Report of two cases with anti-neutrophil cytoplasmic antibodies. Br J Rheumatol 1993;32:640–641
21. Kennerdell JS, Dresner SC. The nonspecific orbital inflammatory syndromes. Surv Ophthalmol 1984;29:93–103
22. Weber AL, Romo LV, Sabates NR. Pseudotumor of the orbit. Clinical, pathologic, and radiologic evaluation. Radiol Clin North Am 1999;37:151–168
23. Olmos PR, Falko JM, Rea GL, et al. Fibrosing pseudotumor of the sella and parasellar area producing hypopituitarism and multiple cranial nerve palsies. Neurosurgery 1993;32:1015–1021
24. Diamond JP, Bloom PA, Ragge N, et al. Localised Wegener's granulomatosis presenting as an orbital pseudotumor with extension into the posterior cranial fossa. Eur J Ophthalmol 1993;3:143–146
25. Takanashi T, Uchida S, Arita M, et al. Orbital inflammatory pseudotumor and ischemic vasculitis in Churg–Strauss syndrome: report of two cases and review of the literature. Ophthalmology 2001;108:1129–1133
26. Lorberboym M, Sacher M. False-positive uptake of TI-201 by an intracranial inflammatory pseudotumor. Clin Nucl Med 1997;22:756–758
27. Char DH, Miller T. Orbital pseudotumor. Fine-needle aspiration biopsy and response to therapy. Ophthalmology 1993;100:1702–1710
28. Mombaerts I, Schlingemann RO, Goldschmeding R, Koornneef L. Are systemic corticosteroids useful in the management of orbital pseudotumor? Ophthalmology 1996;103:521–528
29. Legos B, Fournier P, Chiaroni P, Ritz O. Basal fracture of the skull and lower (IX, X, XI, XII) cranial nerves palsy: four case reports including two fractures of the occipital condyle—a literature review. J Trauma 2000;48:342–348
30. Manni JJ, Scaf JJ, Huygen LM, et al. Hyperostosis cranialis interna. A new hereditary syndrome with cranial nerve entrapment. N Engl J Med 1990;322:450–454
31. Applegate LJ, Applegate GR, Kemp SS. MR of multiple cranial neuropathies in a patient with Camurati–Engelmann Disease: case report. Am J Neurorad 1991;12:557–559
32. Lamabadusuriya SP. Multiple nerve palsies in beta thalassaemia major. Arch Dis Child 1989;64:1060–1061

33. Motamed M, Kalan A. Gradenigo's syndrome. Postgrad Med J 2000;76:559–560

34. Chole RA, Donald PJ. Petrous apicitis. Clinical considerations. Ann Otol Rhinol Laryngol 1983;92:544–545

35. Dave AV, Diaz-Marchan PJ, Lee AG. Clinical and magnetic imaging features of Gradenigo syndrome. Am J Ophthalmol 1997;124:568–570

36. Salvesen R. Raeder's syndrome. Cephalalgia 1999;19: 42–45

37. Schoenhuber R, Vescovin E, Calcaterra S, Merli GA. Temporal bone glioblastoma presenting as Raeder paratrigeminal syndrome. Ital J Neurol Sci 1983;4: 117–119

38. Weinstein JM, Sattler FA, Towfighi J, et al. Optic neuropathy and paratrigeminal syndrome due to *Aspergillus fumigatus*. Arch Neurol 1982;39:582–585

39. Solomon S, Lustig J. Benign Raeder's syndrome is probably a manifestation of carotid artery disease. Cephalalgia 2001;21:1–11

40. Traynor AE, Gertz MA, Kyle RA. Cranial neuropathy associated with primary amyloidosis. Ann Neurol 1991;29:451–454

41. Phanthumchinda K. Multiple cranial nerve palsies as a presenting symptom in primary Sjogren's syndrome. J Med Assoc Thai 1989;72:291–294

42. Agarwal R, Arunachalam PS, Bosman DA. Lemierre's syndrome: a complication of acute oropharyngitis. J Laryngol Otol 2000;114:545–547

43. Panisset M, Eidelman A. Multiple cranial neuropathy as a feature of carotid artery dissection. Stroke 1990; 21:141–147

44. Spillane L, Roberts JR, Meyer AE. Multiple cranial nerve deficits after ethylene glycol poisoning. Ann Emerg Med 1991;20:208–210

45. Nishioka S, Silveira PVP, Ugrinovich R, de Oliveira RB. Scorpion sting with cranial nerve involvement. Toxicon 1992;30:685–686 (edit)

46. Pall JHS, Nightingale S, Clough CG, Spooner D. Progressive multiple cranial neuropathies presenting as a delayed complication of radiotherapy in infancy. Postgrad Med J 1998;64:303–305

47. Patton N, Beatty S, Lloyd IC. Bilateral sixth and fourth cranial nerve palsies in idiopathic intracranial hypertension. J R Soc Med;2000;93:80–81

48. Watters A, MacDonald MJ. Familial recurrent multiple cranial nerve palsies. J Neurol Neurosurg Psychiatry 1994;57:898

49. Balm M, Hammack J. Leptomeningeal carcinomatosis, Presenting features and prognostic factors. Arch Neurol 1996;53:626–632

50. Van Oostenbrugge RJ, Twijnstra A. Presenting features and value of diagnostic procedures in leptomeningeal metastases. Neurology 1999;53:382–385

51. Fouladi M, Gajjar A, Boyett JM, et al. Comparison of CSF cytology and spinal magnetic resonance imaging in the detection of leptomeningeal disease in pediatric medulloblastoma or primitive neuroectodermal tumor. J Clin Oncol 1999;17:3234–3237

52. Glantz MJ, Cole BF, Glantz LK, et al. Cerebrospinal fluid cytology in patients with cancer: minimizing false-negative results. Cancer 1998;82:733–739

53. Gajjar A, Fouladi M, Walter AW, et al. Comparison of lumbar and shunt cerebrospinal fluid specimens for cytologic detection of leptomeningeal disease in pediatric patients with brain tumors. J Clin Oncol 1999; 17:1825–1828

54. Rogers LR, Duchesneau PM, Nunez C, et al. Comparison of cisternal and lumbar CSF examination in leptomeningeal metastasis. Neurology 1992;42:1239–1241

55. Trivedi RA, Nichols P, Coley S, et al. Leptomeningeal glioblastoma presenting with multiple cranial neuropathies and confusion. Clin Neurol Neurosurg, 2000; 102:223–226

56. Fish LA, Friedman DI, Sudun AA. Progressive cranial polyneuropathy caused by primary central nervous system melanoma. J Clin Neuroophth 1990;10:41–44

57. Newman NJ. Multiple cranial neuropathies: presenting signs of systemic lymphoma. Surv Ophthalmol 1992; 37:125–129

58. Perry JR, Fung A, Poon P, Bayer N. Magnetic resonance imaging of nerve root inflammation in the Guillain–Barre syndrome. Neuroradiology 1994;36: 137–140

59. Olivier R, Godfroid E, Heintz R, et al. Lyme Borreliosis in a patient with severe multiple cranial neuropathy. Clin Infect Dis 1995;20:200

60. Mayo DR, Booss J. Varicella-zoster-associated neurologic disease without skin lesions. Arch Neurol 1989; 46:313–315

61. Flanagan P, Hawkings SA, Bryars JH. Infectious mononucleosis with cranial nerve palsies. Ulster Med J 1987;56:69–71

62. Joki-Erkkila VP, Hietaharju A, Numminen J, et al. Multiple cranial nerve palsies as a complication of infectious mononucleosis due to inflammatory lesion in jugular foramen. Ann Otol Rhinol Laryngol 2000; 109: 340–342

63. Maddern BR, Werkhaven J, Wessel HB, Yunis E. Infectious mononucleosis with airway obstruction and multiple cranial nerve palsies. Otolaryngol Head Neck Surg 1991;104:529–532

64. Stern BJ, Krumholz A, Johns C, et al. Sarcoidosis and its neurological manifestations. Arch Neurol 1985;42: 909–917

65. Drachman DA. Neurological complications of Wegener's granulomatosis. Arch Neurol 1963;8:145–155

66. Thajeb P, Tsai JJ. Cerebral and oculorhinal manifestations of a limited form of Wegener's granulomatosis with c-ANCA-associated vasculitis. J Neuroimaging 2001;11:59–63

67. Shuaib A, Becker WJ. Variants of Guillain–Barre syndrome: Miller Fisher syndrome, facial diplegia and multiple cranial nerve palsies. Can J Neurol Sci 1987;14:611–616

68. Saxena A, Sinha S, Tatke M. Intracranial plasma cell granuloma—a case report and review of the literature. Br J Neurosurg 2000;14:492–495

69. Kodsi SR, Younge BR, Leavitt JA, et al. Intracranial plasma cell granuloma presenting as an optic neuropathy. Surv Ophthalmol 1993;38:70–74

70. Steele JC, Vasuvat A. Recurrent multiple cranial nerve palsies: a distinctive syndrome of cranial polyneuropathy. J Neurol Neurosurg Psychiatry 1970;33:828–832

177 Functional Diseases Affecting the Cranial Nerves

James R Keane

"No cases are so well calculated to test the patience and tact of the physician as those of hysteria."[1]

W Hammond, MD (1874)

Overview

A strong case has been made that acute hysteria is a social plea masquerading as a medical condition. So considered, it is not a specific psychiatric illness but rather an attempt to escape from an intolerable situation misdirected to the physician. Acute hysteria may be prolonged or made worse by the attentions of the medical profession and needs to be diagnosed promptly, cured by persuasion if possible, and then, when necessary, followed by sympathetic physicians or a medically sophisticated social agency. As neurological symptoms are the most common and perplexing deficits adopted by hysterics, the neurologist must take the lead in diagnosis and refine his skills of suggestion and persuasion.

The naming of pseudoneurological signs and entities is famously flawed and contentious. Psychiatric classification of hysteria changes with each revision of the *Diagnostic and Statistical Manual*. At present it is classified under somatoform disorders as a "conversion disorder," despite the current disparagement of Breuer and Freud's concept of conversion of psychological conflicts into somatic symptoms.

Although there are many objections to the terms "hysteria," "psychogenic," or "functional," these names continue to be valuable[2,3] and will be used interchangeably in this chapter to indicate mimicry or simulation of neurological disease. Miller Fisher has advanced "neuroreaction" as an umbrella term encompassing medical hysteria and the hysterical phenomena associated with wartime combat and litigation/disability claims.[4] In his view, each of the various pseudoneurological deficits that characterize hysteria can be interpreted as a patient's reaction or response to an emotionally charged state related to need, desire, fear, gain, bewilderment, inability to cope, and fervor.[4] Many neurologists consider simulated neurological signs to be consciously maintained in large part, but, since self-deception is prominent in hysteria and the exact degree of awareness is neither fathomable nor very important, terms such as malingering are best used sparingly, and then usually in a medical-legal context.

Epidemiology

Pseudoneurological attacks are common in the general population but incidence figures are widely disparate and of limited use. Women are affected more often than men (two thirds [313/475] of my patients are women), but hysteria is sufficiently common in men to limit diagnostic value. Older children and young adults are most often affected, but the onset of functional symptoms may occur at any age. The cultural stresses experienced by recent immigrants may predispose them to hysteria, and the presence of language differences interferes with both diagnosis and cure by suggestion.

Certainly, hysteria is a common and challenging part of neurological practice in many cultures throughout the world. Neurological symptoms in 4% of the inpatients I see, 9% of a German general hospital neurological inpatient population,[5] and 4% of a large British neurology outpatient sample[6] had a psychogenic origin. Despite claims of some psychiatrists and many medical historians that classical hysteria has disappeared, it remains a common, and frequently unwelcome, part of neurological practice. Unfortunately, the often difficult diagnosis of hysteria is likely to become more challenging as reliance on computed scans degrades clinical skills.

Etiology and historical context

Hysteria is one of the oldest disorders affecting mankind. Pseudocoma and functional hemiparesis as a response to stress are seen in several animal species and, possibly, the original stress producing pseudoneurological symptoms in man may have been impending ingestion. While the symptoms of seizures, blindness, anesthesia, and paralysis have changed little over millennia, interpretation of the causes has varied with the Zeitgeist.[7]

Religious etiology

Ancient miraculous cures of neurological infirmities must have included many examples of successful treatment of hysteria. In classical Greece, pilgrims to a religious shrine were encouraged to dream of a cure and would often awaken to find their afflictions gone. Alternatively, a replica of the diseased organ could be left at the shrine to facilitate a cure. Identical practices continue to flourish in Latin countries. Metal imprints (milagras) can be seen in many Catholic churches today, left by devout sufferers seeking a cure. Religious cures continue to be a highly effective means of treating hysteria by persuasion, the most dramatic results occurring at public faith-healing sessions. For patients so inclined, a religious referral may be appropriate, following a firm diagnosis.

Wandering uterus

Throughout history, hysteria and seizures have been closely intertwined. The rising epigastric sensation announcing seizures or syncope was interpreted by the ancients as a shift of an unsatisfied uterus toward the diaphragm where "suffocation of the mother" might ensue. A traveling uterus could be returned to its moorings by administering pleasing aromatic substances from below to lure the uterus downward or by inhaling unpleasant odors to drive the uterus back in place. These innocuous treatments probably provided effective suggestion, but when the theory was highjacked in the nineteenth century by a few aggressive surgeons who began to remove offending uteri or ovaries, the cure became considerably worse than the disease.

Witchcraft era

Some witches—probably a minority—were hysterics. Certainly, witch-pricking, the search for localized areas of anesthesia ("the witches claw") as proof of witchcraft, involved suggestibility on the part of the victims as well as obsessive dedication on the part of the witch hunter. The unhappy treatment of hysterical witches marked the nadir of hysteria management.

Physiological causation

The more perceptive of Charcot's contemporaries regarded hysteria as neuromimesis[8] and its symptoms as impairments of the will.[9] While Charcot considered hysteria a psychogenic condition, he never abandoned his belief in an underlying physiological nidus and a hereditary predisposition. While systematically describing the common signs of hysteria, he managed to create a few of the more elaborate hysterical displays. Charcot demonstrated that hysteria occurred in the male and effectively ended the uterine era of hysteria. Unfortunately, he also sponsored such surprisingly primitive treatments as ovarian compression to halt the spread of hysterical seizures. After discovering that symptoms could be induced or removed by the previously discredited tool of hypnotism, he began to consider hypnotism the key to hysteria. Hysterical suggestibility was insufficiently credited as he transferred symptoms from side to side with the aid of giant tuning forks. His pupil Babinski redressed the balance in the next generation by emphasizing suggestibility and treatment by persuasion.

The search for a neurological basis for hysteria, having outlasted the mobile uterus and spells of witchcraft, continues unabated. Gertrude Stein, while a student at Johns Hopkins Medical School, investigated attentional mechanisms in hysteria (but failed to graduate).[10] Each generation seeks a physiological underpinning for hysteria with the latest technological tools. Currently, functional magnetic resonance imaging (MRI) correlates of hysterical deficits are eagerly being sought. Such efforts produce an increasingly sophisticated picture of the physiology of neuroreaction which may ultimately have diagnostic value, but they are bound to be disappointed in the search for a "cause" of hysteria.

Freudian conversion period

Following Freud's brief visit with Charcot, he returned to Vienna enthusiastic about the therapeutic benefits of hypnotism, but soon discovered that free association could reveal the same material. His theory that conversion symptoms represented the physical expression of repressed sexual content held sway in the West for most of the twentieth century, despite the absence of experimental proof or convincing therapeutic benefits. The present emotional backlash against Freud is in the process of removing "conversion reaction" from the lexicon.

Modern social era

More recently, hysteria has been considered a social plea expressed through medical complaints, rather than a psychiatric or medical illness.[11] Seeking the benefits of the sick role is a common human response reified by the award of employee "sick days." The heightened suggestibility of hysterics causes them to enter deeper into the role of a patient and develop enhanced "illness behavior." Dealing with the medical profession reinforces and rewards this sick role and can impede recovery. In this reasonable scheme, recovery is hastened by early dismissal from medical attention. Unfortunately, the hysteric's choice of neurological symptoms requires that the neurologist first undertake the pivotal and often difficult task of establishing a firm diagnosis.

Pathophysiology and pathogenesis

Hysteria is a response to stress manifested by simulation of neurological disease. It has no neuropathological or neurophysiological basis and is not a specific psychiatric disease. Such neuromimicry is best thought of as an inappropriate call for social help through illness behavior.

Genetics

Hysterics are made, not born. Being mildly contagious, functional disease occasionally runs in families.

Clinical features
General approach

The steps to be taken in diagnosing hysteria are:

1. Develop initial suspicion from hysterical signs or an impossible exam
2. Confirm anatomically impossible signs and absence of true neurological signs
3. Judicious use of tests (MRI, others) as needed
4. Remove the hysterical symptoms by persuasion under face-saving cover.

The initial suspicion of functional disease usually surfaces during the neurological examination. Physical signs may be contrary to expectation, or typical signs of simulation may appear.[12] Give-way weakness is common and findings may be inconsistent on testing the same function with different tasks: an inability to stand or walk may be accompanied by normal function while seated or, rarely, the reverse occurs. Optically impossible visual fields (Figure 177.1), pseudoptosis, wrong-way tongue deviation,[12] or any of the signs summarized by Fisher[13] (Table 177.1) may announce the correct diagnosis. At times, the examiner may find himself creating major deficits during the exam for which the history gave no clue. Hysterical signs match the public's concept of neurological disease which, fortunately, departs considerably from reality. Television, for once, serves a useful educational purpose by portraying mostly pseudoneurological illness as a guide for the suggestible patient. As Freud famously noted: "...hysteria behaves as though anatomy did not exist...."[14]

Once suspicion has been raised, the examiner needs to review his findings for any contrary, clearly organic, signs. He should repeat portions of the examination and offer, without strongly suggesting, an opportunity for the patient to display further functional signs (Table 177.1). For example, the visual

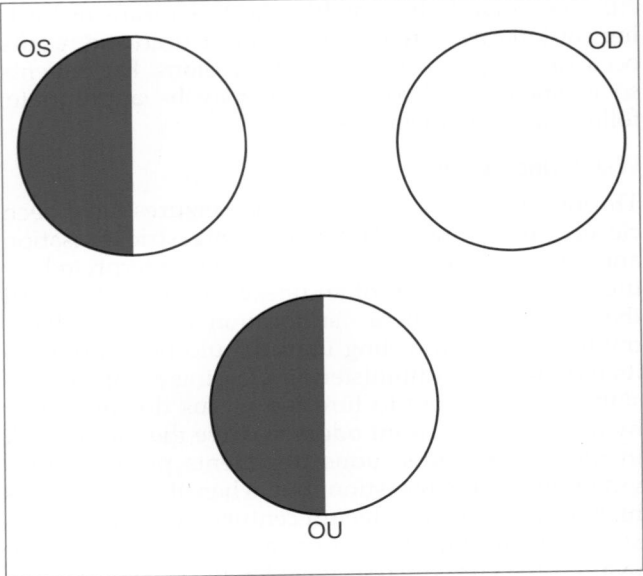

Figure 177.1   The "missing half" hemianopia[23] is the most common functional hemianopia and usually accompanies anesthesia and paralysis on the same side. Full fields in the "good" eye are optically impossible and quickly label the visual field defect as hysterical.

Table 177.1   Common hysterical signs
Give-way weakness
Attributing limitation of movement to pain
Inaccurate finger–nose test becomes finger–cheek
Undue slowness of motor tasks
Apparent great effort on strength tests
Discrepancy in performance for observed versus unobserved tasks
Momentary suspension of a limb when examiner's support suddenly withdrawn
Three finger or pincer grip
Excessive local tenderness
Pain on minimal straight leg excursions
Sensation felt less plainly throughout one side
Inability to feel examiner's touch
Pattern response to multiple stimuli (2 for 3, 2 for 1, etc.)
Patterned incorrect identification of fingers or site touched
Faultless fine manipulation of a small object with failure to identify
Delay in reporting a sensory stimulus
Inconsistencies in timed vibration
Hysterical imbalance with exaggerated wavering
Marked improvement on a test as a result of suggestion
Inconsistency on exam: impaired Romberg test with normal tandem gait
Nonphysiological tremor of the forearm
Weakness in turning the head to the weak side of the body
Deviation of the tongue to the strong side on protrusion
Ability to carry out movements in sleep which are not possible when awake
Unusual responses on memory testing (Ganser syndrome)
Abridged from Fisher[13]

fields should be tested both by simultaneous finger-counting confrontation and centripetal presentation of targets; besides testing each eye separately, a third trial with both eyes open should be conducted.

Simulated disease is difficult to maintain. While apparently testing one function, others can be observed more easily: for example, announcing a test of hand grip will allow you to observe the patient raising his paralyzed arm to help. Observing the sleeping inpatient can be most helpful: seeing a patient move a paralyzed limb, testing lash reflexes in facial anesthesia, or witnessing the deaf respond to loud noises can clinch a diagnosis. Unfortunately, it seems to be a rule that a watched patient never sleeps.

Observation of gait is a critical part of the neurological evaluation in general and is particularly important in hysteria. Walking is such a complicated task that those simulating weakness or ataxia cannot apply their complaints appropriately to this new situation. Clearly, the neurologist diagnosing simulated disease should be experienced and have a thorough knowledge of normal variability as well as an awareness of signs that misleadingly appear functional, such as orthostatic tremor[15] or seizures with maintained consciousness.[16]

Once the diagnosis of a functional etiology is evident, efforts to remove the symptoms should begin promptly, preferably during the initial examination. The patient should be encouraged to perform the apparently limited functions, praised for persistence, and the usual great show of effort (the overflow of effort into unaffected muscles) acknowledged. A prompt cure of the disability is important in confirming the psychogenic etiology: when a patient does even a fair simulation of neurological disease, a cure may be the only way to convince the patient, his family and the referring physician of the nature of the signs. Patients should be a given a face-saving diagnosis such as a fatigue- or stress-induced malfunction, reassured of its temporary nature, and given a face-saving task—usually physical therapy performed with much encouragement—to assist in recovery. Particularly in California, perhaps, alternative medical therapies, such as acupuncture or foot reflexology, or culturally specific therapies delivered by a local curandero, may have great persuasive powers.

Diagnosis of hysteria affecting the cranial nerves

Perhaps the most common sign affecting the cranial nerves is anesthesia of half of the body. In addition to facial hemianesthesia, other cranial nerve sensory functions such as smell, sight, touch, hearing and taste are variably involved. Motor cranial nerve concomitants are unusual in this setting but occasionally gaze to the affected side is avoided and, rarely, facial weakness is simulated. Inasmuch as no organic disease presents in such a nonanatomical fashion, the diagnosis is straightforward.

Blindness of one or both eyes is a common hysterical complaint.[17,18] Simulated complete blindness is easily detected by visual threat or use of a large mirror to elicit following eye movements. Simulation of severe monocular amblyopia is quickly revealed by demonstrating equal optic nerve function with the swinging flashlight test. Partial functional visual loss is more difficult to establish: for monocular loss, the patient can be confused as to which eye is being examined.[19-21] Unilateral or bilateral functional amblyopia can be uncovered by eliciting marked disparities on different tests. Vision can be tested for congruency at varying distances; normal depth perception establishes good vision in each eye[22] and normal color vision testing shows excellent optic nerve function. Color vision test plates are a particularly quick and convincing tool: the large size of the figures can be pointed out to the patient along with the fact that he can hold the pages near his eye and see them easily despite his problem.

The most common pattern of psychogenic visual field loss is severely constricted (tunnel) fields that remain the same size regardless of distance. Most are smaller than five degrees and many are "negative," with objects seen only when moved past fixation from all sides. Spiral fields are tunnel fields with a constantly decreasing radius, often ending at zero. Functional *hemianopias* are common when simultaneous finger-counting confrontation field techniques are employed.[23] Usually associated with ipsilateral monocular visual loss, such fields may present with a complaint of poor vision in one eye or may be "discovered" during examination. Most patients select the optically impossible, "missing field" pattern, in which vision is absent to one side when either the ipsilateral eye or both eyes are tested but full when the "good" eye is examined[24] (Figure 177.1).

Psychogenic diplopia is almost always monocular, and most cases of monocular diplopia seen by neurologists will already have been evaluated for ocular causes.[25] Failure of a pinhole to eliminate monocular diplopia makes a refractive etiology unlikely and reinforces the likelihood of hysterical diplopia. Suggestible patients with true binocular diplopia occasionally will maintain that both images persist monocularly, usually in the eye ipsilateral to the side of diplopia, so it is important not to dismiss monocular diplopia without a careful examination.

Weakness of cranial nerve muscles is usually associated with limb weakness and anesthesia on the same side. Gaze paresis cannot convincingly be sustained and a few minutes of testing will reveal eye movements toward the paralyzed side. Optokinetic nystagmus with symmetric fast and slow phases in forward gaze militates against gaze paralysis. Both organic and hysterical gaze palsies may be accompanied by inability to turn the heard toward the affected side. As is common with simulated neurological deficits, psychogenic head turning difficulty is usually exaggerated so that not only is there a complete inability to move the head past the midline voluntarily, but passive head movement toward that side elicits strong resistance.

Spasm of the near reflex is usually functional[26] but rarely may be due to acute organic disease,[27] sometimes in the pontine tegmentum. Convergence spasm is sometimes confused with bilateral sixth nerve palsy by the inexperienced. However, voluntary convergence cannot be sustained for long and observation will reveal that miosis exactly parallels convergence.

Central nystagmus may result from a wide variety of sedatives and anticonvulsants but true nystagmus cannot be willed.[28] A few gifted individuals can concentrate and converge and make their eyes quiver with high frequency, small amplitude continuous saccades.[29] Such "convergence nystagmus" cannot be sustained for long and its rapid shimmering character is unlike any involuntary eye movement.

Psychogenic ptosis is a red flag which announces that other signs may be simulated as well.[30] Voluntary ptosis results from orbicularis contraction rather than levator relaxation and the patient may actively resist passive opening of the eye. Voluntary ptosis is easily diagnosed by observing that the ipsilateral eyebrow is low (Charcot's sign), rather than the expected elevation needed to overcome a ptotic lid.

While there were reports of hysterical monocular pupillary changes in the last century, such signs undoubtedly represented surreptitious use of mydriatic (rarely miotic) eye drops. Testing with weak (0.1%) pilocarpine eye drops to detect a tonic pupil is then followed by strong (4%) pilocarpine drops which will constrict all except pharmacologically blocked pupils.[31]

Other cranial nerve sensory functions are usually affected together and their disparate anatomical connections make a hysterical diagnosis obvious. Occasionally, the function of one sensory cranial nerve function will be affected selectively. Functional loss of smell and taste are insufficiently dramatic to be seen often by the neurologist, but in one specialized smell clinic, 5% of referrals were judged to have psychogenic anosmia.[32] Acute deafness is uncommon in civilian practice but is sometimes simulated to avoid military service and was a common complaint in World War I combat.[33] Classically, psychogenic deafness is accompanied by anesthesia about the ear, but this probably reflected the expectations of the examiners. Simulated monocular hearing loss, like functional monocular vision loss, can be detected by confusing the patient as to the side being examined. Hearing tests using galvanic skin resistance measurements or auditory evoked potentials will reveal the spurious nature of deafness of one or both ears.

Functional facial anesthesia is rare in the absence of hemianesthesia of the body; a nonanatomical distribution from hairline to jawline is suggestive of a psychogenic origin and recourse to electrical blink reflex testing is rarely needed. Aphonia and mutism are most commonly seen in military practice. Among civilian patients, schizophrenia rather than hysteria is a more likely cause of mutism.[34] Normal whispering indicates that language is unimpaired, and the ability to cough requires functioning vocal cords.

Facial weakness is difficult to simulate or sustain and patients usually adopt an unnatural appearance with tight perioral muscles, partially closed eye and a lowered brow on looking upward. Hysterical tongue weakness almost always has the tongue deviating strongly towards the wrong side, opposite the usual accompanying hemiparesis.[12] Charcot found that simultaneous hysterical facial and lingual involvement usually involved contraction rather than weakness and called that combination "glossolabial hemispasm."

Hysterical elaboration of a structural neurological problem is common and demands that the examiner not construe evidence of suggestibility in one area as proof that all signs are functional. Bell's palsy is a common nidus for functional elaboration.[35] Discovering acute hemifacial weakness, the patient or his associate worry about a stroke. From there, it is only a short step to becoming convinced of ipsilateral weakness. Limb weakness accompanying Bell's palsy almost always disappears with explanation and reassurance. Rarely, however, ipsilateral facial palsy and hemiparesis occur on the basis of multiple organic lesions.

Classification

Hysteria is probably best classified by the neurological function mimicked. The most common varieties (with some overlap) are:

1. Hemisensory defect—which may include cranial nerve dysfunctions
2. Hemiparesis with or without sensory loss
3. Paraparesis with or without sensory loss
4. Monoparesis with or without sensory loss
5. Seizures—alone or with true seizures
6. Gait disorders
   - Hemiparetic
   - Ataxic
   - Unique
7. Movement disorders
   - Cerebelloid
   - Choreiform
   - Parkinsonian
8. Blindness, binocular or monocular
9. Convergence spasm and ptosis
10. Speech disorders and memory loss
11. Face and tongue paralysis
12. "Spread" of organic disease: Bell's palsy with ipsilateral hemiplegia.

Diagnostic criteria

The diagnosis of functional disease is unique in depending upon clinical expertise, aided, when possible, by rapid cure with suggestion. Laboratory and radiological tests offer only negative support. Background features such as hysterical personality, indifference to illness, history of frequent surgery or psychiatric illness, availability of a model for the symptoms, and presence of secondary gain are sufficiently common in patients with organic illness to be unreliable guides to the diagnosis of hysteria.

Differential diagnosis

The diagnostic alternative to a pseudoneurological illness is pseudo-pseudoneurological disease, or misdiagnosis of organic neurological disease. Expert clinical skills and judicious use of laboratory studies should minimize the confusion, but only the inexperienced will think this an easy task.

Treatment

Acute hysteria is a self-limited condition, rather than a disease, and usually causes little long term disability. As its minor variations are sufficiently common to be considered a part of daily life, treatment concerns tend to be overshadowed by diagnostic ones. A large, randomized, controlled treatment trial is unlikely ever to be organized. Not surprisingly, the quality of treatment evidence is poor (grade C, level V), manifested by uncontrolled small case series and, mostly, by unsupported anecdotal testimony such as mine.

Management

The neurological management of hysteria cannot be separated from diagnosis and removal of symptoms. The neurologist's job is to make an accurate diagnosis, using whatever tests are required, and then cure the patient if possible. It is important to enlist the patient's help; confronting him and unmasking his simulation is counterproductive at best, and most unfortunate when the physician is mistaken. It is perfectly reasonable to emphasize that underlying stress might cause such symptoms. Insight into the patient's simulation can be conveyed tacitly by sympathizing with his plight, assuring him that you've dealt with similar problems before, and insisting that a day or two of physical therapy will finish the recovery that has already begun. When the patient is refractory to a cure by suggestion, intervention by social services may assist in alleviating the precipitating stress. Family counseling may be helpful; practical interventions to relieve the precipitating circumstances such as helping the patient change jobs or find a new apartment may appear to reward aberrant behavior but such measures are cheaper and more appropriate than prolonged medical efforts. Acute hysterics at our hospital rarely abuse such assistance and seldom return with new episodes. Certainly, for someone dependent upon government bureaucracy for assistance, acute paralysis is usually more effective than going through channels.

The neurologist's job is reasonably concluded with resolution of symptoms. Usually, a single attack of acute hysterical symptoms resolves promptly without further episodes and the patients manage their lives without evidence of major psychiatric illness. However, depression and anxiety are more common among hysterics than in the general population[36] and some patients benefit from follow-up by a psychiatrically oriented physician. A rare acute hysteric will have severe psychiatric problems, and if the neurologist is not inclined to consider this possibility, regular psychiatric referral is appropriate. Most acute hysterics are happy to talk to a psychiatrist, and such referrals should be offered in the spirit of helping with the associated stress to obviate the patient's later claiming that "the doctors think it's all in my head."

In our hospital, acute hysterical episodes are reversed by suggestion during several days inpatient stay in about half of the patients; perhaps a quarter resolve within the next few weeks, while those with persisting symptoms usually experience little limitation of their normal activities even if blind or paralyzed.[37] Chronic hysteria (Briquet's and Munchausen syndromes) and malingering are refractory to treatment, and management of the occasional patient with these forms of career hysteria is much less satisfactory. While such patients comprise only about 5% of those simulating neurological disease on our wards, their visits are repeated and memorable. Career hysterics are firmly committed to illness behavior and resist change. The neurologist's goal should be to make a firm diagnosis and then attempt to keep the patient and the medical profession from damaging each other. A sympathetic physician should follow such patients at regular intervals and endeavor to keep them out of the emergency department. Munchausen syndrome[38] patients are career hysterics who travel out of town. They tend to dramatize nonmedical elements of their life whereas the Briquet syndrome patient may concentrate on researching and acting out hard-to-disprove medical diseases such as lupus or porphyria. Factitious disease, intentional self-injury with intent to deceive, often accompanies more serious psychiatric disturbance. Factitious damage occurs occasionally in career hysterics (who generally prefer to have the medical profession do the injuring) but is rare among acute hysterics.

The approach to the individual faking neurological symptoms for financial gain or preservation of life is limited to establishing the diagnosis in a manner convincing to the medical and legal professions, and then urging a speedy resolution of the legal or administrative decisions. When the patient faces a stretch in jail or induction into the wartime military, perhaps the best that can be done is to convey to the individual that his performance lacks conviction and he should try another approach to resolving his difficulties. Such situations in which the interests of physicians and patients diverge are uncomfortable for the neurologist, who must walk an ethical tightrope.

Diagnosing and managing the acute hysteric causes anxiety among neurologists who are faced with making a difficult judgement, supported only in a negative way by ancillary testing. Misdiagnosis of hysteria is not appreciated by the patient, his family, his family doctor or his lawyer, and often results in vilification or worse for the diagnostician. Still, for those who are attracted by the detective, problem-solving aspects of neurology, diagnosing hysteria remains one of the last redoubts of pure clinical diagnosis. Where else in neurology can you deal with pleasant patients who are not too bothered by their condition, are generally willing to be cured with alacrity, and often have the good grace to stay cured?

References

1. Hammond W. A treatise on diseases of the nervous system. New York: D Appleton and Company, 1871:634
2. Mace CJ, Trimble MR. "Hysteria," "functional" or "psychogenic"? J R Soc Med 1991;84:471–475
3. Marsden CD. Hysteria—a neurologist's view. Psych Med 1986;16:277–288
4. Fisher CM. Similar disorders viewed with different perspectives (letter). Arch Neurol 1995;52:745
5. Lempert T, Dieterich M, Huppert D, Brandt T. Psychogenic disorders in neurology: frequency and clinical spectrum. Acta Neurol Scand 1990;82:335–40
6. Perkin GD. An analysis of 7836 successive new outpatient referrals. J Neurol Neurosurg Psychiatry 1989; 52:447–448
7. Mills CK. Hysteria. In: Pepper W, Starr I, eds. A System of Practical Medicine. Philadelphia: Lea Bothers, 1886: 205–287
8. Paget J. Clinical lectures on the nervous mimicry of organic diseases. Lancet 1873;2:511–513
9. Reynolds JR. Remarks on paralysis, and other disorders of motion and sensation, dependent on "idea." BMJ 1869;2:483–485
10. Solomons LM, Stein G. Normal motor automatism. Psych Rev 1886;510–512
11. Rabkin R. Conversion hysteria as social maladaptation. Psychiatry 1964;27:349–363
12. Keane JR. Wrong-way deviation of the tongue with hysterical hemiparesis. Neurology 1986;36:1406–1407
13. Fisher CM. Painful states: a neurological commentary. Pain and hysteria. Clin Neurosurg 1984;31:35–39
14. Freud S. Some points for a comparative study of organic and hysterical motor paralysis. In: Strachey J, ed. Pre-psycho-analytic Publications and Unpublished Drafts. Vol 1. Std ed. London: Hogarth Press, 1966:169
15. Wills AJ, Thompson PD, Findley LJ, Brooks DJ. A positron emission tomography study of primary orthostatic tremor. Neurology 1996;46:747–752

16. Ashkenazi A, Kaufman Y, Ben-Hur T. Bilateral focal motor status epilepticus with retained consciousness after stroke. Neurology 2000;54:976–978

17. Parinaud M. The ocular manifestations of hysteria. *In:* Norris WF, Oliver CA, eds. System of Diseases of the Eye. Philadelphia: Lippincott, 1906

18. De Schweinitz GE. Ocular manifestations of hysteria. *In:* Posey WC, Spiller WG, eds. System of Disease of the Eye. Philadelphia: JB Lippincott, 1906:614–695

19. Baudry S. Simulated blindness. *In:* Norris WF, Oliver CA, eds. System of Diseases of the Eye. Philadelphia: Lippincott, 1900

20. Miller BW. A review of practical tests for ocular malingering and hysteria. Surv Ophthalmol 1973;17:241–246

21. Kramer KK, La Piana FG, Appleton B. Ocular malingering and hysteria: diagnosis and management. Surv Opthalmol 1979;24:89–96

22. Levy NS, Glick EB. Stereoscopic perception and Snellen Visual Acuity. Am J Ophthalmol 1974;78:722–724

23. Keane JR. Hysterical hemianopia: the "missing half" field defect. Arch Ophthalmol 1979;97:865–866

24. Keane JR. Patterns of hysterical hemianopia. Neurology 1998;51:1230–1231

25. Records RE. Monocular diplopia. Surv Ophthalmol 1980;24:303–306

26. Cogan DB, Freese CF Jr. Spasm of the near reflex. Arch Ophthalmol 1955;54:752–759

27. Dagi LR, Chrousos CA, Cogan DG. Spasm of the near reflex associated with organic disease. Am J Ophthalmol 1987;103:582–585

28. Luhr AF, Eckel JL. Fixation and voluntary nystagmus: a clinical study. Arch Ophthalmol 1933;9:625–634

29. Shults WT, Stark L, Hoyt WF, Ochs AL. Normal saccadic structure of voluntary nystagmus. Arch Ophthalmol 1977;95:1399–1404

30. Keane JR. Neuro-ophthalmic signs and symptoms of hysteria. Neurology 1982;32:757–762

31. Thompson HS, Newsome DA, Loewenfeld IE. The fixed dilated pupil. Arch Ophthalmol 1971;86:21–27

32. Davidson TM. Anosmia—evaluation and treatment. (Otolaryngology epitome) West J Med 1987;146:219

33. Jones AB, Llewellyn LJ. Malingering or the Simulation of Disease. Philadelphia: P Blakiston's Son, 1917

34. Altshuler LL, Cummings JL, Mills MJ. Mutism: review, differential diagnosis, and report of 22 cases. Am J Psychiatry 1986;143:1409–1414

35. Keane JR. Hysterical hemiparesis accompanying Bell's palsy. Neurology 1993;43:1619

36. Wilson-Barnett J, Trimble MR. An investigation of hysteria using the illness behavior questionnaire. Br J Psychiatry 1985;146:601–608

37. Kathol RG, Cox TA, Corbett JJ, Thompson HS. Functional visual loss: follow-up of 42 cases. Arch Ophthalmol 1983;101:729–735

38. Pankratz L. A review of the Munchausen syndrome. Clin Psychol Rev 1981;1:65–78

XI Peripheral Nerve Disorders (Including Anterior Horn Cell and Autonomic Nervous System)

Section editor: Peter J Dyck

178 Mechanical Nerve Injuries

Robert C Hermann Jr

Introduction

Most peripheral nerve injuries are caused by mild compression or entrapment of the nerve. This chapter considers not only compression and entrapment injuries but also less common injuries from transection, laceration, crush, or severe stretch and the damaging effects of electrical current, extremes of temperature, and radiation.

Classification of nerve injuries

Injuries to peripheral nerves may be categorized by the degree of damage to a single nerve fiber or axon or by the degree of damage to compound nerves containing numerous fascicles, with each fascicle containing many axons and a connective tissue sheath.[1]

The damage to individual axons is of two basic types. Type 1 injury is interruption of conductivity across a segment of the axon without loss of axon continuity (Figure 178.1). Type 2 injury is damage to axonal structures to the degree that the continuity of the axons is interrupted, resulting in degeneration of the axon (wallerian degeneration); the proximal segment of the axon and the cell body of the neuron remain intact. The portion of the neuron proximal to the injury undergoes early and late retrograde alterations that depend partly on whether connectivity is reestablished.

Type 1 axonal injuries are characterized by a failure of conduction of the action potential across the injured segment of the axon, but conduction block is limited only to the region of injury, with conduction being preserved proximally and distally to the focal lesion. In a normal motor unit (i.e., an anterior horn cell, its axon, and the muscle fibers it innervates), the action potentials generated by the muscle fibers are the same regardless of where the axon is stimulated to threshold (Figure 178.2). However, if there is focal conduction block, the muscle action potential will be normal when the axon is stimulated anywhere distal to the point of the block (S1 in Figure 178.3) and absent when the axon is stimulated proximally to the point of the block. In this situation, one assumes that conduction along the axon is intact both proximally and distally to the site of conduction block (S2 in Figure 178.3). In most cases, the disturbance that causes the conduction block is reversible. This type of axonal dysfunction without loss of continuity is called a *neurapractic lesion*. The pathological basis of this type of block is varied and may include the action of a local anesthetic agent, nerve compression, damage to the myelin sheath, or alterations of the function of the axonal cell membrane or its channel proteins.

Type 2 injuries are characterized by axonal interruption, an *axonotmetic lesion* (Figure 178.1). Axonotmetic lesions result in loss of function of the peripheral end organ, as in type 1, or neurapractic, lesions, and also degeneration of the distal axon (wallerian degeneration).[2] Acute and chronic retrograde changes also occur in the proximal axon and cell body; these changes depend partly on whether reconnection of the distal segment is reestablished.

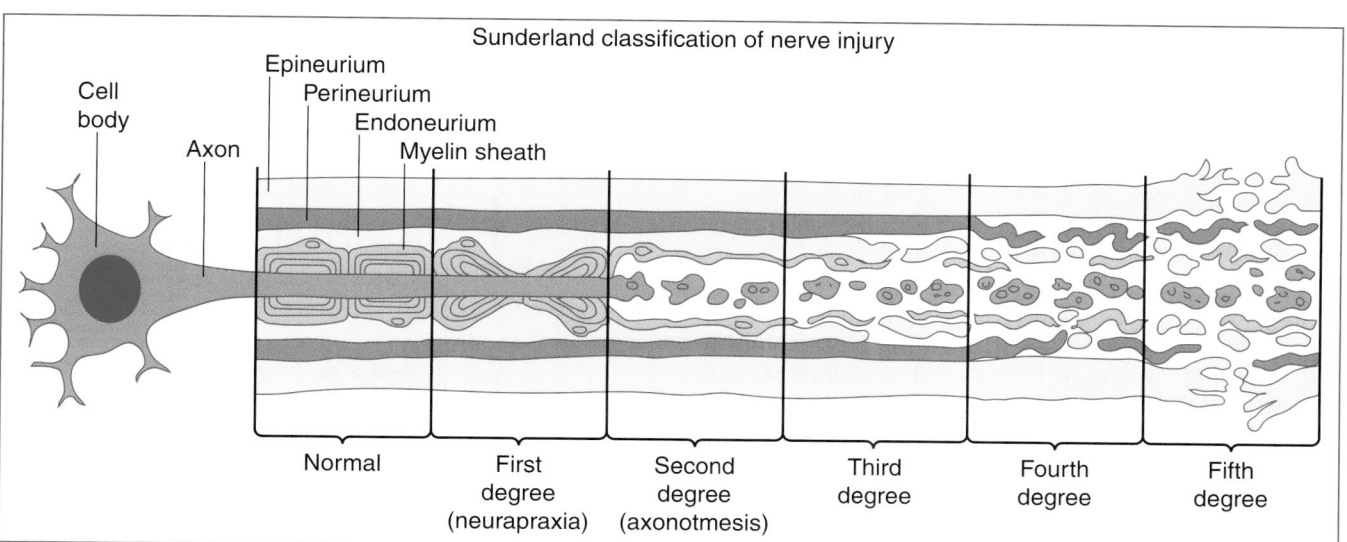

Figure 178.1 Classification of nerve injury by degree of involvement of various neural elements. (From Rayan GM. Compression neuropathies, including carpal tunnel syndrome. Clinical Symposia 1997;49(2):1–32. By permission of *Novartis*.) (See color plate section.)

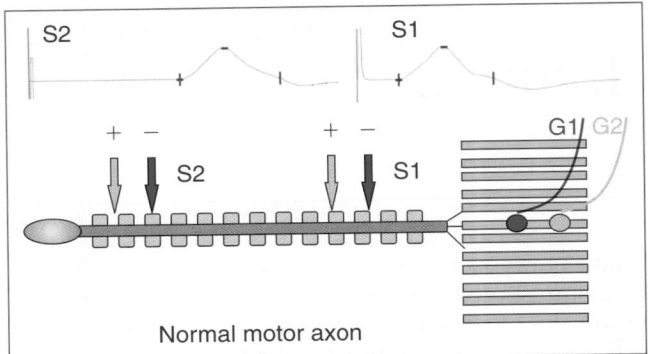

Figure 178.2 Simulation of stimulation and recording from a single normal motor unit. Recording electrodes (G1 and G2) are placed over the muscle fibers innervated by the motor neuron. When the motor neuron axon is stimulated to threshold by an electrical stimulus, an action potential is triggered at the site of the stimulus and conducts down the motor axon to the neuromuscular junctions and generates an action potential in the muscle fibers. The motor axon can be stimulated to threshold at any point along the axon (S1, S2). The latency of the recorded muscle response increases as the distance increases between stimulating electrodes and the muscle.

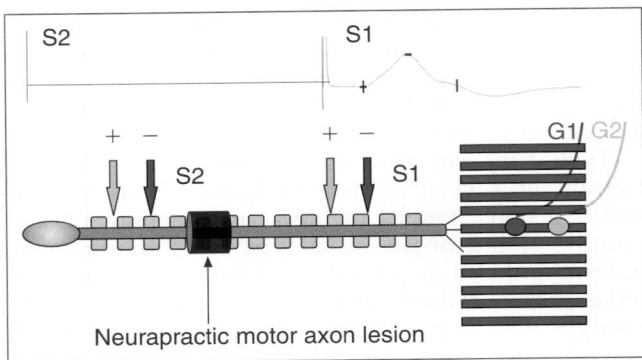

Figure 178.3 Simulation of stimulation and recording from a single motor unit with a neuinapractic motor axon lesion. If a neurapractic, or type 1, lesion occurs along the motor axon and the axon is stimulated distal to the lesion (S1), the action potential will conduct distally to the muscle and produce a recordable muscle response (recorded by electrodes G1 and G2). If the motor axon is stimulated proximal to the lesion (S2), the action potential will conduct to the neurapractic lesion but not across the lesion. Thus, conduction of the action potential will be blocked and the muscle will not respond.

In axonotmetic lesions, electrical stimulation of the initial segment of the axon next to the motor neuron cell body (S2 in Figure 178.4) will generate action potentials that will be conducted along the axon to the point of injury but not across the injured segment. Thus, muscle will not respond. If the distal axon is stimulated electrically distal to the lesion shortly after the injury (S1 in Figure 178.4), the distal segment can generate and conduct action potentials and cause the muscle to contract even though this axonal segment is separated from the neuronal cell body. The response

to electrical stimulation will mimic that of a type 1, or neurapractic, lesion for the first few days. From 3 to 8 days after the injury, the distal segment of the axon degenerates and no response will be obtained from electrical stimulation of the distal segment (Figure 178.5). Thus, after 3 to 8 days, axonotmetic lesions can be distinguished from neurapractic lesions.

In type 2 lesions, the distal segments of sensory axons demonstrate the same basic changes as those of motor axons, but sensory axons separated from the cell body continue to function for 2 or 3 days longer (i.e., for 5 to 11 days) than degenerating motor axons.

It needs to be emphasized that differentiating neurapractic lesions from axonotmetic lesions applies mainly to injuries of individual axons. In a focal nerve

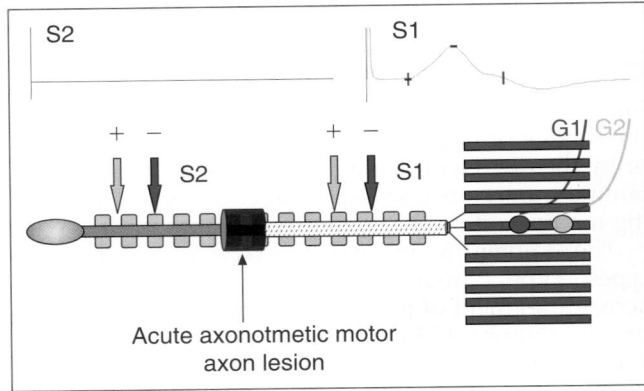

Figure 178.4 Simulation of stimulation and recording from a single motor unit with an acute axonotmetic motor axon lesion. In an axonotmetic, or type 2, lesion, the continuity of the axon at the site of the lesion is disrupted and the distal segment and muscle fibers are separated from the proximal segment and cell body. For the first 3 to 8 days after the lesion, stimulation at the distal site (S1) will produce a muscle response (recorded by electrodes G1 and G2), but the action potential generated by stimulation at the proximal site (S2) will not propagate across the lesion.

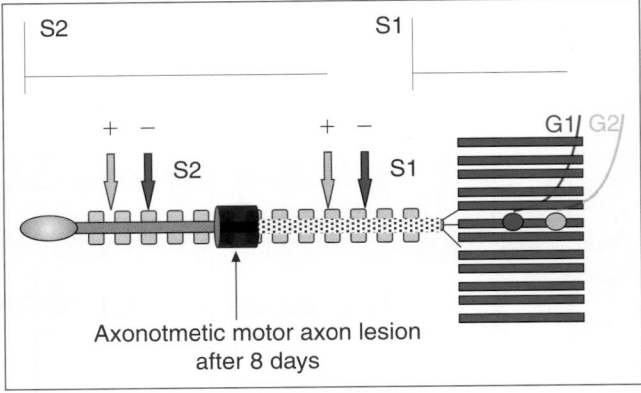

Figure 178.5 Simulation of stimulation and recording from a single motor unit 8 days after an axonotmetic motor axon lesion. After 8 days, the portion of the motor axon distal to the lesion degenerates and no response can be recorded (G1 and G2) from the muscle with stimulation at the distal (S1) or proximal (S2) site.

Table 178.1	Classifications of nerve injuries		
Seddon[3]	**Sunderland[1]**	**Pathology**	**Prognosis for recovery**
Neurapraxia	First-degree	Alterations of myelin sheath or axonal cell membrane	Excellent
Axonotmesis	Second-degree	Axonal loss, with intact endoneurium, perineurium, and epineurium	Good to poor depending on severity of axonal loss, distance to end organ, etc.
Axonotmesis	Third-degree	Axonal loss with disruption of the endoneurium; perineurium and epineurium intact	Moderate Recovery more delayed, incomplete, and usually complicated by aberrant reinnervation
Axonotmesis	Fourth-degree	Axonal loss with disruption of endoneurium and perineurium; epineurium intact	Poor Surgical repair often required
Neurotmesis	Fifth-degree	Axonal loss, with disruption of entire connective tissue sheath and separation of nerve stumps	No or ineffective spontaneous recovery Recovery after surgery depends on many factors

Modified from Dillingham.[5] By permission of the American Association of Electrodiagnostic Medicine.

trunk injury, all the fibers may be transected or they may be compressed but not transected, or various numbers of them may be transected, compressed, or unaffected. The degree and rate of recovery depend also on the disruption of the connective tissue sheaths, the blood supply, and the extent of misconnection of transected axons.

Classifications have been developed to characterize the degree of nerve injury (Table 178.1).[1,3–5]

A more detailed account of nerve injury has been provided by Lundborg.[4]

Long-standing axonotmetic injuries result in retrograde degeneration of the neuronal cell body, preceded by atrophy of the cell body and secondary demyelination of the proximal axon. The number of cell bodies that degenerate after axonotmesis may be as high as 85%, but such severe loss develops over years. The closer the axonal lesion is to the cell body, the more severe the loss of cell bodies. If the entire neuron degenerates, regeneration is not possible.

If the neuron survives, the amount of retrograde change in the axon proximal to the site of the lesion depends on the severity of the injury. The retrograde changes can extend along the axon for 2 cm proximal to the lesion. The axonal stump proximal to the lesion becomes swollen. This swollen area has been attributed to the damming up of materials transported down the axon by anterograde axonal transport. The diameter of the axon proximal to the site of swelling decreases because of the loss of such cytoskeletal elements as neurofilaments.

Transection of peripheral axons causes transitory retrograde changes or central chromatolysis in 10% to 80% of the neuron cell bodies. These changes develop within 6 hours and reach a peak near the end of the first week. The nucleus of the neuron is displaced to the periphery, and the Nissl substance, or endoplasmic reticulum, becomes dispersed and the cell body swells.

The explosion in knowledge about the molecular biology of nerve injury has been reviewed elsewhere.[6,7] Although the details of the processes of neuronal and axonal degeneration and regeneration are not covered in this chapter, excellent reviews are available.[8–12]

Muscle reinnervation occurs by two separate mechanisms: the collateral sprouting mechanism and the axonal regrowth mechanism. If the loss of motor axons to a muscle is incomplete with some motor axons remaining intact, the surviving motor axons generate collateral sprouts from their nerve terminals near the muscle fibers that have lost their innervation (Figure 178.6). These collateral axonal sprouts reinnervate muscle fibers quickly, within days to weeks. However, if all the motor axons to a muscle are severed, reinnervation occurs by regrowth of axonal sprouts from the proximal stump (Figure 178.7). Reinnervation by axonal regrowth takes much longer than

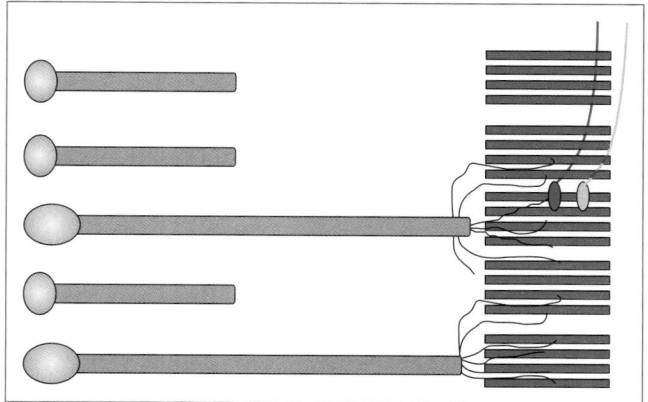

Figure 178.6 Reinnervation of muscle by collateral sprouting after partial axonotmesis.

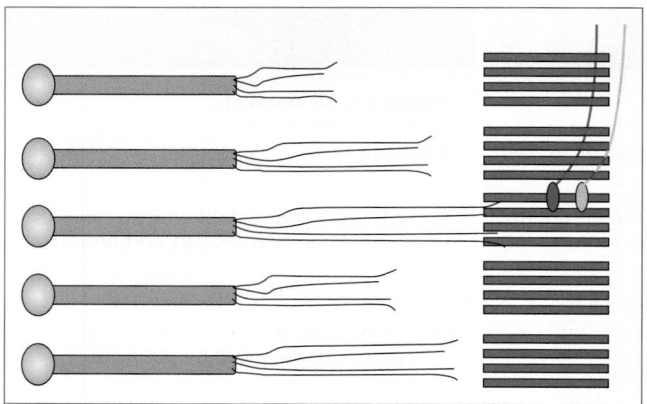

Figure 178.7 Reinnervation of muscle by axonal regrowth after complete axonotmesis.

reinnervation by collateral sprouting. Axonal sprouts grow at a rate of 1 mm per day (approximately 1 inch per month). In the case of complete axonal loss, the time to the beginning of reinnervation is determined primarily by the distance that the axonal sprouts have to travel to reach the muscle, and this takes months to years. This difference between reinnervation by collateral sprouting and reinnervation by axonal regrowth must be considered carefully when informing patients of the chances for improvement and when to expect improvement to occur. Similar mechanisms may apply to sensory reinnervation, but the mechanisms and details are not understood.

Specific types of mechanical nerve damage
Compression and entrapment

Compression and entrapment are frequent causes of mechanical injury to peripheral nerves. The terms have been used in different ways and interchangeably.[13,14] A clear definition of these terms is needed. *Compression* is the act of pressing together or an application of force exerted on the nerve from the outside, so that it is compressed against a rigid underlying structure. Another definition of compression is an action exerted upon a body by an external force that tends to diminish its volume and augment its density. Compression of a peripheral nerve may be a single acute episode, be intermittent but recurrent, or be continuous over a sustained period.

Entrapment neuropathy is an injury that occurs when a nerve passes through an opening that is too small. Entrapment neuropathies are specific forms of compressive neuropathies in which the nerves are normally confined to narrow anatomical passageways and are susceptible to constricting pressure.[15]

The effects of compression depend on many factors, including the magnitude of the force, the rate of change in the deforming force, and the duration and the area over which the force is applied. If the force is applied at a point, nerve fibers and perhaps even the whole nerve may be transected. The larger the area of the nerve subject to the force, the larger the area of damaged nerve. The internal structure of the

nerve, including the number and size of fascicles and the amount of connective tissue, were thought by Sunderland[1] to be important in the susceptibility of nerves to compressive forces. He thought that nerves were more susceptible to compression or pressure when the peripheral nerve was composed of a few large and closely packed fascicles that had little supporting tissue between them.

In an entrapment neuropathy in which the nerve is bound by a closed space, any increase in the volume of any tissue in the compartment will increase the pressure on the nerve. This can include an increase in the volume of the nerve, the blood or blood vessels, bone, tendons, ligaments, connective tissue, or fat.

The fibers most sensitive to compression are the large-diameter myelinated fibers, including afferent fibers conveying touch-pressure, vibration, and proprioception. The largest sensory axons are larger than the motor axons and are usually damaged first by compression. For this reason, sensory nerve conduction studies are often abnormal before motor nerve conduction studies are in compressive lesions.

Acute nerve compression produced by a sphygmomanometer cuff produces a rapidly reversible conduction block that affects the sensory axons conveying touch sensation more than it affects the axons conveying pain sensation.[16–18] This results in a progressive sensory loss that begins distally after 30 to 40 minutes of compression and spreads proximally. It also produces transient paresthesias early in the compression, but more marked paresthesias appear 30 seconds after the cuff has been released, increase for 1 or 2 minutes, and then subside. These sensory phenomena are due to the spontaneous generation of action potentials ectopically in myelinated sensory axons (touch, proprioception, and pressure) in the nerve trunk and in some ways are analogous to fasciculations in motor neurons and their axons.[19] Unmyelinated sensory axons do not appear to generate these ectopic impulses. Continued compression results in loss of function in the form of a neurapractic lesion with conduction block. This form of rapidly reversible conduction block may be the direct result of ischemia, but the mechanism of dysfunction is not clear.[20]

A more persistent acute demyelinating compression block has been produced experimentally by compression of a peripheral nerve with a narrow tourniquet. This produces weakness with relative preservation of sensation. Larger diameter myelinated fibers, particularly motor fibers, appear to be affected more severely. Recovery may begin in days but usually takes 6 to 8 weeks. The conduction block may persist for up to 17 weeks, but persistence longer than 8 weeks suggests other types and degrees of nerve injury. Eventual recovery is good.

Denny-Brown and Brenner[21] investigated acute compression block and found that 1) demyelination occurred focally under the area of compression and 2) recovery was due to remyelination. The primary lesion seems to be the result of displacement of myelin from the area of high pressure under the tourniquet to areas of normal pressure adjacent to the edge of the tourniquet. This causes the myelin internode to cover the node of Ranvier and to be pushed under or to invaginate the next myelin internode. This has been called "sausaging" of the myelin internodes,[22] and it leads to the loss of the edges of the myelin internode, causing paranodal demyelination. Thus, the pathological changes occur primarily at the two edges of the compression rather than under the compression. After longer periods of compression, segmental demyelination, with loss of an entire segment of myelin between two nodes of Ranvier, occurs. Remyelination may occur, but the myelin sheath is thinner and the internodes are shorter, resulting in longer conduction times.

Chronic compression and entrapment neuropathies

In chronic compression and entrapment neuropathies, inspection of the nerve shows thinning of the nerve at the site of compression with enlargement just proximal and, to a lesser degree, distal to the site of compression because of increased endoneurial connective tissue. Microscopically, there is thinning of the axons in the area of compression, demyelination and remyelination, degeneration primarily of large myelinated axons, thickening of perineurial and endoneurial microvessels, and fibrosis. With chronic experimental compression neuropathies, the changes in myelin are found all along the area of compression, unlike in the acute compression model, in which the changes are found at the edges of the areas of compression. The myelin in each internode varies in thickness, with the thin area toward the center of compression and the thick areas toward the edge, creating a "tadpole-like" appearance. The "tadpoles" are arranged so they appear to be swimming away from the center of compression in both directions. The same abnormalities have been found in the few human cases of carpal tunnel syndrome and other common compressive neuropathies that have been examined. This is a mild or early pathological change that is followed sequentially by paranodal and segmental demyelination and then remyelination. In the segment of the axon distal to the compressive lesion, axonal diameter and myelin thickness are decreased.[23]

Friction

Normally, peripheral nerves slide or glide over considerable distances with movement of the body. This gliding movement produces friction with surrounding structures, and rubbing of a nerve against a firm irregular roughened surface induces changes in the connective tissue of the nerve as well as its axons. This is likely to be a problem, particularly in situations in which the nerve moves in a piston-like fashion through a tunnel, there is narrowing of the tunnel, the walls are roughened by osteoarthritic overgrowth, or the nerve is enlarged. Friction is probably a major feature at such common sites where the ulnar nerve enters the cubital tunnel, the common peroneal nerve crosses the neck of the fibula, and the median nerve passes under a supracondylar process. Friction is probably also a factor in some lesions of the median nerve in the carpal tunnel and lesions of the spinal nerves in the intervertebral foramen.

Percussion

Peripheral nerves have been percussed experimentally by hitting the nerve with a weighted object or by dropping a weight on the nerve.[24] Depending on the magnitude of the forces used, percussion causes a transient loss of nerve function that lasts days. Pathologically, the nerve is swollen from edema and the infiltration of cells. The amount of axonal destruction varies. Segmental demyelination and remyelination follow quickly.

Crush

A large force that compresses a peripheral nerve against an unyielding structure such as bone produces an acute nerve crush. Mechanical crush of the nerve fiber forces the axoplasm and the myelin sheath from the area of the lesion. After the injurious force is released, the axoplasm and myelin sheath return and appear relatively normal. Within hours after the crush injury, the endoneurial tube on either side of the crushed region contains mixed axonal and myelin debris. If the blood vessels are damaged at the site of injury, hemorrhage, an early inflammatory reaction, and exudate develop. After 3 days, Schwann cells occupy the endoneurial tube in the crushed region and axonal sprouts begin to appear. Reinnervation is much more effective after a crush injury than after surgical repair of a transected nerve. Hemorrhage, scarring, and disorganization of the endoneurium and perineurium limit recovery.

Stretch and rupture or avulsion

Stretch is the most common mechanism of serious nerve injury. The perineurium provides more elasticity and strength in resistance to stretch to peripheral nerves than does the epineurium. The axons of the nerve roots have less tensile strength and redundancy and are more susceptible to stretch injuries than axons in peripheral nerves.

The impairment of nerve function increases as the magnitude of the deforming force increases. The nerve can be stretched more when the stretch is applied over very long periods. The same amount of stretch applied over a short period causes more severe nerve injury. Although stretching of a compound nerve may result in loss of all function or sensory impairment, it does not seem to result in loss of motor function without loss of sensory function.

During World War II, Highet and Holmes called attention to the problems of nerve stretching at the time of injury and treatment. Experimental studies established that elongation of the nerve by 6% could be tolerated, but elongation of 11% or more caused severe and extensive damage to the nerve.[25] With continued stretch, the perineurium begins to rupture, followed by rupture of axons and then the endoneurial tube. The contents of the fascicles are extruded through the breaks, and the fascicles are torn apart. After the fascicles have been torn, the nerve elongates rapidly, drawing apart the separated ends of the fascicles and leaving only a thin amount of epineurial tissue. This may be termed *avulsion* or *rupture*.

A severe traction injury is a serious problem for several reasons. The rupture of fascicles usually extends over at least 3 to 5 cm of the nerve length. The severity and site of the lesion may be difficult to appreciate by palpation or inspection. The length of the lesion makes the regenerative process less efficient.

Laceration

Seddon[3] collected a series of 385 nerve injuries due to laceration. In 80% of the cases, the laceration was caused by glass, and the rest were caused by knives, sharp metal objects, propeller blades, chainsaws, and animal bites. Nerve lacerations can occur in a closed wound secondary to a bone fracture. Most lacerations are classified as neurotmetic or Sunderland grade five, and the entire nerve is disrupted, with a gap forming between its proximal and distal ends. Severe lesions have little potential for effective regeneration or reinnervation and usually require surgical repair as soon as logistically feasible. The timing of repair after blunt lesions that transect the nerve (e.g., chainsaws) and after similar types of mechanical injuries is less clear.[26] Some favor a delay of 2 to 3 weeks after the injury because then it is easier to tell the difference between damaged but viable nerve tissue and irreparably damaged tissue.

High-velocity missiles

There are 732 civilian shootings daily in the United States.[27] Handguns are involved in 75% of these incidents, rifles in 2%, and shotguns in 4%. The frequency of nerve injuries in different reports has varied widely. Shotgun shootings cause a higher incidence of peripheral nerve injuries and a higher percentage of neurotmetic lesions.[28] Tissue injury is generally more severe with a shotgun blast.

High-velocity missiles such as bullets produce extensive forces when passing through tissue. They produce a shock wave of pressure with rapid expansion, followed by collapse not only in front of the missile but also lateral to the path of the missile. Structures closest to the track of the missile suffer the most, but often structures at considerable distance from the path are also stretched. Nerves are particularly sensitive to such injuries. Nerves directly in the path of the missile are destroyed over long segments. The injuries at a distance from the missile path may be neurapractic or first-degree lesions that are transient or any other degree of severity up to complete separation. Omer[29] reported a spontaneous recovery rate of 69% after a delay of up to 9 months for both low- and high-velocity gunshot wounds during the Vietnam War. Kline and Hudson[30] have recommended that if damaged or severed nerves are identified, their ends be tagged and sutured to the operative bed to avoid retraction and repair be delayed for several weeks. If nerve continuity is more likely or the deficit indicates an incomplete lesion, the injury

should be followed for several months clinically and electrophysiologically. If spontaneous recovery is not evident from either clinical or electromyographic (EMG) testing, exploration and intraoperative recording will probably be required to grade the injury and to determine proper management. According to Kline and Hudson's experience with brachial plexus gunshot injuries, repair of upper or middle trunk components can give good results but repair of lower trunk components gives dismal results.

Injection

Injection injuries most commonly damage the sciatic and radial nerves because the buttocks and upper arm are the usual sites for giving injections. Pain and neurological deficit usually develop immediately after the injection. Onset is delayed in 10% of cases and may indicate a slow-acting agent or the gradual spread of the agent to the nerve from an adjacent injection site.

Injection injuries have been attributed to mechanical needle injury, allergic neuritis, ischemia, and scarring as well as to the direct effect of a neurotoxic substance. Most drugs must be injected directly into the nerve fascicle to cause damage.[31,32] Repeated injections of normal saline into a nerve do not produce injury. Drugs such as diazepam, chlordiazepoxide, chlorpromazine, and benzylpenicillin cause damage even when not injected directly into the nerve. In experimental models, commonly used drugs such as meperidine, diazepam, chlorpromazine, hydrocortisone, triamcinolone, procaine, and tetracaine produce the most severe injury. Gentamicin, cephalothin, methylprednisolone, lidocaine, and bupivacaine produce less severe but pronounced injuries.

Early exploration of the nerve with irrigation to remove the offending agent has not been shown to be helpful. Clinical and electrophysiological examinations should be performed frequently to determine the severity of the injury and to measure any improvement. If the lesion is purely neurapractic, as demonstrated with EMG studies, the prognosis is good. If signs of recovery appear within a few hours or days, the chance of complete recovery is high. However, in 1970, Clark et al.[33] documented complete recovery in only 14% of patients. Partial lesions should be observed unless there is intractable pain or progressive deterioration of function suggesting fibrosis. Kline and Hudson[30] reported that external and internal neurolysis relieved intractable pain in 50% of patients. If the lesion is complete and there is no clinical or electrophysiological recovery of nerve function after 8 to 16 weeks, surgical exploration is usually recommended. In the large series of 80 patients with nerve injection injuries reported by Kline and Hudson,[30] one-half required surgery. The drawback to early exploration of the nerve is that some patients have complete or nearly complete recovery without surgery. Early exploration may cause unnecessary operative damage to the nerve. Also, exploration does not always remove all doubts about what to do at the time of surgery.

Cold

The most common clinical forms of cold injury to peripheral nerve have occurred during major wars and have been nonfreezing nerve injuries called *trench foot* or *immersion foot*. They apparently are more severe not when there is prolonged exposure to cold severe enough to freeze the tissue but when there is recurring cooling and warming. There may or may not be damage to the skin and subcutaneous tissues as well as to nerves. Trench foot is characterized clinically by distal weakness and sensory loss for 2 to 5 hours after removal from the cold. This is followed by severe pain in the affected areas that had become hot and red. Swelling and blistering usually occur. During this stage, the loss of sensory and motor function improves or resolves. The area of sensory loss often is replaced by dysesthetic pain that may persist for years.[34–36] The few electrophysiological studies that have been performed reported decreased amplitude or absence of sensory potentials and slowed motor conduction velocities.[37–39]

Experimental studies on the effects of cold on peripheral nerve fibers suggest that there is considerable variability in the sensitivity of different axons to exposure to cold. Temperatures of 5°C to 9°C produce conduction block in large-diameter, myelinated A fibers.[40] Conduction in small-diameter, unmyelinated C fibers is relatively preserved.[41] In experimental animals, cold exposure decreases blood flow to peripheral nerve by 30% to 80%, and this decrease persists for days.[42] Jia and Pollock[42] found in rats that intermittent cold exposure was more damaging to peripheral nerves than continuous cooling. Others have found that the most severe damage occurs at the transition from normal to cooled nerve.[43] The major effect of cold damage to peripheral nerve is arguably vascular, with resultant ischemia and reperfusion injury, rather than direct damage from the cold. In the more severe lesions, recovery is limited by an increase in interstitial connective tissue and fibrosis.

Ischemia

Peripheral nerves are resistant to ischemia because of the rich anastomotic net of the intrinsic and extrinsic blood supply and the diffusion of oxygen and nutrients from the surrounding structures. Experimentally, it is extremely difficult to damage peripheral nerves by ligation of a single major artery.[44] Blunt[45] was able to produce ischemic damage to the sciatic nerve of rabbits only by the combination of devascularization and wrapping the nerve with a polyethylene film. Hess et al.[46] were able to produce nerve damage by ligating the common, internal, and external iliac arteries. Schmelzer et al.[47] produced temporary ischemia of the rat sciatic nerve. After 30 minutes of ischemia, conduction failure occurred, but it was reversible if the ischemia persisted less than 1 hour. Persistent conduction block developed after 3 hours of ischemia. Nukada and Dyck[48] injected polystyrene microspheres into the major arteries supplying peripheral nerves in the rat and found that the amount of nerve

damaged was related directly to the number of microspheres injected. With injection of a large number of microspheres, the entire nerve became necrotic. Injection of an intermediate number of microspheres caused injury primarily to axons in the center of the fascicles. Only occasionally were wedge-shaped areas of necrosis identified that intuitively would be expected from nerve infarction. The primary injury was to axons, but demyelination was noted at the edges of the most severe damage. McManis and Low[49] demonstrated that the more peripheral fibers were protected from injury by diffusion of oxygen from surrounding tissues. Dyck et al.[50] described the pathological alteration of peripheral nerve due to ischemia in humans. A patchy distribution of nerve fiber degeneration begins in a central fascicular location in watershed zones in the mid upper arm and the mid thigh.

During aortofemoral bypass surgery or peripheral vascular surgery, embolization or graft thrombosis may produce ischemic damage to the distal tibial and peroneal, sciatic, or femoral nerves.[51] Similar complications have been reported after use of transfemoral intra-aortic balloon assist pumps.[52]

Therapeutic or accidental intra-arterial injection of drugs may result in severe arterial spasm and thrombosis, with soft tissue and nerve damage.[53,54] Upper limb ischemia associated with artificial arteriovenous shunts for dialysis has produced ischemic damage to nerves referred to as *ischemic monomelic neuropathy*.[55]

The arterial supply of a nerve may be interrupted by laceration or thrombosis from soft tissue trauma or bone fracture. Typically, this seems to result from bone and arterial lesions near the distal humerus and femur and proximal tibia. The nerves in these areas appear to be unusually vulnerable because long sections of them are dependent on a single nutrient artery. The ischemia resulting from arterial lesions in these areas often affects muscle more than skin and nerve. The ischemia of muscle results in edema that is confined in a closed space or compartment. The swelling causes increased pressure that produces a vicious cycle of decreasing blood supply as pressure increases. These compartment syndromes produce muscle necrosis and secondary nerve damage.[56,57] Volkmann ischemic contracture is the best-understood lesion of this type and frequently occurs after fractures in the region of the elbow. Volkmann ischemic contracture usually results from damage to the brachial artery and results in necrosis, fibrosis, and contractures of the muscles of the hand and flexor aspect of the forearm, and there may be ischemic damage to the nerves, usually the median nerve. It may be difficult to distinguish the relative contributions of nerve and muscle damage to the loss of function. The anterior tibial syndrome is a compartment syndrome in the leg involving the peroneal nerve and muscles of the anterior compartment.

Radiation

The damaging effects of ionizing radiation on peripheral nerves are rare and not fully understood. There may be direct neuronal injury from the radiation or damage to supportive vascular and connective tissue. The cellular damage appears to affect DNA. Cells that have a short cell cycle and frequently divide are more susceptible to radiation damage. The relatively inactive neurons seem to be more resistant. The radiation damage to tissue is generally biphasic, with acute and delayed effects. The acute damage generally is reversible and does not necessarily predict the appearance of late damage. Transient acute radiation injury of peripheral nerves in humans has been described only by Salner et al.[58] who reported on patients who had received radiotherapy for breast cancer and developed paresthesias in the hand and forearm and some pain and weakness that was reversible after weeks or months. The delayed damaging effects of radiation are usually progressive. The late delayed radiation effects probably result from small-vessel injury, with secondary effects on nerve. The damaging effects of radiation generally are more severe with larger total doses, larger fraction sizes, more frequent treatments, and larger volumes of tissue treated.

Most experimental studies that have measured the effects of radiation on peripheral nerves have involved a single large dose of radiation. It should be noted that this generally does not apply to the methods of radiotherapy in humans. Another limitation of many of the studies has been the failure to look for late damaging effects that may occur months to years after radiation. Kinsella et al.[59] concluded from a review of the experimental data that the neuron cell bodies and nerve endings were more sensitive to radiation damage than the axons. Spiess[60] described the changes over a 6-month period after radiation of peripheral nerve. Progressive alterations of the cytoskeleton led to shrinkage and increased density of the axons. The capillary endothelium also underwent progressive pathological change. Eventually, there was axonal destruction. Spiess thought much of the damage was due to direct injury of the axons. Linder[61] concluded that damage to the endothelium of small blood vessels and resultant nerve ischemia was the major problem.

Thomas and Holdorff[16] recommended certain clinical rules for the diagnosis of radiation damage to peripheral nerve. They noted that it was a diagnosis that could be made only after the recurrence of the primary tumor and a radiation-induced sarcoma had been excluded. The damaged nerve must be within the radiation treatment field, and the latent period that follows the treatment should be consistent with that noted in the literature. The dosage of radiation should be in the range that has been found to be neurotoxic. It must be recalled that chemotherapeutic agents and other underlying disease such as diabetes mellitus that also damage nerves and compromise their blood supply may lower the generally accepted safe tolerance limits.

Clinical attention to the damaging effects of radiation has focused on the brachial plexopathy that develops after radiotherapy for breast cancer.[62–65] Stoll and Andrews[66] found that 73% of patients developed neurological symptoms at a dose of 63 Gy compared with only 15% of those who received 58 Gy. This study has been criticized for not clearly distinguishing between radiation damage and metastatic spread of cancer to the brachial plexus. Others have found that complications developed in the brachial plexus in about 1% of cases. Westling et al.[67] reported that the size of the field and the dosage of each fraction influenced the incidence of radiation damage. With a large field and fraction sizes of 4 Gy and a total dose of 64 Gy, 60% of the patients developed neurological problems. Decreasing the fraction size to 3 Gy and the total dose to 44 Gy apparently eliminated neurological complications. Symptoms from radiation damage to the brachial plexus appear anywhere from 5 months to as long as 20 years after radiotherapy. The mean latency is 4 years.

Birch et al.[68] operated on 54 patients with radiation brachial plexopathy. The condition of 10% of patients improved and that of 45% stabilized. According to these authors, there are three indications for surgery: to establish a diagnosis of tumor or radiation damage, to alleviate pain, and the rapid progression of loss of function.

Radiation damage to the lumbosacral plexus has been reported after radiotherapy for testicular tumors and after brachytherapy for gynecological malignancies. The neurological deficits that result suggest damage to the lower motor neurons or motor axons, with relative preservation of autonomic and sensory function. It has been postulated that anterior horn cells in the lower spinal cord are selectively damaged, but the injury may involve motor axons in the roots or lumbosacral plexus.[69] The incidence of neurological damage to lumbosacral anterior horn cells, roots, or plexus appears to be about 1%, and the damage becomes evident 12 to 14 months after radiotherapy.[70]

Electrical

The effects of electrical currents on peripheral nerve are a matter of controversy.[71–75] The majority of these injuries are sustained at the workplace or by the home handyman who makes contact with electrical lines while installing an antenna or using a metal ladder. High-tension electrical currents greater than 1000 V are more injurious than low-tension currents less than 1000 V. It has been difficult to differentiate the damaging effects of heat produced by the electrical current from the effects of the electrical current itself. The electrical current may cause lysis of the neuronal cell membrane by electroporation. In electroporation, the electrical current apparently creates pores in the cell membrane. Another more generally accepted explanation is that the nerve is damaged by the heat produced by the flow of electrical current through the resistance created by body tissues.[76] The location and severity of electrical injuries to peripheral nerves depend on the current pathway, tissue resistance, the amount of current that flows per time, and the duration of the current. These injuries can range from minor to life-threatening and are often associated with extensive soft-tissue injury that leads to amputation of an extremity. The neurological deficits usually occur immediately and involve motor nerves. The neurological dysfunction may resolve in hours or days and has been referred to as "stunning." The nerves that most frequently sustain electrical injury are the median and ulnar nerves in the upper extremity. Pathologically, there is coagulation necrosis of the damaged tissue. Flash thermal burns are generally noted at the entrance and exit sites. The injury may follow the neurovascular bundle from the periphery to the central nervous system, and patchy spinal cord necrosis can result centrally. Scarring is a major problem after the injury. Months to years after the electrical injury, nerve damage may result from vascular damage and progressive perineural fibrosis.

Ferreiro et al.[77] recently reviewed their experience with 59 patients who had high-tension electrical burns. In 74% of patients, the point of entry of the electrical current was in the upper limb, and in 60%, the point of exit was the lower limbs. Nerve lesions developed in 30% of patients, and the median and ulnar nerves were injured most frequently. Ferreiro et al.[77] recommended surgical repair of the nerve in patients with a neurological deficit who had an intact nerve at the time of debridement, no sign of recovery after a maximal observation period of 6 months, and a complete nerve lesion.

Evaluation

A thorough history and technically reliable physical examination, with emphasis on the neurological examination, are most important for successful evaluation and therapy. This includes a careful history of the details of the injury—the extent of motor, sensory, autonomic, and musculoskeletal dysfunction. The temporal profile of the evolution of the different deficits, including attention to the timing of the development of the deficit, is critical. Deficits caused by the injury usually are maximal immediately after the injury and subsequently stabilize or improve. Deficits that develop later, particularly after therapeutic intervention, may be complications of the treatment or may be due to secondary complicating factors such as infection, hemorrhage, or edema. Careful notation of the timing and location of any recovery of function and results of previous therapies is important. The examination must carefully document the location and severity of weakness, atrophy, and sensory and reflex alterations. Nerves and muscles should be palpated and percussed. Soft tissue and bony abnormalities must be noted. The findings must be documented thoroughly and recorded at each examination so that progression or improvement can be determined.

Electrophysiological evaluation including electromyography and nerve conduction studies

Electrophysiological tests can be valuable aids in the evaluation of nerve injuries, but they are not a substitute for a careful clinical evaluation. To understand the usefulness of the test, a basic review may be necessary.[78]

The conduction block produced by neurapractic lesions is demonstrated most easily by motor nerve conduction studies. The motor axons of a nerve are stimulated electrically with recording electrodes placed over a muscle innervated by the nerve. The amplitude and area of the muscle response are good indicators of the amount of functional muscle tissue and, indirectly, of the number of functional motor axons. For example, recording electrodes can be placed over the hypothenar muscles in the hand and the ulnar nerve stimulated at points from the wrist to the supraclavicular fossa (Figure 178.8), and from the wrist stimulation site to the supraclavicular site, little change is found in the amplitude or area. However, in the case of a neurapractic lesion of the ulnar nerve at the elbow, stimulation of the ulnar motor fibers distal to the area of the injury will produce a normal response, but stimulation proximal to the lesion will generate action potentials that are not conducted across the lesion (Figure 178.9). Consequently, a decrease in amplitude and area of the muscle response will occur when stimulating proximal to the lesion compared with the response when stimulating distal to the lesion. If all of the motor axons are involved in a neurapractic lesion of the ulnar nerve at the elbow, a normal response will occur when the stimulation is below the elbow (i.e., distal to the lesion) but no response will occur when the stimulation is above the elbow (i.e., proximal to the lesion). If 50% of the motor axons are injured, then stimulation above the elbow will produce a response 50% less than that elicited with stimulation below the elbow (Figure 178.10). As the injured axons recover, the

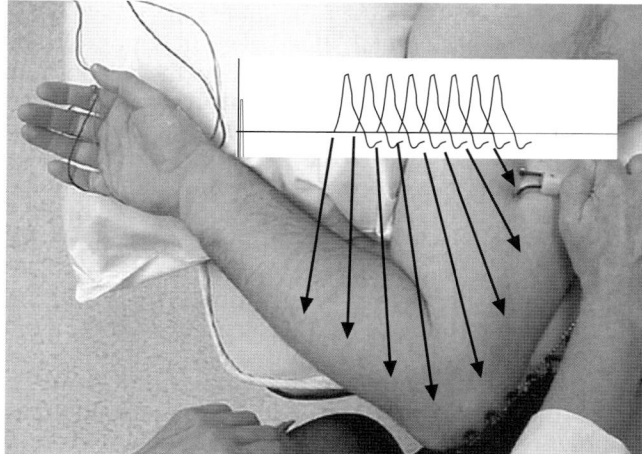

Figure 178.8 Normal ulnar nerve motor conduction study with short segment incremental stimulation ("inching"). Compound muscle action potential (*upper right*) recorded from hypothenar muscles after percutaneous supramaximal stimulation of motor axons along the length of a healthy ulnar nerve beginning at the mid forearm and moving the stimulating site proximally at equally spaced intervals up to the axilla. Note that the amplitude and configuration of the evoked potentials are essentially the same from stimulation at all the levels but the latency from the stimulus becomes progressively longer with more proximal stimulation. (See color plate section.)

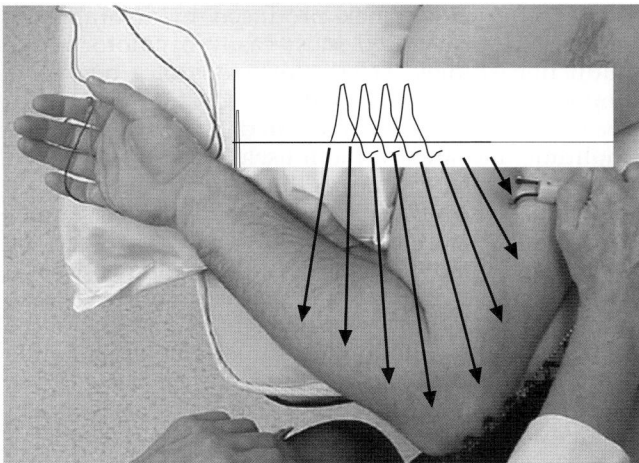

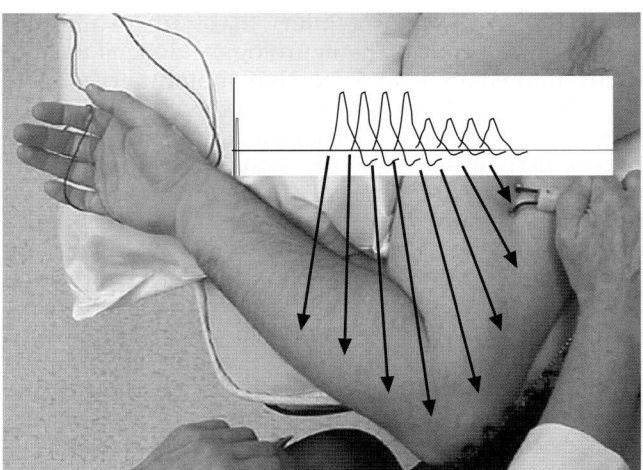

Figure 178.9   Ulnar nerve motor conduction study with short segment incremental stimulation ("inching") in a complete neurapractic lesion at the elbow. The recording of the compound muscle action potential (*upper right*) from hypothenar muscles after percutaneous supramaximal stimulation of motor axons along the length of the ulnar nerve, as described in Figure 178.8. Note that the potentials from stimulation of the four most distal sites (below the elbow) evoke a potential resembling that of a normal subject (Figure 178.8). At and above the elbow, no potential is elicited. These findings would be typical for the first 36 to 48 hours after nerve transection at the elbow or a neurapractic lesion at the elbow. (See color plate section.)

Figure 178.10   Ulnar nerve motor conduction study with short segment incremental stimulation ("inching") in a 50% neurapractic lesion at the elbow. The recording of the compound muscle action potential (*upper right*) from hypothenar muscles after percutaneous supramaximal stimulation of motor axons along the length of the ulnar nerve, as described in Figure 178.8. Note that the potential from stimulation of the four most distal sites (below the elbow) evokes a potential resembling that of a normal subject (Figure 178.8). At and above the elbow, the amplitude of the potential is reduced. These findings are typical of the first 36 to 48 hours after partial nerve transection at the elbow or a partial neurapractic lesion at the elbow. (See color plate section.)

amplitude of the response with stimulation proximal to the lesion will become larger and closer to the value of the response elicited with stimulation distal to the lesion. By using a technique called *inching* or *short segment incremental stimulation*, it is possible to begin stimulating the nerve distal to the lesion and obtain a supramaximal response at one site (Figures 178.8–178.10). At this point, the stimulation site is moved proximally along the nerve in 1-cm or 1-inch increments and the process of supramaximal stimulation is repeated. As the stimulation site is moved proximal to the lesion, the amplitude and area of the response will abruptly decrease.

In axonotmetic lesions, stimulation proximal to the site of injury produces action potentials in the motor axons, and these potentials are conducted along the axons to the site of injury, but they do not conduct across the site of injury. If all the axons are injured, stimulation proximal to the lesion will not produce a response. The complexity arises with stimulation distal to the site of injury. Because distal segments of injured axons continue to conduct action potentials for 3 to 8 days after the injury, stimulation distal to the injury will produce a normal muscle action potential response. The amplitude and area of the compound muscle action potential will be lost or reduced when the stimulation site is more proximal to the lesion. After 3 to 8 days, the distal segments of injured motor axons begin to degenerate and cease to conduct action potentials. At this point, the amplitude and area of the compound muscle action potential begin

to decrease with stimulation distal to the lesion. This phenomenon is important for several reasons. For the first few days after an axonotmetic lesion, the results of motor nerve conduction studies cannot be differentiated from those of a neurapractic lesion and can lead to a falsely optimistic prognosis. However, nerve conduction studies can be useful in precisely localizing the site of the lesion. After 9 days, nerve conduction studies can clearly differentiate a neurapractic lesion from an axonotmetic lesion, but the lesion cannot be localized with this type of motor nerve conduction study.

An injured nerve frequently has a mixture of neurapractic and axonotmetic lesions and the findings are more complex.

Often, a mechanical injury is not severe enough to destroy the axon or to produce conduction block. These milder nerve injuries may damage the myelin sheath or narrow the axon enough to cause focal slowing of conduction across the injured segment. The inching or short segmental incremental stimulation technique can be used to localize precisely an area of focal slowing.

Sensory nerve conduction studies are performed by electrically stimulating peripheral sensory axons at one point and recording their action potentials at another point along the nerve. The response recorded is the summation of the action potentials of the sensory axons; this is the *sensory nerve action potential*. Sensory nerve conduction studies are particularly helpful in distinguishing between lesions that are proximal to a dorsal root ganglion and those distal to the ganglion. Because the dorsal root ganglion is usually located at the intervertebral foramen, lesions proximal to the dorsal root ganglion involve the sensory projections at the root or more central levels. Lesions distal to the dorsal root ganglion involve sensory axons in the spinal nerves, plexuses, or peripheral nerves. If an axonotmetic lesion of sensory axons is distal to the dorsal root ganglion, the distal axons undergo wallerian degeneration and disappear and the sensory nerve action potential is reduced in amplitude or absent. However, if the axonotmetic lesion is proximal to the dorsal root ganglion, the central axons degenerate and disappear. In this case, the distal axons of the dorsal root ganglion are intact and the sensory nerve action potential amplitude is normal. The most striking example of this is a patient who presents with a flail, paralyzed, anesthetic upper extremity after an injury. If the patient has an axonotmetic lesion of the brachial plexus distal to the dorsal root ganglia, the sensory nerve action potentials will be reduced or absent in the anesthetic limb. If the lesion is a root avulsion proximal to the dorsal root ganglion, with no damage to the plexus, the sensory nerve action potentials on nerve conduction studies will be normal in the anesthetic limb.

Electromyography or needle examination Localizing an axonotmetic or neurotmetic lesion with a needle examination can be compared to interpreting a wiring diagram. A muscle is examined, and if the findings are abnormal, the axons in the branch of the nerve to the muscle must be damaged somewhere along their course, either in the branch or proximal to it. The site of the lesion can be determined by examining muscles innervated by more proximal branches of that nerve, part of the plexus, or the nerve root. In partial lesions, the major limitation of this technique is the propensity of partial nerve lesions to involve fascicles to different degrees. At the level of the injury, one fascicle may be injured severely and another relatively spared. This can produce confusing test results. If a muscle is normal on needle examination, it cannot be assumed with certainty that the neural structures in which the axons course proximal to the branch to the muscle are normal. If the needle examination of the muscle is abnormal, the axons to that muscle are damaged somewhere along their course from the anterior horn of the spinal cord. Aside from these limitations, the technique is usually accurate in determining the site of the lesion.

Basic treatment options

The most difficult treatment decisions involving peripheral nerve injuries frequently concern the need for surgical intervention and the timing of surgery. The management of peripheral nerve injuries was reviewed recently.[79–81]

Surgery may be performed either immediately after the injury as primary repair or after 3 to 4 days as delayed primary repair. Secondary repairs may be early at 2 to 4 weeks after the injury, delayed at 3 to 6

months after the injury, or late secondary repairs 1 to 2 years after the injury. Primary or immediate repair appears to be better than secondary repair.[82,83] Immediate primary repair is usually recommended when there has been a clean laceration of the nerve by a sharp object and the nerve endings have not been injured by crush or stretch. If the nerve has been lacerated and not repaired immediately, surgery probably should be performed as soon as possible considering all other variables. Secondary early surgical repair after 2 to 4 weeks usually is recommended for blunt injuries or injuries with extensive soft tissue damage in which the nerve injury appears to be complete or severe. Electrodiagnostic studies can be helpful in determining whether a complete lesion is neurapractic or axonotmetic. Neurapractic lesions should be treated nonsurgically unless they persist longer than expected. If the nerve lesion appears to be complete and axonotmetic, to be due to a traction injury, or to be a grade four or five lesion, surgery is delayed for at most 3 to 6 months. If the nerve is severed or ruptured, surgical repair should be undertaken. Late surgery at 1 to 2 years after the injury generally has not resulted in good recovery of motor function but may be required for pain control or to resect a neuroma.

Surgical repair is usually preceded by exposure and visual inspection and palpation of the nerve, but these techniques are not extremely reliable in determining eventual outcome. If the nerve is intact, the critical question is how much, if any, axonal growth has occurred across the damaged segment. This question can be answered partly with electrophysiological techniques. Resection of scar tissue from around the external surface of the nerve is called external neurolysis and is a low-risk procedure that usually is performed before electrophysiological studies are performed. After the nerve is exposed, it is possible to stimulate the motor axons of a compound nerve above the level of the lesion and to observe the muscles innervated distal to the lesion to document any contraction. A more sensitive electrophysiological technique involves electrical stimulation of the nerve while recording the electrical activity from the muscles innervated distal to the lesion. Electroneurography is another intraoperative technique in which the action potentials of the axons in the nerve are recorded directly from the nerve after stimulating at other points along the nerve. The optimal technique probably is to record from the nerve as far proximally as it is exposed in the operative bed. The nerve is stimulated distally at points separated by 1 cm to 1 inch. If there has not been any growth of the axons across the lesion or if there has been growth of a very small number of axons, stimulation will not produce a response. If a response is obtained with stimulation distal to the lesion, progressively more distal sites can be stimulated to determine how far the axonal sprouts have grown. As the stimulation site is moved more distally, allowance must be made for axons leaving the nerve at branch points along the nerve being stimulated. This type of recording is time-consuming and technically demanding, but it gives a better indication of the amount of axonal regrowth that has occurred in an injured nerve.

Depending on the results of the evaluations at the time of surgical exploration, several surgical options remain, including internal neurolysis, resection and reanastomosis, and resection and grafting.

Internal neurolysis is the surgical technique of opening the epineurium and, under magnification, separating the different fascicles. This procedure risks damage to the blood supply of the nerve and to branches of the fascicles either leaving the nerve or passing from one fascicle to another. The surgeon can inspect the individual fascicles and stimulate and record from them to determine which fascicles are intact and which ones contain regenerating axonal sprouts and which ones do not. One technique of repair is termed fascicular or split repair. This technique follows internal neurolysis. If the fascicles are physically separated, the surgeon attempts to identify the distal and proximal stumps, match up the fascicles, and suture together the distal and proximal stumps of the matching fascicles. If there is no evidence that viable axons cross the injured area of the fascicle, the injured segment is resected as far back as normal-appearing nerve, and an end-to-end repair or graft repair is performed. The risk of this type of fascicular repair is scar and neuroma formation. Also, the constant passage of axons from one fascicle to another suggests that if any length of the fascicle is removed, the axonal content of the proximal and distal portions of the fascicle will be different. This is a greater problem with proximal nerve lesions. Also, it may be difficult to correctly match the individual fascicles. This type of fascicular repair probably works better for median and ulnar nerve lesions at the wrist.[79]

If the nerve is ruptured or severed, the retracted ends must be identified and the surgeon must evaluate the condition of the distal and proximal stumps. The surgeon must determine if the two separated ends of the nerve can be approximated without subjecting the nerve to too much tension or stretch. Then, the surgeon must trim off the damaged portions and attempt to align the fascicles in the proximal stump with those in the distal stump under magnification. The proximal and distal stumps are connected by sutures in either the outer epineurium (epineurial repair) or the interfascicular epineurium (grouped fascicular or fascicular repair) or by using nonsutured techniques. Nonsutured techniques have included wrapping the nerve, gluing the ends together with plasma clot or fibrin glue, or using a carbon dioxide laser to weld the nerve ends together. Suture line tension must be minimized by mobilization of the nerve, positioning, and postoperative immobilization. If the gap is too large and suture line tension is too great, nerve grafting must be considered.

Spinner and Kline[79] have provided general guidelines based on their experience. In their experience, injured nerves with measurable nerve action potentials transmitted across the lesion during intraoperative nerve stimulation have a good recovery of function 90% of the time, and good functional results can be expected in about 70% of end-to-end repairs and 50% of graft repairs. Also, the results are better for patients with short nerve grafts than for those with long grafts, for patients operated on early than for those operated on late, and for young patients than for older ones. The results are worse for proximal lesions than for distal lesions and for lower trunk brachial plexus lesions than for upper trunk lesions. Radial nerve repairs have a better recovery than median nerve repairs, but median nerve repairs have a better recovery than ulnar nerve repairs. In the leg, tibial nerve repairs have better recovery than peroneal nerve repairs.

Primary repair of digital nerves of the hand produces a good or excellent outcome in 45% to 74% of cases.[84] Primary repair of the median and ulnar nerves in the forearm or at the wrist results in excellent sensory recovery in 30% to 60% of cases and in good sensory recovery in 40%. Functionally significant motor recovery occurs in 16% to 90% of cases. Fewer data are available for primary repair of lower extremity nerves, but Roganovic et al.[85] reported good to excellent results in 13% of peroneal nerve repairs. Kline et al.[86] reported on primary repairs of lacerations of the sciatic nerve, and the results were good or better in 90% of tibial repairs and in 80% of peroneal repairs.

Secondary repair 3 weeks to 3 months after sciatic nerve injury resulted in useful motor recovery in the tibial nerve in 83% of cases and in the peroneal nerve in 39%.[87] Useful recovery was achieved in 71% of thigh-level lesions and in only 31% of buttock-level lesions.

If a long segment of the nerve is damaged or a wide gap occurs between the two retracted stumps, an end-to-end repair of the nerve may not be possible. In this case, a nerve graft may be required to bridge the gap. If a nerve graft is placed between the damaged ends of a nerve, the axonal sprouts have to cross two gaps. First, the axons have to grow across the junction of the proximal end of the nerve and the graft, and second, they have to grow through the junction of the distal end of the graft and the nerve. This slows growth, increases the risk of neuroma formation, and increases the risk that the axonal sprouts will not reach the proper end organ. However, grafts up to 20 cm long have been used successfully. The survival and success of the graft depend on the quality of the operative bed and the vascular supply and thickness of the graft. The danger is that the graft will undergo necrosis.

Nerve grafts may be autologous (from the same patient), allografts (from another human), xenografts (from another species), or artificial or man-made.[88] Autologous nerve grafts from a remote donor site are the ones used most commonly for bridging a nerve gap. Autologous nerve grafts have been used successfully, but the removal of a viable nerve from a donor site results in functional impairment and a potentially painful neuroma. Thinner free autologous nerve grafts do better, presumably because of vascularization from the recipient site. Vascularized nerve grafts may be used if a particularly thick or long graft is needed.

Nerve allografts have been performed experimentally but require heavy immunosuppression to avoid rejection. If the allografts are made acellular, they may cause a less severe immune reaction. Tacrolimus (FK506) has been used experimentally to prevent rejection of allografts and has been shown to improve axonal outgrowth.

Silicone tubes have been used to bridge gaps in nerves. Silicone grafts in combination with growth factors, Schwann cells, and basal lamina materials may improve regeneration. Silicone tubes with multiple longitudinal synthetic filaments in the lumen have been effective experimentally.

Collagen-based nerve gap conduits have been used in place of grafts, and it has been suggested that conduits made of laminin, fibronectin, and nerve growth factor may decrease nerve cell body death in dorsal root ganglion neurons and enhance axonal regeneration.

Matsumoto et al.[89] recently reported the results of a study in which an 80-mm gap in the peroneal nerve of dogs was filled with a biodegradable polyglycolic acid-collagen tube containing laminin-coated collagen fibers. When the animals were sacrificed 12 months later, the nerve conduits had been absorbed completely. Compound muscle action potentials could be obtained after 3 months and gradually increased in size until 12 months, but they never reached normal values.

Vanderhooft[90] and Frykman and Gramyk[91] have reviewed the results of nerve grafting. These reviews combined the results from multiple centers because single large series from individual centers are not available. Grafting of digital nerves produced good or better results in 50% of patients. Even with a delay between injury and repair of up to 6 months, 90% of patients had useful recovery. Mackinnon and Dellon[92] performed grafts with polyglycolic tubes in highly selected patients and reported good results in 86%. In median nerve grafts, 81% of patients had fair motor recovery. The success rate for grafts longer than 10 cm was 66%. Good or better sensory recovery was reported in 79% of patients. In ulnar nerve lesions, fair or better motor function was obtained in 63% of patients and good or better sensory results in 75%. Too few series have been reported for conclusions to be drawn about lower extremity nerve grafts.

In nerve injuries in which the proximal segment of the injured nerve cannot be used for grafting, an end-to-side nerve anastomosis has been used.[93,94] The distal segment of the injured nerve is sutured in an end-to-side fashion to an adjacent nerve trunk, usually after an epineurial and sometimes after a perineurial window is formed in the donor nerve. The distal degenerated nerve segment attracts collateral sprouts from the healthy intact axons. Theoretically, the collateral sprouts from the donor nerve should reinnervate the distal segment of the injured nerve.

In the future, tissue engineering, neurotrophic

factors, immunosuppression, and bioimplants may be used to repair peripheral nerves. Neurotrophic factors may help prevent the death of neurons as well as improve axonal regrowth. Nerve allografts may be used successfully with new, more potent, and more tolerable immunosuppressive agents. Either natural or synthetic tubular nerve guidance channels may be alternatives to nerve autografts. Soluble neurotrophic and neurotropic factors can be incorporated directly into nerve guidance conduits to further stimulate nerve regeneration. The inclusion of neural support cells into guidance channels has been attempted. Schwann cells not only provide a substrate on which the axons can elongate but they also provide a source of neurotrophic factors. Fibroblasts can be modified genetically to produce nerve growth factor and basic fibroblast growth factor, which have been used experimentally in the spinal cords of adult rats.

If the nerve injury is so severe that primary repair or grafting is not possible, neurotization may be used. Initially, *neurotization* meant nerve fibers growing into recipient tissue. More recently, the term has been used to describe the anastomosis of one nerve to another. Neurotization is particularly applicable if the damage occurs at the root or proximal spinal nerve level, but it also is considered for proximal nerve injuries at other sites. Neurotization is also useful when a very long segment of nerve has been destroyed. One guide in evaluating the usefulness of neurotization is the "rule of 18." According to this rule, the sum of the number of inches from the site of nerve injury to the supplied muscle plus the number of months the muscle has been denervated should be less than 18 if nerve repair is likely to succeed. If the sum is greater than 18, because of the time between the injury and repair or because of the distance between the site of injury and the muscle, a nerve transfer closer to the muscle can be considered.[95] For example, if the musculocutaneous axons to the biceps muscle are destroyed proximally and the rule of 18 is violated, the chances of primary repair may be poor. In this situation, a portion of the median nerve is divided and connected to the musculocutaneous nerve near the point the musculocutaneous nerve enters the biceps. With this technique, Nath and Mackinnon[95] reported excellent recovery of biceps strength in 20 of 22 patients. Various neural structures such as the cervical plexus, contralateral spinal nerves or components of the brachial plexus, the spinal accessory nerve, phrenic nerve, pectoral nerves, and intercostal nerves have been used. The nerve is severed and the end connected primarily or by graft to a distal nerve such as the musculocutaneous, radial, or median nerve. The interposing nerve graft is usually taken from the sural nerve. More recently, muscles such as the gracilis have been removed from the lower extremity, with particular care to preserve the nerve and vascular supply to the muscle, and transferred to the upper extremity and the nerve connected, usually to an intercostal nerve. This neurotization procedure has produced effective elbow flexion in 25% to 50% of patients. A clinically useful outcome of such reinnervation requires training to produce central motor reorganization.

It generally has been thought that nerve root damage cannot be repaired. Recently, it has been shown experimentally that reimplantation of the ventral roots in rats results in reinnervation of peripheral structures.[96] Chai et al.[96] found in control rats that root avulsion resulted in the death of 35% of the motor neurons at 3 weeks after avulsion and 61% at 6 weeks. With reimplantation of the avulsed ventral roots, nearly 80% to 90% of the motor neurons were alive at 3 or 6 weeks after the injury. Of the surviving motor neurons, 80% were found to regenerate their axons into the reimplanted ventral roots. Recovery after nerve injury may be limited in large part by the loss of the primary neurons. If neuronal survival is not improved, the results of peripheral repair will be limited. Such techniques have been attempted in humans with questionable success.

If the above procedures fail and reinnervation does not occur or many years have elapsed since the injury, other secondary forms of therapy can be attempted. These include tendon transfers and joint stabilization. Physical and occupational therapy are important for preventing contractures or overstretching of muscles and ankylosis of joints and for directing rehabilitation. Other considerations are the optimal use of prostheses, splints, or slings. Protection of skin, muscles, tendons, and joints from secondary complications while awaiting nerve regeneration or recovery is important. Splinting in the best physiological position helps prevent stretching or contractures. Active and passive range of motion exercises must be performed. There should be careful design and timing of exercise programs.

If there are no other useful possibilities, amputation of the extremity may be considered. Amputation should not be performed with the expectation that it will help neuropathic pain.

The role of medical management in peripheral nerve injury is expanding. Recent work has indicated that FK506 and related analogues dose-dependently accelerate the rate of nerve regeneration in the sciatic nerve crush model.[97] The mechanism by which FK506 accelerates nerve regeneration is different from that underlying immunosuppression. However, there are other reasons to suspect that FK506 may be neurotoxic and cause peripheral neuropathy.[98]

As knowledge of the neurotrophic and neurotropic effects of various growth factors expands, systemic or local administration of these agents may enhance neuronal survival and promote regeneration.

References

1. Sunderland S. Nerves and Nerve Injuries. 2nd ed. Edinburgh: Churchill Livingstone, 1978
2. Waller AV. Experiments on the section glossopharyngeal and hypoglossal nerves of the frog and observations of the alterations produced thereby in the structure of their primitive fibres. Philos Trans R Soc Lond B Biol Sci 1850;140:423
3. Seddon H. Surgical Disorders of the Peripheral Nerves. 2nd ed. Edinburgh: Churchill Livingstone, 1975
4. Lundborg G. A 25-year perspective of peripheral nerve surgery: evolving neuroscientific concepts and clinical significance. J Hand Surg [Am] 2000;25:391–414
5. Dillingham TR. Approach to trauma of the peripheral nerves. In: 1998 AAEM Course C: Electrodiagnosis in Traumatic Conditions. AAEM 21st Annual Continuing Education Courses, October 15, 1998, Orlando, Florida. Rochester, MN: American Association of Electrodiagnostic Medicine, 1998:7–12
6. Lodish H, Berk A, Zipursky SL, et al. Molecular Cell Biology. 4th ed. New York: WH Freeman and Company, 2000
7. Goodman SR. Medical Cell Biology. 2nd ed. Philadelphia: Lippincott-Raven, 1998
8. Frostick SP, Yin Q, Kemp GJ. Schwann cells, neurotrophic factors, and peripheral nerve regeneration. Microsurgery 1998;18:397–405
9. Yin Q, Kemp GJ, Frostick SP. Neurotrophins, neurones, and peripheral nerve regeneration. J Hand Surg [Br] 1998;23:433–437
10. Newman JP, Verity AN, Hawatmeh S, et al. Ciliary neurotrophic factor enhances peripheral nerve regeneration. Arch Otolaryngol Head Neck Surg 1996;122:399–403
11. Lewin SL, Utley DS, Cheng ET, et al. Simultaneous treatment with BDNF and CNTF after peripheral nerve transection and repair enhances rate of functional recovery compared with BDNF treatment alone. Laryngoscope 1997;107:992–999
12. Cheng HL, Russell JW, Feldman EL. IGF-I promotes peripheral nervous system myelination. Ann NY Acad Sci 1999;883:124–130
13. Hallett M. Electrophysiologic approaches to the diagnosis of entrapment neuropathies. Neurol Clin 1985;3:531–541
14. Dawson DM, Hallett M, Millender LH. Entrapment Neuropathies. 2nd ed. Boston: Little, Brown and Company, 1990
15. Stewart JD. Compression and entrapment neuropathies. In: Dyck PJ, Thomas PK, Griffin JW, et al., eds. Peripheral Neuropathy. Vol 2, 3rd ed. Philadelphia: WB Saunders Company, 1993:961–979
16. Thomas PK, Holdorff B. Neuropathy due to physical agents. In: Dyck PJ, Thomas PK, Griffin JW, et al., eds. Peripheral Neuropathy. Vol 2, 3rd ed. Philadelphia: WB Saunders Company, 1993:990–1013
17. Gilliatt RW. Physical injury to peripheral nerves: physiologic and electrodiagnostic aspects. Mayo Clin Proc 1981;56:361–370
18. Lewis T, Pickering GW, Rothschild P. Centripetal paralysis arising out of arrested bloodflow to the limb, including notes on form of tingling. Heart 1931;16:1–32
19. Ochoa JL, Torebjork HE. Paraesthesiae from ectopic impulse generation in human sensory nerves. Brain 1980;103:835–853
20. Parry GJ, Linn DJ. Transient focal conduction block following experimental occlusion of the vasa nervorum. Muscle Nerve 1986;9:345–348
21. Denny-Brown D, Brenner C. Paralysis of nerve induced by direct pressure and by tourniquet. Arch Neurol Psychiatry 1944;51:1–26
22. Ochoa J, Fowler TJ, Gilliatt RW. Anatomical changes in peripheral nerves compressed by a pneumatic tourniquet. J Anat 1972;113:433–455
23. Baba M, Fowler CJ, Jacobs JM, Gilliatt RW. Changes in

peripheral nerve fibres distal to a constriction. J Neurol Sci 1982;54:197–208

24. Richardson PM, Thomas PK. Percussive injury to peripheral nerve in rats. J Neurosurg 1979;51:178–187

25. Haftek J. Stretch injury of peripheral nerve: acute effects of stretching on rabbit nerve. J Bone Joint Surg Br 1970;52:354–365

26. Terzis JK, Smith KL. The peripheral nerve: structure, function, and reconstruction. Norfolk, Virginia: Hampton Press; New York: Raven Press, 1990

27. Ordog GJ, Wasserberger J, Balasubramanium S, Shoemaker W. Civilian gunshot wounds—outpatient management. J Trauma 1994;36:106–111

28. Luce EA, Griffen WO. Shotgun injuries of the upper extremity. J Trauma 1978;18:487–492

29. Omer GE Jr. Injuries to nerves of the upper extremity. J Bone Joint Surg Am 1974;56:1615–1624

30. Kline DG, Hudson AR. Nerve Injuries: Operative Results for Major Nerve Injuries, Entrapments, and Tumors. Philadelphia: WB Saunders Company, 1995

31. Gentili F, Hudson AR, Hunter D. Clinical and experimental aspects of injection injuries of peripheral nerves. Can J Neurol Sci 1980;7:143–151

32. Gentili F, Hudson A, Kline DG, Hunter D. Peripheral nerve injection injury: an experimental study. Neurosurgery 1979;4:244–253

33. Clark K, Williams PE Jr, Willis W, McGavran WL III. Injection injury of the sciatic nerve. Clin Neurosurg 1970;17:111–125

34. Altman MI, Hutton SJ. Late neuropathic sequelae of cold injury. J Foot Surg 1987;26:213–216

35. Blair JR, Schatzki R, Orr KD. Sequelae to cold injury in one hundred patients: follow-up study four years after occurrence of cold injury. JAMA 1957;163:1203–1208

36. Shafer JC, Thompson AW. Local cold injury: a report of sequelae. Arch Dermatol 1955;72:335–347

37. Peyronnard JM, Pednault M, Aguayo AJ. Neuropathies due to cold: quantitative studies of structural changes in human and animal nerves. In: den Hartog Jager WA, Bruyn GW, Heijstee APJ, eds. Neurology. Amsterdam: Excerpta Medica, 1978

38. Hanifin JM, Cuetter AC. In patients with immersion foot type of cold injury diminished nerve conduction velocity. Electromyogr Clin Neurophysiol 1974;14:173–178

39. Carter JL, Shefner JM, Krarup C. Cold-induced peripheral nerve damage: involvement of touch receptors of the foot. Muscle Nerve 1988;11:1065–1069

40. Basbaum CB. Induced hypothermia in peripheral nerve: electron microscopic and electrophysiological observations. J Neurocytol 1973;2:171–187

41. Paintal AS. Effects of temperature on conduction in single vagal and saphenous myelinated nerve fibres of the cat. J Physiol 1965;180:20–49

42. Jia J, Pollock M. Cold nerve injury is enhanced by intermittent cooling. Muscle Nerve 1999;22:1644–1652

43. Kennett RP, Gilliatt RW. Nerve conduction studies in experimental non-freezing cold injury: II. Generalized nerve cooling by limb immersion. Muscle Nerve 1991; 14:960–967

44. Chalk CH, Dyck PJ. Ischemic neuropathy. In: Dyck PJ, Thomas PK, Griffin JW, et al., eds. Peripheral Neuropathy. Vol 2, 3rd ed. Philadelphia: WB Saunders Company, 1993:980–989

45. Blunt MJ. Ischemic degeneration of nerve fibers. Arch Neurol 1960;2:528–536

46. Hess K, Eames RA, Darveniza P, Gilliatt RW. Acute ischaemic neuropathy in the rabbit. J Neurol Sci 1979; 44:19–43

47. Schmelzer JD, Zochodne DW, Low PA. Ischemic and reperfusion injury of rat peripheral nerve. Proc Natl Acad Sci USA 1989;86:1639–1642

48. Nukada H, Dyck PJ. Microsphere embolization of nerve capillaries and fiber degeneration. Am J Pathol 1984;115:275–287

49. McManis PG, Low PA. Factors affecting the relative viability of centrifascicular and subperineurial axons in acute peripheral nerve ischemia. Exp Neurol 1988; 99:84–95

50. Dyck PJ, Conn DL, Okazaki H. Necrotizing angiopathic neuropathy: three-dimensional morphology of fiber degeneration related to sites of occluded vessels. Mayo Clin Proc 1972;47:461–475

51. Boontje AH, Haaxma R. Femoral neuropathy as a complication of aortic surgery. J Cardiovasc Surg (Torino) 1987;28:286–289

52. Honet JC, Wajszczuk WJ, Rubenfire M, et al. Neurological abnormalities in the leg(s) after use of intraaortic balloon pump: report of six cases. Arch Phys Med Rehabil 1975;56:346–352

53. Stöhr M, Dichgans J, Dörstelmann D. Ischaemic neuropathy of the lumbosacral plexus following intragluteal injection. J Neurol Neurosurg Psychiatry 1980;43:489–494

54. Castellanos AM, Glass JP, Yung WK. Regional nerve injury after intra-arterial chemotherapy. Neurology 1987;37:834–837

55. Wilbourn AJ, Levin KH. Ischemic neuropathy. In: Brown WF, Bolton CF, eds. Clinical Electromyopathy. 2nd ed. Boston: Butterworth-Heinemann, 1991:369–390

56. Triffitt PD, Konig D, Harper WM, et al. Compartment pressures after closed tibial shaft fracture: their relation to functional outcome. J Bone Joint Surg Br 1992; 74:195–198

57. Mackinnon SE, Dellon AL. Surgery of the Peripheral Nerve. New York: Thieme Medical Publishers, 1988:57

58. Salner AL, Botnick LE, Herzog AG, et al. Reversible brachial plexopathy following primary radiation therapy for breast cancer. Cancer Treat Rep 1981;65: 797–802

59. Kinsella TJ, Weichselbaum RR, Sheline GE. Radiation injury of cranial and peripheral nerves. In: Gilbert HA, Kagan AR, eds. Radiation Damage to the Nervous System: A Delayed Therapeutic Hazard. New York: Raven Press, 1980:145–153

60. Spiess H. Schädigungen am peripheren Nervensystem durch ionisierende Strahlen, mit ausführlich englischer Zusammenfassung. Berlin: Springer-Verlag, 1972

61. Linder E. Über das funktionelle und morphologische Verhalten peripherer Nerven längere Zeit nach Bestrahlung. [Remote effects of radiation on the functional and morphological behavior of the peripheral nerves.] Fortschr Roentgenstrahl 1959;90: 618–624

62. Harper CM Jr, Thomas JE, Cascino TL, Litchy WJ. Distinction between neoplastic and radiation-induced brachial plexopathy, with emphasis on the role of EMG. Neurology 1989;39:502–506

63. Kori SH, Foley KM, Posner JB. Brachial plexus lesions in patients with cancer: 100 cases. Neurology 1981;31: 45–50

64. Thomas JE, Colby MY Jr. Radiation-induced or metastatic brachial plexopathy? A diagnostic dilemma. JAMA 1972;222:1392–1395

65. Maruyama Y, Mylrea MM, Logothetis J. Neuropathy following irradiation: an unusual late complication of radiotherapy. Am J Roentgenol Radium Ther Nucl Med 1967;101:216–219

66. Stoll BA, Andrews JT. Radiation-induced peripheral neuropathy. Br Med J 1966;1:834–837

67. Westling P, Svensson H, Hele P. Cervical plexus lesions following post-operative radiation therapy of mammary carcinoma. Acta Radiol Ther Phys Biol 1972;11:209–216

68. Birch R, Bonney G, Wynn Parry CB. Surgical Disorders of the Peripheral Nerves. Edinburgh: Churchill Livingstone, 1998:326–332

69. Anezaki T, Harada T, Kawachi I, et al. A case of post-irradiation lumbosacral radiculopathy successfully treated with corticosteroid and warfarin [Japanese]. Rinsho Shinkeigaku 1999;39:825–829

70. Ashenhurst EM, Quartey GR, Starreveld A. Lumbosacral radiculopathy induced by radiation. Can J Neurol Sci 1977;4:259–263

71. DiVincenti FC, Moncrief JA, Pruitt BA Jr. Electrical injuries: a review of 65 cases. J Trauma 1969;9:497–507

72. Panse F. Electrical lesions of the nervous system. *In:* Vinken PJ, Bruyn GW, eds. Handbook of Clinical Neurology. Vol 7. Amsterdam: North-Holland Publishing Company, 1970:344–387

73. Solem L, Fischer RP, Strate RG. The natural history of electrical injury. J Trauma 1977;17:487–492

74. Hobby JAE, Laing JE. Electrical injuries of the upper limb. *In:* Tubiana R, ed. The Hand. Vol 3. Philadelphia: WB Saunders Company, 1988:779–787

75. Salzberg CA, Salisbury RE. Thermal injury of peripheral nerve. *In:* Gelberman RH, ed. Operative Nerve Repair and Reconstruction. Vol 1. Philadelphia: JB Lippincott Company, 1991:671–678

76. Danielson JR, Capelli-Schellpfeffer M, Lee RC. Upper extremity electrical injury. Hand Clin 2000;16:225–234

77. Ferreiro I, Melendez J, Regalado J, et al. Factors influencing the sequelae of high tension electrical injuries. Burns 1998;24:649–653

78. Robinson LR. Traumatic injury to peripheral nerves. Muscle Nerve 2000;23:863–873

79. Spinner RJ, Kline DG. Surgery for peripheral nerve and brachial plexus injuries or other nerve lesions. Muscle Nerve 2000;23:680–695

80. Omer GE Jr, Spinner M, Van Beek AL. Management of Peripheral Nerve Problems. 2nd ed. Philadelphia: WB Saunders Company, 1998

81. Birch R, Bonney G, Wynn Parry CB. Surgical Disorders of the Peripheral Nerves. Edinburgh: Churchill Livingstone, 1998

82. Birch R, Raji AR. Repair of median and ulnar nerves: primary suture is best. J Bone Joint Surg Br 1991;73:154–157

83. Vastamaki M, Kallio PK, Solonen KA. The results of secondary microsurgical repair of ulnar nerve injury. J Hand Surg [Br] 1993;18:323–326

84. Allan CH. Functional results of primary nerve repair. Hand Clin 2000;16:67–72

85. Roganovic Z, Savic M, Petkovic S, et al. Results of repair of severed nerves in war injuries [Serbian]. Vojnosanit Pregl 1996;53:463–470

86. Kline DG, Kim D, Midha R, et al. Management and results of sciatic nerve injuries: a 24-year experience. J Neurosurg 1998;89:13–23

87. Taha A, Taha J. Results of suture of the sciatic nerve after missile injury. J Trauma 1998;45:340–344

88. Millesi H. Techniques for nerve grafting. Hand Clin 2000;16:73–91

89. Matsumoto K, Ohnishi K, Kiyotani T, et al. Peripheral nerve regeneration across an 80-mm gap bridged by a polyglycolic acid (PGA)-collagen tube filled with laminin-coated collagen fibers: a histological and electrophysiological evaluation of regenerated nerves. Brain Res 2000;868:315–328

90. Vanderhooft E. Functional outcomes of nerve grafts for the upper and lower extremities. Hand Clin 2000;16:93–104

91. Frykman GK, Gramyk K. Results of nerve grafting. *In:* Gelberman RH, ed. Operative Nerve Repair and Reconstruction. Vol 1. Philadelphia: JB Lippincott Company, 1991:553–567

92. Mackinnon SE, Dellon AL. Clinical nerve reconstruction with a bioabsorbable polyglycolic acid tube. Plast Reconstr Surg 1990;85:419–424

93. Giovanoli P, Koller R, Meuli-Simmen C, et al. Functional and morphometric evaluation of end-to-side neurorrhaphy for muscle reinnervation. Plast Reconstr Surg 2000;106:383–392

94. Rowan PR, Chen LE, Urbaniak JR. End-to-side nerve repair: a review. Hand Clin 2000;16:151–159

95. Nath RK, Mackinnon SE. Nerve transfers in the upper extremity. Hand Clin 2000;16:131–139

96. Chai H, Wu W, So KF, Yip HK. Survival and regeneration of motoneurons in adult rats by reimplantation of ventral root following spinal root avulsion. Neuroreport 2000;11:1249–1252

97. Gold BG, Gordon HS, Wang MS. Efficacy of delayed or discontinuous FK506 administrations on nerve regeneration in the rat sciatic nerve crush model: lack of evidence for a conditioning lesion-like effect. Neurosci Lett 1999;267:33–36

98. Mikol DD, Feldman EL. Neurophilins and the nervous system (editorial). Muscle Nerve 1999;22:1337–1340

Varicella Zoster Virus, Herpes Simplex Virus, Bell's Palsy

Allen J Aksamit

Bell's palsy

Bell's palsy, or idiopathic facial nerve paralysis, has long been suspected of being caused by viral infection. The subacute onset typical of Bell's palsy is consistent with an infectious cause. However, because facial nerve paralysis occurs in many other illnesses, the diagnosis of Bell's palsy depends on typical history and examination findings and the exclusion of other illnesses such as meningeal cancer, tumors involving the cranial nerves, and meningitis. Inflammatory diseases, for example, nervous system Lyme disease and neurosarcoidosis, can present exclusively with facial nerve palsy at the onset. The diagnosis of Bell's palsy is more common than that of any of these other diseases, but diagnosis rests on the clinical exclusion of other causes. Anatomically, Bell's palsy implies isolated involvement of the facial nerve distal to its entry into the internal auditory canal. The findings of magnetic resonance imaging (MRI) of the head are normal, and the cerebrospinal fluid cell count is less than 10/mL.

Ramsay Hunt syndrome

In the early 20th century, the association of facial nerve paralysis with zoster oticus was described and clarified by Ramsay Hunt,[1,2] who through a series of clinical and pathological observations was able to identify the sensory representation of the facial nerve on the pinna of the ear. Ramsay Hunt linked the syndrome of acute facial nerve palsy to cutaneous vesicles on the pinna and external canal and geniculate ganglionitis. Subsequently, virologic techniques confirmed that the syndrome was due to varicella zoster virus (VZV) infection of the facial nerve, with cutaneous VZV eruption involving the pinna.[3] Serological studies showed that antibodies against VZV were increased in infected persons.

Natural history of Bell's palsy

Incidence and natural history studies have not clearly identified a seasonal occurrence of acute idiopathic Bell's palsy.[4] Therefore, a seasonal virus cause is thought unlikely. Also, patients do not usually have an obvious coincident systemic viral syndrome.[4,5] Recovery from Bell's palsy has been suggested to be good, and 85% of patients recover with no "obvious" long-term abnormalities of facial nerve function.[4–7] However, several studies performed in the 1970s suggested that the degree of recovery is correlated with the severity of facial nerve injury at onset.[6,7] These studies suggested that early intervention may have a role in promoting recovery in patients most severely affected at onset.

Data associating herpes simplex virus with Bell's palsy

An increased antibody titer of both herpes simplex virus (HSV) and VZV in serum has been suggested to be associated with Bell's palsy, indicating that these viruses may be an important cause of acute idiopathic facial nerve paralysis.[8] More modern techniques, specifically investigation of ganglia with molecular tools, have confirmed that HSV can reside in the geniculate ganglion of patients with Bell's palsy.[9] Latent HSV type I has been detected by the polymerase chain reaction (PCR) in 70% to 90% of unselected geniculate ganglia collected at autopsy.[10–12] Anecdotal study of patients who have Bell's palsy has isolated HSV by culture when surgical treatment allowed sampling of the perineurium.[13]

More recent molecular studies have suggested an association of HSV with Bell's palsy based on examination of tissue innervated by the facial nerve. Specifically, the basis of these studies was that reactivated HSV in the geniculate ganglion may spread to the skin of the ear, muscle of the face, or saliva in the mouth. The primary study spurring enthusiasm for HSV as a direct cause of Bell's palsy was that of Murakami et al.[14] All the patients had Bell's palsy, and each patient had surgical decompression of the facial nerve. At the time of the decompression, endoneurial fluid and postauricular muscle were examined for the presence of HSV. The endoneurial fluid of 10 of 13 patients and postauricular muscle of 8 of 14 patients were positive for HSV DNA when assayed by sensitive PCR techniques; of 14 patients with Bell's palsy, 11 were HSV-positive. The strength of the study of Murakami et al. was that patients with Ramsay Hunt syndrome were treated the same way and served as controls, and they did not have evidence of HSV. Note, however, that the endoneurial fluid or muscle tissue was sampled from 12 to 87 days after the onset of facial palsy, suggesting that some patients had a prolonged viral infection or false-positive results.

Another study sampled the saliva of patients with Bell's palsy, and 16 of 40 specimens were positive for HSV, but only 3 of 16 patients without Bell's palsy were positive for the virus.[15] The results of this study suggest that some reactivation of HSV is asymptomatic. However, the higher incidence of reactivation associated with Bell's palsy suggests causation. In another PCR study of patients with Bell's palsy, HSV was detected in specimens obtained with a tongue swab.[16]

Data associating varicella zoster virus with Bell's palsy

The above studies that suggested HSV is associated with Bell's palsy also suggested HSV is not present universally among patients with Bell's palsy. These data suggest that PCR or sampling techniques are incompletely sensitive or that another agent may be responsible for causing the palsy. Thus, attention has focused on VZV because of its association with Ramsay Hunt syndrome and because serological studies have shown elevation of VZV in some patients with acute peripheral facial palsy without vesicles.[8,17] Another approach for detecting VZV DNA is to scrape the auricular skin of patients who have acute facial nerve palsy and produce an exudate.[18] Of 19 patients with obvious Ramsay Hunt syndrome who were evaluated in this way, PCR studies were positive for VZV in 17 patients (89%, with 7 patients initially showing no sign of auricular vesicles). In comparison, of 26 patients with Bell's palsy who did not have increased VZV antibody titers serologically, none had VZV detected in the exudate.[18]

Another study used PCR to assay saliva for VZV and coupled this with an assay of serum antibodies in 142 patients who had acute facial nerve palsy. Of 21 patients with clinically diagnosed Ramsay Hunt syndrome, 58% had saliva positive for VZV by PCR and 88% had increased serum antibody titers suggestive of recent activation of VZV.[17] Of the other 121 patients, 29% had saliva positive for VZV by PCR or antibodies against VZV suggestive of recent VZV infection.[17] In this same study, PCR detected HSV in the saliva of 32% of 72 patients with Bell's palsy. Also, antibody studies suggested that the prevalence of HSV antibodies was higher among patients with Bell's palsy (97%) than among controls (59%).[17]

In summary, there is suggestive evidence of reactivation of both HSV and VZV in association with idiopathic Bell's palsy. However, reactivation of virus does not necessarily prove causation, and virus has not been demonstrated directly in the facial nerve. Still, the strong association supports the idea that HSV and VZV have some role in idiopathic Bell's palsy.

Treatment of Bell's palsy

The treatment of Bell's palsy has been debated. Recommendations have included surgical decompression, corticosteroid therapy, and antiviral agents. The issues of treatment have been reviewed recently.[19–21] Most neurologists probably think that surgical decompression of the facial nerve is unproven treatment of Bell's palsy, primarily because no prospective trial has assessed the usefulness of the procedure. Also, the recovery rate associated with no treatment is high. However, at least one author thinks that surgical treatment should be restudied.[21]

Greater controversy surrounds prednisone therapy. Although the effects of prednisone on the outcome of Bell's palsy have been investigated, many of the studies were retrospective, thus introducing bias. Early prospective trials showed no benefit,[22,23] but later prospective studies that compared prednisone and placebo suggested that prednisone was somewhat effective, particularly when applied specifically to patients with complete facial nerve paralysis.[24,25]

A recent meta-analysis of prednisone trials rejected 20 studies because they were retrospective.[26] Of the 27 prospective trials, only 3 stratified outcomes of patients by different degrees of facial paralysis. According to this meta-analysis, treatment of Bell's palsy with prednisone within the first 7 days after onset of facial paralysis had a mild benefit. The authors emphasized the need to direct therapy to patients who have complete facial paralysis and to begin treatment within the first 7 days of symptoms.[26] A recent review for the American Academy of Neurology has led to the recommendation "that steroids are probably effective, and under most circumstances should be considered."[27]

The treatment of Ramsay Hunt syndrome with prednisone is also controversial. Relatively few studies are available, but one retrospective study noted that patients with Ramsay Hunt syndrome who had facial palsy for less than 3 days had greater benefit from treatment with acyclovir and prednisone than patients who began treatment 7 or more days after the onset of facial paralysis.[28]

The assumption that HSV or VZV is an important cause of idiopathic Bell's palsy does not necessarily predict that antiviral therapy effectively restores motor function. Relatively few studies have evaluated acyclovir or other anti-herpesvirus therapy. In a trial that compared acyclovir (400 mg 5 times daily) plus prednisone for 10 days and prednisone alone, significantly more patients in the acyclovir-treated group demonstrated good recovery.[29] Also, fewer patients in the acyclovir-treated group had contracture and synkinesis. In contrast, another trial comparing acyclovir (800 mg 3 times daily for 10 days) and prednisone (for 10 days) with 3 months of follow-up suggested that patients in the prednisone group had greater improvement, with 93% obtaining good improvement (compared with 83% in the acyclovir group).[30] The recovery in the acyclovir group was similar to what has been recorded in natural history studies.

No prospective trial has investigated the treatment of Bell's palsy with oral anti-herpesvirus agents such as famciclovir or valacyclovir. These agents have been shown to be useful in uncomplicated systemic herpes zoster, but it is unclear whether these data can be extrapolated to the treatment of Bell's palsy.

Recommendations

Clear recommendations about the use of prednisone or antiviral agents for the treatment of uncomplicated Bell's palsy are difficult. One set of recommendations from the meta-analysis of prednisone trials is pred-

Table 179.1   Treatment recommendations for acute facial nerve palsy

Clinical circumstance	Suggested treatment	Comment
Bell's palsy onset ≤ 3 days, complete paralysis, immunologically normal	Prednisone 60 mg daily for 5 days and Valacyclovir 1000 mg 3 times daily for 7 days or Famciclovir 500 mg 3 times daily for 7 days	No diabetes or other comorbid condition prohibiting prednisone
Bell's palsy onset ≤ 3 days, incomplete paralysis	Valacyclovir or Famciclovir (doses, as above)	Adjust dose based on renal function and creatinine clearance estimate
Bell's palsy onset ≥ 4 days	No treatment	
Ramsay Hunt syndrome, paresis ≤ 7 days	Acyclovir 800 mg 3 times daily for 10 days or Valacyclovir 1000 mg 3 times daily for 7 days or Famciclovir 500 mg 3 times daily for 7 days	Adjust dose based on creatinine clearance estimate

nisone, 80 mg for 5 days, and famciclovir, 500 mg 3 times daily for 10 days.[26] However, it can be stated that no single regimen has proof of efficacy based on data.

A reasonable recommendation might be as follows. For patients with uncomplicated Bell's palsy and complete facial paralysis who are immunologically normal and within 3 days after the onset of symptoms, combined therapy may be recommended (Table 179.1). Prednisone should be administered 60 to 80 mg daily for 5 days, with a tapering schedule afterward if there are no serious comorbid conditions. This should be combined with antiviral therapy: famciclovir, 500 mg 3 times daily for 7 days, or valacyclovir, 1000 mg 3 times daily for 7 days, or acyclovir, 400 mg 5 times daily for 7 to 10 days. However, until prospective trials have been performed, antiviral and prednisone therapy remain only an opinion-based therapy.

For patients with incomplete paralysis who are within 3 days after the onset of facial palsy, antiviral agents could be offered. These agents are excreted primarily by the kidney and, thus, require adjustments in dose for patients with renal failure. Otherwise, the dose recommendations can be suggested as outlined above. Patients who have had facial palsy longer than 3 days are not likely to benefit from antiviral or prednisone therapy and should be observed.

Uniform treatment recommendations for Ramsay Hunt syndrome are also difficult. For patients with facial paralysis of less than 1 week who can tolerate antiviral therapy, acyclovir, valacyclovir, or famciclovir should be recommended (Table 179.1). However, it is not clear whether antiviral agents given after 3 days of facial paralysis have any effect. More than 7 days after facial palsy, antiviral therapy probably has little or no effect. A more controversial point is whether prednisone should be added to the regimen. Data do not support a clear effect of prednisone therapy added to antiviral therapy. Because there is at least a theoretical risk of VZV dissemina-

tion with prednisone, the current recommendation would be to not prescribe prednisone for Ramsay Hunt syndrome.

Knowledge of the treatment of Bell's palsy is incomplete. However, advances have been made in understanding the association between Bell's palsy and viral infections, and more prospective studies should help to determine the usefulness of antiviral agents in the treatment of this disorder.

References

1. Hunt JR. On herpetic inflammations of the geniculate ganglion: a new syndrome and its complications. J Nerv Ment Dis 1907;34:73–96
2. Hunt JR. The sensory field of the facial nerve: a further contribution to the symptomatology of the geniculate ganglion. Brain 1915;38:418–446
3. Aleksic SN, Budzilovich GN, Lieberman AN. Herpes zoster oticus and facial paralysis (Ramsay Hunt syndrome): clinico-pathologic study and review of literature. J Neurol Sci 1973;20:149–159
4. Hauser WA, Karnes WE, Annis J, Kurland LT. Incidence and prognosis of Bell's palsy in the population of Rochester, Minnesota. Mayo Clin Proc 1971;46:258–264
5. Peitersen E. The natural history of Bell's palsy. Am J Otol 1982;4:107–111
6. Adour KK, Byl FM, Hilsinger RL, Jr, et al. The true nature of Bell's palsy: analysis of 1000 consecutive patients. Laryngoscope 1978;88:787–801
7. May M, Hardin WB, Sullivan J, Wette R. Natural history of Bell's palsy: the salivary flow test and other prognostic indicators. Laryngoscope 1976;86:704–712
8. Hadar T, Tovi F, Sidi J, et al. Specific IgG and IgA antibodies to herpes simplex virus and varicella zoster virus in acute peripheral facial palsy patients. J Med Virol 1983;12:237–245
9. Burgess RC, Michaels L, Bale JF, Jr, Smith RJ. Polymerase chain reaction amplification of herpes simplex viral DNA from the geniculate ganglion of a patient with Bell's palsy. Ann Otol Rhinol Laryngol 1994;103:775–779
10. Furuta Y, Takasu T, Sato KC, et al. Latent herpes simplex virus type 1 in human geniculate ganglia. Acta Neuropathol (Berl) 1992;84:39–44

11. Takasu T, Furuta Y, Sato KC, et al. Detection of latent herpes simplex virus DNA and RNA in human geniculate ganglia by the polymerase chain reaction. Acta Otolaryngol 1992;112:1004–1011

12. Schulz P, Arbusow V, Strupp M, et al. Highly variable distribution of HSV-1-specific DNA in human geniculate, vestibular and spiral ganglia. Neurosci Lett 1998; 252:139–142

13. Mulkens PS, Bleeker JD, Schroder FP. Acute facial paralysis: a virological study. Clin Otolaryngol 1980;5: 303–310

14. Murakami S, Mizobuchi M, Nakashiro Y, et al. Bell palsy and herpes simplex virus: identification of viral DNA in endoneurial fluid and muscle. Ann Intern Med 1996;124:27–30

15. Furuta Y, Fukuda S, Chida E, et al. Reactivation of herpes simplex virus type 1 in patients with Bell's palsy. J Med Virol 1998;54:162–166

16. Bonkowsky V, Kochanowski B, Strutz J, et al. Delayed facial palsy following uneventful middle ear surgery: a herpes simplex virus type 1 reactivation? Ann Otol Rhinol Laryngol 1998;107:901–905

17. Furuta Y, Ohtani F, Kawabata H, et al. High prevalence of varicella-zoster virus reactivation in herpes simplex virus-seronegative patients with acute peripheral facial palsy. Clin Infect Dis 2000;30:529–533

18. Murakami S, Honda N, Mizobuchi M, et al. Rapid diagnosis of varicella zoster virus infection in acute facial palsy. Neurology 1998;51:1202–1205

19. Marra CM. Bell's palsy and HSV-1 infection. Muscle Nerve 1999;22:1476–1478

20. Steiner I, Mattan Y. Bell's palsy and herpes viruses: to (acyclo)vir or not to (acyclo)vir? J Neurol Sci 1999;170: 19–23

21. Friedman RA. The surgical management of Bell's palsy: a review. Am J Otol 2000;21:139–144

22. May M, Wette R, Hardin WB, Jr, Sullivan J. The use of steroids in Bell's palsy: a prospective controlled study. Laryngoscope 1976;86:1111–1122

23. Wolf SM, Wagner JH, Davidson S, Forsythe A. Treatment of Bell palsy with prednisone: a prospective, randomized study. Neurology 1978;28:158–161

24. Austin JR, Peskind SP, Austin SG, Rice DH. Idiopathic facial nerve paralysis: a randomized double blind controlled study of placebo versus prednisone. Laryngoscope 1993;103:1326–1333

25. Shafshak TS, Essa AY, Bakey FA. The possible contributing factors for the success of steroid therapy in Bell's palsy: a clinical and electrophysiological study. J Laryngol Otol 1994;108:940–943

26. Ramsey MJ, DerSimonian R, Holtel MR, Burgess LP. Corticosteroid treatment for idiopathic facial nerve paralysis: a meta-analysis. Laryngoscope 2000;110: 335–341

27. Grogan PM, Gronseth GS. Practice parameter: steroids, acyclovir, and surgery for Bell's palsy (an evidence-based review): report of the Quality Standards Subcommittee of the American Academy of Neurology. Neurology 2001;56:830–836

28. Murakami S, Hato N, Horiuchi J, et al. Treatment of Ramsay Hunt syndrome with acyclovir-prednisone: significance of early diagnosis and treatment. Ann Neurol 1997;41:353–357

29. Adour KK, Ruboyianes JM, Von Doersten PG, et al. Bell's palsy treatment with acyclovir and prednisone compared with prednisone alone: a double-blind, randomized, controlled trial. Ann Otol Rhinol Laryngol 1996;105:371–378

30. De Diego JI, Prim MP, De Sarria MJ, et al. Idiopathic facial paralysis: a randomized, prospective, and controlled study using single-dose prednisone versus acyclovir three times daily. Laryngoscope 1998;108: 573–575

180 Peripheral Nervous System Lyme Disease

Allen J Aksamit

Introduction

The peripheral nervous system complications of Lyme disease include facial nerve palsy, radiculoneuropathy, and peripheral neuropathy.[1-4] Less common peripheral nerve manifestations, for example, mononeuropathies, have been described but are less certain to be caused by Lyme disease.[4] The diagnosis of peripheral nervous system Lyme disease or neuroborreliosis is complicated because of the difficulty interpreting neurological symptoms with relatively few signs and relating them to confirmatory laboratory testing, which is insensitive. Peripheral nerve complications of Lyme disease can be diagnosed confidently by objectively confirming systemic Lyme disease by documenting the skin rash (erythema chronicum migrans) that develops after a tick bite and temporally associating it with a well-recognized neurological syndrome. However, the absence of a tick bite or rash does not exclude Lyme disease.[5]

The most common well-identified clinical syndrome associated with nervous system Lyme disease is facial nerve palsy.[2,4,6-8] Although it usually is unilateral, it can be bilateral in up to 28% of patients.[6] A clue that unilateral facial nerve palsy is associated with Lyme disease is the finding of cerebrospinal fluid (CSF) pleocytosis. However, some authors have used the absence of CSF pleocytosis with facial neuropathy and confirmed Lyme disease to decide among treatment options for nervous system Lyme disease.[7,9] Therefore, the absence of a cell reaction in the CSF of patients with facial nerve palsy does not exclude Lyme disease.

Radiculoneuropathy is the second most common peripheral nerve manifestation of Lyme disease. This is manifested primarily as an asymmetric polyradiculoneuropathy, commonly associated with pleocytosis. The earliest reports of radiculopathy in Lyme disease were from Europe, and the disorder was identified as Bannwarth syndrome.[10-12] This syndrome of ascending, typically asymmetrical, motor greater than sensory polyradiculopathy was linked to Lyme disease about the same time that *Borrelia burgdorferi* was identified as the cause of Lyme disease. This was suggested to be a reversible cause of polyradiculopathy and treatable with antibiotics. Usually both lower extremities are affected, but individual roots can be affected in the upper limb and lower limb simultaneously, spatially separate. The asymmetrical radicular symptoms commonly are painful. Some patients have marked pleocytosis, but this is not found universally.[13] Facial or other cranial neuropathy can occur simultaneously with radiculopathy affecting the limbs.

The motor polyradiculopathy and the more symmetrical diffuse sensory polyneuropathy of Lyme disease[3,13] may have the same mechanism of injury to the nervous system. The distal symmetrical sensory neuropathy can be demonstrated with electromyography (EMG).[13] The diagnosis is established by temporally associating peripheral neuropathy with clinical systemic Lyme disease. Confirmation requires serological or polymerase chain reaction abnormalities in the serum or CSF that show *B. burgdorferi* infection.

Diagnosis

Although normal CSF findings and the absence of serum and CSF antibody responses to *Borrelia* do not entirely exclude the diagnosis of nervous system Lyme disease, they are currently the most sensitive indicators of Lyme disease of the nervous system. Whether Lyme disease is the cause of facial neuropathy, polyradiculopathy, or sensory neuropathy is difficult to determine because of uncertainty about the sensitivity and specificity of serum and CSF abnormalities. The level of CSF total protein in these syndromes ranges from 8 to 400 mg/dl, with mean values in different studies ranging from 42 to 115 mg/dl.[2,14,15] The glucose value is routinely normal, although values as low as 35 mg/dl have been reported.[14] Patients with inflammatory CSF with elevated cell counts are encountered more commonly when headache or other meningeal symptoms and signs are present. However, meningeal symptoms are not required for diagnosis. Among patients with the peripheral nerve syndrome of Lyme disease, pleocytosis is found most frequently in those with polyradiculopathy. When the CSF cell count is elevated, lymphocytes predominate, ranging from 0 to 1830 cells/mm^3, with reported mean values ranging from 11 to 166 cells/mm^3.[2,14-16]

Stereotypical CSF changes indicative of intrathecal antibody synthesis in patients with Lyme disease and peripheral nerve manifestations include an elevated IgG index and IgG synthesis rate and CSF oligoclonal banding.[14] However, the specificity of abnormalities for Lyme disease has not been evaluated prospectively. Facial palsy, polyradiculopathy, or peripheral neuropathy can be caused by other inflammatory diseases (e.g., sarcoidosis), which can nonspecifically increase intrathecal immunoglobulin synthesis, although not against *Borrelia*. The intrathecal synthesis of antibody in Lyme disease is against *B. burgdorferi*.[11,12,17] Assessment is further complicated by the insensitivity of specific antibody assays for Lyme disease in CSF. Nuances in performing the serological tests, with variability between laboratories, make interpretation of negative results difficult.[18,19] Still, paired antibody against *B. burgdorferi* present in the CSF and serum is the best specific test for nervous system Lyme disease.

PCR performed on CSF to confirm the diagnosis of nervous system Lyme disease has had mixed success. Some laboratories have reported high sensitivity for detection of *B. burgdorferi* in inflammatory nervous system Lyme disease.[20] Other laboratories have had less success, with detection rates of 40% to 48%.[21,22] Currently, PCR measurements for Lyme disease in CSF should be regarded as an adjunctive test. When the results are positive, they are helpful and confirmatory, but negative results do not exclude clinically significant disease related to *B. burgdorferi*.

Treatment of nervous system Lyme disease

Early involvement of the nervous system with facial nerve palsy after the onset of clinical acquisition of Lyme disease may be treatable with oral antibiotics (Table 180.1). Current recommendations are to use an oral regimen of doxycycline, 100 mg twice daily, or amoxicillin, 500 mg 3 times daily, for 14 to 21 days.[9] For patients who are unable to tolerate either doxycycline or amoxacillin, cefuroxime axetil, 500 mg twice daily, or a macrolide antibiotic such as azithromycin or clarithromycin may be used. However, these are thought to be less effective than doxycycline or amoxacillin.

However, the treatment for patients who have facial nerve palsy only is debated. Controversy exists about whether facial palsy represents "early" Lyme disease (i.e., disease not affecting the central nervous system) or is an early manifestation of central nervous system invasion, which requires more aggressive intravenous therapy. Some authors have used the presence of CSF pleocytosis as a discriminator to decide whether facial nerve palsy alone due to Lyme disease should be treated with oral or intravenous therapy.[7,9] The intravenous administration of antibiotics is recommended universally if pleocytosis is present.

Most authors agree that if CSF pleocytosis is associated with facial nerve palsy, polyradiculopathy, or polyneuropathy of Lyme disease, the treatment is parenteral antibiotics.[9] The regimen usually recommended is intravenous ceftriaxone, 2 g once daily (Table 180.1). Alternatives are penicillin G, 18 to 24 million units daily divided into every 4-hour dosing, and cefotaxime, 2 g 3 times daily. All these treatment regimens are given for 14 to 28 days. Clearly, patients who have meningitis, encephalopathy, headache, or other central nervous system complications and facial nerve palsy or other peripheral nerve manifestations should receive treatment with parenteral antibiotics. Ceftriaxone is the preferred antibiotic because of its penetration of the CSF and decreased frequency of administration (Table 180.1). Several studies have suggested that, in most cases, these treatments are successful in clearing the peripheral nerve manifestations of Lyme disease.[8,23-25] However, the lack of complete recovery does not indicate persistent infection but may represent residual damage from previous injury.

Lyme disease vaccine has been suggested to be useful in preventing primary Lyme disease; thus, it presumably would be potentially useful in preventing nervous system involvement. There is no published evidence that once neurological disease has occurred, vaccination after infection will boost immune clearing of the agent from the nervous system. Patients who are vaccinated for prevention of Lyme disease require three serial injections. Studies have suggested that the three-injection protocol is approximately 76% effective in preventing postexposure to Lyme disease seroconversion.[26] Also, use of the vaccine does not provide durable protection. It has been estimated that antibodies decrease to near nonprotective levels by 8 months after completing vaccination.[26] A typical regimen for Lyme disease vaccine is vaccination at zero, 1, and 2 to 6 months after the initiation of the vaccine protocol.[27,28] It has been recommended that Lyme disease vaccination be given only in geographically defined high-risk areas, or to people with high-risk behavior.[28] Side effects of the vaccine are soreness at the injection site, generalized myalgias, and a flu-like illness that may last up to 2 to 3 days.

Table 180.1 Recommendations for antimicrobial therapy in neurological Lyme disease

Erythema migrans only	Doxycycline 100 mg orally twice daily *or* Amoxicillin 500 mg orally 3 times daily for 14–21 days
Facial nerve palsy	
Without CSF pleocytosis	Oral regimen above
With CSF pleocytosis	Ceftriaxone 2 g intravenously daily *or* Penicillin G 18–24 million units intravenously daily divided into every 4-hr dosing *or* Cefotaxime 2 g intravenously 3 times daily for 14–28 days
Lyme meningitis, polyradiculopathy, encephalopathy, or peripheral neuropathy	Parenteral regimens above

CSF, cerebrospinal fluid.
Modified from Wormser et al.[9] By permission of the Infectious Diseases Society of America.

References

1. Steere AC, Pachner AR, Malawista SE. Neurologic abnormalities of Lyme disease: successful treatment with high-dose intravenous penicillin. Ann Intern Med 1983;99:767–772
2. Pachner AR, Steere AC. The triad of neurologic manifestations of Lyme disease: meningitis, cranial neuritis, and radiculoneuritis. Neurology 1985;35:47–53
3. Halperin JJ, Little BW, Coyle PK, Dattwyler RJ. Lyme disease: cause of a treatable peripheral neuropathy. Neurology 1987;37:1700–1706
4. Finkel MF. Lyme disease and its neurologic complications. Arch Neurol 1988;45:99–104
5. Reik L, Jr, Burgdorfer W, Donaldson JO. Neurologic abnormalities in Lyme disease without erythema chronicum migrans. Am J Med 1986;81:73–78
6. Dotevall L, Hagberg L. Successful oral doxycycline treatment of Lyme disease-associated facial palsy and meningitis. Clin Infect Dis 1999;28:569–574
7. Albisetti M, Schaer G, Good M, et al. Diagnostic value of cerebrospinal fluid examination in children with peripheral facial palsy and suspected Lyme borreliosis. Neurology 1997;49:817–824
8. Logigian EL, Kaplan RF, Steere AC. Chronic neurologic manifestations of Lyme disease. N Engl J Med 1990;323:1438–1444
9. Wormser GP, Nadelman RB, Dattwyler RJ, et al. Practice guidelines for the treatment of Lyme disease. The Infectious Diseases Society of America. Clin Infect Dis 2000;31(Suppl 1):S1–S14
10. Meyer-Rienecker HJ, Hitzschke B. Lymphocytic meningoradiculitis (Bannwarth's syndrome). In: Vinken PJ, Bruyn GW, eds. Handbook of Clinical Neurology: Infections of the Nervous System: Part II, Vol 34. New York: North-Holland, 1978:571–586
11. Wilske B, Schierz G, Preac-Mursic V, et al. Intrathecal production of specific antibodies against Borrelia burgdorferi in patients with lymphocytic meningoradiculitis (Bannwarth's syndrome). J Infect Dis 1986;153:304–314
12. Henriksson A, Link H, Cruz M, Stiernstedt G. Immunoglobulin abnormalities in cerebrospinal fluid and blood over the course of lymphocytic meningoradiculitis (Bannwarth's syndrome). Ann Neurol 1986;20:337–345
13. Logigian EL, Steere AC. Clinical and electrophysiologic findings in chronic neuropathy of Lyme disease. Neurology 1992;42:303–311
14. Halperin JJ, Volkman DJ, Wu P. Central nervous system abnormalities in Lyme neuroborreliosis. Neurology 1991;41:1571–1582
15. Vallat JM, Hugon J, Lubeau M, et al. Tick-bite meningoradiculoneuritis: clinical, electrophysiologic, and histologic findings in 10 cases. Neurology 1987;37:749–753
16. Weller M, Stevens A, Sommer N, et al. Cerebrospinal fluid interleukins, immunoglobulins, and fibronectin in neuroborreliosis. Arch Neurol 1991;48:837–841
17. Hansen K, Lebech AM. Lyme neuroborreliosis: a new sensitive diagnostic assay for intrathecal synthesis of Borrelia burgdorferi—specific immunoglobulin G, A, and M. Ann Neurol 1991;30:197–205
18. Hedberg CW, Osterholm MT, MacDonald KL, White KE. An interlaboratory study of antibody to Borrelia burgdorferi. J Infect Dis 1987;155:1325–1327
19. Kaiser R, Rauer S. Serodiagnosis of neuroborreliosis: comparison of reliability of three confirmatory assays. Infection 1999;27:177–182
20. Keller TL, Halperin JJ, Whitman M. PCR detection of Borrelia burgdorferi DNA in cerebrospinal fluid of Lyme neuroborreliosis patients. Neurology 1992;42:32–42
21. Lebech AM, Hansen K. Detection of Borrelia burgdorferi DNA in urine samples and cerebrospinal fluid samples from patients with early and late Lyme neuroborreliosis by polymerase chain reaction. J Clin Microbiol 1992;30:1646–1653
22. Pachner AR, Delaney E. The polymerase chain reaction in the diagnosis of Lyme neuroborreliosis. Ann Neurol 1993;34:544–550
23. Dattwyler RJ, Halperin JJ, Pass H, Luft BJ. Ceftriaxone as effective therapy in refractory Lyme disease. J Infect Dis 1987;155:1322–1325
24. Dattwyler RJ, Halperin JJ, Volkman DJ, Luft BJ. Treatment of late Lyme borreliosis—randomised comparison of ceftriaxone and penicillin. Lancet 1988;1:1191–1194
25. Logigian EL, Kaplan RF, Steere AC. Successful treatment of Lyme encephalopathy with intravenous ceftriaxone. J Infect Dis 1999;180:377–383
26. Steere AC, Sikand VK, Meurice F, et al. Vaccination against Lyme disease with recombinant Borrelia burgdorferi outer-surface lipoprotein A with adjuvant. Lyme Disease Vaccine Study Group. N Engl J Med 1998;339:209–215
27. Lyme disease vaccine. Med Lett Drugs Ther 1999;41:29–30
28. Centers for Disease Control. Recommendations for the use of Lyme disease vaccine. Recommendations of the Advisory Committee on Immunization Practices (ACIP). MMWR Recomm Rep 1999;48:1–17, 21–25

181 Diphtheritic Neuropathy

Allen J Aksamit

History

Historical descriptions of diphtheritic neuropathy date to the time of Hippocrates. In a review of its history, McDonald and Kocen[1] noted that the modern name stems from French reports in 1826 and detailed descriptions of diphtheritic paralysis date to 1860. The cause has long been recognized as a bacterial infection, primarily of the oral pharynx, by *Corynebacterium diphtheriae*. When this gram-positive bacillus, by itself benign, contains a lysogenic bacteriophage, it causes clinical diphtheria. It is the exotoxin expressed from the genome of this bacteriophage which is responsible for the toxogenic neurological consequences of the disease, by a similar mechanism of production as botulinum and tetanus toxin.

Clinical

The primary location of infection is oropharyngeal, manifesting as faucial, laryngeal, or nasal disease. Classically, the pharyngitis is manifested as an adherent membranous grayish white exudate involving the mucous membranes. The presence of this pseudomembrane helps to identify the diphtheritic syndrome. Although the bacteria are not invasive and only grow superficially over the involved mucous membranes, the exotoxin produced by the growing bacteria is absorbed and is responsible for the neurological and other systemic manifestations of the disease.

Although the initial manifestations are those of localized pharyngitis, systemic symptoms progress with a generalized disorder of malaise, irritability, anorexia, myalgias, and headache. The degree of oropharyngeal, nasal, and nuchal involvement predicts the severity and often the duration of systemic symptoms, such as the neurological consequences. Assigned degrees of oropharyngeal involvement, graded 1 through 3, have been correlated with worse neurological disease. The degree of neck swelling and induration identifies the assigned degree, with 1 being least and 3, most.[2] Confirmation of the diagnosis in the pharynx can be established by culture of the organism directly. Also, an exotoxin assay is available. Even more sensitive, however, is the ability to perform a polymerase chain reaction (PCR) for the gene of the exotoxin in the bacterial organism.[3,4]

In the most severe cases, symptoms progress with increasing cervical adenopathy, increased temperature, and myocardial involvement, with exotoxin affecting the myocardium. Myocarditis is the most common reason for hemodynamic instability and death.

Diphtheria can arise also in association with wound or cutaneous infection. There is debate about the differences in the neurological manifestations associated with involvement of the limb (discussed below).

Neurological manifestations

Neurological manifestations typically begin as pharyngeal and soft palatal paralysis with dysarthria, hypernasal speech, dysphagia, and nasal regurgitation. This may be the exclusive manifestation of the disease or there may be more widespread involvement of the nervous system.

The frequency of involvement of the nervous system in diphtheria is debated, but in various reviews, the incidence of neuropathy has ranged from 10% to 60%. A 20% incidence has been estimated on the basis of two large series of 2300 cases.[5,6] The incidence of diphtheritic neuropathy in an outbreak of diphtheria in Latvia in the 1990s was 7% (50 of 731 patients), with virtually all the patients presenting with bulbar weakness.[7] The bulbar weakness typically begins 2 to 3 weeks after pharyngitis initially develops, but it may be as late as 6 weeks.

The effects of diphtheria exotoxin on the nervous system include pupillary changes, with symptomatic blurred vision, and changes in accommodation, occasionally with preservation of the light reflex. With severe involvement, these effects can progress to frank ophthalmoplegia, including pupil cycloplegia. The diaphragm can be affected, and involvement of the respiratory muscles can progress to full respiratory embarrassment. Typically in the eighth to twelfth week of illness, general paralysis begins, with mixed sensory and motor symptoms occurring in a distal-to-proximal gradation. This is associated with areflexia. Large sensory fibers are involved more than small sensory fibers. According to a recent review, the bladder was involved in 34% of 50 patients.[7]

In patients with a nonpharyngeal infection, neuropathy has been reported to occur locally first in the limb affected by the wound or cutaneous infection.[8] Older reports, however, suggested that neuropathic symptoms were not expressed focally at the site of the primary cutaneous or wound infection and the neuropathic symptoms were generalized from onset.[9] The average time from cutaneous infection to the onset of neurological illness was 70 days, and patients typically presented with generalized weakness.

Laboratory diagnosis

The clinical association of pseudomembranous pharyngitis, with confirmatory culture or other microbiological studies, helps to identify diphtheria as the cause of progressive paralysis. Diphtheritic neuropathy needs to be distinguished primarily from Guillain-Barré syndrome, which may have similar neuropathic presentation, but Guillain-Barré syndrome is not associated with a pharyngeal infection. Both diphtheritic neuropathy and Guillain-Barré syndrome may produce an ascending paralysis, with a demyelinating polyneuropathy. Electromyography (EMG) shows nerve conduction slowing and other findings of demyelinating neuropathy and does not distinguish between diphtheritic neuropathy and Guillain-Barré syndrome. However, the prominent early involvement of the pharyngeal musculature and systemic manifestations such as myocarditis help to distinguish diphtheria from Guillain-Barré syndrome.

Cerebrospinal fluid (CSF) studies in diphtheritic neuropathy typically show an increase in protein, but the cell count may be normal. This protein–cellular disassociation is similar to that of Guillain-Barré syndrome. However, CSF pleocytosis can be found, more frequently in association with diphtheritic neuropathy, and a recent report includes evidence that a moderate lymphocytic pleiocytosis can occur.[10]

Antibody assay for serological response against the diphtheritic organism can be performed. However, seropositivity does not distinguish between a recent infection and a recent vaccination and does not necessarily indicate neurotoxin-associated disease.

Epidemiology

In developed countries, diphtheria is being eliminated by vaccination of the population. In the United States, the incidence has been estimated at approximately $2/1\,000\,000$ population, with approximately 80% of the population seropositive because of vaccination.[11] However, there is concern about a possible resurgence of the disease in the United States because of an epidemic in Russia and the former Soviet Republics of Ukraine, Georgia, Tajikistan, Azerbaijan, Romania, Lithuania, Latvia, Belarus, and Uzbekistan. For each of these countries, detailed epidemiological studies have been reported recently on this outbreak. The epidemic in the Ukraine, for instance, began in 1991, peaked in 1995, and had declined by 1997.[12] The epidemic had a similar course in Kyrgyzstan[2] and Georgia.[13] These outbreaks have allowed more modern neurological evaluations of patients with diphtheria, including the large group in Latvia referred to above.

Neuropathology

The sensorimotor neuropathy associated with diphtheria is attributed to both segmental and perinodal demyelination.[1] Axonal integrity is maintained. However, in some patients, EMG findings include distal muscle fibrillation that suggests mild axonal degeneration. Associated pathological changes include a proliferation of Schwann cells and macrophages but not infiltration by polymorphonuclear cells or lymphocytes. Remyelination has been correlated with recovery and has been demonstrated experimentally in neurotoxin-induced disease in animals. Sural nerve biopsy specimens have been reported to show segmental demyelination.[14]

Toxin

The neurotoxin is produced by the phage-infected bacteria, originally recognized in 1971. This has been confirmed by studies of the recent epidemic in the former Soviet Republics.[15] Diphtheria toxin has been well studied. It has been characterized as a 62- to 63-kDa protein. The diphtheria toxin catalytically acts as a ribosylating enzyme. It catalytically transfers adenosine diphosphate ribose to a protein called elongation factor. This inhibits the effect of elongation factor and stops protein synthesis. Inactivation of elongation factor in eukaryotic cells has been shown to be critical to the toxicity of diphtheria toxin.

Prognosis

Prognosis is determined primarily by the severity of the initial involvement and the promptness of treatment, particularly with antitoxin. Neurological recovery is slow, usually taking weeks to months, most typically 3 to 6 months.[1] Complete recovery is possible and has been documented.[14] The recent review of the epidemic in Latvia suggested that at 1 year, 6% of patients with diphtheritic neuropathy were unable to walk. Overall mortality was estimated to be 2% to 3%. It was thought that myocardial, rather than neurological, involvement was the primary determinant for mortality. However, neurological impairment was responsible for long-term disability.

Treatment

Treatment centers primarily on the use of antitoxin and antibiotics and particularly prevention in the population by vaccination. Treatment with antitoxin is guided primarily by the extent of involvement at the time of neurological presentation. Antitoxin is most effective if given in the first 48 hours after neurological involvement. However, it should be administered for up to 7 to 10 days after neurological involvement.

The World Health Organization recommends that nasal or laryngeal involvement in isolation be treated with $10\,000$ to $40\,000$ units of antitoxin and the combination of pharyngeal and moderate cervical involvement be treated with $40\,000$ to $60\,000$ units to prevent neurological and cardiac involvement. Patients who present with "severe changes," with profound neck swelling and cervical adenopathy, should be treated with $40\,000$ to $100\,000$ units. On the basis of the recent experience with the epidemics in eastern Europe, it has been suggested that patients with the most toxic involvement, that is, marked neck swelling, should be treated with $100\,000$ to $300\,000$ units.[2] The antitoxin is provided usually in $10\,000$- or $20\,000$-unit vials and should be given by intramuscular injection or slow intravenous infusion. Also, if neurological involvement has been present for more than 3 days, higher doses (from $100\,000$ to $200\,000$ units) are recommended.[2]

Penicillin or erythromycin is recommended for the

treatment of active pharyngitis. A recent trial compared erythromycin and penicillin in treating diphtheria in children and showed that they were equally effective, but penicillin was preferred because intravenous infusion of erythromycin produces phlebitis.[16] This was relevant especially for patients who were unable to take medication orally because of pharyngitis. For adults, the average dose of procaine penicillin is 600 000 to 1.2 million units given intramuscularly daily for 14 days, and of erythromycin, 500 mg daily for 14 days. The suggested pediatric dose for erythromycin is 50 mg/kg for 10 days, and for benzylpenicillin, it is 50 000 U/kg for 5 days intramuscularly and 50 mg/kg orally for an additional 5 days.[16]

Vaccination is the primary means for preventing diphtheria. Neurological side effects associated with the diphtheria vaccine are extremely rare, which distinguishes this vaccine from pertussis vaccine. However, the vaccines are available primarily as combination vaccines, with diphtheria combined with either tetanus alone or, as a trivalent vaccine, also with pertussis vaccine. The trivalent vaccines, the various doses, and the recommendations for use in infants and young children have been reviewed recently; the dose and potency of each commercially available vaccine differ slightly.[17] Vaccination combinations currently available in the United States include Tripedia, ACEL-IMUNE, Infanrix, and Certiva.

Treatment for diphtheritic neuropathy is generally supportive and requires extensive rehabilitation as remyelination occurs. No evidence has been published that immune-modulating medications such as corticosteroids, plasma exchange, or intravenous immunoglobulin promote remyelination, despite the macrophage response found in pathological studies of this disorder.

References

1. McDonald WI, Kocen RS. Diphtheritic neuropathy. In: Dyck PG, Thomas PK, eds. Peripheral Neuropathy. Vol 2, 3rd ed. Philadelphia: WB Saunders Company, 1993: 1412–1417
2. Kadirova R, Kartoglu HU, Strebel PM. Clinical characteristics and management of 676 hospitalized diphtheria cases, Kyrgyz Republic, 1995. J Infect Dis 2000;181(Suppl 1):S110–S115
3. Efstratiou A, Engler KH, Mazurova IK, et al. Current approaches to the laboratory diagnosis of diphtheria. J Infect Dis 2000;181(Suppl 1):S138–S145
4. Kobaidze K, Popovic T, Nakao H, Quick L. Direct polymerase chain reaction for detection of toxigenic Corynebacterium diphtheriae strains from the Republic of Georgia after prolonged storage. J Infect Dis 2000; 181(Suppl 1):S152–S155
5. Rolleston JD, Ronaldson GW. Acute Infectious Diseases: A Handbook for Practitioners and Students. 3rd rev ed. London: Heinemann, 1940
6. Scheid W. Diphtherial paralysis: an analysis of 2292 cases of diphtheria in adults, which included 174 of polyneuritis. J Nerv Ment Dis 1952;116:1095–1101
7. Logina I, Donaghy M. Diphtheritic polyneuropathy: a clinical study and comparison with Guillain-Barré syndrome. J Neurol Neurosurg Psychiatry 1999;67:433–438
8. Walshe FMR. On the pathogenesis of diphtheritic paralysis: II. Clinical observations on the paralysis of facial and extra-facial diphtheria, with an analysis of thirty cases following skin and wound infections. Q J Med 1918–1919;12:14–31
9. Gaskill HS, Korb M. Occurrence of multiple neuritis in cases of cutaneous diphtheria. Arch Neurol Psychiatry 1946;55:559–572
10. Creange A, Meyrignac C, Roualdes B, et al. Diphtheritic neuropathy. Muscle Nerve 1995;18:1460–1463
11. Galazka A. The changing epidemiology of diphtheria in the vaccine era. J Infect Dis 2000;181(Suppl 1):S2–S9
12. Nekrassova LS, Chudnaya LM, Marievski VF, et al. Epidemic diphtheria in Ukraine, 1991–1997. J Infect Dis 2000;181(Suppl 1):S35–S40
13. Quick ML, Sutter RW, Kobaidze K, et al. Epidemic diphtheria in the Republic of Georgia, 1993–1996: risk factors for fatal outcome among hospitalized patients. J Infect Dis 2000;181(Suppl 1):S130–S137
14. Solders G, Nennesmo I, Persson A. Diphtheritic neuropathy, an analysis based on muscle and nerve biopsy and repeated neurophysiological and autonomic function tests. J Neurol Neurosurg Psychiatry 1989;52: 876–880
15. Holmes RK. Biology and molecular epidemiology of diphtheria toxin and the tox gene. J Infect Dis 2000;181(Suppl 1):S156–S167
16. Kneen R, Pham NG, Solomon T, et al. Penicillin vs. erythromycin in the treatment of diphtheria. Clin Infect Dis 1998;27:845–850
17. Centers for Disease Control and Prevention. Pertussis vaccination: use of acellular pertussis vaccines among infants and young children—recommendations of the Advisory Committee on Immunization Practices (ACIP). MMWR 1997;46(No. RR-7):1–25

182 Peripheral Neuropathy and HIV

Nada G Abou-Fayssal and David Simpson

Overview

The introduction of highly active antiretroviral therapy (HAART) in the mid 1990s has led to a reduction in the incidence of opportunistic infections and to longer survival of patients infected with human immunodeficiency virus (HIV). This has also allowed patients to develop late stage neurological disorders. While most central nervous system (CNS) complications, including dementia, toxoplasmosis and lymphoma have declined in the current era of HAART, peripheral neuropathy remains a common complication in this population. The use of neurotoxic antiretroviral therapy, particularly in patients with advanced immunosuppression, has created a pool of long term survivors with increased risk of peripheral neuropathy.

The most common peripheral nerve disorders associated with HIV infection are:

- Distal symmetrical polyneuropathy
  - HIV
  - Neurotoxic
- Inflammatory demyelinating polyneuropathy
  - Autoimmune
  - CMV
- Mononeuropathy multiplex
  - Autoimmune
  - Vasculitis
  - CMV
- Progressive polyradiculopathy
  - CMV
- Autonomic neuropathy
- Diffuse infiltrative lymphocytosis syndrome.

Diagnostic findings and treatment of the HIV-associated neuropathies are summarized in Table 182.1.

Distal symmetrical polyneuropathy

Distal symmetrical polyneuropathy (DSPN) is the most common form of neuropathy associated with HIV infection.[1,2] It occurs in 35% to 50% of patients[3] and is seen more commonly in later stages of the disease when immunosuppression is pronounced.[4,5]

Clinical presentation

Patients with DSPN present with painful dysesthesia and hyperesthesia, initially affecting the lower extremities in a symmetrical fashion, and later involving the hands. Patients often complain of burning pain and uncomfortable tingling in the feet. Physical examination usually reveals symmetrical sensory loss to vibration, pinprick, temperature, and to a lesser degree to joint position sense, in a stocking-and-glove distribution, combined with absent or decreased ankle jerks. Distal weakness develops only late in the course of the disease.[3,6–9] Patients often have a combination of central and peripheral neurological disorders, such as myelopathy, which may confound the diagnosis of DSPN. Thus examination may reveal hyperactive knee reflexes and normal or depressed ankle reflexes.

Diagnosis

The diagnosis of DSPN is predominantly clinical and usually is straightforward with bedside history and neurological examination. However, the diagnosis of peripheral neuropathy in HIV patients is often overlooked or incorrectly assigned. This is particularly true in the context of large antiretroviral studies, in which neurological diagnostic criteria are often imprecise and clinical assessments are usually performed by non-neurological study personnel. Several problems complicate the accurate diagnosis of peripheral neuropathy. Clinicians have difficulty distinguishing the different forms of peripheral neuropathy associated with HIV infection.[2] In an analysis of a large primary antiretroviral trial, Simpson et al. reported that primary HIV site investigators have a high rate of misdiagnosis of DSPN.[10] The distinction between different forms of neuropathy is critical, particularly for toxicity management, since only DSPN may be attributed to the toxic effect of antiretroviral therapy.[11] Electrodiagnostic studies usually show the presence of low amplitude or absent sural nerve action potentials, small tibial and peroneal compound muscle action potential (CMAP) amplitudes, and somewhat preserved nerve conduction velocity (NCV).[5,12] Median and ulnar nerve involvement may be present in advanced stages. Electromyography (EMG) reveals evidence of active or chronic denervation predominantly in distal leg muscles.[9,12]

Sural nerve biopsy confirms the presence of degeneration of myelinated and unmyelinated axons with associated perivascular mononuclear infiltration.[8,13] Blood studies should be performed to exclude other causes of DSPN including diabetes mellitus and vitamin B_{12} deficiency.

Etiology

The pathogenesis of HIV-associated DSPN remains unclear. Postulated mechanisms include cytokine dysregulation and direct viral invasion of peripheral nerves.[14–16] To date, several pathological studies have failed to identify retroviral particles or antigens in nerve roots or dorsal root ganglia, making the theory of direct viral invasion of peripheral nerves

Table 182.1   HIV-associated neuropathies: diagnosis and treatment

Disease	HIV disease stage	Symptoms	Signs	Diagnostic studies	Treatment
Distal symmetrical polyneuropathy	Late	Numbness Pain Paresthesia	Stocking-glove sensory loss Depressed ankle reflexes	*NCS/EMG:* Distal axonopathy *Blood studies:* B$_{12}$, HbA1C, TFT, IPEP	Neurotoxin withdrawal Analgesics Anticonvulsants Opioids Topical agents rhNGF
Inflammatory demyelinating polyneuropathy	Early ≫ late	Ascending weakness Paresthesia	Weakness Mild sensory loss Areflexia.	*CSF:* Mild lymphocytic pleocytosis High protein *NCS/EMG:* Demyelination ± axonopathy	Immunotherapy Corticosteroids (CIDP) Plasmapheresis, IVIg
Mononeuritis multiplex	Early and late	Facial weakness Foot drop Wrist drop	Multifocal cranial and peripheral neuropathies	*NCS/EMG:* Multifocal axonal neuropathy *CSF:* Mononuclear pleocytosis PCR—CMV, HSV, VZV, etc. Cytology—Lymphoma *Blood Studies:* ESR, ANA, cryoglobulin	Early: none, Immunotherapy Late: anti-CMV therapy
Progressive polyradiculopathy	Late	Lower extremity paresthesia and weakness Sphincter dysfunction	Flaccid paraparesis Saddle anesthesia Depressed DTRs Urinary retention	*CSF:* PMN pleocytosis High protein Normal glucose PCR—CMV, HSV, VZV, etc. Cytology— Lymphoma *NCS/EMG:* Polyradiculopathy	Anti-CMV therapy
Autonomic neuropathy	Late > early	Syncope Palpitations Impotence Diarrhea Urinary dysfunction Sweating abnormality	Orthostatic hypotension Resting tachycardia Sweating abnormality	*ECG/Holter:* Arrhythmia *Tilt table:* Orthostatic hypotension *Sweat test* *Stool culture* *Urodynamic studies*	Salt supplement Fludrocortisone Antiarrhythmics Antidiarrheals Neurotoxin withdrawal

Adapted from Simpson DM, Tagliati M. Ann Intern Med 1994;121:769–785
ANA, antinuclear antibodies; CMV, cytomegalovirus; CSF, cerebrospinal fluid; DTRs, deep tendon reflexes; ECG, electrocardiogram; EMG, electromyography; HbA1C, hemoglobin A1C; IPEP, immunoelectrophoresis; IVIg, intravenous immunoglobulin; NCS, nerve conduction studies; PCR, polymerase chain reaction; PMNs, polymorphonuclear leukocytosis; rhNGF, recombinant human nerve growth factor; TFT, thyroid function test.

unlikely.[13,17] Vitamin B$_{12}$ deficiency does not seem to play a major role in DSPN.[12]

Other etiological factors include neurotoxic drugs frequently used in HIV infection such as nucleoside reverse transcriptase inhibitors (NRTIs).[18–20] In early clinical trials, dose-limiting toxicity was described for patients treated with didanosine (ddI), zalcitabine (ddC), and stavudine (d4T).[11] All patients treated with ddC in AIDS Clinical Trial Group (ACTG) Protocol 155 developed peripheral neuropathy, with a mean onset of approximately two months.[21] Most patients enrolled in these early trials had advanced HIV disease, were given high dose NRTIs, and many had had prior antiretroviral therapy. As such, they represent patients with risk factors for the development of HIV-associated neuropathy. In a recent study from the Johns Hopkins AIDS Services, combination therapy of ddI, d4T and hydroxyurea was shown to carry an additive risk for DSPN when compared to ddI or d4T alone.[22] On the other hand, When patients with less advanced immunosuppression and CD4 lymphocyte counts of 200 to 500 cells/mm³ were treated with ddI, ddC and AZT, they showed a lower risk of neurotoxic neuropathy.[10]

While the mechanism of "antiretroviral drug" neuropathy is not proven, it may result from the ability of nucleoside analogs to inhibit mitochondrial gamma DNA polymerase.[23]

Treatment

Treatment of DSPN is problematic and remains mainly supportive. Therapy for painful DSPN is aimed primarily at symptom relief and at improving the quality of life in HIV-infected patients. Breitbart et al. have reported that in 235 patients with AIDS-related pain syndromes, only 16% were prescribed adequate pain relief using the criteria established by the World Health Organization.[24] Treatment of DSPN may vary from the use of nonsteroidal anti-inflammatory drugs (NSAIDs) in mild cases to opiates in severe neuropathy. Despite its widespread use, amitriptyline was not superior to placebo in HIV-associated DSPN.[25,26] Other treatments such as topical capsaicin, mexiletine, peptide T, acupuncture, and vibratory stimulation failed to show significant benefits in controlled studies.[26–29] Lamotrigine, a novel anticonvulsant, has shown promise in a small placebo-controlled study.[30] A larger study of lamotrigine in HIV neuropathy is underway.

A controlled study of recombinant human nerve growth factor (rhNGF), a pathogenesis-based agent meant to regenerate damaged peripheral nerves, revealed significant reduction in pain although evidence of nerve fiber regeneration was not demonstrated.[31] Phase III studies of rhNGF in diabetic neuropathy were negative and future clinical development of rhNGF is uncertain.

Inflammatory demyelinating polyneuropathy

Inflammatory demyelinating polyneuropathy (IDP) occurs usually early in the course of HIV infection and may present in an acute (AIDP) or chronic (CIDP) form.[32,33] AIDP may coincide with HIV seroconversion and can be the initial manifestation of HIV disease.[32,34,35] The prevalence of IDP is not established, with wide ranges reported by different series.[32–34] However, IDP appears to be a relatively infrequent complication of HIV infection.

Clinical features

The clinical features of IDP are indistinguishable between HIV-infected and noninfected patients.[32,37] AIDP presents clinically with rapidly progressive weakness associated with mild sensory deficit and areflexia. In severe cases respiratory failure may occur.[32,38] CIDP has a more chronic course and may be relapsing.[32,33]

Diagnosis

Electrophysiological studies reveal a demyelinating pattern with prolonged distal latencies, prolonged or absent late responses, and reduced CMAP amplitudes as a result of conduction block or secondary axonal degeneration.[32,37]

Cerebrospinal fluid (CSF) in HIV-infected patients with IDP contains high protein with mild lymphocytic pleocytosis in the range of 10 to 50 cells/mm³. This pattern is distinct from the acellular CSF present in HIV-uninfected patients.[32,39] In selected patients CSF should be assayed for cytomegalovirus (CMV) RNA with polymerase chain reaction (PCR).[40] Nerve biopsy in IDP reveals features of demyelination with associated perivascular inflammatory infiltrates, and secondary axonal degeneration. Morgello and Simpson reported autopsy findings in an advanced patient with IDP, revealing primary CMV infection of schwann cells.[41]

Etiology

Autoimmune mechanisms similar to those proposed in HIV-seronegative patients are thought to play a role in IDP associated with early HIV.[2,42,43] An immune-mediated pathogenesis is supported by the presence of increased levels of neopterin and soluble CD8 in the CSF.[44] Furthermore, antiperipheral myelin antibodies have been found in HIV-patients with demyelinating neuropathy.[45] In patients with IDP and advanced immunosuppression (CD4 lymphocyte counts less than 50 to 100 cells/mm³), CMV infection may cause IDP.[43]

Treatment

Despite the lack of controlled trials, case series support the notion that the clinical course and the response to treatment in IDP is similar in HIV-seronegative and seropositive patients. Immunotherapy including plasmapheresis and intravenous immunoglobulins (IVIg) is a potential treatment for AIDP.[32,46] Patients with CIDP may benefit from corticosteroids, but often relapse when treatment with corticosteroids is stopped. Such patients may respond to IVIg or plasmapheresis.[46,47] In severely immunocompromised patients with IDP, particularly when CSF or nerve biopsy shows evidence for CMV infection, antiviral therapy with ganciclovir, foscarnet or cidofovir should be administered.

Mononeuropathy multiplex

Mononeuropathy multiplex (MM) may develop at any stage of HIV infection and, like IDP, may be the initial manifestation of HIV.[12,48,49] MM usually involves one or multiple cranial, spinal and peripheral nerves resulting in multifocal, sensory and motor deficits in the distribution of the involved nerves.[1,9,12] Two distinct entities have been identified: MM, in early HIV disease, may involve the facial or other focal nerves, and usually has a benign and self-limited course. In later stages of HIV, MM has a more rapid course and a poor prognosis.[50]

Diagnosis

Electrophysiological studies in MM reveal axonal degeneration in the distribution of the affected nerves, with reduced CMAP and sensory nerve action potential (SNAP) amplitudes and mild reduction in conduction velocities.[51] EMG reveals evidence of denervation in the muscles innervated by the affected nerve.[9] CSF reveals a mild mononuclear pleocytosis with elevated protein, although these are nonspecific findings in patients with HIV infection.[12] In late stages of HIV, when immunosuppression is advanced, PCR assay of CSF for CMV is indicated, as in IDP.[50]

Nerve biopsy in MM may reveal several patterns. In patients with early HIV disease, axonal degeneration with epineural and endoneural perivascular inflammatory infiltrate has been reported. In late MM, polymorphonuclear infiltrates are present with mixed axonal and demyelinating features and, at times, CMV inclusions.[50]

Etiology

Several mechanisms have been proposed for HIV-associated MM. Early MM is thought to be mediated by autoimmune mechanisms.[48,50] Progressive MM, which usually occurs with severe immunosuppression, is associated with CMV infection.[52] However, other types of infections such as herpes zoster, cryptococcus and toxoplasmosis have been associated with MM. Lymphoma, cryoglobulinemia and vasculitis may also play an etiological role in HIV-associated MM.[12,53,54]

Treatment

Early MM is usually self-limited and tends to remit spontaneously.[48,50] In patients with incomplete recovery or progressive or relapsing MM, uncontrolled case series have reported benefit with immunotherapy such as plasmapheresis, IVIg and corticosteroids.[1] In particular, patients with pathological evidence of vasculitis on nerve biopsy may respond to corticosteroids. When associated with severe immunosuppression, MM is often caused by CMV and should be treated with anti-CMV therapy, as discussed above.[55]

Progressive polyradiculopathy

Progressive polyradiculopathy (PP) was initially reported in 1986[56] and soon was recognized as a life-threatening complication of HIV infection.[57,58] PP is often associated with CMV and usually occurs in late stages of HIV, when immunosuppression is severe.[59] Since the introduction of HAART in the mid 1990s, the incidence of PP has dramatically declined due to immune restoration in most patients. It is possible that with more patients failing all available antiretroviral therapies, the incidence of PP and other late stage neurological disorders may increase.

Patients with PP usually present with a cauda equina syndrome, characterized by painful paresthesias in the legs and rapidly progressing to flaccid paraparesis, areflexia and sphincter dysfunction.[58,60] Upper extremity and cranial involvement is a late finding.[55]

Diagnosis

Electrodiagnostic studies reveal evidence of axonal pathology in lower extremity and lumbar paraspinal muscles with prolonged late responses, low CMAP amplitudes and mildly prolonged conduction velocities.[56] Sural nerve conduction velocities and sensory nerve action potential amplitudes are usually spared unless there is coexistent DSP.[61] The CSF in CMV polyradiculopathy is characteristic and displays marked polymorphonuclear pleocytosis, elevated protein and hypoglycorrhachia.[62,63] However, this pattern has been reported in only about half of the patients with CMV polyradiculopathy. Therefore the absence of a polymorphonuclear reaction should not rule out CMV as the causative agent, but should prompt the consideration of other causes of polyradiculopathy.[62] CSF cultures for CMV are positive in half of the cases of CMV polyradiculopathy. PCR for CMV DNA has proven to be a reliable and sensitive diagnostic assay.[62]

The predominant pathological feature in PP is extensive inflammation and necrosis of dorsal and ventral nerve roots, mainly seen in the lumbosacral region.[56,57] Autopsy reveals evidence of CMV infection including nuclear and cytomegalic inclusions in endothelial, schwann and ependymal cells.[64,65]

Etiology

Numerous series have reported CMV as the most common causative agent associated with PP.[56,65,66] Less common causes of PP include other infectious agents, i.e. *Mycobacterium tuberculosis*,[66] herpes simplex virus (HSV),[67,68] varicella zoster virus (VZV),[69] syphilis,[70,71] and cryptococcus.[66] Noninfectious causes such as lymphomatous infiltration have also been reported.[72]

Treatment

Untreated, PP usually has a rapidly progressive course, with the duration of illness to death ranging from 2 to 30 days. Early diagnosis and initiation of treatment is mandatory in order to avoid irreversible nerve root necrosis, leading to permanent neurological deficits and fatal outcome.

Ganciclovir, foscarnet and cidofovir have proven efficacy in the treatment of HIV-associated CMV disease, and are generally employed in the treatment of CMV polyradiculopathy.[73,74] Early empirical therapy is sometimes necessary as the diagnosis may be delayed or unconfirmed.[75] Since the introduction of HAART and the subsequent improvement in immunocompetence, the prevalence of PP has markedly decreased. A prospective study of antiretroviral therapy for the treatment of HIV-associated PP was suspended due to the failure to accrue subjects in the HAART era.

Autonomic neuropathy

Early anecdotal case series noted the presence of autonomic dysfunction in HIV patients.[76–78] Since then, several investigators have reported dysautonomia to be a common, yet often overlooked complication, occurring more frequently and with greater severity in later stages of HIV infection.[79,80] Clinical dysautonomia occurs mainly in advanced stages of HIV and involves both sympathetic and parasympathetic divisions.[81,82] Parasympathetic dysfunction is manifested by resting tachycardia, impotence and urinary dysfunction. Patients with sympathetic abnormalities present with diarrhea, anhidrosis, syncope and orthostatic hypotension, which may lead at times to cardiorespiratory arrest.[76–78,83]

Diagnosis

The early diagnosis of autonomic dysfunction is important since its presence may increase the risk of cardiorespiratory complications. Cardiovascular reflex function tests (heart rate variability during deep breathing and Valsalva maneuver), blood pressure response to sustained hand-grip test and head-up tilt, QT interval at rest and during Valsalva maneuver and quantitative sudomotor axon reflex test[84–86] are among the available tests used to detect early autonomic involvement. The sensitivity and specificity of such tests have not been established in HIV-infected patients, although several studies report good reliability.[83–86]

Etiology

Autonomic dysfunction in HIV-infected patients is thought to result from central or peripheral nervous system involvement. Abnormalities of the cervical sympathetic ganglia were present at autopsy in six AIDS patients. Investigators have demonstrated the presence of abnormal autonomic axons in small bowel mucosa, and a decrease in oxytocin neurons in the periventricular nucleus of the hypothalamus.[87,88] The pathogenesis of autonomic involvement in HIV infection is uncertain. Villa et al. proposed an autoimmune theory,[84] while other data suggest direct invasion of the virus.[79] Other factors contributing to autonomic dysfunction (mainly manifested by orthostatic hypotension) in HIV infection include iatrogenic causes resulting from drugs such as pentamidine, tricyclic antidepressants and vincristine.[89,90]

Treatment

Treatment of autonomic dysfunction in HIV patients is symptom-oriented, and consists in volume repletion, fludrocortisone for syncope, antiarrhythmic agents for cardiac arrhythmias, and parasympathetic agents for diarrhea. When applicable, removal of the offending medication may be a sufficient step in rendering the patient asymptomatic.

Diffuse infiltrative lymphocytosis syndrome

HIV has been associated with CD8 hyperlymphocytosis, which causes diffuse infiltrative lymphocytosis syndrome (DILS). DILS-associated neuropathy may present as DSPN, IDP or MM.[91] Host inflammatory responses to HIV infection are thought to account for peripheral nerve involvement in DILS.[92]

Conclusion

The science and clinical care of HIV disease is rapidly evolving. The availability of HAART has dramatically improved the prognosis and life span of patients with HIV infection. However, neurological disorders remain common in these patients, particularly as they are living long enough to develop late stage neurological disorders. In the developing world, there is still only limited access to these therapies, and patients often present with neurological disorders as the initial manifestation of HIV disease.

It is therefore incumbent on all clinicians caring for patients with HIV to be familiar with the diagnosis and treatment of these neurological disorders. This is a particular challenge for non-neurologists who care for most patients with HIV. Understanding the neurobiology of HIV disease will provide a foundation for treatment advances in the next decade.

References

1. Miller RG, Parry GJ, Pfaeffl W, et al. The spectrum of peripheral neuropathy associated with ARC and AIDS. Muscle Nerve 1988;11:857–863
2. Simpson DM, Wolfe DE. Neuromuscular complications of HIV infection and its treatment. AIDS 1991;5:917–926
3. So YT, Holtzman DM, Abrams DI, Olney RK. Peripheral neuropathy associated with acquired immunodeficiency syndrome. Prevalence and clinical features from a population-based survey. Arch Neurol 1988;45:945–948
4. Barohn RJ, Gronseth GS, LeForce BR, et al. Peripheral nervous system involvement in a large cohort of human immunodeficiency virus-infected individuals. Arch Neurol 1993;50:167–171
5. Simpson DM, Tagliatti M, Grimmell J, Godbold J. Electrophysiological findings in HIV infection: association with distal symmetrical polyneuropathy and CD4 level (abstract). Muscle Nerve 1994;17:1113–1114
6. Snider WD, Simpson DM, Nielson S, et al. Neurological complications of acquired immune deficiency syndrome: analysis of 50 patients. Ann Neurol 1983;14:403–418
7. Levy RM, Bredesen DE, Rosenblum ML. Neurological manifestations of the acquired immuno-deficiency syndrome (AIDS): experience at UCSF and review of the literature. J Neurosurg 1985;62:475–495
8. De la Monte SM, Gabuzda DH, Ho DD, et al. Peripheral neuropathy in the acquired immunodeficiency syndrome. Ann Neurol 1988;23:485–492
9. Lange DJ, Britton CB, Younger DS, Hays AP. The neuromuscular manifestations of human immunodeficiency virus infections. Arch Neurol 1988;45:1084–1088
10. Simpson DM, Katzenstein DA, Hughes MD, et al. Neuromuscular function in HIV infection: analysis of a placebo-controlled combination antiretroviral trial, AIDS Clinical Group 175/801 Study Team. AIDS 1998;12:2425–2432
11. Simpson DM, Tagliati M. Nucleoside analogue-associated peripheral neuropathy in human immunodeficiency virus infection. J Acquir Immune Defic Syndr Hum Retrovirol 1995;9:153–161
12. Fuller GN, Jacobs JM, Guiloff RJ. Subclinical peripheral nerve involvement in AIDS: an electrophysiological and pathological study. J Neurol Neurosurg Psychiatry 1991;54:318–324
13. Bailey RO, Baltch AL, Venkatesh R, et al. Sensory motor neuropathy associated with AIDS. Neurology 1988;38:886–991
14. Mah V, Vartavarian LM, Akers MA, Vinters HV. Abnormalities of peripheral nerve in patients with

human immunodeficiency virus infection. Ann Neurol 1988;24:713–717

15. Wesselingh SL, Glass J, McArthur JC, et al. Cytokine dysregulation in HIV-associated neurological disease. Adv Neuroimmunol 1994;4:199–206

16. Ho DD, Rota TR, Schooley RT, et al. Isolation of HTLV-III from cerebrospinal fluid and neural tissues of patients with neurologic syndromes related to the acquired immunodeficiency syndrome. N Engl J Med 1985;313:1493–1497

17. Rizzuto N, Cavallaro T, Monaco S. Role of HIV in the pathogenesis of distal symmetrical peripheral neuropathy. Acta Neuropathol (Berl) 1995;90:244–250

18. Grafe MR, Wiley CA. Spinal cord and peripheral nerve pathology in AIDS: the roles of cytomegalovirus and human immunodeficiency virus. Ann Neurol 1989;25:561–566

19. Dubinsky RM, Yarchoan R, Dalakas M, Broder S. Reversible axonal neuropathy from the treatment of AIDS and related disorders with 2',3'-dideoxycytidine (ddC). Muscle Nerve 1989;12:856–860

20. Kieburtz KD, Seidlin M, Lambert JS, et al. Extended follow-up of peripheral neuropathy in patients with AIDS and AIDS-related complex treated with dideoxyinosine. J Acquir Immune Defic Syndr Hum Retrovirol 1992;5:60–64

21. Berger AR, Arezzo JC, Schaumburg HH, et al. 2',3'-dideoxycytidine (ddC) toxic neuropathy: a study of 52 patients. Neurology 1993;43:358–362

22. Moore RD, Wong WM, Keruly JC, McArthur JC. Incidence of neuropathy in HIV-infected patients on monotherapy versus those on combination therapy with didanosine, stavudine and hydroxyurea. AIDS 2000;14:273–238

23. Lewis W, Dalakas MC. Mitochondrial toxicity of antiviral drugs. Nat Med 1995;1:417–422

24. Breitbart W, Rosenfeld BD, Passik SD, et al. The undertreatment of pain in ambulatory AIDS patients. Pain 1996;65:243–249

25. Kieburtz K, Simpson D, Yiannoutsos C. A randomized trial of amitriptyline and mexiletine for painful neuropathy in HIV infection. AIDS Clinical Trial Group 242 Protocol Team. Neurology 1998;51:1682–1688

26. Shlay JC, Chaloner K, Max MB. Acupuncture and amitriptyline for pain due to HIV-related peripheral neuropathy: a randomized controlled trial. Terry Beirn Community Programs for Clinical Research on AIDS. JAMA 1998;280:1590–1595

27. Kemper CA, Kent G, Burton S, Deresinski SC. Mexiletine for HIV-infected patients with painful peripheral neuropathy: a double-blind, placebo-controlled, crossover treatment trial. J Acquir Immune Defic Syndr Hum Retrovirol 1998;19:367–372

28. Paice JA, Ferrans CE, Lashley FR, et al. Topical capsaicin in the management of HIV-associated peripheral neuropathy. J Pain Symptom Manage 2000;19:45–52

29. Paice JA, Shott S, Oldenburg FP, et al. Efficacy of a vibratory stimulus for the relief of HIV-associated neuropathic pain. Pain 2000;84:291–296

30. Simpson D, Olney RK, McArthur JC, et al. A placebo controlled study of lamotrigine in the treatment of painful sensory polyneuropathy associated with HIV infection (abstract). J Neurovirol 1998;4:366

31. McArthur JC, Yiannoutsos C, Simpson DM. A phase II trial of nerve growth factor for sensory neuropathy associated with HIV infection. AIDS Clinical Trials Group Team 291. Neurology 2000;54:1080–1088

32. Cornblath DR, McArthur JC, Kennedy PG, et al. Inflam-

matory demyelinating peripheral neuropathies associated with human T-cell lymphotropic virus type III infection. Ann Neurol 1987;21:32–40

33. Ghika-Schmid F, Kuntzer T, Chave P, et al. Diversite de l'atteinte neuromusculaire de 47 patients infectes par le virus de l'immunodeficience humaine. Schweiz Med Wochenschr 1994;124:791–800

34. Piette AM, Tusseau F, Vignon D. Acute neuropathy coincident with seroconversion for anti-LAV/HTLV-III. Lancet 1986;1:852

35. Cruz Martinez A, Rabano J, Villoslada C, Cabello A. Chronic inflammatory demyelinating polyneuropathy as first manifestation of human immunodeficiency virus infection. Electromyogr Clin Neurophysiol 1990;30:379–383

36. Winer JB, Bang B, Clarke JR. A study of neuropathy in HIV infection. QJM 1992;83:473–488

37. Miller RG, Parry GJ, Pfaeffl W, et al. The spectrum of peripheral neuropathy associated with ARC and AIDS. Muscle Nerve 1988;11:857–863

38. Berger JR, Difini JA, Swerdloff MA, Ayyar DR. HIV seropositivity in Guillain–Barré syndrome (letter). Ann Neurol 1987;22:393–394

39. Dalakas MC. Neuromuscular complications of AIDS. Muscle Nerve 1986;9:92

40. Clifford DB, Buller RS, Mohammed S, et al. Use of polymerase chain reaction to demonstrate cytomegalovirus DNA in CSF of patients with human immunodeficiency virus infection. Neurology 1993;43:75–79

41. Morgello S, Simpson DM. Multifocal cytomegalovirus demyelinative polyneuropathy associated with AIDS. Muscle Nerve 1994;17:176–182

42. Dalakas MC, Pezeshkpour GH. Neuromuscular diseases associated with human immunodeficiency virus infection. Ann Neurol 1988;23(Suppl):S38–S48

43. Hughes RA, Hadden RD, Gregson NA, Smith KJ. Pathogenesis of Guillain–Barré syndrome. J Neuroimmunol 1999;100:74–97

44. Griffin DE, McArthur JC, Cornblath DR. Neopterin and interferon-gamma in serum and cerebrospinal fluid of patients with HIV-associated neurologic disease. Neurology 1991;41:69–74

45. Petratos S, Turnbull VJ, Papadopoulos R, et al. Antibodies against peripheral myelin glycolipids in people with HIV infection. Immunol Cell Biol 1998;76:535–541

46. Cornblath DR, Chaudhry V, Griffin JW. Treatment of chronic inflammatory demyelinating polyneuropathy with intravenous immunoglobulin. Ann Neurol 1991;30:104–106

47. Panicker R, Bloom AL, Compston DA. Inflammatory demyelinating polyneuropathy in a haemophiliac associated with human immunodeficiency virus infection, responding to high dose intravenous immunoglobulin. Postgrad Med J 1988;64:699–700

48. Cornblath DR. Treatment of the neuromuscular complications of human immunodeficiency virus infection. Ann Neurol 1988;23(Suppl):S88–S91

49. Lipkin WI, Parry G, Kiprov D, et al. Inflammatory neuropathy in homosexual men with lymphadenopathy. Neurology 1985;35:1479–1483

50. Harada H, Tamaoka A, Yoshida H, et al. Horner's syndrome associated with mononeuritis multiplex due to cytomegalovirus as the initial manifestation in a patient with AIDS. J Neurol Sci 1998;154:91–93

51. So YT, Olney RK. The natural history of mononeuritis multiplex and simplex in HIV. Neurology 1991;41(Suppl 1):S375

52. Corral I, Quereda C, Casado JL, et al. Acute polyradiculopathies in HIV-infected patients. J Neurol 1997;244:499–504

53. Roullet E, Assueurus V, Gozlan J, et al. Cytomegalovirus multifocal neuropathy in AIDS: analysis of 15 consecutive patients. Neurology 1994;44:2174–2182

54. Brannagan TH III. Retroviral-associated vasculitis of the nervous system. Neurol Clin 1997;15:972–944

55. Stricker RB, Sander KA, Owen WF, et al. Mononeuritis multiplex associated with cryoglobulinemia in HIV infection. Neurology 1992;42:2103–2105

56. Said G, Lacroix C, Chemouilli O, et al. Cytomegalovirus neuropathy in acquired immunodeficiency syndrome: a clinical and pathological study. Ann Neurol 1991;29:139–146

57. Eidelberg JR, Crane LR, Vogel HL, et al. Progressive polyradiculopathy in acquired immune deficiency syndrome. Neurology 1986;36:912–916

58. Behar R, Wiley C, McCutchan JR. Cytomegalovirus polyradiculopathy in AIDS. Neurology 1987;37:557–561

59. de Gans J, Portegies P, Tiessens G, et al. Therapy for cytomegalovirus polyradiculopathy in patients with AIDS. Treatment with Ganciclovir. AIDS 1990;4:421–425

60. Mahieux F, Gray F, Fenelon G, et al. Acute myeloradiculitis due to cytomegalovirus as the initial manifestation of AIDS. J Neurol Neurosurg Psychiatry 1989;52:270–274

61. Matsamoto R, Nakagawa S, Nakayama J, et al. A case of acquired deficiency syndrome presenting acute lumbosacral polyradiculopathy due to opportunistic infection of cytomegalovirus. Rinsho Shinkeigaku 1998;38:653–657

62. So YT, Holtzman DM, Miller RG. Sensory myeloneuropathy in patients with human immunodeficiency virus (HIV) infection. Neurology 1990;40(Suppl):S429

63. Miller RF, Fox JD, Thomas P, et al. Acute lumbosacral polyradiculopathy due to cytomegalovirus in advanced HIV disease: CSF findings in 17 patients. J Neurol Neurosurg Psychiatry 1996;61:456–460

64. Granter SR, Doolittle MH, Renshaw AA. Predominance of neutrophils in the cerebrospinal fluid of AIDS patients with cytomegalovirus radiculopathy. Am J Clin Pathol 1996;105:364–366

65. Mahieux F, Gray F, Fenelon G, et al. Acute myeloradiculitis due to cytomegalovirus as the initial manifestation of AIDS. J Neurol Neurosurg Psychiatry 1989;52:270–274

66. Miller RG, Storey JR, Greco CM. Ganciclovir in the treatment of progressive AIDS-related polyradiculopathy. Neurology 1990;40:569–574

67. Miguelez M, Correa-Nazco VJ, Linares M, et al. Lumbosacral polyradiculomyelitis caused by herpes simplex virus (HSV) in a patient with AIDS. An Med Interna 1999;16:417–419

68. Dahan P, Haettich B, Le Parc JM, Paolaggi JB. Meningoradiculitis due to herpes simplex virus disclosing HIV infection. Ann Rheum Dis 1988;47:440

69. Chretien F, Gray F, Lescs MC, et al. Acute varicella-zoster virus ventriculitis and meningo-myelo-radiculitis in acquired immunodeficiency syndrome. Acta Neuropathol (Berl) 1993;86:659–665

70. Diaz-Villoslada P, Lozano M, Nos C, et al. Syphilitic meningoradiculitis in a patient with HIV. Neurologia 1994;9:253–255

71. Lanska MJ, Lanska DJ, Schmidley JW. Syphilitic polyradiculopathy in an HIV-positive man. Neurology 1988;38:1297–1301

72. Leger JM, Henin D, Belec L, et al. Lymphoma-induced polyradiculopathy in AIDS: two cases. J Neurol 1992;239:132–134

73. Anders HJ, Goebel FD. Neurological manifestations of cytomegalovirus infection in the acquired immunodeficiency syndrome. Int J STD AIDS 1999;10:151–159

74. Cinque P, Cleator GM, Weber T, et al. Diagnosis and clinical management of neurological disorders caused by cytomegalovirus in AIDS patients. European Union Concerted Action on Virus Meningitis and Encephalitis. J Neurovirol 1998;4:120–132

75. Anders HJ, Weiss N, Bogner JR, Goebel FD. Ganciclovir and foscarnet efficacy in AIDS-related CMV polyradiculopathy. J Infect 1998;36:29–33

76. Lin-Greenberg A, Taneja-Uppal N. Dysautonomia and infection with the human immunodeficiency virus. Ann Intern Med 1987;106:167

77. Evenhouse M, Haas E, Snell E, et al. Hypotension in infection with the Human Immunodeficiency Virus. Ann Intern Med 1991;107:598–599

78. Villa A, Foresti V, Confalonieri F. Autonomic neuropathy and HIV. Lancet 1987;2:915

79. Freeman R, Roberts MS, Friedman LS, Broadbridge C. Autonomic function and human immunodeficiency virus infection. Neurology 1990;40:575–580

80. Welby SB, Rogerson SJ, Beeching NJ. Autonomic neuropathy is common in human immunodeficiency virus infection. J Infect 1991;23:123–128

81. Cohen JA, Laudenslager M. Autonomic nervous system involvement in patients with human immunodeficiency virus infection. Neurology 1989;39:1111–1112

82. Becker K, Görlach I, Frieling T, Häussinger D. Characterization and natural course of cardiac autonomic nervous dysfunction in HIV-infected patients. AIDS 1997;11:751–757

83. Craddock C, Pasvol J, Bull R, et al. Cardiorespiratory arrest and autonomic neuropathy on AIDS. Lancet 1987;ii:16–18

84. Villa A, Foresti V, Confalonieri F. Autonomic nervous system dysfunction associated with HIV in intravenous heroin users. AIDS 1992;6:85–89

85. Gordon S, Piaggesi A, Ewing J. Sequential autonomic function tests in HIV infection. AIDS 1990;4:1279–1282

86. Villa A, Forest V, Confalonieri F. Autonomic neuropathy and prolongation of QT interval in human immunodeficiency virus infection. Clin Auton Res 1995;5:48–52

87. Batman PA, Miller ARO, Sedgwick PM, Griffin GE. Autonomic denervation in jejunal mucosa of homosexual men infected with HIV. AIDS 1991;5:1247–1252

88. Purba JS, Hofman MA, Portegies P, et al. Decreased number of oxytocin neurons in the paraventricular nucleus of the human hypothalamus in AIDS. Brain 1993;116:795–805

89. Hemlich CG, Green JK. Pentamidine-associated hypotension and route of administration. Ann Intern Med 1985;103:480

90. Carmichael SM, Engleton L, Ayers CR, et al. Orthostatic hypotension during vincristine therapy. Arch Intern Med 1970;126:290–293

91. Gherardi RK, Chretien F, Delfau-Larue MH, et al. Neuropathy in diffuse infiltrative lymphocytosis syndrome: an HIV neuropathy, not a lymphoma. Neurology 1998;50:1041–1044

92. Price RW. Neuropathy complicating diffuse infiltrative lymphocytosis syndrome. Lancet 1998;35:592–594

183 The Neuropathies of Leprosy

Thomas R Swift and Thomas D Sabin

Overview

The disease leprosy has been known since Biblical times and has been prevalent in many countries of the world, including Northern Europe during the Middle Ages. While usually affecting economically disadvantaged people, it has afflicted kings, princes and national leaders. Some of the well-to-do who have contracted leprosy have written poignant accounts of their long battles with the disease. For over thousands of years there was very little effective treatment for patients with this disorder; instead, society relegated them to be quarantined in leprosaria for long periods of time. These leprosaria are now closing in many countries. Leprosy is worldwide in distribution and at the present time primarily affects poor, tropical and semitropical countries, although it does affect patients in northern countries. When occurring in northern latitudes, the disease may be excessively severe in the face and hands, which are exposed to lower ambient temperatures, since leprosy has a temperature predilection.[1]

Pathogenesis

The etiology of leprosy is quite clear. It is caused by the acid-fast *Mycobacterium leprae* which is similar to tuberculosis. The bacillus reproduces itself slowly (in weeks rather than in hours or days), as with most bacterial pathogens, and therefore the incubation period can be very long. Most people are naturally immune to leprosy, probably about 90%, and even those who are susceptible have varying degrees of immunity which determine the manifestations of the disease they contract.[2] Patients with high resistance to this disease have localized skin lesions in small areas of the body. This is called tuberculoid since it resembles a granuloma such as is seen in tuberculosis. Patients with essentially no resistance to the organism develop lepromatous leprosy which is widespread throughout the body and produces symmetrical deficits due to the constant bloodborne dissemination of organisms. The organism has a predilection to involve peripheral nerve, making it almost unique among bacterial pathogens.[3] In addition, the host's immune response to the presence of the organisms can result in superimposed autoimmune phenomena called reactions. These occur in various forms and can add to the severity of the disease already present. Genetics obviously plays a key role in the determination of susceptibility in individual patients but this is not well understood. Various population groups seem to be relatively immune to this disease whereas other populations or even subpopulations may have very high incidences of leprosy.

Clinical features

The clinical features of leprosy include skin lesions and involvement of upper respiratory tract, peripheral nerves, anterior one third of the eye, and the testes. The disease spares internal organs primarily because they are at a higher temperature; this discourages the growth of leprosy bacilli, which reproduce best at a natural optimum of about 32° Centigrade.[4] In patients with the localized (tuberculoid) form, where some resistance to the disease is present, bacterial organisms tend to be few. There is a vigorous granulomatous response and the patient has one or at most a few skin lesions. Within these skin lesions, nerves are destroyed and the skin lesions are anesthetic (see Figure 183.1) For patients with little immunity to the organism, there is widespread dissemination of organisms. The organisms gain access to the cutaneous nerve endings and cause a gradual destruction of these elements in a temperature-linked pattern so that the coolest areas of the body are the first to be affected and, as the disease progresses, progressively warmer areas are affected (see Figures 183.2 and 183.3). Obviously, the facial promontories, the helices of the ears, the nose, the anterior third of the eyes, testes, and the skin of the extremities are coolest. Organisms rapidly proliferate in these areas. The upper respiratory tract is involved but not the lungs. Patients may have difficulty with nasal breathing and resort to mouth breathing which further increases the coolness of the oral cavity; therefore more proliferation of organisms occurs there. The high resistance form of leprosy, tuberculoid, tends to self-healing with or without treatment. The lower resistance form, lepromatous leprosy, virtually never heals in the absence of effective treatment. In between these two polar extremes is a zone where the patient's resistance to the organism varies from very slight resistance to more vigorous resistance. Such borderline patients can shift back and forth depending on external factors such as the presence of coexistent disease, aging, etc. The classification of leprosy includes high resistance paucibacillary disease, intermediate leprosy, in which the number of bacilli vary from a few to many, and lepromatous leprosy or multibacillary disease.

Diagnosis

Diagnostic criteria for leprosy consist most importantly of the physician considering the diagnosis. In the United States, there are about four thousand patients with leprosy, and worldwide the number is approximately ten million, so that the neurologist is likely to see leprosy much more commonly than some of the rare diseases that so much more is written about. The two diagnostic criteria on clinical examination that are most rewarding to look for are temperature-linked patterns of sensory loss and nerve trunk involvement, and the degree of anesthesia in skin lesions (Figures 183.1 to 183.3). Skin lesions tend to be anesthetic. An unusual form is polyneuritic leprosy, in which nerves are involved but there are few or no skin lesions.[5] These patients, usually in the borderline spectrum, have either mononeuritis multiplex or more rarely a symmetrical neuropathy which is temperature linked. At times, nerve biopsy is necessary to make the diagnosis. Definitive diagnosis in leprosy requires demonstration of organisms in skin or nerve biopsies, or in skin scrapings or nasal secretions. Biopsies can be taken virtually anywhere, from any skin lesion. The organisms are not as acid fast as *Mycobacterium tuberculosis* and can easily be decolorized unless sections are coated with a petroleum product (Fite stain). The organisms are also visible under electron microscopy and there is a specific antibody used for staining the organisms. Recently the entire genome of the leprosy bacillus has been described. There is very little evidence that neuroimaging is useful in the evaluation of leprosy patients. Occasionally, calcification of nerves occurs such as in the ulnar nerve at the elbow, usually the result of resolution of a nerve abscess which can occur in leprosy. However neuroimaging is not ordinarily necessary to make the diagnosis.

Neuropathology

The pathology of leprosy involves looking for acid-fast organisms in tissue sections and tissue smears, particularly where the organisms are found in nerves in the dermis or in nerve biopsies. When present in nerve biopsies, the organisms are almost invariably within Schwann cells rather than axons. Despite this, many of the nerve lesions in leprosy behave as axonal neuropathies. The differential diagnosis includes peripheral neuropathies of other causes; however, if the temperature-linked pattern of leprosy is looked for, the diagnosis can easily be made even in those

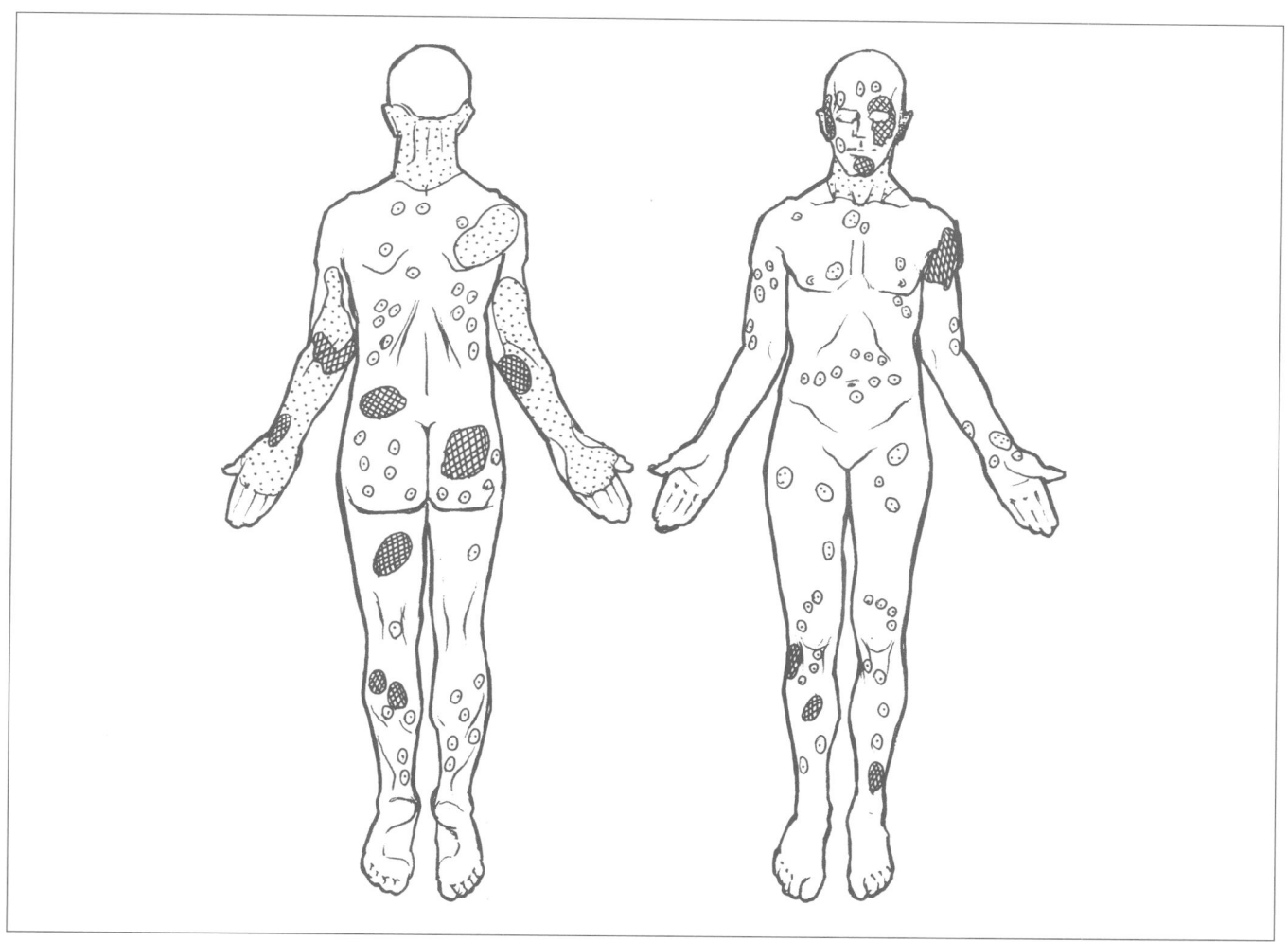

Figure 183.1 Sensory loss to pinprick in a patient with borderline leprosy. The sensory loss tends to be associated with skin lesions. Skin lesions generally occur in cooler areas.

From Sabin TD, Swift TR, Jacobson RR. Ch 74. *In:* Dyck PJ, Thomas PK, eds. Leprosy. Philadelphia: WB Saunders, 1993:1354–1379, with permission.

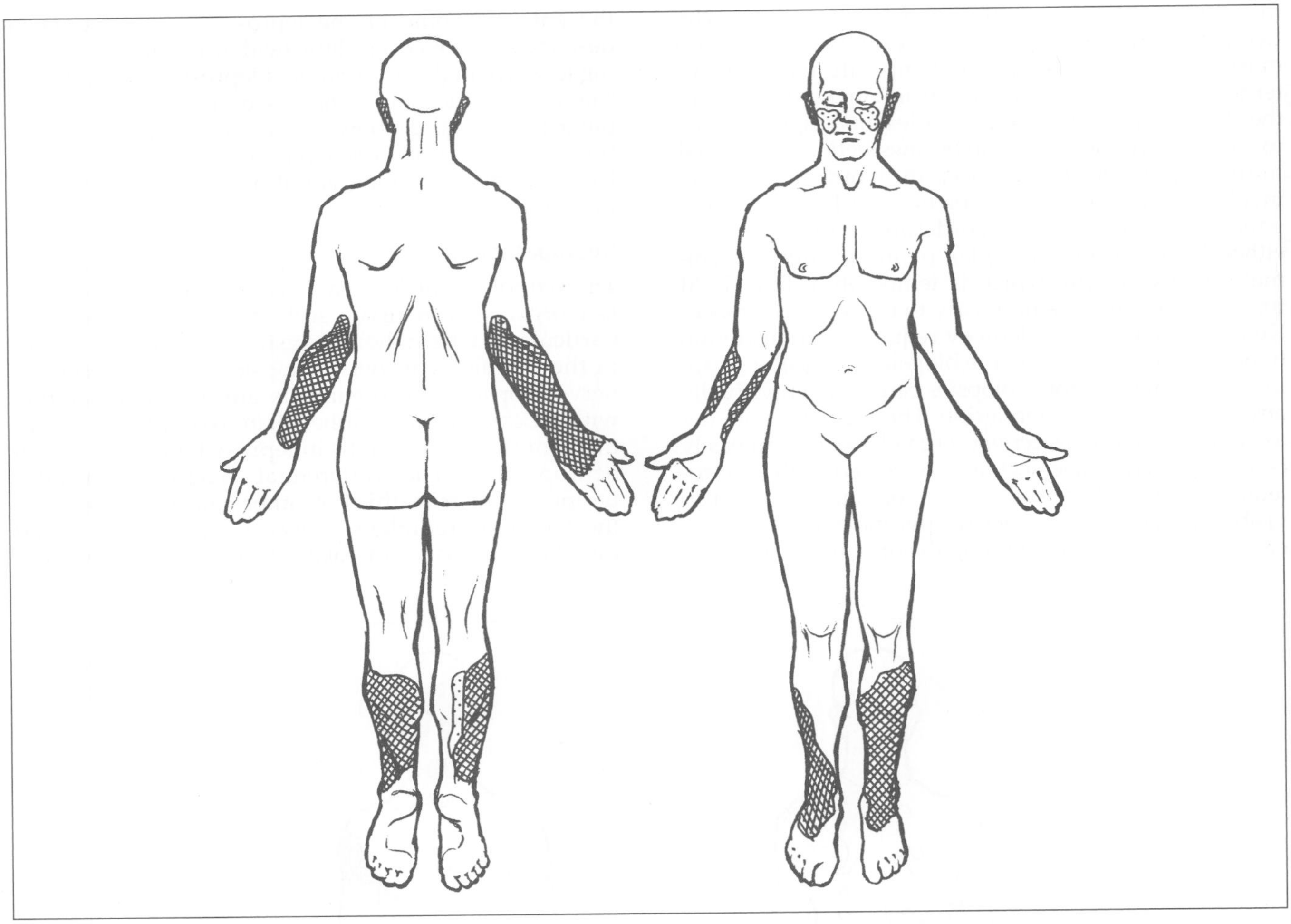

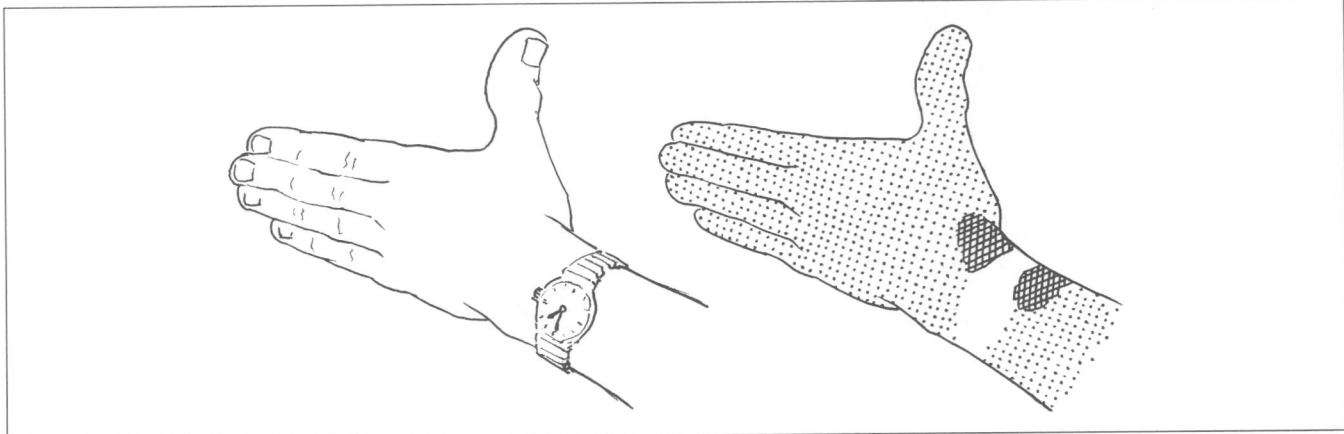

Figure 183.2   A map of sensory loss to pinprick in a patient with lepromatous leprosy. Note the differences between a temperature linked sensory loss and a distal symmetrical neuropathy. Leprosy involves the ears, the malar areas are involved, and there is sparing of the palms and soles. There is also more sensory loss in the extensor surfaces of the forearms than one would expect for the amount of sensory loss in the lower extremities.
     From Sabin TD, Swift TR, Jacobson RR. Ch 74. *In:* Dyck PJ, Thomas PK, eds. Leprosy. Philadelphia: WB Saunders, 1993:1354–1379, with permission.

Figure 183.3   Pinprick loss under a watchband, due to the warmer temperature at that site. This illustrates the thermosensitive growth rate of *M. leprae.* Sensory sparing has also been noted at the site of small cutaneous vascular malformations, and more sensory loss has been seen on the cooler hemiplegic side of the body in other cases of leprosy.
     Drawing by Andrew Swift.

cases where bacilli are no longer present because the disease has been treated or bacilli have been naturally eradicated from tuberculoid lesions. In tuberculoid leprosy where there is a skin lesion, simply testing for sensation over the area of the skin lesion shows sensory loss co-terminal with the skin lesion. At times, an enlarged nerve happens to course directly under a tuberculoid skin lesion.

Differential diagnosis

Most other polyneuropathies tend to produce a glove-stocking distribution of sensory loss, motor weakness and reflex loss. In leprosy, since the major impact of the disease is in the superficial skin which is cool, the deeper modalities are often retained such as the muscle stretch reflexes, vibratory and position sensation, whereas pain and temperature sensation and sweating are lost in the cool areas of the extremities, face and trunk. Very few polyneuropathies involve nerves so short that they could produce sensory loss or motor deficits on the face, but in leprosy these are quite common.[6] Mononeuritis multiplex due to vasculitis, etc., is always a consideration in leprosy since nerve trunk involvement occurs. However, in leprosy, the nerve trunks involved tend to be those in cool locations such as the ulnar nerve at the elbow, the median nerve just proximal to the wrist, the radial nerve at the elbow and the wrist, the peroneal nerve at the knee and at the ankle, the great auricular nerve, and the branches of the facial nerve on the face. These nerves may all be greatly enlarged.

Immune reactions

The management of leprosy requires an understanding of the inflammatory reactions that occur particularly as the disease is treated.[7] In high resistance paucibacillary cases such as tuberculoid and high resistance borderline leprosy, there is a cell-mediated process by which flaring of the lesion takes place, and sometimes additional skin and nerve damage or damage to the anterior third of the eye or testes can occur. In lepromatous leprosy a humoral and cell-mediated process called erythema nodosum leprosum occurs in which the presence of degraded mycobacterial antigen and antibody creates an inflammatory response associated with the infiltration of inflammatory cells, complement, and elevated levels of tumor necrosis factor and other cytotoxic cytokines. This reaction can be very severe and, in the days before effective treatment was available, could go on for months or years. The reaction is so severe that it causes additional damage to the anterior third of the eye, producing iritis, or damage to the nerves producing additional neuritis and further neurological deficits, and can produce painful orchitis. There are skin lesions that resemble erythema nodosum but they are much more extensive and more severe than any other disease producing erythema nodosum. Most of the conditions producing mononeuropathy multiplex involve some form of vasculitis and this is always in the differential diagnosis in patients with polyneuritic leprosy, where it may not be clear from

the beginning if the patient does have leprosy. Of course, the fact that a patient comes from a leprosy-endemic area should provide a clue to the physician.

Pharmacological treatment of leprosy
Antibacterial treatment

The treatment of leprosy has changed drastically in the last ten years and now most patients can be cured with drug therapy. Leprosy is a bacterial infection and, as a consequence, is treated with antibiotics. The first antibiotic to be used in the treatment of leprosy was dapsone, initiated at Carville, Louisiana, in 1940. To some extent, dapsone is still used; however, much more powerful antibiotics are used in addition. The currently used drugs are so effective that therapy does not have to be prolonged as much as in former years. The World Health Organization develops guidelines regarding therapy, the courses of which seem to get shorter every year.[8] A problem for developing countries, where budgets for public health may be small and case-finding is difficult, is that patients may not be treated even though effective antibiotics are available.

In modern times, leprosy does not have such dire consequences as in the pre-antibiotic era and it should be emphasized that with early diagnosis and effective treatment leprosy can be considered almost a trivial infection in most patients. The first order of business is to kill the bacilli. This is effectively accomplished with antibiotics, the exact amounts, combinations, and doses depending upon the nature of the host resistance. For tuberculoid leprosy, which has a tendency to self-healing, a single dose of three antibiotics is enough for cure. This includes rifamycin 600 mg, ofloxacin 400 mg and minocycline 100 mg. Lepromatous leprosy and borderline leprosy with numerous bacilli, both of which are called multibacillary leprosy are also treated with three antibiotics but these are continued for one year: dapsone 50 mg per day, rifamycin 600 mg monthly, and clofazimine 50 mg daily and 300 mg monthly.[2]

Treatment of immunological reactions

Erythema nodosum leprosum or reactions occurring in lepromatous and borderline lepromatous patients must be treated promptly if further disability and disfigurement are to be prevented.[9] Reactions in borderline tuberculoid and tuberculoid leprosy are treated with corticosteroids, for example prednisone in doses of 60 to 80 mg per day. This may need to be continued for varying periods of time depending on the severity of the reaction and the response to treatment. Erythema nodosum leprosum in patients with lepromatous leprosy may also respond to corticosteroids, but an even better drug is thalidomide, which is used in a dose of 300 to 400 mg per day. Thalidomide was originally used for sedation but it was serendipitously found to have very strong effects in erythema nodosum leprosum, where it reduces levels of tumor necrosis factor. Thalidomide causes severe fetal deformities and must never be used by women who are or may become pregnant; if women patients are to be treated, several methods of birth control must be employed as well as careful monitoring for pregnancy. Primary and secondary drug resistance, once feared to be a significant problem in leprosy, seems to be increasingly of less concern. A goal of the World Health Organization is the eradication of leprosy. It is unclear if the infection occurs in woodland animals such as armadillos which can then transmit the infection to humans. It is clear that the prevalence of leprosy tends to diminish as the standard of living goes up.

Treatment of insensitive acral parts

While the bacterial infection is cured, patients have existing nerve damage which does not seem to improve and which continues unchanged throughout the rest of life. Patients who continue to use their limbs without protective pain and temperature sensations will inevitably undergo progressive disabling deformities in the extremities, particularly fingers, toes, feet and hands.[10] While it is not true that digits actually "drop off" in leprosy, reabsorption of soft tissues and bone takes place as a result of repeated injuries to the extremities. Recurrent, often trivial appearing wounds, burns and infections occur over a period of years. A small break in the skin permits entry of common pathogens with development of infection in the fat pads, tendon sheaths and bones of the digits. Since even these infections fail to provoke the self-protective behaviors demanded by pain the process becomes ongoing and over a period of years the fingers are reabsorbed (mitten hands) and the feet are grossly foreshortened. Also, since the autonomic nerves are involved and there is no sweating, the skin becomes brittle and can crack in flexion creases in hands and feet, providing yet another portal of entry for secondary infection. Cigarette smoking is likely to cause "kissing" ulcers on the fingers. The reabsorption of the digits which results is essentially identical to that seen in hereditary sensory neuropathy, syringomyelia (hands only), or diabetic neuropathy. Prevention of absorption requires teamwork in the application of four general principles:

1. The patient must be educated regarding the perils of insensitive limbs. It is amazing how difficult it is to get even very bright patients to acknowledge this without the reinforcing stimulus of pain. The patient must inspect the hands and feet daily for wounds, signs of infection, or tissue stress. A mirror is used to check out the soles. The hands and feet must be hydrated and then the moisture sealed in with a suitable cream.
2. Application of skin moisturizers alone will not suffice because of the loss of sweating due to the autonomic nerve damage. The patient, ideally with the help of an occupational therapist, must learn which other routine activities are dangerous. Simply turning a key in a sticky lock or grasping the cover of a hot saucepan with too small a knob might cause further tissue damage.
3. The limbs must be protected from injury. Special

shoes with individually molded insoles to distribute the forces evenly over the soles may prevent trophic ulcers and loss of digits and eventually the loss of the insensitive feet. Custom-made shoes are very helpful. If there is no leprosy clinic in the area, a diabetic clinic can often provide the necessary care of the feet. The hands are more difficult to protect. Utensils can be modified. Large wooden handles on scissors, keys, cookware and other implements are highly effective.

4. Each wound on the insensitive limb must be treated in ways that simulate the factors which promote healing in the normal individual. There are no mysterious missing trophic substances which impede healing in neuropathic patients. If a wound or burn is treated so as to account for the lack of pain by careful splinting, extra padding and more frequent inspections for early signs of infection, then the injury will heal in the same time as in a normal patient.

The treatment of nerve damage

Nerve damage in leprosy can occur in three ways: first, directly from infiltration by bacilli; second, by the effects of reaction and other immune phenomena taking place in the nerves; and third, by chronic pressure and compression of enlarged nerves. This must be carefully evaluated in individual patients to see if nerve transfer is required or if other protective measures are needed for the nerves. Patients with leprosy are prone to blindness as a result of direct involvement of the anterior third of the eye by leprosy bacilli, by the occurrence of iritis, and by the effects of facial paralysis and insensitivity on the eye which may become scarred and secondarily infected. All these must be guarded against and careful attention must be given by an ophthalmologist.

In future, there might be a vaccine to prevent leprosy, allowing populations at risk to be vaccinated. There was some evidence that patients vaccinated with BCG to prevent tuberculosis had milder forms of leprosy but, at this time, there is no effective leprosy vaccine.[11]

References

1. World Health Organization. Progress towards leprosy elimination. Wkly Epidemiol Rec 1998;73:153–160
2. Jacobson RR, Krahenbuhl JL. Leprosy. Lancet 1999;253:655
3. Weinstein DE, Freedeman VH, Kaplan G. Molecular mechanism of nerve infection in leprosy. Trends Microbiol 1999;(5):185–186
4. Sabin TD. Temperature-linked sensory loss: a unique pattern in leprosy. Arch Neurol 1969;20:257
5. Uplelcar MW, Antia NH. Clinical and histopathological observations on pure neuritic leprosy. Indian J Lepr 1985;48:513
6. Monrad-Krohn GH. The Neurological Aspect of Leprosy. Christiana: Jacob Dybward, 1923
7. Becx-Bleumink M, Bertie D. Occurrence of reactions, their diagnosis and management in leprosy patients treated with multidrug therapy. Lepr Other Mycobact Dis 1992;60:173

8. WHO Expert Committee on Leprosy—World Health Organization. Tech Rep Serv 1998;874:1–43

9. Lockwood DNJ. The management of erythema nodosum leprosum: current and future options. Lepr Rev 1996;67:253–259

10. Brand PW. Deformity in leprosy. *In:* Cochrane RG, Davey TF, eds. Leprosy in Theory and Practice. 2nd ed. Baltimore: Williams and Wilkins, 1964:447

11. Karonga Prevention Trial Group. Randomized controlled trial of single BCG or combined BCG and killed *Mycobacterium leprae* vaccine for prevention of leprosy and tuberculosis in Malawi. Lancet 1996; 348:17–24

184 Peripheral Neuropathies in Chagas Disease

Amilton Antunes Barreira and Osvaldo JM Nascimento

Historical background, epidemiology and transmission

Carlos Chagas identified Chagas disease (CD) in 1909 in the northern region of Minas Gerais State, Brazil. Chagas found a flagellated parasite, which he named *Trypanosoma cruzi* (*T. cruzi*), in the posterior bowel of hematophagous insects. Chagas also found the parasite in the circulating blood of marmosets (*Callithrix penicillata*) and a girl with an acute febrile disease and generalized swollen lymph glands. He later described the acute and chronic forms of the disease as it develops, and the morphology and biology of the hematophagous insect and the parasite.[1] In 1935, Cecilio Romaña described the clinical aspect of the ocular entry door of the parasite that associates unilateral eye edema with regional adenitis and is termed the Romaña sign.[2]

CD is transmitted exclusively in the American hemisphere and has been described from the southern USA to southern Argentina. It is endemic in Latin America. The total number of people infected is about 18 000 000.[3,4] There are about 550 000 new cases and 50 000 deaths reported annually.[5] CD is associated with lack of hygiene and bad living conditions, and transmission mostly occurs in rural areas. In Brazil, the most populous Latin American country with 160 000 000 inhabitants, 6 400 000 people are infected. The number of new cases is diminishing, particularly in the Mercosur trading bloc countries. The complete interruption of vectorial and transfusional transmission in the hemisphere is forecast for the year 2010.[4] The number of infected people living in the USA is calculated to be between 500 000 and 675 000, if we extrapolate from Latin American data and assume that 7.4% are infected among immigrants from those regions to the USA. It is possible that Chagas disease is being underdiagnosed in the USA. The authors were not able to find reports of chagasic megacolon/megaesophagus or of somatic chagasic neuropathy occurring in the USA in recent years. These clinical forms occur in 3% and 10% of patients with Chagas disease, respectively.[6]

T. cruzi is a parasite with different forms and dimensions according to the stage of its life cycle. It is transmitted to man by triatomines. These insects bite vertebrates contaminated with trypomastigotes (circulating forms of *T. cruzi*) (Figure 184.1); the trypomastigotes then undergo morphological changes, multiply, and come to lie in the insect's posterior bowel. When the insect bites people, residual matter containing *T. cruzi* is deposited and penetrates the victim by openings on the skin or in the mucosa. Transmission by the transfusional[7] or transplacental routes,[1] through maternal milk, by laboratory accidents,[8] or during organ transplantation[9] is uncommon.

Pathology, pathogenesis and pathophysiology

Acute phase

After invading the blood stream, the parasites penetrate cells of practically all organs, most frequently striated muscle, heart and smooth muscle; Schwann cells and oligodendroglia and, less frequently, neurons, circulating phagocytes and others may also be infected. The *T. cruzi* aflagellate tissue form (amastigote) (Figure 184.2) multiplies in cycles of about six days, and the host cells suffer massive rupture, allowing the return of parasites to the blood stream as trypomastigotes. These reinfect other cells successively over the next 50 to 60 days, when parasitemia lessens and disappears.[1] In this phase, myocarditis occurs owing to a massive parasitic load in the heart muscle and to inflammatory infiltrates in which neutrophils predominate; this also occurs in other tissues. Meningoencephalitis occurs in a small percentage of patients. This is generally severe and the patient almost always dies. Eventually, trypomastigotes can be found in the cerebrospinal fluid (CSF) in the acute phase.[1,10,11] Chagas[1] refers to the

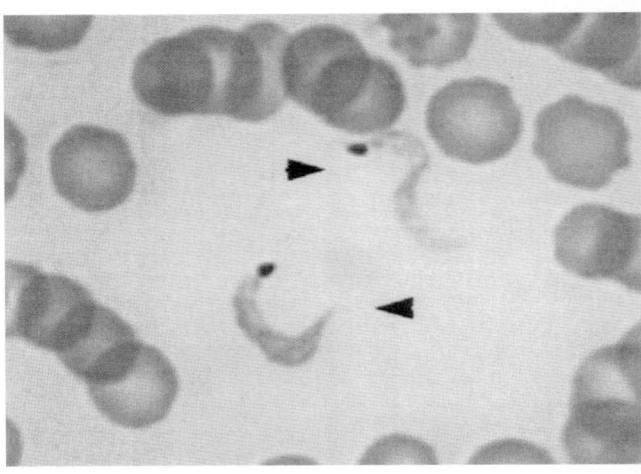

Figure 184.1 Circulating forms of *Trypanosoma cruzi* (trypomastigotes) ×1534. (See color plate section.)

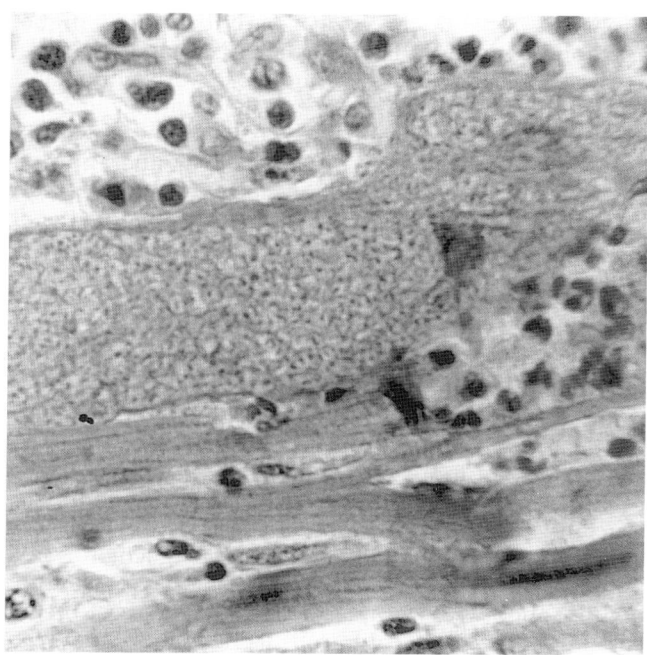

Figure 184.2 Amastigote nest in heart muscle fiber and adjacent inflammatory cells ×661.
Courtesy of Professor Marcos Antonio Rossi.

parasitism of striated muscle that correlates with electromyographic findings in the acute phase.[12,13] However, this is not sufficient to provoke clinical manifestations and is not found during the chronic phase. Peripheral nerves and spinal cord pathology have not been studied in the acute phase.

Indeterminate and chronic phases

After the acute phase, the indeterminate phase occurs. In this phase of the disease serology is always positive but parasitemia is uncommon. There is absence of symptoms and electrocardiogram (EKG), barium enema and esophagogram are normal. The pathogenesis and pathophysiology of the chronic phase are not completely understood. Most likely, the lesions or dysfunctional changes develop progressively during the indeterminate phase until they become symptomatic 20 to 30 years after contamination. Heart disease, with dilatation and cardiac hypertrophy,[14–16] mainly depends on the progressive multifocal, but eventually extensive, chronic infiltrate by lymphocytes and macrophages. However, these lesions are not necessarily associated with the few amastigote nests found in this phase. Inflammation advances during the indeterminate phase and is associated with progressive muscle heart fiber necrosis and substitution by fibrous tissue.[16–19] It is possible that the pathogenic hypothesis proposed below to explain the myocardiopathy might also, in part, explain the involvement of the digestive system's intrinsic innervation and the development of sensorimotor peripheral neuropathy. Antigenic epitopes that cause a cross-reaction between *T. cruzi* and myocardial pro-

teins have been identified, and these could be a stimulus for autoimmune responses by the host.[20] Abnormalities in cardiac microvasculature, described in animal models of *T. cruzi* infections, and demonstrated in cases of Chagas disease, could be responsible for perfusion deficiencies and would explain the EKG alterations observed.[18,21–23] Cardiac autonomic neuronal depopulation with significant nerve degeneration has been documented.[16,24–26] These lesions can progressively cause dilatation in all four chambers, with major functional effects on the right ventricle leading to congestive heart insufficiency, ventricular dysrhythmia and atrioventricular blockades.

Cardiovascular dysfunction secondary to the parasympathetic neuronal loss is considered to be asymptomatic, and presents with great variability on functional and pharmacological testing.[27–34] Neither arterial postprandial hypotension nor postural hypotension has been demonstrated in CD patients,[27,29–31] unlike that seen in cases of multiple system atrophy (MSA),[35] probably because there is preservation of the sympathetic innervation of the vessels in CD. This differs from MSA, in which the central sympathetic control is deranged.[36]

The main reason for gastrointestinal disturbances is the degeneration and loss of neurons from the parasympathetic intramural plexus. This neuronal loss occurs only in the acute phase.[16] The effects of denervation during the indeterminate phase would lead to the following functional and morphological events in the tract: hypermotility, hypertony, aperistalsis, dilatation, muscular hypertrophy, and reduction of the blood flow resulting in excessive hypertrophy, atony and massive dilatation. The pathophysiology of megaesophagus is similar to that of idiopathic achalasia of the inferior sphincter of the esophagus. This constitutes a functional obstacle to the passage of food, playing an important role in the genesis of megaesophagus.[37,38] A dysfunctional rectum resulting from denervation can also constitute a functional obstacle for the progression of the feces. As in the case of achalasia causing megaesophagus, this blockage plays an important role in the genesis of megacolon.[39]

In addition to theories about the pathogenesis of heart disease, there are different hypotheses to explain the loss of neurons. Chagas[40] and Köberle[16] hypothesized that an as yet unidentified neurotoxin could cause degeneration and neuronal loss. Antineuronal antibodies[41] or antibodies against Schwann cells,[42] both encountered in the circulating blood of CD patients, could play a role. It is not known, however, if they are a cause or an effect of the neuronal loss. The systemic injection of CD8 lymphocytes from Chagas-infected to naive mice[43] is associated with endoneural perivascular inflammatory infiltrates and lesions of neighboring fibers. In chronically infected mice, CD4 cells have been detected in the inflammatory infiltrates associated with parasite antigens in tissues, including the brain and sciatic nerves.[44,45] Macrophages could play a role in the pathogenesis of neuronal loss: in rats acutely infected with *T. cruzi*, the loss of neurons in the colon is prevented by daily intraperitoneal injections of Nωnitro L-arginine, an NO-synthase inhibitor.[46] Although this observation opens new perspectives for understanding experimental trypanosomiasis pathogenesis, the role of macrophages or lymphocytes in neuronal loss in patients with CD remains largely unknown.

Because there is no reduction of the amplitude or the conduction velocity, the denervation/reinnervation found at the electrophysiological examination in patients without peripheral polyneuropathy can be attributed to neuronal losses in the ventral horn, followed by axonal sprouting of the preserved axons to the adjacent denervated endplates.[47,48] This view is also supported by the muscle fiber type groupings found in CD muscle biopsies.[49] The sensory component of the discrete or subclinical CD sensorimotor neuropathy could be caused by neuronal loss in the dorsal root ganglia, or by minor lesions of the axons or myelin of the mixed nerves. In two sural nerve biopsies, a moderate reduction of myelinated fiber density was seen, with wallerian degeneration and segmental demyelination.[50] Five biopsies of CD patients, with chronic sensory polyneuropathy with perivascular inflammatory infiltration of mononuclear cells, have been registered.[51,52] These inflammatory infiltrates were not associated with wallerian degeneration or active demyelination. This differs from what occurs in mice infected with *T. cruzi* and is attributed to delayed-type hypersensitivity.[43,53] A mild, predominantly axonal neuropathy was seen in 45 samples of sural nerves from CD necropsies.[54] Thus, there is as yet no plausible explanation for CD neuropathies. They could be sequelae of the neuronal loss occurring during the acute phase of CD.

The HLA-A30 antigen seems to be related to susceptibility to CD, and HLA-DQB1*06 protects against the disease, regardless of the form of presentation, i.e. cardiac or digestive.[55] The relation of these HLA antigens to the somatic neuropathy has not been studied.

Clinical features

Acute phase

The acute phase of Chagas disease starts as a mild febrile and toxemic disease, associated with swollen lymph glands and generalized edema, hepatosplenomegaly, anorexia, nausea, vomiting and diarrhea and, eventually, meningoencephalitis. Clinically evident disease occurs in about 10% of infected patients and is more frequent in children. Mortality varies from 2% to 7%.[56] The most important cause of death in this phase is meningoencephalitis, followed by acute carditis. Pericarditis and myocarditis occur with dilatation of the four cardiac chambers and a significant augmentation in heart volume. There is no study documenting a clinical sensorimotor neuropathy in the acute phase of CD.

Chronic phase

Cardiomyopathy in the chronic phase can be silent, with exclusively regional electrocardiographic alterations. In general, the initial symptoms are fatigue, exertional dyspnea, tachycardia, dizziness, syncope, and thoracic pain due to ventricular dysrhythmia and atrioventricular blockades.[22,57] When cardiac insufficiency arises it is more indicative of systemic congestion than of left heart disease.[25] The liberation of intracardiac thrombi can provoke multiple organ infarction, including strokes.[58,59] The sudden deaths of CD patients may be due to parasympathetic dysfunction and/or to ventricular fibrillation and/or to complete atrioventricular block.[60]

CD patients can also develop swallowing disturbances. In endemic areas, 7% to 10% of patients can have esophageal motility disturbances.[61] The principal complaint of the patients is dysphagia that persists for life. Some patients present persistent dysphagia to solid foods. In more serious cases, food retention and regurgitation occur, with weight loss, odynophagia, eructation, coughing and hiccupping.[60] Although there are no precise data, the occurrence of megacolon is less often diagnosed than megaesophagus, apparently because there is no simple tool for diagnosis of megacolon. The main symptom is constipation that can progress, and, in a few patients, there may be impaction caused by a firm mass of stool or by a true fecaloma, associated with significant abdominal discomfort. At this stage, attacks of relapsing intestinal pseudo-obstruction can take place. More serious and less frequent complications are volvulus, fecaloma-associated stercoral ulceration, "overflow" diarrhea, and ischemic colitis.[61] Sensorimotor peripheral neuropathy, when it occurs, is minor and is seen in about 10% of patients with chronic disease. Hyporeflexia and paresthesia and hypoesthesia to heat and to pain occur; these can involve all four limbs, but more frequently the legs. There are no alterations in motor strength. One third of these patients do not have electromyographic (EMG) changes so the sensory loss could indicate a neuropathy[52] involving nerve fibers with a diameter of 7 μm or less, but there has been no evaluation of sensory loss by computer-assisted systems. It is not known if the CD neuropathy is progressive.

Diagnostic criteria and laboratory investigation

The diagnosis of dilated cardiopathy, as with those of megaesophagus, megacolon and acute meningoencephalitis, in patients living in endemic zones or in patients receiving blood transfusion from donors coming from those regions, requires the search for trypomastigotes in blood smears and the specific serological tests for CD. Motor neuropathy, sensory polyneuropathy and ischemic strokes without any known etiology in people from endemic areas also deserve serological investigation.

The serological tests are very specific for the disease. These include indirect immunofluorescence (human IgG anti-*T. cruzi*); hemagglutination (red blood cells coated with *T. cruzi* antigens that agglutinate when mixed with patients' serum); complement fixation and ELISA (identification of circulating antibodies against *T. cruzi*). The polymerase chain reaction (PCR), using the *T. cruzi* specific primers TCZ-1 and TCZ-2, seems be a more sensitive method for diagnosis of the disease.[62,63] Conduction disturbances, ventricular arrhythmias and altered Q waves suggesting areas of myocardial dysfunction are commonly registered by EKG. The association between right branch blockade and left anterior hemiblockade is very suggestive of CD myocardiopathy. Mural motility abnormalities and thrombi can be documented by echocardiography, ventriculography or by radionuclides.[60] In patients presenting with megaesophagus, barium esophagogram findings are the same as for idiopathic achalasia (Figure 184.3). Manometry and scintillography have the same sensitivity to detect the impaired motility of the CD esophagus.[64] Esophageal endoscopy is only useful for the elimination of other diagnostic possibilities, such as esophageal carcinoma.[65] The barium enema remains the best method for diagnosing megacolon[60] (Figure 184.4). EMG in the acute phase discloses subclinical neuromuscular dysfunction consistent with inflammatory myopathy, peripheral neuropathy and neuromuscular junction dysfunction.[12,13] These EMG alterations can occur singly or may be associated. Evidence of somatic acute denervation can have a transitory character or may be followed by findings of chronic denervation.[66] In the chronic phase, a reduced interference pattern is seen in proximal and distal

muscles and polyphasic or fragmented (some with high amplitude) potentials in others. Motor conduction studies can disclose a prolonged distal latency and/or a mild reduction of the conduction velocity (in general not less than 40 m/s) as with the sensory conduction velocities. One third of the patients present with a mild reduction in the amplitude of compound action motor potentials (CAMP) and sensory amplitude potentials (SAP). Coaxial needle examinations have revealed signs of chronic denervation, predominating in the distal muscles of the inferior limbs[67] or not, confirming previous studies.[47,48,66,68,69]

Differential diagnosis

The differential diagnosis of CD myocardiopathy must be made with rheumatoid cardiopathy, the myocardiopathy secondary to coronary disease and other chronic myocardiopathies borne in mind. This is particularly relevant when there is predominant involvement of the heart muscle in comparison with the involvement of somatic muscles in some muscular dystrophies, and to idiopathic cardiomyopathy. CD megaesophagus must be differentiated from achalasia of the esophagus. CD-associated megacolon must be differentiated from that seen in patients presenting

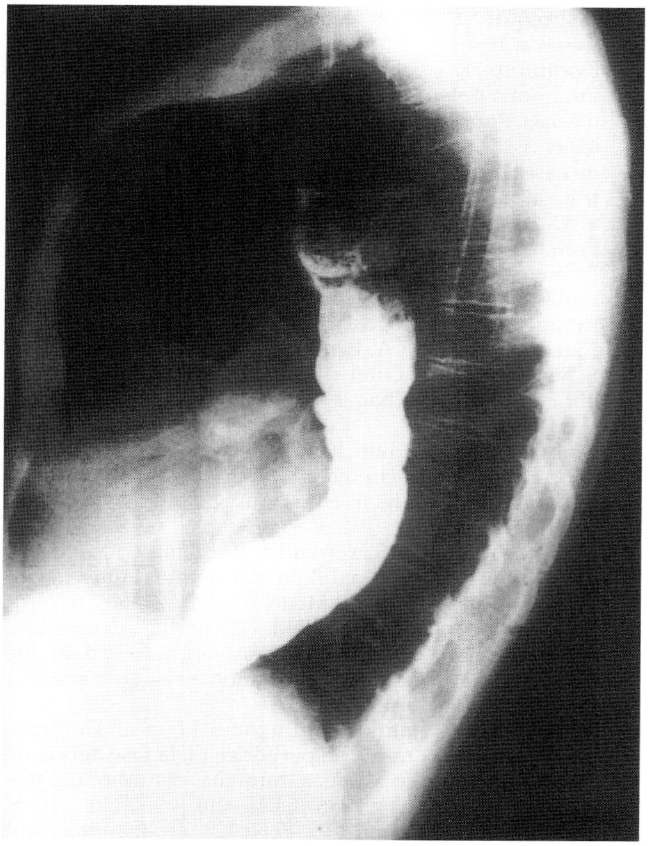

Figure 184.3 Chagasic megaesophagus.

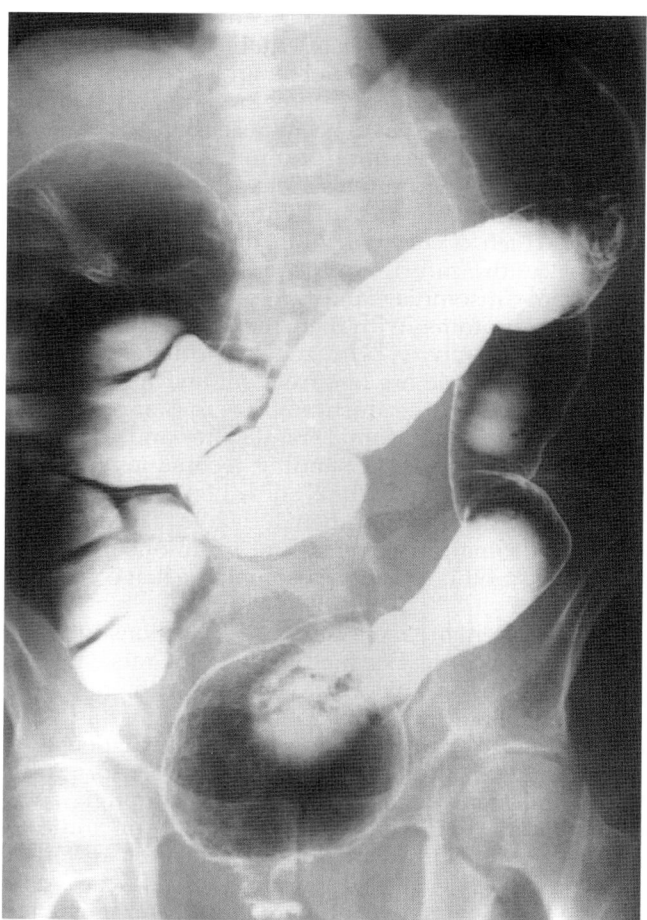

Figure 184.4 Chagasic megacolon.

with psychosis. It must also be distinguished from the megacolon of myxedema and from the megacolon associated with chronic lead intoxication. Mural thickening in patients with scleroderma or amyloidosis can also cause megacolon. Megacolon can also be secondary to the autonomic neuropathy of diabetes mellitus, and severe and long-lasting parkinsonism can be complicated by megacolon. In addition, complete chronic obstruction of the sigmoid colon or rectum and Hirschprung's disease (aganglionosis of distal bowel) can both cause megacolon. CD-related sensorimotor polyneuropathy must be differentiated from that seen in alcoholic and diabetic polyneuropathies. Although there is some overlap between regions endemic for CD and leprosy, it is easy to distinguish the two because leprosy presents as a predominantly sensory multineuropathy or an asymmetric polyneuropathy.

Treatment

There is no specific treatment for CD neuropathies. The parasiticide drugs used for treatment of CD in the acute phase are benznidazole and nifurtimox. Allopurinol or itraconazole can also be effective in treating patients with circulating parasites. One of the restrictions to the treatment with nifurtimox and benznidazole is the variety and intensity of collateral effects, of which the neurologist must be aware. Convulsive seizures, depression, disorientation, reduction of visual acuity, dyspnea, lumbar and precardial pain, psychic excitation, tachycardia, tremor and equilibrium disturbances have been described in patients exclusively treated with nifurtimox. Auditory hallucinations, fatigue and amnesia have been described in patients exclusively treated with benznidazole. Side effects, which occur with both drugs, but are more intense with nifurtimox, are nausea, vomiting, headache, insomnia and polyneuropathy. More intense symptoms with benznidazole are diarrhea and photosensitivity.[70] In general, collateral effects from benznidazole are less frequent and intense than those observed with nifurtimox. There is an increased frequency of chromosomal fragile sites and of micronuclei localized with G banding techniques in 1p31, 2p24, 3p14, 5q34, 6q25, 7q32, 8q24, 14q24, 16q23, Xp22 with nifurtimox, as with benznidazole. These are all in chromosomal areas related to proto-oncogenes or to specific points of chromosomal breakage in neoplasias.[71]

In dogs, benznidazole can produce lesions in cortical and subcortical structures.[72,73] In rats, it can produce arrest of spermatogenesis with complete depletion of germinative cells.[74] In rabbits, as with other nitroarene drugs, there is a high incidence of nonHodgkin lymphomas.[75] In humans, sensorimotor peripheral neuropathy can occur.[76] Although such effects seem to be species dependent or indicate greater susceptibility of some tissues of different animal species to the drug, in humans who have received a heart transplant there is a greater incidence of lymphomas with benznidazole. The collateral effects of both drugs are clearly more intense in adults than in children[77,78] and are dose dependent. The collateral effects of allopurinol are less frequent than those of nitroarenes and occur in about 14% of patients. They include a possible transitory polyneuropathy. Itraconazole does not cause collateral effects involving the nervous system.

Particular attention must be paid to the possibility of overlap between the peripheral neuropathy of CD cases and axonal benznidazole-related neuropathy[76] or nifurtimox- or amiodarone-induced neuropathies; amiodarone is used for the treatment of CD-induced mixed heart arrhythmias. Before starting treatment of CD with these drugs, it is reasonable to perform a neurological examination and EMG study to stage the neuropathy and to provide better further evaluation if overlapping neuropathies provoked by the drugs do occur.

References

1. Chagas C. Nova entidade mórbida do homem—Resumo geral dos estudos etiológicos e clínicos. Mem Inst Oswaldo Cruz 1911;3:219–275
2. Romanã C. Acerca de un síntoma inicial de valor para o diagnóstico de la forma aguda de la enfermedad de Chagas: la conjuntivitis ezquizotripanósica unilateral (hipótesis sobre puerta de entrada conjuntival de la enfermedad). Publicación da le MEPRA 1935;22:16–20
3. Moncayo A. Progress towards the elimination of transmission of Chagas disease in Latin America. World Health Stat Q 1997;50:195–198
4. Anonymous—World Health Organization: Life in the 21st century. A vision for all. The World Health Report, Geneva, 1998
5. Docampo R, Schmuñis GA. Sterol biosynthesis inhibitors: potential chemotherapeutics against Chagas' disease. Parasitol Today 1997;13:129–130
6. Milei J, Mautner B, Storino R, et al. Does Chagas' disease exist as an undiagnosed form of cardiomyopathy in the United States? Am Heart J 1992;123:1732–1735
7. Freitas JLP, Amato Neto V, Nussezveig V, et al. Primeiras verificações de transmissão acidental da moléstia de Chagas ao homem por transfusão de sangue. Rev Paul Med 1952;40:36–42
8. Mazza S, Montana A, Benítez C, et al. Transmission del Schiyzotrypanum cruzi al niño por leche de madre com enfermedad de Chagas. Publicación de la MEPRA 1936;28:41–46
9. Mocelin, AJ, Brandina L, Gordan PA, et al. Immunosuppression and circulating *Trypanosoma cruzi* in a kidney transplant recipient. Transplantation 1977;23(2):1–63
10. Hoff R, Teixeira RS, Carvalho JS, et al. *Trypanosoma cruzi* in the cerebrospinal fluid during the acute stage of Chagas disease. N Engl J Med 1978;298:604–605
11. Jardim E, Takayanagui OM. Chagasic meningoencephalitis with detection of *Trypanosoma cruzi* in the cerebrospinal fluid of an immunodepressed patient. J Trop Med Hyg 1994;97:367–370
12. Benavente OR, Patiñô OL, Lugones H, et al. Compromiso del sistema nervioso periférico en la fase aguda de la enfermedad de Chagas humana. Estudio electromiográfico. Medicina 1986;46:645–646
13. Benavente OR, Patiñô OL, Peña LB, et al. Motor unit involvement in human acute Chagas' disease. Arq Neuropsiquiatr 1989;47:283–286

14. Chagas C, Villela E. Forma cardíaca da tripanosomíase americana. Mem Inst Oswaldo Cruz 1922;14:5–61
15. Laranja FS, Dias E, Nobrega G, et al. Chagas' disease: a clinical, epidemiologic, and pathologic study. Circulation 1956;14:1035–1059
16. Köberle F. Chagas' disease and Chagas' syndrome: the pathology of American trypanosomiasis. Adv Parasitol 1968;6:63–116
17. Teixeira ARL, Teixeira L, Santos-Buch CA. The immunology of experimental Chagas' disease. IV. The production of lesions in rabbits similar to those of chronic Chagas' disease in man. Am J Pathol 1975; 80:163
18. Figueiredo F, Marin-Neto JA, Rossi MA. The evolution of experimental *Trypanosoma cruzi* cardiomyopathy in rabbits: further parasitological, morphological and functional studies. Int J Cardiol 1986;10:277
19. Rossi MA. Patterns of myocardial fibrosis in idiopathic cardiomyopathies and chronic Chagasic cardiopathy. Can J Cardiol 1991;7:287
20. Cunha-Neto EM, Gruber DA, Messias BZI, et al. Autoimmunity in Chagas' disease cardiopathy: biological relevance of a cardiac myosin-specific epitope cross-reactive to an immunodominant *Trypanosoma cruzi* antigen. Proc Natl Acad Sci 1995;92:3541–3545
21. Rossi MA. Microvascular changes as a cause of chronic cardiomyopathy in Chagas' disease. Am Heart J 1990;120:233–236
22. Marin-Neto JA, Marzullo P, Marcassa C. Myocardial perfusion defects in chronic Chagas' disease. Assessment with thallium-201 scintigraphy. Am J Cardiol 1992;69:780–784
23. Torres FW, Acquatella H, Condado J, et al. Coronary vascular reactivity is abnormal in patients with Chagas' heart disease. Am Heart J 1995;129:995–1001
24. Mott KE, Hagstrom JWC. The pathologic lesions of the cardiac autonomic nervous system in chronic Chagas' myocarditis. Circulation 1965;31:273–286
25. Prata A, Andrade A, Guimarães AC. Chagas' heart disease. *In:* Shaper AG, Hutt MSR, Fejfar Z, eds. Cardiovascular Disease in the Tropics. London: British Medical Association, 1974:264–281
26. Lopes ER, Tafuri WL. Involvement of the autonomic nervous system in Chagas' heart disease. Rev Soc Bras Med Trop 1983;16:206
27. Marin-Neto JA, Gallo L Jr, Manço JC, et al. Mechanisms of tachycardia on standing: studies in normal individual and in chronic Chagas' heart patients. Cardiovasc Res 1980;14:541–550
28. Marin-Neto JA, Maciel BC, Gallo L Jr, et al. Effect of parasympathetic impairment on the haemodynamic response to handgrip in Chagas's heart disease. Br Heart J 1986;55:204–210
29. Marin-Neto JA, Bromberg-Marin G, Pazin-Filho A, et al. Cardiac autonomic impairment and myocardial damage involving the right ventricle are independent phenomena in Chagas' disease. Int J Cardiol 1998;65:261–269
30. Amorim DS, Manço JC, Gallo L Jr, et al. Chagas' heart disease as an experimental model for studies of cardiac autonomic function in man. Mayo Clin Proc 1982;57:48–60
31. Amorim DS, Marin-Neto JA. Functional alterations of the autonomic nervous system in Chagas' heart disease. Rev Paul Med 1995;113(2):772–784
32. Gallo L Jr, Morelo-Filho JL, Maciel BC, et al. Functional evaluation of sympathetic and parasympathetic system in Chagas' disease using dynamic exercise. Cardiovasc Res 1987;21:922–927
33. Sousa ACS, Marin-Neto JA, Maciel BC, et al. Cardiac parasympathetic impairment in gastrointestinal Chagas' disease. Lancet 1987;8539:985
34. Emdin M, Marin-Neto JA, Carpeggiani C, et al. Heart rate variability and cardiac denervation in Chagas' disease. J Amb Monit 1992;5(2–3):251–257
35. Hoeldtke RD. Postprandial hypotension. *In:* Low PA, ed. Clinical Autonomic Disorders. Philadelphia: Lippincott-Raven, 1997:737–746
36. Low PA, Bannister RG. Multiple system atrophy and pure autonomic failure. *In:* Low PA, ed. Clinical Autonomic Disorders. Philadelphia: Lippincott-Raven, 1997:555–575
37. Raizman RE, Rezende JM, Neva FA. A clinical trial with pre- and post-treatment manometry comparing pneumatic dilation with bouginage for treatment of Chagas' megaesophagus. Am J Gastroenterol 1980;74:405–409
38. Bettarello A, Pinotti HW. Oesophageal involvement in Chagas' disease. Clin Gastroenterol 1976;5:103–117
39. Cutait DE, Cutait R. Surgery of Chagasic megacolon. World J Surg 1991;15:188–191
40. Chagas C. Processos patogênicos da trypanosomiase americana. Mem Inst Oswaldo Cruz 1916;8:5–39
41. Santos RR, Marquez JO,. Von Gal Furtado CC, et al. Antibodies against neurons in chronic Chagas' disease. Trop Parasitol 1979;30:19–23
42. Khoury EL, Ritacco V, Cosasio PM, et al. Circulating antibodies to peripheral nerve in American trypanosomiasis (Chagas' disease). Clin Exp Immunol 1979;36:8–15
43. Said G, Joskovicz M, Barreira AA, et al. Neuropathy associated with experimental Chagas' disease. Ann Neurol 1985;18:676–683
44. Ben Younes-Chennoufi AB, Said G, Durand A, et al. Cellular immunity to *Trypanosoma cruzi* is mediated by helper T cells (CD4+). Trans R Soc Trop Med Hyg 1988;82:44–47
45. Ben Younes-Chennoufi AB, Hontebeyrie-Joskowicz M, Tricottet V, et al. Persistence of *Trypanosoma cruzi* antigens in the inflammatory lesions of chronically infected mice. Trans R Soc Trop Med Hyg 1988;82:39–43
46. Garcia SB, Paula JS, Givannetti GS, et al. Nitric oxide is involved in the intestinal denervation observed in the acute phase of experimental *Trypanosoma cruzi* infection. Mem Inst Oswaldo Cruz 1996;91(S):43–44
47. Pagano MA, Basso S, Aristimuso GG, et al. Electromyographical findings in human chronic Chagas' disease. Arq Neuropsiquiatr 1978;36:316–318
48. Sanz OP, Aristimuso GG, Ratusnu AF, et al. An electrophysiological investigation of skeletal muscle in human chronic Chagas' disease. Arq Neuropsiquiatr 1978;36:319–326,
49. Taratuto A, Fumo T, Pagano MA, et al. Histological and histochemical changes of the skeletal muscle in human chronic Chagas' disease. Arq Neuropsiquiatr 1978;36:327–331
50. Sica REP. Compromiso del sistema nervioso. *In:* Storino R, Milei J, eds. Enfermidad de Chagas. Buenos Aires: Mosby, 1994:303–320
51. Nascimento OJM, De Freitas MRG, Chimelli LC. Polyneuropathie axonale dans la maladie de Chagas. Rev Neurol (Paris) 1991;147(10):679–681
52. Nascimento OJM, Freitas MRG, Escada TM, et al. Chronic inflammatory polyneuropathy in Chagas' disease. Neurology 1995;45(Suppl):A416
53. Barreira AA, Said G, Krettli AU. Multifocal demyelinative lesions of peripheral nerves in experimental

chronic Chagas' disease. Tran R Soc Trop Med Hyg 1981;75(5):751

54. Chimelli LMC, Schieber MB. The peripheral nerve in Chagas' disease. Morphological findings in the sural nerve of 45 autopsied cases. Brain Pathol 1994;4:560

55. Deghaide NH, Dantas RO, Donadi EA. HLA class I and II profiles of patients presenting with Chagas' disease. Dig Dis Sci 1998;43(2):246–252

56. Rey L. *Trypanosoma cruzi* e Doença de Chagas. *In:* A Doença. Parasitologia. 2nd ed. Rio de Janeiro: Guanabara-Koogan, 1991;138–152

57. Marin-Neto JA, Simões MV, Ayres-Neto EM, et al. Studies of the coronary circulation in Chagas' heart disease. Rev Paul Med 1995;113:826–834

58. Nussenzveig I. Acidentes vasculares cerebrais embólicos na cardiopatia chagásica crônica. Arq Neuropsiquiatr 1953;11:386–402

59. Braga JC, Labrunie A, Villaça F, et al. Tromboembolismo em portadores de cardiopatia chagásica crônica. Rev Soc Card Est São Paulo 1994;4(2):187–191

60. Barreira A, Marin-Neto JA, Oliveira RB. Chagas' Disease. Ch 14. *In:* Appendzeller O, ed. Handbook of Neurology, Amsterdam: Elsevier, 2000;75(31):385–405

61. Rezende JM, Rassi A. Manifestações digestivas na fase aguda da doença de Chagas. *In:* Raia AA, ed. Manifestações digestivas da moléstia de Chagas. São Paulo: Sarvier, 1983;97–107

62. Moser DR, Kirchhoff LV, Donelson JE. Detection of *Trypanosoma cruzi* by DNA amplification using the polymerase chain reaction. J Clin Microbiol 1989; 27(7):1477–1482

63. Kirchhoff LV, Votava JR, Ochs DE, et al. Comparison of PCR and microscopic methods for detecting *Trypanosoma cruzi*. J Clin Microbiol 1996;34(5):1171–1175

64. Oliveira RB, Castillo T, Meneghelli UG, et al. Chagas' disease as a model for the identification of small bowel motor disorders. Gastroenterology 1995;108:A592

65. Rezende JM, Rosa H, Vaz MGM, et al. Endoscopia no megaesôfago. Estudo prospectivo de 600 casos. Arq Gastroenterol 1985;22:53–62

66. DeFaria CR, Melo-Sousa SE, Rassi A. Evidências eletromiográficas de desnervação motora em pacientes na fase crônica da doença de Chagas. Rev Goiania Med 1977;23:125–127

67. Genovese O, Ballario C, Storino R, et al. Clinical manifestations of peripheral nervous system involvement in human chronic Chagas disease. Arq Neuropsiquiat 1996;54(2):190–196,

68. DeFaria CR, Rezende JM, Rassi A. Desnervação periférica nas diferentes formas clínicas da doença de Chagas. Arq Neuropsiquiatr 1988;46:225–237

69. Sanz OP, Sica REP, Baso S, et al. Compromiso del sistema nervioso periferico en la enfermedad de Chagas crônica. Medicina 1980;40:231–233

70. Storino R, Gallerano R, Sosa R. Tratamiento antiparasitario específico. *In:* Storino R, Milei J, eds. Enfermidad de Chagas. Buenos Aires: Mosby, 1994;28:557–568

71. Moya PR, Trombotto GT. Enfermedad de Chagas: efecto clastogenico de nifurtimox y benznidazol em niños. Medicina (B Aires) 1988;48:487–491

72. Flores-Vieira CLL, Barreira AA. Experimental benznidazole encephalopathy: I—Clinical-neurological alterations. J Neurol Sci 1997;150:3–11

73. Flores-Vieira CLL, Chimelli L, Fernandes RMF, et al. Experimental benznidazole encephalopathy: II—Electroencephalographic and morphological alterations. J Neurol Sci 1997;150:13–25

74. Flores-Viera CLLF, Lamano-Carvalho TL, Favaretto ALV, et al. Testes alterations in pubertal benznidazole-treated rats. Braz J Med Biol Res 1989;22:695–698

75. Teixeira ARL, Córdoba JC, Maior IS, et al. Chagas' disease: lymphoma growth in rabbits treated with benznidazole. Am J Trop Med Hyg 1990;42(3):146–158

76. Faria CR, Souza SEM, Rassi A. Polineuropatia periférica induzida por benzonidazol no tratamento da doença de Chagas. Arq Neuropsiquiatr 1986;44:125–129

77. Andrade ALSS, Zicker F, Oliveira RM, et al. Randomised trial of efficacy of benznidazole in treatment of early *Trypanosoma cruzi* infection. Lancet 1996;348: 1407–1413

78. Estani SS, Segura EL, Ruiz AM, et al. Efficacy of chemotherapy with benznidazole in children in the indeterminate phase of Chagas' disease. Am J Trop Med Hyg 1998;59(4):526–529

185 Late Effects of Polio

Anthony J Windebank

Polio epidemics occurred regularly in developed countries during the first half of the twentieth century. Most cases occurred in children in the late summer. Poliovirus is an enterovirus spread by the oral route. The prodromal illness with fever, headache, arthralgia, vomiting, and diarrhea lasted for three or four days. About half of the patients did not have paralytic sequelae. In the other half, paralysis began as the febrile illness was subsiding. Severe back and limb pain, headache, and meningismus developed, accompanied by severe and disabling muscle spasms. Paralysis of individual muscles came on rapidly over days and typically reached a maximum within one week. The virus specifically targeted motor neurons, causing cell death. Any muscle innervated by bulbar or spinal nerves could be affected, although extraocular muscles were spared. Encephalitis occurred in a small proportion of patients and usually resolved within a few days without residua. Paralysis gradually improved over months to years. Recovery depended on collateral sprouting and reinnervation of muscles by surviving motor axons. Residual weakness was permanent in about 50% of survivors. The acute mortality of 10% to 20% was usually due to severe encephalitis or to involvement of respiratory and bulbar muscles. Residual weakness was managed by physical therapy, bracing, and orthopedic procedures to transfer tendons or to stabilize joints. The illness was virtually eliminated from the developed world by immunization programs that began in the mid-1950s. The World Health Organization predicts that global eradication will be accomplished by 2005.

Although the acute disease is now extremely rare, there are 200 000 survivors in the United States with residual weakness.[1] In a population-based study,[2] the mean age, in 1987, of patients with previous paralytic polio was 50 years; the acute illness occurred on average at age 12 years. This population is now 60 to 80 years old. A high incidence of muscle and joint pain, fatigue, and increasing weakness has raised concern about late progression of neurological impairment.[3–5] Population-based studies have demonstrated that neuromuscular function is generally stable in polio survivors.[2,6] There is, however, a significant incidence of joint and muscle pain, which has often been explained by local degenerative joint disease or findings similar to those in fibromyalgia.[6,7] Late progressive muscle weakness occurs in a very small proportion of patients.[4,8,9] It is characterized by focal and very slowly progressive weakness in muscles that were affected by the original disease. Late progression of weakness in patients with non-

paralytic polio probably does not occur. The relationship between polio and amyotrophic lateral sclerosis has been investigated extensively. Antecedent polio does not appear to increase the risk of the development of amyotrophic lateral sclerosis.[9–13]

Treatment of symptoms in a patient with previous polio should be directed by the results of a careful clinical history and examination. History of an illness compatible with acute polio can be obtained from the patient or relatives. In the aging population of polio survivors, other disorders should be identified and treated independently. Degenerative joint disease should be evaluated and treated as for patients without a history of polio. If joint replacement is contemplated, preoperative evaluation of muscle and joint mechanics can guide postoperative physical therapy. Polio survivors with significant residual weakness are prone to pressure injury of nerves because of crutches, braces, and altered anatomy caused by chronic muscle weakness. Muscle and joint pain respond well to physical approaches, with particular attention to gait mechanics or orthotics. The psychological effect of reintroducing braces to a person who put energy into becoming independent must be managed sensitively. Fibromyalgia-like symptoms respond to treatment approaches used in patients without a history of polio.[14] Energy conservation principles benefit fatigue. Pain that does not respond to physical approaches may be helped by nonsteroidal anti-inflammatory agents, cyclooxygenase inhibitors, or tricyclic agents. After careful evaluation, all patients benefit from reassurance that most symptoms have benign underlying causes.

References

1. Feller BA. Prevalence of selected impairments, United States, 1977. Vital and Health Statistics. Series 10, Data from the National Health Survey; no. 134. United States Department of Health and Human Services, Public Health Service, Office of Health Research Statistics, and Technology, National Center for Health Statistics. DHHS Publication No. (PHS) 81–1562, Washington, DC, 1981:15
2. Windebank AJ, Litchy WJ, Daube JR, et al. Late effects of paralytic poliomyelitis in Olmsted County, Minnesota. Neurology 1991;41:501–507
3. Brooke M, Stolov W, Shillam L, Kelly B. The importance of symptom pattern in evaluating post-polio neuromuscular changes. Birth Defects Orig Artic Ser 1987; 23:49–53
4. Dalakas MC, Elder G, Hallett M, et al. A long-term follow-up study of patients with post-poliomyelitis neuromuscular symptoms. N Engl J Med 1986;314: 959–963

5. Halstead LS, Rossi CD. Post-polio syndrome: clinical experience with 132 consecutive outpatients. Birth Defects Orig Artic Ser 1987;23:13–26

6. Windebank AJ, Litchy WJ, Daube JR, Iverson RA. Lack of progression of neurologic deficit in survivors of paralytic polio: a 5-year prospective population-based study. Neurology 1996;46:80–84

7. Trojan DA, Cashman NR. Fibromyalgia is common in a postpoliomyelitis clinic. Arch Neurol 1995;52:620–624

8. Dalakas MC. New neuromuscular symptoms in patients with old poliomyelitis: a three-year follow-up study. Eur Neurol 1986;25:381–387

9. Swanson NR, Fox SA, Mastaglia FL. Search for persistent infection with poliovirus or other enteroviruses in amyotrophic lateral sclerosis-motor neurone disease. Neuromuscul Disord 1995;5:457–465

10. Armon C, Daube JR, Windebank AJ, Kurland LT. How frequently does classic amyotrophic lateral sclerosis develop in survivors of poliomyelitis? Neurology 1990; 40:172–174

11. Brown RH Jr, Weiner HL. The relationship between poliovirus and amyotrophic lateral sclerosis. *In:* Rose FC, ed. Research Progress in Motor Neurone Disease. London: Pitman, 1984:349–359

12. Codd MB, Mulder DW, Kurland LT, et al. Poliomyelitis in Rochester, Minnesota, 1935–1955. Epidemiology and long-term sequelae: a preliminary report. *In:* Halstead LS, Wiechers DO, eds. Late Effects of Poliomyelitis. Miami: Symposia Foundation, 1985:121–134

13. Mulder DW, Rosenbaum RA, Layton DD Jr. Late progression of poliomyelitis or forme fruste amyotrophic lateral sclerosis? Mayo Clin Proc 1972;47:756–761

14. Thompson JM. Tension myalgia as a diagnosis at the Mayo Clinic and its relationship to fibrositis, fibromyalgia, and myofascial pain syndrome. Mayo Clin Proc 1990;65:1237–1248

186 Diabetic Polyneuropathy

Peter J Dyck and Robert A Rizza

Overview

Diabetic neuropathy is not a single entity but has various presentations presumably because of different underlying mechanisms, natural histories, and treatments. Diabetic neuropathy may be categorized as a generalized disorder, diabetic sensorimotor polyneuropathy, or simply diabetic polyneuropathy (DPN). Further categorization includes asymmetric focal or multifocal varieties, that is, lumbosacral radiculoplexus neuropathy, thoracic radiculoneuropathy, diabetic cervical radiculoplexus neuropathy, median neuropathy at the wrist, ulnar neuropathy at the elbow, cranial neuropathy, and autonomic neuropathy.

Early descriptions of diabetic neuritis were published by Marchal de Calvi[1] and Rollo.[2] Loss of knee reflexes was noted by Marinian[3] and Buzzard.[4] The similarity of the clinical findings to those in tabes dorsalis caused Althaus[5] to term some of these disorders *pseudotabes diabetica*. Leyden[6] described three varieties of neuritis: 1) hyperesthetic or neuralgic (painful), 2) paralytic (motor), and 3) ataxic. Pavy[7] emphasized the occurrence of spontaneous pains in the lower limbs especially at night. Rundles[8] noted autonomic involvement in DPN.

Evidence is strong that among diabetic patients the complications of polyneuropathy, retinopathy, and nephropathy are associated.[9,10] Chronic hyperglycemia appears to be the main risk factor for DPN.[11] Average glycosylated hemoglobin levels, duration of diabetes mellitus (DM), age at onset of DM, and type of DM appear to be the most important risk covariates for severity of DPN. Chronic hyperglycemia appears not to be as important a factor in multifocal neuropathies; other mechanisms, notably immune derangement, may be implicated.

Epidemiology

Epidemiological studies can be classified as early descriptions of symptomatic cases, reviews of series of patients with symptomatic diabetic neuropathy, and retrospective or prospective population-based studies of patients with DM. In the last category, Dyck et al.[10] assessed the prevalence and severity (by stages and continuous measures of severity) of varieties of diabetic neuropathies in a prospective cross-sectional and longitudinal study. The survey was based on a prospective assessment of approximately 40% of the patients with diagnosed DM in Rochester, Minn. Coded medical diagnoses were available both for persons agreeing to participate and for those who did not participate, and thus, it was possible to determine whether the patients studied were representative of the diabetic population. At least for patients younger than 70 years, comorbidity was not significantly different for participants and nonparticipants. Therefore, for patients younger than 70 years, by the criterion of comorbidity, the group studied was representative of diabetic patients in Rochester. For patients 70 years or older, the frequency of stroke, heart attack, and other serious illnesses was higher in the group that was not studied. Diabetic patients in Rochester are mainly of northern European extraction, and therefore, the population may not be representative of Native American people, African American people, or Asian American people.

On the prevalence date (January 1, 1986), almost two-thirds of diabetic patients in Rochester had findings of neuropathy, of which the commonest variety (48%) was DPN.[10] Approximately 13% of the patients with DPN had symptoms of polyneuropathy and an even smaller percentage (about 4%) had stage N2b (≥50% weakness of ankle dorsiflexor muscles) (Figure 186.1). The frequency of DPN increased with the duration of DM (Figure 186.2). Univariate analysis generated a list of risk factors associated with severity of DPN. Multivariate analysis, however, indicated that markers of microvessel disease (stage of retinopathy or 24-hour proteinuria), chronic hyperglycemia exposure (glycosylated hemoglobin × duration of DM), and type of DM were the main risk factors for DPN.[11] That chronic hyperglycemia exposure is a major risk factor for DPN also comes from controlled clinical trials discussed in subsequent sections of this chapter.

Etiology, pathophysiology, and pathogenesis

Strong evidence indicates that chronic hyperglycemia is involved in the pathogenesis of DPN. Less clear is the mechanism by which chronic hyperglycemia causes nerve injury. Does hyperglycemia directly cause nerve damage, or does it do so through intermediate steps, e.g., by damaging microvessels? Chronic hyperglycemia is associated with various metabolic alterations of lipids,[12–15] alcohol sugars,[16–21] and *myo*-inositol.[22–24] The glucose, sorbitol, and fructose content of nerves is increased, and *myo*-inositol is decreased in the nerves of animals with untreated experimental diabetes. A statistically significant increase of glucose and fructose levels has also been shown in biopsy specimens of human nerve (Figure 186.3). We found a significant association between fiber loss and severity of increased sorbitol (Figure 186.4). Aldehyde reductase inhibitors, however, have not been as effective in inhibiting or improving neuropathy as

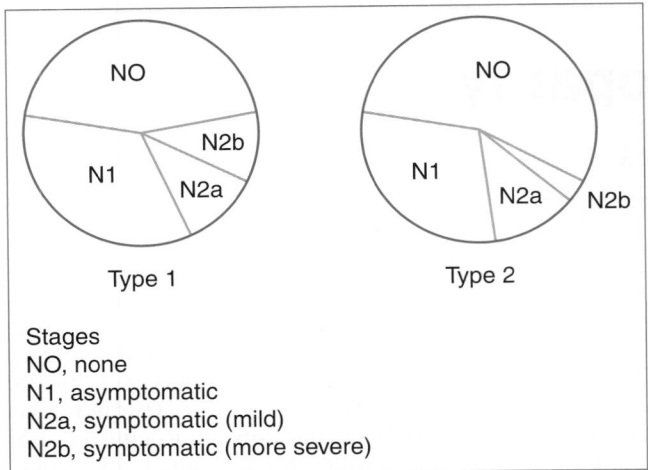

Figure 186.1 In the Rochester Diabetic Neuropathy Study, a cross-sectional and longitudinal community study of patients with diabetes mellitus (DM), mainly of northern European extraction, almost two-thirds of patients had varieties of neuropathy, and diabetic polyneuropathy (DPN) occurred in approximately 50% of the cohort. The figure shows the staged severity of DPN in type 1 (insulin-dependent [IDDM]) and type 2 (non–insulin-dependent [NIDDM]) patients. Whereas DPN occurred in about 50% of patients, stage 2b (impairment sufficient to cause ≥50% weakness of ankle dorsiflexor muscles) occurred in 6% of type 1 patients but in only 1% of type 2 patients. (From Dyck et al.[10] By permission of Lippincott Williams & Wilkins.)

had been hoped.[25] Another putative mechanism is *myo*-inositol deficiency. Although the concentration of *myo*-inositol is decreased in nerves of animals with untreated experimental diabetes, such a decrease has not been demonstrated in conventionally treated diabetic subjects.[26] Also, dietary supplementation with

myo-inositol has been disappointing.[27,28] Another putative metabolic abnormality is the formation of advanced glycation end products (AGE).[29] If AGE could be prevented, perhaps diabetic complications would also be prevented or delayed. Others have postulated an abnormality of phospholipids underlying some functional alterations of nerves.[12–15] Oxidative stress and nitric oxide accumulations have also been considered.[30]

An alternative (to direct injury of nerve fibers or Schwann cells) view is that chronic hyperglycemia or its metabolic counterparts damage microvessels, and their dysfunction affects nerve fibers. Some evidence indicates that chronic hyperglycemia is associated with an alteration of microvessel function and structure and that this alteration may lead to nerve fiber degeneration.[31] Degeneration of pericytes (the cells that form the layer next to endothelial cells of microvessels) and reduplication of basement membranes are typical early morphological changes in diabetic polyneuropathy. The role of pericytes in microvessel well-being is not completely understood. Pericytes may play a role in maintenance of the blood-nerve barrier.

Genetics

Genetic factors are implicated in the development of both type 1 and type 2 DM, but whether they are involved in the different varieties of diabetic neuropathies remains unproved. Since genetic factors regulate various aspects of cellular function and biochemical processes, it is conceivable (and perhaps likely) that they are also implicated in various diabetic neuropathies.

Clinical features

DPN usually begins insidiously with asymptomatic dysfunction of peripheral nerves. In a normative population, an equal percentage of persons is

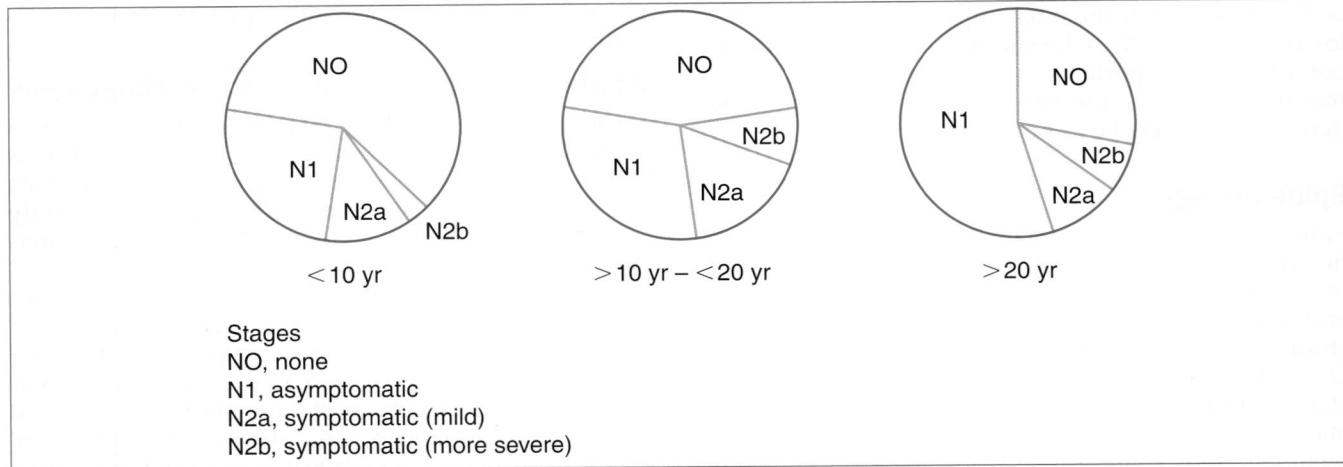

Figure 186.2 Staged severity of diabetic polyneuropathy (DPN) and duration of diabetes mellitus (DM). With increasing duration of DM, the percentage of patients with neuropathy increases: at less than 10 years, about one-third are affected; between 10 and 20 years, slightly more than one-half are affected; and more than 20 years, more than two-thirds are affected. Likewise, the spectrum of staged severity changes with duration of DM. (From Dyck et al.[10] By permission of Lippincott Williams & Wilkins.)

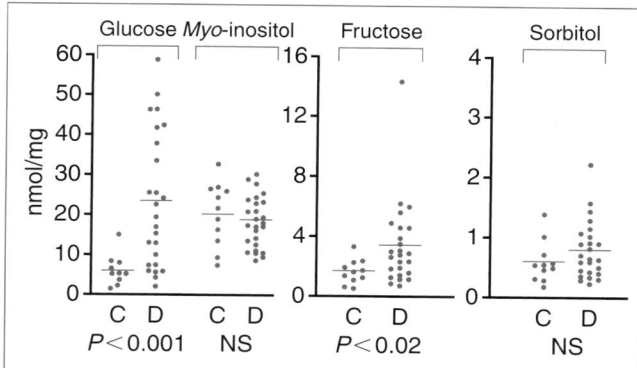

Figure 186.3 Sural nerve glucose, *myo*-inositol, fructose, and sorbitol levels in control subjects (C) and patients with diabetes (D). Bars represent means ±2 SD. Whereas glucose, fructose, and sorbitol are increased in the nerves of diabetic patients, *myo*-inositol is not decreased. (From Dyck et al.[26] By permission of the Massachusetts Medical Society.)

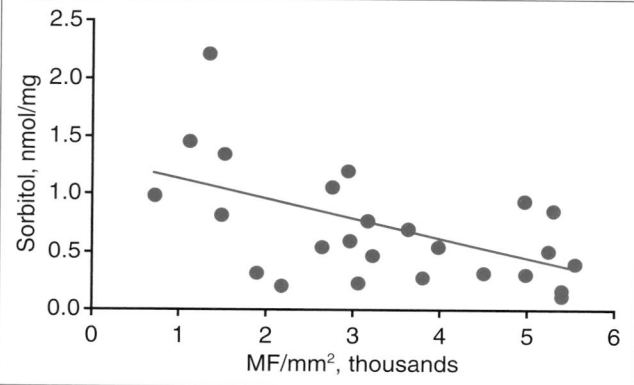

Figure 186.4 Relation of nerve sorbitol level to myelinated fiber (MF) density in sural nerves from 25 patients with diabetes mellitus. The linear regression line was fitted by the method of least squares. The slope is statistically significant ($P = 0.003$). This observation suggests that there may be an association between polyol increase and myelinated fiber decrease (diabetic polyneuropathy). (From Dyck et al.[26] By permission of the Massachusetts Medical Society.)

≥99th percentile for vibration detection threshold. Concurrent with the appearance of abnormal test results, or thereafter, clinical signs develop. These include decrease or loss of ankle reflexes and decrease or loss of vibration sensation of the great toes. With more severe involvement, patients develop variable loss of sensation in the toes, feet, and distal legs; decreased abnormality of muscle stretch reflexes; and autonomic abnormalities and weakness of small foot and ankle dorsiflexor muscles.

The rate and degree of abnormality development vary from patient to patient, presumably depending on applicable risk factors and unknown other factors. Neuropathic symptoms may occur with any degree of severity of neuropathy. Often, symptoms develop only after onset of functional abnormalities and mild clinical impairments. Two kinds of symptoms develop: those caused by hypofunction and those attributable to hyperfunction. Symptoms relating to neural hypofunction include loss of tactile or other mechanoreceptor sensation, sensory ataxia, loss of thermal and pain sensation, autonomic impairment such as impotence, gastroparesis, sudomotor loss, and muscle weakness and atrophy. Symptoms that relate to neural hyperfunction include prickling, a feeling of

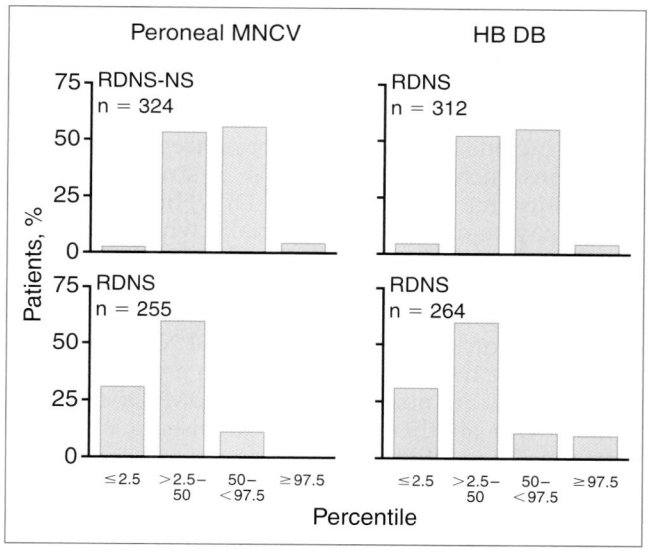

Figure 186.5 The percentage of Rochester Diabetic Neuropathy Study normal subject cohort (RDNS-NS) with peroneal motor nerve conduction velocity (MNCV) or heart beat responses to deep breathing (HB DB) values ≤2.5th, >2.5th to 50th, 50th to <97.5th, and ≥97.5th percentiles. Beneath it are the values for the RDNS patient cohort. Both peroneal MNCV and HB DB have a higher percentage of patients in the >2.5th to 50th percentile than in the 50th to <97.5th percentile. This altered distribution from normal indicates that a shift toward abnormality occurs before the values become unequivocally abnormal (≤2.5th percentile). This result has important implications. First, a subtle abnormality must already be present for some of the patients with "normal values"; and second, a change in a percentile or normal deviate value, even when it occurs in the normal range, may indicate abnormal function. (Data from Dyck et al.[32])

expected to have nerve conduction, vibration detection threshold, and heart pulse response to deep breathing values between the 2.5th and 50th and the 50th and 97.5th percentiles, but this distribution was not found in the Rochester Diabetic Neuropathy Study cohort. In patients with DM without overt neuropathy, considerably more than 50% had values on the abnormal side of the 50th percentile[32] (Figure 186.5). This implies a dysfunction of nerve fibers before the development of overt polyneuropathy.

The first evidence of polyneuropathy is an abnormality evident on functional test results (nerve conduction, vibration detection threshold, or heart pulse with deep breathing), for example, ≤1st or ≤2.5th percentile for conduction velocity or ≥97.5th or

tightness and various pains (e.g., lancinating, surges, burning, freezing, constricting, deep ache). Tenderness on compression of muscles (pressure myalgia) or cramps of the calf may also occur.

Criteria for the diagnosis of DPN are as follows:

1. The patient has DM by American Diabetes Association criteria (two fasting plasma glucose measurements ≥ 126 mg/dL).
2. DM has caused prolonged chronic hyperglycemia. In patients with type 2 DM, the prolonged DM may have been undetected for a long time.
3. The patient has predominantly distal, symmetrical sensory polyneuropathy of the lower limbs.
4. Other causes of neurological disease and sensorimotor polyneuropathy and other varieties of diabetic neuropathy have been excluded as a cause of the polyneuropathy, for example, a broad group of neurological disorders causing sensory symptoms in feet and legs and varieties of diabetic neuropathy other than DPN.
5. Patients usually have some evidence of diabetic retinopathy, nephropathy, or both. Mild degrees of retinopathy can be recognized best by an ophthalmologist with the patient's pupils dilated. A 24-hour urine microalbumin estimation or findings on various renal clearance tests may indicate mild degrees of nephropathy. For more severe involvement, plasma creatinine levels are useful.

The first four criteria should be fulfilled before making the diagnosis of DPN, although not all experts include criterion 2. The presence of the clinical conditions included in criterion 5 strengthens the probability that the diagnosis is DPN, but mild alterations may be overlooked, especially when pupils are not dilated and an ophthalmologist does not perform the examination. Also, use of these criteria may prevent recognition of another, perhaps treatable neurological disorder masquerading as DPN. Perhaps 5% to 10% of the neurological findings in a cohort of diabetic patients are not attributable to DM. Of course, a patient with another neurological disease may also have coexisting DPN.

Quantitating severity of DPN

There are two approaches to quantitate severity of DPN—first is staging or composite scoring of clinical impairment and second, test results.

Staging of DPN may be performed with or without administration of nerve tests, but use of standard clinical instruments and nerve tests improves the accuracy of staging. The clinical nerve tests are the Neuropathy Impairment Score (NIS, which has subscores for lower limbs [NIS LL] and for motor, sensory, and other components); quantitative sensation tests (for vibration, cooling, and heat-pain thresholds); and nerve conduction and quantitative autonomic tests. A combination of nerve conduction, quantitative sensation, and quantitative autonomic tests in the neurological examination improves staging. The staging criteria are given in Table 186.1.

Alternatively, severity of DPN can be expressed as a continuous composite score of points.[33] The procedure to do this is outlined in Table 186.2 This approach has several advantages. First, it permits combining clinical impairments of several kinds and test results and weighs the different components in a standard approach to derive an overall continuous score of severity. Second, it permits the user to set a level of abnormality that may vary with the purpose for which it is to be used, for example, 95th, 97.5th, or 99th percentile. Third, it provides a broad range of abnormalities.

Sensory symptoms and impairments can be divided into two types—large-diameter and small-diameter fiber involvement. There may be hyperfunction or hypofunction in each type. With hypofunction of large sensory fibers, patients may have difficulty recognizing the texture and shape of objects by feel and have sensory ataxia. Hyperfunction of large sensory fibers is not recognizable. Hyperfunction of small sensory fibers may be implicated in the various kinds of pain experienced by patients with DPN. Hypofunction is associated with loss of protective sensation and autonomic dysfunction. Small-fiber sensory loss is obviously a factor in the development of plantar ulcers and Charcot joints. Autonomic nerve fiber dysfunction may be involved in gastroparesis, night diarrhea, rectal and urinary incontinence, sexual impotence, and sudomotor abnormality. Vascular dysfunction may also be involved in the dysfunctions listed above.

Treatment

The emphasis in treatment must first be on prevention of DPN rather than on amelioration of impairments and relief of symptoms. Because the microvascular complications of DM appear to relate most closely to chronic hyperglycemia, the emphasis of treatment must be on trying to achieve near euglycemia from the time of onset of DM.[34] This may be difficult, particularly when DM begins at a young age. Furthermore, low levels of hyperglycemia produce no symptoms and therefore are often ignored by the patient. The risk of hypoglycemia increases as euglycemia is approached. Frequent glucose monitoring is inconvenient, and careful adherence to a structured diet and exercise program is challenging.

Therefore, it is desirable to modulate the adverse metabolic consequences related to chronic hyperglycemia. Conceptually, the metabolic derangement induced by chronic hyperglycemia could be normalized to prevent the complications of retinopathy, neuropathy, and nephropathy. It is still not known, however, whether such normalization of metabolic abnormalities does in fact prevent the deleterious effects of hyperglycemia. Oral supplementation with *myo*-inositol in dosages of 1 gm/d or 3 gm/d does not appear to be efficacious. Administration of aldehyde reductase inhibitors to treat experimental diabetes appears to have beneficial effects on nerve conduction velocity, but they have shown little if any benefit in human studies. Perhaps improved aldehyde reductase inhibitors may be more effective. Similarly, the effec-

Table 186.1   Staging of diabetic polyneuropathy*

Stage	Description	Criteria
N0	No DPN	Test† or clinical‡ Minimal criteria for DPN not fulfilled
N1a	Asymptomatic DPN	No neuropathy symptoms Minimal criteria for DPN fulfilled NIS < 2 points
N1b	Asymptomatic DPN	No neuropathy symptoms Minimal criteria for DPN fulfilled NIS ≥ 2 points
N2a	Symptomatic DPN (mild)	Polyneuropathy symptoms Minimal criteria for neuropathy fulfilled Weakness of ankle dorsiflexion less than 50% bilaterally
N2b	Symptomatic DPN	Polyneuropathy symptoms Minimal criteria for neuropathy fulfilled Weakness of ankle dorsiflexion greater than 50% bilaterally
N3	Disabling DPN	As described in reference 10.

DPN, diabetic polyneuropathy; NIS, Neuropathy Impairment Score.
*As described by Dyck et al.[10]
†Test (minimal) criteria for DPN:
For nerve conduction studies, abnormality (≤1st or ≥99th, or ≤2.5th or ≥97.5th percentile depending on which tail is abnormal and the degree of specificity desired and due to DPN) of at least one attribute of nerve conduction in two separate nerves.
For pulse variation deep breathing (P-DB), abnormality (≤1st or ≤2.5th percentile) of P-DB.
For quantitative sensation tests, vibration detection threshold, cooling detection threshold, or heat-pain 5 at or above the 97.5th percentile.
‡Clinical criteria for DPN:
Unequivocal decrease of ankle reflexes, vibration detection threshold of great toes, or both due to DPN. The decrease should be unequivocally greater than can be accounted for by age, sex, height, and weight. Absence of ankle reflexes is not abnormal when patients are 65 years or older.
Composite score of clinical, test, and combined clinical and test results:
The normal deviates of a group of predetermined tests (e.g., seven, all abnormalities expressed in the upper tail of the distribution) are summed, divided by the number of results needed to provide valid measure (e.g., motor conduction velocity and distal latency cannot be measured when the compound muscle action potential is 0), and the quotient is multiplied by the original number of tests (e.g., seven). A defined level, e.g., at or above the 97.5th percentile, may be used as the minimal criterion for DPN.
No symptoms of polyneuropathy attributable to DPN:
These include symptoms of weakness, sensory symptoms related to hypofunction or hyperfunction (neuropathic-positive sensory symptoms), and autonomic symptoms.

Table 186.2   Calculation of the continuous composite score of DPN severity

Calculate the NIS (LL) + 7 tests (items 17–24, 28–29, and 34–37 of NIS) (normal deviate).
Sum individual scores of the NIS (LL).
Summate normal deviate* for percentile abnormality† of the five attributes of NC of lower limb (peroneal nerve [CMAP, MNCV, and MNDL], tibial nerve [MNDL], and sural [S SNAP]), of VDT, and of HB DB.
Divide by the number of attributes with obtainable values.‡
Multiply by 7 (the number of attributes) and add this number to the global score.

CMAP, compound muscle action potential; DPN, diabetic polyneuropathy; HB DB, heart beat responses to deep breathing; MNCV, motor nerve conduction velocity; MNDL, motor nerve distal latency; NC, nerve conduction; NIS, Neuropathy Impairment Score; NIS (LL), Neuropathy Impairment Score (Lower Limbs); S SNAP, sural nerve action potential; VDT, vibration detection threshold.
*Express all percentile values so that abnormality appears in the upper end of the distribution.
†Express the normal deviate for each percentile value. For tests or NC attributes that are abnormal at low percentile values (e.g., HB DB, NC velocities, and amplitudes), express values as occurring at the high end of the distribution (e.g., 25th becomes 75th percentile, 60th becomes 40th percentile, and 4th becomes 96th percentile).
‡MNCV and MNDL cannot be estimated when CMAP is 0.

tiveness of agents to inhibit glycation of proteins has yet to be demonstrated. Dietary supplementation with an enriched source of the fatty acid linolenic acid (e.g., evening primrose oil) has shown a promising effect, but larger controlled trials are needed. Antioxidants such as vitamin E and alpha-lipoic acid have been tried. In Germany, alpha-lipoic acid, administered intravenously, has been prescribed extensively to treat painful neuropathy, and it was effective in one double-blind trial.[35] Further studies are in progress.

References

1. de Calvi M. Recherches sur les Accidents Diabetiques. Paris, 1864

2. Rollo J. Cases of Diabetes Mellitus. London, 1798

3. Marinian. Contribuzione-allo-studio clinico deiriflessi tendinei. Rivista Clinica di Bologna, 1884

4. Buzzard F. Illustrations of some less known forms of peripheral neuritis, especially alcoholic monoplegia and diabetic neuritis. Br Med J 1890;1:1419

5. Althaus J. On sclerosis of the spinal cord, including locomotor ataxy, spastic spinal paralysis and other system diseases of the spinal cord: their pathology, symptoms, diagnosis, and treatment. London: Green & Company, 1885

6. Leyden E. Die Entzundung der peripheren Nerven. Deut Militar Zeitsch 1887;17:49–100

7. Pavy FW. On diabetic neuritis. Lancet 1904;2:17

8. Rundles RW. Diabetic neuropathy: general review with report of 125 cases. Medicine (Baltimore) 1945;24:111–121

9. Fagerberg S-E. Diabetic neuropathy. A clinical and histological study on the significance of vascular affections. Acta Med Scand 1959;164:1–99

10. Dyck PJ, Kratz KM, Karnes JL, et al. The prevalence by staged severity of various types of diabetic neuropathy, retinopathy, and nephropathy in a population-based cohort: The Rochester Diabetic Neuropathy Study. Neurology 1993;43:817–824

11. Dyck PJ, Davies JL, Wilson DM, et al. Risk factors for severity of diabetic polyneuropathy. Intensive longitudinal assessment of the Rochester Diabetic Neuropathy Study cohort. Diabetes Care 1999;22:1479–1486

12. Randall LO. Changes in lipid composition of nerves from arteriosclerotic and diabetic subjects. J Biol Chem 1938;125:723–728

13. Brown MJ, Iwamori M, Kishimoto Y, et al. Nerve lipid abnormalities in human diabetic neuropathy: a correlative study. Ann Neurol 1979;5:245–252

14. Eliasson SG, Hughes AH. Cholesterol and fatty acid synthesis in diabetic nerve and spinal cord. Neurology 1960;10:143–147

15. Natarajan V, Yao JK, Dyck PJ, Schmid HHO. Early stimulation of phosphatidylcholine biosynthesis during Wallerian degeneration of rat sciatic nerve. J Neurochem 1982;38:1419–1428

16. Brownlee M, Vlassara H, Cerami A. Nonenzymatic glycosylation and the pathogenesis of diabetic complications. Ann Intern Med 1984;101:527–537

17. Pirie A, van Heyningen R. The effect of diabetes on the content of sorbitol, glucose, fructose and inositol in the human lens. Exp Eye Res 1964;3:124–131

18. Kinoshita JH. Cataracts in galactosemia. Invest Ophthalmol 1965;4:786–799

19. Gabbay KH, O'Sullivan JB. The sorbitol pathway: enzyme location and content in normal and diabetic nerve and cord. Diabetes 1968;17:239–243

20. Gabbay KH, Merola LO, Field RA. Sorbitol pathway: presence in nerve and cord with substrate accumulation in diabetes. Science 1966;151:209–210

21. Ward JD, Baker RWP, David BH. Effect of blood sugar control on the accumulation of sorbitol and fructose in nervous tissue. Diabetes 1972;21:1173–1178

22. Daughaday WH, Larner J, Houghton E. The renal excretion of inositol in normal and diabetic human beings. J Clin Invest 1954;33:326–332

23. Clements RS, Reynertson R. Myoinositol metabolism in diabetes mellitus—effect of insulin treatment. Diabetes 1977;26:215–221

24. Greene DA, De Jesus PV Jr, Winegrad AI. Effects of insulin and dietary myoinositol on impaired peripheral motor nerve conduction velocity in acute streptozotocin diabetes. J Clin Invest 1975;55:1326–1336

25. Tomlinson DR. Role of aldose reductase inhibitors in the treatment of diabetic polyneuropathy. In: Dyck PJ, Thomas PK, eds. Diabetic Neuropathy, 2nd ed. Philadelphia: WB Saunders Company, 1999:330–340

26. Dyck PJ, Zimmerman BR, Vilen TH, et al. Nerve glucose, fructose, sorbitol, *myo*-inositol, and fiber degeneration and regeneration in diabetic neuropathy. N Engl J Med 1988;319:542–548

27. Gregersen G, Bertelsen B, Harbo H, et al. Oral supplementation of myoinositol: effects on peripheral nerve function in human diabetics and on the concentration in plasma, erythrocytes, urine and muscle tissue in human diabetics and normals. Acta Neurol Scand 1983;67:164–172

28. Gregersen G, Borsting H, Theil P, Servo C. Myoinositol and function of peripheral nerves in human diabetics: a controlled clinical trial. Acta Neurol Scand 1978;58:241–248

29. Brownlee M. Advanced glycation end products and diabetic peripheral neuropathy. In: Dyck PJ, Thomas PK, eds. Diabetic Neuropathy, 2nd ed. Philadelphia: WB Saunders Company, 1999:353–358

30. Low PA, Nickander KK, Scionti L. Role of hypoxia, oxidative stress, and excitatory neurotoxins in diabetic neuropathy. In: Dyck PJ, Thomas PK, eds. Diabetic Neuropathy, 2nd ed. Philadelphia: WB Saunders Company, 1999:317–329

31. Giannini C, Dyck PJ. Pathologic alterations in human diabetic polyneuropathy. In: Dyck PJ, Thomas PK, eds. Diabetic Neuropathy, 2nd ed. Philadelphia: WB Saunders Company, 1999:279–295

32. Dyck PJ, Dyck PJB, Velosa JA, et al. Patterns of quantitative sensation testing of hypoesthesia and hyperalgesia are predictive of diabetic polyneuropathy: a study of three cohorts. Diabetes Care 2000;23:510–517

33. Dyck PJ, Milton LJ, O'Brien PC, Service FJ. Approaches to improve epidemiological studies of diabetic neuropathy: insights from the Rochester Diabetic Neuropathy Study. Diabetes 1997;46:S5–S8

34. Schade D, Santiago J, Skyler J, et al. Intensive Insulin Therapy. Amsterdam: Excerpta Medica, 1983

35. Ziegler D, Hanefeld M, Ruhnau KJ, et al. Treatment of symptomatic diabetic peripheral neuropathy with the anti-oxidant alpha-lipoic acid. A 3-week multicenter randomized controlled trial (ALADIN Study). Diabetologia 1995;38:1425–1433

This work was supported in part from grants received from the National Institute of Neurologic Disorders and Stroke (NS36797).

Acknowledgments: We gratefully acknowledge the help of JaNean K Engelstad and Mary Lou Hunziker in the preparation of this chapter.

187 Diabetic Radiculoplexus Neuropathies

P James B Dyck

Overview

Since the 19th century, some physicians have known that diabetic neuropathy may be of more than one kind. Leyden[1] divided the neuropathies of diabetes mellitus into "paralytic," "hyperalgesic," and "ataxic." Mulder et al.[2] divided them into "mononeuropathies" and "polyneuropathies," and Asbury[3] distinguished proximal and distal neuropathies. Thomas and Tomlinson[4] classified diabetic neuropathies into "symmetrical," "multifocal," and "mixed polyneuropathies." Taylor and Dyck[5] have used patterns and putative causes as a basis for classification.

The diabetic radiculoplexus neuropathies discussed in this chapter may have a common immunopathological basis. They may be separated into lumbosacral, thoracic, and cervical varieties. The first variety, "diabetic lumbosacral radiculoplexus neuropathy" (DLSRPN),[6] has several names, including "diabetic motor neuropathy,"[1,7] "diabetic amyotrophy,"[8,9] "Bruns-Garland syndrome,"[10,11] "proximal diabetic neuropathy,"[3,12] "diabetic polyradiculopathy,"[13] "diabetic femoral" or "femoral-sciatic neuropathy,"[14,15] "diabetic mononeuritis multiplex,"[16,17] and "diabetic lumbosacral plexus neuropathy."[18] The many names for the same disorder illustrate that various opinions have been held about the underlying pathological mechanisms. The second variety of diabetic radiculoplexus neuropathy is "thoracic radiculoneuropathy," also called "truncal radiculopathy."[19,20] The third variety is "diabetic cervical radiculoplexus neuropathy."[6] It is not clear that cranial neuropathies should be included with diabetic radiculoplexus neuropathy; although in our experience, patients who have one variety of radiculoplexus neuropathy often eventually develop other varieties, including cranial neuropathy (e.g., third-nerve palsy).

Much remains to be learned about diabetic radiculoplexus neuropathies, but the multifocal distribution of lesions in roots, segmental nerves, plexuses, and nerves is known from clinical, electromyographic (EMG), and histopathological study of nerves, at least for DLSRPN.[6] Historically, some cases of DLSRPN were attributed to ischemia (rapid onset, asymmetrical findings)[16,17] and others to metabolic derangement (slow onset, symmetrical findings).[10] In the only case studied postmortem,[16,17] the course was rapid and asymmetrical, with evidence of ischemic injury and an occluded vessel in the obturator nerve. It was unclear whether these subtypes of DLSRPN were separate disease entities or extremes of a continuum.[3] Similarly, there has been disagreement about the role of inflammation. Early investigators[16,17] interpreted inflammatory infiltrates as reactive, whereas more recent ones have thought that some cases were due to vasculitis.[21,22] Our group has found evidence that DLSRPN is a single entity and the ischemic damage is from microvasculitis, which causes both axonal degeneration and segmental demyelination.[6]

Clinical features

Typically, DLSRPN develops in mid or late life in patients with type 2 diabetes mellitus. Symptomatic onset usually begins discretely, and patients often can recall the particular day the symptoms began. This is quite different from diabetic polyneuropathy, which begins insidiously. The typical features are pain, weakness, and paresthesia. The pain usually is of several types—sharp lancinating pain, hurting or deep aching pain, burning pain, and contact allodynia (pain with mild tactile stimuli) are all common and severe. The process begins asymmetrically (usually unilaterally) in the thigh, leg, or buttock. If it begins focally in one of these segments, it usually spreads to unaffected segments of the same side and then to the contralateral side. In our series, the syndrome began unilaterally in 29 of 33 patients and became bilateral in 32.[6] Also, both proximal and distal involvement are common.

Whereas pain may be the most prominent symptom initially, weakness becomes the most severe symptom later. The weakness of DLSRPN is not trivial and half of the patients in our series were wheelchair-dependent at some time during their illness.[6] This often is an incapacitating disorder because the pain and weakness may persist for weeks, months, or even years. With time, the disorder tends to improve spontaneously and, in many cases, almost complete recovery ensues after months to years; however, in our experience, many patients have some degree of residual weakness or pain. Many patients require hospital admission because of the severity of the symptoms and the need for narcotic medications.

Thoracic radiculoneuropathy begins with a band-like pain extending from the back or side of the body to the abdomen or chest. The pain often is associated with a feeling of tightness and "asleep" or "prickling" numbness. Allodynia is common; patients complain that contact with their clothing or belts is painful. The symptoms are usually localized to the abdominal or chest wall. Sometimes, weakness can be recognized by the flaccid outpouching of the abdomen in the region of weak muscles or by EMG findings of paraspinal denervation of affected segmental levels. This disorder is very similar to herpes zoster infection except that a cutaneous eruption does not occur.

In diabetic cervical radiculoplexus neuropathy, the

pain, weakness, and numbness are in the distribution of a portion, if not the entire, brachial plexus. From the clinical and EMG examination, one infers extension into segmental nerves and ganglia and roots and distally into peripheral nerves. These disorders frequently occur together in the same patient, implying that they may have a common underlying mechanism such as microvasculitis.

Epidemiology

In the Rochester Diabetic Neuropathy Study, the prevalence of DLSRPN was approximately 1% of patients with diabetes mellitus,[23] but the incidence has not been determined.

Etiology

The role of chronic hyperglycemic exposure may not be as important as once thought because these disorders appear to occur more frequently in patients with type 2 diabetes mellitus than in those with type 1 who probably have greater hyperglycemic exposure. Furthermore, because these syndromes can also occur in patients without diabetes, it appears that prolonged hyperglycemia is not a prerequisite for the condition. However, because chronic hyperglycemia appears to occur more frequently in patients with diabetes, it is thought to be a risk factor.[24]

The role of inflammation in DLSRPN has been debated. Bradley et al.[18] suggested that in patients with an increased erythrocyte sedimentation rate, DLSRPN was due to an inflammatory or immune cause. Said et al.[21,25] first observed that necrotizing vasculitis could occur in this variety of neuropathy but argued that only some cases were due to vasculitis. Llewelyn et al.[22] confirmed these observations. Study of distal nerve biopsy specimens from 33 prospectively evaluated patients with DLSRPN showed that this syndrome is explained by microvasculitis that causes both axonal degeneration and segmental demyelination.[6] The finding of inflammation, especially in the walls and surrounding tissue of epineurial microvessels, with evidence of ischemic injury (multifocal fiber loss, degeneration of the perineurium, injury neuroma) and previous bleeding (hemosiderin), suggests that an inflammatory or immune process, most likely microvasculitis, contributes to the pathophysiological mechanism of DLSRPN. Frequently, inflammatory infiltrates, often large, involve the walls of microvessels or surround the vessels. We have shown recently that the smooth muscle layers in these nerve microvessels are fragmented in both diabetic and nondiabetic lumbosacral plexopathies (Figure 187.1).[24] Therefore, we suggest that microvasculitis causes the ischemic injury. Studies have not advanced to the point that information is available on the underlying immune mechanisms that lead to this vascular involvement.

Pathogenesis

As noted above, microvasculitis and ischemic injury appear to underlie DLSRPN.[6] Fiber degeneration or loss clearly is multifocal even in distal cutaneous nerves. The most prominent fiber alteration is axonal degeneration. On transverse sections of nerve, one finds axonal enlargements with accumulated organelles; these enlargements have the appearance of axonal stasis of vesicles, mitochondria, and granular material. They are like the axonal enlargements described by Korthals et al.[26,27] and Nukada and Dyck[28,29] as characteristic of the edges of ischemic cores in experimental ischemia. In some places, the perineurium is damaged and the regrowth of neurites into the perineurium and outside the perineurium has formed microfasciculi (injury neuroma), which also has been reported in ischemic injury.[27] Some fibers at the margins of ischemic cores show proximal demyelination at the level of axonal swelling or axonal attenuation and distal axonal degeneration. Also, nerves that show ischemic injury (multifocal fiber loss) are the same ones that have increased frequency of segmental demyelination. Therefore, we think that the process of axonal degeneration and segmental demyelination are linked and perhaps due to ischemia. We did not find evidence of two subtypes of DLSRPN, one demyelinating and one axonal.

Little information is available about the pathological alterations in thoracic radiculoneuropathies, but in a few cases that we have studied, the ganglia have contained prominent inflammatory cell infiltrates (similar to the lumbosacral plexus disorder), suggesting that this is also an immune disorder. There is almost no information on the pathological alterations of cervical radiculoplexus neuropathy, but in several cases of this disorder, we found in biopsy specimens from forearm cutaneous nerves perivascular inflammation causing disruption of vessel walls, multifocal fiber loss, and other changes similar to that of lumbosacral radiculoplexus neuropathy.

Genetics

No information is available about the genetics of diabetic radiculoplexus neuropathies.

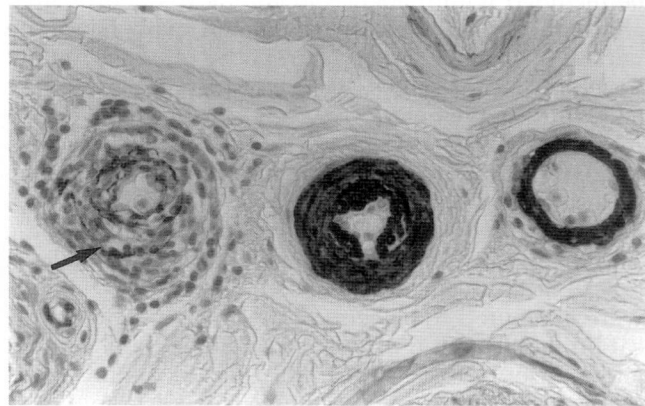

Figure 187.1   Sural nerve from a patient with lumbosacral radiculoplexus neuropathy immunoreacted to smooth muscle actin. The vessel on the left is a thin-walled microvessel with fragmentation of its wall (*arrow*); the fragments are separated by mononuclear cells. The vessels in the middle and on the right are unaffected. (See color plate section.)

Differential diagnosis

Unilateral or asymmetrical involvement of the lumbosacral roots or the lumbar or lumbosacral plexus includes consideration of trauma, retroperitoneal abscess, bleeding or tumor (i.e., lymphoma), radiation injury, inflammatory immune disorders, structural lesions, or other neuropathic processes. Structural lesions have to be excluded by imaging the lumbosacral plexus and cauda equina. Similarly, thoracic radiculoneuropathy raises the question of bony or other structural lesions impinging on roots and nerves or herpes zoster infection. A similar list of conditions needs to be considered for the cervical roots and brachial plexus.

Treatment

Treatment may be divided conveniently into specific treatments, which prevent or ameliorate the disorder, and symptomatic treatments. Currently, only limited information is available on specific treatments for any of these conditions. DLSRPN is probably an immune-mediated neuropathy (as discussed above). Consequently, it is assumed that immunotherapy may be helpful for some patients who have DLSRPN. No controlled studies have been conducted. Said et al.[21] treated two patients, whose nerve biopsy specimens showed vasculitis, with prednisone and reported improvement. In 15 patients, Krendel et al.[30] treated DLSRPN with immunotherapy. Of these 15 patients, 7 received a combination of intravenous immunoglobulin and prednisone; 5, intravenous immunoglobulin alone; 2, a combination of prednisone and cyclophosphamide; and 1, prednisone alone. According to the authors, all patients had improvement and five had marked improvement. Pascoe et al.[31] compared 12 patients with DLSRPN who received treatment (prednisone, intravenous immunoglobulin, or plasma exchange) with 29 who did not. They concluded that most patients had improvement whether treated or not, but the treated group improved to a greater extent and at a faster rate. These results are encouraging that immunomodulating therapies may be helpful in DLSRPN. However, because this is a monophasic illness and spontaneous improvement is usual, these reports of treatment efficacy must be considered preliminary. With this in mind, we are conducting two double-blind placebo-controlled trials. The first compares intravenous immunoglobulin with placebo. Initially, treatment is given several times weekly and then less frequently over 3 months to test whether the infusion of immunoglobulin may be helpful in treating DLSRPN. The second trial compares methylprednisolone and placebo. Large doses of methylprednisolone or placebo are given intravenously, initially several times weekly and then less frequently over 3 months to determine whether treatment alters the course of disease. Because these are ongoing controlled trials, no data about efficacy are available.

Often, the initial symptoms of pain are so severe that lumbosacral radiculoplexus neuropathy, thoracic radiculoneuropathy, and cervical radiculoplexus neuropathy require physician attention and analgesic or perhaps narcotic medication. Occasionally, we have had to admit patients to the hospital to manage the pain. This is not a trivial health problem and needs to be given prompt and vigorous attention. Our group tries to promote good sleep, to reassure patients that the situation ultimately will improve, and to provide sufficient pain relief. Amitriptyline, gabapentin, carbamazepine, and similar agents may provide some degree of pain relief, but narcotics may need to be added to the regimen. Patients should be told that the goal is to improve their pain to a tolerable level, but complete relief may be difficult to obtain without the development of other problems, for example, excessive drowsiness, inability to work, constipation, and difficulty driving. To avoid addiction, defined limits of narcotic use should not be exceeded. Immersing the feet in a cold water bath may be helpful for burning pain. The degree of weakness that ensues may mean that patients need to use a wheelchair or orthotic devices. Physical and occupational therapy may be helpful to strengthen muscles, to encourage better use of limbs in activities of daily living, to prevent contractures, and to improve the patient's mood. It may or may not be possible for patients to continue their usual work for some time. Patients may need to be helped in finding financial support while they are disabled. However, it often is helpful to patients' sense of self-worth if they can continue working, even in some reduced capacity. Patients frequently become depressed, and antidepressant medication should be considered. Our group has seen patients whose weakness has improved markedly, but the depression resulting from the neuropathy has become the main disabling problem that needs treatment. Continuing encouragement is important to reassure patients that their symptoms will improve.

References

1. Leyden E. Beitrag zur Klinik des diabetes mellitus. Wien Med Wochenschr 1893;43:926
2. Mulder DW, Lambert EH, Bastron JA, Sprague RG. The neuropathies associated with diabetes mellitus: a clinical and electromyographic study of 103 unselected diabetic patients. Neurology 1961;11:275–284
3. Asbury AK. Proximal diabetic neuropathy. Ann Neurol 1977;2:179–180
4. Thomas PK, Tomlinson DR. Diabetic and hypoglycemic neuropathy. In: Dyck JP, Thomas PK, Griffin JW, et al., eds. Peripheral Neuropathy. Vol 2, 3rd ed. Philadelphia: WB Saunders Company, 1993:1219–1250
5. Taylor BV, Dyck PJ. Classification of the diabetic neuropathies. In: Dyck PJ, Thomas PK, eds. Diabetic Neuropathy. 2nd ed. Philadelphia: WB Saunders, 1999: 407–414
6. Dyck PJB, Norell JE, Dyck PJ. Microvasculitis and ischemia in diabetic lumbosacral radiculoplexus neuropathy. Neurology 1999;53:2113–2121
7. Bruns L. Ueber neuritsche Lahmungen beim diabetes mellitus. Berlin Klin Wochenschr 1890;27:509
8. Garland H. Diabetic amyotrophy. Br Med J 1955;2: 1287–1290
9. Garland H. Diabetic amyotrophy. Br J Clin Pract 1961; 15:9–13

10. Chokroverty S, Reyes MG, Rubino FA. Bruns-Garland syndrome of diabetic amyotrophy. Trans Am Neurol Assoc 1977;102:173–177

11. Barohn RJ, Sahenk Z, Warmolts JR, Mendell JR. The Bruns-Garland syndrome (diabetic amyotrophy): revisited 100 years later. Arch Neurol 1991;48:1130–1135

12. Williams IR, Mayer RF. Subacute proximal diabetic neuropathy. Neurology 1976;26:108–116

13. Bastron JA, Thomas JE. Diabetic polyradiculopathy: clinical and electromyographic findings in 105 patients. Mayo Clin Proc 1981;56:725–732

14. Skanse B, Gydell K. A rare type of femoral-sciatic neuropathy in diabetes mellitus. Acta Med Scand 1956;155:463–468

15. Calverley JR, Mulder DW. Femoral neuropathy. Neurology 1960;10:963–967

16. Raff MC, Asbury AK. Ischemic mononeuropathy and mononeuropathy multiplex in diabetes mellitus. N Engl J Med 1968;279:17–21

17. Raff MC, Sangalang V, Asbury AK. Ischemic mononeuropathy multiplex associated with diabetes mellitus. Arch Neurol 1968;18:487–499

18. Bradley WG, Chad D, Verghese JP, et al. Painful lumbosacral plexopathy with elevated erythrocyte sedimentation rate: a treatable inflammatory syndrome. Ann Neurol 1984;15:457–464

19. Sun SF, Streib EW. Diabetic thoracoabdominal neuropathy: clinical and electrodiagnostic features. Ann Neurol 1981;9:75–79

20. Kikta DG, Breuer AC, Wilbourn AJ. Thoracic root pain in diabetes: the spectrum of clinical and electromyographic findings. Ann Neurol 1982;11:80–85

21. Said G, Goulon-Goeau C, Lacroix C, Moulonguet A. Nerve biopsy findings in different patterns of proximal diabetic neuropathy. Ann Neurol 1994;35:559–569

22. Llewelyn JG, Thomas PK, King RH. Epineurial microvasculitis in proximal diabetic neuropathy. J Neurol 1998;245:159–165

23. Dyck PJ, Kratz KM, Karnes JL, et al. The prevalence by staged severity of various types of diabetic neuropathy, retinopathy, and nephropathy in a population-based cohort: the Rochester Diabetic Neuropathy Study. Neurology 1993;43:817–824

24. Dyck PJB, Engelstad J, Norell J, Dyck PJ. Microvasculitis in non-diabetic lumbosacral radiculoplexus neuropathy (LSRPN): similarity to the diabetic variety (DLSRPN). J Neuropathol Exp Neurol 2000;59:525–538

25. Said G, Elgrably F, Lacroix C, et al. Painful proximal diabetic neuropathy: inflammatory nerve lesions and spontaneous favorable outcome. Ann Neurol 1997;41:762–770

26. Korthals JK, Wisniewski HM. Peripheral nerve ischemia: part I. Experimental model. J Neurol Sci 1975;24:65–76

27. Korthals JK, Gieron MA, Wisniewski HM. Nerve regeneration patterns after acute ischemic injury. Neurology 1989;39:932–937

28. Nukada H, Dyck PJ. Acute ischemia causes axonal stasis, swelling, attenuation, and secondary demyelination. Ann Neurol 1987;22:311–318

29. Nukada H, Dyck PJ. Microsphere embolization of nerve capillaries and fiber degeneration. Am J Pathol 1984;115:275–287

30. Krendel DA, Costigan DA, Hopkins LC. Successful treatment of neuropathies in patients with diabetes mellitus. Arch Neurol 1995;52:1053–1061

31. Pascoe MK, Low PA, Windebank AJ, Litchy WJ. Subacute diabetic proximal neuropathy. Mayo Clin Proc 1997;72:1123–1132

188 Peripheral Neuropathy Associated With Hypothyroidism and Acromegaly

Caroline M Klein

Hypothyroidism

Overview

Hypothyroidism is a common medical illness in which the circulating levels of thyroid hormone are insufficient. It is often attributed to inadequate dietary intake of iodine. Worldwide, as many as 1 billion people may be at risk for iodine deficiency disorders, including hypothyroidism.[1] Hypothyroidism may also be caused by intrinsic disease of the thyroid gland or, less commonly, may occur as a consequence of pituitary gland or hypothalamic abnormalities.[2] It may occur as a primary idiopathic disease, an autoimmune disorder, Hashimoto thyroiditis, or a drug-induced condition (e.g., with lithium treatment) or after surgical or radioiodine ablation of the thyroid as part of treatment of Graves disease.[2,3]

In 1878, William Ord[4] coined the term *myxedema* to describe the diffuse connective tissue and skin changes he found in patients with hypothyroidism. He was probably the first to associate neurological symptoms with this medical condition. Interestingly, he thought that the diffuse subcutaneous and connective tissue mucoid infiltration he found in these patients might insulate the cutaneous nerve endings from environmental stimuli, thereby interfering with their normal functioning. This would presumably result in diminished sensory input to the central nervous system, leading to lethargy and slowed mentation. In this way, peripheral nerve function may be impaired by virtue of pathological changes in the surrounding connective tissue, not within the nerve itself.

Peripheral neuropathy associated with hypothyroidism is more likely caused by focal nerve entrapment, such as median neuropathy at the wrist or ulnar neuropathy at the elbow, and less likely to be caused by generalized sensorimotor peripheral neuropathy. This seems to be true in spite of findings of more generalized abnormalities on electrophysiological testing that are usually asymptomatic or of doubtful clinical importance. The most common clinical presentation of peripheral nerve involvement in patients with hypothyroidism is paresthesia of the distal extremities, especially the hands, usually caused by median neuropathies at the wrists (Table 188.1). Treatment of the underlying endocrinopathy with hormonal replacement usually relieves these symptoms.

Clinical features

Peripheral neuropathy, diagnosed on the basis of electrophysiological abnormalities, has an estimated prevalence of 718 cases per 1000 patients with hypothyroidism,[5] although in most of these cases it is probably subclinical or asymptomatic.[5–7] Evidence of peripheral neuropathy has been found also in patients with subclinical hypothyroidism.[8–10] Acroparesthesia, or paresthesias of the hands or feet or both, is reported commonly by patients with hypothyroidism;[6,7,9–22] the frequency ranges from 14%[6] to 81%.[7] Thus, focal entrapment neuropathies may be the basis for these symptoms. In fact, median neuropathy at the wrist (carpal tunnel syndrome) occurs frequently in these patients.[3,6,7,10,12,13,15,20,21] Murray and Simpson,[13] in 1958, described some of the earliest cases of median neuropathy at the wrist as an explanation for the acroparesthesias. They found 26 of 35 patients with myxedema had symptoms of tingling paresthesias in the fingers, and 7 of 11 patients evaluated by electromyography (EMG) had electrophysiological abnormalities consistent with median neuropathy at the wrist. A more generalized sensorimotor peripheral neuropathy, with or without median mononeuropathy, has also been described,[3,5,7,14–20,22,23] although much less commonly in patients with hypothyroidism. Scarpalezos and coworkers[6] studied a series of 51 patients with hypothyroidism and found 12 to have abnormal neurological findings and 18 to have

---

Table 188.1 Peripheral neuropathies associated with hypothyroidism or acromegaly

Hypothyroidism
 Focal entrapment mononeuropathies
  Median neuropathy at the wrist (carpal tunnel syndrome)
  Ulnar neuropathy at the elbow (cubital tunnel syndrome)
 Generalized sensorimotor, mixed axonal and demyelinating peripheral neuropathy
 Usually mild or asymptomatic
 Often in association with one or more mononeuropathies

Acromegaly
 Focal entrapment mononeuropathies
  Median neuropathy at the wrist (carpal tunnel syndrome)
 Generalized sensorimotor, demyelinating peripheral neuropathy
  Usually mild or asymptomatic

abnormal EMG findings consistent with a generalized peripheral neuropathy. Similarly, Beghi et al.[5] reported that of 39 consecutive patients with a diagnosis of hypothyroidism, only 33% had a clinical diagnosis of peripheral neuropathy, although 72% had abnormal electrodiagnostic findings.

Less common peripheral or cranial nerve involvement in hypothyroidism includes bilateral phrenic neuropathy[24] and sensorineural hearing loss.[3,12,17,18] Hoarseness (dysphonia) and distortion of speech articulation (dyslalia) are thought to be caused by the mucopolysaccharide infiltration of local tissue in the vocal cords and tongue, respectively, and not involvement of cranial nerve IX, X, or XII.[3,12]

The pathophysiology of peripheral nerve involvement in hypothyroidism is uncertain.[15] Early investigators, such as Nickel et al.,[22] thought that neuropathy was caused by an increase in a basophilic, metachromatic mucoid substance in the endoneurium and perineurium of the nerve, with associated edema, causing interference with normal neuronal metabolic function. Murray and Simpson[13] proposed that in median neuropathy at the wrist, myxedematous tissue within the carpal tunnel caused focal nerve entrapment. Tendon and synovial thickening in the carpal tunnel may contribute to nerve injury,[12,13,15] but such thickening would not explain the pathophysiology of generalized peripheral neuropathy. Others have proposed that deficiency of thyroid hormone may adversely affect the metabolism of either Schwann cells[12,14,17] or neurons,[14,19] resulting in nerve injury by primary demyelination or axonal degeneration, respectively. Thyroid hormone influences cellular respiration and energy expenditure,[2] and the cellular metabolism of nervous tissue, including Schwann cells, may be susceptible to hormone deficiency. Some investigators have found a positive correlation between peripheral neuropathy (its presence and severity) and thyroid hormone deficiency (its severity, duration, or both).[7,8,18,19] Misiunas et al.,[8] in 1995, reported that in patients with early or subclinical hypothyroidism, progression of electrodiagnostic changes correlates with the severity of systemic disease. Other investigators, however, have failed to find a direct correlation.[5,13]

Patients with hypothyroidism and peripheral neuropathy may present with neurological symptoms in addition to systemic symptoms related to thyroid hormone deficiency, which may include fatigue, lethargy, constipation, weight gain, cold intolerance, dry skin, brittle hair and alopecia, brittle nails, and tongue enlargement.[2] However, patients may also present with subclinical hypothyroidism and associated peripheral neuropathy.[8,9,24] Neurological symptoms typically manifest as distal, symmetrical, usually painful paresthesias and may also include distal muscle weakness and depressed or absent deep tendon reflexes,[3,5–7,9–12,14,16–23] although sensory symptoms seem to predominate.[3,5–7,9,11,12,15,17,21,22] Nickel et al.[22] reported that all 25 hypothyroid patients they evaluated described distal extremity paresthesias, but only 15 had objective sensory loss on neurological

examination. With median neuropathy at the wrist, symptoms of carpal tunnel syndrome, including paresthesias and pain in a median nerve distribution with possible weakness or atrophy of thenar muscles, may be seen.[3,12,13,20] Beghi et al.[5] found that of 28 hypothyroid patients with electrodiagnostic findings of peripheral neuropathy, 25 had mild neuropathy and only 3 had moderate to severe neuropathy. In a patient with bilateral phrenic neuropathy reported by Laroche et al.,[24] symptoms of diaphragmatic weakness were the only presenting symptoms of either hypothyroidism or peripheral neuropathy. The natural history of peripheral neuropathy due to hypothyroidism is not well known or well described, because treatment is usually successful.

Diagnosis

Hypothyroidism can be diagnosed on the basis of specific laboratory testing, which includes determining levels of thyroid-stimulating hormone (TSH), serum thyroxine (T_4), and serum triiodothyronine (T_3); calculating the free T_4 index; and testing radioactive iodine uptake. In patients with subclinical hypothyroidism, diagnostic testing may also include measurement of serum TSH levels after administration of thyroid-releasing hormone.[2] A clinical history of previously treated Graves disease or Hashimoto thyroditis, for example, may increase suspicion of hypothyroidism as a cause for median neuropathy at the wrist or generalized peripheral neuropathy in a patient with neuropathic symptoms.

Electrodiagnostic testing can confirm the presence, severity, and characteristics of peripheral neuropathy and document the presence of median neuropathy at the wrist. The most common abnormalities seen on nerve conduction studies are prolonged distal motor latencies, with or without slowing of conduction velocities, and decreased amplitudes, particularly of sensory nerve action potentials.[5–11,14,16–19,23] Dyck and Lambert[14] reported marked temporal dispersion of the ulnar compound muscle action potential with both proximal and distal nerve stimulation in one patient with hypothyroidism (Figure 188.1). Some evidence suggests that the upper extremities may be affected earlier in the course of the peripheral neuropathy.[6,15] Needle examination may show evidence of chronic denervation in distal muscles.[9,10,17,19,22,23] Misiunas and colleagues[8] found that with progression of subclinical hypothyroidism, the amplitudes of both motor and sensory responses in the upper and lower extremities were more likely to be decreased. However, in patients they considered to be at the earliest stage of subclinical hypothyroidism, sensory abnormalities (decreased amplitudes) were confined to the lower extremities, and prolonged motor distal latencies were found in both the upper and lower extremities. The generalized peripheral neuropathy associated with hypothyroidism may be described as symmetrical, distal, and sensorimotor with mixed axonal and demyelinating features electrophysiologically.

In patients with median neuropathy at the wrists,

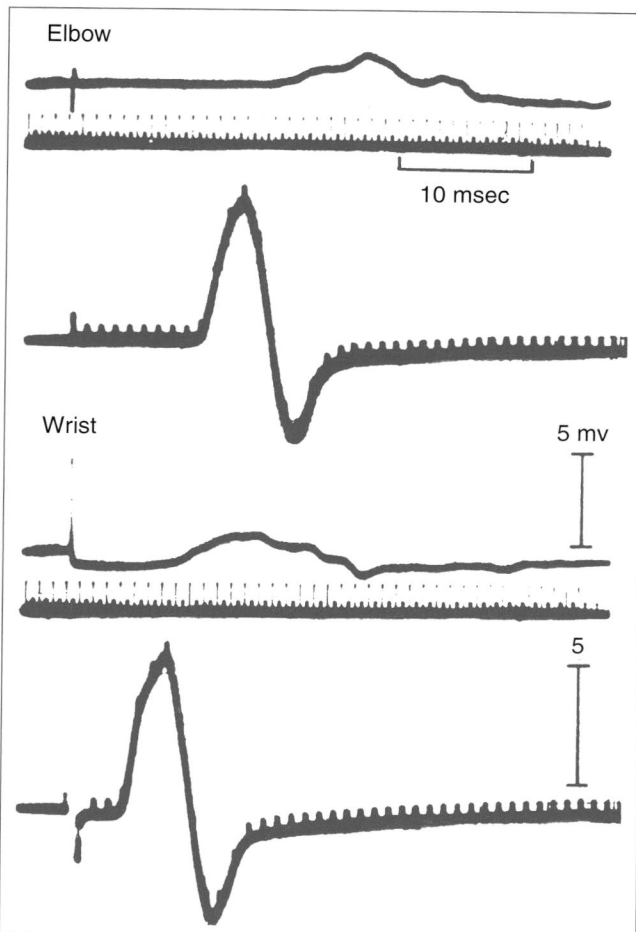

Figure 188.1 Compound muscle action potentials recorded over hypothenar muscles after maximal electrical stimulus of the ulnar nerve at the elbow (upper pair) and wrist (lower pair). Top recording from each pair was obtained before treatment. Bottom recording from each pair was obtained after 9 months of treatment with thyroid hormone. Note longer latency and greater dispersion of the response before treatment and nearly normal response after treatment. (From Dyck and Lambert.[14] By permission of the *Journal of Neuropathology and Experimental Neurology*.)

In addition, lipid droplets, lamellar bodies, and some abnormal-appearing mitochondria were seen in Schwann cells, suggesting a primarily demyelinating process attributable to pathological changes within Schwann cells. However, some pathological findings in axons were also present, suggesting an additional component of axonal degeneration. Other reports of nerve biopsy findings in specimens from hypothyroid patients have confirmed some of these pathological findings,[11,16,17,19,22,23] but some investigators have suggested more strongly that axonal degeneration is the primary pathological process.[11,16,19,22]

The differential diagnosis for generalized peripheral neuropathy associated with hypothyroidism includes other causes of distal, symmetrical, primary demyelinating sensorimotor peripheral neuropathy such as hereditary motor and sensory neuropathies, leprosy, acromegaly, Lyme disease, acquired immunodeficiency syndrome (AIDS)–associated neuropathy, diphtheric neuropathy, acute or chronic inflammatory demyelinating polyradiculoneuropathy (AIDP/CIDP), monoclonal gammopathy, lymphoma, and hereditary neuropathy with liability to pressure palsy (HNPP). The differential diagnosis for carpal tunnel syndrome includes rheumatoid arthritis, diabetes mellitus, pregnancy, occupational overuse, tenosynovitis, eosinophilic fasciitis, or Colles fracture.[25]

Treatment

Treatment of peripheral neuropathy associated with hypothyroidism is thyroid hormone replacement. Possible hormonal formulations used in this treatment include levothyroxine, liothyronine, a combination of these two hormones, or natural thyroid extract. Levothyroxine is the most commonly used and recommended because it results in the most stable serum T_3 concentrations.[2] Recommended initial dosing is 25 µg daily, followed by slow titration to a usual

typical electrodiagnostic features include prolonged distal motor and sensory latencies, reduced amplitudes, and thenar muscle needle examination findings.[6,7,11,13,20,21]

Pathological examination of peripheral nerve from patients with hypothyroidism has been reported. Dyck and Lambert,[14] in 1970, described in detail the findings in sural nerve biopsy specimens from two hypothyroid patients. They found a decreased number of myelinated fibers, segmental demyelination with myelin remodeling, and early onion bulb formation. The amount of mucoid substance within the nerve was increased only slightly compared with that in controls, and no perineurial thickening was seen. Electron microscopic examination showed increased glycogen deposits in both axons and Schwann cells compared with controls (Figure 188.2).

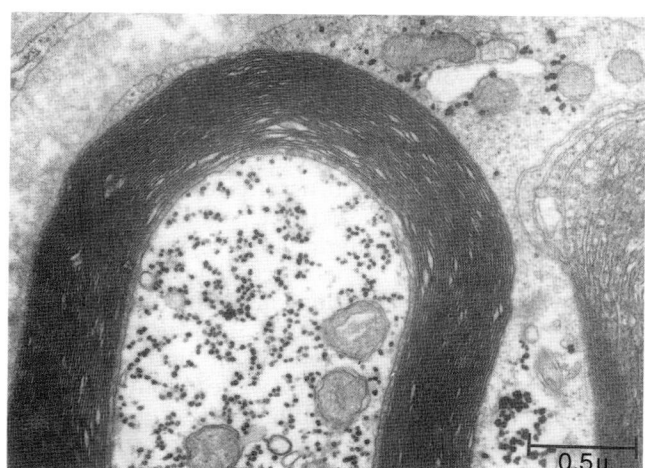

Figure 188.2 Many glycogen granules are present in an axis cylinder of a myelinated fiber with well-preserved myelin. Smaller collections of glycogen granules are seen in the Schwann cell cytoplasm on the right. (From Dyck and Lambert.[14] By permission of the *Journal of Neuropathology and Experimental Neurology*.)

target dose of 1.7 µg/kg of body weight per day.[2] TSH levels should be determined at regular intervals while the patient is receiving hormone replacement therapy. Both symptomatic and electrophysiological improvement in peripheral neuropathy has been reported within weeks to months of thyroid hormone replacement.[9–14,17–19,21–24] Dyck and Lambert[14] reported resolution of neuropathic symptoms and normalization of the neurological findings within 8 months of treatment in one of their patients. Electrophysiologically, conduction velocities, distal latencies, and amplitudes improved dramatically (Figure 188.1). In a single patient with hypothyroid neuropathy, Torres and Moxley[18] described return of sensory nerve action potentials and improved distal latencies on nerve conduction studies after hormonal treatment.

Acromegaly

Overview

Acromegaly, or growth hormone excess, is a relatively uncommon medical condition, with an estimated prevalence of 50 to 70 cases per million population.[26] Peripheral neuropathy as one of the possible systemic manifestations of acromegaly was originally described by Marie and Marinesco,[27] in 1891, and has since been confirmed by others.[12,28–38] Recognition of this association probably began with the often-reported symptoms of acroparesthesias in patients with acromegaly,[29,30,32,37,38] leading to the diagnosis of median neuropathies at the wrists.[30,32,36–39] However, cases of generalized peripheral neuropathy or polyneuropathy have also been reported,[12,29–31,33–36,38] albeit less commonly. The most typical manifestation of peripheral nerve involvement in acromegaly is focal entrapment, such as median neuropathy at the wrist, and not generalized or diffuse sensorimotor peripheral neuropathy (Table 188.1).

Clinical features

The frequency of median neuropathy at the wrists (carpal tunnel syndrome) or generalized peripheral neuropathy among patients with a diagnosis of acromegaly is unclear from the literature. O'Duffy et al.[32] found that 35 of 100 acromegalic patients had bilateral carpal tunnel syndrome, which was graded clinically as mild to moderate in severity. Low et al.[36] studied 11 patients who had acromegaly and found 8 of them had electrophysiological evidence of generalized peripheral neuropathy and 9 had carpal tunnel syndrome, either superimposed on the generalized neuropathy or in isolation. However, comparison of the electrophysiological findings of these 11 patients with similar electrodiagnostic findings in 22 age-matched controls showed marked slowing of motor conduction velocities and reduced sensory nerve action potential amplitudes in the patients with acromegaly. Sural nerve biopsy specimens from asymptomatic acromegalic patients with reportedly normal neurological findings have been found to be abnormal as well,[34] which would corroborate this

finding of subclinical peripheral neuropathy in these patients. Jamal et al.[30] evaluated 24 patients with acromegaly and found 8 with generalized peripheral neuropathy, 4 of whom had superimposed median neuropathies at the wrist, and 6 additional patients with carpal tunnel syndrome alone. Although generalized sensorimotor peripheral neuropathy is thought by some[30] to be common in patients with acromegaly, others[29] believe it to be uncommon. In general, as with patients with hypothyroidism, focal entrapment neuropathies, such as median neuropathy at the wrist, appear to be the most clinically relevant basis for the typical neuropathic symptoms in acromegalic patients (acroparesthesias). Generalized sensorimotor peripheral neuropathy, despite being documented electrophysiologically and pathologically in some of these patients, is likely to remain asymptomatic or subclinical in most patients.

The pathogenesis of either median entrapment neuropathy at the wrist or generalized peripheral neuropathy in acromegaly is uncertain. Of interest, the severity of the peripheral neuropathy does not appear to correlate with growth hormone levels.[30,36,38] Nerve biopsy studies have shown myelinated fiber loss[29,31,33,34,36] and segmental demyelination.[31,33,34,36] The pathological features have been described as "hypertrophic,"[12,29,31] with increased amounts of connective tissue in the endoneurium and perineurium[29,31,33,36,37] as well as increased fascicular size.[36] Onion bulb formation has been reported,[34,36] although it is not always seen,[31,33] perhaps indicating a more advanced or late-stage peripheral nerve injury.[33,34] Based on these pathological findings, the pathogenesis of peripheral nerve injury in acromegaly may be caused by a combination of factors,[12] including stimulation of proliferation of Schwann cells and fibroblasts by growth hormone mediated via insulin-like growth factor 1 (IGF-1),[12,33] leading to locally compressive effects on the neural elements.[12,29] In the case of carpal tunnel syndrome, a possible combination of nerve hypertrophy and bony and soft tissue changes due to growth hormone excess may result in focal median nerve compression.[12,37] These soft tissue changes are presumably the result of alterations in local sodium and water balance caused by growth hormone itself leading to increased extracellular fluid.[12,32,37,38] Dinn and Dinn[34] examined serial sural nerve biopsy specimens from two patients with peripheral neuropathy associated with acromegaly. They found pathological progression in the hypertrophic changes, which they correlated with continued elevated growth hormone levels, suggesting a causal relationship between growth hormone levels and pathological alterations of the peripheral nerve.

The clinical features of this condition include characteristic findings of acromegaly, such as acral enlargement, prognathism, and hyperhidrosis.[25] Neurological symptoms may include mild acral paresthesias in a median nerve distribution as in cases of carpal tunnel syndrome[29,30,32,36–38] or in a more generalized distal extremity distribution.[29,30,36,38] There may be additional symptoms of a more generalized sensorimotor peripheral neuropathy, such as muscle weakness as well as distal to proximal sensory loss and loss of deep tendon reflexes.[29–31,33–36,38] Some authors[30,31,36] have reported that the peripheral nerves of these patients are palpably enlarged, although others[3,38] did not find this to be true. Without treatment, the course of a generalized peripheral neuropathy is most likely to be slowly progressive, although there is at least one report[32] of spontaneous improvement in carpal tunnel syndrome symptoms associated with acromegaly.

Diagnosis

The diagnosis of acromegaly, apart from the clinical features described previously, is based on specific biochemical abnormalities on laboratory testing, including elevated random growth hormone levels (>0.4 μg/L) without suppression (<1.0 to 2.5 μg/L) after an oral glucose tolerance test (OGTT).[26,40,41] Random or baseline measurement of serum growth hormone levels is believed to be too nonspecific to function in isolation as a screening test for the disease.[26] Measuring the growth hormone levels at 60 and 120 minutes after oral administration of 75 to 100 grams of glucose is more useful.[26,40] Serum IGF-1 levels may also be elevated[26,28,40,42,43] and correlate well with disease activity.[26] Because most cases of acromegaly are caused by a growth hormone-secreting pituitary gland tumor, cranial magnetic resonance imaging (MRI) may help confirm the presence of a tumor. Approximately 40% of these growth hormone-secreting tumors are microadenomas (<10 mm in diameter),[28] which may not be visible on neuroimaging. Commonly associated medical conditions include other endocrinopathies such as diabetes mellitus and hypothyroidism.[26]

In a patient with acroparesthesias or clinical features of a sensorimotor peripheral neuropathy, electrodiagnostic testing such as EMG and nerve conduction studies may help confirm the presence of a peripheral neuropathy, demonstrate its distribution, and elucidate its severity. In the case of a generalized sensorimotor peripheral neuropathy, nerve conduction velocities may be slowed,[30,31,33,34,36] and needle examination may reveal chronic denervation changes.[29–31,33,34] The amplitudes of both compound muscle action potentials[31] and sensory nerve action potentials[30,36] have been reported to be low. Distal latencies may be prolonged.[30,31,36] These electrophysiological abnormalities are suggestive of a predominantly demyelinating, sensorimotor peripheral neuropathy.

The differential diagnosis for acromegaly with associated peripheral neuropathy includes other causes of a primarily demyelinating sensorimotor peripheral neuropathy such as AIDP/CIDP, hypothyroidism, AIDS-associated peripheral neuropathy, leprosy, diphtheric neuropathy, Lyme disease, monoclonal gammopathy, lymphoma, drug toxicity, and HNPP. In the case of carpal tunnel syndrome, conditions such as systemic amyloidosis, idiopathic median neuropathy at the wrist, hypothyroidism, wrist trauma, rheumatoid arthritis, diabetes mellitus,[25] and HNPP are considered in the differential diagnosis.

Treatment

Treatment of acromegalic peripheral neuropathy is based on treatment of the underlying growth hormone excess. This approach, in addition to surgical decompression of the carpal tunnel,[32,37] may also be helpful in alleviating acroparesthesias[42] or median neuropathy at the wrist.[32] The goal of treatment of acromegaly is to achieve serum growth hormone levels less than 2.5 μg/L, with suppression of growth hormone levels to less than 1 to 2 μg/L after glucose challenge.[26,28,40–45] Normalization of serum IGF-1 levels for age and sex is another therapeutic goal.[28,40,41,44–47] Treatment of this condition may be surgical, medical, or both if initial attempts are unsuccessful (Figure 188.3). Nonmedical approaches include transsphenoidal resection, direct pituitary irradiation, or gamma knife radiation surgery.[26,28,38,40,41,43,46–52]

The success of pituitary surgery to acromegaly is variable. Jenkins et al.[43] reported a success rate for surgical therapy of 33% when they reviewed outcomes for 89 patients treated over a 10-year period (1963–1973). The important factors related to successful surgical outcome include tumor size, degree of invasiveness, and preoperative growth hormone levels.[40,43,49] Noninvasive microadenomas smaller than 10 mm in patients with growth hormone levels of less than 45 μg/L before surgery have the best surgical outcomes, according to a recent review by Laws et al.[49] Their series of 86 patients undergoing transsphenoidal surgery as initial treatment for acromegaly showed that 67% had normal IGF-1 levels and 52% had growth hormone levels suppressed to less than 1.0 μg/L on an OGTT. Their recurrence rate (defined as elevated growth hormone levels within 10 years after surgery) was only 8% to 10%, and recurrence was seen most frequently in patients who had evidence of tumor invasion at the time of surgery.[49] Although 80% of patients with microadenomas are treated successfully by pituitary surgery, less than 50% of patients with macroadenomas achieve therapeutic criteria of remission with surgery alone,[40,41,46] and the majority of patients with acromegaly have macroadenomas.[41] Complications of transsphenoidal surgery are relatively uncommon and include transient leakage of cerebrospinal fluid, nasal or sinus complications, and transient cranial nerve deficits.[48,49] Less than 1.5% of patients have more serious complications such as carotid artery damage, intracerebral hemorrhage, stroke, visual loss, or hypopituitarism.[43,48,49]

Alternatives to surgical management must be considered if good biochemical results (normal random serum growth hormone level, growth hormone suppression after OGTT, normal serum IGF-1 levels) are not achieved surgically or if the patient refuses pituitary surgery or is a poor surgical candidate. These nonsurgical alternatives include radiotherapy and medical management. No prospective trials have compared surgery with medical management as

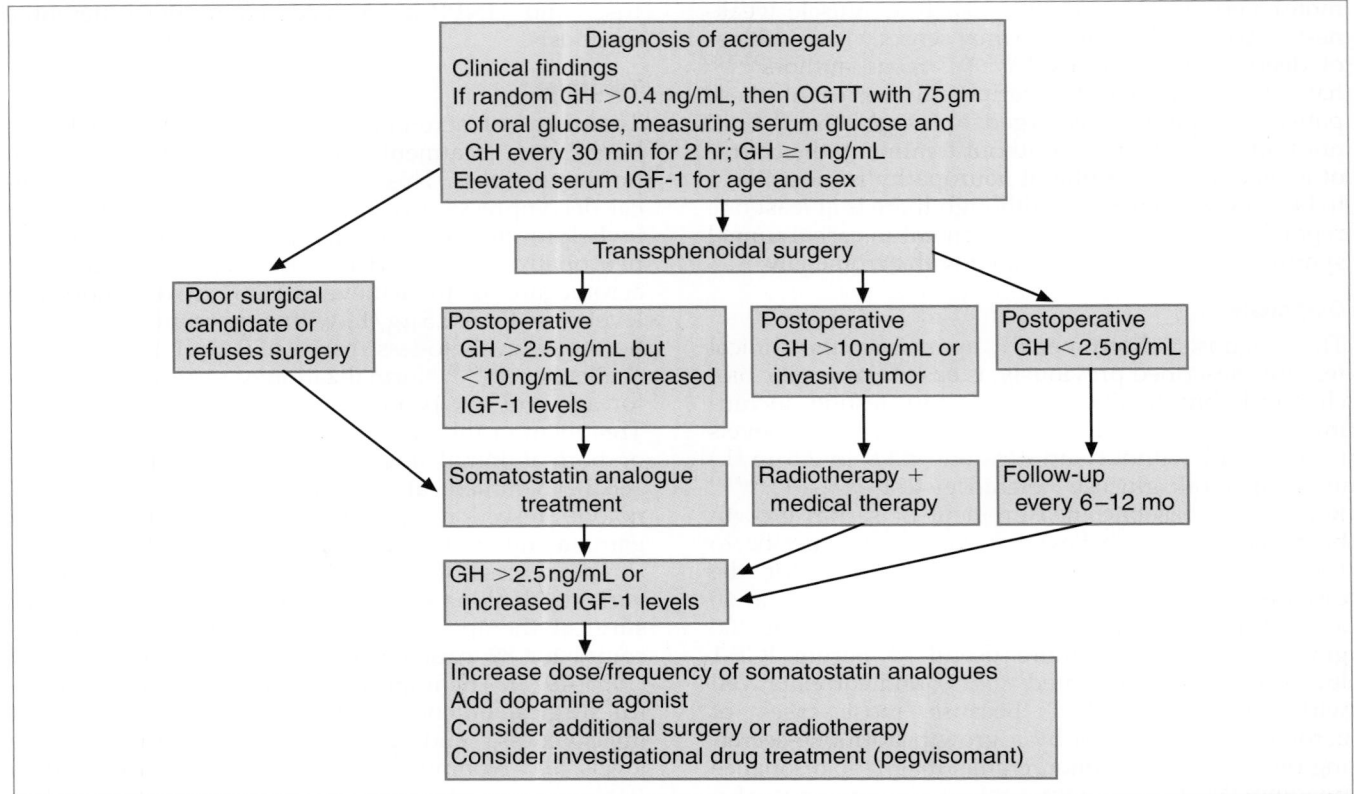

Figure 188.3   Treatment algorithm for acromegaly. GH, growth hormone; IGF-1, insulin-like growth factor 1; OGTT, oral glucose tolerance test.

primary therapy. However, primary medical management instead of surgery or irradiation has been suggested for a subset of acromegalic patients.[45,53] Many surgeons currently recommend adjuvant radiotherapy for patients who have known residual tumor after surgery, an invasive tumor, or persistently elevated levels of growth hormone ($>10\,\mu g/L$) postoperatively.[43,48,49,52]

Radiotherapy, either with external beam or gamma knife radiation, lowers serum IGF-1 and growth hormone levels in patients with acromegaly, but it has not been proven very effective in normalizing these biochemical levels,[41,50,52,53] and the benefits of radiation are typically delayed, sometimes more than 10 years after treatment.[40,41,47,50–52] Barkan et al.[50] reviewed acromegalic patients treated at the University of Michigan between 1975 and 1996 and found that after a mean follow-up of almost 7 years, only 2 of 38 patients had normal serum IGF-1 levels, although growth hormone levels were less than $5\,\mu g/L$ in the majority of these patients. Another study showed that of 46 patients treated with radiotherapy for acromegaly, only 25% had growth hormone levels lower than $2.5\,\mu g/L$ at 5 years.[51] Complications of radiotherapy include panhypopituitarism,[45,51,53] which may develop many years after treatment, affect fertility, and require additional medical treatment.[46] Recent studies have found complications of brain necrosis, optic nerve damage, and increased likelihood of

future malignancy to occur less frequently than previously reported.[41,51,52]

Recent advances in medical management may make radiotherapy a less desirable option for patients requiring additional treatment after surgery. Radiotherapy (and surgery) may have a role in reducing growth hormone levels and decreasing tumor size, leading to improved drug responsiveness.[44,50,53] Because of the long onset of therapeutic benefit from radiotherapy, ongoing medical treatment is usually necessary to lower growth hormone and IGF-1 levels.[41,49] Certainly, if preservation of future fertility is a concern, then limited surgery followed by medical management may be the preferred course of action.[46]

Medical therapy consists of administration of octreotide (a long-acting synthetic somatostatin analogue) or dopamine agonist drugs (bromocriptine, cabergoline) to attempt to suppress growth hormone secretion from the tumor.[26,28,41,42,44,45,47] Standard formulations of octreotide require multiple daily subcutaneous injections; depot formulations of octreotide and lanreotide allow for bimonthly or monthly intramuscular injections.[41,42,44,45] Subcutaneous injections of octreotide are administered at doses of 100 to $200\,\mu g$ three times a day to a maximal total daily dose of $1500\,\mu g$.[26,41,44,45] As primary therapy, subcutaneous octreotide decreases growth hormone levels in up to 50% of patients.[44,45] However, it is probably most effective as adjunctive therapy with surgery or irradiation.[26] Somatostatin analogues, particularly the more recently available long-acting depot formulations, are the drugs of choice for treatment of acromegaly.[41,44–47,54] A recent prospective study of 10 acromegalic patients showed that 80% had growth hormone levels of less than 5 μg/L when receiving depot octreotide or lanreotide.[54] The IGF-1 levels were normalized in 70% and 50% of patients, respectively. Depot octreotide (30 mg intramuscularly every 28 days) produced significantly lower mean growth hormone levels and was more likely to result in lower IGF-1 levels in these patients.[54] The most common adverse effects were transient local injection site discomfort and mild abdominal distress with gastrointestinal upset.[26,41,42,44,45,54] Gallstone formation may increase with these medications because of reduced gallbladder contractility, but the gallstones generally do not cause symptoms.[26,42,44,45,54] These long-acting depot formulations of somatostatin analogues have improved patient comfort and compliance for long-term treatment of acromegaly, and they are more effective than dopamine agonists for lowering patients' growth hormone levels.[41,45,46]

Bromocriptine (20–60 mg/d) is a dopamine agonist that has been used to treat acromegaly, but it may normalize growth hormone levels in less than 10% of patients.[26,41,45] Cabergoline appears to be more effective than bromocriptine for treatment, possibly because of its longer half-life and more specific D_2-receptor binding capacity.[45,55] A recent multicenter, prospective, open-label study found that of 64 patients with acromegaly treated with cabergoline, 39% had IGF-1 levels suppressed to less than 300 μg/L and 46% had growth hormone levels of less than 2 μg/L.[55] The main adverse effects were gastrointestinal symptoms (nausea, vomiting, abdominal pain), orthostatic lightheadedness or hypotension, and nasal congestion.[41,45,55] Although less effective than somatostatin analogues, dopamine agonists may be considered to treat patients who refuse injections, whose growth hormone levels are less than 10 μg/L, or who have either no or suboptimal therapeutic response to somatostatin analogues (approximately 35% of those treated).[45]

The possibility that a combination of somatostatin analogues and dopamine agonists may be beneficial therapeutically was raised in a study of 12 acromegalic patients by Flogstad et al.[56] in 1994. They found that treatment with the combination of bromocriptine and octreotide was more effective in reducing IGF-1 and growth hormone levels than treatment with either drug alone, probably because of increased bioavailability of bromocriptine with this regimen. No further results of combined medical therapy have been published, however. In patients in whom more conventional treatment with single-drug therapy fails, consideration should be given to combination therapy.[41]

The most recently investigated drug for the treatment of acromegaly is pegvisomant, a genetically engineered analogue of growth hormone that acts as a growth hormone receptor antagonist, thus lowering IGF-1 levels.[47,53,57] A 12-week, randomized, double-blind, placebo-controlled trial in 112 patients with acromegaly found a 60% reduction in serum IGF-1 levels in patients who received 20-mg subcutaneous injections daily, with 89% of patients achieving normal IGF-1 levels.[57] Of note, a majority of patients had undergone previous pituitary surgery, radiotherapy, or both. The drug was well tolerated, the most common adverse effect being transient, mild injection site reaction. A single patient had elevated liver enzyme levels, which resolved with discontinuation of the drug but recurred with repeated drug exposure. One concern with this treatment is that the growth hormone levels may increase because of lack of a negative feedback loop and lead to tumor enlargement. A small but nonprogressive increase in growth hormone levels occurred during this 12-week study but was not associated with tumor growth. Development of anti-growth hormone antibodies occurred with low titers in 8 of 80 patients.[57] The long-term effects of this drug vis-à-vis safety and efficacy remain to be determined for the treatment of acromegaly.[47]

Although rapid improvement in symptoms of carpal tunnel syndrome has been reported after surgical removal of the pituitary adenoma,[38] less is known about the effect of surgical or medical treatment of acromegaly on generalized sensorimotor peripheral neuropathy associated with this condition.

References

1. Delange F. The disorders induced by iodine deficiency. Thyroid 1994;4:107–128
2. Wartofsky L. Diseases of the thyroid. In: Isselbacher KJ, Braunwald E, Wilson JD, et al., eds. Harrison's Principles of Internal Medicine. Vol 2, 13th ed. New York: McGraw-Hill, 1994:1930–1953
3. Swanson JW, Kelly JJ Jr, McConahey WM. Neurologic aspects of thyroid dysfunction. Mayo Clin Proc 1981; 56:504–512
4. Ord WM. On myxoedema, a term proposed to be applied to an essential condition in the "cretinoid" affection occasionally observed in middle-aged women. Med Chir Tr 1878;61:57–81
5. Beghi E, Delodovici ML, Bogliun G, et al. Hypothyroidism and polyneuropathy. J Neurol Neurosurg Psychiatry 1989;52:1420–1423
6. Scarpalezos S, Lygidakis C, Papageorgiou C, et al. Neural and muscular manifestations of hypothyroidism. Arch Neurol 1973;29:104–144
7. Fincham RW, Cape CA. Neuropathy in myxedema. A study of sensory nerve conduction in the upper extremities. Arch Neurol 1968;19:464–466
8. Misiunas A, Niepomniszcze H, Ravera B, et al. Peripheral neuropathy in subclinical hypothyroidism. Thyroid 1995;5:283–286
9. Dick DJ, Lane RJ, Nogues MA, Fawcett PR. Polyneuropathy in hypothyroidism. Postgrad Med J 1983;59: 518–519
10. Grabow JD, Chou SM. Thyrotropin hormone deficiency with a peripheral neuropathy. Arch Neurol 1968;19: 284–291
11. Meier C, Bischoff A. Polyneuropathy in hypothyroidism. Clinical and nerve biopsy study of 4 cases. J Neurol 1977;215:103–114

12. Pollard JD. Neuropathy in diseases of the thyroid and pituitary glands. *In:* Dyck PJ, Thomas PK, Griffin JW, et al., eds. Peripheral Neuropathy. Vol 2, 3rd ed. Philadelphia: WB Saunders, 1993:1266–1274

13. Murray IP, Simpson JA. Acroparaesthesia in myxoedema: a clinical and electromyographic study. Lancet 1958;1:1360–1363

14. Dyck PJ, Lambert EH. Polyneuropathy associated with hypothyroidism. J Neuropathol Exp Neurol 1970;29: 631–658

15. Laycock MA, Pascuzzi RM. The neuromuscular effects of hypothyroidism. Semin Neurol 1991;11:288–294

16. Pollard JD, McLeod JG, Honnibal TG, Verheijden MA. Hypothyroid polyneuropathy. Clinical, electrophysiological and nerve biopsy findings in two cases. J Neurol Sci 1982;53:461–471

17. Shirabe T, Tawara S, Terao A, Araki S. Myxoedematous polyneuropathy: a light and electron microscopic study of the peripheral nerve and muscle. J Neurol Neurosurg Psychiatry 1975;38:241–247

18. Torres CF, Moxley RT. Hypothyroid neuropathy and myopathy: clinical and electrodiagnostic longitudinal findings. J Neurol 1990;237:271–274

19. Nemni R, Bottacchi E, Fazio R, et al. Polyneuropathy in hypothyroidism: clinical, electrophysiological and morphological findings in four cases. J Neurol Neurosurg Psychiatry 1987;50:1454–1460

20. Rao SN, Katiyar BC, Nair KR, Misra S. Neuromuscular status in hypothyroidism. Acta Neurol Scand 1980;61: 167–177

21. Golding DN. Hypothyroidism presenting with musculoskeletal symptoms. Ann Rheum Dis 1970;29:10–14

22. Nickel SN, Frame B, Bebin J, et al. Myxedema neuropathy and myopathy. A clinical and pathologic study. Neurology 1961;11:125–137

23. Mohr PD, Heid H. Myeloneuropathy associated with hypothyroidism. Br Med J 1977;1:1005–1006

24. Laroche CM, Cairns T, Moxham J, Green M. Hypothyroidism presenting with respiratory muscle weakness. Am Rev Respir Dis 1988;138:472–474

25. Stevens JC, Beard CM, O'Fallon WM, Kurland LT. Conditions associated with carpal tunnel syndrome. Mayo Clin Proc 1992;67:541–548

26. Daniels GH, Martin JB. Neuroendocrine regulation and diseases of the anterior pituitary and hypothalamus. *In:* Isselbacher KJ, Braunwald E, Wilson JD, et al., eds. Harrison's Principles of Internal Medicine. Vol 2, 13th ed. New York: McGraw-Hill, 1994:1891–1918

27. Marie P, Marinesco G. Sur l'anatomie pathologique de l'acromégalie. Arch de Méd Expér et d'Anat Path 1891; 3:539–565

28. Lamberts SW. Acromegaly and its treatment. J Endocrinol 1997;155(Suppl):S49–S51

29. Stewart BM. The hypertrophic neuropathy of acromegaly: a rare neuropathy associated with acromegaly. Arch Neurol 1966;14:107–110

30. Jamal GA, Kerr DJ, McLellan AR, et al. Generalised peripheral nerve dysfunction in acromegaly: a study by conventional and novel neurophysiological techniques. J Neurol Neurosurg Psychiatry 1987;50:886–894

31. Sandbank U, Bornstein B, Najenson T. Acidophilic adenoma of the pituitary with polyneuropathy. J Neurol Neurosurg Psychiatry 1974;37:324–329

32. O'Duffy JD, Randall RV, MacCarty CS. Median neuropathy (carpal-tunnel syndrome) in acromegaly. A sign of endocrine overactivity. Ann Intern Med 1973;78: 379–383

33. Dinn JJ. Schwann cell dysfunction in acromegaly. J Clin Endocrinol Metab 1970;31:140–143

34. Dinn JJ, Dinn EI. Natural history of acromegalic peripheral neuropathy. Q J Med 1985;57:833–842

35. Lucey C. Neuromuscular involvement in pituitary gigantism. Br Med J 1972;3:49–50

36. Low PA, McLeod JG, Turtle JR, et al. Peripheral neuropathy in acromegaly. Brain 1974;97:139–152

37. Johnston AW. Acroparaesthesiae and acromegaly. Brit Med J 1960;1:1616–1618

38. Pickett JB, Layzer RB, Levin SR, et al. Neuromuscular complications of acromegaly. Neurology 1975;25:638–645

39. Khaleeli AA, Levy RD, Edwards RH, et al. The neuromuscular features of acromegaly: a clinical and pathological study. J Neurol Neurosurg Psychiatry 1984;47: 1009–1015

40. Giustina A, Barkan A, Casanueva FF, et al. Criteria for cure of acromegaly: a consensus statement. J Clin Endocrinol Metab 2000;85:526–529

41. Melmed S, Jackson I, Kleinberg D, Klibanski A. Current treatment guidelines for acromegaly. J Clin Endocrinol Metab 1998;83:2646–2652

42. Sheppard MC, Stewart PM. Treatment options for acromegaly. Metabolism 1996;45:63–64

43. Jenkins D, O'Brien I, Johnson A, et al. The Birmingham pituitary database: auditing the outcome of the treatment of acromegaly. Clin Endocrinol (Oxf) 1995;43: 517–522

44. Stewart PM, James RA. The future of somatostatin analogue therapy. Best Pract Res Clin Endocrinol Metab 1999;13:409–418

45. Newman CB. Medical therapy for acromegaly. Endocrinol Metab Clin North Am 1999;28:171–190

46. Turner HE, Wass JA. Modern approaches to treating acromegaly. QJM 2000;93:1–6

47. Utiger RD. Treatment of acromegaly. N Engl J Med 2000;342:1210–1211

48. Ross DA, Wilson CB. Results of transsphenoidal microsurgery for growth hormone-secreting pituitary adenoma in a series of 214 patients. J Neurosurg 1988;68:854–867

49. Laws ER, Vance ML, Thapar K. Pituitary surgery for the management of acromegaly. Horm Res 2000;53: 71–75

50. Barkan AL, Halasz I, Dornfeld KJ, et al. Pituitary irradiation is ineffective in normalizing plasma insulin-like growth factor I in patients with acromegaly. J Clin Endocrinol Metab 1997;82:3187–3191

51. Thalassinos NC, Tsagarakis S, Ioannides G, et al. Megavoltage pituitary irradiation lowers but seldom leads to safe GH levels in acromegaly: a long-term follow-up study. Eur J Endocrinol 1998;138:160–163

52. Plowman PN. Pituitary adenoma radiotherapy—when, who and how? Clin Endocrinol 1999;51:265–271

53. Parkinson C, Trainer PJ. Growth hormone receptor antagonists therapy for acromegaly. Best Pract Res Clin Endocrinol Metab 1999;13:419–430

54. Turner HE, Vadivale A, Keenan J, Wass JA. A comparison of lanreotide and octreotide LAR for treatment of acromegaly. Clin Endocrinol (Oxf) 1999;51:275–280

55. Abs R, Verhelst J, Maiter D, et al. Cabergoline in the treatment of acromegaly: a study in 64 patients. J Clin Endocrinol Metab 1998;83:374–378

56. Flogstad AK, Halse J, Grass P, et al. A comparison of octreotide, bromocriptine, or a combination of both drugs in acromegaly. J Clin Endocrinol Metab 1994;79: 461–465

57. Trainer PJ, Drake WM, Katznelson L, et al. Treatment of acromegaly with the growth hormone-receptor antagonist pegvisomant. N Engl J Med 2000;342:1171–1177

189 Multiple Endocrine Neoplasia, Type 2B

J Aidan Carney

Overview

Multiple endocrine neoplasia type 2 (MEN 2) is an inherited multitumoral syndrome that has three subtypes: (1) MEN 2A, medullary thyroid carcinoma (MTC), pheochromocytoma, and parathyroid adenoma or hyperplasia; (2) MEN 2B, MTC, pheochromocytoma, ganglioneuromatosis, and various skeletal and connective tissue abnormalities; and (3) familia MTC.

Patients with MEN 2B have a striking facies because of labial enlargement and apparent eyelid eversion, and a marfanoid habitus.[1] The unusual appearance (Figure 189.1) was described by Wagenmann[2] in 1922 and later meticulously detailed by Bazex and Dupré.[3] However, it was not until 1966 that the significance of the physiognomy, namely, its association with two potentially lethal neoplasms (MTC and pheochromocytoma), was recognized by Williams and Pollock.[4]

The designation "MEN 2B" arose as follows. By 1968, it was apparent that there were two distinct familial multiple endocrine neoplasia syndromes. The first one, described by Wermer,[5] was characterized by pituitary, parathyroid, and pancreatic islet tumors; the second, reported by Sipple,[6] included MTC, pheochromocytoma, and parathyroid hyperplasia. To emphasize that these associations were genetically distinct (it had been speculated that they might be related because parathryoid disease occurred in both), Steiner and coworkers[7] suggested that the Wermer and Sipple tumor combinations be designated "multiple endocrine neoplasia type 1 (MEN 1)" and "multiple endocrine neoplasia type 2 (MEN 2)," respectively. Most patients with MEN 2 had a normal appearance, but a small proportion (those discussed in this chapter) had the unusual facial and body appearance mentioned above. To emphasize that the syndromes were genetically different, although they shared the same major endocrine tumors (MTC and pheochromocytoma), Chong and colleagues[8] suggested that the disorders be designated "MEN 2A" and "MEN 2B," the latter referring to the patients with the unusual appearance.

Features

Multiple endocrine neoplasia 2B has a worldwide distribution. The number of sporadic and familial cases is about equal. The disorder is recognizable at a young age because of its striking phenotype. It is due to germline mutation in the *RET* proto-oncogene, which is located in the pericentromeric region of chromosome 10, band q11.2.[9] This gene encodes a member of the receptor tyrosine kinase family of transmembrane receptors. The mutation involves substitution of a threonine for methionine residue in exon 16 (codon 918). The disorder is transmitted as an autosomal dominant trait with parent-of-origin effects.[10] Study of apparent de novo cases has shown that the new mutations are always of male parental origin.[10] The sex ratio in both patients with de novo MEN 2B and the offspring of males transmitting MEN 2B is distorted from the expected. Also, there appears to be a different susceptibility of the *RET* gene to mutation

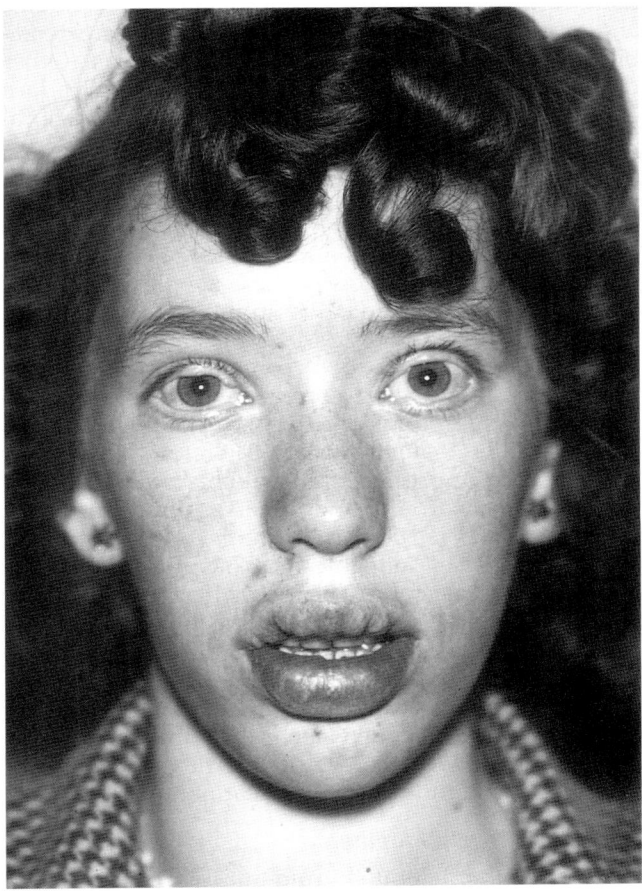

Figure 189.1 Facies of multiple endocrine neoplasia type 2B. Features are elongation of the face, the appearance of eyelid eversion due to thickening of the tarsal plates, a broad nasal root, and nodular (upper lip) and diffuse (lower lip) thickening of the lips. (From Robertson DM, Sizemore GW, Gordon H. Thickened corneal nerves as a manifestation of multiple endocrine neoplasia. Trans Am Acad Ophthalmol Otolaryngol 1975;79:772–787. By permission of Elsevier Science.)

in paternally and maternally derived DNA and a possible role for imprinting of the gene during development.

Face

Patients with MEN 2B have a striking appearance due to diffuse irregular thickening of the lips (bumpy lips), apparent eversion of the eyelids (creating a staring expression), dolichocephaly, and a broad nasal root.[1] Disfiguring deformity of the lips and eyelids may require correction by plastic surgery.

Skeleton

The syndrome includes a series of skeletal and connective tissue abnormalities very similar to those of Marfan syndrome: excessive limb length, loose-jointedness, scoliosis, and pectus excavatum.[1] However, patients with MEN 2B do not exhibit the characteristic ectopia lentis and defective ascending aortic tunica media characteristic of Marfan syndrome. A high-arched palate and prognathism are common. Redundancy and laxity of joint capsules, ligaments, tendons, and fasciae probably are responsible for hyperextensibility of joints, kyphoscoliosis, and hernias. Other common skeletal abnormalities are pes cavus, talipes equinovarus, and genu valgum. Slipped femoral capital epiphysis requires surgical treatment.

Alimentary tract ganglioneuromatosis

The fatal consequences of MEN 2B are usually due to metastatic MTC, less commonly to pheochromocytoma. However, diagnosis of these neoplasms usually is not made in de novo cases until both have become well established. The thyroid neoplasm does not ordinarily cause symptoms or become palpable until it is already metastatic, and correct interpretation of the paroxysmal symptoms produced by the pheochromocytoma tends to be delayed. Therefore, it is very important to appreciate that patients with MEN 2B have serious, chronic, and diverse alimentary tract manifestations, particularly severe constipation and megacolon, that antedate the symptoms of the endocrine neoplasms.[11] These manifestations usually are the presenting complaints of affected patients. The cause of the gastrointestinal disorders is unknown; alimentary tract ganglioneuromatosis has been shown to be associated with poor contractility of the colon, and the association between MTC and diarrhea is well known. Megacolon and diverticular disease of the colon may require surgical treatment.

Medullary thyroid carcinoma

Unilateral or bilateral thyroid masses in the upper portion of the lateral lobes are present in more than half the patients. The tumor cells secrete calcitonin, and the plasma levels of this substance are increased. The neoplasm spreads by the lymphatic and vascular routes. Cervical nodal involvement is common at primary surgery. Blood-borne metastasis occurs to liver, lungs, and bone. The carcinoma is usually but not invariably aggressive:[12,13] approximately 20% of patients die of it. Therefore, it is important to recog-

nize the abnormal phenotype to ensure prompt investigation for and treatment of MTC. Testing for the *RET* proto-oncogene provides an exquisitely sensitive molecular genetic diagnostic test for the tumor.[9] From birth, patients thought to have MEN 2B should have testing for the *RET* mutation.[14]

Treatment of MTC is total thyroidectomy with central lymph node dissection; the parathyroid glands should be preserved.[15] Locally recurrent tumor usually is treated surgically. There is no consensus on management of patients who have increased plasma levels of calcitonin after primary surgery but no clinically detectable disease. Only limited data are available on the effectiveness of chemotherapy for progressive metastasis. The patient's primary relatives should have screening tests for the *RET* mutation and be managed accordingly.

Pheochromocytoma

In at least 50% of patients with MEN 2B, pheochromocytoma is manifested between the ages of 15 and 40 years.[1] One half have the typical paroxysmal symptoms (headaches, sweating, palpitations, dizziness, nervousness, and tremor) and hypertension associated with catecholamine excess. The rest are asymptomatic and normotensive, and the tumor or tumors are detected by measurement of urinary catecholamine content during routine screening in suspected instances. About 10% of the patients die of the neoplasm (because of hypertensive or hypotensive crisis or cardiac arrhythmia). The 24-hour urinary excretion of total and fractionated catecholamines (epinephrine and norepinephrine) and their metabolites (vanillylmandelic acid and metanephrines) should be measured in patients with MEN 2B. The tumor is localized by computed tomography, magnetic resonance imaging, and metaiodobenzylguanidine I^{131} scan. Characteristically, in patients with symptoms, both adrenal glands are replaced by large multinodular pheochromocytomas. In asymptomatic patients, the abnormality may range from diffuse expansion of the medulla with preservation of the shape of the gland (medullary hyperplasia) to small (<1 cm) medullary nodules with or without diffuse enlargement of the medulla.

Treatment of pheochromocytoma is bilateral total adrenalectomy and excision of any extra-adrenal paraganglioma. Bilateral total adrenalectomy is recommended because of the frequency of bilateral adrenal involvement, the possibility of recurrent pheochromocytoma after subtotal adrenalectomy, and the occasional occurrence of malignant disease.[16]

Neurological manifestations

In addition to involvement of the autonomic nervous system (ganglioneuromatosis) mentioned above, somatic motor and sensory neurons may be affected in the syndrome.[1] The nervous system of four Mayo Clinic patients with the syndrome was examined. The results were varied: one patient was poorly muscled but had normal findings on neurological examination; one other had diffuse weakness of all skeletal muscles and hypoactive deep tendon reflexes; another patient had poorly developed musculature and distal muscle weakness; and still another patient had a sensory neuropathy that affected the lower limbs. Similarly inconsistent neurological findings have been described in the literature, ranging from normal findings on examination, through the presence of mild lower limb sensory abnormality, to a decrease or absence of deep tendon reflexes. The nerves in the cubital fossa and neck were enlarged in two patients. A sural nerve biopsy specimen from a patient showed normal myelinated fibers and degeneration and regeneration of unmyelinated nerves, a process that was thought to be responsible for the increase in the size of the nerve. Findings at postmortem examination indicate that certain symptoms can be attributed to a characteristic plaque of tissue composed of hyperplastic, interlacing bands of schwann cells and myelinated fibers overlying the posterior columns of the spinal cord. There is no treatment for neural abnormality.

References

1. Carney JA, Sizemore GW, Hayles AB. Multiple endocrine neoplasia, type 2b. Pathobiol Annu 1978;8:105–153

2. Wagenmann A. Multiple Neurome des Auges und der Zunge. Berl Versamml Dtsch Ophthalmol Gesellsch München 1922;43:282–285

3. Bazex A, Dupré A. Neuromes myéliniques muqueux à localisation centro-faciale et laryngée; neuromes des lèvres, de la langue; des paupières, des narines, du larynx: entité nouvelle? Ann Dermatol Syph Par 1958;85:613–641

4. Williams ED, Pollock DJ. Multiple mucosal neuromata with endocrine tumours: a syndrome allied to von Recklinghausen's disease. J Pathol Bacteriol 1966;91:71–80

5. Wermer P. Genetic aspects of adenomatosis of endocrine glands. Am J Med 1954;16:363–371

6. Sipple JH. The association of pheochromocytoma with carcinoma of the thyroid gland. Am J Med 1961;31:163–166

7. Steiner AL, Goodman AD, Powers SR. Study of a kindred with pheochromocytoma, medullary thyroid carcinoma, hyperparathyroidism and Cushing's disease: multiple endocrine neoplasia, type 2. Medicine (Baltimore) 1968;47:371–409

8. Chong GC, Beahrs OH, Sizemore GW, Woolner LH. Medullary carcinoma of the thyroid gland. Cancer 1975;35:695–704

9. Heshmati HM, Gharib H, Khosla S, et al. Genetic testing in medullary thyroid carcinoma syndromes: mutation types and clinical significance. Mayo Clin Proc 1997;72:430–436

10. Carlson KM, Bracamontes J, Jackson CE, et al. Parent-of-origin effects in multiple endocrine neoplasia, type 2B. Am J Hum Genet 1994;55:1076–1082

11. Carney JA, Go VL, Sizemore GW, Hayles AB. Alimentary-tract ganglioneuromatosis. A major component of the syndrome of multiple endocrine neoplasia, type 2b. N Engl J Med 1976;295:1287–1291

12. Sizemore GW, Carney JA, Gharib H, Capen CC. Multiple endocrine neoplasia type 2B: eighteen-year follow-up of a four-generation family. Henry Ford Hosp Med J 1992;40:236–244

13. Vasen HF, van der Feltz M, Raue F, et al. The natural course of multiple endocrine neoplasia type IIb. A study of 18 cases. Arch Intern Med 1992;152:1250–1252

14. Heshmati HM, Gharib H, van Heerden JA, Sizemore GW. Advances and controversies in the diagnosis and management of medullary thyroid carcinoma. Am J Med 1997;103:60–69

15. Giuffrida D, Gharib H. Current diagnosis and management of medullary thyroid carcinoma. Ann Oncol 1998;9:695–701

16. Dyck PJ, Carney JA, Sizemore GW, et al. Multiple endocrine neoplasia, type 2b: phenotype recognition; neurological features and their pathological basis. Ann Neurol 1979;6:302–314

190 Neuropathies in Liver Disease and Chronic Renal Failure

E Peter Bosch

Peripheral neuropathies in liver disease

Peripheral neuropathies may develop as a direct consequence of acute or chronic liver disease (Table 190.1). These disorders include cryoglobulinemic neuropathy linked to hepatitis C virus infection, neuropathies associated with end-stage liver disease, primary biliary cirrhosis, and vitamin E deficiency in chronic cholestatic liver disease. Viral hepatitis types A, B, and C have been reported as antecedent infections in Guillain–Barré syndrome and cranial neuropathies in anecdotal reports.[1,2] Isolated cases of chronic inflammatory demyelinating polyradiculoneuropathy have been observed in chronic hepatitis B and as a complication after orthotopic liver transplantation.[3,4] There is no need to change the treatment plan (plasmapheresis or immune globulin infusions) for these immune-mediated polyneuropathies because of the underlying liver disease. Systemic disorders affecting both the liver and the peripheral nervous system are discussed elsewhere. Alcoholic liver disease frequently coexists in patients with alcoholic neuropathy. Hepatitis B antigen is found in one-third of patients with polyarteritis nodosa.

Hepatitis C virus infection and mixed cryoglobulinemia

Hepatitis C virus (HCV) infection is associated with various extrahepatic manifestations, including mixed cryoglobulinemia, glomerulonephritis, and porphyria cutanea tarda.[5] Mixed cryoglobulins are cold-precipitable serum proteins consisting of complexes of IgG and monoclonal IgM or polyclonal IgM with rheumatoid factor activity. The detection of anti-HCV antibodies and HCV RNA in serum and cryoprecipitate of most patients with previously so-called essential mixed cryoglobulinemia firmly establishes a causal role for HCV in the formation of cryoglobulins.[6–8] The HCV infection of peripheral blood B-lymphocytes is thought to promote B-cell proliferation and production of immunoglobulins, including rheumatoid factor and cryoglobulins. The cryoglobulins induce cold-dependent activation of complement and hypocomplementemia. This is followed by immune complex-mediated vessel damage leading to vasculitis.[9]

Mixed cryoglobulinemia is a systemic disease characterized by purpura and cutaneous vasculitis, arthralgias, renal dysfunction, and peripheral nerve involvement (Figure 190.1). The reported prevalence of peripheral neuropathy in mixed cryoglobulinemia varies from 37% to 57%, using electrophysiological criteria for confirmation.[10,11] The most common presentation is a painful sensory or sensorimotor polyneuropathy or, less often, mononeuropathy multiplex.[8,10,12] Nerve biopsy specimens confirm necrotizing vasculitis or perivascular inflammation affecting small-sized epineurial vessels together with multifocal or global myelinated fiber loss and acute axonal degeneration.[13] The presence of low serum levels of complement and the demonstration of immunoglobulin deposits of the same composition as the circulating cryoglobulins in the walls of affected vessels suggest

Table 190.1	Neuropathies in liver disease	
Disorder	**Neuropathy**	**Treatment**
Viral hepatitis A, B, C	AIDP, CIDP	IVIG, plasmapheresis
HCV-related mixed cryoglobulinemia	Sensory or sensorimotor polyneuropathy, mononeuropathy multiplex	Plasmapheresis, corticosteroids, cyclophosphamide Interferon alfa and ribavirin
Chronic liver disease	Sensory neuropathy, cardiovagal dysautonomia	Liver transplantation
Primary biliary cirrhosis	Xanthomatous neuropathy, sensory neuronopathy	Plasmapheresis ?
Vitamin E deficiency in cholestatic liver disease	Sensory neuropathy or spinocerebellar syndrome	Vitamin E, TPGS

AIDP, acute inflammatory demyelinating polyradiculoneuropathy; CIDP, chronic inflammatory polyradiculoneuropathy; HCV, hepatitis C virus; IVIG, intravenous immunoglobulin; TPGS, tocopherol polyethylene 1000-glycol succinate.

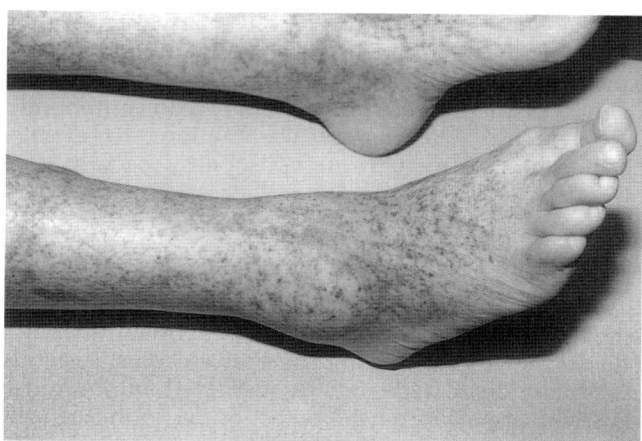

Figure 190.1 Purpura of legs of woman with painful sensorimotor polyneuropathy associated with hepatitis C virus-related mixed cryoglobulinemia. (See color plate section.)

that cryoprecipitable immune complexes are responsible for the disease manifestations.

Treatment There are no clear guidelines to treat HCV-related cryoglobulinemic neuropathy supported by class 1 evidence (e.g. evidence provided by well-designed randomized controlled trials). This is not the case for mixed cryoglobulinemia and chronic hepatitis C. Interferon alfa (given at a dose of 3 megaunits subcutaneously 3 times weekly for 6 months) improves the clinical manifestations of cryoglobulinemia, normalizes the serum level of complement, reduces cryoglobulins, and eliminates HCV RNA levels in 60% of patients (class 1 evidence).[14] However, after the end of this treatment relapse rates are high, up to 85%, and long-term responses are confined to patients who achieve sustained elimination of the HCV RNA.

A more sustained virologic response is seen when patients with chronic hepatitis C are treated with the combination regimen of interferon alfa and ribavirin for 48 weeks compared with interferon alone (class 1 evidence).[15,16] A new formulation called "peginterferon alfa," produced by the addition of a polyethylene glycol molecule to standard interferon, has the advantage of sustained absorption, a slower rate of clearance, a longer half-life, and a protracted antiviral effect permitting once weekly dosing. Peginterferon alfa-2a (180 μg given subcutaneously once a week for 12 months) offers significantly better virologic and biochemical responses than unmodified interferon in patients with chronic hepatitis C.[17] There is reasonable expectation that the combination of peginterferon and ribavirin will further enhance responses, and these studies are under way. An international consensus conference resulted in published guidelines for the treatment of hepatitis C.[18] Uncontrolled case studies have suggested that interferon alfa alone may be efficacious in the treatment of cryoglobulinemic neuropathy, although most patients received either preceding or concurrent immunosuppressive therapy, and treatment responses were poorly defined.[8,12,19,20] One open clinical trial of interferon in cryoglobulinemic

neuropathy reported significant improvement in neuropathic symptoms compared with controls given deflazacort, but differences in nerve conduction variables between the groups were not significant.[21] Other reports have warned about acute worsening of polyneuropathy following initiation of interferon therapy without immunosuppression.[22]

Currently, the treatment of cryoglobulinemic neuropathy rests on evidence provided by expert opinion and uncontrolled reports (i.e. class 3 evidence; Table 190.2). Patients with biopsy-proven vasculitis and progressive severe neurological deficits initially require immunosuppression with either oral cyclophosphamide (2 mg/kg body weight daily) or intravenous cyclophosphamide pulses (0.5–1.0 g/m² every 3 weeks) and corticosteroids.[9,23] Therapeutic plasmapheresis (one calculated plasma volume on alternate days for 2 to 3 weeks) has been recommended for the removal of cryoglobulins during acute exacerbations with rapidly progressive neurological deficits or glomerulonephritis.[24] When clinical remission is achieved, immunosuppressive therapy is tapered, and specific treatment directed against the underlying HCV infection is offered to patients without contraindications to interferon or ribavirin. Before antiviral therapy is commenced, the patient should be referred to a hepatologist for evaluation.

The current recommended treatment regimen consists of interferon alfa (3 megaunits subcutaneously 3 times weekly) in combination with ribavirin (1000–1200 mg daily) for six to twelve months.[18] It is expected that peginterferon alfa will replace unmodified interferon after it has received approval and becomes available. In patients with milder forms of neuropathy, corticosteroids are given without

Table 190.2   Treatment for hepatitis C virus (HCV)-related mixed cryoglobulinemic neuropathy

Supportive
  Avoid cold exposure
  Modify high risk behavior (alcohol, intravenous drug use)
Antiviral
  Consult with hepatologist before treatment
  Obtain serum HCV-RNA level, HIV test, pregnancy test in women, liver biopsy
  Interferon alfa, 3 MU subcutaneously 3 times weekly,* plus riboviriin† for 6 to 12 months
  Peginterferon alfa-2a, 180 μg, subcutaneously once weekly for 12 months†
Immunosuppressive or removal of cryoglobulins
  Plasmapheresis, 3 times weekly for 2 to 3 weeks
  Cyclophosphamide, intravenously 0.5 to 1 g/m² every 3 weeks
  Cyclophosphamide, orally 2 mg/kg daily
  Methylprednisolone, intravenously 500–1000 mg for 3 days, then taper to oral prednisone
  Prednisone, orally 60–80 mg daily, then taper

HIV, human immunodeficiency virus.
*Class 1 evidence for treatment of cryoglobulinemia associated with HCV.[14] †Class 1 evidence for treatment of chronic hepatitis C.[15,17]

cytotoxic agents in combination with interferon or ribavirin (or both).[9] Avoiding exposure to cold is helpful in preventing cutaneous manifestations of cryoglobulinemia. Prospective studies are needed to determine the efficacy and safety of interferon or peginterferon and ribavirin combination therapy in cryoglobulinemic neuropathy.

Chronic liver disease

Peripheral nerve dysfunction is frequently reported in the course of chronic liver disease. Several studies that described relatively small, selected populations of patients with long-standing liver disease found clinical evidence of a mild, predominantly sensory neuropathy in 8% to 68% of patients.[25–29] Electrophysiological abnormalities, consisting mainly of decreased sensory nerve action potentials and mild slowing of motor conduction studies, were present in up to 87% of these patients. The highest frequency of neuropathy by clinical (75%) or electrophysiological criteria (87%) was found among patients who were candidates for liver transplantation for end-stage liver disease.[30] The neuropathy usually is not disabling and often clinically inapparent. Paresthesia in the feet, distal loss of vibratory sense, increased vibratory thresholds of the hallux, and loss of ankle reflexes are the most common findings.

Neuropathological studies of sural nerve specimens show mainly low-grade abnormalities of demyelination and remyelination in teased nerve fiber preparations and a mild decrease in myelinated fiber density.[26,28] Prospective studies of autonomic function have documented a high incidence of autonomic dysfunction in patients with chronic liver disease. Reports have described abnormal cardiovagal reflex tests in 45% of patients with both alcohol-related and non-alcoholic liver disease, with an even higher incidence of 67% among those awaiting liver transplantation.[31–33] Abnormal heart rate variability to deep breathing, in response to the Valsalva maneuver, and abnormal heart rate response to standing were more common than orthostatic hypotension or impaired distal sweating, indicating mainly parasympathetic dysfunction. The prevalence of vagal cardiovascular dysregulation increased with advanced liver disease irrespective of its cause. The presence of autonomic neuropathy boded poorly for the affected patient because a five-fold increase in mortality (30% versus 6% in subjects with normal autonomic studies) was noted over four years of observation.[32] Among patients awaiting liver transplantation, 27% of those with autonomic dysfunction died during a 14-month waiting period, but none without autonomic neuropathy died.[33] The sensory and autonomic neuropathy is believed to be related directly to metabolic changes associated with chronic liver disease, although the precise mechanism is not understood. Alcohol-related liver disease and hemochromatosis may be additional risk factors for the development of neuropathy.

Treatment   No specific treatment is available for the mild neuropathy associated with chronic liver disease. Patients with advanced liver disease awaiting transplantation should be tested for autonomic dysfunction. Consideration should be given for early liver transplantation for patients with autonomic involvement.[33] Preliminary observations have suggested that recovery from neuropathy occurs after orthotopic liver transplantation.[30,34]

Primary biliary cirrhosis

"Primary biliary cirrhosis" is a chronic liver disease that affects mainly middle-aged women and is characterized by inflammatory destruction of intrahepatic bile ducts, which leads to progressive cholestasis and, eventually, liver cirrhosis.[35] A suspected autoimmune cause is supported by the detection of antimitochondrial antibodies and the frequent association with autoimmune diseases. Among the associated autoimmune conditions are sicca syndrome (found in 32% to 67% of patients), followed by Raynaud phenomenon, polyarteritis, scleroderma, and thyroid disorders.[36,37]

The few studies that have been concerned with neuropathy in primary biliary cirrhosis have been limited to case reports or small series of patients. Thomas and Walker[38] described a painful, dysesthetic sensory neuropathy that developed in three women who had advanced primary biliary cirrhosis, strikingly increased serum lipid levels, and cutaneous xanthomas. Sural nerve biopsy specimens from all three women showed perineurial and endoneurial xanthomatous deposits. The authors used the term "xanthomatous neuropathy" and attributed the neuropathy directly to the xanthomatous infiltration of the perineurium. Similar clinical cases of primary biliary cirrhosis with hyperlipidemia and cutaneous xanthomas but without morphological confirmation have been reported. The painful dysesthesia of these patients seemed to respond to plasmapheresis and a decrease in serum lipid levels.[39]

Another distinctive sensory neuronopathy unrelated to lipid abnormalities was described in two women with minimal liver disease.[40,41] Both women presented with an asymmetrical large-fiber sensory syndrome, with loss of proprioception, sensory ataxia, areflexia, and absence of sensory nerve action potentials. Sural nerve biopsy specimens from both women demonstrated loss of large myelinated fibers, which was attributed to an autoimmune process affecting dorsal root ganglia. The prevalence of associated autoimmune disorders is high in primary biliary cirrhosis, most notably keratoconjunctivitis sicca and Sjögren syndrome, which in turn is linked to similar sensory neuropathies.

Clinically significant deficiencies of fat-soluble vitamins A, K, and E are uncommon except in patients with advanced disease. Even though low serum levels of vitamin E were found in 44% of patients with primary biliary cirrhosis, only a few patients with extremely low vitamin E levels had developed a mild sensorimotor neuropathy.[42] A mild or subclinical neuropathy may be more common in primary biliary cirrhosis than the literature seems to indicate. A prospective study using standard autonomic tests and peripheral nerve conduction studies found that 63% of 27 patients with primary biliary cirrhosis had vagal cardiovascular autonomic dysfunction and 41% had minimal symptoms, signs, and neurophysiological abnormalities consistent with neuropathy.[43] The neuropathy correlated with the degree of liver damage but was not associated with either hyperlipidemia or vitamin E deficiency.

Treatment The literature provides no guidance for the management of these rare neuropathies. The underlying disease process in primary biliary cirrhosis can be ameliorated with ursodiol, colchicine, and methotrexate. The only treatment that improves outcome is liver transplantation.[35] Immunosuppressive agents may be justified for patients with disabling sensory neuronopathies associated with sicca syndrome. Glucocorticosteroids should be used with caution because they may worsen underlying osteoporosis. In documented vitamin E deficiency, oral replacement is adequate. It is not known whether therapeutic plasma exchange relieves the painful dysesthesia of xanthomatous neuropathy.

Vitamin E deficiency in cholestatic liver disease

Significant vitamin E deficiency is seen during intestinal fat malabsorption, as occurs in cholestatic liver disease, cystic fibrosis, following extensive small bowel resection, and the inherited disorder of abetalipoproteinemia.[44] The failure to incorporate α-tocopherol in very low-density lipoprotein in the liver is caused by mutations of the α-tocopherol transfer protein gene and leads to low serum levels of vitamin E in the absence of lipid malabsorption in familial isolated vitamin E deficiency.[45] During cholestatic liver disease, bile acid concentrations may fall below the critical level necessary for intestinal intraluminal solubilization, causing malabsorption of fat-soluble vitamins. Prolonged vitamin E deficiency irrespective of its cause may lead to a spinocerebellar syndrome, with large fiber sensory neuropathy, areflexia, proprioceptive loss, ataxia, ophthalmoplegia, and pigmentary retinopathy.[46] In children with cholestatic liver disease, the neurological disorder begins within the first two years of life, and, if left untreated, incapacitating truncal and limb ataxia usually develops by age 10. In adults with chronic cholestasis, it may take two years to deplete vitamin E stores and another five to 10 years for neurological signs to develop.

Vitamin E deficiency is established by low fasting serum levels of vitamin E ($<5\,\mu g/mL$). The ratio of serum vitamin E to total serum lipids has been adopted as a more accurate reflection of the vitamin E status during cholestatic states.[44] Low vitamin E content in sural nerve specimens has been found to precede any morphological change in patients with symptomatic vitamin E deficiency.[47] The mechanism by which vitamin E deficiency causes neurodegeneration is not known, but it may be related to impaired antioxidant defense.

Treatment For all patients with documented vitamin E deficiency, vitamin E supplementation is indicated regardless of the cause. Standard oral forms of vitamin E are given in doses starting at 400 mg twice daily and increased to 100–200 mg/kg daily. If no absorption can be demonstrated after large doses of standard vitamin E, a water-soluble form, tocopheryl polyethylene 1000-glycol succinate (TPGS) in doses of 15–30 IU/kg daily, is recommended.[48] The toxicity of vitamin E is minimal, although large doses in patients who are receiving warfarin have been associated with increased bleeding. Supplementation may result in neurological improvement or cessation of further deterioration.

Neuropathies in chronic renal failure

Uremic polyneuropathy develops in 60% of patients with end-stage renal disease who require dialysis. Most patients have a mild sensory or subclinical neuropathy detected with electrophysiological criteria.[49] Severe uremic neuropathy has become less frequent because of earlier dialysis treatment and renal transplantation. Detailed descriptions of the clinical and electrophysiological aspects of uremic polyneuropathy have been published.[49–53] The main symptoms are restless legs, leg cramps, distal paresthesia, numbness, and burning feet. Neurological signs include distal sensory loss (especially for vibratory sensation), abnormal reflexes, and symmetrical toe extensor weakness. Occasionally, a rapidly progressive, predominantly motor polyneuropathy may develop during the early stages of dialysis.[54] Such a fulminant, severe neuropathy is also seen in the setting of concurrent critical illness or diabetes mellitus.[55,56]

Decreased nerve conduction velocities, prolonged distal latencies, and low amplitudes of muscle and sensory compound potentials often precede symptoms or signs. When the creatinine clearance is less than 10 mL/min, 50% of patients have been found to have abnormal nerve conduction velocities.[51] Needle electromyography shows denervation in distal leg muscles only in moderate or severe cases. Nerve conduction abnormalities persist regardless of the type and duration of dialysis treatment.[51,57,58] The morphological changes of uremic neuropathy include loss of large myelinated axons and segmental demyelination. Morphometric investigations have led to the conclusion that the associated segmental demyelination is due to axonal atrophy.[59,60]

The precise cause of uremic neuropathy is unknown, although several potential neurotoxins, for example, guanidine compounds, *myo*-inositol, parathyroid hormone, and middle molecular weight substances, accumulate in end-stage renal disease.[61]

Treatment

Moderate or severe polyneuropathy in patients receiving chronic dialysis has become rare as a result of earlier initiation of treatment and improved techniques of hemodialysis that use more biocompatible dialyzer membranes and high-flux dialyzers.[62] Attention should be given to avoid or to recognize the

Table 190.3 Mononeuropathies in end-stage renal disease

Type	Mechanism	Treatment
Compression neuropathies: Ulnar nerve at elbow Common peroneal nerve at fibular head	Compression by poor positioning, bedrest	Avoid by proper positioning
Carpal tunnel syndrome	Local edema due to shunt β_2M-associated amyloidosis on long-term hemodialysis	Carpal tunnel release
Ischemic monomelic neuropathy	Acute ischemia of distal median, ulnar, and radial nerves from proximal shunt	Ligation of AV shunt

AV, arteriovenous; β_2M, β_2-microglobulin.

contribution of drugs such as colchicine or nitrofurantoin, which are potentially neurotoxic in renal insufficiency. Numerous investigations have been conducted to assess the long-term effects of hemodialysis on peripheral nerve function. A consensus has emerged that chronic hemodialysis stabilizes uremic neuropathy in the majority of patients. Manipulating the frequency or duration of dialysis may not alter its course.[51,57,58,63] A change from conventional cellulose polymer to synthetic polymer dialyzer membranes, which improve the clearance of middle molecular weight substances, had no effect on nerve conduction velocities in asymptomatic patients.[64] However, Bolton and colleagues[56] reported that three of four patients with subacute motor neuropathy associated with diabetes had improvement by switching from conventional to high-flux hemodialysis.

Chronic ambulatory peritoneal dialysis provides no advantage over hemodialysis.[65] Successful renal transplantation consistently results in clinical, electrophysiological, and structural recovery over a period of three to 12 months.[52,53,66,67] Improvement in nerve conduction velocities may be seen within days after transplantation in asymptomatic to mild cases.[68] However, transplantation seems to have little effect on the course of the neuropathy in diabetic patients with end-stage renal disease. In a well-conducted comparison study, the neuropathy failed to improve in diabetic patients not only after renal transplantation but also in a group of diabetics who had combined renal and pancreas transplants.[69] More recently, investigators reported improvement in nerve conduction velocities but, more importantly, improvement in the quality of life of six patients with successful combined organ transplantation.[70]

Mononeuropathies in end-stage renal disease

Chronic renal failure and the frequently associated malnutrition render peripheral nerves susceptible to compression palsies of the ulnar nerve at the elbow and the fibular nerve at the fibular head (Table 190.3). Proper positioning and padding of pressure points in bedridden patients may avoid such complications. Carpal tunnel syndrome is the most commonly reported compression neuropathy, developing in more than 20% of patients undergoing hemodialysis.[49] Nerve compression from local edema secondary to the forearm arteriovenous shunts and ischemia from a fistula-induced vascular steal syndrome are likely mechanisms in the early course of dialysis. Patients receiving long-term hemodialysis may develop carpal tunnel syndrome because of the deposition of β_2-microglobulin-associated amyloid in the carpal tunnel.[71] Decompression, with sectioning of the flexor retinaculum, is effective.

Ischemic monomelic neuropathy, an acute complication of a more proximal shunt between the cephalic vein and brachial artery, occurs predominantly in diabetic patients with concomitant peripheral vascular disease. It is characterized by abrupt, painful sensory loss of the affected hand and weakness of median-, ulnar-, and radial-innervated distal muscles. Early recognition is critical because prompt ligation of the arteriovenous fistula is required to avoid permanent neurological deficit.[72]

References

1. Tabor E. Guillain–Barré syndrome and other neurologic syndromes in hepatitis A, B, and non-A, non-B. J Med Virol 1987;21:207–216
2. Varona L, Sagasta A, Martin-Gonzalvez JA, et al. Cranial neuropathies and liver failure due to hepatitis A. Neurology 1996;46:1774–1775
3. Inoue A, Tsukada N, Koh CS, Yanagisawa N. Chronic relapsing demyelinating polyneuropathy associated with hepatitis B infection. Neurology 1987;37:1663–1666
4. Taylor BV, Wijdicks EF, Poterucha JJ, Weisner RH. Chronic inflammatory demyelinating polyneuropathy complicating liver transplantation. Ann Neurol 1995;38:828–831
5. Gordon SC. Extrahepatic manifestations of hepatitis C. Dig Dis 1996;14:157–168
6. Agnello V, Chung RT, Kaplan LM. A role for hepatitis C virus infection in type II cryoglobulinemia. N Engl J Med 1992;327:1490–1495
7. Authier FJ, Pawlotsky JM, Viard JP, et al. High incidence of hepatitis C virus infection in patients with cryoglobulinemic neuropathy. Ann Neurol 1993;34:749–750
8. Apartis E, Leger JM, Musset L, et al. Peripheral neu-

ropathy associated with essential mixed cryoglobulinaemia: a role for hepatitis C virus infection? J Neurol Neurosurg Psychiatry 1996;60:661–666

9. Lamprecht P, Gause A, Gross WL. Cryoglobulinemic vasculitis. Arthritis Rheum 1999;42:2507–2516

10. Gemignani F, Pavesi G, Fiocchi A, et al. Peripheral neuropathy in essential mixed cryoglobulinaemia. J Neurol Neurosurg Psychiatry 1992;55:116–120

11. Zaltron S, Puoti M, Liberini P, et al. High prevalence of peripheral neuropathy in hepatitis C virus infected patients with symptomatic and asymptomatic cryoglobulinaemia. Ital J Gastroenterol Hepatol 1998;30: 391–395

12. Tembl JI, Ferrer JM, Sevilla MT, et al. Neurologic complications associated with hepatitis C virus infection. Neurology 1999;53:861–864

13. Nemni R, Corbo M, Fazio R, et al. Cryoglobuinaemic neuropathy. A clinical, morphological and immunocytochemical study of eight cases. Brain 1988;111:541–552

14. Misiani R, Bellavita P, Fenili D, et al. Interferon alfa-2a therapy in cryoglobulinemia associated with hepatitis C virus. N Engl J Med 1994;330:751–756

15. McHutchison JG, Gordon SC, Schiff ER, et al. Interferon alfa-2b alone or in combination with ribavirin as initial treatment for chronic hepatitis C. Hepatitis Interventional Therapy Group. N Engl J Med 1998;339: 1485–1492

16. Poynard T, Marcellin P, Lee SS, et al. Randomised trial of interferon alpha-2b plus ribavirin for 48 weeks or for 24 weeks versus interferon alpha-2b plus placebo for 48 weeks for treatment of chronic infection with hepatitis C virus. International Hepatitis Interventional Therapy Group (IHIT). Lancet 1998;352:1426–1432

17. Zeuzem S, Feinman SV, Rasenack J, et al. Peginterferon alfa-2a in patients with chronic hepatitis C. N Engl J Med 2000;343:1666–1672

18. European Association for the Study of the Liver. EASL International Consensus Conference on Hepatitis C. Paris, 26–28, February 1999, Consensus Statement. J Hepatol 1999;30:956–961

19. Khella SL, Frost S, Hermann GA, et al. Hepatitis C infection, cryoglobulinemia, and vasculitic neuropathy. Treatment with interferon alfa: case report and literature review. Neurology 1995;45:407–411

20. David WS, Peine C, Schlesinger P, Smith SA. Nonsystemic vasculitic mononeuropathy multiplex, cryoglobulinemia, and hepatitis C. Muscle Nerve 1996;19: 1596–1602

21. Ghini M, Mascia MT, Gentilini M, Mussini C. Treatment of cryoglobulinemic neuropathy with alpha-interferon. Neurology 1996;46:588–589

22. Scelsa SN, Herskovitz S, Reichler B. Treatment of mononeuropathy multiplex in hepatitis C virus and cryoglobulinemia. Muscle Nerve 1998;21:1526–1529

23. Siami GA, Siami FS. Plasmapheresis and paraproteinemia: cryoprotein-induced diseases, monoclonal gammopathy, Waldenström's macroglobulinemia, hyperviscosity syndrome, multiple myeloma, light chain disease, and amyloidosis. Ther Apher 1999;3:8–19

24. Misiani R, Bellavita P. Mixed cryoglobulinaemia: a guide to drug treatment. Clin Immunother 1996;5: 115–121

25. Seneviratne KN, Peiris OA. Peripheral nerve function in chronic liver disease. J Neurol Neurosurg Psychiatry 1970;33:609–614

26. Knill-Jones RP, Goodwill CJ, Dayan AD, Williams R. Peripheral neuropathy in chronic liver disease: clinical, electrodiagnostic, and nerve biopsy findings. J Neurol Neurosurg Psychiatry 1972;35:22–30

27. Kardel T, Nielsen VK. Hepatic neuropathy. A clinical and electrophysiological study. Acta Neurol Scand 1974;50:513–526

28. Chari VR, Katiyar BC, Rastogi BL, Bhattacharya SK. Neuropathy in hepatic disorders. A clinical, electrophysiological and histopathological appraisal. J Neurol Sci 1977;31:93–111

29. Fierro B, Raimondo D, Castiglione MG, et al. Peripheral nerve involvement in chronic liver disease. Clinical and electrophysiological study. Ital J Neurol Sci 1986;7: 589–590

30. Iani C, Tisone G, Loberti M, et al. Clinical and neurophysiological evidence of polyneuropathy in liver transplant candidates: preliminary report. Transplant Proc 1999;31:404–405

31. Thuluvath PJ, Triger DR. Autonomic neuropathy and chronic liver disease. Q J Med 1989;72:737–747

32. Hendrickse MT, Thuluvath PJ, Triger DR. Natural history of autonomic neuropathy in chronic liver disease. Lancet 1992;339:1462–1464

33. Fleckenstein JF, Frank S, Thuluvath PJ. Presence of autonomic neuropathy is a poor prognostic indicator in patients with advanced liver disease. Hepatology 1996; 23:471–475

34. Hockerstedt K, Kajaste S, Muuronen A, et al. Encephalopathy and neuropathy in end-stage liver disease before and after liver transplantation. J Hepatol 1992;16:31–37

35. Kaplan MM. Primary biliary cirrhosis. N Engl J Med 1996;335:1570–1580

36. Culp KS, Fleming CR, Duffy J, et al. Autoimmune associations in primary biliary cirrhosis. Mayo Clin Proc 1982;57:365–370

37. Zukowski TH, Jorgensen RA, Dickson ER, Lindor KD. Autoimmune conditions associated with primary biliary cirrhosis: response to ursodeoxycholic acid therapy. Am J Gastroenterol 1998;93:958–961

38. Thomas PK, Walker JG. Xanthomatous neuropathy in primary biliary cirrhosis. Brain 1965;88:1079–1088

39. Turnberg LA, Mahoney MP, Gleeson MH, et al. Plasmaphoresis and plasma exchange in the treatment of hyperlipaemia and xanthomatous neuropathy in patients with primary biliary cirrhosis. Gut 1972;13: 976–981

40. Charron L, Peyronnard JM, Marchand L. Sensory neuropathy associated with primary biliary cirrhosis. Histologic and morphometric studies. Arch Neurol 1980; 37:84–87

41. Illa I, Graus F, Ferrer I, Enriquez J. Sensory neuropathy as the initial manifestation of primary biliary cirrhosis. J Neurol Neurosurg Psychiatry 1989;52:1307

42. Jeffrey GP, Muller DP, Burroughs AK, et al. Vitamin E deficiency and its clinical significance in adults with primary biliary cirrhosis and other forms of chronic liver disease. J Hepatol 1987;4:307–317

43. Hendrickse MT, Triger DR. Autonomic and peripheral neuropathy in primary biliary cirrhosis. J Hepatol 1993;19:401–407

44. Sokol RJ. Fat-soluble vitamins and their importance in patients with cholestatic liver diseases. Gastroenterol Clin North Am 1994;23:673–705

45. Hentati A, Deng HX, Hung WY, et al. Human alpha-tocopherol transfer protein: gene structure and mutations in familial vitamin E deficiency. Ann Neurol 1996;39:295–300

46. Kayden HJ. The neurologic syndrome of vitamin E deficiency: a significant cause of ataxia. Neurology 1993;43:2167–2169

47. Traber MG, Sokol RJ, Ringel SP, et al. Lack of to-
    copherol in peripheral nerves of vitamin E-deficient
    patients with peripheral neuropathy. N Engl J Med
    1987;317:262–265
48. Sokol RJ, Heubi JE, Butler-Simon N, et al. Treatment of
    vitamin E deficiency during chronic childhood
    cholestasis with oral d-alpha-tocopheryl polyethylene
    glycol-1000 succinate. Gastroenterology 1987;93:
    975–985
49. Bolton CF, Young GB. Neurological Complications of
    Renal Disease. Boston: Butterworths, 1990
50. Nielsen VK. The peripheral nerve function in chronic
    renal failure. I. Clinical symptoms and signs. Acta Med
    Scand 1971;190:105–111
51. Nielsen VK. The peripheral nerve function in chronic
    renal failure. VII. Longitudinal course during terminal
    renal failure and regular hemodialysis. Acta Med
    Scand 1974;195:155–162
52. Nielsen VK. The peripheral nerve function in chronic
    renal failure. VIII. Recovery after renal transplantation.
    Clinical aspects. Acta Med Scand 1974;195:163–170
53. Nielsen VK. The peripheral nerve function in chronic
    renal failure. IX. Recovery after renal transplantation.
    Electrophysiological aspects (sensory and motor nerve
    conduction). Acta Med Scand 1974;195:171–180
54. Said G, Boudier L, Selva J, et al. Different patterns of
    uremic polyneuropathy: clinicopathologic study. Neu-
    rology 1983;33:567–574
55. Ropper AH. Accelerated neuropathy of renal failure.
    Arch Neurol 1993;50:536–539
56. Bolton CF, McKeown MJ, Chen R, et al. Subacute
    uremic and diabetic polyneuropathy. Muscle Nerve
    1997;20:59–64
57. Caccia MR, Mangili A, Mecca G, et al. Effects of
    hemodialytic treatment on uremic polyneuropathy. A
    clinical and electrophysiological follow-up study. J
    Neurol 1977;217:123–131
58. Dyck PJ, Johnson WJ, Lambert EH, et al. Comparison of
    symptoms, chemistry, and nerve function to assess ade-
    quacy of hemodialysis. Neurology 1979;29:1361–1368
59. Dyck PJ, Johnson WJ, Lambert EH, O'Brien PC. Seg-
    mental demyelination secondary to axonal degenera-
    tion in uremic neuropathy. Mayo Clin Proc 1971;46:
    400–431
60. Thomas PK, Hollinrake K, Lascelles RG, et al. The
    polyneuropathy of chronic renal failure. Brain 1971;94:
    761–780
61. Galassi G, Ferrari S, Cobelli M, Rizzuto N. Neuromus-
    cular complications of kidney diseases. Nephrol Dial
    Transplant 1998;13(Suppl 7):41–47
62. Pastan S, Bailey J. Dialysis therapy. N Engl J Med
    1998;338:1428–1437
63. Dyck PJ, Johnson WJ, Nelson RA, et al. Uremic neu-
    ropathy. III. Controlled study of restricted protein and
    fluid diet and infrequent hemodialysis versus conven-
    tional hemodialysis treatment. Mayo Clin Proc 1975;50:
    641–649
64. Robles NR, Murga L, Galvan S, et al. Hemodialysis
    with cuprophane or polysulfone: effects on uremic
    polyneuropathy. Am J Kidney Dis 1993;21:282–287
65. Tegner R, Lindholm B. Uremic polyneuropathy: differ-
    ent effects of hemodialysis and continuous ambulatory
    peritoneal dialysis. Acta Med Scand 1985;218:409–416
66. Bolton CF, Baltzan MA, Baltzan RB. Effects of renal
    transplantation on uremic neuropathy. A clinical and
    electrophysiologic study. N Engl J Med 1971;284:
    1170–1175
67. Ahonen RE. Peripheral neuropathy in uremic patients
    and in renal transplant recipients. Acta Neuropathol
    1981;54:43–53
68. Oh SJ, Clements RS Jr, Lee YW, Diethelm AG. Rapid
    improvement in nerve conduction velocity following
    renal transplantation. Ann Neurol 1978;4:369–373
69. Solders G, Wilczek H, Gunnarsson R, et al. Effects of
    combined pancreatic and renal transplantation on dia-
    betic neuropathy: a two-year follow-up study. Lancet
    1987;2:1232–1235
70. Trojaborg W, Smith T, Jakobsen J, Rasmussen K. Effect
    of pancreas and kidney transplantation on the neuro-
    pathic profile in insulin-dependent diabetics with end-
    stage nephropathy. Acta Neurol Scand 1994;90:5–9
71. Ullian ME, Hammond WS, Alfrey AC, et al. Beta-2-
    microglobulin-associated amyloidosis in chronic
    hemodialysis patients with carpal tunnel syndrome.
    Medicine (Baltimore) 1989;68:107–115
72. Riggs JE, Moss AH, Labosky DA, et al. Upper extremity
    ischemic monomelic neuropathy: a complication of vas-
    cular access procedures in uremic diabetic patients.
    Neurology 1989;39:997–998

191 Peripheral Neuropathy Associated with Alcoholism, Malnutrition, and Vitamin Deficiencies

Guillermo A Suarez

Introduction

Peripheral neuropathy due to nutritional disorders is rare in industrialized, or "developed," nations. It is observed in malnourished patients, and although a relationship between nutrition and neuropathy has been postulated, it has been difficult to clarify. These patients often have a primary cause for the malnutrition (e.g., cancer, alcoholism, or malabsorption syndrome) that may contribute to the development of neuropathy, making it difficult to determine a causal relationship. Studies on the association between nutritional deficiency and neuropathy have encountered limitations. Undernourished patients often have multiple nutritional deficiencies and the clinical syndromes overlap (e.g., pellagra, Strachan syndrome, and beriberi have similar clinical features), adding to the difficulty of identifying a specific dietary micronutrient responsible for the illness. Some of the deficiency states have occurred during times of starvation, war, and famine when it has not been possible to study peripheral nerve function. Ethically, it is not acceptable to withhold adequate treatment from a malnourished alcoholic or starved famine patient to make observations while each specific component of the diet is replenished. Furthermore, experimental animal studies have not reproduced such human conditions as alcoholism.

Excellent reviews are available on the central and peripheral complications of nutritional deficiencies.[1,2] This chapter focuses on peripheral nervous system complications associated with alcoholism, malnutrition, and vitamin deficiency.

Alcoholism and neuropathy

Although peripheral neuropathy is a complication of chronic alcoholism, there is considerable debate about the direct role of alcohol in the pathogenesis of neuropathy.[3,4] Some investigators have postulated a nutritional deficiency, whereas others have suggested that alcohol has a toxic effect on nerve function. Nutritional estimates are difficult to ascertain in alcoholic patients because of a memory deficit (Korsakoff syndrome) or because they are unable to provide a reliable history and independent observers are not available.

On the basis of extensive experience with patients who had neuropathy and chronic alcoholism, Victor and Adams[5,6] provided strong evidence in favor of a nutritional cause of alcoholic neuropathy. In their experience, chronic alcohol abuse and dietary deficiencies were closely associated. Patients had major dietary alterations, with prominent weight loss; many patients were 13.5 to 18 kg (30 to 40 lb) below ideal weight. These patients diverted money to buying alcohol and replaced the protein in their diet with simple carbohydrates. This imbalance has been postulated to increase the load on the vitamin B_1 (thiamine) enzymatic system, thus increasing the requirement of vitamin B_1 in the diet. The nutritional hypothesis has been supported by other studies.[3,7–9]

To separate the toxic effects of alcohol from poor nutrition, Behse and Buchtal[10] performed electrophysiological and pathological studies on 37 alcoholics and 6 postgastrectomy Danish patients who had peripheral neuropathy. Of the 37 alcoholic patients, 14 had pronounced nutritional deficiency, and 6 of these patients had a weight loss greater than 10 kg (22.2 lb). All the nonalcoholic postgastrectomy patients had malabsorption and weight loss. The primary source of alcohol consumed by patients was beer, and they drank at least 3 L/day and as many as one-half of them consumed between 5 and 10 L/day. When measured, vitamin levels in these alcoholic patients were normal. The authors attributed this to Danish beer being supplemented with vitamins B_1 and B_6. The clinical features were similar for all patients, whether they were alcoholic with adequate nutrition, alcoholic with poor nutrition, or postgastrectomy patients. The results of electrophysiological and histopathological studies of sural nerve biopsy specimens from alcoholic patients were consistent with axonal loss. The electromyographic (EMG) findings were slightly different for the postgastrectomy group, in whom nerve conduction studies suggested that demyelination was the primary pathological process. This was confirmed with teased fiber preparations. On the basis of these observations, Behse and Buchtal[10] concluded that neuropathy due to malnutrition is different from that associated with alcohol and suggested that alcohol has a toxic effect important in the pathogenesis of alcoholic neuropathy.

Monforte et al.[11] performed detailed autonomic and electrophysiological studies in a group of 107 alcoholic patients and 61 control subjects and found evidence of somatic neuropathy in 36% of alcoholic patients and autonomic neuropathy (mainly cardiovagal) in 24% of alcoholic patients. Malnutrition was not an important factor and was present in only 15 patients. Because no correlation was found between neuropathy and nutritional factors, the authors suggested that alcohol has a direct toxic effect on peripheral nerves.

However, experimental animal studies have failed to demonstrate a direct toxic effect of alcohol on peripheral nerves. Hallett et al.[12] studied the effects of alcohol ingestion on peripheral nerves of monkeys over 3 to 5 years. Electrophysiological and pathological studies were conducted on two groups of animals. Animals fed diets in which 30% to 50% of calories were replaced with alcohol were compared with a control group of animals fed a nutritionally complete diet. The study found no evidence of a toxic effect of alcohol on the nerves of monkeys given the alcohol diet. Bosch et al.[13] studied the effects of rats fed alcohol in their diet. These animals were not nutritionally deficient. Although changes of axonal degeneration were found in one animal, the difference between the control and alcohol-fed groups was not statistical. Other investigators have also failed to provide compelling evidence of a direct toxic effect of alcohol on the peripheral nervous system.[14,15]

In summary, the results of most human and animal studies have suggested that nutritional deficiency rather than a direct toxic effect of alcohol is important in the pathogenesis of alcoholic neuropathy.

Clinical and laboratory features

Alcoholic patients commonly have the features of chronic alcoholism, with the stigmata of liver disease, ataxia, skin changes, and memory impairment, especially in cases of Korsakoff syndrome. The clinical picture is that of chronic sensorimotor neuropathy of insidious onset.[16] The initial symptoms are sensory, with distal symmetrical "burning" or "stabbing" pains of the feet. Sensory symptoms progress to involve the legs and, in severe cases, the hands. Distal leg weakness and wasting accompany the sensory symptoms and affect mainly the lower limbs. Distal sudomotor symptoms such as decreased sweating or hyperhidrosis of the feet and hands with associated skin changes (atrophy, redness) and distal hair loss are consistently present. Orthostatic hypotension and erectile failure may occur in patients with Wernicke-Korsakoff syndrome. Examination findings include gait ataxia, which usually is a combination of midline cerebellar degeneration and sensory ataxia.[17] Deep tendon reflexes are absent or hypoactive in the lower extremities. There are predominantly distal weakness and atrophy of the muscles in the legs, with impairment of all sensory modalities distally. Cranial nerves usually are not affected.

In a subgroup of alcoholic patients, subacute neuropathy may develop, with rapid progression of muscle weakness.[18,19] Patients often exhibit distal pain and calf tenderness. Myoglobinuria has been described in severe cases. The onset appears to be related to bouts of heavy drinking in already malnourished patients.

Because the clinical features of alcoholic neuropathy are not distinctive, it is important to exclude other causes of neuropathy, for example, acquired or inherited, in alcoholic but otherwise well-nourished patients.

Laboratory studies have documented abnormalities consistent with liver disease. Serum levels of transaminases (AST/ALT) are increased, with macrocytosis in the early stages of liver disease. Erythrocyte transketolase is a thiamine-dependent enzyme that may be used as a marker of chronic thiamine deficiency. However, it is not known how frequently this test is abnormal in malnourished alcoholic patients or in those with other deficiency states.

Electrodiagnostic studies have shown the features of a distal, predominantly sensorimotor peripheral neuropathy.[10,18,20] The sensory nerve action potential amplitudes are decreased and conduction velocities are mildly slowed; motor action potentials and conduction velocities have lesser changes. F-wave latencies are preserved, suggesting that proximal conduction is normal. Needle EMG has shown distal denervation. These electrophysiological features are consistent with distal axonal degeneration of sensory and motor nerve fibers.

Agelink et al.[21] evaluated cardiovascular autonomic neuropathy in a group of 35 alcoholic patients and compared the results with 80 healthy controls. They found an association between cardiovascular autonomic neuropathy and somatic neuropathy in 41% of these patients.

The results of cerebrospinal fluid examination are usually negative, although a modest increase in protein concentration may be noted occasionally.

The main pathological finding in sural nerve biopsy specimens is axonal degeneration.[10,18,22] Teased fiber preparations also show axonal degeneration.[23] The percentage of fibers that undergo segmental demyelination is low and not greater than that of control nerves. In studies on transverse sections of epoxy-embedded nerves, the density of myelinated fibers is decreased and the number of fibers undergoing axonal degeneration is increased. Myelinated fibers of all sizes are affected, as are unmyelinated fibers.[24] No interstitial inflammatory changes have been observed. Postmortem studies have disclosed variable degeneration of dorsal root and anterior horn neurons because of distal axonal degeneration. The greater splanchnic nerve is spared, but a loss of parasympathetic and sympathetic ganglia neurons has been reported.[25]

Treatment

The main goals of treatment are abstinence from alcohol and correction of nutritional deficiencies.

For rehabilitation of alcoholic patients, it is important to enlist the advice and help of experts in alcohol rehabilitation and help from the family and close friends. In addition to abstinence from alcohol, the patient needs a balanced diet that is enhanced with vitamins, especially B complex vitamins. Woelk et al.[26] performed a randomized double-blind, placebo-controlled study with a high lipophilic form of thiamine (benfoamine) in 84 patients with chronic alcoholism. Three groups were studied. The first group received benfoamine at a high dose of 320 mg/day for the first 4 weeks, followed by 120 mg/day for an additional 3 weeks. A second group received a combination of vitamin B_6 (720 mg for the first 4 weeks) and B_{12}. A third group received placebo. Clinical symptoms, deficits, and vibration sensation measured at the great toe were used as end points. Benfoamine led to a statistically significant improvement of all the indices. The difference between the placebo and the vitamin B_6 and B_{12} groups was not significant. This latter finding may be related to the high doses of vitamin B_6, which may be toxic.

In addition to vitamin supplementation, symptomatic treatment, especially of pain, may be necessary in the early stages. Nonpharmacological approaches such as soaking the feet in cold tap water or taking simple analgesics such as aspirin and acetaminophen (Tylenol) should be tried first. If these measures are not effective, amitriptyline, starting with 10 mg at bedtime and gradually increasing the dose to 100 mg/day, may be helpful. Gabapentin, starting at 300 mg orally 3 times daily and increasing the dose to 3600 mg/day, is an alternative medication. Tegretol, at a dose of 600 to 1000 mg/day in divided doses, may be useful, especially for lancinating pain.

For patients with mild to moderate alcohol neuropathy who stop drinking and maintain balanced nutrition, the prognosis for recovery of the polyneuropathy is good.[27] However, patients should be informed that the recovery may be slow and usually requires several months. Improvement may depend on the severity and duration of the neuropathy. In a detailed electrophysiological and pathological study, Behse and Buchtal[10] found that sensory symptoms or deficits persisted for 2 or more years in 17 of 18 patients, and this correlated with the lack of significant regeneration observed in sural nerve biopsy specimens. It is uncertain whether this persistence was related to other factors or whether the patients resumed drinking. Johnson and Robinson[28] studied 79 alcoholic patients who had autonomic neuropathy and followed them for up to 7 years. They found that the presence of cardiovagal neuropathy in chronic alcoholics was associated with significantly higher mortality than in the general population.

Vitamin deficiencies

Vitamin B_{12} (cobalamin) deficiency

Vitamin B_{12} (cobalamin) is essential for certain metabolic functions in humans and animals. Pernicious anemia is the most common cause of vitamin B_{12} deficiency, a result of vitamin B_{12} malabsorption. Pernicious anemia is an autoimmune disorder in which intrinsic factor antibodies block the absorption of vitamin B_{12}, which leads to a selective deficiency of the vitamin without deficiency of other vitamins or nutrients. Less common causes of vitamin B_{12} deficiency include strict vegetarian diet, malabsorption

syndromes (including tropical sprue and any disorder that affects the absorption of vitamin B_{12} from the distal ileum), competition for vitamin B_{12} (e.g., parasitic infestation by the fish tapeworm *Diphyllobothrium latum*), and rare congenital enzyme deficiencies.

Vitamin B_{12} is present only in animal products such as meat and dairy foods. The daily requirement for adults is approximately 2 μg.[29] The pathway of vitamin B_{12} absorption, transport, and utilization has been reviewed elsewhere.[30–32] Pernicious anemia occurs more frequently in persons of northern European descent, and the average age at presentation is about 60 years. Estimates of the prevalence of vitamin B_{12} deficiency in the elderly have ranged from 7% to 16%.[33–35]

Pathogenesis   Vitamin B_{12} deficiency alters the function of important enzyme systems, leading to hematological and neurological complications. Megaloblastic anemia is due to diminished DNA synthesis in hematopoietic tissues; however, the biochemical basis of the neurological damage is uncertain. For DNA synthesis, the formation of methionine is the critical step. Methylcobalamin is a cofactor in the conversion of homocysteine to methionine and methyltetrahydrofolate to tetrahydrofolate (THF). This is referred to as the "central reaction." It provides methionine and THF, which are critical for DNA synthesis. Methionine is subsequently adenosylated to S-adenosylmethionine, which is important for transmethylation and polyamine synthesis in the central nervous system. Intermediary byproducts are methylene-THF and formyl-THF, involved in purine synthesis. Methionine facilitates the formation of formyl-THF (Figure 191.1).[30] Vitamin B_{12} deficiency leads to an increase in the serum levels of homocystine and methylmalonic acid, which are useful diagnostic markers. Another enzymatic reaction in which cobalamin is a cofactor involves the mitochondrial conversion of L-methylmalonyl coenzyme A (CoA) to succinyl CoA.[30]

In a recent review of the neurotrophic action of vitamin B_{12}, Scalabrino[31] proposed new perspectives on the pathogenesis of vitamin B_{12} deficiency. He described the role of vitamin B_{12} in the regulation of neurotrophic growth factors and certain cytokines (e.g., tumor necrosis factor α) and their influence on the mechanism of central nervous system degeneration observed in vitamin B_{12} deficiency.

Clinical features   The neurological disorders associated with vitamin B_{12} deficiency have been well described and include myelopathy or subacute combined degeneration of the spinal cord, peripheral neuropathy, and cerebral dysfunction.[36] Lichtheim[37] provided the first adequate clinical description of myelopathy with pathological examination of the spinal cord. Subsequent reports have described the syndrome extensively.[38] Cabot,[39] in a review of 1200 cases of pernicious anemia, noted that paresthesias in the hands and feet were present in almost every patient, even without pathological change in the spinal cord. Woltmann[40] described the neurological

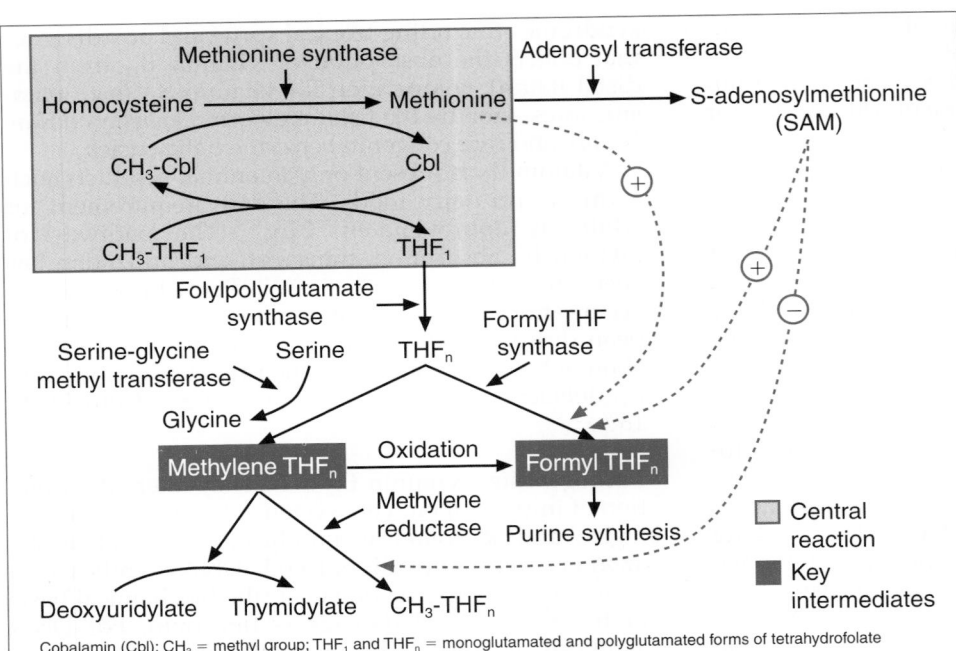

Figure 191.1 Biochemistry of cobalamin (Cbl) deficiency. See text for details. CH$_3$, methyl group; THF$_1$ and THF$_n$, monoglutamated and polyglutamated forms of tetrahydrofolate. (From Tefferi and Pruthi.[30] By permission of Mayo Foundation for Medical Education and Research.)

findings in 150 cases of pernicious anemia and found signs of peripheral neuropathy in approximately 5% of patients, compared with 80% who had spinal cord disease. Healton et al.[41] reported a large series of patients with vitamin B$_{12}$ deficiency evaluated at two university hospitals from 1968 to 1985. Neurological symptoms such as "pins and needles, tingling, and numbness" affecting the feet or the feet and hands were common as initial manifestations, occurring in approximately 70% of patients. Other less frequent symptoms included gait ataxia and weakness. The median duration of symptoms before diagnosis was 4 months. On neurological examination, impairment of vibratory sensation and proprioception in the lower extremities was the most common neurological abnormality. Spasticity, hyperreflexia, and extensor plantar responses were uncommon. This is in contrast with some of the findings of earlier studies. Wilson[42] noted that extensor plantar responses were of early onset and frequent. Other authors have reported uncommon symptoms at the onset, including lightning pains, Lhermitte sign fluttering of the eyelids, and paresthesias of the tongue.[36] The study of Healton et al.[41] could not resolve the longstanding controversy of the contribution of neuropathic deficits versus myelopathy in patients with vitamin B$_{12}$ deficiency. However, two other observations emerged from their study. They found an inverse correlation between hematological findings and neurological deficits: the higher the hematocrit, the worse the neurological impairment. The second observation was related to treatment. Patients in whom vitamin B$_{12}$ deficiency was diagnosed earlier and who had less neurological impairment before treatment had a better outcome after therapy.

Electrophysiological studies have shown decreased sensory nerve action potentials and slow conduction

velocities, consistent with a peripheral neuropathic process. Hemmer et al.[43] recently reviewed the clinical, electrophysiological, and radiological findings in nine patients who had subacute combined degeneration, and in all nine, the clinical and electrophysiological changes were those of posterior column impairment. Somatosensory evoked potentials were abnormal in all nine patients, but nerve conduction studies were only abnormal in five (four with axonal neuropathy and one with demyelinating neuropathy).

The interaction of nitrous oxide with vitamin B$_{12}$ metabolism is important because of a potential clinical presentation. Nitrous oxide, an anesthetic gas, irreversibly oxidizes the cobalt part of methylcobalamin, which leads to a functional deficiency of the vitamin. Layzer[44] and Schilling[45] have reported on patients in whom myeloneuropathy developed after exposure to nitrous oxide. Most cases have occurred in persons who have chronically abused the anesthetic gas for recreational purposes. However, Kinsella and Green[46] and others[47-49] have described patients with unsuspected low or borderline levels of vitamin B$_{12}$ who developed symptoms and deficits after exposure to nitrous oxide for a surgical procedure. This association is important to recognize and should be considered in any patient in whom an acute myeloneuropathy syndrome develops postoperatively.

The results of pathology studies of the peripheral neuropathy associated with vitamin B$_{12}$ deficiency have been inconclusive, and the results of studies in humans and animals have been contradictory. The studies of Pant et al.[50] and Agamanolis et al.[51] failed to provide pathological evidence of peripheral neuropathy. Others have found mild degeneration of peripheral nerve fibers.

In summary, the current evidence indicates that

mild peripheral neuropathy occurs in cobalamin deficiency, but its type and frequency and the stage of disease at which it occurs are unknown. The peripheral neuropathic findings and symptoms are difficult or impossible to differentiate from those of early myelopathy or subacute combined degeneration that generally is responsible for most of the symptoms and signs.

Diagnostic evaluation The range of manifestations of vitamin B_{12} deficiency is wide, and the diagnostic threshold should be low for any patient who presents with a combination of myelopathy and peripheral neuropathy. Patients may not have an associated megaloblastic anemia, and cobalamin deficiency without anemia is not uncommon. The most helpful test is measurement of the serum concentration of

vitamin B_{12}. If the serum level is less than the lower limit of normal, intrinsic factor antibodies are assessed and, if positive, the diagnosis of pernicious anemia is confirmed. However, if the levels of vitamin B_{12} are borderline, the next step is measurement of metabolite levels (homocystine and methylmalonic acid), which are good markers of tissue stores of vitamin B_{12}. Both are increased in vitamin B_{12} deficiency, whereas an increase in homocystine may be seen in folate deficiency. Green and Kinsella[32] have provided a useful algorithm for the diagnosis of vitamin B_{12} deficiency.

Treatment Treatment consists of intramuscular injections of 1000 μg of vitamin B_{12} daily for 5 days to replenish the stores, followed by monthly injections of 500 to 1000 μg indefinitely (Table 191.1). Oral mainte-

Table 191.1 Treatment of neuropathy and associated disorders with vitamins

Vitamin deficiency	Condition	Risk factors	Diagnostic tests	Therapeutic dose
Vitamin B_1 (thiamine)	Beriberi Alcoholic neuropathy	Alcoholism Hyperemesis gravidarum Gastric/intestinal bypass Severe malabsorption Severe malnutrition Prolonged peritoneal or hemodialysis Dietary factors: milled rice without vitamin supplementation	Erythrocyte transketolase activity	Acute deficiency (e.g., beriberi or WKS): 100 mg IV, followed by 100 mg IM daily for 5 days Maintenance: 50 mg/day PO
Vitamin B_{12} (cobalamin)	Pernicious anemia	Autoimmune disorder Malabsorption states Infestation with DL Strict vegetarian diet Nitrous oxide exposure	Vitamin B_{12} level Intrinsic factor antibody Increased homocystine, methylmalonic acid	Vitamin B_{12} IM 1000 μg/day for 5 days, followed by 500–1000 μg IM monthly
Vitamin B_6 (pyridoxine)*	Peripheral neuropathy	General malnutrition Alcoholism Isoniazid and hydralazine	Increased serum cystathionine	50–100 mg/day PO for patients taking isoniazid
Niacin	Pellagra (dementia, diarrhea, dermatitis) Coexisting deficiencies of other vitamins	Severe malnutrition Alcoholism Carcinoid syndrome	—	300–600 mg niacin/day PO for 5 days
Vitamin E (alpha-tocopherol)	Spinocerebellar syndrome Retinitis pigmentosa and acanthocytosis	Fat malabsorption Abetalipoproteinemia (Bassen-Kornsweig disease) Familial vitamin E deficiency	Serum vitamin E levels	For abetalipoproteinemia, vitamin E 100–200 mg/kg daily
Strachan syndrome	Peripheral neuropathy Optic neuropathy Ataxia Dermatitis Myeloneuropathy	Severe malnutrition Multiple vitamin deficiencies	—	Balanced nutritional diet Multivitamin supplementation

DL, *Diphyllobothrium latum*; IM, intramuscularly; IV, intravenously; PO, orally; WKS, Wernicke-Korsakoff syndrome.
*Both deficiency and excess of vitamin B_6 can cause neuropathy.

nance therapy may be an alternative approach after stores have been restocked through intramuscular injections, but the response may be unpredictable.[36] Folic acid may cause temporary remission of the anemia that occurs with vitamin B_{12} deficiency, but it does not prevent the onset of neurological problems (in fact, it may hasten onset).

Beriberi, vitamin B_1 (thiamine) deficiency

The history of beriberi is closely related to the discovery and isolation of vitamins. The introduction of milled white rice (mechanically stripped of the pericarp) with the industrial revolution in the 19th century caused epidemics of beriberi. Thiamine is present in the pericarp of crude rice. By eliminating the thiamine-containing pericarp, mechanically processed rice led to avitaminosis in affected persons. A detailed description of the historic events has been provided by Victor.[6] The neuropathy of beriberi has features similar to those of the neuropathy of chronic alcoholism, suggesting that vitamin B_1 deficiency is common to both of these conditions. Beriberi is rarely seen in isolation in industrialized countries.

The basic mechanism by which thiamine deficiency causes nerve damage is understood only partially. Thiamine is important in the metabolism of carbohydrates. Thiamine pyrophosphate (TPP), the metabolically active form of thiamine, is involved in several enzyme systems, including transketolase, which acts as a coenzyme in the pentose monophosphate pathway and the oxidative decarboxylation of α-ketoacids such as pyruvate and α-ketoglutarate. TPP catalyzes the conversion of pyruvate to acetyl CoA and α-ketoglutarate to succinate in the Krebs cycle[1] (Figure 191.2). Many features of thiamine deficiency result from inhibition of these systems and the accumulation of proximal metabolites. Thiamine also may have a role in neurons, axonal membranes, and transport independently of its function in carbohydrate metabolism. Thiamine is present in many foods, including rice, cereals, yeast, and meats. It does not occur in fats and oils. The recommended daily dietary requirement for adults is 1 to 1.5 mg.[29] The requirement is increased during pregnancy and lactation and in hyperthyroidism. Inadequate intestinal absorption occurs in alcoholism, malabsorption states, and chronic malnutrition. Hemodialysis, peritoneal dialysis, diarrhea, and diuretic therapy can lead to excessive loss of thiamine and, thus, thiamine deficiency.[52]

Clinical features   Wernicke-Korsakoff syndrome (described elsewhere in this book), peripheral neuropathy, and cardiac failure are the clinical features of thiamine deficiency. Polyneuropathy is present in approximately 80% of patients with Wernicke-Korsakoff syndrome. If peripheral neuropathy is the major feature, the condition is referred to as "dry beriberi," and if cardiac failure with edema is superimposed, it is called "wet beriberi." These differences were described more than 100 years ago, but currently, this division is not practical because the wet form may be converted to the dry form after diuresis.

At the onset of symptoms, a slowly progressive neuropathy develops, characterized by painful "burning feet" and calf tenderness. Subsequent progression includes the proximal spread of sensory symptoms, followed by distal muscle weakness and wasting. The skin over the feet and leg becomes dry, hairless, and red, suggesting involvement of sympathetic fibers. Cranial nerve involvement, particularly facial and laryngeal weakness, has been described in cases of nonalcoholic beriberi. Examination demonstrates distal limb weakness with areflexia and impairment of all sensory modalities in a stocking-glove distribution. Subacute visual loss and scotoma have been reported. However, these cases may represent other nutritional deficiencies such as Strachan syndrome. The peripheral neuropathy continues to progress over months until the avitaminosis is corrected.

Evaluation and laboratory studies   This neuropathy has few distinctive clinical features that help neurologists differentiate it from other acquired or inherited neuropathies. Therefore, other causes of distal painful sensorimotor neuropathy should be excluded. It is important to recognize that the deficiency is not limited only to alcoholic patients. Erythrocyte transketolase activity is the most accurate diagnostic test.[53]

Reports of pathology studies of beriberi in nonalcoholic patients are limited.[54] Postmortem studies have shown axonal degeneration in distal nerves. Involvement of the vagus and phrenic nerves has been noted in severe cases, and chromatolysis of dorsal root ganglion neurons and anterior horn cells is likely caused by axonal degeneration. Degeneration in the posterior columns has been observed and attributed to degeneration of dorsal root ganglion neurons. Similar changes have been described in animal models of thiamine deficiency.[55,56]

Treatment   Treatment consists of thiamine supplementation, initially given intravenously, to replenish the stores, followed by oral maintenance therapy with 50 mg of thiamine in addition to a daily multivitamin (Table 191.1).

The best observations on the prognosis and recovery of peripheral nerve function with thiamine supplementation are those of Victor and Adams,[5,6] who described the short-term effect of thiamine on peripheral nerve function in 12 alcoholic patients. Patients were fed a vitamin B-deficient diet for 5 days, with complete abstinence from alcohol. Afterward, thiamine alone was added to the diet, and although symptoms improved in 10 patients, findings on the neurological examination did not change. However, the patients were observed for only 2 weeks. Follow-up of 2 patients who were given maintenance therapy with thiamine and other vitamins of the B group for 8 weeks showed improvement in the neurological findings.

Ohnishi et al.[57] described seven young males who had beriberi as a consequence of eating milled rice without thiamine supplementation. All of them had a

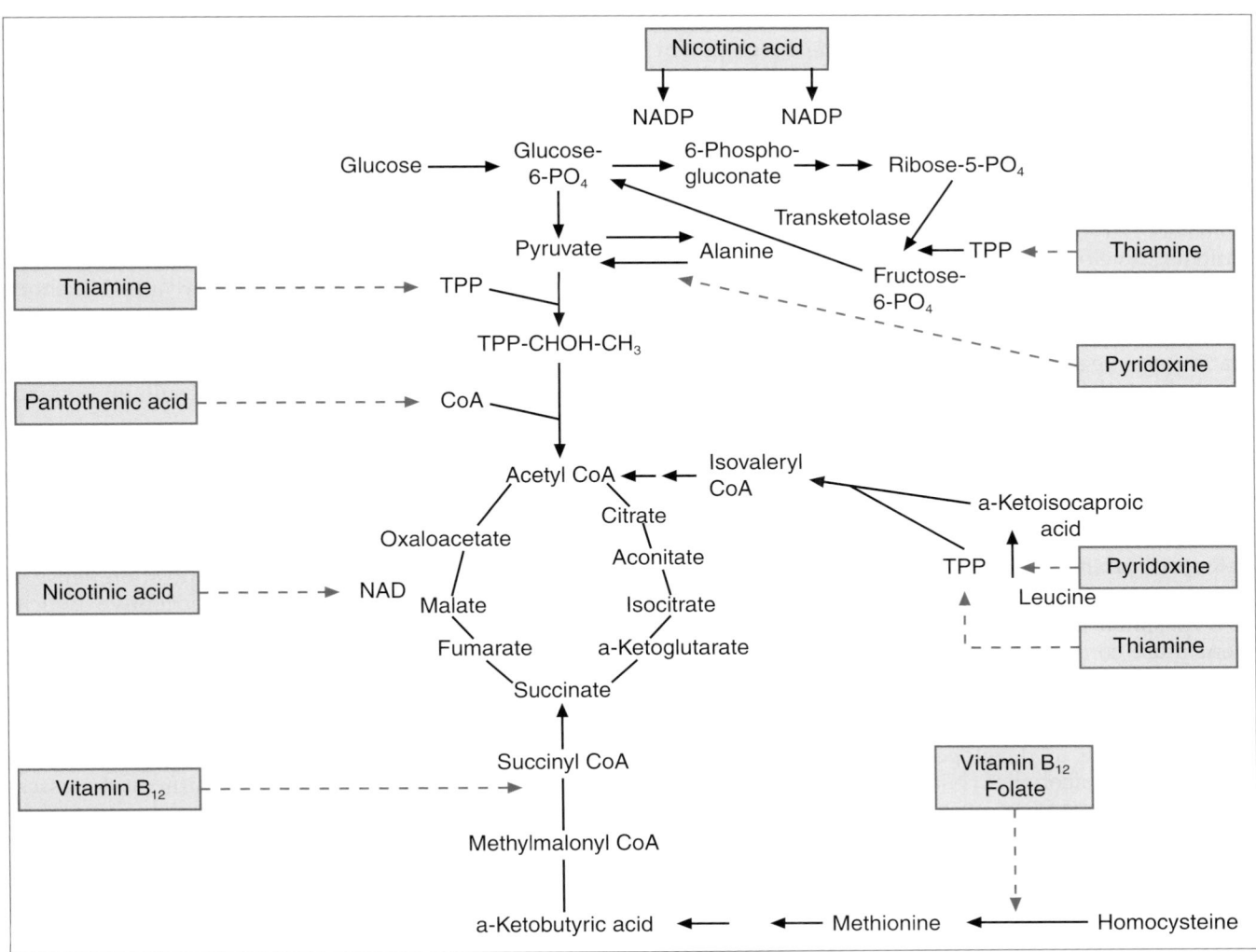

Figure 191.2 Metabolic pathways of thiamine and other vitamins. See text for discussion. CoA, coenzyme A; NAD, nicotinamide adenine dinucleotide; NADP, nicotinamide adenine dinucleotide phosphate; TPP, thiamine pyrophosphate. (From Kinsella and Riley.[1] By permission of WB Saunders Company.)

peripheral neuropathy associated with edema and cardiac enlargement. Axonal degeneration was documented with electrophysiological and morphological studies. For most of them, the edema, cardiac enlargement, and pulse pressure improved dramatically within 1 week after thiamine was added to the diet. The sensorimotor neuropathy improved gradually over several months, indicating axonal degeneration and regeneration.

Vitamin B₆ (pyridoxine) deficiency

Pyridoxal phosphate is the major active metabolite of vitamin B_6, which is a cofactor of many enzymatic reactions of amino acid metabolism, especially tryptophan, glycine, serine, glutamate, and methionine. It also is important for the synthesis of heme precursors. Vitamin B_6 deficiency can produce secondary niacin deficiency because tryptophan is necessary for the synthesis of niacin. Vitamin B_6 is also involved in neurotransmitter metabolism, especially that of γ-aminobutyric acid.

The daily dietary requirement for vitamin B_6 in normal adults is 1.6 to 2 mg.[29] It is present in many foods; for example, cereals, meats, and vegetables are good sources of this vitamin. The daily requirement is increased during pregnancy and with the use of estrogens. Because the vitamin is distributed widely in many foods, deficiency occurs mainly with the use of vitamin B_6 antagonists such as isoniazid (INH), cycloserine, hydralazine, and penicillamine. Dietary excess of vitamin B_6 results in a predominantly sensory peripheral neuropathy or ganglionopathy.[58]

Vilter et al.[59] studied the effects of vitamin B_6 deficiency with the antagonist, desoxypyridoxine. Of the 50 patients studied, 34 developed clinical signs of vitamin B_6 deficiency, including pellagra-like dermatitis, conjunctivitis, anorexia, nausea, glossitis, lethargy, and peripheral neuropathy. Neuropathic symptoms consisted of tingling and numbness in the feet and hands and were progressive in two patients. The neuropathic symptoms and signs rapidly resolved with discontinuation of the antagonist.

After the introduction of isoniazid as an antituberculous drug, several observers noted the development of a peripheral neuropathy characterized by distal and symmetrical tingling and numbness, which could progress rapidly to sensory ataxia and limb weakness.[60,61] Isoniazid promotes the renal excretion of vitamin B_6, resulting in a deficiency state. The incidence of neuropathy has been related to the dose of isoniazid. At doses of 3 to 6 mg/kg daily, 2% of patients developed neuropathy, and when the dose was increased to 16 to 24 mg/kg daily, 44% developed neuropathy.[62]

Pathology studies have shown that axonal degeneration and regeneration affect both myelinated and unmyelinated fibers.[63] Isoniazid-induced neuropathy is reversible by discontinuation of the drug or by supplementation with vitamin B_6. The recommended dose of vitamin B_6 is 50 to 100 mg/day; megadoses greater than 200 mg/day have been associated with sensory neuropathy[58,64] (Table 191.1).

Pellagra (niacin deficiency)

In humans, nicotinic acid, or niacin, is an end product of tryptophan metabolism; thus, the dietary requirement must consider both the tryptophan and niacin content. The dietary daily requirement for adults is 13 to 20 mg of niacin equivalent (1 niacin equivalent = 1 mg of niacin or 60 mg of tryptophan).[29] Pellagra is rare in developed countries, although it still occurs in alcoholics. Niacin deficiency occurs in populations dependent on maize as the main source of carbohydrates. In developed countries, niacin is commonly added as enrichment to bread. Pellagra may be a rare complication of carcinoid syndrome, because of the conversion of tryptophan to serotonin instead of the synthesis of niacin. The three D's—dermatitis, diarrhea, and dementia—characterize the clinical manifestations of pellagra. Peripheral neuropathy occurs in patients with pellagra, but it is clinically indistinguishable from neuropathic beriberi.[65] The neuropathy is due most likely to deficiency of thiamine or other B vitamins, because it does not respond to niacin supplementation alone.[66,67]

Vitamin E deficiency

In humans, alpha-tocopherol is the active form of vitamin E. Vitamin E is absorbed from the gastrointestinal system by a nonenergy-requiring diffusion mechanism. After absorption, it is incorporated into chylomicrons and very low-density lipoprotein and passes from the lymphatic system into the systemic circulation. Alpha-tocopherol transfer protein (alpha-TTP) binds and processes vitamin E in the liver for incorporation into low- and high-density lipoproteins. Next, alpha-tocopherol is transferred from circulating lipoproteins to the cells, where it serves as an antioxidant and free radical scavenger preventing the formation of toxic free radical products. It appears to protect cellular membranes from oxidative stress. The storage of vitamin E in many tissues protects against its deficiency. The daily requirement is 10 to 30 mg.[29]

Causes of vitamin E deficiency   Vitamin E deficiency occurs primarily in association with genetic or acquired lipid malabsorption syndromes. Other causes include decreased intake (rare), dysfunction of the transfer protein, and abetalipoproteinemia.[68–70] An association between fat malabsorption and neurological disorders has been recognized for many years. Vitamin E is hydrophobic and requires solubilization by bile acids before absorption. Therefore, malabsorption results from multiple causes, including cystic fibrosis, chronic cholestasis, biliary atresia, short-bowel syndrome, and other malabsorption syndromes. Harding et al.[71] have described a selective deficiency of vitamin E that is not associated with generalized fat malabsorption but results in a spinocerebellar syndrome.

Clinical features   Several neuromuscular syndromes have been described in association with vitamin E deficiency.[72–74] However, a spinocerebellar syndrome with progressive limb and gait ataxia, areflexia, and impairment of vibration and joint position sense is characteristic of the disease. Proprioceptive deficits may mask cerebellar ataxia, but dysarthria, tremor, and nystagmus are present in some patients and point to involvement of the cerebellum or its pathways. Ophthalmoplegia with ptosis has been observed in some patients. Pigmentary retinopathy may require dilatation of the pupil for confirmation. Proximal muscle weakness is present but difficult to assess because of the ataxia and weight loss due to malabsorption. Pain is not a feature of the syndrome. In chronic vitamin E deficiency, the neurological syndrome develops slowly and insidiously over many years.

In 1950, Bassen and Kornzweig[75] described a distinct syndrome in an 18-year-old girl who presented with diffuse involvement of the central nervous system resembling Friedreich ataxia and accompanied by atypical retinitis pigmentosa and abnormal erythrocytes. Slowly progressive gait and limb ataxia, nystagmus, distal leg weakness and sensory loss, areflexia, and extensor plantar responses developed. A peripheral blood smear showed abnormalities in the shape and size of erythrocytes, which had a crenated appearance; later, these were referred to as "acanthocytes."[75] In 1963, Schwartz et al.[76] recognized the deficiency of β-lipoproteins in the pathogenesis of the syndrome. This autosomal recessive disorder is now referred to as "abetalipoproteinemia," or "Bassen-Kornzweig syndrome," and manifests many of the clinical features of vitamin E deficiency.

Laboratory studies   Electrophysiological studies have shown changes typical of sensory neuropathy, with low-amplitude sensory nerve action potentials, mild slowing of conduction velocities, and preservation of motor responses. Needle EMG has demonstrated only mild distal denervation. Generally, the etiology and duration of the deficiency correlate with the severity of the abnormalities. Somatosensory evoked potentials demonstrate delay in central conduction in symptomatic patients. This delay may occur with tibial somatosensory evoked potentials when median evoked potentials are normal; it usually is not reversed with treatment. Brain auditory evoked potentials have been unremarkable. Cerebrospinal fluid analysis has not demonstrated abnormalities.

Pathology studies Pathology studies in animals and humans have shown degeneration of the rostral segments of the fasciculi gracilis and cuneatus. Why the central projections of the primary afferent neurons are selectively vulnerable in vitamin E deficiency is not known. Sural nerve biopsy specimens have shown loss of myelinated fibers in severe cases.[77] This suggests that the central processes of dorsal root ganglion neurons are more susceptible to damage from vitamin E deficiency.

Diagnosis and treatment The key to the diagnosis of vitamin E deficiency—as for other deficiency states—is a high index of suspicion. Alpha-tocopherol is measured in the serum. The normal range at Mayo Medical Laboratories is 5.5 to 17 mg/L. In patients with vitamin E deficiency and neurological manifestations, the serum levels of vitamin E are undetectable. Hyperlipidemia or hypolipidemia may alter the serum levels of alpha-tocopherol. In this case, serum lipids should be assessed and the ratio between serum vitamin E and total serum lipids should be used as an index of vitamin E status.

Treatment of avitaminosis E requires large doses of the vitamin to prevent further progression of neurological deficits in patients with vitamin E deficiency due to malabsorption states.[78] In patients with abetalipoproteinemia, improvement of neurological function and halting the progression of deficits require high doses of oral vitamin E (100 to 200 mg/kg daily)[79] (Table 191.1). For patients who cannot absorb alpha-tocopherol, an injectable preparation is available.

Other nutritional deficiencies

Strachan syndrome

A distinct syndrome was described by Strachan[80] while working at the Kingston Public Hospital in Jamaica. Large outbreaks of a syndrome characterized by amblyopia, dermatitis, oral ulcerations, ataxia, and painful peripheral neuropathy developed in nutritionally deprived sugar cane workers. Others have described similar findings or parts of the syndrome in prisoners of war and in conditions of nutritional restriction.[81–85]

Patients describe distal burning of their feet, often associated with tingling and numbness. Sensory ataxia with the loss of ankle reflexes is a frequent clinical feature. Pathology studies of Jamaican cane workers and prisoners of war have shown degeneration of fibers and demyelination of the posterior columns of the cervical and thoracic spinal cord and optic nerves.[82] It has been suggested that the clinical features are due to degeneration of both central and peripheral projections of the dorsal root ganglia

neurons. No pathology studies on peripheral nerves of patients with this syndrome have been reported.

Restoration of a normal diet with vitamin supplementation improves the symptoms. In prisoners of war who have long-standing symptoms, the ataxia, neuropathic symptoms, and visual deficits frequently persist despite proper nutrition and vitamin supplementation. This syndrome likely is due to the lack of multiple dietary components, including several B vitamins.

In 1992–1993, an epidemic of optic neuropathy, painful peripheral neuropathy, sensorineural deafness, and myeloneuropathy occurred in Cuba. This epidemic has been reviewed comprehensively by Roman.[86,87] The features were similar to those of Strachan syndrome and beriberi. Persons between 25 and 64 years old were affected predominantly, and a total of 50 862 cases were documented. Pinar del Rio, a rural tobacco-growing province in the western part of the island, sustained the brunt of the epidemic. For epidemiological purposes, cases were classified as "optic forms" (52%) and "peripheral forms" (48%), but combined forms were also frequent.[87] Optic neuropathy was strongly associated with weight loss and smoking. Patients reported visual symptoms and photophobia, with slowly progressive loss of vision. Sadun et al.[88] recognized the typical features of the optic neuropathy with a centrocecal scotoma. Neuropathic symptoms consisted of "burning feet" with superimposed numbness and tingling and, less frequently, painful hands.[89] Nocturnal symptoms often interfered with sleep. Cramps in the feet and calves were also reported. Nerves were painful to touch, with pseudotabetic lancinating pains. Patients noted easy fatigability, but no obvious motor weakness was detected. On examination, deep tendon reflexes were decreased or absent distally, with predominant impairment of vibratory sensation over the feet and also some involvement of light touch, pinprick, and temperature in a stocking-glove distribution. Patients who had myeloneuropathy presented with sensory symptoms similar to neuropathic symptoms but in addition had leg weakness, difficulty walking, increased urinary frequency, and, in men, impotence. These patients had brisk deep tendon reflexes, although extensor plantar responses were infrequently present. Sensorineural deafness with high-pitched tinnitus was often found in association with peripheral neuropathy or optic neuropathy, or both.

Extensive studies of the epidemiology of the Cuban outbreak indicated that nutritional deprivation of vitamins and some amino acids without overt malnutrition was the most likely cause of the epidemic. In support for this theory, children, pregnant women, and the elderly older than 65 years had received nutritional supplementation as part of an ongoing public assistance program and were essentially spared by the epidemic. Also, early treatment of patients with multivitamins, especially of the B group, resulted in remission of the epidemic.[86]

Borrajero et al.[90] described the pathological findings in sural nerve biopsy specimens from 34 patients.

The features were those of axonal neuropathy, with evidence of moderately severe axonal degeneration in 25 patients and endoneurial and perineurial fibrosis and sparse inflammatory cells in the interstitium, without evidence of vasculitis. Myelinated fiber diameter was assessed in 11 patients, and the histogram showed a shift to the right, with a decrease in the number of large myelinated fibers and preservation of small myelinated fibers.

Treatment   Treatment of Strachan syndrome and related conditions consists of nutritional supplementation with multivitamins, especially the B group (Table 191.1). In the Cuban epidemic, treatment with multivitamin supplementation, especially B vitamins, folate, and vitamin A, led to complete remission of the epidemic. However, as in other cases, late treatment of patients with long-standing symptoms produced only partial recovery. No fatal cases related to the epidemic were reported.

Post-gastroplasty neuropathy

Peripheral neuropathy is one of the complications of gastric bypass or bariatric surgery used in the treatment of morbid obesity.

Abarbanel et al.[91] described the neurological complications in 23 patients who had gastric surgery for morbid obesity. Complications occurred 3 to 20 months postoperatively, and all patients had protracted vomiting within the first 3 months after the procedure. Most patients had a subacute symmetrical, predominantly sensory, neuropathy, and two each developed "burning feet syndrome," myelopathy, and Wernicke-Korsakoff encephalopathy. The patients who had burning feet and Wernicke-Korsakoff encephalopathy had remarkable improvement after parenteral thiamine therapy, suggesting they had vitamin B[1] deficiency. In the other cases, no specific cause was found, although complications related to nutritional causes were suspected.

Feit et al.[92] described two patients in whom an unusual neuropathy developed 3 months after gastric surgery for morbid obesity. These patients, as those mentioned above, also had constant vomiting. They had a sensory neuropathy or ganglionopathy with predominant sensory ataxia, areflexia, and marked joint position sense, with pseudoathetosis in the limbs. One patient had quadriparesis after the onset of the sensory symptoms, and the condition improved with aggressive parenteral nutrition. The other patient died of pulmonary embolism, and the autopsy findings showed areas of demyelination in the brachial plexus but no evidence of inflammation and degeneration, with lipid accumulation in the dorsal root ganglion neurons and Schwann cells. Excessive catabolism of fat was postulated as the potential source of the pathological observations. The cases of these two patients may represent the extremes of the spectrum of the clinical syndrome or they may represent entirely separate conditions along the lines of an acquired idiopathic or inflammatory sensory polyganglionopathy.

Other types of neuropathy have been described. A case of lumbosacral plexopathy after bariatric surgery was reported by Harwood et al.[93] A case of thoracic and lumbosacral radiculoplexus neuropathy associated with protracted weight loss after gastric bypass surgery has been observed by the author (unpublished observation). The female patient was morbidly obese and had type 2 diabetes mellitus. Postoperatively, she lost more than 135 kg (300 lb) and the glycemia normalized, but she continued to lose weight. A painful thoracic radiculopathy developed and was accompanied by an intense aching pain in the thigh, followed by leg weakness and asymmetrical knee deep tendon reflexes. This case adds to the spectrum of neuropathic complications associated with gastric surgery for morbid obesity.

The management of the neuropathic complications of bariatric surgery has not been established because the basic mechanism underlying the complications is not known. For patients who continue to lose weight postoperatively, reversal of the procedure is of benefit. However, the outcome of the neuropathy has not been defined entirely. Intuitively, multivitamin and nutritional supplementation seems reasonable, but further study is needed. Patients who have protracted vomiting should receive parenteral thiamine to prevent Wernicke-Korsakoff encephalopathy.

References

1. Kinsella LJ, Riley DE. Nutritional deficiencies and syndromes associated with alcoholism. In: Goetz CG, Pappert EJ, eds. Textbook of Clinical Neurology. Philadelphia: WB Saunders Company, 1999:798–818
2. Windebank AJ. Polyneuropathy due to nutritional deficiency and alcoholism. In: Dyck PJ, Thomas PK, Griffin JW, et al., eds. Peripheral Neuropathy. Vol 2, 3rd ed. Philadelphia: WB Saunders Company, 1993:1310–1321
3. D'Amour ML, Butterworth RF. Pathogenesis of alcoholic peripheral neuropathy: direct effect of ethanol or nutritional deficit? Metab Brain Dis 1994;9:133–142
4. Poupon RE, Gervaise G, Riant P, et al. Blood thiamine and thiamine phosphate concentrations in excessive drinkers with or without peripheral neuropathy. Alcohol Alcohol 1990;25:605–611
5. Victor M, Adams RD. On the etiology of the alcoholic neurologic diseases with special reference to the role of nutrition. Am J Clin Nutr 1961;9:379–397
6. Victor M. Polyneuropathy due to nutritional deficiency and alcoholism. In: Dyck PJ, Thomas PK, Lambert EH, eds. Peripheral Neuropathy. Vol 2. Philadelphia: WB Saunders Company, 1975:1030–1066
7. Fennelly J, Frank O, Baker H, Leevy CM. Peripheral neuropathy of the alcoholic: I, Aetiological role of aneurin and other B-complex vitamins. Br Med J 1964;2:1290–1292
8. Strauss MB. Etiology of "alcoholic" polyneuritis. Am J Med Sci 1935;189:378–382
9. Walsh JC, McLeod JG. Alcoholic neuropathy. Proc Aust Assoc Neurol 1970;7:77–83
10. Behse F, Buchtal F. Alcoholic neuropathy: clinical, electrophysiological, and biopsy findings. Ann Neurol 1977;2:95–110
11. Monforte R, Estruch R, Valls-Sole J, et al. Autonomic and peripheral neuropathies in patients with chronic

alcoholism: a dose-related toxic effect of alcohol. Arch Neurol 1995;52:45–51

12. Hallett M, Fox JG, Rogers AE, et al. Controlled studies on the effects of alcohol ingestion on peripheral nerves of macaque monkeys. J Neurol Sci 1987;80:65–71

13. Bosch EP, Pelham RW, Rasool CG, et al. Animal models of alcoholic neuropathy: morphologic, electrophysiologic, and biochemical findings. Muscle Nerve 1979;2:133–144

14. Juntunen J, Teravainen H, Eriksson K, et al. Peripheral neuropathy and myopathy: an experimental study of rats on alcohol and variable dietary thiamine. Virchows Arch A Pathol Anat Histol 1979;383:241–252

15. Ortiz-Plata A, Palencia G, Garcia E, et al. Ultrastructural changes in limb distal nerves of rats with alcoholism and/or malnutrition before and after dietary correction. J Appl Toxicol 1998;18:89–92

16. Shields RW, Jr. Alcoholic polyneuropathy. Muscle Nerve 1985;8:183–187

17. Scholz E, Diener HC, Dichgans J, et al. Incidence of peripheral neuropathy and cerebellar ataxia in chronic alcoholics. J Neurol 1986;233:212–217

18. Walsh JC, McLeod JG. Alcoholic neuropathy: an electrophysiological and histological study. J Neurol Sci 1970;10:457–469

19. Tabaraud F, Vallat JM, Hugon J, et al. Acute or subacute alcoholic neuropathy mimicking Guillain-Barré syndrome. J Neurol Sci 1990;97:195–205

20. Casey EB, Le Quesne PM. Electrophysiological evidence for a distal lesion in alcoholic neuropathy. J Neurol Neurosurg Psychiatry 1972;35:624–630

21. Agelink MW, Malessa R, Weisser U, et al. Alcoholism, peripheral neuropathy (PNP) and cardiovascular autonomic neuropathy (CAN). J Neurol Sci 1998;161:135–142

22. Tackmann W, Minkenberg R, Strenge H. Correlation of electrophysiological and quantitative histological findings in the sural nerve of man: studies on alcoholic neuropathy. J Neurol 1977;216:289–299

23. Dyck PJ, Gutrecht JA, Bastron JA, et al. Histologic and teased-fiber measurements of sural nerve in disorders of lower motor and primary sensory neurons. Mayo Clin Proc 1968;43:81–123

24. Tredici G, Minazzi M. Alcoholic neuropathy: an electron-microscopic study. J Neurol Sci 1975;25:333–346

25. Low PA, Walsh JC, Huang CY, McLeod JG. The sympathetic nervous system in alcoholic neuropathy: a clinical and pathological study. Brain 1975;98:357–364

26. Woelk H, Lehrl S, Bitsch R, Kopcke W. Benfotiamine in treatment of alcoholic polyneuropathy: an 8-week randomized controlled study (BAP I Study). Alcohol Alcohol 1998;33:631–638

27. Hillbom M, Wennberg A. Prognosis of alcoholic peripheral neuropathy. J Neurol Neurosurg Psychiatry 1984;47:699–703

28. Johnson RH, Robinson BJ. Mortality in alcoholics with autonomic neuropathy. J Neurol Neurosurg Psychiatry 1988;51:476–480

29. Denke M, Wilson JD. Nutrition and nutritional requirements. In: Fauci AS, Braunwald E, Isselbacher KJ, et al., eds. Harrison's Principles of Internal Medicine. Vol 1, 14th ed. New York: McGraw-Hill, 1998:445–447

30. Tefferi A, Pruthi RK. The biochemical basis of cobalamin deficiency. Mayo Clin Proc 1994;69:181–186

31. Scalabrino G. Subacute combined degeneration one century later: the neurotrophic action of cobalamin (vitamin B_{12}) revisited. J Neuropathol Exp Neurol 2001;60:109–120

32. Green R, Kinsella LJ. Current concepts in the diagnosis of cobalamin deficiency. Neurology 1995;45:1435–1440

33. Hanger HC, Sainsbury R, Gilchrist NL, et al. A community study of vitamin B_{12} and folate levels in the elderly. J Am Geriatr Soc 1991;39:1155–1159

34. Pennypacker LC, Allen RH, Kelly JP, et al. High prevalence of cobalamin deficiency in elderly outpatients. J Am Geriatr Soc 1992;40:1197–1204

35. Yao Y, Yao SL, Yao SS, et al. Prevalence of vitamin B_{12} deficiency among geriatric outpatients. J Fam Pract 1992;35:524–528

36. Cole M. Neurological manifestations of vitamin B_{12} deficiency. In: Goetz CG, Aminoff MJ, eds. Handbook of Clinical Neurology, vol 26 (70): Systemic Diseases, Part II. Amsterdam: Elsevier, 1998:367–405

37. Lichtheim L. Zur Kenntniss der perniciösen Anämie. Verh Congr Inn Med 1887;6:84–99

38. Victor M, Lear AA. Subacute combined degeneration of the spinal cord: current concepts of the disease process. Value of serum vitamin B_{12} determinations in clarifying some of the common clinical problems. Am J Med 1956;20:896–911

39. Cabot RC. Pernicious and secondary anaemia, chlorosis, and leukaemia. In: Osler W, McCrae T, eds. Modern Medicine: Its Theory and Practice. Vol 4. Philadelphia, Lea & Febiger, 1908:612–680

40. Woltmann HW. The nervous symptoms in pernicious anemia: an analysis of one hundred and fifty cases. Am J Med Sci 1919;157:400–409

41. Healton EB, Savage DG, Brust JC, et al. Neurologic aspects of cobalamin deficiency. Medicine (Baltimore) 1991;70:229–245

42. Wilson SAK. Neurology. Vol 3, 2nd ed. Baltimore: Williams and Wilkins Company, 1955

43. Hemmer B, Glocker FX, Schumacher M, et al. Subacute combined degeneration: clinical, electrophysiological, and magnetic resonance imaging findings. J Neurol Neurosurg Psychiatry 1998;65:822–827

44. Layzer RB. Myeloneuropathy after prolonged exposure to nitrous oxide. Lancet 1978;2:1227–1230

45. Schilling RF. Is nitrous oxide a dangerous anesthetic for vitamin B_{12}-deficient subjects? JAMA 1986;255:1605–1606

46. Kinsella LJ, Green R. "Anesthesia paresthetica": nitrous oxide-induced cobalamin deficiency. Neurology 1995;45:1608–1610

47. McMorrow AM, Adams RJ, Rubenstein MN. Combined system disease after nitrous oxide anesthesia: a case report. Neurology 1995;45:1224–1225

48. Holloway KL, Alberico AM. Postoperative myeloneuropathy: a preventable complication in patients with B_{12} deficiency. J Neurosurg 1990;72:732–736

49. Flippo TS, Holder WD, Jr. Neurologic degeneration associated with nitrous oxide anesthesia in patients with vitamin B_{12} deficiency. Arch Surg 1993;128:1391–1395

50. Pant SS, Asbury AK, Richardson EP, Jr. The myelopathy of pernicious anemia. A neuropathological reappraisal. Acta Neurol Scand 1968;44(Suppl):1–36

51. Agamanolis DP, Chester EM, Victor M, et al. Neuropathology of experimental vitamin B_{12} deficiency in monkeys. Neurology 1976;26:905–914

52. Jagadha V, Deck JH, Halliday WC, Smyth HS. Wernicke's encephalopathy in patients on peritoneal dialysis or hemodialysis. Ann Neurol 1987;21:78–84

53. Brin M. Erythrocyte transketolase in early thiamine deficiency. Ann NY Acad Sci 1962;98:528–541

54. Wright H. Changes in the neuronal centres in beri-beric neuritis. Br Med J 1901;1:1610–1616

55. Prineas J. Peripheral nerve changes in thiamine-deficient rats: an electron microscope study. Arch Neurol 1970;23:541–548

56. Swank RL. Avian thiamin deficiency: correlation of pathology and clinical behavior. J Exp Med 1940;71:683–702

57. Ohnishi A, Tsuji S, Igisu H, et al. Beriberi neuropathy: morphometric study of sural nerve. J Neurol Sci 1980;45:177–190

58. Schaumburg H, Kaplan J, Windebank A, et al. Sensory neuropathy from pyridoxine abuse: a new megavitamin syndrome. N Engl J Med 1983;309:445–448

59. Vilter RW, Mueller JF, Glazer HS, et al. The effect of vitamin B_6 deficiency induced by desoxypyridoxine in human beings. J Lab Clin Med 1953;42:335–357

60. Gammon GD, Burge FW, King G. Neural toxicity in tuberculous patients treated with isoniazid (isonicotinic acid hydrazide). Arch Neurol Psychiatry 1953;70:64–69

61. Goldman AL, Braman SS. Isoniazid: a review with emphasis on adverse effects. Chest 1972;62:71–77

62. Biehl JP, Nimitz HJ. Studies on the use of a high dose of isoniazid. I. Toxicity studies. Am Rev Tuberc 1954;70:430–441

63. Victor M, Adams RD. The neuropathology of experimental vitamin B_6 deficiency in monkeys. Am J Clin Nutr 1956;4:346–353

64. Parry GJ, Bredesen DE. Sensory neuropathy with low-dose pyridoxine. Neurology 1985;35:1466–1468

65. Spies TD, Chinn AB, McLester JB. Severe endemic pellagra: a clinical study of fifty cases with special emphasis on therapy. JAMA 1937;108:853–857

66. Spies TD, Vilter RW, Ashe WF. Pellagra, beriberi and riboflavin deficiency in human beings: diagnosis and treatment. JAMA 1939;113:931–937

67. Spies TD, Aring CD. The effect of vitamin B_1 on the peripheral neuritis of pellagra. JAMA 1938;110:1081–1084

68. Miller RG, Davis CJ, Illingworth DR, Bradley W. The neuropathy of abetalipoproteinemia. Neurology 1980;30:1286–1291

69. Sokol RJ, Heubi JE, Iannaccone S, et al. Mechanism causing vitamin E deficiency during chronic childhood cholestasis. Gastroenterology 1983;85:1172–1182

70. Sokol RJ. Vitamin E deficiency and neurologic disease. Annu Rev Nutr 1988;8:351–373

71. Harding AE, Muller DP, Thomas PK, Willison HJ. Spinocerebellar degeneration secondary to chronic intestinal malabsorption: a vitamin E deficiency syndrome. Ann Neurol 1982;12:419–424

72. Harding AE, Matthews S, Jones S, et al. Spinocerebellar degeneration associated with a selective defect of vitamin E absorption. N Engl J Med 1985;313:32–35

73. Satya-Murti S, Howard L, Krohel G, Wolf B. The spectrum of neurologic disorder from vitamin E deficiency. Neurology 1986;36:917–921

74. Satya-Murti S. Neurological manifestations of excess and deficiency of vitamin E. In: Goetz CG, Aminoff MJ, eds. Handbook of Clinical Neurology, vol 26 (70): Systemic Diseases, Part II. Amsterdam: Elsevier, 1998:439–453

75. Bassen FA, Kornzweig AL. Malformation of the erythrocytes in a case of atypical retinitis pigmentosa. Blood 1950;5:381–387

76. Schwartz JF, Rowland LP, Eder PA, et al. Bassen-Kornzweig syndrome: deficiency of serum β-lipoprotein. Arch Neurol 1963;8:438–454

77. Sokol RJ, Bove KE, Heubi JE, Iannaccone ST. Vitamin E deficiency during chronic childhood cholestasis: presence of sural nerve lesion prior to 2 1/2 years of age. J Pediatr 1983;103:197–204

78. Sokol RJ, Guggenheim MA, Iannaccone ST, et al. Improved neurologic function after long-term correction of vitamin E deficiency in children with chronic cholestasis. N Engl J Med 1985;313:1580–1586

79. Azizi E, Zaidman JL, Eshchar J, Szeinberg A. Abetalipoproteinemia treated with parenteral and oral vitamins A and E, and with medium chain triglycerides. Acta Paediatr Scand 1978;67:796–801

80. Strachan H. On a form of multiple neuritis prevalent in the West Indies. Practitioner 1897;59:477–484

81. Denny-Brown D. Neurological conditions resulting from prolonged and severe dietary restriction: case reports in prisoners-of-war, and general review. Medicine (Baltimore) 1947;26:41–113

82. Fisher M. Residual neuropathological changes in Canadians held prisoners of war by the Japanese: Strachan's disease. Can Serv Med J 1955;11:157–199

83. Page JA. Painful-feet syndrome among prisoners of war in the Far East. Br Med J 1946;2:260–262

84. Stannus HS. Pellagra and pellagra-like conditions in warm climates. Trop Dis Bull 1936;33:729, 815

85. Cruickshank EK. Painful feet in prisoners-of-war in the Far East: review of 500 cases. Lancet 1946;2:369–372

86. Roman GC. An epidemic in Cuba of optic neuropathy, sensorineural deafness, peripheral sensory neuropathy and dorsolateral myeloneuropathy. J Neurol Sci 1994;127:11–28

87. Roman GC. On politics and health: an epidemic of neurologic disease in Cuba. Ann Intern Med 1995;122:530–533

88. Sadun AA, Martone JF, Muci-Mendoza R, et al. Epidemic optic neuropathy in Cuba: eye findings. Arch Ophthalmol 1994;112:691–699

89. Thomas PK, Plant GT, Baxter P, et al. An epidemic of optic neuropathy and painful sensory neuropathy in Cuba: clinical aspects. J Neurol 1995;242:629–638

90. Borrajero I, Perez JL, Dominguez C, et al. Epidemic neuropathy in Cuba: morphological characterization of peripheral nerve lesions in sural nerve biopsies. J Neurol Sci 1994;127:68–76

91. Abarbanel JM, Berginer VM, Osimani A, et al. Neurologic complications after gastric restriction surgery for morbid obesity. Neurology 1987;37:196–200

92. Feit H, Glasberg M, Ireton C, et al. Peripheral neuropathy and starvation after gastric partitioning for morbid obesity. Ann Intern Med 1982;96:453–455

93. Harwood SC, Chodoroff G, Ellenberg MR. Gastric partitioning complicated by peripheral neuropathy with lumbosacral plexopathy. Arch Phys Med Rehabil 1987;68:310–312

Acute Inflammatory Demyelinating Polyradiculoneuropathy, Acute Motor Axonal Neuropathy and Acute Motor and Sensory Axonal Neuropathy

Richard AC Hughes and David R Cornblath

Overview

Guillain–Barré syndrome (GBS) emerged as a distinct clinical entity after 1916 when Guillain, Barré and Strohl described two soldiers with reversible motor neuropathy associated with an increased CSF protein and normal CSF cell count.[1,2] An extensive clinico-pathological series from the Massachusetts General Hospital in 1969 showed that the underlying pathological basis was usually an acute inflammatory demyelinating polyradiculoneuropathy (AIDP).[3] The past 15 years have seen major advances in understanding GBS. Similar clinical syndromes have distinctive neurophysiological and pathological substrates and are now referred to as acute motor (AMAN) or motor and sensory (AMSAN) axonal neuropathy.[4] Thus, GBS now includes multiple subtypes including AIDP, AMAN, AMSAN, Fisher syndrome (see below), and other rarer variants.[5] Epidemiological studies have revealed the importance of viral and bacterial infections, especially Campylobacter jejuni, in triggering the disease.[6] Immune responses against gangliosides are induced by these infections and have been implicated in pathogenesis, especially of the axonal forms.[7] Randomized controlled trials (RCTs) have shown equivalent benefit from plasma exchange (PE)[8] and intravenous immunoglobulin (IVIg)[9] but not from corticosteroids,[10] while excellent intensive care and rehabilitation have remained paramount.

Epidemiology

The annual incidence of GBS ranges between 0.4 and 4 per 100 000 throughout the world. The variations in reported incidence may only represent differences in case ascertainment. When population based incidence studies have been repeated in the same location no convincing change in incidence has been demonstrated. There is a slight male preponderance and the disease becomes more common with advancing age. There may also be a small peak in the age distribution in young adults.[11] Apart from rare exceptions[12] GBS is sporadic and lacks seasonality. However, in Northern China epidemics of the AMAN form of the disease occur mainly in the summer months and among those from rural districts.[13,14]

Etiology

About two thirds of cases are preceded by symptoms of an upper respiratory or gastrointestinal infection. A wide range of organisms has been blamed; the major culprits for which there is strong evidence of a causal association are:

- Campylobacter jejuni
- Haemophilus influenzae[15]
- Cytomegalovirus
- Epstein–Barr virus
- Mycoplasma pneumoniae
- Rabies vaccine
- "Swine flu vaccine"

Ganglioside injections are a possible cause.[16]
The most commonly identified organisms are Campylobacter jejuni in about 25%, and cytomegalovirus in about 15% of cases.[6,17] There is no tight correlation between one preceding organism and the type of GBS. Thus, although C. jejuni is associated with more severe axonal degeneration, this infection may be followed by any of the different forms of GBS, including Fisher syndrome.[6]

Pathophysiology and pathogenesis

There is a close pathological resemblance between AIDP and experimental autoimmune neuritis (EAN) induced by immunizing laboratory animals with peripheral nerve myelin.[18,19] Immunization with any one of at least three myelin proteins, P0, P2 and PMP22, will induce EAN. Transfer of antimyelin protein T cells alone is sufficient. Attempts to prove that T cell responses to one of these proteins are responsible for AIDP continue but are not yet convincing.[20]

A major thrust of current work centers on the observation that antibodies to gangliosides are commonly found in this group of neuropathies. Antibodies to ganglioside GM1 are present in about 25% of patients with GBS, being more common in patients with preceding C. jejuni infection than those without and somewhat more common in patients with AMAN or AMSAN than in AIDP.[21,22] Attempts to match antibodies to different GBS subtypes and thus explain the pathogenesis are still ongoing but do not yet allow a clear immunological classification of syndromes.[20] Of 132 Dutch patients, 19% had antibodies to the minor ganglioside GM1b and these patients were more likely to have had a preceding *C. jejuni* infection, developed a rapidly progressive, pure motor neuropathy and shown a good response to IVIg but not to PE.[23] In the Chinese patients with AMAN there was a stronger association with antibodies to GD1a than with GM1.[7,24] This observation is of particular interest since monoclonal antibody to GD1a reacts with rat motor but not sensory axons, supporting the hypothesis that antibodies to GD1a could account for AMAN (Lunn, Sheikh and Griffin, personal communication, 2000). *Campylobacter jejuni* carries in its wall sialylated glycoconjugates which resemble gangliosides so that infection might stimulate the production of antibodies.

Genetics

Since only about one person in 1000 with *C. jejuni* infection develops GBS there must be some, presumably immunogenetic, host factor that contributes to pathogenesis. There is an unconfirmed report that HLA DQ1*03 is increased in GBS patients following *C. jejuni* but not in patients with GBS following other infections.[25] Of more importance seems to be the genetics of *C. jejuni*, since there was a striking preponderance of one particular genotype accounting for 9 of 17 cases over a 20-month period in Cape Town.[26] In Japan, when GBS follows *C. jejuni*, the Penner O:19 serotype is usually responsible although this is a rare cause of uncomplicated enteritis.[27,28]

Clinical features

In typical cases the first symptoms are pain, numbness, paresthesiae or weakness, or commonly a combination of all of these. The numbness and paresthesiae usually affect the extremities and spread proximally. The weakness may be initially proximal or distal or a combination of both. The facial nerves are commonly affected and less often the bulbar and ocular motor nerves. In 25% of cases the respiratory muscles become involved, causing respiratory failure and a requirement for artificial ventilation. Autonomic involvement causes retention of urine, ileus, sinus tachycardia, hypertension, cardiac arrhythmia, and postural hypotension. In severe cases muscle wasting becomes evident after about two weeks and may become profound. The disease reaches its nadir in two weeks in most cases and, by an arbitrary but agreed definition, in four weeks in all. After a variable plateau phase, recovery begins with return of proximal followed by distal strength over weeks or months. Between 4% and 15% of patients die, and up to 20% are left dead or disabled after a year despite modern treatment.[29–31] In the survivors fatigue is a common problem.[32]

In children pain is a prominent presenting symptom and may dominate the illness, complicating assessment of weakness. Recovery is more rapid and more likely to be complete.[33]

Classification

Cases of GBS may be classified according to whether the myelin sheaths or axons are affected and whether the motor, sensory or autonomic systems are involved (Table 192.1). In North America and Europe typical cases of GBS usually have AIDP as the underlying substrate and only about 5% of cases have axonal forms of the disease. In northern China, Japan, and Central and South America axonal forms are more common. In AMSAN sensory axons are affected as well as motor. In AMAN the neurological deficit is purely motor. Rare cases of acute transient sensory neuropathy may represent AIDP affecting only sensory nerves or roots but need to be distinguished from acute sensory neuronopathy, which usually leaves persistent deficit. Autonomic involvement is common in GBS, especially in severe cases with respiratory failure, and rare cases of acute dysautonomia without involvement of somatic nerves may be inflammatory and possibly autoimmune.

While in most cases the nerve supply of the limb, cranial and respiratory muscles are diffusely and symmetrically affected, in a minority the neurological deficit is much more focused. The most striking example is the Fisher syndrome, in which the signs are confined to ophthalmoplegia, ataxia and areflexia with some bulbar muscle involvement (see below). Some patients resemble this syndrome at the onset and then develop generalized weakness, the Fisher/GBS overlap syndrome. There is also a rare group who develop bulbar involvement and some of these also develop upper limb involvement. These subgroups are associated, mostly rather loosely, with different patterns of antiganglioside antibodies (Table 192.1).

Diagnostic criteria

The diagnosis of GBS depends on clinical criteria for an acute motor or sensory and motor polyradiculoneuropathy reaching its nadir within four weeks and lacking any other explanation.[34] The finding of an increased CSF protein concentration with a relatively normal CSF cell count is strongly supportive but not mandatory since the CSF is frequently normal during

Table 192.1 Classification of GBS and related disorders and typical antiganglioside antibodies

According to pathology
Acute inflammatory demyelinating polyradiculoneuropathy (AIDP)—GM1 in 25%
Acute motor and sensory axonal neuropathy (AMSAN)
Acute motor axonal neuropathy (AMAN)—GD1a in Chinese, GalNacGD1a in Japanese
Acute sensory neuronopathy
Acute pandysautonomia

Regional variants
Fisher syndrome—GQ1b in 95%
Oropharyngeal—GT1a

Overlap
Fisher/GBS overlap syndrome—GQ1b

Table 192.2   Neurophysiological criteria for AIDP, AMSAN and AMAN

AIDP
At least one of the following in each of at least two nerves, or at least two of the following in one nerve if all others
    inexcitable and dCMAP ≥ 10% LLN
Motor conduction velocity <90% LLN (85% if dCMAP <50% LLN)
Distal motor latency >110% ULN (120% if dCMAP <100% LLN)
pCMAP/dCMAP ratio <0.5 and dCMAP ≥ 20% LLN
F-response latency >120% ULN

AMSAN*
None of the features of AIDP except one demyelinating feature allowed in one nerve if dCMAP <10% LLN
Sensory action potential amplitudes <LLN

AMAN*
None of the features of AIDP except one demyelinating feature allowed in one nerve if dCMAP <10% LLN
Sensory action potential amplitudes >LLN

Inexcitable
dCMAP absent in all nerves or present in only one nerve with dCMAP <10% LLN

After Hadden et al.[35] and Ho et al.[36]
*In the original definitions the difference between AMSAN and AMAN proposed here is implied but not stipulated
dCMAP, compound muscle action potential amplitude after distal stimulation; pCMAP, compound muscle action potential amplitude after proximal stimulation; LLN, lower limit of normal; ULN, upper limit of normal

the first week of the disease. Signs of central nervous system involvement may occur but might indicate another diagnosis. There is debate whether purely sensory forms should be included. The diagnosis should be confirmed and classified into AIDP or AMSAN or AMAN according to neurophysiological criteria (Table 192.2). Most cases of GBS in North America and Europe will conform to the acute inflammatory demyelinating polyneuropathy (AIDP) subtype with smaller numbers of the other subtypes present.[35] In other regions, the proportion of "axonal" subtypes is greater.[4] The subtypes may be identified by electro-diagnosis, but criteria have varied in the reported studies. A single study compared various AIDP criteria in a single patient population, finding that in fact the criteria are similar but not identical in the identification of the AIDP subtype.[37]

Difficulties arise when the electrodiagnostic changes are only minor, as may happen in mild cases, or intermediate, when it may not be possible to assign a patient definitely into one or other category. Particular difficulty arises when nerves are inexcitable because it is then impossible to determine whether the absence of recordable sensory or motor action potentials is due to complete conduction block from demyelination or to axonal degeneration or dysfunction. In this situation the differentiation may perhaps be made by nerve biopsy but such an investigation is rarely necessary except as a research procedure.[38–40]

Differential diagnosis

Although GBS is the most common cause of acute neuromuscular paralysis in most parts of the world, the wide differential diagnosis must not be forgotten (Table 192.3).

Treatment

Early phase

Theoretical considerations and limited empirical evidence suggest that immunotherapy to ameliorate the underlying immunopathogenic disorder should be started early to reduce the amount of demyelination and axonal degeneration. It follows that assessment and establishment of the diagnosis should be conducted

Table 192.3   Differential diagnosis

Acute anterior poliomyelitis
    Caused by poliovirus
    Caused by other neurotropic viruses
Acute myelopathy
    Space-occupying lesions
    Acute transverse myelitis
Peripheral neuropathy
    Guillain–Barré syndromes
    Post-rabies vaccine neuropathy
    Diphtheritic neuropathy
    Heavy metals, biological toxins or drug intoxication
    Acute intermittent porphyria
    Vasculitic neuropathy
    Critical illness neuropathy
    Lymphomatous neuropathy
Disorders of neuromuscular transmission
    Myasthenia gravis
    Biological or industrial toxins
Disorders of muscle
    Hypokalemia
    Hypophosphatemia
    Inflammatory myopathy
    Acute rhabdomyolysis
    Trichinosis
    Periodic paralyses

After Cornblath[41]

rapidly so that treatment can begin before irreversible damage has been done. At the same time regard must be had to the potentially fatal but avoidable complications of the disease—respiratory failure, autonomic complications, especially cardiac arrhythmia, and pulmonary embolism.

The most immediate concern is the possibility of the rapid development of respiratory failure, which occurs in about 25% of patients with Guillain–Barré syndrome. Respiratory failure is more likely in patients with rapid progression, bulbar palsy, upper limb involvement, and autonomic dysfunction. Assessment of the moment when intubation and positive pressure ventilation should be instituted requires frequent examination by an experienced clinician. The over-riding aim is to perform intubation prophylactically under controlled conditions rather than allowing the patient to deteriorate to the point of respiratory and then cardiac arrest. This is the most important message in this chapter. Monitoring vital capacity is the most commonly used and convenient measurement.[42] Values below 20 ml/kg warrant transfer to an intensive therapy unit (ITU) and consideration of intubation and ventilation. Maximum inspiratory pressure less than 30 cm H_2O or maximum expiratory pressure less than 40 cm H_2O are sometimes used as alternative measures.[43] Deteriorating blood gases are a late event and their evaluation is not a satisfactory substitute for careful clinical monitoring. Clinical assessment needs to be global and take into account vital capacity, bulbar palsy, speed of deterioration, respiratory rate, pulse, use of accessory respiratory muscles, distress and fatigue. If tracheostomy is required, the anesthetic agent used during the procedure should not include suxamethonium, which causes dangerous hyperkalemia in the presence of denervating muscle.

Monitoring for possible cardiac arrhythmia should always be undertaken in patients who require or seem likely to require artificial ventilation.[42] Since cardiac arrhythmias may occur before ventilation has started and after it has stopped it is difficult to lay down guidelines for the timing of starting and stopping continuous ECG monitoring which are not unduly restrictive. One suggested plan is to monitor the ECG of all patients who become bed-bound or who have a significant bulbar palsy and continue this monitoring until they are ambulant, the bulbar palsy is virtually recovered, and the tracheostomy tube has been removed if one was inserted. The most dangerous time for arrhythmias is during tracheal suction. The danger may be reduced by hyperoxygenation with 100% oxygen before each suction. Rare patients have recurrent episodes of bradycardia which may require insertion of a pacemaker. There are no useful techniques for predicting the occurrence of cardiac arrhythmias except their occurrence, which makes recurrence more likely. Wide fluctuations of pulse and blood pressure occur in severe cases and may herald serious and sustained autonomic failure.

Other autonomic complications during the early stage include urinary retention, which can be easily managed by catheterization, and paralytic ileus, which is more difficult. Restriction of enteral fluids is only possible as a short term measure because of concerns about malnutrition. Reduction of sedation, opiates and atropine-like drugs, enemas and patience will eventually be rewarded but ileus contributes to the misery of the patient.

Immunotherapy: steroids

Paradoxically, despite the inflammatory and probably immune nature of the underlying pathology, it has not been possible to demonstrate a beneficial effect from steroids. A Cochrane systematic review sought all published and unpublished trials of any form of corticosteroid or adrenocorticotrophic hormone treatment for GBS.[10] Six randomized trials were identified including a total of 195 corticosteroid treated patients and 187 control subjects.[44–48] One trial of intravenous methylprednisolone accounted for 63% of the 382 subjects studied.[47] This trial did not show a significant difference in any disability related outcome between the corticosteroid and placebo groups. The primary outcome measure in the systematic review was the improvement in a seven point disability grade scale 4 weeks after randomization. There was no difference in this outcome between the steroid and no steroid/placebo patients, the weighted mean difference of the three trials being only 0.01 (95% confidence interval [CI] −0.27 to 0.29) grade more in the corticosteroid group. There was also no significant difference between the groups for time to recovery of unaided walking, time to discontinue ventilation in the subgroup who needed ventilation, mortality, death and disability after one year.[10] The conclusion that steroids are not beneficial in GBS may need revision when the results of a large multicenter trial comparing IVIg alone and IVIg with intravenous methylprednisolone become available.[49]

Plasma exchange

By contrast with steroids, plasma exchange has been convincingly shown to be beneficial in patients with GBS so severe that they are unable to walk. A Cochrane systematic review identified six trials which compared plasma exchange alone to supportive care.[50] One trial involving 29 participants only showed a trend towards a more favorable outcome with plasma exchange.[51] The other five showed significantly more improvement in disability grade or more patients improved in disability grade after 4 weeks.[8,52–58] In a meta-analysis of all six studies the proportion of patients on the ventilator 4 weeks after randomization was reduced to 48/321 in the PE group compared to 106/325 in the control group, relative risk 0.56 (95% CI, 0.41 to 0.76, $P = 0.0003$).[50] In a meta-analysis of four studies for which the outcome was available[51,55,56,58] 135/199 PE and 112/205 control patients had recovered full muscle strength after a year, relative risk 1.24 (1.07 to 1.45, $P = 0.005$) in favor of PE.[59] The North American PE trial demonstrated significant benefit from PE given during the first 4 weeks but the benefit was greater when treatment was given during the first week.[8,52] The benefit was less still if patients were treated more than 2 weeks after the onset of neuropathy. It follows from this that patients should be treated as early as possible in the course of their illness.

In one study comparing PE with supportive treatment in Scandinavia[53] the cost of PE was more than offset by the savings in healthcare costs as a result of shorter hospital stay. Similar conclusions have been reached in the UK.[60]

Intravenous immunoglobulin

The report of rapid improvement in six of eight patients with Guillain–Barré syndrome (GBS) treated with IVIg was followed by a randomized controlled trial showing that it was as least as effective as plasma exchange (PE) in hastening recovery.[9,61] A Cochrane systematic review of this and two other RCTs [62,63] has been undertaken.[50] The regimen used in these trials was 0.4 g/kg daily for 5 days, and dose ranging studies have not been done. The mean improvement in disability grade four weeks after randomization was available for two trials.[9,62,63] In a meta-analysis, 204 patients had been treated with IVIg and 194 with PE. The weighted mean difference was 0.11 of a disability grade more improvement in 204 patients treated with IVIg group than in 194 patients treated with PE group, a nonsignificant difference (the 95% CI were −0.14 to 0.37). There was a nonsignificant trend toward faster recovery of unaided walking in both these trials. In the third trial these outcome measures were not available but related measures (proportion of patients improving one grade after 4 weeks and time to recover the ability to do manual work) showed a trend in favor of IVIg compared with PE.[62] There were no significant differences in the meta-analysis of time until discontinuation of mechanical ventilation or the proportions of patients dead or disabled after one year between the IVIg and PE treated groups. In each trial there were more adverse events in the PE than the IVIg group, but because of different definitions of adverse events, a meta-analysis could not be performed. In the two largest trials treatment was much less likely to be discontinued in the IVIg than in the PE treated patients, relative risk 0.11 (95% CI 0.04 to 0.32).

The Cochrane review concluded that IVIg is as effective as PE in hastening recovery from severe GBS when given in the first 2 weeks of the illness in adult patients and the planned dose was much more likely to be administered. In children, one trial did compare IVIg with supportive treatment but it had inadequate allocation concealment and was too small (only 18 patients) to permit robust conclusions. Nevertheless, IVIg is widely used for GBS in pediatric practice and a randomized trial is in progress (Korinthenberg R, personal communication, 2000). In adult practice, IVIg has become the standard treatment for GBS in the UK and most neurology departments in Europe and the USA.

Combination treatments

One large trial comparing IVIg followed by PE with IVIg alone or PE alone showed no significant advantage to the combined regimen in any of the outcomes measured.[63] After 4 weeks there was 0.20 of a grade more improvement in the 128 patients who received both treatments than in the 121 patients who received PE alone but this small difference favoring combined treatment was not significant (95% CI −0.54 to 0.14). The median (inter-quartile range) time to recover unaided walking was 40 (19 to 137) days in the 128 patients who received both treatments and 29 (19 to 148) days in the 121 patients who received PE alone. The difference between these medians was also not significant. There were more complications of treatment in the combined treatment group than in either of the single treatment groups. A small study comparing immunoabsorption with tryptophan polyvinyl exchange alone and immunoabsorption followed by IVIg showed no significant difference between these regimens after one and 12 months.[64] There is therefore no evidence base to support the use of combination treatments.

Treatment of apparently unresponsive patients

A remaining cause of concern is that despite current treatment with IVIg or PE about 20% of patients die or are left disabled. The search for alternative treatments must continue. Particular concern surrounds the treatment options faced by the clinician when the patient fails to improve two or three weeks after initial treatment. A trial is needed to determine whether a further course of IVIg or the use of PE at this stage is beneficial. There is no consensus about the management of this problem. We prefer to give a second course of IVIg[65] because the alternative, plasma exchange, carries more risk and removes the immunoglobulin which had been given as the initial treatment. Other avenues for future consideration include the use of immunomodulatory cytokines and inhibitors of the metalloproteinases which contribute to demyelination.

Plateau phase care

Patients being treated with mechanical ventilation require careful adjustment of the ventilator parameters, chest physiotherapy and tracheal suction to avoid atelectasis. Hyperoxygenation before tracheal suction helps to avoid or minimize the effects of dangerous bradycardia during this powerful vagal stimulus. Most patients who require ventilation come to need tracheostomy, which is best inserted with a percutaneous dilation technique rather than by surgical operation because it leaves a more acceptable long term cosmetic result. We prefer to place a tracheostomy after about five to seven days because it is more comfortable than prolonged oral intubation and may be less traumatic for the vocal cords, but others are prepared to leave an orotracheal tube for up to three weeks.

During the plateau phase excellent general medical

and nursing care are needed for the comfort of the patient and to avoid complications. Regimens of passive movements of all joints through a full range and splinting are used in the often vain attempt to avoid contractures. Since pulmonary embolism causes a small percentage of deaths, prophylaxis should always be considered in patients who are confined to bed. Low dose subcutaneous heparin, either conventional or of low molecular weight, is the conventional treatment. Distressing aching pain occurs in about half of patients and dysesthetic pain in the extremities in 20% and myalgic pain in 10%.[66] Careful positioning, physiotherapy and nonsteroidal anti-inflammatory drugs are often inadequate, and opiates may be required in order to achieve control. Dysesthetic pain may respond to amitriptyline, gabapentin or carbamazepine. The disease is distressing and frightening so that careful and repeated explanation and counseling are important. This may be difficult in the severely paralyzed patient: resort must be made to communicating with letter boards or signing with whatever fragments of movement remain. A visit from a recovered patient can be reassuring and may be arranged through some of the patient support groups (see below).

Nutrition needs to be monitored and maintained. Muscle wasting as a consequence of denervation should not be compounded by iatrogenic starvation. A nasogastric tube is needed in patients with bulbar palsy or respiratory failure, and after two to three weeks we prefer to replace this with a percutaneous gastrostomy which is more comfortable and reduces the risk of sinusitis. The biochemical status requires continued monitoring because of the danger of hyponatremia due to inappropriate secretion of antidiuretic hormone. In adolescents there is also a possibility of dangerous hypercalcemia caused by immobility.

Rehabilitation

A rehabilitation program should be instituted as soon as possible.[67] Occupational and physical therapy should begin during the acute phase, be continued during the plateau phase, and intensified as improvement starts. Therapy practice varies from unit to unit and no randomized trials are available to guide the choice of techniques or of orthoses. It is not clear how soon exercise training should begin and how vigorous it should be. Faced with the inadequacy of the evidence the Delphic oracle's advice, "moderation in all things," is dull but appropriate. Earlier ambulation can be achieved with lightweight customized ankle-foot orthoses and appropriate crutches or canes.

The process of convalescence may be prolonged and needs to be respected because profound fatigue is a common aftermath. Bernsen and colleagues found that 80% of patients[68,69] still had disabling fatigue several years later which interfered with return to work. The reasons for fatigue require careful examination in each individual since they are often not related to conventional measures of residual impairment but to a complex mixture including alterations of mood, differences in coping strategy and other factors which are as yet incompletely understood. Patients often derive benefit from joining a patient support organization such as The Guillain–Barré Syndrome Foundation International (http://www.webmast.com/gbs) in the US and Guillain–Barré Syndrome (http://www.gbs.org.uk/) in the UK.

Acknowledgments

We thank Drs A. Hahn, J. Meythaler, J. Raphael, A. Ropper, F. van der Meché and E. Wijdicks for valuable discussion.

References

1. Guillain G, Barré JA, Strohl A. Sur un syndrome de radiculo-névrite avec hyperalbuminose du liquide cephalo-rachidien sans réaction cellulaire. Remarques sur les caracteres cliniques et graphiques des reflexes tendineux. Bull Soc Méd Hôp Paris 1916;40:1462–1470
2. Hughes RAC. History and Definition. Guillain–Barré Syndrome. Heidelberg: Springer-Verlag, 1990:1–16
3. Asbury AK, Arnason BG, Adams RD. The inflammatory lesion in idiopathic polyneuritis. Its role in pathogenesis. Medicine 1969;48:173–215
4. Griffin JW, Li CY, Ho TW, et al. Guillain–Barré syndrome in northern China. The spectrum of neuropathological changes in clinically defined cases. Brain 1995;118:577–595
5. Ropper AH, Wijdicks EFM, Truax BT. Guillain–Barré Syndrome. Philadelphia: F.A. Davis, 1991
6. Rees JH, Soudain SE, Gregson NA, Hughes RAC. A prospective case control study to investigate the relationship between *Campylobacter jejuni* infection and Guillain–Barré syndrome. N Engl J Med 1995;333:1374–1379
7. Ho TW, Willison HJ, Nachamkin I, et al. Anti-GD1a antibody is associated with axonal but not demyelinating forms of Guillain–Barré syndrome. Ann Neurol 1999;45:168–173
8. The Guillain–Barré Syndrome Study Group. Plasmapheresis and acute Guillain–Barré syndrome. Neurology 1985;35:1096–1104
9. van der Meché FGA, Schmitz PIM, Dutch Guillain–Barré Study Group. A randomized trial comparing intravenous immune globulin and plasma exchange in Guillain–Barré syndrome. N Engl J Med 1992;326:1123–1129
10. Hughes RAC, van der Meché FGA. Corticosteroids for treating Guillain–Barré syndrome (Cochrane Review). *In:* The Cochrane Library, Issue 4, 2000. Oxford: Update Software
11. Hughes RAC, Rees JH. Clinical and epidemiological features of Guillain–Barré syndrome. J Infect Dis 1997;176(Suppl 2):S92–S98
12. Roman GC. Tropical neuropathies. *In:* Hartung H-P, ed. Peripheral Neuropathies: Part 1. London: Baillière Tindall, 1995:469–487
13. McKhann GM, Cornblath DR, Ho TW, et al. Clinical and electrophysiological aspects of acute paralytic disease of children and young adults in northern China. Lancet 1991;338:593–597
14. McKhann GM, Cornblath DR, Griffin JW, et al. Acute motor axonal neuropathy: A frequent cause of acute flaccid paralysis in China. Ann Neurol 1993;33:333–342

15. Mori M, Kuwabara S, Miyake M, et al. *Haemophilus influenzae* infection and Guillain–Barré syndrome. Brain 2000;123:2171–2178

16. Illa I, Ortiz N, Gallard E, et al. Acute axonal Guillain–Barré syndrome with IgG antibodies against motor axons following parenteral gangliosides. Ann Neurol 1995;38:218–224

17. Winer JB, Hughes RAC, Anderson MJ, et al. A prospective study of acute idiopathic neuropathy. II. Antecedent events. J Neurol Neurosurg Psychiatry 1988;51:613–618

18. Lampert PW. Mechanism of demyelination in experimental allergic neuritis. Electron microscopic studies. Lab Invest 1969;20:127–138

19. Prineas JW. Acute idiopathic polyneuritis. An electron-microscope study. Lab Invest 1972;26:133–147

20. Hughes RAC, Gregson NA, Hadden RDM, Smith KJ. Pathogenesis of Guillain–Barré syndrome. J Neuroimmunol 1999;100:74–97

21. Yuki N, Yoshino H, Sato S, Miyatake T. Acute axonal neuropathy associated with anti-GM$_1$ antibodies following Campylobacter enteritis. Neurology 1990;40:1900–1902

22. Rees JH, Gregson NA, Hughes RAC. Anti-ganglioside antibodies in patients with Guillain–Barré syndrome and *Campylobacter jejuni* infection. J Infect Dis 1995;172:605–605

23. Yuki N, Ang CW, Koga M, et al. Clinical features and response to treatment in Guillain–Barré syndrome associated with antibodies to GM1b ganglioside. Ann Neurol 2000;47:314–321

24. Ilyas A, Willison H, Quarles RH, et al. Serum antibodies to gangliosides in Guillain–Barré syndrome. Ann Neurol 1999;23:440–447

25. Rees JH, Vaughan RW, Kondeatis E, Hughes RAC. HLA-Class II alleles in Guillain–Barré syndrome and Miller Fisher syndrome and their association with preceding *Campylobacter jejuni* infection. J Neuroimmunol 1995;62:53–57

26. Lastovica AJ, Goddard EA, Argent AC. Guillain–Barré syndrome in South Africa associated with *Campylobacter jejuni*. J Infect Dis 1997;176(Suppl 2):S139–S143

27. Yuki N, Handa S, Tai T, et al. Ganglioside-like epitopes of lipopolysaccharides from *Campylobacter jejuni* (PEN 19) in three isolates from patients with Guillain–Barré syndrome. J Neurol Sci 1995;130:112–116

28. Yuki N. Molecular mimicry between gangliosides and lipopolysaccharides of *Campylobacter jejuni* isolated from patients with Guillain–Barré syndrome and Miller Fisher syndrome. J Infect Dis 1997;176:S150–S153

29. Prevots DR, Sutter RW. Assessment of Guillain–Barré syndrome mortality and morbidity in the United States: Implications for acute flaccid paralysis surveillance. J Infect Dis 1997;175(Suppl 1):S151–S155

30. Rees JH, Thompson RD, Smeeton NC, Hughes RAC. An epidemiological study of Guillain–Barré syndrome in South East England. J Neurol Neurosurg Psychiatry 1998;64:74–77

31. Van Koningsveld R, van Doorn PA, Schmitz PIM, van der Meché FGA. Changes in referral pattern and its effect on outcome in patients with Guillain–Barré syndrome. Neurology 2001;56:564–566

32. Merkies IS, Schmitz PI, Samijn JP, et al. Fatigue in immune-mediated polyneuropathies. European Inflammatory Neuropathy Cause and Treatment (INCAT) Group. Neurology 1999;53(8):1648–1654

33. Bradshaw DY, Jones HR Jr. Guillain–Barré syndrome in children: Clinical course, electrodiagnosis, and progno-sis. Muscle Nerve 1992;15:500–506

34. Asbury AK, Cornblath DR. Assessment of current diagnostic criteria for Guillain–Barré syndrome. Ann Neurol 1990;27(Suppl):S21–S24

35. Hadden RDM, Cornblath DR, Hughes RAC, et al. Electrophysiological classification of Guillain–Barré syndrome: clinical associations and outcome. Ann Neurol 1998;44:780–788

36. Ho TW, Mishu B, Li CY, et al. Guillain–Barré syndrome in northern China. Relationship to *Campylobacter jejuni* infection and anti-glycolipid antibodies. Brain 1995;118:597–605

37. Alam TA, Chaudhry V, Cornblath D. Electrophysiological studies in the Guillain–Barré syndrome: distinguishing subtypes by published criteria. Muscle Nerve 1998;21:1275–1279

38. Hall SM, Hughes RAC, Payan J, et al. Motor nerve biopsy in severe Guillain–Barré syndrome. Ann Neurol 1992;31:441–444

39. Berciano J, Coria F, Monton F, et al. Axonal form of Guillain–Barré syndrome: evidence for macrophage-associated demyelination. Muscle Nerve 1993;16:744–751

40. Berciano J, Figols J, García A, et al. Fulminant Guillain–Barré syndrome with universal inexcitability of peripheral nerves: A clinicopathological study. Muscle Nerve 1997;20:846–857

41. Cornblath DR (Rapporteur) Acute onset flaccid paralysis. WHO-AIREN/MNH/EPI/93.3, Geneva, 1993

42. Hughes RAC, McLuckie A. Acute neuromuscular respiratory paralysis. *In:* Hughes RAC, ed. Neurological Emergencies. London: BMJ Books, 2000:332–358

43. Lawn ND, Wijdicks EF. Fatal Guillain–Barré syndrome. Neurology 1999;52:635–638

44. Hughes RAC, Newsom-Davis JM, Perkin GD, Pierce JM. Controlled trial of prednisolone in acute polyneuropathy. Lancet 1978;2:750–753

45. Mendell JR, Kissel JT, Kennedy MS, et al. Plasma exchange and prednisone in Guillain–Barré syndrome. A controlled randomised trial. Neurology 1985;35:1551–1555

46. Shukla SK, Agarwal R, Gupta OP, et al. Double blind control trial of prednisolone in Guillain–Barré syndrome—a clinical study. Clinician—India 1988;52:128–134

47. Guillain–Barré Syndrome Steroid Trial Group. Double-blind trial of intravenous methylprednisolone in Guillain–Barré syndrome. Lancet 1993;341:586–590

48. Singh NK, Gupta A. Do corticosteroids influence the disease course or mortality in Guillain–Barré syndrome. J Assoc Physicians India 1996;44:22–24

49. The Dutch Guillain–Barré Study Group. Treatment of Guillain–Barré syndrome with high-dose immune globulins combined with methylprednisolone: a pilot study. Ann Neurol 1994;35:749–752

50. Hughes RAC, Raphael J-C, Swan AV, van Doorn PA. Intravenous immunoglobulin for treating Guillain–Barré syndrome. (Cochrane Review). *In:* The Cochrane Library, Issue 2, 2001. Oxford: Update Software

51. Greenwood RJ, Newsom Davis JM, Hughes RAC, et al. Controlled trial of plasma exchange in acute inflammatory polyradiculoneuropathy. Lancet 1984;1:877–879

52. McKhann GM, Griffin JW, Cornblath DR, et al. Plasmapheresis and Guillain–Barré Syndrome: analysis of prognostic factors and the effect of plasmapheresis. Ann Neurol 1988;23:347–353

53. Osterman PO, Lundemo G, Pirskanen R, et al. Benefi-

cial effects of plasma exchange in acute inflammatory polyradiculoneuropathy. Lancet 1984;2:1296–1299

54. French Cooperative Group on plasma exchange in Guillain–Barré syndrome. Appropriate number of plasma exchanges in Guillain–Barré syndrome. Ann Neurol 1999;41:298–306

55. French Cooperative group in plasma exchange in Guillain–Barré syndrome. Efficiency of plasma exchange in Guillain–Barré syndrome: role of replacement fluids. Ann Neurol 1987;22:753–761

56. French Cooperative Group on plasma exchange in Guillain–Barré syndrome. Plasma exchange in Guillain–Barré syndrome: One-year follow-up. Ann Neurol 1992;32:94–97

57. Farkkila M, Kinnlinen E, Haapanen E, Inanainen M. Guillain–Barré syndrome: quantitative measurement of plasma exchange therapy. Neurology 1987;37:837–840

58. The French Cooperative Group on Plasma Exchange in Guillain–Barré Syndrome. Appropriate number of plasma exchanges in Guillain–Barré syndrome. Ann Neurol 1997;41:298–306

59. Raphael J-C, Chevret S, Hughes RAC. Plasma exchange for treating Guillain–Barré syndrome (Cochrane Review). In: The Cochrane Library, Issue 2, 2001. Oxford: Update Software

60. Tharakan J, Ferner RE, Hughes RAC, et al. Plasma exchange for Guillain–Barré syndrome. J R Soc Med 1989;82:458–461

61. Kleyweg RP, van der Meché FGA, Meulstee J. Treatment of Guillain–Barré syndrome with high dose gammaglobulin. Neurology 1988;38:1639–1642

62. Bril V, Ilse WK, Pearce R, et al. Pilot trial of immunoglobulin versus plasma exchange in patients with Guillain–Barré syndrome. Neurology 1996;46: 100–103

63. Plasma Exchange/Sandoglobulin Guillain–Barré Syndrome Trial Group. Randomised trial of plasma exchange, intravenous immunoglobulin, and combined treatments in Guillain–Barré syndrome. Lancet 1997;349:225–230

64. Haupt WF, Rosenow F, van der Ven C, et al. Sequential treatment of Guillain–Barré syndrome with extracorporeal elimination and intravenous immunoglobulin. J Neurol Sci 1996;137:145–149

65. Farcas P, Avnun L, Herishanu YO, Wirguin I. Efficacy of repeated intravenous immunoglobulin in severe unresponsive Guillain–Barré syndrome. Lancet 1997;350:1747

66. Moulin DE, Hagen N, Feasby TE, et al. Pain in Guillain–Barré syndrome. Neurology 1997;48:328–331

67. Meythaler JM. Rehabilitation of Guillain–Barré syndrome. Arch Phys Med Rehabil 1997;78:872–879

68. Bernsen RAJAM, Jacobs HM, De Jager AEJ, van der Meché FGA. Residual health status after Guillain–Barré Syndrome. J Neurol Neurosurg Psychiatry 1997;62: 637–640

69. Bernsen RAJAM, De Jager AEJ, Schmitz PIM, van der Meché FGA. Residual physical outcome and daily living 3 to 6 years after Guillain–Barré syndrome. Neurology 1999;53:409–410

193 Chronic Inflammatory Demyelinating Polyradiculoneuropathy

Angelika F Hahn

Overview

Chronic inflammatory demyelinating polyradiculoneuropathy (CIDP) is an acquired peripheral nerve disorder of presumed autoimmune etiology. It was Austin[1] and Dyck et al.[2] who first described the characteristic clinical features of this generalized neuropathy that pursues either a relapsing or a chronic progressive course and may be uniquely responsive to corticosteroids. Prineas and McLeod[3] gave a detailed account of the typical electrophysiological findings of marked slowing of motor nerve conductions, and related these to the multifocal, macrophage-mediated segmental demyelination observed in the pathological examination of spinal nerve roots and peripheral nerves. Specific guidelines for the diagnosis of CIDP have now been formulated,[4] based on the analysis of several large patient series.[5-7] Moreover, the natural history of the disease has been carefully delineated, separating CIDP from the acute inflammatory demyelinating neuropathy or Guillain–Barré syndrome (GBS). Both conditions may lead to fairly symmetrical weakness or flaccid limb paralyses, attenuation or loss of deep tendon reflexes, altered sensation and paresthesias. Yet they differ in time course and evolution of clinical signs, and in the tendency of CIDP to follow a chronic progressive or a relapsing course over months to years. Both CIDP and GBS respond favorably to a variety of immune modulatory therapies,[8-12] which lends support for the concept of a shared immunopathogenesis.[13]

Epidemiology

From the few systematic epidemiological studies, the prevalence of CIDP has been estimated at 1.0 to 1.9 per 100 000 population.[14,15] There is a male predominance, and disease onset is most common in the fifth to seventh decade, but may occur at all ages. Patients with relapsing-remitting disease, who make up 40% to 65% of several large case series, tend to have an earlier onset than those with a monophasic and progressive course.[6,7,16,17] As yet, no specific genetic predispositions have been identified. Previous findings of association of CIDP with certain HLA antigens have recently been refuted in a large case study.[18]

Clinical features

In typical CIDP, the motor and sensory deficits develop insidiously over weeks to months (an arbitrarily defined minimum of 8 weeks) or even years, leading eventually to significant disability.[2,7] Occa-

sionally, the presentation may be more acute and not unlike GBS, yet the disease is subsequently shown to assume a relapsing or a progressive course.[19] This is particularly true for children, in whom the onset of symptoms is often more precipitous.[6,20,21] Antecedent infections or other putative triggers such as vaccinations are less commonly identified in CIDP; in fact, it is uncertain whether the reported incidence of 10% to 32%[2,6,22] exceeds that expected by chance alone. However, ascertainment may not be accurate. Patients may simply no longer recall such prodromal events, given the insidious nature of the neuropathy and the common delay in the neurological diagnosis (on average 6 to 12 months from onset of symptoms). The association of CIDP onset or relapse with pregnancy has been noted.[6]

At presentation, most patients report symptoms that reflect a combination of proximal and distal limb muscle weakness and sensory loss. These include gait abnormalities with tendency to trip or fall, difficulty with stairs and with rising from a seated position, weakness and clumsiness of arms and hands, impaired dexterity and inability to identify coins and objects by touch, numbness and paresthesias in the hands or feet and, much more rarely, painful symptoms such as aching or jabbing pains. Consequently, the patient may require ambulatory aids such as a cane or a walker, or may even become wheelchair-dependent or bed-bound.

The examination reveals a variable degree of flaccid weakness in both proximal and distal muscles (100%), usually in a fairly symmetrical distribution. Muscle atrophy is either absent or is of much lesser degree, and deep tendon reflexes are decreased or absent (95%). Facial weakness (15%), ptosis or ophthalmoparesis (5%) and papilledema (7%) are occasionally seen, yet bulbar weakness and respiratory insufficiency are rare. Sensory impairment or loss are common (85%) and are accentuated distally; loss of proprioceptive functions may lead to an irregular postural and action tremor (5%).[2,6,7,16,22]

Disease course and natural history

The clinical course may be stepwise or chronic progressive, or relapsing. Patients with relapsing disease tend to have a more precipitous onset, the disease reaching its nadir commonly within four to eight weeks,[6,22] whereas patients with a monophasic disease form have a more protracted course and their diagnosis is often delayed (mean 4.9 months).[7,17] Spontaneous remissions are rare. The majority of CIDP patients require one or more immunomodulatory therapies to initiate neurological recovery and to bring about long term stabilization. The overall prognosis of CIDP is good. Barohn et al.[7] observed a complete remission in approximately 40% of their patients; most patients required ongoing immunomodulatory therapy and, on long term follow-up, they remained with mild to moderate disability. Outcome and persistent neurological deficits were correlated with electrophysiological and pathological findings of axonal degeneration and nerve fiber loss, a known sequel of the chronically recurring inflammatory demyelination.[23]

Variant forms of CIDP

Rarely, the clinical presentation of CIDP may be purely sensory (in approximately 5%). Such patients have prominent sensory signs and gait ataxia, as well as a large-amplitude action tremor, but little muscle weakness.[16,24,25] However, electrophysiological studies reveal the typical findings of demyelination not only in sensory but also in motor nerves, indicating a more generalized disease process and justifying the diagnosis of CIDP. Conversely, variant forms with pure motor presentations,[2,26] or with focally restricted or asymmetrical disease patterns and regional demyelinating pathology have been described.[27-30] Early in the disease course, such patients may have motor and sensory deficits predominant in the upper limbs, caused by the focal involvement of individual nerves. Yet electrophysiological studies will again show more widespread abnormalities and, on long term follow-up, the condition may evolve into the more typical pattern of a generalized polyradiculoneuropathy.[28,31] The nosological position of rare forms of CIDP, in which there is evidence of multifocal central nervous system (CNS) demyelination, remains uncertain.[32] In studying regular CIDP patients prospectively with magnetic resonance imaging (MRI) of the brain, Feasby et al.[33] found concurrent focal CNS demyelination to be uncommon.

Idiopathic CIDP (CIDP-I) has been differentiated from variant forms of chronic demyelinating neuropathies that occur in association with so-called "monoclonal gammopathies of undetermined significance" (CIDP-MGUS).[17,22,34-36] The latter appear to have a distinct natural history and response to therapy. Yet the clinical presentation of CIDP-MGUS can be remarkably similar, and electrodiagnostic studies may document findings of an acquired demyelinating neuropathy that are indistinguishable from those of CIDP-I.[37] CIDP-MGUS tends to follow a slowly progressive course. It is primarily encountered in older patients (predominantly men), and leads to more pronounced sensory rather than motor deficits. Although current diagnostic criteria distinguish between CIDP-I and CIDP-MGUS, the distinction may turn out to be somewhat arbitrary, since patients with CIDP-I occasionally develop an IgA or IgG monoclonal gammopathy during the course of their illness.[17] Thus, CIDP-MGUS may be part of the CIDP spectrum and contribute to its heterogeneity. It has been suggested that CIDP-IgG/A variants benefit as much as CIDP-I from the current immunomodulatory therapies, while CIDP-IgM is less likely to respond.[34,38,39] The separate classification of the CIDP-IgM variant may thus be justified. These points are set out in a succinct discussion by Dyck and Dyck.[40]

CIDP with concurrent illness

An acquired demyelinating neuropathy, indistinguishable from CIDP-I, may occur in the setting of a variety of disorders:

- HIV infection
- Monoclonal gammopathy
- Chronic active hepatitis
- Inflammatory bowel disease
- Connective tissue disease
- Bone marrow and organ transplants
- Lymphoma
- Melanoma
- Diabetes mellitus
- Thyrotoxicosis
- Nephrotic syndrome
- CNS demyelination.

Although it is important to consider these forms of CIDP in their proper context with the associated disease, the approach to diagnosis and therapy should be the same.

Chronic inflammatory axonal polyneuropathy (CIAP)

Many retrospective series of CIDP contain a variable proportion of cases that are clearly responsive to immunosuppressive drug therapy, but that have clinical, electrophysiological, and pathological features of pure or predominant axonal degeneration.[7,41] Some probably represent very chronic cases of regular CIDP, in whom one may observe a substantial amount of axonal degeneration as a consequence of the chronically recurring inflammatory demyelination.[23] Recently, however, Chroni et al.[42] reported a patient in whom all evidence suggested a primary axonal pathology and who responded favorably to steroid treatment on repeated occasions. The authors therefore considered a possible immune etiology in which the axons rather than the myelin sheath or the Schwann cell were the target of the putative autoimmune responses. A similar pathomechanism has been documented for the rare axonal variant forms of GBS. In analogy, it has been suggested that CIAP may represent an axonal variant form of CIDP. While a few similar patients have been identified,[43,44] on the whole, CIAP is rare and difficult to diagnose with certainty.

Diagnostic criteria and laboratory testing

Criteria for the diagnosis of CIDP are based on four features: the typical clinical symptoms and signs; electrophysiological findings indicative of a predominantly demyelinating neuropathy; lack of pleocytosis and raised protein in the cerebrospinal fluid; and evidence of demyelination and remyelination on nerve biopsy. Accordingly, specific guidelines for the diagnosis of CIDP have been formulated, which also include a set of exclusionary criteria (published in *Neurology* 1991;41:617–618).[4]

The diagnostic work-up requires a detailed electrophysiological study of all four limbs, including the measurement of conduction in proximal nerve segments. Motor conduction velocities are often markedly slow, usually below 80% of normal values; they may be less abnormal early in the disease course, or in cases where demyelination is predominant in spinal nerve roots. In such patients, proximal conductions and F wave latencies will be prolonged. In general, both F wave latencies and distal onset latencies are prolonged. The degree of conduction slowing may vary between nerve segments and between individual nerves. A nonuniform, differential slowing of motor conductions accompanied by conduction block is the hallmark of an acquired demyelinating neuropathy, and permits its differentiation from the most common hereditary neuropathy (CMT Ia).[45] The amplitudes of the compound muscle action potentials (CMAPs) are usually reduced, which is partly due to temporal dispersion of the CMAPs and partly to the loss of motor fibers seen in chronic disease. Accordingly, needle electromyography discloses variable signs of ongoing active denervation. Sensory nerve action potentials (SNAPs) are often not recordable; when measurable, afferent sensory conductions are usually very slow and SNAPs are markedly reduced in amplitude.[46,47]

Examination of the cerebrospinal fluid (CSF) reveals fairly consistently a cell count of less than 10/mm[3] and a raised CSF protein, with average values greater than 600 mg/L (in around 95% of cases). Normal CSF protein levels may be found early in the disease, and therefore do not rule out the diagnosis. A finding of pleocytosis of more than 50 cells/mm[3] should raise suspicion for an associated disorder, such as HIV infection or a hematological malignancy.[48]

Pathological verification of CIDP by nerve biopsy may be required for a definitive diagnosis and is usually mandatory for the inclusion of patients in research studies. In the routine clinical setting, however, results of a sural nerve biopsy were not found to contribute significantly to diagnostic accuracy when the other diagnostic criteria—raised CSF protein and electrophysiological evidence of demyelination—had been met. Therefore, the added diagnostic value of a nerve biopsy has been questioned.[49] A nerve biopsy may be required to exclude other etiologies that may enter the differential diagnosis, such as vasculitis or inherited metabolic disorders. In this case the pathological evaluation will only be fully informative when it includes an analysis of teased fibers, as well as the detailed light microscopic and ultrastructural examination of Epon-embedded nerve sections.

The following laboratory studies should also be done routinely: immune electrophoresis (or immune fixation electrophoresis) of serum and urine in search of a monoclonal protein; a skeletal survey to rule out myeloma; HIV and hepatitis serology, and rheumato-

logical studies; exclusion of diabetes mellitus and hepatic or renal dysfunction. Occasionally, it may be advisable to screen genomic DNA for the exclusion of a hereditary demyelinating neuropathy HMSN type I (Charcot–Marie–Tooth disease; available through Athena Diagnostics).

Magnetic resonance imaging of the lumbar spine may reveal enlarged nerve roots and enhancement of cauda equina after gadolinium injection (69%), indicating very proximal pathology in nerve roots and the disruption of the blood–nerve barrier.[50,51] MRI may thus occasionally be a useful adjunctive test in the diagnosis of CIDP.

Pathogenesis and pathology

Postmortem examinations and the study of nerve biopsies have revealed the characteristic histopathological features of nerve edema, scant lymphocyte infiltrates and macrophage-mediated segmental demyelination and remyelination.[2,3] This was accompanied by an upregulation of MHC class I and II antigens and variable T-cell infiltrates within the nerve fascicles.[52,53] Deposition of immunoglobulin and of activated complement split products have been demonstrated on the outer Schwann cell membranes or the myelin sheaths, thus identifying the target of the immune responses.[16,54,55] The important role for anti-myelin/Schwann cell autoantibodies in the pathogenesis of CIDP was further demonstrated by the successful passive transfer of demyelination with sera and purified IgG from select patients who had improved with plasma exchange therapy.[56] However, the precise neural antigens remain to be identified. Antibodies against myelin protein zero (P0), various glycolipids and against sulfated glucuronyl paragloboside (SGPG) have been found in a small proportion of CIDP patients.[57,97] Their role in the production of specific forms of CIDP remains in debate.[58] The process of segmental demyelination is mediated by activated macrophages, which are observed to infiltrate focally the Schwann cell basement membrane and then to strip and phagocytose the myelin lamellae, while axons remain intact (Figure 193.1).[3] Subsequently, remyelination and repair ensues. Chronic

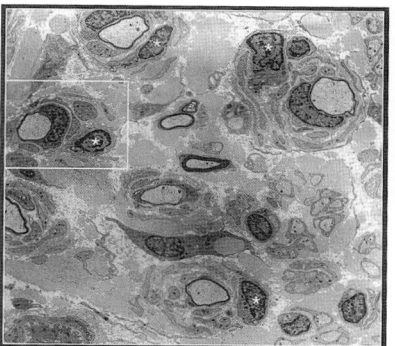
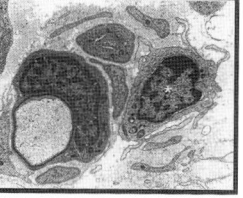

Figure 193.1 Relapsing CIDP sural nerve biopsy: severe chronic demyelination mediated by macrophages (*asterisks* and insert).

disease, with repeated cycles of demyelination and remyelination, may lead to so-called "onion bulb" formations and hypertrophic nerve changes.[2] Such changes are often most prominent in proximal nerve segments, e.g. nerve roots, spinal nerves and major plexuses, but may be observed throughout the peripheral nerves.

Two recent reports have emphasized the prominence of secondary axonal pathology which may be observed with long-standing CIDP and which contributes significantly to functional disability and to the overall prognosis.[23,59] In point of fact, muscle atrophy and dense sensory deficits, the clinical correlates of axon loss, are indicators of poor response to therapy.

Forms of treatment
Background
Current treatments for CIDP assume an immune pathogenesis that, although not yet proven, is well supported by medical evidence. By definition, CIDP is a chronic disorder in which disease activity may persist for years. Treatments are therefore aimed at modulating the abnormal immune responses with the intent of suppressing the disease activity in the long term. This can be achieved by a variety of treatment modalities that are often prescribed individually or in combination.

Following early anecdotal observations of the unique responsiveness of CIDP to corticosteroids,[1–3] prednisone became, and probably still is, the most commonly used therapy for CIDP. To achieve improvement, high doses of prednisone (1 to 1.5 mg/kg) need to be prescribed for several weeks. Subsequent gradual tapering of the dose over months is recommended, since sudden or rapid reduction can lead to a prompt relapse or to an incomplete therapeutic response with the establishment of fixed neurological deficits.[16,23] Benefit from corticosteroids was documented for both adults and children.[60–62] However, the required long term use of steroids can be associated with potentially hazardous and lasting side effects. Therefore, other immune suppressant medications such as azathioprine[7,16] or cyclophosphamide[3,63] have been used concomitantly or alternatively. Observations from controlled trials and from large case series are discussed below.

In the search for alternative treatments, therapeutic plasma exchange (PE) was first used in CIDP in the late 1970s, and found to be of substantial benefit for select patients, particularly those with relapsing CIDP. However, the observed neurological improvements were often not sustained, so that repeat PE treatments were required.[64,65] Thus, PE emerged as useful adjuvant therapy, which was particularly efficacious early on in the disease course, when demyelination was the predominant pathology.[10,66] Moreover, the unique effectiveness of PE provided insights into the pathogenesis, underscoring the importance of humoral factors (antibodies and T-cell-derived cytokines). The value of PE for the treatment of both CIDP and CIDP-MGUS was subsequently confirmed

in several randomized and controlled clinical trials,[9,10,67] that are reviewed below.

More recently, high dose intravenous immunoglobulin (IVIg) was introduced as immunomodulatory therapy for a number of autoimmune disorders, including CIDP. In 1985, Vermeulen et al.[68] summarized the first observations of its use in CIDP, reporting substantial benefit in 13 of 17 (70%) patients with open-label treatment of IVIg (2 g/kg given over 5 days). Neurological function usually began to improve within one week of the infusion, and improvement continued for several weeks. In the majority of patients, however, benefit was not sustained. Instead, they worsened again, but then responded anew and to the same degree with additional IVIg treatments. These observations were confirmed in a number of case series[69–71] and subsequently in several randomized and controlled clinical trials[11,12,72] that will be discussed below. Thus, high dose IVIg can be used effectively and safely in CIDP and will benefit a proportion of patients.

Established therapies
Corticosteroids Steroids (oral prednisone or prednisolone) are considered effective and have become the mainstay of treatment for CIDP. In a randomized and controlled trial of 28 CIDP patients studied for three months, Dyck et al.[5] demonstrated a small but significant and clinically meaningful therapy effect with high dose prednisone. Patients with chronic progressive or relapsing CIDP responded equally well. These observations concur with the retrospective analysis of two large patient series, which documented improvement with corticosteroids in 49 of 76 (65%)[6] and 57 of 59 (95%)[7] CIDP patients, respectively. To achieve this benefit, high doses of prednisone (1 to 1.5 mg/kg per day) had been prescribed for a minimum of four weeks. Thereafter, the medication was gradually tapered over many months. First signs of clinical improvement were observed with a mean delay of 1.9 ± 3.6 months, and maximal benefit was attained only after a mean 6.6 ± 5.4 months.[7] Less than 50% of CIDP patients reached maximal benefit by six months; this was achieved in approximately 95% of patients by 12 months, while 5% were refractory to steroids. On follow-up over 10 years, around 60% of patients with chronically progressive CIDP had achieved full remission, yet only 20% of patients with relapsing CIDP were in remission and not receiving any medication. Benefit from high dose prednisone (1.5 mg/kg per day) has been documented in several uncontrolled studies in children.[61,73] All children improved initially with prednisone; those with a relapsing disease course required a long term prescription and, in addition, other immunomodulatory therapies were used.

Although the prescription of prednisone is convenient and relatively cheap, prolonged use may result in hazardous side effects. Potential complications range from an altered appearance, weight gain, insomnia, mood change, and aggravation of hypertension or of carbohydrate intolerance, to psychosis, peptic ulcers, cataracts, osteoporosis with subsequent vertebral compression fractures and avascular necrosis of the hip. Some of these side effects may be diminished by appropriate countermeasures, such as the prescription of antacids (H2-receptor antagonists); a sodium-restricted, low-carbohydrate and high-protein diet; and osteoporosis prophylaxis with supplemental calcium and bisphosphonates. The potentially serious and lasting complications make steroid therapy less desirable. Nonetheless, use of steroids cannot entirely be avoided, but dose and duration of therapy can now be reduced with the added prescription of other immunomodulatory treatments.

Alternative immunosuppressive medications

Azathioprine In order to reduce long term exposure to high dose prednisone, a combination with azathioprine (2.5 to 3 mg/kg per day) has been advocated.[7,16] Published information is insufficient to judge the potential added benefit. One small study in CIDP, comparing prednisone to the combined therapy of prednisone plus azathioprine (2 mg/kg per day) for nine months, failed to show additional benefit.[74]

Cyclophosphamide Only anecdotal observations are available for the use of cyclophosphamide in relapsing CIDP that could otherwise not be stabilized. Prineas and McLeod[3] were able to induce a sustained remission in 4 of 5 patients with relapsing CIDP with the prescription of oral cyclophosphamide (50 to 150 mg per day). In a recent series of 15 CIDP patients treated with monthly pulses of intravenous cyclophosphamide (1 g/m²) combined with dexamethasone (20 mg) for up to six months, 12 patients showed improved neurological functions and either partial or complete remission.[63] The treatment was well tolerated and improvements developed slowly over an average of 8.5 months (range 1 to 21 months). The three nonresponders in this trial had also been refractory to PE and to high dose IVIg treatments. Benefit from open-label treatments of oral cyclophosphamide and prednisone was reported for patients with CIDP-MGUS.[75]

In view of potentially serious side effects (bone marrow toxicity, azoospermia, and the late development of tumors) the prescription of cyclophosphamide requires careful consideration. Male patients should be offered banking of their sperm prior to therapy.

Cyclosporin A (CsA) CsA has been used with some promise in selected CIDP patients who had failed a variety of other treatments.[76–78] Accordingly, treatments were administered open-label and uncontrolled, and the majority of patients were maintained on a concurrent prescription of prednisone. The most extensive experience with CsA in CIDP has been summarized in a recent paper by Barnett et al.[78] reporting a retrospective analysis of 19 patients (13 with chronic progressive and 6 with relapsing CIDP) who had become refractory to all other therapies. CsA was prescribed with a starting dose of 3 to 7 mg/kg per day; during the course of treatment, the dose was

usually adjusted to 2 to 3 mg/kg and was maintained for a total of six months. Patients were closely monitored for nephrotoxicity and hypertension. Such side effects (dose-dependent and reversible) led to early cessation of treatments in two patients. Significant improvements in scored neurological disability and significant reductions in the mean annual incidence of relapses were observed with CsA. Although such anecdotal reports hold promise, the experience with CsA in CIDP is very limited. The drug is therefore reserved for the exceptional circumstance of therapy-resistant CIDP.

Interferons A small number of anecdotal reports described benefit from interferon beta-1a in selected CIDP patients who had failed all other treatments.[79–81] Short-term improvements were also seen with the use of interferon alfa-2a.[82,83,98] However, a carefully designed, double-blind and controlled trial of interferon beta-1a in 10 CIDP patients, treated for a total of 12 weeks, failed to confirm these results.[84] Moreover, typical CIDP developed in two patients as they were treated with interferon-alfa 2a for their viral hepatitis.[85,86] Use of these medications therefore remains experimental and unproven.

Plasma exchange therapy Dyck and colleagues[9] critically examined the therapy effect of PE in CIDP in a prospective, sham-controlled, double-blind trial of 29 patients with either static or worsening disease. Patients were randomly assigned to receive either six plasma exchange or six sham exchange treatments during three weeks. Significant improvements of scored neurological functions were seen in the PE group, and substantial benefit from PE was recorded in approximately one third of patients with long-standing CIDP. Hahn and coworkers[10] examined the effect of PE in 18 CIDP patients who had not been previously treated, using a similar trial design and a crossover study. Highly significant and large improvements were recorded in all outcome measures, including scores of neurological impairment, grip strength and functional clinical grading. This was corroborated by the electrophysiological studies, which demonstrated among other findings a significant increase of the proximal M-wave amplitudes, thus indicating the reversal of conduction block.[87] Twelve of the 15 patients (80%) who completed the blinded trial experienced substantial benefits, which began usually within days of starting PE. However, the improvements were often not sustained; 8 of 12 patients (66%) relapsed within 7 to 14 days following their last PE. Subsequently, these patients could be stabilized with repeated PE treatments and the more gradual tapering of the exchanges plus the added prescription of either prednisone or cyclophosphamide. PE was considered to be a very effective adjuvant therapy.

PE is remarkably free of complications and may be given on an outpatient basis. In case of poor venous access, a temporary subclavian vein catheter may have to be inserted; this carries a small risk of infection. A major disadvantage of PE is its high cost and limited availability, since it can only be performed in medical centers with such specialized expertise.

Intravenous high dose immunoglobulin (IVIg) The value of IVIg in the treatment of CIDP was underscored by a placebo-controlled, double-blind, crossover trial that confirmed specific and reproducible benefit in a small number of patients, selected for their known response to IVIg. All seven patients improved with IVIg and none responded to placebo.[12] In retrospective analysis of a series of 52 CIDP patients suffering from either chronically progressive or relapsing disease and treated with open-label IVIg over a mean follow-up of four years, van Doorn and colleagues[70] documented benefit with IVIg in 32 patients (62%). Of these, 9 patients (17%) reached a full remission with a single treatment course of IVIg of 2 g/kg, whereas 21 patients (40%) required repeated and ongoing IVIg pulses to maintain the improvements. The following patient characteristics appeared to predict a favorable response to IVIg: disease duration of less than one year; ongoing disease progression; similar weakness in arms and legs; loss of tendon reflexes in the arms; and significant slowing of motor conduction velocities in the median nerve. These parameters define a generalized and progressive demyelinating neuropathy of relatively short duration. The chances of improving with IVIg were estimated at 90% if these parameters were met. In a subsequent analysis of 53 CIDP patients, treated long term with IVIg monotherapy, the authors documented sustained benefit in 41 patients (77%).[88]

Three prospective and randomized trials of IVIg with a double-blind and placebo-controlled design have now been published.[11,89,90] They are summarized in Table 193.1. Surprisingly, the first two-armed trial of 28 patients,[89] carried out in the Netherlands, failed to confirm benefit with IVIg, thus contrasting remarkably with above cited experience with open-label IVIg treatments. On review of the data, it appeared that three patients in the placebo group had improved spontaneously, and that the clinical characteristics defined as predicting a favorable response to IVIg were present in only 6 of the 15 patients randomized to active treatment, whereas they were present in 10 of 13 patients in the placebo group. It is conceivable that these factors could have skewed the result. However, the observations also clearly indicated that

only a subgroup of CIDP patients responded favorably to IVIg. A second controlled, double-blind, crossover study[11] tested IVIg prospectively in 30 CIDP patients who had not previously been treated. Significant improvement was demonstrated in 19 patients (63%): in 9 of 16 patients (56%) with chronic progressive CIDP, and in 10 of 14 patients (71%) with the relapsing form. A comparison of the changes in clinical outcome measures with IVIg versus placebo revealed significant differences in favor of IVIg (improvement in scored neurological disability $P < 0.002$). Moreover, the improvements were comparable to those observed with PE.[10] Neurological improvements usually began within one week of the IVIg infusions and continued to progress until they reached a plateau. In a proportion of patients, the benefits induced were only temporary, lasting a median 6 weeks (range 3 to 22 weeks). However, the beneficial effects were reproduced with repeat open-label treatments, and these patients could eventually be stabilized with IVIg pulse treatments that were given at regular intervals as single-day infusions (IVIg 1 g/kg) before the expected relapse. Six of 11 patients who had failed to respond to IVIg in the controlled trial were subsequently improved with PE and prednisone. This illustrates the importance of trying out the alternative treatments. Five patients (17%) in this trial appeared resistant to all treatment modalities.

Dyck and colleagues[72] compared the therapy effect of IVIg to that of PE in 20 CIDP patients in an observer-blinded, crossover study. The two treatments were found to confer comparable benefits in individual patients, and were thus considered to be equivalent. This finding was confirmed in the retrospective analysis of a large case series.[91] The authors of both reports regarded IVIg as the most convenient first treatment for CIDP. The value of IVIg as first-line therapy was again underscored in a randomized, controlled and double-blind trial of 50 CIDP patients who had not previously been treated.[90]

In view of the ease of its administration, IVIg has become the preferred treatment in children.[73] Its use in this age group has been assessed only anecdotally, yet inferred benefits from IVIg and from PE were also considered to be equivalent. In general, children respond well to these treatments and recover quickly. The rare child may seem relatively refractory to these treatments and may develop a protracted illness, so that other immunomodulatory treatments may be

Table 193.1 Intravenous immunoglobulin G in CIDP: randomized, double-blind, controlled trials

Authors	Trial design		Improvement
Van Doorn et al., 1990[12]	Crossover	7 pts	7/7 (100%)
Vermeulen et al., 1993[89]	Two arm	28 pts	4/15 (27%)
Hahn et al., 1996[11]	Crossover	30 pts	19/30 (63%)
Dyck et al., 1994[72]	Crossover with PE	20 pts	Significant benefit equivalent to PE
Mendell et al., 2000[90]	Untreated CIDP Two arm	50 pts	Significantly improved scored motor functions (76%)

required. The question arises as to whether children may safely receive routine immunizations. A recent study found the risk of relapse of CIDP to be low with booster injections, unless the disease had been originally triggered by a vaccination.[92] In susceptible CIDP patients, booster tetanus immunizations have, on occasion, led to a relapse.[93]

The precise mechanisms by which IVIg exerts its immunomodulatory effects in CIDP are presently not known. Several possible interactions with various steps in the amplification and the effector phases of the immune response are being considered.[94] For a detailed overview and discussion, the reader is referred to an excellent updated review by Dalakas.[95]

For the most part, IVIg is well tolerated, and only minor adverse reactions are seen in less than 10% of patients. Reported adverse reactions include:

Systemic reactions
    headache/nausea
    fever/chills/myalgias
    chest discomfort/shortness of breath
    postinfusion fatigue
Cardiovascular reactions
    hypertension/tachycardia
    cardiac failure
    thromboembolic events
Renal complications
    worsening of kidney failure
    acute renal tubular necrosis
Neurological complications
    migraine
    aseptic meningitis
    reversible encephalopathy/stroke
Hypersensitivity
    anaphylaxis (IgA deficiency)
    hemolytic anemia
    neutropenia
    lymphopenia
    immune complex arthritis
Skin reactions
    urticaria (pruritus)
    petechiae
Effects on serum chemistry
    hyponatremia (artifactual)
    elevated ESR (rouleaux formation)
    decreased hemoglobin (dilutional)
    elevated liver enzymes.

Anaphylactic reactions are very rare, but can occur in patients with selective IgA deficiency (prevalence around 1:1000 population). Serum IgA levels should

therefore be determined prior to treatment; moreover, IVIg infusions should be closely monitored and given in special therapy clinics. The majority of observed side effects are usually improved with either a reduction of the infusion rate or else with symptomatic therapy using acetaminophen or nonsteroidal anti-inflammatory medications. With current safety regulations and the solvent treatment steps in its production, IVIg is considered free of risk of viral transmission, e.g. HIV or hepatitis.

Comparison of plasma exchange, IVIg and prednisone So far, only a few studies have directly compared the effect of various treatments in the same patient. Dyck and colleagues[72] demonstrated that in most responders IVIg and PE were of equivalent value. The trial conducted by Hahn and colleagues[10] provided strong evidence of efficacy of PE in CIDP. The study also showed that the achieved benefits were often not lasting. These patients were shown subsequently to respond favorably to prednisone, albeit with considerable delay. By combining both treatments, the patients were eventually stabilized. Similarly, the beneficial responses induced by IVIg were also often temporary. Stabilization of such patients required continued IVIg pulse therapy and the prescription of prednisone.[11] In a recent randomized controlled cross-over trial IVIg 2 g/kg was found to be equal in effect to a six week course of oral prednisone in most outcome measurements.[96]

A comparison of the three proven treatment modalities is given in Table 193.2. Both IVIg and PE are safe and have fewer side effects, but the treatments are expensive. Moreover, they require commitment in time and travel to specialized centers. By contrast, the prescription of prednisone is convenient and cheap, but the required prolonged prescription of prednisone in high dose may lead to medical complications that are associated with a morbidity of their own. Therefore, the choice of treatment needs to be very carefully considered and tailored to the individual patient.

Approach to the management of CIDP (Figure 193.2)
General remarks. The steps to arrive at a clinical diagnosis of CIDP are outlined in the text and are summarized in the algorithm in Figure 193.2. After the diagnosis of CIDP is confirmed and prior to formulating a treatment plan, it is important to inform the patient thoroughly of the nature of the illness. The discussion should address the heterogeneity and chronicity of the disorder, as well as the possible

Table 193.2   Comparison of prednisone, IVIg and PE for the treatment of CIDP

Treatment	Effective	Estimated % responders	Major side effects	Cost
Prednisone	+	90	Yes	Low
IVIg*	+	66	No	High
Plasma exchange*	+	80	No	High

*May require concurrent immunosuppressive drug therapy.

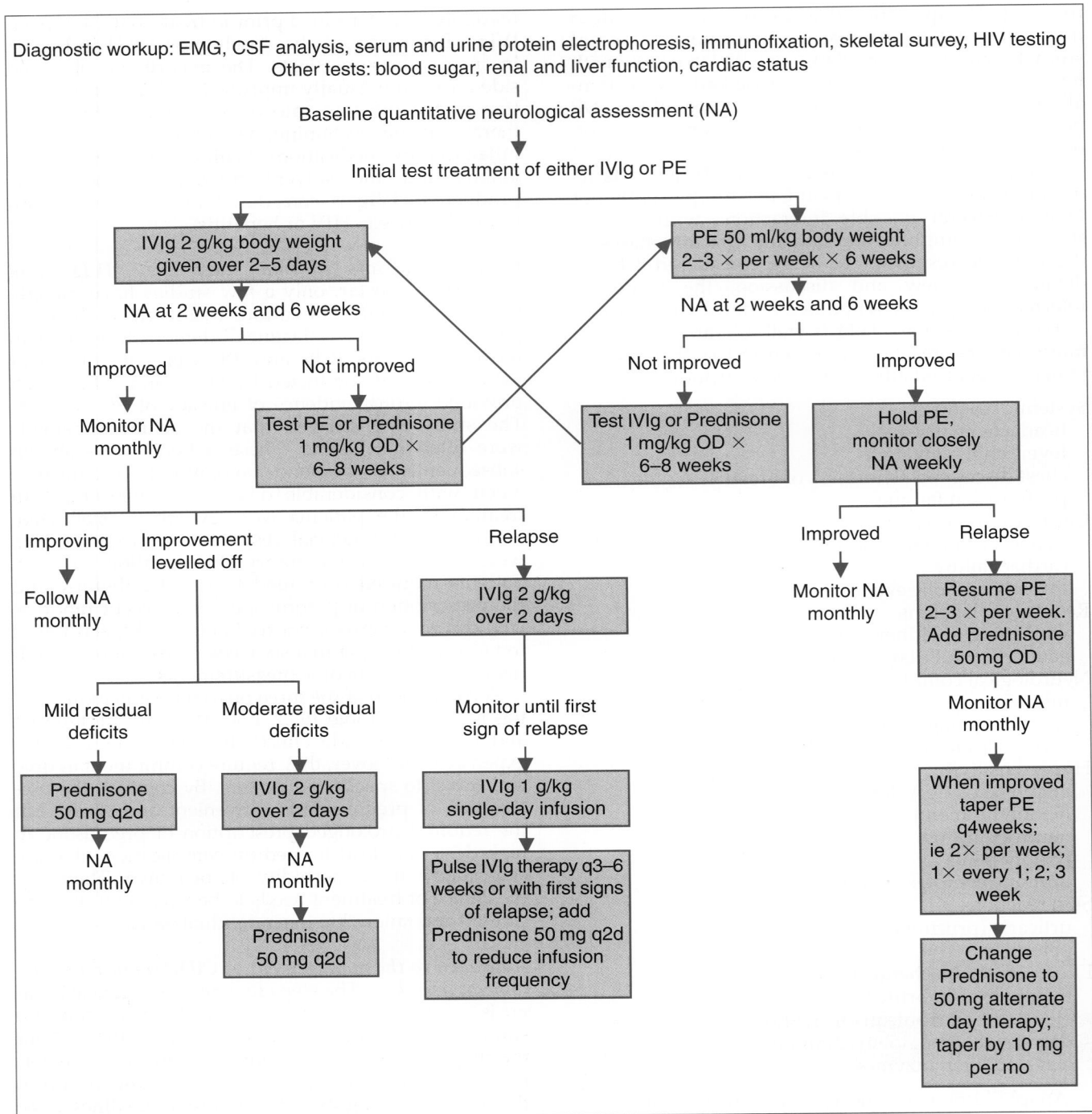

Figure 193.2 Algorithm for the treatment of chronic inflammatory demyelinating polyradiculoneuropathy. EMG = electromyography; CSF = cerebrospinal fluid; IVIg = intravenous immunoglobulin; PE = plasma exchange.

fluctuations in symptoms that may occur and that may have to be addressed by a change or adjustments in the treatments. One needs to emphasize that the therapy, although following a clear plan, will have to be tested and applied to the individual's response. In this way, the patient will be prepared for possible setbacks and will retain trust in the medical management. By definition, CIDP is a chronic disorder in which disease activity may persist for years. Treat-

ments are thus aimed at modulating the abnormal immune responses with the intent of suppressing the ongoing disease activity in the long term. As outlined above, this can be achieved with a variety of modalities, which are prescribed individually or in combination. Discussions about outcome and future function should be guided by cautious optimism. In general, the outlook is favorable, since therapy can lead to restoration of near-normal function in approximately

60% of patients. The risk of relapse remains. Moreover, with long-standing disease, muscle atrophy and weakness, as well as fixed sensory deficits, may develop as a result of secondary axonal loss and are often no longer reversible. Therefore, early and aggressive therapy is advised.

For accurate examination of the treatment response in a given patient, one should use a predetermined scoring system (e.g. assessment of strength in a set of proximal and distal arm and leg muscles, with use of the Medical Research Council scale) to allow for more objective testing of motor and sensory functions, including the recording of tendon reflexes. One may also test specific clinical functions, such as the time required to walk 10 meters, or the measurement of dexterity and hand function by using the Nine-Hole Peg Test. The effort to create a flow chart and to be consistent in the assessment and recording will be essential for judging the effect of therapy.

Initial therapy There are no firm guidelines regarding the choice of the initial therapy. The order of preference may vary from patient to patient and may be dictated, at times, by medical circumstances (steroids are best avoided in menopausal women and in patients with hypertension or diabetes; poor venous access may preclude ready use of PE), or by practical considerations, such as availability of PE or IVIg as well as their high cost. Initially, one should test only one treatment in an adequate dose and for a sufficient length of time to enable accurate judgement of efficacy. During this test period, regular follow-up assessments need to be scheduled. An approach to treatment is outlined in Figure 193.2 and in Table 193.3.

Currently, IVIg is often used in first-line therapy. Efficacy can usually be tested with a single treatment (total dose 2 g/kg given over 2 to 5 days). For a patient with disease of longer standing, an additional one or two IVIg treatments may be required to establish responsiveness, or the lack thereof. Repeat treatments are given at monthly intervals. Predictors that permit assessment of the response to IVIg for a given patient have been formulated by the Dutch group (see

text). On the whole, approximately two thirds of patients can be expected to improve with IVIg. For those patients in whom no clearcut benefit is observed in the test period, the use of IVIg should be abandoned. Comparative studies have shown that, for the most part, IVIg and PE are equivalent in therapeutic effect. However, some of the IVIg nonresponders may clearly benefit from PE; in this circumstance, therefore, it is advisable to test this alternative modality. Again, PE should initially be tested in monotherapy. Once benefit from PE is unequivocally demonstrated, it will be necessary to combine PE with either prednisone or cyclophosphamide to prevent a so-called "rebound relapse" that may follow the long-term use of PE. Until recently, prednisone was often prescribed as first-line therapy and it may still be given preference because of its convenient use and low cost (Table 193.3 sets out a dosing schedule for prednisone). Early signs of improvement with prednisone may be noted within two to three weeks of starting the drug, but full benefit generally requires many months of high dose steroid treatment. Invariably, this will lead to the well-known adverse effects of prednisone. These are usually less prevalent with alternate-day drug scheduling.

Subsequent therapy After the initial test period of six weeks, patients who responded to IVIg should be monitored at monthly intervals. Some may show continued improvement and return to normal function without further IVIg treatments or other drugs. For some patients, improvement may level off at a variable interval. Depending on the degree of residual dysfunction, one may choose to re-treat with IVIg, or, in a case of only mild residual deficits, one may instead use medium doses of prednisone (50 mg on alternate days). This dose is maintained until the patient is further improved. Prednisone is then tapered by 10 mg per month. In our experience, improvement to near-normal function will usually occur within 12 to 18 months of therapy.

In patients with relapsing CIDP, the beneficial effects of IVIg may only be temporary and may last between 3 and 22 weeks (most commonly 6 weeks). The duration of the treatment response needs to be established for each patient, since it will dictate the subsequent treatment intervals. Repeat infusions are given as single-day treatments of IVIg 1 g/kg at regular intervals prior to the expected deterioration or at the earliest signs of a relapse. With this long term IVIg pulse therapy, the patient's improvement can usually be maintained, and neurological functions often continue to improve. One should periodically test whether the IVIg treatment can be stopped. One may also consider adding prednisone at 50 mg on alternate days to reduce the infusion frequency and to assist in achieving stabilization and remission.

If the patient does not respond to IVIg, one should test PE at 50 ml/kg body weight per exchange, scheduled initially at two to three times per week. This exchange frequency should be maintained for 6 weeks, while repeat neurological assessments are carried out at 2 and 6 weeks. Substantial improvements can often be

Table 193.3	Treatment schedule for prednisone
Initial dose	Prednisone 1.0–1.5 mg/kg PO o.d. Maintain dose for 6–8 weeks
Taper off	10 mg on alternate-day dose every two weeks, thus gradually switching to alternate-day treatment
Maintain	Single, high dose (1.0–1.5 mg/kg) on alternate-day treatment for 6–8 weeks
Taper off	If no improvement with prednisone, taper quickly—patient is likely nonresponder
	If improved, taper by 10 mg per month to prednisone 10 mg alternate-day dose
	Then taper by 2.5 mg per month to a maintenance dose of prednisone 5 mg alternate-day dose

seen during this initial trial period: some patients will have stabilized and will not require further exchanges. However, the majority of patients will need ongoing PE treatments. In this case, prednisone should be added at a dose of 50 mg per day for 6 to 8 weeks. Once neurological improvement is established, the PE frequency is tapered off and the prednisone dose is gradually reduced (see Table 193.3). With combined treatment, most patients will return to near-normal function. The occasional patient may require a prescription of oral cyclophosphamide, 75 to 100 mg per day, to achieve full stabilization (guidelines for safety and precautions in the use of this drug are given in the text).

The majority of patients will also respond to prednisone, started at a dose of 1 to 1.5 mg/kg per day (when used in monotherapy) and maintained for 6 to 8 weeks. When improvements have occurred, one begins to taper off the prednisone dose by 10 mg per 2 weeks, while at the same time changing gradually to an alternate-day schedule. This is usually achieved within 10 to 12 weeks (see Table 193.3). A dose of 1.0 to 1.5 mg/kg prednisone on alternate days is then prescribed for 6 to 8 weeks. With this schedule most patients will show adequate improvement. Prednisone is then further tapered off by 10 mg per month to a dose of 10 mg on alternate days. As lower doses are reached, individual adjustments may become necessary. Some patients may relapse when steroids are tapered off and may require a temporary increase in the dose of prednisone. Alternatively, one may choose to add one of the other immunomodulatory therapies. The necessary high doses of steroids render unwanted side effects unavoidable. Calcium supplementation and biphosphonates should be prescribed to prevent osteoporosis. In addition, patients should be involved in regular physical therapy.

Prognosis

The immune modulatory treatments outlined above have considerably improved the prognosis of CIDP, and satisfactory stabilization can be achieved in around 60% of patients. However, the response to treatment with IVIg, PE, corticosteroids or immunosuppressive drugs is difficult to predict. Individual adjustments of therapy will be necessary. It is important to treat aggressively in order to attain an optimal treatment response as soon as possible. The longer the disease persists and smolders, the more it will become refractory to therapy. Chronically recurring inflammatory demyelination will become secondarily accompanied by a loss of axons, which leads to fewer reversible and more fixed neurological deficits, since outcome correlates with the degree of axonal pathology.[23]

References

1. Austin JH. Recurrent polyneuropathies and their corticosteroid treatment. With five-year observations of a placebo-controlled case treated with corticotrophin, cortisone, and prednisone. Brain 1958;81:157–192

2. Dyck PJ, Lais AC, Ohta M, et al. Chronic inflammatory polyradiculoneuropathy. Mayo Clin Proc 1975;50:621–637

3. Prineas JW, McLeod JG. Chronic relapsing polyneuritis. J Neurol Sci 1976;27:427–458

4. Ad Hoc Subcommittee of the American Academy of Neurology AIDS Task Force. Research criteria for diagnosis of chronic inflammatory demyelinating polyneuropathy (CIDP). Neurology 1991;41:617–618

5. Dyck PJ, O'Brien PC, Oviatt KF, et al. Prednisone improves chronic inflammatory demyelinating polyradiculoneuropathy more than no treatment. Ann Neurol 1982;11:136–141

6. McCombe PA, Pollard JD, McLeod JG. Chronic inflammatory demyelinating polyradiculoneuropathy. A clinical and electrophysiological study of 92 cases. Brain 1987;110:1617–1630

7. Barohn RJ, Kissel JT, Warmolts JR, Mendell JR. Chronic inflammatory demyelinating polyradiculoneuropathy. Clinical characteristics, course and recommendations for diagnostic criteria. Arch Neurol 1989;46:878–884

8. Plasma Exchange/Sandoglobulin Guillain–Barré Syndrome Trial Group (1997). Treatment of Guillain–Barré syndrome: comparison of plasma exchange, intravenous immunoglobulin, and plasma exchange followed by intravenous immunoglobulin. Lancet 1997;349:225–230

9. Dyck PJ, Daube J, O'Brien P, et al. Plasma exchange in chronic inflammatory demyelinating polyradiculoneuropathy. N Engl J Med 1986;314:461–465

10. Hahn AF, Bolton CF, Pillay N, et al. Plasma-exchange therapy in chronic inflammatory demyelinating polyneuropathy. A double-blind, sham-controlled, cross-over study. Brain 1996;119:1055–1066

11. Hahn AF, Bolton CF, Zochodne D, Feasby TE. Intravenous immunoglobulin treatment in chronic inflammatory demyelinating polyneuropathy. A double-blind, placebo-controlled, cross-over study. Brain 1996;119:1067–1077

12. van Doorn PA, Brand A, Strengers PFW, et al. High-dose intravenous immunoglobulin treatment in chronic inflammatory demyelinating polyneuropathy: a double-blind, placebo-controlled, cross-over study. Neurology 1990;40:209–212

13. Hartung H-P, Willison H, Jung S, et al. Autoimmune responses in peripheral nerve. Springer Semin Immunopathol 1996;18:97–123

14. Lunn MPT, Manji H, Choudhary PP, et al. Chronic inflammatory demyelinating polyradiculoneuropathy: a prevalence study in south east England. J Neurol Neurosurg Psychiatry 1999;66:677–680

15. McLeod JG, Pollard JD, Macaskill P, et al. Prevalence of chronic inflammatory demyelinating polyneuropathy in New South Wales, Australia. Ann Neurol 1999;46:910–913

16. Dalakas MC, Engel WK. Chronic relapsing (dysimmune) polyneuropathy: Pathogenesis and treatment. Ann Neurol 1981;9(Suppl):134–145

17. Simmons Z, Albers JW, Bromberg MB, Feldman EL. Long-term follow-up of patients with chronic inflammatory demyelinating polyradiculoneuropathy, without and with monoclonal gammopathy. Brain 1995;118:359–368

18. van Doorn PA, Schreuder GMT, Vermeulen M, et al. HLA antigens in patients with chronic inflammatory demyelinating polyneuropathy. J Neuroimmunol 1991;32:133–139

19. Hughes R, Sanders E, Hall S, et al. Subacute idiopathic demyelinating polyradiculoneuropathy. Arch Neurol 1992;49:612–616

20. Simmons Z, Wald JJ, Albers JW. Chronic inflammatory

demyelinating polyradiculoneuropathy in children: 1. Presentation, electrodiagnostic studies, and initial clinical course, with comparison to adults. Muscle Nerve 1997;20:1008–1015

21. Hattori N, Ichimura M, Aoki S, et al. Clinicopathological features of chronic inflammatory demyelinating polyradiculoneuropathy in childhood. J Neurol Sci 1998;154:66–71

22. Simmons Z, Albers JW, Bromberg MB, Feldman EL. Presentation and initial clinical course in patients with chronic inflammatory demyelinating polyradiculoneuropathy: Comparison of patients without and with monoclonal gammopathy. Neurology 1993;43:2202–2209

23. Bouchard C, Lacroix C, Planté V, et al. Clinicopathologic findings and prognosis of chronic inflammatory demyelinating polyneuropathy. Neurology 1999;52:498–503

24. Oh SJ, Joy JL, Kuruoglu R. "Chronic sensory demyelinating neuropathy": chronic inflammatory demyelinating polyneuropathy presenting as a pure sensory neuropathy. J Neurol Neurosurg Psychiatry 1992;55:677–680

25. van Dijk GW, Notermans NC, Franssen H, Wokke JHJ. Development of weakness in patients with chronic inflammatory demyelinating polyneuropathy and only sensory symptoms at presentation: A long-term follow-up study. J Neurol 1999;246:1134–1139

26. Donaghy M, Mills KR, Boniface SJ, et al. Pure motor demyelinating neuropathy: deterioration after steroid treatment and improvement with intravenous immunoglobulin. J Neurol Neurosurg Psychiatry 1994;57:778–783

27. Lewis RA, Sumner AJ, Brown MJ, Asbury AK. Multifocal demyelinating neuropathy with persistent conduction block. Neurology 1982;32:958–964

28. Thomas PK, Claus D, Jaspert A, et al. Focal upper limb demyelinating neuropathy. Brain 1996;119:765–774

29. Saperstein DS, Amato AA, Wolfe GI, et al. Multifocal acquired demyelinating sensory and motor neuropathy: the Lewis–Sumner syndrome. Muscle Nerve 1999;22:560–566

30. Van den Berg-Vos RM, Van den Berg LH, Franssen H, et al. Multifocal inflammatory demyelinating neuropathy. A distinct clinical entity? Neurology 2000;54:26–32

31. Verma A, Tandan R, Adesina AM, et al. Focal neuropathy preceding chronic inflammatory demyelinating polyradiculoneuropathy by several years. Acta Neurol Scand 1990;81:516–521

32. Thomas PK, Walker RWH, Rudge P, et al. Chronic demyelinating peripheral neuropathy associated with multifocal central nervous system demyelination. Brain 1987;110:53–76

33. Feasby TE, Hahn AF, Koopman WJ, Lee DH. Central lesions in chronic inflammatory demyelinating polyneuropathy—An MRI study. Neurology 1990;40:476–478

34. Gosselin S, Kyle RA, Dyck PJ. Neuropathy associated with monoclonal gammopathies of undetermined significance. Ann Neurol 1991;30:54–61

35. Notermans NC, Wokke JHJ, Lokhorst HM, et al. Polyneuropathy associated with monoclonal gammopathy of undetermined significance: a prospective study of the prognostic value of clinical and laboratory abnormalities. Brain 1994;117:1385–1393

36. Notermans NC, Franssen H, Eurelings M, et al. Diagnostic criteria for demyelinating polyneuropathy associated with monoclonal gammopathy. Muscle Nerve 2000;23:73–79

37. Katz JS, Saperstein DS, Gronseth G, et al. Distal acquired demyelinating symmetric neuropathy. Neurology 2000;54:615–620

38. Suarez GA, Kelly JJ Jr. Polyneuropathy associated with monoclonal gammopathy of undetermined significance: further evidence that IgM-MGUS neuropathies are different than IgG-MGUS. Neurology 1993;43:1304–1308

39. Dalakas MC, Quarles RH, Farrer RG, et al. A controlled study of intravenous immunoglobulin in demyelinating neuropathy with IgM gammopathy. Ann Neurol 1996;40:792–795

40. Dyck PJ, Dyck PJ. Atypical varieties of chronic inflammatory demyelinating neuropathies. Lancet 2000;355:1293–1294

41. Gorson KC, Allam G, Ropper AH. Chronic inflammatory demyelinating polyneuropathy: clinical features and response to treatment in 67 consecutive patients with and without a monoclonal gammopathy. Neurology 1997;48:321–328

42. Chroni E, Hall SM, Hughes RAC. Chronic relapsing axonal neuropathy: a first case report. Ann Neurol 1995;37:112–115

43. Julien J, Vital C, Lagueny A, et al. Chronic relapsing idiopathic polyneuropathy with primary axonal lesions. J Neurol Neurosurg Psychiatry 1989;52:871–875

44. Uncini A, Sabatelli M, Mignogna T, et al. Chronic progressive steroid responsive axonal polyneuropathy: a CIDP variant or a primary axonal disorder? Muscle Nerve 1996;19:365–371

45. Lewis RA, Sumner AJ. The electrodiagnostic distinctions between chronic familial and acquired demyelinative neuropathies. Neurology 1982;32:592–596

46. Parry GJ, Aminoff MJ. Somatosensory evoked potentials in chronic acquired demyelinating peripheral neuropathy. Neurology 1987;37:313–316

47. Albers JW, Kelly JJ. Acquired inflammatory demyelinating polyneuropathies. Clinical and electrodiagnostic features. Muscle Nerve 1989;12:435–451

48. Parry GJ. Peripheral neuropathies associated with human immunodeficiency virus infection. Ann Neurol 1988;23:S49–S53

49. Molenaar DSM, Vermeulen M, de Haan R. Diagnostic value of sural nerve biopsy in chronic inflammatory demyelinating polyneuropathy. J Neurol Neurosurg Psychiatry 1998;64:84–89

50. Schady W, Goulding PJ, Lecky BRF, et al. Massive nerve root enlargement in chronic inflammatory demyelinating polyneuropathy. J Neurol Neurosurg Psychiatry 1996;61:636–640

51. Midroni G, Nöel de Tilly L, Gray B, Vajsar J. MRI of the cauda equina in CIDP: clinical correlations. J Neurol Sci 1999;170:36–44

52. Pollard JD, McCombe PA, Baverstock J, et al. Class II antigen expression and T lymphocyte subsets in chronic inflammatory demyelinating polyneuropathy. J Neuroimmunol 1986;13:123–134

53. Schmidt B, Toyka KV, Kiefer R, et al. Inflammatory infiltrates in sural nerve biopsies in Guillain–Barré syndrome and chronic inflammatory demyelinating neuropathy. Muscle Nerve 1996;19:474–447

54. Hays AP, Lee SS, Latov N. Immune reactive C3D on the surface of myelin sheaths in neuropathy. J Neuroimmunol 1988;18:231–244

55. Hafer-Macko CE, Sheikh KA, Li CY, et al. Immune attack on the Schwann cell surface in acute inflammatory demyelinating polyneuropathy. Ann Neurol 1996;39:625–635

56. Yan WX, Taylor J, Andrias-Kauba S, Pollard JD. Passive transfer of demyelination by serum or IgG from chronic inflammatory demyelinating polyneuropathy patients. Ann Neurol 2000;47:765–775

57. Yuki N, Tagawa Y, Handa S. Autoantibodies to peripheral nerve glycosphingolipids SPG, SLPG, and SGPG in Guillain–Barré syndrome and chronic inflammatory demyelinating polyneuropathy. J Neuroimmunol 1996;70:1–6

58. Hartung HP, van der Meche FGA, Pollard JD. Guillain–Barré syndrome, CIDP and other chronic immune-mediated neuropathies. Curr Opin Neurol 1998;11: 497–513

59. Nagamatsu M, Terao S, Misu K, et al. Inflammatory and perikaryal involvement in chronic inflammatory demyelinating polyneuropathy. J Neurol Neurosurg Psychiatry 1999;66:727–734

60. Sladky JT, Brown MJ, Berman PH. Chronic inflammatory demyelinating polyneuropathy of infancy: A corticosteroid-responsive disorder. Ann Neurol 1986;20: 76–81

61. Korinthenberg R. Chronic inflammatory demyelinating polyradiculoneuropathy in children and their response to treatment. Neuropediatrics 1999;30:190–196

62. Molenaar DSM, van Doorn PA, Mermeulen M. Pulsed high dose dexamethasone treatment in chronic inflammatory demyelinating polyneuropathy: a pilot study. J Neurol Neurosurg Psychiatry 1997;62:388–390

63. Good JL, Chehrenama M, Mayer RF, Koski CL. Pulse cyclophosphamide therapy in chronic inflammatory demyelinating polyneuropathy. Neurology 1998;51: 1735–1738

64. Server AC, Lefkowith J, Braine H, McKhann GM. Treatment of chronic relapsing inflammatory polyradiculoneuropathy by plasma exchange. Ann Neurol 1979;6: 258–261

65. Gross MLP, Thomas PK. The treatment of chronic relapsing and chronic progressive idiopathic inflammatory polyneuropathy by plasma exchange. J Neurol Sci 1981;52:69–78

66. Pollard JD, McLeod JG, Gatenby P, Kronenberg H. Prediction of response to plasma exchange in chronic relapsing polyneuropathy. A clinico-pathological correlation. J Neurol Sci 1983;58:269–287

67. Dyck PJ, Low PA, Windebank AJ, et al. Plasma exchange in polyneuropathy associated with monoclonal gammopathy of undetermined significance. N Engl J Med 1991;325(21):1482–1486

68. Vermeulen M, van der Meché FGA, Speelman JD, et al. Plasma and gammaglobulin infusion in chronic inflammatory polyneuropathy. J Neurol Sci 1985;70:317–326

69. Faed JM, Day B, Pollock M, et al. High-dose intravenous human immunoglobulin in chronic inflammatory demyelinating polyneuropathy. Neurology 1989; 39:422–425

70. van Doorn PA, Vermeulen M, Brand A, et al. Intravenous immunoglobulin treatment in patients with chronic inflammatory demyelinating polyneuropathy. Arch Neurol 1991;48:217–220

71. Cornblath DR, Chaudhry V, Griffin JW. Treatment of chronic inflammatory demyelinating polyneuropathy with intravenous immunoglobulin. Ann Neurol 1991; 30:104–106

72. Dyck PJ, Litchy WJ, Kratz KM, et al. A plasma exchange versus immunoglobulin infusion trial in chronic inflammatory demyelination polyradiculoneuropathy. Ann Neurol 1994;36:838–845

73. Simmons Z, Wald JJ, Albers JW. Chronic inflammatory demyelinating polyradiculoneuropathy in children. II. Long-term follow-up, with comparison to adults. Muscle Nerve 1997;20:1569–1575

74. Dyck PJ, O'Brien PC, Swanson C, et al. Combined azathioprine and prednisone in chronic inflammatory demyelinating polyneuropathy. Neurology 1985;35: 1173–1176

75. Notermans NC, Lokhorst HM, Franssen H, et al. Intermittent cyclophosphamide and prednisone treatment of polyneuropathy associated with monoclonal gammopathy of undetermined significance. Neurology 1996;47:1227–1233

76. Tindall RSA. Immunointervention with cyclosporin A in autoimmune neurological disorders. J Autoimmun 1992;5:301–313

77. Mahattanakul W, Crawford TO, Griffin JW, et al. Treatment of chronic inflammatory demyelinating polyneuropathy with cyclosporin-A. J Neurol Neurosurg Psychiatry 1996;60:185–187

78. Barnett MH, Pollard JD, Davies L, McLeod JG. Cyclosporin A in resistant chronic inflammatory demyelinating polyradiculoneuropathy. Muscle Nerve 1998;21:454–460

79. Choudhary PP, Thompson N, Hughes RAC. Improvement following interferon beta in chronic inflammatory demyelinating polyneuropathy. J Neurol 1995; 242:252–253

80. Martina ISJ, van Doorn PA, Schmitz PIM, et al. Chronic motor neuropathies: response to interferon-α1a after failure of conventional therapies. J Neurol Neurosurg Psychiatry 1999;66:197–201

81. Kuntzer T, Radziwill AJ, Lettry-Trouillat R, et al. Interferon-β1a in chronic inflammatory demyelinating polyneuropathy. Neurology 1999;53:1364–1365

82. Sabatelli M, Mignona T, Lippi G, et al. Interferon-alpha may benefit steroid unresponsive chronic inflammatory demyelinating polyneuropathy. J Neurol Neurosurg Psychiatry 1995;58:638–639

83. Gorson KC, Ropper AH, Clark BD, et al. Treatment of chronic inflammatory demyelinating polyneuropathy with interferon-α 2a. Neurology 1998;50:84–87

84. Hadden RDM, Sharrack B, Bensa S, et al. Randomized trial of interferon β-1a in chronic inflammatory demyelinating polyradiculoneuropathy. Neurology 1999;53:57–61

85. Marzo ME, Tintore M, Fabregues O, et al. Chronic inflammatory demyelinating polyneuropathy during treatment with interferon-alpha. J Neurol Neurosurg Psychiatry 1998;65:604–615

86. Meriggioli MN, Rowin J. Chronic inflammatory polyneuropathy after treatment with interferon-α. Muscle Nerve 2000;23:433–435

87. Ashworth NL, Zochodne DW, Hahn AF, et al. Impact of plasma exchange on indices of demyelination in chronic inflammatory demyelinating polyradiculoneuropathy. Muscle Nerve 2000;23:206–210

88. van der Meché FGA, van Doorn PA. The current place of high-dose immunoglobulins in the treatment of neuromuscular disorders. Muscle Nerve 1997;20: 136–147

89. Vermeulen M, van Doorn PA, Brand A, et al. Intravenous immunoglobulin treatment in patients with chronic inflammatory demyelinating polyneuropathy: a double-blind, placebo controlled study. J Neurol Neurosurg Psychiatry 1993;56:36–39

90. Mendell JR, Barohn RJ, Freimer ML, et al. Randomized controlled trial of IVIg in untreated chronic inflammatory demyelinating polyradiculoneuropathy. Neurology 2001;56:445–449

91. Choudhary PP, Hughes RAC. Long-term treatment of chronic inflammatory demyelinating polyradiculoneuropathy with plasma exchange or intravenous immunoglobulin. QJM 1995;88:493–502

92. Hughes RAC, Choudhary PP, Osborn M, et al. Immunization and risk of relapse of Guillain–Barré syndrome or chronic inflammatory demyelinating polyradiculoneuropathy. Muscle Nerve 1996;19:1230–1231

93. Pollard JD, Selby G. Relapsing neuropathy due to tetanus toxoid. J Neurol Sci 1978;37:113–125

94. Stangel M, Tyoka KV, Gold R. Mechanisms of high-dose intravenous immunoglobulins in demyelinating diseases. Arch Neurol 1999;56:661–663

95. Dalakas MC. Intravenous immunoglobulin in the treatment of autoimmune neuromuscular diseases: present status and practical therapeutic guidelines. Muscle Nerve 1999;22:1479–1497

96. Hughes R, Bensa S, Willison H, et al. Randomized controlled trial of intravenous inmmunoglobulin versus oral predinisolone in chronic inflammatory demyelinating polyradiculoneuropathy. Ann Neurol 2001;50: 195–201

97. Yan WX, Archelos JJ, Hartung HP, Pollard JD. P0 protein is a target antigen in chronic inflammatory demyelinating polyradiculoneuropathy. Ann Neurol 2001;50:286–292

98 Vallat JM, Bouche P, Cros D, Hahn H, Leger JM, Magy L, Tabaraud F, Preux PM. Essai multicentrique (phase II) du β-interferon-1a dans les polyradiculonevrites inflammatoires demyelinisantes chroniques: 20 cas. Revue Neurologique 2001;Suppl 1:S29

194 Miller Fisher Syndrome

Hugh J Willison

Overview

Miller Fisher syndrome (MFS), or Fisher syndrome, is a regional variant of Guillain–Barré syndrome (GBS) and was first described in 1956 as the discrete clinical triad of ophthalmoplegia, ataxia, and areflexia.[1] Since the initial description, MFS has evolved as a nosological entity to take into account closely related forme frustes characterized principally by acute cranial neuropathy with ataxia.[2] Bickerstaff[3] described an encephalitic syndrome in which MFS occurs in conjunction with brainstem involvement, comprising pyramidal tract signs and impaired consciousness. In 1992, a major conceptual advance occurred when anti-GQ1b ganglioside antibodies were first identified in MFS,[4] this observation has since been substantiated by other studies. These antibodies are a sensitive and specific marker for MFS and related syndromes and are believed to be the pathophysiological mediators of the disease. In principle, this should direct treatment toward antibody removal or neutralization of effector pathways in the humoral arm of the immune system.

Epidemiology and etiology

MFS occurs worldwide and accounts for 5% to 10% of cases of GBS, the incidence of the latter syndrome being 1 or 2 per 100 000 annually. Like GBS, MFS is an acute postinfectious paralytic syndrome preceded by a diverse range of infections, including upper respiratory tract viral infections and infections with herpes viruses and *Campylobacter jejuni*. The relative frequency of these different types of preceding infections in MFS is unknown and may vary by geographical area, but respiratory viral infections appear to be most common. Irrespective of the preceding infection, anti-GQ1b antibodies are invariably found in the serum of patients with the acute phase of the syndrome.[5]

Pathophysiology and pathogenesis

Currently, a favored model proposes that anti-GQ1b antibodies arise as part of a primary immune response to infectious organisms, including *Campylobacter jejuni*, through molecular mimicry with structurally similar microbial oligosaccharides.[5] Thereafter, anti-GQ1b antibodies are able to gain access to and to bind selectively to GQ1b-enriched sites in the nervous system. Immunocytochemical studies on peripheral nerves indicate that these sites include nodes of Ranvier and terminals of motor nerves innervating extraocular muscles, dorsal root ganglia, and muscle spindles. The discrete distribution of GQ1b is thought

to account for the regionality of the clinical features of the syndrome. GQ1b is also present in the central nervous system, and providing that anti-GQ1b antibodies can cross the blood–brain barrier and access central sites, this could account for the central nervous system features observed in a proportion of patients with MFS. After the anti-GQ1b antibodies bind to neural membranes, they initiate a complement-mediated proinflammatory injury leading to the loss of function expressed clinically as craniobulbar weakness and ataxia. As the primary immune response decays, the syndrome resolves spontaneously provided irreversible axonal injury has not occurred.[6]

Genetics

Some immunogenetic studies have suggested that there may be HLA class 1 and class 2 haplotypes that confer susceptibility to the development of MFS; however, currently, such tests have no clinical use.

Clinical features and natural history, classification, and diagnostic criteria

A history of infection preceding neurological onset by 10 to 20 days is often obtained but is not mandatory. The initial symptoms are usually ocular, comprising diplopia and ptosis.[7] Pupillary paralysis is uncommon but does not exclude the diagnosis. The degree of ophthalmoplegia varies from very minor to complete external paresis and evolves over several days, usually concomitantly with the onset of ataxia and areflexia. Upper limb and gait ataxia may have cerebellar features in addition to sensory ataxia. Sensory symptoms comprising limb and facial paresthesias are common. Typically, facial weakness and bulbar weakness are present to some degree and may be severe.

Some cases of MFS merge into confluent GBS, with respiratory and limb involvement, and similarly, some cases of GBS also evolve to develop an MFS pattern of clinical involvement.[8] Variants include solitary ophthalmoplegia or ataxia and oropharyngeal weakness without ophthalmoplegia. Accompanying coma and other central signs warrant classifying the condition as Bickerstaff encephalitis. Many cases of MFS have evidence of central nervous system involvement affecting the brainstem, cerebellum, and other sites, which have been demonstrated principally with magnetic resonance imaging. If viewed broadly, MFS could be considered a peripheral and central nervous system overlap syndrome with very variable degrees of involvement of particular central or peripheral anatomical sites in individual cases, all permutations being highly associated with anti-GQ1b antibodies.

The clinical course usually evolves over 1 to 2 weeks and is followed by gradual recovery over the following weeks to months. In some recurrent cases, acute episodes occur with full recovery. A chronic relapsing ataxic neuropathy with variable ophthalmoplegia has been reported and closely resembles a chronic MFS-like picture; these patients also have anti-ganglioside antibodies that occur persistently, usually as IgM paraproteins.[9] Cases of chronic "idiopathic" ophthalmoplegia with anti-GQ1b IgG antibodies have also been reported.

In MFS, the results of routine biochemical and hematological tests are normal. The cerebrospinal fluid is acellular and protein concentration is normal or mildly increased. Anti-GQ1b IgG antibodies are increased in more than 90% of cases during the acute phase but may disappear rapidly, often being absent during convalescence. Thus, diagnostic testing should be conducted on serum samples obtained early in the course of the disease. Electrophysiological studies are important to confirm the clinical impression, and they may show reduced sensory nerve action potentials with prolonged latencies. Blink reflexes may be absent or prolonged. Motor studies may be mildly abnormal in the absence of clinical limb weakness. Serological evidence of preceding infection can be sought but does not influence clinical management. Computed tomographic and magnetic resonance imaging of the brainstem and posterior fossa structures do not show abnormality. Occasionally, in Bickerstaff encephalitis, T2-weighted magnetic resonance imaging shows increased signal intensity in the brainstem and cerebellar peduncles, but these findings are neither disease-specific nor always present. The most useful investigation is the anti-GQ1b ganglioside antibody assay, which is positive in more than 90% of cases.

Differential diagnosis

The clinical triad of classic MFS is easily recognized, although forme frustes, including incomplete or evolving syndromes, can cause diagnostic difficulties. Many disorders of the function of axon terminals or peripheral nerves preferentially affect extraocular muscles, including myasthenia gravis, botulism, diphtheria, snake envenomations, metabolic disorders, and drug intoxications. Brainstem syndromes, including encephalitis, basal meningitis, stroke, and Wernicke encephalopathy, also may resemble MFS. Most can be excluded or diagnosed by concomitant clinical features or appropriate tests, and the presence of anti-GQ1b antibodies gives high diagnostic confidence for MFS.

Treatment

No controlled trials have been conducted in MFS, and evidence for therapeutic efficacy of treatments is at best class 3 (i.e., derived from expert opinion and case studies or small series, although such series have not included well-defined historical controls). Because MFS is considered a variant of GBS and an antibody-mediated disease, most expert opinion would follow the class 1 treatment guidelines for GBS, that is, administer plasma exchange (~50 mL/kg of total plasma removed on five occasions over ~7 to 14 days, for a total exchange of 250 mL/kg) or intravenous immunoglobulin (0.4 g/kg daily for 5 days, for a total dose of 2 g/kg). Corticosteroids or other immunosuppressive agents should be avoided. Many case reports or small series of cases of both typical MFS and the Bickerstaff variant have described an apparent benefit from either plasma exchange or intravenous immunoglobulin, based on rapid recovery after treatment; however, in a disease that spontaneously improves after the nadir has been reached, this cannot be construed as definite evidence of efficacy.

Clinical criteria for instituting treatment have not been established formally and need to be judged on a case-by-case basis according to disease severity. Features such as an inability to walk or symptomatic bulbar involvement would certainly be grounds for administering plasma exchange or intravenous immunoglobulin, and it would be prudent to treat patients with lesser symptoms, especially during the phase of disease progression. Because of the rarity of MFS and the widespread acceptance of plasma exchange or intravenous immunoglobulin, no large treatment trials are in progress or have been planned. Immunoadsorption plasmapheresis using a tryptophan-linked gel column is used in Japan to treat MFS and has been shown to selectively remove anti-GQ1b antibodies.[10]

Symptomatic treatment comprises guidelines similar to those used in GBS. Patients bed bound by ataxia or coma require prophylactic treatment for venous thromboembolism. Respiratory and bulbar function require close monitoring in an appropriate intensive setting, especially during periods of clinical evolution in which life-threatening deterioration can be rapid. Bulbar paralysis can readily lead to severe aspiration pneumonia even in the absence of respiratory muscle weakness. Thus, bulbar muscle and respiratory muscle function should be monitored independently. Airway protection by endotracheal intubation may be required, and, if prolonged, it will include temporary tracheostomy. Assisted ventilation may be required in MFS/GBS overlap cases in which respiratory muscle weakness is evident. Clinical judgment on the timing of assisted ventilation is supported by serial measurements of vital capacity and pulse oximetry. Alternate eye patches are used to overcome troublesome diplopia and to protect the cornea from injury. Nutritional and fluid supplementation, communication aids, and other aspects of general medical care require attention. Occasionally, patients may require antimicrobial treatment if the precipitating infection (e.g., *Campylobacter jejuni* enteritis) is still active or if they acquire secondary infections. Physical therapy and speech therapy are needed acutely and during recovery.

References

1. Fisher M. An unusual variant of acute idiopathic polyneuritis (syndrome of ophthalmoplegia, ataxia and areflexia). N Engl J Med 1956;255:57–65

2. Ropper AH. Miller Fisher syndrome and other acute variants of Guillain-Barré syndrome. Baillieres Clin Neurol 1994;3:95–106

3. Bickerstaff ER. Further observations on a grave syndrome with benign prognosis. Br Med J 1957;1: 1384–1387

4. Chiba A, Kusunoki S, Shimizu T, Kanazawa I. Serum IgG antibody to ganglioside GQ1b is a possible marker of Miller Fisher syndrome. Ann Neurol 1992;31:677–679

5. Yuki N. Anti-ganglioside antibody and neuropathy: review of our research. J Periph Nerv Syst 1998;3:3–18

6. Willison HJ, O'Hanlon GM. The immunopathogenesis of Miller Fisher syndrome. J Neuroimmunol 1999; 100:3–12

7. Najim Al-Din AS, Anderson M, Eeg O, Trontelj JV. Neuro-ophthalmic manifestations of the syndrome of ophthalmoplegia, ataxia and areflexia. Observations on 20 patients. Acta Neurol Scand 1994;89:87–94

8. Ter Bruggen JP, van der Meché FGA, De Jager AEJ, Polman CH. Ophthalmoplegic and lower cranial nerve variants merge into each other and into classical Guillain–Barré syndrome. Muscle Nerve 1998;21: 239–242

9. Willison HJ, Paterson G, Veitch J, et al. Peripheral neuropathy associated with monoclonal IgM anti-Pr2 cold agglutinins. J Neurol Neurosurg Psychiatry 1993;56: 1178–1183

10. Yuki N. Tryptophan-immobilised column adsorbs immunoglobulin G anti-GQ1b antibody from Fisher's syndrome: a new approach to treatment. Neurology 1996;46:1644–1651

195 Brachial Plexus Neuropathy

Praful Kelkar and Gareth J Parry

Introduction

Brachial plexus neuropathies have various clinical manifestations depending on the site and extent of the lesion, and they cause various combinations of muscle weakness with atrophy, sensory loss, depressed deep tendon reflexes, and, occasionally, autonomic disturbances of the arm and hand. The etiological classification of these neuropathies is given in Table 195.1.

The discussion in this chapter is restricted to three conditions—idiopathic brachial neuritis (IBN), hereditary neuralgic amyotrophy (HNA), and idiopathic hypertrophic brachial neuritis (IHBN)—and is focused on the therapeutic aspects of these disorders.

Idiopathic brachial neuritis and hereditary neuralgic amyotrophy

IBN has several synonyms, including Parsonage-Turner syndrome, neuralgic amyotrophy, acute shoulder neuritis, acute brachial neuritis, and brachial plexus neuritis. In its typical form, it is a well-defined clinical entity. IBN presents acutely with severe pain in the shoulder that lasts for days to weeks. The severe pain abates as weakness and, later, wasting of muscles develops. Sensory loss is usually mild. IBN usually is unilateral; however, it may be bilateral, but the asymmetry is striking. The weakness has a predilection for shoulder girdle muscles, although forearm and, occasionally, hand muscles may be involved. Caudal cranial nerves and phrenic nerves also may be involved. Occasionally, the weakness is restricted to a single muscle. A highly characteristic feature is the differential involvement of muscles innervated by a single peripheral nerve—a pattern that is seldom seen in other neuropathic disorders. The prognosis for recovery is good for the majority of patients, and relapse is rare.

The cause of IBN is unknown. More than one-half the patients report an antecedent event, such as those listed in Table 195.2. The list suggests that the pathogenesis of IBN may be an immune-mediated attack on the brachial plexus or its branches in the limb. However, this contention is supported by scant pathological or serological evidence.[1] There is a report of four patients whose brachial plexus biopsy specimens showed mononuclear inflammatory infiltrates.[2] Two of these patients had subacute progression of symptoms over several months, which is a much longer progression than usual for IBN. For example, in the large series of 99 patients described by Tsairis and associates,[3] peak motor disability was reached in most patients within 2 to 3 weeks and rarely more than 6 weeks. Furthermore, one of these two patients had a painless course, with a tubular-enhancing region on magnetic resonance imaging of the brachial plexus. These two patients possibly had hypertrophic brachial neuritis (see below) rather than IBN.

Lumbar plexitis, a much less common disorder than IBN, has many striking similarities with IBN. There is asymmetrical pelvic girdle, hip, or buttock pain giving way to weakness and atrophy. Its kinship with IBN is controversial but is supported by the occasional involvement of the lumbosacral plexus in patients with HNA. Inflammatory changes with perivasculitis have been reported in a few cases of lumbar plexitis,[4,5] further supporting an autoimmune inflammatory pathogenesis.

Most cases of brachial neuritis are sporadic. However, some patients have a family history of identical attacks. HNA is an autosomal dominant disorder identical to IBN in almost every respect. The

Table 195.1 Etiological classification of brachial plexus neuropathies

Traumatic
Compressive
   Thoracic outlet syndrome
   Callus from fractures of the clavicle
   Subclavian artery aneurysms
   Neoplasms
      Apical carcinoma of the lung (Pancoast tumor)
      Breast carcinoma
      Other metastatic neoplasms
      Lymphoma

Radiation
Idiopathic (inflammatory)
   Idiopathic brachial neuritis (Parsonage-Turner syndrome)
   Idiopathic hypertrophic brachial neuritis
Inherited
   Acute brachial paralysis in hereditary neuropathy with liability to pressure palsy (HNPP)
   Hereditary neuralgic amyotrophy

Table 195.2 Antecedent illnesses in idiopathic brachial neuritis

Upper respiratory tract infection
Flu-like illness
Pregnancy and parturition
Trauma or surgery at a remote site
Vaccination
Infectious disease—mycoplasma pneumonia, Epstein-Barr virus, brucellosis, human immunodeficiency virus
Intravenous drug abuse
Treatment with interferon

principal difference between the two conditions, other than the hereditary pattern, is the marked tendency for recurrent attacks in HNA. All the antecedent events associated with IBN may cause attacks in patients with HNA. There is a particular propensity for women to have attacks of HNA in relation to parturition. Occasionally, the lower limbs may be involved, which supports the contention that sporadic lumbar plexitis is related to IBN. Some families exhibit a slightly dysmorphic appearance that includes hypotelorism, epicanthic folds, cleft palate, a minor degree of syndactyly (webbing between the 2nd and 3rd toes), primitive pinna with prominent folded helix, long narrow face, facial asymmetry, and short stature[6] (Figure 195.1). This disorder has been linked to 17q24.

Treatment

The treatment of attacks is the same for HNA and IBN. Corticosteroids are often used in the treatment of acute attacks of IBN. There is no evidence that corticosteroids influence the ultimate prognosis, but anecdotal evidence suggests that this treatment leads to a more rapid resolution of the painful phase of the illness, particularly when given early in the course.[7] Typically, oral prednisone is given in a dose of 1 mg/kg (80 mg/day) that is tapered over 2 weeks. There is no demonstrated role for high-dose intravenous gamma globulin treatment, although it has been used empirically.

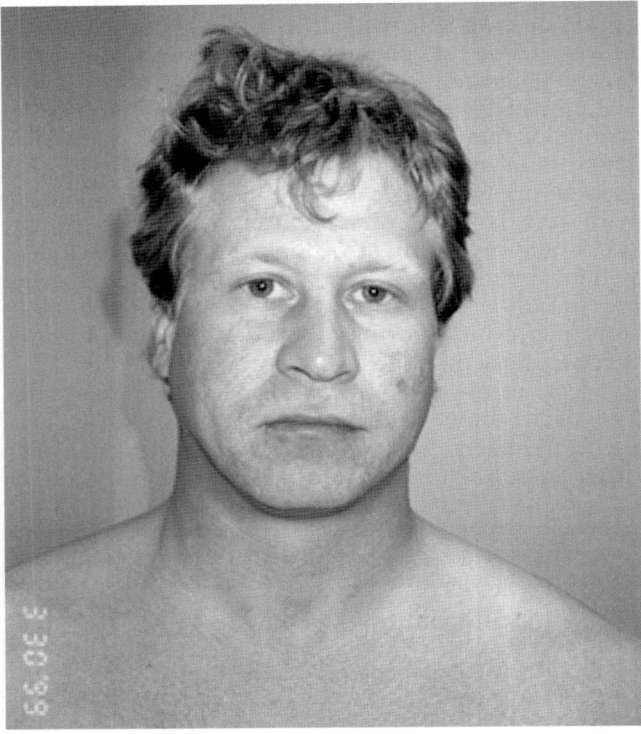

Figure 195.1 A patient with hereditary neuralgic amyotrophy (HMA) showing some dysmorphic features, namely, long narrow face, facial asymmetry, and hypotelorism. (See color plate section.)

In our experience with corticosteroid treatment in a small number of patients with HNA, a high dose of prednisone is effective, particularly if administered very early in the course of the disease. Because these patients and their physicians are familiar with the course of the disease and the earliest symptoms of an attack, treatment usually can be initiated within 24 hours. In some patients, the pain has resolved promptly and weakness has not occurred or has been minimal. Although these observations are uncontrolled, they suggest that corticosteroid treatment may have a beneficial effect. It may be that treatment of sporadic IBN is relatively ineffective because the condition is not recognized promptly, delaying the start of appropriate treatment. We recommend prednisone at a dose of 1 mg/kg daily for 2 weeks and then a tapering dose over the next 2 weeks.

Case presentation

The patient is a 4-year-old girl from a family with HNA. Her older sister, mother, and maternal aunt have all had one or more episodes of acute painful brachial paralysis, and the affected members of the family have the characteristic mild dysmorphic features described above. Because of the familial occurrence, the mother was familiar with the features of the disease, and when her daughter complained of severe arm pain and stopped using the arm, she immediately called her neurologist. Treatment with a high dose of prednisone (25 mg/day) was started within 2 days after the onset of symptoms, and the pain promptly abated. Treatment at full dose was continued for 7 days, and the dose was then tapered over 2 more weeks, without the recurrence of pain. Minimal objective weakness developed. A second similar episode occurred and the response was the same. Episodes in other family members had always been much more protracted, with the development of severe weakness, suggesting that prompt institution of prednisone treatment modified the natural history of the attacks in the young girl.

Pain management and physical therapy

An important aspect of the treatment of IBN is pain management. The pain may be particularly severe, and aggressive treatment may be needed. Acutely, narcotics such as oxycodone hydrochloride or hydromorphone may be required for pain control. Long-term treatment with these medications is to be avoided to minimize the likelihood of habituation and addiction. Some patients may require longer term treatment for pain, for which amitriptyline (75 to 100 mg/day) or gabapentin (2400 to 4800 mg/day in divided doses) may be appropriate. Physical therapy is prescribed to maintain a good range of passive movement at the shoulder to avoid adhesive capsulitis, or "frozen shoulder."

Idiopathic hypertrophic brachial neuritis

IHBN is a rare, predominantly motor disorder affecting the brachial plexus and more distal upper limb nerve trunks. It causes progressive weakness affecting

Table 195.3 Approach to patients with IBN, HNA, or IHBN

Condition	Investigations that may be considered	Management
IBN	EMG MRI—cervical spine, brachial plexus Rule out diabetes mellitus, vasculitis	Oral prednisone (at onset) 60–80 mg/day, taper over 2 weeks Physical therapy Pain management
HNA	If the family history is known, none If family history is not known, same as for IBN	Same as for IBN
IHBN	EMG—particularly looking for conduction block MRI of brachial plexus with gadolinium	IVIG Corticosteroids for some patients

EMG, electromyography; HNA, hereditary neuralgic amyotrophy; IBN, idiopathic brachial neuritis; IHBN, idiopathic hypertrophic brachial neuritis; IVIG, intravenous immunoglobulin; MRI, magnetic resonance imaging.

brachial muscles, and it is characterized by hypertrophy of the components of the brachial plexus. Most commonly, IHBN is a pure motor syndrome that is painless and slowly progressive, although some patients may have pain, sensory abnormalities, or a relapsing-remitting course, with relapses that evolve over long periods. Electrophysiological studies may show conduction block across the brachial plexus.[8,9] Pathological studies in a few patients have shown extensive onion-bulb formation and focal chronic inflammation.[8,10–12] Most likely, IHBN is a localized form of chronic inflammatory demyelinating polyneuropathy or multifocal motor neuropathy. It differs from IBN by its chronic course, absence of pain, and enlargement of the brachial plexus. Many patients have a good response to intravenous immunoglobulin,[8,13] similar to the response reported in patients with multifocal motor neuropathy.[14] Some patients have had a response to corticosteroid treatment[10,15] or cyclophosphamide.[8]

The approach to patients with IBN, HNA, or IHBN is summarized in Table 195.3.

References

1. Sierra A, Prat J, Bas J, et al. Blood lymphocytes are sensitized to brachial plexus nerves in patients with neuralgic amyotrophy. Acta Neurol Scand 1991;83:183–186
2. Suarez GA, Giannini C, Bosch EP, et al. Immune brachial plexus neuropathy: suggestive evidence for an inflammatory-immune pathogenesis. Neurology 1996;46:559–561
3. Tsairis P, Dyck PJ, Mulder DW. Natural history of brachial plexus neuropathy. Report on 99 patients. Arch Neurol 1972;27:109–117
4. Bradley WG, Chad D, Verghese JP, et al. Painful lumbosacral plexopathy with elevated erythrocyte sedimentation rate: a treatable inflammatory syndrome. Ann Neurol 1984;15:457–464
5. Verma A, Bradley WG. High-dose intravenous immunoglobulin therapy in chronic progressive lumbosacral plexopathy. Neurology 1994;44:248–250
6. Keller MP, Chance PF. Inherited neuropathies: from gene to disease. Brain Pathol 1999;9:327–341
7. Sumner AJ. Brachial neuritis. In: Johnson RT, ed. Current Therapy in Neurologic Disease-3. Philadelphia: BC Decker, 1990:374–375
8. Kaji R, Oka N, Tsuji T, et al. Pathological findings at the site of conduction block in multifocal motor neuropathy. Ann Neurol 1993;33:152–158
9. Krarup C, Sethi RK. Idiopathic brachial plexus lesion with conduction block of the ulnar nerve. Electroencephalogr Clin Neurophysiol 1989;72:259–267
10. Bradley WG, Bennett RK, Good P, Little B. Proximal chronic inflammatory polyneuropathy with multifocal conduction block. Arch Neurol 1988;45:451–455
11. Cusimano MD, Bilbao JM, Cohen SM. Hypertrophic brachial plexus neuritis: a pathological study of two cases. Ann Neurol 1988;24:615–622
12. Thomas PK, Claus D, Jaspert A, et al. Focal upper limb demyelinating neuropathy. Brain 1996;119:765–774
13. Van den Bergh PY, Thonnard JL, Duprez T, Laterre EC. Chronic demyelinating hypertrophic brachial plexus neuropathy. Muscle Nerve 2000;23:283–288
14. Parry GJ. Multifocal motor neuropathy: pathology and treatment. In: Kimura J, Kaji R, eds. Physiology of ALS and Related Diseases. Amsterdam: Elsevier, 1997:73–83
15. Adams RD, Asbury AK, Michelsen JJ. Multifocal pseudohypertrophic neuropathy. Trans Am Neurol Assoc 1965;90:30–33

196 Nondiabetic Lumbosacral Radiculoplexus Neuropathy

P James B Dyck

Clinical features and pathophysiology

Diabetic lumbosacral radiculoplexus neuropathy (DLSRPN) (discussed in the section on diabetic neuropathies) is an asymmetrical lower limb syndrome of pain, weakness, paresthesia, and weight loss which usually occurs in patients with mild type 2 diabetes mellitus. Although the condition is severe and debilitating, it usually is monophasic, with the symptoms and deficits expected to resolve in months or years, but improvement is often incomplete.

A similar syndrome of unilateral or asymmetrical lower limb pain, weakness, and paresthesia, that is, lumbosacral radiculoplexus neuropathy (LSRPN), affects nondiabetic patients and is the condition discussed here. LSRPN has been recognized more recently than DLSRPN; the first descriptions were not published until 1981.[1,2] Like its diabetic counterpart, it appears to be a monophasic illness that usually has incomplete recovery.[1,3]

On the basis of our studies, we believe that DLSRPN and LSRPN are essentially alike except for the occurrence of diabetes mellitus in DLSRPN.[3,4] These neuropathies are probably more prevalent in diabetic populations, but the prevalence of the nondiabetic condition is not known. Recently, we completed a study comparing 57 LSRPN patients with 33 DLSRPN patients.[3] Both conditions are characterized by a subacute painful disorder that begins focally in the leg or thigh but becomes more generalized and bilateral with time. Early in the course, pain is the predominant symptom, but late in the course, weakness predominates. Both LSRPN and DLSRPN are associated with an increased concentration of protein in the cerebrospinal fluid, substantial weight loss, abnormalities on quantitative and autonomic testing, and electromyographic features suggestive of patchy but widespread involvement of the lumbosacral roots, plexus, and peripheral nerves.

Until recently, little had been written about the underlying pathological mechanisms in LSRPN. Bradley et al.[5] inferred a possible inflammatory/immune mechanism in three cases of LSRPN and three cases of DLSRPN by showing evidence of ischemic damage (multifocal fiber loss) and perivascular inflammatory cell cuffing. They included only patients with increased erythrocyte sedimentation rates whose biopsy specimens did not show frank necrotizing vasculitis. We have completed a pathological study of nerve biopsy specimens from 47 cases of LSRPN and showed that the main underlying pathological mechanism is ischemic injury from microvasculitis and that both the axonal degeneration and segmental demyelination are due to ischemic injury.[4] Because the vessels involved were small nerve vessels, fibrinoid degeneration of mural elements was not readily appreciated. The pathological findings are the same as those in DLSRPN.[6]

LSRPN has been assumed to be a monophasic illness that resolves with time. However, most of the patients of Evans et al.[1] had incomplete recovery, with long-term morbidity. Similarly, the recovery in our series of LSRPN patients was poor.[3] Although all patients had improvement with time, only 3 of the 42 patients contacted reported that they had recovered completely. Most of the long-term disability involved distal limb structures. Of our 42 patients, 7 had recurrent episodes of lumbosacral plexopathy and only 2 later developed diabetes mellitus.

Treatment

Little is known about the treatment of LSRPN. Bradley et al.[5] reported that four of their six patients had improvement with prednisone. Awerbuch et al.[7] reported that their patient treated with prednisone did not have improvement. Verma and Bradley[8] reported two patients who responded to high-dose intravenous immunoglobulin, and Triggs et al.[9] reported that five patients had improvement with intravenous immunoglobulin.

We conducted an open trial of weekly intravenous infusions of methylprednisolone in 11 LSRPN patients over 8 to 16 weeks.[10] All had marked improvement of pain and many had complete resolution of the pain. All patients had some improvement of weakness, and 9 of the 11 graded this improvement as marked. The median neuropathy impairment score was statistically improved after treatment (Figure 196.1). Before treatment, one-half of the patients were in wheelchairs and all but one used an aid in ambulating. After treatment, only one patient was still in a wheelchair and six walked independently. We consider these treatment data preliminary and not definitive. There were no control patients, and LSRPN can improve spontaneously. However, we believe that the treatment probably was helpful because in all cases the improvement of symptoms began with the initiation of treatment. Placebo-controlled double-blind prospective studies are needed to answer whether immunomodulating therapies are effective in treating LSRPN.

LSRPN is a severe illness with great morbidity.

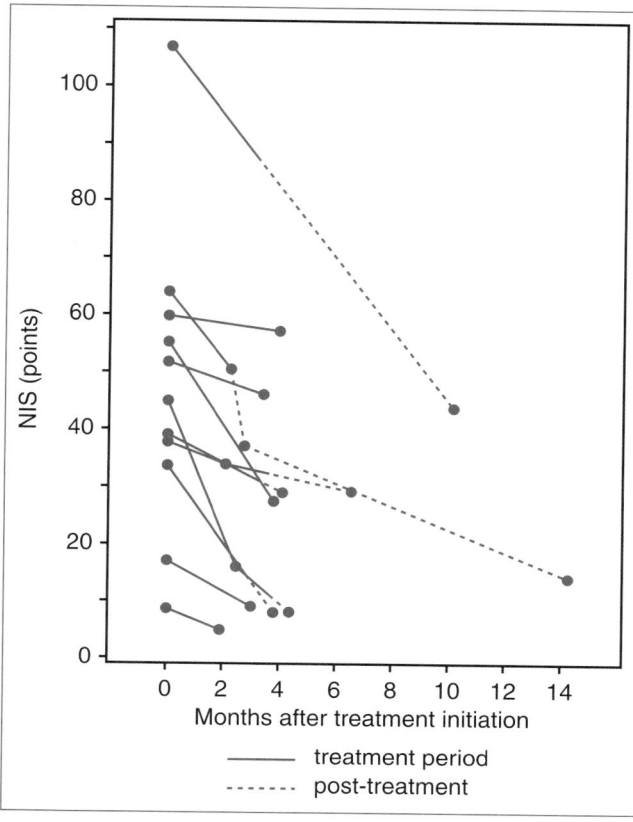

Figure 196.1 Neuropathy impairment score (NIS) of 11 patients with nondiabetic lumbosacral radiculoplexus neuropathy plotted with time after a course of intravenous methylprednisolone therapy. Each line represents a different patient, the dots represent patient evaluations, and the solid lines represent the treatment period. Without exception, the NIS improved (score decreased) during the treatment period, sometimes dramatically (see text for discussion). (From Dyck et al.[10] By permission of the *Canadian Journal of Neurological Sciences*.)

Because it is usually a monophasic illness, physicians often underappreciate the suffering and disability patients experience. Patients frequently are so weak and have such severe pain that they are unable to work; they often require hospitalization to achieve adequate pain control. The pain is severe, and most patients require narcotic medication as well as treatment with other chronic neuropathic pain medicines (for example, tricyclic antidepressants and antiseizure agents). Patients should be warned that it is often impossible to relieve the pain completely and the goal is to make the pain bearable and livable. Almost invariably, patients with LSRPN become depressed because of protracted pain and weakness. These patients usually were healthy, high-functioning persons before they became ill and the illness caused major life changes. They should be warned that although the disease may be monophasic, its course tends to be long and miserable. They should be encouraged to stay involved in hobbies and other interests. Depression should be treated with antidepressant medications. Physical therapy should be used. Their homes should be made as safe as possible, and bracing, such as ankle foot orthoses, should be fitted and used if needed. Physicians need to be aggressive in helping patients with pain control, in being hospitalized, and in obtaining health and disability insurance when needed.

References

1. Evans BA, Stevens JC, Dyck PJ. Lumbosacral plexus neuropathy. Neurology 1981;31:1327–1330
2. Sander JE, Sharp FR. Lumbosacral plexus neuritis. Neurology 1981;31:470–473
3. Dyck PJB, Norell JE, Dyck PJ. Non-diabetic lumbosacral radiculoplexus neuropathy: natural history, outcome and comparison with the diabetic variety. Brain 2001;124:1197–1207
4. Dyck PJ, Engelstad J, Norell J, Dyck PJ. Microvasculitis in non-diabetic lumbosacral radiculoplexus neuropathy (LSRPN): similarity to the diabetic variety (DLSRPN). J Neuropathol Exp Neurol 2000;59:525–538
5. Bradley WG, Chad D, Verghese JP, et al. Painful lumbosacral plexopathy with elevated erythrocyte sedimentation rate: a treatable inflammatory syndrome. Ann Neurol 1984;15:457–464
6. Dyck PJ, Norell JE, Dyck PJ. Microvasculitis and ischemia in diabetic lumbosacral radiculoplexus neuropathy. Neurology 1999;53:2113–2121
7. Awerbuch GI, Nigro MA, Sandyk R, Levin JR. Relapsing lumbosacral plexus neuropathy: report of two cases. Eur Neurol 1991;31:348–351
8. Verma A, Bradley WG. High-dose intravenous immunoglobulin therapy in chronic progressive lumbosacral plexopathy. Neurology 1994;44:248–250
9. Triggs WJ, Young MS, Eskin T, Valenstein E. Treatment of idiopathic lumbosacral plexopathy with intravenous immunoglobulin. Muscle Nerve 1997;20:244–246
10. Dyck PJB, Norell JE, Dyck PJ. Methylprednisolone may improve lumbosacral radiculoplexus neuropathy. Can J Neurol Sci 2001;28:224–227

197 Treatment of Nonmalignant Sensory Ganglionopathies

IA Grant

Overview

Peripheral neuropathies can be classified according to the site of the primary pathological process as neuronopathy, axonopathy, or myelinopathy. Neuronopathies involve motor neurons in the brainstem or spinal cord, primary sensory neurons in dorsal root ganglia or trigeminal ganglia, autonomic neurons, or a combination of these. This chapter discusses diseases of primary sensory neurons, that is, sensory neuronopathies or ganglionopathies.

Cases of pure, progressive sensory loss and sensory ataxia were described in the early 19th century, but relatively recently has it been recognized that this clinical picture may reflect disease of sensory ganglia. In the 19th century, ataxia of the lower limbs typically was ascribed to posterior column degeneration.[1,2] Coexistent degeneration of the posterior columns and peripheral nerves was described in tabes dorsalis by Gowers,[3] although prominent degeneration of peripheral sensory axons would now be considered atypical for that disorder. The concept of primary disease of sensory ganglia was introduced in Denny-Brown's report of two cases of sensory neuropathy associated with lung carcinoma.[4] This landmark report emphasized the contrast between the severe degeneration of dorsal root ganglia neurons, peripheral sensory axons, and dorsal columns and that of other disorders in which degeneration of nerves or tracts is not accompanied by loss of the associated sensory cell bodies. Numerous subsequent reports have defined the clinical, immunological and electrophysiological features of this syndrome, now recognized as a "paraneoplastic syndrome." Although Denny-Brown believed it was a metabolic abnormality, the typically inflammatory nature of the disorder has been demonstrated pathologically in both paraneoplastic[5] and Sjögren syndrome-associated cases.[6,7]

Epidemiology

Epidemiological data are not available for sensory ganglionopathies. No population-based or large cross-sectional or prospective studies have been reported. Because of the inherent difficulty in establishing that the sensory ganglion is the site of the disease process, particularly in mild cases, the prevalence of both paraneoplastic and nonparaneoplastic cases may be underestimated.

Etiology and pathogenesis

Sensory ganglionopathies can occur from various insults, including disturbed immune function, infections, toxins, and inherited disorders (Table 197.1). The discussion in this chapter is limited to the immune-mediated group. Paraneoplastic sensory ganglionopathies are discussed in Chapter 204.

Growing evidence indicates that Sjören syndrome-associated and idiopathic ganglionopathies have an autoimmune cause. However, this is less well understood than it is for paraneoplastic disorder.

In Sjögren syndrome-related cases, an autoimmune cause is assumed partly because of the known autoimmune nature of the associated disease. Limited pathological evidence supports this idea. In a small number of cases, biopsy of dorsal root ganglia has demonstrated mononuclear inflammatory infiltrates,[6–8] composed mainly of T cells, which in one case were chiefly of the cytotoxic subset.[6] A small number of macrophages and plasma cells also were found.[7] Dorsal root ganglia infiltrates are similar but not identical to those found in the salivary glands in Sjögren syndrome, in which helper T cells predominate.[9] Although B cells are present in salivary gland infiltrates, they have not been reported in sensory ganglia.

Serological abnormalities, important in establishing an autoimmune basis for paraneoplastic ganglionopathy, have not been as evident in Sjögren syndrome and idiopathic cases. Nonspecific serological findings such as antinuclear antibodies (ANA) are less common in Sjögren syndrome presenting as sensory neuropathy than in classic Sjögren syndrome.[8] However, Satake[10] identified IgG in the serum and cerebrospinal fluid of a patient with Sjögren syndrome and a hyperalgesic form of ganglionopathy, with immunohistochemical specificity for small dorsal root ganglion neurons. Moll[11] identified antineuronal antibodies in the serum of 10 of 45 patients with Sjögren syndrome. Three patients had an antibody specific for a 38-kd neuronal protein indistinguishable from the anti-Hu (ANNA-1) antibody commonly found in patients with paraneoplastic sensory neuropathy. One of these patients had sensory neuronopathy. These findings raise the possibility that specific antibodies against sensory neurons in patients with Sjögren syndrome may be involved in the pathogenesis of neuropathy.

Increasing evidence suggests that antibodies also may have a role in idiopathic ataxic ganglionopathies. The probable targets in at least some cases are glycolipids located in the plasma membrane. In particular, gangliosides containing disialosyl moities, notably GD1b, appear to be involved. These gangliosides are

Table 197.1   Differential diagnosis of predominantly sensory polyneuropathy

Inherited
  Hereditary sensory and autonomic neuropathies
    (autosomal dominant, autosomal recessive)
  Abetalipoproteinemia (autosomal recessive)
  Spinocerebellar ataxias (autosomal dominant,
    autosomal recessive, X-linked recessive)
  Fabry disease (X-linked recessive)
  Familial amyloid polyneuropathy (autosomal dominant)

Acquired

  Autoimmune
    Inflammatory ganglionopathies
      Paraneoplastic
      Sjögren syndrome/sicca complex
      Idiopathic
    Monoclonal gammopathy
    Acute inflammatory demyelinating polyneuropathy
      Fisher syndrome
      "Sensory Guillain-Barré syndrome"
    Chronic inflammatory demyelinating polyneuropathy
    Primary biliary cirrhosis
    Vasculitis

  Toxic
    Drugs
      Cisplatin
      Metronidazole
      Paclitaxel (Taxol)
      Pyridoxine
      Isoniazid (INH)
      Nucleoside analogues
      Thalidomide
    Heavy metals
      Methyl mercury
      Arsenic
      Thallium
    Others
      Ethanol
      Trichroloethylene
      Polychlorinated biphenyls
      Hexacarbons

  Metabolic
    Diabetes mellitus
    Uremia
    Hypothyroidism

  Deficiency states
    Pyridoxine
    Vitamin E
    Thiamine
    Cobalamin

with other disialosyl-containing gangliosides and this antibody immunolocalized to rodent dorsal root ganglia, motor nerve terminals, muscle spindles, and myelinated fibers. Immunization of rabbits with GD1b leads to the production of anti-GD1b antibodies and, in some animals, to an ataxic ganglionopathy, with degeneration of dorsal root ganglion neurons.[16]

Clinical features

By definition, sensory symptoms and deficits are the major clinical features. The specific symptoms depend on the class of neurons involved. According to the classification of Smith,[17] ganglionopathies can be divided into ataxic, hyperalgesic, and mixed forms. In the ataxic form, loss of large myelinated fibers produces paresthesias, numbness, incoordination, and gait instability, which typically is worse with the removal of visual cues. Examination of these patients demonstrates impairment of vibration and joint position sense, sensory ataxia, pseudoathetosis, and hyporeflexia or areflexia. Strength usually is normal, although minor weakness may be present and related to proprioceptive loss or to true (but generally mild) lower motor neuron involvement. In the hyperalgesic form, dysesthesias and pain (typically burning or lancinating in character) are common, with symptoms related to autonomic involvement in some cases. Examination shows impairment of pain and temperature perception. Accompanying signs of dysautonomia may include tonic pupils, sweating abnormalities, and orthostatic hypotension. Patients with the mixed form have a combination of large- and small-fiber abnormalities.

The distribution of deficits is often distinctive. Findings may be asymmetrical, in some cases involving one limb with complete sparing of the contralateral limb for extended periods. Other findings that suggest the diagnosis include onset in the upper limbs, on the trunk, or in the trigeminal distribution. However, a relatively symmetrical, distal pattern does not exclude the diagnosis, and symmetry becomes more common as the disease progresses.

The course is also highly variable. Acute, subacute, and chronic cases have been described. Several reports have emphasized a distinctive syndrome of acute onset over days, sometimes following an antecedent infectious illness. Chronic ganglionopathies may be more common, but they are less distinctive. After a period of progression, deficits often stabilize for extended periods. However, by this time, patients often are severely disabled. In other patients, the neuropathy remains static or only slowly progressive, with nondisabling deficits, for many years. A stepwise course has also been described.

Windebank[18] described the long-term course in 38 patients with idiopathic sensory ganglionopathy. A monophasic course was observed in 18 patients; an initial period of progression was followed by partial remission in 8 and by a period of stability in 10. In 20 patients, rapid progression was followed by a gradual or stepwise deterioration.

present in the membrane of dorsal root ganglion neurons. Several groups have found circulating IgM directed against GD1b in association with ataxic sensory neuropathies.[12–15] Binding of anti-disialosyl IgM from patients with such neuropathies has been demonstrated on dorsal root ganglion neurons in culture and in tissue sections with the use of immunohistochemical techniques.[14,15] Analyzing an IgM molecule cloned from a patient with a monoclonal gammopathy and chronic ganglionopathy, Willison[15] found that the protein reacted with GD1b as well as

Classification

Several classification schemes have been proposed. Ganglionopathies may be classified according to the size of the affected neurons and fibers, as outlined above. More often, they are classified according to the presence of associated disease as (1) paraneoplastic, (2) Sjögren syndrome- or sicca complex-associated, and (3) idiopathic.

Diagnostic criteria

Laboratory testing

The results of routine blood chemistry and hematological tests usually are normal. The most common laboratory abnormalities are those consistent with an underlying dysimmune process; these depend partly on the presence of associated disease. In Sjögren syndrome-associated cases, serological findings may include ANA, antibodies to extractable nuclear antigens (particularly SS-A), a polyclonal increase in immunoglobulins, and, occasionally, rheumatoid factor.[6,19–21] However, these findings are probably less common than in classical Sjögren syndrome, particularly among patients presenting with ganglionopathy rather than sicca symptoms. In Grant's series,[8] ANA was present in 2 of 11 patients, none of whom had positive rheumatoid factor. Antibodies to extractable nuclear antigens, considered the most specific test for Sjögren syndrome, were also uncommon; SS-A was present in 2 patients and SS-B in 1. These autoantibodies are rare in idiopathic cases.[18,22]

Monoclonal gammopathy is present in a small proportion of idiopathic cases, usually IgM.[13,14,18,22] Because of the absence of associated lymphoproliferative disease, this generally is classified as "monoclonal gammopathy of undetermined significance" (MGUS).

Cerebrospinal fluid (CSF) protein is normal or minimally increased. CSF cell counts nearly always are normal.[18] CSF immunoglobulin levels may be increased.[22] Rarely are oligoclonal bands identified.[10,23]

As noted, antiganglioside antibodies have been identified in individual patients with Sjögren syndrome-associated and idiopathic ataxic ganglionopathies. However, their diagnostic utility in routine practice has not been established, although serology is providing insights into disease mechanisms.

Electrophysiology

Characteristic abnormalities include decrease or absence of sensory nerve action potentials, absence of H reflexes, and absence of somatosensory evoked potentials. Motor nerve conduction studies typically are normal or only mildly abnormal. The most common motor findings are decreased conduction velocities, with occasionally prolonged distal latencies, decreased compound muscle action potential amplitudes, and prolonged F-wave latencies.

The results of needle electromyography usually are normal. In a small proportion of patients, motor unit changes, including long duration units, occur, consistent with low-grade denervation and reinnervation.

Fibrillation potentials in distal muscles are found in some patients, mainly in foot muscles.[18] Impaired motor unit activation is relatively common, presumably as a manifestation of deafferentation.[22]

Imaging studies

Imaging is useful mainly for excluding diseases that may mimic ganglionopathy, such as intrinsic spinal cord disease, and polyradiculopathies due to infectious, inflammatory and neoplastic disorders. Diffuse gadolinium enhancement of the dorsal roots has been described with magnetic resonance imaging of a patient with acute idiopathic ganglionopathy.[23]

Pathology

Sural nerve biopsy generally demonstrates a decrease in the number (density) of myelinated fibers.[18,22] According to some reports, this loss preferentially involves large myelinated fibers,[22] particularly in patients with ataxia. Other findings may include evidence of ongoing axonal degeneration and clusters of regenerating axons. In one series, morphometric studies demonstrated a significantly decreased median axonal area with a preserved median myelin area; in conjunction with evidence of low-grade demyelination and remyelination, this was interpreted to indicate axonal atrophy.[18] Inflammation generally is absent, but occasionally small epineurial infiltrates of mononuclear cells are present. Dorsal root ganglion biopsy findings are discussed above.

Biopsy of minor salivary gland may help establish the presence of Sjögren syndrome.[24] This procedure is well tolerated and is probably underused in the evaluation of sensory ganglionopathies. However, negative biopsy findings do not exclude the Sjögren syndrome, because pathological evidence of sialadenitis is only one of several criteria, which also include ophthalmologic tests for keratoconjunctivitis sicca. Diagnostic criteria have been reviewed elsewhere.[25,26] European Community criteria are summarized in Table 197.2.

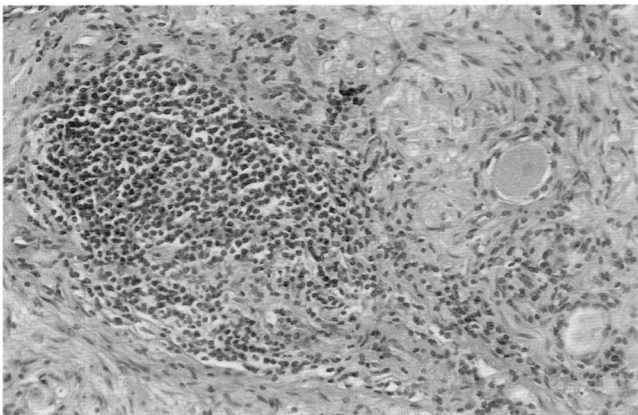

Figure 197.1   Dorsal root ganglion from a patient with sensory ganglionopathy associated with Sjögren syndrome. A mononuclear inflammatory infiltrate is present. Two neuronal cell bodies are seen to right. (Hematoxylin and eosin, ×250.) (See color plate section.)

Table 197.2 European classification criteria for Sjögren syndrome*

I Ocular symptoms: a positive response to at least one of the following three questions:
  1. Have you had daily, persistent dry eyes for more than 3 months?
  2. Do you have a recurrent sensation of sand or gravel in the eyes?
  3. Do you use tear substitutes more than 3 times a day?

II Oral symptoms: a positive response to at least one of the following three questions:
  1. Have you had a daily feeling of dry mouth for more than 3 months?
  2. Have you had recurrently or persistently swollen salivary gland as an adult?
  3. Do you frequently drink liquids to aid in swallowing dry food?

III Ocular signs: objective evidence of ocular involvement defined as a positive result in at least one of the following two tests:
  1. Schirmer I test (≤ 5 mm in 5 minutes)
  2. Rose Bengal score (≥ 4 according to the van Bijsterveld system)

IV Histopathology
  Focus score ≥ 1 in a minor salivary gland biopsy (a focus is defined as an agglomerate of at least 50 mononuclear cells; the focus score is defined by the number of foci in 4 mm^2 of glandular tissue)

V Salivary gland involvement: objective evidence of salivary gland involvement defined as a positive result in at least one of the following three tests:
  1. Salivary scintigraphy
  2. Parotid sialography
  3. Unstimulated salivary flow (≤ 1.5 mL in 15 minutes)

VI Autoantibodies: presence in the serum of the following autoantibodies:
  Antibodies to SS-A, SS-B, or both

*Rules for classification: In patients without any potentially associated disease, the presence of any four of the six items is indicative of primary Sjögren syndrome.
In patients with a potentially associated disease (such as another connective tissue disease) item I or item II plus any two of items III–V is indicative of secondary Sjögren syndrome.

Differential diagnosis

The differential diagnosis of sensory neuropathies is extensive (Table 197.1). Several considerations are important in narrowing the list of possibilities.

It is helpful to distinguish between *purely* sensory neuropathies and those that also have minor motor involvement. Most polyneuropathies encountered in clinical practice present as a predominantly sensory process with minimal or mild motor findings and progress to more obvious motor involvement as the disease worsens. In contrast, the differential diagnosis of a pure sensory neuropathy, with no suggestion of motor involvement on clinical and electrophysiologic grounds, is relatively small. However, as noted above, mild motor changes do not exclude ganglionopathy.

The presence of signs of central nervous system dysfunction is also helpful. Paraneoplastic sensory neuropathies may coexist with brainstem or limbic encephalitis. Long tract signs may suggest vitamin B$_{12}$ deficiency or an inherited process such as spinocerebellar ataxia.

The concept of sensory variants of acute and chronic inflammatory demyelinating polyneuropathies deserves special consideration. Miller-Fisher syndrome is a well-defined variant of Guillain-Barré syndrome and consists of the triad of ophthalmoplegia, ataxia, and areflexia. The presence of eye movement abnormalities should be sought, because they do not occur in sensory ganglionopathies. Several reports have described "sensory Guillain-Barré syndrome" with prominent sensory deficits and areflexia without ophthalmoplegia.[27,28] This diagnosis should be made with caution, because the clinical syndrome of sensory Guillain-Barré syndrome may actually reflect an acute polyganglionopathy. Nerve conduction studies are particularly important, and evidence of segmental demyelination should be sought. The importance of this distinction lays in the clearly treatable nature of Guillain-Barré syndrome and chronic inflammatory demyelinating polyneuropathy (CIDP), in contrast to that of true ganglionopathies (see below).

Treatment

Limited data are available about treatment. No randomized clinical trials have been performed. To date, all the clinical data that have been reported consist of small, retrospective, uncontrolled series (class 3 evidence).

In addition to the lack of clinical trials, several other factors make it difficult to assess the validity of published reports. Study populations have differed widely in age, sex, acuteness of onset, and duration and severity of disease. In contrast to the literature on paraneoplastic ganglionopathies, quantitative methods of assessment have not been used. Thus, an assessment of the response to treatment has often been subjective, with respect to both symptoms and neurological deficits.

Follow-up has varied from a few months to 35

Table 197.3   Studies reporting treatment of idiopathic sensory ganglionopathies

Study	Course	No. of patients	No. of patients treated	Treatment, no. of patients					Reported response
				Corticosteroids	Aza	Chlor	PlEx	IVIg	
Dalakas[22]	Chronic	15	13	13	3*	2*	2*	–	All patients continued to have disease progression
Windebank[18]	Acute	42	14	13	–	–	2†	–	In 10 patients, disease stabilized or improved; and in 4, it progressed†
Sterman[30]	Acute	3	2	2	–	–	–	–	No response
Bang[23]	Acute	1	1	1	–	–	–	1	No response
Hodson[27]	Acute	1	1	–	–	–	1	–	Insufficient treatment period before death to evaluate response

Aza, azathioprine; Chlor, chlorambucil; IVIg, intravenous immunoglobulin, PlEx, plasma exchange.
* Patients also received corticosteroids.
† One patient also received corticosteroids.
‡ In untreated group, disease remained stable or improved in 8 patients and progressed in 20.

years.[18] Because of the very long duration of disease in many patients, including some with acute onset of symptoms, short follow-up may be insufficient to judge treatment effectiveness. In many series, untreated disease has been shown to stabilize spontaneously, with no evidence of progression over a period of years. Thus, a stable clinical course that follows the initiation of treatment may be coincidental.

Because the underlying lesion involves loss of primary sensory neurons, it is likely that an effective treatment may only halt the progression of the disease, that is, reversal of deficits is probably impossible. Some degree of improvement may be possible, for example, if injured but still viable neurons can be "rescued" by treatment so that they regain normal function or if a patient is able to learn to compensate for a new but nonprogressive neurological deficit. Particularly in more severe cases, however, stabilization may be the most realistic treatment objective.

Many reports are difficult to interpret because more than one drug was given concurrently, making it difficult to know which agent was responsible for a putative clinical effect. Assessment of treatment is also difficult because of incomplete information about dosage and duration of treatment.

In regard to the presence of associated disease, it is unclear whether data on the treatment of Sjögren syndrome-associated ganglionopathies are relevant to the treatment of idiopathic cases and vice versa. Critical appraisal of Sjögren syndrome-associated cases is also hampered by the variation in criteria used for the diagnosis of this condition. Finally, among patients with Sjögren syndrome, other inflammatory processes potentially responsive to immunotherapy may coexist with the ganglionopathy. Vasculitis is the major consideration in this regard. If unrecognized vasculitis is present, improvement following treatment may be attributed incorrectly to an effect on the ganglionopathy when the effect actually was due to suppression of vasculitis. This effect is also a concern with respect to an unrecognized inflammatory demyelinating process. Where possible, such cases have been excluded from the review. However, this remains a theoretical possibility in all reported cases.

Studies in which the presence of ganglionopathy can be concluded with reasonable certainty are summarized for idiopathic and Sjögren syndrome-associated cases in Tables 197.3 and 197.4, respectively.

Most authors have reported the use of corticosteroids, either alone or in combination with immunosuppressants, plasma exchange, or intravenous immunoglobulin. Corticosteroid treatment regimens consist mainly of oral prednisone or prednisolone at a dose of 5 to 90 mg daily. The use of pulse-dosed intravenous methylprednisolone has also been reported. In general, these studies have not reported a positive effect. For example, Dalakas[22] treated 13 patients with prednisone (100 mg daily), in some cases in combination with azathioprine, chlorambucil, or plasma exchange. In all patients, the neuropathy continued to progress slowly.

Many of the problems inherent in assessment of treatment are demonstrated by the study of Windebank et al.[18] Among 14 patients with acute-onset idiopathic disease, 13 received corticosteroids using variable regimens. Over extended follow-up, the disease stabilized or improved in 10 patients and continued to progress in 4. However, among 28 patients who received no treatment, 20 had disease progression and 8 had spontaneous improvement or the disease remained stable. Although the difference between the two groups raised the possibility of a treatment effect, the authors pointed out that the

Table 197.4 Studies Reporting Treatment of Sjögren Syndrome-Associated Sensory Ganglionopathies

Study	Course	No. of patients	No. of patients treated	Treatment, no. of patients						Reported response
				Corticosteroids	Aza	Chlor	Pen	PIEx	IVIg	
Griffin[6]	Acute, subacute, chronic	13	10	9	3*	3†	–	1	–	Objective improvement in 1 patient with both oral and intravenous corticosteroids
Kaltreider[31]	Chronic	4‡	4	4	–	–	–	–	–	Reduced trigeminal deficit in 1; no response in trigeminal neuropathy in 3
Font[20]	Chronic	5	3	3	–	–	–	–	–	No response
Gemignani[32]	NR	2	2	2	1	1	–	–	–	Stable or "slight improvement" over 30–36 months
Kennett[21]	Chronic	3	2	2	–	–	–	–	–	No response
Asahina[19]	Chronic	2	2	2§	–	–	2	–	–	Improvement in deficits with subsequent prolonged stability on penicillamine; no response to corticosteroids alone
Molina[29]	Chronic	1	1	1	–	–	–	–	1	Transient response to 5-day course of IVIg on 2 occasions; stable with IVIg every 3 weeks; no clear response to corticosteroids
Pascual[33]	Chronic	1	1	1	–	–	–	–	1	"Subjective and objective response" to prednisone; improved pain with IVIg, with and without prednisone
Hull[34]	Chronic	1	1	1	–	–	–	–	–	Stabilization with low-dose oral corticosteroids
Hankey[35]	Chronic	1	1	1	–	–	–	–	–	No response (continued progression)
Laloux[36]	Chronic	1	1	1	–	–	–	–	–	No response (continued progression)
Malinow[7]	Subacute	1	1	1	–	1	–	–	–	Stabilization of deficits; continued progression of symptoms
Kaplan[37]	Subacute	1	1	1	–	–	–	1	–	Stabilization

Aza, azathioprine; Cyclo, cyclophosphamide; IVIg-intravenous immunoglobulin; NR, not reported; Pen, penicillamine; PlEx, plasma exchange.
*Two patients also received corticosteroids.
†All three patients also received corticosteroids.
‡Trigeminal neuropathy. One patient had biopsy-proven vasculitis of muscle.
§One patient also received cyclosporine.

occurrence of spontaneous improvement in many patients makes it impossible to conclude that the differences were due to treatment.

Griffin[6] reported 13 patients with Sjögren syndrome-associated ganglionopathy, 10 of whom received treatment.[6] Nine patients received corticosteroid therapy, with azathioprine, cyclophosphamide, chlorambucil and plasma exchange also given to a small number. In the majority of patients, the disease had an indolent, slowly progressive course before treatment. One patient appeared to have a response to prednisone (up to 60 mg daily), with improvement in gait ataxia and return of muscle stretch reflexes after 5 weeks of therapy. These deficits recurred when the dose was tapered to 20 mg daily. With re-treatment with intravenous methylprednisolone 1 g daily for 3 days, followed by alternate-day corticosteroid therapy, the diseased again showed objective improvement. However, for the other nine patients given treatment, there was no evidence that treatment altered the course of the disease.

Because of the small number of patients involved, it is impossible to draw conclusions about the effectiveness of other treatment modalities. However, several authors have suggested an effect on the basis of small series. Asahina[19] described two patients with chronic ganglionopathies associated with Sjögren syndrome. In both of them, clinical progression occurred despite oral and intravenous treatment with corticosteroids for 4 weeks. In one patient, the symptoms and deficits clearly improved with treatment with penicillamine, 300 mg daily, in combination with a low dose of prednisolone. Improved joint position sense and sensory ataxia were accompanied by partial recovery in tibial somatosensory evoked potentials. During the subsequent 5 years, the course was stable with continued penicillamine treatment. In the other patient, arrest of progression also coincided with the initiation of penicillamine treatment, followed by "slight amelioration" in subjective sensory loss and ataxia and a stable course over 4 years of treatment.

A possible response to intravenous immunoglobulin treatment was described by Molina[29] in a 60-year-old man with chronic ganglionopathy associated with Sjögren syndrome. After a progressive course, a 5-day course of intravenous immunoglobulin (0.4 g/kg) was followed in 1 week by functional improvement in gait and hand function. This treatment was repeated with the initiation of prednisone (90 mg daily) 3 weeks later. A relapse to the pretreatment state occurred 3 weeks after this second treatment, with an apparent response to another course of intravenous immunoglobulin. The patient's condition reportedly remained stable thereafter with immunoglobulin infusions given every 3 weeks.

Conclusion

To date, effective therapy has not been established for immune-mediated sensory ganglionopathies. Largely anecdotal evidence suggests that corticosteroids, intravenous immunoglobulin, and penicillamine may be of benefit in some patients. However, there is insufficient evidence to permit a general recommendation for therapy. These issues probably will remain unsettled without randomized clinical trials, which will be difficult to perform because of the rarity of the disease, the inherent irreversibility of the underlying process, and the occurrence of spontaneous stabilization and remission. Perhaps future insights into the basic immunological mechanisms of both Sjögren syndrome-associated and non-Sjögren syndrome-associated cases will suggest which of the available agents would be the most rational choice when clinical trials are designed.

References

1. Todd RB. Cyclopaedia of Anatomy and Physiology. London: Longman, Brown, Green, Longmans and Roberts: 1839–1847
2. Stanley E. A case of disease in the posterior columns of the spinal cord. Med Chir Trans 1840;5:80
3. Gowers WR. A Manual of Diseases of the Nervous System. Philadelphia: P Blakiston Son & Co., 1888:311
4. Denny-Brown D. Primary sensory neuropathy with muscular changes associated with carcinoma. J Neurol Neurosurg Psychiatry 1948;11:73–87
5. Horwich MS, Cho L, Porro RS, Posner JB. Subacute sensory neuropathy: a remote effect of carcinoma. Ann Neurol 1977;2:7–19
6. Griffin JW, Cornblath DR, Alexander E, et al. Ataxic sensory neuropathy and dorsal root ganglionitis associated with Sjogren's syndrome. Ann Neurol 1990;27:304–315
7. Malinow K, Yannakakis GD, Glusman SM, et al. Subacute sensory neuronopathy secondary to dorsal root ganglionitis in primary Sjogren's syndrome. Ann Neurol 1986;20: 535–537
8. Grant IA, Hunder GG, Homburger HA, Dyck PJ. Peripheral neuropathy associated with sicca complex. Neurology 1997;48:855–862
9. Dalavanga YA, Drosos AA, Moutsopoulos HM. Labial salivary gland immunopathology in Sjögren's syndrome. Scand J Rheumatol 1986;61Suppl:67–70
10. Satake M, Yoshimura T, Iwaki T, et al. Anti-dorsal root ganglion neuron antibody in a case of dorsal root ganglionitis associated with Sjögren's syndrome. J Neurol Sci 1995;132:122–125
11. Moll JW, Markusse HM, Pijnenburg JJ, et al. Antineuronal antibodies in patients with neurologic complications of primary Sjogren's syndrome. Neurology 1993;43:2574–2581
12. Ilyas AA, Quarles RH, Dalakas MC, et al. Monoclonal IgM in a patient with paraproteinemic polyneuropathy binds to gangliosides containing disialosyl groups. Ann Neurol 1985;18: 655–659
13. Yuki N, Miyatani N, Sato S, et al. Acute relapsing sensory neuropathy associated with IgM antibody against B-series gangliosides containing a Ga1NAc beta 1-4(Gal3-2 alpha NeuAc8-2 alpha NeuAc)beta 1 configuration. Neurology 1992;42:686–689
14. Oka N, Kusaka H, Kusunoki S, et al. IgM M-protein with antibody activity against gangliosides with disialosyl residue in sensory neuropathy binds to sensory neurons. Muscle Nerve 1996;19: 528–530
15. Willison HJ, O'Hanlon GM, Paterson G, et al. A somatically mutated human antiganglioside IgM antibody that induces experimental neuropathy in mice is

encoded by the variable region heavy chain gene, V1-18 (see comments). J Clin Invest 1996;97:1155–1164

16. Kusunoki S, Shimizu J, Ciba A, et al. Experimental sensory neuropathy induced by sensitization with ganglioside GD1b. Ann Neurol 1996;39:424–431

17. Smith BE, Windebank AJ, Dyck PJ. Nonmalignant inflammatory sensory polyganglionopathy. In: Dyck PJ, Thomas PK, eds. Peripheral Neuropathy, 3rd ed. Philadelphia: WB Saunders, 1993:1525–1531

18. Windebank AJ, Blexrud MD, Dyck PJ, et al. The syndrome of acute sensory neuropathy: clinical features and electrophysiologic and pathologic changes (see comments). Neurology 1990;40:584–591

19. Asahina M, Kuwabara S, Nakajima M, Hattori T. D-penicillamine treatment for chronic sensory ataxic neuropathy associated with Sjogren's syndrome. Neurology 1998;51:1451–1453

20. Font J, Valls J, Cervera R, et al. Pure sensory neuropathy in patients with primary Sjogren's syndrome: clinical, immunological, and electromyographic findings. Ann Rheum Dis 1990;49: 775–778

21. Kennett RP, Harding AE. Peripheral neuropathy associated with the sicca syndrome. J Neurol Neurosurg Psychiatry 1986;49:90–92

22. Dalakas MC. Chronic idiopathic ataxic neuropathy. Ann Neurol 1986;19:545–554

23. Bang MS, Han TR, Lim JY. Acute sensory neuronopathy: identified with electrodiagnosis and magnetic resonance imaging. Am J Phys Med Rehabil 1998;77: 494–497

24. Daniels TE. Labial salivary gland biopsy in Sjogren's syndrome. Assessment as a diagnostic criterion in 362 suspected cases. Arthritis Rheum 1984;27(2):147–156

25. Vitali C, Bombardieri S, Moutsopoulos HM, et al. Preliminary criteria for the classification of Sjogren's syndrome. Results of a prospective concerted action supported by the European Community. Arthritis Rheum 1993;36(3): 340–347

26. Fox RI, Saito I. Criteria for diagnosis of Sjogren's syndrome. Rheum Dis Clin North Am 1994;20(2):391–407

27. Hodson AK, Hurwitz BJ, Albrecht R. Dysautonomia in Guillain-Barre syndrome with dorsal root ganglioneuropathy, wallerian degeneration, and fatal myocarditis. Ann Neurol 1984;15:88–95

28. Kanter ME, Nori SL. Sensory Guillain-Barre syndrome. Arch Phys Med Rehabil 1995;76:882–883

29. Molina JA, Benito-Leon J, Bermejo F, et al. Intravenous immunoglobulin therapy in sensory neuropathy associated with Sjogren's syndrome (letter). J Neurol Neurosurg Psychiatry 1996;60: 699

30. Sterman AB, Schaumburg HH, Asbury AK. The acute sensory neuronopathy syndrome: a distinct clinical entity. Ann Neurol 1980;7:354–358

31. Kaltreider HB, Talal N. The neuropathy of Sjogren's syndrome. Trigeminal nerve involvement. Ann Intern Med 1969;70:751–762

32. Gemignani F, Marbini A, Pavesi G, et al. Peripheral neuropathy associated with primary Sjogren's syndrome. J Neurol Neurosurg Psychiatry 1994;57:983–986

33. Pascual J, Cid C, Berciano J. High-dose i.v. immunoglobulin for peripheral neuropathy associated with Sjogren's syndrome (letter; comment). Neurology 1998;51:650–651

34. Hull RG, Morgan SH, Harding AE, Hughes GR. Sjogren's syndrome presenting as a severe sensory neuropathy including involvement of the trigeminal nerve. Br J Rheumatol 1984;23:301–303

35. Hankey GJ, Gubbay SS. Peripheral neuropathy associated with sicca syndrome (letter). J Neurol Neurosurg Psychiatry 1987;50:1085–1086

36. Laloux P, Brucher JM, Guerit JM, et al. Subacute sensory neuronopathy associated with Sjogren's sicca syndrome. J Neurol 1988;235:352–354

37. Kaplan JG, Rosenberg R, Reinitz E, et al. Invited review: peripheral neuropathy in Sjogren's syndrome. Muscle Nerve 1990;13: 570–579

198 Vasculitis of the Peripheral Nervous System

Michael P Collins and John T Kissel

Overview

The term *vasculitis* refers to a pathological process in which blood vessel walls are inflamed and damaged, resulting in ischemic injury to the tissues supplied by those vessels. The clinical manifestations of vasculitis depend on the location, size, and type of involved vessels, underlying pathogenesis, tempo of the disease, and the host's specific immunological responses. Vasculitis may be confined to a single organ, such as the peripheral nervous system (PNS), or affect many tissues simultaneously, with potentially lethal consequences. Systemic vasculitides involving small to medium-sized arteries commonly produce neuropathy because they often affect epineurial arteries. In contrast, vasculitides with mainly microvascular or large vessel involvement infrequently produce neuropathy.

Early pathological descriptions of vasculitis were made possible by advances in histopathological techniques, such as improved embedding and staining procedures and better microscopes, in the latter nineteenth century.[1] The first description of a systemic vasculitis is credited to Kussmaul and Maier, who in 1866 reported a patient with fever, anemia, neuropathy, enteritis, and nephritis, whose autopsy revealed widespread inflammatory lesions of small and medium-sized arteries.[2] They called this condition *periarteritis nodosa*, a term changed to polyarteritis nodosa (PAN) by Ferrari in 1903.[3] Most of the other major vasculitides were subsequently described in the first half of the twentieth century (Table 198.1).

Kernohan and Woltman first drew attention to neuropathy in vasculitis by describing PAN restricted to the PNS.[11] Lovshin and Kernohan made the important observations that vasculitic neuropathy may herald systemic disease, spontaneously regress, and present in a distal, symmetric pattern.[21] The seminal histopathological study of vasculitic neuropathy was published by Dyck and colleagues in 1972.[17] Kissel and colleagues reported one of the first series of vasculitic neuropathy patients in 1985,[22] and nonsystemic vasculitic neuropathy (NSVN) was identified as a unique, PNS-confined form of vasculitis by Dyck and coworkers in 1987.[18]

Classification

Zeek was the first to propose a classification scheme for vasculitic disorders in 1952.[16] Her categorization included periarteritis nodosa, hypersensitivity vasculitis, allergic granulomatous angiitis (Churg–

Table 198.1 Historical milestones in vasculitis and vasculitic neuropathy

Event	Year	Authors
First complete description of systemic vasculitis: "periarteritis nodosa"	1866	Kussmaul and Maier[2]
First report of peripheral nervous system vasculitis in rheumatoid arthritis	1898	Bannatyne[4]
Introduction of term "polyarteritis nodosa"	1903	Ferrari[3]
Patients with temporal arteritis described	1890	Hutchinson[5]
Microscopic polyangiitis distinguished from polyarteritis nodosa	1923	Wohlwill[6]
	1948	Davson et al.[7]
Establishment of Wegener's granulomatosis as a distinct entity	1931	Klinger[8]
	1936	Wegener[9]
	1954	Godman and Churg[10]
First series of patients with peripheral nerve vasculitis reported	1938	Kernohan and Woltman[11]
Hypersensitivity vasculitis distinguished from polyarteritis nodosa	1948	Zeek et al.[12]
Allergic granulomatous angiitis (Churg–Strauss syndrome) identified	1951	Churg and Strauss[13]
Relationship between rheumatoid arthritis and vasculitis firmly established	1951	Sokoloff et al.[14]
	1954	Cruickshank[15]
First published classification system of systemic vasculitis	1952	Zeek[16]
Definitive autopsy study of vasculitic neuropathy	1972	Dyck et al.[17]
Nonsystemic vasculitic neuropathy established as a unique disorder	1987	Dyck et al.[18]
American College of Rheumatology criteria for seven vasculitides published	1990	American College of Rheumatology[19]
Chapel Hill Consensus Conference on Nomenclature of Systemic Vasculitis	1994	Jennette et al.[20]

Strauss syndrome), rheumatic arteritis (associated with rheumatic fever), and temporal arteritis. Wegener's granulomatosis was added in 1954.[10] Many additional classifications have since been proposed based on etiology, size and type of involved vessel, pathology, and clinical features. Most schemes distinguish between *primary* vasculitides, of unknown etiology and with no relationship to other disease processes, and *secondary* vasculitides, which complicate another disease or result from a definable etiology. In 1990, the American College of Rheumatology Subcommittee on Classification of Vasculitis published diagnostic criteria for seven vasculitides— PAN, Churg–Strauss syndrome (CSS), Wegener's granulomatosis (WG), hypersensitivity vasculitis (HSV), Henoch–Schönlein purpura (HSP), temporal (or giant cell) arteritis (TA), and Takayasu's arteritis (TKA).[19] These criteria were based on an analysis of 1000 cases from 48 centers, whereby the clinical findings that best distinguished each form of vasculitis from the other six were selected. While useful for classifying patients for studies, these criteria are not appropriate for diagnosis. For example, one analysis of 198 possible vasculitis patients using this classification found positive predictive values of only 17% to 29% for WG, PAN, TA, and HSV.[23]

The 1994 Chapel Hill Consensus Conference on the Nomenclature of Systemic Vasculitis proposed a classification that has achieved widespread acceptance.[20] The names and definitions for ten vasculitides were selected based on the size and pathology of involved vessels (Table 198.2). This scheme was the first to define microscopic polyarteritis (MPA) as a separate entity—a small-vessel, pauci-immune, nongranulomatous vasculitis with rapidly progressive glomerulonephritis. This system has been criticized for restricting classic PAN to cases affecting small and medium-sized arteries alone, so that otherwise typical PAN with *any* small vessel involvement (e.g. in skin or nerves) is reclassified as MPA; because of this, classic PAN has become rare in recent epidemiological studies (see below).

Vasculitic disorders associated with neuropathy can be divided into five groups, based on the size of

Table 198.2 Names and definitions of vasculitides adopted by the Chapel Hill Consensus Conference on the Nomenclature of Systemic Vasculitis[20]

Large vessel vasculitis	
Giant cell (temporal) arteritis	Granulomatous arteritis of the aorta and its major branches, with a predilection for the extracranial branches of the carotid artery. Often involves the temporal artery. Usually occurs in patients older than 50 and often is associated with polymyalgia rheumatica
Takayasu arteritis	Granulomatous inflammation of the aorta and its major branches. Usually occurs in patients younger than 50
Medium-sized vessel vasculitis	
Polyarteritis nodosa (classic polyarteritis nodosa)	Necrotizing inflammation of medium-sized or small arteries without glomerulonephritis or vasculitis in arterioles, capillaries, or venules
Kawasaki disease	Arteritis involving large, medium-sized, and small arteries, associated with mucocutaneous lymph node syndrome. Coronary arteries are often involved. Aorta and veins may be involved. Usually occurs in children
Small-vessel vasculitis	
Wegener's granulomatosis*	Granulomatous inflammation involving the respiratory tract and necrotizing vasculitis affecting small to medium-sized vessels (e.g. capillaries, venules, arterioles, and arteries). Necrotizing glomerulonephritis is common
Churg–Strauss syndrome*	Eosinophil-rich and granulomatous inflammation involving the respiratory tract and necrotizing vasculitis affecting small to medium-sized vessels, associated with asthma and eosinophilia
Microscopic polyangiitis*	Necrotizing vasculitis, with few or no immune deposits, affecting small vessels (i.e. capillaries, venules, or arterioles). Necrotizing arteritis involving small and medium-sized arteries may be present. Necrotizing glomerulonephritis is very common. Pulmonary capillaritis often occurs
Henoch-Schönlein purpura	Vasculitis with IgA-dominant immune deposits, affecting small vessels (i.e. capillaries, venules, or arterioles). Typically involves skin, gut, and glomeruli, and is associated with arthralgias or arthritis
Essential cryoglobulinemic vasculitis	Vasculitis, with cryoglobulin immune deposits, affecting small vessels (i.e. capillaries, venules, or arterioles), and associated with cryoglobulins in serum. Skin and glomeruli are often involved
Cutaneous leukocytoclastic angiitis	Isolated cutaneous leukocytoclastic angiitis without systemic vasculitis or glomerulonephritis

*Strongly associated with antineutrophil cytoplasmic autoantibodies

Table 198.3   Classification of vasculitides associated with neuropathy

A. Vasculitides resulting from direct infection
  1. Bacterial (e.g. group A β-hemolytic streptococcus, infective endocarditis, Lyme disease)
  2. Viral (e.g. cytomegalovirus, HIV, HTLV-I, varicella zoster virus)
B. Vasculitides resulting from immunological mechanisms
  1. Systemic necrotizing vasculitis
    a. Classic polyarteritis nodosa
    b. Antineutrophil cytoplasmic autoantibody-associated
      (i)   Microscopic polyangiitis
      (ii) Churg–Strauss syndrome
      (iii) Wegener's granulomatosis
    c. Hepatitis B-associated polyarteritis nodosa
    d. Vasculitis with connective tissue disease
      (i)   Rheumatoid arthritis
      (ii) Sjögren's syndrome
      (iii) Systemic lupus erythematosus
      (iv) Mixed connective tissue disease
      (v)   Relapsing polychondritis
  2. Hypersensitivity vasculitis
    a. Henoch–Schönlein purpura
    b. Drug-induced vasculitis (e.g. amphetamines, cocaine)*
    c. Vasculitis associated with infections*
    d. Cryoglobulinemic vasculitis (hepatitis C)*
    e. Vasculitis associated with malignancy*
    f. Diabetic lumbosacral radiculoplexus neuropathy (?)
  3. Giant cell arteritis
    a. Temporal arteritis
  4. Localized vasculitis
    a. Nonsystemic vasculitic neuropathy
  5. Miscellaneous vasculitides
    a. Behçet's disease

*Each of these entities can also produce a systemic necrotizing vasculitis.

involved vessels, presumed immunopathogenesis, and management approaches (Table 198.3). They include: vasculitides from direct vessel infection; systemic necrotizing vasculitides with multiorgan involvement; hypersensitivity vasculitides, with primary cutaneous involvement and an initiating factor triggering an immune complex-mediated process; giant cell arteritides, which affect larger vessels and typically respond to corticosteroids alone; and nonsystemic vasculitic neuropathy (NSVN).

Epidemiology

Two epidemiological studies have determined annual adult incidence rates for vasculitides (Table 198.4).[24,25] Temporal arteritis and cutaneous vasculitides are most common, followed by rheumatoid vasculitis, WG, and MPA. The frequency of vasculitic *neuropathy*, however, is quite different because of the variable prevalence of neuropathy in these conditions and the occurrence of NSVN. In general, neuropathy is common in the systemic necrotizing vasculitides and rare in TA and the predominant skin vasculitides. The relative prevalence of the different types of vasculitic neuropathy is shown in Table 198.5.

Etiology

Most vasculitic neuropathies are presumed to be autoimmune disorders. Rarely, etiological triggers can be identified, such as infections, drugs, or malignancies. The immune mechanisms involved in these cases serve as models for the pathogenesis of the idiopathic vasculitides.

Infections

Virtually any infection can act as an antigenic stimulus for the formation of immune complexes and resulting vasculitis.[26–28] Organisms can also produce vasculitis by direct vascular invasion (e.g. rickettsia), release of toxins acting as superantigens (e.g. staphy-

Table 198.4   Relative annual incidence of systemic vasculitides in adults

Type of vasculitis	Relative annual incidence (percent of all cases)	
	Lugo, Spain[24]	Norwich Health Authority[25] (United Kingdom)
Temporal arteritis	41%	18%
Cutaneous leukocytoclastic angiitis	20%	22%
Microscopic polyangiitis	9.4%	5.0%
Henoch–Schönlein purpura	5.6%	4.8%
Rheumatoid vasculitis	4.5%	18%
Systemic lupus erythematosus	3.7%	5.0%
Wegener's granulomatosis	3.4%	12%
Essential cryoglobulinemic vasculitis	3.4%	1.7%
Malignancy-related vasculitis	3.0%	1.1%
Churg–Strauss syndrome	0.8%	4.6%
Sjögren's syndrome	0.8%	0.0%
Classic polyarteritis nodosa	0.8%	0.0%
Other/unclassified	3.4%	8.4%

Table 198.5   Relative prevalence of vasculitic neuropathy types*

Type of vasculitic neuropathy	Relative prevalence (percent of all reported cases)
Nonsystemic vasculitic neuropathy	30%
Classic polyarteritis nodosa or microscopic polyangiitis	29%
Rheumatoid vasculitis	16%
Connective tissue diseases not otherwise specified	7%
Churg–Strauss syndrome	7%
Lupus vasculitis	3%
Primary Sjögren's syndrome	3%
Malignancy	1%
HIV infection	1%
Wegener's granulomatosis	1%
Miscellaneous (e.g. cryoglobulinemia, temporal arteritis)	2%

*Based on a review of 576 patients in 16 series.

lococci, streptococci), generation of vascular toxins (e.g. pseudomonas), induction of cell-mediated or antibody-mediated immune responses against vascular structures (e.g. ascariasis), and induction of aberrant immunoregulation (e.g. HIV). Viruses with persistent replication, such as hepatitis B, hepatitis C and HIV, have the strongest association with vasculitic neuropathy.[27–29] Other viruses implicated in vasculitis include varicella zoster, herpes simplex, cytomegalovirus (CMV), Epstein–Barr, hepatitis A, parvovirus B19 and hantavirus.

A prototypical infection-related vasculitis is hepatitis B-associated PAN, where immune complex deposition appears to be the primary disease mechanism.[27,29–32] Depending on the population, circulating hepatitis B surface antigen is found in 10% to 55% of patients with classic PAN. The clinical features in these patients are similar to those seen in idiopathic PAN and include renal artery vasculitis, neuropathy, arthralgias, myalgias, fever, weight loss, visceral aneurysms, rashes and gastrointestinal (GI) symptoms. In the largest series of hepatitis B-related PAN, 80% had neuropathy.[32] Chronic hepatitis C (5% to 10% of PAN patients),[33–35] HIV,[36] and parvovirus B19[37] infections are less common causes of a PAN-like illness.

Approximately 2% to 3% of HIV patients develop neuromuscular involvement due to vasculitis.[38–40] This figure likely underestimates the true incidence, however, as HIV patients with painful sensory polyneuropathies are not routinely biopsied, preempting ascertainment of many cases.[41] Vasculitic neuropathies with HIV infection commonly develop during the early symptomatic stage, but can occur in patients with CD4 counts as low as 14/ml.[36] Unlike systemic necrotizing vasculitides, most HIV vasculitis is self-limited and confined to peripheral nerves and muscle.[36,39–42] The pathogenesis of HIV vasculitis is not well understood, although direct infection of endothelial cells by HIV (or other organisms), immune complex deposition, pro-inflammatory cytokine release, and HIV-driven immune dysregulation may

all operate.[39–42] HIV antigens and genomic DNA have been detected in nerve and muscle perivascular cells in biopsies from patients with PNS vasculitis, and HIV replication has been observed in the endoneurial and epineurial inflammatory cell infiltrates.[42–44]

Hepatitis C-associated essential mixed cryoglobulinemia (EMC) is another well-characterized viral vasculitis.[35,45–47] Cryoglobulins are circulating immunoglobulins that precipitate when cooled. There are three types: type I, monoclonal immunoglobulins (or light chains) produced in the setting of various lymphoproliferative diseases; type II, a mixture of monoclonal IgM rheumatoid factors (anti-IgG) and polyclonal IgG; and type III, polyclonal IgM rheumatoid factors and polyclonal IgG. Types II and III are termed mixed cryoglobulins, which can be *essential* or *secondary* to connective tissue diseases, lymphoproliferative disorders, chronic infections, glomerulonephritides, or chronic liver diseases. Approximately 85% of EMC patients suffer from chronic hepatitis C, which leads to lymphoproliferation. The virus chronically infects mononuclear blood and bone marrow cells, especially B lymphocytes, producing a non-neoplastic, oligoclonal B cell expansion, which produces autoantibodies, rheumatoid factors, and cryoglobulins.[48] Mixed cryoglobulins commonly induce immune complex-mediated inflammation of small vessels and a syndrome characterized by palpable purpura and inconstant skin ulcers, urticaria, arthralgias, Raynaud's phenomenon, glomerulonephritis, liver function abnormalities, and adenopathy. Neuropathy from immune complex vasculitis develops in 50% of EMC patients.[49–52] A multifocal neuropathy may occur, but a distal, symmetric, sensorimotor polyneuropathy is more common.

Bacterial vasculitis rarely involves the PNS; exceptional cases have been reported with Group A β-hemolytic streptococcal,[53] *Mycoplasma pneumoniae*,[54] typhoid fever,[55] leptospiral,[56] and *Pseudomonas aeruginosa*[57] infections. Vasculitic neuropathies may also complicate endocarditis and chronic dental infections.[58,59] Although 40% to 60% of Lyme disease patients have PNS manifestations, sural nerve biopsies in these cases usually show epineurial, perivascular inflammation without true vasculitis.[60–62] *Borrelia burgdorferi* DNA has been detected in sural nerve tissue by polymerase chain reaction.[63]

Drugs

A small-vessel vasculitis has been associated with most common pharmacological agents, and as many as 30% to 50% of cases of HSV may be secondary to drugs.[64] Sulfonamides were the first agents recognized to cause vasculitis, but many other drugs have now been implicated.[26,28,64,65] Circulation and deposition of immune complexes is the suspected mechanism in most cases, with the drug acting as a hapten/antigen. However, other types of hypersensitivity reactions can be produced. Most drug-induced vasculitides spare the PNS, but multifocal neuropathies or pathologically proven vasculitic neuropathies have been reported for penicillin,[66] cromolyn,[67] thiouracil,[68] allopurinol,[69] amantadine,[70] and interferon alfa.[71] Drugs of abuse can also cause vasculitis; in particular, amphetamines, cocaine, and heroin.[72] PNS involvement occurs with these agents, but is less common than central nervous system (CNS) vasculitis.[73]

Malignancy

Hypersensitivity vasculitis in the setting of lymphoproliferative disorders is well established.[74] The most frequent neoplasm associated with vasculitis is hairy cell leukemia.[75] Most malignancy-related vasculitides are restricted to the skin, with leukocytoclastic pathology. Vasculitis associated with hairy cell leukemia occasionally has features similar to PAN, but without neuropathy.[75] Lymphocytic lymphomas, chronic lymphocytic leukemia, Hodgkin's disease, angioimmunoblastic lymphadenopathy, and Waldenström's macroglobulinemia are also sometimes responsible for mixed cryoglobulinemic vasculitis, including rare cases of vasculitic neuropathy.[45,46,74,76] Cancer-related PNS vasculitis has been reported more frequently with solid malignancies (prostate, non-small cell lung, colon, renal cell, endometrial, small cell lung, gastric, tongue squamous cell, cervical, bile duct, cholangio and thyroid carcinomas; malignant melanoma) than with hematological disorders (non-Hodgkin lymphoma, chronic lymphocytic leukemia, myelodysplastic syndrome, Hodgkin's disease, and plasmacytoma).[77–81] Most patients present in the sixth to eighth decades, the neuropathy preceding diagnosis of the malignancy in 50%. Most paraneoplastic vasculitides involving the PNS are confined to nerve and muscle, a feature distinguishing them from the primary systemic necrotizing vasculitides.

The mechanisms by which cancers produce vasculitis are unknown.[74,79,82] Tumor antigens may elicit humoral immune responses when circulating in the blood or after implanting on the endothelium, inducing in situ or circulating immune complex formation. Molecular mimicry between antigens on neoplastic and endothelial cells may trigger cross-reacting immune responses. Alternatively, the cancer and the vasculitis may share a common viral etiology, or products from malignant cells may deposit in vessel walls, causing inflammatory reactions. Cancer cells may directly invade or embolize vessel walls.

Pathogenesis

Apart from the infectious and drug-related vasculitides just discussed, the antigens triggering vasculitis are generally unknown. The autoimmune processes resulting in vascular damage are also incompletely understood.[83–85] Typically, more than one mechanism is operating in a given case. All vasculitides are thought to begin with antigen recognition, resulting in a humoral or cellular immune response (or both). Through this process, circulating leukocytes are primed and endothelial cells activated, so that leukocytes adhere to the endothelium and become activated (Figure 198.1).[86–88] This interaction depends on cellular adhesion molecules, cytokines, chemokines, and other inflammatory regulators, which mediate transendothelial migration of leukocytes and recruitment of additional effector cells. Adhesion molecules upregulated in some vasculitides are intercellular adhesion molecule (ICAM)-I, vascular cell adhesion molecule (VCAM)-I, E-selectin, very late antigen (VLA)-4, leukocyte function associated antigen (LFA)-1, and LFA-3. Cytokines associated with vasculitis include tumor necrosis factor (TNF)-α, interleukin (IL)-1, IL-6, IL-8, interferon (INF)-γ, transforming growth factor (TGF)-β1, platelet-derived growth factor (PDGF), and vascular endothelial cell growth factor (VEGF).[86,87]

Immune effector cells damage vessel walls by many mechanisms, including the release of proteolytic enzymes or respiratory burst-associated toxic oxygen free radicals, generation of perforin and complement membrane attack complex that mediate endothelial cell lysis, and possibly enzyme- or Fas ligand-induced apoptosis.[89,90] Intravascular coagulation is also stimulated, along with vessel wall fibrosis, intimal cell proliferation, and development of collateral vessels. Regulatory, anti-inflammatory cytokines (e.g. TGFβ1) eventually downregulate the inflammation and repair gains predominance over destruction.[87] The result is a thickened, fibrosed, and sometimes thrombosed or partially occluded vessel.

At least five primary immune mechanisms mediate vessel injury in the vasculitides. In *immune complex-mediated vasculitis*, antibodies interact with circulating antigens to form antigen–antibody complexes that activate complement and prime leukocytes.[83,91] Immune complexes then deposit in vessel walls and activate more complement, generating chemotactic factors and inflammatory mediators, thereby recruiting neutrophils and other effector cells (Figure 198.1). Immune complex formation underlies most secondary vasculitides related to infections, drugs, malignancy and cryoglobulins, and may be important in connective tissue diseases associated with multiple autoantibodies directed against endogenous antigens.

In *anti-endothelial cell antibody (AECA)-mediated*

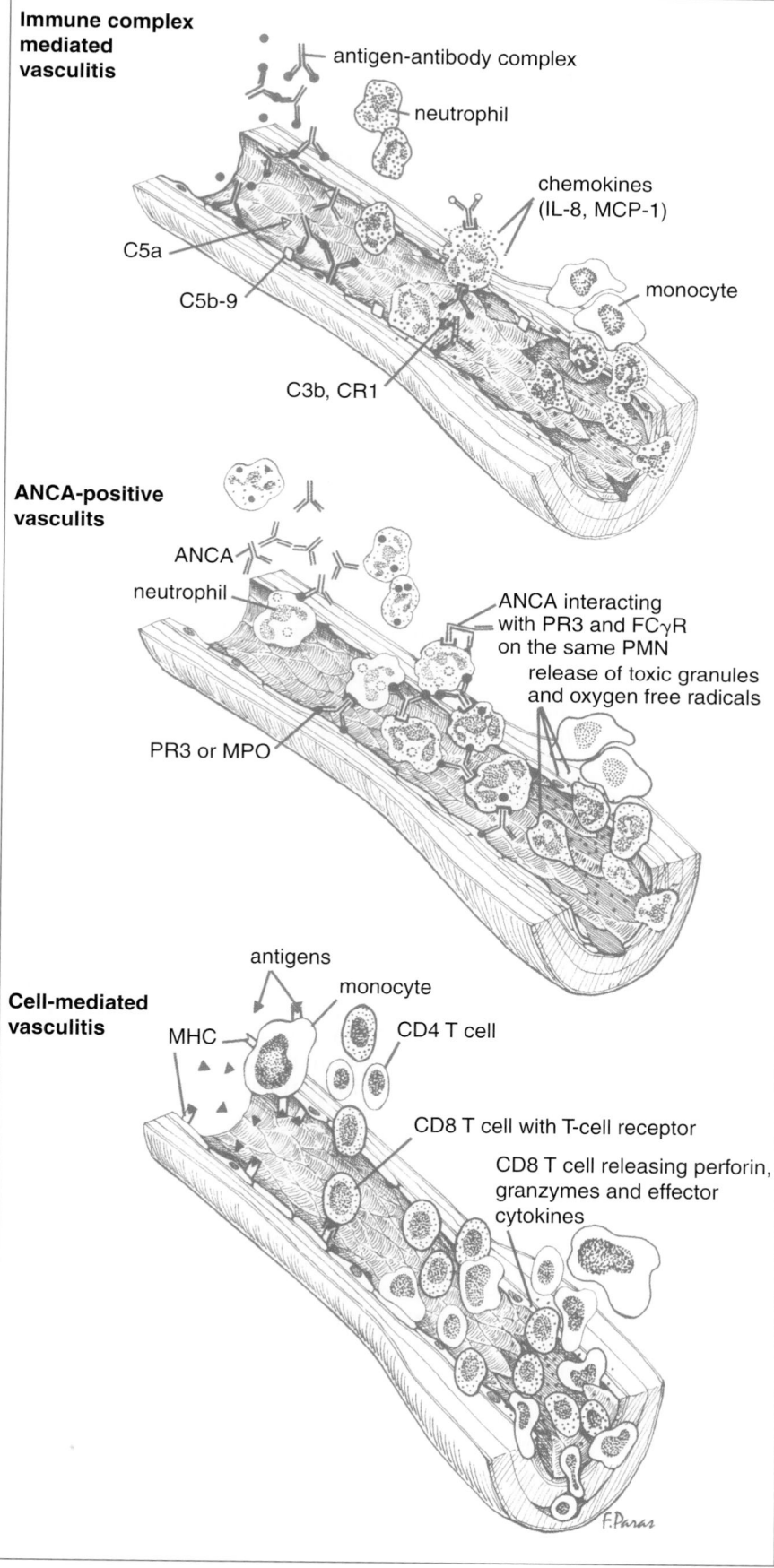

Immune complex mediated vasculitis

- antigen-antibody complex
- neutrophil
- chemokines (IL-8, MCP-1)
- C5a
- C5b-9
- C3b, CR1
- monocyte

ANCA-positive vasculits

- ANCA
- neutrophil
- ANCA interacting with PR3 and FCγR on the same PMN
- release of toxic granules and oxygen free radicals
- PR3 or MPO

Cell-mediated vasculitis

- antigens
- monocyte
- MHC
- CD4 T cell
- CD8 T cell with T-cell receptor
- CD8 T cell releasing perforin, granzymes and effector cytokines

F.Paras

Figure 198.1 *Immune complex-mediated vasculitis* involves antigen–antibody complexes as the initiating immunological event, with neutrophils as the primary effector cells. After the complexes form, they deposit in vessel walls and activate complement proteins, which recruit polymorphonuclear leukocytes. The neutrophils degranulate, liberating proteolytic enzymes, and generate toxic oxygen free radicals. Membranolytic complement membrane attack complex is also produced. *ANCA-mediated vasculitis* also involves antibodies and neutrophils, but not circulating immune complexes. Primed neutrophils express cytoplasmic proteins on their cell surface, including the proteolytic enzymes PR3 and MPO. ANCAs bind to their surface-displayed target antigens and engage Fcγ receptors, triggering neutrophil degranulation and respiratory burst, resulting in damage to the endothelium. Cytokine-activated endothelial cells also express or bind PR3 and MPO that engage ANCAs, thereby enhancing expression of adhesion molecules, promoting chemokine release, and lysing endothelial cells by antibody-dependent cellular cytotoxicity. *Cell-mediated vasculitis* is unique in that the effector cells are primarily cytotoxic T lymphocytes, most likely directed against either endothelial cell antigens or foreign antigens expressed by endothelial cells. These cells release perforin, granzymes (pro-apoptotic proteolytic enzymes), and effector cytokines, which result in cell damage.

vasculitis, circulating antibodies interact with endothelial membrane antigens to form in situ immune complexes that activate complement or result in antibody-dependent cellular cytotoxicity (ADCC).[92,93] AECAs can be detected in 40% to 80% of patients with WG, MPA, TA, TKA, and rheumatoid vasculitis, but there is no convincing evidence to support a primary causal relationship. Although in vitro studies analyzing the ability of AECAs to mediate endothelial cytotoxicity have produced contradictory results, there is compelling evidence that AECAs may sustain vascular inflammation by inducing endothelial cell activation, upregulation of adhesion molecules expression, and secretion of cytokines and chemokines.[94]

Anti-neutrophil cytoplasmic autoantibody (ANCA)-mediated vasculitis may be important in patients with WG, MPA and CSS. ANCAs are autoantibodies directed against cytoplasmic proteins in neutrophils and monocytes (Figure 198.1).[95,96] They are classified as cytoplasmic (c-ANCA), perinuclear (p-ANCA) or atypical (a-ANCA), based on their staining pattern on alcohol-fixed neutrophils. In vasculitis, c-ANCAs usually target proteinase 3 (PR3) while p-ANCAs target myeloperoxidase (MPO), although other antigens have been reported, especially for p-ANCAs. PR3 and MPO are constituents of azurophilic granules in neutrophils and peroxidase-positive lysosomes in monocytes. In vitro, ANCAs activate primed neutrophils and monocytes, causing adherence to endothelial cells, degranulation, and respiratory burst with lysis of endothelial cells.[97,98] PR3 and MPO are also expressed by or bind to activated endothelial cells. ANCA–PR3 or ANCA–MPO complexes on the endothelium upregulate endothelial cell adhesion molecule expression and trigger complement-mediated cell lysis or ADCC. ANCA binding to PR3 might also alter its natural inhibitor, α1-antitrypsin, prolonging this protease's tissue-damaging capability. None of these mechanisms has yet been demonstrated in humans.

In *direct, cellular cytotoxicity-mediated vasculitis*, the effector cells are cytotoxic T cells directed against native or induced endothelial antigens, exogenous antigens processed by endothelial cells, or implanted antigens (Figure 198.1).[85,89] This mechanism is important in vasculitic neuropathies; studies have shown that T cells and macrophages are the predominant cells in epineurial infiltrates in nerve biopsies.[99,102] Both CD4 and CD8 T cells are common, while B cells, NK cells, and neutrophils are rare. Many of the infiltrating T cells express perforin, a cytotoxic T cell effector protein.[99,103] Cytotoxic T cells are activated after major histocompatibility complex (MHC)-restricted binding to antigen-presenting cells. Consistent with this process, patients with vasculitic neuropathy demonstrate mannose receptor upregulation around involved epineurial vessels.[100] Mannose receptors are markers for dendritic cells specialized for antigen capture, processing, and presentation to T cells. Investigations of T cell receptor Vβ gene utilization in nerve biopsies from vasculitic neuropathy patients, however, show no clonally expanded T cells, suggesting that T cells may be nonspecifically recruited to the PNS rather than antigenically selected.[104]

Delayed, cell-mediated hypersensitivity vasculitis is relevant in TA, where vasculitic lesions contain adventitial CD4 T cells clonally expanded in response to an unknown antigen.[87,105] These T cells produce INF-γ, which induces macrophage activation and differentiation, giant cell formation, and the emergence of granulomas near the internal elastic lamina. Macrophages in the media and intima produce cytokines, matrix metalloproteinases, growth factors and reactive oxygen species that damage the vessel and promote intimal proliferation and angiogenesis. In other granulomatous vasculitides (e.g. WG and CSS), similar mechanisms may operate, but immune complexes can also produce granulomas.

Genetics

Although genetic factors may be important in some vasculitides, no genes sufficient to produce vasculitis have yet been identified. Family clusters of vasculitides have been reported for TKA, Behçet's disease, and TA/polymyalgia rheumatica (PMR), and also for WG, PAN, HSP, and MPA.[84,106–113] Most clusters involve siblings or parent–child pairs, making it difficult to exclude environmental factors. Multigeneration pedigrees have also been described.[112] For example, out of 15 PAN and 158 WG patients evaluated at the NIH, only two probands had affected family members,[108] while in TA/PMR, up to 10% of patients have affected first-degree relatives.[110] Familial clustering of NSVN has not been reported.

Most T cell dependent disorders exhibit either a positive or negative association with human leukocyte antigen (HLA) genes. HLA proteins function as antigen-presenting molecules and play an important role in the generation of T cell responses. Strong positive associations have been demonstrated between: (1) TA/PMR and HLA-DRB1;[114,115] (2) Behçet's disease and HLA-B51;[116] (3) TKA and HLA-B52 and -B39.2 (C1-2-A allele);[117] and (4) rheumatoid vasculitis and HLA-DRB1*401.[118] These loci confer increased risk of occurrence in individuals harboring the genotype. Patients with TA, in particular, commonly share a sequence motif spanning amino acid positions 28–31 of the HLA-DRβ1 chain, encoded by the second hypervariable region of the HLA-DRB1 gene.[114] These residues map to the floor of the antigen-binding site of the HLA complex, suggesting an important role for antigen selection and presentation in the pathogenesis of this disease. HLA associations in WG and other ANCA-associated vasculitides are weaker and more heterogeneous, with positive associations demonstrated in some studies for HLA-B7, B8, DR1, DR2, DR4, DR8, DR9, DQw1, and DQw7 and negative associations for HLA-DR3 and DR13DR6.[95,111,119,120] Other studies showed no MHC associations for the same markers.[121,122] This inconsistency suggests that the T cell responses are heterogeneous in these disorders.

Genetic alterations in T cells might also be influential in promoting vasculitis. Depletion of CD8 cytotoxic/suppressor T cells, for example, has been documented in first-degree relatives of patients with TA or PMR compared to controls, suggesting that the low CD8 counts found in patients with TA may represent a genetic trait relevant to pathogenesis.[110] In another study, microsatellite polymorphisms in the cytotoxic T lymphocyte associated antigen (CTLA)-4 gene were associated with WG.[123] Since the CTLA-4 gene product suppresses antigen-driven T cell responses, the association between this antigen and WG implicates uncontrolled antigen-specific T cell activation in the pathogenesis of this disorder.

Another genetic risk factor for ANCA-associated vasculitis is deficiency of α1-antitrypsin (A1AT), the main plasma inhibitor of PR3.[84,95] α1-Antitrypsin is encoded by a polymorphic protease inhibitor (Pi) gene on chromosome 14 with over 75 alleles that define nondeficient and variably deficient phenotypes.[95,124] The PiZ allele, which is the most common allele responsible for reduced plasma A1AT, is overrepresented in patients with ANCA-associated vasculitis. PiZ heterozygosity confers increased risk of fatal outcome in PR3–ANCA positive vasculitis.[124–127] Heritable A1AT deficiencies disrupt the protease/antiprotease balance, favoring ANCA formation due to increased PR3 exposure to immunocompetent cells and enhancing disease activity due to reduced restraint of PR3-mediated proteolysis.[95,128] Another genetic factor in PR3 accessibility is the degree of constitutive PR3 expression on the surface of neutrophils. Patients with a large subset of neutrophils expressing PR3 are at increased risk of developing ANCA-associated systemic vasculitis.[129]

Genetic variation might also modify inflammatory responses to facilitate vasculitis. For example, hereditary complement abnormalities, such as deficiencies of C1q, C2, C3, and C4B, have been associated with vasculitis.[130–133] In addition, TA susceptibility is strongly associated with the TNFa2 polymorphism of the TNFα gene[134] and with a specific polymorphism in the ICAM-I gene.[135] Polymorphisms in the Fcγ receptor (FcγR) genes may also be important. Three classes of FcγR can be distinguished: class I FcγRs are expressed on endothelial cells and class II and III on leukocytes.[136] ANCA activation of neutrophils (which express FcγRIIa and FcγRIIIb) requires cross-linking of surface-expressed ANCA antigens with FcγRs.[95,136] Certain isoforms of the FcγRIIa and FcγRIIIa receptors may be risk factors for disease relapse in WG,[137] but there is no association between polymorphisms of the FcγRIIa and FcγRIIIb genes and the development of ANCA-positive vasculitis.[138,139]

Clinical features

The clinical presentation of a patient with a peripheral nerve vasculitis depends on the distribution of the affected neural vessels, the severity and rate of progression of the vasculitic process, and the spectrum of extraneurological involvement.[18,22,102,140,154] Signs and symptoms of multi-organ involvement should alert the clinician to the likelihood of a systemic vasculitis or underlying connective tissue disease. Commonly affected organs in systemic vasculitis involving the

PNS include the skin, kidneys, joints, liver, gastrointestinal (GI) tract and lungs.[102,140–144,146,148] Patients with NSVN, by definition, have restricted PNS involvement. Constitutional symptoms occur in 75% of patients with systemic vasculitis and 50% of patients with NSVN.[22,141,144,146,147,149,150,154] Fever is more specific, developing in over half of patients with systemic vasculitis and rarely in NSVN. The mean age of onset of vasculitic neuropathy is approximately 60 years in both systemic and nonsystemic cases, with no gender preference.[18,22,102,140–154]

The neuropathy of necrotizing arteritis has a characteristic picture, whether occurring alone or as part of a systemic vasculitis. Although onset is usually over weeks to months, the average delay from symptom onset to diagnosis ranges from 5 to 11 months in various series.[22,153] Some patients present with an acute, severe onset that mimics Guillain–Barré syndrome; others are symptomatic three to five years prior to diagnosis.[155–157] Seventy-five percent of patients experience at least one acute attack and 50% to 60% follow a relapsing course; 25% manifest a chronic, slowly progressive course from onset.[18,154] Multifocal involvement is common and 50% of patients present with a multiple mononeuropathy. In 25%, involvement is extensive and the mononeuropathies "overlap," creating an asymmetric neuropathy that is usually distal predominant. The distribution most difficult to recognize as vasculitic is a distal, symmetric polyneuropathy, which occurs in 25% of patients. This pattern results from extensive, small-vessel ischemia at multiple levels of many nerve trunks. Certain nerves have a propensity to be involved, probably due to poor collateral vascular supplies (Table 198.6). Most patients present with combined motor and sensory deficits; in approximately 10%, findings are purely or predominantly sensory.[152,154] This occurs more commonly in small-vessel vasculitides (e.g. rheumatoid vasculitis, EMC, and HIV infection). The process is usually painful, but approximately 25% of patients are pain free.[22,102,146,148,149,152,154]

Although no systematic analyses have been performed, NSVN appears to have a more benign prognosis than neuropathies in systemic necrotizing vasculitis. Several series suggest that mortality is

Table 198.6 Most commonly involved nerves in vasculitic neuropathies*

Nerve	Frequency of involvement (percent of patients)
Peroneal	91%
Sural	47%
Tibial	44%
Ulnar	43%
Median	30%
Radial	19%

*Based on a review of 411 cases in seven series

approximately 30% in systemic vasculitic neuropathy compared to less than 10% for NSVN.[18,22,140–143,145,148,151,153] Patients with NSVN usually do not relapse or progress to vasculitis in other organs. Neurological morbidity appears to be marginally better in surviving patients with NSVN than in those with systemic vasculitis (e.g. 75% of NSVN patients normal or mildly disabled compared to 65% for patients with systemic vasculitis).[18,102,140,148,153,154] Spontaneous improvement in vasculitic neuropathy is rare.[21]

Diagnostic criteria

In order to diagnose vasculitic neuropathy, detailed electrodiagnostic studies and laboratory testing are required. Bloodwork screens for involvement of other organs and assesses markers of inflammation and autoantibodies seen with a systemic vasculitis or connective tissue disease.[156] In the appropriate setting, leukocytosis, elevated erythrocyte sedimentation rate (ESR), and positive rheumatoid factor are the best laboratory predictors of biopsy-confirmed necrotizing vasculitis. Of these, leukocytosis is the most specific and elevated ESR the most sensitive marker of vasculitic neuropathy.

Electrodiagnostic studies are indispensable for documenting non-length-dependent features of the neuropathy, excluding primary demyelination, and assisting with selection of which nerve to biopsy.[141,157] Electrophysiological findings reflect multifocal axonal damage to motor and sensory fibers. Nerve conduction studies reveal low amplitude or unevocable sensory nerve and compound muscle nerve action potentials. Lower extremity sensory responses are commonly absent. Conduction velocities are normal or mildly reduced, and distal latencies normal or mildly prolonged. Pseudo-conduction block may be demonstrated for 6 to 10 days after ischemic nerve injury, but is transient and disappears as axons degenerate.[158] Persistent partial motor conduction block is rare.[159] A predominance of demyelinating features should always prompt reconsideration of the diagnosis, as biopsy-proven cases of vasculitic neuropathy meeting electrophysiological criteria for a primary demyelinating neuropathy are very rare. Needle electromyography reveals fibrillation potentials in affected muscles in 80% of patients, with decreased recruitment of motor unit action potentials (MUAPs).[154] Long-duration MUAPs are observed in a minority of patients with long-standing disease or a pre-existing PNS condition.[154]

Considering the multiple possible nonvasculitic causes of neuropathy in patients with vasculitis (e.g. entrapment, drug effect, organ failure, critical illness, inflammatory demyelination) and the broad differential diagnosis of asymmetric neuropathy (Table 198.7), most patients with suspected vasculitic neuropathy should undergo nerve biopsy, often in conjunction with muscle biopsy. The sural and superficial peroneal nerves (SPN) are most typically biopsied. A SPN biopsy is usually combined with a peroneus brevis muscle (PBM) biopsy. In patients with sus-

pected vasculitic neuropathy, sural biopsy yields definite pathological evidence of vasculitis in approximately 20% of patients;[157,160,161] the corresponding figure for SPN/PBM biopsy is approximately 30%.[154] Diagnostic criteria for vasculitic neuropathy in patients lacking definitive pathological changes have been proposed (Table 198.8).[154] With application of these criteria, the estimated sensitivity of SPN/PBM biopsy is 60%.[154] Other investigators have determined a similar 50% to 60% sensitivity for sural nerve biopsy.[18,102,157] No study has directly compared these two techniques.

Pathological diagnosis of vasculitis requires inflammation in vessel walls *and* signs of vascular destruction such as fibrinoid necrosis, hemorrhage, or endothelial cell disruption (Figure 198.2).[162] Perivascular or transmural inflammation without structural damage is not sufficient for diagnosis. Many investigators have attempted to enhance pathological sensitivity by defining "suspicious," or "probable" vasculitis categories in specimens lacking frank necrotizing changes.[18,141,152–154,163] Features supporting active or healed vasculitic neuropathy include wallerian-like nerve fiber degeneration, asymmetric fiber loss, perivascular hemosiderin, vessel thrombosis with or without recanalization, luminal narrowing or obliteration, epineurial capillary proliferation, perineurial necrosis, and injury neuroma.[17,18,141,153,163–166] In a cohort of SPN/PBM biopsies performed for suspected vasculitic neuropathy, findings associated with necrotizing vasculitis were wallerian-like degeneration, asymmetric nerve fiber loss, myofiber necrosis and regeneration, and vascular immune deposits of IgM and complement C3.[154,167]

Vasculitis in nerve has a predilection for epineurial vessels with diameters of 75 to 250 µm.[18,148,162] Active lesions are characterized by predominant T cell and macrophage infiltrates, with affected nerves showing reduced myelinated nerve fiber density (with large fibers most susceptible), wallerian-like degeneration, and minimal demyelination/remyelination. Nerve fiber loss is typically asymmetric within and between fascicles. Immunofluorescent staining reveals deposits of IgM, IgG, C3, or C5b-9 membrane attack complex in epineurial vessel walls in 80% of patients.[99,147,148,153,167] Ninety percent of patients have vascular immune deposits in either the SPN or PBM specimens, a finding fairly specific for vasculitis.[167]

Differential diagnosis

Differential diagnosis of vasculitic neuropathy incorporates other asymmetric or multifocal neuropathies (Table 198.7). Common disorders to consider include multifocal sensorimotor demyelinating neuropathy, diabetic (or idiopathic) lumbosacral radiculoplexus neuropathy, multifocal motor neuropathy (MMN), sarcoidosis, Lyme disease, and hereditary neuropathy with liability to pressure palsies (HNPP). The value of nerve biopsy in diagnosing these patients cannot be overemphasized. Electrodiagnostic testing is also crucial in distinguishing the characteristic demyelinating patterns of Lewis–

Table 198.7 Differential diagnosis of vasculitic neuropathy

A. Ischemic neuropathies
   1. Peripheral nerve vasculitis
   2. Diabetes mellitus
      a. Diabetic lumbosacral radiculoplexus neuropathy
      b. Mononeuropathy multiplex (cranial nerve, thoracic, limb)
B. Inflammatory/immune-mediated neuropathies*
   1. Sarcoidosis
   2. Multifocal sensorimotor demyelinating neuropathy (Lewis–Sumner syndrome)
   3. Multifocal motor neuropathy
   4. Multifocal variants of Guillain–Barré syndrome
   5. Idiopathic brachial or lumbosacral plexopathy
   6. Neuropathy with various eosinophilic syndromes
   7. Gastrointestinal conditions (Crohn's, ulcerative colitis, celiac sprue)
C. Infectious neuropathies*
   1. Leprosy
   2. Lyme disease
   3. Viral (HIV, HTLV-I, varicella zoster, cytomegalovirus)
   4. Infective endocarditis
   5. Other (group A β-hemolytic streptococcus, leptospirosis, hepatitis A, *Mycoplasma pneumoniae*, ascaris, *Plasmodium falciparum*)
D. Drug-induced neuropathies*
   1. Prescription drugs (penicillin, cromolyn, thiouracil, allopurinol, amantadine, interferon-α)
   2. Drugs of abuse (amphetamines, cocaine, heroin)
E. Genetic neuropathies
   1. Hereditary neuropathy with liability to pressure palsies
   2. Hereditary neuralgic amyotrophy
   3. Porphyria
   4. Tangier disease
F. Mechanical neuropathies
   1. Multiple peripheral nerve injuries
   2. Multifocal entrapments not related to a genetic disorder
   3. Burns
G. Neuropathies related to malignancy
   1. Direct infiltration of nerves by tumor
   2. Multifocal mass lesions with external compressive effect
   3. Lymphomatoid granulomatosis
   4. Intravascular lymphoma
   5. Neoplastic meningitis
H. Miscellaneous conditions
   1. Sensory perineuritis
   2. Cholesterol emboli syndrome
   3. Idiopathic thrombocytic purpura

*Conditions occasionally associated with vasculitis.

mune small-vessel vasculitis, based on biopsy findings of T cell perivascular inflammation with vascular complement deposits, multifocal nerve fiber loss, and (rarely) necrotizing or leukocytoclastic vasculitis on nerve biopsies.[163,169–172] However, true necrotizing vasculitis is rare in this syndrome[163,169] and spontaneous recovery without treatment is the rule,[168] even in patients with inflammatory nerve lesions.[173] Therefore, if truly vasculitic, the process bears more resemblance to HSV than PAN.

Treatment

The management of a patient with vasculitic neuropathy is often extremely challenging and difficult for both physician and patient. The disorder is relatively uncommon, so that even seasoned neuromuscular specialists often have meager experience in managing these patients. Furthermore, since vasculitis can occur in different settings and present with protean clinical and laboratory manifestations, each patient presents unique and distinctive problems. In many patients, the neuropathy may be a small, insignificant part of the whole clinical picture, so that management of the neuropathy literally takes a "back seat" to more pressing renal, cardiac, or pulmonary concerns. From the neurologist's perspective, it is not unusual for these patients to become "lost to follow-up" after their main care has been assumed by other specialists dealing with some life-threatening complication of the vasculitis.

The treatment of vasculitic neuropathy involves the same basic principles for both primary vasculitides and secondary vasculitides associated with a connective tissue disease or other disorder. The approach can be conceptualized as a series of questions the clinician must address, such as:

- Is it possible to reduce or eliminate antigens perpetuating the immunological processes?
- Is immunosuppressive therapy indicated, and if so, what is the optimum initial regimen?
- Are there alternatives to the standard regimen (prednisone and cyclophosphamide) that are equally effective but less toxic?
- What is the best maintenance regimen?
- How long should treatment be maintained?
- Which agents should be used in refractory patients?
- How can adverse events associated with the therapy be minimized? and
- What supportive/rehabilitative measures are indicated?

Suggested first- and second-line treatment options for the major vasculitides, derived from an evidence-based review of the literature, are developed in the discussion that follows and summarized in Table 198.9.

Antigen removal

Therapy of vasculitic neuropathy must always begin with consideration of whether it is feasible to remove antigens that might be triggering the immunological

Sumner syndrome, MMN, and HNPP from the axonal profile of a vasculitic neuropathy.

Patients with diabetic lumbosacral radiculoplexus neuropathy present subacutely with progressive weakness and pain of the pelvifemoral muscles that is often bilateral but asymmetric.[168] The distal legs and, uncommonly, proximal arms may also be affected. Some have proposed that this condition is an autoim-

Table 198.8 Diagnostic criteria for clinically probable vasculitic neuropathy in patients lacking biopsy-proven necrotizing vasculitis*[154]

1. Clinical presentation typical for a vasculitic neuropathy
   - Asymmetric or multifocal, painful, sensorimotor neuropathy
   - Acute/subacute relapsing, progressive, or relapsing progressive course
   - No spontaneous remission
2. Elevated sedimentation rate or other laboratory evidence of a systemic inflammatory state
3. Electrodiagnostic evidence of an active, asymmetric, axonal, sensorimotor neuropathy
4. Suggestive neuromuscular pathology
   - Vascular thickening, narrowing or obliteration of the vascular lumen, thrombosis, periadventitial capillary proliferation, hemosiderin deposits, asymmetric nerve fiber loss, or wallerian-like degeneration
5. Clinical response to immunosuppressive therapy
6. Clinicopathological evidence of a systemic/secondary etiology
   - Concurrent condition known or suspected to predispose to vasculitis (connective tissue diseases, certain infections, certain drugs, malignancies/paraproteinemias, cryoglobulinemia)
   - Simultaneous multi-organ, non-peripheral nerve involvement
   - Biopsy-proven vasculitis in other tissues

*Diagnosis requires at least three of the first five criteria for nonsystemic vasculitic neuropathy; criterion six also mandatory for systemic vasculitis.

response. Unfortunately, this approach is possible only in vasculitides arising secondary to drug exposures, malignancy, or an infection. Identification of a drug-induced vasculitis usually mandates discontinuation of the drug, although if the vasculitis is severe enough, additional immunosuppressive therapy is indicated (see above).

As expected for such an uncommon entity, no class 1 or 2 treatment trials have been reported for paraneoplastic vasculitis, so that treatment must be based on anecdotal case reports (class 3). There are at least 20 biopsy-substantiated cases of paraneoplastic vasculitic neuropathy for which treatment information is available.[77–81,174–186] These reports reveal a high response rate (80%), irrespective of treatment (class 3). Cancer-related vasculitic neuropathies may improve with anticancer therapy alone (be it surgery, radiation, or chemotherapy), presumably by reducing tumor antigen load.[78,81,178,182] In patients for whom cancer therapy is not indicated, or for patients failing antineoplastic measures, trials with prednisone alone or prednisone combined with cyclophosphamide are indicated (class 3).

Of the infectious vasculitides, antigen removal is especially important for those due to chronic viral infections, since immunosuppressive treatment alone in these patients may enhance the infection and worsen the prognosis.[29] For example, many studies have shown that corticosteroid therapy in patients with chronic hepatitis B (HBV) infection activates viral replication, increases serum HBV-DNA levels, amplifies expression of HBV genome and gene products, predisposes to chronic active hepatitis, and accelerates hepatic damage and eventual mortality.[30,32,187–190] The cornerstone of treatment for these patients, therefore, involves antiviral agents, often coupled with plasma exchange to remove circulating immune complexes, with short courses of corticosteroids as necessary for severe, life-threatening vasculitis (class 3). Vidarabine, the antiviral agent

initially used in these protocols, has been largely replaced by interferon-alfa (3 million units three times per week). Lamivudine and famciclovir have also been used in this setting, but with somewhat mixed results.[191–193] The French Vasculitis Study Group is currently assessing the effectiveness of lamivudine in place of interferon-alfa in an open-label trial.[194]

Interferon-alfa also successfully treats vasculitis related to hepatitis C virus (HCV)-associated essential mixed cryoglobulinemia (EMC).[45–47] Approximately 85% of EMC cases are caused by chronic HCV infection; conversely, 10% to 55% with chronic hepatitis C develop EMC.[45,195] Five unblinded randomized controlled trials of INF-α in patients with symptomatic EMC have shown initial response rates of 60% to 90%, with significantly higher rates in the INF-α treated patients (class 1).[196–200] Unfortunately, relapses occur in up to 85% of patients after INF-α is discontinued.[196,197,200,201] This situation mirrors that for the treat-

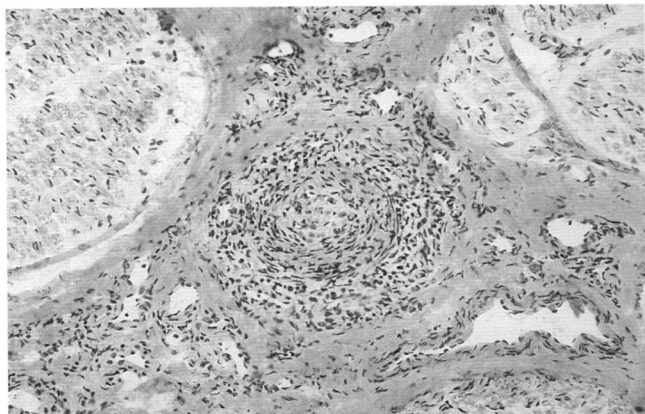

Figure 198.2 This superficial peroneal nerve biopsy specimen shows a necrotic epineurial blood vessel destroyed by a marked perivascular and transmural inflammatory cell infiltration. (See color plate section.)

ment of chronic hepatitis C itself, where INF-α for six months produces a 40% to 50% short term hepatitis remission rate and a 10% to 15% sustained response. Treatment for 12 to 24 months increases the sustained response rate to 25%.[202] Combining INF-α with ribavirin and treating for at least 48 weeks yields the highest long term response rate, up to 50%.[203-205] Adding ribavirin to INF-α also enhances the response of HCV-related cryoglobulinemic vasculitis.[206] However, the neuropathy with mixed cryoglobulinemia is more refractory to therapy than other manifestations; and only 30% to 40% of neuropathies improve with INF-α.[35,196,201,207,208]

To further complicate matters, INF-α itself can exacerbate pre-existing vasculitic neuropathy or produce a new neuropathy.[209] INF-α has been implicated in a wide variety of neuropathies, including sensorimotor, multifocal neuropathies typical of vasculitis;[71,210] distal, axonal, sensorimotor polyneuropathies;[211] an acute, diffuse, axonal motor neuropathy;[212] a chronic inflammatory demyelinating disorder;[213] an acute autonomic and sensory neuropathy;[214] and a trigeminal sensory neuropathy.[215] These neuropathies have occurred from two weeks to several months after the commencement of therapy.

In view of the limited efficacy of INF-α in treating cryoglobulinemic neuropathies and its potential for causing PNS complications, immunosuppressive therapy with corticosteroids, cyclophosphamide, and plasma exchange (see below) should be considered if INF-α does not immediately stabilize the neuropathy. This regimen was standard (class 3) for severe EMC prior to the discovery of the HCV association in the 1990s[45,46,216] and is often effective in relieving PNS manifestations.[217]

Vasculitis occurring with HIV infection may also respond to attempts to reduce antigen load. This vasculitis may arise from the HIV organism itself, immune complex deposition, altered immune responses, or opportunistic agents, especially CMV.[218] For treatment of CMV, an initial three-week course of ganciclovir 5 mg/kg IV every 12 hours or foscarnet 90 mg/kg IV every 12 hours is followed by lifelong suppressive therapy with lower doses of these drugs (class 3). Treatment regimens in HIV vasculitis similar to those used in hepatitis B-associated PAN have been proposed, employing antiviral therapy (zidovudine) combined with plasma exchanges (class 3).[40] There are no data on the use of highly active antiretroviral therapy in patients with HIV-associated vasculitis. To the extent that case reports mirror clinical practice, prednisone monotherapy is the most commonly utilized therapeutic modality in HIV vasculitis, with an 80% response rate.[36,41,219-223] However, interpretation of this class 3 data is confounded by the tendency of many HIV vasculitic neuropathies to remit spontaneously.[217,224]

Immunosuppressive therapy

Despite the intuitive appeal of reducing the antigen load to treat vasculitis, most vasculitides (including NSVN) are truly idiopathic in that no inciting antigen

can be identified. The majority of patients, therefore, including many with causative infections (e.g. HIV), require immunosuppressive treatment. Traditional recommendations for therapy have been grounded on the results of retrospective studies and case series (class 3) employing nonstandardized protocols and definitions of disease. Fortunately, this situation has changed over the last ten years. New therapeutic strategies have evolved due to the development of uniformly applied classification schemes, improved knowledge of disease pathogenesis, identification of prognostic factors, and the formation of multicenter collaborative groups (e.g. the European Vasculitis Study Group [EUVAS] and the International Network for the Study of the Systemic Vasculitides [INSSYS]).[225,227] As a result, randomized controlled trials (RCTs) have appeared, providing guidance for the rational treatment of various vasculitic disorders.[228]

Unfortunately, treatment of vasculitic *neuropathy* (including NSVN) has not yet been approached with the same investigatory rigor. Aside from a single, small, class 2 study of pulse corticosteroid therapy,[102] there are no controlled (class 1 or 2) data relevant to the treatment of vasculitic neuropathy, nor are there any large case series with detailed analyses of therapeutic responses. Recommendations for managing vasculitic neuropathy, therefore, depend mainly on clinical experience and extrapolations from systemic vasculitis trials. This approach, however, may not always be valid, since a therapy shown to be effective for one type of vasculitis (e.g. PAN) may not necessarily be applicable to other vasculitides. As in any vasculitis, immunosuppressive therapy in vasculitic neuropathy demands balance between adequate suppression of the pathogenic autoimmune processes and avoidance of serious drug toxicity.

Standard combination therapy The traditional regimen used for treating primary or secondary systemic necrotizing vasculitides (with or without neuropathy) involves a combination of corticosteroids (CS) and cyclophosphamide (CYC). The origins of this combination date to the early 1950s when the first reports of cortisone for treating PAN and WG appeared.[229,230] Corticosteroids alone were of limited value in the treatment of WG,[231,232] but did significantly improve survival in patients with PAN (class 2).[233,234] The first reported use of alkylating agents (nitrogen mustard) in WG was by Fahey and associates in 1954.[235] Many favorable reports ensued involving a variety of cytotoxic agents, alone or in combination with CS.[231] A seminal contribution was Fauci and Wolff's 1973 observations on 15 patients with WG treated with cytotoxic therapy, usually low-dose oral CYC.[236] Although 3 patients died, the remaining 12 achieved complete remissions for up to 63 months.

In the course of managing 85 patients with WG over the next ten years, Fauci and coworkers refined this combination regimen into the "standard therapy" for WG, a regimen now also commonly employed for vasculitic neuropathy.[237,238] Although "standard," the protocol was never validated in a RCT. Treatment is initiated with oral CYC 2 mg/kg/day and prednisone 1 mg/kg/day. In patients with fulminant, rapidly progressive disease, higher doses of CYC (4 to 5 mg/kg/day), prednisone (2 mg/kg/day), or intravenous methylprednisolone (15 mg/kg or 1 g/day) are employed for the first three to five days of treatment.[237,239] Limited class 3 evidence, including personal observations of the authors and other neuromuscular clinicians, indicates that approximately 80% of vasculitic neuropathies show an initial response to pulse methylprednisolone.[239,240] On the other hand, one class 2 study of 28 patients with CSS-associated neuropathy treated with prednisone, eight of whom also received pulse methylprednisolone 1000 mg/day for three days, showed that the early (four week) response and long term neurological outcome were unaffected by the use of intravenous methylprednisolone.[102] Nevertheless, intravenous steroid pulses remain a first-line option for patients with vasculitic neuropathies exhibiting rapid evolution, profound motor deficits, or associated kidney, heart, lung, gastrointestinal tract, or CNS involvement.

In the standard regimen, daily prednisone is continued for two to four weeks and then gradually converted to alternate day dosing (1 mg/kg q.o.d.) over one to two months. In patients with vasculitic neuropathy, conversion to alternate day prednisone can usually be abruptly accomplished, without risk of disease exacerbation (class 3). The every other day regimen is maintained until the neuropathy stabilizes and control of non-neurological manifestations is assured, a process that typically takes two to three months. Depending on disease control and patient tolerance, corticosteroids are then gradually tapered by 5 mg every two to three weeks. Tapering is usually completed in 6 to 12 months. Relapse during the tapering process usually requires repeat pulsing with intravenous methylprednisolone or oral prednisone; alternatively, the CYC dose may be increased. Cyclophosphamide is continued for one year after the patient has achieved complete remission and then stopped or tapered by 25 mg decrements every two to three months until the patient is off all medications. In NSVN, CYC can sometimes be safely discontinued after six months (class 3).

Although no studies of this protocol have been performed in vasculitic neuropathy, the superiority of the combination regimen to CS monotherapy has now been confirmed in a cohort survey of patients with ANCA-associated vasculitides (primarily MPA) (class 2).[241,242] In this study, patients treated with CS alone had a significantly lower remission rate and higher relapse rate compared with patients on combined therapy. Moreover, the risk of death was decreased by a factor of 5.56 in the CS/CYC cohort.

The necessity of cytotoxic therapy in PAN and CSS is less clear. Many patients with these conditions are effectively managed with CS alone.[243] Class 1 and 2 studies have shown no overall difference in survival

and relapse rate between PAN and CSS patients treated with (1) prednisone alone, or (2) prednisone plus CYC.[244–246] However, when stratified into poor- and good-prognosis groups according to a Five-Factor Score (FFS) (serum creatinine above 1.58 mg/dl, proteinuria more than 1 g/day, gastrointestinal tract involvement, CNS involvement, cardiomyopathy), survival *is* significantly prolonged in poor-prognosis patients (FFS greater than or equal to 2) treated with combined CYC and CS.[246] Therefore, the initial treatment for patients with severe vasculitis should include both CYC and CS (class 2). Cyclophosphamide is also beneficial for patients with corticosteroid-refractory disease.[247]

The French Vasculitis Study Group is currently investigating appropriate indications for CS and other immunosuppressive agents in CSS and PAN as a function of visceral involvement assessed by the FFS.[194,227] Prior to enrolment, patients are classified into good and bad prognostic groups according to the FFS. Patients with poor prognostic signs at the time of diagnosis are treated with combined CS and pulse CYC (0.6 g/m^2), with randomization to either 6 or 12 monthly CYC pulses. An analysis of the preliminary data showed a relapse rate of 17% for the 12-month group and 41% for the 6-month group. In patients with a good prognosis (FFS less than or equal to 1), treatment is initiated with prednisolone alone. Patients failing CS monotherapy are randomized to receive either azathioprine or CYC.

There are other vasculitides, such as TA, for which CS alone remain the mainstay of therapy.[248–251] Corticosteroids provide rapid control of the most common symptoms (headache, stiffness, polymyalgia rheumatica (PMR) pain) of TA within 24 to 72 hours. The efficacy of CS in preventing blindness is also well established (class 2, 3).[252,253] No RCT has investigated the proper starting dose of prednisone in TA. There is emerging class 2 evidence that doses less than 60 mg/day, and possibly as low as 20 mg/day, may be sufficient for disease control in patients free of visual loss, CNS symptoms, and other significant organ dysfunction.[254–256] Most experts now recommend an initial prednisone dose of 0.5 to 1 mg/kg/day in uncomplicated cases.[248–251] Patients with visual symptoms, CNS disease, or other serious manifestations are conventionally (class 3) treated with higher prednisone (60 to 80 mg/day). Available class 2 evidence suggests that intravenous pulse CS are no more effective than high dose prednisone in preserving or improving visual function.[257,258] Although no large series or controlled study has addressed treatment of TA-related neuropathies, the available case reports and series (class 3) indicate that more than 90% of these neuropathies respond to CS monotherapy.[259–263]

Methotrexate (MTX) may be used as an alternative to CYC for induction of remission in patients with "non-life-threatening" WG (e.g. no acute renal failure or pulmonary hemorrhage). Based on three open uncontrolled (class 3) studies enrolling a total of 68 patients, it can be concluded that MTX in doses of 15 to 25 mg/week, combined with prednisone in doses of 20 to 60 mg/day, is effective in inducing remission in patients with non-life-threatening WG (75% to 80% remission rate), but with a high (57% to 58%) relapse rate.[264-267] A European (EUVAS) RCT assessing the efficacy of MTX versus CYC for induction and maintenance therapy of patients with WG lacking renal involvement is ongoing.[225,227]

Despite the effectiveness of the combination regimen in controlling the inflammatory processes associated with vasculitis, long term surveillance reveals that standard therapy-treated WG is a chronic, relapsing disease, necessitating long term exposure to pharmacological therapy and engendering considerable risk for serious drug-related toxicity.[268,269] In one series, relapses occurred in 50% of patients at periods of three months to 16 years after onset of the remission and permanent disease-related morbidity evolved in 86% of patients, including 42% with chronic renal failure.[268] Significant treatment-associated side effects in this series included steroid-induced cataracts (21%), fractures (11%), diabetes (8%), and avascular necrosis (3%) and cyclophosphamide-induced ovarian failure (57%), hemorrhagic cystitis (43%), bladder cancer (3%), and myelodysplasia (2%); 46% of patients experienced one or more serious infections. Compared with the general population, there was a 2.4-fold increased malignancy rate in the treated patients, a 33-fold increase in bladder cancers, and an 11-fold increase in lymphomas. In another prospective study of standard therapy in 23 patients with WG, 70% of patients had infectious complications, including an alarming 30% incidence of *Pneumocystis carinii* pneumonia.[270]

Variations on the standard combination regimen
The need for less toxic therapeutic regimens is apparent and has led to modifications of the standard protocol. In order to minimize exposure to CYC and the bladder toxicity associated with continuous oral use of this agent, intravenous pulses have been tried in different dosing regimens, usually 0.35 to 1.0 g/m² body surface area (or 15 mg/kg) every one to four weeks for periods up to two years.[271] Several class 1[270,272,274] and 2[242,275,276] studies suggest that pulse CYC is as effective as continuous oral CYC in inducing remission in patients with primary systemic vasculitides, with similar mortality rates but lower cumulative doses, resulting in fewer infections and drug-related side effects. On the other hand, pulse intravenous CYC is probably less effective than continuous oral regimens in *maintaining* remissions. One way to circumvent this problem may be to administer more frequent pulses or more sustained therapy (i.e. over one year), tactics that are the focus of ongoing investigations. The largest RCT of continuous versus pulse CYC in the treatment of ANCA-associated systemic vasculitis is currently ongoing, sponsored by the EUVAS.[227] At this time, however, pulse CYC is not routinely recommended for patients with vasculitic neuropathy.

A second approach to reducing complications from standard therapy involves switching from oral CYC to an alternative immunosuppressive agent once remission is achieved, typically in three to six months.[228] Azathioprine (AZA) is the most widely utilized remission-maintaining drug, at doses ranging from 1 to 2 mg/kg/day. Many class 3 studies have documented its efficacy in maintaining remission in patients with WG, MPA, and PAN.[269,272,277,278] The overall relapse rate for patients maintained on AZA and CS in these series is 40%, a figure that compares favorably with the 50% relapse rate for WG patients treated with standard therapy. A recently completed, 18-month, European RCT (class 1) compared CYC with AZA for maintenance of remission in 141 patients with ANCA-associated systemic vasculitis. The study revealed no differences between the two groups in relapse rate (17%), disease activity, cumulative organ damage, and incidence of severe adverse effects (28%).[279] The investigators concluded that AZA was as effective as continued CYC in maintaining remission in ANCA-associated vasculitis. Recent data suggest that prolonging AZA maintenance from one to two years may reduce the relapse rate even further, from 30% to 10% (class 3).[280] Although there is no information on AZA in vasculitic neuropathies, the preceding class 1 and 3 evidence supporting its use as a remission-maintaining agent in ANCA-associated systemic vasculitides suggests that it may have similar efficacy in maintenance therapy of PNS vasculitis. It is a particularly appealing option for patients poorly tolerant of maintenance CYC.

Studies on MTX as a CYC-sparing drug for maintenance therapy of systemic vasculitis have focused on WG. Two uncontrolled class 3 series involving 64 patients suggested that patients with WG can be maintained on weekly MTX (15 to 25 mg or 0.3 mg/kg per week) after remission is induced with CS and CYC.[281,282] Relapse rates in these studies (15%) were similar to those seen with 18 to 24 months of AZA. The role of MTX for maintenance in other vasculitides is less clear; more controlled data on this important question are needed. At present, MTX, like AZA, appears to be a reasonable alternative to CYC for maintenance therapy in patients with vasculitic neuropathy.

Data are sparse on the use of other agents for maintenance of remission in systemic vasculitis, and there are no data on their use in vasculitic neuropathy. Several small class 2 and 3 studies, mainly in ANCA-associated vasculitides, suggest that cyclosporine,[283,284] mycophenolate mofetil,[285] and leflunomide[286] may be as effective as AZA in maintaining remissions. Randomized, controlled trials comparing these agents with CYC, AZA, and MTX are needed to determine optimum maintenance therapy for vasculitis.[227]

One interesting and unique approach to limiting immunosuppressive therapy concerns the use of trimethoprim–sulfamethoxazole (TMP/SMX) in WG. Initial trials with this agent were prompted by the theory that respiratory tract infections trigger relapses in WG. DeRemee and colleagues in 1985 were the first to report a series of WG patients with positive responses to the drug.[287] Their study proved influential, spawning many additional case reports and series (class 3) over the next ten years.[232,288,291] In these studies, TMP/SMX was most commonly used as an initial remission induction agent for patients with *limited* (i.e. nonrenal) WG, alone or combined with CS. Reported response rates were widely divergent, with approximately 60% of patients improving and approximately 25% relapsing.[232,287,291] In a more recent analysis of 20 such patients, remission was induced in 85%, but 50% relapsed after a median follow-up of 14 months.[292] One randomized, double-blind, placebo-controlled (class 1) trial of TMP/SMX for *maintenance* of remission in WG has been reported.[293] In this trial, patients receiving TMP/SMX had significantly fewer upper airway relapses than patients receiving placebo. Therefore, TMP/SMX appears to be a reasonable alternative for initial (class 3) or maintenance (class 1) therapy of limited WG, with or without CS. There is no information on the response of vasculitic neuropathies to TMP/SMX.

Another strategy for minimizing drug toxicity during maintenance therapy of systemic vasculitis is the institution of more rapidly tapering courses of corticosteroids (class 3). Modified corticosteroid dosing regimens have been published, but none is the focus of an ongoing RCT. The EUVAS is currently investigating multiple protocols for treatment of ANCA-associated vasculitis. In all of these protocols, prednisolone is begun at 1 mg/kg/day and then rapidly reduced to 0.75 mg/kg/day after 1 week, 0.4 mg/kg/day after 4 weeks, 0.25 mg/kg/day after 8 weeks, 15 mg/day total after 6 months, and then more gradually tapered up to 18 months.[225,227] Another variation involves starting prednisone at 1 mg/kg/day for the first month and then tapering the alternate-day dose on alternate days by 10 mg/week until the patient reaches a dose of 1 mg/kg every other day. Tapering then continues at the same rate until prednisone is completely stopped by the end of the fourth or fifth month.[294] How useful these differing protocols will prove to be in patients with various types of vasculitic neuropathy remains to be determined. Currently, however, it seems reasonable to employ them in patients intolerant of prednisone, especially if the neuropathy is relatively mild and remission has been induced by the initial treatment.

A final way to limit drug toxicity related to immunosuppressive therapy is to eliminate the cytotoxic drug altogether and treat with CS monotherapy. Although previous studies (discussed above) have shown that CS monotherapy is not as effective as the combination regimen for many types of systemic vasculitis, NSVN can sometimes be treated with CS alone, especially if the neuropathy is predominantly sensory or the motor involvement is restricted and stable.[153,295] These patients, however, must be followed closely with detailed motor and sensory examinations. The clinician must be prepared to add a second agent (usually CYC) at the first indication that the disease is becoming refractory to CS, spreading to other organs (uncommon in patients with NSVN), or

recurring as the CS are tapered. As already noted, there is some class 2 and class 1 evidence that cytotoxic agents may not always be necessary in PAN patients, especially if the disease is limited. Several studies have established that multiple mononeuropathy is not an adverse prognostic factor for survival in PAN,[245,296,297] suggesting that combination therapy is not mandatory in these patients.

Other immunosuppressive strategies

The search for less toxic therapies for the vasculitides led to a consideration of nonpharmacological modalities such as plasma exchange (PE) and intravenous immunoglobulin (IVIg). These techniques held special interest for those vasculitides posited to depend on humoral immunopathogenic mechanisms (e.g. immune complexes and ANCAs). Efficacy has been demonstrated in some, but not all, forms of systemic vasculitis. The focus has recently shifted to organ-specific responses, including the ability of PE and IVIg to improve vasculitic neuropathies.

Plasma exchange Plasma exchange has been utilized for various vasculitides since the mid 1970s, theoretically to remove potentially pathogenic circulating immune complexes, antibodies (including ANCAs), inflammatory mediators, and soluble cellular adhesion molecules.[228,298] The procedure has been investigated as an initial remission-inducing intervention, both alone and in combination with other immunosuppressive agents, and in patients with severe, refractory disease. Although the literature is replete with descriptions of PE for *induction* therapy in patients with vasculitis, almost all are uncontrolled case reports, opinions, or small series. Only a few, unblinded RCTs have been performed. Two studies conducted by the French Vasculitis Study Group involved 140 patients with PAN, MPA, or CSS randomized to treatment with drug therapy alone (prednisone or prednisone and intravenous CYC) or drug therapy with PE.[299,300] Both studies revealed no significant difference between the two groups in initial response rate, relapse rate, long term recovery, or long term survival. Despite the negative outcomes of these two investigations, PE is still used in severe cases of systemic vasculitis, especially with significant renal involvement or pulmonary hemorrhage.[294,301] One class 1 study showed that dialysis-dependent patients with rapidly progressive glomerulonephritis secondary to ANCA-associated vasculitides were more likely to recover if treated with PE.[302]

There is extensive class 3 evidence (case reports and series from the 1970s and 1980s) favoring the use of PE in patients with mixed cryoglobulinemic vasculitis. The treatment effect in this condition is probably mediated by a reduction in the cryocrit. Pooled results from multiple reports and small series in which PE was used alone or combined with low doses of CS reveal an 80% response rate,[303–309] which includes the PNS manifestations.[307,309,310] Mixed cryoglobulinemic patients have also been successfully treated with PE in combination with prednisone, immunosuppressive agents, and antiviral drugs.[35,45,46,216,217,308] Rheumatoid vasculitis is another disorder that has been treated with PE in class 3 trials, almost always combined with prednisone and other immunosuppressive drugs.[311,313] There are rare anecdotal reports of PE used as initial *monotherapy* of CSS-associated multiple mononeuropathy,[314] HIV-related vasculitic neuropathy,[315] hepatitis B-associated PAN,[316] PAN-induced visual loss,[317] and severe HSP.[318] Harder to interpret is class 3 evidence of PE efficacy in combination with other modalities for initial treatment of HBV-associated PAN,[32] HIV-associated vasculitis,[40] and HSV.[319]

Plasma exchange is also a class 3 therapeutic option for patients refractory to standard therapy. Plasma exchange has never been studied in a prospective, controlled manner in these refractory patients, but there are scattered reports of successful add-on or mono-therapy in PAN,[320] systemic rheumatoid vasculitis,[312] WG,[321] cutaneous vasculitis,[322] CSS,[323] and lupus-associated vasculitic neuropathy.[324]

In summary, PE is not recommended as initial monotherapy for any form of vasculitis, with or without neuropathy. However, it is a reasonable adjunctive intervention for dialysis-dependent patients with rapidly progressive glomerulonephritis (class 1) and for patients with alveolar hemorrhage due to small vessel vasculitis, chronic viral-induced vasculitis, mixed cryoglobulinemic vasculitis, severe rheumatoid vasculitis, severe hypersensitivity vasculitides, threatened visual loss from vasculitis, or almost any treatment-refractory systemic vasculitis (class 3). Vasculitic neuropathies associated with these conditions generally improve hand-in-hand with the non-neurological manifestations. There are no data on the use of PE in NSVN, precluding an evidence-based treatment recommendation.

Intravenous immunoglobulins In vasculitis, intravenous immunoglobulin (IVIg) therapy has been studied almost exclusively as rescue therapy for patients with refractory or relapsing disease. Most reports have described single cases or small series of patients (class 3) with a variety of vasculitides refractory to CS monotherapy or the combination CS/CYC regimen.[37,223,325,330] Most studies describe positive responses to IVIg, with approximately 80% of patients improving and 50% achieving a complete remission (Table 198.10). Although some patients have gone into remission for up to four years after a single 2 g/kg course of IVIg,[37,327] scheduled follow-up doses may be important in minimizing the relapse rate.[326,329,330] The only RCT of IVIg in vasculitis involved 34 patients with ANCA-associated vasculitides who had failed therapy with prednisone and CYC or AZA.[331] Patients receiving IVIg (0.4 mg/kg/day for five days) had an initial response rate of 82% compared to 35% for the placebo group, a significant difference. Neuropathies improved in five of seven IVIg-treated patients. However, the effect was transient, with 36% of responders relapsing after three months, indicating that repeated dosing may be

necessary. There are limited data on IVIg in previously untreated patients; several case reports and small series (class 3) suggest that IVIg may induce remission in at least some treatment-naïve patients.[325,332] More evidence is needed before IVIg can be recommended as a first-line treatment for patients with vasculitic neuropathy. However, it may be employed as a second-line option in patients refractory to standard therapy.

Other agents for refractory patients

Cyclosporine has been used successfully in patients with vasculitis unresponsive to or intolerant of conventional therapy, but the evidence is confined to a few case reports and one small series (class 3). Most patients had WG,[321,333,334] but positive responses were also observed in CSS,[335] mixed cryoglobulinemia,[336] and HSP.[337] Etoposide (VP-16) may be another highly effective agent in patients with WG who have failed treatment with CS and CYC.[338,339]

Lymphocyte depletion using monoclonal antibodies (mAbs) or antithymocyte globulin (ATG) is a newer therapeutic alternative, having produced long-term remissions in several patients with resistant disease. The mAb studies utilized a humanized anti-CD52 mAb (CAMPATH-1H), whose major immunological effect is to produce a prolonged depletion of both CD4 and CD8 T cells.[340,341] Humanized anti-CD4 mAbs were used adjunctively in relapsing patients. Almost all patients treated with these antibodies achieved remission. Relapses were common, but retreatment was uniformly successful. A second strategy for reducing autoreactive T cell activity in vasculitis is the use of rabbit ATG. Two series have been reported, describing 15 treatment-refractory patients with WG.[342,343] Thirteen of the 15 patients improved, 11 partially and 2 completely, with no relapses observed. The EUVAS is currently conducting an open, multicenter, pilot study of ATG in patients with progressive or relapsing ANCA-associated vasculitis despite treatment with conventional regimens.[227]

Many other investigational approaches have benefited small numbers of patients with refractory vasculitis in preliminary reports, including mycophenolate mofetil,[344] 15-deoxyspergualin (gusperimustrihydrochloride),[345] etanercept,[346] autologous hematopoietic stem cell transplantation,[347] semi-specific tryptophan immunoabsorption,[348] and humanized mAbs against CD18 (β_2-integrin).[349] Whether these or any other investigational agents will prove useful in patients with vasculitic neuropathy remains to be determined.

Duration of therapy

In addition to which immunosuppressive regimen to use, another important question facing the clinician concerns the duration of therapy. As outlined above, the standard combination regimen usually entails at least one year of treatment with CS and an additional year of CYC therapy. During this time, it is crucial for the clinician to follow patients closely, with visits every four to six weeks. At these visits, detailed motor

Table 198.9 Summary of treatment options in major vasculitides

Vasculitis type	First-line treatment (level of evidence)	Second-line options for refractory patients (level of evidence)
Nonsystemic vasculitic neuropathy (NSVN) Severe (rapid evolution; major motor deficits)	Induction (standard therapy): IV MP 15 mg/kg (1.0 g)/day for 3–5 days Oral CYC 2.0 mg/kg/day PRD 1.0 mg/kg/day, switched to q.o.d. after 2–4 weeks Maintenance (after remission): Continue CYC for 6–12 months Taper PRD over 6–12 months (class 3)	(1) MTX 15–25 mg oral or IV q. week for 18–24 months PRD 1.0 mg/kg/day, tapered as above (class 3) (2) IVIg 0.5 g/kg/day × 4 days, then 0.5 g/kg/day q. 3–4 weeks × 6–12 months (class 3)
Mild (slow evolution; sensory predominant)	PRD 1.0 mg/kg/day, tapered as above (class 3)	
ANCA-associated vasculitis (WG, MPA)	Induction (standard therapy): IV MP, CYC, and PRD as for NSVN (class 3) Maintenance (after remission): (1) Continue CYC 2 mg/kg/day × 12 months, then taper by 25 mg q. 2–3 months (class 3); or (2) Switch CYC to AZA 1.5–2.0 mg/kg/ day × 18–24 months (class 3); or (3) Switch to CYC to MTX 15–25 mg PO or IV q. week × 18–24 months (class 3)	(1) Replace oral CYC with pulse IV CYC 0.5 to 1.0 g/m² q. 3–4 weeks × 12–24 months (class 1, 2) (2) Replace CYC with MTX 15–25 mg oral or IV q. week × 24 months (class 3) (3) IVIg (see NSVN) (class 1, 3) (4) PE 6–12 × (class 3)
c-PAN and CSS	(1) Patients with ≥2 poor-prognostic factors (creatinine >1.58 mg/dl, proteinuria >1 g/day; CNS, GI, or cardiac involvement): treat as ANCA-associated vasculitis (class 1, 2) (2) Patients with ≤1 poor-prognostic factors: PRD alone as in standard therapy (class 2)	See ANCA-associated vasculitides INF-α in treatment-refractory CSS (class 3)
HBV-associated PAN	PRD 1 mg/kg/day × 2 weeks; PE 2–3/week × 10 weeks; INF-α 3 million U t.i.w. until HBeAb seroconversion or ×12 months (class 3)	(1) Higher doses of INF-α (as in hepatitis B): 10 million U t.i.w. or 5 million U/day (class 3) (2) Lamivudine 100 mg/day with/without INF-α (class 3)
HCV-associated cryoglobulinemic vasculitis	INF-α 3 million U t.i.w. and ribavirin 1000–1200 mg/day × 12 months (class 1) PE 1–3/week × 9 weeks (class 3)	Induction: Oral CYC 2 mg/kg/day PRD 1.0 mg/kg/day, changing to q.o.d. after 2–4 weeks and then tapering; PE 1–3/week × 9 weeks (class 3) Maintenance (after remission): INF-α and ribavirin × 6 to 12 months (class 1)
HIV-associated vasculitic neuropathy CMV-positive vasculitis	Ganciclovir (class 3 for this indication) Induction—5 mg/kg IV q. 12 hours × 3 weeks Maintenance—1000 mg PO	Foscarnet (class 3) Induction—90 mg/kg IV q. 12 hours × 3 weeks Maintenance—90 mg/kg/day IV
CMV-negative vasculitis	Start or maximize antiretroviral therapy (class 3)	(1) PRD 0.5–1.0 mg/kg/day, tapered over 6–12 months (2) PE 1–3/week for 10 weeks (3) IVIg (see NSVN) (All class 3)
Cancer-associated vasculitic neuropathy	Treat malignancy (class 3)	(1) Standard therapy with PRD and CYC (see ANCA-associated vasculitis) (class 3) (2) IVIg (see NSVN) (class 3)
Temporal arteritis	PNS, CNS, or visual symptoms: PRD 1 mg/kg/day (60–80 mg/day) with slow taper after 4 weeks (class 2, 3) No serious manifestations: PRD 0.5–1.0 mg/kg/day (20–60 mg/day) with slow taper after 2–4 weeks (class 2, 3)	(1) IV MP 500–2000 mg/day × 2–5 days (class 3) (2) MTX 15 mg q. week added to PRD (class 1)

ANCA, antineutrophil cytoplasmic autoantibody; AZA, azathioprine; CMV, cytomegalovirus; CNS, central nervous system; CSS, Churg–Strauss syndrome; CYC, cyclophosphamide; GI, gastrointestinal; HbeAb, hepatitis B e antibody; HBV, hepatitis B virus; HCV, hepatitis C virus; HIV, human immunodeficiency virus; INF-α, interferon alfa; IV, intravenous; IVIg, pooled intravenous immunoglobulins; MPA, microscopic polyangiitis; MP, methylprednisolone; MTX, methotrexate; NSVN, nonsystemic vasculitic neuropathy; c-PAN, classic polyarteritis nodosa; PE, plasma exchange; PNS, peripheral nervous system; PRD, prednisone; q.o.d., every other day; t.i.w., three times per week; WG, Wegener's granulomatosis.

Table 198.10 Treatment trials of intravenous immunoglobulin (IVIg) in systemic vasculitis

Reference	No. patients	Follow-up (months)	Controls	Vasculitis type	IVIg regimen	Initial response rate	Long-term (≥6 months) remission rate	Relapse rate
325	26	12	None	ANCA-associated (WG, MPA, RV)	0.4 g/kg/day × 5 days	26/26 (100%)	18/26 (69%)	6/26 (23%)
328	15	1–3	None	WG	30 g/day × 5 days	7/15 (47%)	—	—
329	7	12	None	c-PAN (ANCA-negative)	0.25 g/kg/day × 4 days	7/7 (100%)	6/7 (86%)	0/7 (0%)
330	10	1–6	None	WG, CSS, undifferentiated	0.5 g/kg q. 4 weeks × 6–12 0.4 g/kg/day × 5 days	6/10 (60%)	—	—
331	34	12	Placebo (randomized)	ANCA-associated (WG, MPA)	0.4 g/kg/day × 5 days	14/17 (82%)	9/17 (53%)	5/7 (71%)
Total	**92**					**60/75 (80%)**	**33/50 (66%)**	**11/40 (28%)**

ANCA, antineutrophil cytoplasm autoantibody; CSS, Churg–Strauss syndrome; MPA, microscopic polyangiitis; c-PAN, classic polyarteritis nodosa; q., every; RV, rheumatoid vasculitis; WG, Wegener's granulomatosis.

testing using a reproducible grading scale and careful sensory testing must be performed and recorded to document whether or not the patient is developing new deficits as a result of continued ischemic nerve injury. In equivocal situations, periodic quantitative sensory testing (as with the CASE IV system) and quantitative motor testing (using any of a number of computerized testing systems) are sometimes helpful in following a patient's clinical course. Such testing may be particularly important in patients with significant pain, since patients (and clinicians) often erroneously assume that a vasculitis is inactive if the patient is pain free.

New motor or sensory deficits occurring during treatment are usually an indication to alter the doses of the current regimen or change to another agent. However, it is important to keep in mind that vasculitic nerve injury is predominantly axonal, so that recovery depends to a great extent on axonal regeneration, which is not necessarily promoted or accelerated by immunosuppressive therapy. Neurological improvement may, therefore, be extremely slow, depending on where along the nerve's course the vasculitic injury occurred. In fact, it is somewhat unusual to document any objective improvement in the first few weeks or months of therapy. More commonly, patients initially simply stop progressing (i.e. develop no new motor or sensory problems), true improvement in strength or sensation not becoming evident until several months of therapy. During this early phase of treatment, it is crucial that the regimen not be altered or abandoned before adequate control of vascular inflammation has occurred.

Limitation of adverse events

An important, and frequently overlooked, aspect of the management of patients with vasculitic neuropathy concerns the need for an aggressive program to limit adverse events associated with the commonly used immunosuppressive drugs. Nothing is more frustrating to both patient and physician than to achieve an excellent subjective and objective response to an immunosuppressive regimen, only to have the recovery delayed by treatment-related morbidity such as medication toxicity, opportunistic infection, or malignancy. Unfortunately, this situation develops in up to 70% of vasculitis patients treated with the traditional combination regimen.[268,270]

The main side effects of prednisone that need to be addressed *as soon as therapy is initiated* include weight gain, hypertension, glucose intolerance, electrolyte imbalance, cataracts, glaucoma, mood alterations, osteoporosis, steroid myopathy and avascular necrosis of the femoral head and other bones (Table 198.11).[350] All patients should be placed on a strict low calorie, reduced sodium, low-simple sugar diet, with tracking of weight and blood pressure at every visit. Serum electrolyte and glucose determinations are critical during the early phases of treatment, but should be monitored periodically throughout the treatment course. Ocular examinations, to include intraocular pressure checks, should be performed every 6 to 12

months, with therapy initiated immediately for elevated intraocular pressures. The judicious use of antidepressants and short term sedative hypnotics can prove invaluable in managing mood swings and insomnia, which, if severe enough, can interfere with patient compliance.

Osteoporosis is the most insidious and serious complication of steroid treatment and also one of the most difficult to treat once it develops.[351,353] Most patients on chronic steroids develop some degree of bone loss beginning within the first few months of treatment.[354] Reduced mobility due to motor impairment, encountered in many patients with vasculitic neuropathy, may also contribute to bone loss. Fifteen percent of all patients and 20% of postmenopausal women suffer a vertebral compression fracture within one year of starting CS therapy.[355,356] Bone density should be determined by dual energy x-ray absorptiometry (DEXA) before therapy is begun and at least yearly for as long as therapy continues.[351,353] If bone loss occurs at a rate greater than 3% per year, osteoporosis treatment will need to be instituted or augmented.[353] Laboratory tests to exclude secondary causes of osteoporosis are recommended (Table 198.11).[351,352] Supplementation with calcium (1000 to 1500 mg/day) and vitamin D (800 to 1000 IU/day) or calcitriol (0.25 to 0.50 µg/day) should be started immediately in all patients.[357] Postmenopausal women should begin estrogen replacement under the direction of their primary physician, gynecologist, or endocrinologist, provided there are no contraindications. Similarly, testosterone replacement therapy should be considered in hypogonadal men. Bisphosphonates such as etidronate (given in cycles of 400 mg/day for 14 days repeated every 3 months), alendronate (5 to 10 mg/day or 50–70 mg once weekly), or residronate (5 mg/day) inhibit bone resorption and have been shown in many RCTs (class 1) to both prevent and treat CS-induced osteoporosis.[352,353,355,356] Bisphosphonates are the only osteoporosis medications demonstrated in a RCT to reduce CS-related vertebral fractures.[356] They should be considered first-line therapy for the prevention and treatment of CS-induced osteoporosis. Activity as tolerated by the patient's overall status and, in particular, exercise producing intermittent axial loading help to limit osteoporosis and reduce the risk of fracture.[358]

The principal side effects associated with chronic CYC include bone marrow suppression, opportunistic infections, bladder toxicity, gonadal failure, and increased risk of malignancy (Table 198.12).[268] A complete blood count should be obtained at least monthly during the early phases of treatment and at least every three months for as long as treatment persists. Patients should undergo tuberculin skin testing before therapy is begun; positive responders must be started on antituberculous therapy. The risk of bladder toxicity, which presents as hemorrhagic cystitis in 40% of patients, can be reduced by periodic urinalyses and encouraging patients to drink at least two quarts of water a day and void frequently.[268] These

Table 198.11   Adverse effects and management: corticosteroids

Side effects

Common (>10%)
Osteoporosis/fractures
Fluid retention/edema
Hypertension
Hyperglycemia
Menstrual irregularities
Growth suppression
Increased appetite; weight gain
Suppression of hypothalamic–pituitary–adrenal axis
Hirsutism
Skin atrophy; bruising
Impaired wound healing
Acne
Cataracts
Moon facies; truncal adiposity
Susceptibility to infections
Insomnia
Psychiatric reactions
Nausea

Uncommon (<10%)
Avascular necrosis of hips and other joints
Tendon rupture
Epidural lipomatosis
Myopathy
Hypokalemia
Glaucoma
Opportunistic infections
Bowel perforation
Encephalopathy

Monitoring

Baseline
CBC, electrolytes, glucose, glycated hemoglobin
Blood pressure
Eye examination
PPD, chest x-ray, hepatitis B, hepatitis C, HIV
Osteoporosis risk assessment
- Calcium, phosphorus, creatinine, alkaline phosphatase, 25-OH vitamin D, testosterone level, TSH, serum protein electrophoresis, 24-hour urinary calcium
- Bone densitometry

Follow-up
CBC, electrolytes, glucose
Blood pressure
Eye examination (yearly)
Bone densitometry (yearly)

Preventative measures

Diet
Calorie-restricted, low sodium, low
   simple sugar
Adequate calcium
Eliminate tobacco and alcohol

Osteoporosis prophylaxis
Regular weightbearing, resistance exercises

Calcium 1000–1500 mg/day
Vitamin D 800–1000 IU/day or calcitriol
   0.25–0.50 μg/day
Thiazide diuretics if urinary calcium
   >300 mg/day
Consider hormone replacement in
   postmenopausal women
Consider testosterone replacement in
   hypogonadal men
Bisphosphonates
- Cyclic etidronate 400 mg/day × 2 weeks
     q. 3 months; or
- Alendronate 5–10 mg/day (or 50–70 mg/
     week); or
- Risedronate 5 mg/day

Infections
No live vaccines

Give influenza and pneumococcal vaccines
Pneumocystis carinii prophylaxis
(W/concomitant immunosuppressives)
- Trimethoprim/sulfamethoxazole
     160/800 mg t.i.w.

measures also help to reduce the risk of bladder cancer, which occurs in 16% of patients within 15 years of first exposure to CYC.[359] There is a significantly increased risk of *Pneumocystis carinii* pneumonia in patients on combination CS/CYC therapy, and prophylaxis using TMP/SMX is recommended.[270,360,361] The main side effects of other medications used in treating vasculitis are listed in Tables 198.13 to 198.15.

Symptomatic and supportive care

Supportive care of the patient with vasculitic neuropathy involves pain management, rehabilitation concerns, and counseling and patient education. High dose corticosteroids are often effective in reducing the neuropathic pain associated with nerve ischemia. For many patients, however, pain persists despite adequate immunosuppression, and additional therapy is needed with tricyclic antidepressants, carbamazepine, gabapentin, mexiletine, clonazepam, tramadol, topical capsaicin or lidocaine, or one of the other medications used for neuropathic pain.[362] In some patients, proceeding directly to scheduled narcotics provides more rapid and effective pain relief than that afforded by sequential trials on multiple less effective agents. With rare exceptions, pain control alone is not a sufficient reason to keep a patient on high dose corticosteroids.

Rehabilitation issues can usually be only addressed after the patient's pain is reduced, neurological status stabilized, and non-neurological complications controlled. Physical therapy is indispensable in patients with motor impairments to maintain strength and range of motion, limit contractures, and reduce the likelihood of developing steroid-induced muscle weakness. The value of exercise in limiting osteoporosis has already been mentioned. Patients with profound weakness may benefit from appropriate bracing and walking aids (e.g. cane, wheeled walker, or crutches). A manual or power wheelchair may be required to maintain mobility. Occupational therapy helps maximize function and assists in activity-of-daily-living skills, particularly in patients with significant arm weakness.

The value of counseling and psychological support for patients with vasculitic neuropathy cannot be overemphasized. Physicians need to clearly inform patients about the chronic nature of their disease,

including the fact that improvement may not occur for weeks to months after therapy has begun. Patients must also understand the side effects of their medications and be made aware of the dire consequences of suddenly stopping high-dose corticosteroid therapy and the possible need for increased corticosteroid dosing with any physiological stress (trauma, infection or surgery). Patients should obtain a medication necklace or bracelet, clearly identifying that they are on corticosteroid and cytotoxic medication. Patients also need to be aware of the need for close medical follow-up with their primary care physicians, especially for assessment of any opportunistic infections.

The motor impairments associated with many cases of vasculitic neuropathy, frequent medication side effects, inevitably prolonged rehabilitation and recovery, and uncertain prognosis place patients with vasculitic neuropathy at high risk for depression and other psychological reactions.[363] Elderly individuals treated with high doses of corticosteroids are particularly susceptible to psychiatric complications. Although there are no hard data on the incidence of depression in patients with vasculitic neuropathy, the treating physician must maintain a high index of suspicion and be willing and able to provide appropriate pharmacological and psychological support for patients who do become depressed. In some instances, this requires psychiatric referral for more intensive therapy.

Table 198.12   Adverse effects: cyclophosphamide

Side effects
Infertility
- Oligo/aspermia 50–90%
- Amenorrhea 30–60%
Bone marrow suppression 30–50%
Susceptibility to infection 30–50%
Hemorrhagic cystitis 10–50%
GI distress (nausea, diarrhea) 20–45%
Alopecia 15–35%
Rash 1–5%
Malignancy
- Bladder 16% at 15 years
- Myelodysplastic syndrome 2–8%
- Lymphoid cancer 1–2%
- Skin (rare)

Monitoring
Baseline
CBC, liver functions, urinalysis
Creatinine (reduced dosing in renal failure)
Chest x-ray, PPD, hepatitis B, hepatitis C, HIV

Preventative measures
Hemorrhagic cystitis
Oral dosing
- Administer as single morning dose
- Frequent voiding
- Consume 2–3 L fluids per day
Intravenous (IV) dosing
- IV fluids 1–1.5 L before and after infusion
- IV mesna 60–100% of cyclophosphamide dose

Follow-up
CBC
Urinalysis (including q. 6 months after therapy)
Cystoscopy q. 1–2 years (if history of hemorrhagic cystitis)

Infections
No live vaccines
Give influenza and pneumococcal vaccines
Pneumocystis carinii prophylaxis (see Table 198.11)
Neutropenia
- Neutropenic precautions
- Consider recombinant human granulocyte colony stimulating factor

Table 198.13 Adverse effects: methotrexate

Side effects
Bone marrow suppression 5–25%
• Leukopenia > anemia, thrombocytopenia
Susceptibility to infection 1–10%
Hepatotoxicity
• Liver function abnormalities 10–35%
• Cirrhosis 1–3%
GI distress (nausea, abdominal pain) 5–20%
Mucositis 5–10%
Impaired wound healing
Pneumonitis 1–7%
Alopecia 1–10%
Nodulosis 5–10%
Hyperhomocysteinemia (precise incidence unknown)
• ? Accelerated atherosclerosis
Malignancy (rare)
• Reversible Epstein–Barr virus-associated lymphoma

Monitoring
Baselines
CBC, liver functions, albumin
Creatinine (avoid in renal failure)
Folate, vitamin B_{12}
Pulmonary functions
Chest x-ray, PPD, hepatitis B, hepatitis C, HIV

Follow-up
CBC, liver functions, albumin
Creatinine
Liver biopsy if persistently abnormal liver functions

Preventative measures
Folate supplementation
Rationale
• Reduce hematological, GI, mucositic, alopecic side effects
• Reduce hyperhomocysteinemia
• ? Reduce hepatotoxicity
Folic acid 1–5 mg/day; or
Folinic acid 2.5–5 mg q. week on day after MTX

Infections
No live vaccines
Give influenza and pneumococcal vaccines
Pneumocystis carinii prophylaxis (with corticosteroids)
(See Table 198.11)

Table 198.14 Adverse effects: azathioprine

Side effects
Bone marrow suppression 5–30%
• Leukopenia > anemia, thrombocytopenia
Susceptibility to infection 1–10%
GI distress (nausea, diarrhea) 5–20%
Hepatotoxicity 5–10%
• Cirrhosis <1%
Pancreatitis 5%
Impaired wound healing
Hypersensitivity reaction 1–10%
Mucositis 1–10%
Alopecia 1–10%
Malignancy (rare)
• Reversible Epstein–Barr virus-associated lymphoma
• Lymphoproliferative disorders, skin cancer

Monitoring
Baseline
CBC
Liver functions
Chest x-ray, PPD, hepatitis B, hepatitis C, HIV

Follow-up
CBC
Liver functions

Preventative measures
GI Prophylaxis
Administer in divided doses with food

Infections
No live vaccines
Give influenza and pneumococcal vaccines
Pneumocystis carinii prophylaxis (with corticosteroids)
(See Table 198.11)

Table 198.15   Adverse effects: intravenous immunoglobulin (IVIg)

Side effects
Headache (including migraine) 25–50%
Fever, chills 10–30%
Immediate systemic symptoms 5–15%
- Chills, myalgias, back pain, chest tightness, arthralgias, nausea, abdominal pain, anxiety, flushing, dyspnea, mild hypotension

Aseptic meningitis 5–10%
Rash 3–7%
Transient leukopenia 5%
Thromboembolic events 4%
- Myocardial infarction, stroke, venous thrombosis
- ? Due to hyperviscosity

Acute renal failure 1–2%
- Risk factors: pre-existing renal dysfunction, diabetes mellitus, volume depletion, age >65, sepsis, paraproteinemia, sucrose-containing IVIg

Transmission of infectious agents (rare)
Anaphylaxis in IgA-deficient patients (rare)

Monitoring

Baseline	Follow-up
CBC, BUN, creatinine	CBC
Quantitative immunoglobulins	BUN, creatinine
Consider lipids, serum protein electrophoresis, cryoglobulins, viscosity	

Preventative measures

Headache and systemic symptoms	Nephrotoxicity (high risk patients)	Migraine
Temporarily hold or reduce rate of infusion	IV fluids 1.0–1.5 L before and after infusion	Pharmacological prophylaxis
		• Propranolol and others
Consider premedication	Use minimum IVIg concentration	
• Acetaminophen 1000 mg	Avoid products with sucrose stabilizers	
• Diphenhydramine 25–50 mg	Infuse at slow rate (<2 mg/kg/min)	
• Hydrocortisone IV 1–2 mg/kg		
• Prednisone 100 mg		

References

1. Crissey JT, Parish LC. Vasculitis: The historical development of the concept. Clin Dermatol 1999;17:493–497
2. Kussmaul A, Maier R. Ueber eine bisher nicht beschriebene eigenthumliche Arterien-erkrankung (Periarteritis nodosa), die mit Morbus Brightii und rapid fortschreitender allgemeiner Muskellahmung einhergeht. Dtsch Arch Klin Med 1866;1:484–518
3. Ferrari E. Ueber polyarteritis acuta nodosa (sogenannte Periarteritis nodosa) und ihre Beziehungen zur Polymyositis und Polyneuritis acuta. Beitr Pathol Anat 1903;34:350–386
4. Bannatyne GA. Rheumatoid Arthritis: Its Pathology, Morbid Anatomy and Treatment. 2nd ed. Bristol, UK: John Wright & Sons, 1898
5. Hutchinson J. Diseases of the arteries. On a peculiar form of thrombotic arteritis of the aged which is sometimes productive of gangrene. Arch Surg (Lond) 1890;1:323–329
6. Wohlwill F. Uber die nur Mikroskopisch erkenbarre Form der Perarteritis nodosa. Arch Pathol Anat 1923;246:377–411
7. Davson J, Ball J, Platt R. The kidney in periarteritis nodosa. QJM 1948;17:175–202
8. Klinger H. Grenzformen der Periarteritis nodosa. Frankfurt Z Pathol 1931;42:455–480
9. Wegener F. Uber generalisierte, septische Gefasserkrankungen. Verh Dtsch Pathol Ges 1936;29:202–209
10. Godman GC, Churg J. Wegener's granulomatosis. Pathology and review of the literature. Arch Pathol 1954;58:533–553
11. Kernohan JW, Woltman HW. Periarteritis nodosa: a clinicopathological study with special reference to the nervous system. Arch Neurol Psychiatry 1938;39:655–686
12. Zeek PM, Smith CC, Weeter JC. Studies on periarteritis nodosa. III. The differentiation between the vascular lesions of periarteritis nodosa and of hypersensitivity. Am J Pathol 1948;24:889–917
13. Churg J, Strauss L. Allergic granulomatosis, allergic angiitis, and periarteritis nodosa. Am J Pathol 1951;27:277–301
14. Sokoloff L, Wilens SL, Bunim JJ. Arteritis of striated muscle in rheumatoid arthritis. Am J Pathol 1951;27:157–173
15. Cruickshank B. The arteritis of rheumatoid arthritis. Ann Rheum Dis 1954;13:136–145

16. Zeek PM. Periarteritis nodosa: a critical review. Am J Clin Pathol 1952;22:777–790

17. Dyck PJ, Conn DL, Ozaki H. Necrotizing angiopathic neuropathy: three-dimensional morphology of fiber degeneration related to sites of occluded vessels. Mayo Clin Proc 1972;47:461–475

18. Dyck PJ, Benstead TJ, Conn DL, et al. Nonsystemic vasculitic neuropathy. Brain 1987;110:843–854

19. Hunder GG, Arend WP, Bloch DA, et al. The American College of Rheumatology 1990 criteria for the classification of vasculitis: introduction. Arthritis Rheum 1990;33:1101–1107

20. Jennette JC, Falk AJ, Andrassy K, et al. Nomenclature of systemic vasculitides: proposal of an international consensus conference. Arthritis Rheum 1994;37:187–192

21. Lovshin LL, Kernohan JW. Peripheral neuritis in periarteritis nodosa. A clinicopathologic study. Arch Intern Med 1948;82:321–338

22. Kissel JT, Slivka AP, Warmolts JR, Mendell JR. The clinical spectrum of necrotizing angiopathy of the peripheral nervous system. Ann Neurol 1985;18: 251–257

23. Rao JK, Allen NB, Pincus T. Limitations of the 1990 American College of Rheumatology classification criteria for the diagnosis of vasculitis. Ann Intern Med 1998;129:345–352

24. Gonzalez-Gay MA, Garcia-Porrua C. Systemic vasculitis in adults in northwestern Spain, 1988–1997. Clinical and epidemiological aspects. Medicine 1999;78:292–308

25. Watts RA, Scott DG. Classification and epidemiology of the vasculitides. Baillieres Clin Rheumatol 1997;11:191–217

26. Somer T, Finegold SM. Vasculitides associated with infections, immunization, and antimicrobial drugs. Clin Infect Dis 1995;20:1010–1036

27. Mandell BF, Calabrese LH. Infections and systemic vasculitis. Curr Opin Rheumatol 1998;10:51–57

28. Del Rosso A, Generini S, Pignone A, Matucci-Cerinic M. Vasculitides secondary to systemic diseases. Clin Dermatol 1999;17:533–547

29. Guillevin L, Lhote F, Gherardi R. The spectrum and treatment of virus-associated vasculitides. Curr Opin Rheumatol 1997;9:31–36

30. Sergent JS, Lockshin MD, Christial CL, Gocke DJ. Vasculitis with hepatitis B antigenemia: long-term observations in nine patients. Medicine 1976;55:1–18

31. Guillevin L, Lhote F, Jarrousse B, et al. Polyarteritis related to hepatitis B virus. A retrospective study of 66 patients. Ann Med Interne (Paris) 1992;143(Suppl 1): 63–74

32. Guillevin L, Lhote F, Cohen P, et al. Polyarteritis nodosa related to hepatitis B virus: a prospective study with long-term observation of 41 patients. Medicine 1995;74:238–253

33. Quint L, Deny P, Guillevin L, et al. Hepatitis C virus in patients with polyarteritis nodosa. Prevalence in 38 patients. Clin Exp Rheumatol 1991;9:253–257

34. Carson CW, Conn DL, Czaja AJ, et al. Frequency and significance of antibodies to hepatitis C virus in polyarteritis nodosa. J Rheumatol 1993;20:304–309

35. Cacoub P, Maisonobe T, Thibault V, et al. Systemic vasculitis in patients with hepatitis C. J Rheumatol 2001;28:109–118

36. Font C, Miro O, Pedrol E, et al. Polyarteritis nodosa in human immunodeficiency virus infection: report of four cases and review of the literature. Br J Rheumatol 1996;35:796–799

37. Finkel TH, Torok TJ, Ferguson PJ, et al. Chronic parvovirus B19 infection and systemic necrotizing vasculitis: opportunistic infection or aetiological agent? Lancet 1994;343:1255–1258

38. Fuller GN, Jacobs JM, Guiloff RJ. Nature and incidence of peripheral nerve syndromes in HIV infection. J Neurol Neurosurg Psychiatry 1993;56:372–381

39. Brannagan TH. Retroviral-associated vasculitis of the nervous system. Neurol Clin 1997;15:927–944

40. Gisselbrecht M, Cohen P, Lortholary O, et al. Human immunodeficiency virus-related vasculitis. Clinical presentation of and therapeutic approach to eight cases. Ann Med Interne (Paris) 1998;149:398–405

41. Bradley WG, Verma A. Painful vasculitic neuropathy in HIV-1 infection: relief of pain with prednisone therapy. Neurology 1996;47:1446–1451

42. Gherardi R, Belec L, Mhiri C, et al. The spectrum of vasculitis in human immunodeficiency virus-infected patients. Arthritis Rheum 1993;36:1164–1174

43. Gherardi R, Lebargy F, Gaulard C, et al. Necrotizing vasculitis and HIV replication in peripheral nerves (letter). N Engl J Med 1989;321:685–686

44. Gherardi RK, Mhiri C, Baudrimont M, et al. Iron pigment deposits, small vessel vasculitis, and erythrophagocytosis in the muscle of human immunodeficiency virus-infected patients. Hum Pathol 1991;22:1187–1194

45. Dispenzieri A, Gorevic PD. Cryoglobulinemia. Hematol Oncol Clin North Am 1999;13:1315–1349

46. Lamprecht P, Gause A, Gross WL. Cryoglobulinemic vasculitis. Arthritis Rheum 1999;42:2507–2516

47. Ramos-Casals M, Trejo O, Garcia-Carrasco M, et al. Mixed cryoglobulinemia: new concepts. Lupus 2000;9: 83–91

48. De Vita S, De Re V, Gasparotto D, et al. Oligoclonal non-neoplastic B cell expansion is the key feature of type II mixed cryoglobulinemia. Arthritis Rheum 2000;43:94–102

49. Garcia-Bragado F, Fernandez JM, Navarro C, et al. Peripheral neuropathy in essential mixed cryoglobulinemia. Arch Neurol 1988;45:1210–1214

50. Ferri C, LaCivita L, Cirafisi C, et al. Peripheral neuropathy in mixed cryoglobulinemia: clinical and electrophysiologic investigations. J Rheumatol 1992;19: 889–895

51. Gemignani F, Pavesi G, Manganelli P, et al. Peripheral neuropathy in essential mixed cryoglobulinemia. J Neurol Neurosurg Psychiatry 1992;55:116–120

52. Zaltron S, Puoti M, Liberini P, et al. High prevalence of peripheral neuropathy in hepatitis C virus infected patients with symptomatic and asymptomatic cryoglobulinemia. Ital J Gastroenterol Hepatol 1998;30: 391–395

53. Traverso F, Martini F, Banchi L, et al. Vasculitic neuropathy associated with beta-hemolytic streptococcal infection: a case report. Ital J Neurol Sci 1997;18: 105–107

54. Kidron D, Barron SA, Mazliah J. Mononeuritis multiplex with brachial plexus neuropathy coincident with *Mycoplasma pneumoniae* infection. Eur Neurol 189;29: 90–92

55. Ozen H, Cemeroglu P, Ecevit Z, et al. Unusual neurologic complications of typhoid fever (aphasia, mononeuritis multiplex, and Guillain-Barre syndrome): a report of two cases. Turk J Pediatr 1993;35: 141–144

56. Hancox RJ, Karalus N, Singh V. Mononeuritis multiplex in leptospirosis (letter). Scand J Infect Dis 1991; 23:395–396

57. Tanaka E, Tada K, Amitani R, Kuze F. Systemic hypersensitivity vasculitis associated with bronchiectasis. Chest 1992;102:647–649

58. Pamphlett R, Walsh J. Infective endocarditis with inflammatory lesions in the peripheral nervous system. Acta Neuropathol 1989;78:101–104

59. Cacoub P, Sbai A, Gatel A, et al. Vascularites systemiques post-infectieuses: guerison sans corticotherapie. J Mal Vasc 1997;22:29–34

60. Meier C, Grahmann F, Engelhardt A, Dumas M. Peripheral nerve disorders in Lyme-borreliosis. Nerve biopsy studies from eight cases. Acta Neuropathol 1989;79:271–278

61. Halperin J, Luft BJ, Volkman DJ, Dattwyler RJ. Lyme neuroborreliosis: peripheral nervous system manifestations. Brain 1990;113:1207–1221

62. Kindstrand E, Nilsson BY, Hovmark A, et al. Polyneuropathy in late Lyme borreliosis—a clinical, neurophysiological and morphological description. Acta Neurol Scand 2000;101:47–52

63. Maimone D, Villanova M, Stanta G, et al. Detection of Borrelia burgdorferi DNA and complement membrane attack complex deposits in the sural nerve of a patient with chronic polyneuropathy and tertiary Lyme disease. Muscle Nerve 1997;20:969–975

64. Dubost JJ, Souteyrand P, Sauvezie B. Drug-induced vasculitides. Baillieres Clin Rheumatol 1991;5:119–138

65. Merkel PA. Drugs associated with vasculitis. Curr Opin Rheumatol 1998;10:45–50

66. Schrier RW, Bulger RJ, VanArsdel PP. Nephropathy associated with penicillin and homologues. Ann Intern Med 1966;64:116–127

67. Rosenberg JL, Edlow D, Sneider R. Liver disease and vasculitis in a patient taking cromolyn. Arch Intern Med 1978;138:989–991

68. Dalgleish PG. Polyarteritis nodosa after thiouracil. Lancet 1952;2:319–320

69. Berbegaal J, Morera J, Andrada E, et al. Sindrome de hipersensibilidad al allopurinol. Aportacion de un nuevo caso y revision de la literatura esponola. Med Clin (Barc) 1994;102:178–180

70. Shulman LM, Minagar A, Sharma K, Weiner WJ. Amantadine-induced peripheral neuropathy. Neurology 1999;53:1862–1865

71. Pateron D, Fain O, Sehonnou J, et al. Severe necrotizing vasculitis in a patient with hepatitis C virus infection treated with interferon. Clin Exp Rheumatol 1996;14:79–81

72. Mockel M, Kampf D, Lobeck H, Frei U. Severe panarteritis associated with drug abuse. Intensive Care Med 1999;25:113–117

73. Stafford CR, Bogdanoff BM, Green L, Spector HB. Mononeuropathy multiplex as a complication of amphetamine angiitis. Neurology 1975;25:570–572

74. Wooten MD, Jasin HE. Vasculitis and lymphoproliferative diseases. Semin Arthritis Rheum 1996;26:564–574

75. Hasler P, Kistler H, Gerber H. Vasculitides in hairy cell leukemia. Semin Arthritis Rheum 1995;25:134–142

76. Prior R, Schober R, Scharffetter K, Wechsler W. Occlusive microangiopathy by immunoglobulin (IgM-kappa) precipitation: pathogenetic relevance in paraneoplastic cryoglobulinemic neuropathy. Acta Neuropathol 1992;83:423–426

77. Johnson PC, Rolak LA, Hamilton RH, Laguna JF. Paraneoplastic vasculitis of nerve: a remote effect of cancer. Ann Neurol 1979;5:437–444

78. Vincent D, Dubas F, Hauw JJ, et al. Nerve and muscle microvasculitis in peripheral neuropathy: a remote effect of cancer? J Neurol Neurosurg Psychiatry 1986;49:1007–1010

79. Kurzrock R, Cohen PR, Markowitz A. Clinical manifestations of vasculitis in patients with solid tumors: a case report and review of the literature. Arch Intern Med 1994;154:334–340

80. Oh SJ. Paraneoplastic vasculitis of the peripheral nervous system. Neurol Clin 1997;15:849–863

81. Blumenthal D, Schochet S, Gutmann L, et al. Small-cell carcinoma of the lung presenting with paraneoplastic peripheral nerve microvasculitis and optic neuropathy (letter). Muscle Nerve 1998;21:1358–1359

82. Greer JM, Longley S, Edwards NL, et al. Vasculitis associated with malignancy: experience with 13 patients and literature review. Medicine 1988;67:220–230

83. Sneller MC, Fauci AS. Pathogenesis of vasculitic syndromes. Med Clin North Am 1997;81:221–242

84. Nowack R, Flores-Suarez LF, van der Woude FJ. New developments in pathogenesis of systemic vasculitis. Curr Opin Rheumatol 1998;10:3–11

85. Moore PM. Vasculitic neuropathies (editorial). J Neurol Neurosurg Psychiatry 2000;68:271–276

86. Kevil CG, Bullard DC. Roles of leukocyte/endothelial cell adhesion molecules in the pathogenesis of vasculitis. Am J Med 1999;106:677–687

87. Sundy JS, Haynes BF. Cytokines and adhesion molecules in the pathogenesis of vasculitis. Curr Rheumatol Rep 2000;2:402–410

88. Zlotnik A, Morales J, Hedrick JA. Recent advances in chemokines and chemokine receptors. Crit Rev Immunol 1999;19:1–47

89. Shresta S, Pham CT, Thomas DA, et al. How do cytotoxic lymphocytes kill their targets? Curr Opin Immunol 1998;10:581–587

90. Sabelko KA, Russell JH. The role of Fas ligand in vivo as a cause and regulator of pathogenesis. Curr Opin Immunol 2000;12:330–335

91. Mannik M. Serum sickness and pathophysiology of immune complexes. In: Rich RR, Fleisher TA, Schwartz BD, et al., eds. Clinical Immunology. Principles and Practice. St. Louis: Mosby, 1996:217–230

92. Meroni PL, Del Papa N, Raschi E, et al. Is there any pathogenic role for the anti-endothelial cell antibodies (AECA) in autoimmune vasculitis? J Biol Regul Homeostat Agents 1997;11:127–132

93. Praprotnik S, Rozman B, Blank M, Shoenfeld Y. Pathogenic role of anti-endothelial cell antibodies in systemic vasculitis. Wien Klin Wochenschr 2000;112:660–664

94. Carvalho D, Savage C, Isenberg D, Pearson J. IgG anti-endothelial cell autoantibodies from patients with systemic lupus erythematosus or systemic vasculitis stimulate the release of two endothelial cell-derived mediators, which enhance adhesion molecule expression and leukocyte adhesion in an autocrine manner. Arthritis Rheum 1999;42:631–640

95. Harper L, Savage CO. Pathogenesis of ANCA-associated systemic vasculitis. J Pathol 2000;190:349–359

96. Schultz DR, Diego JM. Antineutrophil cytoplasm antibodies (ANCA) and systemic vasculitis: update of assays, immunopathogenesis, controversies, and report of a novel de novo ANCA-associated vasculitis after kidney transplantation. Semin Arthritis Rheum 2000;29:267–285

97. Radford DJ, Lord JM, Savage CO. The activation of the neutrophil respiratory burst by anti-neutrophil cytoplasm autoantibody (ANCA) from patients with sys-

temic vasculitis requires tyrosine kinases and protein kinase C activation. Clin Exp Immunol 1999;118: 171–179

98. Radford DJ, Savage CO, Nash GB. Treatment of rolling neutrophils with antineutrophil cytoplasm antibodies causes conversion to firm integrin-mediated adhesion. Arthritis Rheum 2000;43:1337–1345

99. Kissel JT, Riethman JL, Omerza J, et al. Peripheral nerve vasculitis: immune characterization of the vascular lesions. Ann Neurol 1989;25:291–297

100. Khalili-Shirazi A, Gregson NA, Londei M, et al. The distribution of CD1 molecules in inflammatory neuropathy. J Neurol Sci 1998;158:154–163

101. Satoi H, Oka N, Kawasaki T, et al. Mechanisms of tissue injury in vasculitic neuropathies. Neurology 1998;50:492–496

102. Hattori N, Ichimura M, Nagamatsu M, et al. Clinicopathological features of Churg–Strauss syndrome-associated neuropathy. Brain 1999;122:427–439

103. Stepp SE, Mathew PA, Bennett M, et al. Perforin: more than just an effector molecule. Immunol Today 2000;21:254–256

104. Bosboom WM, Van den Berg LH, Mollee I, et al. Sural nerve T-cell receptor Vβ gene utilization in chronic inflammatory demyelinating polyneuropathy and vasculitic neuropathy. Neurology 2001;56:74–81

105. Weyand CM, Goronzy JJ. Arterial wall injury in giant cell arteritis. Arthritis Rheum 1999;42:844–853

106. Levy M. Familial cases of Berger's disease and anaphylactoid purpura; more frequent than previously thought (letter). Am J Med 1989;87:246–248

107. Akpolat T, Koc Y, Yeniay I, et al. Familial Behçet's disease. Eur J Med 1992;1:391–395

108. Rottem M, Cotch MF, Fauci AS, Hoffman GS. Familial vasculitis: report of 2 families. J Rheumatol 1994;21: 561–563

109. Numano F, Kobayashi Y, Maruyama Y, et al. Takayasu arteritis: clinical characteristics and the role of genetic factors in its pathogenesis. Vasc Med 1996;1:227–233

110. Johansen M, Elling P, Elling H, Olsson A. A genetic approach to the aetiology of giant cell arteritis: depletion of the CD8+ T-lymphocyte subset in relatives of patients with polymyalgia rheumatica and arteritis temporalis. Clin Exp Rheumatol 1995;13:745–748

111. Nowack R, Lehmann H, Flores-Suarez LF, et al. Familial occurrence of systemic vasculitis and rapidly progressive glomerulonephritis. Am J Kidney Dis 1999; 34:364–373

112. Rotenstein D, Gibbas DL, Majmudar B, Chastain EA. Familial granulomatous arteritis with polyarthritis of juvenile onset. N Engl J Med 1982;306:86–90

113. Kone-Paut I, Geisler I, Wechsler B, et al. Familial aggregation in Behçet's disease: high frequency in siblings and parents of pediatric probands. J Pediatr 1999; 35:89–93

114. Weyand CM, Hicok KC, Hunder GG, Goronzy JJ. The HLA-DRB1 locus as a genetic component in giant cell arteritis. Mapping of a disease-specific motif to the antigen binding site of the HLA-DR molecule. J Clin Invest 1992;90:2355–2361

115. Rauzy O, Fort M, Nourhashemi F, et al. Relation between HLA DRB1 alleles and corticosteroid resistance in giant cell arteritis. Ann Rheum Dis 1998; 57:380–382

116. Mizuki N, Ota M, Katsuyama Y, et al. Association analysis between the MIC-A and HLA-B alleles in Japanese patients with Behçet's disease. Arthritis Rheum 1999;42:1961–1966

117. Kimura A, Ota M, Katsuyama Y, et al. Mapping of the HLA-linked genes controlling the susceptibility to Takayasu's arteritis. Int J Cardiol 2000;75(Suppl 1): S105–S110

118. Perdriger A, Chales G, Semana G, et al. Role of HLA-DR-DR and DR-DQ associations in the expression of extraarticular manifestations and rheumatoid factor in rheumatoid arthritis. J Rheumatol 1997;24:1272–1276

119. Papiha SS, Murty GE, Ad'Hia A, et al. Association of Wegener's granulomatosis with HLA antigens and other genetic markers. Ann Rheum Dis 1992;51: 246–248

120. Griffith ME, Pusey CD. HLA genes in ANCA-associated vasculitides. Exp Clin Immunogenet 1997;14: 196–205

121. Murty GE, Mainss BT, Middleton D, et al. HLA antigen frequencies and Wegener's granulomatosis. Clin Otolaryngol 1991;16:448–451

122. Zhang L, Jayne DR, Zhao MH, et al. Distribution of MHC class II alleles in primary systemic vasculitis. Kidney Int 1995;47:294–298

123. Huang D, Giscombe R, Zhou Y, Lefvert AK. Polymorphisms in CTLA-4 but not tumor necrosis factor-alpha or interleukin 1beta genes are associated with Wegener's granulomatosis. J Rheumatol 2000;27: 397–401

124. Esnault VL, Testa A, Audrain M, et al. Alpha 1-antitrypsin genetic polymorphism in ANCA-positive systemic vasculitis. Kidney Int 1993;43:1329–1332

125. Elzouki AN, Segelmark M, Wieslander J, Eriksson S. Strong link between the alpha 1-antitrypsin PiZ allele and Wegener's granulomatosis. J Intern Med 1994;236:543–548

126. Callea F, Gregorini G, Sinico A, et al. Alpha 1-antitrypsin (AAT) deficiency and ANCA-positive systemic vasculitis: genetic and clinical implications. Eur J Clin Invest 1997;27:696–702

127. Segelmark M, Elzouki AN, Wieslander J, Eriksson S. The PiZ gene of alpha 1-antitrypsin as a determinant of outcome in PR3-ANCA-positive vasculitis. Kidney Int 1995;48:844–850

128. Esnault VL, Audrain MA, Sesboue R. Alpha-1-antitrypsin phenotyping in ANCA-associated diseases: one of several arguments for protease/antiprotease imbalance in systemic vasculitis. Exp Clin Immunogenet 1997;14:206–213

129. Witko-Sarsat V, Lesavre P, Lopez S, et al. A large subset of neutrophils expressing membrane proteinase 3 is a risk factor for vasculitis and rheumatoid arthritis. J Am Soc Nephrol 1999;10:1224–1233

130. Minta JO, Winkler CJ, Biggar WD, Greenberg M. A selective and complete absence of C1q in a patient with vasculitis and nephritis. Clin Immunol Immunopathol 1982;22:225–237

131. Gelfand EW, Clarkson JE, Minta JO. Selective deficiency of the second component of complement in a patient with anaphylactoid purpura. Clin Immunol Immunopathol 1975;4:269–276

132. Roord JJ, Daha M, Kuis W, et al. Inherited deficiency of the third component of complement associated with recurrent pyogenic infections, circulating immune complexes, and vasculitis in a Dutch family. Pediatrics 1983;71:81–87

133. Ault BH, Stapleton FB, Rivas ML, et al. Association of Henoch-Schonlein purpura glomerulonephritis with C4B deficiency. J Pediatr 1990;117:753–755

134. Mattey DL, Hajeer AH, Dababneh A, et al. Association of giant cell arteritis and polymyalgia rheumatica with

different tumor necrosis factor microsatellite polymorphisms. Arthritis Rheum 2000;43:1749–1755

135. Salvarini C, Casali B, Boiardi L, et al. Intercellular adhesion molecule 1 gene polymorphisms in polymyalgia rheumatica/giant cell arteritis: association with disease risk and severity. J Rheumatol 2000;27:1215–1221

136. van der Pol W, van de Winkel JG. IgG receptor polymorphisms: risk factors for disease. Immunogenetics 1998;48:222–232

137. Dijstelbloem HM, Scheepers RH, Oost WW, et al. Fcgamma receptor polymorphisms in Wegener's granulomatosis: risk factors for disease relapse. Arthritis Rheum 1999;42:1823–1827

138. Tse WY, Abadeh S, McTiernan A, et al. No association between neutrophil FcgammaRIIa allelic polymorphism and anti-neutrophil cytoplasm antibody (ANCA)-positive vasculitis. Clin Exp Immunol 1999;117:198–205

139. Tse WY, Abadeh S, Jefferis R, et al. Neutrophil FcgammaRIIIb allelic polymorphism in anti-neutrophil cytoplasm antibody (ANCA)-positive systemic vasculitis. Clin Exp Immunol 2000;119:574–577

140. Moore PN, Fauci AS. Neurologic manifestations of systemic vasculitis: a retrospective study of the clinicopathologic features and responses to therapy in 25 patients. Am J Med 1981;71:517–524

141. Wees SJ, Sunwoo IN, Oh SJ. Sural nerve biopsy in systemic necrotizing vasculitis. Am J Med 1981;71:525–532

142. Castaigne P, Brunet P, Hauw JJ, et al. Systeme nerveux peripherique et panarterite noueuse: revue de 27 cas. Revue Neurol (Paris) 1984;140:343–352

143. Chang RN, Bell CC, Hallett M. Clinical characteristics and prognosis of vasculitic mononeuropathy multiplex. Arch Neurol 1984;41:618–621

144. Bouche P, Leger JM, Travers MA, et al. Peripheral neuropathy in systemic vasculitis: clinical and electrophysiologic study of 22 patients. Neurology 1986;36:1598–1602

145. Harati Y, Niakan E. The clinical spectrum of inflammatory-angiopathic neuropathy. J Neurol Neurosurg Psychiatry 1986;49:1313–1316

146. Said G, LaCroix-Ciaudo C, Fujimura H, et al. The peripheral neuropathy of necrotizing arteritis: a clinicopathological study. Ann Neurol 1988;23:461–465

147. Panegyres PK, Blumbergs PC, Leong AS-Y, Bourne AJ. Vasculitis of peripheral nerve and skeletal muscle: clinicopathological correlation and immunopathogenic mechanisms. J Neurol Sci 1990;100:193–202

148. Hawke SHB, Davies L, Pamphlett R, et al. Vasculitic neuropathy: a clinical and pathological study. Brain 1991;114:2175–2190

149. Nicolai A, Bonetti B, Lazzarino LG, et al. Peripheral nerve vasculitis: a clinico-pathological study. Clin Neuropathol 1995;14:137–141

150. Puechal X, Said G, Hilliquin P, et al. Peripheral neuropathy with necrotizing vasculitis in rheumatoid arthritis. A clinicopathologic and prognostic study of thirty-two patients. Arthritis Rheum 1995;38:1618–1629

151. Singhal BS, Khadilkar SV, Gursahani RD, Surya N. Vasculitic neuropathy: profile of twenty patients. J Assoc Physicians India 1995;43:459–461

152. Chia L, Fernandez A, LaCroix C, et al. Contribution of nerve biopsy findings to the diagnosis of disabling neuropathy in the elderly: a retrospective review of 100 consecutive patients. Brain 1996;119:1091–1098

153. Davies L, Spies JM, Pollard JD, McLeod JG. Vasculitis

confined to peripheral nerves. Brain 1996;119:1441–1448

154. Collins MP, Mendell JR, Periquet MI, et al. Superficial peroneal nerve/peroneus brevis muscle biopsy in vasculitic neuropathy. Neurology 2000;55:636–643

155. Bosch X, Navarro M, Lopez-Soto A, et al. Primary polyarteritis nodosa presenting as acute symmetric quadriplegia. Clin Exp Rheumatol 1999;17:232–234

156. Cuellar ML, Espinoza LR. Laboratory testing in the evaluation and diagnosis of vasculitis. Curr Rheumatol Rep 2000;2:417–422

157. Claussen GC, Thomas TD, Goyne C, et al. Diagnostic value of nerve and muscle biopsy in suspected vasculitis cases. J Clin Neuromusc Dis 2000;1:117–123

158. McCluskey L, Feinberg D, Cantor C, Bird S. "Pseudo-conduction block" in vasculitic neuropathy. Muscle Nerve 1999;22:1361–1366

159. Jamieson PW, Guiliani MJ, Martinez AJ. Necrotizing angiopathy presenting with multifocal conduction blocks. Neurology 1991;41:442–444

160. Hellman DB, Laing TJ, Petri M, et al. Mononeuritis multiplex: the yield of evaluations for occult rheumatic diseases. Medicine 1988;67:145–153

161. Rappaport WD, Valenti J, Hunter GC, et al. Clinical utilization and complications of sural nerve biopsy. Am J Surg 1993;166:252–256

162. Midroni G, Bilbao JM. Biopsy Diagnosis of Peripheral Neuropathy. Boston: Butterworth-Heinemann, 1995:241–265

163. Dyck PJ, Norell JE, Dyck PJ. Microvasculitis and ischemia in diabetic lumbosacral radiculoplexus neuropathy. Neurology 1999;53:2113–2121

164. Adams CW, Buk SJ, Hughes RA, et al. Perls' ferrocyanide test for iron in the diagnosis of vasculitic neuropathy. Neuropathol Appl Neurobiol 1989;15:433–439

165. Fujimura H, LaCroix C, Said G. Vulnerability of nerve fibers to ischaemia: a quantitative light and electron microscopic study. Brain 1991;114:1929–1942

166. Schutz G, Schroder JM. Number and size of epineurial blood vessels in normal and diseased human nerves. Cell Tissue Res 1997;290:31–37

167. Collins MP, Mendell JR, Periquet MI, et al. Immunostaining in vasculitic neuropathy: sensitivity and specificity of findings (abstract). Ann Neurol 1997;42:415

168. Barohn RJ, Sahenk Z, Warmolts JR, Mendell JR. The Bruns-Garland syndrome (diabetic amyotrophy) revisited 100 years later. Arch Neurol 1991;48:1130–1135

169. Said G, Goulon-Goeau C, Lacroix C, Moulonguet A. Nerve biopsy findings in different patterns of proximal diabetic neuropathy. Ann Neurol 1994;35:559–569

170. Younger DS, Rosoklija G, Hays AP, et al. Diabetic peripheral neuropathy: a clinicopathologic and immunohistochemical analysis of sural nerve biopsies. Muscle Nerve 1996;19:722–727

171. Llewelyn JG, Thomas PK, King RH. Epineurial microvasculitis in proximal diabetic neuropathy. J Neurol 1998;245:159–165

172. Kelkar P, Masood M, Parry GJ. Distinctive pathologic findings in proximal diabetic neuropathy (diabetic amyotrophy). Neurology 2000;55:83–88

173. Said G, Elgrably F, LaCroix C, et al. Painful proximal diabetic neuropathy: inflammatory nerve lesions and spontaneous favorable outcome. Ann Neurol 1997;41:762–770

174. Levine GB, Mills PE Jr, Epstein WV. Circulating IgG globulin anti-IgG globulin complex in a patient with carcinoma of the lung and severe neuromyopathy. J Lab Clin Med 1967;69:749–757

175. Torvik A, Berntzen AE. Necrotizing vasculitis without visceral involvement. Postmortem examination of three cases with affection of skeletal muscles and peripheral nerves. Acta Med Scand 1968;184:69–77

176. Tassin S, Ferriere G, Laterre EC. Mononevrite multiple dans un cas de macroglobulinemia de Waldenstrom. Acte Neurol Belg 1980;80:287–297

177. Cupps TR, Fauci AS. Neoplasm and systemic vasculitis: a case report. Arthritis Rheum 1082;25:475–476

178. Gherardi RK, Amiel H, Martin-Mondiere C, et al. Solitary plasmacytoma of the skull revealed by a mononeuritis multiplex associated with immune complex mediated vasculitis. Arthritis Rheum 1989;32:1470–1473

179. Oh SJ, Slaughter R, Harrell. Paraneoplastic vasculitic neuropathy: a treatable neuropathy. Muscle Nerve 1991;14:152–156

180. Hughes RA, Britton T, Richards M. Effects of lymphoma on the peripheral nervous system. J R Soc Med 1994;87:526–530

181. Matsumuro K, Izumo S, Umehara F, et al. Paraneoplastic vasculitic neuropathy: immunohistochemical studies on a biopsied nerve and post-mortem examination. J Intern Med 1994;236:225–230

182. Younger DS, Dalmau J, Inghirami G, et al. Anti-Hu-associated peripheral nerve and muscle microvasculitis. Neurology 1994;44:181–183

183. Hatzis GS, Papachristodoulou A, Delladetsima IK, Moutsopoulos HM. Polyarteritis nodosa associated with cholangiocarcinoma. Lupus 1998;7:301–306

184. Antoine J-C, Mosnier J-F, Absi L, et al. Carcinoma associated paraneoplastic peripheral neuropathies in patients with and without anti-onconeural antibodies. J Neurol Neurosurg Psychiatry 1999;67:7–14

185. Aslangul-Castier E, Papo T, Amoura Z, et al. Systemic vasculitis with bilateral perirenal haemorrhage in chronic myelomonocytic leukaemia. Ann Rheum Dis 2000;59:390–393

186. Hamidou MA, Koiri DE, Audrain M, Grolleau J-Y. Systemic antineutrophil cytoplasm antibody vasculitis associated with lymphoid neoplasia. Ann Rheum Dis 2001;60:293–295

187. Lam KC, Lai CL, Trepo C, Wu PC. Deleterious effect of prednisolone in HBsAg-positive chronic active hepatitis. N Engl J Med 1981;304:380–386

188. Scullard GH, Smith CI, Merigan TC, et al. Effects of immunosuppressive therapy on viral markers in chronic active hepatitis B. Gastroenterology 1981; 81:987–991

189. Lau JY, Bird GL, Alexander GJ, Williams R. Effects of immunosuppressive therapy on hepatic expression of hepatitis B viral genome and gene products. Clin Invest Med 1993;16:226–236

190. Fei GZ, Sylvan SP, Yao GB, Hellstrom UB. Quantitative monitoring of serum hepatitis B virus DNA and blood lymphocyte subsets during combined prednisolone and interferon-alpha therapy in patients with chronic hepatitis B. J Viral Hepat 1999;6:210–227

191. Kruger M, Boker KH, Zeidler H, Manns MP. Treatment of hepatitis B-related polyarteritis nodosa with famciclovir and interferon alfa-2b. J Hepat 1997; 26:935–939

192. Wicki J, Olivieri J, Pizzolato G, et al. Successful treatment of polyarteritis related to hepatitis B virus with a combination of lamivudine and interferon alpha (letter). Rheumatology 1999;38:183–185

193. Maclachlan D, Battegay M, Jacob AL, Tyndall A. Successful treatment of hepatitis B-associated polyarteritis nodosa with a combination of lamivudine and conventional immunosuppressive therapy: a case report (letter). Rheumatology 2000;39:106–108

194. Guillevin L. Polyarteritis nodosa and Churg–Strauss angiitis. Clin Exp Immunol 2000;120(Suppl 1):33–35

195. Cacoub P, Renou C, Rosenthal E, et al. Extrahepatic manifestations associated with hepatitis C virus infection. A prospective multicenter study of 321 patients. Medicine 2000;79:47–56

196. Ferri C, Marzo E, Longombardo G, et al. Interferon-alpha in mixed cryoglobulinemia patients: a randomized, crossover-controlled trial. Blood 1993;81: 1132–1136

197. Dammacco F, Sansonno D, Han JH, et al. Natural interferon-α versus its combination with 6-methylprednisolone in the therapy of type II mixed cryoglobulinemia: a long-term, randomized, controlled study. Blood 1994;84:3336–3343

198. Misiani R, Bellavita P, Fenili D, et al. Interferon alfa-2a therapy in cryoglobulinemia associated with hepatitis C virus. N Engl J Med 1994;330:751–756

199. Lauta VM, De Sangro MA. Long-term results regarding the use of recombinant interferon alpha-2b in the treatment of II type mixed essential cryoglobulinemia. Med Oncol 1995;12:223–230

200. Mazzaro C, Laccin T, Moretti M, et al. Effects of two different alpha-interferon regimens on clinical and virological findings in mixed cryglobulinemia. Clin Exp Rheumatol 1995;13(Suppl 13):S181–S185

201. Adinolfi LE, Utili R, Zampino R, et al. Effects of long-term course of alpha-interferon in patients with chronic hepatitis C associated to mixed cryoglobulinaemia. Eur J Gastroenterol Hepatol 1997;9:1067–1072

202. Hoofnagle JH, Di Bisceglie AM. The treatment of chronic viral hepatitis. N Engl J Med 1997;336:347–356

203. Davis GL, Esteban-Mur R, Rustgi V, et al. Interferon alfa-2b alone or in combination with ribavirin for the treatment of relapse of chronic hepatitis C. N Engl J Med 1998;339:1493–1499

204. McHutchison JG, Gordon SC, Schiff ER, et al. Interferon alfa-2b alone or in combination with ribavirin as initial treatment for chronic hepatitis C. N Engl J Med 1998;339:1485–1492

205. Poynard T, Marcellin P, Lee SS, et al. Randomized trial of interferon α2b plus ribavirin for 48 weeks or 24 weeks versus interferon α2b plus placebo for 48 weeks for treatment of chronic infection with hepatitis C virus. Lancet 1998;352:1426–1432

206. Zuckerman E, Keren D, Slobodin G, et al. Treatment of refractory, symptomatic, hepatitis C virus related mixed cryoglobulinemia with ribavirin and interferon-α. J Rheumatol 2000;27:2172–2178

207. Casato M, Lagana B, Antonelli G, et al. Long-term results of therapy with interferon-alpha for type II essential mixed cryoglobulinemia. Blood 1991;78: 3142–3147

208. Ghini M, Mascia MT, Gentilini M, Mussini C. Treatment of cryoglobulinemic neuropathy with α-interferon (letter). Neurology 1996;46:588–589

209. Scelsa SN, Herskovitz S, Reichler B. Treatment of mononeuropathy multiplex in hepatitis C virus and cryglobulinemia. Muscle Nerve 1998;21:1526–1529

210. Sakajiri K, Takamori M. Multiple mononeuropathy during recombinant interferon-alpha 2a therapy for chronic hepatitis C [in Japanese]. Rinsho Shinkeigaku 1992;32:1041–1043

211. Quattrini A, Comi G, Nemni R, et al. Axonal neuropathy associated with interferon-α treatment for hepatitis

C: HLA-DR immunoreactivity in Schwann cells. Acta Neuropathol 1997;94:504–508

212. Negoro K, Fukusako T, Morimatsu M, Liao C. Acute axonal polyneuropathy during interferon-α-2a therapy for chronic hepatitis C (letter). Muscle Nerve 1994;17:1351–1352

213. Marzo ME, Tintore M, Fabregues O, et al. Chronic inflammatory demyelinating polyneuropathy during treatment with interferon-alpha (letter). J Neurol Neurosurg Psychiatry 1998;65:604

214. Irioka T, Yamada M, Yamawaki M, et al. Acute autonomic and sensory neuropathy after interferon α-2b therapy for chronic hepatitis C (letter). J Neurol Neurosurg Psychiatry 2001;70:408–410

215. Read SJ, Crawford DH, Pender MP. Trigeminal sensory neuropathy induced by interferon-alpha therapy (letter). Aust N Z J Med 1995;25:54

216. Geltner D. Therapeutic approaches to mixed cryoglobulinemia. Springer Semin Immunopathol 1988;10:103–113

217. Valbonesi M, Montani F, Mosconi L, et al. Plasmapheresis and cytotoxic drugs for mixed cryoglobulinemia. Haematologia 1984;17:341–451

218. Roullet E, Assuerus V, Gozlan J, et al. Cytomegalovirus multifocal neuropathy in AIDS: analysis of 15 consecutive cases. Neurology 1994; 44:2174–2182

219. Lipkin WI, Parry G, Kiprov D, Abrams D. Inflammatory neuropathy in homosexual men with lymphadenopathy. Neurology 1985;35:1479–1483

220. Valeriano-Marcet J, Ravichandran L, Kerr LD. HIV associated systemic necrotizing vasculitis. J Rheumatol 1990;17:1091–1093

221. Chamouard JM, Smadja D, Chaunu MP, Bouche P. Neuropathie par vasculite necrosanta au cours de l'infection par le VIH1. Rev Neurol (Paris) 1993:358–361

222. Massari M, Salvarani C, Portioli I, et al. Polyarteritis nodosa and HIV infection: no evidence of a direct pathogenic role of HIV. Infection 1996:24:159–161

223. Schifitto G, Barbano RL, Kieburtz KD, et al. HIV related vasculitic mononeuropathy: a role for IVIg? (letter). J Neurol Neurosurg Psychiatry 1997;63:255–256

224. So YT, Olney RK. The natural history of mononeuropathy multiplex and simplex in patients with HIV infection (abstract). Neurology 1991;41(Suppl 1):375

225. Jayne DR, Rasmussen N. Treatment of antineutrophil cytoplasm autoantibody-associated systemic vasculitis: initiatives of the European Community Systemic Vasculitis Clinical Trials Study Group. Mayo Clin Proc 1997;72:737–747

226. Rasmussen N, Hoffman GS. Collaborative studies in Europe and the USA: where to go? Clin Exp Immunol 2000;120(Suppl 1):17

227. Jayne D. Update on the European Vasculitis Study Group trials. Curr Opin Rheumatol 2001;13:48–55

228. Jayne D. Evidence-based treatment of systemic vasculitis. Rheumatology 2000;39:585–595

229. Baggenstoss, AH, Shick RM, Polley HF. The effect of cortisone on the lesions of periarteritis nodosa. Am J Pathol 1951;27:537–559

230. Stratton HJ, Price TM, Skelton MO. Granuloma of the nose and periarteritis nodosa. BMJ 1953;1:127–130

231. Hollander D, Manning RT. The use of alkylating agents in the treatment of Wegener's granulomatosis. Ann Intern Med 1967:67:393–398

232. Hoffman GS. Immunosuppressive therapy is always required for treatment of Wegener's granulomatosis. Sarcoidosis Vasc Diffuse Lung Dis 1996;13:249–252

233. Frohnert PP, Sheps SG. Long-term follow-up study of periarteritis nodosa. Am J Med 1967;43:8–14

234. Leib ES, Restivo C, Paulus HE. Immunosuppressive and corticosteroid therapy of polyarteritis nodosa. Am J Med 1979;67:941–947

235. Fahey J, Leonard E, Churg J, Godman G. Wegener's granulomatosis. Am J Med 1954;17:168–179

236. Fauci AS, Wolff SM. Wegener's granulomatosis: studies in eighteen patients and a review of the literature. Medicine 1973;52:535–561

237. Fauci AS, Haynes BF, Katz P, et al. Wegener's granulomatosis: prospective and therapeutic experience with 85 patients for 21 years. Ann Intern Med 1983;98:76–85

238. Kissel JT, Collins MP, Mendell JR. Vasculitic neuropathy. In: Mendell JR, Kissel JT, Cornblath DR, eds. Diagnosis and Management of Peripheral Nerve Disorders. New York: Oxford University Press, 2001:202–232

239. Guillevin L, Rosser J, Cacoub P, et al. Methylprednisolone in the treatment of Wegener's granulomatosis, polyarteritis nodosa and Churg–Strauss angiitis. APMIS Suppl 1990;19:52–53

240. Lino AM, Hirata MT, Baeta AM, et al. Terapeutica intravenosa com metilprednisolona e ciclofosfamida na vasculite do sistema nervoso periferico. Avaliacao de oito pacientes. Arq Neuropsiquiatr 1998;56:274–280

241. Hogan SL, Nachman PH, Wilkman AS, et al. Prognostic markers in patients with antineutrophil cytoplasmic autoantibody-associated microscopic polyangiitis and glomerulonephritis. J Am Soc Nephrol 1996;7:23–32

242. Nachman PH, Hogan SL, Jennette JC, Falf RJ. Treatment response and relapse in antineutrophil cytoplasmic autoantibody-associated microscopic polyangiitis and glomerulonephritis. J Am Soc Nephrol 1996;7:33–39

243. Langford CA. Treatment of polyarteritis nodosa, microscopic polyangiitis, and Churg–Strauss syndrome: where do we stand? (editorial). Arthritis Rheum 2001;44:508–512

244. Guillevin L, Jarrousse B, Lok C, et al. Long-term follow-up after treatment of polyarteritis nodosa and Churg–Strauss angiitis with comparison of steroids, plasma exchange and cyclophosphamide to steroids and plasma exchange. A prospective randomized trial of 71 patients. J Rheumatol 1991;18:567–574

245. Cohen RD, Conn DL, Ilstrup DM. Clinical features, prognosis, and response to treatment in polyarteritis. Mayo Clin Proc 1980;55:146–155

246. Gayraud M, Guillevin L, le Toumelin P, et al. Long-term followup of polyarteritis nodosa, microscopic polyangiitis, and Churg–Strauss syndrome: analysis of four prospective trials including 278 patients. Arthritis Rheum 2001;44:666–675

247. Fauci AS, Katz P, Haynes BF, Wolff SM. Cyclophosphamide therapy of severe systemic necrotizing vasculitis. N Engl J Med 1979;301:235–238

248. Wilke WS. Large vessel vasculitis (giant cell arteritis, Takayasu arteritis). Baillieres Clin Rheumatol 1997;11:285–313

249. So YT. Giant cell arteritis, polymyalgia rheumatica and Takayasu arteritis. In: Aminoff MJ, Goetz CG, eds. Handbook of Clinical Neurology. Vol 27 (71): Systemic Diseases, Part III. New York: Elsevier Science, 1998:191–207

250. Evans JM, Hunder GG. Polymyalgia rheumatica and giant cell arteritis. Rheum Dis Clin North Am 2000;26:493–515

251. Langford CA. Takayasu's arteritis, giant cell arteritis, and polymyalgia rheumatica. In: Weisman MH, Wein-

blatt ME, Louie JS, eds. Treatment of the Rheumatic Diseases. Companion to Kelley's Textbook of Rheumatology. Philadelphia: WB Saunders, 2001:353–363

252. Birkhead NC, Wagener HP, Shick RM. Treatment of temporal arteritis with adrenal corticosteroids: results in fifty-five cases in which lesion was proved at biopsy. JAMA 1957;163:821–827

253. Russell RW. Giant-cell arteritis. A review of 35 cases. QJM 1959;28:471–489

254. Behn AR, Perera T, Myles AB. Polymyalgia rheumatica and corticosteroids: how much for how long? Ann Rheum Dis 1983;42:374–378

255. Myles AB, Perera T, Ridley MG. Prevention of blindness in giant cell arteritis by corticosteroid treatment. Br J Rheumatol 1992;31:103–105

256. Nesher G, Rubinow A, Sonnenblick M. Efficacy and adverse effects of different corticosteroid dose regimens in temporal arteritis: a retrospective study. Clin Exp Rheumatol 1997;15:303–306

257. Gonzalez-Gay MA, Blanco R, Rodriguez-Valverde V, et al. Permanent visual loss and cerebrovascular accidents in giant cell arteritis. Arthritis Rheum 1998;41:1497–1504

258. Kupersmith MJ, Langer R, Mitnick H, et al. Visual performance in giant cell arteritis (temporal arteritis) after 1 year of therapy. Br J Ophthalmol 1999;83:796–801

259. Golbus J, McCune WJ. Giant cell arteritis and peripheral neuropathy: a report of 2 cases and review of the literature. J Rheumatol 1987;14:129–134

260. Nesher G, Rosenberg P, Shorer Z, et al. Involvement of the peripheral nervous system in temporal arteritis-polymyalgia rheumatica. Report of 3 cases and review of the literature. J Rheumatol 1987;14:358–360

261. Caselli RJ, Daube JR, Hunder GG, Whisnant JP. Peripheral neuropathic syndromes in giant cell (temporal) arteritis. Neurology 1988;38:685–689

262. Rivest D, Brunet D, Desbiens R, Bouchard J-P. C-5 radiculopathy as a manifestation of giant cell arteritis. Neurology 1995;45:1222–1224

263. Fishel B, Zhukovsky G, Alon M, et al. Peripheral neuropathy associated with temporal arteritis. Clin Rheumatol 1998;17:163–165

264. Sneller MC, Hoffman GS, Talar-Williams C, et al. An analysis of forty-two Wegener's granulomatosis patients treated with methotrexate and prednisone. Arthritis Rheum 1995;38:608–613

265. Langford CA, Fauci AS, Talar-Williams C, Sneller MC. Treatment of Wegener's granulomatosis with methotrexate and glucocorticoids: update on rate of relapse (abstract). Arthritis Rheum 1996;39(Suppl): S211

266. de Groot K, Muhler M, Reinhold-Keller E, et al. Induction of remission in Wegener's granulomatosis with low dose methotrexate. J Rheumatol 1998;25:492–495

267. Stone JH, Tun W, Hellman DB. Treatment of non-life threatening Wegener's granulomatosis with methotrexate and daily prednisone as the initial therapy of choice. J Rheumatol 1999;26:1134–1139

268. Hoffman GS, Kerr GS, Leavitt RY, et al. Wegener granulomatosis: an analysis of 158 patients. Ann Intern Med 1992;116:488–498

269. Gordon M, Luqmani RA, Adu D, et al. Relapses in patients with a systemic vasculitis. QJM 1993;86: 779–789

270. Guillevin L, Cordier J-F, Lhote F, et al. A prospective, multicenter, randomized trial comparing steroids and pulse cyclophosphamide versus steroids and oral cyclophosphamide in the treatment of generalized Wegener's granulomatosis. Arthritis Rheum 1997;40:2187–2198

271. Richmond R, McMillan TW, Luqmani RA. Optimisation of cyclophosphamide therapy in systemic vasculitis. Clin Pharmacokinet 1998;34:79–90

272. Adu D, Pall A, Luqmani RA, et al. Controlled trial of pulse versus continuous prednisolone and cyclophosphamide in the treatment of vasculitis. QJM 1997; 90:401–409

273. Gayraud M, Guillevin L, Cohen P, et al. Treatment of good-prognosis polyarteritis nodosa and Churg–Strauss syndrome: comparison of steroids and oral or pulse cyclophosphamide in 25 patients. French Cooperative Study Group for Vasculitides. Br J Rheumatol 1997;36:1290–1297

274. Haubitz M, Schellong S, Gobel U, et al. Intravenous pulse administration of cyclophosphamide versus daily oral treatment in patients with antineutrophil cytoplasmic antibody-associated vasculitis and renal involvement. Arthritis Rheum 1998;41:1835–1844

275. Nachman PH, Hogan SL, Dooley MA, et al. Remission, relapse and side effects in patients with ANCA-small vessel vasculitis (SVV) treated with intravenous (IV) versus oral (PO) cyclophosphamide (CYP) (abstract). J Am Soc Nephrol 1997;8:94A

276. Aasarod K, Iversen BM, Hammerstrom J, et al. Wegener's granulomatosis: clinical course in 108 patients with renal involvement. Nephrol Dial Transplant 2000;15:611–618

277. Jayne DR, Gaskin G, Pusey CD, Lockwood CM. ANCA and predicting relapse in systemic vasculitis. QJM 1995;88:127–133

278. Westman KW, Bygren PG, Olsson H, et al. Relapse rate, renal survival, and cancer morbidity in patients with Wegener's granulomatosis or microscopic polyangiitis with renal involvement. J Am Soc Nephrol 1998;9:842–852

279. Jayne D, Gaskin G. Randomized trial of cyclophosphamide versus azathioprine during remission in ANCA-associated vasculitis (CYCAZAREM) (abstract). J Am Soc Nephrol 1999;10:105A

280. Pusey CD. Microscopic polyangiitis. Clin Exp Immunol 2000;120(Suppl 1):32

281. de Groot K, Reinhold-Keller E, Tatsis E, et al. Therapy for the maintenance of remission in sixty-five patients with generalized Wegener's granulomatosis. Methotrexate versus trimethoprim/sulfamethoxazole. Arthritis Rheum 1996;39:2052–2061

282. Langford CA, Talar-Williams C, Barron KS, Sneller MC. A staged approach to the treatment of Wegener's granulomatosis. Induction of remission with glucocorticoids and daily cyclophosphamide switching to methotrexate for remission maintenance. Arthritis Rheum 1999;42:2666–2673

283. Haubitz M, Koch KM, Brunkhorst R. Cyclosporin for the prevention of disease reactivation in relapsing ANCA-associated vasculitis. Nephrol Dial Transplant 1998;13:2074–2076

284. Nachman PH, Segelmark M, Westman K, et al. Recurrent ANCA-associated small vessel vasculitis after transplantation; a pooled analysis. Kidney Int 1999;56:1544–1550

285. Nowack R, Gobel U, Klooker P, et al. Mycophenolate mofetil for maintenance therapy of Wegener's granulomatosis and microscopic polyangiitis: a pilot study in 11 patients with renal involvement. J Am Soc Nephrol 1999;10:1965–1971

286. Metzler C, Low-Friedrich I, Reinhold-Keller E, et al.

Leflunomide, a new, promising agent in maintenance of remission in Wegener's granulomatosis (abstract). Clin Exp Immunol 1998;112(Suppl 1):56

287. DeRemee RA, McDonald TJ, Weiland LH. Wegener's granulomatosis: observations on treatment with antimicrobial agents. Mayo Clin Proc 1985;60:27–32

288. Israel HL. Sulfamethoxazole-trimethoprim therapy for Wegener's granulomatosis. Arch Intern Med 1988;148:2293–2295

289. Boudes P. Wegener's granulomatosis and trimethoprim/sulfamethoxazole treatment (letter). Arthritis Rheum 1989;32:1052

290. Rasmussen N, Petersen J, Remvig L, Andersen V. Treatment of Wegener's granulomatosis with trimethoprim-sulfamethoxazole. APMIS Suppl 1990; 19:61–62

291. Reinhold-Keller E, de Groot K, Rudert H, et al. Response to trimethoprim/sulfamethoxazole in Wegener's granulomatosis depends on the phase of disease. QJM 1996;89:15–23

292. Cohen Tervaert JW, Stegeman CA, Kallenberg CG. Novel therapies for anti-neutrophil cytoplasmic antibody-associated vasculitis. Curr Opin Nephrol Hypertens 2001;10:211–217

293. Stegeman CA, Cohen Tervaert JW, de Jong PE, Kallenberg CG. Trimethoprim-sulfamethoxazole (co-trimazole) for the prevention of relapses of Wegener's granulomatosis. N Engl J Med 1996;335:16–20

294. Falk RJ, Nachman PH, Hogan SL, Jennette JC. ANCA glomerulonephritis and vasculitis: A Chapel Hill perspective. Semin Nephrol 2000;20:233–243

295. Collins MP, Kissel JT, Mendell JR. Vasculitic neuropathies. In: Antel J, Birnbaum G, Hartung H-P, eds. Clinical Neuroimmunology. Malden, MA: Blackwell Science, 1998:316–339

296. Fortin PR, Larson MG, Watters K, et al. Prognostic factors in systemic necrotizing vasculitis of the polyarteritis nodosa group—a review of 45 cases. J Rheumatol 1995;22:78–84

297. Guillevin L, Lhote F, Gayrand M, et al. Prognostic factors in polyarteritis nodosa and Churg–Strauss syndrome: a prospective study in 342 patients. Medicine 1996;75:17–28

298. Tesar V, Jelinkova E, Masek E, et al. Influence of plasma exchange on serum levels of cytokines and adhesion molecules in ANCA-positive renal vasculitis. Blood Purif 1998;16:72–80

299. Guillevin L, Fain O, Lhote F, et al. Lack of superiority of steroids plus plasma exchange to steroids alone in the treatment of polyarteritis nodosa and Churg–Strauss syndrome. A prospective, randomized trial in 78 patients. Arthritis Rheum 1992;35:208–215

300. Guillevin L, Lhote F, Cohen P, et al. Corticosteroids plus pulse cyclophosphamide and plasma exchanges versus corticosteroids plus pulse cyclophosphamide alone in the treatment of polyarteritis nodosa and Churg–Strauss syndrome patients with factors predicting poor prognosis. Arthritis Rheum 1995;38:1638–1645

301. Gianviti A, Trompeter RS, Barrat TM, et al. Retrospective study of plasma exchange with idiopathic rapidly progressive glomerulonephritis and vasculitis. Arch Dis Child 1996;75:186–190

302. Pusey CD, Rees AJ, Evans DJ, et al. Plasma exchange in focal necrotizing glomerulonephritis without anti-GBM antibodies. Kidney Int 1991;40:757–763

303. Berkman EM, Orlin JB. Use of plasmapheresis and partial plasma exchange in the management of

patients with cryoglobulinemia. Transfusion 1980; 20:171–178

304. Gorevic PD, Kassab HJ, Levo Y, et al. Mixed cryoglobulinemia: clinical aspects and long-term follow-up of 40 patients. Am J Med 1980;69:287–308

305. McLeod BC, Sassetti RJ. Plasmapheresis with return of cryoglobulin-depleted autologous plasma (cryoglobulinpheresis) in cryoglobulinemia. Blood 1980; 55:866–870

306. Sinico RA, Fornasieri A, Fiorini G, et al. Plasma exchange in the treatment of essential mixed cryoglobulinemia nephropathy. Long-term follow up. Int J Artif Organs 1984;8(Suppl 2):15–18

307. Ferri C, Gremignai G, Bombardieri S, et al. Plasma-exchange in mixed cryoglobulinemia. Effects on renal, liver and neurological involvement. La Ricerca Clin Lab 1986;16:403–411

308. Frankel AH, Singer DR, Winearls CG, et al. Type II essential mixed cryoglobulinemia: presentation, treatment and outcome in 13 patients. QJM 1992;82:101–124

309. Apartis E, Leger J-M, Musset L, et al. Peripheral neuropathy associated with essential mixed cryoglobulinemia: a role for hepatitis C virus infection? J Neurol Neurosurg Psychiatry 1996;60:661–666

310. Murai H, Inaba S, Kira J, et al. Hepatitis C virus associated cryoglobulinemic neuropathy successfully treated with plasma exchange. Artif Organs 1995;19:334–338

311. Scott DG, Bacon PA, Bothamley JE, et al. Plasma exchange in rheumatoid vasculitis. J Rheumatol 1981;8:433–439

312. Roux H, Gaborit P, Bonnefoy-Cudraz M, et al. Echanges plasmatiques et polyarthrites rhumatoides avec vascularite. A propos de six observations. Rev Rhum Mal Osteoartic 1983;50:105–109

313. Winkelstein A, Starz TW, Agarwal A. Efficacy of combined therapy with plasmapheresis and immunosuppressants in rheumatoid vasculitis. J Rheumatol 1984;11:162–166

314. Iwamoto Y, Okuda B, Tachibana H, Sugita M. A case of allergic granulomatous angiitis with beneficial effects of plasma exchange [in Japanese]. Rinsho Shinkeigaku 1997;37:115–118

315. Strickler RB, Sanders KA, Owen WF, et al. Mononeuritis multiplex associated with cryoglobulinemia in HIV infection. Neurology 1992;42:2103–2105

316. Chalopin JM, Rifle G, Turc JM, et al. Immunological findings during successful treatment of HBsAg-associated polyarteritis nodosa by plasmapheresis alone. Br Med J 1980;280:368

317. Saraux H, Le Hoang P, Laroche L. Neuropathie optique ischeemique aigue anterieure et posterieure au cours d'une peri-arterite noueuse. Traitement par plasmapherese. J Fr Ophtalmol 1982;5:55–61

318. Hattori M, Ito K, Konomoto T, et al. Plasmapheresis as the sole therapy for rapidly progressive Henoch-Schonlein purpura nephritis in children. Am J Kidney Dis 1999;33:427–433

319. Wysenbeek AJ, Calabrese LH, Mandel DR, Clough JD. Limited plasmapheresis in fulminant leukocytoclastic vasculitis. J Rheumatol 1982;9:315–318

320. Bletry O, Bussel A, Badelon I, et al. Interet des echanges plasmatiques au cours des angeites necrosantes. 11 cas. Nouv Presse Med 1982;11:2827–2831

321. Georganas C, Ioakimidis D, Iatrou C, et al. Relapsing Wegener's granulomatosis: successful treatment with cyclosporin-A. Clin Rheumatol 1996;15:189–192

322. Turner AN, Whittaker S, Banks I, et al. Plasma

exchange in refractory cutaneous vasculitis. Br J Dermatol 1990;122:411–415

323. Fregoni V, Perseghin P, Epsis R, et al. Churg–Strauss syndrome with peripheral polyneuropathy refractory to steroidal and immunosuppressive therapy successfully treated with plasma exchange. Recenti Prog Med 1995;86:353–354

324. Hughes RA, Cameron JS, Hall SM, et al. Multiple mononeuropathy as the initial presentation of systemic lupus erythematosus—nerve biopsy and response to plasma exchange. J Neurol 1982;228: 239–247

325. Jayne DR, Lockwood CM. Pooled intravenous immunoglobulin in the management of systemic vasculitis. Adv Exp Med Biol 1993;336:469–472

326. Boman S, Ballen JL, Seggev JS. Dramatic responses to intravenous immunoglobulin in vasculitis. J Intern Med 1995;238:375–377

327. Gedalia A, Correa H, Kaiser M, Sorensen R. Case report: steroid sparing effect of intravenous gamma globulin in a child with necrotizing vasculitis. Am J Med Sci 1995;309:226–228

328. Richter C, Schnabel A, Csernok E, et al. Treatment of anti-neutrophil cytoplasmic antibody (ANCA)-associated vasculitis with high-dose intravenous immunoglobulin. Clin Exp Immunol 1995;101:2–7

329. Altmeyer P, Seifarth D, Bacharach-Muhles M. Hochdosierte intravenose Immunglobulin (IVIG)-Therapie bei therapieresistenter ANCA-negativer, nekrotisierender Vaskulitis. Hautarzt 1999;50:853–858

330. Levy Y, Sherer Y, George J, et al. Serologic and clinical response to treatment of systemic vasculitis and associated autoimmune disease with intravenous immunoglobulin. Int Arch Allergy Immunol 1999; 119:231–238

331. Jayne DR, Chapel H, Adu D, et al. Intravenous immunoglobulin for ANCA-associated systemic vasculitis with persistent disease activity. QJM 2000; 93:433–439

332. Uziel Y, Silverman ED. Intravenous immunoglobulin therapy in a child with cutaneous polyarteritis nodosa. Clin Exp Rheumatol 1998;16:187–189

333. Schollmeyer P, Grotz W. Ciclosporin in the treatment of Wegener's granulomatosis (WG) and related diseases. APMIS Suppl 1990;19:54–55

334. Allen NB, Caldwell DS, Rice JR, McCallum RM. Cyclosporin A therapy for Wegener's granulomatosis. Adv Exp Med Biol 1993;336:473–476

335. McDermott EM, Powell RJ. Cyclosporin in the treatment of Churg–Strauss syndrome (letter). Ann Rheum Dis 1998;57:258–259

336. Ballare M, Bobbio F, Poggi S, et al. A pilot study on the effectiveness of cyclosporine in type II mixed cryoglobulinemia. Clin Exp Rheumatol 1995;13(Suppl 13):S201–S203

337. Schmaldienst S, Winkler S, Breiteneder S, Horl WH. Severe nephrotic syndrome in a patient with Henoch-Schonlein purpura: complete remission after cyclosporine A. Nephrol Dial Transplant 1997;12: 790–792

338. Papo T, Le Thi Huong D, Wiederkehr JL, et al. Etoposide in Wegener's granulomatosis (letter). Rheumatology 1999;38:473–475

339. Morton SJ, Lanyon PC, Powell RJ. Etoposide in Wegener's granulomatosis (letter). Rheumatology 2000;39:810–811

340. Lockwood CM, Thiru S, Stewart S, et al. Treatment of refractory Wegener's granulomatosis with humanized monoclonal antibodies. QJM 1996;89:903–912

341. Lockwood CM. Refractory Wegener's granulomatosis: a model for shorter immunotherapy of autoimmune diseases. J R Coll Physicians Lond 1998;32:473–478

342. Hagen EC, de Keizer RJ, Andrassy K, et al. Compassionate treatment of Wegener's granulomatosis with rabbit anti-thymocyte globulin. Clin Nephrol 1995;43:351–359

343. Van der Woude FJ, Schmitt WH, Birck R, et al. New immunomodulating concepts in ANCA-associated disease. Clin Exp Immunol 2000;120(Suppl 1):16

344. Nachman PH, Joy MS, Hogan SL, et al. Mycophenolate mofetil (MMF): preliminary results of a feasibility trial in relapsing ANCA small vessel vasculitis (abstract). Clin Exp Immunol 2000;120(Suppl 1):72

345. Birck R, Warnatz K, Lorenz HM, et al. Successful treatment of refractory ANCA-associated vasculitis (mostly Wegener's granulomatosis) with 15-deoxyspergualin (abstract). Arthritis Rheum 2000;43(Suppl):S367

346. Stone JH, Uhlfelder MI, Hellman DB, et al. Etanercept in Wegener's granulomatosis: a six-month open-label trial to evaluate safety (abstract). Arthritis Rheum 2000;43(Suppl):S404

347. Tyndall A, Fassas A, Passweg J, et al. Autologous haematopoietic stem cell transplants for autoimmune disease—feasibility and transplant-related mortality. Bone Marrow Transplant 1999;24:729–734

348. Elliot JD, Lockwood CM, Hale G, Waldmann H. Semi-specific immuno-absorption and monoclonal antibody therapy in ANCA positive vasculitis: experience in four cases. Autoimmunity 1998;28:163–171

349. Lockwood CM, Elliot JD, Brettman L, et al. Anti-adhesion molecule therapy as an interventional strategy for autoimmune inflammation. Clin Immunol 1999; 93:93–106

350. Boumpas DT. Glucocorticoid therapy for immune diseases: basic and clinical correlates. Ann Intern Med 1993;119:1198–1208

351. Hochberg MC, Prashker MJ, Greenwald M, et al. Recommendations for the prevention and treatment of glucocorticoid-induced osteoporosis (American College of Rheumatology Task Force on Osteoporosis Guidelines). Arthritis Rheum 1996;39:1791–1801

352. Eastell R, Reid DM, Compston J, et al. A UK Consensus Group on management of glucocorticoid-induced osteoporosis: an update. J Intern Med 1998;244:271–292

353. Adachi JD, Olszynski WP, Hanley DA, et al. Management of corticosteroid-induced osteoporosis. Semin Arthritis Rheum 2000;29:228–251

354. Buckley LM. Clinical and diagnostic features of glucocorticoid-induced osteoporosis. Clin Exp Rheumatol 2000;18(Suppl 21):S41–S43

355. Adachi JD, Bensen WG, Brown J, et al. Intermittent etidronate therapy to prevent corticosteroid-induced osteoporosis. N Engl J Med 1997;337:382–387

356. Wallach S, Cohen S, Reid DM, et al. Effects of risedronate treatment on bone density and vertebral fracture in patients on corticosteroid therapy. Calcif Tissue Int 2000;67:277–285

357. Amin S, LaValley MP, Simms RT, Felson DT. The role of vitamin D in corticosteroid-induced osteoporosis. A meta-analytic approach. Arthritis Rheum 1999;42: 1740–1751

358. Dalsky GP, Stocke KS, Ehsani AA, et al. Weight-bearing exercise training and lumbar bone mineral content in postmenopausal women. Ann Intern Med 1988;108:824–828

359. Talar-Williams C, Hijazi YM, Walther MM, et al. Cyclophosphamide-induced cystitis and bladder

cancer in patients with Wegener granulomatosis. Ann Intern Med 1996;124:477–484

360. Ognibene FP, Shelhaamer JH, Hoffman GS, et al. *Pneumocystis carinii* pneumonia: a major complication of immunosuppressive therapy in patients with Wegener's granulomatosis. Am J Respir Crit Care Med 1995;151:795–799

361. Chung JB, Armstrong K, Schwartz JS, Albert D. Cost-effectiveness of prophylaxis against *Pneumocystis*

carinii pneumonia in patients with Wegener's granulomatosis undergoing immunosuppressive therapy. Arthritis Rheum 2000;43:1841–1848

362. Sindrup SH, Jensen TS. Pharmacologic treatment of pain in polyneuropathy. Neurology 2000;55:915–920

363. Koutantji M, Pearce S, Harrold E. Psychological aspects of vasculitis (editorial). Rheumatology 2000;39:1173–1179

The Treatment of Multifocal Motor Neuropathy with Conduction Block (MMN-CB)

Bruce V Taylor

Overview and historical points

Multifocal motor neuropathy with conduction block (MMN-CB) is a rare, focal, motor predominant mononeuropathy multiplex. It was first recognized as an entity in 1982.[1] In 1988, Pestronk described five additional patients with conduction block neuropathy, serum antiganglioside antibodies and a therapeutic response to immunomodulating therapy with cyclophosphamide.[2] Subsequently, numerous small series of patients and small treatment trials have been published.[3–5] It is clear that MMN-CB is not a new disorder as most patients had previously received the diagnosis of focal motor neuron disease or monomelic amyotrophy, or had multiple nerve decompressions for presumed entrapment neuropathies.

Epidemiology

MMN-CB is an uncommon entity with less than 200 cases presented in the world literature. It has been estimated that in major centers 10 patients will be seen with motor neuron disease (the major differential diagnosis of MMN-CB) for every case of MMN-CB.[6] MMN-CB is usually seen in patients older than 18 years of age and generally has its onset before the age of 45. There is a slight male to female preponderance of 1.5:1.[7]

Etiology

There are few etiological clues as to the cause of MMN-CB. An association with prior campylobacter infection has been suggested.[8] Several acute postinfectious cases of motor conduction block neuropathy have been reported following acute, well-documented campylobacter enteritis.[9,10] An association with antiganglioside antibodies and a response to immunomodulating therapy in a majority of cases may suggest an underlying abnormality of autoimmunity.

Pathophysiology and pathogenesis

Understanding of the underlying pathophysiology of MMN-CB has been hampered by the lack of pathological studies of mixed nerves at the site of conduction block. Evidence for both demyelination with inflammation[11] and axonal loss[12] has been reported. Minor changes of demyelination in the sural nerves of patients with MMN-CB have been noted.[13] A lack of clear diagnostic criteria has hampered the investiga-

tion of the pathological basis of the disorder. Electrophysiological studies have demonstrated significant generalized demyelination with conduction block,[14,15] while others have emphasized axonal loss as the principal electrophysiological substrate of the condition.[7] An autoimmune etiology for MMN-CB is supported by the presence of high titer antibodies directed at ganglioside epitopes in a significant proportion of cases.[16] Additional evidence is provided by induction of conduction block by in vivo antibody transfer in some studies.[17–19] but not in others.[20,21] An antibody mediated process centered on the nodes of Ranvier and in particular the axolemma at this site would explain many of the observed features.[22]

Genetics

There is currently no evidence that MMN-CB is a genetic illness.

Clinical features

MMN-CB is an upper limb predominant, generally asymmetric motor mononeuropathy multiplex.[4,7] The cardinal symptom is painless weakness often involving the small muscles of the hands. Onset is usually over months to years but can be more rapid. Wasting frequently occurs, particularly late in the course of the disease, but is present in up to 50% of cases at diagnosis. Cramps and fasciculations are seen in less than a third of cases. Cranial motor nerves are rarely if ever involved,[23] similarly the phrenic nerves are only rarely affected.[24] Reflexes are usually depressed in affected limbs and are therefore often asymmetrical. The presence of upper motor neuron signs or more than minimal sensory symptoms and signs should raise significant diagnostic doubt. Autonomic symptoms and pain are not seen. The electrophysiological hallmark of this condition is the presence of focal conduction block of motor fibers in mixed nerves, not at common sites of compression and without significant temporal dispersion. In the majority of cases the disease progresses slowly: no deaths directly attributable to MMN-CB have been recorded. The natural history of MMN-CB is of slow progression over many years with hand function frequently being disproportionately affected. Nearly all patients retain their ability to live independently and to care for themselves and the majority remain at work although with some modification of the work environment.[7]

Classification

Attempts at defining subgroups on the basis of severity of conduction block, presence of serum ganglioside antibodies, elevated CSF protein or response to immunomodulating therapy have not proved successful.

Diagnostic criteria

These are shown in Table 199.1.

Differential diagnosis

In general, MMN-CB is a unique neuropathic process, easily distinguishable from its major differential diagnoses. Confusion occurs when the diagnostic criteria are not met or there are confounding variables. The presence of an added sensory neuropathy such as diabetic distal sensory polyneuropathy may make for difficulty in arriving at the correct diagnosis. The principal differentials include the recently described Lewis–Sumner syndrome,[25] motor predominant chronic inflammatory demyelinating polyradicu-loneuropathy (CIDP), monomelic motor neuron disease, progressive muscular atrophy, and hereditary neuropathy with pressure palsy. The eponymous term Lewis–Sumner syndrome was coined recently to describe a group of patients with motor predominant conduction block neuropathy, significant generalized peripheral nerve demyelination and a good response to immunomodulating therapy.[25] Most authors feel that the Lewis–Sumner syndrome is a variant of CIDP and is clearly clinically and electrophysiologically distinct from MMN-CB.

Treatment

One of the principal reasons for the significant research and clinical interest in MMN-CB has been the awareness that a significant proportion of patients will respond to the use of immunomodulating therapy. Certainly, the initial reports in 1988 by Pestronk et al. of a response to cyclophosphamide in two patients raised much interest.[2] Since then there have been a number of reports dealing with various immunomodulating therapies for treatment of MMN-CB. Most interest has centered on the use of high dose human intravenous immunoglobulin (IVIg) or cyclophosphamide, both intravenously and oral, either as a sole treatment or in combination with IVIg. Corticosteroids have been tried in a number of patients with little success; in some cases they actually worsened the condition.[26–28] Plasma exchange has been demonstrated to be beneficial in a small proportion of cases but there have been reports of patients worsening during treatment with plasma exchange.[29,30] Attempts at treatment with interferon beta-1a have shown some improvement in longstanding cases where other therapies have been unsuccessful[31] but in other reports deterioration in a significant proportion of patients has been noted.[32] Cerebrospinal fluid (CSF) filtration and immunoabsorption have not produced significant responses.[33,34]

In 1992, Charles et al. produced the first case report of the use of IVIg in the treatment of MMN-CB, reporting a patient who, after five days of 0.2 g/kg of intravenous immunoglobulin, noted a striking improvement in muscle strength that lasted 6 to 7 weeks.[35] Shortly afterwards, Kermode et al. produced a second positive report of IVIg in the treatment of MMN-CB, documenting the results of the initial treatment of five patients.[36] Over the next several years multiple small trials describing the beneficial effects of IVIg as treatment for MMN-CB appeared.[4,37,38] All these reports were of short term treatment with IVIg in high dosages. Two small, short, double-blind trials of IVIg therapy have been published. Both demonstrated a clear initial benefit with IVIg therapy.[5,39] Recently, three reports of longer term treatment of patients with IVIg have been published.[4,5,40] Azulay et al. in 1997 reported the treatment of 18 patients with IVIg, followed for 9 to 48 months.[5] They noted a clinical improvement in 67% of patients; however, they noted that the response was transitory. Van den Berg et al. in 1998 reported the long term effect of IVIg in 6 MMN-CB patients, followed for 24

Table 199.1   Based on an assessment of 46 patients with MMN-CB followed longitudinally

CRITERIA FOR THE DIAGNOSIS OF MULTIFOCAL MOTOR NEUROPATHY WITH CONDUCTION BLOCK (MMN-CB)

- Patients have a motor predominant peripheral neuropathy or multiple mononeuropathies without upper motor neuron signs. Minor sensory symtoms are permitted but overt sensorimotor neuropathies are excluded.
- On EMG/NCS persisting motor conduction block must be present not at common sites of compression.

  Minimum criteria for CB
  - A greater than 30% reduction in negative peak area or amplitude between distal and proximal stimulation sites of all motor nerves except the tibial nerve. A greater than 50% reduction in negative peak area and/or amplitude between ankle and knee sites is required for diagnosis of CB in the tibial nerve. In the absence of significant temporal dispersion.
  - CB cannot be assessed on nerves where the distal CMAP amplitude is less than 1 mV.
  - Abnormal temporal dispersion is defined as a >25% increases in the negative peak duration of the proximally evoked CMAP, as compared to that evoked with distal stimulation.
- Diffuse demyelination is absent outside areas of CB.
- Needle examination reveals evidence of active and/or chronic denervation in muscles supplied by nerves with CB.
- Other causes of motor predominant neuropathy must be excluded on clinical, electrophysiological and laboratory criteria. Particulary inherited motor neuropathies or neuronopathies, hereditary neuropathy with liability to pressure palsy, motor neuron disease and chronic or acute inflammatory demyelinating polyneuropathies.

to 48 months.[40] One of the clearest findings was that treatment with IVIg produced an initial good response that lasted for up to a year in one patient, but generally lasted less than 12 weeks in the other five patients. During follow-up, despite regular weekly infusions of immunoglobulin, there was clear evidence of disease progression with loss of muscle power, development of new sites of conduction block, and worsening of some existing sites of conduction block. This suggests that IVIg probably does not specifically alter the underlying pathological process but may slow or partially control it. Bouche et al., in 1995, also demonstrated this finding in 19 patients treated with IVIg. One third responded well to the use of IVIg.[4] However, the response was not sustained and there was clear evidence of disease progression with the development of new sites of conduction block despite continuing therapy with IVIg.

Of the other immunosuppressive agents used, the only modality to have any real success has been the chemotherapeutic alkylating agent cyclophosphamide. Individual case reports have reported stabilization with azathioprine.[4] However, the earliest reports of successful treatment for MMN-CB were with intravenous cyclophosphamide.[2] In 1991, Feldman et al. reported the use of an intensive regimen of $3 g/m^2$ of intravenous cyclophosphamide given over 8 days, followed by the institution of oral cyclophosphamide 2 mg/kg one month later with a significant improvement in the patients studied.[26]

In 1994, Tan reported the benefit of cyclophosphamide using $3 g/m^2$ intravenously, followed by oral cyclophosphamide, and noted that five of the 11 patients with conduction block responded.[41] Oral cyclophosphamide by itself has not been shown to be effective.[23]

Recently, authors have advocated the use of a combination of IVIg and oral cyclophosphamide that allows for a gradual reduction in the frequency of the IVIg infusions.[42] However, the long term effectiveness of this therapy in modifying the underlying disease process is unknown. The use of cyclophosphamide is controversial in this condition as many of the patients are young and have a very slowly progressive disorder which is not life threatening and does not necessarily lead to significant impairment. Cyclophosphamide is associated with the development of secondary tumors, particularly transitional cell cancer of the bladder and lymphoma, hemorrhagic cystitis and liver dysfunction, and does expose the patient to the development of neutropenia.[43–45] There has been one report of the development of acute myelogenous leukemia following prolonged intravenous cyclophosphamide therapy for MMN-CB.[46] The use of oral or intravenous cyclophosphamide should always be accompanied by adequate pre- and post-dosage hydration to prevent the development of hemorrhagic cystitis. The use of the bladder protective agent mesna is not advocated for the dosages of cyclophosphamide utilized to treat MMN-CB provided there is no pre-existing bladder condition and appropriate hydration

is undertaken. A record of the total cumulative dosage of cyclophosphamide should be kept, as there is evidence that the risk of development of secondary tumors is greater once the total administered dosage reaches 85 g.[47] Monitoring patients for the presence of microscopic nonglomerular hematuria may alert the clinician to those patients more likely to develop transitional cell cancers of the bladder.

All patients should receive an initial course of therapy with IVIg. An exception is the unusual situation of a patient with established severe stable atrophy, with no evidence of involvement of nerves elsewhere, in whom observation can be employed.

The most efficacious dosage regimen for IVIg has not been established. Generally, two regimens are used for initiating therapy; they are probably of similar efficacy. The first involves the use of a loading dose of 0.4 g/kg of IVIg daily for 5 days, and the second the use of IVIg 0.4 g/kg once weekly for 6 weeks. Generally, the maximum clinical response is seen 3 weeks following the first regimen and at the end of the 6 week cycle. At this point most neuromuscular physicians will reassess and make a decision as to whether therapy has been successful. Occasionally patients are seen in whom the initial loading dosage may produce a response lasting longer than one year. Maintenance therapy is almost invariably required and the most appropriate maintenance regimen is controversial. Some authors advocate repeating the loading dosage of IVIg for 3 to 5 days monthly or at other intervals depending on the patient's response. Others prefer a decreasing regimen of weekly infusions, initially 0.2 g/kg once weekly for 6 weeks and, if this maintains the patient, then second weekly with gradual reductions in dosage and lengthening of the interval until the minimum dosage of IVIg required is found. In many countries IVIg is in scarce supply, and the second regimen is probably more useful as less IVIg is generally used. Most patients, despite appropriate therapy will progress with the development of new sites of conduction block and increasing weakness and muscle atrophy. Intensifying the regimen of IVIg infusions does not appear to be of benefit, and adjuvant therapy with cyclophosphamide is often considered.

Oral cyclophosphamide can be used in combination with IVIg infusions at a dosage of 2 mg/kg lean body weight orally daily with oral hydration prior to the dosage. Treatment should be limited if possible to one year of therapy or a cumulative dose of less than 85 g of cyclophosphamide. The combination of intravenous cyclophosphamide given at monthly intervals at a dosage of $1 g/m^2$ of body surface area and IVIg has not been studied formally. It may have an advantage over regular oral cyclophosphamide, however, as a lower overall dosage of cyclophosphamide is required. Patients treated with intravenous cyclophosphamide must be well hydrated (e.g. 2 to 3 liters 24 hours before and 48 hours after each infusion) to reduce the risk of hemorrhagic cystitis but do not require continued oral hydration between doses.

All current data on the treatment of MMN-CB are

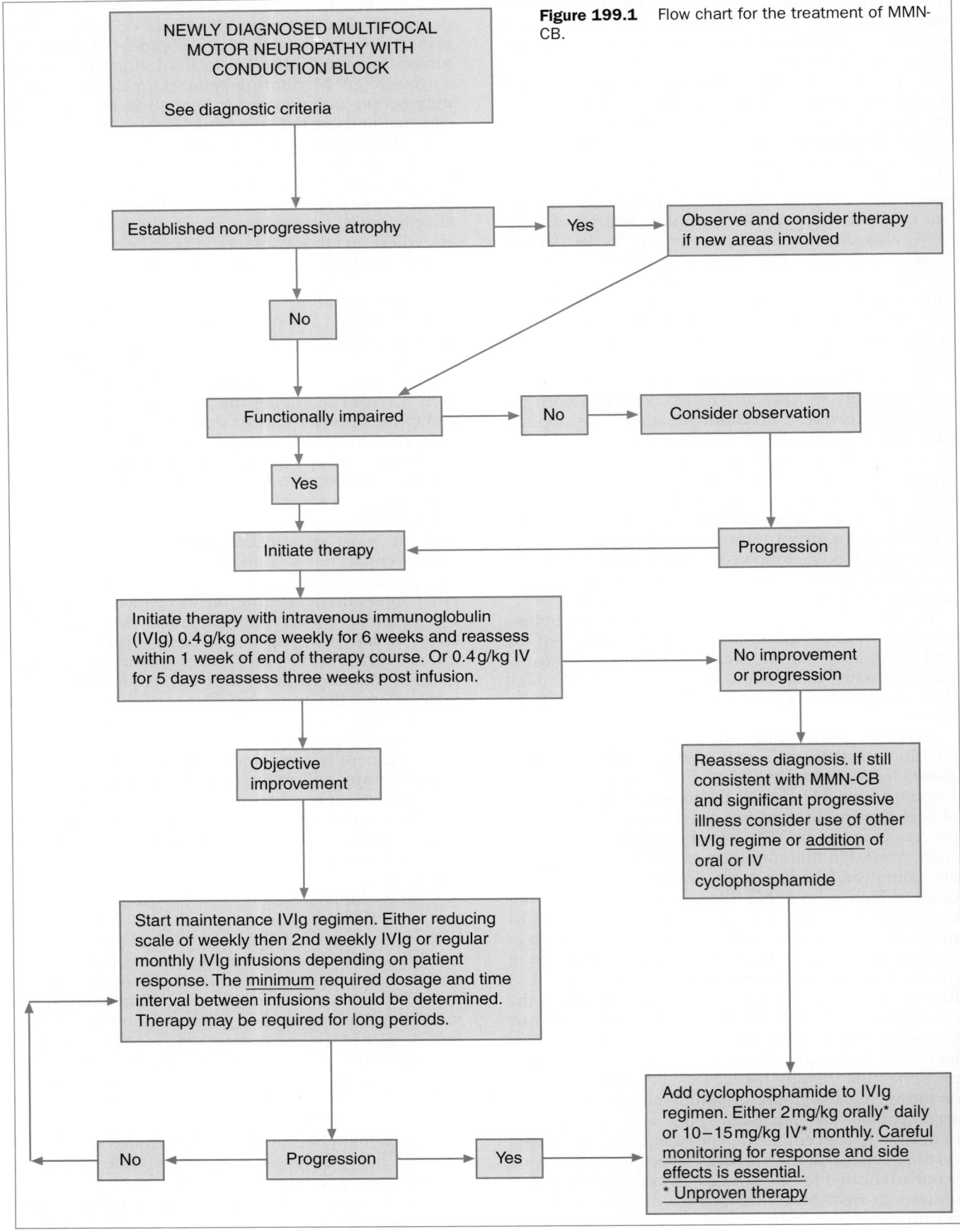

Figure 199.1   Flow chart for the treatment of MMN-CB.

observational, and only two small double-blind trials exist. More information from controlled double-blind large multicenter trials is clearly required but may prove difficult due to the rareness of the condition. It is also clear that different and novel approaches to therapy are required as the current treatment options are not curative and clear disease progression occurs despite seemingly adequate therapy. Additionally, cyclophosphamide has significant side effects and there is no clear risk to benefit analysis for treatment with this medication. Consequently, treatment decisions need to be made on an individual basis. Careful monitoring of objective as well as subjective responses to therapy is highly desirable, particularly when the use of cyclophosphamide is considered. A flow chart for treatment of MMN-CB is presented in Figure 199.1.

References

1. Lewis RA, Sumner AJ. The electrodiagnostic distinctions between chronic familial and acquired demyelinative neuropathies. Neurology 1982;32:592–596
2. Pestronk A, Cornblath DR, Ilyas AA, et al. A treatable multifocal motor neuropathy with antibodies to GM1 ganglioside. Ann Neurol 1988;24:73–78
3. Parry GJ, Clarke S. Multifocal acquired demyelinating neuropathy masquerading as motor neuron disease. Muscle Nerve 1988;11:103–107
4. Bouche P, Moulonguet A, Younes-Chennoufi AB, et al. Multifocal motor neuropathy with conduction block: a study of 24 patients. J Neurol Neurosurg Psychiatry 1995;59:38–44
5. Azulay JP, Rihet P, Pouget J, et al. Long term follow up of multifocal motor neuropathy with conduction block under treatment. J Neurol Neurosurg Psychiatry 1997;62:391–394
6. Chaudhry V. Multifocal motor neuropathy. Semin Neurol 1998;18:73–81
7. Taylor BV, Wright RA, Harper CM, Dyck PJ. Natural history of 46 patients with multifocal motor neuropathy with conduction block. Muscle Nerve 2000;23: 900–908
8. Taylor B, Speed B, et al. Serological evidence for prior infection with the bacterium campylobacter jejuni/coli in multifocal motor neuropathy. J Clin Neurosci 1998;5:33–35
9. Sugie K, Murata K, Ikoma K, et al. A case of acute multifocal motor neuropathy with conduction block after *Campylobacter jejuni* enteritis. Rinsho Shinkeigaku 1998;38:142–145
10. White JR, Sachs GM, Gilchrist JM. Multifocal motor neuropathy with conduction block and *Campylobacter jejuni*. Neurology 1996;46:562–563
11. Kaji R, Oka N, Tsuji T, et al. Pathological findings at the site of conduction block in multifocal motor neuropathy. Ann Neurol 1993;33:152–158
12. Grant I, Gruener G, et al. Focal fibre loss and axonal regeneration is prominent in multifocal motor neuropathy with conduction block. Can J Neurol Sci 1996(Suppl 1):7 (Abstract)
13. Corse AM, Chaudhry V, Crawford TO, et al. Sensory nerve pathology in multifocal motor neuropathy. Ann Neurol 1996;39:319–325
14. Chaudhry V, Corse AM, Comblath DR, et al. Multifocal motor neuropathy: electrodiagnostic features. Muscle Nerve 1994;17:198–205
15. Katz JS, Wolfe GI, Bryan WW, et al. Electrophysiologic findings in multifocal motor neuropathy. Neurology 1997;48:700–707
16. Taylor, BV, Gross L, Windebank AJ. The sensitivity and specificity of anti-GM1 antibody testing. Neurology 1996;47:951–955
17. Santoro M, Uncini A, Corbo M, et al. Experimental conduction block induced by serum from a patient with anti-GM1 antibodies. Ann Neurol 1992;31:385–390
18. Uncini A, Santoro M, Corbo M, et al. Conduction abnormalities induced by sera of patients with multifocal motor neuropathy and anti-GM1 antibodies. Muscle Nerve 1993;16:610–615
19. Roberts M, Willison HJ, Vincent A, Newsom-Davis J. Multifocal motor neuropathy human sera block distal motor nerve conduction in mice. Ann Neurol 1995;38:111–118
20. Harvey GK, Toyka KV, Zielasek J, et al. Failure of anti-GM1 IgG or IgM to induce conduction block following intraneural transfer. Muscle Nerve 1995;18:388–394
21. Hirota N, Kaji R, Bostock H, et al. The physiological effect of anti-GM1 antibodies on saltatory conduction and transmembrane currents in single motor axons. Brain 1997;(120 Pt 12):2159–2169
22. Takigawa T, Yasuda H, Kikkawa R, et al. Antibodies against GM1 ganglioside affect K+ and Na+ currents in isolated rat myelinated nerve fibers. Ann Neurol 1995;37:436–442
23. Kaji R, Shibasaki H, Kimura J. Multifocal demyelinating motor neuropathy: cranial nerve involvement and immunoglobulin therapy. Neurology 1992;42(3 Pt 1): 506–509
24. Beydoun SR, Copeland D. Bilateral phrenic neuropathy as a presenting feature of multifocal motor neuropathy with conduction block. Muscle Nerve 2000;23:556–559
25. Saperstein DS, Amato AA, Wolfe GI, et al. Multifocal acquired demyelinating sensory and motor neuropathy: the Lewis-Sumner syndrome. Muscle Nerve 1999;22:560–566
26. Feldman, EL, Bromberg MB, Albers JW, Pestronk A. Immunosuppressive treatment in multifocal motor neuropathy. Ann Neurol 1991;30:397–401
27. Van den Berg LH, Lokhorst H, Wokke JH. Pulsed high-dose dexamethasone is not effective in patients with multifocal motor neuropathy. Neurology 1997;48:1135
28. Donaghy M, Mills K, Boniface SJ, et al. Pure motor demyelinating neuropathy: deterioration after steroid treatment and improvement with intravenous immunoglobulin. J Neurol Neurosurg Psychiatry 1994; 57:778–783
29. Elliott JL, Pestronk A. Progression of multifocal motor neuropathy during apparently successful treatment with human immunoglobulin. Neurology 1994;44: 967–968
30. Carpo M, Cappellari A, Mora G, et al. Deterioration of multifocal motor neuropathy after plasma exchange. Neurology 1998;50:1480–1482
31. Martina I, Doorn PV, Schmitz PI, et al. Chronic motor neuropathies: response to interferon-beta1A after failure of conventional therapies. J Neurol Neurosurg Psychiatry 1999;66:197–201
32. VandenBerg-Vos R, Van den Berg LH, Franssen H, et al. Treatment of multifocal motor neuropathy with interferon-beta1A. Neurology 2000;54:1518–1521
33. Finsterer J, Schwerer B, Bittner BS, Mamoli B. Cerebrospinal fluid filtration and immunoglobulins in multifocal motor neuropathy. Clin Neuropathol 1999;18: 31–36

34. Finsterer J, Derfler K. Immunoadsorption in multifocal motor neuropathy. J Immunother 1999;22:441–442
35. Charles N, Benoit P, Vial C, et al. Intravenous immunoglobulin treatment in multifocal motor neuropathy. Lancet 1992;340:182
36. Kermode AG, Laing BA, Carroll WM, Mastaglia FL. Intravenous immunoglobulin for multifocal motor neuropathy. Lancet 1992;340:920–921
37. Chaudhry V, Corse AM, Comblath DR, et al. Multifocal motor neuropathy: response to human immune globulin. Ann Neurol 1993;33:237–242
38. Nobile-Orazio E, Meucci N, Barbieri S, et al. High-dose intravenous immunoglobulin therapy in multifocal motor neuropathy. Neurology 1993;43(3 Pt 1):537–544
39. Van den Berg LH, Kerkhoff H, Oey PL, et al. Treatment of multifocal motor neuropathy with high dose intravenous immunoglobulins: a double blind, placebo controlled study. J Neurol Neurosurg Psychiatry 1995;59:248–252
40. Van den Berg LH, Franssen H, Wokke JH. The long-term effect of intravenous immunoglobulin treatment in multifocal motor neuropathy. Brain 1998;(121 Pt 3):421–428
41. Tan E, Lynn J, Amato AA, et al. Immunosuppressive treatment of motor neuron syndromes. Arch Neurol 1994;51:194–200
42. Meucci N, Cappellari A, Barbieri S, et al. Long term effect of intravenous immunoglobulins and oral cyclophosphamide in multifocal motor neuropathy. J Neurol Neurosurg Psychiatry 1997;63:765–769
43. Ortmann R, Klippel J. Update on cyclophosphamide for systemic lupus erythematosus. Rheum Dis Clin North Am 2000;26:363–375
44. Baker G, Kahl L, Schumacher HR Jr, et al. Malignancy following treatment of rheumatoid arthritis with cyclophosphamide. Long term case controlled follow-up study. Am J Med 1987;83:1–9
45. Pederson-Bjergaard J, Ersboll J, Hansen VL, et al. Carcinoma of the urinary bladder after treatment with cyclophosphamide for non-hodgkins lymphoma. N Engl J Med 1988;318:1028–1032
46. Chaudhry V, Corse A, et al. Maintainance immune-globulin therapy for multifocal motor neuropathy. Ann Neurol 1996;40:513–514
47. Talar-Williams C, Hijazi YM, Walther MM. Cyclophosphamide induced cystitis and bladder cancer in patients with Wegners granulomatosis. Ann Intern Med 1996;124:477–484

200 Sarcoidosis and Peripheral Neuropathy

Caroline M Klein

Overview

Sarcoidosis is a multisystem granulomatous disease that may involve the nervous system in a small percentage of cases. Affected components of the nervous system may include cranial, spinal, and peripheral nerves. Probably the earliest report of nerve involvement was in 1909 with Heerfordt's[1] description of cranial and spinal nerve deficits in a case of "uveoparotid fever." A subsequent case reported by MacBride in 1923[2] included peripheral neuropathy as well as multiple cranial neuropathies in association with "uveoparotitis," which was recognized later as a manifestation of sarcoidosis.

The most common manifestation of sarcoidosis affecting the peripheral nervous system is cranial neuropathy, whereas generalized sensorimotor peripheral neuropathy or polyradiculopathy occurs much less frequently. As described below, multiple cranial neuropathies may develop either sequentially or simultaneously. Spontaneous remission is possible, particularly with isolated cranial nerve involvement. When treatment is required, response is generally good. Generalized sensorimotor peripheral neuropathy, which is more uncommon, is more likely to occur in the context of chronic systemic or multisystem sarcoidosis and is less likely to remit spontaneously or to respond favorably to available immunomodulating therapies. Treatment regimens, including prolonged corticosteroid therapy, followed by or in conjunction with other immunomodulating agents such as cytotoxic agents or antimalarial drugs, have had limited and variable success. Treatment protocols for more diffuse or generalized peripheral nerve involvement are not well established, particularly because few patients have peripheral nervous system involvement exclusively, but also usually have central nervous system (CNS) lesions that complicate the response to any therapy. Because peripheral or cranial neuropathy due to sarcoidosis has no distinguishing clinical or electrophysiological features, it is important to document evidence of systemic disease or to obtain positive nervous tissue biopsy evidence of sarcoidosis to establish this association.

Clinical features

The frequency of clinical involvement of the nervous system with sarcoidosis has been estimated to be about 5% (range, 3.5% to 16%),[3–12] with a higher percentage (up to 27%) seen in autopsy cases.[13] Because the data about this condition are based on case reports or retrospective reviews of cases, the actual frequency of neurosarcoidosis is unknown. A smaller number of cases has included involvement of cranial, spinal, or peripheral nerves alone or in addition to CNS disease. The most commonly involved nerves are the cranial nerves, reported in 24% to 73% of cases,[3–7,14–16] and peripheral neuropathy has been reported in 6% to 40%.[3–7,14–18] In one large series of 537 patients with sarcoidosis, James and Sharma[7] found 1.3% with peripheral neuropathy and 4.7% with cranial neuropathy. The exact frequency of peripheral nerve involvement in sarcoidosis is probably unknown, because many asymptomatic patients may have sensory nerve conduction abnormalities when specifically tested.[19] As many as one-third of patients with neurological manifestations of sarcoidosis have multiple neurological symptoms in various combinations, without a specific or characteristic pattern (Table 200.1).[4,14]

In many patients, neurological symptoms may be the initial symptoms of the disease.[3,6,9,14,16,20–24] A retrospective review of 25 patients with neurosarcoidosis followed for an average of 10 years at Johns Hopkins Hospital identified neurological symptoms as the initial presenting clinical feature in only 56%, although 88% had systemic sarcoidosis at the time of diagnosis and all eventually developed multisystem disease.[24]

Although neurological manifestations may occur early in the course of this systemic disease, usually within the first 2 years,[3,4,12,22,24–26] some neurological manifestations may be chronic. In particular, peripheral nerve involvement is thought more likely to

---

Table 200.1 Patterns of peripheral nervous system involvement in systemic sarcoidosis

Cranial neuropathy
  Most common
  Cranial nerves II and VII frequently affected
  May occur sequentially or simultaneously

Generalized axonal peripheral neuropathy
  Multiple mononeuropathies
  Symmetric
    Primarily sensory
    Primarily motor
    Mixed sensorimotor (most common)

Polyradiculopathy
  Thoracolumbar levels (most common)
  Multiple cervical levels
  Single or multiple (cauda equina) lumbosacral levels

Acute inflammatory demyelinating polyradiculoneuropathy
  (AIDP); Guillain-Barré syndrome
  Least common

occur in conjunction with chronic systemic disease.[10,17,27] Less commonly, neurological disease is the only manifestation of sarcoidosis.[9,12,15,21,22] At diagnosis, the average age, sex, and race of these patients has not been found to differ from those of the general population of patients with sarcoidosis, the majority of whom are young (30–50 years), female, and African-American.[4,6,7,12] Of interest is that one series reported more cardiac and eye involvement in patients with neurosarcoidosis than in patients with other systemic disease.[12] This association provides insight on prognosis and mortality, because cardiac arrhythmias and sudden cardiac death are common manifestations of cardiac sarcoidosis.[28]

The cause of the neurological manifestations of sarcoidosis is unknown, just as the cause of the disorder itself is as yet undetermined.[29,30] Formation of noncaseating granulomas in various tissues, including nerve, appears to reflect locally enhanced cellular immunity precipitated by an unknown trigger or antigen.[29–31] Various infectious organisms, including cell wall-deficient mycobacteria, noninfectious or environmental agents, and autoimmune antigens, have been proposed as possible triggers for granuloma formation, but none have been proven to be the cause.[30–33]

Pathological examination of peripheral nerves from patients with sarcoid neuropathy has identified inflammatory cells surrounding epineurial blood vessels[33–37] and typical noncaseating granulomas located in the epineurium, perineurium,[34,35,37,38] and, in some cases, the endoneurium.[35,36] Axonal degeneration and demyelination are most likely caused by axonal loss.[35,36] Unmyelinated fibers are usually spared,[34] although their loss in addition to that of myelinated fibers has been reported.[33] The mechanism of nerve injury may be either local compression from granulomas[35,37] or vascular inflammation leading to nerve ischemia.[33] The exact pathophysiological mechanism of nerve fiber degeneration is unclear.[34,39]

Patterns of peripheral nerve involvement in sarcoidosis include multiple mononeuropathies (either cranial or peripheral nerves), polyneuropathy (pure sensory, pure motor, sensorimotor), or polyradiculopathy (Table 200.1).[39] Onset of symptoms may be acute or subacute, including cases that appear clinically similar to Guillain-Barré syndrome[14,17,40,41] ("acute inflammatory demyelinating polyradiculoneuropathy").

Cranial neuropathies

In patients with sarcoidosis, cranial nerve involvement is common and can potentially involve any cranial nerve, but the most frequent form is facial nerve palsy, either unilateral or bilateral.[6,9,12,14,16,21] The optic nerve is the second most commonly affected cranial nerve.[9,42] Trigeminal nerve involvement is generally limited to sensory fibers.[6,21,43] Multiple cranial neuropathies in an individual patient may occur sequentially in a multiple mononeuropathy pattern[44] or simultaneously. Cranial neuropathies usually develop acutely or subacutely[21] and may

spontaneously resolve or respond favorably to treatment.[6,9,12,14,24,45] However, residual facial weakness with aberrant reinnervation occurs occasionally.[7,21,38]

Peripheral neuropathy

Peripheral neuropathy may present as multiple mononeuropathies[3,14,21,36,40] or as symmetrical sensory,[18,21,27,40,46] motor,[5,21] or mixed sensorimotor[5,16,21,40] peripheral neuropathy. Slowly progressive sensorimotor peripheral neuropathy is probably the most common presentation of peripheral nerve disease caused by sarcoidosis.[39,40] A pattern of polyradiculopathy is less common[38,47] but most likely to involve the thoracolumbar levels.[47] Typically, a patchy pattern of nerve root involvement, with sensory changes on the trunk, is associated with mild weakness and asymmetrical deep tendon reflexes.[39,47] Isolated cases of unilateral multiple cervical radiculopathies[48] or single[46] or multiple (cauda equina)[49] lumbosacral root lesions have been reported. Peripheral neuropathy is more likely than cranial neuropathy to occur in chronic systemic sarcoidosis,[9,10,14,40] but cranial neuropathies are often seen in patients with peripheral neuropathy due to sarcoidosis.[5,36,40,42] The clinical course is variable, from acute to chronic to relapsing.[20,21,24,40]

Prognostic factors for patients with neurosarcoidosis, including those with peripheral nerve involvement, are difficult to define because of the small number of patients with this condition and commonly concomitant multisystem disease (Table 200.2). In a retrospective study at Johns Hopkins Hospital of 25 patients with neurosarcoidosis, 90% of the neurological manifestations remitted or improved, but one-third of the patients had a relapsing course.[24] Luke et al.[24] estimated that two-thirds of patients with neurosarcoidosis have a single episode and a good prognosis. However, others suggest that the presence of neurological involvement signifies a poorer outcome.[17,50] Patients with isolated cranial neuropathy have been found to have the best prognosis overall.[24,26,50] CNS lesions (e.g., spinal cord, cerebral, or brainstem mass lesions), optic neuritis, and hydrocephalus are all associated with a much poorer long-term prognosis,[24,26] and patients with any of these conditions are much more likely to experience relapse.[24] In a recent report from Queens Square in London, more than 70% of 15 patients with spinal cord disease consisting of intramedullary tumor or meningitic-radicular disease had clinical deterioration over an 18-month follow-up period.[50] Peripheral nerve disease caused by sarcoidosis, excluding cranial neuropathies, probably has an intermediate prognosis, depending on the extent of associated CNS disease. Polyneuropathy that occurs in conjunction with chronic systemic sarcoidosis seems least likely to improve,[17,21] whereas patients with acute or subacute peripheral neuropathy (without significant CNS involvement) may have a better prognosis, either with or without treatment.[6,21,22,24,39–41,45]

Limited data are available on mortality associated with neurosarcoidosis. One retrospective study of 37

Table 200.2 Prognostic factors in patients with neurosarcoidosis

Good
   Isolated cranial neuropathy
   Mild peripheral neuropathy
Poor
   Hydrocephalus
   Spinal cord lesion (intramedullary mass or meningitic-radicular involvement)
   Cerebral mass lesion
   Epilepsy
   Brainstem mass lesion
   Encephalopathy
   Optic nerve involvement (neuritis)

patients followed over 30 years (1965–1995) reported deaths from complications of sarcoidosis in 18%, half of whom (3 patients, only 1 given a treatment regimen—prednisone) had an acute inflammatory demyelinating polyradiculoneuropathy (similar to Guillain-Barré syndrome).[17]

Diagnosis

Diagnosis of cranial or peripheral neuropathy due to sarcoidosis is relatively straightforward in patients with a prior diagnosis of systemic sarcoidosis in whom other causes of peripheral neuropathy can be excluded. However, as noted above, neurological symptoms may be the initial presentation of the disease, which makes the diagnostic process more challenging. If sarcoidosis is suspected as the underlying cause of peripheral neuropathy in a patient without a systemic diagnosis, careful evaluation for systemic disease may yield evidence of a multisystem disorder in many cases.[51] Frequently, evidence of

intrathoracic disease, as well as ocular abnormalities such as uveitis or iridocyclitis, can be demonstrated, leading to the diagnosis of sarcoidosis.[3,4,6,7,15–17,21,22,47] Approximately 80% to 90% of patients with sarcoidosis, including those with neurological involvement, have intrathoracic disease.[11,17,26,30,51]

Diagnostic evaluation to obtain evidence of systemic sarcoidosis begins with a careful clinical history and a general physical examination (Table 200.3). Specific questioning of the patient about possible occupational or environmental exposures may yield important information. Laboratory evaluation includes routine blood work, urinalysis, and serological testing for Lyme disease, HIV, syphilis, and autoimmune disease, including vasculitis and tuberculin skin testing with cutaneous anergy panel. Plain chest radiography and pulmonary function testing are needed to investigate for pulmonary disease. A baseline electrocardiogram (ECG) and slit-lamp examinations are also recommended. If ECG abnormalities are found, further testing with 24-hour Holter monitoring and echocardiography are warranted.[28] If the chest radiograph is normal, a high-resolution chest CT scan, bronchoscopy, or gallium-67 body scan may yield additional findings.[10,17,50] Some investigators do not recommend gallium 67 for routine clinical use because of the extent of radiation exposure, the scan's lack of spcificity, and the poor correlation between this scan and the clinical course of sarcoidosis.[51] Biopsy of specific tissues is necessary to establish the presence of sarcoidosis in at least 2 different organ systems. Biopsies may be made of lymph nodes, skin lesions, lung, conjunctiva, minor salivary glands (e.g., lower lip), or nasal mucosa, depending on clinical suspicion and abnormal findings on laboratory tests. All biopsy specimens must be examined histologically

Table 200.3 Suggested diagnostic evaluation for peripheral neuropathy due to sarcoidosis

Establish diagnosis of systemic sarcoidosis
  Clinical history, including occupational and environmental exposures
  Physical examination (general, neurological)
  Laboratory examination
    Complete blood count; routine chemistry panel; serum calcium; serum angiotensin-converting enzyme; serological testing for Lyme disease, HIV, syphilis, and autoimmune diseases, including vasculitis
    24-Hour urinary calcium concentration, routine urinalysis
    Plain chest radiography (if negative, consider CT scan of chest, bronchoscopy, gallium-67 body scan)
    Pulmonary function tests
    Electrocardiogram (ECG) (if abnormal, conduct 24-hour ECG monitoring, echocardiography)
    Tuberculin skin test, including cutaneous anergy panel
    Slit-lamp examination
    Biopsy of suspected involved organs (e.g., transbronchial lung, skin lesions, lymph nodes, conjuctiva, minor salivary glands [e.g., lower lip], nasal mucosa)
    Consider rhinoscopy (if history of recurrent acute or chronic sinusitis)
Investigate neurological involvement
  Electrodiagnostic testing with nerve conduction studies, electromyography
  Cerebrospinal fluid examination, including cell count, protein and glucose concentrations, fungal-mycobacterial testing, and bacterial stains and cultures
  Magnetic resonance imaging with contrast medium (gadolinium) of brain and/or spinal cord and nerve roots
  Biopsy of involved peripheral sensory nerve or nerve root
  Consider visual evoked potentials and/or additional neuro-ophthalmological evaluation, including fluorescein angiography

for the presence of noncaseating granulomas and tested specifically for fungal or mycobacterial infectious organisms.

Additional laboratory testing may measure increased serum concentrations of angiotensin-converting enzyme (ACE), which have been found in 30% to 70% of patients with neurosarcoidosis.[10,17,21,45,52] With this relatively nonspecific test,[30] concentrations tend to be increased in patients with pulmonary disease.[10] Even when increased, serum ACE does not appear correlated with the course of neurological disease due to sarcoidosis.[3,45] However, some investigators have suggested serial monitoring of serum ACE in individual patients to document response to therapeutic interventions.[10,11]

Although not considered very sensitive,[39] and currently used in only a small number of centers,[11,30,50,51] the Kveim test may help confirm the diagnosis of systemic sarcoidosis.[16,30,50,53] In this test, intradermal injection of homogenized spleen or lymph node tissue from a patient with sarcoidosis is followed by biopsy of the resulting skin papule 4 to 6 weeks later.[51,53] The Kveim antigen is not commercially available[11,51,53] nor is it approved by the U.S. Food and Drug Administration for routine clinical use in patients, most likely because of concern about the potential transmission of infectious agents such as HIV.[10,51] The widespread availability of other tests that lead more quickly to the diagnosis of sarcoidosis has caused the Kveim test to be used mainly for its historical or research value.

Neurological evaluation also may include examination of cerebrospinal fluid (CSF). Elevated CSF ACE, although highly specific, is relatively insensitive and therefore not considered a reliable diagnostic test.[17,21,39,45,52,54] Additional CSF analysis may or may not reveal abnormalities,[21,27,37,52] such as lymphocytic pleocytosis, elevated protein, and low glucose levels.[5,6,14,16,38,39,42,45,47,52] A decreased level of CSF glucose is more common in patients with more central, particularly meningeal, lesions than in those with isolated peripheral nerve involvement.[14,38,39]

Imaging studies such as magnetic resonance imaging (MRI) of the spine with contrast medium may provide evidence of nerve root enlargement or focal infiltration,[46–49] although this finding is not specific for sarcoidosis. Because the presence of peripheral nerve involvement in systemic sarcoidosis does not exclude the possibility of CNS lesions, which may be relatively asymptomatic, examination of the brain with contrast-enhanced (e.g., gadolinium) MRI must be considered. Electrodiagnostic testing can be used to demonstrate electrophysiological evidence of neuropathy, either cranial or peripheral, and can further characterize the pattern of the abnormality and its severity, including whether it involves multiple mononeuropathies, polyneuropathy (sensory, motor, or sensorimotor), polyradiculopathy, cranial neuropathy, or any combination of these. Both axonal and demyelinating changes may be seen,[15,20,21,34–37,40] but nerve conduction studies may be normal, particularly with patchy or polyradicular involvement only.[43]

Positive nerve or root biopsy for noncaseating granulomas of a clinically involved nerve provides the most conclusive diagnostic evidence of sarcoidosis[33–39,46,49,55] (Figure 200.1). To characterize the pathology adequately and to rule out infectious causes, nerve biopsy should be performed only at a medical center able to conduct a broad array of histological and histochemical analyses. Other causes of granulomatous nerve disease, including tuberculosis, parasitic or fungal disease, and lepromatous disease, should be excluded, if possible.

The differential diagnosis for peripheral neuropathy due to sarcoidosis would include other granulomatous conditions, such as tuberculosis, leprosy, and spirochetal, fungal, or parasitic infection.[55] In addition to conditions identifiable through tissue diagnosis, other causes for the patterns of peripheral neuropathy seen in sarcoidosis, such as systemic or nonsystemic vasculitis, diabetes mellitus, acute or chronic inflammatory demyelinating polyradicu-

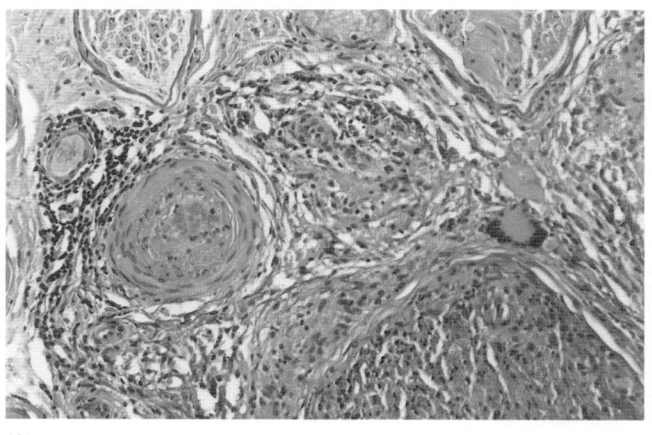
(A)

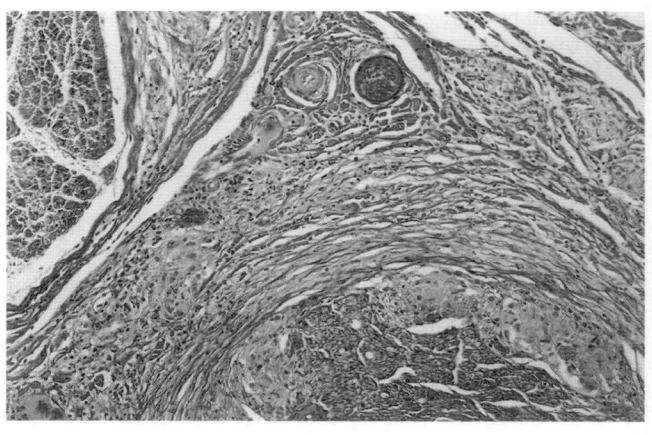
(B)

Figure 200.1   Transverse, paraffin-embedded tissue sections of a sural nerve biopsy from a patient with sarcoidosis. Hematoxylin-eosin stain (A) and Masson stain with trichrome (B) of tissue sections show multinucleated giant cells, epithelioid granuloma, and mononuclear inflammatory cell infiltrates associated with nerve fascicles. (Courtesy of PJ Dyck and J Englestad, Mayo Clinic, Rochester, Minnesota.) (See color plate section.)

lopathy, lymphoma, and meningeal carcinomatosis, should be considered.

Treatment

Patients with peripheral neuropathy due to sarcoidosis have been treated primarily with corticosteroids, which corresponds to the standard clinical management of systemic or pulmonary sarcoidosis.[31,51,56–58] There have been no controlled clinical trials evaluating the efficacy of steroids or any other specific treatments for patients with this condition.[3,16,20,57] This lack of clinical trials is probably due, in part, to the relative rarity of peripheral nerve manifestations in sarcoidosis and also due, in part, to the likelihood that these patients would already be receiving other medical treatment for systemic, particularly pulmonary, manifestations of sarcoidosis. In some cases, the natural history of the disease has been found to include spontaneous remission,[5,16,21,22,24,57] which raises the question of whether treatment is even necessary.[5,6,57] In 1 series of 50 patients, the clinical course of treated patients compared with untreated patients was not found to be clearly different.[14]

Most authors would recommend a course of medical treatment, particularly when neurological involvement is clinically significant[5,10,11,30,45,47,51,58] (Figure 200.2, Table 200.4). Treatment of patients with a high dose of corticosteroids (orally or intravenously), followed by a slow taper, may lead to rapid[3,5,12,23,24,27,35,40,50] but perhaps only minimal or partial[15,21,34,40,50] improvement in neurological symptoms. General recommendations are for treatment with oral prednisone, starting at a dosage of 40 to

Table 200.4 Treatment of peripheral neuropathy due to sarcoidosis	
Drug	**Dosage/administration**
Prednisone/ prednisolone	40–60 mg/d, po[4,10,11,16,17,21,24,38,49,57,58] *or* pulse IV 1000 mg[43,50] *or* 0.5–1 mg/kg[51] *or* 3 g/d for 3 d[10]
Azathioprine	2–3 mg/kg/d, po[56,57,59]
Methotrexate	7.5–25 mg/wk po *or* IM[10,50,56,57,59–61]
Chloroquine/ hydroxychloroquine	250 mg bid *or* 200 mg qd bid *or* qod po[10,17,18,50,51,56,57,59]
Cyclophosphamide	50–150 mg/d po[56,57,59] *or* 0.5–0.75 g/m^2 q mo IV[56,57] *or* 500–2000 mg IV q 2 wk[59]
Chlorambucil	2–8 mg/d po[56,57,59]
Cyclosporine	3–10 mg/kg/d po[56,57,59,62]

bid, twice daily; IM, intramuscular; IV, intravenous; po, oral; q, each, every; qd, every day; qod, every other day.

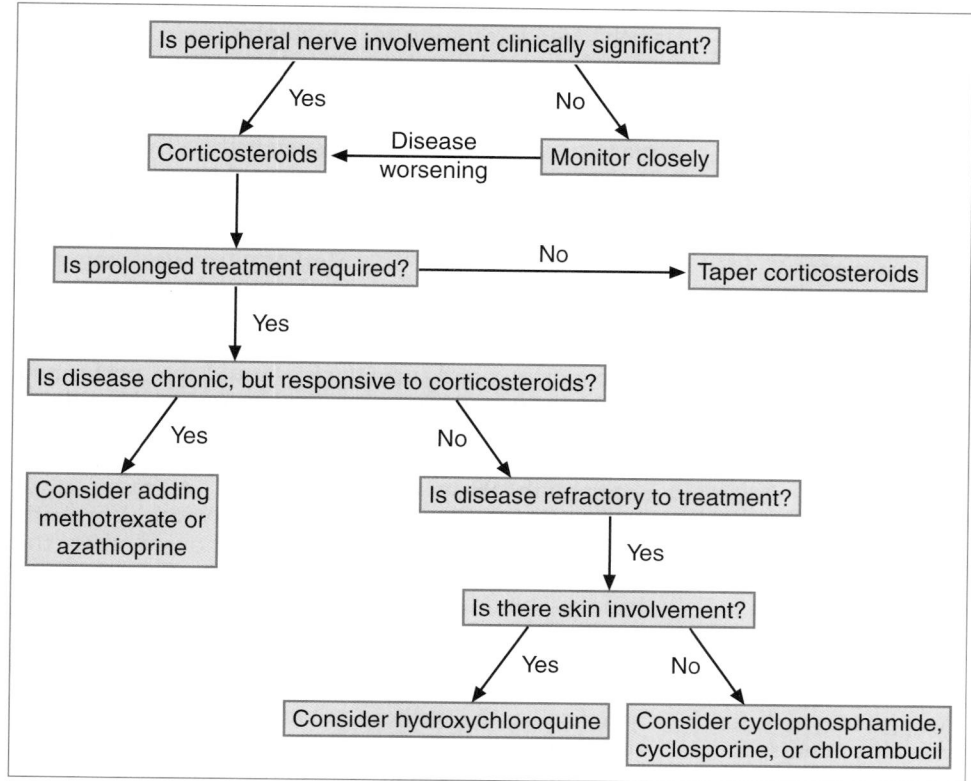

Figure 200.2 Suggested treatment algorithm for peripheral neuropathy in sarcoidosis.

60 mg daily or every other day.[4,10,11,16,17,21,24,38,49,57,58] The course of the peripheral or cranial neuropathy may become relapsing as the immunosuppressive therapy is tapered,[27,44] which may require increasing the dose of prednisone or adding treatment with intravenous corticosteroids.[10,21,43,51] To lessen the chance of relapse, Matthews[44] has suggested continuing steroid treatment for several months after resolution of neurological symptoms. Chronic prednisone therapy, at low dosages such as 10 to 15 mg daily, may be needed if a relapsing course evolves.[10,24] Zajicek et al.[50] used a corticosteroid regimen starting with pulse doses of methylprednisolone (1 g intravenously daily for 3 days) given with 25 mg daily of oral prednisolone or its equivalent and then repeating the intravenous bolus weekly while tapering the oral dose.

If the side effects or complications of steroid therapy become intolerable, if the response to corticosteroids is poor, or if a prolonged course of steroid treatment is anticipated, alternative immunosuppressive treatments should be considered (Figure 200.2). These include cytotoxic agents, such as azathioprine,[21,23,25,47,51,56,57,59] chlorambucil,[21,25,51,56,57,59] methotrexate,[10,12,17,21,25,50,56,57,59–61] cyclophosphamide,[12,25,50,51,56,57,59] and cyclosporine,[21,25,56,57,59,62] or the antimalarial drugs chloroquine and hydroxychloroquine[10,17,18,50,51,59] (Table 200.4). Whether a patient has a response to corticosteroid therapy should be evident in most cases within 1 to 3 months.[57] Sharma[17,18] described good results and no major side effects with the use of chloroquine (250 mg bid) and hydroxychloroquine (200 mg bid) in patients with neurosarcoidosis who could not tolerate treatment with corticosteroids. Stern et al.[62] used a combination of cyclosporine and prednisone in 6 patients with refractory neurosarcoidosis, including 1 patient with peripheral neuropathy. Although this combination was found to be safe and effective, and allowed reduction of the prednisone to 30% to 60% of the initial dose, clinical deterioration occurred in 4 of 6 patients, 1 of whom died. Thus, cyclosporine was found to have minimal treatment benefit apart from its steroid-sparing effect.[62]

A review by Agbogu et al.[25] of multiple alternative immunosuppressive treatments in patients with refractory neurosarcoidosis suggested an algorithm of cyclosporine or azathioprine in combination with corticosteroids when there is inadequate response to steroids alone, followed by chlorambucil, methotrexate, or cyclophosphamide, until the clinical course is stabilized. They recommended an alternative immunosuppressive therapy for patients who develop corticosteroid side effects or require large doses of corticosteroids to control neurological symptoms. Another treatment algorithm suggests azathioprine or methotrexate (alone or in combination with prednisone) or chloroquine or hydroxychloroquine as second-line agents after corticosteroids, with cytotoxic agents such as cyclophosphamide, chlorambucil, and cyclosporine being reserved for chronic, progressive, and refractory cases because of their greater risk for complications and side effects.[57] For all patients, the dose and duration of any medical therapy should be individualized and adjusted according to response and side effects[56,57] (Figure 200.2).

Side effects from prednisone treatment include diabetes mellitus, posterior subcapsular cataracts, hypertension, avascular necrosis, osteoporosis, gastritis, weight gain, tremor, mental status changes, insomnia, and peripheral edema.[63] Patients should be monitored closely for these complications and given appropriate treatment.[56,57,63] Alternate-day prednisone therapy, given as a single dose at 8 AM, may help reduce the likelihood of complications.[63] In the event of trauma, surgery, or intercurrent severe illness, patients receiving long-term corticosteroid therapy should be instructed to take stress-dose hydrocortisone (100–400 mg/d, in divided doses) to minimize medical complications due to adrenal suppression.[51,63] Female patients older than 40 years should have their bone density measured before initiation of corticosteroid therapy.[51,63] Low-risk patients whose degree of bone loss at baseline is not severe are unlikely to need corticosteroids long-term or become immobilized, but should be given estrogen, vitamin D, and calcium supplementation. In contrast, when bone loss is severe, the patients who have a history of vertebral compression fractures or who are likely to be immobilized or need long-term corticosteroid therapy should be given alendronate (5 mg orally daily). Postmenopausal patients not receiving hormone replacement therapy also should be prescribed alendronate (10 mg orally daily).[63] Gastrointestinal complications from corticosteroid therapy may be minimized by instructing patients to take their medication with food and to avoid the use of nonsteroidal anti-inflammatory drugs.[63]

If used, additional immunosuppressive therapy, such as azathioprine, methotrexate, cyclophosphamide, cyclosporine, or chlorambucil, requires monitoring of the patient's complete blood count and liver function tests to check for toxic effects on bone marrow and the liver, respectively (Table 200.5). Patients taking methotrexate should be scheduled for liver biopsies after each 1000 mg to monitor for hepatotoxicity, which cannot be detected necessarily from routine blood tests.[51,59,61] Methotrexate use may also lead to mucositis, which can usually be treated with oral folate (1 mg orally daily).[61] In addition, renal function should be monitored in patients taking cyclosporine, and urinalysis should be performed regularly in patients receiving cyclophosphamide to monitor for hemorrhagic cystitis.[56,57,59] Long-term increased risk of hematological malignancy may also occur with these cytotoxic agents. A case-control study of 119 patients who had rheumatoid arthritis treated with cyclophosphamide showed that the treated group had a higher incidence of cancer (e.g., urinary, bladder, skin, and hematological malignancies) than the controls.[64] The mean total dose and mean duration of cyclophosphamide treatment were the most significant risk factors for future malignancy. Specifically, the authors recommend routine screening with cystoscopy for patients receiving a cumulative dose greater than 85 g.[64]

Table 200.5   Most common potential treatment complications

Drug	Complication	Possible intervention
Cyclophosphamide	Hemorrhagic cystitis Nausea Carcinogenicity Hematological Teratogenicity Gonadal dysfunction	Increased oral fluid intake Antiemetic with IV therapy Intermittent IV dosing vs. oral dosing CBC q mo Appropriate contraception Possible use of long-acting gonadotropin-releasing hormone analogues*
Methotrexate	Hepatotoxicity Mucositis Teratogenicity Hematological Renal toxicity	Liver biopsy after each 1-g cumulative dose Folate 1 mg po qd Appropriate contraception CBC q mo Avoid if creatinine >0.3 mg/dL Limited use of nonsteroidal anti-inflammatory medications Renal function monitoring
Hydroxychloroquine	Retinal toxicity Nausea	Eye exam q 6 mo Take with meals
Azathioprine	Hematological Nausea Teratogenicity	CBC q mo Divided dosing Appropriate contraception
Cyclosporine	Hypertension Renal toxicity Hematological malignancies	Frequent monitoring Renal function monitoring CBC during and after treatment
Chlorambucil	Hematological Teratogenicity Carcinogenicity	CBC q mo Appropriate contraception Frequent monitoring

CBC, complete blood count; IV, intravenous; po, oral; q, each, every; qd, every day.
*Effectiveness not proven. See Conclusion of this chapter.
Data from Baughman and Lower.[59]

In both male and female patients of childbearing age, possible teratogenic side effects of these medications should be avoided with proper contraceptive use.[51,56,57] Before initiating treatment, patients should be counseled about their potential risk for infertility and other gonadal dysfunction. In general, alkylating agents such as cyclophosphamide have a greater likelihood of causing gonadal toxicity than do antimetabolites such as methotrexate.[65-67] The patient's age at initiation of treatment, the medication dose, and the duration of treatment are also important factors in determining the risk of gonadal toxicity.[65-69] For both men and women, increasing age is generally inversely correlated to the dose of cytotoxic agent leading to clinically significant gonadal dysfunction.[65] Sperm cryopreservation before treatment (given normal sperm count and motility) is a good option for male patients.[65] Female patients may wish to consider embryo cryopreservation (which can be time-consuming and expensive) or even oocyte or ovarian tissue cryopreservation, which may be possible in the future.[67,70] Women older than 30 years may develop primary ovarian failure due to treatment with cytotoxic agents such as cyclophosphamide, resulting in early menopausal symptoms and increased risk of osteoporosis and cardiovascular disease.[65,69] Sequential hormonal replacement with estrogen and progestin is required to alleviate this complication.[65,69]

These patients typically need a higher dose of estrogen (1.25 mg conjugated estrogen) than do women with natural menopause.[69] Currently, no known treatment is effective for infertility from primary ovarian failure, but a 5% to 10% chance of pregnancy has been reported notwithstanding.[69] Some authors have also suggested potential protection of gonadal function during chemotherapy with the use of long-acting gonadotropin-releasing hormone analogues that suppress gonadal activity,[65,66,68] but this approach remains unproven.[70]

Chloroquine and hydroxychloroquine have known ocular toxicities that should be monitored with regular ophthalmological examinations.[18,56] Prolonged treatment with chloroquine has been shown to lead to additional possible complications, such as toxic myopathy, cardiopathy, peripheral neuropathy, and neuropsychiatric disturbances.[18] Hydroxychloroquine may help reduce hyperglycemia in patients who also have diabetes mellitus or steroid-induced hyperglycemia that limits their treatment with corticosteroids.[18] Both drugs have been used safely in patients with neurosarcoidosis to stabilize symptoms successfully, either continuously for as long as 21 months or intermittently for more than 3 years.[18] However, all patients on immunosuppressive treatment should be carefully monitored for infectious complications.

Conclusion

Overall, the prognosis is good for improvement or recovery in patients with peripheral or cranial neuropathy due to sarcoidosis.[4,21,24] Peripheral neuropathy in the context of chronic systemic sarcoidosis is most likely to have a chronic course and to be more challenging therapeutically (Figure 200.2).

Although the etiological agent responsible for sarcoidosis has not been identified, further investigation into the immune response involved in this condition may lead to more specific treatments.[30] In particular, the development of agents that inhibit the steps leading to T-cell activation and cytokine release seen in sarcoidosis holds promise for future therapeutic options.[30,31] One area of recent investigation has focused on drugs known to inhibit the activity of tumor necrosis factor alpha, such as thalidomide and pentoxifylline.[30,51,71,72] Thus far, thalidomide has been reported to be of benefit only for treatment of cutaneous sarcoidosis.[30,59,71,73,74] However, a major potential side effect of this medication, in addition to its teratogenicity,[71,75] is sensory peripheral neuropathy,[71,73,75,76] which makes it an unlikely candidate for treatment of peripheral nerve disease due to sarcoidosis. Treatment of pulmonary sarcoidosis with pentoxifylline monotherapy or combination therapy with corticosteroids has demonstrated benefits in terms of stabilizing or improving the condition of patients with pulmonary disease or of producing a steroid-sparing effect.[72] To date, pentoxifylline has not been used specifically to treat peripheral nerve disease in sarcoidosis.

References

1. Heerfordt CT. Uber eine Febris uveo-parotidea sub-chronica, an der Glandula parotis und der uvea der Auges lokalisiert und haufig mit Paresen cerebrospinaler Nerven kompliziert. Graefes Arch Ophthal 1909;70:94–254

2. MacBride HJ. Uveoparotitic paralysis. J Neurol Psychopathol 1923;4:242

3. Chen RC, McLeod JG. Neurological complications of sarcoidosis. Clin Exp Neurol 1989;26:99–112

4. Stern BJ, Krumholz A, Johns CJ. Neurosarcoidosis: presentation and management. Ann N Y Acad Sci 1986; 465:722–730

5. Silverstein A, Feuer MM, Siltzbach LE. Neurologic sarcoidosis. Arch Neurol 1965;12:1–11

6. Wiederholt WC, Siekert RG. Neurological manifestations of sarcoidosis. Neurology 1965;15:1147–1154

7. James DG, Sharma OP. Neurosarcoidosis. Proc R Soc Med 1967;60:1169–1170

8. Mayock RL, Bertrand P, Morrison CE, Scott JH. Manifestations of sarcoidosis: analysis of 145 patients, with a review of nine series selected from the literature. Am J Med 1963;35:67–89

9. Delaney P. Neurologic manifestations in sarcoidosis: review of the literature, with a report of 23 cases. Ann Intern Med 1977;87:336–345

10. Belfer MH, Stevens RW. Sarcoidosis: a primary care review. Am Fam Physician 1998;58:2041–2050, 2055–2056

11. DeRemee RA. Sarcoidosis. Mayo Clin Proc 1995;70: 177–181

12. Lower EE, Broderick JP, Brott TG, Baughman RP. Diag-nosis and management of neurological sarcoidosis. Arch Intern Med 1997;157:1864–1868

13. Manz HJ. Pathobiology of neurosarcoidosis and clinico-pathologic correlation. Can J Neurol Sci 1983;10:50–55

14. Oksanene V. Neurosarcoidosis: clinical presentations and course in 50 patients. Acta Neurol Scand 1986;73: 283–290

15. Wells CE. The natural history of neurosarcoidosis. Proc R Soc Med 1967;60:1172–1174

16. Stern BJ, Krumholz A, Johns C, et al. Sarcoidosis and its neurological manifestations. Arch Neurol 1985;42: 909–917

17. Sharma OP. Neurosarcoidosis: a personal perspective based on the study of 37 patients. Chest 1997;112: 220–228

18. Sharma OP. Effectiveness of chloroquine and hydroxy-chloroquine in treating selected patients with sarcoidosis with neurological involvement. Arch Neurol 1998; 55:1248–1254

19. Challenor YB, Felton CP, Brust JC. Peripheral nerve involvement in sarcoidosis: an electrodiagnostic study. J Neurol Neurosurg Psychiatry 1984;47:1219–1222

20. Scott TF. Neurosarcoidosis: progress and clinical aspects. Neurology 1993;43:8–12

21. Chapelon C, Ziza JM, Piette JC, et al. Neurosarcoidosis: signs, course and treatment in 35 confirmed cases. Medicine (Baltimore) 1990;69:261–276

22. Oksanen V, Gronhagen-Riska C, Fyhrquist F, Somer H. Systemic manifestations and enzyme studies in sarcoidosis with neurologic involvement. Acta Med Scand 1985;218:123–127

23. Elkin R, Willcox PA. Neurosarcoidosis: a report of 5 cases. S Afr Med J 1985;67:943–946

24. Luke RA, Stern BJ, Krumholz A, Johns CJ. Neurosarcoidosis: the long-term clinical course. Neurology 1987; 37:461–463

25. Agbogu BN, Stern BJ, Sewell C, Yang G. Therapeutic considerations in patients with refractory neurosarcoidosis. Arch Neurol 1995;52:875–879

26. Neville E, Walker AN, James DG. Prognostic factors predicting the outcome of sarcoidosis: an analysis of 818 patients. Q J Med 1983;52:525–533

27. Payne CR, Tait D, Batten JC. Sarcoidosis and chronic sensory neuropathy. Postgrad Med J 1980;56:781–782

28. Mitchell DN, du Bois RM, Oldershaw PJ. Cardiac sarcoidosis (editorial). BMJ 1997;314:320–321

29. Moller DR. Etiology of sarcoidosis. Clin Chest Med 1997;18:695–706

30. Muller-Quernheim J. Sarcoidosis: immunopathogenetic concepts and their clinical application. Eur Respir J 1998;12:716–738

31. Agostini C, Costabel U, Semenzato G. Sarcoidosis news: immunologic frontiers for new immunosuppressive strategies. Clin Immunol Immunopathol 1998;88: 199–204

32. Jones RE, Chatham WW. Update on sarcoidosis. Curr Opin Rheumatol 1999;11:83–87

33. Vital C, Aubertin J, Ragnault JM, et al. Sarcoidosis of the peripheral nerve: a histological and ultrastructural study of two cases. Acta Neuropathol (Berl) 1982;58: 111–114

34. Galassi G, Gibertoni M, Mancini A, et al. Sarcoidosis of the peripheral nerve: clinical, electrophysiological and histological study of two cases. Eur Neurol 1984;23: 459–465

35. Oh SJ. Sarcoid polyneuropathy: a histologically proved case. Ann Neurol 1980;7:178–181

36. Nemni R, Galassi G, Cohen M, et al. Symmetric sarcoid

polyneuropathy: analysis of a sural nerve biopsy. Neurology 1981;31:1217–1223

37. Gainsborough N, Hall SM, Hughes RA, Leibowitz S. Sarcoid neuropathy. J Neurol 1991;238:177–180
38. Scott TS, Brillman J, Gross JA. Sarcoidosis of the peripheral nervous system. Neurol Res 1993;15:389–390
39. Matthews WB. Sarcoid neuropathy. In: Dyck PJ, Thomas PK, Griffin JW et al., eds. Peripheral Neuropathy. Vol 2, 3rd ed. Philadelphia: WB Saunders, 1993: 1418–1423
40. Zuniga G, Ropper AH, Frank J. Sarcoid peripheral neuropathy. Neurology 1991;41:1558–1561
41. Strickland GT Jr, Moser KM. Sarcoidosis with a Landry-Guillain-Barre syndrome and clinical response to corticosteroids. Am J Med 1967;43:131–135
42. Colover J. Sarcoidosis with involvement of the nervous system. Brain 1948;71:451–475
43. Allen RK, Merory J. Intravenous pulse methyl prednisolone in the successful treatment of severe sarcoid polyneuropathy with pulmonary involvement. Aust N Z J Med 1985;15:45–46
44. Matthews WB. Sarcoidosis of the nervous system. J Neurol Neurosurg Psychiat 1965;28:23–29
45. Lynch JP III, Sharma OP, Baughman RP. Extrapulmonary sarcoidosis. Semin Respir Infect 1998;13: 229–254
46. Baron B, Goldberg AL, Rothfus WE, Sherman RL. CT features of sarcoid infiltration of a lumbosacral nerve root. J Comput Assist Tomogr 1989;13:364–365
47. Koffman B, Junck L, Elias SB, et al. Polyradiculopathy in sarcoidosis. Muscle Nerve 1999;22:608–613
48. Atkinson R, Ghelman B, Tsairis P, et al. Sarcoidosis presenting as cervical radiculopathy: a case report and literature review. Spine 1982;7:412–416
49. Campbell JN, Black P, Ostrow PT. Sarcoid of the cauda equina: case report. J Neurosurg 1977;47:109–112
50. Zajicek JP, Scolding NJ, Foster O, et al. Central nervous system sarcoidosis—diagnosis and management. QJM 1999;92:103–117
51. Johns CJ, Michele TM. The clinical management of sarcoidosis: a 50-year experience at the Johns Hopkins Hospital. Medicine (Baltimore) 1999;78:65–111
52. Oksanen V. New cerebrospinal fluid, neurophysiological and neuroradiological examinations in the diagnosis and follow-up of neurosarcoidosis. Sarcoidosis 1987; 4:105–110
53. James DG, Williams WJ. Kveim-Siltzbach test revisited. Sarcoidosis 1991;8:6–9
54. Dale JC, O'Brien JF. Determination of angiotensin-converting enzyme levels in cerebrospinal fluid is not a useful test for the diagnosis of neurosarcoidosis (letter). Mayo Clin Proc 1999;74:535
55. Williams WJ. The identification of sarcoid granulomas in the nervous system. Proc R Soc Med 1967;60: 1170–1172
56. Baughman RP, Lower EE. Steroid-sparing alternative treatments for sarcoidosis. Clin Chest Med 1997;18: 853–864
57. Baughman RP, Sharma OP, Lynch JP III. Sarcoidosis: is therapy effective? Semin Respir Infect 1998;13:255–273
58. Turiaf J, Johns CJ, Terstein AS, et al. The problem of the

treatment of sarcoidosis: report of the Subcommittee on Therapy. Ann N Y Acad Sci 1976;278:743–751
59. Baughman RP, Lower EE. Alternatives to corticosteroids in the treatment of sarcoidosis. Sarcoidosis Vasc Diffuse Lung Dis 1997;14:121–130
60. Soriano FG, Caramelli P, Nitrini R, Rocha AS. Neurosarcoidosis: therapeutic success with methotrexate. Postgrad Med J 1990;66:142–143
61. Lower EE, Baughman RP. Prolonged use of methotrexate for sarcoidosis. Arch Intern Med 1995;155:846–851
62. Stern BJ, Schonfeld SA, Sewell C, et al. The treatment of neurosarcoidosis with cyclosporine. Arch Neurol 1992; 49:1065–1072
63. Gorroll AH, Mulley AG Jr. Primary Care Medicine. 4th ed. Philadelphia: Lippincott Williams and Wilkins, 2000: 660–666
64. Baker GL, Kahl LE, Zee BC, et al. Malignancy following treatment of rheumatoid arthritis with cyclophosphamide: long-term case-control follow-up study. Am J Med 1987;83:1–9
65. Chapman RM. Gonadal injury resulting from chemotherapy. Am J Ind Med 1983;4:149–161
66. Waxman J. Chemotherapy and the adult gonad: a review. J R Soc Med 1983;76:144–148
67. Reichman BS, Green KB. Breast cancer in young women: effect of chemotherapy on ovarian function, fertility, and birth defects. J Natl Cancer Inst Monogr 1994;16:125–129
68. Rivkees SA, Crawford JD. The relationship of gonadal activity and chemotherapy-induced gonadal damage. JAMA 1988;259:2123–2125
69. Kalantaridou SN, Nelson LM. Premature ovarian failure is not premature menopause. Ann N Y Acad Sci 2000;900:393–402
70. Meirow D. Ovarian injury and modern options to preserve fertility in female cancer patients treated with high dose radio-chemotherapy for hemato-oncological neoplasias and other cancers. Leuk Lymphoma 1999;33: 65–76
71. Tseng S, Pak G, Washenik K, et al. Rediscovering thalidomide: a review of its mechanism of action, side effects, and potential uses. J Am Acad Dermatol 1996; 35:969–979
72. Zabel P, Entzian P, Dalhoff K, Schlaak M. Pentoxifylline in treatment of sarcoidosis. Am J Respir Crit Care Med 1997;155:1665–1669
73. Lee JB, Koblenzer PS. Disfiguring cutaneous manifestation of sarcoidosis treated with thalidomide: a case report. J Am Acad Dermatol 1998;39:835–838
74. Rousseau L, Beylot-Barry M, Doutre MS, Beylot C. Cutaneous sarcoidosis successfully treated with low doses of thalidomide (letter). Arch Dermatol 1998;134: 1045–1046
75. Powell RJ, Gardner-Medwin JM. Guideline for the clinical use and dispensing of thalidomide. Postgrad Med J 1994;70:901–904
76. Ochonisky S, Verroust J, Bastuji-Garin S, et al. Thalidomide neuropathy incidence and clinico-electrophysiologic findings in 42 patients. Arch Dermatol 1994;130: 66–69

201 Neuropathy Associated with the Monoclonal Gammopathies

Robert A Kyle

Brief overview

The presence of monoclonal protein (IgG, IgA, or IgM) in the serum of a patient with peripheral neuropathy should raise suspicion of primary amyloidosis (AL) or POEMS syndrome (osteosclerotic myeloma) as well as Waldenström's macroglobulinemia, other lymphoproliferative disorders, or multiple myeloma. If these diseases are excluded by appropriate diagnostic studies, the patient may have monoclonal gammopathy of undetermined significance (MGUS) ("benign" monoclonal gammopathy) with associated neuropathy. Not all neuropathies in patients with MGUS are related to the presence of MGUS. Therefore, it is necessary to consider other causes of neuropathy by evaluating the pattern, course, electrophysiological features, cerebrospinal fluid (CSF) findings, and other features of the neuropathy to decide whether it is likely to be related to MGUS.

Monoclonal gammopathy of undetermined significance

Monoclonal gammopathy of undetermined significance is characterized by the presence of M monoclonal (M) protein in persons without evidence of multiple myeloma, macroglobulinemia, amyloidosis, or other related disorders. The term "benign monoclonal gammopathy" is misleading because one does not know at the time of diagnosis whether the M protein will remain stable and benign or progressively increase and the patient develop symptomatic multiple myeloma, macroglobulinemia, or amyloidosis.

The disorder is characterized by the presence of a serum M-protein concentration less than 3 g/dl, less than 10% plasma cells in the bone marrow, no or only a small amount of M protein (light chain, Bence Jones protein) in the urine, and the absence of lytic bone lesions. Furthermore, anemia, hypercalcemia, and renal insufficiency are absent. Most important, stability of the M protein and failure of development of other abnormalities during long-term follow-up are necessary for the diagnosis of MGUS.

Almost two thirds of patients at the Mayo Clinic with newly detected M protein have MGUS.[1] The disorder is found in 3% of patients older than 70 years in Sweden,[2] in the United States,[3] and in France.[4] An M protein is found in approximately 1% of persons older than 50 years.

It is important for both the patient and the physician to determine whether the M protein remains stable and benign or whether symptomatic multiple myeloma, amyloidosis, or macroglobulinemia will develop. At the Mayo Clinic, we have followed 241 patients who had monoclonal gammopathy diagnosed before January 1, 1971, but who had no evidence of multiple myeloma or related disorders at the time the M protein was detected.[1] After follow-up of 24 to 38 years, the number of patients still alive and with a stable M protein (i.e. a benign condition) was 25 (10%) (Table 201.1). The M protein had increased to 3 g/dl or greater in 26 patients (11%), and 127 died of unrelated causes (53%). Multiple myeloma, macroglobulinemia, or a related lymphoproliferative process or primary amyloidosis developed in 63 patients (26%).[5] Of these 63 patients, 43 (68%) had

Table 201.1 Course of 241 patients with monoclonal gammopathy of undetermined significance

Group	Description	At follow-up after 24–38 years	
		No. of patients	%
1	No substantial increase of serum or urine monoclonal protein (benign)	25	10
2	Monoclonal protein ≥3.0 g/dl but no myeloma or related disease	26	11
3	Died of unrelated cause	127	53
4	Development of myeloma, macroglobulinemia, amyloidosis, or related disease	63	26
Total		241	100

From Kyle and Rajkumar.[5] By permission of WB Saunders Company.

This is supported in part by CA62242 from the National Cancer Institute.

multiple myeloma, 8 had primary amyloidosis (AL), 7 had Waldenström's macroglobulinemia, and 5 had malignant lymphoproliferative disease (Table 201.2). The time from recognition of the M protein to the diagnosis of serious disease ranged from 2 to 29 years (median, 10 years). It is obvious that patients with a benign gammopathy must be followed indefinitely because serious disease can develop 30 or more years after M protein is detected. The pertinent features of MGUS, multiple myeloma, primary amyloidosis, and POEMS syndrome (osteosclerotic myeloma) are given in Table 201.3.

Association of monoclonal gammopathy of undetermined significance with peripheral neuropathy

Kahn et al.[6] detected 58 cases of monoclonal gammopathy without evidence of multiple myeloma or related disorders in 1400 serum samples from patients admitted to a large neurological referral hospital. Of the 58 patients, 16 had peripheral neuropathy. Nine of the 16 patients had slow nerve conduction velocities, and 7 of the 9 had an IgM κ monoclonal protein. In another series of 132 patients with monoclonal gammopathy, 4 had peripheral neuropathy, of whom 3 had an IgM κ monoclonal protein.[7]

Table 201.2 Development of myeloma or related diseases in 63 patients with monoclonal gammopathy of undetermined significance

Diseases	No. of patients	%	Interval to diagnosis in years	
			Median	Range
Multiple myeloma	43	68	10	2–29
Macroglobulinemia	7	11	8.5	4–20
Amyloidosis	8	13	9	6–19
Lymphoproliferative	5	8	10.5	6–22
Total	63	100		

From Kyle and Rajkumar.[5] By permission of WB Saunders Company.

Table 201.3 Clinical and laboratory features of MGUS, multiple myeloma, primary amyloidosis, and POEMS syndrome

Feature	MGUS	Multiple myeloma	Primary amyloidosis	POEMS syndrome
Symptoms	Asymptomatic	Bone pain, fatigue	Edema, fatigue, dyspnea, paresthesias	Paresthesias
Peripheral neuropathy	No	No	Yes (15%*)	Yes (90 + %*)
Serum M protein, median, g/dl	1.1	3	1.2	1.1
Size of serum M spike, g/dl	≤3	>3	<3 (93%*)	<3
BMPC, %	≤10	>10	<20	<10
Hemoglobin	Normal	<12 g/dl (65%*)	Normal	Normal or ↑
Serum creatinine	Normal	>2 mg/dl (20%*)	>2 mg/dl (20%*)	Normal
Urine, nephrotic	No	No	Yes (30%*)	No
Skeletal X-ray	Normal	Lytic or fracture	Normal	Sclerotic
Diagnosis	M protein <3 g/dl BMPC < 10% No features of myeloma	BMPC > 10% M protein serum and/or urine (98%*)	Amyloid in tissue: subcutaneous fat (70%*), BM (55%*)	Biopsy of sclerotic lesion
Therapy	None	Autol PBSCT Melphalan/prednisone	Melphalan/prednisone Autol PBSCT	Radiation to lesion If disseminated, melphalan/ prednisone or autol PBSCT

Autol, autologous; BM, bone marrow; BMPC, bone marrow plasma cells; M, monoclonal; MGUS, monoclonal gammopathy of undetermined significance; PBSCT, peripheral blood stem cell transplant.
*Percentage values in parentheses refer to percentage of patients.

During 1 year in the electromyography laboratory at the Mayo Clinic, a clinically apparent neuropathy was identified in 692 patients. Of these patients, 358 had an associated systemic disease (e.g. diabetes mellitus, alcoholism, or connective tissue disorder) known to cause neuropathy and the other 334 had no apparent associated systemic condition. Of these 334 patients, 279 had serum protein electrophoresis, which demonstrated M protein in 28 (10%). The associated diseases were MGUS in 16 patients, primary amyloidosis in 7, myeloma in 3, Waldenström's macroglobulinemia in 1, and γ heavy chain disease in 1 (Table 201.4). Kelly et al.[8] showed a statistically significant increase in the prevalence of M proteins in patients with peripheral neuropathy compared with the normal population in Minnesota, France, and Sweden. Peripheral neuropathy was diagnosed clinically in this group of patients, and the incidence would have been greater if the diagnosis had been based only on electrophysiological evidence.

Etiology and pathogenesis

The cause of peripheral neuropathy associated with monoclonal gammopathy is unknown. In some instances, there may be a genetic factor. A mother and son were reported to have IgM M protein and peripheral neuropathy.[9] In another report, a brother and sister had IgM M protein and demyelinating peripheral neuropathy.[10]

Purified monoclonal IgG from patients with polyneuropathy associated with myeloma or monoclonal gammopathy was injected daily into mice, and the mice developed demyelinating peripheral neuropathy with slowed nerve conduction velocity. Injection of Fab fragments from monoclonal IgG produced a similar demyelination.[11] An IgM protein reacting with myelin-associated glycoprotein (MAG) in three patients with peripheral neuropathy was injected intraneurally in the sciatic nerve of cats and produced demyelination, and the M protein and complement on the surface of the myelin sheaths suggested to Dalakas et al.[12] that the M protein reacted with an epitope of myelin. In contrast, injection of serum from three patients with M proteins and chronic sensorimotor polyneuropathy into rat sciatic nerves showed no evidence of demyelination or nerve conduction abnormalities.[13] The relationship between M protein and demyelinating neuropathy is unclear, but most reports suggest that the immunoglobulin has a role in demyelination. Many investigators believe that the neuropathy in MGUS is due to a demyelinating disorder rather than an axonal one, but this has not been established.

Clinical features

Typically, MGUS neuropathy has the following features: 1) M protein occurs in the serum; 2) amyloidosis, POEMS syndrome (osteosclerotic myeloma), or related disorders are not present; 3) a symmetrical sensorimotor polyradiculopathy or neuropathy occurs, usually beginning insidiously in the toes and extending to the feet and legs; the lower extremities

Table 201.4 Associated diseases in 28 patients with sensorimotor peripheral neuropathy and M protein*	
	No. of patients
MGUS	16
Primary amyloidosis	7
Myeloma	3
Macroglobulinemia	1
Heavy chain disease	1

M, monoclonal; MGUS, monoclonal gammopathy of undetermined significance.
*Serum electrophoresis showed M protein in samples from 28 of 279 patients with neuropathy demonstrated electromyographically.

are involved in 90% of patients and muscle stretch reflexes are decreased or absent; 4) it occurs in the sixth or seventh decades of life; 5) males are affected more frequently than females; 6) paresthesias, ataxia, and pain may be prominent; and 7) cranial nerves are not involved. IgM is the most frequent monoclonal gammopathy, followed by IgG and IgA. The association of neuropathies and monoclonal gammopathies has been reviewed elsewhere.[14–16]

Pathology

The IgM M protein associated with anti-MAG activity and peripheral neuropathy binds to myelin sheaths.[17] Direct electron microscopic immunochemistry studies with colloidal gold show deposition of IgM within the myelin and extending throughout the compact myelin in both large and small myelinated fibers. This finding suggests that the deposition of the IgM M protein has a role in pathogenesis. However, whether IgM initiates the myelin damage or precipitates it in an already damaged nerve has not been determined.

In nine patients with M protein and peripheral neuropathy, endothelial proliferation produced thickening of the vessel walls in the vasa nervorum. These microvascular changes possibly caused ischemia and loss of axons.

Single-fiber preparations may show swelling of internodal myelin. Localization of myelin thickening and widening of myelin lamellae suggest a link between the two abnormalities.[18]

Electromyographic studies

Nerve conduction is characteristically abnormal in motor and sensory fibers in both the upper and lower extremities. Conduction velocity of motor fibers is approximately 20% below the normal range.[19] Smith et al.[19] emphasized the decrease in motor nerve conduction velocity in 12 patients with neuropathy with an IgM M protein. The amplitude of the compound muscle action potential is severely decreased in the lower limb nerves. Frequently, responses cannot be elicited from sensory fibers in upper and lower limb nerves. Needle electromyography shows denervation in 80% of patients. Both demyelination and denervation may be present.[20] The sural nerve usually is involved more severely than the median nerve.

IgM monoclonal proteins and peripheral neuropathy

In 1980, Latov et al.[21] described a patient with sensorimotor peripheral neuropathy and an IgM M protein. The M protein was directed against peripheral nerve myelin, as documented by complement fixation and immunoabsorption. Myelin-associated glycoprotein has a molecular weight of approximately 100 000 and consists of 30% carbohydrate. The IgM M protein binds to a carbohydrate moiety in MAG.[22]

Approximately one half of patients with peripheral neuropathy and IgM M protein have IgM antibodies that bind to MAG.[23–26] This binding is specific because it can be blocked completely by MAG isolated from human myelin.[27] The anti-MAG IgM titers in 16 patients with peripheral neuropathy and IgM M protein reacting with MAG ranged from 1:12 800 to 1:100 000. Low antibody titers to MAG (1:400 or less) were found in 8 of 24 patients with an IgM M protein without neuropathy. Very low titers (1:200 or less) were found in 17% of control patients without monoclonal gammopathy.[28]

The IgM proteins do not bind to *de*glycosylated MAG, which suggests that the reactive determinants contain carbohydrate moieties.[29] It has been shown also that *de*glycosylation of MAG abolishes the recognition of MAG by the patient's IgM protein.[30]

In a review of 40 patients with polyneuropathy associated with an IgM gammopathy, all but one had symmetrical polyneuropathy. It was predominantly sensory in 13 and purely sensory in 17 others. Electrophysiological studies demonstrated demyelination in 83% of patients and axonal degeneration in 6%. Anti-MAG antibodies were found in 65% of patients and were associated only with demyelinating polyneuropathies.[31]

In a series of 52 patients with symptomatic IgM monoclonal gammopathy, symptomatic neuropathy occurred in 3 of 4 patients with a high anti-MAG titer and in 3 of 21 with a low anti-MAG titer.[32] This suggests that anti-MAG activity correlates with peripheral neuropathy.

Reaction of M proteins with components other than MAG

In addition to the MAG determinants, other antigens such as glycolipids have been found.[33] Freddo et al.[34] reported that IgM M protein from 16 patients with anti-MAG activity bound to two glycolipids in the peripheral nerve. Anti-glycolipid antibodies have been associated with IgM neuropathies, Guillain–Barré syndrome, and multifocal neuropathies.[35]

Gangliosides represent other target antigens.[36] Ilyas et al.[37] reported that an IgM M protein from three patients with peripheral neuropathy bound to the carbohydrate portion of MAG and also to a single ganglioside of sciatic nerve. High titers of anti-GD_{1a} ganglioside antibodies were reported in 5% of patients with chronic inflammatory demyelinating polyneuropathy (CIDP), in 18% with multifocal motor neuropathy, in 3.8% with lower motor neuron

disease, and in 1.8% with amyotrophic lateral sclerosis. Some decrease in antibody titer was noted when patients had clinical improvement.[38]

The IgM M protein may be reactive with chondroitin sulfate and produce axonal rather than myelin damage. Clusters of thinly myelinated fibers consistent with regeneration after axonal degeneration were seen in one patient. Others have reported binding of the IgM M protein to chondroitin sulfate C.[39,40] A predominantly sensory neuropathy has been described in association with monoclonal or polyclonal IgM antibodies directed against sulfatide. Ilyas et al.[41] reported reaction with antibody to GD_{1b} or disialosyl gangliosides. Motor neuropathy with anti-G_{M1b} is associated with motor neuropathy.

An extensive review of antibodies associated with peripheral neuropathy was published in 1999.[42]

Differential diagnosis

Neuropathy in MGUS must be distinguished from CIDP, amyloidosis, osteosclerotic myeloma (POEMS syndrome) and multiple myeloma, T-cell and B-cell lymphomatosis involvement, and paraneoplastic neuropathies as well as metabolic and toxic neuropathies.

Chronic inflammatory demyelinating polyneuropathy may occur at any age. In a comparison of 45 patients with CIDP and 15 with MGUS-associated neuropathy, the authors noted that the latter had less severe weakness, greater imbalance, ataxia, loss of vibratory sensation in the hands, and absence of median and ulnar sensory potentials.[43] In another study, the clinical course was progressive in most patients with MGUS, whereas those with CIDP were more likely to have a relapsing course. Impairment appeared to develop more slowly in the patients with MGUS, who also had less severe functional impairment and a lesser degree of weakness as well as sensory changes.[44] In contrast, Maisonobe et al.[45] noted no significant clinical or electrophysiological differences between patients with CIDP and those with CIDP with monoclonal gammopathy. They reported that patients with anti-MAG antibody had more pronounced slowing of the peroneal motor nerve conduction velocity, a lower frequency of conduction block, and a distal accentuation of conduction slowing.[45]

In summary, CIDP may occur at any age. Motor symptoms tend to predominate over sensory symptoms, and there is a greater tendency for the course to be relapsing. M proteins are not found.

Gosselin et al.[46] reviewed their experience with 65 patients with MGUS and sensorimotor peripheral neuropathy: 31 had IgM, 24 had IgG, and 10 had IgA M proteins. Those with an IgM M protein had 1) sensory ataxia, 2) decreased nerve conduction, and 3) more frequent dispersion of the compound muscle action potential. Patients with IgM were overrepresented in the neuropathy group.

In a comparison of 19 patients with IgM MGUS and 15 with IgG MGUS, Simovic et al.[47] noted prolongation of distal latencies of the median and ulnar motor nerves in the IgM MGUS group as well as greater slowing of peroneal nerve conduction velocity and more severe demyelination. Anti-MAG antibodies failed to distinguish a subgroup of patients with IgM MGUS neuropathy.

Neuropathies associated with MGUS differ from those associated with primary amyloidosis in the following respects: 1) in MGUS, the lower limbs are preferentially affected, but upper and lower limbs tend to be affected to a greater degree in amyloidosis; 2) the course in amyloidosis is always slowly progressive; 3) although amyloidosis may present as a sensorimotor neuropathy, autonomic features (postural hypotension, sphincter dysfunction, and anhydrosis) and organ (heart or kidney) failure are often seen. Such autonomic features and organ failure do not occur in MGUS neuropathy.

Treatment

Treatment of patients with peripheral neuropathy and monoclonal gammopathy has shown promise. Plasma exchange produced improvement of neuropathy in 6 of 10 patients with polyneuropathy and monoclonal gammopathy. Three others had stabilization of their neuropathy. After cessation of plasma exchange, the neuropathy progressed.[48] In a randomized trial, 39 patients with MGUS and peripheral neuropathy were assigned to receive either plasma exchange twice weekly or sham plasma exchange in a double-blind trial. Patients who initially had sham plasma exchange subsequently received plasma exchange in an open trial. The average neuropathy disability score improved by 2 points in the sham exchange group and by 12 points in the plasma exchange group. In the open trial in which patients who initially had sham exchange received plasma exchange, the neuropathy disability score, weakness score, and summed compound muscle action potentials improved more with plasma exchange than with sham exchange. In both the double-blinded and open trials, IgG or IgA gammopathy had a better response to plasma exchange than IgM gammopathy.[49] In another study, 8 of 13 patients with monoclonal gammopathy and peripheral neuropathy obtained benefit with plasma exchange.[50]

In a prospective study of 44 patients with an IgM M protein and peripheral neuropathy, patients were randomly assigned to either chlorambucil (0.1 mg/kg daily) orally or chlorambucil plus 15 courses of plasma exchange during the first 4 months of treatment. No difference was found between the two treatment groups, suggesting that plasma exchange conferred no additional benefit to chlorambucil therapy.[51] In a prospective study of 16 patients with monoclonal gammopathy (IgM in 11 and IgG in 5) and sensorimotor peripheral neuropathy, cyclophosphamide plus prednisone treatment produced improvement in 8 and stabilization of the neuropathy in 6 others.[52]

Fludarabine, a purine analog, produced clinical and neurophysiological improvement in 3 of 4 patients with an IgM M protein and peripheral neuropathy.[53] Another study also reported that 7 of 10 patients with an IgM M protein and neuropathy had a response to fludarabine, and 7 of the 8 patients had anti-MAG antibodies.[54]

Rituximab produced improvement in all 5 patients with neuropathy and IgM antibody to MAG or G_{M1} ganglioside. Rituximab is a monoclonal antibody directed against CD20, which is a common surface membrane marker in lymphoma. The patients received 4 weekly infusions of rituximab without major side effects. Plasma exchange and cyclophosphamide had previously been successful in all 5 patients, but they had relapse.[55]

We also have prescribed chlorambucil for patients with IgM monoclonal gammopathy and melphalan for those with IgG and IgA monoclonal gammopathies and peripheral neuropathy. The responses to therapy have been gratifying in some of these patients. Kelly et al.[56] reported that 9 of 10 patients with peripheral neuropathy and an IgM M protein had a response to prednisone, cyclophosphamide, chlorambucil, azathioprine, or plasmapheresis.

Intravenous administration of gamma globulin has been beneficial in some patients with CIDP, but it has been disappointing for patients with peripheral neuropathy associated with a monoclonal gammopathy. A randomized study comparing intravenous immunoglobulin with placebo and followed by crossover showed improved strength in 2 of the 11 patients and improved sensory neuropathy in 1 other. Antibody titers to MAG or gangliosides did not change. Thus, only 27% of patients had any benefit.[57]

Monoclonal gammopathy and motor neuron diseases

Although several patients who had both monoclonal gammopathy and motor neuron disease have been reported, there is little evidence for a causal relationship. Rowland et al.[58] reported on a patient with an IgM κ M protein and amyotrophic lateral sclerosis and reviewed the published cases of 14 other patients with motor neuron disease and monoclonal gammopathy. Patten[59] described 4 patients with amyotrophic lateral sclerosis and IgG monoclonal gammopathy. In a literature review, Latov[60] found 19 cases of motor neuron disease and monoclonal gammopathy. Merlini et al.[61] reported on 3 patients with amyotrophic lateral sclerosis, 2 of whom had an IgG monoclonal protein and 1, biclonal gammopathy (IgG κ/IgA λ).

Multiple myeloma

Multiple myeloma is characterized by bone pain, weakness, and fatigue. Renal insufficiency and hypercalcemia frequently occur, and almost every patient has anemia. An M protein is found in the serum or urine of 98% of patients at the time of diagnosis. Radiographs show such abnormalities as lytic lesions, osteoporosis, or fractures in 80% of patients. Diagnosis is made by the demonstration of an increased number of plasma cells in the bone marrow.

Neurological involvement is manifested most often by nerve root pain. Compression of the spinal cord or cauda equina, usually caused by myeloma arising in the marrow cavity of a vertebral body and extending to the extradural space, occurs in about 5% of patients and may produce severe back pain with radicular features, weakness, or paralysis of the lower extremities as well as bowel or bladder incontinence. Peripheral neuropathy is uncommon, but when present, it usually is associated with amyloidosis.

Silverstein and Doniger[62] detected peripheral neuropathy in 10 (3.5%) of 277 hospitalized patients with multiple myeloma, and 3 of the 10 patients had amyloidosis. Davison and Balser[63] reported a patient who had peripheral neuritis of the upper extremities and multiple myeloma. At autopsy, demyelination was found, but there was no evidence of myelomatous invasion of the nerves. In a series of 23 patients with multiple myeloma, 3 had clinical neuropathy and 6 had electrophysiological evidence of peripheral neuropathy.[64]

The author of this chapter identified 10 patients who had typical multiple myeloma and peripheral neuropathy, 4 of whom had systemic amyloidosis. Four of the other 6 patients presented with peripheral neuropathy, and myeloma was discovered during evaluation of the neuropathy. Four patients had a relatively mild sensorimotor neuropathy that involved the lower extremities and was slowly progressive. There was no evidence of improvement from chemotherapy for myeloma. Another patient had a predominantly sensory neuropathy, and still another had severe muscle weakness and facial palsy bilaterally as well as respiratory insufficiency.

Delauche et al.[65] reported on 3 patients who had multiple myeloma and progressive sensorimotor polyneuropathy; the demyelinating neuropathy did not respond to melphalan and prednisone. The presence of a λ light chain within neurons has been reported in a patient with multiple myeloma.[66]

Solitary plasmacytoma

Solitary plasmacytoma of bone may be associated with peripheral neuropathy. In one report, a sacral plasmacytoma produced severe peripheral neuropathy, which improved after surgical removal and irradiation.[67] Read and Warlow[68] reported on solitary myeloma and peripheral neuropathy in 3 patients and reviewed the reported cases of 13 others.

Waldenström macroglobulinemia

Waldenström macroglobulinemia is the result of an uncontrolled proliferation of lymphocytes and plasma cells in which a large IgM M protein is produced. Neuropathy associated with a modest-sized IgM M protein is described above. Weakness, fatigue, and symptoms of hyperviscosity syndrome, including oronasal bleeding, blurred vision, dizziness, and dyspnea, may occur. Pallor, hepatosplenomegaly, and lymphadenopathy may be found on physical examination. Funduscopic examination shows dilatation of retinal vessels and hemorrhages. The sensorimotor peripheral neuropathy in macroglobulinemia does not differ from that in patients with MGUS of the IgM type.

Normocytic normochromic anemia is usually found. Serum protein electrophoresis demonstrates a tall, narrow peak or dense band that represents the IgM M protein; 75% of these proteins have a κ light chain. A small monoclonal light chain is found in the urine of 80% of patients. The bone marrow contains an increase in lymphocytes and plasma cells. Lytic bone lesions occur in fewer than 5% of patients.

POEMS syndrome (osteosclerotic myeloma)

POEMS syndrome is characterized by **p**olyneuropathy, **o**rganomegaly, **e**ndocrinopathy, **M** protein, and **s**kin changes.[69] Osteosclerotic lesions are seen on the radiographs of more than 90% of patients.

Clinical features

POEMS syndrome occurs in about 2% of patients with multiple myeloma, and they are about a decade younger than the average age of myeloma patients. Symptoms of peripheral neuropathy usually dominate the clinical picture. The duration of symptoms is usually 1 to 2 years but may be longer. Symptoms begin in the feet and consist of the feeling of tingling, pins and needles, and coldness. Motor involvement follows the sensory symptoms. Both are distal, symmetrical, and progressive, gradually spreading proximally. Severe weakness occurs in more than one half of the patients and results in their inability to climb stairs, arise from a chair, or grip objects firmly with the hands. The course is usually slowly progressive, and patients may be confined to a wheelchair. Autonomic symptoms are not a feature, but impotence is common. In contrast to multiple myeloma, bone pain and fractures rarely occur.

Physical examination shows asymmetrical, sensorimotor neuropathy involving the extremities. It is worse distally. Muscle weakness is more marked than sensory loss. More than one half of patients have severe muscle weakness with areflexia. Touch-pressure, vibratory, and joint position sensations are usually affected. Loss of temperature discrimination and nociception is less frequent. Cranial nerves are not involved except for papilledema.

Hepatomegaly occurs in almost one half of patients, but splenomegaly and lymphadenopathy are found in a small proportion. Although hyperpigmentation is common, it frequently is not recognized. Hypertrichosis is characterized by development of stiff, coarse, black hair on the extremities. Gynecomastia and testicular atrophy may be seen. Pitting edema of the lower extremities is common. Occasionally, ascites and pleural effusion occur. Angiomas of the skin may be prominent.

Pulmonary hypertension may be associated with POEMS syndrome. In the series of Lesprit et al.,[70] 5 of 20 patients with POEMS syndrome had pulmonary hypertension. All the patients had dyspnea and pulmonary artery systolic pressure ranging from 50 to 65 mm Hg.

Laboratory features

In contrast to multiple myeloma, anemia is not a feature of POEMS syndrome. Hemoglobin concentration may be increased, causing confusion with polycythemia. Thrombocytosis is found in more than one half of patients.[71] In contrast to multiple myeloma, hypercalcemia and renal insufficiency are rarely present. The bone marrow usually contains fewer than 5% plasma cells. An M protein is found in the serum of almost 90% of patients. The size of the M protein is small (median, 1.1 g/dl) and rarely more than 3 g/dl. The M protein usually is IgG or IgA and almost always the λ type.[72] The presence of Bence Jones proteinuria is infrequent.

Endocrine findings

Diabetes mellitus and gonadal dysfunction are the most common endocrinopathies. Diabetes is often mild. Gonadal dysfunction usually is associated with increased serum levels of luteinizing hormone and follicle-stimulating hormone, indicative of primary failure.

Hyperprolactinemia may account for hypogonadism or galactorrhea. The cause of hyperprolactinemia is not apparent. Gynecomastia is common and probably related, in the majority of cases, to increased levels of estrogen. Hypothyroidism is not uncommon but is usually mild; it is associated with low thyroxine levels and increased levels of thyroid-stimulating hormone.

Skin change

Hyperpigmentation is the most common skin change in POEMS syndrome. In some instances, it may be due to excessive melanocyte-stimulating hormone from the pituitary. Thickening of the skin has been reported, as have Raynaud's phenomenon and clubbing. Angiomas of the skin may be prominent.

Radiographic findings

Osteosclerotic lesions are the hallmark of POEMS syndrome and occur in approximately 90% of patients. Almost one half have a solitary sclerotic lesion and about one third have many sclerotic lesions. The lesions often are modest in size and misinterpreted as benign bony sclerosis. However, they may produce a striking ivory (sclerotic) vertebral body (Figure 201.1). Oftentimes both osteosclerotic and osteolytic lesions are found. A small sclerotic rim surrounding a large lytic lesion can easily be overlooked. Computed tomography may be helpful in identifying the lesions. The pelvis, spine, ribs, and proximal extremities are most often involved. Driedger and Pruzanski[73] estimated that one half of patients with plasma cell dyscrasia and osteosclerotic lesions had peripheral neuropathy.

Pathogenesis

The relationship between multiple myeloma and osteosclerotic myeloma is not clear. Waldenström et al.[74] questioned whether patients with osteosclerotic myeloma in fact had multiple myeloma. The term "myeloma" may be a misnomer because these patients differ in many ways from those with typical multiple myeloma. Patients with osteosclerotic myeloma are at least a decade younger than those with multiple myeloma. Patients with multiple myeloma often present with bone pain, weakness, or fatigue, whereas peripheral neuropathy is a cardinal feature of osteosclerotic myeloma. In contrast, peripheral neuropathy is rarely seen in multiple myeloma and, when it does occur, it usually is due to amyloidosis. Factors differentiating the two disorders are: the infrequency of anemia, hypercalcemia, renal insufficiency, and bone pain; the rarity of fractures; the low levels of M protein in the serum and urine; and the small number of plasma cells in the bone marrow of patients with osteosclerotic myeloma (POEMS syndrome). The clinical features of POEMS syndrome—

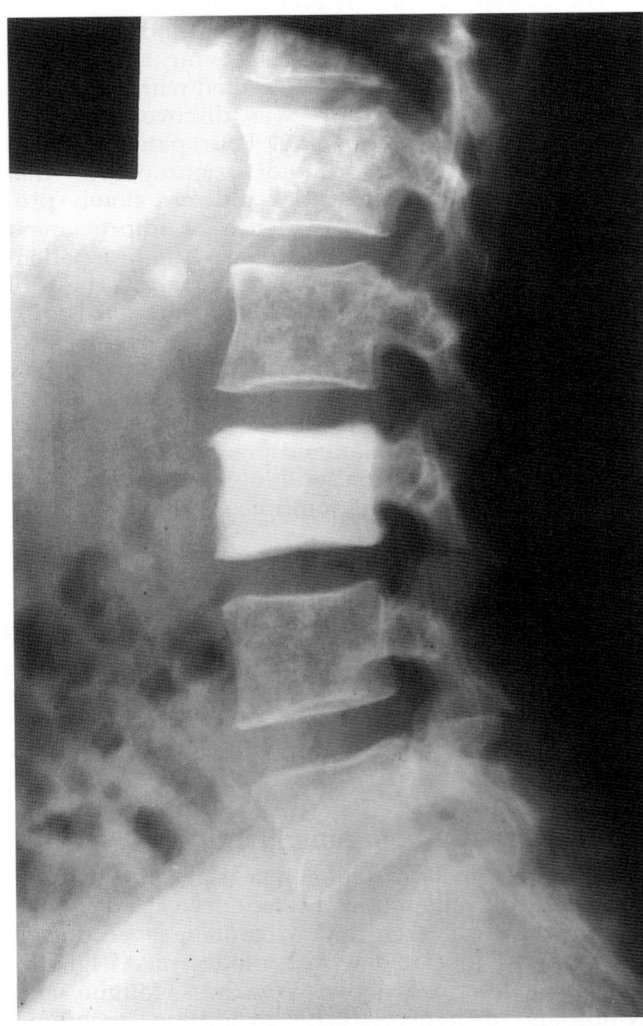

Figure 201.1   Ivory (sclerotic) vertebra in a patient with osteosclerotic myeloma. (From Kyle RA, Dyck PJ. Osteosclerotic myeloma [POEMS syndrome]. *In:* Dyck PJ, Thomas PK, Griffin JW, et al., eds. Peripheral Neuropathy. Vol 2, 3rd ed. Philadelphia: WB Saunders Company, 1993:1288–1293. By permission of the publisher.)

such as sensorimotor peripheral neuropathy, osteosclerotic bone lesions, endocrine features, hepatosplenomegaly, and skin changes—all help to distinguish between the two entities. Furthermore, patients with POEMS syndrome do not have renal insufficiency or multiple fractures. They rarely, if ever, die of multiple myeloma.

The cause of POEMS syndrome is unknown. The patients have higher levels of interleukin-1β, interleukin-6, and tumor necrosis factor α than patients with multiple myeloma; consequently, these cytokines and lymphokines have an important role in pathogenesis.[75] Increased levels of vascular endothelial growth factor are frequent in POEMS syndrome, and the levels often decrease with successful treatment of the syndrome.[76]

Human herpesvirus type 8 (HHV-8) DNA sequences were found in 7 of 13 patients with POEMS syndrome.[77] Two thirds of the tested samples of patients with POEMS syndrome and multicentric Castleman's disease were positive for HHV-8. Antibodies to HHV-8 were found in 78% of patients with POEMS syndrome and Castleman's disease and 22% of those with POEMS syndrome without multicentric Castleman's disease. Five of 14 patients with POEMS syndrome had increased levels of interleukin-6.[78] Two patients were studied serially and showed an increase in interleukin-6 levels antedating exacerbations of their symptoms. The levels decreased following treatment with high-dose methylprednisolone.

The plasma cells may secrete an immunoglobulin or another substance that is toxic to peripheral nerves. It is tempting to speculate that λ light chains are involved in the pathogenesis of the syndrome, because of their unexpected frequency.

Electromyography

Nerve conduction studies show moderate slowing of conduction velocity, with prolonged distal latencies and progressive dispersion of the compound muscle action potentials as the stimulating electrodes are moved proximally. The slowing of motor conduction is proportionately greater than the decrease in the amplitude of the compound muscle action potential. Distal fibrillation potentials are found on needle electromyography. The findings suggest polyneuropathy with prominent demyelination as well as features of axonal degeneration.

Cerebrospinal fluid

The protein concentration in the cerebrospinal fluid is increased in virtually all patients. More than one half of our patients had a protein value greater than 100 mg/dl.[20] The cell count almost always is normal. Plasma cells are not present in the cerebrospinal fluid.

Histological features

Biopsy of the sural nerve usually shows both axonal degeneration and demyelination. In a study of five patients with osteosclerotic myeloma, Ono et al.[79] found a loss of myelinated fibers and an increased frequency of axonal degeneration in teased fibers. The

peaks of histograms of myelinated nerve fibers were displaced to smaller categories, suggesting fiber atrophy or fiber degeneration. There was a lack of an increased number of demyelinated axons. Cellular infiltration is minimal, and amyloid deposits are not found.

Association with Castleman disease

Castleman disease (giant lymph node hyperplasia, angiofollicular lymph node hyperplasia) and osteosclerotic myeloma have been reported.[80] Kobayashi et al.[81] reported a patient with peripheral neuropathy and osteosclerotic myeloma who had lymphadenopathy and involvement of the salivary glands, with an angiofollicular lymphoid lesion. Gherardi et al.[82] found angiofollicular lymph node hyperplasia in two of three patients with POEMS syndrome. In our experience, about 15% of patients with POEMS syndrome also have Castleman disease.

Diagnosis

The diagnosis of POEMS syndrome depends on the demonstration of an increased number of abnormal plasma cells in a biopsy specimen from the osteosclerotic lesion. Plasma cells stain with a single class of heavy chain and a single type of light chain. POEMS syndrome is a monoclonal plasma cell proliferative disorder.

Patients with POEMS syndrome usually present with sensorimotor peripheral neuropathy. A metastatic bone survey must be done to detect osteosclerotic lesions. These lesions can be subtle and easily confused with benign fibrous dysplasia or a vertebral hemangioma. The M protein in the serum and urine is small and may easily be overlooked unless immunofixation is performed.

Course

Patients with POEMS syndrome have a chronic course. They survive for years, in contrast to those with multiple myeloma, whose median survival is approximately 3.5 years. The cause of death in POEMS syndrome is not excessive proliferation of plasma cells and large tumor mass. The natural history is that of progressive peripheral neuropathy until the patient is bedridden. Death usually results from inanition or terminal bronchopneumonia.

Treatment

Single or multiple osteosclerotic lesions in a limited area should be treated with radiation in the tumoricidal dosage range of 40 to 50 cGy. The neuropathy improves substantially in more than one half of the patients. This improvement may be very slow and not apparent for the first 6 months. We have had patients who have continued to have improvement for 2 to 3 years after irradiation.[20]

If the patient has widespread osteosclerotic lesions, systemic therapy is necessary. Kuwabara et al.[83] reported that five of six patients given melphalan and prednisone had various degrees of improvement in their neuropathy and other symptoms. We prefer melphalan (0.15 mg/kg daily) plus prednisone (20 mg 3 times daily) for 7 days every 6 weeks. Lymphocyte and platelet counts should be made every 3 weeks, and the dosage of melphalan altered so that there is some cytopenia at midcycle. An H_2 antagonist should be given with the prednisone. We usually treat patients for 1 year and then discontinue treatment if the clinical condition is stable. There is risk of myelodysplasia or acute leukemia with continued therapy. Others also have reported benefit with melphalan and prednisone.[84,85]

Although corticosteroids occasionally may produce a response, they generally are ineffective.[86] Plasma exchange may be helpful in some patients, but it usually is of little benefit.[20] Autologous stem cell transplantation following high-dose melphalan is a consideration for younger patients with widespread osteosclerotic lesions. The stem cells should be collected before the patient is exposed to alkylating agents, because these agents will reduce the hematopoietic stem cells. Currently, the mortality of the procedure is only 2%.

References

1. Kyle RA. "Benign" monoclonal gammopathy—after 20 to 35 years of follow-up. Mayo Clin Proc 1993;68:26–36
2. Axelsson U, Bachmann R, Hällen J. Frequency of pathological proteins (M-components) in 6995 sera from an adult population. Acta Med Scand 1966;179:235–247
3. Kyle RA, Finkelstein S, Elveback LR, Kurland LT. Incidence of monoclonal proteins in a Minnesota community with a cluster of multiple myeloma. Blood 1972;40:719–724
4. Saleun JP, Vicariot M, Deroff P, Morin JF. Monoclonal gammopathies in the adult population of Finistèr, France. J Clin Pathol 1982;35:63–68
5. Kyle RA, Rajkumar SV. Monoclonal gammopathies of undetermined significance. Hematol Oncol Clin North Am 1999;13:1181–1202
6. Kahn SN, Riches PG, Kohn J. Paraproteinaemia in neurological disease: incidence, associations, and classification of monoclonal immunoglobulins. J Clin Pathol 1980;33:617–621
7. Johansen P, Leegaard OF. Peripheral neuropathy and paraproteinemia: an immunohistochemical and serologic study. Clin Neuropathol 1985;4:99–104
8. Kelly JJ Jr, Kyle RA, Miles JM, et al. The spectrum of peripheral neuropathy in myeloma. Neurology 1981; 31:24–31
9. Busis NA, Halperin JJ, Stefansson K, et al. Peripheral neuropathy, high serum IgM, and paraproteinemia in mother and son. Neurology 1985;35:679–683
10. Jønsson V, Schrøder HD, Stachelin JT, et al. Autoimmunity related to IgM monoclonal gammopathy of undetermined significance, peripheral neuropathy and connective tissue sensibilization caused by IgM M-protein. Acta Med Scand 1988;223:255–261
11. Besinger UA, Toyka KV, Anzil AP, et al. Myeloma neuropathy: passive transfer from man to mouse. Science 1981;213:1027–1030
12. Dalakas MC, Flaum MA, Rick M, et al. Treatment of polyneuropathy in Waldenström's macroglobulinemia: role of paraproteinemia and immunologic studies. Neurology 1983;33:1406–1410
13. Bosch EP, Ansbacher LE, Goeken JA, Cancilla PA.
14. Peripheral neuropathy associated with monoclonal gammopathy: studies of intraneural injections of monoclonal immunoglobulin sera. J Neuropathol Exp Neurol 1982;41:446–459
14. Latov N. Pathogenesis and therapy of neuropathies associated with monoclonal gammopathies. Ann Neurol 1995;37(Suppl 1):S32–S42
15. Kissel JT, Mendell JR. Neuropathies associated with monoclonal gammopathies. Neuromusc Disord 1995;6: 3–18
16. Ropper AH, Gorson KC. Neuropathies associated with paraproteinemia. N Engl J Med 1998;338:1601–1607
17. Dellagi K, Dupouey P, Brouet JC, et al. Waldenström's macroglobulinemia and peripheral neuropathy: a clinical and immunologic study of 25 patients. Blood 1983; 62:280–285
18. Rebai T, Mhiri C, Heine P, et al. Focal myelin thickenings in a peripheral neuropathy associated with IgM monoclonal gammopathy. Acta Neuropathol 1989;79: 226–232
19. Smith IS, Kahn SN, Lacey BW, et al. Chronic demyelination neuropathy associated with benign IgM paraproteinaemia. Brain 1983;106:169–195
20. Kelly JJ Jr. The electrodiagnostic findings in peripheral neuropathy associated with monoclonal gammopathy. Muscle Nerve 1983;6:504–509
21. Latov N, Sherman WH, Nemni R, et al. Plasma-cell dyscrasia and peripheral neuropathy with a monoclonal antibody to peripheral-nerve myelin. N Engl J Med 1980;303:618–621
22. Nobile-Orazio E, Hays AP, Latov N, et al. Specificity of mouse and human monoclonal antibodies to myelin-associated glycoprotein. Neurology 1984;34:1336–1442
23. Latov N, Hays AP, Sherman WH. Peripheral neuropathy and anti-MAG antibodies. Crit Rev Neurobiol 1988;3:301–332
24. Lieberman F, Marton LS, Stefansson K. Pattern reactivity of IgM from the sera of eight patients with IgM monoclonal gammopathy and neuropathy with components of neural tissues: evidence for interaction with more than one epitope. Acta Neuropathol 1985;68: 196–200
25. O'Shannessy DJ, Ilyas AA, Dalakas MC, et al. Specificity of human IgM monoclonal antibodies from patients with peripheral neuropathy. J Neuroimmunol 1986;11:131–136
26. Seligmann M, Brouet J-C, Dellagi K. Antibody activities of human monoclonal gammopathies with special emphasis on monoclonal IgM in patients with peripheral neuropathy. In: Radl J, Hijmans W, Van Camp B, eds. Proceedings of the EURAGE Symposium on Monoclonal Gammopathies, Clinical Significance and Basic Mechanisms. Brussels, Belgium, September 19–20, 1985: 49–55
27. Steck AJ, Murray N, Meier C, et al. Demyelinating neuropathy and monoclonal IgM antibody to myelin-associated glycoprotein. Neurology 1983;33:19–23
28. Nobile-Orazio E, Francomano E, Daverio R, et al. Antimyelin-associated glycoprotein IgM antibody titers in neuropathy associated with macroglobulinemia. Ann Neurol 1989;26:543–550
29. Shy ME, Vietorisz T, Nobile-Orazio E, Latov N. Specificity of human IgM M-proteins that bind to myelin-associated glycoprotein: peptide mapping, deglycosylation, and competitive binding studies. J Immunol 1984;133:2509–2512
30. Frail DE, Edwards AM, Braun PE. Molecular characteristics of the epitope in myelin-associated glycoprotein

that is recognized by a monoclonal IgM in human neuropathy patients. Mol Immunol 1984;21:721–725

31. Chassande B, Leger JM, Younes-Chennoufi AB, et al. Peripheral neuropathy associated with IgM monoclonal gammopathy: correlations between M-protein antibody activity and clinical/electrophysiological features in 40 cases. Muscle Nerve, 1998;21:55–62

32. Meucci N, Baldini L, Cappellari A, et al. Anti-myelin-associated glycoprotein antibodies predict the development of neuropathy in asymptomatic patients with IgM monoclonal gammopathy. Ann Neurol 1999;46:119–122

33. Kusunoki S, Kohriyama T, Pachner AR, et al. Neuropathy and IgM paraproteinemia: differential binding of IgM M-proteins to peripheral nerve glycolipids. Neurology 1987;37:1795–1797

34. Freddo L, Ariga T, Saito M, et al. The neuropathy of plasma cell dyscrasia: binding of IgM M-proteins to peripheral nerve glycolipids. Neurology 1985;35:1420–1424

35. Fredman P. The role of antiglycolipid antibodies in neurological disorders. Ann NY Acad Sci 1998;845:341–352

36. Steck AJ, Murray N, Dellagi K, et al. Peripheral neuropathy associated with monoclonal IgM autoantibody. Ann Neurol 1987;22:764–767

37. Ilyas AA, Quarles RH, MacIntosh TD, et al. IgM in a human neuropathy related to paraproteinemia binds to a carbohydrate determinant in the myelin-associated glycoprotein and to a ganglioside. Proc Natl Acad Sci USA 1984;81:1225–1229

38. Carpo M, Nobile-Orazio E, Meucci N, et al. Anti-GD$_{1a}$ ganglioside antibodies in peripheral motor syndromes. Ann Neurol 1996;39:539–543

39. Sherman WH, Latov N, Hays AP, et al. Monoclonal IgM kappa antibody precipitating with chondroitin sulfate C from patients with axonal polyneuropathy and epidermolysis. Neurology 1983;33:192–201

40. Yee WC, Hahn AF, Hearn SA, Rupar AR. Neuropathy in IgM lambda paraproteinemia: immunoreactivity to neural proteins and chondroitin sulfate. Acta Neuropathol 1989;78:57–64

41. Ilyas AA, Quarles RH, Dalakas MC, et al. Monoclonal IgM in a patient with paraproteinemic polyneuropathy binds to gangliosides containing disialosyl groups. Ann Neurol 1985;18:655–659

42. Quarles RH, Weiss MD. Autoantibodies associated with peripheral neuropathy. Muscle Nerve 1999;22:800–822

43. Gorson KC, Allam G, Ropper AH. Chronic inflammatory demyelinating polyneuropathy: clinical features and response to treatment in 67 consecutive patients with and without a monoclonal gammopathy. Neurology 1997;48:321–328

44. Simmons Z, Albers JW, Bromberg MB, Feldman EL. Long-term follow-up of patients with chronic inflammatory demyelinating polyradiculoneuropathy, and without and with monoclonal gammopathy. Brain 1995;118:359–368

45. Maisonobe T, Chassande B, Vérin M, et al. Chronic dysimmune demyelinating polyneuropathy: a clinical and electrophysiological study of 93 patients. J Neurol Neurosurg Psychiatry 1996;61:36–42

46. Gosselin S, Kyle RA, Dyck PJ. Neuropathy associated with monoclonal gammopathies of undetermined significance. Ann Neurol 1991;30:54–61

47. Simovic D, Gorson KC, Ropper AH. Comparison of IgM-MGUS and IgG-MGUS polyneuropathy. Acta Neurol Scand 1998;97:194–200

48. Sherman WH, Olarte MR, McKiernan G, et al. Plasma exchange treatment of peripheral neuropathy associated with plasma cell dyscrasia. J Neurol Neurosurg Psychiatry 1984;47:813–819

49. Dyck PJ, Low PA, Windebank AJ, et al. Plasma exchange in polyneuropathy associated with monoclonal gammopathy of undetermined significance. N Engl J Med 1991;325:1482–1486

50. Mazzi G, Raineri A, Zucco M, et al. Plasma-exchange in chronic peripheral neurological disorders. Int J Artif Organs 1999;22:40–46

51. Oksenhendler E, Chevret S, Leger JM, et al. Plasma exchange and chlorambucil in polyneuropathy associated with monoclonal IgM gammopathy. IgM-associated Polyneuropathy Study Group. J Neurol Neurosurg Psychiatry 1995;59:243–247

52. Notermans NC, Lokhorst HM, Franssen H, et al. Intermittent cyclophosphamide and prednisone treatment of polyneuropathy associated with monoclonal gammopathy of undetermined significance. Neurology 1996;47:1227–1233

53. Wilson HC, Lunn MP, Schey S, Hughes RA. Successful treatment of IgM paraproteinaemic neuropathy with fludarabine. J Neurol Neurosurg Psychiatry 1999;66:575–580

54. Sherman WH, Latov N, Lange D, et al. Fludarabine for IgM antibody-mediated neuropathies (abstract). Ann Neurol 1994;36:326–327

55. Levine TD, Pestronk A. IgM antibody-related polyneuropathies: B-cell depletion chemotherapy using Rituximab. Neurology 1999;52:1701–1704

56. Kelly JJ Jr, Adelman LS, Berkman E, Bhan I. Polyneuropathies associated with IgM monoclonal gammopathies. Arch Neurol 1988;45:1355–1359

57. Dalakas MC, Quarles RH, Farrer RG, et al. A controlled study of intravenous immunoglobulin in demyelinating neuropathy with IgM gammopathy. Ann Neurol 1996;40:792–795

58. Rowland LP, Defendini R, Sherman W, et al. Macroglobulinemia with peripheral neuropathy simulating motor neuron disease. Ann Neurol 1982;11:532–536

59. Patten BM. Neuropathy and motor neuron syndromes associated with plasma cell disease. Acta Neurol Scand 1984;70:47–61

60. Latov N. Plasma cell dyscrasia and motor neuron disease. Adv Neurol 1982;36:273–279

61. Merlini G, Rutigliano L, Masnaghetti S, et al. Neuromuscular disorders associated with monoclonal immunoglobulins (abstract). In: International Conference on Multiple Myeloma. Biology, Pathophysiology, Prognosis and Treatment. Abstracts. Bologna, Italy, June 19–22, 1989:215

62. Silverstein A, Doniger DE. Neurologic complications of myelomatosis. Arch Neurol 1963;9:534–544

63. Davison C, Balser BH. Myeloma and its neural complications. Arch Surg 1937;35:913–936

64. Walsh JC. The neuropathy of multiple myeloma: an electrophysiological and histological study. Arch Neurol 1971;25:404–414

65. Delauche MC, Clauvel JP, Seligmann M. Peripheral neuropathy and plasma cell neoplasias: a report of 10 cases. Br J Haematol 1981;48:383–392

66. Borges LF, Busis NA. Intraneuronal accumulation of myeloma proteins. Arch Neurol 1985;42:690–694

67. Davidson S. Solitary myeloma with peripheral polyneuropathy—recovery after treatment. Calif Med 1972;116:68–71

68. Read D, Warlow C. Peripheral neuropathy and solitary plasmacytoma. J Neurol Neurosurg Psychiatry 1978;41:177–184

69. Bardwick PA, Zvaifler NJ, Gill GN, et al. Plasma cell dyscrasia with polyneuropathy, organomegaly, endocrinopathy, M protein, and skin changes: the POEMS syndrome. Report on two cases and a review of the literature. Medicine (Baltimore) 1980;59:311–322

70. Lesprit P, Godeau B, Authier FJ, et al. Pulmonary hypertension in POEMS syndrome: a new feature mediated by cytokines. Am J Respir Crit Care Med 1998;157:907–911

71. Kelly JJ Jr, Kyle RA, Miles JM, Dyck PJ. Osteosclerotic myeloma and peripheral neuropathy. Neurology 1983;33:202–210

72. Takatsuki K, Sanada I. Plasma cell dyscrasia with polyneuropathy and endocrine disorder: clinical and laboratory features of 109 reported cases. Jpn J Clin Oncol 1983;13:543–555

73. Driedger H, Pruzanski W. Plasma cell neoplasia with osteosclerotic lesions: a study of five cases and a review of the literature. Arch Intern Med 1979;139:892–896

74. Waldenström JG, Adner A, Gydell K, Zettervall O. Osteosclerotic "plasmacytoma" with polyneuropathy, hypertrichosis, and diabetes. Acta Med Scand 1978;203:297–303

75. Gherardi RK, Belec L, Soubrier M, et al. Overproduction of proinflammatory cytokines imbalanced by their antagonists in POEMS syndrome. Blood 1996;87:1458–1465

76. Watanabe O, Maruyama I, Arimura K, et al. Overproduction of vascular endothelial growth/vascular permeability factor is causative in Crow-Fukase (POEMS) syndrome. Muscle Nerve 1998;21:1390–1397

77. Belec L, Mohamed AS, Authier FJ, et al. Human herpesvirus 8 infection in patients with POEMS syndrome-associated multicentric Castleman's disease. Blood 1999;93:3643–3653

78. Hitoshi S, Sato K, Susuki K, et al. The role of interleukin-6 in Crowe-Fukase syndrome [Japanese]. Rinsho Shinkeigaku 1992;32:577–582

79. Ono K, Ito M, Hotchi M, et al. Polyclonal plasma cell proliferation with systemic capillary hemangiomatosis, endocrine disturbance, and peripheral neuropathy. Acta Pathol Jpn 1985;35:251–267

80. Bitter MA, Komaiko W, Franklin WA. Giant lymph node hyperplasia with osteoblastic bone lesions and the POEMS (Takatsuki's) syndrome. Cancer 1985;56:188–194

81. Kobayashi H, Ii K, Sano T, et al. Plasma-cell dyscrasia with polyneuropathy and endocrine disorders associated with dysfunction of salivary glands. Am J Surg Pathol 1985;9:759–763

82. Gherardi R, Baudrimont M, Kujas M, et al. Pathological findings in three non-Japanese patients with the POEMS syndrome. Virchows Arch [A] Path Anat Histopathol 1988;413:357–365

83. Kuwabara S, Hattori T, Shimoe Y, Kamitsukasa I. Long term melphalan-prednisolone chemotherapy for POEMS syndrome. J Neurol Neurosurg Psychiatry 1997;63:385–387

84. Donofrio PD, Alpers JW, Greenberg HS, Mitchell BS. Peripheral neuropathy in osteosclerotic myeloma: clinical and electrodiagnostic improvement with chemotherapy. Muscle Nerve 1984;7:137–141

85. Parra R, Fernandez JM, Garcia-Bragado F, et al. Successful treatment of peripheral neuropathy with chemotherapy in osteosclerotic myeloma. J Neurol 1987;234:261–263

86. Tobin MJ, Fitzgerald MX. The Japanese plasma cell dyscrasia syndrome: case report and theory of pathogenesis. Postgrad Med J 1982;58:786–789

202 Amyloidosis

Robert A Kyle and Angela Dispenzieri

Brief overview

Early in the 18th century, Wainewright described amyloid involving the liver. The term "amyloid" was coined by Schleiden, the German botanist, in 1838 to describe a normal amylaceous constituent of plants. The terms "waxy" and "lardaceous" were used to describe the substance. In the 1840s, Budd recognized that the substance was albuminous rather than fatty. Virchow observed that the cerebral corpora amylacea had the staining properties of starch and named it "amyloid" (i.e., cellulose-derived).[1] Wilks reported a case of lardaceous viscera that was unrelated to infection, and this may have been the first report of primary amyloidosis (AL) (amyloid light chain). Bennhold, in 1922, introduced Congo red as a diagnostic test and subsequently as a histological stain. Six years later, Divry and Florkin reported that amyloid stained with Congo red showed green birefringence when viewed under polarized light. Cohen and Calkins demonstrated that all forms of amyloid have a nonbranching, fibrillar ultrastructure.

Amyloid appears homogeneous when viewed under the light microscope, and it stains pink with hematoxylin and eosin. The amyloid fibril consists of two to five filaments arranged in a cross-β-pleated sheet configuration. The fibrils are insoluble and resist proteolytic digestion.

Classification of amyloidosis

Although all types of amyloid appear the same with light and electron microscopy, the fibrils consist of different types of protein (Table 202.1). The fibrils in AL consist of monoclonal κ or λ light chains. Rarely, monoclonal heavy chains are responsible. The major component of the amyloid fibril in secondary amyloidosis (AA) is protein A. It has a molecular weight of 8.5 kDa, contains 76 amino acids, and is derived from serum amyloid A (SAA), which is an acute-phase protein. The level of SAA is increased in patients with rheumatoid arthritis and Crohn's disease. There are several types of familial amyloidosis (AF), with different precursor proteins forming the fibrils. The most common precursor proteins are variants of the transthyretin molecule. The Portuguese, Swedish, and Japanese variants are characterized by the substitution of methionine for valine at residue 30 (Met 30) of the transthyretin molecule, and the predominant manifestation is sensorimotor peripheral neuropathy.

Cardiomyopathy from a transthyretin (TTR) mutation has been reported in Denmark (Met 111) and from the Appalachian area of the United States (Ala 60). Familial renal amyloid from mutations of the fibrinogen Aα chain (Leu 554 or Glu 526) or mutations of lysozyme have been recognized. Amyloid associated with familial Mediterranean fever consists of protein A. Hereditary cerebral hemorrhage with amyloidosis (HCHWA) has been recognized in Iceland and the

Table 202.1 Classification of amyloidosis

Amyloid protein	Syndrome	Precursor
AL	Primary (includes multiple myeloma)	κ or λ light chain
AA	Secondary	Protein A
ATTR	Neuropathic—Portuguese, Japanese, Swedish, etc.	Transthyretin mutant
AApo A-I	Iowa kindred	Apolipoprotein A-I
	Cardiopathic—Danish, Appalachian	Transthyretin (prealbumin) mutant
	Nephropathic—FMF	Protein A
AGEL	Corneal lattice dystrophy	Gelsolin
AFIB	Nephropathic	Fibrinogen α chain
	Hereditary cerebral hemorrhage with amyloidosis, Icelandic (HCHWA-I)	Cystatin C
Aβ	Hereditary cerebral hemorrhage with amyloidosis, Dutch (HCHWA-D)	Aβ
AS	Senile systemic amyloidosis (cardiac)	Transthyretin (prealbumin) normal
Aβ$_2$M	Dialysis arthropathy	β$_2$-Microglobulin

AA, amyloid protein A; AApo A-I, amyloid apolipoprotein A-I; Aβ, amyloid β protein; Aβ$_2$M, amyloid β$_2$-microglobulin; AFIB, amyloid fibrinogen α chain; AGEL, amyloid gelsolin; AL, amyloid light chain; AS, amyloid senile systemic amyloidosis; ATTR, amyloid transthyretin; FMF, familial Mediterranean fever.

This was supported in part by CA 62242 from the National Cancer Institute.

Netherlands. The amyloid in the Icelandic form consists of a mutant cystatin C, whereas the Dutch form consists of β protein identical to that seen in Alzheimer disease except for a mutation in which glutamine instead of glutamic acid is present at residue 22 of Aβ. Senile systemic amyloidosis involving the heart is another rare form of amyloid. It results from the deposition of apparently normal transthyretin. $β_2$-Microglobulin amyloidosis can occur in patients undergoing long-term dialysis.

This chapter is limited to AL and AF because neurological involvement is rare in AA and dialysis-associated amyloidosis. In the author's practice, currently 88% of patients have AL and only 1% have AF.

Primary amyloidosis

Epidemiology

The overall incidence rate of AL is 0.9 per 100 000/year, which means there are approximately 2500 new cases in the United States annually.[2] The median age at onset of AL is approximately 65 years; only 1% of patients are younger than 40 years. Men are affected more frequently than women. The cause of AL is not known. There is no distinct genetic influence.

Pathophysiology and pathogenesis

The fibrils in AL consist of monoclonal κ or λ light chains. Rarely, monoclonal heavy chains are responsible. Repeated injections of monoclonal light chains from patients with AL can produce amyloidosis in mice.[3] The light chain (κ/λ) ratio is 1:2, which is the reverse of that in multiple myeloma (2:1). All $λ_{VI}$ proteins have been associated with amyloidosis. Patients whose clones derived from $λ_{VI}$ usually present with prominent renal involvement, whereas those with $V_λ$ or unknown donors often have dominant cardiac or other organ involvement. There appear to be important associations of $V_λ$ gene utilization and clinical manifestations.[4] Amyloid P component and glycosaminoglycans are present in amyloid deposits, but their role is unknown. Little is known about the catabolism of amyloid fibrils.

Clinical features

Weakness or fatigue and weight loss are the most frequent initial symptoms. Weight loss occurs in more than one half of patients, with a median loss of approximately 20 lb. Purpura, particularly in the periorbital and facial areas, occurs in about 15% of patients. Paresthesias, light-headedness, and syncope are often noted in patients with peripheral neuropathy or autonomic neuropathy. Dyspnea and pedal edema are frequent in patients with congestive heart failure. The liver is palpable in about one fourth of patients and the spleen, in only 5%. Approximately 10% of patients have macroglossia.

Peripheral neuropathy is the major manifestation of AL in about one sixth of patients. Most commonly, the initial symptoms are sensory and consist of loss of sensation, altered sensation, prickling, numbness, and pain. The pain may be burning or lancinating. The neuropathy usually is distal, symmetrical, and progressive. Dysesthetic numbness may be severe. The lower extremities are involved earlier and more severely than the upper extremities. Muscle weakness develops later. The symptoms usually are present for at least a year before the diagnosis is made. Autonomic symptoms—light-headedness, orthostatic hypotension, or decreased sweating—occur in about two thirds of patients with neuropathy.[5]

The possibility of amyloidosis must be considered in any patient with a sensorimotor peripheral neuropathy. Sural nerve biopsy is the only certain way to exclude the possibility of amyloidosis. In 26 patients with sural nerve biopsy-proven amyloid neuropathy and M protein in the serum or urine, 81% had paresthesias, 65% had muscle weakness, and 58% had numbness.[6] The median duration of symptoms before diagnosis was 29 months. At the time of diagnosis, 17 patients had symptoms of autonomic neuropathy. The neuropathy was chronic and progressive. Twenty-two patients died, and the median survival was 25 months. Progressive amyloidosis was the cause of death in most patients. Rajani et al.[7] reported that 1.2% of 1098 sural nerve biopsy specimens were positive for amyloid deposition. Neuropathy was predominantly sensory in 6 patients, motor in 2, and mixed in 5. The endoneurium was involved in 12 patients and the epineurium in 9. Axonal loss was moderate or severe in 12 of the 13 patients. Axonal degeneration predominated over demyelination in 8 of 10 cases that were evaluated.[7]

Orthostatic hypotension is found in about 10% of patients with AL. It usually is caused by involvement of the autonomic nervous system. Orthostatism may be severe enough to produce light-headedness and syncope that prevent ambulation. Cranial neuropathy is rare but may be the initial finding.[8] Impotence frequently occurs. The neuropathy is progressive, but death usually occurs from cardiac or renal amyloid.

Carpal tunnel syndrome is present in about one fifth of patients. The symptoms consist of paresthesias in the distribution of the median nerve, which supplies the skin of the first three fingers and the lateral half of the fourth finger. The symptoms frequently are worse at night, and the paresthesias or pain may awaken the patient. Later, the thenar muscles may atrophy. Electromyography is helpful for differentiating carpal tunnel syndrome from a cervical root lesion.

More than one fourth of patients with AL present with nephrotic syndrome or renal failure, and approximately 15% have congestive heart failure at the time of diagnosis. The frequency of amyloid syndromes at diagnosis is shown in Figure 202.1. No reason is known for amyloid involving the heart in one person and the peripheral nerves in another.

Anemia is not a prominent feature unless the patient has renal failure, multiple myeloma, or gastrointestinal tract bleeding. Thrombocytosis occurs in 10% of patients. Renal insufficiency is found in almost 50% of patients at diagnosis, and the serum concen-

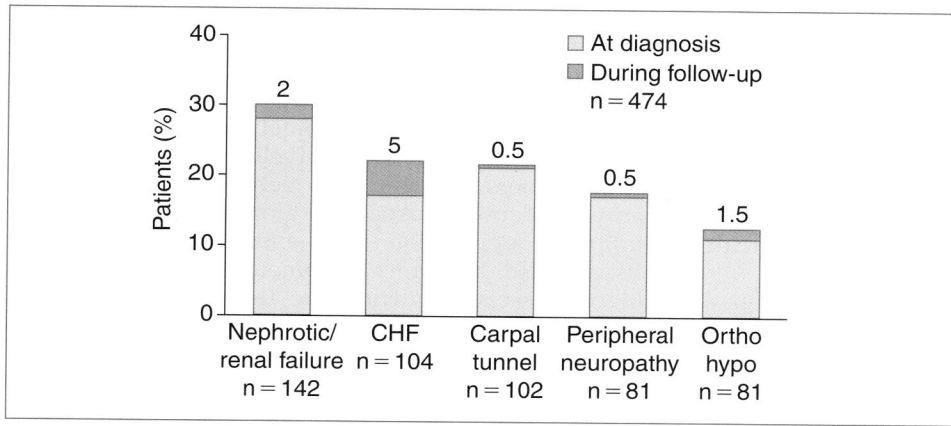

Figure 202.1 Frequency of amyloid syndromes at diagnosis of primary amyloidosis. CHF, congestive heart failure; ortho hypo, orthostatic hypotension. (From Kyle and Gertz.[5] By permission of WB Saunders Company.)

tration of creatinine is greater than 2.0 mg/dl in about 20%.

The serum protein electrophoretic pattern shows a localized band or spike in one half of patients, but the size of the M spike is modest (median, 1.4 g/dl). Hypogammaglobulinemia is seen in 20% of patients, and immunoelectrophoresis or immunofixation of the serum shows a monoclonal protein in about 70%, with IgG being the most common, followed by IgA. Approximately 25% of patients have only free monoclonal light chains. Thirty-six percent of patients have a urine protein value of 3 g/24 hr or higher. It consists mainly of albumin, but three fourths of patients have a small monoclonal light chain. λ-Light chains are twice as common as κ chains. Immunoelectrophoresis or immunofixation of the serum and urine shows an M protein in almost 90% of patients with AL. Approximately one fifth of patients have bone marrow plasmacytosis of 20% or more (median, 7%).

The electrocardiogram shows low voltage in the limb leads or loss of anterior septal forces, mimicking the findings of myocardial infarction. The echocardiogram is abnormal in two thirds of patients at diagno-

sis. An increase in septal thickness is associated with shorter survival. Characteristically, restrictive cardiomyopathy is found.

The median survival of 474 patients with AL evaluated within 1 month after diagnosis was 13.2 months, and for those presenting with overt congestive heart failure, median survival was 4 months (Figure 202.2). In about one half of patients, death is attributed to cardiac involvement from congestive heart failure or arrhythmias.

Diagnostic criteria

The possibility of AL must be considered in every patient who has M protein in the serum or urine and who also has unexplained nephrotic syndrome or renal insufficiency, congestive heart failure, sensorimotor peripheral neuropathy, carpal tunnel syndrome, hepatomegaly, or idiopathic malabsorption. In fact, the presence of a monoclonal light chain in the urine of a patient with nephrotic syndrome is almost always due to AL or light-chain deposition disease.

The diagnosis of AL requires the demonstration of amyloid deposits in tissue. Generally, AL amyloid is

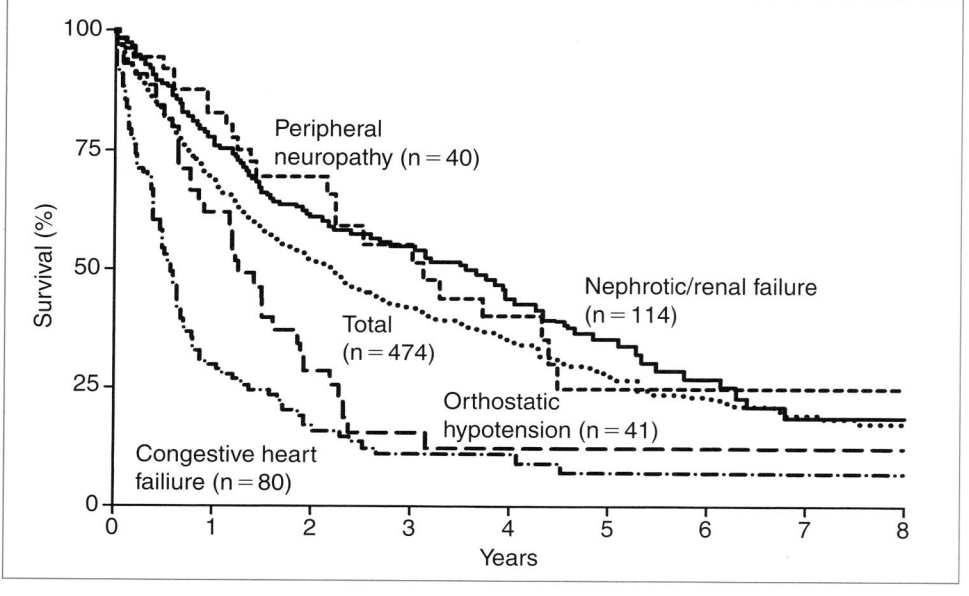

Figure 202.2 Survival in primary amyloidosis, by syndrome, arranged hierarchically. (From Kyle and Gertz.[5] By permission of WB Saunders Company.)

resistant to potassium permanganate exposure, whereas AA amyloid loses its affinity for Congo red, but this is not reliable. The use of antisera to κ, λ, protein A, transthyretin, and β_2-microglobulin is the best approach for diagnosis and proper classification.[9] In some patients, the results of staining with Congo red are negative, but electron microscopy shows typical amyloid fibrils. Electron microscopy is not practical as a routine approach, because it is difficult and expensive.

Initially, a bone marrow aspirate and biopsy should be performed to determine the number of plasma cells and whether they are monoclonal. The bone marrow biopsy specimen should be stained for amyloid, because it is positive in more than 50% of patients. An abdominal fat aspirate is positive in 70% to 80%. The specimen must be stained properly with Congo red and interpreted by an experienced pathologist. The results of bone marrow or subcutaneous fat biopsy are positive in almost 90% of patients with AL. If the results are negative, rectal biopsy, including the submucosa, is recommended. If these sites are negative for disease but the physician still suspects amyloidosis, tissue should be obtained from the organ suspected to be involved (Figure 202.3).

[123]I-labeled serum amyloid P component, a nuclear scan, can be used to identify and monitor the extent of systemic amyloidosis.[10] However, it is not readily available. Increased uptake of technetium 99m pyrophosphate is not reliable for diagnosis.

Motor nerve conduction velocities usually are just below normal value, with decreased or absent compound muscle action potential amplitudes. Distal motor latencies tend to be normal. The amplitude of sensory nerve action potentials is more frequently abnormal than that of compound muscle action potentials. In most cases, sensory nerve action potentials cannot be recorded. In most patients, needle electromyography shows fibrillation and neurogenic motor potentials.

Axonal degeneration, sometimes with predominant involvement of small myelinated and nonmyelinated fibers, occurs. In peripheral neuropathy, amyloid deposits, usually in globular or diffuse form, infiltrate epineurial and endoneurial connective tissue. Also, the walls of epineurial and endoneurial blood vessels frequently are thickened by amyloid deposits. There is a gross loss of myelin fibers, which usually show signs of active axonal degeneration. Marked loss of unmyelinated fibers usually is seen on electron microscopy. Teased-fiber studies show a preponderance of axonal degeneration. The amyloid deposits react with antisera to κ or λ light chains. Electron microscopy shows bundles of immunogold-labeled amyloid fibrils in coated and uncoated single membrane-bound vesicles of endoneurial macrophages. Schwann cells do not contain intracellular amyloid.

Differential diagnosis

Patients with AL can be classified into those with and those without associated multiple myeloma. This distinction is based on the percentage of plasma cells in the bone marrow, the size of the M protein in the serum and urine, and the skeletal survey. In both groups, the fibril protein is a product of the plasma cells, and in many patients it is difficult to determine whether multiple myeloma is present. However, the presence of multiple myeloma has no effect on survival during the first year after diagnosis. In practice, it is better to think of AL and multiple myeloma as part of a continuous spectrum of plasma cell proliferation.

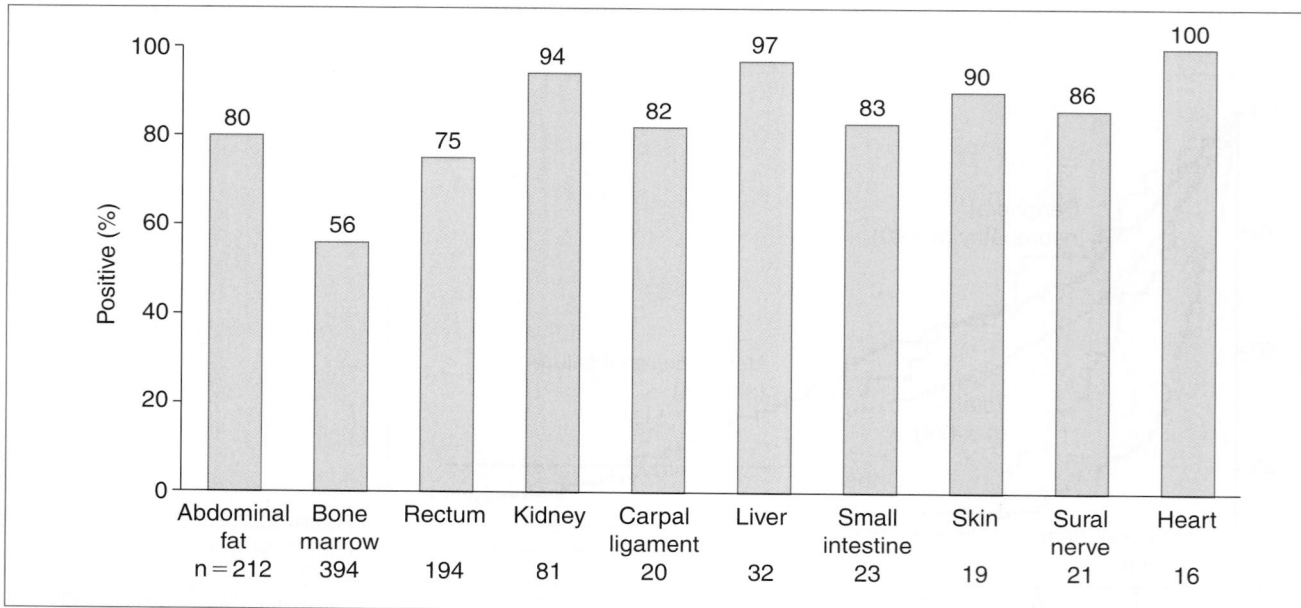

Figure 202.3   Results of biopsy in primary amyloidosis. (From Kyle and Gertz.[5] By permission of WB Saunders Company.)

If the patient has no M protein in the serum or urine and no monoclonal plasma cells in the bone marrow, the possibility of familial amyloidosis must be considered even if there is no positive family history. Immunohistochemical staining must be done to determine the type of amyloid. If transthyretin is detected, a search for a mutation must be performed.

Treatment

Because amyloid fibrils consist of monoclonal light chains, treatment with alkylating agents effective against plasma cell neoplasms is warranted. In a placebo-controlled, double-blind study of 55 patients with AL, patients randomly assigned to melphalan and prednisone continued treatment longer and received larger doses than did those in the placebo group. Proteinuria decreased more than 50% in 10 of 24 patients in the melphalan and prednisone group.[11] In a prospective study of 220 patients with biopsy-proven AL, patients were randomly assigned to receive 1) colchicine, melphalan, and prednisone, 2) melphalan and prednisone, or 3) colchicine alone. They were stratified according to major clinical manifestations: renal disease (105 patients), cardiac involvement (46 patients), peripheral neuropathy (19 patients), or other (50 patients). The median duration of survival after randomization was 8.5 months for the colchicine group (Figure 202.4), 18 months for the melphalan and prednisone group, and 17 months for the melphalan, prednisone, and colchicine group ($P < 0.001$).[12] To determine whether more intensive chemotherapy is beneficial, 101 patients were randomly assigned to receive either melphalan and prednisone or a combination of drugs: vincristine, BCNU, melphalan, cyclophosphamide, and prednisone (VBMCP). Therapy with multiple alkylating agents did not result in a higher response rate or longer survival time than standard therapy with melphalan and prednisone.[13] However, treatment with alkylating

agents may be associated with myelodysplastic syndrome or acute leukemia.[14]

High-dose chemotherapy has shown promise in destroying the light-chain-producing plasma cells. Of 25 patients with AL given melphalan ($200\,mg/m^2$) followed by infusion of previously collected peripheral blood stem cells, 62% experienced a hematological response of the clonal plasma cell disorder and 11 of 17 survivors had amyloid-related organ improvement.[15] Patients must be selected carefully for high-dose therapy. For example, patients with major cardiac involvement have a higher mortality and, at this time, should not receive high-dose chemotherapy.

Colchicine, vitamin E, and α_2-interferon have all been disappointing treatments. Gianni et al.[16] reported the use of 4'-iodo-4'-deoxydoxorubicin for AL. This agent has an affinity for amyloid deposits and may help dissolve them. It appears to be less effective for patients with visceral involvement than those with soft tissue deposits. This drug is currently being evaluated in the United States, but the initial results have been disappointing.

General treatment

Treatment of peripheral neuropathy with standard chemotherapy generally is ineffective. Comenzo et al.[15] have reported neurological improvement after peripheral stem cell transplantation in four of five patients. Dysesthesias tend to disappear as sensory involvement worsens. Analgesics and sedatives may be helpful depending on the type and severity of symptoms. Amitriptyline, gabapentin, and fluphenazine have been of benefit in some patients. The dysesthesias may be sufficiently distressing to require narcotics for control. Codeine is useful, and the long-term risks of habituation and tolerance are modest.

Treatment of orthostatic hypotension is challenging. Patients should rise slowly and sit on the edge of

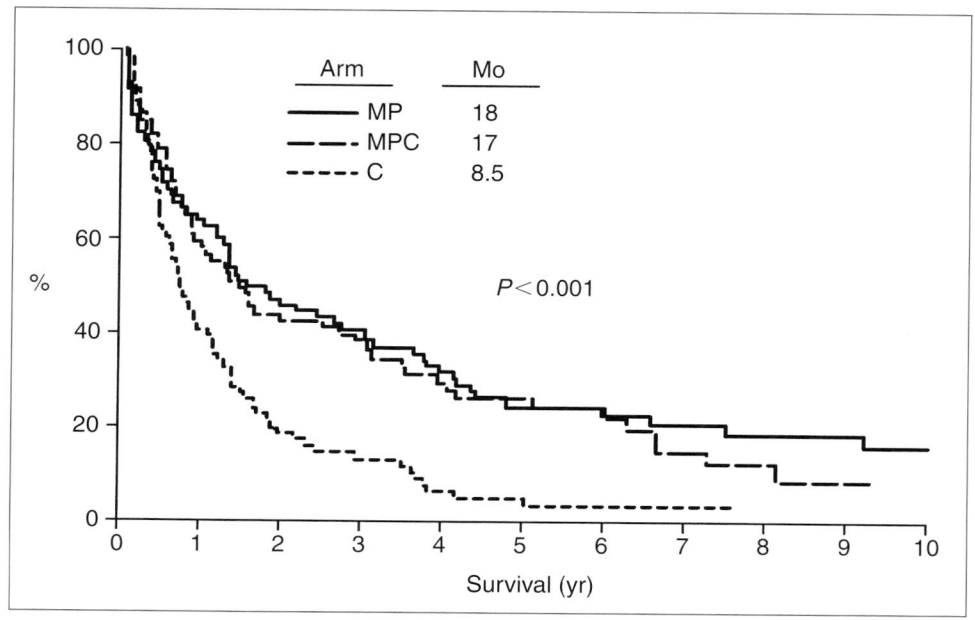

Figure 202.4 Median survival after randomization in 220 cases of primary amyloidosis (AL). Treatment arms included colchicine (C), melphalan and prednisone (MP), and melphalan, prednisone, and colchicine (MPC). (From Kyle RA, Gertz MA. Amyloidosis. *In:* Schrier RW, Klahr S, eds. Atlas of Diseases of the Kidney. Vol 4. Philadelphia: Current Medicine, 1999;3.1–3.15. By permission of the publisher.)

the bed for a few minutes before assuming an upright position. Elastic support extending to the waist (leotards) may be helpful. Fludrocortisone is often associated with increased fluid retention. Midodrine or L-threo-3,4-dihydroxyphenylserine (L-threo-DOPS) may be of some benefit. Octreotide may help in the management of both autonomic-induced diarrhea and orthostatic hypotension. Decompression of the carpal ligament relieves the pain of carpal tunnel syndrome, but residual sensory loss is frequent.

Familial amyloidosis

In 1952, Andrade[17] described a Portuguese family from Porto who had lower extremity neuropathy, followed by muscle weakness. Subsequently, autonomic neuropathy manifested by impotence, incontinence, and diarrhea occurred. Involvement of the heart and kidney was not prominent. Symptoms began in the third decade of life, and death occurred within 10 years after onset of symptoms. Vitreous opacities were infrequent.

Epidemiology

The greatest number of patients (more than 1000) have been reported from the Porto, Portugal, region. Andersson[18] reported familial amyloidosis in northern Sweden that was clinically similar to the Portuguese type except that the average age at onset was 55 years and it was more often associated with cardiac conduction abnormalities, malabsorption, and peptic ulcer. Familial amyloid polyneuropathy has been reported among residents of Kumamoto and Nagano prefectures in Japan. The clinical features are similar to those of the Portuguese patients, but they usually are later in onset. Familial amyloid polyneuropathy has been reported from many parts of the world. Of 13 European families with amyloid polyneuropathy, 10 carried the TTR Met 30 mutation found in the Portuguese, Swedish, and Japanese patients.[19] Familial amyloidosis accounts for less than 5% of the cases of amyloidosis examined at the Mayo Clinic.

Pathogenesis

The amyloid fibrils of the Portuguese, Japanese, and Swedish types of familial amyloidosis all consist of transthyretin (prealbumin),[20] with methionine substituted for valine at position 30 (TTR Met 30).[21] However, more than 80 transthyretin mutations have been reported.[22,23] The genetic code for transthyretin is on human chromosome $18q11.2 \rightarrow 18q12.1$. Transthyretin, a transport molecule for thyroxin and retinol, is a tetramer consisting of four identical noncovalently associated subunits. Each monomer consists of 127 amino acid residues and has a molecular weight of 14 000. Conformational changes due to amino acid substitutions are thought to destabilize the structure, causing aggregation and the formation of amyloid fibrils. The structural changes of transthyretin in the formation of amyloid have been reviewed by Kelly et al.[24] Cohorts of familial amyloid arising from mutations in the apoliproprotein A-I

molecule, α-fibrinogen, gelsolin, lysozyme, and cystatin C have also been described.

Clinical features

Clinical features include paresthesias and loss of pain and temperature in the lower extremities, followed by muscular weakness. Autonomic involvement is prominent and is manifested as orthostatic hypotension or motility disturbances of the gastrointestinal tract, including alternating severe constipation and diarrhea. Other features are nausea, vomiting, and loss of weight. Autonomic involvement of the bladder may produce incomplete emptying or incontinence. Cranial nerve involvement is uncommon. Electrocardiographic abnormalities often consist of low voltage and conduction disturbances.

Rukavina et al.[25] described a family of Swiss origin who lived in Indiana. Carpal tunnel syndrome developed in family members in the fifth decade of life and was followed by a sensorimotor peripheral neuropathy that often involved the lower extremities. Many affected members survived into the sixth and seventh decades. Autonomic involvement was not a feature, and nephropathy and cardiac involvement were not prominent. The transthyretin variant consisted of a substitution of serine for isoleucine at amino acid residue 84 (TTR Ser 84).

A large family of German-English ancestry living in Texas had sensorimotor peripheral neuropathy of all extremities. Other features included cardiomyopathy and orthostatic hypotension. Symptoms usually began in the sixth or seventh decade. Affected members had a variant of transthyretin, with a tyrosine for serine substitution at amino acid 77.[26]

Congestive heart failure from amyloid deposition was found in 5 of 12 siblings in a Danish family.[27] The amyloid in the heart consisted of transthyretin, with a methionine substitution in position 111.[28]

Familial amyloidosis has been recognized in persons from the Appalachian region of the United States. They frequently have sensorimotor peripheral neuropathy and carpal tunnel syndrome, but the major manifestation is cardiac. An Ala 60 mutation of transthyretin has been identified.[29]

A large kindred in Iowa with neuropathy affecting all four extremities and renal involvement has been described.[30] Neuropathy began in the fourth decade of life. The average survival was 12 years after diagnosis, with death due to renal failure. The amyloid fibrils consisted of apolipoprotein A-I (ApoA-I), in which there was an arginine for glycine substitution at position 26.[31] ApoA-I mutations may also be responsible for amyloid nephropathy, hepatopathy, and cardiomyopathy.[32]

Patients with familial amyloidosis may present with hypertension and mild renal insufficiency that progresses to end-stage renal failure. The onset is in the fifth to seventh decade of life. Four mutations of α-fibrinogen have been recognized.[32,33]

Most commonly, familial amyloidosis due to mutations in the gelsolin molecules is associated with type II lattice corneal dystrophy, but neuropathy, nephropathy, and cardiomyopathy have also been described. Unique to this form of amyloidosis, the cranial nerves are preferentially involved over the sensory nerves.[32]

Diagnosis

The diagnosis depends on the demonstration of amyloid in tissue. Subcutaneous fat aspirate or sural nerve biopsy is suitable for this purpose. Immunohistochemical staining shows transthyretin in the majority of specimens. Mutations of fibrinogen, apolipoprotein A-I, gelsolin, lysozyme, and cystatin C have also been recognized.

Screening for a transthyretin variant using polyacrylamide gel electrophoresis (PAGE), followed by isoelectric focusing under partially denaturing conditions, detected 74 of 77 (96%) variants with a specificity of 100%. No false-positive results were obtained, and only 4% were false-negative.[34] Restriction fragment length polymorphism analysis may also be used for diagnosis. DNA is extracted from whole blood and digested with a restriction enzyme. Electrophoresis in agarose is performed, and the gel is subjected to Southern blot transfer. Autoradiography is performed after hybridization with a DNA probe labeled with p32Dc TP13. This permits recognition of the disease in asymptomatic children of affected parents.

Histological examination shows selective loss of unmyelinated and small myelinated fibers of the sural nerve (both usually are involved; Figure 202.5). Teased-fiber studies show linear rows of myelin ovoids characteristic of degenerating axons. The largest and most numerous deposits of amyloid are within fascicles. In some cases, nodules of amyloid indent myelinated fibers, producing large sacculations of the fiber on both sides of the compression.[35] Said et al.[36] reported distortion of the myelin sheaths, segmental demyelination, and wallerian degeneration adjacent to amyloid deposits.

Differential diagnosis

The incidence of biopsy specimens positive for familial amyloidosis is similar to that for AL. The presence

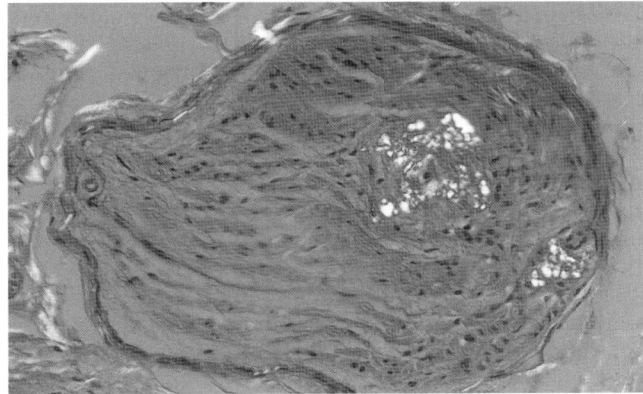

Figure 202.5 Congo red stain of sural nerve viewed under polarizing light showing selective loss of unmyelinated and small myelinated fibers in a patient with familial amyloidosis. (See color plate section.)

of a monoclonal protein in the serum or urine is strong evidence of AL. Patients with secondary amyloidosis (AA) have rheumatoid arthritis, a variant of Crohn's disease, or chronic infection. A positive family history of amyloidosis is very useful, but in our experience approximately one half of patients with familial amyloidosis have a negative family history until after amyloidosis is diagnosed. Almost one third of the patients with familial amyloidosis evaluated at our institution initially had been thought to have AL and some had inappropriately been given chemotherapy.[37] The major features of AL and TTR amyloidosis are compared in Table 202.2.

Treatment

Liver transplantation has been introduced as a treatment for familial amyloidosis with transthyretin mutations.[38] Because transthyretin is synthesized in the liver, orthotopic liver transplantation (OLT) is a reasonable intervention. The same case can be made for patients with fibrinogen Aα amyloidosis. In contrast, this intervention is not justified with apolipoprotein A-I amyloid because this protein is synthesized in both the intestine and the liver.

Table 202.2 Comparison of the major features of primary and familial amyloidosis

Amyloidosis	Clinical features	Diagnostic studies	Therapy
Primary (AL)	Nerves (peripheral and autonomic neuropathy, carpal tunnel) Heart (CHF, arrhythmias) Renal proteinuria, insufficiency	Subcutaneous fat aspirate Bone marrow aspirate and biopsy Immunofixation (serum and urine) Sural nerve biopsy Immunohistochemical staining	Alkylating agents Autologous stem cell transplant
Familial (ATTR)	Nerves (peripheral sensorimotor neuropathy) Heart (CHF, arrhythmias)	Subcutaneous fat aspirate Immunofixation (serum and urine) for exclusion Sural nerve biopsy Immunohistochemical staining	Liver transplant

CHF, congestive heart failure.

Similarly, OLT has no role in the treatment of amyloid due to gelsolin (synthesized in the skeletal muscle and macrophages) or cystatin C (synthesized in neutrophils, macrophages, and other cell types).

A review of the first 20 patients in Sweden who had OLT for familial amyloidosis due to transthyretin mutations showed that 14 (70%) were alive 10 to 52 months after transplantation. Nutritional status, ambulation, and gastrointestinal and urinary symptoms were improved.[39] Amyloid deposits in the spleen, kidneys, and adrenals were reduced in 5 of 8 patients who received ^{123}I-SAP after liver transplantation.[40] However, 5 of 11 patients had increased left ventricular thickening after liver transplantation. Congestive heart failure developed in one patient and sudden cardiac death occurred in another. Four of the 5 patients had a Glu 42 Gly mutation and the fifth had an Ala 36 Pro variant.[41] Stangou et al.[42] also described 3 patients with progression of cardiac amyloidosis after OLT. In another series, 3 of 13 patients who had liver transplantation for familial amyloidosis died because of amyloid deposition in the conduction system of the heart.[43] In yet another patient, cardiomyopathy and neuropathy developed after OLT.[44]

In a group of patients with familial amyloidosis who had OLT, survival was improved if the patient had a good nutritional state at the time of operation. Gastric retention and malabsorption were adverse prognostic features.[45] Despite clinical improvement in autonomic symptoms, Suhr et al.[46] found no statistically significant improvement in sympathetic or parasympathetic effects on heart rate variability. In one patient, the number of myelinated fibers in the sural nerve was markedly increased 3 years after liver transplantation, but amyloid deposits were still present.[47] In a quality-of-life evaluation after liver transplantation, the Swedish investigators reported that 10 of 12 patients had improvement.[48] Because of the shortage of liver donors in Japan, left lobar grafts from family members were performed in 6 patients with familial amyloidosis and were successful.[49]

Flufenamic acid inhibits the conformational changes of transthyretin associated with amyloid fibril formation.[50] An effort is being made to design new compounds that bind to transthyretin with high affinity and thus prevent amyloid formation through stabilization of the normally folded form of transthyretin.

A selective transthyretin adsorption column has been used in the treatment of familial amyloidosis. An ion-exchange resin made of porous beads of polyvinyl alcohol gel covalently bound with dimethylaminoethanol decreased the concentrations of both normal and variant transthyretin to about half of the preabsorption levels.[51] However, whether this will decrease amyloid deposition remains to be determined.

Orthostatic hypotension is a major problem in familial amyloidosis. L-threo-DOPS, a synthetic precursor of norepinephrine, eliminated symptoms of orthostatic hypotension in 8 of 9 patients. The side effects included tachycardia and nausea.[52] Carvalho et al.[53] reported improvement in all 20 patients with orthostatic hypotension who were given L-threo-DOPS. Double-blind, randomized, placebo-controlled studies with a larger number of patients and a longer follow-up are necessary. Two multicenter European trials are under way.[54]

Other forms of familial amyloidosis

Hereditary cerebral hemorrhage with amyloidosis (HCHWA) has been recognized in Iceland and the Netherlands. In the Icelandic form, symptoms develop in the third or fourth decade of life. The condition is characterized by cerebral hemorrhage, usually before the age of 40, that can cause immediate death. Some patients have repeated strokes. Amyloid deposits are most common in the basal ganglia but also occur in the small arteries and arterioles, meninges, and brain. The amyloid consists of a mutant cystatin C (leu 68 Gln)[55,56] and has been designated as "hereditary cystatin C amyloid angiopathy" (HCCAA). It can be diagnosed with a polymerase chain reaction-based assay to detect the mutation in DNA from a sample of the patient's blood.[57]

In the Dutch form of HCHWA (HCHWA-D), repeated cerebral hemorrhages occur at intervals of days to years. Dementia develops in 75% of patients. Amyloid involves the cortical arterioles as well as the arachnoid vessels. Plaque-like lesions are found in the cortical gray matter.[58] The amyloid consists of β protein identical to that seen in senile dementia of Alzheimer's type except for a mutation in which glutamine instead of glutamic acid is present at residue 22 of Aβ.[58]

Type II corneal lattice dystrophy has been noted in a large Finnish kindred and is associated with cranial neuropathy, leonine facies, mild peripheral neuropathy, and systemic amyloidosis.[59] Spinal, cerebral, and meningeal amyloid angiopathy with deposition of gelsolin-related amyloid is found.[60] Renal involvement manifested as nephrotic syndrome and subsequently end-stage renal failure has been reported. Cardiac failure is uncommon. A mutant gelsolin gene producing a protein with asparginine in place of aspartic acid at position 187 has been found. It is thought that symptoms are due to the accumulation of amyloid derived from plasma gelsolin in the tissues.[61]

References

1. Virchow R. Cited by Schwartz P. Amyloidosis: Cause and Manifestation of Senile Deterioration. Springfield, Illinois: Charles C Thomas, 1970
2. Kyle RA, Linos A, Beard CM, et al. Incidence and natural history of primary systemic amyloidosis in Olmsted County, Minnesota, 1950 through 1989. Blood 1992;79:1817–1822
3. Solomon A, Weiss DT, Pepys MB. Induction in mice of human light-chain associated amyloidosis. Am J Pathol 1992;140:629–637
4. Comenzo RL, Wally J, Kica G, et al. Clonal immunoglobulin light chain variable region germline gene use in AL amyloidosis: association with dominant amyloid-related organ involvement and survival after

stem cell transplantation. Br J Haematol 1999;106:744–751

5. Kyle RA, Gertz MA. Primary systemic amyloidosis: clinical and laboratory features in 474 cases. Semin Hematol 1995;32:45–59

6. Rajkumar SV, Gertz MA, Kyle RA. Prognosis of patients with primary systemic amyloidosis who present with dominant neuropathy. Am J Med 1998;104:232–237

7. Rajani B, Rajani V, Prayson RA. Peripheral nerve amyloidosis in sural nerve biopsies. Arch Pathol Lab Med 2000;124:114–118

8. Traynor AE, Gertz MA, Kyle R. Cranial neuropathy associated with primary systemic amyloidosis. Ann Neurol 1991;29:451–454

9. Linke RP, Nathrath WBJ, Eulitz M. Classification of amyloid syndromes from tissue sections using antibodies against various amyloid fibril proteins: report of 142 cases. In: Glenner GG, Osserman EF, Bendett EP, et al., eds. Amyloidosis. New York: Plenum Press, 1986:599–605

10. Hawkins PN, Lavender JP, Pepys MB. Evaluation of systemic amyloidosis by scintigraphy with ^{123}I-labeled serum amyloid P component. N Engl J Med 1990;323:508–513

11. Kyle RA, Greipp PR. Primary systemic amyloidosis: comparison of melphalan and prednisone versus placebo. Blood 1978;52:818–827

12. Kyle RA, Gertz MA, Greipp PR, et al. A trial of three regimens for primary amyloidosis: colchicine alone, melphalan and prednisone, and melphalan, prednisone and colchicine. N Engl J Med 1997;336:1202–1207

13. Gertz MA, Lacy MQ, Lust JA, et al. Prospective randomized trial of melphalan and prednisone versus vincristine, carmustine, melphalan, cyclophosphamide, and prednisone in the treatment of primary systemic amyloidosis. J Clin Oncol 1999;17:262–267

14. Gertz MA, Kyle RA. Acute leukemia and cytogenetic abnormalities complicating melphalan treatment of primary systemic amyloidosis. Arch Intern Med 1990;150:629–633

15. Comenzo RL, Falk R, Reisinger J, et al. Dose-intensive melphalan with blood stem-cell support for the treatment of AL (amyloid light-chain) amyloidosis: survival and responses in 25 patients. Blood 1998;91:3662–3670

16. Gianni L, Bellotti V, Gianni AM, Merlini G. New drug therapy of amyloidoses: resorption of AL-type deposits with 4'-iodo-4'-deoxydoxorubicin. Blood 1995;86:855–861

17. Andrade C. A peculiar form of peripheral neuropathy; familial atypical generalized amyloidosis with special involvement of the peripheral nerves. Brain 1952;75:408–427

18. Andersson R. Familial amyloidosis with polyneuropathy: a clinical study based on patients living in northern Sweden. Acta Med Scand Suppl 1976;590:1–64

19. Holt IJ, Harding AE, Middleton L, et al. Molecular genetics of amyloid neuropathy in Europe. Lancet 1989;1:524–526

20. Costa PP, Figueira AS, Bravo FR. Amyloid fibril protein related to prealbumin in familial amyloidotic polyneuropathy. Proc Natl Acad Sci U S A 1978;75:4499–4503

21. Saraiva MJ, Costa PP, Goodman DS. Genetic expression of a transthyretin mutation in typical and late-onset Portuguese families with familial amyloidotic polyneuropathy. Neurology 1986;36:1413–1417

22. Planté-Bordeneuve V, Lalu T, Misrahi M, et al. Genotypic-phenotypic variations in a series of 65 patients with familial amyloid polyneuropathy. Neurology 1998;51:708–714

23. Connors LH, Richardson AM, Theberge R, Costello CE. Tabulation of transthyretin (TTR) variants as of 1/1/2000. Amyloid 2000;7:54–69

24. Kelly JW, Colon W, Lai Z, et al. Transthyretin quaternary and tertiary structural changes facilitate misassembly into amyloid. Adv Protein Chem 1997;50:161–181

25. Rukavina JG, Block WD, Jackson CE, et al. Primary systemic amyloidosis: a review and an experimental, genetic, and clinical study of 29 cases with particular emphasis on the familial form. Medicine (Baltimore) 1956;35:239–334

26. Libbey CA, Rubinow A, Shirahama T, et al. Familial amyloid polyneuropathy. Demonstration of prealbumin in a kinship of German/English ancestry with onset in the seventh decade. Am J Med 1984;76:18–24

27. Frederiksen T, Gotzsche H, Harboe N, et al. Familial primary amyloidosis with severe amyloid heart disease. Am J Med 1962;33:328–348

28. Nordlie M, Sletten K, Husby G, Ranlov PJ. A new prealbumin variant in familial amyloid cardiomyopathy of Danish origin. Scand J Immunol 1988;27:119–122

29. Benson MD, Wallace MR, Tejada E, et al. Hereditary amyloidosis: description of a new American kindred with late onset cardiomyopathy. Appalachian amyloid. Arthritis Rheum 1987;30:195–200

30. Van Allen MW, Frolich JA, Davis JR. Inherited predisposition to generalized amyloidosis. Clinical and pathological study of a family with neuropathy, nephropathy, and peptic ulcer. Neurology 1969;19:10–25

31. Nichols WC, Dwulet FE, Liepnieks J, Benson MD. Variant apolipoprotein AI as a major constituent of a human hereditary amyloid. Biochem Biophys Res Commun 1988;156:762–768

32. Benson MD. Familial amyloidosis: variations on a theme by Andrade. In: Kyle RA, Gertz MA, eds. Amyloid and Amyloidosis 1998. New York: Parthenon Publishing, 1999:230–234

33. Benson MD, Liepnieks J, Uemichi T, et al. Hereditary renal amyloidosis associated with a mutant fibrinogen alpha-chain. Nat Genet 1993;3:252–255

34. Connors LH, Ericsson T, Skare J, et al. A simple screening test for variant transthyretins associated with familial transthyretin amyloidosis using isoelectric focusing. Biochim Biophys Acta 1998;1407:185–192

35. Dyck PJ, Lambert EH. Dissociated sensation in amyloidosis. Compound action potential, quantitative histologic and teased-fiber, and electron microscopic studies of sural nerve biopsies. Arch Neurol 1969;20:490–507

36. Said G, Ropert A, Faux N. Length-dependent degeneration of fibers in Portuguese amyloid polyneuropathy: a clinicopathologic study. Neurology 1984;34:1025–1032

37. Gertz MA, Kyle RA, Thibodeau SN. Familial amyloidosis: a study of 52 North American-born patients examined during a 30-year period. Mayo Clin Proc 1992;67:428–440

38. Holmgren G, Ericzon BG, Groth CG, et al. Clinical improvement and amyloid regression after liver transplantation in hereditary transthyretin amyloidosis. Lancet 1993;341:1113–1116

39. Suhr OB, Holmgren G, Steen L, et al. Liver transplantation in familial amyloidotic polyneuropathy. Transplantation 1995;60:933–938

40. Rydh A, Suhr O, Hietala S-O, et al. Serum amyloid P component scintigraphy in familial amyloid polyneu-

ropathy: regression of visceral amyloid following liver transplantation. Eur J Nucl Med 1998;25:709–713

41. Dubrey S, Davidoff R, Skinner M, et al. Progression of ventricular wall thickening after liver transplantation for familial amyloidosis. Transplantation 1997;64:74–80

42. Stangou AJ, Hawkins PN, Heaton ND. Progressive cardiac amyloidosis following liver transplantation for familial amyloid polyneuropathy. Transplantation 1998;66:229–233

43. Pomfret E, Lewis WD, Jenkins RL, et al. Effect of orthotopic liver transplantation on the progression of familial amyloidotic polyneuropathy. Transplantation 1998;65:918–925

44. García-Herola A, Prieto M, Pascual S, et al. Progression of cardiomyopathy and neuropathy after liver transplantation in a patient with familial amyloidotic polyneuropathy caused by tyrosine-77 transthyretin variant. Liver Transplant Surg 1999;5:246–248

45. Suhr O, Danielsson A, Rydh A, et al. Impact of gastrointestinal dysfunction on survival of liver transplantation for familial amyloidotic polyneuropathy. Dig Dis Sci 1996;41:1909–1914

46. Suhr OB, Wiklund U, Ando Y, et al. Impact of liver transplantation on autonomic neuropathy in familial amyloidotic polyneuropathy: an evaluation by spectral analysis of heart rate variability. J Intern Med 1997;242:225–229

47. Ikeda S-I, Takei Y-I, Yanagisawa N, et al. Peripheral nerves regenerated in familial amyloid polyneuropathy after liver transplantation. Ann Intern Med 1997;127:618–620

48. Jonsen E, Suhr O, Athlin E, Wikström L. Quality of life after liver transplantation in patients with familial amyloidotic polyneuropathy. Amyloid 1996;3:124–129

49. Kawasaki S, Makuuchi M, Matsunami H, et al. Living related liver transplantation in adults. Ann Surg 1998;227:269–274

50. Peterson SA, Klabunde T, Lashuel HA, et al. Inhibiting transthyretin conformational changes that lead to amyloid fibril formation. Proc Natl Acad Sci USA 1998;95:12956–12960

51. Tokuda T, Kondo T, Hanaoka N, et al. A selective transthyretin-adsorption column for the treatment of

patients with familial amyloid polyneuropathy. Amyloid 1998;5:111–116

52. Wikstrom L, Bjerle P, Boman K, et al. L-threo-DOPS treatment of orthostatic hypotension in Swedish patients with familial amyloidotic polyneuropathy (TTR-met[30]). Amyloid 1996;3:162–166

53. Carvalho MJ, van den Meiracker AH, Boomsma F, et al. Improved orthostatic tolerance in familial amyloidotic polyneuropathy with unnatural noradrenaline precursor L-threo-3,4-dihydroxyphenylserine. J Auton Nerv Syst 1997;62:63–71

54. de Freitas F. Treatment of orthostatic hypotension with L-threo-DOPS in familial amyloidotic polyneuropathy (editorial). Amyloid 1996;3:212–213

55. Jensson O, Gudmundsson G, Arnason A, et al. Hereditary cystatin C (gamma-trace) amyloid angiopathy of the CNS causing cerebral hemorrhage. Acta Neurol Scand 1987;76:102–114

56. Wang ZZ, Jensson O, Thorsteinsson L, Vinters HV. Microvascular degeneration in hereditary cystatin C amyloid angiopathy of the brain. APMIS 1997;105:41–47

57. Abrahamson M. Molecular basis for amyloidosis related to hereditary brain hemorrhage. Scand J Clin Lab Invest 1996;56(Suppl 226):47–56

58. Bornebroek M, Westendorp RGJ, Haan J, et al. Mortality from hereditary cerebral hemorrhage with amyloidosis—Dutch type. The impact of sex, parental transmission and year of birth. Brain 1997;120:2243–2249

59. Meretoja J. Familial systemic paramyloidosis with lattice dystrophy of the cornea, progressive cranial neuropathy, skin changes and various internal symptoms. A previously unrecognized heritable syndrome. Ann Clin Res 1969;1:314–324

60. Kiuru S, Salonen O, Haltia M. Gelsolin-related spinal and cerebral amyloid angiopathy. Ann Neurol 1999;45:305–311

61. Kangas H, Ulmanen I, Paunio T, et al. Functional consequences of amyloidosis mutation for gelsolin polypeptide—analysis of gelsolin-actin interaction and gelsolin processing in gelsolin knock-out fibroblasts. FEBS Lett 1999;454:233–239

203 Peripheral Neuropathy in the Lymphomas and Leukemias

Thomas M Habermann

To appreciate the scope of peripheral neuropathy in lymphoma and leukemia requires understanding the broad spectrum of these hematological malignancies.[1] The most important issue is the classification of the underlying disease process. Drugs are the most significant cause of peripheral neuropathy in leukemia and lymphoma. Age-related changes in pharmacokinetics are important in the development of peripheral neuropathy,[2] and other factors also contribute (Table 203.1). Neuropathies associated with hematological malignancies may be classified as "axonopathy" (most characteristically due to drugs), "demyelinating disease" (more characteristically related to dysproteinemia or disease), or "neuronopathy."[3]

Peripheral neuropathy may occur at presentation, as a manifestation of the disease, as a complication of therapy or other supportive treatment, or as a complication of survival. The neuropathy may be a polyradiculoneuropathy, multiple mononeuropathy, sensorimotor polyneuropathy, sensory polyneuropathy, or a mononeuropathy. The presentation may be acute or chronic.

Frequently, the reports are clinical descriptions, and the findings are not documented by a neurologist or by electromyographic (EMG) studies. The variability in incidence is multifactorial.[4] Some reports include electrophysiological evidence of peripheral neuropathy and others do not. Some series have included patients who had electrophysiological evidence of peripheral neuropathy without clinical symptoms. Grading the severity of chemotherapy-induced peripheral neuropathy according to the World Health Organization (WHO), Eastern Cooperative Oncology Group (ECOG), and National Cancer Institute of Canada has pitfalls because of variations among the classifications and interobserver agreement.[5] Caution is needed in interpreting results across studies that used different scales for grading neurotoxicity in peripheral neuropathy. The recently developed Common Toxicity Grading System should be used in clinical trials to grade peripheral neuropathy related to toxicities of treatment (Table 203.2).

Table 203.1 Factors important in the development of peripheral neuropathy in hematological malignancies

Age-related changes in pharmacokinetics of drugs
Functional reserve of target organs
Complications of unrelated diseases
Therapeutic interventions
Dose-related treatment-related toxicities
Preceding treatments that predispose to development of peripheral neuropathy
Preexisting peripheral neuropathy

Table 203.2 United States of America National Cancer Institute Common Toxicity Criteria: neurology

Neuropathy	0	1	2	3	4
Motor	Normal	Subjective weakness, but no objective findings	Mild objective weakness interfering with function but not with activities of daily living	Objective weakness interfering with activities of daily living	Paralysis
Sensory	Normal	Loss of deep tendon reflexes or paresthesia (including tingling) but no interference with function	Objective sensory loss or paresthesia (including tingling) interfering with function, but not with activities of daily living	Sensory loss or paresthesia interfering with activities of daily living	Permanent sensory loss interfering with function

From the National Cancer Institute Cancer Therapy Evaluation Program, Common Toxicity Criteria, Version 2.0, published April 30, 1999. Retrieved May 9, 2002, from the World Wide Web: http://ctep.cancer.gov/forms/CTCv20_4-30-992.pdf

Peripheral neuropathy in non-Hodgkin lymphoma

Non-Hodgkin lymphoma (NHL) constitutes a diverse group of disorders that vary in their histological, immunophenotypic, and genotypic criteria; natural history; response to treatment; and survival rates. Peripheral neuropathy may complicate the clinical course of lymphoma. Various classifications of lymphoma have been proposed; the most recent is the WHO classification, which is a modification of the Revised European American Lymphoid Neoplasms Classification[1,6] (Table 203.3). Treatment varies according to the histological classification, type of presentation, and whether the disease is newly diagnosed or a relapse. The numerous treatment options have been reviewed recently by Habermann.[7]

Classification of peripheral neuropathy

A classification should be comprehensive and aid physicians in the evaluation and management of patients. Several classifications have been reported.[4,8,9] The one presented in Table 203.4 is a modification of previous classifications. It provides a framework to aid in the formulation of a differential diagnosis and in the diagnostic work-up. Menigoradicular localizations are central (vs. peripheral)[10] and may or may not be included in different series.[4] Thus, because leptomeningeal lymphomas are not considered peripheral, they are not included in this classification. From a neurological perspective, the clinical presentation of peripheral neuropathy is not unique in most cases and usually does not provide specific information. The most essential element of the clinical history of

---

Table 203.3   Proposed World Health Organization classification of lymphoid neoplasms

B-cell neoplasms

I.   Precursor B-cell neoplasm: precursor B-lymphoblastic leukemia/lymphoma
II. Peripheral B-cell neoplasms
    1. B-cell chronic lymphocytic leukemia/prolymphocytic leukemia/small lymphocytic lymphoma
    2. Lymphoplasmacytoid lymphoma/immunocytoma
    3. Mantle cell lymphoma
    4. Follicle center lymphoma, follicular
       Provisional cytologic grades: I (small cell), II (mixed small and large cell), III (large cell)
    5. Marginal zone B-cell lymphoma
       Extranodal (MALT-type) with or without monocytoid B cells
    6. Provisional entity: splenic marginal zone lymphoma (with or without villous lymphocytes)
    7. Hairy cell leukemia
    8. Plasmacytoma/plasma cell myeloma
    9. Diffuse large B-cell lymphoma
   10. Burkitt lymphoma
   11. Provisional entity: high-grade B-cell lymphoma, Burkitt-like

T-cell and putative natural killer (NK)-cell neoplasms

I.   Precursor T-cell neoplasm: precursor T-lymphoblastic lymphoma/leukemia
II. Peripheral T-cell NK-cell neoplasms
    1. T-cell chronic lymphocytic leukemia/prolymphocytic leukemia
    2. Large granular lymphocytic leukemia
       T-cell type
       NK-cell type
    3. Mycosis fungoides/Sézary syndrome
    4. Peripheral T-cell lymphoma, unspecified
       Provisional cytological categories: medium-sized cell, mixed medium and large cell, large cell, lymphoepithelioid cell
       Provisional subtype: hepatosplenic γδ T-cell lymphoma
       Provisional subtype: subcutaneous panniculitic T-cell lymphoma
    5. Angioimmunoblastic T-cell lymphoma
    6. Angiocentric lymphoma
    7. Intestinal T-cell lymphoma (with or without enteropathy associated)
    8. Adult T-cell lymphoma/leukemia
    9. Anaplastic large-cell lymphoma (ALCL), CD30+, T and null-cell types
   10. Provisional entity: anaplastic large-cell lymphoma, Hodgkin-like

Hodgkin disease

I.   Lymphocyte predominance
II. Nodular sclerosis
III. Mixed cellularity
IV. Lymphocyte depletion
V.   Provisional entity: lymphocyte-rich classic Hodgkin disease

---

MALT, mucosa-associated lymphoid tissue. Modified from Harris et al.[1] By permission of the American Society of Clinical Oncology.

Table 203.4   Differential diagnosis of peripheral neuropathy in lymphoma

Chemotherapy-related neurotoxicity
   Vinca alkaloids: vincristine, vinblastine, vindesine,
      vinorelbine
   Cisplatin, carboplatin
   Taxanes: paclitaxel (Taxol), docetaxel
   Cytarabine
   Procarbazine
   Etoposide (VP-16)
   Interferon alpha and alfa recombinant
   Adenosine deaminase inhibitors
      (2-chlorodeoxyadenosine, fludarabine)
   Thalidomide
   Others
Directly related to malignant cells in peripheral nervous
   system
   B-cell
      Tumor proliferation
      Intravascular lymphomatosis
      Peripheral neuropathy due to nerve infiltration by
         lymphoma in AIDS
   T-cell
      Distal root involvement
      Subacute polyradiculoneuritis associated with
         lymphomatous infiltrates of epineurium
IgM monoclonal protein with antimyelin activity
Other peripheral nervous system disorders whose
   occurrence is enhanced by dysimmune status of the
   patient
   Lymphoma-associated vasculitis
   Guillain–Barré syndrome
   Chronic inflammatory demyelinating polyneuropathy
Autoimmune
   Lymphoma-associated vasculitis
   Guillain–Barré syndrome
   Chronic inflammatory demyelinating polyneuropathy
Related to bone marrow/peripheral stem cell
   transplantation
   Unrelated donor, allogeneic, autologous
   Chemotherapy conditioning regimens: VP-16, cisplatin
   Graft-vs.-host disease prophylaxis: cyclosporine,
      FK506
   Graft-vs.-host disease management: thalidomide,
      interferon alpha
   Chronic graft-vs.-host disease with vasculitis
   Chronic illness polyneuropathy
   Chronic inflammatory demyelinating polyneuropathy
Paraneoplastic
   Subacute motor mononeuropathy
   Neuromyotonia
Compression by tumor
Radiation-induced
Secondary complications of disease
   Infectious: Herpes zoster
   Cachexia and nutritional deficiencies associated with
      malignancy
Cause undetermined

AIDS, acquired immunodeficiency syndrome.

the disease and its management is to define special therapeutic interventions and the unique complications of specific lymphoma histologies.

General issues of treatment

Follicular lymphomas and diffuse large cell B-cell lymphomas account for about 70% of all lymphomas. The paradox of NHLs is that the follicular and diffuse low-grade types have long survival but generally are not curable, even though they are responsive to initial uncomplicated and relatively nontoxic therapy. In contrast, B-cell diffuse large cell lymphoma, peripheral T-cell NLH, and other intermediate lymphomas are potentially curable but have short survival if complete clinical remission is not achieved with initial treatment. For most cases of NHL, chemotherapy is the primary treatment. In two randomized trials of diffuse large cell lymphoma (stage I or II disease) treated with chemotherapy followed by radiotherapy or observation, the Southwestern Oncology Group and the ECOG showed that the addition of radiotherapy is beneficial.[11]

CHOP (cyclophosphamide, doxorubicin [hydroxydaunomycin], vincristine [oncovin], and prednisone) chemotherapy for six to eight cycles is the treatment of choice for diffuse large cell NHL.[12] The reported complete remission rates in several series range from 50% to 70%, with relapse rates of 7% for years two to five. Cure rates are 30% to 40%. Prognostic factors have been identified.[13,14] Extranodal disease is an adverse prognostic factor, but lymphomatous involvement of the peripheral nervous system is rare and has not been found to be a worse prognostic factor than involvement of other extranodal sites. Disease relapse is treated with more aggressive regimens such as DHAP (dexamethasone, cytosine arabinoside, and cisplatin). If there is evidence of a response to treatment, then high doses of chemotherapy with drug regimens that include cyclophosphamide and etoposide (VP-16) with or without radiotherapy are administered, followed by peripheral blood or autologous bone marrow transplantation.[15,16]

Low-grade NHL and "diffuse" low-grade NHL (small lymphocytic lymphoma, lymphoplasmacytic lymphoma, mantle cell lymphoma, nodal marginal zone lymphoma, low-grade B-cell lymphomas of mucosa-associated lymphoid tissue [MALT], and splenic marginal zone lymphoma) are frequently treated with CVP (cyclophosphamide, vincristine, and prednisone) or CHOP at presentation or relapse. With these regimens, the reported response rates are 57% to 80%, with five-year disease-free survival of 18% to 60% and overall five-year survival rates of 49% to 67%. The median disease-free interval is 17 months. Disease relapse is treated with various programs, including interferon and nucleoside adenosine deaminase inhibitors (pentostatin, fludarabine, and cladribine).

Peripheral neuropathy due to chemotherapy

The most common cause of peripheral neuropathy in NHL and Hodgkin disease is chemotherapy. The drugs that most commonly cause this are vinca alkaloids.[17] Vincristine causes a symmetrical mild axonal peripheral neuropathy that usually is reversible. This occurs in most patients who have received vincristine therapy and is the dose-limiting toxicity of the drug. The severity varies greatly. The onset is insidious and characterized by myalgias, progressive decrease or loss of deep tendon reflexes of the ankle, decreased vibratory sensation, decreased light touch or pinprick sensation, distal paresthesias affecting the hands before the feet, foot drop, wrist drop, weakness (which may appear rapidly), and motor disability (difficulty walking and muscle atrophy).[18–20] The muscles affected most frequently in the upper extremity are the extensor muscles of the wrist and fingers. As the cumulative dose increases, so does the frequency of neurotoxicity.[21] Deep tendon reflexes are usually lost after three or more weekly doses.[22] This toxic effect is essentially dose-dependent.[19] Toxicity grading and dose reductions have been standardized. The standard dose of vincristine is $1.4\,mg/m^2$; however, a significant number of patients do not receive full doses of vincristine. Enhanced neurotoxic effects have been described with cyclosporine,[23] dexamethasone and doxorubicin,[24] and isoniazid.[25] Of patients treated with vincristine and hematopoietic colony-stimulating factors, 22% developed pain and motor weakness in the legs only, both of which are unusual features of classic vincristine neuropathy.[26] Also, the risk of neurotoxic effects is enhanced with liver dysfunction, because inactivation of the drug is impaired. Distal extremity weakness typically improves after treatment with the drug has been discontinued; however, ankle deep tendon reflexes do not return. In most cases, the peripheral neuropathy is reversible.[27] Autonomic neuropathy characterized by constipation and urinary retention and cranial neuropathies may be a complication of these therapies. The initial sequelae of the accidental intrathecal administration of vincristine may include peripheral neuropathy, and it may result in devastating neurological toxicities.[28,29] An emergent treatment protocol includes drainage of the cerebrospinal fluid, ventriculolumbar perfusion with 2.5% lactated Ringer solution, and intravenous administration of glutamic acid.[30] Liposomal vincristine also causes peripheral neuropathy and does not appear to have any therapeutic advantage.[31]

In other malignancies, vinorelbine, a semisynthetic vinca alkaloid, is associated with mild-to-moderate sensorimotor distal symmetrical axonal neuropathy.[32] Vindesine and vinblastine are less neurotoxic than vincristine.

Vinca alkaloids interact with the microtubular protein tubulin,[33] thus preventing formation of microtubules, which inhibits the movement of mitotic spindles. The microtubular system of peripheral nerves is essential to axonal transport.

Cisplatin is associated with peripheral neuropathy.[34,35] The association between the risk of peripheral neuropathy and hypomagnesemia with cisplatin is significant.[36] Symptoms are common at cumulative doses of $300\,mg/m^2$ and universal at $500\,mg/m^2$, doses rarely achieved in lymphoproliferative disorders. In the rat model, cisplatin neurotoxicity affects primarily dorsal root ganglia, with mild structural changes in peripheral nerves.[37] In testicular cancer, a synthetic ACTH analogue, Org 2766, ameliorated but did not completely prevent cisplatin neuropathy.[38] Less toxicity has been reported with the analogue carboplatin.[39]

Etoposide and teniposide may cause a mild sensorimotor peripheral neuropathy.[40] High-dose cytarabine therapy has been associated with sensory peripheral neuropathy.[41] Procarbazine may cause a mild peripheral neuropathy, with paresthesias and loss of deep tendon reflexes.[42]

Fludarabine is being incorporated into the initial treatment and management of patients with relapse of a follicular low-grade lymphoma. In a phase II study, two of 44 patients were reported to have peripheral neuropathy.[43] Peripheral neuropathy related to 2-chlorodeoxyadenosine developed in a patient with a paraneoplastic neurological syndrome associated with lymphoma.[44]

Other new drugs have been evaluated in lymphomatous disorders. The main toxic effect associated with paclitaxel given at standard doses is peripheral neuropathy, and doses greater than or equal to $250\,mg/m^2$ cause predominantly sensory or sensorimotor polyneuropathy. Neurotoxic complications affect motor fibers and small and large sensory fibers. The effect is moderate, reversible, and not dose-limiting.[45,46] Painful proximal muscle weakness may develop.[47] The neuropathy may progress after treatment with paclitaxel has been discontinued.[48] Docetaxel (Taxotere), a semi-synthetic analogue of paclitaxel, inhibits tubulin depolymerization. In a unique report, serial neurological examinations performed on 186 patients were followed by quantitative sensory and motor nerve conduction studies. In 11% of patients, a small-fiber sensorimotor peripheral neuropathy developed at cumulative doses of 50 to $750\,mg/m^2$ and at dose levels of 10 to $115\,mg/m^2$. Proximal and distal extremity weakness developed in 10 patients.[49] Quantitative sensory testing with current perception threshold was not as useful as the clinical features or nerve conduction studies in detecting neuropathy. Peripheral neuropathy rates of up to 49% have been reported in patients treated with docetaxel.[50] Vibration perception did not correlate with clinical signs and symptoms. Platinum and oxaliplatin are associated with reversible peripheral neuropathy.[51]

The role of interferon alpha in follicular NHL is debated.[7] A mild distal, reversible sensorimotor neuropathy may be a complication of this therapy.

Thalidomide is being studied in clinical trials as an antiangiogenesis agent; it has a role in the management of acute and chronic graft-versus-host disease in allogeneic bone marrow transplantation.[52–54] It is associated with a predominantly sensory peripheral neuropathy, with painful symmetrical distal paresthesias, but muscle weakness may occur.[55,56] In a prospective study of nine patients, three had clinical and electrophysiological alterations and two others had only electrophysiological alterations consistent with early neuropathy at three months. There is a possible relationship with slow acetylators.[57] Recovery may be slow, and this complication may not be reversible. Further progression of the neuropathy after discontinuation of the treatment has been reported.[58] Neuronal or axonal degeneration without significant peripheral demyelination characterizes this complication. An extensive degeneration of sensory fibers, including the central branches in the posterior columns of the spinal cord, have been documented at autopsy.[59]

The management of chemotherapy-induced peripheral neuropathy

Preexisting peripheral neuropathy is a relative contraindication for treatment with drugs associated with peripheral neuropathy. Preexisting hereditary and acquired peripheral nervous system disorders predispose patients to a more severe neuropathy of earlier onset. Patients receiving chemotherapy must be followed and evaluated before each cycle. Peripheral neuropathy should be graded according to the Common Toxicity scale, and dose alterations should be prescribed. The development of a moderate degree of muscle weakness is an indication to discontinue therapy until the weakness disappears. This is not an absolute contraindication to future therapy. Peripheral neuropathies associated with chemotherapy usually improve after treatment with the implicated drug has been discontinued, although it may take months. Amifostine significantly reduced peripheral neuropathy in a series of patients with ovarian carcinoma.[60] Further randomized studies in lymphoma will be essential before incorporating this as a standard of prophylaxis. Liposomal vincristine also causes peripheral neuropathy and does not appear to have a therapeutic advantage. Neurotrophic factors (nerve growth factor, glial cell line-derived neurotrophic factor, and insulin-like growth factor) are potential new agents to test in managing chemotherapy-induced peripheral neuropathy.[61]

Peripheral neuropathy secondary to lymphoma

Peripheral neuropathy as a direct manifestation of lymphoma is unusual,[31] but it can occur from compression (epidural lesions or masses) or infiltration by malignant lymphoma, so-called neurolymphomatosis. B-cell NHL, T-cell NHL, and intravascular malignant lymphomatosis are the histological types involved in peripheral neuropathy secondary to lymphoma. The neuropathy should be described with this terminology. The term "neurolymphomatosis" should not be incorporated routinely into the diagnostic vernacular of lymphoma directly involving the peripheral nervous system. Peripheral neuropathy by infiltration may be present at the initial presentation; however, it is more often a complication of relapse. The lymphoma may be a B-cell or peripheral T-cell NHL and may involve the roots and plexuses.[8] T-cell lymphomas may involve

the distal parts of nerves and are associated with subacute polyradiculoneuritis.[62] Symptomatic remitting and relapsing or progressive peripheral neuropathy due to direct tumor infiltration of peripheral nerves by T-cell NHL is rare.[63,64] The lesion has angiotropic features, with wallerian degeneration of the myelinated fibers. Solitary primary lymphoma of the sciatic nerve has also been reported.[65]

Intravascular lymphomatosis NHL may involve the peripheral nervous system. Cells plug the vasa nervorum (capillaries, arterioles, and venules).[66,67] This is followed by ischemia of nerve fibers or by demyelination.[68,69] Neurologically, the most common presentation is characterized by mental status changes and pyramidal tract signs. Intravascular lymphomatosis may also involve other organs such as the lung and skin.[66,67] Often, the diagnosis may not be established until at autopsy.[70] Fever, weight loss, and other systemic symptoms may complicate the disease.[71] The neuropathy is sensorimotor and axonal and presents as a mononeuropathy or mononeuropathy complex.[8,72] The incidence of peripheral neuropathy is unknown in intravascular lymphomatosis. Peripheral nerve may be a source of biopsy specimens in this extranodal lymphoma. Patients may have a response to chemotherapy.[73]

Immunoglobulins that react against myelin-associated glycoprotein (MAG), IgM anisulfatide antibodies, may be associated with a mixed sensory and motor peripheral neuropathy in NHL and are associated with low-grade lymphoplasmacytic NHL. Preliminary trials are evaluating the role of rituximab (Rituxan), an anti-CD20 monoclonal antibody that has been approved by the United States Food and Drug Administration (FDA) for the management of NHL. Demyelinating neuropathies caused by an immunoglobulin reaction against MAG, but not axonal peripheral neuropathies, may respond to this treatment.

Peripheral nerve injury in the brachial or lumbosacral plexus may occur from compression due to invasion by the tumor or from radiotherapy. Tumor invasion or radiotherapy injuries are likely caused by injury to the endothelium and microvasculature. Differentiating the cause of these injuries later in the course of the patient history may not be possible. Electromyographic evidence of myokymia is more characteristic of radiation injury but may occur in inflammatory polyradiculopathy.[74]

Radiotherapy may produce neurological deficits, especially of the brachial or lumbosacral plexus. This complication characteristically occurs after a latent period of at least six months. Pain is prominent in brachial plexopathies but not in lumbosacral plexopathies, because sensory and autonomic fibers are spared. In most cases, the plexopathy is progressive.

Bone marrow transplantation or peripheral blood transplantation has become the standard of care in different histologic subsets of NHL relapse. Peripheral neuropathy associated with bone marrow transplantation has been reported to be related to different types of transplants (unrelated greater than allogeneic, which is greater than autologous), conditioning regimens, graft-versus-host disease, prophylaxis and management of graft-versus-host disease, critical illness polyneuropathy, and complications of preexisting demyelinating neuropathy. As a post-transplantation complication, motor disability may be associated with significant morbidity and mortality. The majority of these neuropathies have demyelinating features. Openshaw[75] recommended that neuropathies likely to be immunologically mediated be managed empirically with immunosuppressive therapy. However, experience is too limited to suggest specific regimens.

Previous chemotherapy regimens that a patient has received are an important factor in peripheral neuropathies that complicate bone marrow transplantation. From two to eight weeks after receiving etoposide (60 mg/kg intravenously) and melphalan (140 to 160 mg/m² intravenously), six of 142 patients developed a new sensorimotor polyneuropathy.[76] All six patients had previously received vincristine. Sixty months after transplantation, three patients had EMG evidence of a distal sensory polyneuropathy. The manifestations are: (1) a motor axonal neuropathy that resolves after the treatment is discontinued or the dose is decreased or (2) a sensorimotor multifocal demyelinating neuropathy that improves after plasma exchange or intravenous immunoglobulin treatment.[77,78]

A patient who presents with NHL may also have Guillain–Barré syndrome.[8,79,80] This disorder has been associated with relapse of lymphoma.[81] Chronic inflammatory demyelinating polyneuropathy has many of the clinical and electrophysiological features of Guillain–Barré syndrome[82] and has been reported to be a post-transplantation complication in NHL.[83]

Radiation may induce peripheral neuropathy. Nerve roots are relatively resistant to radiation side effects. Rarely, a lower motor neuron syndrome affecting the legs may develop after irradiation of the distal spinal cord and cauda equina. Its pathogenesis is unclear.[84] The usual course is progressive deterioration, occasionally with one to two years of stable neurological symptoms.

Herpes varicella zoster is the most common cause of peripheral nervous system involvement in NHL.[79,85] However, this involvement is not formally considered a peripheral neuropathy. It is associated with advanced disease, chemotherapy, splenectomy, and radiotherapy.[79]

Some patients do not exhibit lymphomatous infiltrates in the peripheral nerves, but perivascular infiltrates are seen in the perineurium of biopsy specimens.[8,86,87] Vital et al.[8] suggested that these infiltrates probably have the same mechanism of action as those in paraneoplastic syndromes that occur in carcinoma. Not all patients have inflammatory cells in peripheral nerves.[88]

Hodgkin lymphoma

The spectrum of peripheral neuropathy in Hodgkin lymphoma is similar to that of NHL. The characteristic paraneoplastic manifestation of Hodgkin lymphoma is cerebellar degeneration related to anti-Tr antibodies and not peripheral neuropathy.[89] Paraneoplastic brachial neuropathy has been reported in Hodgkin lymphoma.[90,91] The most common causes of brachial plexopathy are tumor infiltration and radiation damage.[92] Prednisolone therapy produced complete recovery in a patient with Hodgkin lymphoma in complete remission.[90] According to subsequent reports, peripheral neuropathy has not improved with corticosteroid therapy.[91]

Subacute motor mononeuropathy is a remote effect in Hodgkin lymphoma, and Guillain–Barré syndrome may be a complication of the disease.[93,94] Peripheral neuropathy is a complication after autologous bone marrow transplantation in Hodgkin disease.[95]

Chronic lymphocytic leukemia

Chronic lymphocytic leukemia is the most common leukemia in the Western world. Most cases are B-cell in immunophenotype. The disease is not curable but is responsive to chemotherapy. The treatments of choice include chlorambucil; chlorambucil and prednisone; cyclophosphamide, vincristine, and prednisone; and fludarabine. Other purine nucleoside analogues have been evaluated but are not important therapeutically. Treatment-related side effects are mainly autoimmune phenomena in patients with untreated disease and infectious complications in those with treated disease.

The purine analogues fludarabine, cladribine, and pentostatin are associated with sporadic neurotoxicity.[96] At recommended doses, each agent induced neurotoxicity, mostly mild and reversible, in approximately 15% of patients.[97]

Sensorimotor polyneuropathy associated with chronic lymphocytic leukemia and IgM antiganglioside antibody has been reported.[98,99] Vasculitic mononeuropathy and inflammatory demyelinating neuropathy may be associated with chronic lymphocytic leukemia.[100] Malignant B-cells have been identified at autopsy in the endoneurium, dorsal root ganglia, and peripheral nerves.[101,102]

Chronic myelogenous leukemia

Chronic myelogenous leukemia is a myeloproliferative disorder characterized by a specific chromosome abnormality: the 9;22 translocation. As in other malignant hematological disorders, peripheral neuropathy is related predominantly to treatment or disease relapse. Also, vasculitic neuropathy is associated with chronic graft-versus-host disease.[103] Chronic inflammatory demyelinating polyneuropathy has been reported after bone marrow transplantation in patients with chronic myelogenous leukemia.[104–106] A response to plasma exchange and to the discontinuation of cyclosporine therapy has been reported.[106] Acute inflammatory demyelinating polyneuropathy has been noted in chronic myeloid leukemia.[105,107,108] Interferon may cause peripheral neuropathy in patients with chronic myelogenous leukemia.[109–111]

Table 203.5   Major clinical and laboratory features of lymphomas and leukemias associated with peripheral neuropathy

Disease	Key clinical presentation features with peripheral neuropathy	Immunohistochemical diagnosis of the disorder	Histological features of nerve biopsy
Peripheral B-cell diffuse large cell lymphoma Secondary	Chemotherapy Radiotherapy Peripheral stem cell or bone marrow transplant Guillain–Barré syndrome	No evidence of lymphoma	No evidence of lymphoma
Primary	Lymphadenopathy	CD19$^+$, CD20$^+$, κ/λ light chain restriction	Morphologic and immunohistochemical evidence of lymphoma
Peripheral T-cell lymphoma Secondary	Chemotherapy Peripheral stem cell or bone marrow transplant	No evidence of lymphoma	No evidence of lymphoma
Primary	Lymphadenopathy, extranodal involvement	Aberrant T-cell expression, CD3$^+$, CD7$^+$, CD5$^+$, CD2$^+$	Evidence of lymphoma: immunologic, morphologic
Intravascular malignant lymphomatosis	Mental status changes Pyramidal tract signs Lung lesions Skin lesions	CD20$^+$	Evidence of lymphoma: morphologic, immunologic
Peripheral B-cell lymphoplasmacytoid lymphoma	Lymphadenopathy	Immunoglobulin against MAG IgM antisulfatide antibodies	
Hodgkin lymphoma–secondary	Chemotherapy	Nondiagnostic	No evidence of Hodgkin lymphoma
Chronic lymphocytic leukemia–secondary	Chemotherapy Vasculitic	Nondiagnostic Inflammatory	Nondiagnostic Inflammatory
Chronic lymphocytic leukemia–primary	Lymphocytosis, lymphadenopathy, splenomegaly IgM antiganglioside antibody	CD20$^+$, CD5$^+$, CD23$^+$, dim monoclonal light chain restriction	CD20$^+$, CD5$^+$, CD23$^+$, dim monoclonal light chain restriction
Chronic myelogenous leukemia	Chemotherapy Disease relapse Vasculitis Postperipheral blood or bone marrow transplant	Not applicable; the key diagnostic feature is cytogenetic: t(9,22)	Leukemic Nonspecific vasculitis
Hairy cell leukemia	Chemotherapy Vasculitis	Tartrate-resistant acid phosphatase, CD20$^+$, CD11c$^+$, CD5$^-$, CD25$^+$, CD103$^+$	Nonspecific vasculitis
Acute myelogenous leukemia	Chemotherapy Infiltrative disease: M7 and M5 types Disease relapse Peripheral stem cell/bone marrow transplant	M5:CD11b$^+$, My8$^+$, CD14$^+$ M7:factor VIII antigen+ CD42$^+$	Leukemic infiltrate in M5 and M7 with positive immunohistochemical stains
Acute lymphocytic leukemia	Increased peripheral blood blast count	Early preB: CD19$^+$, CD20$^+$ PreB: surface immunoglobulin positive (clg+) B cell: surface immunoglobulin-positive T cell: CD3$^+$, CD7$^+$, CD5$^+$, CD2$^+$	If leukemic infiltrate positive: morphologic and immunohistochemical stains positive
Myelodysplastic syndrome	Cytopenias	Nonspecific	If leukemic infiltrate positive: morphologic immunohistochemical stains positive

MAG, myelin-associated glycoprotein.

Hairy cell leukemia

Hairy cell leukemia is an uncommon leukemia for which three therapies have been approved by the FDA: alfa recombinant interferon, pentostatin (2'-deoxycoformycin), and 2-chlorodeoxyadenosine. Vasculitis is a rare complication of hairy cell leukemia.

Pentostatin is not associated with peripheral neuropathy, which may develop as a complication of interferon treatment.[109–111]

Acute myelogenous leukemia

Peripheral neuropathy in acute myelogenous leukemia is related to the type of leukemia (M5, M7 [megakaryoblastic]), the therapy (primary, relapse, or transplantation), and the complications of disease. Diffuse peripheral polyneuropathy and infiltrative neuropathy have been documented in acute monoblastic leukemia.[112–114] High-dose cytosine arabinoside therapy is a well-documented cause of peripheral neuropathy.[115–117] Diffuse peripheral neuropathy can be a presenting feature of patients with relapse of acute leukemia.[118] New programs for management of relapse of acute leukemia are evaluating fludarabine. Peripheral neuropathy is associated with fludarabine and cytosine arabinoside chemotherapy for acute leukemia.[119,120] Sensorimotor peripheral neuropathy developed in two of five patients who received 2-chlorodeoxyadenosine at a dose of $19 \, mg/m^2$ daily and in all four patients who received a dose of $20 \, mg/m^2$ daily.[121] Isolated infiltration of the sciatic nerve by chloroma has been reported.[122] Peripheral neuropathy is a complication of bone marrow transplantation and may be associated with cyclosporine therapy.[123]

Acute lymphocytic leukemia

The causes of peripheral neuropathy in acute lymphocytic leukemia are similar to those in acute myelogenous leukemia.

Myelodysplastic syndromes

Chronic myelomonocytic leukemia may be associated with acute demyelinating peripheral neuropathy.[124] Peripheral sensorimotor polyneuropathy, with an IgA paraprotein, responsive to prednisone has been reported.[125]

Conclusion

Hematological malignances are a complex group of disorders, and the causes of peripheral neuropathy associated with them are diverse. The initial evaluation requires a detailed history, a complete physical examination, and a detailed neurological examination. The history and review of systems must inquire about other diseases associated with peripheral neuropathy. A detailed drug history must be obtained. Further diagnostic evaluation and management depend on these details. The clinical and pathological associations of hematological malignances and peripheral neuropathy are summarized in Table 203.5. The most common causes are related to the treatment of these diseases. Currently, the therapeutic management of the associated neuropathy frequently includes altering drug doses or discontinuing treatment with the drug. If the cause is related directly to infiltration by the underlying disease, chemotherapy or radiotherapy may be required. Additional basic research into the pathogenesis and molecular mechanisms should lead to new therapeutic interventions.

References

1. Harris NL, Jaffe ES, Diebold J, et al. World Health Organization Classification of Neoplastic Diseases of the Hematopoietic and Lymphoid Tissues: report of the Clinical Advisory Committee meeting-Airlie House, Virginia, November 1997. J Clin Oncol 1999;17:3835–3849
2. Balducci L, Mowry K. Pharmacology and organ toxicity of chemotherapy in older patients. Oncology (Huntingt) 1992;6(Suppl):62–68
3. Apfel SC, Kessler JA. Neurotrophic factors in the treatment of peripheral neuropathy. Ciba Foundation Symposium 1996;196:98–119
4. Vallat JM, De Mascarel HA, Bordessoule D, et al. Non-Hodgkin malignant lymphomas and peripheral neuropathies—13 cases. Brain 1995;118:1233–1245
5. Postma TJ, Heimans JJ, Muller MJ, et al. Pitfalls in grading severity of chemotherapy-induced peripheral neuropathy. Ann Oncol 1998;9:739–744
6. Harris NL, Jaffe ES, Stein H, et al. A revised European-American classification of lymphoid neoplasms: a proposal from the International Lymphoma Study Group. Blood 1994;84:1361–1392
7. Habermann TM. State-of-the-art treatments in non-Hodgkin's lymphoma. Cancer Res Ther Control 1999;9:303–314
8. Vital C, Vital A, Julien J, et al. Peripheral neuropathies and lymphoma without monoclonal gammopathy: a new classification. J Neurol 1990;237:177–185
9. Hughes RA, Britton T, Richards M. Effects of lymphoma on the peripheral nervous system. J R Soc Med 1994;87:526–530
10. Henson RA, Urich H, eds. Cancer and the Nervous System: The Neurological Manifestations of Systemic Malignant Disease. Oxford: Blackwell Scientific Publications, 1982:368–405
11. Miller TP, Dahlberg S, Cassady JR, et al. Chemotherapy alone compared with chemotherapy plus radiotherapy for localized intermediate- and high-grade non-Hodgkin's lymphoma. N Engl J Med 1998;339:21–26
12. Fisher RI, Gaynor ER, Dahlberg S, et al. Comparison of a standard regimen (CHOP) with three intensive chemotherapy regimens for advanced non-Hodgkin's lymphoma. N Engl J Med 1993;328:1002–1006
13. The International Non-Hodgkin's Lymphoma Prognostic Factors Project. A predictive model for aggressive non-Hodgkin's lymphoma. N Engl J Med 1993;329:987–994
14. Shipp MA. Prognostic factors in aggressive non-Hodgkin's lymphoma: who has "high-risk" disease? Blood 1994;83:1165–1173
15. Philip T, Armitage JO, Spitzer G, et al. High-dose therapy and autologous bone marrow transplantation after failure of conventional chemotherapy in adults with intermediate-grade or high-grade non-Hodgkin's lymphoma. N Engl J Med 1987;316:1493–1498

16. Gianni AM, Bregni M, Siena S, et al. High-dose chemotherapy and autologous bone marrow transplantation compared with MACOP-B in aggressive B-cell lymphoma. N Engl J Med 1997;336:1290–1297

17. Legha SS. Vincristine neurotoxicity. Pathophysiology and management. Med Toxicol 1986;1:421–427

18. Sandler SG, Tobin W, Henderson ES. Vincristine-induced neuropathy. A clinical study of fifty leukemic patients. Neurology 1969;19:367–374

19. Casey EB, Jellife AM, Le Quesne PM, Millett YL. Vincristine neuropathy. Clinical and electrophysiological observations. Brain 1973;96:69–86

20. Rosenthal S, Kaufman S. Vincristine neurotoxicity. Ann Intern Med 1974;80:733–737

21. Desai ZR, Van den Berg HW, Bridges JM, Shanks RG. Can severe vincristine neurotoxicity be prevented? Cancer Chemother Pharmacol 1982;8:211–214

22. MacDonald DR. Neurotoxicity of chemotherapeutic agents. In: Perry MC, ed. The Chemotherapy Source Book. Baltimore: Williams & Wilkins, 1992:666–679

23. Bertrand Y, Capdeville R, Balduck N, Philippe N. Cyclosporin A used to reverse drug resistance increases vincristine neurotoxicity. Am J Hematol 1992;40:158–159

24. Weber DM, Dimopoulos MA, Alexanian R. Increased neurotoxicity with VAD-cyclosporin in multiple myeloma. Lancet 1993;341:558–559

25. Hildebrand J, Kenis Y. Additive toxicity of vincristine and other drugs for the peripheral nervous system. Three case reports. Acta Neurol Belg 1971;71:486–491

26. Weintraub M, Adde MA, Venson DJ, et al. Severe atypical neuropathy associated with administration of hematopoietic colony-stimulating factors and vincristine. J Clin Oncol 1996;14:935–940

27. Nowacki P, Dolinska D, Stankiewicz J, Grzelec H. Impairment of peripheral nervous system in patients with non-Hodgkin's lymphomas treated with CBVPM/AVBP and CHOP schedules. Acta Haematol Pol 1992;23:111–116

28. Manelis J, Freudlich E, Ezekiel E, Doron J. Accidental intrathecal vincristine administration. Report of a case. J Neurol 1982;228:209–213

29. Zaragoza MR, Ritchey ML, Walter A. Neurourologic consequences of accidental intrathecal vincristine: a case report. Med Pediatr Oncol 1995;24:61–62

30. Dyke RW. Treatment of inadvertent intrathecal injection of vincristine. N Engl J Med 1989;321:1270–1271

31. Gelmon KA, Tolcher A, Diab AR, et al. Phase I study of liposomal vincristine. J Clin Oncol 1999;17:697–705

32. Pace A, Bove L, Nistico C, et al. Vinorelbine neurotoxicity: clinical and neurophysiological findings in 23 patients. J Neurol Neurosurg Psychiatry 1996;61:409–411

33. Green LS, Donoso JA, Heller-Bettinger IE, Samson FE. Axonal transport disturbances in vincristine-induced peripheral neuropathy. Ann Neurol 1977;1:255–262

34. Roelofs RI, Hrushesky W, Rogin J, Rosenberg L. Peripheral sensory neuropathy and cisplatin chemotherapy. Neurology 1984;34:934–938

35. Thompson SW, Davis LE, Kornfeld M, et al. Cisplatin neuropathy. Clinical, electrophysiologic, morphologic, and toxicologic studies. Cancer 1984;54:1269–1275

36. Ashraf M, Scotchel PL, Krall JM, Flink EB. cis-Platinum-induced hypomagnesemia and peripheral neuropathy. Gynecol Oncol 1983;16:309–318

37. Barajon I, Bersani M, Quartu M, et al. Neuropeptides and morphological changes in cisplatin-induced dorsal root ganglion neuronopathy. Exp Neurol 1996;138:93–104

38. van Gerven JMA, Hovestadt A, Moll JWB, et al. The effects of an ACTH (4–9) analogue on development of cisplatin neuropathy in testicular cancer: a randomized trial. J Neurol 1994;241:432–435

39. van Glabbeke M, Renard J, Pinedo HM, et al. Iproplatin and carboplatin induced toxicities: overview of phase II clinical trial conducted by the EORTC Early Clinical Trials Cooperative Group (ECTG). Eur J Cancer Clin Oncol 1988;24:255–262

40. O'Dwyer PJ, Leyland-Jones B, Alonso MT, et al. Etoposide (VP-16-213). Current status of an active anticancer drug. N Engl J Med 1985;312:692–700

41. Russell JA, Powles RL. Neuropathy due to cytosine arabinoside (letter). Br Med J 1974;4:652–653

42. Weiss HD, Walker MD, Wiernik PH. Neurotoxicity of commonly used antineoplastic agents. N Engl J Med 1974;291:75–81

43. Solal-Celigny P, Brice P, Brousse N, et al. Phase II trial of fludarabine monophosphate as first-line treatment in patients with advanced follicular lymphoma: a multicenter study by the Groupe d'Etude des Lymphomes de l'Adulte. J Clin Oncol 1996;14:514–519

44. Warzocha K, Krykowksi E, Gora-Tybor J, et al. Fulminant 2-chlorodeoxyadenosine-related peripheral neuropathy in a patient with paraneoplastic neurological syndrome associated with lymphoma. Leuk Lymphoma 1996;21:343–346

45. Iniguez C, Larrode P, Mayordomo JI, et al. Reversible peripheral neuropathy induced by a single administration of high-dose paclitaxel. Neurology 1998;51:868–870

46. Goss P, Stewart AK, Couture F, et al. Combined results of two phase II studies of Taxol (paclitaxel) in patients with relapsed or refractory lymphomas. Leuk Lymphoma 1999;34:295–304

47. Freilich RJ, Balmaceda C, Seidman AD, et al. Motor neuropathy due to docetaxel and paclitaxel. Neurology 1996;47:115–118

48. van den Bent MJ, van Raaij-van den Aarssen VJ, Verweij J, et al. Progression of paclitaxel-induced neuropathy following discontinuation of treatment. Muscle Nerve 1997;20:750–752

49. New PZ, Jackson CE, Rinaldi D, et al. Peripheral neuropathy secondary to docetaxel (Taxotere). Neurology 1996;46:108–111

50. Hilkens PH, Verweij J, Stoter G, et al. Peripheral neurotoxicity induced by docetaxel. Neurology 1996;46:104–108

51. Germann N, Brienza S, Rotarski M, et al. Preliminary results on the activity of oxaliplatin (L-OHP) in refractory/recurrent non-Hodgkin's lymphoma patients. Ann Oncol 1999;10:351–354

52. Vogelsang GB, Hess AD, Gordon G, Santos GW. Treatment and prevention of acute graft-versus-host disease with thalidomide in a rat model. Transplantation 1986;41:644–647

53. McCarthy DM, Kanfer E, Taylor J, Barrett AJ. Thalidomide for graft-versus-host disease. Lancet 1988;2:1135

54. Heney D, Norfolk DR, Wheeldon J, et al. Thalidomide treatment for chronic graft-versus-host disease. Br J Haematol 1991;78:23–27

55. Gibbels E. Toxic injuries in thalidomide medication [German]. Forschr Neurol Psychiatr Grenzgeb 1967;35:393–411

56. Clemmensen OJ, Olsen PZ, Andersen KE. Thalidomide neurotoxicity. Arch Dermatol 1984;120:338–341

57. Hess CW, Hunziker T, Kupfer A, Ludin HP. Thalidomide-induced peripheral neuropathy. A prospective clinical, neurophysiological and pharmacogenetic evaluation. J Neurol 1986;233:83–89

58. Hafström T. Polyneuropathy after neurosedyn (thalidomide) and its prognosis. Acta Neurol Scand 1967;43(Suppl 32):1–41

59. Klinghardt GW. Arzneimittelschadigungen des peripheren Nervensystems unter besonderer Berucksichtigung der Polyneuropathie durch Isonicotinsaurchydrazid (experimentelle und human pathologische Untersuchungen). In: Proceedings of the V International Congress of Neuropathology. Amsterdam: Excerpta Medica Foundation, 1965:292–301

60. Rose PG. Amifostine cytoprotection with chemotherapy for advanced ovarian carcinoma. Semin Oncol 1996;23(Suppl 8):83–89

61. Apfel SC. Managing the neurotoxicity of paclitaxel (Taxol) and docetaxel (Taxotere) with neurotrophic factors. Cancer Invest 2000;18:564–573

62. Vital C, Bonnaud E, Arne L, et al. Polyneuritis in chronic lymphoid leukemia. Ultrastructural study of the peripheral nerve [French]. Acta Neuropathol (Berl) 1975;32:169–172

63. Leblond V, Raphael M, et al. Lymphomes maligns non-Hodgkiniens (LMNH) de type peripherique avec atteinte cutanee et neurologique (abstract). Nouv Rev Fr Hematol 1984;26:110

64. Gherardi R, Gaulard P, Prost C, et al. T-cell lymphoma revealed by a peripheral neuropathy. A report of two cases with an immunohistologic study on lymph nodes and nerve biopsies. Cancer 1986;58:2710–2716

65. Pillay PK, Hardy RW Jr, Wilbourn AJ, et al. Solitary primary lymphoma of the sciatic nerve: case report. Neurosurgery 1988;23:370–371

66. Pfleger L, Tappeiner J. Zur Kenntnis der systemisierten Endotheliomatose der cutanen Blutgefässe (Reticuloendotheliose?). Hautarzt 1959;10:359

67. Glass J, Hochberg FH, Miller DC. Intravascular lymphomatosis. A systemic disease with neurologic manifestations. Cancer 1993;71:3156–3164

68. Gemignani F, Marchesi G, Di Giovanni G, et al. Low-grade non-Hodgkin B-cell lymphoma presenting as sensory neuropathy. Eur Neurol 1996;36:138–141

69. Levin KH, Lutz G. Angiotropic large-cell lymphoma with peripheral nerve and skeletal muscle involvement: early diagnosis and treatment. Neurology 1996; 47:1009–1011

70. Domizio P, Hall PA, Cotter F, et al. Angiotropic large cell lymphoma (ALCL): morphological, immunohistochemical and genotypic studies with analysis of previous reports. Hematol Oncol 1989;7:195–206

71. Dubas F, Saint-Andre JP, Pouplard-Barthelaix A, et al. Intravascular malignant lymphomatosis (so-called malignant angioendotheliomatosis): a case confined to the lumbosacral spinal cord and nerve roots. Clin Neuropathol 1990;9:115–120

72. Pellicone JT, Goldstein HB. Pulmonary malignant angioendotheliomatosis. Presentation with fever and syndrome of inappropriate antidiuretic hormone. Chest 1990;98:1292–1294

73. Legerton CW III, Sergent JS. Intravascular malignant lymphoma mimicking central nervous system lupus. Arthritis Rheum 1993;36:135

74. Thomas JE, Cascino TL, Earle JD. Differential diagnosis between radiation and tumor plexopathy of the pelvis. Neurology 1985;35:1–7

75. Openshaw H. Peripheral neuropathy after bone marrow transplantation. Biol Blood Marrow Transplant 1997;3:202–209

76. Imrie KR, Couture F, Turner CC, et al. Peripheral neuropathy following high-dose etoposide and autologous bone marrow transplantation. Bone Marrow Transplant 1994;13:77–79

77. Ayres RC, Bousset B, Wixon S, et al. Peripheral neurotoxicity with tacrolimus. Lancet 1994;343:862–863

78. Wilson JR, Conwit RA, Eidelman BH, et al. Sensorimotor neuropathy resembling CIDP in patients receiving FK506. Muscle Nerve 1994;17:528–532

79. Correale J, Monteverde DA, Bueri JA, Reich EG. Peripheral nervous system and spinal cord involvement in lymphoma. Acta Neurol Scand 1991;83:45–51

80. Sumi SM, Farrell DF, Knauss TA. Lymphoma and leukemia manifested by steroid-responsive polyneuropathy. Arch Neurol 1983;40:577–582

81. Phan TG, Manoharan A, Pryor D. Relapse of central nervous system Burkitt's lymphoma presenting as Guillain–Barré syndrome and syndrome of inappropriate ADH secretion. Aust N Z J Med 1998;28:223–224

82. Dalakas MC. Advances in chronic inflammatory demyelinating polyneuropathy: disease variants and inflammatory response mediators and modifiers. Curr Opin Neurol 1999;12:403–409

83. Griggs JJ, Commichau CS, Rapoport AP, Griggs RC. Chronic inflammatory demyelinating polyneuropathy in non-Hodgkin's lymphoma. Am J Hematol 1997;54: 332–334

84. Bowen J, Gregory R, Squier M, Donaghy M. The post-irradiation lower motor neuron syndrome: neuronopathy or radiculopathy? Brain 1996;119:1429–1439

85. Currie S, Henson RA, Morgan HG, Poole AJ. The incidence of the non-metastatic neurological syndromes of obscure origin in the reticuloses. Brain 1970;93:629–640

86. Johnson PC, Rolak LA, Hamilton RH, Laguna JF. Paraneoplastic vasculitis of nerve: a remote effect of cancer. Ann Neurol 1979;5:437–444

87. Vesterby A, Reske-Nielsen E, Kristensen IB, et al. Late nervous system disorders in cured malignant lymphoma: a clinical and neuropathological study. Clin Neuropathol 1988;7:134–138

88. Walsh JC. Neuropathy associated with lymphoma. J Neurol Neurosurg Psychiatry 1971;34:42–50

89. Trotter JL, Hendin BA, Österland CK. Cerebellar degeneration with Hodgkin disease. An immunological study. Arch Neurol 1976;33:660–661

90. Lachance DH, O'Neill BP, Harper CM Jr, et al. Paraneoplastic brachial plexopathy in a patient with Hodgkin's disease. Mayo Clin Proc 1991;66:97–101

91. Symonds RP, Hogg RB, Bone I. Paraneoplastic neurological syndromes associated with lymphomas. Leuk Lymphoma 1994;15:487–490

92. Williams HM, Diamond HD, Craver LF, Parsons H. Neurological Complications of Lymphomas and Leukemias. Springfield, Illinois: Charles C Thomas, 1959

93. Cameron DG, Howell DA, Hutchinson JL. Acute peripheral neuropathy in Hodgkin's disease: report of a fatal case with histologic features of allergic neuritis. Neurology 1958;8:575–577

94. Lisak RP, Mitchell M, Zweiman B, et al. Guillain–Barré syndrome and Hodgkin's disease: three cases with immunological studies. Ann Neurol 1977;1:72–78

95. Snider S, Bashir R, Bierman P. Neurologic complications after high-dose chemotherapy and autologous bone marrow transplantation for Hodgkin's disease. Neurology 1994;44:681–684

96. Cheson BD, Vena DA, Foss FM, Sorensen JM. Neurotoxicity of purine analogs: a review. J Clin Oncol 1994;12:2216–2228

97. Stelitano C, Morabito F, Kropp MG, et al. Fludarabine treatment in B-cell chronic lymphocytic leukemia: response, toxicity and survival analysis in 47 cases. Haematologica 1999;84:317–323

98. Mitsui Y, Kusunoki S, Hiruma S, et al. Sensorimotor polyneuropathy associated with chronic lymphocytic leukemia, IgM antigangliosides antibody and human T-cell leukemia virus I infection. Muscle Nerve 1999;22:1461–1465

99. Jonsson V, Svendsen B, Vorstrup S, et al. Multiple autoimmune manifestations in monoclonal gammopathy of undetermined significance and chronic lymphocytic leukemia. Leukemia 1996;10:327–332

100. Creange A, Theodorou I, Sabourin JC, et al. Inflammatory neuromuscular disorders associated with chronic lymphoid leukemia: evidence for clonal B cells within muscle and nerve. J Neurol Sci 1996;137:35–41

101. Thomas FP, Vallejos U, Foitl DR, et al. B cell small lymphocytic lymphoma and chronic lymphocytic leukemia with peripheral neuropathy: two cases with neuropathological findings and lymphocyte marker analysis. Acta Neuropathol 1990;80:198–203

102. Grisold W, Jellinger K, Lutz D. Human neurolymphomatosis in a patient with chronic lymphatic leukemia. Clin Neuropathol 1990;9:224–230

103. Gabriel CM, Goldman JM, Lucas S, Hughes RA. Vasculitic neuropathy in association with chronic graft-versus-host disease. J Neurol Sci 1999;168:68–70

104. Bashir RM, Bierman P, McComb R. Inflammatory peripheral neuropathy following high dose chemotherapy and autologous bone marrow transplantation. Bone Marrow Transplant 1992;10:305–306

105. Johnson NT, Crawford SW, Sargur M. Acute acquired demyelinating polyneuropathy with respiratory failure following high-dose systemic cytosine arabinoside and marrow transplantation. Bone Marrow Transplant 1987;2:203–207

106. Liedtke W, Quabeck K, Beelen DW, et al. Recurrent acute inflammatory demyelinating polyradiculitis after allogeneic bone marrow transplantation. J Neurol Sci 1994;125:110–111

107. Eliashiv S, Brenner T, Abramsky O, et al. Acute inflammatory demyelinating polyneuropathy following bone marrow transplantation. Bone Marrow Transplant 1991;8:315–317

108. Silber E, Lane RJ, Hopkinson NS. Demyelinating polyneuropathy in a patient with chronic myeloid leukemia. Muscle Nerve 1998;21:974–975

109. Weiss K. Safety profile of interferon-alpha therapy. Semin Oncol 1998;25(Suppl 1):9–13

110. Vial T, Descotes J. Clinical toxicity of the interferons. Drug Saf 1994;10:115–150

111. Bernsen PL, Wong Chung RE, Vingerhoets HM, Janssen JT. Bilateral neuralgic amyotrophy induced by interferon treatment. Arch Neurol 1988;45:449–451

112. Lin KP, Yeh TP, Wang S, et al. Polyneuropathy associated with acute monoblastic leukemia: a case report. Chung Hua I Hsueh Tsa Chih (Taipei) 1996;58:435–438

113. Krendel DA, Albright RE, Graham DG. Infiltrative polyneuropathy due to acute monoblastic leukemia in hematologic remission. Neurology 1987;37:474–477

114. Nishi Y, Yufu Y, Shinomiya S, et al. Polyneuropathy in acute megakaryoblastic leukemia. Cancer 1991;68:2033–2036

115. Powell BL, Capizzi RL, Lyerly ES, Cooper MR. Peripheral neuropathy after high-dose cytosine arabinoside, daunorubicin, and asparaginase consolidation for acute non-lymphocytic leukemia. J Clin Oncol 1986;4:95–97

116. Nevill TJ, Benstead TJ, McCormick CW, Hayne OA. Horner's syndrome and demyelinating peripheral neuropathy caused by high-dose cytosine arabinoside. Am J Hematol 1989;32:314–315

117. Paul M, Joshua D, Rahme N, et al. Fatal peripheral neuropathy associated with axonal degeneration after high-dose cytosine arabinoside in acute leukaemia. Br J Haematol 1991;79:521–523

118. Lekos A, Katirji MB, Cohen ML, et al. Mononeuritis multiplex. A harbinger of acute leukemia in relapse. Arch Neurol 1994;51:618–622

119. Kornblau SM, Cortes-Franco J, Estey E. Neurotoxicity associated with fludarabine and cytosine arabinoside chemotherapy for acute leukemia and myelodysplasia. Leukemia 1993;7:378–383

120. Estey E, Plunkett W, Gandhi V, et al. Fludarabine and arabinosylcytosine therapy of refractory and relapsed acute myelogenous leukemia. Leuk Lymphoma 1993;9:343–350

121. Vahdat L, Wong ET, Wile MJ, et al. Therapeutic and neurotoxic effects of 2-chlorodeoxyadenosine in adults with acute myeloid leukemia. Blood 1994;84:3429–3434

122. Stillman MJ, Christensen W, Payne R, Foley KM. Leukemic relapse presenting as sciatic nerve involvement by chloroma (granulocytic sarcoma). Cancer 1988;62:2047–2050

123. Lind MJ, McWilliam L, Jip J, et al. Cyclosporin associated demyelination following allogeneic bone marrow transplantation. Hematol Oncol 1989;7:49–52

124. Konstadoulakis MM, Papasavvas P, Bitsaktis A, et al. Acute demyelinating peripheral neuropathy in a patient with double monoclonal gammopathy and chronic myelomonocytic leukemia. Muscle Nerve 1993;16:431–432

125. Maeda T, Ashie T, Kikuiri K, et al. Chronic myelomonocytic leukemia with polyneuropathy and IgA-paraprotein. Jpn J Med 1989;28:709–716

204 Paraneoplastic Neuropathy Syndromes: Principles and Treatment

Alan Pestronk

Paraneoplastic neurological syndromes

General principles

A paraneoplastic neurological syndrome (PNS) is temporally associated with, but anatomically remote from, a neoplasm.[1–9] The *temporal relationship* of a PNS to the associated neoplasm is variable. The PNS may precede, or follow, the identification of a neoplasm by weeks, months, or occasionally years. *Clinical features* of PNS are often distinctive. The presence of a typical clinical PNS indicates that the occurrence of its associated neoplasms is likely. In some PNS, such as the sensory neuronopathy associated with anti-Hu antibodies, the association with neoplasm is very strong.[10] The detection of anti-Hu or other such antibodies is an indication to search vigorously for a related neoplasm both at the time of initial evaluation and during subsequent evaluations.[8,9] The *malignancy of PNS-associated neoplasms* varies considerably. Neoplasms associated with the PNS necrotic myopathy can be life threatening.[11] The responsiveness of the tumor to treatment often determines survival. In other PNS long term prognosis depends on therapy of the neurological disorder, because the tumor either remains small or is often effectively treated. Thymomas with associated myasthenia gravis are an example of this category.[12] The *strength* and *specificity of association* of neoplasms and a PNS vary and depend on the specific PNS, other related clinical factors and the type of neoplasm. Disorders that are clinically identical to a PNS can occur in the absence of cancer. Lambert–Eaton myasthenic syndrome is associated with neoplasm in about 50% of patients,[13] but the relationship is probably much more consistent in older adults with a history of smoking. Some types of neoplasms are associated with several different PNS. Small cell lung cancers can be related to Lambert–Eaton myasthenia, autonomic neuropathy, sensory neuronopathy, myelopathy, cerebellar ataxia, opsoclonus-myoclonus, and limbic encephalitis syndromes. The *prevalence* of PNS is variable. A neuromyopathy with distal sensory loss and proximal weakness is very common in patients with neoplasms who have lost more than 15% of their body weight. In contrast, disabling PNS, with distinctive clinical features that involve selective regions of the nervous system, are less common or rare. The prevalence of PNS in the setting of specific neoplasms ranges from 30% for thymoma patients with myasthenia gravis to less than 1% for neoplasms associated with some central nervous system disorders.[9]

PNS can be classified according to their underlying etiologies, including immune, metabolic and endocrine, vascular with clotting disorders, and infectious. Immune PNS are commonly associated with humoral mechanisms. They can be subdivided into groups, based on the features of their associated autoantibodies (Table 204.1). One category includes disorders in which both the neoplasm and the diseased tissue contain a protein that is an antigenic target. This category is further divided into two groups of PNS that depend on the subcellular location of the autoantigen: surface membrane, or intracellular. A third group of PNS is associated with secretion of an autoantibody by the neoplasm. These three groups have distinctive clinical, pathological and immune characteristics and responses to treatment (Tables 204.1 and 204.2).

The responses to treatment of immune PNS, and other neuromuscular disorders, fall into general patterns based on their classification according to features of their associated immune disorders (Tables 204.1 and 204.2).

1. When the antigenic target is a surface membrane molecule, typically a receptor or ion channel, the associated PNS often responds to a wide variety of immunotherapies directed at T or B cell function. Examples of these syndromes include myasthenia gravis with IgG antibodies to nicotinic acetylcholine receptors, Lambert–Eaton myasthenic syndrome (LEMS) with IgG antibodies to voltage gated calcium channels, and Isaac's syndrome with IgG antibodies to voltage gated potassium channels.

2. When the antigenic target is located intracellularly, the rule is a poor response of the associated PNS to any immunomodulating treatment. The paraneoplastic subacute sensory neuronopathy with IgG antibodies to the neuronal nuclear antigen Hu has features that are typical of this group.

3. When the neoplasm synthesizes a disease-associated IgM antibody, the associated PNS syndromes typically respond to a limited repertoire of cytotoxic immunotherapies that are directed at B cells or plasma cells. Effective immunomodulating treatment usually only occurs when levels of autoantibodies are substantially reduced for prolonged periods (months to years). This group of disorders includes several syndromes with serum monoclonal IgM antibodies that are often directed against a carbohydrate epitope on a glycolipid or

Table 204.1 General features of paraneoplastic neurological syndromes

Features of syndrome		Tumor protein is antigenic target		Neoplasm produces antibody
		Intracellular antigen	Surface membrane antigen	
Clinical	Lesion locations	Central nervous system Occasionally peripheral NS	Nerve or muscle Rare central NS	Common: peripheral nerve Occasional: muscle Damage to axons or myelin
	Cellular pathology	Neural cell death	Membrane dysfunction Focal damage to nerve or muscle cell	
	Time course of disease	Subacute onset → plateau	Subacute onset → plateau	Chronic progressive
	Typical syndromes	Sensory neuronopathy (Hu) Cerebellar ataxia (Yo; CV2) Limbic encephalitis (Hu; Ma2)	Myasthenia gravis Lambert–Eaton syndrome Neuromyotonia (Isaac's) ? CIDP	Neuropathies: multifocal motor (IgM) MAG sensory-motor (IgM) POEMS (IgG or IgA) cryoglobulinemia amyloidosis axonal sensory
Neoplasm	Specific types	Small cell lung Gynecological Testicular	Small cell lung Thymoma Lymphoma	MGUS Lymphoma
	Frequency	Nearly always: 80% to 95%	Common: 10% to 70%	Nearly always
Antigen	Types	RNA binding proteins Golgi-related proteins	Transmitter receptors Ion channels	Glycolipids Glycoproteins
	Location	Tissue: disease; neoplasm Cell: nucleus, or cytoplasm	Tissue: disease; neoplasm Cell: Surface membrane	Tissue: disease Cell: surface
Antibody	Location	Serum CSF	Serum Usually not CSF	Serum
	Type	Polyclonal IgG	Polyclonal IgG	Monoclonal IgM: known target (60%) IgG or IgA: no known target
	Pathogenic	Rarely	Often	Probably
Commonly effective treatments		Rare	Corticosteroids Immunomodulation T cell immunosuppression Plasma exchange ? Intravenous immunoglobulin	Immunomodulation Cytotoxic ? Rituximab (IgM M-proteins)

NS, nervous system; MAG, myelin-associated glycoprotein; CIDP, chronic immune demyelinating polyneuropathy; POEMS, Polyneuropathy, Organomegaly, Endocrine, M-protein, Skin changes; MGUS, Monoclonal Gammopathy of Unknown Significance.

glycoprotein. Specific examples include motor neuropathies with IgM binding to GM1 ganglioside and sensory-motor demyelinating neuropathies with IgM binding to myelin-associated glycoprotein (MAG).

4. When a demyelinating neuropathy syndrome is associated with motor conduction block on electrodiagnostic testing, strength often improves within a few weeks of treatment using intravenous immunoglobulin. This group of syndromes includes chronic immune demyelinating polyneuropathy (CIDP) and multifocal motor neuropathy (MMN). Demyelinating neuropathies without conduction block only rarely show functionally useful benefit after intravenous immunoglobulin treatment.

The spectrum of responses of different PNS to treatments is wide, and the possible treatments often have prominent side effects or high cost, therefore an accurate, well-documented diagnosis is important

before embarking on therapy. The rarity of paraneoplastic syndromes means that there are few large, controlled trials of long term therapy. Most of the treatment strategies discussed in this chapter are based on small, uncontrolled, patient series, anecdotal reports and personal experience.

Characteristic syndromes (Tables 204.3 and 204.4)

Paraneoplastic subacute sensory neuronopathy (SSN) is associated with an immune response (anti-Hu antibodies; ANNA I) directed against an intracellular nuclear antigen that is present in both neural tissue and the associated neoplasm (Tables 204.1 and 204.4).[1-10] SSN presents clinically with numbness and pain progressing over one to eight weeks. A history of smoking is found in most patients. Examination shows asymmetric sensory loss that typically involves the face, trunk, and proximal, as well as distal, regions of the arms and legs. All sensory modalities

Table 204.2   Chronic immune-mediated neuromuscular disorders: general treatment strategies based on diagnostic test results

	Features of diagnostic testing		Disease examples	Commonly effective treatment
Nerve conduction	Conduction block		MMN CIDP	IVIg
EMG	Thoracic paraspinous denervation		Motor neuropathy	None
Antibodies	IgM monoclonal	Target antigen: carbohydrate Antibody location: serum	MMN MAG neuropathy Sulfatide neuropathy GALOP syndrome	Cyclophosphamide ? Rituximab Not corticosteroids
	IgG polyclonal	Target antigen: membrane protein Antibody location: serum	Myasthenia gravis Lambert–Eaton Neuromyotonia ? CIDP	Corticosteroids Immunomodulation T cell immunosuppression Plasma exchange ? Intravenous immunoglobulin
		Target antigen: intracellular protein Antibody location: serum + CSF	Anti-Hu ganglionopathy	None
		Target antigen: carbohydrate Antibody location: serum	Acute motor neuropathy	IVIg
	IgG monoclonal	Target antigen: unknown Antibody location: serum	POEMS	Uncertain

are affected. Patients may become disabled by the severe sensory ataxia and pseudoathetosis resulting from the deafferentation. Strength is usually normal. Tendon reflexes are diffusely diminished or absent. Nerve conduction studies show diminished or absent sensory responses with normal motor studies. SSN may occur as an isolated clinical syndrome, but is more commonly associated with central nervous system signs, ranging from mild nystagmus to cerebellar ataxia or limbic encephalopathy. Cerebrospinal fluid (CSF) commonly shows a mild pleocytosis and elevated protein. Serum and CSF IgG antibodies that bind to the Hu family of 35 to 40 kDa nuclear proteins are characteristic of SSN. Measurement of anti-Hu antibodies is a useful diagnostic test in patients with sensory neuronopathy syndromes, but not in distal sensory neuropathies. The antigenic Hu proteins have specificity for neurons, but are also found in cells of small cell lung cancers (SCLC), the most commonly associated neoplasm. SSN with anti-Hu antibodies is almost always associated with a neoplasm, especially SCLC, but neoplasm is found at initial evaluation in only 50% of cases. Evaluation of patients with a clinical SSN syndrome but no known cancer should include: (1) a careful and complete general physical examination, including breast and lymph nodes; (2) imaging of the chest and abdomen by computed tomography or magnetic resonance imaging (CT, MRI); (3) evaluation of the CSF for IgG and oligoclonal bands, cells and cytology; (4) measurement of anti-Hu antibodies in serum (and possibly CSF). If a malignancy is not found on the initial evaluation, periodic re-evaluation is recommended every one or two years, especially if anti-Hu antibodies are detected, or the CSF shows abnormal immunoglobu-

lins or cells. The malignancy of SCLC may be lower in the setting of anti-Hu antibodies. Treatment of SSN consists of therapy for the associated neoplasm. There is almost never improvement in the SSN syndrome after treatment; however, physical therapy may allow the patient, over time, to compensate partially for the sensory loss. Long term survival depends on the malignancy of the associated neoplasm and the degree of CNS involvement. The differential diagnosis of SSN includes Sjögren's syndrome and drug toxicity from *cis*-platinum or pyridoxine.

Demyelinating neuropathy with serum IgM binding to anti-myelin-associated glycoprotein (MAG) is associated with IgM antibodies that are produced by a neoplasm (monoclonal gammopathy of unknown significance [MGUS]) (Table 204.1).[14–16] Anti-MAG syndromes present clinically with distal, symmetric pansensory loss in the feet. With progression of the syndrome, sensory loss in the hands may occur. Weakness is typically mild and is most prominent distally in the legs. Gait ataxia and intention tremor are also clinically important symptoms that often produce significant disability. The anti-MAG neuropathy is typically slowly progressive over a period of years, but eventually becomes disabling in some patients, especially due to the gait disorder or hand tremor. The earliest signs of demyelination on nerve conduction studies are prolonged distal motor latencies. Motor conduction velocities eventually become slowed, and compound muscle action potentials may be dispersed, but there is no conduction block. Sensory nerve action potentials are small or absent. A serum IgM M-protein is found in 85% of patients by testing with immunofixation methodology. If an IgM

Table 204.3   Paraneoplastic demyelinating polyneuropathy syndromes

Neuropathy syndrome	Features	Electrophysiology	Antibody and target	M-protein type and frequency	Treatment
Chronic immune demyelinating polyneuropathy (CIDP)	Motor > sensory Weakness: proximal + distal symmetric Sensory loss: distal Onset: 1 to 80 years Chronic or relapsing	Motor + sensory NCV: slow conduction block Distal latency: long F-waves: abnormal	Antibody targets: β-tubulin heparan sulfate Antibody class: IgM or IgG Frequency: 20%	IgG 15%	T-cell suppression: prednisone cyclosporin A methotrexate IVIg Plasma exchange
Multifocal motor neuropathy (MMN)	Motor only: distal >Proximal asymmetric arms > legs Onset: 25 to 60 years Slowly progressive	Motor only: conduction block axonal loss EMG: no paraspinous denervation	Antibody target: GM1 ganglioside Antibody class: IgM	IgM 20%	IVIg B cell suppression PE + cyclophosphamide ? Rituximab
Anti-MAG neuropathy	Sensory > motor: distal symmetric Gait disorder Tremor Onset: >50 years Slowly progressive	Motor + sensory Distal latency: long NCV: slow No conduction block Axonal loss	Antibody target: myelin-associated glycoprotein (MAG) Antibody class: IgM Frequency: 100%	IgM 85%	B cell suppression PE + cyclophosphamide ? Rituximab
Antisulfatide neuropathy	Sensory > motor distal symmetric, sensory Onset: >45 years	Prolonged distal Latency Slow NCV Axonal loss	Antibody target: sulfatide Antibody class: IgM	IgM 90%	IVIg B cell suppression PE + cyclophosphamide
GALOP syndrome	Gait disorder Sensory > motor Distal Symmetric Tremor Onset: >50 years	Motor + sensory Distal latency: long NCV: Slow No conduction block Axonal loss	Antibody target: sulfatide in lipid membrane Antibody class: IgM	IgM 80%	IVIg B cell suppression PE + cyclophosphamide
Anti-GM2 and GalNAc-GD1a and neuropathy	Sensory > motor Ataxia: limb and gait Distal Symmetric or asymmetric Onset: adult Slowly progressive	Slow NCV	Antibody target: GM2 GalNAc-GD1a Antibody class: IgM	IgM Common	IVIg
Polyneuropathy Organomegaly Endocrinopathy M-protein Skin changes	Sensory and motor Symmetric Onset: 25 to 60 years Progressive	Slow NCV Axonal loss	?	IgA or IgG 90%	? Cyclophosphamide

M-protein is detected, our procedure is to perform a skeletal survey. We examine the bone marrow for evidence of neoplasm if the results of the skeletal survey are abnormal, levels of total serum IgM are very high (greater than 2 g/dl), or levels of total IgG or IgA are below normal limits.

Anti-MAG polyneuropathies may respond to combined therapy with plasma exchange and cyclophosphamide.[17] Therapeutic regimens should aim to utilize sufficient cyclophosphamide treatments to reduce anti-MAG antibody titers by 60% or more. We use 6 monthly treatments with intravenous cyclophosphamide (1 g/m^2), each preceded by two

plasma exchanges. A specific detailed protocol for this procedure is maintained on our website (http://www.neuro.wustl.edu/neuromuscular/anti body/ctxrx.html). Intravenous cyclophosphamide is probably equally effective to oral dosing, has fewer adverse effects, and utilizes a 50% to 70% lower cumulative dose of drug. This regimen produces a sustained reduction in titers of serum anti-MAG antibodies in approximately 60% to 80% of patients. Most patients in whom antibody titers are reduced show functional benefit. Improvement typically begins after 3 to 6 months, continues for 6 to 18 months, and may persist for 2 to 6 years after treatment. As cytotoxic drugs have prominent possible side effects, a judgment must be made, in each individual case, whether disability from the sensory loss, gait disorder, tremor or weakness is sufficiently severe to justify the possible risks involved.

Rituximab (Rituxan), a monoclonal antibody directed against the CD20 antigen on B cells, is currently under investigation for treatment of IgM antibody-related neuropathies.[18] The drug rapidly eliminates B cells from the circulation. Rituximab appears to have relatively few short term side effects. Preliminary studies suggest that improvement in disabling symptoms, especially the gait disorder, may occur beginning 3 to 6 months after treatment. A specific, detailed, and updated protocol for this procedure is maintained on our website (http://www.neuro.wustl.edu/neuromuscular/antibody/rituxan.htm).

There is no improvement in features of anti-MAG neuropathy after treatment with intravenous immunoglobulin (IVIg), or with drugs, such as corticosteroids, azathioprine, cyclosporin A, or methotrexate, that produce immunosuppression mainly through effects on T cells.

Multifocal motor neuropathy (MMN) is another syndrome that can be associated with IgM antibodies produced by a neoplasm (MGUS) (Table 204.1).[19–21] MMN typically presents with asymmetric weakness at a wrist or in the intrinsic muscles of one hand. MMN is a multifocal demyelinating neuropathy characterized by a slowly progressive, predominantly distal, asymmetric weakness with no sensory symptoms or signs. There are no upper motor neuron signs. Electrodiagnostic studies show evidence of demyelination, especially conduction block, selectively involving motor axons. High titer IgM anti-GM1 ganglioside antibodies can be found in about 80% of patient serums.[22] About 20% of patients have a serum IgM M-protein on immunofixation testing. Numerous controlled and uncontrolled clinical studies have demonstrated that strength in MMN often improves after short term treatment with IVIg. This therapeutic response to IVIg is typical of

Table 204.4   Paraneoplastic axonal polyneuropathy syndromes

Neuropathy syndrome	Features	Electrophysiology	Antibody and target	Neoplasm	Treatment
Axonal neuropathies					
Sensory-motor neuropathy	Sensory > motor Symmetric Common Systemic: >15% weight loss	Axonal loss	None	Many neoplasms	Nutrition Identify and treat neoplasm
Mononeuritis multiplex	Motor + sensory Asymmetric Distribution: multiple nerves Onset: acute to subacute	Axonal loss Asymmetric	Hepatitis C Rheumatoid factor Cryoglobulinemia Distribution: serum	Leukemia Lymphoma	Identify and treat neoplasm or Infection Immunosuppression
Neuromyotonia (Isaac's syndrome)	Weakness: distal and proximal stiffness	Fasciculations	K⁺ channels Voltage gated Antibody Class: IgG Distribution: serum	Thymoma	Symptomatic Carbamazepine Phenytoin Plasma exchange ? Prednisone
CV2	Sensory > Motor Axonal loss CNS: cerebellar; encephalopathy Eye: optic neuritis; uveitis	Axonal loss	66 kDa protein Oligodendrocytes Antibody Class: IgG Distribution: serum + CSF	SCLC	Identify and treat neoplasm
CRMP-5	Sensory > motor, autonomic CNS: cerebellar; encephalopathy	Axonal loss	CRMP-5 Synaptic regions Antibody Class: IgG Distribution: serum + CSF	SCLC	Identify and treat neoplasm
M-protein	Sensory > motor Axonal loss	Axonal loss	Monoclonal IgM, IgG or IgA No defined antigenic target	Myeloma Lymphoma MGUS	Identify and treat neoplasm

continued

Table 204.4 *continued*

Neuropathy syndrome	Features	Electrophysiology	Antibody and target	Neoplasm	Treatment
Autonomic neuropathies					
Enteric neuropathy	Gastroparesis Intestinal pseudo-obstruction Esophageal achalasia Dysphagia		Hu antibody Class: IgG Distribution: serum + CSF	Thymoma SCLC	Identify and treat neoplasm
Amyloid neuropathy	Sensory loss: distal; symmetric axonal loss: small > large Autonomic	Axonal loss Carpal tunnel	Target: not known Antibody Class: IgG, IgM Distribution: serum	Multiple myeloma	Identify and treat neoplasm
Neuronopathies					
Sensory neuronopathy	Onset: subacute Sensory loss: diffuse, asymmetric numbness/ paresthesias dysesthesias/pain sensory ataxia CNS: limbic encephalitis cerebellar syndrome	Absent sensory nerve action potentials (SNAPs)	Hu antibody Class: IgG Distribution: serum + CSF	SCLC (90%) Breast Ovary prostate	Identify and treat neoplasm
Motor neuronopathy	Onset: subacute Weakness: arms > legs usually asymmetric mild	Small CMAPs	Not known	Lymphoma	Identify and treat neoplasm
Motor neuronopathy	Onset: subacute Weakness: arms + legs onset asymmetric severe	Small CMAPs	βIV spectrin	Breast Ductal adenocarcinoma	Identify and treat neoplasm

MGUS, monoclonal gammopathy of undetermined significance; SCLC, small cell lung cancer.

demyelinating neuropathies that have motor conduction block as a characteristic feature (Table 204.2). However, it remains to be seen whether IVIg, a very expensive treatment that probably has no effect on the underlying immune process, prevents the progressive axonal loss that can occur in MMN over time. Other treatment responses in MMN are similar to those in neuropathies with IgM anti-MAG antibodies. When the response to IVIg is not sufficient, or wanes with time, therapy of MMN with combined plasma exchange and cyclophosphamide may be followed by improvement in strength. Preliminary studies suggest that rituximab may be effective in the treatment of this IgM antibody-associated neuropathy.[18] Corticosteroid (prednisone or methylprednisolone) treatment is rarely helpful in MMN and may often exacerbate weakness.

Several other *demyelinating neuropathy syndromes* (Table 204.3) are associated with M-proteins. Demyelinating neuropathies are associated with IgM M-proteins that bind to sulfatide,[23] GALOP[24] antigen, β-tubulin,[25] or GM2 ganglioside.[26] Treatment for these

syndromes is based on sparse anecdotal evidence, but therapeutic trials are typically based on strategies employed for MMN and anti-MAG neuropathies, as outlined above. About 15% of patients with chronic immune demyelinating polyneuropathy (CIDP) have serum IgG M-proteins. Treatment strategies for these patients are generally similar to those for CIDP without M-proteins.

POEMS syndrome (Polyneuropathy, Organomegaly, Endocrinopathy or edema, M-protein and Skin changes), also known as Crow–Fukase syndrome, is a multisystem disorder that is associated with a chronic demyelinating polyneuropathy.[27] The syndrome is somewhat more common in males, and appears to be more prevalent in Japan. Organomegaly may involve liver, spleen or lymph nodes. Optic disk swelling may occur in a majority of patients. Edema may be very severe and develop into anasarca. Endocrine disorders may include glucose intolerance and hypothyroidism. Other endocrine-related systemic disorders can include gynecomastia, amenorrhea and impotence. Most POEMS patients have an IgA or IgG λ monoclonal gammopathy. As the levels of the M-protein are often low, the most sensitive testing method, immunofixation, should always be utilized. POEMS is associated with high levels of vascular endothelial growth factor (VEGF) in the serum. Osteosclerotic myeloma is commonly associated with POEMS and should be sought on a skeletal survey. This x-ray evaluation will detect osteoblastic lesions that may be missed on bone scans. Bone lesions are more common with IgG than IgA M-proteins. Multiple myeloma (lytic), MGUS, and multicentric Castleman's disease also occur with POEMS. Disseminated Castleman's disease presents with lymphadenopathy. The disorder is often accompanied by hepatosplenomegaly, anemia, polyclonal hypergammaglobulinemia and overproduction of interleukin 6, possibly associated with human herpesvirus 8. The POEMS neuropathy presents with paresthesias and coldness in the feet. Sensory loss and weakness progress from distal to proximal regions over a period of one to two years and may become severely disabling. Electrodiagnostic studies in POEMS show demyelination without conduction block. Nerve pathology may include axonal loss, segmental demyelination and uncompacted myelin. The POEMS neuropathy often responds to treatment when a localized osteosclerotic myeloma is identified. In POEMS with MGUS or myeloma, only occasional patients improve with systemic therapy of the neoplasm.

Distal axonal sensory-motor neuropathy (Table 204.4) a mild to moderately severe, is frequently associated with neoplasms.[8,9] This syndrome is especially common with weight loss of more than 15%, and with chronicity of the tumor. The neuropathy is characterized by distal, symmetric sensory loss and paresthesias, with weakness and wasting that is especially prominent in the legs. An accompanying myopathy with atrophy of type II muscle fibers produces proximal weakness. Axonal loss is seen with low amplitude sensory and motor amplitudes and normal conduction velocities on electrophysiological studies. This neuromyopathy has been described in association with a variety of solid tumors (lung, breast, stomach), lymphoma, and plasma cell dyscrasia. The pathogenesis of this disorder is probably metabolic, and not immune. Treatment of the neoplasm often results in resolution of the neuromyopathy.

Several axonal neuropathies may be immune-mediated PNS. Primary acquired *amyloidosis* (AL) may present with carpal tunnel syndrome or a small fiber neuropathy involving selective loss of pain and temperature sensory modalities.[28] When amyloid neuropathy is suspected, biopsy of tissue, especially both muscle and nerve, is indicated. Amyloid is detected in the biopsied tissue by staining with Congo red. Treatment strategies are typically aimed at the neoplasm producing the associated M-protein.

Peripheral nerve vasculitis producing mononeuritis multiplex or asymmetric sensory-motor polyneuropathy, has been reported with lymphomas, leukemias, or carcinoma of the lung, prostate, kidney or stomach.[29] Treatment strategies include therapy for the neoplasm and additional regimens similar to those used generally for vasculitis. Corticosteroids, with or without cyclophosphamide, are commonly employed. Mononeuritis multiplex appearing in the setting of lymphoma may also result from direct tumor infiltration of peripheral nerves.[30] Polyneuropathy, presenting either with a subacute mononeuritis multiplex or a slowly progressive distal symmetric sensorimotor polyneuropathy, occurs in approximately 20% of patients with *cryoglobulinemia*.[31] Treatment strategies for cryoglobulinemia include therapy for any associated infections (interferon alfa-2a for hepatitis C) or neoplasms, and combinations of corticosteroids, immunosuppression and plasma exchange for the vasculopathic neuropathy.[32]

Axonal, predominantly sensory polyneuropathies may be associated with *serum M-proteins* of IgM, IgG or IgA class. Typically, in these neuropathies, no antigenic target of the M-protein is found, especially with IgG or IgA antibodies. Sensory loss is usually panmodal, symmetric and distal. It can be severe enough to produce a sensory gait ataxia. Weakness is mild, and most often confined to the feet or toes. Treatment with immunomodulating drugs or plasma exchange does not commonly produce useful long term functional benefit.

Two rare PNS syndromes with central nervous system disorders and mild, predominantly axonal, sensory greater than motor neuropathies have been described in association with serum and CSF IgG antibodies to *CV2* and *CRMP-5 antigens*.[8,33,34] No treatments have been described.

Two paraneoplastic *lower motor neuron syndromes* have been described. Mild asymmetric weakness may occur in association with lymphomas and myeloproliferative disorders.[35] Weakness develops progressively and then stabilizes or improves. Treatment is directed at the associated neoplasm. A more severe lower motor neuron syndrome developing over a period of months has been described in association with ductal adenocarcinoma of the breast.[36] Serum antibodies bind to βIV spectrin that is present at axon initial segments and nodes of Ranvier. There was no response to immunomodulating therapies. Partial improvement in strength occurred after the neoplasm was surgically removed.

Neuromyotonia (Isaac's syndrome) is associated with an immune response (IgG binding to voltage-gated potassium channels) directed against a cell surface neural antigen that is present both in neural tissue and the associated neoplasm.[37] Clinically, patients present with muscle stiffness and cramps that may be exacerbated by exercise. Some patients have symptoms of a sensory neuropathy with paresthesias or numbness. Associated neoplasms include lung, thymus and Hodgkin's lymphoma. Evaluation for associated neoplasms includes a complete general physical examination, including breast and lymph nodes, and CT imaging of the chest. Common symptomatic treatments for neuromyotonia include carbamazepine (200 to 600 mg/day) or phenytoin (200 to 400 mg/day). Plasma exchange may be effective in patients who fail to respond to symptomatic treatment. Reports are varied regarding the efficacy of corticosteroids.

References

1. Pestronk A. Paraneoplastic syndromes. Neuromuscular Disease Center at Washington University in Saint Louis. http://www.neuro.wustl.edu/neuromuscular 2001

2. Grisold W, Drlicek M. Paraneoplastic neuropathy. Curr Opin Neurol 1999;12:617–625

3. Giometto B, Taraloto B, Graus F. Autoimmunity in paraneoplastic neurological syndromes. Brain Pathol 1999;9:261–273

4. Scaravilli F, An SF, Groves M, Thom M. The neuropathology of paraneoplastic syndromes. Brain Pathol 1999;9:251–260

5. Rees J. Paraneoplastic syndromes. Curr Opin Neurol 1998;11:633–637

6. Newsom-Davis J. Paraneoplastic neurological disorders. J R Coll Physicians Lond 1999;33:225–227

7. Dropcho EJ. Neurological paraneoplastic syndromes. J Neurol Sci 1998;153:264–278

8. Rudnicki SA, Dalmau J. Paraneoplastic syndromes of the spinal cord, nerve and muscle. Muscle Nerve 2000; 23:1800–1818

9. Posner JB. Neurologic Complications of Cancer. Philadelphia: FA Davis, 1995:353–385

10. Lucchinetti CF, Kimmel DW, Lennon VA. Paraneoplastic and oncologic profiles of patients seropositive for type 1 antineuronal nuclear autoantibodies. Neurology 1998;50:652–657

11. Levin MI, Mozaffar T, Al-Lozi MT, Pestronk A. Paraneoplastic necrotizing myopathy: Clinical and pathological features. Neurology 1998;50:764–767

12. Penn AS. Thymectomy for myasthenia gravis. In: Lisak RP, ed. Handbook of Myasthenia Gravis and Myasthenic Syndromes. New York: Marcel Dekker, 1994: 321–339

13. Newsome-Davis J, Lang B. The Lambert–Eaton myasthenic syndrome. In: Engel AG, ed. Myasthenia Gravis and Myasthenic Disorders. New York: Oxford University Press, 1999:205–228

14. Pestronk A. Chronic immune polyneuropathies and serum autoantibodies. Neuroimmunology for the Clinician. Boston: Butterworth-Heinemann, 1997:237–251

15. Nobile-Orazio. Neuropathies associated with anti-MAG antibodies and IgM monoclonal gammopathies. In: Latov N, Wokke JHJ, Kelly JJ Jr, eds. Immunology and Infectious Diseases of the Peripheral Nerves. Cambridge UK: Cambridge University Press, 1998:168–189

16. Ropper AH, Gorson KC. Neuropathies associated with paraproteinemia. N Engl J Med 1998;338:1601–1607

17. Blume G, Pestronk A, Goodnough LT. Anti-MAG antibody associated polyneuropathies: improvement following immunotherapy with monthly plasma exchange and intravenous cyclophosphamide. Neurology 1995;45:1577–1580

18. Levine TD, Pestronk A. IgM antibody-related polyneuropathies: Treatment with B-cell depletion chemotherapy using rituximab. Neurology 1999;52:1701–1704

19. Pestronk A. Multifocal motor neuropathy: Diagnosis and treatment. Neurology 1998;51:S22–S24

20. Parry G. AAEM case report#30: Multifocal motor neuropathy. Muscle Nerve 1996;19:269–276

21. Nobile-Orazio E. Multifocal motor neuropathy. J Neuroimmunol 2001;115:4–18

22. Pestronk A, Choksi R. Multifocal motor neuropathy. Serum IgM anti-GM1 ganglioside antibodies in most patients detected using covalent linkage of GM1 to ELISA plates. Neurology 1997;49:1289–1292

23. Lopate G, Parks BJ, Goldstein JM, et al. Polyneuropathies associated with high titre antisulphatide antibodies: characteristics of patients with and without serum monoclonal proteins. J Neurol Neurosurg Psychiatry 1997;62:581–585

24. Pestronk A, Choksi R, Bieser K, et al. Treatable gait disorder and polyneuropathy associated with high titer serum IgM binding to antigens that copurify with myelin-associated glycoprotein. Muscle Nerve 1994; 17:1293–1300

25. Connolly AM, Pestronk A, Mehta S, et al. Serum IgM monoclonal autoantibody binding to the 301 to 314 amino acid epitope of beta-tubulin: clinical association with slowly progressive demyelinating polyneuropathy. Neurology 1997;48:243–248

26. Lopate G, Choksi R, Pestronk A. Serum IgM binding to gangliosides GalNAc-GD1a and GM2: Association with a chronic demyelinating sensory > motor polyneuropathy. Neurology 2000;54 S3:A369

27. Kelly JJ Jr. Polyneuropathies associated with myeloma, POEMS, and non-malignant IgG and IgA monoclonal gammopathies. In: Latov N, Wokke JHJ, Kelly JJ Jr, eds. Immunology and Infectious Diseases of the Peripheral Nerves. Cambridge UK: Cambridge University Press, 1998:225–237

28. Kyle RA, Dyck PJ. Amyloidosis and neuropathy. In: Dyck PJ, Thomas PK, eds. Peripheral Neuropathy. 3rd ed. Philadelphia: WB Saunders, 1993:1294–1303

29. Matsumuro K, Izumo S, Umehara F, et al. Paraneoplastic vasculitic neuropathy: immunohistochemical studies on a biopsied nerve and post-mortem examination. J Intern Med 1994;236:225–230

30. Kuntzer T, Lobrinus JA, Janzer RC, et al. Clinicopathological and molecular biological studies in a patient with neurolymphomatosis. Muscle Nerve 2000;23: 1604–1609

31. Thomas FP, Lovelace RE, Ding XS, et al. Vasculitic neuropathy in a patient with cryoglobulinemia and anti-MAG IGM monoclonal gammopathy. Muscle Nerve 1992;15:891–898

32. Cacoub P, Maisonobe T, Thibault V, et al. Systemic vasculitis in patients with hepatitis C. J Rheumatol 2001; 28:109–118

33. de la Sayette V, Bertran F, Honnorat J, et al. Paraneoplastic cerebellar syndrome and optic neuritis with anti-CV2 antibodies: clinical response to excision of the primary tumor. Arch Neurol 1998;55:405–408

34. Yu Z, Kryzer TJ, Griesmann GE, et al. CRMP-5 neuronal autoantibody: marker of lung cancer and thymoma-related autoimmunity. Ann Neurol 2001;49: 146–154

35. Bir LS, Keskin A, Yaren A, et al. Lower motor neuron disease associated with myelofibrosis. Clin Neurol Neurosurg 2000;102:109–112

36. Berghs S, Ferracci F, Maksimova E, et al. Autoimmunity to beta IV spectrin in paraneoplastic lower motor neuron syndrome. Proc Natl Acad Sci USA 2001;98: 6945–6950

37. Hart I, Vincent A, Willison H. Neuromyotonia and antiganglioside-associated neuropathies. In: Engel AG, ed. Myasthenia Gravis and Myasthenic Disorders. New York: Oxford University Press, 1999:229–239

205 Inherited Neuropathies With Known Metabolic Derangement

Ted M Burns

Overview

Many of the inherited disorders discussed in this chapter have been classified historically as inborn errors of metabolism. These inherited disorders associated with peripheral neuropathy are of autosomal recessive or X-linked inheritance. These disorders are rare, but need to be recognized because many require specific therapy, for example enzyme replacement therapy or bone marrow transplantation. In addition to any specific therapy, treatment of an inborn error of metabolism must include genetic counseling, prognostic advice, and supportive therapy to improve quality of life and to prevent and treat premature complications.

This chapter is organized into two sections: those inborn errors of metabolism that frequently present with peripheral neuropathy, and those disorders that usually present with other clinical features but may have concomitant clinical or subclinical peripheral neuropathy. In the latter category, peripheral neuropathy may rarely be the presenting feature.

The clinical and laboratory features, and treatment (where available) of those diseases is summarized in Table 205.1.

Inborn errors of metabolism that often present clinically as peripheral neuropathy

Fabry disease

The first report of Fabry disease was in 1898 by the dermatologist W. Anderson.[1] Anderson described his findings to J. Fabry, who reported a similar case that same year.[2] Proteinuria and skin changes were described, and Anderson and Fabry termed the condition "angiokeratoma corporis diffusum."

Fabry disease is a rare X-linked recessive disorder of glycosphingolipid metabolism caused by deficient activity of lysosomal α-galactosidase A.[3–5] α-Galactosidase A is encoded on the long arm of the X chromosome (Xq22). Twenty-five to 35% of cases of Fabry disease may be due to spontaneous mutations.[6] Its incidence has been estimated at 1:117000 births.[7] Cleavage of the terminal galactose unit of glycosphingolipid is impaired, resulting in accumulation of globotriaosylceramide (Gb$_3$) and other glycosphingolipids in many cells, including vascular endothelial cells and smooth muscle cells, and many cell types in the kidneys, heart, eyes and nerves.[8–11]

The clinical hallmarks of Fabry disease are attacks of neuropathic pain, angiokeratomas of skin, and progressive kidney disease. Clinical onset is typically in childhood or adolescence. Recurrent episodes of disabling neuropathic pain in the extremities is an early complaint. Pain may be precipitated by physical activity or febrile illness.[12] Anhidrosis is common, probably from damage to unmyelinated nerve fibers. The angiokeratomas of skin are telangiectasias of the epidermis associated with proliferation of keratin and epidermal cells. Angiokeratomas appear before the end of the first decade as blood-filled papules over the umbilical area, loins, penis and scrotum. Other common stigmata are tortuous conjunctival vessels and corneal and lenticular opacities. Accumulation of Gb$_3$ causes proteinuria, progressive kidney failure, hypertrophic cardiomyopathy, cardiac conduction disturbances, and strokes. Most heterozygous females have corneal epithelial dystrophy, and some may suffer the same symptoms and complications as affected males. Complications of renal, cardiac and cerebrovascular disease usually cause death in untreated patients in the fourth or fifth decade.

Diagnosis is made by enzyme assay of α-galactosidase A activity in leukocytes or plasma, or increased levels of galactosylceramide in plasma or urinary sediment. Hemizygous males have very low or absent levels of α-galactosidase A activity, while heterozygous female carriers have an intermediate level of enzymatic activity. Prenatal diagnosis is possible using enzyme assay of α-galactosidase A activity in chorionic villi or amniotic cells. Sensory nerve action potentials in Fabry disease may be normal.[11] Mild abnormalities of motor conduction have been reported in some cases, usually occurring in only one or two nerves studied.[13] Histopathological studies of peripheral nerves have shown preferential loss of small myelinated and unmyelinated fibers and dorsal root ganglion cell bodies.[11]

Two recent studies have demonstrated efficacy of enzyme replacement.[8,9] Schiffmann et al. reported, in a double-blind, placebo-controlled trial, improvement in neuropathic pain in patients treated with recombinant α-galactosidase A (Transkaryotic Therapies, Inc, Cambridge, Mass) at a dose of 0.2 mg/kg intravenously over 40 minutes administered every other week for 6 months.[9] Patients were 18 years or older, with a median age of 34 years, and had median symptom duration of between 12 and 13 years. The primary end-point of "pain at its worst" without pain medications as measured by the Brief Pain Inventory (BPI) short form was statistically significantly better in the treatment group.[14] Other BPI measures were also significantly better in the treatment group. Four

Table 205.1 Inborn errors of metabolism associated with peripheral neuropathy

Disease	Clinical peripheral neuropathy	Common clinical features	Laboratory features	Treatment (see text for details)
Fabry	Episodic painful sensory symptoms, anhidrosis	Kidney disease (e.g. proteinuria), angiokeratomas	Reduced α-galactosidase A activity (<6% in males, 10% to 50% in women)	Intravenous α-galactosidase A (see text for dose)
Tangier	Syringomyelia-like or relapsing multifocal neuropathies	Large, lobulated, orange or yellow-gray tonsils, splenomegaly, corneal deposits	Very low apo A-I, apo A-II, VLDL. Low cholesterol. Normal or mildly elevated TG	No specific pharmacological therapy
Abetalipoproteinemia	Areflexia, reduced or absent joint position, vibration sensation	Steatorrhea and intermittent diarrhea, progressive ataxia, retinitis pigmentosa	Low cholesterol and TG; absent apo B, LDL, VLDL, chylomicrons; acanthocytes	Vitamin E 200–300 IU/kg per day, vitamin A 200–400 IU/kg per day; vitamin K 5–10 mg/day
Refsum	Charcot–Marie–Tooth phenotype	Retinitis pigmentosa, cerebellar ataxia and elevated CSF protein	Increased serum levels of phytanic acid	Dietary avoidance of phytanic acid
Globoid cell leukodystrophy	Yes, but often overshadowed	Dementia, hypertonicity, spastic quadriplegia, visual loss	Reduced galactocerebrosidase activity	Bone marrow transplantation, including childhood, juvenile and adult-onset cases, and early infantile-onset cases
Metachromatic leukodystrophy	Yes, but often overshadowed	Dementia, hypertonicity, dysarthria, spastic quadriplegia, visual loss	Reduced arylsulfatase A activity	Bone marrow transplantation, including early juvenile, late juvenile and adult-onset cases, and presymptomatic siblings of children with late infantile onset
ALD, AMN	Rare as dominant feature	ALD: mental retardation, seizures, spasticity; AMN: paraparesis, adrenal insufficiency	Elevated VLCFA in tissue and body fluids	Bone marrow transplantation, including early symptomatic childhood-onset cerebral ALD. Currently not recommended for AMN without cerebral involvement
Cerebrotendinous xanthomatosis	Overshadowed by CNS disease	Mental retardation, ataxia, spasticity, dysarthria	Elevated plasma cholestanol	Chenodeoxycholic acid 250 mg PO t.i.d.; consider HMG-CoA reductase inhibitors
Mitochondrial neuropathy	Prevalence approx. 25%, clinical or subclinical	Encephalomyopathy (e.g. MELAS), MERFF, Leigh syndrome, NARP, sensory ataxia	Elevated blood lactate, pyruvate, alanine; elevated CSF lactate, pyruvate	Consider CoQ_{10} 300 mg/day, L-carnitine 1–3 g/day b.i.d or t.i.d. with meals, vitamin C, riboflavin, thiamine, menadione/vitamin K_3
Cockayne syndrome	Overshadowed by CNS disease	Mental retardation, growth failure, microcephaly, skin photosensitivity, senile appearance, hearing loss	Fibroblast studies of low UV survival dose and impaired excision repair	No specific pharmacological therapy
Adult polyglucosan body disease	Progressive sensorimotor polyneuropathy	Upper motor neuron involvement, neurogenic bladder, dementia	Intra-axonal polyglucosan bodies, decreased GBE activity	No specific pharmacological therapy

of 11 patients in the treatment group taking pain medication at the beginning of the trial were able to discontinue pain medications, whereas none of the 11 patients in the placebo group taking pain medications was able to do so. Improvements in renal pathology, renal function and cardiac conduction were also observed in the treatment group. Eng et al. recently reported results of a double-blind, placebo-controlled trial of recombinant α-galactosidase A (Genzyme, Cambridge, Mass.) at a dose of 1 mg/kg intravenously administered every other week for 20 weeks.[8] Only 9 of 29 patients in the treatment group had renal microvascular endothelial deposits of Gb_3 compared to 29 of 29 patients in placebo group after 20 weeks. Microvascular endothelial deposits were also decreased in the skin and heart of patients in the treatment group. Eng et al. were not able to show a significant difference in neuropathic pain between the treatment and placebo groups as measured by the McGill Pain Questionnaire as statistically significant decreases in scores were observed in both groups at week 20.[8] Recombinant α-galactosidase A was reported to be well tolerated and safe in both studies. Myalgias, fever and rigors were more frequent in the α-galactosidase A groups. IgG seroconversion was common, but did not affect end-points in either study. Thus, enzyme replacement therapy has recently been shown to be efficacious in Fabry disease and appears to be the first line of treatment in affected individuals. At the time of this writing, recombinant α-galactosidase A treatment is under FDA review in the United States.

Other treatment options have included kidney transplantation[15] and symptomatic pain relief with carbamazepine and phenytoin.[16]

Tangier disease

Tangier disease was named after Tangier Island, Virginia, in the Chesapeake Bay, home of the first two reported cases.[17] Tangier disease is a very rare autosomal recessive disorder characterized by very low or absent serum high density lipoproteins (HDL) and their constituent apolipoproteins A-I (apo A-I) and A-II (apo A-II). The molecular defect in Tangier disease is a mutation in the ATP-binding cassette (ABC) transporter 1 gene (ABC1) that encodes a cholesterol efflux regulatory protein (CERP).[18–20] ABC transporters are membrane proteins that translocate substrates across cellular membranes.[21] There are 48 or so ABC transporters of human cells.[21] In normal cells, ABC1 helps cholesterol exit the cell, where it combines with lipid-poor apo A-I to form HDL. In Tangier disease, ABC1 mutations cause cholesterol to accumulate within the cell.[20]

The clinical hallmarks of Tangier disease are peripheral neuropathy and large, lobulated orange or yellow-gray tonsils. Cholesterol esters accumulate in tonsils and other tissues, including the liver, spleen, lymph nodes, cornea and peripheral nerves.[22] Splenomegaly and corneal deposits are other important clinical clues.

Peripheral neuropathy occurs in approximately half of patients.[23–25] The peripheral neuropathy presents as one of two distinct syndromes which never coexist in the same patient: as a multifocal neuropathy more frequent in the first two decades of life, or as a slowly progressive symmetrical neuropathy in a syringomyelia-like distribution affecting adults.[23,25,26] The presentation of the multifocal form may be as multiple mononeuropathies or asymmetric polyneuropathies occurring over years. The symptoms are predominantly weakness of subacute onset, sometimes associated with numbness and tingling. Resolution of weakness within weeks or months is common, but the weakness may be progressive. The syringomyelia-like presentation begins with dissociated sensory loss to pain and temperature and progressive weakness and wasting in the face, arms and upper trunk.[23,25,26] Attacks of lancinating pain may occur.

Tangier homozygotes present with low total plasma cholesterol levels and normal-to-high plasma triglyceride levels.[25,27,28] HDL cholesterol is very low or absent. Apo A-I, the principal apoprotein of HDL, is markedly reduced to approximately 1% to 3% of normal values, and apo A-II is 5% to 10% of normal values. Apo-B levels are normal.[22,25] In abetalipoproteinemia, another peripheral neuropathy with hypocholesterolemia, triglycerides and apo B levels are markedly decreased. Nerve conduction studies generally show only mild abnormalities in the relapsing mononeuropathy form, while sensory potentials are often absent in the syringomyelia-like form.[12,23,25]

There is currently no specific pharmacological treatment for Tangier disease. The current emphasis is on genetic counseling and supportive therapy.

Abetalipoproteinemia (Bassen–Kornzweig syndrome) and hypolipoproteinemia

Abetalipoproteinemia is an autosomal recessive disorder first described by Bassen and Kornzweig in 1950.[29] Atypical retinitis pigmentosa, ataxia and abnormal erythrocyte morphology with a crenated appearance and variation in size (acanthocytes) were described in an 18-year-old girl with consanguineous parents. In 1957, Jampel and Falls observed that serum cholesterol was very low in affected individuals.[30] The absence of plasma lipoproteins containing apolipoprotein B (apo B) was recognized in 1960.[31,32]

Abetalipoproteinemia is due to the absence of the microsomal triglyceride transfer protein (MTP), which is necessary for the assembly of the VLDL particle.[33–36] The lack of MTP results in failure to produce apo B-containing lipoproteins for secretion. In the enteric cell, chylomicrons are not produced because of the MTP absence, and thus dietary lipids and fat-soluble vitamins A, D, E and K are not absorbed in the intestine and transported into the circulation.[37]

The main clinical features are steatorrhea and intermittent diarrhea, progressive peripheral neuropathy and ataxia, and impaired night vision secondary to retinitis pigmentosa.[29,37–39] Clinical onset is the first or second decade,[38] and one third of affected children have neurological problems during the first year of life.[28] The clinical features are usually the result of malabsorption of lipids, including the fat-soluble vitamins, resulting in poor weight gain and growth retardation. The peripheral neuropathy usually predates the clinical onset of retinitis pigmentosa and sometimes predates ataxia, and thus may be the first symptom or sign. The progressive ataxia is due to spinocerebellar and cerebellar degeneration. Patients may be unable to walk by the mid 20s. Atypical retinitis pigmentosa may be a relatively late finding although electroretinography may show low amplitudes earlier.[38]

The diagnosis may be made in infants with fat malabsorption or fat intolerance with total cholesterol levels between 20 and 50 mg/dl and triglyceride levels less than 20 mg/dl. Apo-B, low density lipoproteins (LDL), very low density lipoproteins (VLDL) and chylomicrons are absent. Vitamin E and other fat-soluble vitamin levels will be low. Prothrombin levels may be increased because of low vitamin K stores. Mild to moderate anemia is common with abnormal erythrocyte morphology (acanthocytes). Nerve conduction studies reveal low sensory action potential amplitudes with slight slowing of sensory conduction velocities. Motor nerve conduction studies are usually normal.[12]

Many of the complications of abetalipoproteinemia result from poor absorption of the fat-soluble vitamins, and patients should be treated with oral vitamins E, A and K.[37,39,40] Oral vitamin E doses should be 200 to 300 IU/kg per day (equivalent to 150 to 200 mg/kg per day). Adults may require up to 30 000 IU/day of vitamin E. Plasma vitamin E levels cannot be monitored.[37] Oral vitamin A is recommended at a dose of 200 to 400 IU/kg per day.[37,39,40] Plasma levels of vitamin A should be monitored; however, plasma vitamin A levels do not reflect tissue stores and patients should be monitored for vitamin A toxicity.[37] Vitamin K (5 to 10 mg/day) can normalize the prothrombin time. Plasma vitamin D levels should be assessed, but usually patients do not need vitamin D supplementation.[37] Restriction of dietary fat may control steatorrhea, and most patients learn to consume a diet that minimizes malabsorption symptoms.[37]

Familial hypolipoproteinemia is a rare syndrome that differs from abetalipoproteinemia on a molecular basis, but homozygotes are phenotypically indistinguishable from abetalipoproteinemia. Many gene mutations have been described.[28,41] Homozygotes have a similar pattern of plasma apoproteins and lipoproteins. However, the ratio of free to esterified cholesterol in plasma is normal in hypolipoproteinemia and elevated in abetalipoproteinemia. Heterozygotes have apo B and LDL levels about 50% of normal. They are usually asymptomatic, but may have diminished or absent deep tendon reflexes and ataxia.[42,43] Treatment is similar to that of abetalipoproteinemia.

Refsum disease

In 1945, Sigveld Refsum reported five patients suffering from a disorder that he first named heredoataxia hemeralopica polyneuritiformis.[44] The term Refsum's disease was proposed in 1947 by H. Viets.[45] In 1963, high concentrations of phytanic acid were found in postmortem tissues from a 7-year-old girl who had suffered from Refsum disease.[46]

Refsum disease is an autosomal recessively inherited disorder of lipid metabolism. This rare disease may be more prevalent in Scandinavian countries, northern France, the British Isles and Ireland.[47] Refsum disease is caused by a deficiency of phytanoyl-CoA hydroxylase (PhyH), a peroxisomal protein that catalyzes the first step in phytanic acid alpha oxidation. Deficiency of PhyH leads to the accumulation of phytanic acid, a 20-carbon branched-chain fatty acid, which is exclusively derived from exogenous sources. Mutations in the phytanoyl-CoA hydroxylase gene have been identified.[48,49] Refsum disease differs from infantile Refsum disease, which is a peroxisomal disorder and variant of Zellweger's syndrome.

The clinical tetrad is retinitis pigmentosa, demyelinating peripheral neuropathy, cerebellar ataxia and elevated CSF protein, but the tetrad is not observed in all patients. Clinical onset of Refsum disease is between early childhood and the fourth decade. Most patients have clinical manifestations by age 20.[50] Impaired night vision usually is the first manifestation, and retinal pigmentary changes are an obligatory finding.[47] Electroretinography is diagnostically useful in the early stages. Peripheral neuropathy is often not observed at the onset of disease manifestations, but is present in most patients later in the disease, often as a demyelinating Charcot–Marie–Tooth phenotype. The neuropathy is usually chronic progressive, but may be episodic in the early stages, especially in the setting of illness, surgery or during pregnancy.[47,51] In other cases, however, the neuropathy may be absent or mild. Cerebellar ataxia is a less frequent finding.[47] Other clinical clues include progressive hearing loss, cataracts, cardiomyopathy, skeletal abnormalities and anosmia. Skin changes include dry skin, palmar hyperkeratosis, and ichthyosis. Short metatarsal bones, especially the third and fourth metatarsals, are found in many cases.[47] Pyramidal signs do not occur and intelligence is not affected.

The diagnosis is supported by increased serum levels of phytanic acid. The identification by gas chromatography of the phytanic acid peak from closely positioned fatty acid peaks sometimes leads to false identification of Refsum disease, and confirmation by an expert may be necessary. Motor conduction velocities may be markedly slow in the primarily demyelinating range, sometimes even less than 10 m/s. Sensory nerve conduction is also impaired. Onion bulbs are prominent histological findings on nerve biopsy.[52,53] The pathogenesis of peripheral nerve demyelination is unknown.

Dietary avoidance of foods that contain phytanic acid is recommended. Phytanic acid is found in dairy products, beef, lamb, and some seafood. Dietary restriction has been successful in lowering phytanic acid levels, leading to improvement in nerve conduction studies, ataxia, strength, and skin changes.[54] Specific pharmacotherapy for Refsum disease is currently not available. The current emphasis is on dietary restriction, genetic counseling and supportive therapy.

Inborn errors of metabolism in which peripheral neuropathy is often overshadowed by other presenting clinical features

Globoid cell leukodystrophy

Beneke, in 1908, and Krabbe, in 1916, described the pathological features of globoid cell leukodystrophy (GLD).[55,56] GLD is a very rare autosomal recessive lysosomal storage disorder caused by a deficiency of the enzyme galactocerebrosidase.[57] At least 60 mutations have been reported in the GALC gene, and the gene is located at 14q24.3–q32.1.[58,59] The enzyme cleaves galactose from galactocerebroside. Other substrates, such as psychosine, are important in the pathogenesis.[60,61] Deficiency of the enzyme results in storage of galactocerebroside galactosylceramide in central nervous system (CNS) white matter and other organs. The prevalence is 1:67 000 live births.[62]

The clinical manifestations result from progressive CNS and peripheral nervous system (PNS) demyelination. The disorder most often presents in the "classical" form (Krabbe disease) between 3 and 8 months of age with motor retardation, seizures, hypertonicity and optic atrophy.[63] The infant usually is hyperirritable, startles easily and is sensitive to light. Seizures, vomiting and fevers may be prominent features. The peripheral neuropathy is demyelinating and is usually overshadowed by other clinical features. Later, opisthotonic posturing, deafness and blindness develop. Children rarely live beyond 2 years.[64]

Although a less common presentation, a prolonged floppy infant variant with a clinically predominant demyelinating peripheral neuropathy is reported.[63] Infants often assume a characteristic flaccid frog position. CSF protein is normal or only slightly elevated. An acute polyneuropathy variant has been reported in a 1½-year-old girl.[64,65] This clinical presentation is exceedingly rare, however.

Late-onset cases are less common and typically present between the ages of 2 and 6 years. Clinical symptoms and signs may differ, even between cases in the same family. Peripheral neuropathy is sometimes present. In time, the clinical picture becomes more uniform and the dominant features become dementia, optic atrophy, cortical blindness and spastic quadriplegia. Adolescent and adult onset cases have been reported, with age of onset between 10 and 35 years. Mental retardation, pyramidal signs, loss of vision and a demyelinating peripheral neuropathy occur. GLD may present as polyneuropathy in this age group.[66]

Enzyme activity may be assayed in leukocytes or serum, and chorionic villus assay allows prenatal diagnosis. An abnormal myelin pattern is found on head CT or MRI.[67,68] Nerve conduction studies reveal a widespread, uniform demyelinating polyneuropathy[69] in the majority of early-onset cases and in many of the later-onset variants.[70] The characteristic histopathological feature is the presence of multinucleated globoid cells which contain PAS-positive material. Electron-dense granules and inclusions are seen by electron microscopy in the globoid cell cytoplasm. Sural nerve biopsy reveals evidence of segmental demyelination and occasional onion bulb formation. Inclusions in the schwann cells and macrophages can be observed with electron microscopy.

Bone marrow transplantation (BMT) should be considered for childhood, juvenile or adult-onset cases with neurological manifestations.[62,71] Clinical remissions have been reported in these patients. BMT may also be beneficial for early-onset GLD (Krabbe disease).[62,72]

Krivit et al. reported the results of five affected children treated with hematopoietic stem-cell transplantation.[72] Four patients received marrow from an HLA-identical sibling, and the fifth patient was treated with unrelated umbilical cord blood with one HLA-DR mismatch. Age at transplantation ranged from 2 months to 11.1 years. After transplant, two patients with late-onset disease had resolution of neurological disability, including gait dysfunction, ataxia, tremors and motor incoordination. In three patients, cognition, language and memory continued to develop normally. One infant transplanted at 2 months was reported at 18 months to have language development and to be ambulating.[71,72] Nerve conduction studies showed markedly improved median motor nerve conduction velocities in one child, but no significant differences in two others. Serial MRI scans showed smaller areas of signal intensity in two children and no significant changes in two. Grade I or II graft-versus-host disease of the skin occurred in three patients.

Intrauterine transplantation for fetal onset GLD has been unsuccessful. One fetus who underwent intrauterine transplantation died in utero. In two others, engraftment following intrauterine transplantation could not be demonstrated. Consequently both underwent postnatal BMT, but died of complications.[71,73] Neonatal hematopoietic stem cell transplantation, performed within weeks of birth, appears promising as an alternative to intrauterine transplantation.[62]

Metachromatic leukodystrophy

In 1910, Alzheimer and Nissl described the first cases of diffuse sclerosis with accumulation in the central nervous system of "prelipoid substances."[74,75] The term metachromatic leukodystrophy (MLD) was first used by Einarson and Neel in 1938 to emphasize the histological finding of granular lipid substances that stain metachromatically with acid aniline dyes.[56] MLD is a rare autosomal recessively inherited disease with an incidence of 1 in 40 000 in Washington state and 1 in 50 000 in Sweden.[76,77]

MLD is caused by a deficiency of arylsulfatase A or its activator protein. Arylsulfatase A is involved in sulfated glycolipid degradation, including cerebroside 3-sulfate, a lipid that makes up 3% to 4% of myelin membrane lipids. Arylsulfatase A is assisted by small acidic protein, SAP or saposin B, during the metabolism of these lipids.[78] The human arylsulfatase A gene is located on the long arm of chromosome 22. The mutation has been identified in 60% to 70% of the arylsulfatase A genes in MLD populations studied.[79]

MLD usually presents in infancy (i.e. late-infantile form) with rapid motor regression and the development of spasticity, dysarthria, dementia and ataxia.[64,80–82] Death usually occurs before age 10 years.[84] A juvenile form manifests between ages 4 and 16 years, with behavioral abnormalities, intellectual deterioration, gait disturbance, ataxia, blindness and peripheral neuropathy.[82] An adult form has clinical onset between the second and seventh decade and is dominated by dementia and behavioral disturbances. The type and course are similar in affected family members.[83]

MLD may rarely present with peripheral neuropathy as the dominant feature.[84–88] In the early phase, the presentation may be of a pure peripheral neuropathy, with the subsequent development of CNS involvement.[85,88,89] Nerve conduction velocities are in the demyelinating range.[85–88]

The diagnosis is made by arylsulfatase A enzyme assay of leukocytes. Prenatal diagnosis may be made by assay of enzyme activity of cultured amniotic fluid or chorionic villus cells. Pseudodeficiency is present in 1% of the normal population.[71] CSF protein is usually elevated.[82,85,86,88] MRI demonstrates CNS demyelination. The pathological features are destruction of central and peripheral myelin, gliosis, ballooned macrophages, and metachromatic staining of accumulated sulfatides with toluidine blue and cresyl violet in macrophages and in schwann cell cytoplasm.[84–86,90]

Bone marrow transplantation (BMT) should be considered for presymptomatic siblings of children with late infantile MLD and for children in the early stages of juvenile MLD.[81,91–97] Case reports of early juvenile MLD patients with affected siblings suggest stabilization of CNS deterioration and normalization of enzyme levels.[62,93,95] Other good candidates for BMT are patients with late juvenile and adult MLD.[95] This is because the progression of disease is slow in these later-onset cases. BMT has been accomplished in more than 50 patients, including one patient with normalization of enzyme activity for at least 14 years.[62] In the late-infantile form, rapidly progressing symptoms by the time of diagnosis may limit the benefit from BMT. Sufficient time, perhaps one year after BMT, is needed for donor-derived microglial cells to enter the CNS and provide enzyme.[62,95]

Patients with more advanced disease at the time of BMT appear to continue to deteriorate despite treatment. Malm et al. reported results of allogenic BMT in four children with MLD. Two children were classified as late infantile and two as juvenile MLD.[81] Two children with stage II MLD progressed markedly following BMT. A child with stage I–II juvenile MLD had progression the first two years following BMT, but then seemed to stabilize. A fourth child with stage I late infantile MLD continued to worsen two years following BMT, but the course of disease was more prolonged than that of a brother who had earlier died. The authors recommend that BMT only be considered for presymptomatic siblings of children with late infantile MLD and mildly affected juvenile MLD children.[81]

In another study, of three patients with late infantile MLD and clinical findings of ataxia and gait dysfunction, two patients progressed to a vegetative state and one patient to tetraparesis and optic atrophy, despite BMT.[98] Three other children with juvenile MLD were transplanted between the ages of 8 and 14. They were severely disabled before BMT, and cognitive decline and progression of symptoms worsened following BMT. MRI of the six MLD patients showed progression of central nervous system demyelination in four and stabilization in two.

Adrenoleukodystrophy and adrenomyeloneuropathy

The first description of a male with adrenoleukodystrophy (ALD) was by Schilder in 1913. The first description of the association of adrenal insufficiency and diffuse cerebral sclerosis was by Siemerling and Creutzfeldt in 1923.[59,99,100] The minimum total frequency of males with ALD in the United States population has been estimated to be 1:42 000, and the minimum combined frequency of ALD hemizygotes and heterozygotes has been estimated to be 1:16 800.[101] Prevalence estimates are similar in Europe.[102,103]

ALD and adrenomyeloneuropathy (AMN) are variants of an X-linked recessive peroxisomal disorder characterized by abnormally high concentrations of very long chain fatty acids (VLCFA) (C > 22) in tissues and body fluids.[104,105] The mutated gene encodes the ALD protein (ALDP), which is an ATP-binding cassette (ABC) protein.[106] Specifically, ALDP is one of four homologous human peroxisomal membrane ABC "half-transporter" proteins (ABCD1.[107] Human peroxisomal "half-transporter" proteins probably dimerize with partners to determine transporter substrate.[108] ALDP is required for the peroxisomal localization of VLCFA-CoA synthetase enzyme, and without normal localization to the peroxisome the enzyme may not function.[109] VLCFA must be converted to VLCFA-CoA by VLCFA-CoA synthetase so that the VLCFA can be oxidized in the beta-oxidation pathway.[110] Consequently, ALD/AMN patients have decreased peroxisomal beta oxidation associated with reduced activity of the VLCFA-CoA synthetase enzyme. The gene encoding the ALDP is localized to Xq28.[106] More than 340 mutations have been identified, which do not correlate with the phenotype (see http://x-ald.nl/).[101,111–113]

The childhood cerebral form of ALD is characterized by childhood onset of progressive cerebral and cerebellar degeneration of white matter leading to blindness, quadriparesis, dementia, ataxia and death by the second decade of life. In childhood cerebral ALD, peripheral nerve abnormalities are minimal relative to the progressive cerebral involvement. The phenotypic variant AMN is usually a slowly progressive myelopathy with clinical onset beginning in the third or fourth decade for men, and the fourth or fifth decade for women. Severe spastic paraparesis, sphincter disturbances and sensory loss in the lower extremities develop over a period of 5 to 15 years.[114] AMN may rarely present in childhood.[115] About 70% of patients with AMN develop adrenal insufficiency with attacks of nausea and vomiting, generalized weakness, skin hyperpigmentation, and weight loss. Adult-onset hypogonadism and erectile dysfunction may occur. At least half of heterozygous women develop milder neurological disease in middle age or later.[105,116,117]

Diagnosis in males is reliably made by measuring plasma VLCFA levels.[118] In females, the VLCFA gives false-negative results in 15% of heterozygous women.[111] Immunofluorescence assays and mutation analysis may help to identify heterozygous women.[119–121] MRI demonstrates CNS demyelination. Nerve conduction studies often suggest a mixed neuropathic pattern of multifocal demyelination and axonal loss.[122,123] Peroneal F wave latency is most often abnormal, followed by peroneal motor conduction velocity.[122] The demyelinating changes are not uniform along the length of nerve. Sural nerve biopsy may show a reduction in small and large myelinated fiber density and onion bulb formations.[114]

Bone marrow transplantation (BMT) has demonstrated efficacy in early symptomatic cases of childhood onset cerebral ALD.[62,71,92,105,124,125] Aubourg et al. first reported benefit from BMT in an 8-year-old boy with early symptomatic cerebral ALD.[125] The patient had disappearance of symptoms and resolution of multifocal brain lesions previously detected on MRI. Since then, over 100 patients with cerebral ALD have been treated with BMT.[62,71,124] The 5-year actuarial probability of survival following BMT is 62% by Kaplan–Meier analysis.[62,71] In contrast, almost all boys with MRI showing abnormality who did not undergo BMT died secondary to disease progression.[62,71,74] Long term clinical stabilization and in some cases improvement has been documented, including a 5- to 10-year follow-up study of transplanted ALD children.[124] An IQ score of 80 or better appears to best define the early cerebral ALD group of patients with the best prognosis.[62,74] BMT is not recommended for patients with advanced stage cerebral disease because of high morbidity and mortality rates. BMT has been unsuccessful and may have accelerated neurological deterioration in such cases.[126]

A major clinical challenge is differentiating asymptomatic patients who will develop the cerebral form of ALD and die within years from those patients who will develop the more benign adult form of AMN.

BMT is not indicated for patients in whom there is no clinical or radiological evidence of CNS involvement because more than half of such patients do not develop the childhood cerebral form of disease.[101] Surveillance by MRI and neuropsychological testing every 6 months is recommended for asymptomatic boys. Brain MRI changes precede clinical manifestations and aid in predicting clinical course.[62,71] Magnetic resonance spectroscopy may be more sensitive and should be considered if available. Patients with an increased MR severity score, occipital involvement and age less than 8 years are particularly prone to rapid loss of function and should be considered for immediate transplantation.

Currently, there is no evidence that BMT is of benefit for AMN.[101] Neither of two AMN patients treated with BMT had clinical remission.[62] The recommendation is to follow the clinical course without intervention as the disease may progress slowly over decades. As many as 35% of patients with AMN develop cerebral disease, usually after many years, and transplantation should be considered for adult disease with early cerebral involvement.[62]

Some authors recommend that in preparation for BMT such patients should be placed on dietary restrictions and given Lorenzo's oil (glycerol trioleate oil [GTO] and glycerol trioleate [GTE]) to lower VLCFA levels. Anecdotal evidence suggests that the outcome of BMT may be better when VLCFA levels are normalized prior to BMT.[62,71] It is also recommended that total parental nutrition be without lipid emulsions.[62,71] A special total body irradiation preparative with sparing of the brain has recently been advocated.[62,71]

Despite early promise, the results of dietary therapy have been disappointing. VLCFA are derived from diet and from endogenous synthesis that elongates long-chain fatty acids. Dietary restriction of VLCFA has not resulted in clinical improvement.[127] Dietary trials using glycerol trioleate oil (GTO) plus dietary restriction decreased plasma levels of VLCFA but there was no clinical benefit.[116,128] An open dietary trial using a combination of GTO and GTE (Lorenzo's oil) plus dietary restriction of VLCFA normalized plasma levels of VLCFA, but did not improve the clinical course for symptomatic AMN patients.[129] In this study, the mean Expanded Disability Status Scale (EDSS) and ambulation-index score worsened for symptomatic AMN men during the treatment trial. There was no significant change for symptomatic AMN women and preclinical boys. Thrombocytopenia was common, but none of the patients had abnormal bleeding. Asymptomatic neutropenia occurred in three patients.

It is unknown whether AMN women and asymptomatic AMN boys develop a less severe course if placed on GTE and GTO oils. The results of dietary therapy of 12 months or more for 86 asymptomatic patients were inconclusive.[130] The patients were followed for a mean of 33 months (12 to 84 months). Fifty-six percent of the patients remained well, 14% had equivocal worsening of MRI or behavior, and the remainder had unequivocal neurological, behavioral and/or neuroradiological worsening. Kaplan–Meier estimator techniques were used to compare these results with historical controls and suggested that dietary therapy in this subset of patients may perhaps be beneficial.

Immunosuppressive therapies have been evaluated because of the intense lymphocytic infiltration observed in brain parenchyma at autopsy, but failed to prevent progression of disease.[128,131,132]

Cerebrotendinous xanthomatosis

Cerebrotendinous xanthomatosis (CTX) is a rare, autosomal recessive lipid storage disease first described in 1937.[133,134] CTX is caused by a deficiency of the mitochondrial enzyme 27-sterol hydroxylase (CYP-27).[135] Over 30 mutations have been described in the CYP 27 gene in CTX patients.[136] The CYP-27 deficiency results in large amounts of cholesterol and the 5-α-reduced form of cholesterol, cholestanol, being produced and accumulating in eye lenses, muscle tendons, CNS and PNS.[137–140] Bile acid synthesis is impaired,[141,142] resulting in the absence of chenodeoxycholic acid in the bile and the excretion of large amounts of bile alcohols in bile and urine.[143–145]

CTX is characterized clinically by tendinous xanthomas, progressive cerebellar ataxia, pyramidal paresis, dementia, cataracts, premature atherosclerosis, endocrine hypofunction and pulmonary dysfunction. Onset is usually by the end of the first or second decade, and progression is usually slow.[136] Pyramidal tract signs are present in 67%, cerebellar signs in 60%, low intelligence in 57%, and peripheral neuropathy and epilepsy in 24%. Bilateral premature cataracts are present in 90%, tendon xanthomas in 45%, and intractable diarrhea in 33%.[136] Tendinous xanthomas may not develop until the third or fourth decade. Peripheral neuropathy is not a predominant clinical feature.[133,136,139,146,147]

The diagnosis is confirmed by identification of cholestanol in serum, urine and bile. Cholesterol levels in serum are usually normal. Peripheral nerve conduction velocities may be slow with prolonged distal latencies, especially in the lower extremities.

Chenodeoxycholic acid (CDCA) given orally can supplement the enterohepatic bile acid pool and thereby inhibit abnormal endogenous bile acid synthesis.[133] Berginer et al. treated 17 symptomatic patients with oral chenodeoxycholic acid 750 mg per day, in three divided doses, for at least one year.[133] Most patients on CDCA therapy showed reversal of neurological disability. Dementia, pyramidal tract signs and cerebellar ataxia improved in the majority of patients. Peripheral sensory loss was reported to improve in six of seven patients. Plasma cholestanol concentrations declined markedly, and CDCA became a major component of bile acid with suppression of endogenous bile acid synthesis. Oral CDCA was well tolerated in this study. Other reports support the efficacy of CDCA in CTX.[148–152] The electrophysiological results of five CTX patients treated with CDCA 750 mg/day in three oral doses for 11 years were also encouraging, with persistent improvement in nerve conduction studies and evoked potential latencies.[153]

At the present time, chenodeoxycholic acid is distributed to CTX patients in the United States under IND #46209 from the Food and Drug Administration, and Institutional Review Board approval from the UMDNJ Medical School, Newark, New Jersey, and VA Medical Center, East Orange, New Jersey.[154]

HMG-CoA reductase inhibitors in combination with CDCA may also be helpful.[151,152,155–157] HMG-CoA reductase inhibitors may lower further the serum cholestanol concentrations.[156] Moreover, HMG-CoA reductase inhibitors reduce LDL cholesterol levels, lowering the risk of premature atherosclerosis in CTX patients.[152,156]

Mitochondrial disorders

Leigh first reported a case of subacute necrotizing encephalomyelopathy in a 7-month-old boy in 1951.[158] Many enzyme deficiencies and nuclear and mitochondrial DNA mutations have been discovered for the subacute necrotizing encephalomyelopathy phenotype and other mitochondrial phenotypes.

Mitochondria are devoted to the production of adenine triphosphate (ATP), and mitochondrial dysfunction with cellular energy failure may lead to cell death. Mitochondria play a critical role in apoptotic cell death via energy failure and other mechanisms, including release of caspase-activating proteins, alterations in cellular reduction-oxidation state, and production of reactive oxygen species.[159]

The reported incidence of clinical or subclinical peripheral neuropathy in mitochondrial disease is near 25%.[159–164] Peripheral neuropathy may be a clinical feature of various mitochondrial syndromes, including mitochondrial myopathy, mitochondrial encephalomyopathy lactic acidosis and stroke-like episodes (MELAS), myoclonus epilepsy with ragged-red fibers (MERFF), Kearns–Sayre syndrome, and Leigh syndrome.[161–169] Peripheral neuropathy may be a relatively dominant feature in some cases, for example in neuropathy, ataxia and retinitis pigmentosa (NARP), sensory ataxic neuropathy and mitochondrial neurogastrointestinal encephalomyopathy.[159] Leigh disease has been reported to present with a Guillain–Barré-like syndrome in a 4-year-old girl.[165]

Diagnosis is aided by elevated blood or CSF lactate and pyruvate, as well as elevated blood alanine. A generalized aminoaciduria, organic aciduria or low blood carnitine may also be seen in mitochondrial disease.[159] Nerve conduction studies are usually consistent with an axonal neuropathy, although demyelinating neuropathies in mitochondrial disease have been reported.[162,163,167–174] Neuroimaging may reveal CNS involvement. Muscle biopsy frequently aids diagnosis, and ragged red fibers are the hallmark of mitochondrial dysfunction. Genetic testing is also commercially available for many mutations.

Therapy includes monitoring for complications and supportive care. For example, cardiac pacing may be necessary for patients with cardiac conduction defects. Intraocular lens replacement in an individual with cataracts may be necessary. Aerobic exercise training appears beneficial, and may increase mitochondrial number and enzyme activity.[175,176] Valproate should be avoided because it inhibits oxidative phosphorylation.[159,177]

Coenzyme Q_{10} (CoQ_{10}) has been effective in cases of isolated coenzyme Q_{10} deficiency,[178] and there are many anecdotal reports of clinical benefit of CoQ_{10} in various mitochondrial disorders.[179–184] However, the results were disappointing for CoQ_{10} supplements in a double-blind multicenter study.[185] Nonetheless, CoQ_{10} at a dose of 300 mg/day is generally well tolerated and commonly prescribed. L-carnitine (1 to 3 g/day, b.i.d. or t.i.d. with meals) is often used in conjunction with CoQ_{10}. Other supplements that target the respiratory chain include vitamin C (1 g q.i.d.), riboflavin (100 to 300 mg/day), thiamine (300 mg/day) and menadione/vitamin K_3 (10 mg q.i.d.). Efficacy is also not proved although there are anecdotal reports of improvement in some patients.[159,177,181,186–188]

Dichloroacetate (DCA) has been shown to lower concentrations of lactic acid, perhaps by promoting the flux of pyruvate into the citric acid cycle.[189,190] Consequently, there has been interest in DCA therapy in mitochondrial disorders. Improvement in peripheral neuropathy has been anecdotally reported.[191,192] However, a recent study of 27 individuals with congenital lactic acidemia treated for one year with DCA (generally 50 mg/kg per day divided into two oral doses, plus oral thiamine 100 mg/day) reported that 12 patients whose nerve conduction studies (NCS) were normal at baseline developed NCS abnormalities within one year. Two patients had NCS abnormality at baseline, and NCS parameters worsened in both patients during treatment. Symptoms of neuropathy were reported by only three patients, however. The authors' conclusion was that peripheral neuropathy appears to be a common side effect of chronic DCA therapy, and NCS should be monitored during DCA treatment. Other side effects of DCA include sedation, transient elevation of liver transaminases, headache and dizziness.[190]

Cockayne syndrome

Cockayne syndrome (CS) is a very rare autosomal recessive disorder first described by Cockayne in 1936.[193] Individuals with CS have a defect in transcription-coupled DNA repair.[194,195] Two complement group proteins (CS-A and CS-B) have been identified, and the majority of CS patients have been assigned to the CS-B complementation group.[194,195] Cells with mutations in CS-A and CS-B fail to ubiquitinate RNA polymerase II.[194] CS cells exhibit high sensitivity to ultraviolet (UV) light and delayed RNA synthesis recovery after UV irradiation.[196]

The clinical hallmarks of CS are postnatal growth failure and progressive neurological dysfunction.[197–199] The children are of normal size at birth. Growth failure is reported in all patients, and weight is more affected than length (i.e. "cachectic dwarfism"). Microcephaly is common. Delayed psychomotor development, often severe, is an almost constant feature. Other common features are sensorineural hearing loss, skin photosensitivity, senile appearance, optic atrophy, sensorimotor peripheral neuropathy, ataxia, dental caries, corneal opacities and arrested facies with large ears, deep set eyes and large aquiline nose.[197,199,200]

The peripheral neuropathy of CS is common but usually not a presenting or prominent clinical feature. Reduced deep tendon reflexes and distal amyotrophy may be present.[200] The peripheral neuropathy is demyelinating with slow nerve conduction velocities.[197,199–202] Segmental demyelination and remyelination with onion bulb formation and a moderate decrease in density of myelinated fibers are observed on sural nerve biopsy.[200–202]

Diagnosis is based on clinical features and fibroblast studies showing low UV survival dose and impaired excision repair. Current treatment of CS includes supportive care and management of complications, including intraocular lens replacement for cataracts and appropriate dental care.[203,204]

Adult polyglucosan body disease

Adult polyglucosan body disease (APBD) is a very rare autosomal recessive glycogen storage disease characterized by progressive upper and lower motor neuron dysfunction, sensory loss in the lower extremities, sphincter dysfunction, and sometimes dementia.[205–213] Symptom onset is usually in the fifth to seventh decade.[205,211] In a subgroup of patients, usually of Ashkenazi Jewish origin, APBD is an allelic variant of glycogen storage disease type IV (GSD IV) caused by glycogen branching enzyme (GBE) deficiency.[212–215] Non-Ashkenazi APBD patients are found less frequently to have GBE deficiency, and thus other biochemical defects may also cause APBD.[214,215] GBE gene mutations have recently been described.[213,215] In APBD, polyglucosan bodies are widely distributed in peripheral nerve axons, CNS neurons and astrocytes, heart, skeletal and smooth muscles.[205,209]

On nerve biopsy, PAS-positive polyglucosan bodies are found in both myelinated and unmyelinated axons and in schwann cells.[205–212,214,215] Electrodiagnostic studies usually suggest an axonal sensorimotor polyneuropathy,[205,211,212] although demyelinating features have been described.[206,207,212] MRI reveals atrophy of the cervical spinal cord and diffuse white matter signal abnormalities in the periventricular white matter and subcortical regions.[211,212,215] Somatosensory evoked potential studies may reveal prolonged interpeak latencies.[205,211] The diagnosis may be confirmed by a skin biopsy from the axilla showing inclusions in myoepithelial cells of apocrine glands.[216] GBE activity in leukocytes is markedly reduced in some patients, especially patients of Ashkenazi origin.[212–215]

There is no specific pharmacological therapy for APBD, and the current emphasis is on supportive care.

References

1. Anderson W. A case of "angeio-keratoma". Br J Dermatol 1898;10:113–117

2. Fabry J. Ein Beitrag zur Kenntnis der purpura haemorrhagica nodularis (purpura papulosa haemorrhagica hebrae). Arch Dermatol Syph Berlin 1898;43:187–200

3. Brady RO. Medical progress: the sphingolipidoses. N Engl J Med 1966;275:312–318

4. Brady RO, Gal AE, Bradley RM, et al. Enzymatic defect in Fabry's disease: ceramidetrihexosidase deficiency. N Engl J Med 1967;276:1163–1167

5. Kornreich R, Desnick RJ, Bishop DF. Nucleotide sequence of human α-galactosidase A gene. Nucleic Acids Res 1989;17:3301–3302

6. Brady RO. Fabry disease. In: Dyck PJ, Thomas PK, eds. Peripheral Neuropathy. Vol 2. 3rd ed. Philadelphia: WB Saunders, 1993:1169–1178

7. Miekle PJ, Hopwood JJ, Clague AE, Carey WF. Prevalence of lysosomal storage disorders. JAMA 1999;281:249–254

8. Eng CM, Guffon N, Wilcox WR, et al., for the International Collaborative Fabry Disease Study Group. Safety and efficacy of recombinant human alpha galactosidase A replacement therapy in Fabry's disease. N Engl J Med 2001;345:9–16

9. Schiffmann R, Kopp JB, Austin HA, et al. Enzyme replacement therapy in Fabry disease. JAMA 2001; 285:2743–2749

10. Kahn P. Anderson-Fabry disease: a histopathological study of three cases with observations on the mechanism of production of pain. J Neurol Neurosurg Psychiatry 1973;36:1053–1062

11. Ohnishi A, Dyck PJ. Loss of small peripheral sensory neurons in Fabry disease. Arch Neurol 1974;31: 120–127

12. Ouvrier RA, McLeod JG, Pollard JD. Neuropathies in metabolic and degenerative disorders. In: Ouvrier RA, McLeod JG, Pollard JD, eds. Peripheral Neuropathy in Childhood. 2nd ed. London: Mac Keith Press, 1999: 172–200

13. Sheth KJ, Swick HM. Peripheral nerve conduction in Fabry disease. Ann Neurol 1980;7:319–323

14. Cleeland CS, Gonin R, Hatfield AK, et al. Pain and its treatment in outpatients with metastatic cancer. N Engl J Med 1994;330:592–596

15. Bühler FR, Thiel G, Dubach UC, et al. Kidney transplantation in Fabry's disease. Br Med J 1973;3:28–29

16. Lockman LA, Hunninghake DB, Krivit W, Desnick RJ. Relief of pain of Fabry's disease by diphenylhydantoin. Neurology 1973;28:871–875

17. Fredrickson DS, Altrocchi PH, Avioli LV, et al. Tangier disease–combined clinical staff conference at the National Institutes of Health. Ann Intern Med 1961;55:1016–1031

18. Brooks-Wilson A, Marcil M, Clee SM, et al. Mutations in ABC1 in Tangier disease and familial high density lipoprotein deficiency. Nat Genet 1999;22:336–345

19. Remaley AT, Rust S, Rosier M, et al. Human ATP-binding cassette transporter 1 (ABC1): genomic organization and identification of the genetic defect in the original Tangier disease kindred. Proc Natl Acad Sci USA 1999;96:12685–12690

20. Young SG, Fielding CJ. The ABCs of cholesterol efflux. Nat Genet 1999;22:316–318

21. Higgins CF, Linton KJ. The xyz of ABC transporters. Science 2001;293:1782–1784

22. Yao JK, Herbert PN. Lipoprotein deficiency and neuromuscular manifestations. In: Dyck PJ, Thomas PK, eds. Peripheral Neuropathy. Vol 2. 3rd ed. Philadelphia: WB Saunders, 1993:1179–1194

23. Pollock M, Nukada H, Frith RW, et al. Peripheral neuropathy in Tangier disease. Brain 1983;106:911–928

24. Suarez BK, Schonfeld G, Sparkes RS. Tangier disease: heterozygote detection and linkage analysis. Hum Genet 1982;60:150–156

25. Pietrini V, Rizzuto N, Vergani C, et al. Neuropathy in Tangier disease: a clinicopathologic study and review of the literature. Acta Neurol Scand 1985;72:495–505

26. Dyck PJ, Ellefson RD, Yao JK, Herbert PN. Adult onset of Tangier disease. 1. Morphometric and pathological studies suggesting delayed degradation of neutral lipids after fiber degeneration. J Neuropathol Exp Neurol 1978;37:119–137

27. Gilbert-Barness E, Barness LA, Olson RE. Disorders of lipid metabolism. In: Metabolic Diseases: Foundations of Clinical Management, Genetics and Pathology. Vol 1. Natick, MA: Eaton Publishing, 2000:297–298

28. Yao JK, Herbert PN, Fredrickson DS, et al. Biochemical studies in a patient with a Tangier syndrome. J Neuropathol Exp Neurol 1978;37:138–154

29. Bassen FA, Kornzweig AL. Malformation of erythrocytes in a case of atypical retinitis pigmentosa. Blood 1950;5:381–387

30. Jampel RS, Falls HF. Atypical retinitis pigmentosa, acanthocytosis and heredodegenerative neuromuscular disease. Arch Ophthalmol 1958;59:818–820

31. Marbry CC, Di George AM, Auerbach VH. Studies concerning the defect in a patient with acanthocytosis. Clin Res 1960;8:371

32. Salt HB, Wolff OH, Lloyd JK, et al. On having no beta-lipoprotein: a syndrome comprising abetalipoproteinemia, acanthocytosis, and steatorrhea. Lancet 1960;2: 325–329

33. Sharp D, Blinderman L, Combs KA, et al. Cloning and gene defects in microsomal triglyceride transfer protein associated with abetalipoproteinemia. Nature 1993;365:65–69

34. Wetterau JR, Aggerbeck LP, Bouma M-E, et al. Absence of microsomal triglyceride-transfer protein in individuals with abetalipoproteinemia. Science 1992; 258:999–1001

35. Ricci B, Sharp D, O'Rourke E, et al. A 30-amino acid truncation of the microsomal triglyceride transfer protein large subunit disrupts its interaction with protein disulfide-isomerase and causes abetalipoproteinemia. J Biol Chem 1995;270:14281–14285

36. Ohashi K, Ishibashi S, Osuga J, et al. Novel mutations in the microsomal triglyceride transfer protein gene causing abetalipoproteinemia. J Lipid Res 2000;41: 1199–1204

37. Rader DJ, Brewer HP. Abetalipoproteinemia. New insights into lipoprotein assembly and vitamin E metabolism from a rare genetic disease. JAMA 1993; 270:865–869

38. Wichman A, Buchthal F, Pezeshkpour GH, Gregg RE. Peripheral neuropathy is abetalipoproteinemia. Neurology 1985;35:1279–1289

39. Illingworth RD, Connor WE, Miller RG. Abetalipoproteinemia: report of two cases and review of therapy. Arch Neurol 1980;37:659–662

40. Muller DPR, Lloyd JK, Bird AC. Long-term management of abetalipoproteinemia: possible role for vitamin E. Arch Dis Child 1977;52:209–214

41. Young SG, Hubl ST, Smith RS, et al. Familial hypobetalipoproteinemia caused by a mutation in the apolipoprotein B gene that results in a truncated

species of apolipoprotein B (B-31). J Clin Invest 1990; 85:993–942

42. Ross RS, Gregg RE, Law SW, et al. Homozygous hypo-betalipoproteinemia: a disease distinct from abeta-lipoproteinemia at the molecular level. J Clin Invest 1988;81:590–595

43. Mawatari S, Iwashita H, Kuroiwa Y. Familial hypo-B-lipoproteinemia. J Neurol Sci 1972;16:93–101

44. Refsum S. Heredo-ataxia hemeralopica polyneuriti-formis—familial syndrome not previously described; preliminary report. Nord Med 1945;28:2682–2685

45. Viets HR. Refsum's disease. N Engl J Med 1947;236:996

46. Klenk E, Kahike W. Über das Vorkommen der 3,7,11,15-tetramethylhexadecansäure (Phytansäure) in den Cholesterinestern und anderen Lipoidfraktionen der Organe bei einem Krankheits-Fall unbekannter Genese (Verdacht auf Heredopathia atactica polyneu-ritiformis [Refsum-Syndrom]). Hoppe Seylers Z Physiol Chem 1963;333:133–139

47. Skjeldal OH, Stokke O, Refsum S. Phytanic acid storage disease. In: Dyck PJ, Thomas PK, eds. Periph-eral Neuropathy. Vol 2. 3rd ed. Philadelphia: WB Saunders, 1993:1149–1160

48. Jansen GA, Ofman R, Ferdinandusse S, et al. Refsum disease is caused by mutations in the phytanoyl-CoA hydroxylase gene. Nat Genet 1997;17:190–193

49. Milhalik SJ, Morrell JC, Kim D, et al. Identification of PAHX, a Refsum disease gene. Nat Genet 1997;17: 185–189

50. Skjeldal OH, Stokke O, Refsum S, et al. Clinical and biochemical heterogeneity in conditions with phytanic acid accumulations. J Neurol Sci 1987;77:87–96

51. Veltema AN, Verjaal A. Sur un cas d'hérédopathie ataxique polynévritique: maladie de Refsum. Rev. Neurol 1961;104:15

52. Cammermeyer J. Neuropathological changes in hered-itary neuropathies: manifestation of the syndrome heredopathia atactica polyneuritiformis in the pres-ence of interstitial hypertrophic polyneuropathy. J Neuropathol Exp Neurol 1956;15:340–361

53. Thomas PK. Pathology of Refsum's disease. In: Dyck PJ, Thomas PK, eds. Peripheral Neuropathy. Vol 2. 3rd ed. Philadelphia: WB Saunders, 1993:1154–1160

54. Stokke O, Eldjarn L. Biochemical and dietary aspects of Refsum's disease. In: Dyck PJ, Thomas PK, Lambert EH, Bunge R, eds. Peripheral Neuropathy. 2nd ed. Philadelphia: WB Saunders 1984:1684–1693.

55. Krabbe KH. A new familial infantile form of diffuse brain sclerosis. Brain 1916;39:74–114

56. Thomas PK. Other inherited neuropathies. In: Dyck PJ, Thomas PK, eds. Peripheral Neuropathy. Vol 2. 3rd ed. Philadelphia: WB Saunders, 1993:1194–1218.

57. Suzuki K, Suzuki Y. Globoid cell leucodystrophy (Krabbe's disease): deficiency of galactocerebroside beta-galactosidase. Proc Natl Acad Sci USA 1970; 66:302–309

58. Suzuki K, Suzuki Y, Suzuki K. Galactoylceramide lipi-dosis: globoid-cell leukodystrophy (Krabbe disease). In: Scriver CR, Beaudet AL, Sly WS, Valle D, eds. The Metabolic Basis of Inherited Disease. 7th ed. New York: McGraw-Hill, 1995:2671

59. Kaye EM. Update on genetic disorders affecting white matter. Pediatr Neurol 2001;24:11–24

60. Igisu H, Suzuki K. Progressive accumulation of toxic metabolite in a genetic leukodystrophy. Science 1984;224:753–755

61. Svennerholm L, Vanier MT, Mansson JE. Krabbe disease: a galactosylsphingosine (psychosine) lipido-sis. J Lipid Res 1980;21:53–64

62. Krivit W, Aubourg P, Shapiro E, Peters C. Bone marrow transplantation for globoid cell leukodystro-phy, adrenoleukodystrophy, metachromatic leukodys-trophy, and Hurler syndrome. Curr Opin Hematol 1999;6:377–382

63. Hagberg B. Krabbe's disease: clinical presentation of neurological variants. Neuropediatr 1984;15(Suppl): S11–S15

64. Hagberg B. The clinical diagnosis of Krabbe's infantile leucodystrophy. Acta Paediatr Scand 1963;52:213

65. Lyon G. Four cases of late-onset Krabbe disease. Pre-liminary report. International Symposium on Recent Progress in Neurolipidoses and Allied Disorders. Lyon, May 3–June 2, 1983

66. Marks HG, Scavina MT, Kolodny EH, et al. Krabbe's disease presenting as a peripheral neuropathy. Muscle Nerve 1997;20:1024–1028

67. Sasaki M, Sakuragawa N, Takashima S, et al. MRI and CT findings in infantile Krabbe disease. Pediatr Neurol 1991;7:283–288

68. Zafeiriou DI, Michelakaki EM, Anastasiou AL, et al. Serial MRI and neurophysiological studies in late-infantile Krabbe disease. Pediatr Neurol 1996;15: 240–244

69. Hogan GR, Gutmann L, Chou SM. The peripheral neu-ropathy of Krabbe's (globoid) leukodystrophy. Neu-rology 1969;19:1093–1097

70. Lyon G, Jardin L, Aicardi J. Etude au microscope élec-tronique d'un nerf périphérique dans un cas de leu-codystrophie de Krabbe. J Neurol Sci 1971;12:263–274

71. Krivit W, Peters C, Shapiro EG. Bone marrow trans-plantation as effective treatment of central nervous system disease in globoid cell leukodystrophy, metachromatic leukodystrophy, adrenoleukodystro-phy, mannosidosis, fucosidosis, aspartylglucosamin-uria, Hurler, Maroteaux-Lamy, and Sly syndromes, and Gaucher disease type III. Curr Opin Neurol 1999;12:167–176

72. Krivit W, Shapiro EG, Peters C, et al. Hematopoietic stem-cell transplantation in globoid-cell leukodystro-phy. N Engl J Med 1998;338:1119–1126

73. Bambach BJ, Moser HW, Blakemore K, et al. Engraft-ment following in utero bone marrow transplantation for globoid cell leukodystrophy. Bone Marrow Trans-plant 1997;19:399–402

74. Alzheimer A. Beiträge zur Kenntnis der pathologis-chen Neuroglia und ihre Beziehungen zu den Abbau-vorgängen im Nervengewebe. In: Alzheimer A, Nissl F, eds. Histologische und histopathologische Arbeiten uber die Grosshirnrinde mit Besonderer Berucksichtigung der Pathologischen Anatomie der Geisteskrankheiten. Vol III. Jena: Gustav Fischer, 1910:401

75. Nissl F. Encyclopädie der mikroskopischen Technik. In: Ehrlich P, Krause R, Mosse M, et al., eds. Nerven-system. 2nd ed. Berlin: Urban and Schwarzenberg, 1910:284

76. Farrell DF. Heterozygote detection in MLD. Allelic mutations at the ARA locus. Hum Genet 1981;59: 129–134

77. Gustavsom KH, Hagberg B. The incidence and genet-ics of metachromatic leukodystrophy in Northern Sweden. Acta Paediatr Scand 1971;60:585–590

78. Inui K, Emmett M, Wenger DA. Immunological evid-ence for a deficiency in an activator protein for sul-fatide sulfatase in a variant of metachromatic leukodystrophy. Proc Natl Acad Sci USA 1983;80: 3074–3077

79. Gieselmann A, Polten J, Kreysing J, von Figura K. Molecular genetics of metachromatic leukodystrophy. J Inherit Metab Dis 1994;17:500–509

80. McKhann GM. Metachromatic leukodystrophy: clinical and enzymatic parameters. Neuropediatrics 1984; 15(Suppl):4–10

81. Malm G, Ringén O, Winiarski J, et al. Clinical outcome in four children with metachromatic leukodystrophy treated by bone marrow transplantation. Bone Marrow Transplant 1996;17:1003–1008

82. MacFaul R, Cavanagh N, Lake BD, et al. Metachromatic leukodystrophy: review of 38 cases. Arch Dis Childhood 1982;57:168–175

83. Polten A, Fluharty AL, Fluharty CB, et al. Molecular basis of different forms of metachromatic leukodystrophy. N Engl J Med 1991;324:18–22

84. Hagberg B, Sourander P, Thoren L. Peripheral nerve changes in the diagnosis of metachromatic leucodystrophy. Acta Paediatrica 1962;51(Suppl 135):63–71

85. de Silva KL, Pearce J. Neuropathy of metachromatic leukodystrophy. J Neurol Neurosurg Psychiatry 1973; 36:30–33

86. Aziz H, Pearce J. Peripheral neuropathy in metachromatic leukodystrophy. BMJ 1968;4:300

87. Fullerton PM. Peripheral nerve conduction in metachromatic leucodystrophy (sulfatide lipidosis). J Neurol Neurosurg Psychiatry 1964;27:100–105

88. Yudell A, Gomez MR, Lambert EH, Dockerty MB. The neuropathy of sulfatide lipidosis (metachromatic leukodystrophy). Neurology 1967;17:103–111, 127

89. Tasker W, Chutorian AM. Chronic polyneuritis of childhood. J Pediatr 1969;74:699–708

90. Webster H deF. Schwann cell alterations in metachromatic leucodystrophy: Preliminary phase and electron microscopic observations. J Neurol Neurosurg Psychiatry 1962;21:534–554

91. Krivit W, Shapiro EG. Bone marrow transplantation for storage diseases. In: Forman SJ, Blume KG, Thomas ED, eds. Bone Marrow Transplantation. Oxford: Blackwell Scientific Publication, 1994:883–893

92. Krivit W, Lockman LA, Watkins PA, et al. The future for treatment by bone marrow transplantation for adrenoleukodystrophy, globoid cell leukodystrophy and Hurler syndrome. J Inherit Metab Dis 1995;18:398–412

93. Krivit W, Lipton ME, Lockman LA. Prevention of deterioration in metachromatic leukodystrophy by bone marrow transplantation. Am J Med Sci 1987;294: 80–85

94. Shapiro EG, Lipton ME. White matter dysfunction and its neurophysiological correlates: a longitudinal study of a case of metachromatic leukodystrophy by bone marrow transplantation. J Clin Exp Neuropsychol 1992;14:610–624

95. Shapiro EG, Lockman LA, Balthazor M, Krivit W. Neuropsychological outcomes of several storage diseases with and without bone marrow transplantation. J Inher Metab Dis 1995;18:413–429

96. Kaye EM. Lysosomal storage diseases. Curr Treat Opin Neurol 2001;3:249–256

97. Pridjian G, Humbert J, Willis J, Shapira E. Presymptomatic late-infantile metachromatic leukodystrophy treated with bone marrow transplantation. J Pediatr 1994;125:755–758

98. Hoogerbrugge PM, Brouwer OF, Bordigoni P, et al., for the European Group for Bone Marrow Transplantation. Allogeneic bone marrow transplantation for lysosomal storage diseases. Lancet 1995;345:1398–1402

99. Siemerling E, Creutzfeldt HG. Bronzekrankheit und sklerosierende encephalomyelitis. Arch Psychiatr Nervenkr 1923;68:217–244

100. Poser CM, Goutieres F, Carpentier MA, Aicardi J. Schilder's myelinoclastic diffuse sclerosis. Pediatrics 1986;77:107–112

101. Bezman L, Moser AB, Raymond GV, et al. Adrenoleukodystrophy: Incidence, new mutation rate, and results of extended family screening. Ann Neurol 2001;49:512–517

102. Sereni C, Paturneau-Jouas M, Aubourg P, et al. Adrenoleukodystrophy in France: an epidemiological study. Neuroepidemiology 1993;12:229–233

103. van Geel BM, Assies J, Weverling GJ, Barth PG. Predominance of the adrenomyeloneuropathy phenotype of X-linked adrenoleukodystrophy in the Netherlands: a survey of 30 kindreds. Neurology 1994;44:2343–2346

104. Moser HW, Moser AB, Frayer KK, et al. Adrenoleukodystrophy: increased plasma content of saturated very long chain fatty acids. Neurology 1981; 31:1241–1249

105. Moser HW, Moser AB, Smith KD, et al. Adrenoleukodystrophy: phenotypic variability and implications for therapy. J Inherit Metab Dis 1992;15: 645–664

106. Mosser J, Douar AM, Sarde CO, et al. Putative X-linked adrenoleukodystrophy gene shares unexpected homology with ABC transporters. Nature 1993;361:726–730

107. Liu LX, Janvier K, Berteaux-Lecellier V, et al. Homo- and heterodimerization of peroxisomal ATP-binding cassette half-transporters. J Biol Chem 1999;274: 32738–32743

108. Ewart GD, Cannell D, Cox GB, Howells AJ. Mutational analysis of the traffic ATPase (ABC) transporters involved in uptake of eye pigment precursors in Drosophila melanogaster. Implications for structure-function relationships. J Biol Chem 1994;269: 10370–10377

109. Yamada T, Taniwaki T, Shinnoh N, et al. Adrenoleukodystrophy protein enhances association of very long-chain acyl-coenzyme A synthetase with the peroxisome. Neurology 1999;52:614–616

110. Steinberg SJ, Kemp S, Braiterman LT, Watkins PA. Role of very-long-chain acyl-coenzyme A synthetase in X-linked adrenoleukodystrophy. Ann Neurol 1999;46: 409–412

111. Berger J, Moser HW, Forss-Petter S. Leukodystrophies: recent developments in genetics, molecular biology, pathogenesis and treatment. Curr Opin Neurol 2001;14:305–312

112. O'Neill GN, Aoki M, Brown RH. ABCD1 translation-initiator mutation demonstrates genotype-phenotype correlation for AMN. Neurology 2001;57:1956–1962

113. Smith KD, Kemp S, Braiterman LT, et al. X-linked adrenoleukodystrophy: Genes, mutations, and phenotypes. Neurochem Res 1999;24:521–535

114. Griffin JW, Goren E, Schaumburg H, et al. Adrenomyeloneuropathy: A probable variant of adrenoleukodystrophy. I. Clinical and endocrinologic aspects. Neurology 1977;27:1107–1113

115. Rosen NL, Lechtenberg R, Wisniewski K, et al. Adrenomyeloneuropathy with onset in early childhood. Annals Neurol 1985;17:311–312

116. Moser HW, Moser AB, Naidu S, Bergin A. Clinical aspects of adrenoleukodystrophy and adrenomyeloneuropathy. Dev Neurosci 1991;13:254–261

117. Restuccia D, Di Lazzaro V, Valeriani M, et al. Neurophysiological abnormalities in adrenoleukodystrophy

carriers: evidence of different degrees of central nervous system involvement. Brain 1997;120: 1139–1148

118. Moser AB, Kreiter N, Bezman L, et al. Plasma very long chain fatty acids in 3000 peroxisome disease patients and 29 000 controls. Ann Neurol 1999;45: 100–110

119. Boehm CD, Cutting GR, Lachtermacher MB, et al. Accurate DNA-based diagnostic and carrier testing for X-linked adrenoleukodystrophy. Mol Genet Metab 1999;66:128–136

120. Feigenbaum V, Lombard-Platet G, Guidoux S, et al. Mutational and protein analysis of patients and heterozygous women with X-linked adrenoleukodystrophy. Am J Hum Genet 1996;58:1135–1144

121. Watkins PA, Gould SJ, Smith MA, et al. Altered expression of ALDP in X-linked adrenoleukodystrophy. Am J Hum Genet 1995;57:292–301

122. Chaudhry V, Moser HW, Cornblath DR. Nerve conduction studies in adrenomyeloneuropathy. J Neurol Neurosurg Psychiatry 1996;61:181–185

123. van Geel BM, Koelman J, Bath PG, Ongerboer de Visser BW. Peripheral nerve abnormalities in adrenomyeloneuropathy: A clinical and electrodiagnostic study. Neurology 1996;46:112–118

124. Shapiro E, Krivit W, Lockman L, et al. Long-term beneficial effect of bone-marrow transplantation of childhood-onset cerebral X-linked adrenoleukodystrophy. Lancet 2000;356:713–718

125. Aubourg P, Blanche S, Jambaqué I, et al. Reversal of early neurologic and neuroradiologic manifestations of X-linked adrenoleukodystrophy by bone marrow transplantation. N Engl J Med 1990;322:1860–1866

126. Moser HW, Tutschka PJ, Brown FR III, et al. Bone marrow transplant in adrenoleukodystrophy. Neurology 1984;34:1410–1417

127. Brown FR, Van Duyn MA, Moser AB, et al. Adrenoleukodystrophy: effects of dietary restriction of very long chain fatty acids and of administration of carnitine and clofibrate on clinical status and plasma fatty acids. Johns Hopkins Med J 1982;151:164–173

128. Moser HW, Naidu S, Kumar AJ, Rosenbaum AE. The adrenoleukodystrophies. Crit Rev Neurobiol 1987;3: 29–88

129. Aubourg P, Adamsbaum C, Lavallard-Rousseau MC, et al. A two-year trial of oleic and erucic acids ("Lorenzo's") as treatment for adrenomyeloneuropathy. N Engl J Med 1993;329:745–752

130. Moser HW, Kok F, Neumann S, et al. Adrenoleukodystrophy update: Genetics and effect of Lorenzo's oil therapy in asymptomatic patients. Int Pediatr 1994;9:196–204

131. Stumpf DA, Hayward A, Haas R, et al. Adrenoleukodystrophy: failure of immunosuppression to prevent neurological progression. Arch Neurol 1981; 38:48–49

132. Naidu S, Bresnan MJ, Griffin D, et al. Childhood adrenoleukodystrophy: failure of intensive immunosuppression to arrest neurologic progression. Arch Neurol 1988;45:846–848

133. Berginer VM, Salen G, Shefer S. Long term treatment of cerebrotendinous xanthomatosis with chenodeoxycholic acid. N Engl J Med 1984;311:1649–1652

134. Van Bogaert L, Scherer HJ, Froelich A, Epstein E. Une deuxieme observation de cholesterinose tendineuse symetrique avec symptomes cerebraux. Ann de Med 1937;42:69–101

135. Cali JJ, Hsieh C-L, Francke U, Russell DW. Mutations

in the bile acid biosynthetic enzyme sterol 27-hydroxylase underlie cerebrotendinous xanthomatosis. J Biol Chem 1991;266:7779–7783

136. Verrips A, Hoefsloot LH, Steenbergen GCH, et al. Clinical and molecular genetic characteristics of patients with cerebrotendinous xanthomatosis. Brain 2000;123:908–919

137. Menkes J, Schimshock JR, Swanson PD. Cerebrotendinous xanthomatosis: the storage of cholestanol within the nervous system. Arch Neurol 1969;19:47–53

138. Salen G. Cholestanol deposition in cerebrotendinous xanthomatosis: a possible mechanism. Ann Intern Med 1971;75:843–851

139. Katz DA, Scheinberg L, Horoupian DS, Salen G. Peripheral neuropathy in cerebrotendinous xanthomatosis. Arch Neurol 1984;42:1008–1010

140. Voiculescu V, Alexianu M, Popescu-Tismana G, et al. Polyneuropathy with lipid deposition in Schwann cells and axonal degeneration in cerebrotendinous xanthomatosis (abstract). Muscle Nerve (Suppl) 1986:129

141. Salen G, Grundy SM. The metabolism of cholestanol, cholesterol, and bile acids in cerebrotendinous xanthomatosis. J Clin Invest 1973;52:2822–2835

142. Setoguchi T, Salen G, Tint GS, Mosbach EH. A biochemical abnormality in cerebrotendinous xanthomatosis: impairment of bile acid biosynthesis associated with incomplete degradation of the cholesterol side chain. J Clin Invest 1974;53:1393–1401

143. Shefer S, Dayal B, Tint GS, et al. Identification of pentahydroxy bile alcohols in cerebrotendinous xanthomatosis: characterization of 5β-cholestane-3α, 7α, 12α, 24ξ, 25-pentol and 5β-cholestane-3α, 7α, 12α, 24ξ, 25-pentol. J Lipid Res 1975;16:280–286

144. Hoshita T, Yasuhara M, Une M, et al. Occurrence of bile alcohol glucuronides in bile of patients with cerebrotendinous xanthomatosis. J Lipid Res 1980;21: 1015–1021

145. Wolthers BG, Volmer M, van der Molen J, et al. Diagnosis of cerebrotendinous xanthomatosis (CTX) and effect of chenodeoxycholic acid therapy by analysis of urine using capillary gas chromatography. Clin Chim Acta 1983;131:52–65

146. Ohnishi A, Mitsudome A, Murai Y. Primary segmental demyelination in the sural nerve in Cockayne's syndrome. Muscle Nerve 1987;10:163–167

147. Kuritzky A, Berginer VM, Korczyn AD. Peripheral neuropathy in cerebrotendinous xanthomatosis. Neurology 1979;29:880–881

148. Donaghy M, King RHM, McKeran RO, et al. Cerebrotendinous xanthomatosis: clinical, electrophysiological and nerve biopsy findings, and response to treatment with chenodeoxycholic acid. J Neurol 1990;237:216–219

149. Pedley TA, Emerson RG, Warner CL, et al. Treatment of cerebrotendinous xanthomatosis with chenodeoxycholic acid. Ann Neurol 1985;18:517–518

150. Waterreus RJ, Koopman BJ, Wolthers BG, Oosterhuis HJGH. Cerebrotendinous xanthomatosis (CTX): a clinical survey of the patient population in the Netherlands. Clin Neurol Neurosurg 1987;89:169–175

151. Nakamura T, Matsuzawa Y, Takemura K, et al. Combined treatment with chenodeoxycholic acid and pravastatin improves plasma levels associated with marked regression of tendon xanthomas in CTX. Metabolism 1991;40:741–746

152. Kuriyama M, Tokimura Y, Fujiyama J, et al. Treatment of cerebrotendinous xanthomatosis: effects of chenodeoxycholic acid, pravastatin, and combined use. J Neurol Sci 1994;125:22–28

153. Mondelli M, Sicurelli F, Scarpini C, et al. Cerebrotendinous xanthomatosis: 11-year treatment with chenodeoxycholic acid in five patients. An electrophysiological study. J Neurol Sci 2001;190:29–33

154. Salen G. Chenodeoxycholic treatment of cerebrotendinous xanthomatosis (reply to letter). Neurology 2001;56:695

155. Salen G, Batta AK, Tint GS, Shefer S. Comparative effects of lovastatin and chenodeoxycholic acid on plasma cholestanol levels and abnormal bile acid metabolism in cerebrotendinous xanthomatosis. Metabolism 1994;43:1018–1022

156. Verrips A, Wevers RA, Van Engelen BGM, et al. Effect of simvastatin in addition to chenodeoxycholic acid in patients with cerebrotendinous xanthomatosis. Metabolism 1999;48:233–238

157. Peynet J, Laurent A, De Liege P, et al. Cerebrotendinous xanthomatosis: treatment with simvastatin, lovastatin, and chenodeoxycholic acid in 3 siblings. Neurology 1991;41:434–436

158. Leigh D. Subacute necrotizing encephalomyelopathy in an infant. J Neurol Neurosurg Psychiatry 1951;14:216–221

159. Nardin RA, Johns DR. Mitochondrial dysfunction and neuromuscular disease. Muscle Nerve 2001;24:170–191

160. Eymard B, Penicaud A, Leger JM, et al. Peripheral nerve in mitochondrial disease: clinical and electrophysiological data. A study of 28 cases. Rev Neurol (Paris) 1991;147:508–512

161. Petty RK, Harding AE, Morgna-Hughes JA. The clinical features of mitochondrial myopathy. Ann Neurol 1980;7:262–268

162. Chu CC, Huang CC, Fang W, et al. Peripheral neuropathy in mitochondrial encephalomyopathies. Eur Neurol 1997;37:110–115

163. Yiannikas C, McLeod JG, Pollard JD, Baverstock J. Peripheral neuropathy associated with mitochondrial myopathy. Ann Neurol 1986;20:249–257

164. Mizusawa H, Ohkoshi N, Watanabe M, Kanazawa I. Peripheral neuropathy of mitochondrial myopathies. Rev Neurol (Paris) 1991;147:501–507

165. Coker SB. Leigh disease presenting as Guillain–Barré syndrome. Pediatr Neurol 1993;9:61–69

166. Torbergsen T, Stalberg E, Bless JK. Nerve-muscle involvement in a large family with mitochondrial cytopathy: electrophysiological studies. Muscle Nerve 1991;14:35–41

167. Rusanen H, Majamaa K, Tolonen U, et al. Demyelinating polyneuropathy in a patient with the tRNA (Leu) (UUR) mutation at base pair 3243 of the mitochondrial DNA. Neurology 1995;45:1188–1192

168. Pezeshkpour G, Krarup C, Buchtal F, et al. Peripheral neuropathy in mitochondrial disease. J Neurol Sci 1987;77:285–304

169. Peyronnard JM, Charron L, Bellavance A, Marchand L. Neuropathy and mitochondrial myopathy. Ann Neurol 1980;7:262–268

170. Teener JW, Sladky JT. Demyelinating neuropathy as a feature of mitochondrial encephalomyopathy. Ann Neurol 1994;34:508–509

171. Fang W. Polyneuropathy in the mtDNA base pair 3243 point mutation. Neurology 1996;46:1494–1495

172. Fang W, Huang CC, Lee CC, et al. Ophthalmologic manifestations in MELAS syndrome. Arch Neurol 1993;50:977–980

173. Threlkeld AB, Miller NR, Golnik KC, et al. Ophthalmic involvement in myo-neuro-gastrointestinal encephalopathy syndrome. Am J Ophthalmol 1992;114:322–328

174. Uncini A, Serridei S, Silvestri G, et al. Ophthalmoplegia, demyelinating neuropathy, leukoencephalopathy, myopathy and gastrointestinal dysfunction with multiple deletions of mitochondrial DNA: A mitochondrial multisystem disorder in search of a name. Muscle Nerve 1994;17:667–674

175. Brierly EJ, Johnson MA, James OF, Turnbull DM. Effects of physical activity and age on mitochondrial function. QJM 1996;89:251–258

176. Cox MH. Exercise training programs and cardiorespiratory adaptation. Clin Sports Med 1991;10:19–32

177. Taylor RW, Chinnery PF, Clark KM, et al. Treatment of mitochondrial disease. J Bioenerg Biomembr 1997;29:195–205

178. Ogasahara S, Nishikawa Y, Yorifuji S, et al. Treatment of Kearns-Sayre syndrome with coenzyme Q10. Neurology 1986;36:45–53

179. Bendahan D, Desnuelle C, Vanuxem D, et al. 31P NMR spectroscopy and ergometer exercise test as evidence for muscle oxidative performance improvement with coenzyme Q in mitochondrial myopathies. Neurology 1992;42:1203–1208

180. Ihara Y, Namba R, Kuroda S, et al. Mitochondrial encephalomyopathy (MELAS): pathological study and successful therapy with coenzyme Q10 and idebenone. J Neurol Sci 1989;90:263–271

181. Matthews PM, Ford B, Dandurand RJ, et al. Coenzyme Q10 with multiple vitamins is generally ineffective in treatment of mitochondrial disease. Neurology 1993;43:884–890

182. Yamamoto M, Sato T, Anno M, et al. Mitochondrial myopathy, encephalopathy, lactic acidosis, and stroke-like episodes with recurrent abdominal symptoms and coenzyme Q10 therapy. J Neurol Neurosurg Psychiatry 1987;50:1475–1481

183. Yamanaka N, Kimura K, Yi S, et al. A case of motor and sensory neuropathy with elevated serum lactate and pyruvate which responded to large dose of coenzyme Q10 therapy. Rinsho Shinkegaku 1989;29:885–889

184. Zierz S, Jahns G, Jerusalem F. Coenzyme Q in serum and muscle of 5 patients with Kearns-Sayre syndrome and 12 patients with ophthalmoplegia plus. J Neurol 1989;236:97–101

185. Bresolin N, Bet L, Binda A, et al. Clinical and biochemical correlations in mitochondrial myopathies treated with coenzyme Q10. Neurology 1988;38:892–899

186. Eleff S, Kennaway NG, Buist NR, et al. 31P NMR study of improvement in oxidative phosphorylation by vitamins K3 and C in a patient with a defect in electron transport at complex III in skeletal muscle. Proc Natl Acad Sci USA 1984;81:3529–3533

187. Argov Z, Bank WJ, Maris J, et al. Treatment of mitochondrial myopathy due to complex III deficiency with vitamins K3 and C: a 31P-NMR follow-up study. Ann Neurol 1986;19:598–602

188. Calvani M, Koverech A, Caruso G. Treatment of mitochondrial diseases. In: DiMauro S, Wallace DC, eds. Mitochondrial DNA in Human Pathology. New York: Raven Press, 1993:173–198

189. Robinson BH, Chun K, MacKay N, et al. Isolated and combined deficiencies of the alpha-keto acid dehydrogenase complexes. Ann NY Acad Sci 1989;573:337–346

190. Stacpoole PW. The pharmacology of dichloroacetate. Metabolism 1989;38:1124–1144

191. Stacpoole PW, Moore GW, Kornhauser DM. Toxicity of chronic dichloroacetate. N Engl J Med 1979;300:372

192. Kurlemann G, Paetzke I, Möller H, et al. Therapy of

complex I deficiency: peripheral neuropathy during dicholoroacetate therapy. Eur J Pediatr 1995;154: 928–932

193. Cockayne EA. Dwarfism with retinal atrophy and deafness. Arch Dis Child 1936;11:1–8

194. Cleaver JE, Thompson LH, Richardson AS, States JC. A summary of mutations in the UV-sensitive disorders: xeroderma pigmentosum, Cockayne syndrome, and trichothiodystrophy. Hum Mutat 1999;14:9–22

195. Mallery DL, Tanganelli B, Colella S, et al. Molecular analysis of mutations in the CSB (ERCC6) gene in patients with Cockayne syndrome. Am J Hum Genet 1998;62:77–85

196. Mayne LV, Lehmann AR. Failure of RNA synthesis to recover after UV irradiation: an early defect in cells from individuals with Cockayne's syndrome and xeroderma pigmentosum. Cancer Res 1982;42:1473–1478

197. Nance MA, Berry SA. Cockayne syndrome: review of 140 cases. Am J Med Genet 1992;42:68–84

198. Cantani A, Bamonte G, Bellioni P. Rare syndromes I. Cockayne syndrome: a review of the 129 cases so far reported in the literature. Eur Rev Med Pharm Sci 1987;9:9–17

199. Özdirim E, Topcu M, Özön A, Cila A. Cockayne syndrome: review of 25 cases. Pediatr Neurol 1996;15: 312–316

200. Vos A, Gabreëls-Festen A, Joosten E, et al. The neuropathy of Cockayne syndrome. Acta Neuropathol (Berl) 1983;61:153–156

201. Ohnishi A, Mitsudome A, Murai Y. Primary segmental demyelination in the sural nerve in Cockayne's syndrome. Muscle Nerve 1987;10:163–167

202. Moosa A, Dubowitz V. Peripheral neuropathy in Cockayne's syndrome. Arch Dis Child 1970;45:674–677

203. McElvanney AM, Wooldridge WJ, Khan AA, Ansons AM. Ophthalmic management of Cockayne's syndrome. Eye 1996;10:61–64

204. Sorin MS. Cockayne's syndrome: dental findings and management. J Clin Pediatr Dent 1994;18:299–302

205. Cafferty, MS, Lovelace RE, Hays AP, et al. Polyglucosan body disease. Muscle Nerve 1991;14:102–107

206. Gray F, Gherardi R, Marshall A, et al. Adult polyglucosan body disease (APBD). J Neuropathol Exp Neurol 1988;47:459–474

207. Matsumuro K, Izumo S, Minauchi Y, et al. Chronic demyelinating neuropathy and intra-axonal polyglucosan bodies. Acta Neuropathol 1993;86:95–99

208. Vos AJM, Joosten EMG, Gabreëls-Festen AAWM. Adult polyglucosan body disease: clinical and nerve biopsy findings in two cases. Ann Neurol 1983;13: 440–444

209. Robitaille Y, Carpenter S, Karpati G, DiMauro S. A distinct form of adult polyglucosan body disease with massive involvement of central and peripheral neuronal processes and astrocytes. A report of four cases and a review of the occurrence of polyglucosan bodies in other conditions such as Lafora's disease and normal aging. Brain 1980;103:315–336

210. Okamoto K, Llena JF, Hirano A. A type of adult polyglucosan body disease. Acta Neuropathol 1982; 58:73–77

211. Klein CK, Bosch EP, Dyck PJ. Probable adult polyglucosan body disease. Mayo Clin Proc 2000;75:1327–1331

212. Lossos A, Barash V, Soffer D, et al. Hereditary branching enzyme dysfunction in adult polyglucosan body disease: a possible metabolic cause in two patients. Ann Neurol 1991;30:655–662

213. Lossos A, Meiner Z, Barash V, et al. Adult polyglucosan body disease in Ashkenazi Jewish patients carrying the Tyr329Ser mutation in the glycogen-branching enzyme gene. Ann Neurol 1998; 44:867–872

214. Bruno C, Servidei S, Shanske S, et al. Glycogen branching enzyme deficiency in adult polyglucosan body disease. Ann Neurol 1993;33:88–93

215. Ziemssen F, Sindern E, Schroder JM, et al. Novel missense mutations in the glycogen-branching enzyme gene in adult polyglucosan body disease. Ann Neurol 2000;47:536–540

216. Milde P, Guccion JG, Kelly J, et al. Adult polyglucosan body disease. Arch Pathol Lab Med 2001;125:519–522

206 Porphyria

Anthony J Windebank

Introduction

Abnormalities in porphyrin metabolism cause organic psychoses and peripheral neuropathy. Although the underlying enzyme abnormality is always present, neurological manifestations occur episodically as acute attacks. Drug ingestion or hormonal changes usually precipitate the attacks.

Pathogenesis of neurological porphyrias

Porphyrins are intermediates in the synthesis of heme. The heme ring is chelated with iron and bound to various apoproteins to form hemoglobin and the cytochromes. All cells synthesize heme, but the most important tissues are liver and bone marrow. Nervous system complications are associated only with abnormalities of liver heme metabolism. Three disorders are associated with neurological porphyria: acute intermittent porphyria, hereditary coproporphyria, and variegate porphyria. The major steps in heme synthesis are shown in Figure 206.1, together with the more common enzyme abnormalities that lead to porphyria.

Inheritance

The genetic defect underlying acute intermittent porphyria is inherited as an autosomal dominant abnormality of porphobilinogen deaminase activity (Figure 206.1).[1–5] Estimates of gene prevalence vary but are on the order of 1 to 10 000 to 1 to 100 000. The true incidence is difficult to assess because the disease is recognized only in persons who have acute attacks of neurological disease. Family members of affected persons may have low levels of porphobilinogen deaminase, but they do not have clinically overt disease. Acute attacks are precipitated by drug ingestion (Table 206.1), hormonal changes, and nutritional deprivation. Attacks rarely occur before puberty and are more frequent in women than men, particularly in the luteal phase of the menstrual cycle.

Hereditary coproporphyria was first recognized as a distinct genetic entity in 1955.[6] It has an autosomal dominant pattern of inheritance.[7,8] The gene probably occurs less frequently than that for acute intermittent porphyria, although because the disease is milder and more likely to occur in latent form,[9] the true frequency is difficult to assess. Patients with this disorder present either with the skin manifestations or the acute attacks of neurological disease, which are similar to but usually less severe than those occurring with acute intermittent porphyria. Attacks are more common in women than men and are usually drug-induced.[10]

Variegate porphyria is also dominantly inherited and occurs most frequently in Dutch South Africans. The incidence has been estimated at 1 in 3000 of this group. Most patients in South Africa have had their inheritance traced to a single Boer couple in the late seventeenth century.[11,12] This form of porphyria may

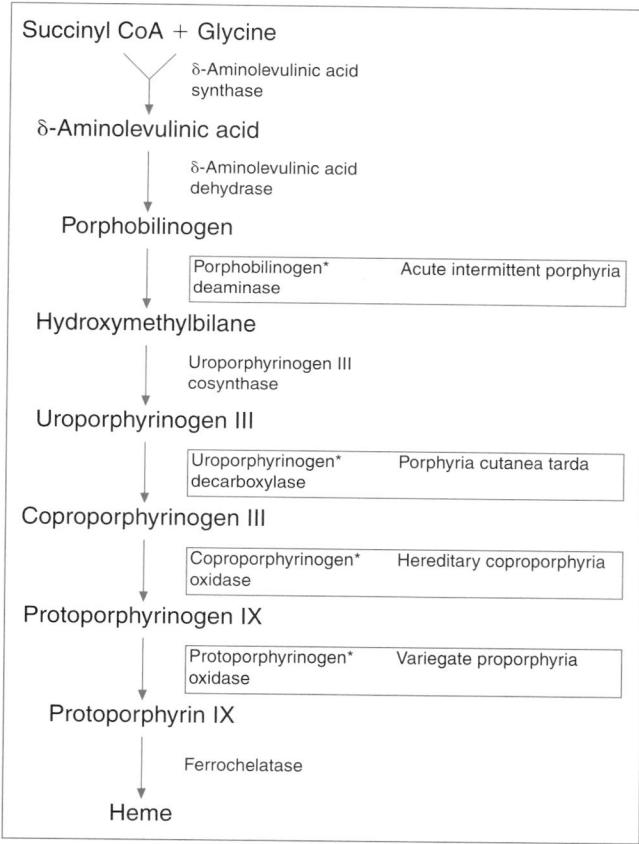

Figure 206.1 The metabolic pathway of hepatic heme synthesis. Deficiency of the enzymes in boxes are responsible for the clinical types of porphyria. Porphobilinogen deaminase (uroporphyrinogen I synthase), coproporphyrinogen oxidase, and protoporphyrinogen oxidase are usually deficient on a genetic basis and associated with acute attacks of neurological disease. Uroporphyrinogen decarboxylase deficiency may be on a genetic basis or occur from toxic (usually alcohol-induced) liver disease. Porphyria cutanea tarda is not associated primarily with neurological disease. CoA, coenzyme A. *Enzymes that may be assayed in reference laboratories. From Windebank AJ, Bonkowsky HL: Porphyric neuropathy. *In*: Dyck PJ, Thomas PK, Griffin JW, et al., eds. Peripheral Neuropathy. Vol 2, 3rd ed. Philadelphia, WB Saunders, 1993:1161–1168. By permission of the publisher.

Table 206.1   Drugs and chemicals in acute hepatic porphyrias*

Reported to exacerbate disease	Theoretically risky†	Believed to be safe
Barbiturates	Alcuronium	Aspirin
Bemegride	Allyl-containing compounds	Atropine
Chloramphenicol	Bupivacaine	Bromides
Chlordiazepoxide	Clonazepam (large doses)	Calcium salts
Chloroquine	Clonidine	Chloral hydrate
Chlorpropamide	Etidocaine	Chlorpromazine
Danazol	Hydralazine	Corticosteroids
Diazepam	Lidocaine	Cyclopropane
Ergot preparations	Mepivacaine	Dicumarol
Estrogens	Methyclothiazide	Droperidol
Ethanol excess	Pargyline	Ether
Eucalyptol (in mouthwash)	Phenoxybenzamine	Fentanyl
Glutethimide	Prilocaine	Gallamine
Griseofulvin	Pyrrocaine	Guanethidine
Halothane	Spironolactone	Mefenamic acid
Hydantoins		Meperidine
Imipramine		Methadone
Ketamine		Morphine
Meprobamate		Neostigmine
Methyldopa		Nitrous oxide
Methyprylon		Pancuronium
Methsuximide		Paraldehyde
Nikethamide		Penicillin
Oral contraceptives		Pentamethonium
Pentazocine		Procaine
Phensuximide		Promazine
Phenylbutazone		Promethazine
Progestagens		Propoxyphene
Pyrazinamide		Propranolol
Pyrazolone derivatives		Reserpine
Sulfonamides		Succinylcholine
Theophylline derivatives		Tetracycline
Tolbutamide		Tubocurarine
Troxidone		Vitamins A, B, C, D, and E
Valproate		

*Among agents reported to exacerbate disease, those in italic type are incriminated most often. Those listed as theoretically risky have not been incriminated clearly in humans, but experimental studies indicate they have potential for damage. Those believed to be safe have been used in humans without ill effects, are not theoretically risky, and have not been reported to exacerbate porphyria.

†All agents known to induce cytochrome P-450 or to increase heme turnover in the liver are theoretically risky.

From Windebank AJ, Bonkowsky HL: Porphyric neuropathy. *In*: Dyck PJ, Thomas PK, Griffin JW, et al., eds. Peripheral Neuropathy. Vol 2, 3rd ed. Philadelphia, WB Saunders, 1993:1161–1168. By permission of the publisher.

have been responsible for the mental illness of George III.[13] The name *variegate porphyria* is used because patients may have acute neurological attacks only, skin manifestations only, a combination of both, or neither. The acute attacks are precipitated by the same factors as those in acute intermittent porphyria and hereditary coproporphyria.

Metabolic abnormalities underlying acute episodes

The metabolic changes are best understood for acute intermittent porphyria and have been reviewed recently in detail.[14] The disease was rare before the advent of modern pharmaceuticals. Virtually all drugs that induce the hepatic microsomal cytochrome P-450 system may induce attacks of acute intermittent porphyria. In affected persons, the residual activity of porphobilinogen deaminase is sufficient for normal rates of heme synthesis to occur. When the

cytochrome P-450 system is activated by a drug, there is increased incorporation of heme into cytochrome P-450 and a decrease in the pool of free heme. This induces increased synthesis of δ-aminolevulinic acid (ALA) synthase. The underactive porphobilinogen deaminase then becomes the rate-limiting step in heme synthesis, and the preceding substrates ALA and porphobilinogen rapidly accumulate. Because they are not metabolized further, they leak out of hepatocytes, are taken up into other tissues, and excreted in the urine. The accumulation of ALA and porphobilinogen are thought to cause disease manifestations.

Heme synthesis is also influenced by hormonal changes and blood glucose levels. Progesterone, estrogen, and testosterone induce ALA synthase. This may explain why attacks of acute intermittent porphyria do not occur before puberty in men or women and are most likely to occur in women in the luteal phase of the menstrual cycle.[3] Starvation induces ALA synthase. The mechanism for this is not known, but it is thought to be a direct consequence of low intracellular levels of glucose. This is the rationale for the administration of glucose in the treatment of acute intermittent porphyria.

Mechanism of cell injury

There are two types of neurological abnormality. The first involves physiological changes with psychiatric disturbances, seizures, disorders of consciousness, and autonomic changes. These are rapidly reversed when the metabolic changes return to normal. Porphobilinogen mimics the action of serotonin and may act as a false neurotransmitter. Other potential effects include inhibition of transmitter release at neuromuscular junctions and interaction of ALA with receptors for γ-aminobutyric acid (GABA), a major inhibitory neurotransmitter. ALA is related structurally to GABA and is a partial GABA agonist. Transient dysfunction of the central nervous system in acute porphyria, particularly the development of delirium and seizures, may be explained on the basis of ALA blocking normal GABA neurotransmission.[15,16]

Structural neuronal damage in the peripheral nervous system may be caused by several mechanisms. Because of the enzyme defect, the production of heme-containing proteins for oxygen transport and electron transport is deficient. This may lead to decreased energy metabolism and cell death. It is also possible that the metabolites ALA and porphobilinogen, which are known to accumulate in attacks of porphyria, are directly neurotoxic. Mice with a targeted mutation in the porphobilinogen deaminase gene develop a motor neuropathy, providing strong evidence that altered porphyrin metabolism causes the damage in the peripheral nervous system.[17]

Pathological changes in porphyria

Wallerian degeneration in the peripheral nervous system has been described.[18] It is not clear whether the axon or the Schwann cell is the primary target for damage in porphyria.[19] The most detailed pathological[20] and electrophysiological[21] studies suggest that the neuron or axon is the major target. It is likely that segmental demyelination[22,23] and slowed nerve conduction[24] found in some cases reflect demyelination due to axonal changes resulting from repeated or chronic insults. Autonomic disturbances are a prevalent feature of attacks of acute intermittent porphyria,[1] but pathological studies of the autonomic nervous system have been limited.

Clinical features of porphyria

The hepatic porphyrias—acute intermittent porphyria, hereditary coproporphyria, and variegate porphyria—are associated with neurological disease. The erythropoietic porphyrias cause photosensitivity but not neurological disease. The enzyme defects producing hepatic porphyria are illustrated in Figure 206.1. Acute intermittent porphyria is associated with acute attacks of severe neurological dysfunction induced by drugs or hormonal changes. Skin changes do not occur. Similar but less severe neurological manifestations occur with hereditary coproporphyria and variegate porphyria. In both, the inherited enzyme defect occurs after the condensation of the tetrapyrrole porphyrin ring and, thus, porphyrins may accumulate in the skin and cause photosensitivity. In all types, attacks may be precipitated by drugs, hormonal changes, starvation, or other severe stress. Porphyria cutanea tarda or symptomatic porphyria is usually associated with decreased activity of uroporphyrinogen decarboxylase (either genetic or acquired) and is associated with iron overload and liver disease often related to ethanol abuse. These patients do not have acute attacks of neuropathy due to porphyria.

During acute attacks, excess tetrapyrroles are excreted in the urine. The colorless porphyrinogens are excreted but are oxidized readily to the intensely colored corresponding porphyrin, causing the urine to turn red or purple. This is most apparent if the urine is exposed to light and air. In acute intermittent porphyria, large excesses of porphyrins are not excreted, but the high concentrations of porphobilinogens in the urine may result in nonenzymatic condensation producing the same urine color changes. In addition, porphobilinogen may polymerize to form a nonporphyrin polymer, porphobilin, which is black. Patients often present with acute, colicky abdominal pain that mimics acute bowel perforation or renal colic. Sedation or anesthesia for laparotomy may promote progression of the attack. Constipation and tachycardia further simulate an acute abdominal emergency. It is not known whether abdominal symptoms are due to a local effect of heme precursors or heme deficiency on muscle or nerves of the gastrointestinal tract or to acute autonomic neuropathy.

Psychiatric symptoms involve restlessness, agitation, and nightmares that may progress to frank psychosis with delirium, hallucinations, coma, and seizures. All these events and progression to neuropathy are accelerated if inappropriate sedating drugs are administered.

Neuropathy develops within 2 or 3 days after the onset of abdominal and psychiatric symptoms. It may resemble acute inflammatory polyradiculoneuropathy (Guillain-Barré syndrome). Motor symptoms are the earliest and most prominent clinical manifestations. Asymmetrical weakness may begin in the upper limbs or with cranial nerves; facial weakness and difficulty swallowing are common. Proximal and distal muscles are affected. Sensory symptoms of migratory, unpleasant paresthesias are less prominent. Maximal weakness usually is reached within a few days, although it may occur in a stepwise, progressive fashion over several weeks.[19,25] Sympathetic hyperactivity with pupil dilatation, tachycardia, hypertension, hesitancy of micturition, and constipation is common. Weakness may progress to respiratory failure. A characteristic feature is patchy weakness with prominent proximal weakness and distal sparing or weakness of selected muscle groups.[19] Reflexes are usually lost in propor-

Table 206.2   Quantitative porphyrin and enzyme levels in porphyrias associated with neuropathy

	Urine				Fecal			Erythrocyte	
	ALA	PBG	Uro	Copro	Uro	Copro	Proto	PBG deaminase*	Coproporphyrinogen oxidase
Acute intermittent porphyria									
Latent	N or ↑	N or ↑	N or ↑	N or ↑	N	N	N	↓ (or N)	N
Active	↑↑†	↑↑†	↑†	↑†	N or ↑	N or ↑	N or ↑	↓† (or N)	N
Hereditary coproporphyria									
Latent	N or ↑	N or ↑	N or ↑	↑↑	N	↑†	N or ↑	N	↓ (or N)
Active	↑↑	↑↑	↑	↑↑	N or ↑	↑↑	↑	N	↓ (or N)
Variegate porphyria									
Latent	N	N	N	↑	N	↑	↑	N	N
Active	↑↑†	↑↑†	↑†	↑↑†	N or ↑	↑	↑↑	N	N

ALA, δ-aminolevulinic acid; Copro, coproporphyrin; N, normal; PBG, porphobilinogen; Proto, protoporphyrin; Uro, uroporphyrin; ↑, mild or moderate increase; ↑↑, markedly increased; ↓, decreased activity.
*Also known as uroporphyrinogen I synthase or hydroxymethylbilane synthase.
†The most reliable indicators of disease.
From Windebank AJ, Bonkowsky HL: Porphyric neuropathy. *In*: Dyck PJ, Thomas PK, Griffin JW, et al., eds. Peripheral Neuropathy. Vol 2, 3rd ed. Philadelphia, WB Saunders, 1993:1161–1168. By permission of the publisher.

tion to the degree of muscle weakness. Atrophy appears early and may be severe. Comparatively mild sensory loss may produce a symmetrical glove-and-stocking loss or a patchy proximal loss involving predominantly the upper limbs and trunk.[25]

The prognosis for recovery from an individual attack depends on severity. Mortality from acute attacks of porphyria was about 30% before the advent of hematin therapy and modern intensive care techniques.[1,25] Now it is less than 10%.[4,9] Recovery from the psychiatric and autonomic features is usually rapid. Recovery from the neuropathic damage depends on the severity of axonal and neuronal loss during the acute attack. Good functional recovery is the rule, although recovery may be prolonged and incomplete, as would be expected for a process involving axonal degeneration.[26,27]

Diagnosis

The differential diagnosis of acute or subacute, predominantly motor, neuropathy associated with gastrointestinal disturbance includes Guillain-Barré syndrome and acute intoxication, especially by metals. The gastrointestinal disturbance of porphyria is generally more severe than that of Guillain-Barré syndrome. Psychiatric manifestations and seizures do not occur with Guillain-Barré syndrome. Arsenic or thallium poisoning should be suspected in all cases of acute neuropathy preceded by severe nausea, vomiting, and abdominal pain. The metals may also cause psychiatric changes and, occasionally, seizures. History of urine color change should raise the suspicion of porphyria. Similarly, the association of chronic photosensitivity should alert the physician to the possibility of hereditary coproporphyria or variegate porphyria. The only reliable way to distinguish between

acute metal poisoning and porphyria is to make the appropriate measurements in blood or urine.

Measurement of relevant enzyme levels and porphyrin levels in blood, urine, and stool are the most important diagnostic tools (Table 206.2). In all acute attacks of porphyria, the urinary excretion of ALA is markedly increased. In symptomatic acute intermittent porphyria, increases in urinary porphyrins are modest and fecal porphyrins are normal or slightly increased. In contrast, in symptomatic hereditary coproporphyria, there are marked increases in urinary and fecal coproporphyrin excretion, and in variegate porphyria, fecal protoporphyrin excretion is increased. Increases in urinary or fecal excretions of coproporphyrin are modest in variegate porphyria.

Diagnosis is more difficult if patients are not experiencing acute symptoms. In latent acute intermittent porphyria, measurement of porphobilinogen deaminase activity will identify most asymptomatic patients (Table 206.2). Direct gene testing is possible but not yet commercially available. In hereditary coproporphyria, urine and fecal coproporphyrin levels are usually increased between attacks. In comparison, with a drug-induced increase in coproporphyrin levels, only urine levels are increased. In hereditary coproporphyria, coproporphyrinogen oxidase activity in erythrocytes is usually but not invariably decreased. Therefore, to make a reliable diagnosis, urine and fecal levels of porphyrin should be quantified. Latent variegate porphyria usually is accompanied by normal urine levels of porphyrin or a moderate increase in the levels of coproporphyrin. It usually is suspected on the basis of skin photosensitivity, especially in those of Afrikaner heritage. In the feces, coproporphyrin and protoporphyrin levels generally are increased between attacks. Currently,

Table 206.3   Treatment of porphyria

	Acute intermittent porphyria	Hereditary coproporphyria	Variegate porphyria
Latent or inactive			
Drugs	Avoid porphyrinogenic drugs	Avoid porphyrinogenic drugs	Avoid porphyrinogenic drugs
Skin protection	None necessary	Avoid sun exposure	Avoid sun exposure
Diet	Avoid prolonged carbohydrate deprivation	Avoid prolonged carbohydrate deprivation	Avoid prolonged carbohydrate deprivation
Acute episode			
Pain	Meperidine or morphine	Meperidine or morphine	Meperidine or morphine
Seizures	Treat only if repetitive	Treat only if repetitive	Treat only if repetitive
Nutrition	Glucose 3–500 g/24 hours IV	Glucose 3–500 g/24 hours IV	Glucose 3–500 g/24 hours IV
Hematin	2–5 mg/kg daily by IV infusion over 60 minutes	2–5 mg/kg daily by IV infusion over 60 minutes	2–5 mg/kg daily by IV infusion over 60 minutes

IV, intravenous.

protoporphyrinogen oxidase levels are not measured routinely.

Increased urinary levels of porphyrin are often discovered during laboratory testing for undiagnosed neuropathy. Drugs that induce the cytochrome P-450 system in liver microsomes, even in normal subjects, may induce ALA synthase activity and increase urine levels of coproporphyrin. In these cases, fecal porphyrin excretions of coproporphyrin and protoporphyrin should be normal. Finally, if treatment with all medications is stopped and the patient does not ingest alcohol for 2 weeks, urine coproporphyrin excretion should return to normal. This laboratory observation of increased urinary coproporphyrin is not associated directly with neurological disease.

Electrophysiological studies demonstrate features consistent with axonal degeneration; compound muscle action potentials are decreased in proportion to the degree of muscle weakness. Slowing and dispersion are more apparent during recovery when axons are regenerating and when they may be thinly myelinated before they are fully regenerated.[21] Sensory conduction may be well preserved if patients do not have prominent sensory involvement. Needle electromyography shows changes typical of denervation. During the recovery phase, changes typical of reinnervation occur. Because of the possible patchy nature of muscle involvement, it is important to examine clinically the muscles involved.

Treatment

Treatment is summarized in Table 206.3. Avoidance of acute attacks is the major goal of treatment. It depends almost entirely on the avoidance of drugs that induce cytochrome P-450 (Table 206.1). In most cases, it is safest to avoid administering all drugs to patients who have porphyria. If drugs are necessary, only those that are known to be safe should be used. Many new drugs have not been available long enough to know whether they have the potential to induce porphyria.

The three forms of neuropathic porphyrias are dominantly inherited. Relatives who are at risk should have screening tests for latent disease (Table 206.2) and be instructed in drug avoidance strategies if appropriate.

Because a decreased supply of glucose to the liver may increase ALA synthase activity, as mentioned above, patients with known acute porphyria should be advised to avoid periods of prolonged starvation or excessive physical stress without carbohydrate loading.

Therapy for acute attacks

All drugs that may further exacerbate the disease should be avoided. Chlorpromazine is useful for managing agitation and anxiety. Meperidine or morphine may be given for pain relief. Seizures occur in fewer than 5% of patients with acute intermittent porphyria[28] but are difficult to manage. Commonly prescribed parenteral anticonvulsants (barbiturates and hydantoins) are potent inducers of porphyria. Anecdotal reports suggest that gabapentin[29] and clonazepam[30] may be taken safely, although both clonazepam and valproic acid have been shown to be porphyrinogenic in experimental systems and may exacerbate acute intermittent porphyria.[31] Older drugs such as the bromides and paraldehyde may be used, although their absorption from intramuscular injection is quite variable. Paraldehyde is no longer available for clinical use in the United States. Thus, bromides may be the therapy of choice. For patients who have an occasional and nonrepetitive seizure, it probably is safest not to treat the seizures directly but to concentrate on management of the underlying porphyria. Acute infection and hyponatremia should be treated aggressively. The hyponatremia should be corrected gradually to minimize the risk of development of central pontine myelinolysis.

Maintenance of blood and tissue glucose levels is important. Glucose is infused to provide 3 g to 500 g per 24 hours.[9]

Intravenous administration of heme is the most direct and effective therapy for acute porphyria.[32–34] This has been reviewed recently.[14] The drug is given in the hydroxylated form as hematin (Panhematin,

Abbott Laboratories, Highland Park, IL). A daily intravenous dose of 2 to 5 mg/kg is given over 30 to 60 minutes and repeated daily for 3 to 14 days. The 24-hour cumulative dose should not exceed 6 mg/kg. Solutions of hematin are unstable, and the dissolved preparation should be given within 1 hour after reconstitution. Because the final solution is not transparent, it is recommended that filters be used in the intravenous line to avoid infusion of particulate material. Higher doses have been implicated in causing renal damage.[35] Bonkowsky[9] has suggested that hematin is more stable when reconstituted with albumin in a 1:1 molar ratio (1 mg hematin:100 mg albumin). This forms methemalbumin, which is stable in solution for up to 24 hours and has been shown by Bonkowsky[9] to inhibit production of ALA and porphobilinogen. Infusion of hematin early in an acute attack appears to produce a rapid and reproducible remission of symptoms.[36] Because heme is presumed to act by suppressing the induction of ALA synthase and is rapidly cleared by the liver, it is possible for the attack to recur rapidly after cessation of therapy. If therapy is discontinued during an acute attack, ALA and porphobilinogen levels in serum may increase rapidly and require additional infusion of hematin for suppression.[37] Hematin is effective in the management of all three types of neuropathic porphyria.

Acknowledgments

The helpful comments of Dr. Gregory D Cascino and the expert secretarial assistance of Jane M Meyer are most gratefully acknowledged.

References

1. Goldberg A. Acute intermittent porphyria: a study of 50 cases. Q J Med 1959;28:183–209
2. Hierons R. Changes in the nervous system in acute porphyria. Brain 1957;80:176–192
3. Kappas A, Sassa S, Anderson KE. The porphyrias. In: Stanbury JB, Wyngaarden JB, Fredrickson DW, et al., eds. The Metabolic Basis of Inherited Disease. 5th ed. New York: McGraw-Hill, 1983:1301–1384
4. Stein JA, Tschudy DP. Acute intermittent porphyria: a clinical and biochemical study of 46 patients. Medicine (Baltimore) 1970;49:1–16
5. Wetterberg L. A Neuropsychiatric and Genetical Investigation of Acute Intermittent Porphyria. Thesis, Uppsala Universitet. Norstedts, Sweden: Svenska Bokförlaget, 1967
6. Berger H, Goldberg A. Hereditary coproporphyria. Br Med J 1955;2:85–88
7. Connon JJ, Turkington V. Hereditary coproporphyria. Lancet 1968;2:263–264
8. Goldberg A, Rimington C, Lochhead AC. Hereditary coproporphyria. Lancet 1967;1:632–636
9. Bonkovsky HL. Porphyrin and heme metabolism and the porphyrias. In: Zakim D, Boyer TD, eds. Hepatology: A Textbook of Liver Disease. Vol 1, 2nd ed. Philadelphia: WB Saunders Company, 1990:378–424
10. Brodie MJ, Thompson GG, Moore MR, et al. Hereditary coproporphyria: demonstration of the abnormalities in haem biosynthesis in peripheral blood. Q J Med 1977;46:229–241
11. Dean G. The Porphyrias: A Story of Inheritance and Environment. 2nd ed. Philadelphia: JB Lippincott Company, 1971
12. Eales L, Day RS, Blekkenhorst GH. The clinical and biochemical features of variegate porphyria: an analysis of 300 cases studied at Groote Schuur Hospital, Cape Town. Int J Biochem 1980;12:837–853
13. Macalpine I, Hunter R. George III and the Mad-Business. London: Allen Lane, 1969
14. Windebank AJ, Bonkowsky HL. Porphyric neuropathy. In: Dyck PJ, Thomas PK, Griffin JW, et al., eds. Peripheral Neuropathy. 4th ed. Philadelphia: WB Saunders, 2002:1161–1168
15. Bonkowsky HL, Schady W. Neurologic manifestations of acute porphyria. Semin Liver Dis 1982;2:108–124
16. Yeung Laiwah AC, Moore MR, Goldberg A. Pathogenesis of acute porphyria. Q J Med 1987;63:377–392
17. Lindberg RL, Porcher C, Grandchamp B, et al. Porphobilinogen deaminase deficiency in mice causes a neuropathy resembling that of human hepatic porphyria. Nat Genet 1996;12:195–199
18. Erbslöh W. Zur Pathologie und pathologischen Anatomie der toxischen Polyneuritis nach Sulfonalgebrauch. Dtsch Z Nervenheilkd 1903;23:197–204
19. Ridley A. Porphyric neuropathy. In: Dyck PJ, Thomas PK, Lambert EH, Bunge R, eds. Peripheral Neuropathy. Vol 2, 2nd ed. Philadelphia: WB Saunders Company, 1984:1704–1716
20. Cavanagh JB, Mellick RS. On the nature of the peripheral nerve lesions associated with acute intermittent porphyria. J Neurol Neurosurg Psychiatry 1965;28:320–327
21. Albers JW, Robertson WC, Jr, Daube JR. Electrodiagnostic findings in acute porphyric neuropathy. Muscle Nerve 1978;1:292–296
22. Anzil AP, Dozic S. Peripheral nerve changes in porphyric neuropathy: findings in a sural nerve biopsy. Acta Neuropathol (Berl) 1978;42:121–126
23. Thomas PK. The morphological basis for alterations in nerve conduction in peripheral neuropathy. Proc R Soc Med 1971;64:295–298
24. Mustajoki P, Seppalainen AM. Neuropathy in latent hereditary hepatic porphyria. Br Med J 1975;2:310–312
25. Ridley A. The neuropathy of acute intermittent porphyria. Q J Med 1969;38:307–333
26. Bosch EP, Pierach CA, Bossenmaier I, et al. Effect of hematin in porphyric neuropathy. Neurology 1977;27:1053–1056
27. Sorensen AW, With TK. Persistent pareses after porphyric attacks. S Afr Med J 1971, Sept 25:101–103
28. Bylesjo I, Forsgren L, Lithner F, Boman K. Epidemiology and clinical characteristics of seizures in patients with acute intermittent porphyria. Epilepsia 1996;37:230–235
29. Zadra M, Grandi R, Erli LC, et al. Treatment of seizures in acute intermittent porphyria: safety and efficacy of gabapentin. Seizure 1998;7:415–416
30. Magnessen CR, Doherty JM, Hess RA, Tschudy DP. Grand mal seizures and acute intermittent porphyria: the problem of differential diagnosis and treatment. Neurology 1975;25:121–125
31. Bonkowsky HL, Sinclair PR, Emery S, Sinclair JF. Seizure management in acute hepatic porphyria: risks of valproate and clonazepam. Neurology 1980;30:588–592
32. Bonkowsky HL, Tschudy DP, Collins A, et al. Repression of the overproduction of porphyrin precursors in acute intermittent porphyria by intravenous infusions of hematin. Proc Natl Acad Sci USA 1971;68:2725–2729
33. Lamon JM, Frykholm BC, Hess RA, Tschudy DP. Hematin therapy for acute porphyria. Medicine (Baltimore) 1979;58:252–269

34. Watson CJ. Editorial: hematin and porphyria. N Engl J Med 1975;293:605–607

35. Dhar GJ, Bossenmaier I, Petryka ZJ, et al. Effects of hematin in hepatic porphyria: further studies. Ann Intern Med 1975;83:20–30

36. Pierach CA. Hematin therapy for the porphyric attack. Semin Liver Dis 1982;2:125–131

37. Bonkowsky HL, Sinclair PR, Sinclair JF. Hepatic heme metabolism and its control. Yale J Biol Med 1979;52:13–37

207 Hereditary Sensory and Autonomic Neuropathies

Peter J Dyck and Christopher J Klein

Disorders included in hereditary sensory and autonomic neuropathies

The four characteristics that set hereditary sensory and autonomic neuropathies (HSANs) apart from other neuropathies and system atrophies are the following: 1) a genetic basis, 2) selective and predominant involvement of primary sensory, with or without autonomic, neurons (axons), 3) liability to acral (distal limb) tissue injury and mutilation, and 4) separation from genetic disorders with selective involvement of mainly large-diameter afferent neurons (axons), with or without spinocerebellar and cerebellar neuron involvement. Many chronic sensorimotor neuropathies must be differentiated from HSANs. An algorithm that may be used to do this is provided in Figure 207.1.

Epidemiology

The frequency of cases with congenital onset is very rare, and the prevalence has not been determined with accuracy. Also, the frequency of autosomal dominant forms of HSAN, especially by various clinical syndromes, is unknown.

Differential diagnosis and classification

HSANs may be categorized mainly by the age at onset, the nature of mendelian inheritance, the populations of sensory and autonomic neurons (axons) affected, and the molecular genetic mechanisms. Currently, the molecular genetic information is insufficient for adequate categorization.

An algorithm that can be used to differentiate HSANs from, on the one hand, spinocerebellar degeneration disorders and, on the other hand, from acquired sensorimotor polyneuropathies is given in Figure 207.1. An important initial point of distinction is between disorders that are congenital or recognized during infancy and disorders that develop later. Generally, the congenital disorders are recessive, whereas most HSANs that develop later are autosomal dominant. Distinguishing between autosomal dominant sensory neuropathies and acquired sensorimotor neuropathies is easy when there is a family history of a similar disorder, but when there is not, a series of steps might be considered. The 10-step approach we advocate includes the following: 1) characterize the anatomical-pathological pattern of involvement, 2) confirm this pattern with electrophysiological and other tests, 3) infer the pathological site and mechanism of nerve fiber alterations, 4) consider

the onset and course, 5) decide whether the disorder is likely to be acquired or inherited, 6) look for associations between past and present disease, 7) perform hematological, biochemical, serological, imaging, and other tests, 8) consider evaluation of kin, 9) consider obtaining tissue for pathology studies (skin, nerve, and other specimens), and 10) consider performing a

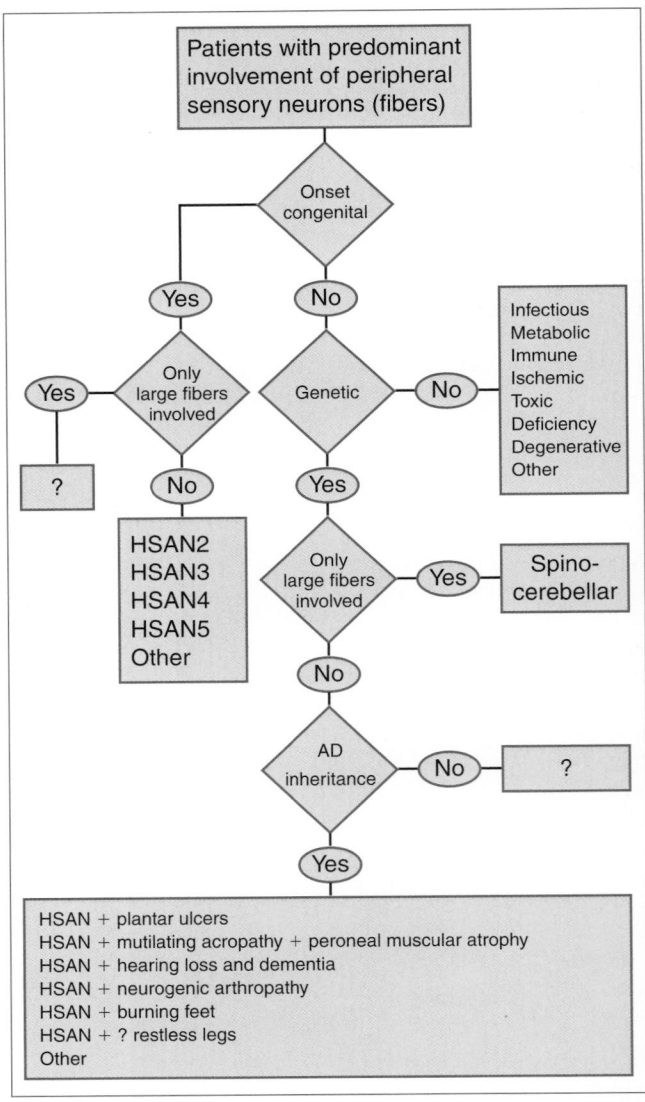

Figure 207.1 Diagnostic algorithm helpful in distinguishing among disorders of patients with predominant involvement of peripheral sensory neurons. AD, autosomal dominant; HSAN, hereditary sensory and autonomic neuropathy.

therapeutic trial.[1] In the diseases considered here, steps 1–5 and 8 might be the most important ones and the other steps may not apply. Actual evaluation of kin (step 8) is often needed because of the mildness or misinterpretation of the symptoms and findings in relatives. Within a few years, it will be possible to diagnose varieties of HSAN with specific DNA tests.

Distinguishing between autosomal dominant HSANs and spinocerebellar degeneration disorders is not always easy because the latter often begin with symptoms attributable to primary sensory neuron (fiber) involvement. Several varieties of spinocerebellar degeneration are autosomal recessive, for example, Friedreich ataxia. Early large-fiber dysfunction and loss of large-diameter peripheral sensory neurons are typical of spinocerebellar degeneration but not of HSANs. Generally, large-diameter sensory fibers convey information from mechanoreceptors (i.e., tactile sensation, two-point discrimination, hair displacement, vibratory sensation, and joint position and motion). Reduced amplitudes of sensory nerve action potentials are also an indication of the involvement of large-diameter sensory fibers. Therefore, in spinocerebellar degeneration, some of these functions may be abnormal, but spontaneous pain and loss of thermal or pain sensation (evidence of involvement of small fibers) do not typically occur, as they do in disorders of small sensory fiber involvement, for example, HSANs. Loss of pain and thermal sensation is typical of HSANs. Locomotor and cerebellar ataxia is typical of spinocerebellar degeneration but not of HSANs. Molecular genetic markers are available for identifying many of the spinocerebellar degeneration disorders.

Autosomal dominant HSANs

Historical

Many names have been given to this group of disorders: "mal perforant du pied,"[2] "singular affection of os pied,"[3] "familial symmetric gangrene with arthropathy,"[4] "familial neural trophic disturbances of lower extremity,"[5] "hereditary perforating ulcers,"[6] "lumbosacral syringomyelia,"[7] "ulcerative and mutilating acropathy,"[8] "hereditary sensory radicular neuropathy,"[9] "familial and sporadic neurogenic acro-osteolysis,"[10] "acrodystrophic neuropathy,"[11] and "hereditary sensory neuropathy type 1"[12] or "hereditary sensory and autonomic neuropathy type 1" (HSAN1).[13] Mutations in *SPTLC1*, encoding serine palmitoyltransferase, long-chain base subunit-1, located at chromosome 9q22.1-22.3, are responsible for HSAN1 in some families. These mutations are associated with increased de novo synthesis of ceramide, which causes premature neuronal apoptosis.[14,15]

Classification

We think it is unlikely that a single molecular genetic mechanism underlies the different autosomal dominant syndromes that have been described because considerable clinical heterogeneity distinguishes them. However, this is not to say that each of the syndromes listed here will be found to have a unique and different molecular genetic mechanism.

The syndromes described here as HSAN1 have the following features in common: 1) autosomal dominant inheritance, 2) a predominance of sensory (and autonomic) symptoms and findings and, when present, tissue injury that is greatest in the acral regions of the lower limbs, 3) system atrophy of classes of sensory and autonomic fibers, 4) insidious onset in the second or later decades, and 5) slow progression.

Tissue injury (plantar ulcers and stress fractures) and neurogenic arthropathy or infection (cellulitis, lymphangitis, or osteomyelitis) are not primary events directly attributable to the genetic abnormality. They result from the loss of protective sensation and other factors (Figure 207.2). These tissue complications are not inevitable. They probably can be averted with prevention of injury, limb care, and treatment. In several kindreds we have studied, the degree of sensory loss appeared to be related to acral mutilation, but other factors (injury, neglect of injury, excessive use of insensitive parts of the body, inadequate or faulty treatment, and indifference to health care) contributed.

The occurrences of tissue injury (e.g., plantar ulcers or neurogenic arthropathy) are not reliable markers of varieties of HSAN.

Although direct inheritances from generation to generation (with male-to-male transmission) is expected in autosomal dominant HSAN,[3,4,6] siblings may be affected without their parents being affected, raising questions about the mode of inheritance, parentage, and perhaps other mechanisms.

HSAN ± plantar ulcers An extensively studied kinship is that of Hicks.[16] The stereotypic features are 1) autosomal dominant inheritance, 2) onset in second or later decades, 3) panmodality sensory loss in toes, feet, or distal legs, with very slow progression to involve more proximal segments of the lower limbs and distal segments of the upper limbs, 4) a variable degree of lancinating or other pain that typically occurs in clusters and in the affected limb segments, usually without paresthesia and asleep numbness, 5) a variable degree of pes cavus deformity, 6) callus formation especially over the plantar surface of the first and second metatarsal heads, 7) development of necrotic tissue and ulceration at the site of callus formation, 8) episodic cellulitis, lymphangitis, and osteomyelitis that lead to extrusion of sequestered bone and shortening of the foot, 9) some degree of leg muscle weakness and atrophy, and 10) a low number of myelinated and unmyelinated fibers in the sural nerve undergoing distal axonal atrophy and degeneration.

HSAN ± mutilating acropathy and peroneal muscle atrophy Affected persons in kindreds with this phenotype[17–19] have all the features outlined in the syndrome described above, but they have a pronounced degree of muscle weakness and atrophy in the distal lower limb. The similarity of this syndrome with hereditary motor and sensory neuropathy 2 (Charcot-

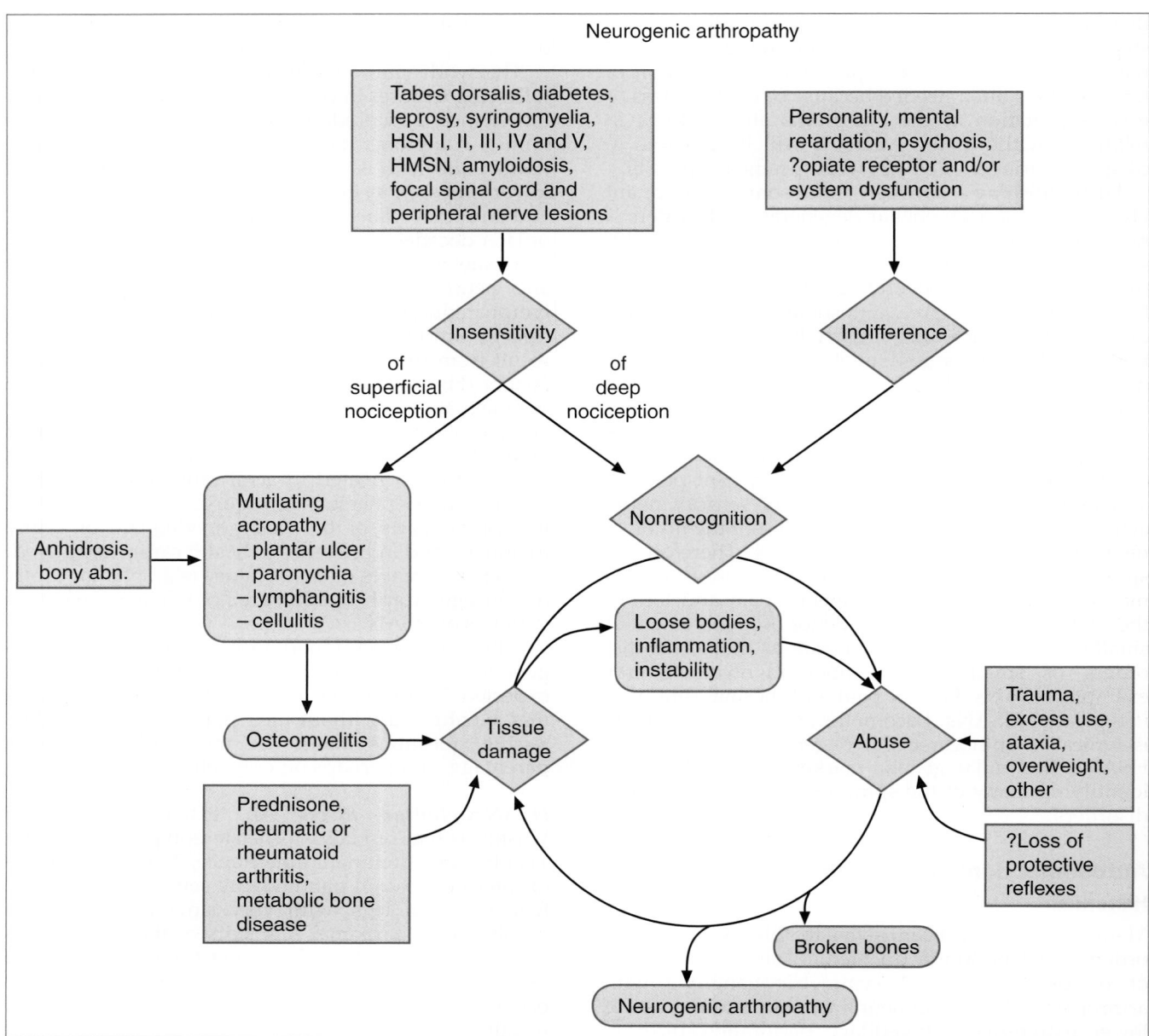

Figure 207.2 Hypothetical algorithm of diseases and risk factors leading to neurogenic arthropathy. abn., abnormality; HMSN, hereditary motor and sensory neuropathy; HSN, hereditary sensory neuropathy. (From Dyck et al.[21] By permission of the American Academy of Neurology.)

Marie-Tooth [CMT] 2) is striking, but linkage to CMT2A and CMT2B appears to have been excluded.[19]

HSAN ± mutilating acropathy ± hearing loss ± dementia We studied a unique kindred with this syndrome.[20] It has similarities and dissimilarities with the kindred described by Hicks[16] and subsequently by Denny-Brown.[9] The Hicks' kindred had progressive sensory neuropathy and sensorineural hearing loss but probably did not have a dementing illness. One of the subjects was reported to have "subnormal memory and intelligence."

HSAN ± neurogenic arthropathy We described a unique syndrome of patients with neurogenic

arthropathy (especially of the knees, elbows, and shoulders), subclinical neuropathy, and a family history of arthropathy in seven kindreds.[21] The natural history of this syndrome is quite different from that of the syndromes described above. Studies of the patients' bones did not indicate decreased bone strength under tension or abnormal structure.

HSAN ± burning feet We reported the case of a young woman with burning pain on the soles of her feet. This pain was aggravated by warmth and relieved by cooling. The only evidence of neuropathy was subtle change in teased fibers of the sural nerve.[22] Other kin were discovered who also had burning pain

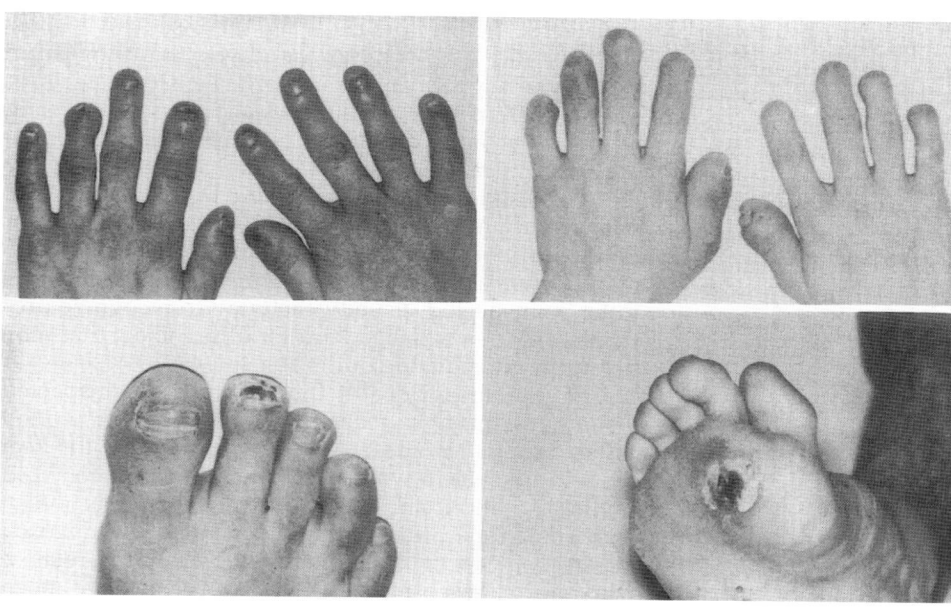

Figure 207.3   Hands and feet of two teenage boys showing the typical mutilating acropathy of hereditary sensory and autonomic neuropathy 2. (From Dyck et al.[12] By permission of the publisher.)

on the soles of the feet, and some of the examined relatives had a low-grade polyneuropathy. We inferred that a low-grade sensory neuropathy accounted for the burning pain and suggested that HSAN may manifest itself mainly as burning pain, restless legs, lancinating pain, or other neuropathic positive sensory symptoms (N-PSS). Linkage analysis, however, in at least one large German family with burning pain of the feet and autosomal dominant inheritance did not show association with HSAN1 on chromosome 9q22 or CMT2B at 3q13-q22.[23]

HSAN ± restless legs   This association is less well documented (see preceding syndrome).

Congenital recessively inherited HSANs

These disorders are characterized by 1) congenital or infantile or early childhood onset, 2) sporadic or sibling occurrence—recessive inheritance, 3) relatively static neuropathic impairment of selected classes of sensory or autonomic neurons (axons), and 4) mutilation of soft and bony tissues because of insensitivity and other factors. These rare disorders are described only briefly here; they have been reviewed in detail elsewhere.[24]

HSAN2

Varieties of HSAN2 probably were described as "Morvan's disease," "painless whitlows,"[25] "syringomyelia of infancy,"[26,27] "familial neuropathy of unknown etiology resembling Morvan's disease,"[28] "hereditary sensory neuropathy,"[29–31] "congenital sensory neuropathy,"[32–34] "progressive sensory neuropathy,"[35] "syndrome of the neural crest,"[36] and "acrodystrophic neuropathy."[11] Because we recognized that it was a variety of hereditary sensory neuropathies (now HSANs), we call it *HSAN2*.

The hallmarks of HSAN2 are 1) sporadic or sibship occurrence suggesting autosomal recessive inheritance; 2) onset of symptoms in infancy or early child-

hood suggesting congenital onset; 3) occurrence of paronychia; whitlows; ulcers of the fingers (Figure 207.3); plantar ulcers; unrecognized fractures of the foot, hand, and, less commonly, limb bones; and Charcot joints; 4) sensory loss that affects all modalities and affects the lower and upper limbs and perhaps the trunk; 5) absence or diminution of tendon reflexes, usually in all limbs; 6) sweating loss, especially over acral parts, but without postural hypotension, sphincter disturbance, or impotence in males; 7) absence of sensory nerve action potentials; and 8) virtual absence of myelinated fibers, with a decreased number of unmyelinated fibers in the sural nerves. Chromosomal localization has not been established.

HSAN3

This is usually called *familial dysautonomia* or *Riley-Day syndrome*. Characteristic features are 1) sporadic or sibship occurrence suggesting recessive inheritance, 2) congenital occurrence or onset in infancy, 3) occurrence predominantly in Ashkenazi Jews, 4) predominant involvement of peripheral sensory (all classes) and autonomic neurons (axons), lesser involvement of motor neurons (axons), and possible involvement of other classes of central nervous system neurons, 5) history of poor sucking and repeated episodes of fever, 6) blotchy skin, 7) absence of fungiform papillae on the tongue, and 8) dry eyes.

Mutations in the *IKBKAP* gene (inhibitor of kappa light polypeptide gene enhancer in B cells, kinase-associated protein) located at 9q31[37] are thought to cause HSAN3. Two mutations have been identified, and both are thought to disrupt phosphorylation (*IKBKAP*, IVS20DS, T-C, +6; ARG696PRO). Why such a defect would lead to dysautonomia and sensory neuropathy is not known. Genetic testing for the two mutations will allow for ease of carrier and affected assessment in a population (Ashkenazi Jews) in which a strong founder effect accounts for the limited responsible mutation.

HSAN4

The characteristic features of HSAN4 are 1) congenital or infantile onset, 2) sporadic or sibling occurrence—probably recessively inherited, 3) repeated high fevers that may cause death, 4) decreased pain sensation and absence of sweating, 5) mental retardation in some patients, and 6) virtual absence of unmyelinated fibers in sural nerve and genetic abnormality of *trkA* receptor gene. The initial consideration of this gene located at 1q21-22 as a candidate for HSAN4 came from a mouse mutant with a similar phenotype.[38] Subsequent human work has identified multiple mutations, including deletion, splice site mutations, and missense mutations—all in the tryosine kinase domain of *trkA*.[39] Other mutations in separate families are noted for causing disruption of extracellular domain involved in nerve growth factor binding.[40] Some of these patients were found to have more than one mutation within the *trkA* gene. The gene is thought important for inducing neurite outgrowth and promoting embryonic sensory and sympathetic neuron outgrowth.

HSAN5

Low et al.[41] reported on a 4-year-old child who had selective loss of pain sensation that affected the extremities. The number of small myelinated fibers (Aδ) of the sural nerve was selectively decreased compared with that of controls. Other similar patients were reported by Donaghy et al.[42] A Pakistani patient has been identified to have exon 8 tyrosine 359 cysteine *NTRK 1* mutation predicted to yield partial loss of gene function.[43] Others with the HSAN5 phenotype will need to be identified before firm conclusions can be made about the allelic nature of HSAN4 and HSAN5.

Treatment

Gene therapy is not available for any inherited sensory neuropathy. Also, there is no evidence that any of the growth factors are useful. Because genetic abnormalities of the trkA receptor appear to be involved in some congenital varieties of HSAN and nerve growth factor and trkA receptor are involved in development of sympathetic nerve fibers and dorsal root C fibers, trials of nerve growth factor administered at very early times (perhaps even in utero) may be considered a potential treatment. Currently, the emphasis must be on avoidance of injury and prevention of acral mutilation and the treatment of N-PSS.

Prevention of acral mutilation is particularly challenging, especially in congenital sensory neuropathy. As soon as the problem of sensation is recognized, special steps should be taken to try to prevent injury. The temperature of the hot water heater for the home should be turned down (e.g., to 42°C) so the person will not be scalded even when only the hot water is turned on. Stops may be affixed to drawers and doors so they cannot be slammed shut on insensitive acral parts of the body. Measures may need to be taken so that hands cannot be placed on the hot burners of stoves. It is difficult to prevent a child from hurting himself or herself by chewing on insensitive areas such as the lips, tongue, or cheek; jumping from excessive heights; or damaging insensitive parts to spite a parent or guardian. Ideally, the supervising adult will be able to set physical limits without resorting to physical punishment. Visual inspection of the feet and hands and good judgment by the patient and parents are needed to avoid excessive activity or damage. Shoes must be long and wide enough to avoid callus and skin breakdown. The inside of shoes must be inspected visually each day to recognize protruding nails, a retained sock, or other object that may be unrecognized and could cause injury.

The plantar surface of the feet must be inspected visually each day to recognize a blackened or eroded callus or plantar ulcer. We advise soaking the feet daily in lukewarm water to hydrate the skin, to avoid callus formation, and to ensure regular inspection of feet. The temperature of the water must be judged by a sensitive part of the patient's body or by a relative with normal sensation. After the feet have been soaked, a light coat of petroleum jelly is applied. Shoes should be worn at all times. If ulcers develop, weight bearing should be stopped or severely curtailed until the ulcer has healed. Debridement of the ulcer and antibiotic treatment with development of cellulitis may be needed for infected ulcers. Because of repeated infection (e.g., osteomyelitis), some patients may lose the structure of the forefoot, in which case, amputation may be needed. Patients with neurogenic arthropathy may be able to continue to walk with degenerating joints, but they will want to limit their physical activity or activities that cause additional damage. We think that patients will want to modify their life style, physical activities, and medical care to preserve damaged acral parts. Avoiding excessive weight is important. Injury, repeated injury, neglect of injury or infection, lack of concern, and excessive surgical treatment can lead to spiraling acral mutilation.

Neuropathic symptoms may be divided into negative (related to neurological impairments) and positive N-PSS. The latter include prickling sensation, pain (lancinating, burning, freezing, deep-ache, allodynia [pain caused by mechanical stimuli usually insufficient to cause pain]), asleep-numbness (like that induced by a local anesthetic, tight, constricted), and related symptoms. These symptoms may be improved by good sleep, relief of anxiety or depression, and physical treatment (e.g., cold soaks and pharmacological treatment).

Acknowledgment

We gratefully acknowledge the help of JaNean K. Engelstad and Mary L. Hunziker in the preparation of this chapter.

References

1. Dyck PJ, Grant IA, Fealey RD. Ten steps in characterizing and diagnosing patients with peripheral neuropathy. Neurology 1996;47:10–17
2. Granger ME. Sensory neuropathy with ulcerative

mutilating acropathy: an isolated case. Neurology 1960; 10:725–734

3. Nélaton M. Affection singulière des os du pied. Gaz Hôp Civils et Militaires 1852;4:13–14

4. Bruns O. Aus den Gesellschaften. Neurol Centralbl 1903;22:598

5. Gobell R, Runge W. Zeir Fälle von familiärer Trophoneurose der unteren Extremitäten. München Med Wschr 1914;61:102

6. Schultze F. Familiär auftrendes Malumperforans der Füsse (familiäre lumbale Syringomyelie?). Dtsch Med Wschr 1917;43:69–71

7. Van Epps C, Kerr HD. Familial lumbosacral syringomyelia. Radiology 1940;35:160–173

8. Thévenard A. L'acropathie ulcéro-mutilante familiale. Rev Neurol (Paris) 1942;74:193–203

9. Denny-Brown D. Hereditary sensory radicular neuropathy. J Neurol Neurosurg Psychiatry 1951;14:237–252

10. Fogelson MH, Rorke LB, Kaye R. Spinal cord changes in familial dysautonomia. Arch Neurol 1967;17:103–108

11. Spillane JD, Wells CEC. Acrodystrophic neuropathy: a critical review of the syndrome of trophic ulcers, sensory neuropathy, and bony erosion, together with an account of 16 cases in South Wales. London: Oxford University Press, 1969

12. Dyck PJ, Ohta M. Neuronal atrophy and degeneration predominantly affecting peripheral sensory neurons. In: Dyck PJ, Thomas PK, Lambert EH, eds. Peripheral Neuropathy. 1st ed. Philadelphia: WB Saunders Company, 1975:791–824

13. Dyck PJ. Neuronal atrophy and degeneration predominantly affecting peripheral sensory and autonomic neurons. In: Dyck PJ, Thomas PK, Lambert EH, Bunge R, eds. Peripheral Neuropathy. 2nd ed. Philadelphia: WB Saunders Company, 1984:1557–1599

14. Dawkins JL, Hulme DJ, Brahmbhatt SB, et al. Mutations in SPTLC1, encoding serine palmitoyltransferase, long chain base subunit-1, cause hereditary sensory neuropathy type I. Nat Genet 2001;27:309–312

15. Bejaoui K, Wu C, Scheffler MD, et al. SPTLC1 is mutated in hereditary sensory neuropathy, type 1. Nat Genet 2001;27:261–262

16. Hicks EP. Hereditary perforating ulcer of the foot. Lancet 1922;1:319–321

17. England AC, Denny-Brown D. Severe sensory changes, and trophic disorder, in peroneal muscular atrophy (Charcot-Marie-Tooth Type). Arch Neurol Psychiatry 1952;67:1–22

18. Dyck PJ, Kennel AJ, Magal IV, Kraybill EN. A Virginia kinship with hereditary sensory neuropathy: peroneal muscular atrophy and pes cavus. Mayo Clin Proc 1965;40:685–694

19. Dubourg O, Barhoumi C, Azzedine H, et al. Phenotypic and genetic study of a family with hereditary sensory neuropathy and prominent weakness. Muscle Nerve 2000;23:1508–1514

20. Wright A, Dyck PJ. Hereditary sensory neuropathy with sensorineural deafness and early-onset dementia. Neurology 1995;45:560–562

21. Dyck PJ, Stevens JC, O'Brien PC, et al. Neurogenic arthropathy and recurring fractures with subclinical inherited neuropathy. Neurology 1983;33:357–367

22. Dyck PJ, Low PA, Stevens JC. "Burning feet" as the only manifestation of dominantly inherited sensory neuropathy. Mayo Clin Proc 1983;58:426–429

23. Stogbauer F, Young P, Kuhlenbaumer G, et al. Autosomal dominant burning feet syndrome. J Neurol Neurosurg Psychiatry 1999;67:78–81

24. Dyck PJ. Neuronal atrophy and degeneration predominantly affecting peripheral sensory and autonomic neurons. In: Dyck PJ, Thomas PK, Griffin JW, et al., eds. Peripheral Neuropathy. Vol 2, 3rd ed. Philadelphia: WB Saunders Company, 1993;1065–1093

25. Head H. Morvan's disease. London Hosp Gaz, Clin Suppl 1903;10:5–7

26. Bousquet D. Un cas de syringomyélie chez l'enfant. Ann Med Chir Infant Paris 1906;10:673–679

27. Cruchet R, Petges G, Joulia M. Un cas de maladie de Morvan chez un enfant de sept ans. Bull Mem Soc Med Chir Bordeaux 1920;282–290

28. Ogryzlo MA. A familial peripheral neuropathy of unknown etiology resembling Morvan's disease. Can Med Assoc J 1946;54:547–553

29. Heller IH, Robb P. Hereditary sensory neuropathy. Neurology 1955;5:15–29

30. Hould F, Verret S. Hereditary radicular neuropathy with sensory loss: study of a French-Canadian family [French]. Laval Med 1967;38:454–459

31. Schoene WC, Asbury AK, Astrom KE, Masters R. Hereditary sensory neuropathy: a clinical ultrastructural study. J Neurol Sci 1970;11:463–487

32. Pinsky L, DiGeorge AM. Congenital familial sensory neuropathy with anhidrosis. J Pediatr 1966;68:1–13

33. Wadia NH, Dastur DK. Congenital sensory neuropathy. World Neurol 1960;1:409–421

34. Winkelmann RK, Lambert EH, Hayles AB. Congenital absence of pain: report of a case and experimental studies. Arch Dermatol 1962;85:325–339

35. Johnson RH, Spalding JM. Progressive sensory neuropathy in children. J Neurol Neurosurg Psychiatry 1964;27:125–130

36. Brown JW, Podosin R. A syndrome of the neural crest. Arch Neurol 1966;15:294–301

37. Blumenfeld A, Slaugenhaupt SA, Axelrod FB, et al. Localization of the gene for familial dysautonomia on chromosome 9 and definition of DNA markers for genetic diagnosis. Nat Genet 1993;4:160–164

38. Smeyne RJ, Klein R, Schnapp A, et al. Severe sensory and sympathetic neuropathies in mice carrying a disrupted Trk/NGF receptor gene. Nature 1994;368; 246–249

39. Indo Y, Tsuruta M, Hayashida Y, et al. Mutations in the TRKA/NGF receptor gene in patients with congenital insensitivity to pain with anhidrosis. Nat Genet 1996;3: 485–488

40. Mardy S, Miura Y, Endo F, et al. Congenital insensitivity to pain with anhidrosis: novel mutations in the TRKA (NTRK1) gene encoding a high-affinity receptor for nerve growth factor. Am J Hum Genet 1999;64: 1570–1579

41. Low PA, Burke WJ, McLeod JG. Congenital sensory neuropathy with selective loss of small myelinated fibers. Ann Neurol 1978;3:179–182

42. Donaghy M, Hakin RN, Bamford JM, et al. Hereditary sensory neuropathy with neurotrophic keratitis: description of an autosomal recessive disorder with a selective reduction of small myelinated nerve fibres and a discussion of the classification of the hereditary sensory neuropathies. Brain 1987;110:563–583

43. Houlden H, King RH, Hashemi-Nejad A, et al. A novel TRK A (NTRK1) mutation associated with hereditary sensory and autonomic neuropathy type V. Ann Neurol 2001;49:521–525

208 Hereditary Motor Neuropathies

Michel Melanson

Overview

Hereditary motor neuropathies (HMN) are a heterogeneous group of disorders predominantly affecting the motor neuron and its axon. Some of these have been covered in other chapters, including the autosomal recessive spinal muscular atrophies (SMA) and X-linked Kennedy's disease. These disorders have been classified according to the pattern of muscle weakness, inheritance and age of onset (Table 208.1). Genetic linkage analysis has added a new dimension to the classification of inherited motor neuropathies. This chapter will also review the topic of late onset hexosaminidase deficiency presenting as motor neuron disease.

Distal hereditary motor neuropathies

Case reports and series of patients with distal HMN are found in the literature under a variety of names including distal spinal muscular atrophy,[1,2] peroneal muscular atrophy[3] and spinal Charcot–Marie–Tooth. In Pearn and Hudgson's study of North East England,[4] this form of HMN accounts for approximately 10% of all cases of spinal muscular atrophy. The clinical presentation is usually before the second decade but onset ranging from childhood to late adulthood has been reported. A review of 34 cases by Harding and Thomas[5] reported distal muscle weakness and wasting in the legs in all cases with additional involvement of the upper limbs in one quarter. In some cases weakness can begin in the upper extremities[1] or remain confined to the hands.[6] Inheritance is usually autosomal dominant, although recessive and sporadic cases have been described.[7]

Timmerman et al.[8,9] found genetic linkage to chromosome 12q24 in an autosomal dominant kindred of distal HMN II. The mean age of onset was 21.6 years, patients presenting with slowly progressive distal leg muscle weakness with less severe weakness in the arms. A clinically distinct congenital, nonprogressive form of spinal muscular atrophy restricted to the lower limbs also maps to the same region.[10] Linkage to chromosome 12q was also found in a kindred with scapuloperoneal spinal muscular atrophy.[11] Despite their similar genetic loci, these three disorders are not believed to be allelic since they share very few clinical similarities.

The distinction between hereditary motor and hereditary sensory-motor neuropathies relies on the presence or absence of sensory symptoms and signs. Overt sensory loss is frequently absent in patients with type II hereditary sensory-motor neuropathy[7] and requires the presence of abnormal sensory action potentials in order to make the distinction from HMN. Recently, Sambuughin et al.[12] reported a Mongolian kindred of distal HMN in which some members had evidence of sensory involvement. They found linkage to the same locus as Charcot–Marie–Tooth type 2D[13] on chromosome 7p15, suggesting that these are allelic disorders. Christodoulou et al.[14] reported a Bulgarian family with an autosomal dominant, juvenile onset spinal muscular atrophy with predominant upper limb involvement that also links to chromosome 7p. Recessive forms of distal HMN also exist, including an infantile onset spinal muscular atrophy with diaphragm paralysis[15] for which linkage was found in one family to chromosome 11q13.[16] More recently, a novel form of distal hereditary motor neuronopathy has been described in seven consanguineous families from Jordan.[17] The age of onset ranges from 6 to 10 years of age, beginning with distal lower extremity weakness and muscle atrophy. Pyramidal signs are frequently encountered early in the course while upper limb weakness is generally a later feature. Inheritance is autosomal recessive with genetic linkage to chromosome 9p21.

Scapuloperoneal and proximal hereditary motor neuronopathies

Scapuloperoneal distribution weakness can be the result of a myopathic or neurogenic process. Davidenkow[7] described an autosomal dominant form of neurogenic scapuloperoneal syndrome (scapuloperoneal hereditary motor neuropathy type I).[18] The age of onset was in the second or third decade of life with either distal leg weakness or shoulder girdle weakness. The prognosis is generally good with a slowly progressive course. Some of these resemble the cases described by DeLong and Siddique.[18] This New England kindred with progressive scapuloperoneal atrophy, laryngeal palsy and congenital absence of muscles shows a dominant pattern of inheritance for which genetic linkage has been found on chromosome 12q.[11] The more common form of scapuloperoneal motor neuropathy appears to be recessively inherited.[7] These type II inherited scapuloperoneal motor neuropathies begin at an earlier age and are frequently accompanied by skeletal deformities such as talipes equinovarus and joint contractures. The prognosis is not well established but at least some appear to have a nonprogressive disorder. Proximal motor neuropathies, including the spinal muscular atrophies, are the topic of another chapter.

Table 208.1 Classification of hereditary motor neuropathy

Distribution/type	Alternative titles	Inheritance	Linkage	Age of onset	Clinical features	Progression
Distal						
HMN type I	Spinal form of Charcot–Marie–Tooth (distal hereditary motor neuronopathy)	AD		2–20 years	Symmetrical distal weakness and atrophy	No bulbar signs Slowly progressive
HMN type II	Spinal form of Charcot–Marie–Tooth	AD	12q24	20–40 years	Begins with toe, foot extensor weakness Legs weaker than arms	Slowly progressive
HMN type III	Mild juvenile form	AR		2–10 years		
HMN type IV	Severe juvenile form	AR		4 months–20 years	Unable to walk after 30 years	
HMN type V	SMA type V SMA with upper limb predominance	AD	7p15 ?allelic to CMT2D	Mean 17 years	Weakness in hands Leg involvement in half Pyramidal signs in some	Very slow progression
HMN type VI	Severe infantile form	AR		Infancy	Never able to walk	
HMN type VII		AD			Vocal cord paralysis	
Distal HMN–Jerash type	Jerash hereditary motor neuronopathy	AR	9p21	6–10 years	Weakness begins in legs Pyramidal signs	Slowly progressive
Distal infantile SMA with diaphragm paralysis	SMARD1	AR	11q13	1–2 months	Weakness predominantly in distal upper limbs, diaphragm	Death by 3 months Respiratory failure
Scapuloperoneal						
Type I	Scapuloperoneal amyotrophy (neurogenic type)	AD	12q24 ?allelic to HMN II	Usually adult (4–70)	Laryngeal palsy Absence of muscles	Variable Worse in males
Type II	Kaeser/Stark–Kaeser syndrome	AR		Early childhood Adolescence	Talipes equinovarus Joint contractures	? Nonprogressive
Proximal						
Type I	SMA type I Werdnig–Hoffmann disease	AR	5q	In utero–6 months	Severe, hypotonic at birth	Death usually by 18 months
Type II	SMA type II Kugelberg–Welander disease	AR	5q	3 months–15 years	Never stand	Death 18 months–40 years
Type III	SMA type III Kugelberg–Welander disease	AR	5q	15–60 years	Can stand independently	Variable, normal life expectancy
Type IV	Juvenile SMA	AD		6 months–5 years	Rare bulbar involvement	Slowly progressive
Type V	SMA type IV Adult onset spinal muscular atrophy	AD		25–65 years	Bulbar symptoms more frequent than type IV	More rapid progression than type IV Death 2–3 decades after diagnosis
Bulbar						
Type I	Vialetto–van Laere syndrome	?AR		Second decade	Deafness Limb weakness later	Respiratory failure Death in third to fourth decade
Type II	Fazio–Londe	AR		Early childhood		Death in 50% by 18 months

AD, autosomal dominant; AR, autosomal recessive; HMN, hereditary motor neuropathy; SMA, spinal muscular atrophy.

Bulbar hereditary motor neuronopathies

Fazio and later Londe[7] reported cases of progressive bulbar palsy with onset in childhood or early adulthood. Inheritance is autosomal recessive or more rarely dominant. The symptoms include excessive drooling, stridor and frequent respiratory infections followed by dysphagia, facial weakness and extraocular palsy. Limb weakness is rare and death occurs within 18 months of onset in about half of patients reported. Brown–Vialetto–van Laere syndrome[7] presents with dysphagia, dysarthria, facial weakness and sensorineural deafness in the first or second decade of life followed by limb weakness in some. Familial and sporadic cases have been described.[19]

Adult hexosaminidase deficiency

Hydrolysis of the ganglioside GM2 requires the lysosomal isoenzyme hexosaminidase A (Hex A) and the GM2 activator. Hex A is composed of two subunits, α and β. Defects in the genes coding for these subunits or the activator may lead to GM2 gangliosidosis. The phenotypic expression appears to depend on residual Hex A activity. In the more common presentation, Tay–Sachs disease, there is profound Hex A deficiency leading to an early onset, rapidly progressive neurodegenerative disease. This is associated with homozygous or compound heterozygous mutations in the HEX A gene which codes for the α subunit. A similar clinical presentation can result from mutations in the β subunit gene (HEX B) which cause Sandhoff's disease. A number of reports describe hexosaminidase deficiency presenting in adolescents or adults with progressive muscle weakness and atrophy.[20–22] Weakness tends to be symmetric and more pronounced proximally. Some of these cases resemble juvenile onset spinal muscular atrophy with predominant involvement of spinal motor neurons.[21–24] Although relatively pure motor neuron involvement does occur with late onset hexosaminidase deficiency,[23] most patients eventually develop varying degrees of multisystem degeneration. Upper motor neuron involvement is noted in some,[20] frequently accompanied by cognitive decline, cerebellar ataxia and peripheral sensory nerve involvement. Nerve conduction velocities are typically normal, however there is evidence of chronic active denervation on electromyography (EMG). Membranous cytoplasmic bodies in the myenteric plexus are seen on rectal biopsy but diagnosis can be made with an enzymatic assay. The later onset and slower course of the disease are likely due to residual ganglioside GM2 hydrolyzing activity.[25] Most adult onset patients with Tay–Sachs disease, including those with a motor neuron disease phenotype, are compound heterozygotes harboring a HEX A gene point mutation resulting in a Gly269Ser substitution and one of the two Ashkenasi infantile Tay–Sachs alleles.[26] The adult form of Sandhoff's disease presenting with a motor neuronopathy has been associated with compound heterozygote mutations in the HEX B gene, including an individual with a A619G/A1367C

genotype[27] and a more recently described C1214T transition in compound heterozygosity with a Δ5′ mutation.[28]

Therapeutic considerations

With the exception of hexosaminadase deficiency, specific gene mutations for the inherited motor neuropathies have not yet been found. Therefore, treatment is generally rehabilitative rather than directed toward the underlying genetic defect. Such therapies are individualized and aim to improve mobility and preserve range of motion. A variety of passive stretch exercises can be carried out by patients or their caregivers. These exercises can prevent contractures which most commonly involve the finger flexors, hip and knee flexors and foot plantar flexors. Heating by ultrasound can enable more effective stretching since collagen fibers are more easily elongated at temperatures between 40 and 43 degrees Celsius.[29] Two sessions of five repetitions are carried out twice a day depending on the site and degree of weakness and contractures. A therapist can assist in re-educating patients with fixed and progressive muscle weakness. Exercises directed at improving strength and endurance are tailored according to the patient's needs. This is supplemented with education regarding transfers and other activities of daily living.

Assistive devices are often required in patients with progressive muscle weakness. When involvement is primarily distal in the upper extremities, dorsal wrist and hand orthoses can improve mobility. With distal lower limb weakness, leaf-spring ankle-foot orthoses are used to prevent foot drop. More proximal involvement such as quadriceps weakness may require knee bracing in order to prevent genu recurvatum. Surgical procedures are generally not recommended in patients with progressive muscular weakness such as the inherited motor neuropathies. A triple arthrodesis has long been used for ankle and foot paralysis. This procedure involves fusion of the subastragalar, calcaneocuboid and talonavicular joints. Wetmore et al.[30] published their experience with triple arthrodesis in 16 patients with distal lower extremity weakness due to Charcot–Marie–Tooth disease. They found unsatisfactory long term results in most of their patients, likely due to the dynamic changes encountered with progressive neuropathies. Similar limitations would also apply to tendon transfer surgery.

Several therapeutic approaches are currently under study for the treatment of hexosaminidase deficiency. Adenoviral gene transfer in hexosaminidase A-deficient knock-out mice has been shown to lead to restoration of enzymatic activity in peripheral tissues.[31] Another approach is to decrease production of the substrate GM2. The glycosphingolipid synthesis inhibitor N-butyldeoxynojirimycin can reduce GM2 accumulation in brains of Tay–Sachs mice.[32] Enzyme replacement therapies have been successful in some forms of sphingolipidosis[33] but a major limiting factor in Tay–Sachs is delivery of the enzyme to the appropriate tissues. With improvement of delivery systems for both enzyme and genes, specific therapeutic interventions may soon be available for patients with both early and adult onset hexosaminidase deficiencies.

References

1. Meadows JC, Marsden CD. A distal form of chronic spinal muscular atrophy. Neurology 1969;19:53–58
2. McLeod JG, Prineas JW. Distal type of chronic spinal muscular atrophy—clinical, electrophysiological and pathological studies. Brain 1971;94:703–714
3. Dyck PJ, Lambert EH. Lower motor and primary sensory neuron diseases with peroneal muscular atrophy. II. Neurological, genetic and electrophysiologic findings in various neuronal degenerations. Arch Neurol 1968;18:619–625
4. Pearn JH, Hudgson P. Distal spinal muscular atrophy—a clinical and genetic study of 8 kindreds. J Neurol Sci 1979;43:183–191
5. Harding AE, Thomas PK. Hereditary distal spinal muscular atrophy—a report on 34 cases and review of the literature. J Neurol Sci 1980;45:337–348
6. O'Sullivan DG, McLeod JG. Distal chronic spinal muscular atrophy involving the hands. J Neurol Neurosurg Psychiatry 1978;41:653–658
7. Harding AE. Inherited neuronal atrophy and degeneration predominantly of the lower motor neurons. *In:* Dyck PJ, Thomas PK, Griffin JW, et al., eds. Peripheral Neuropathy. 3rd ed. Philadelphia: WB Saunders, 1993: 1051–1064
8. Timmerman V, Raeymaekers P, Nelis E, et al. Linkage analysis of distal hereditary motor neuropathy type II (distal HMN II) in a single pedigree. J Neurol Sci 1992; 109:41–48
9. Timmerman V, De Jonghe P, Simokovic S, et al. Distal hereditary motor neuropathy type II (distal HMN II): mapping of a locus to chromosome 12q24. Hum Mol Genet 1996;5:1065–1069
10. van der Vleuten AJ, van Ravenswaaij-Arts CM, Frijns CJ, et al. Localization of the gene for a dominant congenital spinal muscular atrophy predominantly affecting the lower limbs to chromosome 12q23–24. Eur J Hum Genet 1998;6:376–382
11. Isozumi K, DeLong R, Kaplan J, et al. Linkage of scapuloperoneal spinal muscular atrophy to chromosome 12q24.1-q24.31. Hum Mol Genet 1996;5:1377–1382
12. Sambuughin N, Sivakumar K, Selenge B, et al. Autosomal dominant distal spinal muscular atrophy type V (dSMA-V) and Charcot–Marie–Tooth disease type 2D (CMT2D) segregate within a single large kindred and map to a refined region on chromosome 7p15. J Neurol Sci 1998;161: 23–28
13. Ionasescu V, Searby C, Sheffield VC, et al. Autosomal dominant Charcot–Marie–Tooth axonal neuropathy mapped on chromosome 7p (CMT2D). Hum Mol Genet 1996;5:1373–1375
14. Christodoulou K, Kyriakides T, Hristova AH, et al. Mapping of a distal form of spinal muscular atrophy with upper limb predominance to chromosome 7p. Hum Mol Genet 1995;4:1629–1632
15. Bertini E, Gadisseux JL, Palmieri G, et al. Distal infantile spinal muscular atrophy associated with paralysis of the diaphragm: a variant of infantile spinal muscular atrophy. Am J Med Genet 1989;33:328–335
16. Grohmann K, Wienker TF, Saar K, et al. Diaphragmatic spinal muscular atrophy with respiratory distress is heterogeneous, and one form is linked to chromosome 11q13-q21. Am J Hum Genet 1999;65:1459–1462
17. Christodoulou K, Zamba E, Tsingis M, et al. A novel form of distal hereditary motor neuronopathy maps to chromosome 9p21.1-p12. 2000;48:877–884
18. DeLong R, Siddique T. A large New England kindred with autosomal dominant neurogenic scapuloperoneal amyotrophy with unique features. Arch Neurol 1992;49:905–908
19. Megarbane A, Desguerres I, Rizkallah E, et al. Brown-Vialetto-Van Laere syndrome in a large inbred Lebanese family: Confirmation of autosomal recessive inheritance? Am J Med Genet 2000;92:117–121
20. Mitsumoto H, Sliman RJ, Schafer IA, et al. Motor neuron disease and adult hexosaminidase-A deficiency in two families: evidence for multisystem degeneration, Ann Neurol 1985;17:378–385
21. Parnes S, Karpati G, Carpenter S, et al. Hexosaminidase-A deficiency presenting as atypical juvenile-onset spinal muscular atrophy. Arch Neurol 1985; 24:1176–1180
22. Johnson WG, Wigger HJ, Karp HR, et al. Juvenile spinal muscular atrophy: a new hexosaminidase deficiency phenotype. Ann Neurol 1982;11:11–16
23. Dale AJD, Engel AG, Rudd NL. Familial hexosaminidase-A deficiency with Kugelberg–Welander phenotype and mental change (abstract). Ann Neurol 1983;14:109
24. Jellinger K, Anzil AP, Seemann D, Bernheimer H. Adult GM2 gangliosidosis masquerading as slowly progressive muscular atrophy: motor neuron disease phenotype. Clin Neuropathol 1982;1:31–44
25. Gravel RA, Clarke JTR, Kaback MM, et al. The Gm2 gangliosidoses. *In:* Shriver CR, Beaudet AL, Sly WS, eds. The Metabolic and Molecular Basis of Inherited Diseases. 7th ed. New York: McGraw-Hill, 1995: 2839–2879
26. Navon R, Proia RL. The mutations in Ashkenazi Jews with adult Gm2 gangliosidosis, the adult form of Tay–Sachs disease. Science 1989;243:1471–1474
27. Banerjee P, Siciliano L, Oliveri D, et al. Molecular basis of an adult form of β-hexosaminidase B deficiency with motor neuron disease. Biochem Biophys Res Commun 1991;181:108–115
28. Gomez-Lira M, Sangalli A, Motters M, et al. A common β hexosaminidase gene mutation in adult Sandhoff disease patients. Hum Genet 1995;96: 417–422
29. Stillwell KG, Thorsteinsson G. Rehabilitation procedures. *In:* Dyck PJ, Thomas PK, Griffin JWF, et al., eds. Peripheral Neuropathy. 3rd ed. Philadelphia: WB Saunders, 1993:1692–1708
30. Westmore RS, Drennan JC. Long-term results of triple arthrodesis in Charcot–Marie–Tooth disease. J Bone Joint Surg Am 1989;71:417–422
31. Guidotti JE, Mignon A, Haase G, et al. Adenoviral gene therapy of the Tay–Sachs disease in hexosaminidase-A deficient knock-out mice. Hum Mol Genet 1999;8: 831–838
32. Platt FM, Neises GR, Reinkensmeir G, et al. Prevention of lysosomal storage in Tay–Sachs mice treated with N-butyldeoxynojirimycin. Science 1997;276:428–431
33. Barton NW, Brady RO, Dambrosia JM, et al. Replacement therapy for inherited enzyme deficiency—macrophage-targeted glucocerebrosidase for Gaucher's disease. N Engl J Med 1991;324:1464–1470

209 Hereditary Neuropathy With Liability to Pressure Palsy

Jan Meuleman and Phillip F Chance

Overview

Hereditary neuropathy with liability to recurrent pressure-sensitive palsies (HNPP; also called tomaculous neuropathy) is an autosomal dominant disorder that produces a painless episodic, recurrent, focal demyelinating neuropathy. HNPP generally develops during adolescence, and may cause attacks of numbness, muscular weakness, and atrophy. Peroneal palsies, carpal tunnel syndrome and other entrapment neuropathies may be frequent manifestations of HNPP. Motor and sensory nerve conduction velocities may be reduced in clinically affected patients, as well as in asymptomatic gene carriers. The histopathological changes observed in peripheral nerves of HNPP patients include segmental demyelination and tomaculous or "sausage-like" formations. Mild overlap of clinical features with Charcot–Marie–Tooth disease type 1 (CMT1) may lead HNPP patients to be misdiagnosed as having CMT1. HNPP and CMT1 are both demyelinating neuropathies, however their clinical, pathological and electrophysiological features are quite distinct. A brachial plexus neuropathy is sometimes the only clinical sign of HNPP, and it may sometimes be misdiagnosed as hereditary neuralgic amyotrophy (HNA), the second autosomal dominant recurrent focal neuropathy. However, HNPP and HNA are clinically and genetically distinct. Genetically, HNPP is mostly caused by a 1.5 megabase pair (Mb) deletion on chromosome 17p11.2–12. A duplication of this 1.5 Mb region leads to CMT1A. Both HNPP and CMT1A phenotypes are caused by a dosage effect of the PMP22 gene, which is contained within this deleted/duplicated region. This is reflected in reduced mRNA and protein levels in sural nerve biopsy samples from HNPP patients. The identification of a 2-basepair deletion and early termination codon within exon 1 of *PMP22* in an HNPP family without the deletion further supports this theory. At this moment, the sole treatment for HNPP consists of preventative and symptom easing measures. Further studies focusing on the precise role of the PMP22 protein and its surrounding pathway might elucidate future therapeutic possibilities.

Clinical features

Hereditary neuropathy with liability to pressure palsies (HNPP and McKusick No. 162500) is an autosomal dominant disorder which typically leads to episodic, painless, recurrent, focal motor and sensory peripheral neuropathies. First described by De Jong in 1947, HNPP is an entrapment or compressive neuropathy: many episodes are preceded by a minor compression or trauma of the affected peripheral nerve. The most vulnerable sites are the wrist, elbow, knee and shoulder, affecting the median, ulnar and peroneal nerve and brachial plexus respectively.[1] A history of limb trauma or prolonged positioning of the limb may be obtained in some cases. The onset of HNPP is usually in childhood or adolescence, with a high degree of penetrance; however, clinically asymptomatic obligate gene carriers are sometimes noted. When palsies occur they may be debilitating in that they may last for days to weeks and may require installation of a lower limb brace or ankle-foot orthosis in the cases of prolonged peroneal palsies. Hypoactive deep tendon reflexes and mild *pes cavus* may be observed in clinically asymptomatic patients. The spectrum of clinical presentation in HNPP is broad and may range from clinically asymptomatic or subclinical to, more typically, recurrent palsies and in some advanced cases progressive residual deficits mimicking indolent forms of CMT1.[2–5] Guidelines for the diagnosis of HNPP have been reported previously.[6]

In an analysis of 39 HNPP patients from 16 unrelated pedigrees, two thirds of patients had the typical presentation of acute mononeuropathy and the remaining subjects were thought to have features consistent with a more long-standing polyneuropathy. Furthermore, it was noted that over 40% of affected persons were unaware of their illness and 25% of patients were essentially symptom free at the time of observation.[7] More recently, the spectrum of clinical and neurophysiological findings in 99 patients with HNPP was documented.[8] The majority of patients in this survey (70%) presented with a typical history of a single, focal episode of neuropathy, however there were patients with short term or chronic sensory syndromes, as well as asymptomatic gene carriers. The clinical findings in a subset of patients with the classical presentation of HNPP are shown in Table 209.1. Rarely, patients with HNPP may present with a more fulminant course in which palsies affecting more than one limb are seen.[9] Other rare associations with HNPP include a report of central nervous system demyelination.[10]

Very few studies have addressed the epidemiology of HNPP; one such study from Western Finland reported a prevalence of 16 per 100 000.[11]

Table 209.1 Clinical findings in 70 patients with typical HNPP	
Feature	
Total no. of patients	70 (40M/30F)
Age at examination (mean, range)	38 (14–73)
Age at onset (mean, range)	23 (7–73)
Acute nerve palsies	70 (100%)
Positional sensory symptoms	8 (11%)
Painless symptoms	70 (100%)
History of compression	46 (65%)
Pes cavus	13 (18%)
Generalized areflexia	9 (12%)
Absent ankle jerks	26 (37%)
Neurological sequelae	9 (15%)

From Mouton et al.[8]

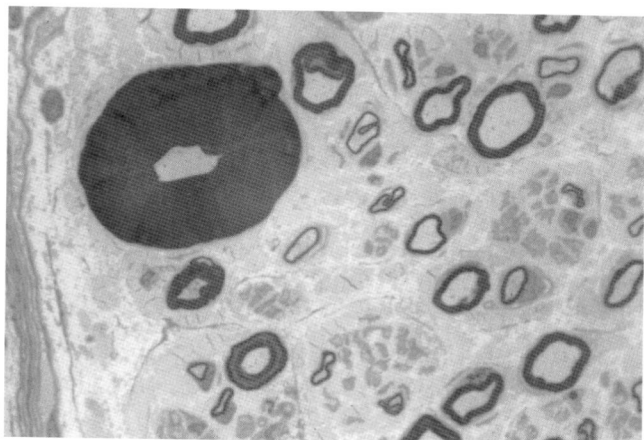

Figure 209.1 Cross-section of a sural nerve biopsy from a patient with HNPP showing a tomaculum. Thinly myelinated axons are also seen. One-micron section prepared from plastic embedded specimen, toluidine blue staining. Original magnification ×400. (See color plate section.)
Courtesy of Dr. Zarife Sahenk, Dept. of Neurology, Ohio State University, Columbus, Ohio.

Histopathological features

In 1972, Behse et al. documented the pathological features of HNPP.[12] Histological assessment of sural nerve biopsies reveals segmental de- and re-myelination. The presence of tomaculi or "sausage" shaped structures is the pathological signature of HNPP. They consist of massive redundancy or overfolding of variable thickness layers in the myelin sheath.[13] It should be noted that tomaculi are likely not a pathological feature of HNPP. They may also be seen in Charcot–Marie–Tooth neuropathy type 4B (with myelin outfolding), IgM paraproteinemic neuropathy, chronic inflammatory demyelinating polyneuropathy and Dejerine–Sottas disease.[14] Tomaculi have also been observed in cases of Charcot–Marie–Tooth neuropathy types 1 and 8 (associated with extrapyramidal syndrome), neurogenic scapuloperoneal syndrome and multiple sclerosis.[15,16] While tomaculi are generally considered an important diagnostic feature of HNPP (see Figure 209.1), rare patients showing axonal regeneration and lacking tomaculi have been observed.[17]

Electrophysiological features

The abnormal neurophysiological features of HNPP were described by Earl et al.[18] and are consistent with demyelination, showing mildly prolonged motor and sensory nerve conduction velocities in a symmetrical, generalized pattern. Conduction blocks are characteristic of affected segments in symptomatic nerves, especially over entrapment sites. Mildly reduced nerve conduction velocities and prolonged distal motor latencies are not restricted to those nerves affected by a palsy, but are found in a generalized pattern, even in asymptomatic gene carriers. While slowing of motor and sensory nerve conduction velocities is commonly observed in hereditary demyelinating neuropathies, the nerve conduction velocities of patients with HNPP are typically normal or only slightly prolonged. In HNPP the parameters most commonly affected include: (1) increased distal motor latencies in the median nerves; (2) slowed sensory nerve conduction velocities in median nerves at the wrists; and (3) increased distal motor latencies and mild slowing of nerve conduction velocities in the peroneal nerves.[8]

Genetic basis

The genetic locus for HNPP maps to chromosome 17p11.1–12, where it is most commonly associated with a large, 1.5 Mb (megabase pair) DNA deletion.[19] A duplication of exactly this 1.5 Mb region had previously been shown to be detrimental in Charcot–Marie–Tooth neuropathy type 1A, the most common form of CMT1.[20,21] In a study of 156 patients with HNPP, 84% were found to have the associated 1.5 Mb DNA deletion.[22] HNPP deletions and CMT1A duplications of a different size have been observed, although they are very rare.[23] The 1.5 Mb region as well as the deletions and duplications of "aberrant" size harbor the peripheral myelin protein-22 (PMP22) gene. The PMP22 gene encodes a 160-amino acid membrane-associated protein with a predicted molecular weight of 18 kDa that is increased to 22 kDa by glycosylation.[24] The PMP22 protein is localized to the compact portion of peripheral nerve myelin,[25] contains four putative transmembrane domains, and is highly conserved in evolution.[26] Two different tissue-specific transcripts (neural and non-neural) of PMP22 arise through two alternatively used promoters.[27]

Furthermore, nine mutations have been reported in HNPP: two 2-basepair (bp) deletions, one single bp deletion, a single bp insertion, three point mutations, and two splice site mutations.[28-37]

Three important questions emerge from the knowledge of the genetic basis of HNPP: first, how exactly do the HNPP deletion and CMT1A duplication arise; second, what exactly causes the HNPP phenotype;

and, third, how can we prevent or cure this phenotype?

Origin of the HNPP deletion

The mechanism underlying the generation of the CMT1A DNA duplication and HNPP deletion has been the subject of numerous investigations. Since the vast majority of the duplications and deletions in unrelated patients and in *de novo* duplication/deletion patients are the exact same size, it is hypothesized that a precise, recurring mechanism may account for the generation of the duplicated CMT1A chromosome and the deleted HNPP chromosome.[19,21,38,39] As depicted in Figure 209.2, it was proposed that the deleted chromosome in HNPP and the duplicated chromosome in CMT1A are the reciprocal products of unequal crossing over, a likely mechanism for generating the DNA duplication and the deletion.[19] A low-copy number repeat sequence (CMT1A-REP element) was identified flanking the 1.5 Mb segment on chromosome 17p11.2–p12.[40] The CMT1A-REP sequence, which is an intrinsic structural property of a normal chromosome 17, appears to mediate misalignment of homologous chromosomal segments during meiosis, with subsequent crossing over to produce the CMT1A duplication or HNPP deletion.

Analysis of *de novo* rearrangements leading to either the CMT1A duplication or the HNPP deletion suggests that this process may be sex dependent. Most *de novo* CMT1A duplications appear to be the result of unequal crossing over between homologous chromosomes occurring during spermatogenesis. However, analysis of *de novo* HNPP deletions suggests that they are generated by unequal sister chromatid exchange during oogenesis.[41,42]

The origin of the CMT1A-REP repeat has been investigated through an analysis of homologous sequences in nonhuman primates. The CMT1A-REP repeat arose during primate evolution. Southern blot analysis indicated that the chimpanzee has two copies of a CMT1A-REP-like sequence, whereas the gorilla, orangutan, and gibbon have a single copy.[43] These observations suggest that the CMT1A-REP sequence appeared as a repeat before the divergence of chimpanzee and human, but after gorilla and human around six to seven million years ago.

Genetic defects and their results/effects

In order to elucidate the exact cause of the HNPP phenotype, several facts have to be taken into account, the first of which is the 1.5 Mb deletion on chromosome 17p11.2–p12. Since the majority of the HNPP patients carry this deletion, they are haploinsufficient at this locus. They are therefore predicted to have only 50% of the normal expression of the PMP22 gene in peripheral nerves, while CMT1A patients, carrying the 1.5 Mb duplication, would have a 50% increase in PMP22 expression. Indeed, various sural nerve biopsy studies showed that PMP22 mRNA levels are increased/decreased in CMT1A/HNPP patients respectively, in comparison to unaffected persons.[44,45] An interesting question is whether PMP22 is the only gene within this 1.5 Mb segment of which the dosage effect is contributing to the HNPP/CMT1A phenotype. A first hint was provided by the deletions and duplications of aberrant size which did still include PMP22.[23] However, the different PMP22 mutations in patients without the HNPP deletion are the best proof of the critical, detrimental character of PMP22 in the HNPP phenotype. A 1-basepair insertion, as well as a 1-basepair and two different 2-basepair deletions in PMP22 cause a frameshift, leading to an altered, nonfunctional protein.[28,33–35,37] Two point mutations create an early stop codon, leading to a truncated protein.[32,36] Two splice mutations are predicted to cause exon skipping, also resulting in an altered, nonfunctional protein.[29,31] The pathogenic mechanism of these PMP22 mutations is hypothesized to be that they either mimic the dosage effect of the HNPP deletion by creation of a null allele, or dominant negatively interfere with the function of the remaining normal PMP22 protein. So far, only one point mutation has been reported to cause an amino acid substitution. This Val30Met is predicted to occur at the border of the first transmembrane domain and the extracellular loop. Patient nerve xenografts onto mice sciatic nerve showed a marked delay in the onset of myelination with an impairment of regenerative capacity and an increased neurofilament density, in comparison with nerve xenografts from unaffected individuals. These observations demonstrated the effect of the HNPP point mutation on the ability of schwann cells to

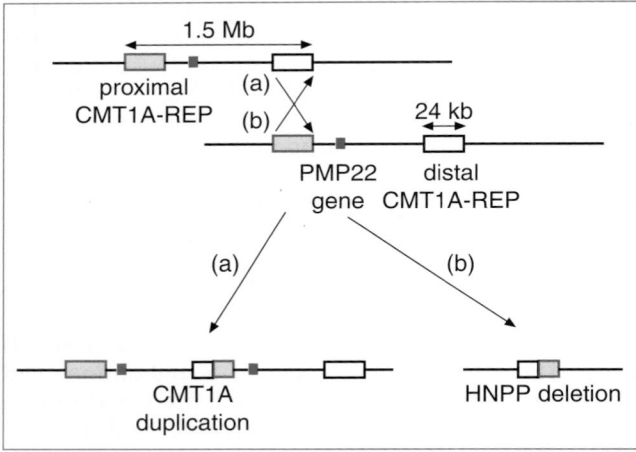

Figure 209.2 Proposed mechanism of unequal crossing-over, leading to the CMT1A duplication and the HNPP deletion on chromosome 17p11.2–p12. The proximal (shaded) and distal (unshaded) copies of the CMT1A-REP repeats have 99% sequence identity and may mediate misalignment of the chromosome 17 homologs during meiosis (top). One recombination pathway leads to the CMT1A tandem duplication (a) and the reciprocal recombination pathway leads to the HNPP deletion (b). Note that the CMT1A duplication chromosome has gained a 1.5 Mb segment and harbors two copies of the PMP22 gene. Conversely, the HNPP deleted chromosome has lost a 1.5 Mb segment from chromosome 17, including a copy of the PMP22 gene.

myelinate axons and pointed to perturbations in the axonal cytoskeleton resulting from a hypothesized interaction between the mutant schwann cells and their axons. The function of PMP22 will need to be clarified in order to reconcile the various mutational mechanisms involving this myelin component in HNPP and other associated peripheral neuropathies.

Genesis of the HNPP phenotype

Several attractive hypotheses for the function of PMP22 have evolved from observations on the structure and expression of this critical myelin component. The PMP22 gene is specifically expressed in schwann cells and is identical to a growth arrest-specific gene, gas3.[24,46–48] A direct role in schwann cell mitosis is suggested by the observation of impaired differentiation of schwann cells in transgenic mice carrying increased copies of PMP22 as well as the observation that in NIH-3T3 cells an apoptotic phenotype may be induced through increased expression of PMP22.[49,50] Furthermore, a role in cell adhesion may be suggested since the PMP22 protein is known to carry an L2/HNK-1 carbohydrate adhesion epitome.[51] Unfolded separation of the inner myelin lamellae in HNPP may also suggest decreased cell adhesion when PMP22 is partially deficient.[52]

Animal models for HNPP

A powerful tool to obtain more information on the pathomechanism of a disease is the study of animal models. Several animal models are available involving PMP22. According to the hypothesis that the pathomechanism of HNPP is a dosage effect, one might predict that the total absence of the *PMP22* gene would also cause demyelinating neuropathy, likely more severe than HNPP. Such patients have not yet been described, but a murine model with this genotype has been described.[53] Homozygous deletion *(PMP22$^{-/-}$)* "knock-out" mice develop a severe demyelinating neuropathy with very slow conduction velocities (7 m/sec) and striking demyelination on pathological examination, including the evolution of demyelinated axons in *pmp22$^{-/-}$* mice, as tomaculous myelin sheaths are replaced by thin to absent ones. Heterozygous deletion *(pmp22$^{+/-}$)* mice are less affected, with minimal slowing of conduction velocities and little evidence of demyelination in biopsies, although numerous tomaculi eventually develop in affected nerve. These data confirm that the loss of the *pmp22* gene, and not another gene in the 1.5 Mb deletion, is detrimental for HNPP. The precise mechanism of demyelination in *pmp22$^{+/-}$* mice is unknown. It can be speculated that these mice synthesize only half as much PMP22 and protein as their wildtype counterparts, thereby altering the stoichiometry of the proteins in compact myelin, which in turn leads to demyelination.

A naturally occurring bovine illness appears to resemble HNPP. This bovine neuropathy shows tomaculous neuropathy with the clinical features of weak shuffling gait, dysphagia and chronic rumenal bloat.[54]

Differential diagnosis of HNPP versus hereditary neuralgic amyotrophy (HNA)

HNPP may be clinically confused with HNA (familial brachial plexus neuropathy). As mentioned before, a brachial plexus neuropathy is sometimes the only clinical sign of HNPP.[55] Approximately 10% of HNPP patients have had involvement of the brachial plexus, and in some patients a brachial plexopathy is the initial or only expression of HNPP. Furthermore, both diseases were earlier speculated to represent the same condition, or allelic variants of the same locus,[13,56,57] justifying the need for differential diagnostic tools to distinguish between HNPP and HNA.

HNA is an autosomal dominant disorder causing episodes of paralysis and muscle weakness initiated by severe pain.[4] Episodes are often triggered by infections, immunizations, the puerperium and stress.[58] Electrophysiological studies in HNA show normal or mildly prolonged motor nerve conduction velocities distal to the brachial plexus. A generalized neuropathy is not present in HNA. Pathological studies have found axonal degeneration in nerves examined distal to the plexus abnormality.[59] In some HNA pedigrees there are mild dysmorphic features of hypotelorism and short stature.[60] The prognosis for recovery of normal function of affected limbs in HNA is good, although recurrent episodes can cause residual deficits. HNA is genetically linked to chromosome 17q25,[61–63] although genetic heterogeneity has been reported.[64–66] The underlying pathogenesis of HNA is unknown.

Two studies have shown that HNPP and HNA are two distinct clinical, electrophysiological, and genetic diseases.[67–69] Diagnostic guidelines for both HNPP and HNA have been published.[6,70] The main differential criteria are summarized in Table 209.2.

Therapy

At the time of writing, there is no specific treatment for HNPP. The current therapy consists of conservative management and symptom easing measures. The first, and perhaps most important, element of the treatment is early detection and diagnosis of the disease. The knowledge that HNPP is often triggered by compression or trauma of the peripheral nerves gives the patient the possibility to avoid those movements or joint positions that most often evoke an HNPP episode. As mentioned above, diagnostic guidelines have been reported previously.[6] Furthermore, several genetic tools have been designed for a reliable diagnosis.[38,71,72] These techniques have even been used for the prenatal diagnosis of CMT1A[73,74] and could therefore eventually also be used in genetically diagnosed HNPP patients.

The second element of the treatment is conservative management to avoid evoking HNPP episodes.[75] Overall, two basic rules apply: (1) excessive force or repetitive movements should be reduced to a minimum; (2) extreme, awkward or static joint positions should be avoided. Since the wrist, elbow, knee and shoulder are the most vulnerable sites, special

Table 209.2 Differential criteria for HNPP and HNA.

	HNPP	HNA
Neuropathy	Generalized with focal episodes	Focal episodes, not generalized
Localization	Mainly entrapment sites	Brachial plexus
Phenotype	Painless	Painful
Preceding events	Compression/trauma	Infections, immunizations, puerperium, stress, exercise
Electrophysiology	Slowed nerve conduction velocities, conduction block over entrapment sites, also measurable in unaffected nerves	Normal to slightly reduced nerve conduction velocities in affected nerves, normal elsewhere
Histopathology	Tomacula De- and re-myelination	Minor, focal axonal degeneration distal to affected brachial plexus, normal elsewhere
Genetics	1.5 Mb deletion at 17p11.2–p12 or deletion of aberrant size mutations in PMP22	Linked to 17q25 Genetic heterogeneity

management rules can be considered. At the wrist (carpal tunnel), episodes are mostly caused by forceful gripping, repetitive movements or extreme wrist bending. Tools and gloves can be used to improve grip, and wrist splints can prevent extreme wrist bend during the night. At the elbow, episodes are mostly triggered by repetitive or sustained bending and by habitual leaning on the elbows. Management consists of elbow pads to reduce pressure, a headset for use during long telephone conversations, and eventually an elbow splint during the night. The most frequent trigger at the knee is habitual crossing of the legs. A lower leg brace can stabilize ankles in case this causes recurrent stretch injury at the knee. The complexity of the brachial plexus means that many factors can evoke an HNPP episode at the shoulder. Avoiding overhead work or sleeping with the arms overhead, and maintaining a good posture can reduce the risk.

A single case report mentions surgery to reduce pressure on the ulnar nerve, however a follow-up study is not yet available.[76] Although various surgical treatments of carpal tunnel syndrome (CTS) exist,[77] no reports have been published on such surgery in HNPP patients. Given the vulnerability of the peripheral nerves in HNPP patients, surgery is generally considered unfavorable.

Since HNPP is mainly caused by the dosage effect of PMP22 due to the 1.5 Mb deletion on chromosome 17p11.2–p12, one could reason that increasing the gene dosage might rescue the defect. The reverse would be true for the CMT1A patients carrying a duplication increasing the PMP22 expression. However, several hurdles have to be overcome. First of all, increasing PMP22 expression requires either the stimulation of the endogenous PMP22 or a gene transfer introducing another copy of the PMP22 gene. Further study of the PMP22 promoters and the recent discovery of a positive regulatory element of PMP22[78] could provide a future avenue for therapeutic research. A gene transfer to correct the shortage of PMP22 has the difficulty of the limited accessibility of the peripheral nerves. Furthermore, this strategy would need to correct the PMP22 expression without increasing the dosage too much, which would lead to the CMT phenotype. Although several animal models are available to study the possibilities of gene therapy, it might take years before a safe and efficient therapy became available.

References

1. De Jong JGY. Over families met hereditaire dispositie tot het optreden van neuritiden gecorreleered met migraine. Psychiatr Neurol B (Amst) 1947;50:60
2. Chance PF. Inherited demyelinating neuropathy: Charcot–Marie–Tooth disease and related disorders. In: Rosenberg RN, Prusiner SB, DiMauro S, et al., eds. The Molecular and Genetic Basis of Neurological Disease. Oxford: Butterworth-Heinemann, 1996:807–816
3. Dyck PJ, Chance P, Lebo R, et al. Hereditary motor and sensory neuropathies. In: Dyck PJ, Thomas PK, Griffin JW, et al., eds. Peripheral Neuropathy. 3rd ed. Philadelphia: WB Saunders, 1993:1094–1136
4. Windebank AJ. Inherited recurrent focal neuropathies. In: Dyck PJ, Thomas PK, Griffin JW, et al., eds. Peripheral Neuropathy. 3rd ed. Philadelphia: WB Saunders, 1993:1137–1148
5. Kumar N, Muley S, Pakim AS, et al. Phenotypic variability in hereditary neuropathy with liability to pressure palsy (HNPP) (abstract). Neurology 1998;50:A73
6. Dubourg O, Mouton P, Brice A, et al. Guidelines for diagnosis of hereditary neuropathy with liability to pressure palsies. Neuromuscul Disord 2000;10:206–208
7. Pareyson D, Scaioli V, Taroni F, et al. Phenotypic heterogeneity in hereditary neuropathy with liability to pressure palsies associated with chromosome 17p11.2–12 deletion. Neurology 1996;46:1133–1137
8. Mouton P, Tardieu BS, Gouider R, et al. Spectrum of clinical and electrophysiological features in HNPP patients with the 17p11.2 deletion. Neurology 1999;52:1440–1446
9. Crum BA, Sorenson EJ, Abad GA, Dyck PJB. Fulminant case of hereditary neuropathy with liability to pressure palsy. Muscle Nerve 2000;23:979–983
10. Amato AA, Barohn RJ. Hereditary neuropathy with liability to pressure palsies: association with central nervous

system demyelination. Muscle Nerve 1996;19: 770–773

11. Meretoja P, Silander K, Kalimo H, et al. Epidemiology of hereditary neuropathy with liability to pressure palsies (HNPP) in south western Finland. Neuromuscul Disord 1997;8:529–532

12. Behse F, Buchthal F, Carlsen F, Knappeis GG. Hereditary neuropathy with liability to pressure palsies: electrophysiological and histopathological aspects. Brain 1972;95:777–794

13. Madrid R, Bradley WG. The pathology of neuropathies with focal thickening of the myelin sheath (tomaculous neuropathy): Studies on the formation of the abnormal myelin sheath. J Neurol Sci 1975;25:415–448

14. Sander S, Ouvrier RA, McLeod JG, et al. Clinical syndromes associated with tomacula or myelin swellings in sural nerve biopsies. J Neurol Neurosurg Psychiatry 2000;68:483–488

15. Alexianu M, Macovei M, Alexianu ME, et al. Tomaculous neuropathy with unusual clinical aspects. Rom J Neurol Psychiatry 1995;33:229–235

16. Drulovi J, Dozic S, Levic Z, et al. Unusual association of multiple sclerosis and tomaculous neuropathy. J Neurol Sci 1998;7:217–222

17. Sessa M, Nemni R, Quattrini A, et al. Atypical hereditary neuropathy with liability to pressure palsies (HNPP): the value of direct DNA diagnosis. J Med Genet 1997;34:889–892

18. Earl CJ, Fullerton PM, Wakefield GS, et al. Hereditary neuropathy with liability to pressure palsies. QJM 1964; 33:481–498

19. Chance P, Alderson MK, Leppig KA, et al. DNA deletion associated with hereditary neuropathy with liability to pressure palsies. Cell 1993;72:143–151

20. Lupski JR, et al. DNA duplication associated with Charcot–Marie–Tooth disease type 1A. Cell 1991;66: 219–232

21. Raeymaekers P, Timmerman V, Nelis E, et al. Duplication in chromosome 17p11.2 in Charcot–Marie–Tooth neuropathy type 1A (CMT 1A). Neuromuscul Disord 1991;1:93–97

22. Nelis E, van Broeckhoven C, De Jonghe P, et al. Estimation of the mutation frequencies in Charcot–Marie–Tooth disease type 1 and hereditary neuropathy with liability to pressure palsies: a European collaborative study. Eur J Hum Genet 1996;4:25–33

23. Chapon F, Diraison P, Lechevalier B, et al. Hereditary neuropathy with liability to pressure palsies with a partial deletion of the region often duplicated in Charcot–Marie–Tooth disease, type 1A. J Neurol Neurosurg Psychiatry 1996;61:535–536

24. Manfioletti G, Ruaro ME, Del Sal G, et al. A growth arrest-specific (gas) gene codes for a membrane protein. Mol Cell Biol 1990;10:2924–2930

25. Snipes GJ, Suter U, Welcher AA, Shooter EM. Characterization of a novel peripheral nervous system myelin protein (PMP-22/SR13). J Cell Biol 1992;117:225–238

26. Patel PI, Roa BB, Welcher AA, et al. The gene for the peripheral myelin protein PMP-22 is a candidate for Charcot–Marie–Tooth disease type 1A. Nat Genet 1992; 1:157–165

27. Suter U, Snipes GJ, Schoener-Scott R, et al. Regulation of tissue-specific expression of alternative peripheral myelin protein-22 (PMP22) gene transcripts by two promoters. J Biol Chem 1994;26:25795–25808

28. Nicholson GA, Valentijn LJ, Cherryson AK, et al. A frame shift mutation in the PMP22 gene in hereditary neuropathy with liability to pressure palsies. Nat Genet 1994;6:263–266

29. Bort S, Nelis E, Timmerman V, et al. Mutational analysis of the MPZ, PMP22 and Cx32 genes in patients of Spanish ancestry with Charcot–Marie–Tooth disease and hereditary neuropathy with liability to pressure palsies. Hum Genet 1997;99:746–754

30. Sahenk Z, Chen L, Freimer M. A novel PMP22 point mutation causing HNPP phenotype: studies on nerve xenografts. Neurology 1998;5:702–707

31. Meuleman J, Pou-Serradell A, Lofgren A, et al. A novel 3′-splice site mutation in peripheral myelin protein 22 causing hereditary neuropathy with liability to pressure palsies. Neuromuscul Disord 2001;11:400–403

32. Haites NE, Nelis E, Van Broekhoven C, et al. 3rd workshop of the European CMT consortium: 54th ENMC international workshop on genotype/phenotype correlations in Charcot–Marie– Tooth type 1 and hereditary neuropathy with liability to pressure palsies, 28–30 November 1997, Naarden, The Netherlands. Neuromuscul Disord 1998;8:591–603

33. Young P, Wiebusch H, Stogbauer F, et al. A novel frameshift mutation in PMP22 accounts for hereditary neuropathy with liability to pressure palsies. Neurology 1997;48:450–452

34. Lenssen PP, Gabreels-Festen AA, Valentijn LJ, et al. Hereditary neuropathy with liability to pressure palsies. Phenotypic differences between patients with the common deletion and a PMP22 frame shift mutation. Brain 1998;121:1451–1458

35. Bissar-Tadmouri N, Parman Y, Boutrand L, et al. Mutational analysis and genotype/phenotype correlation in Turkish Charcot–Marie–Tooth Type 1 and HNPP patients. Clin Genet 2000;58:396–402

36. Pareyson D, Taroni F. Deletion of the PMP22 gene and hereditary neuropathy with liability to pressure palsies. Curr Opin Neurol 1996;9:348–354

37. Taroni F, Bottis S, Sghirlanzoni A, et al. A nonsense mutation in the PMP22 gene in hereditary neuropathy with liability to pressure palsies (HNPP) not associated with the 17p11.2 deletion. Am J Hum Genet 1995;57:A229

38. Raeymaekers P, Timmerman V, Nelis E, et al. Estimation of the size of the chromosome 17p11.2 duplication in Charcot–Marie–Tooth neuropathy type 1a (CMT1a). HMSN Collaborative Research Group. J Med Genet 1992;29:5–11

39. Wise CA, Garcia CA, Davis SN, et al. Molecular analyses of unrelated Charcot–Marie–Tooth (CMT) disease patients suggest a high frequency of the CMTIA duplication. Am J Hum Genet 1993;53:853–863

40. Pentao L, Wise CA, Chinault AC, et al. Charcot–Marie–Tooth type 1A duplication appears to arise from recombination at repeat sequences flanking the 1.5 Mb monomer unit. Nat Genet 1992;2:292–300

41. Lopes J, Ravise N, Vandenberghe A, et al. Fine mapping of de novo CMT1A and HNPP rearrangements within CMT1A-REPs evidences two distinct sex-dependent mechanisms and candidate sequences involved in recombination. Hum Mol Genet 1998;7:141–148

42. Lopes J, Vandenberghe A, Tardieu S, et al. Sex-dependent rearrangements resulting in CMT1A and HNPP. Nat Genet 1997;17:136–137

43. Kiyosawa H, Chance PF. Primate origin of the CMT1A-REP repeat and analysis of a putative transposon-associated recombinational hotspot. Hum Mol Genet 1996; 5:745–753

44. Yoshikawa H, Nishimura T, Nakatsuji Y, et al. Elevated expression of messenger RNA for peripheral myelin protein 22 in biopsied peripheral nerve of patients

Charcot–Marie–Tooth disease type 1A. Ann Neurol 1994;35:445–450

45. Schenone A, Nobbio L, Mandich P, et al. Under expression of messenger RNA for peripheral myelin protein 22 in hereditary neuropathy with liability to pressure palsies. Neurology 1997;48:445–449

46. Suter U, Welcher AA, Ozcelik T, et al. Trembler mouse carries a point mutation in a myelin gene. Nature 1992;356:241–244

47. Spreyer P, Kuhn G, Hanemann CO, et al. Axon-regulated expression of a Schwann cell transcript that is homologous to a "growth arrest-specific" gene. EMBO J 1991;10:3661–3668

48. Welcher AA, Suter U, De Leon M, et al. A myelin protein is encoded by the homolog of a growth arrest-specific gene. Proc Natl Acad Sci USA 1991;88:7195–7199

49. Magyar JP, Martini R, Ruelicke T, et al. Impaired differentiation of Schwann cells in transgenic mice with increased PMP22 gene dosage. J Neurosci 1996;16:5351–5360

50. Fabbretti E, Edomi P, Brancolini C, et al. Apoptotic phenotype induced by overexpression of wild-type gas3/PMP22: its relation to the demyelinating peripheral neuropathy CMT1A. Genes Dev 1995;9:1846–1856

51. Snipes GJ, Suter U, Shooter EM. Human peripheral myelin protein-22 carries the L2/HNK-1 carbohydrate adhesion epitope. J Neurochem 1994;61:1961–1964

52. Yoshikawa H, Dyck PJ. Uncompacted inner myelin lamellae in inherited tendency to pressure palsy. J Neuropathol Exp Neurol 1991;50:649–657

53. Adlkofer K, Martini R, Aguzzi A, et al. Hypermyelination and demyelinating peripheral neuropathy in Pmp22-deficient mice. Nat Genet 1995;11:274–280

54. Hill BD, Prior H, Blakemore WF, Black PF. A study of pathology of a bovine primary peripheral neuropathy with features of tomaculous neuropathy. Acta Neuropathol 1996;91:545–548

55. Ørstavik K, Skard Heier M, Young P, Stogbauer F. Brachial plexus involvement as the only expression of hereditary neuropathy with liability to pressure palsies. Muscle Nerve 2001;24:1093–1096

56. Bradley WG, Madrid R, Thrush DC, Campbell MJ. Recurrent brachial plexus neuropathy. Brain 1975;98:381–398

57. Martinelli P, Fabbri R, Moretto G, et al. Recurrent familial brachial plexus palsies as the only clinical expression of "tomaculous" neuropathy. Eur Neurol 1989;29:61–66

58. Meuleman J, Timmerman V, Van Broeckhoven C, De Jonghe P. Hereditary neuralgic amyotrophy. Neurogenetics 2001;3:115–118

59. Tsairis P, Dyck PJ, Mulder DW. Natural history of brachial plexus neuropathy. Report on 99 patients. Arch Neurol 1972;127:109–117

60. Jacob JC, Andermann F, Robb J, et al. Heredofamilial neuritis with brachial predilection. Neurology 1961;11:1025–1033

61. Pellegrino JE, Rebbeck TR, Brown MJ, et al. Mapping of hereditary neuralgic amyotrophy (familial brachial plexus neuropathy) to distal chromosome 17q. Neurology 1996;46:1128–1132

62. Wehnert M, Timmerman V, Spoelders P, et al. Further evidence supporting linkage of hereditary neuralgic amyotrophy to chromosome 17q. Neurology 1997;48:1719–1721

63. Stogbauer F, Young P, Timmerman V, et al. Refinement of the hereditary neuralgic amyotrophy (HNA) locus to chromosome 17q24–q25. Hum Genet. 1997;99:685–687

64. Van Alfen N, van Engelen BG, Reinders JW, et al. The natural history of hereditary neuralgic amyotrophy in the Dutch population: two distinct types? Brain 2000;123:718–723

65. Watts G, O'Briant KC, Borreson TE, et al. Evidence for genetic heterogeneity in hereditary neuralgic amyotrophy. Neurology 2001;13:675–678

66. Kuhlenbaumer G, Meuleman J, De Jonghe P, et al. Hereditary Neuralgic Amyotrophy (HNA) is genetically heterogeneous. J Neurol 2001;248:861–865

67. Chance PF, Lensch MW, Lipe H, et al. Hereditary neuralgic amyotrophy and hereditary neuropathy with liability to pressure palsies: two distinct genetic disorders. Neurology 1994;44:2253–2257

68. Gouider R, Le Guern E, Emile J, et al. Hereditary neuralgic amyotrophy and hereditary neuropathy with liability to pressure palsies: two distinct clinical, electrophysiologic, and genetic entities. Neurology 1994;44:2250–2252

69. Windebank AJ, Schenone A, Dewald GW. Hereditary neuropathy with liability to pressure palsies and inherited brachial plexus neuropathy—two genetically distinct disorders. Mayo Clin Proc 1995;70:743–746

70. Kuhlenbaumer G, Stogbauer F, Timmerman V, De Jonghe P. Diagnostic guidelines for hereditary neuralgic amyotrophy or heredofamilial neuritis with brachial plexus predilection. On behalf of the European CMT Consortium. Neuromuscul Disord 2000;10:515–517

71. LeGuern E, Ravise N, Gouider R, et al. Microsatellite mapping of the deletion in patients with hereditary neuropathy with liability to pressure palsies (HNPP): new molecular tools for the study of the region 17p12→p11 and for diagnosis. Cytogenet Cell Genet 1996;72:20–25

72. Shaffer LG, Kennedy GM, Spikes AS, Lupski JR. Diagnosis of CMT1A duplications and HNPP deletions by interphase FISH: implications for testing in the cytogenetics laboratory. Am J Med Genet 1997;69:325–331

73. Kashork CD, Chen KS, Lupski JR, Shaffer LG. Prenatal diagnosis of Charcot–Marie–Tooth disease type 1A by interphase fluorescence in situ hybridization. Prenat Diagn 1999;19:446–449

74. Navon R, Timmerman V, Lofgren A, et al. Prenatal diagnosis of Charcot–Marie–Tooth disease type 1A (CMT1A) using molecular genetic techniques. Prenat Diagn 1995;15:633–640

75. Liebelt J, Parry G. Conservative management of hereditary neuropathy with liability to pressure palsies. http://www.hnpp.org/index.htm

76. Taggart TF, Allen TR. Surgical treatment of a tomaculous neuropathy. J R Coll Surg Edinb 2001;46:240–241

77. Gerritsen AA, Uitdehaag BM, van Geldere D, et al. Systematic review of randomized clinical trials of surgical treatment for carpal tunnel syndrome. Br J Surg 2001;88:1285–1295

78. Hai M, Bidichandani SI, Patel PI. Identification of a positive regulatory element in the myelin-specific promoter of the PMP22 gene. J Neurosci Res 2001;65:508–519

210 Hereditary Spinocerebellar Degeneration

John L Goudreau

Introduction

The inherited spinocerebellar ataxias are a heterogeneous group of disorders characterized by progressive cerebellar dysfunction associated with the loss of neurons in the cerebellum and its connections. Although manifestations of cerebellar disease predominate, there is often clinical and neuropathological evidence for involvement of the brainstem, spinal cord, basal ganglia, retina, and peripheral nervous system. Most adult-onset spinocerebellar ataxias are inherited in an autosomal dominant fashion and demonstrate considerable phenotypic variation among families. Ataxia due to autosomal recessive transmission, infection, toxins, and metabolic disorders is discussed elsewhere.

Adult-onset ataxia syndromes have been recognized as a distinct entity since Pierre Marie applied the term "hérédo-ataxie cérébelleuse" in 1893 to describe a group of cases that differed from Friedreich ataxia and demonstrated later onset, autosomal dominant inheritance, increased muscle stretch reflexes, and increased occurrence of ophthalmoplegia.[1] Various classification schemes, mainly pathological,

have been proposed and have created a confusing terminology, including Marie ataxia, cerebellar-olivary degeneration, olivopontocerebellar atrophy, and spinocerebellar atrophy.

Harding[2] proposed a cogent classification scheme for adult-onset autosomal dominant cerebellar ataxias (ADCAs). Patients with ADCA have in common the clinical manifestations of progressive cerebellar degeneration but are separated into ADCA types I, II, and III on the basis of other distinct clinical features. Additional features of supranuclear ophthalmoplegia, optic atrophy, extrapyramidal symptoms, dementia, and peripheral neuropathy or amyotrophy characterize ADCA-I. All cases of ADCA-II have associated retinal degeneration. ADCA-III comprises cases of pure cerebellar degeneration.

More recently, families with adult-onset ataxia have been recognized in terms of their specific genetic locus and identified as numerical subtypes of spinocerebellar ataxia (SCA) according to the order of gene discovery.[3,4] Currently, 16 subtypes of SCA are recognized (Table 210.1), with more likely to be identified in the future.[5] Although genetic classification is

Table 210.1   Genetic classification of autosomal dominant ataxias

SCA type	Gene locus	Gene product	Mutation	Allele size		Prevalence in ADCA, %
				Normal	Disease	
1	6p23	Ataxin-1	CAG expansion	6–36	42–81	3–15
2	12q24.1	Ataxin-2	CAG expansion	14–31	36–64	6–15
3	14q32.1	Ataxin-3	CAG expansion	13–41	61–85	30–40
4	16q22.1	Unknown	Unknown	NA	NA	7 families
5	11cen	Unknown	Unknown	NA	NA	2 families
6	19p13	Ca^{+2} channel	CAG expansion	6–20	21–30	5–15
7	3p12–13	Ataxin-7	CAG expansion	4–19	37–200+	2–5
8	13q21	Unknown	CTG expansion	16–37	100–152	1 family
10	22q13	Unknown	ATTCT expansion	10–22	1000–4500	5 families
11	15q14–21.3	Unknown	Unknown	NA	NA	1 family
12	5q31–33	PPP2R2B	CAG expansion	7–28	66–78	1 family
13	19q	TATA box binding protein	Unknown	NA	NA	1 family
14	19q	Unknown	Unknown	NA	NA	1 family
16	12p	Unknown	Unknown	NA	NA	1 family
DRPLA	12p13.31	Atrophin-1	CAG expansion	7–23	49–75	<1
EA-1	12p13	K$^+$ channel	Point	NA	NA	NA
EA-2	19p13	Ca^{+2} channel	Missense/truncate	NA	NA	NA

ADCA, autosomal dominant cerebellar ataxia; DRPLA, dentatorubropallidoluysian dystrophy; EA, episodic ataxia; PPP2R2B, brain-specific regulatory subunit of protein phosphatase 2 A; SCA, spinocerebellar ataxia.

Table 210.2   Causes of progressive cerebellar ataxia and potential diagnostic tests

Category/disease	Potential diagnostic test
Structural lesions	MRI
Stroke, AVM, primary and secondary	
neoplasm, foramen magnum compression	
Demyelinating disease	MRI, CSF analysis
Infectious/parainfectious	CSF analysis, viral serological testing
Rubella, CJD	
Immune-mediated	CSF analysis
Paraneoplastic	Purkinje cell; CRMP-5 and GAD-65 antibodies; systemic cancer work-up
Gluten-associated	Anti-gliadin antibodies, small-bowel biopsy
Metabolic	
Vitamin E deficiency	Vitamin E
Vitamin B_{12} deficiency	Vitamin B_{12}, CBC, peripheral blood smear
Hypothyroidism	TSH, free T_4
Inherited	
Autosomal recessive	
Friedreich ataxia	EMG/NCS, ECG, specific gene test
Wilson disease	Ceruloplasmin, urine copper, slit-lamp exam
Ataxia-telangiectasia	Alpha-fetoprotein, IgA
Refsum disease	Phytanic acid
GM_2 gangliosidosis	Hexosaminidase A
Xeroderma pigmentosum	
Cockayne syndrome	
Mitochondrial	EMG, lactic acid, muscle biopsy, mitochondrial DNA testing
Drugs/toxins	Toxicology screen
Chronic alcohol, anti-epileptic drugs, thallium	

AVM, arteriovenous malformation; CBC, complete blood count; CJD, Creutzfeldt-Jakob disease; CRMP-5, collapsin-response mediator protein-5; CSF, cerebrospinal fluid; ECG, electrocardiography; EMG, electromyography; MRI, magnetic resonance imaging; NCS, nerve conduction study; T_4, thyroxine; TSH, thyroid-stimulating hormone.

the "gold standard," this approach has practical limitations. Specifically, there is substantial overlap between the SCA phenotypes and often striking heterogeneity of symptoms among family members with identical genetic mutations.

Although the clinical ADCA scheme and genetic SCA scheme are not completely coherent, there are some common threads. For example, features of SCAs 1, 2, 3, and 4 correspond to the clinical category of ADCA-I. In addition, all ADCA-II families with pigmentary retinal degeneration carry the SCA-7 mutation. Finally, SCAs 5, 6, and perhaps 11 present with an almost pure cerebellar syndrome, which would be classified as ADCA-III. The other SCA phenotypes are too variable or have not been characterized to the extent that would allow the assignment of a corresponding clinical ADCA type.

Epidemiology

Ataxia is a common neurological presenting symptom and has an extensive list of potential causes (Table 210.2). Familial adult-onset spinocerebellar degeneration is less common than sporadic ataxia, with an estimated incidence of 5 in 100 000.[2,6] However, apparent sporadic cases may have a genetic basis due to spontaneous mutations, subclinical disease in ancestors, or an incomplete or inaccurate family history (e.g., adoption, nonpaternity). Genetic mutations are found in as many as 19% of patients with adult-onset ataxia

without a family history of the disease.[7] SCA-3 is the most common spinocerebellar degeneration syndrome, comprising approximately one-third of dominantly inherited cases (Table 210.1). SCA-2 is the second most common spinocerebellar degenerative disorder and accounts for about 12% of familial cases.[8] The prevalence seems to parallel the relative size of the normal allele range in a population, suggesting that a large normal allele is a risk factor for further expansion of trinucleotide repeats (TNRs).[9]

Pathophysiology and genetics

Varying degrees of cerebellar, brainstem, and spinocerebellar tract atrophy are observed in all cases of spinocerebellar degeneration. The regional distribution of atrophy typically corresponds to the clinical manifestations.[10] The combination of cerebellar degeneration with prominent loss of neurons in the pons and inferior olivary nucleus defines the pathological subtype of olivopontocerebellar atrophy. Other forms of spinocerebellar degeneration demonstrate atrophy and cell loss within the basal ganglia, brainstem motor nuclei, spinal cord, and retina. Gliosis and neuronal loss, particularly of cerebellar Purkinje cells, are common histopathological findings. Intranuclear and cytoplasmic inclusion bodies may be observed (Figure 210.1).

Many of the dominantly inherited SCA syndromes are associated with expansion of a TNR motif, often

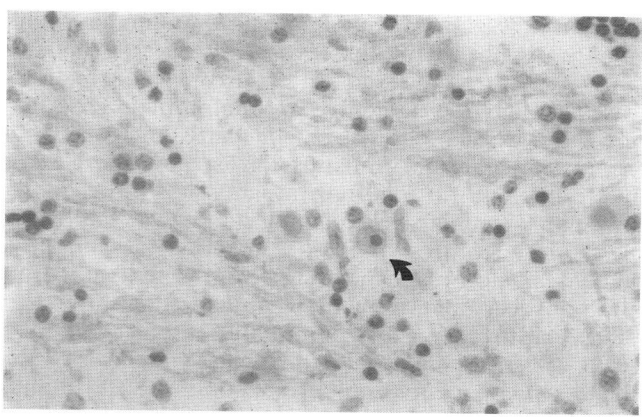

Figure 210.1 Histopathological findings in spinocerebellar ataxia-3. Note neuronal loss, gliosis, and ubiquitin-immunoreactive neuronal intranuclear inclusion body (*arrow*). (Basal pons immunostained with anti-ubiquitin antibody and counterstained with hematoxylin-eosin; ×100.) (Courtesy of Brent Clark, M.D., University of Minnesota.) (See color plate section.)

within the 5' coding region of a gene (Table 210.1). A wide variety of disparate SCA genes, of largely unknown function, harbor DNA sequences prone to expansion. Expansion of the CAG triplet, which codes for the amino acid glutamine, is the mutation seen in many SCAs. Disease occurs when the TNR expansion in the mutated allele exceeds that of the normal range.[11] The mechanism underlying TNR expansion is not completely understood, but it is thought to involve abnormal secondary structures in DNA sequences containing TNRs (e.g., hairpin loops and triplexes) in combination with resultant problems with gap and mismatch repair systems.[12,13]

A clearer understanding of the cascade of pathological events leading from TNR expansion to disease is evolving. In the case of CAG repeats, the expanded polyglutamine tract is clearly involved in toxicity. Polyglutamine regions, especially when increased in size, self associate and begin to form insoluble aggregates. These aggregates are found in the neuronal nuclear and cytoplasmic inclusions seen in pathologically affected areas of the brain. Polyglutamine aggregation could cause disease by sequestering critical cytoplasmic or nuclear targets.[14] Alternatively, the "toxic peptide" hypothesis proposes that cleavage of the expanded polyglutamine regions releases pathogenic peptide fragments that initiate the pathways leading to cell death.[15]

TNR expansion is often associated with the phenomenon of genetic anticipation, in which successive generations develop a more severe disease phenotype at an earlier age at onset (Figure 210.2).[16,17] In this non-mendelian form of inheritance, the number of repeats is unstable and can increase with subsequent generations. As the TNR number grows, the increased size of the gene product confers greater aberrant pathological properties, resulting in accelerated cell death. There is a correlation between the number of TNRs and the age at onset as well as phenotypic severity.

The length of TNRs accounts for only part of the variability, and other modifying genes and environmental factors must also have a role. Thus, the number of repeats cannot accurately predict disease onset or severity in a particular patient.

The frequency and degree of expansion are often greater when the disease allele is transmitted from the father to offspring. The exact mechanism of this paternal effect is not known but may be due to meiotic instability of TNR during gametogenesis.[12]

Clinical features

SCA-1 often presents in adulthood (fourth to fifth decades) with dysarthria, ataxia of gait and limbs, and variable muscle wasting of the lower extremities. In patients with SCA-1, Orr et al.[18] identified an expanded CAG repeat motif on chromosome 6p23 that encodes for a novel protein designated ataxin-1. Additional signs of pyramidal tract involvement, including hyperreflexia, extensor plantar responses, and increased muscle tone, may be present in the lower extremities. Late manifestations include dystonia, choreoathetosis, and mild sensory deficits such as reduced proprioception. Magnetic resonance imaging (MRI) of the brain typically shows cerebellar cortical and vermian atrophy, with mild occasional brainstem atrophy.[19]

The average age at onset of SCA-2 is 30 years (range, 16 to 58 years).[20] The common clinical features include truncal ataxia, dysarthria, slow saccades, supranuclear ophthalmoparesis, and optic nerve atrophy. Peripheral sensory neuropathy, fasciculations of facial muscles, dysphagia, dystonia, dementia, pyramidal tract signs, or decreased muscle stretch reflexes have been noted in fewer than 50% of patients. MRI findings are similar to those of SCA-1, and pathology studies in both SCA-1 and SCA-2 demonstrate severe loss of cerebellar Purkinje cells and degeneration of the olivocerebellar pathways.[19]

SCA-3 presents with gait and limb ataxia, along

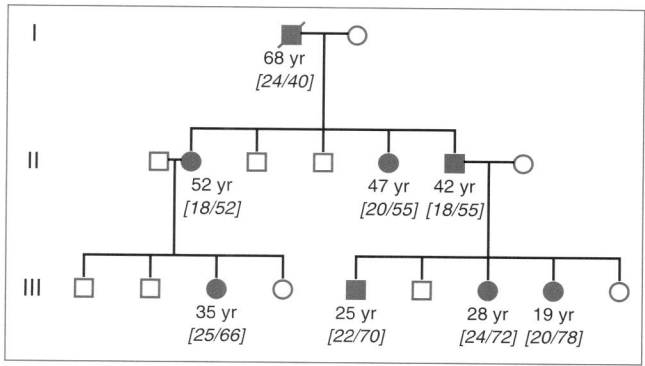

Figure 210.2 Autosomal dominant pedigree demonstrating genetic anticipation and repeat expansion. A representative three-generation pedigree is shown for a family with spinocerebellar ataxia. Squares, males; circles, females. Filled symbols represent affected individuals. Age at symptom onset in years; number of trinucleotide repeat units for each allele are in brackets.

with dysarthria and gaze palsy. This disorder was first described in a family that emigrated to the United States from the Portuguese Azores and was initially identified as Machado-Joseph disease (MJD), after the family name.[21] SCA-3 and MJD are allelic, meaning that both disorders result from expansion of CAG repeats in the 3' end of the ataxin-3 gene located on chromosome 14q32.1.[22] The clinical manifestations and age at onset of SCA-3/MJD are variable and depend on the size of TNR expansion. Patients with repeat lengths greater than 74 have early onset of disease (before age 30) and have additional features of pyramidal and extrapyramidal involvement. Patients with repeat lengths of less than 71 have later onset of disease (after age 40) and have signs of peripheral neuropathy.[19,23] The MJD phenotype may have distinct features of dystonia, facial and lingual fasciculations, and lid retraction.

SCA-4 was described in a large kindred presenting with progressive ataxia beginning in the fourth to fifth decades. Additional features include extensor plantar responses, decreased muscle stretch reflexes, and peripheral sensory neuropathy. Dysarthria or oculomotor dysfunction develops in less than half of the affected family members. The causative gene for SCA-4 is localized to chromosome 16q22.1, but the precise nature of the mutation is not known.[24]

SCA-5 and SCA-6 present with an almost pure cerebellar syndrome characterized by gait and limb ataxia, nystagmus, and dysarthria. Disease onset in SCA-5 varies between 10 and 68 years. Bulbar involvement has been noted in two cases. The gene for SCA-5 has been localized to the pericentromeric region of chromosome 11, but no candidate gene has been identified.[25]

The relatively late onset of progressive ataxia and dysarthria seen in SCA-6 is distinct (mean age at onset, 52 years). Otherwise, the clinical features are similar to those of SCA-5, but patients occasionally have additional features of posterior column and pyramidal tract involvement. The frequency of SCA-6 may be increased in Japanese populations, but it has been documented in various other populations, too. A relatively short CAG expansion in the coding region of the voltage-gated calcium channel has been identified in families with SCA-6.[26] Mutations in this same gene have been identified in familial hemiplegic migraine and episodic ataxia type 2.[27] The CAG repeat in SCA-6 appears to be relatively stable and less prone to further expansion. As a result, anticipation is not a common feature of SCA-6. Sporadic cases have been documented, and the frequency of SCA-6 mutations in cases of ataxia without a family history is significant. Therefore, SCA-6 should be considered in sporadic cases of late-onset ataxia.[7]

CAG expansion in exon 3 of the SCA-7 gene, located on chromosome 3q12–13, is found in all families with the ADCA-II phenotype. The clinical onset, usually with progressive loss of vision, can occur at any age between birth and 65 years. Progressive retinal degeneration and pigmented macular dystrophy are distinguishing features of SCA-7 and are typically followed by ataxia of gait, limb movements, and speech. With early onset cases, decreased muscle stretch reflexes and sensory loss can develop. Rare cases can include dementia, ophthalmoplegia, nystagmus, dyskinesia, chorea, or spasticity. Increased frequency of maternal transmission is a unique genetic feature of SCA-7. Paternal transmission, however, is associated with larger expansions and anticipation.[28]

Clinical features of SCA-8 include gait and limb ataxia, ataxic or spastic dysarthria, and nystagmus, with onset of symptoms between ages 18 and 65. In a single family, SCA-8 is potentially associated with a CTG expansion in the 3' untranslated region of the ataxin-8 gene located on chromosome 13q21.[29] Symptomatic carriers in this family have CTG expansions in a range (107 to 127 repeats) and demonstrate contraction of repeat size with paternal transmission, along with a bias toward expansion with maternal transmission. These features are similar to those of myotonic dystrophy, a disorder that is also associated with a CTG expansion. SCA-8, however, does not have the myriad of systemic symptoms observed in myotonic dystrophy.

An autosomal dominant ataxia, primarily in several Mexican families, has been localized to chromosome 22q13 and identified as SCA-10. The clinical phenotype is predominantly signs and symptoms of cerebellar dysfunction. Several patients with SCA-10 experienced seizures, but it is unclear if this is part of the disease process or is due to other causes. The age at onset is 26 to 45 years, and there is clinical and genetic evidence for anticipation. Expansion of a unique pentanucleotide repeat-containing sequence (ATTCT) has been identified in intron 9 of the SCA-10 gene in these families.[30]

SCA-11, a relatively benign autosomal dominant ataxia, has been linked to chromosome 15q14–21.3 in one British family. Affected individuals show an isolated, slowly progressive ataxic syndrome similar to SCA-5 and SCA-6, with disease onset from age 15 to 55 and a normal lifespan.[31]

SCA-12 exhibits onset of symptoms in the fourth decade of life (range, 8 to 55 years). This disease has been described in a single large family and is likely a very rare cause of spinocerebellar degeneration. Initial symptoms include postural tremor, ataxia of gait and limb movement, and nystagmus. Other features include ophthalmoparesis and increased muscle stretch reflexes. This disorder results from a CAG expansion in the 5' promoter region of a gene that encodes for a brain-specific regulatory subunit of protein phosphatase 2A (PPP2R2B).[32]

Four other novel autosomal dominant spinocerebellar degeneration syndromes have been described recently in Japanese families. SCA-13, SCA-14, and SCA-16 have been localized to chromosomes 19q, 19q13.4-qter, and 8q22.1–24.1, respectively. The specific mutation or causative genes have not been identified. SCA-13 presents with cerebellar ataxia in combination with mental retardation.[33] Patients with late-onset (older than 39 years) SCA-14 have a pure cerebellar syndrome, whereas those with early onset (younger than 27 years) have intermittent axial myoclonus, followed by cerebellar ataxia.[34] Patients with SCA-16 have cerebellar ataxia plus head tremor, with onset of disease from 20 to 66 years.[35]

Dentatorubropallidoluysian atrophy (DRPLA) can also present as spinocerebellar degeneration but often in combination with dementia, parkinsonism, chorea, and myoclonic epilepsy, with disease onset in young patients. This disorder is more common in patients of Asian/Japanese descent, accounting for as many as 20% of cases of autosomal dominant ataxia.[9] DRPLA has also been identified in other populations, for example, the Haw River syndrome in North America.[36] A CAG expansion in the atrophin gene located on chromosome 12 has been identified in patients with DRPLA.[37]

Episodic ataxias may sometimes present as a progressive spinocerebellar degeneration syndrome in the context of acute exacerbations of ataxia. Two forms of episodic ataxia have been identified, each with unique clinical and genetic features.[38] Type 1 presents with episodic, brief ataxia, and dysarthria, often precipitated by exercise or startle. Myokymia of the face or hands may be present interictally or during attacks. Patients harbor point mutations in the voltage-gated potassium channel gene located on chromosome 12p13.[39] Type 2 can present with intermittent ataxia, dysarthria, vertigo, diplopia, and oscillopsia lasting from a few minutes up to 72 hours and may be precipitated by emotional stress and exercise. Gaze-evoked nystagmus is frequently observed between attacks in type-2 episodic ataxia. A missense or truncating mutation in the voltage-gated calcium channel is found in patients with type-2 episodic ataxia. As noted above, mutations in this same calcium channel gene are found in SCA-6 and familial hemiplegic migraine.[27] Unlike other spinocerebellar ataxias, the condition of patients with type-1 or type-2 episodic ataxia may improve with phenytoin or acetazolamide, respectively.[40,41]

Diagnostic process and criteria and differential diagnosis

Initially, MRI of the brain and testing for other causes of spinocerebellar degeneration should be pursued (Table 210.2). The history and physical examination provide the focus and direction for the work-up. For example, subacute onset of ataxia and weight loss should direct the clinician toward possible paraneoplastic causes. If no cause is uncovered, genetic testing is warranted, especially in patients with a positive family history. Genetic testing should also be considered when the family history is unavailable or ambiguous. If there is no clear family history, then testing for Friedreich ataxia and SCA-6 (when commercially available) could be considered. Nerve conduction studies and electromyography may provide useful clues when there is evidence for involvement of peripheral motor or sensory nerves.

The intrafamilial heterogeneity and overlap of symptoms between the SCA genotypes pose considerable problems for differentiating or classifying the various SCAs on the basis of clinical or laboratory findings.[19,42,43] Genetic testing for the specific mutation, where available, is the optimal approach to make a specific diagnosis. Although a positive finding on gene testing yields an unequivocal diagnosis, a negative test result has little value beyond exclusion of the specific SCA entity. A single SCA diagnostic test costs approximately $300, and tests are commercially available for SCA-1, 2, 3, 4, 6, 7, and 8 and DRPLA (see www.genetests.org for latest test availability). The cost of individual tests may be less if run on a panel. However, blanket testing for all available gene mutations in every patient with spinocerebellar degeneration may not be feasible or cost-effective.

Clinical clues may suggest a specific genotype and guide selection of specific genetic tests rather than testing an entire panel (Table 210.3).[44,45] Prominent visual loss and retinopathy suggest SCA-7. Nearly pure cerebellar syndromes and absence of other features are seen in SCA-5, 6, 8, and 11. Onset at age older than 50 and normal lifespan are characteristic of SCA-6 and SCA-11. Prominent ocular motility problems are observed in SCA-1, 2, 3, and 7, with bulging eyes and lid retraction in the MJD phenotype of SCA-3. Prominent sensory neuropathy is seen in SCA-4 and amyotrophy can be seen in SCA-1, 2, and 3. Decreased muscle stretch reflexes are seen in SCA-2, 3, and 4, whereas increased reflexes or other pyramidal tract signs are present in SCA-1, 3, and 12. Dementia may be observed in SCA-2 and SCA-7, and mental retardation is notable in SCA-13. Chorea and myoclonus may suggest DRPLA. Seizures may be seen in DRPLA and perhaps SCA-7 and 10. An algorithm for choosing genetic tests is presented in Figure 210.3.

Genetic counseling is an important component of the diagnostic process when inherited ataxias are considered. With the wide range of onset for most of the autosomal dominant ataxias, the risk for offspring of affected individuals does not diminish until late in life. Also, no effective disease-modifying treatment is available. Thus, many at-risk patients will contemplate life and childbearing decisions before they can be certain whether they will be affected by the disease. With these issues in mind, genetic testing should be offered to adults in the context of formal genetic counseling or a presymptomatic testing program. Typically, these approaches are carried out over several sessions and include genetic counseling, psychological assessments, and follow-up. Discussions should include issues of job and insurance discrimination, confidentiality, and possible psychological reactions to either positive or negative test results.

Treatment

Currently, no definitive treatment is available to alter the natural history of inherited spinocerebellar degeneration. Therapeutic modalities are focused on supportive care and physical rehabilitation of symptoms. However, several potential disease-modifying treatments are being considered on the basis of advances

Table 210.3   Clinical and diagnostic clues to spinocerebellar ataxia genotypes

Clinical feature	Suggested genotype	Diagnostic features	Suggested genotype
Age at onset		**MRI features**	
Child (<10 years)	7, 13, DRPLA	Cerebellar + olivopontine atrophy	1, 2
Young (<20 years)	1, 2, 3	Cerebellar + brainstem atrophy	3, 7
Old (>55 years)	6	Pure cerebellar atrophy	5, 6, 8, 11
Prominent anticipation	7, DRPLA		
Normal lifespan	6, 11		
Retinopathy	7	**Neurophysiological features**	
Slow saccades/ophthalmoplegia		Decreased NCV	1, 2, 3, rarely 6
Early	2, 7	Reduced SNAP	1, 2, 3, rarely 6
Late	1, 3	Absent SNAP	4
Lid retraction/bulging eyes	2, 3		
Sensory neuropathy	4		
Reduced muscle stretch reflexes	2, 3, 4		
Amyotrophy	1, 2, 3		
Pyramidal signs	1, 3, 12		
Extrapyramidal signs	1, 3, 7, 12 (rarely 2, 6, 8)		
Chorea	2, DRPLA		
Dementia	2, 7, DRPLA		
Mental retardation	13		
Seizure	7, 10, DRPLA		
Postural tremor	12, 16		
Myoclonus	2, 14, DRPLA		

DRPLA, dentatorubropallidoluysian atrophy; MRI, magnetic resonance imaging; NCV, nerve conduction velocity; SNAP, sensory nerve action potential.

in the understanding of the molecular pathology of spinocerebellar degeneration (Table 210.4). Testing of any potential intervention will be fostered by the development of a unified clinical rating scale for ataxia.[46]

The strong dependence of disease character on repeat length has raised the possibility of stopping expansion at the DNA level as an effective therapeutic strategy. Recent animal studies suggest that age-dependent expansion occurs in somatic tissues, particularly the brain.[47] This raises the possibility that ongoing, age-dependent TNR expansion may be responsible for disease progression. Therefore, one approach would be to target the DNA polymerases and repair proteins believed to be involved in DNA expansion. If successful, prevention of further expansion could prevent disease progression and diminish severity.

Mutation analysis and transgenic animal models have unequivocally identified the expanded polyglutamine protein as a key to the disease process.[17] Targeting the expanded polyglutamine protein and inhibition of the downstream cascade of pathological events offer further avenues for intervention. Prevention of protein aggregation or methods to increase proteosomal clearance of expanded polyglutamines could significantly alter the degenerative process. Also, several downstream cellular processes are suspected to be altered by polyglutamine-dependent aggregation and could be used as therapeutic targets. Potential strategies include the following: 1) replenishing mitochondrial energy metabolism lost because of oxidative stress (creatine, coenzyme Q_{10}),[48] 2) inhibiting glutamate-mediated excitotoxicity (lamotrigine, remacemide, riluzole),[49] 3) inhibiting apoptosis

Table 210.4   Potential therapeutic interventions in spinocerebellar ataxia

Proposed pathological mechanism	Target or specific intervention
DNA expansion	DNA polymerases and repair proteins
DNA expression	Promoter antisense oligonucleotides
Polyglutamine aggregation	Polyglutamine antibodies, anti-aggregation factors
Mitochondria energy defects	Creatine, coenzyme Q_{10}
Excitotoxicity	Glutamate receptor or release antagonists
Apoptosis	Caspase inhibitors
Growth factors	Recombinant growth factors (BDNF, CNTF)
Calcium channelopathies (SCA-6, EA-2)	Phenytoin, acetazolamide, flunarizine

BDNF, brain-derived neurotrophic factor; CNTF, ciliary neurotrophic factor; EA, episodic ataxia; SCA, spinocerebellar ataxia.

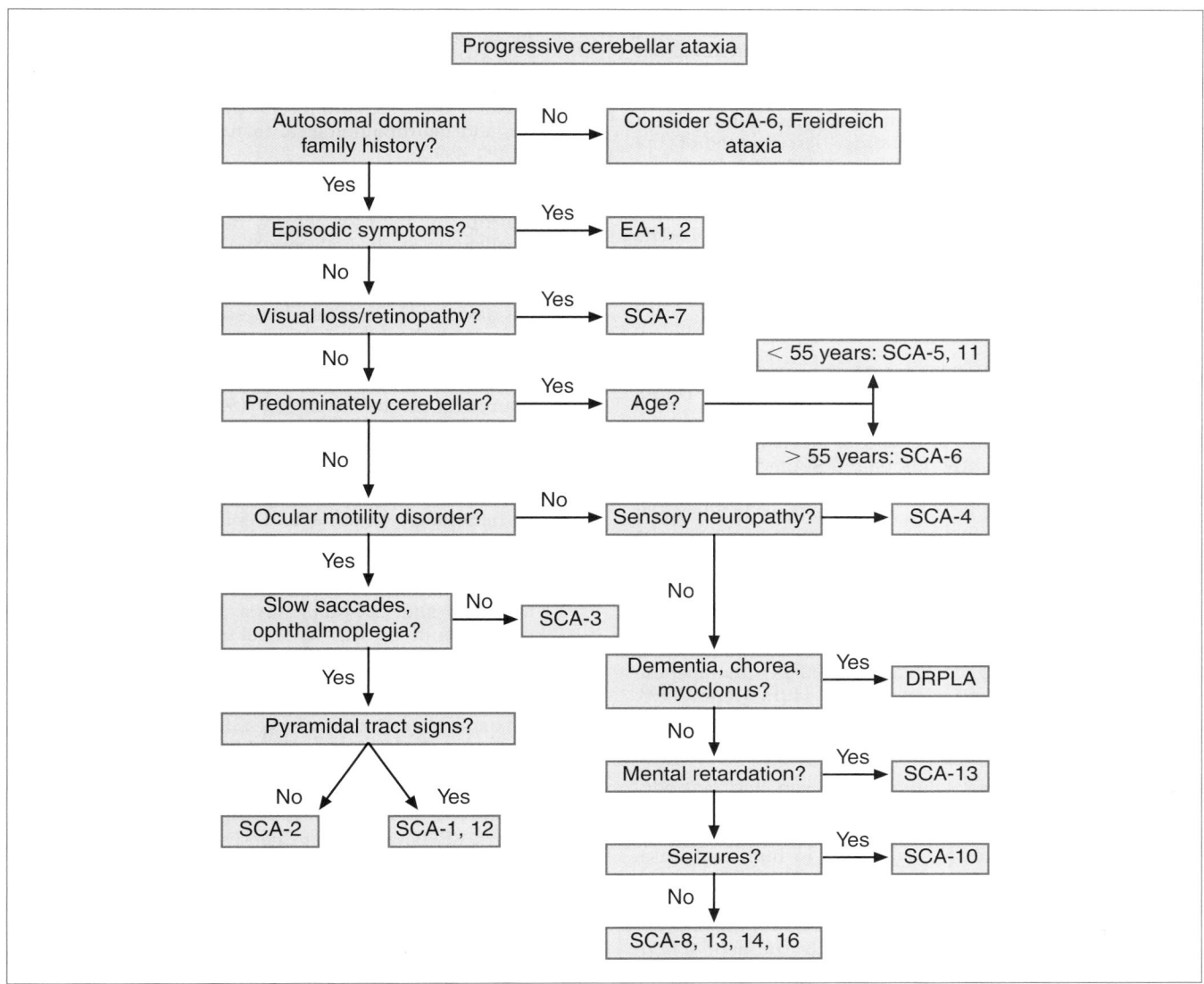

Figure 210.3 Algorithm for selecting specific spinocerebellar ataxia (SCA) subtypes on the basis of clinical features. DRPLA, dentatorubropallidoluysian atrophy; EA-1 and EA-2, episodic ataxia types 1 and 2.

and caspases (minocycline),[50] and 4) supplementing nerve growth factors (brain-derived neurotrophic factor).[51,52] Although appealing from a theoretical standpoint, the effectiveness of the above approaches has not been evaluated in controlled clinical trials.

An ideal approach might seek to eliminate entirely the expression of the mutant protein before any toxicity occurs by using a compound that inhibits protein expression from the mutant allele. This strategy would need to target selectively the mutant allele, because the normal allele is often necessary for cell survival. Attempts at antigene treatments using antisense oligonucleotides have been limited to cell cultures.[53,54] Although gene therapy is immature, recent studies in an animal model of Huntington disease demonstrated that selective inhibition of polyglutamine protein expression from a mutant, expanded allele can reverse the pathological phenotype present in mutant animals.[55] This provides proof of the prin-

ciple that specific inhibition of an expanded TNR allele can reverse the disease process. This antigene strategy has not been reproduced in animal models of spinocerebellar degeneration, and human trials are in the distant future, at best. The identification and delivery of a small molecule that can effectively and specifically inhibit the expanded TNR allele in vivo remain a daunting task.

In most cases, carriers of the expanded TNR alleles encountered in spinocerebellar degeneration can be identified long before clinical symptoms develop. Early detection and relatively late onset of disease render patients with inherited spinocerebellar degeneration particularly suitable for disease-modifying intervention. Although definitive therapy is not yet possible, the rapid advance in the understanding of basic disease mechanisms is leading to expanded approaches to effective therapy for spinocerebellar degeneration.

References

1. Marie P. Sur l'hérédo-ataxie cérébelleuse. Semaine Méd Paris 1893;13:444–447
2. Harding AE. The clinical features and classification of the late onset autosomal dominant cerebellar ataxias: a study of 11 families, including descendants of the "Drew family of Walworth." Brain 1982;105:1–28
3. Evidente VG, Gwinn-Hardy KA, Caviness JN, Gilman S. Hereditary ataxias. Mayo Clin Proc 2000;75:475–490
4. Klockgether T, Wullner U, Spauschus A, Evert B. The molecular biology of the autosomal-dominant cerebellar ataxias. Mov Disord 2000;15:604–612
5. Subramony SH, Filla A. Autosomal dominant spinocerebellar ataxias ad infinitum? (Editorial). Neurology 2001;56:287–289
6. Konigsmark BW, Weiner LP. The olivopontocerebellar atrophies: a review. Medicine (Baltimore) 1970;49:227–241
7. Schols L, Szymanski S, Peters S, et al. Genetic background of apparently idiopathic sporadic cerebellar ataxia. Hum Genet 2000;107:132–137
8. Moseley ML, Benzow KA, Schut LJ, et al. Incidence of dominant spinocerebellar and Friedreich triplet repeats among 361 ataxia families. Neurology 1998;51:1666–1671
9. Takano H, Cancel G, Ikeuchi T, et al. Close associations between prevalences of dominantly inherited spinocerebellar ataxias with CAG-repeat expansions and frequencies of large normal CAG alleles in Japanese and Caucasian populations. Am J Hum Genet 1998;63:1060–1066
10. Gilman S. The spinocerebellar ataxias. Clin Neuropharmacol 2000;23:296–303
11. Zoghbi HY, Orr HT. Glutamine repeats and neurodegeneration. Annu Rev Neurosci 2000;23:217–247
12. McMurray CT. DNA secondary structure: a common and causative factor for expansion in human disease. Proc Natl Acad Sci USA 1999;96:1823–1825
13. McMurray CT. Huntington's disease: new hope for therapeutics. Trends Neurosci 2001;24(Suppl):S32–S38
14. Takahashi J, Tanaka J, Arai K, et al. Recruitment of nonexpanded polyglutamine proteins to intranuclear aggregates in neuronal intranuclear hyaline inclusion disease. J Neuropathol Exp Neurol 2001;60:369–376
15. Gusella JF, MacDonald ME. Molecular genetics: unmasking polyglutamine triggers in neurodegenerative disease. Nat Rev Neurosci 2000;1:109–115
16. Zoghbi HY. Spinocerebellar ataxias. Neurobiol Dis 2000;7:523–527
17. Orr HT. Beyond the Qs in the polyglutamine diseases. Genes Dev 2001;15:925–932
18. Orr HT, Chung MY, Banfi S, et al. Expansion of an unstable trinucleotide CAG repeat in spinocerebellar ataxia type 1. Nat Genet 1993;4:221–226
19. Schols L, Amoiridis G, Buttner T, et al. Autosomal dominant cerebellar ataxia: phenotypic differences in genetically defined subtypes? Ann Neurol 1997;42:924–932
20. Geschwind DH, Perlman S, Figueroa CP, et al. The prevalence and wide clinical spectrum of the spinocerebellar ataxia type 2 trinucleotide repeat in patients with autosomal dominant cerebellar ataxia. Am J Hum Genet 1997;60:842–850
21. Nakano KK, Dawson DM, Spence A. Machado disease: a hereditary ataxia in Portuguese emigrants to Massachusetts. Neurology 1972;22:49–55
22. Twist EC, Casaubon LK, Ruttledge MH, et al. Machado

Joseph disease maps to the same region of chromosome 14 as the spinocerebellar ataxia type 3 locus. J Med Genet 1995;32:25–31
23. Durr A, Stevanin G, Cancel G, et al. Spinocerebellar ataxia 3 and Machado-Joseph disease: clinical, molecular, and neuropathological features. Ann Neurol 1996;39:490–499
24. Flanigan K, Gardner K, Alderson K, et al. Autosomal dominant spinocerebellar ataxia with sensory axonal neuropathy (SCA4): clinical description and genetic localization to chromosome 16q22.1. Am J Hum Genet 1996;59:392–399
25. Ranum LP, Schut LJ, Lundgren JK, et al. Spinocerebellar ataxia type 5 in a family descended from the grandparents of President Lincoln maps to chromosome 11. Nat Genet 1994;8:280–284
26. Zhuchenko O, Bailey J, Bonnen P, et al. Autosomal dominant cerebellar ataxia (SCA6) associated with small polyglutamine expansions in the alpha 1A-voltage-dependent calcium channel. Nat Genet 1997;15:62–69
27. Ophoff RA, Terwindt GM, Vergouwe MN, et al. Familial hemiplegic migraine and episodic ataxia type-2 are caused by mutations in the Ca^{2+} channel gene CACNL1A4. Cell 1996;87:543–552
28. David G, Durr A, Stevanin G, et al. Familial hemiplegic migraine and episodic ataxia type-2 are caused by mutations in the Ca^{2+} channel gene CACNL1A4. Hum Mol Genet 1998;7:165–170
29. Koob MD, Moseley ML, Schut LJ, et al. An untranslated CTG expansion causes a novel form of spinocerebellar ataxia (SCA8). Nat Genet 1999;21:379–384
30. Matsuura T, Yamagata T, Burgess DL, et al. Large expansion of the ATTCT pentanucleotide repeat in spinocerebellar ataxia type 10. Nat Genet 2000;26:191–194
31. Worth PF, Giunti P, Gardner-Thorpe C, et al. Autosomal dominant cerebellar ataxia type III: linkage in a large British family to a 7.6-cM region on chromosome 15q14–21.3. Am J Hum Genet 1999;65:420–426
32. O'Hearn E, Holmes SE, Calvert PC, et al. SCA-12: tremor with cerebellar and cortical atrophy is associated with a CAG repeat expansion. Neurology 2001;56:299–303
33. Herman-Bert A, Stevanin G, Netter JC, et al. Mapping of spinocerebellar ataxia 13 to chromosome 19q13.3-q13.4 in a family with autosomal dominant cerebellar ataxia and mental retardation. Am J Hum Genet 2000;67:229–235
34. Yamashita I, Sasaki H, Yabe I, et al. A novel locus for dominant cerebellar ataxia (SCA14) maps to a 10.2-cM interval flanked by D19S206 and D19S605 on chromosome 19q13.4-qter. Ann Neurol 2000;48:156–163
35. Miyoshi Y, Yamada T, Tanimura M, et al. A novel autosomal dominant spinocerebellar ataxia (SCA16) linked to chromosome 8q22.1–24.1. Neurology 2001;57:96–100
36. Burke JR, Wingfield MS, Lewis KE, et al. The Haw River syndrome: dentatorubropallidoluysian atrophy (DRPLA) in an African-American family. Nat Genet 1994;7:521–524
37. Nagafuchi S, Yanagisawa H, Sato K, et al. Dentatorubral and pallidoluysian atrophy expansion of an unstable CAG trinucleotide on chromosome 12p. Nat Genet 1994;6:14–18
38. Brandt T, Strupp M. Episodic ataxia type 1 and 2 (familial periodic ataxia/vertigo). Audiol Neurootol 1997;2:373–383
39. Browne DL, Gancher ST, Nutt JG, et al. Episodic

ataxia/myokymia syndrome is associated with point mutations in the human potassium channel gene, *KCNA1*. Nat Genet 1994;8:136–140

40. Vaamonde J, Artieda J, Obeso JA. Hereditary paroxysmal ataxia with neuromyotonia. Mov Disord 1991;6: 180–182

41. Koller W, Bahamon-Dussan J. Hereditary paroxysmal cerebellopathy: responsiveness to acetazolamide. Clin Neuropharmacol 1987;10:65–68

42. Klockgether T, Dichgans J. Genotype-phenotype correlation in spinocerebellar ataxias (SCA). Electroencephalogr Clin Neurophysiol Suppl 1999;50:195–201

43. Schelhaas HJ, Ippel PF, Beemer FA, Hageman G. Similarities and differences in the phenotype, genotype and pathogenesis of different spinocerebellar ataxias. Eur J Neurol 2000;7:309–314

44. Subramony SH, Vig PJ, McDaniel DO. Dominantly inherited ataxias. Semin Neurol 1999;19:419–425

45. Tan EK, Ashizawa T. Genetic testing in spinocerebellar ataxias: defining a clinical role. Arch Neurol 2001;58: 191–195

46. Trouillas P, Takayanagi T, Hallett M, et al. International Cooperative Ataxia Rating Scale for pharmacological assessment of the cerebellar syndrome. The Ataxia Neuropharmacology Committee of the World Federation of Neurology. J Neurol Sci 1997;145:205–211

47. Kovtun IV, McMurray CT. Trinucleotide expansion in haploid germ cells by gap repair. Nat Genet 2001;27: 407–411

48. Ferrante RJ, Andreassen OA, Jenkins BG, et al. Neuroprotective effects of creatine in a transgenic mouse model of Huntington's disease. J Neurosci 2000;20: 4389–4397

49. Kieburtz K. Antiglutamate therapies in Huntington's disease. J Neural Transm Suppl 1999;55:97–102

50. Chen M, Ona VO, Li M, et al. Minocycline inhibits caspase-1 and caspase-3 expression and delays mortality in a transgenic mouse model of Huntington disease. Nat Med 2000;6:797–801

51. Perez-Navarro E, Canudas AM, Akerund P, et al. Brain-derived neurotrophic factor, neurotrophin-3, and neurotrophin-4/5 prevent the death of striatal projection neurons in a rodent model of Huntington's disease. J Neurochem 2000;75:2190–2199

52. Zuccato C, Ciammola A, Rigamonti D, et al. Loss of Huntington-mediated BDNF gene transcription in Huntington's disease. Science 2001;293:493–498

53. Haque N, Isacson O. Antisense gene therapy for neurodegenerative disease? Exp Neurol 1997;144:139–146

54. Boado RJ, Kazantsev A, Apostol BL, et al. Antisense-mediated down-regulation of the human huntingtin gene. J Pharmacol Exp Ther 2000;295:239–243

55. Yamamoto A, Lucas JJ, Hen R. Reversal of neuropathology and motor dysfunction in a conditional model of Huntington's disease. Cell 2000;101:57–66

211 Motor Neuron Diseases

Anthony J Windebank

Introduction

Several diseases are characterized by the selective and progressive loss of upper or lower motor neurons. Although the clinical presentation and age at onset vary, they form various characteristic patterns. The clinical features and pattern of inheritance have determined the classification of the disorders. In most cases, the pathological features are not distinctive. There is simple loss of motor neurons, and the pathological features have not been used extensively as a basis for classification. Several potential mechanisms for motor neuron loss have been proposed recently.

Pathogenesis of motor neuron diseases

The mechanism of cell loss in motor neuron disease is not known. Evidence from tissue culture, transgenic mouse, and human models indicates that three abnormalities may converge and result in motor neuron death: glutamate toxicity, disordered neurofilament structure, and oxidative stress. Other potential mechanisms include loss of trophic factor function, DNA damage, and disruption of energy metabolism in motor neurons.

Rothstein et al.[1] demonstrated specific loss of the glial glutamate transporter (GLT-1 or GLAST) in the brains and spinal cords of patients with amyotrophic lateral sclerosis (ALS). This observation was confirmed by others.[2] Drugs that block glutamate toxicity (riluzole and gabapentin) have produced small benefit in ALS[3,4] and in animal models.[5,6]

A role for oxidative stress in familial ALS was suggested when a linked mutation in copper-zinc superoxide dismutase (SOD) was identified by Rosen et al.[7] Many other mutations have now been identified in SOD,[8] and overexpression of this mutation in mice produces a motor neuron disease with features resembling those of human ALS. The mechanism by which this mutation leads to motor neuron death is debated but probably involves a toxic gain of function. This may result in hydroxyl radical formation, nitration of protein tyrosine residues, protein aggregation, or copper-zinc toxicity. There is evidence for all of these occurring in the animal model.[9] Increased formation of 3-nitrotyrosine has been demonstrated in the cerebrospinal fluid (CSF) and spinal cords of ALS patients[10-12] and G73R SOD mutant mice.[13] However, Bruijn et al.[13] did not find increased levels of protein-bound nitrotyrosine in the spinal cords of either mutant mice or humans with sporadic ALS. There also is evidence that oxidative stress occurs in sporadic ALS. Protein carbonyl levels reportedly are increased significantly in the brains and spinal cords of patients with sporadic ALS.[14,15]

Neurofilament abnormalities were described first in sporadic and familial ALS by Hirano et al.[16,17] With electron microscopy, they determined that hyaline inclusion bodies in proximal motor axons consisted of accumulated neurofilaments. This was confirmed by others.[18-20] In addition, the accumulation of neurofilaments was demonstrated in the corticospinal tract.[21] A potential pathogenic role for abnormal neurofilament accumulation has been demonstrated in human and animal genetic studies. Figlewicz et al.[22] identified a series of novel mutations in neurofilament genes associated with ALS. In transgenic mouse models, overexpression of human neurofilament genes leads to premature motor neuron degeneration.[23]

There is evidence that each of these processes may have a primary role in initiating motor neuron death in different models. There also is evidence from human autopsy studies that all these processes may be involved in the disease process. Downstream consequences of these processes include disordered mitochondrial function, impaired axonal transport, abnormal intracellular calcium handling, and DNA or protein damage. The final step may involve initiation of cell death pathways, apoptosis, or necrosis (Figure 211.1). Models that take into account all these factors may lead to broader therapeutic strategies than those targeted to block a single primary pathogenic insult. For this strategy to be successful, individual components of the neuronal death process in human or closely related animal models must be identified.

Clinical forms of motor neuron disease

Motor neuron diseases usually are categorized according to the anatomy of motor neuron loss, heredity, and age at onset. This practical classification scheme is summarized in Table 211.1.

Generalized motor neuron diseases

ALS is the commonest form of motor neuron disease, with an incidence in developed countries of 1 to 5/100 000 population.[24-29] There is a slight overrepresentation of men in many epidemiological studies. The pattern of disease has remained remarkably stable over many years, and the overall incidence has not changed with time.[30] The risk of developing ALS increases with age. Rarely, patients in the third and fourth decades of life present with classic ALS. The clinical manifestations result from the loss of upper and lower motor neurons. The death of lower motor neurons is accompanied by muscle atrophy, fasciculations, and weakness. Sensory and autonomic

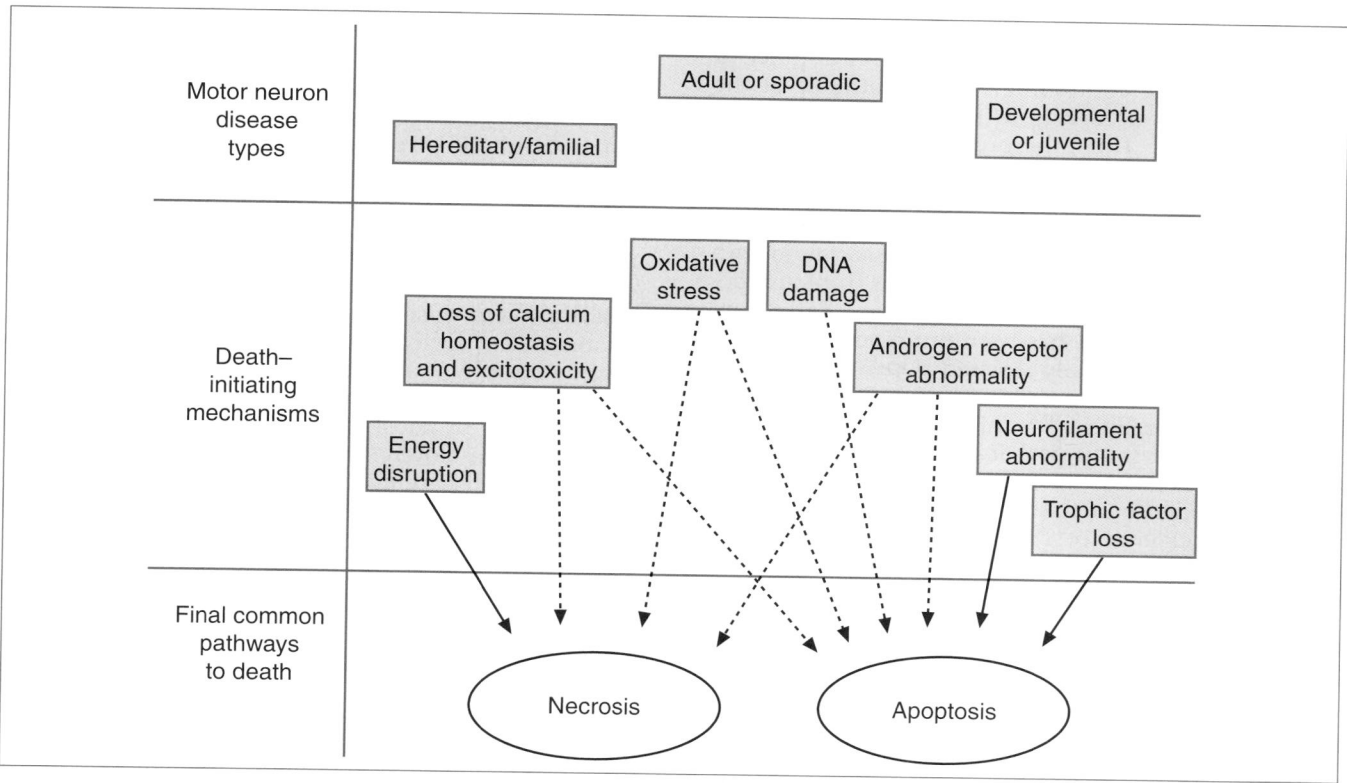

Figure 211.1 Several cellular mechanisms have been proposed to explain cell death in motor neuron disease. In most forms of the disease, evidence indicates that multiple pathways are involved in cell death. In human sporadic amyotrophic lateral sclerosis, there is clear evidence that glutamate excitotoxicity and neurofilament abnormalities are important. In different familial forms of motor neuron disease, there are mutations of the superoxide dismutase (*SOD*) gene, in neurofilament proteins, and in the androgen receptor. Mechanisms may be interconnected. In transgenic animal models in which the mutated human *SOD* gene is overexpressed, abnormal accumulations of neurofilaments occur. In most human forms of motor neuron disease, it is not known whether the final pathway to death involves necrosis or apoptosis. It also is not known why motor neurons are selectively vulnerable to most of these disturbances. The implication for treatment is that it is likely that combinations of therapeutic agents may be needed to arrest disease progression. (*Solid lines*, experimentally established mechanisms; *dotted lines*, hypothetical mechanisms.)

Table 211.1 Anatomical classification of motor neuron diseases

Generalized motor neuron disease
  Sporadic ALS
  Familial ALS
  ALS-Parkinson-dementia complex
Lower motor neuron disease (or SMA)
  Sporadic SMA
  Childhood SMA
  Inherited SMA
    Dominant
    Recessive
    X-linked
    Bulbospinal muscular atrophy
Upper motor neuron disease
  Primary lateral sclerosis
  Progressive pseudobulbar palsy
Focal motor neuron disease
Disorders mimicking motor neuron disease

ALS, amyotrophic lateral sclerosis; SMA, spinal muscular atrophy.

functions are well preserved, although specialized testing may reveal mild deficits of both.[31,32] Slowness and incoordination of movement result from upper motor neuron loss. Deep tendon reflexes may be increased, normal, or reduced depending on the balance of upper and lower motor neuron loss of a particular reflex arc. Functional loss typically begins in one limb or in bulbar-innervated muscles and becomes multifocal as the disease progresses. Trunk and breathing muscles become involved, and respiratory failure is the usual cause of death. Extraocular muscles and sacrally innervated sphincter muscles are rarely involved.

About 5% of patients with classic ALS report a positive family history. The familial form of the disease is not clinically distinct from the sporadic form,[33] although some kinships may show more posterior column sensory involvement.[34] The inherited form of ALS has provided new insights into underlying disease mechanisms. As discussed above, 20% to 30% of familial cases are associated with mutations in the copper-zinc *SOD* gene. Currently, this is the only mutation of use clinically. The identification of the mutation in affected families may have adjunctive benefit in genetic counseling. The penetrance of the many mutations occurring in the *SOD* gene has not been established. Thus, the presence of the mutation in an individual patient does not indicate a 100% risk of developing the disease. Absence of the mutation excludes any increased risk of developing ALS.

Motor neuron disease may occur in association with other neurodegenerative diseases such as frontotemporal dementia[35] and Parkinson disease. Parkinson-dementia-ALS complex has been prominent in a small number of geographically isolated populations. Up to 10% of the Chomorro people of Guam were found to have an ALS-like illness.[20,22] This was identified shortly after World War II but probably had been present for many generations. As the population became westernized, the incidence of the ALS-like disease decreased, while the incidence of Parkinson-dementia complex increased. This strongly suggests an environmental influence, but none has been identified.

Lower motor neuron diseases

Diseases associated with progressive lower motor neuron degeneration may be congenital disorders or present in childhood or adulthood. These diseases usually are referred to as the spinal muscular atrophies (SMAs). Typically, severity is linked to age at onset. The most severe cases present as congenital or early childhood disorders: Werdnig-Hoffmann disease (or SMA1). More benign forms present in adolescence or early adulthood: Kugelberg-Welander disease (or SMA3). Intermediate forms are designated SMA2 and adult-onset forms as SMA4. Inheritance may be recessive or X-linked. Adult forms frequently appear to be sporadic.

Major advances have been made in the last 10 years in understanding the genetics of SMA. Most cases are associated with mutations in the *SMN1* gene on chromosome 5q13. Severity of disease is attributed to mutations or deletions of additional closely linked genes including the *SMN2* and neuronal apoptosis inhibitor protein (*NAIP*) genes.[36] The X-linked form of the disease may be associated with signs of androgen insufficiency, including gynecomastia. It is associated with a triplet repeat expansion in the androgen receptor gene. In the classic form, or Kennedy disease, bulbar and lumbosacral spinal motor neurons are preferentially involved. However, as genetic diagnosis has become more widespread, atypical asymmetric forms have been recognized.

Infantile and childhood forms may present as decreased fetal movements, floppy infant syndrome, failure to meet early motor milestones, or loss of ability to walk. Cases of later onset present with proximal or distal limb weakness associated with atrophy and hyporeflexia. In adults, especially those with later onset, disease is slowly progressive, with the gradual loss of limb function over many years. The life expectancy of patients with adult-onset SMA3 is normal.[37]

Upper motor neuron diseases

Primary lateral sclerosis and progressive pseudobulbar palsy involve predominantly the degeneration of upper motor neurons. Both disorders typically begin in late adult life. Primary lateral sclerosis presents with insidiously progressive lower limb spasticity. Over many years, this progresses to involve the upper limbs but rarely bulbar muscles. Respiratory function usually is not compromised. Progressive bulbar or pseudobulbar palsy presents with progressive dysarthria and dysphagia. Careful examination often demonstrates signs of both lower motor neuron (tongue atrophy and fasciculations) and upper motor neuron (increased jaw or palmomental reflexes) involvement. In most patients, the dysphagia and dysarthria are slowly progressive. In most of these patients, the disease eventually progresses to a generalized motor neuron disease resembling ALS.

Focal motor neuron diseases

A rare form of focal motor neuron disease, initially described in young Japanese men,[38] may present in young adults. It has been named focal or segmental motor neuron disease, monomelic amyotrophy, and Sobue disease. It has been observed in all races.[39] Patients present with onset of weakness in the distribution of a single nerve root, most frequently C7 or C8 and rarely in L5.[40] Painless weakness and atrophy often develop over several months to a year and then remain stable for many years. There is often mild or subclinical involvement in the distribution of the contralateral root. An important characteristic is that, although weakness and atrophy may be quite profound in the distribution of the affected root, the rest of the clinical and electromyographic findings are normal.

Differential diagnosis of motor neuron disease

The diagnosis of motor neuron disease is based on the history and clinical examination findings. The presence of upper motor neuron features is established by clinical examination. In some cases, imaging may be required to eliminate a structural lesion as the cause of upper motor neuron signs. Magnetic resonance imaging in ALS shows characteristic mild changes in the corticospinal tracts.[41,42] Electromyography is used to confirm the presence and distribution of lower motor neuron loss. A few conditions mimic the clinical features of ALS. Laboratory testing may be required to rule out other causes of weakness.

Cervical spinal cord lesions

Cervical spinal cord lesions may produce lower motor neuron signs in the arms and upper motor neuron signs in the legs. However, sensory loss and loss of sphincter control commonly occur with spinal cord compression and rarely occur in ALS. In doubtful cases, imaging of the cervical spinal cord is appropriate.

Chronic inflammatory demyelinating polyradiculoneuropathy

Chronic inflammatory demyelinating polyradiculoneuropathy can occur in a motor predominant form. Reflexes are almost always decreased or absent. Electrophysiological testing shows widespread slowing of nerve conduction, which would not be present in motor neuron disease. Malignant or inflammatory infiltration of roots may produce multisegmental weakness and atrophy. It is almost always accompanied by severe pain, whereas motor neuron diseases are painless. The CSF is usually normal in ALS, although the protein concentration may be increased slightly. In chronic inflammatory demyelinating polyradiculoneuropathy, the CSF protein is significantly increased. Malignant or inflammatory pleocytosis characterizes infiltrative root disease.

Myopathy

Myopathies may produce painless weakness and atrophy with preserved reflexes and sensation. Inclusion body myositis causes multifocal, asymmetrical weakness and atrophy in older persons. In inclusion body myositis, electromyography demonstrates myopathic changes. Occasionally muscle biopsy is necessary to confirm or to rule out myopathy.

Focal or multifocal peripheral nerve disease

Focal or multifocal peripheral nerve disease may produce weakness and atrophy that mimic motor neuron disease. Most peripheral nerve compression syndromes produce sensory loss or pain in the distribution of the nerve. The anterior interosseous branch of the median nerve, the posterior interosseous branch of the radial nerve, and the deep motor branch of the ulnar nerve may be subject to compression or injury and produce weakness without sensory loss.[43] The clinical and electromyographic distribution of involvement in a single peripheral nerve distribution should always raise the question of local injury rather than a generalized motor neuron disease.

Multifocal motor neuropathy is a rare immune-mediated disorder that produces multifocal asymmetrical weakness and atrophy with preserved reflexes. Upper motor neuron signs of spasticity, pathological reflexes, and bulbar signs are not present in this disorder. It typically begins in the upper limbs and progresses insidiously.[44] The diagnosis is established by nerve conduction studies that demonstrate the presence of multiple areas of conduction block at sites not usually associated with compression. The upper limbs are affected preferentially.[44] In about 50% of patients, the titer of antibodies directed against ganglioside epitopes is increased.[45] It is important to identify this disorder because it may respond to immune-modulating therapy.[45]

Treatment of motor neuron disease
Pharmacological therapies

Many trials of drug therapy have been completed. Most have not demonstrated a treatment benefit.

These include trials of corticosteroids, other forms of immunosuppression,[46] chelation therapy,[47] antiglutamatergic drugs such as gabapentin,[48] and neuronal growth factors, including ciliary neuronotrophic factor[49] and brain-derived neurotrophic factor.[50] None have shown a benefit. Insulin-like growth factor-1 did show a small benefit in slowing disease progression in a single randomized, placebo-controlled trial.[51] This study is being repeated to determine whether the drug may be approved for general clinical use.

Riluzole prevents the presynaptic release of glutamate and has been shown to slow disease progression in ALS.[3,48,52] Studies have suggested that an oral dose of 50 mg twice daily provided the best balance between side effects and benefit. More than 1100 patients were involved in clinical trials, which had similar results. The chances of survival were increased in patients in the treatment group. The practical benefit was a slowing of disease progression so that tracheostomy-free survival was extended by about 3 months. Nausea, fatigue, and elevated liver function tests occurred in about 10% of patients[9] and significant abnormalities of liver function, in about 3%. Riluzole is recommended for the treatment of patients with ALS;[53] liver function tests should be repeated at 3-month intervals. About 20% to 30% of patients stop taking the drug because of expense, lack of perceived benefit, or adverse events.

None of the agents mentioned above have been evaluated in any other form of motor neuron disease.

Supportive therapy in ALS

Supportive and symptomatic therapy is critically important for patients with all forms of motor neuron disease, especially ALS (Table 211.2). Important elements include management of respiratory function, depression, diet, swallowing, and communication. Educating and engaging the support of family and friends are of great benefit. Also, the patient needs to be provided with access to physical medicine, occupational therapy, social service, support group, and hospice resources. This is often best administered in the environment of an ALS or neuromuscular clinic where these resources can be brought to the patient in one location instead of involving multiple prolonged visits to the medical center. The best care is delivered when there is close cooperation between an engaged family or general physician and the specialized team at the medical center.

Management of diet in ALS

Patients with bulbar involvement usually develop dysarthria and dysphagia in concert. The initial swallowing difficulty usually involves slowing of tongue movements, so that it is difficult to move food around in the mouth and difficult to move food to the back of the mouth to initiate swallowing. This may be helped by adjustment of posture during eating and by modifying the consistency of food. As the swallowing difficulty worsens, patients have more difficulty with controlling food, so that it enters the esophagus rather than the airway. Again, modifying the consistency of

Table 211.2 Treatment of motor neuron disease by symptom

Symptom	Treatment First line	Second line	Comments
Progression of weakness	Riluzole—50 mg twice daily	Vitamin E—2000 units daily	Riluzole is only drug approved for prevention of progression of weakness in ALS
Spasticity	Physical measures—stretching Baclofen—5–20 mg orally every 6 hr	Tizanidine—2 mg orally 3 or 4 times daily (gradually increased; maximum, 36 mg/day) Clonazepam—0.5–1.0 mg orally at bedtime for nocturnal spasms Combination of baclofen & tizanidine	Frequent dosage adjustments required; avoid using medications in the setting of leg weakness (falls) Baclofen withdrawal must be gradual (seizures, encephalopathy)
Weight loss due to inadequate caloric intake	Modify consistency of foods; use food blender; add thickening agents to liquids; calorie supplements	PEG	PEG placement recommended before VC falls below 50%, to minimize respiratory complications
Fatigue	Optimize sleep hygiene	Modafinil—200 mg AM	Consider contributing factors (depression, nocturnal hypoventilation)
Drooling	Low-dose anticholinergic antidepressants (e.g., amitriptyline—25 mg daily or twice daily)	Scopolamine patch changed every 3 days	Avoid overtreatment so that secretions do not become sticky and difficult to handle
Upper respiratory tract infections	Early use of antibiotics if any suggestion of bronchitis or pneumonia	Home supply of antibiotics to use at first sign of upper respiratory tract infection	
Constipation	Maintain good fluid input; fruit and vegetables in diet; high fiber intake	Stool softeners, suppositories	Constipation may be exacerbated by drugs used to treat depression or drooling
Communication disorders	Speech therapy to help early dysarthria	Writing tablets; pointing boards; electronic communication aids	
Nocturnal hypoventilation	Nocturnal nasal positive pressure ventilation; BiPAP	Supplementary oxygen by nasal cannula unless hypercapnia present	Should monitor initial use of BiPAP with oximetry to ensure effectiveness
Respiratory failure	Intermittent BiPAP; supplemental oxygen	Tracheostomy and positive pressure ventilation	Patients may require sedation or anxiolytics during terminal respiratory failure
Depression	Treat as depression associated with other chronic diseases; tricyclics	SSRIs	Use anticholinergic effects of antidepressant to reduce drooling
Emotional incontinence	Tricyclics	SSRIs	Low doses often sufficient
Inability to perform activities of daily living	Home modifications with help of occupational therapist	Engage social services	Support groups may be helpful for some patients and their families

ALS, amyotrophic lateral sclerosis; BiPAP, biphasic positive airway pressure; PEG, percutaneous endoscopic gastrostomy; SSRIs, selective serotonin reuptake inhibitors; VC, vital capacity.

food may be helpful. Patients tend to have most difficulty with hard or crumbly solids or with thin liquids. The use of a food blender or the addition of liquid thickening agents may make food and liquids easier to manage. The expert help of a speech pathologist or physical therapist with an interest in swallowing is very useful. A video swallowing X-ray study may provide additional information to aid in management. The major practical difficulty for patients is that meals become very slow and choking occurs frequently. Weight loss occurs as a result of both decreased caloric intake and loss of muscle mass due to disease. It is beneficial to limit weight loss due to starvation, which may accelerate disease progression.

The most widespread intervention for swallowing difficulty in ALS is percutaneous endoscopic gastrostomy (PEG). A tube is placed directly from the outer abdominal wall into the stomach under endoscopic control. This can be used for direct placement of fluids, medications, or liquid dietary supplements. The advantage of gastrostomy is that it can be used to supplement oral intake while some swallowing function is retained. It reduces the effort involved in meals while maintaining caloric intake and retaining the pleasure of eating. It does not protect against gastric reflux and aspiration. There has been an ongoing debate about the timing of PEG placement. There is a balance between early placement, allowing for maintenance of weight before respiratory complications begin, and the patient's willingness to accept invasive maintenance measures before they are absolutely necessary. Patients may accept PEG placement more readily if it is perceived as a measure to increase comfort by decreasing the amount of effort required for maintaining caloric and fluid intake. In our practice, we start to talk to patients about PEG as soon as they experience early symptoms of dysphagia. The final decision about placement involves discussion among the patient and family, the nutrition team, gastroenterologists, and pulmonologists. Careful education after PEG placement is essential for successful outcome.

Dysphagia rarely occurs in other forms of motor neuron disease. When it does occur, it is managed as it is in ALS.

Management of respiration in ALS

Most patients with ALS die of the complications of progressive respiratory failure. Management requires a sensitive approach that considers the wishes of the patient and family, pulmonary function, and the social support for the maintenance and expense of interventions. Respiratory failure occurs gradually over months, so that graded discussions and interventions can occur as the disease progresses.

Patient education is critical to management of respiratory failure. Soon after ALS is diagnosed, most patients are aware that respiratory failure is the usual cause of death, but it is difficult to accept this until symptoms of respiratory failure become apparent. Thus, decisions about life support may change as the disease evolves. In the early stages, denial is common and many patients decide that they will not accept mechanical ventilatory support. As the reality approaches, some change their mind. The medical support team must be aware of this possibility and not hold patients to decisions made early in the disease. Assuring the patient that there are graded levels of intervention and that the symptoms of terminal respiratory failure are manageable for patients with ALS is helpful. Patients with neuromuscular failure do not suffer from the type of air hunger or gasping experienced by those with primary lung disease. It is appropriate to seriously engage patients in discussions about respiratory support as soon as signs of respiratory failure appear.

Standard pulmonary function tests are helpful for following respiratory function in patients with ALS. These include vital capacity, maximal voluntary ventilation in 2 minutes, and maximal inspiratory and expiratory pressures. These should be completed regularly at 3 or 6 monthly clinic visits. Early in the disease, they provide a baseline for monitoring later change. Early symptoms of respiratory failure usually include difficulty with sleep breathing. They are more likely to occur in patients with bulbar and upper limb involvement. Breathing difficulties may first become apparent as disturbed sleep or with more insidious symptoms of daytime sleepiness, morning confusion, or headache. When symptoms develop or pulmonary function test values deteriorate, overnight oximetry becomes useful. The oximeter is available as a portable machine that the patient takes home. It noninvasively measures and records peripheral blood oxygenation. If nocturnal hypoventilation is pronounced, such measures as changing sleep position or supplemental oxygen may be helpful. If these do not resolve the hypoventilation or symptoms, noninvasive mechanical ventilation should be considered. Nasal positive pressure ventilation, similar to that used with obstructive sleep apnea, can alleviate symptoms. Optimal treatment involves overnight admission to a sleep-monitoring facility to ensure proper fitting of equipment and improvement of hypoxia. Nocturnal nasal ventilation, which improves comfort, provides a link to invasive mechanical ventilation with tracheostomy. Many patients accept the help of nasal ventilation but then elect for symptomatic relief of respiratory symptoms rather than tracheostomy. Use of anxiolytics or small doses of narcotics ensure comfort during the terminal phase of the disease.

Respiratory failure is rare in primary lateral sclerosis and occurs late in the course of SMA. Discussions about ventilatory support are tempered in patients with SMA by the knowledge that prolonged survival with a well-maintained quality of life is possible.

Management of communication in ALS

Dysarthria is caused by upper and lower motor neuron involvement of bulbar muscles and is usually associated with dysphagia. Loss of respiratory force and spasticity produce slurred, slowed speech with low volume. Speech pathologists or therapists initially concentrate on teaching patients to slow their speech and to exaggerate articulation to improve intelligibility. If intelligibility is lost but hand function is retained, writing or computer-assisted communication devices are helpful. The latter are particularly useful for computer-literate patients. Sophistication and miniaturization of speech synthesizers have markedly improved, and their cost has decreased substantially. Illustrated pointing boards may help severely impaired patients. It is critical for physicians and caregivers to remember that a severely dysarthric or anarthric person with ALS usually has normal hearing and intellect. There is a natural tendency to assume that a person who cannot speak cannot understand spoken language.

Mild to moderate dysarthria is common in primary lateral sclerosis but rare in lower motor neuron diseases or SMA. When present, it should be managed as it is in ALS.

Role of physical and occupational therapy in motor neuron disease

The physiatrist and occupational therapist are key members of the medical support team. Exercise does not improve muscle strength in motor neuron diseases. However, mild to moderate exercises maintain muscle and joint flexibility. They improve comfort and prevent contractures and frozen joints for patients with severe weakness. Stretching exercises also reduce cramps in patients with upper motor neuron limb weakness. Physical and occupational therapists work together to provide assistive devices and to educate the patient and caregivers in their use. These include aids for walking, mobility, transferring, toilet use, bathing, dressing, and eating.

The course of ALS is relatively short, and rapid transitions occur between stages of mobility and independence. The cost and effort of providing a particular type of assistance must be balanced against the time that it is likely to be useful. In more slowly progressive forms of motor neuron disease such as primary lateral sclerosis or SMA, assistive interventions may provide benefit for many years.

Role of social support services in motor neuron disease

In many countries, financial support from the state or from health insurance is not optimal for patients with chronic, progressive, disabling diseases. This becomes important for providing in-home or residential nursing care and for purchasing or supporting assistive devices. Medical and community social workers are trained to help clients gain full access to benefits. In some cases, voluntary organizations provide additional important support, including financial resources, provision of assistive devices, and participation in support groups.

General medical management of ALS

The care team is usually centered in a medical center.

For many patients, this may be distant from their home. Participation of the family or general physician is necessary for management of other medical problems that occur between clinic visits. Good communication between the family physician and the specialized team enhances overall care. Prompt treatment of respiratory infections may preempt pneumonia. Many patients benefit from having a supply of antibiotics so treatment can be started at the first sign of an upper respiratory tract infection. Decubiti and deep venous thrombosis are uncommon in ALS. Prophylactic anticoagulation is not indicated unless there are additional risk factors for clotting.

In summary, motor neuron diseases, including ALS, do not usually present problems in diagnosis. Although they are not curable, new treatments are becoming available to slow disease progression. In all cases, the quality of life can be improved by an attentive care team that addresses all aspects of the patient's symptoms and environment.

Acknowledgments

Review of the manuscript by members of the ALS team at Mayo Clinic including Julie Haubenschild, RN, Eric Sorenson, MD, Timothy Aksamit, MD, Katherine Stolp-Smith, MD, and Adele Neven improved this review. The skillful secretarial assistance of Jane Meyer was much appreciated. The Mayo ALS team is supported by the ALS Association and by the Muscular Dystrophy Association.

References

1. Rothstein JD, Dykes-Hoberg M, Pardo CA, et al. Knockout of glutamate transporters reveals a major role for astroglial transport in excitotoxicity and clearance of glutamate. Neuron 1996;16:675–686
2. Fray AE, Ince PG, Banner SJ, et al. The expression of the glial glutamate transporter protein EAAT2 in motor neuron disease: an immunohistochemical study. Eur J Neurosci 1998;10:2481–2489
3. Bensimon G, Lacomblez L, Meininger V. A controlled trial of riluzole in amyotrophic lateral sclerosis. ALS/Riluzole Study Group. N Engl J Med 1994;330:585–591
4. Miller RG, Moore D, Young LA, et al. Placebo-controlled trial of gabapentin in patients with amyotrophic lateral sclerosis. WALS Study Group. Western Amyotrophic Lateral Sclerosis Study Group. Neurology 1996;47:1383–1388
5. Gurney ME, Cutting FB, Zhai P, et al. Benefit of vitamin E, riluzole, and gabapentin in a transgenic model of familial amyotrophic lateral sclerosis. Ann Neurol 1996;39:147–157
6. Gurney ME, Fleck TJ, Himes CS, Hall ED. Riluzole preserves motor function in a transgenic model of familial amyotrophic lateral sclerosis. Neurology 1998;50:62–66
7. Rosen DR, Siddique T, Patterson D, et al. Mutations in Cu/Zn superoxide dismutase gene are associated with familial amyotrophic lateral sclerosis. Nature 1993;362:59–62
8. Radunovic A, Leigh PN. Cu/Zn superoxide dismutase gene mutations in amyotrophic lateral sclerosis: correlation between genotype and clinical features. J Neurol Neurosurg Psychiatry 1996;61:565–572

9. Cookson MR, Shaw PJ. Oxidative stress and motor neurone disease. Brain Pathol 1999;9:165–186

10. Abe K, Pan LH, Watanabe M, et al. Upregulation of protein-tyrosine nitration in the anterior horn cells of amyotrophic lateral sclerosis. Neurol Res 1997;19:124–128

11. Beal MF, Ferrante RJ, Browne SE, et al. Increased 3-nitrotyrosine in both sporadic and familial amyotrophic lateral sclerosis. Ann Neurol 1997;42:644–654

12. Tohgi H, Abe T, Yamazaki K, et al. Remarkable increase in cerebrospinal fluid 3-nitrotyrosine in patients with sporadic amyotrophic lateral sclerosis. Ann Neurol 1999;46:129–131

13. Bruijn LI, Beal MF, Becher MW, et al. Elevated free nitrotyrosine levels, but not protein-bound nitrotyrosine or hydroxyl radicals, throughout amyotrophic lateral sclerosis (ALS)-like disease implicate tyrosine nitration as an aberrant in vivo property of one familial ALS-linked superoxide dismutase 1 mutant. Proc Natl Acad Sci USA 1997;94:7606–7611

14. Bowling AC, Schulz JB, Brown RH Jr, Beal MF. Superoxide dismutase activity, oxidative damage, and mitochondrial energy metabolism in familial and sporadic amyotrophic lateral sclerosis. J Neurochem 1993;61:2322–2325

15. Shaw PJ, Ince PG, Falkous G, Mantle D. Oxidative damage to protein in sporadic motor neuron disease spinal cord. Ann Neurol 1995;38:691–695

16. Hirano A, Nakano I, Kurland LT, et al. Fine structural study of neurofibrillary changes in a family with amyotrophic lateral sclerosis. J Neuropathol Exp Neurol 1984;43:471–480

17. Hirano A, Donnenfeld H, Saski S, Nakano I. Fine structural observations of neurofilamentous changes in amyotrophic lateral sclerosis. J Neuropathol Exp Neurol 1984;43:461–470

18. Munoz DG, Greene C, Perl DP, Selkoe DJ. Accumulation of phosphorylated neurofilaments in anterior horn motoneurons of amyotrophic lateral sclerosis patients. J Neuropathol Exp Neurol 1988;47:9–18

19. Sasaki S, Maruyama S, Yamane K, et al. Ultrastructure of swollen proximal axons of anterior horn neurons in motor neuron disease. J Neurol Sci 1990;97:233–240

20. Sobue G, Hashizume Y, Yasuda T, et al. Phosphorylated high molecular weight neurofilament protein in lower motor neurons in amyotrophic lateral sclerosis and other neurodegenerative diseases involving ventral horn cells. Acta Neuropathol 1990;79:402–408

21. Okamoto K, Hirai S, Shoji M, et al. Axonal swellings in the corticospinal tracts in amyotrophic lateral sclerosis. Acta Neuropathol 1990;80:222–226

22. Figlewicz DA, Krizus A, Martinoli MG, et al. Variants of the heavy neurofilament subunit are associated with the development of amyotrophic lateral sclerosis. Hum Mol Genet 1994;3:1757–1761

23. Julien JP, Cote F, Collard JF. Mice overexpressing the human neurofilament heavy gene as a model of ALS. Neurobiol Aging 1995;16:487–490

24. Yoshida S, Mulder DW, Kurland LT, et al. Follow-up study on amyotrophic lateral sclerosis in Rochester, Minn., 1925 through 1984. Neuroepidemiology 1986;5:61–70

25. Incidence of ALS in Italy: evidence for a uniform frequency in Western countries. Neurology 2001;56:239–244

26. Dietrich-Neto F, Callegaro D, Dias-Tosta E, et al. Amyotrophic lateral sclerosis in Brazil: 1998 national survey. Arq Neuropsiquiatr 2000;58:607–615

27. Preux PM, Druet-Cabanac M, Couratier P, et al. Estimation of the amyotrophic lateral sclerosis incidence by capture-recapture method in the Limousin region of France. J Clin Epidemiol 2000;53:1025–1029

28. Wiederholt WC. Neuroepidemiologic research initiatives on Guam: past and present. Neuroepidemiology 1999;18:279–291

29. Traynor BJ, Codd MB, Corr B, et al. Incidence and prevalence of ALS in Ireland, 1995–1997: a population-based study. Neurology 1999;52:504–509

30. Sorenson EJ, Stalker AP, Kurland LT, Windebank AJ. Amyotrophic lateral sclerosis in Olmsted County, Minnesota, 1925 to 1998. Neurology 2002;59:280–282

31. Mulder DW, Bushek W, Spring E, et al. Motor neuron disease (ALS): evaluation of detection thresholds of cutaneous sensation. Neurology 1983;33:1625–1627

32. Daube JR, Litchy WJ, Low PA, Windebank AJ. Classification of ALS by autonomic abnormalities. Excerpta Medica International Congress Series 1988;No. 769:189–191

33. Mulder DW, Kurland LT, Offord KP, Beard CM. Familial adult motor neuron disease: amyotrophic lateral sclerosis. Neurology 1986;36:511–517

34. Hirano A, Kurland LT, Sayre GP. Familial amyotrophic lateral sclerosis: a subgroup characterized by posterior and spinocerebellar tract involvement and hyaline inclusions in the anterior horn cells. Arch Neurol 1967;16:232–243

35. Caselli RJ, Windebank AJ, Petersen RC, et al. Rapidly progressive aphasic dementia and motor neuron disease. Ann Neurol 1993;33:200–207

36. Schmalbruch H, Haase G. Spinal muscular atrophy: present state. Brain Pathol 2001;11:231–247

37. Zerres K, Rudnik-Schoneborn S, Forrest E, et al. A collaborative study on the natural history of childhood and juvenile onset proximal spinal muscular atrophy (type II and III SMA): 569 patients. J Neurol Sci 1997;146:67–72

38. Sobue I, Saito N, Iida M, Ando K. Juvenile type of distal and segmental muscular atrophy of upper extremities. Ann Neurol 1978;3:429–432

39. De Freitas MR, Nascimento OJ. Benign monomelic amyotrophy: a study of twenty-one cases. Arq Neuropsiquiatr 2000;58:808–813

40. Munchau A, Rosenkranz T. Benign monomelic amyotrophy of the lower limb—case report and brief review of the literature. Eur Neurol 2000;43:238–240

41. Hecht MJ, Fellner F, Fellner C, et al. MRI-FLAIR images of the head show corticospinal tract alterations in ALS patients more frequently than T2-, T1- and proton-density-weighted images. J Neurol Sci 2001;186:37–44

42. Comi G, Rovaris M, Leocani L. Review neuroimaging in amyotrophic lateral sclerosis. Eur J Neurol 1999;6:629–637

43. Stewart JD. Compression and entrapment neuropathies. In: Dyck PJ, Thomas PK, Griffin JW, et al., eds. Peripheral Neuropathy. Vol. 2, 3rd ed. Philadelphia: WB Saunders Company, 1993;961–979

44. Taylor BV, Wright RA, Harper CM, Dyck PJ. Natural history of 46 patients with multifocal motor neuropathy with conduction block. Muscle Nerve 2000;23:900–908

45. Taylor BV, Gross L, Windebank AJ. The sensitivity and specificity of anti-GM1 antibody testing. Neurology 1996;47:951–955

46. Griggs RC. Perspectives on the treatment of neuromuscular disease. Adv Neurol 1977;17:1–12

47. Conradi S, Ronnevi LO, Nise G, Vesterberg O. Long-

time penicillamine-treatment in amyotrophic lateral sclerosis with parallel determination of lead in blood, plasma and urine. Acta Neurol Scand 1982;65:203–211

48. Miller RG, Moore DH II, Gelinas DF, et al. Phase III randomized trial of gabapentin in patients with amyotrophic lateral sclerosis. Neurology 2001;56:843–848

49. A double-blind placebo-controlled clinical trial of subcutaneous recombinant human ciliary neurotrophic factor (rHCNTF) in amyotrophic lateral sclerosis. ALS CNTF Treatment Study Group. Neurology 1996;46: 1244–1249

50. A controlled trial of recombinant methionyl human BDNF in ALS: The BDNF Study Group (Phase III). Neurology 1999;52:1427–1433

51. Lai EC, Felice KJ, Festoff BW, et al. Effect of recombinant human insulin-like growth factor-I on progression of ALS. A placebo-controlled study. The North America ALS/IGF-1 Study Group. Neurology 1997;49: 1621–1630

52. Lacomblez L, Bensimon G, Leigh PN, et al. Dose-ranging study of riluzole in amyotrophic lateral sclerosis. Amyotrophic Lateral Sclerosis/Riluzole Study Group II. Lancet 1996;347:1425–1431

53. Practice advisory on the treatment of amyotrophic lateral sclerosis with riluzole: report of the Quality Standards Subcommittee of the American Academy of Neurology. Neurology 1997;49:657–659

212 Neurotoxic Metals

Russell A Wilke and Thomas P Moyer

Introduction

General toxicity

Heavy metals have been recognized as toxins for centuries. Recently, it has been estimated that approximately 0.6% of the North American population has an exposure history or examination findings that warrant further study for possible heavy-metal intoxication.[1] Laboratory data suggest that approximately 0.05% of this population will have abnormal findings on metal analysis.[2]

The overall pathophysiological effect of any metal exposure is determined by the condition of the host, the dose and route of exposure, and the specific chemical form of the metal involved. Toxic metals occur in various forms. Some are elemental, others are inorganic salts, and still others are constituents of complex organic molecules. The relative toxicity of each of these forms varies.

Neurotoxicity

Most heavy metals are not neurotoxic. For example, antimony, barium, beryllium, bismuth, boron, gallium, germanium, indium, molybdenum, rubidium, strontium, tin, and vanadium have little or no direct effect on the nervous system.

Although some heavy metals are capable of causing neuronal injury, they are characterized primarily by their damage to other organ systems. These include aluminum (osteomalacia),[3,4] cadmium (renal tubular damage),[5] chromium (carcinogenesis), cobalt (cardiomyopathy), copper (hepatocellular injury), iron (gastrointestinal necrosis), nickel (pulmonary edema), selenium (cardiomyopathy), silicon (pneumoconiosis), silver (skin changes and liver necrosis), gold (exfoliative dermatitis), and zinc (gastrointestinal disturbances).

The few metals that are considered primarily neurotoxic[6] include arsenic, lead, lithium (discussed elsewhere in this book), manganese, mercury, platinum, and thallium. The focus of this chapter is the diagnosis and treatment of clinical syndromes associated with these neurotoxic metals.

Specific neurotoxic metals

Arsenic

Arsenic exists in several chemical forms.[7,8] Arsine gas is the most toxic form. It is formed when arsenic-containing metal alloys are exposed to acids. This rarely occurs outside the smelting of various ores. Inorganic arsenic salts, however, are considerably more common and are found in several household products (particularly rodenticides and insecticides), and tea-spoonful amounts can cause marked systemic toxicity. Organic derivatives of arsenic are commonly found in seafood; they are relatively nontoxic.

Arsenic salts exist primarily in trivalent (As_2O_3) and pentavalent (As_2O_5) states. Both are highly reactive in biological systems. These molecules combine rapidly with sulfhydryl groups, disrupt protein structure, and alter enzyme activity. Trivalent arsenic also uncouples oxidative phosphorylation and can function as a direct metabolic poison. Generally, arsenic salts are highly corrosive, and acute exposures are associated with marked gastrointestinal symptoms. This radiopaque metal usually can be visualized on abdominal radiographs as patchy infiltrates, but this finding is not diagnostic. Repeated exposure also leads to skin changes, including hyperpigmentation and desquamation. The presence of nail thickening and Mees lines (broad white lines) of fingernails and toenails is highly suggestive of arsenic toxicity.

Acute arsenic ingestion induces, within a few days, vomiting and watery diarrhea that may persist for 36 to 48 hours and typically is followed by prickling and asleep numbness and pain of the toes, feet, and distal legs and distal muscle weakness. Typically, the hands are affected less than the feet. With intermittent or chronic ingestion, the gastrointestinal and polyneuropathy symptoms may be more protracted. Occasionally, a symmetric polyradiculoneuropathy pattern develops not unlike that of Guillain-Barré syndrome. A scaly rash of the skin with darkening may occur with prolonged use. The diagnosis is made by finding increased levels of inorganic arsenic in the plasma and urine of a patient with a characteristic syndrome and broad white lines of the fingernails (Mees lines). Hair and nail clippings may need to be analyzed. Homicidal or suicidal attempts have to be considered. A degree of psychopathy is often present.

In suspected cases, the aim should be to prevent further exposure to the metal. Also, the use of chelating agents should be considered, and rehabilitation should be instituted. When it is suspected or known that arsenic intoxication is likely, the patient must be informed and proper precautions must be taken to prevent further exposure. Because the poison may be given by a close relative, it may be necessary to isolate and protect the patient and to inform the appropriate police and legal authorities. Chelating agents may be given as treatment, but their value has not been firmly established. Because recovery may be prolonged and incomplete, physical medicine and rehabilitation must be emphasized.

Lead

Currently, lead is the only heavy metal whose screening is recommended by the United States Preventive Services Task Force. It can be found in the environment in three forms: elemental (metallic lead), inorganic (lead salts), and organic (gasoline additives such as tetraethyl lead). If ingested, adults absorb approximately 10%. The absorption rate is higher in children. Thus, attention has been given to minimizing pediatric exposure, as occurs with the ingestion of lead paint.

Chronic exposure to lead affects the bone marrow (sideroblastic anemia), kidneys (renal tubular damage), and nervous system.[9] Abdominal pain, or lead colic, can also occur. Although chronic lead exposure has been linked to an asymmetrical peripheral neuropathy with predominantly motor features (e.g., wrist drop), the central effects of lead toxicity are more devastating.[10] Early symptoms include headache, irritability, insomnia, and ataxia. As encephalopathy develops, the patient may exhibit alternating periods of excitement and lethargy, occasionally accompanied by tonic-clonic seizure. The preponderance of this problem in children has led the Centers for Disease Control and Prevention to establish fairly aggressive guidelines for the treatment of lead intoxication.[10,11] Children whose blood lead concentration is greater than 20 μg/dL are candidates for chelation therapy (outlined below), which also is indicated for any person whose blood level of lead is greater than 45 μg/dL. There is concern that low-level lead exposure, for example, by infants or young children picking and eating lead paint from walls or from breathing petroleum fumes containing lead, leads to improper mental development.

Manganese

Manganese is an essential trace element. Although present in urban air and in most water supplies, the normal physiological route of uptake for this metal is through the ingestion of manganese-containing food. Within the intestinal mucosa, manganese uses the same transport protein as iron. Thus, its absorption is increased during states of iron deficiency. Because manganese is excreted primarily in the bile, patients with hepatobiliary disease can also have increased levels of manganese.

The primary target of manganese toxicity is the central nervous system (CNS).[12,13] As a divalent cation, manganese readily crosses the blood-brain barrier. It is concentrated in the striatum of the brain. The diagnostic hallmark of CNS manganese toxicity is degeneration of the globus pallidus, with relative sparing of the substantia nigra. The result is a Parkinson-like dystonic syndrome characterized by tremor and severe retropulsion. Some patients with extensive striatal degeneration also develop a peculiar high-stepped gait sometimes referred to as a cock-walk.

Because manganese-induced parkinsonism is relatively selective for the globus pallidus, the dopaminergic neurons of the substantia nigra appear to be spared. Thus, the role of L-dopa in treating this syndrome is controversial.[14] Although patients with manganese toxicity appear to have fewer medication-related side effects such as dyskinesias and the on-off phenomenon, they have tended to respond less well to L-dopa than patients with idiopathic Parkinson disease.

Mercury

Mercury is found in the environment in three forms: elemental (thermometers), inorganic (mercury salts), and organic (fungicides). The toxicity of each form is extremely variable. Elemental mercury is relatively nontoxic unless biologically organified in the environment. Mercury salts are particularly corrosive. Mercuric salts are more toxic than mercurous salts. Organic mercurials are less corrosive but more toxic than salts. Approximately 90% of methylmercury ingested is absorbed by the gastrointestinal mucosa, in comparison with 10% of a soluble mercury salt. Organic mercurials also cross the blood-brain barrier and placenta.

Alkyl mercury species, such as methylmercury (CH_3Hg^+), are very toxic and highly selective for lipid-rich tissues. The nervous system is their primary target. In the case of methylmercury, peripheral symptoms appear when circulating levels of the substance begin to approach the high nanomolar range. Paresthesias are caused by a predominantly sensory peripheral neuronopathy. At higher concentrations of methylmercury, length-dependent axonal damage can lead to proprioceptive changes and ataxia. Marked exposure also leads to CNS toxicity (tremor, dysarthria, and death).

Platinum

Organic platinum complexes are highly toxic, and several of these agents have been developed for use as antineoplastic agents. One agent, cis-diamminedichloroplatinum (II), has been shown to be highly efficacious in the treatment of tumors of epithelial (germ cell) and neuroendocrine (oat cell) lineage. The common name for this drug is cisplatin. Its primary dose-limiting side effects are ototoxicity, nephrotoxicity, and neurotoxicity.[15] Although central neurotoxicity is rare, sensory peripheral neuropathy occurs quite often. This effect is related to cumulative drug dose and may progress for several months after therapy has been discontinued.[16]

Cisplatin induces predominantly a sensory peripheral neuropathy. Because this agent does not cross the blood-brain barrier, cell bodies of motor neurons and other CNS neurons are not exposed directly to toxic levels. Conversely, the primary sensory neurons of the dorsal root ganglia are exposed to serum levels of the drug.[17] The majority of patients who receive more than 500 mg cisplatin/m² develop distal paresthesias.

Thallium

Thallium is a byproduct of lead smelting. It is also present in agricultural pesticides. Although a few rodenticides are still thallium-based, insecticides containing thallium essentially have been replaced by newer synthetic organic compounds. Therefore, thallium neuropathy is seen infrequently. It is accompanied usually by alopecia.[18]

Like inorganic arsenic, thallium salts are highly reactive with sulfhydryl groups on essential cellular proteins. Thus, thallium exposure produces a syndrome very similar to arsenic neuropathy. Most patients develop a length-dependent sensorimotor axonopathy. Because of its structural similarity to essential monovalent cations, thallium is also able to gain access to the CNS. Patients exposed to large amounts of thallium (>1 g) can develop seizures.

General diagnostic considerations

Neurotoxic symptoms attributable to heavy metal toxicity can manifest as changes in the CNS or peripheral nervous system. Acute encephalopathy is quite rare. However, chronic low-level exposure to neurotoxic metals is often associated with diffuse central changes (e.g., lead encephalopathy). Focal changes can also occur (e.g., manganese and striatal toxicity).

Distal axonopathy is the most common type of peripheral neuropathy in neurotoxic syndromes. Neurotoxic syndromes tend to be length-dependent and to occur at lower doses of toxic metal than the CNS changes. Because the cell bodies of the dorsal root ganglia are outside the blood-brain barrier, peripheral sensory neuronopathy can also occur (e.g., dorsal root ganglion damage induced by methylmercury). Other variants of peripheral neuropathy typically encountered in neurological practice (mononeuritis, ischemic neuropathy, and demyelinating disease) are relatively uncommon in cases of metal toxicity.

Laboratory analysis

Generally, the diagnosis of heavy metal toxicity requires demonstration of three features: 1) a source of exposure, 2) relevant signs and symptoms, and 3) an abnormal concentration of the metal in the appropriate tissue.[2] If one of these features is absent, the diagnosis of metal toxicity cannot be made. Thus, laboratory testing has a key role in making the diagnosis. Appropriate specimen collection and accurate analytic technique can have an important effect on diagnosis.

Arsenic

Arsenobetaine and arsenocholine are the two organic forms of arsenic commonly found in food.[19] They are relatively nontoxic. The toxic forms of this chemical are the inorganic species As^{+3}, or As(III), and As^{+5}, or As(V),[7] with As^{+3} being more toxic than As^{+5}. Detoxification occurs as As^{+3} is oxidized to As^{+5} and then methylated by the liver to monomethylarsine (MMA) and dimethylarsine (DMA). As^{+3} and As^{+5} may be found in the urine shortly after ingestion.[20] Urinary As^{+3} and As^{+5} concentrations peak at approximately 10 hours and return to normal after 30 hours. At 24 hours, MMA and DMA are the predominate species. The biological half-life of inorganic arsenic is 4 to 6 hours; the biological half-life of the methylated metabolites is 20 to 30 hours.

To distinguish among toxic inorganic species and nontoxic organic species of arsenic of seafood origin, clinical laboratories have developed techniques to distinguish the various species of arsenic in biological fluids and tissues.[8,20,21] Normally, total arsenic is excreted in the urine at a rate less than 120 μg/24 hours. After a seafood meal, the arsenic concentration may reach 350 μg/24 hours. However, the major species present will be arsenobetaine or arsenocholine.

Hair analysis is sometimes used to document the chronicity of exposure. Arsenic circulating in the blood binds to protein and forms a covalent complex with sulfhydryl groups on cysteine residues. Arsenic has a high affinity for keratin (with its high cysteine content), and the concentration of arsenic in hair or fingernails is higher than in other tissues. Because hair grows at a rate of approximately 0.5 cm/month, hair collected from the nape of the neck can be used to document recent exposure. Axillary or pubic hair is used to document long-term (6 to 12 months) exposure. Hair arsenic content greater than 1 μg/g dry weight indicates excessive exposure.

Serum is the least useful specimen for identifying arsenic exposure. Serum concentrations of inorganic arsenic remain elevated for only a short time after exposure. Arsenic rapidly disappears into the large body pool of phosphates (arsenic and phosphorus share several chemical properties, reflected by their similar positions in the periodic table).

Lead

Although a considerable fraction of absorbed lead is incorporated rapidly into bone and erythrocytes, lead ultimately is distributed among all body tissues. Lipid-dense tissues such as the CNS are particularly sensitive to organic forms of lead. Ultimately, all lead is excreted in the bile or urine. Turnover of lead in the soft tissue occurs within approximately 120 days.[2]

Measurement of lead in whole blood has been declared by the Centers for Disease Control to be the best test for detecting lead exposure. Concentrations less than 10 μg/dL are considered normal. Concentrations greater than 45 μg/dL usually require chelation therapy (see below). Measurement of urine excretion rates either before or after chelation therapy can be used as an indicator of lead exposure.[22] Typical baseline urine lead concentrations before chelation are in the range of 10 to 120 μg/L. Following chelation, it is normal for urine output of lead to increase approximately fourfold; typical urine concentrations of lead after chelation are in the range of 40 to 480 μg/L. Significant body burden of lead is indicated if the post chelation concentration exceeds baseline by more than sixfold. Erythrocyte protoporphyrin concentration is not a sensitive indicator of low-level lead exposure, but it can be used as an indicator of lead overdose.[23] Normally, the lead content of hair is less than 5 μg/g; a concentration greater than 25 μg/g indicates severe lead exposure.

Manganese

Blood and urine manganese concentrations are both good indicators of exposure. Normal manganese concentrations in the serum range from 0.3 to 0.9 ng/mL. Normal urinary excretion ranges from 0.2 to 0.5 µg/day. Manganese-containing dust is common, and contamination of urine can easily occur. Thus, special attention must be paid to specimen collection to avoid contamination.[2]

Mercury

Analysis for mercury in blood, urine, and hair can be used to determine exposure. The quantity of mercury in blood and urine correlates with the degree of toxicity, and hair analysis can be used to determine the chronicity of exposure.[24] In whole blood, the concentration of mercury is normally less than 10 µg/L. Persons who have mild occupational exposure (e.g., dentists) may routinely have whole blood levels approaching 15 µg/L. Significant exposure is indicated by a whole blood level greater than 50 µg/L (if exposure is to alkyl mercury) or greater than 200 µg/L (if exposure is to mercury salts). The World Health Organization has noted that daily urine excretion exceeding 50 µg/day indicates significant exposure. The hair content of mercury is normally less than 1 µg/g; greater amounts indicate increased exposure.

Measurement of urine excretion rates either before or after chelation therapy can be used as an indicator of mercury exposure. Typical baseline urine mercury concentrations before chelation are in the range of 1 to 10 µg/L. After chelation, the urine output of mercury normally increases by about fourfold; typical urine mercury concentrations after chelation are in the range of 4 to 40 µg/L. Significant body burden of mercury is indicated if the post chelation concentration exceeds baseline by more than sixfold.

Thallium

Normal serum concentrations of thallium are less than 10 ng/mL. Normal urinary excretion is less than 10 µg/L. Exposed patients can have serum levels as high as 50 µg/mL, with urine output in excess of 500 mg/L.[21]

Chelation therapy

Chelation involves the formation of a molecular complex in which a metal ion is associated with a larger electron donor (referred to as a ligand). Chelating agents are used sometimes in the treatment of metal toxicity, but it should be emphasized that this represents only a secondary form of treatment.[25,26] Chelation therapy can be associated with transient worsening of symptoms, attributable to the initial mobilization of the toxic metal. The primary treatment of metal toxicity consists of defining and eliminating the source of exposure.

Chelating agents vary in their specificity for individual metals. Generally, they are water soluble and have a relatively low affinity for essential metals such as calcium. Some of the more commonly used chelating agents are discussed below.

Dimercaprol

Dimercaprol (2,3-dimercaptopropanol) was the first clinically useful chelating agent.[26] It is also called British Anti-Lewisite (BAL). This agent was designed during World War II to treat soldiers exposed to an arsenic-containing gas called Lewisite. Dimercaprol chelates arsenic through an interaction with its two sulfhydryl moieties. Dimercaprol is also effective at chelating other heavy metals, including inorganic mercury. Thus, it is a satisfactory second choice for chelation therapy of mercury toxicity. However, it should not be used in the treatment of selenium or tellurium toxicity, because it has been shown to increase the toxicity of these agents.

EDTA

The calcium disodium ($CaNa_2$) salt of ethylenediaminetetraacetic acid (EDTA) will chelate any metal that has a higher binding affinity for EDTA than calcium.[26] Because lead has an affinity for EDTA which is more than a million times greater than that of calcium, EDTA is often used to treat acute lead toxicity. Its benefits, however, must be weighed carefully against the risk of using this drug. Intravenous administration of $CaNa_2$EDTA can be associated with renal damage. EDTA has a high affinity for cadmium, but it is contraindicated for treating cadmium overdose because too much cadmium will be mobilized, causing renal damage. Before initiating EDTA therapy, one should confirm that the patient does not have an excessive body burden of cadmium (measure the blood or urine concentration).

Succimer

Succimer (2,3-dimercaptosuccinic acid) is chemically similar to dimercaprol.[26] It is more water soluble than dimercaprol and less toxic. Succimer easily crosses the gastrointestinal mucosa and, thus, is well absorbed orally. Because it can induce lead diuresis, succimer is a first-line therapy in most cases of chronic lead toxicity (when blood levels exceed 45 µg/dL).[27] It also has proved to be useful in treating inorganic mercury toxicity.

Penicillamine

Penicillamine is a derivative of penicillin. It not only has anti-inflammatory activity but can also chelate various metal ions. It is commonly used to chelate copper in patients with Wilson disease and is sometimes used to reduce the body burden of other potentially toxic metals (e.g., arsenic, lead, and mercury). However, approximately 25% of the patients who take this drug have to stop taking it because of adverse effects. Penicillamine has been associated with skin rashes, renal function changes, bone marrow suppression, and drug-induced lupus. It also chelates various essential metals, including cobalt and zinc.

Screening, prevention, and occupational monitoring

The incidence of heavy metal poisoning in industrial countries is similar to that of common inborn errors of metabolism (e.g., neonatal hypothyroidism and phenylketonuria). Currently, lead is the only heavy metal whose screening is recommended by the United States Preventive Services Task Force[28] and the Centers for Disease Control and Prevention.[29]

Lead is commonly found in our environment. Inorganic lead is present in ceramics, crystal, and paint (up to 35%, wt/wt).[30] Water transported through lead-soldered pipes can contain lead. Other potential sources include leaded gasoline, bootleg liquor products (distilled in lead-containing automobile radiators), and traditional home medicines. Before the 1970s, high concentrations of this metal were found in soil adjacent to homes painted with lead-based paints and on highways where organic lead derivatives had accumulated from the use of leaded gasoline in automobiles. Several regulatory policy changes have since been implemented to address this problem. All fuel used in personal automobiles must now contain unleaded gasoline. The lead content of paint intended for household use has also been restricted; it must now be less than 0.5% (wt/wt). Ambient lead levels have begun to decline, and screening for lead toxicity is indicated only for selected high-risk populations (e.g., children residing in older houses).[29]

Except for arsenic, lead, and mercury, environmental exposure to neurotoxic metals is fairly uncommon in the general population.[31–33] (Mercury is present in some seafood products; fish considered safe for consumption contain $<0.3\,\mu g/g$.) In comparison, occupational exposure to heavy metals is common, particularly in the process of smelting various ores. The levels of heavy metals in employees working in such an environment should be monitored frequently.[33] The most common form of monitoring involves measuring airborne metal concentrations during production. To ensure worker safety, the National Institute for Occupational Safety and Health (NIOSH) has established threshold limit values (TLVs) for airborne concentrations and timed interval exposure limits. The condition of workers may also be monitored by measurement of biological samples.

References

1. Centers for Disease Control. NIOSH Criteria Documents/Occupational Hazard Assessments/Special Hazard Reviews/Joint Occupational Health Documents: Publications Containing Occupational Safety and Health Recommendations. National Institute for Occupational Safety and Health, 2000. Retrieved 7–16–02 from the World Wide Web: http://www.cdc.gov/niosh/critdoc2.html
2. Moyer TP. Toxic metals. In: Burtis CA, Ashwood ER, eds. Tietz Textbook of Clinical Chemistry. 3rd ed. Philadelphia: WB Saunders Company, 1999:982–998
3. Bushinsky DA, Sprague SM, Hallegot P, et al. Effects of aluminum on bone surface ion composition. J Bone Miner Res 1995;10:1988–1997
4. Erasmus RT, Savory J, Wills MR, Herman MM. Aluminum neurotoxicity in experimental animals. Ther Drug Monit 1993;15:588–592
5. Viaene MK, Roels HA, Leenders J, et al. Cadmium: a

possible etiological factor in peripheral polyneuropathy. Neurotoxicology 1999;20:7–16
6. Spencer PS, Schaumburg HH, eds. Experimental and Clinical Neurotoxicology. 2nd ed. New York: Oxford University Press, 2000
7. Hindmarsh JT, McCurdy RF. Clinical and environmental aspects of arsenic toxicity. Crit Rev Clin Lab Sci 1986;23:315–347
8. Moyer TP. Testing for arsenic. Mayo Clin Proc 1993;68:1210–1211
9. Royce SE, Needleman HL, eds. Lead Toxicity. Atlanta, Georgia: United States Department of Health & Human Services, Public Health Service, Agency for Toxic Substances and Disease Registry, 1990
10. Pocock SJ, Smith M, Baghurst P. Environmental lead and children's intelligence: a systematic review of the epidemiological evidence. BMJ 1994;309:1189–1197
11. Binder S, Falk H, eds. Strategic Plan for the Elimination of Childhood Lead Poisoning. Atlanta, Georgia: United States Department of Health and Human Services, Public Health Service, Centers for Disease Control, 1991
12. Calne DB, Chu NS, Huang CC, et al. Manganism and idiopathic parkinsonism: similarities and differences. Neurology 1994;44:1583–1586
13. Mergler D, Huel G, Bowler R, et al. Nervous system dysfunction among workers with long-term exposure to manganese. Environ Res 1994;64:151–180
14. Graham DG. Catecholamine toxicity: a proposal for the molecular pathogenesis of manganese neurotoxicity and Parkinson's disease. Neurotoxicology 1984;5:83–95
15. Gamelin E, Allain P, Maillart P, et al. Long-term pharmacokinetic behavior of platinum after cisplatin administration. Cancer Chemother Pharmacol 1995;37:97–102
16. Jacobs JM, Le Quesne PM. Toxic disorders. In: Adams JH, Duchen LW, eds. Greenfield's Neuropathology. 5th ed. New York: Oxford University Press, 1992:881–987
17. Windebank AJ. Metal neuropathy. In: Dyck PJ, Thomas PK, eds. Peripheral Neuropathy. Vol 2, 3rd ed. Philadelphia: WB Saunders Company, 1993:1549–1570
18. Meggs WJ, Hoffman RS, Shih RD, et al. Thallium poisoning from maliciously contaminated food. J Toxicol Clin Toxicol 1994;32:723–730
19. Lawrence JF, Michalik P, Tam G, Conacher HBS. Identification of arsenobetaine and arsenocholine in Canadian fish and shellfish by high-performance liquid chromatography with atomic absorption detection and confirmation by fast atom bombardment mass spectrometry. J Agriculture Food Chem 1981;34:315–319
20. Nixon DE, Moyer TP. Arsenic analysis II: rapid separation and quantification of inorganic arsenic plus metabolites and arsenobetaine from urine. Clin Chem 1992;38:2479–2483
21. Nixon DE, Moyer TP. Routine clinical determination of lead, arsenic, cadmium, and thallium in urine and whole blood by inductively coupled plasma mass spectrometry. Spectrochimica Acta Part B Atomic Spectroscopy 1996;51:13–25
22. Berger OG, Gregg DJ, Succop PA. Using unstimulated urinary lead excretion to assess the need for chelation in the treatment of lead poisoning. J Pediatr 1990;116:46–51
23. Nixon DE, Moyer TP, Windebank AJ, et al. Lack of correlation of low levels of whole blood and serum lead in humans: an experimental evaluation of this relationship in animals. Trace Substances Environ Health 1985;19:248–256
24. Nixon DE, Mussmann GV, Moyer TP. Inorganic,

organic, and total mercury in blood and urine: cold vapor analysis with automated flow injection sample delivery. J Anal Toxicol 1996;20:17–22

25. Gossel TA, Bricker JD. Principles of Clinical Toxicology. 3rd ed. New York: Raven Press, 1994

26. Goyer RA. Toxic effects of metals. *In:* Klaassen CD, ed. Casarett & Doull's Toxicology: The Basic Science of Poisons. 5th ed. New York: McGraw-Hill, 1996:691–736

27. Graziano JH, Lolacono NJ, Meyer P. Dose-response study of oral 2,3-dimercaptosuccinic acid in children with elevated blood lead concentrations. J Pediatr 1988;113:751–757

28. U.S. Preventive Services Task Force. Guide to Clinical Preventive Services. 2nd ed. Alexandria, Virginia: International Medical Publishing, 1996

29. Centers for Disease Control. Preventing Lead Poisoning in Young Children: A Statement. 4th rev ed. Atlanta, Georgia: United States Department of Health and Human Services, Public Health Service, 1991

30. Chadzynski L. Manual for the Identification and Abatement of Environmental Lead Hazards. United States Public Health Service, 1986

31. Echeverria D, Heyer NJ, Martin MD, et al. Behavioral effects of low-level exposure to elemental Hg among dentists. Neurotoxicol Teratol 1995;17:161–168

32. Stopford W. Industrial exposure to mercury. *In:* Nriagu JO, ed. The Biogeochemistry of Mercury in the Environment. New York: Elsevier/North-Holland, 1979: 367–397

33. Tsalev DL, Zaprianov ZK. Atomic Absorption Spectrometry in Occupational and Environmental Health Practice. Boca Raton, Florida: CRC Press, 1983

213 Critical Illness Polyneuropathy

Charles F Bolton

Brief overview

Critical illness polyneuropathy (CIP) was described and named more than 15 years ago.[1,2] Since then, cases have been reported from the United States, France, the Netherlands, Austria, Germany, and Spain.[3,4] Although CIP is a common occurrence in the intensive care unit (ICU), it is rarely diagnosed in most ICUs because of the lack of knowledge, difficulties in clinical assessment, and failure to perform electrophysiological studies. Nonetheless, CIP is a significant cause of difficulty in weaning patients from the ventilator and of long-term morbidity among survivors.[5] Critical illness polyneuropathy is one of several nervous system complications of sepsis and multiple organ failure[6] (Figure 213.1)—the combination of sepsis and multiple organ failure is now designated as systemic inflammatory response syndrome (SIRS)—induced by trauma as well as by infection. Although there is no specific treatment, diagnosis is important for prognosis and the institution of various nonspecific treatments. Moreover, research is needed to achieve a better understanding of the pathophysiology of the condition and, hence, a more specific treatment. This chapter emphasizes the nature of critical illness, the possible pathophysiology, the clinical and electrophysiological features of CIP, and the differential diagnosis (see Chapter 105 for management of generalized weakness in the ICU). Nonspecific and potential specific treatments also are discussed.

Epidemiology

Critical illness polyneuropathy occurs in 50% to 70% of patients who have sepsis and multiple organ failure,[5,7,8] and sepsis and multiple organ failure occur in 50% of patients in the medical and surgical ICUs of major medical centers.[9]

Etiology

Retrospective[2] and prospective[8] studies have failed to implicate several potential causes of CIP, including types of primary illness or injury, Guillain–Barré syndrome, medications (e.g. aminoglycoside antibiotics and neuromuscular blocking agents), and specific nutritional deficiencies. On the supposition that CIP may have an immune-mediated basis, Wijdicks and Fulgham[10] administered immunoglobulins intravenously to three patients but without any beneficial effect. Zochodne et al.[2] and Witt et al.[8] have speculated that SIRS (sepsis) is the cause. The severity of the polyneuropathy can be quantified from electrophysiological data.[8] It tends to be more severe with the length of stay in the ICU, increasing blood

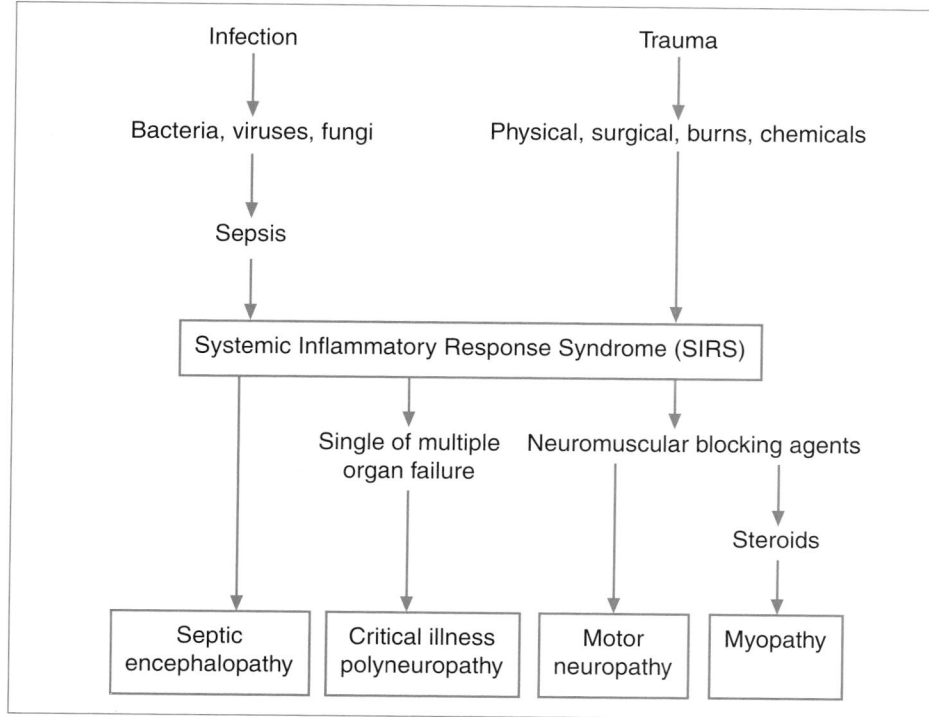

Figure 213.1 The various factors associated with the development of the systemic inflammatory response syndrome (SIRS) and its nervous system complications. (Modified from Bolton CF. Critical illness polyneuropathy. *In*: Asbury AK, Thomas PK, eds. Peripheral Nerve Disorders. Oxford: Butterworth-Heinemann, 1995:262–280. By permission of the publisher.)

concentration of glucose, and decreasing serum concentration of albumin. All these factors are recognized manifestations of sepsis and multiple organ failure syndrome.[11] Hund et al.[12] isolated a humoral factor from the sera of patients with CIP, but the precise nature of the toxin has not been identified.

Pathophysiology and pathogenesis

The morphological features of CIP have been demonstrated through biopsy of peripheral nerve and muscle and comprehensive autopsy study of both the central and peripheral nervous systems of nine patients.[2] The motor and sensory fibers of peripheral nerves show primary axonal degeneration but no evidence of inflammation, as may be seen in Guillain–Barré syndrome. Muscle specimens show scattered atrophic fibers in acute denervation and grouped atrophy in chronic denervation. Occasional necrotic muscle fibers suggest an associated primary myopathy. The only central nervous system manifestation is central chromatolysis of anterior horn cells and loss of dorsal root ganglion cells due to axonal damage in peripheral nerves. No changes appear distinctive for CIP. In the well-designed prospective study of Latronico et al.,[13] in which electrophysiological studies and biopsies of peripheral nerve and muscle were performed, primary effects on both nerve and muscle were reported. Importantly, in some patients, the electrophysiological findings were abnormal but the results of biopsy study of nerve and muscle were normal. This suggests that a functional disturbance of the peripheral nervous system precedes structural change. This functional disturbance also probably involves the central nervous system because the brains of patients with severe septic encephalopathy may not have any pertinent morphological abnormality at autopsy.[14]

With current knowledge of the general effects of sepsis on the human body and the pathophysiology of human peripheral nerve, it is possible to speculate on the pathophysiology of CIP. The microcirculation is disturbed in sepsis[6] (Figure 213.2). Blood vessels supplying peripheral nerves normally lack autoregulation, rendering them susceptible to such disturbances.[15] Moreover, the cytokines secreted in sepsis have histamine-like properties that may increase microvascular permeability.[2] The resulting endoneural edema could induce hypoxia through an increase in intercapillary distance and other mechanisms. Severe energy deficits would result and induce a primary axonal degeneration, most likely distally if highly energy-dependent systems involving axonal transport of structural proteins are involved. The predominantly distal involvement may explain why recovery in some patients can be unexpectedly short, conforming to the short length of nerve along which axonal regeneration occurs. Also, cytokines themselves possibly have a direct toxic effect on peripheral

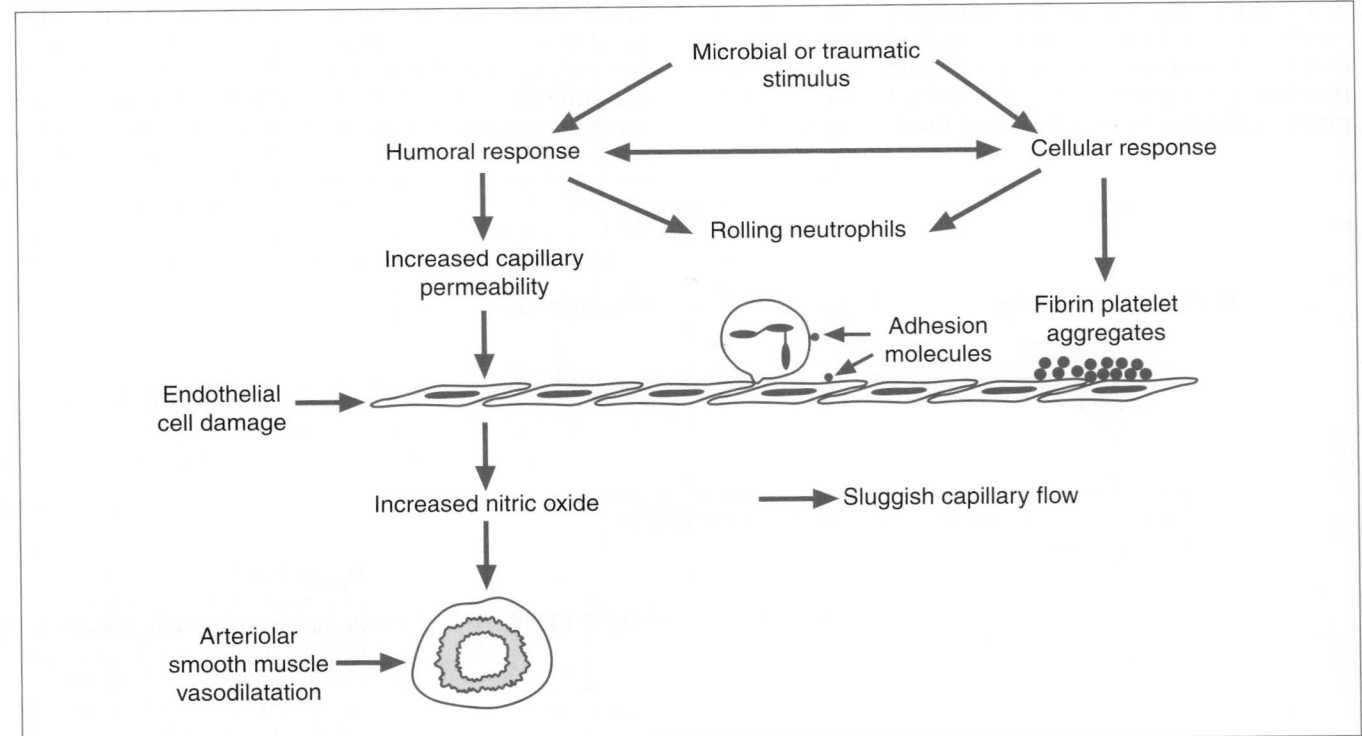

Figure 213.2   Possible mechanisms of disturbance of the microcirculation in systemic inflammatory response syndrome (sepsis). The end result is sluggish capillary flow due to vasodilatation and neutrophil and platelet aggregation. Thus, essential substances are blocked from entering the parenchyma of the organ. Increased capillary permeability promotes tissue edema and passage of potentially toxic substances. (From Bolton CF. Critical illness polyneuropathy. *In*: Asbury AK, Thomas PK, eds. Peripheral Nerve Disorders. Oxford: Butterworth-Heinemann, 1995:262–280. By permission of the publisher.)

nerve. To the author's knowledge, such an effect has not been demonstrated in humans, but in laboratory animals tumor necrosis factor (TNF) decreases the resting transmembrane potential of skeletal muscle fibers in vitro[16] and induces muscle proteolysis.[17]

Disturbances of the microcirculation to nerve and muscle also may explain the effects of neuromuscular blocking agents and corticosteroids. Through increased capillary permeability induced by sepsis, neuromuscular blocking agents, notably vecuronium or its metabolite 3-desacetyl-vecuronium,[18] could have a direct toxic effect on peripheral nerve axons. These neuromuscular blocking agents also may cause functional denervation through prolonged neuromuscular blocking action.[19] The result would be denervation atrophy of muscle. When patients who have asthma or transplant surgery develop acute myopathy after treatment with neuromuscular blocking agents and corticosteroids,[20] the author suspects that they also have SIRS, because infection is often a precipitating event in asthma and transplant surgery is a major traumatic event. Animal experiments by Karpati et al.[21] have shown that if muscle is denervated by nerve transection and corticosteroids are administered, a thick-filament myopathy occurs, similar to myopathy in humans. Thus, in humans, CIP and the additional effects of neuromuscular blocking agents would denervate muscle and corticosteroid treatment would then induce a thick-filament myopathy. These and other mechanisms are discussed by Lacomis et al.[20] (see Chapter 105).

Despite the above considerations, it must be recognized that the exact cause of CIP is unknown. Also unknown is why the effects on the peripheral nervous system may vary widely in both site and severity, with many patients having various combinations of effects on peripheral nerve motor fibers, sensory fibers, and muscle.[6] This led Op de Coul et al.[22] to propose the term "critical illness polyneuromyopathy." Additional investigations are needed, for example, biopsy examination of the distal motor axon and neuromuscular junction and further studies of the toxin found in the blood of patients with CIP.

Genetics

Critical illness polyneuromyopathy has no apparent familial tendency. Possible changes in DNA have not been investigated.

Clinical features

Critical illness polyneuromyopathy is a complication of the septic syndrome, SIRS,[6] which is identified in a patient who has a severe infective or traumatic insult and is manifested by a temperature higher than 38°C or lower than 36°C, heart rate faster than 90 beats/minute, respiratory rate greater than 20 breaths/minute or $PaCO_2$ less than 32 mm Hg (<4.3 kPa), and a leukocyte count greater than 12×10^9/L or less than 4×10^9/L or 10% immature forms. Typically, as SIRS becomes more severe, episodes of septic shock occur and evidence of multiple organ failure develops.[11]

Difficulty in weaning the patient from the ventilator and, less commonly, limb weakness are noted after the first week in the ICU.[4] Deep tendon reflexes are depressed in only half of the patients; hence, electrophysiological studies are necessary to establish the diagnosis. A more severe polyneuropathy can be suspected when, with deep painful stimulation of the distal extremities, limb movements seem weak despite strong grimacing of facial musculature. Rarely, CIP may occur in children.[6]

The earliest electrophysiological sign of CIP is a decrease in the amplitude of compound muscle action potentials, with a minor change in latency.[6] These changes are typical of axonal damage. Fibrillation potentials and positive sharp waves may not appear in muscle until 3 weeks after such damage. Motor unit potentials, if they can be activated voluntarily by the patient (but may not be activated because of sedation or septic encephalopathy), often appear normal or somewhat low in amplitude and polyphasic, suggesting an associated primary involvement of muscle by sepsis. These electrophysiological changes also could be due to primary myopathy. Thus, it is important to demonstrate depression of the amplitude of sensory compound action potentials before a firm electrophysiological diagnosis of polyneuropathy can be made.[4] Repetitive nerve stimulation studies also should be performed to demonstrate a defect in neuromuscular transmission. This defect does not occur in sepsis but is present if neuromuscular blocking agents have been administered. The effects of these agents may persist from several hours to days if the patient has kidney or liver failure. The technique of direct electrical stimulation of muscle developed by Rich et al.[23] may prove valuable in distinguishing between CIP and critical illness myopathy and in demonstrating abnormalities of the muscle membrane. Also, phrenic nerve conduction studies and needle electromyography of the chest wall and diaphragm are important in establishing that the difficulty in weaning the patient from the ventilator in fact is due to CIP.[24]

Classification

Critical illness polyneuropathy should be classified as a toxic–metabolic polyneuropathy, an axonal motor and sensory polyneuropathy that is reversible.

Diagnostic criteria

The diagnostic criteria for CIP are listed in Table 213.1.

Differential diagnosis

The approach to patients in the ICU who have weakness of limb and respiratory muscles should be systematic. Investigations may include magnetic resonance imaging of the spinal cord, neurophysiological studies, measurement of creatine kinase concentration, and muscle biopsy. There are two main categories of patients with CIP. The first category consists of patients in whom paralysis develops rapidly before admission to the ICU. Because of the acuteness

Table 213.1 Diagnostic criteria for critical illness polyneuropathy*

Patient has sepsis and multiple organ failure (SIRS)
Difficulty weaning patient from ventilator after non-neuromuscular causes such as heart and lung disease have been excluded
Possible limb weakness
Electrophysiological evidence of axonal motor and sensory polyneuropathy
Near-normal levels of creatine phosphokinase

*These diagnostic criteria are now well established, but in certain circumstances, other acute axonal polyneuropathies, such as thiamine deficiency, porphyria, etc., should be excluded.

of the situation, there is not sufficient time to investigate the underlying cause until after the patient's condition has been stabilized. Conditions to be considered are high cervical spinal cord lesion due to trauma, neoplasm or infection, motor neuron disease in which the respiratory muscles are affected before other muscles, Guillain–Barré syndrome, and other acute polyneuropathies such as porphyria and the acute axonal forms of Guillain–Barré syndrome, including the pure motor variety particularly common in northern China.[25] Axonal forms of Guillain–Barré syndrome may be difficult to distinguish from CIP if the onset occurs after the patient has been admitted to the ICU for severe infection. Yuki and Hirata[26] have suggested that measurement of certain IgG class autoantibodies may be used to differentiate the two conditions. Mild, chronic polyneuropathies such as diabetic polyneuropathy may affect predominantly the nerves of respiration, or after admission to the ICU, sepsis may worsen a preexisting polyneuropathy. Occasionally, defects in neuromuscular transmission, myasthenia gravis, and Lambert–Eaton myasthenic syndrome present with primary respiratory failure. Finally, healthy persons or those who have a long-standing myopathy, such as muscular dystrophy, may receive various insults, mechanical, toxic, infective, etc., which induce an acute myopathy ranging from mild to severe, with myoglobinuria and muscle necrosis. Although these patients will require treatment in an ICU, they may have a good outcome, except in unusually severe forms.

The second category is patients who have been admitted to the ICU for a severe primary illness or trauma in whom neuromuscular disease later develops. Ischemic myelopathy, which affects mainly anterior horn cells, may result from cardiac arrest, atherosclerosis, a surgical procedure on the aorta, or severe pulmonary disease. A prime consideration is CIP.

In the ICU, neuromuscular transmission disorders most frequently are due to noncompetitive neuromuscular blocking agents administered to lower metabolic demands, to prevent shivering or fighting with the ventilator, to improve chest compliance, or to decrease intracranial pressure. If used briefly, for less than 48 hours, these agents do not cause a problem.

However, if the patient has kidney or liver failure, even short-acting agents such as vecuronium may cause neuromuscular blockage for as long as 2 weeks.[18] This blockage can be detected with repetitive nerve stimulation. Sepsis itself does not induce neuromuscular transmission defects.[6]

In the ICU, limb weakness that develops suddenly has been called acute quadriplegic myopathy.[27] Other terms that have been used[20] include acute myopathy of intensive care, critical care myopathy, acute illness myopathy, critical illness myopathy, acute myopathy with selective lysis of myosin filaments, and acute necrotizing myopathy of intensive care.[28] Acute quadriplegic myopathy often occurs in association with the use of neuromuscular blocking agents and corticosteroids, which are given to treat acute severe asthma or to manage patients in the post-transplant state. The clinical signs are purely motor, with deep tendon reflexes decreased or absent. Electrophysiological testing suggests myopathy. Creatine phosphokinase levels vary, but they are usually normal or mildly increased except in acute necrotizing myopathy. Muscle biopsy shows a distinctive loss of thick myosin filaments and various degrees of muscle fiber atrophy and necrosis. Early recovery can be anticipated except if necrosis is severe. However, some patients with myopathic features may have a distal motor axonopathy that may induce "myopathic"-appearing motor unit potentials and may be difficult to distinguish from a primary myopathy.

The high prevalence of myopathy (39 of 92 patients) reported by Lacomis et al.[29] may reflect the large number of post-transplantation patients receiving high doses of corticosteroids in the ICU, in contrast to the much lower incidence of myopathy (5%) in the London, Canada, ICU, which does not manage post-transplantation patients. In prospective studies of CIP by Witt et al.,[8] Berek et al.,[7] and Leijten and De Weerd[3] and studies of critical illness myopathy and neuropathy by Latronico et al.,[13] no correlation was found between the administration of these agents and neuromuscular disease. These conditions likely represent a spectrum of disorders, to which sepsis (SIRS) induced by a major surgical procedure such as transplantation or infections associated with ICU care are underlying factors and neuromuscular blocking agents and corticosteroids are contributing factors. Critical illness myopathy probably is an appropriate term to cover these various conditions.

Table 213.2 outlines how these various neuromuscular complications of sepsis may be differentiated. Cachectic myopathy is difficult to identify by clinical and electrophysiological assessment, but it may be inferred by the nonspecific muscle biopsy finding of type II fiber atrophy.

Prevention

Because CIP is a complication of SIRS, methods to avoid the development of SIRS must be considered. This is not normally possible before admission to the ICU, but preventive measures should be considered after the patient has been admitted to the ICU. Such

Table 213.2 Comparison of various neuromuscular complications of sepsis

Condition	Antecedent illness	Clinical features	Electrophysiology	Morphology	Treatment	Prognosis
Critical illness polyneuropathy	SIRS	Absent or signs of polyneuropathy	Consistent with primary axonal degeneration of motor and sensory fibers	Primary axonal degeneration of nerve, denervation atrophy of muscle	Treat SIRS	Good in 40% who survive organ failure
Axonal motor neuropathy	SIRS, neuromuscular blocking agents and neuropathy	Acute quadriplegia	Neuromuscular transmission defect and/or axonal motor neuropathy	Denervation atrophy on muscle biopsy	Treat SIRS. Stop steroids and neuromuscular blocking agents	Good
Critical illness myopathy	SIRS, neuromuscular blocking agents, corticosteroids	Acute quadriplegia	Neuromuscular transmission defect and/or myopathy	Thick myosin filament loss or necrosis on muscle biopsy	Treat SIRS. Stop steroids and neuromuscular blocking agents	Good
Acute necrotizing myopathy of intensive care	Transient infection, trauma, etc.	Severe muscle weakness, increased serum creatine kinase, often myoglobinuria	Positive sharp waves and fibrillation potentials on needle electromyography	Panfascicular muscle fiber necrosis	Treat SIRS, hemodialysis for myoglobinuria	May be poor
Cachectic myopathy	Severe systemic illness, prolonged recumbency	Diffuse muscle wasting	Normal	Normal or type II fiber atrophy	Physiotherapy, improved nutrition	Good

SIRS, systemic inflammatory response syndrome.

measures include scrupulous aseptic techniques, constant surveillance for infecting organisms, and avoidance of surgical procedures whenever possible. Corticosteroids and neuromuscular blocking agents may contribute to critical illness myopathy; they therefore should be avoided or given at the lowest possible dosage and for as short a time as possible.

Nonspecific treatment of critical illness polyneuropathy

After the diagnosis of CIP has been made, treatment is overseen by a specialist in critical care medicine. The broad areas are 1) treatment of sepsis and multiple organ failure; 2) management of difficulty in weaning the patients from the ventilator; 3) physiotherapy and rehabilitation. The literature in these areas of treatment is extensive, and despite many studies, varying from class 1 to class 3, the value of the treatment is still not proven.[11] Thus, only general principles are described in the following discussion.

Treatment of sepsis and multiple organ failure

The initial insult should be identified if possible and treated. Antibiotics should be administered appropriate to the organism, if isolated. If a septic focus can be identified, it should be drained surgically. Episodes of septic shock should be treated vigorously. Low volume should be treated with fluid replacement and various inotropes and other drugs. Any coagulopathy should be corrected. Cardiac arrhythmias are common in shock and should be corrected.

If there is upper respiratory insufficiency, the airway should be protected by intubation and adequate amounts of oxygen delivered, although adequate oxygen may not reach the parenchyma because of the severe oxygen debt due to dysfunction of the microcirculation. This early and progressive treatment may prevent the development of multiple organ failure, but when it does develop, various treatments are instituted for each organ, with varying results. These may be directed specifically at the dysfunction of certain organs. For example, dysfunction of the gut may be prevented by early use of enteral feedings; if rest periods between enteral feedings are used, this may allow acidity to return to the stomach, thus killing bacteria and decreasing the incidence of nosocomial infection in the gut. In the kidney, fluid resuscitation and the use of inotropes and diuretic drugs may prevent renal failure.

Despite these measures, the mortality rate for sepsis and multiple organ failure in the ICU is approximately 50%.[11]

Difficulty in weaning from the ventilator

Patients with CIP typically have a period of difficulty in being weaned from the ventilator. This usually occurs after sepsis and multiple organ failure have been controlled and there is no apparent cardiac or pulmonary cause for difficulty in weaning. At this point, neurological examination, electrophysiological tests, measurement of creatine phosphokinase concentration, and, if necessary, muscle biopsy are per-

formed to define any neuromuscular cause for difficulty in weaning. The author believes that the use of phrenic nerve conduction and needle electromyography of the chest wall and diaphragm is valuable in proving that the cause for the respirator insufficiency is neuromuscular.[24] After a neuromuscular cause has been established, it will be noted that weaning fails because when ventilator support is discontinued, the respiratory rate becomes unacceptably high (<35/min), tidal volumes become unacceptably low (<5 ml/kg), and respiratory acidosis develops. Several types of ventilators, ventilator settings, and other measures may be used. Weaning is considered successful if breathing becomes spontaneous without ventilator support after 2 days. Measurements such as vital capacity, ratio of respiratory rate to tidal volume, peak negative inspiratory pressure, maximal voluntary ventilation, or occlusion pressure are useful for assessing respiratory function before, during, and after weaning.

The author believes there is confusion surrounding the management of some aspects of difficulty in weaning. If the patient has been shown to have CIP, muscle-strengthening exercises are unlikely to be helpful until after the respiratory muscles have been reinnervated. However, if there is little evidence of CIP and the cause of the respiratory weakness is disuse atrophy of the diaphragm, muscle-strengthening exercises are of value. Finally, if the patient is thought to have diaphragmatic fatigue, which in clinical situations is almost impossible to prove, then theoretically the best method of management is to continue ventilatory support, resting of the diaphragm, and gradual attempts at weaning, without the use of vigorous muscle-training exercises.

Physiotherapy and rehabilitation

Initially, CIP may be identified while the patient is in the ICU or after he or she has been transferred to a general medical ward, where weakness of the limbs prevents sitting or walking, feeding, and dressing. In either circumstance, formal consultation with physiotherapy and rehabilitation should be arranged. Initially, only light exercises to promote muscle strength, to maintain joint mobility, and to prevent contracture should be instituted. As the patient becomes stronger, greater strengthening exercises should be used. The program of rehabilitation may be lengthy and involve consultation with occupational medicine and the use of various assistive devices.

Specific treatment of critical illness polyneuropathy

The rationale for the treatment of CIP is to treat SIRS. Retrospective and prospective studies (class 3) have shown a strong association between CIP and SIRS.[2,4,5,7,8] It has been observed that if the above-described nonspecific methods of treatment are successful, CIP improves in a matter of weeks in mild cases and in months in severe cases.[2,5,8] The results of clinical and electrophysiological studies should indicate whether there is progressive reinnervation of muscle and restoration of sensory function. However, in extremely severe cases of critical illness polyneuropathy, a rare circumstance, recovery may not occur.[8]

Specific treatment of systemic inflammatory response syndrome

Much research, in many cases with carefully controlled trials (class 1 to class 2), has centered on the treatment of gram-negative sepsis, with a "magic bullet" to interrupt the septic cascade in its early stages. Attempts at treatment have included monoclonal and polyclonal antibodies directed against bacterial endotoxin, monoclonal antibodies to TNF-α, fusion protein constructs of soluble TNF receptors, interleukin-1 receptor antagonists, platelet-activating factor receptor antagonist, BN5202, and N-acetylcysteine (a drug that acts as an oxygen radical scavenger). So far, none has been effective.[6,30] A review by Vincent and Tielemans[31] of various hemofiltration techniques and plasma exchange indicated that these forms of treatment have not been effective. A novel approach with detoxification plasma filtration, which clears several cytokines from the plasma, has shown promise in a small preliminary trial.[32]

Treatment of critical illness polyneuropathy with intravenous immunoglobulins

Intravenously administered immunoglobulin (IVIg) has been widely used as a supplemental treatment for sepsis, septic shock, and systemic inflammation in critically ill patients.[33] Although IVIg is not a "magic bullet" and its effectiveness has not clearly been proved, it shows promise in decreasing the morbidity associated with sepsis. In an open trial including three patients, Wijdicks and Fulgham[10] did not show improvement in CIP after IVIg. However, in a more extensive, albeit retrospective (class 3), study of 33 patients, early treatment of gram-negative sepsis with IVIg may have prevented the development of CIP.[34]

Role of total parenteral and enteral nutrition

On the basis of clinical observation, Waldhausen et al.[35] have proposed that enteral nutrition may cause CIP. They surmised that in critical illness the enzyme activity for the oxidation of glucose is decreased through the metabolism of fats and conversion by oxidation to ketone bodies. With the accumulation of glucose, phosphorylated glycolytic intermediates accumulate and block the energy cascade, hence causing axonal degeneration in peripheral nerves. Marino and Millili[36] have theorized that with total parenteral nutrition and enteral nutrition, polyunsaturated fatty acids, which are oxidized more readily in sepsis, may damage the vascular endothelium and various cell membranes, including those of the nervous system, and may increase the production of inflammatory cytokines. All these effects would tend to cause CIP. However, Bolton and Young[37] and Leijten et al.[38] have argued that prospective studies (class 3)[8,38] have shown no statistical relationship between the administration of enteral or parenteral nutrition and the development of CIP. Moreover, the author believes that many of the nutrients in these treatments are essential for the health of the nervous system, notably the various B vitamins and vitamin E. Thus, it would seem unwise to limit the use of whatever currently accepted methods are necessary to improve nutrition in critically ill patients.

Acknowledgment

The author is grateful to Ms. Andrea Gross for her work on the manuscript.

References

1. Bolton CF, Gilbert JJ, Hahn AF, Sibbald WJ. Polyneuropathy in critically ill patients. J Neurol Neurosurg Psychiatry 1984;47:1223–1231
2. Zochodne DW, Bolton CF, Wells GA, et al. Critical illness polyneuropathy. A complication of sepsis and multiple organ failure. Brain 1987;110:819–841
3. Leijten FSS, De Weerd AW. Critical illness polyneuropathy. A review of the literature, definition and pathophysiology. Clin Neurol Neurosurg 1994;96:10–19
4. Zifko UA, Zipko HT, Bolton CF. Clinical and electrophysiological findings in critical illness polyneuropathy. J Neurol Sci 1998;159:186–193
5. Leijten FSS, Harinck-de Weerd JE, Poortvliet DCJ, de Weerd AW. The role of polyneuropathy in motor convalescence after prolonged mechanical ventilation. JAMA 1995;274:1221–1225
6. Bolton CF. Sepsis and the systemic inflammatory response syndrome: neuromuscular manifestations. Crit Care Med 1996;24:1408–1416
7. Berek K, Margreiter J, Willeit J, et al. Polyneuropathies in critically ill patients: a prospective evaluation. Intensive Care Med 1996;22:849–855
8. Witt NJ, Zochodne DW, Bolton CF, et al. Peripheral nerve function in sepsis and multiple organ failure. Chest 1991;99:176–184
9. Tran DD, Groeneveld AB, van der Meulen J, et al. Age, chronic disease, sepsis, organ system failure, and mortality in a medical intensive care unit. Crit Care Med 1990;18:474–479
10. Wijdicks EF, Fulgham JR. Failure of high dose intravenous immunoglobulins to alter the clinical course of critical illness polyneuropathy (letter). Muscle Nerve 1994;17:1494–1495
11. Baue AE, Berlot G, Gullo A, eds. Sepsis and Organ Dysfunction: Epidemiology and Scoring Systems: Pathophysiology and Therapy. Milan, Italy: Springer-Verlag, 1998
12. Hund E, Herkert M, Becker CM, Hacke W. A humoral neurotoxic factor in sera of patients with critical illness polyneuropathy (abstract). Ann Neurol 1996;40:539
13. Latronico N, Fenzi F, Recupero D, et al. Critical illness myopathy and neuropathy. Lancet 1996;347:1579–1582
14. Young GB, Bolton CF, Austin TW, et al. The encephalopathy associated with septic illness. Clin Invest Med 1990;13:297–304
15. Low PA, Tuck RR, Takeuchi M. Nerve microenvironment in diabetic neuropathy. In: Dyck PJ, Thomas PK, Asbury AK, et al., eds. Diabetic Neuropathy. Philadelphia: WB Saunders, 1987:266–278
16. Tracey KJ, Lowry SF, Beutler B, et al. Cachectin/tumor necrosis factor mediates human muscle denervation: topical 31-P spectroscopy studies. Magn Reson Med 1988;7:373–383

17. Fong Y, Moldawer LL, Marano M, et al. Cachectin/TNF or IL-alpha induces cachexia with redistribution of body proteins. Am J Physiol 1989;256:R659–R665

18. Segredo V, Caldwell JE, Matthay MA, et al. Persistent paralysis in critically ill patients after long-term administration of vecuronium. N Engl J Med 1992;327:524–528

19. Wernig A, Pecot-Dechavassine M, Stover H. Sprouting and regression of the nerve at the frog neuromuscular junction in normal conditions after prolonged paralysis with curare. J Neurocytol 1980;9:278–303

20. Lacomis D, Giuliani MJ, Van Cott A, Kramer DJ. Acute myopathy of intensive care: clinical, electromyographic, and pathological aspects. Ann Neurol 1996;40:645–654

21. Karpati G, Carpenter S, Eisen AA. Experimental core-like lesions and nemaline rods. A correlative morphological and physiological study. Arch Neurol 1972;27:237–251

22. Op de Coul AA, Verheul GA, Leyten AC, et al. Critical illness polyneuromyopathy after artificial respiration. Clin Neurol Neurosurg 1991;93:27–33

23. Rich MM, Bird SJ, Raps EC, et al. Direct muscle stimulation in acute quadriplegic myopathy. Muscle Nerve 1997;20:665–673

24. Bolton CF. Clinical neurophysiology of the respiratory system. AAEM Minimonograph #40. Muscle Nerve 1993;16:809–818

25. McKhann GM, Cornblath DR, Griffin JW, et al. Acute motor axonal neuropathy: a frequent cause of acute flaccid paralysis in China. Ann Neurol 1993;33:333–342

26. Yuki N, Hirata K. Relation between critical illness polyneuropathy and axonal Guillain–Barré syndrome (letter). J Neurol Neurosurg Psychiatry 1999;67:128–129

27. Hirano M, Ott BR, Raps EC, et al. Acute quadriplegic myopathy: a complication of treatment with steroids, nondepolarizing blocking agents, or both. Neurology 1992;42:2082–2087

28. Zochodne DW, Ramsay DA, Saly V, et al. Acute necrotizing myopathy of intensive care: electrophysiological studies. Muscle Nerve 1994;17:285–292

29. Lacomis D, Petrella FT, Giuliani MJ. Causes of neuromuscular weakness in the intensive care unit: a study of ninety-two patients. Muscle Nerve 1998;21:610–617

30. Opal SM, Yu RL Jr. Antiendotoxin strategies for the prevention and treatment of septic shock. New approaches and future directions. Drugs 1998;55:497–508

31. Vincent JL, Tielemans C. Continuous hemofiltration in severe sepsis: is it beneficial? J Crit Care 1995;10:27–32

32. Levy H, Ash SR, Knab W, et al. Systemic inflammatory response syndrome treatment by powdered sorbent pheresis: the BioLogic-Detoxification Plasma Filtration System. ASAIO J 1998;44:M659–M665

33. Werdan K. Supplemental immune globulins in sepsis. Clin Chem Lab Med 1999;37:341–349

34. Mohr M, Englisch L, Roth A, et al. Effects of early treatment with immunoglobulin on critical illness polyneuropathy following multiple organ failure and gram-negative sepsis. Intensive Care Med 1997;23:1144–1149

35. Waldhausen E, Mingers B, Lippers P, Keser G. Critical illness polyneuropathy due to parenteral nutrition (letter). Intensive Care Med 1997;23:922–923

36. Marino PL, Millili JJ. Possible role of dietary lipids in critical illness polyneuropathy (letter). Intensive Care Med 1998;24:87

37. Bolton CF, Young GB. Critical illness polyneuropathy due to parenteral nutrition (letter). Intensive Care Med 1997;23:924–925

38. Leijten FSS, De Weerd AW, Harinck-De Weerd JE, et al. Critical illness polyneuropathy due to parenteral nutrition (letter). Intensive Care Med 1997;23:925

214 Paresthesias and Pain

Rose M Dotson

Brief overview

The International Association for the Study of Pain has defined pain as a subjective sensory and emotional experience that is unpleasant and associated with actual or potential tissue damage.[1] Pain is frequently a prominent and distressing symptom for patients who have a peripheral neuropathy or nerve injury. Many patients who have neuropathic pain also experience *paresthesias*, spontaneous or evoked abnormal sensations that are not unpleasant, and *dysesthesias*, unpleasant spontaneous or evoked sensations. Dysesthesias include both *allodynia*, pain due to a non-noxious stimulus that normally is nonpainful, and *hyperalgesia*, increased pain perception in response to a stimulus that usually produces pain.[1-4]

Research conducted in the last 20 years has resulted in an exponential increase in the understanding of the complex mechanisms that result in neuropathic pain associated with trauma or disease affecting peripheral nerves. The focus of this chapter is on the pharmacological treatment of pain that occurs in disorders of peripheral nerves. The discussion includes a brief review of the epidemiology, etiology, and pathophysiology of neuropathic pain and useful diagnostic tests.

Epidemiology

Pain has considerable emotional and social impact on our society because it is one of the most common reasons for patients to seek medical care. For example, peripheral neuropathy develops in 50% of all persons who have diabetes mellitus, and 10% of them have neuropathic pain.[5] Paresthesias and pain are common symptoms in acquired chronic sensory-predominant polyneuropathies, which have a prevalence greater than 3% in the population, and 10% to 30% of these cases are idiopathic.[4,6-9] In a recent report of 402 patients with peripheral neuropathy, 23% had chronic cryptogenic sensory polyneuropathy (CCSP).[3] Pain was a presenting complaint in 72% of the patients with CCSP, and 62% of these patients reported having paresthesias along with the pain. Pain may be an important symptom at the time of clinical presentation in 55% to 85% of patients with acute inflammatory demyelinating polyradiculoneuropathy (Guillain–Barré syndrome).[10,11]

Etiology

Neuropathic pain occurs when disease or injury alters the function of peripheral nerves. This is in contrast to nociceptive pain, which is perceived because of impending or actual tissue damage.[1,2] Several diseases may cause peripheral neuropathy with pain and paresthesias (discussed below). Also, nerve injuries due to entrapment, compression, crush, transection, or traction of the nerve may cause neuropathic pain.

Pathophysiology and pathogenesis

Both noninflammatory and, less commonly, inflammatory dysfunction of the peripheral nervous system that produces mononeuropathy or polyneuropathy can cause neuropathic pain. Several underlying mechanisms that affect large or small nerve fibers or both may result in neuropathic pain (Table 214.1).

Lesions at the level of the primary afferent neuron (PAN) may result in pain and paresthesias. One possibility is a direct attack on the nerve trunk that may activate the nervi nervorum and the primary nociceptive fibers within the nerve bundles. Activated macrophages that release inflammatory mediators (prostaglandin E2, serotonin, bradykinin, epinephrine, adenosine) and cytokines such as tumor necrosis factor-α can produce sensitization and ectopic discharges of PANs.[2,12] Ectopic firing of nerve fibers that causes pain and paresthesias may also be due to areas

Table 214.1 Potential mechanisms of neuropathic pain
Direct attack on nerve trunk that causes activation of nervi nervorum
Inflammatory mediators and cytokines sensitize PANs, causing ectopic discharges
Demyelination or damage to nerve fibers or terminals, causing ectopic nerve discharges
Up-regulation of PN3/SNS sodium channels
Neurogenic inflammation
Sympathetic–sensory nerve interactions
Secondary messengers, immediate early genes causing prostaglandin production and PAN sensitization
Ephaptic transmission
Loss of A fibers that inhibit pain in the CNS
Phenotypic switch in A fibers
NGF-induced nerve sprouting at DRG and redistribution of sodium channels on nerves
Ectopic activity in deafferented spinal nociceptive neurons
WDR neurons in lamina V showing windup phenomenon
NMDA up-regulation in the spinal cord resulting in central sensitization
PANs release tachykinins that increase intracellular calcium, NMDA receptor activity
Neuroanatomical reorganization in the spinal cord

CNS, central nervous system; DRG, dorsal root ganglion; NGF, nerve growth factor; PAN, primary afferent neuron; SNS, sensory neuron-specific; WDR, wide dynamic range.

of demyelination or damaged nerve fibers or terminals.[13,14] Tetrodotoxin-resistant voltage-gated sodium channels (PN3/sensory-neuron specific) are up-regulated after nerve injury, resulting in a lowered threshold for nerve activation and spontaneous activity in PANs following injury.[15,16] Nerve growth factors may contribute to this and to abnormal sprouting of terminal nerve fibers, which may also cause neuropathic pain.[17]

Neurogenic inflammation occurs when unmyelinated nerve fibers antidromically release various peptides, substance P, calcitonin gene-related peptide, and neurokinins. The neurogenic flare response and hyperalgesia are the result of this secretory activity of nociceptors.[18,19]

Partial nerve injury can cause PANs that normally are unresponsive to catecholamines to express functional adrenergic receptors on their membrane and to develop catecholamine sensitivity. Ephaptic transmission may occur between C nociceptive fibers and sympathetic postganglionic fibers when nerve fibers are regenerating. This may explain the rare clinical occurrence of sympathetically maintained pain in nerve lesions.[20,21] Also, sympathetic terminals at the site of injury or inflammation release serotonin, bradykinins, and prostaglandin, with the potential to sensitize PANs.[22] The release of tachykinins (substance P, neurokinin A) and NMDA up-regulation may lead to calcium release and increased cell excitability. Prostaglandin production due to second messengers (nitric oxide, protein kinase C, phospholipase C) and immediate early gene expression (c-fos, c-jun, NFκB) contribute to the sensitization process.[23,24]

According to the gate control theory, involvement of primarily large fibers can result in the loss of central pain inhibition by large myelinated axons.[2] In addition, A-beta fibers may transmit nociceptive information in the setting of peripheral nerve injury or inflammation. Animal studies have shown that some of these nerve fibers make a phenotypic switch and may begin to express substance P, neuropeptide Y, and calcitonin gene-related peptide, similar to normal nociceptor PANs.[25,26]

Experimental nerve injury results in altered α_2-receptor expression at the level of the dorsal root ganglion and sprouting of sympathetic vasomotor fibers around large primary afferent cell bodies. These nerve sprouts may spontaneously synapse on satellite cells and provide the neural substrate for sympathetic and norepinephrine activation of ectopic activity in afferent cells.[2,22] However, the degree of sympathetic fiber sprouting in the dorsal root ganglion after peripheral nerve injury does not necessarily correlate with the amount of apparent sympathetically maintained mechanical and cold allodynia.[27]

Nociceptive neurons in the spinal cord that are deafferented can generate spontaneous activity from hyperexcitability. The windup phenomenon, that is, incomplete repolarization with repetitive stimulation, occurs in wide dynamic range neurons located in lamina V. These are the only neurons in this lamina that receive direct input from PANs and C-fiber afferents that can generate long excitatory postsynaptic potentials (A fibers generate shorter excitatory postsynaptic potentials). This means that a barrage of PAN impulses can partially depolarize the resting membrane potential of the wide dynamic range neurons and cause magnesium ions to leave their normal sites in the channels of NMDA receptors, which are then activated. Peripheral nerve injury and deafferentation result in the release of substance P, neurokinins, and excitatory neurotransmitters (e.g., glutamate and aspartate) that activate NMDA receptors. This allows calcium ions to rush in and trigger a cascade of intracellular events that result in neuropathic pain and central sensitization.[2,28–30]

Nerve injury can cause long-term neuroanatomical reorganization at the level of the spinal cord, with many large myelinated sensory axons sending sprouts into lamina II instead of their usual targets in laminae I, III, IV, and V. The sprouting of A-beta fibers into spinal areas where postsynaptic targets normally receive input from only small afferent fibers may result in allodynia and a "nonanatomical" pain distribution.[31]

Genetics

Several hereditary neuropathies are associated with neuropathic pain. These disorders and the known genetic features are discussed in other chapters in this Section. Studies of "knockout" mice have helped to substantiate that the PN3/sensory neuron-specific sodium channel on sensory neurons has a role in chronic neuropathic pain.[15] Mice with these null mutations for protein kinase C-gamma, the second messenger molecule of interneurons in the substantia gelatinosa, have less thermal and mechanical allodynia despite normal acute pain in response to nerve injury.[23] Gene deletion studies have implicated even nicotinic receptors in nociceptive processing.[32] Through studies of "knockout" mice, knowledge has been gained about neuronal plasticity that occurs in injury and the development of various types of nociceptors.[33,34]

Clinical features

Patients with neuropathic pain frequently report spontaneous and stimulus-induced pain along with other disturbances of sensation that may be worse at night. They commonly describe the spontaneous pains as "burning," "electric shock-like," "sharp," "shooting," "deep aching," or "raw sensations" that occur simultaneously or consecutively. Other common sensory symptoms include numbness, with reduced sensation to mechanical and thermal stimuli. Painful peripheral neuropathies are not uncommonly associated with hyperalgesia and allodynia.

Patients who have primarily axonal peripheral neuropathies frequently report the onset of symptoms in the distal and plantar surfaces of the toes and feet which gradually progress over months to years to involve more proximal portions of the extremities. In many patients, symptoms are noted eventually in the distal upper extremities at the time they reach the proximal lower extremities.

Autonomic nerve fibers are commonly affected in polyneuropathies with prominent involvement of small fibers. In these patients, symptoms include excessive or reduced sweating and skin temperature, alterations in skin color (paleness or redness), and alopecia of the extremities, frequently in areas corresponding to the areas of sensory disturbance. Patients may also complain of dry eyes and mouth, reduced pupillary adjustments to changes in ambient light, early satiety, constipation, diarrhea, orthostatic or postprandial lightheadedness, urinary retention, or impairment of sexual function. Physical examination may show dry, cold, discolored hairless skin of the extremities and orthostatic hypotension without an appropriate tachycardic response.

Pain may also occur in patients who have primarily demyelinating polyneuropathies. Most commonly, this is moderate-to-severe deep aching or throbbing low back pain that radiates into the lower extremities, sometimes as distally as the calves. The second most common type of pain in these patients is dysesthetic pain of the lower and, less frequently, upper extremities. A smaller, but still considerable, number of patients with acute inflammatory demyelinating polyradiculoneuropathy report aching or cramping pain in the extremities, with local muscle tenderness and joint stiffness. Activation of nociceptors in muscles that are becoming paralyzed, inflammation of nerve roots, and irritation of the nervi nervorum innervating nerve trunks may be the underlying causes of pain in this syndrome.[10,11]

Multiple mononeuropathies may be painful and can appear confluent by the time the patient presents for evaluation. Careful attention to the history of the onset and progression of symptoms will uncover evidence for symptoms attributable to mononeuropathies occurring in a stepwise fashion. This is important because the evaluation for an underlying cause can be influenced by this finding.

Erythromelalgia that results in red, hot, burning, swollen feet and, sometimes, hands may occur in polyneuropathy. Typically, these patients have heat and mechanical hyperalgesia, and cooling of the involved skin temporarily relieves the spontaneous and stimulus-induced pain. However, erythromelalgia may also occur in myeloproliferative disorders, central nervous system diseases (stroke, multiple sclerosis, autonomic disorders), collagen vascular disease, infectious diseases (influenza, infectious mononucleosis), or in response to medications (bromocriptine, nifedipine, hepatitis B vaccination).[35]

Also, some patients with peripheral neuropathy present with cold painful skin, cold hyperalgesia, and cold hypesthesia. They have increased thresholds for cold perception, and the first sensation perceived with a cold stimulus is in fact burning pain.[36]

Diagnostic criteria

Patients with neuropathic pain may have large-fiber sensory involvement, with abnormalities of light touch, vibration, or proprioception detected on physical examination. Abnormalities of small fibers detected on examination may include disturbances of pain and temperature in the form of reduced sensation or hypersensitivity. Quantitative sensory testing of vibration, cooling, pressure, heat pain, and cold pain may help to quantify deficits or provide documentation of allodynia and hyperalgesia due to involvement of large and small fibers.[37,38] Patients may also have motor nerve fiber disease, as evidenced by muscle weakness, atrophy, and, in some cases, fasciculations. Initially, deep tendon reflexes may be decreased distally and then proximally when the afferent or efferent limb of the reflex arc is affected by the neuropathy.[18]

Nerve conduction studies and electromyography may provide evidence for axonal polyneuropathy in the form of sensory nerve action potentials, fibrillation potentials, poorly recruited large motor unit potentials, and decreased amplitudes of compound muscle action potentials. Demyelinating neuropathies may show prolonged distal latencies or slowed conduction velocities, temporal dispersion, or conduction block on nerve conduction studies.[37,38]

Autonomic laboratory testing may confirm and quantify autonomic neuropathy in patients who have a painful polyneuropathy that affects small nerve fibers. The sympathetic skin response (which can easily be performed in an electromyography laboratory), quantitative sudomotor axon reflex test, and thermoregulatory sweat test are useful in the evaluation of sudomotor function. Cardiovagal impairment can be documented by measuring the variation in heart rate in response to deep breathing. Measurement of heart rate and beat-to-beat blood pressure while the patient performs the Valsalva maneuver is useful in assessing cardiovagal, peripheral adrenergic, and cardiac adrenergic function. Monitoring the patient's blood pressure and heart rate in the supine and upright tilt or standing positions allows confirmation of orthostatic intolerance or hypotension, further confirming impairment of adrenergic function.[37,38]

Classification

Pain conditions are classified as "neuropathic" or "nociceptive" according to the definitions noted above. Also, they frequently are classified according to the underlying cause.

Differential diagnosis

Several diagnostic possibilities need to be considered for patients who present with a major complaint of pain in the setting of a peripheral neuropathy (Table 214.2). Factors that may help determine the cause of a painful neuropathy include the severity and quality of pain; associated sensory, motor, or autonomic symptoms; onset and progression of symptoms; laboratory investigations for underlying diseases; and neurodiagnostic tests (nerve conduction studies, electromyography, quantitative sensory testing, autonomic testing, and nerve biopsy).[38]

Treatment

Several options are available for the treatment of neuropathic pain; however, they may provide no more

Table 214.2   Painful polyneuropathies

Metabolic
  Diabetic
    Chronic: SFN
              LFN and SFN
              LFN, SFN, and autonomic neuropathy
    Acute: Distal sensory
            Lumbar radiculoplexoneuropathy
            Brachial radiculoplexoneuropathy
  Acute or chronic alcoholic
  Uremic
  Hypothyroid
  Niacin deficiency (pellagra)
  Thiamine deficiency (beriberi)
  Multiple deficiencies: thiamine, niacin, riboflavin,
    pyridoxine (Strachan syndrome: amblyopia, painful
    neuropathy, orogenital dermatitis)
  Amyloid
HIV-related neuropathy
Acute inflammatory demyelinating polyradiculoneuropathy
  (Guillain–Barré syndrome)
Toxins/drugs—arsenic, mercury, perhexiline, thallium,
  isoniazid, cisplatin, vincristine, nitrofurantoin,
  disulfiram
Idiopathic small-fiber neuropathy
Cryptogenic sensorimotor neuropathy
Hereditary
  Hereditary sensory neuropathy type 1
  Fabry disease
  Burning feet syndrome
  Hereditary autonomic sensory neuropathies
Vasculitic neuropathy
  Large epineurial vessel involvement
    Rheumatoid arthritis
    Wegener granulomatosis
    Polyarteritis nodosa
    Churg-Strauss syndrome
  Small epineurial vessel involvement
    Sjögren syndrome
    Systemic lupus erythematosus
    Nonsystemic peripheral nerve vasculitis
Acute porphyria
Paraneoplastic sensory neuronopathy or peripheral
  neuropathy
Nonfreezing cold injury

HIV, human immunodeficiency virus; LFN, large-fiber neuropathy;
SFN, small-fiber neuropathy.

than partial pain relief for only some patients. Therefore, every effort should made early in the course of the neuropathy to determine the cause and, if possible, to treat the underlying cause (disease-specific treatments are discussed elsewhere in the text). The major categories of symptomatic treatment include physical measures, topical agents, oral medications, intrathecal drugs, neurostimulators, neuroablative procedures, and alternative therapies. The available oral agents include antidepressants (especially tricyclics), antiepileptic drugs, non-narcotic analgesics, antiarrhythmics, and narcotic analgesics (Tables 214.3 and 214.4).[39,40]

Physical measures should be considered the first-line symptomatic treatment for neuropathies. These may include soaking the painful area of skin in warm/cold water, followed by massage with lotion or petroleum jelly and the application of menthol- or aspirin-containing creams, lotions, or salves. Patients should carefully inspect their feet daily, wear thick cotton socks, and select roomy, well-fitted shoes. A regular exercise program, including aerobic activity that may result in the release of pain-relieving endorphins, is helpful. The physician should encourage patients to maintain work, hobbies, and interests outside the home as much as possible to help distract them from the pain. Some patients find that support groups allow them to better understand and cope with chronic neuropathic pain. Also, patients may be instructed in desensitization therapy by physical therapists so that they may practice this daily at home.[40]

Reports are contradictory about the use of topical capsaicin cream for painful polyneuropathy. However, some patients derive partial benefit from this treatment after they get past the initial few days to weeks of C-nociceptor sensitization that causes burning discomfort.[39,41–43] Studies have shown that epidermal nerve fibers and the subepidermal neural plexus degenerate with repeated application of capsaicin to the skin. After this treatment is discontinued, the epidermis is gradually reinnervated and nociceptive sensation returns to the treated area of skin.[44,45] Capsaicin cream (0.025% and 0.075%) may be applied initially at the lower concentration and then applied at the higher concentration after the patient is able to tolerate the increased dose. Patients should be instructed to apply a thin film of the cream to the affected area three or four times daily for up to 3 weeks before determining that the treatment is not effective.

Lidocaine, in a gel, cream, or patch formulation, may also be considered for the treatment of peripheral neuropathic pain.[39,46] Studies of patients with postherpetic neuralgia have shown that a patch containing 5% lidocaine provides substantial pain relief without causing systemic side effects.[47,48] This treatment may be considered for neuropathic pain due to other causes, especially if the patient has rather focal areas of more severe spontaneous pain or allodynia. A thin film of 2% to 5% lidocaine cream or gel may be applied three times daily to the painful area or the

Table 214.3   Pharmacological agents used systemically to treat neuropathic pain

Tricyclic antidepressants—amitriptyline, nortriptyline,
  imipramine, desipramine, clomipramine
Antiepileptic drugs—gabapentin, carbamazepine,
  lamotrigine
Non-narcotic/combination action analgesics—
  acetaminophen, nonsteroidal anti-inflammatory drugs,
  tramadol
Local anesthetics/antiarrhythmics—mexiletine (oral)
Selective serotonin reuptake inhibitors—fluoxetine,
  paroxetine
Narcotic analgesics—oxycodone, morphine sulfate,
  methadone, fentanyl

Table 214.4	Non-narcotic medications for neuropathic pain: doses and adverse reactions	
Medication	**Recommended doses**	**Adverse reactions**
First-line agents		
Acetaminophen	650–1000 mg bid/tid	Hepatotoxicity (to avoid, limit daily dose to 4000 mg)
Nonsteroidal anti-inflammatory drugs	Depends on medication prescribed	Nausea, abdominal pain, gastric ulcers, headache, edema, dizziness
Capsaicin cream	0.025% initially, 0.075% later Apply thin film to skin tid/qid	Local skin irritation, burning sensation for up to first 2–3 weeks
Lidocaine patch, cream, or solution	Apply 1–3 patches to painful area for 12 h, q 24–72 h Apply thin film of cream or solution tid	Local skin irritation
Tricyclic antidepressants – amitriptyline, nortriptyline, imipramine, desipramine, clomipramine	10–25 mg po at bedtime (desipramine may be taken every morning) May titrate by 10–25 mg/day weekly to 75–150 mg daily	Dry mouth, constipation, urinary retention, sedation, orthostatic hypotension, tachycardia, weight gain, seizures Contraindicated with some cardiac disease Insomnia with desipramine
Second-line agents		
Gabapentin	100 mg po tid, 300 mg daily or 300 mg tid May titrate by 100–300 mg/day weekly to 1600 mg tid 900–1200 mg tid for elderly Lower doses in renal impairment	Somnolence, ataxia, dizziness, nausea, vomiting, fatigue
Carbamazepine (first-line agent for trigeminal neuralgia)	100 mg po bid May titrate by 100 mg/day every 3 days to 200–500 mg bid/tid	Dizziness, sedation, nausea, vomiting, ataxia, bone marrow suppression, SIADH, elevated liver function studies, cardiac arrhythmias
Tramadol	25 mg po daily May titrate by 25 mg/day every 3 days to 25 mg qid, then titrate by 50 mg/day to 100 mg qid	Nausea, vomiting, constipation, dizziness, headache, somnolence, seizures
Third-line agents		
Lamotrigine	25 mg po bid May titrate by 50 mg/day every 2 weeks to 250–350 mg bid	Rash, sedation, fatigue, dizziness, headache, Stevens-Johnson syndrome/toxic epidermal necrolysis
Mexiletine	150 mg po at bedtime May titrate by 150 mg/day weekly to 300–400 mg tid	Nausea, fatigue, dizziness, headache, tremor, sleep disturbance, chest pain, tachycardia, palpitations
Paroxetine	10–20 mg po daily or 25 mg daily sustained-release May titrate by 10–20 mg/day weekly to 20–60 mg daily	Sedation, dry mouth, headache, insomnia, dizziness
Fluoxetine	20 mg po daily May titrate by 20 mg/day weekly to 80 mg daily	Asthenia, tremor, headache, insomnia, gastrointestinal symptoms

bid, twice daily; po, orally; qid, four times daily; SIADH, syndrome of inappropriate antidiuretic hormone; tid, three times daily.

lidocaine patch may be applied for 12 hours every 24 to 72 hours for pain as an adjunct to other forms of therapy.

Chronic low-intensity neuropathic pain that requires an oral medication may be treated initially with nonprescription analgesics such as aceta-minophen, enteric-coated salicylates, or other nonsteroidal anti-inflammatory drugs. Commonly, patients start by taking a dose of the medication in late afternoon and repeating the dose at bedtime, because neuropathic pain frequently is more intense in the evening and at night.

For most patients with neuropathic pain, the first-line prescription oral agent should be a tricyclic anti-depressant (TCA): amitriptyline, nortriptyline, imipramine, or desipramine. TCAs have several mechanisms of action, including central blockade of norepinephrine reuptake (desipramine) or central blockade of serotonin and norepinephrine reuptake (amitriptyline, nortriptyline, and imipramine) that may influence the brainstem–dorsal horn nociceptive modulating system. Other mechanisms of action include sodium and calcium channel blocking, weak NMDA receptor blocking, and binding to histaminergic, adrenergic, and cholinergic receptor sites. All these mechanisms may have a role in providing pain relief and producing the side effects caused by TCAs.[39,46,49–51]

TCAs should be started at a low dose of 25 mg/day, or 10 mg/day for patients who are older or have a tendency to drug intolerance or an illness that may make them prone to side effects. The dose should be titrated up by 10- to 25-mg/day increments weekly to the lowest dose that produces the greatest benefit with tolerable side effects. This slow titration minimizes side effects and allows for evaluation of a beneficial effect. It may take 1 to 2 weeks, with a peak at up to 6 weeks, to achieve a beneficial effect.[49] Most patients who benefit from TCAs require a dose of 75 to 150 mg/day. TCAs may help to alleviate all types of neuropathic pain, but studies have indicated that only about 30% of patients obtain more than a 50% reduction in pain.[49–51]

The side effects that usually are the most limiting are those due to the action of TCAs at cholinergic receptors. These include dry mouth, constipation, urinary retention (especially in males with prostate enlargement), blurred vision, sedation, mild cognitive impairment, and tachycardia. Patients with a history of seizures or those taking other medications that may lower the threshold for seizures are at greater risk for having additional seizure episodes. Cardiac contraindications for the use of TCAs include recent myocardial infarction (within 6 months), unstable angina, congestive heart failure, frequent premature ventricular contractions, history of sustained ventricular arrhythmias, long QT syndrome, or marked conduction block (bifascicular or trifascicular).[52] The action of TCAs at adrenergic receptors may cause orthostatic hypotension, especially in elderly patients or those with underlying autonomic neuropathy. This usually occurs early in the course of treatment with an excessive initial dose or with rapid titration upward. Sedation is a TCA side effect that may be used to the patient's benefit by timing the daily dose 1 to 2 hours before bedtime. Both sedation and weight gain are side effects that are due to the action of TACs at histamine receptors.[51]

Studies of selective serotonin reuptake inhibitors have shown that this family of medications is much less effective in the treatment of neuropathic pain than TCAs. Fluoxetine and paroxetine may be effective for depression associated with pain and minimally beneficial for neuropathic pain.[50,51]

Antiepileptic drugs (AEDs) are useful neuromodulating medications that may provide relief from neuropathic pain. Of AEDs, gabapentin is commonly used as a first-line agent for neuropathic pain because its effectiveness may be noted within 1 to 2 weeks after treatment is initiated. Gabapentin was developed to mimic the effect of γ-aminobutyric acid (GABA), to which it is structurally related. However, because gabapentin does not bind to GABA receptors, the exact mechanism by which it relieves neuropathic pain is not certain. Gabapentin has several pharmacological actions: it alters the synthesis and release of GABA in the brain, interacts with the system L-amino acid transporter, alters monoamine neurotransmitter release and blood serotonin levels, and inhibits voltage-activated sodium channels.[39,53] A central mechanism of action is suggested by the findings that gabapentin binds to the $\alpha_2\delta$ subunit of a voltage-dependent calcium channel and calcium has an important role at the NMDA receptor in central sensitization following peripheral nerve injury.[54]

Two multicenter double-blind, placebo-controlled clinical trials have shown that gabapentin is helpful for the treatment of pain due to postherpetic neuralgia and diabetic peripheral neuropathy.[55,56] Compared with placebo, gabapentin was more effective in relieving pain and sleep interference and had a more positive effect on the patient's quality of life and mood. The dose may be started at 300 mg three times daily for patients who tolerate medications well. However, for those who are usually intolerant of medications, are elderly, or have renal insufficiency, a dose of 100 mg three times daily or 300 mg at bedtime is preferred.[57] Patients should increase the dose as needed and tolerated by 100 or 300 mg/day each week, up to a maximal dose of 4800 mg/day in three divided doses for young healthy patients. Healthy elderly patients usually should titrate up to a dose of only 2700 to 3600 mg/day. Patients who have renal impairment, especially a creatinine clearance less than 60 mL/minute, require lower doses because gabapentin is excreted unchanged by the kidneys. The slow rate of titration may allow patients to determine the lowest beneficial dose and, thus, avoid taking excessive amounts of medication. Because gabapentin is not lipid-bound and does not affect the levels or effectiveness of other medications, it may be given without dose modification in conjunction with other agents to treat neuropathic pain.[55,56]

Gabapentin has several relatively common side effects, including somnolence, fatigue, ataxia, dizziness, nausea, and vomiting, which may cause a patient to discontinue taking the medication. This may be avoided by initiating treatment at a low dose and using the slow titration schedule noted above, because the adverse reactions of sedation, dizziness, and ataxia have been shown to be dose-dependent.[55,56]

There is evidence that carbamazepine is helpful for the treatment of pain due to postherpetic neuralgia, diabetic neuropathy, or trigeminal neuralgia. Its mechanism of action likely occurs at voltage-dependent sodium channels to stabilize the membranes of nerve fibers in the nociceptive system. Also, carbamazepine is structurally similar to TCAs and may have some of the same sites of action in the nervous system.[58]

More than 30 years ago, studies of 151 patients established that carbamazepine was the initial treatment of choice for trigeminal neuralgia.[59–62] These double-blind, placebo-controlled, crossover studies used a categorical scale for measurement of pain relief and showed pain improvement of 56% to 75% when patients were given carbamazepine versus 0% to 26% when they were given placebo. However, 30% to 40% of patients in the trials experienced tolerance or intolerable adverse reactions that caused them to discontinue taking the medication. Daily carbamazepine doses of 400 to 1000 mg produced a serum concentration of carbamazepine of 6 to 10 mg/L that corresponded to good pain relief.[60]

Two other placebo-controlled crossover studies performed 25 to 30 years ago demonstrated that painful diabetic peripheral neuropathy also responded to carbamazepine therapy.[63,64] A total of 40 study patients received a median daily carbamazepine dose of 600 mg and experienced more improvement in pain, sleep, and ability to walk than with placebo.

The preferred method for giving carbamazepine to treat painful peripheral neuropathy is to start with 100 mg twice daily. This is increased by 100-mg/day increments every 3 to 5 days to reach the point of adequate pain relief or intolerable side effects, usually 400 to 1000 mg/day in two or three divided doses. Adverse reactions that cause patients to discontinue taking carbamazepine include dizziness, sedation, nausea, vomiting, ataxia, bone marrow suppression, hyponatremia due to inappropriate antidiuretic hormone, and, rarely, elevated liver function tests or cardiac arrhythmias. Thus, liver function tests, a complete blood count, and the serum level of sodium should be determined immediately before starting treatment and periodically during treatment. Because carbamazepine induces liver enzymes, it may interact with many drugs, and this should always be considered if patients are taking other medications.

Lamotrigine, a newer AED, acts as an antagonist at sodium channels of PANs and may provide relief from neuropathic pain. This drug stabilizes slow, inactivated conformation of type IIA neuronal sodium channels, thus inhibiting repetitive firing of action potentials despite sustained neuronal depolarization.[65,66] In animal models, lamotrigine has been shown to decrease the amplitude of action potentials in presynaptic terminals, resulting in a decrease in the amount of transmitter, primarily glutamate, released from the axon. It also appears to relieve pain of prostaglandin E_2-induced hyperalgesia and streptozocin-induced diabetic neuropathy in rats.[67,68]

There are anecdotal reports and limited placebo-controlled trials demonstrating the benefits of lamotrigine in patients with neuropathic pain.[66,69–72] A 31-day double-blind, placebo-controlled crossover study of 14 patients with refractory trigeminal neuralgia treated with a steady dose of phenytoin or carbamazepine showed that adding a 400-mg maintenance dose of lamotrigine had superior antineuralgic properties compared with placebo ($P = 0.011$).[69] Although adverse events, most commonly dizziness, constipation, and nausea, were reported, this did not result in withdrawal from the trial. Also, because of only moderate binding to plasma proteins, lamotrigine did not alter the plasma concentration of carbamazepine. Baseline measures of hemoglobin, platelet count, leukocyte count, creatinine, and liver function tests were also stable during treatment. In contrast, a randomized, double-blind, placebo-controlled trial that evaluated the effect of 200 mg of lamotrigine in 100 patients with neuropathic pain measured total pain, pain character, sensitivity, numbness, paresthesia, sleep, mobility, mood, quality of life, and analgesic consumption. This lower dose of lamotrigine did not substantially alter any of the study variables.[70]

The dosage of lamotrigine used to treat neuropathic pain is similar to that for treating epilepsy, starting at 25 mg twice daily and increasing by 50 mg/day at 2-week intervals to 500 mg/day in two divided doses. In epilepsy trials, some patients were given the maximal dose of 700 mg/day. However, because the addition of valproic acid inhibits the clearance of lamotrigine and may increase its steady-state concentration slightly more than twofold, patients who take both medications usually require lower doses of lamotrigine.[73] Slow titration lessens the likelihood of side effects, especially serious skin rash, Stevens-Johnson syndrome, or toxic epidermal necrolysis.[73]

Tramadol, a non-narcotic centrally acting synthetic analgesic, should be considered as a second-line agent in the treatment of neuropathic pain. This drug relieves neuropathic pain by two mechanisms: as a weak mu-opioid agonist and as an inhibitor of serotonin and norepinephrine uptake. Tramadol has been shown in randomized, double-blind, placebo-controlled trials to produce marked relief of spontaneous pain and mechanical allodynia in patients with pain due to polyneuropathy.[74,75] One study has indicated there are long-term benefits for patients with painful diabetic neuropathy treated with tramadol for 6 months.[76]

Because the adverse events reported most commonly with tramadol are nausea, vomiting, constipation, dizziness, headache, and somnolence, it should be prescribed with caution for patients taking medications (TCAs, AEDs) that have a similar side-effect profile. Patients who are taking other medications that increase the possibility of seizures (TCAs, opioids) or who have a past history of seizures are at risk for having increased seizure activity. A slow titration rate of tramadol starting at 25 mg/day and increasing by 25-mg increments every 3 days up to 100 mg/day has been shown to lessen the occurrence of nausea or vomiting, which causes patients to discontinue taking this drug.[77] Thereafter, dosage increases may be made in 50-mg/day increments to reach the maximal recommended dosage of 400 mg/day in four divided doses.

Mexiletine, an oral antiarrhythmic agent that is a sodium channel antagonist and structurally related to lidocaine, may relieve symptoms of neuropathic pain. The results of several randomized, placebo-controlled trials that evaluated the use of this drug in treating painful diabetic neuropathy have indicated that doses of 300 to 675 mg/day may reduce subjective pain ratings.[78–82] In one study, mexiletine also substantially improved the quality of sleep and relieved nocturnal, but not daytime, pain. Adverse events, most commonly nausea and other gastrointestinal symptoms, occurred in 13.5% to 50% of the patients. Thus, taking mexiletine with food or antacids may be useful for some patients. Less frequent adverse events included fatigue, dizziness, headache, tremor, and sleep disturbance. Although some patients experience chest pain, transient tachycardia, and palpitations, no serious cardiac arrhythmias have been reported in patients taking mexiletine for painful neuropathy. A baseline electrocardiogram is important because mexiletine can worsen cardiac arrhythmias or cardiac conduction block.[82]

Several factors have to be considered because mexiletine is metabolized in the liver. Thus, liver function tests should be performed before mexiletine therapy is initiated, because lower doses may be needed for patients with impaired liver function. With the rare occurrence of impaired liver function among patients taking mexiletine, periodic monitoring of liver function tests seems appropriate. Although some patients are "extensive metabolizers" who have cytochrome P-450 2D6, others are "poor metabolizers" who lack this isoenzyme. The extensive metabolizers are susceptible to drug interactions between mexiletine and quinidine and metoprolol, which are metabolized by cytochrome P-450 2D6, and theophylline, which is metabolized by cytochrome P-450 1A2. Mexiletine dosage may need to be adjusted for patients who take phenytoin and rifampicin concomitantly because these drugs induce metabolism of mexiletine. Additional monitoring should include baseline and periodic complete blood counts because leukopenia and thrombocytopenia are rare occurrences with mexiletine therapy.[81]

The limited evidence for efficacy and the marked potential for adverse events render mexiletine a third-line agent for treatment of neuropathic pain. To improve patient tolerance, it may be started at 150 mg at bedtime and increased in 150-mg/day increments on a weekly basis up to 300 mg three times daily or if necessary to the maximal recommended daily dosage of 1200 mg.[81,82]

Although the use of opioids in the treatment of neuropathic pain is controversial, these types of medications may be useful for neuropathic pain. Opioids that act at the mu-receptor, for example, morphine, fentanyl, methadone, and oxycodone, lessen the pain of postherpetic neuralgia and other neuropathic pain syndromes (Table 214.5).[39,83] The pain of some patients may respond well to oral narcotics, for example, oxycodone or morphine, and the clinician may want to consider this early in the course of treatment of neuropathic pain. Some patients find that a small dose of

a short-acting narcotic, for example, 5 to 10 mg of oxycodone or 5 to 30 mg of morphine sulfate taken immediately before going to bed may be helpful at night. In some cases, the patient may be allowed to take the short-acting narcotic dose as needed to determine the total daily dosage requirements that provide pain relief. The amount taken each day should be titrated upward over 48 hours or more to minimize side effects (usually constipation, sedation, and nausea). The next step is to replace this medication with an extended-release narcotic formulation at a dose that is usually about 30 mg twice daily of oxycodone or 150 mg/75 kg body weight twice daily of morphine sulfate.

Methadone, a much less expensive lipophilic narcotic medication than oxycodone or morphine sulfate, can be administered by multiple routes, has a relatively long half-life (30.4 ± 16.3 hours), and is a consideration for patients whose pain responds to narcotic analgesics.[83–85] Also, methadone is a noncompetitive NMDA antagonist, with an affinity for this receptor that is similar to that of ketamine, a drug whose clinical usefulness is limited because of its prominent side effects.[86] Another benefit of methadone in the treatment of pain is its lack of active metabolites, commonly a limiting factor in the use of other opioids such as morphine, hydromorphone, meperidine, and fentanyl. Because methadone shows incomplete cross-tolerance, it may be prescribed when intolerable side effects limit the use of other narcotics.[85] This also means that the dosage of methadone administered to patients must be carefully individualized. Studies have shown that 4 to 35 mg of methadone every 8 hours is necessary initially for opioid-naïve pain patients versus a fixed methadone dose that is 10% to 50% of the previous morphine dose for patients previously given narcotics.[84,85] Patients may need additional doses for breakthrough pain that occurs between the scheduled doses.

Patients who take narcotic analgesics should be instructed to follow directions carefully and to practice a bowel program consisting of adequate fluid and fiber intake. Some pain medicine specialists enter into a written or oral agreement with the patient to use narcotic medications prescribed only by one clinician and to stay within the prescribed limit each month. Narcotic medications should be prescribed even more cautiously for patients who have a history of addictive behavior. The physician and patient should keep in mind that the need for narcotic medications may be lessened considerably by the upward titration and eventual benefit of so-called neuromodulating medications, for example, TCAs and AEDs.

A patient with neuropathic pain may require treatment with a combination of some of the above medications. If a medication is only partially beneficial, the addition of a second medication that has another mechanism of action may provide additional pain relief. The physician should try to avoid starting treatment with more than one medication simultaneously because this makes it difficult to determine which drug causes any adverse events that may occur. Also,

Table 214.5   Opioid analgesics for neuropathic pain: doses and adverse reactions

Medication	Recommended doses	Adverse reactions
Oxycodone	5–10 mg po at bedtime, may titrate by 5–10 mg/day every 2–7 days to 30 mg every 4–6 h or higher if necessary For long-term use, divide total daily amount for every 12 h dosing of long-acting formulation Alternatively, may start long-acting drug initially at 10 mg every 12 h and increase by 10 mg/dose every 2–7 days Allow 5–10 mg bid of short-acting drug for breakthrough pain	Dizziness, sedation, nausea, vomiting, constipation, urinary retention, respiratory depression, circulatory depression, headache, dry mouth, sweating
Morphine sulfate	5–30 mg po at bedtime, may titrate by 5–15 mg/day every 2–7 days to 30 mg every 4–6 h or higher if necessary Reduce dose if side effects warrant For long-term use, divide total daily dose amount for every 12 h or every 8 h dosing of long-acting drug Allow 5–15 mg bid of short-acting drug for breakthrough pain	Similar to oxycodone
Fentanyl	25 μg/h transdermal patch every 72 h; may increase by 25 μg/h every 72 h for every 90 mg/24 h of short-acting morphine sulfate or equianalgesic dose of another opioid after 3 days initially and then every 6 days if necessary to 300 μg/h every 72 h or, if necessary, every 48 h Allow use of short-acting oral opioid as above for breakthrough pain	Similar to oxycodone
Methadone	2.5–10 mg po every 3–4 h PRN until stable daily dose achieved, then divide total daily amount for bid dosing Allow use of short-acting oral opioid as above for breakthrough pain	Similar to oxycodone Accumulation over days may increase toxicity, especially in elderly or those with organ failure

bid, twice daily; po, orally; PRN, as needed.

a patient may end up taking more medication than necessary for appropriate pain relief.

In summary, the complex mechanisms underlying chronic neuropathic pain are at least partially understood and this information can be used to choose more rationally treatment options for these patients. Currently, the clinician should strive to treat the underlying cause of neuropathic pain whenever possible in the hope of preventing or eliminating the neuropathic lesion. Otherwise, only symptomatic physical or pharmacological measures of pain control are recommended.

References

1. Merskey H, Bogduk N, eds. Classification of Chronic Pain: Descriptions of Chronic Pain Syndromes and Definitions of Pain Terms. 2nd ed. Seattle, Washington: IASP Press, 1994
2. Woolf CJ, Mannion RJ. Neuropathic pain: aetiology, symptoms, mechanisms, and management. Lancet 1999;353:1959–1964
3. Wolfe GI, Baker NS, Amato AA, et al. Chronic cryptogenic sensory polyneuropathy: clinical and laboratory characteristics. Arch Neurol 1999;56:540–547
4. Dyck PJ. Cryptogenic sensory polyneuropathy. Arch Neurol 1999;56:519–520
5. Dyck PJ, Kratz KM, Karnes JL, et al. The prevalence by staged severity of various types of diabetic neuropathy, retinopathy, and nephropathy in a population-based cohort: the Rochester Diabetic Neuropathy Study. Neurology 1993;43:817–824
6. Italian General Practitioner Study Group (IGPSG). Chronic symmetric symptomatic polyneuropathy in the elderly: a field screening investigation in two Italian regions. I. Prevalence and general characteristics of the sample. Neurology 1995;45:1832–1836
7. McLeod JG, Tuck RR, Pollard JD, et al. Chronic polyneuropathy of undetermined cause. J Neurol Neurosurg Psychiatry 1984;47:530–535
8. Grahmann F, Winterholler M, Neundorfer B. Cryptogenic polyneuropathies: an out-patient follow-up study. Acta Neurol Scand 1991;84:221–225
9. Hopf HC, Althaus HH, Vogel P. An evaluation of the course of peripheral neuropathies based on clinical and

neurographical re-examinations. Eur Neurol 1973;9: 90–104

10. Moulin DE, Hagen N, Feasby TE, et al. Pain in Guillain–Barré syndrome. Neurology 1997;48:328–331

11. Ropper AH, Shahani BT. Pain in Guillain–Barré syndrome. Arch Neurol 1984;41:511–514

12. Woolf CJ, Salter MW. Neuronal plasticity: increasing the gain in pain. Science 2000;288:1765–1769

13. Ochoa J, Cline M, Dotson R, Marchettini P. Pain and paresthesias provoked mechanically in human cervical root entrapment (sign of Spurling). Single sensory unit antidromic recording of ectopic bursting, propagated nerve impulse activity. *In*: Pubols LM, Sessle BJ, eds. Effects of Injury on Trigeminal and Spinal Somatosensory Systems. New York: Liss, 1987;389–397

14. Campero M, Serra J, Marchettini P, Ochoa JL. Ectopic impulse generation and autoexcitation in single myelinated afferent fibers in patients with peripheral neuropathy and positive sensory symptoms. Muscle Nerve 1998;21:1661–1667

15. Akopian AN, Souslova V, England S, et al. The tetrodotoxin-resistant sodium channel SNS has a specialized function in pain pathways. Nat Neurosci 1999;2:541–548

16. Waxman SG, Cummins TR, Dib-Hajj S, et al. Sodium channels, excitability of primary sensory neurons, and the molecular basis of pain. Muscle Nerve 1999;22: 1177–1187

17. McMahon SB, Bennett DLH. Growth factors and pain. *In*: Dickenson A, Besson JM, eds. The Pharmacology of Pain. New York: Springer, 1997;135–165

18. Kumazawa T. Primitivism and plasticity of pain—implication of polymodal receptors. Neurosci Res 1998;32:9–31

19. Kumazawa T. The polymodal receptor: bio-warning and defense system. Prog Brain Res 1996;113:3–18

20. Sato J, Perl ER. Adrenergic excitation of cutaneous pain receptors induced by peripheral nerve injury. Science 1991;251:1608–1610

21. Perl ER. Cutaneous polymodal receptors: characteristics and plasticity. Prog Brain Res 1996;113:21–37

22. Jänig W, Levine JD, Michaelis M. Interactions of sympathetic and primary afferent neurons following nerve injury and tissue trauma. Prog Brain Res 1996;113: 161–184

23. Malmberg AB, Chen C, Tonegawa S, Basbaum AI. Preserved acute pain and reduced neuropathic pain in mice lacking PKCγ. Science 1997;278:279–283

24. Zigmond MJ, Bloom FE, Landis SC, et al, eds. Fundamental Neuroscience. San Diego: Academic Press, 1999

25. Neumann S, Doubell TP, Leslie T, Woolf CJ. Inflammatory pain hypersensitivity mediated by phenotypic switch in myelinated primary sensory neurons. Nature 1996;384:360–364

26. Wakisaka S, Youn SH, Kato J, et al. Neuropeptide Y-immunoreactive primary afferents in the dental pulp and periodontal ligament following nerve injury to the inferior alveolar nerve in the rat. Brain Res 1996;712:11–18

27. Kim HJ, Na HS, Sung B, Hong SK. Amount of sympathetic sprouting in the dorsal root ganglia is not correlated to the level of sympathetic dependence of neuropathic pain in a rat model. Neurosci Lett 1998;245:21–24

28. Coderre TJ, Katz J, Vaccarino AL, Melzack R. Contribution of central neuroplasticity to pathological pain: review of clinical and experimental evidence. Pain 1993;52:259–285

29. Dickenson AH. Spinal cord pharmacology of pain. Br J Anaesth 1995;75:193–200

30. Davies SN, Lodge D. Evidence for involvement of N-methylaspartate receptors in "wind-up" of class 2 neurones in the dorsal horn of the rat. Brain Res 1987;424:402–406

31. Woolf CJ, Shortland P, Coggeshall RE. Peripheral nerve injury triggers central sprouting of myelinated afferents. Nature 1992;355:75–78

32. Marubio LM, del Mar Arroyo-Jimenez M, Cordero-Erausquin M, et al. Reduced antinociception in mice lacking neuronal nicotinic receptor subunits. Nature 1999;398:805–810

33. Silos-Santiago I, Fagan AM, Garber M, et al. Severe sensory deficits but normal CNS development in newborn mice lacking TrkB and TrkC tyrosine protein kinase receptors. Eur J Neurosci 1997;9:2045–2056

34. Liebl DJ, Tessarollo L, Palko ME, Parada LF. Absence of sensory neurons before target innervation in brain-derived neurotrophic factor-neurotrophin 3-, and TrkC-deficient embryonic mice. J Neurosci 1997;17:9113–9121

35. Davis MD, O'Fallon WM, Rogers RS III, Rooke TW. Natural history of erythromelalgia: presentation and outcome in 168 patients. Arch Dermatol 2000;136: 330–336

36. Ochoa JL, Yarnitsky D. The triple cold syndrome. Cold hyperalgesia, cold hypoaesthesia and cold skin in peripheral nerve disease. Brain 1994;117:185–197

37. Dotson RM. Clinical neurophysiology laboratory tests to assess the nociceptive system in humans. J Clin Neurophysiol 1997;14:32–45

38. Sandroni P, Dotson R. Neurological assessment and workup of the patients with neuropathic pain. Curr Anesthesiol Rep 2000;2:207–213

39. Sindrup SH, Jensen TS. Efficacy of pharmacological treatments of neuropathic pain: an update and effect related to mechanism of drug action. Pain 1999;83:389–400

40. Low PA, Dotson RM. Symptomatic treatment of painful neuropathy. JAMA 1998;280:1863–1864

41. Low PA, Opfer-Gehrking TL, Dyck PJ, et al. Double-blind, placebo-controlled study of the application of capsaicin cream in chronic distal painful polyneuropathy. Pain 1995;62:163–168

42. The Capsaicin Study Group. Treatment of painful diabetic neuropathy with topical capsaicin. A multicenter, double-blind, vehicle-controlled study. Arch Intern Med 1991;151:2225–2229

43. Culp WJ, Ochoa J, Cline M, Dotson R. Heat and mechanical hyperalgesia induced by capsaicin. Cross modality threshold modulation in human C nociceptors. Brain 1989;112:1317–1331

44. Simone DA, Nolano M, Johnson T, et al. Intradermal injection of capsaicin in humans produces degeneration and subsequent reinnervation of epidermal nerve fibers: correlation with sensory function. J Neurosci 1998;18:8947–8959

45. Nolano M, Simone DA, Wendelschafer-Crabb G, et al. Topical capsaicin in humans: parallel loss of epidermal nerve fibers and pain sensation. Pain 1999;81:135–145

46. Kingrey WS. A critical review of controlled clinical trials for peripheral neuropathic pain and complex regional pain syndromes. Pain 1997;73:123–139

47. Galer BS, Rowbotham MC, Perander J, Friedman E. Topical lidocaine patch relieves postherpetic neuralgia more effectively than a vehicle topical patch: results of an enriched enrollment study. Pain 1999;80:533–538

48. Kanazi GE, Johnson RW, Dworkin RH. Treatment of

postherpetic neuralgia: an update. Drugs 2000;59: 1113–1126

49. Max MB, Culnane M, Schafer SC, et al. Amitriptyline relieves diabetic neuropathy pain in patients with normal or depressed mood. Neurology 1987;37:589–596

50. Max MB, Lynch SA, Muir J, et al. Effects of desipramine, amitriptyline, and fluoxetine on pain in diabetic neuropathy. N Engl J Med 1992;326:1250–1256

51. McQuay HJ, Tramer M, Nye BA, et al. A systematic review of antidepressants in neuropathic pain. Pain 1996;68:217–227

52. Roose SP, Laghrissi-Thode F, Kennedy JS, et al. Comparison of paroxetine and nortriptyline in depressed patients with ischemic heart disease. JAMA 1998;279: 287–291

53. Taylor CP, Gee NS, Su TZ, et al. A summary of mechanistic hypotheses of gabapentin pharmacology. Epilepsy Res 1998;29:233–249

54. Gee NS, Brown JP, Dissanayake VU, et al. The novel anticonvulsant drug, gabapentin (neurontin), binds to the $\alpha_2\delta$ subunit of a calcium channel. J Biol Chem 1996;271:5768–5776

55. Rowbotham M, Harden N, Stacey B, et al. Gabapentin for the treatment of postherpetic neuralgia: a randomized controlled trial. JAMA 1998;280:1837–1842

56. Backonja M, Beydoun A, Edwards KR, et al. Gabapentin for the symptomatic treatment of painful neuropathy in patients with diabetes mellitus: a randomized controlled trial. JAMA 1998;280:1831–1836

57. Dyck PJ, Litchy WJ, Lehman KA, et al. Variables influencing neuropathic endpoints: the Rochester Diabetic Neuropathy Study of Healthy Subjects. Neurology 1995;45:1115–1121

58. Swerdlow M. Anticonvulsant drugs and chronic pain. Clin Neuropharmacol 1984;7:51–82

59. Campbell FG, Graham JG, Zilkha KJ. Clinical trial of carbamazepine (Tegretol) in trigeminal neuralgia. J Neurol Neurosurg Psychiatry 1966;29:265–267

60. Killian JM, Fromm GH. Carbamazepine in the treatment of neuralgia. Use of side effects. Arch Neurol 1968;19:129–136

61. Nicol CF. A four year double-blind study of Tegretol in facial pain. Headache 1969;9:54–57

62. Tomson T, Tybring G, Bertilsson L, et al. Carbamazepine therapy in trigeminal neuralgia: clinical effects in relation to plasma concentration. Arch Neurol 1980;37:699–703

63. Rull JA, Quibrera R, Gonzalez-Millan H, Lozano Castaneda O. Symptomatic treatment of peripheral diabetic neuropathy with carbamazepine (Tegretol): double blind crossover trial. Diabetologia 1969;5: 215–218

64. Wilton TD. Tegretol in the treatment of diabetic neuropathy. S Afr Med J 1974;48:869–872

65. Leach MJ, Lees G, Riddall DR. Lamotrigine: mechanisms of action. In: Levy RH, Mattson RH, Meldrum BS, eds. Antiepileptic Drugs. 4th ed. New York: Raven Press, 1995:861–869

66. Nakamura-Craig M, Follenfant RL. Lamotrigine and analgesia; a new treatment for chronic pain. In: Gebhart GF, Hammond DL, Jensen TS. Proceedings of the 7th World Congress on Pain. Seattle, Washington: IASP Press, 1994:725–730

67. Nakamura-Craig M, Follenfant RL. Effect of lamotrigine in the acute and chronic hyperalgesia induced by PGE2 and in the chronic hyperalgesia in rats with streptozotocin-induced diabetes. Pain 1995;63:33–37

68. Xie X, Lancaster B, Peakman T, Garthwaite J. Interaction of the antiepileptic drug lamotrigine with recombinant rat brain type IIA Na+ channels and with native Na+ channels in rat hippocampal neurones. Pflugers Arch 1995;430:437–446

69. Zakrzewska JM, Chaudhry Z, Nurmikko TJ, et al. Lamotrigine (Lamictal) in refractory trigeminal neuralgia: results from a double-blind placebo controlled crossover trial. Pain 1997;73:223–230

70. McCleane G. 200 mg daily of lamotrigine has no analgesic effect in neuropathic pain: a randomised, double-blind, placebo controlled trial. Pain 1999;83:105–107

71. Devulder J, De Laat M. Lamotrigine in the treatment of chronic refractory neuropathic pain. J Pain Symptom Manage 2000;19:398–403

72. Simpson DM, Olney R, McArthur JC, et al. A placebo-controlled trial of lamotrigine for painful HIV-associated neuropathy. Neurology 2000;54:2115–2119

73. Kanner AM, Frey M. Adding valproate to lamotrigine: a study of their pharmacokinetic interaction. Neurology 2000;55:588–591

74. Harati Y, Gooch C, Swenson M, et al. Double-blind randomized trial of tramadol for the treatment of the pain of diabetic neuropathy. Neurology 1998;50:1842–1846

75. Sindrup SH, Andersen G, Madsen C, et al. Tramadol relieves pain and allodynia in polyneuropathy: a randomised, double-blind controlled trial. Pain 1999;83: 85–90

76. Harati Y, Gooch C, Swenson M, et al. Maintenance of the long-term effectiveness of tramadol in treatment of the pain of diabetic neuropathy. J Diabetes Complications 2000;14:65–70

77. Petrone D, Kamin M, Olson W. Slowing the titration rate of tramadol HCl reduces the incidence of discontinuation due to nausea and/or vomiting: a double-blind randomized trial. J Clin Pharm Ther 1999;24: 115–123

78. Stracke H, Meyer UE, Schumacher HE, Federlin K. Mexiletine in the treatment of diabetic neuropathy. Diabetes Care 1992;15:1550–1555

79. Wright JM, Oki JC, Graves L III. Mexiletine in the symptomatic treatment of diabetic peripheral neuropathy. Ann Pharmacother 1997;31:29–34

80. Oskarsson P, Ljunggren JG, Lins PE. Efficacy and safety of mexiletine in the treatment of painful diabetic neuropathy. The Mexiletine Study Group. Diabetes Care 1997;20:1594–1597

81. Jarvis B, Coukell AJ. Mexiletine. A review of its therapeutic use in painful diabetic neuropathy. Drugs 1998; 56:691–707

82. Anonymous. Drugs for cardiac arrhythmias. Med Lett Drugs Ther 1989;31:35–40

83. Portenoy RK. Current pharmacotherapy of chronic pain. J Pain Symptom Manage 2000;19 Suppl:S16–S20

84. Fainsinger R, Schoeller T, Bruera E. Methadone in the management of cancer pain: a review. Pain 1993;52: 137–147

85. Mercadante S, Casuccio A, Calderone L. Rapid switching from morphine to methadone in cancer patients with poor response to morphine. J Clin Oncol 1999;17:3307–3312

86. Ebert B, Andersen S, Krogsgaard-Larsen P. Ketobemidone, methadone and pethidine are non-competitive N-methyl-D-aspartate (NMDA) antagonists in the rat cortex and spinal cord. Neurosci Lett 1995;187:165–168

215 Treatment of Sexual Dysfunction and Cystopathy in Peripheral Nerve Disorders

Jay C Lee and Claire C Yang

Peripheral nerve disorders can impair both sexual function and bladder function. The most common form of male neuropathic sexual dysfunction, erectile dysfunction, can be due to disruption of the pudendal (genital) somatosensory tracts or the autonomic innervation to the penis mediating the hemodynamics of erection. Other causes of erectile dysfunction include vascular, psychological, endocrine, and penile structural problems. One or more of these may be etiologic factors in combination with neurological disease. The study of the neurophysiology of female sexual dysfunction is still relatively new; thus, not all the causative factors have been elucidated.

Cystopathy that results from peripheral nerve disorders is manifested as autonomic denervation of the detrusor, resulting in urinary retention, or as loss of sensation, resulting in bladder overdistention. With chronic overdistention, the bladder secondarily loses its motor function. In both instances, failure of the bladder to empty completely leads to voiding symptoms and incontinence and increases the risk of infection, stone formation, and renal failure.

The standard treatments for sexual dysfunction and cystopathy include both medical and surgical options. In erectile dysfunction, the goal of treatment is to restore an erection rigid enough for intercourse. Treatment of cystopathy is aimed at maintaining social continence, having efficient bladder drainage at regular intervals, minimizing urinary symptoms, and avoiding infection. Treatment of genitourinary complications due to peripheral nerve disorders should take into consideration the patient's physical and cognitive limitations.

Treatment of male sexual dysfunction: erection

On the basis of the cause of sexual dysfunction and the treatment goals, appropriate therapy can be instituted (Table 215.1). Special considerations for patients with neuropathy must be taken into account. Rarely do the treatments for sexual dysfunction improve sensory loss or hyperesthesia. With the more invasive treatments such as intracavernosal injection or penile prosthesis, sensory problems may be aggravated.

Psychological counseling and sexual therapy

The majority of studies investigating erectile dysfunction and neuropathy have examined patients with diabetes mellitus, because it is a common cause of neuropathy. According to reports of comprehensive psychological and physiological testing, approximately 10% of males with diabetes who complain of impotence have primary psychogenic impotence.[1,2] On psychological assessment, affective factors have been found in 50% of impotent men with diabetes.[3] Psychological treatment for these men and their partners can be helpful in their regaining sexual health. Even if a psychogenic cause cannot be elucidated, studies have demonstrated that psychosocial support is a synergistic adjunct to other therapies.[4,5] A description of psychological methods is beyond the scope of this chapter, and the reader is referred to other sources.[6-8]

Medical treatment

Many medications are known to cause or exacerbate erectile dysfunction (Table 215.2).[9] High blood pressure medications are the most common type of drugs associated with impotence. Changing from one class of drug to another may improve the symptoms. Also, antidepressants such as selective serotonin reuptake inhibitors are associated with impotence. Switching antidepressant medications to trazodone has demonstrated efficacy in restoring erectile function.[10] If a temporal association can be identified between treatment with a particular medication and the onset of sexual dysfunction, a change in the patient's drug regimen should be attempted in consultation with the patient's primary physician.

The most commonly used systemic medications for the treatment of erectile dysfunction are testosterone

Table 215.1 Treatment options for male sexual dysfunction

Psychosocial
   Psychotherapy
   Sex/couples therapy
Medical treatment
   Medication changes
   Hormone replacement
   Oral medications
Vacuum constriction device
Penile injection therapy
Penile prosthesis

Table 215.2 Common drugs that cause sexual dysfunction

Drug	Examples, generic name (brand name)	Effect
Tricyclic antidepressants (TCA)	Amitriptyline (Elavil)	Decreased libido, impotence, delayed ejaculation/orgasm
	Imipramine (Tofranil)	
Selective serotonin reuptake inhibitors (SSRI)	Fluoxetine (Prozac)	Delayed ejaculation/orgasm, decreased libido
	Sertraline (Zoloft)	
Monoamine oxidase inhibitors (MAOI)	Phenelzine (Nardil)	Impotence, delayed ejaculation/orgasm
	Isocarboxazid (Marplan)	
Sedatives	Alprazolam (Xanax)	Decreased libido, delayed ejaculation/orgasm
	Diazepam (Valium)	
Antipsychotics	Haloperidol (Haldol)	Impotence, delayed or painful ejaculation/orgasm
	Thioridazine (Mellaril)	
Diuretics	Thiazide diuretics	Impotence, decreased libido
	Spironolactone (Aldactone)	
Centrally acting sympatholytics	Clonidine (Catapres)	Impotence, delayed or retrograde ejaculation
	Methyldopa (Aldomet)	
β-Blockers	Propranolol (Inderal)	Impotence, loss of libido
	Atenolol (Tenormin)	
	Metoprolol (Lopressor)	
Antiarrhythmics	Digoxin (Lanoxin)	Decreased libido, impotence
	Amiodarone (Cordarone)	
Histamine (H_2)-blockers	Ranitidine (Zantac)	Impotence, decreased libido
	Famotidine (Pepcid)	
	Cimetidine (Tagamet)	
Antiepileptics	Barbiturates	Decreased libido, impotence
	Carbamazepine (Tegretol)	
	Phenytoin (Dilantin)	
Anti-Parkinson	Doxepin (Sinequan)	Decreased libido, ejaculatory dysfunction
Antiandrogens	Leuprolide (Lupron)	Impotence, decreased libido
	Goserelin (Zoladex)	

and sildenafil (Viagra). The primary effect of testosterone replacement therapy on sexual function in a hypogonadal male is to improve libido and, secondarily, to improve potency.[11] Testosterone replacement therapy should be instituted only in patients who have documented hypogonadism. These patients will have low serum levels of testosterone and may have increased levels of lutenizing hormone. Testosterone enanthate, 200 mg intramuscularly every 2 to 3 weeks, is one of the most commonly used preparations. New transdermal forms of testosterone are now available (Testoderm TTS 5 mg/day or Androderm 5 mg/day). Oral formulations are not well absorbed from the gastrointestinal tract, and they are associated with liver enzyme abnormalities. The risk of increasing the incidence of prostate disease in patients receiving testosterone replacement therapy has not been substantiated;[12,13] however, a serum prostate-specific antigen test and a digital rectal examination are recommended for older men before and during replacement therapy.

Sildenafil is a selective inhibitor of phosphodiesterase type 5, which acts to decrease the degradation of cyclic guanosine monophosphate. Inhibition of this enzyme enhances the effects of neurotransmitters such as nitric oxide to cause relaxation of the penile sinusoidal tissue, resulting in tumescence.[14] Doses of 50 to 100 mg have been used with success in 65% to 80% of patients.[15] The medication must be taken approximately 1 hour before attempted sexual activity. Without sexual stimulation, no erection results. The most serious side effect of sildenafil is profound hypotension when taken in conjunction with nitrates. Sildenafil is contraindicated for patients taking nitrates of any form. If there is any concern about cardiac tolerance, sildenafil should not be prescribed. Other side effects include headache, flushing, dyspepsia, rhinitis, and visual disturbances. Priapism is very rare and has been documented only in patients who received sildenafil in combination with other therapies such as intracavernosal injections. All side effects are self-limited.

Apomorphine is a dopaminergic agonist with centrally acting effects that result in erection.[16,17] Preliminary studies have demonstrated an improvement in erectile dysfunction due to psychogenic impotence with one sublingual dose of 3 or 4 mg.[18] The most common side effect is nausea.

Other medications currently being investigated include new phosphodiesterase inhibitors with fewer side effects than sildenafil and topical preparations of currently available oral medications. Combination therapy with medications and other forms of treatment is also being studied.

Vacuum constriction device

The vacuum constriction device (VCD) is a noninvasive mechanical apparatus used to create an erect penis (Fig. 215.1). The device consists of a plastic cylinder, a vacuum pump, and an elastic constriction band. The cylinder is placed over the penis, and the pump is used to produce a vacuum within the cylinder which acts to draw blood into the erectile tissue. The pump is either hand- or battery-operated. When maximal penile engorgement is achieved, the constriction band is transferred to the base of the erect penis, holding blood in the corpora to maintain the erection. The vacuum device then is slipped off. Because constriction of blood flow results in penile ischemia, the band may not be left on longer than half an hour. The device can be reused after detumescence.

The VCD is successful for the majority of impotent men and, when used appropriately, has minimal side effects. It is not effective for obese men who have a substantial suprapubic fat pad that buries the penis or for those with limited manual dexterity. Overall satisfaction has been reported to be 60% to 70% among men using the device.[19,20] Those who have been unsatisfied with the VCD have cited ecchymosis, lack of spontaneity, and awkwardness of use as reasons for discontinuing treatment. Penile injury has been described in men with insensate genitals who have left the constriction band on for extended periods.

Penile injection therapy

Penile injection therapy, or intracorporeal therapy, has been used widely since the mid-1980s.[21] The medications are vasoactive substances that increase blood flow within the penile erectile tissue by decreasing vascular resistance.[15] Intracorporeal injections work best in men with neurological or psychogenic impotence. This type of treatment is not recommended for men with severe psychiatric disease, poor manual dexterity or eyesight, or morbid obesity. It is contraindicated for men with an existing penile prosthesis.

The most commonly used vasoactive substances are prostaglandin E_1 (PGE_1) (alprostadil), papaverine, and phentolamine.[15,22] The first two have been given individually, and all three have been given in various combinations. Combination use was introduced to decrease the amount of individual medication needed, thus avoiding some of the toxicity of each drug. In 1998, the FDA approved PGE_1 for penile injection therapy. The safety profile of PGE_1 has made it the first-line drug for injection therapy, as recommended by the American Urological Association Clinical Guidelines Panel.[20]

The medication is delivered through a 27-gauge needle similar to that used for administering insulin. The appropriate dose is determined through titration to achieve a rigid erection that is adequate for intercourse and lasts 30 to 60 minutes. Men with primarily neurogenic impotence, such as young men with diabetes, typically require less medication than those with vasculogenic impotence. The injection is made at the base of the penis on the lateral aspect to avoid nerves and vessels (Fig. 215.2). An erection develops within 5 to 10 minutes. Alternate sides of the penis are used with each injection, and this treatment should be limited to twice a week to avoid intracorporeal fibrosis.

Long-term follow-up has demonstrated that patient satisfaction with penile injection therapy is good. Although the initial acceptance rate for the treatment is 50%,[23] up to 80% of patients have continued treatment. Reasons for dissatisfaction include pain, inconvenience, loss of efficacy, and lack of sexual interest.

The side effects of penile injection therapy include penile pain, priapism, and plaque formation (fibrosis); the incidence varies for each medication. Penile pain is the most common side effect[24] and may occur at the injection site or along the shaft of the penis after an erection begins. Priapism is a prolonged erection and occurs in 1% to 4% of all men receiving the treatment.[23] It should be treated within 4 to 6 hours by placing a butterfly catheter within the corpora and irrigating the stagnant blood to relieve intracorporeal

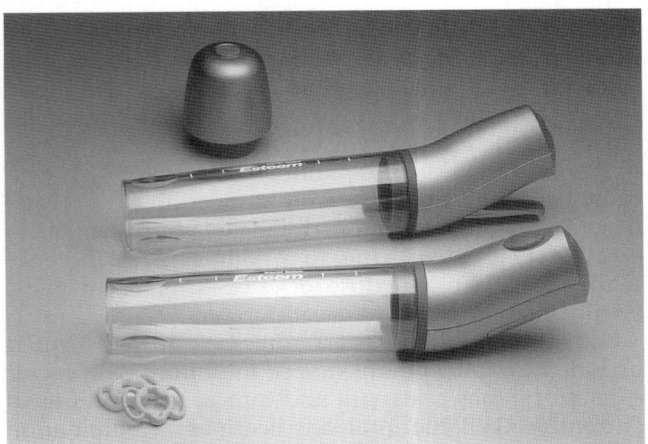

Figure 215.1 Vacuum constriction device. (Photograph courtesy of Timm Medical Technologies, Inc., Eden Prairie, MN). (See color plate section.)

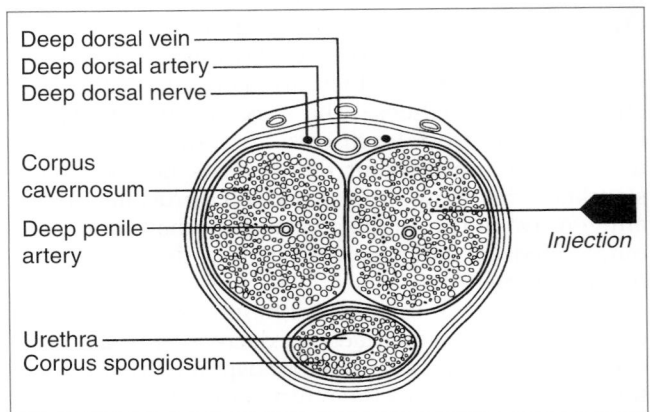

Figure 215.2 Cross-sectional view of the penis, demonstrating intrapenile administration of prostaglandin E_1

pressure. Subsequent infusion of sympathomimetic agents induces vasoconstriction and detumescence. Plaque formation is scarring that occurs in response to the trauma of the injection as well as to the medication itself. The duration of treatment is related directly to the incidence of fibrosis.[25] Plaque formation is a relative indication to discontinue treatment. A case of penile necrosis due to fulminant infection of the corpora has been reported in a man with diabetes.[26] Patients receiving anticoagulation may experience local hematoma formation.

Because the dosing must be titrated carefully to produce the desired effects without priapism, all men considering this mode of therapy should be referred to a urologist for teaching and monitoring.

Intraurethral therapy

The FDA recently approved the use of intraurethral PGE_1, which delivers active drug via absorption across the urethral mucosa into the corpora. Its overall efficacy is questionable, and it is not commonly prescribed.

Penile prosthesis

Penile prostheses were used initially in the 1960s and have since been a standard treatment option for erectile dysfunction. The first penile prosthetic devices were rigid and semirigid devices; the first inflatable models were introduced in 1973.[27] Many modifications made in the last 2 decades have resulted in improved durability and biocompatibility. With the current array of nonsurgical options, a surgical implant generally is reserved for men in whom other less invasive treatments have failed, because placement of a prosthetic device permanently precludes other forms of treatment.

The semirigid prostheses are solid silicone cylinders containing a metal or plastic interlocking component system. The interlocking design allows the penis to be malleable and yet maintain a fixed position. The cylinders are placed within the corpora cavernosa after the spongy erectile tissue has been obliterated. The patient bends his penis downward when its not in use and straightens it for sexual activity. The inflatable models consist of a pump, a reservoir, and inflatable rods that are interconnected by tubing (Fig. 215.3). Fluid is transferred from the reservoir to the rods to achieve erection. The pump is placed in the scrotum, and the reservoir is placed behind the rectus muscle. Some models have a combination pump and reservoir that are placed in the scrotum.

From 70% to 90% of men and 50% to 80% of their partners report satisfaction with all types of prostheses.[28–30] Reasons for dissatisfaction include inadequate penile length or girth, change in sensation, and lack of concealment.

Complications of implants, including mechanical failure, infection, and erosion, can be significant. When they occur, removal or replacement of the device is warranted. The incidence of mechanical failure has decreased with improvements in the design of the prostheses. Failure rates are lower with

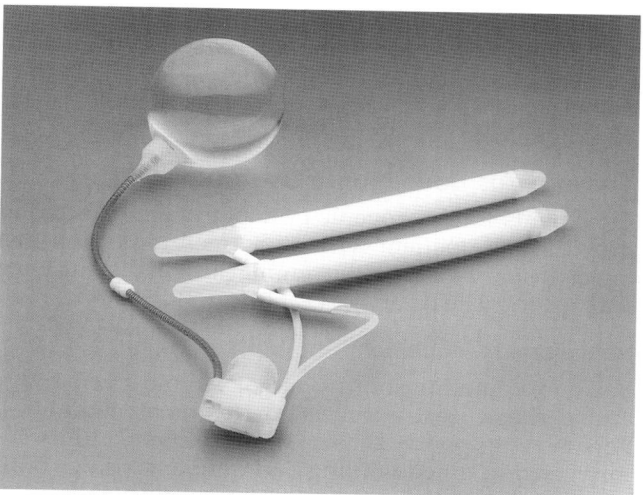

Figure 215.3 700 Ultrex Plus Penile Prosthesis. (Photograph courtesy of American Medical Systems, Inc., Minnetonka, Minnesota)

the semirigid devices, but they are still prone to erosion. The incidence of long-term mechanical failure with current prostheses is estimated to be 5%, with the majority of reoperations occurring within the first 5 years after implantation.[28,30] Men with insulin-dependent diabetes who have a history of urinary tract infections or other infections or those with poor glucose control[31] have been identified as a high-risk population for prosthetic infection. With stringent patient selection, men with diabetes in general have not been found, in several large series of implants, to have a higher reoperation rate than men without diabetes;[32–34] however, the most severe complications have been reported in men with diabetes.[35] Erosion of part of the device can occur through infection or ischemia. The sites of erosion include the urethra, because of prolonged catheterization, and the glans.[36] Several months after a prosthesis has been removed, it may be replaced after the corpora has healed.

The most common causes of impotence in men are neurological, vascular, psychological, and endocrine. Frequently, the dysfunction has more than one cause. With organic impotence, there also may be an important psychological overlay to the patient's situation, and this should be addressed.

Female sexual dysfunction

Female sexual dysfunction includes disorders of arousal and orgasm, decreased desire, and pain with sexual activity.[37] To date, the neurophysiology of female sexual dysfunction has not been well defined. Treatments that may be most applicable to women with peripheral nerve disease include over-the-counter topical lubricants (e.g., K-Y jelly) or hormone replacement therapy for vaginal dryness, vibrator use for decreased genital sensation, testosterone supplementation for decreased libido,[38] and sex therapy. Before effective treatments can be instituted, research is needed to determine the normal physiology and pathophysiology of female sexual dysfunction. Current clinical trials include the use of sildenafil,[39] but sildenafil has not been approved by the FDA for treating female sexual dysfunction.

Therapy for neurogenic cystopathy

Treatments for neurogenic cystopathy are directed at providing the patient with a continent, infection-free lower urinary tract with minimal urinary symptoms and appropriate drainage (Table 215.3).

Behavioral management

Behavioral modification is one of the most important and perhaps least appreciated treatment modalities. Persons with poorly sensate or insensate bladders are instructed in timed voiding and double voiding. With timed voiding, patients are told to attempt urination every 4 to 6 hours regardless of the urge to void. Double voiding is a maneuver in which patients with large post-void residual volumes are advised to reattempt urination 3 to 5 minutes after initially voiding. Both these techniques are used to prevent the accumulation of large volumes or urine, to avoid overdistention, and possibly to preserve detrusor contractility when sensation is decreased. The use of Valsalva maneuver to empty the bladder should not be encouraged because it can contribute to relaxation of the pelvic floor, with subsequent bladder, uterine, and enteric prolapse in women and the development of inguinal hernia in men. After overflow incontinence has been ruled out, physical therapy to strengthen pelvic floor muscles can be helpful in men and women with symptoms of stress urinary incontinence.[40]

Clean intermittent catheterization

Clean intermittent catheterization (CIC) was popularized by Lapides et al.[41] in 1972 and is now a common and indispensable tool in bladder hygiene. The concept of CIC is based on the importance of efficient bladder emptying, despite possible bacterial admission. It maintains low bladder pressure, allows total evacuation of bladder contents, gives the patient voluntary control of urination, and bypasses the sequelae of chronic catheterization. Commencement of CIC often results in improvement in the symptoms of irritative voiding (e.g., frequency, nocturia, incontinence) caused by large residual urine volumes. Patients are instructed to catheterize on a schedule that drains volumes between 400 and 500 mL. Anticholinergic medications usually are not needed to suppress residual detrusor activity in patients with peripheral neuropathy. These medications can be implemented if patients have persistent irritative symptoms even with dedicated CIC. Low-dose anticholinergic agents such as oxybutinin, 5 mg orally twice daily, or tolteradine, 2 mg orally twice daily, may be prescribed for residual detrusor hyperreflexia. Infectious, inflammatory, and neoplastic processes should be ruled out if severe irritative symptoms persist. This requires referral to a urologist. Most patients can perform CIC, presuming that they have adequate cognition and the manual dexterity or physical agility to perform the catheterization. Catheter care consists of cleaning the reusable catheters with soap and water after each use, followed by air-drying. Maintaining clean technique is the objective, because sterile procedure generally is not feasible.

A few complications are associated with CIC, for example, occasional urinary tract infections, urinary tract trauma during catheterization, and bladder stone formation, resulting from the introduction of foreign bodies such as lint or hair into the bladder. Bacteriuria and pyuria are common but generally should not be treated unless the patient has symptoms (e.g., fever, dysuria/pain, or incontinence). Suppressive antibiotic treatment for patients who perform CIC has failed to demonstrate any benefit.[42] Frequent urinary tract infections can be due to improper catheterization technique or other problems, such as urolithiasis.

Urine collection devices

For men who are unable to perform CIC, condom catheters are often used to collect urine. For the catheters to be effective, the patient's bladder must evacuate reasonably well, which often is not so in cystopathy. Despite the theoretical benefit of being external, chronic bacteriuria still exists because of the high concentration of organisms at the urethral meatus.[43] Patients with a poorly emptying bladder, such as those with severe neuropathy, who use condom catheters are at risk for recurrent infections.

Patients with neuropathy in urinary retention or those who are unable to care for themselves can use indwelling catheters (suprapubic or urethral) for urine drainage. Many patients tolerate them well, despite the known complications of chronic catheterization. Catheter care includes changing the catheter monthly, securing the catheter to the patient's leg to avoid unnecessary movement or traction, and a one-way valve on the drainage bag to prevent the reflux of drained urine. Copious intake of fluid is recommended to minimize the accumulation of sediment in the bladder. Treatment should be started with

Table 215.3 Treatment options for neurogenic cystopathy

Behavioral management
    Timed voiding
    Double voiding
    Physical therapy
Clean intermittent catheterization
Urine collection devices
    Condom catheters
    Indwelling catheters
Pharmacological management
    α-Adrenergic blocking agents
    Anticholinergic agents
Surgical procedures
    Bladder outlet procedures
    Implanted nerve stimulators

Table 215.4 α-Adrenergic antagonists

Drug	Maximal dosage	Titration
Terazosin	10 mg orally qhs	1 mg orally qhs × 1 wk, then 2 mg orally qhs × 1 wk, then 5 mg orally qhs
Doxazosin	8 mg orally qhs	1 mg orally qhs × 1 wk, then 2 mg orally qhs × 1 wk, then 4 mg orally qhs
Tamsulosin	0.4 mg orally daily	Not needed

qhs = at bedtime

indwelling Foley catheterization, because the insertion of suprapubic tubes is more difficult and has greater risks (e.g., bleeding, perforation, and risk to surrounding viscera). If the patient tolerates the indwelling Foley catheter and remains dry, then a suprapubic catheter should be considered. Long-term urethral catheterization can cause erosion of the urethra and periurethral skin. Thus, for patients requiring long-term indwelling catheterization, a suprapubic catheter is preferable. Also, the care of suprapubic tubes generally is easier because of their more accessible location.

Pharmacological agents

Patients with only mild cystopathy and intact sensation should receive treatment for urinary symptoms according to the same guidelines as for patients without neuropathy. However, the physician must be aware of the possibility of progression of the neurological process, and surveillance to assess bladder emptying must be maintained.

In men, decreasing outlet resistance with the use of α-adrenergic blocking agents can diminish the symptoms of obstructive and irritative voiding. Some of these agents require titration because of the side effect of orthostatic hypotension (Table 215.4).

There is evidence in humans that detrusor contraction is mediated cholinergically. Bethanechol, a cholinergic agonist,[44] has been used to treat detrusor areflexia. A daily dose of several hundred milligrams orally has been suggested. However, the absence of randomized trials, the deficiency of drug metabolism data, and the impression that bethanechol lacks efficacy[45] have discouraged treatment with this drug. Currently, no other medications are available to resuscitate the denervated bladder.

Surgical management

Transurethal prostatectomy can be performed in men with mild forms of cystopathy who also have evidence for bladder outlet obstruction due to benign prostatic hyperplasia. This method of decreasing outlet resistance may allow the patient to empty his bladder more effectively, but detrusor contractility must be confirmed with cystometry preoperatively or the patient may experience retention postoperatively. Other therapies for obstruction due to benign prostatic hyperplasia include transurethral needle ablation of the prostate and urethral stents.[46,47] A relatively new therapeutic option for selected patients with urinary retention is a surgically implanted sacral

nerve root stimulator that triggers contraction of the denervated detrusor muscle.[48]

Conclusions

Standard management options for the genitourinary sequelae of peripheral neuropathy provide patients with a functional substitute for diminished sexual or urinary capacity. Development of new treatments for peripheral neuropathy—the primary cause of these problems—may improve or reverse the dysfunction. Continued research in the area of genitourinary innervation, particularly using electrophysiological techniques to identify neuropathy in the genitourinary tract, will contribute to improve our understanding and treatment of the neuropathological causes of sexual dysfunction and cystopathy.

References

1. Sarica K, Arikan N, Serel A, et al. Multidisciplinary evaluation of diabetic impotence. Eur Urol 1994;26: 314–318
2. Veves A, Webster L, Chen TF, et al. Aetiopathogenesis and management of impotence in diabetic males: four years experience from a combined clinic. Diabet Med 1995;12:77–82
3. Buvat J, Lemaire A, Buvat-Herbaut M, et al. Comparative investigations in 26 impotent and 26 nonimpotent diabetic patients. J Urol 1985;133:34–38
4. Rosen RC, Leiblum SR. Treatment of sexual disorders in the 1990s: an integrated approach. J Consult Clin Psychol 1995;63:877–890
5. Kaplan HS. The combined use of sex therapy and intrapenile injections in the treatment of impotence. J Sex Marital Ther 1990;16:195–207
6. Osborne D. Psychologic evaluation of impotent men. Mayo Clin Proc 1976;51:363–366
7. Tiefer L, Schuetz-Mueller D. Psychological issues in diagnosis and treatment of erectile disorders. Urol Clin North Am 1995;22:767–773
8. Wylie KR. Treatment outcome of brief couple therapy in psychogenic male erectile disorder. Arch Sex Behav 1997;26:527–545
9. Drugs that cause sexual dysfunction: an update. Med Lett 1992;34:73–78
10. Nelson RP. Nonoperative management of impotence. J Urol 1988;139:2–5
11. Kwan M, Greenleaf WJ, Mann J, et al. The nature of androgen action of male sexuality: a combined laboratory-self report study on hypogonadal men. J Clin Endocrinol Metab 1983;57:557–562
12. Cooper CS, MacIndoe JH, Perry PJ, et al. The effect of exogenous testosterone on total and free prostate specific antigen levels in healthy young men. J Urol 1996;156:438–441

13. Douglas TH, Connelly RR, McLeod DG, et al. Effect of exogenous testosterone replacement on prostate-specific antigen and prostate-specific membrane antigen levels in hypogonadal men. J Surg Oncol 1995;59: 246–250

14. Boolell M, Gepi-Attee S, Gingell JC, Allen MJ. Sildenafil, a novel effective oral therapy for male erectile dysfunction. Br J Urol 1996;78:257–261

15. Lue TF, Tanagho EA. Physiology of erection and pharmacological management of impotence. J Urol 1987; 137:829–836

16. Lal S, Laryea E, Thavundayil JX, et al. Apomorphine-induced penile tumescence in impotent patients—preliminary findings. Prog Neuropsychopharmacol Biol Psychiatry 1987;11:235–242

17. Segraves RT, Bari M, Segraves K, Spirnak P. Effect of apomorphine on penile tumescence in men with psychogenic impotence. J Urol 1991;145:1174–1175

18. Heaton JP, Morales A, Adams MA, et al. Recovery of erectile function by the oral administration of apomorphine. Urology 1995;45:200–206

19. Baltaci S, Aydos K, Kosar A, Anafarta K. Treating erectile dysfunction with a vacuum tumescence device: a retrospective analysis of acceptance and satisfaction. Br J Urol 1995;76:757–760

20. Montague DK, Barada JH, Belker AM, et al. Clinical Guidelines Panel on Erectile Dysfunction: summary report on the treatment of organic erectile dysfunction. The American Urological Association. J Urol 1996; 156:2007–2011

21. Virag R. Intracavernous injection of papavarine for erectile failure (letter). Lancer 1982;2:938

22. Porst H. The rationale for prostaglandin E_1 in erectile failure: a study of worldwide experience. J Urol 1996; 155:802–815

23. Fallon B. Intracavernous injection therapy for male erectile dysfunction. Urol Clin North Am 1995;22:833–845

24. Lugg J, Rajfer J. Drug therapy for erectile dysfunction. AUA Update Series 1996;15:290

25. Lakin MM, Montague DK, VanderBrug-Medendorp S, et al. Intracavernous injection therapy: analysis of results and complications. J Urol 1990;143:1138–1141

26. Schwarzer JU, Hofmann R. Purulent corporeal cavernositis secondary to papavarine-induced priapism. J Urol 1991;146:845–846

27. Scott FB, Bradley WE, Timm GW. Management of erectile impotence. Use of implantable inflatable prosthesis. Urology 1973;2:80–82

28. Lewis RW. Long-term results of penile prosthetic implants. Urol Clin North Am 1995;22:847–856

29. Porena M, Mearini L, Mearini E, et al. Penile prosthesis implantation and couple's satisfaction. Urol Int 2000;63: 185–187

30. Kabalin JN, Kuo JC. Long-term followup of and patients satisfaction with the Dynaflex self-contained inflatable penile prosthesis. J Urol 1997;158:456–459

31. Bishop JR, Moul JW, Sihelnik SA, et al. Use of glycosylated hemoglobin to identify diabetics at high risk for penile periprosthetic infections. J Urol 1992;147:386–388

32. Montague DK. Periprosthetic infections. J Urol 1987; 138:68–69

33. Radomski SB, Herschorn S. Risk factors associated with penile prosthesis infection. J Urol 1992;147:383–385

34. Wilson SK, Delk JR II. Inflatable penile implant infection: predisposing factors and treatment suggestions. J Urol 1995;153:659–661

35. Bejany DE, Perito PE, Lustgarten M, Rhamy RK. Gangrene of the penis after implantation of penile prosthesis: case reports, treatment recommendations and review of the literature. J Urol 1993;150:190–191

36. McClellan DS, Masih BK. Gangrene of the penis as a complication of penile prosthesis. J Urol 1985;133: 862–863

37. Basson R, Berman J, Burnett A, et al. Report of the International Consensus Development Conference on Female Sexual Dysfunction: definitions and classifications. J Urol 2000;163:888–893

38. Redmond GP. Hormones and sexual function. Int J Fertil Womens Med 1999;44:193–197

39. Basson R, McInnes R, Smith MD, et al. Efficacy and safety of sildenafil in estrogenized women with sexual dysfunction associated with female sexual arousal disorder. Obstet Gynecol 2000;95 Suppl 1:S54

40. Kegel AH. Physiologic therapy for urinary stress incontinence. JAMA 1951;146:915

41. Lapides J, Diokno AC, Silber SJ, Lowe BS. Clean, intermittent self-catheterization in the treatment of urinary tract disease. J Urol 1972;107:458–461

42. Mohler JL, Cowen DL, Flanigan RC. Suppression and treatment of urinary tract infection in patients with an intermittently catheterized neurogenic bladder. J Urol 1987;138:336–340

43. Golji H. Complications of external condom drainage. Paraplegia 1981;19:189–197

44. Barrett DM. The effect of oral bethanechol chloride on voiding in female patients with excessive residual urine: a randomized double-blind study. J Urol 1981;126:640–642

45. Wein AJ, Malloy TR, Shofer F, Raezer DM. The effects of bethanechol chloride on urodynamic parameters in normal women and in women with significant residual urine volumes. J Urol 1980;124:397–399

46. Badlani GH. Role of permanent stents. J Endourol 1997;11:473–475

47. Kletscher BA, Oesterling JE. Prostatic stents. Current perspectives for the management of benign prostatic hyperplasia. Urol Clin North Am 1995;22:423–430

48. Hohenfellner M, Schultz-Lampel D, Dahms S, et al. Bilateral chronic sacral neuromodulation for treatment of lower urinary tract dysfunction. J Urol 1998;160: 821–824

216 Gastrointestinal Dysmotility and Sphincter Dysfunction

Adil E Bharucha and Michael Camilleri

Overview

Gastrointestinal (GI) motility is regulated by the intrinsic or enteric nervous system, which contains the same number ($\approx$100 million) of neurons as the spinal cord and is organized into myenteric and submucous plexuses. In addition to neurons and nerve fibers, these plexuses also contain interstitial cells of Cajal, which probably serve as pacemakers and conductors of electrical activity and mediate neurotransmission from enteric neurons.[1] The myenteric plexus is primarily responsible for controlling motility, whereas the submucous plexus regulates mucosal absorption. These functions involve responding to sensory input from the lumen (via chemo- or osmoreceptors) or the wall (via mechanoreceptors) and integration at a local level (e.g., peristaltic reflex) or over longer distances (e.g., the interdigestive migrating motor complex that spreads from the stomach to the ileum [Figure 216.1]). Extrinsic sympathetic and parasympathetic pathways modulate the enteric nervous system. Afferent signals course along these nerves from the gut to the central nervous system (CNS; Figure 216.2, Table 216.1). Disorders of the autonomic nervous system manifest primarily as abnormalities in motor or sensory function; less frequently, absorption, secretion, or other digestive processes may be abnormal.

Table 216.1 Principles of modulation of gut motility and sensation by the extrinsic nervous system

Has most pronounced effects on skeletal muscle portions (i.e., upper esophageal sphincter and external anal sphincter). With regard to gut smooth muscle, the influence on stomach and distal colon is greater than on the small bowel.

Primarily integrates activity in widely separated regions, often through reflexes that have synapses in prevertebral ganglia; GI smooth muscle functions reasonably well without extrinsic nerves.

Comprises parasympathetic and sympathetic pathways, which have opposing effects. Parasympathetic pathways are excitatory to smooth muscle while inhibiting sphincters. Sympathetic input inactivates intrinsic excitatory cholinergic neural circuits, but does not directly innervate muscle. Reduced sympathetic inhibitory input ("the brake") may lead to excessive or uncoordinated phasic pressure activity in the gut.

Conveys afferent input from the gut to the central nervous system via a classic three-neuron pathway to the brainstem reticular formation or the thalamus. These afferents are predominantly unmyelinated C fibers that respond to low-threshold, polymodal stimulation and accompany splanchnic sympathetic fibers to the central nervous system. Pain perception depends on higher intensity stimulation of naked nerve endings that act as mechanoreceptors. Descending pathways serve to modulate incoming afferent signals by inhibiting or facilitating dorsal horn neurons.

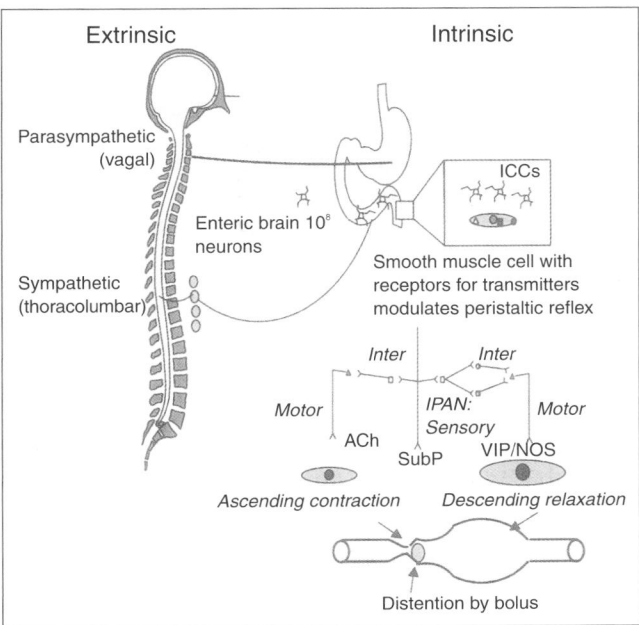

Figure 216.1 Interactions between extrinsic neural pathways and the "enteric brain" (i.e., the intrinsic nervous system) modulate contractions of GI smooth muscle. Interactions between transmitters (e.g., peptides, amines) and receptors alter muscle membrane potentials by stimulating bidirectional ion fluxes. In turn, membrane characteristics dictate whether or not the muscle cell contracts. ACh, acetylcholine; CVA, cerebrovascular accident; ICCs, interstitial cells of Cajal; inter, interneuron; IPAN, intestinal primary afferent neurons; NOS, nitric oxide synthase; SubP, substance P; VIP, vasoactive intestinal polypeptide. (Modified from Camilleri M, Phillips SF. Disorders of small intestinal motility. Gastroenterol Clin North Am 1989;18:405–424. By permission of WB Saunders Company.)

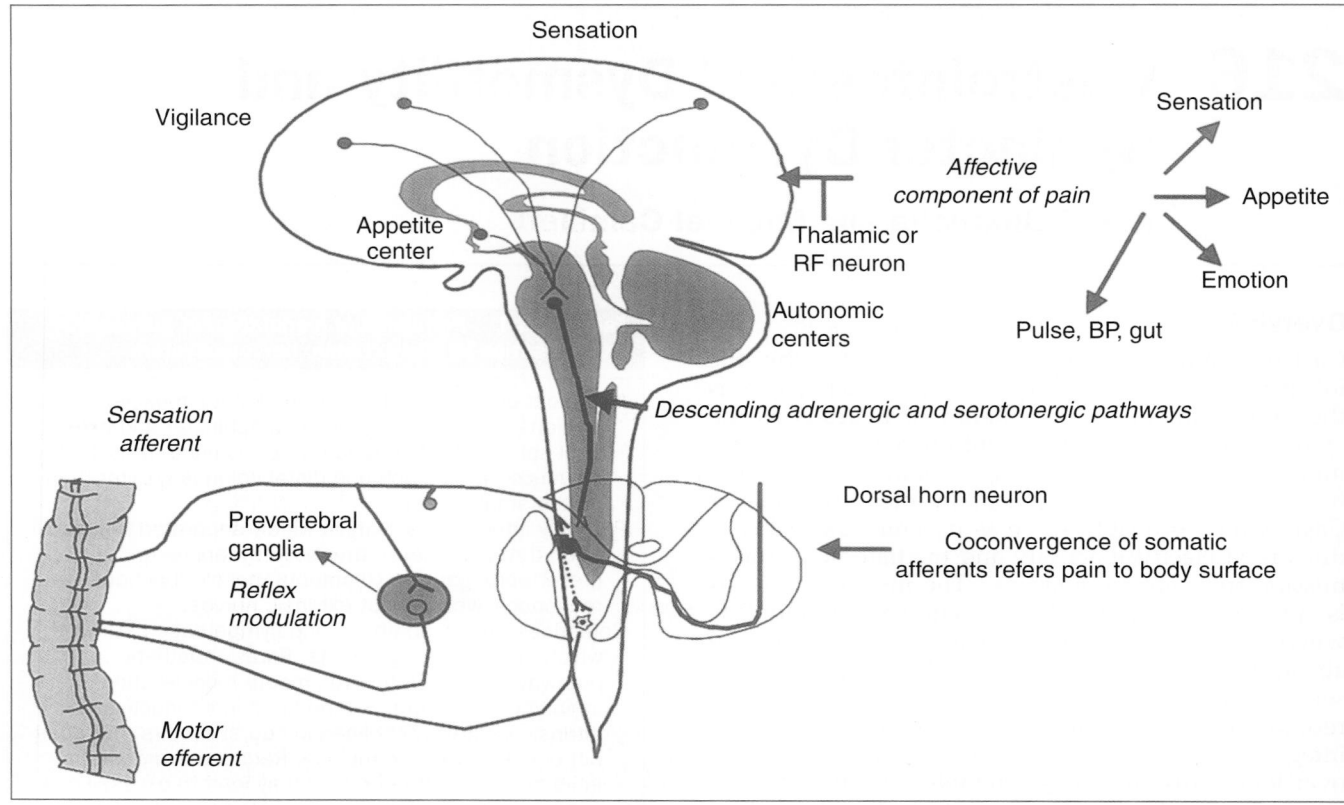

Figure 216.2   Pathways involved in visceral sensation. As with somatic sensation, a three-neuron chain links the gut to conscious perception. Sensation leads to reflex modulation of gut function, and descending spinal pathways reduce afferent signals conveyed through the dorsal horn neuron. BP, blood pressure; RF, reticular formation. (Modified from Camilleri M, Saslow SB, Bharucha AE. Gastrointestinal sensation: mechanisms and relation to functional gastrointestinal disorders. Gastroenterol Clin North Am 1996;25:247–258. By permission of WB Saunders Company.)

Gastrointestinal manifestations

Disorders at several levels of the neural axis (e.g., dysautonomias or autonomic neuropathies affecting peripheral pathways, spinal cord transection, multiple sclerosis, or strokes) may alter sensory or motor function in the GI tract. Tables 216.2 to 216.5 summarize the pathophysiology, clinical features, and evaluation of the four common manifestations of neurological disorders (i.e., dysphagia, gastroparesis and chronic intestinal pseudo-obstruction, constipation, and fecal incontinence).

Extrinsic neurological disorders causing gut dysmotility

This review concentrates on neurological diseases of extrinsic neural control and smooth muscle that affect gut motility.

Autonomic epilepsy and migraine

Infrequent causes of nausea, vomiting, or abdominal pain may include autonomic epilepsy and migraine.

Postpolio dysphagia

Patients who have postpolio syndrome with bulbar involvement frequently have dysphagia and aspira-

tion. Attention to the position of the patient's head during swallowing can decrease the incidence of choking and aspiration, as can changing food consistency to semisolids.

Brainstem tumors

Brainstem lesions can present with isolated GI motor dysfunction. In the absence of increased intracranial pressure, symptoms likely result from direct effects of a mass in the brainstem, with distortion of the vomiting center on the floor of the fourth ventricle. Motor dysfunction is typically evident on manometric or radionuclide studies of the stomach and small bowel.[8] Although most reports are associated with vomiting, patients with colonic or anorectal dysfunction have also been described.[9] The presence of autonomic neuropathy in a patient with a motility disorder necessitates a search for a structural CNS lesion, particularly if tests suggest a preganglionic sympathetic lesion. Magnetic resonance imaging (MRI) is considered preferable to computed tomography (CT) for detecting brainstem lesions.[8]

Parkinson disease

GI symptoms occurring commonly in patients with Parkinson disease include abnormal salivation,

Table 216.2 Oropharyngeal dysphagia

Definition.—Difficulty in swallowing, with a holdup in the cervical area. However, even patients with distal esophageal obstruction may experience sensation of cervical holdup.

Etiology.—Usually attributable to a disease, often systemic, affecting any level of the swallowing pathway, rather than an oropharyngeal disorder.

Clinical features.—Symptoms of *oral* dysfunction include drooling from the mouth, inability to chew or propel the bolus from the mouth, sialorrhea or xerostomia, difficulty initiating swallowing, piecemeal swallowing, and dysarthria. Symptoms of *pharyngeal* dysfunction include an immediate sense of bolus holdup localized to the neck, nasal regurgitation, the need to swallow repeatedly to clear food or fluid from the pharynx, coughing or choking during meals, gurgly voice, and dysphonia. Physical findings relate to the underlying neurological disorder (i.e., cranial nerve dysfunction, neuromuscular disease, cerebellar dysfunction, or movement disorder). The gag reflex does not predict severity of pharyngeal dysfunction or aspiration risk; the reflex is absent in 20% to 40% of healthy adults.

Evaluation.—Nasoendoscopy of the oropharynx can be used to evaluate for malignancy and may provide clues to a neurogenic or myogenic etiology of swallowing dysfunction. Findings from videofluoroscopic swallowing study may provide additional clues about the cause of dysfunction, particularly in patients with upper esophageal sphincter dysfunction (e.g., Zenker's diverticulum), quantify severity of swallowing dysfunction, and suggest which compensatory swallowing maneuvers will compensate for dysfunction. Videofluoroscopy is the only way to be certain whether a dysphagic patient is aspirating. Presence of aspiration probably predicts risk of pneumonia.

Principles of management.—In addition to an assessment of severity of swallowing dysfunction with videofluoroscopy, other factors guide the decision to institute nonoral feeding (e.g., the likelihood that therapeutic maneuvers will compensate for dysfunction, the natural history and prognosis of the underlying illness, and the patient's cognitive ability). Because swallowing may improve considerably in the first 2 weeks after a stroke, long-term decisions should be delayed for that period.

Table 216.3 Gastroparesis and chronic intestinal pseudo-obstruction

Definition.—Clinical syndromes result from deranged gastric or small intestinal motility rather than from mechanical obstruction. Megacolon refers to fecal dilatation greater than 12 cm and sigmoid colonic dilatation greater than 6.5 cm at the pelvic brim.

Etiology.—Includes extrinsic neurological diseases that occur at any level of the brain-neural axis, neuronal dysfunction in the myenteric plexus,[2] or degeneration of smooth muscle. Common causes may include autonomic neuropathies such as diabetes mellitus.[2] Phenothiazines, antihypertensive agents such as clonidine, tricyclic antidepressants that have anticholinergic effects, and calcium channel blockers also impair motility. Colonic dilatation or megacolon may be acute (Ogilvie syndrome), chronic, or toxic.[3] Acute megacolon is attributed to a sympathetically mediated reflex response to several serious medical or surgical conditions in elderly patients, often after orthopedic fractures or operations. Chronic megacolon may be congenital (Hirschsprung disease) or it may represent the end stage of any form of refractory constipation. Toxic megacolon is caused by underlying colonic inflammation, such as in ulcerative or infectious colitis.

Clinical features.—Symptoms range from vague postprandial abdominal discomfort to recurrent postprandial emesis resulting in weight loss and malnutrition. Bowel habits range from constipation to diarrhea; the latter suggests bacterial overgrowth. A succussion splash may be detected on physical examination. Patients with acute megacolon are often relatively asymptomatic, despite marked abdominal distention and percussion tympany.

Evaluation.—When the diagnosis is in doubt, gastric outlet or mechanical small intestinal obstruction should be excluded by a barium study or gastroscopy. Impaired emptying can be documented by scintigraphy. Intubated studies of pressure profiles by manometric transducers in the distal stomach and small bowel identify motor dysfunction (Figure 216.3), differentiate neuropathic from myopathic processes (Figure 216.3), and exclude mechanical obstruction that may have been missed on previous radiography of the small bowel. Autonomic function tests are abnormal in patients with extrinsic nerve dysfunction, but normal in patients with intrinsic nerve dysfunction. Brain imaging is indicated if there is no obvious cause for dysmotility, particularly if autonomic tests suggest a central lesion. In smokers, the presence of paraneoplastic antibodies may lead to chest computed tomography that reveals a small cell lung cancer.[4] The diagnosis of megacolon is established by plain abdominal radiographs or a contrast enema demonstrating colonic dilatation; distal colonic obstructive lesion should be excluded by a contrast enema or flexible endoscopy before administering neostigmine.

Principles of management.—Treatment approaches include dietary measures, venting or decompression if necessary, and treatment and prophylaxis for bacterial overgrowth (see Tables 216.7 and 216.8). In addition, pharmacological agents that enhance gastrointestinal contractility are useful in the acute condition. Intravenous erythromycin can be used for 48–72 hours in gastroparesis, and intravenous neostigmine can be used in acute colonic pseudo-obstruction. Neostigmine also enhances contractility of the small bowel, and case reports suggest it may temporarily relieve distention in acute or chronic intestinal pseudo-obstruction.

Table 216.4   Constipation

Definition.—A common symptom, perceived by the patient as infrequent, incomplete evacuation or excessively hard stools.

Etiology.—One or more factors may cause constipation: inadequate fiber intake, lack of exercise, a direct consequence of a disorder, or medications. Autonomic neuropathies may be associated with impaired colonic propulsion, impaired pelvic floor function, and diminished rectal sensation; consequently, patients may not experience the urge to defecate. In patients with Parkinson disease, Lewy bodies have been found in the enteric nervous system, the pelvic floor may not relax normally during defecation, and anticholinergic agents may delay transit. In addition to impaired colonic transit or pelvic floor function or both, paraplegic patients may lack the ability to increase intra-abdominal pressure during expulsion.

Clinical features.—A digital rectal examination may disclose impacted stool and provide insights into abnormal pelvic floor function, which may be manifested as paradoxical contraction of the puborectalis or as inadequate or excessive perineal descent during simulated defecation.

Evaluation.—Consider the possibility of and, if necessary, exclude an obstructing lesion by barium radiography or colonoscopy, particularly if patients are anemic or have blood in the stool. Assess colonic transit by radiopaque markers or scintigraphic techniques. Assess pelvic floor dysfunction by anorectal manometry with balloon expulsion and by pelvic floor imaging during defecation by scintigraphic or barium defecography, if clinically indicated. Delayed colonic transit does not necessarily indicate colonic motor dysfunction because the delay may be caused by pelvic floor dysfunction.

Principles of management.—Fiber intake from foods and supplements should be given twice daily with fluids or meals and increased gradually over several weeks to the target of 12–14 g fiber per day.[5] Increased bloating with fiber supplements may subside after several weeks or necessitate switching to another preparation, such as methylcellulose (e.g., Citrucel). The next step is to add an inexpensive saline agent, such as milk of magnesia, titrated to produce soft but not liquid stools. If necessary, stimulant laxatives such as bisacodyl (e.g., Dulcolax) or polyethylene glycol should be considered. Other "colonic prokinetics" are in development; the use of prostaglandins and colchicine to treat constipation is not recommended. Disordered evacuation responds poorly to laxatives, but often ($\approx$75%) responds well to biofeedback therapy.[6]

Table 216.5   Fecal incontinence

Definition.—Involuntary leakage of stool from the anus.

Etiology.—In the absence of neurological disease, idiopathic fecal incontinence is frequently due to anal sphincter weakness resulting from sphincter defects caused by obstetric trauma, aggravated by stretch-induced pudendal nerve injury; the latter is often attributable to prolonged straining in constipated patients or to obstetric trauma. Common neurological disorders associated with fecal incontinence include multiple sclerosis, Parkinson disease, multiple system atrophy, Alzheimer disease, strokes, diabetic neuropathy, and spinal cord lesions.

Clinical features.—External sphincter weakness often manifests as urge incontinence or as stress incontinence during coughing, sneezing, or laughing. Internal anal sphincter weakness, as in diabetic autonomic neuropathy or systemic sclerosis, often manifests as nocturnal incontinence, or "passive" incontinence (i.e., without prior warning). Diminished rectal sensation may impair ability to distinguish between flatus and stool in rectum. Inspection of the anus with and without straining in the lateral decubitus and seated positions will detect rectal prolapse; a digital rectal exam can assess resting and squeeze tone in the anal canal and can exclude impaction.

Evaluation.[7]—Proctoscopy and barium enema or colonoscopy may exclude mucosal lesions; if unrevealing, assess anorectal function with manometry to measure anal canal pressures, rectal sensation of balloon distention, defecation process by ability to expel a balloon from the rectum, anorectal angle, and defecating proctography. The identification of pudendal neuropathy by pudendal nerve latencies is suboptimal because the technique lacks sensitivity and specificity for identifying pudendal nerve damage. Needle electromyography of the external sphincter provides a sensitive measure of denervation (fibrillation potentials) and can usually identify myopathic (small polyphasic motor unit potentials), neurogenic (large polyphasic motor unit potentials), or mixed injury.

Principles of management.—Treatment includes care of the perianal skin and use of incontinence pads. Regularization of bowel habits may be achieved with fiber supplements and judicious use of laxatives for constipated patients, and with antidiarrheal agents such as loperamide (Imodium) for those with diarrhea. Biofeedback therapy can be used to enhance anal sphincter tone and modulate rectal sensation. However, patients who have severe weakness or lack rectal sensation, and in whom little can be achieved with medical or biofeedback therapy, may require colostomy for a more manageable solution to chronic incontinence. The role of other surgical approaches (e.g., anal sphincter or pelvic floor repair, creation of a new anal sphincter with or without electrical stimulation) for fecal incontinence is unclear. No randomized trials have compared surgical intervention to nonsurgical approaches.

dysphagia, nausea, constipation, and defecatory dysfunction.[10] The prevalence of these symptoms appears correlated with the duration and severity of Parkinsons, not with diet or treatment. Dysphagia is frequently associated with choking and disordered salivation and may be attributable to direct involvement of oropharyngeal and upper esophageal sphincter muscles by the primary disease process. Constipation often manifests not by decreased stool frequency but by disturbed stool consistency and excessive straining suggestive of defecatory dysfunction resulting from paradoxical puborectalis contraction during defecation. Degeneration of dopaminergic neurons in the myenteric plexus is considered important in the

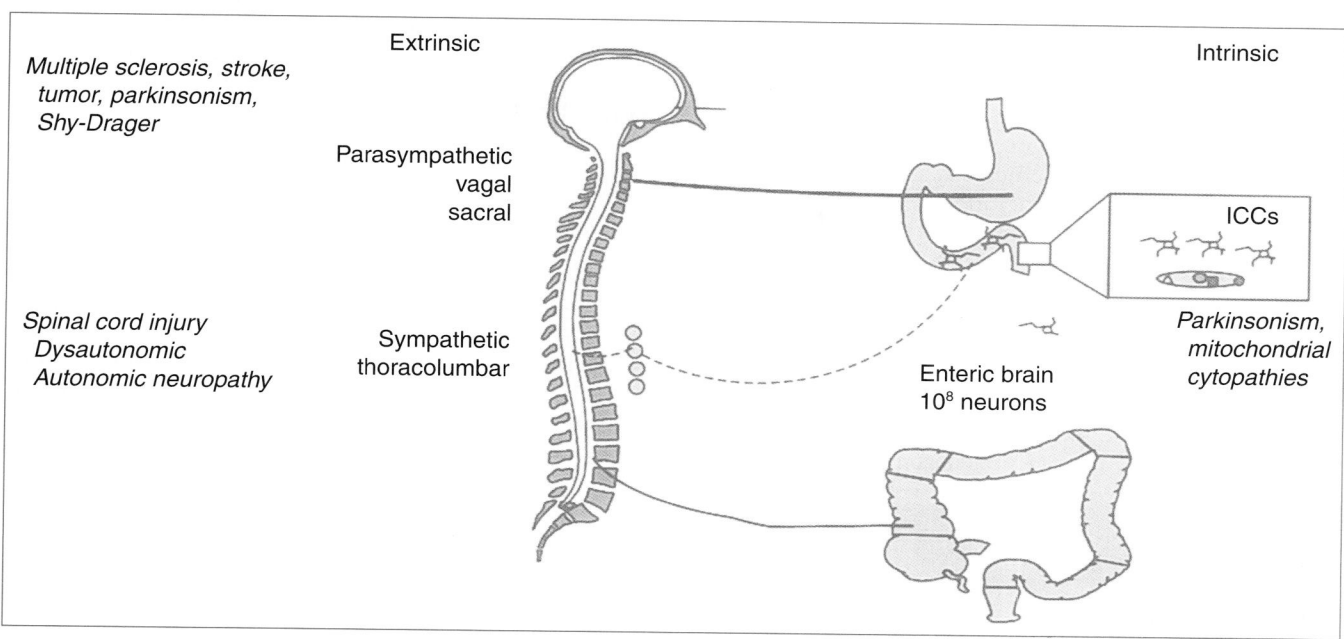

Figure 216.3   Various neurological diseases affect extrinsic and intrinsic gut neuromuscular function.

pathogenesis of constipation related to Parkinson disease (Figure 216.4).[11]

Autonomic system degeneration

Pandysautonomia   or   selective   dysautonomias
Pandysautonomia is characterized by preganglionic or postganglionic lesions affecting both sympathetic and parasympathetic nerves. Vomiting, paralytic ileus, constipation, or a chronic pseudo-obstruction syndrome has been reported in patients with acute, subacute, or familial dysautonomias. Motor dysfunctions have been documented in the esophagus, the stomach, and the small bowel. Selective cholinergic dysautonomia affects parasympathetic nerves and sympathetic nerves to sweat glands and may also impair both upper and lower GI motor activity. These disorders may follow a viral infection, such as infectious mononucleosis.[12]

Idiopathic orthostatic hypotension   Idiopathic orthostatic hypotension is sometimes associated with motor dysfunction of the gut, such as esophageal dysmotility, gastric stasis, alteration in bowel movements, and fecal incontinence.[13] Cardiovascular abnormalities usually precede gut involvement. The precise site of the lesion causing the gut dysmotility is unknown.

Multiple system atrophy   The condition known as "multiple system atrophy" (MSA) has been associated with esophageal dysmotility, pseudo-obstruction, constipation, and fecal incontinence.[14] In contrast to what happens in amyotrophic lateral sclerosis (ALS), the anterior horn cells supplying the urethral and anal sphincters, termed "Onuf's nucleus," are often affected early in the course of MSA, causing urinary and bowel dysfunction. In one study, results of elec-

tromyographic study of the anal sphincter were abnormal in 82% of patients with MSA.[15]

Peripheral neuropathy

Acute peripheral neuropathy   Autonomic dysfunction is associated with nausea, vomiting, abdominal cramps, constipation, Guillain-Barré syndrome, herpes zoster, Epstein-Barr virus, botulism from type B exotoxin, or cytomegalovirus (CMV). Human immunodeficiency virus (HIV)-induced diarrhea may be another manifestation of autonomic dysfunction (see below).

Chronic peripheral neuropathy   Chronic peripheral neuropathy is the most commonly encountered extrinsic neurological disorder that results in GI motor dysfunction.

Diabetes mellitus   Diabetic autonomic neuropathy of the gut has been studied extensively and has been reviewed elsewhere.[16] The occurrence and spectrum of GI symptoms in middle-aged community subjects with insulin- and noninsulin-dependent diabetes mellitus do not differ from those of the general population,[17] except for constipation in persons with insulin-dependent diabetes mellitus.[18] Gastroparesis is most consistent with disease-related vagal dysfunction; hyperglycemia delays gastric emptying. During the early stages of diabetes, gastric emptying of liquids is accelerated, but this has little impact on glycemic control.

Constipation   A frequent, although often unreported, symptom in patients with diabetes is constipation. It is associated with an absent myoelectric response of the colon to meal ingestion, slow colonic transit, and abnormal rectal evacuation. In many diabetic patients, constipation is associated with medication (e.g., calcium channel blockers).[18]

Diarrhea   Fecal incontinence or diarrhea, or both, may result from several mechanisms (reviewed in detail elsewhere). These include dysfunction of the anorectal sphincter or abnormal rectal sensation, steatorrhea due to bacterial overgrowth, or rapid transit from uncoordinated small-bowel motor activity. Rarely, an associated gluten enteropathy or pancreatic exocrine insufficiency may be present.

Paraneoplastic neuropathy   GI symptoms (from

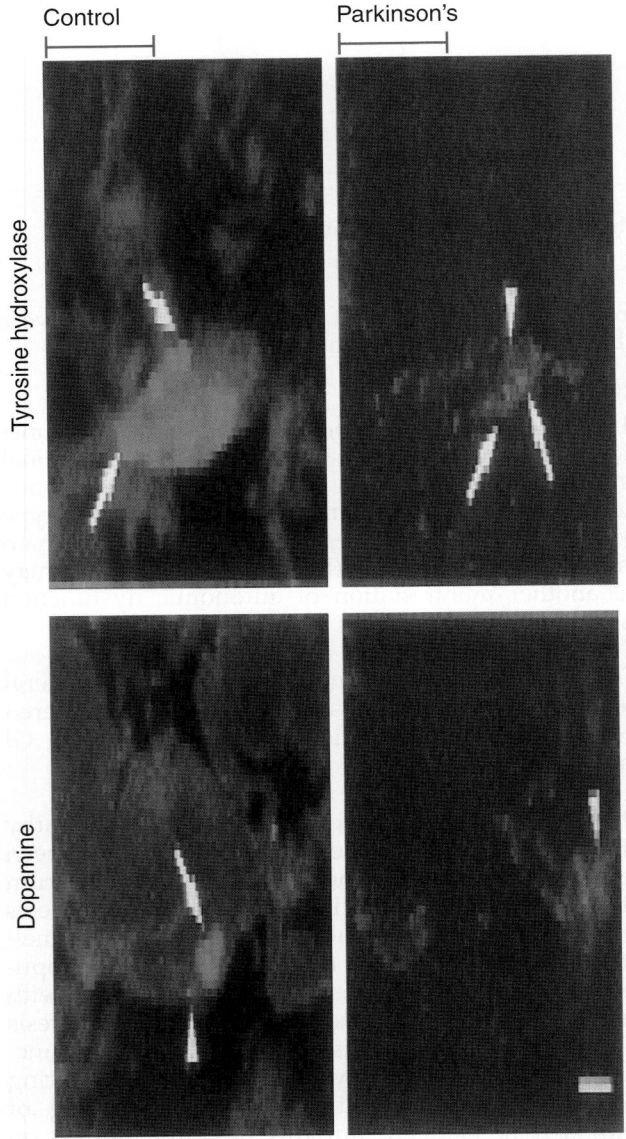

Figure 216.4   Immunohistochemistry of myenteric plexus showing positively stained neurons (*arrows*) in healthy control and patient with Parkinson disease; bar = 1 μm. Note the significantly greater reduction in dopamine (*arrows*) compared to tyrosine hydroxylase neurons. (From Singaram et al.[11] By permission of Lancet Ltd.) (See color plate section.)

achalasia to pseudo-obstruction) have been reported in association with small cell carcinoma of the lung (>95% of cases), kidney cancer, and pulmonary carcinoid.[19] A circulating IgG antibody (called "ANNA-1" or "anti-Hu") directed against enteric neuronal nuclei[20] has been detected, suggesting that the enteric plexus is the major target of this immune paraneoplastic process. Several patients also have shown evidence of extrinsic visceral neuropathies,[19,21] suggesting a more extensive neuropathological process. Chest radiographic findings are frequently negative and chest CT is indicated when the syndrome is suspected, typically in middle-aged smokers with recent onset of nausea, vomiting, or intolerance to food. ANNA-1 is associated with paraneoplastic neuropathies, 14% of which are restricted to GI manifestations.[4]

Amyloid neuropathy   Familial or acquired amyloid neuropathy may lead to constipation, diarrhea, or steatorrhea. Intestinal myoelectric disturbances in amyloidosis[13] mimic those of ganglionectomy.[22]

Chronic sensory and autonomic neuropathy of unknown cause   The rare, nonfamilial form of slowly progressive neuropathy referred to as chronic sensory and autonomic neuropathy of unknown cause affects several autonomic functions. Patients may have only a chronic autonomic disturbance (e.g., abnormal sweating or blood pressure control or GI dysfunction) for many years before peripheral sensory symptoms become apparent. One review from the Mayo Clinic of 27 patients with idiopathic autonomic neuropathy identified GI involvement in 19.[23]

Porphyria   Acute intermittent porphyria (AIP) and hereditary coproporphyria may present with abdomi-

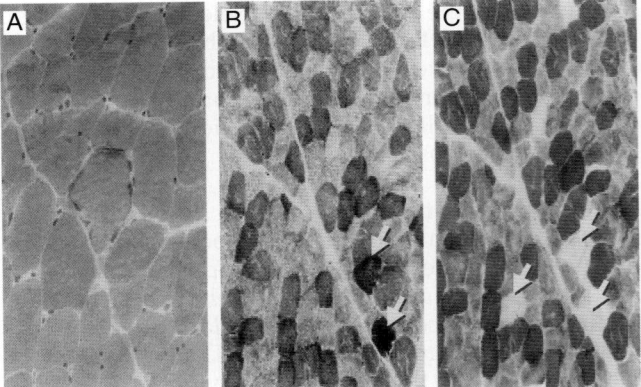

Figure 216.5   Mitochondrial cytopathy in mitochondrial neurogastrointestinal encephalomyopathy. *A,* Note the ragged red fibers on modified Gomori stain reflecting a few muscle fibers with prominent subsarcolemmal mitochondria. *B,* In contrast, ragged blue fibers indicate succinate dehydrogenase positive fibers (*arrow*) are *C,* cytochrome c oxidase-negative, indicating the mitochondrial enzyme deficiency (*arrow*). (From Mueller et al.[29] By permission of American Gastroenterological Association.) (See color plate section.)

Table 216.6   Management of dysphagia[31]

Intervention	Rationale	Evidence	Trade-off between benefit and harms
Nonoral feeding	Reduces risk of aspiration and pneumonia	Aspiration and pneumonia risks are higher in patients who have feeding tubes	Aspiration of oral secretions may occur despite feeding tube placement; cuffed tracheostomy may be more effective
Dietary modification* Thickened liquids	Thick liquids are less likely to spill over tongue base	Reduces risk of pneumonia in dysphagic patients after stroke	
Swallowing therapy Postural manipulation* Strengthening exercises or thermal stimulation[†]	Reduces radiographic aspiration; effect on bolus unclear	No evidence for long-term benefit or improved oral intake	
Cricopharyngeal myotomy[†] for neuropathic or myopathic dysphagia	Relieves dysphagia, especially in patients with functional and structural abnormalities	Limited data support efficacy	
Specific therapy for primary disease	Improves neuromuscular coordination	Possibly no improvement after specific therapy for Parkinson disease or myasthenia gravis, but anecdotal favorable reports in thyrotoxicosis and myopathies	

*Grade B therapeutic option (supported by at least one randomized controlled trial or one high-quality study of nonrandomized cohorts).
[†]Grade C therapeutic option (supported by expert opinions generally derived from basic research, applied physiological evidence, or first principles, but not necessarily based on controlled or randomized trials).

nal pain, nausea, vomiting, and constipation. Dilation and impaired motor function may also occur in any part of the intestinal tract. These symptoms result from extrinsic autonomic dysfunction or intrinsic neuromyopathy.

HIV infection   Neurological disease may manifest at any phase of the infection with HIV-1. Autonomic dysfunction may be associated with chronic diarrhea, possibly as a result of increased extrinsic parasympathetic activity of the gut[24] or damage to the enteric plexuses.[25]

Spinal cord injury   Ileus is a frequent but transient complication after spinal cord injury. With chronic spinal cord injury, disorders of upper GI motility are uncommon. In contrast, colonic and anorectal dysfunction are common and result from interruption of supraspinal control of the sacral parasympathetic supply to the colon, pelvic floor, and anal sphincters.[26,27]

The loss of voluntary control of defecation may be the most significant disturbance in patients who rely on reflex rectal stimulation for stool evacuation. Loss of control of the external anal sphincter with fecal incontinence is the most common chronic GI problem in patients with spinal cord injury. It can usually be managed with a combination of bulk agents and scheduled enemas.

Multiple sclerosis   Severe constipation frequently accompanies urinary bladder dysfunction in patients with advanced multiple sclerosis.[28] To date, studies have not been sufficiently detailed to assess the relative contributions of the sympathetic and parasympathetic denervation. Pelvic colon dysfunction is probably due to impaired supraspinal or spinal control, affecting the sacral parasympathetic supply to the colon. The mechanism of impaired gut transit in multiple sclerosis is incompletely understood.

Myasthenia gravis

Dysphagia occurs in 30% to 60% of patients with myasthenia gravis, is noted at diagnosis in ≈20% of patients, and may not be associated with typical ocular signs. Therefore, edrophonium (Tensilon) testing and EMG should be considered in the appropriate clinical setting.

Mitochondrial cytopathies

Organ disturbances in mitochondrial cytopathies reflect the importance of mitochondria in the normal function of skeletal muscle and the nervous system (Figure 216.5). The mitochondrial disorder affecting

Table 216.7   Management of gastroparesis

Intervention	Rationale	Evidence	Benefit vs. harm
Dietary modification Reduce dietary fiber and fat content*	Antral hypomotility impairs digestion of dietary fiber; lipids delay gastric emptying by inducing CCK release	No clinical trials	No side effects
Venting gastrostomy[32†] and feeding jejunostomy[†]	Permits gastric decompression and enteral feeding	Provides symptom relief Maintains nutritional status	Maintains nutrition without complications of parenteral nutrition
Prokinetic agents Cisapride[†] 10–20 mg ac tid and hs[33]	Stimulates serotonin 5-HT$_4$ receptors to ↑ acetylcholine release from enteric nervous system, facilitating antro-pyloroduodenal contraction	At 6 wk: Symptoms ≡ placebo ↑ GE for solids At 1 yr (open trial): ↓ symptoms and ↑ GE for liquids only	Risk of ↑ QT interval and life-threatening ventricular arrhythmias (use restricted to company-sponsored research protocols)
Erythromycin (motilin receptor agonist)[†] 3 mg/kg IV q 8 hr for 72 hr[34]	Stimulates motilin receptors to dose-dependent ↑ gastric antral motility	Acute exacerbation of gastroparesis (↑ GE for solids and ↓ symptoms)	Vomiting and abdominal cramps may occur Risk of ↑ QT interval with certain drugs Prolonged (i.e., ≥1 mo) oral therapy not effective
Antiemetic agents[†] Metoclopramide (Reglan), 10–15 mg ac Trimethobenzamide (Tigan)	Central and peripheral dopamine D$_2$ receptor antagonist	↓ Symptoms (1 mo) Unknown effect on GE	Extrapyramidal side effects may be irreversible Hyperprolactinemia
Domperidone (Motilium)[†] 20 mg qid—not available in U.S.	Dopaminergic D$_2$ receptor antagonist; doesn't cross blood–brain barrier; central antiemetic effect	↓ Symptoms (up to 2 mo); ↑ GE for liquids only	Extrapyramidal side effects rare Can ↑ prolactin by blocking D$_2$ receptors in posterior pituitary
Gastric electrical stimulation*	↑ GE by electrical stimulation	↓ Symptoms and ↑ GE in open-label studies	

ac, before meals; CCK, cholecystokinin; GE, gastric emptying; hs, at bedtime; IV, intravenous; q, each, every; qid, four times a day; tid, three times a day; ≡, defined as; ↑, increase; ↓, decrease.
*Grade C therapeutic option (supported by expert opinions generally derived from basic research, applied physiological evidence, or first principles, but not necessarily based on controlled or randomized trials).
†Grade B therapeutic option (supported by at least one randomized controlled trial or one high-quality study of nonrandomized cohorts).
‡Grade A therapeutic option (same level of support as for Grade B).

the gut is called "mitochondrial neurogastrointestinal encephalomyopathy" (MNGIE), but it is also referred to as "oculogastrointestinal muscular dystrophy" (OGIMD), or "familial visceral myopathy type II." This autosomal recessive condition with GI and liver manifestations may present at any age—typically with hepatomegaly or hepatic failure in the neonate, seizures or diarrhea in infancy, and liver failure or chronic intestinal pseudo-obstruction in children or adults.

MNGIE is characterized clinically by severe GI dysmotility, external ophthalmoplegia, ptosis, peripheral neuropathy, and leukoencephalopathy. The small intestine is dilated or has multiple diverticula, and the amplitude of contractions is typical of a myopathic disorder.[29] Some patients have a combination of intestinal dysmotility with Kearns-Sayre syndrome or transfer dysphagia due to abnormal coordination and propagation of the swallow through the pharynx and

the skeletal muscle portion of the esophagus, possibly reflecting cranial nerve disorders. This combination of conditions becomes even more devastating when the smooth muscle portion of the esophagus is affected by the associated MNGIE.

Apart from the obvious external ophthalmoplegia, these patients manifest skeletal muscle pain and cramps and systemic (lactic) acidosis. Circulating muscle enzyme levels (e.g., creatine kinase, aspartate aminotransferase, aldolase) are elevated, and modified Gomori staining of muscle biopsy specimens shows characteristic ragged red fibers. This appearance results from the hypertrophy of mitochondria in the subsarcolemmal position in a few muscle fibers and the lack of mitochondria in other muscle fibers. In the intestine, there is hypertrophy of the circular muscle layer, atrophy of the longitudinal muscle, and megamitochondria in myenteric neurons and muscle cells.[30]

Table 216.8	**Management of intestinal pseudo-obstruction**
Intervention	**Comments**
Maintain nutrition and hydration*	Oral or enteral route preferred Liquids or homogenized solids preferred Supplement vitamins and trace elements
Stimulate organized motility	Neostigmine*—inhibits cholinesterase, facilitating cholinergic neurotransmission in the myenteric plexus and neuromuscular junction; an initial dose of 1–2 mg IV, administered with monitoring of heart rate and BP, is effective in acute colonic pseudo-obstruction; case reports support its efficacy in acute exacerbations of chronic intestinal pseudo-obstruction. Cholinergic side effects (e.g., abdominal pain, excessive salivation, vomiting, bradycardia, and syncope) can be reversed if necessary by atropine Cisapride†—improves gastric emptying for solids, but not symptoms in patients with chronic intestinal pseudo-obstruction Octreotide†—induces small intestinal activity fronts that may accelerate transit if propagated; in an uncontrolled study, octreotide (50 µg qhs) improved GI symptoms in scleroderma
Suppress bacterial overgrowth*	Rotating course of antibiotics for 7 days q mo. Options include norfloxacin (400 mg bid), amoxicillin-clavulanic acid (500 mg tid), doxycycline (100 mg bid), and metronidazole (250 mg tid)
Relieve distention*	Venting gastrostomy or jejunostomy can be placed surgically or by endoscopy. Before neostigmine, colonoscopic tube decompression was the preferred approach for Ogilvie syndrome
Surgical therapy*	Selective indications: Failure of nonoperative palliative management Severe persistent intestinal distention (venting, enterostomy) Localized pseudo-obstruction (resection, bypass) Enteral nutritional support (when possible)

bid, two times per day; BP, blood pressure; GI, gastrointestinal; IV, intravenous; qhs, at bedtime; qid, four times per day; tid, three times per day.
*Grade A therapeutic option (supported by at least one randomized controlled trial or one high-quality study of nonrandomized cohorts).
†Grade B therapeutic option (supported by expert opinions generally derived from basic research, applied physiological evidence, or first principles, but not necessarily based on controlled or randomized trials).

Management of gastrointestinal dysmotilities in neurological disorders

Tables 216.6–216.10 summarize the therapeutic modalities for dysphagia, gastroparesis, chronic intestinal pseudo-obstruction, constipation, and fecal incontinence. These therapeutic options have been graded from class A to C on the basis of the quality of the supporting evidence for their use. Recommendations graded as A or B are supported by at least one randomized controlled trial or one high-quality study of nonrandomized cohorts. Grade C recommendations are expert opinions generally derived from basic research, applied physiological evidence, or first principles, but not necessarily based on controlled or randomized trials.

Table 216.9   Management of constipation

Type, name, dosage	Mechanism of action	Time to onset	Side effects
Fiber* 　Bran (1 cup/d) 　Psyllium (Metamucil, 1 tsp 　　up to tid) 　Methylcellulose (Citrucel, 　　1 tsp up to tid)	↓ Stool bulk, ↑ colonic transit time, 　↑ GI motility	Weeks	Bloating, flatulence, iron and calcium malabsorption (methylcellulose may cause less bloating); increase dose gradually
Stool softener† 　Docusate sodium (Colace, 　　100 mg bid)		12–72 hr	Ineffective for constipation
Hyperosmolar agents* 　Sorbitol (15–30 mL qd or bid) 　Lactulose (Chronulac, 　　15–30 mL qd or bid)	Nonabsorbable disaccharides ↑ osmolality and are metabolized by colonic bacteria into short-chain fatty acids that accelerate colonic transit	24–48 hr	Transient abdominal cramps, flatulence; sweet-tasting (lactulose)
Polyethylene glycol 　　(Miralax, 17 g/d)	Osmotically ↑ intraluminal fluids	0.5–1 hr	Incontinence due to potency
Suppository† 　Glycerin (up to daily) 　Bisacodyl (Dulcolax, 　　10 mg daily)	Evacuation induced by local rectal stimulation	0.25–1 hr 0.25–1 hr	Rectal irritation Rectal irritation
Oral stimulant 　Bisacodyl (Dulcolax, 　　10 mg po up to 3 times/wk)	Similar to senna (see anthraquinones)	6–8 hr	Incontinence, hypokalemia, abdominal cramps
Anthraquinones (senna, cascara) 　Senokot (2 tab qd to 4 tab bid) 　Perdiem (plain, 1–2 tsp qd) 　(Peri-Colace, 1–2 tabs qd)	Electrolyte transport altered by ↑ intraluminal fluids; myenteric plexus stimulated; motility ↑	8–12 hr	Degeneration of Meissner plexus and Auerbach plexus (unproven), malabsorption, abdominal cramps, dehydration, melanosis coli
Saline laxative 　Magnesia 　Milk of magnesia (15–30 mL 　　qd or bid)	Fluid osmotically drawn into small bowel lumen; CCK-stimulated; colon transit time ↓	1–3 hr 1–3 hr	Magnesium toxicity, dehydration, abdominal cramps, incontinence; avoid in renal failure
Lubricant 　Mineral oil (15–45 mL)	Stool lubricant	6–8 hr	Lipid pneumonia, fat-soluble vitamin malabsorption, dehydration, incontinence
Enemas (all per rectum) 　Mineral oil retention 　　(100–250 mL qd) 　Tap water (500 mL) 　Phosphate (Fleet, 1 unit) 　Soapsuds (1500 mL)	Stool softened and lubricated (mineral oil), evacuation induced by distended colon; mechanical lavage (others)	6–8 (mineral oil) 5–15 min (others)	Incontinence, mechanical trauma Hyperphosphatemia
Biofeedback therapy†	Restores anal sphincter and puborectalis relaxation during defecation; improves rectal sensation	NA	None; intensive and often expensive treatment

bid, two times per day; CCK, cholecystokinin; GI, gastrointestinal; po, orally; qd, every day; qid, four times per day; tab, tablet; tid, three times per day; ↑, increase; ↓, decrease.
*Grade A therapeutic option (supported by at least one randomized controlled trial or one high-quality study of nonrandomized cohorts).
†Grade C therapeutic option (supported by expert opinions generally derived from basic research, applied physiological evidence, or first principles, but not necessarily based on controlled or randomized trials).
†Grade B therapeutic option (same level of support as for Grade A).

Table 216.10 Management of fecal incontinence			
Intervention	**Side effects**	**Comments**	**Mechanism of action**
Incontinence pads*[35] Disposable bodyworns (largest category of containment product) Reusable bodyworns Disposable underpads Reusable underpads	Skin irritation	Disposable products provide skin protection superior to that of nondisposable products. Underpad products are slightly cheaper than bodyworn products	Provides skin protection and prevents soiling of linen Polymers conduct moisture away from skin
Antidiarrheal agents* Loperamide (Imodium, up to 16 mg/d in divided doses) Diphenaxylate (5 mg qid)	Constipation		↑ Fecal consistency ↓ Urgency ↑ Anal sphincter tone
Enemas[†]	(See Table 216.1)	Rectal evacuation decreases likelihood of fecal incontinence	
Biofeedback therapy using anal canal pressure or surface EMG sensors[†][36]		Limited efficacy in cognitively impaired or significantly depressed patients	↑ Anal sphincter tone Improved rectal sensation
Sphincteroplasty for sphincter defects[†][37]	Wound infection	Restricted to isolated sphincter defects without denervation	Restores sphincter integrity
Sacral nerve stimulation[†]	Infection	Preliminary uncontrolled trials are promising	Unclear; possibly modulates deranged rectal sensitivity or increases anal sphincter pressure
Artificial sphincter[†]	Device erosion, failure, and infection	Either artificial device or gracilis transposition with or without electrical stimulation; available in selected centers only	

qid, four times per day; ↑, increase; ↓, decrease.
*Grade A therapeutic option (supported by at least one randomized controlled trial or one high-quality study of nonrandomized cohorts).
[†]Grade B therapeutic option (same level of support as for Grade A).
[†]Grade C therapeutic option (supported by expert opinions generally derived from basic research, applied physiological evidence, or first principles, but not necessarily based on controlled or randomized trials).

References

1. Sanders KM. A case for interstitial cells of Cajal as pacemakers and mediators of neurotransmission in the gastrointestinal tract. Gastroenterology 1996;111: 492–515

2. Colemont LJ, Camilleri M. Chronic intestinal pseudo-obstruction: diagnosis and treatment. Mayo Clin Proc 1989;64:60–70

3. Bharucha AE, Phillips SF. Megacolon: acute, toxic, and chronic. Curr Treat Options Gastroenterol 1999;2: 517–523

4. Lucchinetti CF, Kimmel DW, Lennon VA. Paraneoplastic and oncologic profiles of patients seropositive for type 1 antineuronal nuclear autoantibodies. Neurology 1998;50:652–657

5. Locke GR III, Pemberton JH, Phillips SF. AGA technical review on constipation: American Gastroenterological Association. Gastroenterology 2000:119:1766–1778

6. Enck P. Biofeedback training in disordered defecation: a critical review. Dig Dis Sci 1993;38:1953–1960

7. Diamant NE, Kamm MA, Wald A, Whitehead WE. AGA technical review on anorectal testing techniques. Gastroenterology 1999;116:735–760

8. Wood JR, Camilleri M, Low PA, Malagelada JR. Brainstem tumor presenting as an upper gut motility disorder. Gastroenterology 1985;89:1411–1414

9. Weber J, Denis P, Mihout B, et al. Effect of brain-stem lesion on colonic and anorectal motility: study of three patients. Dig Dis Sci 1985;30:419–425

10. Edwards LL, Pfeiffer RF, Quigley EM, et al. Gastrointestinal symptoms in Parkinson's disease. Mov Disord 1991;6:151–156

11. Singaram C, Ashraf W, Gaumnitz EA, et al. Dopaminergic defect of enteric nervous system in Parkinson's disease patients with chronic constipation. Lancet 1995; 346:861–864

12. Vassallo M, Camilleri M, Caron BL, Low PA. Gastrointestinal motor dysfunction in acquired selective cholinergic dysautonomia associated with infectious mononucleosis. Gastroenterology 1991;100:252–258

13. Camilleri M, Malagelada JR, Stanghellini V, et al. Gastrointestinal motility disturbances in patients with orthostatic hypotension. Gastroenterology 1985;88: 1852–1859

14. Shy GM, Drager GA. A neurological syndrome associated with orthostatic hypotension: a clinical-pathologic study. Arch Neurol 1960;2:511–527

15. Palace J, Chandiramani VA, Fowler CJ. Value of

sphincter electromyography in the diagnosis of multiple system atrophy. Muscle Nerve 1997;20:1396–1403

16. von der Ohe M, Camilleri M, Zimmerman BR. Management of diabetic enteropathy. Endocrinologist 1993;3: 400–408

17. Janatuinen E, Pikkarainen P, Laakso M, Pyorala K. Gastrointestinal symptoms in middle-aged diabetic patients. Scand J Gastroenterol 1993;28:427–432

18. Maleki D, Locke GR III, Camilleri M, et al. Gastrointestinal tract symptoms among persons with diabetes mellitus in the community. Arch Intern Med 2000;160: 2808–2816

19. Chinn JS, Schuffler MD. Paraneoplastic visceral neuropathy as a cause of severe gastrointestinal motor dysfunction. Gastroenterology 1988;95:1279–1286

20. Lennon VA, Sas DF, Busk MF, et al. Enteric neuronal autoantibodies in pseudoobstruction with small-cell lung carcinoma. Gastroenterology 1991;100:137–142

21. Sodhi N, Camilleri M, Camoriano JK, et al. Autonomic function and motility in intestinal pseudoobstruction caused by paraneoplastic syndrome. Dig Dis Sci 1989; 34:1937–1942

22. Marlett JA, Code CF. Effects of celiac and superior mesenteric ganglionectomy on interdigestive myoelectric complex in dogs. Am J Physiol 1979;237:E432–E443

23. Suarez GA, Fealey RD, Camilleri M, Low PA. Idiopathic autonomic neuropathy: clinical, neurophysiologic, and follow-up studies on 27 patients. Neurology 1994;44:1675–1682

24. Coker RJ, Horner P, Bleasdale-Barr K, et al. Increased gut parasympathetic activity and chronic diarrhoea in a patient with the acquired immunodeficiency syndrome. Clin Auton Res 1992;2:295–298

25. Griffin GE, Miller A, Batman P, et al. Damage to jejunal intrinsic autonomic nerves in HIV infection. AIDS 1988;2:379–382

26. Stone JM, Nino-Murcia M, Wolfe VA, Perkash I. Chronic gastrointestinal problems in spinal cord injury patients: a prospective analysis. Am J Gastroenterol 1990;85:1114–1119

27. Sun WM, Read NW, Donnelly TC. Anorectal function in incontinent patients with cerebrospinal disease. Gastroenterology 1990;99:1372–1379

28. Weber J, Grise P, Roquebert M, et al. Radiopaque markers transit and anorectal manometry in 16 patients with multiple sclerosis and urinary bladder dysfunction. Dis Colon Rectum 1987;30:95–100

29. Mueller LA, Camilleri M, Emslie-Smith AM. Mitochondrial neurogastrointestinal encephalomyopathy: manometric and diagnostic features. Gastroenterology 1999; 116:959–963

30. Perez-Atayde AR, Fox V, Teitelbaum JE, et al. Mitochondrial neurogastrointestinal encephalomyopathy: diagnosis by rectal biopsy. Am J Surg Pathol 1998;22: 1141–1147

31. Cook IJ, Kahrilas PJ. AGA technical review on management of oropharyngeal dysphagia. Gastroenterology 1999;116:455–478

32. Kim CH, Nelson DK. Venting percutaneous gastrostomy in the treatment of refractory idiopathic gastroparesis. Gastrointest Endosc 1998;47:67–70

33. Camilleri M. Appraisal of medium- and long-term treatment of gastroparesis and chronic intestinal dysmotility. Am J Gastroenterol 1994;89:1769–1774

34. Janssens J, Peeters TL, Vantrappen G, et al. Improvement of gastric emptying in diabetic gastroparesis by erythromycin: preliminary studies. N Engl J Med 1990; 322:1028–1031

35. Shirran E, Brazzelli M. Absorbent products for the containment of urinary and/or faecal incontinence in adults. Cochrane Database Syst Rev 2000;2:CD001406

36. Norton C, Hosker G, Brazzelli M. Biofeedback and/or sphincter exercises for the treatment of faecal incontinence in adults. Cochrane Database Syst Rev 2000;2: CD002111

37. Bachoo P, Brazelli M, Grant A. Surgery for faecal incontinence in adults. Cochrane Database Syst Rev 2000;2: CD001757

217 Neurogenic Orthostatic Hypotension

Phillip A Low

The term neurogenic orthostatic hypotension is used to distinguish between orthostatic hypotension that results from pharmacological agents and orthostatic hypotension that can affect otherwise normal persons under extreme circumstances. Neurogenic orthostatic hypotension results from a lesion in the central, preganglionic, or postganglionic autonomic pathways.

Definition of orthostatic hypotension

A consensus conference convened on November 16, 1995, in Phoenix, Arizona, sponsored by the American Autonomic Society and co-sponsored by the American Academy of Neurology, defined orthostatic hypotension as a reduction of systolic blood pressure of at least 20 mmHg or diastolic blood pressure of at least 10 mmHg within three minutes after standing up.[1] The use of a tilt table in the head-up position at an angle of at least 60 degrees was accepted as an alternative. The consensus conference recommended that the confounding variables of food ingestion, time of day, state of hydration, ambient temperature, recent recumbency, postural deconditioning, hypertension, medications, sex, and age be considered. Orthostatic hypotension may be symptomatic or asymptomatic. If the patient has symptoms suggestive of but does not have documented orthostatic hypotension, blood pressure measurements should be repeated.

The values chosen are reasonable screening values but are associated with 5% false-positive values. A value of 30-mmHg decrease in systolic blood pressure would reduce the frequency of false-positive values to 1%.[2] Preferably, an autonomic laboratory study should be performed to confirm the presence of adrenergic failure. A formal grading scale can be generated (Table 217.1).[3] The grade is based on the components of (1) frequency and severity of symptoms, (2) standing time before the onset of symptoms and presyncope, (3) influence on activities of daily living, and (4) blood pressure data.

Epidemiology

The prevalence of orthostatic hypotension is not known with certainty. If orthostatic hypotension associated with aging is included, the prevalence is quite high among subjects older than 70 years. Prevalences (as prevalence in the population and as percentage of the population affected with orthostatic hypotension) that are best estimates based on current data are provided in Table 217.2. For adults who have diabetes mellitus (combined type 1 and type 2 diabetes), the percentage of patients with orthostatic hypotension evaluated from 1987 to 1997 was 10%. The mean age

Table 217.1 Symptom grade of orthostatic intolerance

Grade I
1. Orthostatic symptoms that are infrequent, inconstant, or only under conditions of increased orthostatic stress
2. Standing time >15 min
3. Unrestricted activities of daily living
4. Blood pressure indices may or may not be abnormal

Grade II
5. Orthostatic symptoms that are frequent, developing at least once a week; orthostatic symptoms commonly develop with orthostatic stress
6. Standing time >5 min on most occasions
7. Some limitation in activities of daily living
8. Some change in cardiovascular indices; these may be orthostatic hypotension, decrease in pulse pressure by >50%, or excessive oscillations in blood pressure

Grade III
9. Orthostatic symptoms develop on most occasions and are regularly unmasked by orthostatic stresses
10. Standing time >1 min on most occasions
11. Marked limitation in activities of daily living
12. Orthostatic hypotension is present >50% of the time, recorded on different days

Grade IV
13. Orthostatic symptoms consistently present
14. Standing time <1 min on most occasions
15. Patient is seriously incapacitated, being bed- or wheelchair-bound because of orthostatic intolerance; syncope/presyncope are common if patient attempts to stand
16. Orthostatic hypotension is consistently present

Table 217.2 Estimated prevalence of orthostatic hypotension in different autonomic disorders

Disorder	Prevalence	Reference
Aging	14% to 20%	Low[4]
Diabetes mellitus	10%*	
Other autonomic neuropathies	10 to 50 per 100 000	
Multiple system atrophy	5 to 15 per 100 000	
Pure autonomic failure	10 to 30 per 100 000	

*Prevalence for adult combined type 1 and type 2 diabetes mellitus for the Rochester Diabetic Cohort for 1997 (PI: PJ Dyck).

of the Rochester Diabetic Cohort over this decade was 60.6 ± 11.7 years.

Causes

The causes of neurogenic orthostatic hypotension are listed in Table 217.3. The most important causes are multiple system atrophy, pure autonomic failure, diabetic autonomic neuropathy, idiopathic (presumed immune-mediated) neuropathy, and paraneoplastic autonomic neuropathy; in some practices, tetraplegia is a common cause. In a prospective study of 90 consecutive patients who were referred for suspected orthostatic hypotension and were evaluated in the Mayo Autonomic Laboratory and confirmed to have orthostatic hypotension, the diagnoses were pure autonomic failure in 33%, multiple system atrophy/Shy-Drager syndrome in 26%, autonomic neuropathy in 17%, diabetic autonomic neuropathy in 14%, olivopontocerebellar atrophy in 2%, and miscellaneous in 8%.

Table 217.3   Causes of neurogenic orthostatic hypotension

Autonomic disorders *without* CNS or PNS involvement
  Pure autonomic failure

Autonomic disorders with brain involvement
  Multiple system atrophy
  Wernicke-Korsakoff syndrome
  Posterior fossa tumors
  Baroreflex failure
  Olivopontocerebellar atrophy

Autonomic disorders with spinal cord involvement
  Traumatic tetraplegia
  Syringomyelia
  Subacute combined degeneration
  Multiple sclerosis
  Spinal cord tumors

Autonomic neuropathies
  Acute autonomic neuropathies
    Acute panautonomic neuropathy (pandysautonomia)
    Acute paraneoplastic autonomic neuropathy
    Guillain–Barré syndrome
    Botulism
    Porphyria
    Drug-induced acute autonomic neuropathies
    Toxic acute autonomic neuropathies
  Chronic peripheral autonomic neuropathies
    Pure adrenergic neuropathy
    Combined sympathetic and parasympathetic failure
      (autonomic dysfunction clinically *important*)
      Amyloidosis
      Diabetic autonomic neuropathy
      Paraneoplastic autonomic (including
        panautonomic) neuropathy
      Sensory neuronopathy with autonomic failure
        (most commonly associated with Sjögren
        syndrome)
      Familial dysautonomia (Riley-Day syndrome)
      Immune-mediated
      Dysautonomia of old age

Clinical manifestations

Orthostatic hypotension is relatively common but usually asymptomatic. In fact, most patients with "asymptomatic" orthostatic hypotension have symptoms, albeit subtle, under certain conditions of orthostatic stress. The symptoms vary by age. A distribution of symptoms based on a prospective study of 90 consecutive patients with confirmed orthostatic hypotension is given in Table 217.4.[5] Lightheadedness was common, as expected. However, about half the patients had difficulty in concentrating and thinking, and for those older than 70, this may be the most common symptom, which, although subtle, seriously impairs quality of life. Palpitations, tremulousness, anxiety, and nausea are symptoms of autonomic overaction and occur in younger patients and those who have only partial autonomic failure, typically autonomic neuropathy.

Symptoms typically are worse in the early morning, after meals, with an increase in core temperature, with prolonged standing, and with activity. The early morning severity of orthostatic hypotension is related to the nocturnal diuresis that many patients have.[6] Postprandial worsening is almost the rule, occurring within 30 minutes after a meal and lasting about an hour. Patients commonly recognize that they have more orthostatic symptoms after a hot bath or hot tub or on a hot day. Indeed, any stress that results in vasodilatation of skin vessels worsens symptoms. Patients who get up in the middle of the night out of a warm bed have vasodilatation and, thus, worse orthostatic hypotension. Similarly, symptoms may be worse after ingestion of alcohol because of vasodilatation. Orthostatic hypotension is also worse with physical activity sufficient to cause muscle vasodilatation. These symptoms are due to cerebral hypoperfusion. When orthostatic hypotension is severe and sustained, syncope occurs. After the diagnosis is made, syncope tends to be relatively uncommon because patients learn to recognize the symptoms of orthostatic hypotension and to take corrective steps.

On examination, orthostatic hypotension is confirmed. Patients who have partial preservation of baroreflexes may have marked tachycardia (Figure 217.1, *top*), indicating that the vagal component of the

Table 217.4   Symptoms of orthostatic intolerance in 90 consecutive patients

Symptom	Patients, %
Lightheadedness (dizziness)	88
Weakness or tiredness	72
Cognitive (thinking/concentrating)	47
Blurred vision	47
Tremulousness	38
Vertigo	37
Pallor	31
Anxiety	29
Palpitations	26
Clammy feeling	19
Nausea	18

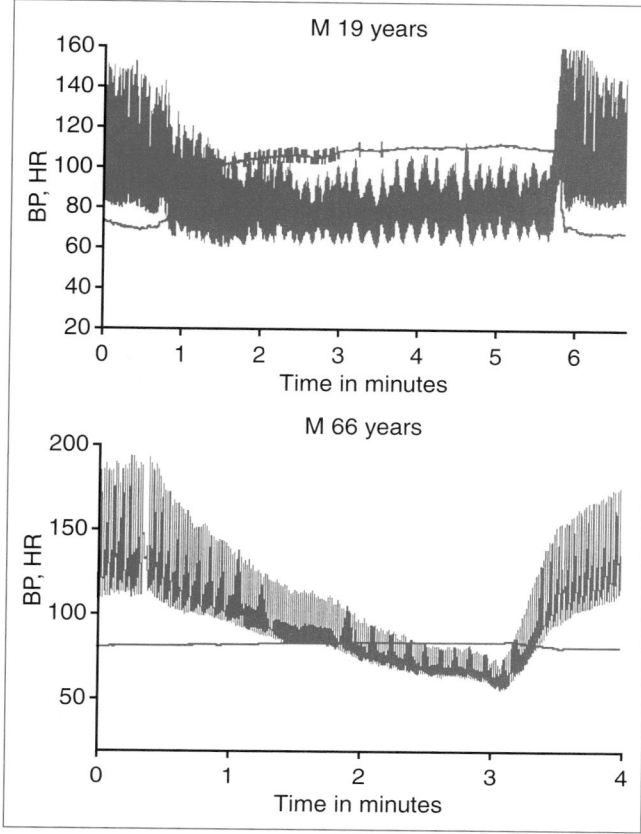

Figure 217.1 Blood pressure (BP) and heart rate (HR) responses to head-up tilt. *Top*, A 19-year-old man with idiopathic length-dependent autonomic neuropathy shows orthostatic hypotension with compensatory tachycardic response. *Bottom*, Orthostatic hypotension with fixed heart rate, indicative of more complete baroreflex failure, in a 66-year-old man.

baroreflex is intact. Note the prominent oscillations in blood pressure at baroreflex loop frequency, with some modest improvement in blood pressure over time. With generalized and more complete autonomic failure, orthostatic hypotension is associated with a fixed heart rate (Figure 217.1), indicating that both the cardiovagal and peripheral adrenergic limbs of the baroreflex have failed.

Patients note that certain maneuvers reduce orthostatic hypotension.[7] For example, it is less when they pace than when they stand perfectly still. Muscle contraction results in a pumping action that increases venous return. Patients also notice that certain physical maneuvers, such as bending forward, crossing the legs, and performing a toe rise, alleviate symptoms. These physical countermaneuvers are considered below (see "Treatment").

Course and prognosis

The prognosis depends on the specific disorders. Patients with classic multiple system atrophy have a median survival of about seven years from the time of diagnosis.[8] Wenning et al.,[9] however, reported a median survival of 9.5 years, calculated by Kaplan-Meier analysis. Similar results have been reported,[10] and patients with sporadic olivopontocerebellar atrophy have been suggested to have longer survival than those with striatonigral degeneration.[10] The differences reported in survival are likely related to the criteria used to define multiple system atrophy. The downhill course is marked by increasing rigidity, urinary incontinence, and, sometimes, marked stridor, which may require tracheotomy. Death frequently is due to respiratory obstruction or failure after worsening rigidity, akinesia, and bladder disorder. With the appreciation of the spectrum of severities, an attempt has been made to relate the severity and distribution of autonomic and nonautonomic involvement to outcome. Sandroni et al.[11] reviewed the clinical and autonomic features of all patients with extrapyramidal and cerebellar disorders studied in the Mayo Autonomic Reflex Laboratory from 1983 to 1989. Orthostatic blood pressure reduction, percentage of anhidrosis on the thermoregulatory sweat test, quantitative sudomotor axon reflex test, and forearm response and heart rate response to deep breathing strongly regressed with the severity of clinical involvement. The severity and distribution of autonomic failure at the time of the first evaluation were predictive of a greater rate of progression two years later. Saito et al.[10] came to the same conclusion. Sandroni et al.[11] concluded that the earlier and the more severe the involvement of the autonomic nervous system and, to a lesser extent, the striatonigral system, the poorer the prognosis.

Information on the clinical features, progression, and outcome in pure autonomic failure is limited. Some patients with this condition are relatively free of symptoms for many years, with standing blood pressure near 80 mmHg. The natural history of pure autonomic failure is that of a slow progression occurring over 10 to 15 years.[8] The percentage of cases of pure autonomic failure that evolve into multiple system atrophy is probably about 10%.

The development of orthostatic hypotension worsens the prognosis. Ewing et al.[12] reported a mortality rate of 50% at 2.5 years for patients with symptomatic diabetic autonomic neuropathy. However, these patients had long-standing clinical autonomic neuropathy and died of renal failure. Subsequent studies have suggested that autonomic failure worsens the prognosis, but the prognosis is less dismal than originally thought.[13]

The clinical and laboratory features of 229 patients with primary systemic amyloidosis evaluated at the Mayo Clinic were reviewed, and the authors concluded that the median survival from the time of diagnosis for patients with peripheral neuropathy, carpal tunnel syndrome, orthostatic hypotension, or cardiac failure was 60, 45, 9.5, and 6.5 months, respectively.[14]

The Mayo experience is that idiopathic immune-mediated autonomic neuropathy has a chronic debilitating course, with the majority of patients having marked residual deficits. Patients appear to have substantial improvement over the first year, followed by a slower rate of improvement over the subsequent four years.[15] Overall, approximately one in three patients has good functional recovery.

Pathophysiology and pathogenesis

The maintenance of postural normotension without an excessive heart rate increment depends on an adequate blood volume and the integration of many reflex and humoral systems and several key vascular beds, including the striated muscle, splanchnic-mesenteric, and cerebrovascular beds.

An adequate blood volume is essential. Hypovolemia regularly causes orthostatic hypotension, even if vascular reflexes are intact. Hypovolemia can also be relative. Denervation decreases vascular tone and increases vascular capacity. Patients who have adrenergic failure will be relatively hypovolemic, although plasma volume is normal. Their orthostatic intolerance can improve if the plasma volume is expanded, hence the importance of volume expansion in the treatment of orthostatic hypotension. A decreased red cell mass or normocytic, normochromic anemia of chronic autonomic failure aggravates orthostatic hypotension. Correcting anemia with erythropoietin improves orthostatic intolerance.[16,17]

Two sets of baroreflexes, the arterial (or high-pressure) and venous (or low-pressure) baroreflexes, are mainly responsible for the reflex control of blood pressure and the circulation. When systemic pulse pressure or mean arterial pressure decreases, baroreceptors are unloaded in the carotid sinus and aortic arch.[18] These are arterial baroreceptors. Afferent impulses from the carotid sinus travel via the glossopharyngeal nerves and impulses from the carotid arch travel via the vagus nerves to synapse in the nucleus of the tractus solitarius. From this nucleus, a polysynaptic cardiovagal pathway travels to the nucleus ambiguus and dorsal motor nucleus of the vagus and, thence, via the vagus nerve to the sinoatrial node. Sympathetic function is regulated by the rostroventrolateral nucleus of medulla, which projects to the intermediolateral column of the thoracic spinal cord that, in turn, provides sympathetic innervation to the heart and periphery (arterioles and venules).[19] In addition to arterial baroreceptors, there are low-pressure baroreceptors. The effective stimulus is a decrease in central venous pressure, that is, these receptors are responsive to changes in volume. Cardiopulmonary receptors in the heart and lungs send mainly nonmyelinated vagal fibers to the nucleus of the tractus solitarius. The central pathways and efferents are the same as for arterial baroreceptors.

The splanchnic-mesenteric capacitance bed is a large-volume, low-resistance system of great importance in the maintenance of postural normotension in humans. It constitutes 25% to 30% of the total blood volume.[20] Unlike muscle veins, splanchnic veins have an abundance of smooth muscle and a rich sympathetic innervation. The mesenteric capacitance bed is markedly responsive to both arterial and venous baroreflexes. Venoconstriction is mediated by α-adrenergic receptors.[21] The nerve supply to the mesenteric bed is mostly from preganglionic axons in the greater splanchnic nerve, with cell bodies in the intermediolateral column (mainly T4 to T9), that synapse in the celiac ganglion, from whence postganglionic adrenergic fibers supply effector cells. Considerable clinical and research evidence supports the importance of splanchnic outflow in the maintenance of postural normotension in humans. Postural hypotension occurs regularly after bilateral splanchnic neurectomy, but neither bilateral lumbar sympathectomy nor cardiac denervation alone causes it.[22,23] In patients with complete spinal cord lesions, postural hypotension is most pronounced when the splanchnic outflow is affected (above T6). Abnormalities in the splanchnic autonomic outflow have been found in human diabetic neuropathy, indicating that preganglionic fibers can be affected.[24]

Cerebral vasoregulation is important for ensuring adequate and stable flow to the brain in spite of changing systemic blood pressure. The maintenance of constant blood flow in spite of variations in blood pressure is termed autoregulation.[25] Within a mean blood pressure range of approximately 50 to 150 mmHg, a change in blood pressure produces insignificant change in cerebral perfusion. Previous studies of patients with orthostatic hypotension demonstrated an expansion of the autoregulated range at both the upper and lower limits, so that cerebral perfusion remained relatively constant with the patient supine (when supine hypertension might be present) and in response to standing (when orthostatic hypotension occurs).[26–28]

Treatment

The treatment of orthostatic hypotension has four goals. The first is to improve orthostatic blood pressure without excessive supine hypertension. The second is to improve standing time. The third is to relieve orthostatic symptoms. The fourth goal, related to the second goal, is to improve the patient's ability to perform orthostatic activities of daily living.

Although the symptoms of orthostatic hypotension can always be relieved, it is more difficult to do so without unacceptable supine hypertension, because patients with generalized autonomic failure have baroreflex failure, and a regular component of this failure is the loss of postural regulation of blood pressure. A reasonable practical goal is a regimen that relieves symptoms most of the day with supine blood pressure that does not usually exceed 180/110 mmHg. Patients with neurogenic orthostatic hypotension have greater fluctuations than normal (loss of baroreflexes or "buffer nerves") and often have supine hypertension. The 180/110 mmHg value is quite acceptable, because patients are taught to avoid lying flat.

Patients who have asymptomatic orthostatic hypotension do not require treatment. However, this needs to be qualified because most patients with orthostatic hypotension do have symptoms at some time. The orthostatic stresses may be time of day (early morning), a meal, an increase in core

Table 217.5   Standard initial treatment of orthostatic hypotension

Patient education
High salt diet (10–20 g/day)
High fluid intake (20 oz/day); coffee or tea beneficial
Elevate head of bed four inches
Correct anemia
Maintain postural stimuli
Physical countermaneuvers

temperature, physical activity, or reduced salt or fluid intake. Older patients may become symptomatic after a period of bed rest or after taking a diuretic. It is necessary to recognize patients who have iatrogenic orthostatic hypotension. Common drugs include antihypertensive agents and calcium channel entry blocking drugs. Insulin, levodopa, or tricyclic antidepressants can also cause vasodilatation and orthostatic hypotension in predisposed subjects. The first-line treatment of orthostatic hypotension is outlined in Table 217.5.

Nonpharmacological management

Patient education   Patient education is critically important, and its lack is probably the single-most important factor in the relatively poor control of orthostatic hypotension. The twin elements of switching to a patient-centered decision-making model and a dynamic model of management require detailed patient education. The patient should understand in simple terms the maintenance of postural normotension and its practical implications (importance of blood volume and activation of the humoral mechanism by postural training). They need to understand the orthostatic stressors and their mechanisms. After these stressors have been explained, patients have no difficulty recognizing them.

Suggestions about modifications in the activities of daily living include how to handle early morning and postprandial orthostatic hypotension. In a patient-centered management plan, the patient will discover additional useful modifications. Patients should be shown how to keep a blood pressure log. This is extremely useful when there is a change in management, when there is worsening of symptoms, and when blood pressure management is fine-tuned. Oftentimes, it is uncertain whether the worsening of symptoms is related to worsening orthostatic hypotension or to some other mechanism. The patient or preferably the spouse or other support person should use an automated sphygmomanometer to measure the blood pressure with the patient supine and after standing for one minute. Recordings should be taken on awakening, after a meal, during a time of maximal orthostatic tolerance, during a time of poor orthostatic tolerance, and before and one hour after medication.

Patients need to understand the sodium content of common food items and to be educated about high sodium intake. Daily salt intake should be between 150 and 250 mEq of sodium (10 to 20 g of salt). The

relationship between salt intake and blood pressure is close. Some patients are intensely sensitive to salt intake and can fine-tune their plasma volume and blood pressure control with salt intake alone. Foods with a high salt content include fast foods such as hamburgers, hot dogs, chicken pieces, French fries, and fish fries. Canned soups, chili, ham, bacon, sausage, additives such as soya sauce, and commercially processed canned products also have a high sodium content. Patients should have at least one glass or cup of fluid with meals and at least two glasses at other times each day to obtain 2 to 2.5 L of fluid daily.

Patients need to have a high potassium diet because of the combination of high sodium intake and fludrocortisone. Fruits, especially bananas, and vegetables have high potassium content. Patients should have a snack with more fluids at night. Postprandial orthostatic hypotension reduces some of the nocturnal hypertension.

Educating patients how to manage situations of increased orthostatic stress is important. After patients discover their ability to cope with these situations—typically more effectively than most physicians can manage—they develop a great sense of empowerment.

Physical countermaneuvers are helpful in prolonging the time a patient can remain upright. These include such maneuvers as toe-raise, crossing the legs, contracting the thigh muscles, and bending at the waist.[29,30]

Volume expansion   All patients with neurogenic orthostatic hypotension require the standard treatment for orthostatic hypotension aimed at expanding blood volume. Generous fluid intake is critically important and often neglected in the elderly, who need five to eight 8-oz glasses of fluid each day. Salt supplementation is essential. Most patients manage with added salt with their meals. Occasionally, patients prefer to use salt tablets (available as 0.5- and 1-g tablets). It is important to recognize that vasoconstrictors are ineffective when plasma volume is substantially decreased. Many patients who have inadequate control of orthostatic hypotension have inadequate salt intake. This can be verified by checking the 24-hour urinary concentration of sodium. Patients who have a value less than 170 mmol/24 hours can be given supplemental sodium, 1 to 2 g three times daily. Their weight, symptoms, and urinary concentration of sodium should be checked one or two weeks later.[31]

Postural adjustment   The head of the bed is elevated four inches for two reasons. First, it reduces nocturia, probably by stimulating renin release. Second, it reduces supine hypertension. During the day, it is important to maintain adequate orthostatic stress. If patients are tilted up repeatedly, orthostatic hypotension gradually attenuates. This likely results from the release of renin and arginine vasopressin, which requires more sustained or repetitive orthostatic stress. Another mechanism that has been suggested is extravasated plasma around veins providing a vascular cuff, increasing venomotor tone.

Compression garments   For some patients, wearing a tightly fitting body stocking ameliorates orthostatic hypotension and associated symptoms. These stockings have to be well-fitted and put on before arising. They work by reducing the venous capacitance bed. Their disadvantages are the cumbersome application and discomfort in hot weather. Some available sources are Jobst (800-537-1063), Barton-Carey (800-421-0444), Sigvaris (800-322-7744), and Camp (800-492-1088). A measured Jobst stocking is especially useful. Some subjects find that a tightly fitting girdle or abdominal binder is as helpful.

Physical countermaneuvers   Physical countermaneuvers that involve the contraction of certain muscle groups of the lower extremities decrease venous capacitance and increase venous return.[30] These maneuvers, which once learned can substantially prolong standing time, include crossing of the legs and contracting the leg muscles of one leg against the other, slow stepping or marching on the spot, propping the leg up on a chair, or contraction of the thigh muscles.[29]

Pharmacological management

Drug treatment is an important part of the overall therapeutic regimen and, if used well, greatly enhances blood pressure control.[32] The main drugs are fludrocortisone and midodrine.

Midodrine and fludrocortisone   The optimal approach, with the availability of midodrine, is to expand plasma volume modestly without inducing marked supine hypertension and to add midodrine during the waking period to reduce orthostatic hypotension. The safest approach to volume expansion is oral salt supplementation. The minimal effective dose of midodrine is 5 mg. Most patients respond best to 10 mg. The duration of action is between two and four hours, corresponding to the blood levels of midodrine and its active metabolite desglymidodrine.[33] The onset of action is between 30 minutes and one hour. In some patients, the duration of action of midodrine is short, less than four hours. Because one of the mechanisms of hypertensive swings is severe hypotension, it is best to increase the frequency of dosing to every three hours during the period of maximal orthostatic stress. Patients should generally avoid midodrine after 6 pm.

For patients who cannot take enough salt or who do not have an adequate response to midodrine, fludrocortisone, 0.1 mg once or twice daily, can be added to provide volume expansion and to sensitize vascular smooth muscle. This approach of reducing dependence on fludrocortisone and avoiding nocturnal midodrine substantially reduces supine hypertension.

Uncommonly, the dose of fludrocortisone may be increased to 0.4 or 0.6 mg daily for patients with refractory orthostatic hypotension. Because the regulatory reflexes are greatly impaired, it is necessary to overexpand the plasma volume slightly in these patients. A reasonable clue for adequate volume expansion is a weight gain of 3 to 5 lb. Mild dependent edema is to be expected. The potential risks are congestive heart failure and excessive supine hypertension. Two weeks after starting treatment with fludrocortisone, patients should have their blood pressure checked while supine and standing.

Treatment for periods of orthostatic decompensation

Patients who have restricted autonomic neuropathy and associated postural tachycardia have periods of orthostatic decompensation. Patients with generalized autonomic failure also have episodes of apparent decompensation when they have greater orthostatic hypotension or less response to pressor agents. These patients need to be evaluated for a cause of decompensation. The causes include fluid deficit, hypokalemia, anemia, deconditioning related to a recent period of recumbency, and another illness (including pump [cardiac] failure). Often, however, no cause is found. The patient appears to respond to management with volume expansion. The first approach is the "bouillon treatment." The patient makes one of these extremely salty soups and drinks about five 8-oz servings in half a day. An alternative is supplemental sodium chloride, 2 g three times daily, and a minimum of eight 8-oz servings of fluids daily for two days. If the patient does not have improvement with this regimen or reports that fluid is not being retained, desmopressin, one puff each nostril at bedtime, is taken for one week. The dose of vasoconstrictor can be adjusted upward. This is when a tight-fitting body stocking (e.g. Jobst) can be beneficial. Fludrocortisone, 0.2 mg three times daily, can be taken for one week. The drug is traditionally considered to be slowly cumulative in its action; however, recent studies have suggested that it also has a rapid mode of action. If all these measures are unsuccessful, the treatment is isotonic saline, 1 to 2 L, given intravenously.

Hospital management of severe orthostatic hypotension

Some patients with severe orthostatic hypotension need acute hospital management. In addition to a search for the cause of orthostatic hypotension and specific treatment, management is aimed at improving orthostatic tolerance to the degree that subsequent management can be continued on an outpatient basis. A regimen of treatment extending over approximately three days is suggested. These patients are volume-depleted, either absolutely or relatively (because of increased capacity due to denervation). Intravenous infusion of 1 to 2 L of isotonic saline is needed to expand plasma volume. Early volume expansion is critically important because hypovolemia greatly reduces the effectiveness of vasoconstrictors in increasing blood pressure, markedly affecting the sensitivity of cardiopulmonary but not carotid-cardiac baroreflex responses to α-agonists.[34] In elderly patients, care needs to be exercised to avoid heart failure. Postural training is needed. The head of the bed is elevated four inches or at an angle of 10 to 30 degrees. The patient spends an increasing period of time seated and standing. Treatment with fludrocortisone, 0.2 mg/day, is commenced, as is sodium chloride, 1 g three times daily, and high fluid intake. During this time, the patient is educated about dietary salt content, maintenance of postural normotension, physical countermaneuvers, management of periods of increased orthostatic stress, and supine hypertension. Blood pressure is measured with the patient supine and standing one minute before and one hour after 10 mg of midodrine, and the supine and standing values are recorded hourly to establish the optimal dose and duration of action.

Treatment of early morning orthostatic hypotension

The most common time of day that orthostatic hypotension is worse is on awakening. In some patients, this occurs because of excessive nocturia. For many patients, the situation is improved by sleeping with the head of the bed elevated (reducing nocturia). A common routine is to drink two cups of strong coffee (250 mg caffeine), to take vasoconstrictors, and to read the newspaper before getting up.

Treatment of postprandial orthostatic hypotension

Patients often have postprandial accentuation of orthostatic hypotension. This can occur with any type of neurogenic orthostatic hypotension but is particularly common with diabetic autonomic neuropathy. It often occurs on the background of gastrointestinal autonomic neuropathy, highlighting the great importance of the splanchnic-mesenteric bed in orthostatic blood pressure control. This is a large-volume (20% to 30% of total blood volume) capacitance bed that, unlike other venous beds, is exquisitely baroreflex responsive. Some patients with mild postprandial orthostatic hypotension discover that the worsening can be reduced by frequent small meals, and some find that certain foods are most troublesome and should be avoided. Some patients report that hot drinks or hot food need to be avoided. Carbohydrates are especially troublesome.

Ibuprofen, 400 to 800 mg, or indomethacin, 25 to 50 mg, with the meal is well tolerated and should be tried. The next step is the administration of a vasoconstrictor such as midodrine, 10 mg. A problem with vasoconstrictors is the aggravation of gastroparesis. Rarely, symptoms suggestive of gut ischemia may occur.

If all the approaches are inadequate, the somatostatin analogue octreotide can be administered with the meal. The dose is 25 μg by subcutaneous injection. The dose can be increased if necessary to 100 to 200 μg. This is the most efficacious agent but requires parenteral administration.

Treatment of nocturnal hypertension

Normal subjects have a diurnal variation in blood pressure, with lower nocturnal blood pressure. Patients with neurogenic orthostatic hypotension have nocturnal hypertension. To minimize the problems of nocturnal hypertension, pressor medications should not be taken after 6 pm. The head of the bed should be elevated, resulting in lower intracranial blood pressure. A nighttime snack with a glass of fluids (not coffee or tea) results in some postprandial hypotension and can be used to increase fluid intake and decrease nocturnal hypertension. Patients who enjoy a glass of wine should drink it at this time for its vasodilator effect.

Occasionally, it is not possible to control orthostatic hypotension without marked nocturnal hypertension. For these patients, hydralazine (Apresoline), 25 mg, can be given at night. Because this drug has sodium-retaining properties, it is especially suitable. Alternatives include the angiotensin-converting enzyme inhibitor nifedipine (Procardia), 10 mg, or a nitroglycerin patch.

Erythropoietin

Mild-to-moderate normocytic, normochromic anemia is not uncommon. After it has been determined that iron stores are adequate, the patient can be given erythropoietin. The anemia may be due to renal denervation, resulting in a decrease in renin.[16] A typical dose of erythropoietin, administered subcutaneously three times weekly, is 50 U/kg until reticulocytosis and an increase in the hematocrit occur.[17,35] The duration of treatment is three to 10 weeks.

References

1. The consensus committee of the American Autonomic Society and the American Academy of Neurology. Consensus statement on the definition of orthostatic hypotension, pure autonomic failure, and multiple system atrophy. Neurology 1996;46:1470
2. Low PA, Denq JC, Opfer-Gehrking TL, et al. Effect of age and gender on sudomotor and cardiovagal function and blood pressure response to tilt in normal subjects. Muscle Nerve 1997;20:1561–1568
3. Low PA, ed. Clinical Autonomic Disorders: Evaluation and Management. 2nd ed. Philadelphia: Lippincott-Raven, 1997:179–208
4. Low PA, ed. Clinical Autonomic Disorders: Evaluation and Management. 2nd ed. Philadelphia: Lippincott-Raven, 1997:161–175
5. Low PA, Opfer-Gehrking TL, McPhee BR, et al. Prospective evaluation of clinical characteristics of orthostatic hypotension. Mayo Clin Proc 1995;70:617–622
6. Bannister R. Multiple-system atrophy and pure autonomic failure. In: Low PA, ed. Clinical Autonomic Disorders: Evaluation and Management. Boston: Little, Brown and Company, 1993:517–525
7. Denq JC, Opfer-Gehrking TL, Giuliani M, et al. Efficacy of compression of different capacitance beds in the amelioration of orthostatic hypotension. Clin Auton Res 1997;7:321–326
8. Low PA, Bannister R. Multiple system atrophy and pure autonomic failure. In: Low PA, ed. Clinical Autonomic Disorders: Evaluation and Management. 2nd ed. Philadelphia: Lippincott-Raven, 1997:555–575

9. Wenning GK, Ben Shlomo Y, Magalhaes M, et al. Clinical features and natural history of multiple system atrophy. An analysis of 100 cases. Brain 1994;117:835–845

10. Saito Y, Matsuoka Y, Takahashi A, Ohno Y. Survival of patients with multiple system atrophy. Intern Med 1994;33:321–325

11. Sandroni P, Ahlskog JE, Fealey RD, Low PA. Autonomic involvement in extrapyramidal and cerebellar disorders. Clin Auton Res 1991;1:147–155

12. Ewing DJ, Campbell IW, Clarke BF. The natural history of diabetic autonomic neuropathy. Q J Med 1980;49:95–108

13. Hilsted J, Low PA. Diabetic autonomic neuropathy. In: Low PA, ed. Clinical Autonomic Disorders: Evaluation and Management. 2nd ed. Philadelphia: Lippincott-Raven, 1997:487–507

14. Kyle RA, Greipp PR. Amyloidosis (AL). Clinical and laboratory features in 229 cases. Mayo Clin Proc 1983;58:665–683

15. Suarez GA, Fealey RD, Camilleri M, Low PA. Idiopathic autonomic neuropathy: clinical, neurophysiologic, and follow-up studies on 27 patients. Neurology 1994;44:1675–1682

16. Biaggioni I, Goldstein DS, Atkinson T, Robertson D. Dopamine-beta-hydroxylase deficiency in humans. Neurology 1990;40:370–373

17. Hoeldtke RD, Streeten DH. Treatment of orthostatic hypotension with erythropoietin. N Engl J Med 1993;329:611–615

18. Auer RN, Coulter KC. The nature and time course of neuronal vacuolation induced by the N-methyl-D-aspartate antagonist MK-801. Acta Neuropathol 1994;87:1–7

19. Joyner MJ, Shepherd JT. Autonomic control of circulation. In: Low PA, ed. Clinical Autonomic Disorders: Evaluation and Management. Boston: Little, Brown and Company, 1993:55–67

20. Rowell LB, Detry JM, Blackmon JR, Wyss C. Importance of the splanchnic vascular bed in human blood pressure regulation. J Appl Physiol 1972;32:213–220

21. Thirlwell MP, Zsoter TT. The effect of propranolol and atropine on venomotor reflexes in man. Venous reflexes—effect of propranolol and atropine. J Med 1972;3:65–72

22. White JC, Smithwick RH. The Autonomic Nervous System; Anatomy, Physiology, and Surgical Application. 2nd ed. New York: The Macmillan Company, 1941

23. Wilkins RW, Culbertson JW, Ingelfinger FJ. The effect of splanchnic sympathectomy in hypertensive patients upon estimated hepatic blood flow in the upright as contrasted with the horizontal position. J Clin Invest 1951;30:312–317

24. Low PA, Walsh JC, Huang CY, McLeod JG. The sympathetic nervous system in diabetic neuropathy. A clinical and pathological study. Brain 1975;98:341–356

25. Symon L. Pathological regulation in cerebral ischemia. In: Wood JH, ed. Cerebral Blood Flow: Physiologic and Clinical Aspects. New York: McGraw-Hill Book Company, 1987:413–424

26. Eldar M, Battler A, Neufeld HN, et al. Transluminal carbon dioxide-laser catheter angioplasty for dissolution of atherosclerotic plaques. J Am Coll Cardiol 1984;3:135–137

27. Depresseux JC, Rousseau JJ, Franck G. The autoregulation of cerebral blood flow, the cerebrovascular reactivity and their interaction in the Shy-Drager syndrome. Eur Neurol 1979;18:295–301

28. Brooks DJ, Redmond S, Mathias CJ, et al. The effect of orthostatic hypotension on cerebral blood flow and middle cerebral artery velocity in autonomic failure, with observations on the action of ephedrine. J Neurol Neurosurg Psychiatry 1989;52:962–966

29. Bouvette CM, McPhee BR, Opfer-Gehrking TL, Low PA. Role of physical countermaneuvers in the management of orthostatic hypotension: efficacy and biofeedback augmentation. Mayo Clin Proc 1996;71:847–853

30. Ten Harkel AD, van Lieshout JJ, Wieling W. Effects of leg muscle pumping and tensing on orthostatic arterial pressure: a study in normal subjects and patients with autonomic failure. Clin Sci (Colch) 1994;87:553–558

31. El-Sayed H, Hainsworth R. Salt supplement increases plasma volume and orthostatic tolerance in patients with unexplained syncope. Heart 1996;75:134–140

32. Fealey RD, Robertson D. Management of orthostatic hypotension. In: Low PA, ed. Clinical Autonomic Disorders: Evaluation and Management. Boston: Little, Brown and Company, 1993:731–743

33. Low PA, Gilden JL, Freeman R, et al. Efficacy of midodrine vs placebo in neurogenic orthostatic hypotension. A randomized, double-blind multicenter study. Midodrine Study Group. JAMA 1997;277:1046–1051

34. Thompson CA, Tatro DL, Ludwig DA, Convertino VA. Baroreflex responses to acute changes in blood volume in humans. Am J Physiol 1990;259:R792–R798

35. Perera R, Isola L, Kaufmann H. Effect of recombinant erythropoietin on anemia and orthostatic hypotension in primary autonomic failure. Clin Auton Res 1995;5:211–213

218 Orthostatic Intolerance

Phillip A Low

Definitions

Orthostatic intolerance is defined as symptoms of cerebral hypoperfusion or autonomic overaction which develop while the subject is standing but are relieved by recumbency. Symptoms of hypoperfusion include lightheadedness, dizziness, diminished concentration, and syncope; those of autonomic overaction include palpitations, tremulousness, nausea, and syncope. *Postural tachycardia syndrome* (POTS) is defined as the development of orthostatic symptoms associated with a heart rate increment of 30 beats/minute or greater and an absolute rate greater than 120 beats/minute. The classification of orthostatic intolerance is given in Table 218.1. At one extreme is neurocardiogenic syncope, in which blood pressure and heart rate to head-up tilt is normal (for most of the time). Mild orthostatic intolerance and POTS are associated with an excessive increase in heart rate without orthostatic hypotension. At the other extreme is neurogenic orthostatic hypotension, in which there is an excessive decrease in blood pressure (this is discussed in Chapter 217).

Table 218.1	Classification of orthostatic intolerance
Neurocardiogenic (vasovagal) syncope
Mild orthostatic intolerance
Postural tachycardia syndrome (POTS)
Neurogenic orthostatic hypotension

We chose these practical and reasonable criteria rather than requiring an increment that is related to our normative data by age and sex. Because the age range of most patients with POTS is 15 to 40 years, an increment of 30 beats/minute exceeds the 99th percentile of 271 Mayo control subjects who were 10 to 83 years old.[1] Some patients may have a heart rate increment of 30 beats/minute with a standing heart rate less than 120 beats/minute, criteria that we would previously have accepted.[2,3] These patients are best considered to have mild orthostatic intolerance, which tends to be more heterogeneous in etiology. Causes include mild hypovolemia and deconditioning with prolonged bed rest; reduced orthostatic tolerance is sometimes associated with mitral valve prolapse and certain phases of the menstrual cycle.

There is considerable confusion about terminology. Terms such as "effort syndrome," "neurasthenia," "idiopathic hypovolemia,"[4] and "sympathotonic orthostatic hypotension," which emphasize sympathetic overactivity,[5] and "mitral valve prolapse syndrome"[6] exemplify a focus on particular aspects of the patient's disease. Most patients with mitral valve prolapse do not have florid dysautonomia,[7] and the "dysautonomic" patients with mitral valve prolapse are indistinguishable from those with similar complaints and normal echocardiographic findings;[8] thus, the implication that mitral valve prolapse is somehow mechanistically involved with POTS is questionable. Some patients with chronic fatigue syndrome have orthostatic intolerance with tilt-induced syncope, and a subset has a response to treatment directed at syncope;[9] however, most patients with chronic fatigue syndrome do not have POTS.

Prevalence

The prevalence of these conditions is not known precisely. Syncope is common. From 10% to 20% of the population have had a syncopal episode at some time.[10,11] The prevalence of mild orthostatic intolerance and POTS is known even less well; it probably is about five times that of neurogenic orthostatic hypotension. Orthostatic intolerance is underrecognized and typically misdiagnosed.

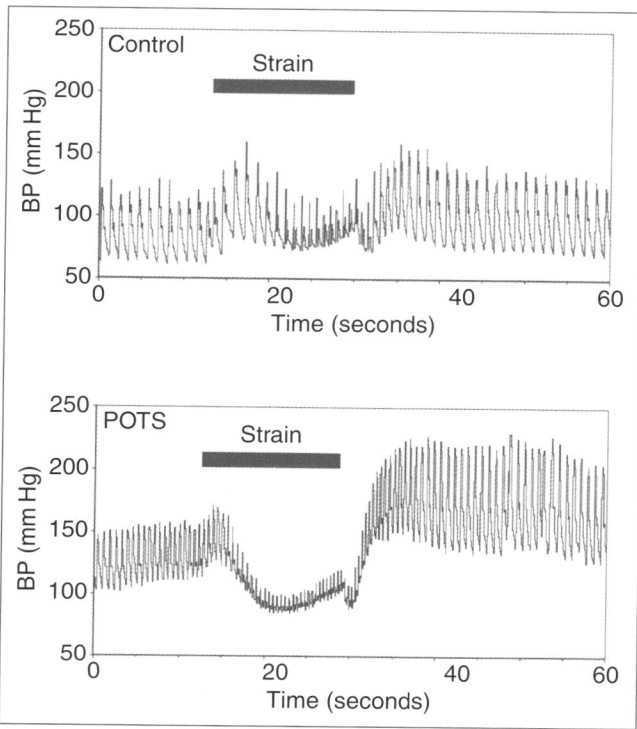

Figure 218.1 Valsalva maneuver of a 40-year-old female control subject and an age-matched female patient with postural tachycardia syndrome (POTS). The latter has compression of pulse pressure and an exaggerated blood pressure overshoot. Filled bar indicates duration of Valsalva maneuver.

Clinical features

The age at presentation most commonly is between 15 and 50 years.[12] Most patients that we have evaluated have had the symptoms for about 1 year. The orthostatic symptoms consist of lightheadedness, visual blurring or tunneling, palpitations, tremulousness, and weakness (especially of the legs). Less frequent symptoms are those of hyperventilation, anxiety, chest wall pain, nausea, acral coldness or pain, and headaches. The symptoms these patients experience differ from those of patients with orthostatic hypotension in that there are pronounced symptoms of sympathetic activation (Table 218.2). Unlike patients with neurogenic orthostatic hypotension, symptoms are not generally worse in the early morning. Also, the relationship between a meal and the symptoms is less consistent. Symptoms are worse with activity, heat, and high altitude. Postprandial bloating or nausea is relatively common. There may be an overrepresentation of migraine and sleep disorders.[3] The overrepresentation of women is clear. We have found a consistent female:male ratio of 5:1.[12]

Approximately one-half of the patients have an antecedent, presumably viral, illness.[2,3] Some patients with POTS have a cyclical exacerbation of symptoms. The symptoms deteriorate considerably in some women at certain stages of the menstrual cycle associated with marked weight and fluid changes. Typically, these patients have large fluctuations in their weight, sometimes up to 5 lb. Others have cycles of several days of intense orthostatic intolerance, followed by a similar period when the symptoms are less. Patients may have episodic symptoms at rest associated with changes in blood pressure and heart rate unrelated to arrhythmias. Typically, the heart rate alteration is sinus tachycardia, although bradycardia may occur. Fatigue can be a problem during these episodes. Some patients describe periods when they have trouble retaining fluid in spite of large

intake. Fluid balance and antidiuretic hormone levels are not well documented. Orthostatic intolerance with low blood pressure that requires repeated visits to the emergency department for intravenous infusions of saline is uncommon but not rare. The relationship of orthostatic intolerance to anxiety and panic is complex. Patients with typical anxiety-panic disorder are easy to differentiate from those with POTS, and the orthostatic "anxiety" symptoms are easy to differentiate from an anxiety disorder in most patients. However, the relationship can be more complicated because many of the symptoms of anxiety are mediated by the autonomic nervous system. Orthostatic stress can evoke anxiety-panic symptoms in predisposed subjects. Patients with panic disorders and those with POTS share such clinical features as discomfort at the onset of symptoms, shortness of breath with hyperventilation, dizziness or faintness, palpitations, trembling, numbness or tingling sensations,

Table 218.2 Frequency of orthostatic symptoms in patients with postural tachycardia syndrome (POTS) and in those with neurogenic orthostatic hypotension

Symptom	% of patients	
	POTS	Neurogenic orthostatic hypotension
Dizziness	100	100
Blurred vision	80	82
Tiredness	80	91
Nausea	66	18
Palpitations	60	9
Tremulousness	47	18
Breathing difficulties	40	0
Sweating	27	9
Anxiety	20	18
Gastrointestinal	20	36
Vasomotor	13	0

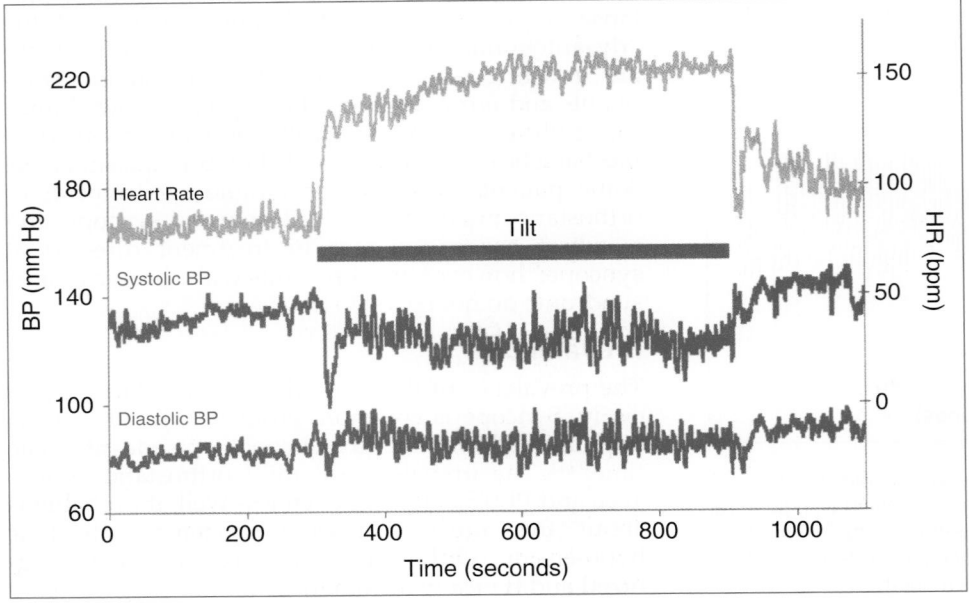

Figure 218.2 Exaggerated heart rate response in a patient with postural tachycardia syndrome without orthostatic hypotension in response to head-up tilt. Filled bar indicates period of tilt. BP, blood pressure.

flushes or chills, chest pain, and generalized weakness. In a small proportion of patients, the two disorders appear to coexist. The proposed central mechanisms for POTS and panic disorders may overlap. The noradrenergic system is involved in both disorders.[13] Other central neurotransmitters that potentially affect the production of panic disorders include γ-aminobutyric acid,[14] serotonin,[15] and adenosine.[16] Their role in POTS needs to be evaluated. Also, both conditions currently have certain treatments in common, including treatment with phenobarbital, benzodiazepines, β-blockers,[17] and clonidine.[18]

Clinical examination demonstrates an excessive heart rate increment. Pulse pressure may be excessively reduced. One clinical correlate is the difficulty in palpating the radial pulse with continued standing of the patient or with the performance of a Valsalva maneuver (Flack sign). Another clinical sign is the development of acral coldness. With continued standing, there may be venous prominence, resulting in a blueness and even swelling of the feet.[19]

Etiology

The etiology and pathophysiology of POTS appear to be heterogeneous. Some patients clearly have an idiopathic autonomic neuropathy. Evidence for autonomic neuropathy includes the following features. Patients typically develop the disorder after an infection, presumably viral. They have sudomotor denervation as indicated by the absence of distal responses on the quantitative sudomotor axon reflex test (QSART) and anhidrosis on the thermoregulatory sweat test.[2,20] Also, they have evidence of peripheral adrenergic denervation, with cardiovascular changes of absent late phase II, failure of systemic peripheral resistance to increment on head-up tilt,[3] and reduced norepinephrine release in the lower as compared with the upper extremity. *Secondary POTS* refers to patients who have a known autonomic disorder with peripheral denervation and relative preservation of the autonomic innervation of the heart. Causes include autonomic neuropathies (e.g., diabetic, amyloid, idiopathic); less commonly, it is a stage in the evolution of pure autonomic failure or multiple system atrophy.

Another mechanism is hypovolemia, reported by some investigators[4,21,22] but not others. Venous pooling in the limbs[3,19,23] or splanchnic-mesenteric bed[24] is another abnormality. Either or both of these mechanisms result in reduced preload and a secondary excessive increase in norepinephrine levels, typically to levels greater than 600 pg/mL,[25] resulting in a hyperadrenergic state.

Many patients appear to have β-receptor supersensitivity. The excessive heart rate response to isoproterenol correlates with the heart rate response to head-up tilt.[12] Another mechanism is central (presumably brainstem) dysfunction. These patients have spontaneous episodes of tachycardia, and on head-up tilt, they have an exaggerated diastolic blood pressure response (an increase >20 mmHg). Their 24-hour blood pressure recordings are characterized by large oscillations in blood pressure.

Diagnosis

The diagnosis of POTS is based on the presence of orthostatic symptoms associated with unexplained excessive orthostatic tachycardia. Thus, conditions that can result in tachycardia, such as thyrotoxicosis, cardiac rhythm abnormalities, pheochromocytoma, hypoadrenalism, dehydration, and medications (vasodilators, diuretics, β-agonists), need to be excluded. The presence of a defined autonomic neuropathy (diabetes, amyloidosis, inherited) also needs to be excluded. The role of the laboratory is to confirm orthostatic intolerance and to demonstrate evidence of autonomic denervation. Approximately one-half of the patients have a restricted autonomic neuropathy, typically a length-dependent type.[2,3] *Length-dependent neuropathy* refers to a neuropathy in which the ends of the longer fibers are affected before the shorter fibers. In the autonomic nervous system, the postganglionic sympathetic adrenergic fibers to the limbs and splanchnic-mesenteric bed are the longest fibers; next are the vagal fibers to the heart, which have a long preganglionic path. The cardiac adrenergic fibers, in contrast, are relatively short.

The anhidrosis on QSART and the thermoregulatory sweat test has a neuropathic distribution. Sweating is impaired in the lower extremities to varying degrees: the feet typically are anhidrotic and the legs are involved to different extents. The distribution of anhidrosis can be patchy or more widespread. Khurana[22] reported segmental or patchy anhidrosis in six of the eight patients studied. Skin potential abnormalities, with a loss of skin potentials in the lower extremity, have also been described.[26] The heart rate response to deep breathing and the Valsalva ratio are usually normal and often large.[3,22,27]

The beat-to-beat blood pressure responses to the Valsalva maneuver are abnormal in about two-thirds of patients.[3,27] The pulse pressure often decreases by more than 50%. Early phase II is exaggerated, and late phase II may be reduced or absent. Phase IV is normal but, more often, excessively large (Fig. 218.1). The cardiovascular responses to tilt-up are abnormal. The heart rate response varies from 120 to 170 beats/minute on head-up tilt typically by 2 minutes. The heart rate response may oscillate excessively; in patients with marked peripheral denervation, the variability may be reduced. The blood pressure responses occur in several patterns. Patients who have prominent venous pooling may have an excessive decrease in pulse pressure. Some have a prominent hypertensive response, with increases in diastolic blood pressure by up to 50 mmHg, with large fluctuations. Some patients have relatively normal blood pressure responses but have tachycardia and symptoms (Fig. 218.2). The pattern of responses with peripheral sudomotor deficits, absent late phase II with intact phase IV, and normal forced respiratory sinus arrhythmia are consistent with length-dependent autonomic neuropathy. Patients

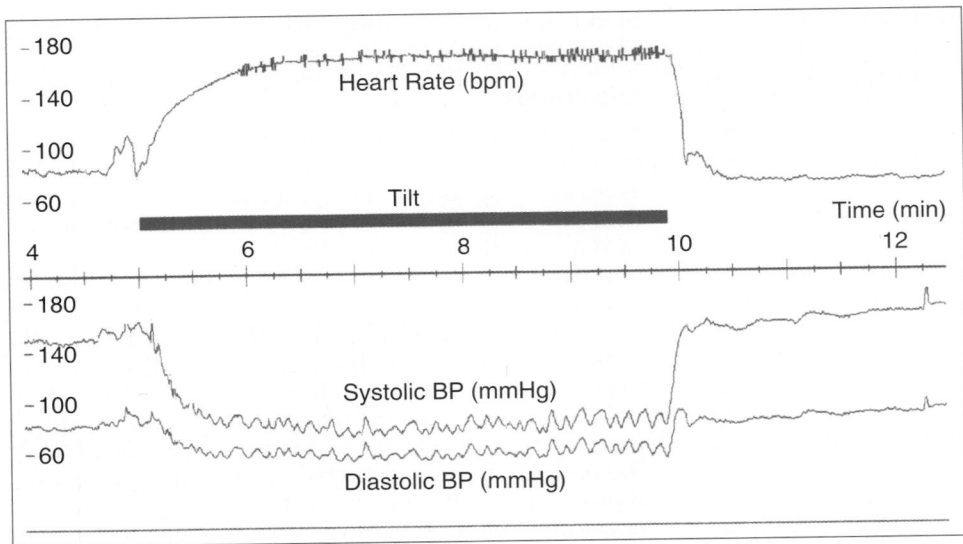

Figure 218.3 Exaggerated heart rate response in a patient with postviral autonomic neuropathy, orthostatic hypotension, and orthostatic tachycardia. Filled bar indicates duration of head-up tilt.

with secondary POTS can have orthostatic hypotension and POTS (Fig. 218.3). The plasma level of norepinephrine is normal with the patient supine and excessive with the patient erect,[23,27] likely because of increased baroreceptor unloading.

Differential diagnosis

The main differential diagnosis of POTS includes neurogenic orthostatic hypotension, other causes of orthostatic intolerance, and anxiety-panic attacks (Table 218.3). Differentiating POTS from neurogenic orthostatic hypotension is straightforward and summarized in Table 218.2. The symptoms of orthostatic hypotension are similar, but symptoms of sympathetic overactivity, such as tremulousness, anxiety, nausea, sweating, and acral vasoconstriction, occur in POTS and not in neurogenic orthostatic hypotension (Table 218.4). In the latter, orthostatic hypotension and evidence of generalized autonomic failure (cardiovagal, adrenergic, sudomotor) are found (Table 218.4). It is more difficult to differentiate POTS from other causes of orthostatic intolerance. Mild orthostatic intolerance due to an illness that requires prolonged bed rest, dehydration, hypovolemia, or a medication effect usually is readily recognized. A related condition is constitutional orthostatic intolerance. Patients with this always had some degree of orthostatic intolerance. In their youth, they may have had syncopal episodes in response to prolonged standing or syncope in response to pain or the sight of blood. They may have had transient lightheadedness on standing up suddenly. These patients are more prone to develop a greater degree of orthostatic intolerance after a period of bed rest or a viral illness. The condition may be familial. Conditions that deserve special attention are chronic fatigue syndrome and mitral valve prolapse. POTS is differentiated from chronic fatigue syndrome by the predominance of orthostatic symptoms. Chronic fatigue affects the sexes less unevenly, is dominated by nonorthostatic

symptoms, and has many quasi-infectious symptoms. However, some of the patients have orthostatic intolerance, including tachycardia. In both POTS and chronic fatigue syndromes, patients have marked worsening of symptoms after syncope or presyncope, perhaps because nonorthostatic symptoms are a continuation of postsyncopal symptoms. We recommend that when the feature of fatigue predominates, the condition should be designated as *POTS associated with chronic fatigue syndrome*. Similarly, orthostatic intolerance should not be considered an integral part of mitral valve prolapse. When orthostatic intolerance is a feature of mitral valve prolapse, the condition should be recognized as orthostatic intolerance or *POTS associated with mitral valve prolapse*. Chronic fatigue syndrome and mitral valve prolapse are described in greater detail below.

Chronic fatigue syndrome

Currently, chronic fatigue syndrome is defined by the Centers for Disease Control and Prevention as fatigue of at least 6 months' duration seriously interfering with the patient's life and without evidence of various organic or psychiatric illnesses that can produce chronic fatigue. The criteria include myalgias, postexertional malaise, headaches, and a group of infectious-type symptoms (chronic fever and chills, sore throat, lymphadenopathy). These criteria appear to distinguish patients with chronic fatigue syndrome from healthy control subjects and from the comparison groups with multiple sclerosis and depression.[28] In addition to chronic fluctuating fatigue, patients have somatic, cognitive, depressive, and sleep dysfunction. The patients often are separated into those with postviral and those with nonpostviral fatigue syndrome. The relationship to orthostatic intolerance is inconstant. Patients may have orthostatic intolerance and some amelioration of their symptoms with treatment of orthostatic intolerance.[9]

Table 218.3   Comparison of vasovagal syncope, postural tachycardia syndrome (POTS), and neurogenic orthostatic hypotension

Variable	Vasovagal syncope	POTS & MOI	Neurogenic orthostatic hypotension
HR, supine	Normal	Mild ↑	Normal
BP, supine	Normal	Normal	
HR, HUT	Normal until presyncope	↑	↑
BP, HUT	Normal until presyncope	Normal, pulse pressure ↓	↓
Symptoms, HUT	Nil	Present	Present, usually
Syncope	Yes (↓ HR & BP)	Yes (↓ HR & BP)	Yes (↓ BP, fixed HR)

BP, blood pressure; HR, heart rate; HUT, head-up tilt; MOI, mild orthostatic intolerance.

Table 218.4   Comparison of patients with generalized autonomic neuropathy and those with postural orthostatic tachycardia syndrome (POTS)

Variable	Neurogenic orthostatic hypotension	POTS
Orthostatic dizziness	Variably present	Present
Orthostatic tremulousness	Absent	Common
Orthostatic palpitations	Absent	Common
Orthostatic hypotension	Consistent	Usually absent
Orthostatic tachycardia	Reduced	Exaggerated
Supine norepinephrine	Usually reduced	Normal or increased
Standing norepinephrine	Reduced	Increased
HR response to deep breathing	Reduced	Normal
Valsalva ratio	Reduced	Normal or increased
BP$_{BB}$ to Valsalva maneuver		
Early phase II	Markedly increased	Increased
Late phase II	Absent	Normal or reduced
Phase IV	Absent	Increased

BP$_{BB}$, beat-to-beat blood pressure; HR, heart rate.

Mitral valve prolapse

Mitral valve prolapse, the commonest human abnormality of heart valves, affects about 4% of the population.[7] The term *mitral valve prolapse syndrome* is applied loosely to patients who have several somatic and autonomic symptoms. The autonomic symptoms described in the literature are those of POTS in patients with mitral valve prolapse. Whether patients with mitral valve prolapse are excessively prone to the development of POTS is not known.

Prognosis of POTS

Little information is available on prognosis. Our own early experience has been analyzed.[29] We used a structured questionnaire focused on autonomic status at follow-up: the ability to remain on the feet, degree of improvement, standing time, ability to work at the patient's occupation or at home, ability to withstand orthostatic stressors, weight gain or loss, and most beneficial treatment. Follow-up (mean, 67 ± 52 months) has been completed for 40 patients. Overall, at follow-up, 80% of patients had improvement and 60% were functionally back to normal; 67% were able to stand for longer than 30 minutes without symptoms, and 90% were able to work. However, these

patients were not entirely asymptomatic. Symptoms may be provoked by meals (30% of patients), exercise (69% of patients), and heat exposure (77% of patients). Patients with an antecedent event appeared to have a better response than those with spontaneous POTS (90% vs. 70% had improvement; 84% vs. 50% were able to stand >30 minutes). Most commonly, patients continued salt supplementation. Among medications, β-blockers were the most efficacious. Khurana[22] reported on the follow-up of six patients 8 to 17 years after autonomic evaluation: two patients had spontaneous and complete improvement, one had partial improvement, and three had persistence of symptoms.

Management
Step 1

On the basis of a detailed history, examination, and general medical evaluation, including electrocardiography (ECG), it should be possible to determine whether further evaluation is warranted. Patients who have POTS (standing heart rate >120 beats/minute, orthostatic symptoms, marked impairment in the ability to perform activities of daily living) should be evaluated further and treated. Many patients with mild orthostatic intolerance have a recognizable mechanism for orthostatic deconditioning (e.g., confined to bed for more than a few days, debilitating illness, hypovolemia) and may not need an extensive evaluation.

Step 2

After the decision has been made to evaluate the patient, the study should include cardiac and autonomic laboratory evaluations. The cardiac evaluation usually includes a cardiac interview and examination, ECG, chest radiography, and 24-hour Holter monitoring, and the decision is made whether to perform cardiac electrophysiological studies. Electrophysiological testing is most useful in patients with heart disease manifested as 1) abnormal ventricular function (decreased ejection fraction), 2) abnormal ECG (conduction defect, ischemia, arrhythmia, multifocal ventricular ectopic beats), and 3) cardiac arrhythmia on Holter monitoring.[30]

As true for patients with syncope, it is likely that electrophysiological studies will be least useful in patients without heart disease, with an ejection fraction greater than 40%, and with normal findings on ECG and Holter monitoring.[11]

Step 3

The neurological evaluation comprises a neurologic history, examination, and tests seeking evidence for autonomic neuropathy. The autonomic laboratory evaluation follows and comprises a modified (10 minutes or longer head-up tilt) autonomic reflex screen and thermoregulatory sweat test. The 24-hour urinary sodium concentration should be measured. Normal subjects should excrete more than 170 mmol/24 hours.[31] Plasma catecholamines should be measured; they typically have an orthostatic value greater than 600 pg/mL.

Step 4

The findings of the cardiac and autonomic evaluations are synthesized, and treatment is planned. POTS is best considered a syndrome of orthostatic intolerance rather than a disease sui generis. It is reasonable to document the presence and severity of POTS and to seek evidence of associated autonomic neuropathy, mitral valve prolapse, deconditioning, or history of vasovagal syndrome. The severity of POTS, the plasma volume, the degree of vagotonia (degree and duration of reflex bradycardia with the Valsalva maneuver and tilt back, Valsalva ratio, and heart rate range), β-adrenergic supersensitivity (heart rate increment, anxiety, tremor, and reduction of muscle peripheral resistance), and central integration (blood pressure and heart rate oscillations) are determined. The patient's disorder is classified according to the pathophysiologic mechanism, and treatment is individualized.

A patient with deconditioning and hypovolemia should sleep with the head of the bed elevated 4 inches. Also, the plasma volume should be expanded with generous intake of salt and fludrocortisone

(sleeping with the head of the bed elevated may expand plasma volume). The salt intake should be between 150 and 250 mEq of sodium (10 to 20 g of salt). Patients who are intensely sensitive to salt intake can fine-tune their plasma volume and blood pressure control with salt intake alone. Foods that have a high salt content include fast foods such as hamburgers, hot dogs, chicken pieces, french fries, and fish fries. Canned soup, chili, ham, bacon, sausage, additives such as soya sauce, and commercially processed canned products also have a high sodium content. The patient should have at least one glass or cup of fluids at mealtime and at least two at other times each day to obtain 2 to 2.5 L/day. Fludrocortisone, 0.1 to 0.4 mg/day, can be prescribed if salt supplementation alone is ineffective.

A different approach to treatment is needed for patients who have venous pooling. Body stockings may be beneficial as a temporary measure. Several approaches appear to be effective for some of these patients, including physical countermaneuvers[32,33] and a 3-month program of graduated training. Resistance training may be more beneficial than endurance training.[34]

The best treatment for patients who have peripheral adrenergic failure manifested as a loss of late phase II or frank orthostatic hypotension is fludrocortisone and an α-agonist. Midodrine appears to have the best absorption, predictable duration of action, and lack of central nervous system side effects.

Patients with florid POTS who have β-receptor supersensitivity tend to have a response to β-antagonists, but they sometimes are exquisitely sensitive to these agents. At conventional doses, fatigue is a major problem. We prescribe propranolol (Inderal), which may be more efficacious than β-selective nonlipophilic agents at a dose of 10 mg/day, increasing the dose over 2 to 3 weeks to 30 to 60 mg/day. The aim is to maintain the heart rate increment at about 50% of the pretreatment level. For patients with bronchospasm, a β-selective lipophilic agent such as metoprolol (Lopressor) can be given at a beginning dose of 25 mg/day and increased to the typical dose of 50 mg twice daily. For patients who have central side effects, including lethargy or depression, a nonlipophilic agent is preferred. Nadolol, at a beginning dose of 10 mg/day and increased to 40 mg as needed, is a useful nonselective agent. β-Selective agents such as atenolol (Tenormin), betaxolol (Kerlone), and acebutolol (Sectral) can be prescribed. The beginning doses of atenolol, betaxolol, and acebutolol are 25 mg, 10 mg, and 200 mg, respectively.

Treatment is particularly difficult if patients have unstable hypertensive responses to tilt. Some of these patients have a blood pressure response as high as 250/150 mm Hg on standing. In some of these patients, the autonomic instability responds to oral phenobarbital, with a beginning dose of 60 mg at night and 15 mg every morning. An alternative treatment is clonidine or another α2-agonist. Clonidine is given at a dose of 0.1 mg twice daily and increased to the maximally tolerated dose. Autonomic instability reportedly responds to microvascular decompression of the brainstem, but the role of surgical therapy has not been defined.

Occasionally, patients are evaluated during the acute postviral phase of the illness. For these patients, treatment with plasma exchange or intravenous gammaglobulin may be considered, especially if there is additional evidence of acute autonomic neuropathy. Recently, dramatic improvement in autonomic function has been reported following intravenous immunoglobulin treatment.[35–37] Autonomic recovery was well documented in the case of Smit et al.[35] Improvement has also been reported in a case associated with a lung carcinoma.[38]

References

1. Low PA, Denq JC, Opfer-Gehrking TL, et al. Effect of age and gender on sudomotor and cardiovagal function and blood pressure response to tilt in normal subjects. Muscle Nerve 1997;20:1561–1568

2. Schondorf R, Low PA. Idiopathic postural orthostatic tachycardia syndrome: an attenuated form of acute pandysautonomia? Neurology 1993;43:132–137

3. Low PA, Opfer-Gehrking TL, Textor SC, et al. Comparison of the postural tachycardia syndrome (POTS) with orthostatic hypotension due to autonomic failure. J Auton Nerv Syst 1994;50:181–188

4. Fouad FM, Tadena-Thome L, Bravo EL, Tarazi RC. Idiopathic hypovolemia. Ann Intern Med 1986;104:298–303

5. Hoeldtke RD, Dworkin GE, Gaspar SR, Israel BC. Sympathotonic orthostatic hypotension: a report of four cases. Neurology 1989;39:34–40

6. Coghlan HC, Phares P, Cowley M, et al. Dysautonomia in mitral valve prolapse. Am J Med 1979;67:236–244

7. Devereux RB, Kramer-Fox R, Kligfield P. Mitral valve prolapse: causes, clinical manifestations, and management. Ann Intern Med 1989;111:305–317

8. Taylor AA, Davies AO, Mares A, et al. Spectrum of dysautonomia in mitral valvular prolapse. Am J Med 1989;86:267–274

9. Bou-Holaigah I, Rowe PC, Kan J, Calkins H. The relationship between neurally mediated hypotension and the chronic fatigue syndrome. JAMA 1995;274:961–967

10. Allen SC, Taylor CL, Hall VE. A study of orthostatic insufficiency by the tiltboard method. Am J Physiol 1945;143:11–20

11. Shen W-K, Gersh BJ. Syncope: mechanisms, approach, and management. In: Low PA, ed. Clinical Autonomic Disorders: Evaluation and Management. Boston: Little, Brown and Company, 1993:605–640

12. Low PA, Schondorf R, Novak V, et al. Postural tachycardia syndrome. In: Low PA, ed. Clinical Autonomic Disorders: Evaluation and Management. 2nd ed. Philadelphia: Lippincott-Raven, 1997:681–697

13. Uhde TW, Tancer M. Chemical models of panic: a review and critique. In: Tyrer P, ed. Psychopharmacology of Anxiety. Oxford: Oxford University Press, 1988:110–131

14. Insel TR, Ninan PT, Aloi J, et al. A benzodiazepine receptor-mediated model of anxiety. Studies in nonhuman primates and clinical implications. Arch Gen Psychiatry 1984;41:741–750

15. Wise CD, Berger BD, Stein L. Benzodiazepines: anxiety-reducing activity by reduction of serotonin turnover in the brain. Science 1972;177:180–183

16. Boulenger JP, Uhde TW, Wolff EA III, Post RM. Increased sensitivity to caffeine in patients with panic disorders. Preliminary evidence. Arch Gen Psychiatry 1984;41:1067–1071

17. Tyrer P. Current status of beta-blocking drugs in the treatment of anxiety disorders. Drugs 1988;36:773–783

18. Uhde TW, Stein MB, Vittone BJ, et al. Behavioral and physiologic effects of short-term and long-term administration of clonidine in panic disorder. Arch Gen Psychiatry 1989;46:170–177

19. Streeten DHP. Orthostatic Disorders of the Circulation, Mechanisms, Manifestations and Treatment. New York: Plenum Medical Book Company, 1987

20. Schondorf R, Low PA. Idiopathic postural tachycardia syndrome. In: Low PA, ed. Clinical Autonomic Disorders: Evaluation and Management. Boston: Little, Brown and Company, 1993:641–652

21. Rosen SG, Cryer PE. Postural tachycardia syndrome. Reversal of sympathetic hyperresponsiveness and clinical improvement during sodium loading. Am J Med 1982;72:847–850

22. Khurana RK. Orthostatic intolerance and orthostatic tachycardia: a heterogeneous disorder. Clin Auton Res 1995;5:12–18

23. Streeten DH, Anderson GH Jr, Richardson R, Thomas FD. Abnormal orthostatic changes in blood pressure and heart rate in subjects with intact sympathetic nervous function: evidence for excessive venous pooling. J Lab Clin Med 1988;111:326–335

24. Tani H, Singer W, McPhee BR, et al. Splanchnic and systemic circulation in the postural tachycardia syndrome (abstract). Clin Auton Res 1999;9:231–232

25. Jacob G, Biaggioni I, Mosqueda-Garcia R, et al. Relation of blood volume and blood pressure in orthostatic intolerance. Am J Med Sci 1998;315:95–100

26. Hoeldtke RD, Davis KM. The orthostatic tachycardia syndrome: evaluation of autonomic function and treatment with octreotide and ergot alkaloids. J Clin Endocrinol Metab 1991;73:132–139

27. Low PA, Gilden JL, Freeman R, et al. Efficacy of midodrine vs placebo in neurogenic orthostatic hypotension. A randomized, double-blind multicenter study. Midodrine Study Group. JAMA 1997;277:1046–1051

28. Komaroff AL, Fagioli LR, Geiger AM, et al. An examination of the working case definition of chronic fatigue syndrome. Am J Med 1996;100:56–64

29. Sandroni P, Opfer-Gehrking TL, McPhee BR, Low PA. Postural tachycardia syndrome: clinical features and follow-up study. Mayo Clin Proc 1999;74:1106–1110

30. Kapoor WN, Hammill SC, Gersh BJ. Diagnosis and natural history of syncope and the role of invasive electrophysiologic testing. Am J Cardiol 1989;63:730–734

31. El-Sayed H, Hainsworth R. Salt supplement increases plasma volume and orthostatic tolerance in patients with unexplained syncope. Heart 1996;75:134–140

32. van Lieshout JJ, ten Harkel AD, Wieling W. Physical manoeuvres for combating orthostatic dizziness in autonomic failure. Lancet 1992;339:897–898

33. Bouvette CM, McPhee BR, Opfer-Gehrking TL, Low PA. Role of physical countermaneuvers in the management of orthostatic hypotension: efficacy and biofeedback augmentation. Mayo Clin Proc 1996;71:847–853

34. Hakkinen K, Hakkinen A. Neuromuscular adaptations during intensive strength training in middle-aged and elderly males and females. Electromyogr Clin Neurophysiol 1995;35:137–147

35. Smit AAJ, Vermeulen M, Koelman JHTM, Wieling W. An unusual recovery in a patient with acute pandysautonomia after intravenous immunoglobulin therapy (abstract). Clin Auton Res 1995;5:323A

36. Heafield MT, Gammage MD, Nightingale S, Williams AC. Idiopathic dysautonomia treated with intravenous gammaglobulin. Lancet 1996;347:28–29

37. Mericle RA, Triggs WJ. Treatment of acute pandysautonomia with intravenous immunoglobulin. J Neurol Neurosurg Psychiatry 1997;62:529–531

38. Bohnen NI, Cheshire WP, Lennon VA, Van Den Berg CJ. Plasma exchange improves function in a patient with ANNA-1 seropositive paraneoplastic autonomic neuropathy (abstract). Neurology 1997;48:A131

219 Treatment of Central Autonomic Disorders

Eduardo E Benarroch

Central autonomic disorders may manifest either as autonomic failure or autonomic hyperactivity. Autonomic failure is a prominent manifestation of central neurodegenerative disorders. Shy and Drager[1] first described the syndrome of autonomic failure due to degeneration of preganglionic neurons in the intermediolateral cell columns in association with other neurological manifestations. This syndrome is now referred to as *multiple system atrophy* (MSA).[2] The syndrome of central autonomic hyperactivity in association with brain tumors and hydrocephalus was described by Penfield[3] in 1929 as "diencephalic autonomic epilepsy."

Epidemiology and etiology

The most common causes of generalized central autonomic failure are MSA and Parkinson disease. The most common causes of autonomic hyperactivity, particularly the hypersympathetic state, are acute neurological catastrophes such as head trauma and subarachnoid hemorrhage generally associated with acute hydrocephalus or increased intracranial pressure and autonomic dysreflexia in patients with spinal cord lesions above level T5. Iatrogenic causes include neuroleptic malignant syndrome and serotonin syndrome. Autonomic hyperactivity may also be a prominent manifestation of stroke, seizures, and mass lesions involving midline diencephalic or brainstem structures. For example, strokes involving the insular cortex may produce hemianhidrosis or cardiac arrhythmias, and seizures arising from the medial temporal lobe or anterior cingulate gyrus may produce syncope, tachyarrhythmias, vomiting, piloerection, or other autonomic manifestations.[4]

Pathophysiology and pathogenesis

Autonomic failure in MSA and Parkinson disease reflects primarily a loss of sympathetic preganglionic neurons.[5] In MSA, there is also loss of autonomic neurons in the ventrolateral medulla,[6] and in Parkinson disease, there is evidence of involvement of the sympathetic ganglia.[7] The mechanisms of autonomic hyperactivity are not understood completely. Acute hypertension in neurological catastrophes has been attributed classically to the Cushing response.[8] This response is thought to reflect excitation of hypoxia-sensitive sympathoexcitatory neurons of the rostral ventrolateral medulla in reaction to brainstem ischemia produced by an acute increase in intracranial pressure, as in acute hydrocephalus, severe head injury, or mass lesion. Distortion of the brainstem may cause hypertension in patients with cerebellar hemorrhage or infarct, and baroreflex failure causes fluctuating hypertension in patients with medullary lesions that involve the nucleus tractus solitarius bilaterally.[9]

Clinical features

The manifestations of central autonomic failure include orthostatic hypotension, anhidrosis, gastrointestinal dysmotility, impotence, and neurogenic bladder. The prognosis of MSA is poor and is determined not by the severity of autonomic failure but by the progressive motor disability and development of laryngeal stridor and sleep apnea. Autonomic failure in Parkinson disease is milder and occurs later in the course of the disease.

The most common manifestations of autonomic hyperactivity are related to the sympathetic system and include hypertension, arrhythmias, hyperhidrosis, peripheral vasoconstriction, hyperthermia or hypothermia, and mydriasis. Generally, central types of autonomic hyperactivity tend to begin abruptly after the onset of acute injury and then to fluctuate and only persist for several hours or days. However, peripheral dysautonomia is more often paroxysmal and recurs over longer periods.[10] The massive sympathoexcitation that occurs in the setting of subarachnoid hemorrhage or other neurological catastrophes may produce severe hypertension and tachyrhythmias, electrocardiographic changes and increased serum levels of creatine kinase suggestive of cardiac ischemia, and neurogenic pulmonary edema. Less commonly, autonomic hyperactivity involves the parasympathetic system and manifests with bradyarrhythmia (including bradycardia, sinus arrest, and atrioventicular block), hypotension, and sialorrhea or bronchorrhea.

Diagnosis and differential diagnosis

Autonomic failure is diagnosed on the basis of the clinical history, physical examination, and autonomic function tests. In MSA, the earliest manifestations include erectile dysfunction and urinary frequency, but the most disabling manifestations are orthostatic hypotension and urinary retention and incontinence. Orthostatic hypotension with blunted compensatory heart rate response is detected clinically and documented with beat-to-beat measurements of arterial pressure and heart rate during head-up tilt or active standing. Impaired thermoregulatory sweating with preserved sudomotor axon reflex is characteristic of

MSA. Impaired heart rate variability during deep breathing reflects cardiovagal failure. Indices of adrenergic failure include not only orthostatic hypotension but an exaggerated decrease in arterial pressure in late phase II and absence of overshoot in phase IV of the Valsalva maneuver and impaired increase of plasma norepinephrine levels upon standing. Impaired cardiac uptake of levodopa indicates involvement of the cardiac sympathetic ganglia and is seen in Parkinson disease but not in MSA. Hypotonic bladder, electromyographic evidence of denervation of the external sphincters, and magnetic resonance imaging findings of involvement of the putamen, pons, or cerebellum occur in MSA but not Parkinson disease.

The diagnosis of autonomic hyperactivity is clinical. Neuroimaging studies, particularly magnetic resonance imaging, identify strokes, acute hydrocephalus, or mass lesions responsible for this syndrome.

Treatment of autonomic failure

Other chapters in this book consider the treatment of the manifestations of autonomic failure, including orthostatic hypotension, neurogenic bladder and sexual dysfunction, and gastrointestinal dysmotility. Only the salient aspects are discussed below.

Orthostatic hypotension

The principles of management of orthostatic hypotension are patient education, adjustments in the diet, physical maneuvers, and drug therapy.[11,12] Most patients benefit from postural maneuvers such as leg crossing or squatting, increased daily intake of salt (10 to 20 g) and water (a minimum of 2 to 2.5 L), avoidance of large carbohydrate-rich meals and alcohol, and mild exercise. Sleeping with the head of the bed elevated by 15 to 30 cm prevents supine hypertension and decreases nocturnal diuresis and natriuresis, thus ameliorating the orthostatic intolerance in early morning hours.

Drugs used to treat orthostatic hypotension are summarized in Table 219.1. Fludrocortisone acetate (Florinef) is the drug of choice for treatment of neurogenic orthostatic hypotension. Its full pressor action, which depends on its mineralocorticoid effect, appears in 1 to 2 weeks. Treatment begins with a dose of 0.1 mg taken orally before noon and then increased slowly at 0.1-mg increments at 1- to 2-week intervals. Few patients require more than 0.4 mg/day. Potential side effects are congestive heart failure, supine hypertension, hypokalemia (in 50% of patients), hypomagnesemia (in about 5% of patients), and headache, particularly in young patients.

Currently, midodrine (ProAmatine) is the vasoconstrictor drug of choice. It is transformed in the liver to desglymidodrine, a potent α_1-adrenoreceptor agonist in arteries and veins. It is absorbed almost completely (93%) after oral administration, and its active metabolite has a predictive peak plasma concentration (1 hour) and half-life (approximately 3 hours). Treatment is started usually at a dose of 2.5 mg at breakfast and lunch and increased in 2.5-mg steps daily until a satisfactory response occurs or a dosage of 30 to 40 mg daily is achieved. Almost all patients experience piloerection, paresthesia in the scalp, and pruritus, which are generally mild and rarely lead to discontinuation of the treatment. To avoid supine hypertension, midodrine should not be taken after 4 or 5 PM, and patients should be instructed never to lie flat.

Recombinant human erythropoietin (epoetin alfa [Epogen], 25 to 75 U/kg subcutaneously 3 times weekly for 3 weeks, followed by a maintenance dose of 25 U/kg 3 times weekly) may be helpful for patients with primary autonomic failure and anemia in whom other measures are insufficient. Desmopressin acetate (DDAVP), a synthetic vasopressin analogue with antidiuretic effects via activation of V2 receptors, may be administered to patients with severe nocturia. It is administered in a single intranasal dose (5 to 40 μg) at night. Because of the risk of development of hyponatremia, treatment is always initiated with the patient hospitalized. Octreotide ([Sandostatin] 50 to 100 μg 1 or 2 times daily) is an analogue of somatostatin that inhibits the release of vasodilator gastrointestinal peptides; its main indication is treatment of severe postprandial hypotension.

Neurogenic bladder

Therapy of voiding dysfunction is best initiated only after a thorough urodynamic evaluation.[13] Detrusor hyperreflexia without outlet obstruction frequently occurs in patients with Parkinson disease and during the initial phases of MSA. Management includes the use of anticholinergic drugs such as oxybutynin ([Ditropan] 2.5 to 5 mg 3 or 4 times daily) or tolterodine tartrate ([Detrol] 1 or 2 mg twice daily). Timed voiding and moderate fluid restriction are helpful in reducing frequency, urgency, and urge incontinence; DDAVP can be useful in patients who have marked incontinence and nocturia. Detrusor hyperreflexia and detrusor-sphincter dyssynergy are frequent manifestations of spinal cord involvement by trauma or multiple sclerosis. The most reasonable management for these patients is anticholinergic treatment in combination with intermittent self-catheterization. Alpha$_1$-antagonists such as prazosin or terazosin may help relax the internal sphincter, and baclofen or dantrolene may relax the external sphincter. In patients with MSA, hypotonic bladder and detrusor areflexia eventually develop because of involvement of the sacral parasympathetic nuclei and the nucleus of Onuf. The most effective treatment is intermittent self-catheterization. Patients who are unable to perform intermittent self-catheterization because of motor difficulties may require an indwelling catheter or suprapubic diversion.[13,14]

Gastrointestinal dysmotility

The principles of management of any gastrointestinal motility disorder include 1) restoration of hydration and nutrition by the oral, enteral, or parenteral route, 2) suppression of bacterial overgrowth, and 3) use of prokinetic agents or stimulating laxatives. The first

Table 219.1	Drugs for management of orthostatic hypertension			
Drug	**Action**	**Dose**	**Rationale**	**Side effects**
Fludrocortisone (Florinef)	Mineralocorticoid	Initial—0.1 mg po Increase by 0.1 mg every 1–2 wk up to 0.4 mg daily	Volume expansion; use after appropriate dietary salt (10–20 g/day) and water (2-2.5 L) intake	Edema (mild pedal edema is desirable), congestive heart failure, supine hypertension, hypokalemia, hypomagnesemia
Midodrine (ProAmatine)	Prodrug, transformed in liver to desglymidodrine (α_1-receptor agonist in arteries and veins)	Initial—2.5 mg PO at breakfast and lunch Increase by 2.5 mg up to 10 mg qid if needed. Do not take after 4–5 PM to avoid supine hypertension	Vasoconstriction, increase in venous return and total peripheral resistance Has more predictable intestinal absorption, peak plasma levels, and half-life than other vasoconstrictor drugs	Piloerection, scalp pruritus, supine hypertension
Erythropoietin (recombinant human Epogen)	Stimulates erythropoiesis	25–75 U/kg daily for 3 wk Maintenance dose 25 mg/kg 3 times weekly Needs iron supplementation	Increase volume in patients with mild hypochromic anemia	High cost Risk of venous thrombosis
Desmopressin (DDAVP)	Synthetic agonist of V2 vasopressin receptor in renal tubules	5–50 µg single intranasal dose	Antidiuretic effect Indicated for patients with severe polyuria	Hyponatremia Start treatment with patient hospitalized
Octreotide (Sandostatin)	Somatostatin analogue	50–100 µg	Inhibits release of vasodilator gut peptides Indicated for patients with severe postprandial hypotension	Nausea, abdominal pain, fat malabsorption

PO, orally; qid, 4 times daily.

line of treatment of bowel hypomotility is an increase in dietary fiber (up to 25 g daily) with water (300 to 400 mL 4 times daily) and exercise.[14,15] Psyllium (up to 30 g daily) or methylcellulose (up to 6 g daily) with a concomitant increase in fluid intake may further increase stool bulk. If these measures are ineffective, stool softeners (e.g., docusate sodium, 100 to 500 mg daily) or lubricants (e.g., mineral oil) may be used in conjunction with an osmotic agent (e.g., Milk of Magnesia). Glycerine suppositories or sodium phosphate enemas promote fluid retention in the rectum and stimulate evacuation. The contact cathartics such as bisacodyl should be used sparingly because excessive use may damage the myenteric plexus. Metoclopramide (5 to 20 mg orally, 30 minutes before meals and at bedtime) has a direct central antiemetic effect via blockade of D_2 receptors in the area postrema and an indirect prokinetic effect via release of acetylcholine from intramural cholinergic neurons. Metoclopramide may worsen parkinsonism, and long-term treatment poses the risk of tardive dyskinesia. Cisapride ([Propulsid] 20 mg 3 times daily and at bedtime) increases upper gastrointestinal tract motility by enhancing the release of acetylcholine from neurons of the myenteric plexus. Cisapride may produce prolongation of the QT interval, predisposing to torsades de pointes, ventricular tachycardia, and ventricular fibrillation.

Management of autonomic hyperactivity

Acute autonomic emergencies generally should be managed in an intensive care unit with continuous monitoring of cardiovascular, respiratory, and renal function in addition to neurological and, in some cases, intracranial pressure monitoring.[10] The basic management of autonomic hyperactivity usually is the same regardless of the primary cause. Adequate hydration and prevention, recognition, and management of triggering factors such as pain, infection, or reflex stimuli are critically important. Unlike autonomic failure, autonomic hyperactivity commonly reflects potentially preventable or treatable mechanisms. For example, paroxysms of hypertension in patients with mass lesions can be prevented by close monitoring and stabilization of intracranial pressure, by avoiding bladder distension and other reflexogenic stimuli in patients with spinal cord trauma and autonomic dysreflexia, and by treating pain in patients with Guillain-Barré syndrome. Some conditions such as alcohol withdrawal and neuroleptic malignant syndrome may require specific drug therapy. Neurogenic hypertension and other autonomic manifestations of neurological catastrophes are discussed in detail in other chapters. Some general principles and management of less common central autonomic disorders are considered below. Drugs used in the treatment of central autonomic hyperactivity are summarized in Table 219.2.

Neurogenic hypertension and cardiac arrhythmias in acute neurological catastrophes

In most cases, hypertension in acute central nervous system lesions is reversible, and blood pressure normalizes 24 hours after the acute event. After excluding confounding factors such as pain or agitation, pharmacological treatment could be considered (Table 219.3).[16] Increased blood pressure after acute stroke or head injury probably should be left untreated except in patients with impending congestive heart failure, computed tomographic evidence of rapidly worsening cerebral edema, or extreme surges of blood pressure or in patients who are candidates for thrombolytic therapy. It is reasonable to administer antihypertensive drugs when the mean arterial pressure (MAP) is 130 mmHg or higher in previously normotensive patients or 150 mmHg or higher in chronically hypertensive patients or when the cerebral perfusion pressure (CPP) is higher than 85 mmHg. These variables can be calculated as follows:

$$\text{MAP} = \text{Diastolic Pressure} + (\text{Systolic Pressure} - \text{Diastolic Pressure})/3$$
$$\text{CPP} = \text{MAP} - \text{Intracranial Pressure}$$

Labetalol hydrochloride (Normodyne, Trandate), a selective α_1- and nonselective β-adrenergic antagonist, is administered as a 20-mg bolus in 5 minutes, followed by 20 to 40 mg every 15 min up to a total of 300 mg. Esmolol hydrochloride (Brevibloc) is a cardioselective β-blocker that has a rapid onset of action (1 or 2 min) and short half-life (10 to 20 min); the loading dose is 500 µg/kg in a 1-minute bolus; maintenance doses may range from 50 µg/kg per minute to 200 µg/kg per minute to control hypertensive episodes. Both labetalol and esmolol are contraindicated in patients with chronic obstructive pulmonary disease or congestive heart failure. Enalapril (Vasotec) is an angiotensin-converting enzyme inhibitor that, unlike other vasodilators, does not produce reflex sympathetic stimulation and resets the autoregulatory curve to lower pressure levels, decreasing the risk of cerebral ischemia with the lowering of blood pressure. The starting dose is 1 to 5 mg, followed by repeat doses every 6 hours. The main disadvantage of enalapril is its slow onset of action (15 to 30 min) and peak effect (3 to 4 hours). Sodium nitroprusside (Nipride) has an immediate onset of action and may be the last resort when other medications fail; it is still the drug of choice for treatment of patients with hypertension due to abuse of sympathomimetic drugs who are admitted for closed head injury. Clonidine has been administered to patients who have subarachnoid hemorrhage and may have a role in the treatment of hypertension related to opiate or alcohol withdrawal.

Arrhythmias in acute neurological disorders generally are caused by exaggerated sympathetic activity. They range from sinus tachycardia (the most common) to potentially serious ventricular arrhythmias. Most cardiac arrhythmias are transient and do not require treatment. Sinus tachycardia is the most common arrhythmia in patients with acute neurological disease and may cause a substantial decrease in cardiac output when the frequency reaches more than 200 beats/min. Myocardial ischemia may develop. Treatment is with β-blockers such as esmolol (500 µg/kg intravenously in 1 minute, followed by 50 to 200 µg/kg per minute as maintenance dose) or metoprolol (5 to 15 mg intravenously). Other supraventricular tachyarrhythmias such as atrial fibrillation, atrial flutter, or multifocal atrial tachycardia are treated with verapamil (2.5- to 5-mg intravenous bolus, followed by another 2.5 to 5 mg after 15 minutes) or β-blockers (e.g., metoprolol, 2 mg intravenously). Severe sinus bradycardia commonly develops in patients with acute lesions in the posterior fossa or rapidly progressive herniation from a supratentorial lesion; it also can occur after taking morphine for pain control or as a manifestation of vagovagal reflexes in patients with Guillain-Barré syndrome or acute spinal cord injury. Atropine (0.5- to 1-mg bolus) is given to prevent these episodes. Atropine also is indicated for management of accelerated junctional rhythm. Atrioventricular block requires cardiac pacing. Ventricular tachycardia is treated with lidocaine (200-mg bolus over 20 minutes, followed by an infusion of 2 to 4 mg/min) in patients with normal blood pressure or with cardioversion in patients with pronounced hypotension. Torsades de pointes, which occasionally occurs in patients with subarachnoid hemorrhage, is a form of ventricular tachycardia that has a characteristic polymorphic morphology and is associated with a prolonged QT interval. Its treatment includes overdrive pacing, magnesium sulphate, or isoproterenol.

Autonomic hyperactivity associated with acute head injury with decortication may respond to morphine and bromocriptine.[17] In some cases, treatment with anticonvulsants may be helpful when other measures have failed. In acute hydrocephalus, autonomic hyperactivity resolves rapidly after drainage of the hydrocephalus.

Hyperhidrosis

Hyperhidrosis may be a manifestation of sympathetic hyperactivity during diencephalic paroxysms that

Table 219.2 Drugs for treatment of central autonomic hyperactivity

Drug and mechanism of action	Dose	Indications	Precautions
Central imidazoline I(1) and α_2-receptor agonist Clonidine	0.1 mg bid, up to 0.3 mg tid Patch 0.1, 0.2, or 0.3 mg/day for 7 days	Baroreflex failure Paroxysmal hyperhidrosis Autonomic dysreflexia Opioid withdrawal Alcohol withdrawal	Sedation, dry mouth Rebound hypertension if abruptly discontinued Bradycardia Local skin reactions with patch
5-HT_2 and H_1 receptor antagonist Cyproheptadine	4–20 mg daily divided every 8 hr	Paroxysmal hyperhidrosis Serotonin syndrome	Sedation Appetite stimulation, dry mouth
D_2 receptor agonist Bromocriptine	2.5–10 mg tid via nasogastric tube	Neuroleptic malignant syndrome Sympathetic hyperactivity in head trauma	Hypotension, vomiting, exacerbation of psychosis
mu-Type opioid receptor agonist Morphine sulphate	10–30 mg every 4 hr via nasogastric tube 2.5–20 mg im or iv every 4 hr as needed	Pain-induced sympathetic hyperactivity Sympathetic hyperactivity in head trauma	Central nervous system depression
Positive modulators of GABA A receptors Chlordiazepoxide Lorazepam Clonazepam	50–100 mg q 4–6 hr 0.5–2 mg q 4–6 hr 0.5 mg tid up to 20 mg/day	Alcohol withdrawal	Central nervous system depression
α_1-Blockers Phenoxybenzamine Doxazosin Terazosin Prazosin	10–20 mg tid 1–20 mg once daily 2.5–5 mg once daily 3 mg tid	Hypertension in autonomic dysreflexia	Hypotension Fluid retention
β-Adrenergic blockers Labetalol (selective α_1, nonselective β) Esmolol (β_1) Propranolol (β_1 and β_2, crosses BBB) Metoprolol (β_1)	See Table 219.3 See Table 219.3 10–80 mg/dose every 6–8 hr po 50 mg bid, increase at weekly intervals up to 100–450 mg/d in 2–3 divided doses	Hypertension in neurological catastrophes Supraventricular arrhythmias Alcohol withdrawal Hyperhidrosis	Bradycardia, bronchospasm, Raynaud phenomenon Contraindicated in CHF and COPD
Muscarinic antagonists Atropine sulphate Oxybutynin Glycopyrrolate	0.5–1-mg bolus 2.5–5 mg tid 1–2 mg tid	Severe bradycardia Hyperhidrosis	Tachycardia, dry mouth, dry skin, urinary retention Contraindicated in patients with narrow-angle glaucoma and obstructive uropathy
Calcium channel blockers Verapamil Nifedipine	2.5–5-mg bolus 10 mg sublingual	Supraventricular tachyarrhythmias Autonomic dysreflexia	Hypotension, bradycardia, AV block Constipation Flushing, hypotension, angina
ACE inhibitors Enalapril Captopril Lisinopril	1–5 mg q 6 hr 12.5 mg qhs 10 mg qhs	Hypertension in neurological catastrophes Severe supine hypertension in patients with autonomic failure	Hypotension, edema, hyperkalemia

ACE, angiotensin-converting enzyme; AV, atrioventricular; BBB, blood-brain barrier; bid, 2 times daily; CHF, congestive heart failure; COPD, chronic obstructive pulmonary disease; im, intramuscularly; iv, intravenously; po, orally; q, every; qhs, at bedtime; qid, 4 times daily; tid, 3 times daily.

Table 219.3   Drugs for management of hypertension in neurological catastrophes

Drug	Mechanism of action	Dose	Onset of action	Duration of action	Disadvantages/ side effects
Labetalol (Normodyne, Trandate)	α- and β-Blocker	20–mg bolus in 5 min, repeat 20–40-mg bolus every 15 min up to 300 mg	5–10 min	3–6 hr	Nausea, vomiting, scalp tingling, burning throat, dizziness, heart block, bronchospasm
Esmolol (Brevibloc)	Cardioselective β-blocker	Loading—500 µg/kg in 1-min bolus Maintenance— 50–200 µg/kg per min	1–2 min	10–20 min	Administered in D_5W, thus risk of free water load Contraindicated in COPD and CHF
Enalapril	ACE inhibitor	1–5 mg, repeated every 6 hr	15–30 min	3–4 hr	Slow onset of action
Nitroprusside (Nipride)	Direct vasodilator	Start at 0.25 µg/kg per min; titrate up to 10 µg/kg per min	Immediate	1–2 min	Nausea, vomiting, muscle twitching, thiocyanate-cyanide intoxication

ACE, angiotensin-converting enzyme; CHF, congestive heart failure; COPD, chronic obstructive pulmonary disease; D_5W, dextrose in 5% water.

occur in severe head trauma or other neurological catastrophes. Paroxysmal hyperhidrosis with hypothermia is also a rare manifestation of agenesis of the corpus callosum (Shapiro syndrome). Sometimes, these episodes can be prevented with clonidine (0.1 to 0.3 mg orally up to 3 times daily or in a transdermal patch delivering 0.1, 0.2, or 0.3 mg daily for a week) or cyproheptadine (starting with 4 to 8 mg at bedtime and increasing up to 4 to 8 mg 4 times daily). In addition, peripheral muscarinic antagonists such as oxybutynin or glycopyrrolate ([Robinul] 1 or 2 mg 2 or 3 times daily) may prevent both hyperhidrosis and hypothermia in these patients.[18]

In most cases, however, hyperhidrosis is a chronic, benign, and, occasionally, familial disorder (i.e., essential hyperhidrosis). Patients with essential hyperhidrosis may benefit from treatment with anticholinergic drugs such as glycopyrrolate (1 or 2 mg orally 3 times daily) or propantheline (15 mg orally 3 times daily). Classic treatments for regional (axillary, palmar, or plantar) hyperhidrosis include tap water iontophoresis, local application of aluminum chloride or chloral hydrate, and surgical or endoscopic thoracic or lumbar sympathectomy.[19] Most recently, botulinum toxin administered intracutaneously has been proved effective in treating regional hyperhidrosis, including palmar and axillary hyperhidrosis and gustatory sweating. The beneficial effect may last 4 to 8 months in axillary hyperhidrosis and up to 12 months in palmar hyperhidrosis.[20]

Autonomic dysreflexia

Autonomic dysreflexia is a dramatic manifestation of traumatic spinal cord injury above the level of T5. Its main pathophysiological feature is a generalized and unpatterned reflex sympathetic (and parasympathetic) activation triggered by various visceral or somatic noxious or innocuous stimuli below the level of the spinal cord lesion.[21] Its most common triggering factor is bladder distension, and its most serious manifestation is severe hypertension, which may produce hypertensive encephalopathy or intracranial, subarachnoid, or retinal hemorrhage. The combination of parasympathetic and sympathetic stimulation may cause potentially dangerous supraventricular and ventricular arrhythmias. Autonomic dysreflexia may be prevented by appropriate medical care of patients with spinal cord injury, including bowel and bladder programs and skin care. Both the patient and family should be educated about possible causes, prevention, presentation, and first aid measures.

In the acute setting, placing the patient upright and removing the precipitating stimulus (including tight clothing), inserting a catheter under local anesthesia to relieve bladder distension, or treating fecal impaction may resolve the episode without the need for drug therapy. When hypertension persists despite these measures, antihypertensive treatment is indicated. Alpha-adrenergic blockers such as phenoxybenzamine (10 to 20 mg 3 times daily), prazosin (3 mg 3 times daily), doxazosin (1 to 20 mg once daily), or terazosin (2.5 to 5 mg once daily) have proved to be superior to placebo in reducing the severity and duration of episodes of autonomic dysreflexia without a marked lowering of resting arterial pressure or erectile function. A potential advantage of these drugs is they relax the internal urethral sphincter. Clonidine, an imidazoline I(1) and α_2-receptor agonist that acts primarily at the medullary level, has been given prophylactically because it may prevent hypertension in tetraplegic

Table 219.4   Clinical Institute Withdrawal Assessment (CIWA)

Nausea and vomiting (Ask: "Do you feel sick to your stomach?")
0 no nausea and no vomiting
1 mild nausea with no vomiting
2
3
4 intermittent nausea with dry heaves
5
6
7 constant nausea, frequent dry heaves, and vomiting

Tremor (arms extended and fingers spread apart)
0 no tremor
1 no tremor visible, but can feel fingertip to fingertip
2
3
4 moderate, with patient's arm extended
5
6
7 severe, even with arms not extended

Paroxysmal sweats
0 no sweat visible
1 barely perceptible sweating, palm moist
2
3
4 beads of sweat obvious on the forehead
5
6
7 drenching sweats

Anxiety (Ask: "Do you feel nervous?")
0 no anxiety, at ease
1 mildly anxious
2
3
4 moderately anxious, or guarded, so anxiety is inferred
5
6
7 equivalent to acute panic states as seen in severe delirium or acute schizophrenic reaction

Agitation
0 normal activity
1 somewhat more than normal activity
2
3
4 moderately fidgety and restless
5
6
7 paces back and forth during most of the interview, or constantly thrashes about

Tactile disturbances (Ask: "Have you any itching, pins and needles sensation, any burning, and numbness, or do you feel bugs crawling under your skin?")
0 none
1 very mild itching, pins and needles, burning or numbness
2 mild itching, pins and needles, burning or numbness
3 moderate itching, pins and needles, burning or numbness
4 moderately severe hallucinations
5 severe hallucinations
6 extremely severe hallucinations
7 continuous hallucinations

Auditory disturbances (Ask: "Are you more aware of sounds around you? Are they harsh? Do they frighten you? Are you hearing anything that is disturbing you? Are you hearing things you know are not there?")
0 not present
1 harshness or ability to frighten
2 mild harshness or ability to frighten
3 moderate harshness or ability to frighten
4 moderately severe hallucinations
5 severe hallucinations
6 extremely severe hallucinations
7 continuous hallucinations

Visual disturbances (Ask: "Does the light appear too bright? Is its color different? Does it hurt your eyes? Are you seeing anything that is disturbing to you? Are you seeing things you know are not there?")
0 not present
1 very mild sensitivity
2 mild sensitivity
3 moderate sensitivity
4 moderately severe sensitivity
5 severe hallucinations
6 extremely severe hallucinations
7 continuous hallucinations

Headache. Fullness in head (Ask: "Does your head feel different? Does it feel like there is a band around your head? Do not rate for dizziness or lightheadedness. Otherwise, rate severity.")
0 not present
1 very mild
2 mild
3 moderate
4 moderately severe
5 severe
6 very severe
7 extremely severe

Orientation and clouding of sensorium (Ask: "What day is this? Where are you? Who am I?")
0 oriented and can do serial additions
1 cannot do serial additions or is uncertain about date
2 disoriented for date by 1 or 2 calendar days
3 disoriented for date by 3 or more calendar days
4 disoriented for place and/or person

Call physician if
    Pulse >120/min
    Systolic BP >160 or <100, diastolic BP >100 or <60
    Respirations >30/min or <10/min
    Temperature >38.5°C
    Vomiting blood/coffee grounds
    Passing bloody/tarry stools
    Seizure activity
    Stuporous (difficult to arouse) or comatose (unable to arouse)
    CIWA score increase is more than 10 over previous measurement
    Cumulative dose during the first 24 hours of either 400 mg of chlordiazepoxide po, lorazepam 8 mg iv, or lorazepam 16 mg po

BP, blood pressure; iv, intravenously; po, orally.

patients during bladder stimulation. Nifedipine, 10 mg sublingually, is given for procedural prophylaxis and initial treatment of acute episodes of hypertension.[21] Anticholinergic drugs such as glycopyrrolate, oxybutynin, and propantheline may control excessive sweating during the episodes but may worsen urinary retention.[21,22] Any surgical, urological, obstetrical, or radiological procedures may precipitate an episode of autonomic dysreflexia. Anesthetic techniques to prevent these episodes include topical anesthesia for cystoscopic procedures, general anesthesia, or epidural anesthesia.

Neuroleptic malignant syndrome

Neuroleptic malignant syndrome is the most severe complication of neuroleptic treatment, which blocks D_2 receptors, and may be life-threatening. Early recognition and management are essential for recovery. Treatment includes discontinuation of the dopaminergic (D_2) antagonist drug, fluid replacement, antipyretics, use of a cooling blanket, and cardiovascular stabilization. Bromocriptine is given orally or through a nasogastric tube at doses of 2.5 to 10 mg 3 times daily up to 20 mg 4 times daily in some cases. Rigidity responds within the first day and hyperthermia over several days. Side effects include nausea, hypotension, delirium, and exacerbation of the psychotic illness. There may be recrudescence of the symptoms if bromocriptine treatment is discontinued prematurely. Dantrolene sodium (1 or 2 mg/kg daily up to 10 mg/kg daily intravenously), an antagonist of the muscle ryanodine receptor, can control hyperthermia and prevent rhabdomyolysis.[23] Dantrolene may produce an increase in liver function tests, posing the risk of hepatitis.

Lorazepam may be useful in controlling agitation and catatonia. Amantadine and memantine block glutamate NMDA (N-methyl-D-aspartate) receptors and have been proposed as an alternative treatment for neuroleptic malignant syndrome. This proposal is based on experimental evidence of an antagonistic balance between dopamine and excitatory neurotransmission in the basal ganglia.

Delirium tremens

Delirium tremens is the most severe manifestation of the alcohol withdrawal syndrome and constitutes a medical emergency. It is characterized by extreme autonomic hyperactivity with tachycardia, fever, diaphoresis, flushing, and hypertension in conjunction with anxiety, insomnia, tremor, visual or tactile hallucinations, and fluctuating levels of psychomotor activity. The development of profuse diarrhea and hyperpyrexia precedes vascular collapse and death. The best treatment is prevention. The main treatment for patients who are withdrawing from alcohol and exhibit any withdrawal phenomenon (e.g., tachycardia, anxiety, tremor, seizures) is a benzodiazepine such as chlordiazepoxide (50 to 100 mg, repeated every 2 to 4 hours if needed) or lorazepam (0.5 to 2.0 mg every 4 to 6 hours as needed). Many consider lorazepam the drug of choice because it undergoes

glucuronization and has an intermediate half-life. A randomized double-blind trial compared the effects of the administration of chlordiazepoxide in response to signs or symptoms of withdrawal (i.e., symptom-triggered therapy) with the effects of administration according to a fixed schedule (e.g., 50 to 100 mg orally every 4 hours, with additional doses as needed).[24] Symptom-triggered therapy decreased the duration of treatment (median, 9 vs. 68 hours) and the amount of benzodiazepine administered; furthermore, it was as efficacious as the fixed-schedule therapy in preventing seizures or delirium tremens during alcohol withdrawal.[24] Clonidine and propranolol can reduce the autonomic manifestations of delirium tremens but should only be given together with benzodiazepines. The management of delirium tremens is based on the Clinical Institute Withdrawal Assessment (CIWA) protocol. This includes the assessment of 10 clinical variables; 9 of them (nausea and vomiting, tremor, paroxysmal sweats, anxiety, agitation, tactile disturbances, auditory disturbances, visual disturbances, and headache/fullness in the head) are each graded in severity from 0 (absent) to 7 (most severe); orientation and clouding of sensorium are graded from 0 to 4 (Table 219.4).

References

1. Shy GM, Drager GA. A neurological syndrome associated with orthostatic hypotension: a clinical-pathologic study. Arch Neurol 1960;2:511–527
2. Consensus statement on the definition of orthostatic hypotension, pure autonomic failure, and multiple system atrophy. J Neurol Sci 1996;144:218–219
3. Penfield W. Diencephalic autonomic epilepsy. Arch Neurol & Psychiat 1929;22:358–374
4. Benarroch EE, Chang F-LF. Central autonomic disorders. J Clin Neurophysiol 1993;10:39–50
5. Oppenheimer DR. Lateral horn cells in progressive autonomic failure. J Neurol Sci 1980;46:393–404
6. Benarroch EE, Smithson IL, Low PA, Parisi JE. Depletion of catecholaminergic neurons of the rostral ventrolateral medulla in multiple systems atrophy with autonomic failure. Ann Neurol 1998;43:156–163
7. Goldstein DS, Holmes C, Cannon RO III, et al. Sympathetic cardioneuropathy in dysautonomias. N Engl J Med 1997;336:696–702
8. Cushing H. Concerning a definite regulatory mechanism of the vaso-motor centre which controls blood pressure during cerebral compression. Bull Johns Hopkins Hosp 1901;12:290–292
9. Biaggioni I, Whetsell WO, Jobe J, Nadeau JH. Baroreflex failure in a patient with central nervous system lesions involving the nucleus tractus solitarii. Hypertension 1994;23:491–495
10. Ropper AH. Acute autonomic emergencies and autonomic storm. In: Low PA, ed. Clinical Autonomic Disorders: Evaluation and Management. Boston: Little, Brown and Company, 1993:747–760
11. Low PA. Neurogenic orthostatic hypotension. In: Johnson JT, Griffith JW, eds. Current Therapy in Neurologic Disease. 4th ed. St. Louis: Mosby-Year Book, 1993:21–26
12. Robertson D, Davis TL. Recent advances in the treatment of orthostatic hypotension. Neurology 1995; 45(Suppl 5):S26–32

13. Chancellor MB, Blaivas JG. Urological and sexual problems in multiple sclerosis. Clin Neurosci 1994;2:189–195

14. Freeman R, Miyawaki E. The treatment of autonomic dysfunction. J Clin Neurophysiol 1993;10:61–82

15. Camilleri M. Disorders of gastrointestinal motility in neurologic diseases. Mayo Clin Proc 1990;65:825–846

16. Tietjen CS, Hurn PD, Ulatowski JA, Kirsch JR. Treatment modalities for hypertensive patients with intracranial pathology: options and risks. Crit Care Med 1996;24:311–322

17. Bullard DE. Diencephalic seizures: responsiveness to bromocriptine and morphine. Ann Neurol 1987;21: 609–611

18. LeWitt PA, Newman RP, Greenberg HS, et al. Episodic hyperhidrosis, hypothermia, and agenesis of corpus callosum. Neurology 1983;33:1122–1129

19. Khurana RK. Paraneoplastic autonomic dysfunction. In:

Low PA, ed. Clinical Autonomic Disorders: Evaluation and Management. 2nd ed. Philadelphia: Lippincott-Raven, 1997:545–554

20. Odderson IR. Hyperhidrosis treated by botulinum A exotoxin. Dermatol Surg 1998;24:1237–1241

21. Mathias CJ, Frankel HL. Cardiovascular control in spinal man. Annu Rev Physiol 1988;50:577–592

22. Trop CS, Bennett CJ. Autonomic dysreflexia and its urological implications: a review. J Urol 1991;146: 1461–1469

23. Ebadi M, Pfeiffer RF, Murrin LC. Pathogenesis and treatment of neuroleptic malignant syndrome. Gen Pharmacol 1990;21:367–386

24. Saitz R, Mayo-Smith MF, Roberts MS, et al. Individualized treatment for alcohol withdrawal: a randomized double-blind controlled trial. JAMA 1994;272:519–523

XII Muscle Disease

Section editor: Andrew G Engel

220 Principles of Muscle Disorders

Brenda L Banwell

Muscle diseases arise from abnormal development of the muscle fibers, loss of the structural integrity of muscle fibers, or dysfunction of the biochemical pathways operating within the fibers.

Muscle anatomy and function

Skeletal muscle is the major organ responsible for locomotion; it is also the source of carbohydrate-derived energy during anaerobic physical activity as well as the major source of amino acids mobilized during catabolic stress for hepatic gluconeogenesis and direct oxidation. Each muscle is composed of myriad muscle fibers. The mature muscle fiber is a multinucleated, postmitotic cell enveloped by plasma membrane, the sarcolemma, which is surrounded by basal lamina and endomysial connective tissue. Groups of muscle fibers, or fascicles, are surrounded by the perimysium, and the entire muscle is enveloped by a collagenous epimysium. Nerve branches, blood vessels, muscle spindles, and fat cells lie within the perimysium.[1]

Each muscle fiber is composed of a large number of myofibrils. The striated appearance of the muscle fiber is due to repeating structural units, or "sarcomeres," within the myofibrils. Each sarcomere is limited by Z disks. Emanating from the Z disk are thin filaments, composed of actin, troponin, and tropomyosin. The thin filaments interdigitate with other fine filaments and intracellular proteins to form an intricate scaffolding associated with the normal Z disk. The structural integrity of the myofiber is further supported by the association of myofibrils with sarcolemma-spanning proteins (α-, β-, δ-, and γ-sarcoglycan, β-dystroglycan, α7β1 integrin), subsarcolemmal proteins (dystrophin, plectin), and nuclear membrane-associated proteins (lamin A/C, lamin B, emerin). An ordered array of cytoskeletal proteins is also important for the normal positioning of subcellular organelles, such as mitochondria, the sarcoplasmic reticulum, and the transverse tubule system.

Each muscle fiber is innervated by one branch of a motor neuron. Neural input is required for coordinated muscle contraction, and it provides trophic support to the muscle fiber. The motor neuron and the group of muscle fibers innervated by its terminal branches constitute a "motor unit." All muscle fibers within a motor unit have a similar histochemical profile. Muscle fibers from varying motor units intermingle randomly, resulting in a checkerboard arrangement of the different histochemical fiber types. Type 1 fibers are rich in oxidative enzymes but low in glycolytic enzymes, resulting in a slow-twitch,

fatigue-resistant phenotype. Type 2B fast-twitch fibers are rich in glycolytic enzymes but low in oxidative enzymes and, thus, fatigue quickly. Type 2A fibers have features intermediate between those of type 1 and type 2B.

The nerve-muscle junction comprises the nerve terminal separated by a synaptic space from a specialized, infolded segment of the sarcolemma, the postsynaptic membrane. The postsynaptic membrane is enriched with acetylcholine receptors (AChRs) and various transmembrane and subsarcolemmal proteins whose expression is restricted to, or markedly enhanced in, this region. Nerve stimulation results in the release of quantal packets of acetylcholine from the nerve terminal. The neurotransmitter traverses the synaptic space, binds to AChR, and generates an end plate potential. When the end plate potential exceeds the threshold for activation of the perijunctional voltage-sensitive sodium channels, it generates a muscle fiber action potential. The action potential is propagated into the interior of the muscle fiber through the transverse tubular system, which then effects the release of calcium from the sarcoplasmic reticulum. The release of calcium triggers a coordinated series of events leading to the coupling of excitation to contraction.[2] Calcium binds to troponin on the thin filaments, resulting in a conformational change in tropomyosin which then allows repeated binding of myosin cross-bridges to the actin filaments, accompanied by a conformational change in the cross-bridges. This results in shortening of the sarcomere. The cycle is reversed and muscle relaxation occurs as calcium is actively pumped back into the sarcoplasmic reticulum and the interaction of the cross-bridges with the thin filaments ceases.[2]

Types of muscle diseases

Muscle disease can result from any pathological process that affects the structure or function of any muscle fiber component or the supporting connective tissue, vascular elements, and nerve supply. Diseases of the central nervous system also can alter the function of nerve and muscle, and some metabolic diseases cause dysfunction of the central nervous system and muscle simultaneously.

The term "myopathy" refers to any pathological process involving muscle. Some forms of myopathy, such as severe inflammatory myopathies and muscular dystrophies, are relentlessly progressive, causing the replacement of contractile elements with fatty and fibrous connective tissue. Mutations in genes encoding sarcolemma-associated proteins cause various forms of muscular dystrophy.[3–7] The putative proteins include components of the basal lamina (laminin α-2, and the α1-, α2-, and α3-subunits of type VI collagen),[8,9] integral membrane-spanning protein components of the sarcolemma (α, β, δ, and γ-sarcoglycans, and integrin α7),[3–5,10] and structural proteins associated with the cytoplasmic face of the sarcolemma (dystrophin, caveolin-3, plectin).[11–13] Mutations in sarcolemma-associated proteins result in muscle fiber necrosis, suggesting that the support provided by these proteins is critical for the structural integrity of contracting muscle fiber. Not all forms of muscular dystrophy, however, involve sarcolemma-associated proteins,[14–16] and in some forms of muscular dystrophy, the putative proteins have yet to be identified.

The most common acquired inflammatory myopathies are dermatomyositis, polymyositis, and inclusion body myositis. Muscle inflammation can also occur with acute viral or parasitic infections and in patients with acquired immunodeficiency syndrome. Dermatomyositis may present in children or adults with muscle pain, weakness, violaceous discoloration of the eyelids, erythematous skin lesions over extensor surfaces of the joints, malar rash, percutaneous calcium deposits (pediatric cases), and mild to markedly increased serum levels of creatine kinase (CK). In adults, dermatomyositis may be associated with malignancy. Polymyositis usually presents with symmetrical proximal weakness. Muscle pain, dysphagia, respiratory muscle weakness, and cardiac involvement also may occur, but skin rash is absent. Polymyositis is rare in childhood. Inclusion body myositis is the most common form of inflammatory myopathy in late adulthood and presents as an insidiously progressive, painless muscle weakness. Immunosuppressant therapies are often successful in treating dermatomyositis, variably successful for polymyositis, and have little efficacy in inclusion body myositis.

Structurally distinct myopathies have unique pathological hallmarks, such as nemaline bodies, single or multiple cores devoid of oxidative enzyme activity, centrally placed nuclei, or abnormal cytoplasmic inclusions (fingerprint bodies, spheroid bodies). Weakness generally is present in childhood and is usually nonprogressive, but late progression can occur in congenital nemaline myopathy, or clinical deterioration may occur in any of the structurally distinct congenital myopathies with intercurrent pulmonary infections or with development of notable scoliosis.

Myopathies associated with impaired metabolism of glycogen or lipid or impaired mitochondrial function are termed "metabolic myopathies." These disorders as well as acquired myopathies associated with specific medications, toxins, or nutritional deficiencies are discussed in the chapter on metabolic myopathies.

In all forms of muscle disease, individual muscles are affected with variable severity. Although the pattern of muscle involvement is often useful for clinical classification, the mechanism whereby some muscles are preferentially affected and neighboring muscles are spared is not known.

The diagnosis of muscle diseases

The diagnosis of muscle disease requires a careful history and thorough neurological examination. Clinical findings are further clarified with electromyographic (EMG) studies that include nerve conduction studies and repetitive nerve stimulation, muscle biopsy, muscle imaging, and, in selected diseases, biochemical or genetic analysis.

Clinical history

The history must be recorded chronologically and should establish the age at the onset of symptoms, the rate of disease progression, and the nature of the symptoms. Neonatal onset myopathies are often associated with reduced fetal movement in utero and may be associated with breech delivery and polyhydramnios. At birth, the affected infants feed poorly, have a weak cry, and are at risk for recurrent aspiration pneumonia. Childhood-onset myopathies present with delayed acquisition of motor milestones or loss of previously acquired motor skills.

Genetic history

A detailed family pedigree should be established. Consanguineous marriages or marriages within isolated communities raise the possibility of an autosomal recessive disease. Myopathies with prominent manifestations in affected males, with little or minimal symptoms in heterozygote females, and transmitted only maternally point to X-linked inheritance. Increasingly severe manifestations in subsequent generations suggest genetic anticipation due to a progressive expansion, from generation to generation, of trinucleotide repeats in an unstable gene. A negative family history does not exclude autosomal recessive inheritance, a new mutation, or unrecognized subtle manifestations in affected relatives. Whenever possible, parents and siblings should be examined.

Symptoms of muscle diseases

Symptoms of muscle disease include localized or diffuse weakness, reduced exercise tolerance, muscle pain, and abnormal spontaneous muscle activity. Muscle fatigue that develops with mild exertion is common in congenital or acquired myasthenic conditions and in some mitochondrial myopathies. Muscle fatigue (often associated with muscle pain and electrically silent muscle cramps) that develops shortly after the onset of strenuous exertion occurs with different glycolytic enzyme deficiencies or with muscle ischemia due to vascular insufficiency. Symptoms that develop minutes to hours after exercise or during sustained exercise suggest a defect of fatty acid oxidation. Muscle pain at rest occurs in patients with inflammatory myopathies, dermatomyositis, vasculitis, viral or parasitic myositis, or polymyalgia rheumatica.

Abnormal muscle activity may manifest as muscle

cramps, fasciculations, myotonia, or tetany. "Muscle cramps" are involuntary painful contractions that last seconds to minutes.[17] Cramps may occur in healthy persons after strenuous exertion. Dehydration, renal failure, and electrolyte imbalance also can produce muscle cramps.[17] "Fasciculations" are caused by spontaneous activation of motor units.[17] They may occur in normal persons, often during times of stress or after consumption of caffeine. Fasciculations in patients with progressive muscle atrophy and weakness suggest anterior horn cell disease. Infants with spinal muscular atrophy may have fasciculations of the tongue. "Myotonia," often described as muscle stiffness, is due to tetanic activation of individual muscle fibers; repetitive muscle fiber depolarizations produce discharges that wax and wane in amplitude and frequency. Patients with myotonic dystrophy may be minimally affected by myotonia,[18] whereas the myotonia associated with sodium and chloride channelopathies can be disabling. The most severe form of abnormally sustained muscle contraction is tetany. Tetany occurs in patients with hypocalcemia, hypomagnesemia, or metabolic alkalosis or in patients exposed to the exotoxin elaborated by the organism *Clostridium tetani*.

Clinical examination

Inspection

Muscles should be inspected for symmetry and focal or generalized hypertrophy (increased bulk of a strong muscle), pseudohypertrophy (increased bulk of a weak muscle), or atrophy. Pseudohypertrophy of the calf muscles occurs in dystrophinopathies, in juvenile onset spinal muscular atrophy, in partially denervated muscles due to radiculopathy, and in childhood acid maltase deficiency.[17] Inspection also should include a search for fasciculations, myokymia, and clinical and percussion myotonia.

Weakness of the shoulder girdle muscles results in scapular displacement, or "winging."[17] Muscle atrophy occurs in chronic myopathies or neuropathies, and it also is prominent in patients with disuse due to spinal cord injury. Weakness of axial muscles results in flexible or fixed spinal deformities. The spine should be inspected with the patient standing and seated. Patients with weakness of the neck extensor muscles have a "dropped head" appearance or they may support their chin in their hand. Patients with paraspinal weakness have flexible or fixed spinal curvatures or an exaggerated lumbar lordosis, and those with fatiguable weakness have flexible scoliosis that worsens with prolonged standing. Contractures of the spine, termed "rigid spine syndrome," occur in some congenital myopathies, in Emery–Dreifuss muscular dystrophy, and in some forms of merosin-positive congenital muscular dystrophy.[19] Limb muscle weakness may result in flexion contractures of individual joints; weakness of the small muscles of the feet can cause foot deformities. The patient's gait should be observed. Gait abnormalities can be associated with proximal or distal lower extremity weakness, loss of proprioception, ataxia or dystonia, or spasticity. Weakness of the pelvic muscles results in a waddling gait; weakness of the ankle dorsiflexors causes a footdrop gait.

Inspection of the face should document the position of the eyelids and ocular globes. Ptosis, or closure of the lid over the superior portion of the iris, is characteristic of congenital and autoimmune myasthenic disorders, mitochondrial myopathies, and oculopharyngeal dystrophy and occurs in some patients with myotubular myopathy. Fluctuating extraocular palsies associated with diplopia occur in autoimmune myasthenia gravis. Isolated extraocular muscle palsies, often manifesting as diplopia, are not a feature of myopathies or myasthenia gravis. Ocular palsies *without* diplopia occur in oculopharyngeal dystrophy, mitochondrial myopathies, and congenital myasthenic syndromes. Elongated facies with poor oral closure, persistent drooling, and inability to drink from a straw or to whistle indicate facial muscle weakness. A high arched palate suggests tongue or facial muscle weakness present in utero or during early childhood. Clinical features common to specific neuromuscular disorders are listed in Table 220.1.

Palpation

Muscles should be palpated for tenderness, focal nodules (sarcoid), or for increased density (fibrotic muscle in Duchenne dystrophy). Muscle tone should be assessed by moving each limb. Hypotonia in infancy manifests as pronounced head lag when the infant is pulled gently into a seated position, by the ability to adduct the arm fully across the chest (scarf sign), by an abducted posture of the legs or "frog-leg" position, and by a tendency of the infant to slip through the examiner's fingers when lifted under the arms.[17] Hypotonia also occurs in infants with cerebellar lesions, during the acute phase of severe anoxic brain injury or sepsis, in some genetic syndromes (Prader–Willi syndrome), in peroxisomal or metabolic disorders, and in severe hypothyroidism.[17]

Manual muscle strength testing

Muscle strength traditionally is graded using the 5-point British Medical Council scale as follows: 0, no contraction; 1, flicker or trace contraction; 2, active movement with gravity eliminated; 3, active movement against gravity; 4, active movement against gravity and resistance; and 5, normal power. In young children, observation of the child at play and noting how the child rises from a lying position, walks, and climbs onto the examination table is more informative than formal manual muscle testing. Patients with significant torso and proximal lower extremity weakness exhibit Gowers sign when asked to rise from a recumbent position. The patient will perform a series of maneuvers in which he or she rolls onto the side, sits up, transfers from a seated position to a four-point stance, and then extends the knees, places the hands on the thighs, and moves the hands up the legs until becoming upright.

Table 220.1   Common features of neuromuscular disease*

Finding	Seen in	Comments
Muscle hypertrophy†	Myotonia congenita	Patients typically have a generalized increase in muscle bulk, often with prominent hypertrophy of neck muscles
Muscle pseudohypertrophy‡	DMD/BMD SMA-juvenile AMD Partially denervated muscle	In boys with DMD, calf muscle pseudohypertrophy is an early feature but not detectable late in the disease
Ptosis	MG CMS Mt OPMD MM	The degree of ptosis may be fixed (OPMD, MM, Mt) or fluctuate throughout the day (MG, CMS). Fatiguable ptosis, which improves with administration of edrophonium, suggests defect of neuromuscular transmission (MG, CMS)
Ophthalmoplegia	MG CMD Mt	
Bulbar muscle weakness	MG CMS OPMD IBM ALS SMA	
Action/percussion myotonia	Myotonia congenita Paramyotonia congenita MD Hypothyroidism	In children with congenital MD, myotonia is rarely detectable before age 8 years
Hearing impairment	Congenital variant of FSHD Mt	
Skin involvement	Dermatomyositis EBS-MD	
Respiratory failure	MG CMS Congenital MD AMD DMD Nemaline myopathy Myotubular myopathy	Although respiratory muscle weakness may be noted in any patient with severe myopathy, the disorders listed are those in which respiratory involvement is prominent
Cardiac involvement	EDMD DMD/BMD MD MG	Cardiac arrhythmias pose significant risk to patients with EDMD and MD and to dystrophinopathy patients during or following surgery; patients with BMD may develop cardiomyopathy even with only moderate limb weakness; clinically symptomatic cardiomyopathy occurs in terminal phase of DMD; rarely, patients with MG may develop cardiomyopathy during myasthenic crisis

ALS, amyotrophic lateral sclerosis; AMD, acid maltase deficiency; BMD, Becker MD; CMS, congenital myasthenic syndromes; DMD, Duchenne MD; EBS-MD, epidermolysis bullosa simplex MD; EDMD, Emery–Dreifuss MD; FSHD, fascioscaphulohumeral MD; IBM, inclusion body myositis; MD, muscular dystrophy; MG, myasthenia gravis; MM, myotubular myopathy; Mt, mitochondrial myopathies; OPMD, oculopharyngeal MD; SMA-juvenile, spinal muscular atrophy, juvenile onset
*Clinical features common to specific neuromuscular disorders are described. The table is meant as a general guide rather than an exhaustive list.
†Hypertrophy refers to enlargement of a clinically strong muscle.
‡Pseudohypertrophy refers to enlargement of a clinically weak muscle.

Percussion

Tendon reflexes should be elicited by percussion and enhanced by reinforcement if necessary. In newborn infants, the tendon reflexes at the ankle and triceps may be difficult or impossible to elicit.[17] In selected patients, percussion of the tongue, finger extensors, and thenar eminence may elicit myotonia. Percussion over injured or regenerating peripheral nerves may elicit pain (Tinel sign).

General physical examination

Examination of the skin and hair may aid in the diagnosis of muscle disease. Premature frontal balding is associated with myotonic dystrophy. A purple skin rash on the face and exposed skin surfaces and peri-ungal erythema point to dermatomyositis. All patients with muscle disease should have an electro-cardiographic study, and any patient with muscular dystrophy should also have an echocardiographic study to exclude a concomitant cardiomyopathy.

Investigation of patients with muscle disease

Laboratory tests

An increase in the serum level of CK, or more specifically the muscle-derived CK isoform (CK-MM), occurs in many myopathies. CK is markedly increased in dystrophinopathies, in the more severe forms of sarcoglycanopathies, and in patients with metabolic, traumatic, or anesthetic-induced rhab-domyolysis. A mild increase in CK also occurs in some patients with peripheral neuropathy or anterior horn cell disease. The blood lactate level may be increased in patients with mitochondrial myopathy, but a normal value does not exclude this diagnosis. Exercise testing may aid in the investigation of disorders of muscle energy metabolism.[20] In patients with acute muscle pain or weakness, electrolyte and endocrine disorders should be excluded, and treatment with medications known to cause muscle damage[21] should be discontinued. Commercially available molecular genetic studies for myotonic dystrophy and mutations in dystrophin may be diagnostic in some patients. Many recently described genetic loci for various myopathies[7] are being studied in research centers and are not yet available for clinical diagnosis.

Electromyography

EMG consists of nerve conduction studies, repetitive nerve stimulation, and needle examination of selected muscles. The purpose of EMG studies is to (1) localize the cause of weakness to muscle, neuromuscular junction, motor nerves, or anterior horn cells, (2) evaluate the severity of the disorder, (3) delineate the pattern of muscle or nerve involvement, and (4) judge the response to therapy.[22]

Nerve conduction velocities are normal in patients with myopathy. A needle examination of muscle is performed with the muscle at rest, during slight voluntary activation, and during strong voluntary contraction. Individual motor units within a muscle vary slightly in size and shape. Normal motor unit potentials have an initial positive phase, followed by a negative phase and ending with a positive phase. In myopathies, motor unit potentials are often complex with five or more phases and are termed "polyphasic."[22] The amplitude of motor unit potentials is often decreased in myopathies and increased with anterior horn cell disease or reinnervation. When muscle contracts against a force, an increasing number of motor units are recruited. In patients with myopathy, weakness of individual motor units leads to early and rapid recruitment of additional motor units. In normal resting muscle, there is a brief burst of activity after the EMG needle is inserted, but the muscle is otherwise silent.[22] In both myopathies and neuropathies, abnormal spontaneous fibrillation potentials and positive sharp waves are recorded.[22] Fibrillations and positive waves indicate loss of innervation due to neuropathy, segmental muscle necrosis, or regenerating fibers that have not yet been innervated.[22] The degree of fibrillation is a useful index of disease activity in inflammatory myopathies.[23]

Muscle imaging

Muscles may be imaged with ultrasonography, computed tomography (CT), and magnetic resonance imaging (MRI). In children with the clinical features of dermatomyositis, confirmatory findings on MRI may obviate muscle biopsy.[24] In patients with muscular dystrophy, ultrasonography may show increased tissue density and MRI demonstrate muscle replacement by fatty tissue.[25] MRI findings in inflammatory myopathies include muscle edema, muscle calcification, and fatty infiltration. MRI scans can be performed serially to evaluate disease progression or response to therapy.[26]

Muscle biopsy

Muscle biopsy is a key component in the diagnosis of most muscle diseases. Biopsy should be performed on an affected but not too severely involved limb muscle. Whenever possible, biopsy of the gastrocnemius muscle should be avoided, because this muscle is prone to show myopathic changes when partially denervated. Muscles that have been injected or examined recently by EMG are unsuitable for diagnosis. The quality of the biopsy depends on excision of a well-oriented, noncauterized specimen that is flash-frozen and processed with conventional histochemical techniques. Marked myopathic alterations may not be detected in paraffin-embedded tissue.[27] Immunocytochemical localization of specific proteins can be performed for the diagnosis of some forms of muscular dystrophy, specific enzyme histochemistry may be used to identify some glycolytic enzyme defects, and detailed analysis of mitochondrial function can be performed in specialized laboratories.

Management

The management of specific muscle disorders is discussed in subsequent chapters in this section. For many patients, the following general principles apply: (1) mechanical function of weak muscles should be maintained as long as possible, often with the use of bracing or ambulatory aids, (2) early referral should be made to physical and occupational therapy for proper seating and chest physiotherapy and to orthopedics for scoliosis management, (3) homes should be modified for safety (handrails in the bathroom, raised toilet seats, wall-to-wall carpeting),[16] and (4) the psychological and psychosocial impact of the disease on the patient and family must be addressed and appropriate support provided by the treating medical team, with referral to specified patient support groups when available.

References

1. Sanes JR. The extracellular matrix. *In*: Engel AG, Franzini-Armstrong C, eds. Myology. Vol 1, 2nd ed. New York: McGraw-Hill, 1994:242–260

2. Homsher E. The cross-bridge cycle and the energetics of contraction. *In*: Engel AG, Franzini-Armstrong C, eds. Myology. Vol 1, 2nd ed. New York: McGraw-Hill, 1994:375–390

3. Straub V, Campbell KP. Muscular dystrophies and the dystrophin-glycoprotein complex. Curr Opin Neurol 1997;10:168–175

4. Lim LE, Campbell KP. The sarcoglycan complex in limb-girdle muscular dystrophy. Curr Opin Neurol 1998;11:443–452

5. Bushby KM. Making sense of the limb-girdle muscular dystrophies. Brain 1999;122:1403–1420

6. Ozawa E, Noguchi S, Mizuno Y, et al. From dystrophinopathy to sarcoglycanopathy: evolution of a concept of muscular dystrophy. Muscle Nerve 1998;21:421–438

7. Kaplan JC, Fontaine B. Neuromuscular disorders: gene location. Neuromuscul Disord 2000;10:I-XV

8. Cohn RD, Herrmann R, Sorokin L, et al. Laminin alpha2 chain-deficient congenital muscular dystrophy: variable epitope expression in severe and mild cases. Neurology 1998;51:94–100

9. Speer MC, Tandan R, Rao PN, et al. Evidence for locus heterogeneity in the Bethlem myopathy and linkage to 2q37. Hum Mol Genet 1996;5:1043–1046

10. Rutherford SL, Zuker CS. Protein folding and the regulation of signaling pathways. Cell 1994;79:1129–1132

11. Banwell BL, Russel J, Fukudome T, et al. Myopathy, myasthenic syndrome, and epidermolysis bullosa simplex due to plectin deficiency. J Neuropathol Exp Neurol 1999;58:832–846

12. Miller RG, Hoffman EP. Molecular diagnosis and modern management of Duchenne muscular dystrophy. Neurol Clin 1994;12:699–725

13. Kunkel L. Caveolin-3 deficiency as a cause of limb-girdle muscular dystrophy. J Child Neurol 1999;14:33–34

14. Bione S, Maestrini E, Rivella S, et al. Identification of a novel X-linked gene responsible for Emery–Dreifuss muscular dystrophy. Nat Genet 1994;8:323–327

15. Bonne G, Di Barletta MR, Varnous S, et al. Mutations in the gene encoding lamin A/C cause autosomal dominant Emery-Dreifuss muscular dystrophy. Nat Genet 1999;21:285–288

16. Pizzuti A, Friedman DL, Caskey CT. The myotonic dystrophy gene. Arch Neurol 1993;50:1173–1179

17. Gomez MR. The clinical examination. *In*: Engel AG, Franzini-Armstrong C, eds. Myology. Vol 1, 2nd ed. New York: McGraw-Hill, 1994:746–763

18. Harper PS, Rüdel R. Myotonic dystrophy. *In*: Engel AG, Franzini-Armstrong C, eds. Myology. Vol 2, 2nd ed. New York: McGraw-Hill, 1994:1192–1219

19. Flanigan KM, Kerr L, Bromberg MB, et al. Congenital muscular dystrophy with rigid spine syndrome: a clinical, pathological, radiological, and genetic study. Ann Neurol 2000;47:152–161

20. Haller RG, Bertocci LA. Exercise evaluation of metabolic myopathies. *In*: Engel AG, Franzini-Armstrong C, eds. Myology. Vol 1, 2nd ed. New York: McGraw-Hill, 1994:807–821

21. Pascuzzi RM. Drugs and toxins associated with myopathies. Curr Opin Rheumatol 1998;10:511–520

22. Stalberg E, Falck B. The role of electromyography in neurology. Electroecephalogr Clin Neurophysiol 1997;103:579–598

23. Daube JR. Electrodiagnosis of muscle disorders. *In*: Engel AG, Franzini-Armstrong C, eds. Myology. Vol 1, 2nd ed. New York: McGraw-Hill, 1994:764–794

24. Keim DR, Hernandez RJ, Sullivan DB. Serial magnetic resonance imaging in juvenile dermatomyositis. Arthritis Rheum 1991;34:1580–1584

25. Scheuerbrandt G. First meeting of the Duchenne Parent Project in Europe: Treatment of Duchenne Muscular Dystrophy. 7–8 November 1997, Rotterdam, The Netherlands. Neuromuscul Disord 1998;8:213–219

26. Adams EM, Chow CK, Premkumar A, Plotz PH. The idiopathic inflammatory myopathies: spectrum of MR imaging findings. Radiographics 1995;15:563–574

27. Engel AG. The muscle biopsy. *In*: Engel AG, Franzini-Armstrong C, eds. Myology. Vol 1, 2nd ed. New York: McGraw-Hill, 1994:822–831

221 Congenital Myopathies

Kathryn N North

The congenital myopathies are a heterogeneous group of neuromuscular conditions which are defined by distinctive histochemical or ultrastructural changes in muscle. This group of disorders typically present in infancy or early childhood with hypotonia and muscle weakness. There is wide variation in clinical severity within each group and marked clinical overlap with other neuromuscular disorders including the muscular dystrophies, metabolic myopathies, and spinal muscular atrophy. Therefore accurate diagnosis requires the combined evaluation of the clinical data, the electromyogram (EMG), and the histopathological findings.

The first report of a congenital myopathy was that by Shy and Magee in 1956.[1] They described a hereditary, non-progressive disorder that subsequently became known as central core disease. Prior to this, the spinal muscular atrophies were the only well defined neuromuscular disorder of infancy and childhood. Most patients with congenital myopathies were confusingly classified under such descriptive terms as "amyotonia congenita" or "benign congenital hypotonia." In 1969, Dubowitz clarified the classification of these disorders with his delineation of the "new myopathies,"[2] later termed "congenital myopathies." The congenital myopathies are rare disorders. In a series of 250 patients with severe neonatal hypotonia 34 out of the 250 (14%) were diagnosed as having a congenital myopathy;[3] eight of these (3% of the total) had nemaline myopathy which is perhaps the most common type.

Clinically, the congenital myopathies have a number of common features: early onset with generalized weakness, hypotonia and hyporeflexia, poor muscle bulk, dysmorphic features secondary to the myopathy (pectus carinatum, scoliosis, foot deformities, a high arched palate, elongated facies), and a distinguishing but not specific morphological feature on muscle biopsy. Apart from the specific morphologic abnormality, the muscle does not usually demonstrate necrosis or fibrosis and there is no glycogen or lipid storage. Serum creatine kinase (CK) is usually normal or mildly elevated, and EMG is either normal or myopathic.

Over the past three decades, the number of morphologically distinct congenital myopathies has grown rapidly, paralleling the advent and refinement of myopathological techniques such as electron microscopy, enzyme histochemistry and immunocytochemistry and, more recently, molecular genetic techniques. Certain congenital myopathies are well defined clinically, morphologically and genetically (Table 221.1). These "classical" congenital myopathies are central core disease, nemaline myopathy, myotubular myopathy, and the myofibrillar (or desmin-related) myopathies. In addition, there are a number of myopathies defined by specific structural abnormalities that have not yet been proven by genetic studies to represent distinct entities (Table 221.2).

Table 221.1 Congenital myopathies with identified gene loci

Disorder	Inheritance	Protein and gene (Symbol)	Chromosome localization	References
Nemaline myopathy (NEM)	AD AR	α-Tropomyosin$_{SLOW}$ (NEM1: *TPM3*)	1q22-q23	Laing et al., 1995[4] Tan et al., 1999[5]
	AR AD AR sporadic	Nebulin (NEM2) Skeletal muscle α-actin (*ACTA1*) *Expand (see below)	2q21.2-2q22 1q42.1	Pelin et al., 1999[6] Nowak et al., 1999[7]
Central core disease	AD sporadic	Ryanodine receptor (CCD: *RYR1*)	19q13.1	Zhang et al., 1993[8] Quane et al., 1993[9]
Myotubular myopathy	X-linked	Myotubularin (*MTMX*)	Xq28	Laporte et al., 1996[10]
Myofibrillar myopathy (MFM) or desmin-related myopathy (DRM)	AD	αB-Crystallin *(CRYAB)*	11q22	Vicart et al., 1998[11]
	AD and AR AD AD	Desmin (*DES*) ? ?	2q35 2q24-31 10q22.3	Goldfarb et al., 1998[12] Nicolao et al., 1999[13] Melberg et al., 1999[14]
Multiminicone disease	AR	Selenoproton	1p36	Ferreiro et al., 2002[7C]
	*EXPAND Nemdine myopathy AD AR	β-tropomyosin troporin I	9p13.2 19q13.4	Donner et al., 2002[7A] Johnston et al., 2000[7B]

Table 221.2   Other structural congenital myopathies: nosological entities

Probable: some familial cases	Possible: several sporadic cases	Doubtful nosology or single sporadic cases

Congenital fibre type disproportion
Cylindrical spirals myopathy
Fingerprint body myopathy
Tubular aggregate myopathy
Vacuolar myopathy
Hyaline body myopathy
	Reducing body myopathy
	Sarcotubular myopathy
	Myopathy with hexagonally
	   cross-linked tubular arrays
		Lamellar body myopathy
		Zebra body myopathy
		Broad A band myopathy
		Cop disease
		Myopathy with mosaic fibres and interlocking
		   sarcomeres

Modified from Goebel and Anderson 1999,[15] 56th European Neuromuscular Centre (ENMC) workshop: structural congenital myopathies. Neuromuscular Disorders 1999;9:50–57. See also Fardeau and Tome[3] for more detail about the individual disorders.

Nemaline myopathy

Specific clinical features

The clinical phenotype of nemaline myopathy is extremely heterogenous,[16] with five subgroups currently identified, based on clinical severity and age of onset. These subgroups include congenital-onset (subdivided into severe, intermediate, and "typical" forms based on presence or absence of antigravity movements at birth, the degree of respiratory involvement, and presence or absence of contractures), childhood-onset, and adult-onset forms. The "typical congenital" form of nemaline myopathy usually presents at birth or during the first year of life with hypotonia, weakness, and feeding difficulties. Some cases present later with delayed attainment of motor milestones, a waddling gait, or speech abnormalities. Facial weakness is common. There is often distal as well as proximal weakness, and some patients have initially been thought to have peroneal paresis because of their foot drop. The respiratory muscles are always involved, although hypoventilation may not be clinically obvious; cardiac involvement is rare. The course of the disease is often static or only very slowly progressive, and most patients will be able to lead an active life. Others may experience deterioration during the prepubertal period of rapid growth and some will start using a wheelchair at this time.[17] The severe-congenital form of nemaline myopathy presents at birth with severe hypotonia and muscle weakness, little spontaneous movement, difficulties with sucking and swallowing, gastro-oesophageal reflux and respiratory insufficiency. Death due to respiratory insufficiency or recurrent pneumonia is common during the first weeks or months of life. However, even severely hypotonic patients with lack of spontaneous respiration at birth have been known to survive, some of them with little residual disability.[18–20]

The inheritance of nemaline myopathy can be autosomal dominant, autosomal recessive or sporadic (including new dominant mutations). In the last 7 years, mutations in five genes have been identified in a subset of patients with nemaline myopathy. These genes all encode protein components of the thin filament of muscle: α-tropomyosin$_{slow}$, nebulin, skeletal α-actin, β-tropomyosin, tropanin I (Table 221.1).

Pathological features

The diagnostic feature of nemaline myopathy is the presence of distinct rod-like inclusions, nemaline bodies, in the skeletal muscle fibers of affected patients (Figure 221.1). The rods are not visible on hematoxylin and eosin (H&E) staining, but appear as red or purple structures against the blue-green myofibrillar background with the modified Gomori trichrome stain. The number of rods in a muscle specimen does not appear to correlate with disease severity. The rods are considered to be derived from the lateral expansion of the Z-line, based on their structural continuity with Z-lines and electron density using electron microscopy (EM), and positive staining with antibodies to α-actinin which is a major component of the Z-line in skeletal muscle.[21,22] Additional pathological features include type I fiber predominance, as well as fibre atrophy and/or fiber hypertrophy.[23,24]

Central core disease (CCD)

Specific clinical features

The original case report of Shy and Magee[1] exemplifies the typical clinical manifestations of CCD. The disorder usually presents in infancy with weakness and hypotonia. Motor milestones are delayed; many patients do not walk until three to four years of age. Muscle weakness is symmetrical and mild; active movement of all muscle groups against gravity and resistance is usually present and most patients achieve ambulation. Weakness is more severe in the lower limbs and preferentially affects proximal musculature. Usually patients are only mildly disabled, and weakness is non-progressive or only slowly progressive. Most patients have poor muscle bulk, but muscle atrophy is not conspicuous. Mild weakness of facial and neck muscles can occur but the extraocular muscles are spared. Musculoskeletal deformities such as kyphoscoliosis, congenital dislocation of the hip, pes cavus, pes planus and thoracic deformities, occur frequently. The severity of the deformity often does not correlate with the degree of muscle weakness; in some individuals, skeletal deformities are the sole manifestation of disease. Significant respiratory insufficiency is unusual, cardiac abnormalities occur rarely, and intellectual performance is not impaired.[25]

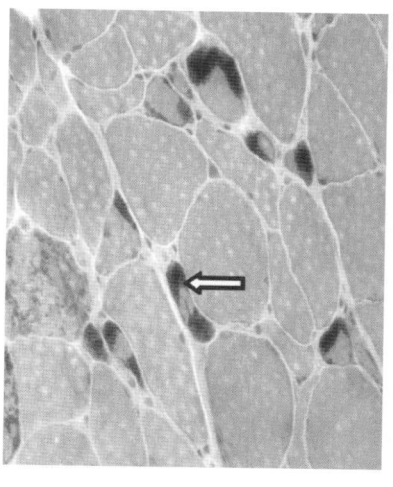

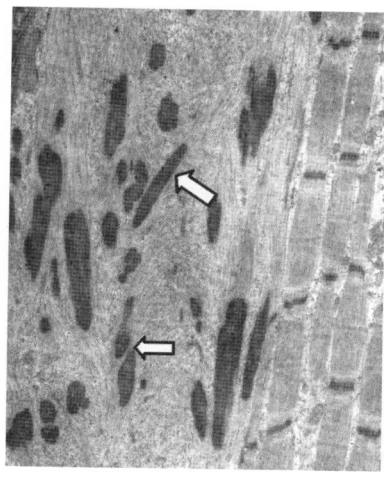

Figure 221.1 Nemaline myopathy A. Gomari trichrome stain shows collections of rods at the periphery of most muscle fibers (arrow) B. Electron micrograph, longitudinal section of demonstrating rods parallel to the long axis of the muscle fiber (arrow). Rods have the same electron density as the 2-lines of adjacent sarcomeres.

(A)

(B)

Although the majority of patients reported display the "typical" clinical phenotype, central cores may be found in individuals who are asymptomatic, in patients with mild weakness or skeletal deformity, and in patients with raised serum CK as their only manifestation of the disorder.[25,26] Central core disease is associated with an increased risk of malignant hyperthermia (MH) (see below). The CK elevation correlates with concomitant susceptibility to MH, but not all patients with susceptibility to MH and CCD have an elevated CK.[25] Rarely patients with CCD have more severe muscle weakness and motor impairment.[25,27,28]

Central core disease is inherited in an autosomal dominant fashion with variable expression and incomplete penetrance in most families. Patients with CCD may be asymptomatic or only mildly affected, and thus muscle biopsy may be the only way to identify an affected family member. Disease-causing mutations have been identified in the ryanodine receptor-1 gene (RYR-1) in patients with central core disease and susceptibility to MH.[8,9] To date, the proportion of patients with CCD due to RYR1 mutations is not known. Both CCD and MH are considered to be genetically heterogeneous, but additional candidate genes for CCD have not yet been identified (Table 221.1).

Pathological features

The characteristic abnormality of CCD is the presence of a single, well-circumscribed circular region in the center of the majority of type 1 fibers, the central core (Figure 221.2). The cores consist of a zone of reduced oxidative enzyme activity that stains negatively for phosphorylase and glycogen.[29,30] On electron microscopy, the cores are devoid of mitochondria and sarcoplasmic reticulum.[30] In some cores the integrity of the myofibrils is preserved (structured cores); other cores display focal myofibrillar degeneration (unstructured cores). In longitudinal sections, the cores extend the entire length of the muscle fiber. The non-core areas of the fiber appear normal by histo-

chemical criteria. In the majority of cases there is a type 1 fiber predominance.

Myotubular (centronuclear) myopathy
Specific clinical features

There are three groups of myotubular (centronuclear) myopathies based on clinical and genetic features.[31] The X-linked recessive form is the best-defined clinically and genetically. Onset is commonly in utero and the pregnancy is complicated by polyhydramnios. There may be a history of miscarriages and neonatal deaths of male infants in the maternal line. Affected males present at birth with severe floppiness and weakness, facial diplegia, and difficulties with respiration and feeding. Additional features include thin ribs, contractures of the hips and knees, puffy eyelids, ophthalmoplegia and cryptorchidism. Many affected males die in the neonatal period. The gene for X-linked myotubular myopathy has been identified as MTM1 on Xq28[10] and is thought to be involved in a signal transduction pathway necessary for late myogenesis (Table 221.1). The major differential diagnosis is congenital myotonic dystrophy, which needs to be excluded by molecular genetic methods.

The autosomally inherited forms of myotubular myopathy are extremely rare with only a few reported confirmed familial cases. The autosomal recessive type usually presents in infancy or early childhood with respiratory distress, hypotonia, a weak cry and difficulty sucking. Ophthalmoplegia, ptosis and facial diplegia are common. The clinical course is characterized by delay in motor milestones, slowly progressing weakness, and development of scoliosis; by adolescence many patients are confined to a wheelchair.[31,32] The autosomal dominant and sporadic forms usually present in adulthood with a much milder phenotype.[33,34] The chromosomal loci for the autosomal forms of myotubular myopathy are not known and therefore genetic diagnosis is not possible. Myotonic dystrophy is the major differential diagno-

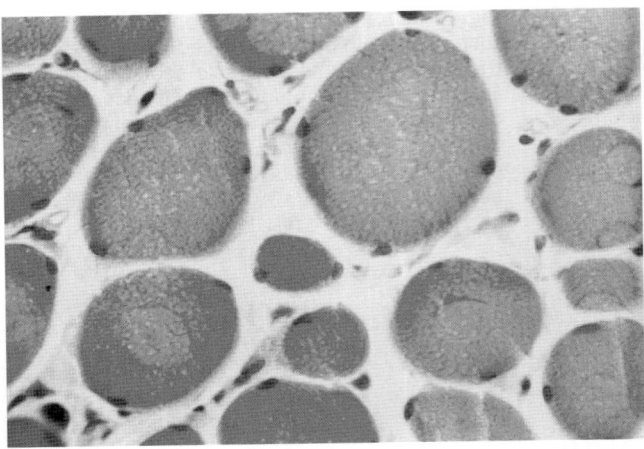
(A)

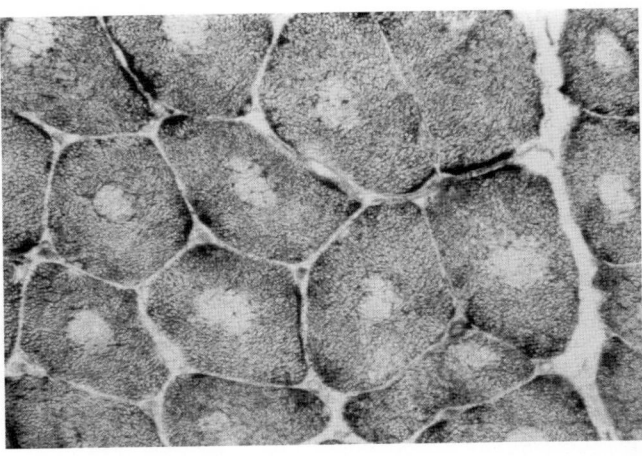
(B)

Figure 221.2   Central Core Disease A. The cores are not apparent on haematoxylin endcosin staining. B. Transverse sections stained for NADH show absence of enzyme activity in single large central cores. (See color plate section.)

sis of patients with muscle weakness and centrally placed nuclei on muscle biopsy.

Pathological features

The characteristic histological feature is the predominance of small type 1 fibers with centrally placed nuclei resembling fetal myotubes. There is usually an aggregation of mitochondria in the center of the muscle fiber, associated with dense oxidative enzyme staining and a lack of staining with myosin adenosine triphosphatase (ATPase). Obligate carriers of the X-linked form of myotubular myopathy are usually asymptomatic, but approximately 50% may have their carrier status verified by muscle biopsy.[31]

Myofibrillar (desmin-related) myopathies
Specific clinical features

The desmin-related myopathies are a clinically and genetically heterogeneous group of disorders defined by the presence of desmin-positive myofibrillar aggregates on muscle biopsy.[35–37] The age of onset ranges from early childhood to middle age. Weakness is most commonly distal, or may be more diffuse, and bulbar or respiratory involvement occurs in some families. Cardiac symptomatology may dominate the clinical picture, particularly hypertrophic cardiomyopathy or atrioventricular conduction block.[38] Lens opacities and neuropathic features have also been reported in some families. Inheritance is usually autosomal dominant, although recessive and X-linked cases have also been reported. Disease-causing mutations in α-B crystallin, and in desmin itself have recently been identified.[11,12] In addition, at least two and probably not fewer than four additional chromosomal loci have been identified by linkage analysis (see Table 221.1)

Pathological features

The common pathological feature in this group of myopathies is the activation of a degradative process that primarily affects the myofibrils. The lytic lesions become depleted of actin, α-actinin, and occasionally of titin, nebulin and myosin. Compacted and degraded myofibrillar components accumulate in hyaline spheroidal structures that react intensely for actin. Desmin, accumulates in some but not all, abnormal fiber regions, together with many other proteins: e.g., lamin B, αB-crystallin, gelsolin, ubiquitin, α1-antichymotrypsin, dystrophin, γ-sarcoglycan, large deposits of congophilic amyloid material and neural cell adhesion molecule (NCAM), a marker of regeneration. Because desmin is not the only abnormal material that accumulates, because the common denominator is myofibrillar degradation, and because of genetic heterogeneity, the noncommital term of *myofibrillar myopathy* was proposed as a substitute for "desmin storage myopathy" and "desmin related myopathy."[36,37]

Treatment of congenital myopathies

There is currently no curative treatment available for patients with congenital myopathy. Nevertheless, a multidisciplinary approach to the management of the individual patient will greatly improve quality of life, and can even influence survival. The therapeutic approach to this group of patients should be considered in the following four areas:

* **prevention:** genetic counselling and prenatal diagnosis
* **monitoring:** developing a plan for the prospective detection of complications
* **risk management:** special care during surgical procedures, anaesthetics and childbirth
* **symptomatic therapy and rehabilitation:** physical and occupational therapy, orthopaedic inter-

vention, respiratory care and management of feeding difficulties.

Prevention

Genetic counselling and prenatal diagnosis Genetic counselling and prediction of genetic risk for future offspring for families with congenital myopathies can be challenging—even for those disorders in which disease genes have been identified and molecular genetic testing is available. For example, nemaline myopathy is the best characterized of the myopathies at the molecular level but is genetically heterogeneous. Five disease-genes have been identified but mutations have been identified only in the minority of cases (<30%) and it is likely that a number of other disease gene mutations can result in the same clinical and pathological phenotype. In addition, for those genes that have been identified, inheritance may be autosomal dominant, sporadic (new dominant), or autosomal recessive; and an unaffected parent may have more than one affected offspring due to mosaicim for a disease-causing mutation in their germ-cells (ova or sperm; so-called *germline mosaicism*). Therefore definitive genetic counselling and prenatal diagnosis can only be offered when a disease-causing mutation has been identified and prenatal diagnosis is performed on tissue from the unborn fetus (by chorionic villus biopsy or amniocentesis). In some cases, linkage analysis may also be possible for prenatal diagnosis.

When only one person in a family is affected by a specific congenital myopathy, determining the mode of inheritance can be a problem. Clinical evaluation of both parents is necessary to rule out minor muscle weakness. Muscle biopsy of parents may be useful, but interpretation of abnormal findings can be difficult. For example if a clinically healthy parent has abnormalities on muscle biopsy, it may not be possible to distinguish whether they are a manifesting heterozygote for a recessive gene, or whether the disorder is dominant and they have no clinical manifestations (incomplete penetrance). If one parent shows overt disease clinically and typical histological abnormalities on muscle biopsy, while the other parent is healthy and shows normal findings on muscle biopsy, the likely mode of inheritance is autosomal dominant. If both parents are clinically healthy and show no abnormality on muscle biopsy, dominant transmission from one of the parents is unlikely, leaving the possibility of a new dominant mutation in the child (with minimal risk to future offspring), germline mosaicism in one of the parents (with low but significant risk to future offspring) or recessive inheritance with a 25% recurrence risk. As the molecular genetics of these disorders are clarified, some of these diagnostic issues may be resolved.

Monitoring

Prospective detection of medical complications The congenital myopathies are clinically heterogeneous in terms of age of onset, rate of progression and the sever-

ity of respiratory, cardiac, bulbar and skeletal muscle involvement. The mainstay of therapy for patients with congenital myopathy is *early detection* of disease manifestations and complications, and early referral to a *multidisciplinary team* of health care professionals for ongoing assessment and intervention. The clinical status and therapeutic needs of each patient must be assessed at regular intervals by a coordinating physician who then makes the appropriate referrals. The "coordinating physician" may be a paediatrician, neurologist or geneticist. The involvement of a Rehabilitation Specialist may also greatly assist in the coordination and appropriate timing of many of the interventions. The checklist in Table 221.3 provides a useful guide to the possible needs of this patient group. The timing of each assessment or referral, and the frequency of follow-up assessments is at the discretion of the coordinating physician. However it is anticipated that all congenital onset myopathy patients will require *at least* ongoing input from a physiotherapist and occupational therapist and possibly a speech pathologist, regular monitoring of pulmonary function, a baseline sleep study and screening for scoliosis.

Risk management

Surgical procedures and anesthetic risks Central core disease is associated with an increased risk of MH.[25,39,40] However, since the diagnosis is unknown in many patients undergoing muscle biopsy, MH precautions should be taken prior to a definitive diagnosis. Malignant hyperthermia is an autosomal dominant disorder characterized by an increase in skeletal muscle metabolism in response to certain inhalation narcotics (particularly halothane) and depolarizing muscle relaxants (particularly succinylcholine). The disorder is thought to be due to an abnormality of calcium metabolism. The triggering agent increases the myoplasmic calcium concentration resulting in an increased production of heat. The major symptom is general hyperthermia and it may be fatal if untreated. Malignant hyperthermia is still considered to be the most frequent cause of death during anesthesia. At present, the susceptibility to MH can only be diagnosed by an in vitro pharmacological contracture test.[41] Triggering anaesthetic agents should be avoided in susceptible individuals. As the first exposure to the trigger substances elicits an event in only 50% of MH susceptible patients, a previous history of tolerance of halothane or succinylcholine does not ensure that these agents can be used safely in the future anesthetics. If any surgery is planned in a patient with central core disease, or in an individual who may be at risk of MH, the anesthetist should be aware of the patient's diagnosis. Malignant hyperthermia has not been clearly associated with other congenital myopathies, although one report describes three children with nemaline myopathy in whom the heart rate decreased during induction of anesthesia for cardiac surgery, and body temperature increased during or after surgery.[42]

In general, patients with congenital myopathy

Table 221.3   Management of patients with congenital myopathy

Problem identified	Referral	Possible interventions
Skeletal muscle involvement – hypotonia – weakness – contractures	Physiotherapy Occupational therapy	Objective testing of muscle strength Regular exercise program Active and passive stretching Standing frame Orthotics/splinting—upper and lower limb Serial plaster casting Enhance mobility—walking frames or wheelchair Liaise with local services
Respiratory muscle involvement – reduced respiratory capacity – recurrent chest infections – aspiration – nocturnal hypoxia – respiratory failure	Physiotherapy Lung function tests Sleep study Respiratory physician Occupational therapy	Breathing exercises Chest physiotherapy to clear secretions Seating assessment Influenza vaccination Aggressive management of acute infections including antibiotic therapy Nocturnal ventilation Assisted ventilation Liaise with local services
Bulbar involvement – feeding and swallowing difficulties – failure to thrive	Speech pathologist Dietitian Gastroenterologist	Speech therapy Modified barium swallow Caloric supplementation/thickened feed Gavage feeding or gastrostomy feeding
Bulbar involvement – dysarthria – excessive drooling	Speech pathologist Surgeon	Speech therapy Anti-cholinergic medications Pharyngoplasty Salivary duct surgery
Developmental or psychosocial delay	Occupational therapy Physiotherapy Speech pathology Psychologist Developmental physician	Assessment Advice re: appropriate intervention/liaise with local services Developmental stimulation Home programs Reassessment if deterioration
Scoliosis	Physiotherapy Orthopaedic surgeon	Baseline assessment including spinal X-ray Monitoring of degree of curve Bracing Corrective surgery
Foot deformities	Physiotherapy Orthopaedic surgeon	Splinting/serial casting Corrective surgery
Cardiac involvement – conduction defects – cardiomyopathy – cor pulmonale	Cardiologist	ECG, Holter monitor, cardiac echo Medication if indicated
Inability to perform activities of daily living (ADL) – inability to achieve independence with bathing, toiletting, dressing, feeding – difficulties with access – handwriting difficulties	Occupational therapy Community nurse	Aides for individual ADL Wheelchair assessment Home nursing assistance Home visit and modifications School visit and modifications Typing and computer programs Car modifications Liaise with local services
Excessive weight gain – limits mobility and exacerbates weakness	Dietitian Physiotherapy	Calorie-controlled diet Exercise program
Inability to participate in sport/leisure activities	Physiotherapy Occupational therapy	Liaise with/visit schools Contact with sporting organizations for people with disabilities Hydrotherapy

Table 221.3 *continued*

Problem identified	Referral	Possible interventions
Constipation	Dietitian Physician Gastroenterologist	High fiber diet Laxatives/enemas
Depression or behavioral problems	Psychologist	Individual or family therapy Medication
Family financial and social difficulties	Social work Muscular Dystrophy Association Government Assistance Bodies	Disability allowance/pension Carers allowance Support groups Financial assistance with equipment and home modifications Transport and travel assistance
Planning future pregnancies	Geneticist Genetic counselor	Genetic counselling Planning prenatal diagnosis
Planning surgery	Consult with anesthetist Respiratory physician	Malignant hyperthermia precautions Lung function tests and physiotherapy pre-surgery
Planning future employment	Vocational counseling service Occupational therapy	Planning school studies Vocational planning Work experience Training, work placement and support
Coordination of care	Paediatrician or "subspecialist with an interest" e.g Neurologist, Geneticist, or Rehabilitation Specialist	Contact with General Practitioner via telephone and letter Liaison with local services Copy of all correspondence to key persons and family Arrange case conferences when necessary Determine timing of respiratory, orthopedic and palliative interventions

tolerate surgical procedures and general anesthetics well. However respiratory complications may occur. In our series of 143 patients with nemaline myopathy,[43] five patients had unexpected post-operative respiratory failure which necessitated prolonged ventilatory support in three patients and resulted in the death of another. Another child had an unexpected respiratory arrest 24 hours after fundoplication, and one developed persisting post-operative lobar atelectasis. Therefore, preoperative assessment of respiratory status, and performance of serial pulmonary function tests may be useful to guide timing of surgical intervention. In addition, prolonged immobility may exacerbate or worsen muscle weakness, so that patients should be mobilized as soon as possible after a surgical procedure.

Obstetric complications In general, adult females with congenital myopathies tolerate childbirth well, however there is a high incidence of obstetric complications associated with the delivery of a child with congenital myopathies presenting in the newborn period. In our series of 65 cases of neonatal onset nemaline myopathy,[43] obstetric complications were recorded in 31 cases (48%). Problems included polyhydramnios (19 cases), decreased fetal movements (24 cases), and delivery complicated by an abnormal presentation, fetal distress or failure to progress (30 cases). Eleven of 65 infants were premature, whilst 26 children were delivered by Caesarian section for unstable lie or breech presentation.

Symptomatic therapy and rehabilitation

Table 221.3 provides an overview of possible interventions necessary in the rehabilitation and ongoing patient with congenital myopathy. The main factors influencing prognosis are respiratory capacity and the development of scoliosis.[44,45] Thus the monitoring of respiratory function and the spine are essential elements in the ongoing care of these patients.

Respiratory care Respiratory problems are a common feature of congenital myopathies, and are the primary cause of death, not only in the neonatal period but throughout life. Respiratory failure can occur at any age and the degree of skeletal muscle weakness does not necessarily reflect the degree of respiratory muscle involvement.[46] Respiratory compromise occurs secondary to involvement of the intercostals and diaphragm in combination with weakening of the abdominal muscles and/or progressive scoliosis. Bulbar involvement increases the risk of aspiration, and poor nutritional status may increase susceptibility to respiratory infection.

Most patients will show restriction of their respiratory capacity on testing, even if they are symptom-free. In addition patients with congenital myopathy run a great risk of insidious nocturnal hypoxia. Symptoms include sleep disturbance, nightmares, morning headache, daytime tiredness and weight loss. However nocturnal hypoxia may occur even in the absence of morning symptoms, and several patients have experienced sudden respiratory failure.[44,45,47]

All patients with congenital myopathy should have at least baseline evaluation of their respiratory status, with frequency of re-evaluation depending on the patient's clinical status. Investigations include, lung function testing (vital capacity, forced expiratory volume in one second [FEV1], and maximal inspiratory and expiratory pressures), oximetry, evaluation of CO_2 during waking and asleep, and an assessment of bulbar function. The timing of intervention will depend on the clinical status of the patient; however any patient with a vital capacity of less than 50% of predicted value should be evaluated at least annually. Postural drainage, regular chest physiotherapy and a manually assisted cough may assist respiratory toilet in patients with bulbar weakness, reduced vital capacity and recurrent aspiration. Any respiratory infections should be treated early and aggressively, including intravenous antibiotics. Some children will require short-term assisted ventilation during intercurrent illness. The patient and their family should be provided with information and education concerning the possibility of respiratory insufficiency and the options for home mechanical ventilation. In addition, they should meet with a physician and other patients who have experience with home mechanical ventilation so that informed choices can be made, if and when ventilation is necessary.[48]

Indications for ventilatory support include CO_2 retention ($pCO_2 > 50$ mmHg), chronic hypoxia ($pO_2 < 90$ mmHg), vital capacity of less than 1 L, and recurrent pneumonia. The options for the preferred method of home mechanical ventilation will depend on the clinical status of the patient, the rate of progression and the natural history of the underlying disorder, and should be determined in conjunction with an experienced physician, the patient and their family. Options include bilevel positive airway pressure by nasal mask and tracheostomal ventilation if non-invasive means are not feasible.[48,49] Oxygen is rarely indicated, but may be necessary if oxygen saturation remains less than 90% once hypoventilation has been corrected.

The institution of home ventilation requires a large and ongoing support network for the patient and their families, and may not be appropriate for some cases of congenital myopathy. For example, some patients with severe neonatal onset congenital myopathies (for example some cases of nemaline myopathy and X-linked myotubular myopathy) require ventilation from birth and never achieve the ability to breathe independently. In such cases, it may be more appropriate to counsel families for conservative management.[16] Aggressive management is more appropriate for the older child, for whom assisted ventilation will result in marked improvement in quality of life.

Feeding difficulties Feed intolerance occurs commonly in patients with congenital myopathy presenting in the newborn period. In addition, bulbar dysfunction can result in chewing and swallowing difficulties, recurrent aspiration, gastroesophageal reflux and poor nutritional status at any age. Feeding problems in the newborn period often necessitate commencement of gavage feeds. Approximately half of these infants will improve and will come to tolerate bottle feeds and soft solids.[43] However insertion of a gastrostomy tube with or without fundoplication should be considered if problems persist after the first few months of life. Those children with relatively mild neonatal symptoms tend improve with increasing age, ultimately tolerating a full oral diet with few complications. Bulbar dysfunction, in combination with facial weakness, can also result in dysarthria, poor articulation, poor control of secretions and recurrent aspiration.

Joint contractures and scoliosis

While there is little published data on the approach to orthopaedic problems in children with specific congenital myopathies, there are many useful studies focussing on the management of patients with muscular dystrophy and other neuromuscular disorders which are of relevance to this patient population.[50,51] This section summarizes the approach to joint contractures and scoliosis used in our Neuromuscular Service.

The physiotherapist and orthopaedic surgeon play an essential role in the ongoing care of children with congenital myopathy (Table 221.3). A regular program of muscle stretches and exercise will help to prevent or minimize joint contractures and promote cardiorespiratory health. Ideally, the majority of such "therapies" should take place at home and become integrated into the child's day-to-day activities. Orthotics, splinting and serial plaster casting may be necessary particularly in the treatment of a tight Achilles tendon. Surgical release is indicated for contractures that do not respond to aggressive physiotherapy—particularly if such surgery will result in improved function, or will facilitate activities of daily living.

All patients with congenital myopathy should be monitored for the development of scoliosis, kyphosis or kyphoscoliosis. Once a curve is detected, the child should be referred to an orthopaedic surgeon and have serial spinal X-rays. Progressive spinal deformity can lead to pain and difficulty in standing, walking, sitting, or balancing. There may be deterioration in motor function and independence, and more importantly, respiratory function may be further compromised with the development of restrictive lung disease. Regular pulmonary function studies allow the clinician to establish a profile for the individual patient, and to guide the timing of intervention. Treatment options include bracing and spinal fusion (arthrodesis). Spinal bracing may be an alternative to surgery in children who are unable to walk—while it does not correct, prevent or reverse the curvature, it may improve sitting stability. Scoliosis may be difficult to treat in the child who can walk, but has significant proximal weakness. This group of patients often rely on lumbar lordosis and a side-to-side waddle to walk. Bracing or spinal arthrodesis may limit the compensatory waddle and lordosis, resulting in deterioration in gait.

Operative stabilization can be effective in halting the progression of spinal deformity. Surgery is indicated if the curve is progressing, pulmonary function is impaired, and spinal fusion is unlikely to impair motor function. The introduction of segmental spinal instrumentation with sublaminar wire fixation (incorporating Luque rods), has greatly eased post-operative management. The posterior surgical approach is considered the best way to prevent progression of spinal deformity, and to maintain correction. An anterior surgical approach in patients who rely greatly on the anterior abdominal muscles and diaphragm for respiration can lead to respiratory difficulty post-operatively and to major long-term diminution of respiratory function. The most important factors related to the timing of surgery are a high degree of flexibility of the spine and a pulmonary forced vital capacity that is reasonably stable and more than 30% predicted value. When rigidity develops, the correction of the curve is minimized and the value of the intervention is decreased.

Exercise

There is a paucity of literature concerning the risks and benefits of exercise in children with neuromuscular disorders. The only studies performed have been with Duchenne muscular dystrophy, which has limited relevance to children with less severe and non-progressive congenital myopathies. The ultimate cause of physical impairment in neuromuscular disorders is loss of normally functioning muscle fibers. While 30–40% of muscle tissue can be lost before clinical weakness is appreciated, exercise performance may be compromised at an earlier stage. Submaximal strengthening exercises with frequent rest periods are recommended for patients with neuromuscular disorders, although exercising to the point of exhaustion should be avoided.[52] Regular enjoyable low-impact activities, such as cycling or swimming, are ideal, with supervision to monitor for excessive fatigue or increased weakness.

Although no direct medical benefits have been scientifically demonstrated in children with muscle disorders, regular exercise promotes cardiovascular well-being and general fitness. Anecdotally, it has been noted that some patients with nemaline myopathy achieve significant improvement with a regular exercise regime, probably due to compensatory hypertrophy of a subset of muscle fibers (North, unpublished observations). Conversely, some patients become significantly weaker after prolonged periods of immobilization, suggesting poor recovery from disuse atrophy. In some patients, a component of their weakness and poor endurance may be due to non-myopathic disuse atrophy and, at least, this component of the problem should respond to exercise. Any exercise program should also include regular stretches to help maintain joint range of motion. Participation in regular group activities can be beneficial in terms of improved socialization, self-esteem and independence, limiting isolation and loneliness.

Future prospects

Over the next few years, it is likely that the genetic loci for the majority of congenital myopathies will be identified. The completion of the Human Genome Project, and the development of technologies for rapid automated detection of mutations (e.g. DNA micro-array) will greatly enhance our ability to provide accurate genetic counseling and prenatal diagnosis for patients and families with congenital myopathy. The identification of disease-causing mutations is the first step towards a better understanding of the pathogenesis of this group of disorders, and the development of "curative" rather than symptomatic therapies.

References

1. Shy GM, Magee KR. A new congenital non-progressive myopathy. Brain 1956;79:610–621
2. Dubowitz V. The "new" myopathies. Neuropediatrics 1969;1:137–148
3. Fardeau M, Tome FMS. Congenital myopathies. *In:* Engel AG, Franzini-Armstrong C, eds. Myology. 2nd ed. New York: McGraw-Hill, 1994:1487–1533
4. Laing NG, Wilton SD, Akkari PA, et al. A mutation in the α tropomyosin gene *TPM3* associated with autosomal dominant nemaline myopathy. Nature Genet 1995; 9:75–79
5. Tan P, Briner J, Boltshauser E, et al. Homozygosity for a nonsense mutation in the alpha-tropomyosin gene TPM3 in a patient with severe congenital nemaline myopathy. Neuromusc Disord 1999;9:573–579
6. Pelin K, Hilpela P, Donner K, et al. Mutations in the nebulin gene associated with autosomal recessive nemaline myopathy. Proc Natl Acad Sci 1999;96: 2305–2310
7. Nowak KJ, Wattanasirichaigoon D, Goebel HH, et al. Mutations in the skeletal muscle α-actin gene in patients with actin myopathy and nemaline myopathy. Nature Genetics 1999;23:208–212
7A Donner K, Ollikainen M, Ridanpaa M et al. Mutations in the β-tropomyosin (TPM2) gene – a rare cause of nemaline myopathy. Neuromusc Disord 2002;12:151–158
7B Johnston JJ, Kelley RI, Crowford TO et al. A novel nemaline myopathy in the Amish caused by a mutation in Troporin TI. Am J Human Genet 2000;67:814
7C Ferreiro A, Ouijano-Roy S, Picheraw C, et al. Mutations in the selenoprotein N gene, 21 which is implicated in rigid spine muscular dystrophy, cause the classical phenotype of mutliminicore disease Am J Hum Genet 2002;71:739–749

8. Zhang Y, Chen HS, Khanna VK, et al. A mutation in the human ryanodine receptor gene associated with central core disease. Nature Genet 1993;5:46–50

9. Quane KA, Healy JMS, Keating KE, et al. Mutations in the ryanodine receptor gene in central core disease and malignant hyperthermia. Nature Genet 1993;5:46–50

10. Laporte J, Hu L-J, Kretz C, et al. A gene mutated in X-linked myotubular myopathy defines a new putative tyrosine phosphatase family conserved in yeast. Nature Genet 1996;13:175–182

11. Vicart P, Caron A, Guicheney P, et al. A missense mutation in αB-crystallin chaperone gene causes a desmin-related myopathy. Nature Genetics 1998;20:92–95

12. Golfarb LG, Park K-Y, Cervenakova L, et al. Missense mutations in desmin associated with familial cardiac and skeletal myopathy. Nature Genetics 1998;19:402–403

13. Nicolao P, Xiang F, Gunnarson L-G, et al. Autosomal dominant myopathy with muscle weakness and early respiratory muscle involvement maps to chromosome 2q. Am J Hum Genet 1999;64:788–792

14. Melberg A, Oldfors A, Blomstrom-Lundquist C, et al. Autosomal dominant myofibrillar myopathy with arrhythmogenic right ventricular cardiomyopathy linked to chromosome 10q. Ann Neurol 1999;46:684–692

15. Goebel HH, Andersen JR. Structural congenital myopathies. 56th ENMC-sponsored International Workshop. Neuromusc Disord 1999;9:50–57

16. North KN, Laing N, Wallgren-Pettersson C. Nemaline myopathy: current concepts. J Med Genet 1997;34:705–713

17. Wallgren-Pettersson C, Clarke A. The congenital myopathies. In: Rimoin DL, Connor JM, Pyeritz RE, Emery AEH, eds. Emery and Rimoin's Principles and Practice of Medical Genetics. 3rd ed. Churchill Livingstone, 1996

18. Roig M, Hernandez MA, Salcedo S. Survival from symptomatic nemaline myopathy in the newborn period. Pediat Neurosci 1987;13:95–97

19. Banwell BL, Singh NC, Ramsay DA. Prolonged survival in neonatal nemaline myopathy. Pediatr Neurol 1994;10:335–337

20. Wallgren-Pettersson C. Congenital nemaline myopathy: a clinical follow-up study of twelve patients. J Neurol Sci 1989;89:1–14

21. Jockusch BM, Veldman H, Griffiths G, et al. Immunofluorescence microscopy of a myopathy. α-Actinin is a major constituent of nemaline rods. Exp Cell Res 1980;127:409–420

22. Wallgren-Pettersson C, Jasani B, Newman GR, et al. α-Actinin in nemaline bodies in congenital nemaline myopathy: immunological confirmation by light and electron microscopy. Neuromusc Disord. 1995;5:93–104

23. Volpe P, Damiani E, Margreth A. Fast to slow change of myosin of nemaline myopathy: electrophoretic and immunologic evidence. Neurology 1982;32:37–41

24. Miike T, Ohtani Y, Tamari H, et al. Muscle fiber type transformation in nemaline myopathy and congenital fiber type disproportion. Brain Dev 1986;8:526–532

25. Shuaib A, Paasuke RT, Brownell AKW. Central core disease. Clinical features in 13 patients. Medicine 1987;66:389–396

26. Byrne E, Blumbergs PC, Hallpike JF. Central core disease. Study of a family with five affected generations. J Neurol Sci 1982;53:77–83

27. Manzur AY, Sewry CA, Ziprin J, et al. A severe clinical and pathological variant of central core disease with possible autosomal recessive inheritance. Neuromuscular Disorders 1998;8:467–473

28. Lynch PJ, Tong J, Lehane M, et al. A mutation in the transmembrane/luminal domain of the ryanodine receptor is associated with abnormal Ca^{2+} release channel function and severe central core disease. Proc Natl Acad Sci 1999:96:4164–4169

29. Seitelberger F, Wanko T, Gavin MA. The muscle fibre in central core disease: histochemical and electron microscopic observations. Acta Neuropathol 1961;1:223–237

30. Hayashi K, Miller RG, Brownell AKW. Central core disease: ultrastructure of the sarcoplasmic reticulum and T-tubules. Muscle Nerve 1989;12:95–102

31. Wallgren-Pettersson C, Clarke A. Myotubular myopathy. In: Emery AEH, ed. Neuromuscular disorders: clinical and molecular genetics. John Wiley and Sons Ltd, 1998:263–276

32. Wallgren-Pettersson C, Thomas NST. Report of the 20th ENMC sponsored international workshop: myotubular/centronuclear myopathy. Neuromusc Disord 1994;4:71–74

33. McLeod JG, Baker W, Lethlean AK, Shorey CD. Centronuclear myopathy with autosomal dominant inheritance. J Neurol Sci 1972;15:375–387

34. Wallgren-Pettersson C, Clarke A, Samson F, et al. The myotubular myopathies: differential diagnosis of the X-linked recessive, autosomal dominant and autosomal recessive forms and present state of DNA studies. J Med Genet 1995;32:673–679

35. Goebel HH, Fardeau M. Desmin in myology. Neuromusc Disord 1995;5:161–166

36. Goebel HH, Fardeau M. Familial desmin-related myopathies and cardiomyopathies—from myopathology to molecular and clinical genetics. Neuromusc Disord 1996;6:383–388

37. Engel AG. Myofibrillar myopathy. Ann Neurol 1999;46:681–682

38. Dalakas MC, Park K-Y, Semino-Mora C, et al. Desmin myopathy; a skeletal myopathy with cardiomyopathy caused by mutations in the desmin gene. New Engl J Med 2000;342:770–779

39. Denborough MA, Dennett XK, Anderson RM. Central core disease and malignant hyperthermia. Br Med J 1973;1:272

40. Wedel DJ. Malignant hyperthermia and neuromuscular disease. Neuromusc Disord 1992;2:157–164

41. European Malignant Hyperpyrexia Group. A protocol for the investigation of malignant hyperpyrexia susceptibility. Br J Anaesth 1984;56:1267–1269

42. Asai T, Fujise K, Uchida M. Anaesthesia for cardiac surgery in children with nemaline myopathy. Anaesthesia 1992;47:405–408

43. Ryan MM, Schnell C, Strickland C, et al. Nemaline myopathy: a clinical study of 143 cases. Ann Neurol 2001;50:312–320

44. Howard RS, Wiles CM, Hirsch NP, Spencer GT. Respiratory involvement in primary muscle disorders: assessment and management. Q Journal Med 1993;86:175–189

45. Sasaki M, Yoneyama H, Nonaka I. Respiratory muscle involvement in nemaline myopathy. Pediatr Neurol 1990;6:425–427

46. Gilgoff I. Pulmonary management. In: Therapy for Childhood Neuromuscular Diseases. San Diego, 1994

47. Heckmatt JZ, Loh L, Dubowitz V. Night-time nasal ventilation in neuromuscular disease. Lancet 1990;335:579–582

48. Rutgers M, Lucassen H, Kesteren RV, Leger P. Respiratory insufficiency and ventilatory support. 39th ENMC

International workshop, Naarden, The Netherlands, 26–28 January 1996. Neuromusc Disord 1996;6:431–435

49. Guilleminault C, Phillip P, Robinson A. Sleep and neuromuscular disease: bilevel positive airway pressure by nasal mask as a treatment for sleep disordered breathing in patients with neuromuscular disease. J Neurol Neurosurg Psychiatr 1998;65:225–232

50. Shapiro F, Specht L. The diagnosis and orthopaedic treatment of childhood spinal muscular atrophy, peripheral neuropathy, Friedreich ataxia and arthrogryposis. J Bone Joint Surgery 1993;75:1699–1714

51. Hsu JD. The development of current approaches to the management of spinal deformity for patients with neuromuscular disease. Seminars in Neurology 1995;15:24–28

52. Kilmer DD, McDonald CM. Childhood progressive neuromuscular disease. In: Goldberg B, ed. Sports and exercise for children with chronic health conditions. Champaign IL, USA: Human Kinetics Publishers, 1995: 109–121

222 Muscular Dystrophies

Brenda L Banwell

Historical overview

Descriptions of boys with progressive motor paralysis (now known as "Duchenne muscular dystrophy") date back to reports by Dr. Charles Bell in 1830.[1] Dr. Edward Meryon, in his book *Practical and Pathological Researches on the Various Forms of Paralysis* published in 1864, described the clinical and pathological findings in eight affected boys from three families. He was the first to recognize the maternal inheritance of this disorder.[1] In his report he stated that "fibers were found to be completely destroyed, the sarcous element being diffused, and in many places converted into oil globules and granular matter, whilst the sarcolemma and tunic of the elementary fiber was broken down and destroyed."[1]

Over the next 100 years, genetic and phenotypically distinct forms of muscular dystrophy were recognized. In the late 1970s, genetic studies linked the Duchenne gene to chromosome Xp21, and the cDNA and protein product, dystrophin, were discovered in 1987.[2,3] Many other genes encoding structural proteins associated with the sarcolemma, nuclear membrane proteins, and proteins involved in myofiber metabolism have now been sequenced and mutations ascribed to specific forms of dystrophy. The genes for other dystrophies have yet to be discovered.

This chapter discusses the management of patients with muscular dystrophy and highlights issues pertinent to specific forms of dystrophy. Even with the best current management, the inexorable downhill progression of the dystrophic process cannot be arrested. The recent rapid advances in gene therapy, however, hold promise that the course of these diseases eventually may be mitigated.

Epidemiology

The incidence of several forms of muscular dystrophy is listed in Table 222.1. Some dystrophies show regional variability due to founder effects or the relative frequency of consanguineous marriages. The incidence of milder forms of dystrophy, mild variants of more severe dystrophies, and severe forms of dystrophy that result in death before diagnosis is likely underestimated.

Etiology

The genetically distinct forms of muscular dystrophy that have been recognized result from mutations in genes encoding integral structural proteins of the sarcolemmal membrane (α, β, γ, and δ sarcoglycan, integrin $\alpha7$) and structural proteins associated with the inner (dystrophin, plectin) or outer (laminin $\alpha2$, collagen type VI) or specialized regions of the sarcolemma (caveolin 3), with the inner nuclear membrane (emerin, lamin A/C, plectin), with muscle-specific protein kinases (myotonic dystrophy protein kinase), with muscle-specific proteases (calpain), and with proteins whose function remains to be defined (dysferlin). The distribution within muscle of proteins implicated in the various muscular dystrophies is outlined schematically in Figure 222.1. In dystrophinopathies, ultrastructural studies have shown focal loss of the sarcolemma[4] and increased calcium in the muscle fiber regions underlying the sarcolemmal defects.[5] A similar loss of sarcolemmal integrity likely underlies the pathological changes of the limb-girdle dystrophies associated with sarcoglycan mutations.[6] The defects in sarcolemmal-associated proteins likely predisposes the fiber to damage during contraction. How deficiency of proteins not associated with the

Table 222.1 Incidence and prevalence of common muscular dystrophies

Disease	Incidence/prevalence	Reference
Duchenne muscular dystrophy	1/3300	5
Becker muscular dystrophy	1/18 000–1/31 000	5
Female dystrophinopathy carriers	40/100 000	5
Manifesting female dystrophinopathy carriers	1/100 000	5
Emery–Dreifuss muscular dystrophy	1/100 000	87
Myotonic dystrophy	1/8000	53
Oculopharyngeal muscular dystrophy	1/200 000	70
Fascioscapulohumeral muscular dystrophy	1/20 000	74
Muscle–eye–brain disease	1/50 000 (Finland) and isolated cases elsewhere	98
Fukuyama congenital muscular dystrophy	7–12/100 000 (Japan)	97

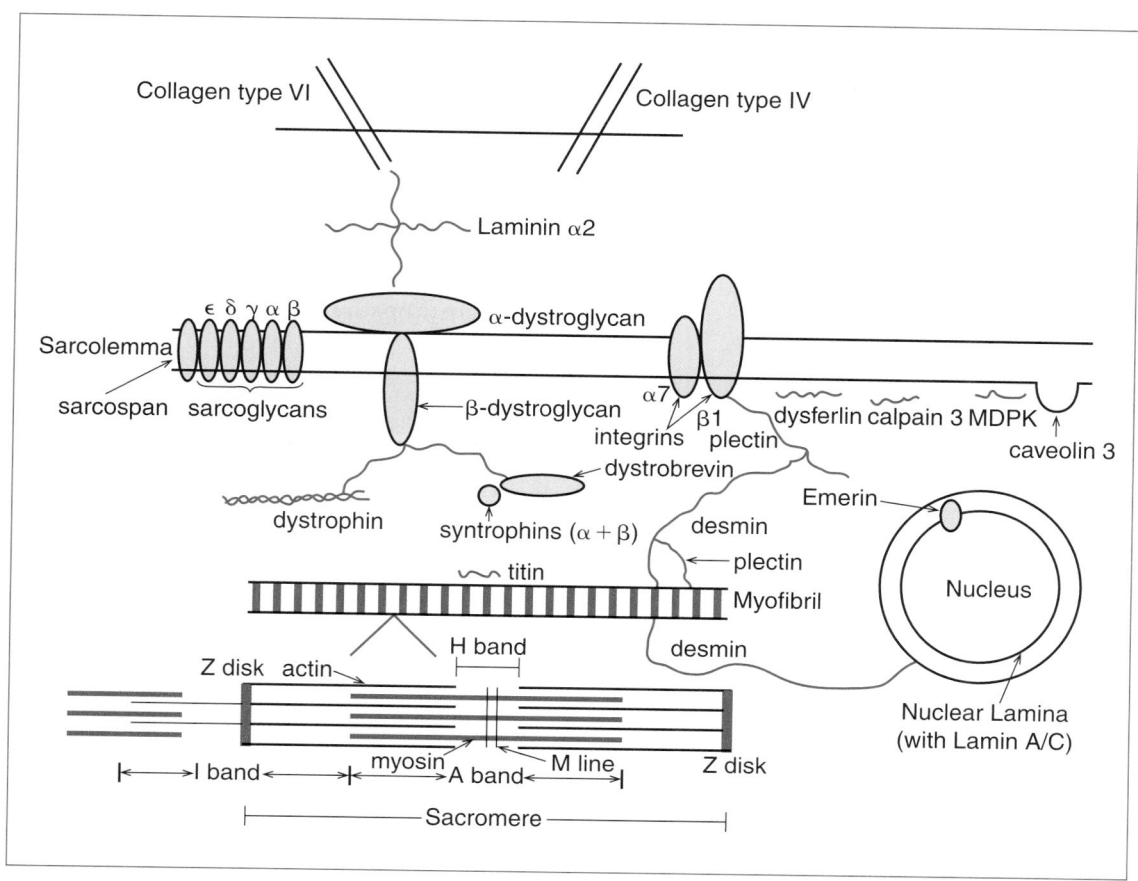

Figure 222.1 Representation of various proteins implicated in muscle disease and their distribution within the myofiber. (Only proteins discussed in the chapter are shown.) Collagen type IV and type VI, laminin α2, and α-dystroglycan are components of the basement membrane surrounding muscle; α-, β-, γ-, δ-, and ε-sarcoglycan, sarcospan, β-dystroglycan, and α7- and β1-integrins span the sarcolemma, and caveolin 3 exists in specialized regions of the sarcolemma termed "caveolae." Emerin is located in the inner nuclear membrane, and lamin A/C is a component of the inner nuclear lamina. Proteins localized to the subsarcolemmal region include dystrophin, α- and β-syntrophin, and dystrobrevin. Desmin and plectin are concentrated at the region of the Z-disk and also form important cross-linkages throughout the cytosol. The cellular distribution of dysferlin, calpain 3, and MDPK (myotonic dystrophy protein kinase) have not been fully elucidated; for convenience, these proteins are depicted in the cytosol near the sarcolemmal membrane. In the lower part of the figure, the contractile apparatus of the myofiber, the "sarcomere," is outlined. As shown, electron-dense bands termed "Z-disks" delineate the sarcomere. Thin filaments emanate from the Z-disk, forming the I band on either side of the Z-disk. The thin filaments are joined together at the Z-disk by the protein α-actinin (not shown). The I band is composed of thin filaments that extend from the Z-disk to intersect with thick filaments of the A band, troponin and tropomyosin (not shown), which form a complex important for contractile regulation, and a large intermediate filament protein, nebulin. The A band is composed of thick filaments interlaced with thin filaments for part of its length and a central region devoid of thin filaments. Thick filaments are composed primarily of myosin as well as C protein, H protein, X protein, AMP deaminase, creatine kinase, M protein, and myomesin (not shown) and are associated along their length with the giant protein titin. The midpoint of the A band is termed the "H band," which is of lower density owing to the absence of thin filaments in this region. The midpoint of the H band is termed the "M line."

sarcolemma results in disease is unknown. Why are only some forms of dystrophy manifest at birth? Why is there regional muscle involvement in most forms of dystrophy, with severely affected muscles immediately adjacent to muscles showing minimal disease? The answers to these questions await better understanding of the function, regulation, and interactions of the mutant proteins.

Genetic classification

The current classification of the muscular dystrophies

and the available genetic information are listed in Tables 222.2 to 222.5.

Diagnosis

The clinical manifestations of the muscular dystrophies vary with the age of the patient and the type of dystrophy. Features common to childhood-onset dystrophies include neonatal hypotonia, generalized muscle weakness, recurrent aspiration, weak cry, prominent head lag, decreased muscle bulk, reduced or absent tendon reflexes, and delayed acquisition of motor milestones. Later onset dystrophies present with generalized or regional muscle weakness and atrophy and reduced exercise tolerance. Patients may report symptoms of cardiac or respiratory failure (described below). The family history may document relatives who have muscle disease, cardiac disease, sudden death, reactions to anesthesia, recurrent fetal loss, or neonatal deaths. Examination of family members is important, especially in myotonic dystrophy or fascioscapulohumeral dystrophy in which mildly affected persons are often unaware of their disease.

Laboratory investigation of patients, and occasionally also of family members, includes determination of the serum level of creatine kinase (CK), electromyography (EMG) studies, electrocardiography, muscle biopsy, and genetic studies. The serum level of CK is increased in most forms of muscular dystrophy, but it also is increased in other metabolic and acquired muscle diseases. EMG demonstrates myopathic features (short-duration polyphasic motor unit potentials and, often, fibrillation potentials), and differentiates myopathy from neuropathy. Imaging studies, including

Table 222.2   Autosomal recessive dystrophies[106]

Disease	Locus	Gene Product	Gene
LGMD 2A	15q15	calpain 3	CAPN3
LGMD 2B	2p13	dysferlin	DYSF
LGMD 2C	13q12	γ-sarcoglycan	SGCG
LGMD 2D	17q12-21.33	α-sarcoglycan	SGCA
LGMD 2E	4q12	β-sarcoglycan	SGCB
LGMD 2F	5q33-q34	δ-sarcoglycan	SGCD
LGMD 2G	17q11-12	telethonin	
LGMD 2H	9q31-q34.1	E3-ubiquinone ligase	TRIM32
LGMD 2I	19q13.3	fukutin-related protein	FKRP
LGMD 2J	2q31	titin	TTN
Distal myopathy with rimmed vacuoles	9p1-q1		
Miyoshi myopathy	2q12-14	dysferlin	DYSF
Hereditary inclusion body myopathy	9p1-q1	GNE*	GNE
Epidermolysis bullosa simplex with muscular dystrophy	8q24	plectin	PLEC1

*GNE= UDP-N-acetylglucosamine 2-epimerase/N-acetylmannosamine kinase

Table 222.3   Autosomal dominant dystrophies

Disease	Locus	Gene product	Gene
LGMD 1A	5q22-q34	myotilin	MYOT
LGMD 1B	1q11-21	lamin A/C	LMNA
LGMD 1C	3p25	caveolin	CAV3
LGMD 1D	6q23		
LGMD 1E	7q		
Fascioscapulohumeral dystrophy	4q35		
Facioscapulohumeral dystrophy type 2			
Myotonic dystrophy	19q13	myotonin-protein kinase	
Myotonic dystrophy type 2	3q21	zinc finger 9	ZNF9
Oculopharyngeal muscular dystrophy	14q11.2-q13	poly(A) binding protein 2	PABP2
Bethlem myopathy	21q22.3	collagen type VI a1 or a2 subunit	COL6A1
COL6A2			
Bethlem myopathy	2q37	collagen type VI a3 subunit	COL6A3
Emery-Dreifuss-autosomal dominant type	1q11-q23	lamin A/C	LMNA
Myofibrillar Myopathy*	11q22		
2q35		αB-crystallin	
desmin		CRYAB	
DES			
Tibial muscular dystrophy	2q	titin	TTN
Autosomal dominant distal myopathy	14		
Welander's distal myopathy			
Familial Dilated Cardiomyo-pathy with conduction defect and muscular dystrophy	6q23		

* Genetically heterogeneous

Table 222.4 X-Linked dystrophies

Disease	Locus	Gene product	Gene
Duchenne dystrophy	Xp21.2	dystrophin	DYS
Becker dystrophy	Xp21.2	dystrophin	DYS
Emery-Dreifuss	Xq28	emerin	EMD
X-linked myopathy with excessive autophagy	Xq28		

Table 222.5 Congenital dystrophies[106]

Inheritance	Symbol	Disease	Locus	Gene Product	Gene
AR	MDC1A	Congenital muscular dystrophy with merosin deficiency*	6q2	laminin-α2 chain	LAMA2
AR	MDC1B	Congenital muscular dystrophy with secondary merosin deficiency			
AR	MDC1C	Congenital muscular dystrophy 1C	19q1	fukutin-related protein	FKRP
AR		Congenital muscular dystrophy with integrin deficiency	12q13	integrin-α7	ITGA7
AR	RSMD1	Congenital muscular dystrophy with rigid spine	1p35-36	selenoprotein N	SEPN1
AR	FCMD	Fukuyama muscular dystrophy	9q31-q33	fukutin	
AR	MEB	Muscle-eye-brain disease	1p32-p34	POMGnT1	
AR	WWS	Walker Warburg Syndrome			
AR	UCMD	Ullrich syndrome	21q2	collagen VI	COL6A1
			21q2		COL6A2
			2q3		COL6A3

* late onset variants exist

computed tomography (CT), magnetic resonance imaging (MRI), and ultrasonography of muscle may be useful. In Duchenne dystrophy, ultrasonographic examination is very sensitive for detecting fibrosis.[7] In other diseases, such as Miyoshi distal dystrophy, CT of the lower limbs shows a characteristic pattern of muscle involvement.[8] For most dystrophies, muscle biopsy is still the cornerstone of diagnosis. Appropriately stained or reacted frozen sections typically show myopathic features—that is, necrotic and regenerating fibers, fiber size variation, fiber splitting, internalized nuclei, and endomysial and perimysial fibrosis—as well as disease-specific features described below. Immunocytochemistry using the currently available antibodies may be diagnostic for dystrophinopathies, sarcoglycanopathies, and the dystrophies caused by deficiency of laminin α2 (merosin), emerin, integrin α7, or plectin. Commercially available genetic studies alone can be used to diagnose myotonic dystrophy or dystrophinopathy.

It is important to exclude an acquired myopathy from genetically determined dystrophy. Inflammatory myopathy, viral or parasitic myositis, toxic myopathy due to exposure to toxins or certain medications, or metabolic myopathy may present with weakness and increased serum levels of CK. The absence of previous neuromuscular complaints, a history of recent illness, onset of illness with exposure to a new medication, and rapid progression suggest an acquired process. Severe muscle pain favors an inflammatory or metabolic disorder. There are exceptions to these generalizations. Muscle pain is a frequent symptom of Becker dystrophy, and the progression of some inflammatory myopathies can be insidious. Moreover, some dystrophies appear to present more acutely either because of concomitant illness or because early symptoms were not recognized.

Management and treatment: general considerations

General health

Avoidance of obesity is extremely important for all patients with muscular dystrophy because excess weight increases the work that muscles must perform for ambulation, compromises seating, exacerbates respiratory insufficiency, and hinders self or assisted transfer.[5] The total caloric requirements vary with lean body mass, decreasing by at least 10% in nonambulatory patients even if the lean body mass remains unchanged. A well-balanced high-fiber diet is essential to prevent constipation, a problem that can be very serious in nonambulatory patients. Patients should consume adequate fluids, both to reduce constipation and to help keep respiratory secretions thin. A urine specific gravity between 1.010 and 1.015 is ideal. Dependent peripheral edema develops in many nonambulatory patients. Edema results in increased weight and decreased mobility, and it predisposes to skin ulcers and infection. Elevating the legs periodically, maximizing mobility, performing range of motion exercises, reducing dietary sodium, and the judicious use of diuretics may be helpful. Any patient in whom edema develops should be examined for signs of cardiomyopathy, respiratory insufficiency, and cor pulmonale. Certain medications, namely β-blockers, nonsteroidal anti-inflammatory agents, and calcium channel blockers, can also cause dependent edema and should be avoided if possible.

Physical and occupational therapy

The goal of physical therapy is to prolong ambulation and to prevent contractures.[7] Muscle fibrosis and imbalance between flexor and extensor muscles can result in hip, knee, or ankle contractures.[5] Passive range-of-motion exercises, performed after a brief warm-up, for approximately 30 minutes daily delay or even prevent contractures and improve ambulation.[7] Excessive exercise, indicated by muscle pain after exertion, should be avoided because it may increase muscle damage.[5] As disability proceeds, individualized aids may be of enormous benefit. Door handle modifications, handrails in the bathroom, computers, and companion dogs are a few examples. The overall goal is to increase independence and to allow patients to pursue educational, vocational, and leisure activities. *Muscular Dystrophy: The Facts*[9] and numerous publications by the Muscular Dystrophy Association of the United States and of Great Britain contain further information.

Orthopedic management

The development of contractures impedes ambulation and function of patients with muscular dystrophy.[10,11] Flexion contractures of the knees and hips produce hyperlordosis of the lower spine, and Achilles tendon contractures produce toe-walking.[10]

The surgical management of contractures is individualized but may include one or more of the following: release of flexion contractures of the hips, release of the tensor fasciae latae to correct abduction contractures, and tenotomy of the Achilles tendon combined with a posterior tibial-tendon transfer to allow dorsiflexion and eversion rather than excessive plantar flexion and inversion.[11] If performed while the patient is still ambulatory but already showing gait impairment, contracture release may prolong ambulation by 1 to 3 years.[11] However, lengthening already severely weakened muscles may further decrease strength, and intervention to restore walking after a patient has been nonambulatory for more than 3 to 6 months is of no benefit.[11] The orthopedic management of scoliosis is described below in the section on Duchenne dystrophy.

As with any operative procedure, appropriate anesthesia must be used (see below), and cardiac and respiratory function must be investigated and monitored carefully. Early and active physiotherapy is crucial in the postoperative period, and immobilization must be minimized.[10]

Respiratory care

Respiratory compromise in patients with muscular dystrophy may be associated with intercurrent chest infection or may develop as a chronic component of the underlying muscle disease.[12–17]

Respiratory management, outlined in Figure 222.2, includes the following preventive measures: avoidance of smoking or exposure to second-hand smoke, annual influenza vaccination, early and aggressive recognition and treatment of pulmonary infections, avoidance of large evening meals, and avoidance of cough suppressants and nocturnal sedatives.[7] A high protein, low calorie diet sufficient to maintain ideal body weight is recommended because obesity increases the risk of obstructive sleep apnea and further compromises respiratory function.[18]

One of the earliest symptoms of respiratory failure is exertional dyspnea.[17] Baseline pulmonary function studies should be performed on all patients at the time muscular dystrophy is diagnosed and then performed routinely with a frequency dictated by the type of dystrophy and the rate of disease progression. Weakness of the respiratory muscles results in a restrictive ventilatory defect and eventual hypercapnia.[7] Maximal inspiratory (P_{Imax}) and expiratory (P_{Emax}) pressures are often reduced by more than 50%.[7] Subsequently, the patient's vital capacity and forced expiratory volume in 1 second (FEV_1) decrease. Reduction of the vital capacity closely reflects the degree of general disability[18] and predicts the need for artificial ventilation.[19] A vital capacity less than 1.5 L, especially in combination with hypercarbia ($PaCO_2 > 45$ mm Hg) or hypoxemia ($PaO_2 < 75$ mm Hg), indicates that ventilatory support is needed.[7] As P_{Emax} decreases below 40 cm H_2O, cough becomes ineffective, causing mucous plugging and microatelectasis, which will eventually decrease O_2 diffusing capacity and lead to hypoxemia. During the period of intercostal and accessory muscle atonia associated with REM sleep, ventilation is supported by movements of the diaphragm muscle. Diaphragmatic weakness, particularly prominent in Duchenne dystrophy, results in orthopnea, and REM-sleep associated hypoventilation.[12] Paradoxical inward movement of the abdominal muscles during inspiration and more than 20% decrease in vital capacity on lying down from sitting also indicate diaphragmatic weakness. Chest wall deformities caused by shortening or fibrosis of intercostal and accessory muscles or by progressive scoliosis decrease chest wall compliance and further compromise respiratory function.[18]

Many patients with relatively static forms of dystrophy have nocturnal hypoxemia and complain of symptoms related to nocturnal hypoventilation.[20] Poor sleep, frequent nocturnal awakenings, night terrors or nightmares, nocturnal seizures, morning

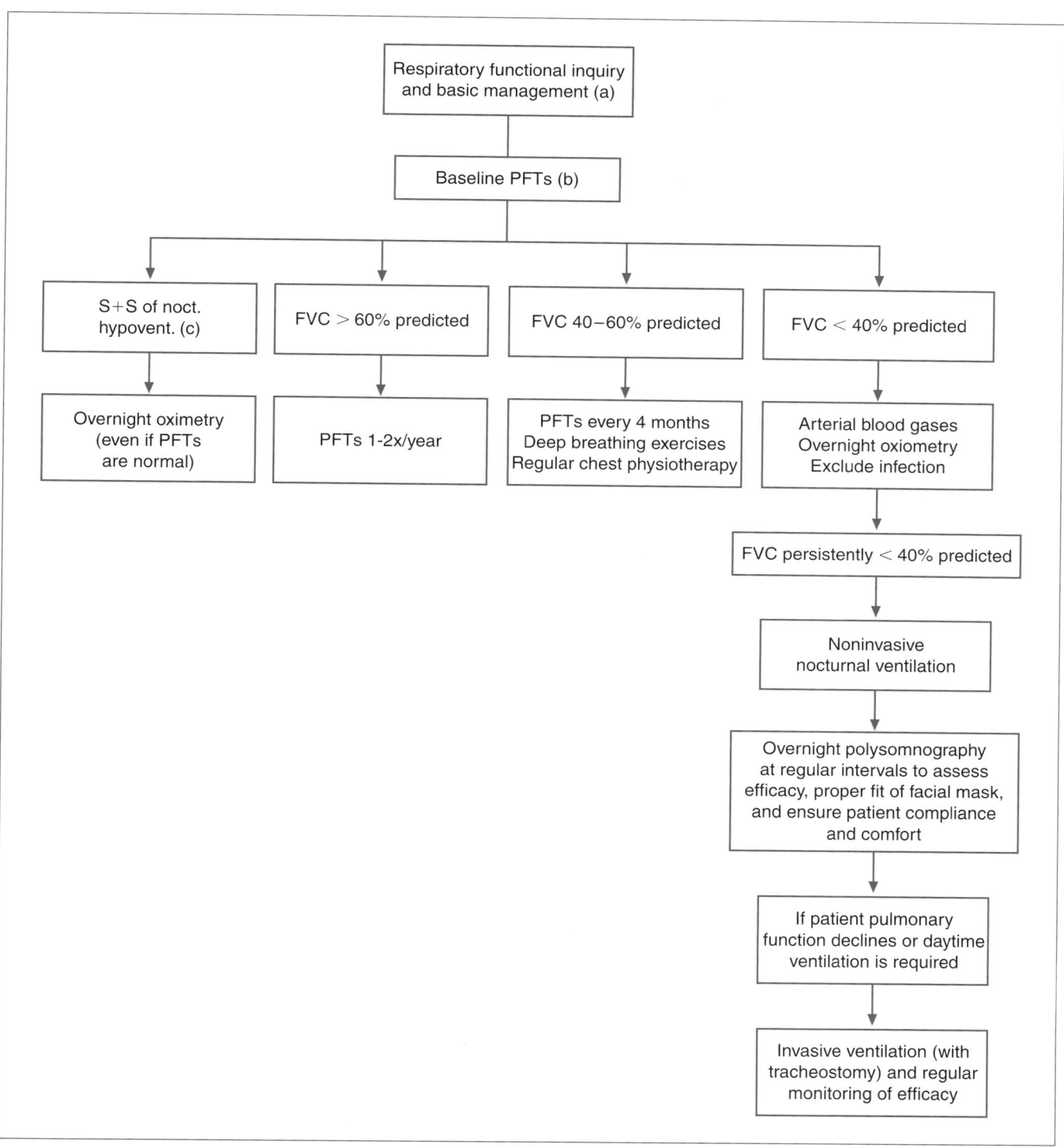

Figure 222.2   A general guide for the respiratory management of patients with neuromuscular disease. The suggested pulmonary function variables are similar to those outlined by the Muscular Dystrophy Association in its pamphlet, "Breathe Easy." The importance of general health maintenance and careful inquiry into clinical features of nocturnal hypoventilation are stressed. (a) Basic respiratory management of all patients with marked muscle weakness includes healthy diet with adequate protein, avoidance of obesity, scoliosis screening and management, early recognition and treatment of chest infection (chest physiotherapy, postural drainage, adequate hydration to thin secretions, antibiotics), and annual influenza vaccination. (b) Patients should be encouraged to exert their maximal effort, testing mask or tubing should be properly fitted for the patient, and intercurrent or recent illness should be noted. (c) Symptoms of nocturnal hypoventilation: daytime hypersomnolence, morning headache, poor or declining school/work performance, excessive fatigue, unexplained weight loss, or failure to gain weight (infant or child). FVC, forced vital capacity; noct. hypovent., nocturnal hypoventilation; PFTs, pulmonary function tests; S+S, symptoms and signs.

headaches, reduced school performance, and daytime hypersomnolence are symptoms of nocturnal hypoventilation.[7,12,13] In these patients, routine daytime pulmonary function tests may fail to detect the degree of respiratory compromise. Polysomnography in combination with oximetry and transcutaneous CO_2 measurements are required for adequate assessment.[13] For these patients, long-term nocturnal ventilation at home can dramatically improve the quality of life.[17] Biphasic positive airway pressure (BiPAP) delivered via nasal mask is well tolerated. It rapidly improves nocturnal hypoxemia, restores normal sleep patterns, eliminates morning headaches, reduces daytime somnolence, and prevents cor pulmonale.[20] Assisted ventilation is discussed further in the section on Duchenne muscular dystrophy.

Cardiovascular management

Involvement of cardiac muscle can be prominent in patients and manifesting carriers of dystrophinopathies and in patients with Emery–Dreifuss muscular dystrophy or myotonic dystrophy.[21–24] Rarely, heart disease develops in patients with fascioscapulohumeral,[23] congenital muscular dystrophy associated with merosin deficiency,[25] or sarcoglycanopathies.[26,27] Syncope or palpitations should prompt immediate cardiac assessment. Additional studies, including Holter monitoring, His bundle electrocardiograms, or echocardiography, should be performed on symptomatic patients under the guidance of a cardiologist.[22]

Anesthetic issues

Anesthetic complications can occur in patients with muscular dystrophy, particularly in those with dystrophinopathies[5] or myotonic dystrophy.[24] The complications include tachycardia, atrial and ventricular fibrillation, a malignant hyperthermia-like reaction, and, rarely, cardiac arrest.[1] These complications occur even in the absence of overt cardiomyopathy.[1] Postoperatively, a marked increase in the CK level and myoglobinuria may occur in Duchenne patients.[1] Anesthetists should avoid the use of nondepolarizing blocking agents and be alert to the risk of complications in any patient with muscular dystrophy.

Psychological issues

The diagnosis of a progressive neuromuscular disorder has an enormous impact on the psychological well-being of the patient and the patient's family. Both the patient and the family should be provided with information about local and national support groups and be offered specific counseling as needed. Because the psychological effects of a chronic disease may not be manifested immediately, it is important to periodically ask the patient and family about their emotional well-being. Many parents are reluctant to ask for help because they feel that this reflects a lack of compassion or commitment to their child. It is crucial that parents spend time together as a couple and have time to focus attention on their other children. The incidence of marital discord is greater than 50% and the divorce rate is higher than 25% for couples with a chronically ill child.[9] Many communities have a local Muscular Dystrophy Association chapter that enables parents to derive support from other parents and allows affected children to spend time with other similarly affected children. Summer camp programs provide invaluable independence and recreation for children as well as respite for families. In the case of an affected adult, a few hours each day of in-home nursing services provides relief for the spouse or care-giver.

Whenever a specific dystrophy is diagnosed, the initial discussion should occur when both parents are present. The decision to include the child in the initial discussion depends on the age and cognitive maturity of the child. Open, accurate, and honest discussions with the child over time increase understanding of the disease and encourage discussion of frustrations, fears, and expectations. It is important to encourage independence and to recognize a child's need for privacy. In late adolescence, these issues become pressing, as the teenager attempts to form peer and sexual relationships, establish educational and vocational goals, and achieve independent living arrangements. Independent living or group home arrangements can be achieved in many cases by careful planning and with home assessment by an occupational therapist.

Gene therapy

Despite reasons for optimism, numerous hurdles remain before gene therapy can be realized for muscular dystrophy.[28] Trials of dystrophin replacement using local intramuscular injections of paternally derived myoblasts failed to result in long-term dystrophin expression in mature muscle fibers and did not improve muscle strength or patient outcome in boys with Duchenne muscular dystrophy.[29]

In a recent review, Karpati[28] proposed five strategies for gene therapy: (1) specifically designed pharmacotherapy, (2) protein replacement (not applicable for structural proteins), (3) upregulation of a functional protein analogue, (4) RNA repair, and (5) somatic gene replacement. Of these strategies, the latter three hold the most promise. Utrophin, a protein encoded on chromosome 6, has 80% sequence homology to dystrophin.[30] In mature muscle, utrophin is localized to the postsynaptic sarcolemma of the neuromuscular junction.[31,32] In fetal muscle, utrophin is also expressed at the extrajunctional sarcolemma.[32] In the dystrophin-deficient (mdx) mouse and in muscle from patients with Duchenne muscular dystrophy, utrophin expression resembles the fetal pattern.[30] However, this naturally occurring up-regulation of utrophin is not sufficient to prevent ongoing muscle damage in patients with Duchenne muscular dystrophy.[5] The mdx mouse, a murine model for Duchenne muscular dystrophy, has absence of dystrophin expression in muscle, increased levels of CK, pathological features of mild dystrophy in selected muscles, and mild weakness.[5] In recent studies, mdx mice genetically engineered to overexpress a truncated utrophin minigene or full-length utrophin showed improved mechanical strength, normal or minimally increased serum levels of CK, and little or no dystrophic changes in muscle.[30,33,34] A search for methods to up-regulate utrophin expression in humans is under way.

RNA repair involves the use of targeted antisense oligonucleotides designed to bind to mutated RNA regions, change the reading frame, and bypass the original mutation.[28] It is postulated that RNA repair occurs spontaneously in the small number of dystrophin-positive (revertant) fibers found in muscle of patients with Duchenne muscular dystrophy. Early studies of this technique are also under way.

Somatic gene cell replacement for muscular dystrophy holds great promise, but numerous methodological issues remain to be solved. In general terms, replacement of a defective gene requires the following:

- Knowledge of the target gene and its promoters
- The ability to construct a full-length gene, or a functional "minigene"
- The ability to insert the gene or minigene into a vector
- Creation of a vector large enough to receive the insert, small enough to infect the tissue of interest, and modified enough to prevent vector-related disease or malignancy
- Delivery of the vector (with the inserted gene) to a significant proportion of affected muscles
- Failure of the vector to disrupt other proteins
- Processing of the newly inserted gene by the host cell must lead to continual expression and appropriate cellular localization of the target protein
- The ability of the newly expressed protein to associate with its appropriate binding partners
- Tolerance of the patient's immune system to both the vector and the newly expressed protein

Several dystrophin minigenes have been engineered successfully into viral vectors, but human trials must await the development of safe and efficient delivery systems.

Disease-specific management issues

Duchenne and Becker muscular dystrophies

Dystrophin is a large cytoskeletal protein (427 kDa) expressed in many tissues.[5] It is particularly important at the sarcolemma of skeletal muscle, where it forms a complex with a group of membrane-associated glycoproteins.[35,36] In general, frame-shifting deletions cause a virtual absence of dystrophin expression in muscle and result in the Duchenne muscular dystrophy phenotype, whereas in-frame deletions or missense mutations with attenuated dystrophin expression produce the milder Becker muscular dystrophy phenotype.[5]

Clinical features Boys with Duchenne muscular dystrophy present around the age of 3 years with a clumsy gait, frequent falls, and toe walking. The disease progresses such that ambulation is typically lost by age 13 years, and death ensues in the second or third decade. Patients with Becker muscular dystrophy may present similarly but retain the ability to walk past age 13 years, or they may be mildly affected and not present until adulthood. Some patients with Becker muscular dystrophy, and some female carriers of dystrophin mutations, present with an isolated cardiomyopathy.[5,23]

Diagnosis The diagnosis of either Duchenne or Becker muscular dystrophy rests on the history, physical examination, serum level of CK (increased), muscle biopsy findings, and genetic studies. The serum level of CK is elevated 10- to 50-fold at age 3 years and declines by approximately 20% per year thereafter.[37] Because of the enormous size of the dystrophin gene, only certain regions are screened by commercially available molecular DNA studies. Large scale deletions are detected in only 60% to 70% of affected patients.[7] It is important to recognize that a Duchenne or Becker muscular dystrophy phenotype cannot be predicted reliably on the basis of the type of mutation alone.[37] In families in which no mutation is found, linkage analysis looking for markers that cosegregate with the X-chromosome of a patient with Duchenne muscular dystrophy can be performed provided a sufficient number of family members are available. Muscle biopsy studies using antibodies directed against the carboxyl and amino termini and rod domain of dystrophin can be helpful in distinguishing Duchenne from Becker muscular dystrophy and for establishing the diagnosis of a dystrophinopathy in the 30% to 40% of such patients in whom no mutation was found.[5] Most patients with Duchenne muscular dystrophy show absence of dystrophin immunoreactivity in all but a few "revertant" fibers.[5] However, patients with partially preserved dystrophin expression cannot be guaranteed to have a Becker muscular dystrophy phenotype. Western blot analysis of the muscle shows decreased dystrophin content and an abnormal size of the mutated protein.[7] Muscle biopsy specimens may show patchy dystrophin immunoreactivity in manifesting female carriers or in unaffected mothers.[5] Because only 70% of female carriers have increased serum levels of CK, this test alone is not sufficient to exclude carrier status.[37]

Genetic counseling Genetic counseling should be provided to parents and siblings of patients with Duchenne or Becker muscular dystrophy. Female carriers have a 50% chance of producing an affected son, and 50% of female offspring will be carriers. Not all cases of dystrophinopathy are familial, because of the high spontaneous mutation rate in the dystrophin gene. The risk in these families for a subsequently affected son is approximately 7%.[37]

Prenatal diagnosis of dystrophin deficiency can be performed on amniocytes or chorionic villus samples.[37] Preimplantation diagnosis performed after a single cell biopsy at the blastomere stage before in vitro fertilization is available for families with known mutations.[38] Needle biopsy specimens from a limb muscle of an at-risk fetus can be analyzed with dystrophin antibodies, but there is a 3% to 5% miscarriage rate with the procedure.[39] Specialized techniques, such as transfection studies of fetal amniocytes or chorionic villus cells using the muscle promoter myoD with analysis of dystrophin expression in transfected cells, are performed at a few research centers.[40] Fetuses with absent dystrophin expression can then be detected.

Treatment   Despite reasons for optimism about the future of genetic therapies, current treatment for boys with Duchenne or Becker muscular dystrophy revolves around the prevention or limitation of secondary complications and maximizing the quality of life.

1. *Physical therapy*: Parents and caregivers need to be taught by an experienced therapist the appropriate techniques to prevent contractures. Range of motion exercises may cause minor discomfort. If pain is elicited, the exercise should be stopped and the child examined for fracture or joint injury. Physical therapy in combination with appropriate surgical intervention may prolong ambulation for 1 to 5 years.[7] Therapy should consist of range of motion exercises, passive stretching, and participation in enjoyable exercises and sports in the early phase (age 2 to 8 years) and continuation of stretching and participation in concentric exercises such a supervised swimming in the intermediate phase (age 8 to 12 years).[7] The use of long-leg orthotics (Dubowitz braces) may prolong the ability to stand by up to 3.9 years.[7] Fitting of these braces may require release of existing ankle and hip contractures.

2. *Scoliosis*: The development of scoliosis is invariant in Duchenne muscular dystrophy but is delayed if ambulation is prolonged into adolescence.[41] The scoliotic curve progresses at a rate of 1 to 2 degrees per month after ambulation is lost.[42] Bracing and proper seating (narrow width chair, proper back support) slow the progression of scoliosis, but surgical intervention is eventually required. Surgical intervention is indicated when the spinal curvature reaches 40 degrees or if it is rapidly progressive.[5] Spinal stabilization using the sublaminar wire technique (Luque instrumentation) and spinal arthrodesis decreases spinal curvature by approximately 50% and results in substantial improvement in seating, comfort, cosmetic appearance, and quality of life.[42] Respiratory function is not markedly improved with spinal stabilization.[11,42]

   As with any operative procedure, appropriate anesthesia must be administered (see below), and cardiac and respiratory function should be investigated and monitored carefully. Patients with dystrophin deficiency also have platelet dysfunction, despite normal bleeding time, and may require extensive blood replacement during a spinal operation.[7] Early and active physiotherapy are crucial postoperatively, and immobilization must be minimized.

3. *Corticosteroids*: Ambulation is prolonged in patients with Duchenne muscular dystrophy treated with corticosteroids.[43–46] The beneficial effects of corticosteroids may be due to increased muscle mass (decreased protein catabolism or increased protein synthesis), sarcolemmal membrane stabilization, or suppression of the immune response directed against degenerating fibers.[47] The best results are achieved with prednisone at a dose of 0.75 mg/kg daily.[43] Improvement in strength testing is noted by 10 days and becomes maximal by 2 months.[45] The subsequent rate of decline in muscle strength is decreased in comparison with that of untreated historical controls, and this effect is sustained for at least 3 years.[43] These benefits must be weighed against the potentially severe side effects of long-term prednisone administration (weight gain, cushingoid appearance, avascular necrosis of the femoral head, osteopenia, hyperglycemia, cataracts, and gastrointestinal distress). Treatment with an equivalent anti-inflammatory dose of deflazacort produces benefits similar to those observed with prednisone.[48] In the initial trial, patients given deflazacort had less weight gain but developed significantly more cataracts than patients given prednisone.[48] Immunosuppression with azathioprine (Imuran) alone or in combination with prednisone was found to be of no value.[46] A 3-month pilot trial using the anabolic steroid oxandrolone (0.1 mg/kg daily) showed statistically significant improvement in muscle strength scores comparable to the results achieved in the corticosteroid trials.[49] No side effects were reported.

4. *Respiratory management*: Seventy percent of deaths in Duchenne muscular dystrophy are respiratory.[18] Mechanical ventilation of patients with a progressive disability raises numerous ethical, financial, emotional, and practical issues for affected boys and their families. These issues must be discussed openly and, preferably, well before respiratory intervention has to be considered. In Japan, nearly all affected boys offered assisted ventilation chose to pursue this option.[19]

   Respiratory assessment requires detailed pulmonary function studies. Baseline studies should be performed shortly after diagnosis and then repeated every 6 to 12 months. After ambulation has been lost, pulmonary function must be monitored more frequently. The first stage of respiratory failure, due to a weak cough, results in accumulated secretions and microatelectasis.[50] Incentive spirometry, used before a marked decline in pulmonary function, may help reduce atelectasis. However, the use of spirometry to improve respiratory muscle strength is of no benefit.[51] Intermittent use of an Emerson In-Exsufflator, a small electrical machine that pushes a fixed volume of air into the lungs and then forcefully withdraws air and mucus, may be helpful in patients with a weak cough, especially during intercurrent pulmonary infections. The second stage of ventilatory failure relates to nocturnal hypoventilation.[50] At this point, the vital capacity is usually less than 30% of predicted and polysomnography demonstrates hypoxemia that is most prominent during REM sleep.

When vital capacity decreases to 10% to 20% of predicted or is less than 1 L, assisted ventilation should be considered.[19] The use of assisted ventilation can prolong life by as much as 10 years.[52] Both negative and positive pressure ventilation systems are available for nocturnal or full-time ventilation. Negative pressure ventilation, initially pioneered as the iron lung and now as the cuirass tank or wrap (poncho), provides ventilatory support using negative pressure to expand the chest. Although used extensively in Japan until 1992, use of this system is waning, largely because of its lack of portability, discomfort (skin abrasions, coldness), difficulty in fitting the device to the chest wall leading to air leaks, and, most importantly, increased episodes of obstructive apnea.[52] For those who use this form of ventilation, additional nasal continuous positive airway pressure is advocated to decrease the risk of upper airway obstruction.[7] Positive airway pressure ventilation can be provided using nasal or facial masks or via tracheostomy. For many patients, therapy is initiated with noninvasive nasal or facial masks, and when ventilatory requirements increase, tracheostomy is performed. Tracheostomy provides access for suction and improved pulmonary toilet. The use of a Passy–Muir valve allows enough air to pass around the tracheostomy cannula to permit speech. All patients with tracheostomies need humidified O_2 to reduce thickening of secretions. Safety measures must be observed: a back-up ventilator must be present if the patient is ventilator-dependent, ventilator maintenance must be performed routinely, caregivers must be adept at cannula replacement, and alarm systems (including chest wall apnea monitors) must be used.[7] A helpful booklet, *Breathe Easy—Respiratory Care for Children With Muscular Dystrophy*, is distributed by the Muscular Dystrophy Association.

5. *Cardiac management*: Essentially all patients with Duchenne muscular dystrophy will show signs of cardiac disease by their 18th birthday. Changes in the electrocardiogram (ECG), including conduction defects and sinus tachyarrhythmias,[37] are present by age 10 years but are of limited value in predicting marked cardiac compromise. Patients should be followed by a cardiologist after 8 years of age and should have echocardiography annually beginning at age 10.[7] Cardiac failure may be helped by treatment with angiotensin-converting enzyme inhibitors. Digoxin may cause severe arrhythmias and must be used with extreme caution.[7]

6. *Gastrointestinal management*: Dystrophin is also expressed in smooth muscle.[5] Many patients with Duchenne muscular dystrophy have impaired gastric motility and can present with severe gastric distention and intestinal pseudo-obstruction.[37] Acute abdominal pain should receive immediate medical attention.

7. *Education*: Although the role of dystrophin in the central nervous system is unknown, a functional role is suggested by the fact that the average intelligence quotient of boys with Duchenne muscular dystrophy is 1 standard deviation below the mean (even in comparison with siblings),[37] and 30% of the boys have significant learning disabilities or are mentally retarded. Educational needs must be assessed and modified if required.

Myotonic dystrophy

"Myotonic dystrophy" is the most common form of muscular dystrophy in adults.[53]

Genetics The myotonic dystrophy gene localizes to chromosome 19q13.3. The genetic defect results from a trinucleotide (CTG) expansion in the 3′ noncoding region of the myotonic dystrophy protein kinase (*DMPK*) gene.[54] The number of (CTG) repeats correlates positively with disease severity.[55] Patients with minimally expanded repeats $(CTG)_{38-60}$ may be asymptomatic and have normal findings on electromyography.[56] Genetic anticipation, the tendency for disease severity (and number of expanded repeats) to increase in subsequent generations, occurs and is especially likely when the mother is the affected parent.[24] DMPK is a transmembrane protein localized to the sarcoplasmic reticulum and appears to be expressed predominantly in type I fibers, at the neuromuscular junction, and in intrafusal fibers of the muscle spindle.[54] The function of DMPK and the mechanism whereby expansion in the noncoding region of the protein results in disease are not understood. Recent studies have shown a reduction in expression of DMPK in muscle specimens from affected patients, suggesting a dominant negative effect of the trinucleotide expansion at the RNA level.[57] Alternatively, the expanded region may disrupt function of a contiguous gene, such as the myotonic dystrophy-associated homeobox gene (*DMAHP*).[58]

Clinical features

Myotonic dystrophy is a multisystem disorder of variable severity, and many mildly affected patients are unaware of their diagnosis. Affected patients have weakness of facial (ptosis, long myopathic facies), jaw (temporomandibular dislocations), distal limb, and, to a lesser degree, proximal muscles of the shoulder and pelvic girdle.[24] Limb weakness is usually mild and progresses slowly. Weakness of ankle dorsiflexion as well as more proximal weakness necessitates use of a cane or wheelchair by more severely affected patients.[24] "Action myotonia" is often described by patients as difficulty in releasing their grip or in initiating voluntary movements. "Percussion myotonia" is best demonstrated in the tongue, hand, or finger extensor muscles by firmly tapping the muscle with a reflex hammer.

Cardiac manifestations, including conduction block and tachyarrhythmias due to degeneration of the cardiac conducting system, can occur in otherwise mildly affected patients. More than 90% of patients with myotonic dystrophy show gradually progressive ECG abnormalities, which may require His-bundle as well as routine ECG recordings for diagnosis.[24] Sudden death is well documented.

The diaphragm is often involved, resulting in nocturnal respiratory compromise and manifesting as daytime hypersomnolence.[59] Although weakness of respiratory and facial muscles and craniofacial abnormalities, including micrognathia, predispose to respiratory compromise, an additional defect in central respiratory drive has also been suggested.[13]

The involvement of smooth muscle causes disturbed swallowing, constipation, weakness of the anal sphincter (especially notable in affected children and often mistaken for abuse), and delayed gallbladder emptying, with an increased incidence of gallstones.[24]

Cataracts develop in most patients with myotonic dystrophy, and retinal degeneration also can occur. Examination with a slit lamp to look for multicolored subcapsular cataracts and a detailed retinal examination should be performed annually.[24]

Endocrine manifestations include testicular atrophy, reduced fertility, hyperglycemia with increased insulin resistance (true diabetes is rare), and early-onset frontal balding.[24,53]

The combination of effects on the uterine smooth muscle and the endocrine system results in a high incidence of pregnancy complications, including fetal loss, hydramnios, prolonged labor, retained placenta, postpartum hemorrhage, and an increased risk of premature delivery.[24]

A more severe form of myotonic dystrophy occurs in congenitally affected neonates. Affected infants have severe bifacial weakness with a "tented mouth," poor feeding, diffuse hypotonia, thin ribs, elevated diaphragms, and respiratory failure often requiring artificial ventilation. Some infants also have arthrogryposis and hydrocephalus.[24,60] Neonatal mortality is high. In one study, all infants who required ventilation for more than 4 weeks eventually succumbed, even if they were weaned successfully from ventilatory support.[61] In less severely affected infants, motor development is delayed but ambulation eventually is achieved.[60] Cognition is significantly impaired in at least two-thirds of affected children, and few are of normal intelligence.[24]

Diagnosis   Serum CK levels are normal or minimally increased.[24] Muscle biopsy findings include increased central nuclei, ringed fibers, type I fiber atrophy, sarcoplasmic masses, and a variable degree of fibrosis.[24] EMG studies show electrical myotonia consisting of discharges that wax and wane in frequency and amplitude as well as positive sharp waves, fibrillation potentials, and myopathic motor units. EMG studies rarely show myotonia until late childhood. The presence of myotonia early in life suggests the diagnosis of a nondystrophic myotonic disorder.[24] Because many mildly affected women are unaware of their condition until the birth of an affected child, EMG should be performed on all mothers of severely hypotonic neonates.

Management

1. *Myotonia*: Unlike other myotonic disorders, the myotonia of myotonic dystrophy is rarely disabling.[24] In the few patients with marked myotonia, phenytoin (100 mg 3 times daily) may be of benefit. Women must be warned about the risk of teratogenesis, and phenytoin therapy should be stopped before conception. Medications such as tocainide, procainamide, and quinidine used to treat other myotonic disorders may exacerbate cardiac arrhythmias and should be avoided.[24]

2. *Anesthesia*: A malignant hyperthermia-like reaction, postulated to be due to abnormal calcium influx from the extracellular space, may occur with depolarizing muscle relaxants and neostigmine.[24] It is critical that anesthetists be aware of the diagnosis of myotonic dystrophy preoperatively. A medic alert bracelet is advised.

3. *Cardiac*: Signs of progressive conduction defects or symptoms of syncope or palpitations should prompt immediate cardiac assessment and Holter monitoring. Pacemaker insertion may be required.[53]

4. *Respiratory*: Hypersomnia may be improved but not entirely reversed by nocturnal assisted ventilation. In these patients, methylphenidate may enhance alertness.[13,59] Respiratory muscle training can improve respiratory strength.[62] Opiates, barbiturates, and benzodiazepines can cause marked respiratory depression and should be prescribed with caution. Nocturnal sedatives should be avoided.[24]

Patients with an autosomal dominant disorder that shares many of the features of myotonic dystrophy but without an expanded trinucleotide repeat on chromosome 19 have been reported.[63–66] The disorder is genetically and clinically heterogeneous. The terms "proximal myotonic dystrophy" and "myotonic dystrophy type 2" have been applied and some kindreds have been linked to chromosome 3q.[7,66–68]

Oculopharyngeal muscular dystrophy

Genetics   Genetic studies show an expanded (GCG) repeat from $(GCG)_6$ to $(GCG)_{8-13}$ in the amino terminus of the poly(A) binding protein 2 gene (*PABP2*) located on chromosome 14q11.[69] Inheritance in these families follows an autosomal dominant pattern. Two percent of the normal population harbor a single copy of an alternative $(GCG)_7$ allele, which when combined with an expanded $(GCG)_{8-13}$ allele produces a particularly severe phenotype. Patients homozygous for the $(GCG)_7$ allele are mildly symptomatic, and these kindreds show an autosomal recessive pattern of inheritance.[69] Although the function of the *PABP2* gene has yet to be elucidated, it is postulated that expansions of the polyalanine tract may cause aggregation and possibly defective degradation of the poly(A) binding protein. These abnormal aggregates may correspond to the filamentous 7- to 10-nm nuclear inclusions that are the pathological signature of the disease.[70]

Clinical features   Oculopharyngeal muscular dystrophy presents in the 5th to 6th decade of life with progressive dysphagia, ptosis, and proximal muscle weakness.[69,70] When ptosis is severe, the patient tilts the head back and contracts the frontalis muscle in order to see.[70]

Diagnosis The serum levels of CK usually are normal, and EMG studies show a myopathic pattern.[70] Increased serum levels of IgA and IgG were reported in French-Canadian pedigrees, but this could have been related to intercurrent pulmonary infections due to chronic aspiration.[70] Muscle biopsy specimens show atrophic fibers, rimmed vacuoles (especially in atrophic fibers), scattered ragged red fibers, and degenerating fibers.[70] Intranuclear inclusions consisting of 7- to 10-nm filaments are demonstrated by electron microscopy.[70]

In the presence of a strong family history of late-onset ptosis and dysphagia, the diagnosis of oculopharyngeal muscular dystrophy is straightforward. Mitochondrial myopathy and myasthenia gravis are the main differential diagnoses. Short stature, deafness, central nervous system involvement, increased serum levels of lactate, pigmented retinopathy and night blindness, onset before age 20 years, and a maternal pattern of inheritance suggest a mitochondrial disorder. The presence of circulating acetylcholine receptor antibodies, a decremental response to repetitive stimulation during EMG, and a history of fatiguable weakness point to a myasthenic disorder.

Treatment
1. *Dysphagia*: Patients with oculopharyngeal muscular dystrophy have dysfunction of the striated muscle of the upper one-third of the esophagus (cricopharyngeal achalasia). The failure of the cricopharyngeal muscles to contract properly results in pooling of secretions and food in the hypopharynx and predisposes to aspiration.[71] Severe difficulty with swallowing leads to reduced oral intake and subsequent malnutrition. Patients who require more than 7 seconds to drink 80 mL of ice water are likely to have significant achalasia, and formal swallowing studies should be performed.[72] Cricopharyngomyotomy provides dramatic relief of the obstruction.[73]
2. *Ptosis*: Ptosis, defined as a palpebral fissure width less than 8 mm,[73] may be improved with the use of lid crutches or may be corrected with blepharoplasty.[70]

Fascioscapulohumeral muscular dystrophy

Genetics Fascioscapulohumeral muscular dystrophy is an autosomal dominant disorder, with 10% of cases due to spontaneous mutations.[74,75] The most severely affected patients are more likely to have spontaneous mutations or to have inherited the disorder from their mother.[76] The genetic locus for this condition is at the telomeric region 4q35 and is associated with deletion of an integral number of tandemly arrayed 35- to 300-kb repeats.[77] This likely exerts an adverse effect on upstream genes (position effect variegation), but the genes whose functions are altered have not been discovered.[77] There is a direct correlation between the number of deleted repeats and the severity of disease.[76]

Clinical features Fascioscapulohumeral muscular dystrophy is characterized by weakness of the facial, upper limb, and shoulder girdle muscles, with later involvement of lower extremity muscles in about 20% of cases.[74] Weakness of the anterior tibial muscles produces a footdrop gait, which can become disabling for some patients.[78] Weakness of the shoulder girdle results in scapular instability, marked limitation in arm abduction, and the characteristic "scapular winging."[79] Hearing loss and retinal venous anomalies are common but may be subclinical.[78] The risk of Coats disease (retinal telangiectasias, exudate, and retinal detachment) is increased.[78]

A more severe congenital variant presents with one or more of the following: severe facial diplegia, marked sensorineural hearing loss, Coats disease, and weakness that may progress to wheelchair dependence in the second decade of life.[80,81]

Diagnosis Pathological changes in muscle are variable and reflect the regional and asymmetrical distribution of the disease. A biopsy specimen from a mild to moderately affected muscle shows increased fiber size variation, increased central nuclei, occasional necrotic fibers, fibers with a lobulated distribution of oxidative enzymes, and increased endomysial and perimysial connective tissue.[78] In some cases, small perivascular, endomysial, or perimysial collections of mononuclear cells are also present.[78] Approximately 60% to 80% of patients with fascioscapulohumeral muscular dystrophy have a modest increase in the serum level of CK, and EMG demonstrates a myopathic pattern.[78]

Treatment Many patients with fascioscapulohumeral muscular dystrophy are affected only mildly and require no specific treatment.

1. *Scapular arthrodesis*: For patients with severe limitation of arm abduction, scapular arthrodesis can be considered. Scapular arthrodesis involves the use of an iliac crest bone graft and wiring to fix the scapula to the thoracic rib cage.[79] The procedure offers long-lasting improvement in shoulder movement, but it is associated with the risk of perioperative pneumothorax and pulmonary atelectasis.[79]
2. *Medications*: Treatment with corticosteroids does not increase a patient's strength.[82] A pilot trial of the β_2-agonist albuterol showed a 12% improvement in muscle strength over 3 months.[83]
3. *Ophthalmology*: Visual loss due to Coats disease may be prevented by early diagnosis and therapeutic photocoagulation of abnormal vessels.[80]
4. *Audiology*: The sensorineural hearing loss in congenitally affected patients may be improved with hearing aids. Early recognition and intervention are important for language development.

Emery–Dreifuss muscular dystrophy

Genetics Two phenotypically similar diseases are termed "X-linked" and "autosomal dominant" Emery–Dreifuss muscular dystrophy. The X-linked form is due to mutations in the nuclear membrane-associated protein emerin.[84] The gene for the autosomal dominant form encodes the nuclear lamina-associated protein lamin A/C[85] and appears to be an allelic disorder to the autosomal dominant limb girdle dystrophy associated with cardiac involvement (LGMD 1B).[86] How mutations in these genes result in muscular dystrophy is not understood.

Clinical features Both forms of Emery–Dreifuss muscular dystrophy are characterized by the early onset of elbow, neck, and Achilles tendon contractures, slowly progressive wasting and weakness of the proximal muscles, and potentially lethal cardiac conduction block and cardiomyopathy.[85]

Diagnosis The serum level of CK is moderately increased, and EMG shows myopathic features with rare fasciculations.[87] Muscle biopsy studies demonstrate myopathic features and angulated atrophic type I fibers.[87] In the X-linked form of the disease, immunostains for the nuclear lamina-associated protein emerin show reduced or absence of nuclear membrane staining. Emerin is also expressed in skin, and the diagnosis of an affected male or a carrier female can be made by immunostaining skin biopsy specimens.[88]

Treatment Treatment in Emery–Dreifuss muscular dystrophy is aimed at preventing the cardiac complications of the disease. Up to 40% of the patients die suddenly, most without preceding cardiac symptoms.[89] Thus, early diagnosis of the disease is essential. All patients should be monitored closely by a cardiologist. Timely insertion of a cardiac pacemaker is lifesaving.[87]

Congenital muscular dystrophy

Genetics Congenital muscular dystrophies are degenerative disorders of muscle with in utero or early infantile onset. "Merosin-deficient congenital muscular dystrophy" is associated with mutations in the *LAMA2* gene encoding the laminin α2 chain (merosin), a component of the basement membrane surrounding muscle.[90–92] Congenital muscular dystrophy with preserved laminin α2 expression and without severe structural abnormalities of the central nervous system is likely a genetically heterogeneous disorder.[91] A small number of these patients have been reported to have mutations in the integrin α7 gene.[93]

Prenatal diagnosis of merosin-deficient congenital muscular dystrophy can be performed on trophoblast tissue obtained from chorionic villus sampling.[94] This test is reliable only in families with a complete absence of laminin α2 (merosin). Confirmatory linkage analysis should also be performed.[94]

Three forms of congenital muscular dystrophy are associated with severe central nervous system anomalies.[95] "Fukuyama congenital muscular dystrophy" is the second commonest form of muscular dystrophy in Japan,[96] but it is not restricted to the Asian population. It is an autosomal recessive disorder due to mutations in the protein fukutin encoded on chromosome 9q31.[97] The function of fukutin, a secreted protein, is unknown.[97] "Muscle–eye–brain disease" has been reported predominantly in Finland and is linked to chromosome 1p32–p34.[98] The third and most severe form is Walker–Warburg syndrome. The locus for this disorder has not been mapped.[99]

Clinical features Neonates have marked hypotonia, weakness, increased serum levels of CK, and delayed motor development. Many also have or develop contractures and have marked respiratory and feeding difficulties.[91,100]

Patients with merosin-deficient congenital muscular dystrophy have severe nonprogressive weakness; they are able to sit by age 3 years but have poor head control and most remain wheelchair-dependent. Rarely, patients with partial merosin deficiency present with a limb-girdle distribution of weakness,[101] which may manifest in adulthood.[102] Cognition is usually normal in congenital or late-onset cases, despite MRI scans that demonstrate abnormally high T2 signal in the white matter.[95] However, a seizure disorder develops in up to 30% of patients.[103] Merosin is also expressed in Schwann cells, and merosin-deficient patients have a mild demyelinating peripheral neuropathy.[91] Rarely, there is cardiac involvement.[25]

Congenital muscular dystrophy associated with normal cognition, normal findings on neuroimaging, and preserved merosin expression is termed "merosin-positive," or "pure," congenital muscular dystrophy. These children usually are affected less severely than those with merosin-negative congenital muscular dystrophy, and ambulation may eventually be achieved.[91]

Fukuyama congenital muscular dystrophy, muscle–eye–brain disease, and Walker–Warburg syndrome are associated with severe central nervous system malformations (one or more of the following: lissencephaly, polymicrogyria, polymacrogyria, hydrocephalus, encephalocele, malformations of the cerebellum and midline structures, and abnormal white matter) and ocular manifestations (retinal detachment, severe myopia, macrocornea).[91,99,100,104,105]

Patients with Fukuyama congenital muscular dystrophy are weak and few attain ambulation. Most are mentally retarded, with IQ scores between 20 and 90, and 20% have epilepsy.[91] Ocular abnormalities may be present, but most patients have some functional vision.[91] Survival is into the second decade of life.[91]

Muscle–eye–brain disease is associated with facial dysmorphism (prominent forehead, narrow temporal areas) and severe central nervous system and ocular malformations. Patients may survive into late adulthood but are severely retarded.[98]

Patients with Walker–Warburg syndrome typically

die within the first 6 months of life, have brain and ocular malformations, and are clinically blind.[99]

Diagnosis Muscle biopsy findings in all the forms of congenital muscular dystrophy show prominent fiber size variation and fibrosis. Necrotic fibers are rare and help to differentiate congenital muscular dystrophy from Duchenne dystrophy.[106] Antibodies directed against the laminin α2 chain are attenuated or absent in muscle and skin in merosin-deficient patients; thus, biopsy of either tissue may be useful.[91] It is important to note that some merosin-deficient patients have attenuated reactivity only with antibodies directed against the 300-kD fragment that contains the N terminal region of the laminin α2 chain and preserved reactivity with antibodies directed against the 80-kD isoform that contains the C terminal end of the molecule.[91] Thus, both antibodies should be used if merosin deficiency is suspected.

Treatment Management of children with congenital muscular dystrophy centers on prevention of contractures and scoliosis and requires close monitoring of respiratory function. Seizures should be treated with conventional anticonvulsant agents.

Summary

This chapter highlights specific issues in the management of the more common forms of muscular dystrophy. As the disease loci are mapped, the candidate genes sequenced, and the physiological function and cellular localization of the putative proteins discovered, specific therapies and possibly cures for these debilitating conditions may emerge.

References

1. Emery A. Duchenne Muscular Dystrophy. 2nd edn. Oxford: Oxford University Press, 1993
2. Koenig M, Hoffman EP, Bertelson CJ, et al. Complete cloning of the Duchenne muscular dystrophy (DMD) cDNA and preliminary genomic organization of the DMD gene in normal and affected individuals. Cell 1987;50(3):509–517
3. Hoffman EP, Brown RH Jr, Krunkel LM. Dystrophin: the protein product of the Duchenne muscular dystrophy locus. Cell 1987;51(6):919–928
4. Mokri B, Engel AG. Duchenne dystrophy: electron microscopic findings pointing to a basic or early abnormality in the plasma membrane of the muscle fiber. Neurology 1975;25(12):1111–1120
5. Engel AG, Yamamoto M, Fischbeck KH. Dystrophinopathies. In: Engel AG, Franzini-Armstrong C, eds. Myology. New York: McGraw-Hill, 1994: 1133–1187
6. Holt KH, Lim LE, Straub V, et al. Functional rescue of the sarcoglycan complex in the BIO 14.6 hamster using delta-sarcoglycan gene transfer. Mol Cell 1998;1(6):841–848
7. Scheuerbrandt G. First meeting of the Duchenne Parent Project in Europe: Treatment of Duchenne Muscular Dystrophy. 7–8 November 1997, Rotterdam, The Netherlands. Neuromuscul Disord 1998;8(3–4):213–219
8. Barohn RJ, Amato AA, Griggs RC. Overview of distal myopathies: from the clinical to the molecular. Neuromuscul Disord 1998;8(5):309–316
9. Emery A. Muscular Dystrophy—The Facts. Oxford: Oxford University Press, 1994
10. Goertzen M, Baltzer A, Voit T. Clinical results of early orthopaedic management in Duchenne muscular dystrophy. Neuropediatrics 1995;26(5):257–259
11. Shapiro R, Specht L. The diagnosis and orthopaedic treatment of inherited muscular diseases of childhood [see comments]. J Bone Joint Surg Am 1993; 75(3):439–454
12. Barbe F, Quera-Salva MA, McCann C, et al. Sleep-related respiratory disturbances in patients with Duchenne muscular dystrophy. Eur Respir J 1994;7(8):1403–1408
13. Barthlen GM. Nocturnal respiratory failure as an indication of noninvasive ventilation in the patient with neuromuscular disease [see comments]. Respiration 1997;64 Suppl 1:35–38
14. Birnkrant DJ, Pope JF, Eiben RM. Management of the respiratory complications of neuromuscular diseases in the pediatric intensive care unit. J Child Neurol 1999;14(3):139–143
15. Howard RS, Wiles CM, Hirsch NP, Spencer GT. Respiratory involvement in primary muscle disorders: assessment and management. Q J Med 1993; 86(3):175–189
16. Kelly BJ, Luce JM. The diagnosis and management of neuromuscular diseases causing respiratory failure. Chest 1991;99(6):1485–1494
17. Polkey MI, Lyall RA, Moxham J, Leigh PN. Respiratory aspects of neurological disease. J Neurol Neurosurg Psychiatry 1999;66(1):5–15
18. Smith PE, Calverley PM, Edwards RH, et al. Practical problems in the respiratory care of patients with muscular dystrophy. N Engl J Med 1987;316(19):1197–1205
19. Fukunaga H, Okubo R, Moritoyo T, et al. Long-term follow-up of patients with Duchenne muscular dystrophy receiving ventilatory support. Muscle Nerve 1993;16(5):554–558
20. Heckmatt JZ, Loh L, Dubowitz V. Nocturnal hypoventilation in children with nonprogressive neuromuscular disease. Pediatrics 1989;83(2):250–255
21. Ortiz-Lopez R, Li H, Su J, et al. Evidence for a dystrophin missense mutation as a cause of X-linked dilated cardiomyopathy [see comments]. Circulation 1997;95(10):2434–2440
22. Stollberger C, Finsterer J, Keller H, et al. Progression of cardiac involvement in patients with myotonic dystrophy, Becker's muscular dystrophy and mitochondrial myopathy during a 2-year follow-up. Cardiology 1998;90(3):173–179
23. de Visser M, de Voogt WG, la Riviere GV. The heart in Becker muscular dystrophy, facioscapulohumeral dystrophy, and Bethlem myopathy. Muscle Nerve 1992; 15(5):591–596
24. Harper PS, Rudel R. Myotonic dystrophy. In: Engel AG, Franzini-Armstrong C, eds. Myology. New York: McGraw-Hill Inc., 1994:1192–1219
25. Spyrou N, Philpot J, Foale R, et al. Evidence of left ventricular dysfunction in children with merosin-deficient congenital muscular dystrophy. Am Heart J 1998;136(3):474–476
26. Melacini P, Fanin M, Duggan DJ, et al. Heart involvement in muscular dystrophies due to sarcoglycan gene mutations. Muscle Nerve 1999;22(4):473–479
27. Mascarenhas DAN, Spodick DH, Chad DA, et al. Cardiomyopathy of limb-girdle muscular dystrophy. J Am Coll Cardiol 1994;24:1328–1333
28. Karpati G, Pari G, Molnar MJ. Molecular therapy for genetic muscle diseases—status 1999. Clin Genet 1999;55(1):1–8

29. Karpati G, Ajdukovic D, Arnold D, et al. Myoblast transfer in Duchenne muscular dystrophy [see comments]. Ann Neurol 1993;34(1):8–17

30. Deconinck N, Tinsley J, De Backer F, et al. Expression of truncated utrophin leads to major functional improvements in dystrophin-deficient muscles of mice. Nat Med 1997;3(11):1216–1221

31. Gramolini AO, Jasmin BJ. Duchenne muscular dystrophy and the neuromuscular junction: the utrophin link. Bioessays 1997;19(9):747–750

32. Gramolini AO, Dennis CL, Tinsley JM, et al. Local transcriptional control of utrophin expression at the neuromuscular synapse. J Biol Chem 1997; 272(13):8117–8120

33. Tinsley JM, Potter AC, Phelps SR, et al. Amelioration of the dystrophic phenotype of mdx mice using a truncated utrophin transgene [see comments]. Nature 1996;384(6607):349–353

34. Tinsley J, Deconinck N, Fisher R, et al. Expression of full-length utrophin prevents muscular dystrophy in mdx mice. Nat Med 1998;4(12):1441–1444

35. Ozawa E, Noguchi S, Mizuno Y, et al. From dystrophinopathy to sarcoglycanopathy: evolution of a concept of muscular dystrophy. Muscle Nerve 1998; 21(4):421–438

36. Ohlendieck K, Matsumura K, Ionasescu VV, et al. Duchenne muscular dystrophy: deficiency of dystrophin-associated proteins in the sarcolemma. Neurology 1993;43(4):795–800

37. Miller RG, Hoffman EP. Molecular diagnosis and modern management of Duchenne muscular dystrophy. Neurol Clin 1994;12(4):699–725

38. Holding C, Bentley D, Roberts R, et al. Development and validation of laboratory procedures for preimplantation diagnosis of Duchenne muscular dystrophy. J Med Genet 1993;30(11):903–909

39. Benzie RJ, Ray P, Thompson D, et al. Prenatal exclusion of Duchenne muscular dystrophy by fetal muscle biopsy. Prenat Diagn 1994;14(4):235–238

40. Sancho S, Mongini T, Tanji K, et al. Analysis of dystrophin expression after activation of myogenesis in amniocytes, chorionic-villus cells, and fibroblasts. A new method for diagnosing Duchenne's muscular dystrophy. N Engl J Med 1993;329(13):915–920

41. Rodillo EB, Fernandez-Bermejo E, Heckmatt JZ, Dubowitz V. Prevention of rapidly progressive scoliosis in Duchenne muscular dystrophy by prolongation of walking with orthoses. J Child Neurol 1988: 3(4):269–274

42. Granata C, Merlini L, Cervellati S, et al. Long-term results of spine surgery in Duchenne muscular dystrophy [see comments]. Neuromuscul Disord 1996; 6(1):61–68

43. Fenichel GM, Mendell JR, Moxley RT, III, et al. A comparison of daily and alternate-day prednisone therapy in the treatment of Duchenne muscular dystrophy. Arch Neurol 1991;48(6):575–579

44. Fenichel GM, Florence JM, Pestronk A, et al. Long-term benefit from prednisone therapy in Duchenne muscular dystrophy. Neurology 1991;41(12):1874–1877

45. Griggs RC, Moxley RT, III, Mendell JR, et al. Prednisone in Duchenne dystrophy. A randomized, controlled trial defining the time course and dose response. Clinical Investigation of Duchenne Dystrophy Group. Arch Neurol 1991;48(4):383–388

46. Griggs RC, Moxley RT, III, Mendell JR, et al. Duchenne dystrophy: randomized, controlled trial of prednisone (18 months) and azathioprine (12 months) [see comments]. Neurology 1993;43(3 Pt 1):520–527

47. Dubrovsky AL, Angelini C, Bonifati DM, et al. Steroids in muscular dystrophy: where do we stand? Neuromuscul Disord 1998;8(6):380–384

48. Reitter B. Deflazacort vs. prednisone in Duchenne muscular dystrophy: trends of an ongoing study. Brain Dev 1995;17Suppl:39–43

49. Fenichel G, Pestronk A, Florence J, et al. A beneficial effect of oxandrolone in the treatment of Duchenne muscular dystrophy: a pilot study. Neurology 1997; 48(5):1225–1226

50. Lyager S, Steffensen B, Juhl B. Indicators of need for mechanical ventilation in Duchenne muscular dystrophy and spinal muscular atrophy. Chest 1995; 108(3):779–785

51. Rodillo E, Noble-Jamieson CM, Aber V, et al. Respiratory muscle training in Duchenne muscular dystrophy. Arch Dis Child 1989;64(5):736–738

52. Yasuma F, Sakai M, Matsuoka Y. Effects of noninvasive ventilation on survival in patients with Duchenne's muscular dystrophy [letter]. Chest 1996; 109(2):590

53. Barnes PR. Clinical and genetic aspects of myotonic dystrophy [see comments]. Br J Hosp Med 1993; 50(1):22–30

54. Ueda H, Shimokawa M, Yamamoto M, et al. Decreased expression of myotonic dystrophy protein kinase and disorganization of sarcoplasmic reticulum in skeletal muscle of myotonic dystrophy. J Neurol Sci 1999;162:38–50

55. Pizzuti A, Friedman DL, Caskey CT. The myotonic dystrophy gene. Arch Neurol 1993;50(11):1173–1179

56. Reardon W, Harley HG, Brook JD, et al. Minimal expression of myotonic dystrophy: a clinical and molecular analysis. J Med Genet 1992;29(11):770–773

57. Timchenko LT, Miller JW, Timchenko NA, et al. Identification of a (CUG)n triplet repeat RNA-binding protein and its expression in myotonic dystrophy. Nucleic Acids Res 1996;24(22):4407–4414

58. Kleser TR, Otten AD, Bird TD, Tapscott SJ. Trinucleotide repeat expansion at the myotonic dystrophy locus reduces expression of DMAHP. Nat Genet 1997;16(4):402–406

59. van der Meche FG, Boogaard JM, van den Berg BB. Treatment of hypersomnolence in myotonic dystrophy with a CNS stimulant. Muscle Nerve 1986;9(4):341–344

60. Harper PS. Congenital myotonic dystrophy in Britain. I. Clinical aspects. Arch Dis Child 1975;50(7):505–513

61. Rutherford MA, Heckmatt JZ, Dubowitz V. Congenital myotonic dystrophy: respiratory function at birth determines survival. Arch Dis Child 1989;64(2): 191–195

62. Abe K, Matsuo Y, Kadekawa J, et al. Respiratory training for patients with myotonic dystrophy. Neurology 1998;51:641–642

63. Ricker K, Grimm T, Koch MC, et al. Linkage of proximal myotonic myopathy to chromosome 3q [see comments]. Neurology 1999;52(1):170–171

64. von zur Muhlen F, Klass C, Kreuzer H, et al. Cardiac involvement in proximal myotonic myopathy. Heart 1998;79(6):619–621

65. Udd B, Krahe R, Wallgren-Pettersson C, et al. Proximal myotonic dystrophy—a family with autosomal dominant muscular dystrophy, cataracts, hearing loss and hypogonadism: heterogeneity of proximal myotonic syndromes? Neuromuscul Disor 1997;7(4):217–228

66. Day JW, Roelofs R, Leroy B, et al. Clinical and genetic characteristics of a five-generation family with a novel form of myotonic dystrophy (DM2). Neuromuscul Disord 1999;9(1):19–27

67. Ranum LP, Rasmussen PF, Benzow KA, et al. Genetic

mapping of a second myotonic dystrophy locus. Nat Genet 1998;19(2):196–198

68. Ricker K. Myotonic dystrophy and proximal myotonic myopathy. J Neurol 1999;246(5):334–338

69. Brais B, Bouchard JP, Xie YG, et al. Short GCG expansions in the PABP2 gene cause oculopharyngeal muscular dystrophy [published erratum appears in Nat Genet 1998 Aug;19(4):404]. Nat Genet 1998; 18(2):164–167

70. Tome FMS, Fardeau M. Oculopharyngeal Muscular Dystrophy. In: Engel AG, Franzini-Armstrong C, eds. Myology. New York: McGraw-Hill, 1994:1233–1245

71. Cook IJ, Kahrilas PJ. AGA technical review on management of oropharyngeal dysphagia. Gastroenterology 1999;116:455–478

72. Bouchard JP, Marcoux S, Gosselin F, et al. A simple test for the detection of the dysphagia in members of families with oculopharyngeal muscular dystrophy (OPMD). Can J Neurol Sci 1992;19:296–297

73. Grewal RP, Cantor R, Turner G, et al. Genetic mapping and haplotype analysis of oculopharyngeal muscular dystrophy. Neuroreport 1998;9(6):961–965

74. Fisher J, Upadhyaya M. Molecular genetics of facioscapulohumeral muscular dystrophy (FSHD). Neuromuscul Disord 1997;7(1):55–62

75. Griggs RC, Tawil R, Storvick D, et al. Genetics of facioscapulohumeral muscular dystrophy: new mutations in sporadic cases. Neurology 1993;43(11): 2369–2372

76. Zatz M, Marie SK, Cerqueira A, et al. The facioscapulohumeral muscular dystrophy (FSHD1) gene affects males more severely and more frequently than females. Am J Med Genet 1998;77(2):155–161

77. Lemmers RJ, van der Maarel SM, van Deutekom JC, et al. Inter- and intrachromosomal sub-telomeric rearrangements on 4q35: implications for facioscapulohumeral muscular dystrophy (FSHD) aetiology and diagnosis. Hum Mol Genet 1998;7(8):1207–1214

78. Munsat TL. Facioscapulohumeral Disease and the Scapuloperoneal Syndrome. In: Engel AG, Franzini-Armstrong C, eds. Myology. New York: McGraw-Hill, 1994:1220–1232

79. Andrews CT, Taylor TC, Patterson VH. Scapulothoracic arthrodesis for patients with facioscapulohumeral muscular dystrophy. Neuromuscul Disord 1998;8(8):580–584

80. Taylor DA, Carroll JE, Smith ME, et al. Facioscapulohumeral dystrophy associated with hearing loss and Coats syndrome. Ann Neurol 1982;12(4):395–398

81. Okinaga A, Matsuoka T, Umeda J, et al. Early-onset facioscapulohumeral muscular dystrophy: two case reports. Brain Dev 1997;19(8):563–567

82. Tawil R, McDermott MP, Pandya S, et al. A pilot trial of prednisone in facioscapulohumeral muscular dystrophy. FSH-DY Group. Neurology 1997;48(1):46–49

83. Kissel JT, McDermott MP, Natarajan R, et al. Pilot trial of albuterol in facioscapulohumeral muscular dystrophy. FSH-DY Group. Neurology 1998;50(5):1402–1406

84. Bione S, Maestrini E, Rivella S, et al. Identification of a novel X-linked gene responsible for Emery-Dreifuss muscular dystrophy. Nat Genet 1994;8(4):323–327

85. Bonne G, Di Barletta MR, Varnous S, et al. Mutations in the gene encoding lamin A/C cause autosomal dominant Emery-Dreifuss muscular dystrophy. Nat Genet 1999;21(3):285–288

86. Muchir A, Bonne G, van der Kooi AJ, et al. Identification of mutations in the gene encoding lamin A/C in the autosomal dominant form of limb-girdle muscular dystrophy with cardiac involvement (LGMD1B) (abst). Neuromuscul Disord 1999;9:500

87. Grimm T, Janka M. Emery-Dreifuss muscular dystrophy. In: Engel AG, Franzini-Armstrong C, eds. Myology. New York: McGraw-Hill, 1994:1188–1191

88. Mora M, Cartegni L, Di Blasi C, et al. X-linked Emery-Dreifuss muscular dystrophy can be diagnosed from skin biopsy or blood sample. Ann Neurol 1997; 42(2):249–253

89. Merlini L, Granata C, Dominici P, Bonfiglioli S. Emery-Dreifuss muscular dystrophy: report of five cases in a family and review of the literature. Muscle Nerve 1986;9(6):481–485

90. Muntoni F, Sewry CA. Congenital muscular dystrophy: from rags to riches [editorial comment]. Neurology 1998;51(1):14–16

91. Voit T. Congenital muscular dystrophies: 1997 update. Brain Dev 1998;20(2):65–74

92. Naom IS, D'Alessandro M, Topaloglu H, et al. Refinement of the laminin alpha2 chain locus to human chromosome 6q2 in severe and mild merosin deficient congenital muscular dystrophy. J Med Genet 1997; 34(2):99–104

93. Hayashi YK, Chou FL, Engvall E, et al. Mutations in the integrin alpha7 gene cause congenital myopathy. Nat Genet 1998;19(1):94–97

94. Voit T, Fardeau M, Tome FM. Prenatal detection of merosin expression in human placenta [letter]. Neuropediatrics 1994;25(6):332–333

95. Barkovich AJ. Neuroimaging manifestations and classification of congenital muscular dystrophies [see comments]. AJNR Am J Neuroradiol 1998;19(8):1389–1396

96. Toda T, Yoshioka M, Nakahori Y, et al. Genetic identity of Fukuyama-type congenital muscular dystrophy and Walker-Warburg syndrome. Ann Neurol 1995; 37(1):99–101

97. Kobayashi K, Nakahori Y, Miyake M, et al. An ancient retrotransposal insertion causes Fukuyama-type congenital muscular dystrophy. Nature 1998;394(6691): 388–392

98. Cormand B, Avela K, Pihko H, et al. Assignment of the muscle-eye-brain disease gene to 1p32–p34 by linkage analysis and homozygosity mapping. Am J Hum Genet 1999;64(1):126–135

99. Dobyns WB, Pagon RA, Armstrong D, et al. Diagnostic criteria for Walker-Warburg syndrome [see comments]. Am J Med Genet 1989;32(2):195–210

100. Fukuyama Y, Osawa M, Saito K. Congenital Muscular Dystrophies. 1st edn. Tokyo: Elsevier Science BV, 1997

101. Martinello F, Angelini C, Trevisan CP. Congenital muscular dystrophy with partial merosin deficiency and late onset epilepsy. Eur Neurol 1998;40(1):37–45

102. Tan E, Topaloglu H, Sewry C, et al. Late onset muscular dystrophy with cerebral white matter changes due to partial merosin deficiency. Neuromuscul Disord 1997;7(2):85–89

103. Voit T. Congenital muscular dystrophies: 1997 update. Brain Dev 1998;20(2):65–74

104. Haltia M, Leivo I, Somer H, et al. Muscle-eye-brain disease: a neuropathological study. Ann Neurol 1997; 41(2):173–180

105. Valanne L, Pihko H, Katevuo K, et al. MRI of the brain in muscle-eye-brain (MEB) disease. Neuroradiology 1994;36(6):473–476

106. Banker BQ. The congenital muscular dystrophies. In: Engel AG, Franzini-Armstrong C, eds. Myology. New York: McGraw-Hill, 1994:1275–1289

107. Kaplan JC, Fontaine B. Neuromuscular disorders: gene location [In Process Citation]. Neuromuscul Disord 1999;9(8):I–VIII

223 Inflammatory Myopathies

FL Mastaglia, BA Phillips and PJ Zilko

Since the definitive monograph on polymyositis by Walton and Adams in 1958[1] the inflammatory myopathies have come to be recognized as a clinically and etiologically diverse group of disorders, which may result from autoimmune mechanisms directed against the skeletal muscle or its microvasculature, or invasion of muscle by a wide range of microorganisms. The three most common forms of inflammatory myopathy encountered in clinical practice are polymyositis, dermatomyositis, and inclusion body myositis (Table 223.1). Yunis & Samaha[2] first introduced the term inclusion body myositis with reference to cases with distinctive muscle fibre inclusions.[3] It is now known that this condition has characteristic clinical and histopathological features which distinguish it from the other inflammatory myopathies and that it accounts for up to one-third of cases of inflammatory myopathy referred to a neuromuscular clinic.[4]

Table 223.1 Classification of inflammatory myopathies

Microbial
  Viral (influenza A and B; adenovirus; Coxsackie; HIV; HTLV-1)
  Bacterial (acute suppurative myositis; pyomyositis)
  Fungal (candidiasis; amebiasis)
  Parasitic (trichinosis; toxoplasmosis; cysticercosis)

Immune-mediated
  Dermatomyositis
    Isolated
      Malignancy
      Vasculitis
      Connective tissue diseases
  Polymyositis
    Isolated
      Connective tissue diseases
      Other autoimmune diseases
      HIV/HTLV-I infection
      Drugs (e.g. D-penicillamine)
  Inclusion body myositis
    Isolated
      Other autoimmune diseases
      Connective tissue diseases
      HIV infection

Miscellaneous
  Granulomatous myositis
  Vasculitic myositis
  Localized forms
  Eosinophilic syndromes
  Macrophagic myofasciitis
  Congenital and infantile forms

Epidemiology

Epidemiological studies have shown a combined annual incidence of polymyositis and dermatomyositis of 2.18 cases per million in Israel,[5] 5.5 cases per million in the USA[6] and 7.6 cases per million in Sweden.[7] The incidence is higher in females than males and, in the USA is highest in black females. The prevalence of inclusion body myositis has been estimated to be 9.3 per million in Western Australia with an age-adjusted prevalence of 35.3 per million over the age of 50 years.[8] A prevalence figure of 4.3 per million in the Netherlands was considered to represent an under-estimate.[9]

Aetiopathogenesis

The majority of cases of inflammatory myopathy encountered in neurological practice are immune-mediated and may occur in isolation, or in association with a systemic connective tissue disease or other autoimmune disorder, a retroviral infection (e.g. HIV or HTLV1) or malignancy in the case of dermatomyositis (Table 223.1).[4,10] It is now known that different immune mechanisms are involved in the pathogenesis of the three major forms of inflammatory myopathy. In dermatomyositis, a complement-dependent humoral attack on vascular endothelial cells is thought to be responsible and to lead to a depletion of the muscle capillary bed and ischemic muscle damage.[11–13] On the other hand, in polymyositis and inclusion body myositis, cytotoxic muscle fibre necrosis occurs as a result of invasion of muscle fibres by $CD8^+$ T cells and macrophages.[14,15] In inclusion body myositis there is also a progressive vacuolo-filamentous degeneration of muscle fibres and deposition of amyloid and other associated proteins, whose relationship to the T cell mediated inflammatory process remains uncertain.[16,17] The pathogenesis of the rarer eosinophilic and granulomatous forms of myositis is less well understood.

Genetics

With the exception of rare familial cases of inflammatory myopathy,[18] the vast majority of cases are sporadic. There is, however, evidence of genetic predisposition to the development of the immune-mediated inflammatory myopathies which is thought to be multifactorial.[19,20] The strongest link is with the major histocompatibility complex antigens B8 and DR3 which, in Caucasoids, have been associated with each of the major subgroups of inflammatory myopathy, and especially with inclusion body myositis.[21]

Clinical features

In polymyositis and dermatomyositis there is usually diffuse muscle weakness which is more severe proximally, whereas in inclusion body myositis there is characteristically a more selective pattern of involvement of the quadriceps femoris in the lower limbs and the forearm flexor muscles in the upper limbs, although other muscle groups are also affected as the disease progresses. The onset is usually more acute and the rate of progression more rapid in dermatomyositis than in polymyositis, while in inclusion body myositis the tempo of the condition is much slower. Dysphagia, due to involvement of the esophageal or pharyngeal musculature, may occur in each of the three major forms of myositis. When present, the characteristic skin changes of dermatomyositis are diagnostic, but they may be inconspicuous or absent at the time of presentation. Raynaud's phenomenon, articular symptoms, and other systemic features are more likely to occur in patients with dermatomyositis or with an associated connective tissue disease (overlap syndrome).

Without treatment, the clinical course is usually progressive in each of the major forms of myositis. Most patients with polymyositis or dermatomyositis respond to treatment and may make a full or virtually full recovery.[22] However, spontaneous relapses may occur at any time, particularly in patients with dermatomyositis.[23] Adverse prognostic factors include advanced age, long delay to diagnosis and commencement of treatment, the presence of certain myositis-specific auto-antibodies, and associated vasculitis, malignancy or other systemic disease.[24,25]

Classification

A working classification of the inflammatory myopathies is given in Table 223.1. The classification of the non-infective varieties remains somewhat arbitrary given the incomplete state of understanding of the aetiopathogenesis of a number of these disorders.

Diagnostic process

The diagnosis of an inflammatory myopathy is based initially upon a detailed clinical evaluation, with particular attention to the pattern of muscle involvement, and inspection for the characteristic skin changes of dermatomyositis on the face, hands, and trunk. Elevation of the serum creatine kinase (CK) level supports the diagnosis of an inflammatory myopathy but the CK level may be normal or only mildly elevated, particularly in dermatomyositis and inclusion body myositis. Electromyography will usually confirm the diagnosis of a primary myopathic disorder and will often also show prominent spontaneous muscle fiber potentials in patients with active myositis, but the changes may be patchy. Mixed myopathic and neuropathic features may be found in patients with inclusion body myositis. Muscle biopsy is the definitive diagnostic procedure and should always be performed before starting treatment to confirm the inflammatory nature and type of myopathy and to allow recognition of rarer forms such as eosinophilic, granulomatous, and parasitic myositis. Muscle imaging with computerized tomography (CT) or magnetic resonance (MRI) may be helpful particularly in the investigation of focal forms of myositis and inclusion body myositis, and in selecting an appropriate muscle for biopsy.

Differential diagnosis

The inflammatory myopathies must be distinguished from drug-induced and metabolic myopathies such as McArdle's disease, lipid storage, mitochondrial, hypokalemic and endocrine myopathies. In addition, when muscle pain is a feature, fibromyalgia and polymyalgia rheumatica need to be considered. In the more chronic inclusion body myositis the major differential diagnoses are motor neuron disease, late-onset forms of muscular dystrophy and mitochondrial myopathies.

Treatment

The treatment of the autoimmune inflammatory myopathies is largely empirical and has traditionally relied upon the use of glucocorticoids and other forms of immunosuppressive therapy (Tables 223.2 and 223.3). Because of their known efficacy in the treatment of polymyositis and dermatomyositis, glucocorticoids have never been subjected to controlled clinical trials, nor has the relative efficacy of the other immunosuppressive agents in glucocorticoid-resistant cases been formally evaluated. The most important recent advance has been the introduction of high-dose intravenous immunoglobulin therapy for the treat-

Table 223.2 Treatment options for inflammatory myopathies
First-line
Glucocorticoids
Second-line
Methotrexate
Azathioprine
Intravenous immunoglobulin*
Third-line
Intravenous immunoglobulin
Cyclosporine
Cyclophosphamide
Plasmapheresis
Last option
Whole body/lymphoid irradiation
Thoracic duct drainage
Thymectomy
Emerging therapies
Newer immunosuppressive agents (e.g. tacrolimus, mycophenolate mofetil)
Cytokine-based therapies (e.g. TNF-α blockers, interferon β)
Hemopoietic stem cell transplantation
*In patients who are immunodeficient or have other contraindications to the use of cytotoxic agents

Table 223.3   Details of major therapies for inflammatory myopathies

Therapeutic agent	Indication	Route	Dose	Adverse effects (major)	Precautions	Monitoring for toxicity	Monitoring disease activity
Prednisone	First-line	Oral	Initially ~1 mg/kg; gradual taper >4–6 weeks and conversion to alt die regimen	Cushingoid features; hypertension; fluid retention; diabetes mellitus; infections; cataracts; glaucoma; osteoporosis; aseptic bone necrosis; steroid myopathy	Elderly patients and post-menopausal females (calcium supplements plus calcitriol or a bisphosphonate if high fracture risk). Diabetics. Previous or active peptic ulcer (H_2 receptor blocker). Active infection. Old tuberculosis (commence anti-TB therapy before prednisone). Severe immunodeficiency (trimethoprim for pneumocystis prophylaxis)	Regular clinical and ophthalmic assessments. Monitor growth in children. Plasma glucose and electrolytes. Bone density measurement in females	MRC grading, quantitative muscle assessment and serum CK every 1–3 months
Methylprednisolone	Severe PM or DM	IV	1000 mg/day for 3 days	As for prednisone	As for prednisone	As for prednisone	As for prednisone
Methotrexate	Second-line	Oral	7.5–15 mg/once weekly	Bone marrow depression; gastrointestinal symptoms; hepatic and renal dysfunction; pneumonitis	Reduce alcohol intake. Contraindicated in pregnancy, hepatic disease, renal failure, blood dyscrasia, and active peptic ulcer. Use with caution in patients with diabetes, alcoholism, and severe obesity. Administer folic acid 5 mg/week to reduce risk of bone marrow depression	Monitor blood count and liver function studies every 4–8 weeks	As for prednisone
Azathioprine	Second-line	Oral	2–3 mg/kg/day in divided doses	Transient leucopenia; macrocytosis; idiosyncratic hypersensitivity reaction with fever, myalgia, rash; hepatotoxicity; pancreatitis. Risk of malignancy low with treatment <5 years	Contraindicated in pregnancy and if hypersensitivity reaction occurs. Reduce dose to one quarter if patient is on a xanthine oxidase inhibitor (e.g. allopurinol)	Monitor blood count and liver function studies every 4–8 weeks	As for prednisone

Table 223.3 *continued*

Therapeutic agent	Indication	Route	Dose	Adverse effects (major)	Precautions	Monitoring for toxicity	Monitoring disease activity
Cyclophosphamide	Third-line	Oral IV	2–2.5 mg/kg/d 500–1000 mg pulse dose every 2–4 weeks	Transient leucopenia; bone marrow depression; alopecia; hemorrhagic cystitis; infertility; increased risk of malignancy (especially vesical)	Contraindicated in pregnancy, bone marrow depression, untreated infection, and recent surgery. Allopurinol increases risk of marrow depression. Avoid bladder toxicity with high fluid intake (2–3 L/day) while on oral therapy or 2-mercaptoethane Na sulphonate with pulse doses	Monitor blood count, urinalysis monthly	As for prednisone
Cyclosporine	Third-line	Oral	2–3 mg/kg/day in divided doses	Hypertension; renal toxicity; hepatic dysfunction; skin rashes; pancreatitis; neurotoxicity	Contraindicated in renal failure, poorly controlled hypertension, infection, and immunodeficiency. Many drugs affect blood level of cyclosporine; avoid nephrotoxic drugs	Monitor blood pressure and serum creatinine levels monthly. Monitoring of plasma levels of cyclosporine only necessary with higher doses	As for prednisone
Immunoglobulin	Third-line*	IV	0.4 g/kg/day for 5 days in initial course followed by monthly 3 day courses for 3–6 months	Headache; anaphylactic reactions (especially if IgA deficient); aseptic meningitis; acute renal failure; thromboembolic events	Contraindicated in IgA deficiency, hyperviscosity syndromes, renal insufficiency, and severe vascular disease. Use with caution in the elderly and patients with history of vascular disease. Risk of adverse reactions is reduced by slow infusion rate especially in the initial course	Clinical evaluation during course of treatment. Monitor renal function	As for prednisone

*Second-line in patients with immunodeficiency.

ment of patients who fail to respond adequately to glucocorticoids and immunosuppressive agents or who are unable to tolerate these drugs. In general, the available forms of treatment all have non-selective effects on the immune system and the possibility of more specific immunotherapy awaits the identification of the target antigens against which the autoimmune process is directed and a more complete understanding of the immune effector mechanisms in the different types of inflammatory myopathy.

Assessing the response to treatment

Evaluating the response to treatment in patients with inflammatory myopathies requires reliable clinical and laboratory criteria and should include quantitative measures of muscle performance which are sufficiently sensitive to detect significant changes with time.[26,27] Conventional manual muscle testing and Medical Research Council [UK] (MRC) grading of muscle groups is of limited value for the serial assessment of muscle function because of the subjectivity of the technique and lack of sensitivity to change. For these reasons, myometry using the Penny and Giles hand-held myometer or similar instrument, or isokinetic dynamometry, which allows measurement of muscle torque through a range of motion, are preferable for the serial assessment of muscle function. In addition, functional scales and timed tests should be included in the assessment protocol as they provide information which pertains to the patient's ability to perform everyday activities. Functional assessment of the respiratory muscles should also be performed in patients with severe myositis who may have respiratory muscle weakness.

The serum CK level is the most reliable biochemical indicator of disease activity in the individual patient, provided that it is elevated initially.[26] The serum CK should be monitored at regular intervals after the initiation of treatment and a rise may be the first indication of reactivation of the myositis. However, it is important that other causes of an elevated CK level such as strenuous exercise, muscle trauma, intramuscular injections, myotoxic drugs and metabolic disorders such as hypokalemia and hypothyroidism should first be excluded. Conversely, glucocorticoids may lead to a non-specific reduction in serum CK levels, which may be misleading in assessing the response to treatment if it is not accompanied by an improvement in muscle performance.

Dermatomyositis and polymyositis
Glucocorticoid therapy

Glucocorticoids remain the standard first-line treatment for patients with clinically significant myositis because of their combined anti-inflammatory and immunosuppressive actions.[28,29] Treatment is usually commenced with oral prednisolone in a dose of ~1 mg/kg/day in a single or divided doses. Higher doses have been advocated by some workers, but in our experience do not confer additional benefit and increase the likelihood of developing a steroid myopathy and other side effects. High-dose alternate-

day oral therapy and pulse therapy with intravenous methylprednisolone have also been advocated as first-line therapy (Class 3)[30,31] but have not been formally evaluated. In patients with very severe myositis treatment may be commenced with intravenous methylprednisolone (1000 mg daily for three consecutive days; or three doses on alternate days) followed by oral prednisolone. A lower starting dose may be necessary in patients with a high risk of developing steroid side-effects (for example the elderly; postmenopausal females with osteoporosis; diabetics); combined therapy with prednisolone and a second-line agent such as methotrexate or azathioprine may be used in such cases. Combined therapy with prednisone and azathioprine was shown to be associated with a better long-term outcome in a double-blind controlled trial performed at the Mayo Clinic (Class 2)[32,33] and has been advocated for patients with severe myositis, or when the diagnosis has been delayed (Class 3).[27] Combined initial therapy also appears to be associated with a lower relapse rate.[34,35]

The initial dose of prednisolone should be continued for a period of four to six weeks during which clinical improvement usually commences and the serum CK level falls. Improvement in muscle strength may however lag behind the fall in CK level. The rate of reduction is individualized taking into account the degree of clinical improvement and concern regarding steroid side effects in each particular patient. In general, it is possible to reduce the dose of prednisolone by 5–10 mg/week during the second month of treatment and to then change to an alternate day regimen to reduce the degree of adrenal suppression and steroid side-effects. Treatment should be continued for at least 12 months after muscle function recovers and the serum CK level returns to normal, preferably using a maintenance dose of prednisolone of <10 mg/day (or <20 mg on alternate days) to reduce the risk of steroid myopathy. Muscle strength and serum CK should continue to be monitored during conversion from daily to alternate day therapy.

Steroid myopathy should be suspected when there is persisting or increasing weakness, particularly of the proximal lower limb muscles, after the serum CK level has returned to normal. A gradual reduction in the dose of prednisolone, or conversion to an alternate day regimen, will usually lead to a progressive improvement in muscle function. At times it is difficult to know whether deteriorating muscle function is due to active myositis or to steroid myopathy and in some patients it may be necessary to repeat the electromyography and muscle biopsy. A regular exercise program and administration of B group vitamins may help to prevent or reverse steroid myopathy (Class 2).[36,37]

Patients taking corticosteroids should be assessed regularly for adverse effects, particularly infections, hypertension, diabetes mellitus, cataracts, glaucoma, osteoporosis, aseptic necrosis of the hip and shoulder joints. Serum electrolytes and glucose levels should be monitored every one to two months. Calcium supplements (1–1.5 g/day) should be administered routinely. In addition, in post-menopausal females with a reduced bone density and high fracture risk further bone loss may be prevented by administering a vitamin D preparation (such as calcitriol) or one of the bisphosphonate drugs (such as etidronate or alendronate) which also reduce the risk of fractures (Class 2).[38,39] In patients with a history of peptic ulceration an H_2-receptor blocker should be administered to prevent reactivation of the ulcer. Particular caution should be exercised in patients with a history or chest X-ray changes of past tuberculosis who should be commenced on anti-tuberculous therapy prior to the initiation of prednisolone because of the risk of re-activating the infection and inducing miliary tuberculosis. In patients with HIV infection and immunodeficiency trimethoprim is administered for prophylaxis against pneumocystis pneumonia.

Steroid-resistant cases

While most patients with dermatomyositis or polymyositis are satisfactorily controlled with prednisolone and achieve a complete or worthwhile remission, in some cases there is continued deterioration and it is necessary to introduce a second-line agent. In addition, in a significant proportion of cases relapses occur during withdrawal of steroid therapy or, more often, during a period of stable maintenance therapy.[23] It is preferable to introduce a second-line agent at a relatively early stage as it will allow a more rapid reduction in the dose of prednisolone and thereby make it less likely that a steroid myopathy or other steroid side-effects will develop (Class 3).[40]

The choice of a second-line agent is largely empirical. In general, methotrexate or azathioprine are preferred, while in patients who are immunodeficient or have an adverse reaction to these drugs, intravenous immunoglobulin is regarded as the treatment of choice. Although there have been no comparative trials of methotrexate and azathioprine, our preference is for methotrexate which can be administered in a single weekly oral dose and is considered to have a lower risk of inducing malignancy than azathioprine.[41] In a small group of patients who fail to respond to these second-line modalities of treatment it may be necessary to consider a trial of another immunosuppressive agent such as cyclophosphamide or cyclosporine.

In patients who relapse during steroid therapy it may suffice to increase the dose of prednisolone (for example, up to 50 mg/day) or, in more severe relapses, it may be necessary to add a second-line agent such as methotrexate or azathioprine or to use intravenous immunoglobulin therapy (see below).

Immunosuppressive agents

Methotrexate The drug interferes with DNA synthesis in proliferating lymphocytes and their precursors by competitively inhibiting the enzyme tetrahydrofolic acid reductase, which converts folic acid to tetrahydrofolate. Although it has not been tested in controlled clinical trials, retrospective studies have indicated that methotrexate can be beneficial and may be more effective than azathioprine in some groups of patients (Class 3).[42] The drug is usually administered orally in a starting dose of 7.5–10 mg once weekly, increasing if necessary by 2.5 mg/week/month to a maximum dose of 20 mg/week. Higher doses of up to 30–40 mg/week may be used but are more likely to cause gastrointestinal side-effects and are best given by the intramuscular or intravenous route (Class 3).[43] A folic acid supplement (5 mg of folic acid) is administered once weekly, four days after the dose of methotrexate, to reduce the risk of bone marrow depression.

Other side effects are uncommon and include fever, pruritus, skin rash, ulcerative stomatitis, diarrhea, hepatic and renal toxicity and interstitial pneumonitis.[42] The blood count and liver function tests should be monitored on a monthly basis. The drug is contraindicated in patients with hepatic disease, renal failure, or blood dyscrasia and during pregnancy and should be used with caution in diabetics, alcoholics, the elderly and in patients with infection, active peptic ulcer or severe obesity. Patients should be advised to avoid alcohol or reduce their intake to a minimum. Although there are no controlled human data, methotrexate does not appear to have carcinogenic effects, at least with short to medium term administration.

Azathioprine The drug is a sulfide analogue of hypoxanthine, which is converted to 6-mercaptopurine and inhibits DNA and RNA synthesis in lymphocytes that are proliferating and differentiating. While the major effect is on T cells, azathioprine may also be effective in antibody-mediated disorders, which are T cell dependent. The only controlled clinical trial has been in combination with prednisolone as first-line therapy showing no additional benefit at three months but a better long-term outcome than with prednisolone alone (Class 2).[32,33] Administration is by the oral route in a dose of 2–3 mg/kg/day in divided doses with food. Side effects are uncommon but occasional patients may have an idiosyncratic reaction with fever, rash, myalgia, abdominal pain, and vomiting. Transient leucopenia and macrocytosis occur in about 20% of patients. Individuals with mutations in the thiopurine methyltransferase gene are prone to develop severe reactions including hemopoietic toxicity when taking azathioprine and can be identified by genotyping if the test is available.[45] Other uncommon side-effects include hepatotoxicity and pancreatitis. The blood count and liver function should be monitored at least monthly. The risk of malignancy is considered to be low with periods of administration less than five years.[46]

Cyclophosphamide The drug undergoes conversion in the liver to its active form which acts as an alkylating agent and causes lymphopenia with depletion particularly of B cells.[47] Cyclophosphamide is therefore better suited for the treatment of antibody-mediated disorders such as dermatomyositis, particularly if there is an associated vasculitis (Class

3).[48] There are, however, few reports of the use of cyclophosphamide in inflammatory myopathies and no controlled clinical trials (Class 3).[49,50] The drug can be administered orally in a dose of 2–2.5 mg/kg/day or intravenously as a pulse dose of 500–1000 mg every two to four weeks, the latter being associated with fewer adverse effects in our experience.

The drug usually induces a transient neutropenia and need not be discontinued or reduced in dose unless the white cell count remains below 3×10^3/L or other hematological complications such as thrombocytopenia, anemia or pancytopenia develop. Other adverse effects include alopecia, gastrointestinal symptoms, hemorrhagic cystitis, infertility, and an increased incidence of malignancies, particularly bladder cancer. It is usually possible to avoid bladder toxicity by maintaining a high fluid intake (two to three liters per day) during oral therapy, or by administering intravenous 2-mercaptoethane sodium sulphonate (MESNA) in patients having pulse therapy.[51,52] In males of reproductive age storage of sperm in a sperm bank is recommended prior to commencement of therapy. In females of childbearing age an ovarian wedge biopsy may be performed for long-term storage of ova and subsequent in vitro fertilization.

Cyclosporine The drug has a more selective effect on the immune system than the other immunosuppressive agents, inhibiting T cell activation and the secretion of cytokines by helper-inducer T cells.[53] Although there have not been any published controlled trials, a number of reports have indicated that low-dose cyclosporine can be beneficial particularly in resistant cases of juvenile dermatomyositis (Class 3)[54,55] as well as some adult cases of polymyositis and dermatomyositis (Class 3).[56] The drug has also been reported to be effective as first-line therapy in some patients with early dermatomyositis (Class 3).[57] It is given orally in a starting dose of 3 mg/kg/day in divided doses. The dose is then adjusted according to the clinical response and occurrence of side-effects and should ideally be kept in the range of 2–3 mg/kg/day to reduce side-effects. Routine monitoring of plasma levels is not necessary when using doses in this range.

The most important side effects are hypertension and nephrotoxicity, the occurrence of which is indicated by an elevation of the serum creatinine level. Other adverse effects include headache, hirsutism, gingival hypertrophy, tremor, fatigue, gastrointestinal symptoms, pancreatitis, thrombocytopenia and hemolytic anemia.

Intravenous immunoglobulin therapy

High dose intravenous immunoglobulin therapy (IVIG) has been shown to be effective in patients with drug-resistant dermatomyositis in a double-blind crossover trial (Class 2)[58] and a number of uncontrolled studies have also demonstrated its efficacy as add-on therapy in patients with polymyositis, dermatomyositis and overlap syndromes (Class 3).[59,60]

However, IVIG therapy was not found to be effective when used as first-line therapy in polymyositis or dermatomyositis (Class 3).[61]

The doses of IVIG and regimens used have varied in different studies and there are at present no reliable guidelines as to the most effective regimen. Current practice is to administer a dose of 2 g/kg body weight over a five-day period (i.e. 0.4 g/kg/day) in the initial course and to follow this with monthly three or five day courses for a period of three to six months (Class 3).[60] In our experience improvement usually begins after the first or second course of treatment and if there is no improvement after the third course it is reasonable to discontinue therapy (Class 3).[60] Further controlled trials are required to determine the optimal administration regimen and minimal effective dose of this expensive form of treatment.

Adverse reactions are usually minor and include headache, nausea, fever, itching, and myalgia. More serious complications are uncommon and include aseptic meningitis, thromboembolic events, acute renal failure, and anaphylactic reactions, particularly in patients with immunoglobulin A (IgA) deficiency. The risk of headache and more serious adverse reactions may be reduced by a slow rate of IVIG infusion, particularly for the first dose (over two to three hours). Hepatitis C infection was associated with the use of certain brands of immunoglobulin in the USA[62] but there is no longer considered to be a significant risk of transmission of viral infections with current serum screening procedures and preparative techniques. Immunoglobulin therapy is contraindicated in patients with IgA deficiency, hyperviscosity syndromes, renal insufficiency, and severe vascular disease and should be used with caution in the elderly.

Immunoglobulin therapy may exert its effect in a number of ways. In dermatomyositis improvement has been shown to correlate with a reduction in intercellular adhesion molecule-1 (ICAM-1) expression and dissolution of C5b-9 deposits in muscle capillaries and it has been suggested that IVIG blocks the formation of the membrane attack complex of complement.[58,63] Other possible mechanisms of action include binding of anti-idiotypic antibodies to circulating auto-antibodies or B cells, suppression of T cell mediated responses, inhibition of cytokines and blockade of macrophage Fc receptors.[64,65]

Plasmapheresis

Uncontrolled studies suggested that plasmapheresis could be effective in combination with glucocorticoid and immunosuppressive therapy in drug-resistant cases of polymyositis or dermatomyositis (Class 3),[66] but this was not confirmed in a subsequent double-blind randomized trial comparing plasma exchange, leukapheresis and sham apheresis after discontinuation of immunosuppressive drugs (Class 2).[67] It may therefore be that, as has been postulated with IVIG therapy,[60] plasmapheresis is more effective in patients who are on concurrent immunosuppressive therapy. Intravenous immunoglobulin therapy is now preferred to plasmapheresis because of its greater ease of administration, and appears to be of equal or greater benefit although there have not been any comparative studies of these two forms of treatment.

Other forms of treatment

A number of other forms of treatment have been reported to be effective in some cases of refractory polymyositis or dermatomyositis, but their efficacy has not been proven in controlled clinical trials (Table 223.2). The alkylating agent chlorambucil (4 mg/day) has been reported to be beneficial in some patients with recalcitrant dermatomyositis (Class 3)[68] but is thought to be associated with a higher risk of leukemia than the other cytotoxic agents.[69] Low-dose whole-body X irradiation has been reported to induce a sustained remission in some refractory cases (Class 3),[70,71] while lymphoid irradiation has also been reported to be effective (Class 3).[72] Benefit has been reported in some refractory cases with thoracic duct drainage or thymectomy (Class 3).[73]

Physical exercise and therapy

Patients with inflammatory myopathies should be encouraged to undertake regular physical activity. In the early stages after commencement of treatment, and during relapses, patients should be instructed to simply carry out range of motion exercises to prevent the development of contractures. Once the activity of the disease has been controlled, an isometric exercise program for key muscle groups, such as quadriceps, followed by a lightweight isotonic program to build up muscle strength may be introduced.[74] Resistive exercise has been shown to improve muscle strength in patients with polymyositis or dermatomyositis (Class 2)[75] and a regular isokinetic training program has been shown to help reverse steroid myopathy (Class 2).[36] At a later stage, a low intensity aerobic exercise program (e.g. bicycle, step or pool) can be recommended and has been shown to improve muscle performance (Class 2).[76]

Juvenile dermatomyositis

In most cases of juvenile dermatomyositis the disease is satisfactorily controlled with glucocorticoids and goes into remission within the first two years (Class 3).[77] Both high (2 mg/kg/day) and low doses (1 mg/kg/day) of prednisone have been advocated, but the latter is usually effective, and is preferable as it is less likely to cause serious side-effects such as growth retardation, osteoporosis and gastrointestinal perforation (Class 3).[78] However, there have not been any comparative trials of the two regimens. Combined therapy with prednisone and azathioprine or methotrexate has been advocated as a means of allowing earlier prednisone withdrawal (Class 3).[79] Pulse therapy with intravenous methylprednisolone (30 mg/kg/day for three days followed by weekly or twice-weekly pulses) has been reported to be effective as initial therapy and to result in complete remission in some cases (Class 3).[30]

In patients who are not adequately controlled with glucocorticoids other options include additional immunosuppression with azathioprine, methotrexate, cyclosporine or cyclophosphamide, or intravenous immunoglobulin therapy, but none of these have undergone controlled evaluation. In an uncontrolled trial of cyclosporine in 26 patients with juvenile dermatomyositis who were not controlled with glucocorticoids and immunosuppressive agents, a full functional recovery occurred in 22 cases and it was possible to discontinue glucocorticoids in 24 cases (Class 3).[55] Immunoglobulin therapy has been reported to be effective in a small uncontrolled study (Class 3).[80]

Hydroxychloroquine has been reported to improve both the skin rash and the weakness in patients who respond incompletely or relapse while on glucocorticoid therapy (Class 3).[81] Various forms of treatment including topical and systemic glucocorticoids, diltiazem, colchicine, diphosphonates, probenecid, aluminium hydroxide and low dose warfarin have been recommended for the subcutaneous calcinosis which develops in many patients with juvenile dermatomyositis but none of these are uniformly effective and none has been formally evaluated in a controlled clinical trial.[82]

Inclusion body myositis

In contrast to other inflammatory myopathies, inclusion body myositis (IBM) is usually resistant to glucocorticoids and other forms of treatment and the condition continues to progress.[83] However, in occasional cases the condition stabilizes or may improve after commencement of treatment (Class 3).[84–86] These include patients with an associated connective tissue disease in some of whom there is a good response to glucocorticoid therapy at least initially. In a study in which muscle biopsies were performed before and after glucocorticoid therapy, continued clinical deterioration was found to occur in spite of a reduction in inflammation and numbers of muscle fibers invaded by T cells, whereas the numbers of vacuolated fibers and fibers with amyloid deposits increased.[17]

Intravenous immunoglobulin therapy has been evaluated in a number of small open studies and two larger double-blind studies. Improvement in muscle strength and functional abilities was reported in three of four patients in one study (Class 3)[87] while in another study of five patients there was no improvement in MRC grades or functional scales but improvement in myometric scores occurred in some less severely affected muscles in one case (Class 3).[60] In the other open study of nine patients none showed any clinical improvement (Class 3).[88] In a double-blind placebo-controlled cross-over study involving 19 patients there was no statistically significant improvement in overall muscle strength although there was minor functional benefit in some patients and nine patients chose to continue IVIG therapy after the trial (Class 2).[89] In another placebo-controlled study of 22 patients, stabilization of the condition or mild improvement was also reported (Class 2).[90] Because of the very modest benefits and the expensive nature of this form of treatment, IVIG therapy is not currently recommended for routine use in patients with inclusion body myositis.

Our current approach, once the diagnosis has been established, and provided that the patient's general condition is satisfactory, is to recommend a three month trial of oral prednisolone (~1 mg/kg/day), alone or in combination with a steroid-sparing agent such as methotrexate (starting with 7.5 mg/week) or azathioprine (1.5–2.5 mg/kg/day) if there is particular concern about steroid side-effects. If there is evidence of continued deterioration over a three to six month period with quantitative muscle testing, treatment is discontinued. On the other hand, if muscle strength improves or stabilizes, the dose of prednisolone is gradually reduced to a maintenance level, as in the treatment of polymyositis or dermatomyositis (see above), and continued in combination with methotrexate or azathioprine.

Patients with IBM should be instructed to undertake regular physical exercise, including an isometric exercise program, which has been shown to improve muscle strength (Class 3).[91] Non-steroidal anabolic agents, such as clenbuterol, may help to preserve muscle strength in patients who continue to deteriorate (Class 3) and warrant further evaluation in a controlled trial. Other forms of treatment which have been suggested on empirical grounds but which have not been formally evaluated include L-carnitine, coenzyme Q, testosterone and anti-oxidants.[92] Cricopharyngeal myotomy may be helpful in patients with severe dysphagia.[93]

Eosinophilic myositis

Eosinophilic polymyositis

The clinical picture in this condition is indistinguishable from that of the more usual form of polymyositis but the muscle biopsy shows a predominance of eosinophils in the inflammatory infiltrate.[94] In some cases, the myositis is part of a systemic hypereosinophilic syndrome characterized by eosinophilia, anemia, cardiac and pulmonary involvement, skin changes, peripheral neuropathy and encephalopathy.[95,96]

Patients with the isolated form of polymyositis have been reported to do well with glucocorticoid therapy using conventional doses of prednisone (Class 3).[94] Some patients with the hypereosinophilic syndrome have a good response to glucocorticoid therapy while others fail to respond.[95] Leukaphoresis may be beneficial in resolving the systemic symptoms (Class 3).[95]

Eosinophilic perimyositis and fasciitis

These conditions are characterized by widespread muscle pain and stiffness. In eosinophilic fasciitis (Shulman's syndrome), there is also thickening and induration of the skin of the extremities. The muscle biopsy findings include a mixed eosinophil and mononuclear cell infiltrate in the perimysium and fascia, and perifascicular fiber necrosis or atrophy in the underlying muscle tissue.[10] Most patients respond to treatment with glucocorticoids (Class 3).[97]

Eosinophilia-myalgia syndrome

This syndrome, which was associated with the ingestion of contaminated preparations of L-tryptophan during the late 1980s, was associated with severe myalgia, skin rashes and oedema, arthralgia, dyspnoea, weight loss, peripheral neuropathy and a scleroderma-like infiltration and thickening of the skin.[98,99] Muscle biopsy showed fiber atrophy, and a mixed perivascular and perimysial infiltrate of lymphocytes, macrophages and eosinophils.[100] Treatment with prednisone in the early stages of the condition led to improvement in the myalgia and skin changes, but did not produce complete resolution of the illness nor prevent the development of later manifestations in many patients (Class 3).[98,101]

HIV-related myositis and myopathies

A symptomatic myopathy develops in up to 30% of patients with HIV infection.[102,103] The myopathy may develop at any stage of the infection and may be related to the effects of the infection itself, of the antiretroviral agent zidovudine (AZT) which is known to cause a mitochondrial myopathy, or to an opportunistic muscle infection (Table 223.4).[102] HIV myopathy is characterized by the sub-acute onset of proximal muscle weakness which may be accompanied by myalgia, although this is less frequent than in the AZT-induced myopathy.[104] Muscle biopsy shows similar changes to those in non-HIV associated polymyositis with muscle fiber necrosis, a mixed infiltrate of lymphocytes and macrophages, and CD8+ T cells surrounding and invading muscle fibers.[102] In some cases rod-bodies or cytoplasmic bodies are prominent and the inflammatory changes are inconspicuous.[105] A progressive muscle wasting syndrome of uncertain pathogenesis commonly occurs in patients with more advanced HIV infection.[106]

Table 223.4   HIV-related muscle diseases

HIV myopathy
  Inflammation (HIV polymyositis)
  Necrosis with minimal inflammation
  Rod bodies

Subclinical neuromuscular involvement
  Inflammation
  Denervation
  Type II fibre atrophy

HIV wasting syndrome
  Type II fibre atrophy

Rhabdomyolysis

Myasthenia gravis

Opportunistic muscle infections

Modified from Dalakas.[102]

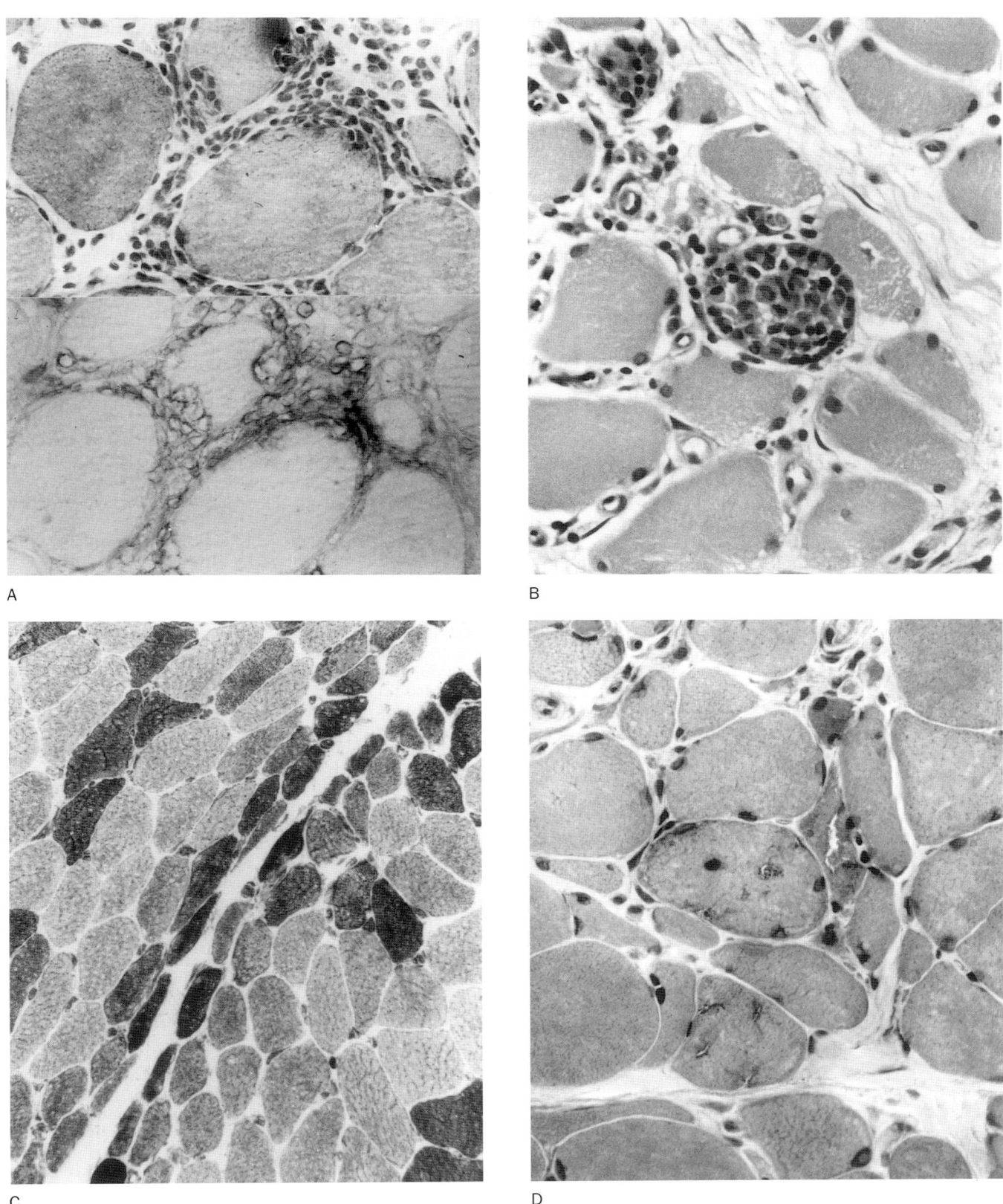

Figure 223.1 *A.* Endomysial inflammatory infiltrate with predominance of CD8+ lymphocytes surrounding and focally invading muscle fibers in a case of polymyositis (anti-CD8+ antibody). Courtesy of Dr. AG Engel. *B.* Single muscle fiber necrosis and myophagia in a case of polymyositis (hematoxylin and eosin). *C.* Perifascicular muscle fiber atrophy in a case of dermatomyositis (NADH tetrazolium reductase stain). *D.* Muscle fibers containing basophilic-rimmed vacuoles in a case of inclusion body myositis (hematoxylin and eosin).

Treatment with prednisone, using a similar regimen as in non-HIV associated myositis (see above), has been found to be effective in improving muscle strength in patients with HIV myopathy in uncontrolled case studies and in a prospective placebo-controlled study (Class 2).[107] Prednisone has also been reported to be effective in some cases with prominent rod-bodies and minimal inflammatory changes (Class 3),[105] and in the HIV-associated muscle wasting syndrome (Class 3).[106] Although it has not been subjected to a controlled clinical trial, intravenous immunoglobulin therapy has been recommended as the treatment of choice for patients with HIV myopathy as it avoids steroid side-effects and further immunosuppression and, in particular, the risk of activating latent opportunistic infections (Class 3).[102] In patients who develop symptoms of myopathy while taking AZT, a muscle biopsy may help to determine whether the myopathy is inflammatory or drug-related. However, if the patient is unwilling to undergo biopsy, or if the biopsy is inconclusive, the drug should be withdrawn while continuing other anti-retroviral treatment. If there is no improvement after a period of four to eight weeks a short course of prednisone or IVIG therapy should be considered (Class 3).[102] Non-steroidal anti-inflammatory drugs may provide symptomatic relief in patients with severe myalgia (Class 3).[102] In patients with an opportunistic muscle infection, the appropriate anti-microbial therapy should be administered once the organism has been identified.

Parasitic myositis

Many parasites may cause muscle infestation and result in a focal or diffuse inflammatory myopathy.[108,109] The conditions most commonly encountered in neurological practice are trichinosis, cysticercosis and toxoplasmosis, which is more common in immunodeficient patients. A parasitic disorder should be considered in patients with diffuse myalgia and muscle tenderness, which are common during the stage of muscle invasion by a number of parasites. Other clues include a history of overseas travel, the ingestion of raw or inadequately cooked pork or other meat products, and an eosinophilia in the peripheral blood. In trichinosis, facial erythema, periorbital edema and skin rash may occur during the systemic phase of the illness and the clinical picture may closely resemble that of dermatomyositis. On the other hand, the encysted phase of certain parasites such as cysticercus may give rise to single or multiple calcified nodules, which may be visible on plain radiographs, or to painless muscle swelling.[108]

The current treatment of choice for trichinosis is albendazole in a dose of 400 mg twice daily for 14 days or, alternatively, merbendazole 5 mg/kg twice daily for the same period.[110] Concomitant glucocorticoid therapy (prednisone 40–60 mg/day) is recommended to counter any systemic hypersensitivity reaction associated with death of the worms. While anti-helminthic therapy will eliminate adult worms from the gut, it has no effect on muscle larvae or on the course of the disease in established cases.[108] Albendazole may also be used for the treatment of cysticercosis, or, alternatively, praziquantel 50 mg/kg/day for five days.[110]

Toxoplasmosis is usually an acute self-limiting disease in immunocompetent individuals and anti-microbial therapy is not necessary. However, treatment may be required if there is evidence of persisting myositis, particularly in immunodeficient individuals. Recommended treatment consists of a combination of sulphadiazine 1–1.5 g/day in four divided doses and pyrimethamine starting with a loading dose of 200 mg in two divided doses on day one followed by a daily dose of 25–50 mg/day in immunocompetent patients and 75–100 mg/day in patients with immunodeficiency.[110] Folinic acid 5–10 mg/day should also be administered to counteract the anti-metabolite action of pyrimethamine on normal tissues.

References

1. Walton JN, Adams PD. Polymyositis. Edinburgh and London: Livingstone, 1958
2. Yunis EJ, Samaha FJ. Inclusion body myositis. Lab Invest 1971;25:240–248
3. Adams RD, Samaha FJ, Kakulas BA. A myopathy with cellular inclusions. Trans Amer Neurol Assoc 1965; 90:213–216
4. Dalakas MC. Polymyositis, dermatomyositis and inclusion body myositis. New Engl J Med 1991;325: 1487–1498
5. Benbasset J, Geffel D, Zlotnick A. Epidemiology of polymyositis-dermatomyositis in Israel, 1960–76. Isr J Med Sci 1980;16:197–200
6. Oddis CV, Conte CG, Steen VD, Medsger TA. Incidence of polymyositis-dermatomyositis: a 20-year study of hospital diagnosed cases in Allegheny County, PA. J Rheumatol 1990;17:1329–1334
7. Weitoft T. Occurrence of polymyositis in the county of Gavleborg, Sweden. Scan J Rheumatol 1997;26:104–106
8. Phillips BA, Zilko P, Mastaglia FL. Prevalence of sporadic inclusion body myositis in Western Australia. Muscle & Nerve 2000;23:970–973
9. Badrising UA. Maat-Schieman M, Van Duinen SG, et al. Epidemiology of inclusion body myositis in the Netherlands. Neuromusc Disord 1997;6/7:463–464
10. Mastaglia FL, Ojeda VJ. Inflammatory myopathies: part I. Ann Neurol 1985;17:215–227
11. Whitaker JN, Engel WK. Vascular deposits of immunoglobulin and complement in idiopathic inflammatory myopathy. N Engl J Med 1972;286: 333–338
12. Kissel JT, Mendell JR, Rammohan KW. Microvascular deposition of complement membrane attack complex in dermatomyositis. N Engl J Med 1986;314:329–334
13. Emslie-Smith AM, Engel AG. Microvascular changes in early and advanced dermatomyositis: a quantitative study. Ann Neurol 1990;27:343–356
14. Engel AG, Arahata K. Mononuclear cells in myopathies. Hum Pathol 1986;17:704–721
15. Goebels N, Michaelis D, Engelhardt M, et al. Differential expression of perforin in muscle-infiltrating T cells in polymyositis. J Clin Invest 1996;97:2905–2910
16. Garlepp MJ Mastaglia FL. Inclusion body myositis. J Neurol Neurosurg Psychiatry 1996;60:251–255
17. Barohn RJ, Amato AA, Sahenk Z, et al. Inclusion body

myosis: explanation for poor response to immuno-suppressive therapy. Neurology 1995;45:1302–1306

18. Garcia-de-la Torre I, Ramirez-Cassilas A, Hernandez-Vazquez L. Acute familial myositis with a common autoimmune response. Arthritis Rheum 1991;34:744–750

19. Garlepp MJ. Genetics of the idiopathic inflammatory myopathies. Curr Opin Rheumatol 1996;8:514–520

20. Rider LG, Gurley RC, Pandey JP, et al. Clinical, serologic, and immunogenetic features of familial idiopathic inflammatory myopathy. Arthritis Rheum 1998;41:710–719

21. Garlepp MJ, Laing B, Zilko PJ, et al. HLA associations with inclusion body myositis. Clin Exp Immunol 1994;98:40–45

22. DeVere R, Bradley WG. Polymyositis: its presentation, morbidity and mortality. Brain 1975;98:637–666

23. Phillips BA, Zilko P, Garlepp MJ, Mastaglia FL. Frequency of relapses in patients with polymyositis and dermatomyositis. Muscle Nerve 1998;21:1668–1672

24. Henriksson KG, Sandstedt P. Polymyositis—treatment and prognosis: a study of 107 patients. Acta Neurol Scandinav 1982;65:280–300

25. Lilley H, Dennett X, Byrne E. Biopsy proven polymyositis in Victoria 1982–1987: analysis of prognostic factors. J Roy Soc Med 1994;87:323–326

26. Mastaglia FL, Laing BA, Zilko P. Treatment of inflammatory myopathies. Bailliere's Clinical Neurology 1993;2:717–740

27. Mastaglia FL, Phillips BA, Zilko PJ. Treatment of inflammatory myopathy. Muscle Nerve 1997;20:651–664

28. Auphan N, DiDonato JA, Rosette C, et al. Immunosuppression by glucocorticoids: Inhibition of NF-kB activity through induction of IkB synthesis. Science 1995;270:286–290

29. Horst HJ, Flad HD. Corticosteroid-interleukin 2 interactions: inhibition of binding of interleukin 2 to interleukin 2 receptors. Clin Exp Immunol 1987;68:156–161

30. Laxer RM, Stein LD, Petty RE. Intravenous pulse methylprednisolone treatment of juvenile dermatomyositis. Arthritis Rheum 1987;30:328–334

31. Matsubara S, Sawa Y, Takamori M, et al. Pulsed intravenous methylprednisolone combined with oral steroids as the initial treatment of inflammatory myopathies. J Neurol Neurosurg Psychiatry 1994;7:1008

32. Bunch TW, Worthington JW, Combs JJ, et al. Azathioprine with prednisone for polymyositis. A controlled, clinical trial. Ann Int Med 1980;92:365–369

33. Bunch TW. Prednisone and azathioprine for polymyositis: long-term follow-up. Arthritis Rheum 1981;24:45–48

34. Miro O, Laguno M, Grau JM, et al. Relapses in idiopathic inflammatory myopathies. Muscle Nerve 1999;22:1159–1160

35. Mastaglia FL, Phillips BA, Zilko P, et al. Relapses in idiopathic inflammatory myopathies. Muscle Nerve 1999;22:1160–1161

36. Horber FF, Schiedegger JR, Grunig BE, Frey FJ. Thigh muscle mass and function in patients treated with glucocorticoids. Eur J Clin Invest 1985;15:302–307

37. Sakai Y, Kobayashi K, Iwata N. Effects of an anabolic steroid and vitamin B complex upon myopathy induced by corticosteroids. Eur J Pharmacol 1978;52:353–359

38. Adachi JD, Benson WG, Brown J, et al. Intermittent etidronate therapy to prevent corticosteroid-induced osteoporosis. N Engl J Med 1997;337:382–387

39. Saag KG, Emkey R, Schnitzer TJ, et al. Alendronate for the prevention and treatment of glucocorticoid-induced osteoporosis. N Engl J Med 1998;339:292–299

40. Zilko PJ, Mastaglia FL, Phillips BA. Idiopathic inflammatory myopathies. Biodrugs 1997;7:262–272

41. Kremer JM. Is methotrexate oncogenic in patients with rheumatoid arthritis? Semin Arthritis Rheum 1997;26:785–787

42. Joffe MM, Love LA, Leff RL, et al. Drug therapy of the idiopathic inflammatory myopathies: predictors of response to prednisolone, azathioprine and methotrexate and a comparison of their efficacy. Amer J Med 1993;94:379–387

43. Oddis CV. Therapy for myositis. Curr Opin Rheumatol 1991;3:919–924

44. Conaghan PG, Brooks PM, Quinn DI, Day RO. Hazards of low dose methotrexate. Aust N Z J Med 1995;25:670–673

45. Black AJ, McLeod HL, Capell HA, et al. Thiopurine methyltransferase genotype predicts therapy-limiting severe toxicity from azathioprine. Ann Intern Med 1998;129:716–718

46. Confraveaux C, Saddier P, Grimaud J, et al. Risk of cancer from azathioprine therapy in multiple sclerosis: a case-control study. Neurology 1996;46:1607–1612

47. Turk L, Poulter LW. Selective depletion of lymphoid tissue by cyclophosphamide. Clin Exp Immunol 1972;10:285–296

48. Griggs RC, Karpati G. The pathogenesis of dermatomyositis. Arch Neurol 1991;48:21–22

49. Cronin ME, Miller FW, Hicks JE, et al. The failure of intravenous cyclophosphamide therapy in refractory idiopathic myopathy. J Rheumatol 1989;16:1225–1228

50. Haga HJ, D'Cruz D, Asherson R, Hughes GR. Short term effects of intravenous pulses of cyclophosphamide in the treatment of connective tissue disease crises. Ann Rheum Dis 1992;51:885–888

51. Freedman A, Ehrlich RM, Ljung BM. Prevention of cyclophosphamide cystitis with 2-mercaptoethane sodium sulfonate: a histologic study. J Urol 1984;132:580–582

52. Radis CD, Kahl LE, Baker GL, et al. Effects of cyclophosphamide on the development of malignancy and on long term survival of patients with rheumatoid arthritis. Arthritis Rheum 1995;38:1120–1127

53. Elliott JF, Lin Y, Mizel SB, et al. Induction of interleukin 2 messenger RNA inhibited by cyclosporin A. Science 1984;226:1439–1441

54. Heckmatt J, Saunders C, Peters AM, et al. Cyclosporin in juvenile dermatomyositis. Lancet 1989;i:1063–1066

55. Mansur AY, Topaloglu H, Jungbluth H, et al. Cyclosporin treatment in juvenile dermatomyositis: a review of 26 cases. Muscle Nerve 1998(Suppl 7):S150

56. Leuck CJ, Trend PT, Swash M. Cyclosporin in the management of polymyositis and dermatomyositis. J Neurol Neurosurg Psychiatry 1991;54:1007–1008

57. Grau JM, Herrero C, Casademont J, et al. Cyclosporin A as first choice for dermatomyositis. J Rheumatol 1994;21:381–382

58. Dalakas MC, Illa I, Dambrosia JM, et al. A controlled trial of high-dose intravenous immune globulin infusions as treatment for dermatomyositis. N Engl J Med 1993;329:1993–2000

59. Cherin P, Herson S, Wechsler B, et al. Efficacy of intravenous gammaglobulin therapy in chronic refractory polymyositis and dermatomyositis: an open study with 20 adult patients. Am J Med 1991;91:162–168

60. Mastaglia FL, Phillips BA, Zilko PJ. Immunoglobulin

therapy in inflammatory myopathies. J Neurol Neurosurg Psychiatry 1998;65:107–110

61. Cherin P, Piette JC, Wechsler B, et al. Intravenous gamma globulin as first line therapy in polymyositis and dermatomyositis: an open study in 11 adult patients. J Rheumatol 1994;21:1092–1097

62. Bertorini TE, Nance AM, Horner LH, et al. Complications of intravenous gammaglobulin in neuromuscular and other diseases. Muscle Nerve 1996;19:388–391

63. Basta M, Dalakas MC. High-dose intravenous immunoglobulin exerts its beneficial effect in patients with dermatomyositis by blocking endomysial deposition of activated complement fragments. J Clin Invest 1994;94:1729–1735

64. Dwyer JM. Manipulating the immune system with immune globulin. New Engl J Med 1992;326:107–116

65. Dalakas MC. Intravenous immune globulin therapy for neurologic diseases. Ann Intern Med 1997;126: 721–730

66. Dau PC. Plasmapheresis in idiopathic inflammatory myopathy. Arch Neurol 1981;38:544–552

67. Miller FW, Leitman SF, Cronin ME, et al. Controlled trial of plasma exchange and leukapheresis in polymyositis and dermatomyositis. New Engl J Med 1992;326:1380–1384

68. Sinoway PA, Callen JP. Chlorambucil: an effective corticosteroid sparing agent for patients with recalcitrant dermatomyositis. Arthritis Rheum 1993;43:876–879

69. Kahn MF, Arlet J, Bloch-Michel H, et al. Acute leukaemia's after treatment using cytotoxic agents for rheumatological purpose. Nouvell Presse Medicale 1979;8:1393–1397

70. Engel WK, Lighter AS, Galdi AP. Polymyositis: remarkable response to total body irradiation. Lancet 1981;i:658

71. Morgan SH, Bernstein RM, Coppen J, et al. Total body irradiation and the course of polymyositis. Arthritis Rheum 1985;28:831–835

72. Rosenberg NL, Ringel SP. Adult polymyositis and dermatomyositis. In: Mastaglia FL, ed. Inflammatory Diseases of Muscle. Oxford: Blackwell Scientific Publications, 1988:87–106

73. Lane RJM, Hudgson P. Thymectomy in polymyositis. Lancet 1984;i:626

74. Hicks JE. Role of rehabilitation in the management of myopathies. Curr Opin Rheumatol 1998;10:548–555

75. Escalante A, Miller L, Beardmore TD. Resistive exercise in the rehabilitation of polymyositis/dermatomyositis. J Rheumatol 1993;20:1340–1344

76. Wiesinger GR, Quittan M, Aringer M, et al. Improvement of physical fitness and muscle strength in polymyositis/dermatomyositis patients by a training programme. Br J Rheumatol 1998;37:196–200

77. Malleson P. Juvenile dermatomyositis: a review. J Roy Soc Med 1982;75:33–37

78. Miller G, Heckmatt JZ, Dubowitz V. Drug treatment of juvenile dermatomyositis. Arch Dis Child 1983;58: 445–450

79. Sarnat HB. Juvenile dermatomyositis. In: Mastaglia FL, ed. Inflammatory Diseases of Muscle, Oxford: Blackwell Scientific Publications, 1988:71–86

80. Sansome A, Dubowitz V. Intravenous immunoglobulin in juvenile dermatomyositis: four year review of nine cases. Arch Dis Child 1995;72:24–28

81. Olson NY, Lindsley CB. Adjunctive use of hydroxychloroquine in childhood dermatomyositis. J Rheumatol 1989;16:1545–1547

82. Spiera R, Kagen L. Extramuscular manifestations in idiopathic inflammatory myopathies. Curr Opin Rheumatol 1998;10:556–561

83. Lotz BP, Engel AG, Nishino H, et al. Inclusion body myositis. Brain 1989;112:727–747

84. Leff RL, Miller FW, Hicks J, et al. The treatment of inclusion body myositis: a retrospective review and a randomized, prospective trial of immunosuppressive therapy. Medicine 1993;72:225–235

85. Lindberg C, Persson LC, Björkaader J, Oldfors A. Inclusion body myositis: clinical, morphological, physiological and laboratory findings in 18 cases. Acta Neurol Scand 1994;89:123–131

86. Sayers ME, Chou SM, Calabrese LH. Inclusion body myositis: analysis of 32 cases. J Rheumatol 1992;19: 1385–1389

87. Soueidan SA, Dalakas MC. Treatment of inclusion body myositis with high-dose intravenous immunoglobulin. Neurology 1993;43:876–879

88. Amato AA, Barohn RJ, Jackson CE, et al. Inclusion body myositis: treatment with intravenous immunoglobulin. Neurology 1994;444:1516–1518

89. Dalakas MC, Sonies B, Dambrosia J, et al. Treatment of inclusion body myositis with IVIg: a double-blind placebo-controlled study. Neurology 1997;48: 712–716

90. Walter MC, Lochmuller H, Toepfer M, et al. High-dose immunoglobulin therapy in sporadic inclusion body myositis: a double-blind placebo-controlled study. J Neurol 2000;247:22–28

91. Spector SA, Lemmer JT, Koffman BM, et al. Safety and efficacy of strength training in patients with sporadic inclusion body myositis. Muscle Nerve 1997;20: 1242–1248

92. Engel WK, Askanas V. Treatment of inclusion-body myositis and hereditary inclusion body myopathy with reference to pathogenic mechanisms. In: Askanas V, Serratrice G, King Engel W, eds. Inclusion-body Myositis and Myopathies, Cambridge: Cambridge University Press, 1998:351–382

93. Danon MJ, Friedman M. Inclusion body myositis associated with progressive dysphagia: treatment with cricopharyngeal myotomy. Can J Neurol Sci 1989; 16:436–439

94. Kumamoto T, Ueyama H, Fujimoto S, et al. Clinicopathologic characteristics of polymyositis patients with numerous tissue eosinophils. Acta Neurol Scand 1996;94:110–114

95. Layzer RB, Shearn MA, Satya-Murti S. Eosinophilic polymyositis. Ann Neurol 1977;1:65–71

96. Pickering MC, Walport MJ. Eosinophilic myopathic syndromes. Curr Opin Rheumatol 1998;10:504–510

97. Simon DB, Sufit RL. Clinical spectrum of fascial inflammation. Muscle Nerve 1982;5:525–531

98. Silver RM, Heyes MP, Maize JC, et al. Scleroderma, fasciitis and eosinophilia associated with the ingestion of tryptophan. New Engl J Med 1990;322:874–881

99. Belongia EA, Hedberg CW, Gleich GJ, et al. An investigation of the cause of the eosinophilia-myalgia syndrome associated with tryptophan use. New Engl J Med 1990;323:357–365

100. Emslie-Smith AM, Engel AG, Duffy J, Bowles CA. Eosinophilia myalgia syndrome: 1. Immunocytochemical evidence for a T cell-mediated immune effector response. Ann Neurol 1991;29:524–528

101. Culpepper RC, Williams RG, Mease PJ, et al. One-year outcome in the eosinophilia-myalgia syndrome. Ann Intern Med 1991;115:437–442

102. Dalakas MC. Retroviruses and inflammatory

myopathies in humans and primates. Bailliere's Clinical Neurology 1993;2:659–691

103. Lange DJ. AAEM Minimonograph #41: neuromuscular diseases associated with HIV-1 infection. Muscle Nerve 1994;17:16–30

104. Simpson DM, Citak KA, Godfrey E, et al. Myopathies associated with human immunodeficiency virus and zidovudine: can their effects be distinguished? Neurology 1993;43:971–976

105. Gonzales MF, Olney RK, So YT, et al. Sub acute structural myopathy associated with human immunodeficiency virus infection. Arch Neurol 1988;45:585–587

106. Simpson DM, Bender AN, Farraye J, et al. Human immunodeficiency virus wasting syndrome may rep-resent a treatable myopathy. Neurology 1990;40: 535–538

107. Simpson DM, Tagliati M. Neurologic manifestations of HIV infection. Ann Intern Med 1994;121:769–785

108. Grove DI. Parasitic and fungal infections of muscle. *In:* Mastaglia FL, ed. Inflammatory Diseases of Muscle. Oxford: Blackwell Scientific Publications, 1988:164–184

109. Pallis CA, Lewis PD. Involvement of human muscle by parasites. *In:* Walton JN, Karpati G, Hilton Jones D, eds. Disorders of Voluntary Muscle. Edinburgh: Churchill Livingstone, 1994:743–759

110. Gilbert DN, Moellering RC, Sande M. The Guide to Antimicrobial Therapy. Merck-Sharp & Dohme. Virginia, USA: Antimicrobial Therapy Incorporated, 1998

224 Metabolic Myopathies

Deborah L Renaud and Joe TR Clarke

Muscle weakness and hypotonia are common findings in many inborn errors of metabolism, and in some, frank myopathy dominates the clinical manifestations of the disease. Myopathy is particularly prominent in primary disorders of energy metabolism, including many disorders of carbohydrate metabolism, fatty acid oxidation disorders, and mitochondrial electron transport defects. Drugs and toxic substances that interfere with energy production or utilization may also produce acute or chronic myopathies. Any of these disorders may precipitate life-threatening rhabdomyolysis. The early recognition and aggressive management of acute rhabdomyolysis can be life saving. Prevention is based primarily on the identification of the predisposing underlying metabolic defect or exogenous precipitant. This chapter will outline the management of the inherited and acquired defects in metabolism that result in myopathy and the treatment of rhabdomyolysis.

General overview[1,2]

Resting muscle derives most of its energy from fatty acid oxidation. The pattern of muscle fuel utilization during exercise is determined by the type, intensity, and duration of the activity. At the onset of exercise, local stores of adenosine triphosphate (ATP), as well as ATP derived predominantly from the hydrolysis of phosphocreatine, are sufficient to sustain exercise for only a few seconds. Adenosine triphosphate produced by the anaerobic oxidation of local glycogen-derived glucose to lactate provides most of the energy required in the first 30 seconds of sustained exercise. This is followed by a transition to aerobic oxidative phosphorylation, the principal mechanism for energy production during sustained exercise. Intramuscular glycogen is the primary source of oxidative fuel for the first 30 to 90 minutes of sustained exercise. As muscle glycogen stores are depleted, free fatty acids and glucose produced in the liver become the primary substrates for oxidative energy production. The supply of free fatty acids, derived from triglycerides stored as adipose tissue, is virtually limitless, allowing for prolonged exercise. The shift to free fatty acid oxidation and increased blood flow to muscle during sustained exercise underlie the "second wind" phenomenon experienced by patients with inherited disorders of carbohydrate metabolism.

Approach to the diagnosis of metabolic myopathy

History

The age of onset, distribution and course of the muscle weakness, and associated signs of multisystem involvement are all important elements of the history of metabolic myopathy. The onset of weakness may occur at any age, and the course may be chronically progressive or episodic, or both. The effect of exercise is a particularly important discriminating feature of the various metabolic causes of myopathy. Exercise intolerance in mitochondrial disorders is characterized by easy fatigability and tends to be severe. On the other hand, patients with disorders of carbohydrate metabolism complain of muscle fatigue and painful muscle cramping with strenuous exercise. They often report that the muscle power improves and the cramping pain resolves with sustained exercise, the so-called "second wind" phenomenon. In contrast to patients with defects in carbohydrate metabolism, those with fatty acid oxidation defects tend to develop cramps late in the course of prolonged exercise, or even some hours after the cessation of the exercise. A history of pigmenturia, suggesting rhabdomyolysis, is typical, though not invariably present, in patients with defects in muscle energy metabolism.

A history of developmental delay or regression in a child may indicate that the myopathy is associated with central nervous system (CNS) involvement. However, it is important to distinguish gross motor developmental delay caused by muscle weakness from global developmental disabilities resulting from effects of the disease on the CNS. Central nervous system involvement, including hearing or visual impairment, is common in patients with mitochondrial myopathies. Cardiomyopathy is a prominent feature of some of the disorders of carbohydrate metabolism, especially Pompe disease (glycogen storage disease, type 2). It is also a typical clinical characteristic of some of the fatty acid oxidation defects and disorders of mitochondrial electron transport. Cyclic vomiting and failure to thrive are often seen in children with fatty acid oxidation defects. A history of medication for some pre-existing condition, or a history of substance abuse, is an important clue to the possibility of drug-induced myopathy.

A history of myopathy in relatives of the patient is obviously important in identifying patients who might have inherited metabolic disorders. Many of the conditions are transmitted as autosomal recessive disorders, and there may be a history of parental consanguinity. On the other hand, the absence of a family history does not rule out the possibility of an inherited metabolic myopathy. In the case of mitochondrial myopathies, the patient may have a family history of conditions, such as sudden unexpected death in infancy, cardiomyopathy, hepatopathy, deafness, diabetes or recurrent hypoglycemia, migraine, seizures or ophthalmoplegia, in which the skeletal myopathy may be subtle.

Physical examination

The examination of the muscular system is described in detail in the first chapter of this section. In addition to signs referable to the muscular system, patients with inherited metabolic myopathies often exhibit clinical evidence of involvement of other elements of the nervous system and to non-neurological systems, especially the heart. Some of the more common or characteristic non-muscular and non-neurological physical findings are shown in Table 224.1.

Routine laboratory studies

Creatine kinase (CK) levels are generally increased in disorders of carbohydrate metabolism, but may be normal in other metabolic myopathies in the absence of acute rhabdomyolysis. Plasma lactate levels are often, but not always, elevated in patients with mito-chondrial myopathies or disorders of gluconeogenesis. Lactate levels in CSF are also often elevated, even when the plasma lactate concentration may be normal. Lactate may be spuriously elevated if processing of the blood sample is delayed. The lactate-to-pyruvate (L/P) ratio in plasma is normally less than 20. In primary disorders of pyruvate metabolism, the L/P ratio remains normal, even when lactate levels are very high. In contrast, it is generally increased in patients with mitochondrial respiratory chain defects. It is also elevated in patients with lactic acidosis caused by circulatory failure or poor tissue perfusion, sometimes making the discrimination between primary and secondary causes of lactic acidosis difficult. Lactic acidemia is associated with an elevation in plasma alanine concentrations.[3]

Electromyography abnormalities are generally nonspecific in the majority of metabolic myopathies. Nerve conduction studies are useful for confirming the presence of peripheral nerve involvement, which

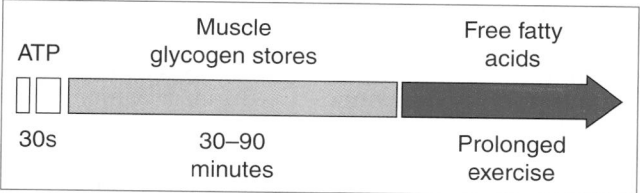

Figure 224.1 Energy utilization during exercise in normal muscle.

may not be obvious in the presence of the weakness. Peripheral neuropathy is an important feature of some of the metabolic myopathies (Table 224.1).

Specific studies

Urinary organic acid analysis is often useful in the diagnosis of primary metabolic myopathies. In patients with defects in fatty acid β-oxidation, organic acid analysis often shows the presence of intermediates of β-oxidation, such as short- and medium-chain dicarboxylic acids, especially during acute illness with metabolic decompensation. Any of the disorders of mitochondrial energy metabolism may be associated with increased excretion of tricarboxylic acid cycle intermediates, and boys with Barth syndrome typically excrete increased amounts of 3-methylgluta-conic acid in the urine. In contrast, organic acid analysis is usually normal in patients with carnitine cycle defects.

Total and free carnitine levels in plasma are markedly decreased in patients with primary muscle carnitine deficiency caused by defects in the plasmalemmal carnitine transporter. They are also usually mildly to moderately decreased in other fatty acid oxidation disorders, except in carnitine palmitoyl transferase I deficiency in which they may be elevated. The difference between the total and free carnitine concentrations represents the acylcarnitine fraction. An increase in the ratio of acylcarnitine to free carnitine in plasma, normally less than 0.4, is a

Table 224.1 Physical findings in patients with inherited metabolic myopathies

Physical findings	Mitochondrial myopathies	Fatty acid oxidation defects	Glycogen storage diseases
Neurological signs			
Mental deficiency, dementia	+++	±[1]	0
Ptosis, external ophthalmoplegia	+++	0	0
Retinal dystrophy	++	+	0
Ataxia	++[2]	+	0
Acute encephalopathy	+	+++[3]	0
Visual impairment	++	±	0
Deafness	++	0	0
Peripheral neuropathy	++	++	+
Non-neurological signs			
Hepatomegaly	+	++	++[4]
Cardiomyopathy	++	++	++[5]

[1]Usually secondary to acute metabolic decompensation; [2]Often intermittent; [3]Intermittent, associated with acute illness, hepatopathy, hyperammonemia; [4]GSD types III, IV, VIII (Table 224.2); [5]Especially GSD type II, but also types III, IV, and VIII.

common feature of disorders of fatty acid oxidation. The acylcarnitine fraction is also increased by administration of certain drugs, such as valproic acid. Analyses of acylcarnitines in urine, plasma, tissue extracts, or cultured skin fibroblasts usually show characteristic patterns in cases of fatty acid oxidation.[4] Fasting plasma free fatty acid concentrations are disproportionately increased, relative to ketone levels, in fatty acid oxidation disorders, producing elevated free fatty acid-to-3-hydroxybutyrate ratios, normally less than two.[3]

Imaging and spectroscopy

Conventional magnetic resonance imaging (MRI) of muscle is of little help in the diagnosis of primary metabolic myopathies. However, MRI studies of the brain may show characteristic changes, particularly in the basal ganglia, in patients with mitochondrial respiratory chain defects. In addition, a lactate peak on proton MR spectroscopy of the brain is often present.[5]

Near-infrared spectroscopy   Near-infrared spectroscopy of muscle provides a dynamic, noninvasive means by which to measure oxygenation of blood hemoglobin and muscle myoglobin.[6–8] In normal muscle, a shift from oxygenated to deoxygenated hemoglobin and myoglobin is seen at the onset of exercise owing to increased utilization of oxygen by mitochondria. This normal early deoxygenation of myoglobin is not seen in patients with myophosphorylase and phosphofructokinase deficiencies. However, if the exercise is sustained, late deoxygenation occurs, coinciding with the development of the clinical "second wind" phenomenon. Patients with mitochondrial respiratory chain defects, who have impairment in oxygen utilization, show an increase in relative blood oxygenation in muscle with exercise. By contrast, patients with disorders of fatty acid metabolism show a normal deoxygenation response to exercise.[2]

[31]P magnetic resonance spectroscopy (P-MRS)   P-MRS is another non-invasive technique for the detection and monitoring of metabolites of oxidative phosphorylation during rest, exercise and recovery. Seven spectral peaks can normally be recorded from normal muscle: three from ATP and one each from phosphocreatine (PCr), inorganic phosphate (Pi), phosphomonoesters (PME), and phosphodiesters (PDE). At rest, patients with mitochondrial oxidative phosphorylation defects show elevated Pi concentrations, which may be accompanied by low levels of PCr. During exercise, these patients show a further rise in Pi and concomitant fall in PCr, accompanied by a fall in muscle intracellular pH. Post-exercise recovery is also impaired. In muscles in which glycolysis or glycogenolysis is impaired, a paradoxical increase in pH is seen owing to impaired production of lactic acid. [31]P magnetic resonance spectroscopy is useful to distinguish between these two groups of disorders since impairment of glycolysis results in the accumulation of glycolytic metabolites resulting in an increased PME peak.[9]

Provocative testing

The forearm ischemic exercise test   This test is useful in the investigation of energy production by anaerobic glycolysis (lactate production) and the integrity of the purine nucleotide cycle (ammonia production). With a blood pressure cuff inflated above the elbow in order to produce ischemia, serial blood samples are drawn from the forearm of the patient during rapid, repetitive opening and closing of the fist. In a normal individual, plasma lactate and ammonia concentrations both increase at least three- to four-fold above resting levels during ischemic exercise, then return to baseline within 10 to 15 minutes after cessation of the exercise and restoration of the circulation. Defects of carbohydrate metabolism, such as McArdle disease (myophosphorylase deficiency) produce a normal rise in ammonia, but a blunted lactate response. Insufficiency of the ammonia response alone is typical of myoadenylate deaminase deficiency. This test requires patient cooperation; failure of both lactate and ammonia responses is suggestive of poor effort.[1,3,10]

Dynamic exercise testing   Dynamic exercise testing, using a treadmill or stationary cycle, is useful to test the integrity of the oxidative pathways. Expired gas is collected during exercise in order to measure maximum oxygen consumption (VO_{2max}). Oxygen consumption is often decreased in patients with myophosphorylase or phosphofructokinase deficiency because of decreased availability of glucose as a substrate for oxidative phosphorylation.[2] The impairment of VO_{2max} is even greater in patients with hereditary defects of mitochondrial respiration;[11] in patients with a fatty acid oxidation defect, carnitine palmitoyl transferase II (CPT II) deficiency, VO_{2max} was normal.[12]

Monitored prolonged starvation   The metabolic response to fasting is useful in the evaluation of patients with suspected primary disorders of energy metabolism, especially inherited fatty acid oxidation defects.[13] Care must be taken to monitor patients closely and to terminate testing at the first clinical or biochemical evidence of hypoglycemia. Patients with fatty acid oxidation defects tolerate fasting poorly. After several hours of starvation, they generally develop hypoglycemia, often quite suddenly, and analyses of plasma free fatty acids, 3-hydroxybutyrate, and acylcarnitines, as well as urinary organic acids, show abnormalities typical of the diseases. Children with disorders of carbohydrate metabolism also tolerate fasting poorly, tending also to become hypoglycemic. However, ketogenesis is generally intact, and analyses of plasma and urinary metabolites may show only increased ketone concentrations.

Muscle biopsy

Open muscle biopsy is preferred to needle biopsies for the evaluation of metabolic myopathy in order to obtain sufficient tissue for histology, histochemistry, and electron microscopy, as well as for enzyme assays. Histochemical panels for muscle customarily include stains for adenosine triphosphatase (ATPase), nicotinamide adenine dinucleotide-tetrazolium reductase (NADH-TR), succinate dehydrogenase (SDH), cytochrome oxidase, acid phosphatase, myophosphorylase, phosphofructokinase, and myoadenylate deaminase, as well as Gomori trichrome, periodic-acid Schiff (PAS) and oil red O (ORO) stains. The contents of vacuoles in sections prepared from unfixed, frozen tissue can be determined to be glycogen (PAS positive) or lipid (ORO positive), and lysosomal vacuoles are identifiable by their increased staining for acid phosphatase. Ragged-red fibers, which are typical of most of the mitochondrial myopathies, are identifiable in sections stained with Gomori trichrome stain. Electron microscopic examination is particularly useful for the demonstration of ultrastructural abnormalities associated with lysosomal accumulation of glycogen, in GSD type II, or complex lipid. It will also reveal characteristic mitochondrial abnormalities, such as paracrystalline inclusions, in patients with mitochondrial myopathies. More subtle mitochondrial ultrastructural abnormalities, accompanied by excessive neutral lipid storage, may be seen in fatty acid oxidation defects.[10] Enzyme assays and polarigraphic studies on fresh muscle are particularly useful for the specific diagnosis of defects of mitochondrial respiration.[14]

Molecular studies

Commercial molecular testing is readily available for the common mutations associated with medium chain acyl-CoA dehydrogenase (MCAD) deficiency, long-chain 3-hydroxyacyl-CoA dehydrogenase deficiency (LCHAD) deficiency and some of the common mitochondrial DNA mutations. Molecular analyses for most other disorders are available on an individual basis in research laboratories.

Disorders of carbohydrate metabolism

Brief overview[15,16]

Glycogen is utilized by skeletal muscle as a short-term, high-energy fuel for muscle contraction. The production of glucose by the phosphorolytic degradation of cytosolic glycogen occurs in a stepwise fashion. Phosphorylase catalyzes the sequential cleavage of α1,4-linked glucose molecules from the non-reducing end of the polymer, producing glucose-1-phosphate. At least three tissue-specific isoenzymes of phosphorylase exist, in brain, liver and muscle. Phosphorylase *b* kinase catalyzes the activation of inactive phosphorylase *b* to active phosphorylase *a* by phosphorylation of the enzyme protein, stimulating glycogen breakdown. Complete glycogen breakdown requires the removal of the branch points in the polymer. This reaction is catalyzed by a debranching enzyme, which has two separate catalytic activities. When α1,6-linked branches of the polymer have been shortened, by the action of phosphorylase, to four glucose residues, the three terminal residues are transferred and linked α1,4 to the end of the linear core of the polymer in a reaction catalyzed

by the transferase part of the enzyme. The remaining α1,6-linked glucose residue is hydrolyzed by the amylo-1,6-glucosidase part of the enzyme. Hydrolytic glycogen degradation occurs in lysosomes in a reaction catalyzed by acid α-glucosidase (acid maltase), which has both α1,4 and α1,6-glucosidase activities. The product of the reaction is free glucose. The physiological role of lysosomal glycogen is unclear; it does not appear to be a quantitatively important source of substrate glucose for energy production.

Classification

The disorders of carbohydrate metabolism causing myopathy are classified according to the metabolic process disrupted by the enzyme defect (Table 224.2). The numerical classification is included primarily for historical reasons only, for the majority of disorders of carbohydrate metabolism are, in fact, not associated with abnormal storage of glycogen, as suggested by the way they were previously labeled.

Clinical features

Defects of glycogenolysis[16-18]

- *McArdle disease, (GSD V)* The cardinal clinical feature of this disorder, caused by deficiency of muscle phosphorylase, is exercise intolerance, accompanied by muscle cramps associated with vigorous exercise. Most patients describe a "second wind" phenomenon described above. Approximately half the patients with the disease develop myoglobinuria after exercise. Eventually, most patients develop mild fixed proximal muscle weakness. Diagnosis is generally made in the second or third decade of life, although a history of exercise intolerance in childhood is often present.

- *Cori-Forbes disease, (GSD III)* This disease, which is caused by deficiency of debrancher enzyme, occurs in two forms. In GSD IIIa, both liver and muscle debrancher isozymes are deficient. In GSD IIIb, the defect is confined to liver, without any muscle involvement. In both forms, patients generally present in infancy or early childhood with hepatomegaly and fasting hypoglycemia, accompanied by failure to thrive. Slowly progressive weakness usually develops in early adulthood, although gross motor milestones may be delayed in up to a third of patients, and some children develop severe myopathy long before puberty. Weakness and atrophy affects primarily the distal extremities and hands, but it may be generalized in some cases. Patients with distal myopathy may have an associated peripheral neuropathy. Exercise intolerance and myoglobinuria are uncommon. Hypertrophic cardiomyopathy may occur. This is generally mild, though it may progress to become life threatening in rare cases.[19,20]

- *Phosphorylase b kinase (PBK) deficiency, (GSD VIII)* At least four clinically distinct phenotypes have been described with PBK deficiency, two of them involving skeletal muscle. One form of the disease presents with hepatomegaly and a non-progressive myopathy. In another form, only

Table 224.2   Classification of disorders of carbohydrate metabolism associated with myopathy

	Enzyme defect	Inheritance	Gene locus	Clinical features
Defects of glycogenolysis				
McArdle disease, GSD V	Myophosphorylase	AR	11q13	Myopathy, exercise intolerance, rhabdomyolysis
Cori-Forbes disease, GSD III	Debrancher enzyme	AR	1p21	Myopathy, cardiomyopathy, hepatomegaly, liver disease, hypoglycemia
PBK deficiency, GSD VIII	Phosphorylase *b* kinase	AR	16q12–q13?	Myopathy, exercise intolerance, rhabdomyolysis, hepatomegaly
Defects of glycolysis				
Tarui disease, GSD VII	Muscle phosphofructokinase	AR	12q13.3	Myopathy, exercise intolerance, rhabdomyolysis, hemolytic anemia
PGK deficiency, GSD IX	Phosphoglycerate kinase	XR	Xq13	Myopathy, rhabdomyolysis, hemolytic anemia, psychomotor retardation
PGM deficiency, GSD X	Muscle phosphoglycerate mutase	AR	7p13–p12.3	Myopathy, exercise intolerance, rhabdomyolysis
LDH-M deficiency, GSD XI	Lactate dehydrogenase	AR	11p15.4	Myopathy, exercise intolerance, rhabdomyolysis
Defects of glycogen synthesis				
Andersen disease, GSD IV	Glycogen branching enzyme	AR	3p12	Myopathy, cardiomyopathy, hepatomegaly, liver disease, hypoglycemia
Lysosomal glycogenoses				
Pompe disease, GSD IIa	Lysosomal α-glucosidase (Acid maltase)	AR	17q25.2–q25.3	Myopathy, cardiomyopathy
Danon disease, GSD IIb	LAMP-2 (lysosome-associated membrane protein-2)	AD, AR, XLD	Xq24	Myopathy, cardiomyopathy, psychomotor retardation

muscle is involved, and the disease presents in a manner similar to McArdle disease, with exercise intolerance and myoglobinuria.

Defects of glycolysis

- *Tarui disease (GSD VII)* The muscle symptoms of Tarui disease, caused by deficiency of muscle phosphofructokinase, are indistinguishable from those of McArdle disease. Unlike the latter, however, exercise intolerance is made worse by high dietary carbohydrate consumption. Hemolytic anemia resulting in mild jaundice may occur. Myogenic hyperuricemia may result in gouty arthritis. An early-onset, severe myopathic variant has been described.
- *Phosphoglycerate kinase deficiency (GSD IX)* In this very rare disorder, myopathy is accompanied by hemolytic anemia, and it may be associated with CNS symptoms, including developmental disability, seizures and behavioral disturbances. An isolated myopathic form with exercise intolerance and myoglobinuria has also been described.

- *Phosphoglycerate mutase deficiency (GSD X)* This disorder presents as a pure myopathy, characterized by exercise intolerance, cramps and recurrent myoglobinuria.
- *Lactate dehydrogenase-M deficiency (GSD XI)* This disorder may be asymptomatic or present with exercise intolerance, cramps and recurrent myoglobinuria. An eczematous rash is often seen as an accompanying feature.
- *Aldolase A deficiency* A single patient has been described who presented with hemolytic anemia, mild developmental delay, myopathy, exercise intolerance and recurrent myoglobinuria during febrile illnesses.[21]

Defects of glycogen synthesis

- *Andersen disease (GSD IV)* Four clinically distinct forms of branching enzyme deficiency have been described. The most common presents as rapidly progressive liver dysfunction resulting in death, from cirrhosis, by five years of age. Hypoglycemia may occur as a result of cirrhosis. Hypotonia,

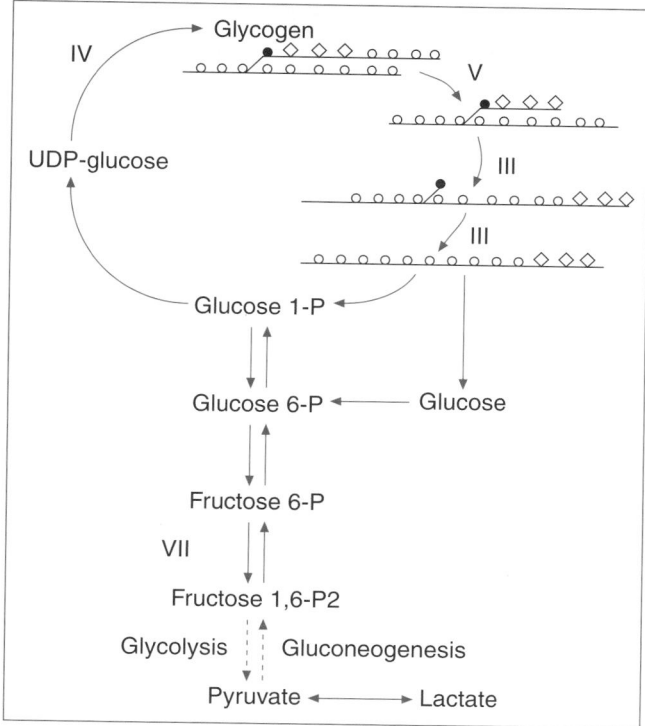

Figure 224.2 Major pathways of glycogenolysis and glycogen synthesis. Roman numerals refer to the following enzymes: III, debranching enzyme; IV, branching enzyme; V, phosphorylase; VII phosphofructokinase.

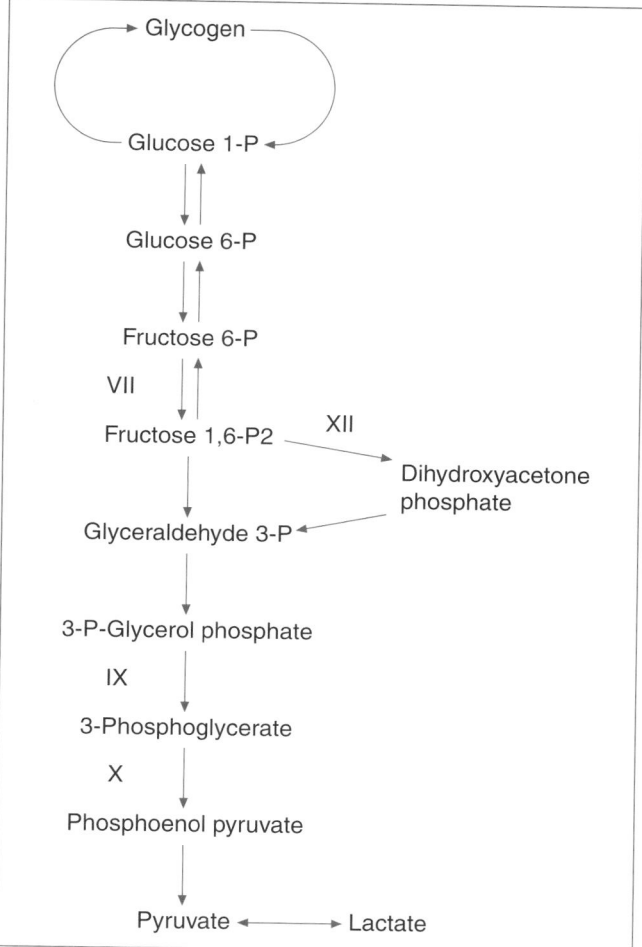

Figure 224.3 Major pathways of glycolysis. Roman numerals refer to the following enzymes: VII. phosphofructokinase; IX, phosphoglycerate kinase; X, phosphoglycerate mutase; XII aldolase.

muscle weakness and atrophy are generally overshadowed by the severity of the liver disease. The neuromuscular form consists of slowly progressive muscle weakness and atrophy, but without exercise intolerance. In the third form, cardiomyopathy may be the most predominant feature. The fourth form, also called adult polyglucosan body disease, presents with progressive upper and lower motor neuron involvement, loss of sensory nerve function, bladder and sphincter dysfunction and dementia.[16,17,20]

Lysosomal glycogenoses

- *Acid maltase deficiency (GSD IIa)* Three clinical presentations of acid maltase deficiency have been described, all caused by deficiency of lysosomal acid α-glucosidase. The infantile form, or Pompe disease, presents early in infancy with profound hypotonia and skeletal muscle weakness, along with a rapidly progressive hypertrophic cardiomyopathy, resulting in death within the first two years of life. Enlargement of the tongue and feeding difficulties are frequently seen. In the childhood form, onset occurs in late infancy or early childhood with predominantly skeletal myopathy. Cardiomyopathy is unusual. Motor milestones are delayed and progressive proximal and respiratory muscle weakness develops. Death in the second decade is usually secondary to respiratory failure. The adult form of the disease, typically with onset after 20 years of age, presents as a slowly progressive myopathy, which mimics polymyositis or limb-girdle myopathy. Up to a third of patients present initially with respiratory failure, which is also the most common cause of death in these patients. Electron microscopic examinations of skeletal muscle biopsies from patients with all forms of GSD II show intralysosomal accumulation of glycogen, although much of the glycogen accumulation is actually cytosolic.[20,22]

- *Danon disease (GSD IIb)* Lysosomal glycogen storage disease with normal acid maltase (Danon disease) presents with the clinical triad of proximal muscle weakness, hypertrophic cardiomyopathy and developmental disability.[23] Two forms of the disease have been described.[20] The late-onset cardiomusculoskeletal "pseudo-Pompe" form appears to be either autosomal dominant or X-linked dominant based on family studies. Patients present with a progressive hypertrophic cardiomyopathy, often associated with arrhythmias and conduction block.

Table 224.3 Treatment of disorders of carbohydrate metabolism

Treatment	Classification of recommendation	Quality of evidence	References
Maintenance of normoglycemia (Debranching enzyme deficiency)	A	II-3, III	16, 24
High-protein diet (McArdle disease, Pompe disease)	C	II-3	16, 20
Branched-chain amino acid supplementation (McArdle disease)	D	II-1	25
Vitamin B$_6$ supplementation (McArdle disease)	B	II-3	26, 27
Carbohydrate loading prior to exercise (McArdle disease)	B	II-3	16
(Tarui disease)	D	II-3	16

Table 224.4 Classification of recommendations and grades of quality of evidence

Categories for strength of each recommendation

Category	Definition
A	Good evidence to support a recommendation for use
B	Moderate evidence to support a recommendation for use
C	Poor evidence to support a recommendation for or against use
D	Moderate evidence to support a recommendation against use
E	Good evidence to support a recommendation against use

Categories for quality of evidence on which recommendations are made

Grade	Definition
I	Evidence from at least one properly randomized, controlled trial
II	Evidence from at least one well-designed clinical trial without randomization, from cohort or case-controlled analytic studies, preferably from more than one center, from multiple time series, or from dramatic results in uncontrolled experiments
III	Evidence from opinions of respected authorities on the basis of clinical experience, descriptive studies, or reports of expert committees

From MacPherson DW. Evidence-based medicine. Canada Communicable Disease Report 1994;20–17:145–147.

Varying degrees of muscle involvement and the absence of diaphragmatic involvement are typical. Most patients have borderline to severe mental retardation. Males usually present earlier, in the second or third decades of life, and are more severely affected than females with the disease. The rare early-onset form of Danon disease presents in early infancy, with marked hypotonia and hypertrophic cardiomyopathy, associated with global developmental delay. Electron microscopic findings are similar to those found in classical Pompe disease, except for the presence of sarcolemmal indentations reminiscent of X-linked recessive vacuolar myopathy.

Treatment of disorders of carbohydrate metabolism

A summary of the treatment of disorders of carbohydrate metabolism is shown in Table 224.3, and a classification of the quality of the evidence supporting the treatment is shown in Table 224.4. In many instances, treatment of metabolic myopathy is primarily supportive. Patients with respiratory muscle weakness may benefit from continuous positive airway pressure and other forms of ventilatory support, particularly during sleep. Cardiac insufficiency, when present, often responds, at least temporarily, to aggressive therapy. Patients who are prone to hypoglycemia should avoid fasting prior to surgical procedures and should receive continuous glucose infusions throughout the operative and early post-operative periods. No specific anesthetics are known to interact with these disorders. Genetic counseling and screening of family members permits the avoidance of precipitating factors for recurrent rhabdomyolysis and the resultant permanent muscle weakness and renal impairment which may occur in some patients.

Dietary manipulation Maintenance of normoglycemia in debranching enzyme deficiency is achieved by the avoidance of fasting coupled with the administration of frequent high-carbohydrate feeds. Supplementations with uncooked cornstarch and nocturnal nasogastric or gastric continuous feeds are often important in order to prevent nocturnal hypoglycemia.[16,24] High-protein diets have been reported to produce some improvement in endurance in individual patients with McArdle or Pompe disease; however, the long-term benefit of this treatment remains controversial.[16,20] Dietary supplementation with branched-chain amino acids for the treatment of McArdle disease has also shown mixed results. A recent study found decreased exercise capacity in five of six patients with McArdle disease following ingestion of a solution of branched-chain amino acids. This was associated with a lowering of peak free fatty acid levels.[25]

Vitamin supplements Vitamin B$_6$ (pyridoxine) is a cofactor for myophosphorylase. Patients with McArdle disease do not show overt signs of vitamin B$_6$ deficiency. However, they show evidence of subclinical deficiency on the stimulated erythrocyte aspartate aminotransferase assay (an index of vitamin B$_6$ status). Vitamin B$_6$ supplementation in four patients with McArdle disease resulted in improved exercise tolerance. Withdrawal of vitamin therapy in one patient was accompanied by deterioration of exercise tolerance and the development of muscle cramping.[26,27]

Exercise management Avoidance of strenuous exercise prevents symptoms of exercise intolerance and decreases the need for specific treatment. Exercise tolerance is improved in McArdle disease by oral glucose or fructose or by injection of glucagon prior to exercise whereas carbohydrates significantly worsen exercise tolerance in Tarui disease.[16]

Enzyme replacement The intravenous injection of purified acid α-glucosidase has been shown to result in dose-dependent clinical, biochemical and histopathological improvement in acid maltase deficient quail.[28] This approach to the treatment of Pompe disease is currently under active investigation.

Disorders of fatty acid metabolism

Brief overview

At least 21 separate enzymes and transporters are involved in the oxidative metabolism of fatty acids in mitochondria, many of them associated with distinct clinical disorders, including acute and chronic myopathies. The importance of recognition of these clinical entities lies in the fact that most of these potentially fatal disorders are treatable.

Whereas short- and medium-chain fatty acids enter mitochondria directly, long-chain fatty acids are dependent upon esterification with carnitine, by the carnitine cycle, for transport into mitochondria. Free long-chain fatty acids are initially esterified with coenzyme A (CoA) in the outer mitochondrial membrane by the enzyme, long-chain acyl-CoA synthetase. A second enzyme, carnitine palmitoyl transferase I (CPT I), located on the inner aspect of the outer mitochondrial membrane, catalyzes the transesterification of long-chain acyl-CoAs to long-chain acylcarnitines, with the release of free coenzyme A. This permits transport of long-chain fatty acyl groups across the mitochondrial membrane. A plasmalemmal carnitine transporter facilitates entry of free carnitine into cells. In a transport process catalyzed by carni-

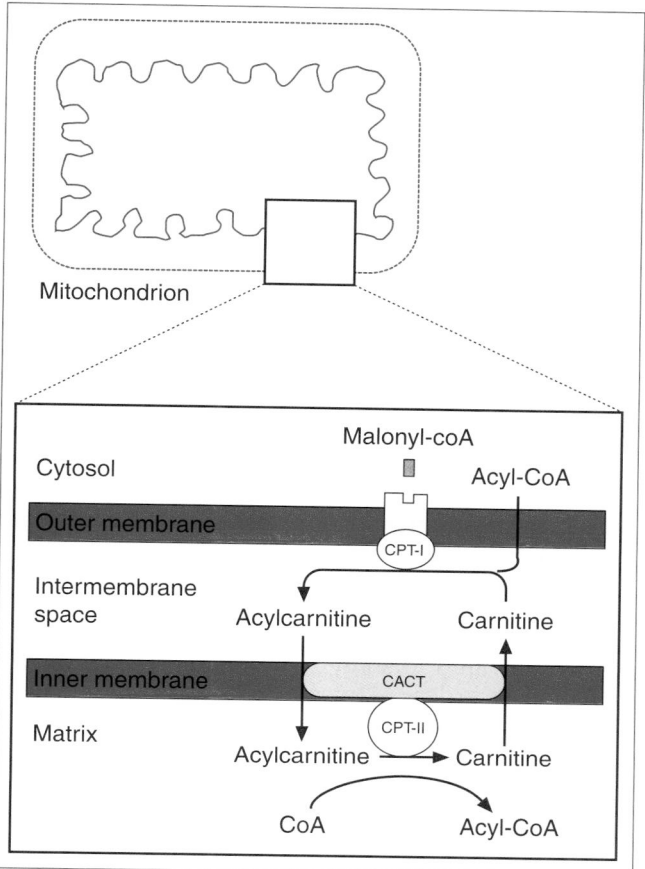

Figure 224.4   The carnitine shuttle. CPT, carnitine palmitoyltransferase; CACT, carnitine/acylcarnitine translocase.

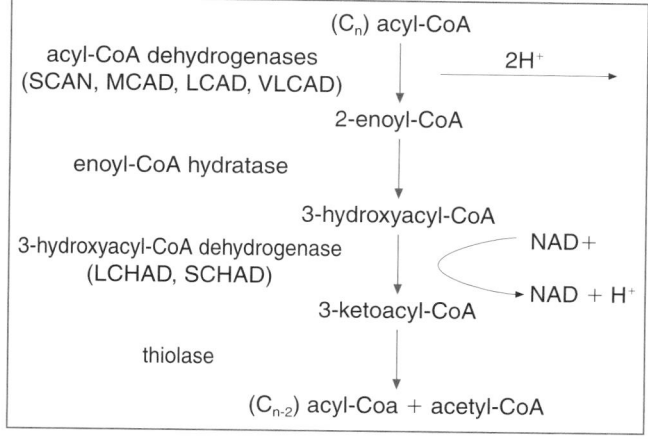

Figure 224.5   Schematic representation of intramitochondrial fatty acid β-oxidation. SCAD, short-chain acyl-CoA dehydrogenase; MCAD, medium-chain acyl-CoA dehydrogenase; LCAD, long-chain acyl-CoA dehydrogenase; VLCAD, very-long-chain acyl-CoA dehydrogenase; LCHAD, long-chain-3-hydroxyacyl-CoA dehydrogenase; SCHAD, short-chain-3-hydroxyacyl-CoA dehydrogenase. (C$_n$) represents number of carbons in acyl-CoA.

tine-acylcarnitine translocase, the acylcarnitines shuttle across the inner mitochondrial membrane in exchange for free carnitine. Carnitine palmitoyl transferase II (CPT II), located in the inner aspect of the inner mitochondrial membrane, transfers the acyl moiety from carnitine to CoA, restoring the acyl-CoAs and releasing free carnitine. Intramitochondrial fatty acyl CoAs undergo repeated cycles of β-oxidation. Each turn of the cycle involves four consecutive enzymatic reactions, catalyzed by acyl-CoA dehydrogenase, enoyl-CoA hydratase, 3-hydroxyacyl-CoA dehydrogenase and finally a thiolase. This results in shortening of the fatty acid chain by two carbons and the production of a single molecule of acetyl-CoA. Acetyl-CoA is further oxidized in the tricarboxylic acid cycle to CO_2 and water, with the production of ATP. Accumulation of acetyl-CoA, resulting from accelerated fatty acid oxidation during starvation, causes the formation of the "ketones," acetoacetate and 3-hydroxybutyrate.

Classification

The disorders of fatty acid metabolism are generally subdivided into disorders involving the carnitine cycle and disorders of intramitochondrial β-oxidation of fatty acids (Table 224.5).

Clinical features

Hereditary defects of fatty acid oxidation may present in a variety of ways. The most common and probably the most widely recognized presentation is as recurrent acute metabolic decompensation, associated with hypoketotic hypoglycemia, following prolonged fasting or some febrile intercurrent illness. In contrast to all the others, two of the disorders, short-chain acyl-CoA dehydrogenase (SCAD) and short-chain hydroxyacyl-Co A dehydrogenase (SCHAD) deficiencies, are characterized by hypoglycemia accompanied by increased, rather than inappropriately decreased, ketosis. Acute metabolic decompensation, including hepatic encephalopathy, is often superimposed on evidence of chronic abnormalities of fatty acid oxidation-dependent tissues, such as liver, heart and muscle. The liver is usually enlarged and shows micovesicular steatosis on biopsy. Hypertrophic or dilated cardiomyopathy may be prominent and complicated by life-threatening cardiac arrhythmias. In some patients, the cardiac involvement dominates the clinical presentation. Generalized and relatively non-specific hypotonia and weakness may be the only indication of skeletal muscle involvement. However, in some patients, chronic proximal myopathy, associated with recurrent myoglobinuria precipitated by febrile illness, drugs or prolonged exercise, may be the dominant presenting problem. Central nervous system involvement is rare and is usually attributable to episodes of acidosis or hypoglycemia. Sudden death has been reported, often mislabeled as sudden infant death syndrome. A recent retrospective review of liver samples from non-accidental sudden infants deaths demonstrated that 6.5% of these deaths might be attributable to underlying fatty acid oxidation defects.[29]

Carnitine cycle disorders[30,31]

- *Plasma membrane carnitine transporter deficiency* Proximal myopathy and progressive hypertrophic or dilated cardiomyopathy associated with markedly reduced plasma and tissue carnitine concentrations are the hallmarks of this disorder.[32] Hypoketotic hypoglycemia, hepatocellular dysfunction, and sudden death have also been described.
- *Carnitine palmitoyl transferase I (CPT I) deficiency* Classical infantile "hepatic" CPT I deficiency presents in the first year of life with hypoketotic hypoglycemia, encephalopathy and hepatomegaly and little or no skeletal or cardiac muscle involvement.
- *Carnitine palmitoyl transferase II (CPT II) deficiency* Three distinct forms of this disorder have been described. A rare neonatal form presents with severe hypoketotic hypoglycemia and generalized steatosis associated with dysmorphic features and multiple malformations. Patients with the infantile hepatomuscular form of CPT II deficiency develop cardiomyopathy and arrhythmias associated with hypotonia, hepatomegaly and episodes of hypoketotic hypoglycemia. The most common form of CPT II deficiency, the adult myopathic form, generally presents in adolescence or later with recurrent episodes of rhabdomyolysis and myoglobinuria precipitated by prolonged fasting, intercurrent illness or prolonged exercise.
- *Carnitine-acylcarnitine translocase deficiency* Most patients with this disorder present acutely in the neonatal period with hyperammonemia, hypoglycemia, cardiac arrhythmias, and profound hypotonia. Survival beyond the newborn period is unusual.

Fatty acid oxidation disorders Patients with intramitochondrial fatty acid oxidation defects may be difficult to differentiate clinically from those with carnitine cycle defects (Table 224.5). However, some exhibit distinguishing clinical features.
- *Short-chain acyl-CoA dehydrogenase (SCAD) deficiency* Patients with SCAD deficiency may present in the newborn period with metabolic acidosis, vomiting and poor feeding. Developmental delay, seizures, severe skeletal myopathy and failure to thrive generally develop subsequently. One case of SCAD deficiency was recently reported in which the patient presented with congenital multicore myopathy and progressive external ophthalmoplegia.[33] In contrast to other fatty acid oxidation defects, SCAD deficiency is characterized by hyperketotic, rather than hypoketotic, hypoglycemia, and the urine contains excess ethylmalonic and methylsuccinic acids.
- *Multiple acyl-CoA dehydrogenase deficiency (glutaric aciduria type II)* The neonatal form of this disorder is characterized by profound hypotonia, hepatomegaly, hypoglycemia, metabolic acidosis and sweaty-feet odor. Neonatal presentation may be associated with facial dysmorphism and multiple congenital anomalies. Patients surviving the

Table 224.5   Classification of disorders of fatty acid oxidation

	Enzyme defect	Inheritance	Gene locus	Clinical features
Carnitine cycle disorders				
Plasma membrane carnitine transporter deficiency	Sodium ion-dependent carnitine transporter (OCTN2)	AR	5q33.1	Myopathy, rhabdomyolysis, cardiomyopathy, hypoglycemia, hepatomegaly, sudden death
CPT I deficiency	Carnitine palmitoyltransferase I	AR	L-CPT I, 11q13 M-CPT I, 22q13.3	Hepatomegaly, hypoglycemia, encephalopathy BUT NO myopathy or cardiomyopathy
CPT II deficiency	Carnitine palmitoyltransferase II	AR	1p32	Myopathy, exercise intolerance, rhabdomyolysis (cardiomyopathy/ arrythmias)
Carnitine-acylcarnitine translocase deficiency	Carnitine-acylcarnitine translocase	AR	3p21.31	Hyperammonemia, hypoglycemia, cardiac arrythmias, hypotonia
Fatty acid oxidation disorders				
VLCAD deficiency	Very long-chain acyl-CoA dehydrogenase	AR	17p11.2–p11.1	Myopathy, rhabdomyolysis, cardiomyopathy, hepatomegaly, hypoglycemia
LCAD deficiency	Long-chain acyl-CoA dehydrogenase	AR	2q34–q35	Myopathy, rhabdomyolysis, cardiomyopathy, hypoglycemia
MCAD deficiency	Medium-chain acyl-CoA dehydrogenase	AR	1p31	Hypoketotic hypoglycemia, Reye's-like episodes, sudden death BUT NO myopathy
SCAD deficiency	Short-chain acyl-CoA dehydrogenase	AR	12q22-qter	Myopathy, failure to thrive, acidosis, progressive developmental delay
Multiple acyl-CoA dehydrogenase deficiency (glutaric aciduria type II)	Electron transfer flavoprotein (ETF) or ETF-coenzyme Q oxidoreductase (ETF-Qo)	AR	15q23–q25 19q13.3 4q32-qter	Myopathy, hepatomegaly, hypoglycemia, acidosis, facial dysmorphism, multiple congenital abnormalities, cardiomopathy
Trifunctional protein/ LCHAD deficiency	Trifunctional protein/ long-chain hydroxyacyl-CoA dehydrogenase	AR	2p23	Myopathy, rhabdomyolysis, cardiomyopathy, hepatic dysfunction, hypoglycemia, neuropathy, pigmentary retinopathy
SCHAD deficiency	Short-chain hydroxyacyl-CoA dehydrogenase	AR	4q22–26	Myopathy, cardiomyopathy, sudden death ketotic hypoglycemia, hepatic dysfunction

newborn period develop rapidly progressive cardiomyopathy. An adult form of the disease, with myopathy and exertional myalgias, has also been described. These patients may variably experience vomiting, hypoglycemia or hepatomegaly, in addition to myopathy. Urinary organic acid analysis shows the presence of excess ethylmalonic and adipic acids.

- *Trifunctional protein/long-chain 3-hydroxyacyl-CoA dehydrogenase (LCHAD) deficiency* Like other fatty acid oxidation defects, this disorder often presents as hypoketotic hypoglycemia with liver dysfunction, or sudden, unexpected death, usually in infancy. However, cardiomyopathy is more common and generally more severe than in the other fatty acid oxidation disorders. Hypotonia is a

Table 224.6   Treatment of disorders of fatty acid oxidation

Treatment	Classification of recommendation	Quality of evidence

Dietary manipulation
  High-carbohydrate, low-fat diet
  Avoidance of fasting
	A	II-3, III

Carnitine supplementation		
Carnitine transporter deficiency	A	II-3
Other fatty acid oxidation disorders	C	III
Riboflavin supplementation		
MADD, SCAD deficiency	B	II-3, III

MADD, multiple acyl-CoA dehydrogenase deficiency; SCAD, short-chain acyl-CoA dehydrogenase.

common initial feature, and progressive myopathy may develop. Peripheral sensorimotor neuropathy and pigmentary retinopathy are common features of LCHAD deficiency, setting this disorder apart from other fatty acid oxidation defects.

Treatment of disorders of fatty acid metabolism

A summary of the treatment of disorders of fatty acid metabolism is shown in Table 224.6.

Dietary manipulation Avoidance of prolonged fasting is by far the most important aspect of dietary management of fatty acid oxidation defects. Most patients with disorders of fatty acid oxidation do better on a high-carbohydrate, low-fat diet, supplemented with fat-soluble vitamins and small amounts of essential fatty acids. Uncooked cornstarch drinks at bedtime and during febrile illnesses, when fasting may occur, helps to provide a long-lasting source of carbohydrate to minimize the need to utilize free fatty acids for energy production. Medium-chain triglyceride (MCT) oil is used as the source of dietary fat for patients with disorders of long-chain fatty acid metabolism. Essential fatty acid supplementation is particularly important in patients receiving most of the fat in their diets as MCT. Medium-chain triglyceride oil is specifically and absolutely contraindicated in patients with medium-chain acyl-CoA dehydrogenase deficiency.

Medications and dietary supplements Carnitine supplementation (100 mg/kg/day) may be life saving in plasma membrane carnitine transporter deficiency. Its usage in other disorders of fatty acid metabolism remains controversial. Long-chain acylcarnitines may be arrhythmogenic. Riboflavin (100 mg/day) may be beneficial in multiple acyl-CoA dehydrogenase deficiency and in some patients with SCAD deficiency.

Exercise management Avoidance of prolonged exercise decreases the risk of acute rhabdomyolysis. Exercise tolerance might theoretically be improved by the consumption of cornstarch drinks prior to the initiation of exercise, although this has not been specifically studied.

Treatment of acute decompensation During episodes

of acute metabolic decompensation, intravenous glucose delivered at a rate of 8–10 mg/kg/min should be initiated in order to maintain normoglycemia and to shut down fatty acid oxidation. This may require the co-administration of insulin, a powerful inhibitor of the hormone-sensitive lipase in adipose tissue. Hyperglycemia may exacerbate lactic acidosis. Once the patient is stable and the plasma ammonium has returned to normal, free amino acids (1 g/kg/24 h) may be added to the intravenous, or delivered by nasogastric tube. A high-carbohydrate, low-fat diet is added once recovery has begun. Cardiomyopathy and cardiac arrhythmias often require ongoing therapy and monitoring.

Anesthesia Prolonged fasting should be avoided prior to surgical procedures, and patients should receive continuous glucose infusions throughout the operative and immediate post-operative periods. No specific anesthetics are known to interact with these disorders.

Drug–drug and drug–metabolite interactions Acute episodes of rhabdomyolysis may be precipitated by drugs. Aspirin, which has been historically associated with Reye's syndrome, is specifically contraindicated in patients with fatty acid oxidation disorders. Valproic acid has been shown to interfere with fatty acid metabolism; long-term administration of the drug may cause carnitine depletion.

Genetic counseling All the disorders of fatty acid metabolism causing myopathy are inherited as autosomal recessive disorders. Potentially fatal attacks of metabolic decompensation are preventable. Screening of family members of patients with a history of sudden unexplained death often results in the detection of affected siblings at risk for sudden death. Early initiation of treatment may be life saving.

Mitochondrial disorders

Brief overview

Mitochondria are the principal source of metabolic energy in all cells, except for erythrocytes. Their double-membrane structure consists of a smooth

Table 224.7   Classification of mitochondrial disorders

	Inheritance	Clinical phenotypes
mtDNA defects		
Large scale rearrangements (deletions/duplications)	Sporadic	Kearns-Sayre syndrome, CPEO, Pearson's syndrome, myopathy, diabetes mellitus, deafness
Point mutations	Maternal	MELAS, MERRF, LHON, NARP, Leigh's disease
nDNA defects		
Defects of genes encoding enzymatic or structural proteins	Mostly AR, except PDH deficiency (XLR)	Disorders of pyruvate metabolism; defects of the tricarboxylic acid cycle; defects of the respiratory chain; Luft's Disease (OXPHOS coupling abnormality)
Defects of translocases	AR	Adenine nucleotide translocator porin (voltage-dependent anion channel)
Defects of protein importation	AR or AD	HSP60 deficiency, leader peptide mutations
Defects of intergenomic signaling	AR or AD	mtDNA depletion syndrome, multiple mtDNA deletions

outer membrane and an invaginated inner membrane enclosing the matrix space. The outer membrane contains a number of important proteins involved in energy metabolism, including long-chain acyl-CoA synthetase and CPT I, as well as proteins required for importation of nuclear encoded components of the mitochondrial electron transport chain. The multi-subunit complexes of the respiratory chain and oxidative phosphorylation are located within the inner mitochondrial membrane. The intramitochondrial matrix is the site of pyruvate oxidation, fatty acid β-oxidation and the tricarboxylic acid cycle, and it is also the site of synthesis of urea, ketones, various amino acids, nucleotides, and heme. The processing and assembly of imported mitochondrial proteins also occurs within the intramitochondrial matrix.

Mitochondria contain approximately 1000 gene products—only 37 are encoded by mitochondrial DNA (mtDNA) and synthesized within mitochondria; all the rest are encoded by nuclear DNA (nDNA) and synthesized in the cytosol. The mitochondrial genome is a double-stranded circular structure consisting of 16 569 base pairs of DNA. It encodes two ribosomal RNAs (rRNA), 22 transfer RNAs (tRNA) and 13 polypeptides that form part of the respiratory chain complex. Nuclear-encoded polypeptides are synthesized on cytoplasmic polyribosomes. They are imported and sorted within mitochondria in a complex series of steps. Chaperone proteins, called heat-shock proteins, hsp70 and hsp60, respectively, mediate the unfolding of cytoplasmic polypeptides prior to importation and the subsequent folding and assembly of imported proteins.

The respiratory chain/oxidative phosphorylation system comprises five multiunit complexes, complexes I to V. Electrons produced by the oxidative catabolism of fats, proteins and carbohydrates, are transferred sequentially from complexes I and II to coenzyme Q_{10}, then to complexes III and IV, with oxygen as the final electron acceptor. Energy derived from electron transfer is used by complexes I, III, and IV to pump protons from the matrix to the space between the inner and outer mitochondrial membranes, producing a proton gradient across the inner

membrane. Protons are then transported back into the matrix by complex V with the generation of ATP.[34–37]

Classification

Disorders of mitochondrial respiration may result from defects in either nuclear or mitochondrial genes affecting the synthesis, importation, or assembly of components of the respiratory chain or of the enzymes involved in energy production (Table 224.7).

Clinical features

Genetic disorders of mitochondrial respiration may present at virtually any age in a wide variety of ways.[36–42] Although most present with some degree of myopathy, the clinical spectrum includes multiple organ systems, in a variety of combinations. Hypotonia and delayed gross motor development are often early indications of generalized myopathy. Muscle weakness is usually generalized in the more severe disorders; it may be proximal in milder forms. Exercise intolerance generally presents as premature fatigue, often with hyperpnoea secondary to lactic acidosis. Later in the course of the disease, this may be followed by fixed muscle weakness. Unlike disorders

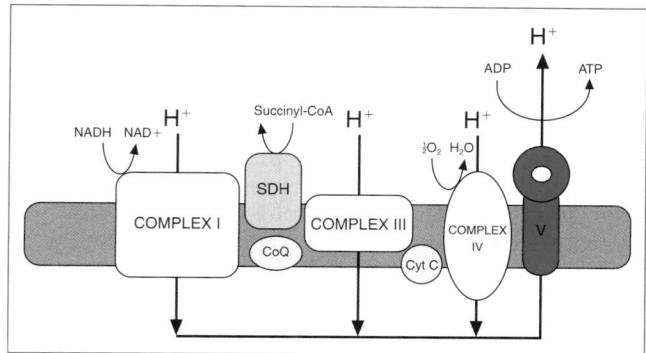

Figure 224.6   Schematic representation of the mitochondrial respiratory chain. Complex I, NADH dehydrogenase; Complex II, Succinate dehydrogenase (SDH); Complex III, CoQH2-cytochrome c reductase; Complex IV, cytochrome c oxidase; Complex V, ATP synthase.

of carbohydrate and fatty acid metabolism, mitochondrial myopathies are often associated with chronic encephalopathy and other neurological symptoms. Ocular abnormalities, particularly ptosis, chronic progressive external ophthalmoplegia (CPEO), optic atrophy and retinopathy are common. Deafness is particularly prominent in maternally inherited disorders of mtDNA. Other neurological features of specific disorders may include any combination of seizures, ataxia, movement disorders, stroke-like episodes, or peripheral neuropathy. Non-neurological involvement may include various combinations of cardiomyopathy, cardiac arrhythmias, diabetes mellitus, pancreatic insufficiency, hepatopathy, bone marrow dysfunction, and nephropathy.

Defects of mitochondrial DNA (mtDNA) Mitochondria, and therefore mtDNA defects, are inherited maternally. When a cell, which contains up to several hundred mitochondria, contains two different mitochondrial genotypes, because of the presence of some mitochondria containing mtDNA mutations, the cell is said to be heteroplasmic. The age of onset, tissues and organs affected, and the clinical severity of a disorder caused by a mtDNA mutation are related to the degree of heteroplasmy, that is, the proportion of abnormal mtDNA within each cell. Although specific clinical entities have been associated with certain types of mtDNA mutations, the overlap between them is considerable (Table 224.7).

- *Large scale rearrangements (deletions/duplications)* Kearns-Sayre syndrome is a multisystem disorder characterized by early onset (before age 20) progressive external ophthalmoplegia and pigmentary retinopathy associated with at least one of the following: heart block, cerebellar ataxia, or cerebrospinal fluid protein above 1 g/L. Proximal muscle weakness, sensorineural hearing loss, dementia, and endocrine abnormalities including diabetes mellitus are also relatively common additional features of the disease. The prognosis is poor, with death often occurring in the third or fourth decade. Chronic progressive external ophthalmoplegia (CPEO) may present as an isolated entity or associated with the appearance of typical ragged-red fibers in the histopathology of Gomori trichrome-stained muscle biopsies. Chronic progressive external ophthalmoplegia association with ragged-red fiber myopathy presents in adolescence or young adulthood with ptosis, ophthalmoplegia and proximal limb muscle weakness. The course of this disorder is relatively benign, with a normal life expectancy. Pearson syndrome usually presents in infancy with refractory sideroblastic anemia, pancytopenia, and exocrine pancreatic dysfunction. Patients surviving beyond early childhood may experience regression of the hematological condition and develop features of Kearns-Sayre syndrome. Maternally inherited diabetes mellitus and deafness have been described secondary to either

mtDNA deletions/duplications or point mutations in mitochondrially encoded tRNAs or rRNA.
- *Point mutations* More than 50 distinct point mutations in the mitochondrial DNA have been described. Although a number of apparently distinct clinical entities have been described, there is considerable overlap between them, and specific point mutations may be associated with different clinical phenotypes. Mitochondrial encephalomyopathy, lactic acidosis and stroke-like episodes (MELAS) are the most common of those presenting in late childhood and early adulthood. Generalized seizures, recurrent migraine-like headaches and dementia also occur in this disease. Myopathy is associated with ragged-red fibers on muscle biopsy. This pathological feature is also one of the hallmarks of myoclonic epilepsy with ragged-red fibers (MERRF), which presents clinically with myoclonic epilepsy, cerebellar ataxia, and myopathy, along with various other common features of mitochondrial disorders. The syndrome of neuropathy, ataxia, retinitis pigmentosa (NARP), associated with ATPase 6 deficiency, and Leber's hereditary optic neuropathy (LHON) present in early adulthood and are usually not associated with ragged-red fibers on muscle biopsy.

Defects of nuclear DNA (nDNA)
- *Defects of genes encoding enzymatic or structural proteins* Disruption of any one of the vast number of nuclear genes encoding polypeptides required for pyruvate metabolism or respiration may result in mitochondrial myopathy. The most common disorder of pyruvate metabolism, caused by mutations affecting the E1 component of the pyruvate dehydrogenase (PDH) complex, results in three main clinical syndromes. The severe neonatal form presents in the first few days of life with hypotonia, lethargy, seizures, failure to thrive, agenesis of the corpus callosum, and lactic acidosis. Death usually occurs by six months of age. A less severe, but clinically similar form associated with optic atrophy and ophthalmoplegia, presents in the first six months of life and generally causes death by age three years. The benign form, with normal psychomotor development, presents in late infancy with intermittent ataxia and exercise intolerance. Defects of the tricarboxylic acid cycle are extremely rare, probably because complete deficiency of any of the enzymes involved would likely be incompatible with life. Disorders of the respiratory chain comprise those defects involving complexes I–V as well as coenzyme Q_{10} deficiency. In general, these disorders present with either severe progressive infantile myopathy, benign infantile myopathy, or late-onset myopathy with exercise intolerance. Encephalopathy is often a prominent feature of defects of the respiratory chain, and multisystem involvement is common. Luft's disease, caused by loose coupling of oxidative phosphorylation, is unique in its clinical presentation. Euthyroid hypermetabolism, manifested as heat intolerance,

Table 224.8   Treatment of mitochondrial disorders

Treatment	Classification of recommendation	Quality of evidence	References
Ketogenic diet	C	II-3	47–49
Thiamine, lipoic acid (PDH deficiency)	C	III	50–52
Coenzyme Q supplementation	C	II-3	54–60
Other vitamins and free radical scavengers	C	III	
Creatine	B	II-1	65
Dichloroacetate (for lactic acidosis)	B	II-3, III	69–81
Aerobic training	B	II-3	83

PDH, pyruvate dehydrogenase

hyperhidrosis, polyphagia, and polydipsia, is accompanied by mild to moderate muscle weakness and exercise intolerance.

- *Defects of translocases* A number of translocases are required for the movement of metabolites across the inner mitochondrial membrane. However, clinical diseases have been associated with only a small number. Carnitine-acylcarnitine translocase deficiency is discussed above with the carnitine cycle disorders. Deficiency of the adenine nucleotide translocator (ANT) results in dysfunction of the respiratory chain presenting as mitochondrial myopathy. Deficiency of porin, a voltage-dependent anion channel in the outer mitochondrial membrane, has been described presenting as hypotonia, developmental delay, seizures, hydrocephalus and dysmorphic features.[38,39]

- *Defects of protein importation* Patients with deficiency of heat shock protein 60 (hsp60) have been reported presenting as severe encephalomyopathy with multisystem involvement. Multiple mitochondrial enzyme deficiencies occur secondary to impairment of folding and assembly of imported peptides.[40,41] Leader peptide mutations may cause single enzyme defects resulting from faulty importation of the polypeptide into the mitochondria.[38]

- *Defects of intergenomic signaling* MtDNA depletion syndrome, a quantitative defect of mtDNA, is characterized clinically by myopathy and less commonly hepatopathy or cardiomyopathy. The severe congenital form presents soon after birth and results in death within the first year of life. The late-onset form, resulting from less marked depletion of mtDNA, presents in infancy or childhood and is associated with a longer survival.[42] Multiple mtDNA deletions are the consequence of a disruption of intergenomic signaling. These patients may present with isolated chronic progressive external ophthalmoplegia or may have associated weakness, exercise intolerance or cardiomyopathy.[38] Mitochondrial neurogastrointestinal encephalomyopathy (MNGIE) is a disorder characterized clinically by generalized myopathy, ptosis, CPEO, gastrointestinal dysmotility, peripheral neuropathy, leukoencephalopathy and lactic acidosis presenting in the second to fifth decades of life. The finding of either multiple mtDNA deletions or

mtDNA depletion in this disorder appears to be related to mutations in the nuclear gene encoding thymidine phosphorylase.[43]

Treatment of mitochondrial disorders

With some notable exceptions, efforts to improve the muscle weakness and exercise intolerance associated with the various defects in mitochondrial respiration by dietary manipulation, vitamin supplements, drugs, or physical therapy have been disappointing (Table 224.8). The rarity of the conditions, the multisystem involvement, marked clinical heterogeneity, variability of the course of the diseases in individual patients, and relative lack of sensitive means for assessment of the outcome of therapy have made the evaluation of various treatments difficult. Anecdotal accounts have appeared of "improvement" in patients with mitochondrial myopathies treated with various combinations of vitamins, drugs, and chemicals. However, few have withstood critical evaluation or efforts to duplicate the experience under rigorous clinical trial conditions.

Dietary manipulation Boys with the relatively benign form of pyruvate dehydrogenase complex (PDH) deficiency have been reported to respond well to treatment with a ketogenic diet, with improvement in exercise tolerance and chronic ataxia and decreased frequency of metabolic decompensation, particularly if therapy is instituted early.[44,45] The results of treating patients with severe PDH deficiency by the same dietary manipulation have been disappointing, although there has been at least one report of clinical improvement in an infant with Leigh disease treated with a ketogenic diet.[46] In patients with mitochondrial respiratory chain defects, a high carbohydrate intake may exacerbate the lactic acidosis and cause clinical deterioration. However, apart perhaps from decreasing the frequency of acute metabolic decompensation, they do not appear to derive significant long-term benefit from dietary carbohydrate restriction or a ketogenic diet.

Medications, vitamins and other supplements

- *Vitamins and related supplements* Thiamine and lipoic acid are integral cofactors of the E1 and E3 components, respectively, of the normal PDH complex. Individual patients with PDH deficiency have been reported who have responded well to treatment with thiamine[47,48] or lipoic acid.[49] However, the majority of patients with PDH deficiency show no clinically significant response to treatment with high doses of these vitamins. The role of vitamin therapy of mitochondrial respiratory chain defects is also unclear. Coenzyme Q_{10} (ubiquinone) plays a pivotal role in mitochondrial electron transport.[50] The reported response of patients with mitochondrial respiratory chain defects to treatment with coenzyme Q_{10} or related compounds has been variable. A number of reports of small series of patients with mitochondrial cytopathies showing improvement with coenzyme Q_{10} therapy have been published,[51–55] including at least one double-blind, crossover study.[56] However, other studies failed to show significant clinical or metabolic improvement in patients with mitochondrial diseases receiving coenzyme Q_{10}, along with vitamins K3 and C, riboflavin, thiamine and niacin.[57] No patient has shown dramatic and sustained clinical improvement on coenzyme Q_{10} therapy. Even in those studies reporting beneficial responses to treatment, the number of patients in each study was small, and only some of the patients showed improvement. The clinical improvements, though statistically significant in some cases, were only modest. All were of short duration; the long-term effectiveness of coenzyme Q_{10} therapy is still uncertain. Many primary and secondary mitochondrial diseases, including age-related degenerative disorders, are thought to result from accumulation of oxygen free radicals, suggesting the possibility that treatment with free radical scavengers, such as vitamin E, dimethyl-glycine, menadione, selenium, or ascorbic acid, may be beneficial.[58] The results of studies on cultured fibroblasts have confirmed the presence of increased free radical formation in patients with complex I deficiency.[59] This and other observations prompted several attempts to influence the course of the disease in individual patients with mitochondrial myopathies. However, no systematic trials to evaluate the efficacy of the treatment have yet been done. No patient with a mitochondrial myopathy has shown dramatic or sustained improvement on treatment with anti-oxidants. Creatine supplementation has been suggested to improve athletic performance by its effect on skeletal muscle.[60,61] In a randomized crossover study of the treatment of mitochondrial myopathies with creatine monohydrate, significantly increased high-intensity, isometric, anaerobic and aerobic muscle power was reported in seven patients with severe exercise tolerance.[62] This short-term observation on a small number of patients warrants further investigation.

• *Medications* The activity of the PDH complex is regulated by a phosphorylation (inactivation)–dephosphorylation (activation) cycle catalyzed by PDH kinase and PDH phosphatase, respectively.

Dichloroacetic acid (DCA) activates PDH by inhibiting PDH kinase and maintaining the enzyme complex in the active, non-phosphorylated state.[63] It also appears to stabilize the E1 component of the PDH complex in patients with E1α mutations.[64,65] Treatment with the drug has been reported to produce decreased blood and cerebrospinal fluid (CSF) lactate levels, with improvement in clinical symptoms, in patients with mitochondrial encephalomyopathies.[66–74] The results of other studies are not so encouraging.[75–77] Most of the reported experience with DCA treatment of mitochondrial disorders is anecdotal, involving short-term studies of small numbers of patients. Some patients appear to benefit from therapy, at least with respect to muscle or brain energy metabolism. However, treatment does not appear to have had a dramatic or sustained clinical effect on the course of the disease in any.[78] Elucidation of the potential short- and long-term beneficial effects of drug treatment of mitochondrial myopathies clearly requires further investigation. Another aspect of this complex class of metabolic disorders calling for caution and further investigation is the potential for adverse drug reactions in patients in whom mitochondrial respiration is impaired. The metabolism of many xenobiotics is dependent on energy derived from mitochondrial respiration, and some drugs, such as the barbiturates, are known to impair mitochondrial energy metabolism. Although anesthetics have been used safely in patients with mitochondrial disorders, theoretical risks may exist when combinations of barbiturates, narcotics, benzodiazepines and nitrous oxide are used. It is unclear whether patients with mitochondrial myopathies may be at increased risk of developing malignant hyperthermia.[79]

Physical therapy Although exercise tolerance is limited in patients with mitochondrial myopathies, aerobic training may reverse the effects of deconditioning and improve exercise tolerance.[80]

Drug-induced myopathy

Brief overview[81–83]

More than 200 drugs have been reported to be associated with acute or chronic myopathy or rhabdomyolysis. Any drug, whether prescribed, over-the-counter, natural or illicit, is a potential cause of acquired myopathy. In the majority of cases, removal of the offending drug results in resolution of symptoms of myopathy.

Classification

Generalized drug-induced myopathies may be classified according to clinical features as painful, or painless, and with or without neuropathy. A classification of toxic myopathy based on the underlying pathogenetic mechanisms, in so far as it is known, is presented in Table 224.9. Focal myopathies may also

Table 224.9   Major drug-induced myopathies

Corticosteroid-induced myopathy
Necrotizing
  Lovastatin, pravastatin, simvastatin
  Clofibrate, gemfibrozil
  ε-Aminocaproic acid
  Ethanol abuse
  Hypervitaminosis E
  Etretinate, isotretinoin

Hypokalemic
  Diuretics
  Laxatives
  Licorice
  Amphotericin B
  Ethanol abuse

Lysosomal storage
  Chloroquine or hydroxychloroquine
  Amiodarone
  Other amphiphilic cationic drugs

Antimicrotubular
  Colchicine
  Vincristine

Inflammatory
  D-Penicillamine
  Procainamide
  Cimetidine

Mitochondrial
  Zidovudine
  Germanium

Myasthenic syndromes
  D-Penicillamine
  Chloroquine
  Antibiotics
  β-Blockers

Others
  Cyclosporine
  Emetine, ipecac syrup
  L-Tryptoph

occur as a result of intramuscular injections, particularly with the administration of antibiotics, lidocaine, diazepam, pentazocine and meperidine.[81,83,84]

Pathophysiology and pathogenesis

Little is known about the specific pathophysiology of most drug-induced myopathies. Clinically and pathologically, the myopathy may classify as a necrotizing, hypokalemic, lysosomal storage, inflammatory, or a mitochondrial myopathy. Necrotizing myopathy presents with acute or sub-acute onset of myalgia, tenderness and weakness associated with muscle fiber necrosis and regeneration. Rhabdomyolysis may result from continued use of the responsible drug. Hypokalemia may lead to a severe, painless, generalized or proximal weakness associated with vacuolar myopathy and fiber necrosis on muscle biopsy. Repletion of potassium reverses the clinical and pathological features. Drug-induced lysosomal storage myopathy, now known to result from the administration of one of more than 50 amphiphilic drugs,[84] will be discussed in further detail in relation to anti-malarials. Drug-induced inflammatory myopathy mimics idiopathic polymyositis both clinically and pathologically. Steroid administration may be required in addition to withdrawal of the toxic drug in order to induce remission. Mitochondrial myopathy, with ragged-red fibers and mitochondrial biochemical and ultrastructural abnormalities on muscle biopsy, has been described with zidovudine (AZT) treatment of HIV (human immunodeficiency virus) infection. Zidovudine may act as a false substrate for the mitochondrial DNA polymerase.[84] Impairment of respiratory chain oxidative capacity, as well as depletion of mitochondrial DNA, without uncoupling of oxidative phosphorylation, has been demonstrated in AZT-treated rats.[85] Myasthenic syndromes may result from the production of anti-acetylcholine-receptor antibodies (D-penicillamine) or interference with neuromuscular transmission, either in the presynaptic region (lithium, sedatives), in the postsynaptic region (tetracyclines, emetine, morphine, phenothiazines), or both (aminoglycosides, polymyxins, β-blockers, chlorpromazine).[81]

Some specific drug-induced myopathies

Corticosteroids

- *Acute corticosteroid-associated critical care myopathy* Severe generalized weakness or paralysis associated with prolonged dependence on ventilatory assistance is characteristic of acute corticosteroid myopathy. The myopathy is generalized, involving both proximal and distal muscles. Deep tendon reflexes may be decreased or absent. Sensation, cranial nerve function and cognition are generally unaffected. A delayed rise in creatine kinase (CK) is seen. Neuroimaging, analysis of cerebrospinal fluid and electrocardiogram are normal. The main finding on electromyographic (EMG) studies is a marked decrease in compound motor action potential amplitudes.[86,87] The use of neuromuscular junction blocking medications, muscle disuse and sepsis may potentiate the effects of high dose corticosteroids.[86] Acute corticosteroid myopathy has also been described in patients receiving sedatives (propofol and benzodiazepines), rather than neuromuscular junction blockers, during ventilation.[87] Muscle biopsies typically show features of an acute necrotizing myopathy. Electron microscopy reveals loss of thick filaments with decreased A-band density and absent M-lines, indicating depletion of myosin filaments. Thin actin filaments are well preserved.[87] Quantitative analyses of skeletal muscle from patients with acute corticosteroid-associated myopathy have demonstrated a general decrease in myofibrillar proteins with a specific loss of myosin and myosin-associated proteins. Myosin mRNA was found to be absent in patient samples. In addition, impaired force-generating capacity was noted. Clinical recovery is associated with reversal of the pathological changes.[86] Disuse and cytokine production in the critical care setting may potentiate protein loss. Apart from withdrawal of high-dose corticosteroid therapy, the treatment is mainly supportive. Residual weakness may be present for up to six months or longer. Intensive physiotherapy and rehabilitation is necessary for full recovery.

- *Chronic corticosteroid myopathy* Chronic corticosteroid myopathy is characterized by the gradual onset of symmetrical, painless muscle weakness, involving primarily the hip muscles and, to a variable extent, the shoulder and proximal limb muscles. Reflexes are usually preserved. Plasma creatine kinase levels are typically normal. Electromyographic studies show non-specific myopathic changes, with low-amplitude, short-duration motor unit potentials. Muscle biopsies show selective type 2 fiber atrophy, without necrosis or regeneration. Subsarcolemmal lipid droplets may be prominent. Electron microscopy may reveal mitochondrial aggregation and vacuolar changes.[81,88–90] No consistent relationship has been observed between the dose or the duration of corticosteroid therapy and the onset of muscle weakness.[81,89] The risk of developing myopathy is increased by the administration of fluorinated glucocorticoids.[90] The pathogenic mechanisms underlying the development of chronic corticosteroid myopathy are uncertain. Enhanced protein catabolism and inhibition of protein synthesis are felt to be contributing factors.[90] The roles of glucocorticoid-induced insulin resistance and drug-induced alterations in carbohydrate metabolism are uncertain. Inhibition of the mitochondrial matrix acyl-CoA dehydrogenases (LCAD, MCAD, SCAD), resulting in impairment of β-oxidation of medium and short-chain fatty acids, has been demonstrated in mouse liver in response to corticosteroids.[91] Drug-induced impairment of fatty acid oxidation in muscle could mimic the myopathy seen in inherited disorders of fatty acid oxidation. In some cases, corticosteroid-induced hypokalemia may play a role in the pathogenesis of myopathy.[90] The pathogenesis of chronic myopathy related to corticosteroid administration is likely multifactorial. Glucocorticoids exert their therapeutic effects via both genomic and non-genomic mechanisms. The genomic actions are mediated by the binding of glucocorticoids to a cytosolic glucocorticoid receptor. This generates a conformational change permitting the complex to be translocated to the nucleus where it interacts with specific glucocorticoid-responsive elements in the DNA. The interaction promotes the initiation of transcription of some genes and suppresses the transcription of others. Non-genomic effects are less well understood. They appear to be mediated by two different mechanisms. The first involves the presumed activation of second messenger systems by the binding of glucocorticoids to steroid-selective membrane receptors. The second appears to involve the dissolution of the glucocorticoid within the plasma membrane; resulting in a physicochemical change that stabilizes the membrane and alters the activities of membrane-associated proteins.[92] Corticosteroid-induced myopathies are reversible on reduction of the dosage of the drug. Safe tapering may require the addition of corticosteroid-sparing drugs, such as methotrexate. A change to alternate day dosing or to a non-fluorinated glucocorticoid may be beneficial. Optimization of nutritional status and protein supplementation may minimize further protein catabolism and promote recovery. Since resolution of the muscle weakness often takes several months, even when corticosteroids have been withdrawn completely, physiotherapy and exercise are critical to full recovery of muscle strength. During this time, other drugs that may result in myopathy are best avoided.[88]

Anti-malarials Myopathy is a rare complication of treatment with the anti-malarial drugs, chloroquine and hydroxychloroquine. Slowly progressive proximal muscle weakness, involving the lower extremities followed by the upper extremities, is typical. In some patients, decreased tendon reflexes and mild sensory abnormalities signal the presence of a peripheral neuropathy. The skeletal myopathy may be accompanied by myocardial involvement with congestive heart failure; in some patients cardiomyopathy is the presenting problem. Electromyography often shows both myopathic and neuropathic changes.

Muscle biopsies in chloroquine-treated patients show vacuolization and swelling of myocytes. Myonecrosis may be present. Electron microscopy reveals curvilinear bodies, myeloid bodies and myelin figures, as well as glycogen accumulation. Similar findings are present in endomyocardial biopsies, in the presence of cardiomyopathy. Sural nerve biopsies show evidence of both segmental demyelination and axonopathy. Myeloid bodies and myelin figures can be demonstrated in Schwann cells by electron microscopy, and curvilinear bodies are seen in pericytes. Pathological findings in patients receiving hydroxychloroquine are similar but less severe.[93]

The mechanism by which chloroquine and hydroxychloroquine produce muscle weakness is unclear. The pathological features are presumed to result from the inactivation or inhibition of acid-dependent lysosomal enzymes by the accumulation of the basic drug within the lysosome. Tau and β-amyloid protein precursor have been shown to accumulate in chloroquine myopathy, secondary to impaired degradation within the lysosome. The authors postulate that that the degradation of other cytosolic proteins, including Alzheimer-related proteins, may also be impaired in chloroquine myopathy.[94] In similar fashion, the degradation of other substances by the lysosomes may be impaired.

Most patients receiving long-term treatment with anti-malarial drugs have underlying connective tissue diseases. The clinical differentiation of a toxic myopathy from polymyositis or muscle involvement associated with the underlying disorder, such as systemic lupus erythematosis, may be difficult. In addition, many of these patients receive concurrent treatment with corticosteroids. Muscle biopsy may be required to distinguish between these entities. Curvilinear bodies will only be present in patients with myopathy associated with chloroquine and hydroxychloroquine.[93] Discontinuation of anti-malarial treatment results in a gradual improvement in clinical symptoms and pathological findings.

Statin lipid-lowering drugs The statins are selective inhibitors of 3-hydroxy-3-methylglutaryl-CoA (HMG-CoA) reductase, the rate-limiting reaction in cholesterol biosynthesis. Mevalonic acid, the product of the reaction, is required for the biosynthesis of ubiquinone, isoprenoids, dolichols and prenylated proteins, in addition to cholesterol. This class of drugs, which includes lovastatin, pravastatin, simvastatin, fluvastatin, atorvastatin and cerivastatin, are highly effective for the treatment of hypercholesterolemia. Asymptomatic elevation of serum creatine kinase levels appears to be a relatively common finding in patients receiving statin treatment, though the levels were not significantly higher than with placebo in most studies.[95] An acute necrotizing myopathy with myalgia, proximal muscle weakness and elevated plasma creatine kinase may occur in up to 0.5% of patients on monotherapy.[84]

The risk of myopathy is increased by the concurrent administration of erythromycin, cyclosporine, niacin, gemfibrozil, fibrates or azole antifungals.[95,96] The majority of these adverse drug interactions are mediated by inhibition of the cytochrome P450 3A4 isoenzyme, causing increased plasma levels of the statin drug.[96,97] The mechanism by which combination lipid-lowering regimens, using niacin, gemfibrozil or fibrates, result in an increased risk of myopathy is not known. Hepatic insufficiency, cholestasis, alcohol abuse and other risk factors for rhabdomyolysis may also contribute to increased risk.[98]

The primary mechanism underlying the muscle damage seen with the administration of statins is not known. Ubiquinone (coenzyme Q_{10}) is an important component of the mitochondrial respiratory chain. Coenzyme Q_{10} levels in blood, liver and heart are decreased by lovastatin treatment in rats.[99] Cardiac patients and a healthy volunteer with hypercholesterolemia showed both decreased blood levels of coenzyme Q_{10} and a measurable decrease in cardiac function when treated with lovastatin. Supplementation with coenzyme Q_{10} in these patients resulted in an improvement in cardiac function. A decrease in ubiquinone plasma levels was also demonstrated in 40 patients treated with statins when compared to untreated hypercholesterolemic patients. An elevation of lactate/pyruvate ratios, suggestive of possible mitochondrial dysfunction, was also seen in treated patients. However, no correlation could be demonstrated between ubiquinone levels and lactate/pyruvate ratios in individual patients. The possible relationship between impaired ubiquinone synthesis, mitochondrial dysfunction and myopathy

---

Table 224.10   Causes of rhabdomyolysis

Associated with inherited disorders
Disorders of carbohydrate metabolism
Myophosphorylase deficiency (McArdle's Disease, GSD V)
   Muscle phosphofructokinase deficiency (Tarui's Disease, GSD VII)
   Debrancher enzyme deficiency (Cori-Forbes Disease, GSD III)
   Phosphorylase b kinase deficiency
   Phosphoglycerate kinase deficiency
   Muscle Phosphoglycerate Mutase Deficiency
   Lactate Dehydrogenase Deficiency
Mitochondrial disorders
Carnitine palmitoyltransferase deficiency
Fatty acid oxidation disorders
Myoadenylate deaminase deficiency
Malignant hyperthermia
Muscular dystrophies

Environmental
Physical trauma
Excessive exercise
Extremes in body temperature
   Hyperthermia
   Hypothermia
Electrical shock/lightning strike

Salt and water imbalances (endocrine causes)
Hypokalemia
   Renal tubular acidosis
   Hyperaldosteronism
   Drug-Induced
   Licorice ingestion
Hypernatremia
Water intoxication
Hypophosphatemia
Hyperosmolar nonketotic coma
Diabetic ketoacidosis
Myxedema
Thyroid storm

Infectious
Bacterial
Viral
Richettsial
Fungal

Associated with other medical conditions
Autoimmune/inflammatory
   Polymyositis/dermatomyositis
   Systemic lupus erythematosis
   Polyarteritis nodosum
   Vasculitis
Generalized status epilepticus
Ischemic
   Arterial or venous occlusion
   Air embolism
   Sickle cell disease
   Compartment syndrome

Drugs, Toxins and Venoms
Pharmaceutical Agents
   (see Table 9 and reference 82)
Alcohol abuse
Illicit drugs
   Cocaine
   Heroin
   Amphetamine
   Phencyclidine
Natural products
   containing natural derivatives of drugs/toxins known to be associated with rhabdomyolysis
Toxins
Venoms/poisons

related to statin administration has not been specifically examined.

Discontinuation of statin administration at the onset of symptoms including muscle pain, tenderness or weakness may prevent more serious muscle damage and progression to rhabdomyolysis. Periodic monitoring of plasma creatine kinase activities does not necessarily prevent or predict the onset of myopathy or rhabdomyolysis. Treatment is mainly supportive. Clinical studies have not been performed to determine the efficacy of coenzyme Q_{10} (ubiquinone) administration in the prevention of statin-induced myotoxicity.

Rhabdomyolysis

Brief overview

Rhabdomyolysis usually presents as a clinical syndrome with myalgia, which may be accompanied by muscle weakness. Examination of the patient may reveal swelling and tenderness of the involved muscles. Damage to muscle cells results in leakage of cellular contents, including muscle enzymes, myoglobin, salts (especially potassium and phosphates), carnitine and creatine.[100] Elevation of creatine kinase is a key diagnostic feature. Large quantities of myoglobin are rapidly cleared by the kidneys, producing dark brown to mahogany-colored urine.[101] A vast array of etiological factors, both endogenous and exogenous, have been associated with rhabdomyolysis (Table 224.10).

Pathophysiology and pathogenesis

Abnormalities in muscle metabolism, whether inherited or acquired, may result in impairment in ATP production or ATP depletion.[82,100,102] Excessive energy utilization, leading to ATP depletion in otherwise normal muscle, may result from excessive exercise, involuntary prolonged muscle contraction (status epilepticus, dystonia, rigidity) or hyperthermia. Energy derived from ATP is used not only for muscle contraction, but also for the maintenance of homeostatic ion-gradients across the cell membrane, involving primarily sodium, potassium and calcium. Ion imbalance leads to loss of integrity of the cell membrane (sarcolemma) and leakage of cellular contents from muscle cells.[82] The abnormal distribution of salts and water across the muscle sarcolemma, regardless of the etiology, may precipitate an episode of rhabdomyolysis in a similar fashion.

The final common pathway for muscle cell necrosis likely results from the influx of calcium from the extracellular space because of loss of sarcolemmal integrity. This results in maximal contraction of contractile elements further depleting ATP. The inability to pump calcium ions back into the sarcoplasmic reticulum results in sustained muscle fiber contraction. Calcium entering the mitochondria uncouples oxidative phosphorylation and further impairs energy production. Furthermore, the excessive intracellular calcium activates calcium-dependent proteases and stimulates the release of autolytic enzymes from lyso-

somes leading to cell destruction.[101] The mechanisms by which infectious agents cause muscle cell death are less clear, but they are postulated to involve direct invasion of myocytes and toxin generation.[103]

Diagnosis

A thorough clinical history will often reveal the potential etiology of rhabdomyolysis. Extremes of temperature, physical trauma or excessive exercise are usually obvious in the history. The recent ingestion of any drug, whether prescribed, over-the-counter, natural or illicit, must be considered to be potentially causative. Alcohol, a commonly abused drug, is one of the more common causes of toxic myopathy. The absence of a provocative agent increases the likelihood that a primary muscle disorder exists. Furthermore, a history of preceding exercise intolerance may point to an underlying metabolic defect. Drugs may precipitate an acute decompensation in metabolically vulnerable muscle. The clinical clues associated with inflammatory disorders and medical conditions predisposing to imbalances of water and electrolytes may be subtler. Risk factors for HIV and symptomatology suggestive of an infectious etiology need to be specifically explored.

The ortho-toluidine (dipstick) test will detect both myoglobin and hemoglobin in the urine. Although this test is sensitive for the presence of myoglobinuria, it may be negative even in the presence of significant muscle breakdown. Immunochemical methods and electrophoresis are required for definite distinction between hemoglobin and myoglobin.[82]

Table 224.11   Treatment of acute rhabdomyolysis

1. Stop ongoing rhabdomyolysis
   a) Remove the causative agent when possible
   b) Control excessive muscle activity and maintain normothermia

2. Maintain urine production and adequate blood pressure to prevent renal failure
   a) Correct hypovolemia with isotonic saline (up to 150 mL/kg may be required) and maintain hydration
   b) Force diuresis with mannitol as a single dose (1 g/kg, up to 25 g) or as a continuous infusion
   c) Alkalinize the urine using intravenous sodium bicarbonate

3. Treat hyperkalemia aggressively.
   a) Intravenous insulin and glucose may be required.
   b) Rarely, dialysis must be considered if persistent

4. Monitor cardiac rhythm closely
5. Monitor calcium levels but treat hypocalcemia only if symptomatic
6. Monitor intracompartmental tissue pressure to prevent compartment syndrome and compression neuropathy

Pyomyositis resulting in fever and muscle tenderness can be distinguished from rhabdomyolysis on CT scan/MRI by the absence in the latter of abscess formation associated with myonecrosis.[103] It is important to distinguish myoglobinuria secondary to rhabdomyolysis from other forms of pigmenturia. Multiple causes of hemoglobinuria and hematuria exist and these may also present with acute renal failure making the distinction from myoglobinuria invaluable. Other forms of pigmenturia, usually resulting in red urine, include porphyrins (porphyria), pyrazolons (drugs), phenolphthalein (chemicals) and beets (nutritional).[104]

By far the most serious and life-threatening complication of rhabdomyolysis is acute renal failure. Evidence of acute tubular necrosis is often present. Oliguria is generally associated with elevation of plasma creatinine out of proportion to the increase in blood urea nitrogen (BUN) (i.e. low BUN-to-creatinine ratio) owing to release of creatinine from damaged muscle cells.[100] Renal failure, when it develops, further exacerbates the hyperkalemia and hyperphosphatemia associated with rhabdomyolysis.

Initial hypocalcemia may result from sequestration of calcium by damaged muscle. Patients who develop acute renal failure may subsequently develop hypercalcemia during the diuretic phase. This is felt to result from mobilization of calcium from muscle and the effects of hyperphosphatemia. Large quantities of intracellular potassium released from injured myocytes leads to hyperkalemia. The combination of hyperkalemia and hypocalcemia may precipitate life-threatening cardiac arrhythmias.[102] Swelling of injured muscle can lead to elevated pressures within the fascial compartments with eventual compartment syndrome and muscle ischemia. Compression neuropathies due to immobilization or the development of compartment syndrome may be irreversible.[82]

Treatment

Acute treatment The first step in the immediate treatment of an episode of rhabdomyolysis is removal of any suspected etiological agent. Secondly, aggressive monitoring and treatment of the associated complications of muscle necrosis and myoglobinuria may prevent renal failure and other secondary effects of ion imbalance. Maintenance of passive mobility beyond the initial rest period is important in the prevention of contractures. A treatment protocol is outlined in Table 224.11.

Anticipatory treatment Prevention of recurrent episodes of rhabdomyolysis relies on the identification of underlying precipitating factors accounting for the problem in the individual patient. Appropriate treatment of patients identified with specific inherited disorders of muscle energy metabolism is particularly important for the prevention of recurrence of rhabdomyolysis. Drugs known to interfere with the specific metabolic pathway involved should be avoided since these may precipitate decompensation in an otherwise well-controlled patient. When a specific

medication or toxin has been identified as the precipitating agent, avoidance of chemically related drugs or those that produce similar biochemical disturbances is advisable. Athletes should be counseled regarding appropriate exercise protocols and cautioned regarding the usage of "natural" products that interfere with energy metabolism and may result in muscle breakdown during exercise.

References

1. Martin A, Haller RG, Barohn R. Metabolic myopathies. Curr Opin Rheumatol 1994;6:552–558

2. Taivassalo T, Reddy H, Matthews PM. Muscle responses to exercise in health and disease. Neurol Clin 2000;18:15–34

3. Zschocke J, Hoffman GF. Vademecum metabolicum: manual of metabolic pediatrics. Friedrichsdorf: Schattauer, 1999

4. Shen JJ, Matern D, Millington DS, et al. Acylcarnitines in fibroblasts of patients with long-chain 3-hydroxy-acyl-CoA dehydrogenase deficiency and other fatty acid oxidation disorders. J Inherit Metab Dis 2000;23:27–44

5. Gadian DG, Leonard JV. The role of magnetic resonance spectroscopy in the investigation of lactic acidosis and inborn errors of energy metabolism. J Inherit Metab Dis 1996;19:548–552

6. Ferrari M, Binzoni T, Quaresima V. Oxidative metabolism in muscle. Philos Trans R Soc Lond B Biol Sci 1997;352:677–683

7. Ozawa T, Sahashi K, Nakase Y, Chance B. Extensive tissue oxygenation associated with mitochondrial DNA mutations. Biochem Biophys Res Commun 1995;213:432–438

8. Bank W, Park J, Lech G, Chance B. Near-infrared spectroscopy in the diagnosis of mitochondrial disorders. Biofactors 1998;7:243–245

9. Argov Z, Arnold DL. MR spectroscopy and imaging in metabolic myopathies. Neurol Clin 2000;18:35–52

10. Pourmand R. Metabolic myopathies. A diagnostic evaluation. Neurol Clin 2000;18:1–13

11. Elliot DL, Buist NR, Goldberg L, et al. Metabolic myopathies: evaluation by graded exercise testing. Medicine 1989;68(3):163–272

12. Lewis SF, Vora S, Haller RG. Abnormal oxidative metabolism and O_2 transport in muscle phosphofructokinase deficiency. Journal of Applied Physiology 1991;70(1):391–398

13. Bonnefont JP, Specola NB, Vassault A, et al. The fasting test in paediatrics: application to the diagnosis of pathological hypo- and hyperketotic states. Eur J Pediatr 1990;150:80–85

14. Zheng XX, Shoffner JM, Voljavec AS, Wallace DC. Evaluation of procedures for assaying oxidative phosphorylation enzyme activities in mitochondrial myopathy muscle biopsies. Biochim Biophys Acta 1990;1019:1–10

15. Brown DH. Glycogen metabolism and glycolysis in muscle. In: Engel AG, Franzini-Armstrong C, eds. Myology. New York: McGraw-Hill Inc., 1994:648–664

16. Chen Y-T, Burchell A. Glycogen storage disorders. In: Scriver CR, Beaudet AL, Sly CS, Valle D, eds. The metabolic and molecular bases of inherited disease. 7th ed. New York: McGraw-Hill, 1995:935–965

17. DiMauro S, Servidei S, Tsujino S. Disorders of carbohydrate metabolism: glycogen storage diseases. In: Rosenberg RN, Prusiner SB, DiMauro S, Barchi RL,

eds. The molecular and genetic basis of neurological disease. Boston: Butterworth-Heinemann, 1997: 1067–1097

18. Tsujino S, Nonaka I, DiMauro S. Glycogen storage myopathies. Neurol Clin 2000;18:125–150

19. Kiechl S, Kohlendorfer U, Thaler C, et al. Different clinical aspects of debrancher deficiency myopathy. J Neurol Neurosurg Psychiatry 1999;67:364–368

20. Amato AA. Acid maltase deficiency and related myopathies. Neurol Clin 2000;18:151–65

21. Kreuder J, Borkhardt A, Repp R, et al. Inherited metabolic myopathy and hemolysis due to a mutation in aldolase A. N Engl J Med 1996;334:1100–1104

22. Engel AG, Hirschhorn R. Acid maltase deficiency. In: Engel AG, Franzini-Armstrong C, eds. Myology. New York: McGraw-Hill Inc., 1994:1533–1553

23. Danon MJ, Oh SJ, DiMauro S, et al. Lysosomal glycogen storage disease with normal acid maltase. Neurology 1981;31:51–57

24. Gremse DA, Bucuvalas JC, Balistreri WF. Efficacy of cornstarch therapy in type III glycogen-storage disease. Am J Clin Nutr 1990;52:671–674

25. MacLean D, Vissing J, Vissing SF, Haller RG. Oral branched-chain amino acids do not improve exercise capacity in McArdle disease. Neurology 1998;51: 1456–1459

26. Beynon RJ, Bartram C, Hopkins P, et al. McArdle's disease: molecular genetics and metabolic consequences of the phenotype. Muscle Nerve 1995;3: S18–S22

27. Phoenix J, Hopkins P, Bartram C, et al. Effect of vitamin B_6 supplementation in McArdle's disease: a strategic case study. Neuromuscul Disord 1998;8: 210–212

28. Kikuchi T, Yang HW, Pennybacker M, et al. Clinical and metabolic correction of Pompe disease by enzyme therapy in acid maltase-deficient quail. J Clin Invest 1998;101:827–833

29. Boles RG, Buck EA, Blitzer MG, et al. Retrospective biochemical screening of fatty acid oxidation disorders in postmortem livers of 418 cases of sudden death in the first year of life. J Pediatr 1998;132:924–933

30. Pons R, De Vivo DC. Primary and secondary carnitine deficiency syndromes. J Child Neurol 1995;10(Suppl 2):S8–S24

31. Brivet M, Boutron A, Slama A, et al. Defects in activation and transport of fatty acids. J Inherit Metab Dis 1999;22:428–441

32. Tein I, De Vivo DC, Bierman F, et al. Impaired skin fibroblast carnitine uptake in primary systemic carnitine deficiency manifested by childhood carnitine-responsive cardiomyopathy. Pediatr Res 1990;28: 247–255

33. Tein I. Neonatal metabolic myopathies. Semin Perinatol 1999;23:125–151

34. Schon EA. The mitochondrial genome. In: Rosenberg RN, Prusiner SB, DiMauro S, Barchi RL, eds. The molecular and genetic basis of neurological disease. Boston: Butterworth-Heinemann, 1997:189–200

35. Lee CP, Martens ME. Mitochondrial respiration and energy metabolism in muscle. In: Engel AG, Franzini-Armstrong C, eds. Myology. New York: McGraw-Hill Inc., 1994:624–647

36. Morgan-Hughes JA. Mitochondrial diseases. In: Engel AG, Franzini-Armstrong C, eds. Myology. New York: McGraw-Hill Inc., 1994:1610–1660

37. Shoffner JM. Mitochondrial myopathy diagnosis. Neurol Clin 2000;18:105–123

38. DiMauro S, Bonilla E, Davidson M, et al. Mitochondria in neuromuscular disorders. Biochim Biophys Acta 1998;1366:199–210

39. Sue CM, Hirano M, DiMauro S, De Vivo DC. Neonatal presentations of mitochondrial metabolic disorders. Semin Perinatol 1999;23:113–124

40. Briones P, Vilaseca MA, Ribes A, et al. A new case of multiple mitochondrial enzyme deficiencies with decreased amount of heat shock protein 60. J Inherit Metab Dis 1997;20:569–577

41. Agsteribbe E, Huckriede A, Veenhuis M, et al. A fatal, systemic mitochondrial disease with decreased mitochondrial enzyme activities, abnormal ultrastructure of the mitochondria and deficiency of heat shock protein 60. Biochem Biophys Res Commun 1993;193: 146–154

42. Vu TH, Sciacco M, Tanji K, et al. Clinical manifestations of mitochondrial DNA depletion. Neurology 1998;50:1783–1790

43. Nishino I, Spinazzola A, Hirano M. Thymidine phosphorylase gene mutations in MNGIE, a human mitochondrial disorder. Science 1999;283:689–692

44. Falk RE, Cederbaum SD, Blass JP, et al. Ketonic diet in the management of pyruvate dehydrogenase deficiency. Pediatrics 1976;58:713–721

45. Wexler ID, Hemalatha SG, McConnell J, et al. Outcome of pyruvate dehydrogenase deficiency treated with ketogenic diets. Studies in patients with identical mutations. Neurology 1997;49:1655–1661

46. Wijburg FA, Barth PG, Bindoff LA, et al. Leigh syndrome associated with a deficiency of the pyruvate dehydrogenase complex: results of treatment with a ketogenic diet. Neuropediatrics 1992;23:147–152

47. Pastoris O, Savasta S, Foppa P, et al. Pyruvate dehydrogenase deficiency in a child responsive to thiamine treatment. Acta Paediatr 1996;85:625–628

48. Naito E, Ito M, Yokota I, et al. Thiamine-responsive lactic acidaemia: role of pyruvate dehydrogenase complex. Eur J Pediatr 1998;157:648–652

49. Matalon R, Stumpf DA, Michals K, et al. Lipoamide dehydrogenase deficiency with primary lactic acidosis: favorable response to treatment with oral lipoic acid. J Pediatr 1984;104:65–69

50. Nohl H, Gille L, Staniek K. The biochemical, pathophysiological, and medical aspects of ubiquinone function. Ann NY Acad Sci 1998;854:394–409

51. Chan A, Reichmann H, Kogel A, et al. Metabolic changes in patients with mitochondrial myopathies and effects of coenzyme Q_{10} therapy. J Neurol 1998; 245:681–685

52. Ihara Y, Namba R, Kuroda S, et al. Mitochondrial encephalomyopathy (MELAS): pathological study and successful therapy with coenzyme Q_{10} and idebenone. J Neurol Sci 1989;90:263–271

53. Argov Z, Bank WJ, Maris J, et al. Treatment of mitochondrial myopathy due to complex III deficiency with vitamins K3 and C: a ^{31}P-NMR follow-up study. Ann Neurol 1986;19:598–602

54. Ikejiri Y, Mori E, Ishii K, et al. Idebenone improves cerebral mitochondrial oxidative metabolism in a patient with MELAS. Neurology 1996;47:583–585

55. Abe K, Matsuo Y, Kadekawa J, et al. Effect of coenzyme Q_{10} in patients with mitochondrial myopathy, encephalopathy, lactic acidosis, and stroke-like episodes (MELAS): evaluation by noninvasive tissue oximetry. Journal of The Neurological Sciences 1999;162(1):65–68

56. Chen RS, Huang CC, Chu NS. Coenzyme Q_{10} treatment in mitochondrial encephalomyopathies.

Short-term double-blind, crossover study. European Neurology 1997;37(4):212–218

57. Matthews PM, Ford B, Dandurand RJ, et al. Coenzyme Q_{10} with multiple vitamins is generally ineffective in treatment of mitochondrial disease. Neurology 1993; 43:884–890

58. Luft R. The development of mitochondrial medicine. Proc Natl Acad Sci USA 1994;91:8731–8738

59. Luo X, Pitkänen S, Kassovska-Bratinova S, et al. Excessive formation of hydroxyl radicals and aldehydic lipid peroxidation products in cultured skin fibroblasts from patients with complex I deficiency. J Clin Invest 1997;99:2877–2882

60. Williams MH, Branch JD. Creatine supplementation and exercise performance: an update. J Am Coll Nutr 1998;17:216–234

61. Juhn MS, Tarnopolsky M. Oral creatine supplementation and athletic performance: a critical review. Clin J Sport Med 1998;8:286–297

62. Tarnopolsky MA, Roy BD, MacDonald JR. A randomized, controlled trial of creatine monohydrate in patients with mitochondrial cytopathies. Muscle Nerve 1997;20:1502–1509

63. Stacpoole PW. The pharmacology of dichloroacetate. Metabolism: Clinical and Experimental 1989;38: 1124–1144

64. Morten KJ, Beattie P, Brown GK, Matthews PM. Dichloroacetate stabilizes the mutant E1alpha subunit in pyruvate dehydrogenase deficiency. Neurology 1999;53:612–616

65. Morten KJ, Caky M, Matthews PM. Stabilization of the pyruvate dehydrogenase E1alpha subunit by dichloroacetate. Neurology 1998;51:1331–1315

66. Saijo T, Naito E, Ito M, et al. Therapeutic effect of sodium dichloroacetate on visual and auditory hallucinations in a patient with MELAS. Neuropediatrics 1991;22:166–167

67. Saitoh S, Momoi MY, Yamagata T, et al. Effects of dichloroacetate in three patients with MELAS. Neurology 1998;50:531–534

68. Pavlakis SG, Kingsley PB, Kaplan GP, et al. Magnetic resonance spectroscopy: use in monitoring MELAS treatment. Arch Neurol 1998;55:849–852

69. Taivassalo T, Matthews PM, De Stefano N, et al. Combined aerobic training and dichloroacetate improve exercise capacity and indices of aerobic metabolism in muscle cytochrome oxidase deficiency. Neurology 1996;47:529–534

70. Kimura S, Osaka H, Saitou K, et al. Improvement of lesions shown on MRI and CT scan by administration of dichloroacetate in patients with Leigh syndrome. J Neurol Sci 1995;134:103–107

71. Kuroda Y, Ito M, Naito E, et al. Concomitant administration of sodium dichloroacetate and vitamin B_1 for lactic acidemia in children with MELAS syndrome. J Pediatr 1997;131:450–452

72. Kuroda Y, Ito M, Toshima K, et al. Treatment of chronic congenital lactic acidosis by oral administration of dichloroacetate. J Inherit Metab Dis 1986;9: 244–252

73. Kimura S, Ohtuki N, Nezu A, et al. Clinical and radiologic improvements in mitochondrial encephalomyelopathy following sodium dichloroacetate therapy. Brain Dev 1997;19:535–540

74. De Stefano N, Matthews PM, Ford B, et al. Short-term dichloroacetate treatment improves indices of cerebral metabolism in patients with mitochondrial disorders. Neurology 1995;45(6):1193–1198

75. Stacpoole PW, Barnes CL, Hurbanis MD, et al. Treatment of congenital lactic acidosis with dichloroacetate. Arch Dis Child 1997;77:535–541

76. Takanashi J, Sugita K, Tanabe Y, et al. Dichloroacetate treatment in Leigh syndrome caused by mitochondrial DNA mutation. J Neurol Sci 1997;145:83–86

77. Tulinius MH, Eriksson BO, Hjalmarson O, et al. Mitochondrial myopathy and cardiomyopathy in siblings. Pediatr Neurol 1989;5:182–188

78. Walker UA, Byrne E. The therapy of respiratory chain encephalomyopathy: a critical review of the past and current perspective. Acta Neurol Scand 1995;92: 273–280

79. Cohen BH, Shoffner J, DeBoer G. Anesthesia and mitochondrial cytopathies. Mitochondrial News 1998;3:1–6

80. Taivassalo T, De Stefano N, Argov Z, et al. Effects of aerobic training in patients with mitochondrial myopathies. Neurology 1998;50:1055–1060

81. Le Quintrec JS, Le Quintrec JL. Drug-induced myopathies. Baillieres Clin Rheumatol 1991;5:21–38

82. Curry SC, Chang D, Connor D. Drug- and toxin-induced rhabdomyolysis. Ann Emerg Med 1989;18: 1068–1084

83. George KK, Pourmand R. Toxic myopathies. Neurol Clin 1997;15:711–730

84. Victor M, Sieb JP. Myopathies due to drugs, toxins, and nutritional deficiency. In: Engel AG, Fransini-Armstrong C, eds. Myology. New York: McGraw-Hill Inc., 1994: 1697–1725

85. Masini A, Scotti C, Calligaro A, et al. Zidovudine-induced experimental myopathy: dual mechanism of mitochondrial damage. J Neurol Sci 1999;166:131–140

86. Larsson L, Li X, Edstrom L, et al. Acute quadriplegia and loss of muscle myosin in patients treated with non-depolarizing neuromuscular blocking agents and corticosteroids: mechanisms at the cellular and molecular levels. Crit Care Med 2000;28:34–45

87. Hanson P, Dive A, Brucher JM, et al. Acute corticosteroid myopathy in intensive care patients. Muscle Nerve 1997;20:1371–1380

88. Anagnos A, Ruff RL, Kaminski HJ. Endocrine neuromyopathies. Neurol Clin 1997;15:673–696

89. Nesbitt LT, Jr. Minimizing complications from systemic glucocorticosteroid use. Dermatol Clin 1995;13: 925–939

90. Dukes MNG. Corticotrophins and corticosteroids. In: Dukes MNG, ed. Meyler's side effects of drugs. Amsterdam: Elsevier Science B.V., 1996:1189–1209

91. Letteron P, Brahimi-Bourouina N, Robin MA, et al. Glucocorticoids inhibit mitochondrial matrix acyl-CoA dehydrogenases and fatty acid β-oxidation. Am J Physiol 1997;272:G1141–G1150

92. Buttgereit F, Wehling M, Burmester GR. A new hypothesis of modular glucocorticoid actions: steroid treatment of rheumatic diseases revisited [see comments]. Arthritis Rheum 1998;41:761–767

93. Estes ML, Ewing-Wilson D, Chou SM, et al. Chloroquine neuromyotoxicity. Clinical and pathologic perspective. Am J Med 1987;82:447–455

94. Oyama F, Murakami N, Ihara Y. Chloroquine myopathy suggests that tau is degraded in lysosomes: implication for the formation of paired helical filaments in Alzheimer's disease. Neurosci Res 1998;31:1–8

95. Hsu I, Spinler SA, Johnson NE. Comparative evaluation of the safety and efficacy of HMG-CoA reductase inhibitor monotherapy in the treatment of primary hypercholesterolemia. Ann Pharmacother 1995;29: 743–759

96. Corsini A, Bellosta S, Baetta R, et al. New insights into the pharmacodynamic and pharmacokinetic properties of statins. Pharmacol Ther 1999;84:413–428

97. Herman RJ. Drug interactions and the statins. Can Med Assoc J 1999;161:1281–1286

98. Moghadasian MH. Clinical pharmacology of 3-hydroxy-3-methylglutaryl coenzyme A reductase inhibitors. Life Sci 1999;65:1329–1337

99. Folkers K, Langsjoen P, Willis R, et al. Lovastatin decreases coenzyme Q levels in humans. Proc Natl Acad Sci USA 1990;87:8931–8934

100. Penn AS. Myoglobinuria. *In:* Engel AG, Franzini-Armstrong C, eds. Myology. New York: McGraw-Hill Inc., 1994:1679–1696

101. Brumback RA, Feeback DL, Leech RW. Rhabdomyolysis in childhood. A primer on normal muscle function and selected metabolic myopathies characterized by disordered energy production. Pediatr Clin North Am 1992;39:821–858

102. David WS. Myoglobinuria. Neurol Clin 2000;18:215–243

103. Singh U, Scheld WM. Infectious etiologies of rhabdomyolysis: three case reports and review. Clin Infect Dis 1996;22:642–649

104. Blau N, Duran M, Blaskovics ME. Physician's guide to the laboratory diagnosis of metabolic diseases. New York: Chapman & Hall, 1996

225 Myotonia and Periodic Paralysis: Disorders of Voltage-Gated Ion Channels

Stephen C Cannon

Overview

Electrical signaling in skeletal muscle, heart, and nerve evolved as a means of transmitting information rapidly over long distances. In skeletal muscle, contraction is initiated by the release of calcium ions from the sarcoplasmic reticulum, which in turn is triggered by depolarization of the transverse tubule (T tubule) by an action potential propagated from the motor end plate. The fidelity and high speed of this signaling pathway depend on the coordinated actions of several classes of voltage-sensitive ion channels. Mutations in voltage-gated ion channel genes cause several heritable disorders in humans.[1,2] These so-called ion channelopathies tend to produce paroxysmal symptoms: myotonia or periodic paralysis of skeletal muscle; epilepsy, migraine, or episodic ataxia with central nervous system (CNS) involvement; and repolarization defects with an increased susceptibility to tachyarrhythmias in cardiac disorders. Defective voltage-gated ion channels may pathologically increase the electrical excitability of a cell, reduce excitability, or even cause a complete loss of excitability. In skeletal muscle, periodic paralysis results from a loss of electrical excitability, whereas myotonia is a state of enhanced excitability in which self-sustained bursts of discharges impair relaxation after voluntary contraction.

The myotonias and periodic paralyses constitute a diverse group of rare inherited disorders of skeletal muscle.[3-5] In all these disorders, the primary abnormality is an alteration in the electrical excitability of the muscle fiber. The excitability changes lead to intermittent defects in electrical signaling that are manifest clinically as transient myotonic stiffness or episodic attacks of weakness. Myotonia is usually worst with the first few contractions after a period of rest and resolves with repeated muscular activity ("warm-up phenomenon"). In contrast, the stiffness paradoxically worsens with ongoing activity in paramyotonia. The electromyogram (EMG) shows runs of repetitive discharges elicited by percussing the muscle or by voluntary contraction. The discharges vary in amplitude and frequency and are not abolished by nondepolarizing blockers of neuromuscular transmission, such as curare, which demonstrates that the spikes are generated autonomously by the muscle fiber. Periodic paralysis presents as episodic attacks of generalized weakness, with no regular periodicity, that vary in severity from mild to flaccid paralysis. The diaphragm and intercostal muscles usually are spared, so that hypoventilation and respiratory failure are exceedingly rare. Also, the extraocular muscles characteristically are unaffected. Attacks may last from hours to a day or longer. Rest after exercise, emotional stress, cooling, and variations in carbohydrate intake or potassium may precipitate attacks. Between attacks muscle function is typically normal, although some patients develop a late-onset, mildly progressive proximal myopathy. In some families affected persons have only myotonia or only periodic paralysis, but in other families myotonia and periodic paralysis may occur alternately in the same person.

Several clinical disorders have been delineated along the spectrum of altered excitability from myotonia to periodic paralysis (Figure 225.1). Myotonia congenita (MC) is characterized by myotonia that is present at birth or within the first decade, is nonprogressive, and is not associated with dystrophy. A dominantly inherited form was first described in 1876

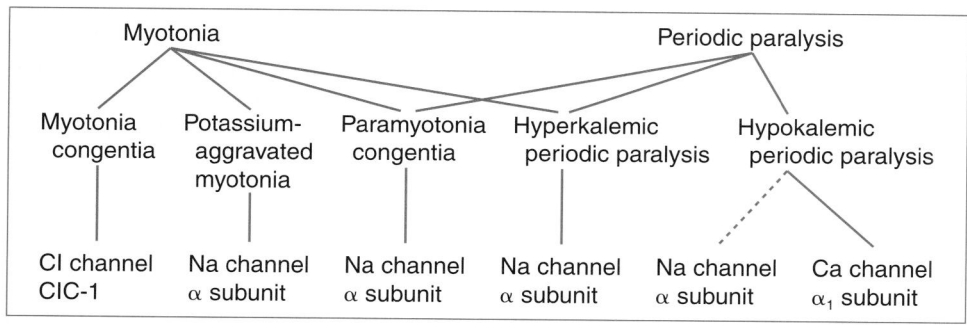

Figure 225.1 Clinical spectrum of the non-dystrophic myotonias and periodic paralyses. Myotonia predominates in disorders further to the left in this spectrum, and periodic paralysis is the major symptom for those toward the right. The underlying molecular genetic defects in each disorder are mutations in voltage-gated ion channel genes (bottom row). Ca, calcium; Cl, chloride; ClC-1, skeletal muscle chloride channel; Na, sodium.

Table 225.1   Clinical features of non-dystrophic myotonias and periodic paralyses

Feature	Myotonia congenita		Potassium-aggravated myotonia*	Paramyotonia congenita	Hyperkalemic periodic paralysis	Hypokalemic periodic paralysis
Inheritance	Dominant	Recessive	Dominant	Dominant	Dominant	Dominant
Penetrance	High	High	High	High	High	Reduced for females
Age of onset	Congenital	1st decade	1st decade	1st decade	1st decade	2nd decade (puberty)
Myotonia						
Stiffness	Moderate	Severe	Mild–severe	Moderate	Mild	None
Distribution	Generalized	Generalized, legs	Variable	Hands, face	Hands, face	—
Special features	Improves with warm-up	Improves with warm-up	Fluctuates, aggravated by K, pain with stiffness	Paramyotonia, aggravated by cold	Aggravated by K	—
EMG	3+	3+	2+–3+	2+–3+	0–2+	0
Episodic weakness						
Severity	None	Mild	None	Mild–severe	Moderate–severe	Severe (when present)
Distribution	—	Legs or arms	—	Regional or generalized	Regional or generalized	Generalized
Duration	—	Transient (seconds)	—	Minutes to 1 day	Minutes to 1 day	Hours to days
Provocation	—	Forceful effort after rest	—	Cold, rest after exercise	K, rest after exercise, fasting	Rest after exercise, carbohydrates
Permanent weakness	None	None	None	None	Variable late-onset proximal weakness	Prominent late-onset proximal weakness

EMG, electromyography: K, potassium.
*Includes myotonia fluctuans, myotonia permanens, and acetazolamide-responsive myotonia.

by Thomsen,[6] whose family had the disorder (Thomsen disease). Eighty years later, Becker[7] recognized that the most common inheritance pattern of MC is recessive. At the other end of the spectrum, hypokalemic periodic paralysis (HypoPP) presents with attacks of flaccid paralysis in association with hypokalemia, but no myotonia. Inheritance is autosomal dominant, with reduced penetrance in women. In 1951, Tyler et al.[8] described a family with autosomal dominant periodic paralysis and hyperkalemia. Hyperkalemic periodic paralysis (HyperPP) can occur without myotonia, with myotonia, or with paramyotonia. Paramyotonia congenita (PMC) is a related disorder first described by Eulenberg[9] in 1886, in which cold-exacerbated paramyotonia is the predominant symptom but prolonged attacks of weakness may also occur. With the advent of molecular genetic testing, many forms of dominantly inherited myotonia without periodic paralysis or dystrophy were found to be allelic to HyperPP and PMC (i.e., different mutations in the same gene cause all three disorders). In comparison with MC, the myotonia is usually worsened by cooling or administration of potassium, and this syndrome has been named "potassium-aggravated myotonia" (PAM).[10]

The molecular genetic defects have been identified as mutations in voltage-gated ion channel genes for each of the clinically delineated forms of non-dystrophic myotonia and periodic paralysis (Figure 225.1). Mutations in a skeletal muscle chloride channel gene on chromosome 7, CLCN-1, cause either

dominant or recessive MC.[11] HypoPP is caused by missense mutations in the α subunit gene of the skeletal muscle L-type calcium channel on chromosome 1.[12–14] Mutations in the skeletal muscle isoform of the sodium channel α subunit on chromosome 17 may give rise to myotonia without weakness ("potassium-aggravated myotonia"),[10] to paramyotonia with intermittent weakness (PMC)[15], to periodic paralysis and mild myotonia in association with an increased serum potassium (HyperPP)[16], or periodic paralysis with hypokalemia and no myotonia (HypoPP)[38]. The most common cause of HypoPP, however, is missense mutations in the α1 subunit gene of the skeletal muscle L-type calcium channel on chromosome 1.

Chloride channel disorders: dominant and recessive myotonia congenita

Clinical features

MC may be inherited in either a dominant (Thomsen disease) or recessive (Becker generalized myotonia) pattern. In both forms, generalized myotonic stiffness is the predominant symptom and periodic paralysis does not occur (Table 225.1). Stiffness worsens with the first few contractions after rest and then resolves with continued activity. In contrast to HyperPP and PMC, the myotonia is not aggravated by cold. Often, stiffness is most pronounced in the legs, and children may present with frequent falls. Strength is preserved, although myotonic stiffness may be followed by transient weakness. Myotonia may be congenital or appear in the first decade, it otherwise is non-progressive. In comparison with dominant MC, the recessive form usually has a later onset of 10 to 15 years, greater severity of myotonic stiffness, more pronounced muscular hypertrophy (especially of the thigh and gluteal muscles) with associated lordosis, and transient weakness with initial forceful effort.[17] Both the recessive and the dominant forms of MC are rare disorders. Recessive MC has a prevalence of about 1:50 000, and there is no apparent ethnic or geographic clustering. Dominant MC is much rarer than first reported because most cases of dominantly inherited myotonia without periodic paralysis were subsequently found to be due to sodium channel mutations and, are thus, forms of PAM, not MC.

Molecular genetics

Dominant MC and recessive MC are both caused by mutations in CLCN-1, the gene coding for the predominant chloride channel expressed in skeletal muscle.[11] The gene spans 40 kb on chromosome 7q35, contains 22 introns, and codes for a 988-amino-acid protein.[18] More than 40 different mutations have been identified in CLCN-1 in families with MC.[2] Neither the location nor the type of mutation allows an a priori prediction of whether the phenotype will be dominant or recessive. In general, dominant MC is associated with missense mutations or premature stops near the carboxyl terminus. The mutation in Thomsen's family has been identified as a proline to leucine substitution at position 480.[19] Mutations associated with recessive MC are more varied, and include deletions, insertions, and splicing defects as well as missense and nonsense mutations. Most patients with recessive MC are compound heterozygotes with a different recessive mutation in each CLCN-1 allele, rather than arising from homozygous mutations in consanguineous marriages. Thus far, the diversity of mutations associated with MC and the size of the CLCN-1 gene have precluded the development of a commercially available genetic test for MC mutations.

Pathophysiology and pathogenesis

The first insights into the pathophysiology of myotonia came from microelectrode studies of muscle fibers from myotonic goats. In a classic series of experiments,[20,21] Bryant and colleagues found that the input resistance of myotonic fibers was increased because of a severe decrease in the resting conductance to chloride ions. Hereditary myotonia in goats most closely resembles dominant MC in humans. Decreased chloride conductance was found in human fibers from patients with either dominant or recessive MC.[22] The chloride hypothesis of myotonia was supported by the observation that normal fibers became myotonic either in chloride-free solution or in the presence of chloride channel blockers (anthracene-9-carboxylic acid). Drug-induced myotonia has occurred with agents developed to reduce hypercholesterolemia (clofibrate or 20–25 diazocholesterol) by decreasing the chloride conductance.[23,24]

The resting chloride conductance of skeletal muscle is notably high ($130\,\mu$Siemen/cm^2 at -80 mV) and helps maintain the membrane potential at its resting value. About two-thirds of the total conductance in resting fibers is contributed by the chloride channel ClC-1; the rest is due to potassium-selective channels. The reversal potential for ClC-1 is approximately equal to the normal resting potential. If the membrane potential varies from its resting value, large chloride currents flow to re-establish the resting potential. This electrical buffering is particularly important for skeletal muscle in which trapping of potassium in the T tubules tends to depolarize the fiber. With each action potential, the T tubular potassium concentration increases transiently because of the egress of potassium ions from inside the fiber into the long narrow diffusion-limited tubules. The increased potassium concentration in the T tubule (extracellular space) depolarizes the fiber. Current flow though chloride channels normally opposes this depolarization, so that each action potential causes a transient afterdepolarization of only 0.1 mV. In myotonic muscle, the same T tubular accumulation of potassium depolarizes the fiber by about 1 mV after each action potential. With progressive accumulation of potassium, this afterdepolarization is sufficient to generate self-sustained bursts of myotonic discharges.[25]

The chloride conductance must be severely decreased for a muscle fiber to exhibit myotonia. Pharmacological models have shown that myotonia occurs only after more than 70% of the normal chloride conductance is lost.[26] This observation and the dimeric structure of the chloride channel explain why mutations in the same channel gene may cause either dominant or recessive MC.[27] Mutations that cause a total loss of ClC-1 function result in recessive MC. The reduced channel density from haploinsufficiency does not decrease the chloride conductance sufficiently to cause myotonia. This suggests that severely truncated ClC-1 and other recessive mutations do not interfere with the assembly and function of wild type ClC-1 channels expressed by the normal allele. In contrast, expression of mutant ClC-1 channels associated with dominant MC results in functional homodimeric chloride channels, but the voltage-dependence of opening is shifted far toward depolarized potentials. Coexpression of mutant and wild type channels results in heterodimeric channels whose voltage-dependence of opening is also dramatically shifted toward depolarized potentials.[28] Thus, the dominant MC mutations exert a dominant-negative effect on the resting chloride conductance by shifting the voltage-dependence of activation.

Diagnosis

The clinical hallmarks of MC (Table 225.1) were recognized in the initial report by Thomsen:[6] generalized myotonic stiffness, non-progressive course, absence of muscular dystrophy, and heritability (dominant for Thomsen disease and a later-recognized recessive form). The inheritance is mendelian, with high penetrance and equal frequency in males and females, although females often have milder symptoms. Laboratory investigations are most notable for the presence of myotonic discharges detected on EMG in virtually every muscle tested. There are no distinguishing EMG features of myotonic discharges in MC in comparison with other myotonic disorders, aside from the high prevalence and generalized distribution. Heterozygous carriers of recessive MC are asymptomatic, but about two-thirds of them have latent myotonia detected with EMG.[29] Muscle biopsy specimens show fiber hypertrophy, central nuclei, and a decreased number of type 2 fibers, but these changes are non-specific. The serum level of creatine kinase usually is normal or increased two- to threefold. Molecular genetic screening for mutations in *CLCN-1* is not available commercially.

In the differential diagnosis of myotonia, the most crucial obligation is to exclude myotonic dystrophy (or dystrophia myotonica, DM). Often, the distinction is easily made on clinical grounds. DM is a multisystem disorder for which progressive distal and bulbar muscular dystrophy usually is more disabling than the mild distal myotonia. Additional organ system involvement in DM includes the eyes (cataract, retinal degeneration, ptosis), brain (mental retardation, hypersomnia), heart (conduction defects, arrythmias, cardiomyopathy), endocrine system (testicular atrophy), skin (alopecia), and smooth muscle (dysphagia, gut dysmotility, megacolon). Inheritance in DM is always dominant with high penetrance, and successive generations are affected more severely (genetic anticipation), particularly with maternal transmission. The genetic defect in DM is an expanded trinucleotide repeat (CTG) in the 3'-untranslated region of the myotonic protein kinase gene (*DMPK*) on chromosome 19q13.3.[30] Normals have 5 to 40 CTG repeats, whereas those with DM have 50 to more than 2000. Higher numbers of repeats are correlated with earlier onset and greater severity of symptoms. Molecular genetic screening for the number of CTG repeats in the *DMPK* gene has provided a sensitive and specific test for DM.

Proximal myotonic myopathy (PROMM or DM2) is a dominantly inherited multisystem disorder with features similar to DM, but there is no pathological expansion of the CTG repeat in the *DMPK* gene.[31] The myotonia in PROMM is typically mild and fluctuating, and EMG invariably shows myotonic discharges. Associated features include proximal (hip and neck) weakness, cataracts, episodic muscle pain (thigh, upper arm, shoulder), action tremor, and hypogonadism; cerebral white matter abnormalities are seen on magnetic resonance imaging (MRI). Unlike DM, PROMM is not associated with mental deficiency or with progressive dystrophy of distal muscles. PROMM is caused by an expansion of CCTG repeats in intron on a zinc finger gene (ZNF9) on chromosone 3q.[32]

The distinction between MC and PAM or PMC can be more problematic. However, this is largely an academic exercise because all three disorders have a benign course and respond similarly to therapeutic

intervention. The distinguishing features of MC, PAM, and PMC are listed in Table 225.1. Paramyotonia of the hands, face, and tongue that is worsened by cooling and may be associated with prolonged attacks of weakness is pathognomonic for PMC. The importance of distinguishing PMC from MC is that the weakness in PMC can be treated effectively with carbonic anhydrase inhibitors. PAM may be impossible to distinguish clinically from dominant MC. In fact, most published "cases" of Thomsen disease have been discovered to have sodium channel mutations and thus are cases of PAM, not dominant MC. In PAM, the severity of myotonia fluctuates more than in MC. Another distinguishing feature is that cooling or ingestion of foods high in potassium often worsens myotonia dramatically in PAM but has little effect in MC. Provocative clinical testing with potassium loading is not recommended, because patients with PAM may experience a prolonged and intense bout of myotonia with considerable discomfort.

Treatment

The pharmacological treatment of myotonia is similar for all the myotonic disorders regardless of the underlying ion channel defect (Table 225.2). Myotonia responds best to drugs that decrease the electrical excitability of the sarcolemma by blocking voltage-dependent sodium channels in a use-dependent fashion (local anesthetics, antiarrhythmics, and antiepileptic agents). The preferred drug is mexiletine, starting at 200 mg 3 times daily. Elderly patients or those with heart disease should consult a cardiologist before treatment with mexiletine is initiated. Tocainide, another anti-arrhythmia agent, is no longer recommended because of rare instances of blood dyscrasias and pulmonary fibrosis. Anecdotally, the antiepileptic agents carbamazepine and phenytoin are thought to be less effective than mexiletine,[3] but controlled comparisons have not been performed.

On the basis of the pathophysiology of MC, a rational treatment approach would be to pharmacologically increase the chloride conductance of skeletal muscle. Taurine and the R-(+) isomer of clofibric acid produce measurable increases in the resting chloride conductance of skeletal muscle. However, the changes are modest and not sufficient to prevent myotonia.[33]

The response to therapy can be assessed objectively with a simple stair-climbing test.[34] First, the patient rests quietly for 15 minutes on a chair at the foot of the stairs. Next, he or she climbs 10 steps as fast as possible. Healthy persons make the climb in about 3 seconds, whereas those with myotonia may require several tens of seconds. Improvement with warm-up can be measured with repeated trials.

Most patients with MC do not require medication or prefer not to take it. Instead, patients learn from experience how to minimize their myotonia. Typical maneuvers include slowly increasing the level of muscular exertion to "warm-up" after periods of rest and avoiding exacerbating conditions such as hypocalcemia or drugs such as clofibrate or inhibitors of cholesterol synthesis.

Myotonia and Periodic Paralysis: Disorders of Voltage-Gated Ion Channels

Table 225.2 Treatment of myotonia and periodic paralysis

Symptom	Disorder	First-line treatment	Alternative treatment
Myotonia	MC (AD or AR) PAM PMC	Mexiletine 600–1200 mg/day in 3 doses	Phenytoin 300 mg/day Carbamazepine 400 to 1200 mg/day
Periodic paralysis Acute attack	HyperPP	Glucose 100 g PO or carbohydrate-rich food	Hydrochlorothiazide 25 mg
		Acetazolamide 125 mg (if not used prophylactically)	Albuterol 2 puffs, repeat as needed
	HypoPP	Acetazolamide 125 mg (if not used prophylactically) KCl 20–120 mEq PO	For severe attacks with impaired swallowing and respiratory compromise, intravenous KCl 50 mEq/L in 5% mannitol infused at 250 mL/hr
Prophylaxis	PMC	Avoid cold environment Acetazolamide 125–1500 mg/day*	Mexiletine 600 to 1200 mg/day
	HyperPP	Frequent carbohydrate-rich meals Limit K⁺ intake "Warm-down" after exercise Acetazolamide 125–1500 mg/day	Dichlorphenamide 25–100 mg/day Hydrochlorothiazide 25–50 mg/day
	HypoPP	High potassium diet Avoid carbohydrate-rich meals Avoid strenuous exercise Acetazolamide 125–1500 mg/day	Dichlorphenamide 25–100 mg/day KCl 10–40 mEq/day Spironolactone 100 mg/day†

AD, autosomal dominant; AR, autosomal recessive; HyperPP, hyperkalemic periodic paralysis; HypoPP, hypokalemic periodic paralysis; KCl, potassium chloride; MC, myotonia congenita; PAM, potassium-aggravated myotonia; PMC, paramyotonia congenita; PO, orally.
*In some patients with PMC, acetazolamide may induce weakness.
†Spironolactone and KCl supplements should not be taken concurrently.

Sodium channel disorders: hyperkalemic periodic paralysis, paramyotonia congenita, potassium-aggravated myotonia

Clinical features

Missense mutations of the skeletal muscle sodium channel α subunit may cause dominantly inherited myotonia, periodic paralysis, or both. The sodium channelopathies have been delineated clinically into four allelic disorders that lie in the middle of spectrum of altered membrane excitability (Figure 225.1).

HyperPP presents with recurrent episodes of weakness that are often associated with an increased venous concentration of potassium (>5.0 mmol/L). Hyperkalemia may cause T-wave changes in the electrocardiogram, but life-threatening cardiac arrhythmias do not occur. The serum level of potassium may be normal during an attack, and a more consistent finding in HyperPP is a provocation of weakness with the administration of potassium. Attacks of weakness begin in childhood and often increase in frequency to weekly or, in severe cases, even daily episodes. During a severe attack, affected muscles are flaccid and electrically inexcitable. Recovery occurs spontaneously, usually within an hour, but full strength may not return for days. Attacks of weakness often occur within minutes of resting after exercise or in the morning before breakfast. Weakness is worsened or provoked by a potassium-rich diet, cold ambient temperatures, fasting, emotional stress, and pregnancy. An incipient attack may be aborted by exercise or carbohydrate ingestion. In HyperPP, myotonia or paramyotonia may occur, especially near the time of a paralytic attack, but recurrent weakness is always the predominant symptom. After the third decade, the frequency of attacks decreases and a mildly progressive proximal myopathy may develop .

PMC is characterized by myotonic stiffness that paradoxically worsens with repeated contractions (paramyotonia) and is aggravated by cold temperatures.[4] The muscles of the hands and face are affected most commonly. Episodic weakness may occur, either spontaneously or with prolonged exposure to cold, and may be as severe as in periodic paralysis. Paramyotonia is present at birth and persists throughout life. Attacks of weakness typically occur during adolescence. Inheritance is dominant, with high penetrance. Variants of PMC have been reported in which paramyotonia occurs even in a warm environment or cooling provokes attacks of weakness without stiffness or cold-induced paramyotonia occurs without weakness.[4]

PAM presents as dominantly inherited myotonia of variable severity and the absence of weakness or dystrophy.[10] Before molecular genetic testing was available, most of the patients were thought to have dominant MC. In contrast to MC, the myotonia of

PAM fluctuates from day to day and may be aggravated by rest several minutes after exercise or by potassium ingestion.[35] A rare form of PAM, myotonia permanens, has been described in which severe persistent myotonia is debilitating to the point of impeding respiration.[10] In other families, PAM presents as painful myotonia[36] or myotonia that is responsive to acetazolamide.[37]

HypoPP has also been observed in association with mutations in SCN4A.[38] The clinical features are episodes of generalized weakness and hypokalemia, often after exercise or upon awakening in the morning. Sodium channel mutations are an infrequent cause of HypoPP, accounting for only about 10% of cases, whereas calcium channel mutations are found in about 70% of affected families.[68] As in the Ca-channel based HypoPP, myotonia does not occur in HypoPP due to Na channel mutations.

Molecular genetics

Electrophysiological studies by Lehmann-Horn et al.[39,40] in the 1980s implicated the skeletal muscle sodium channel as a candidate disease gene in HyperPP and PMC. Subsequently, both disorders were found to be genetically linked to SCN4A, the gene for the α subunit of the adult skeletal muscle isoform of the sodium channel on chromosome 17q23–q25.[16,41] SCN4A spans 35 kb, contains 24 exons, and codes for the 1836-amino-acid α subunit of the skeletal muscle sodium channel (SkM1).[42,43] To date, 31 different mutations in SCN4A have been identified in families with HyperPP, PMC, PAM, and HypoPP. In skeletal muscle, the voltage-gated sodium channel is a heterodimer of the pore-forming α subunit and an accessory β1 subunit. SkM1 is expressed selectively in innervated skeletal muscle; therefore, mutations in SCN4A do not cause CNS dysfunction or cardiac arrhythmia. The β1 subunit is expressed in skeletal muscle, heart, and brain. A mutation in the β1 subunit has been associated, with dominantly inherited febrile seizures,[44] but no neuromuscular disorder has been attributed to a β1 defect.

All the mutations identified in SCN4A lead to missense substitutions in which one conserved amino acid is replaced by another residue.[45] Each mutation usually produces a consistent phenotype (HyperPP, PMC, PAM or HypoPP), although phenotypic variability is found both within a family and between unrelated families with the same mutation.[46] Some mutations occur more frequently than others. Of the ten mutations associated with HyperPP, Thr-704-Met is found in 60% of families and Met-1592-Val in 32%; the other mutations have been identified in only one or two families. Haplotype analysis suggests that common mutations have arisen independently in unrelated families.[47] Eleven mutations have been identified in PMC, with the most common ones being Thr-1313-Met (45%) and Arg-1448-Cys (35%). Several PMC mutations are clustered in a voltage-sensor domain of the channel, with four different substitutions at Arg-1448. Seven mutations have been reported in PAM. Three of these are in the fast inacti-

vation gate at Gly-1306, and the clinical severity of myotonia increases with the size of the residue substituted for glycine: Ala < Val < Glu.[10] Four SCN4A missense mutations have been identified in HypoPP, all of which are in voltage-sensing regions of the channel.

Molecular genetic screening for mutations in SCN4A is not available commercially.

Pathophysiology and pathogenesis

Most of the missense mutations in SkM1 produces gain-of-function defects by altering the open-closed transitions of the channel in response to membrane voltage. Heterologous expression studies have shown that the most common defect is an impairment of inactivation.[45] Some mutations disrupt the completeness of inactivation, so that on average 2% to 5% of channels remain open. Others slow the rate of inactivation, shift its voltage dependence, or accelerate the rate of recovery from inactivation. Also, some mutations enhance activation by causing channels to open for smaller depolarizations from the resting potential. The inactivation and activation defects both result in a larger inward sodium current flowing through mutant channels than for wild type ones. This aberrant inward current may either trigger the afterdischarges underlying myotonia or depolarize the resting potential, which results in a loss of excitability and flaccid paralysis.

Model systems have been used to explore how the gating defects identified in mutant channels cause myotonia or paralysis. These investigations have also provided a basis for understanding why the functional defects of one mutation may lead to depolarization-induced weakness (HyperPP), whereas channel defects of another mutation cause myotonic discharges but no paralysis (PAM).

The first observation was that even a subtle disruption of sodium channel inactivation is sufficient to produce myotonia.[48] Inactivation was rendered partially incomplete (2% of the sodium current failed to inactivate within 100 milliseconds) by applying sea anemone toxin (ATXII) to rat skeletal muscle in vitro. Toxin-exposed fibers had myotonic afterdischarges, and the relaxation in twitch force was slowed by an order of magnitude. This sodium channel-based myotonia shares a mechanistic feature with myotonia caused by decreased chloride conductance in MC. In both cases, mechanical disruption of the T tubules abolishes the afterdischarges.[25,48] Activity-dependent accumulation of potassium in the T tubules initiates the afterdischarges in both forms of myotonia. With a severely decreased chloride conductance, the accumulated potassium ions cause a larger depolarization of the resting potential, which may trigger afterdischarges. With inactivation-deficient sodium channels, the modest depolarization induced by potassium ion accumulation is sufficient to activate a substantial sodium current, which further depolarizes the fiber and elicits an action potential. In agreement with the toxin studies, computer-based simulations of a model fiber have demonstrated that even a modest disruption of sodium current inactivation (0.8% to 2%) causes myotonic afterdischarges.[49]

The computational model predicts that a slightly more severe defect of sodium channel inactivation or augmented activation will produce depolarization-induced paralysis. In the simulation, if 3% or more of the sodium current fails to inactivate or activation is shifted toward depolarized voltages by more than 10 mV, the afterdischarges dissipate and the membrane potential settles to an aberrantly depolarized value of -40 mV, compared to the normal resting value of -90 mV. From this depolarized potential, most (97%) sodium conductance is inactivated, so the system is refractory from generating any additional discharges and flaccid paralysis ensues. Thus, the dominant negative effect of mutant sodium channels is exerted through their effect on membrane potential. In agreement with these simulations, heterologous expression studies have shown that mutations associated with HyperPP have more severe defects in sodium channel gating than those in PAM.

Another form of sodium channel inactivation opposes the chronic depolarization-induced paralysis produced by an anomalously persistent sodium current. In addition to fast inactivation, which occurs within 1 millisecond and limits the firing rate and action potential duration, sodium channels undergo an independent slow inactivation process during maintained depolarizations of seconds or longer. Slow inactivation will attenuate the persistent sodium current and might thereby prevent an attack of paralysis.[50] This prediction was borne out in experimental studies. The two most common causes of HyperPP (Thr-704-Met and Met-1592-Val) and a rarer mutation (Ile-693-Thr) all have disrupted slow inactivation.[51,52] However, not all HyperPP mutations have slow inactivation defects. Slow inactivation is too sluggish to prevent transient myotonic discharges, and no defects in slow inactivation have been observed for mutations associated with myotonia without weakness.[52] These observations have led to the proposal that defects of slow inactivation greatly increase the propensity for periodic paralysis and suggest that slow inactivation normally may protect the fiber from prolonged episodes of depolarization-induced weakness.

Diagnosis

The distinctive clinical features of the syndromes within the HyperPP–PMC–PAM spectrum and the different treatment strategies justify retaining this diagnostic scheme (Table 225.1) rather than combining these disorders into a single class of sodium channelopathy. In exemplary cases, the diagnosis is unambiguous. However, many clinical variants with overlapping symptoms and laboratory findings have been described. The differential diagnosis among these entities is made on clinical grounds for two reasons: 1) the genotype-phenotype correlations are still being defined, so in many cases the identification of a specific mutation provides supportive rather than definitive data; and 2) molecular genetic testing is not yet widely available.

The diagnosis of HyperPP is readily established when episodes of periodic paralysis are associated with serum potassium levels greater than 4.5 mmol/L and the inheritance pattern is dominant. A normal potassium level does not exclude the diagnosis, and rebound hypokalemia may occur during recovery. Interictally, potassium levels are normal. Myotonia may occur in HyperPP, but the predominant symptom is episodic weakness. Paradoxical or cold-induced myotonia in association with periodic paralysis is diagnostic of PMC rather than HyperPP. Not all patients with HyperPP have myotonia, but its presence excludes the diagnosis of HypoPP.

Histological examination often shows myopathic changes that range from abnormal variation in fiber size and central nuclei to necrosis and vacuolated fibers.[53] Ultrastructural studies have shown proliferation and dilatation of the sarcoplasmic reticulum and T tubular systems. However, biopsy specimen from affected muscle may not show any abnormality, which implies that the alteration in electrical excitability can occur without morphological changes in the fiber. These pathological changes occur in both HypoPP and HyperPP.

Provocative testing can be used to support a suspected diagnosis of HyperPP. A simple noninvasive test is to monitor the response to vigorous exercise.[54] The subject exercises on a treadmill or stationary bicycle for 30 minutes, with the heart rate increased above 120 beats/minute, and then rests motionlessly in bed. The serum level of potassium will increase during exercise and then quickly decrease to baseline levels. After 15 to 30 minutes of rest, patients with HyperPP have a secondary increase in the serum level of potassium that does not occur in normal subjects.[55] Coincident with hyperkalemia, the compound muscle action potential (CMAP) amplitude decreases dramatically[54] and the patient may become weak. If the distinction between HyperPP and HypoPP is not clear, potassium challenge may be necessary. Severe renal disease or adrenal insufficiency is a contraindication to potassium challenge. Continuous cardiac monitoring should be performed, and resuscitation equipment and personnel must be readily available. The test is most sensitive when performed with the patient in the fasting state, after a period of exercise. From 40 to 120 mmol of potassium chloride is administered orally in an unsweetened solution. An attack usually occurs within 1 to 2 hours, as evidenced by a marked decrease in muscle strength or a decrease in CMAP amplitude.[56]

PMC should be suspected in patients with dominantly inherited exercise- or cold-induced myotonic stiffness, especially of the hands and face. Paramyotonia is the predominant symptom, but spontaneous or cold-induced attacks of weakness may occur and do not exclude the diagnosis of PMC. Myotonic discharges are detected in virtually every muscle examined, even at warm ambient temperatures. Muscle cooling is used as a provocative test to confirm the diagnosis of PMC.[57] Baseline CMAP amplitude, maximal isometric force, and relaxation time of the finger flexor muscles are measured, and then the forearm is immersed in chilled water (15°C) for 30 minutes. On repeat testing of the cooled limb, patients with PMC have decreased CMAP amplitude and dramatic slowing of relaxation time. In many patients, the maximal isometric force is less than 50% of the baseline value. If cold worsens the myotonia but does not cause weakness, the patient may have PMC or PAM.[58]

The clinical presentation of PAM overlaps considerably with that of dominant MC and PMC (Table 225.1). The core features of PAM are generalized myotonia that often fluctuates spontaneously over the course of days or in relation to activity, dominant inheritance, and no episodic attacks of weakness. Cooling does not aggravate myotonia in chloride-channel-based MC, but often worsens the stiffness in PAM. The activity-dependent variation in myotonia differs between PAM and PMC. In PMC, paramyotonic stiffness increases over seconds to minutes of continued muscular activity. The exercise-induced worsening of myotonia in PAM usually occurs with a longer delay, often after a period of rest, and may persist for several hours. The other major distinction between PMC and PAM is that attacks of weakness exclude the diagnosis of PAM. An oral potassium challenge results in marked worsening of myotonia in PAM,[58] but provocative testing generally is not advisable because patients may experience severe myotonic stiffness and muscle pain for several hours to a day or longer.

Treatment

Pharmacological therapy for the HyperPP–PMC–PAM spectrum is directed toward ameliorating myotonia or periodic paralysis (Table 225.2). As with chloride-channel-based MC, the preferred drugs for preventing myotonia and paramyotonia in the sodium channel disorders are use-dependent sodium channel blockers. Mexiletine, 200 mg 3 times daily, is effective for both cold- and exercise-induced stiffness in PMC and PAM.[58] Tocainide is also effective, but it is not recommended because of the risk of blood dyscrasias. In some patients, myotonia is not markedly affected by sodium channel blockers. The carbonic anhydrase inhibitor acetazolamide has had a beneficial effect in some cases of PAM,[37] but it may induce weakness in patients with PMC.[59] The use of chronic medication must be tailored to the patient's needs. Patients with the severe myotonia permanens variant of PAM require life-long mexiletine therapy. Some patients with PMC take mexiletine only during the winter months when cold aggravates the myotonia. However, the majority of patients with PAM or PMC do not require pharmacological treatment of myotonia; instead they learn how to avoid exacerbating factors such as cold, vigorous exercise, and potassium-rich foods.

The pharmacological management of periodic paralysis differs from the approaches used to treat myotonia. Despite myotonia and periodic paralysis both being due to gain-of-function defects in SkM1,

use-dependent sodium channel blockers are effective against stiffness but much less effective for preventing weakness, perhaps because weakness results from a loss of channel availability due to voltage-dependent inactivation in the depolarization-induced paralytic state, whereas myotonia is caused by excessive sodium channel activity. Block by mexiletine, which is more potent for depolarized channels, in principle could aggravate weakness.

Carbonic anhydrase inhibitors are the preferred prophylactic agents for periodic paralysis, both HyperPP and HypoPP.[60,61] Acetazolamide treatment should be started at low doses, 125 mg/day, and then gradually increased to 1500 mg/day until a favorable response is obtained. Virtually all patients complain of paresthesias and a distaste for carbonated beverages while receiving acetazolamide treatment. The other major side effect of chronic acetazolamide treatment is the development of renal calculi. In some patients with PMC, acetazolamide may induce attacks of weakness.[62] A more potent carbonic anhydrase inhibitor, dichlorphenamide, has been shown to be more effective than placebo in a double-blind crossover study.[63] The relative efficacy of acetazolamide and dichlorphenamide has not been tested in a controlled trial. The mechanism by which carbonic anhydrase inhibitors prevent periodic paralysis has not been firmly established. One hypothesis is that the mild metabolic acidosis induced by these drugs is protective against depolarization-induced paralysis.[64] The other common prophylactic medication is a thiazide diuretic given to promote kaliuresis.[60,65] Low dosages usually are sufficient (25 mg hydrochlorothiazide daily) and the serum level of potassium should not be decreased below 3.3 mmol/L. Patients learn to reduce the risk of attacks by avoiding exposure to cold or strenuous exercise, "warming down" after exercise, maintaining a low potassium diet, and eating frequent carbohydrate-rich meals.

In most cases, no intervention is required during an attack of weakness in HyperPP or PMC. Patients recover spontaneously over minutes to hours. Often, recovery is hastened by eating carbohydrate-rich foods, drinking carbonated beverages, or exercising lightly. Other patients find that an attack can be aborted with an oral dose of a thiazide diuretic or acetazolamide or by inhalation of a β-adrenergic agonist.[66]

Calcium channel disorders: hypokalemic periodic paralysis

Clinical features

HypoPP is the most common form of dominantly inherited periodic paralysis. The clinical hallmarks of HypoPP are episodic weakness in association with hypokalemia and the absence of myotonia (Table 225.1).[4] Hypokalemia is observed consistently during attacks of weakness in HypoPP, in contrast to the more varied serum levels found in attacks of HyperPP. Symptoms begin around puberty or later, with episodic attacks of weakness that may be mild or cause severe quadriparesis with decreased vital capacity and hypoventilation. Attacks often occur during the night or upon awakening and are precipitated by carbohydrate-rich meals or strenuous activity the preceding day. In comparison with HyperPP, the episodes of weakness in HypoPP are more severe and of longer duration. Persistent interictal weakness may fluctuate slowly over weeks.[61] The episodic attacks diminish in frequency in the third or fourth decade, and a fixed proximal myopathy eventually develops in most patients. Penetrance of the episodic attacks is reduced in females, and some affected women present with late-onset proximal myopathy in the absence of any clinically recognized attacks of paralysis. Life-expectancy is not foreshortened by HypoPP.

Molecular genetics

A molecular defect in HypoPP was first identified by genetic linkage analysis. Using a genome-wide search with polymorphic dinucleotide repeats, Fontaine et al.[12] mapped the HypoPP locus to chromosome 1q21-31.[12] The gene encoding the α subunit of the L-type calcium channel of skeletal muscle, CACNL1A3, had previously been mapped to this region and was screened as a candidate disease gene. Three missense mutations in CACNL1A3 have been identified in families with HypoPP.[13,14] All three involve substitutions at positively charged arginine residues in the proposed voltage-sensing regions of the channel. The incomplete penetrance in females is unique to the Arg-528-His mutation, which occurs in about 50% of families with HypoPP.[67] The Arg-1239-His mutation accounts for most of the other cases of HypoPP in which a genetic defect has been identified, whereas the Arg-1239-Gly mutation has been identified in only one family.[13] On the basis of haplotype analysis of affected families and the occurrence of de novo mutations, the high prevalence of the Arg-528-His and Arg-1239-His mutations does not appear to be due to a founder effect.[67] In about 10% of HypoPP families, the causative mutation is in the Na channel gene, SCN4A. Four mutations have been identified, occurring at one of the two arginines in voltage-sensing regions of the channel.[68]

Pathophysiology and pathogenesis

During an attack of weakness, affected fibers are depolarized and electrically inexcitable because of the normal inactivation of sodium channels. The cause of the aberrant depolarization in the resting potential has not been established. In vitro studies on uncut fibers dissociated from open biopsy specimens have shown that decreasing the potassium concentration to 1 mM depolarizes HypoPP fibers by about 20 mV, whereas the same maneuver causes normal fibers to hyperpolarize by 10 mV.[69] The role of insulin in provoking attacks of weakness is most likely related to promoting a shift of extracellular potassium ions into muscle.[69] Early reports of altered insulin release or responsiveness of peripheral tissues have been disproved by more sensitive in vivo glucose-clamp

studies.[70] Under basal conditions (3.5 mM [K+]) the resting potential of HypoPP fibers is depolarized (−76 mV) compared with normals (−86 mV). The aberrant depolarization is not blocked by tetrodotoxin[69] or nitrendipine,[71] which excludes voltage-dependent sodium or L-type calcium channels as the source of the depolarizing current. Voltage-clamp studies have suggested an abnormally reduced inwardly rectifying potassium current in HypoPP fibers.[71] Patch recordings from fibers carrying the Arg-528–His mutation have demonstrated an impairment of the adenosine triphosphate (ATP)-sensitive potassium channel.[72] The inwardly rectifying potassium current carried by these channels was reduced because of a decrease in the tendency of channels to open in response to high intracellular [Mg-ADP]/[ATP] and because the ability of potassium ions to pass through the open channel was impaired.

Generally, a pathological decrease in the permeability of a cell to potassium results in depolarization of the resting potential, as occurs in HypoPP. For an inwardly rectifying potassium channel, the permeability defect could be compounded by lowering the extracellular potassium concentration. However, the precise mechanism by which HypoPP fibers depolarize while normal ones hyperpolarize in low external potassium concentrations and the pathogenic link between a missense mutation in the L-type calcium channel and the ATP-sensitive potassium channel defect remain to be established. Functional studies of mutant HypoPP calcium channels in heterologous expression systems have demonstrated that all three mutations reduce the calcium current density, slow the rate of channel opening, and enhance the rate of closing.[73–75] The net result is predicted to be a decrease in activity-dependent calcium entry in HypoPP fibers.

The pathomechanism of the late-onset proximal myopathy is even less well understood. The age at onset, rate of progression, and maximal degree of impairment are not well correlated with the frequency or severity of the episodic attacks of weakness,[76] although the relation between periodic paralysis and fixed myopathy is still a source of controversy.[77] Histological studies have shown vacuolated fibers, increased variation in fiber size, and central nuclei.[53] These changes usually are more prominent in HypoPP than in HyperPP and correlate with the clinical severity of the myopathy. Ultrastructural examination has demonstrated a spectrum of pathological changes involving the sarcoplasmic reticulum and T tubules and vacuoles in different stages of evolution arising from lakes of degraded membranous material.

Diagnosis

The diagnosis of HypoPP should be considered whenever episodic attacks of weakness occur in association with hypokalemia. The serum potassium level returns to normal between attacks, and a persistently low potassium concentration suggests a secondary cause of periodic paralysis, such as renal or gastrointestinal potassium wastage. The lack of an autosomal dominant inheritance pattern does not exclude the diagnosis because sporadic cases are well known and females with the Arg-528–His mutation often do not have clinically evident attacks of paralysis. Abnormalities in muscle fiber conduction velocity may help identify asymptomatic patients in a family known to have HypoPP.[78] Most attention in HypoPP has focused on the episodic attacks of paralysis. However, the late-onset myopathy with permanent weakness may be a more consistent feature; the expression of periodic paralysis is more variable.[77] Myotonia is not a feature of HypoPP and, if present, suggests the diagnosis of HyperPP or PMC.

In the differential diagnosis of HypoPP, it is imperative to exclude thyrotoxic periodic paralysis. The two disorders have many clinical similarities.[79] Distinguishing features of the thyrotoxic form include a strong male predominance, nearly 75% of cases occur in Asians, weakness rarely occurs before age 20, laboratory evidence of thyrotoxicosis (either triiodothyroxine [T_3] or thyroxine [free T_4] levels may be increased and decreased thyroid-stimulating [TSH] is the most sensitive test[80]), and symptoms resolve with return of the euthyroid state. In the Japanese population, nearly 2% of patients with hyperthyroidism have at least one episode of periodic paralysis. Despite this ethnic bias, the family history is usually negative and genetic linkage analysis has failed to identify a susceptibility locus.

Laboratory studies can be used to distinguish between HyperPP without myotonia and HypoPP in cases for which the serum concentration of potassium could not be measured during an attack or when the value was equivocal. The simplest approach is to induce an attack by exercise and carbohydrate ingestion. On the first hospital day, the patient exercises vigorously for at least 30 minutes on a treadmill or stationary bicycle and is then fed a high carbohydrate dinner such as pasta. Strength, CMAP amplitude, and the serum concentration of potassium are assessed the next morning. If this simple test fails to provide a definitive diagnosis, provocative testing with glucose loading or glucose plus insulin is performed.[4] Provocative testing must be performed only in an inpatient setting, with monitoring of the serum concentration of potassium and glucose and continuous electrocardiographic monitoring. An oral glucose load of 2 g/kg body weight is given in the morning. In patients with HypoPP, weakness, decreased CMAP amplitude, and hypokalemia usually occur within a few hours. Negative test results do not exclude the diagnosis of HypoPP. Further provocation can be performed with the administration of 10 U of insulin subcutaneously at the time of the oral glucose load. If positive results for HypoPP are still not apparent, the test can be repeated another day with 2 g of glucose per kilogram of body weight given intravenously over 60 minutes in combination with insulin up to 0.1 U/kg at 30 and 60 minutes into the infusion.[81] Even under such demanding conditions, weakness may not develop in some patients with HypoPP.

Thus, a positive test result is more informative than the lack of a response.

A highly reliable, but somewhat invasive, test for HypoPP is intra-arterial epinephrine challenge.[82] This test must be performed in a critical care suite by physicians experienced with intra-arterial catheter placement. Epinephrine is infused into the brachial artery at 2 µg/min for 5 minutes. A decrease in the CMAP amplitude of more than 30% within 10 minutes in the hypothenar or adductor pollicis muscle or a decrease in isometric tension of the adductor pollicis is considered a positive result.

EMG findings are informative only in that the presence of myotonia excludes the diagnosis of HypoPP. Muscle biopsy results may provide supportive evidence in that large central vacuoles are more prominent in HypoPP than in other forms of periodic paralysis, but the presence of vacuoles is not specific for HypoPP.

Treatment

As with other forms of periodic paralysis and myotonia, many patients with HypoPP do not require pharmacological intervention. Patients learn to minimize the occurrence of episodic attacks by avoiding strenuous exercise, consuming fruits or juices high in potassium, and limiting carbohydrate intake.[4] If an attack of weakness occurs, recovery may be hastened by ingesting 20 to 120 mEq of potassium chloride in an unsweetened solution (Table 225.2). Strength usually improves dramatically within an hour. Even large doses of potassium taken orally are usually ineffective at preventing attacks of weakness. Care must be taken to prevent patients from escalating the dosage and becoming psychologically "potassium dependent." Rarely, potassium may be needed to be given intravenously for a severe acute attack. Potassium chloride (50 mEq/L) should be infused at 250 mL/hr in a 5% solution of mannitol because potassium chloride mixed in a 5% solution of glucose has been associated with worsening of muscle strength and failure of the serum concentration of potassium to normalize.[83]

The treatment of HypoPP improved considerably with the discovery that carbonic anhydrase inhibitors decrease the frequency and severity of the episodic attacks of weakness and improve muscle strength between attacks.[61] The most commonly prescribed medication is acetazolamide, starting at 125 mg/day and gradually increasing the dosage as needed to a maximum of 1500 mg/day. As described above for HyperPP, the most common side effect is paresthesias and chronic treatment may lead to the development of renal calculi. Some patients benefit by taking supplemental potassium concurrently with acetazolamide. Drugs that decrease urinary excretion of potassium, such as triamterene (150 mg/day) or the aldosterone antagonist spironolactone (100 mg/day), may also improve symptoms, but they are contraindicated if the patient is taking potassium supplements. Patients with attacks refractory to acetazolamide may benefit from the more potent carbonic anhydrase inhibitor dichlorphenamide, 50 to 300 mg/day.[63] It has not been established whether a reduction in the acute attacks of weakness with carbonic anhydrase inhibitors has any effect on the development of late-onset proximal myopathy in HypoPP.

Additional forms of intervention are still being explored because some attacks are refractory to acetazolamide or the patient cannot tolerate the side effects. A trial of verapamil, a dihydropyridine-type calcium channel blocker, showed no benefit in patients with HypoPP.[84] This finding is consistent with the expression studies that have shown that mutant calcium channels conduct less current than normal.[75] Because membrane inexcitability during an attack of paralysis is due to a pathological depolarization of the resting potential,[69] an alternative treatment strategy has been to use drugs that open potassium channels, thereby repolarizing the membrane.[85] *In vitro* studies of human HypoPP fibers have shown that cromakalim, which promotes opening of the ATP-sensitive potassium channel, is able to repolarize the membrane potential and to restore twitch force.[86] Fiber repolarization is also augmented by pinacidil, another ATP-sensitive potassium channel opener. Diazoxide, which is a more potent opener of ATP-sensitive potassium channels in pancreatic β cells than in skeletal muscle, was initially effective in preventing attacks of weakness in HypoPP, but after a few months of therapy the paralytic episodes returned.[87] The clinical use of these agents has been limited by the side effects of hypotension and hyperglycemia. The cloning of ATP-sensitive potassium channels and the discovery of distinct isoforms in skeletal muscle, smooth muscle, and pancreas offer the possibility for developing drugs that act selectively on the skeletal muscle ATP-sensitive potassium channel.[85] If found, these agents likely will prove beneficial in the prophylactic management of paralytic attacks in both HypoPP and HyperPP and in suppressing myotonia arising from sodium or chloride channel defects.[88]

References

1. Ashcroft FM. Ion Channels and Disease: Channelopathies. San Diego: Academic Press, 2000
2. Lehmann-Horn F, Jurkat-Rott K. Voltage-gated ion channels and hereditary disease. Physiol Rev, 1999;79: 1317–1372
3. Rüdel R, Lehmann-Horn F, Ricker K. The nondystrophic myotonias. *In:* Engel AG, Franzini-Armstrong C, eds. Myology: Basic and Clinical. 2nd ed. Vol. 2. New York: McGraw-Hill, 1994:1291–1302
4. Lehmann-Horn F, Engel AG, Ricker K, Rüdel R. The periodic paralyses and paramyotonia congenita. *In:* Engel AG, Franzini-Armstrong C, eds. Myology: Basic and Clinical. 2nd ed. Vol. 2. New York: McGraw-Hill, 1994:1303–1334
5. Cannon SC. Ion channel defects in the hereditary myotonias and periodic paralyses. *In:* Martin JB, ed. Molecular Neurology. New York: Scientific American, 1998:257–277
6. Thomsen J. Tonische Krämpfe in willkürlich beweglichen Muskeln in Folge von ererbter psychischer Disposition. Arch Psychiatr Nervenkr 1876;6:702–718
7. Becker P. Zur Frage der Heterogenie der erblichen

Myotonien. Nervenarzt 1957;28:455–460
8. Tyler FH, Stephens FE, Gunn FD, Perkoff GT. Studies in disorders of muscle. VII. Clinical manifestations and inheritance of a type of periodic paralysis without hypopotassemia. J Clin Invest 1951;30:492–502
9. Eulenberg A. Über eine familiäre, durch 6 Generationen verfolgbare Form congenitaler Paramyotonie. Neurol Zentralkl 1886;5:265–272
10. Lerche, H, Heine R, Pika U, et al. Human sodium channel myotonia: slowed channel inactivation due to substitutions for a glycine within the III–IV linker. J Physiol 1993;470:13–22
11. Koch MC, Steinmeyer K, Lorenz C, et al. The skeletal muscle chloride channel in dominant and recessive human myotonia. Science 1992;257:797–800
12. Fontaine B, Vale-Santos J, Jurkat-Rott K, et al. Mapping of the hypokalaemic periodic paralysis (HypoPP) locus to chromosome 1q31-32 in three European families. Nature Genetics 1994;6:267–272
13. Ptacek LJ, Tawil R, Griggs RC, et al. Dihydropyridine receptor mutations cause hypokalemic periodic paralysis. Cell 1994:77:863–868
14. Jurkat-Rott K, Lehmann-Horn F, Elbaz A, et al. A calcium channel mutation causing hypokalemic periodic paralysis. Hum Mol Gen 1994;3:1415–1419
15. Koch MC, Ricker K, Otto M, et al. Linkage data suggesting allelic heterogeneity for paramyotonia congenita and hyperkalemic periodic paralysis on chromosome 17. Hum Genet 1991;88:71–74
16. Fontaine B, Khurana TS, Hoffman EP, et al. Hyperkalemic periodic paralysis and the adult muscle sodium channel alpha-subunit gene. Science 1990;250:1000–1002
17. Deymeer F, Cakirkaya S, Serdaroglu P, et al. Transient weakness and compound muscle action potential decrement in myotonia congenita. Muscle Nerve 1998; 21:1334–1337
18. Lorenz C, Meyer-Kleine C, Steinmeyer K, et al. Genomic organization of the human muscle chloride channel ClC-1 and analysis of novel mutations leading to Becker-type myotonia. Hum Mol Genet 1994;3: 941–946
19. Steinmeyer K, Lorenz C, Pusch M, et al. Multimeric structure of ClC-1 chloride channel revealed by mutations in dominant myotonia congenita (Thomsen). EMBO J 1994;13:737–743
20. Bryant SH, Morales-Aguilera A. Chloride conductance in normal and myotonic muscle fibres and the action of monocarboxylic acids. J Physiol 1971;219:367–383
21. Bryant SH. Cable properties of external intercostal muscle fibres from myotonic and nonmyotonic goats. J Physiol 1969;204:539–550
22. Lipicky RJ, Bryant SH, Salmon JH. Cable parameters, sodium, potassium, chloride, and water content, and potassium efflux in isolated external intercostal muscle of normal volunteers and patients with myotonia congenita. J Clin Invest 1971;50:2091–2103
23. Winer N, Martt JM, Somers JE, et al. Induced myotonia in man and goat. J Lab Clin Med 1965;66:758–769
24. Kwiecinski H, Lehmann-Horn F, Rüdel R. Drug-induced myotonia in human intercostal muscle. Muscle Nerve 1988;11:576–581
25. Adrian RH, Bryant SH. On the repetitive discharge in myotonic muscle fibres. J Physiol 1974;240:505–515
26. Furman RE, Barchi RL. The pathophysiology of myotonia produced by aromatic carboxylic acids. Ann Neurol 1978;4:357–365
27. Jentsch TJ, Friedrich T, Schriever A, Yamada H. The ClC chloride channel family. Pflugers Arch 1999;437: 783–795

28. Pusch M, Steinmeyer K, Koch MC, Jentsch TJ. Mutations in dominant human myotonia congenita drastically alter the voltage dependence of the ClC-1 chloride channel. Neuron 1995;15:1455–1463

29. Deymeer F, Lehmann-Horn F, Serdaroglu P, et al. Electrical myotonia in heterozygous carriers of recessive myotonia congenita. Muscle Nerve 1999;22:123–125

30. Brook JD, McCurrach ME, Harley HG, et al. Molecular basis of myotonic dystrophy: expansion of a trinucleotide (CTG) repeat located at the 3′ end of a transcript encoding a protein kinase family member. Cell 1992;68:799–808

31. Ricker K, Koch MC, Lehmann-Horn F, et al. Proximal myotonic myopathy: a new dominant disorder with myotonia, muscle weakness, and cataracts. Neurology 1994;44:1448–1452

32. Liquori CL, Ricker K, Moseley ML, Jacobsen JF, Kress W, Naylor SL, Day JW, Ranum L. Myotonic dystrophy type 2 caused by a CCTG expansion in intron 1 of ZNF9. Science 2001;293:864–867.

33. Bryant SH, Conte-Camerino D. Chloride channel regulation in the skeletal muscle of normal and myotonic goats. Pflugers Arch 1991;417:605–610

34. Birnberger KL, Rüdel R, Struppler A. Clinical and electrophysiological observations in patients with myotonic muscle disease and the therapeutic effect of N-propyl-ajmalin. J Neurol 1975;210:99–110

35. Ricker K, Lehmann-Horn F, Moxley RT III. Myotonia fluctuans. Arch Neurol 1990;47:268–272

36. Rosenfeld J, Sloan-Brown K, George AL Jr. A novel muscle sodium channel mutation causes painful congenital myotonia. Ann Neurol 1997;42:811–814

37. Ptacek LJ, Tawil R, Griggs RC, et al. Sodium channel mutations in acetazolamide-responsive myotonia congenita, paramyotonia congenita, and hyperkalemic periodic paralysis. Neurology 1994;44:1500–1503

38. Bulman DE, Scoggan KA van Oene MD, et al. A novel sodium channel mutation in a family with hypokalemic periodic paralysis. Neurology 1999;53: 1932–1936

39. Lehmann-Horn F, Rüdel R, Dengler R, et al. Membrane defects in paramyotonia congenita with and without myotonia in a warm environment. Muscle Nerve 1981;4:396–406

40. Lehmann-Horn F, Rüdel R, Ricker K, et al. Two cases of adynamia episodica hereditaria: in vitro investigation of muscle cell membrane and contraction parameters. Muscle Nerve 1983;6:113–121

41. Ebers GC, George AL, Barchi RL, et al. Paramyotonia congenita and hyperkalemic periodic paralysis are linked to the adult muscle sodium channel gene. Ann Neurol 1991;30:810–816

42. McClatchey AI, Lin CS, Wang J, et al. The genomic structure of the human skeletal muscle sodium channel gene. Hum Mol Genet 1992;1:521–527

43. George AL Jr, Komisarof J, Kallen RG, Barchi RL. Primary structure of the adult human skeletal muscle voltage-dependent sodium channel. Ann Neurol 1992;31:131–137

44. Wallace RH, Wang DW, Singh R, et al. Febrile seizures and generalized epilepsy associated with a mutation in the Na$^+$-channel beta$_1$ subunit gene SCN1B. Nat Genet 1998;19:366–370

45. Cannon SC. Spectrum of sodium channel disturbances in the nondystrophic myotonias and periodic paralyses. Kidney Int 2000;57:772–779

46. Rüdel R, Ricker K, Lehmann-Horn F. Genotype-phenotype correlations in human skeletal muscle sodium channel diseases. Arch Neurol 1993;50:1241–1248

47. Plassart E, Reboul J, Rime CS, et al. Mutations in the muscle sodium channel gene (SCN4A) in 13 French families with hyperkalemic periodic paralysis and paramyotonia congenita: phenotype to genotype correlations and demonstration of the predominance of two mutations. Eur J Hum Genet 1994;2:110–124

48. Cannon SC, Corey DP. Loss of Na$^+$ channel inactivation by anemone toxin (ATX II) mimics the myotonic state in hyperkalaemic periodic paralysis. J Physiol 1993;466:501–520

49. Cannon SC, Brown RH Jr, Corey DP. Theoretical reconstruction of myotonia and paralysis caused by incomplete inactivation of sodium channels. Biophys J 1993;65:270–288

50. Ruff RL. Slow Na$^+$ channel inactivation must be disrupted to evoke prolonged depolarization-induced paralysis. Biophys J 1994;66:542–545

51. Cummins TR, Sigworth FJ. Impaired slow inactivation in mutant sodium channels. Biophys J 1996;71:227–236

52. Hayward LJ, Sandoval GM, Cannon SC. Defective slow inactivation of sodium channels contributes to familial periodic paralysis. Neurology 1999;52:1447–1453

53. Engel AG. Hypokalemic and hyperkalemic periodic paralyses. In: Goldensohn ES, Apfel SH, eds. Scientific Approaches to Clinical Neurology. Philadelphia: Lea & Febiger, 1977:1742–1765

54. McManis PG, Lambert EH, Daube JR. The exercise test in periodic paralysis. Muscle Nerve 1986;9:704–710

55. Ricker K, Camacho LM, Grafe P, et al. Adynamia episodica hereditaria: what causes the weakness? Muscle Nerve 1989;12:883–891

56. Streib EW. Differential diagnosis of myotonic syndromes. Muscle Nerve 1987;10:603–615

57. Subramony SH, Malhotra CP, Mishra SK. Distinguishing paramyotonia congenita and myotonia congenita by electromyography. Muscle Nerve 1983;6:374–379

58. Ricker K, Moxley RT III, Heine R, Lehmann-Horn F. Myotonia fluctuans. A third type of muscle sodium channel disease. Arch Neurol 1994;51:1095–1102

59. Riggs JE. The periodic paralyses. Neurol Clin 1988;6:485–498

60. McArdle B. Adynamia episodica hereditaria and its treatment. Brain 1962;85:121–148

61. Griggs RC, Engel WK, Resnick JS. Acetazolamide treatment of hypokalemic periodic paralysis. Prevention of attacks and improvement of persistent weakness. Ann Intern Med 1970;73:39–48

62. Riggs JE, Griggs RC, Moxley RT III. Acetazolamide-induced weakness in paramyotonia congenita. Ann Intern Med 1977;86:169–173

63. Tawil R, McDermott MP, Brown R Jr, et al. Randomized trials of dichlorphenamide in the periodic paralyses. Working Group on Periodic Paralysis. Ann Neurol 2000;47:46–53

64. Lehmann-Horn F, Kuther G, Ricker F, et al. Adynamia episodica hereditaria with myotonia: a non-inactivating sodium current and the effect of extracellular pH. Muscle Nerve 1987;10:363–374

65. Ricker K, Bohlen R, Rohkamm R. Different effectiveness of tocainide and hydrochlorothiazide in paramyotonia congenita with hyperkalemic episodic paralysis. Neurology 1983;33:1615–1618

66. Wang P. Clausen T. Treatment of attacks in hyperkalaemic familial periodic paralysis by inhalation of salbutamol. Lancet 1976;1:221–223

67. Elbaz A, Vale-Santos J, Jurkat-Rott K, et al. Hypokalemic periodic paralysis and the dihydropyridine

receptor (CACNL1A3): genotype/phenotype correlations for two predominant mutations and evidence for the absence of a founder effect in 16 Caucasian families. Am J Hum Genet 1995;56:374–380

68. Sternberg D, Maisonobe T, Jurkat-Rott K, Nicole S, Launay E, Chauveau D, Tabti N, Lehmann-Horn F, Hainque B, Fontaine B. Hypokalaemic periodic paralysis type 2 caused by mutations at codon 672 in the muscle sodium channel gene SCN4A. Brain 2001;124:1091–1099.

69. Rüdel R, Lehmann-Horn K, Ricker K, Kuther G. Hypokalemic periodic paralysis: in vitro investigation of muscle fiber membrane parameters. Muscle Nerve 1984;7:110–120

70. Ligtenberg JJ, Van Haeften TW, Van Der Kolk Le, et al. Normal insulin release during sustained hyperglycaemia in hypokalaemic periodic paralysis: role of the potassium channel opener pinacidil in impaired muscle strength. Clin Sci (Lond), 1996;91:583–589

71. Ruff RL. Insulin acts in hypokalemic periodic paralysis by reducing inward rectifier K^+ current. Neurology 1999;53:1556–1563

72. Tricarico D, Servedei S, Tonali P, et al. Impairment of skeletal muscle adenosine triphosphate-sensitive K^+ channels in patients with hypokalemic periodic paralysis. J Clin Invest 1999;103:675–682

73. Lapie P, Goudet C, Nargeot J, et al. Electrophysiological properties of the hypokalaemic periodic paralysis mutation (R528H) of the skeletal muscle alpha 1s subunit as expressed in mouse L cells. FEBS Lett 1996;382:244–248

74. Jurkat-Rott K, Uetz U, Pika-Hartlaub U, et al. Calcium currents and transients of native and heterologously expressed mutant skeletal muscle DHP receptor alpha1 subunits (R528H). FEBS Lett 1998;423:198–204

75. Morrill JA, Cannon SC. Effects of mutations causing hypokalaemic periodic paralysis on the skeletal muscle L-type Ca^{2+} channel expressed in *Xenopus laevis* oocytes. J Physiol (Lond) 1999;520(2):321–336

76. Buruma OJ, Bots GT. Myopathy in familial hypokalaemic periodic paralysis independent of paralytic attacks. Acta Neurol Scand 1978;57:171–179

77. Links TP, Zwarts MJ, Wilmink JT, et al. Permanent muscle weakness in familial hypokalaemic periodic paralysis. Clinical, radiological and pathological aspects. Brain 1990;113:1873–1889

78. Zwarts MJ, van Weerden TW, Links TP, et al. The muscle fiber conduction velocity and power spectra in familial hypokalemic periodic paralysis. Muscle Nerve 1988;11:166–173

79. Engel AG. Thyroid function and periodic paralysis. Am J Med 1961;30:327–333

80. Griggs RC, Bender AN, Tawil R. A puzzling case of periodic paralysis. Muscle Nerve 1996;19:362–364

81. Riggs JE, Griggs RC. Diagnosis and treatment of the periodic paralyses. Clin. Neuropharmacol 1979;4:123–138

82. Engel AG, Lambert EH, Rosevear JW, Tauxe WN. Clinical and electromyographic studies in a patient with primary hypokalemic periodic paralysis. Am J Med 1965;38:626–640

83. Griggs RC, Resnick J, Engel WK. Intravenous treatment of hypokalemic periodic paralysis. Arch Neurol 1983;40:539–540

84. Links TP, Arnoldus EP, Wintzen AR, et al. The calcium channel blocker verapamil in hypokalemic periodic paralysis [letter]. Muscle Nerve 1998;21:1564–1565

85. Lawson K. Potassium channel openers as potential therapeutic weapons in ion channel disease. Kidney Int 2000;57:838–845

86. Grafe P, Quasthoff F, Strupp M, Lehmann-Horn F. Enhancement of K^+ conductance improves in vitro the contraction force of skeletal muscle in hypokalemic periodic paralysis. Muscle Nerve 1990;13:451–457

87. Johnsen T. Trial of the prophylactic effect of diazoxide in the treatment of familial periodic hypokalemia. Acta Neurol Scand 1977;56:525–532

88. Quasthoff S, Spuler A, Spittelmeister W, et al. K^+ channel openers suppress myotonic activity of human skeletal muscle in vitro. Eur J Pharmacol 1990;186:125–128

Myasthenia Gravis and Myasthenic Syndromes

Andrew G Engel

Historical overview

Thomas Willis is credited with the first clinical description of myasthenia gravis (MG). In 1672, he described a patient with weakness of limb muscles that became worse during the day and was associated with weakness of the tongue provoked by "long, hasty, or laborious speaking." During the last quarter of the 19th century, Wilks, Erb, Goldflam, and Jolly described the major clinical features of MG. In 1895, Jolly also reported progressive decrease in the strength of tetanically stimulated muscles that recovered with rest and suggested treatment of MG with physostigmine. In 1900, Campbell and Bramwell emphasized that disease especially involved the most constantly used muscles and the symptoms fluctuated. In 1901, Laquer and Weigert detected thymoma in a patient with MG, and in 1905, Buzzard described lymphoid hyperplasia of the myasthenic thymus. In 1940, Blalock noted that thymectomy is beneficial in MG. In 1934, Walker noted the similarity of curare poisoning to MG and again suggested physostigmine for therapy for MG. Neostigmine has been used since 1935 to treat MG; pyridostigmine became available two decades later.

An autoimmune etiology of MG was first proposed by Simpson.[1] In 1973, Patrick and Lindstrom[2] reported myasthenic symptoms in rabbits immunized with eel acetycholine receptor (AChR). In the same year, Fambrough et al.[3] showed a reduced amount of AChR at the MG end plate (EP). By 1977, the autoimmune origin of the disease was firmly established by animal models of AChR-induced MG,[4] demonstration of anti-AChR antibodies in nearly 90% of MG patients,[5] passive transfer of MG from human to mouse,[6] and localization of IgG and complement at the MG EP.[7] These findings provided a rational basis for immunotherapy of MG with plasmapheresis,[8] prednisone,[9] and intravenous immunoglobulin (IVIG).[10]

Epidemiology

Recent estimates of the annual incidence of MG range from 6 to 11 per million.[11–13] Estimates of prevalence range from 118 to 150 per million.[11,13] The female incidence peaks in the third decade and the male incidence in the sixth or seventh decade of life.[14] Grob[15] has estimated that mortality of MG fell tenfold in the past century and threefold since 1960. A recent estimate of the death rate of MG is ~1 per million per year.[13]

Etiology

In most patients with MG, the disease stems from an autoimmune response against AChR. Consistent with this, 80% to 90% of MG patients have circulating antibodies against AChR.[5,16] A recent report that 17 of 24 MG patients without anti-AChR antibodies have a significant titer of antibodies against MuSK, a muscle-specific tyrosine kinase that has a role in the aggregation of AChR at the EP, implies that MG can also arise from an autoimmune response against MuSK.[17]

Pathophysiology and pathogenesis

The basic event that breaks tolerance to self-AChR remains unknown, but three predisposing conditions are now well established: treatment with penicillamine,[18] treatment with α- or β-interferon,[19,20] and bone marrow transplantation.[21] As in other autoimmune diseases, the afferent limb of the immune response involves presentation of processed antigen (peptide fragments of AChR) by histocompatibility complex (HLA) class II-positive antigen-presenting cells to specific autoreactive CD4$^+$ T helper cells, which in turn stimulate production by B cells and plasma cells of antibodies that recognize specific epitopes of AChR. The thymus gland is likely involved in autoimmunity to MG for the following reasons: it contains epithelial cells (known as myoid cells) that express AChR; the myasthenic thymus harbors lymph nodes with germinal centers that contain AchR-specific B cells that secrete anti-AChR antibodies; the gland is hyperplastic in ~70% of patients and harbors epithelial tumors in ~15% of patients.[22] These findings suggest that a thymic abnormality could result in recognition of self-AChR components as nonself and thereby trigger the afferent limb of the immune response.

The efferent limb of the autoimmune response is mediated by anti-AChR antibodies that decrease the number of EP AChRs by antibody-dependent complement-mediated lysis of the junctional folds,[23,24] accelerated internalization and destruction AChRs (antigenic modulation),[25] and blocking of the binding of acetylcholine (ACh) to AChR.[26,27] The AChR deficiency decreases the amplitude of the miniature EP potential (MEPP) and hence that of the EP potential (EPP), which in turn reduces the safety margin of neuromuscular transmission.

The basic event that breaks tolerance to self-MuSK is also unknown. Anti-MuSK antibodies inhibit agrin-induced clustering of extrajunctional AChRs

Table 226.1   Clinical features of autoimmune myasthenia gravis

Abnormal weakness and fatigability of some or all voluntary muscles
Weakness increases with repeated or sustained exertion and in the course of the day
Menses, viral or other infections, and emotional upsets can worsen the symptoms
Symptoms respond to anticholinesterase drugs
External ocular muscles are affected initially in ~50% of patients and eventually in ~90%
Voluntary muscles innervated by cranial nerves (facial, masticatory, lingual, pharyngeal, and laryngeal muscles) and cervical, pectoral girdle, and hip flexor muscles are also frequently affected; proximal limb muscles usually are affected more severely than distal ones
Brisk or normally active tendon reflexes that may diminish if repeatedly elicited; reflexes can be absent from muscles that cannot be activated by voluntary effort
No objective sensory deficits
Symptoms can fluctuate from day to day, week to week, or over longer periods of time
Spontaneous remissions lasting for varying periods; long and complete remissions are rare; most spontaneous remissions occur during the first 3 years of the disease
In patients with progression from mild to more severe disease, the weakness tends to spread from ocular to facial to lower bulbar muscles and then to truncal and limb muscles. However, this sequence may vary and different muscles may be affected either together or in succession
The disease is initially ocular in ~40% of patients but remains confined to the ocular muscles in only ~15%. Close to 90% of the generalizations occur within 13 months after onset
Thymic lymphofollicular hyperplasia occurs in ~70% of patients and thymoma in ~15%
Association with other autoimmune disease(s) in ~25% of patients

expressed by myotubes;[17] this suggests that they also decrease the density of AChRs at the EP. Studies of MuSK-antibody-positive MG, however, are still incomplete: the number of AChRs per EP has not been determined, no immune deposits have been demonstrated at the EP, EP fine structure has not been analyzed, and electrophysiological studies of patient EPs have not been performed. Thus, the pathogenesis MuSK-antibody-positive MG is less well understood than that of AChR-antibody-positive MG.

The pathogenesis of MG in patients with neither anti-AChR nor anti-MuSK antibodies is unclear. Some seronegative patients with ocular MG test positively for AChR antibodies when their disease becomes generalized;[16] other seronegative patients may have a genetically determined congenital myasthenic syndrome.

Genetics

Autoimmune MG is an acquired disease, but susceptibility to develop MG depends on AChR epitope presentation to particular major HLA proteins whose expression on immune cells is genetically determined. This is reflected in the higher incidence of HLA-A1, -B8, and -DR3 determinants in young Caucasian MG patients and of different HLA determinants in other age and racial groups. Involvement of the AChR α subunit gene in susceptibility to MG has also been proposed.[28] Other susceptibility genes in MG include those encoding cytotoxic lymphocyte-associated antigen, interleukin-1β, interleukin-1 receptor antagonist, and tumor necrosis factor α and β (reviewed in [29]). There are few reports of MG in adults in a familial setting[30] or transmission of seropositive MG by recessive[31] or dominant[29,32] inheritance. No defined candidate gene loci could be identified in these families.

Clinical features

MG can occur as an acquired disease after infancy or in a transient neonatal form. The clinical features of acquired MG are summarized in Table 226.1.

Transient neonatal MG occurs in 10% to 20% of infants born to myasthenic women[33] and is due to transplacental transfer of anti-AChR antibodies from mother to fetus. Symptoms consisting of feeding and respiratory difficulty, ptosis, feeble cry, and facial or generalized weakness appear in the first few hours after birth and last a mean duration of 18 days.[33] Some infants whose mothers carry antibodies with specificities against fetal AChR that contains the γ instead of the ε subunit are born with arthrogryposis as well as myasthenic symptoms.[34]

Classification

The classification of MG based on clinical status proposed by Osserman and Genkins in 1971[14] is still useful: group 1, ocular; group 2A, mild generalized; group 2B, moderately severe generalized; group 3, acute fulminating; and group 4, late severe.

Diagnosis

The diagnosis of MG is based on the clinical history, physical findings, pharmacological tests (see section on Edrophonium below), electromyographic (EMG) investigations (conventional needle EMG, study of the decremental response, and, in some cases, single fiber recordings), and tests for anti-AChR antibodies that bind, modulate, or block AChR. Tests for modulating and blocking antibodies are needed only when the test for binding antibodies is negative. A typical history is one of acquired weakness and fatigability increased by exertion and have generalized disease which also involves the external ocular muscles, a positive anticholinesterase (AchE) drug test, and a decremental

Table 226.2 Differential diagnosis of autoimmune myasthenia gravis	
Disorder	Diagnostic clues (in addition to absence of anti-AChR antibodies)
Neurasthenia	Giving way on muscle testing, negative pharmacological tests, no EMG decrement
Oculopharyngeal muscular dystrophy	Nonfluctuating symptoms, no diplopia, no EMG decrement, muscle biopsy findings, molecular genetic tests
Mitochondrial myopathy	Diplopia unusual, lactacidemia, multisystem features, muscle biopsy findings, no EMG decrement
Intracranial compressive lesion	Initially only one cranial nerve involved, no EMG decrement, MRI
Lambert-Eaton syndrome	Cranial nerves tend to be spared, hyporeflexia, autonomic symptoms, characteristic EMG findings, association with lung cancer or other malignancies in a high proportion of cases
Congenital myasthenic syndromes	Onset in infancy in most, similarly affected relatives, specific EMG findings in some syndromes, intracellular microelectrode and morphological studies of EP, genetic analysis
Organophosphate intoxication	History of exposure, CNS symptoms, low serum butyrylcholinesterase level; repetitive CMAPs on EMG
Botulism	In infants: constipation, hypotonia, multiple cranial nerve palsies, descending weakness. Detection of toxin in feces
	In adults: prodromal gastrointestinal symptoms, dry painful throat, blurred vision, cycloplegia, dilated pupil, early cranial nerve involvement and then descending weakness, detection of toxin in serum or feces
Miller-Fisher syndrome	Ataxia, altered reflexes, cerebrospinal fluid examination
Guillain-Barré syndrome	Loss of reflexes, sensory symptoms, cerebrospinal fluid examination, nerve conduction studies
Periodic paralysis	Cranial muscles spared, potassium levels, reflexes lost during attacks, often family history

AChR, acetylcholine receptor; CMAP, compound muscle fiber action potential; CNS, central nervous system; EMG, electromyogram; EP, end plate; MRI, magnetic resonance imaging.

EMG response are usually sufficient to confirm the diagnosis. A positive test for AChR antibodies supports the diagnosis, but a negative test does not exclude it. In a large study, the test was positive in 100% of adults with moderately severe or severe MG, in 80% with mild generalized MG, in 50% with ocular MG, and in 25% of those in remission.[35] Other studies have shown seropositivity in up to 80% of patients with ocular MG.[16] There are also patients who have congenital symptoms, or no involvement of the external ocular muscles, or symptoms that are confined to the external ocular muscles and do not fluctuate, or atypical associated neurological findings, or a history compatible with MG but no weakness on examination. Such patients may or may not have a decremental EMG response or a positive AChE drug response and may or may not have MG. In these patients, determination of the anti-AChR antibody titer is especially helpful. If negative, then more specialized electrophysiological and morphological studies of the EP are required to confirm or to exclude the diagnosis of MG (see section below on the diagnosis of congenital myasthenic syndromes). For a detailed discussion of the relative usefulness of the different diagnostic tests, the reader is referred to a recent review by Seybold.[16]

Striated muscle antibodies that recognize myosin, actin, titin, and the calcium release channel of the sarcoplasmic reticulum also occur in MG patients. Their role in the disease remains unknown, but they are a sensitive marker for thymoma in younger patients. These antibodies were present in 84% of patients with thymoma. In patients without thymoma, they were present in 5% with onset before age 40 and in 47% with onset after age 40.[36]

Once the diagnosis of MG is established, all patients should have computed tomography (CT) of the chest for detection of thymoma or to document thymic enlargement.

Differential diagnosis

The differential diagnosis of autoimmune MG and clues that help to differentiate other disorders from MG are listed in Table 226.2.

Treatment

AChE drugs, which increase the synaptic response to ACh, and manipulation of the immune response by alternate-day prednisone therapy, immunosuppressants other than prednisone, plasmapheresis, and IVIG are currently acceptable forms of therapy for MG. There is general agreement on four principles of therapy.

Table 226.3   Equivalent dosages, routes of administration, and duration of action of anti-AChE drugs

Drug	Single dose in adults (single dose in children)			Onset	Usual duration
	Oral	Intravenous	Intramuscular of subcutaneous		
Pyridostigmine bromide (Mestinon)	60–90 mg* (1–2 mg/kg)†,‡	2 mg	2 mg (0.05–0.15 mg/kg)	10–45 min	3–6 hr
Slow-release pyridostigmine bromide (Mestinon Timespan)	90–180 mg	—	—	1 hr	6–10 hr
Neostigmine bromide	15 mg (0.5 mg/kg)	—	—	—	2–3 hr
Neostigmine methylsulfate	—	0.5 mg	0.5–1.5 mg (0.01–0.04 mg/kg)	<10–30 min	1–2 hr
Ambenonium chloride (Mytelase)	10 mg	—	—	60 min	6–8 hr

AChE, acetylcholinesterase.
*Total daily dose in adults should not exceed 600 mg.
†Total daily dose in children should not exceed 7 mg/kg.
‡Available as syrup, 12 mg/ml, for pediatric use.

1. Anti-AChE drugs are first-line agents for treating all forms of MG.
2. Anti-AChE drugs are the mainstay of therapy for ocular MG.
3. Plasmapheresis and IVIG have only transient effects and do not confer greater long-term protection than immunosuppressants alone.
4. Thymoma is an absolute indication for thymectomy.

Despite these principles, there are no universally accepted criteria for the timing, sequence, or combination of thymectomy, prednisone, and other immunosuppressants in the management of different grades of MG. Adequately controlled clinical trials in MG were carried out in only a few instances. These pertained to the use of cyclosporine,[37] prednisone with or without azathioprine,[38] prednisone vs. azathioprine,[39] and pulsed intravenous methylprednisolone.[40] However, the relative risks and benefits of the various modalities of treatment are reasonably well defined and allow rational management of most patients. Recent excellent reviews describe the pros and cons of different therapeutic modalities in MG and suggest useful approaches to managing patients with different grades of disease.[41,42]

Anti-AChE drugs[43]

Anti-AChE medications provide symptomatic relief without suppressing the underlying immune process that causes and perpetuates MG. Moreover, because of their side effects, doses employable in clinical practice mitigate rather than eliminate the myasthenic symptoms. Patients who require more than recommended doses for adequate relief of their symptoms are candidates for other modalities of treatment. Recommended dosages, routes of administration, and duration of action of currently used anti-AChE drugs are summarized in Table 226.3.

Anti-AChE drugs act by increasing the lifetime of ACh in the synaptic space; this increases the number of AChRs reached by ACh and allows individual ACh molecules to bind to AChRs repeatedly. These effects enhance the synaptic response to ACh and, hence, the safety margin of neuromuscular transmission.

Side effects of anti-AChE drugs result from parasympathetic overactivity, indicated by increased tearing, salivation, and bronchial secretions; enhanced gastrointestinal tract motility with diarrhea and abdominal cramps; meiosis; bradycardia; and hypotension. Rare patients carrying a polymorphism in the promoter region of the gene that encodes the catalytic subunit of AChE show acute exaggerated sensitivity to conventional doses of anti-AChE medications.[44] The side effects can be mitigated by concurrently administered oral or subcutaneous doses of atropine, 0.5 to 1 mg in adults and 0.01 mg/kg in children, or by glycopyrrolate (Robinul), 1 to 2 mg for adults and 0.04 to 0.1 mg/kg for children. Patients with persistent diarrhea can be treated with 5 mg diphenoxylate (Lomotil) once or twice daily.[41]

Higher than recommended doses of anti-AChE drugs can result in desensitization of AChRs, producing increasing weakness and, ultimately, a cholinergic crisis. Moreover, there is experimental evidence that long-term high-dose exposure to anti-AChE drugs causes degeneration of the junctional folds, loss of postsynaptic AChRs, and decreased MEPP amplitude.[45] These alterations are similar to those caused by MG itself.

Pyridostigmine bromide is generally preferred to the shorter acting neostigmine bromide. Pyridostigmine is available in 60-mg tablets, in 180-mg slow-release ("timespan") tablets, and as a syrup containing 12 mg of the medication per milliliter. The drug acts within 45 minutes, and its effects last from 3 to 6 hours. It is less likely to cause muscarinic side effects and may be more effective in controlling bulbar weakness than neostigmine.[46] The dose in adults may range from 30 mg taken every 6 hours to 90 mg taken every 3 hours. The timespan preparation is taken at bedtime because its effects last through the night. The syrup is useful in children and patients requiring nasogastric feeding. The total daily dose should not exceed 600 mg daily in adults and 7 mg/kg daily in children. Pyridostigmine bromide is also available for intramuscular or intravenous administration in the form in 2-mL ampules, with each milliliter containing 5 mg of the drug. Approximately 1/30th of the oral dose of the drug may be given parenterally for an equivalent effect. Parenteral administration of the drug is useful postoperatively or in other situations when patients cannot take medications orally.

Neostigmine bromide (Prostigmin) is available in 15-mg tablets, and one tablet is equivalent to a 60-mg tablet of pyridostigmine bromide. Orally administered neostigmine acts within 30 minutes and its effects last for 2 to 3 hours. In adults, the dose may range from 7.5 to 30 mg taken every 3 to 4 hours. In infants and children, the recommended dose is 2 mg/kg daily. Muscarinic side effects, especially abdominal cramps and diarrhea, are mitigated by concurrent administration of atropine or glycopyrrolate. Neostigmine methylsulfate is administered intramuscularly or intravenously, and 1 mg of the parenterally administered drug is equivalent to 15 mg of the oral medication. For children, the recommended parenteral dose is 0.01 to 0.04 mg/kg every 2 to 3 hours. Intranasal therapy with 9 to 14 mg of neostigmine methylsulfate is also effective.[47]

Ambenonium chloride is available in 10-mg tablets. It is seldom used because of its long duration of action and greater tendency to accumulate. However, it is the anti-AChE medication of choice for patients who develop sensitivity to the bromide ion.

Edrophonium chloride (Tensilon) is used intravenously as an adjunct to diagnosis, but not for treatment, of MG. The drug acts in 1 to 3 minutes, and its effects last for 5 to 10 minutes. In adults, 2 mg is injected over 20 seconds. If no response occurs after 45 seconds, an additional 8 mg is given. Atropine should be available for parenteral administration for the rare case in which edrophonium causes severe bradycardia, cardiac arrhythmia, or hypotension. For children who weigh less than 34 kg, the maximal dose of edrophonium is 1 mg; and for those weighing more than 34 kg, the dose should be limited to 2 mg. For details concerning the usefulness and evaluation of the edrophonium test, the reader is referred to reference 16.

In using anti-AChE drugs, the physician needs to determine the optimal dose and interdose interval for each patient. Once this is established and after patients fully understand the potential side effects of the medication, they are encouraged to adjust the dose and interdose intervals without exceeding the maximal recommended daily dose, so that the regimen is appropriately tailored to the their level of activity.

Corticosteroid therapy

Alternate-day prednisone therapy is a relatively safe and reliable form of treatment of MG.[48,49] It is indicated for disabling disease not responding adequately to anti-AChE drugs.[50] The medication is more effective in patients with disease onset after the age of 40 than in younger patients.[50]

Prednisone may affect MG by altering the functional properties of T cells and macrophages or the secretion of cytokines and other immune mediators.[51] Corticosteroids also stimulate the synthesis of junctional AChRs in innervated cultured human muscle;[52] therefore, they could increase the synthesis of AChRs at the EP in vivo. That the drug modifies the immune response to AChR is evidenced by decrease of the AChR antibody titer in patients responding to therapy.[53,54]

Various treatment regimens have been advocated, but no consensus has emerged on optimal therapy for patients with different grades of MG. Because high initial doses of corticosteroids can transiently worsen MG, the regimen recommended by Seybold and Drachman[48] that increases the dose gradually has been widely adopted. An initial alternate-day dose of 25 mg is raised in 12.5-mg steps every 6 days until either 100 mg or maximal benefit is reached. Complete remission attributed to alternate-day prednisone therapy has been reported in 37% to 69% of patients and significant improvement, in 17% to 42%.[48,55,56] In one study, the average time for significant improvement was 4.9 months and the average dosage was 68 mg on alternate days.[57] The time required for depression of the antibody titer varies, but the most striking decreases are usually the most rapid and occur in less than 3 months.[53]

In patients with moderately severe MG or exacerbation of generalized MG, intravenous "pulse" methylprednisolone (2 g daily at 5-day intervals × 3 or 2 g on 2 consecutive days) produces satisfactory improvement within 2 to 3 days for a mean period of 8 weeks with minimal side effects. After improvement, oral prednisone therapy is used to maintain improvement.[10,40]

From 30% to 60% of patients receiving long-term alternate-day prednisone therapy develop significant side effects.[9,50] These include cushingoid appearance, weight gain, hypertension, peptic ulcers causing gastrointestinal hemorrhage, aseptic necrosis of the femoral head, osteoporosis causing vertebral collapse and long-bone fractures, posterior subcapsular cataracts, infection, and diabetes mellitus. Cataracts, infection, and bone changes are especially frequent in patients older than 50 years. When the dose of the drug is decreased, about one-fifth of patients develop short-lasting withdrawal symptoms consisting of arthralgias, myalgias, fever, and sterile joint effusions.[9] There is general agreement that patients receiving long-term prednisone therapy should be monitored closely for development of hypertension, hypokalemia, hyperglycemia, and osteoporosis. Patients are advised to avoid extra salt in their diet and to take antacids and supplemental calcium (1 g daily) with vitamin D. Potassium supplements should be taken by patients who develop hypokalemia. Tuberculin-positive patients should receive prophylactic antituberculosis therapy. Postmenopausal women should be offered estrogen therapy. Patients receiving moderate doses of corticosteroids should be treated with trimethoprim-sulfamethoxazole (Bactrim), one double strength tablet three times per week, to reduce the likelihood of *Pneumocystis carinii* pneumonia.[58]

Azathioprine

Azathioprine is converted in the body to mercaptopurine, which is converted into mercaptopurine-containing nucleotides that interfere with DNA and RNA synthesis. This inhibits the division of rapidly proliferating cells and reduces counts of both T cells and B cells.

Azathioprine therapy in doses of 2 to 3 mg/kg daily results in remission or significant improvement in 70% to 90% of patients.[59,60] The minimal time for improvement is 3 months. About one-half of the patients have relapse after treatment is stopped.[59]

The use of azathioprine in combination with alternate-day prednisone (or prednisolone) is associated with fewer treatment failures, longer remissions, and fewer side effects than when either drug is used alone.[38] Moreover, the most severe forms of MG, often resistant to either drug alone, benefit from the combination of both drugs.[61] However, the full therapeutic and corticosteroid-sparing effects of azathioprine become apparent only during the second and third years of combined therapy.[38]

Among 271 MG patients treated with azathioprine, the side effects included myelosuppression indicated by leukopenia, thrombocytopenia, and, less frequently, anemia (18%); serious infection (7%); gastrointestinal tract irritation (8%); and signs of hepatotoxicity (6%) (pooled results of studies by Mertens[59] and others[60,62]). Long-term monitoring of the complete blood count (weekly for 4 weeks, then biweekly for 1 month, and monthly thereafter) and liver function tests every 6 months are advisable for patients receiving azathioprine. The drug is potentially teratogenic, and its long-term use in patients with organ transplants carries an increased risk of neoplasia, especially lymphoma. The risk of neoplasia in MG patients treated with azathioprine is likely small and has not been assessed.

Thiopurine methyltransferase (TPMT) is a polymorphic enzyme important in the catabolism of 6-mercaptopurine. Assay of TPMT in erythrocytes indicates that 0.3% of the population is homozygous and 11% heterozygous for polymorphisms that decrease TPMT activity. In those with a homozygous defect, azathioprine treatment can induce fatal bone marrow toxicity.[63,64] Therefore, erythrocyte TPMT assay is advisable for patients who are to receive azathioprine treatment. Homozygous TPMT deficiency is a contraindication to azathioprine treatment; heterozygous TPMT deficiency dictates extra caution in using the drug.

Cyclophosphamide

This drug, like azathioprine, interferes with DNA synthesis. The oral dose of the drug is 1 to 2 mg/kg daily. Pooled results of two studies show that cyclophosphamide therapy improved MG in 84% of patients.[65,66] Despite these reports, the drug is seldom used because of its toxicity (severe bone marrow depression, hemorrhagic cystitis, bladder tumors, hair loss, anovulation, azoospermia). Moreover, its therapeutic effect is not significantly greater than that of azathioprine.

Cyclosporine

Cyclosporine interferes with signaling pathways required for the clonal expansion of lymphocytes. The drug prevents T-cell proliferation by reducing the expression of cytokine genes (e.g., the gene coding for interleukin-2) required for T-cell activation and proliferation[51] and is widely used for immunosuppression in transplant recipients.

In 1987, a controlled clinical trial of 20 MG patients showed that cyclosporine has beneficial effects in MG.[37] Pooled results of uncontrolled studies since then have demonstrated that the drug produced significant clinical improvement in 64 of 91 patients with disease refractory to other forms of immunotherapy.[67-70] In a study of 57 patients who took cyclosporine for a median of 3.5 years, the median time to clinical response was 7 months, with some patients having a response as early as 1 week. The initial dose was 5 mg/kg daily divided into two doses taken 12 hours apart. The dose was subsequently adjusted to maintain trough blood levels of 100 to 150 ng/L, and later on the basis of serum creatinine levels and clinical improvement. After maximal improvement, the dose was decreased to the minimum needed to maintain improvement. Nephrotoxicity was detected in close to one-third of patients, most of them elderly, and in five, this prompted withdrawal of the medication. Six patients developed cancer: skin cancer in four, B-cell lymphoma in one, and adenocarcinoma of the uterus in one.[70] The usefulness of cyclosporine in MG is limited by its cost, nephrotoxicity, and hypertension during long-term therapy and by risk of malignancy.

Tacrolimus and rapamycin (sirolimus) affect T-cell proliferation in a manner similar to that of cyclosporine. Their safety and efficacy in the treatment of MG have not been evaluated.

Mycophenolate mofetil (CellCept)

This drug exerts a cytostatic effect on both T cells and B cells by inhibiting inosine monophosphate dehydrogenase, a rate-limiting enzyme in the de novo synthesis of guanosine nucleotides. It also induces apoptosis of activated T cells, limits recruitment of immune cells into sites of graft rejection, and decreases peroxynitrite-mediated tissue damage.[71] The pooled results of four open-label clinical studies of mycophenolate mofetil in 45 patients with MG inadequately controlled by other medications indicate that 69%

improved significantly and without appreciable side effects.[72–75] The dose of the drug is 1 g every 12 hours. Improvement begins 2 weeks to 2 months after the start of therapy. Known side effects of the drug include mild gastrointestinal discomfort, sometimes with diarrhea, and dose-dependent leukopenia.[75,76] Therefore, the complete blood count should be monitored the same way as for patients treated with azathioprine. Cytomegalovirus infection and activation of latent tuberculosis were reported in transplant recipients exposed to multiple immunosuppressants.[77,78]

Plasmapheresis

Plasmapheresis removes circulating anti-AChR antibodies, but it is a complicated and costly procedure that should be used only as a life-saving measure in severe generalized or fulminating MG refractory to all other forms of readily available therapy. Usually 1 to 1.5 plasma volumes are removed at each procedure in exchange for saline containing albumin or plasma protein fractions. Regional anticoagulation with citrate is used during the exchange.[79] There are no absolute rules about the number of exchanges or the interval between the exchanges, but daily exchanges are more effective than alternate-day exchanges,[80] and three to five exchanges are usually required to obtain a satisfactory clinical response. Objective improvement typically appears after a delay of a few days and correlates with a decrease of the AChR antibody titer. When treatment is stopped, the antibody titer increases again, and the symptoms recur unless other immunosuppressants are used. Thus, plasmapheresis itself does not confer greater long-term protection than immunosuppressant therapy alone.[81] Risks of the procedure include hypocalcemia due to anticoagulation with citrate salts, hypotension, and infection from intravenous manipulations. If a central venous catheter needs to be placed, then the risks also include pneumothorax and thrombosis.[79]

Selective immunoadsorption of plasma with tryptophan-linked polyvinylalcohol gels is an alternative to plasmapheresis. Because this decreases plasma albumin only modestly, there is no need for protein replacement.[82]

Intravenous immunoglobulin therapy

Like plasmapheresis, IVIG provides a costly temporary beneficial effect in MG. The exact mechanism of action of IVIG is still unclear. IVIG is usually infused at 400 mg/kg on each of 5 consecutive days, or at 1 g/kg on 2 consecutive days, but neither the minimal effective dose nor the optimal dosing schedule has been determined for MG[83] or for other autoimmune diseases.

Among 48 patients severely affected by MG, 70% had a favorable response to IVIG, with improvement occurring within 2 to 3 weeks from the start of therapy. The mean duration of the response was 64 days for those also receiving corticosteroids and 35 days for those who were not.[84] It has not been established that IVIG therapy is superior to plasmapheresis. According to one study, IVIG provided less improvement in ventilatory status than plasmapheresis 2 weeks after therapy.[85]

Adverse reactions to IVIG occur in about 5% of recipients.[83,86] These include low-grade fever, myalgias, headache, and vasomotor reactions that can be mitigated by premedication with antihistamines and by slowing the rate of infusion.[83,87] More serious complications related to blood hyperviscosity or hyperosmolarity include deep venous thrombosis, renal insufficiency, aseptic meningitis, and cerebral infarction. Patients with selective IgA deficiency, agammaglobulinemia, or severe hypogammaglobulinemia may experience an anaphylactic reaction with repeated infusions. Therefore, serum levels of IgA, IgG, and IgM should be determined for all patients before IVIG therapy is stated.[41,83]

Thymectomy

That the thymus gland has a role in the pathogenesis of MG is generally accepted (see section above on Pathogenesis and Pathophysiology). This, as well as the reports in the 1940s and 1950s on the usefulness of thymectomy in MG,[88–90] provided the rationale for its subsequent use. The following views have evolved during the past 50 years:

1. Neither duration of illness nor sex contraindicate thymectomy in MG
2. The percentage of remissions after thymectomy continues to increase with time
3. Females with shorter duration of disease, hyperplastic glands, and high antibody titer improve more rapidly than males, but after 10 years the results tend to equalize
4. From 7 to 10 years after thymectomy, the remission rate is of the order of 40% to 60% in all categories of cases except for ones with thymoma[91–95]
5. Thymectomy is also effective in children with autoimmune MG, but it should be avoided during the first 5 years of life because of the risk of immunodeficiency.[96,97]
6. Although thymectomy can be effective in ocular MG and may prevent generalization of the disease,[98] it is not recommend for ocular symptoms only[99]
7. Older patients are more responsive to medical therapy,[50] have higher surgical morbidity, and may not realize the full benefits of the procedure in their lifetime.[99] Therefore, thymectomy is seldom recommended after the age of 65
8. Thymoma is an absolute indication for thymectomy at any age
9. Transcervical thymectomy may miss ectopic thymic tissue; therefore transsternal thymectomy combined with a search for thymic tissue in the cervical region is required for complete thymectomy[100,101]

Despite these generalizations, some cautionary voices have been heard. Grob[15] has counseled that therapeutic measures, including thymectomy, must be evaluated in relation to the natural course of MG.

In most patients, the disease reaches its maximal severity within 3 years and is then followed by a chronic phase that tends to diminish in severity. Moreover, in recent decades, a similar proportion of thymectomized and nonthymectomized patients had similar improvement a mean of 12 years after onset.[15] Similar conclusions were reached by other investigators.[102] Also, in 2000, the Quality Standards Subcommittee of the American Academy of Neurology failed to determine whether the observed association between thymectomy and improved outcome of MG resulted from thymectomy or multiple differences in baseline characteristics between surgical and nonsurgical groups. Therefore, it did not consider the benefit of thymectomy in nonthymomatous MG as conclusively established.[103] The controversy will not be resolved until a large-scale, long-term, prospective, controlled clinical trial has been conducted on thymectomy versus conservative therapy. Meanwhile, thymectomy remains part of the armamentarium for treatment of generalized MG.

Management of different grades and types of myasthenia gravis

Transient neonatal MG Anti-AChE medications are given at 2- to 4-hour intervals orally when symptoms are mild and parenterally if there is feeding difficulty. The appropriate pediatric dosages are indicated in Table 226.3. Severely ill infants may require respiratory support, plasmapheresis, or exchange transfusions.[41]

Ocular MG Therapy begins with anti-AChE drugs. In refractory cases, ptosis can be relieved with lid-crutches and diplopia, with an eye patch or an occluding contact lens.[104] Disabling ptosis not responding to drug therapy also can be treated surgically.[105,106] Patients become candidates for alternate-day prednisone therapy only after the above measures fail to produce a response.

There is evidence that treatment of ocular MG with alternate-day prednisone or azathioprine (or both) can prevent generalization of the disease.[107,108] Because a high proportion of patients with ocular MG develop generalized disease within 2 years after onset,[109] treatment of recent-onset ocular MG with alternate-day prednisone or azathioprine (or both) is a justifiable option.[108,110]

Mild generalized MG All patients are treated with pyridostigmine, with careful titration of the dose to obtain maximal relief of symptoms, but not exceeding 600 mg daily for adults and 7 mg/kg daily for children. Patients without an adequate response are candidates for alternate-day prednisone therapy. If prednisone fails to provide adequate relief or more than 20 to 30 mg of prednisone is required on alternate days to control symptoms, azathioprine is added as a third medication. Thymectomy is an elective procedure for patients between the ages of 5 and 65 years.

Moderately severe to severe MG The initial approach is treatment with pyridostigmine in combination with alternate-day prednisone and azathioprine. Thymectomy is recommended as an elective procedure for patients between the ages of 5 and 65. Patients who do not have a response to combined therapy with prednisone and azathioprine are treated with prednisone in combination with mycophenolate mofetil or cyclosporine.

Fulminating MG and myasthenic crisis The approach advocated here is based largely on that recommended by Keesey.[42] Patients who are unable to swallow or who require respiratory support are candidates for admission to an intensive care unit and treatment with one or more courses of plasmapheresis or IVIG and high-dose corticosteroids. Corticosteroid therapy is initiated with intravenous "pulse" methylprednisolone, 2 g on two consecutive days, followed by 60 to 100 mg of prednisone given orally daily until improvement occurs. With this regimen, 85% of the patients have improvement within 21 days, and all have improvement after 2 months. When the patient can be weaned from respiratory support and is able to swallow, prednisone is tapered by 10 mg weekly to 50 mg daily; alternate-day therapy is then initiated by increasing the dose 1 day by 5 mg and decreasing it on the other day by 5 mg, until the dose is 100 mg on alternate days.[42] After several months of high-dose alternate-day prednisone treatment, the dose is tapered very slowly, with careful monitoring of the patient's clinical status and antibody titer, to the lowest level required to control the disease.

Pregnancy and MG Pyridostigmine and corticosteroids can be administered, but treatment with azathioprine and other cytotoxic medications should be discontinued several months before pregnancy is contemplated. The dose of anti-AChE drugs needs to be adjusted because of altered rates of intestinal absorption and renal excretion.[41] Plasmapheresis and IVIG are options for critically ill patients.

Seronegative MG The clinical features of seronegative and seropositive MG are similar,[111–113] but patients with seronegative MG seldom have thymic hyperplasia and do not harbor thymoma; therefore, thymectomy is generally avoided in these patients. Otherwise, management is the same as for seropositive MG.[111–113]

Drugs with adverse effects on MG Aminoglycoside antibodies block presynaptic calcium currents,[114] which decreases the number of ACh quanta released by a nerve impulse,[115] hence, decreasing the safety margin of neuromuscular transmission. Therefore, streptomycin, dihydrostreptomycin, polymyxin, colistin, neomycin, kanamycin, and gentamicin should be avoided or used with great caution in MG. Ampicillin,[116] erythromycin,[117] chlorpromazine, morphine, procainamide, quinine, quinidine, chloroquine and other quinoline drugs,[118–120] β-adrenergic blockers,[121,122] gabapentin,[123] calcium channel blockers, and phenothiazine can also worsen neuromuscular transmission and should be avoided or used with caution. The contrast agent for magnetic resonance imaging, gadolinium diethylenetriamine pentaacetic acid, also decreases quantal release and can worsen MG.[124] Neuromuscular blocking agents should be avoided in myasthenic patients undergoing surgery. Treatment with D-penicillamine[18] or with interferon-α or -β[19,20] should also be avoided because these drugs can induce or abet the immune response to AChR. For a more detailed review of adverse drug effects in MG, the reader is referred to reference 125.

Lambert-Eaton myasthenic syndrome

Historical overview

In 1951, Anderson et al.[126] observed a patient who had a bronchial neoplasm and "an unusual form of peripheral neuropathy, possibly similar to myasthenia gravis." In 1956, Lambert, Eaton, and Rooke[127] and, in 1957, Eaton and Lambert[128] described the essential clinical and EMG features of the syndrome in six patients: five of the six were men; two patients had carcinoma of the lung, two had suspected carcinoma of the lung, one had reticulum cell sarcoma of the lung, and one had cerebellar ataxia without carcinoma. They all had weakness and abnormal fatigability on exertion, but the distribution of the weakness, the EMG findings, and the response to anti-AChE drugs were different from those observed in MG. Subsequently, the syndrome was referred to as the Lambert-Eaton myasthenic syndrome (LEMS). In 1968, Elmqvist and Lambert[129] showed that LEMS is associated with markedly decreased quantal release by nerve impulses. In 1981, Lang, Newsom-Davis, and Wray[130] obtained strong evidence for an autoimmune cause of the disease by transferring the electrophysiological features of LEMS from humans to mice with IgG. In the following year, Fukunaga et al[131] showed with freeze-fracture electron microscopy that the motor nerve terminal of patients with LEMs is depleted of voltage-gated calcium channels (VGCCs), thereby implicating these channels as the target of LEMS antibodies.

Epidemiology

The precise incidence or prevalence of LEMS in the general population is not known, but the incidence of neoplastic LEMS is linked to that of small cell lung carcinoma (SCLC): 3% of all patients with SCLC are estimated to have LEMS.[132] Conversely, ~42% of those with LEMS have SCLC, and ~5% have other carcinomas.[133,134] Neoplastic LEMS is uncommon in people younger than 40 years and affects men more frequently than women, probably because of the different smoking habits of the two sexes. Nonneoplastic LEMS can occur at any age. It can be associated with other autoimmune diseases such as pernicious anemia, hypothyroidism, hyperthyroidism, Sjögren syndrome, vitiligo, celiac disease, or juvenile-onset diabetes mellitus. Subacute cerebellar degeneration

Table 226.4   Clinical features of Lambert-Eaton myasthenic syndrome

Weakness and fatigability of proximal limb and truncal muscles. Lower limbs more affected than upper limbs
Hyporeflexia or areflexia involving some or all tendon reflexes
Strength and reflexes facilitate after sustained exertion
Mild or transient ocular symptoms in 70% of patients
Dysautonomic symptoms (decreased salivation and sweating, orthostatism, abnormal pupillary light reflex, and impotence) in 80% of patients
Myalgias, chiefly of thigh muscles, and paresthesias in some patients
Severe respiratory muscle involvement is uncommon
Slight or no response to anti-AChE drugs
Associations with malignancy, especially SCLC, in ~45% of patients

AChE, acetylcholinesterase; SCLC, small cell lung carcinoma.

occurs with both neoplastic and nonneoplastic LEMS (reviewed in reference 135).

Etiology

Neoplastic LEMS likely results from sensitization to epitopes shared between VGCCs expressed by carcinoma cells and those present in motor nerve terminals, cerebellum, and autonomic ganglia.[132] Nonneoplastic LEMS also stems from autoimmunity-directed VGCCs, but the mechanism that instigates loss of tolerance to the self-VGCC is not understood.

Pathophysiology and pathogenesis

The binding of antibodies to VGCCs on the presynaptic membrane results in their aggregation and accelerated internalization.[131,136,137] Depletion of the presynaptic VGCCs curtails calcium ingress into the nerve terminal when the terminal is depolarized by nerve impulses. This decreases the number of quanta released by a nerve impulse and compromises the safety margin of neuromuscular transmission.[138] High-frequency stimulation of motor nerves or sustained voluntary effort results in the gradual accumulation of calcium in the nerve terminal; this facilitates evoked quantal release and mitigates the defect. The frequent dysautonomic features of LEMS are attributed to anti-VGCC antibodies recognizing VGCCs in autonomic ganglia.[139]

Clinical features

The frequent association of LEMS with carcinoma is discussed above. The other clinical features of LEMS are summarized in Table 226.4.

Diagnosis

The diagnosis rests on the clinical findings, EMG features, and detection of anti-VGCC antibodies. The EMG features consist of an abnormally low-amplitude initial compound muscle-action potential (CMAP) that facilitates more than 100% after a few seconds of tetanic stimulation or maximal voluntary contraction. Low-frequency (2 to 3 Hz) stimulation of rested muscle further decreases the CMAP amplitude, but recovery begins after the fourth to eighth stimulus. Anti-VGCC antibodies of the P/Q type are detected in 85% of LEMS patients in a radio-immunoassay that uses VGCCs extracted from small cell carcinomas labeled with ^{125}I-ω-conotoxin MVIIC derived from *Conus magus*.[140] Once the diagnosis of LEMS is established, all patients must be evaluated for an underlying lung carcinoma.

Differential diagnosis

This includes MG, Guillain-Barré syndrome, peripheral neuropathy, polymyositis, botulinum poisoning, magnesium intoxication, and, in younger patients, congenital myasthenic syndromes.

The distribution of the weakness, the edrophonium test, EMG studies, and tests for circulating AChR antibodies distinguish MG from LEMS. Rare patients have both LEMS and MG by clinical, EMG, and serological criteria.[141] The distribution of the weakness and the hyporeflexia may suggest the diagnosis of Guillain-Barré syndrome. However, LEMS has a more insidious onset, and the increase of strength during voluntary contraction, the normal cerebrospinal fluid examination, and the EMG findings should point to the diagnosis of LEMS. The hyporeflexia and occasional peripheral paresthesia in LEMS may suggest a peripheral neuropathy. However, sensory and motor nerve conduction velocities are normal, fibrillation potentials are absent, and nerve stimulation studies show the typical features of LEMS. Both botulinum poisoning[142] and magnesium intoxication[143] decrease the quantal content of the EPP and can closely mimic the clinical and EMG features of LEMS. However, the onset of these syndromes is more abrupt than that of LEMS. Magnesium intoxication can arise from accidental poisoning or after abuse of magnesium-containing cathartics.[144] The history and determination of the serum level of magnesium will establish the correct diagnosis.

Treatment

Anticancer therapy, pharmacological agents, and immunosuppression are used in the treatment of LEMS.

Anticancer therapy In neoplastic LEMS, the neuromuscular transmission defect may improve when chemotherapy or radiotherapy (or both) induces tumor regression,[132] but the response is transient and LEMS recurs when the tumor recurs.

Pharmacological agents Anticholinesterase drugs have only a slight effect in LEMS[145,146] and are used only when other measures fail or are contraindicated.

Guanidine increases evoked quantal release and has a beneficial effect in LEMS,[147] but it is seldom used because of its undesired side effects, which include ataxia, paresthesias, gastrointestinal distress, confusion, dry skin, atrial fibrillation, hypotension, bone marrow depression, and nephritis.[148–150]

The drug of choice is 3,4-diaminopyridine (3,4-DAP). This medication prolongs the duration of the presynaptic action potential by blocking the outward potassium current.[151,152] This increases calcium entry into the nerve terminal, which in turn increases quantal release. The medication is effective in relieving both the motor and autonomic symptoms of LEMS.[153–156] The recommended dose is up to 1 mg/kg daily in divided doses. The drug is well tolerated, with generally only mild side effects. These include peripheral and perioral paresthesias, adrenergic side effects (palpitation, sleeplessness, ventricular extrasystoles), and cholinergic side effects (increased bronchial secretions, cough, and diarrhea). Higher doses are not recommended because of possible seizures.[154,157] The drug has not been approved for clinical use by the U.S. Food and Drug Administration, but it can be obtained as an investigational drug and used under the auspices of Institutional Review Boards.

Immunosuppression Plasmapheresis is effective in LEMS,[158] but its beneficial effects appear more slowly than in MG. Therapy with IVIG can also induce a temporary remission.[159] These modalities of treatment should be used only in severely ill patients and when 3,4-DAP is unavailable.

Either azathioprine or corticosteroids can improve LEMS. The two drugs act synergistically with each other, but not with plasma exchange.[158] Optimal treatment of nonneoplastic LEMS consists of modest doses of alternate-day prednisone and 1.5 to 2 mg/kg daily of azathioprine. In neoplastic LEMS, antitumor therapy may be combined with alternate-day prednisone treatment. Either form of LEMS is also treated with 3,4-DAP. After clinical improvement, which is usually gradual, the prednisone dose can be decreased gradually over many months to establish the minimal maintenance requirement. In some patients, immunotherapy improves the condition to the extent that 3,4-DAP treatment can also be withdrawn.

Congenital myasthenic syndromes
Historical overview

In 1937, Rothbart[160] described four brothers younger than 2 years who had a myasthenic disorder, and by 1972, Bundey[161] had collected 97 familial cases of myasthenia with onset before the age of 2. After the discovery of the autoimmune origin of MG in the 1970s and of LEMS in the 1980s, it became apparent that myasthenic disorders occurring in a familial or congenital setting have a different etiology. Subsequent investigation of patients with congenital myasthenic syndromes (CMS) by ultrastructural, in vitro electrophysiological, and molecular genetic methods showed several distinct syndromes stemming from presynaptic, synaptic, and postsynaptic defects (reviewed in reference 162).

Epidemiology

No reliable information is available on the incidence and prevalence of CMS. These syndromes are not uncommon but are frequently misdiagnosed or go undiagnosed for a number of reasons: CMS can closely mimic other disorders (see section on differential diagnosis below); physicians are less familiar with CMS than with other neurological disorders; and the correct diagnosis of some CMS requires specialized methods of investigation currently available at only a few medical centers. It is now known, however, that some CMS are endemic in the Near East where closed communities and consanguineous marriages are relatively frequent.[163,164]

Etiology and pathogenesis

The CMS represent a heterogeneous group of inherited disorders arising from presynaptic, synaptic, or postsynaptic defects. In each syndrome, the safety margin of neuromuscular transmission is compromised by one or more specific mechanisms. The safety margin of neuromuscular transmission is defined as the difference between the amplitude of the EPP and the amplitude of the depolarization required to trigger a muscle fiber action potential. Mechanisms that impair the safety margin of neuromuscular transmission involve the synthesis or packaging of ACh quanta into synaptic vesicles, the calcium-dependent evoked release of ACh quanta from the nerve terminal, and the efficiency of released quanta in generating a postsynaptic depolarization. Quantal efficiency depends on the geometry of the EP, the density and functional state of AChE in the synaptic space, and the density and kinetic properties of the AChR. (Also see section on classification of the CMS below).

Genetics

The postsynaptic slow-channel CMS is caused by dominantly inherited gain-of-function mutations in different AChR subunits. All other CMS are caused by recessive loss-of-function mutations in EP-specific proteins.

Clinical features

A typical clinical history for CMS is one of myasthenic symptoms since infancy or early childhood, normal or delayed motor milestones, sometimes progression of symptoms during adolescence or adult life, and negative tests for anti-AChR antibodies. Some syndromes (e.g., the slow-channel syndrome[165]) may not present until the second or third decade of life, and in the CMS caused by a defect in choline acetyltransferase, the symptoms can be episodic.[166] Some CMS have special clinical features (see section on diagnosis below).

Classification of the CMS

A site-of-defect-based classification of CMS based on 155 kinships investigated at Mayo Clinic is given in Table 226.5. The classification is still tentative because additional CMS might yet be discovered and because in some incompletely studied disorders, for example, limb-girdle CMS[167] and CMS associated with facial malformation in Iranian Jews,[168] the site of the defect is not known.

Inspection of Table 226.5 shows that most postsynaptic syndromes stem from a kinetic abnormality or

Table 226.5   Classification of congenital myasthenic syndromes (CMS) based on 142 kinships investigated at Mayo Clinic

Defect	No. of kinships
Presynaptic	
Choline acetyltransferase deficiency (CMS with episodic apnea)	6
Paucity of synaptic vesicles associated with reduced quantal release	1
Lambert-Eaton syndrome-like	1
Other presynaptic defects	4
Synaptic	
End plate AChE deficiency	24
Postsynaptic	
Kinetic abnormality with/without AChR deficiency	37
AChR deficiency, with/without minor kinetic abnormality*	67
Rapsyn deficiency	14
Plectin deficiency	1
Total	**155**

AChE, acetylcholinesterase; AChR, acetylcholine receptor.
*The high frequency of this group is due in part to 52 kinships being of Mediterranean/Near Eastern or Gypsy origin who frequently carry homozygous low-expressor mutations in the AChR ε subunit.

deficiency of AChR. Two major kinetic types of CMS have been identified: slow-channel CMS and fast-channel CMS. The slow-channel syndrome is associated with slow-decaying EP currents, destabilization of the closed channel state, prolonged activation episodes of AChR, and an EP myopathy caused by cationic overloading of the postsynaptic region. The fast-channel syndrome is associated with fast-decaying EP currents, destabilization of the open channel state, abnormally brief activation episodes of AChR, and no anatomical footprint.[162]

Diagnosis

The clinical features from which a generic diagnosis of a CMS can be made as well as phenotypic clues pointing to specific types of CMS are listed in Table 226.6. In many patients, however, the phenotypic features do not point to a specific diagnosis. In these patients, specialized morphological, electrophysiological, and molecular genetic studies are required for a specific diagnosis.

Differential diagnosis

The differential diagnosis of the CMS is listed in Table 226.7.

Treatment

Pharmacological therapy is dictated by the defect underlying a given CMS. Moreover, drugs beneficial in some CMS are contraindicated in others. Therefore, a specific diagnosis is essential for rational therapy.

In general terms, CMS either decrease or increase the synaptic response to ACh. When a CMS decreases

Table 226.6 Diagnosis of a congenital myasthenic syndrome (CMS)

Generic diagnosis
Fatigable weakness involving ocular, bulbar, and limb muscles since infancy or early childhood
Similarly affected relative
Decremental EMG response at 2- to 3-Hz stimulation
Negative tests for anti-AChR antibodies

Exceptions and caveats
In some CMS, onset is delayed
There may be no similarly affected relatives
EMG abnormalities may not be present in all muscles or are present only intermittently
Weakness can be restricted to selected muscles

Clues pointing to a specific diagnosis
EP AChE deficiency[169]
Repetitive CMAPs
Refractoriness to cholinesterase inhibitors
Delayed pupillary light reflexes
Slow-channel CMS[165]
Repetitive CMAPs
Selectively severe involvement of cervical and wrist and finger extensor muscles in most patients
Dominant inheritance
EP choline acetyltransferase deficiency (CMS with episodic apnea)[166]
Recurrent apneic episodes, spontaneous or with fever, vomiting, or excitement
No or variable myasthenic symptoms between acute episodes; eye movements may be spared
Stimulation at 10 Hz for 5 min causes marked decrease of CMAP followed by slow recovery; EMG decrement at 2 Hz absent at rest, appears after stimulation at 10 Hz for 5 min, then disappears slowly

AChE, acetylcholinesterase; AChR, acetylcholine receptor; CMAP, compound muscle fiber action potential; EMG, electromyogram; EP, end plate.

Table 226.7 Differential diagnosis of congenital myasthenic syndromes

Neonatal period, infancy, childhood
Spinal muscular atrophy
Morphologically distinct congenital myopathies (central core disease, nemaline myopathy, myotubular myopathy)
Congenital muscular dystrophies
Infantile myotonic dystrophy
Mitochondrial myopathy
Brainstem anomaly
Möbius syndrome
Infantile botulism
Autoimmune myasthenia gravis*

Older patients
Motor neuron disease
Radial nerve palsy[†]
Peripheral neuropathy[†]
Limb-girdle or facioscapulohumeral muscular dystrophy
Mitochondrial myopathy
Chronic fatigue syndrome
Seropositive and seronegative autoimmune myasthenia gravis

*Not reported in the first year of life.
[†]This diagnosis was suspected in some cases of slow-channel congenital myasthenic syndrome.

cated because it may further deplete the store of synaptic vesicles available for release.

LEMS-like CMS Hypothetically, this disorder should respond to 3,4-DAP, but in one patient observed by the author, 3,4-DAP was ineffective.

EP AChE deficiency There is no satisfactory drug therapy for this disease. Anti-AChE drugs have no effect on neuromuscular transmission and can cause excessive muscarinic side effects. Some patients report subjective improvement from taking ephedrine sulfate, 25 mg 2 to 3 times daily, but two patients observed by the author did not have improvement with ephedrine. Alternate-day prednisone therapy had a slight beneficial effect in two patients but was ineffective in one and appeared to worsen the symptoms in another. In a severely ill respirator-dependent infant, improvement occurred by intermittent blockade of AChR by atracurium, an agent that protects AChR from overexposure to ACh, allowing for temporary withdrawal of respiratory support.[171]

Slow-channel CMS Specific therapy for this syndrome exists in the form of quinidine. This drug is a long-lived, open-channel blocker of AChRs that shortens the duration of channel opening events in a concentration-dependent manner.[170] Quinidine, 5 μM/L, decreases the duration of slow-channel opening events severalfold to that of wild-type, but reduces wild-type channel opening events only by ~50%.[170]

Adult slow-channel CMS is treated with 200 mg quinidine sulfate 3 times daily for 1 week; the dose is then increased gradually to maintain a serum level of 1

the synaptic response, anti-AChE drugs, which increase the number of AChRs activated by each quantum, and 3,4-DAP, which increases the number of quanta released by a nerve impulse, are used. When a CMS increases the synaptic response because of a slow-channel-type molecular defect, quinidine is used because it acts as a long-lived open-channel blocker of AChRs.[170] However, quinidine is contraindicated in all other types of CMS, and anti-AChE drugs and 3,4-DAP are potentially harmful in the slow-channel CMS.

Management of different types of CMS
Choline acetyltransferase deficiency (CMS with episodic apnea) Treatment consists of prophylactic use of pyridostigmine. Because apneic attacks can occur suddenly, the parents should be provided with an inflatable rescue bag and a fitted mask, should be instructed in the intramuscular injection of neostigmine methylsulfate, and be advised to install an apnea monitor in the home.

Paucity of synaptic vesicles associated with reduced quantal release This disorder responds partially to anticholinesterase medications. 3,4-DAP is contraindi-

to 2.5 µg/mL (3 to 7.5 µM/L). After a satisfactory serum level is established, equivalent doses of Quinidex, a slow-release form of quinidine sulfate, can be given. The doses for children are 15 to 60 mg/kg daily of quinidine sulfate in four to six divided doses, or Quinidex, 10 to 15 mg/kg daily in three divided doses. With this regimen, patients have improvement in their endurance and EMG tests over many months.[172]

Quinidine is contraindicated in CMS other than the slow-channel syndrome. Untoward effects of quinidine include gastrointestinal reactions with diarrhea and cinchonism. Hypersensitivity to the drug can result in drug fever, abnormal liver function tests, hemolytic anemia, agranulocytosis, thrombocytopenic purpura, and toxic drug rash. Quinidine also worsens atrioventricular conduction defects and can aggravate a prolonged QT interval, which predisposes to ventricular arrythmias. Quinidine also inhibits cytochrome P-450IIDA and thereby impairs the metabolism of codeine, tricyclic antidepressants, other antiarrhythmic drugs, and digoxin. Administration of verapamil, cimetidine, and agents that alkalize urine may augment the serum level of quinidine, and quinidine potentiates the anticoagulant effects of warfarin.[43]

Slow-channel CMS patients who are unable to tolerate quinidine can be treated with fluoxetine in gradually increasing doses until a total daily dose of 100 mg is attained. Fluoxetine is a less effective long-lived open-channel blocker of the AChR channel than quinidine, and its beneficial effects develop even more slowly than those of quinidine (AG Engel and T Fukudome, unpublished observations, 1999). Adverse effects of fluoxetine include mild nausea, nervousness, insomnia, sexual dysfunction, and hyponatremia in the elderly.[43]

Fast-channel CMS   Fast-channel CMS patients respond well to combined therapy with pyridostigmine, in doses similar to those used in autoimmune MG, and 3,4-DAP, 1 mg/kg daily in divided doses.[173] Patients without concomitant EP AChR deficiency respond better than those in whom the fast-channel mutation also reduces expression of AChR. The mode of action and potentially adverse effects of 3,4-DAP are discussed above (see treatment of the Lambert-Eaton syndrome).

EP AChR deficiency with or without minor kinetic abnormality   Most patients have a favorable but incomplete response to cholinesterase inhibitors. The additional use of 3,4-DAP, 1 mg/kg daily in divided doses, results in further significant improvement in about one-third of patients.[173] A favorable response to 3,4-DAP combined with pyridostigmine in unselected CMS patients was reported previously,[174] but in an another clinical trial, CMS patients with predominantly ocular symptoms showed little response to 3,4-DAP.[175] In our experience, 3,4-DAP increases endurance and reduces lid ptosis, but external ocular muscles respond less than limb muscles, and in some patients, the medication becomes less effective with continued use.

General measures   Severely affected CMS patients are born with or develop a restrictive ventilatory defect, cannot swallow, and develop progressive spinal deformities. Some CMS infants are unable to breathe at birth but can be weaned off the respirator after a few months. Ventilatory defects that develop later in life initially require nocturnal and, later, daytime ventilatory support. Spinal deformities must be monitored carefully; if they are progressive and significant, corrective surgery is indicated. Surgery is best performed in the early teens, after vertebral growth has ceased. Severe dysphagia requires feeding via a gastrostomy tube. With early specific diagnosis and therapy, the above life-threatening consequences of the CMS can be mitigated or obviated.

References

1. Simpson JA. Myasthenia gravis: a new hypothesis. Scott Med J 1960;5:419–436
2. Patrick J, Lindstrom J. Autoimmune response to acetylcholine receptor. Science 1973;180:871–872
3. Fambrough DM, Drachman DB, Satyamurti S. Neuromuscular junction in myasthenia gravis: decreased acetylcholine receptors. Science 1973;182:293–295
4. Lindstrom JM. Experimental autoimmune myasthenia gravis: Induction and treatment. *In:* Engel AG, ed. Myasthenia Gravis and Myasthenic Disorders. New York: Oxford University Press, 1999:111–130
5. Lindstrom JM, Seybold ME, Lennon VA, et al. Antibody to acetylcholine receptor in myasthenia gravis. Prevalence, clinical correlates, and diagnostic value. Neurology 1976;26:1054–1059
6. Toyka KV, Drachman DB, Griffin DE, et al. Myasthenia gravis. Study of humoral immune mechanisms by passive transfer to mice. N Engl J Med 1977;296:125–131
7. Engel AG, Lambert EH, Howard FM. Immune complexes (IgG and C3) at the motor end-plate in myasthenia gravis: ultrastructural and light microscopic localization and electrophysiologic correlations. Mayo Clin Proc 1977;52:267–280
8. Pinching AJ, Peters DK. Remission of myasthenia gravis following plasma-exchange. Lancet 1976;ii:1373–1376
9. Brunner NG, Berger CL, Namba T, Grob D. Corticotropin and corticosteroids in generalized myasthenia gravis: comparative studies and role in management. Ann NY Acad Sci 1976;274:577–595
10. Arsura E, Brunner NG, Namba T, Grob D. High-dose intravenous methylprednisolone in myasthenia gravis. Arch Neurol 1985;42:1149–1153
11. Robertson NP, Deans J, Compston DA. Myasthenia gravis: a population based epidemiological study in Cambridgeshire, England. J Neurol Neurosurg Psychiatry 1998;65:492–496
12. Poulas K, Tsibri E, Papanastasiou D, et al. Equal male and female incidence of myasthenia gravis. Neurology 2000;54:1202–1203
13. Guidetti D, Sabadini R, Bondavalli M, et al. Epidemiological study of myasthenia gravis in the province of Reggio Emilia, Italy. Eur J Epidemiol 1998;14:381–387
14. Osserman KE, Genkins G. Studies in myasthenia gravis: review of a twenty-year experience in over 1200 patients. Mt Sinai J Med 1971;38:497–537
15. Grob D. Natural history of myasthenia gravis. *In:* Engel AG, ed. Myasthenia Gravis and Myasthenic

Disorders. New York: Oxford University Press, 1999: 131–145

16. Seybold ME. Diagnosis of myasthenia gravis. *In:* Engel AG, ed. Myasthenia Gravis and Myasthenic Disorders. New York: Oxford Univeristy Press, 1999:146–166

17. Hoch W, McConville J, Helms S, et al. Auto-antibodies to the receptor tyrosine kinase MuSK in patients with myasthenia gravis without acetylcholine receptor antibodies. Nat Med 2001;7:365–368

18. Fawcett PR, McLachlan SM, Nicholson LV, et al. D-Penicillamine-associated myasthenia gravis: immunological and electrophysiological studies. Muscle Nerve 1982;5:328–334

19. Gurtubay IG, Morales G, Arechaga O, Gallego J. Development of myasthenia gravis after interferon alpha therapy. Electromyogr Clin Neurophysiol 1999;39:75–78

20. Harada J, Tamaoka A, Kohno Y, et al. Exacerbation of myasthenia gravis in a patient after interferon-β treatment for chronic active hepatitis C. J Neurol Sci 1999; 165:182–183

21. Batocchi AP, Evoli A, Servidei S, et al. Myasthenia gravis during interferon alfa therapy. Neurology 1995; 45:382–383

22. Hohlfeld R, Wekerle H. The immunopathogenesis of myasthenia gravis. *In:* Engel AG, ed. Myasthenia Gravis and Myasthenic Disorders. New York: Oxford University Press, 1999:87–110

23. Sahashi K, Engel AG, Lambert EH, Howard FM Jr. Ultrastructural localization of the terminal and lytic ninth complement component (C9) at the motor endplate in myasthenia gravis. J Neuropathol Exp Neurol 1980;39:160–172

24. Nakano S, Engel AG. Myasthenia gravis: quantitative immunocytochemical analysis of inflammatory cells and detection of complement membrane attack complex at the end-plate in 30 patients. Neurology 1993;43:1167–1172

25. Stanley EF, Drachman DB. Effect of myasthenic immunoglobulin on acetylcholine receptors of intact mammalian neuromuscular junctions. Science 1978; 200:1285–1287

26. Drachman DB, Adams RN, Josifek LF, Self SG. Functional activities of autoantibodies to acetylcholine receptors and the clinical severity of myasthenia gravis. N Engl J Med 1982;307:769–775

27. Jahn K, Franke C, Bufler J. Mechanism of block of nicotinic acetylcholine receptor channels by purified IgG from seropositive patients with myasthenia gravis. Neurology 2000;54:474–479

28. Garchon HJ, Djabiri F, Viard JP, et al. Involvement of human muscle acetylcholine receptor alpha-subunit gene (CHRNA) in susceptibility to myasthenia gravis. Proc Natl Acad Sci USA 1994;91: 4668–4672

29. Li F, Szobor A, Croxen R, et al. Dominantly inherited familial myasthenia gravis as a separate genetic entity without involvement of defined candidate gene loci. Int J Mol Med 2001;7:289–294

30. Marrie RA, Sahlas DJ, Bray GM. Familial autoimmune myasthenia gravis: four patients involving three generations. Can J Neurol Sci 2000;27:307–310

31. Bergoffen J, Zmijewski CM, Fischbeck KH. Familial autoimmune myasthenia gravis. Neurology 1994;44: 551–554

32. Szobor A. Familial myasthenia gravis: nine patients in two generations. Acta Med Hung 1991;48:145–149

33. Namba T, Brown SB, Grob D. Neonatal myasthenia gravis: report of two cases and review of the literature. Pediatrics 1970;45:488–504

34. Riemersma S, Vincent A, Beeson D, et al. Association of arthrogryposis multiplex congenita with maternal antibodies inhibiting fetal acetylcholine receptor function. J Clin Invest 1996;98:2358–2363

35. Tindall RS. Humoral immunity in myasthenia gravis: biochemical characterization of acquired antireceptor antibodies and clinical correlations. Ann Neurol 1981; 10:437–447

36. Limburg PC, The TH, Hummel-Tappel E, Oosterhuis HJ. Anti-acetylcholine receptor antibodies in myasthenia gravis. Part 1. Relation to clinical paramters in 250 patients. J Neurol Sci 1983;58:357–370

37. Tindall RS, Rollins JA, Phillips JT, et al. Preliminary results of a double-blind, randomized, placebo-controlled trial of cyclosporine in myasthenia gravis. N Engl J Med 1987;316:719–724

38. Palace J, Newsom-Davis J, Lecky B. A randomized double-blind trial of prednisolone alone or with azathioprine in myasthenia gravis. Myasthenia Gravis Study Group. Neurology 1998;50:1778–1783

39. Bromberg MB, Wald JJ, Forshew DA, et al. Randomized trial of azathioprine or prednisone for initial immunosuppressive treatment of myasthenia gravis. J Neurol Sci 1997;150:59–62

40. Lindberg C, Andersen O, Lefvert AK. Treatment of myasthenia gravis with methylprednisolone pulse: a double blind study. Acta Neurol Scand 1998;97:370–373

41. Seybold ME. Treatment of myasthenia gravis. *In:* Engel AG, ed. Myasthenia Gravis and Myasthenic Disorders. New York: Oxford University Press, 1999: 167–201

42. Keesey J. A treatment algortihm for autoimmune myasthenia in adults. Ann NY Acad Sci 1998;841:753–768

43. Drug Evaluations Annual. Milwaukee, Wisconsin: American Medical Association, 1995

44. Shapira M, Tur-Kaspa I, Bosgraaf L, et al. A transcription-activating polymorphism in the ACHE promoter associated with acute sensitivity to anti-acetylcholinesterases. Hum Mol Genet 2000;9:1273–1281

45. Engel AG, Lambert EH, Santa T. Study of long-term anticholinesterase therapy. Effects on neuromuscular transmission and on motor end-plate fine structure. Neurology 1973;23:1273–1281

46. Osserman KE. Symposium on myasthenia gravis: Progress report on mestinon bromide (pyridostigmine bromide). Am J Med 1955;19:737–739

47. Sghirlanzoni A, Pareyson D, Benvenuti C, et al. Efficacy of intranasal administration of neostigmine in myasthenic patients. J Neurol 1992; 239:165–169

48. Seybold ME, Drachman DB. Gradually increasing doses of prednisone in myasthenia gravis. Reducing the hazards of treatment. N Engl J Med 1974;290:81–84

49. Engel WK, Festoff BW, Patten BM, et al. Myasthenia gravis. Ann Intern Med 1974;81:225–246

50. Sghirlanzoni A, Peluchetti D, Mantegazza R, et al. Myasthenia gravis: prolonged treatment with steroids. Neurology 1984;34:170–174

51. Manipulation of the immune response. *In:* Janeway CA Jr, Travers P, Walport M, Capra JD, eds. Immunobiology: The Immune System in Health and Disease. 4th ed. New York: Elsevier, 1999:537–578

52. Kaplan I, Blakely BT, Pavlath GK, et al. Steroids induce acetylcholine receptors on cultured human muscle: implications for myasthenia gravis. Proc Natl Acad Sci 1990;87:8100–8104

53. Seybold ME, Lindstrom JM. Patterns of acetylcholine receptor antibody fluctuation in myasthenia gravis. Ann NY Acad Sci 1981;377:292–306

54. Oosterhuis HJ, Limburg PC, Hummel-Tappel E, The TH. Anti-acetylcholine receptor antibodies in myasthenia gravis. Part 2. Clinical and serological follow-up of individual patients. J Neurol Sci 1983;58:371–385

55. Evoli A, Batocchi AP, Palmisani MT, et al. Long-term results of corticosteroid therapy in patients with myasthenia gravis. Eur Neurol 1992;32:37–43

56. Cosi V, Citterio A, Lombardi M, et al. Effectiveness of steroid treatment in myasthenia gravis: a retrospective study. Acta Neurol Scand 1991;84:33–39

57. Tindall RS. Humoral immunity in myasthenia gravis: effect of steroids and thymectomy. Neurology 1980;30: 554–557

58. Yale SH, Limper AH. Pneumocystis carinii pneumonia in patients without acquired immunodeficiency syndrome: associated illness and prior corticosteroid therapy. Mayo Clin Proc 1996;71:5–13

59. Mertens HG, Hertel G, Reuther P, Ricker K. Effect of immunosuppressive drugs (azathioprine). Ann NY Acad Sci 1981;377:691–699

60. Mantegazza R, Antozzi C, Peluchetti D, et al. Azathioprine as a single drug or in combination with steroids in the treatment of myasthenia gravis. J Neurol 1988;235:449–453

61. Myasthenia Gravis Clinical Study Group. A randomised clinical trial comparing prednisone and azathioprine in myasthenia gravis. Results of the second interim analysis. J Neurol Neurosurg Psychiatry 1993;56:1157–1163

62. Hohlfeld R, Michels M, Heininger K, et al. Azathioprine toxicity during long-term immunosuppression of generalized myasthenia gravis. Neurology 1988;38: 258–261

63. Lennard L, Van Loon JA, Weinshilboum RM. Pharmacogenetics of acute azathioprine toxicity: relationship to thiopurine methyltransferase genetic polymorphism. Clin Pharmacol Ther 1989;46:149–154

64. Vuchetich JP, Weinshilboum RM, Price RA. Segregation analysis of human red blood cell thiopurine methyltransferase activity. Genet Epidemiol 1995;12: 1–11

65. Perez MC, Buot WL, Mercado-Danguilan C, et al. Stable remissions in myasthenia gravis. Neurology 1981;31:32–37

66. Niakan E, Harati Y, Rolak LA. Immunosuppressive drug therapy in myasthenia gravis. Arch Neurol 1986;43:155–156

67. Nyberg-Hansen R, Gjerstad L. Myasthenia gravis treated with cyclosporin. Acta Neurol Scand 1988;77: 307–313

68. Goulon M, Elkharrat D, Gajdos P. Treatment of severe myasthenia gravis with cyclosporin. A 12-month open trial [French]. Presse Med 1989;18:341–346

69. Bonifati DM, Angelini C. Long-term cyclosporine treatment in a group of severe myasthenia gravis patients. J Neurol 1997;244:542–547

70. Ciafaloni E, Nikhar NK, Massey JM, Sanders DB. Retrospective analysis of the use of cyclosporine in myasthenia gravis. Neurology 2000;55:448–450

71. Allison AC, Eugui EM. Mycophenolate mofetil and its mechanisms of action. Immunopharmacology 2000;47: 85–118

72. Hauser RA, Malek AR, Rosen R. Successful treatment of a patient with severe refractory myasthenia gravis using mycophenolate mofetil. Neurology 1998;51: 912–913

73. Ciafaloni E, Massey JM, Tucker-Lipscomb B, Sanders DB. Mycophenolate mofetil for myasthenia gravis: an open-label pilot study. Neurology 2001;56:97–99

74. Meriggioli MN, Rowin J. Treatment of myasthenia gravis with mycophenolate mofetil: a case report. Muscle Nerve 2000;23:1287–1289

75. Chaudhry V, Cornblath DR, Griffin JW, et al. Mycophenolate mofetil: a safe and promising immunosuppressant in neuromuscular diseases. Neurology 2001;56:94–96

76. Simmons WD, Rayhill SC, Sollinger HW. Preliminary risk-benefit assessment of mycophenolate mofetil in transplant rejection. Drug Saf 1997;17:75–92

77. Waiser J, Schotschel R, Budde K, Neumayer HH. Reactivation of tuberculosis after conversion from azathioprine to mycophenolate mofetil 16 years after renal transplantation. Am J Kidney Dis 2000;35:E12

78. Moreso F, Seron D, Morales JM, et al. Incidence of leukopenia and cytomegalovirus disease in kidney transplants treated with mycophenolate mofetil combined with low cyclosporine and steroid doses. Clin Transplant 1998;12:198–205

79. Report of the Therapeutics and Technology Assessment Subcommittee of the American Academy of Neurology. Assessment of plasmapheresis. Neurology 1996;47:840–843

80. Yeh JH, Chiu HC. Plasmapheresis in myasthenia gravis. A comparative study of daily versus alternately daily schedule. Acta Neurol Scand 1999;99:147–151

81. Hawkey CJ, Newsom-Davis J, Vincent A. Plasma exchange and immunosuppressive drug treatment in myasthenia gravis: no evidence for synergy. J Neurol Neurosurg Psychiatry 1981;44:469–475

82. Grob D, Simpson D, Mitsumoto H, et al. Treatment of myasthenia gravis by immunoadsorption of plasma. Neurology 1995;45:338–344

83. Howard JF Jr. Intravenous immunoglobulin for the treatment of acquired myasthenia gravis. Neurology 1998;51(Suppl 5):S30–S36

84. Arsura E. Experience with intravenous immunoglobulin in myasthenia gravis. Clin Immunol Immunopathol 1989;53:S170–S179

85. Qureshi AI, Choudhry MA, Akbar MS, et al. Plasma exchange versus intravenous immunoglobulin treatment in myasthenic crisis. Neurology 1999;52:629–632

86. Brannagan TH 3rd, Nagle KJ, Lange DJ, Rowland LP. Complications of intravenous immune globulin treatment in neurologic disease. Neurology 1996;47:674–677

87. Stangel M, Hartung HP, Marx P, Gold R. Intravenous immunoglobulin treatment of neurological autoimmune diseases. J Neurol Sci 1998;153:203–214

88. Blalock A. Thymectomy in the treatment of myasthenia gravis: Report of 20 cases. J Thorac Surg 1944;13: 316–339

89. Schwab RS, Leland CC. Sex and age in myasthenia gravis as critical factors in incidence and remission. JAMA 1953;153:1270–1273

90. Eaton LM, Clagett OT. Symposium on myasthenia gravis: present status of thymectomy in treatment of myasthenia gravis. Am J Med 1955;19:703–717

91. Horowitz SH, Genkins G, Papatestas AE, Kornfeld P. Electrophysiologic evaluations of thymectomy in myasthenia gravis. Preliminary findings. Neurology 1976;26:615–619

92. Penn AS, Jaretzki A 3rd, Wolff M, et al. Thymic abnormalities: antigen or antibody? Response to thymectomy in myasthenia gravis. Ann NY Acad Sci 1981;377: 786–804

93. Papatestas AE, Genkins G, Kornfeld P, et al. Effects of thymectomy in myasthenia gravis. Ann Surg 1987;206: 79–88

94. Mulder DG, Graves M, Herrmann C. Thymectomy for myasthenia gravis: recent observations and comparisons with past experience. Ann Thorac Surg 1989;48: 551–555

95. Evoli A, Batocchi AP, Provenzano C, Taylor WF. Thymectomy in the treatment of myasthenia gravis: report of 247 patients. J Neurol 1988;235:272–276

96. Rodriguez M, Gomez MR, Howard FM Jr, Taylor WF. Myasthenia gravis in children: long-term follow-up. Ann Neurol 1983;13:504–510

97. Batocchi AP, Evoli A, Palmisani MT, et al. Early-onset myasthenia gravis: clinical characteristics and response to therapy. Eur J Pediatr 1990;150:66–68

98. Schumm F, Wietholter H, Fateh-Moghadam A, Dichgans J. Thymectomy in myasthenia with pure ocular symptoms. J Neurol Neurosurg Psychiatry 1985;48: 332–337

99. Lanska DJ. Indications for thymectomy in myasthenia gravis. Neurology 1990;40:1828–1829

100. Jaretzki A 3rd, Penn AS, Younger DS, et al. "Maximal" thymectomy for myasthenia gravis. Results. J Thorac Cardiovasc Surg 1988;95:747–757

101. Bulkley GB, Bass KN, Stephenson GR, et al. Extended cervicomediastinal thymectomy in the integrated management of myasthenia gravis. Ann Surg 1997;226: 324–334

102. Werneck LC, Cunha FM, Scola RH. Myasthenia gravis: a restrospective study comparing thymectomy to conservative treatment. Acta Neurol Scand 2000;101: 41–46

103. Gronseth GS, Barohn RJ. Practice parameter: thymectomy for autoimmune myasthenia gravis (an evidence-based review): Report of the Quality Standards Subcommittee of the American Academy of Neurology. Neurology 2000;55:7–15

104. Daroff RB. Ocular myasthenia: diagnosis and therapy. In: Glaser J, ed. Neuro-Opthalmology. St. Louis: C.V. Mosby, 2001:62–71

105. Castronuovo S, Krohel GB, Kristan RW. Blepharoptosis in myasthenia gravis. Ann Opthalmol 1983;15: 751–754

106. Bradley EA, Bartley GB, Chapman KL, Waller RR. Surgical correction of blepharoptosis in patients with myasthenia gravis. Trans Am Ophthalmol Soc 2000;98:173–180

107. Kupersmith MJ, Moster M, Bhuiyan S, et al. Beneficial effects of corticosteroids on ocular myasthenia gravis. Arch Neurol 1996;53:802–804

108. Sommer N, Sigg B, Melms A, et al. Ocular myasthenia gravis: response to long-term immunosuppressive treatment. J Neurol Neurosurg Psychiatry 1997;62:156–162

109. Grob D, Brunner NG, Namba T. The natural course of myasthenia gravis and effect of therapeutic measures. Ann NY Acad Sci 1981;377:652–669

110. Evoli A, Batocchi AP, Minisci C, et al. Therapeutic options in ocular myasthenia gravis. Neuromuscul Disord 2001;11:208–216

111. Soliven BC, Lange DJ, Penn AS, et al. Seronegative myasthenia gravis. Neurology 1988;38:514–517

112. Verma PK, Oger JJ. Seronegative generalized myasthenia gravis: low frequency of thymic pathology. Neurology 1992;42:586–589

113. Evoli A, Batocchi AP, Lo Monaco M, et al. Clinical heterogeneity of seronegative myasthenia gravis. Neuromuscul Disord 1996;6:155–161

114. Redman RS, Silinsky EM. Decrease in calcium currents induced by aminoglycoside antibiotics in frog motor nerve endings. Br J Pharmacol 1994;113:375–378

115. Elmqvist D, Josefsson JO. The nature of the neuromus-

116. Argov Z, Brenner T, Abramsky O. Ampicillin may aggravate clinical and experimental myasthenia gravis. Arch Neurol 1986;43:255–256

117. May EF, Calvert PC. Aggravation of myasthenia gravis by erythromycin. Ann Neurol 1990;28:577–579

118. Osserman KE. Myasthenia Gravis. New York: Grune & Stratton, 1958.

119. Kornfeld P, Horowitz SH, Genkins G, Papatestas AE. Myasthenia gravis unmasked by antiarrhythmic agents. Mt Sinai J Med 1976;43:10–14

120. Sieb JP, Milone M, Engel AG. Effects of the quinoline derivatives quinine, quinidine, and chloroquine on neuromuscular transmission. Brain Res 1996;712:179–189

121. Herishanu Y, Rosenberg P. Letter: beta-blockers and myasthenia gravis. Ann Intern Med 1975;83:834–835

122. Confavreux C, Charles N, Aimard G. Fulminant myasthenia gravis soon after initiation of acebutolol therapy. Eur Neurol 1990;30:279–281

123. Boneva N, Brenner T, Argov Z. Gabapentin may be hazardous in myasthenia gravis. Muscle Nerve 2000; 23:1204–1208

124. Nordenbo AM, Somnier FE. Acute deterioration of myasthenia gravis after intravenous administration of gadolinium-DTPA. Lancet 1992;340:1168

125. Wittbrodt ET. Drugs and myasthenia gravis. An update. Arch Intern Med 1997;157:399–408

126. Anderson HJ, Churchill-Davidson HC, Richardson AT. Bronchial neoplasm with myasthenia: prolonged apnoea after administration of succinylcholine. Lancet 1953;ii:1291–1293

127. Lambert EH, Eaton LM, Rooke ED. Defect of neuromuscular transmission associated with malignant neoplasm. Am J Physiol 1956;187:612–613

128. Eaton LM, Lambert EH. Electromyography and electric stimulation of nerves in diseases of motor unit: observations on myasthenic syndrome associated with malignant tumors. JAMA 1957;163:1117–1124

129. Elmqvist D, Lambert EH. Detailed analysis of neuromuscular transmission in a patient with the myasthenic syndrome sometimes associated with bronchogenic carcinoma. Mayo Clin Proc 1968;43:689–713

130. Lang B, Newsom-Davis J, Wray D, et al. Autoimmune aetiology for myasthenic (Eaton-Lambert) syndrome. Lancet 1981;ii:224–226

131. Fukunaga H, Engel AG, Lang B, et al. Passive transfer of Lambert-Eaton myasthenic syndrome with IgG from man to mouse depletes the presynaptic membrane active zones. Proc Natl Acad Sci USA 1983;80: 7636–7640

132. Newsom-Davis J, Lang B. The Lambert-Eaton myasthenic syndrome. In: Engel AG, ed. Myasthenia Gravis and Myasthenic Disorders. New York: Oxford University Press, 1999:205–228

133. O'Neill JH, Murray NM, Newsom-Davis J. The Lambert-Eaton myasthenic syndrome. A review of 50 cases. Brain 1988;111:577–596

134. Gutmann L, Phillips LH 2nd. Trends in the association of Lambert-Eaton myasthenic syndrome with carcinoma. Neurology 1992;42:848–850

135. Engel AG. Myasthenic syndromes. In: Engel AG, Franzini-Armstrong C, eds. Myology. Vol 2, 2nd ed. New York: McGraw-Hill, 1994:1798–1835

136. Fukuoka T, Engel AG, Lang B, et al. Lambert-Eaton myasthenic syndrome: II. Immunoelectron microscopy localization of IgG at the mouse motor end-plate. Ann Neurol 1987;22:200–211

137. Nagel A, Engel AG, Lang B, et al. Lambert-Eaton myasthenic syndrome IgG depletes presynaptic membrane active zone particles by antigenic modulation. Ann Neurol 1988;24:552–558

138. Lambert EH, Elmqvist D. Quantal components of endplate potentials in the myasthenic syndrome. Ann NY Acad Sci 1971;183:183–199

139. Waterman SA, Lang B, Newsom-Davis J. Effect of Lambert-Eaton myasthenic syndrome antibodies on autonomic neurons in the mouse. Ann Neurol 1997;42:147–156

140. Motomura M, Johnston I, Lang B, et al. An improved diagnostic assay for Lambert-Eaton myasthenic syndrome. J Neurol Neurosurg Psychiatry 1995;58:85–87

141. Newsom-Davis J, Leys K, Vincent A, et al. Immunological evidence for the co-existence of the Lambert-Eaton myasthenic syndrome and myasthenia gravis in two patients. J Neurol Neurosurg Psychiatry 1991;54:452–453

142. Cull-Candy SG, Lundh H, Thesleff S. Effects of botulinum toxin on neuromuscular transmission in the rat. J Physiol 1976;260:177–203

143. del Castillo J, Engbaek L. The nature of neuromuscular block caused by magnesium. J Physiol (Lond) 1954;124:370–384

144. Swift TR. Weakness from magnesium-containing cathartics: electrophysiologic studies. Muscle Nerve 1979;2:295–298

145. Lambert EH, Rooke ED, Eaton LM, Hodgson CH. Myasthenic syndrome occasionally associated with bronchial neoplasm: neurophysiologic studies. In: Viets HR, ed. Proceedings: International Symposium on Myasthenia Gravis. Springfield, IL: Charles C. Thomas, 1961:362–410

146. Kamenskaya MA, Elmqvist D, Thesleff S. Guanidine and neuromuscular transmission. II. Effect on transmitter release in response to repetitive nerve stimulation. Arch Neurol 1975;32:510–518

147. Lambert EH, Rooke ED. Myasthenic state and lung cancer. In: Brain WR, Norris FH Jr, eds. The Remote Effects of Cancer on the Nervous System. New York: Grune & Stratton, 1965:67–80

148. Minot AS, Dodd K, Riven SS. Use of guanidine hydrochloride in the treatment of myasthenia gravis. JAMA 1939;113:553–559

149. Norris FH Jr, Calanchini PR, Fallat RJ, et al. The administration of guanidine in amyotrophic lateral sclerosis. Neurology 1974;24:721–728

150. Cherington M. Guanidine and germine in Eaton-Lambert syndrome. Neurology 1976;26:944–946

151. Maeno T. Kinetic analysis of a large facilitatory action of 4-aminopyridine on the motor nerve terminal of the neuromuscular junction. Proc Jpn Acad 1980;56:241–245

152. Saint DA. The effects of 4-aminopyridine and tetraethylammonium on the kinetics of transmitter release at the mammalian neuromuscular synapse. Can J Physiol Pharmacol 1989;67:1045–1050

153. Lundh H, Nilsson O, Rosen I. Treatment of Lambert-Eaton syndrome: 3,4-diaminopyridine and pyridostigmine. Neurology 1984;34:1324–1330

154. McEvoy KM, Windebank AJ, Daube JR, Low PA. 3,4-Diaminopyridine in the treatment of Lambert-Eaton myasthenic syndrome. N Engl J Med 1989;321:1567–1571

155. Lundh H, Nilsson O, Rosen I, Johansson S. Practical aspects of 3,4-diaminopyridine treatment of the Lambert-Eaton myasthenic syndrome. Acta Neurol Scand 1993;88:136–140

156. Sanders DB, Massey JM, Sanders LL, Edwards LJ. A randomized trial of 3,4-diaminopyridine in Lambert-Eaton myasthenic syndrome. Neurology 2000;54:603–607

157. Sanders DB, Howard JF Jr, Massey JM. 3,4-Diaminopyridine in Lambert-Eaton myasthenic syndrome and myasthenia gravis. Ann NY Acad Sci 1993;681:588–590

158. Newsom-Davis J, Murray NM. Plasma exchange and immunosuppressive drug treatment in the Lambert-Eaton myasthenic syndrome. Neurology 1984;34:480–485

159. Bird SJ. Clinical and electrophysiologic improvement in Lambert-Eaton syndrome with intravenous immunoglobulin therapy. Neurology 1992;42:1422–1423

160. Rothbart HB. Myasthenia gravis in children: its familial incidence. JAMA 1937;108:715–717

161. Bundey S. A genetic study of infantile and juvenile myasthenia gravis. J Neurol Neurosurg Psychiatry 1972;35:41–51

162. Engel AG, Ohno K, Sine SM. Congenital myasthenic syndromes. In: Engel AG, ed. Myasthenia Gravis and Myasthenic Disorders. New York: Oxford University Press, 1999:251–297

163. Ohno K, Anlar B, Ozdirim E, et al. Myasthenic syndromes in Turkish kinships due to mutations in the acetylcholine receptor. Ann Neurol 1998;44:234–241

164. Middleton L, Ohno K, Christodoulou K, et al. Chromosome 17p-linked myasthenias stem from defects in the acetylcholine receptor epsilon-subunit gene. Neurology 1999;53:1076–1082

165. Engel AG, Lambert EH, Mulder DM, et al. A newly recognized congenital myasthenic syndrome attributed to a prolonged open time of the acetylcholine-induced ion channel. Ann Neurol 1982;11:553–569

166. Ohno K, Tsujino A, Brengman JM, et al. Choline acetyltransferase mutations cause myasthenic syndrome associated with episodic apnea in humans. Proc Natl Acad Sci USA 2001;98:2017–2022

167. McQuillen MP. Familial limb-girdle myasthenia. Brain 1966;89:121–132

168. Goldhammer Y, Blatt I, Sadeh M, Goodman RM. Congenital myasthenia associated with facial malformations in Iraqi and Iranian Jews. A new genetic syndrome. Brain 1990;113:1291–1306

169. Hutchinson DO, Walls TJ, Nakano S, et al. Congenital endplate acetylcholinesterase deficiency. Brain 1993;116:633–653

170. Fukudome T, Ohno K, Brengman JM, Engel AG. Quinidine normalizes the open duration of slow-channel mutants of the acetylcholine receptor. Neuroreport 1998;9:1907–1911

171. Breningstall GN, Kurachek SC, Fugate JH, Engel AG. Treatment of congenital endplate acetylcholinesterase deficiency by neuromuscular blockade. J Child Neurol 1996;11:345–346

172. Harper CM, Engel AG. Quinidine sulfate therapy for the slow-channel congenital myasthenic syndrome. Ann Neurol 1998;43:480–484

173. Harper CM, Engel AG. Treatment of 31 congenital myasthenic syndrome (CMS) patients with 3,4-diaminopyridine (DAP) (abstract). Neurology 2000;54(Suppl 3): A395

174. Palace J, Wiles CM, Newsom-Davis J. 3,4-Diaminopyridine in the treatment of congenital (hereditary) myasthenia. J Neurol Neurosurg Psychiatry 1991;54:1069–1072

175. Anlar B, Varli K, Ozdirim E, Ertan M. 3,4-Diaminopyridine in childhood myasthenia: double-blind, placebo-controlled trial. J Child Neurol 1996;11:458–461

227 Malignant Hyperthermia

Denise J Wedel

History

Early historical descriptions of conditions consistent with the diagnosis of malignant hyperthermia (MH) can be found in the literature. In 1929, a French pathologist described postoperative pallor and hyperthermia associated with high mortality in children. However, these findings were not linked with a genetic trait.[1] In 1960, Denborough and Lovell[2] first reported deaths that occurred during general anesthesia and had a familial association. A young man with a rugby-induced tibial fracture that required open reduction expressed fear about ether anesthesia because several members of his family had died during surgery. He was reassured that ether would be avoided; instead, he was anesthetized with the newly available volatile gas anesthetic halothane. The patient developed fulminant MH, but with symptomatic therapy, he survived. In retrospect, his survival was fortuitous, because before the use of dantrolene, the mortality of fulminant MH was approximately 70% to 80%.

In 1969, Kalow et al.[3] studied a small community in Wisconsin where an unusually high number of anesthetic-related deaths associated with hyperthermia occurred. They reported a metabolic error of muscle metabolism associated with decreased threshold contracture responses in skeletal muscle samples from patients who had recovered from episodes of MH. This discovery formed the basis of diagnostic contracture testing, still the "gold standard" for MH diagnosis.

In 1975, Harrison[4] reported the efficacy of dantrolene in treating porcine MH. Dantrolene sodium was approved by the United States Food and Drug Administration (FDA) in the early 1980s and is the mainstay in MH treatment. Its efficacy when given early has been reviewed by Kolb et al.[5]

Incidence and mortality

MH is an inherited disorder of skeletal muscle that affects humans and certain strains of animals, primarily swine. The reported incidence of MH ranges from 1:4500 anesthetics (when succinylcholine is used) to 1:60 000 anesthetics involving MH triggers. The incidence varies depending on the prevalence of the gene(s) for MH in a geographic area, but MH is reported worldwide and affects all racial groups.

MH is rare in infants, and the incidence decreases after age 50 years. Most cases occur in children and young adults, and males are affected more frequently than females. Neonatal piglets have a lower frequency of halothane-triggered MH than 4-week-old and older piglets according to in vivo and in vitro (muscle

strips) studies.[5] The reason for this age-related difference in sensitivity is not understood.

MH is associated with central core disease and King-Denborough syndrome (short stature, musculoskeletal abnormalities, and mental retardation). Whether it is associated with other myopathies such as Duchenne muscular dystrophy is more controversial. Evidence for an association with congenital muscular defects, sudden infant death syndrome, neuroleptic malignant syndrome, or sudden death in adults is weak or nonexistent.[6]

Before the introduction of dantrolene, the mortality rate was approximately 80%, but this has decreased to about 10%. Most fatal cases are either extremely fulminant or MH is diagnosed too late for dantrolene to be effective. Many hospitals, free-standing ambulatory centers, and office-based practices still do not stock intravenous dantrolene.

Approximately 50% of MH-susceptible persons have had a previous triggering anesthetic without MH developing.[7] In an animal model, several factors prevent or delay MH triggering, including cool ambient temperatures in the operating room, use of nontriggering agents that delay onset of MH (e.g., sodium pentothal, narcotics, or nondepolarizing muscle relaxants), and short anesthetic exposure.[8,9] Individual responses may be affected by variable gene penetrance and other undetermined genetic or environmental factors.[10,11] Also, a previous occurrence of MH may have been overlooked because of inadequate monitoring or nonfulminant clinical expression.

Pathophysiology

In humans, MH is a subclinical myopathy that manifests on exposure to triggering agents. When this occurs, there is uninhibited release of free ionized calcium from the sarcoplasmic reticulum, the main intracellular storage site, into the myofilament space. Aerobic and anaerobic metabolism increase, thus providing ATP to fuel the pumps that maintain calcium balance and resulting in increased heat production. Moreover, the high intracellular levels of calcium uncouple oxidative phosphorylation, resulting in uncontrolled thermogenesis. The rigidity associated with MH results from high levels of myofibrillar calcium reaching contracture threshold. The sarcoplasmic reticulum, and more specifically its calcium release channel (also referred to as the ryanodine receptor), has been studied extensively to identify more precisely the mechanism that triggers MH. However, the varied clinical syndrome and complex genetic inheritance suggest that a simple solution is unlikely. More recently, the role of second messengers and modulators of calcium release have been implicated, and there is evidence that the sodium channel may contribute to the pathophysiological mechanism of MH. The physiology and structure of the sarcoplasmic reticulum calcium release channel has been reviewed elsewhere.[12,13]

Genetics

In humans, MH is transmitted by autosomal dominant inheritance with variable expression. However, MH-susceptible swine have an autosomal recessive pattern of inheritance. The rate of spontaneous mutation is unknown. Studies of large MH-affected populations have indicated that several mutations of the gene encoding the ryanodine receptor (*RYR1* on chromosome 19q12-13.2) and genes on chromosomes 17, 1, 3, and 7 can result in MH. This may explain why the expression of MH is so variable.[14]

The initial reports that identified a specific base pair alteration (Arg615Cys) in *RYR1* of swine raised hope that a specific DNA test would be available for diagnosing human MH,[15–17] but this mutation is now known to occur in fewer than 10% of human MH families.[17] Several different mutations of *RYR1* (more than 20 by recent count) have been demonstrated in humans, some affecting only one family, but these mutations do not account for the majority of persons affected with MH. In studies of 109 persons from 25 families affected with *RYR1* mutations, the concordance between genetic testing and in vitro contracture responses was excellent (98.5% sensitivity, 81.8% specificity).[18] Although the genotypic variability is discouraging, it is not unexpected because of the clinical variability of MH and the complexity of intracellular calcium control.

In summary, MH is a heterogeneous genetic disorder with a highly variable clinical presentation. Hence, the prospect of a widely, clinically applicable DNA test for MH in the near future is unlikely.

Clinical presentation

MH is characterized by a hypermetabolic response to triggering anesthetic agents. Although the reaction can be variable in onset and severity, increased carbon dioxide production, increased oxygen consumption, acid-base disturbance (combined metabolic and respiratory acidosis), and rhabdomyolysis are present to some degree.

The onset of MH can be acute and fulminant or delayed and covert. It can occur at any time during the anesthesia and even as late as 24 hours postoperatively. A subacute episode may regress with discontinuation of the anesthetic, but even in this case, dantrolene therapy is advisable because of possible recrudescence.[19]

Trismus provoked by succinylcholine is observed less frequently than previously because it is used less often in children during induction of volatile gas anesthesia. Of the patients in whom trismus or masseter muscle rigidity develops, 50% test positively on the in vitro contracture test for MH.[20–22] Although trismus usually does not progress to fulminant MH,

Table 227.1 Signs and symptoms of malignant hyperthermia

Increased end-tidal CO_2
Tachypnea
Muscle rigidity
Rhabdomyolysis
Hyperthermia
Sympathetic hyperactivity
    Tachycardia
    Dysrhythmias
    Sweating
    Hypertension
Late complications
    Muscle edema
    Cerebral edema
    Cardiac arrest
    Renal failure

patients in whom trismus develops must be observed closely for evidence of hypermetabolism as well as rhabdomyolysis, which can be severe. Despite reports of safely continuing triggering anesthesia after trismus, the risk of fulminant MH developing after trismus is significant. Therefore, the triggering agent should be stopped when trismus occurs.

The rare occurrence of life-threatening hyperkalemia after the administration of succinylcholine in young males with undiagnosed Duchenne muscular dystrophy led to the 1992 FDA recommendation that succinylcholine be avoided in children unless specifically indicated. When cardiac arrest occurs after the administration of succinylcholine in a male child, hyperkalemia should be assumed and treated along with MH. If possible, a muscle sample should be obtained for histological examination and dystrophin studies.[23]

Follow-up for trismus or succinylcholine-induced rhabdomyolysis of any cause should include serial measurements of creatine kinase (CK) levels every 6 hours for up to 48 hours or until the levels begin to decrease. There is a high correlation with positive results on subsequent muscle contracture testing when the peak CK (usually at 12 to 18 hours) exceeds 20 000 IU/L.[24] These patients can have pronounced rhabdomyolysis, with increased urine and serum levels of myoglobin, and can require vigorous treatment with hydration and diuresis to prevent renal complications. Whether dantrolene should be administered when there are no signs of MH is a matter of controversy.

Signs and symptoms of MH reflect a state of highly increased metabolism (Table 227.1). Hyperthermia is often delayed; its absence should not delay treatment when other clinical signs are present. The earliest signs of MH include increased end-tidal levels of carbon dioxide, tachycardia, and tachypnea. Laboratory testing is essential to confirm the diagnosis (Table 227.2). Although arterial blood gas analysis usually is sufficient, comparison of arterial and mixed venous gases is preferred because the mixed venous sample reflects muscle effluent. The widening gap between venous and arterial carbon dioxide pressure

Table 227.2   **Supportive laboratory tests for confirmation of diagnosis of malignant hyperthermia**

Blood gas analysis
   Arterial
   Mixed venous
Serum creatine kinase every 6 hr for 24 hr
Myoglobin—serum and urine
Serum potassium, calcium, lactate
Prothrombin time, activated partial thromboplastin time,
   fibrin split products

during the early stages of MH is an early indication of the metabolic derangement occurring in skeletal muscle. Initially, oxygen consumption and cardiac output are increased in a healthy person because the metabolic rate is increased. In an untreated episode of MH, the process eventually outpaces the ability of the system to compensate, resulting ultimately in cardiac arrest with subsequent organ failure.

Other conditions that have hypermetabolism as an underlying mechanism can mimic MH. These include pheochromocytoma, hyperthyroidism, cocaine intoxication, and sepsis. The action of dantrolene is not well understood, and the response to treatment alone will not necessarily distinguish between these conditions and MH. Careful analysis of clinical signs and laboratory test results usually indicates the diagnosis, although this analysis is sometimes best done after the episode has been treated and the patient's status is stable clinically.

Triggers

An acute MH episode depends on three variables: 1) genetic predisposition, 2) presence of a triggering agent, and 3) absence or overriding of inhibitory factors. The only anesthetic agents known to trigger MH are the potent inhalation agents, including the newer agents sevoflurane and desflurane, and succinylcholine. Anesthetic and resuscitative agents safe to use in MH-susceptible patients are listed in Table 227.3. Controversy about the administration of catecholamines in MH-susceptible patients has been resolved, and these agents may also be included in the management of these patients.[25]

Treatment

The treatment plan recommended for incipient MH during general anesthesia is given in Table 227.4.

Table 227.3   **Safe anesthetic agents and resuscitative drugs for malignant hyperthermia-susceptible persons**

Barbiturates
Narcotics
Etomidate
Propofol
Ketamine
Nondepolarizing muscle relaxants
Nitrous oxide
Local anesthetics
Epinephrine and norepinephrine

Table 227.4   **Treatment plan for incipient malignant hyperthermia (MH) during general anesthesia**

An "MH cart" should be accessible in a central area (e.g., recovery room) and should contain dantrolene, sterile water for mixing, blood gas kits, resuscitation drugs, and other items such as laboratory order forms and MH protocol
Discontinue triggers and hyperventilate patient with 100% oxygen while instituting symptomatic treatment (Table 227.5)
When MH is suspected, give dantrolene early and rapidly. Initial dose, 2.5 mg/kg, can be repeated as needed until signs of MH abate. The recommended total dose is 10 mg/kg, but it can be exceeded safely.[26] If patient does not respond after receiving recommended maximal dose, consider alternative diagnoses
Avoid overcooling the patient. Usually, administration of dantrolene promptly decreases core temperature, so external cooling efforts must be monitored closely
After successful treatment, give dantrolene intravenously, 1 mg/kg every 6 hr for 24 hr. Observe patient's condition with appropriate laboratory testing for at least 24 to 48 hr after MH episode. Calcium channel blockers should not be given concomitantly with dantrolene because of the risk of life-threatening hyperkalemia and cardiovascular collapse[27,28]

Table 227.5   **Symptomatic treatment of malignant hyperthermia**

Cooling
   Surface (ice, cooling blanket)
   Central
      Intravenous iced saline
      Nasogastric and rectal lavage
      Intra-abdominal lavage
      Cardiac bypass
Sodium bicarbonate for metabolic acidosis
Antiarrhythmics
Management of hyperkalemia—insulin/glucose
Diuretics—mannitol, furosemide (dantrolene contains
   3 g mannitol per bottle)

Symptomatic treatment of MH is outlined in Table 227.5.

Dantrolene, a hydantoin derivative with a half-life of about 10 hours, is safe when administered intravenously in the recommended doses.[29–32] Side effects include nausea, malaise, light-headedness, muscle weakness, and irritation at the site of administration because of the high pH of the drug. Muscle weakness is usually peripheral and does not markedly affect respiration, although it may be a problem in newborns or debilitated patients. If possible, dantrolene should be avoided during obstetrical labor and delivery. Dantrolene contains a large amount of mannitol, which should be considered when treating patients with diuretics.

After the patient's condition is stable, genetic counseling should be offered to the family. Materials describing MH, contracture testing, safe anesthetic management in the operating room and the dental office, and patient support information are available from the Malignant Hyperthermia Association of the United States (MHAUS). Medical records should be marked clearly to avoid future exposure to triggering anesthetics, and the patient should be instructed to wear a medic alert bracelet or tag indicating susceptibility to MH. It is especially important that the familial nature of MH be explained to the patient and immediate family so that information about the reaction can be disseminated to other family members.

Anesthesia for patients known to be susceptible to malignant hyperthermia

Treatment with intravenous dantrolene is no longer recommended before the induction of anesthesia. Nontriggering anesthesia without pretreatment has not been associated with MH episodes. The anesthesia machine can be prepared by removing or completely draining all vaporizers, replacing rubber hoses and soda lime, and flushing with high-flow oxygen or air (10 L/min) for 10 minutes. If vaporizers are drained and left in place, the dials should be taped securely as a reminder that inhalation agents should not be delivered.

The standard intraoperative monitors, including end-tidal carbon dioxide and core temperature, are recommended for all patients.[33] Arterial and central venous monitoring are added as indicated by the surgical procedure or medical condition. Regional anesthesia is an excellent alternative when appropriate to the procedure, and all local anesthetics are safe. Exposure to potential contamination in the recovery room can be avoided by isolating the patient or by having the patient recover in the operating room before being taken directly to the ward, although these precautions may be unnecessarily conservative.

MH-susceptible patients can be managed as outpatients if the usual precautions are observed. Ambulatory centers should have dantrolene available in dosages sufficient to treat a fulminant episode in an adult. Postoperative observation can be managed according to the hospital protocol.

Evaluation of susceptibility

A patient with the diagnosis of possible MH susceptibility should be questioned carefully about any unexplained intraoperative deaths of family members, unexpected adverse events under anesthesia, heat stroke or heat intolerance, exercise-induced rhabdomyolysis, associated myopathies, a family or personal history of heavy musculature or muscle cramping, and minor muscle abnormalities such as ptosis, strabismus, or scoliosis.

Serum CK testing is nonspecific and insensitive. However, the serum level of CK is increased in 70% of MH-susceptible patients, a finding that is often consistent within a family. Although CK testing is not a good screening test, it can be of use in some situations. The test should be conducted with the patient fasting and without a history of recent muscle trauma. According to a recent study, 50% of patients with persistently increased serum levels of CK and no per-

sonal or family history of MH have a positive in vitro contracture test.[34] The authors recommended that these patients receive nontriggering anesthesia.

In vitro contracture testing with halothane, caffeine, and ryanodine on fresh muscle from the vastus lateralis is the only test currently accepted for diagnosis of MH susceptibility. The sensitivity is greater than 95% and the specificity is 80% to 85%. The muscle sample must be harvested at a biopsy center, of which there are fewer than 10 in North America. The North American biopsy centers have agreed to a standardized protocol.[35] Muscle from MH-susceptible persons is more sensitive to caffeine and develops larger contractures to halothane and ryanodine than that of normal persons. The addition of ryanodine contracture responses appears to add further sensitivity to the testing. The North American Malignant Hyperthermia Registry was created as a repository for patient and control data and is supported by the North American biopsy centers, general donations, and MHAUS.

Several tests have been proposed for MH susceptibility, but they have not been standardized or confirmed. These include histological examination of muscle without contracture testing, electromyography, skinned fiber testing, platelet ATP depletion, and calcium uptake from muscle strips.

Information sources

MHAUS is a lay organization that provides support for patients, physicians, and other health care providers. It publishes books, pamphlets, and a quarterly newsletter and sponsors a 24-hour hotline for assisting health care workers treating acute MH episodes and providing information to patients and health care workers about MH (Malignant Hyperthermia Association of the United States, 32 South Main Street, PO Box 1069, Sherburne, NY 13815, Phone 1-800-98-MHAUS [1-800-986-4287]). A fax-on-demand system has been introduced recently (1-800-440-9990). The MH hotline number is 1-800-MH-HYPER (1-800-644-9737). Current information on MH is available on the Internet at http://www.mhaus.org.

References

1. Ombrédanne L. De l'influence de l'anesthesique employé dans la genèse des accidents post-opératoires de pâleur-hyperthermie observés chez les nourrissons. Rev Med Fr 1929;10:617
2. Denborough MA, Lovell RRH. Anaesthetic deaths in a family (letter to the editor). Lancet 1960;2:45
3. Kalow W, Britt BA, Terreau ME, Haist C. Metabolic error of muscle metabolism after recovery from malignant hyperthermia. Lancet 1970;2:895–898
4. Harrison GG. Control of the malignant hyperpyrexic syndrome in MHS swine by dantrolene sodium. Br J Anaesth 1975;47:62–65
5. Kolb ME, Horne ML, Martz R. Dantrolene in human malignant hyperthermia. Anesthesiology 1982;56:254–262
6. Wedel DJ. The effect of age on the development of MH in susceptible piglets (abstract). Anesthesiology 1994;81:A426

7. Wedel DJ. Malignant hyperthermia and neuromuscular disease. Neuromuscul Disord 1992;2:157–164

8. Halsall PJ, Cain PA, Ellis FR. Retrospective analysis of anaesthetics received by patients before susceptibility to malignant hyperpyrexia was recognized. Br J Anaesth 1979;51:949–954

9. Nelson TE. Porcine malignant hyperthermia: critical temperatures for in vivo and in vitro responses. Anesthesiology 1990;73:449–454

10. Gronert GA, Milde JH. Variations in onset of porcine malignant hyperthermia. Anesth Analg 1981;60:499–503

11. Ellis FR, Cain PA, Harriman DGF. Multifactorial inheritance of malignant hyperthermia susceptibility. *In:* Aldrete JA, Britt BA eds., Malignant Hyperthermia. New York: Grune & Stratton, 1978, 329–338

12. Zucchi R, Ronca-Testoni S. The sarcoplasmic reticulum Ca^{2+} channel/ryanodine receptor: modulation by endogenous effectors, drugs and disease states. Pharmacol Rev 1997;49:1–51

13. Mickelson JR, Louis CF. Malignant hyperthermia: excitation-contraction coupling, Ca^{2+} release channel, and cell Ca^{2+} regulation defects. Physiol Rev 1996;76:537–592

14. Levitt RC, Nouri N, Jedlicka AE, et al. Evidence for genetic heterogeneity in malignant hyperthermia susceptibility. Genomics 1991;11:543–547

15. MacLennan DH, Duff C, Zorzato F, et al. Ryanodine receptor gene is a candidate for predisposition to malignant hyperthermia. Nature 1990;343:559–561

16. Fujii J, Otsu K, Zorzato F, et al. Identification of a mutation in porcine ryanodine receptor associated with malignant hyperthermia. Science 1991;253:448–451

17. McCarthy TV, Healy JM, Heffron JJ, et al. Localization of the malignant hyperthermia susceptibility locus to human chromosome 19q12-13.2. Nature 1990;343:562–564

18. Brandt A, Schleithoff L, Jurkat-Rott K, et al. Screening of the ryanodine receptor gene in 105 malignant hyperthermia families: novel mutations and concordance with the in vitro contracture test. Hum Mol Genet 1999;8:2055–2062

19. Short JA, Cooper CM. Suspected recurrence of malignant hyperthermia after post-extubation shivering in the intensive care unit, 18 h after tonsillectomy. Br J Anaesth 1999;82:945–947

20. Ellis FR, Halsall PJ. Suxamethonium spasm. A differential diagnostic conundrum. Br J Anaesth 1984;56:381–384

21. Flewellen EH, Nelson TE. Halothane-succinylcholine induced masseter spasm: indicative of malignant hyperthermia susceptibility? Anesth Analg 1984;63:693–697

22. Schwartz L, Rockoff MA, Koka BV. Masseter spasm with anesthesia: incidence and implications. Anesthesiology 1984;61:772–775

23. Farrell PT. Anaesthesia-induced rhabdomyolysis causing cardiac arrest: case report and review of anaesthesia and the dystrophinopathies. Anaesth Intensive Care 1994;22:597–601

24. Larach MG, Rosenberg H, Larach DR, Broennle AM. Prediction of malignant hyperthermia susceptibility by clinical signs. Anesthesiology 1987;66:547–550

25. Maccani RM, Wedel DJ, Hofer RE. Norepinephrine does not potentiate porcine malignant hyperthermia. Anesth Analg 1996;82:790–795

26. DeRuyter ML, Wedel DJ, Berge KH. Hyperthermia requiring prolonged administration of high-dose dantrolene in the postoperative period. Anesth Analg 1995;80:834–836

27. Flewellen EH, Nelson TE. Prophylactic and therapeutic doses of dantrolene for malignant hyperthermia. Anesthesiology 1984;61:477

28. Flewellen EH, Nelson TE, Jones WP, et al. Dantrolene dose response in awake man: implications for management of malignant hyperthermia. Anesthesiology 1983;59:275–280

29. Morgan KG, Bryant SH. The mechanism of action of dantrolene sodium. J Pharmacol Exp Ther 1977;201:138–147

30. Wedel DJ, Quinlan JG, Iaizzo PA. Clinical effects of intravenously administered dantrolene. Mayo Clin Proc 1995;70:241–246

31. Gronert GA, Ahern CP, Milde JH, White RD. Effect of CO_2, calcium, digoxin, and potassium on cardiac and skeletal muscle metabolism in malignant hyperthermia susceptible swine. Anesthesiology 1986;64:24–28

32. Saltzman LS, Kates RA, Corke BC, et al. Hyperkalemia and cardiovascular collapse after verapamil and dantrolene administration in swine. Anesth Analg 1984;63:473–478

33. Baumgarten RK, Reynolds WJ. Early detection of malignant hyperthermia. Anesthesiology 1985;63:123

34. Weglinski MR, Wedel DJ, Engel AG. Malignant hyperthermia testing in patients with persistently increased serum creatine kinase levels. Anesth Analg 1997;84:1038–1041

35. Larach MG. Standardization of the caffeine halothane muscle contracture test. North American Malignant Hyperthermia Group. Anesth Analg 1989;69:511–515

228 Stiff-Man Syndrome

Kathleen M McEvoy

Introduction

In 1956, Moersch and Woltman[1] described a syndrome of progressive muscular rigidity with superimposed painful spasms. They had observed 14 such cases at Mayo Clinic over 34 years and dubbed it "the stiff-man syndrome" (SMS). This term aptly described the clinical presentation of their patients as well as the predominant sex. Subsequent recognition of the higher proportion of females afflicted and the trend toward sex-neutral language have led many to adopt the less mellifluous term "stiff-person syndrome."

For many years the existence of SMS as a distinct clinical entity was doubted by many who believed that the symptoms were purely psychogenic. In 1988, Solimena et al.[2] published their report of glutamic acid decarboxylase (GAD) autoantibodies in a patient with SMS, diabetes mellitus, and epilepsy. With this, the recognition of SMS as an autoimmune neurological condition was established. The pathogenesis of SMS and the mechanism of action of these antibodies have been subjects of speculation and investigation.[3,4] In some cases SMS-like syndromes may be inflammatory,[5,6] paraneoplastic,[7,8] or congenital.[9]

Before the discovery of effective treatment, SMS could be incapacitating and even devastating. The "herculean" muscle spasms have been documented to fracture bones and to bend orthopedic pins. In 1963, Howard[10] discovered that diazepam, then newly available, remarkably reduced the muscular spasms and rigidity. The next major step in therapy followed the recognition of autoimmunity. Immunotherapy has proven in most cases to moderate but not to eliminate symptoms,[11,12] and other symptomatic measures remain an essential part of treatment.

Epidemiology

Documented SMS is rare, but the condition often goes unrecognized. Typically, diagnosis is delayed despite multiple medical evaluations, and the true prevalence is not known. By 1990, approximately 100 well-documented cases had been reported in the world literature. As with other autoimmune disorders, females are afflicted more often than males. The average age at onset is about 40 years, but SMS has been found in the pediatric age group. There appears to be no specific racial or geographic predominance.

Etiology

Typical SMS is thought to be autoimmune-mediated and to be associated with the tendency to organ-specific polyendocrine autoimmunity. The triggering agent for the autoimmune response is unknown, and there is little evidence for inflammation. Stiff-man variants may be paraneoplastic, and symptoms may result at least in part from encephalomyelitis rather than a specific pathogenetic immune attack. A congenital form of SMS has been described.[9]

Pathophysiology and pathogenesis

The pathogenesis of SMS is not clearly understood. It is tempting to postulate that GAD antibodies are pathogenetic, because theoretically they might interfere with the production of γ-aminobutyric acid (GABA), an inhibitory neurotransmitter. This has been shown to occur in vitro.[4] Because GAD is a cytoplasmic enzyme, the mechanism of antibody access is uncertain, but several groups have shown that antibodies may penetrate living cells, including neurons.[13] However, in one patient, GAD antibody levels remained elevated during successful immunosuppressive therapy, while T-cell reactivity diminished in correlation with the patient's symptoms.[14] This finding suggests that cell-mediated immunity may be pathogenetic.

The clinical manifestations of SMS are consistent with a disturbance in inhibitory neurotransmission in either the spinal cord or supraspinal regulatory pathways. Histopathological studies have shown reduced GABA in the brain and spinal cord.[15] Physiological studies in SMS patients have shown that the functioning of some GABA-ergic inhibitory circuits in the brain and spinal cord are impaired, but others may be spared.[16] In some systems, sparing may be due to colocalization of glycine, also an inhibitory neurotransmitter, but in other systems, it may reflect differing immunological specificities or accessibility of GAD to the antibody.

Like GAD, amphiphysin is a cytoplasmic enzyme in the nerve terminal. It may be involved in endocytosis of synaptic vesicles. In cases of paraneoplastic SMS, antibodies to amphiphysin may be pathogenetic. However, they have been described in paraneoplastic cases with other neurological manifestations but without rigidity.[17] Autoimmunity in many paraneoplastic syndromes may be cell-mediated, perhaps triggered by antibody-specific T-cell responses.[18] Pathology studies of cases of paraneoplastic SMS have demonstrated inflammation (paraneoplastic encephalomyelitis),[19] and the associated neuronal cell loss may represent the actual pathogenetic mechanism. Indeed, the pathology findings in paraneoplastic encephalomyelitis are similar to those of progressive encephalomyelitis with rigidity.[15,19]

Progressive encephalomyelitis with rigidity

generally has not been recognized to be paraneoplastic. Most cases that have been described have been fairly rapidly fatal, and no underlying tumor has been noted at autopsy. Inflammation and neuronal loss are particularly prominent in the brainstem and spinal cord. The rigidity may be due to depletion of spinal inhibitory interneurons or to cell loss in inhibitory centers in the brainstem. A few cases have prolonged survival, are tumor-free, and may develop brainstem myoclonus, so-called jerking stiff-man.[5]

Genetics

Patients with SMS often have a personal and family history of organ-specific autoimmune disorders and the associated autoantibodies. The predisposition to type 1 diabetes mellitus is especially strong. The *DQB1*0201* allele, a known susceptibility allele for type 1 diabetes mellitus and other autoimmune disorders, is present in 72% of SMS patients (versus 38% of controls).[20] The additional presence of *0602*-related alleles in some patients may protect them from the development of diabetes.

Clinical features

Axial muscular rigidity with secondary spinal deformity, usually lumbar hyperlordosis, is typically the initial feature, with subsequent development of superimposed painful spasms and muscular hypertrophy.[1] Less commonly, symptoms may begin in one limb and, after months or years, spread to the trunk. Onset is usually insidious, and the progression of symptoms is fairly gradual over months or years, typically reaching a plateau. Spontaneous flares or remissions do not occur, although exogenous factors may exacerbate symptoms.

Patients complain mainly of axial stiffness and aching, difficulties with gait and mobility, and painful muscle spasms. The spasms are often startle-induced in response to an unexpected noise or touch or they may be triggered by a sudden movement. They produce widespread stiffness, sometimes spasmodic. Because they render the person totally unable to call upon compensatory postural reflexes, falls with injuries are common. Emotional stimuli and cold exposure typically aggravate stiffness and spasms. Alcohol consumption may reduce symptoms.

Untreated SMS may be devastating. Even with aggressive treatment, many patients are markedly limited in their mobility and lifestyle, but most remain ambulatory and lifespan is not curtailed.

Muscular rigidity produces hypertrophy of paraspinal and abdominal muscles, with exaggerated lumbar lordosis (or a "hunching" of the shoulders in the upper axial form of the disease). This deformity tends to be fixed, even with the person supine, and may be present during sleep, despite cessation of muscle activity. Spinal motion is severely limited, so that bending occurs exclusively at the hips. Arising from a supine or sitting position is slow and ungainly, and getting up off the floor is nearly if not entirely impossible. Volitional movement is difficult. Gait is characteristically stiff, slow, and robotic. Fear of

falling, although well founded, often adds to the limitation.

Apart from these findings directly related to muscular hyperactivity, the findings on neurological examination are usually normal, although hyper-reflexia is common, and extensor toe signs may be seen occasionally. Cerebellar findings are sometimes present in otherwise typical SMS. A pure cerebellar syndrome has been described in association with GAD antibodies,[21] suggesting that there may be a common pathogenesis.

Classification

SMS remains a clinical diagnosis. The typical (truncal) form has been strictly defined.[22] Until the pathophysiological mechanisms are completely understood and diagnosis is made on this basis, there will be some blurring of the distinction between subtypes of SMS and other disorders that may simulate SMS.

Disorders in the SMS spectrum may be classified as typical SMS, focal SMS (stiff-limb syndrome), paraneoplastic stiff-man, or progressive encephalomyelitis with rigidity. The term *stiff-man plus* has been used to describe patients with additional neurological signs or focal manifestations.[23] It might best be used to describe patients with typical SMS plus signs that may be thought to result directly from the GAD antibodies, such as cerebellar signs. It seems erroneous to use it for conditions thought to have an altogether different underlying pathophysiological mechanism or for what might be considered partial, focal manifestations of otherwise typical SMS ("stiff-man minus"?).

Because of the high rate of antibody negativity in some series,[24,25] it has been suggested that there is an "idiopathic" form of typical SMS, which may not be immune-mediated. Diagnostic details are not always clear, however, and in some series with a uniform in-house clinical assessment, antibody positivity exceeds 90%.[6,26] Furthermore, "antibody-negative" forms of other autoimmune diseases are well recognized. Thus, it is not clear that there is an etiologically separate non-autoimmune or idiopathic form of typical SMS.

There is overlap among the above-described types. For example, many cases of paraneoplastic SMS present with a stiff upper limb[8,27] and pathologically show encephalomyelitic abnormalities.[7] Some stiff-limb cases have high titers of GAD antibodies and respond well to typical SMS therapy.[28] These cases may represent a subtype of typical SMS. Other stiff-limb cases are antibody-negative, fluctuate greatly in severity, and progress to greater disability than typical SMS, showing a poor response to treatment.[6] These may be pathogenetically distinct.

Cases of paraneoplastic and encephalomyelitic SMS tend to show focal neurological abnormalities not seen in typical SMS, such as lower motor neuron signs, sensory abnormalities, or brainstem deficits, which presumably result from the inflammatory process itself rather than from organ-specific autoimmunity. GAD antibodies have been detected in some cases of progressive encephalomyelitis with rigidity and paraneoplastic stiffness with amphiphysin antibodies, leading to speculation that the syndromes may be related pathogenetically to typical SMS. Although this may be true, it should be noted that 8% of healthy control subjects were positive for GAD65 antibodies in one study,[26] and the coexistence of these antibodies, particularly in patients with other antibodies, does not prove causation.

Diagnostic criteria

Lorish et al.[22] refined the diagnostic criteria for typical SMS. The criteria include 1) a prodrome of axial muscle stiffness and rigidity in axial muscles, 2) slow progression of stiffness resulting in impaired ambulation, 3) fixed deformity of the spine (in general, pronounced lordosis), 4) presence of superimposed episodic spasms precipitated by sudden movement, noise, or emotional upset, 5) normal motor and sensory findings on neurological examination, 6) continuous motor unit activity on electromyography abolished by diazepam given intravenously or a positive therapeutic response to oral diazepam, and 7) normal intellect. The diagnosis of SMS is outlined in Table 228.1.

Table 228.1   Diagnosis of stiff-man syndrome

History
  Temporal profile of development of symptoms—typically subacute
  Presence of startle-induced spasms
  Absence of complaints of weakness or sensory disturbance

Examination
  Distribution of stiffness—axial versus appendicular, symmetry
  Characteristic spinal deformity
  Cerebellar or long-tract signs?
  Response to startle (benzodiazepines may suppress this)

Laboratory testing
  Routine electromyography
    Normal except for inability to suppress firing
    Benzodiazepines may suppress this finding
    Primarily helpful to rule out conditions that simulate stiff-man syndrome
  Other electrophysiological testing
    Look for disorders of hyperexcitability of lower motor neurons
    Surface electromyography to assess pattern of involvement, startle response
  Serological testing
    GAD65 antibodies in typical stiff-man syndrome
    Amphiphysin antibodies in some paraneoplastic syndromes
    Potassium channel antibodies in Isaacs syndrome
    Ganglionic acetylcholine receptor antibodies in some cramp/spasm disorders
  MRI
    Typically, normal findings
  Cerebrospinal fluid
    Typically, normal findings

The "board-like" rigidity of the abdominal and paraspinal muscles and the hypertrophy of paraspinal muscles are very helpful in diagnosis. The absence of startle-induced spasms in an untreated patient casts doubt on the diagnosis, but modest doses of agents that promote GABA transmission are effective in controlling these spasms despite persisting rigidity in many partially treated cases.

Some of the conditions commonly associated with SMS may result directly from GAD autoimmunity. About 30% of patients with SMS have type 1 diabetes mellitus, presumably reflecting the action of GAD antibodies. Psychiatric disturbances, including anxiety, depression, and substance abuse, are common[29,30] and may also relate to impaired GABA metabolism. Although epilepsy has been thought to be associated with SMS, a review of the literature does not clearly indicate that the overall incidence is higher than in the general population. GAD antibodies have been reported in refractory epilepsy without SMS.[31] As noted above, cerebellar signs without SMS have been reported in non-SMS patients who have GAD antibodies.[21] GAD antibodies from SMS patients but not from diabetic patients have been shown to decrease GABA production in crude rat cerebellar extracts,[32] and nuclear magnetic resonance spectroscopy has demonstrated decreased brain levels of GABA in SMS patients.[3]

Several other associations have been described with typical SMS, including myasthenia gravis,[33,34] immune-mediated retinopathy,[35] Graves disease (personal observation), and dysphagia with gastrointestinal dysmotility.[36] These may only reflect an underlying autoimmune diathesis, because patients with SMS clearly have an increased prevalence of autoantibodies generally and often have polyendocrine failure. Thyroid autoantibodies are particularly common in antibody-positive SMS.[26]

Laboratory testing

The majority of patients with typical SMS have antibodies to GAD65 in high titer, and some have antibodies to GAD67. In series that adhere to strict diagnostic criteria, seropositivity approaches 90% to 98%.[6,26] Lower titers of GAD antibody (less than 20 nmol/L) are prevalent in the diabetic population without SMS and may be found in normal subjects.[26] Occasionally, higher titers may be detected in polyendocrine autoimmunity without SMS. Other organ-specific autoantibodies are often present in SMS. In many cases, the cerebrospinal fluid findings have been normal, but in some series a high rate of elevated IgG synthesis and oligoclonal banding have been found.[37] Routine electromyography (EMG) is notable for continuous activation of otherwise normal motor unit activity, which patients are unable to suppress voluntarily but which is suppressed by diazepam.[22] Specialized electrophysiological testing demonstrates abnormal antagonist co-contraction and exaggerated startle responses, which fail to habituate.[16,24]

Imaging

Magnetic resonance imaging (MRI) of the neuraxis typically does not show any abnormality, but areas of increased T_2 signal in the brain and cervical cord have been reported in isolated cases, some of which clearly are not cases of typical SMS.[38–40]

Pathology

Few pathology studies have been conducted in patients with typical SMS, and neuropathological analysis has been of little help in elucidating the pathogenesis of the syndrome. Some autopsy reports of "stiff-man syndrome" are cases of encephalomyelitis with rigidity.[15] Minor abnormalities, without marked inflammation, have been described in several cases of typical SMS.[15] Findings of GABA-ergic cell loss in the cerebellum and decreased size of Renshaw cells in the spinal cord support the hypothesis that GAD antibodies may be pathogenetic.[41] Other reports have shown structural changes in large spinal motor neurons[42,43] and loss of smaller alpha and gamma motor neurons.[42]

Differential diagnosis

Clinical acumen is key to the diagnosis. Although the recognition of SMS by neurologists and psychiatrists is improving, SMS undoubtedly is still underdiagnosed in general practice. SMS is frequently misdiagnosed and, thus, treated inadequately or inappropriately.

Stiff-limb syndrome

Although distal extremity involvement without axial rigidity may occur in antibody-positive and otherwise typical SMS,[27] it may be a distinct clinical syndrome in some cases, as mentioned above.[6,23] Isolated lower extremity posturing and stiffness could represent an extrapyramidal, dystonic condition. Isolated upper extremity involvement should raise suspicion of an underlying malignancy, even if GAD antibodies are present.

Progressive encephalomyelitis with rigidity

This condition appears to be primarily inflammatory. It begins in the brainstem with bulbar signs and spreads quickly to the spinal cord, causing progressive and widespread neurological deficits. In the reported cases, death ensues, sometimes within weeks. Pathological examination shows encephalomyelitis, with inflammatory infiltrates in the gray matter of the brainstem and spinal cord.[15] Rarely, patients survive what appears to have been an attack of this condition and persist with a chronic form of muscular rigidity (personal observation), sometimes with associated myoclonic-like spasms (jerking stiff-man syndrome).[5]

Paraneoplastic stiff-man syndromes

A clinical syndrome that resembles SMS is associated with malignancy and antibodies directed against amphiphysin. This has been described primarily in patients with small cell lung carcinoma or carcinoma of the breast.[7,44] The upper extremities are often involved. Pathology studies and imaging findings often suggest encephalomyelitis. Successful treatment of the tumor may induce some remission of symptoms.[8] In a patient who had SMS-like symptoms and amphiphysin antibodies, no tumor had been detected after 3 years, suggesting possible primary autoimmunity.[39] Immunosuppression was effective in controlling the symptoms.

Other causes of muscular rigidity

Isaacs syndrome can be differentiated from SMS by the following features:[45] 1) generally, distal and focal limb involvement, 2) persistence of activity despite sleep or general anesthesia, 3) characteristic abnormalities on clinical electrophysiological testing (neuromyotonia), 4) response to carbamazepine or phenytoin, and 5) in some cases, the presence of anti-voltage-gated potassium channel or antineuronal nicotinic acetylcholine receptor antibodies.

There appears to be a spectrum of neuromuscular hyperexcitability pathogenetically related to Isaacs syndrome, with voltage-gated potassium channel antibodies or antineuronal nicotinic acetylcholine receptor antibodies but without neuromyotonia.[46]

Chronic tetany is extremely rare and should produce trismus and risus sardonicus. Psychogenic contraction may be more variable and should not produce prominent hypertrophy.

Other causes of startle-induced spasms

Hereditary hyperekplexia should not produce sustained rigidity between startle. Also, it is familial. Normal hypervigilance or psychogenic startle should be distinguishable on motor reflex testing and should habituate. Startle-induced spasms may be seen in association with rigidity in focal spinal cord lesions such as syringomyelia or tumor, perhaps because of the loss of interneurons. Associated motor and sensory deficits and abnormal imaging findings should distinguish these conditions from SMS.

Treatment

Advances in management of SMS have paralleled the understanding of the pathophysiology of the disorder. Before the discovery in 1963 that diazepam effectively suppresses spasms and decreases rigidity in SMS,[10] the condition was medically untreatable. Reported cases were dramatic, severe, and incapacitating. The efficacy of diazepam led investigators to focus on deficiency of GABA-ergic transmission as a key factor in the pathogenesis. Over the years, other agents that increase GABA-ergic transmission, including benzodiazepines, baclofen, vigabatrin, and tiagabine, have proved effective to various degrees. Perhaps many patients had long before discovered and relied on the ameliorating effects of ethyl alcohol, an over-the-counter enhancer of GABA-ergic transmission.

The association of SMS with endocrine disorders and autoimmunity had been noted, but it was not

Table 228.2   Treatment of stiff-man syndrome

Pharmacological
  First line—oral neuromodulation
    Benzodiazepines
    • Diazepam—5 mg 2–3 times daily, maximum >300 mg/day
    • Clonazepam—0.25 mg 2–3 times daily, maximum 20 mg/day
    Antispasticity agents
    • Baclofen—10 mg 2–3 times daily, maximum 80–120 mg/day
    • Tizanidine—4 mg 2–3 times daily, maximum 36 mg/day
    Anticonvulsants
    • Divalproex—250 mg 2–3 times daily, maximum 3000 mg/day
    • Tiagabine—4 mg 2–4 times daily, maximum 56 mg/day
  Second line—immunosuppression/modulation
    Corticosteroids
      Oral prednisone, initially 60 mg/day (or up to 1 mg/kg daily) for 2 months
      Switch to every other day and then taper dose
      Monitor for multiple side effects
      Effective but complications with long-term use
    Azathioprine (see Table 228.3)
      First, check thiopurine methyltransferase if available
      Titrate dose up over 4 weeks from 50 mg/day
      Target dose: 2–2.5 mg/kg daily in divided doses
      Monitor blood count and liver enzymes
      Suitable for long-term use
      If tapered, taper slowly, e.g., 25 mg every 6 months, to avoid relapse
    Other immunosuppressive agents—efficacy unknown, should help if antibodies are pathogenetic
    • Mycophenolate mofetil—presumably same doses as for myasthenia gravis
    • Rituximab
    Intravenous immunoglobulin
      1.0 g/kg per infusion on two consecutive days, each month; may increase interval between treatments as tolerated
    Plasma exchange
      Total plasma exchange, 4–6 treatments over 4–14 days, then increase interval between treatments as tolerated
  Third line—intrathecal baclofen pump

Nonpharmacological
  Exercise
    Emphasis on flexibility, stretching, and balance
    Yoga, t'ai chi chuan
    Slow and sustained activity rather than rapid repetitive activity
  Modalities
    Heat and gentle massage may be helpful
    Cold often aggravates muscle spasms
  Behavioral therapies
    Relaxation tapes
    Biofeedback training
    Cognitive behavioral strategies

until 1988, when Solimena et al.[2] published their report of GAD antibodies in SMS, that immunosuppressive treatment gained a foothold. The results have been mixed, but overall favorable, with generally better responses to oral immunosuppression than to plasma exchange.[12] The response to immunosuppression usually is less than complete, and modifiers of GABA-ergic transmission as well as behavioral and supportive therapies continue to be important.

The interplay between psychiatric and neurological symptoms poses special challenges in the management of SMS. Tinsley et al.[29] noted five possible interactions: 1) psychiatric symptoms may exacerbate stiffness, 2) SMS may contribute to the development of psychiatric symptoms (e.g., simple phobia after a traumatic fall), 3) treatment for SMS (e.g., diazepam

or prednisone) may produce psychiatric symptoms, 4) there may be a concurrent but unrelated disorder, and 5) concurrent and related syndromes such as anxiety, depression, or alcoholism—all of which represent dysfunction of the GABA system—may exist. Psychiatric input is often helpful in the management of patients with SMS.

Pharmacological treatment

Pharmacotherapy has been effective in many reported cases of SMS and is warranted in most patients by the time they come to medical attention (Table 228.2). Options include enhancement of GABA-ergic neurotransmission with oral agents, immunotherapy, and intrathecal administration of baclofen. Treatment approaches have been rational and based on an understanding of the pathophysiological mechanisms, but because of the rarity of the disorder, treatment experience is essentially anecdotal. Because randomized, placebo-controlled trials with statistically meaningful numbers of comparable patients are not feasible, the therapy literature is dominated by case reports. In many cases, the responses are obvious.

Generally, the first line of therapy is agents that enhance GABA-ergic transmission, such as benzodiazepines or baclofen. The response is often dramatic, especially the suppression of spasms. The dose may be titrated upward as needed. Very large doses are often required: typically 50 to 70 mg daily, sometimes more than 100 mg daily, and in rare cases, more than 300 mg daily. Although these agents generally are well tolerated, sedation and depression may be a problem for some patients. Contrary to a popularly held notion, SMS patients may abuse benzodiazepines. Baclofen, vigabatrin, and tiagabine are preferable in this regard but are somewhat less effective in tolerated doses. They may be prescribed in addition to benzodiazepines as "sparing agents," allowing improved control of SMS symptoms without the risk of escalating the use or abuse of benzodiazepines. Clinicians must also be alert to the concomitant use of alcohol, which many patients use to ameliorate symptoms.[29] Behavioral and physical therapy may reduce the need for increasing doses of medications.

Although GABA-ergic agents do not usually eliminate symptoms, failure of the disease to respond or to have a minimal response to these agents may signify an erroneous diagnosis. However, a response to treatment cannot be taken as diagnostic of SMS, because other conditions such as psychogenic or upper motor neuron disorders may also be expected to show improvement.

If satisfactory control cannot be achieved with GABA-ergic agents and additional supportive therapy, immunosuppression should be considered. Before embarking on this therapy, the diagnosis of an immune-mediated form of stiffness should be reasonably secure. A high titer of GAD antibodies is strong evidence in the appropriate clinical setting. There undoubtedly are antibody-negative cases that are actually autoimmune as well and may be related to undetected GAD antibodies, other pathogenetic antibodies, or cell-mediated mechanisms. A typical clinical presentation for SMS, without confounding abnormalities on examination or laboratory testing, especially if there is evidence for a predisposition to organ-specific autoimmunity, may be considered as probable autoimmune SMS. These patients may be appropriate candidates for a trial of immunosuppression. The same may be true for atypical antibody-negative patients, for example, those with stiff-limb syndromes or brainstem signs, but in these patients, the suspicion of underlying malignancy should be high. Occasionally, the severity of the condition and the lack of response to any palliative therapy leaves the compassionate physician little choice but to try

immunotherapy, however atypical the presentation or meager the evidence for autoimmunity.

The options for immunotherapy are several (Table 228.2). Oral prednisone in moderately high doses is effective fairly rapidly, and a pronounced response often develops within several weeks. Thus, prednisone is often a good first choice, especially as a diagnostic or therapeutic trial. For diabetic patients, the potential short-term complication is obvious, but it usually can be managed with adjustments of the insulin dose. Longer-term treatment with corticosteroids has the usual multiple risks in any patient and requires appropriate prophylaxis, patient education, and medical monitoring. Osteoporosis and bone fragility are of particular concern in this patient population prone to injurious falls.

The response to total plasma exchange (TPE) generally has been disappointing;[12,47–50] intravenous immunoglobulin (IVIG) appears to be more effective.[11,49,51–56] However, the small number of patients who have been treated and possible variations in patient presentation and diagnosis make meaningful comparison and predictions difficult. Delakis et al.[56] have shown in a double-blind, placebo-controlled, crossover trial in 16 patients that monthly infusions of IVIG, 2 g/kg, divided in two daily doses, provides marked relief of symptoms. The cost of the drug averages more than $10 000 per month. These treatments provide only transient benefit at best and generally are not feasible for long-term management. They may be indicated for patients with severe SMS requiring rapid rescue from symptoms, as diagnostic trials for patients with moderately severe SMS to determine whether longer-term immunosuppression is warranted, or as an occasional booster treatment.

Azathioprine has been effective in long-term management of SMS symptoms, in some cases allowing prednisone to be tapered off and the dose of GABA-ergic agents to be decreased.[12] Dosages in the range of 2 to 2.5 mg/kg daily may be required, at least initially. The onset of action is slow, requiring 4 to 6 months to become apparent and even longer to reach maximal benefit. The offset of action is also slow, and thus tapering off of medication should be gradual, titrating to the lowest effective dose over many months to avoid relapse. The drug is well tolerated by most patients. The incidence of side effects is low, but some are severe, so cautious introduction and close long-term monitoring are required (Table 228.3). If liver toxicity develops, it usually does so within weeks. Occasionally, suppression of the leukocyte count may be early and devastating (sometimes after the first dose), but it may develop after months or even years of treatment, underscoring the need for ongoing follow-up. A genetically determined low level of thiopurine methyltransferase in erythrocytes (rbc TPMT) may be a predictor of reduced azathioprine metabolism; with severe (homozygous) deficiency, azathioprine should probably not be used at all.[57]

A recent epidemiological analysis in Europe demonstrated that patients with rheumatological disease treated with azathioprine or other immunosup-

Table 228.3   Azathioprine in stiff-man syndrome

Indications
  Gait and mobility impairment despite maximal
    conservative therapy
  Excessive side effects with required doses of
    nonimmunosuppressive agents

Contraindications
  Relative
    Heterozygous low rbcTPMT
    Low-normal leukocyte count
    History of malignancy
    History of taking alkylating agents
  Absolute
    Known intolerance of azathioprine
    Leukopenia
    Concomitant treatment with allopurinol, ACE
      inhibitors
    Pregnancy

Dosage
  50 mg/day for 1 week; 50 mg 2 times daily for 1 week;
    50 mg 3 times daily for 1 week
  Then 2 to 2.5 mg/kg daily in divided doses

Monitoring
  CBC and liver enzymes weekly for 1 month, monthly for
    1 year
  Quarterly thereafter unless dose increased or lab
    abnormalities

Dose adjustments
  Leukocytes $<2.8 \times 10^9$/L
    Halve dose, recheck lab values in 1 week
    Continue at half dose if counts rebound
    Consider cautious increase
  Leukocytes $<2.5 \times 10^9$/L
    Hold dose and recheck in 1 week
    Resume at half dose if counts rebound

Response
  Elevated MCV reflects metabolic effect of drug
  Onset of clinical effect is delayed (4 to 6 months or
    longer)
  Offset is also delayed, taper should be slow

ACE, angiotensin-converting enzyme; CBC, complete blood count; MCV, mean corpuscular volume; rbcTPMT, erythrocyte thiopurine methyltransferase.

pressive agents (methotrexate, cyclophosphamide, and chlorambucil) have an increased risk of developing malignancy of the immune system, skin, or bladder (incidence rate ratio of approximately 3.7).[58] The observed effect was related to the duration of exposure to immunosuppressive drugs. Whether similar risks apply to patients with neurological disease is not known, but the possibility must be discussed with patients when immunosuppressive treatment is offered.

The efficacy of immunosuppressive agents other than prednisone and azathioprine in SMS is not known. Potential risks of treatment must be balanced against the risks of inadequate management. With advances in understanding of the immunological pathogenetic mechanisms in SMS and the development of new, more specific, and less toxic immuno-

suppressive agents, this balance may swing toward treatment.

Intrathecal baclofen is effective and may be considered when oral GABA-ergic agents and immunotherapy fail or are not tolerated.[59-61] With normal underlying muscle strength, SMS seems an ideal condition for this treatment because decreased tone will not unmask weakness, a risk in most spastic disorders. Oral baclofen should be kept readily available, however, to prevent acute ventilatory restriction by muscular rigidity and spasms in the event of sudden pump failure, and intravenous diazepam may be needed emergently in such an event. One patient died because of pump failure.[60] Intrathecal baclofen treatment is not a small undertaking, initially or in the long term. Surgical pump placement, titration of dosing, frequent refill visits, and management of the not-infrequent pump and catheter complications require major financial and time investments as well as emotional flexibility and stability of the patient. This treatment option is generally impractical for patients who do not live near a major center where it is available.

Botulinum toxin may be used to improve muscle spasms and rigidity in SMS and related disorders[62] (personal observation).

Symptomatic treatments

Management of patients with SMS should include evaluation of lifestyle factors and other medical issues that may contribute to the symptoms. Appropriate treatment of anxiety, depression, phobias, and substance abuse will improve the neuromuscular response to treatment, and psychiatric consultation is often required. Often, behavioral therapy techniques are helpful. Sertraline may aggravate SMS in some patients, despite its beneficial effect on mood and attitude (personal observation).

The altered body mechanics and persistent muscular activation in patients with SMS predispose them to muscle strains and pain, which in turn aggravates the muscle spasms. Formal physical therapy and exercise programs, including slow gentle stretches, such as yoga and t'ai chi chuan, may be helpful.

As with any medical condition, patient education is essential. Knowledge and understanding lead to improved insight and a sense of control. Interaction with other SMS patients may help to relieve the feelings of isolation and hopelessness that often develop after diagnosis of a rare disorder. Long-distance communication is usually necessary because SMS patients tend to be few and far between.

References

1. Moersch FP, Woltman HW. Progressive fluctuating muscular rigidity and spasm ("stiff-man" syndrome): report of a case and some observations in 13 other cases. Proc Staff Meet Mayo Clin 1956;31:421–427
2. Solimena M, Folli F, Denis-Donini S, et al. Autoantibodies to glutamic acid decarboxylase in a patient with stiff-man syndrome, epilepsy, and type I diabetes mellitus. N Engl J Med 1988;318:1012–1020

3. Levy LM, Dalakas MC, Floeter MK. The stiff-person syndrome: an autoimmune disorder affecting neurotransmission of gamma-aminobutyric acid. Ann Intern Med 1999;131:522–530

4. Dinkel K, Meinck HM, Jury KM, et al. Inhibition of gamma-aminobutyric acid synthesis by glutamic acid decarboxylase autoantibodies in stiff-man syndrome. Ann Neurol 1998;44:194–201

5. Leigh PN, Rothwell JC, Traub M, Marsden CD. A patient with reflex myoclonus and muscle rigidity: "jerking stiff-man syndrome." J Neurol Neurosurg Psychiatry 1980;43:1125–1131

6. Barker RA, Revesz T, Thom M, et al. Review of 23 patients affected by the stiff man syndrome: clinical subdivision into stiff trunk (man) syndrome, stiff limb syndrome, and progressive encephalomyelitis with rigidity. J Neurol Neurosurg Psychiatry 1998;65:633–640

7. Bateman DE, Weller RO, Kennedy P. Stiffman syndrome: a rare paraneoplastic disorder? J Neurol Neurosurg Psychiatry 1990;53:695–696

8. Rosin L, DeCamilli P, Butler M, et al. Stiff-man syndrome in a woman with breast cancer: an uncommon central nervous system paraneoplastic syndrome. Neurology 1998;50:94–98

9. Sander JE, Layzer RB, Goldsobel AB. Congenital stiff-man syndrome. Ann Neurol 1980;8:195–197

10. Howard FM Jr. A new and effective drug in the treatment of the stiff-man syndrome: preliminary report. Proc Staff Meet Mayo Clin 1963;38:203–212

11. Amato AA, Cornman EW, Kissel JT. Treatment of stiff-man syndrome with intravenous immunoglobulin. Neurology 1994;44:1652–1654

12. McEvoy KM. Stiff-man syndrome. In: Feske S, Samuels M, eds. Office Practice of Neurology. New York: Churchill Livingstone, 1996:691–695

13. Alarcon-Segovia D, Ruiz-Arguelles A, Llorente L. Broken dogma: penetration of autoantibodies into living cells. Immunol Today 1996;17:163–164

14. Hummel M, Durinovic-Bello I, Bonifacio E, et al. Humoral and cellular immune parameters before and during immunosuppressive therapy of a patient with stiff-man syndrome and insulin dependent diabetes mellitus. J Neurol Neurosurg Psychiatry 1998;65:204–208

15. Simonati A, Rizzuto N. Neuropathology of the stiff-man syndrome. In: Layzer RB, Sandrini G, Piccolo G, Martinelli P, eds. Motor Unit Hyperactivity States. New York: Raven Press, 1993:89–99

16. Floeter MK, Valls-Sole J, Toro C, et al. Physiologic studies of spinal inhibitory circuits in patients with stiff-person syndrome. Neurology 1998;51:85–93

17. Antoine JC, Ábsi L, Honnorat J, et al. Antiamphiphysin antibodies are associated with various paraneoplastic neurological syndromes and tumors. Arch Neurol 1999;56:172–177

18. Jaeckle KA. Autoimmunity in paraneoplastic neurological syndromes: closer to the truth? Ann Neurol 1999;45:143–145

19. Armon C, Swanson JW, McLean JM, et al. Subacute encephalomyelitis presenting as stiff-person syndrome: clinical, polygraphic, and pathologic correlations. Mov Disord 1996;11:701–709

20. Pugliese A, Solimena M, Awdeh ZL, et al. Association of HLA-DQB1*0201 with stiff-man syndrome. J Clin Endocrinol Metab 1993;77:1550–1553

21. Abele M, Weller M, Mescheriakov S, et al. Cerebellar ataxia with glutamic acid decarboxylase autoantibodies. Neurology 1999;52:857–859

22. Lorish TR, Thorsteinsson G, Howard FM Jr. Stiff-man syndrome updated. Mayo Clin Proc 1989;14:629–636

23. Brown P, Marsden CD. The stiff man and stiff man plus syndromes. J Neurol 1999;246:648–652

24. Meinck HM, Ricker K, Hulser PJ, Solimena M. Stiff man syndrome: neurophysiological findings in eight patients. J Neurol 1995;242:134–142

25. Grimaldi LM, Martino G, Braghi S, et al. Heterogeneity of autoantibodies in stiff-man syndrome. Ann Neurol 1993;34:57–64

26. Walikonis JE, Lennon VA. Radioimmunoassay for glutamic acid decarboxylase (GAD65) autoantibodies as a diagnostic aid for stiff-man syndrome and a correlate of susceptibility to type 1 diabetes mellitus. Mayo Clin Proc 1998;73:1161–1166

27. Silverman IE. Paraneoplastic stiff limb syndrome. J Neurol Neurosurg Psychiatry 1999;67:126–127

28. Saiz A, Graus F, Valldeoriola F, et al. Stiff-leg syndrome: a focal form of stiff-man syndrome. Ann Neurol 1998;43:400–403

29. Tinsley JA, Barth EM, Black JL, Williams DE. Psychiatric consultations in stiff-man syndrome. J Clin Psychiatry 1997;58:444–449

30. Black JL, Barth EM, Williams DE, Tinsley JA. Stiff-man syndrome: results of interviews and psychologic testing. Psychosomatics 1998;39:38–44

31. Peltola J, Kulmala P, Isojarvi J, et al. Autoantibodies to glutamic acid decarboxylase in patients with therapy-resistant epilepsy. Neurology 2000;55:46–50

32. Helfgott SM. Stiff-man syndrome: from the bedside to the bench. Arthritis Rheum 1999;42:1312–1320

33. Nicholas AP, Chatterjee A, Arnold MM, et al. Stiff-persons' syndrome associated with thymoma and subsequent myasthenia gravis. Muscle Nerve 1997;20:493–498

34. Aso Y, Sato A, Narimatsu M, et al. Stiff-man syndrome associated with antecedent myasthenia gravis and organ-specific autoimmunopathy. Intern Med 1997;36:308–311

35. Steffen H, Menger N, Richter W, et al. Immune-mediated retinopathy in a patient with stiff-man syndrome. Graefes Arch Clin Exp Ophthalmol 1999;237:212–219

36. Soykan I, McCallum RW. Gastrointestinal involvement in neurologic disorders: stiff-man and Charcot-Marie-Tooth syndromes. Am J Med Sci 1997;313:70–73

37. Solimena M, Folli F, Aparisi R, et al. Autoantibodies to GABA-ergic neurons and pancreatic beta cells in stiff-man syndrome. N Engl J Med 1990;322:1555–1560

38. Meinck HM, Ricker K, Hulser PJ, Solimena M. Stiff man syndrome: neurophysiological findings in eight patients. J Neurol 1995;242:134–142

39. Schmierer K, Valdueza JM, Bender A, et al. Atypical stiff-person syndrome with spinal MRI findings, amphiphysin autoantibodies, and immunosuppression. Neurology 1998;51:250–252

40. Mitsumoto H, Schwartzman MJ, Estes ML, et al. Sudden death and paroxysmal autonomic dysfunction in stiff-man syndrome. J Neurol 1991;238:91–96

41. Warich-Kirches M, Von Bossanyi P, Treuheit T, et al. Stiff-man syndrome: possible autoimmune etiology targeted against GABA-ergic cells. Clin Neuropathol 1997;16:214–219

42. Ishizawa K, Komori T, Okayama K, et al. Large motor neuron involvement in stiff-man syndrome: a qualitative and quantitative study. Acta Neuropathol (Berl) 1999;97:63–70

43. Saiz A, Minguez A, Graus F, et al. Stiff-man syndrome

with vacuolar degeneration of anterior horn motor neurons. J Neurol 1999;246:858–860

44. Dropcho EJ. Antiamphiphysin antibodies with small-cell lung carcinoma and paraneoplastic encephalomyelitis. Ann Neurol 1996;39:659–667

45. Isaacs HA. A syndrome of continuous muscle-fibre activity. J Neurol Neurosurg Psychiatry 1961;24:319–325

46. Vernino S, Auger RG, Emslie-Smith AM, et al. Myasthenia, thymoma, presynaptic antibodies, and a continuum of neuromuscular hyperexcitability. Neurology 1999;53:1233–1239

47. Harding AE, Thompson PD, Kocen RS, et al. Plasma exchange and immunosuppression in the stiff man syndrome. Lancet 1989;2:915

48. Karlson EW, Sudarsky L, Ruderman E, et al. Treatment of stiff-man syndrome with intravenous immune globulin. Arthritis Rheum 1994;37:915–918

49. Nakamagoe K, Ohkoshi N, Hayashi A, et al. Marked clinical improvement by plasmapheresis in a patient with stiff-man syndrome: a case with a negative anti-GAD antibody. Rinsho Shinkeigaku 1995;35:897–900

50. Vicari AM, Folli F, Pozza G, et al. Plasmapheresis in the treatment of stiff-man syndrome. N Engl J Med 1989;320:1499

51. Brashear HR, Phillips LH II. Autoantibodies to GABAergic neurons and response to plasmapheresis in stiff-man syndrome. Neurology 1991;41:1588–1592

52. Khanlou H, Eiger G. Long-term remission of refractory stiff-man syndrome after treatment with intravenous immunoglobulin. Mayo Clin Proc 1999;74:1231–1232

53. Sevrin C, Moulin T, Tatu L, et al. "Stiff-man" syndrome treated with intravenous immunoglobulins. Rev Neurol (Paris) 1998;154:431

54. Barker RA, Marsden CD. Successful treatment of stiff man syndrome with intravenous immunoglobulin. J Neurol Neurosurg Psychiatry 1997;62:426–427

55. Vieregge P, Branczyk B, Barnett W, et al. Stiff-man syndrome: report of 4 cases. Nervenarzt 1994;65:712–717

56. Dalakas MC, Fujii M, Li M, et al. High-dose intravenous immune globulin for stiff-person syndrome. N Engl J Med 2001;345:1870–1876

57. Naughton MA, Battaglia E, O'Brien S, et al. Identification of thiopurine methyltransferase (TPMT) polymorphisms cannot predict myelosuppression in systemic lupus erythematosus patients taking azathioprine. Rheumatology (Oxford) 1999;38:640–644

58. Asten P, Barrett J, Symmons D. Risk of developing certain malignancies is related to duration of immunosuppressive drug exposure in patients with rheumatic diseases. J Rheumatol 1999;26:1705–1714

59. McEvoy KM, Silbert PL, Stolp-Smith KA, et al. A double-blind, placebo-controlled trial of intrathecal baclofen therapy in stiff-man syndrome. Ann Neurol 1994;36:317

60. Meinck HM, Tronnier V, Rieke K, et al. Intrathecal baclofen treatment for stiff-man syndrome: pump failure may be fatal. Neurology 1994;44:2209–2210

61. Stayer C, Tronnier V, Dressnandt J, et al. Intrathecal baclofen therapy for stiff-man syndrome and progressive encephalomyelopathy with rigidity and myoclonus. Neurology 1997;49:1591–1597

62. Liguori R, Cordivari C, Lugaresi E, Montagna P. Botulinum toxin A improves muscle spasms and rigidity in stiff-person syndrome. Mov Disord 1997;12:1060–1063

229 Cramps and Myalgias

C Michel Harper Jr

Introduction

Muscle pain is a common symptom, which in isolation is nonspecific. Myalgias may be a prominent complaint in systemic infections, in hematological, rheumatological, and endocrine disorders, in central nervous system diseases, and in peripheral neuropathies, neuromuscular junction disorders, and myopathies. Even after extensive testing, most patients with isolated myalgias (with or without fatigue) do not have an identifiable disease.[1] Many of these patients are given the diagnosis of fibromyalgia, a clinical syndrome defined by diffuse pain and tenderness on digital palpation of at least 11 of 18 anatomically defined trigger points.[2] Fibromyalgia frequently responds to symptomatic therapy with tricyclic antidepressants, nonsteroidal anti-inflammatory agents, and physical therapy.

When muscle pain is associated with involuntary muscle shortening, the differential diagnosis is confined to disorders of the central and peripheral nervous systems (Table 229.1). Disorders of the central nervous system, myotonia, and metabolic muscle diseases that can be associated with pain and stiffness are discussed in other chapters. This chapter focuses on disorders associated with hyperexcitability of the motor axon or nerve terminal (i.e., cramps, symptomatic tetany, cramp-fasciculation syndrome, and Isaacs syndrome) and a rare disorder of muscle (rippling muscle disease). Many of these disorders respond symptomatically to membrane-stabilizing drugs. Isaacs syndrome, many cases of cramp-fasciculation syndrome, and some cases of rippling muscle disease are autoimmune in origin and may respond to immunotherapy.

Fibromyalgia

Epidemiology

The estimated prevalence of fibromyalgia in the general population is approximately 2%.[3] It is more common among women and increases in frequency with age.

Etiology and pathophysiology

The cause of fibromyalgia is unknown. Because it is defined by clinical criteria, multiple causative factors likely exist. By definition, the results of tests for chronic systemic and neuromuscular disorders are negative. Psychological factors are often implicated as a cause or as an exacerbating factor of fibromyalgia syndrome. Many patients have features in common with those of other chronic pain syndromes, including indirect evidence of an up-regulation of central pain mechanisms.[4]

Clinical features

Chronic diffuse pain and tenderness over muscles, joints, and tendinous insertions are cardinal manifestations. Fatigue, morning stiffness, and insomnia are common. Patients frequently have multiple nonspecific somatic complaints. The neurological and general physical examination findings are normal except for multiple trigger points that are tender to palpation. By definition, the condition is chronic, lasting 3 months or longer.[2] Complete resolution of the symptoms is unusual; however, the results of long-term follow-up studies have indicated substantial improvement in two-thirds of patients up to 10 years after the diagnosis.[5]

The diagnostic criteria for fibromyalgia are listed in Table 229.2.[2] Objective abnormalities found on physical or laboratory examination that suggest peripheral nerve, neuromuscular junction, muscle, or rheumatological disease exclude the diagnosis of primary fibromyalgia.

Table 229.1 Causes of muscle stiffness and spasms

Central nervous system
  Upper motor neuron
    Spasticity
  Basal ganglia
    Rigidity
    Dystonia
    Choreoathetosis
    Ballismus
  Lower motor neuron
    Stiff-man syndrome
    Paraneoplastic encephalomyelitis
    Tetanus
    Strychnine intoxication

Peripheral nervous system
  Motor axon/nerve terminal
    Cramps (simple and pathological)
    Symptomatic tetany
    Cramp-fasciculation syndrome
    Isaacs syndrome (neuromyotonia)
  Neuromuscular junction
    Cholinesterase inhibition (drugs, toxins)

Muscle
  Myotonia (sarcolemmal channelopathies)
  Muscle contracture (metabolic muscle disease)
  Rippling muscle disease

Table 229.2 Diagnostic criteria for fibromyalgia

A. Widespread pain involving both sides of body, including areas above and below waist as well as axial skeleton (of at least 3 months' duration)

B. Pain on digital palpation of at least 11 of 18 tender points:
   Anterior aspect transverse process C5–7
   Anterior surface second rib, near costochondral junction
   Elbow region, 2 cm distal to lateral epicondyle
   Knee, medial aspect, just proximal to joint line
   Occiput, at insertion of occipital muscles
   Trapezius, midportion of upper border
   Supraspinatus, near medial border of scapula
   Upper outer quadrant of gluteal region
   Greater trochanter of femur

Modified from Wolfe et al.[2] By permission of the American College of Rheumatology.

Table 229.3 Differential diagnosis of fibromyalgia

Chronic infections—hepatitis, human immunodeficiency virus infection, syphilis, Lyme disease, Whipple disease, toxoplasmosis, trichinosis, brucellosis, subacute bacterial endocarditis, occult abscess

Systemic inflammatory disorders—vasculitis, sarcoidosis, paraneoplastic disorders, connective tissue diseases, Behçet disease, inflammatory bowel disease

Occult malignancy

Metabolic disorders—thyroid or adrenal disease; chronic heart, pulmonary, liver, or kidney disease; vitamin deficiencies; intoxications

Hematological disorders—anemia, myeloproliferative disease

Central nervous system disorders—multiple sclerosis, mitochondrial cytopathies, chronic meningitis or encephalitis, stiff-man syndrome, paraneoplastic encephalomyeloradiculopathy with rigidity, tetanus, strychnine poisoning

Peripheral nervous system disorders—cramps (benign or pathological), symptomatic tetany, cramp-fasciculation syndrome, clinical neuromyotonia (Isaacs syndrome), polyradiculoneuropathy, metabolic and inflammatory myopathies, neuromuscular junction disease (myasthenia gravis or Lambert-Eaton syndrome)

Laboratory testing

There is no diagnostic or contributory laboratory test for fibromyalgia. The erythrocyte sedimentation rate, serum level of creatine kinase, serological testing for connective tissue and other inflammatory diseases, serum level of lactate, and electromyographic (EMG) and muscle biopsy findings are all normal.

Differential diagnosis

Disorders that affect multiple organ systems can produce symptoms similar to idiopathic fibromyalgia (Table 229.3). Chronic systemic infections or inflammatory diseases, occult malignancy, metabolic disorders, and hematological disorders should all be considered. Neurological diseases that affect the central nervous system, peripheral nerve, neuromuscular junction, or muscle can also produce symptoms similar to those of fibromyalgia (Table 229.3). Complete neurological and general physical examinations as well as basic laboratory tests, including complete blood count, kidney and liver function tests, creatine kinase, erythrocyte sedimentation rate, antinuclear antibodies, extractable nuclear antigen, anti-neutrophil cytoplasmic antibody, thyroid studies, and chest radiography serve as adequate screening studies. Additional studies such as EMG, cerebrospinal fluid (CSF) analysis, magnetic resonance imaging (MRI) of the central nervous system, and muscle biopsy are required in selected cases.

Treatment

Treatment strategies for fibromyalgia have included various traditional and alternative forms of therapy. Many patients try dietary supplements, biofeedback, hypnosis, acupuncture, and massage therapy. No objective data support the usefulness of alternative therapies. Corticosteroids, sedatives, and phenothiazines have also been tried, with little objective benefit.

There is class 1 evidence (randomized controlled trials) to support the usefulness of amitriptyline[6,7] and cyclobenzaprine[8] in the treatment of idiopathic fibromyalgia (Table 229.4). Amitriptyline treatment is initiated at a dose of 10 to 25 mg at bedtime and is gradually increased by 25 mg every 2 to 4 weeks to a dose of 75 to 100 mg daily. Slow titration of the dose is important to minimize side effects such as sedation and dry mouth. Other side effects include loss of concentration, nocturnal myoclonus, nightmares, urinary retention, and constipation. Nortriptyline is an alternative to amitriptyline for patients who are intolerant of the anticholinergic side effects. The dose and titration schedule are identical for nortriptyline and amitriptyline. Cyclobenzaprine is used in doses of 10 to 30 mg daily. Side effects are similar to those of the tricyclic antidepressants, with sedation, light-headedness, and dry mouth being most common.

There is class 3 evidence (case reports and uncontrolled series) to suggest that gabapentin, fluoxetine, and nonsteroidal anti-inflammatory agents are beneficial in fibromyalgia.[9–12] Gabapentin treatment is started at a dose of 300 mg 3 times daily and increased as tolerated up to 600 to 900 mg 3 times daily. Sedation, dizziness, poor concentration, and impaired memory are common side effects of gabapentin. Fluoxetine is given in doses of 10 to 20 mg daily. The drug is administered in the morning so it does not aggravate the insomnia associated with fibromyalgia. Nonsteroidal anti-inflammatory drugs are frequently beneficial but should only be used for short intervals

Table 229.4 Medications used to treat fibromyalgia

Medication	Dose	Contraindications	Common adverse effects
Amitriptyline or nortriptyline	10–100 mg at bedtime, lower dose in liver disease	Post acute myocardial infarction, MAO inhibitors	Sedation, dry mouth, constipation, urinary retention
Cyclobenzaprine	10 mg 3 times daily	MAO inhibitors	Sedation, dry mouth, dizziness
Gabapentin	300–600 mg 3 times daily	Allergy to drug	Sedation, light-headedness, ataxia, weight gain
Fluoxetine	10–20 mg every morning, lower dose in liver disease	MAO inhibitors	Insomnia, tremor, nervousness, GI upset
Nonsteroidal anti-inflammatory drugs	Variable, depending on specific agent	Allergy to aspirin or nonsteroidal anti-inflammatory drugs, active peptic ulcer or recent GI tract bleeding	GI upset, constipation, tinnitus, edema, renal toxicity with long-term use

GI, gastrointestinal; MAO, monoamine oxidase.

because of the potential for kidney dysfunction when used chronically. Other antidepressants and psychotherapy are used when symptoms of depression are prominent. Physical therapy with emphasis on daily stretching and graded aerobic exercise is effective for most patients, especially if incorporated into the patient's daily routine and continued indefinitely.[13]

All the therapies currently available for fibromyalgia are more effective when given in combination with patient education and reassurance. Patients are often relieved to know that they do not have a serious life-threatening disease and that they have "a name" attached to their condition, especially when convinced that the physician is supportive and willing to re-examine them if and when symptoms change.

Common cramps, symptomatic tetany, and cramp-fasciculation syndrome

Epidemiology

A muscle cramp is characterized by the sudden onset of a painful muscle contraction that is often precipitated by muscle shortening and relieved by muscle stretch. Cramps occur in normal persons, especially after exercise or the use of caffeine or other stimulants, or in association with metabolic disturbances. They are confined usually to lower extremity muscles but occasionally involve upper limb, axial, or cranial muscles. Common or benign cramps are not associated with other symptoms or signs of neurological disease (except fasciculations) and respond to simple treatment measures (i.e., replacement of fluid and electrolytes, correction of other metabolic disturbances, regular stretching exercises, avoidance of caffeine and other stimulants, or treatment with calcium, magnesium, or quinine). Pathological cramps occur during intoxication with acetylcholinesterase inhibitors (e.g., organophosphates and pyridostig-

mine), in cramp-fasciculation syndrome, and in diseases that damage or cause degeneration of the anterior horn cell or peripheral motor axon (Table 229.5). Pathological cramps are often associated with weakness, muscle atrophy, and other manifestations of damage to the motor unit.

"Symptomatic tetany" describes a state of widespread, frequent, and disabling cramps associated with severe fluid or electrolyte (or both) disturbances. In tetany, cramps are associated with widespread fasciculations and are triggered by hyperventilation, percussion of a nerve (e.g., Chvostek sign), or partial limb ischemia (e.g., Trousseau carpopedal spasm). By definition, the cramps and fasciculations resolve when the underlying metabolic disturbance is corrected. Cramp-fasciculation syndrome is similar to symptomatic tetany except that no underlying

Table 229.5 Disorders associated with muscle cramps

Benign or simple cramps

Symptomatic tetany
  Fluid and electrolyte imbalance, kidney or liver failure, hemodialysis, pregnancy, hypothyroidism, adrenal insufficiency or hypercortisonism (endogenous or exogenous)

Disorders affecting anterior horn cells
  Amyotrophic lateral sclerosis, spinal muscular atrophy, poliomyelitis (including old polio), focal motor neuron disease, structural lesions of spinal cord (syrinx, arteriovenous malformation, tumor, myelitis)

Disorders of motor axon or nerve terminal
  Mono- or polyradiculopathy, diffuse or focal peripheral neuropathy, cramp-fasciculation syndrome, Isaacs syndrome (clinical neuromyotonia), cholinesterase inhibitor intoxication

metabolic disorder can be identified. Patients complain of widespread, frequent, and disabling cramps that are spontaneous or triggered by voluntary muscle activation. Cramp-fasciculation syndrome and Isaacs syndrome have clinical and electrophysiological similarities, including serological evidence of circulating antibodies to potassium channels or, in some patients, neuronal ganglionic-type acetylcholine receptors.[14,15]

Etiology and pathophysiology

Most evidence suggests that cramps arise from the distal intramuscular portion of the motor axon at the nerve terminal or just proximal to it.[16] During initiation of a cramp, action potentials arise in one or more nerve terminals and spread rapidly to adjacent nerve terminals of the same and nearby motor units. This explains the characteristic buildup of high-amplitude and high-frequency motor unit potentials (MUPs) on EMG recordings during cramps as well as the occurrence of numerous fasciculations immediately preceding and following the cramp discharge. Changes in the microenvironment of the intramuscular nerve terminals caused by axonal degeneration, demyelination, immune-mediated channelopathies, or metabolic disturbances increase the tendency for cramp discharges to occur. Drugs that block ion channels and stabilize neuronal membranes reduce the development and propagation of cramp discharges. In some cases of cramp-fasciculation syndrome, there is clinical or electrophysiological evidence (or both) of a peripheral neuropathy, but in the majority, there is no other obvious peripheral nerve lesion. Electrophysiological studies in cramp-fasciculation syndrome show evidence of peripheral nerve hyperexcitability. Repetitive firing of F waves can occur, and repetitive stimulation frequently produces persistent MUP activity or cramp discharges.[17,18] Needle EMG demonstrates frequent fasciculation potentials, MUPs that fire in doublets or triplets, and frequent cramp discharges.[18] The cramp discharges occur spontaneously or are provoked by hyperventilation or limb ischemia (or both). Electrolytes and laboratory measures of kidney, liver, and endocrine function are normal.

Many cases of cramp-fasciculation syndrome have an autoimmune pathogenesis.[14,15] Cramp-fasciculation syndrome may be preceded by an acute infection, occur in association with other autoimmune diseases (e.g., myasthenia gravis, connective tissue disease, autoimmune thyroid disease), or occur as a paraneoplastic syndrome.

Clinical features and classification

Cramps are preceded by fasciculations and an ill-defined subjective tightening of the affected muscle. Shortly thereafter, the cramp is initiated with an explosive palpable contraction that usually can be aborted by passive stretching of the muscle. Prolonged, severe, or recurrent cramps leave residual tenderness and swelling of the muscle and can produce an increase in serum levels of creatine kinase.

Table 229.6 Diagnostic criteria for cramps and related syndromes

Cramp
- Sudden onset of painful muscle contraction associated with visible and palpable shortening of muscle
- Precipitated by muscle contraction, relieved by passive muscle stretch
- Preceded and followed by frequent fasciculations of affected muscle
- Associated with high-frequency discharge of otherwise normal MUPs on EMG recordings that characteristically build to a crescendo over 10–30 seconds at onset of cramp

Common cramp
- Isolated to 1 or 2 distal muscles
- Infrequent, related to exercise or minor metabolic disturbances
- No other manifestations of peripheral nerve hyperexcitability or degeneration

Symptomatic tetany
- Widespread, frequent severe cramps and fasciculations
- Paresthesias and other manifestations of peripheral nerve excitability (e.g., Chvostek or Trousseau sign)
- Significant metabolic disturbance (most commonly hypocalcemia or hypomagnesemia, also liver, kidney, thyroid, and adrenal dysfunction)

Cramp-fasciculation syndrome
- Widespread, frequent severe cramps and fasciculations
- Paresthesias and other manifestations of peripheral nerve excitability
- Absence of significant metabolic disturbance
- Other signs of autoimmunity common (including antibodies to potassium channels or presynaptic neuronal acetylcholine receptors)

EMG, electromyography; MUPs, motor unit potentials

Individual cramps are confined to one muscle or even a portion of a muscle, but multiple muscles can be involved simultaneously.

The diagnostic criteria for cramps and related syndromes are listed in Table 229.6. Cramps that occur independently of other diseases are referred to as "common," "benign," or "idiopathic cramps" (Table 229.5). Common cramps typically are infrequent, short-lived, and isolated to a single muscle or region of the body (usually the calf or foot).

"Symptomatic tetany" describes the syndrome of widespread frequent cramps, fasciculations, paresthesias, and other manifestations of peripheral nerve excitability (e.g., Chvostek and Trousseau signs) associated with a well-defined metabolic disturbance such as hypocalcemia or hypomagnesemia. When the manifestations of tetany occur in the absence of a well-defined metabolic disturbance, the most likely diagnosis is cramp-fasciculation syndrome. Clinically, the patients complain of constant but fluctuating myalgias, muscle stiffness, fasciculations, and frequent muscle cramps that affect unusual muscles (e.g., of the hands, abdominal wall, or thigh or paraspinal muscles) and occur with sufficient frequency and severity to be disabling. Patients often complain of migratory paresthesias, which likely represent hyperexcitability of peripheral sensory neurons. Some authors combine cramp-fasciculation syndrome and Isaacs syndrome under the generic classification of "continuous muscle fiber activity" caused by generalized hyperexcitability of the peripheral nervous system.[19]

Laboratory studies

Laboratory studies are normal in simple cramps. In symptomatic tetany, abnormalities such as hypocalcemia, hypomagnesemia, hyponatremia, or hypokalemia are noted on one or more metabolic tests or on kidney, liver, or endocrine function tests. These test results are normal in cramp-fasciculation syndrome, but some patients have increased antibody titers to voltage-gated potassium channels or neuronal-ganglionic-type acetylcholine receptor antibodies.[14] These antibody assays are not routinely available in all centers but can be obtained through the Neuroimmunology Laboratory at Mayo Medical Reference Laboratories.

Nerve conduction studies may show evidence of a sensorimotor peripheral neuropathy in some patients with cramp-fasciculation syndrome. In cases of symptomatic tetany or cramp-fasciculation syndrome, manifestations of peripheral nerve hyperexcitability are present on electrophysiological studies. These include repetitive firing of F waves, abnormal strength-duration curves, and cramps or other forms of continuous muscle fiber activity induced by repetitive stimulation, exercise, ischemia, or hyperventilation.

Differential diagnosis

Cramps must be differentiated from other disorders that produce painful shortening of the muscle. Central lesions such as focal task-specific or segmental dystonia can simulate cramps. "Dystonia" is characterized by cocontraction of agonist-antagonist muscle groups producing stereotypical movements or fixed postures. EMG recordings show normal-appearing MUPs firing at physiological firing rates. "Contracture" describes a state of muscle shortening that is unaccompanied by detectable electrical muscle activity on standard EMG recordings. Contractures are characteristic of disorders of glycogen metabolism (e.g., myophosphorylase deficiency). These occur during intense exercise and produce painful shortening of the muscle that is electrically silent. The exact mechanism of contracture in glycolytic disorders is not known, but presumably it is related to the acute deficiency of ATP that accompanies the block in glycogen metabolism. Myalgias, stiffness, and, in some cases, myoglobinuria can also occur in disorders of lipid metabolism (primary and secondary carnitine deficiencies or defects of fatty acid oxidation) or in mitochondrial myopathies. "Myotonia" describes involuntary shortening and delayed relaxation of muscle that occurs in association with characteristic waxing-and-waning myotonic discharges on EMG. Muscle pain is particularly common and disabling in myotonia associated with proximal myotonic myopathy. Rippling muscle disease is associated with a wave of partial contraction that is transmitted slowly through the body of the muscle, which in most cases is electrically silent. "Neuromyotonia" (Isaacs syndrome) is associated with diffuse stiffness and hypertrophy of muscles clinically and waning bursts of MUPs firing at very high frequencies (>200 Hz). Isaacs syndrome has also been referred to as the "syndrome of continuous muscle activity"[20] because of various other spontaneous discharges seen on EMG, including myokymic discharges, fasciculations, doublets, triplets, and cramps. Isaacs syndrome and cramp-fasciculation syndrome may have a similar pathophysiological mechanism and represent a spectrum of disorders characterized by continuous muscle activity caused by hyperexcitability of the terminal portion of the motor axon. In addition to true neuromyotonic discharges, classic Isaacs syndrome is frequently associated with symptoms and signs of hypermetabolism such as fever and diaphoresis.[20]

Treatment Simple cramps respond to stretching in combination with fluid and electrolyte supplementation, especially when cramps occur in association with exercise or dehydration. Warming of the distal lower extremities is beneficial in some persons. Tetany resolves after the precipitating metabolic disturbance has been corrected. If cramps are severe, as in cramp-fasciculation syndrome (or, occasionally, motor neuron disease, peripheral neuropathy, radiculopathy, or refractory simple cramps), symptomatic pharmacological treatment is indicated (Table 229.7).

A calcium or magnesium supplement taken orally may be beneficial even when the serum levels of calcium and magnesium are within normal limits. Zinc sulfate has been reported to alleviate frequent cramps associated with liver cirrhosis.[21] If supplementation is unsuccessful, quinine is the traditional drug of choice for treating simple cramps. There is evidence from clinical trials that quinine decreases the frequency of muscle cramps.[22,23] Tinnitus is the most frequent side effect of quinine, but more serious adverse reactions such as acute allergic reactions (including hepatitis), hemolytic anemia, and immune thrombocytopenia can also occur. Membrane-stabilizing drugs and benzodiazepines are used to treat refractory simple cramps or disabling cases of cramp-fasciculation syndrome. Only anecdotal evidence is available with regard to the symptomatic treatment of cramp-fasciculation syndrome.[18,19,24–28] Most of the available data are from opinion, case reports, or small uncontrolled series. Drugs that have been reported to be of benefit include carbamazepine, gabapentin, clonazepam, valproic acid, lamotrigine, phenytoin, and mexiletine. Botulinum toxin has been used to treat severe recurrent cramps refractory to other treatments.[29] Immunomodulating therapy (e.g.,

Table 229.7 Symptomatic drug therapy for cramps and syndromes of continuous muscle activity

Name and indication	Dose	Contraindications	Common adverse effects
Calcium carbonate C, CMA	500 mg twice daily, reduce in kidney impairment	Hypercalcemia	Constipation, hypertension
Magnesium C, CMA	50–100 mg 3 times daily, reduce in kidney impairment	Heart block	Diarrhea
Zinc sulfate C, CMA	200 mg twice daily	None	Metallic taste, GI upset, headache
Quinine C, CMA	260 mg once or twice daily, reduce in liver disease	Allergy to quinine, myasthenia gravis	Tinnitus, thrombocytopenia, hemolytic uremia syndrome, allergic reactions
Carbamazepine C, CMA	100–200 mg twice or 3 times daily	Allergy to drug	Sedation, light-headedness, ataxia, diplopia, blood dyscrasias
Gabapentin C, CMA	300–600 mg 3 times daily	Allergy to drug	Sedation, light-headedness, ataxia, weight gain
Clonazepam C, CMA	0.5–2 mg twice daily, reduce in liver disease	Narrow-angle glaucoma	Sedation, light-headedness, ataxia
Valproic acid (divalproex sodium) C, CMA	250 mg twice or 3 times daily	Liver disease	GI upset, sedation, light-headedness, tremor, weight gain
Baclofen CMA	5–30 mg 3 times daily, reduce in kidney impairment	Allergy to drug	Sedation, light-headedness, ataxia, constipation
Tizanidine hydrochloride CMA	4–8 mg 3 times daily	Allergy to drug	Sedation, light-headedness, dry mouth
Phenytoin CMA	100–300 mg daily	Allergy to drug	Ataxia, gum hypertrophy, blood dyscrasias, peripheral neuropathy
Lamotrigine CMA	50 mg daily initially, then up to 250 mg twice daily	Allergy to drug	Allergic reactions (including Stevens-Johnson syndrome), sedation, headache
Mexiletine CMA	150–300 mg 3 times daily, reduce in liver disease	Drug allergy, 2nd- or 3rd-degree heart block	Ataxia, tremor, arrhythmias, hypotension
Dantrolene sodium CMA	25 mg daily initially, then up to 100 mg twice or 3 times daily	Liver disease	Sedation, GI upset, liver dysfunction
Prednisone CMA	30–60 mg daily	Diabetes mellitus, osteoporosis, obesity	Cataracts, weight gain, hypertension, hyperglycemia, osteoporosis, glaucoma, thinning of skin
IVIG or plasma exchange CMA	400 mg/kg, give infusion (or exchange) once or twice weekly for 4 weeks, then reassess	Kidney failure, active coronary artery disease	IVIG: allergic reactions, headache, renal dysfunction Plasma exchange: hypotension, complications of venous access

C, benign or simple cramps; CMA, continuous muscle activity, including cramp-fasciculation syndrome and Isaacs syndrome (clinical neuromyotonia); GI, gastrointestinal; IVIG, intravenous immunoglobulin.

prednisone, plasma exchange, or intravenous immunoglobulin) may be of benefit in selected cases of cramp-fasciculation syndrome.[14,19,30–32] However, only single case reports or small uncontrolled series have been reported. Immunotherapy is reserved for patients with disabling symptoms that are refractory to symptomatic therapy and have evidence of an autoimmune pathogenesis (i.e., serum antibodies to potassium channels or neuronal acetylcholine receptors or a personal history of other autoimmune diseases).

Isaacs syndrome (clinical neuromyotonia)

Epidemiology In 1961 and 1967, Isaacs[20,33] described

the clinical and electrophysiological features of three patients who had generalized muscle stiffness and excessive sweating caused by hyperexcitability of peripheral nerves. The condition responded to treatment with either phenytoin or carbamazepine.[24,33] Unique high-frequency bursts of EMG activity called "neuromyotonic discharges" were observed in these original cases of "Isaacs syndrome," in addition to fasciculations, cramps, doublets, triplets, and myokymic discharges. The spontaneous activity disappeared with neuromuscular blockade but not with peripheral nerve block or general anesthesia, suggesting that the nerve terminal is the site of origin. Subsequently, similar cases were described under various terms, including "continuous muscle fiber activity," "quantal squander," "generalized idiopathic myokymia," "cramp-fasciculation syndrome," "normocalcemic tetany," and "neuromyotonia." However, not all cases of "neuromyotonia" described in the literature have neuromyotonic discharges on EMG. The disorders lumped under these general terms share features of muscle stiffness, cramps, clinical myokymia, and EMG evidence of peripheral nerve hyperactivity. These disorders may represent a continuous spectrum of the same process, with mild cases of "cramp-fasciculation syndrome" at one end and "clinical neuromyotonia" or classical "Isaacs syndrome" at the other. However, there is evidence that the peripheral nerve hyperexcitability that characterizes these disorders arises from different regions of the motor axon and through different mechanisms.[19] Until the exact pathogenesis is known, there will continue to be confusion and controversy over the nomenclature used to describe these syndromes.

Etiology and pathophysiology Some cases of clinical neuromyotonia (Isaacs syndrome) are associated with a generalized peripheral neuropathy (inherited or acquired), whereas others result from exposure to various neurotoxins (organophosphates, mercury, gold, snake venom, or penicillamine) (Table 229.8). Most idiopathic cases of neuromyotonia appear to be autoimmune in origin. This is supported by the association with other autoimmune disorders, occurrence as a paraneoplastic syndrome, finding of serum antibodies to various ion channels on the nerve terminal, passive transfer experiments, and improvement with immunomodulating therapy.[14,19,32]

The mechanism of peripheral nerve hyperexcitability in clinical neuromyotonia varies. Evidence from animal models indicates that neuromyotonia associated with peripheral neuropathies (inherited or acquired) arises from ephaptic transmission between axons in the proximal motor nerve or hyperexcitability of the motor neuron cell body within the spinal cord.[32] Toxins may have a direct effect on ion channels or indirect effects by altering axonal myelination or inducing autoimmune reactions to axonal or nerve terminal antigens. In some idiopathic autoimmune and paraneoplastic cases, antibodies to voltage-gated potassium channels on motor nerve terminals led to prolonged repolarization and repetitive discharge of

the axon.[31] Antibodies to presynaptic neuronal ganglionic-type acetylcholine receptors located on the motor nerve terminal may also lead to peripheral nerve hyperexcitability in classic Isaacs syndrome and cramp-fasciculation syndrome.[34]

Clinical features Classic Isaacs syndrome is characterized by the insidious onset and progression of generalized muscle stiffness. Other common features include muscle cramps, fasciculations, clinical myokymia, excessive sweating, and generalized muscle hypertrophy. Involvement of cranial muscles may lead to various symptoms, including dysarthria, dysphagia, dysphonia, and difficulty chewing. An unusual generalized slowness of movement often gives the false impression of a psychogenic illness. Some patients describe transient paresthesias and myalgias, but pain is not usually a prominent feature. Some patients have evidence of a peripheral neuropathy, but weakness is rare, particularly in idiopathic or autoimmune types. The disease may begin at any time after the first decade. In most cases, the disease progresses slowly; however, spontaneous and activity-related fluctuation is common. As noted above, less severe forms of clinical neuromyotonia have been described under various names. The clinical manifestations are similar to those of classic Isaacs syndrome, although most lack cranial involvement, excessive sweating, and generalized muscle hypertrophy. Frequent and severe cramps, especially in unusual locations, are usually classified under the heading of "cramp-fasciculation syndrome" (Table 229.6).

Laboratory testing The findings on serum antibody testing in classic Isaacs syndrome are similar to those mentioned above for cramp-fasciculation syndrome, except that a higher percentage of patients with Isaacs syndrome have increased serum titers of voltage-gated potassium channel antibodies.[14,31,32] Also, electrophysiological studies have shown similarities between the two syndromes, with repetitive firing of F waves, abnormal strength-duration curves, and continuous muscle fiber activity induced by repetitive nerve stimulation.[35] In contrast to the cramp-fasciculation syndrome, classic Isaacs syndrome tends to have

Table 229.8 Classification of clinical neuromyotonia

Inherited
    Spinal muscular atrophy
    Inherited neuropathy (CMT1)

Acquired
    Peripheral neuropathy (usually demyelinating)
    Neurotoxin exposure (organophosphates, mercury, gold, snake venom, and so forth)

Autoimmune
    Idiopathic
    Paraneoplastic (especially thymoma, small cell lung carcinoma)

35. Maddison P, Newsom-Davis J, Mills KR. Strength-
    duration properties of peripheral nerve in acquired
    neuromyotonia. Muscle Nerve 1999;22:823–830

41. Stephan DA, Hoffman EP. Physical mapping of the rip-
    pling muscle disease locus. Genomics 1999;55:268–274

42. Ansevin CF, Agamanolis DP. Rippling muscles and

230 Overview of Movement Disorders

Stanley Fahn

Introduction

Movement disorders can be defined as neurological syndromes in which there is either an excess of movement or a paucity of voluntary and automatic movements, unrelated to weakness or spasticity (Table 230.1). The former are commonly referred to as hyperkinesias (excessive movements), dyskinesias (unnatural movements), and abnormal involuntary movements. The term dyskinesias is usually used, but all are interchangeable. The five major categories of dyskinesias, in alphabetical order, are: chorea, dystonia, myoclonus, tics and tremor. Table 230.1 presents the complete list.

The paucity of movement group can be referred to as hypokinesia (decreased amplitude of movement), but bradykinesia (slowness of movement) and akinesia (loss of movement) are reasonable alternative names. The parkinsonian syndromes are the most common cause of such paucity of movement; other hypokinetic disorders represent only a small group of patients. Basically, movement disorders can be conveniently divided into parkinsonism and all other types; there is about an equal number of patients in each of these two groups.

Table 230.1   List of movement disorders

I. *Hypokinesias*
A. Akinesia/bradykinesia (parkinsonism)
B. Apraxia
C. Blocking (holding) tics
D. Cataplexy and drop attacks
E. Catatonia, psychomotor depression, and obsessional slowness
F. Freezing phenomenon
G. Hesitant gaits
H. Hypothyroid slowness
I. Rigidity
J. Stiff-muscles

II. *Hyperkinesias*

A. Abdominal dyskinesias	L. Jumpy stumps
B. Akathitic movements	M. Moving toes/fingers
C. Asynergia/ataxia	N. Myoclonus
D. Athetosis	O. Myokymia
E. Ballism	P. Myorhythmia
F. Chorea	Q. Paroxysmal dyskinesias
G. Dysmetria	R. Restless legs
H. Dystonia	S. Stereotypy
I. Hemifacial spasm	T. Tics
J. Hyperekplexia	U. Tremor
K. Hypnogenic dyskinesias	

The origins of abnormal movements

Most movement disorders are associated with pathological alterations in the basal ganglia or their connections. The basal ganglia are a group of gray matter nuclei lying deep within the cerebral hemispheres (caudate, putamen, and pallidum), the diencephalon (subthalamic nucleus), and the mesencephalon (substantia nigra). There are some exceptions to this general rule. Pathology of the cerebellum or its pathways typically results in impairment of coordination (asynergy, ataxia), misjudgment of distance (dysmetria) and intention tremor. Myoclonus and many forms of tremors do not appear to be related primarily to basal ganglia pathology, and often arise elsewhere in the central nervous system, including the cerebral cortex (cortical reflex myoclonus), brainstem (cerebellar outflow tremor, reticular reflex myoclonus, hyperekplexia, and rhythmical brainstem myoclonus such as palatal myoclonus and ocular myoclonus), and spinal cord (rhythmical segmental myoclonus and non-rhythmic propriospinal myoclonus). Moreover, many myoclonic disorders are associated with diseases in which the cerebellum is involved, such as those causing the Ramsay Hunt syndrome of progressive myoclonic ataxia. It is not known for certain which part of the brain is associated with tics, although the basal ganglia and the limbic structures have been implicated. Certain localizations within the basal ganglia are classically associated with specific movement disorders: substantia nigra—bradykinesia and rest tremor; subthalamic nucleus—ballism; caudate nucleus—chorea; and putamen—dystonia. Finally, there is a growing body of evidence supporting the notion that some movement disorders are peripherally induced.[1,2]

Epidemiology

Movement disorders are common neurological problems, and epidemiological studies are available for some of them (Table 230.2).[3–17] There have been several studies for Parkinson's disease (PD), and these have been carried out in a number of countries.[3]

Genetics

A large number of movement disorders are genetic in etiology, and some of the diseases have now been mapped to specific regions of the genome, and some have even been localized to a specific gene (Table 230.3).[19–145] For example, seven genetic loci have so far been identified with Parkinson's disease (PD) or variants of classical PD. Several of them have been identified with a specific gene and protein. A

Table 230.2   Prevalence of movement disorders

Disorder	No. per 100 000	Reference
Restless legs	9800*	3
Essential tremor	415	4
Parkinson's disease	187	5
Tourette's syndrome	29–1052	6, 7
	2990	8
Primary torsion dystonia	33	9
Hemifacial spasm	7.4–14.5	10
Hereditary ataxia	6	11
Huntington's disease	2–12	12, 13
Wilson's disease	3	14
Progressive supranuclear palsy	2	15
	6.4	16
Multiple system atrophy	4.4	16

*For restless legs, the rate cited is in a population >65 years. For Parkinson's disease, the rate is 347 per 100 000 for ages over 40 years.[17]

comprehensive list of movement disorders whose genes have been mapped or identified are listed in Table 230.3. Several inherited movement disorders are due to expanded repeats of the trinucleotide cytosine-adensosine-guanosine (CAG), and Friedreich's ataxia by the expanded trinucleotide repeat of guanosine-adensosine-adenosine (GAA). Normal individuals contain an acceptable number of these trinucleotide repeats in their genes, but these triplicate repeats are unstable and, when expanded, lead to disease (Table 230.4).[62,146] Neurogenetics is one of the fastest moving research areas in neurology, so the list in Table 230.3 keeps expanding rapidly.

Differential diagnosis of hypokinesias

Akinesia/bradykinesia

Akinesia, bradykinesia, and hypokinesia literally mean absence, slowness, and decreased amplitude of movement, respectively. The three terms are commonly grouped together for convenience and usually referred to under the term of bradykinesia. These phenomena are a prominent and most important feature of parkinsonism, and are often equated as a *sine qua non* for parkinsonism. Although akinesia means lack of movement, the label is often used to indicate a very severe form of bradykinesia. Brady-kinesia is mild in early Parkinson's disease, and becomes more severe in advanced Parkinson's disease and other forms of parkinsonism. The primary parkinsonism disorder known as Parkinson's disease, also referred to as idiopathic parkinsonism, is the most common type of parkinsonism encountered by the neurologist. However, drug-induced parkinsonism is probably the most common form of parkinsonism since neuroleptic drugs (dopamine receptor blocking agents), which cause drug-induced parkinsonism, are widely prescribed for treating psychosis.

Bradykinesia is a cardinal symptom of all types of parkinsonism.

Akinesia/bradykinesia/hypokinesia is manifested *cranially* by masked facies (hypomimia), decreased frequency of blinking, impaired upgaze and convergence of the eyes, soft speech (hypophonia) with loss of inflection (aprosody), and drooling of saliva due to decreased spontaneous swallowing; *in the arms* by slowness in raising the shoulder and the arm, loss of spontaneous movement such as gesturing, smallness and slowness of handwriting (micrographia), difficulty with hand dexterity for shaving, brushing teeth, and putting on make-up; *in the legs* by a short-stepped, shuffling gait with decreased armswing; and *in the trunk* by difficulty arising from a chair, getting out of automobiles; and turning in bed. Bradykinesia thus encompasses a loss of automatic movements as well as slowness in initiating movement on command and reduction in amplitude of the voluntary movement. An early feature of reduction of amplitude is the decrementing of the amplitude with repetitive finger tapping or foot tapping, which also manifests impaired rhythm of the tapping. Carrying out two activities simultaneously is impaired,[147] and this difficulty may represent bradykinesia as well.[148] With the stimulation of a sufficient sensory input, bradykinesia, hypokinesia and akinesia can be temporarily overcome.

Apraxia

Apraxia is traditionally defined as a disorder of voluntary movement that cannot be explained by weakness, spasticity, rigidity, sensory loss, or cognitive impairment. It can exist and be tested for in the presence of a movement disorder provided that akinesia, rigidity, or dystonia is not so severe that voluntary movement cannot be executed. The concepts of apraxia are being refined into more discrete identifiable syndromes as knowledge of the functions of the cortical systems controlling voluntary movement advances.[149] A quick, convenient method for testing for apraxia at the bedside is to ask patients to copy a series of hand postures shown to them by the examiner.

Apraxias are found in a number of movement disorders, for example *cortical-basal* ganglionic degeneration (CBGD) and progressive supranuclear palsy. A number of other phenomena reflecting cerebral cortex dysfunction may be seen in such patients. The alien limb phenomenon, also seen in CBGD, consists of involuntary, spontaneous movements of an arm or leg, which curiously and spontaneously moves to adopt odd postures quite beyond the control or understanding of the patient. Intermanual conflict is another such phenomenon; one hand irresistibly and uncontrollably begins to interfere with the voluntary action of the other. The abnormally behaving limb may also show forced grasping of objects, such as blankets or clothing. Such patients often exhibit other frontal lobe signs, such as a grasp reflex or utilization behavior, in which they compulsively pick up objects presented to them and begin to employ them. For

Table 230.3 Gene localization of movement disorders

Category	Pattern of inheritance	Chromosome region	Name of gene	Gene identified	Triplet repeat	Name of protein	Function	References
Parkinson's disease								
Familial								
Parkinson's disease	Autosomal dominant	4q21-q22	PARK1	Yes	No	Alpha-synuclein	synaptic	19–21
Young-onset Parkinson's disease	Autosomal recessive	6q25.2-q27	PARK2	Yes	No	Parkin	Ubiquitin-protein ligase	22–26
Susceptibility locus	Autosomal dominant	2p13	PARK3	No	N/I	N/I	N/I	27
Parkinson's disease with essential tremor	Autosomal dominant	4p	PARK4	No	N/I	N/I	N/I	28
Familial Parkinson's disease	Autosomal recessive	4p15	PARK5	Yes	No	Ubiquitin carboxylase Terminal hydrolase L1	Hydrolase ubiquitin	29
Familial Parkinson's disease	Mitochondrial	Mitochondrial	N/I	No	No	N/I	Complex I	30
Familial Parkinson's disease	Mitochondrial gene	Mitochondrial	ND4	Yes	No	N/I	Complex I	31
Parkinson-plus syndromes								
Fronto-temporal dementia	Autosomal dominant	17q21-q23	Tau	Yes	No	Tau	N/I	32–34
Pick's disease	?	17q21-q23	Tau	Yes	No	Tau	N/I	35
PSP and CBGD	Susceptibility locus	17q21-q23	Tau	Yes	No	Tau	N/I	36–42
MSA	?	3P21	ZNF231	Yes	No	Zinc finger protein	Nuclear protein	43
Parkinson's MELAS syndrome	Mitochondrial gene	Mitochondrial	Cytochrome b	Yes	No	Cytochrome b	Complex IIIb	44
Familial ALS	Autosomal dominant	21q	SOD1	Yes	No	Cu/Zn superoxide dismutase	Convert superoxide to H_2O_2	45
Ataxia syndromes								
Friedreich ataxia	Autosomal recessive	9q13-q21.1	X25	Yes	GAA	Frataxin	Phospho-inositide/Fe homeostasis in mitochondria	46
Early onset cerebellar ataxia	Autosomal recessive	13q11-12	No	No	N/I	N/I	N/I	47, 48

continued

Table 230.3 *Continued*

Category	Pattern of inheritance	Chromosome region	Name of gene	Gene identified	Triplet repeat	Name of protein	Function	References
X-linked congenital ataxia	X-linked recessive	X	No	No	N/I	N/I	N/I	49
Ataxic cerebral palsy	Autosomal recessive	9p12-q12	No	No	N/I	N/I	N/I	50
Posterior column ataxia with retinitis pigmentosa	Autosomal recessive	1q31-q32	AXPC 1	No	No	N/I	N/I	51
Adult-onset ataxia with tocopherol deficiency	Autosomal recessive	8q13.1-13.3	α-TTP	Yes	No	α-Tocopherol transfer protein gene	Transfers α-T to mitochondria	52
Ataxia-telangiectasia	Autosomal recessive	11q22-q23	ATM	Yes	No	PI-3 kinase	DNA repair	53, 54
SCA-1	Autosomal dominant	6p22-p23	SCA1	Yes	CAG	Ataxin-1	N/I	55
SCA-2	Autosomal dominant	12q23-24.1	SCA2	Yes	CAG	Ataxin-2	N/I	56
SCA-3 (Machado–Joseph disease)	Autosomal dominant	14q32.1	SCA3	Yes	CAG	Ataxin-3	N/I	57
SCA-4	Autosomal dominant	16q22.1	SCA4	No	N/I	N/I	N/I	58, 59
SCA-5	Autosomal dominant	11cent	SCA5	No	N/I	N/I	N/I	60
SCA-6	Autosomal dominant	19p13	CACNL1A4	Yes	CAG	–	Ca²⁺ channel	61, 62
SCA-7	Autosomal dominant	3q12-13	SCA7	Yes	CAG	N/I	N/I	63–65
SCA-8	Autosomal dominant	13q21	SCA8	Yes	CTG	N/I	N/I	66
SCA-10	Autosomal dominant	22q13	SCA10	No	N/I	N/I	N/I	67, 68
SCA-12	Autosomal dominant	5q31-q33	PPP2R2B	Yes	CAG	Phosphatase 2A	N/I	69, 70
SCA-13	Autosomal dominant	19q13.3-q13.4	SCA13	No	N/I	N/I	N/I	71
SCA-14	Autosomal dominant	19q13.4-qter	SCA13	No	N/I	N/I	N/I	72

Table 230.3 *Continued*

Category	Pattern of inheritance	Chromosome region	Name of gene	Gene identified	Triplet repeat	Name of protein	Function	References
Choreic syndromes								
Huntington's disease	Autosomal dominant	4p16.3	IT15	Yes	CAG	Huntington	N/I	73
Huntington-like disease	Autosomal dominant	20p	N/I	No	No	N/I	N/I	74
Huntington-like disease	Autosomal recessive	4p15.3	N/I	No	No	N/I	N/I	75
Neuro-acanthocytosis	Autosomal recessive	9q21	—	No	N/I	N/I	N/I	76, 77
Benign hereditary chorea	Autosomal dominant	14q	No	No	N/I	N/I	N/I	78
Choreoathetosis								
Choreoathetosis and mental retardation	X-linked recessive	Xp11	N/I	N/I	N/I	N/I	N/I	79
Lesch–Nyhan syndrome	X-linked recessive	Xq26-q27.2	HPRT	Yes	No	Hypoxanthine-guanine-phosphoribosyl transferase		80
Dystonia								
Oppenheim's torsion dystonia	Autosomal dominant	9q34	DYT1	Yes	No, GAG deletion	Torsin A	ATP binding	81, 82
Lubag (X-linked dystonia-parkinsonism)	X-linked recessive	Xq13.1	DYT3	No	N/I	N/I	N/I	83, 84
Dopa-responsive dystonia	Autosomal dominant	14q22.1-q22.2	DYT5	Yes	No	GTP cyclo-hydrolase 1	Synthesis of BH4	85, 86
Cranio-cervical dystonia	Autosomal dominant	8p21-q22	DYT6	No	N/I	N/I	N/I	87
Familial torticollis	Autosomal dominant	18p?	DYT7	N/I	N/I	N/I	N/I	88
Myoclonus-dystonia	Autosomal dominant	7q21-q31	DYT11	Yes	No	Epsilon-sarcoglycan	N/I	89, 90

continued

Table 230.3 *Continued*

Category	Pattern of inheritance	Chromosome region	Name of gene	Gene identified	Triplet repeat	Name of protein	Function	References
Rapid-onset dystonia-parkinsonism	Autosomal dominant	19q13	DYT12	N/I	N/I	N/I	N/I	91, 92
Cervical-cranial-brach.	Autosomal dominant	1p36.13-p36.32	DYT13	No	N/I	N/I	N/I	93
Deafness-dystonia-optic atrophy	X-linked recessive	X	DDP	Yes	No	DDP	Intermembrane protein transport in mitochondria	94–97
Dystonic lipidosis (Niemann–Pick type C)	Autosomal recessive	18q11-12	NPC1	Yes	No	—	Esterification of LDL derived cholesterol	98
Neuro degeneration with iron deposition	Autosomal recessive	20p12.3-p13	PANK 2	N/I	N/I	N/I	Panto thenate kinase	99, 100
Hyperekplexia Hereditary hyperekplexia	Autosomal dominant	5q34-q35	STHE	Yes	No	GLRA1	Glycine receptor	101
Myoclonus Unverricht–Lundborg disease	Autosomal recessive	21q22.3	EPM1	No	N/I	Cystatin B	Cysteine protease inhibitor	102, 103
Lafora body disease	Autosomal recessive	6q24	EPM2A	Yes	No	Laforin	Tyrosine phosphatase	104–106
Progressive myoclonus epilepsy	Mitochondrial gene	Mitochondrial	tRNA (Ser (UCN))	Yes	No	N/I	N/I	107
Familial adult myoclonus epilepsy	Autosomal dominant	8q23.3-q24.1	FAME	No	No	N/I	N/I	
Familial Creutzfeldt-Jakob disease	Autosomal dominant	20pter-p12	PRNP	Yes	No	Prion protein	N/I	108

Table 230.3 *Continued*

Category	Pattern of inheritance	Chromosome region	Name of gene	Gene identified	Triplet repeat	Name of protein	Function	References
Dentatorubral-pallidoluysian atrophy	Autosomal dominant	12p12-ter	—	Yes	CAG	Atrophin	N/I	109, 110
Paroxysmal dyskinesias								
Episodic ataxia-1/myokymia	Autosomal dominant	12p13	Kv1.1	Yes	No	KCNA1	K$^+$ channel	111,112
Episodic ataxia-2/vestibular	Autosomal dominant	19p13	CACN L1A4	Yes	No	CACNL 1A4	Ca^{2+}	113, 114
Paroxysmal kinesigenic dyskinesia (PKD)	Autosomal dominant	16p11.2-q11.2	—	No	N/I	N/I	N/I	115, 116
Paroxysmal kinesigenic dyskinesia (PKD)	Autosomal dominant	16q13-q22.1	EKD2	No	N/I	N/I	N/I	117
Paroxysmal nonkinesigenic dyskinesia (PKND) (Mount–Reback syndrome)	Autosomal dominant	2q34	FPD1	No	N/I	N/I	N/I	118–123
Paroxysmal dyskinesia and spasticity	Autosomal dominant	1p	CSE	No	N/I	N/I	N/I	124
Paroxysmal dyskinesia and infantile convulsions and childhood exercise-induced dyskinesia	Autosomal recessive	16p12-q11.2	N/I	No	N/I	N/I	N/I	125–128

continued

Table 230.3   *Continued*

Category	Pattern of inheritance	Chromosome region	Name of gene	Gene identified	Triplet repeat	Name of protein	Function	References
Familial hypnogenic seizures/ dystonia	Autosomal dominant	20q12.2-13.3	CHRN A4	Yes	No	CHRNA4	Nicotinic Ach receptor	129, 130
Tics								
Tourette syndrome	Autosomal dominant	11q23	—	No	N/I	N/I	N/I	131
Stereotypies								
Rett syndrome	X-linked dominant	Xq28	MECP2	Yes	No	Methyl-CpG-binding protein	Binds CpG proteins	132, 133
Tremor								
Familial essential tremor	Autosomal dominant	2p22-p25	ETM	N/I	N/I	N/I	N/I	134
Familial essential tremor	Autosomal dominant	3q1	FET1	N/I	N/I	N/I	N/I	135
Hereditary geniospasm	Autosomal dominant	9q13-q21	—	N/I	N/I	N/I	N/I	136
Roussy–Lévy syndrome	Autosomal dominant	17p11.2	CMT-1B	Yes	No	Peripheral myelin protein	Myelin	137
A variety of movements								
Wilson's disease	Autosomal recessive	13q14.3	ATB7B	Yes	No	Cu-ATPase	Copper transport	138, 139
Neuronal ceroid lipofuscinoses (Batten's disease):								
Infantile	Autosomal recessive	1p32	CLN1	Yes	No	Palmitoyl protein thioesterase	Lysosomal proteolysis	140, 141
Late-infantile-classical	Autosomal recessive	9q13-q21	CLN2	Yes	No	Pepstatin-insensitive protease	Lysosomal proteolysis	142

Table 230.3 *Continued*

Category	Pattern of inheritance	Chromosome region	Name of gene	Gene identified	Triplet repeat	Name of protein	Function	References
Finnish late infantile	Autosomal recessive	13q22	CLN5	Yes	No	Unnamed membrane protein	Lysosomal proteolysis	143
Variant late infantile	Autosomal recessive	15q21-23	CLN6	No	N/I	N/I	N/I	142
Variant late infantile	Autosomal recessive	N/I	CLN7	No	N/I	N/I	N/I	144
Variant late infantile	Autosomal recessive	1p32	CLN1	Yes	N/I	Palmitoyl protein thioesterase	Lysosomal proteolysis	145
Juvenile	Autosomal recessive	16p12	CLN3	Yes	No	Battenin	Lysosomal proteolysis	144, 146, 147
Variant juvenile	Autosomal recessive	1p32	CLN1	Yes	N/I	Palmitoyl protein thioesterase	Lysosomal proteolysis	145

N/I, not yet identified; CAG, cytosine-adenosine-guanosine trinucleotide; GAA, guanosine-adenosine-adenosine; BH4, tetrahydrobiopterin.

Table 230.4   Size of trinucleotide repeats

Disease	Type of nucleotide	In normals	In disease
Huntington disease	CAG	11–34	37–121
SCA-1	CAG	19–36	42–81
SCA-2	CAG	15–29	35–59
SCA-3 (Machado–Joseph)	CAG	12–40	66 > 200
SCA-6	CAG	4–16	21–28
SCA-7	CAG		estimated 64
DRPLA	CAG	7–34	49–83
Friedreich's ataxia	GAA	7–22	120–1700

Data in part from Brooks and Fischbeck[46] and Riess et al.[62]
SCA, spinocerebellar degeneration; DRPLA, dentatorubral-pallidoluysian atrophy.

example, if a pen is presented with no instructions, they pick it up and write.

Blocking (holding) tics

Blocking (or holding) is a motor phenomenon that is seen occasionally in patients with tics and is characterized as a brief interference of social discourse and contact. There is no loss of consciousness and, although patients do not speak during these episodes, they are fully aware of what has been spoken. The tics appear in two situations: 1) as an accompanying feature of some prolonged tics, such as during a protracted dystonic tic or during tic status; and 2) as a specific tic phenomenon in the absence of an accompanying obvious motor or vocal tic. The latter occurrences have the abruptness and duration of a dystonic tic or a series of clonic tics, but they do not occur during an episode of an obvious motor tic.

Although both types can be called blocking tics, the first type can be considered "intrusions" because the interruption of activity is due to a positive motor phenomenon (i.e., severe, somewhat prolonged motor tics) that interferes with other motor activities. An example is a burst of tics that is severe enough to interrupt ongoing motor acts, including speech.

The second type, i.e. inhibition of ongoing motor activity without an obvious "active" tic, can be considered as a negative motor phenomenon, i.e. a "negative" tic. The negative type of blocking tics should be differentiated from absence seizures or other paroxysmal episodes of loss of awareness. There is never loss of awareness with blocking tics. Individuals with intrusions and negative blocking recognize that they have these interruptions of normal activity, and are fully aware of the environment during them, even if they are unable to speak at that time.

Cataplexy and drop attacks

Drop attacks can be defined as sudden falls with or without loss of consciousness, due either to collapse of postural muscle tone or to abnormal muscle contractions in the legs. About two-thirds of cases are of unknown etiology.[150] There are many neurological and non-neurological causes of symptomatic drop attacks. Neurological disorders include leg weakness, sudden falls in parkinsonian syndromes including those due to freezing, transient ischemic attacks, epilepsy, myoclonus, startle reactions, paroxysmal dyskinesias, structural CNS lesions, and hydrocephalus. Syncope and cardiovascular disease account for non-neurological causes. Idiopathic drop attacks usually appear between the ages of 40 and 59 years, with the prevalence increasing with advancing age,[151] and are a common cause of falls and fractures in the elderly.[152,153] A review of drop attacks has been provided by Lee and Marsden.[154]

Cataplexy is another cause of symptomatic drop attacks that does not fit the categories listed above. Patients with cataplexy fall suddenly without loss of consciousness, but with inability to speak during an attack. There is a precipitating trigger, usually laughter or a sudden emotional stimulus. The patient's muscle tone is flaccid and remains this way for many seconds. Cataplexy is usually just one feature of the narcolepsy syndrome, which also include sleep paralysis and hypnagogic hallucinations, in addition to the characteristic feature of uncontrollable falling asleep. A review of cataplexy has been provided by Guilleminault.[155]

Catatonia, psychomotor depression, and obsessional slowness

Gelenberg[156] defined catatonia as a syndrome characterized by catalepsy (abnormal maintenance of posture or physical attitudes), waxy flexibility (retention of the limbs for an indefinite period of time in the positions in which they are placed), negativism, mutism, and bizarre mannerisms. Patients with catatonia can remain in one position for hours, and move exceedingly slowly to commands, usually requiring the examiner to push them along. However, when moving spontaneously they move quickly, such as when scratching themselves. In contrast to patients with parkinsonism, there is no concomitant cogwheel rigidity, freezing, or loss of postural reflexes. Classically, catatonia is a feature of schizophrenia, but it can occur with severe depression. Gelenberg also stated that catatonia can appear with conversion hysteria, dissociative states, and with organic brain disease.

However, this author believes that his organic syndromes of akinetic mutism, abulia, encephalitis etc. should be distinguished from catatonia, and prefer that catatonia be considered a psychiatric disorder.

Depression is commonly associated with a general slowness of movement as well as thinking, so-called psychomotor retardation, and catatonia can be considered an extreme case of this problem. Although depressed patients are widely recognized to manifest slowness in movement, some (particularly children) may not have the more classical symptoms of low mood, dysphoria, anorexia, insomnia, somatizations, and tearfulness. In this situation, slowness due to depression can be difficult to distinguish from the bradykinesia of parkinsonism; like catatonia, lack of rigidity and preservation of postural reflexes may help differentiate psychomotor slowness from parkinsonism. However, there can be loss of facial expression and decreased blinking in both catatonia and depression. Lack of Myerson's sign, snout reflex, and palmomental reflexes are the rule, all of which are usually present in parkinsonism. In children with psychomotor depression and motor slowness, the differential diagnosis is that of juvenile parkinsonism, including Wilson's disease and the akinetic form of Huntington's disease.

Some patients with obsessive–compulsive disorder (OCD) may present with extreme slowness of movement, so-called obsessional slowness. Hymas et al.[157] evaluated 17 such patients, out of 59 admitted to hospital with OCD. These patients had difficulty initiating goal-directed action, and had many suppressive interruptions and perseverative behavior. Besides slowness, some patients had cogwheel rigidity, decreased armswing when walking, decreased spontaneous movement, hypomimia and flexed posture. However, there was no decrementing of either amplitude or speed with repetitive movements, no tremor and no micrographia. Also there was no freezing or loss of postural reflexes. Like other forms of OCD, this is a chronic illness. Fluorodopa PET scans revealed no abnormality of dopa uptake, thereby clearly distinguishing this disorder from Parkinson's disease.[158] However, there is hypermetabolism in orbital, frontal, premotor, and midfrontal cortex, suggesting excessive neural activity in these regions.

Freezing

Freezing refers to transient periods, usually lasting several seconds, in which the motor act is halted and the patient is "stuck in place." It commonly develops in parkinsonism, both primary and atypical.[159] The freezing phenomenon has also been called motor blocks.[160] The terms "pure akinesia"[161–163] and "gait ignition failure"[164,165] refer to syndromes in which freezing is the predominant clinical feature, with only minimal other features of parkinsonism.

In freezing the voluntary motor activity being attempted is halted because agonists and antagonist muscles are simultaneously and isometrically contracting,[166] preventing normal execution of voluntary movement. The motor blockage, therefore, is not one

of lack of muscle tone or flaccidity, but rather is analogous to being glued to a position forcing the patient to make an increased effort to overcome being "stuck." With freezing of gait, by far the most common form of the freezing phenomenon, as the patient attempts to move the feet, short, incomplete steps are attempted but the feet tend to remain in the same place ("glued to the ground"). After a few seconds the freezing clears spontaneously, and the patient is able to move at a normal pace again, until the next freezing episode develops. Often patients learn some trick maneuver to terminate the freezing episode sooner. Stepping over an "inverted cane" when the legs begin to freeze is one method by which they can manage to ambulate.

Although freezing most often affects walking, it can manifest in other ways. Speech can be "arrested," with the patient repeating a sound until it finally becomes unstuck and speech then continues. This can be considered a severe form of parkinsonian palilalia, which usually refers to a repetition of the first syllable of the word. Parkinsonian palilalia differs from the palilalia seen in patients with Tourette syndrome, in which there is repetition of entire words or a string of words.

Freezing of the arms, such as during handwriting or teeth-brushing, has also been reported.[161] Difficulty opening the eyes can be another kind of freezing. Eyelid freezing was originally called "apraxia of eyelid opening," which is a misnomer because the problem is not an apraxia. Eyelid freezing has also been called "levator palpebrae inhibition"[167] and even a form of dystonia. Although previously unrecognized as a freezing phenomenon, and usually considered a form of body bradykinesia, difficulty in arising from a chair may be due to freezing in some patients. Patients use many tricks to overcome freezing, but these may not always be successful. An update on the freezing phenomenon is provided in a review by Fahn.[168]

As discussed above, the freezing phenomenon occurs in parkinsonism, whether it be primary (Parkinson's disease),[160] secondary (such as vascular parkinsonism) or Parkinson-plus syndromes, such as progressive supranuclear palsy and multiple system atrophy. It can also appear as an idiopathic freezing gait without other features of parkinsonism, except for loss of postural reflexes and mild bradykinesia.[164,169] In some patients it may be an early sign of impending progressive supranuclear palsy[170] or due to nigropallidal degeneration.[171]

Hesitant gaits

Hesitant gaits or uncertain gaits are seen in a number of syndromes. The cautious gait seen in some elderly people is slow on a wide base with short steps, and superficially may resemble that of parkinsonism except there are no other parkinsonian features. Fear of falling, either because of perceived instability or actual loss of postural righting reflexes, produces an inability to walk independently without holding onto people or objects. Because this abnormal gait disappears when the person walks holding onto someone, it is often considered to be a psychiatric disorder, a phobia of open spaces (i.e. agoraphobia). However, because previous falls usually play a role in patients developing this disorder, the current author believes it to be a true fear of falling, distinguishable from agoraphobia, which is a separate syndrome. Fear of falling should be differentiated from other types of psychogenic gait disorders. A cautious gait may be superimposed upon any other gait disorder.

The senile gait disorder (or gait disorder of the elderly) is a poorly understood condition that comprises a number of different syndromes.[165] In gait ignition failure,[164] also called primary freezing gait,[169] the problem is one of getting started. Once underway, such patients walk fairly briskly, and equilibrium is preserved. In the frontal gait disorders, there is also start-hesitation, and walking is with slow, small, shuffling steps, similar to that in Parkinson's disease. However, there are few other signs of parkinsonism, and equilibrium is preserved. Such a gait can occur with frontal lobe tumors, cerebrovascular disease and hydrocephalus, all causing frontal lobe damage. This pattern has been incorrectly called frontal ataxia or gait apraxia in the older literature.

Other hesitant gaits are those due to severe disequilibrium. These types of gait have been associated with frontal cortex and deep white matter lesions (frontal disequilibrium) or thalamic and midbrain lesions (subcortical disequilibrium).[165]

Hypothyroid slowness

Along with decreased metabolic rate, cool temperature, bradycardia, myxedema, loss of hair, hoarseness and myotonia, severe hypothyroidism can also feature motor slowness, weakness, and lethargy. These signs could be mistaken for the bradykinesia of parkinsonism, but the combination of the other signs of hypothyroidism, along with lack of rigidity and loss of postural reflexes, should aid the correct diagnosis.

Rigidity

Rigidity is characterized as increased muscle tone to passive motion. It is distinguished from spasticity in that it is present equally in all directions of the passive movement, equally in flexors and extensors, and throughout the range of motion, and it does not exhibit the clasp-knife phenomenon. Rigidity can be smooth (lead-pipe) or jerky (cogwheel). Cogwheeling occurs in the same range of frequencies as action and resting tremor[172] and appears to be due to superimposition of a tremor rhythm.[173] Cogwheel rigidity is more common than the lead-pipe variety in parkinsonism (nigral lesion), and lead-pipe rigidity can be caused by a number of other central nervous system lesions,[174] including those involving corpus striatum (hypoxia, vascular, neuroleptic malignant syndrome), midbrain (decorticate rigidity), medulla (decerebrate rigidity), and spinal cord (tetanus).

An increase in passive muscle tone can sometimes lead to impaired motor performance or even immobil-ity. Before there was a clear understanding of bradykinesia, rigidity was considered to be responsible for the paucity of movement in parkinsonism. However, rigidity is clearly distinct from bradykinesia; the former is more easily treated by levodopa therapy or by stereotactic thalamotomy and can then be relieved, while bradykinesia with residual paucity of movement persists. When rigidity is extremely severe so that the examiner can barely move the limbs, as in patients with neuroleptic malignant syndrome, the patient is virtually unable to move. The extended neck occasionally seen in progressive supranuclear palsy (Steele–Richardson–Olszewski syndrome) may be due to rigidity (vs. dystonia); the neck can be immobile in this disorder, and axial muscles are also rigid.

Rigidity is one part of the neuroleptic malignant syndrome (NMS), which is an idiosyncratic adverse effect of dopamine receptor blocking agents, usually antipsychotic drugs,[175,176] but it has also been reported to occur on sudden discontinuation of levodopa therapy.[177,178] The clinical features of the syndrome are the abrupt onset of a combination of rigidity/dystonia, fever with other autonomic dysfunctions such as diaphoresis and dyspnea, and an altered mental state including confusion, stupor, or coma. The level of serum creatine kinase activity is usually elevated. The dopamine receptor blocking agents may have been administered at therapeutic, not toxic, dosages. There does not seem to be any relationship with the duration of therapy. It can develop soon after the first dose or anytime after prolonged treatment. This is a potentially lethal disorder unless treated; up to 25% of cases die.[179] NMS is sometimes called malignant catatonia,[180] and needs to be distinguished from malignant hyperthermia.

Stiff muscles

Stiff muscles are produced by continuous muscle firing without muscle disease, and are not due to rigidity or spasticity. Briefly, there are four major categories of stiff-muscle syndromes: continuous muscle fiber activity or neuromyotonia, encephalomyelitis with rigidity, the stiff-limb syndrome, and the stiff-person syndrome.[181] Neuromyotonia is a syndrome of myotonic failure of muscle relaxation plus myokymia and fasciculations. Clinically it manifests as continuous muscle activity causing stiffness and cramps. The best known neuromyotonic disorder is Isaacs syndrome.

Stiff-person syndrome refers to a rare disorder[182] in which many somatic muscles are continuously contracting isometrically, resembling "chronic tetanus," in contrast to dystonic movements, which produce abnormal twisting and patterned movements and postures. The contractions of stiff-person syndrome are usually forceful and painful and most frequently involve the trunk and neck musculature. The proximal limb muscles can also be involved, but rarely does the disorder first affect the distal limbs. Benzodiazepines and valproate are usually somewhat effective. Withdrawal of these agents results in an increase of painful spasms. This disorder has now been recognized to be an autoimmune disease, with circulating antibodies against the GABA-synthesizing enzyme, glutamic acid decarboxylase, and also other types of antibodies, including against insulin.[183–185] Diabetes is a common accompanying disorder. The diagnosis can now be aided by laboratory testing for these antibodies. The syndrome of interstitial neuronitis, also called encephalomyelitis with rigidity and myoclonus, is a more acute variant of the stiff-person syndrome. The so-called stiff-baby syndrome is actually due to infantile hyperekplexia, in which the muscles continue to fire repeatedly and so frequently that the muscles appear to contract continuously.

Evaluation of a dyskinesia

The first question to be answered when seeing a patient for the possible presence of abnormal movements is whether or not involuntary movements are actually present. It must be considered whether the suspected abnormal movements might be purposeful voluntary movements, such as exaggerated gestures, mannerisms or compulsive movements, or if sustained contracted muscles might be "involuntary" muscle tightness to reduce pain (so-called guarding). It should be noted that as a general rule abnormal involuntary movements are exaggerated with anxiety and diminish during sleep. They may or may not lessen with amobarbital or with hypnosis.

Once it has been decided that abnormal movements are present, the next question is to determine the category of the involuntary movement, such as chorea, dystonia, myoclonus, tics, and tremor—i.e. determine the nature of the involuntary movements. To do so, it is important to note features such as rhythmicity, speed, duration, pattern (e.g. repetitive, flowing, continual, paroxysmal, diurnal), induction (i.e. stimuli-induced, action-induced, exercise-induced), complexity of the movements (complex vs. simple), suppressibility by volitional attention or by sensory tricks, and whether the movements are accompanied by sensations such as restlessness or the urge to make a movement that can release a built up tension. In addition, the examiner must determine which body parts are involved. The evaluation for the type of dyskinesia is the major subject of the next section in this chapter.

The third task is to determine the etiology of the abnormal involuntary movements. Is the disorder hereditary, sporadic, or symptomatic of some known neurological disorder? As a general rule, the etiology can be ascertained on the basis of the history and judicially selected laboratory tests.

The final question is how best to treat the movement disorder. Treatments of the various movement disorders are covered in the appropriate chapters of this book.

Differential diagnosis of dyskinesias

The differential diagnosis of movement disorders depends primarily on their clinical features. It is important to observe and describe the nature of the involuntary movements as mentioned above. In addition, examination for postural changes, alteration of muscle tone, loss of postural reflexes, motor impersistence, and any other neurological abnormalities on the general neurological examination, is performed. A list of abnormal involuntary movements is presented alphabetically in Table 230.1. A brief description of each of these is now presented, along with its major recognizable and differentiating features.

Abdominal dyskinesias

Abdominal dyskinesias are continuous movements of the abdominal wall or sometimes the diaphragm. The movements persist, and their sinuous, rhythmic nature has led to their being called belly dancer's dyskinesia.[186] They may be associated with abdominal trauma in some cases, and a common result is segmental abdominal myoclonus.[187] Another common cause is tardive dyskinesia. Hiccups, which is regularly recurring diaphragmatic myoclonus, does not move the abdomen and umbilicus in a sinewy fashion, but with sharp jerks and typically with noises, as air is expelled by the contractions.

Akathitic movements

Akathisia (from the Greek, meaning unable to sit still) refers to a feeling of inner, general restlessness, which is reduced or relieved by moving about. The typical akathitic patient, when sitting, may caress the scalp, cross and uncross the legs, rock the trunk, squirm in the chair, get out of the chair often to pace back and forth, and even make noises such as moaning. Carrying out these motor acts brings temporary relief from the sensations of akathisia. Akathitic movements are complex and usually stereotyped, with the same type of movements being employed over and over. Other movement disorders showing complex movements are tics, compulsions, mannerisms, and the stereotypies associated with mental retardation, autism, or psychosis.

Akathisia does not necessarily have to affect the whole body; an isolated body part can be affected. Focal akathisia often produces a sensation of burning or pain, again relieved by moving that body part. Common sites for focal akathisia are the mouth and vagina.[188]

Akathisia may be expressed by vocalizations, such as continual moaning, groaning, or humming. Other movement disorders associated with moaning sounds or humming are tics, oromandibular dystonia, Huntington's disease, and parkinsonian disorders.[189,190]

Akathitic movements and vocalizations can be transiently suppressed by the patient if he or she is asked to do so.

The most common cause of akathisia is iatrogenic. It is a frequent complication of antidopaminergic drugs, including those that block dopamine receptors (such as antipsychotic drugs and certain antiemetics) and those that deplete dopamine (such as reserpine and tetrabenazine). Akathisia can occur when drug therapy is initiated (acute akathisia), subsequently with the emergence of drug-induced parkinsonism, or after chronic treatment (tardive akathisia). Acute akathisia is eliminated upon withdrawal of the medication. Tardive akathisia is usually associated with the syndrome of tardive dyskinesia. Like tardive dyskinesia, tardive akathisia is aggravated by discontinuing the neuroleptic, and it is usually relieved by increasing the dose of the offending drug which masks the movement disorder. When associated with tardive dyskinesia, the akathitic movements can be rhythmic, such as body rocking, or marching in place. In this situation it is difficult to be certain if such rhythmic movements are due to akathisia or to tardive dyskinesia.

The exact mechanism of akathisia is not known, but it seems that the dopamine systems are involved, possibly in the limbic system or frontal cortex. It is of interest that akathisia, both generalized and regional, can be present in patients with Parkinson's disease.

Asynergia/ataxia/dysmetria

Asynergia or dyssynergia refers to decomposition of movement due to breakdown of normal coordinated execution of a voluntary movement. It is one of the cardinal clinical features of cerebellar disease or of lesions involving the pathways to or from the cerebellum. Asynergia of a limb results in a decomposition of movement instead of a smooth, continuous movement; it is associated with a tendency to miss the target and worsens when approaching a target. Limb asynergia is also manifested by dysdiadochokinesia, which refers to the break-up and irregularity that occurs when the limb is attempting to carry out rapid alternating movements. Because of its association with cerebellar disease, limb asynergia is frequently accompanied by dysmetria (the misjudging of distance) with its characteristic overshooting (hypermetria) and undershooting (hypometria) the target, and occasionally by intention (or terminal) tremor (see tremor, below). In addition, asynergia is usually associated with hypotonia, loss of check (when a voluntary ballistic movement is unable to stop precisely on target when the limb reaches its destination), and rebound (when sudden displacement of a limb results in excessive over correction to return to the baseline position). Asynergia is seen only during voluntary movement, and is not appreciated when the limb is at rest. Ataxia of gait is typified by unsteadiness with a wide base, the body swaying, and an inability to walk on tandem (heel-to-toe).

Athetosis

Athetosis has been used in two senses: 1) to describe a class of slow, writhing, continuous, involuntary movements; and 2) to describe the syndrome of athetoid cerebral palsy. This syndrome commonly occurs as a result of injury to the basal ganglia in the prenatal or perinatal period or during infancy. Athetoid movements affect the limbs, especially distally, but can also involve axial musculature, including the neck, face, and tongue. When not present in certain body parts at rest, it can often be brought out

by having the patient carry out voluntary motor activity elsewhere on the body; this phenomenon is known as overflow. For example, speaking can induce increased athetosis in the limbs, neck, trunk, face, and tongue. Athetosis often is associated with sustained contractions producing abnormal posturing. In this regard, athetosis blends with dystonia. However, the speed of these involuntary movements can sometimes be faster and blend with those of chorea, for which the term choreoathetosis is used. Athetosis resembles "slow" chorea in that the direction of movement changes randomly and in a flowing pattern.

Pseudoathetosis refers to distal athetoid movements of the fingers and toes owing to loss of proprioception, which can be due to sensory deafferentation (sensory athetosis) or to central loss of proprioception.[191]

Ballism

Ballism refers to very large amplitude choreic movements of the proximal parts of the limbs, causing flinging and flailing limb movements. Ballism is most frequently unilateral, which is referred to as hemiballism. This is often the result of a lesion in the contralateral subthalamic nucleus or its connections, or to multiple small infarcts (lacunes) in the contralateral striatum. In rare instances ballism occurs bilaterally (biballism) due to bilateral lacunes in the basal ganglia.[192] Like chorea, ballism can sometimes occur as a result of overdosage of levodopa.

Chorea

Chorea refers to involuntary, irregular, purposeless, non-rhythmic, abrupt, rapid, unsustained movements that seem to flow from one body part to another. A characteristic feature of chorea is that the movements are unpredictable in timing, direction, and distribution (i.e. are random). Although some neurologists erroneously label almost all non-rhythmic, rapid involuntary movements as choreic, many in fact are not. Non-choreic rapid movements can be tics, myoclonus, and dystonia; in these conditions, the movements repeat themselves in a set distribution of the body (i.e. are patterned) and do not have the changing, flowing nature of choreic movements that travel around the body. In rapid dystonic movements there is a recognizable repetitive pattern to the movements in the affected body parts, unlike the random nature of chorea. The prototypical choreic movements are those seen in Huntington's disease, in which the brief and rapid movements are irregular and occur randomly as a function of time. In Sydenham's chorea and in the withdrawal emergent syndrome, the flowing choreic movements have a restless-like appearance.

When choreic movements are infrequent, they appear as isolated, small amplitude, brief movements, somewhat slower than myoclonus, but sometimes difficult to distinguish from it. When chorea is more pronounced the movements occur almost continually, presenting as involuntary movements flowing from one site to another of the body.

Choreic movements can be partially suppressed, and the patient can often camouflage some of the movements by incorporating them into semipurposeful movements, known as parakinesia. Chorea is usually accompanied by motor impersistence ("negative chorea"), the inability to maintain a sustained contraction. A common symptom of motor impersistence is the dropping of objects. Motor impersistence is detected by examining for the inability to keep the tongue protruded and by the presence of the "milkmaid" grip due to the inability to keep the fist in a sustained tight grip.

Dystonia

Dystonia refers to twisting movements that tend to be sustained at the peak of the movement, are frequently repetitive, and often progress to prolonged abnormal postures. In contrast to chorea, dystonic movements repeatedly involve the same group of muscles (i.e. they are patterned). Agonist and antagonist muscles contract simultaneously (co-contraction) to produce the sustained quality of dystonic movements. The speed of the movement varies widely from slow (athetotic dystonia) to shock-like (myoclonic dystonia). When the contractions are very brief, e.g. less than a second, they are referred to as dystonic spasms; when they are sustained for several seconds they are called dystonic movements; and when they last minutes to hours, they are known as dystonic postures. When present for weeks or longer, the postures can lead to permanent fixed contractures.

When dystonia first appears, the movements typically occur when the affected body part is carrying out a voluntary action (action dystonia) and are not present when the body part is at rest. With progression of the disorder, dystonic movements can appear at distant sites when other parts of the body are voluntarily moving (overflow), such as occurs also in athetosis and in dopa-induced dyskinesias. With further progression dystonic movements become present when the body is "at rest." Even at this stage, dystonic movements are usually made more severe with voluntary activity. Whereas primary dystonia often begins as action dystonia and may persist as the kinetic (clonic) form, symptomatic dystonia often begins as fixed postures (tonic form).

When a single body part is affected, the condition is referred to as focal dystonia. Common forms of focal dystonia are spasmodic torticollis (cervical dystonia), blepharospasm (upper facial dystonia), and writer's cramp (hand dystonia). Involvement of two or more contiguous regions of the body is referred to as segmental dystonia. Generalized dystonia indicates involvement of one or both legs, the trunk, and some other part of the body. Multifocal dystonia involves two or more regions, not conforming to segmental or generalized dystonia. Hemidystonia refers to involvement of the arm and leg on the same side.

One type of focal dystonia requires special mention, namely sustained contractions of ocular muscles, resulting in tonic ocular deviation—usually upward gaze. This was referred to as oculogyric crisis when such sustained ocular deviation was encountered in victims of encephalitis lethargica, and later in those survivors who developed post-encephalitic parkinsonism. Primary torsion dystonia does *not* involve the ocular muscles, hence oculogyria is not truly a feature of dystonia syndromes. Rather, it is more common today as a complication of dopamine receptor blocking agents. It also occurs in drug-induced parkinsonism or other parkinsonian syndromes such as juvenile parkinsonism and the parkinsonism associated with the degenerative disease known as neuronal intranuclear inclusion disease,[193,194] and with the biochemical deficiency of monoamines in the metabolic disorders of aromatic amino acid decarboxylase deficiency[195] and pterin deficiencies.[196] There has been a case report of oculogyric crises in a patient with dopa-responsive dystonia[197] and its phenocopy, tyrosine hydroxylase deficiency. Paroxysmal tonic upgaze has also been seen in infants and children. It eventually subsides,[198] but may be a forerunner of developmental delay, intellectual disability or language delay indicating impaired corticomesencephalic control of vertical eye movements.[199]

Although classical torsion dystonia may appear initially only as an action dystonia, it usually progresses to manifest as continual contractions. In contrast to this continual type of classical torsion dystonia, a variant of dystonia also exists in which the movements occur in attacks, with a sudden onset and limited duration—known as paroxysmal kinesigenic dyskinesias and paroxysmal non-kinesigenic dyskinesias. These are categorized among the paroxysmal disorders. Among the other disorders to be differentiated from dystonia are tonic tics (also called dystonic tics), which also appear as sustained contractions.

Hemifacial spasm

Hemifacial spasm, as the name indicates, refers to unilateral facial muscle contractions. Generally these are continual rapid, brief, repetitive spasms, but can also be more prolonged sustained tonic spasms mixed with periods of quiescence. Often the movements can be brought out when the patient voluntarily and forcefully contracts the facial muscles; when the patient then relaxes the face, the involuntary movements appear. Hemifacial spasm usually affects both upper and lower parts of the face, but patients are commonly more concerned about closure of the eyelid than of the contractions of the cheek or at the corner of the mouth. The eyebrow tends to elevate with the facial contractions owing to being pulled upwards by the forehead muscles. The disorder is believed to involve the facial nerve, and sometimes it is due to compression of the nerve by an aberrant blood vessel.[200] Hemifacial spasm is an example of a peripherally induced movement disorder.

It can be easily distinguished from blepharospasm, since the latter involves the face bilaterally and often the dystonic contractions spread to contiguous structures, such as oromandibular and nuchal muscles. Rarely is blepharospasm due to dystonia unilateral. In such a circumstance, it can be difficult clinically to distinguish it from hemifacial spasm. In contrast to hemifacial spasm, blepharospasm tends to pull the eyebrow down because of contraction of the procerus muscle in addition to the orbicularis oculi. Another condition that has been confused with hemifacial spasm is repetitive facial myoclonus seen with Whipple's disease. In this disorder the myoclonic jerks tend to be fairly rhythmical, the contractions usually involve the other side of the face to some extent, and the movements are not sustained. Electromyography may be of assistance since hemifacial spasm is associated with high frequency repetitive discharges, and sometimes with evidence of facial nerve denervation and ephaptic transmission. The contractions in both hemifacial spasm and blepharospasm are intermittent, but both can be sustained.

Hyperekplexia

Hyperekplexia ("startle disease") is an excessive startle reaction to a sudden, unexpected stimulus.[201-203] The startle response can be either a short "jump" or a more prolonged tonic spasm causing falls. This condition can be familial or sporadic. It may be related to jumping disorders, and other similar conditions like latah and myriachit, but all of these appear to be influenced by social and group behavior. After the initial jump to the unexpected stimulus, there is automatic speech or behavior, such as striking out. In some of these, there is automatic obedience to words as "jump" or "throw."[203]

Hypnogenic dyskinesias

Most dyskinesias disappear during deep sleep, although they may emerge during light sleep. The major exception is symptomatic rhythmical oculopalatal myoclonus, which persists during sleep, in addition to being present while the patient is awake.[204] There are, however, a few movement disorders that are present only when the patient is asleep. The most common hypnogenic dyskinesia is the condition known as periodic movements in sleep,[205-208] formerly referred to as nocturnal myoclonus.[209] The latter term is unacceptable because the movements are not shock-like, but in fact are rather slow. They appear as flexor contractions of one or both legs, with dorsiflexion of the big toe and the foot, and flexion of the knee and hip. They occur in intervals, approximately every 20 seconds, and hence have been given its new, more acceptable name.[205] Periodic movements in sleep are a frequent component of the restless legs syndrome. In addition to periodic movements in sleep, this syndrome also is associated with myoclonic- and dystonic-like movements during sleep and while the patient is drowsy.[208]

Another rare nocturnal dyskinesia is hypnogenic paroxysmal dystonia or other dyskinesias that occur only during sleep. Hypnogenic dystonia can be complex and with sustained contractions, similar to that occurring in torsion dystonia. As depicted in its name, such movements occur as a paroxysm during sleep and last only a few minutes. They may or may not awaken the patient. Some may be frontal lobe seizures.[210]

Jumpy stumps

Jumpy stumps are uncontrollable and sometimes exhausting chaotic movements of the stump remaining from amputated limbs. When they occur, it is after a delayed period of time after the amputation.[211]

Moving toes and fingers

The painful legs, moving toes syndrome refers to a disorder in which the toes of one foot or both feet are in continual flexion–extension with some lateral motion, associated with a deep pain in the ipsilateral leg.[212] The constant movement has a sinusoidal quality. The movements and pain are continuous and both occur even during sleep, though they may be reduced, and the normal sleep pattern may be altered.[213] The leg pain is much more troublesome to the patient than are the constant movements. In some patients with this disorder there is evidence for a lesion in the lumbar roots or in the peripheral nerves.[213-215] An analogous disorder, "painful arm, moving fingers," has also been described.[216]

Myoclonus

Myoclonic jerks are sudden, brief, shock-like involuntary movements caused by muscular contractions (positive myoclonus) or inhibitions (negative myoclonus). The most common form of negative myoclonus is asterixis, which frequently accompanies various metabolic encephalopathies. In asterixis, the brief flapping of the outstretched limbs is due to transient inhibition of the muscles that maintain posture of those extremities. Unilateral asterixis has been described with focal brain lesions of the contralateral medial frontal cortex, parietal cortex, internal capsule and ventrolateral thalamus.[217]

Myoclonus can appear when the affected body part is at rest or when it is performing a voluntary motor act, so-called action myoclonus. Myoclonic jerks are usually irregular (arrhythmic), but can be rhythmical (such as in palatal myoclonus or in ocular myoclonus, with a rate of approximately 2 Hz). Rhythmical ocular myoclonus due to a lesion in the dentato-olivary pathway needs to be distinguished from arrhythmic and chaotic opsoclonus, or dancing eyes. Rhythmic myoclonus is typically due to a structural lesion of the brainstem or spinal cord (and is therefore also called segmental myoclonus), but not all cases of segmental myoclonus are rhythmic, and some types of cortical epilepsia partialis continua can be rhythmic. Oscillatory myoclonus is depicted as rhythmic jerks that occur in a burst and then fade. Spinal myoclonus, in addition to presenting as segmental and rhythmical, can also present as flexion axial jerks triggered by a distant stimulus, that is, travels via a slow conducting spinal pathway, and called propriospinal myoclonus.[218]

Myoclonic jerks occurring in different body parts are often synchronized, a feature that may be specific for myoclonus. The jerks can often be triggered by sudden stimuli such as sound, light, visual threat, or movement (reflex myoclonus). Myoclonus has a relationship to seizures in that both seem to be the result of hyperexcitable neurons.

Cortical reflex myoclonus usually presents as a focal myoclonus and is triggered by active or passive muscle movements of the affected body part. It is associated with high amplitude ("giant") somatosensory evoked potentials and with cortical spikes observed by computerized back averaging, time-locked to the stimulus.[219] Spread of cortical activity within the hemisphere and via the corpus callosum can produce generalized cortical myoclonus or multifocal cortical myoclonus.[220] Reticular reflex myoclonus[221] is more often generalized or spreads along the body away from the source in the brainstem in a timed-related sequential fashion.

The fact that rhythmical myoclonus consists of contractions of agonists rather than alternating agonist–antagonist contractions, and that those in one body part are synchronized with contractions elsewhere, are strong arguments for categorizing rhythmical myoclonus as a myoclonic disorder and not a type of tremor. Furthermore, rhythmical myoclonias tend to persist during sleep, whereas tremors usually disappear during sleep.

Action or intention myoclonus is often encountered after cerebral hypoxia-ischemia (Lance–Adams syndrome) and with certain degenerative disorders, such as progressive myoclonus epilepsy (Unverricht–Lundborg disease) and progressive myoclonic ataxia (Ramsay Hunt syndrome). Usually action myoclonus is more disabling than rest myoclonus. Negative myoclonus also occurs in the Lance–Adams syndrome. When it involves the thigh muscles while the patient is standing, it manifests as bouncy legs. In the opsoclonus–myoclonus syndrome, originally described by Kinsbourne[222] and subsequently called both "dancing eyes, dancing feet" and "polymyoclonia" by Dyken and Kolar,[223] the amplitude of the myoclonus is usually very tiny, resembling irregular tremors. Because of the small amplitudes of the continuous, generalized myoclonus, we prefer the term minipolymyoclonus, a term originally used by Spiro[224] to describe small amplitude movements in childhood spinal muscular atrophy, and also used by Wilkins et al.[225] for the type of myoclonus seen in primary generalized epileptic myoclonus.

Myokymia and synkinesis

Myokymia is a fine persistent quivering or rippling of muscles (sometimes called "live flesh" by patients). The term has evolved since first used,[226] when it described benign fasciculations. Although some may still refer to the benign fasciculations that frequently occur in orbicularis oculi as myokymia, Denny-Brown and Foley[227] distinguished between myokymia and benign fasciculations based on electromyography (EMG). In myokymia, the EMG reveals regular groups of motor unit discharges, especially doublets and triplets, occurring with a regular rhythmic discharge. Myokymia occurs most commonly in facial

muscles. Most facial myokymias are due to pontine lesions, particularly multiple sclerosis,[228,229] and less often due to pontine glioma. When due to multiple sclerosis, facial myokymia tends to abate after weeks or months. When due to a pontine glioma, facial myokymia may persist indefinitely and can be associated with facial contracture. Myokymia is also a feature of neuromyotonia (see stiff muscles, above). Myokymia can persist during sleep. Continuous facial myokymia in multiple sclerosis has been found by MRI to be caused by a pontine tegmental lesion involving the postnuclear, postgenu portion of the facial nerve.[230]

Aberrant reinnervation of the facial nerve following denervation, such as from Bell's palsy, is manifested by synkinesis, which is the occurrence of involuntary movements in one part of the face accompanying voluntary contraction of another part. For example, moving the mouth in a smile may cause the eyelid to close.

In this section, to be complete, fasciculations are mentioned—the small amplitude contractions of muscles innervated by a motor unit. This is seen predominantly with disease of the anterior horn cells, and presents as low amplitude intermittent twitching of muscles due to motor unit discharges, usually not strong enough to move a joint although this can occur, particularly in children.

Myorhythmia

The term, myorhythmia, has been used in different ways over time. Herz[231,232] used it to refer to the somewhat rhythmical movements seen in patients with torsion dystonia. Today these are simply called dystonic movements, and there is no distinction between the movements that are repetitive and those that are not. Dystonic myorhythmia should not be confused with dystonic tremor, which strongly resembles other tremors but is due to dystonia. Monrad-Krohn and Refsum[233] used the term "myorhythmia" to label what is today called palatal myoclonus or other rhythmical myoclonias. This meaning of myorhythmia has also been adopted by Masucci et al.[234] The present author would use the term to represent a low frequency (<3 Hz), prolonged, rhythmical or repetitive movement in which the movement does not have the sharp square wave appearance of a myoclonic jerk. As such the term would not apply it to palatal myoclonus, nor to the sinusoidal cycles of most tremors (parkinsonian, essential, cerebellar) because the frequency of these tremors is faster than that defined for myorhythmia.

The most typical disorder in which the term myorhythmia is applied is Whipple's disease, in which there are slow-moving, repetitive, synchronous, rhythmical contractions in ocular, facial, masticatory, and other muscles—so-called oculo-facio-masticatory myorhythmia.[235–237] There is often also vertical supranuclear ophthalmoplegia. Ocular myorhythmia is manifested as continuous, horizontal, pendular, vergence oscillations of the eyes, usually of small amplitude, occurring about every second. They may be asymmetrical and may continue in sleep. They never diverge beyond the primary position, and divergence and convergence are at the same speed. They are not accompanied by pupillary miosis. The movements in the face, jaw and skeletal muscles are about the same frequency, but may be somewhat quicker and be more like rhythmical myoclonus. The abnormal movements of facial and masticatory muscles can also persist in sleep, as seen also with palatal myoclonus.

Sometimes the term myorhythmia may be applied to slow, undulating, rhythmic movements of muscles, unrelated to Whipple's disease. Perhaps some of these types of movements are part of the spectrum of complex tics, while in others they may represent psychogenic movements.

Paroxysmal dyskinesias

The paroxysmal dyskinesias represent various types of dyskinetic movements, particularly choreoathetosis and dystonia, that occur "out-of-the-blue" and then disappear after being present for seconds, minutes or hours. The patient can remain normal for months between attacks, or there can be many attacks per day.

Paroxysmal kinesigenic dyskinesia (PKD) is the best described and easiest to diagnose because it is characteristically triggered by a sudden movement; the abnormal movements last seconds to a few minutes. PKD can be hereditary or symptomatic, and usually is successfully treated with anticonvulsants. The abnormal movements easily habituate, i.e. they fail to recur if the inciting trigger is immediately repeated. These movements can be dystonic, ballistic, or choreic. There may be many brief paroxysmal bursts of movements each day.

Paroxysmal non-kinesigenic dyskinesia (PNKD) is often familial, is triggered by stress, fatigue, caffeine, or alcohol, and can last minutes to hours. It is more difficult to treat than the kinesigenic variety, but it sometimes responds to clonazepam or other benzodazepines, and to acetazolamide. PNKD can be familial or sporadic. Sporadic PNKD, in the author's experience, is more often a psychogenic movement disorder, particularly if it is a combination of both paroxysmal and continual dystonias. Episodic ataxias and tremors are also part of the paroxysmal dyskinesia spectrum. They are usually familial, and may include vestibular signs and symptoms.

Restless legs

The term restless legs syndrome refers to more than just the phenomenon of restless legs, where the patient has unpleasant crawling sensations in the legs, particularly when sitting and relaxing in the evening, and which then disappear on walking.[238] The complete syndrome consists of several parts, of which one or more may be present in any individual. While the unpleasant dysesthesias in the legs are the most common symptom, as mentioned above in the discussion on hypnogenic dyskinesias, the clinical spectrum may also include periodic movements in sleep, myoclonic jerks, more sustained dystonic movements, or stereotypic movements that occur while the patient is awake, particularly in the late evening.[239] Other movement disorders associated with a sensory phenomenon are akathisia (feeling of inner restlessness) and tics (feeling of relief of tension or sensory urges upon producing a tic).

Stereotypy

Stereotypy refers to coordinated movements that repeat themselves continually and identically. However, there may be long periods of minutes between movements, or they may be very frequent. When they occur at irregular intervals, stereotypies may not always be easily distinguished from motor tics, compulsions, gestures, and mannerisms.[240] In their classic monograph on tics, Meige and Feindel[241] distinguished between stereotypies and motor tics by describing the latter as acts that are impelling but not impossible to resist, whereas the former, while illogical, are without an irresistible urge. Tics almost always occur intermittently and not continuously, i.e. they occur paroxysmally out of a background of normal motor behavior. Although stereotypies can also be bursts of repetitive movements emerging out of a background of normal motor activity, they often repeat themselves in a uniform repetitive fashion for long periods of time.[242] Stereotypies typically occur in patients with tardive dyskinesia, and with schizophrenia, mental retardation, and autism, which assists in separating these from motor tics.[243] Stereotypies apparently occur in Asperger's syndrome, a form of mild autism. They have been seen in patients with the Kluver–Bucy syndrome, and in children left alone and when not in contact with other people.

Although motor tics are often considered to be stereotypic, when a tic bursts out it is not necessarily a repetition of the previous tic movement. Thus, tics are usually not repetitive from one burst to the next. However, the same type of tic movement will usually recur after some period of time passes, which provides their stereotypic nature. The diversity of motor tics is one feature that sets their phenomenology apart from stereotypies. Tics are rarely continuously repetitive, and when this occurs the term "tic status" can be applied. As will be pointed out below, tics have many other features that aid in the diagnosis, such as their suppressibility, their accompaniment by an underlying urge or compulsion to make the movement, their variability, their migration from one body part to another part, their abruptness, their brevity, and the repetitiveness, rather than randomness, of the particular body part affected by the movements.[244] Therefore, while tics have an element of stereotypy, this type of stereotypy, which can be considered paroxysmal, intermittent, or at most continual (meaning with interruptions), needs to be distinguished from continuous (uninterrupted) involuntary movements that repeat themselves over and over again unceasingly. The latter type of continuous stereotypy is what distinguishes the disorders known as stereotypies and is the hallmark of abnormal movements in patients with classical tardive dyskinesia, which is called tardive stereotypy,[245] the most common type of stereotypy seen in movement disorder clinics.

Compulsions are repetitive, purposeless, usually complex movements seen in patients with obsessive–compulsive disorder (OCD). They are associated with an irresistible urge to make the movement, and patients realize they are making the movements in response to this "need to do so." In this respect compulsions resemble tics and not stereotypies, which are not accompanied by any urge. In fact, some patients with Tourette syndrome also have OCD, and in this situation it may be impossible to distinguish between tics and compulsions. Like stereotypies, compulsions could be carried out in a uniform repetitive fashion for long periods of time, but do so at the expense of all other activities because compulsions may be impossible to stop. In contrast, stereotypies can usually be stopped on command, and the patient will have normal motor behavior until they start up again, usually as soon as the patient is no longer paying attention to the command.

Gestures are culturally developed, expressive, voluntary movements calculated to indicate a particular state of mind, and which may also be used as a means of adding emphasis to oratory.[242] Mannerisms are sets of movements that include gestures, plus more peculiar and individualistic movements not considered as bothersome. Mannerisms can be considered to represent a type of motor signature that individualizes a person. Sometimes mannerisms can be bizarre, and these could be considered tics or on the borderline with tics. Because gestures and mannerisms rarely continually repeat themselves, they are not likely to be confused with stereotypies but there may be a problem at times in distinguishing them from tics.

From the above description, stereotypies can be divided into two phenomenologically distinct groups. One type is that in which the stereotypy, though repetitive for prolonged periods, occurs intermittently, with normal motor activity being the general background. It is this type that can be difficult to distinguish from tics and compulsions. The second type is that in which the repetitive movements are virtually always there, with less time spent without them. The most common of this type of continuous stereotypy is that of classical tardive dyskinesia (TD). The movements seen in classical TD are rhythmical and continuously repetitive complex chewing movements (oral–buccal–lingual dyskinesia). Often this tardive stereotypy will appear together in the same patient with different motor phenomena that comprise the tardive dyskinesia syndromes.

Tics

Tics consist of abnormal movements (motor tics) or abnormal sounds (phonic tics). When both types of tics are present, the designation of Gilles de la Tourette syndrome or Tourette syndrome is commonly applied. Tics frequently vary in severity over time, and can have remissions and exacerbations.

Motor and phonic tics can be simple or complex, and occur abruptly for brief moments from a background of normal motor activity. Thus they are paroxysmal in occurrence unless so severe as to be continual. A single simple motor tic may be impossible to distinguish from a myoclonic or choreic jerk; each of these is an abrupt, sudden, isolated movement. Examples include a shoulder shrug, head jerk, blink, dart of the eyes, and twitch of the nose. Most of the time such simple tics are repetitive, such as a run of eye blinking or a sequence of several simple tics in a row. In this pattern, tics can be easily distinguished from the other hyperkinesias. Even when tics are simple jerks, more complex forms of tics may also be present in the same patient, allowing the diagnosis to be established by "the company it keeps." One type of simple tic is quite distinct, namely ocular. Eye movements are not a feature of chorea or myoclonus, but are common in tics.[246]

Complex motor tics are very distinct, consisting of coordinated patterns of sequential movements that can appear in different parts of the body and are not necessarily identically from occurrence to occurrence in the same body part. Examples of complex tics include such acts as touching the nose, touching other people, head shaking with shoulder shrugging, kicking of legs, and jumping. Obscene gesturing (copropraxia) is another example.

Like akathitic movements, tics are usually preceded by an uncomfortable feeling or sensory urge that is relieved by carrying out the movement—i.e. like "scratching the itch." Thus, the movements and sounds can be considered "unvoluntary." Unless very severe, tics can be voluntarily suppressed for various periods of time; however, when suppressed, inner tension builds up and is only relieved by an increased burst of more tics.

In addition to being as rapid as myoclonic jerks, tics can also be sustained contractions, resembling dystonic movements. The complex sequential pattern of muscular contractions in dystonic tics makes the diagnosis obvious in most cases. Moreover, torsion dystonia is a continual hyperkinesia, whereas tics are paroxysmal bursts of varying duration.

Involuntary ocular movements can be an important feature for differentiating tics from other dyskinesias. Whether a brief jerk of the eyes or more sustained eye deviation, ocular movements can occur as a manifestation of tics. Very few other dyskinesias involve ocular movements. The exceptions are: 1) opsoclonus (dancing eyes), which is a form of myoclonus; 2) ocular myoclonus (rhythmic vertical oscillations at a rate of 2 Hz) that often accompanies palatal myoclonus; 3) ocular myorhythmia, a slow horizontal oscillation; and 4) oculogyric spasms (a sustained deviation of the eyes, thus a dystonia) associated with dopamine receptor blocking drugs or as a consequence of encephalitis lethargica or other parkinsonian disorders (such as neuronal intranuclear hyaline inclusion disease and aromatic amino acid decarboxylase deficiency).

Phonic tics can range from simple throat-clearing sounds or grunts to verbalizations and the utterance of obscenities (coprolalia). Sniffing can also be a phonic tic, involving nasal passages rather than the vocal apparatus. Like motor tics, phonic tics can also be divided into simple and complex tics. Throat-clearing and sniffing represent simple phonic tics, whereas verbalizations are considered complex phonic tics.

Involuntary phonations occur in only a few other neurological disorders beside tics. These include the moaning in akathisia and in parkinsonism; the brief sounds in oromandibular dystonia and Huntington's disease; and the sniffing, spitting, groaning, or singing occasionally encountered in Huntington's disease and neuroacanthocytosis.

Tremor

Tremor is an oscillatory, usually rhythmical and regular, movement affecting one or more body parts, such as the limbs, neck, tongue, chin, or vocal cords. Jerky, irregular "tremor" is usually a manifestation of myoclonus. Tremor is produced by rhythmic alternating or simultaneous contractions of agonists and antagonists. The rate, location, amplitude, and constancy vary depending on the specific type of tremor and its severity. It is helpful to determine whether the tremor is present at rest (with the patient sitting or lying in repose), with posture-holding (with the arms or legs extended in front of the body), with action (such as writing or pouring water), or with intention maneuvers (such as bringing the finger to touch the nose). Tremors can then be classified as tremor at rest, postural tremor, action tremor or intention tremor, respectively. Some tremors may be present only during a specific task (such as writing) or with a specific posture, such as standing, as in orthostatic tremor. These are called task-specific or position-specific tremors, respectively, and may overlap with task-specific and position-specific action dystonias, which may also appear as tremors (dystonic tremor). Etiologies and treatment of tremors differ according to the type of tremor phenomenology. It is important to realize that wing-beating and other bizarre tremors can be a manifestation of Wilson's disease. A combination of rest tremor and a worse intention tremor may indicate a lesion in the midbrain, commonly called and mislabeled as "rubral" tremor (which should be more appropriately called midbrain tremor).

References

1. Jankovic J. Post-traumatic movement disorders: central and peripheral mechanisms. Neurology 1994;44: 2006–2014
2. Marsden CD. Peripheral movement disorders. *In:* Marsden CD, Fahn S, eds. Movement Disorders 3. Oxford: Butterworth-Heinemann, 1994:406–417
3. Rothdach AJ, Trenkwalder C, Haberstock J, et al. Prevalence and risk factors of RLS in an elderly population—The MEMO Study. Neurology 2000;54: 1064–1068
4. Haerer AF, Anderson DW, Schoenberg BS. Prevalence of essential tremor. Results from the Copiah County study. Arch Neurol 1982;39:750–751
5. Kurland LT. Epidemiology: incidence, geographic distribution and genetic considerations. *In:* Fields WS, ed. Pathogenesis and Treatment of Parkinsonism. Springfield, IL: Charles C Thomas, 1958:5–49.
6. Caine ED, McBride MC, Chiverton P, et al. Tourette's syndrome in Monroe County school children. Neurology 1988;38:472–475
7. Comings DE, Himes JA, Comings BG. An epidemiologic study of Tourette's syndrome in a single school district. J Clin Psychiatry 1990;51:463–469
8. Mason A, Banerjee S, Eapen V, et al. The prevalence of Tourette syndrome in a mainstream school population. Dev Med Child Neurol 1998;40:292–296
9. Nutt JG, Muenter MD, Aronson A, et al. Epidemiology of focal and generalized dystonia in Rochester, Minnesota. Mov Disord 1988;3:188–194
10. Auger RG, Whisnant JP. Hemifacial spasm in Rochester and Olmsted County, Minnesota, 1960 to 1984. Arch Neurol 1990;47:1233–1234
11. Schoenberg BS. Epidemiology of inherited ataxias. *In:* Kark RAP, Rosenberg RN, Schut LJ, eds. The Inherited Ataxias. Adv Neurol 1978;21:15–32
12. Harper PS. The epidemiology of Huntington's disease. Hum Genet 1992;89:365–376
13. Kokmen E, Ozekmekci S, Beard CM, et al. Incidence and prevalence of Huntington's disease in Olmstead County, Minnesota (1950–1989). Arch Neurol 1994;51: 696–698
14. Reilly M, Daly L, Hutchinson M. An epidemiological study of Wilson's disease in the Republic of Ireland. J Neurol Neurosurg Psychiatry 1993;56:298–300
15. Golbe LI. The epidemiology of PSP. J Neural Transm 1994;42:263–273
16. Schrag A, Ben-Shlomo Y, Quinn NP. Prevalence of progressive supranuclear palsy and multiple system atrophy: a cross-sectional study. Lancet 1999;354: 1771–1775
17. Schoenberg BS, Anderson DW, Haerer AF. Prevalence of Parkinson's disease in the biracial population of Copiah County, Mississippi. Neurology 1985;35: 841–845
18. Tanner CM. Pathological clues to the cause of Parkinson's disease. *In:* Marsden CD, Fahn S, eds. Movement Disorders 3. Oxford: Butterworth-Heinemann, 1994: 124–146
19. Polymeropoulos MH, Higgins JJ, Golbe LI, et al. Mapping of a gene for Parkinson's disease to chromosome 4q21-q23. Science 1996;274:1197–1199
20. Polymeropoulos MH, Lavedan C, Leroy E, et al. Mutation in the alpha-synuclein gene identified in families with Parkinson's disease. Science 1997;276:2045–2047
21. Kruger R, Kuhn W, Muller T, et al. Ala30Pro mutation in the gene encoding alpha-synuclein in Parkinson's disease. Nat Genet 1998;18:106–108
22. Matsumine H, Yamamura Y, Kuzuhara S, et al. A gene for autosomal recessive form of early onset parkinsonism maps to chromosome 6q. Neurology 1997;48:A394
23. Matsumine H, Yamamura Y, Hattori N, et al. A microdeletion of D6S305 in a family of autosomal recessive juvenile Parkinsonism (PARK2). Genomics 1998;49:143–146
24. Kitada T, Asakawa S, Hattori N, et al. Mutations in the parkin gene cause autosomal recessive juvenile parkinsonism. Nature 1998;392:605–608
25. Abbas N, Lucking CB, Ricard S, et al. A wide variety

of mutations in the parkin gene are responsible for autosomal recessive parkinsonism in Europe. Hum Mol Genet 1999;8:567–574

26. Shimura H, Hattori N, Kubo S, et al. Familial Parkinson disease gene product, parkin, is a ubiquitin-protein ligase. Nat Genet 2000;25:302–305

27. Gasser T, Mullermyhsok B, Wszolek ZK, et al. A susceptibility locus for Parkinson's disease maps to chromosome 2p13. Nat Genet 1998;18:262–265

28. Farrer M, Gwinn-Hardy K, Muenter M, et al. A chromosome 4p haplotype segregating with Parkinson's disease and postural tremor. Hum Mol Genet 1999;8:81–85

29. Leroy E, Boyer R, Auburger G, et al. Polymeropoulos MH. The ubiquitin pathway in Parkinson's disease. Nature 1998;395:451–452

30. Swerdlow RH, Parks JK, Davis JN, et al. Matrilineal inheritance of complex I dysfunction in a multigenerational Parkinson's disease family. Ann Neurol 1998;44:873–881

31. Simon DK, Pulst SM, Sutton JP, et al. Familial multisystem degeneration with parkinsonism associated with the 11778 mitochondrial DNA mutation. Neurology 1999;53:1787–1793

32. Lynch T, Sano M, Marder KS, et al. Clinical characteristics of a family with chromosome 17-linked disinhibition dementia parkinsonism amyotrophy complex. Neurology 1994;44:1878–1884

33. Foster NL, Wilhelmsen K, Sima AAF, et al. Frontotemporal dementia and parkinsonism linked to chromosome 17: a consensus conference. Ann Neurol 1997;41:706–715

34. Hutton M, Lendon CL, Rizzu P, et al. Association of missense and 5'-splice-site mutations in tau with the inherited dementia FTDP-17. Nature 1998;393:702–705

35. Pickering-Brown S, Baker M, Yen SH, et al. Pick's disease is associated with mutations in the tau gene. Ann Neurol 2000;48:859–867

36. Baker M, Litvan I, Houlden H, et al. Association of an extended haplotype in the tau gene with progressive supranuclear palsy. Hum Mol Genet 1999;8:711–715

37. Morris HR, Janssen JC, Bandmann O, et al. The tau gene A0 polymorphism in progressive supranuclear palsy and related neurodegenerative diseases. J Neurol Neurosurg Psychiat 1999;66:665–667

38. Bugiani O, Murrell JR, Giaccone G, et al. Frontotemporal dementia and corticobasal degeneration in a family with a P301S mutation in tau. J Neuropathol Exp Neurol 1999;58:667–677

39. Delisle MB, Murrell JR, Richardson R, et al. A mutation at codon 279 (N279K) in exon 10 of the Tau gene causes a tauopathy with dementia and supranuclear palsy. Acta Neuropathol 1999;98:62–77

40. Higgins JJ, Adler RL, Loveless JM. Mutational analysis of the tau gene in progressive supranuclear palsy. Neurology 1999;53:1421–1424

41. Spillantini MG, Yoshida H, Rizzini C, et al. A novel tau mutation (N296N) in familial dementia with swollen achromatic neurons and corticobasal inclusion bodies. Ann Neurol 2000;48:939–943

42. Stanford PM, Halliday GM, Brooks WS, et al. Progressive supranuclear palsy pathology caused by a novel silent mutation in exon 10 of the tau gene—expansion of the disease phenotype caused by tau gene mutations. Brain 2000;123:880–893

43. Hashida H, Goto J, Zhao ND, et al. Cloning and mapping of ZNF231, a novel brain-specific gene encoding neuronal double zinc finger protein whose expression is enhanced in a neurodegenerative disorder, multiple system atrophy (MSA). Genomics 1998;54:50–58

44. De Coo IFM, Renier WO, Ruitenbeek W, et al. A 4-base pair deletion in the mitochondrial cytochrome b gene associated with parkinsonism/MELAS overlap syndrome. Ann Neurol 1999;45:130–133

45. Rosen DR, Siddique T, Patterson D, et al. Mutations in Cu/Zn superoxide dismutase gene are associated with familial amyotrophic lateral sclerosis. Nature 1993;362:59–62

46. Pandolfo M, Munaro M, Cocozza S, et al. A dinucleotide repeat polymorphism (d9s202) in the Friedreich's ataxia region on chromosome-9q13-q21.1. Hum Mol Genet 1993;2:822

47. Bouchard et al. 1998

48. Mrissa N, Belal S, BenHamida C, et al. Linkage to chromosome 13q11-12 of an autosomal recessive cerebellar ataxia in a Tunisian family. Neurology 2000;54:1408–1414

49. Bertini E, des Portes V, Zanni G, et al. X-linked congenital ataxia: a clinical and genetic study. Am J Med Genet 2000;92:53–56

50. McHale DP, Jackson AP, Campbell DA, et al. A gene for ataxic cerebral palsy maps to chromosome 9p12-q12. Eur J Human Genet 2000;8:267–272

51. Higgins JJ, Morton DH, Loveless JM. Posterior column ataxia with retinitis pigmentosa (AXPC1) maps to chromosome 1q31-q32. Neurology 1999;52:146–150

52. Gotoda T, Arita M, Arai H, et al. Adult-onset spinocerebellar dysfunction caused by a mutation in the gene for the α-tocopherol-transfer protein. N Engl J Med 1995;333:1313–1318

53. Ambrose HJ, Byrd PJ, McConville CM, et al. Physical map across chromosome 11q22-q23 containing the major locus for ataxia telangiectasia. Genomics 1994;21:612–619

54. Savitsky K, Bar-Shira A, Gilad S, et al. A single ataxia telangiectasia gene with a product similar to PI-3 kinase. Science 1995;268:1749–1753

55. Banfi S, Servadio A, Chung MY, et al. Identification and characterization of the gene causing type 1 spinocerebellar ataxia. Nat Genet 1994;7:513–520

56. Lopes-Cendes I, Andermann E, Attig E, et al. Confirmation of the SCA-2 locus as an alternative locus for dominantly inherited spinocerebellar ataxias and refinement of the candidate region. Am J Hum Genet 1994;54:774–781

57. Kawaguchi Y, Okamoto T, Taniwaki M, et al. CAG expansions in a novel gene for Machado–Joseph disease at chromosome 14q32.1. Nat Genet 1994;8:221–228

58. Lopes-Cendes I, Andermann E, Rouleau GA. Evidence for the existence of a fourth dominantly inherited spinocerebellar ataxia locus. Genomics 1994;21:270–274

59. Flanigan K, Gardner K, Alderson K, et al. Autosomal dominant spinocerebellar ataxia with sensory axonal neuropathy (SCA4): clinical description and genetic localization to chromosome 16q22.1. Am J Hum Genet 1996;59:392–399

60. Ranum LPW, Schut LJ, Lundgren JK, et al. Spinocerebellar ataxia type 5 in a family descended from the grandparents of President Lincoln maps to chromosome 11. Nat Genet 1994;8:280–284

61. Zhuchenko O, Bailey J, Bonnen P, et al. Autosomal dominant cerebellar ataxia (SCA6) associated with small polyglutamine expansions in the alpha 1A-voltage-dependent calcium channel. Nat Genet 1997;15:62–69

62. Riess O, Schols L, Bottger H, et al. SCA6 is caused by moderate CAG expansion in the alpha(1A)-voltage-dependent calcium channel gene. Hum Mol Genet 1997;6:1289–1293

63. Lindblad K, Savontaus ML, Stevanin G, et al. An expanded CAG repeat sequence in spinocerebellar ataxia type 7. Genome Res 1996;6:965–971

64. David G, Abbas N, Coullin P, et al. The gene for autosomal dominant cerebellar ataxia type II is located in a 5-cM region in 3p12-p13: genetic and physical mapping of the SCA7 locus. Am J Hum Genet 1996; 59:1328–1336

65. David G, Abbas N, Stevanin G, et al. Cloning of the SCA7 gene reveals a highly unstable CAG repeat expansion. Nat Genet 1997;17:65–70

66. Koob MD, Moseley ML, Schut LJ, et al. An untranslated CTG expansion causes a novel form of spinocerebellar ataxia (SCA8). Nat Genet 1999;21:379–384

67. Zu L, Figueroa KP, Grewal R, Pulst SM. Mapping of a new autosomal dominant spinocerebellar ataxia to chromosome 22. Am J Hum Genet 1999;64:594–599

68. Matsuura T, Achari M, Khajavi M, et al. Mapping of the gene for a novel spinocerebellar ataxia with pure cerebellar signs and epilepsy. Ann Neurol 1999;45: 407–411

69. O'Hearn E, Holmes SE, Calvert PC, et al. SCA-12: Tremor with cerebellar and cortical atrophy is associated with a CAG repeat expansion. Neurology. 2001; 56:287–289

70. Fujigasaki H, Verma IC, Camuzat A, et al. SCA12 is a rare locus for autosomal dominant cerebellar ataxia: a study of an Indian family. Ann Neurol 2001;49:117–121

71. Herman-Bert A, Stevanin G, Netter JC, et al. Mapping of spinocerebellar ataxia 13 to chromosome 19q13.3-q13.4 in a family with autosomal dominant cerebellar ataxia and mental retardation. Amer J Hum Genet 2000;67:229–235

72. Yamashita I, Sasaki H, Yabe I, et al. A novel locus for dominant cerebellar ataxia (SCA14) maps to a 10.2-cM interval flanked by D19S206 and D19S605 on chromosome 19q13.4-qter. Ann Neurol 2000 Aug;48(2): 156–163

73. Huntington's Disease Collaborative Research Group. A novel gene containing a trinucleotide repeat that is expanded and unstable on Huntington's disease chromosome. Cell 1993;72:971–983

74. Xiang FQ, Almqvist EW, Huq M, et al. A Huntington disease-like neurodegenerative disorder maps to chromosome 20p. Am J Hum Genet 1998;63:1431–1438

75. Kambouris M, Bohlega S, Al-Tahan A, Meyer BF. Localization of the gene for a novel autosomal recessive neurodegenerative Huntington-like disorder to 4p15.3. Amer J Hum Genet 2000;66:445–452

76. Rubio JP, Danek A, Stone C, et al. Chorea-acanthocytosis: genetic linkage to chromosome 9q21. Am J Hum Genet 1997;61:899–908

77. Rubio JP, Levy ER, Dobson-Stone C, Monaco AP. Genomic organization of the human G alpha 14 and G alpha q genes and mutation analysis in chorea-acanthocytosis (CHAC). Genomics 1999;57:84–93

78. deVries BBA, Arts WFM, Breedveld GJ, et al. Benign hereditary chorea of early onset maps to chromosome 14q. Am J Hum Genet 2000;66:136–142

79. Reyniers E, Van Bogaert P, Peeters N, et al. A new neurological syndrome with mental retardation, choreoathetosis, and abnormal behavior maps to chromosome Xp11. Am J Hum Genet 1999;65:1406–1412

80. Sege-Peterson K, Nyhan WL, Page T. Lesch–Nyhan disease and HPRT deficiency. *In:* Rosenberg RN, Prusiner SB, DiMauro S, et al., eds. The Molecular and Genetic Basis of Neurological Disease. Stoneham, MA: Butterworth-Heinemann, 1993:241–260

81. Kramer PL, Heiman GA, Gasser T, et al. The DYT1 gene on 9q34 is responsible for most cases of early limb-onset idiopathic torsion dystonia in non-Jews. Am J Hum Genet 1994;55:468–475

82. Ozelius LJ, Hewett JW, Page CE, et al. The early-onset torsion dystonia gene (DYT1) encodes an ATP binding protein. Nat Genet 1997;17:40–48

83. Wilhelmsen KC, Weeks DE, Nygaard TG, et al. Genetic mapping of "lubag" (X-linked dystonia-parkinsonism) in a Filipino kindred to the pericentromeric region of the X chromosome. Ann Neurol 1991;29:124–131

84. Müller U, Haberhausen G, Wagner T, et al. DXS106 and DXS559 flank the X-linked dystonia-parkinsonism syndrome locus (DYT3). Genomics 1994;23:114–117

85. Nygaard TG, Wilhelmsen KC, Risch NJ, et al. Linkage mapping of dopa-responsive dystonia (DRD) to chromosome 14q. Nat Genet 1993;5:386–391

86. Ichinose H, Ohye T, Takahashi E, et al. Hereditary progressive dystonia with marked diurnal fluctuation caused by mutations in the GTP cyclohydrolase I gene. Nat Genet 1994;8:236–242

87. Almasy L, Bressman SB, Raymond D, et al. Idiopathic torsion dystonia linked to chromosome 8 in two Mennonite families. Ann Neurol 1997;42:670–673

88. Leube B, Rudnicki D, Ratzlaff T, et al. Idiopathic torsion dystonia: assignment of a gene to chromosome 18p in a German family with adult onset, autosomal dominant inheritance and purely focal distribution. Hum Mol Genet 1996;5:1673–1677

89. Nygaard TG, Raymond D, Chen C, et al. Localization of a gene for myoclonus-dystonia to chromosome 7q21-q31. Ann Neurol 1999 Nov;46(5):794–798

90. Zimprich A, Grabowski M, Asmus F, et al. Mutations in the gene encoding epsilon-sarcoglycan cause myoclonus-dystonia syndrome. Nat Genet 2001;29: 66–69

91. Kramer PL, Mineta M, Klein C, et al. Rapid-onset dystonia-parkinsonism: linkage to chromosome 19q13. Ann Neurol 1999;46:176–182

92. Pittock SJ, Joyce C, O'Keane V, et al. Rapid-onset dystonia-parkinsonism—a clinical and genetic analysis of a new kindred. Neurology 2000;55:991–995

93. Valente EM, Bentivoglio AR, Cassetta E, et al. DYT13, a novel primary torsion dystonia locus, maps to chromosome 1p36.13–36.32 in an Italian family with cranial-cervical or upper limb onset. Ann Neurol 2001; 49:362–366

94. Koehler CM, Leuenberger D, Merchant S, et al. Human deafness dystonia syndrome is a mitochondrial disease. Proc Natl Acad Sci USA 1999;96:2141–2146

95. Jin H, Kendall E, Freeman TC, et al. The human family of deafness/dystonia peptide (DDP) related mitochondrial import proteins. Genomics 1999;61:259–267

96. Tranebjaerg L, Hamel BCJ, Gabreels FJM, et al. A de novo missense mutation in a critical domain of the X-linked DDP gene causes the typical deafness-dystonia-optic atrophy syndrome. Eur J Human Genet 2000;8: 464–467

97. Rothbauer U, Hofmann S, Muhlenbein N, et al. Role of the deafness dystonia peptide 1 (DDP1) in import of human Tim23 into the inner membrane of mitochondria. J Biol Chem 2001;276:37327–37334

98. Lossos A, Schlesinger I, Okon E, et al. Adult-onset Niemann–Pick type C disease: clinical, biochemical, and genetic study. Arch Neurol 1997;54:1536–1541

99. Taylor TD, Litt M, Kramer P, et al. Homozygosity mapping of Hallervorden–Spatz syndrome to chromosome 20p12.3-p13. Nat Genet 1996;14:479–481

100. Zhou B, Westaway SK, Levinson B, et al. A novel pantothenate kinase (PANK2) is defective in Hallervorden–Spatz syndrome. Nat Genet 2001;28:350–354

101 Shiang R, Ryan SG, Zhu YZ, et al. Mutations in the alpha I subunit of the inhibitory glycine receptor cause the dominant neurologic disorder, hyperekplexia. Nat Genet 1993;5:351–358

102. Lehesjoki AE, Koskiniemi M, Norio R, et al. Localization of the EPM1 gene for progressive myoclonus epilepsy on chromosome 21: linkage disequilibrium allows high resolution mapping. Hum Mol Genet 1993;2:1229–1234

103. Lehesjoki AE, Koskiniemi M. Clinical features and genetics of progressive myoclonus epilepsy of the Unverricht–Lundborg type. Ann Med 1998;30:474–480

104. Maddox LO, Descartes M, Collins J, et al. Identification of a recombination event narrowing the Lafora disease gene region. J Med Genet 1997;34:590–591

105. Minassian BA, Lee JR, Herbrick JA, et al. Mutations in a gene encoding a novel protein tyrosine phosphatase cause progressive myoclonus epilepsy. Nat Genet 1998;20:171–174

106. Serratosa JM, Gomez-Garre P, Gallardo ME, et al. A novel protein tyrosine phosphatase gene is mutated in progressive myoclonus epilepsy of the Lafora type (EPM2). Hum Mol Genet 1999;8:345–352

107. Jaksch M, Klopstock T, Kurlemann G, et al. Progressive myoclonus epilepsy and mitochondrial myopathy associated with mutations in the tRNA(Ser(UCN)) gene. Ann Neurol 1998;44:635–640

108. Prusiner SB. Genetic and infectious prion diseases. Arch Neurol 1993;50:1129–1153

109. Nagafuchi S, Yanagisawa H, Sato K, et al. Dentatorubral and pallidoluysian atrophy expansion of an unstable CAG trinucleotide on chromosome-12p. Nat Genet 1994;6:14–18

110. Koide R, Ikeuchi T, Onodera O, et al. Unstable expansion of CAG repeat in hereditary dentatorubral-pallidoluysian atrophy (DRPLA). Nat Genet 1994;6:9–13

111. Browne DL, Gancher ST, Nutt TG, et al. Episodic ataxia/myokymia syndrome is associated with point mutations in the human potassium channel gene, KCNA1. Nat Genet 1994;8:136–140

112. Litt M, Kramer P, Browne D, et al. A gene for episodic ataxis/myokymia maps to chromosome 12p13. Am J Hum Genet 1994;55:702–709

113. Vahedi K, Joutel A, van Bogaert P, et al. A gene for hereditary paroxysmal cerebellar ataxia maps to chromosome 19p. Ann Neurol 1995;37:289–293

114. von Brederlow B, Hahn A, Koopman WJ, et al. Mapping the gene for acetazolamide responsive hereditary paroxysmal cerebellar ataxia to chromosome 19p. Hum Mol Genet 1995;4:279–284

115. Tomita H, Nagamitsu S, Wakui K, et al. Paroxysmal kinesigenic choreoathetosis locus maps to chromosome 16p11.2-q12.1. Am J Hum Genet 1999;65:1688–1697

116. Bennett LB, Roach ES, Bowcock AM. A locus for paroxysmal kinesigenic dyskinesia maps to human chromosome 16. Neurology 2000;54:125–130

117. Valente EM, Spacey SD, Wali GM, et al. A second paroxysmal kinesigenic choreoathetosis locus (EKD2) mapping on 16q13-q22.1 indicates a family of genes which give rise to paroxysmal disorders on human chromosome 16. Brain 2000;123:2040–2045

118. Fouad GT, Servidei S, Durcan S, et al. A gene for familial paroxysmal dyskinesia (FPD1) maps to chromosome 2q. Am J Hum Genet 1996;59:135–139

119. Fink JK, Rainier S, Wilkowski J, et al. Paroxysmal dystonic choreoathetosis: tight linkage to chromosome 2q. Am J Hum Genet 1996;59:140–145

120. Fink JK, Hedera P, Mathay JG, Albin RL. Paroxysmal dystonic choreoathetosis linked to chromosome 2q: clinical analysis and proposed pathophysiology. Neurology 1997;49:177–183

121. Hofele K, Benecke R, Auburger G. Gene locus FPD1 of the dystonic Mount–Reback type of autosomal–dominant paroxysmal choreoathetosis. Neurology 1997;49:1252–1257

122. Jarman PR, Wood NW, Davis MT, et al. Hereditary geniospasm: linkage to chromosome 9q13-q21 and evidence for genetic heterogeneity. Am J Hum Genet 1997;61:928–933

123. Raskind WH, Bolin T, Wolff J, et al. Further localization of a gene for paroxysmal dystonic choreoathetosis to a 5-cM region on chromosome 2q34. Hum Genet 1998;102:93–97

124. Auburger G, Ratzlaff T, Lunkes A, et al. A gene for autosomal dominant paroxysmal choreoathetosis spasticity (CSE) maps to the vicinity of a potassium channel gene cluster on chromosome 1p, probably within 2 cM between D1S443 and D1S197. Genomics 1996;31:90–94

125. Szepetowski P, Rochette J, Berquin P, et al. Familial infantile convulsions and paroxysmal choreoathetosis: a new neurological syndrome linked to the pericentromeric region of human chromosome 16. Am J Hum Genet 1997;61:889–898

126. Lee WL, Tay A, Ong HT, et al. Association of infantile convulsions with paroxysmal dyskinesias (ICCA syndrome): confirmation of linkage to human chromosome 16p12-q12 in a Chinese family. Hum Genet 1998;103:608–612

127. Carelli V, Ghelli A, Bucchi L, et al. Biochemical features of mtDNA 14484 (ND6/M64V) point mutation associated with Leber's hereditary optic neuropathy. Ann Neurol 1999;45:320–328

128. Guerrini R, Bonanni P, Nardocci N, et al. Autosomal recessive rolandic epilepsy with paroxysmal exercise-induced dystonia and writer's cramp: delineation of the syndrome and gene mapping to chromosome 16p12-11.2. Ann Neurol 1999;45:344–352

129. Oldani A, Zucconi M, Asselta R, et al. Autosomal dominant nocturnal frontal lobe epilepsy—a video-polysomnographic and genetic appraisal of 40 patients and delineation of the epileptic syndrome. Brain 1998;121:205–223

130. Nakken KO, Magnusson A, Steinlein OK. Autosomal dominant nocturnal frontal lobe epilepsy: an electroclinical study of a Norwegian family with ten affected members. Epilepsia 1999;40:88–92

131. Merette C, Brassard A, Potvin A, et al. Significant linkage for Tourette syndrome in a large French Canadian family. Am J Hum Genet 2000;67:1008–1013

132. Sirianni N, Naidu S, Pereira J, et al. Rett syndrome: confirmation of X-linked dominant inheritance, and localization of the gene to Xq28. Am J Hum Genet 1998;63:1552–1558

133. Amir RE, Vanden-Veyver IB, Wan M, et al. Rett syndrome is caused by mutations in X-linked MECP2, encoding methyl-CpG-binding protein 2. Nat Genet 1999;23:185–188

134. Higgins JJ, Pho LT, Nee LE. A gene (ETM) for essential

tremor maps to chromosome 2p22-p25. Mov Disord 1997;12:859-864

135. Gulcher JR, Jonsson D, Kong A, et al. Mapping of a familial essential tremor gene, FET1, to chromosome 3q13. Nat Genet 1997;17:84–87

136. Jarman PR, Davis MB, Hodgson SV, et al. Paroxysmal dystonic choreoathetosis—genetic linkage studies in a British family. Brain 1997;120:2125–2130

137. Planté-Bordeneuve V, Guiochon-Mantel A, Lacroix C, et al. The Roussy–Levy family: from the original description to the gene. Ann Neurol 1999;46:770–773

138. Tanzi RE, Petrukhin K, Chernov I, et al. The Wilson disease gene is a copper transporting ATPase with homology to the Menkes disease gene. Nat Genet 1993;5:344–350

139. Bull PC, Thomas GR, Rommens JM, et al. The Wilson disease gene is a putative copper transporting P-type ATPase similar to the Menkes gene. Nat Genet 1993; 5:327–337

140. Jarvela I, Schleutker J, Haataja L, et al. Infantile form of neuronal ceroid lipofuscinosis (CLN1) maps to the short arm of chromosome 1. Genomics 1991;9:170–173

141. Vesa J, Hellsten E, Verkruyse LA, et al. Mutations in the palmitoyl protein thioesterase gene causing infantile neuronal ceroid lipofuscinosis. Nature 1995;376: 584–587

142. Sharp JD, Wheeler RB, Lake BD, et al. Loci for classical and a variant late infantile neuronal ceroid lipofuscinosis map to chromosomes 11p15 and 15q21-23. Hum Mol Genet 1997;6:591–596

143. Savukoski M, Klockars T, Holmberg V, et al. CLN5, a novel gene encoding a putative transmembrane protein mutated in Finnish variant late infantile neuronal ceroid lipofuscinosis. Nat Genet 1998;19:286–288

144. Mole SE. Batten disease: four genes and still counting. Neurobiol Disease 1998;5:287–303

145. Das AK, Becerra CHR, Yi W, et al. Molecular genetics of palmitoyl-protein thioesterase deficiency in the US. J Clin Invest 1998;102:361–370

146. Brooks BP, Fischbeck KH. Spinal and bulbar muscular atrophy; a trinucleotide-repeat expansion neurodegenerative disease. Trends Neurosci 1995;18:459–461

146. Jarvela I, Autti T, Lamminranta S, et al. Clinical and magnetic resonance imaging findings in Batten disease: analysis of the major mutation (1.02-kb deletion). Ann Neurol 1997;42:799–802

147. Michalewski MP, Kaczmarski W, Golabek AA, et al. Evidence for phosphorylation of CLN3 protein associated with Batten disease. Biochem Biophys Res Commun 1998;253:458–462

147. Schwab RS, Chafetz ME, Walker S. Control of two simultaneous voluntary motor acts in normal and in parkinsonism. Arch Neurol Psychiat 1954;72:591–598

148. Fahn S. Akinesia. In: Berardelli A, Benecke R, Manfredi M, Marsden CD, eds. Motor Disturbances. II. London: Academic Press, 1990:141–150

149. Pramstaller PP, Marsden CD. The basal ganglia and apraxia. Brain 1996 Feb;119(Pt 1):319–340

150. Meissner I, Wiebers DO, Swanson JW, O'Fallon WM. The natural history of drop attacks. Neurology 1986; 36:1029–1034

151. Stevens DL, Matthews WB. Cryptogenic drop attacks: an affliction of women. Br Med J 1973;1:439–442

152. Sheldon JH. On the natural history of falls in old age. Br Med J 1960;2:1685–1690

153. Nickens H. Intrinsic factors in falling among the elderly. Arch Int Med 1985;145:1089–1093

154. Lee MS, Marsden CD. Drop attacks. In: Fahn S, Hallett

MH, Lueders HO, Marsden CD, eds. Negative Motor Phenomena. New York: Lippincott-Raven, 1995:41–52

155. Guilleminault C, Gelb M. Clinical aspects and features of cataplexy. In: Fahn S, Hallett MH, Lueders HO, Marsden CD, eds. Negative Motor Phenomena. New York: Lippincott-Raven, 1995:65–77

156. Gelenberg AJ. The catatonic syndrome. Lancet 1976; 1:1339–1341

157. Hymas N, Lees A, Bolton D, et al. The neurology of obsessional slowness. Brain 1991;114:2203–2233

158. Sawle GV, Hymas NF, Lees AJ, Frackowiak RSJ. Obsessional slowness—functional studies with positron emission tomography. Brain 1991;114: 2191–2202

159. Giladi N, Kao R, Fahn S. Freezing phenomenon in patients with parkinsonian syndromes. Mov Disord 1997;12:302–305.

160. Giladi N, McMahon D, Przedborski S, et al. Motor blocks in Parkinson's disease. Neurology 1997;42: 333–339

161. Narabayashi H, Imai H, Yokochi M, et al. Cases of pure akinesia without rigidity and tremor and with no effect by L-DOPA therapy. In: Birkmayer W, Hornykiewicz O, eds. Advances in Parkinsonism. Basle: Editiones Roche, 1976:335–342

162. Narabayashi H, Kondo T, Yokochi F, Nagatsu T. Clinical effects of L-threo-3,4-dihydroxyphenylserine in cases of parkinsonism and pure akinesia. Adv Neurol 1986;45:593–602

163. Imai H, Narabayashi H, Sakata E. "Pure akinesia" and the later added supranuclear ophthalmoplegia. Adv Neurol 1986;45:207–212

164. Atchison PR, Thompson PD, Frackowiak RSJ, Marsden CD. The syndrome of gait ignition failure: a report of six cases. Mov Disord 1993;8:285–292

165. Nutt JG, Marsden CD, Thompson PD. Human walking and higher-level gait disorders, particularly in the elderly. Neurology 1993;43:268–279

166. Andrews CJ. Influence of dystonia on the response to long-term L-dopa therapy in Parkinson's disease. J Neurol Neurosurg Psychiatry 1973;36:630–636

167. Lepore FE, Duvoisin RC. "Apraxia" of eyelid opening: an involuntary levator inhibition. Neurology 1985; 35:423–427

168. Fahn S. The freezing phenomenon in parkinsonism. In: Fahn S, Hallett M, Lueders HO, Marsden CD, eds. Negative Motor Phenomena. New York: Lippincott-Raven, 1995:53–63

169. Achiron A, Ziv I, Goren M, et al. Primary progressive freezing gait. Mov Disord 1993;8:293–297

170. Riley DE, Fogt N, Leigh RJ. The syndrome of "pure akinesia" and its relationship to progressive supranuclear palsy. Neurology 1994;44:1025–1029

171. Katayama S, Watanabe C, Khoriyama T, et al. Slowly progressive L-DOPA nonresponsive pure akinesia due to nigropallidal degeneration: a clinicopathological case study. J Neurol Sci 1998;161:169–172

172. Lance JW, Schwab RS, Peterson EA. Action tremor and the cogwheel phenomenon in Parkinson's disease. Brain 1963;86:95–110

173. Denny-Brown D. The Basal Ganglia and their Relation to Disorders of Movement. London: Oxford University Press, 1962:75

174. Fahn S. Clinical aspects and treatment of rigidity and dsytonia. In: Benecke R, Conrad B, Marsden CD, eds. Motor Disturbances I. London: Academic Press, 1987: 101–110

175. Smego RA Jr, Durack DT. The neuroleptic malignant syndrome. Arch Int Med 1982;142:1183–1185

176. Kurlan R, Hamill R, Shoulson I. Neuroleptic malignant syndrome. Clin Neuropharmacol 1984;7:109–120

177. Friedman JH, Feinberg SS, Feldman RG. A neuroleptic malignant-like syndrome due to levodopa therapy withdrawal. JAMA 1985;254:2792–2795

178. Keyser DL, Rodnitzky RL. Neuroleptic malignant syndrome in Parkinson's disease after withdrawal or alteration of dopaminergic therapy. Arch Intern Med 1991;151:794–796

179. Henderson VW, Wooten GF. Neuroleptic malignant syndrome: a pathogenetic role for dopamine receptor blockade. Neurology 1981;31:132–137

180. Boeve BF, Rummans TA, Philbrick KL, Callahan MJ. Electrocardiographic and echocardiographic changes associated with malignant catatonia. Mayo Clin Proc 1994;69:645–650

181. Thompson PD. Stiff people. In: Marsden CD, Fahn S, eds. Movement Disorders 3. Oxford: Butterworth-Heinemann, 1994:373–405

182. Spehlmann R, Norcross K. Stiff-man syndrome. Clin Neuropharmacol 1979;4:109–121

183. Solimena M, Folli F, Denis-Donini S, et al. Autoantibodies to glutamic acid decarboxylase in a patient with stiff-man syndrome, epilepsy, and type I diabetes mellitus. N Engl J Med 1988;318:1012–1020

184. Solimena M, Folli F, Aparisi R, et al. Autoantibodies to GABAergic neurons and pancreatic beta cells in stiff-man syndrome. N Engl J Med 1990;322:1555–1560

185. Blum P, Jankovic J. Stiff-person syndrome: an autoimmune disease. Mov Disord 1991;6:12–20

186. Iliceto G, Thompson PD, Day BL, et al. Diaphragmatic flutter, the moving umbilicus syndrome, and belly dancers dyskinesia. Mov Disord 1990;5:15–22

187. Kono I, Ueda Y, Araki K, et al. Spinal myoclonus resembling belly dance. Mov Disord 1994;9:325–329

188. Ford B, Greene P, Fahn S. Oral and genital tardive pain syndromes. Neurology 1994;44:2115–2119

189. Micheli F, Fernandez Pardal M, Giannaula R, Fan S. What is it? Case 3, 1991: Moaning in a man with parkinsonian signs. Mov Disord 1991;6:376–378

190. Friedman JH. Involuntary humming in autopsy-proven Parkinson's disease. Mov Disord 1993;8:401–402

191. Sharp FR, Rando TA, Greenberg SA, et al. Pseudo-choreoathetosis—movements associated with loss of proprioception. Arch Neurol 1994;51:1103–1109

192. Sethi KD, Nichols FT, Yaghmai F. Generalized chorea due to basal ganglia lacunar infarcts. Mov Disord 1987;2:61–66

193. Kilroy AW, Paulsen WA, Fenichel GM. Juvenile parkinsonism treated with levodopa. Arch Neurol 1972;27:350

194. Funata N, Maeda Y, Koike M, et al. Neuronal intranuclear hyaline inclusion disease: report of a case and review of the literature. Clin Neuropathol 1990;9(2):89–96

195. Hyland K. Surtees RAH, Rodeck C, Clayton PT. Aromatic L-amino acid decarboxylase deficiency: clinical features, diagnosis, and treatment of a new inborn error of neurotransmitter amine synthesis. Neurology 1992;42:1980–1988

196. Hyland K, Arnold LA, Trugman JM. Defects of biopterin metabolism and biogenic amine biosynthesis: clinical, diagnostic, and therapeutic aspects. In: Fahn S, Marsden CD, DeLong MR, eds. Dystonia 3. Adv Neurol 1998;78:301–308

197. Lamberti P, Demari M, Iliceto G, et al. Effect of L-dopa on oculogyric crises in a case of dopa-responsive dystonia. Mov Disord 1993;8:236–237

198. Ouvrier RA, Billson MD. Benign paroxysmal tonic upgaze of childhood. J Child Neurol 1988;3:177–180

199. Hayman M, Harvey AS, Hopkins IJ, et al. Paroxysmal tonic upgaze: a reappraisal of outcome. Ann Neurol 1998;43:514–520

200. Jannetta PJ. Surgical approach to hemifacial spasm: microvascular decompression. In: Marsden CD, Fahn S, eds. Movement Disorders. London: Butterworth Scientific, 1982:330–333

201. Andermann F, Andermann E. Excessive startle syndromes: startle disease, jumping, and startle epilepsy. Adv Neurol 1986;43:321–338

202. Brown P, Rothwell JC, Thompson PD, et al. The hyperekplexias and their relationship to the normal startle reflex. Brain 1991;114:1903–1928

203. Matsumoto J, Hallett M. Startle syndromes. In: Marsden CD, Fahn S, eds. Movement Disorders 3. Oxford: Butterworth-Heinemann, 1994:418–433

204. Deuschl G, Mischke G, Schenck E, et al. Symptomatic and essential rhythmic palatal myoclonus. Brain 1990;113:1645–1672

205. Coleman RM, Pollack CP, Weitzman ED. Periodic movements in sleep (nocturnal myoclonus): relation to sleep disorders. Ann Neurol 1980;8:416–421

206. Lugaresi E, Cirignotta F, Montagna P, Coccagna G. Myoclonus and related phenomena during sleep. In: Chase M, Weitzman ED, eds. Sleep Disorders: Basic and Clinical Research. New York: Spectrum, 1983:123–127

207. Lugaresi E, Cirignotta F, Coccagna G, Montagna P. Nocturnal myoclonus and restless legs syndrome. Adv Neurol 1986;43:295–307

208. Hening W, Walters A, Kavey N, et al. Dyskinesias while awake and periodic movements in sleep in restless legs syndrome: treatment with opioids. Neurology 1986;36:1363–1366

209. Symonds CP. Nocturnal myoclonus. J Neurol Neurosurg Psychiatry 1953;16:166–171

210. Fish DR, Marsden CD. Epilepsy masquerading as a movement disorder. In: Marsden CD, Fahn S, eds. Movement Disorders 3. Oxford: Butterworth-Heinemann, 1994:346–358

211. Marion MH, Gledhill RF, Thompson PD. Spasms of amputation stumps: a report of 2 cases. Mov Disord 1989;4:354–358

211. Spillane JD, Nathan PW, Kelly RE, Marsden CD. Painful legs and moving toes. Brain 1971;94:541–556

213. Montagna P, Cirignotta F, Sacquegna T, et al. "Painful legs and moving toes" associated with polyneuropathy. J Neurol Neurosurg Psychiatry 1983;46:399–403

214. Nathan PW. Painful legs and moving toes: evidence on the site of the lesion. J Neurol Neurosurg Psychiatry 1978;41:934–939

215. Dressler D, Thompson PD, Gledhill RF, Marsden CD. The syndrome of painful legs and moving toes. Mov Disord 1994;9:13–21

216. Verhagen WIM, Horstink MWIM, Notermans SLH. Painful arm and moving fingers. J Neurol Neurosurg Psychiatry 1985;48:384–389

217. Obeso JA, Artieda J, Burleigh A. Clinical aspects of negative myoclonus. In: Fahn S, Hallett M, Luders HO, Marsden CD, eds. Negative Motor Phenomena. Adv Neurol 1995;67:1–7

218. Brown P, Thompson PD, Rothwell JC, et al. Axial myoclonus of propriospinal origin. Brain 1991;114:197–214

219. Obeso JA, Rothwell JC, Marsden CD. The spectrum of

cortical myoclonus: from focal reflex jerks to spontaneous motor epilepsy. Brain 1985;108:193–224

220. Brown P, Day BL, Rothwell JC, et al. Intrahemispheric
and interhemispheric spread of cerebral cortical
myoclonic activity and its relevance to epilepsy. Brain
1991;114:2333–2351

221. Hallett M, Chadwick D, Adam J, Marsden CD. Reticular reflex myoclonus: a physiological type of human
post-hypoxic myoclonus. J Neurol Neurosurg Psychiatry 1977;40:253–264

222. Kinsbourne M. Myoclonic encephalopathy of infants.
J Neurol Neurosurg Psychiatry 1962;25:271–279

223. Dyken P, Kolar O. Dancing eyes, dancing feet: Infantile polymyoclonia. Brain 1968;91:305–320

224. Spiro AJ. Minipolymyoclonus: a neglected sign in
childhood spinal muscular atrophy. Neurology 1970;
20:1124–1126

225. Wilkins DE, Hallett M, Erba G. Primary generalized
epileptic myoclonus: a frequent manifestation of
minipolymyoclonus of central origin. J Neurol Neurosurg Psychiatry 1985;48:506–516

226. Schultze F. Beitrage zur Muskelpathologie. I.
Myokymie (Muskelwogen) besonders an den Unterex-
tremitaten. Dtsch Z Nervenheilk 1895;6:65–70

227. Denny-Brown D, Foley JM. Myokymia and the benign
fasciculations of muscular cramps. Trans Ass Am Phys
1948;61:88–96

228. Andermann F, Cosgrove JBR, Lloyd-Smith DL, et al.
Facial myokymia in multiple sclerosis. Brain 1961;84:
31–44

229. Matthews WB. Facial myokymia. J Neurol Neurosurg
Psychiatry 1966;29:35–39

230. Jacobs L, Kaba S, Pullicino P. The lesion causing continuous facial myokymia in multiple sclerosis. Arch
Neurol 1994;51:1115–1119

231. Herz E. Die amyostatischen Unruheerscheinungen.
Klinisch kinematographische Analyse ihrer Kennze-
ichen und Beleiterscheinungen. J Psychologie Neurologie 1931;43:146–163

232. Herz E. Dystonia. I. Historical review: analysis of dystonic symptoms and physiologic mechanisms
involved. Arch Neurol Psychiatry 1944;51:305–318

233. Monrad-Krohn GH, Refsum S. The Clinical Examination of the Nervous System, 11th ed. New York: Paul
B. Hoeber, 1958:96

234. Masucci EF, Kurtzke JF, Saini N. Myorhythmia: a
widespread movement disorder. Clinicopathological
correlations. Brain 1984;107:53–79

235. Schwartz NA, Selhorst JB, Ochs AL, et al. Oculomasticatory myorhythmia: a unique movement disorder
occurring in Whipple's disease. Ann Neurol 1986;20:
677–683

236. Hausser-Hauw C, Roullet E, Robert R, Marteau R.
Oculo-facio-skeletal myorhythmia as a cerebral complication of systemic Whipple's disease. Mov Disord
1988;3:179–184

237. Tison F, Louvetgiendaj C, Henry P, et al. Permanent
bruxism as a manifestation of the oculo-facial syndrome related to systemic Whipple's disease. Mov
Disord 1992;7:82–85

238. Ekbom KA. Restless legs syndrome. Neurology 1960;
10:868–873

239. Walters AS, Hening WA, Chokroverty S. Review and
videotape recognition of idiopathic restless legs syndrome. Mov Disord 1991;6:105–110

240. Tan A, Salgado M, Fahn S. The characterization and
outcome of stereotypic movements in nonautistic children. Mov Disord 1997;12:47–52

241. Meige H, Feindel E. Tics and their treatment (trans.
Wilson SAK). London: Appleton, 1907:57–58

242. Lees AJ. Tics and Related Disorders. Edinburgh:
Churchill Livingstone, 1985

243. Shapiro AK, Shapiro ES, Young JG, Feinberg TE. Gilles
de la Tourette Syndrome, 2nd ed. New York: Raven
Press, 1988

244. Fahn S. Motor and vocal tics. In: Kurlan R, ed. Handbook of Tourette's Syndrome and Related Tic and
Behavioral Disorders. New York: Marcel Dekker,
1993:3–16

245. Jankovic J. Stereotypies. In: Marsden CD, Fahn S, eds.
Movement Disorders 3. Oxford: Butterworth-Heinemann, 1994:503–517

246. Frankel M, Cummings JL. Neuro-ophthalmic abnormalities in Tourette's syndrome: functional and
anatomic implications. Neurology 1984;34:359–361

231 Medical Treatment of Parkinson's Disease and its Complications

Stanley Fahn and Blair Ford

Introduction

In his brief monograph *An Essay on the Shaking Palsy* published in 1817, the English physician and geologist James Parkinson provided the first clear description of the disease that now bears his name.[1] Parkinson's seminal observations were based on a sample of six patients, but give as complete and eloquent a depiction of the clinical features and natural history of this disease as has ever been written. Over the course of the nineteenth century many other clinicians added to the description of Parkinson's disease (PD), including Charcot, who first treated the disease using the anticholinergic agent belladonna.

Little was known about the cause of PD for 100 years after the original description. The encephalitis of von Economo, striking Europe in 1915, caused a flu-like illness followed by somnolence and parkinsonism, and providing evidence of a viral cause for the syndrome.[2] The first anatomical clues as to the seat of the disorder were provided by a case of hemiplegic parkinsonism caused by a tuberculoma of the right cerebral peduncle, destroying the substantia nigra.[3] In a careful pathological series of 54 patients, including nine cases of PD, Tretiakoff discovered that degeneration of the substantia nigra was a consistent feature of the disorder.[4] Tretiakoff also discovered eosinophilic neuronal inclusions, previously described by Lewy in 1913,[5] in the surviving cells of the substantia nigra.

Pathological observations in PD were not linked to a deficit in dopamine for another 50 years. In 1957, Montagu discovered that dopamine was present in the mammalian brain.[6] Carlsson showed that the depletion of striatal dopamine could induce a state of parkinsonism, reversible by injections of levodopa.[7] Subsequently, Carlsson and Hornykiewicz suggested that levodopa could be used to treat Parkinson's disease. Cotzias, using large doses of racemic DL-dopa (up to 16 g daily), was the first to bring about a complete disappearance of symptoms in patients with PD.[8] Subsequently, levodopa became the standard treatment for Parkinson's disease. Through the 1970s and 1980s, newer dopamine agonists were added to the therapeutic armamentarium.

Surgical treatments of Parkinson's disease began in the 1940s but fell into disuse with the introduction of levodopa in the late 1960s. When it became clear in the 1980s that medication treatment was frequently complicated by intractable dyskinesias and "wearing-off" motor fluctuations, stereotactic posteroventral medial pallidotomy re-emerged as a treatment for advanced PD. In the 1990s, deep brain stimulation was developed as a treatment for medication-refractory tremor, and with time replaced all previous lesion-based surgical treatments for PD.

The treatment of PD has evolved rapidly over the last three decades. Advances in molecular biology have opened the prospect of treating PD using nerve growth factors, implantable dopamine-producing cells derived from stem cells, and gene therapy—all therapeutic approaches that are under development. This chapter provides a discussion of the currently available medical treatment for PD and its complications.

Epidemiology

The prevalence of Parkinson's disease is estimated to be between 0.1% and 0.5%, with approximately a million Americans affected by the disorder. The true prevalence of PD remains unknown, however. Estimates of disease prevalence vary widely around the world, ranging between 31 per 100 000 to 328 per 100 000.[9]

The most important risk factor for Parkinson's disease appears to be age. Parkinson's disease has a median onset at about 56 years, and is rare before the age of 30. In most studies, Parkinson's disease prevalence does not differ between the genders. Approximately 13% of patients seen in a hospital clinic give a history of an affected first degree relative. A cluster of parkinsonism in young narcotic addicts exposed to intravenous MPTP (1-methyl-4-phenyl-1,2,3,6-tetrahydropyridine) suggested that exposure to an environmental toxin could cause Parkinson's disease in some cases. Epidemiological studies have shown a higher incidence of Parkinson's disease in rural communities, and among populations that use well water or who are exposed to herbicides and pesticides.[9] Trauma is often listed as a risk factor for Parkinson's disease, based on retrospective case control studies. Cigarette smoking appears to have an inverse correlation with the subsequent development of Parkinson's disease.

Clinical manifestations

Parkinsonism is a syndrome characterized by any combination of five cardinal features: tremor at rest, rigidity, bradykinesia, loss of postural reflexes and gait freezing. Parkinsonism is caused most frequently by idiopathic ("classic") Parkinson's disease, as described by James Parkinson, but it may be caused by a large list of other diseases, including vascular parkinsonism, drug-induced parkinsonism, other neurodegenerative disorders, trauma, brain tumors, hydrocephalus and others.

Several diagnostic criteria have been developed for Parkinson's disease, but the diagnostic gold standard remains the postmortem evaluation. Two separate clinical pathological series concluded that only 76% of patients with a clinical diagnosis of PD actually met pathological criteria for PD, while the remaining 24% had other causes of parkinsonism.[10,11] Even among experts in PD, an analysis of autopsy data, imaging studies, response to levodopa and atypical clinical features indicated an 8.1% error rate in the initial diagnosis.[12]

The manifestations of Parkinson's disease may vary from a barely perceptible tremor to severe generalized akinetic-rigid parkinsonism at the end stage of the disease. Bradykinesia, the most characteristic clinical sign of Parkinson's disease, correlates well with the striatonigral deficit of the disease.[13] Bradykinesia may be initially manifested by a subtle lack of spontaneous or adventitious movements. Patients sit unnaturally still, like a statue, and have a paucity of facial expressiveness ("facial masking"). Bradykinesia also produces slowness of movement, with a characteristic decrement in the amplitude of all repetitive movements. In addition to whole body slowness and impairment in fine motor movements, other consequences of bradykinesia include drooling due to a lack of spontaneous swallowing, soft monotonous speech, a reduced arm swing when walking, and short, sometimes shuffling, steps.

The rest tremor is perhaps the most obvious feature of Parkinson's disease and is considered by some to be the best clinical correlate of idiopathic Parkinson's disease on postmortem analysis. The tremor readily disappears with posture-holding or during manual activities, in contrast to the tremor of essential tremor, which is an action tremor. However, only 75% of patients with idiopathic Parkinson's disease have a tremor at rest, and sometimes this can disappear during the course of the illness.

Rigidity is demonstrated by passively flexing, extending and rotating body parts, and has a cogwheeling aspect, especially if there is an associated tremor. At times, rigidity can cause discomfort and pain, especially around the shoulder. PD typically begins asymmetrically, involving the arm or hand. The classic presentation of the disease is the gradual development of an intermittent rest tremor in one hand, accompanied by slight bradykinesia and rigidity.

One of the most disabling symptoms of Parkinson's disease is gait freezing, also referred to as gait ignition failure or a magnetic gait. Freezing is the transient inability to take a step, and usually afflicts people as they are beginning to walk, when they pivot on turning, as they go through a doorway or narrow space, in crowded situations, or as they approach a chair or other target. At times, freezing can be so disabling that patients are unable to walk. Disorders associated with prominent and early-onset freezing include progressive supranuclear palsy (PSP), multiple system atrophy (MSA), and vascular parkinsonism.

Loss of postural reflexes, or postural instability, the most dangerous of motor impairments in PD, is tested by an abrupt pull backwards. When combined with axial rigidity and bradykinesia, the loss of postural reflexes places an individual at extreme risk of falling. Falling often results in fractures, and is the cause of severe morbidity and mortality in PD.

Non-motor symptoms of Parkinson's disease include a number of neurobehavioral disturbances, such as depression, anxiety, dementia, sleep disorders, and psychosis. Olfactory function is typically impaired in Parkinson's disease, even in very early stages. Drooling (sialorrhea) is one of the most socially disabling symptoms of Parkinson's disease. Autonomic disturbances, including orthostatic hypotension, constipation, excessive sweating, bladder control abnormalities, and sexual dysfunction also occur frequently in patients with PD.

Although therapeutic advances have a major positive impact on the quality of life, epidemiological studies have not been able to demonstrate that levodopa, the most effective treatment for PD, significantly prolongs life. Several studies, however, have concluded that PD patients have a nearly normal life expectancy. In a prospective study of 800 patients followed from the early stages of disease for an average of 8.2 years, the overall death rate was 2.1% per year, similar to that of an age and gender matched US population without PD. The most frequent cause of death in Parkinson's disease is pneumonia.

Differential diagnosis

Parkinson's disease is the primary disorder causing parkinsonism, but the differential diagnosis includes many secondary causes (Table 231.1). Features found particularly useful in differentiating PD from other neurodegenerative forms of parkinsonism (known as Parkinson-plus syndromes, and discussed in Chapter 232) include: the absence of tremor, early gait abnormality, early postural instability, pyramidal tract findings, and a poor response to levodopa (Table 231.2). Taken together these clinical features cast doubt on the diagnosis of idiopathic PD, and suggest a Parkinson-plus syndrome. Other causes of parkinsonism include drugs, trauma, vascular disease, hydrocephalus, and Wilson disease; a complete list is provided in the table.

There is no blood test or other diagnostic marker that conveniently confirms the diagnosis of Parkinson's disease, but advanced neuroimaging techniques may be helpful in demonstrating a dopaminergic deficit in selected cases. 18-fluorodopa positron emission tomography (PET) imaging typically reveals a reduction in fluorodopa uptake, particularly in the putamen, in the brains of patients with PD, even in early stages.[14] Involvement of the postsynaptic, striatal dopamine receptor containing neurons in atypical parkinsonism syndromes is a useful diagnostic clue. Using ^{11}C-raclopride, patients with untreated Parkin-

Table 231.1   Classification of parkinsonism*

I. Primary (idiopathic) parkinsonism
Parkinson's disease
Juvenile parkinsonism

II. Multisystem degenerations ("Parkinsonism-plus")
Progressive supranuclear palsy (PSP),
    Steele–Richardson–Olszewski disease (SRO)
Multiple system atrophy (MSA)
 • Striatonigral degeneration (SND or MSA-P)
 • Olicopontocerebellar atrophy (OPCA or MSA-C)
 • Shy–Drager syndrome (SDS)
Lytico–Bodig or Parkinsonism–Dementia–ALS complex
    of Guam (PDACG)
Cortical-basal ganglionic degeneration (CBGD)
Progressive pallidal atrophy
Parkinsonism–dementia complex
Pallidopyramidal disease

III. Heredodegenerative parkinsonism
Hereditary juvenile dystonia-parkinsonism
Autosomal dominant Lewy body disease
Huntington disease
Wilson disease
Hereditary ceruloplasmin deficiency
Hallervorden–Spatz disease
Olivopontocerebellar and spinocerebellar degenerations
Machado–Joseph disease
Familial amyotrophy–dementia–parkinsonism
Disinhibition–dementia–parkinsonism–amyotrophy
    complex
Gerstmann–Strausler–Scheinker disease
Familial progressive subcortical gliosis
Lubag (X-linked dystonia-parkinsonism)
Familial basal ganglia calcification
Mitochondrial cytopathies with striatal necrosis
 • Ceroid lipofuscinosis
Familial parkinsonism with peripheral neuropathy
Parkinsonian–pyramidal syndrome
Neuroacanthocytosis
Hereditary hemochromatosis

IV. Secondary (acquired, symptomatic) parkinsonism
Infectious postencephalitic, AIDS, subacute sclerosing
            panencephalitis, Creuzfeldt–Jakob
            disease, prion diseases
Drugs   dopamine receptor blocking drugs
            (antipsychotic, antiemetic drugs),
            reserpine, tetrabenazine, alpha-methyl-
            dopa, lithium, flunarizine, cinnarizine
Toxins   MPTP, CO, Mn, Hg, CS_2, cyanide, methanol,
            ethanol
Vascular   multi-infarct, Binswanger disease
Trauma   pugilistic encephalopathy
Other   parathyroid abnormalities, hypothyroidism,
            hepatocerebral degeneration, brain
            tumor, paraneoplastic, normal pressure
            hydrocephalus, non-communicating
            hydrocephalus, syringomesencephalia,
            hemiatrophy-hemiparkinsonism,
            peripherally-induced tremor and
            parkinsonism, psychogenic, psychomotor
            retardation

Table 231.2   NINDS diagnostic criteria for Parkinson's disease

Group A features: characteristic of PD
1. Resting tremor
2. Bradykinesia
3. Rigidity
4. Asymmetric onset

Group B features; suggestive of alternative diagnoses
1. Features unusual early in the clinical course
    a. Prominent postural instability in the first 3 years
       after symptom onset
    b. Freezing phenomenon in the first 3 years
    c. Hallucinations unrelated to medications in the first
       3 years
    d. Dementia preceding motor symptoms or in the first
       year
2. Supranuclear gaze palsy (other than restriction of
   upward gaze) or slowing of vertical saccades
3. Severe, symptomatic dysautonomia unrelated to
   medications
4. Documentation of condition known to produce
   parkinsonism and plausibly connected to the
   patient's symptoms (such as suitably located focal
   brain lesions or neuroleptic use within the past 6
   months)

son's disease are shown to have well-preserved striatal D2 receptors, while patients with atypical parkinsonism have a decrease in D2 receptor density.[15] Similarly, SPECT imaging shows decreased striatal binding of IBZM, a D2 receptor ligand,[16] and a decrease in presynaptic dopamine reuptake of I-123 beta-CIT, a dopamine transporter ligand.[17] In addition to reduced density of dopamine receptors, patients with atypical parkinsonism have decreased striatal metabolism, as demonstrated by deoxyglucose PET scans.[18]

In the absence of a specific biological marker, the diagnosis of PD can be made with certainty only at autopsy. PD is pathologically defined as a neurodegenerative disorder with (1) depigmentation of the substantia nigra, associated with degeneration of melanin and dopamine containing neurons, especially in the pars compacta of SN, and (2) the presence of Lewy bodies in the SN pars compacta and other brain regions.

Etiology

The cause of Parkinson's disease remains unknown. The selective loss of dopaminergic neurons in the substantia nigra underlies the main motor features of the disorder, but the degeneration of these cells is not understood. Proposed mechanisms of pathogenesis include genetic defects, oxidative stress, mitochondrial dysfunction, excitotoxicity, trauma, viral infection and other environmental factors. To date, no unified theory of pathogenesis accounting for sporadic and genetic PD has been established. Hereditary factors are more likely to play a role in young-onset cases than in patients developing PD over the age of 60.

Sporadic parkinsonism is common, accounting for 90% of cases, but in a small number of families PD is clearly inherited as a genetic disorder. Autosomal-recessive juvenile parkinsonism (AR-JP) is caused by mutations of a gene on chromosome 6q, encoding for the protein designated *parkin*.[19] Parkin gene mutations have been identified as a major cause of familial young onset PD, but also occur in cases of late onset familial PD that resemble classic idiopathic PD.[20,21] Parkin and its mRNA are widely distributed in peripheral tissues and in nervous tissue, with especially high levels in the substantia nigra.[22] The role of parkin is unknown but the protein appears to act as a ligase in the polyubiquitination of an unknown substrate, named protein X, prior to proteolysis.[23] The sequence of pathogenesis is not worked out, but parkin mutations seem to result in a loss of ligase activity, preventing the degradation of protein X, which in turn may be cytotoxic. It has been proposed that ubiquitin protein ligases play a role in regulating apoptotic cell death, and that genetic defects interrupting this process underlie the neuronal degeneration in PD.

Several genes are associated with PD, and more will likely be identified. In a large Italian family, PD with Lewy body pathology and levodopa-responsiveness was linked to an Ala53Thr mutation in the alpha synuclein gene on chromosome 4q21-q23.[24,25] The same gene mutation was found in several other unrelated Greek families, and a second alpha synuclein mutation was discovered in German families.[26] The normal function of alpha synuclein remains unknown, but the protein is abundantly expressed in brain, including within the substantia nigra. Alpha synuclein is also present within Lewy bodies. Alpha synuclein mutations are not responsible for most cases of familial Parkinson's disease, however, and do not appear to occur in sporadic PD or Parkinson's plus syndromes.

Other mutations in adult onset PD have been described, and may be important in the concept of cell death in PD. PD has been associated with mutation in the gene encoding for UCH-L1, an enzyme responsible for removing the ubiquitin from protein fragments following proteolysis.[27] As with the parkin mutation, a genetic defect that relates to ubiquitination supports the notion that the dopaminergic cell loss in PD may result from a disturbance of intracellular protein processing.

In non-genetic cases, accounting for the majority of PD, it has been proposed that the disease results from a combination of an environmental injury plus normal aging. In normal individuals at birth, the substantia nigra contains approximately 400 000 cells. By age 60, approximately 250 000 cells remain. Why the substantia nigra loses neurons as part of the normal aging process is not clear, but some have hypothesized the presence of an endogenous toxin. A number of different schemes have been proposed to explain the selective nigral cell death in PD, including oxidant stress, mitochondrial dysfunction, excitotoxic injury, nitric oxide, intracellular accumulation of calcium, defective iron metabolism and inflammatory processes.

Several lines of evidence suggest that the substantia nigra is selectively exposed to oxidative stress.[28] Dopamine metabolism by monoamine oxidase forms the free radicals superoxide and hydrogen peroxide. Excess iron in the substantia nigra further promotes the formation of the hydroxyl radical from hydrogen peroxide. Dopamine auto-oxidation in the presence of iron forms several other reactant species that could induce oxidative stress. In the brain, the major pathway for scavenging hydrogen peroxide involves glutathione and glutathione peroxidase. Levels of glutathione in the substantia nigra are profoundly depleted in Parkinson's disease, and may reflect a failure of antioxidant mechanisms in PD.

Mitochondrial dysfunction in the brain of PD has been proposed as a cause of PD.[29] Complex I activity of the mitochondrial respiratory chain in the substantia nigra pars compacta is reduced by 35% in PD. Impaired energy metabolism due to a Complex I defect could enhance the susceptibility of neurons to exogenous or endogenous mitochondrial toxins. In experimental models of PD, the complex I toxin rotenone, a commonly used herbicide, leads to selective loss of dopaminergic neurons and the presence of ubiquitin and alpha-synuclein positive inclusions.

The mechanism of dopaminergic cell death in MPTP exposure involves complex I toxicity. MPTP is converted to the active metabolite MPP^+ by monoamine oxidase. MPP^+ enters neurons and accumulates within mitochondria, where it inhibits complex I, leading to defective ATP production, increased free radical production, and increased susceptibility to excitotoxic injury by extracellular glutamate.[30] Most cases of PD are clearly not caused by rotenone or MPTP, but the mechanisms of toxicity provide insight into the vulnerability of the dopamine-containing neurons of the substantia nigra.

Medical treatment of PD

General principles of treatment

Keep the patient functioning independently as long as possible Since PD is a progressive disease and since no medications to date have been shown to stop the progression of the disease, the long-term goal in treating PD is to keep the patient functioning independently for as long as possible. Clearly, if medications could provide persisting symptomatic relief without adverse effects, no additional therapy for PD would be needed. The difficulty is that 75% of patients have serious complications after 6 years of levodopa therapy (Table 231.3).[31] Younger patients (less than 60 years of age) are particularly prone to develop the motor complications of fluctuations and dyskinesias.[32–35] Some physicians therefore recommend utilizing dopamine agonists in younger patients, rather than levodopa, when beginning therapy, in an attempt to delay the onset of these problems.[36,37] Controlled clinical trials comparing dopamine agonists and levodopa as the initial therapeutic agent have found that motor complications are less likely to occur with dopamine agonists.[38–40] But each of these

Table 231.3 Five major responses to >5 years of levodopa therapy (n = 330 patients)[31]

	n	%
1. Smooth, good response	83	25
2. Troublesome fluctuations	142	43
3. Troublesome dyskinesias	67	20
4. Toxicity at therapeutic or subtherapeutic dosages	14	4
5. Total or substantial loss of efficacy	27	8

studies also showed that levodopa was more effective in improving parkinsonian symptoms and signs as measured quantitatively by the Unified Parkinson's Disease Rating Scale (UPDRS). At all stages of disease, the goal of therapy is not to suppress all symptoms of parkinsonism but to maintain the patient's ability to be functional.

Individualize therapy The treatment of PD needs to be individualized. Each patient presents with a unique set of symptoms, signs, response to medications, and a host of social, occupational, and emotional problems that need to be addressed. The goal is to keep the patient functioning independently as long as possible. It is important to consider the patient's symptoms, the degree of functional impairment, and the expected benefits and risks of available therapeutic agents. It is essential to find out what troubles the patient the most. Keep in mind that younger patients are more likely to develop motor fluctuations and dyskinesias; while older patients are more likely to develop confusion, sleep–wake alterations, and psychosis.

Neuroprotective therapy If any drug could slow the progression of the disease process, it would make sense to use it as soon as the disease is diagnosed. As of this writing, no proven protective or restorative effect of a drug has been demonstrated with certainty. But studies are in progress looking at various agents to determine if they have such an effect.

When used early in PD, selegiline can delay the need for levodopa by an average of 9 months.[41–44] Because it has a mild symptomatic effect that is long lasting,[42] its ability to delay progression of disability can be explained entirely by this symptomatic effect. In favor of some neuroprotective effect is that after 2 months of washout of the drug, patients had slightly milder PD than did those on placebo.[42] However, because selegiline has a very long duration of action as an inhibitor of MAO type B,[45] this observation could represent an insufficient washout period. Furthermore, selegiline's benefit in delaying the introduction of levodopa gradually diminishes over time,[42] with the best results occurring in the first year of treatment. Additional long-term follow-up of DATATOP subjects showed that placebo-treated subjects fared better than selegiline-subjects when the drug was reintroduced after a 2-month washout period and that the two groups were identical in developing levodopa complications.[46,47] The net effect is that there is no convincing evidence that selegiline delayed the need for levodopa because of a protective effect; all results could be those of a drug with mild symptomatic benefit. Tocopherol (Vitamin E), a fat-soluble antioxidant, was independently evaluated as a neuroprotective agent in PD, but no beneficial effect was detected.[48]

Patients should be encouraged to remain active and mobile PD leads to decreased motivation and increased passivity. An active exercise program, even early in the disease, can combat this. Furthermore, such a program involves patients in their own care, allows muscle stretching and full range of joint mobility, and enhances a better mental attitude towards fighting the disease. By encouraging the patient to take responsibility for fighting the devastations of the disease, he or she becomes an active participant. Physical therapy, which can be implemented in the form of a well-constructed exercise program, is useful in all stages of the disease. For physical benefit, exercise aids the patient by stretching joints that tend to be utilized in PD with a reduced range of motion; it tones up muscles; and builds up strength. In advanced stages of PD, physical therapy may be even more valuable by keeping joints from becoming frozen, and providing guidance on how best to remain independent in mobility. It has been shown that PD patients who exercise intensively and regularly have better motor performance.[49,50] If exercise is not maintained, the benefit is lost.[51]

Medications for PD

Dopaminergic agents A great many drugs have been developed for PD, and Tables 231.4 and 231.5 classify them according to their mechanisms of action. Selection of the most suitable drugs for the individual patient and deciding when to utilize them in the course of the disease is a challenge to the treating clinician. In many of the Parkinson-plus disorders the

Table 231.4 Dopaminergic agents

Dopamine precursor	Levodopa
Decarboxylase inhibitor	Carbidopa, benserazide
Dopamine agonists	Bromocriptine, pergolide, pramipexole, ropinirole, apomorphine, cabergoline, lisuride, piribedil
Catechol-O-methyltransferase inhibitors	Entacapone, tolcapone
Dopamine releaser	Amantadine
Dopamine receptor blocker	Domperidone
MAO type B inhibitor	Selegiline, lazabemide, rasagiline
MAO type A&B inhibitor	Tranylcypromine, phenelzine

Table 231.5   Non-dopaminergic agents for motor symptoms

Antimuscarinics	Trihexyphenidyl, benztropine, ethopropazine
Antihistaminics	Diphenhydramine, orphenadrine
Antiglutamatergics	Amantadine, dextromethorphan, riluzole
Muscle relaxants	Cyclobenzaprine, diazepam, baclofen
Antioxidant vitamins	Ascorbate, tocopherol
Mitochondrial enhancer	Coenzyme Q10
Adenosine A$_{2A}$ receptor antagonists (in clinical trials)	
Neurotrophins	Neuroimmunophylins (in clinical trials), GDNF (in clinical trial)

response to treatment is not satisfactory, but the same general principles for treating PD are the basis for treating these disorders as well. Because PD is a chronic progressive disease, patients require lifelong treatment. Medications and their doses will change over time as adverse effects and new symptoms are encountered.

Because most of the motor symptoms of PD are related to striatal dopamine deficiency,[52] dopamine replacement therapy is the major medical approach to treating the disease. Table 231.4 lists these dopaminergic drugs. The most powerful drug is levodopa. It is usually administered with a peripheral decarboxylase inhibitor. In Table 231.4, both carbidopa and benserazide are listed as peripheral dopa decarboxylase inhibitors, although in the US only carbidopa is available. In many other countries benserazide is also available. Carbidopa/levodopa is marketed as Sinemet or generic; the combination is available in standard (e.g., Sinemet standard) and controlled-release (e.g. Sinemet CR) formulations. The former allows a more rapid onset, and the latter allows for a slightly longer plasma half-life. Benserazide/levodopa is marketed as standard Madopar and Madopar HBS (for slow release). These agents potentiate levodopa, allowing about a four-fold reduction in dosage to obtain the same benefit. Moreover, by preventing the formation of peripheral dopamine that can act at the area postrema (vomiting center), they block the development of nausea and vomiting. If additional carbidopa is needed for patients in whom nausea persists, it can be prescribed and patients can obtain it from their pharmacy; the additional peripheral decarboxylase inhibitor may overcome the nausea.

Besides being metabolized by aromatic amino acid decarboxylase, levodopa is also metabolized by catechol-O-methyltransferase (COMT) to form 3-O-methyldopa. Two COMT inhibitors are currently available; tolcapone and entacapone. These agents extend the plasma half-life of levodopa without increasing its peak plasma concentration, and can thereby prolong the duration of action of each dose of levodopa. The net effect with multiple dosings a day, though, is to elevate the average plasma concentration but smooth out the variations in the concentration. Tolcapone has two potential adverse effects that need to be explained to the patient. A small percentage will develop elevated liver transaminases, and patients need to have baseline and follow-up liver function tests. Death has occurred in three patients who had no liver function surveillance.[53] Entacapone has not shown these hepatic changes. With tolcapone, a small percentage of patients will develop diarrhea that doesn't appear for about 6 weeks after starting the drug. The diarrhea can be explosive, so the patient may not have any warning. Entacapone appears not to have these adverse effects.

The next most powerful drugs, after levodopa, in treating PD symptoms are the dopamine agonists. Of those listed in Table 231.4, bromocriptine, pergolide, pramipexole and ropinirole are available in the United States, and these are discussed below. Lisuride, cabergoline, piribedil and apomorphine are marketed in some countries. Lisuride has considerable 5-HT agonist activity. Cabergoline is the longest acting, and could be taken just once a day,[54,55] which is potentially helpful in preventing or reducing the "wearing-off" effect. Piribedil is relatively weak, but has been touted as having an anti-tremor effect. Apomorphine, being water soluble, is usually employed as a rapidly acting dopaminergic to overcome "off" states, i.e. provide a rescue. It is either injected subcutaneously or applied intranasally. Because of its emesis-producing propensity, the patient must be pretreated with an antinauseant such as domperidone. Apomorphine and lisuride (also water soluble) may be used by continuous subcutaneous infusion to provide a smooth response for patients who fluctuate between dyskinetic and "off" states. Apomorphine may be the most powerful dopamine agonist, and activates both the dopamine D1 and D2 receptors.

Bromocriptine is the least potent of the available oral dopamine agonists. Pergolide, pramipexole and ropinirole are comparably effective in clinical practice, but some patients will respond better to one than the others. Only pergolide has agonist activity at the D1 receptor (modest). The activation of the D2 receptor is known to be important in obtaining an anti-PD response, whereas it is unknown how important D3 receptor activation is for improving the anti-PD response. Bromocriptine, pergolide, pramipexole and ropinirole activate the dopamine D3 as well as the D2 receptor, but their ratios of affinities for these two receptors are different.[56] All dopamine agonists are less likely to induce dyskinesias compared to levodopa.[57] The agonists can be used as adjuncts to levodopa therapy[58,59] or as monotherapy.[60–65]

All dopamine agonists can induce confusion and hallucinations in elderly patients. Leg edema occurs in some patients. Pramipexole and ropinirole, and other dopaminergics as well (but with probably less frequency) can cause sleepiness and sleep attacks. This can be dangerous for the patient who drives an automobile, and motor vehicle accidents have occurred with patients falling asleep at the wheel.[66–69]

Amantadine has several actions. It activates release of dopamine from nerve terminals, blocks dopamine re-uptake into the nerve terminals, has antimuscarinic effects, and blocks glutamate receptors. Its dopaminergic actions make it a useful drug in about two-thirds of patients, but it can induce livedo reticularis, ankle edema, visual hallucinations, and confusion.

Domperidone is a peripherally-active dopamine receptor blocker, and is useful in preventing gastrointestinal upset from levodopa and the dopamine agonists. Although it doesn't enter the CNS it can still block the dopamine receptors in the area postrema, thereby preventing nausea and vomiting. By not penetrating the CNS it does not block the dopamine receptors in the striatum, thus not interfering with the action of dopamine or dopamine agonists. Domperidone is not yet marketed in the United States, but patients can obtain it from Canada.

Monoamine oxidase (MAO) inhibitors offer mildly effective symptomatic benefit. MAO type B inhibitors eliminate concern about the "cheese effect" with type A inhibitors. Although there is debate about possible protective benefit with selegiline, long-term use indicates it predominantly has symptomatic effects.[46,47] Selegiline has a slight ameliorating effect for mild "wearing-off" from levodopa.[70] Lazabemide is another type B MAOI, but is a reversible inhibitor. It shows the same symptomatic effect in PD as does selegiline.[71] It is not known whether it has a neuronal rescue effect. Rasagiline is another MAO type B irreversible inhibitor, like selegiline. It is currently undergoing clinical trials in patients with PD and has been reported to reduce the severity of PD.[72] Neither lazabemide nor rasagiline is commercially available. In contrast to selegiline, neither of them is metabolized to methamphetamine. Similarly to selegiline, both drugs do not require a tyramine-restricted diet.

Non-dopaminergic agents Non-dopaminergic agents (Table 231.5) are also useful to treat PD symptoms, particularly antimuscarinic drugs, commonly referred to as anticholinergics. These agents have been widely used since the 1950s but date back to the nineteenth century, when Charcot treated patients with PD using belladonna. Antimuscarinic drugs may reduce all symptoms of PD, but they have found special favor in treating tremor. However, because of their propensity to cause memory impairment and hallucinations in the elderly population, anticholinergics should be avoided in patients over the age of 70 years. The antihistaminics, tricyclics and cyclobenzaprine (Flexeril) have milder anticholinergic properties that make them useful in PD, particularly in the older patient who should not take the stronger anticholinergics.

Amantadine, listed in Table 231.4 as a dopaminergic agent, is listed also in Table 231.5 because it has antiglutamatergic effects; this property might account for its usefulness in reducing choreic dyskinesias induced by levodopa.[73,74] Dextromethorphan is another antiglutamatergic agent that may reduce the severity of dyskinesias by 50%.[74] Another useful class of drugs is the benzodiazepines, which reduce anxiety and thereby decrease parkinsonian tremor that is exacerbated by stress. Diazepam is usually well tolerated and does not exacerbate parkinsonian symptoms, whereas chlordiazepoxide can.[75] Lorazepam and alprazolam are other useful benzodiazepine agents. The muscle relaxants listed in Table 231.5 might help in treating "off" and peak-dose dystonias. Because oxidative stress may play a role in the pathogenesis of PD, high doses of antioxidant vitamins are reasonable therapeutic choices for patients with PD. The DATATOP study showed that tocopherol by itself has no effect, but the combination of ascorbate and tocopherol may be more effective than either of these two vitamins alone.[76,77]

Agents for non-motor complications of PD

Many non-motor problems are commonly present in patients with Parkinson's disease, occasionally overshadowing the motor symptoms of the disorder (Table 231.6). Drugs available to improve memory in Alzheimer's disease may be tried in patients with Parkinson's disease who have dementia, whether from diffuse Lewy body disease or from concomitant Alzheimer's disease. These drugs are centrally active cholinesterase inhibitors, donepezil and rivastigmine. Initial concern that they may worsen tremor and bradykinesia has not been a problem, perhaps because dopaminergic agents are also being given in these patients.

Because depression is common in patients with PD, this symptom needs to be vigorously attacked if present; otherwise it is difficult to reduce parkinsonian symptoms. The tricyclics and selective serotonin reuptake inhibitors are useful antidepressants in PD. It is not certain if one type of antidepressant class of compounds is superior to the other in treating the depression accompanying PD. The selective serotonin re-uptake inhibitors may aggravate parkinsonism if antiparkinsonian drugs are not being utilized concurrently. If insomnia is a problem for the patient, using an antidepressant at bedtime that is also a soporific, such as amitriptyline, can be doubly advantageous. Amitriptyline has considerable somnolence-inducing effect. The MAO-B inhibitor selegiline is not effective as an antidepressant. The inhibitors of both types A and B MAO are very effective, but they cannot be given in the presence of levodopa because of swings in blood pressure.

Psychosis induced by levodopa and the dopamine agonists can often be controlled by clozapine or quetiapine without worsening the parkinsonism. Clozapine is a dibenzodiazepine antipsychotic drug. It is called an atypical neuroleptic because it rarely causes drug-induced parkinsonism. Clozapine is primarily a selective D4 receptor antagonist, and can treat levodopa-induced psychosis without worsening parkinsonism.[78–89] Weekly monitoring of white blood cells is necessary to prevent irreversible agranulocytosis by allowing the discontinuation of this drug if a drop in leukocyte count is observed. Because of this need for weekly blood counts, olanzapine and quetiapine may be useful substitutes; however, the dose of

Table 231.6	**Non-dopaminergic agents for non-motor symptoms**
Behavioral	
Dementia	Donepezil, rivastigmine
Depression	Selective serotonin reuptake inhibitors, tricyclics, ECT
Psychosis	Clozapine, quetiapine, olanzapine, ziprasidone
Stress/anxiety	Benzodiazepines; diazepam, lorazepam, alprazolam
Apathy	Methylphenidate
Fatigue	Modafinil
Sleep-related	
Daytime sleepiness	Modafinil
Insomnia	Quetiapine, zolpidem, benzodiazepine
REM-sleep behavior disorder	Clonazepam
Restless legs	Opioids (e.g., propoxyphene, oxycodone)
Autonomic	
Orthostasis	Fluodrocortisone, midodrine (ProAmantine)
Urinary urgency	Oxybutynin (Ditropan), tolterodine (Detrol)
Impotence	Sildenafil
Gastrointestinal	
Constipation	High fiber diet, psyllium, polyethylene glycol (MiraLax)
Nausea	Trimethobenzamide (Tigan), domperidone, ondansetron (Zofran)
Sialorrhea	Propantheline

olanzapine needs to be kept small because it is a D2 antagonist and can worsen PD.[90]

Stress, excitement and anxiety make parkinsonian symptoms worse, especially tremor. In fact, tremor that is otherwise well controlled can re-emerge under stress. The benzodiazepines, by reducing anxiety, can partially offset this worsening of tremor. Apathy and fatigue are common in Parkinson's disease, and no medication as yet has been found satisfactory. Antidepressants and stimulants may help apathy, but no systemic studies have been reported. Similarly, stimulants (including caffeine) and modafinil may help fatigue and drowsiness, including medication-induced sedation by levodopa and dopamine agonists.

Various sleep problems are commonly encountered in PD. Nocturnal insomnia needs to be treated because the quality of life will otherwise suffer, and excessive daytime sleepiness may ensue, giving the diurnal sleep reversal pattern. Hypnotics, such as zolpidem and benzodiazepines can be safely used in PD. Quetiapine and clozapine often allow a good night's sleep, and can be utilized even in the absence of psychosis. Acting out dreams, so-called REM-sleep behavior disorder, is not uncommon and is usually avoided with clonazepam at bedtime. Restless legs syndrome and periodic movements in sleep are quite common in patients with PD, usually responding to dopamine agonists, or an opioid such as propoxyphene and oxycodone can be effective. They should be administered an hour or so before the usual onset of these symptoms.

Orthostatic hypotension is not a common feature in PD except as a complication of dopaminergic or other medications. Severe othostasis, especially as a presenting sign of parkinsonism, suggests a diagnosis of multiple systems atrophy (MSA). Fluodrocortisone to increase salt retention and midodrine as an alpha-1 adrenergic receptor agonist can be effective in preventing syncope.

Dyssynergia of the bladder sphincters can be a problem, and relief can be obtained with peripheral antimuscarinics. Oxybutynin (Ditropan) and tolterodine (Detrol) are commonly used for this condition. Difficulty obtaining erections can occur in patients with PD, and these men have reported benefit with sildenafil.

One of the most common complaints by patients with PD is constipation. This symptom can be a factor of both the disease and the medications used to treat PD. High fiber diet, including bran or dried fruits, or bulk forming agents (Metamucil), are often sufficient to relieve constipation. If dietary modification is not effective, one can try the standard laxatives or polyethylene glycol (MiraLax).

Nausea can be a complication of dopamine agonists and levodopa. Domperidone, a peripheral dopamine receptor blocker is effective. Because it is not available in the US, trimethobenzamide (Tigan) can be tried. Sialorrhea is due to infrequent and inadequate spontaneous swallowing of saliva. Peripherally active antimuscarinics such as propantheline can be quite effective. Injecting botulinum toxin into the parotid glands may benefit some patients.

Treatment of mild PD

The earliest stage of PD begins when the symptoms are first noticed and the diagnosis is made. At this point, there is no threat to the patient's activity of daily living capacity. The designation of "early stage" lasts until the symptoms begin to become troublesome. There is a general consensus that in the early stage of PD when the symptoms are noticed but not troublesome, symptomatic treatment with levodopa or other drugs is not necessary. All symptomatic drugs can induce side effects, and if a patient is not

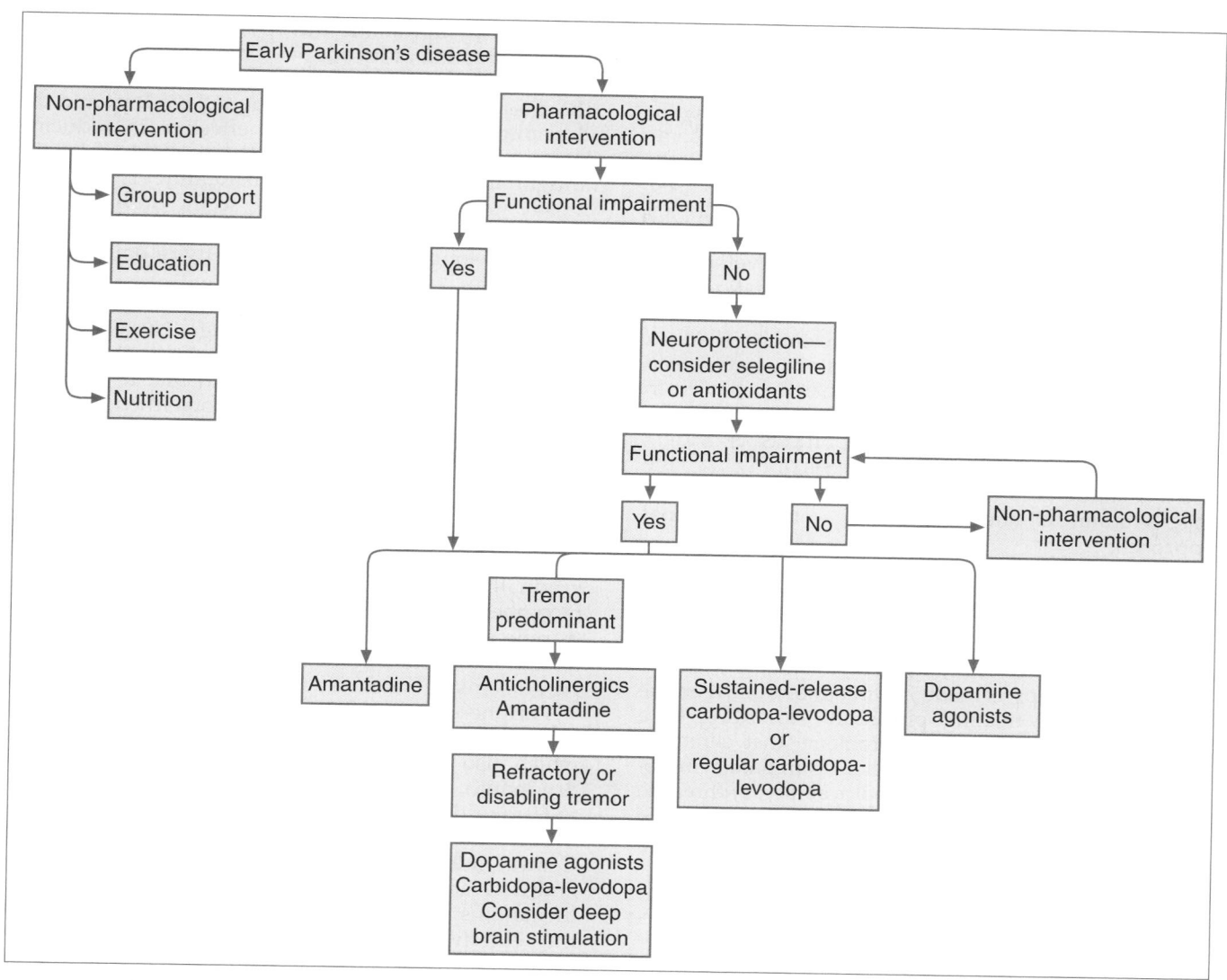

Figure 231.1   Algorithm for treating early or mild Parkinson's disease.

troubled by mild symptoms socially or occupationally, the introduction of these drugs can be delayed until symptoms become more pronounced. The clinician needs to discuss this choice with the patient, each will have to make a decision. Most neurologists do not use levodopa or other potent antiparkinson agents when the diagnosis is first established and the disease presents with no threat to physical, social, or occupational activities.[91–93] An algorithm for the treatment of mild PD is provided in Figure 231.1.

Because symptomatically beneficial medications are not needed, patients in the early, recently diagnosed stage of PD are excellent candidates for participating in a clinical trial in which a placebo is one of the treatment arms. Another elective option is to use an MAOI or a dopamine agonist in the hope that they might have some neuroprotective effect, without proof, while providing mild symptomatic effect and delaying the introduction of levodopa needs to be discussed. The dopamine agonists have been shown to

have some antioxidant properties *in vitro* and in some animal models.[94–100]

As discussed above, selegiline is a relatively selective inhibitor of the enzyme MAO-B. Unlike MAO-A inhibitors, which can induce a hypertensive crisis if the patient ingests tyramine-containing foods (the "cheese effect"), selegiline is free of this risk if the dose is not increased beyond 10 mg per day. Selegiline has a mild symptomatic benefit (about 10%)[101] and is metabolized to methamphetamine and amphetamine. When given early in the course of the disease, selegiline can extend the duration of the need of levodopa by an average of 9 months. There is controversy whether selegiline has some neuroprotective action in addition to its mild symptomatic one, and some physicians will use this drug in this early phase although long-term follow-up indicates that discontinuing selegiline will bring back the same degree of parkinsonian symptoms as in a control group of non-treated patients.[46] The dose of selegiline should not exceed 5 mg twice daily because its specificity as a selective type B inhibitor of MAO is lost, and it will also inhibit MAO-A at higher doses. Because of its long half-life many physicians believe that a much smaller dose could be equally effective, although this has not been tested. If insomnia develops, 5 mg in the morning (avoiding later doses) can usually correct this. When selegiline is used in the presence of levodopa, it potentiates levodopa's effect and lower doses of levodopa can usually be achieved. Selegiline does not prevent the development of levodopa-induced complications of fluctuations and dyskinesias.[47] Selegiline decreases the risk of patients developing freezing of gait.[102] Interestingly, MAO-A inhibitors, but not MAO-B inhibitors, have been shown to reduce stress-induced freezing behavior in rats.[103]

Because the oxidant stress hypothesis is widely held as a likely one in the pathogenesis of PD,[104–117] the use of a combination of antioxidants, including selegiline, vitamin C and vitamin E seems a rational approach.

Treatment of mild to moderate PD

When PD becomes more severe the signs and symptoms of the illness begin to interfere with daily activities and quality of life. The judgment to initiate symptomatic drug therapy is made in discussions between the patient and the treating physician. According to a survey,[101] the most common problems that clinicians consider important for the decision to initiate symptomatic agents are: 1) threat to employability; 2) threat to ability to handle domestic, financial, or social affairs; 3) threat to handling activities of daily living; and 4) appreciable worsening of gait or balance.

The choice of drugs is wide, and there is no single treatment algorithm that has been shown to be superior to any other. The concept of a "dopa-sparing" strategy means that levodopa, the most potent antiparkinsonian agent, is used as the drug of last resort, after trials of agonists and other agents. Studies have shown that such an approach will delay the development of levodopa-induced motor fluctuations and dyskinesias, but patients on dopamine agonists experience less relief of parkinsonism than those on levodopa. A reasonable approach is to consider the patient's age, life demands and need for suppression of parkinsonism. If the symptoms are not severe enough to require levodopa and the patient is younger than 60, a dopa-sparing strategy seems appropriate. Younger patients (less than 60 years of age) are particularly prone to developing the motor complications of fluctuations and dyskinesias.[32–35] For patients older than 70 or those with cognitive decline, levodopa is the preferred first-line therapy. Not only is there less need for a dopa-sparing strategy in these elderly patients, but they are also more susceptible to confusion, psychosis, or drowsiness from other antiparkinson drugs, including dopamine agonists. Levodopa provides the greatest benefit for the lowest risk of these adverse effects. A list of medications for PD is provided in Tables 231.7 and 231.8.

Amantadine can be useful, not only in the early phases of symptomatic therapy, thereby forestalling the introduction of levodopa or reducing the required dosage of levodopa, but also in the advanced stage of the disease as an adjunctive drug to levodopa and the dopamine agonists. It is also effective in reducing levodopa-induced dyskinesias,[73,74] probably from its antiglutamatergic activity. Amantadine is excreted mostly unchanged in the urine, so the dose needs to be reduced in patients with renal impairment. The half-life is long, about 28 hours, so twice daily dosing is adequate.

The anticholinergics are less effective antiparkinson agents than the dopamine agonists. The anticholinergics are estimated to improve parkinsonism by about 20%. Many clinicians find that if tremor is not relieved by an agonist or levodopa, then the addition of an anticholinergic drug is often effective. Commonly used anticholinergics are trihexyphenidyl (Artane) and benztropine mesylate (Cogentin); but there are many others. To minimize adverse effects, start with low doses (trihexyphenidyl 1 mg twice daily; benztropine 0.5 mg twice daily) and increase gradually to 2 mg three times daily for trihexyphenidyl and 1 mg three times daily for benztropine. As would be expected, if anticholinergics lessen parkinsonism, cholinergic agents aggravate parkinsonism,[118] including nicotine.[119]

Peripheral anticholinergic adverse effects include blurred vision (treated with pilocarpine eye drops, which also must be utilized if glaucoma is present), dry mouth, and urinary retention. Pyridostigmine, up to 60 mg tid if necessary, can sometimes be helpful in overcoming dry mouth and urinary difficulties. Central side effects are predominantly forgetfulness and decreased short-term memory. Occasionally hallucinations and psychosis can occur, particularly in the elderly. Powerful anticholinergics should be avoided in patients older than 70 years of age. If tremor persists in this age range despite the presence of levodopa or dopamine agonists, utilize drugs with a weaker anticholinergic effect, such as diphenhydramine (Benadryl), orphenadrine (Norflex), cyclobenzaprine (Flexeril) and amitriptyline (Elavil). Diphenhydramine and amitriptyline can cause drowsiness; therefore they can also be used as a hypnotic. For tremor control, the dose should be increased gradually until at least 50 mg 3 times daily is reached for diphenhydramine and orphenadrine; 20 mg 3 times daily for cylclobenzaprine; and 25 mg 3 times daily for amitriptyline.

When using dopamine agonists, it is best to start with a tiny dose (bromocriptine 1.25 mg before bed; pergolide 0.05 mg hs; pramipexole 0.125 mg before bed; ropinirole 0.25 mg-hs) for the first 3 days, and then switch from bedtime to daytime dosing for the remainder of the first week. Ropinirole can be started at 0.25 mg tid for the first week. The daily dose can be increased gradually (bromocriptine 1.25 mg per day every week; pergolide 0.125 mg per day weekly; pramipexole 0.125 mg q 2 days for 10 days, then 0.125 mg per day weekly; ropinirole 0.5 mg per day twice weekly), building the dosage up on a four times

Table 231.7 Symptomatic agents for Parkinson's disease

Agent	Tablet size	Dosing	Actions	Indications	Adverse effects
Amantadine (Symmetrel)	100 mg Syrup—50 mg/5 ml	100 mg tid to qid	Dopamine agonist Anticholinergic-like NMDA inhibitor	Monotherapy in early or mild PD; More effective for tremor than bradykinesia or rigidity; Adjuvant agent for use with dopamine agonists or levodopa; anti-dyskinesia agent	Dry mouth, urinary retention constipation, confusion, hallucinations, depression, ankle edema, livedo reticularis, insomnia or somnolence
Bromocriptine (Parlodel)	2.5 mg, 5 mg	2.5 mg tid to 10 mg qid	Ergot alkaloid derivative that is D2 agonist and weak D1 antagonist	Monotherapy in early PD, or adjuvant therapy in advanced PD Also effective in prolactinoma and hyperprolactinemia	Headache, nausea, anorexia, dyspepsia, dizziness, orthostatic hypotension, ankle edema, mottled skin rash, nasal congestion, somnolence, dyskinesias, vivid dreams and hallucinations, behavioral changes, confusion, fatigue
Pergolide (Permax)	0.05 mg, 0.25 mg, 1.0 mg	Up to 6 mg/d	Ergot alkaloid derivative that is potent D2 agonist and weak D1 agonist	Monotherapy in early PD, or adjuvant therapy in advanced PD	Headache, nausea, dyspepsia, ankle edema, dizziness, orthostatic hypotension, somnolence, dyskinesias, vivid dreams and hallucinations, behavioral changes, confusion, fatigue
Pramipexole (Mirapex)	0.125 mg, 0.25 mg, 0.5 mg, 1.0 mg, and 1.5 mg	Up to 1.5 mg tid	Non-ergoline dopamine agonist; Binding affinity for D3, D2, and D4 receptor family	Monotherapy in early PD, or adjuvant therapy in advanced PD	Nausea, dizziness, orthostatic hypotension, somnolence, dyskinesias, vivid dreams and hallucinations, behavioral changes, confusion, fatigue
Ropinirole (Requip)	0.25 mg, 0.5 mg 1.0 mg, 2.0 mg 5.0 mg	1 mg tid to 5 mg 5 times a day	Non-ergoline dopamine agonist; Binding affinity for D3, D2, and D4 receptor family	Monotherapy in early PD, or adjuvant therapy in advanced PD	Nausea, dizziness, orthostatic hypotension, somnolence, dyskinesias, vivid dreams and hallucinations, behavioral changes, confusion, fatigue
Levodopa (Larodopa) Carbidopa/ levodopa (Sinemet) (Sinemet CR)	Levodopa—100 mg, 250 mg, 500 mg Carbidopa/Levodopa 10/100 mg, 25/100 mg, 25/250 mg Controlled release carbidopa/ levodopa 25/100 mg, 50/200 mg	300 to 1500 mg/d of levodopa component	L-dopa is the precursor of dopamine: In presence of peripheral gut dopa decarboxylase taken into the bloodstream, crosses the blood–brain barrier, and is centrally decarboxylated to dopamine	Symptomatic treatment of PD Drug is regarded as the most potent agent for most cardinal and secondary symptoms of PD: tremor, bradykinesia, rigidity, gait freezing, inhibitor, L-dopa is effective postural instability or cognitive for deterioration	Nausea, anorexia, vomiting, confusion, drowsiness, hallucinations, psychosis, behavioral changes, postural hypotension, dyskinesias hypomimia, and micrographia; not

Table 231.8   Adjuvant agents for Parkinson's disease

Agent	Tablet size	Dosing	Actions	Indications	Adverse effects
Selegiline (Eldepryl) (Deprenyl)	5 mg	5 mg bid	Selective irreversible inhibitor of monoamine oxidase B (MAOB)	Role is not defined but agent is used as a mild antioxidant to delay progression of mild PD and need for other symptomatic treatment; mild symptomatic effect	Insomnia, nightmares, and exacerbation of all potential dopaminergic adverse effects (see Table 231.7)
Domperidone (Motilium)	10 mg	10 mg tid 20 mg qid	Peripheral dopamine receptor antagonist with no central DA blockade	Levodopa-induced nausea in Parkinson's disease	Galactorrhea, gynecomastia, dry mouth, headaches, abdominal cramping
Entacapone (Comtan)	200 mg	1 tablet taken up to 8 times a day	Highly selective reversible peripherally-acting COMT inhibitor in gut, rbc and liver	Wearing-off motor fluctuations in PD: prevents metabolism of levodopa, allowing it to act longer	Diarrhea, nausea, urine discoloration, prolongation and increase in all levodopa-induced adverse effects, including dyskinesias
Tolcapone (Tasmar)	100 mg, 200 mg	100 mg tid to 200 mg tid	Selective, reversible peripherally and centrally acting COMT inhibitor	Wearing-off motor fluctuations in PD: prevents metabolism of levodopa, allowing it to act longer	Diarrhea, nausea, urine discoloration, prolongation, and increase in all levodopa-induced adverse effects, including dyskinesias. Linked to rare cases of hepatic failure; use of tolcapone requires chronic monitoring of liver transaminases
Apomorphine	Injectable solution, available in ampules to fill pre-calibrated syringe	Usually 1 mg to 5 mg sc	Potent direct-acting dopamine agonist with affinity for D1 and D2 receptors	Unpredictable wearing off motor fluctuations in PD: gives fast-acting dopaminergic stimulation, enabling patient quick onset during a wearing off episode	Nausea, vomiting (requires pre-treatment with domperidone), sedation, confusion, hallucinations, hypotension, dyskinesias

a day dosing schedule until benefit or a dose around 40 mg/day (bromocriptine), 4–6 mg/day (pergolide and pramipexole), or 24 mg/day (ropinirole) is reached. Use the lowest dose that provides adequate benefit.

If levodopa is used in the mild stage disease, there is evidence to suggest keeping the dose as low as possible.[120,121] One strategy is to build the dosage to carbidopa/levodopa 25/100 to 50/200 mg tid and then add a dopamine agonist if the patient needs more symptomatic relief. If a patient's disability is beyond the scope of efficacy of dopamine agonists, amantadine, anticholinergics and selegiline, treatment with levodopa becomes necessary to control symptoms.

Levodopa is usually given combined with a peripheral decarboxylase inhibitor (carbidopa (Sinemet and generics) or benserazide (Madopar) to prevent the formation of dopamine peripherally, thereby usually avoiding the otherwise common peripheral adverse effects of anorexia, nausea and vomiting. Many patients require at least 50–75 mg of carbidopa a day for adequate inhibition of peripheral dopa decarboxylase. If the dose of levodopa is less than 300 mg per day, then the 25/100 mg strength tablets should be used and not the 10/100 mg tablets. In some patients even 75 mg per day of carbidopa is inadequate, and nausea, anorexia or vomiting still occur. In such patients, higher doses of carbidopa are required; carbidopa tablets (Lodosyn) can be obtained by special request from Sinemet's distributor (DuPont Pharma).

Carbidopa/levodopa is marketed in both standard release (Sinemet and generics) and sustained-release (Sinemet CR) tablets, the latter of which provides a longer plasma half-life and lower peak plasma levels of levodopa than standard Sinemet. Unfortunately, Sinemet CR has not been shown to prevent the development of response fluctuations. A 5-year study in 618 dopa-naive patients compared Sinemet CR and standard Sinemet therapy, and there was no difference between the two groups in the development of either fluctuations or dyskinesias.[122,123] An Italian study found that using small, divided doses during the day is more likely to lead to loss of the long duration response.[124]

A pre-bedtime dose of Sinemet CR may allow the patient some mobility during the night. Disadvantages of Sinemet CR are the lack of a rapid response with each dose and a delayed response that can be excessive, resulting in sustained severe dyskinesias that cannot be controlled except by sedating the patient. Moreover, the response to individual doses of Sinemet CR is less predictable than standard Sinemet. It is complicated to use both standard Sinemet and Sinemet CR to smooth out fluctuations, but this is often necessary. Finally, it should be remembered that not all of the carbidopa/levodopa in Sinemet CR is absorbed because some of the medication may have reached the large intestine before all of it was absorbed in the small intestine. A dose of Sinemet CR is equal to about two-thirds to three-quarters of an identical dose of standard Sinemet.

On the other hand, Sinemet CR is useful as a first-line drug in patients older than age 70 to slow the rate of absorption and lower the peak plasma level of levodopa, making it less likely for the patient to develop peak dose drowsiness or confusion. For younger patients, in whom cognitive adverse effects are less likely to occur, standard carbidopa/levodopa is preferred in order to observe the response and better monitor the effectiveness of the drug.

Sinemet CR is available in two strengths, a carbidopa/levodopa 50/200 mg tablet that is scored and can be broken in half, and a 25/100 mg unscored tablet. Crushing either tablet loses the slow-release property because the matrix is no longer intact. When Sinemet CR is added to a patient taking a dopamine agonist, a dose of 25/100 mg 3 times daily (built up gradually by 25/100 mg weekly) often suffices. When used alone, it often is necessary to use these dosages after meals to reduce initial nausea and vomiting; the dose can later be increased to 50/200 mg 3 or 4 times daily. If greater relief is required, a dopamine agonist should then be added.

Standard carbidopa/levodopa is available in 10/100, 25/100, and 25/250 mg tablets. Because of the desire to have at least 75 mg per day of carbidopa, the 25/100 mg tablets should be used when the drug is introduced. An increase of 25/100 mg per day per week until 3 times daily dosing is achieved is often

adequate. Not every symptom of PD responds equally well. Bradykinesia and rigidity respond best, while tremor can be more resistant. If a response is seen, but with symptoms later returning or worsening, increasing to 50/200 mg 3 times daily is a reasonable goal before adding a dopamine agonist. If agonists are already being taken and there is still an inadequate response, the dosage of levodopa should be increased gradually, switching to the 25/250 mg tablets as necessary. A dose of 25/250 mg 4 times daily may be required. A reasonably high dose before concluding that levodopa is ineffective is 2000 mg of levodopa per day.

A patient's response or lack of response to levodopa is a very important piece of information to help differentiate PD from Parkinsonism-plus syndromes. If the response to a large daily dose of levodopa (in the order of 2000 mg) is negligible, it is most likely that the disorder is not PD.[125] However, an adequate response does not insure the diagnosis of PD. All cases of presynaptic disorders (e.g., reserpine-induced, MPTP-induced, post-encephalitic parkinsonism) will respond to levodopa. Also, patients in the early stages of multiple system atrophy and progressive supranuclear palsy may improve with levodopa; later in these diseases, when dopamine receptors are lost, the response is lost. Some patients with Shy–Drager syndrome and olivopontocerebellar atrophy may continue to have intact dopamine receptors in the striatum and continue to respond to levodopa. The only effective drugs in situations where levodopa is not effective are the anticholinergics and amantadine, even though only mildly so.

As PD progresses, the duration of effect of a dose of levodopa becomes shorter.[126] The effective half-life of a dose of levodopa declines in relation to both worsening of symptoms and duration of disease. The half-life declines from a mean of 262 min in Stage I patients, to 142 min in Stage II, to 54 min in Stage III. The rate of decline becomes smaller as the disease progresses. The mean annual reduction of the effective half-life slows down as the disease worsens, dropping by 37 minutes/year in Stage I patients and by 6.5 minutes/year in Stage III, and is about 17% per year of the disease.

It is important to avoid sudden withdrawal of levodopa; a "neuroleptic" malignant syndrome can ensue, with fever, rigidity, and incoherence.[127,128] Tapering levodopa over 3 days appears to be safe.

Treatment of advanced PD

Advanced Parkinson's disease (PD) is that stage of the disease when there is at least one of the following conditions: 1) sufficient disability to interfere with independence despite levodopa therapy; 2) sufficient loss of postural reflexes so that the patient must be cautious when walking; 3) the presence of the freezing phenomenon to make walking difficult; 4) pronounced postural deformity; or 5) when complications of medical treatment (fluctuations, dyskinesias, psychosis) from levodopa have developed. Reducing the complications of medical

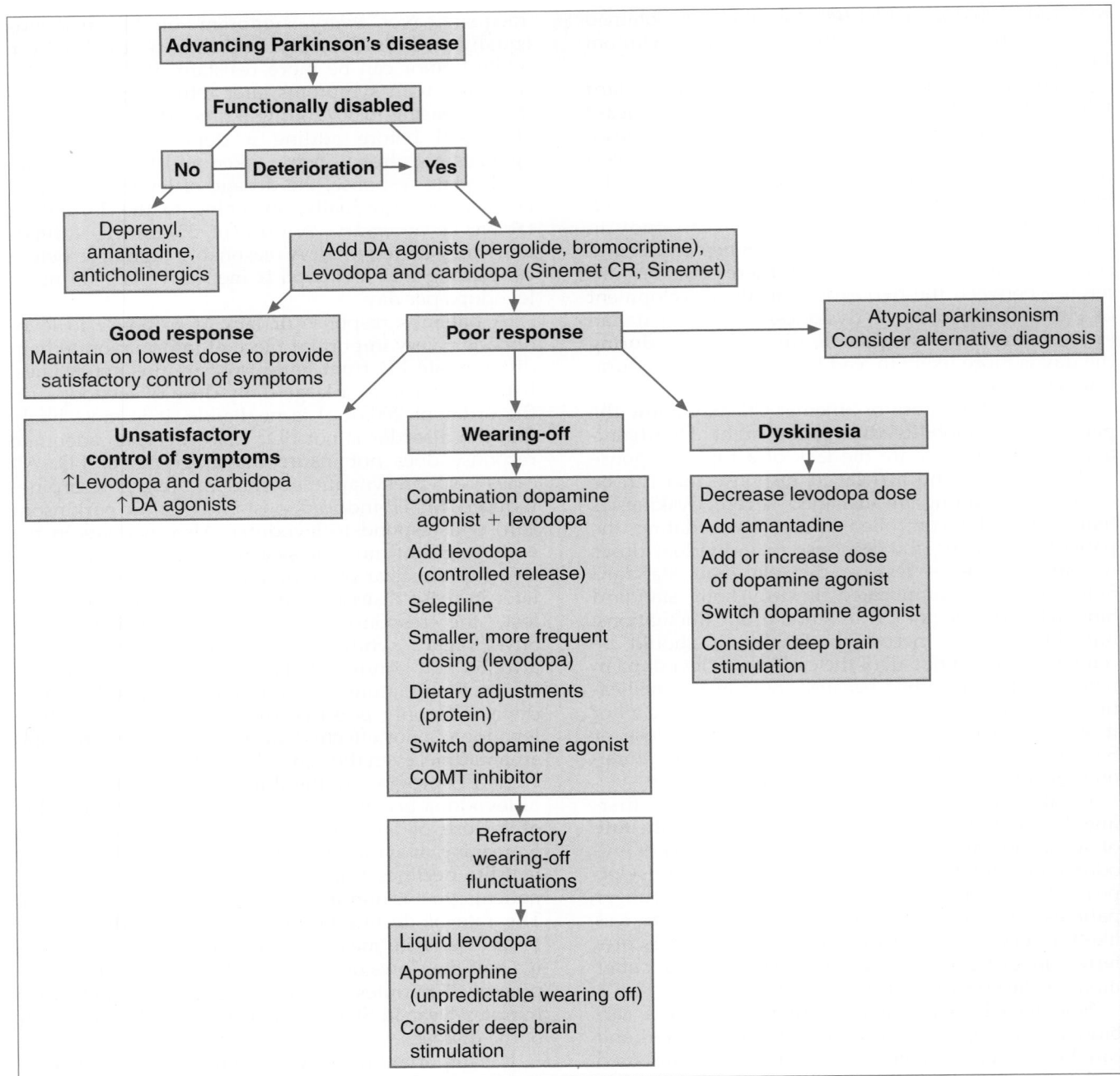

Figure 231.2   Algorithm for treating advanced Parkinson's disease.

treatment can become a central goal of therapy for advanced PD. In advanced PD, because of the severity of the clinical situation, all patients should be receiving levodopa therapy or at least have had a trial of this drug even if not able to remain on it because of disabling adverse effects. An algorithm for the treatment of advanced PD is provided in Figure 231.2.

Motor complications   The motor complications can be divided into two categories, fluctuations ("off" states) and dyskinesias. These are subdivided by their

temporal relationship with each dose of levodopa, and the associated clinical motor and sensory phenomena (Table 231.8). The "off" state usually consists of a return of parkinsonian symptoms and signs, such as bradykinesia, tremor, rigidity, immobility and freezing (so-called "off freezing"). There are also other features of "off" states in many patients. "Off dystonia" is the presence of sustained contractions and spasms, often painful, and most common early in the morning on arising and involving the feet. So-called "sensory offs" or equivalently "behavioral offs"

Table 231.9 Dopaminergic complications and treatment

Complications of dopaminergic agents	Intervention
Predictable end-of-dose wearing-off	Shorten dosing interval Using long-acting levodopa Add selegiline or dopamine agonist Add COMT inhibitor
Sudden or unpredictable wearing-off	Add agonist Administer doses of liquid levodopa Apomorphine
Delayed therapeutic response following each dose of levodopa	Use larger dose Take levodopa on empty stomach Liquid levodopa Avoid long-acting levodopa preparation
Poor therapeutic response following each dose of levodopa	Increase levodopa dose Use regular levodopa preparation Use liquid levodopa Add dopamine agonist Avoid large protein intake
Dyskinesias	Decrease levodopa dose Take small individual doses of levodopa more frequently Use liquid levodopa frequently administered Add dopamine agonist Consider stereotactic neurosurgery

COMT, catechol-O-methyltransferase.

are the sensory and behavioral phenomena that may accompany motor (parkinsonian) "off" states, or may be present as an "off" in the absence of severe parkinsonian signs. Sensory "offs" consist of pain, akathisia, depression, anxiety, dysphoria, or panic, and usually a mixture of more than one of these. Sensory "offs," like dystonic "offs," are extremely poorly tolerated. It is often the presence of these sensory and behavioral phenomena—more so than parkinsonian or dystonic "offs"—that drives patients to take more and more levodopa, turning them into "levodopa addicts." Table 231.9 provides a list of dopaminergic complications and their treatment.

Response fluctuations usually begin as mild wearing off (end-of-dose failure). Wearing off can be determined when an adequate dosage of levodopa does not last 4 hours. Typically, in the first couple of years of treatment, there is a long-duration response.[129] As the disease progresses or as levodopa treatment continues, the long-duration response fades and the short-duration response becomes predominant, leading to the wearing-off effect. The "offs" tend to be mild at first, but over time often become deeper with more severe parkinsonism; simultaneously, the duration of the "on" response becomes shorter. Eventually, many patients develop sudden "offs" in which the deep state of parkinsonism develops over minutes rather than tens of minutes. Sudden "offs" are less predictable in terms of timing with the dosings of levodopa. Many patients who develop response fluctuations also develop abnormal involuntary movements, i.e. dyskinesias.

Levodopa-induced dyskinesias appear to be related to the degree of dopamine receptor denervation supersensitivity. It is difficult to induce dyskinesias in normal animals or people, but with a high-enough dose this has been achieved in monkeys.[130] With increasing denervation, resulting in increased receptor sensitivity, there is more likelihood of developing choreic dyskinesias at a lower dose of levodopa.[131] Dystonic reactions (forceful sustained contractions) may evolve over time in patients who earlier had choreic dyskinesias. However, some patients develop peak-dose dystonia at relatively low dosages; these may be patients with multiple system atrophy.[36] The major risk factor for peak-dose dyskinesia appears to be severity of the disease.[131]

Chase[132] and Metman et al.[133] summarized their views on the mechanisms leading to the development of fluctuations from levodopa therapy. They believe that the fluctuations are related to altered dopaminergic mechanisms at both the presynaptic and postsynaptic levels. Wearing-off phenomena initially reflect the loss of dopamine storage capacity of the degenerating nigrostriatal system. Then, with increasing degeneration of the nigrostriatal system, swings in plasma levodopa concentrations associated with standard dosage regimens produce non-physiological fluctuations in intrasynaptic dopamine. As a result of long-term discontinuous stimulation, secondary changes occur at sites downstream from the dopamine system and appear to underlie the progressive worsening of wearing-off phenomena as well as the eventual appearance of other response complications.

Chronic intermittent stimulation of normally tonically active dopaminergic receptors activates specific signaling cascades in striatal dopaminoceptive medium spiny neurons. This evidently results in long-term potentiation of the synaptic efficacy of glutamate receptors of the N-methyl-D-aspartate (NMDA) subtype on these GABAergic efferents, due to increased phosphorylation of the serine and tyrosine moieties in these receptors. As a consequence of their increasing sensitivity to excitation by cortical glutamatergic projections, it would appear that medium spiny neuron function changes to favor the appearance of response fluctuations of the "on–off" type and peak-dose dyskinesias. The inability of standard levodopa treatment to restore striatal dopaminergic function in a more physiological manner clearly contributes to the appearance of motor complications. Continuous dopaminergic replacement not only reverses these complications in parkinsonian patients but also prevents their development in animal models of Parkinson's disease.

There are many choices available to control wearing off. When mild, it may be ameliorated with the addition of selegiline[70] (introduced as 2.5 mg daily, and increasing to 5 mg twice daily, as necessary). Selegiline potentiates the action of levodopa, but its introduction can induce confusion and psychosis (particularly in the elderly) and dyskinesias. A lower dose of levodopa may be necessary. Shortening the dose interval of carbidopa-levodopa may improve wearing-off fluctuations. Long acting carbidopa-levodopa ("controlled release" Sinemet CR) can also be effective in patients with mild wearing-off.[55,134,135] It is possible gradually to switch from standard carbidopa/levodopa to Sinemet CR, beginning with the last dose of the day and working forward each day. Because it takes over an hour for slow-release medication to become effective, most patients will also require supplemental standard carbidopa/levodopa to obtain an adequate response.

Direct-acting dopamine agonists, which have a longer biological half-life than levodopa, can also be used in combination with standard Sinemet or Sinemet CR.[136] As a general rule, dopamine agonists are useful to improve the severity of the "off" state, but can also reduce the amount of "off" time per day. Pergolide, pramipexole and ropinirole are more effective than bromocriptine and are preferred. These drugs in combination with levodopa can increase dyskinesias while reducing the severity of the "offs." In this situation the levodopa dosage needs to be reduced. Because of its long half-life, cabergoline can be effective even with once-a-day dosing.[137,138]

COMT inhibitors have an advantage because if effective, they are effective immediately. They increase the amount of "on" time by about an hour per day.[139–141] Entacapone has a shorter duration of action than tolcapone and its 200 mg tablet needs to be given simultaneously with carbidopa/levodopa, working with that dose only. Thus, if only one or two doses of levodopa result in wearing off, then entacapone can be given just with those doses. Enta-

capone does not require any precautions for assessing liver function, whereas tolcapone does. Tolcapone can produce fulminant hepatitis; this is rare, but it has caused death.[53,142] Therefore, patients should not be given tolcapone unless the wearing off is a great problem and other medications have failed to relieve the clinical fluctuations. Patients need a baseline liver transaminase profile, which should be followed biweekly. Discontinuing tolcapone if a rise in transaminase activity is seen should be sufficient to reverse the hepatic change. Patients should also be warned that diarrhea, including explosive diarrhea, could develop in 6–8 weeks on tolcapone. Entacapone causes less of a problem with diarrhea, but it turns the urine a yellow-orange. Tolcapone comes in 100 and 200 mg tablets, and patients should start with 100 mg once daily increasing fairly rapidly to thrice daily dosing. If not effective, they can switch to the 200 mg tablets.

Patients with a deep "off" may benefit from a rescue dose of anti-PD medication. Dissolving levodopa in carbonated water and drinking it usually provides a response in about 10–15 minutes. Subcutaneous or intranasal apomorphine injections provides a similar response.[143] Levodopa ethylester appears to provide an equally rapid response.[144]

The "sudden off" phenomenon is a more difficult problem to overcome. It is now clear that direct-acting dopamine agonists, slow release levodopa, amantadine, and selegiline are ineffective for this problem. Subcutaneous injection of the dopamine agonist, apomorphine, is effective in turning the patient back "on" quickly,[145] as is an oral administration of dissolved Sinemet. In order to block nausea and vomiting by apomorphine, the peripheral dopamine receptor antagonist, domperidone, also needs to be taken. Increasingly severe on-phase dyskinesias and postural instability mar the long-term therapeutic response of apomorphine in many patients.

Failure of the patient to respond to each dose of levodopa is sometimes related to poor gastric emptying.[146,147] A radionuclide gastric emptying study showed that PD patients had prolonged gastric emptying compared with the normal control subjects, and that this was increased in fluctuating patients with dose failures compared to non-fluctuators.[148] The problem of dose failures can be overcome by dissolving levodopa in liquid prior to ingesting it. For this situation, individual doses of Sinemet can be liquefied whenever needed. It dissolves readily in carbonated water because of the acidity of the water and the bubbles. When a dose failure occurs, the patient can take dissolved Sinemet and will usually respond in 10 to 15 minutes. Another approach is to use apomorphine injections[149] or levodopa ethyl ester injections.[148]

Melamed and Bitton[150] reported that patients with fluctuations often also have a problem in getting an "on" effect with the first dose in the morning. These patients tend to have a longer delay with this dose than non-fluctuators. The mechanism is not clear, but it may have to do with obtaining adequate plasma levels. Many patients need a larger dosage of levodopa as their first dose of the day in order to "kick in" a response to the medication. Since the first dose is often accompanied by a higher plasma level of levo-dopa than later doses,[151,152] the problem may not be entirely pharmacokinetic; rather, it is possible that the dopamine receptors are in a low-affinity state and require more dopamine agonism to activate them. To treat the delayed "on" by obtaining a higher plasma level of levodopa sooner, the patient should dissolve Sinemet before swallowing.

Ingested protein may interfere with levodopa absorption. In some patients, competition with other amino acids in the diet can interfere with transport of levodopa across the intestinal mucosa and across the blood–brain barrier.[153,154] Only rarely does this competition with other amino acids pose a serious difficulty for patients. This problem can be helped by having non-protein meals at breakfast and lunch, and a higher protein intake at dinner.

The freezing phenomenon[155] is often listed as a type of fluctuation because the patient transiently has difficulty initiating movement. However, this phenomenon probably should be considered distinct and separate from the other types of fluctuations. Freezing takes many forms, and these have different names, such as start hesitation, target hesitation, turning hesitation, startle (fearfulness) hesitation, and sudden transient freezing. It is not clear if any of these types has a different pathophysiological mechanism. Of major importance is the need to distinguish between "off freezing" and "on freezing." "Off freezing" is best explained as a feature of PD, and its treatment is to keep the patient from going "off." "On freezing" remains an enigma, and this problem tends to be aggravated by increasing the dosage of levodopa. It is not benefited by adding direct-acting dopamine agonists; rather, it is lessened by reducing the dosage of levodopa. Both the "on" and "off" types of freezing appear to correlate with duration of illness and duration of levodopa therapy.[156] Although Narabayashi et al.[157] reported benefit with L-threo-dops, supposedly a precursor of brain norepinephrine, the current authors have not seen any benefit with this drug in the treatment of "on freezing," nor any evidence that this drug increases norepinephrine in rat brain or human cerebrospinal fluid.

Treatment of dyskinesias associated with levodopa therapy Peak-dose dyskinesias are due to too much dopaminergic stimulation. Reducing the individual dose of levodopa can resolve this problem. Another method to reduce peak-dose dyskinesia is to substitute higher doses of a dopamine agonist while lowering the dose of levodopa. Dopamine agonists are less likely to cause dyskinesias, and therefore can usually be used in this situation quite safely. If lowering the dose of Sinemet results in more severe "off" states, then the agonists become more important. Sinemet CR can help some patients by keeping the peak plasma levels of levodopa at a lower level. However, there is also the danger of increased dyskinesias at the end of the day as the blood levels become sustained from frequent

dosing. Once dyskinesias appear with Sinemet CR, they last for a considerable duration of time because of the slow decay in the plasma drug level.

Amantadine has been found to be a useful antidyskinetic agent,[73,74,158–160] aside from its dopaminergic effect. Its antidyskinetic effect is dose dependent, and patients often require 400 mg/day.

Another approach is to use clozapine, the atypical neuroleptic that does not aggravate parkinsonism. Clozapine can suppress dopa-induced dyskinesias, while simultaneously increasing "on" time without dyskinesias.[161–164] Adverse effects consist of sedation, sialorrhea, and orthostatic hypotension.

Increasing serotonin activity in the substantia nigra could induce or worsen parkinsonism, as is sometimes seen with fluoxetine treatment. A trial of fluoxetine, a selective serotonin uptake inhibitor, was shown to reduce dyskinesias induced by apomorphine treatment,[165] suggesting that it be considered in levodopa-induced dyskinesias. Propranolol is another drug reported to reduce dyskinesias.[166] Buspirone appears to be somewhat effective in reducing the severity of dyskinesias,[167] but because buspirone has resulted in aggravating tardive dyskinesia,[168] it may have some dopamine receptor blocking activity.

Dystonic spasms are not always a sign of levodopa overdosage. This is particularly true in many instances of painful sustained contractions. Painful dystonic cramps most often occur when the plasma level of levodopa is low, particularly in the early morning.[169] A survey of 383 patients with PD revealed that 16% had experienced early morning dystonia.[170] However, this type of dystonia can occur at any time the patient goes "off."[171] Early morning dystonia is a form of "off" dystonia, albeit the most common form. In this sense, "off" dystonia is a pharmacokinetic problem, and it has been correlated with low plasma levels of levodopa after an intravenous infusion was discontinued.[172] Preventing "offs" is the best way to control "off" dystonia. If patients with "off" dystonia are given a drug holiday from levodopa, after a few days the painful dystonia will disappear and the patient will be left with a baseline parkinsonian state, and without painful dystonia (unpublished observations).

Combination of fluctuations and dyskinesias Many patients with advanced PD have both clinical fluctuations ("wearing off" or "on–off") and dyskinesias (usually peak-dose and sometimes end-of-dose). Most patients are more troubled by the "off" states, when they are fully or partially immobile, than they are from dyskinesias. In other words, they prefer having the dyskinesias rather than being unable to move freely. As a result of their discomfort with the "off" states, patients tend to overdose themselves, resulting in alternating "offs" and dyskinesias. In the extreme form of this situation, patients experience only "off" states or generalized dyskinesias, but have no normal motor function during the day.

A cumbersome but sometimes effective approach to the combination of "wearing off" and dyskinesias is liquefied Sinemet, taken in small doses throughout the day.[173] A simple method of preparation is to dissolve 10 tablets of 25/100 mg strength tablets in a liter of acidified solution (dietetic soda, seltzer or other carbonated water, or ascorbic acid solution) with vitamin C 1000 mg. The ascorbate is required to stabilize the solution, which should be refrigerated and kept in a dark environment to prevent oxidation of levodopa. Liquefied Sinemet has been found to improve the amount of "on" time[174–176] and can also reduce dyskinesias. A more heroic approach is to administer an infusion of levodopa via an intraduodenal pump[177–181] or subcutaneous infusions of apomorphine.[182]

The treatment considerations described above may be helpful, but often pharmacological interventions prove ineffective. Reducing the medication helps the dyskinesias but produces intolerable parkinsonism, whereas treatment of the parkinsonism exacerbates the dyskinesias. In this setting, a neurosurgical treatment such as bilateral deep brain stimulation of the subthalamic nuclei or globus pallidus should be considered.

Falling Falling is a common feature of Parkinson's disease as the illness progresses and there is increasing loss of postural reflexes. Since this particular cardinal sign of Parkinson's disease is little benefited by levodopa therapy,[183] the risk of falling persists and worsens despite pharmacotherapy.[184] Because levodopa may allow patients to be more mobile, such as allowing them to rise more easily from a chair and walk independently, the persistence of postural instability increases the likelihood of falling. Thus, this complication of levodopa therapy in this particular subpopulation of patients with PD is technically not a true adverse effect of the medication, but a complication of the improvement in mobility in a patient at risk for falling. In this situation the patient should use physical assistance, such as a walker. An alternative approach is to keep the patient sufficiently parkinsonian so mobility-associated falling is limited.

Intractable tremor Persistent tremor, i.e. rest tremor that has been resistant to antiparkinsonian medication, may sometimes respond to clozapine.[78,185] If unresponsive to any medications, deep brain stimulation of the thalamus or subthalamic nucleus should be considered.

Non-motor complications of Parkinson's disease

While the motor symptoms of Parkinson's disease dominate the clinical picture—and even define the parkinsonian syndrome—many patients with PD have other complaints. Sensory symptoms, including pain, may occur, as do symptoms of autonomic dysfunction including syncope. Problems with bladder and bowel control, and sexual dysfunction, are common. Changes in mood, slowness in thinking (bradyphrenia) and a declining cognitive capacity are frequent causes for concern. Helping patients with PD to cope with these difficulties is just as important as

Table 231.10   Sensory symptoms in Parkinson's disease
Pain
Paresthesiae
Numbness
Burning
Akathisia
Restless legs syndrome

manipulating therapy to provide control of their motor symptoms. In addition, antiparkinsonian drugs commonly induce unwanted non-motor effects and aggravate such complaints. So-called sensory "offs" are often under appreciated, but are usually a greater source of discomfort than motor "offs." Table 231.10 provides a list of sensory symptoms in PD.

Sensory symptoms Many text books do not list pain and the other sensory complaints in Table 231.10 as a part of PD. Unpleasant sensations are often not considered as a symptom of the disease, but this is not the case.[186–190] A constant, boring pain in the initially affected limb may be the first complaint of PD. Aching in the shoulder and arm is often attributed to bursitis or a frozen shoulder, or in the hip and leg to arthritis. That such pain is due to the PD is shown by its relief with antiparkinsonian medication. Once adequate dosing is achieved, whether or not mobility is restored, such pain commonly abates. Of course patients with PD may also have coincidental joint disease, so if the pain persists, they require appropriate investigation.

Another initial complaint, particularly in younger patients, may be painful dystonic foot cramps, especially on walking. Rarely, a similar painful cramp may occur in the hands. An extended big toe or curling of small toes may be seen with the cramping. When patients with PD develop fluctuations and dyskinesias, pain may become a major feature. "Off-period" dystonia often is painful, and may manifest as early morning painful cramps, particularly affecting the feet.[169] Similar painful dystonic cramps may emerge during "off" periods during the day, and can be very distressing.[171] Some patients may experience more generalized excruciating pain during "off" periods, often a deep-seated aching, but sometimes with a more superficial burning quality. Again, such pains disappear when the patient is switched "on" by appropriate medication to regain mobility. "Off-period" pain may be an indication for the use of rapidly-acting water-soluble preparations of levodopa or apomorphine rescue injections.

Other specific sensory symptoms, such as burning, numbness and paresthesia, are less common in PD. However, some patients may describe rather non-specific paresthesia in the affected limbs, but objective sensory signs are not evident.[186,187] A rare patient may have sensory complaints from levodopa therapy, unaccompanied by dystonia. Electroconvulsive therapy (ECT) can be effective in alleviating the problem. If parkinsonian pain occurs during an "off"

Table 231.11	Autonomic dysfunction in Parkinson's disease
Bladder problems
Sexual dysfunction
Hypotension
Gastrointestinal
Seborrhea
Sweating

or due to parkinsonism, medications should be increased to avoid "offs." (Sensory "offs" are considered later in this chapter.) If pain occurs during peak-dose dystonia, the dose should be lowered. If pain is secondary to levodopa or dopamine agonists, the causal agent must be reduced or eliminated. Occasionally the ergot dopamine agonists, bromocriptine and pergolide, cause a burning pain with inflammatory skin on parts of the body, known as St Anthony's fire. The agonist needs to be discontinued.

A more common sensory symptom is akathisia or a sense of inner restlessness. This is sometimes focused on the legs, with uncomfortable paresthesiae and the need to move them to gain relief, in which case it may be termed a true restless legs syndrome.[191] More often, there is a sense of generalized inner restless discomfort, demanding walking for relief, when akathisia is the more appropriate description.[192] Akathisia may be a presenting feature of PD. The symptoms of both restless legs and akathisia may respond to dopamine replacement therapy. Akathisia may also occur during the "off" period.[193]

Bladder and sexual problems The autonomic dysfunctions in patients with PD can be segregated into urogenital problems and those that affect other functions, such as blood pressure, the gastrointestinal tract and skin (Tables 231.11 and 231.12).

Urinary frequency and urgency, with nocturia, are common complaints in PD.[194] Of course PD patients are of an age when prostatic problems in the male and stress incontinence in the female commonly occur, but PD itself affects bladder control, due to detrusor hyperreflexia. As a result, premature uninhibited bladder contractions cause frequency and urgency, which can be particularly troublesome at night and during "off" periods. Araki and Kuno[195] assessed voiding dysfunction in 203 consecutive PD patients, and found that 27% had symptomatic voiding dysfunction. Its severity correlated with the severity of PD, and not with disease duration, age, or gender.

Prostatic outflow obstruction can add to the problem in the male. Incontinence not explained by immobility when taken by the urge to micturate, or by retention with overflow, is not, however, a part of PD. True neurogenic incontinence in someone with parkinsonism suggests a diagnosis of multiple system atrophy,[196] in which case, anal sphincter EMG studies may reveal signs of denervation due to involvement of Onuf's nucleus in the sacral spinal cord, which does not occur in PD.

The diagnosis of significant prostate enlargement in PD is difficult, and prostatectomy by the unwary often leads to disaster. Prostatectomy should only be considered in those with proven outflow obstruction. A simple screening test in patients with PD is non-invasive ultrasonic estimation of post-micturition residual volume, and simple mechanical measurement of urinary flow rate. If there is significant residual volume after urination ($>100 \, \text{mL}$) or if the flow rate is reduced there may be bladder outlet obstruction. Further investigation by more extensive urody-

Table 231.12	Management approach to autonomic and medical problems in Parkinson's disease	
Symptom	**Evaluation and management approach**	**Treatment agents**
Orthostatic hypotension	Restrict concurrent antihypertensive medications Encourage salt and fluid intake Antigravity support stockings	Fludrocortisone Midodrine
Urinary incontinence	Reduce fluid intake in the evenings Bladder training and voiding schedules Urological evaluation to exclude prostatic hypertrophy as a cause of urgency in men Urodynamic evaluation	Oxybutynin Propanetheline Hyoscyamine sulfate Nocturnal desmopressin intranasal spray
Constipation	Dietary modification—increase fiber content Increase physical activity Avoid anticholinergic medication	Stool softeners, bulk forming agents, laxatives Cisapride Enemas
Sexual dysfunction	Review medications Medical and urological evaluation for men with impotence	Psychological evaluation Erectile agents Treatment of depression

Dysphagia	Swallowing evaluation
	Soft or puréed diet
		Optimize antiparkinsonian medications and
		  plan to eat during periods of most
		  favorable treatment effect
		Feeding gastrostomy

namic studies and other urological testing is required. If there is no significant residual volume or reduction of flow rate, urinary frequency and urgency may be helped by a peripheral antimuscarinic drug such as oxybutynin (Ditropan), 5 to 10 mg at night or 5 mg tid. Fluid intake should be reduced at night. A tricyclic antidepressant with anticholinergic properties, such as amitriptyline, may help sleep not only through its sedative actions but also by reducing bladder irritability. Intranasal DDAVP (desmopressin) at night also may reduce nocturia.

Impotence in the male patient with PD causes distress to both partners. PD itself does not normally cause impotence, although this is a common early complaint in multiple system atrophy. Loss of libido and failure to gain or sustain erections may have some other cause in this age group, be it psychological, vascular, hormonal or neurogenic, and appropriate investigation is warranted. Some antidepressant drugs, monoamine oxidase inhibitors, and antihypertensive medications may impair sexual performance. Failure of erection can be overcome by a variety of intrapenile or oral medications such as sildenafil (Viagra).[197] Parkinsonian symptoms are not affected, but a side benefit of reduced dyskinesias has been reported.[198] Hypersexuality, particularly in the male, is a rare and unacceptable side-effect of dopamine replacement therapy in PD, and usually requires reduction of antiparkinsonian medication.

Other autonomic disturbances   Lewy body degeneration affects the autonomic nervous system in PD. Both sympathetic ganglion neurons and parasympathetic myenteric and cardiac plexi can be involved.[199–201] In addition, central autonomic nuclei, such as those of the hypothalamus and dorsal motor nucleus of the vagus, can show Lewy body degeneration.[202]

Control of blood pressure may be compromised by sympathetic failure with impaired vasoconstriction and inadequate intravascular volume. Faintness on standing (pre-syncope) and frank loss of consciousness on standing (postural syncope) can occur due to postural hypotension. Orthostatic hypotension may also cause posturally-induced fatigue and weakness, blurring of vision, and "coat-hanger" neck and shoulder aching. Hypotension also may occur postprandially due to gastrointestinal vasodilatation. Levodopa and dopamine agonist drugs may aggravate postural hypotension. Prominent early symptoms of postural hypotension are, of course, one of the hallmarks of multiple system atrophy (MSA), so such complaints may raise concern over the diagnosis of PD. The severity of postural hypotension in PD is rarely as severe as that seen in MSA. Nevertheless, treatment may be required. A selective peripheral dopamine antagonist such as domperidone sometimes helps, as does increasing fluid and salt intake, with head-up tilt at night, which reduces nocturnal polyuria. Intranasal DDAVP (desmopressin) (5–40 μg) at night also reduces nocturnal polyuria, but can cause hypona-

tremia. However, a small dose of fludrocortisone (0.1 to 0.5 mg) to promote salt retention, or midodrine (Pro-Amantine; a selective α-agonist) (2.5 to 5 mg tid), may be required to maintain adequate blood pressure.

Gastrointestinal problems cause significant disability in PD.[203,204] Dysphagia is mainly due to poor masticatory and oropharyngeal muscular control making it difficult to chew and propel the bolus of food into the pharynx and esophagus.[205,206] Soft food is easier to eat, and antiparkinsonian medication improves swallowing.

Parasympathetic failure may contribute to gastrointestinal problems in PD, causing delay in esophageal and gastric motility. A sense of bloating, indigestion and gastric reflux are common in PD.[204] Many factors contribute to delayed gastric emptying, including immobility, parasympathetic failure, constipation and antiparkinsonian drugs (both anticholinergic and dopamine agonists). Levodopa is absorbed in the upper small bowel, so gastric stasis may slow or prevent levodopa assimilation, leading to "delayed on" dose failures after single oral doses (either there is an excessive interval before the drug works, or it does not work at all).

Constipation is another frequent complaint in PD,[204,206] and is multifactorial. Again, immobility, drugs, reduced fluid and food intake, as well as parasympathetic involvement prolonging colonic transit time may all contribute. In addition, malfunction of the striated muscles of the pelvic floor due to the PD itself may make evacuation of the bowels difficult.[207,208] Constipation may exacerbate gastric stasis. Anticholinergic drugs should be stopped and physical exercise increased. The role of levodopa in causing or treating constipation is uncertain; this drug usually does not relieve the problem, and some patients believe it makes it worse. Constipation is helped by adequate fluid intake, fruit, vegetables, fiber and lactulose (10–20 g per day) or other mild laxatives. This "rancho recipe," provided by Dr Cheryl Waters, has been found useful for many patients: mix together one cup each of bran, applesauce and prune juice, take two tablespoons every morning, refrigerate for 1 week, then discard. Polyethylene glycol powder (marketed as MiraLax) can be effective to overcome constipation; the usual dose is 17 g/day dissolved in a glass of water at bedtime. Refractory constipation may be helped by apomorphine injections to assist defecation.[209,210]

For patients who have abdominal bloating due to suppression of peristalsis when they are "off," keeping them "on" with levodopa or other dopaminergics is beneficial.

Excessive sebum (seborrhea) is probably due more to facial immobility than to overproduction of oil. The greasy skin contributes to seborrheic dermatitis and dandruff. Medicated soaps and shampoos help. Blepharitis also is common, due in part to reduced blinking, and artificial teardrops may help.

Excessive sweating can be a problem, particularly in the form of sudden drenching sweats (sweating crises). Sage and Mark[211] showed that drenching sweats is usually an "off" phenomenon, and found treatment with dopamine agonists to be effective.

Excessive salivation is due more to failure to swallow than to over production.[212] Drooling of saliva can be helped by chewing gum or by peripherally-acting anticholinergic drugs. If these are unsuccessful, intraparotid injections of botulinum toxin A or B can sometimes be effective in reducing salivary secretions and drooling.[213]

Respiratory distress Respiratory distress such as dyspnea can occur as a symptom of PD in some patients, including during the "off" period.[214] In addition, it can also occur as a complication of dystonia, usually peak-dose dystonia[215] and with some dopamine agonists, particularly pergolide. Removing the offending drug is required. "Off" period dyspnea is difficult to treat, other than attempting to keep the patient "on." Despite the sensation of dyspnea, oxygen saturation is not affected because the patient will have a voluntary sigh or transient deep breathing when feeling short of breath. Some Parkinson-plus syndromes may have an accompanying apnea that is life-threatening, such as postencephalitic parkinsonism,[216,217] frontotemporal dementia,[218] multiple system atrophy,[219,220] Joseph disease (SCA-3),[221] and other familial parkinsonian syndromes.[222]

Sleep disturbances PD patients often have troubled nights for many reasons (Table 231.13).[223–226] The major problem is difficulty with sleep maintenance (sleep fragmentation). Frequent awakenings may be caused by tremor re-appearing in the lighter stages of sleep, difficulty turning in bed due to nocturnal akinesia as the effects of day time administration of dopaminergic drugs wear off at night, and nocturia. In addition, periodic leg movements in sleep (sometimes associated with restless legs), nocturnal myoclonus, sleep apnea, REM sleep behavioral disorders (intense dream-like motor and behavioral problems) and parasomnias (nocturnal hallucinations and nocturnal wandering with disruptive behavior) may all disrupt sleep in PD. Reversal of sleep rhythm with sundowning also is common in PD.[226] Many of these conditions probably occur more frequently in PD than in other aged populations, and as a result PD patients and their care-givers face disrupted nights, which lead to poor quality of life and worse parkinsonism the next day. In fact, along with depression, poor sleep is a major factor in a PD patient's assessment of having a poor quality of life.[227] A good night's sleep reduces the severity of daytime parkinsonism, and many patients comment on sleep benefit, describing better mobility the morning after a restful night. Indeed, patients with marked sleep benefit may not require antiparkinsonian medication for some hours after they awake, and some PD patients find that a day time nap "charges the batteries." These may be the young-onset PD patients with mutations in the parkin gene, for they typically show sleep benefit.[228]

The reasons for the various causes of disturbed

Table 231.13 Sleep problems in Parkinson's disease
Sleep fragmentation
REM sleep behavior disorder
Excessive daytime sleepiness
Altered sleep–wake cycle
Drug-induced sleep attacks

sleep are multiple. Nocturnal tremor, akinesia and nocturia are often due to the PD itself. Depression, which is common in PD, may cause insomnia, and drugs given to treat PD symptoms may interfere with sleep. PD pathology may also contribute to REM sleep behavioral disorders and parasomnias, especially in those with incipient or frank dementia. The animal model of REM sleep without atonia indicates that lesions to the perilocus ceruleus disrupt the excitatory connection to the nucleus reticularis magnocellularis in the descending medullary reticular formation, and disable the hyperpolarization of the alpha spinal motoneurons.[229]

The treatment of sleep disorders in PD is important. Attention to sleep hygiene by avoiding alcohol, caffeine and nicotine, and excessive fluid intake at night is helpful. Deprenyl (selegiline), which is metabolized to methamphetamine, should not be given at night. Treatment of depression may be required. A sedative antidepressant such as amitriptyline (10 to 25 mg at night) can be very useful, not only to induce and maintain sleep but also to reduce urinary frequency. A dose of a long-acting levodopa preparation last thing at night may improve nocturnal akinesia,[230,231] but levodopa given at night may provoke excessive dreaming and disrupted sleep in some patients.[232] A benzodiazepine, especially clonazepam, may lessen REM sleep behavior disorders. Propoxyphene is useful for periodic leg movements of sleep and restless legs.[233] A small bedtime dose of clozapine[85] or quetiapine may be very effective in improving sleep.

Excessive daytime sleepiness (EDS) occurs in about 15% of patients with PD, and is associated with more severe PD. In those with cognitive decline,[234] EDS is determined by short sleep latency and sleep-onset REM periods. EDS was found not to correlate with disease severity, total sleep time or sleep stage percentages, but rather to primary impairments of waking arousal and REM-sleep expression.[235]

Some patients who sleep a lot during the daytime may have a problem related to drowsiness following a dosage of levodopa. This phenomenon usually occurs in patients with developing or more pronounced dementia. With post-levodopa drowsiness, patients can sleep for much of the daytime, and are then up at night. This altered sleep–wake cycle makes life unbearable for the care-giver, who requires adequate sleep at night. If a patient becomes drowsy after each dose of medication, this may be a sign of overdosage. Reducing the dosage can correct this problem. Sometimes, substituting Sinemet CR for standard Sinemet may help, because this provides a slower rise in plasma and brain levels of levodopa.

For those with excessive daytime sleepiness, the antisoporific agent modafinil can sometimes be beneficial. If the patient's sleep problem has advanced to that of an altered sleep–wake cycle, it is important to get the patient onto a sleep–wake schedule that fits with the rest of the household. To correct the problem it may be necessary to use a combination of approaches. Efforts must be made to stimulate the patient physically and mentally during the daytime and force wakefulness otherwise there will be difficulty in sleeping at night. At night the patient should then be drowsy enough so that he or she can sleep. If this fails, it may be necessary to use stimulants in the morning and sedatives at night in order to reverse the altered state. This should be done in addition to keeping the patient awake during the day. Drugs such as methylphenidate and amphetamine are usually well tolerated by patients with Parkinson's disease, and a 10 mg dose of either of these two drugs, repeated once if necessary, may be helpful. To encourage sleep at night, a hypnotic may be necessary in addition to using daytime stimulants. It should be noted that strong sedatives, such as barbiturates, are poorly tolerated by patients with Parkinson's disease. Milder hypnotics, such as benzodiazepines, are usually taken without difficulty. Short-acting benzodiazepines are preferable, but if the patient awakens too early a longer-acting one may need to be used.

Falling asleep while driving and without warning is a serious problem that has been encountered with dopaminergic agents, and seems more likely to occur with pramipexole and ropinirole, although it is not limited to these drugs.[66–69] Once sleep attacks have occurred, the patient should not drive, except on short trips, or the medication should be changed. Fortunately, modafinil has been reported to be helpful in preventing sleep attacks.[236]

Fatigue Although fatigue can be a symptom of sleepiness or depression, it is also a symptom unassociated with these other states. In patients with PD, fatigue is often a complaint during the earliest phase of the disease, before motor symptoms (such as stiffness and slowness) become prominent. As these other features of PD develop, with their important contribution to disability, they became more of a complaint than fatigue. However, when specifically asked, patients commonly cite fatigue as an important problem. In a community study of elderly people in Norway, 44% of PD patients and 18% of healthy controls reported fatigue.[237] Treating depression and daytime sleepiness can be helpful, but when fatigue is an independent symptom, no treatment has been found satisfactory. Despite the claimed benefit of amantadine in treating fatigue in multiple sclerosis, neither this drug nor the monoamine oxidase inhibitor, selegiline, have been found particularly beneficial in treating fatigue in PD.

Depression and anxiety It is common in patients

Table 231.14   Disturbances of personality and behavior in Parkinson's disease

Depression
Fearfulness
Anxiety
Loss of assertive drive
Passivity
Dependency
Inability to make decisions
Loss of motivation, apathy
Abulia

with PD to find a change in personality (Table 231.14). Such a change may precede motor symptoms but usually develops and worsens over the course of PD. Executives with decision-making tasks may find their duties so difficult that they are unable to continue in their work. Passivity, dependency and lack of motivation are often more troublesome for the spouse than for the patient. Abulia is a severe form of apathy, both mental and motor, with not only a loss of initiative and drive but also a general restriction of activities, including reticence in speaking. Abulia is a recognized clinical syndrome due to caudate and prefrontal dysfunction, so may well feature in the overall symptomatology of PD. In its milder form (i.e. apathy), the loss of initiative, both mental and motor, is often commented upon by the spouse or close relatives, who perceive a change in personality. Spouses particularly complain about lack of desire in the patient to socialize with friends and communicate freely. Such alterations in activity may be due to depression, but not infrequently there is no change in mood. The personality alterations do not respond to dopamine replacement therapy in the way the motor problems of PD do, nor antidepressants, unless depression is present and is itself the cause of the apathy.

Depression is common in PD, with at least a third of patients exhibiting significant depressive symptoms in cross-sectional surveys.[238,239] However, it often is difficult to distinguish true depression from the apathy (abulia) associated with PD, especially in the presence of the characteristic expressionless face, bowed posture and slowed movement, which resemble the psychomotor retardation of a primary depressive illness. The critical factor is whether the patient has a true disturbance of mood (dysphoria), with low spirits, loss of interest, bleak outlook, typical depressive sleep disturbance, paranoid ruminations and sometimes suicidal thoughts.

The reasons for depression in PD are debated. On the one hand, depressive symptoms are not surprising in vulnerable individuals faced with the disabilities and handicaps imposed by PD, with reduced activity and independence, and the prospect of a chronic incurable condition. Such reactive depression certainly contributes to the problem. However, there is also the probability that the pathology of PD in itself may predispose to depression, especially that involving serotonergic and noradrenergic systems, which have been implicated in the neurochemical basis of primary depressive illnesses. The substantia nigra itself is implicated by the report that deep brain stimulation of this structure in a patient with PD induced acute severe depression.[240]

The recognition and treatment of depression in PD may have a major impact on the overall disability imposed by the illness. Most antidepressant drugs can be used safely in PD. However, non-selective monoamine oxidase inhibitors are contraindicated in those on levodopa because of potential pressor reactions. There also have been concerns over the use of selective serotonin re-uptake inhibitors (SSRIs), which in a few cases have been reported to interact with levodopa to induce the "serotonin syndrome" (confusion, myoclonus, rigidity and restlessness) and to worsen PD symptoms. Despite these worries, many depressed patients with PD have been treated safely and successfully with SSRIs, for example fluoxetine or paroxetine (20 to 40 mg daily). By enhancing serotonergic "tone" and thereby potentially inhibiting dopaminergic neurons in the substantia nigra, there is the potential, especially in the absence of dopaminergic drug treatment, that SSRIs may increase parkinsonian symptoms, but such events are rare.[241–245] The traditional tricyclic antidepressants also can be employed, although their sedative and anticholinergic properties may be detrimental in the aged. If a severely depressed patient with PD fails to respond to antidepressant drug treatment, electroconvulsive therapy (ECT) can be used.[246] Indeed, ECT in itself can temporarily improve mobility in PD.

Anxiety and panic can be major difficulties in PD.[247] Many patients, even early in the illness, complain of loss of confidence. In particular they fear social occasions and public display at work, and they tend to withdraw from outside life. In part, this is due to anxiety over their friends and acquaintances perceiving that they have PD, and to their loss of mobility and their non-verbal emotional responses to social interactions. However, some also develop a generalized and disturbing anxiety state, which may require psychotherapy and anxiolytic drug treatment. Those in the more advanced stages of the illness may experience profound anxiety and even terror during "off" periods.[248]

Often anxiety can be relieved by effective antiparkinsonian drug therapy, but if uncontrolled and pervasive it may require an antidepressant and, if dysphoria is present, a benzodiazepine (e.g. lorazepam 0.5 to 2 mg tid) or buspirone. However, all these drugs can increase confusion in those who are cognitively impaired.

Many patients have sensory or behavioral "off" periods, either accompanying or instead of a motor "off." The behavioral symptoms can consist of depression, anxiety, dysphoria and panic; the sensory consist mainly of pain. These sensory or behavioral "offs" are most distressing to the patient. Whereas motoric "offs" represent insufficient dopaminergic "tone" in the neostriatum, the behavioral and sensory "offs" probably represent insufficient dopaminergic "tone" in the limbic dopaminergic areas of the brain, such as the nucleus accumbens, amygdala, and cingulate cortex.

Cognitive problems If specifically looked for, about two-thirds of patients with early PD will show abnormalities of cognitive function on formal neuropsychological testing.[249–252] In particular, such patients are weak in performance of tests sensitive to frontal lobe dysfunction, such as verbal fluency, the Wisconsin card sorting test, the Tower of London test and its variants, and tests of working memory. Poor performance on tests such as these suggests abnormalities of frontal lobe executive functions, which may be due to defective input from non-motor basal ganglia regions (via thalamus) into prefrontal cerebral cortical areas. Thus, some patients with early PD may exhibit a fronto-striatal cognitive syndrome, sometimes rather inaccurately described as a subcortical dementia, in the absence of any major defects in language, episodic memory, or visuospatial functions. The pathological substrate of such a fronto-striatal cognitive syndrome in PD is debatable. Dopamine deficiency in the non-motor regions of the striatum, especially the caudate nucleus (which receives from and projects to prefrontal cerebral cortex), loss of dopamine projections from the midbrain ventral tegmental area to the frontal lobes, loss of cortical cholinergic projections from the substantia innominata, loss of cortical noradrenergic projections from the locus ceruleus, and cortical Lewy body degeneration may all contribute.

The clinical question is to what extent such neuropsychological defects intrude into everyday life in patients with PD. In this context two clinical features of PD deserve further comment, namely bradyphrenia and abulia

Bradyphrenia, or slowness of thought, probably is a real component of PD in many patients. For example, patients may comment on a slowing of mental processing and memory retrieval, and examination of neuropsychological test performance may show delay in deciding on choices although the final decisions are correct. Finding the right word or the answer to a question may be slow. The "tip of the tongue" problem refers to patients knowing the word they want, but being unable to say it at that moment, a problem often encountered in PD.[253] Some patients with PD spontaneously volunteer the observation that they have less ability to deal with mental problems, particularly multiple tasks at the same time. However, the extent to which depression may contribute to such problems is controversial. The general concept of bradyphrenia could be considered in the wider issue of abulia.

The overall impression of cognitive dysfunction in non-demented patients with PD may be summarized as follows:

1. Many, but not all patients with early PD, may exhibit subtle frontostriatal cognitive impairments. In early stage PD, these do not necessarily intrude into everyday life.

2. A substantial number of patients with early PD do

complain of some cognitive change, in particular a slowing of thought, a difficulty or delay in memory retrieval, and problems in handling multiple tasks.

3. Such cognitive impairments may be due to depression, when there is a change in mood, but often there is no dysphoria.

Unfortunately, these selective cognitive impairments do not seem to respond to dopamine replacement therapy in the way the motor problems of PD do, nor do they respond to antidepressants, unless depression is present and is itself the cause of the slowness of thinking. It is important to assess and treat any concurrent depression, and also to review current drug therapy. Anticholinergics, amantadine, dopamine agonists and even levodopa in excess may well impair cognitive function, especially in the elderly PD patient. Whether these cognitive difficulties are the precursor to frank dementia is uncertain, but obviously they raise such concern.

Unfortunately, a sizable proportion of those with PD eventually develop a multifocal, pervasive dementia. This typically occurs in the elderly patient. Cross-sectional studies suggest that in those with PD aged over 65 years, some 20% will be demented, as opposed to 10% of non-PD individuals in this age group.[250] Prospective longitudinal studies suggest that up to 40% of those with PD will dement as they age.[254–256] Correlations for developing dementia are older age, greater severity and longer duration of PD, and male gender.

Concurrent Alzheimer's disease, probably coincidental, obviously accounts for some of the dementia in PD.[257] However, in recent years it has become apparent that widespread Lewy body degeneration is another common cause of dementia,[258] second in frequency to Alzheimer's disease. Such dementia with Lewy bodies, as it is now known,[259] may coexist with the pathological changes of Alzheimer's disease, particularly with amyloid plaques rather than neurofibrillary tangles. One hypothesis is that the two pathologies, Lewy body degeneration in cerebral cortex and the cholinergic substantia innominata, and Alzheimer's disease changes, coexist by chance but summate to cause dementia. Another hypothesis is that the one predisposes to the other, and it is intriguing that α-synuclein is a component of both plaques (the non-amyloid component) and Lewy bodies. Whatever the pathogenic mechanism, this combination (which some have called the Lewy body variant of Alzheimer's disease) is a common cause of dementia in PD. Pure dementia with Lewy bodies is probably less common, but it has been shown pathologically that cortical Lewy bodies can be associated with cognitive impairment independent of AD-type pathology.[260]

Thus, there are at least three common substrates for dementia in PD: Alzheimer's disease, Alzheimer's disease with Lewy bodies, and diffuse Lewy body disease (also called dementia with Lewy bodies). A fourth possibility is dementia with basal ganglia pathology of PD; whether such dementia in patients with PD occurs without the spread of Lewy bodies into the cortex is uncertain. It addition, all the other causes of dementia may occur in patients with PD, including cerebrovascular disease, rarer degenerations such as frontotemporal dementia and Pick's disease, cerebral tumors and other intracranial mass lesions, hydrocephalus, metabolic, endocrine and nutrional disorders.

Accordingly, the first step in assessment of a patient with PD who is dementing is to undertake the usual investigations for known causes, especially those that are treatable. Depression causing a pseudo-dementia must also be carefully assessed.

Having excluded such symptomatic causes of dementia, the clinical picture may give important clues as to the underlying degenerative condition causing the dementia. Prominent early memory difficulties with language, praxis and visuospatial problems pointing to temporo-parietal dysfunction suggest Alzheimer's disease. A variable, fluctuating dementia with prominent hallucinations (especially visual), confusion and an unusual susceptibility to neuroleptics may indicate dementia with Lewy bodies,[259,261] i.e. diffuse Lewy body disease. Prominent behavioral, speech and memory difficulties may point to frontotemporal dementia or Pick's disease.

FDG PET scans were correlated with the dementia score on the UPDRS. A deficit in glucose utilization was found with left limbic structures such as the cingulate gyrus, parahippocampal gyrus, and medial frontal gyrus.[262]

Whatever the pathological substrate of dementia in PD, the syndrome poses formidable management problems. The challenge is to maintain mobility using adequate doses of antiparkinsonian medication without exacerbating the mental and behavioral problems. Behavioral disturbances, including verbal and physical aggression, wandering, agitation, inappropriate sexual behavior, uncooperativeness, and urinary incontinence, cause major difficulties. General structured care in a familiar environment is essential. Judicious use of day-care facilities and home assistants may be necessary. Drug therapy should be simplified, removing selegiline, anticholinergic agents, amantadine and dopamine agonists. Depression may require specific treatment, preferably avoiding antidepressants with marked anticholinergic properties. Nocturnal sedation may require quetiapine, which provides both sedation and antihallucinatory effects. Clozapine does the same, but requires weekly ascertainment for neutropenia. Other bedtime hypnotics, such as benzodiazepines and zolpidem, can be effective. Donepezil (Aricept), which provides modest, usually transient benefit in Alzheimer's disease, may sometimes help those with PD who are demented, but the value of this treatment is uncertain, and the cholinergic property may aggravate motoric symptoms of PD. Rivastigmine, an other centrally active cholinesterase inhibitor, was found to provide some improvement in apathy, anxiety, delusions and hallucinations.[263]

Dementia, with or without a frank confusional

state, is the commonest cause of final nursing home placement in those with PD, and shortens life expectancy.[264]

Psychosis Hallucinations occur in a significant proportion of those with PD, especially in the aged. In a community study in Norway, 10% of PD patients had hallucinations with insight retained, and another 6% had more severe hallucinations or delusions.[265] Psychotic features appear to be due to a complex interaction between the progressive and widespread pathology of the illness (diffuse cortical Lewy body degeneration, concurrent Alzheimer plaques and tangles, and cortical cholinergic, noradrenergic and serotonergic denervation), the unwanted effects of drugs (anticholinergics, levodopa and dopamine agonists), and intercurrent illness (such as infections or metabolic disturbances).

Isolated visual hallucinations are fairly common.[266,267] Auditory hallucinations are very uncommon.[268] Visual hallucinations often take the form of familiar humans or animals, which the patients know are false (pseudo-hallucinations). Such hallucinations may progress to a delusional paranoid state (often concerning infidelity) or a frank confusional state with impairment of attentiveness and disorientation.

Faced with such symptoms, although antiparkinsonian drug therapy is the most likely cause it is wise first to search for some intercurrent illness, such as a stroke or intracranial mass lesion, a chest or urinary infection, disturbance of electrolytes, renal or hepatic function, anemia, or endocrine dysfunction. Psychosis due to antiparkinsonian medications can usually be counteracted by atypical antipsychotics, drugs that usually do not aggravate parkinsonism at a dosage that therapeutic benefit for the psychosis is encountered. Start with quetiapine (Seroquel) because this drug does not cause agranulocytosis and does not require blood count monitoring.[269] A dose of 25 to 50 mg at night may control confusion and psychosis without worsening the parkinsonism. Because of the potential for drowsiness, it is best initially to use a small dose of such drugs at night, thereafter gradually increasing the dose to that required to control the confusion without worsening the parkinsonism. The benefit of aiding sleep at night is an advantage, but try to avoid a dose that might extend the drowsiness to daytime. If quetiapine is ineffective or produces too much daytime drowsiness or other adverse effects, including worsening of parkinsonism, clozapine (Clozaril) should be tried next, starting with 12.5 at night to avoid daytime drowsiness, and increasing the dose until benefit or adverse effects are encountered. It is probably more effective than quetiapine, but its use requires regular monitoring of blood counts to prevent the 1 to 2% risk of agranulocytosis).[78–89,270,271]

Other so-called atypical antipsychotics appear to be so designated for marketing purposes. Olanzapine can be effective, but easily increases parkinsonism so needs to be used in small doses to avoid a worsening of parkinsonism,[90,272–274] and is therefore relegated to

third choice. Risperidone more closely resembles a typical, rather than an atypical antipsychotic, and worsens PD. Molindone, pimozide or other relatively weak antipsychotics might also be considered.

If psychosis continues without adequate benefit from the antipsychotics, selegiline, anticholinergics and amantadine should be withdrawn. The need for anxiolytics and antidepressants should be reconsidered. If the symptoms persist, dopamine agonists should be reduced or stopped. If necessary, the dose of levodopa should be tapered. However, more often than not, as drugs are reduced to improve the mental state mobility deteriorates. A brittle balance is reached in which the patient is either mobile but confused, paranoid or hallucinating, or is mentally clear but immobile. More dopamine replacement therapy is required to maintain mobility, but causes a recurrence of the confusion, and it is very difficult to achieve a compromise. In this situation, a limited drug holiday, withdrawing dopaminergic drugs for 1 to 2 days each week, may help to dispel psychotoxicity, allowing a reasonable dose of medication to maintain mobility on other days. Sustained withdrawal of levodopa provokes unacceptable parkinsonism and, sometimes, particularly if withdrawn suddenly, a "neuroleptic" malignant syndrome.[127,128] When it comes to balancing between drug-induced psychosis and parkinsonism, it is essential to keep in mind that intact mental function is more important than intact motor function.

References

1. Parkinson J. An Essay on the Shaking Palsy. London: Sherwood, Neely and Jones, 1817
2. Von Economo C. Encephalitis Lethargica, its Sequelae and Treatment. (trans. KO Newman). London: Oxford, 1931
3. Blocq P, Marinesco G. Sur un cas de tremblement parkinsonien hemiplegique symptomatique d'une tumeur du pedoncle cerebral. Comptes Rendus Hebd Seances et Memoires Soc Boil 1893;5:105–111
4. Tretiakoff C. Contribution a l'etude de l'anatomie pathologique du locus niger de Soemmering avec quelques deductions relatives a le pathogenie des troubles du tonius musculaire et de la maladie de Parkinson. Doctoral Thesis, University of Paris, Paris, 1919
5. Lewy FH. Zur patholoischen anatomie der Paralysis Agitans. Zeitschr Nervenheilk 1913;50:50–55
6. Montagu KA. Catechol compounds in rat tissues and in brains of different animals. Nature 1957;180:244
7. Carlsson A, Lindquist M, Magnusson T. 3,4-dihydroxy-phenylalanine and 5-hydroxytryptophan as reserpine antagonists. Nature 1957;180:200
8. Cotzias GC, van Woert MH, Schiffer LM. Aromatic amino acids and modification of parkinsonism. New Engl J Med 1967;276:374–379
9. Tanner CM. Epidemiology of Parkinson's disease. Neurol Clin North Am 1992;10:317–329
10. Rajput AH,, Rozdilsky B, Rajput A. Accuracy of clinical diagnosis in parkinsonism—a prospective study. Can J Neurol Sci 1991;18:275–278
11. Hughes AJ, Daniel SE, Kilford L, Lee AJ. Accuracy of clinical diagnosis of idiopathic Parkinson's disease: a clinicopathologic study. J Neurol Neurosurg Psychiatr 1992;55:181–184

12. Jankovic J, Rajput AH, McDermott MP, Perl DP. The evolution of diagnosis in early Parkinson's disease. Arch Neurol 2000;57:369–372

13. Vingerhoets FJG, Schulzer M, Calne DB, et al. Which clinical sign of Parkinson's disease best reflects the nigrostriatal lesion? Ann Neurol 1997;41:58–64

14. Brooks DJ. PET: its clinical role in neurology. J Neurol Neurosurg Psychiatr 1991;54:1–4

15. Brooks DJ, Ibanez V, Sawle GV, et al. Striatal D2 receptor status in patients with Parkinson's disease, striatonigral degeneration, and progressive supranuclear palsy, as measured with 11C-raclopride and positron emission tomography. Ann Neurol 1992;31:184–191

16. Schwarz J, Tatsch K, Arnold G, et al. ^{123}I-iodobenzamide-SPECT predicts dopaminergic responsiveness in patients with de novo parkinsonism. Neurology 1992;42:556–561

17. Marek KL, Seibyl JP, Zoghbi SS, et al. [123]I beta-CIT SPECT imaging demonstrates bilateral loss of dopamine transporters in hemi-Parkinson's disease. Neurology 1996;46:231–237

18. Eidelberg D, Takikawa S, Moeller JR, et al. Striatal hypometabolism distinguishes striatonigral degeneration form Parkinson's disease. Ann Neurol 1993;33:518–527

19. Kitada T, et al. Mutations in the parkin gene cause autosomal recessive juvenile parkinsonism. Nature 1998;392:605–608

20. Klein C, Pramstaller PP, Kis B. Ann Neurol 2000;48:65–71

21. Lucking CB, Durr A, Bonifati V, et al. The French Parkinson's Disease Genetics Study Group. Association between early-onset-Parkinson's disease and mutation in the parkin gene. New England J Med 2000;342:1560–1567

22. Horowitz JM, Myers J, Stachowiak MK and Torres G. Identification and distribution of parkin in rat brain. NeuroReport 1999;10:3393–3397

23. Shimura H, Hattori N, Kubo S-I, et al. Familial Parkinson disease gene product, parkin, is a ubiquitin-protein ligase. Nature Genet 2000;25:302–305.

24. Polymeropoulos MH, Higgins JJ, Golbe LI, et al. Mapping of a gene for Parkinson's disease to chromosome 4q21-q23. Science 1996;274:1197–1199

25. Polymeropoulos MH, Lavedan C, Leroy E, et al. Mutation in the alpha-synuclein gene identified in families with Parkinson's disease. Science 1997;276:2045–2047

26. Kruger R, Kuhn W, Muller T, et al. Ala30Pro mutation in the gene encoding alpha-synuclein in Parkinson's disease. Nature Genet 1998;18:106–108

27. Leroy E, Boyer R, Auberger G, et al. The ubiquitin pathway in Parkinson's disease. Nature 1998;394:451–452

28. Jenner P, Olanow CW. Oxidative stress and the pathogenesis of Parkinson's disease. Neurology 47 1996;S161–S170

29. Schapira AH, Cooper JM, Dexter D, et al. Mitochondrial complex I deficiency in Parkinson's disease. J Neurochem 54 1990a;823–827

30. Tipton KF, Singer TP. Advances in our understanding of the mechanisms of the neurotoxicity of MPTP and related compounds. J Neurochem 1993;61:1191–1206

31. Fahn S. Adverse effects of levodopa. In: Olanow CW, Lieberman AN, eds. The Scientific Basis for the Treatment of Parkinson's Disease. Carnforth: Parthenon Publishing Group, 1992:89–112

32. Quinn N, Critchley P, Marsden CD. Young-onset Parkinson's disease. Mov Disord 1987;2:73–91

33. Kostic V, Przedborski S, Flaster E, Sternic N. Early development of levodopa-induced dyskinesias and response fluctuations in young-onset Parkinson's disease. Neurology 1991;41:202–205

34. Gershanik OS. Early-onset parkinsonism. In: Jankovic J, Tolosa E, eds. Parkinson's Disease and Movement Disorders, 2nd ed. Baltimore: Williams & Wilkins, 1993:235–252

35. Wagner ML, Fedak MN, Sage JI, Mark MH. Complications of disease and therapy: a comparison of younger and older patients with Parkinson's disease. Ann Clin Lab Sci 1996;26:389–395

36. Quinn N. Multiple system atrophy. In: Marsden CD, Fahn S, eds. Movement Disorders 3. Oxford: Butterworth-Heinemann, 1994:262–281

37. Fahn S. Parkinsonism. In: Rakel RE, ed. Conn's Current Therapy. Philadelphia: WB Saunders, 1998;944–953

38. Rascol O, Brooks DJ, Korczyn AD, et al. A five-year study of the incidence of dyskinesia in patients with early Parkinson's disease who were treated with ropinirole or levodopa. N Engl J Med 2000;342:1484–1491

39. Parkinson Study Group. Pramipexole vs levodopa as initial treatment for Parkinson disease—a randomized controlled trial. JAMA 2000;284:1931–1938

40. Oertel WH. Pergolide vs. L-dopa (PELMOPET) Mov Disord 2000;15(Suppl 3):5

41. Parkinson Study Group. Effect of deprenyl on the progression of disability in early Parkinson's disease. N Engl J Med 1989a;321:1364–1371

42. Parkinson Study Group. Effects of tocopherol and deprenyl on the progression of disability in early Parkinson's disease. N Engl J Med 1993;328:176–183

43. Myllyla VV, Sotaniemi KA, Vuorinen JA, Heinonen EH. Selegiline as initial treatment in de novo parkinsonian patients. Neurology 1992;42:339–343

44. Palhagen S, Heinonen EH, Hagglund J, et al. Selegiline delays the onset of disability in de novo parkinsonian patients. Neurology 1998;51:520–525

45. Parkinson Study Group. Cerebrospinal fluid homovanillic acid in the DATATOP study on Parkinson's disease. Arch Neurol 1995;52:237–245

46. Parkinson Study Group. Impact of deprenyl and tocopherol treatment on Parkinson's disease in DATATOP subjects not requiring levodopa. Ann Neurol 1996;39:29–36

47. Parkinson Study Group. Impact of deprenyl and tocopherol treatment on Parkinson's disease in DATATOP patients requiring levodopa. Ann Neurol 1996;39: 37–45

48. Parkinson Study Group. Mortality in DATATOP: a multicenter trial in early Parkinson's disease. Ann Neurol 1998;43:318–325

49. Reuter I, Engelhardt M, Stecker K, Baas H. Therapeutic value of exercise training in Parkinson's disease. Med Sci Sport Exercise 1999;31:1544–1549

50. Behrman AL, Cauraugh JH, Light KE. Practice as an intervention to improve speeded motor performance and motor learning in Parkinson's disease. J Neurol Sci 2000;174:127–136

51. Lokk J. The effects of mountain exercise in Parkinsonian persons—a preliminary study. Arch Gerontol Geriatr 2000;31:19–25

52. Hornykiewicz O. Dopamine (3-hydroxytyramine) and brain function. Pharmacol Rev 1966;18:925–964

53. Watkins P. COMT inhibitors and liver toxicity. Neurology 2000;55(Suppl 4):S51–S52

54. Ahlskog JE, Wright KF, Muenter MD, Adler CH. Adjunctive cabergoline therapy of Parkinson's disease: comparison with placebo and assessment of dose responses and duration of effect. Clin Neuropharmacol 1996;19:202–212

55. Hutton JT, Morris JL. Long-acting carbidopa-levodopa in the management of moderate and advanced Parkinson's disease. Neurology 1992;42(Suppl 1):51–56

56. Perachon S, Schwartz JC, Sokoloff P. Functional potencies of new antiparkinsonian drugs at recombinant human dopamine D-1, D-2 and D-3 receptors. Eur J Pharmacol 1999;366:293–300

57. Schrag AE, Brooks DJ, Brunt E, et al. The safety of ropinirole, a selective nonergoline dopamine agonist, in patients with Parkinson's disease. Clin Neuropharmacol 1998;21:169–175

58. Lieberman A, Olanow CW, Sethi K, et al. A multicenter trial of ropinirole as adjunct treatment for Parkinson's disease. Neurology 1998;51:1057–1062

59. Pinter MM, Pogarell O, Oertel WH. Efficacy, safety, and tolerance of the non-ergoline dopamine agonist pramipexole in the treatment of advanced Parkinson's disease: a double blind, placebo controlled, randomised, multicentre study. J Neurol Neurosurg Psychiat 1999;66:436–441

60. Kieburtz K, Shoulson I, McDermott M, et al. Parkinson Study Group. Safety and efficacy of pramipexole in early Parkinson disease: A randomized dose-ranging study. JAMA 1997;278:125–130

61. Brooks DJ, Abbott RJ, Lees AJ, et al. A placebo-controlled evaluation of ropinirole, a novel D2 agonist, as sole dopaminergic therapy in Parkinson's disease. Clin Neuropharmacol 1998 Mar–Apr;21(2):101–107

62. Sethi KD, O'Brien CF, Hammerstad JP, et al. Ropinirole for the treatment of early Parkinson disease: A 12-month experience. Arch Neurol 1998;55:1211–1216

63. Rinne UK. Early dopamine agonist therapy in Parkinson's disease. Mov Disord 1989;4(Suppl 1):S86–S94

64. Rinne UK. Lisuride, a dopamine agonist in the treatment of early Parkinson's disease. Neurology 1989;39:336–339

65. Kulisevsky J, Lopez-Villegas D, Garcia-Sanchez C, et al. A six-month study of pergolide and levodopa in de novo Parkinson's disease patients. Clin Neuropharmacol 1998;21:358–362

66. Frucht S, Rogers JD, Greene PE, et al. Falling asleep at the wheel: motor vehicle mishaps in persons taking pramipexole and ropinirole. Neurology 1999;52:1908–1910

67. Hoehn MM. Falling asleep at the wheel: motor vehicle mishaps in people taking pramipexole and ropinirole. Neurology 2000;54:275

68. Schapira AHV. Sleep attacks (sleep episodes) with pergolide. Lancet 2000;355:1332–1333

69. Ferreira JJ, Galitzky M, Montastruc JL, Rascol O. Sleep attacks and Parkinson's disease treatment. Lancet 2000;355:1333–1334

70. Golbe LI, Lieberman AN, Muenter MD, et al. Deprenyl in the treatment of symptom fluctuations in advanced Parkinson's disease. Clin Neuropharmacol 1988;11: 45–55

71. Parkinson Study Group. A controlled trial of lazabemide (RO19-6327) in untreated Parkinson's disease. Ann Neurol 1993;33:350–356

72. Rabey JM, Sagi I, Huberman M, et al. Rasagiline mesylate, a new MAO-B inhibitor for the treatment of Parkinson's disease: A double-blind study as adjunctive therapy to levodopa. Clin Neuropharmacol 2000; 23:324–330

73. Rajput A, Wallukait M, Rajput AH. 18 month prospective study of amantadine (Amd) for dopa (LD) induced dyskinesias (DK) in idiopathic Parkinson's disease. Can J Neurol Sci 1997;24:S23

74. Metman LV, Del Dotto P, van den Munckhof P, et al. Amantadine as treatment for dyskinesias and motor fluctuations in Parkinson's disease. Neurology 1998;50:1323–1326

75. Schwartz GA, Fahn S. Newer medical treatment in parkinsonism. Med N Am 1970;54:773–777

76. Fahn S. A pilot trial of high-dose alpha-tocopherol and ascorbate in early Parkinson's disease. Ann Neurol 1992;32:S128–S132

77. Yoshikawa T. Free radicals and their scavengers in Parkinson's disease. Eur Neurol 1993;33:60–68

78. Friedman JH, Lannon MC. Clozapine in idiopathic Parkinson's disease. Neurology 1990;40:1151–1152

79. Pfeiffer RF, Kang J, Graber B, et al. Clozapine for psychosis in Parkinson's disease. Mov Disord 1990;5: 239–242

80. Kahn N, Freeman A, Juncos JL, et al. Clozapine is beneficial for psychosis in Parkinson's disease. Neurology 1991;41:1699–1700

81. Factor SA, Brown D. Clozapine prevents recurrence of psychosis in Parkinson's disease. Mov Disord 1992;7: 125–131

82. Greene P, Cote L, Fahn S. Treatment of drug-induced psychosis in Parkinson's disease with clozapine. Adv Neurol 1993;60:703–706

83. Pinter MM, Helscher RJ. Therapeutic effect of clozapine in psychotic decompensation in idiopathic Parkinson's disease. J Neural Transm-Parkinsons 1993; 5:135–146

84. Factor SA, Brown D, Molho ES, Podskalny GD. Clozapine: A 2-year open trial in Parkinson's disease patients with psychosis. Neurology 1994;44:544–546

85. Rabey JM, Treves TA, Neufeld MY, et al. Low-dose clozapine in the treatment of levodopa-induced mental disturbances in Parkinson's disease. Neurology 1995; 45:432–434

86. Diederich N, Keipes M, Grass M, Metz H. Use of clozapine for psychiatric complications of Parkinson's disease. Rev Neurol 1995;151:251–257

87. Ruggieri S, Depandis MF, Bonamartini A, et al. Low dose of clozapine in the treatment of dopaminergic psychosis in Parkinson's disease. Clin Neuropharmacol 1997;20:204–209

88. Factor SA, Friedman JH. The emerging role of clozapine in the treatment of movement disorders. Mov Disord 1997;12:483–496

89. Friedman J, Lannon M, Comella C, et al. Low-dose clozapine for the treatment of drug-induced psychosis in Parkinson's disease. N Engl J Med 1999;340: 757–763

90. Jimenez-Jimenez FJ, Tallon-Barranco A, Orti-Pareja M, et al. Olanzapine can worsen parkinsonism. Neurology 1998;50:1183–1184

91. Fahn S. Consensus? How to proceed in treatment today. Conclusions. In: Rinne UK, Nagatsu T, Horowski R, eds. International Workshop Berlin Parkinson's Disease. Bussum: Medicom Europe, 1991: 368–371

92. Fahn S. Is levodopa toxic? Neurology 1996;47: S184–S195

93. Fahn S. Parkinson disease, the effect of levodopa, and the ELLDOPA trial. Arch Neurol 1999;56:529–535

94. Felten DL, Felten SY, Fuller RW, et al. Chronic dietary pergolide preserves nigrostriatal neuronal integrity in

aged-Fischer-344 rats. Neurobiol Aging 1992;13:339–351

95. Carvey PM, Pieri S, Ling ZD. Attenuation of levodopa-induced toxicity in mesencephalic cultures by pramipexole. J Neural Transm 1997;104:209–228

96. Gassen M, Gross A, Youdim MBH. Apomorphine enantiomers protect cultured pheochromocytoma (PC12) cells from oxidative stress induced by H_2O_2 and 6-hydroxydopamine. Mov Disord 1998;13:242–248

97. Sawada H, Ibi M, Kihara T, et al. Dopamine D2-type agonists protect mesencephalic neurons from glutamate neurotoxicity: mechanisms of neuroprotective treatment against oxidative stress. Ann Neurol 1998;44:110–119

98. Zou LL, Jankovic J, Rowe DB, et al. Neuroprotection by pramipexole against dopamine- and levodopa-induced cytotoxicity. Life Sci 1999;64:1275–1285

99. Iida M, Miyazaki I, Tanaka K, et al. Dopamine D2 receptor-mediated antioxidant and neuroprotective effects of ropinirole, a dopamine agonist. Brain Res 1999;838:51–59

100. Vu TQ, Ling ZD, Ma SY, et al. Pramipexole attenuates the dopaminergic cell loss induced by intraventricular 6-hydroxydopamine. J Neural Transm 2000;107:159–176

101. Parkinson Study Group. DATATOP: a multicenter controlled clinical trial in early Parkinson's disease. Arch Neurol 1989b;46:1052–1060

102. Giladi N, McDermott MP, Fahn S, et al. Freezing of gait in PD: prospective assessment in the DATATOP cohort. Neurology 2001;56:1712–1721

103. Maki Y, Inoue T, Izumi T, et al. Monoamine oxidase inhibitors reduce conditioned fear stress-induced freezing behavior in rats. Eur J Pharmacol 2000;406:411–418

104. Graham DG, Tiffany SM, Bell WR, Gutknecht WF. Autooxidation versus covalent binding of quinone as the mechanism of toxicity of dopamine, 6-hydroxydopamine and related compounds toward C1300 neuroblastoma cells in vitro. Mol Pharmacol 1978;14:644–653

105. Cohen G. The pathobiology of Parkinson's disease: biochemical aspects of dopamine neuron senescence. J Neural Transm 1983;(Suppl 19):89–103

106. Cohen G. Monoamine oxidase, hydrogen peroxide, and Parkinson's disease. Adv Neurol 1986;45:119–125

107. Fahn S. The endogenous toxin hypothesis of the etiology of Parkinson's disease and a pilot trial of high dosage antioxidants in an attempt to slow the progression of the illness. Ann NY Acad Sci 1989;570:186–196

108. Fornstedt B, Pileblad E, Carlsson A. In vivo autoxidation of dopamine in guinea pig striatum increases with age. J Neurochem 1990;55:655–659

109. Olanow CW. Oxidation reactions in Parkinson's disease. Neurology 1990;40(Suppl 3):32–37

110. Olanow CW. An introduction to the free radical hypothesis in Parkinson's disease. Ann Neurol 1992;32:S2–S9

111. Jenner P. Oxidative stress as a cause of Parkinson's disease. Acta Neurol Scand 1991;84:6–15

112. Jenner P, Dexter DT, Sian J, et al. Oxidative stress as a cause of nigral cell death in Parkinson's disease and incidental Lewy body disease. Ann Neurol 1992;32:S82–S87

113. Jenner P, Schapira AHV, Marsden CD. New insights into the cause of Parkinson's disease. Neurology 1992;42:2241–2250

114. Fahn S, Cohen G. The oxidant stress hypothesis in Parkinson's disease: evidence supporting it. Ann Neurol 1992;32:804–812

115. Zigmond MJ, Hastings TG, Abercrombie ED. Neurochemical responses to 6-hydroxydopamine and L-dopa therapy: implications for Parkinson's disease. Ann NY Acad Sci 1992;648:71–86

116. Spencer JPE, Jenner P, Halliwell B. Superoxide-dependent depletion of reduced glutathione by L-DOPA and dopamine. Relevance to Parkinson's disease. Neuroreport 1995;6:1480–1484

117. Alam ZI, Jenner A, Daniel SE, et al. Oxidative DNA damage in the parkinsonian brain: An apparent selective increase in 8-hydroxyguanine levels in substantia nigra. J Neurochem 1997;69:1196–1203

118. Duvoisin RC. Cholinergic–anticholinergic antagonism in parkinsonism. Arch Neurol 1967;17:124–136

119. Ebersbach G, Stock M, Muller J, et al. Worsening of motor performance in patients with Parkinson's disease following transdermal nicotine administration. Mov Disord 1999;14:1011–1013

120. Poewe WH, Lees AJ, Stern GM. Low-dose L-dopa therapy in Parkinson's disease: a 6-year follow-up study. Neurology 1986;36:1528–1530

121. Lesser RP, Fahn S, Snider SR, et al. Analysis of the clinical problems in parkinsonism and the complications of long-term levodopa therapy. Neurology 1979;29:1253–1260

122. Block G, Liss C, Reines S, et al. Comparison of immediate-release and controlled release carbidopa/levodopa in Parkinson's disease—a multicenter 5-year study. Eur Neurol 1997;37:23–27

123. Koller WC, Hutton JT, Tolosa E, Capilldeo R. Immediate-release and controlled-release carbidopa/levodopa in PD—A 5-year randomized multicenter study. Neurology 1999;53:1012–1019

124. Zappia M, Oliveri RL, Bosco D, et al. The long-duration response to L-dopa in the treatment of early PD. Neurology 2000;54:1910–1915

125. Marsden CD, Fahn S. Problems in Parkinson's disease. In: Marsden CD, Fahn S, eds. Movement Disorders. London: Butterworth Scientific, 1982:1–7

126. Contin M, Riva R, Martinelli P, et al. A levodopa kinetic-dynamic study of the progression in Parkinson's disease. Neurology 1998;51:1075–1080

127. Friedman JH, Feinberg SS, Feldman RG. A neuroleptic malignantlike syndrome due to levodopa therapy withdrawal. JAMA 1985;254:2792–2795

128. Hirschorn KA, Greenberg HS. Successful treatment of levodopa-induced myoclonus and levodopa withdrawal-induced neuroleptic malignant syndrome: a case report. Clin Neuropharmacol 1988;2:278–281

129. Muenter MD, Tyce GM. L-dopa therapy of Parkinson's disease: Plasma L-dopa concentration, therapeutic response, and side effects. Mayo Clin Proc 1971;46:231–239

130. Sassin JF, Taub S, Weitzman ED. Hyperkinesia and changes in behavior produced in normal monkeys by L-dopa. Neurology 1972;22:1122–1125

131. Cedarbaum JM, Gandy SE, McDowell FH. Early initiation of levodopa treatment does not promote the development of motor response fluctuations, dyskinesias, or dementia in Parkinson's disease. Neurology 1991;41:622–629

131. Horstink MWIM, Zijlmans JCM, Pasman JW, et al. Severity of Parkinson's disease is a risk factor for peak-dose dyskinesia. J Neurol Neurosurg Psychiatry 1990;53:224–226

132. Chase TN. The significance of continuous dopaminer-

gic stimulation in the treatment of Parkinson's disease. Drugs 1998;55:1–9

133. Metman LV, Konitsiotis S, Chase TN. Pathophysiology of motor response complications in Parkinson's disease: hypotheses on the why, where, and what. Mov Disord 2000;15:3–8

134. Bush DF, Liss CL, Morton A, Sinemet CR. Multicenter Study Group. An open multicenter long-term treatment evaluation of Sinemet CR. Neurology 1989; 39(Suppl 2):101–104

135. Pahwa R, Busenbark K, Huber SJ, et al. Clinical experience with controlled-release carbidopa/levodopa in Parkinson's disease. Neurology 1993;43: 677–681

136. Parkinson Study Group. Safety and efficacy of pramipexole in early Parkinson disease: A randomized dose-ranging study. JAMA 1997;278:125–130

137. Geminiani G, Fetoni V, Genitrini S, et al. Cabergoline in Parkinson's disease complicated by motor fluctuations. Mov Disord 1996;11:495–500

138. Inzelberg R, Nisipeanu P, Rabey JM, et al. Double-blind comparison of cabergoline and bromocriptine in Parkinson's disease patients with motor fluctuations. Neurology 1996;47:785–788

139. Adler CH, Singer C, O'Brien C, et al. Randomized, placebo-controlled study of tolcapone in patients with fluctuating Parkinson disease treated with levodopa-carbidopa. Arch Neurol 1998;55:1089–1095

140. Kieburtz K, Shoulson I, Fahn S, et al. Parkinson Study Group. Entacapone improves motor fluctuations in levodopa-treated Parkinson's disease patients. Ann Neurol 1997;42:747–755

141. Rinne UK, Bracco F, Chouza C, et al. Early treatment of Parkinson's disease with cabergoline delays the onset of motor complications: Results of a double-blind levodopa controlled trial. Drugs 1998;55:23–30

142. Assal F, Spahr L, Hadengue A, et al. Tolcapone and fulminant hepatitis. Lancet 1998;352:958

143. Dewey RB, Maraganore DM, Ahlskog JE, Matsumoto JY. A double-blind, placebo-controlled study of intranasal apomorphine spray as a rescue agent for off-states in Parkinson's disease. Mov Disord 1998;13: 782–787

144. Djaldetti R, Melamed E. Levodopa ethylester: a novel rescue therapy for response fluctuations in Parkinson's disease. Ann Neurol 1996;39:400–404

145. Hughes AJ, Bishop S, Kleedorfer B, et al. Subcutaneous apomorphine in Parkinson's disease: response to chronic administration for up to five years. Mov Disord 1993;8:165–170

146. Rinne UK, Larsen JP, Siden A, Worm-Petersen J. Nomecomt Study Group. Entacapone enhances the response to levodopa in parkinsonian patients with motor fluctuations. Neurology 1998;51:1309–1314

147. Fahn S. Episodic failure of absorption of levodopa: a factor in the control of clinical fluctuations in the treatment of parkinsonism. Neurology 1977;27:390

148. Djaldetti R, Baron J, Ziv I, Melamed E. Gastric emptying in Parkinson's disease: patients with and without response fluctuations. Neurology 1996;46:1051–1054

149. Ostergaard L, Werdelin L, Odin P, et al. Pen injected apomorphine against off phenomena in late Parkinson's disease: a double blind, placebo controlled study. J Neurol Neurosurg Psychiatry 1995;58:681–687

150. Melamed E, Bitton V. Delayed onset of responses to individual doses of L-dopa in parkinsonian fluctuators: an additional side effect of long-term L-dopa therapy. Neurology 1984;34(Suppl 2):270

151. Shoulson I, Glaubiger GA, Chase TN. "On–off" response: clinical and biochemical correlations during oral and intravenous levodopa administration. Neurology 1975;25:1144–1148

152. Fahn S. Fluctuations of disability in Parkinson's disease: pathophysiological aspects. In: Marsden CD, Fahn S, eds. Movement Disorders. London: Butterworth Scientific, 1982:123–145

153. Muenter MD, Sharpless NS, Tyce GM. Plasma 3-O-methyldopa in L-dopa therapy of Parkinson's disease. Mayo Clin Proc 1972;47:389–395

154. Nutt JG, Woodward WR, Hammerstad JP, et al. The "on–off" phenomenon in Parkinson's disease. N Engl J Med 1984;310:483–488

155. Fahn S. The freezing phenomenon in parkinsonism. Adv Neurol 1995;67:53–63

156. Giladi N, McMahon D, Przedborski S, et al. Motor blocks in Parkinson's disease. Neurology 1992;42: 333–339

157. Narabayashi H, Kondo T, Yokochi F, Nagatsu T. Clinical effects of L-threo-3,4-dihydroxyphenylserine in cases of parkinsonism and pure akinesia. Adv Neurol 1986;45:593–602

158. Metman LV, Del Dotto P, LePoole K, et al. Amantadine for levodopa-induced dyskinesias—A 1-year follow-up study. Arch Neurol 1999;56:1383–1386

159. Snow BJ, Macdonald L, Mcauley D, Wallis W. The effect of amantadine on levodopa-induced dyskinesias in Parkinson's disease: a double-blind, placebo-controlled study. Clin Neuropharmacol 2000;23:82–85

160. Luginger E, Wenning GK, Bosch S, Poewe W. Beneficial effects of amantadine on L-dopa-induced dyskinesias in Parkinson's disease. Mov Disord 2000;15: 873–878

161. Bennett JP, Landow ER, Schuh LA. Suppression of dyskinesias in advanced Parkinson's disease. 2. Increasing daily clozapine doses suppress dyskinesias and improve parkinsonism symptoms. Neurology 1993;43:1551–1555

162. Bennett JP, Landow ER, Dietrich S, Schuh LA. Suppression of dyskinesias in advanced Parkinson's disease: moderate daily clozapine doses provide long-term dyskinesia reduction. Mov Disord 1994;9:409–414

163. Durif F, Vidailhet M, Assal F, et al. Low-dose clozapine improves dyskinesias in Parkinson's disease. Neurology 1997;48:658–662

164. Pierelli F, Adipietro A, Soldati G, et al. Low dosage clozapine effects on L-dopa induced dyskinesias in parkinsonian patients. Acta Neurol Scand 1998;97: 295–299

165. Durif F, Vidailhet M, Bonnet AM, et al. Levodopa-induced dyskinesias are improved by fluoxetine. Neurology 1995;45:1855–1858

166. Carpentier AF, Bonnet AM, Vidailhet M, Agid Y. Improvement of levodopa-induced dyskinesia by propranolol in Parkinson's disease. Neurology 1996;46: 1548–1551

167. Bonifati V, Fabrizio E, Cipriani R, et al. Buspirone in levodopa-induced dyskinesias. Clin Neuropharmacol 1994;17:73–82

168. LeWitt PA, Walters A, Hening W, McHale D. Persistent movement disorders induced by buspirone. Mov Disord 1993;8:331–334

169. Melamed E. Early-morning dystonia: a late side effect of long-term levodopa therapy in Parkinson's disease. Arch Neurol 1979;36:308–310

170. Currie LJ, Harrison MB, Trugman JM, et al. Early morning dystonia in Parkinson's disease. Neurology 1998;51:283–285

171. Ilson J, Fahn S, Cote L. Painful dystonic spasms in Parkinson's disease. Adv Neurol 1984;40:395–398

172. Bravi D, Mouradian MM, Roberts JW, et al. End-of-dose dystonia in Parkinson's disease. Neurology 1993; 43:2130–2131

173. Metman LV, Hoff J, Mouradian MM, Chase TN. Fluctuations in plasma levodopa and motor responses with liquid and tablet levodopa/carbidopa. Mov Disord 1994;9:463–465

174. Kurth MC, Tetrud JW, Irwin I, et al. Oral levodopa/cardibopa solution versus tablets in Parkinson's patients with severe fluctuations—a pilot study. Neurology 1993;43:1036–1039

175. Pappert EJ, Buhrfiend C, Lipton JW, et al. Levodopa stability in solution: time course, environmental effects, and practical recommendations for clinical use. Mov Disord 1996;11:24–26

176. Pappert EJ, Goetz CG, Niederman F, et al. Liquid levodopa/carbidopa produces significant improvement in motor function without dyskinesia exacerbation. Neurology 1996;47:1493–1495

177. Sage JI, McHale DM, Sonsalla P, et al. Continuous levodopa infusions to treat complex dystonia in Parkinson's disease. Neurology 1989;39:888–891

178. Sage JI, Trooskin S, Sonsalla PK, Heikkila RE. Experience with continuous enteral levodopa infusions in the treatment of 9 patients with advanced Parkinson's disease. Neurology 1989;39(Suppl 2):60–63

179. Bredberg E, Nilsson D, Johansson K, et al. Intraduodenal infusion of a water-based levodopa dispersion for optimisation of the therapeutic effect in severe Parkinson's disease. Eur J Clin Pharmacol 1993;45:117–122

180. Kurth MC, Tetrud JW, Tanner CM, et al. Double-blind, placebo-controlled, crossover study of duodenal infusion of levodopa carbidopa in Parkinson's disease patients with on–off fluctuations. Neurology 1993;43: 1698–1703

181. Nilsson D, Hansson LE, Johansson K, et al. Long-term intraduodenal infusion of a water based levodopa-carbidopa dispersion in very advanced Parkinson's disease. Acta Neurol Scand 1998;97:175–183

182. Colzi A, Turner K, Lees AJ. Continuous subcutaneous waking day apomorphine in the long term treatment of levodopa induced interdose dyskinesias in Parkinson's disease. J Neurol Neurosurg Psychiatry 1998;64: 573–576

183. Klawans HL. Individual manifestations of Parkinson's disease after ten or more years of levodopa. Mov Disord 1986;1:187–192

184. Agid Y, Graybiel AM, Ruberg M, et al. The efficacy of levodopa treatment declines in the course of Parkinson's disease: do nondopaminergic lesions play a role? Adv Neurol 1990;53:83–100

185. Jansen ENH. Clozapine in the treatment of tremor in Parkinson's disease. Acta Neurol Scand 1994;89: 262–265

186. Snider SR, Fahn S, Isgreen WP, Cote LJ. Primary sensory symptoms in parkinsonism. Neurology 1976; 26:423–429

187. Koller WC. Sensory symptoms in Parkinson's disease. Neurology 1984;34:957–959

188. Quinn NP, Koller WC, Lang AE, Marsden CD. Painful Parkinson's disease. Lancet 1986;1:1366–1369

189. Goetz CG, Tanner CM, Levy M, et al. Pain in Parkinson's disease. Mov Disord 1986;1:45–49

190. Ford B, Louis ED, Greene P, Fahn S. Oral and genital pain syndromes in Parkinson's disease. Mov Disord 1996;11:421–426

191. Lang AE. Restless legs syndrome and Parkinson's disease: insights into pathophysiology. Clin Neuropharmacol 1987;10:476–478

192. Lang AE, Johnson K. Akathisia in idiopathic Parkinson's disease. Neurology 1987;37:477–481

193. Lang AE. Withdrawal akathisia: case reports and a proposed classification of chronic akathisia. Mov Disord 1994;9:188–192

194. Fitzmaurice H, Fowler CJ, Rickards D, et al. Micturition disturbance in Parkinson's disease. Br J Urol 1985 Dec;57(6):652–656

195. Araki I, Kuno S. Assessment of voiding dysfunction in Parkinson's disease by the international prostate symptom score. J Neurol Neurosurg Psychiat 2000;68: 429–433

196. Stocchi F, Carbone A, Inghilleri M, et al. Urodynamic and neurophysiological evaluation in Parkinson's disease and multiple system atrophy. J Neurol Neurosurg Psychiatry 1997;62:507–511

197. Zesiewicz TA, Helal M, Hauser RA. Sildenafil citrate (Viagra) for the treatment of erectile dysfunction in men with Parkinson's disease. Mov Disord 2000;15: 305–308

198. Swope DM. Preliminary report: use of sildenafil to treat dyskinesias in patients with Parkinson's disease. Neurology 2000;54(Suppl 3):A90–A91

199. Qualman SJ, Haupt HM, Yang P, Hamilton SJ. Esophageal Lewy bodies associated with ganglion cell loss in achalasia. Similarity to Parkinson's disease. Gastroenterology 1984;87:848–856

200. Kupsky WJ, Grimes MM, Sweeting J, et al. Parkinson's disease and megacolon: Concentric hyaline inclusions (Lewy bodies) in enteric ganglion cells. Neurology 1987;37:1253–1255

201. Wakabayashi K, Takahashi H, Takeda E, et al. Parkinson's disease: the presence of Lewy bodies in Auerbach's and Meissner's plexuses. Acta Neuropathol 1988;76:217–221

202. Eadie MJ. The pathology of certain medullary nuclei in parkinsonism. Aust Ann Med 1963;86:781–792

203. Edwards LL, Pfeiffer RF, Quigley EMM, et al. Gastrointestinal symptoms in Parkinson's disease. Mov Disord 1991;6:151–156

204. Edwards LL, Quigley EMM, Pfeiffer RF. Gastrointestinal dysfunction in Parkinson's disease–frequency and pathophysiology. Neurology 1992;42:726–732

205. Bushmann M, Dobmeyer SM, Leeker L, Perlmutter JS. Swallowing abnormalities and their response to treatment in Parkinson's disease. Neurology 1989;39: 1309–1314

206. Edwards LL, Quigley EM, Harned RK, et al. Characterization of swallowing and defecation in Parkinson's disease. Am J Gastroenterol 1994;89:15–25

207. Mathers SE, Kempster PA, Swash M, Lees AJ. Constipation and paradoxical puborectalis contraction in anismus and Parkinson's disease: a dystonic phenomenon. J Neurol Neurosurg Psychiatry 1988;51:1503–1507

208. Mathers SE, Kempster PA, Law PJ, et al. Anal sphincter dysfunction in Parkinson's disease. Arch Neurol 1989;46:1061–1064

209. Edwards LL, Quigley EMM, Harned RK, et al. Defecatory function in Parkinson's disease: response to apomorphine. Ann Neurol 1993;33:490–493

210. Merello M, Leiguarda R. Adynamic bowel syndrome in Parkinson's disease with dramatic response to apomorphine. Clin Neuropharmacol 1994;17:574–577

211. Sage JI, Mark MH. Drenching sweats as an off phenomenon in Parkinson's disease: Treatment and

relation to plasma levodopa profile. Ann Neurol 1995;37: 120–122

212. Bateson MC, Gibberd FB, Wilson RSE. Salivary symptoms in Parkinson's disease. Arch Neurol 1973;29: 274–275

213. Pal PK, Calne DB, Calne S, Tsui JKC. Botulinum toxin A as treatment for drooling saliva in PD. Neurology 2000;54:244–247

214. Ilson J, Braun N, Fahn S. Respiratory fluctuations in Parkinson's disease. Neurology 1983;33(Suppl 2):113

215. Braun AR, Tanner CM, Goetz CG, Klawans HL. Respiratory distress due to pharyngeal dystonia: a side effect of chronic dopamine agonism. Neurology 1983; 33(Suppl 2):220

216. Efthimiou J, Ellis SJ, Hardie RJ, Stern GM. Sleep apnea in idiopathic and postencephalitic parkinsonism. Adv Neurol 1987;45:275–276

217. Strieder DJ, Baker WG, Baringer JR, Kazemi H. Chronic hypoventilation of central origin. A case with encephalitis lethargica and Parkinson's syndrome. Am Rev Resp Dis 1967;96:501–507

218. Lynch T, Sano M, Marder KS, et al. Clinical characteristics of a family with chromosome 17-linked disinhibition dementia parkinsonism amyotrophy complex. Neurology 1994;44:1878–1884

219. Chester CS, Gottfried SB, Cameron DI, Strohl KP. Pathophysiological findings in a patient with Shy–Drager and alveolar hypoventilation syndromes. Chest 1988;94:212–214

220. Salazar-Grueso EF, Rosenberg RS, Roos RP. Sleep apnea in olivopontocerebellar degeneration: treatment with trazodone. Ann Neurol 1988;23:399–401

221. Kitamura J, Kubuki Y, Tsuruta K, et al. A new family with Joseph disease in Japan. Homovanillic acid, magnetic resonance, and sleep apnea studies. Arch Neurol 1989;46:425–428

222. Perry TL, Wright JM, Berry K, et al. Dominantly inherited apathy, central hypoventilation, and Parkinson's syndrome: clinical, biochemical, and neuropathologic studies of 2 new cases. Neurology 1990;40:1882–1887

223. Factor SA, McAlarney T, Sanchez-Ramos JR, Weiner WJ. Sleep disorders and sleep effect in Parkinson's disease. Mov Disord 1990;4:280–285

224. Askenasy JJM. Sleep in Parkinson's disease. Acta Neurol Scand 1993;87(Suppl 3):167–170

225. Van Hilten B, Hoff JI, Middelkoop HAM, et al. Sleep disruption in Parkinson's disease—assessment by continuous activity monitoring. Arch Neurol 1994;51: 922–928

226. Bliwise DL, Watts RL, Watts N, et al. Disruptive nocturnal behavior in Parkinson's disease and Alzheimer's disease. J Geriatr Psychiatry Neurol 1995; 8:107–110

227. Karlsen KH, Larsen JP, Tandberg E, Maeland JG. Influence of clinical and demographic variables on quality of life in patients with Parkinson's disease. J Neurol Neurosurg Psychiat 1999;66:431–435

228. Elibol B, Hattori N, Atac FB, et al. Distinguishing clinical features in patients with parkin mutations. Neurology 2000;54(Suppl 3):A444

229. Ferini-Strambi L, Zucconi M. REM sleep behavior disorder. Clin Neurophysiol 2000;111:S136–S140

230. Lees AJ. A sustained-release formulation of L-dopa (Madopar HBS) in the treatment of nocturnal and early-morning disabilities in Parkinson's disease. Eur Neurol 1987;27(Suppl 1):126–134

231. Laihinen A, Alihanka J, Raitasuo, et al. Sleep movements and associated autonomic nervous activities in patients with Parkinson's disease. Acta Neurol Scand 1987;76:64–68

232. Nausieda PA, Weiner WJ, Kaplan LR, et al. Sleep disruption in the course of chronic levodopa therapy: an early feature of the levodopa psychosis. Clin Neuropharmacol 1982;5:183–194

233. Hening W, Walters A, Kavey N, et al. Dyskinesias while awake and periodic movements in sleep in restless legs syndrome: Treatment with opioids. Neurology 1986;36:1363–1366

234. Tandberg E, Larsen JP, Karlsen K. Excessive daytime sleepiness and sleep benefit in Parkinson's disease: a community-based study. Mov Disord 1999;14:922–927

235. Rye DB, Bliwise DL, Dihenia B, Gurecki P. Daytime sleepiness in Parkinson's disease. J Sleep Res 2000; 9:63–69

236. Hauser RA, Wahba MN, Zesiewicz TA, Anderson WM. Modafinil treatment of pramipexole-associated somnolence. Mov Disord 2000;15:1269–1271

237. Karlsen K, Larsen JP, Tandberg E, Jorgensen K. Fatigue in patients with Parkinson's disease. Mov Disord 1999;14:237–241

238. Brown RG, MacCarthy B, Gotham AM, et al. Depression and disability in Parkinson's disease: a follow-up of 132 cases. Psychol Med 1988;18:49–55

239. Dooneief G, Chen J, Mirabello E, et al. An estimate of the incidence of depression in idiopathic Parkinson's disease. Arch Neurol 1992;49:305–307

240. Bejjani BP, Damier P, Arnulf I, et al. Transient acute depression induced by high-frequency deep-brain stimulation. N Engl J Med 1999;340:1476–1480

241. Jansen Steur ENH. Increase of Parkinson disability after fluoxetine medication. Neurology 1993;43: 211–213

242. Jimenez-Jimenez FJ, Tejeiro J, Martinez-Junquero G, et al. Parkinsonism exacerbated by paroxetine. Neurology 1994;44:2406

243. Richard IH, Maughn A, Kurlan R. Do serotonin reuptake inhibitor antidepressants worsen Parkinson's disease? A retrospective case series. Mov Disord 1999; 14:155–157

244. Ceravolo R, Nuti A, Piccinni A, et al. Paroxetine in Parkinson's disease: effects on motor and depressive symptoms. Neurology 2000;55:1216–1218

245. Tesei S, Antonini A, Canesi M, et al. Tolerability of paroxetine in Parkinson's disease: a prospective study. Mov Disord 2000;15:986–989

246. Douyon R, Serby M, Klutchko B, Rotrosen J. ECT and Parkinson's disease revisited: a "naturalistic" study (see comments). Am J Psychiatry 1989;146:1451–1455

247. Stein MB, Heuser IJ, Juncos JL, Uhde TW. Anxiety disorders in patients with Parkinson's disease (see comments). Am J Psychiatry 1990;147:217–220

248. Nissenbaum H, Quinn NP, Brown RG, et al. Mood swings associated with the "on–off" phenomenon in Parkinson's disease. Psychol Med 1987;17:899–904

249. Lees AJ, Smith E. Cognitive defects in the early stages of Parkinson's disease. Brain 1983;106:257–270

250. Brown RG, Marsden CD. Cognitive function in Parkinson's disease: from description to theory. Trends Neurosci 1990;13:21–29

251. Levin BE, Llabre MM, Weiner WJ. Cognitive impairment associated with early Parkinson's disease. Neurology 1989;39:557–561

252. Cooper JA, Sagar HJ, Jordan N, et al. Cognitive impairment in early, untreated Parkinson's disease and its relationship to motor disability. Brain 1991;114: 2095–2122

253. Matison R, Mayeux R, Rosen J, Fahn S. "Tip-of-the-

tongue" phenomenon in Parkinson disease. Neurology 1982;32:567–570

254. Biggins CA, Boyd JL, Harrop FM, et al. A controlled, longitudinal study of dementia in Parkinson's disease. J Neurol Neurosurg Psychiatry 1992;55:566–571

255. Mayeux R, Chen J, Mirabello E, et al. An estimate of the incidence of dementia in idiopathic Parkinson's disease. Neurology 1990;40:1513–1517

256. Hughes TA, Ross HF, Musa S, et al. A 10-year study of the incidence of and factors predicting dementia in Parkinson's disease. Neurology 2000;54:1596–1602

257. Boller F, Mizutani T, Roessmann U, Gambetti P. Parkinson disease, dementia, and Alzheimer disease: clinicopathological correlations. Ann Neurol 1980;7: 329–335

258. Byrne EJ, Lennox G, Lowe J, Godwin-Austen RB. Diffuse Lewy body disease: clinical features in 15 cases. J Neurol Neurosun Ps 1989;52:709–717

259. McKeith IG, Galasko D, Kosaka K, et al. Consensus guidelines for the clinical and pathological diagnosis of dementia with Lewy bodies: report of the consortium on DLB International Workshop. Neurology 1996;47:113–124

260. Mattila PM, Rinne JO, Helenius H, et al. Alpha-synuclein-immunoreactive cortical Lewy bodies are associated with cognitive impairment in Parkinson's disease. Acta Neuropathol 2000;100:285–290

261. McKeith IG, Perry EK, Perry RH. Report of the second dementia with Lewy body international workshop—diagnosis and treatment. Neurology 1999;53:902–905

262. Wu JC, Iacono R, Ayman M, et al. Correlation of intellectual impairment in Parkinson's disease with FDG PET scan. Neuroreport 2000;11:2139–2144

263. McKeith IG, Grace JB, Walker Z, et al. Rivasitigmine in the treatment of dementia with Lewy bodies: preliminary findings from an open trial. Int J Geriatr Psychiatr 2000;15:387–392

264. Goetz CG, Stebbins GT. Risk factors for nursing home placement in advanced Parkinson's disease. Neurology 1993;43:2227–2229

265. Aarsland D, Larsen JP, Cummings JL, Laake K. Prevalence and clinical correlates of psychotic symptoms in Parkinson disease—a community-based study. Arch Neurol 1999;56:595–601

266. Naimark D, Jackson E, Rockwell E, Jeste DV. Psychotic symptoms in Parkinson's disease patients with dementia. J Am Geriatr Soc 1996;44:296–299

267. Sanchez-Ramos JR, Ortoll R, Paulson GW. Visual hallucinations associated with Parkinson's disease. Arch Neurol 1996;53:1265–1268

268. Inzelberg R, Kipervasser S, Korczyn AD. Auditory hallucinations in Parkinson's disease. J Neurol Neurosurg Psychiatry 1998;64:533–535

269. Fernandez HH, Friedman JH, Jacques C, Rosenfeld M. Quetiapine for the treatment of drug-induced psychosis in Parkinson's disease. Mov Disord 1999;14: 484–487

270. Scholz E, Dichgans J. Treatment of drug-induced exogenous psychosis in parkinsonism with clozapine and fluperlapine. Eur Arch Psychiatry Neurol Sci 1985; 235:60–64

271. Wolters EC, Hurwitz TA, Mak E, et al. Clozapine in the treatment of parkinsonian patients with dopaminomimetic psychosis. Neurology 1990;40: 832–834

272. Wolters EC, Jansen ENH, Tuynman-Qua HG, Bergmans PLM. Olanzapine in the treatment of dopaminomimetic psychosis in patients with Parkin-son's disease. Neurology 1996;47:1085–1087

273. Friedman J. Olanzapine in the treatment of dopaminomimetic psychosis in patients with Parkin-son's disease. Neurology 1998;50:1195–1196

274. Goetz CG, Blasucci LM, Leurgans S, Pappert EJ. Olanzapine and clozapine—comparative effects on motor function in hallucinating PD patients. Neurology 2000; 55:789–794

Further reading

Aaltonen H, Kilkku O, Heinonen E, Makilkola O. Effect of adding selegiline to levodopa in early, mild Parkinson's disease—evidence is insufficient to show that combined treatment increases mortality. Br Med J 1998;317:1586–1587

Acuff RV, Thedford SS, Hidiroglou NN, et al. Relative bioavailability of RRR- and all-rac-alpha-tocopherol acetate in humans: studies using deuterated compounds. Am J Clin Nutr 1994;60:397–402

Agid Y, Ahlskog E, Albanese A, et al. Levodopa in the treatment of Parkinson's disease: A consensus meeting. Mov Disord 1999;14:911–913

Agid Y, Bonnet AM, Signoret JL, Lhermitte F. Clinical, pharmacological, and biochemical approach of "onset- and end-of-dose" dyskinesias. Adv Neurol 1979;24: 401–410

Agid Y. Levodopa: is toxicity a myth? Neurology 1998;50: 858–863

Antonini A, Schwarz J, Oertel WH, et al. Long-term changes of striatal dopamine D-2 receptors in patients with Parkinson's disease: A study with positron emission tomography and [C-11]Raclopride. Mov Disord 1997;12:33–38

Asin KE, Domino EF, Nikkel A, Shiosaki K. The selective dopamine D1 receptor agonist A-86929 maintains efficacy with repeated treatment in rodent and primate models of Parkinson's disease. J Pharmacol Exp Ther 1997;281:454–459

Ballard PA, Tetrud JW, Langston JW. Permanent human parkinsonism due to 1-methyl-4-phenyl-1,2,3,6-tetrahydropyridine (MPTP): seven cases. Neurology 1985;35:949–956

Barbato L, Stocchi F, Monge A, et al. The long-duration action of levodopa may be due to a postsynaptic effect. Clin Neuropharmacol 1997;20:394–401

Ben-Shlomo Y, Churchyard A, Head J, et al. Investigation by Parkinson's disease Research Group of United Kingdom into excess mortality seen with combined levodopa and selegiline treatment in patients with early, mild Parkinson's disease: further results of randomised trial and confidential inquiry. Br Med J 1998;316:1191–1196

Berger K, Breteler MMB, Helmer C, et al. Prognosis with Parkinson's disease in Europe: A collaborative study of population-based cohorts. Neurology 2000;54(Suppl 5):S24–S27

Bernheimer H, Birkmayer W, Hornykiewicz O, et al. Brain dopamine and the syndromes of Parkinson and Huntington. J Neurol Sci 1973;20:415–455

Blanchet PJ, Allard P, Gregoire L, et al. Risk factors for peak dose dyskinesia in 100 levodopa-treated parkinsonian patients. Can J Neurol Sci 1996;23:189–193

Blanchet PJ, Papa SM, Metman LV, et al. Modulation of levodopa-induced motor response complications by NMDA antagonists in Parkinson's disease. Neurosci Biobehav Rev 1997;21:447–453

Blin J, Bonnet A-M, Agid Y. Does levodopa aggravate Parkinson's disease? Neurology 1988;38:1410–1416

Bravi D, Mouradian MM, Roberts JW, et al. Wearing-off fluctuations in Parkinson's disease: contribution of postsynaptic mechanisms. Ann Neurol 1994;36:27–31

Brown RG, Marsden CD. How common is dementia in Parkinson's disease? Lancet 1984;2:1262–1265

Burns RS, Chiueh CC, Markey SP, et al. A primate model of parkinsonism: selective destruction of dopaminergic neurons in the pars compacta of the substantia nigra by N-methyl-4-phenyl-1,2,3,6-tetrahydropyridine. Proc Natl Acad Sci USA 1983;80: 4546–4550

Calne DB, Stern GM, Laurence DR, et al. L-Dopa in postencephalitic parkinsonism. Lancet 1969;1:744–746

Canesi M, Antonini A, Mariani CB, et al. An overnight switch to ropinirole therapy in patients with Parkinson's disease. J Neural Transm 1999;106:925–929

Caraceni T, Scigliano G, Musicco M. The occurrence of motor fluctuations in parkinsonian patients treated long term with levodopa: role of early treatment and disease progression. Neurology 1991;41:380–384

Chase TN, Mouradian MM, Engber TM. Motor response complications and the function of striatal efferent systems. Neurology 1993;43(Suppl 6):S23–S27

Chase TN, Oh JD, Blanchet PJ. Neostriatal mechanisms in Parkinson's disease. Neurology 1998;51:S30–S35

Chase TN, Oh JD, Konitsiotis S. Antiparkinsonian and antidyskinetic activity of drugs targeting central glutamatergic mechanisms. J Neurol 2000;247:36–42

Clarke CE. Does levodopa therapy delay death in Parkinson's disease? A review of the evidence. Mov Disord 1995;10:250–256

Clough CG, Bergmann KJ, Yahr MD. Cholinergic and dopaminergic mechanisms in Parkinson's disease after long-term L-DOPA administration. Adv Neurol 1984; 40:131–140

Colosimo C, Merello M, Hughes AJ, et al. Motor response to acute dopaminergic challenge with apomorphine and levodopa in Parkinson's disease: implications for the pathogenesis of the on-off phenomenon. J Neurol Neurosurg Psychiatry 1996;60: 634–637

Contin M, Riva R, Martinelli P, et al. Effect of meal timing on the kinetic-dynamic profile of levodopa/carbidopa controlled release in parkinsonian patients. Eur J Clin Pharmacol 1998;54:303–308

Crystal HA, Dickson DW, Lizardi JE, et al. Antemortem diagnosis of diffuse Lewy body disease. Neurology 1990;40:1523–1528

Dave M. Clozapine-related tardive dyskinesia. Biol Psychiatry 1994;35:886–887

Davis GC, Williams AC, Markey SP, et al. Chronic parkinsonism secondary to intravenous is injection of meperidine analogues. Psychiatry Research 1979;1: 249–254

de Jong GJ, Meerwaldt JD, Schmitz PIM. Factors that influence the occurrence of response variations in Parkinson's disease. Ann Neurol 1987;22:4–7

de Yebenes JG, Vazquez A, Martinez A, et al. Biochemical findings in symptomatic dystonias. Adv Neurol 1988;50:167–175

Direnfeld LK, Feldman RG, Alexander MP, Kelly-Hayes M: Is L-dopa drug holiday useful? Neurology 1980;30:785–788

Donnan PT, Steinke DT, Stubbings C, et al. Selegiline and mortality in subjects with Parkinson's disease—a longitudinal community study. Neurology 2000;55: 1785–1789

Duvoisin RC, Antunes JL, Yahr MD. Response of patients with postencephalitic parkinsonism to levodopa. J Neurol Neurosurg Psychiatry 1972;35:487–495

Duvoisin RC. Hyperkinetic reactions with L-DOPA. In; Yahr MD, ed. Current Concepts in the Treatment of Parkinsonism. New York: Raven Press, 1974:203–210

Duvoisin RC. Variations in the "on–off" phenomenon. Adv Neurol 1974;5:339–340

Ehringer H, Hornykiewicz O. Verteilung von Noradrenalin und Dopamin (3-Hydroxytryamin) im Gehirn des Menschen und ihr Verhalten bei Erkrankungen des extrapyramidalen Systems. Klin Wschr 1960;38: 1238–1239

Eichhorn TE, Brunt E, Oertel WH. Ondansetron treatment of L-dopa-induced psychosis. Neurology 1996;47:1608–1609

Fabbrini G, Juncos J, Mouradian MM, et al. Levodopa pharmacokinetic mechanisms and motor fluctuations in Parkinson's disease. Ann Neurol 1987;21:370–376

Fabbrini G, Mouradian MM, Juncos JL, et al. Motor fluctuations in Parkinson's disease: Central pathophysiological mechanisms, Part I. Ann Neurol 1988;24: 366–371

Factor SA. The initial treatment of Parkinson's disease. Mov Disord 2000;15:360–361

Fahn S, Barrett RB. Increase of parkinsonian symptoms as a manifestation of levodopa toxicity. Adv Neurol 1979;24:451–459

Fahn S, Chouinard S. Experience with tranylcypromine in early Parkinson's disease. J Neural Transm 1998;(Suppl)52:49–61

Fahn S, Isgreen WP. Long-term evaluation of amantadine and levodopa combination in parkinsonism by double-blind crossover analyses. Neurology 1975;25: 695–700

Fahn S, Rudolph A, Parkinson Study Group. Neurologists' treatment patterns for Parkinson's disease (PD). Mov Disord 1996;11:595

Fahn S, Togasaki D, Chouinard S. MAO-A and -B inhibition with tranylcypromine in early Parkinson's disease: clinical and CSF effects. Mov Disord 1998;13: 148

Fahn S. "On–off" phenomenon with levodopa therapy in parkinsonism: clinical and pharmacologic correlations and the effect of intramuscular pyridoxine. Neurology 1974;24:431–441

Fahn S. The spectrum of levodopa-induced dyskinesias. Ann Neurol 2000;47(Suppl 1):S2–S11

Fahn S. Welcome news about levodopa, but uncertainty remains. Ann Neurol 1998;43:551–554

Fernandez HH, Friedman JH. Punding on L-dopa. Mov Disord 1999;14:836–838

Fox MW, Ahlskog JE, Kelly PJ. Stereotactic ventrolateralis thalamotomy for medically refractory tremor in post-levodopa era Parkinson's disease patients. J Neurosurg 1991;75:723–730

Frankel JP, Lees AJ, Kempster PA, Stern GM. Subcutaneous apomorphine in the treatment of Parkinson's disease. J Neurol Neurosurg Psychiatry 1990;53: 96–101

Friedman JH. Akathisia with clozapine. Biol Psychiatry 1993;33:852–853

Furuya R, Hirai A, Andoh T, et al. Successful perioperative management of a patient with Parkinson's disease by enteral levodopa administration under propofol anesthesia. Anesthesiology 1998;89:261–263

Galvez-Jimenez N, Lang AE. Perioperative problems in Parkinson's disease and their management: Apomorphine with rectal domperidone. Can J Neurol Sci 1996;23:198–203

Gardner DM, Tailor SA, Walker SE, Shulman KI. The making of a user friendly MAOI diet. J Clin Psychiatry 1996;57(3):99–104

Glozman JM, Bicheva KG, Fedorova NV. Scale of quality of life of caregivers (SQLC). J Neurol 1998;245:S39–S41

Growdon JH, Kieburtz K, McDermott MP, et al. Parkinson Study Group. Levodopa improves motor function without impairing cognition in mild non-demented Parkinson's disease patients. Neurology 1998;50:1327–1331

Hamilton ITJ, Gilmore WS, Benzie IFF, et al. Interactions between vitamins C and E in human subjects. Br J Nutr 2000;84:261–267

Hardie RJ, Lees AJ, Stern GM. On–off fluctuations in Parkinson's disease. Brain 1984;107:487–506

Hershey T, Black KJ, Stambuk MK, et al. Altered thalamic response to levodopa in Parkinson's patients with dopa-induced dyskinesias. Proc Natl Acad Sci USA 1998;95:12016–12021

Hillen ME, Sage JI. Nonmotor fluctuations in patients with Parkinson's disease. Neurology 1996;47: 1180–1183

Hoehn MM. Levodopa-induced postural hypotension. Arch Neurol 1975;32:50–51

Horstink MWIM, Zijlmans JCM, Pasman JW, et al. Which risk factors predict the levodopa response in fluctuating Parkinson's disease. Ann Neurol 1990;27:537–543

Hutton JT, Koller WC, Ahlskog JE, et al. Multicenter, placebo-controlled trial of cabergoline taken once daily in the treatment of Parkinson's disease. Neurology 1996;46:1062–1065

Jacobs H, Vieregge A, Vieregge P. Sexuality in young patients with Parkinson's disease: a population based comparison with healthy controls. J Neurol Neurosurg Psychiat 2000;69:550–552

Kagan VE, Fabisiak JP, Quinn PJ. Coenzyme Q and vitamin E need each other as antioxidants. Protoplasma 2000;214:11–18

Kastrup O, Gastpar M, Schwarz M. Acute dystonia due to clozapine. J Neurol Neurosurg Psychiatry 1994; 57:119

Kelly PJ, Ahlskog JE, Goerss SJ, et al. Computer-assisted stereotactic ventralis lateralis thalamotomy with microelectrode recording control in patients with Parkinson's disease. Mayo Clin Proc 1987;62: 655–664

Klawans HL, Goetz C, Bergen D. Levodopa-induced myoclonus. Arch Neurol 1975;32:331–334

Koller WC. Sensory symptoms in Parkinson's disease. Neurology 1984;34:957–959

Kujawa K, Leurgans S, Raman R, et al. Acute orthostatic hypotension when starting dopamine agonists in Parkinson's disease. Arch Neurol 2000;57:1461–1463

Lai CT, Yu PH. Dopamine and L-beta-3,4-dihydroxy-phenylalanine hydrochloride (L-DOPA)-induced cytotoxicity towards catecholaminergic neuroblastoma SH-SY5Y cells—effects of oxidative stress and antioxidative factors. Biochem Pharmacol 1997;53:363–372

Lang AE, Hobson DE, Martin W, Rivest J. Excessive daytime sleepiness and sudden onset sleep in Parkinson's disease: a survey from 18 Canadian movement disorders clinics. Neurology 2001;56(Suppl 3):A307

Langston JW, Ballard P, Tetrud JW, Irwin I. Chronic parkinsonism in humans due to a product of meperidine-analog synthesis. Science 1983;219:979–980

Langston JW, Ballard PA. Parkinsonism induced by 1-methyl-4-phenyl-1,2,5,6-tetrahydropyridine: Implications for treatment and the pathophysiology of Parkinson's disease. Can J Neurosci 1984;11:160–165

Langston JW, Forno LS, Rebert CS, Irwin I. 1-Methyl-4-phenyl-1,2,5,6-tetrahydropyridine causes selective damage to the zona compacta of the substantia nigra in the squirrel monkey. Brain Res 1984;292:390–394

Lees AJ. Comparison of therapeutic effects and mortality data of levodopa and levodopa combined with selegi-line in patients with early, mild Parkinson's disease. Br Med J 1995;311:1602–1607

Lhermitte F, Agid Y, Signoret JL. Onset and end-of-dose levodopa-induced dyskinesias. Arch Neurol 1978;35:261–262

Ling LH, Ahlskog JE, Munger TM, et al. Constrictive pericarditis and pleuropulmonary disease linked to ergot dopamine agonist therapy (cabergoline) for Parkinson's disease. Mayo Clin Proc 1999;74:371–375

Luquin MR, Scipioni O, Vaamonde J, et al. Levodopa-induced dyskinesias in Parkinson's disease: clinical and pharmacological classification. Mov Disord 1992;7: 117–124

Mally J, Stone TW. Improvement in Parkinsonian symptoms after repetitive transcranial magnetic stimulation. J Neurol Sci 1999;162:179–184

Maricle RA, Nutt JG, Valentine RJ, Carter JH. Dose–response relationship of levodopa with mood and anxiety in fluctuating Parkinson's disease: A double-blind, placebo-controlled study. Neurology 1995;45:1757–1760

Marsden CD, Parkes JD, Quinn N. Fluctuations of disability in Parkinson's disease—clinical aspects. In: Marsden CD, Fahn S, eds. Movement Disorders. London: Butterworth Scientific, 1982:96–122

Martinez-Martin P. An introduction to the concept of "quality of life in Parkinson's disease." J Neurol 1998; 245:S2–S6

McDowell FH, Sweet RD. The "on–off" phenomenon. In: Birkmayer W, Hornykiewicz O, eds. Advances in Parkinsonism. Basle: Editiones Roche, 1976:603–612

Melamed E, Bitton V, Zelig O. Episodic unresponsiveness to single doses of L-dopa in parkinsonian fluctuators. Neurology 1986;36:100–103

Mena MA, Pardo B, Paino CL, de Yebenes JG. Levodopa toxicity in foetal rat midbrain neurones in culture—modulation by ascorbic acid. Neuroreport 1993;4:438–440

Merims D, Ziv I, Djaldetti R, Melamed E. Riluzole for levodopa-induced dyskinesias in advanced Parkinson's disease. Lancet 1999;353:1764–1765

Metman LV, Del Dotto P, Blanchet PJ, et al. Blockade of glutamatergic transmission as treatment for dyskinesias and motor fluctuations in Parkinson's disease. Amino Acids 1998;14:75–82

Metman LV, Del Dotto P, Natte R. Dextromethorphan improves levodopa-induced dyskinesias in Parkinson's disease. Neurology 1998;51:203–206

Metman LV, Locatelli ER, Bravi D, et al. Apomorphine responses in Parkinson's disease and the pathogenesis of motor complications. Neurology 1997;48:369–372

Metman LV, van den Munckhof P, Klaassen AAG, et al. Effects of supra-threshold levodopa doses on dyskinesias in advanced Parkinson's disease. Neurology 1997;49:711–713

Montastruc JL, Rascol O, Senard JM, Rascol A. A randomised controlled study comparing bromocriptine to which levodopa was later added, with levodopa alone in previously untreated patients with Parkinson's disease: a five-year follow up. J Neurol Neurosurg Psychiatry 1994;57:1034–1038

Montastruc JL, Rascol O, Senard JM. Treatment of Parkinson's disease should begin with a dopamine agonist. Mov Disord 1999;14:725–730

Mouradian MM, Heuser IJE, Baronti F, Chase TN. Modification of central dopaminergic mechanisms by continuous levodopa therapy for advanced Parkinson's disease. Ann Neurol 1990;27:18–23

Mouradian MM, Heuser IJE, Baronti F, et al. Pathogenesis of dyskinesias in Parkinson's disease. Ann Neurol 1989;25:523–526

Mouradian MM, Juncos JL, Fabbrini G, Chase TN. Motor fluctuations in Parkinson's disease. Ann Neurol 1989;25:633–634

Mouradian MM, Juncos JL, Fabbrini G, et al. Motor fluctuations in Parkinson's disease: central pathophysiological mechanisms, Part II. Ann Neurol 1988;24: 372–378

Muenter MD, Sharpless NS, Tyce GM, Darley FL. Patterns of dystonia ("I-D-I" and "D-I-D") in response to L-dopa therapy of Parkinson's disease. Mayo Clin Proc 1977;52:163–174

Murata M, Kanazawa I. Repeated L-dopa administration reduces the ability of dopamine storage and abolishes the supersensitivity of dopamine receptors in the striatum of intact rat. Neurosci Res 1993;16:15–23

Murata M, Mizusawa H, Yamanouchi H, Kanazawa I. Chronic levodopa therapy enhances dopa absorption: contribution to wearing-off. J Neural Transm 1996;103: 1177–1185

Myllyla VV, Sotaniemi KA, Hakulinen P, et al. Selegiline as the primary treatment of Parkinson's disease—A long-term double-blind study. Acta Neurol Scand 1997;95:211–218

Mytilineou C, Han SK, Cohen G. Toxic and protective effects of L-dopa on mesencephalic cell cultures. J Neurochem 1993;61:1470–1478

Narabayashi H. Surgical approach to tremor. In: Marsden CD, Fahn S, eds. Movement Disorders. London: Butterworth Scientific, 1982:292–299

Nutt JG, Carter JH, Lea ES, Woodward WR. Motor fluctuations during continuous levodopa infusions in patients with Parkinson's disease. Mov Disord 1997; 12:285–292

Nutt JG, Carter JH, Woodward W, et al. Does tolerance develop to levodopa? Comparison of 2-H and 21-H levodopa infusions. Mov Disord 1993;8:139–143

Nutt JG, Woodward WR, Anderson JL. The effect of carbidopa on the pharmacokinetics of intravenously administered levodopa: the mechanism of action in the treatment of parkinsonism. Ann Neurol 1985;18: 527–543

Nutt JG. On–off phenomenon: relation to levodopa pharmacokinetics and pharmacodynamics. Ann Neurol 1987;22:535–540

Obeso JA, Grandas F, Vaamonde J, et al. Motor complications associated with chronic levodopa therapy in Parkinson's disease. Neurology 1989b;39(Suppl 2): 11–19

Obeso JA, Vaamonde J, Grandas F, et al. Overcoming pharmacokinetic problems in the treatment of Parkinson's disease. Mov Disord 1989;4(Suppl 1):S70–S85

Olanow CW, Fahn S, Langston JW, Godbold J. Selegiline and mortality in Parkinson's disease. Ann Neurol 1996;40:841–845

Olanow CW, Myllyla VV, Sotaniemi KA, et al. Effect of selegiline on mortality in patients with Parkinson's disease: a meta-analysis. Neurology 1998;51:825–830

Onofri M, Paci C, Thomas A. Sudden appearance of invalidating dyskinesia-dystonia and off fluctuations after the introduction of levodopa in two dopaminomimetic drug naive patients with stage IV Parkinson's disease. J Neurol Neurosurg Psychiatry 1998;65:605–606

Papa SM, Engber TM, Kask AM, Chase TN. Motor fluctuations in levodopa treated parkinsonian rats: relation to lesion extent and treatment duration. Brain Res 1994;662:69–74

Pardo B, Mena MA, Casarejos MJ, et al. Toxic effects of L-

dopa on mesencephalic cell cultures: Protection with antioxidants. Brain Res 1995;682:133–143

Pardo B, Mena MA, Fahn S, De Yebenes JG. Ascorbic acid protects against levodopa-induced neurotoxicity on a catecholamine-rich human neuroblastoma cell line. Mov Disord 1993;8:278–284

Pearce RKB, Banerji T, Jenner P, Marsden CD. De novo administration of ropinirole and bromocriptine induces less dyskinesia than L-dopa in the MPTP-treated marmoset. Mov Disord 1998;13:234–241

Pederzoli M, Girotti F, Scigliano G, et al. L-Dopa long-term treatment in Parkinson's disease: age-related side effects. Neurology 1983;33:1518–1522

Pfitzenmeyer P, Foucher P, Dennewald G, et al. Pleuropulmonary changes induced by ergoline drugs. Eur Resp J 1996;9:1013–1019

Pfutzner W, Przybilla B. Malignant melanoma and levodopa: is there a relationship? Two new cases and a review of the literature. J Am Acad Dermatol 1997; 37:332–336

Piercey MF, Hoffmann WE, Smith MW, Hyslop DK. Inhibition of dopamine neuron firing by pramipexole, a dopamine D-3 receptor-preferring agonist, comparison to other dopamine receptor agonists. Eur J Pharmacol 1996;312:35–44

Poewe W. Adjuncts to levodopa therapy: Dopamine agonists. Neurology 1998;50 (Suppl 6):S23–S26

Przuntek H, Welzel D, Gerlach M, et al. Early institution of bromocriptine in Parkinson's disease inhibits the emergence of levodopa-associated motor side effects. Long-term results of the PRADO study. J Neural Transm 1996;103:699–715

Rinne UK, Koskinen V, Lonnberg P. Neurotransmitter receptors in the parkinsonian brain. In: Rinne UK, Klingler M, Stamm G, eds. Parkinson's Disease: Current Progress, Problems and Management. Amsterdam: Elsevier/North-Holland Biomedical Press, 1980:93–107

Rivera-Calimlin L, Dujovne CA, Morgan JP, et al. L-Dopa treatment failure: explanation and correction. Br Med J 1970;4:93–94

Rodriguez M, Lera G, Vaamonde J, et al. Motor response to apomorphine and levodopa in asymmetric Parkinson's disease. J Neurol Neurosurg Psychiatry 1994;57: 562–566

Roos RAC, Vredevoogd CB, Vandervelde EA. Response fluctuations in Parkinson's disease. Neurology 1990;40:1344–1346

Sacks OW, Kohl M, Schwartz W, Messeloff C. Side-effects of L-dopa in postencephalic parkinsonism. Lancet 1970;1:1006

Sacks OW. Awakenings. Garden City, NY; Doubleday & Co., 1974

Safferman AZ, Lieberman JA, Pollack S, Kane JM. Akathisia and clozapine treatment. J Clin Psychopharmacol 1993;13:286–287

Sage JI, Duvoisin RC. Sudden onset of confusion with severe exacerbation of parkinsonism during levodopa therapy. Mov Disord 1986;1:267–270

Saunders-Pullman R, Gordon-Elliott J, Parides M, et al. The effect of estrogen replacement on early Parkinson's disease. Neurology 1999;52:1417–1421

Schrag A, Jahanshahi M, Quinn N. How does Parkinson's disease affect quality of life? A comparison with quality of life in the general population. Mov Disord 2000;15:1112–1118

Schuh LA, Bennett JP. Suppression of dyskinesias in advanced Parkinson's disease. 1. Continuous intravenous levodopa shifts dose–response for production of dyskinesias but not for relief of parkinsonism in patients with advanced Parkinson's disease. Neurology 1993:43:1545–1550

Shaunak S, Wilkins A, Pilling JB, Dick DJ. Pericardial, retroperitoneal, and pleural fibrosis induced by pergolide. J Neurol Neurosurg Psychiat 1999;66:79–81

Steele TD, Hodges DB, Levesque TR, Locke KW. D-1 agonist dihydrexidine releases acetylcholine and improves cognitive performance in rats. Pharmacol Biochem Behav 1997;58:477–483

Tan EK, Ondo W. Clinical characteristics of pramipexole-induced peripheral edema. Arch Neurol 2000;57: 729–732

Targum SD, Abbott JL. Efficacy of quetiapine in Parkinson's patients with psychosis. J Clin Psychopharmacol 2000;20:54–60

Tatton WG. Selegiline can mediate neuronal rescue rather than neuronal protection. Mov Disord 1993; 8:S20–S30

Thomas P, Lalaux N, Vaiva G, Goudemand M. Dose-dependent stuttering and dystonia in a patient taking clozapine. Am J Psychiatry 1994;151:1096

Torstenson R, Hartvig P, Langstrom B, et al. Differential effects of levodopa on dopaminergic function in early and advanced Parkinson's disease. Ann Neurol 1997;41:334–340

Turjanski N, Lees AJ, Brooks DJ. In vivo studies on striatal dopamine D1 and D2 site binding in L-dopa-treated Parkinson's disease patients with and without dyskinesias. Neurology 1997;49:717–723

Weiner WJ, Factor SA, Sanchez-Ramos JR, et al. Early combination therapy (bromocriptine and levodopa) does not prevent motor fluctuations in Parkinson's disease. Neurology 1993;43:21–27

Weiner WJ, Koller WC, Perlik S, et al. Drug holiday and management of Parkinson disease. Neurology 1980;30:1257–1261

Weiner WJ. The initial treatment of Parkinson's disease should begin with levodopa. Mov Disord 1999; 14:716–724

Yahr MD. Evaluation of long-term therapy in Parkinson's disease: mortality and therapeutic efficacy. In: Birkmayer W, Hornykiewicz O, eds. Advances in Parkinsonism. Basle: Editiones Roche, 1976:444–455

Zoldan J, Friedberg C, Livneh M, Melamed E. Psychosis in advanced Parkinson's disease: Treatment with ondansetron, a 5-HT3 receptor antagonist. Neurology 1995;45:1305–1308

Parkinsonism Plus Disorders

Madhavi Thomas and Joseph Jankovic

The term "parkinsonism" is used to describe neurological disorders characterized by the presence of cardinal features of tremor, rigidity and bradykinesia in addition to loss of postural reflexes and freezing. The most common cause of parkinsonism is Parkinson's disease (PD), an idiopathic form of parkinsonism caused by degeneration of the substantia nigra. Disorders such as progressive supranuclear palsy (PSP), multiple system atrophy (MSA), corticobasal degeneration (CBD), vascular parkinsonism, and pallidal degeneration have been collectively termed "parkinsonism plus disorders" or "atypical parkinsonism," due to the presence of parkinsonism combined with additional neurological deficits.

Progressive supra nuclear palsy

Definition and history

Progressive supranuclear palsy (PSP) also known as "Steele-Richardson-Olszewski syndrome" is a multisystem degenerative disease characterized by progressive postural instability, falls, vertical and horizontal supranuclear gaze palsy, rigidity, bradykinesia, pseudobulbar palsy and subcortical dementia. Although there were prior reports by Posey (1904) and Spiller (1905), Steele, Richardson and Olszewski first used the term "progressive supranuclear palsy" in 1963 and the following year published nine cases of PSP, including the clinical and pathological findings.[1,2]

Epidemiology, incidence, and age at onset

There are a limited number of epidemiological studies of PSP, but the reported estimated annual incidence rate is 1.39 per 100 000 and prevalence is 0.3 cases per 100 000 population.[3] A study estimating the incidence of PSP in Olmsted county Minnesota found an average incidence rate (new cases per 100 000 person years) of 5.3 for ages 50–99 years. The incidence increased from 1.7 at 50–59 years to 14.7 at age 80–99 years.[4] A large population-based study using currently accepted diagnostic criteria for PSP conducted in the London area found prevalence rates of 6.4 per 100 000.[5] A recent study carried out in UK using a "Russian doll model" of analysis including national, regional and community levels of population survey showed a prevalence range of 1.0 to 6.5 per 100 000 cases for PSP.[6]

Progressive supranuclear palsy is more common in men than women with a sex ratio of 2:1. Age at onset is usually between 55–70 years (mean 63) with the earliest onset being at 45. Interval of progression from onset of illness to assisted walking is 3.1 years, and from onset to chair or bed confinement is 8.2 years.[3]

The mean survival rate is 5.9–6.9 years and the usual cause of death is pulmonary embolism, pneumonia or renal failure.[7] Progressive supranuclear palsy is a disorder of unknown etiology, which is usually sporadic, but can rarely occur as a familial form.[8–10]

Pathology

On autopsy, gross examination of the brain shows normal cortex, atrophy of globus pallidus, thalamus, pontine tegmentum and midbrain. There is evidence of degeneration of substantia nigra, red nucleus, subthalamic nucleus, locus ceruleus and globus pallidus. Pathological studies show characteristic changes with variable neuronal loss and gliosis in association with neurofibrillary tangles and/or neuropil threads. Neuronal degeneration is seen in the basal nucleus of Meynert, mesencephalic tegmentum, locus ceruleus, red nucleus, globus pallidus (both internum and externum), putamen, caudate, subthalamic nucleus, substantia nigra, reticular formation, brainstem-basis pontis, superior colliculi, periaqueductal gray mater, occulomotor nuclei, vestibular nuclei, cerebellum and spinal cord.[1,11–13] Pathological criteria were proposed by Hauw et al.,[14] and the validity and reliability were studied by Litvan et al.[15]

Microscopic examination of the affected regions in the brain of PSP patient shows neurofibrillary tangles (NFT), granulovacuolar degeneration (GVD), gliosis and rare Lewy bodies.[16] Calbindin-D_{28k} immunoreactivity is reduced in the neurons in globus pallidus of patients with PSP and in substantia nigra pars reticulata of patients with striatonigral degeneration[17] which indicates a role for calcium induced cytotoxicity.

Abnormal tau containing astrocytic inclusions are present in basal ganglia and brain stem in patients with PSP.[18–20] Conrad et al., first suggested that changes in tau gene may serve as a genetic marker for PSP and showed that 95% patients were homozygous for the A0/A0 allele with the dinucleotide polymorphism in intron 9 of the tau gene.[18] The A0 allele is seen in 91% patients and the A0/A0 genotype is seen in 84% patients with PSP and in asymptomatic relatives of PSP patients.[19] Extended 5′ tau haplotype with four single nucleotide polymorphisms (SNP's) in tau exons 1, 4A and 8 have 98% sensitivity and 67% specificity, suggesting this is a sensitive marker for sporadic PSP.[20]

Biochemical changes

Biochemical changes in PSP involve dopaminergic, cholinergic, and aminergic systems. There is loss of nigral dopaminergic neurons, decrease in striatal dopamine, decreased dopamine receptor density ($D_2 > D_1$ receptors), decreased cholineacetyl transferase activity, and loss of nicotinic cholinergic receptors in basal forebrain in PSP.[21–26] A 50–60% decrease in neurons expressing GAD-65 (glutamic acid decarboxylase epitope 65) mRNA is seen in caudate, ventral striatum, and both segments of globus pallidus.[24] GABAergic (gamma aminobutyric acid) medium spiny neurons are unaffected in PSP. There is increased glutamate in striatum, pallidum, nucleus accumbens, and in occipital and temporal cortex. Glutathione is increased in substantia nigra of patients with PSP.[25] Cholinergic neurons degenerate in the Edinger Westphal nucleus, rostral interstitial nucleus of Cajal, medial longitudinal fasciculus, superior colliculus, medial dorsal nucleus of thalamus and pedunculopontine nucleus.[21,26] There is slight reduction in the substance-P levels within the substantia nigra. Reduced adenosine triphosphate (ATP) production rate in the mitochondria was shown in a study of muscle mitochondrial function in patients with PSP.[27]

Clinical features

Clinical presentation of PSP is very unique with an immutable stare and rigid "arc de cercle" gait which has also been described as the gait of a "dancing bear" or a "Frankenstein gait." The cardinal clinical manifestations of PSP include supranuclear gaze palsy, pseudobulbar palsy, neck dystonia, parkinsonism, poor equilibrium, falls and subcortical dementia.[1,2,28–30] Patients have a characteristic facial expression with a worried or astonished look.[30] In a review of 126 patients unsteadiness of gait, frequent falling, monotonous speech, loss of eye contact, slowness of movement and mentation, sloppy eating habits, and non-specific visual difficulty were the most typical presenting features.[28] Early onset, presence of falls, slowness, and early downward gaze palsy correlate with rapid progression.[31]

Gait is stiff and broad based. Falls occur especially when PSP patients pivot and lose balance instead of turning en-bloc. Some patients with PSP may present with the syndrome of "pure akinesia" and gait ignition failure. Uncompensated loss of postural reflexes and freezing especially while turning, associated with a peculiar lack of insight into the difficulties with equilibrium (possibly secondary to frontal lobe dysfunction) lead to frequent falling. Litvan et al.,[29] showed that 63% of PSP patients report falls as their initial symptom; dysarthria is the second most common symptom (40% in the first year), and bradykinesia is the third most common problem (22% during the first year).

Visual disturbances include diplopia, blurred vision, burning eyes, and light sensitivity.[32] Patients often lose their ability to read and become sloppy eaters because they cannot see below horizontal level. Some patients also have trouble maintaining eye contact. Impairment of saccades and vertical optokinetic nystagmus (OKN), mild limitation of voluntary down gaze, inability to converge and the presence of square wave jerks are some of the early ocular findings. Initially, the ophthalmoparesis can be overcome by the oculocephalic maneuver but with disease progression and brain stem involvement, vestibuloocular reflexes may be lost suggesting additional nuclear involvement. Involuntary ocular fixation is a rarely mentioned, but typical feature of PSP. This is often manifested when patients walk and change direction. The eyes and head often remain fixated in the original direction while the body is facing in a different direction. Marked reduction of blink rate is also characteristic of PSP.[32,33] Bilateral impairment of the antisaccade task (looking in the direction opposite to a visual stimulus) correlates well with frontal lobe dysfunction in PSP.[34]

Apraxia of eyelid opening, also termed lid freezing can be defined, as a non-paralytic inability to open the eyes at will in the absence of visible contraction of orbicularis oculi. The inability to open eyes may follow either voluntary or involuntary eye closure. Apraxia of eyelid opening is frequently associated with blepharospasm which is the most common form of dystonia (29%) in PSP cases and more than 1/3 cases have apraxia of eyelid opening.[33,35]

Pseudobulbar symptoms are characterized by dysarthria, dysphagia and emotional lability. Dysphagia is seen in 18% of patients within the two years after onset of disease and in 45% of patients by five years.[36] Speech is characterized by spastic, hypernasal, hypokinetic, ataxic, monotonous, and low pitched dysarthria.[37] Some patients have continuous involuntary vocalizations including loud, groaning, moaning or humming sounds.[28]

Axial dystonia is seen in 56% cases and was initially described as "truncal apraxia" but some authors feel that the posturing lacks typical features of a dystonia.[38] Neck extension is felt to be uncommon despite traditional reports in the literature, and occasionally neck flexion is seen. Limb dystonia, oromandibular dystonia, and blepharospasm are some of the manifestations of dystonia seen in PSP patients.[39]

Up to 52% patients have cognitive or behavioral changes in the first year, but rarely at the onset of disease (8%). Cognitive abnormalities typically include relative preservation of short-term memory, cognitive slowing, impairment of executive functioning, subcortical dementia with deficits in tasks requiring sequential movements, conceptual shifts, and rapid retrieval of verbal knowledge. Apathy, disinhibition, dysphoria, anxiety and irritability are the behavioral abnormalities commonly seen in PSP patients.[40–42]

Other clinical features include normal olfaction,[43] tremor (12–16% patients), and rarely arm levitation.[44] Seizures were reported only in one study.[45] Patients have rapid eye movement (REM) sleep abnormalities secondary to loss of 60–80% of the cell bodies within the pedunculopontine tegmental nucleus. Patients with PSP have REM sleep abnormalities including increased latency to the first REM period and a great reduction in duration of REM sleep. Stage II sleep is devoid of sleep spindles and slow wave sleep is accompanied by atonia.[46,47]

Litvan et al.,[48–50] have proposed clinical criteria in 1996. Clinical criteria include possible, probable and definite PSP. The classification is based onset, postural instability, saccadic and eye movement abnormalities and definite PSP can be confirmed only after histopathological examination. They have also identified several exclusionary and inclusionary criteria.[48–50]

Differential diagnosis

The differential diagnosis of PSP includes other neurodegenerative disorders such as PD, MSA, corticobasal ganglionic degeneration (CBD), progressive pallidal degeneration, Lewy-body dementia, and Creutzfeld-Jacob disease. Other disorders such as Wilson's disease, Whipple's disease, and Neimann-Pick disease type C also have some features similar to Parkinson plus syndromes. Features of vascular PSP secondary to multi-infarct state are prior strokes,[51] focal dystonia, and asymmetric and predominantly lower body involvement, cortical and pseudobulbar signs, dementia, bowel and bladder incontinence.[52] In one study, about 81% patients with PSP had hypertension.[53]

Laboratory tests and investigations

Laboratory investigations are rarely helpful in confirming the diagnosis of PSP. Electro-encephalography (EEG) may show variable degree of slowing in the frontal areas. Polysomnography shows lack of sleep spindles and increased latency to first REM period.[46,47] Electro-oculography (EOG) is useful in distinguishing PSP from other parkinsonian diseases; in PSP there is decreased horizontal saccade amplitude and velocity, but normal latency.[54] Acoustic startle responses are abnormal in PSP (but normal in MSA).[55,56] Slow movement and information processing can be evaluated by cortical evoked potentials. Sensory evoked potentials are abnormal.[57] Progressive supranuclear palsy patients have remarkable delayed latencies of P2 and P300 components. Central motor conduction could be impaired in up to 40% patients with PSP in the absence of sensory changes and there is evidence for depression of N30 SEP (Somatosensory evoked potentials) wave in patients with PSP, which is thought to be due to malfunction of cortico-striato-cortical loop.[57,58]

Computed tomography (CT) scans and magnetic resonance imaging (MRI) of the brain show atrophy of midbrain and region around third ventricle in more than half of PSP patients. Thinning of quadrigeminal plate particularly in the superior part on the sagittal MRI, and increased signal in periaqueductal region on proton density MRI support diagnosis of PSP. There is widening of third ventricle with atrophy of mid brain "Eye of the tiger sign," similar to that seen in neurodegeneration with brain iron accumulation type-1 (NBIA-1) is rare.[59,60] Magnetic resonance (MR) spectroscopy findings in patients with PSP are reduced NAA/Cr (N-acetyl aspartate/creatine ratio) in the brain stem, centrum semiovale, and frontal and precentral cortex and reduced NAA/Cho (choline) in the lentiform nucleus. These findings demonstrate the pattern of cortical and subcortical involvement.

[18]F-fluorodopa positron emission tomography (PET) and single photon emission computed tomography (SPECT) scans show reduced uptake in the frontal areas, also seen in other parkinsonian disorders, but in contrast to PD in which the reduced uptake is largely confined to the putamen, the entire striatum (putamen and caudate) are affected in PSP. Also, in contrast to PD, striatal dopamine D_2 receptor density using ligands such as [76]BR bromospiperone or [11]raclopride are also markedly decreased on PET scans.[61] Glucose hypometabolism in the frontal cortex indicates a more widespread degeneration in PSP that extends beyond the nigrostriatal dopaminergic system.[60–65] [123]I Beta carbomethoxy-3-beta-(4-iodophenyl)-tropane (β-CIT) Single photon emission computerized tomography (β-CIT SPECT) findings also support the involvement of the presynaptic nigrostriatal system.[66]

Treatment

Treatment of PSP has been disappointing. No definitive therapies are available. There were several reviews of various medications used in PSP.[67–69] Dopaminergic therapies, such as levodopa and dopamine agonists, are usually transiently or mildly effective in patients with PSP, partly because of loss of postsynaptic dopamine receptors and partly due to involvement of the non-dopaminergic neurotransmitter systems. In a retrospective analysis[67] improvement was seen in about 56% of patients and the rest showed no benefit. The dosage in these studies varied from 1.5–9 gm of levodopa and 750–1500 mg of carbidopa/levodopa. Major adverse events reported were hallucinations secondary to the stimulation of intact mesolimbic and mesocortical pathways. In the absence of more effective therapies patients should undergo at least a two-month therapeutic trial with 1500 mg of levodopa (with carbidopa) per day in three divided doses. Levodopa induced chorea or other forms of dyskinesias are rare, but dystonia may occur. Although bradykinesia may improve slightly, there is usually little or no improvement in balance, ophthalmoparesis, and other features of PSP.

Deprenyl, a selective monoamine oxidase type B inhibitor was studied in small number of patients with no benefit.[67] Amantadine with dopaminergic and anti-glutaminergic properties has been reported to be minimally effective.[67,69] Some patients were reported to have improvement of parkinsonian features and pseudobulbar signs and others had improvement of extra ocular motility. When administered to 46 PSP patients amantadine produced transient therapeutic response in 15%.[67–70]

There are several studies using dopamine agonists for the treatment of PSP. There was no meaningful response to bromocriptine, a D_2 receptor agonist, even at dosages of up to 70 mg in one study. The lack of response has been attributed to the loss of D_2 receptors. Pergolide, a potent D_2, and to a lesser extent D_1 receptor agonist, produced marginal improvement in gait, dysarthria, reduction in overall disability and motor impairment at a dosage of 4 mg per day in a controlled study with three PSP patients.[71] Pergolide is fairly well tolerated but some patients experience postural hypotension, mental status changes, nausea and nasal stuffiness. There was a recent report of use of pramipexole in PSP in six patients with no measurable benefit.[72] Lisuride hydromaleate, a semi-synthetic ergot alkaloid which is a more potent D_2 receptor agonist than bromocriptine and has a serotonin agonist effect, was found ineffective and caused hallucinations in patients with PSP.[73]

Antidepressants have been tried in several studies. Amitryptiline is a potent inhibitor of serotonin uptake and has anticholinergic effects. Overall 28 PSP patients were treated with amitryptiline and 13 were reported to have transient improvement of parkinsonian symptoms and three had improvement of ophthalmoparesis. Amitriptyline is useful for emotional incontinence and has been shown to improve gait and rigidity (three patients had some improvement in gait and rigidity). Amitryptiline has been found to be more beneficial than the less anticholinergic tricyclics like imipramine and desipramine. Fluoxetine and trazodone had no effects on motor function.[74,75]

Methysergide, which is an anti-serotonergic drug with mild dopamine agonist activity, has been reported initially as being helpful with improvement in a few patients. These results were not consistent. Methysergide offered mild benefit for cognitive dysfunction.[76]

Cholinergic approaches were tried because of the relatively selective lesions in the mediodorsal and forebrain cholinergic nuclei and the expected outcome was an improvement in memory. RS-86, a cholinergic agonist, was tried in order to check for beneficial effects on cognitive function. RS-86 is a directly acting mixed M1/M2 muscarinic agonist and neither presynaptic mechanisms nor preformed acetylcholine are needed for its action. RS-86 shortens REM sleep latency and prolongs the duration of REM sleep. There were no effects on motor symptoms or cognitive functions in PSP patients who were treated with RS-86.[77,78]

Physostigmine is a cholinesterase inhibitor and has been shown to improve long term verbal memory and visuospatial attention slightly but worsens gait. This drug has been tried to evaluate response with respect to cognition, spatial attention and dysphagia. Motor function did not change unlike the response noted in PD. There was marginal improvement in cognition, but no beneficial effects on motor function. There was inconsistent improvement in long-term memory. There was no improvement in swallowing with use of physostigmine in an independent study.[79–81] While there is no observed benefit from cholinergic agents, anticholinergics may worsen mental status and gait in PSP. Recently donepezil was tried without any benefit.[82]

Noradrenergic therapies have also been tried with no benefit. Idazoxan is a presynaptic α_2-receptor blocker and was reported to improve gait and postural instability. Overall, effect of idazoxan is to increase norepinephrine (NE) transmission thereby stimulating α-receptors in the sensory motor cortex, cerebellum, brain stem and spinal cord. Idazoxan administered at a dose of 40 mg three times a day

improved mobility, balance and gait but the magnitude of change in Unified Parkinson Disease Rating Scale (UPDRS) scale was small. There was no effect on cognitive function. Side effects consisted mainly of action tremor and transient hypertension and tachycardia, but these were not severe enough to withdraw the medication. Though there was mild benefit from the medication the results of this study are not significant enough to use idazoxan as a treatment option.[83]

Efaroxan is a potent selective α_2-antagonist, the overall effect of which is to increase noradrenaline release from central and post-ganglionic nerve endings. Efaroxan, used in a controlled study involving 16 PSP patients, produced no improvement at a dose of 2 mg three times a day. Furthermore, some patients experienced sympathetic side effects in the form of anxiety and hypertension.[84]

Milacemide (2-n-pentalineaminoacetamide) is a prodrug of glycine. It is metabolized by monoamine oxidase B (MAO-B) to glycineamide and then to glycine. The drug was found to be of no benefit in patients with PSP (and in patients with myoclonus).[85] Nalaxone, given at a dose of 1.2 mg intravenously dissolved in normal saline over one hour, was reported to have nearly abolished the symptoms of dizziness for about two hours in two patients with PSP.[86]

Aniracetam is a cerebral metabolic activator that presumably improves synaptic transmitter efficacy and has acetylcholine like effect. In a trial with two patients with PSP aniracetam was reported to have improved intellectual function in one patient and dystonia in a second patient.[87] There was also some improvement in the speed of volitional movement and balance. Zolpidem was also tried, but no benefit has been observed.[88] Agitation associated with PSP may be at least partially controlled with thiothixine, carbamazepine and trazodone.[89]

Electroconvulsive therapy (ECT) increases the responsiveness of postsynaptic dopamine receptors. When administered to PSP patients there was worsening of symptoms in the first week, but during the second week there was some improvement of motor symptoms with some worsening of cognitive and bulbar function and painful limb dystonia.[90]

Botulinum toxin blocks acetylcholine from presynaptic terminal at the neuromuscular junction and as such it causes local chemodenervation. It has been used successfully in the treatment of dystonia and other conditions associated with involuntary muscle spasms. When injected into the pre-tarsal portion of the orbicularis oculi of the upper eyelid and also in the lower lid it can effectively treat PSP related blepharospasm and even apraxia of eyelid opening. Eyelid crutches may be helpful for patients with poor response to botulinum toxin injections. There are also some surgical options such as orbicularis myectomy, reinsertion of levator aponeurosis, and frontalis suspension. Prisms are useful for diplopia related to dysconjugate gaze, but have not been found helpful in patients with down gaze palsy due to PSP. Artificial tears like methylcellulose eyedrops or polyvinyl eye drops and petrolatum-based ointment at night are helpful in preventing exposure conjunctivitis and keratitis.

Multiple system atrophy

Definition and history

Multiple system atrophy (MSA) is a term used to define an adult onset progressive disorder of unknown etiology clinically characterized by a variable combination of autonomic dysfunction, parkinsonism, cerebellar ataxia, and pyramidal signs.[91] There are three clinical syndromes included under MSA: (1) Shy-Drager syndrome when autonomic dysfunction predominates (MSA-A), (2) striatonigral degeneration when parkinsonian features predominate (MSA-P), and (3) olivopontocerebellar atrophy when cerebellar features predominate (MSA-C).[95]

Historically, the first case of MSA may have been the description of a patient with autonomic symptoms in the 1817 Essay on the Shaking Palsy by James Parkinson. Menzel originally described clinical features in 1891 and Dejerine and Thomas coined the term "Olivopontocerebellar atrophy" in 1900. In the 1950s the term "Shy-Drager syndrome" was used and in the 1960s Adams et al., introduced the term "Striatonigral degeneration."[91] In 1969 Graham and Oppenheimer proposed the term "Multiple System Atrophy."[92]

Etiology of MSA is not known. Multiple system atrophy is usually sporadic and genetic causes are unlikely. An etiological role of environmental toxins like formaldehyde, malathion, and diazinon n-hexane, benzene, methyl-isobutyl-ketone, and pesticides has been suggested in some patients, one with typical pathological features of MSA.[93] Similar to PD, an inverse relationship to smoking has been demonstrated in MSA.[94]

Epidemiology, incidence, and age at onset

Average annual incidence rate is estimated to be three new cases per 100000 person years,[4] and the age adjusted prevalence is estimated to be 4.4 per 100000.[5] MSA affects both men and women equally, though one study showed a slight male preponderance. The age at onset is between 33–76 years (mean 53) with a progressive course resulting in disability within five years; the median survival is 9.5 years.[95] The survival was poorest in MSA-A followed by MSA-P and MSA-C in one study.[96] Ben-Shlomo et al.,[97] found survival to range from 0.5 to 24 years (mean: 6.2); cerebellar features were associated with a marginally better survival. There is a direct correlation between severity of disease and nigro striatal cell loss.[98] Despite marked degeneration in the olivopontocerebellar system, particularly the cerebellar vermis, the cerebellar pathology does not correlate with the presence of cerebellar signs. Some investigators have suggested that an earlier and more severe involvement of the autonomic nervous system indicates poor prognosis.[96]

Pathology

Pathologically, MSA is characterized by selective neuronal loss, gliosis and demyelination affecting substantia nigra, putamen, inferior olives, pons, locus ceruleus, dorsal motor nucleus of vagus, Purkinje cells of cerebellum, intermediolateral cell column and Onuf's nucleus in spinal cord. Both sympathetic and parasympathetic systems are involved. Involvement of at least three areas including the putamen and substantia nigra is required for the pathological diagnosis of MSA.[99,100] The brunt of pathology is in the dorsolateral portion of the striatum, ventrolateral portion of the globus pallidus, and in the substantia nigra.[101] Degeneration of the catecholaminergic neurons in the intermediate reticular formation of the rostral ventrolateral medulla correlates well with autonomic failure in patients with MSA.[102,103] The medial spiny neurons that give rise to both the direct pathway from the striatum to the internal segment of the globus pallidus (GPi), and the indirect pathway from the striatum to the external segment of the globus pallidus (GPe), are affected. Gliosis seems to be much more prevalent in GPe than GPi.

Oligodendroglial cytoplasmic inclusions (GCI), argyrophilic and halfmoon, oval or conical in shape, constitute a subcellular pathological hallmark of MSA.[104,105] Oligodendroglial cytoplasmic inclusions are distributed primarily in the putamen, pallidum, supplementary and primary motor cortex, the reticular formation, basis pontis, the middle cerebellar peduncle, and the cerebellar white matter.[106] Oligodendroglial cytoplasmic inclusions consist of filaments that are 20–30 nm in diameter and contain the classical cytoskeletal antigens ubiquitin, mitogen activated protein kinase (MAP-5), β-crystallin, α-synuclein and tau. The tau profile is different from other disorders like PSP, AD and CBD.[104,106] Oligodendroglial cytoplasmic inclusions are also seen in PSP and CBD, but they are more numerous and more widely distributed in MSA.[107] Recently p39 immunoreactive GCIs have been reported as the pathological hallmark of MSA.[108] A cdk5 (cyclin dependent kinase) activator in oligodendrocytes, p39 induces formation of GCI in the oligodendrocytes. Midkine a neurotrophic factor has also been identified in the GCI indicating a rescue of neurons via oligodendrocyte-axon interaction.[109] Multiple system atrophy lacks the features such as ballooned neurons, NFT, and neuropil threads. Lewy bodies have been seen in about 10% patients with MSA but GCIs are not a feature of PD.[110] α-Synuclein, a 140 amino acid presynaptic protein that is affected by point mutations in some families with PD and is present in Lewy bodies, is also present in GCIs in MSA.[111] α-Synuclein is abundantly expressed in the brain, typically enriched at the presynaptic terminals, and might be implicated in lifelong learning, and memory functions.[112] In mutant mice α-synuclein is shown to be a presynaptic, activity dependent, negative regulator of dopamine transmission.[113] No mutations were identified in α-synuclein in MSA,[114] but α-synuclein in MSA has been shown to be more soluble in detergent compared to other synucleinopathies, which indicates that highly aggregated species are not essential for pathogenesis.[115]

Biochemical changes

Neurochemical changes in MSA involve loss of tyrosine hydroxylase and tetrahydrobiopterin, a co-factor for TH. Concentrations of homovanillic acid (HVA) are decreased in CSF post-synaptic dopamine receptors are lost. Norepinephrine (NE) levels are decreased in locus ceruleus and hypothalamus. There are low levels of 3-MHPG, a major metabolite of NE in cerebrospinal fluid (CSF). Serotonin is decreased in brain and spinal cord and 5-HIAA (5-hydroxy indole acetic acid) is decreased in CSF. Cholineacetyl transferase and acetylcholinesterase are decreased in the cerebral cortex, cerebellar cortex, basis pontis, inferior olive and CSF. Substance P is decreased in both CSF and spinal cord. Low levels of serum erythropoietin have been shown in MSA patients with anemia suggesting that this may be a future therapeutic option.[116]

Clinical features

The following clinical features are felt to be the best predictors of MSA: dysautonomia, poor response to levodopa, speech or bulbar dysfunction, falls and absence of dementia, and of levodopa induced confusion and oromandibular dystonia. Impotence is the most common presenting symptom in men; in women the most common symptom is urinary incontinence.[95]

Parkinsonism is seen in 81% patients with MSA-P subtype. Parkinsonian features, such as bradykinesia and rigidity, are described as symmetric, but some degree of asymmetry may be present. Cerebellar signs are found in about 44% of patients and usually start with limb and gait ataxia with a progression to include other features of cerebellar disease.[117]

Extraocular movement abnormalities include slowing of volitional saccades and some abnormalities of pursuit. Iris atrophy was originally described by Shy and Drager. In a large Japanese family with MSA-C the following neuro-ophthalmologic findings were noted: limitation of upgaze, horizontal gaze impairment, sparing of pupillary reactivity, convergence spasm and loss of vestibulo-ocular reflexes.[118]

Autonomic failure occurs in 78% patients with MSA. Major problems in this category include orthostatic hypotension, bladder and bowel dysfunction, sexual impotence, hyperhidrosis and hypohidrosis. Cognitive dysfunction, consistent with subcortical dementia, is noted in about 25% of patients with MSA; frontal executive dysfunction and emotional lability are also relatively frequent.[119] Multiple system atrophy patients often have a disabling dysarthria, dysphonia and dysphagia. Respiratory problems secondary to laryngeal involvement can occur and the time of onset of this symptom can be variable. Vocal cord paralysis, sleep apnea, and cardiac arrhythmias increase the risk of sudden death.[120] Inspiratory stridor and sighing are very common, particularly in the MSA-P. Sleep disturbance in the form of REM behavior disorder is seen in up to 90% patients with MSA. Snoring, severe obstructive sleep apnea, and oxygen desaturation necessitate aggressive treatment to prevent long-term complications.

Other features suggestive of MSA include early postural instability, hyperactive deep tendon reflexes, anterocollis, and facial dystonia resulting from levodopa therapy. Other movement disorders noted in patients with MSA include rest and action tremor, dystonia, cortical myoclonus, stimulus sensitive focal reflex myoclonus, and hemiballism and chorea, unrelated to dopaminergic therapy.[121]

Diagnostic criteria for MSA have been adapted from consensus statement on diagnosis of MSA.[122] In a review of 188 pathologically proven cases of MSA, 28% patients had all four systems (parkinsonism, cerebellar dysfunction, corticospinal signs, and dysautonomia) involved; 18% had the combination of parkinsonism, pyramidal and autonomic findings, 11% had parkinsonian, cerebellar and autonomic findings, another 11% had parkinsonism and dysautonomia, 10% had only parkinsonism, and parkinsonism was absent in 11% of all cases.[100,122–124] When patients present with parkinsonism alone, without other evidence of MSA, they may be difficult to differentiate from PD during the first six years.[125] Evidence of orthostatic hypotension was present in 68% of patients, but severe orthostatic hypotension was noted in only 15%. Patients with MSA usually develop symptomatic orthostatic hypotension within the first year after onset of symptoms[117] and urinary dysfunction may occur even earlier. In another study of 16 autopsy-proven cases of MSA, Litvan et al.,[125] identified early severe autonomic failure, absence of cognitive impairment, early cerebellar symptoms, and early gait problems as the best predictors of the diagnosis of MSA. In a study designed to validate the clinical criteria for MSA, the accuracy was best when at least six of eight of the following features were present: sporadic adult onset, dysautonomia, parkinsonism, pyramidal signs, cerebellar signs, no levodopa response, no cognitive dysfunction, or no downward gaze palsy.[125]

Differential diagnosis

Differential diagnosis of MSA includes other parkinsonism plus syndromes such as PSP and CBD that have certain specific features that help identify the disease. Other diseases like spinocerebellar ataxia could be difficult to distinguish especially when dealing with olivopontocerebellar atrophy (OPCA). Genetic testing and other features of MSA like autonomic involvement and cognitive dysfunction would be helpful.

Laboratory tests and investigations

Investigations for MSA include neuroimaging studies and tests for autonomic dysfunction. Several diagnostic tests for autonomic dysfunction are used to help in the diagnosis of MSA. Liquid meal, consisting chiefly of glucose and milk, markedly reduces blood pressure in patients with MSA but not in those with PD.[126–129] In addition to the tests of autonomic function, patterns of plasma levels of catecholamines and their metabolites may be helpful in differentiating the various forms of autonomic failures.[129–133] Tilt table testing is very useful in detecting early autonomic dysfunction. There is minimal or absent NE (norepinephrine) despite drop of blood pressure after tilting head-up or upright on the tilt test in patients with MSA. Clonidine increases growth hormone (GH) levels in normal controls and in those with primary autonomic failure, but this is not seen in patients with MSA. The reliability of the clonidine-GH test, however, has not been fully assessed.[133] Patterns of plasma catecholamine levels and their metabolites may be helpful in differentiating various forms of autonomic failure.

Studies primarily designed to localize the site of autonomic impairment include investigation of neurogenic bladder,[134,135] sphincter electromyography (EMG) and other investigations designed to test the integrity of the autonomic nervous system. Neurogenic sphincter EMG, however, can be also seen in other disorders, including PD, PSP, Huntington's disease and a variety of common urological problems. Sphincter EMG is a useful ancillary study in MSA and denervation and reinnervation are recorded in the external urethral and rectal sphincter on EMG.[136]

In a study comparing polysomnograms of seven patients with MSA-A to seven control patients, significant obstructive sleep apnea without oxygen desaturation was seen in four of the five non-tracheotomized MSA-A patients; three of these patients later died suddenly during sleep.[137] In a more recent study, Plazzi et al.,[138,139] demonstrated that 90% of MSA patients experience some form of REM sleep behavioral disorder. While somatosensory, visual, and auditory evoked responses are often abnormal, motor evoked potentials are usually normal.[140]

Magnetic resonance imaging in patients with MSA sometimes reveals areas of hypointensity in the striatum and linear hypertensity along the lateral border of the posterolateral putamen on T2-weighted images. The increased signal on T2 may correspond to activated microglia. Hyperintense signal is also frequently present in the pons and is known as the "hot-cross bun sign." Computed tomography and MRI scans in patients with MSA-C typically show pancerebellar and brainstem atrophy, enlarged fourth ventricle and cerebellopontine angle cisterns, and demyelination of transverse pontine fibers on T2-weighted MRI images. Using volumetric MRI atrophy related changes in basal ganglia, brainstem and cerebellum have been quantified and patients with MSA-P can be distinguished from idiopathic PD.[141–144]

Using proton magnetic resonance spectroscopy, Davie et al.,[145] showed a significant reduction in the N-acetylaspartate (NAA)/creatine ratio from the lentiform nucleus in six of seven patients with SND and in only one of nine with PD. Similar abnormalities were also found in some patients with OPCA and most likely reflect regional neuronal loss. Further

studies are needed to determine whether this technique can reliably differentiate between MSA and Parkinson's disease. Single photon emission computed tomography (SPECT) studies including [123]I β-CIT SPECT and IBZM-SPECT show decreased striatal binding, but are not helpful in identifying patients with early MSA. The reduced ^{11}C-diprenorphine uptake suggests that, in addition to involvement of the nigrostriatal projection, some MSA patients have a loss of intrinsic striatal neurons that contain pre- and post-synaptic mu, kappa, and delta opioid receptors.[66,146]

Positron emission tomography scanning has revealed decreased striatal and frontal lobe metabolism and a reduction in D2 receptor density in the striatum.[147–150] Using ^{18}F fluorodeoxyglucose (FDG), ^{18}F fluorodopa (FDOPA) and ^{11}C raclopride (RACLO) PET scans, the combination of FDG and RACLO is felt to reliably differentiate between MSA and PD, but PET scans alone cannot distinguish between the different forms of parkinsonism.[152] There is significant reduction of specific binding to the type 2 vesicular monoamine transporter (VMAT2) with PET and ^{11}C dihydrotetrabenazine as a VMAT2 ligand in striatal monoaminergic pre-synaptic terminal of patients with MSA.[146–153]

Recently cardiac MIBG [^{123}I-metaiodobenzoguanidine] scintigraphy was shown to be unaffected with a normal heart/mediastinum ratio in patients with MSA compared to patients with idiopathic PD.[154] Using PET scan technology to measure 6-[^{18}F] fluorodopamine-derived radioactivity in myocardium, Goldstein et al.,[155] found normal rates of cardiac spillover of norepinephrine and normal production of levodopa, dihydroxyphenyl-glycol, and dihydroxyphenylacetic acid suggestive of intact cardiac sympathetic terminals in patients with SDS (Shy-Drager syndrome). This is in contrast to absent radioactivity in patients with PAF (primary autonomic failure), indicating loss of postganglionic sympathetic terminals in this peripheral autonomic disorder. The value of this test in diagnosing SDS, however, has been questioned since both sympathetic and parasympathetic failure have been associated with MSA-A.[156]

Treatment

Non-pharmacological Several pharmacological and physiological methods are available for symptomatic treatment in patients with MSA. There are various precipitating factors for orthostatic hypotension including sudden head up posture change, warm weather, hot bath, straining at micturition and defecation, exercise, postprandial state, especially after a heavy carbohydrate meal, alcohol and medications like antihypertensives.

Avoidance of extreme heat (air and water temperature), alcohol, large meals, getting up rapidly and straining excessively and increase sodium and fluid intake are measures patients can follow at home. Use of compressive stockings (patient's may find this uncomfortable) and sleeping in a reverse Trendelenburg position to increase renin secretion is useful but may be uncomfortable. Patients should be advised to take small frequent meals, have a regular exercise program utilizing the horizontal position like swimming or rowing. Elastic stockings and modified abdominal binders are uncomfortable and patient compliance tends to be a problem with these measures.[156] Patients should be encouraged to use walkers and wheelchairs in order to prevent falls.

Pharmacological   There are several medications that are available for treatment of autonomic dysfunction (Table 232.1). Fludrocortisone is the first medication which is useful and its side effects are few at low doses. It expands plasma volume and sensitizes vascular receptors to NE. It is used in a dose of 0.1–0.3 mg at night. Ephedrine may also be used in a dose of 15–45 mg three times daily, but when taken late in the day it may cause insomnia. Side effects are tremor, decreased appetite, and urinary retention.[156] Indomethacin has been used with success at dosages of 50 mg three times a day, but its mechanism in the treatment of orthostatic hypotension is not well understood. Desmopressin is given as a nasal spray and it acts on renal tubular vasopressin-2 receptors and is useful in nocturnal hypotension and nocturnal

polyuria in patients with autonomic dysfunction. It is given intranasally at 10-40 mcg or orally at a dose of 100–400 mcg per day. Side effects of this medication include hyponatremia and water intoxication. Yohimbine, another α_2 agonist that increases plasma catecholamines and blocks peripheral presynaptic α_2 receptors, has been shown to be useful in MSA.[156]

Of the various agents used in the treatment of orthostatic hypotension, midodrine has been best studied. Midodrine has an active metabolite desglymidodrine, which is an α_1 agonist and a vasoconstrictor with an excellent safety profile and without CNS or cardiac effects. Beneficial effects of the drug may be due to reduction of venous pooling in the legs; it has no effect on splanchnic circulation.[157,158] Used in a dosage of 5–10 mg three time per day it effectively controls orthostatic hypotension. Side effects include pruritus of the scalp, urinary hesitancy and retention. Octreotide, a medication initially used for postprandial hypotension, has been shown to be more helpful when used in combination with midodrine in treating orthostatic hypotension. Octreotide is used at a dose of 25–50 mcg subcutaneously and is injected half an hour before meals. When used in combination, midodrine is taken 1–2 hours before giving the octreotide

Table 232.1   Medications for autonomic dysfunction in MSA[156]

Medication and category	Additional mechanism of action
I. Fluid and sodium retention, and sensitization of alpha adrenergic receptors	Fludrocortisone and prednisone also inhibit extraneuronal catecholamine uptake and indomethacin also blocks presynaptic inhibitory adrenergic receptor and decreases circulatory vasodilator proteins
Fludrocortisone	
Prednisone	
Indomethacin	
II. Alpha agonists	
Ephedrine	Indirectly acting sympathomimetic
Amphetamine	Sympathomimetic, and CNS stimulant
Midodrine	None
Clonidine	None
Methylphenidate	CNS stimulant
Phenylephrine	No additional mechanism
III. Blockade of presynaptic adrenergic receptor	
Mianserin	Blockade of neuronal uptake
Yohimbine	None
IV. Beta blockers	
Propranolol	Blockade of neuronal uptake
Pindolol	Intrinsic sympathomimetic activity
V. Increase norepinephrine synthesis	
L-threo-DOPS	None
VI. Noradrenergic vasoconstrictor	
Dihydroergotamine	None
Vasopressin	None
VII. Ganglionic stimulation	
Caffeine	CNS stimulant
VIII. Dopamine receptor blocker	
Metoclopramide	None

Medications are categorized based on their primary mechanism of action. Additional mechanisms are listed for each medication. CNS, central nervous system.

injection. Octreotide is a splanchnic and systemic vasoconstrictor which increases cardiac output. Octreotide does not suppress orthostatic hypotension but increases duration of upright posture maintenance. Both midodrine and octreotide act synergistically in postprandial and postural hypotension. Side effects of octreotide include loose bowel movements or diarrhea, decreased pancreatic enzyme function. Patients who take octreotide need to be on pancreatic enzyme supplements.[159,160] 3,4 DL threo DOPS, a synthetic NE precursor, increases NE levels and thus increases blood pressure. Initially studied in postprandial hypotension 3,4 DL threo DOPS was found to be useful by increasing systolic and diastolic blood pressure in supine and upright positions and preventing fall in blood pressure in response to tilting. At a dose of 1000 mg per day no side effects were observed in the study except for supine hypertension.[161,162] This drug, however, is not yet readily available in the USA.

Levodopa has been used in several MSA patients in an attempt to treat parkinsonian features. Three types of levodopa responsiveness were noted in MSA: a short duration motor improvement with associated "on" period dyskinesias, dyskinesias without any motor improvement, and a delayed deterioration of motor status over several weeks after withdrawal of levodopa including bulbar dysfunction. In this group of patients there was a rapid restoration of motor function following re-introduction of levodopa. This variable pattern of response to levodopa is unlike the response seen in PD. Over 90% fail to maintain symptomatic benefit from levodopa into the advances stages of the disease. Orofacial dyskinesias, usually in a form of oromandibular dystonia, were seen in 50% patients treated with levodopa. One possible explanation for this poor responsiveness is that striatal degeneration results in loss of postsynaptic dopamine receptors. In addition to nigrostriatal degeneration, there is also involvement of putaminal output pathway to globus pallidus and substantia nigra. This pathway is a common component of both the motor loop of the corticobasal circuit and the lateral nigrostriatal loop.

Dopamine agonists have not been well studied in MSA.[163–167] Yohimbine, an α_2 agonist that increases plasma catecholamines and blocks peripheral presynaptic α_2 receptors, has been shown to be useful in MSA.[168] Amantadine has been studied in patients with OPCA at a dosage of 200 mg per day with mixed results.[169]

On urodynamic testing patients with MSA have three types of urinary dysfunction. They have defects in filling phase (63–74%), voiding phase (27–79%) and post-void residuals (74%). There are α-adrenergic receptors in bladder neck and posterior urethra. Impaired sphincter relaxation at this location may be responsible for voiding difficulties and large amount of residuals. Prazosin and moxisylate are specific antagonists of these α-adrenergic receptors. In a controlled study done in 49 patients there was improvement in symptoms in 47.6% in prazosin group and

53.6% in the moxisylate group. Orthostatic hypotension was seen in about 23% in prazosin group and 11% in moxisylate group. More than 35% patients had reduction in residual volume and there was improvement in urinary urgency, frequency and incontinence. The dosage used was prazosin 1 mg and moxisylate 10 mg three times a day in an oral form.[170] Patients have detrusor hyperreflexia due to loss of inhibition of input into the pontine micturition center. Management of detrusor hyperreflexia is difficult but it may be managed by intermittent catheterization either by the patient or his or her caregiver.[171] Botulinum toxin injections into the bladder wall may provide relaxation of the bladder and an increase in the bladder capacity.[172] Oxybutynin is also useful in this situation. Measurement of post void residual is recommended before starting an anticholinergic agent. If there is a poor response to medication, urological evaluation for urinary stones or some other structural lesion must be considered. Frequent findings in patients with MSA are early onset of anorectal dysfunction and low resting anal pressure, decreased voluntary contractility, paradoxical anal contraction or insufficient relaxation. Patients benefit from a regular bowel regimen.

Patients with MSA with voice change or difficulties with breathing must have a thorough ear, nose and throat (ENT) evaluation. Vocal cord paralysis may result from involvement of nucleus accumbens but has not been pathologically proven. Vocal cord palsy with resultant laryngeal stridor is a potential complication for patients with MSA. There are several procedures which can be used instead of tracheostomy and its complications for patients who have vocal cord abductor paralysis. The procedures available are arytenoidectomy, cordectomy, cord lateralization, laryngeal re-innervation. Eventually patients may require a tracheostomy.[173–174] Recently carbon dioxide laser arytenoidectomy has been reported as a treatment in a patient with MSA (Shy-Drager syndrome).[175]

Atrial pacemakers have been tried in a few patients, but have not been found to be very effective. A bionic baroreflex system has been studied to be useful in animal models of baroreflex failure and hopefully may undergo further studies in future for autonomic dysfunction refractory to medical management.[176]

Corticobasal ganglionic degeneration
Definition and history

Corticobasal ganglionic degeneration or corticobasal degeneration (CBD) is a term used to describe a syndrome with marked asymmetry of involvement, focal rigidity, dystonia, ideomotor apraxia, gait and speech apraxia, coarse rest and action tremor, cortical myoclonus, cortical sensory deficit and parkinsonism. Rebeiz, Kolodny, and Richardson[177,178] first described CBD in three patients with asymmetric akinetic-rigid syndrome with a dystonic and apraxic arm with tremor and myoclonus. In addition, the patients also had sensory symptoms and sensory findings in the form of absence of position sense in the affected limb. These patients were found at autopsy to have "corticodentatonigral degeneration with neuronal achromasia." Pathologically they had frontoparietal atrophy, neuronal loss, gliosis and achromasia of neurons (swelling of neurons with resistance to staining). Gibb and co-workers[179] described similar cases and coined the term corticobasal degeneration. In their description three patients had a progressive disease with clinical resemblance to progressive supranuclear palsy and pathological features of Pick's disease. They identified neuronal inclusions which were named corticobasal inclusions. Both these classic descriptions identify similarities to other disorders most importantly Pick's disease and PSP. Corticobasal degeneration is also known as cortical-basal ganglionic degeneration[180] and cortico-nigral degeneration with neuronal achromasia.[181]

Epidemiology, incidence, and age at onset

Corticobasal degeneration is a rare disorder with age at onset being 60.9 ± 9.7 years (range 40–76).[182] In a study by Riley et al.,[180] mean age of onset was 60 years (range 51–71). In a study of 14 patients the age of onset was 63 ± 7.7 years.[183] The youngest patient reported is 40 years for a clinically diagnosed case and 45 years for a pathologically diagnosed case. Men and women are both affected and an increased incidence ratio in men and women of 3:2 was noted[184] while others reported a female preponderance. Corticobasal degeneration follows a progressive course with death at 5–10 years (7.9 ± 2.6) after onset.[183] There are no studies to assess the incidence of this disease but a calculated incidence was suggested to be 0.62–0.92 per 100 000 per year.[185] Corticobasal degeneration is a sporadic disease, but there may be a certain genetic predisposition in the tau gene. Other risk factors such as toxins have not been investigated to date.

Pathology and biochemical findings

Gross pathological examination in CBD brain shows asymmetric narrowing of cortical gyri most marked in the parasaggital regions. Superior frontal gyrus is more involved than middle and inferior frontal gyri. Temporal and occipital lobes are spared.[184,186] There is thinning of anterior part of corpus callosum and attenuation of anterior limb of internal capsule, degeneration of the basal ganglia, including the substantia nigra (SN). There is loss of neuromelanin in substantia nigra and atrophy of midbrain tegmentum, with attenuation of medial third of cerebral peduncles.[179,187–189] Rarely hydrocephalus ex-vacuo, dilatation of aqueduct of sylvius, atrophy of corpus callosum are noted on autopsy.[190]

Pathological diagnosis of CBD is based on the following microscopic features which include cortical degeneration with tau positive and ubiquitin negative intraneuronal inclusions, but without neuritic plaques or NFT in pyramidal neurons layers 4 and 5. Presence of numerous ballooned achromatic neurons, but no evidence of Pick bodies, and presence of glial cell

cytoplasmic inclusions. There is severe substantia nigra cell loss with pale inclusions and occasional basophilic inclusions, but no Lewy bodies or neurofibrillary tangles (NFT). The residual neurons show globose NFT, which are called "corticobasal bodies." But there is no clear difference between NFT and corticobasal bodies. Ballooned neurons (chromatolytic, achromasic) are seen in anterior cingulate gyrus, insular cortex, amygdala, claustrum, thalamus, subthalamic nucleus, and red nucleus.[184,186] Ballooned neurons are immunopositive for phosphorylated neurofilaments, anti-β crystallin, HSP 27 (heat shock protein), ubiquitin but negative for α-synuclein.[177,186,191] While ballooned neurons are not specific for CBD, tau-containing distal astrocytic processes producing "astrocytic plaques" have been suggested by Feany and Dickson[188] to be a distinctive pathological feature of CBD. Ballooned neurons are also found in Pick's disease, PSP, Alzheimer's dementia (AD), Creutzfeldt-Jacob disease (CJD), and amyotrophic lateral sclerosis (ALS).[1,191]

These cortical plaques, which are amyloid and microglia-negative, represent clusters of miliary-like tau positive structures within the distal processes of the astrocytes. Neurofibrillary tangles in this disorder are identical to those seen in AD and PSP.[192–194] Neuropil contains assortment of tau immunoreactive cell processes. Oligodendroglial cytoplasmic inclusions (GCI) are negative for tau, but positive for ubiquitin, α-synuclein. Coiled bodies, which are found in oligodendroglia, are positive for tau.[195] Biochemical findings include normal acetyl transferase unlike Alzheimer's dementia.

Abnormal phosphorylation of tau is not specific for CBD; it can be seen in a variety of neurodegenerative disorders. In the CBD brain, however, tau accumulates as two polypeptides of 64 and 68 kDA which are not recognized by antibodies specific to the adult tau sequences encoded by exons 3 and 10 of the tau gene.[189,196,197] Tau immunostains usually show granular neuronal deposits, neuropil threads, and glial inclusions.[192,195] Di Maria et al.,[199] investigated the role of tau gene in CBD and were unable to identify any mutations. However, there was an over expression of the A0 allele in the CBD cases compared to controls and the haplotype H1 was found in 91% cases of CBD. These results indicate that tau gene plays an important role in pathogenesis of sporadic forms of CBD similar to PSP.

A relationship between CBD, Pick's disease and PSP is suggested by the presence of ballooned neurons and nigral basophilic inclusions, usually present in all three disorders. Though clinically and pathologically similar, there are some distinguishing pathological features.[200] Families with clinical features of Pick's disease and the pathological picture of CBD have been described.[201] Some patients with clinical presentation consistent with frontotemporal dementia (FTD) have been found to have CBD at autopsy.[202] The overlap in clinical and pathological features between CBD, PSP and Pick's disease has been a topic of recent reviews.[184,203,204]

Dopamine concentration is reduced in the CBD brains throughout the striatum and SN when compared to age-matched controls.[205] Dopamine is decreased in basal ganglia. It is unknown if any other neurotransmitter abnormalities are involved in this disease.

Clinical features

Typical clinical presentation of CBD is in the sixth or seventh decade with a slowly progressive unilateral jerky or tremulous, akinetic-rigid, dystonic or alien limb with dementia. The most striking features of CBD include marked asymmetry of involvement, focal rigidity and dystonia with contractures, hand, gait and speech apraxia, coarse rest and action tremor, cortical myoclonus, cortical sensory deficit and parkinsonism.[196,197] Other features include language disturbances and early speech alterations, frontal lobe symptomatology, depression, apathy, irritability and agitation.[206] Riley and Lang[204,205] proposed diagnostic criteria for clinical diagnosis of CBD based on predominance of pyramidal and basal ganglia signs.

The asymmetric onset differentiates CBD from most other neurodegenerative disorders. Asymmetric hand clumsiness was the most common presenting symptom, noted at onset in 50% of the patients.[183] At the time of the first neurological visit, about three years after the onset, the following signs were present: unilateral limb rigidity (79%), bradykinesia (71%), ideomotor apraxia (64%), postural imbalance (45%), unilateral limb dystonia (43%), and cortical dementia (36%). In a series of 147 cases collected from eight centers, the following features were most common: parkinsonism (100%), higher cortical dysfunction (93%), dyspraxia (82%), gait disorder (80%), dystonia (71%), tremor (55%), myoclonus (55%), alien limb (42%), cortical sensory loss (33%), and dementia (25%).[206,207]

In CBD the common movement disorders are akinesia, rigidity, postural instability, limb dystonia, cortical myoclonus, and postural/intention tremor. Cortical signs, such as cortical sensory loss, apraxias (ideational and ideomotor), and the "alien limb" phenomenon have been well described.[205] Ideomotor apraxia, possibly secondary to involvement of the supplementary motor area (SMA), is the most typical form of apraxia.[205,206] Limb contractures, often preceded by the "alien" hand phenomenon, are common.[208–210] The anterior or motor alien hand syndrome must be differentiated from sensory or posterior syndrome associated with a lesion in the thalamus, splenium of corpus callosum, and temporal-occipital lobe. In some cases of CBD alien hand phenomenon is associated with spontaneous arm levitation.

Best predictors for early diagnosis of CBD are asymmetric limb dystonia, parkinsonism, ideomotor apraxia, and absence of balance or gait abnormalities.[211,212] During the later stages of the illness the features which are predictive are delayed onset of balance and gait disturbances, ideomotor apraxia, early cognitive disturbance and focal myoclonias.

Stimulus sensitive myoclonus and moderate frontal subcortical deterioration are characteristic of CBD.

Tremor is mainly a postural and intention tremor and irregular and jerky with a frequency of 6–8 Hz. It may evolve into stimulus sensitive myoclonus. Focal myoclonus, usually involving one arm, present at rest and exacerbated by voluntary movement or in response to sensory stimulation, resembles typical cortical myoclonus, but differs in several features. In contrast to the typical reflex cortical myoclonus which is characterized by long latency (50 msec in hand), enlarged somatosensory evoked responses (SEP) and cortical discharge preceding the movement the reflex myoclonus associated with CBD is usually not associated with enlarged SEP and has shorter duration (40 msec).[213–215] This suggests that the characteristic short-latency reflex myoclonus in CBD represents enhancement of a direct sensory-cortical pathway, whereas the more typical reflex cortical myoclonus involves abnormal sensory-motor cortical relays.[216]

Patients with CBD have asymmetric limb dystonia with the arm more frequently affected. Head, neck, trunk or lower extremity dystonia is less common. Dystonia is associated with rigidity, apraxia, alien limb phenomenon and cortical sensory loss in the affected limb. As dystonia advances patients develop fixed postures or contractures. Dystonia of the upper extremity shows flexion at the hand and forearm, adduction at the shoulder, flexion of the fingers at the metacarpophalangeal joints, extended or flexed at the proximal and distal interphalangeal joints, and variable degrees of postures with or without associated contractures. Pain with dystonia is seen in approximately 40% cases and is associated with contractures.[186,217,218] Akinesia, rigidity and apraxia are the most common findings during the course of CBD occurring in over 90% cases within the first three years of illness.[189,205] Rigidity can reach extreme proportions. Usually arms are more affected than legs. In milder forms rigidity is indistinguishable from dystonic rigidity seen in PD.[182,205] Less frequently patients can present with combined arm and leg involvement, gait disorder with postural instability, dysarthria, dysphasia, orofacial dyspraxia, loss of facial expression, unilateral painful paresthesias, cortico spinal tract signs, and behavioral problems.[182,184,186] Apraxia is usually in the form of ideomotor, ideational or limb kinetic apraxia. Ideational apraxia is observed in the later stages of the disease or in patients with dementia and language dysfunction at presentation.[208,209]

Cognitive problems show a pattern different from that seen in AD. Patients have sparing of consolidation processes of explicit memory, which is normally controlled by the hippocampus. They have dramatic impairment of performance on motor and gesture organization. Overall, cognitive abnormalities follow a subcortico-frontal pattern of dementia associated with gesture disorders and this is considered to be relatively specific for CBD.[219,220] Other neuropsychological problems like depression, apathy, irritability, agitation and frontal lobe-like behavior are seen in these patients and some patients have obsessive compulsive disorder.[219] A recent study showing dementia as a common presentation of CBD[221] is contrary to our clinical observation of dementia as a relatively late manifestation. The neuropsychological studies show a pattern of deficits different from that seen in PSP or AD. Corticobasal ganglionic degeneration patients perform better on tests of immediate and delayed recall of verbal material and poorly on tests of praxis, finger tapping speed, and motor programming.[222] The CBD patients have prominent deficits on tests of sustained attention/mental control and verbal fluency, and mild deficits on confrontation naming similar to AD.[223] The spectrum of neuropsychological deficits in CBD is broadening.[196] Depression occurs in 73% patients, 40% patients have apathy, irritability is seen in 20% and agitation in 20% patients diagnosed with CBD.[223]

Many patients with CBD have aphasia in the form of anomic, Broca's, and transcortical motor aphasia.[224,225] Patients have swallowing difficulties and dysarthria, oral apraxia and apraxia of speech. Patients with CBD have a pattern of better response to non-respiratory oral gestures than respiratory oral gestures. Patients also exhibit oculomotility disturbance particularly manifested by impaired convergence and vertical and horizontal gaze.[226] In contrast to PSP, the vertical saccades are only slightly impaired in CBD and usually only involve upward gaze; furthermore, there is a marked increase in horizontal saccade latency in CBD which correlates well with an "apraxia score."[226]

Differential diagnosis

Differential diagnosis of CBD is mainly PSP, PD, and FTDP-17. Usually a family history of a similar disorder and autosomal dominant inheritance would suggest FTDP-17. There are clinical and pathological similarities between PSP and CBD, the CBD patients, however, have much more marked asymmetry in their motor deficits, less severe ophthalmoparesis, and more prominent apraxia and myoclonus. A combination of dementia with an apractic limb and involuntary movements should prompt the clinician to seek further supportive evidence for the diagnosis of CBD.

Laboratory tests and investigations

Computed tomography scans show asymmetrical parietal lobe atrophy or asymmetric frontoparietal atrophy lobe atrophy corresponding to the most affected side which helps to differentiate CBD from PSP.[205,227] Magnetic resonance imaging scans may show "eye of tiger" signs, which is more typically seen in NBIA-1 (neurodegeneration with brain iron accumulation type-1).[228] There is atrophy of the mid-portion of corpus callosum, which correlates with cognitive impairment and abnormalities on PET scans. In a clinical-radiological study of eight patients with CBD compared to 36 controls, Yamauchi et al.,[229] found atrophy of the corpus callosum, especially the middle portion, which correlated with cognitive impairment and cerebral cortical metabolism measured by ^{18}F-fludeoxyglucose PET. The PET scans show reduced ^{18}[F] fluorodopa uptake in the caudate and putamen, and markedly asymmetrical cortical hypometabolism especially in the superior temporal and inferior parietal lobe.[230–232] Corticobasal ganglionic degeneration patients have been shown to have a global reduction of oxygen and glucose metabolism (fluorodeoxyglucose) most prominent in the cerebral cortex contralateral to the most affected limb and a decrease in metabolism in the thalamus.[233] There is corresponding reduction in the cerebral blood flow (CBF) most evident in the frontoparietal, medial frontal and temporoparietal regions.[234–241] Fluorodopa PET scans show reduced uptake in caudate, putamen and asymmetric cerebral cortical hypometabolism in the superior temporal and inferior parietal lobe and in putamen and thalamus.[230,235]

Neurophysiological studies are consistent with cortical myoclonus except in some unusual cases where there is either parietal atrophy or pathological hyperexcitability of the motor cortex. In two CBD patients with myoclonus SEP showed reduced $N_2 0$ amplitudes but without giant SEP.[242] Although the other neurophysiological studies were consistent with cortical reflex myoclonus, the unusual absence of SEP may be explained by either cortical parietal atrophy or by pathological hyperexcitability of the motor cortex due to a loss of inhibitory input from the sensory cortex.[243]

Treatment

Unfortunately no definitive treatments are available for CBD. In a study with review of treatment of 147 patients with CBD, 92% patients were tried on dopaminergic agents and 87% were on a combination of levodopa and carbidopa; 25% received a dopamine agonist and 20% received selegiline, which is a MAO-B inhibitor, and 16% patients were on amantadine. Other medications used included benzodiazepines, anticholinergics, baclofen, antidepressants, neuroleptics, propranolol, anticonvulsants, and botulinum toxin injections.[244,245] Levodopa has been shown to be of some benefit with about 24% patients showing some improvement in a retrospective analysis. No improvement was seen in 71%, and 5% had side effects with worsening of parkinsonian features, dystonia, myoclonus or gait disturbance. Dosage was between 100–2000 mg of levodopa with a mean dosage of 300 mg per day of levodopa. Combination of levodopa-carbidopa produced improvement in about 26% patients. No patient experienced drug related worsening of higher cortical functions. Bradykinesia and rigidity improved the most. Dyskinesias are not a major problem in patients even when high dose levodopa was used. Most frequent adverse effects from levodopa are gastrointestinal (GI) complaints and confusion, somnolence, dizziness and hallucinations. Dopamine agonists like bromocriptine have been tried with very little improvement (6%). Dopamine agonist use causes side effects of GI symptoms, confusion and dizziness. Selegiline showed mild benefit in 10%. Amantadine had benefit in 13% patients with improvement in gait, rigidity and tremor.

Clonazepam is very helpful in treating myoclonus. Up to 40% patients showed benefit with benzodiazepines. Other agents such as baclofen and anticholinergics do not show any benefit. Patients also benefit from botulinum toxin injections for dystonia which clearly improves the pain component of the rigid-dystonic limb. Antidepressants such as tricyclic antidepressants, selective serotonin reuptake inhibitors (SSRI), and bupropion were given in 16 patients with improvement in one patient who received fluoxetine. Benzodiazepines and anticonvulsants caused a side effect of sedation in the study. Anticonvulsants and propranolol were helpful for tremor. Although our experience has been extremely disappointing, controlled studies are needed to evaluate the efficacy of dopaminergic drugs and other agents in this disorder.

For treatment of neuropsychological problems such as depression initial choice would be an SSRI like citalopram or sertraline, paroxetine, fluoxetine or fluoxamine. If patients are unresponsive or intolerant to this group of medications tricyclic antidepressants, such as nortriptyline or desipramine may be useful. For severe depression ECT may be considered, although there are no studies to evaluate response of patients to ECT.

For speech and swallowing problems patients need early evaluation and measures, including percutaneous endoscopic gastrostomy (PEG) tube placement depending on the severity of symptoms. To date, no effective treatment has been found, although myoclonus may improve with clonazepam, and painful rigidity and dystonia both upper limb and in the form of blepharospasm improves with botulinum toxin injections.[217,218] Ideomotor apraxia may improve with tactile stimulation, such as the use of the appropriate tool.[246] Patients have a progressive course and death is secondary to aspiration pneumonia or due to other causes of long term disability.

Vascular parkinsonism

Definition

Vascular parkinsonism (VP) is a term applied to patients with clinical symptoms of "lower body parkinsonism," multiple cerebral infarctions in the basal ganglia or white matter or both, with or without dementia in the absence of any prior neurodegenerative disease or medications that can cause parkinsonism, and with an insufficient response to dopaminergic medications.[247–249]

History

In 1929 Critchley[247] defined atherosclerotic parkinsonism as being characterized by rigidity, masked face, and short-stepped gait in an elderly hypertensive person and proposed that multiple vascular insults of the basal ganglia were related to the core symptoms. There was no neuropathological correlation of these findings. In the London Parkinson's disease brain bank study[250] three out of 100 patients clinically diagnosed as having PD were found to have VP.

Pathology

Yamanouchi and Nagura[251] reported a clinicopathological study of 24 patients who were diagnosed with VP (17 men and 7 women). Most neuropathologically confirmed patients showed short-stepped gait, lead pipe rigidity, symmetry of rigidity, absence of resting tremor and poor response to antiparkinsonian drugs. Half or more patients had pseudobulbar palsy and pyramidal tract signs. There is preservation of pigmented neurons in the substantia nigra in VP and Binswanger disease. Presence of Lewy bodies is an exclusionary criteria for these patients. There were vascular lesions extending throughout less than one third of basal ganglia structure, pallor in area occupying more than two thirds of frontal white matter, mamillary body, and some amount of pallor in occipital white matter (less than that seen in patients with Binswangers disease). Mechanisms proposed for pathogenesis include impairment of long loop reflexes traversing the white matter thereby leading to disruption of sensorimotor integration leading to parkinsonism. Diffuse vascular lesions disrupt interconnecting fiber tracts between basal ganglia and motor cortex.[251]

Clinical features

Vascular parkinsonism can be divided into two subgroups. Possible VP in patients who with vascular lesions on MRI and history of stroke and probable VP in patients with onset of parkinsonism shortly after acute stroke. There are several types of parkinsonism associated with cerebrovascular disease: (1) parkinsonism indistinguishable from idiopathic PD, (2) PSP that is clinically identical to the idiopathic variety of PSP, (3) lower body parkinsonism, and (4) other parkinsonian gait disorders.[252]

Clinical features of patients with VP include older age at onset with average age of 71.3 as compared to 62.7 in idiopathic PD. There is a slight preponderance in men compared to women (57.9% vs. 50%).[252] Vascular parkinsonism patients have higher frequency of dementia, prior strokes, and vascular risk factors; 25% patients present with clinical features of parkinsonism within one month after a stroke. Patients with VP are older, more likely to present with gait difficulty rather than tremor, and less likely to respond to levodopa as compared to patients with idiopathic PD. Vascular parkinsonism patients are also more likely to have predominant lower body involvement, postural instability,[249,250] falls, dementia, corticospinal findings, incontinence, and pseudobulbar affect. The severity of lower body parkinsonism correlates with the severity of chronic subcortical ischemia.[253]

"Lower body" parkinsonism, a condition in which upper body motor function is relatively preserved while gait is markedly impaired, has been previously linked to multiple lacunar infarcts.[253,254] Binswanger's disease, a form of leukoencephalopathy caused by hypoxia-ischemia of distal watershed periventricular territories associated with aging, hyperviscosity and increased fibrinogen levels,[255,256] can rarely present as levodopa-responsive parkinsonism.[257] About 10% of patients with small deep infarcts and white matter lesions, have been found to have a parkinsonian syndrome.[258] It is possible that some of the familial forms of vascular parkinsonism represent the entity CADASIL, a cerebral autosomal dominant arteriopathy associated with stroke and dementia, caused by a mutation in the Notch 3 gene.[259]

Laboratory tests and investigations

Investigations in patients with VP must include MRI of the brain and studies to evaluate risk factors for stroke including laboratory investigations and cardiac work up for cardioembolic source. The MRIs of the brain show TI and T2 changes, consistent with subcortical ischemic changes in basal ganglia and white matter. The numbers of ischemic lesions on the MRI are greater in patients with VP than in controls with hypertension and PD.[249,256] Location of the infarcts in the basal ganglia seems to correlate well with VP.[260] TRODAT-1 is a cocaine analog that can bind to the dopamine transporter sites at the presynaptic neuron membrane and can easily be labeled with Tc[99m]. ^{99m}Tc-TRODAT-1 has been shown to have bilaterally symmetric uptake in the striatum of VP patients. The uptake of ^{99m}Tc-TRODAT-1 does not correlate with the severity of parkinsonism or the extent of lesions of cerebral infarcts in the basal ganglia in VP. In patients with PD there is an asymmetry in the uptake of ^{99m}Tc-TRODAT-1 in addition to preferentially decreased uptake in the putamen in the contralateral side.[261] Similar findings were reported in the 2β-carboxymethoxy-3β 4-^{123}I-iodophenyl tropane ([123]I β-CIT) SPECT studies on VP patients.[262] These results are consistent with the pathological finding in VP patients that chronic subcortical ischemia is induced by the total extent of lesions in the basal ganglia, caused by multiple infarctions or hemorrhage, but not due to damage to dopaminergic neurons. On a proton spectroscopy study Zijmens et al.,[263] have shown that dopamine neurons in striatum are preserved in VP (vascular parkinsonism).

Treatment

Treatment for VP is difficult. It is unclear if stroke prevention therapies halt the progression. Patients should be on antiplatelet therapy, and, if clinically indicated, anticoagulation may be needed for stroke prevention depending on the risk factors identified. These patients show an overall lack of responsiveness to levodopa. There was response to levodopa in 24.6% patients in one study.[252,253] An appropriate dose adjustment depending on the response would be ideal. There are no studies on dopamine agonists for treatment of VP.

Pallidal degeneration

Definition

Pallidal degeneration and variants represent a group of rare autosomal recessive or sporadic neurodegenerative disorders with significant pathological and clinical overlap and atrophy of various parts of the pallidoluysionigral system. Clinical presentation is in the form of dystonia, choreoathetosis, rigid akinesia, oculomotor gait disorders and pseudobulbar palsy.

Clinical features and pathology

Included in this category are: (1) pallidal degeneration with atrophy of globus pallidus with gliosis and degeneration of efferent pallidal fibers, (2) pallidoluysian atrophy a disorder with bilateral atrophy and gliosis of external pallidum and subthalamic nucleus, (3) pallidonigral and pallidonigroluysian degeneration with involvement of pallidum, subthalamic nucleus, and substantia nigra with associated fiber systems, occasional involvement of ventromedial thalamic nucleus and deposition of iron in the degenerate nuclei, and (4) pallidal degeneration with polyglucosan bodies is a progressive choreiform or dystonic disorder or presenting with non-progressive cerebral palsy. Autopsy in the latter disorder shows symmetric degeneration globus pallidus externum, or status marmoratus of basal ganglia, associated with polyglucosan bodies in neuronal perikarya, axons and dendrites (Bielschowsky bodies).[264]

Dentatorubro-pallidoluysian atrophy (DRPLA) is a rare autosomal dominant neurodegenerative disorder with three clinical phenotypes: (1) ataxo-choreoathetoid, (2) pseudo-Huntington, and (3) myoclonus epilepsy type with considerable intrafamilial variations.[265] This disorder appears to be more common in Japan and Europe, although there are some families reported from North America.[266] Neuropathology shows multiple system degeneration with involvement of dentatorubral and pallidofugal systems, subthalamic nucleus, spinocerebellar and motor systems. There are some intaneuronal inclusions seen that are thought to be related to pathogenesis in polyglutamine expansion. DRPLA has a polyglutamine repeat (CAG) on the short arm of chromosome 12p 13.31. Polyglutamine repeat length correlates with the age of onset of the disease.[265,267]

Japanese investigators have described pure pallidal degeneration with adult onset presentation manifested chiefly by slowness of eye movement, slow speech, mild dysphagia, bilateral Babinski sign, and wide based and unsteady gait. Usual age of pure pallidal degeneration is 5–14 years with slow relentless duration. Torsion dystonia, choreoathetosis were observed from an early stage and akinesia was noted late in disease. Rigidity is not severe. There is one case report of pure pallidal degeneration with adult onset.[264,268]

Investigations should include MRI scans to identify any lesions in the globus pallidum in pallidal degeneration cases. In DRPLA patients MRI shows cerebellar atrophy with dilatation of the fourth ventricle. There is atrophy of the tegmentum, and midbrain with dilatation of aqueduct. T2-weighted images show hyperintensity of cerebral white matter.[264–268]

Patients with pallidal degeneration do not show response to dopaminergic agents. In cases with clinical features involving chorea, medications such as haloperidol or fluphenazine can be used. Dopamine

Table 232.2   Treatment of various symptoms in parkinsonism plus syndromes

Symptoms	Treatment
Ocular problems	
Dry eyes	Artificial tears
Ocular apraxia	Botulinum toxin injections
Diplopia	Prisms
Psychiatric and behavioral	
Depression	SSRI's or tricyclic antidepressants
Emotional lability	Amitryptiline
Agitation	Trazodone
Dystonia	
Dystonia	Botulinum toxin injection to affected area
Blepharospasm	Botulinum toxin injections
Parkinsonism	
Bradykinesia and rigidity	Carbidopa/levodopa dosage of up to 2 gm per day for at least two months
Urinary dysfunction	Self intermittent catherization and anticholinergics
Gait and balance	Physical therapy, walkers, gait training and training while turning and educate about falls
Speech and swallowing	
Dysphagia	Speech pathologist and soft/pureed diet and consider PEG
Dysarthria	Speech therapy and communication devices
Drooling	Cautious use of anticholinergics
Sleep	
Snoring, sleep apnea	CPAP
REM sleep behavior disorder	Clonazepam

CPAP, continuous positive airway pressure; SSRI, selective serotonin reuptake inhibitors.

depleting agents such as reserpine and tetrabenazine may be helpful. For focal dystonia botulinum toxin injections may be helpful.

Supportive treatment for parkinsonism plus disorders

We will now discuss management of some of the common problems associated with parkinsonism plus disorders such as sleep disorders, aspects of rehabilitation and future therapies in parkinsonism plus disorders (see Table 232.2).

Sleep problems are seen in several neurodegenerative disorders. Sleep disturbance is present in almost all cases of PSP and MSA. Treatment involves general measures such as reduction or withdrawal of medications contributing to sleep problems, regular sleep schedules, sleep hygiene, avoidance of caffeine or alcohol in the evenings. Use of hypnotics not more than two to three times a week, avoidance of daytime naps and treatment of associated depression or anxiety is helpful. For patients with obstructive sleep apnea nasal CPAP (continuous positive airway pressure) is very useful. This helps to improve sleep quality and reduction of daytime somnolence. Severe respiratory dysfunction and hypoxia in the presence of laryngeal stridor may need emergency tracheostomy. In patients with REM sleep behavior disorders or nocturnal hallucinations, clonazepam at a dose of 0.5–1 mg at night is useful.[46,47,137,138]

Rehabilitation in patients with parkinsonism plus disorders may need measures that are similar to those used in patients with PD. Fiber supplements help with constipation. Physical therapy must involve a regular exercise program of one hour per day three times a week. Range of motion exercises, flexibility and balancing exercises are the most important components of gait training. Truncal exercises, clasping hands behind one's back help to improve posture in patients with parkinsonian features. Patients and families must understand the need for a regular exercise program. In advanced cases stretching and support to avoid contractures are important. Speech therapists can help patients with voice treatment programs to increase voice intensity and phonation and vocal volume. In some patients who have significant difficulty, communication aids and training the caretaker are very helpful to patient.

Swallowing problems are commonly seen. Patients must have an early evaluation by speech therapist. Modified barium swallow is very helpful in evaluating the phase of swallowing that is affected. Patients can be taught certain techniques such as modification of the supraglottic swallow, which can help prevent aspiration. For advanced cases evaluation for gastrostomy tube placement is needed. For constipation, patients need to have a regular bowel regimen and laxatives.

Neuroprotective therapies have not been studied in any of the above disorders. It is unclear if antioxidants such as vitamin E, coenzyme Q_{10}, or selegiline may favorably alter the natural history of the disease. Future therapies may involve trophic factors including GDNF (glial derived growth factor) and antiglutaminergic agents. Gene therapy may be useful in patients with familial forms of these syndromes. Stem cell transplantation may also be an option in future. In addition to all the above measures, patient and family education about the disease and expectations must be given utmost importance. Participation in patient support groups must be encouraged.

References

1. Steele JC, Richardson JC, Olszewski J. Progressive supranuclear palsy: a heterogeneous degeneration involving the brainstem, basal ganglia and cerebellum with vertical gaze and pseudobulbar palsy, nuchal dystonia and dementia. Arch Neurol 1964;10:333–359

2. Steele JC. Historical notes. J Neural Transm Suppl 1994;42:3–14

3. Golbe LI. Epidemiology of progressive supranuclear palsy. J Neural Trans Suppl 1994;42:213–273

4. Bower JH, Maraganore DM, McDonnell SK, Rocca WA. Incidence of progressive supranuclear palsy and multiple system atrophy in Olmsted county, Minnesota 1976–1990. Neurology 1997;49:1284–1288

5. Schrag A, Ben-Shlomo Y, Quinn NP. Prevalence of progressive supranuclear palsy and multiple system atrophy: a cross-sectional study. Lancet 1999;354:1771–1775

6. Nath U, Ben-Shlomo Y, Thomson RG, et al. The prevalence of progressive supranuclear palsy (Steele-Richardson-Olszewski syndrome) in the UK. Brain 2001;124(Pt 7):1438–1449

7. Litvan I, Mangone CA, McKee A, et al. Natural history of progressive supranuclear palsy (Steele-Richardson-Olszewski syndrome) and clinical predictors of survival: a clinicopathological study. J Neurol Neurosurg Psychiatry 1996;60:615–620

8. Brown J, Lantos P, Stratton M, et al. Familial progressive supranuclear palsy. J Neurol Neurosurg Psychiatry 1993;56:473–476

9. de Yebenes JG, Sarasa JL, Daniel SE, Lees AJ. Familial progressive supranuclear palsy. Description of a pedigree and review of literature. Brain 1995;118:1095–1104

10. Tetrud JW, Golbe LI, Forno LS, Farmer PM. Autopsy-proven progressive supranuclear palsy in two siblings. Neurology 1996;46:931–934

11. Lantos PL. The neuropathology of progressive supranuclear palsy. J Neural Trans Suppl 1994;42: 132–152

12. Hardman CD, Halliday GM, McRitchie DA, Morris JGL. The subthalamic nucleus in Parkinson's disease and progressive supranuclear palsy. J Neuropath Exp Neurol 1997;56:132–142

13. Jellinger KA. Neurodegenerative disorders with extrapyramidal features: a neuropathological overview. J Neural Transm Suppl 1995;46:33–57

14. Hauw JJ, Daniel SE, Dickson D, et al. Preliminary NINDS neuropathologic criteria for Steele-Richardson-Olszewski syndrome. Neurol 1994;44:2015–2019

15. Litvan I, Hauw JJ, Bartko JJ, et al. Validity and reliability of the preliminary NINDS neuropathological criteria for progressive supranuclear palsy and related disorders. J Neuopathol Exp Neurol 1996;55:97–105

16. De Bruin VM, Lees AJ. Subcortical neurofibrillary degeneration presenting as Steele-Richardson-Olszewski and other related syndromes: a review of 90 pathologically verified cases. Mov Disord 1994;9(4):381–389

17. Ito H, Goto S, Sakamoto S, Hirano A. Calbindin-D$_{28k}$ in the basal ganglia of patients with parkinsonism. Ann Neurol 1992;32:543–550

18. Conrad C, Andreadis A, Trojanowski JQ, et al. Genetic evidence for the involvement of tau in progressive supranuclear palsy. Ann Neurol 1997;41:277–281

19. Hoenicka J, Perez M, Perez-Tur J, et al. The tau gene A0 allele and progressive supranuclear palsy. Neurology 1999;53:1219–1225

20. Higgins JJ, Golbe LI, De Biase A, et al. An extended 5'-tau susceptibility haplotype in progressive supranuclear palsy. Neurol 2000;55(9):1364–1367

21. Young A. Progressive supranuclear palsy: postmortem chemical analysis. Ann Neurol 1985;18:521–522

22. Pierot L, Desnos L, Blin J, et al. D$_1$ and D$_2$-type dopamine receptors in patients with Parkinson's disease and progressive supranuclear palsy. J Neurol Sci 1988;86:291–306

23. Pascual J, Berciano J, Grijalba B, et al. Dopamine D$_1$ and D$_2$ receptors in progressive supranuclear palsy: an autoradiographic study. Ann Neurol 1992;32:703–707

24. Levy R, Ruberg M, Herrero MT, et al. Alterations of GABAergic neurons in the basal ganglia of patients with progressive supranuclear palsy: an in situ hybridization study of GAD$_{67}$ messenger RNA. Neurol 1995;45:127–134

25. Perry TL, Hansen S, Jones K. Brain amino acids and glutathione in progressive supranuclear palsy. Neurol 1988;38:943–946

26. Shinotoh H, Namba H, Yamaguchi M, et al. Positron emission tomographic measurement of acetylcholinesterase activity reveals differential loss of ascending cholinergic systems in Parkinson's disease and progressive supranuclear palsy. Ann Neurol 1999;46: 62–69

27. Di Monte DA, Harati Y, Jankovic J, et al. Muscle mitochondrial ATP production in progressive supranuclear palsy. J Neurochem 1994;62:1631–1634

28. Jankovic J, Friedman DI, Pirozzolo FJ, McCrary JA. Progressive supranuclear palsy: motor, neurobehavioral, and neuro-ophthalmic findings. Adv Neurol 1990;53:293–304

29. Litvan I. Diagnosis and management of progressive supranuclear palsy. Semin Neurol 2001;21(1):41–48

30. Jankovic J. Progressive supranuclear palsy. clinical and pharmacologic update. Neurol Clin 1984;2(3):473–486

31. Santacruz P, Uttl B, Litvan I, Grafman J. Progressive supranuclear palsy: a survey of disease course. Neurol 1998;59(6):1637–1647

32. Friedman DI, Jankovic J, McCrary JA. Neuro-ophthalmic findings in progressive supranuclear palsy. J Clin Neuroophthalmol 1992;12(2):104–109

33. Rivaud-Pechoux S, Vidailhet M, Gallouedec G, et al. Longitudinal ocular motor study in corticobasal degeneration and progressive supranuclear palsy. Neurol 2000;54(5):1029–1032

34. Vidailhet M, Rivaud S, Gouider-Khouja N, et al. Eye movements in parkinsonian syndromes. Ann Neurol 1994;35:420–426

35. Grandas F, Esteban A. Eyelid motor abnormalities in progressive supranuclear palsy. J Neural Transm Suppl 1994;42:33–41

36. Litvan I, Sastry N, Sonies BC. Characterizing swallowing abnormalities in progressive supranuclear palsy. Neurol 1997;48(6):1654–1662

37. Kluin K, Gilman S, Foster N, et al. Neuropathological correlates of dysarthria in progressive supranuclear palsy. Arch Neurol 2001;58(2):265–269

38. Rivest J, Quinn N, Marsden CD. Dystonia in Parkinson's disease, multiple system atrophy, and progressive supranuclear palsy. Neurol 1990;40:1571–1578

39. Daniel SE, de Bruin VMS, Lees AJ. The clinical and pathological spectrum of Steele-Richardson-Olszewski syndrome (progressive supranuclear palsy): a reappraisal. Brain 1995;118:759–770

40. Pillon B, Dubois B. Cognitive and behavioral impairments. *In:* Litvan I, Agid Y, eds. Progressive supranuclear palsy. Clinical and research approaches. Oxford: Oxford University Press, 1992:223–239

41. Litvan I. Cognitive disturbances in progressive supranuclear palsy. J Neural Transm Suppl 1994;42:69–78

42. Litvan I, Mega MS, Cummings JL, Fairbanks L. Neuropsychiatric aspects of progressive supranuclear palsy. Neurol 1996;47(5):1184–1189

43. Doty RL, Golbe LI, McKeown DA, et al. Olfactory testing differentiates between progressive supranuclear palsy and idiopathic Parkinson's disease. Neurol 1993;43:962–965

44. Barclay CL, Bergeron C, Lang AE. Arm levitation in progressive supranuclear palsy. Neurology 1999;52:879–882

45. Nygaard TG, Duvoisin RC, Manocha M, Chokroverty S. Seizures in progressive supranuclear palsy. Neurol 1989;39:138–140

46. Aldrich MS, Foster NL, White RF, et al. Sleep abnormalities in progressive supranuclear palsy. Ann Neurol 1989;25(6):577–581

47. Montplaisir J, Petit D, Decary A, et al. Sleep and quantitative EEG in patients with progressive supranuclear palsy. Neurol 1997;49:999–1003

48. Litvan I., Agid Y, Calne D, et al. Clinical research criteria for the diagnosis of progressive supranuclear palsy. Neurol 1996;47:1–9

49. Litvan I, Agid Y, Jankovic J, et al. Accuracy of clinical criteria for the diagnosis of progressive supranuclear palsy (Steele-Richardson-Olszewski syndrome). Neurol 1996;46(4):922–930

50. Litvan I, Agid Y, Calne D, et al. Clinical research criteria for the diagnosis of progressive supranuclear palsy (Steele-Richardson-Olszewski syndrome): report of the NINDS-SPSP international workshop. Neurol 1996;47(1):1–9

51. Winikates J, Jankovic J. Vascular PSP. J Neural Transm Suppl 1994;42:189–201

52. Dubinsky RM, Jankovic J. Progressive supranuclear palsy and a multi-infarct state. Neurol 1987;37:570–576

53. Ghika J, Bogousslavsky J. Presymptomatic hypertension is a major feature in the diagnosis of progressive supranuclear palsy. Arch Neurol 1997;54:1104–1108

54. Vidailhet M, Rivaud S, Gouider-Khouja N, et al. Saccades and antisaccades in parkinsonian syndromes. Adv Neurol 1999;80:377–382

55. Vidailhet M, Rothwell JC, Thompson PD, et al. The auditory startle response in the Steele-Richardson-Olszewski syndrome and Parkinson's disease. Brain 1992;115(Pt 4):1181–1192

56. Rothwell JC, Vidailhet M, Thompson PD, et al. The auditory startle response in progressive supranuclear palsy. J Neural Transm Suppl 1994;42:43–50

57. Abruzzese G, Tabaton M, Morena M, et al. Motor and sensory evoked potentials in progressive supranuclear palsy. Mov Disord 1991;6(1):49–54

58. Johnson R, Jr. Event-Related Potentials. *In:* Litvan I, Agid Y, eds. Progressive supranuclear palsy clinical and research approaches. Oxford: Oxford University Press, 1992:122–154

59. Soliveri P, Monza D, Paridi D, et al. Cognitive and magnetic resonance imaging aspects of corticobasal degeneration and progressive supranuclear palsy. Neurol 1999;53:502–507

60. Schrag A, Good CD, Miszkiel K, et al. Differentiation of atypical parkinsonian syndromes with routine MRI. Neurol 2000;54:697–702

61. Burn DJ, Sawle GV, Brooks DJ. Differential diagnosis of Parkinson's disease, MSA and Steele-Richardson-Olszewski syndrome: discriminant analysis of F-dopa PET data. J Neurol Neurosurg Psych 1994;5:278–284

62. Brooks DJ. PET studies in progressive supranuclear palsy. J Neural Transm Suppl 1994;42:119–134

63. Santens P, De Reuck J, Crevits L, et al. Cerebral oxygen metabolism in patients with progressive supranuclear palsy: a positron emission tomography study. Eur Neurol 1997;37(1):18–22

64. Foster NL, Minoshima S, Johanns J, et al. PET measures of benzodiazepine receptors in progressive supranuclear palsy. Neurol 2000;54(9):1768–1773

65. Ilgin N, Zubieta J, Reich SG, et al. PET imaging of the dopamine transporter in progressive supranuclear palsy and Parkinson's disease. Neurol 1999;52(6):1221–1226

66. Pirker W, Asenbaum S, Bencsits G, et al. [^{123}I] β-CIT SPECT in multiple system atrophy, progressive supranuclear palsy, and corticobasal degeneration. Mov Disord 2000;15(6):1158–1167

67. Neiforth KA, Goelbe LI. Retrospective study of drug response in 87 patients with progressive supranuclear palsy. Clin Neuropharm 1993;16(4):338–346

68. Cole DG, Growdon GH. Therapy for progressive supranuclear palsy: past and future. J Neural Transm Suppl 1994;42:283–290

69. Kompoliti K, Goetz CG, Litvan I, et al. Pharmacological therapy in PSP. Arch Neurol 1998;55:1099–1102

70. Jackson JA, Jankovic J, Ford J. Progressive supranuclear palsy: clinical features and response to treatment in 16 patients. Ann Neurol 1983;13(3):273–278

71. Jankovic, J. Controlled trial of pergolide mesylate in Parkinson's disease and progressive supranuclear palsy. Neurol 1983;33:505–507

72. Weiner WJ, Minager A, Shulman M. Pramipexole in progressive supranuclear palsy. Neurol 1999;62:873–874

73. Neophytides A, Lieberman AN, Goldstein M, et al. The use of lisuride a potent dopamine and serotonin agonist, in the treatment of progressive supranuclear palsy. J Neurol Neurosurg Psych 1982;45:261–263

74. Litvan I, Chase TN. Traditional and experimental therapeutic approaches. *In:* Litvan I, Agid Y, eds. Progressive supranuclear palsy clinical and research approaches. Oxford: Oxford University Press, 1992:254–269

75. Newman GC. Treatment of progressive supranuclear palsy with tricyclic antidepressants. Neurol 1985;35:1189–1192

76. Rafal RD, Grimm RJ. Progressive supranuclear palsy: functional analysis of the response of methysergide and antiparkinsonian agents. Neurol 1981;31:1507–1518

77. Litvan I, Blesa R, Clark K, et al. Pharmacological evaluation of the cholinergic system in progressive supranuclear palsy. Ann Neurol 1994;36(1):55–61

78. Foster NL, Aldrich MS, Bluemlein L, et al. Failure of cholinergic agonist RS-86 to improve cognition and movement in PSP despite effects on sleep. Neurol 1989;39:257–261

79. Kertzman C, Robinson DL, Litvan I. Effects of physostigmine on spatial attention in patients with progressive supranuclear palsy. Arch Neurol 1990;47:1346–1350

80. Frattali CM, Sonies BC, Chi-Fishman G, Litvan I. Effects of physostigmine on swallowing and oral

motor functions in patients with progressive supranuclear palsy: a pilot study. Dysphagia 1999;14:165–168

81. Litvan I, Gomez C, Atak JR, et al. Physostigmine treatment of progressive supranuclear palsy. Ann Neurol 1989;26(3):404–407

82. Fabbrini G, Barbanti P, Bonifati V, et al. Donepzil in the treatment of progressive supranuclear palsy. Acta Neurol Scand 2001;103;123–125

83. Ghika J, Tennis M, Hoffman E, et al. Idazoxan treatment in progressive supranuclear palsy. Neurol 1991; 41:986–990

84. Rascol O, Sieradzan K, Saint-Paul H, et al. Efaroxan, an α_2 antagonist, in the treatment of progressive supranuclear palsy. Mov Disord 1998;13(4):673–676

85. Gordon MF, Diaz-Olivo R, Hunt AL, Fahn S. Therapeutic trial of milacemide in patients with myoclonus and other intractable movement disorders. Mov Disord 1993;8(4):484–488

86. Sandyk R, Iacono RP. Naloxone ameliorates presyncopial sensations in progressive supranuclear palsy. Int J Neurosci 1987;35:89–90

87. Takamura N, Shinji T, Akiyoshi A, et al. Aniracetam for treatment of patients with progressive supranuclear palsy. Eur Neurol 1997;37:195–198

88. Daniele A, Moro E, Bentivoglio AR. Zolpidem in progressive supranuclear palsy. NEJM 1999;341(7):543

89. Schneider LS, Gleason RP, Chui HC. Progressive supranuclear palsy with agitation: response to trazodone but not to thoithixine or carbamazepine. J Geri Psych Neurol 1989;2:109–113

90. Hauser RA, Trehan R. Initial experience with electroconvulsive therapy for progressive supranuclear palsy. Mov Disord 1994;9(4):467–469

91. Wenning GK, Seppi K, Scherfler C. Multiple system atrophy. Sem Neurol 2001;12(1):33–40

92. Graham JG, Oppenheimer DR. Orthostatic hypotension and nicotinic sensitivity in a case of multiple system atrophy. J Neurol Neurosurg Psych 1969;32:28–34

93. Hanna P, Jankovic J, Kilkpatrick J. Multiple system atrophy: the putative causative role of environmental toxins. Arch Neurol 1999;56:90–94

94. Vanacore N, Bonifati V, Fabbrini G, et al. Smoking habits in multiple system atrophy and progressive supranuclear palsy. Neurol 2000;54(1):114–119

95. Wenning GK, Shlomo YB, Magalhaes M, et al. Clinical features and natural history of multiple system atrophy. An analysis of 100 cases. Brain 1994;117:835–845

96. Saito Y, Matsuoka Y, Takahashi A, Ohno Y. Survival of patients with multiple system atrophy. Int Med 1994;33:321–325

97. Ben-Shlomo Y, Wenning GK, Tison F, Quinn NP. Survival of patients with pathologically proven multiple system atrophy: a meta-analysis. Neurol 1997;48: 484–493

98. Wenning GK, Ben-Shlomo Y, Magalhaes M, et al. Clinicopathological study of 35 cases of multiple system atrophy. J Neurol Neurosurg Psych 1995;58:160–166

99. Gilman S, Low PA, Quinn N, et al. Consensus statement on the diagnosis of multiple system atrophy. J Auto Nerv Syst 1998;74:189–192

100. Quinn N. Multiple system atrophy. In: Marsden CD, Fahn S. eds. Movement Disorders 3. Oxford: Butterworth-Heinemann, 1994:262–281

101. Ito H, Kusaka H, Matsumoto S, Imai T. Striatal efferent involvement and its correlation to levodopa efficacy in patients with multiple system atrophy. Neurol 1996;47: 1291–1299

102. Benarroch EE, Smithson IL, Low PA, Parisi JE. Deple-

tion of catecholaminergic neurons of the rostral ventrolateral medulla in multiple system atrophy with autonomic failure. Ann Neurol 1998;43:156–163

103. Benarroch EE, Schmeichel AM, Parisi JE. Involvement of the ventrolateral medulla in parkinsonism with autonomic failure. Neurol 2000;54:963–968

104. Papp MI, Khan JE, Lantos PL. Glial cytoplasmic inclusions in the CNS of patients with multiple system atrophy (striatonigral degeneration, olivopontocerebellar atrophy and Shy-Drager syndrome). J Neurol Sci 1989;94:79–100

105. Papp M, Lantos P. Accumulation of tubular structures in oligodendroglial and neuronal cells as the basic alteration in multiple system atrophy. J Neurol Sci 1992;107:172–182

106. Cairns NJ, Atkinson PF, Hanger DP, et al. Tau protein in glial cytoplasmic inclusions of multiple system atrophy can be distinguished from abnormal tau in Alzheimer's disease. Neurosci Lett 1997;230:49–52

107. Gilman S, Quinn NP. The relationship of multiple system atrophy to sporadic olivopontocerebellar atrophy and other forms of idiopathic late-onset cerebellar atrophy. Neurol 1996;46:1197–1199

108. Honjyo Y, Kawamuto Y, Nakamura S, et al. P39 immunoreactivity in glial cytoplasmic inclusions in brains with multiple system atrophy. Acta Neuropathol 2001;101:190–194

109. Kato S, Shinozawa T, Takikawa, et al. Midkine, a neurotrophic factor is present in glial cytoplasmic inclusions of the multiple system atrophy brains. Acta Neuropathol 2000;100:481–489

110. Litvan I, Goetz C, Jankovic J, et al. What is the accuracy of the clinical diagnosis of multiple system atrophy? A clinicopathological study. Arch Neurol 1997;54:937–944

111. Arima K, Ueda K, Sunohara N, et al. NACP/alpha-synuclein immunoreactivity in fibrillary components of neuronal and oligodendroglial cytoplasmic inclusions in the pontine nuclei in multiple system atrophy. Acta Neuropathol (Berl) 1998;96(5):439–444

112. Clayton DF, George JM. Synucleins in synaptic plasticity and neurodegenerative disorders. J Neurosci Res 1999;58:120–129

113. Abeliovich A, Schmitz, Farinas I, et al. Mice lacking alpha synuclein display functional deficits in the nigro striatal dopamine system. Neuron 2000;25:239–252

114. Ozawa T, Takano H, Onodera O, et al. No mutation in the entire coding region of the alpha-synuclein gene in pathologically confirmed cases of multiple system atrophy. Neurosci Lett 1999;270:110–112

115. Campbell BCV, Mclean CA, Culvenor JG, et al. The solubility of alpha-synuclein in multiple system atrophy differs from that of dementia with Lewy bodies and Parkinson's disease. J Neurochem 2001;76: 87–96

116. Winkler AS, Marsden J, Parton M, et al. Erythropoietin deficiency and anaemia in multiple system atrophy. Mov Disord 2001;16(2):233–239

117. Wenning GK, Tison F, Shlomo BY, et al. Multiple system atrophy: a review of 203 pathologically proven cases. Mov Disord 1997;12:133–147

118. Vidailhet M, Rivaud S, Gouider-Khouja N, et al. Eye movements in parkinsonian syndromes. Ann Neurol 1994;35:420–426

119. Litvan I. Parkinsonism-dementia syndromes. In: Jankovic J, Tolosa E, eds. Parkinson's disease and movement disorders. 3rd ed. Baltimore, Maryland: Williams and Wilkins, 1998:819–836

120. Isozaki E, Naito A, Horichuchi S, et al. Early diagnosis and stage classification of vocal cord abductor paralysis in patients with multiple system atrophy. J Neurol Neurosurg Psych 1996;60:399–402

121. Salazar G, Valls-Sole J, Marti MJ, et al. Postural and action myoclonus in patients with parkinsonian type multiple system atrophy. Mov Disord 2000;15(1):77–83

122. The Consensus Committee of the American Autonomic Society and the American Academy of Neurology. Consensus statement on the definition of orthostatic hypotension, pure autonomic failure, and multiple system atrophy. Neurol 1996;46(5):1470

123. Gilman S, Low PA, Quinn N, et al. Consensus statement on the diagnosis of multiple system atrophy. J Aut Nerv Syst 1998;74:189–192

124. Albanese A, Colosimo C, Bentivoglio AR, et al. Multiple system atrophy presenting as parkinsonism: clinical features and diagnostic criteria. J Neurol Neurosurg Psych 1995;59:144–151

125. Litvan I, Booth V, Wenning GK, et al. Retrospective application of a set of clinical diagnostic criteria for the diagnosis of multiple system atrophy. J Neural Transm 1998;105:217–227

126. Thomaides T, Chaudhuri RK, Maule S, et al. Growth hormone response to clonidine in central and peripheral primary autonomic failure. Lancet 1992;340:263–266

127. Thomaides T, Bleasdale-Barr K, Chaudhuri KR, et al. Cardiovascular and hormonal responses to liquid food challenge in idiopathic Parkinson's disease, multiple system atrophy, and pure autonomic failure. Neurol 1993;43:900–904

128. Cohen J, Low P, Fealey R, et al. Somatic and autonomic function in progressive autonomic failure and multiple system atrophy. Ann Neurol 1987;22:692–699

129. Goldstein DS, Polinsky RJ, Garty M, et al. Patterns of plasma levels of catechols in neurogenic orthostatic hypotension. Ann Neurol 1989;26:558–563

130. Goldstein DS, Holmes C, Cannon RO, et al. Sympathetic cardio-neuropathy in dysautonomias. N Engl J Med 1997;336:696–702

131. Mathias CJ. Orthostatic hypotension: causes, mechanisms, and influencing factors. Neurol 1995;45(Suppl 5):S6–S11

132. Mathias CJ. Autonomic disorders and their recognition. N Engl J Med 1997;336:721–724

133. Kimber J, Watson L, Mathias CJ. Abnormal suppression of arginine-vasopressin by clonidine in multiple system atrophy. Clin Auton Res 1999;9(5):271–274

134. Fowler CJ. Investigation of neurogenic bladder. J Neurol Neurosurg Psych 1996;60(1):6–13

135. Stocchi F, Carbone A, Inghiller M, et al. Urodynamic and neurophysiologic evaluation in Parkinson's disease and multiple system atrophy. J Neurol Neurosurg Psych 1997;62:507–511

136. Schwarz J, Kornhuber M, Bischoff C, Straube A. Electromyography of the external anal sphincter in patients with Parkinson's disease and multiple system atrophy: frequency of abnormal spontaneous activity and polyphasic motor unit potentials. Muscle Nerve 1997;20(9):1167–1172

137. Munschauer FE, Loh L, Bannister R, Newsom-Davis J. Abnormal respiration and sudden death during sleep in multiple system atrophy with autonomic failure. Neurol 1990;40(4):677–679

138. Plazzi G, Corsini R, Provini F, et al. REM sleep behavior disorders in multiple system atrophy. Neurol 1997;48(4):1094–1097

139. Plazzi G, Cortelli P, Montagna P, et al. REM sleep behaviour disorder differentiates pure autonomic failure from multiple system atrophy with autonomic failure. J Neurol Neurosurg Psych 1998;64(5):683–685

140. Abele M, Schulz JB, Burk K, et al. Evoked potentials in multiple system atrophy (MSA). Acta Neurol Scand 2000;101(2):111–115

141. Pastakia B, Polinsky R, Di Chiro G, et al. Multiple system atrophy (Shy-Drager syndrome): MR imaging. Radiology 1986;159(2):499–502

142. Schrag A, Kingsley D, Phatouros C, et al. Clinical usefulness of magnetic resonance imaging in multiple system atrophy. J Neurol Neurosurg Psych 1998;65(1):65–71

143. Konagaya M, Konagaya Y, Iida M. Clinical and magnetic resonance imaging study of extrapyramidal symptoms in multiple system atrophy. J Neurol Neurosurg Psych 1994;57(12):1528–1531

144. Schulz JB, Skalej M, Wedekind D, et al. Magnetic resonance imaging-based volumetry differentiates idiopathic Parkinson's syndrome from multiple system atrophy and progressive supranuclear palsy. Ann Neurol 1999;45(1):65–74

145. Davie CA, Wenning GK, Barker GJ, et al. Differentiation of multiple system atrophy from idiopathic Parkinson's disease using proton magnetic resonance spectroscopy. Ann Neurol 1995;37(2):204–210

146. Schulz JB, Klockgether T, Petersen D, et al. Multiple system atrophy: natural history, MRI morphology, and dopamine receptor imaging with [123]IBZM-SPECT. J Neurol Neurosurg Psych 1994;57(9):1047–1056

147. Bhatt MH, Snow BJ, Martin WRW, et al. Positron emission tomography in Shy-Drager syndrome. Ann Neurol 1990;28:101–103

148. Schrag A, Rinne JO, Burn DJ, et al. Olivopontocerebellar atrophy and multiple system atrophy: clinical follow-up of 10 patients studied with PET. Ann Neurol 1998;44(1):151–152

149. Gilman S, Frey KA, Koeppe RA, et al. Decreased striatal monoaminergic terminals in olivopontocerebellar atrophy and multiple system atrophy demonstrated with positron emission tomography. Ann Neurol 1996;40:885–892

150. Rinne JO, Burn DJ, Mathias CJ, et al. Positron emission tomography studies on the dopaminergic system and striatal opioid binding in the olivopontocerebellar atrophy variant of multiple system atrophy. Ann Neurol 1995;37:568–573

151. Antonini A, Leenders KL, Vontobel P, et al. Complementary PET studies of striatal neuronal function in the differential diagnosis between multiple system atrophy and Parkinson's disease. Brain 1997;120(Pt 12):2187–2195

152. Brooks DJ, Ibanez V, Sawle GV, et al. Differing patterns of striatal ^{18}F-dopa uptake in Parkinson's disease, multiple system atrophy, and progressive supranuclear palsy. Ann Neurol 1990;28(4):547–555

153. Brooks DJ, Salmon EP, Mathias CJ, et al. The relationship between locomotor disability, autonomic dysfunction, and the integrity of the striatal dopaminergic system in patients with multiple system atrophy, pure autonomic failure, and Parkinson's disease, studied with PET. Brain 1990;113(Pt 5):1539–1552

154. Braune S, Reinhardt M, Schnitzer R, et al. Cardiac uptake of [123I] MIBG separates Parkinson's disease from multiple system atrophy. Neurology 1999;53(5):1020–1025

155. Goldstein DS, Holmes C, Li ST, et al. Cardiac sympa-

thetic denervation in Parkinson disease. Ann Intern Med 2000;133(5):338–347

156. Mathias CJ, Kimber JR. Treatment of postural hypotension. J Neurol Neurosurg Psych 1998;65(3):285–289

157. Jankovic J, Hiner BC, Brown DC, Rubin M. Neurogenic orthostatic hypotension: a double blind placebo-controlled study with midodrine. Am J Med 1993;95:38–48

158. Wright RA, Kaufman HC, Perera R, et al. A double blind, dose-response study of midodrine in neurogenic orthostatic hypotension. Neurol 1998;51(1):120–126

159. Bordet R, Benhadjali J, Destee A, et al. Octreotide effects on orthostatic hypotension in patients with multiple system atrophy: a controlled study of acute administration. Clin Neuropharm 1995;18(1):83–89

160. Hoeldtke RD, Horvath GG, Bryner KD, Hobbs GR. Treatment of orthostatic hypotension with midodrine and octreotide. J Clin Endocr Med 1998;83(2):339–343

161. Freeman R, Young J, Landsberg L, Lipstiz L. The treatment of postprandial hypotension in autonomic failure with 3,4-threoDOPS. Neurol 1996;47(6):1414–1420

162. Freeman R, Landsberg L, Young J. The treatment of neurogenic orthostatic hypotension with 3,4,DL-threo-DOPS. Neurol 1999;53(1):2151–2157

163. Hidefumi I, Hirofumi K, Sadayuki M, Terukini I. Striatal efferent involvement and its correlation to levodopa efficacy in patients with multisystem atrophy. Neurol 1996;47(5):1291–1299

164. Hughes AJ, Colosimo C, Kleedorfer B, et al. The dopaminergic response in multiple system atrophy. J Neurol Neurosurg Psych 1992;55(11):1009–1013

165. Kimber JR, Watson L, Mathias CJ. Neuroendocrine responses to levodopa in multiple system atrophy. Mov Disord 1999;14(6):981–987

166. Parati EA, Fentoni V, Geminiani GC, et al. Response to L-dopa in multiple system atrophy. Clin Neuropharm 1993;16(2):139–144

167. Polinsky RJ. Multiple system atrophy clinical aspects, pathophysiology and treatment. Neurol Clin 1984;2(3):487–498

168. Senard JM, Rascol O, Durrieu G, et al. Effects of Yohimbine on plasma catecholamine levels in orthostatic hypotension related to Parkinson's disease or multiple system atrophy. Clin Neuropharm 1993;16(1):70–76

169. Botez MI, Botez-Marquard T, Elie R, et al. Amantadine hydrochloride treatment in olivopontocerebellar atrophy: a long-term follow up study. Eur Neurol 1999;41:212–215

170. Sakakibara R, Hattori T, Uchiyama T, et al. Are alpha-blockers involved in lower urinary tract dysfunction in multiple system atrophy? A comparison of prazosin and moxisylate. J Aut Nerv Syst 2000;79:191–195

171. Miller M. Nocturnal polyuria in older people: pathophysiology and implications. J Am Geriatric Soc. 2000;48(10):1321–1329

172. Dykstra DD. Effects of botulinum toxin type A on detrusor-sphincter dyssenergia in spinal cord injury patients. In: Jankovic J, Hallett M, eds. Therapy with botulinum toxin. New York, NY: Marcel Dekker, Inc, 1994:535–541

173. Hayashi M, Isozaki E, Oda M, et al. Loss of large myelinated nerve fibers of the recurrent laryngeal nerve in patients with multiple system atrophy and vocal cord palsy. J Neurol Neurosurg Psych 1997;62(3):234–238

174. Isozaki E, Tanabe H. Early diagnosis and stage classification of vocal cord abductor paralysis in patients with multiple system atrophy. J Neurol Neurosurg Psych 1996;60(4):399–402

175. Umeno H, Ueda H, Mori K, et al. Management of impaired vocal fold movement during sleep in a patient with shy-drager syndrome. Am J Otolaryngol 2000;21(5):344–348

176. Takayuki S, Toru K, Toshiaki S, et al. Novel therapeutic strategy against central baroreflex failure a bionic baro reflex system. Circulation 1999;20:299–304

177. Rebeiz JJ, Kolodny EH, Richardson EP. Corticodentatonigral degeneration with neuronal achromasia: a progressive disorder of late adult life. Trans Am Neurol Assoc 1967;92:23–26

178. Rebeiz JJ, Kolodny EH, Richardson EP. Corticodentatonigral degeneration with neuronal achromasia. Arch Neurol 1968;18:20–23

179. Gibb WR, Luthert PJ, Marsden CD. Clinical and pathological features of corticobasal degeneration. Adv Neurol 1990;53:51–54

180. Riley DE, Lang AE, Lewis A, et al. Cortical-basal ganglionic degeneration. Neurology 1990;40:1203–1212

181. Paulus W, Selim M. Corticonigral degeneration with neuronal achromasia and basal neurofibrillary tangles. Acta Neuropath 1990;81:89–94

182. Rinne JO, Lee MS, Thompson PD, Marsden CD. Corticobasal degeneration: a clinical study of 36 cases. Brain 1994;117:1183–1196

183. Wenning GK, Litvan I, Jankovic J, et al. Natural history and survival of 14 patients with corticobasal degeneration confirmed at postmortem examination. J Neurol Neurosurg Psychiatry 1998;64:184–189

184. Schneider JA, Watts RL, Gearing M, et al. Corticobasal degeneration: neuropathologic and clinical heterogeneity. Neurology 1997;48:959–969

185. Togasaki DM, Tanner CM. Epidemologic aspects. In: Litvan I, Goetz C, Lang AE, eds. Advances in Neurology. Corticobasal degeneration and related disorders. London: Lippincott Williams and Wilkins, 2000;82:53–60

186. Watts R, Brewer RP, Schneider JA, Mirra SS. Corticobasal degeneration. In: Watts RL, Koller WC, eds. Movement disorders: neurologic principles and practice. New York: McGraw Hill, 1997:611–621

187. Lippa CF, Cohen R, Smith TW, Drachman DA. Primary progressive aphasia with focal neuronal achromasia. Neurol 1991;41:882–886

188. Lowe J, Errington DR, Lenox G, et al. Ballooned neurons in several neurodegenerative diseases and stroke contain B crystallin. Neuropathology Applied Neurobiol 1992;18:341–350

189. Kumar R, Bergeron C, Pollanen MS, Lang AE. Cortical-basal ganglionic degeneration. In: Jankovic J, Tolosa E, eds. Parkinson's disease and movement disorders. 3rd ed. Baltimore, Maryland: Williams and Wilkins, 1998:297–316

190. Yamauchi H, Fukuyama H, Nagahama Y, et al. Atrophy of the corpus callosum, cortical hypometabolism, and cognitive impairment in corticobasal degeneration. Arch Neurol 1998;55(5):609–614

191. Smith TW, Lippa CF, de Girolama U. Immunocytochemical study of ballooned neurons in cortical degeneration with neuronal achromasia. Clin Neuropathol 1992;11:28–35

192. Feany MB, Dickson DW. Widespread cytoskeletal pathology characterizes corticobasal degeneration. Am J Pathol 1995;146(6):1388–1396

193. Delacourte A, Buee L. Normal and pathological tau

proteins as factors for microtubule assembly. Int Rev Cytol 1997;171:167–224

194. Dickson DW. Neurodegenerative diseases with cytoskeletal pathology: a biochemical classification. Ann Neurol 1997;42:541–544

195. Dickson DW, Anderton B, Morris H, et al. International medical workshop covering progressive supranuclear palsy, multiple system atrophy and cortico basal degeneration. Mov Disord 2001;16(2): 382–395

196. Bergeron C, Pollanen MS, Weyer L, Lang AE. Cortical degeneration in progressive supranuclear palsy. a comparison with cortical-basal ganglionic degeneration. J Neuropathol Exp Neurol 1997;56(6):726–734

197. Bergeron C, Davis A, Lang AE. Corticobasal ganglionic degeneration and progressive supranuclear palsy presenting with cognitive decline. Brain Pathol 1998;8(2):355–365

198. Dickson DW. Neuropathologic differentiation of progressive supranuclear palsy and corticobasal degeneration. J Neurol 1999;246(Suppl 2):II6–II15

199. Di Maria E, Tabaton M, Vigo T, et al. Corticobasal degeneration shares a common genetic background with progressive supranuclear palsy. Ann Neurol 2000;47(3):374–377

200. Growdon JH, Primavera JM. Case 11-2000. N Engl J Med 2000;342:1110–1117

201. Brown J, Lantos PL, Roques P, et al. Familial dementia with swollen achromatic neurons and corticobasal inclusion bodies: a clinical and pathological study. J Neurol Sci 1996;135:21–30

202. Mathuranath PS, Xuereb JH, Bak T, Hodges JR. Corticobasal ganglionic degeneration and/or frontotemporal dementia? A report of two overlap cases and review of literature. J Neurol Neurosurg Psychiatry 2000;68:304–312

203. Lang AE, Bergeron C, Pollanen MS, Ashby P. Parietal pick's disease mimicking cortical-basal ganglionic degeneration. Neurology 1994;44:1436–1440

204. Boeve BF, Maraganore DM, Parisi JE, et al. Pathologic heterogeneity in clinically diagnosed corticobasal degeneration. Neurology 1999;53(4):795–800

205. Riley DE, Lang AE, Lewis A, et al. Cortical-basal ganglionic degeneration. Neurology 1990;40:1203–1212

206. Litvan I, Cummings JL, Mega M. Neuropsychiatric features of corticobasal degeneration. J Neurol Neurosurg Psychiatry 1998;65(5):717–721

207. Kompoliti K, Goetz CG, Boeve BF, et al. Clinical presentation and pharmacological therapy in corticobasal degeneration. Arch Neurol 1998;55(7):957–961

208. Leiguarda R, Lees AJ, Merello M, et al. The nature of apraxia in corticobasal degeneration. J Neurol Neurosurg Psychiatry 1994;57(4):455–459

209. Leiguarda R, Merello M, Balej J. Apraxia in corticobasal degeneration. Adv Neurol 2000;82:103–121

210. Doody RS, Jankovic J. The alien hand and related signs. J Neurol Neurosurg Psych 1992;55:806–810

211. Litvan I, Agid Y, Goetz C, et al. Accuracy of clinical diagnosis of corticobasal degeneration: a clinicopathological study. Neurol 1997;48:119–125

212. Litvan I, Grimes DA, Lang AE. Phenotypes and prognosis: clinicopathologic studies of corticobasal degeneration. Adv Neurol 2000;82:183–196

213. Thompson PD, Day BL, Rothwell JC, et al. The myoclonus in corticobasal degeneration: evidence for two forms of cortical reflex myoclonus. Brain 1994; 117(Pt 5):1197–1207

214. Thompson PD. Myoclonus in corticobasal degeneration. Clin Neurosci 1995;3(4):203–208

215. Thompson PD, Shibasaki H. Myoclonus in corticobasal degeneration and other neurodegenerations. Adv Neurol 2000;82:69–81

216. Strafella A, Ashby P, Lang AE. Reflex myoclonus in cortical-basal ganglionic degeneration involves a transcortical pathway. Mov Disord 1997;12:360–369

217. Vanek Z, Jankovic J. Corticobasal degeneration. dystonia in corticobasal degeneration. Adv Neurol 2000;82: 61–67

218. Vanek Z, Jankovic J. Dystonia in corticobasal degeneration. Mov Disord 2001;16(2):252–257

219. Pillon B, Blin J, Vidailhet M, et al. The neuropsychological pattern of corticobasal degeneration: comparison with progressive supranuclear palsy and Alzheimer's disease. Neurology 1995;45(8):1477–1483

220. Pillon B, Dubois B. Memory and executive processes in corticobasal degeneration. Adv Neurol 2000;82:91–101

221. Grimes DA, Lang AE, Bergeron CB. Dementia as the most common presentation of cortical-basal ganglionic degeneration. Neurology 1999;53:1969–1974

222. Massman PJ, Kreiter KT, Jankovic J, Doody RS. Neuropsychological functioning in cortico-basal ganglionic degeneration: differentiation from Alzheimer's disease. Neurology 1996;36:720–726

223. Cummings JL, Litvan I. Neuropsychiatric aspects of corticobasal degeneration. Adv Neurol 2000;82: 147–152

224. Frattali CM, Grafman J, Patronas N, et al. Language disturbances in corticobasal degeneration. Neurology 2000;54(4):990–992

225. Frattali CM, Sonies BC. Speech and swallowing disturbances in corticobasal degeneration. Adv Neurol 2000;82:153–160

226. Vidailhet M, Rivaud-Pechoux S. Eye movement disorders in corticobasal degeneration. Adv Neurol 2000; 82:161–167

227. Soliveri P, Monza D, Paridi D, et al. Cognitive and magnetic resonance imaging aspects of corticobasal degeneration and progressive supranuclear palsy. Neurology 1999;53(3):502–507

228. Molinuevo JL, Munoz E, Valldeoriola F, Tolosa E. The eye of the tiger sign in cortico-basal ganglionic degeneration. Mov Disord 1999;14:169–171

229. Yamauchi H, Fukuyama H, Nagahama Y, et al. Atrophy of the corpus callosum, cortical hypometabolism, and cognitive impairment in corticobasal degeneration. Arch Neurol 1998;55:609–614

230. Sawle GV, Brooks DJ, Marsden CD, Frackowiak SJ. Corticobasal degeneration. Brain 1991;114:541–556

231. Eidelberg D, Dhawan V, Moeller JR, et al. The metabolic landscape of cortico-basal ganglionic degeneration: regional asymmetries studied with positron emission tomography. J Neurol Neurosurg Psych 1991; 54:856–862

232. Blin J, Vidailhet MJ, Pillon B, et al. Corticobasal degeneration: decreased and asymmetrical glucose consumption as studied with PET. Mov Disord 1992;7: 348–354

233. Brooks DJ. Corticobasal degeneration: functional imaging studies in corticobasal degeneration. Adv Neurol 2000;82:209–215

234. Okuda B, Tachibana H. The nature of apraxia in corticobasal degeneration. J Neurol Neurosurg Psych 1994; 57(12):1548–1549

235. Okuda B, Tachibana H. Cerebral blood flow in corticobasal degeneration. Mov Disord 1995;10(6):803

236. Okuda B, Tachibana H, Kawabata K, et al. Cerebral blood flow correlates of higher brain dysfunctions in

corticobasal degeneration. J Geriatr Psychiatry Neurol 1999;12(4):189–193

237. Okuda B, Kodama N, Tachibana H, et al. Visuomotor ataxia in corticobasal degeneration. Mov Disord 2000; 15(2):337–340

238. Okuda B, Tachibana H, Kawabata K, et al. Cerebral blood flow in corticobasal degeneration and progressive supranuclear palsy. Alzheimer Dis Assoc Disord 2000;14(1):46–52

239. Okuda B, Tachibana H, Kawabata K, et al. Comparison of brain perfusion in corticobasal degeneration and Alzheimer's disease. Dement Geriatr Cogn Disord 2001;12(3):226–231

240. Laureys S, Salmon E, Garraux G, et al. Fluorodopa uptake and glucose metabolism in early stages of corticobasal degeneration. J Neurol 1999;246(12):1151–1158

241. Garraux G, Salmon E, Peigneux P, et al. Voxel-based distribution of metabolic impairment in corticobasal degeneration. Mov Disord 2000;15(5):894–904

242. Brunt ER, van Weerden TW, Pruim J, Lakke JW. Unique myoclonic pattern in corticobasal degeneration. Mov Disord 1995;10(2):132–142

243. Lu CS, Ikeda A, Terada K, et al. Electrophysiological studies of early stage corticobasal degeneration. Mov Disord 1998;13(1):140–146

244. Kompoliti K, Goetz CG, Boeve BF, et al. Clinical presentation and pharmacological therapy in corticobasal degeneration. Arch Neurol 1998;55(7):957–961

245. Kompoliti K, Goetz CG. Therapeutic approaches. Adv Neurol 2000;82:217–222

246. Graham NL, Zeman A, Young AW, et al. Dyspraxia in a patient with corticobasal degeneration: the role of visual and tactile inputs to action. J Neurol Neurosurg Psychiatry 1999;67(3):334–344

247. Critchley M. Atherosclerotic parkinsonism. Brain 1929; 52–53

248. Eadie MJ, Sutherland JM, Atherosclerosis in parkinsonism. J Neurol Neurosurg Psychiatry 1964;27: 237–240

249. Parkes JD, Marsden CD, Rees JE, et al. Parkinson's disease, cerebral atherosclerosis and senile dementia. Q J Med 1974;43:49–61

250. Daniel SE, Lees AJ. Parkinson's disease society brain bank, London: overview and research. J Neural Transm 1993;39:165–172

251. Yamanouchi H, Nagura H. Neurological signs and frontal white matter lesions in vascular parkinsonism. A clinicopathologic study. Stroke 1997;28(5):965–969

252. Winikates J, Jankovic J. Clinical correlates of vascular parkinsonism. Arch Neurol 1999;56:98–102

253. Trenkwalder C, Paulus W, Krafeczyc S, et al. Postural stability differentiates "lower body" from idiopathic parkinsonism. Acta Neurol Scan 1995;91:444–452

254. Fitzgerald PM, Jankovic J. Lower body parkinsonism: evidence for vascular etiology. Mov Disord 1989;4: 249–260

255. Thompson PD, Marsden CD. Gait disorder of subcortical arteriosclerotic encephalopathy: Binswanger disease. Mov Disord 1987;2:1–8

256. Roman GC. New insight into Binswanger disease. Arch Neurol 1999;56:1061–1106

257. Mark MH, Sage JI, Walters AS, et al. Binswanger's disease presenting as levodopa-responsive Parkinson's disease: clinicopathological study of three cases. Mov Disord 1995;10:450–454

258. Van Zagten M, Lodder J, Kessels F. Gait disorder and parkinsonian signs in patients with stroke related to small deep infarcts and white matter lesions. Mov Disord 1998;13:89–95

259. Joutel A, Dodick DD, Parisi JE, et al. De novo mutation in the Notch3 gene causing CADASIL. Ann Neurol 2000;47:388–391

260. Zijlmans JC, Thikssen HO, Vogels OJ, et al. MRI in patients with suspected vascular parkinsonism. Neurol 1995;45:2183–2188

261. Tzen KY, Lu CS, Yen TC, et al. Differential diagnosis of Parkinson's disease and vascular parkinsonism by ^{99m}Tc-TRODAT-1. J Nuclear Med 2001;42(3):408–413

262. Bencsits G, Pirker W, Asenbaum S, et al. Comparison of the ^{123}I beta-CIT snf SPECT in lower body parkinsonism and Parkinson's disease [Abstract]. Mov Disord 1998;13(Suppl):106

263. Zijlmans JC, de Koster A, van't Hof MA, et al. Proton magnetic resonance spectroscopy in suspected vascular parkinsonism. Acta Neurol Scand 1994;90:405–411

264. Aizawa H, Kwak T, Shimuzu T, et al. A case of adult onset pure pallidal degeneration: clinical manifestations and neuropathological observations. J Neurol Sci 1991;102:76–82

265. Becher MW, Rubinzstein DC, Leggo JC, et al. Dentatorubro-pallidoluysian atrophy (DRPLA): clinical and neuropathological findings in genetically confirmed North American and European pedigrees. Mov Disord 1997;12(4):519–530

266. Thomas M, Jankovic J. Dentatorubro-pallidoluysian atrophy (DRPLA) in North American families. Abstract accepted for ANA Oct 2001

267. Kanazawa I. Molecular Pathology of Dentatorubral-pallidoluysian atrophy. Philos Trans R Soc Lon B Biol Sci 1999;354(1386):1069–1078

268. Aizawa H, Kwak S, Shimizu T, et al. A case of adult onset pure pallidal degeneration. II. Analysis of neurotransmitter markers, with special reference to the termination of pallidothalamic tract in human brain. J Neurol Sci 1991 Mar;102(1):83–91

233 Surgical Treatment of Parkinson's Disease

Anthony E Lang and Galit Kleiner-Fisman

Surgery for Parkinson's disease dates back to the late 1930s when excision of parts of the cerebral cortex was used to treat dystonia and tremor. These procedures and subsequent lesions of the internal capsule and cerebral peduncle regularly produced hemiparesis in addition to reducing tremor. In the early 1940s, Meyers[1] introduced open surgery of the basal ganglia including pallidotomy. Although this did result in significant relief of tremor and rigidity, mortality was extremely high. An important turning point in this field was the introduction of stereotactic techniques in the 1950s by Spiegel and Wycis[2,3] who used coagulation to lesion the globus pallidus and ansa lenticularis of parkinsonian patients. Cooper[4,5] championed a number of techniques to lesion various regions of the basal ganglia in parkinsonian patients. These included inflating small balloons within the target in an attempt to predict subsequent responses (and complications) and the use of alcohol injections and lesioning with cyroprobes. Hassler[6] introduced surgery of the ventrolateral thalamus based on knowledge of the anatomic connections between the pallidum and this region. Using micro-recording techniques, Narabayashi[7,8] defined the importance of the ventral intermediate (Vim) nucleus of the thalamus as the specific target for tremor. Much later he also emphasized the need for larger more anteriorly expanded lesions to control levodopa-induced dyskinesias.[9] Neurosurgery for Parkinson's disease reached a peak in the 1960s, however, the subsequent introduction of levodopa resulted in a marked decline in its use. Until recently, "functional neurosurgery" (which was almost exclusively thalamotomy) was used in a small subgroup of patients who were considered to have drug resistant "tremor dominant" Parkinson's disease.

Recently there has been a resurgence in the use of surgical treatment for Parkinson's disease.[10] There are a variety of reasons for this renewed interest. Although levodopa and other newer drugs may be extremely effective in lessening the disability of Parkinson's disease, a number of problems arise particularly motor fluctuations and dyskinesias. These may be the most disabling features of the illness in the later stages. There have been major advances in our understanding of the functional interactions of the basal ganglia, particularly in the parkinsonian state. It is now known that the dopamine deficiency of Parkinson's disease results in hyperactivity of the outflow regions of the basal ganglia, the internal segment of the globus pallidus (GPi) and the

substantia nigra reticulata (SNr), in part driven by over activity of the subthalamic nucleus (STN). The over-activity of the GPi and SNr results in excessive inhibition (GABA) of their downstream targets, the motor thalamus and brainstem locomotor areas, which results in reduced activation of pre-motor cortical regions (Figure 233.1). Stereotactic techniques have also improved in recent years particularly with the introduction of magnetic resonance imaging and modern computer technology. Another factor that has encouraged the resurgence in neurosurgical therapies for Parkinson's disease (PD) is the rapidly developing field of neural transplantation and regeneration. Indeed, the modern era of functional neurosurgery for PD was initiated in the 1980s by the use of adrenal medullary transplantation, which has since been abandoned due to poor efficacy and high morbidity. It should be emphasized that despite the pronounced increased utilization of functional neurosurgical therapy for PD, it has been almost exclusively based on Class III evidence. Until very recently[11,12] no randomized controlled clinical trials existed in this field.

General considerations

Before a patients' surgical candidacy can be considered, certain general issues applicable to most surgical therapies for Parkinson's disease need to be addressed. Indications for surgery are summarized in Table 233.1. The underlying diagnosis must be carefully considered. Some of the most disabled patients sent for surgical opinion, especially those with a relatively short history of disease do not have Parkinson's disease. The currently available neurosurgical treatments are generally ineffective for other diseases such as multiple system atrophy, progressive supranuclear palsy and corticobasal degeneration.

Table 233.1 Indications for Parkinson's disease surgery

Diagnosis of idiopathic PD (other less common forms of L-dopa responsive parkinsonism may also be appropriate)

Clear response to L-dopa (generally >30%)

Severe PD (minimal score of 30 points on the motor portion of the UPDRS when the patient has been without medications for at least 12 hours)

Motor complications that cannot be controlled by pharmacologic therapy or intolerance to higher doses of dopaminergic drugs (caution if psychiatric side-effects are the principal dose-limiting factor)

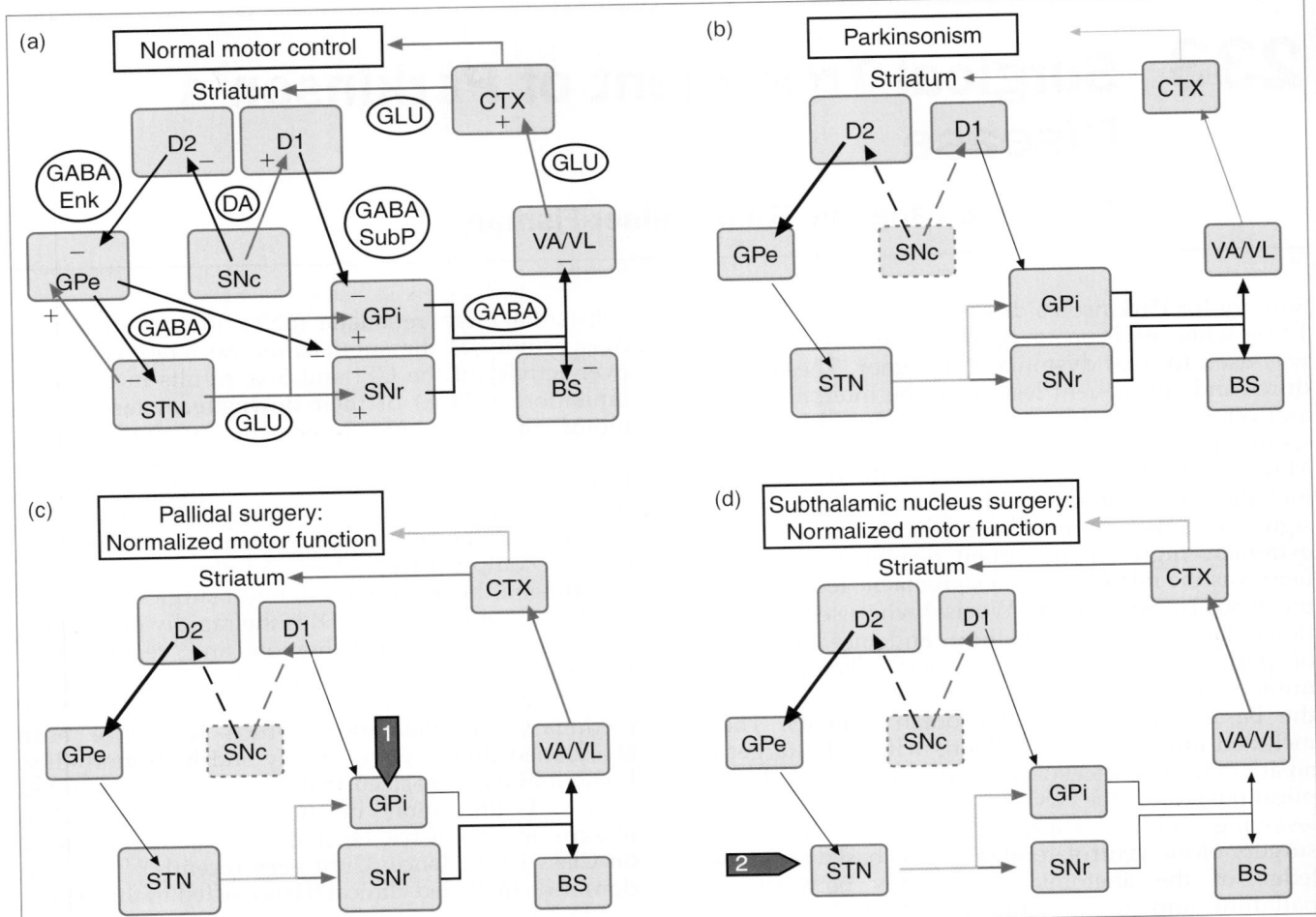

Figure 233.1 Schematic representation of basal ganglia function in (a) Normal motor control (b) Parkinsonism (c) Pallidal surgery (d) Subthalamic nucleus surgery. Gpe, globus pallidus externa; Gpi, globus pallidus interna; STN, subthalamic nucleus; SNr, substantia nigra reticulata; SNc, substantia nigra compacta; BS, brain stem; VA/VL, ventral anterior and ventral lateral nucleus of thalamus; CTX, cortex; GABA, gamma amino butyric acid; DA, dopamine; Enk, enkephalin; Glu, glutamate; SubP, substance P; + (blue arrows), excitatory; − (black arrows), inhibitory. *These pathways are left out of the subsequent figures in the interest of simplicity.

Underlying cognitive dysfunction is common in Parkinson's disease, frequently increases following neurosurgery and when prominent should serve as an absolute contraindication to surgery. Age may have a negative impact on outcome and so neurosurgery should be undertaken quite cautiously in the elderly. Exclusion criteria for surgery are detailed in Table 233.2. An understanding of the "target symptoms" is critical in choosing between surgical techniques. For example, Vim thalamotomy is almost exclusively effective for tremor. Lesions are generally poorly tolerated when applied bilaterally and if this is to be done, a long hiatus should be planned between lesioning the two sides. For this reason, if the patient suffers from severe bilateral disability, bilateral STN or GPi deep brain stimulation (DBS) or a unilateral lesion followed by contralateral DBS should be considered. Optimum benefit from STN DBS often requires a reduction in dopaminergic medication doses to diminish stimulation/drug-induced dyskinesias. Therefore, the patient with severe bilateral disability should probably not be considered for unilateral STN stimulation. The same may apply to combining STN stimulation with a contralateral GPi procedure since the latter usually requires continued use of medication at the preoperative level. The relative merits of individual targets and approaches are outlined in Table 233.3.

Aside from drug-resistant tremor, there is no convincing evidence available to indicate that symptoms

Table 233.2 Exclusion criteria for Parkinson's disease surgery

Major psychiatric illness
Cognitive impairment
Other substantial medical co-morbidities
Presence of cardiac pacemaker (DBS)
Parkinsonism due to causes other than idiopathic Parkinson's disease (levodopa resistant)
Symptoms not responsive to dopaminergic agents
Advanced age (relative contra-indication)

Table 233.3 Relative merits of surgical approaches

Surgical procedure	Advantages	Disadvantages
Unilateral	Decreased risk of complications compared to bilateral surgery	Suboptimal effect for bilateral disease and axial symptomatology
Bilateral	Effective for bilateral limb and axial symptoms	Increased risk of surgical morbidity; increased risk of adverse effects due to surgery
Lesion	One time intervention without need for close monitoring, programming or adjusting	Irreversible; if lesion is suboptimal with respect to location or size, may need second procedure
Deep brain stimulation	Adjustable, reversible	Battery needs to be replaced every 3–5 years; potential for hardware related complications such as infection, breakage or erosion of skin over wire; time and labor-consuming programming and monitoring
Thalamus	Effective for drug-resistant tremor	Minimal or no effect on bradykinesia, mild reduction of rigidity; if bilateral, risk of hypophonia and dysarthria
Globus pallidus pars interna	Effective for bradykinesia, rigidity, tremor; decreased drug-induced dyskinesia	No change in medication dose; little evidence that persistent on-period symptoms (e.g. postural instability, falls, dysarthria and on-period freezing) are improved
Subthalamic nucleus	Effective for bradykinesia, rigidity, tremor; decreased drug-induced dyskinesia; decrease in medication requirements	Little evidence that persistent on-period symptoms (e.g. postural instability, falls, dysarthria and on-period freezing) are improved
Adrenal medulla transplant	Some modest, questionable improvement in severity of off-period parkinsonism;	High incidence of neurological and cardiopulmonary complications; deemed unacceptable therapy by Therapeutics and Technology Assessment Subcommittee of the American Academy of Neurology
Human fetal mesencephalic transplant	Evidence for long-term survival of implanted tissue; improvement in off-period parkinsonism; modest benefit in most patients <60	No benefit in patients >60 in one study; delayed increase in dyskinesia some patients developed spontaneous dyskinesia independent of dopaminergic therapy in one study; remains investigational

resistant to levodopa respond to any of the currently available surgical techniques. These include on-period ambulatory dysfunction such as freezing and falls, as well as dysarthria. It is therefore critical to determine the extent to which the patient's disability relates to symptoms that are levodopa-resistant and for the patient and family to have a realistic understanding of the limitations (as well as the potential complications) of surgery.

Ablative lesions/deep brain stimulation

The role of surgical technical factors remains controversial with respect to outcome and complication rate. Some authorities strongly believe that the use of microelectrode recording both enhances the successful localization of the lesion or electrode placement and reduces complications while others, who utilize macro-stimulation only, argue that the clinical outcome is no better with micro-recording, the technique adds unnecessarily to the duration of the procedure and that the complication rate is higher given the number of needle electrode passes necessary for the micro-recording. Unfortunately there is little hard evidence available to support either view, however, most authorities do acknowledge the importance of having some form of electrophysiological guidance in addition to anatomical imaging. The risk of a significant cerebral hemorrhage is present with any stereotactic procedure and is estimated at between 2–5%. There is no convincing evidence that this is higher with micro-recording techniques.

It is widely recognized that initial clinical benefit from lesion procedures is sometimes lost very early in the postoperative period (in the first three months). Generally, when this occurs the lesion was either too small or sub-optimally placed and usually a repeat procedure is required. The advantage of DBS is that the stimulation is titratable and can be adjusted in order to recapture lost initial benefit, however, some patients do require electrode repositioning if the initial response is found to be sub-optimal.

The deep brain stimulation "hardware" consists of a quadripolar electrode implanted in the target site in the brain (Figure 233.2) connected to a neurostimulator (pulse generator) that is implanted subcutaneously in the chest wall. The neurostimulator can be turned on and off externally by a "therapy controller" used with the most common Medtronic models, the Kinetra and Soletra. Its parameters such as electrode polarity, amplitude, pulse width and frequency are adjusted by this external programmer to optimize clinical effect and minimize unwanted side effects.

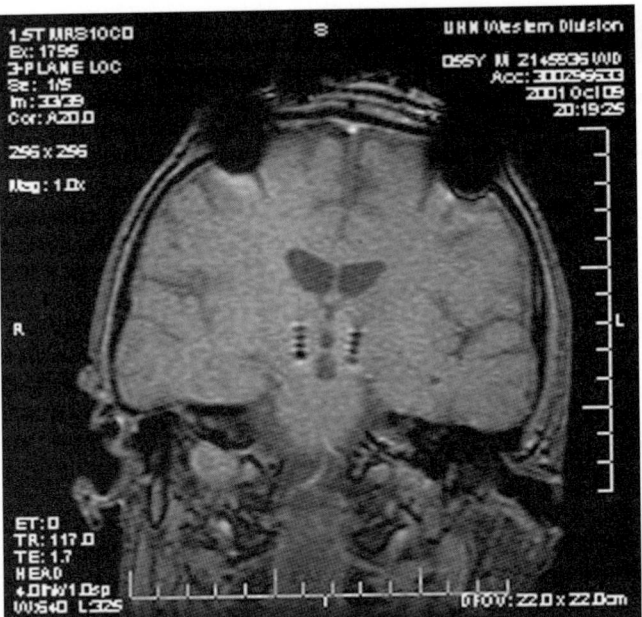

Figure 233.2   TI coronal MRI image showing quadripolar electrodes implanted in bilateral sub-thalamic nuclei.

Some of the initial clinical benefit obtained with DBS procedures comes from a so-called micro-lesion effect due to the trauma of the procedure itself. Most studies have shown that this effect dissipates in the majority of patients in the first few weeks following surgery. Safety (generally no permanent lesion, safer for bilateral procedures) and efficacy (especially related to the titratability) are often cited as major advantages of DBS over lesions. However, it should be acknowledged that there are a variety of complications unique to DBS, which are not uncommon and must be factored into any decision to proceed with this therapy. These include skin erosion, infection, fracture of electrodes, migration of leads, and the inevitable eventual battery failure with the requirement for further surgical replacement. In addition, optimization of stimulation parameters, especially in the GPi and STN often requires a great deal of time and effort on the part of the patient and the medical staff.

The mechanism of action of DBS is poorly understood. It is known that the effects are not due to destruction of the region of stimulation (i.e. not a method of chronically lesioning the brain).[13] Since the clinical effects essentially mimic those of lesioning the same regions of the brain it has been argued that this constitutes an electrical neuronal blockade. However, it is known that the effects of stimulation are much greater on axons than neural cell bodies and especially on large axons running parallel to the plane of stimulation. Therefore, it is possible that beneficial results of DBS derive from the stimulation of inhibitory circuits. It is also possible that the mechanism of action differs depending upon the region being stimulated. More work is required to enhance our understanding of the physiological mechanisms underlying DBS and to improve the technology utilized to apply this novel therapy.

Thalamus

Thalamotomy   Currently most surgeons place thalamic lesions in the Vim nucleus, which is believed to be the recipient of cerebellar input. However, there is still some variability in the target site for thalamotomy;[14] less commonly chosen sites still include the subthalamic region (not the subthalamic nucleus), the zona incerta and fields of Forel, and the medial thalamic nuclear complex. Thalamotomy is indicated for medication-resistant, disabling, preferably asymmetrical tremor. Rigidity may also be reduced and when present, pain and parkinsonian dystonia may also be improved. These latter effects and the effect on levodopa-induced dyskinesias may be dependent upon expansion of the lesion anteriorly from the Vim into the region of the thalamus receiving afferents from the medial pallidum.[9,15] Bradykinesia (and all its attendant disability, including writing disturbance) is not improved and speech and gait dysfunction may even worsen. The ideal patient will have little in the way of other features of PD resulting in any disability. It should be emphasized that such "tremor dominant" patients are uncommon especially after several years of disease (possibly accounting for less than 5% of the patient population). More often, tremor is not a major source of disability and other symptoms, particularly bradykinesia and gait dysfunction, eventually supervene even in those classified as tremor-dominant earlier in the course of their disease. Because thalamotomy is ineffective for other features of PD, tremor reduction due to surgery may not necessarily translate into reduction in level of disability or improved function.

Microelectrode or semi-microelectrode recording and stimulation define the presence of cells firing in synchrony with the tremor ("tremor cells"). The response of cells to active and passive movement, and sensory input, as well as the location of nearby structures such as the internal capsule laterally and sensory thalamus posteriorly, also contribute to defining the optimal location for lesioning. Electro-coagulation is the most common method of performing lesions currently.

Most evidence for the efficacy of thalamotomy is Class III with one recent comparison between thalamotomy and thalamic DBS utilizing a randomized controlled trial study design.[11] Moderate to good reduction in contralateral tremor is evident in approximately 80% of cases.[16] This benefit may be sustained for many years.[17] Contralateral thalamotomy probably has an equal chance of improving tremor in the opposite limbs, however, the risk of adverse effects, most notably permanent speech dysfunction and cognitive decline is considerable and most authorities now recommend thalamic DBS if the opposite side is to be considered for surgery.

Transient complications (lasting up to three months) are common after unilateral thalamotomy. Between a third and two thirds of patients may experience contralateral weakness, sensory complaints, ataxia, dystonia, apraxia, or inattention, confusion, aphasia, or dysarthria. Up to 25% of patients experience more persistent or permanent complications[16] including death (generally from intracerebral hemorrhage at the time of the procedure although delayed deaths may occur from myocardial infarction, pulmonary embolus or aspiration pneumonia). A recently published randomized comparison between thalamotomy and thalamic DBS found that the efficacy of the two procedures was roughly equivalent, however, thalamic DBS was associated with fewer important adverse effects.[11]

Gamma knife thalamotomy has been reported in individual cases and small poorly controlled case series.[18,19] Generally this has been reserved for treatment of patients considered poor operative risks or where the technology and expertise for conventional stereotactic neurosurgery are unavailable. Not surprisingly (especially considering the predominance of case reports), effective control of contralateral tremor has been reported with this technique. However, adverse effects due to spread of the lesion beyond the confines of the Vim thalamus have been commonly described. A number of published studies involving conventional stereotactic ablative procedures have documented the common need to change the final site of lesioning from that predicted by imaging alone based on information obtained during intra-operative electrophysiological assessment.[20–22] Obviously, this is not possible with gamma knife treatment and will always represent a significant limitation to the efficacy of this approach. More recently, long-term results from 158 patients who underwent gamma knife thalamotomy for tremor of various etiologies were reported.[23] Contrary to previous reports, this study suggests that gamma knife Vim thalamotomy is an effective treatment for tremor with a superior safety profile compared to deep brain stimulation and radio-frequency lesioning. Despite this positive report, the general consensus of experts in the field is that the role of gamma knife treatment of Parkinson's disease and other movement disorders is extremely limited. Even when benefit is obtained, there is the potential for late and progressive neurological deficits, an issue that may be under-represented in the literature.

Thalamic deep brain stimulation The principle advantages of DBS are that it is titratable, based on both efficacy and side effects, and that permanent complications are less common than with lesions, particularly when bilateral procedures are preformed. The indications for thalamic DBS are similar to those for thalamotomy with the additional option of performing bilateral procedures including implantation contralateral to a previous thalamotomy. As indicated above, the short-term efficacy of thalamic stimulation is equivalent to that of thalamotomy, however, DBS appears to be better tolerated and is now becoming the treatment of choice unless there are clear contraindications or strong arguments against this option. Available studies have provided randomized double-blind evaluations of stimulation on *vs.* off demonstrating marked (even complete) contralateral tremor suppression in 80–90% of patients. This has been variably associated with alterations in functional abilities.[24,25] One randomized study of 68 patients receiving either thalamotomy or thalamic DBS reported equally effective suppression of drug-resistant tremor after six months, but patients treated with stimulation were found to have improved functional status with fewer adverse events.[11] Generally, thalamic DBS has been ineffective in reducing levodopa-induced dyskinesias although one study has suggested a pronounced effect with more posterior, medial and deeper placement of the electrodes (possibly in the region of the center median-parafascicular nuclear complex).[26] Due to the limitations of thalamic surgery with respect to symptoms of PD other than tremor and the clear efficacy of surgical procedures involving the globus pallidus and STN for these features, the role of thalamic DBS in PD will become rather limited as other surgical procedures become more widely adopted.

Globus pallidus

Pallidotomy Laitinen "reintroduced" posteroventral medial pallidotomy (PVMP) for Parkinson's disease in 1992.[27] Renewed interest in pallidotomy relates to the greater clinical benefit to parkinsonism obtained with localization of the lesion in the sensorimotor GPi in contrast to the older, more anterior lesions, and the striking ameliorative effect of PVMP on levodopa-induced dyskinesias (which were not an issue in the earlier pre-levodopa era of functional neurosurgery for Parkinson's disease).

Unilateral pallidotomy is primarily indicated for advanced levodopa-responsive PD with motor fluctuations manifested by disabling off periods and drug-induced dyskinesias.[28] The benefit is largely experienced on the side contralateral to the lesion although mild but transient improvement may be seen on the ipsilateral side and in axial features (e.g. postural stability and gait disorder). Contralateral drug-induced dyskinesias respond to a greater extent than other features, improving by between 80–95%. Ipsilateral dyskinesias may improved by 40–50% however we have found that this response is lost between the first and second post-operative year.[29] Total off-period motor and activities of daily living (ADL) scores improve by 25–30% with reductions in contralateral parkinsonism including tremor, rigidity and bradykinesia accounting for much of this change. On-period scores change very little except as explained by reduction in disabling dyskinesias (i.e. manifest by improvement in ADL scores). Generally, the doses of anti-Parkinson's medications change very little in response to pallidotomy or pallidal DBS.

There is very little long-term follow-up data available to establish the duration of benefit from PVMP. One prospective study[30] reported sustained reduction in limb dyskinesia and off state tremor score on the side contralateral to pallidotomy after three years, however, all other measures deteriorated and ADL's continued to worsen. We have reported evidence that those who obtain an initial good response may sustain benefit in all aspects of contralateral parkinsonism and dyskinesias for up to 5.5 years, however, contralateral bradykinesia and total motor scores demonstrated some loss of original benefit and total ADL scores were no longer significantly improved compared to the baseline preoperative state.[31]

Despite its widespread application, support for the use of pallidotomy in PD is almost exclusively based on evidence derived from uncontrolled case series. Two groups have recently confirmed the significant beneficial effects of pallidotomy to both off-period parkinsonism and levodopa-induced dyskinesias in randomized controlled clinical trials. The first, a multi-center study from the Netherlands[12,32] and the second, a single center trial from Emory University in the US.[33] This second group followed patients for four years and found that they showed sustained improvements in contralateral tremor, akinesia, and drug-induced dyskinesia. Another study from Argentina demonstrated similar benefits in those undergoing unilateral pallidotomy one year earlier in contrast to an unoperated control group who lacked necessary financial support.[34]

There have been several attempts to predict who might benefit most from PVMP.[28,35] Younger patients may do better than older ones, although age has not been a universal predictor in all studies. A good sustained response to levodopa is generally felt to be an important and useful predictive factor. Motor fluctuations with dyskinesia and precise lesion placement predicted a good response to unilateral pallidotomy. Positron emission tomography evidence of hypermetabolism of the globus pallidus is not a practical predictive factor given the limited availability of positron emission tomography (PET) scanning.

Adverse effects of pallidotomy are common. Overall, most studies (commonly reporting their initial experiences with this new procedure; i.e. at the outset of the learning curve) report 10–15% incidence of persistent adverse effects with unilateral pallidotomy. The majority of these complications are mild and well tolerated and appear to be outweighed by the motor benefits of the surgery. The close proximity of the posteroventral medial pallidum to the optic tract and internal capsule, account for visual field defects and contralateral weakness (especially involving the face) following pallidotomy. The incidence of these complications has declined from initial reports as surgical groups have become more experienced with the procedure. Weight gain is an extremely common "complication" of successful pallidotomy.[36,37] This probably occurs on a multifactorial basis largely, but not exclusively, due to the reduction in drug-induced dyskinesias. Weight gain is now recognized as a feature of all successful pallidal and STN procedures.

Neuropsychological evaluations have demonstrated quite variable consequences of pallidotomy. Most patients experience either little or no functional decline, although, persistent verbal fluency deficits are common after left-sided lesions. Behavioral changes may develop in a small proportion of patients. Patients with pre-existing cognitive dysfunction commonly experience transient post-operative confusion as well as persistent worsening of cognitive function. Careful neuropsychological screening should be performed in patients being considered for pallidotomy and significant cognitive deficits are considered a contraindication to the procedure.

There are no reliable data to support the safety and efficacy of bilateral pallidotomy. Claims vary widely ranging from pronounced benefit in selected patients, (beyond that obtained with a unilateral procedure) and little or no additional risk[38,39] to variable additional benefits but with a high incidence of complications[42] particularly with respect to speech,[40] cognition and behavior.[41] In one study of staged bilateral pallidotomy,[42] it was noted that after the second procedure several months after the first, there were further modest improvements in some symptoms, but the patients were less responsive to levodopa. When bilateral procedures are deemed necessary, deep brain stimulation should usually be considered a more appropriate alternative.

There is limited experience with gamma knife pallidotomy. Although one group has claimed comparable benefit to radiofrequency lesioning[43] (not supported in a comparison of their data to reports on the effects of pallidotomy from other groups), others report limited benefit and substantial complications.[44,45] As with gamma knife thalamotomy, this method cannot be recommended for the treatment of Parkinson's disease at the present time.

Pallidal deep brain stimulation   Preliminary results of pallidal DBS are extremely promising but limited. Unilateral pallidal DBS may provide benefit equivalent to that obtained with unilateral pallidotomy.[46] Unilateral pallidal DBS may be applied very successfully in patients who have undergone previous contralateral pallidotomy.[47] Recently, 38 patients with medically intractable PD undergoing bilateral pallidal stimulation have been reported. At three months, double blind cross-over evaluations revealed significant improvement in off-period parkinsonian features as well as suppression of on-period drug-induced dyskinesias.[48] Continuous stimulation (usually applied around the clock) can result in a marked reduction in the amount of time spent in the off-period with a concomitant significant increase in the time spent on without dyskinesias. The GPi is a relatively large nuclear structure compared to the Vim thalamus and subthalamic nucleus. This may account for variable responses reported for dyskinesias and parkinsonian features depending upon exact site of stimulation.[49,50] Adverse effects are similar to those seen with pallidotomy. Although it is generally believed that DBS is safer than lesioning, comparative data are not available. The few available reports certainly seem to indicate that bilateral pallidal stimulation is much better tolerated (with respect to adverse effects) than bilateral pallidotomy. Stimulation often results in acute adverse effects (usually experienced during the programming period) such as tonic contraction of contralateral muscles and visual disturbances (phosphenes) due to spread of current to the internal capsule or optic tract respectively. These resolve with adjustments in stimulation parameters. As mentioned earlier in the general comments section, complications of DBS include infection, breakage and failure of the "hardware."

In contrast to the Vim thalamus, programming of pallidal DBS (as well as STN DBS—see below) can be complex and time-consuming. The effects of DBS need to be assessed in detail in both the off and on states. Drug dosage changes may be required (less frequently with pallidal than with STN stimulation). Thus, this treatment should only be offered by groups with considerable experience in the post-operative management of these various treatment factors.

Subthalamic nucleus

Lesions of the subthalamic nucleus "Subthalamic" lesions were not uncommonly used in the treatment of Parkinson's disease in the pre-levodopa era. However, this term referred to the immediate subthalamic region involving afferent input to the thalamus rather than the subthalamic nucleus, which surgeons attempted to avoid at all costs for fear of causing hemiballism. With advances in our understanding of the role of the subthalamic nucleus in the pathogenesis of parkinsonism and observations that STN DBS and even spontaneous lesions of the STN (e.g. infarcts) may result in striking improvements in parkinsonism, subthalamic nucleotomy is being investigated in a small number of centers[51,52] with promising preliminary results. Until further reports are forthcoming, this procedure should only be applied by experienced academic centers involved in carefully evaluating its safety and efficacy.

Deep brain stimulation of the subthalamic nucleus As with pallidal stimulation, experience with stimulation of the STN is quite limited. Most studies have evaluated bilateral STN DBS as opposed to unilateral procedures. Generally, in contrast to pallidal stimulation, reduction in drug-induced dyskinesias with STN DBS requires a concomitant reduction in dopaminergic medication.[53,54] In patients with significant bilateral disability there is a concern that this reduction in medication may not be tolerated by the unoperated side if they were to undergo only a unilateral procedure. A similar concern applies to the combination of unilateral STN DBS with contralateral pallidal DBS or lesioning.[55] However, these issues require further intensive evaluation.

Double-blind evaluation of the effects of bilateral STN DBS[56,48] has confirmed the significant beneficial effects reported in open studies. All features of off-period parkinsonism have been shown to respond to an extent roughly equivalent to the benefit obtained with levodopa.[53,57] On-period features may also improve although it is not clear that STN stimulation results in benefit beyond that obtained with a "supermaximal" dose of levodopa. Off-period dystonia generally responds extremely well. As mentioned above, peak-dose dyskinesias also improve although largely due to the concomitant reduction in dopaminergic drug dosages. The latter may also result in some improvement in so-called "on-period freezing." As described with pallidal stimulation, diary evaluations in patients treated with continuous STN stimulation demonstrate a pronounced reduction in the proportion of the day spent in the off state (this combined with the significant reduction in the severity of the off periods may result in patients having difficulty determining whether they are off or on) with a concomitant increase in time "on without dyskinesias."

Subthalamic nucleus stimulation is generally well tolerated although a variety of complications are possible. Transient confusion is relatively common in the immediate postoperative period in patients undergoing bilateral implantation. Elderly patients may experience more persistent cognitive impairment.[58] Even younger patients with no pre-procedure cognitive dysfunction may show slight degradation in executive function although it is arguable whether this is clinically significant.[59,60] As with all stereotactic procedures, intracranial hemorrhage during surgery may result in permanent neurological deficits (depending on where along the needle/electrode tract the hemorrhage is located). "Eyelid-opening apraxia" may occur in a small proportion of patients; botulinum toxin may be effective in controlling this complication. Excessive reduction in levodopa dosage may result in hypophonia or changes in behavior that respond to a slight increase in dopaminergic drugs. Stimulation-related complications, due to spread of the current to nearby structures (which resolve on changing stimulation parameters) include contralateral tonic muscle contraction (pyramidal tract), diplopia (fascical of the third nerve) and contralateral paraesthesiae (medial lemniscus). Unusual behavioral changes directly due to stimulation have included profound depression[61] as well as laughter and mirth.[62,63] Hardware complications (e.g. infection, breakage) remain an ongoing potential risk in patients with DBS of any sort.

The relative efficacy of GPi *vs.* STN stimulation is unknown. Uncontrolled, non-randomized studies have suggested that DBS in the STN may be more effective than GPi DBS with the additional advantages of allowing lower doses of anti-Parkinson medications and lower voltages of stimulation (resulting in longer battery life). However, in the only available small pilot study published to date, patients randomized to GPi ($n = 4$) or STN ($n = 5$) stimulation obtained equivalent benefit.[64] A retrospective study of patients treated with STN or GPi DBS found equal efficacy with respect to "off" period motor symptoms, dyskinesias and fluctuations. Subthalamic nucleus stimulation DBS patients had substantial reduction in their anti-parkinsonian medications and required much less electrical power, however, they also required more intensive postoperative monitoring and had a higher incidence of adverse events such as dysarthria, anhedonia and depression, that were related to levodopa withdrawal.[65] Further studies evaluating this important question are awaited with interest.

Neurotransplantation

Adrenal medullary transplantation As mentioned in the introduction, adrenal transplantation led the resurgence of interest in neurosurgery for Parkinson's disease. However, this treatment has been essentially abandoned because of limited efficacy and high morbidity and mortality. It involved a combination of two surgical procedures, adrenalectomy (transabdominal or retroperitoneal) and craniotomy for tissue implantation (some were performed using an open technique and others stereotactically). The dissected adrenal medullary tissue was implanted unilaterally, generally into the caudate head on the non-dominant side. The few reports of pathological examination of patients treated in this fashion revealed no or very few surviving cells.[66] Subsequent to the initial trials, attempts to improve tissue viability and outcomes included special perfusion techniques and the addition of trophic[67] factors or peripheral nerve cografts[68] as well as the use of fetal adrenal medullary cells. No controlled studies were performed. Most open studies showed some improvement in the severity of off-period parkinsonism and increased number of hours on.[69] However, the high incidence of neurological and cardiopulmonary complications encouraged a Therapeutics and Technology Assessment Subcommittee of the American Academy of Neurology to designate this an unacceptable therapy.[70]

Human fetal mesencephalic cell transplantation Despite very encouraging preliminary reports, this treatment still requires further investigation in the treatment of Parkinson's disease. To date, only Class III evidence is available involving very small numbers of patients. The publication of results from two large controlled trials are awaited with great interest (see below). There are numerous variables to consider in evaluating the available reports including number of sides implanted (unilateral *vs.* bilateral), location of the implants (caudate, putamen, both), the extent of the host striatum that is targeted, preparation of the tissue (blocks of tissue *vs.* cell suspensions), tissue storage techniques, screening of tissue for infectious agents, testing of tissue for dopamine production and viability, fetal donor age (varies between five and 17 weeks although after 10 weeks cells may be largely differentiated and have sent out neuritic processes), number of fetuses used (one to four per side), and the nature and duration of immunosuppression used (nil *vs.* short term low dose cyclosporin *vs.* more complete and prolonged immunosuppression). Positron emission tomography studies have provided evidence for survival of the implanted tissue as long as 10 years following the original surgery.[71] Postmortem studies of two patients from a single center 18 and 19 months after surgery demonstrated large numbers of surviving transplanted dopaminergic neurons extensively reinnervating the host striatum in a patch-matrix configuration.[72,73]

Most clinical reports have described improvement in off-period parkinsonism and time in the on state. However, an NIH funded sham-surgery controlled clinical trial from New York and Denver showed only modest benefits in most patients under the age of 60 (with tremor and gait not responding), although some were able to discontinue dopaminergic medications, and no significant benefit in patients over the age of 60 years.[74] The response of dyskinesias to fetal transplants has varied. Some studies report pronounced reduction in time on with dyskinesias.[75] However, others have reported a delayed increase in dyskinesias and a small number of the younger patients participating in the New York/Denver study have developed spontaneous dyskinesias occurring independent of dopaminergic therapy.[74] This latter experience raises grave concerns, at least for the transplantation technique used in this study. Otherwise, in contrast to adrenal transplantation, morbidity and mortality have been quite low with this procedure, generally related to the expected complications of stereotactic surgery and to immunosuppressive therapy when used in higher doses for prolonged periods.

As stated, this approach remains investigational and may never be applied on a large scale in view of many important outstanding issues including opposition on ethical grounds and the impracticality of numbers of fetuses that may be necessary to fully reinnervate the parkinsonian striatum (up to four on each side). Some of these problems may be resolved if effective neuro-transplantation can be performed using other sources of tissue.

Transplantation using other sources of tissue Experimental studies have implanted a variety of tissues in parkinsonian animal models including carotid body, genetically manipulated cells (altered to produce dopamine or trophic factors), stem cells, cells encapsulated in polymeric capsules in order to prevent rejection, and xenotransplants. Only the latter has been applied to a limited number of patients to date using porcine fetal mesencephalic cells. Preliminary data suggests that patients have shown mild benefit, no evidence of porcine endogenous retroviral infection,[76] and a single postmortem study did show a small number of viable transplanted dopaminergic neurons in the transplant sites.[77] However, a preliminary report of a randomized, double blind trial of porcine fetal mesencephalic transplantation indicated that grafted patients improved no more than sham-operated control subjects.[78]

Other surgical approaches to neuroregeneration

Surgery may be utilized in order to provide access to the brain for trophic substances that cannot be taken systemically either due to inability to cross the blood-brain barrier or to systemic toxicity. Trophic factors could be infused into the cerebrospinal fluid (CSF) or the brain parenchyma, intermittently or continuously. Alternatively, a source of trophic factor production could be implanted into the brain such as cells genetically modified to produce one or more trophic substances. To date the only attempt to apply this form of treatment was a multi-center placebo controlled trial of intracerebroventricular injections of glial derived neurotrophic factor (GDNF). This trial was halted prematurely due to lack of efficacy and side effects. Given the efficacy of GDNF in restoring the function of dopaminergic neurons in animal models of parkinsonism,[79,80] there is still hope that it could be effective in human Parkinson's disease possibly via a different method of administration (e.g. intraparenchymal infusion).

Conclusions

This is an exciting time in the management of Parkinson's disease. After a prolonged period of inactivity following the introduction of levodopa, an important role has once again been established for surgical therapies. As biological and technological advances occur, it is likely that the role of neurosurgical therapy will continue to evolve. The multifaceted nature of modern functional neurosurgery predicts a very active role for these techniques in managing Parkinson's disease for the foreseeable future.

References

1. Meyers R. Surgical interruption of the pallidofugal fibres. Its effect on the syndrome of paralysis agitans and technical considerations in its application. NY State J Med 1942;42:317–325
2. Spiegel EA, Wycis HT, Marks M, Lee AJ. Stereotaxic apparatus for operations on the human brain. Science 1946;106:349–350
3. Spiegel EA, Wycis HT. Ansotomy in paralysis agitans. Arch Neurol Psychiat (Chic) 1954;71:598–614
4. Cooper IS. Involuntary movement disorders. New York: Hoeber, 1969
5. Cooper IS. Intracerebral injection of procaine into the globus pallidus in hyperkinetic disorders. Science 1954;119:417–418
6. Hassler R. The influence of stimulations and coagulations in the human thalamus on the tremor at rest and its physiopathologic mechanism. Excerpta Medica 1955;(Second International Congress of Neuropathology, Excerpta Medica Foundation. Amsterdam):637–642
7. Narabayashi H, Ohye C. Parkinsonian tremor and nucleus ventralis intermedius on the human thalamus. In: Desmedt JE, ed. Physiological tremor. Pathological tremors and clonus. Basal: S. Karger, 1978:165–172
8. Narabayashi H. Surgical approach to tremor. In: Marsden CD, Fahn S, eds. Movement disorders. London: Butterworth Scientific, 1982:292–299
9. Narabayashi H, Yokochi F, Nakajima Y. Levodopa-induced dyskinesia and thalamotomy. J Neurol Neurosurg Psychiatry 1984;47:831–839
10. Speelman JD, Bosch DA. Resurgence of functional neurosurgery for Parkinson's disease: a historical perspective. Mov Disord 1998;13(3):582–588
11. Schuurman PR, Bosch DA, Bossuty PMM, et al. A comparison of continuous thalamic stimulation and thalamotomy for suppression of severe tremor. N Engl J Med 2000;342:461–468
12. De Bie RM, De Haan RJ, Nijssen PC, et al. Unilateral pallidotomy in Parkinson's disease: a randomized, single-blind, multicentre trial. Lancet 1999;354(9191):1665–1669
13. Caparros-Lesebvre D, Ruchoux MM, Blond S, et al. Long-term thalamic stimulation in Parkinson's disease: postmortem anatomoclinical study. Neurology 1994;44:1856–1860
14. Laitinen LV. Brain targets in surgery for Parkinson's disease. J Neurosurg 1985;62:349–351
15. Page RD, Sambrook MA, Crossman AR. Thalamotomy for the alleviation of levodopa-induced dyskinesia: experimental studies in the 1-methyl-4-phenyl-1,2,3,6-tetrahydropyridine-treated parkinsonian money. Neuroscience 1993;55:147–165
16. Jankovic J, Cardoso F, Grossman RG, Hamilton WJ. Outcome after stereotactic thalamotomy for parkinsonian, essential, and other types of tremor. Neurosurgery 1995;37:680–686
17. Diederich N, Goetz CG, Stebbins GT, et al. Blinded evaluation confirms long-term asymmetric effect of unilateral thalamotomy or subthalamotomy on tremor in Parkinson's disease. Neurology 1992;42:1311–1314
18. Young RF, Shumway-Cook A, Vermeulen SS, et al. Gamma knife radiosurgery as a lesioning technique in movement disorder surgery. J Neurosurg 1998;89(2):183–193
19. Duma CM, Jacques DB, Kopyov OV, et al. Gamma knife radiosurgery for thalamotomy in parkinsonian tremor: a five-year experience. J Neurosurg 1998;88(6):1044–1049
20. Kirschman DL, Milligan B, Wilkinson S, et al. Pallidotomy microelectrode targeting: neurophysiology-based target refinement. Neurosurgery 2000;46(3):613–622
21. Guridi J, Gorospe A, Ramos E, et al. Stereotactic targeting of the globus pallidus internus in Parkinson's disease: imaging versus electrophysiological mapping. Neurosurgery 1999;45(2):278–287
22. Gross RE, Lombardi WJ, Hutchison WD, et al. Variability in lesion location after microelectrode-guided pallidotomy for Parkinson's disease: anatomical, physiological, and technical factors that determine lesion distribution. J Neurosurg 1999;90(3):468–477
23. Young RF, Jacques S, Mark R, et al. Gamma knife thalamotomy for treatment of tremor: long-term results. J Neurosurg 2000;93:128–135
24. Koller W, Pahwa R, Busenbark K, et al. High-frequency unilateral thalamic stimulation in the treatment of essential and parkinsonian tremor. Ann Neurol 1997;42(3):292–299
25. Limousin P, Speelman JD, Gielen F, Janssens M. Multicentre European study of thalamic stimulation in parkinsonian and essential tremor. J Neurol Neurosurg Psychiatry 1999;66(3):289–296
26. Caparros-Lefebvre D, Blond S, Feltin MP, et al. Improvement of levodopa induced dyskinesias by thalamic deep brain stimulation is related to slight variation in electrode placement: possible involvement of the centre median and parafascicularis complex. J Neurol Neurosurg Psychiatry 1999;67(3):308–314
27. Laitinen LV, Bergenheim AT, Hariz MI. Leksell's posteroventral pallidotomy in the treatment of Parkinson's disease. J Neurosurg 1992;76:53–61
28. Lang AE, Duff J, Saint-Cyr JA, et al. Posteroventral medial pallidotomy in Parkinson's disease. J Neurol 1999;246(21):II/28–II/42
29. Lang AE, Lozano AM, Montgomery E, et al. Posteroventral medial pallidotomy in advanced Parkinson's disease. N Engl J Med 1997;337:1036–1042

30. Pal PK, Samii A, Kishore A, et al. Long-term outcome of unilateral pallidotomy: follow up of 15 patients for three years. J Neurol Neurosurg Psychiatry 2000;69(3): 337–344

31. Fine J, Duff J, Chen R, et al. Long-term follow-up of unilateral pallidotomy in advanced Parkinson's disease. N Engl J Med 2000;342(23):1708–1714

32. De Bie RMA, Schuurman PR, Bosch DA, et al. Outcome of unilateral pallidotomy in advanced Parkinson's disease: cohort study of 32 patients. J Neurol Neurosurg Psychiatry 2001;71(3):375–382

33. Baron MS, Vitek JL, Bakay RAE, et al. Treatment of advanced Parkinson's disease by unilateral posterior GPi pallidotomy: four-year results of a pilot study. Mov Disord 2000;15(2):230–237

34. Merello M, Nouzeilles MI, Cammarota A, et al. Comparison of one-year follow-up evaluations of patients with indication for pallidotomy who did not undergo surgery versus patients with Parkinson's disease who did undergo pallidotomy: a case control study. Neurosurgery 1999;44(3):461–467

35. Van Horn G, Hassenbusch SJ, Zouridakis G, et al. Pallidotomy: a comparison of responders and nonresponders. Neurosurgery 2001;48(2):263–271

36. Lang AE, Lozano A, Tasker R, et al. Neuropsychological and behavioural changes and weight gain after medial pallidotomy. Ann Neurol 1997;41:834–835

37. Ondo WG, Ben-Aire L, Jankovic J, et al. Weight gain following unilateral pallidotomy in Parkinson's disease. Acta Neurol Scand 2000;101(2):79–84

38. Iacono RP, Lonser RR, Kuniyoshi S. Unilateral versus bilateral simultaneous posteroventral pallidotomy in subgroups of patients with Parkinson's disease. Stereotact Funct Neurosurg 1995;65(1–4):6–10

39. Counihan TJ, Shinobu LA, Eskandar EN, et al. Outcomes following staged bilateral pallidotomy in advanced Parkinson's disease. Neurology 2001;56(6): 799–802

40. Scott R, Gregory R, Hines N, et al. Neuropsychological, neurological and functional outcome following pallidotomy for Parkinson's disease. A consecutive series of eight simultaneous bilateral and twelve unilateral procedures. Br 1998;121(4):659–675

41. Ghika J, Ghika-Schmid F, Fankhauser H, et al. Bilateral contemporaneous posteroventral pallidotomy for the treatment of Parkinson's disease: neuropsychological and neurological side effects. Report of four cases and review of the literature. J Neurosurg 1999;91(2):313–321

42. Intemann PM, Masterman D, Subramanian I, et al. Staged bilateral pallidotomy for treatment of Parkinson disease. J Neurosurg 2001;94(3):437–444

43. Young RF, Vermeulen S, Posewitz A, Shumway-Cook A. Pallidotomy with the gamma knife: a positive experience. Stereotact Funct Neurosurg 1998;70:218–228

44. Friedman JH, Epstein M, Sanes JN, et al. Gamma knife pallidotomy in advanced Parkinson's disease. Ann Neurol 1996;39(4):535–538

45. Duma CM, Jacques DB, Kopyov O, et al. Gamma knife radiosurgery for the treatment of movement disorders. Prog Neurol Surg 1998;14:195–211

46. Merello M, Nouzeilles MI, Kuzis G, et al. Unilateral radiofrequency lesion versus electrostimulation of posteroventral pallidum: a prospective randomized comparison. Mov Disord 1999;14(1):50–56

47. Gálvez-Jiménez N, Lozano A, Tasker R, et al. Pallidal stimulation in Parkinson's disease patients with a prior unilateral pallidotomy. Can J Neurol Sci 1998;25(4): 300–305

48. Obeso JA, Guridi J, Rodriguez-Oroz MC, et al. Deep-brain stimulation of the subthalamic nucleus or the pars interna of the globus pallidus in Parkinson's disease. N Engl J Med 2001;345(13):956–963

49. Krack P, Pollak P, Limousin P, et al. Opposite motor effects of pallidal stimulation in Parkinson's disease. Ann Neurol 1998;43(2):180–192

50. Bejjani B, Damier P, Arnulf I, et al. Pallidal stimulation for Parkinson's disease: two targets? Neurology 1997;49(6):1564–1569

51. Gill SS, Heywood P. Bilateral dorsolateral subthalamotomy for advanced Parkinson's disease. Lancet 1997; 350:1224

52. Alvarez L, Macias R, Guridi J, et al. Dorsal subthalamotomy for Parkinson's disease. Mov Disord 2001;16(1): 72–78

53. Limousin P, Krack P, Pollak P, et al. Electrical stimulation of the subthalamic nucleus in advanced Parkinson's disease. N Engl J Med 1998;339(16):1105–1111

54. Krack P, Pollak P, Limousin P, et al. From off-period dystonia to peak-dose chorea. The clinical spectrum of varying subthalamic nucleus activity. Br 1999;122(6): 1133–1146

55. Merello M. Subthalamic stimulation contralateral to a previous pallidotomy: an erroneous indication? Mov Disord 1999;14(5):890–890

56. Kumar R, Lozano AM, Kim YJ, et al. Double-blind evaluation of subthalamic nucleus deep brain stimulation in advanced Parkinson's disease. Neurology 1998; 51(3):850–855

57. Krack P, Pollak P, Limousin P, et al. Subthalamic nucleus or internal pallidal stimulation in young onset Parkinson's disease. Br 1998;121(3):451–457

58. Saint-Cyr JA, Trépanier LL, Kumar R, et al. Neuropsychological consequences of chronic bilateral stimulation of the subthalamic nucleus in Parkinson's disease. Br 2000;123(10):2091–2108

59. Dujardin K, Defebvre L, Krystkowiak P, et al. Influence of chronic bilateral stimulation of the subthalamic nucleus on cognitive function in Parkinson's disease. J Neurol 2001;248(7):603–611

60. Strafella AP, Paus T, Barrett J, Dagher A. Repetitive transcranial magnetic stimulation of the human prefrontal cortex induces dopamine release in the caudate nucleus. J Neurosci 2001;21(15):NIL7–NIL10

61. Bejjani BP, Damier P, Arnulf I, et al. Transient acute depression induced by high-frequency deep-brain stimulation. N Engl J Med 1999;340(19):1476–1480

62. Krack P, Kumar R. Mirthful laughter induced by STN stimulation. Mov Disord 2001;16(5):867–875

63. Kumar R, Krack P, Pollak P. Transient acute depression-induced by high-frequency deep-brain stimulation [letter]. N Engl J Med 1999;341:1003–1004

64. Burchiel KJ, Anderson VC, Favre J, Hammerstad JP. Comparison of pallidal and subthalamic nucleus deep brain stimulation for advanced Parkinson's disease: results of a randomized blinded pilot study. Neurosurgery 1999;45:1375–1384

65. Volkmann J, Allert N, Voges J, et al. Safety and efficacy of pallidal or subthalamic nucleus stimulation in advanced PD. Neurology 2001;56(4):548–551

66. Jankovic J, Grossman R, Goodman C, et al. Clinical, biochemical, and neuropathologic findings following transplantation of adrenal medulla to the caudate nucleus for treatment of Parkinson's disease. Neurology 1989;39:1227–1234

67. Olson L, Backlund E-O, Edendal T, et al. Intraputaminal infusion of nerve growth factor to support adrenal

medullary autographs in Parkinson's disease. Arch Neurol 1991;48:373–381

68. Watts RL, Subramanian T, Freeman A, et al. Effect of stereotaxic intrastriatal co-grafts of autologous adrenal medulla and peripheral nerve in Parkinson's disease: two-year follow-up study. Exp Neurol 1997;147(2): 510–517

69. Goetz GC, Olanow WC, Koller W. Multicenter study of autologous adrenal medullary transplantation to the corpus striatum in patients with advanced Parkinson's disease. N Engl J Med 1989;320:337–341

70. Hallet M, Litvan I, the Task Force on Surgery for Parkinson's disease. Evaluation of surgery for Parkinson's disease: a report of the Therapeutics and Technology Assessment Subcommittee of the American Academy of Neurology. Neurology 1999;53:1910–1921

71. Piccini P, Brooks DJ, Björklund A, et al. Dopamine release from nigral transplants visualized in vivo in a Parkinson's patient. Nat Neurosci 1999;2(12):1137–1140

72. Kordower JH, Freeman TB, Snow BJ, et al. Neuropathological evidence of graft survival and striatal reinnervation after the transplantation of fetal mesencephalic tissue in a patient with Parkinson's disease. N Engl J Med 1995;332:1118–1124

73. Kordower JH, Freeman TB, Chen EY, et al. Fetal nigral grafts survive and mediate clinical benefit in a patient with Parkinson's disease. Mov Disord 1998;13(3): 383–393

74. Freed CR, Greene PE, Breeze RE, et al. Transplantation of embryonic dopamine neurons for severe Parkinson's disease. N Engl J Med 2001;344(10):710–719

75. Hauser RA, Freeman TB, Snow BJ, et al. Long-term evaluation of bilateral fetal nigral transplantation in Parkinson disease. Arch Neurol 1999;56(2):179–187

76. Schumacher JM, Ellias SA, Palmer EP, et al. Transplantation of embryonic porcine mesencephalic tissue in patients with PD. Neurology 2000; 54(5):1042–1050

77. Deacon T, Schumacher J, Dinsmore J, et al. Histological evidence of fetal pig neural cell survival after transplantation into a patient with Parkinson's disease. Nature Med 1997;3(3):350–353

78. Hauser RA, Watts RL, Freeman TB, et al. A double-blind randomized controlled, multi-center clinical trial of the safety and efficacy of transplanted fetal procine ventral mesencephalic cells versus imitation surgery in patients with PD. Mov Disord 2001;16(5):983–984

79. Gash DM, Zhang ZM, Ovadia A, et al. Functional recovery in parkinsonian monkeys treated with GDNF. Nature 1996;380(6571):252–255

80. Lapchak PA, Gash DM, Collins F, et al. Pharmacological activities of glial cell line-derived neurotrophic factor (GDNF): preclinical development and application to the treatment of Parkinson's disease. Exp Neurol 1997;145(2 Pt 1):309–321

234 The Diagnosis and Treatment of Normal Pressure Hydrocephalus

Steven J Frucht and Robert R Goodman

Introduction

In 1965, Adams, Fisher, Hakim, Ojemann and Sweet described a new syndrome in patients with hydro-cephalus. Patients displayed the clinical triad of gait disturbance, urinary incontinence and cognitive impairment.[1] Intracranial pressures were normal ($<20\,cm\ H_2O$), and patients improved clinically after placement of a ventriculo-peritoneal shunt. Unlike other causes of gait disturbance and cognitive impairment in the elderly, normal pressure hydrocephalus (NPH) is potentially reversible if diagnosed and treated in a timely fashion. The disorder is often considered in the evaluation of the older patient who presents with a gait disorder. However, the clinical uncertainty surrounding the diagnosis is further hampered by the lack of a reliable test to forecast who will benefit from placement of a shunt. This chapter reviews the clinical features and diagnosis of NPH and summarizes recent advances in treatment.

Epidemiology

The incidence and prevalence of NPH are unknown. In one multicenter retrospective study of 166 consecutive NPH patients in Amsterdam undergoing shunt placement, only one third improved clinically. The incidence of shunt-responsive NPH was only 2.2 per million per year in this study,[2] suggesting that shunt-responsive NPH is a rare condition. At the opposite end of the spectrum, a door-to-door survey of parkinsonism in individuals over age 65 living in two German villages unexpectedly revealed 4 of 982 inhabitants (0.41%) with NPH.[3] The true incidence and prevalence of NPH probably lies somewhere in between these two values, although the disorder is probably over-diagnosed by neurologists searching for a treatable cause of gait disturbance and cognitive decline.

Etiology

Symptomatic NPH follows subarachnoid hemorrhage, meningitis or trauma, and is distinct from idiopathic NPH. Symptomatic NPH occurs when there is an extraventricular obstruction to CSF flow at the level of the arachnoid villi. There is no evidence that idiopathic NPH results from a similar mechanism. Twenty-seven patients who underwent shunt placement for NPH also had a parenchymal and lepto-meningeal biopsy during the procedure. There was no correlation between clinical outcome and the presence of arachnoid fibrosis in the biopsies.[4]

Pathophysiology and pathogenesis

More recent studies suggest that NPH may result from ischemic periventricular white matter disease.[5] Subcortical infarcts change the tensile strength of the lateral wall of the ventricles, leading to ventricular dilatation.[6] In a case-controlled study of 65 patients with NPH, there was a significant association between NPH and hypertension, cardiac and cerebral atherosclerotic disease.[7] The severity of clinical symptoms also correlated with the presence of hypertension. Further, measurements of regional cerebral blood flow using technetium-99m HMPAO SPECT have demonstrated that patients with NPH have deficits in subcortical white matter blood flow, and that these deficits improve after shunting.[8–10] This suggests that prominent cerebral ventricles are a symptom of the underlying disorder and not the primary cause.

Genetics

There are no known genetic causes of symptomatic or idiopathic NPH.

Clinical features

Miller Fisher elegantly summarized the clinical features of NPH.[11] Gait disturbance occurs early. Patients complain of imbalance and difficulty climbing stairs, and they may unexpectedly fall. On examination, rapid alternating movements of the feet and toe tapping are slow, and the tone in the legs is often increased. The patient's inability to arise and walk is frequently more severe than would be expected by the deficits present in other parts of the neurological examination.

A major source of confusion for neurologists is that the spectrum of NPH gaits is broad. Classically the step is shortened, wide-based and magnetic, with the feet barely leaving the floor. Imbalance on turns and impaired recovery on the pull test are near-constant findings. The term "lower-body parkinsonism" does not do full justice to the gait and balance impairment that characterize the condition.

Cognitive impairment is a frequent finding in NPH, but this classically follows the change in gait. In the authors' experience and in the original descriptions of NPH, patients with early cognitive impairment or in whom cognitive deficits overshadow the gait disturbance are unlikely to have shunt-responsive NPH. Affected patients are apathetic and passive, and Miller Fisher characterized the disturbance in mentation as a mild abulia. Unlike patients with Alzheimer's disease, verbal performance is preserved while non-verbal tasks such as performing calculations and figure copying are often impaired.

Urinary incontinence is common and is usually a late development. In its full-blown state, patients may be unconcerned about urinating in front of others. However, most NPH patients only have mild urinary symptoms by the time the diagnosis is considered.

Differential diagnosis

Gait disorders are common in older individuals, and are a major source of morbidity and even mortality.[12] A disturbance anywhere within the neuraxis may manifest as a gait disturbance, and the differential diagnosis of the older individual with an abnormal gait is broad. However, when vestibular dysfunction, sensory neuropathy, compressive myelopathy and cerebellar disturbances can be excluded, there remain a group of disorders that produce "lower-body parkinsonism." These include vascular parkinsonism, progressive supranuclear palsy (PSP), NPH, and the poorly defined entity "gait disorder of the elderly."

First described by Critchley, vascular (or arteriosclerotic) parkinsonism is a contested clinical entity. Many patients with significant subcortical ischemia have normal gaits, and conversely, patients with lower-body parkinsonism who have normal saccadic eye movements and normal-sized ventricles may have no evidence of ischemic burden. The gait disorder of vascular parkinsonism may be indistinguishable from that of NPH.[13] However patients with vascular parkinsonism often have associated neurological abnormalities that are not seen in NPH. In a case-control study of 24 patients with pathologically proven vascular parkinsonism,[14] half had pyramidal tract signs or pseudobulbar palsy.

Early falling is a common symptom in PSP, often bringing the patient to medical attention. Falls may be serious, resulting in fractures, and patients may be unaware of their risk for falling. The presence of square wave jerks, impaired vertical saccadic eye movements and depressed optico-kinetic nystagmus suggests PSP. One variant of PSP with normal or nearly normal eye movements may present with an isolated gait disorder.[15,16] First described in Japan, the syndrome of pure akinesia is pathologically identical to PSP and is usually resistant to treatment.

Occasionally, evaluation of an elderly patient with a gait disorder does not reveal a likely cause for disability. These patients are often diagnosed with a "senile gait disorder" or "gait disorder of the elderly." These terms should be abandoned, as they do not add any useful information and give the false impression that these patients share an underlying common pathology or mechanism. In truth, gait disorder of the elderly simply means that an older person has a gait disturbance, and that the neurologist has no idea why.

Diagnostic criteria

What is the single best diagnostic test for NPH, and how can neurologists predict which patients will improve with a shunt? In standard clinical practice neurologists often perform serial lumbar punctures in hospital, removing a large volume of CSF ($>30\,cm^3$) and assessing the patient's gait and mentation. Interpreting the results of the "tap test" is difficult for several reasons. This technique is particularly prone to false positives, as patients are motivated to get better, particularly if they are subjected to something as unpleasant as repeated spinal taps. Even if a large volume of CSF is removed with each tap, the change in tensile forces on the lateral walls of the ventricle may be insufficient to result in clinical benefit. If improvements do occur, they may be delayed until after the patient has left the hospital. In at least one study, the CSF tap test was not found to be useful in evaluating eventual response to shunting.[17]

Other investigators have attempted to measure outflow resistance to CSF to predict response to shunting.[18] Although patients with a resistance greater than or equal to $18\,mmHg/mL$ per minute were likely to improve with a shunt, the test was not helpful if resistance was lower than this value. Hyperdynamic CSF flow in the aqueduct was thought to be highly suggestive of NPH,[19,20] but is no longer considered useful in the diagnosis.

The most useful diagnostic test to predict outcome after shunt surgery is controlled CSF drainage by a lumbar subarachnoid catheter.[21] Removing CSF at $10\,cm^3$/hour ($240\,cm^3$/day) approximates, as closely as possible, the change in CSF dynamics that will occur with a shunt. At Columbia-Presbyterian Medical Center, patients are routinely admitted to the hospital for placement of a lumbar drain and videotaping of their examinations over 3 days. If there is absolutely no improvement in gait with CSF drainage, it is hard to justify placing a shunt in these patients.

Treatment

The most universally accepted criterion for the diagnosis of NPH is a significant and prolonged improvement of gait/balance after creation of an extracranial shunt. However, since there is a significant risk of serious morbidity and a small risk of mortality associated with the surgical creation of a shunt, it is of utmost importance to shunt only patients with a substantial chance of clinical benefit. In the authors' experience, the appropriate clinical history, neurological examination and brain MRI (or CT) findings and a clear gait improvement with continuous lumbar spinal drainage have predicted a greater than 90% chance of persistent improvement with shunting.[22] Many series have reported a significantly lower chance of lasting clinical improvement (64% to 87%) with similar selection criteria.[23–25] While one explanation for a lack of benefit with shunting is improper diagnosis, another significant possibility is that the patient is "under-shunted." Also, the single greatest morbidity of shunting this patient population is "over-shunting" (i.e. excessive reduction of ventricular size) with the development of a subdural hygroma or hematoma (3% to 23% of patients).[23,25–27] A variety of shunt systems have been available for the treatment of hydrocephalus since the 1950s.[28]

There are essentially three components to a shunt: a ventricular catheter, a one-way pressure or flow-regulated valve, and a distal catheter. The most popular valves are the Hakim ball valve type (Codman/J&J) and the PS Medical delta valve (a membrane pressure valve in series with a siphon control mechanism; Medtronic Corp.). Recently, both these valve types have become available with externally adjustable closing pressures (Hakim programmable valve, Codman; PS Medical Strata valve, Medtronic Corp.). Although a variety of shunt options exists, and these have been applied to NPH (e.g. ventriculoperitoneal, ventriculoatrial, ventriculopleural and lumboperitoneal), ventriculoperitoneal shunting is the generally preferred method. The surgical procedure for shunt creation is relatively straightforward, but meticulous technique, attention to detail and the use of a familiar shunt system are the keys to obtaining a high rate of success and low complication rate. In addition to the problems of "under-shunting" and "over-shunting" that are prominent concerns in NPH patients (mentioned above), the surgeon is concerned with the usual risks of shunting patients with hydrocephalus. These include particularly the risks of shunt malfunction (requiring re-operation) and infection (requiring removal of shunt hardware and antibiotic treatment). Large series of adult patients have been reported, with a 28.7% rate of re-operation for malfunction[29] and an approximately 8% infection rate.[30]

The most important innovation in shunt technology, particularly for patients with presumed NPH, has been the development of externally adjustable valves. Some experience with these valves has suggested that they provide an improved outcome (versus the non-adjustable valves) for NPH patients.[31] Since these have been in use at the Columbia-Presbyterian Center (1998), the approach has been to start with the valve set at a closing pressure close to the patient's starting intracranial pressure and then gradually to lower the valve setting until significant clinical improvement is seen.[22] In a reported series of 20 patients[22] this yielded clinical improvement in all patients at the time of last available follow-up, and there was no morbidity in the series. Additional experience in similar patients (unpublished observations) has led to one patient with a subdural hematoma requiring evacuation (with full recovery) and several patients (<10%) with lack or loss of clinical improvement. One of the greatest challenges in the care of NPH patients is to determine the goal of shunting, and there is significant controversy regarding this issue. With non-adjustable shunt valve systems, patients without clinical improvement are often told that they do not have reversible symptoms or that they do not actually have NPH. Some surgeons feel that the goal must be to achieve a significant reduction in ventricular size, even in one report advocating aggressive negative pressure drainage to reduce ventricular size (in selected patients).[32] The authors have been very reluctant to pursue this as a goal, because of the concern of producing morbidity with subdural hygromas or hematomas. Their approach, with gradual valve setting lowering until clinical improvement, has been associated with a small (but measurable) reduction of ventricular volume, once significant clinical improvement has occurred.[22] The bulk of their clinical experience has been with the programmable Hakim valve, and it is not yet clear whether the PS Medical Strata valve will yield similar results.

NPH patients represent a clinical challenge from both a diagnostic and a treatment perspective, however it is critical for clinicians to understand that many of these patients obtain dramatic improvement to their quality of life with effective shunting.

References

1. Adams RD, Fischer CM, Hakim S, et al. Symptomatic occult hydrocephalus with "normal" cerebrospinal fluid pressure. New Engl J Med 1965;273:117–126
2. Vanneste J, Augustijn P, Dirven C, et al. Shunting normal-pressure hydrocephalus: do benefits outweigh the risks? A multicenter study and literature review. Neurology 1992;42:54–59
3. Trenkwalder C, Schwarz J, Gebhard J, et al. Starnberg trial on epidemiology of parkinsonism and hypertension in the elderly. Prevalence of Parkinson's disease and related disorders assessed by a door-to-door survey of inhabitants older than 65 years. Arch Neurol 1995;52:1017–1022
4. Bech RA, Waldemar G, Gjerris F, et al. Shunting effects in patients with idiopathic normal pressure hydrocephalus; correlation with cerebral and leptomeningeal biopsy findings. Acta Neuochir (Wien) 1999;141:633–639
5. Penar PL, Lakin WD, Yu J. Normal pressure hydrocephalus: an analysis of aetiology and response to shunting based on mathematical modeling. Neurol Res 1995;17:83–88
6. Tanaka K, Yonekawa Y, Miyake H, et al. Idiopathic normal pressure hydrocephalus in elderly patients: its pathophysiology and diagnosis. No Shinkei Geka 1993;21:403–408
7. Krauss JK, Regel JP, Vach W, et al. Vascular risk factors and arteriosclerotic disease in idiopathic normal pressure hydrocephalus of the elderly. Stroke 1996;27:24–29
8. Waldemar G, Schmidt JF, Delecluse F, et al. High resolution SPECT with 99m-Tc-d,l-HMPAO in normal pressure hydrocephalus before and after shunt operation. J Neurol Neurosurg Psychiatry 1993;56:655–664
9. Larsson A, Bergh A, Bilting M, et al. Regional cerebral blood flow in normal pressure hydrocephalus: diagnostic and prognostic aspects. Eur J Nucl Med 1994;21:118–123
10. Shih W, Tasdemiroglu E. Reversible hypoperfusion of the cerebral cortex in normal pressure hydrocephalus on technetium-99m-HMPAO brain SPECT images after shunt operation. J Nucl Med 1995;36:470–473
11. Fisher CM. The clinical picture in occult hydrocephalus. Clin Neurosurg 1977;24:270–284
12. Sudarsky L. Geriatrics: gait disorders in the elderly. New Engl J Med 1990;322:1441–1446
13. Thompson PD, Marsden CD. Gait disorder of subcortical arteriosclerotic encephalopathy: Binswanger's disease. Mov Disord 1987;2:1–8

14. Yamanouchi H, Nagura H. Neurological signs and frontal white matter lesions in vascular parkinsonism; a clinicopathologic study. Stroke 1997;28:965–969

15. Matsuo H, Takashima H, Kishikawa M, et al. Pure akinesia: an atypical manifestation of progressive supranuclear palsy. J Neurol Neurosurg Psychiatry 1991;54:397–400

16. Riley DE, Fogt N, Leigh RJ. The syndrome of "pure akinesia" and its relationship to progressive supranuclear palsy. Neurology 1994;44:1025–1029

17. Malm J, Kristensen B, Karlsson T, et al. The predictive value of cerebrospinal fluid dynamic tests in patients with the idiopathic adult hydrocephalus syndrome. Arch Neurol 1995;52:783–789

18. Boon AJW, Tans JTJ, Delwel EJ, et al. Dutch normal pressure hydrocephalus study: prediction of outcome after shunting by resistance to outflow of cerebrospinal fluid. J Neurosurg 1997;87:687–693

19. Hakim R, Black PM. Correlation between lumbo-ventricular perfusion and MRI-CSF flow studies in idiopathic normal pressure hydrocephalus. Surg Neurol 1998;49:14–20

20. Kim MH, Shin KM, Song JH. Cine MR CSF flow study in hydrocephalus: what are the valuable parameters? Acta Neuochir (Suppl) 1998;71:343–346

21. Williams MA, Razumovsky AY, Hanley DF. Comparison of Pcsf monitoring and controlled CSF drainage diagnose normal pressure hydrocephalus. Acta Neurochir (Suppl) 1998;71:328–330

22. Anderson RC, Grant JJ, De La Paz R, et al. Volumetric measurements in the detection of reduced ventricular volume in patients with normal-pressure hydrocephalus whose clinical condition improved after ventriculoperitoneal shunt placement. J Neurosurg 2002;97:73–79

23. Black PM. Idiopathic normal pressure hydrocephalus. Results of shunting in 62 patients. J Neurosurg 1980;53:371–377

24. McQuarrie IG, Saint-Louis L, Scherer PB. Treatment of normal pressure hydrocephalus with low versus medium pressure cerebrospinal fluid shunt. Neurosurgery 1984;15:484–488

25. Petersen RC, Mokri B, Laws ER. Response to shunting procedure in idiopathic normal pressure hydrocephalus. Ann Neurol 1982;12:99

26. Greenberg JO, Shenkin HA, Adam R. Idiopathic normal pressure hydrocephalus: a report of 73 patients. J Neurol Neurosurg Psychiatry 1977;40:336–341

27. McCullough DC, Fox JL. Negative intracranial pressure hydrocephalus in adults with shunts and its relationship to the production of subdural hematoma. J Neurosurg 1974;40:372–375

28. Pudenz R. The surgical treatment of hydrocephalus—an historical review. Surg Neurol 1980;15:15–26

29. Puca A, Anile C, Maira G, Rossi G. Cerebrospinal fluid shunting for hydrocephalus in the adult: factors related to shunt revision. Neurosurgery 1991;29:822–826

30. Renier D, Lacombe J, Pierre-Kahn A. Factors causing acute shunt infection. Computer analysis of 1174 operations. J Neurosurg 1984;61:1072–1078

31. Miyake H, Ohta T, Kajimoto Y, et al. New concept for the pressure setting of a programmable pressure valve and measurement of in vivo shunt flow performed using a microflowmeter. Technical note. J Neurosurg 2000;92:181–187

32. Beneficial effect of siphoning in treatment of adult hydrocephalus. Arch Neurol 1999;56:1224–1229

235 Syringomyelia

William E Krauss

Introduction

Syringomyelia is the presence of a fluid-filled cavity within the spinal cord. *Syringobulbia* often refers to the extension of syringomyelia into the brainstem. *Hydromyelia* and *syringohydromyelia* are abnormal enlargement of the central canal of the spinal cord. In 1546, Esteinne provided the first pathological description of syringomyelia, and in 1892, Abbe and Coley[1] first described the surgical treatment of syringomyelia.

Despite clear definitions, syringomyelia and related disorders defy simple classification. Syringomyelia usually signifies the result of several different disease processes. Except for idiopathic syringomyelia, it is inaccurate to classify syringomyelia as a distinct disease, rather it is a secondary manifestation of another primary disease process.

In a discussion of therapeutics, it is necessary to distinguish between syringomyelia and hydromyelia on the basis of the cause and pathophysiological mechanism. To treat syringomyelia, the underlying cause must be identified. The pathophysiological mechanism and treatment varies for each type (Table 235.1).

Etiology and epidemiology

Syringomyelia is rare. Because of its numerous causes, it is difficult to present meaningful data about its epidemiology. The major causes are Chiari malformation and foramen magnum obstruction, communicating hydrocephalus, trauma, spinal cord tumor, infection, inflammation, cervical spondylosis, and idiopathic. Epidemiology is related directly to the primary disease process. For example, spinal cord injury is a disease of young males. Thus post-traumatic syringomyelia has a male predominance, with a mean age at onset in the early fourth decade. Syringomyelia is found in 4% to 5% of persons who have severe spinal cord injury,[2,3] and the onset can be several years after the injury.

In one series of Chiari I malformations, syringomyelia developed in 32% of cases;[4] the incidence in Chiari II malformations is even higher.[5] Syringomyelia is found in 45% of cases of intramedullary spinal cord tumor.[6] Syrinxes have been described in association with spinal cord astrocytomas, ependymomas, and hemangioblastomas. Meaningful demographic data are not available about postinfectious and postinflammatory syringomyelia.

Pathophysiology

No theory adequately explains the pathophysiological mechanism of syringomyelia. A common feature in many forms of syringomyelia is a derangement or obstruction in the normal circulation of the cerebrospinal fluid (CSF) at or below the foramen magnum.

In Chiari malformations, the disruption occurs at the foramen magnum. Several theories have been proposed about syringomyelia due to Chiari malformation. Heiss et al.[7] have demonstrated the presence of pressure waves in the upper cervical subarachnoid space that may lead to progressive syringomyelia. According to these authors, the cerebellar tonsils occlude the foramen magnum and act as a piston on the CSF in the upper cervical subarachnoid space during systole. This squeezes the upper cervical cord and underlying syrinx. Fluid is forced to the poles of the syrinx and propagates it (Figure 235.1).

Communicating intracranial hydrocephalus may lead to progressive syringomyelia through direct transmission of increased intracranial pressure to the central canal of the spinal cord. This rare cause of syringomyelia requires a connection between the fourth ventricle and central canal, but this connection usually is obliterated in adults. In post-traumatic, postinfectious, or postinflammatory syringomyelia, the derangement occurs below the foramen magnum in the spinal canal. Several authors have proposed that obliteration of the subarachnoid space by post-traumatic, postinfectious, or postinflammatory scarring alters local CSF hydrodynamics and tethers the spinal cord.[8-13] In post-traumatic syringomyelia, bone fragments may project directly into the spinal canal and alter normal spinal CSF hydrodynamics, leading to the local development of a syrinx, possibly by bulk CSF inflow through the Virchow-Robin spaces.[12]

Tumor-associated syrinxes may develop directly from the neoplasm, with transudation of protein-

Table 235.1. Causes of syringomyelia
Foramen magnum obstruction—Chiari malformation, basilar invagination
Spinal cord tumor—astrocytoma, ependymoma, hemangioblastoma
Post-traumatic, postinfectious, postinflammatory
Intracranial communicating hydrocephalus
Cervical spondylosis
Myelomalacia and loss of spinal cord parenchyma
Idiopathic

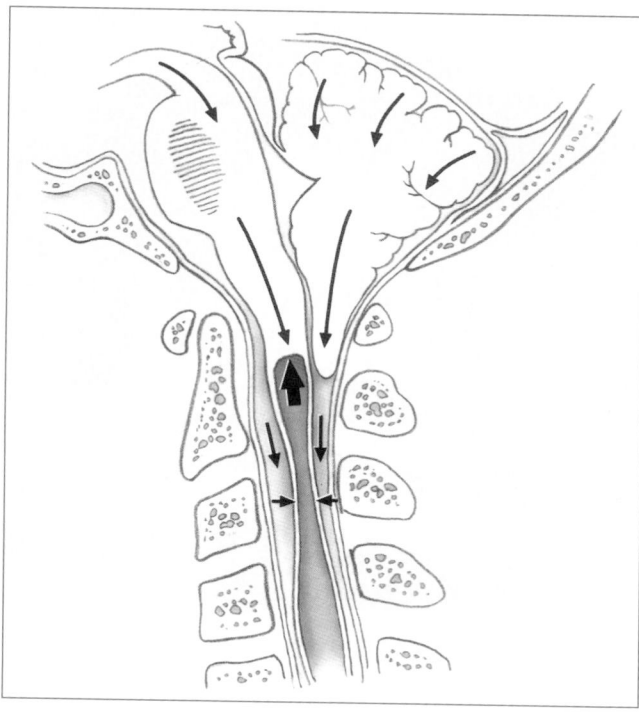

Figure 235.1 Schematic depiction of syrinx propagation related to hindbrain herniation (Chiari malformation). Pressure waves develop at the foramen magnum from periodic downward displacement of the cerebellar tonsils during systole. This results in compression of the syrinx, which elongates. (Modified from Heiss et al.[7] By permission of the *Journal of Neurosurgery*.)

Symptom/sign	Incidence, %
Pain (dysesthetic)	68–80 (37)
Spasticity	70
Gait disturbance	53
Nystagmus*	30
Horner syndrome	8
Bladder involvement	12
Increased motor deficit[†]	86
Increased sensory deficit[†]	87

Table 235.2 Incidence of symptoms and signs of syringomyelia

*With Chiari malformation.
[†]Without Chiari malformation.
Modified from Williams B. Syringomyelia. Neurosurg Clin N Am 1990 (July);1:653-685. By permission of WB Saunders Company.

aceous fluid by tumor blood vessels leading to cavity formation. The loss of spinal cord parenchyma after a severe insult to the cord may lead to syrinx formation. In these cases, small irregular syrinxes form in areas of myelomalacia. In all types, neurological dysfunction may be caused by ischemia or mechanical disruption of axons.[12]

Clinical features

Symptoms and signs

The classic presentation of syringomyelia is progressive bilateral brachial amyotrophy and dissociated sensory loss with a cape-like distribution. Currently, this classic presentation is rarely seen because of early diagnosis with magnetic resonance imaging (MRI). Patients may present with symptoms and signs related to a Chiari malformation, syrinx, or both. Brainstem dysfunction, upper and lower motor neuron signs, lower cranial neuropathies, cerebellar signs, pain, and sensory disturbances may occur in various combinations. As the size of the syrinx and intraluminal pressure increase, progressive myelopathy ensues. Some of the more common clinical features are summarized in Table 235.2.

Natural history

If untreated, syringomyelia is a slowly progressive

process in more than 50% of patients who have the disorder.[14] Disease progression leads to progressive motor, sensory, and sphincter dysfunction. Ultimately, complete loss of spinal cord function is possible. Extension of the syrinx into the medulla may fatally disrupt cardiorespiratory centers. Also, progressive sensory involvement may lead to severe intractable dysesthetic pain.

Diagnostic criteria

Imaging

Plain radiography Plain radiographs may provide evidence of conditions that may lead to syringomyelia. Fractures, basilar invagination, congenital vertebral anomalies, and spinal canal enlargement caused by tumor may all be seen on plain radiographs. However, plain radiographs are not necessary or especially useful in establishing the diagnosis.

Computed tomography and myelography Myelography with computed tomography (CT) was the standard diagnostic study during the 1980s. Spinal cord enlargement or dye blockage provides indirect evidence of syringomyelia. Delayed filling of the syrinx cavity provides direct evidence of a syrinx. In rare circumstances, this test is still necessary when MRI is not possible because the patient has a pacemaker or metallic implants or is claustrophobic.

Magnetic resonance imaging MRI with T_1- and T_2-weighted imaging is the study of choice. Multiplanar imaging demonstrates the cavity clearly in all cases. Gadolinium contrast can identify associated tumors. An associated Chiari malformation can be identified with visualization of the foramen magnum. Associated communicating hydrocephalus can be identified with imaging of the ventricular system. The signal of syrinx fluid is similar to that of CSF on T_1 (low) and T_2 (high) images. Diagnosis and proper treatment planning depend on good MRI studies (Figures 235.2, 235.3, and 235.4).

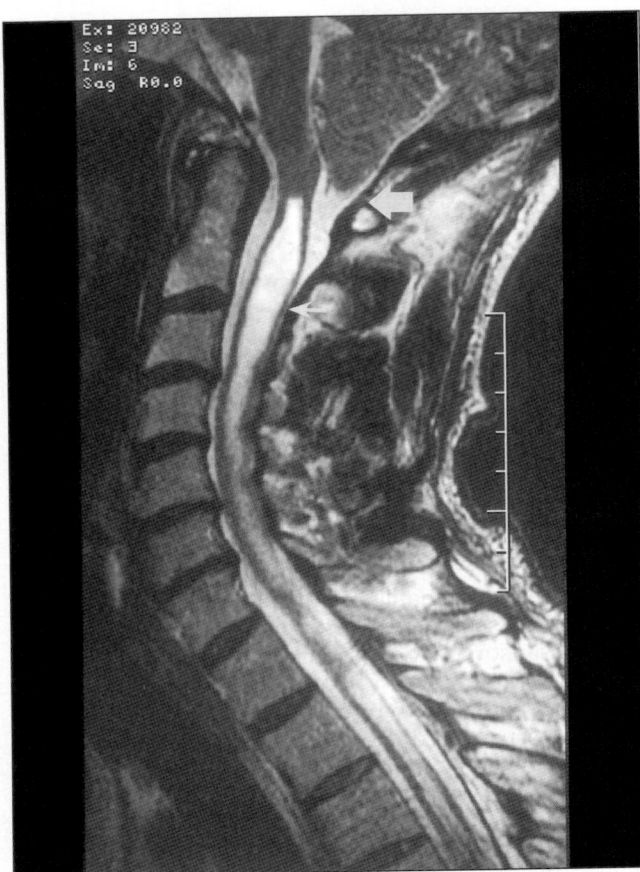

Figure 235.2 A typical syrinx (*small arrow*) associated with a Chiari I malformation (*large arrow*). In most cases, the syrinx resolves completely after posterior fossa decompression and duraplasty.

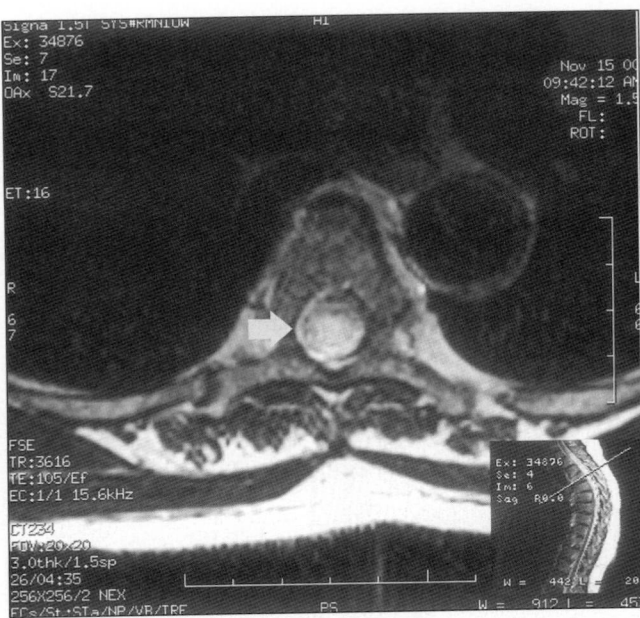

Figure 235.3 A syrinx (*arrow*) associated with obliteration of the normal subarachnoid space of the spinal cord. This is seen in post-traumatic, postinfectious, and postinflammatory settings. The treatment of choice is reconstruction of the subarachnoid space, which may entail bony decompression, lysis of adhesions, and duraplasty.

Differential diagnosis

The differential diagnosis of syringomyelia includes demyelinating disease, motor neuron disease, combined systems disease, cervical spondylotic myelopathy, and neurosyphilis. These various conditions usually are readily distinguished with MRI.

Treatment

Challenges

No simple treatment is available for syringomyelia. All effective treatments are surgical and entail considerable perioperative risk. For many syrinxes, treatment is directed at the underlying lesion and is relatively straightforward. Treatments for post-traumatic, postinfectious, postinflammatory, and idiopathic syrinxes are limited by the poor understanding of their pathophysiological mechanisms.

Because the risk-to-benefit ratio is relatively high for most surgical treatments, the challenge is deciding who should have treatment. Syrinxes can range from being asymptomatic or mildly symptomatic to being relentlessly progressive. The mere presence of a syrinx is not an indication for surgery.

Most of the surgical treatments have a high long-term failure rate. Recurrent scarring, shunt failure, and tumor recurrence are major causes of disease progression despite treatment. The durability of surgical treatment is especially a problem in syringomyelia (post-traumatic, postinfectious, postinflammatory) associated with subarachnoid scarring.

Evidence

The literature on surgical treatment consists of case series in which a specific surgical technique and treatment outcomes were examined (class 3 evidence) (Table 235.3). No randomized trials, case-control, or cohort studies have been conducted.

First-line treatments

The first-line treatments for various causes of syringomyelia are listed in Figure 235.5. Suboccipital craniectomy with duraplasty (foramen magnum decompression) is the treatment of choice for Chiari-associated syrinxes (Figure 235.6a) (Maher CPM, Krauss W, unpublished data).[5] The surgical goal is to open the subarachnoid space at the foramen magnum. By removing the posterior rim of the foramen magnum and augmenting the dural tube, the surgeon reestablishes the subarachnoid space. The associated syringomyelia resolves in more than 70% of patients, and symptoms improve in up to 70%

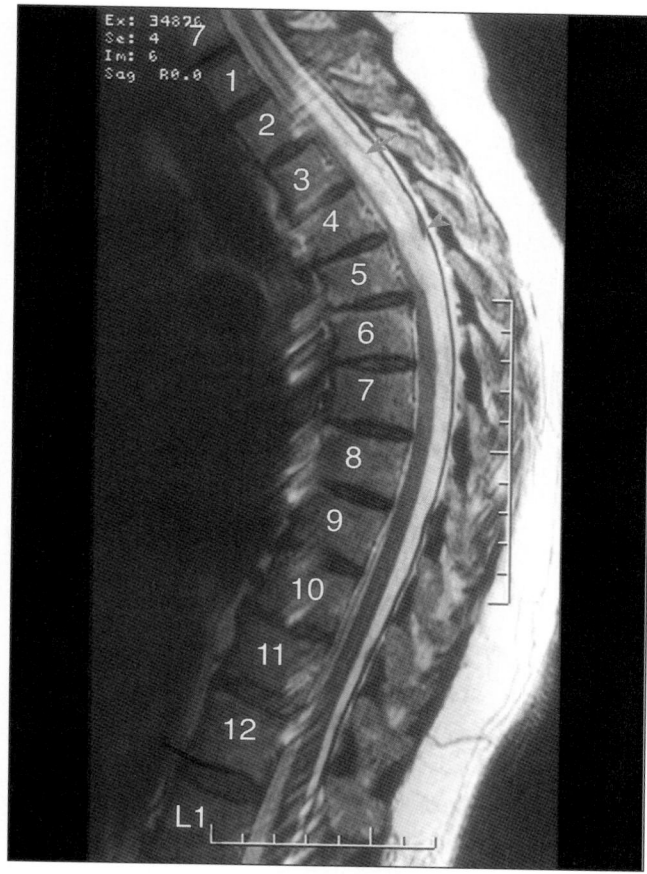

Figure 235.4 A T$_2$-weighted sagittal magnetic resonance image demonstrating a syrinx (*arrow*) from T1 to T6. The syrinx was caused by dural calcification (*arrowhead*) at the inferior pole of the syrinx. After removal of the dural calcification, the syrinx resolved.

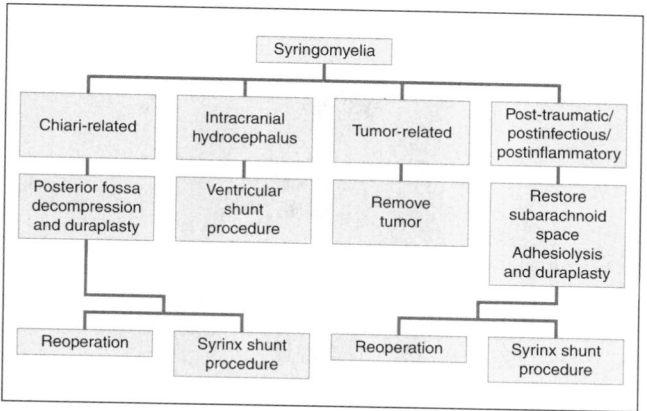

Figure 235.5 Algorithm for the treatment of syringomyelia.

(Maher CPM, Krauss W, unpublished data). Syrinx shunting and obex plugging are unnecessary adjuncts to this first-line treatment. The surgical risk of mortality is small, but the risk of significant morbidity is 5% to 8%.

A ventriculoperitoneal shunt procedure is excellent for treating syringomyelia associated with intracranial hydrocephalus. In more than 90% of patients, the syrinx and associated symptoms resolve.

Restoration of the spinal subarachnoid space is the first-line treatment for a post-traumatic, postinfectious, or postinflammatory syrinx (Figure 235.6b). The general concept of this treatment is simple, but the application is not. In some cases of post-traumatic syringomyelia, removal of a compressive lesion (bone or soft tissue), correction of a spinal deformity, or indirect decompression via laminectomy (or a combi-

Table 235.3 Outcomes of surgical treatment

Series	Cause	Treatment	Stable neurological condition, % patients	Follow-up, years
Sgouros and Williams[9]	Varied	Shunting	50	10
Vernet et al.[15]	Varied	Shunting	100	2
Milhorat et al.[16]	Varied	CVD and shunting	70	3
Samii and Klekamp[6]	Tumor	Tumor removal	75	> 1 (good preoperative neurological status)
			32	> 1 (poor preoperative neurological status)
Klekamp et al.[10]	Postinfectious, post-traumatic, postinflammatory	Laminectomy, adhesiolysis, duraplasty	83	2.5
Maher CPM, Krauss W (unpublished data)	Chiari	CVD ± syringo-subarachnoid shunt	70	1[†]

CVD, cranioverteberal decompression.
*Predominantly Chiari malformation and post-traumatic-associated.
[†]No statistical difference with or without shunting.

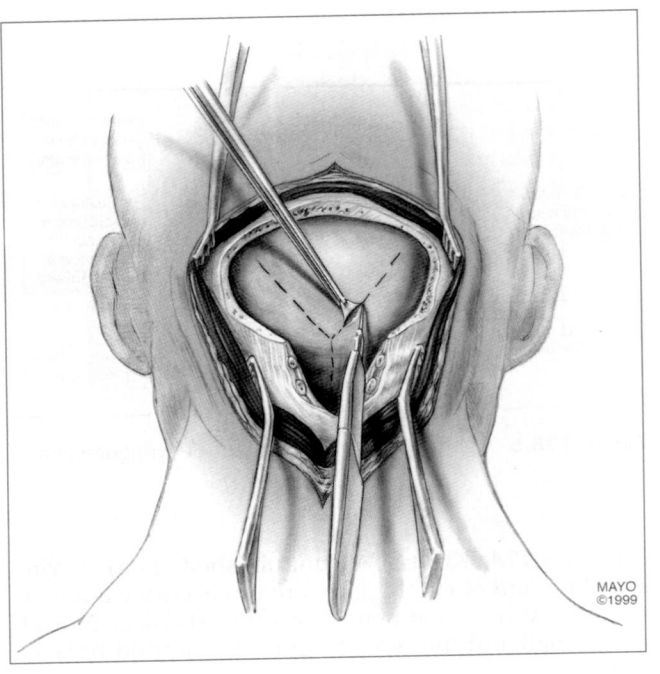 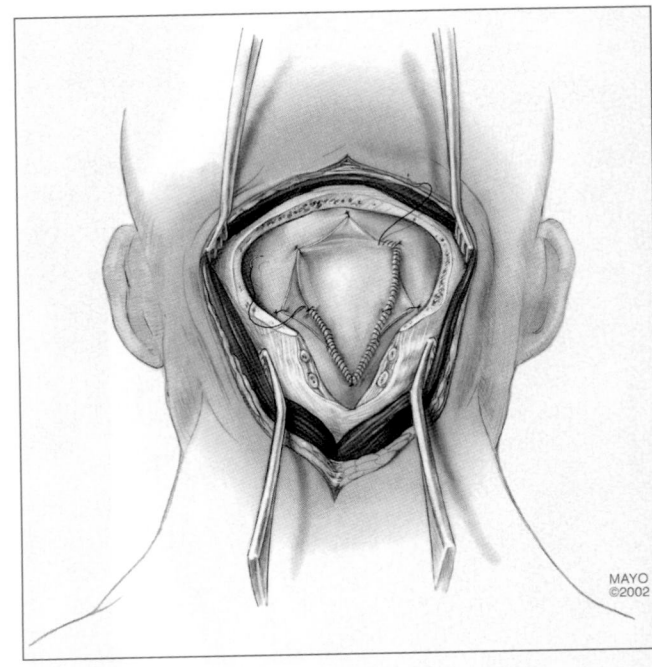

(a)

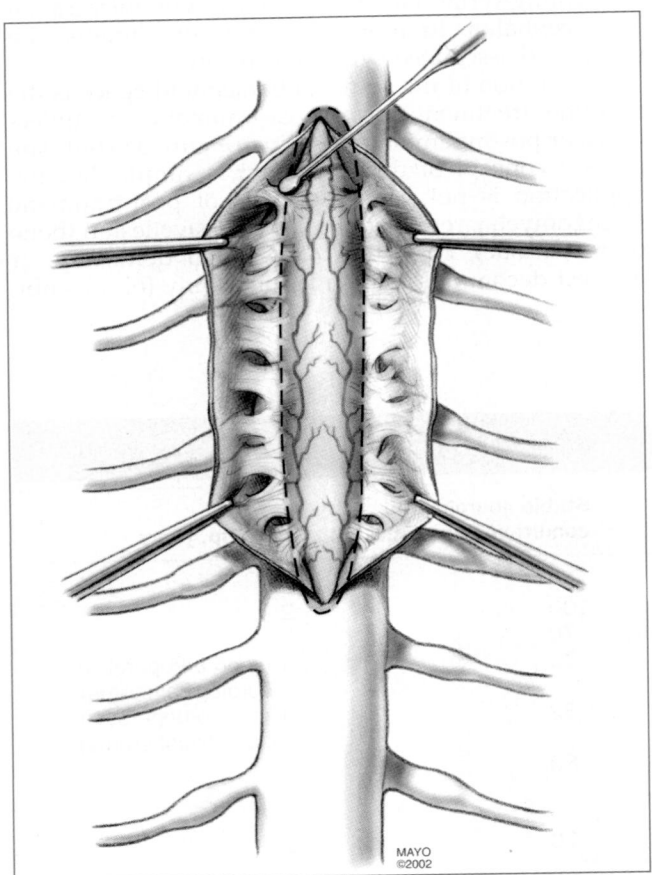 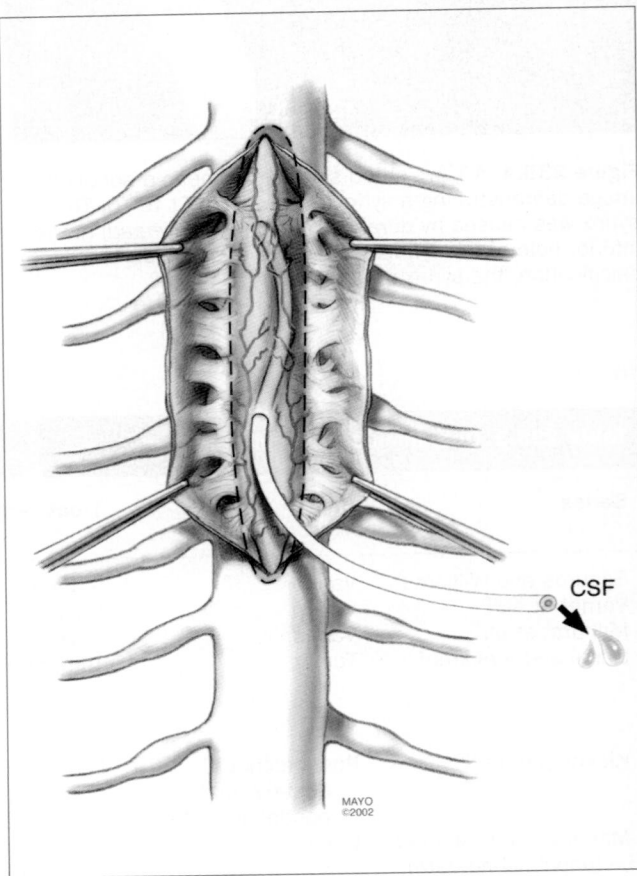

(b)

Figure 235.6 Various treatments for syringomyelia. (a), Treatment of Chiari-related syringomyelia with posterior fossa decompression (*left*) and duraplasty (*right*). (b), Treatment of adhesion-related syringomyelia with adhesiolysis and duraplasty (*left*) and shunting (*right*). (By permission of Mayo Foundation.)

nation of these) may reconstruct the subarachnoid space. In addition, some authors have advocated opening the dura mater and lysing subarachnoid adhesions to normalize spinal CSF dynamics. Often, duraplasty is performed to create more space around the spinal cord.[9,10] In cases of postinfectious or postinflammatory syringomyelia, treatment is more difficult. Identification of the compromised subarachnoid space may be impossible or subarachnoid adhesions may be so extensive that the surgical procedure is not practical. However, for patients in whom treatment is possible, the neurological status stabilizes in more than 80%.[10]

Tumor removal is the treatment of choice for tumor-associated syrinxes.[6] To classify this as a treatment for syringomyelia is misleading because the goal is successful treatment of the tumor. Syringomyelia is an attendant phenomenon that ceases to be a problem after successful resection of the tumor.

Syrinxes due to myelomalacia usually do not require treatment. Idiopathic syrinxes usually are treated with shunting, as discussed below.

Second-line treatments

The second-line treatment for all types is placement of a syrinx shunt. Enthusiasm for this procedure has waned with the growing realization that most shunts ultimately have mechanical failure.[9,10] When a shunt fails, the disease progresses. Because of the need to perform myelotomy in a compromised spinal cord, the risk-to-benefit ratio of the procedure is high. Significant perioperative complications occur in at least 15% of patients.[10] However, long-term neurological stabilization is achieved in approximately 50% of patients. Data suggest that placing the distal end of the shunt in the pleural space is more effective than placing it in the subarachnoid space.[15]

Other treatments

Painful dysesthesias and spasticity are associated with syringomyelia. Gabapentin and tricyclic antidepressants have been useful in treating dysesthesias and baclofen, in treating spasticity. In extreme cases of spasticity, a baclofen drug delivery system has had to be implanted.

Monitoring treatment

Clinical outcome is the most relevant and sensitive indicator of efficacy. Serial neurological examinations are necessary to document neurological stabilization. Most surgical treatments have a short-term (less than 5 years) success rate of 70% or better. Because any surgical treatment may fail ultimately, long-term surveillance is necessary. New neurological progression usually signals disease recurrence. In most cases, recurrent scarring has occurred or the shunt has failed. In these cases, revision surgery may be necessary.

Serial MRI studies are useful in documenting the size of the syrinx. Although a decrease in syrinx size is desirable, clinical stabilization or improvement is not always associated with radiographic evidence of shrinkage of the syrinx. This may be related to decreased compliance of the spinal cord from chronic syringomyelia.

Complications

All the surgical treatments have considerable risk of perioperative morbidity. The dreaded complication is neurological worsening as a direct result of surgical manipulation. Lysing spinal cord adhesions, correcting post-traumatic spinal deformities, and performing myelotomy for shunt placement all have a 10% to 15% risk of causing a new neurological deficit.[9,10]

Conclusions

Proper treatment of syringomyelia depends on accurately identifying its cause. For Chiari-, tumor-, or hydrocephalus-associated syringomyelia, treatments that have excellent efficacy and durability are available. For post-traumatic, postinfectious, or postinflammatory syringomyelia, treatment is a short-term measure; this reflects the limited understanding of the pathophysiological mechanisms of these types of syringomyelia.

References

1. Abbe R, Coley WB. Syringomyelia, operation; exploration of cord; withdrawal of fluid. J Nerv Ment Disorders 1892;19:512–520
2. Schurch B, Wichmann W, Rossier AB. Post-traumatic syringomyelia (cystic myelopathy): a prospective study of 449 patients with spinal cord injury. J Neurol Neurosurg Psychiatry 1996;60:61–67
3. Kramer KM, Levine AM. Posttraumatic syringomyelia: a review of 21 cases. Clin Orthop 1997;334:190-199
4. Paul KS, Lye RH, Strang FA, Dutton J. Arnold-Chiari malformation: review of 71 cases. J Neurosurg 1983;58:183–187
5. Rauzzino M, Oakes WJ. Chiari II malformation and syringomyelia. Neurosurg Clin N Am 1995;6:293–309
6. Samii M, Klekamp J. Surgical results of 100 intramedullary tumors in relation to accompanying syringomyelia. Neurosurgery 1994;35:865–873
7. Heiss JD, Patronas N, DeVroom HL, et al. Elucidating the pathophysiology of syringomyelia. J Neurosurg 1999;91:553–562
8. el Masry WS, Biyani A. Incidence, management, and outcome of post-traumatic syringomyelia. J Neurol Neurosurg Psychiatry 1996;60:141–146
9. Sgouros S, Williams B. A critical appraisal of drainage in syringomyelia. J Neurosurg 1995;82:1–10
10. Klekamp J, Batzdorf U, Samii M, Bothe HW. Treatment of syringomyelia associated with arachnoid scarring caused by arachnoiditis or trauma. J Neurosurg 1997;86:233–240
11. Perrouin-Verbe B, Lenne-Aurier K, Robert R, et al. Post-traumatic syringomyelia and post-traumatic spinal canal stenosis: a direct relationship: review of 75 patients with a spinal cord injury. Spinal Cord 1998;36:137–143
12. Milhorat TH, Capocelli AL Jr, Anzil AP, et al. Pathological basis of spinal cord cavitation in syringomyelia: analysis of 105 autopsy cases. J Neurosurg 1995;82:802–812

13. Caplan LR, Norohna AB, Amico LL. Syringomyelia and arachnoiditis. J Neurol Neurosurg Psychiatry 1990; 53:106–113

14. Boman K, Iivanainen M. Prognosis of syringomyelia. Acta Neurol Scand 1967;43:61–68

15. Vernet O, Farmer JP, Montes JL. Comparison of syringopleural and syringosubarachnoid shunting in the treatment of syringomyelia in children. J Neurosurg 1996;84:624–628

16. Milhorat TH, Kotzen RM, Mu HT, et al. Dysesthetic pain in patients with syringomyelia. Neurosurgery 1996;38:940–946

236 Focal Dystonias: Blepharospasm, Cervical Dystonia, Spasmodic Dysphonia, Writer's Cramp

Cynthia Comella, Christy Ludlow and Mark Hallett

Focal dystonia, the most common form of the disorder, may affect many different parts of the body. Generally, it presents in adult life while generalized dystonia presents in childhood. Dystonia may begin as focal and then spread contiguously to affect more of the body. The most frequently occurring forms are discussed here.

Blepharospasm

Brief overview

Blepharospasm is a focal dystonia involving the periocular muscles (Figure 236.1A). Clinical manifestations include increased blinking and spasms of involuntary eye closure. Involvement of the lower face or jaw in association with blepharospasm is referred to as Meige's syndrome. Essential blepharospasm can cause significant disability by interfering with vision.

Epidemiology

Blepharospasm has an estimated incidence of 4.6 per million and prevalence of 17 per million according to an epidemiological survey conducted in Rochester, Minnesota.[1] The Epidemiologic Study of Dystonia in Europe (ESDE) found that 22% of the 957 dystonia patients identified had blepharospasm.[2]

Etiology

Most cases of blepharospasm appear to be sporadic, although some may well be hereditary based on a genetic factor with reduced penetrance. In many circumstances, there are ocular symptoms at onset, but whether they indicate an etiological role for ocular pathology is uncertain. Blepharospasm can result from focal lesions in the basal ganglia and brainstem, and can be a feature of basal ganglia disorders such as Parkinson's disease.[3]

Pathophysiology and pathogenesis

In blepharospasm, there is a loss of brainstem inhibition as demonstrated by diminution of the normal inhibition of the R2 following paired stimulation, suggesting a loss of brainstem inhibitory mechanisms.[3-7] Transcranial magnetic stimulation (TMS) of the vertex showed a reduction of the silent period (SP) recorded in contracting upper and lower facial muscles in blepharospasm patients when compared to normal controls, reflecting reduced excitability of cortical inhibitory neurons.[8]

Sensory and motor systems are both implicated in the pathogenesis of blepharospasm as determined by PET measurements of regional blood flow.[9] A reduction of dopamine D_2-like binding in the putamen suggests alterations of basal ganglia function.[10]

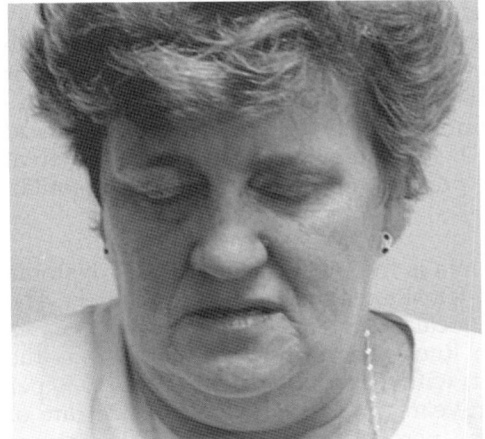
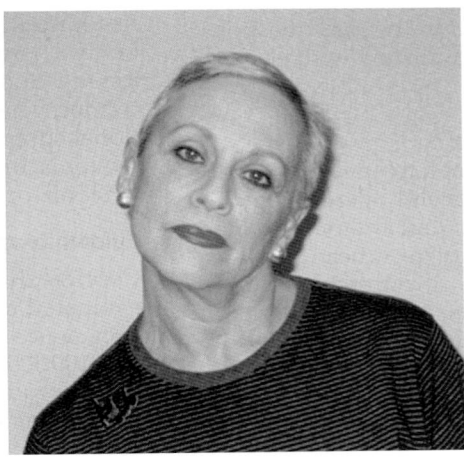

Figure 236.1 *A*, Patient with blepharospasm. *B*, Patient with cervical dystonia, manifested mainly by left laterocollis. (See color plate section.)

Genetics

Thirty-six percent of blepharospasm patients report at least one first or second degree family member with a movement disorder.[11] Clinical evidence of genetic anticipation in primary cranial dystonia further suggests a genetic factor in some families. As with other forms of familial dystonia, blepharospasm is a heterogeneous disorder that may be autosomal dominant with a reduced penetrance.[12] No gene, however, has yet been identified.

Clinical features

Primary blepharospasm typically begins in adulthood, with an average age of onset of 59 years. Women are affected more than men in a 2.3:1 ratio.[2] The onset of blepharospasm is gradual, with symptoms of increased blinking often preceding more frank spasms. The onset of blepharospasm is usually bilateral but may be unilateral in 20% of patients.[13] Blepharospasm is an involuntary eye closure, with contractions of the orbicularis oculi muscle. Many patients report sensations of grittiness, photophobia and eye irritation occurring at onset of symptoms,[3] but most patients have no demonstrable ocular pathology. Intrinsic visual acuity remains intact, although there may be functional blindness due to the involuntary eye closure in as many as 66% of patients.[13] Exacerbating factors for blepharospasm include bright light, wind and stress. These factors may make it impossible for the patient to perform tasks such as driving a car. Blepharospasm symptoms may be improved by a variety of "tricks" such as talking, singing, pulling on the upper eyelid, yawning or chewing gum.

Classification

Blepharospasm may be a primary or secondary dystonia. Primary blepharospasm occurs in the absence of other neurological abnormalities and has no discoverable etiology. Secondary blepharospasm arises from a number of underlying etiologies.[3] Coexistent lower facial and jaw dystonia is the most frequent concomitant problem and is called Meige's syndrome.

Diagnostic criteria

Blepharospasm is a clinical diagnosis based primarily on the appearance of the patient. In the rare questionable case, the diagnosis can be confirmed with electrophysiology.

Differential diagnosis

The nondystonic causes of blepharospasm include local eye pathology, apraxia of eyelid opening, myasthenia gravis, hemifacial spasm, and motor tics. Blepharospasm can occur secondary to other disorders including Parkinson's disease, progressive supranuclear palsy, multiple systems atrophy and other parkinsonian disorders. It has also been described in patients with Huntington's disease.

Treatment

Prior to the introduction of botulinum toxin injections, the treatment of blepharospasm was problematic. Anticholinergic drugs are generally considered the first choice, but the experience of many clinicians is that chronic administration of anticholinergic drugs improves symptoms in fewer than 20% to 25%, often with intolerable side effects.[14,15] Other oral drugs have been assessed in uncontrolled trials. There may be a "good" response in up to 50% of the patients, but it tends to be transient.

The introduction of botulinum toxin as a therapeutic agent was a major milestone in the clinical management of blepharospasm, and it is regarded by most clinicians as the treatment of choice for blepharospasm.[16,17] Numerous studies, mostly observational, show successful control of facial spasm in 75% to 100% of patients. Onset of action following injections occurs within 2 to 3 days, maximal effect is at 2 weeks, and duration of effect is from 2 to 6 months with the average being approximately 3 to 4 months. Side effects from botulinum toxin injection include diplopia, ptosis, dry eyes, photophobia, lid entropion, and epiphora.

Surgical interventions are viewed as an alternative when other modes of therapy have been unsuccessful in alleviating disability due to blepharospasm. Partial blepharoplasty and myectomy involves stripping portions of the orbicularis oculi muscle, in particular the pretarsal, preseptal and preorbital regions. It has been variably successful, with complications including forehead numbness, ptosis and cosmetic problems.[13] For patients with suboptimal response to botulinum toxin, blepharoplasty and limited myectomy may enhance the effects of the injection and prolong the interval between botulinum toxin injections by as much as 2 to 3 months.[18]

Cervical dystonia

Brief overview

Cervical dystonia (CD) was originally called spasmodic torticollis. Until a few decades ago, CD was often considered to be a psychiatric disorder. The condition is defined as a focal dystonia involving the cervical musculature causing abnormal postures of the head, neck and shoulders (Figure 236.1B). There may be overlying muscle spasms causing quick, repetitive jerking movements, which may be mistaken for tremor. The distinguishing feature of CD is the directional preponderance of the movements. Cervical dystonia may be a part of generalized or segmental dystonia or be present in isolation as a focal dystonia.

Epidemiology

Cervical dystonia is the most common focal dystonia evaluated in referral movement disorders centers. The prevalence of focal dystonia is estimated at 33 cases per 100 000 in Rochester, Minnesota, and CD is the most frequent with a crude incidence of 10.9 per million person-years, and a crude prevalence rate of 88.6 per million persons.[1] A cross-sectional study of dystonia conducted by the Epidemiologic Study of Dystonia in Europe found that CD constituted almost half of the cases of focal dystonia identified.[2] The disorder typically begins in the fifth decade, affecting women about twice as often as men.[2]

Etiology

In the absence of other neurological or medical conditions, CD is categorized as a primary dystonia. Although trauma, immunological disorders, and vestibular dysfunction have all been suggested as possible causative factors, none of these has been proven. Familial CD is reported, but no gene has been identified.

Pathophysiology and pathogenesis

The pathophysiology of cervical dystonia is not known. Electrophysiological tests have demonstrated abnormalities in blink reflex recovery and exteroceptive silent periods, suggesting a loss of central inhibitory mechanisms.[5–7]

Genetics

Although most cases of cervical dystonia appear to be sporadic, clinical investigations have suggested that an autosomal dominant genetic mutation with reduced penetrance is responsible for cervical dystonia in many patients. The DYT1 gene has been excluded as a cause of familial CD. Both DYT6[19] and DYT7[20] have been identified as possible loci in large families with cervical dystonia. As with other focal dystonias, CD is likely, however, to be genetically heterogeneous.[21]

Clinical features

The salient feature of CD is the involuntary movements of the head, neck and shoulders, causing sustained abnormal postures occasionally with overlying spasms. Approximately 60% of CD patients experience pain in the neck region. Pain may be a mild discomfort or may be so severe as to be the major disabling feature.[22] Pain may primarily arise from muscle spasm in CD, but there may also be other coexistent disorders, including cervical arthritis, radiculopathy and occipital neuralgia.

Cervical dystonia is a lifelong disorder that fluctuates in severity and intensity over its course. From 10% to 20% of patients will have a partial or complete remission.[23] Remissions most commonly occur within the first year after symptom onset and are more frequent in younger patients. Most remissions are transient, lasting from weeks to years. The frequency of permanent remission is unknown, but estimated to be less than 1%. Maximum disability usually occurs within 5 years of onset.[23] Factors observed to worsen symptoms include stress, exercise, and particular postures. Sensory tricks (gestes antagonistes) such as a touch to the cheek or to the back of the head, may improve symptoms dramatically.

Approximately 25% of patients with torticollis will have spread of symptoms beyond the neck. The mean time for onset to spread is 6 to 7 years. Most patients will only experience spread to one or two contiguous body areas. Only 6% will develop generalized dystonia.[24]

Classification

The terminology applied to CD describes the abnormal postures of the head and neck observed. Torticollis is a horizontal rotation of the head, retrocollis is an extension of the head, anterocollis is a forward flexion of the head with flexion of the chin, and latercollis is a lateral tilting of the head toward the shoulder. Lateral or sagittal shift refers to the movement of the neck on the shoulders. The head and neck postures of cervical dystonia are often complex, combining movements in several axes. Isolated head tremor, in the horizontal axis (no-no) or with a directional preference, may be the only manifestation of CD.

Diagnostic criteria

Cervical dystonia is a clinical diagnosis defined as a focal dystonia involving muscles of the neck.

Differential diagnosis

The differential diagnosis of nondystonic torticollis is broad and varies with the age of the patient. Primary cervical dystonia is rare in infancy and childhood. The most common cause of torticollis in infants is congenital muscular torticollis with shortening of a sternocleidomastoid muscle causing a head tilt. Other causes of torticollis developing in infancy include intrauterine crowding, malformations of the cervical spine, and Arnold–Chiari malformations. Torticollis in childhood is usually due to either cervical abnormalities or rotational atlanto-axial subluxation. Nasopharyngeal infections, posterior fossa and cervical cord lesions are other local causes of torticollis. Abnormal posturing of the head may occur to compensate for visual disturbances, such as diplopia or congenital nystagmus. Sandifer's syndrome arising from gastro-esophageal reflux and esophagitis should also be considered. Adulthood onset cervical dystonia is common, and is rarely secondary to underlying pathology. Adults with torticollis of sudden onset with a restricted range of movement in whom the posture is unchanged by sleep should be evaluated for underlying structural lesions.

Treatment

Current treatments for cervical dystonia are symptomatic. No curative therapies are available. Treatment options include oral medications, chemodenervation and surgical management.

Anticholinergic drugs offer the greatest possibility of benefit. A retrospective analysis of 71 CD patients reported that 39% had a good response to anticholinergic agents, with women faring better than men.[25] Peripheral side effects such as dry mouth, blurred vision, and urinary retention are frequent, but may be reversed using a peripheral cholinesterase inhibitor (glycopyrrolate). The central side effects are dose limiting, and include memory loss and sedation.

Other drugs that may be helpful in some patients

include carbidopa/levodopa, clonazepam, and baclofen. Although also reported to be sometimes helpful, dopamine receptor blocking agents are discouraged. Tetrabenazine can be useful, but is currently not generally available in the USA.

Botulinum toxin type A has shown benefit in both double-blind and open-label studies. The percentage of patients improving ranges from 60% to 85%.[16,26] Approximately 30% of patients experience adverse effects, the most common being dysphagia and neck weakness. A small percentage of patients receiving repeated injections develop resistance to the effect of botulinum toxin type A. The development of new types of botulinum toxin provides an alternative for CD patients with resistance to type A. Controlled clinical trials using botulinum toxin type B, for example, show significant improvement in patients with and without resistance to type A.[27,28]

Surgical treatments for CD are reserved for patients with disabling symptoms who fail drug treatments. Peripheral procedures include peripheral denervation, rhizotomy and myectomy, but only peripheral denervation has been promising. This involves a specific lesion of the branch of the spinal accessory nerve to the sternocleidomastoid muscle and a selective ramisectomy of the branches serving the posterior neck muscles.[29] Following surgery, the recovery time is prolonged, requiring a period of rehabilitation. The success rate in carefully selected patients operated on by experienced surgeons is over 80% and the complication rate is low. Central nervous system surgery would be considered a last resort, especially in patients with CD, where there are virtually no data available.

Spasmodic dysphonia

Brief overview

Spasmodic dysphonia, originally called spastic dysphonia, is characterized by spasmodic interruptions in the voice. In the adductor type (ADSD), intermittent hyperadductions of the vocal folds shut off the voice for short periods. In the abductor type (ABSD), the voice breaks are breathy due to intermittent prolonged openings of the vocal folds during voiceless consonants. Both were originally thought to be functional voice disorders, due either to misuse or to a form of hysterical dysphonia. This was first challenged when ADSD patients were shown to have neurological disorders.[30] The disorder became classified as an organic dysphonia when a unilateral nerve section was found helpful.[31] In the 1980s the name was changed to denote the spasmodic intermittent quality of the voice symptoms. The disorder was finally classified as a task-specific focal dystonia, sometimes referred to as laryngeal dystonia with the advent of botulinum toxin therapy.[32]

Epidemiology

Little information is available on the epidemiology of ADSD due to poor recognition of the disorder. Based on estimates from one population study,[1] there may be 15 000 cases in the USA today.

Etiology

The etiology is unknown and almost all cases are sporadic. One third of cases report onset following an upper respiratory infection or nerve injury. Laryngeal nerve demyelination was first reported by Dedo et al.,[33] but this has been both supported and refuted by others. Although ADSD occurs in some families with idiopathic torsion dystonia, few sporadic cases report association with other focal dystonias.

Pathophysiology and pathogenesis

Voice breaks in ADSD are coincident with spasmodic bursts in the thyroarytenoid muscle, although bursts in other muscles can occur.[34] When voice breaks are absent, however, muscle activation is normal in both adductor and abductor laryngeal muscles.[35] In ABSD, the prolonged voiceless consonants are assumed to be due to spasmodic bursts in the posterior cricoarytenoid muscle, the only laryngeal abductor muscle. Electromyographic studies thus far, however, have not supported this assumption.[35] In voice tremor, often associated with either ADSD or ABSD, a variety of muscles are affected across patients.[36] Abnormalities in blink reflex conditioning were found in some ADSD cases. The conditioning of laryngeal long latency responses is altered in both ADSD and ABSD,[37] indicating that the central suppression of laryngeal sensory–motor responses is affected in these disorders.

Genetics

No linkage studies have been conducted, and fewer than 1 per 100 patients have other family members affected with spasmodic dysphonia. No cases of spasmodic dysphonia have been reported with the *DYT1* gene GAG deletion.

Clinical features

The disorder usually begins in middle age with a gradual increase in symptom frequency, severity and consistency over 1 to 2 years, with symptoms rarely remitting after this time. The disorder is specific to speech; other aspects of laryngeal function such as laughter, crying and singing are not as affected, if at all.

Classification

Adductor type spasmodic dysphonia affects 85% of patients; the other 15% have ABSD. An associated vocal tremor is present in at least one third of both types. In ADSD, voice breaks occur during vowels resulting in prolonged glottal stops or intermittent periods of a strained or strangled voice quality. In ABSD, voiceless consonants (p, t, k, f, s, h) are prolonged and perceived as breathy breaks. Both types of patients complain of increased effort associated with speech production.

Differential diagnosis

There is no biological marker for this disorder, and identification is based on symptom characteristics. A multidisciplinary team is recommended for diagnosis

Table 236.1   Treatments for spasmodic dysphonia

Type of disorder	Treatment approach	Percent of patients with benefit	Degree of symptom remission	Period of benefit	Side effects
ADSD	BOTOX® in the thyroarytenoid muscle; 2 units bilaterally or 12 units unilaterally	90%	90%	3–4 months	Dysphagia 3–5 days Transient breathiness for ~2 weeks
ABSD	BOTOX® in the posterior cricoarytenoid muscle; 5 units bilaterally or 12 units unilaterally	66%	50%	2–3 months	Stridor ~2 weeks
ABSD	BOTOX® in the cricothyroid muscles; 5 units bilaterally	60%	50%	2–3 months	Dysphagia ~1 week
ADSD	Recurrent laryngeal nerve avulsion	90%	90%	3–7 years	Dysphagia 2 weeks Breathy or hoarse voice may persist
ADSD	Selective denervation and reinnervation (bilateral)	70%	70%	2 years	Breathy for 3–6 months Aspiration for 1–2 months

ABSD, abductor spasmodic dysphonia; ADSD, adductor spasmodic dysphonia.

of spasmodic dysphonia including an otolaryngologist, speech-language pathologist, neurologist and psychiatrist.[38] Other idiopathic voice disorders, such as muscular tension dysphonia, do not involve intermittent spasmodic changes in the voice. In muscular tension dysphonia, abnormal hypertense laryngeal postures are consistent during voice production and patients respond to manual laryngeal manipulation (use of massage to stretch the strap muscles and adjust the level of the thyroid cartilage in the throat) to reduce tension.[39] Confusion occurs in diagnosis when patients with spasmodic dysphonia also develop increased muscle tension in an effort to overcome vocal instability, resulting in symptoms of both disorders. Disorders such as a vocal fold paralysis or weakness, gastroesophageal reflux, vocal fold nodules/polyps and cysts must be ruled out by laryngeal examination. A psychiatric evaluation may be required if a psychogenic voice disorder is suspected.[38]

Benign essential tremor can also produce voice breaks and occurs more often in women, sometimes with an associated head tremor. Such patients may also develop muscular tension dysphonia in an effort to overcome vocal tremor.

Treatment

Only symptomatic treatments aimed at reducing the occurrence of voice breaks are currently available (Table 236.1). Initially, unilateral section of the recurrent laryngeal nerve, resulting in a unilateral paralysis of the adductor and abductor muscles, reduces voice breaks.[31] With time, however, symptoms recur as a result of reinnervation.[40] Botulinum toxin type A (BOTOX®) injection produces a partial temporary chemodenervation for up to 4 months, either by small injections of 1 to 2.5 units into both of the thyroarytenoid muscles[32] or a unilateral injection of 12 to 15 units in ADSD.[41] Spasmodic bursts are reduced in

both treated and untreated muscles[34] and relate to voice improvement. This therapy is effective in at least 90% of ADSD patients based on one small randomized controlled class I trial[42] and multiple case series class III reports.[32,41] A recent large series reported that patients continue to show benefit for up to 10 years with repeated injections.[43] Botulinum toxin type A is less effective in ABSD. When patients with only cricothyroid muscle spasms are injected, significant improvements occur,[44] while up to two thirds of ABSD patients injected in the posterior cricoarytenoid muscle receive some degree of benefit.[45]

Surgical attempts at prolonged symptom control have, in the past, been relatively short-lived, for 1 to 3 years. Recent approaches aimed at preventing reinnervation by the original axons to the thyroarytenoid muscle extend the benefit period. Extensive recurrent nerve avulsion maintains symptom control in 78% of patients for 3 to 7 years.[46] In another technique, the portion of the recurrent laryngeal nerve that innervates the thyroarytenoid muscle is selectively denervated and reinnervated with branches of the ansa cervicalis nerve.[47] A total of 21 patients have been followed for up to 36 months with good benefit. Detrimental effects on voice quality, breathing and/or swallowing may resolve or require further surgery. Many patients, however, seem willing to accept some deficit in voice quality in exchange for less effort and reduced numbers of voice breaks. Both the etiology of the disorder and the pathogenesis of symptoms must be understood before optimal long-term effective treatments can be developed.

Writer's cramp
Brief overview

Writer's cramp is the most common form of task-specific focal hand dystonia. Many other repetitive hand activities can lead to dystonia, and the general term "occupational cramp" is often used. Other common forms are pianist's cramp, guitar player's cramp and typist's cramp. In the earlier or mildest form, the disorder affects the specific task, but not other tasks using the same muscles. In more severe forms, multiple tasks may be affected. While the disorder has been recognized for many years, the medical profession has oscillated between believing it was an organic disease of the nervous system or a psychiatric disorder. In modern times, it was the paper of Sheehy and Marsden that convinced neurologists that writer's cramp was a dystonia by demonstrating its relationship to other dystonias.[48]

Epidemiology

There are no definitive epidemiological studies. Focal hand dystonia turns up in surveys of dystonia, and, like other focal dystonias, appears sporadic.[1] Considering all focal dystonias together, however, the familial incidence is increased and is consistent with autosomal dominant inheritance with very low penetrance.[49,50] The other striking feature is that the disorder almost always is seen in the setting of repetitive use of the hand for many years.

Etiology

The etiology is unknown, but it would seem likely that the disorder is the consequence of repetitive activity on the background of a genetic predisposition.[6,7] The proportion of these two components may vary. Certain patients have only little repetitive use, and, of course, there are many unaffected persons who have just as much use, or more, than that of patients. An animal model of blepharospasm demonstrates how it may take two factors to produce dystonia, in that situation a dopamine deficiency and a facial palsy.[51]

Pathophysiology and pathogenesis

Extensive studies have been done and are summarized elsewhere.[5-7] Electromyography studies show lack of appropriate reciprocal inhibition and overflow into extraneous muscles. Spinal and brainstem reflexes show loss of inhibition. Extensive studies of cortical physiology with electroencephalography (EEG), neuroimaging and transcranial magnetic stimulation mapping suggest also a loss of cortical inhibition in generating the neural command. While no overt pathology has been demonstrated in the basal ganglia, by analogy to other dystonias the fundamental disturbance is likely to be there. Since the basal ganglia can regulate inhibition, this seems reasonable. One study that directly implicates the basal ganglia shows a reduction of D_2 binding in the striatum.[10]

Genetics

As noted under Epidemiology, while the disorder may be autosomal dominant with low penetrance, no gene has as yet been found or linked.

Clinical features

The hand will not obey the will in carrying out skilled tasks and assumes abnormal postures. The problem can affect just a single digit or the whole arm. In most cases this occurs without pain, although muscle aching can occur if there have been many prolonged spasms. At least at first, no other skilled task of the hand is affected. Usually these disorders do not progress beyond the focal, task-specific problem, although sometimes they do generalize to other tasks or other parts of the body. Typically, the problem is chronic.

Classification

Each disorder is named by the specific task affected. The terms "simple writer's cramp" and "dystonic writer's cramp" can be used to refer to complete task specificity and some generalization, respectively.[48]

Diagnostic criteria

The diagnosis is purely clinical and no tests are ordinarily done. Patients will show abnormalities of physiological investigations such as reciprocal inhibition,[52] but these are not generally carried out in practice.

Differential diagnosis

When someone presents with hand dysfunction, there are generally three diagnostic considerations: 1) musculoskeletal disorders including the overuse syndrome; 2) nerve entrapment; 3) focal dystonia. In the large experience of Lederman with 672 musicians with upper extremity symptoms, 64% had musculoskeletal disorders including overuse, 7% had dystonia, and 22.5% had a peripheral nerve disorder.[53]

Overuse, also known as repetition strain injury or RSI, is due to the cumulative effect on tissue of repeated physical stress.[54] The pathology is not clear, and differentiation from inflammatory conditions such as tendinitis and tenosynovitis has sometimes been difficult and confusing. The principal symptom is that of pain—in the muscle, muscle–tendon region, or ligaments—that is precipitated by playing the instrument. As the disorder progresses the pain lasts longer after stopping playing and may even become continuous. Symptoms of nerve injury include weakness, loss of sensation, paresthesias and pain.[54]

Treatment

In many situations, patients are able to accomplish their tasks with their other hand or in some other way and never seek treatment. For writing, for example, patients may switch to their other hand, or type. Sometimes alteration of technique may be sufficient to change the movement to a different task; shifting to mostly proximal arm muscles in order to write may be effective. There are also writing aids and tricks such as altering the size of the pen. Physical therapy, in general, has not been effective, but a new method has been suggested with positive early results.[55]

Oral therapy has generally not been useful although individual patients might respond. The most successfully used agent is trihexyphenidyl. Since it has been shown that rare cases of dopa-responsive dystonia present as focal dystonia in adult life,[56] a case could be made for trying levodopa.

The most successful treatment has been focal injections of botulinum toxin. Toxin is injected into the overactive muscles. This can significantly improve the dystonia although it does not, in general, return function to a normal level. Several small double-blind studies have been done,[57] and long term follow-up shows the possibility of benefit continuing over many years.[58] The satisfaction of the patient depends on his or her need and expectation. Professional musicians, for example, would be less likely to be pleased given their need for exquisite motor control.[59]

References

1. Nutt JG, Muenter MD, Aronson A, et al. Epidemiology of focal and generalized dystonia in Rochester, Minnesota. Mov Disord 1988;3:188–194

2. Epidemiologic Study of Dystonia in Europe (ESDE) Collaborative Group. Sex-related influences on the frequency and age of onset of primary dystonia. Neurology 1999;53:1871–1873

3. Hallett M, Daroff RB. Blepharospasm: report of a workshop. Neurology 1996;46:1213–1218

4. Berardelli A, Rothwell JC, Day BL, Marsden CD. Pathophysiology of blepharospasm and oromandibular dystonia. Brain 1985;108:593–608

5. Berardelli A, Rothwell JC, Hallett M, et al. The pathophysiology of primary dystonia. Brain 1998;121:1195–1212

6. Hallett M. The neurophysiology of dystonia. Arch Neurol 1998;55:601–603

7. Hallett M. Physiology of dystonia. In: Fahn S, Marsden CD, DeLong M, eds. Dystonia 3. Advances in Neurology. Vol 78. Philadelphia: Lippincott-Raven, 1998:11–18

8. Curra A, Romaniello A, Berardelli A, et al. Shortened cortical silent period in facial muscles of patients with cranial dystonia. Neurology 2000;54:130–135

9. Feiwell RJ, Black KJ, McGee-Minnich LA, et al. Diminished regional cerebral blood flow response to vibration in patients with blepharospasm. Neurology 1999;52:291–297

10. Perlmutter JS, Stambuk MK, Markham J, et al. Decreased [18F]spiperone binding in putamen in idiopathic focal dystonia. J Neurosci 1997;17:843–850

11. Defazio G, Livrea P, Guanti G, et al. Genetic contribution to idiopathic adult-onset blepharospasm and cranial cervical dystonia. Eur Neurol 1993;33:345–350

12. Waddy HM, Fletcher NA, Harding AE, Marsden CD. A genetic study of idiopathic focal dystonias. Ann Neurol 1991;29:320–324

13. Grandas F, Elston J, Quinn N, Marsden CD. Blepharospasm, a review of 264 patients. J Neurol Neurosurg Psychiatry 1988;51:767–772

14. Nutt JG, Hammerstad JP, deGarmo P, Carter J. Cranial dystonia: double-blind crossover study of anticholinergics. Neurology 1984;34:215–217

15. Lang AE, Sheehy MP, Marsden CD. Anticholinergics in adult-onset focal dystonia. Can J Neurol Sci 1982;9:313–319

16. Hallett M. One man's poison—clinical applications of botulinum toxin [editorial]. N Engl J Med 1999;341:118–120

17. Elston JS. Botulinum toxin for blepharospasm. In: Jankovic J, Hallett M, eds. Therapy with Botulinum Toxin. New York: Marcel Dekker, 1994:191–197

18. Mauriello JA Jr, Keswani R, Franklin M. Long-term enhancement of botulinum toxin injections by upper-

eyelid surgery in 14 patients with facial dyskinesias. Arch Otolaryngol Head Neck Surg 1999;125:627–631

19. Almasy L, Bressman SB, Raymond D, et al. Idiopathic torsion dystonia linked to chromosome 8 in two Mennonite families. Ann Neurol 1997;42:670–673

20. Leube B, Hendgen T, Kessler KR, et al. Evidence for DYT7 being a common cause of cervical dystonia (torticollis) in Central Europe. Am J Med Genet 1997;74:529–532

21. Jarman PR, del Grosso N, Valente EM, et al. Primary torsion dystonia: the search for genes is not over. J Neurol Neurosurg Psychiatry 1999;67:395–397

22. Chan J, Brin MF, Fahn S. Idiopathic cervical dystonia: clinical characteristics. Mov Disord 1991;6:119–126

23. Lowenstein DH, Aminoff MJ. The clinical course of spasmodic torticollis. Neurology 1988;38:530–532

24. Greene P, Kang UJ, Fahn S. Spread of symptoms in idiopathic torsion dystonia. Mov Disord 1995;10:143–152

25. Greene P, Shale H, Fahn S. Experience with high dosages of anticholinergic and other drugs in the treatment of torsion dystonia. Adv Neurol 1988;50:547–556

26. Comella CL, Buchman AS, Tanner CM, et al. Botulinum toxin injection for spasmodic torticollis: increased magnitude of benefit with electromyographic assistance. Neurology 1992;42:878–882

27. Brashear A, Lew MF, Dykstra DD, et al. Safety and efficacy of NeuroBloc (botulinum toxin type B) in type A-responsive cervical dystonia. Neurology 1999;53:1439–1446

28. Brin MF, Lew MF, Adler CH, et al. Safety and efficacy of NeuroBloc (botulinum toxin type B) in type A-resistant cervical dystonia. Neurology 1999;53:1431–1438

29. Bertrand CM. Selective peripheral denervation for spasmodic torticollis: surgical technique, results, and observations in 260 cases. Surg Neurol 1993;40:96–103

30. Aminoff MJ, Dedo HH, Izdebski K. Clinical aspects of spasmodic dysphonia. J Neurol Neurosurg Psychiatry 1978;41:361–365

31. Dedo HH. Recurrent laryngeal nerve section for spastic dysphonia. Ann Otol Rhinol Laryngol 1976;85:451–459

32. Blitzer A, Brin MF. Laryngeal dystonia: A series with botulinum toxin therapy. Ann Otol Rhinol Laryngol 1991;100:85–89

33. Dedo HH, Townsend JJ, Izdebski K. Current evidence for the organic etiology of spastic dysphonia. Otolaryngol Head Neck Surg 1978;86:875–880

34. Bielamowicz S, Ludlow CL. Effects of botulinum toxin on pathophysiology in adductor spasmodic dysphonia. Ann Otol Rhinol Laryngol 2000;109:194–203

35. Van Pelt F, Ludlow CL, Smith PJ. Comparison of muscle activation patterns in adductor and abductor spasmodic dysphonia. Ann Otol Rhinol Laryngol 1994;103:192–200

36. Koda J, Ludlow CL. An evaluation of laryngeal muscle activation in patients with voice tremor. Otolaryngol Head Neck Surg 1992;107:684–696

37. Deleyiannis F, Gillespie M, Yamashita T, et al. Laryngeal long-latency response conditioning in abductor spasmodic dysphonia. Ann Otol Rhinol Laryngol 1999;108:612–619

38. Morrison M, Rammage L, Nichol H, et al. The management of voice disorders. San Diego, California: Singular Publishing Group, 1994

39. Roy N, Ford CN, Bless DM. Muscle tension dysphonia and spasmodic dysphonia: the role of manual laryngeal tension reduction in diagnosis and management. Ann Otol Rhinol Laryngol 1996;105:851–856

40. Fritzell B, Hammarberg B, Schiratzki H, et al. Long-term results of recurrent laryngeal nerve resection for adductor spasmodic dysphonia. J Voice 1993;7:172–178

41. Ludlow CL, Naunton RF, Sedory SE, et al. Effects of botulinum toxin injections on speech in adductor spasmodic dysphonia. Neurology 1988;38:1220–1225

42. Truong DD, Rontal M, Rolnick M, et al. Double-blind controlled study of botulinum toxin in adductor spasmodic dysphonia. Laryngoscope 1991;101:630–634

43. Blitzer A, Brin MF, Stewart CF. Botulinum toxin management of spasmodic dysphonia (laryngeal dystonia): a 12-year experience in more than 900 patients. Laryngoscope 1998;108:1435–1441

44. Ludlow CL, Naunton RF, Terada S, Anderson BJ. Successful treatment of selected cases of abductor spasmodic dysphonia using botulinum toxin injection. Otolaryngol Head Neck Surg 1991;104:849–855

45. Blitzer A, Brin M, Stewart C, et al. Abductor laryngeal dystonia: a series treated with botulinum toxin. Laryngoscope 1992;102:163–167

46. Weed DT, Jewett BS, Rainey C, et al. Long-term follow-up of recurrent laryngeal nerve avulsion for the treatment of spastic dysphonia. Ann Otol Rhinol Laryngol 1996;105:592–601

47. Berke GS, Blackwell KE, Gerratt BR, et al. Selective laryngeal adductor denervation-reinnervation: a new surgical treatment for adductor spasmodic dysphonia. Ann Otol Rhinol Laryngol 1999;108:227–231

48. Sheehy MP, Marsden CD. Writers' cramp—a focal dystonia. Brain 1982;105:461–480

49. Stojanovic M, Cvetkovic D, Kostic VS. A genetic study of idiopathic focal dystonias. J Neurol 1995;242:508–511

50. Leube B, Kessler KR, Goecke T, et al. Frequency of familial inheritance among 488 index patients with idiopathic focal dystonia and clinical variability in a large family. Mov Disord 1997;12:1000–1006

51. Schicatano EJ, Basso MA, Evinger C. Animal model explains the origins of the cranial dystonia benign essential blepharospasm. J Neurophysiol 1997;77:2842–2846

52. Panizza ME, Hallett M, Nilsson J. Reciprocal inhibition in patients with hand cramps. Neurology 1989;39:85–89

53. Lederman RJ. AAEM minimonograph #43: neuromuscular problems in the performing arts. Muscle Nerve 1994;17:569–577

54. Dawson DM, Hallett M, Wilbourn AJ, eds. Entrapment Neuropathies. 3rd ed. Philadelphia: Lippincott-Raven, 1999

55. Candia V, Elbert T, Altenmuller E, et al. Constraint-induced movement therapy for focal hand dystonia in musicians [letter]. Lancet 1999;353:42

56. Steinberger D, Topka H, Fischer D, Muller U. GCH1 mutation in a patient with adult-onset oromandibular dystonia. Neurology 1999;52:877–879

57. Cole R, Hallett M, Cohen LG. Double-blind trial of botulinum toxin for treatment of focal hand dystonia. Mov Disord 1995;10:466–471

58. Karp BI, Cole RA, Cohen LG, et al. Long-term botulinum toxin treatment of focal hand dystonia. Neurology 1994;44:70–76

59. Cole RA, Cohen LG, Hallett M. Treatment of musician's cramp with botulinum toxin. Med Prob Perform Artists 1991;6:137–143

237 Generalized Torsion Dystonia

Michele Tagliati, Kyra Blatt and Susan B Bressman

Dystonia is a movement disorder characterized by sustained, involuntary muscle contractions generating twisting and repetitive movements or abnormal postures.[1] Different muscle groups can be involved with variable extent and severity, ranging from intermittent contractions limited to single body region (focal dystonia) to generalized dystonia involving the axial and limb muscles (Table 237.1).

Oppenheim first used the term dystonia in 1911, when he described a childhood-onset syndrome that he called *dystonia musculorum deformans*.[2] Now, almost 100 years later, many different causes of dystonia are recognized. Although a detailed discussion of the numerous forms of dystonia goes beyond the scope of this chapter, characterization of the cause and clinical features of dystonia is a fundamental step before planning any treatment. Decision regarding treatment is linked to the classification of dystonia (primary or

Table 237.1   Classification of dystonia

1. By age at onset
    1.1 Early onset (<26 years): First symptoms in a leg or arm with frequent progression to involve other limbs and the trunk.
    1.2 Late onset (>26 years): First symptoms affecting the neck, cranial muscles including vocal cords or arm; tends to remain localized with restricted spread to adjacent muscles.
2. By distribution
    2.1 Focal: A single area is involved.
         Upper face (blepharospasm)
         Oromandibular
         Vocal cords (spasmodic dysphonia)
         Neck (spasmodic torticollis)
    2.2 Segmental: Two or more contiguous areas are affected.
         Cranial (face + jaw + tongue + vocal cords)
         Cranial + cervical + brachial
         Bibrachial
         Axial (neck + trunk).
    2.3 Multifocal: Two or more noncontiguous body regions are involved.
         One or both arms + one leg and
         Cranial muscle involvement (e.g. blepharospasm) + leg dystonia.
         Hemidystonia is a type of multifocal dystonia.
         Generalized: Both legs +/− trunk are involved and at least one other region.
3. By cause
    3.1 Primary: Dystonia only sign and evaluation does not reveal an identifiable exogenous cause or other inherited or degenerative disease.
         3.1.1 DYT1 or TOR1A: Early limb onset
         3.1.2 DYT6: Mixed phenotype in two Mennonite families.
         3.1.3 DYT7: Late onset cervical.
         3.1.4 DYT13: Early and adult onset cranial cervical brachial. Other loci to be identified
    3.2 Secondary:
         3.2.1 Inherited non-degenerative (Dystonia Plus)
                a. Dopa-Responsive-Dystonia (DRD): due to DYT5 and other genetic defects
                b. Myoclonus-Dystonia: due to DYT11 and possibly other genetic defects
                c. Rapid-Onset Dystonia-Parkinsonism due to DYT12.
         3.2.2 Inherited degenerative
                AD, AR, X-linked (DYT3), mitochondrial
         3.2.3 Degenerative disorders of unknown etiology
                Parkinson's disease (PD), Progressive Supranuclear Palsy (PSP), Cortico basal ganglionic degeneration (CBGD)
         3.2.4 Acquired
                Drugs (DA receptor blockers), trauma, hypoxia, infections, tumors
         3.2.5 Other movement disorders with dystonic phenomenology
                Tics, paroxysmal dyskinesias (DYT8, 9, 10)

AD, autosomal dominant; AR, autosomal recessive; DA, dopamine.

secondary), age of onset, duration, extent of muscle involvement and disability. The identification, when possible, of a specific cause of dystonia may suggest a treatment directed at the particular etiology.

Two broad etiologic categories are defined: primary, or idiopathic; and secondary, or symptomatic.[1] Abnormal postures and movements are the only neurological abnormality in primary dystonia, where no consistent pathological changes are found and diagnostic studies are unrevealing. Although it may be difficult to estimate because of the variable expression resulting in missed or under diagnosis, prevalence for generalized dystonia in Rochester, Minnesota was calculated to be 3.4 per 100 000.[3] Primary dystonia may be inherited, and several genes or gene loci have been identified.[4] Many adult onset cases, however, are sporadic, and the genetic contribution remains to be clarified. There is a bimodal distribution in the age at onset of primary dystonia with modes at ages nine (early-onset) and 45 (late-onset) years and a nadir at 27 years.[5] Early-onset dystonia usually first involves a leg or arm, and less commonly starts in the neck or vocal cords.[6,7] The majority of early-onset patients beginning with leg or arm dystonia progress to involve more than one limb and about 50% eventually generalize. Conversely, almost all patients with generalized primary dystonia have onset in childhood. Late-onset primary dystonia commonly affects the neck or cranial muscles and less frequently involves an arm at onset. Moreover, late-onset primary dystonia tends to remain localized as focal or segmental dystonia.

Usually dystonia is present continually throughout the day, whenever the affected body part is in use or, in more severe cases, at rest; it disappears with deep sleep. Remissions are rare in early-onset generalized dystonia. Complete remissions may occur in patients with cervical dystonia[8,9] and rarely a patient with generalized dystonia may have a partial remission.[10] Pain rarely occurs with dystonia in most parts of the body, with the notable exception of cervical dystonia, where 75% of patients complain of pain.[11]

Secondary forms of dystonia can result from an assortment of lesions, many involving the basal ganglia and/or dopamine synthesis, that are either inherited (e.g. dopa-responsive dystonia [DRD], Wilson's disease, gangliosidoses), or due to exogenous factors (e.g. perinatal injury, infections, neuroleptic medications). Clinical abnormalities other than dystonia (e.g. parkinsonism, dementia, ataxia, optic atrophy) are frequently present in symptomatic dystonias, imaging studies often reveal changes involving the basal ganglia and other laboratory findings usually help in diagnosis. The relationship between age-onset and signs of dystonia is somewhat different for the symptomatic dystonias. Unlike primary dystonia, symptomatic dystonia beginning in adults is more likely to generalize. Another major distinction between primary and symptomatic dystonias is that a much higher proportion of patients with symptomatic dystonia develop hemidystonia.[12]

With the cloning of the DYT1 gene[13] it is now possible to diagnose a leading cause of generalized primary dystonia. About 90% of generalized primary dystonias in Ashkenazi Jews and 50% of generalized primary dystonia in other populations are due to the same recurring mutation, a GAG deletion.[14] This mutation results in the loss of a glutamic acid in the translated protein, Torsin A.[13] Because almost all cases of primary dystonia due to DYT1 have the same mutation, screening is relatively easy and commercially available.[15] A detailed discussion of the diagnostic workup in dystonia goes beyond the purpose of this chapter. Diagnostic guidelines are summarized in Table 237.2.

Regardless of etiology, age at onset, or distribution

Table 237.2   Diagnostic evaluation of dystonia

1. Exam shows only typical dystonia (Primary Dystonia):
   1.1 Onset <26 years or older if there is a relative with early onset:
       a. DYT1 test with genetic counselling
          If negative
       b. Levodopa trial to rule out DRD
          If negative
       c. Ceruloplasmin levels, slit lamp to rule out Wilson's disease
   1.2 Onset >26 years
       a. Ceruloplasmin levels
       b. Brain MRI

2. Exam shows dystonia with other signs and/or history suggests exogenous factor (Secondary Dystonia):
   2.1 If history suggests tardive dystonia
       Ceruloplasmin levels, slit lamp to rule out Wilson's disease
   2.2 If history and exam suggest structural lesion
       Imaging studies and other appropriate laboratory studies (e.g. CSF)
   2.3 If history and exam suggest metabolic or other inherited disease
       Levodopa trial, ceruloplasmin, slit lamp, MRI and, as per diagnostic likelihood: blood smear for acanthocytes, antiphospholipid antibodies, genetic testing (HD, SCA3, mitochondrial), lysosomal analysis, alphafetoprotein, lactate/pyruvate, amino acids in serum and urine, urine organic acids, skin, muscle, nerve, bone marrow biops, CSF analysis, EMG/NCV, EEG.

DRD, dopa-responsive dystonia; MRI, magnetic resonance imaging; CSF, cerebro-spinal fluid; HD, Huntington's disease; SCA, spino-cerebellar atrophy; EMG, electromyography; NCV, nerve conduction velocities; EEG, electroencephalogram.

of the dystonic movements, relatively little is known about their pathophysiology. Neurophysiological studies show a variety of motor and sensory abnormalities that can be explained by a loss of inhibitory control at the segmental (spinal cord, brainstem) or cortical level. Convincing evidence shows that the basic disorder is most likely to be found in the supraspinal command signal.[16] Results obtained with several experimental modalities have demonstrated that patients with dystonia have less efficient cortical inhibition than normal subjects.[17] A lack of inhibition, likely mediated by a dysfunction within the basal ganglia, would lead to excessive cortical activity and abnormal movements. The role of the basal ganglia and defective dopamine neurotransmission is supported by evidence in primary and secondary dystonias. Many secondary dystonias are caused by pathological lesions in the basal ganglia.[18] Positron emission tomography (PET) and intraoperative neurophysiological studies have documented abnormalities of basal ganglia physiology in both primary and secondary forms of dystonia.[19–21] In an attempt to organize these findings, current models of basal ganglia circuitry, based primarily on the study of Parkinson's disease (PD), have been adapted to dystonia. According to these models, the discharge pattern and rate of the internal part of the globus pallidus (GPi) is the key factor associated with hypokinetic and hyperkinetic movements disorders. Increased inhibitory influence of the GPi on the thalamocortical pathway will lead to hypokinetic disorders such as PD, while decreased and irregular GPi activity will cause hyperkinetic disorders such as hemiballismus and dystonia. As we will see, many of the medical and particularly surgical therapies currently used in generalized dystonia are presumed to target this abnormal basal ganglia output.

Treatment

In a small minority of patients with symptomatic generalized dystonia specific treatment can be instituted (e.g. DRD, Wilson's disease, psychogenic dystonia). Therefore, the investigation of all children and adolescents with uncomplicated "pure" dystonia must include exclusion of Wilson's disease by measurement of serum ceruloplasmin, slit lamp examination for Kayser-Fleischer rings, and magnetic resonance imaging (MRI). The specific diagnosis and treatment of DRD will be discussed in detail in another chapter.

For the great majority of patients with dystonia, treatment is aimed at controlling symptoms rather than cause. In rare cases of "dystonic storm," prompt treatment can be life-saving.[22] Three main symptomatic treatment options can be devised: (1) physical and supportive therapy, (2) pharmacotherapy, and (3) surgical procedures.

Physical and supportive therapy

The role of patient and caregiver education and supportive care cannot be emphasized enough for a comprehensive approach to the management of patients with dystonia. In addition to the classical role of the physician and other healthcare providers, the Internet era is contributing new and powerful resources for continuing patient education and emotional support. Websites like *WeMove* (www.wemove.org) or the *Dystonia Medical Research Foundation* (www.dystonia-foundation.org) provide information services edited by medical experts, including educational tools, lists of advocacy and support organizations around the world.

Physical therapy and orthopedic devices can improve forced postures and prevent muscle contractures. As dystonia is a central problem of motor control, physical therapy programs for dystonia usually focus on enhancing the patient's ability to compensate for the abnormal muscle tone as well as trying to utilize alternative brain pathways to relieve the dystonia. Moreover, the use of orthopedic devices (bracing) may play a role in the treatment of dystonia. As many patients have "sensory tricks" (*geste antagonistique*) that can control the dystonic posture and favor a return of the body part to a more normal position, braces can be custom-made to reproduce the sensory trick. Another important function of orthopedic braces is to prevent muscle contractures, in addition to range of motion exercises to maintain limb mobility. Unfortunately, bracing can be uncomfortable, is usually bulky and is often poorly tolerated, especially by children.[23]

There is currently little published about physical therapy techniques specifically targeted to dystonia. In a small study including five musicians with focal hand dystonia (secondary to repetitive rigorous usage), Candia et al.,[24] used magnetic source imaging to show increased cortical somatosensory representation of the dystonic digits. They used constraint-induced therapy, a technique involving the immobilization by splint(s) of one or more of the digits other than the focal dystonic finger. The focal dystonic finger was then required to carry out repetitive exercises for 1.5–2.5 h daily over a period of eight consecutive days under therapist supervision. The authors demonstrated improvement in all patients at nine months with two musicians resuming concert performances.[24] Using subthreshold repetitive transcranial magnetic stimulation (rTMS), Siebner et al.,[25] reported transient handwriting improvement in patients with writer's cramp, associated with normalization of cortico-cortical inhibition. Further investigation of rTMS in larger patient groups will help clarifying the role of this type of therapy as well as other "alternative" non-pharmacological practices, including sensory feedback, muscle relaxation and meditation techniques, which may reveal to be useful additions to conventional medical and surgical therapies.

Pharmacotherapy

Pharmacotherapy can be divided into two categories, including local injections of botulinum toxin into dystonic muscles (mostly limited to the treatment of focal dystonias), and systemic administration of medications with several effects on the central nervous

Table 237.3   Treatment of dystonia

Generic name	Trade name	Daily dosage (mg)	Mechanism of action
Trihexyphenidyl	Artane	6–40	Anticholinergic
Benztropoine	Cogentin	4–15	Anticholinergic
Orphenadrine	Norflex	200–800	Anticholinergic
Cyclobenzaprine	Flexeril	20–60	Anticholinergic
Clonazepam	Klonopin	1–12	GABA Agonist
Lorazepam	Ativan	1–16	GABA Agonist
Diazepam	Valium	10–100	GABA Agonist
Chlodiazepoxide	Librium	10–100	GABA Agonist
Baclofen	Lioresal	40–120	Presynaptic GABA Agonist substance-P antagonist
Tizanidine	Zanaflex	4–32	Alpha 2 adrenergic agonist
Carbamazepine	Tegretol	1600–1600	Na$^+$ channel blocker
Levodopa/Carbidopa	Sinemet (CR)	75/300–200/2000	Dopamine precursor
Tetrabenazine	Nitoman	50–300	Monoamine depleter and blocker
Botulinum Toxin A	BOTOX	5–400 units	Ach release blockade
Botulinum Toxin B	Myobloc	250–20 000 units	Ach release blockade
Triple Combination	Tetrabenazine 75 mg/day, Pimozide 6–25 mg/day and Trihexyphenidyl 6–30 mg/day		

GABA, gamma-aminobutyric acid; Na$^+$, sodium; DBS, deep brain stimulation.
Surgical procedures: Pallidal DBS, Thalamotomy, Pallidotomy, Peripheral Denervation, Myectomy.

system (CNS) (Table 237.3). Many drugs have been reported to be of some benefit in patients with dystonia,[26,27] but no single pharmacological agent has been found to consistently produce improvement, despite a number of drug studies in fairly large series of patients.[28] These large studies and other limited series have provided enough data to draw some general conclusions.

At the present time, mostly due to our limited knowledge of the biochemical alterations in primary dystonia, pharmacological treatment of dystonia is based on empirical rather than scientific rationale. Over the next paragraphs, we will review pharmacotherapy available for the treatment of generalized dystonia and its proposed rationale. Most of the drugs currently used are effective on the principal neurotransmitters within the basal ganglia: acetylcholine, gamma-aminobutyric acid (GABA) and dopamine.

Cholinergic drugs The influence of cholinoactive substances upon motor activity has traditionally been attributed to the well-established cholinergic innervation of the striatum.[29] Clinical evidence shows that cholinergic agents tend to produce tremor, whereas anticholinergic agents are quite effective for treating the rigidity and bradykinesia of parkinsonism.[30] However, it is unclear why anticholinergics are effective in the treatment of dystonia and acute dystonic reactions due to antipsychotic drugs. The physiological effect of acetylcholine is exceedingly complex. The major effect of acetylcholine is to cause a relatively prolonged reduction of potassium conductance that makes target cortical neurons more susceptible to other excitatory inputs.[31] In the striatum, cholinergic interneurons regulate the activity of GABAergic projections to the GPi. It has been suggested that decreased levels of norepinephrine[32,33] lead to

increased cholinergic activity in the brain of patients with primary dystonia.[32] It is unknown whether large doses and a long time are required to achieve the maximum central anticholinergic effect, or whether other changes, such as adaptation of receptors or alterations of other central neurotransmitters, are necessary.[34]

- *Anticholinergics* Despite their unclear mechanism of action, anticholinergic drugs have become one of the mainstays of pharmacological treatment of dystonia. Double-blind studies[35] and other open-label trials on large numbers of patients[36,37] have supported the efficacy of these drugs. Approximately 50% of children and 40% of adults with primary dystonia report moderate to dramatic benefit from high-dose anticholinergics. Triexyphenidyl is the best-studied agent. Other compounds reported to be beneficial in dystonia include benztropine, biperiden, atropine, procyclidine, orphenadrine, scopolamine and ethopropazine.[28] The therapeutic dose can vary considerably. Customarily, the starting dose of triexyphenidyl is 1–2.5 mg/day, which can be increased weekly on a three- or four-times-a-day schedule until benefits or side effects are encountered. Doses as high as 120–180 mg/day can be attained in children, with an average of 20–40 mg/day. Adults rarely tolerate very high doses without side effects. It is not clear why high doses are often required and why it may take some weeks or months for greatest benefit to be obtained. Dose-limiting problems experienced with anticholinergic therapy can be divided into peripheral and central adverse effects. Peripheral side effects include constipation, dry mouth, urinary retention and blurred vision, which can often be avoided using peripherally acting anticholinesterase drugs (e.g. pyridostigmine) or muscarinic agonists (e.g. pilocarpine, usually in eye drops form). Central adverse effects, such as forgetfulness, confusion, restlessness, hallucinations or psychosis warrant a reduction of the anticholinergic dose, with consequent reduced effectiveness on dystonic symptoms. Central adverse effects are more common in adults than in children. This finding could explain, at least in part, the lower percentage of adults who respond compared to children. Nevertheless, the effects on intellect, memory and school performance in children should always be monitored; if memory is affected, daily dose should be reduced. Despite the very high doses of anticholinergic drugs employed in patients with dystonia, little or no long-term difficulties have been reported. Greene et al.,[38] reviewed the long-term response to anticholinergics in 227 patients with dystonia and reported that more than 50% of patients with childhood onset responded with moderate to marked improvement, and approximately 40% of adult-onset patients also responded. While factors such as severity of dystonia, gender, ethnic background, and previous thalamotomy did not correlate with therapeutic response to anticholinergics, improvement was statistically more likely if the medication was begun within five years of onset. This finding suggests that delay of treatment may result in an unfavorable response, although this point has never been systematically studied. The pharmacokinetics of trihexyphenidyl show an initial rapid distribution phase and a later, slower elimination phase. This pattern does not change between short-term and long-term treatment. Serum levels of trihexyphenidyl do not correlate with therapeutic response or toxicity.[39]

GABAergic drugs Gamma-aminobutyric acid (GABA) is an abundant and ubiquitous inhibitory neurotransmitter in the CNS. Therefore, GABAergic mechanisms can modulate the abnormal motor behavior characteristic of dystonia at several levels. Impairment of GABAergic transmission may be involved in the pathophysiology of dystonia in a genetic animal model for primary dystonia.[40]

Most of the intrinsic circuitry as well as the main output of the basal ganglia is GABAergic. Results obtained with several experimental modalities have demonstrated that patients with dystonia have less efficient cortical inhibition than normal subjects.[17] In particular, reduced intracortical paired-pulse inhibition in dystonia[41] is thought to reflect defective activation of inhibitory GABAergic interneurons. A lack of inhibition, likely mediated by a dysfunction within the basal ganglia, would lead to excessive cortical activity and abnormal movements in dystonia.

- *Benzodiazepines* Benzodiazepines act on high affinity binding sites, which are part of the benzodiazepine receptor complex. This structure also includes a GABA recognition site and a chloride membrane channel; it is thought that benzodiazepine

and GABA agonists ultimately enhance chloride ion flow, resulting in hyperpolarization and decreased cell firing. Even though they have been used in the treatment of dystonia for many years, there are no controlled studies documenting the effects of benzodiazepines, but only anecdotal reports.[42] Benzodiazepines may provide additional benefit for patients with inadequate response to anticholinergics. Clonazepam and diazepam are the compounds generally used to treat dystonia, but there is no conclusive evidence of superiority of any one benzodiazepine. Approximately 15% of 177 patients with primary dystonia responded positively to clonazepam in one study.[38] In particular, clonazepam is sometimes beneficial for Meige syndrome and myoclonic dystonia.[22,43] As with all drugs in this family, clonazepam is slowly titrated up to a tolerated maximum (10–20 mg/day) and high dosages are often employed. Dose-limiting side effects include sedation, ataxia, irritability and confusion. If benzodiazepines need to be discontinued, doses should be tapered out slowly in order to avoid withdrawal symptoms including worsening of dystonia. The same holds true for all pharmacological therapy of dystonia.

- *Baclofen* Baclofen (chemically known as 4-amino-3-(4-chlorophenol) butanoic acid) is structurally similar to the naturally occurring inhibitory neurotransmitter gamma-aminobutyric acid (GABA). Acting as a GABAb autoreceptor agonist, baclofen increases threshold for excitation of primary afferent nerves and decreases the release of excitatory amino acids from presynaptic sites in the dorsal horn of the spinal cord and thalamus. As a consequence, baclofen inhibits monosynaptic extensor and polysynaptic flexor reflexes, suppressing the effects of muscle stretching and cutaneous stimulation on the development of spasticity and dystonia. Baclofen also produces CNS depressant effects including sedation, somnolence, ataxia and respiratory and cardiovascular depression. After oral administration, baclofen is rapidly and extensively absorbed. Due to its muscle relaxant and antispastic properties, baclofen in high dosage has emerged as an important drug for the treatment of dystonia. Initially found to be beneficial in patients with blepharospasm,[44,45] baclofen was later studied in other types of dystonia.[46] Baclofen is currently one of the first oral therapeutic choices in particular for focal oromandibular dystonia and it is also used, often as an adjunct to anticholinergics, for generalized dystonia.[22,46] Moderate to marked benefit was reported by 20% of 108 adult patients with several forms of primary dystonia treated with baclofen.[46] Similar to that observed with anticholinergics, high dosages (40–120 mg/day) are needed, adult-onset focal dystonia are less likely to benefit than childhood-onset primary dystonia; patients who had dystonia for less than five years tend to have a more favorable response than those with longer-duration disease.[47] Occasionally, a very dramatic response to baclofen occurs in children with primary generalized dystonia, but it may not be sustained. At the high dose necessary in dystonia, baclofen can produce CNS adverse effects before being beneficial. This finding has promoted the use of intrathecal infusion of baclofen, a method that allows the continuous administration of minimal doses of drugs in the cerebrospinal fluid.[48] Test doses of baclofen are routinely injected into the lumbar sac before the implant. Only patients with positive baclofen tests undergo the surgical placement of a pump through which the baclofen is slowly administered in the CSF. Intrathecal baclofen infusions have been shown to be an effective therapy for spasticity[49] and dystonia.[50–52] Both primary and secondary types of dystonia may benefit from this procedure, but it is unclear if the etiology of dystonia and DYT1 status predict clinical response.[51] Intrathecal baclofen may benefit more leg and trunk involvement than arm, neck or cranial dystonia.[12] Secondary dystonia, especially when there is associated spasticity,[50] and tardive dystonia have shown impressive improvement in some reports[51,53] but the proportion of patients showing sustained improvement is not large. Only two of fourteen patients with primary or secondary dystonia showed unequivocal clinical benefit in a recent series.[51] Moreover, equipment-related complications are fairly common and potentially serious.[51,54]

Dopaminergic drugs   Dopamine is a neurotransmitter affecting brain processes that control movement, emotional response, and ability to experience pleasure and pain. The best-studied function of dopamine is its regulation of basal ganglia activity. The striatum, major input complex of the basal ganglia, receives dopaminergic input from the substantia nigra pars compacta (SNc) and projects to the internal segment of the globus pallidus (Gpi), the major output site of the basal ganglia, via the complementary activity of "direct" and "indirect" pathways.[16] There is evidence that in dystonia, in contrast to Parkinson's disease, the direct, D1 receptor mediated pathway is overactive, whereas the indirect, D2 receptor mediated pathway is underactive.[55,56] This finding may explain why both dopaminergic agonists and antagonists have been found to be potentially beneficial in patients with dystonia.

• *Dopamine agonists*   Shortly after the introduction of levodopa for Parkinson's disease, the dopamine precursor was also tried in patients with torsion dystonia. Some initial, anecdotal case reports were encouraging,[57,58] while others failed to report benefit from levodopa[59,60] or reported worsening symptoms after an initial improvement.[61] In a survey of 39 dystonic patients who had received levodopa, 5% reported lasting improvement, while 39% showed only initial short-lived benefit; symptoms were worse in another 34% of patients.[62] As discussed in another chapter, patients with dopa-responsive dystonia (DRD) obtain a dramatic

response to low-dosage levodopa or dopamine agonists.[63–66] This may explain the finding of occasional impressive responses to dopaminergic agents in reports antedating the understanding of DRD as a distinct pathological entity. Those patients with primary and other secondary forms of dystonia who respond to levodopa generally need higher doses than those used for DRD.[67,68] Only a small percentage of patients with non-DRD forms of dystonia have shown a favorable response to dopamine agonists[69,70] with approximately the same efficacy as levodopa.[71–74] Although the response to these drugs has been quite disappointing, no studies have compared the results of different dopamine agonists with those obtained with levodopa and anticholinergics. In one study, levodopa and dopamine agonists were used in patients who had failed to respond to anticholinergics.[38] Only 12% of 41 patients tested with dopamine agonist therapy had a favorable response. On the other hand, several patients who had failed previous trials of levodopa responded to anticholinergic therapy. Therefore, it seems that less patients with dystonia respond to dopaminergic therapy as compared to anticholinergics.

• *Dopamine antagonists*   While only a small fraction of patients with dystonia responds to dopaminergic drugs, a larger subset (approximately 25%) responds favorably to dopamine antagonists, including dopamine receptor blockers and dopamine storage depletors.[46,70,75,76] A common explanation to this paradox is that torsion dystonia is due to more than one pathophysiologic mechanism; therefore, patients with different types of dystonia may respond to different classes of drugs. Consistent with this hypothesis is the fact that there are no reports of patients responding to both dopamine agonists and antagonists. There is evidence that different pathways regulated by dopamine in the basal ganglia may be simultaneously over- and under active in patients with dystonia.[16,55,56] Phenothiazines, haloperidol, tetrabenazine, and pimozide have been the most frequently used dopamine antagonists in the treatment of dystonia. However, the results of studies using these compounds have been highly variable. The frequency of response to these drugs varied from 0% to 78% in generalized and segmental dystonia.[70] In an analysis of open-label trials of antidopaminergics in patients with primary dystonia, 35% of 26 patients treated with dopamine receptor blockers and 25% of 44 patients treated with dopamine depletors showed moderate to marked benefit.[38] It must be noted that most of these patients were also taking anticholinergics. The combination of a dopamine depletor (tetrabenazine), a dopamine receptor blocker (pimozide), and an anticholinergic (trihexyphenidyl) was reported to exert synergistic benefit in some patients with dystonia.[36] This classic "cocktail" was created empirically. Tetrabenazine was kept at a relatively low dose

(75–150 mg/day) in order to avoid depression. In fact, tetrabenazine depletes the brain not only of dopamine, but also of norepinephrine and serotonin, which may be involved with the pathophysiology of depression. Pimozide (or haloperidol) was added to increase dopamine antagonism, while trihexyphenidyl was included to prevent drug-induced parkinsonism and for its effect on dystonia. It is not clear whether both the dopamine receptor blocker and the dopamine depletor are necessary in combination or whether a higher dosage of either one drug would be equally effective. Tetrabenazine alone has been found helpful in the treatment of some patients with dystonia, in particular those with tardive dystonia.[23,77] However, tetrabenazine is not available in the USA and needs to be ordered by prescription in other countries including Canada and Great Britain. The atypical antipsychotic medication clozapine, a D4 dopamine receptor blocker with low affinity for D2 receptors, appears to improve tardive dystonia,[78] generalized dystonia and Meige syndrome.[79] Side effects, such as sedation and orthostatic hypotension can be treatment limiting. Moreover, the need for weekly blood-drawings to monitor for aganulocytosis is a practical limitation for the use of this drug. The role of other atypical antipsychotics in the treatment of dystonia is currently unclear.

Other pharmacological agents Initial reports documented the effectiveness of carbamazepine in dystonia,[80,81] but they could not be reproduced by subsequent studies showing only a small percentage of successful treatments.[82] In a large study of 67 patients treated with carbamazepine, only 11% obtained moderate or greater benefit.[38] Nygaard et al.,[83] reported a good initial response to carbamazepine in a few patients with DRD; however, clinical benefit was not sustained.

Alcohol is effective in patients with hereditary myoclonic dystonia[84] as well as in some cases of cervical dystonia, but it has little or no effect in patients with cranial or generalized dystonia.[85] Greene et al.,[38] reported that 7% of 14 patients treated with lithium had a favorable response, as did 4% of 25 patients treated with tricyclic antidepressants. Clonidine is not effective in patients with generalized dystonia.[38,86]

Central cannabinoid receptors are densely located in the output nuclei of the basal ganglia.[87] Moreover, there is evidence that endogenous cannabinoid transmission affects other transmitter systems within the basal ganglia by increasing GABAergic transmission, inhibiting glutamate release and affecting dopaminergic uptake.[88] If an endogenous cannabinoid tone plays a role in the mechanisms of motor control,[89,90] the central cannabinoid system may be involved in the pathophysiology of several movement disorders. There is some evidence from uncontrolled studies that cannabinoids are of therapeutic value in the treatment of several movement disorders including some forms of dystonia.[91,92] However, a recent randomized,

placebo-controlled study failed to show significant improvement of dystonia following treatment with the cannabinoid agonist Nabilone.[93]

Botulinum toxin Besides pharmacological therapy, patients with generalized dystonia may require injections of botulinum toxin to treat focal problems.[94] Botulinum toxin A is considered the treatment of choice for many focal dystonias including blepharospasm, spasmodic dysphonia and torticollis.[94–97] Recently, botulinum toxin serotype B has been approved for treatment of cervical dystonia.[98] When injected into a muscle, botulinum toxin produces transient local paralysis by preventing the release of acetylcholine and interfering with neuromuscular transmission. Interestingly, botulinum toxin may also exert central effects. A recent study showed that botulinum toxin could transiently alter the excitability of the cortical motor areas by reorganizing the inhibitory and excitatory intracortical circuits.[99] Such cortical changes probably originate through peripheral mechanisms and may explain the beneficial effects of botulinum toxin injections that outlast or lack correlation with motor weakness.

Because most patients with early-onset dystonia generally have widespread abnormalities with the involvement of many muscle groups, limited local injections are usually not useful. Moreover, extensive injections and the use of higher dosages predispose the patient to the risks of unwarranted weakness and the formation of blocking antibodies. Nevertheless, in some patients with generalized dystonia botulinum toxin injections may be used to treat a particular body region that is more severely involved or may not respond adequately to systemic medications.

Surgical therapy

Peripheral procedures Peripheral denervation procedures were extensively used prior to the advent of botulinum toxin (BTX) therapy with some positive results, mainly in the treatment of cervical dystonia. These include (1) extradural selective sectioning of posterior (dorsal) rami (posterior ramisectomy); (2) intradural sectioning of anterior cervical roots (anterior cervical rhizotomy); and (3) microvascular decompression of the spinal accessory nerve.[22] Although the first procedure[100] was considered the procedure of choice, no study has compared the different surgical approaches. Following cervical muscle denervation, pain has been described to improve more than the abnormal neck posture. In one series of 40 patients with cervical dystonia, 38% experienced a significant reduction of the neck pain or improvement in the ability to control their head, while 10% noted worsening after the surgery.[101] Other complications included local numbness, neck weakness and stiffness, and dysphagia.

Spinal cord stimulation for cervical dystonia, has been shown to be ineffective by a controlled trial,[102] while selective sensory stimulation of the accessory nerve can beneficially modify cervical dystonia in some patients.[103]

Central procedures   The better understanding of basal ganglia physiology and the unexpected finding that pallidotomy improves levodopa-induced dystonia in PD[104–106] have renewed interest in the surgical treatment of dystonia. Stereotactic surgery is generally reserved for severely affected individuals who do not respond to medication or botulinum toxin injections.

Although several surgical procedures have been employed, only two have shown some degree of success in the treatment of dystonia: thalamotomy and pallidotomy. Thalamotomy was long favored as the operation to relieve Parkinson's disease symptoms, and subsequently primary and secondary dystonia. The results of thalamotomy in dystonia have been inconsistent, with some patients showing impressive improvement and others failing to show immediate or enduring benefit.[107] Cooper[108] performed ventrolateral cryothalamotomy on 226 patients operated on between 1955–1974 and reported that 25% had a marked improvement, 45% improved moderately, 18% had no change and 12% worsened. Other surgical series present less favorable results, ranging from 25% to 50% success rate.[109,110] It is generally agreed that thalamotomy is more effective for limb compared to axial dystonia. Moreover, patients with hemidystonia requiring unilateral thalamotomy do better than patients with generalized dystonia requiring bilateral procedures. Dysarthria occurred in 11% of patients who had unilateral lesions and 56% with bilateral procedures in one study.[110] Because of the high incidence of speech abnormalities, bilateral surgery is usually avoided.

Although thalamotomy has played a major role in the treatment of generalized dystonia in the past, experience in Parkinson's disease has shown that bilateral pallidotomy may be a safer and more effective treatment of movement disorders including dystonia. There are very few data concerning pallidotomy since the development of imaging and microelectrode recording techniques that allow precise lesion localization. In the largest series of 37 patients, eight of 10 patients with bilateral primary dystonia improved, whereas five of 10 patients with bilateral secondary dystonia, six of eight patients with focal secondary dystonia, and four of seven patients with primary spasmodic torticollis also improved after pallidotomy.[111] A few more cases of successful pallidotomy have been recently reported in primary generalized dystonia,[112,113] spurring further interest in this form of treatment. Pallidotomy would exert its therapeutic effect by disrupting abnormal patterns of discharge within the GPi and thus restoring or releasing the normal function to basal ganglia circuits.[21]

The use of pallidotomy in patients with dystonia is limited by several problems. Unilateral pallidotomy may not be successful in axial disease,[21] and more data comparing unilateral and bilateral procedures are needed. Similar to thalamotomy, bilateral pallidotomy carries more risk for complications, including confusion, dysarthria, dysphagia, and limb weakness. In general, as genetic, molecular biology and neuro-

physiological research advance our understanding of the causes and pathophysiology of dystonia, there is growing concern about the use of ablative neurosurgical techniques.

Deep brain stimulation (DBS) may effectively overcome some of these problems. Deep brain stimulation was first used in the 1970s for the treatment of chronic pain, but over the last 15 years it has been progressively applied to the surgical approach of parkinsonism and other movement disorders. In fact, DBS is currently applied to the GPi and the subthalamic nucleus (STN) with significant results. There are significant theoretical advantages of DBS over neuroablative techniques. The effects of DBS are reversible and patients remain eligible for future therapies. Because the DBS lead is left in place, physicians have on-going access to the site, allowing them to adjust stimulation parameters in response to changes in the patient's illness. Deep brain stimulation also allows surgeons to intervene at targets that cannot, or should not be lesioned. In addition, DBS stimulation provides unique approach to the study of pathophysiology of basal ganglia in humans. High cost and need for maintenance of the device are the main disadvantages of DBS.

Initial reports describing the use of pallidal DBS in dystonia have been positive. Kumar et al.,[114] reported that GPi DBS in a patient with severe primary generalized dystonia resulted in immediate improvement of all aspects of dystonia. Clinical improvement was confirmed by reduced PET activation bilaterally in the primary motor, lateral premotor, supplementary motor, anterior cingulate, and prefrontal areas and ipsilaterally in the lentiform nucleus. The authors concluded that altering basal ganglia function with GPi DBS reverses the over activity of certain motor cortical areas present in dystonia. Tronnier et al.,[115] described three patients with generalized dystonia who underwent implantation of bilateral pallidal stimulation electrodes, with follow-up at 6–18 months. Two had primary dystonia, one DYT1(−) and one DYT1(+), and the third had secondary dystonia (birth asphyxia). The DYT1(−) patient experienced dramatic improvement, with Burke-Fahn Movement Scale score falling from 84 to 34.5. Score for Patient 2 (secondary dystonia) fell only from 70 to 60, although the patient reported greater subjective benefit. Score for the DYT1(+) patient fell from 77 to 55.5. The authors report that after switching off the stimulation in one patient at the one year-follow-up, it took two days for dystonic symptoms to return, suggesting possible plastic changes or reorganization of somatosensory input to the GPi neurons. Coubes et al.,[116] reported positive results of bilateral DBS of the GPi in 15 patients (mean age 14.2 years) with severe early onset generalized dystonia. Mean Burke-Fahn-Marsden Dystonia Rating Scale score was reduced from 69.5 to 11.1. Improvement was greatest for the seven DYT1(+) individuals, who improved a mean of 90.3%. Thirteen patients could walk without aids, including several that were confined to bed before surgery. Patients reported rapid and complete disappearance of pain, and medications were reduced.

In our experience, pallidal DBS is a safe and effective therapy in selected patients with medically intractable generalized dystonia. At the Beth Israel Medical Center in New York, we have recently implanted bilateral DBS leads in the GPi of six patients (four females and two males, age range 13–63) with medically intractable primary dystonia and one 18-year-old girl with dystonia secondary to ischemic encephalopathy. Four patients with primary dystonia tested positive for the DYT1 gene defect. Deep brain stimulation settings were slowly and systematically increased to achieve best clinical effect. We used large pulse width (210–400 microsec) and high frequency (130 Hz) stimulation. We observed near-complete resolution of symptoms in two patients and significant improvement in five out of six with primary dystonia. Clinical improvement was progressive and most evident 6–12 months after surgery. Secondary dystonia showed less impressive but subjectively satisfactory results. Clinically, muscle spasms and dyskinetic movements showed a more rapid improvement, while resolution of dystonic postures had a slower time course and was only partial in some cases. We observed no major complications in any of the patients.

Conclusion

Dystonia comprises a heterogeneous group of disorders, which can have a variety of etiologies. Primary childhood dystonia may be inherited and several genes or gene loci have been identified. However, inheritance patterns are not always obvious because of reduced penetrance. Most adult cases are sporadic. Numerous degenerative, acquired and toxic disorders can also cause dystonia. This heterogeneity and the fact that dystonia is a relatively rare disease, which is not commonly seen by most physicians including primary care doctors, may cause misdiagnosis, delay in proper treatment and persistent suffering. Pharmacological treatment usually provides some benefit in patients with dystonia, but no single pharmacological agent has been found to consistently produce improvement. Botulinum toxin injections have revolutionized the treatment of focal dystonias, but have limited use in the most severe forms of generalized dystonia. Pallidotomy and pallidal deep brain stimulation are showing encouraging results in selected patients with intractable dystonia. Advance in genetic research and improved understanding of the pathophysiology of dystonia are needed to provide better care for this disabling neurological condition.

References

1. Fahn S, Marsden CD, Calne DB. Classification and investigation in dystonia. In: Marsden CD, Fahn S, eds. Movement disorders 2. London: Buttersworth, 1987: 332–358
2. Oppenheim H. Uber eine eigenartige Krampfkrankheit des kindlichen und jugendlichen Alters (Dysbasia lordotica progressiva, Dystonia musculorum deformans). Neurol Centrabl 1911;30:1090–1107
3. Nutt JG, Muenter MD, Aronson A, et al. Epidemiology of focal and generalized dystonia in Rochester, Minnesota. Mov Disord 1988;3:188–194
4. Bressman SB. Dystonia. Curr Opin Neurol 1998;11: 363–372
5. Bressman SB, de Leon D, Brin MF, et al. Idiopathic torsion dystonia among Ashkenazi Jews: evidence for autosomal dominant inheritance. Ann Neurol 1989;26: 612–620
6. Bressman SB, de Leon D, Kramer PL, et al. Dystonia in Ashkenazi Jews: clinical characterization of a founder mutation. Ann Neurol 1994;35:771–777
7. Greene P, Kang UJ, Fahn S. Spread of symptoms in idiopathic torsion dystonia. Mov Disord 1995;10: 143–152
8. Jayne D, Lees AJ, Stern GM. Remission in spasmodic torticollis. J Neurol Neurosurg Psychiatry 1984;47: 1236–1237
9. Friedman A, Fahn S. Spontaneous remissions in spasmodic torticollis. Neurology 1986;36:398–400
10. Eldridge R, Ince SE, Chernow B, et al. Dystonia in 61-year-old identical twins: observations over 45 years. Ann Neurol 1984;16:356–358
11. Chan J, Brin MF, Fahn S. Idiopathic cervical dystonia: clinical characteristics. Mov Disord 1991;6:119–126
12. Bressman SB, Fahn S. Childhood dystonia. In: Watts RL, Koller WC, eds. Movement disorders: neurologic principles and practice. New York: McGraw Hill, 1997: 419–428
13. Ozelius LJ, Hewett JW, Page C, et al. The early-onset torsion dystonia gene (DYT1) encodes an ATP-binding protein. Nat Genet 1997;17:40–48
14. Bressman SB, Sabatti C, Raymond D, et al. The DYT1 phenotype and guidelines for diagnostic testing. Neurology 2000;54:1746–1752
15. Klein C, Friedman J, Bressman S, et al. Genetic testing for early-onset torsion dystonia (DYT1): introduction of a simple screening method, experiences from testing of a large patient cohort, and ethical aspects. Genet Test 1999;3:323–328
16. Hallett M. The neurophysiology of dystonia. Arch Neurol 1998;55:601–603
17. Berardelli A, Rothwell JC, Hallett M, et al. The pathophysiology of primary dystonia. Brain 1998;121: 1195–1212
18. Bhatia KP, Marsden CD. The behavioural and motor consequences of focal lesions of the basal ganglia in man. Brain 1994;117:859–876
19. Karbe H, Holthoff VA, Rudolf J, et al. Positron emission tomography demonstrates frontal cortex and basal ganglia hypometabolism in dystonia. Neurology 1992;42:1540–1544
20. Eidelberg D, Dhawan V, Takikawa S, et al. Regional metabolic covariation in idiopathic torsion dystonia: [18F]flurorodeoxyglucose PET studies. Mov Disord 1992;7:297
21. Vitek JL, Chockkan V, Zhang JY, et al. Neuronal activity in the basal ganglia in patients with generalized dystonia and hemiballismus. Ann Neurol 1999;46: 22–35
22. Jankovic J. Treatment of dystonia. In: Watts RL, Koller WC, eds. Movement disorders: neurologic principles and practice. New York: McGraw Hill, 1997:443–454
23. Jankovic J, Beach J. Long-term effects of tetrabenazine in hyperkinetic movement disorders. Neurology 1997; 48:358–362
24. Candia V, Elbert T, Altenmuller E, et al. Constraint-induced movement therapy for focal hand dystonia in musicians. The Lancet 1999; 353:42–43

25. Siebner HR, Tormos JM, Ceballos-Baumann AO, et al. Low-frequency repetitive transcranial magnetic stimulation of the motor cortex in writer's cramp. Neurology 1999;52:529–537

26. Eldridge R. The torsion dystonias: literature review and genetic and clinical studies. Neurology 1970;20:1–78

27. Goetz CG, Horn SS. Treatment of tremor and dystonia. Neurol Clin 2001;19:129–144

28. Bressman SB, Greene P. Dystonia. Curr Treat Options Neurol 2000;2:275–285

29. Mesulam MM, Mash D, Hersh L, et al. Cholinergic innervation of the human striatum, globus pallidus, subthalamic nucleus, substantia nigra and red nucleus. J Comp Neurol 1992;323:252–268

30. Penney JB, Young AB. Speculations on the functional anatomy of basal ganglia disorders. Annu Rev Neurosci 1983;6:73–94

31. McCormick DA. Cellular mechanisms of cholinergic control of neocortical and thalamic neuronal excitability. In: Steriade M, Biesold D, eds. Brain cholinergic systems. New York: Oxford University Press, 1990;236–264

32. Hornykiewicz O, Kish SJ, Becker LE, et al. Brain neurotransmitters in dystonia musculorum deformans. N Engl J Med 1986;315:347–353

33. Jankovic J, Svendsen CN, Bird ED. Brain neurotransmitters in dystonia. N Engl J Med 1987;316:278–279

34. Burke RE. The relative selectivity of anticholinergic drugs for the M1 and M2 muscarinic receptor subtypes. Mov Disord 1986;1:135–144

35. Burke RE, Brin MF, Fahn S, et al. Analysis of the clinical course of non-Jewish, autosomal dominant torsion dystonia. Mov Disord 1986;1:163–178

36. Marsden CD, Marion M-H, Quinn N. The treatment of severe dystonia in children and adults. J Neurol Neurosurg Psychiatry 1984;47:1166–1173

37. Lang AE. High dose anticholinergic therapy in adult dystonia. Canad J Neurol Sci 1986;13:42–46

38. Greene PE, Shale H, Fahn S. Analysis of open-label trials in torsion dystonia using high dosages of anticholinergics and other drugs. Mov Disord 1988;3:46–60

39. Burke RE, Fahn S. Pharmacokinetics of trihexyphenidyl after short-term and long-term administration to dystonic patients. Ann Neurol 1985;18:35–40

40. Fredow G, Loscher W. Effects of pharmacological manipulation of GABAergic neurotransmission in a new mutant hamster model of paroxysmal dystonia. Eur J Pharmacol 1991;192:207–219

41. Ridding MC, Sheean G, Rothwell JC, et al. Changes in the balance between motor cortical excitation and inhibition in focal, task specific dystonia. J Neurol Neurosurg Psychiatry 1995;59:493–498

42. Ziegler DK. Prolonged relief of dystonic movements with diazepam. Neurology 1981;31:1457–1458

43. Jankovic J, Ford J. Blepharospasm and orofacial-cervical dystonia: clinical and pharmacological findings in 100 patients. Ann Neurol 1983;13:402–411

44. Gollomp SM, Fahn S, Burke RE, et al. Therapeutic trials in Meige syndrome. Adv Neurol 1983;37:207–213

45. Fahn S, Hening WA, Bressman S, et al. Long-term usefulness of baclofen in the treatment of essential blepharospasm. Advances in Ophthalmic Plastic & Reconstructive Surgery 1985;4:219–226

46. Greene P. Baclofen in the treatment of dystonia. Clin Neuropharmacol 1992;15:276–288

47. Greene PE, Fahn S. Baclofen in the treatment of idiopathic dystonia in children. Mov Disord 1992;7:48–52

48. Narayan RK, Loubser PG, Jankovic J, et al. Intrathecal baclofen for intractable axial dystonia. Neurology 1991; 41:1141–1142

49. Penn RD, Savoy SM, Corcus D, et al. Intrathecal baclofen for severe spinal spasticity. N Eng J Med 1989;320:1517–1521

50. Ford B, Greene PE, Louis ED, et al. Intrathecal baclofen in the treatment of dystonia. Adv Neurol 1998;78: 199–210

51. Walker RH, Danisi FO, Swope DM, et al. Intrathecal baclofen for dystonia: benefits and complications during six years of experience. Mov Disord 2000;15: 1242–1247

52. Jaffe MS, Nienstedt LJ. Intrathecal baclofen for generalized dystonia: a case report. Arch Phys Med Rehabil 2001;82:853–855

53. Dressler D, Oeljeschlager RO, Ruther E. Severe tardive dystonia: treatment with continuous intrathecal baclofen administration. Mov Disord 1997;12:585–587

54. Teddy P, Jamous A, Gardner B, et al. Complications of intrathecal baclofen delivery. Br J Neurosurg 1992;6: 115–118

55. Perlmutter JS, Tempel LW, Black KJ, et al. MPTP induces dystonia and parkinsonism. Clues to the pathophysiology of dystonia. Neurology 1997;49: 1432–1438

56. Eidelberg D, Moeller JR, Antonini A, et al. Functional brain networks in DYT1 dystonia. Ann Neurol 1998;44: 303–312

57. Chase TN. Biochemical and pharmacologic studies of dystonia. Neurology 1970;20:122–130

58. Coleman M. Preliminary remarks on the L-dopa therapy of dystonia. Neurology 1970;20:114–121

59. Barrett RE, Yahr MD, Duvoisin RC. Torsion dystonia and spasmodic torticollis—results of treatment with L-dopa. Neurology 1970;20:122–130

60. Mandell S. The treatment of dystonia with L-dopa and haloperidol. Neurology 1970;20:103–106

61. Cooper IS. Levodopa-induced dystonia. Lancet 1972;2:1317–1318

62. Eldridge R, Kanter W, Koerber T. Levodopa in dystonia. Lancet 1973;2:1027–1028

63. Deonna T. DOPA-sensitive progressive dystonia of childhood with fluctuations of symptoms: Segawa's syndrome and possible variants. Neuropediatrics 1986; 17:81–85

64. Rondot P, Ziegler M. Dystonia—L-dopa responsive or juvenile parkinsonism? J Neural Transm 1983;19: 273–281

65. Allen N, Knopp W. Hereditary parkinsonism—dystonia with sustained control by L-dopa and anticholinergic medication. Adv Neurol 1976;14:201–213

66. Segawa M, Hosaka A, Miyagawa F, et al. Hereditary progressive dystonia with marked diurnal fluctuation. Adv Neurol 1976;14:215–233

67. Hunt AL, Giladi N, Bressman S, Fahn S. L-dopa treatment in idiopathic torsion dystonia. Neurology 1991;41(Suppl 1):293

68. Fletcher NA, Thompson PD, Scadding JW, Marsden CD. Successful treatment of childhood onset symptomatic dystonia with levodopa. J Neurol Neurosurg Psychiatry 1993;56:865–867

69. Lang AE. Dopamine agonists in the treatment of dystonia. Clin Neuropharmacol 1985;8:38–57

70. Lang AE. Dopamine agonists and antagonists in the treatment of idiopathic dystonia. Adv Neurol 1988;50: 561–570

71. Newman RP, LeWitt PA, Shults C, et al. Dystonia: treatment with bromocriptine. Clin Neuropharmacol 1985;8:328–333

72. Nutt JG, Hammerstad JP, Carter JH, deGarmo PL.

Lisuride treatment of focal dystonias. Neurology 1985; 35:1242–1243

73. Quinn NP, Lang AE, Sheehy MP, Marsden CD. Lisuride in dystonia. Neurology 1985;35:766–769

74. Stahl SM, Berger PA. Bromocriptine, physostigmine, and neurotransmitter mechanisms in the dystonias. Neurology 1982;32:889–892

75. Jankovic J. Treatment of hyperkinetic movement disorders with tetrabenazine: a double-blind crossover study. Ann Neurol 1982;11:41–47

76. Lang AE, Marsden CD. Alphamethylparatyrosine and tetrabenazine in movement disorders. Clin Neuropharmacol 1982;5:375–387

77. Jankovic J, Orman J. Tetrabenazine therapy of dystonia, chorea, tics, and other dyskinesias. Neurology 1988;38:391–394

78. Trugman JM, Leadbetter R, Zalis ME, et al. Treatment of severe axial tardive dystonia with clozapine: case report and hypothesis. Mov Disord 1994;9:441–446

79. Karp BI, Goldstein SR, Chen R, et al. An open trial of clozapine for dystonia. Mov Disord 1999;14:652–657

80. Geller M, Kaplan B, Christoff N. Dystonic symptoms in children: treatment with carbamazepine. JAMA 1974;229:1755–1757

81. Geller M, Kaplan B, Christoff N. Treatment of dystonic symptoms with carbamazepine. Adv Neurol 1976;14:403–410

82. Isgreen WP, Fahn S, Barrett RE, et al. Carbamazepine in torsion dystonia. Adv Neurol 1976;14:411–416

83. Nygaard TG, Marsden CD, Fahn S. Dopa-responsive dystonia: long-term treatment response and prognosis. Neurology 1991;41:174–181

84. Quinn NP, Rothwell JC, Thompson PD, Marsden CD. Hereditary myoclonic dystonia, hereditary torsion dystonia and hereditary essential mycolonus: an area of confusion. Adv Neurol 1988;50:391–401

85. Biary N, Koller W. Effect of alcohol on dystonia. Neurology 1985;35:239–240

86. Riker DK, Hurtig H, Lake CR, et al. Open trial of clonidine in dystonia musculorum deformans. Soc Neurosci Abstracts 1982;8:563

87. Pertwee RG. Pharmacology of cannabinoid CB1 and CB2 receptors. Pharmacol Ther 1997;74:129–180

88. Sullivan JM. Cellular and molecular mechanisms underlying learning and memory impairments produced by cannabinoids. Learn Mem 2000;7:132–139

89. Rodriguez de Fonseca F, Del Arco I, Martin-Calderon JL, et al. Role of the endogenous cannabinoid system in the regulation of motor activity. Neurobiol Dis 1998; 5:483–501

90. Sanudo-Pena MC, Tsou K, Walker JM. Motor actions of cannabinoids in the basal ganglia output nuclei. Life Sci 1999;65:703–713

91. Consroe P. Brain cannabinoid systems as targets for the therapy of neurological disorders. Neurobiol Dis 1998;5:534–551

92. Muller-Vahl KR, Kolbe H, Schneider U, Emrich HM. Cannabis in movement disorders. Forsch Komplementarmed 1999;6(Suppl 3):23–27

93. Fox SH, Kellett M, Moore AP, Crossman AR, Brotchie JM. Randomized, double-blind, placebo-controlled trial to assess the potential of cannabinoid receptor stimulation in the treatment of dystonia. Mov Disord 2002;17:145–149

94. Cardoso F, Jankovic P. Clinical use of botulinum neurotoxins. In: Montecucco C, ed. Clostridial neurotoxins. Berlin: Springer, 1995:123–141

95. Greene P, Kang U, Fahn S, et al. Double-blind, placebo-controlled trial of botulinum toxin injections for the treatment of spasmodic torticollis. Neurology 1990;40:1213–1218

96. Brin MF. Interventional neurology: treatment of neurological conditions with local injection of botulinum toxin. Arch Neurobiol 1991;54:173–189

97. Jankovic J, Brin MF. Therapeutic uses of botulinum toxin. N Engl J Med 1991;324:1186–1194

98. Lew MF, Brashear A, Factor S. The safety and efficacy of botulinum toxin type B in the treatment of patients with cervical dystonia: summary of three controlled clinical trials. Neurology 2000;55(12 Suppl 5):S29–S35

99. Gilio F, Curra A, Lorenzano C, et al. Effects of botulinum toxin type A on intracortical inhibition in patients with dystonia. Ann Neurol 2000;48:20–26

100. Bertrand CM, Molina-Negro P. Selective peripheral denervation in 111 cases of spasmodic torticollis: rationale and results. Adv Neurol 1988;50:637–643

101. Jankovic J, Leder S, Warner D, Schwartz K. Cervical dystonia: clinical findings and associated movement disorders. Neurology 1991;41:1088–1091

102. Goetz CG, Penn RD, Tanner CM. Efficacy of cervical cord stimulation in dystonia. Adv Neurol 1988;50: 645–649

103. Leis AA, Dimitrijevic MR, Delapasse JS, Sharkey PC. Modification of cervical dystonia by selective sensory stimulation. J Neurol Sci 1992;110:79–89

104. Laitinen LV, Bergenheim AT, Hariz MI. Ventroposterolateral pallidotomy can abolish all parkinsonian symptoms. Stereotact Funct Neurosurg 1992;58:14–21

105. Dogali M, Fazzini E, Kolodny E, et al. Stereotactic ventral pallidotomy for Parkinson's disease. Neurology 1995;45:753–761

106. Lozano AM, Lang AE, Galvez-Jimenez N, et al. Effect of GPi pallidotomy on motor function in Parkinson's disease. Lancet 1995;346:1383–1387

107. Tasker RR. Ablative procedures for dystonia. In: Germano IM, ed. Neurosurgical treatment of movement disorders. Park Ridge, IL: The American Association of Neurological Surgeons, 1998:255–266

108. Cooper IS. Twenty-year follow-up study of the neurosurgical treatment of dystonia musculorum deformans. Adv Neurol 1976;14:423–452

109. Mundinger F, Riechert T, Disselhoff J. Long term results of stereotaxic operations on extrapyramidal hyperkinesia (excluding parkinsonism). Confin Neurol 1970;32:71–78

110. Andrew J, Fowler CJ, Harrison MJG. Stereotaxic thalamotomy in 55 cases of dystonia. Brain 1983;106: 981–1000

111. Burzaco J. Stereotactic pallidotomy in extrapyramidal disorders. Appl Neurophysiol 1985;48:283–287

112. Iacono RP, Kuniyoshi SM, Lonser RR, et al. Simultaneous bilateral pallidoansotomy for idiopathic dystonia musculorum deformans. Pediatr Neurol 1996;14: 145–148

113. Lozano AM, Kumar R, Gross RE, et al. Globus pallidus internus pallidotomy for generalized dystonia. Mov Disord 1997;12:865–870

114. Kumar R, Dagher A, Hutchison WD, et al. Globus pallidus deep brain stimulation for generalized dystonia: clinical and PET investigation. Neurology 1999;53: 871–874

115. Tronnier VM, Fogel W. Pallidal stimulation for generalized dystonia. Report of three cases. J Neurosurg 2000;92:453–456

116. Coubes P, Roubertie A, Vayssiere N, et al. Early-onset generalized dystonia: neurosurgical treatment by continuous bilateral stimulation of the internal globus pallidus in 15 patients. Neurology 2000;54(Suppl 3):A220

238 Dopa-Responsive Dystonia

Michele Tagliati, Erin Elmore and Susan B Bressman

In 1976, Segawa and his colleagues provided the first detailed description of dopa-responsive dystonia (DRD), a disease characterized by the onset of progressive dystonia, initially and most severely affecting the lower limbs, often marked by diurnal variations, features of parkinsonism, hyperreflexia and a dramatic and sustained response to low-dose levodopa therapy.[1] This disorder displays genetic and phenotypic heterogeneity and is inherited as an incompletely penetrant autosomal dominant trait in the majority of cases.[2,3] Segregation analysis suggests a higher penetrance in women as compared to men although it is unclear whether the severity of the disorder differs between the sexes.[3,4] There is no known ethnic predilection with the prevalence in both England and Japan estimated at 0.5 per million.[2] and it is thought to comprise approximately 5% of all childhood dystonias not associated with an obvious etiology. The average age of onset is 6.1 years and there is a 2–3:1 female to male predominance. Although most commonly diagnosed in younger patients, DRD can occur in adult patients with the onset most resembling a form of non-progressive idiopathic Parkinson's disease (PD).

Clinical features

Typically, DRD presents in mid-childhood (5–6 years) and an infantile onset with a picture mimicking cerebral palsy has been reported.[5] In children the history is usually one of an abnormal gait with leg and foot posturing, which worsens as the day progresses. The legs may assume various sustained postures including plantar flexion, inversion, and eversion positions. The arm and trunk muscles often become involved; less commonly retrocollis or torticollis may develop.[6] Parkinsonian features include hypomimia, bradykinesia with progressive slowing and reduced dexterity of fine movements, rigidity and postural instability. Presenting signs and symptoms can be difficult to distinguish from primary torsion dystonia and juvenile PD.

In about 25% of cases, hyperreflexia occurs, particularly in the legs occasionally with associated plantar extensor signs. The presence of hyperreflexia and dystonia can lead to the erroneous diagnosis of diplegic cerebral palsy.[5] Diurnal fluctuations occur in the majority of cases with symptoms worsening through the day and dramatic improvement or complete resolution after a period of sleep. Fluctuations of symptoms have also been noted during menses and in the first month of pregnancy in older patients.

Over the years the clinical spectrum of this disorder has broadened to include focal cervical dystonia,[6] adult-onset parkinsonism,[7,8] adult-onset oromandibular dystonia,[9] spontaneously remitting dystonia,[10] developmental delay and spasticity mimicking cerebral palsy,[11] postural tremor[6] and limb dystonia that is not only diurnal but clearly related to exercise.[12]

Pathogenesis

Since its earliest description, the pathogenesis of DRD was believed to involve a defect in the dopamine synthetic pathway with evidence from genetic, biochemical, imaging and pathological studies. Over the last decade the cause for most DRD cases has been elucidated and is constituted by a number of heterozygous mutations in the GTP-cyclohydrolase I (GCHI) gene located chromosome 14 (DYT 5).[13–16] New mutations appear to be a common occurrence.[17] GCHI is the first and rate-limiting enzyme in the synthesis of tetrahydrobiopterin, which is an essential cofactor for tyrosine (but also phenylalanine and tryptophan) hydroxylase and thus dopamine synthesis.[13,14] It is now evident that some cases of DRD are due to compound heterozygous mutations in GCHI.[18] Moreover, homozygous mutations in other enzymes involved in dopamine synthesis including tyrosine hydroxylase,[19–21] and the 6-pyruvoyltetrahydropterin synthase (6-PTS)[22] can cause DRD; however, the clinical picture is often more severe in these homozygous conditions and includes signs other than dystonia (such as hypotonia, severe bradykinesia, drooling, and ptosis).

Decreased levels of tetrahydrobiopterin and homovanillic acid (a major metabolite of dopamine) in the cerebrospinal fluid were historically the first clue to a defect in dopamine synthesis.[23–25] Fluorodopa-uptake positron emission tomography (PET) scans are virtually normal indicating that the nigrostriatal pathway and dopamine storage are structurally intact.[26] On the other hand, results obtained with [^{11}C]-raclopride PET showed elevated dopamine D_2 receptor binding in the striatum of DRD patients, presumably caused by dopaminergic deficiency.[27,28] Interestingly, upregulation of D_2 binding sites has been described in both dystonic and asymptomatic DRD carriers, suggesting that the input of other compensatory mechanisms must play a role in determining the clinical expression of DRD.[27]

A detailed postmortem study found a normal number of nigral dopamine neurons with normal tyrosine hydroxylase activity. No inclusion bodies or evidence of gliosis or degeneration were described in the striatum. However, nigral dopamine cells were hypopigmented, dopamine levels were decreased in the substantia nigra and striatum, while tyrosine hydroxylase activity was reduced in the stiatum.[29]

These findings suggest limited if any degenerative changes in the setting of this biopterin deficiency state.

Diagnosis

In order to confirm the diagnosis of DRD (and to distinguish its specific genetic etiology) various imaging and biochemical tests have been investigated since genetic analysis is complex. The multiple mutations that have been discovered are spread over the six exon-containing coding regions for GTP cyclohydrolase (GTPCH). This mutational heterogeneity presents a challenge for genetic testing. Since no common mutation in GCHI has been found, sequencing of all six exons may be necessary. Even with sequencing, a proportion of cases have no, as yet, identified mutation.[13,30]

One sensitive and specific test for both affected and non-manifesting GCHI gene carriers is phenylalanine loading.[31] Biopterin is necessary for the hydroxylation of phenylalanine to tyrosine in the liver. As DRD patients have normal baseline levels of phenylalanine and tyrosine, a phenylalanine challenge results in abnormal elevations of serum phenylalanine, decreased tyrosine, and elevated phenylalanine/tyrosine ratios at one, two, and four hours post-load. Phenylalanine loading, however, does not distinguish DRD from phenylketoneuria (PKU) carriers. In this case, either measurement of biopterin (which is decreased in DRD) or repeating the challenge after giving biopterin (which corrects the defect in DRD) will define the diagnosis.

GCPCH activity can be decreased to less than 20% of normal in lymphocytes of patients with DRD, suggesting a useful assay in detecting the genetic defect.[32] In addition, it was recently suggested that measuring intracellular neopterin and biopterin (BH_4 metabolic products) concentrations and GTPCH activity in cultured skin fibroblasts could be another useful aid in diagnosing BH_4 deficiency syndromes and DRD.[33]

Among the conditions that need to be distinguished from DRD are DYT1 dystonia and juvenile parkinsonism due to homozygous or compound heterozygous parkin gene mutations.[6] Generally the occurrence of early and prominent parkinsonism and severe dyskinesias with levodopa treatment favors parkin mutations. One test that has been used to distinguish DRD from juvenile parkinsonism is fluorodopa PET, which is normal in DRD. Similarly, single-photon emission tomography using [^{123}I]β-CIT, a sensitive marker of dopamine uptake sites, is also normal in DRD.[34] Table 238.1 summarizes the principal clinical and diagnostic findings in DRD, juvenile parkinsonism and childhood-onset primary dystonia.

Treatment

Levodopa

A dramatic and sustained response of dystonic and parkinsonian symptoms to low-dosage levodopa is the hallmark feature for DRD. On rare occasions, response may be less than complete and higher doses may be needed,[6] especially for those patients with compound heterozygous mutations and adult-onset cases.[9,17]

Initial response occurs within hours to days following the start of dopaminergic therapy and maximal benefit is usually achieved within weeks to months.[1,5,35–37] Nygaard and colleagues reported that even patients who had remained untreated for years showed a dramatic response to levodopa therapy.[38] Because of the remarkable and long-lasting response, levodopa therapy is the initial recommended treatment in all pediatric cases of dystonia which lack any other clear cut etiology.

The recommended daily dose of carbidopa/levodopa 25/100 in DRD is half a tablet (50 mg of levodopa) to start, with a gradual increase over time. Some patients may show benefit with less than 100 mg of levodopa a day; higher doses can result in drug-induced dyskinesias.[39] Important drug interactions concern those patients being treated with nonselective monoamine oxidase inhibitors. Side effects of levodopa include nausea, though this is uncommon with the low dosages of combined levodopa/carbidopa employed. Additional carbidopa can be given to relieve this symptom. Confusion, constipation, urinary retention and constipation although rare, may also occur and will most likely be resolved with a dose reduction.

Levodopa-induced dyskinesias may occasionally occur,[5,6] but typical complications of long-term levodopa therapy such as disabling response fluctuations as observed in adult and juvenile PD have not been reported in DRD patients. Only five of 66 patients with presumed DRD experienced "wearing off" two to four hours after taking levodopa, while other response fluctuations such as "freezing" or "on-off" phenomenon were not reported.[5] In addition, 10 patients reported dyskinesias during the initiation of therapy that disappeared with a dose reduction and did not reappear with dose elevations. These patients were described as having more prolonged and severe disease.

Other agents

It is unclear if other agents, including anticholinergics and dopamine agonists, should be used instead or more likely in addition to levodopa. Because of the excellent and sustained response to levodopa, few other agents have been systematically studied. It is known that anticholinergics can also be very effective in DRD and indeed occult cases of DRD have been diagnosed after a dramatic response to low-dose triexyphenidyl.[18] Carbamazepine is another agent reported to be effective in DRD,[5] but this effect was not maintained over time. Finally, in our experience dopaminergic agonists can provide further benefit as add-on therapy when signs of disease re-emerge after several years of successful levodopa treatment (Bressman, unpublished observation).

Table 238.1   Differential diagnosis of dopa-responsive dystonia (DRD)

	DRD	Childhood-onset primary dystonia	Juvenile parkinsonism
Average age of onset	Early childhood (range infancy to 50s)	Late childhood (range 4–44)	Adolescence (range 7–58)
Gender	Female > Male	Male = Female	Male > Female
Initial signs	Leg dystonia Stiffed-leg gait	Limb dystonia Rarely neck or voice	Foot dystonia Parkinsonism
Diurnal fluctuations	Frequent	Rare	Rare
Bradykinesia	Yes	No	Yes
Postural instability	Yes	No	Yes
Response to L-dopa Initial Long-term	Excellent at low dose Stable	None or slight	Good at moderate dose Fluctuations with dyskinesias
CSF studies HVA biopterin neopterin	⇓ ⇓⇓ ⇓⇓	= = =	⇓ ⇓ ⇓
Functional imaging F-dopa PET	Normal	Normal	Decreased
Inheritance	AD (reduced penetrance)	AD (reduced penetrance)	AR
Gene	Heterozygous GTPCH mutation in most patients	Heterozygous DYT1 GAG deletion in many patients	Homozygous or compound heterozygous *Parkin* mutation in most patients
Genetic testing	Research only	Commercial	Research only
Prognosis	Excellent with therapy	Progressive at first then stabilizes	Moderate progression despite therapy

Adapted from Bressman and Fahn, 1997.[40] HVA, homovanillic acid; AD, autosomal dominant; AR, autosomal recessive.

References

1. Segawa M, Hosaka A, Miyagawa F, et al. Hereditary progressive dystonia with marked diurnal fluctuation. Adv Neurol 1976;14:215–233
2. Nygaard TG, Wilhelmsen KC, Risch NJ, et al. Linkage mapping of dopa-responsive dystonia (DRD) to chromosome 14q. Nature Genetics 1993a;5:386–391
3. Nygaard TG. An analysis of North American families with dopa-responsive dystonia. In: Segawa, ed. Hereditary progressive dystonia with marked diurnal fluctuation. Carnforth: Parthenon Publishing, 1993b:97–104
4. Louis E, Lynch T, Bressman SB, et al. Gender differences in dopa-responsive dystonia. Neurology 1994;44:A368–A369
5. Nygaard TG, Marsden CD, Fahn S. Dopa-responsive dystonia: long-term treatment response and prognosis. Neurology 1991;41:174–181
6. Tassin J, Durr A, Bonnet AM, et al. Levodopa-responsive dystonia. GTP cyclohydrolase I or parkin mutations? Brain 2000;123:1112–1121
7. Nygaard TG, Takahashi H, Heiman GA, et al. Long-term treatment response and fluorodopa positron emission tomographic scanning of parkinsonism in a family with dopa-responsive dystonia. Ann Neurol 1992;32:603–608
8. Harwood G, Hierons R, Fletcher NA, Marsden CD. Lessons from a remarkable family with dopa-responsive dystonia. J Neurol Neurosurg Psychiatry 1994;57:460–463
9. Steinberger D, Topka H, Fischer D, Muller U. GCH1 mutation in a patient with adult-onset oromandibular dystonia. Neurology 1999;52:877–879
10. Di Capua M, Bertini E. Remission in dihydroxyphenylalanine-responsive dystonia. Mov Disord 1995;10:223
11. Nygaard TG, Waran SP, Levine RA, et al. Dopa-responsive dystonia simulating cerebral palsy. Pediatr Neurol 1994;11:236–240
12. Deonna T, Roulet E, Ghika J, Zesiger P. Dopa-responsive childhood dystonia: a forme fruste with writer's cramp, triggered by exercise. Dev Med Child Neurol 1997;39:49–53
13. Ichinose H, Ohye T, Takahashi E, et al. Hereditary progressive dystonia with marked diurnal fluctuations caused by mutations in the GTP-cyclohydrolase 1 gene. Nature Genetics 1994;8:236–242
14. Furukawa Y, Shimadzu M, Rajput AH, et al. GTP-cyclohydrolase I gene mutations in hereditary progressive and dopa-responsive dystonia. Ann Neurol 1996;39:609–617
15. Ichinose H, Suzuki T, Inagaki H, et al. Molecular genetics of dopa-responsive dystonia. Biol Chem 1999;380:1355–1364
16. Ichinose H, Inagaki H, Suzuki T, et al. Molecular

mechanisms of hereditary progressive dystonia with marked diurnal fluctuation, Segawa's disease. Brain Dev 2000;22(Suppl 1):S107–S110

17. Furukawa Y, Kish SJ, Bebin EM, et al. Dystonia with motor delay in compound heterozygotes for GTP-cyclohydrolase I gene mutations. Ann Neurol 1998;44:10–16

18. Jarman PR, Bandmann O, Marsden CD, Wood NW. GTP-cyclohydrolase I mutations in patients with dystonia responsive to anticholinergic drugs. J Neurol Neurosurg Psychiatry 1997;63:304–308

19. Knappskog PM, Flatmark T, Mallet J, et al. Recessively inherited L-dopa-responsive dystonia caused by a point mutation (Q381K) in the tyrosine hydroxylase gene. Hum Mol Genet 1995;4:1209–1212

20. Lüdecke B, Dworniczak B, Bartholome K. A point mutation in the tyrosine hydroxylase gene associated with Segawa's syndrome. Hum Genet 1995;95:123–125

21. van den Heuvel LP, Luiten B, Smeitink JA, et al. A common point mutation in the tyrosine hydroxylase gene in autosomal recessive L-dopa-responsive dystonia in the Dutch population. Hum Genet 1998;102:644–646

22. Hanihara T, Inoue K, Kawanishi C, et al. 6-Pyruvoyl-tetrahydropterin synthase deficiency with generalized dystonia and diurnal fluctuation of symptoms: a clinical and molecular study. Mov Disord 1997;12:408–411

23. Williams A, Eldridge R, Levine R, et al. Low CSF hydroxylase cofactor (tetrahydrobiopterin) levels in inherited dystonia. Lancet 1979;2:410–411

24. LeWitt PA, Miller LP, Levine RA, et al. Tetrahydrobiopterin in dystonia: identification of abnormal metabolism and therapeutic trials. Neurology 1986;36:760–764

25. Furukawa Y, Nishi K, Kondo T, et al. CSF biopterin levels and clinical features of patients with juvenile parkinsonism. Adv Neurol 1993;60:562–567

26. Snow BJ, Nygaard TG, Takahashi H, Calne DB. Positron emission tomographic studies of dopa-responsive dystonia and early-onset idiopathic parkinsonism. Ann Neurol 1993;34:733–738

27. Kishore A, Nygaard TG, de la Fuente-Fernandez R, et al. Striatal D2 receptors in symptomatic and asymptomatic carriers of dopa-responsive dystonia measured with [11C]-raclopride and positron-emission tomography. Neurology 1998;50:1028–1032

28. Kunig G, Leenders KL, Antonini A, et al. D2 receptor binding in dopa-responsive dystonia. Ann Neurol 1998;44:758–762

29. Rajput AH, Gibb WRG, Zhong XH, et al. Dopa-responsive dystonia: pathologic and biochemical observations in a case. Ann Neurol 1994;35:396–462

30. Bandmann O, Nygaard TG, Surtees R, et al. Dopa-responsive dystonia in British patients: new mutations of the GTP-cyclohydrolase I gene and evidence for genetic heterogeneity. Hum Mol Genet 1996;5:403–406

31. Hyland K, Fryburg JS, Wilson WG, et al. Oral phenylalanine loading in dopa-responsive dystonia: a possible diagnostic test. Neurology 1997;48:1290–1297

32. Nagatsu T, Ichinose H. GTP-cyclohydrolase I gene, dystonia, juvenile parkinsonism, and Parkinson's disease. J Neural Transm Suppl 1997;49:203–209

33. Bonafe L, Thony B, Leimbacher W, et al. Diagnosis of dopa-responsive dystonia and other tetrahydrobiopterin disorders by the study of biopterin metabolism in fibroblasts. Clin Chem 2001;47:477–485

34. Naumann M, Pirker W, Reiners K, et al. [123I]beta-CIT single-photon emission tomography in dopa-responsive dystonia. Mov Disord 1997;12:448–451

35. Deonna T. Dopa-sensitive progressive dystonia of childhood with fluctuations of symptoms: Segawa's syndrome and possible variants. Neuropediatrics 1986;17:81–85

36. Rondot P, Ziegler M. Dystonia-L-dopa responsive or juvenile parkinsonism? J Neural Transm 1983;(Suppl 19):273–281

37. Allen N, Knopp W. Hereditary parkinsonism-dystonia with sustained control by L-dopa and anticholinergic medication. Adv Neurol 1976;14:201–213

38. Nygaard TG, Marsden CD, Duvoisin RC. Dopa-responsive dystonia. Adv Neurol 1988;50:377–384

39. Bressman SB, Greene PE. Dystonia. Curr Treat Options Neurol 2000;2:275–285

40. Bressman SB, Fahn S. Childhood dystonia. In: Watts RI, Koller WC eds. Movement Disorders: neurologic principles and practice. New York: McGraw Hill, 1997:419–428

239 Huntington's Disease

Joseph Jankovic and Tetsuo Ashizawa

In 1872 George Huntington, at the age of 22 and only one year after graduating from Columbia College of Physicians and Surgeons, published his assay "On Chorea" in the Philadelphia journal "The Medical and Surgical Reporter".[1] Although he wrongly assumed that the disease existed exclusively on the east end of Long Island where he practiced with his father, he is appropriately credited for drawing attention to this heredodegenerative disorder and for describing the cardinal features of the disease: inherited, progressive, and manifested by chorea, cognitive impairment and depression. Since there are many other manifestations of the disease and chorea may not even be present, the term "Huntington's disease" (HD) rather than "Huntington's chorea" seems more appropriate.[2,3] Although chorea (known as "the dancing mania") has been recognized since the middle ages, the origin of the affected families described by Huntington, was traced to the early 17th century in the village of Bures in South-East England. The inhabitants of this area later migrated to various parts of the world accounting for the marked variation in the regional prevalence of HD. While the estimated prevalence of HD in the US is 2–10 per 100 000 people, in certain regions of the world the prevalence is as high as 52 (Lake Maracaibo, Venezuela) and 560 (Moray Firth, Scotland) per 100 000.[4]

Clinical aspects

In a study involving 1901 patients with HD, the following were considered the most frequent presenting symptoms in descending order: chorea, trouble walking, unsteadiness, irritability, depression, clumsiness, speech difficulty, memory loss, dropping of objects, lack of motivation, paranoia, intellectual decline, sleep disturbance, hallucination, weight loss and sexual problems.[5] Besides chorea, other motor symptoms typically affecting patients with HD include dysarthria, dysphagia, aerophagia, postural instability, ataxia, dystonia, bruxism, myoclonus, and tics.[6–8] Impairment of fine motor movements and of rapid eye saccades has been found to be among the earliest manifestation of the disease.

In addition to chorea, the other two components of the HD triad include cognitive decline and various psychiatric symptoms.[9] While some studies showed that cognitive deficits correlated with the number of CAG repeats in asymptomatic carriers of the HD gene,[10] other studies found no correlation between cognitive decline and CAG repeats in symptomatic patients with HD.[11] The neurobehavioral symptoms typically consist of personality changes, agitation, irritability, anxiety, apathy, social withdrawal, impul-siveness, depression, mania, paranoia, delusions, hostility, hallucinations, psychosis, and various sexual disorders. In a study of 52 patients with HD, Paulsen et al.,[12] found the following neuropsychiatric symptoms in descending order of frequency: dysphoria, agitation, irritability, apathy, anxiety, disinhibition, euphoria, delusions, and hallucinations.[12] Behaviors such as agitation, anxiety and irritability have been related to hyperactivity of the medial and orbitofrontal cortical circuitry.[13]

Cognitive changes, manifested chiefly by loss of recent memory, poor judgment, impaired concentration and acquisition, occur in nearly all patients with HD; but some patients with late-onset chorea never develop dementia.[14] In one study, dementia was found in 66% of 35 HD patients.[15] Tasks requiring psychomotor or visuospatial processing, such as skills required by the Trail Making B and Stroop Interference Test, are impaired early in the course of the disease and deteriorate at a more rapid rate than memory impairment.[16] Although neurobehavioral symptoms may precede motor disturbances in some cases, de Boo et al., showed that motor symptoms are more evident than cognitive symptoms in early stages of HD.[17] Most studies have found that neuropsychological tests do not differentiate between presymptomatic persons who are positive for the HD gene from those who are negative,[17] but some studies have found that cognitive changes may be the first symptoms of HD.[18] In a longitudinal study by the Huntington Study Group of 260 persons considered "at risk" for HD, Paulsen et al., found that this group had worse scores on the cognitive section of the Unified Huntington's Disease Rating Scale (UHDRS) at baseline, an average two years before the development of motor manifestations of the disease.[9] High suicidal ideation has been found in HD gene carriers as compared to non-carriers.[19] In another study of 171 presymptomatic gene carriers compared to 414 non-gene carriers, Kirkwood et al. found that the carriers performed significantly worse on the digit symbol, picture arrangement and arithmetic subscales of the revised Wechsler Adult Intelligence Scale (WAIS-R) and various movement and choice time measures.[20] An adjustment to the results of testing appears to depend more on psychological make-up of the individual before the testing than on the testing itself.[21] Nevertheless, because of ethical and legal implications for positive identification of a gene carrier, predictive testing should be performed by a team of clinicians and geneticists who are not only knowledgeable about the disease and the genetic techniques, but who are also sensitive to the psychosocial and ethical issues associated with such testing.

About 10% of HD cases have their onset before age 20, but the typical peak age at onset is in the fourth and fifth decade. Young-onset patients usually inherit the disease from their father while older-onset patients are more likely to inherit the gene from their mother. Juvenile HD (onset of symptoms before 20 years) typically presents with the combination of progressive parkinsonism, dementia, ataxia, and seizures. In contrast, adult HD usually presents with the insidious onset of clumsiness and adventitious movements which may be wrongly attributed to simple nervousness. Bradykinesia is usually evident in patients with the rigid form of HD, but when it co-exists with chorea it may not be fully appreciated on a routine examination.[22] Bradykinesia in HD may be an expression of "post-synaptic parkinsonism" and it may explain why a reduction in chorea with anti-dopaminergic drugs rarely improves overall motor functioning and indeed may cause an exacerbation of the motor impairment.[23,24]

In addition to motor, cognitive and behavioral abnormalities, most patients with HD lose weight during the course of their disease despite increased appetite. The pathogenesis of weight loss in HD is unknown, but one study showed that patients with HD have a 14% higher sedentary energy expenditure than controls and that this appears to be correlated with the severity of the movement disorder.[25]

Because of the rich clinical expression of HD, the severity of the disease and its impact on daily functioning is difficult to measure and express in quantitative terms. This is important not only in following patients as they progress through the natural course of the disease but also in assessing their response to therapeutic interventions. The UHDRS, developed by The Huntington Study Group, has been used to assess various clinical features of HD, specifically motor function, cognitive function, behavioral abnormalities, and functional capacity.[26,27] In addition, an assessment protocol has been developed to evaluate various neurological and behavioral features in HD patients undergoing striatal grafting.[28] Reilman et al., showed that variability in isometric grip forces while grasping an object correlates well with UHDRS and progressive motor deficits associated with HD.[29]

The natural course of HD varies, but on average the duration of illness from onset to death is about 15 years for adult HD; it is about 4–5 years shorter for the juvenile variant. Patients with juvenile onset (<20 years) and with late onset (>50 years) of symptoms have the shortest duration of the disease.[5] Progressive motor dysfunction, dementia, dysphagia, and incontinence not only impact adversarially on the quality of life, but eventually lead to institutionalization and death from aspiration, infection, and poor nutrition.[30]

Genetics

Huntington's disease is regarded as truly an autosomal dominant disease in that homozygotes do not appear to differ clinically from typical heterozygotes. Localization of a gene marker near the tip of the short arm of chromosome 4 in 1983 initiated an intensive search for the abnormal gene, which was finally cloned 10 years later.[31] Mutation responsible for the disease consists of an unstable expansion of the CAG repeat sequence in the 5' end of a large (210 kb) gene, IT15. This gene, located at 4p16.3, contains 67 exons and encodes a 348 kilodalton protein, called "huntingtin". The expanded CAG repeat, located in exon 1, alters huntingtin by elongating a polyglutamine segment near its NH_2-terminus. Huntingtin is associated with vesicle membranes and microtubules and as such probably has a role in endocytosis, intracellular trafficking and membrane recycling. N-terminal mutant huntingtin binds to synaptic vesicles and inhibits their glutamate uptake in vitro.[32] Analyzing DNA for the expansion of respective trinucleotide repeats utilizing polymerase chain reaction (PCR) and Southern blotting has provided means for a reliable diagnostic test. Such a test is helpful not only in confirming the diagnosis in index cases, but also in clarifying the diagnosis in atypical cases and in asymptomatic at-risk individuals.

Whereas the number of repeats varies between 10 and 29 copies in unaffected individuals, the HD gene contains more than 36 such repeats. The intermediate-sized CAG repeats range from 27 to 35. Although these individuals are usually asymptomatic this CAG repeat may spontaneously expand in successive generations resulting in so-called "sporadic" HD. Several studies have demonstrated that the number of repeats inversely correlates with the age at onset ("anticipation").[33–35] The Huntington Study Group is currently conducting The Pilot Huntington At Risk Observational Study (PHAROS) to prospectively characterize the transition from health to illness ("phenoconversion"). Although some studies suggest possible correlation between the length of CAG repeats and the rate of progression,[36] other studies have found no correlation between the CAG repeats and the progression or the age at onset and the progression of disease.[37–40] The rate of disease progression is generally faster in paternally transmitted HD independent of the CAG repeat length. The trinucleotide repeat is relatively stable over time in lymphocyte DNA, but is unstable in sperm DNA. This appears to account for the marked increase in the number of trinucleotide repeats to offspring by affected fathers, leading to a 10:1 ratio of juvenile HD with the affected parent being the father.

Because of the poor correlation between the number of CAG repeats and the rate of progression some investigators have argued that the number of CAG repeats should not be disclosed to the patient or even to the physician. We, however, believe that the following guidelines are appropriate and prudent: (1) the CAG repeat size should be disclosed to appropriately informed physicians and counselors who take care of the patient, (2) an appropriate training should be provided to inform physicians and counselors about the implications of the CAG repeat size in HD, and (3) information regarding the CAG repeat size should be disclosed to patients upon the patient's request, given that appropriate counseling is made available to the patient.[2]

Neuroimaging

Except for striatal atrophy, particularly involving the putamen, magnetic resonance imaging (MRI) is unremarkable.[41] This suggests that the putamen is underdeveloped in HD or that it is one of the earliest structures to atrophy. Striatal volume loss correlates with length CAG repeats.[41] Several MRI volumetric and single photon emission computed tomography (SPECT) blood flow studies have shown that basal ganglia volume and blood flow are reduced even before individuals become symptomatic with HD.[42] In addition to striatal atrophy shown by neuroimaging studies, a variety of techniques, such as positron emission tomography (PET) scans of ^{18}F-2-fluoro-2-deoxyglucose uptake and SPECT, have been used to demonstrate hypometabolism and reduced regional cerebral blood flow in the basal ganglia and the cortex.[42] Abnormalities in striatal metabolism measured by PET scans may precede caudate atrophy.[43] Regional cerebral metabolic rate of glucose consumption has been found to be decreased by 62% in the caudate, 56% in the lenticular nucleus and by 17% in the frontal cortex.[44] Bilateral reduction in the uptake of technetium-99m HM-PAO (hexamethyl-propylene-amine-oxime) and iodine-123 IMP (inosine 5'-monophosphate) in the caudate and putamen has been demonstrated by SPECT in patients with HD.[45] Using PET and [11C]Flumazenil binding to gamma amino butyric acid (GABA) receptors in the striatum, Künig et al., found marked reduction in the caudate (but not in the putamen) of HD patients as compared to normal controls.[46] The authors interpreted these findings as indicative of compensatory GABA receptor upregulation in the striatal (putamen) GABAergic medium spiny neurons projecting to the pallidum. None of the imaging studies, however, including PET scans are sensitive enough to reliably detect evidence of disease in truly pre-symptomatic persons.

Neuropathology and neurochemistry

Postmortem changes in HD brains include neuronal loss and gliosis in the cortex and the striatum, particularly in the caudate nucleus. Morphometric analysis of the prefrontal cortex in HD patients reveals loss of cortical pyramidal cells, particularly in layers III, V, and VI.[47] Chorea seems to be related to the loss of medium spiny striatal neurons projecting to the lateral pallidum (GPe), whereas rigid-akinetic symptoms correlate with the additional loss of striatal neurons projecting to the substantia nigra compacta (SNc) and medial pallidum (GPi).[48] Pathological studies have suggested that the earliest changes associated with HD consist of degeneration of the striato-substantia nigra zona reticulata (SNr) neurons followed by striato-GPe and striato-SNr neurons, and finally striato-GPi neurons. There appears to be a correlation between the number of CAG repeats and the severity of pathology; longer trinucleotide repeat length is associated with greater neuronal loss in the

caudate and putamen.[49] Increased density of oligondendrogliocytes and intranuclear inclusions were found in the tail of the caudate nucleus among presymptomatic HD gene carriers, suggesting that pathological changes occur long before the onset of symptoms.[50]

Huntingtin, the product of the HD gene, is expressed throughout the brain in both affected and unaffected regions and, therefore, its contribution to neurodegeneration in HD is unclear. Since the mutated huntingtin is not limited to vulnerable neurons, other factors besides mutated huntingtin must play a role in the neuronal degeneration associated with HD.[51] An immunohistochemical study showed that neuronal staining for huntingtin is reduced in the striatal medium-sized spiny neurons, but the large striatal neurons that are spared in HD retain normal levels of huntingtin.[52] Surprisingly, however, huntingtin staining was markedly reduced in both segments of the globus pallidus. This suggests a postsynaptic response to a reduction in striatal inputs; or it may indicate that the globus pallidus is for some as yet unknown reason preferentially involved in HD.

The finding of neuronal intranuclear inclusions (NII) and dystrophic neurites in the two regions that are most affected in HD, the cortex and striatum, has revolutionized our understanding of the genetic-pathological mechanisms of this heredodegenerative disorder.[53] Using an antiserum against the NH₂-terminal of huntingtin, DiFiglia et al.,[53] found intense labeling localized to neuronal intranuclear inclusions in the brains of three juvenile and six adult cases of HD. These inclusions had an average diameter of 7.1 μ and were almost twice as large as the nucleolus. The neurons with these inclusions were found in all cortical layers and the medium-sized neurons of the striatum, but not in the globus pallidus or the cerebellum. They were more frequent in the juvenile HD and in these cases the inclusions were found not only in the nuclei, but also in the cytoplasm. These inclusions are composed of granules, straight and tortuous filaments and fibrils and they are not membrane bound. Since the aggregates in the nucleus consist mostly of N-terminal fragments of the whole huntingtin protein, it has been postulated that the protein has to be cleaved before it enters the nucleus. Mutant huntingtin fragments accumulate in axon terminals and interfere with glutamate uptake.[54,55]

While some studies have shown a moderate (40%) degree of neuronal degeneration in the substantia nigra, particularly noticeable in the medial and lateral thirds,[56] this is probably not sufficient to cause bradykinesia either in the choreic or the rigid-akinetic HD patients.[57] Measurements of brain dopamine concentrations and cerebrospinal fluid (CSF) homovanillic acid (HVA) levels have yielded conflicting results. In one study, CSF HVA was normal in 51 patients with early HD and there was no correlation between HVA levels and the degree of parkinsonism.[58] Dopamine, acetylcholine, and serotonin receptors are decreased in the striatum. Using PET imaging of dihydrotetrabenazine as a marker of striatal vesicular monoamine transporter type-2 (VMAT2), Bohnen found reduced binding particularly in the posterior putamen, similar to Parkinson's disease (PD), particularly in patients with akinetic-rigid HD.[59]

Postsynaptic loss of dopamine receptors may be responsible for the parkinsonian findings in some HD patients.[22] Using PET to measure binding of specific D_1 and D_2 receptor ligands in the striatum, several studies found that these two receptors are markedly decreased in individuals who have the HD mutation, but are still presymptomatic.[60,61] Loss of the medium-sized spiny neurons, which normally constitute 80% of all striatal neurons, is associated with a marked decrease in GABA and enkephalin levels. In contrast, the cholinergic and somatostatin striatal interneurons seem to be relatively spared in HD. Other neuropeptide alterations in HD include a decrease in substance-P, cholecystokinin, and met-enkephalin and an increase in somatostatin, thyrotropin-releasing hormone, neurotensin and neuropeptide Y.

Pathogenesis

The finding that N-methyl-D-aspartate (NMDA) receptors are markedly reduced in the putamen and cerebral cortex was the first clue that suggested an NMDA mediated excitotoxicity as a mechanism of neuronal degeneration in HD.[62] In support of the excitotoxic theory is the observation that certain excitatory neurotoxins produce useful animal models of HD. Intrastriatal injections of quinolinic acid preferentially damage the medium-sized spiny neurons containing calbindin Dk28, enkephalin, and substance P, the very same neurons that degenerate in HD.[63]

Another postulated mechanisms of cell death in HD is that a defect in mitochondrial energy metabolism makes certain neurons more vulnerable to the excitotoxic effects of endogenous glutamate. Defects in mitochondrial oxidative phosphorylation have been postulated to decrease cellular adenosine triphosphate (ATP) production resulting in a concomitant decrease in sodium-potassium ATPase activity and partial membrane depolarization. Under normal circumstances the NMDA receptor-associated channels are blocked by a voltage-dependent Mg^{2+} system that pumps Mg^{2+} out of the cell. As a result of decreased ATPase activity, caused by the inhibition of oxidative phosphorylation, the normal resting potential cannot be maintained resulting in the opening of the channel and influx of calcium. This triggers a cascade of events leading to a production of free radicals and associated oxidative damage to various cellular elements. Thus, as a result of inhibition of oxidative phosphorylation, even low levels of excitatory amino acids become toxic, a process referred to as "slow excitotoxicity". Intrastriatal injections of inhibitors of oxidative phosphorylation, such as aminooxyacetic acid or 1-methyl-y-phenylpyridium (MPP$^+$), or a systemic administration of 3-nitropropionic acid (3-NP), a mitochondrial poison, into animals produce a syndrome with striking resemblance to HD.[64,65] Severe defects have been demonstrated in the

activities particularly of complexes II and III in the caudate nuclei of HD patients.[62] Dichloroacetate, which stimulates pyruvate dehydrogenase complex, has been found to increase survival and improve motor function and prevent striatal atrophy in R6/2 and N171–82Q transgenic mouse models of HD.[66] The mutant huntingtin may contribute to the apoptotic cell death in HD via caspase activation through mitochondrial cytochrome c release.[67,68]

The obvious question still to be answered is how the mutation in the HD gene leads to selective damage of certain neuronal populations. The huntingtin mutation could cause a loss of function or a gain of function of huntingtin. A loss of physiological function of the mutant huntingtin would result in haploinsufficiency because HD is an autosomal dominant disorder and heterozygous HD patients should express normal huntingtin from the normal gene. For most proteins, cells can function normally if there is 50% of the normal amount, and this is true for huntingtin. Patients with the Wolf-Hirschhorn deletion syndrome, in which a chromosome 4p region containing the entire HD gene is deleted, do not show signs of HD.[69] To study the effect of loss of function, huntingtin deficiency was created in mice by inactivating the Hdh gene, the mouse ortholog of the human HD gene (knockout mice).[70] Mice homozygous for the knockout gene showed embryonic lethality; however, heterozygous mice were normal without signs of HD phenotype. These data suggest that a loss of normal function of huntingtin is not sufficient to cause HD. Thus, gain-of-function mechanisms have become the central hypothesis of HD pathogenesis. Then, the next question is what function the mutant huntingtin gains.

Huntingtin is cleaved in vitro by caspase 3, which is a pro-apoptotic cysteine protease also known as apopain, and the cleavage is more efficient when the polyglutamine tract is expanded.[67] The products of this cleavage include a truncated N-terminal fragment that contains the polyglutamine tract. Experiments in cell culture models showed that the N-terminal fragment preferentially enters the nucleus and increases caspase-1 transcription, which leads to caspase-3 activation, cytochrome c release, disruption of mitochondrial membrane potential, and subsequent apoptosis.[54,68] Transgenic mice that express an N-terminal fragment of human mutant huntingtin developed progressive neurological abnormalities resembling features of HD, including choreiform-like movements, involuntary stereotypic movements, tremor, epileptic seizures, and weight loss.[71] These mice developed pronounced neuronal intranuclear inclusions, containing huntingtin N-terminus and ubiquitin, prior to the development of the neurological phenotype. In human HD brains, the N-terminal fragment of mutant huntingtin was also localized to neuronal intranuclear inclusions and dystrophic neurites in the cortex and striatum, and polyglutamine length showed a positive correlation with the extent of huntingtin accumulation in these structures.[53] As in the transgenic mice, ubiquitin was found in the neuronal intranuclear inclusions and dendritic neurites, which suggest that abnormal huntingtin is targeted for proteolysis but is resistant to removal. Electron micrographs of these aggregates revealed a fibrillar or ribbon-like morphology, reminiscent of scrapie prions and beta-amyloid fibrils in Alzheimer's disease.

Although multiple processes have been postulated to relate CAG expansion to neurodegeneration there is a growing body of evidence to suggest that the expansion leads to protein aggregation.[32,55,72] Aggregation is proportional to polyglutamine repeat length and no aggregation can be induced in experimental models for repeat lengths of 27 or fewer glutamines. This may in part explain the inverse correlation of repeat length and age at onset. Various transgenic murine models of HD have been developed, but the R6/2 transgenic mouse line has been studied most extensively.[73,74] These mice develop normally until 5–7 weeks of age when they start manifesting irregular gait, abrupt shuddering movements, resting tremors, followed by epileptic seizures, muscle wasting and premature death at 14–16 weeks. Striatal neurons show ubiquinated neuronal inclusions, similar to human HD. Analysis of glutamate receptors in symptomatic 12-week-old R6/2 mice revealed decreases compared with age-matched littermate controls.[75] Other neurotransmitter receptors known to be affected in HD were found decreased in R6/2 mice, including dopamine and muscarinic cholinergic, but not GABA receptors. D_1-like and D_2-like dopamine receptor binding was drastically reduced to one-third of control in the brains of 8- and 12-week-old R6/2 mice. Altered expression of neurotransmitter receptors precedes clinical symptoms in R6/2 mice and may contribute to subsequent pathology. Biochemical analysis at 12 weeks shows a marked reduction in striatal aconitase[76] indicative of damage by superoxide (O_2^-.) and peroxynitrite ($ONOO^-$), similar to human HD.[62] In addition, the R6/2 transgenic mouse has a marked reduction in striatal and cortical mitochondrial complex IV activity and increased immunostaining for inducible NO synthase and nitrotyrosine.[76] Since these changes occur before evidence of neuronal death the above findings suggest that mitochondrial dysfunction and free radical damage play an important role in the pathogenesis of HD.

Important insights into the potential function of huntingtin has been gained by the study of various mouse models in which the HD homolog gene was inactivated ("knock-out" models)[70] or expanded CAG repeats are introduced into the mouse hypoxanthine phosphoribosyltransferase gene ("knock-in" models).[77] Homozygous inactivation resulted in embryonic death suggesting that huntingtin is critical for early embryonic development. Since this model does not mimic adult HD and homozygote individuals apparently are indistinguishable from heterozygotes, it suggests that the HD gene mutation involves "gain" rather than "loss" in function. This hypothesis, however, has been challenged because the earlier studies suggesting no phenotypic difference between heterozygous and homozygous HD were based on linkage studies and focused predominantly on the age at onset.[78] Furthermore, homozygous transgenic mice expressing mutant huntingtin cDNA have a shorter life spans compared with heterozygous mice. This suggests that either a double-dose of mutant huntingtin or loss of the normal allele (loss of function) contributes to the disease. Either wild-type or mutant huntingtin is needed for normal brain development. Thus HD appears to result from a new toxic property of the mutant protein (gain of function) and loss of neuroprotective activity of the normal huntingtin (loss of function).[78]

Full-length huntingtin, when expressed in transgenic mice, does not appear to produce neurological disease, but only the shortened or truncated form of the protein appears to be toxic to neuronal cells. Mutant huntingtin causes cell toxicity through different mechanisms including the formation of inclusions and aggregates and by decreasing transcriptional activation by cyclic adenosine monophosphate responsive element-binding (CREB) protein (CBP), a mediator of cell survival signals containing a short polyglutamine stretch.[79] By recruiting CREB into cellular aggregates, the mutant huntingtin prevents it from participating as a co-activator in CREB-mediated transcription, supporting the toxic "gain-of-function" mechanism of cell death in HD. The polyglutamine-containing domain of abnormal huntingtin protein directly binds the acetyltransferase domains of CBP and p300/CBP-associated factor (P/CAF).[80] This reduces acetyltransferase activity and decreases acetylation of histones H_3 and H_4, proteins that package DNA. This in turn resulted in a decrease in gene transcription, suggesting that histone-deacetylase inhibitors could prevent HD related neurodegeneration.

Although the aggregates are histological hallmarks of HD neuropathology, there is no direct evidence that the aggregates themselves are toxic to the cells. Available data provide evidence that aggregate formation precedes cell death; however, these data do not necessarily indicate that the aggregates cause cell death. Evidence for the toxicity of aggregates comes from experimental data obtained in cell culture models of HD and dentatorubral-pallidoluysian atrophy (DRPLA), which shares clinical, histological and molecular similarities to HD. In these cells, inhibition of transglutamination, which is considered to be a key step for aggregate formation, prevented apoptosis.[81] It has been postulated that the aggregates of mutant huntingtin cannot be properly removed from the cell and thus may interfere with the metabolic activities of the affected neurons.[53] The aggregates do not only contain the mutant huntingtin but also normal huntingtin, ubiquitin, and some of the huntingtin-interacting proteins.[77] The function of some of the interacting proteins may be compromised by sequestration of these proteins into the aggregates.[82] Since ubiquitin is important in protein degradation and this process requires energy, the cells that are most vulnerable to the accumulation of the ubiquitin-huntingtin aggregates are those whose metabolic function has been already compromised, possibly as a result of toxins that interfere with oxidative phosphorylation. This concept then may link this new finding of region-selective accumulation of huntingtin aggregates and inclusions[53] with the theories of regional impairment of energy metabolism.[83]

However, there is also evidence suggesting that aggregates are products of a cell's detoxification efforts possibly as a result of impaired ubiquitin-proteasomal processing.[84] Deficiency of E6-AP ubiquitin ligase reduces nuclear inclusion frequency while accelerating polyglutamine-induced pathology in a transgenic mouse model of spinocerebellar ataxia type 1 (SCA1), another disease caused by CAG-polyglutamine expansion.[85] E6-AP ubiquitin ligase is essential for ubiquitination of huntingtin, which precedes the aggregate formation. Thus, it has been postulated that the aggregate formation represents a protective function of the cells instead of pathogenic toxicity.[86,87] However, further studies are needed to settle these two opposing views of polyglutamine-containing aggregates.

Experimental data have suggested that huntingtin interacts with other cellular proteins, including huntingtin associated protein 1 (HAP-1),[88] glyceraldehyde-3-phosphate dehydrogenase (GAPDH),[89] apopain[67] and ubiquitin conjugating enzyme (hE2–25K).[90] In the presence of calcium, huntingtin also interacts indirectly with calmodulin.[91] Among all these interactions, HAP-1, and apopain show huntingtin-specific interactions, while GAPDH interacts with other molecules containing a polyglutamine tract. The interactions of HAP-1, GAPDH, apopain and calmodulin with huntingtin are stronger when the polyglutamine tract is longer, whereas the huntingtin-E2–25K interaction is not obviously dependent on the CAG length. Expanded huntingtin also interacts with p53 and represses transcription of the p53-regulated genes, p21WAF1/CIP1 and MDR-1.[92] However, there are a new group of interacting proteins that appear to have direct relevance to the HD pathogenesis. For example, proteins containing a WW domain interact with huntingtin, and these WW domain proteins include splisosome proteins and transcription factors.[93] The expression of another transcriptional activator, CA150, which contains an imperfect glutamine-alanine repeat, is increased and co-localized in the neuronal huntingtin-ubiquitine aggregates in HD brains.[94] Thus, altered transcription regulation may play a major pathogenic role in HD. Huntingtin also interacts with chaperone proteins that unfold the expanded mutant huntingtin protein, preventing the aggregate formation in a cell culture model.[95] Studies have shown that processing of polyglutamine-containing proteins by proteases (such as caspases) liberates truncated fragments with expanded polyglutamine tracts that can form aggregates through hydrogen bonding or transglutaminase activity and may be toxic to the cell. Abnormalities in proteasome function are associated with altered expression of stress-response proteins or heat shock proteins that function as chaperons. The chaperons normally maintain proteins in an appropriate conformation and renature misfolded proteins (aggregates).[96] Over expression of these chaperone proteins protects cells from toxicity induced by huntingtin with expanded polyglutamines.[95–97] It has been postulated that the mutant huntingtin with an expanded polyglutamine tract, which is resistant to proteasome-mediated protein processing, overloads the proteasome machinery, enhancing the pathogenic effects of mutant huntingtin. Since truncated proteins that contain the expanded polyglutamine tract appear to be more toxic than the full-length protein, blocking proteolytic processing, aggregation, and nuclear uptake may be reasonable therapeutic strategies.

Since all these proteins are expressed not only in the striatum but also in other parts of the brain, regional distributions of these proteins are an unlikely cause of the selective neuronal death in HD. In HD transgenic mice, aggregation of N-terminal huntingtin fragments also preferentially occurs in HD-affected neurons and their processes and axonal terminals.[32,55] We must postulate another tissue-specific variable to explain why the medium-sized spiny neurons are selectively vulnerable. The WW domain proteins are of particular interest because they have been shown to specifically bind to soluble, aberrantly migrating, forms of full-length mutant huntingtin specific to HD target tissue.[98] Another potential explanation comes from differential somatic instability of the expanded CAG repeat in the HD gene. In striatum of transgenic HD mice, the CAG repeat shows age-dependent expansions resulting in the repeat size exceeding 250 CAGs in some striatal cells, which are substantially greater than the repeat size range found in other tissues.[99]

Although overwhelming evidence supports the gain-of-function mechanism of HD, contribution of pathophysiological mechanisms involving proteins that bind to CAG repeats within the huntingtin RNA has also been postulated.[100] A loss of function of huntingtin may contribute to HD pathophysiology through defective ability of expanded huntingtin to up-regulate transcription of brain-derived neurotrophic factor (BDNF), a pro-survival factor produced by cortical neurons that is necessary for survival of striatal neurons in the brain.[101,102]

Differential diagnosis

Discussion of differential diagnosis of chorea and HD is beyond the scope of this chapter. Several neurodegenerative disorders, some with expanded trinucleotide repeats, have been reported as phenocopies of HD, including the spinocerebellar atrophy, particularly SCA2 and SCA3 and DRPLA.[103,104] Unstable CAG expansion has been identified as the mutation in a gene on chromosome 12.[105,106] An autosomal dominant HD-like neurodegenerative disorder, now classified as Huntington's disease-like 1 (HDL1), was mapped to chromosome 20p.[107] Another disorder, termed Huntington's disease-like 2 or HDL2, is characterized by onset in the fourth decade, involuntary movements such as chorea and dystonia as well as other movement disorders (bradykinesia, rigidity, tremor), dysarthria, hyperreflexia, gait abnormality, psychiatric symptoms, weight loss, and dementia with progression from onset to death in about 20 years.[108] The neuroimaging and neuropathological findings are very similar to those in HD. Unlike the family linked to chromosome 20p, seizures are not present in this latter family. All 10 affected family members had a CAG repeat expansion of 50 to 60 triplets, but linkage to known loci on chromosome 4p and 20p was excluded. While the majority of genetic forms of chorea are inherited in an autosomal dominant pattern, a novel autosomal recessive neurodegenerative Huntington-like disorder has been described.[109] Beginning at 3–4 years of age and manifested by chorea, dystonia, ataxia, gait disorder, spasticity, seizures, mutism, intellectual impairment, and bilateral frontal and caudate atrophy, this neurodegenerative disorder has been linked to 4p15.3, different from the 4p16.3 HD locus. This disorder has now been classified as HDL3.

Treatment

Huntington's disease is one of few neurodegenerative diseases in which the diagnosis can be made long before the onset of clinical symptoms. This offers an opportunity to intervene in the earliest stages of the neurodegenerative cascade, perhaps even before the disease-related cell loss is initiated.[110] Furthermore, studies on human HD and mouse models of HD suggest that the CNS phenotype appears before neuronal loss. Furthermore, in a HD mouse model in which expression of mutant huntingtin can be controlled (conditional transgenic mouse model), neurobehavioral and neuropathological changes were reversed after shutting off the transgene expression.[111] These findings suggest that a continuous influx of the mutant protein is required to maintain inclusions and symptoms, raising the possibility that HD may be reversible. Thus HD is an excellent model for testing early neuroprotective treatments. As noted earlier, the HD mouse models can be used to test some novel neuroprotective strategies.

Based on our current understanding of the mechanisms of neurodegeneration in HD, the rational approach would be: (1) to eliminate the mutant huntingtin protein or (2) to prevent the mutant huntingtin protein from producing the gain-of-function effects. In HD, the expanded CAG repeat in the gene is transcribed into an expanded CAG repeat in the mRNA, which is then translated into an expanded glutamine repeat in the huntingtin protein. At present, selective inhibition of the mutant HD gene transcription and translation is not feasible in patients. However, sequence-specific cleavage of huntingtin mRNA by catalytic DNA, an oligodeoxynucleotide with RNA-cleaving enzymatic activity, has been demonstrated in a mammalian cell culture model.[112] This resulted in significant reduction of huntingtin protein expression. Ribozyme, RNA with RNA-cleaving enzymatic activity, may also be of interest in this strategy.[113]

However, a more practical approach is to prevent the mutant huntingtin protein from producing the gain-of-function effects. We now know that the huntingtin protein interacts to other proteins. Thus, modulators of such interactions may decrease the gain-of-function effect, leading to therapeutic benefits. One example involves interaction of caspase-1 and caspase-3 (apopain) with huntingtin. Caspases are important for induction of apoptosis. Caspase-3 is also involved in N-terminal cleavage of huntingtin, which is an important step for the gain of function mechanism. Chen et al.,[114] found that minocycline delays disease progression, possibly by reducing the production of caspase-1 and caspase-3, and by decreasing inducible nitric oxide synthetase (iNOS) activity in R6/2 mice. Another caspase inhibitor with potential neuroprotective effects, currently tested in patients with HD, is ethyl eicosapentaenoate (LAX101). Pure fatty acid, highly concentrated in fish oil, has also been found to be effective in some pilot trials in HD and schizophrenia. These important observations, of course, have obvious therapeutic implications and suggest that caspase inhibitors may play a role in the treatment of HD and related neurodegenerative disorders.[110,115] Human trials of minocycline are underway.

Over expression of chaperone proteins that interact with huntingtin may also have therapeutic effects. Although abnormal protein aggregation has been postulated to play an important role in the pathogenesis of HD, DiFiglia and her colleagues showed that aggregation was not intimately involved in cell death.[116] While general inhibitors of caspases prolonged cell life they did not alter aggregation, whereas specific caspase-3 inhibitors inhibited aggregation but had no effect on survival. However, if mutant huntingtin aggregates play an important disease-causing role in HD, preventing the formation of aggregations by intracellular antibodies or chemical reagents may be used as a treatment strategy. Transglutaminase inhibitors, such as cystamine and monodansyl cadaverine, reduce aggregate formation and as such may be potential therapeutic agents in diseases caused by CAG-repeat expansion.[81,117] Interestingly, antibodies against polyglutamines also prevent huntingtin aggregation in vitro and in cell culture model.[118,119] Inhibitors of pathogenic interactions between huntingtin and some of the other proteins may also prove important for treatment of HD. Another approach is to offset the consequence of abnormal interaction between the mutant huntingtin and transcription co-repressors by histone deacetylase inhibitors, such as phenylbutyrate, suberoylanilide hydroxamic acid (SAHA) and pyroxamide, to arrest polyglutamine-dependent neurodegeneration.[80,120] However, encouraging results have been obtained, so far, only in a Drosophila model of HD.[80] Transgenic animal models and cell culture models are being used to screen candidate pharmacological agents for treatment of HD.

Yet, another therapeutic approach is to intervene in the final pathway of cell degeneration. CoQ10

Table 239.1	Treatment of Huntington's disease

Adequate nutrition

Physical, speech and occupational therapy

Treat/prevent aspiration, fecal impaction, incontinence

Support
    Life-planning, disability benefits, household help,
      home equipment, supervise smoking, child care,
      day care, institutional care, hospice

Care-giver support

Anxiolytics
    benzodiazepines, propranolol, clonidine

Antidepressants
    tricyclics (nortriptyline, amitriptyline, imipramine)
    SSRIs (fluoxetine, sertraline, fluvoxamine, paroxetine,
      venlafaxine, citalopram)

DA receptor blocking drugs or DA depleting drugs for
severe chorea, psychosis
    quetiapine, olanzapine, ziprasidone, clozapine,
      fluphenazine, risperidone, haloperidol,
      tetrabenazine

Glutamate release inhibitors and receptor blockers
(remacemide, riluzole)

Mitochondrial electron transport enhancers and free
radical scavengers
    CoQ10, nicotinamide, creatine

Caspase and iNOS inhibitors
    minocycline, ethyl eicosapentaenoate or ethyl-EPA,
    LAX-101

Histone deacetylase inhibitors

Trophic factors

Fetal transplants

(ubiquinone) carries electrons from complexes I and II to complex II of the mitochondrial electron transport chain and as such, it can act as an antioxidant or as a pro-oxidant, depending on the cell's redox potential.[121] A clinical trial conducted by the Huntington Study Group, comparing CoQ10 and remacemide, an NMDA ion channel blocker, showed a 13% slowing in total functional capacity decline with CoQ10, but this difference failed to reach statistical significance.[122] Behavioral treatment may also have some benefit. Using the HD mouse models, several studies have shown that the onset of neurological deficit was significantly delayed if the mice were raised in an enriched and stimulating environment.[123,124]

Until effective neuroprotective therapy is found the management of patients with HD will focus primarily on relief of symptoms designed to improve their quality of life. Psychosis, one of the most troublesome symptoms, usually improves with neuroleptics, such as haloperidol, pimozide, fluphenazine and thioridazine. These drugs, however, can induce tardive dyskinesia and other adverse effects and, therefore, they should be used only if absolutely needed to control symptoms. Clozapine (Clozaril), an atypical antipsychotic drug that does not cause tardive dyskinesia, may be a useful alternative to the typical neuroleptics, but its high cost, risk of agranulocytosis, and other potential side effects may limit its use.[125] It is likely that the other atypical anti-psychotics, such as olanzapine (Zyprexa) and quetiapine fumarate (Seroquel), will also provide beneficial effects. Anxiolytics and antidepressants also may be useful in some patients with psychiatric problems.

Monoamine depleting drugs such as reserpine and tetrabenazine may not only help to control psychotic symptoms, but more importantly these monoamine depleters relieve chorea. Although tetrabenazine can cause or exacerbate depression, sedation, akathisia and parkinsonism, in our experience it is clearly the most effective anti-chorea drug.[126] Paradoxically, some patients with HD benefit from dopaminergic drugs, particularly when the disease is associated with parkinsonism.[127] A novel dopaminergic modulator OSU6162 has been reported to improve chorea in a patient with HD,[128] but further studies on the pharmacology and clinical efficacy of the drug are needed. Whether blocking glutamate release from the presynaptic terminals by drugs such as riluzole or lamotrigine or whether other antiglutamatergic drugs will be effective in slowing down the otherwise inexorable progression of the disease awaits further studies. Dystonia and bruxism, occasionally present in patients with HD, can be effectively treated with local injections of botulinum toxin.[8] Pallidotomy, known to be effective in the treatment of levodopa-induced dyskinesias in patients with Parkinson's disease, has also been found to be useful in the treatment of dystonia associated with HD.[129]

Following up on some encouraging results from animal studies, the delivery of trophic factors, such as nerve growth factor (NGF) and ciliary neutrophic factor (CNTF) by genetically modified cells, into the striatum of patients with HD has become a reachable goal.[130,131] Implantation of NF-producing fibroblasts into the rat striatum appeared to protect these animals against neurotoxic effects of excitatory amino acids quinolate and quisqualate.[132] Whether intrastriatal implantations of genetically engineered cells designed to produce trophic factors, such CNTF[130,133] or fetal cells will be useful in the treatment of HD awaits the results of further animal and clinical studies.[134] No change in functional status or hyperkinetic movements were observed in 12 HD patients treated with transplantation of fetal porcine striatal cells,[135] but in another study,[136] motor and cognitive improvement was noted in three of five patients after staged grafting of both striatal areas with human fetal neuroblasts. The observation that implanted fetal neuronal cells survive in the HD brain and reconstitute damaged neuronal connections, suggests that the host HD disease process does not affect the grafted tissue.[134]

References

1. Huntington G. On chorea. Medical and Surgical Reporter 1872;26:320–321

2. Jankovic J, Ashizawa T. Huntington's disease. *In:* Appel SH, ed. Current Neurology. Vol 15. Chicago: Mosby Year Book, 1995:29–60a

3. Penney JB, Young AB. Huntington's disease. *In:* Jankovic J, Tolosa E, eds. Parkinson's Disease and Movement Disorders. 3rd ed. Baltimore: Williams and Wilkins, 1998:341–356

4. Harper PS. The epidemiology of Huntington's disease. Hum Gen 1992;89:365–376

5. Foroud T, Gray J, Ivashina J, Conneally PM. Differences in duration of Huntington's disease based on age at onset. J Neurol Neurosurg Psychiatry 1999;66: 52–56

6. Ashizawa T, Jankovic J. Cervical dystonia as the initial presentation of Huntington's disease. Mov Disord 1996;11:457–459

7. Louis ED, Lee P, Quinn L, Marder K. Dystonia in Huntington's disease: prevalence and clinical characteristics. Mov Disord 1999;14:95–101

8. Tan E-K, Jankovic J, Ondo W. Bruxism in Huntington's disease. Mov Disord 2000;15:171–173

9. Paulsen JS, Zhao H, Staout JC, et al. Clinical markers of early disease in persons near onset of Huntington's disease. Neurology 2001;57:658–662

10. Foroud T, Siemers E, Kleindorfer D, et al. Cognitive scores in carriers of Huntington's disease gene compared to noncarriers. Ann Neurol 1995;37:657–664

11. Zappacosta B, Monza D, Meoni C, et al. Psychiatric symptoms do not correlate with cognitive decline, motor symptoms, or CAG repeat length in Huntington's disease. Arch Neurol 1996;53:493–497

12. Paulsen JS, Ready RE, Hamilton JM, et al. Neuropsychiatric aspects of Huntington's disease. J Neurol Neurosurg Psychiatry 2001;71:310–314

13. Litvan I, Paulsen JS, Mega MS, Cummings JL. Neuropsychiatric assessment of patients with hyperkinetic and hypokinetic movement disorders. Arch Neurol 1998;55:1313–1319

14. Britton JW, Uiti RJ, Ahlskog JE, et al. Hereditary late-onset chorea without significant dementia: genetic evidence for substantial phenotypic variation in Huntington's disease. Neurology 1995;45:443–447

15. Pillon B, Dubois B, Ploska A, Agid Y. Severity and specificity of cognitive impairment in Alzheimer's, Huntington's, and Parkinson's diseases and progressive supranuclear palsy. Neurology 1991;41:634–643

16. Bamford KA, Caine ED, Kido DK, et al. A prospective evaluation of cognitive decline in early Huntington's disease. Neurology 1995;45:1867–1873

17. de Boo GM, Tibben A, Lanser JB, et al. Early cognitive and motor symptoms in identified carriers of the gene for Huntington's disease. Arch Neurol 1997;54: 1353–1357

18. Hahn-Barma V, Deweer B, Dürr A, et al. Are cognitive changes the first symptoms of Huntington's disease? A study of gene carriers. J Neurol Neurosurg Psychiatry 1998;64:172–177

19. Robins Wahlin T-B, Bäckman L, Haegermark A, et al. High suicidal ideation in persons testing for Huntington's disease. Acta Neurol Scand 2000;102:150–161

20. Kirkwood SC, Siemers E, Hodes ME, et al. Subtle changes among presymptomatic carriers of the Huntington's disease gene. J Neurol Neurosurg Psychiatry 2000;69:773–779

21. Meiser B, Dunn S. Psychological impact of genetic testing for Huntington's disease: an update of the literature. J Neurol Neurosurg Psychiatry 2000;69:574–578

22. Sánchez-Pernaute R, Künig G, del Barrio Albe A, et al. Bradykinesia in early Huntington's disease. Neurology 2000;54:119–125

23. Berardelli A, Noth J, Thompson PD, et al. Pathophysiology of chorea and bradykinesia in Huntington's disease. Mov Disord 1999;14:398–403

24. Reuter I, Hu MTM, Andrews TC, et al. Late onset levodopa responsive Huntington's disease with minimal chorea masquerading as Parkinson plus syndrome. J Neurol Neurosurg Psychiatry 2000;68:238–241

25. Pratley RE, Salbe AD, Ravussin E, Caviness JN. Higher sedentary energy expenditure in patients with Huntington's disease. Ann Neurol 2000;47:64–70

26. Huntington Study Group. Unified Huntington's Disease Rating Scale: reliability and consistency. Mov Disord 1996;11:136–142

27. Siesling S, van Vugt JPP, Zwinderman KAH, et al. Unified Huntington's Disease Rating Scale: a follow up. Mov Disord 1998;13:915–919

28. CAPIT-HD Committee. Core assessment program for intracerebral transplantation in Huntington's disease (CAPIT-HD). Mov Disord 1996;11:143–150

29. Reilmann R, Kirsten F, Quinn N, et al. Objective assessment of progression in Huntington's disease: a 3-year follow-up study. Neurology 2001;57:920–924

30. Helder DI, Kaptein AA, van Kempen GMJ, et al. Impact of Huntington's disease on quality of life. Mov Disord 2001;16:325–330

31. The Huntington's Disease Collaborative Research Group. A novel gene containing a trinucleotide repeat that is expanded and unstable on Huntington's disease chromosomes. Cell 1993;72:971–983

32. Li H, Li SH, Johnston H, Shelbourne PF, et al. Aminoterminal fragments of mutant huntingtin show selective accumulation in striatal neurons and synaptic toxicity. Nat Genet 2000;25:385–389

33. Gusela JF, MacDonald ME. Huntington's disease: CAG genetics expands neurobiology. Curr Opin Neurobiol 1995;5:656–662

34. Nance MA, and the US Huntington Disease Genetic Testing Group. Genetic testing of children at risk for Huntington's disease. Neurology 1997;49:1048–1053

35. Brinkman RR, Mezei MM, Theilmann J, et al. The likelihood of being affected with Huntington disease by a particular age, for a specific CAG size. Am J Hum Genet 1997;60:1201–1210

36. Antonini A, Leenders KL, Eidelberg D. [11C] Raclopride-PET studies of the Huntington's disease rate of progression: relevance of the trinucleotide repeat length. Ann Neurol 1998;43:253–255

37. Ashizawa T, Wong L-JC, Richards CS, et al. CAG repeat size and clinical presentation in Huntington's disease. Neurology 1994;44:1137–1143

38. Claes S, Zand KV, Legius E, et al. Correlations between triplet repeat expansion and clinical features in Huntington's disease. Arch Neurol 1995;113:749–753

39. Kieburtz K, MacDonald M, Shih C, et al. Trinucleotide repeat length and progression of illness in Huntington's disease. J Med Genet 1994;31:872–874

40. Feigin A, Kieburtz K, Bordwell K, et al. Functional decline in Huntington's disease. Mov Disord 1995;10: 211–214

41. Rosas HD, Goodman J, Chen YI, et al. Striatal volume loss in HD as measured by MRI and the influence of CAG repeat. Neurology 2001;57:1025–1028

42. Harris GJ, Codori AM, Lewis RF, et al. Reduced basal ganglia blood flow and volume in pre-symptomatic, gene-tested persons at-risk for Huntington's disease. Brain 1999;122:1667–1678

43. Grafton ST, Mazziotta JC, Pahl JJ, et al. A comparison of neurological, metabolic, structural, and genetic evaluations in persons at risk for Huntington's disease. Ann Neurol 1990;28:614–621

44. Kuwert T, Lange HW, Langen K-J, et al. Cortical and subcortical glucose consumption measured by PET in patients with Huntington's disease. Brain 1990;113:1405–1423

45. Nagel JS, Ichise M, Holman BL. The scintigraphic evaluation of Huntington's disease and other movement disorders using single photon emission computed tomography perfusion brain scans. Sem Nucl Med 1991;21:11–23

46. Künig G, Leenders KL, Sanchez-Pernaute R, et al. Benzodiazepine receptor binding in Huntington's disease: [^{11}C]Flumazenil uptake measured using positron emission tomography. Ann Neurol 2000;47:644–648

47. Sotrel A, Paskevich PA, Kiely DK, et al. Morphometric analysis of the prefrontal cortex in Huntington's disease. Neurology 1991;41:1117–1123

48. Albin RL. Selective neurodegeneration in Huntington's disease. Ann Neurol 1995;38:835–836

49. Furtado S, Suchowersky O, Rewcastle NB, et al. Relationship between trinucleotide repeats and neuropathological changes in Huntington's disease. Ann Neurol 1996;39:132–136

50. Gómez-Tortosa E, MacDonald M, Friend JC, et al. Quantitative neuropathological changes in presymptomatic Huntington's disease. Ann Neurol 2001;49:29–34

51. Gourfinkel-An I, Cancel G, Trottier Y, et al. Differential distribution of the normal and mutated forms of huntingtin in the human brain. Ann Neurol 1997;42:712–719

52. Sapp E, Schwartz C, Chase K, et al. Huntingtin localization in brains of normal and Huntington's disease patients. Ann Neurol 1997;42:604–612

53. DiFiglia M, Sapp E, Chase KO, et al. Aggregation of huntingtin in neuronal intranuclear inclusions and dystrophic neurites in brain. Science 1997;277:1990–1993

54. Li SH, Lam S, Cheng AL, Li XJ. Intranuclear huntingtin increases the expression of caspase-1 and induces apoptosis. Hum Mol Genet. 2000;9:2859–2867

55. Li H, Li SH, Johnston H, et al. Amino-terminal fragments of mutant huntingtin show selective accumulation in striatal neurons and synaptic toxicity. Nat Genet 2000;25:385–389

56. Oyanagi K, Takeda S, Takashi H, et al. A quantitative investigation of the substantia nigra in Huntington's disease. Ann Neurol 1989;26:13–19

57. Albin RL, Young AB, Penney JB, et al. Abnormalities of striatal projection neurons and N-methyl-D-aspartate receptors in presymptomatic Huntington's disease. N Engl J Med 1990;332:1293–1298

58. Kurlan R, Goldblatt D, Zaczek R, et al. Cerebrospinal fluid homovanillic acid and parkinsonism in Huntington's disease. Ann Neurol 1988;24:282–284

59. Bohnen NI, Koeppe RA, Meyer P, et al. Decreased striatal monoaminergic terminals in Huntington disease. Neurology 2000;54:1753–1759

60. Weeks RA, Piccini P, Harding AE, Brooks DJ. Striatal D$_1$ and D$_2$ dopamine receptor loss in asymptomatic mutation carriers of Huntington's disease. Ann Neurol 1996;40:49–54

61. Andrews TC, Weeks RA, Turjanski N, et al. Huntington's disease progression. PET and clinical observations. Brain 1999;122:2353–2363

62. Tabrizi SJ, Cleeter MWJ, Xuereb J, et al. Biochemical abnormalities and excitotoxicity in Huntington's disease brain. Ann Neurol 1999;45:25–32

63. Ferrante RJ, Kowall NW, Cipolloni PB, et al. Excitotoxin lesions in primates as a model for Huntington's disease: histopathological and neurochemical characterization. Exp Neurology 1993;119:46–71

64. Beal MF, Brouillet E, Jenkins BG, et al. Neurochemical and histologic characterization of striatal excitotoxic lesions produced by the mitochondrial toxin 3-nitropropionic acid. J Neurosci 1993;13:4181–4192

65. Brouillet E, Jenkins BG, Hyman BT, et al. Age-dependent vulnerability of the striatum to the mitochondrial toxin 3-nitropropionic acid. J Neurochemistry 1993;60:356–359

66. Andreassen OA, Ferrante RJ, Huang H-M, et al. Dichloroacetate exerts therapeutic effects in transgenic models of Huntington disease. Ann Neurol 2001;50:112–117

67. Goldberg YP, Nicholson DW, Rasper DM, et al. Cleavage of huntingtin by apopain, a proapoptotic cystein protease, is modulated by the polyglutamine tract. Nat Genet 1996;13:442–449

68. Jana NR, Zemskov EA, Wang GH, Nukina N. Altered proteasomal function due to the expression of polyglutamine-expanded truncated N-terminal huntingtin induces apoptosis by caspase activation through mitochondrial cytochrome c release. Hum Mol Genet 2001;10:1049–1059

69. Judge CG, Garson OM, Pitt DB, Sutherland GR. A girl with Wolf-Hirschorn syndrome and mosaicism 46,XX-46,XX,4p-. J Ment Defic Res 1974;18:79–85

70. Duyao MP, Auerbach AB, Ryan A, et al. Inactivation of the mouse Huntington's disease gene homolog Hdh. Science 1995;269:407–410

71. Mangiarini L, Sathasivam K, Seller M, et al. Exon 1 of the HD gene with an expanded CAG repeat is sufficient to cause a progressive neurological phenotype in transgenic mice. Cell 1996;87:493–506

72. Perutz MF, Windle AH. Cause of neural death in neurodegenerative diseases attributable to expansion of glutamine repeats. Nature 2001;412:143–144

73. Ona VO, Li M, Vonsattel JPG, et al. Inhibition of caspase-1 slows disease progression in a mouse model of Huntington's disease. Nature 1999;399:263–267

74. Mangiarini L, Sathasivam K, Bates GP. Molecular pathology of Huntington's disease: animal models and nuclear mechanisms. Neuroscientist 1999;5:383–391

75. Cha JH, Kosinski CM, Kerner JA, et al. Altered brain neurotransmitter receptors in transgenic mice expressing a portion of an abnormal human huntington disease gene. Proc Natl Acad Sci 1998;95:6480–6485

76. Tabrizi SJ, Workman J, Hart PE, et al. Mitochondrial dysfunction and free radical damage in the Huntington R6/2 transgenic mouse. Ann Neurol 2000;47:80–86

77. Reddy PH, Williams M, Tagle DA. Recent advances in understanding the pathogenesis of Huntington's disease. TINS 1999;22:248–255

78. Cattaneo E, Rigamonti D, Coffredo D, et al. Loss of normal huntingtin function: new developments in Huntington's disease research. TINS 2001;24:182–188

79. Nucifora FC, Sasaki M, Peters MF, et al. Interference by huntingtin and atrophin-1 with CBP-mediated transcription leading to cellular toxicity. Science 2001;291:2423–2428

80. Steffan JS, Bodai L, Pallos J, et al. Histone deacetylase inhibitors arrest polyglutamine-dependent neurodegeneration in Drosophila. Nature 2001;413:739–743

81. Igarashi S, Koide R, Shimohata T, et al. Suppression of aggregate formation and apoptosis by transglutaminase inhibitors in cells expressing truncated DRPLA proteins with an expanded polyglutamine stretch. Nat Genet 1998;18:111–117

82. Preisinger E, Jordan BM, Kazantsev A, Housman D. Evidence for a recruitment and sequestration mechanism in Huntington's disease. Philos Trans R Soc Lond B Biol Sci 1999;354:1029–1034

83. Beal MF, Henshaw DR, Jenkins BG, et al. Coenzyme Q10 and nicotinamide block striatal lesions produced by the mitochondrial toxin malonate. Ann Neurol 1994;36:882–888

84. Chung KKK, Dawson VL, Dawson TM. The role of the ubiquitin-protasomal pathway in Parkinson's disease and other neurodegenerative disorders. TINS 2001;24(Suppl):S7–S14

85. Cummings CJ, Reinstein E, Sun Y, et al. Mutation of the E6-AP ubiquitin ligase reduces nuclear inclusion frequency while accelerating polyglutamine-induced pathology in SCA1 mice. Neuron 1999;24:879–892

86. Kuemmerle S, Gutekunst CA, Klein AM, et al. Huntington aggregates may not predict neuronal death in Huntington's disease. Ann Neurol 1999;46:842–849

87. Klement IA, Zoghbi HY, Orr HT. Pathogenesis of polyglutamine-induced disease: a model for SCA1. Mol Genet Metab 1999;66:172–178

88. Li XJ, Li SH, Sharp AH, et al. A huntingtin-associated protein enriched in brain with implications for pathology. Nature 1995;378:398–402

89. Burke JR, Enghild JJ, Martin ME, et al. Huntingtin and DRPLA proteins selectively interact with the enzyme GAPDH. Nat Med 1996;2:347–350

90. Kalchman MA, Graham RK, Xia G, et al. Huntingtin is ubiquitinated and interacts with a specific ubiquitin-conjugating enzyme. J Biol Chem 1996;271: 19385–19394

91. Bao J, Sharp AH, Wagster MV, et al. Expansion of polyglutamine repeat in huntingtin leads to abnormal protein interactions involving calmodulin. Proc Natl Acad Sci USA 1996;93:5037–5042

92. Steffan JS, Kazantsev A, Spasic-Boskovic O, et al. The Huntington's disease protein interacts with p53 and CREB-binding protein and represses transcription. Proc Natl Acad Sci USA 2000;97:6763–6768

93. Passani LA, Bedford MT, Faber PW, et al. Huntingtin's WW domain partners in Huntington's disease postmortem brain fulfill genetic criteria for direct involvement in Huntington's disease pathogenesis. Hum Mol Genet 2000;9:2175–2182

94. Holbert S, Denghien I, Kiechle T, et al. The Gln-Ala repeat transcriptional activator CA150 interacts with huntingtin: neuropathologic and genetic evidence for a role in Huntington's disease pathogenesis. Proc Natl Acad Sci USA 2001;98:1811–1816

95. Jana NR, Tanaka M, Wang GH, Nukina N. Polyglutamine length-dependent interaction of Hsp40 and Hsp70 family chaperones with truncated N-terminal huntingtin: their role in suppression of aggregation and cellular toxicity. Hum Mol Genet 2000;9:2009–2018

96. Kobayashi Y, Sobue G. Protective effects of chaperons on polyglutamine diseases. Brain Research Bull 2001; 56:165–168

97. Carmichael J, Chatellier J, Woolfson A, et al. Bacterial and yeast chaperones reduce both aggregate formation and cell death in mammalian cell models of Huntington's disease. Proc Natl Acad Sci USA 2000;97: 9701–9705

98. Wheeler VC, White JK, Gutekunst CA, et al. Long glutamine tracts cause nuclear localization of a novel form of huntingtin in medium spiny striatal neurons in HdhQ92 and HdhQ111 knock-in mice. Hum Mol Genet 2000;9:503–513

99. Kennedy L, Shelbourne PF. Dramatic mutation instability in HD mouse striatum: does polyglutamine load contribute to cell-specific vulnerability in Huntington's disease? Hum Mol Genet 2000;9:2539–2544

100. McLaughlin BA, Spencer C, Eberwine J. CAG trinucleotide RNA repeats interact with RNA-binding proteins. Am J Hum Genet 1996;59:561–569

101. Dragatsis I, Levine MS, Zeitlin S. Inactivation of Hdh in the brain and testis results in progressive neurodegeneration and sterility in mice. Nat Genet 2000;26: 300–306

102. Zuccato C, Ciammola A, Rigamonti D, et al. Loss of huntingtin-mediated BDNF gene transcription in Huntington's disease. Science 2001;293:493–498

103. Rosenblatt A, Ranen NG, Rubinsztein DC, et al. Patients with features similar to Huntington's disease, without CAG expansion in huntingtin. Neurology 1998;51:215–220

104. Thomas M, Jankovic J. Dentatorubral-pallidoluysian atrophy in North American families. Ann Neurol 2001;50(Suppl 1):S65

105. Koide R, Ikeuchi T, Onodera O, et al. Unstable expansion of CAG repeat in hereditary dentatorubral-pallidoluysian atrophy (DRPLA). Nature Genetics, 1994;6: 9–13

106. Komure O, Sano A, Nishino N, et al. DNA analysis in hereditary dentatorubral-pallidoluysian atrophy: correlation between CAG repeat length and phenotypic variation and the molecular basis anticipation. Neurology 1995;45:143–149

107. Xiang F, Almqvist EW, Huq M, et al. A Huntington disease-like neurodegenerative disorder maps to chromosome 20p. Am J Hum Genet 1998;63:1431–1438

108. Margolis RL, O'Hearn E, Rosenblatt A, et al. A disorder similar to Huntington's disease is associated with a novel CAG repeat expansion. Ann Neurol 2001; 50:373–380

109. Kambouris M, Bohlega S, Al-Tahan A, Meyer BF. Localization of the gene for a novel autosomal recessive neurodegenerative Huntington-like disorder to 4p15.3. Am J Hum Genet 2000;66:445–452

110. McMurray CT. Huntington's disease: new hope for therapeutics. TINS 2001;24(Suppl):S32–S37

111. Yamamoto A, Lucas JJ, Hen R. Reversal of neuropathology and motor dysfunction in a conditional model of Huntington's disease. Cell. 2000;101:57–66

112. Yen L, Strittmatter SM, Kalb RG. Sequence-specific cleavage of huntingtin mRNA by catalytic DNA. Ann Neurol 1999;46:366–373

113. Phylactou LA, Darrah C, Wood MJ. Ribozyme-mediated trans-splicing of a trinucleotide repeat. Nat Genet 1998;18:378–381

114. Chen M, Ona VO, Li M, Ferrante RJ, et al. Minocycline inhibits caspase-1 and caspase-3 expression and delays mortality in a transgenic mouse model of huntington disease. Nat Med 2000;6:797–801

115. Friedlander RM. Role of caspase-1 in neurologic disease. Arch Neurol 2000;57:1273–1276

116. Kim M, Lee HS, LaForet G, et al. Mutant huntingtin expression in clonal striatal cells: dissociation of

inclusion formation and neuronal survival by caspase inhibition. J Neurosci 1999;19:964–973

117. Violante V, Luongo A, Pepe I, et al. Transglutaminase-dependent formation of protein aggregates as possible biochemical mechanism for polyglutamine diseases. Brain Research Bull 2001;56:169–172

118. Heiser V, Scherzinger E, Boeddrich A, et al. Inhibition of huntingtin fibrillogenesis by specific antibodies and small molecules: implications for Huntington's disease therapy. Proc Natl Acad Sci USA 2000;97:6739–6744

119. Lecerf JM, Shirley TL, Zhu Q, et al. Human single-chain Fv intrabodies counteract in situ huntingtin aggregation in cellular models of Huntington's disease. Proc Natl Acad Sci USA 2001;98:4764–4769

120. Marks PA, Richon VAM, Breslow R, Rifkind RA. Histone deactylase inhibitors as new cancer drugs. Curr Opin Oncologe 2001;13:377–483

121. Shults CW, Schapira AHV. A cue to queue for CoQ? Neurology 2001;57:375–376

122. Huntington Study Group. A randomized, placebo-controlled trial of coenzyme Q10 and remacemide in Huntington's disease. Neurology 2001;57:397–404

123. Van Dellen A, Blakemore C, Deacon R, et al. Delaying the onset of Huntington's in mice. Nature 2000;404:721–722

124. Carter RJ, Hunt MJ, Morton AJ. Environmental stimulation increases survival in mice transgenic for exon 1 of the Huntington's disease gene. Mov Disord 2000;15:925–937

125. Bonuccelli U, Ceravolo R, Maremmani C, et al. Clozapine in Huntington's chorea. Neurology 1994;44:821–823

126. Jankovic J, Beach J. Long-term effects of tetrabenazine in hyperkinetic movement disorders. Neurology 1997;48:358–362

127. Racette BA, Perlmutter JS. Levodopa responsive parkinsonism in an adult with Huntington's disease. J Neurol Neurosurg Psychiatry 1998;65:577–579

128. Tedroff J, Ekesob A, Sonesson C, et al. Long-lasting improvement following (-)-OSU6162 in a patient with Huntington's disease. Neurology 1999;53:1605–1606

129. Cubo E, Shannon KM, Penn RD, Kroin JS. Internal globus pallidotomy in dystonia secondary to Huntington's disease. Mov Disord 2000;15:1248–1251

130. Kordower JH, Isacson O, Emerich DF. Cellular delivery of trophic factors for the treatment of Huntington's disease: is neuroprotection possible? Exp Neurol 1999;159:4–20

131. Mittoux V, Joseph JM, Conde F, et al. Restoration of cognitive and motor functions by ciliary neurotrophic factor in a primate model of Huntington's disease. Human Gene Therapy 2000;11:1177–1187

132. Schumacher JM, Short MP, Hyman BT, et al. Intracerebral implantation of nerve growth factor-producing fibroblasts protects striatum against neurotoxic levels of excitatory amino acids. Neuroscience 1991;45:561–570

133. Emerich DF, Winn SR, Hantraye PM, et al. Protective effect of encapsulated cells producing neurotrophic factor CNTF in a monkey model of Huntington's disease. Nature 1997;386:395–399

134. Freeman TB, Cicchetti F, Hauser RA, et al. Transplanted fetal striatum in Huntington's disease: phenotypic development and lack of pathology. Proc Natl Acad Sci USA 2000;97:13877–13882

135. St. Hillaire M, Shannon K, Schumacher J, et al. Transplantation of fetal porcine striatal cells in Huntington's disease: preliminary safety and efficacy results. Neurology 1998;50:A80–A81

136. Bachoud-Levi A-C, Remy P, Nguyen J-P, et al. Motor and cognitive improvements in patients with Huntington's disease after neural transplantation. Lancet 2000;356:1975–1979

240 Neuroacanthocytosis

Madhavi Thomas and Joseph Jankovic

"Acantho" is a term derived from a Greek word used to describe "thorns", and acanthocytes are abnormally shaped red blood cells that appear "thorny". Although up to 3% of acanthocytes in the blood may be considered normal, various neurological syndromes have been described with a considerably higher percentage of these abnormal red cells.

Familial neuroacanthocytosis (NA), named by Yamamoto et al.,[1] in 1982, was defined by Spitz et al., in 1985 as a rare neurodegenerative disorder characterized by acanthocytes in the peripheral smear, motor neuron disease, and movement disorder, manifested by chorea, tongue and lip biting, parkinsonism, orofacial dyskinesias, and vocal or facial tics.[2]

The association between acanthocytosis and movement disorders was initially reported in 1968 in two separate North American kindreds by Critchley et al.,[3] and Levine et al.,[4] and the syndrome was named the "Levine-Critchley syndrome" or "Chorea-acanthocytosis". Estes et al.,[5] however, recognized the genetic nature of this disorder even before the initial reports in a family with autosomal dominant form of NA reported in 1967.

Neuroacanthocytosis is classified into four categories: (1) NA with normal serum lipoproteins, (2) NA with hypobetalipoproteinemia, (3) NA with abetalipoproteinemia, and (4) X-linked NA or McLeod syndrome.[2] In a review by Stevenson and Hardie neurological disorders with acanthocytes are classified into the following three categories: (1) NA with normal lipoproteins (2) abetalipoproteinemia, familial hypobetalipoproteinemia and hypoprebetalipoproteinemia and (3) McLeod syndrome.[6]

Epidemiology, incidence and age at onset

Neuroacanthocytosis is a rare disorder, described in families in Europe, North America, Scandinavia, Mexico and Japan. There is a reported 3:1 male preponderance in Japanese cases.[7] Although the series of 19 cases by Hardie et al.,[8] from the UK had a relatively equal gender distribution (10 men and 9 women), there was an overall 2:1 male preponderance in reported European cases.[9] Age at onset is variable with a range of 8 to 62 years (mean age 32).[7,8] The disease progresses over 7 to 10 years and death results from aspiration and other complications of long-standing disability. However, in some patients the course may stabilize with only slight or no progression for several years.

Inheritance

In 15 cases of 40 patients reported from Japan and in 7 of 19 patients from the UK no family history could be identified.[7,8] Most cases, however, are inherited in an autosomal dominant or autosomal recessive pattern. The X-linked form of NA is referred to as the McLeod syndrome. In the autosomal dominant and recessive NA a linkage has been localized by positional cloning to the 6cM region of chromosome 9 q21.[10,11] Candidate genes in the G protein α subunit family, particularly the G-αq that is expressed in the brain and in mature erythrocytes have been cloned, but no mutations have been identified.[12] Recently, Ueno et al. carried out a linkage free analysis in the region of chromosome 9q21 in the Japanese population and identified a 260bp deletion in the EST (expressed sequence tags) region K1AA0986 in exon 60, 61 which was homozygous in patients with NA and heterozygous in their parents. Further sequencing has identified a polyadenylation site with a protein with 3096 amino acid residues, which has been named "Chorein" by the authors. This deletion is not found in normal Japanese and European population.[13] In another study by Rampoldi et al. in European patients a novel gene encoding a 3174 amino acid protein on chromosome 9q21 with 73 exons was identified. They identified 16 mutations in the CHAC (chorea-acanthocytosis) gene. These mutations were identified in various exons. They suggested that CHAC encodes an evolutionarily conserved protein involved in protein sorting.[14] The gene responsible for McLeod syndrome has been identified at the chromosome Xp21 locus designated as XK. Mutations identified by various authors include frame shift mutations in exon 2 at codon 151, deletion at codon 90 in exon 2, and at codon 408 in exon 3, and splicing mutations in intron 2 of the XK gene.[15–22] The etiology of sporadic cases of NA is unknown.

Pathology

Pathological changes of NA include neuronal loss and gliosis in the caudate nucleus, putamen, medial thalamus, globus pallidus, and ventrolateral substantia nigra and rarely in the anterior horn cells of spinal cord.[23–25] There is no involvement of cortex, cerebellum, subthalamic nucleus, and brain stem, which distinguishes NA pathologically from Huntington's disease (HD) and dentatorubropallidoluysian atrophy (DRPLA).[26–28] There is degeneration and dysfunction of the connecting pathways between the caudate nucleus and the frontal cortex in NA.[24] Despite the loss of neurons in the caudate nucleus, there is normal activity of GAD (glutamic acid decarboxylase) and acetyl cholinesterase, unlike HD.[29] Some studies have found a decrease in substance P, increase in NE (norepinephrine) in the CSF (cerebrospinal fluid), putamen, globus pallidus and a reduction of 5-HT (5-hydroxytryptophan), GABA (gamma amino butyric acid) and substance P in the basal ganglia.[25,30]

Biochemical changes

The diagnostic hallmark of NA is abnormally shaped erythrocytes. Under certain conditions of physiological stress, otherwise normal erythrocytes may undergo morphological transformation into acanthocytes or Burr cells (cells with rounded projections). Normal individuals have less than 2% acanthocytes in the peripheral smear; the presence of more than 3% acanthocytes is considered abnormal.[8] Acanthocytes are sometimes absent early but appear later in the course of the disease.[24,31] Spectrin and ankyrin are erythrocyte membrane proteins, which have been localized to various tissues including the neurons. Both the erythrocyte and neuronal spectrin may arise from alternative mRNA transcription of the same gene. Abnormalities in ankyrin and spectrin binding alter the conformation of the erythrocyte and make it more self-digestible.[32-34] Erythrocyte membrane abnormalities can be induced by in vitro stress.[35-38] Membrane protein anion transporter defects and alterations of band-3 related senescent cell antigens in erythrocytes have been studied in patients with NA.[39-41] There is evidence of decreased linoleic acid and stearic acid, but palmitic acid appears to be increased in the erythrocytes.[42] All these changes may be responsible for the alteration in stability of erythrocytes, but the cause for neuronal loss remains unknown.

In McLeod's syndrome, ultrastructural findings of membrane skeletal changes are similar to those found in NA. Membrane protrusions depend on irregular distribution of the membrane skeletons and abnormal function of the Kx and Kell erythrocyte proteins. Kx protein is thought to interact with and stabilize the Kell protein, which is associated with the underlying membrane skeleton of the erythrocyte. Defects in the Kx and Kell protein have been thought to lead to changes in the organization of membrane skeletal networks resulting in the formation of acanthocytes.[35,43]

Clinical features

There is a broad spectrum of clinical findings in patients with NA and they are summarized in Table 240.1.[7,8] Sakai et al. proposed clinical criteria as follows: adult onset of symptoms, progressive orofacial dyskinesia and choreic movements of extremities, tongue or lip biting, denervation, erythrocytic acanthocytosis, and an increased level of serum CPK (creatine phosphokinase).[44,45]

Involuntary movements described in patients with NA range from chorea to phonic and motor tics, dystonia, and a variety of stereotypic dyskinesias.[6,46-48] Involuntary movements in NA are suppressible by performing mental calculations and by voluntarily sustained muscle contractions in patients with NA.[49,50] Chorea is one of the most commonly reported clinical finding and is seen in up to 58% patients with NA. Patients with chorea secondary to NA are often misdiagnosed as having Huntington's disease. Chorea is seen in the extremities and trunk. Orofacial dyskinesias are more prominent than choreiform movements in the extremities in patients with NA unlike the pattern in Huntington's disease. Orofacial dyskinesias are often associated with tongue biting and mutilation of the lips. The orofacial stereotypy consists of repetitive movement of the tongue and protrusion out of the mouth. The tongue often tends to push food out of the mouth when attempting to eat. This "feeding dystonia" interferes with chewing and swallowing.[1,6] Electromyography (EMG) of the tongue while feeding showed inappropriate contractions of masseter

Table 240.1   Clinical features of neuroacanthocytosis

	European patients Hardie et al.[8]	Japanese patients Kuroiwa et al.[7]
Chorea	58%	58%
Orofacial dyskinesia	53%	88%
Lip and tongue biting	16%	83%
Dysarthria	74%	13%
Absent/depressed DTRs	68%	20%
Dementia	63%	23%
Seizures	42%	28%
Muscle weakness and wasting	16%	58%
Dystonia	47%	N/A
Vocalizations	47%	N/A
Tics	42%	N/A
Parkinsonism	34%	N/A
Psychiatric problems	58%	N/A
Limb dyskinesia	N/A	90%
Hypotonia	N/A	55%
Gait disturbance	N/A	18%
Increased muscle CPK	58%	N/A

N/A, data not available; DTR, deep tendon reflexes; CPK, creatine phospho kinase.

muscles when the tongue was stuck out. When the patient attempted to eat there were contractions of the genioglossus muscle. When the masseter was used for chewing there were excessive contractions of genioglossus resulting in the food being pushed out and tongue biting.[1] Dystonia in the limbs, face and bulbar muscles may be the presenting and most striking movement disorder of NA.[8] Dystonia can also be responsible for the frequently observed dysarthria, which can progress to virtual anarthria in some patients.

The hyperkinetic movement disorder can be gradually replaced by parkinsonism which may emerge later in the course of the disease as the dominant feature.[2,7,8,27–29,51] Bostantjopolou et al. have described a patient with atypical familial parkinsonism manifested by gait instability, hypomimia, hypometric vertical and horizontal saccades, memory difficulties and caudate atrophy on magnetic resonance imaging (MRI) with acanthocytosis.[51] Neuroacanthocytosis related parkinsonism has a variable severity and is manifested chiefly by rigidity, bradykinesia, hypomimia, and gait difficulties. A supination and pronation tremor at a frequency of 3–4 Hz, which later generalized, was noted in the patient described by Spitz et al.[2] That patient also had vertical ophthalmoparesis similar to progressive supranuclear palsy. Patients with NA and parkinsonism usually respond poorly to levodopa.

Motor and phonic tics as well as other features of Tourette syndrome have been well described in NA.[1–3,8,30] Phonic tics include grunting, sucking, sighing, blowing, gasping or monosyllabic utterances but not recognizable words often accompanied by belching, sniffing, spitting or clicking.[8] Additionally, the patients described by Spitz et al., had coprolalia.[2] Neuroacanthocytosis should always be considered in the differential diagnosis of adult onset tourettism, particularly when it is associated with other neurological disorders such as motor neuron disease, dystonia or parkinsonism. Although generalized tonic, clonic and other seizures usually occur late in the course, they may be the initial presentation of NA.[52,53]

Behavioral abnormalities including cognitive changes, obsessive-compulsive disorder, depression, anxiety, and paranoid delusions, are seen to a variable degree in most patients with NA. Patients are often described as easily distractable and neglectful of their personal appearance and social skills resulting in an inability to work. Cognitive impairment is in the form of subcortical dementia associated with impaired frontal executive function. Some patients have impulsivity, distractibility, preservative behavior, as well as planning and organizational difficulties.[54] The pattern of neuropsychiatric features observed in patients with NA is very similar to that of Huntington's disease and dentatorubral-pallidoluysian atrophy (DRPLA).

Neurological examination usually shows involuntary movements, typically chorea, stereotypy, tics, or dystonia, as well as hypotonia, muscle wasting and weakness. The posture and gait are often quite peculiar, resembling a "rubber man" with exaggerated extensor posturing of the trunk. The reflexes are usually depressed or absent.[1–8,55–58]

In addition to the neurological features, NA patients also have hemolytic anemia[59] and sometimes cardiomyopathy, more common in the McLeod syndrome.[60] Clinical features of McLeod syndrome are similar to NA, but patients have a higher incidence of myopathy, cardiomyopathy and hemolytic state. Patients with McLeod syndrome show abnormal Kell blood group antigen (antigen to Kell protein) and areflexia, myopathy, cardiomyopathy, chorea, seizures, cognitive impairment and a permanent hemolytic state associated with high muscle creatine phosphokinase (CPK).[61–65]

Differential diagnosis

Differential diagnosis of NA includes all the disorders listed in Table 240.2. The overlap in clinical features between NA and Huntington's disease makes this differentiation particularly important. The predominance of oral dyskinesias and bulbar dysfunction at onset with relatively less neuropsychiatric abnormalities, however, would be more suggestive of NA.[6–9] Neuroacanthocytosis differs from Bassen-Kornzweig disease by the absence of defect in the serum lipoprotein profile and normal lipid absorption. Bassen-Kornzweig syndrome presents in childhood with pigmentary retinopathy, ataxia, sensory disturbances, visual field defects and fatty diarrhoea. There are reports of a late infantile form of "neurodegeneration with brain iron accumulation type-1" (NBIA-1 or eponym Hallervorden-Spatz disease) in association with acanthocytes in the peripheral smear.[66] HARP syndrome (hypobetalipoproteinemia, acanthocytosis, retinitis pigmentosa and pallidal degeneration) shared clinical features with both NA and NBIA-1 (Hallervoden-Spatz disease). The onset of neurological symptoms in HARP is usually in pre-school age and death occurs before adulthood.[67,68] As noted before NA is an important cause of secondary tourettism.[69]

Table 240.2   Differential diagnosis of NA

Neurological disorders with acanthocytosis
Bassen-Kornzweig syndrome
Hypobetalipoproteinemia and acanthocytosis
Chorea-acanthocytosis
McLeod syndrome
NBIA-1 (Neurodegeneration with brain iron deposition type 1)
HARP syndrome (hypobetalipoproteinemia, acanthosytosis, retinitis pigmentosa and pallidal degeneration)

Neurological disorders without acanthocytosis
Huntington's disease
Wilson's disease
Pallidal degeneration

Laboratory tests and investigations

Laboratory tests should include complete blood count, peripheral smear including examination of erythrocytes after subjecting them to in vitro stress such as incubation with saline, ethylenediamine tetraacetic acid (EDTA), or carbon dioxide. In addition, quick freeze-deep etching method and self-forming percoll gradients have been used to increase diagnostic accuracy. Electron microscopy (EM) is occasionally needed to reveal abnormal acanthocytes in the circulating blood.[35] Kell antigens (to identify a McLeod phenotype) and genetic testing for CAG triplet repeat expansion associated with Huntington's disease and DRPLA should be performed to exclude these phenocopies. Since the NA gene and mutations on chromosome 9q21 have been identified, routine testing for the various mutations may soon be possible. Creatine phosphokinase is usually elevated but liver panel, lipoprotein assay, and serum ceruloplasmin are normal. Anti-GM1 (ganglioside) antibody has been shown to be associated with NA and may contribute to peripheral nerve demyelination and should be checked, particularly in patients with peripheral neuropathy.[70,71]

Neuroimaging studies in NA show atrophy of the caudate with computed tomography (CT) and prolonged signal intensity in the atrophic basal ganglia with MRI.[47,72–74] Fluorodopa positron emission tomography (PET) scans show decreased uptake in the caudate nucleus.[75,76] A marked reduction in striatal [^{11}C] raclopride (D_2) receptor binding was noted in the study by Brooks et al.[77] Iodobenzamide (IBZM-SPECT) scans in McLeod's syndrome shows decreased striatal D_2 receptor binding indicating dysfunction or reduction of cells in the striatum.[78] Electroencephalography (EEG) is usually normal but may show slight slowing of background activity or an epileptiform focus. Back averaging studies show a pre movement potential (*Bereitschafts potential*) prior to an "involuntary movement" suggesting a "voluntary" component, similar to tics associated with Tourette syndrome[49]. Electromyography in patients with NA usually shows evidence of chronic denervation, with giant motor units because of collateral reinnervation. Most patients have sensorimotor polyneuropathy with more pronounced involvement of the distal parts of the nerve. Muscle biopsy shows both neurogenic and myopathic changes, type 2 fiber atrophy, targetoid fibers and angulated fibers, fiber splitting and central nucleation.[7,23,26,47,48,73,79–83] Sural nerve biopsy shows changes suggestive of degeneration and regeneration with shortened internodes and giant axonal changes indicative of a defect in axonal transport.[7,23,26,47,79,83]

Treatment

Medications

Management of the patient with NA is difficult; the mainstay is symptomatic treatment and supportive care (Table 240.3). Due to the rarity of the disease, there are no prospective or controlled studies in NA.

Table 240.3 Symptomatic treatment and supportive care for patients with NA

Parkinsonism	Levodopa
Dysphagia	Early swallow evaluation and consideration of PEG (percutaneous enteric gastrostomy)
Chorea	Tetrabenazine, reserpine, fluphenazine, haloperidol, clonazepam
Seizures	Phentoin, tegretol, phenobarbital, valproic acid
Behavioral changes	SSRIs (serotonin reuptake inhibitors), nortryptiline, olanzapine, quetiapine
Dystonia	Botulinum toxin injections
Physical therapy	Gait training and stretching exercises
Genetic counseling	For family members

Management of chorea is similar to that in Huntington's disease. High potency neuroleptics such as haloperidol and fluphenazine may suppress the chorea, but they are frequently associated with side effects including rigidity, sedation, apathy and risk of tardive dyskinesia. If tetrabenazine[84–86] (see below), which has a much lower risk of tardive complications, is not available, a dose of about 0.5–1 mg per day of haloperidol or fluphenazine may be initiated, but the patient has to be followed carefully for any signs of tardive dyskinesia. Chlorpromazine enters the lipid bilayer and reverses echinocytic changes and has been studied not only as a symptomatic drug but also as a potential neuroprotective agent. In various case reports chlorpromazine had no effect on the course or symptoms of the disease.[1,3,26,36,56]

Dopamine depletors such as tetrabenazine and reserpine may be used to treat chorea in patients with NA. Reserpine and tetrabenazine deplete dopamine and serotonin from neuronal terminals; tetrabenazine also blocks the D_2 receptor. The usual dose of reserpine is 0.25–1 mg per day.[29,56] Tetrabenazine is given at a dose of 25 mg twice a day and increased to 50 mg three to four times a day as needed and as tolerated. Potential side effects of dopamine depleters include depression, sleepiness, gastrointestinal disturbance and a dose dependent parkinsonism.[84–86]

In NA patients with parkinsonian features dopaminergic agents such as levodopa may be beneficial, but the loss of dopamine receptors as indicated by pathologic and PET studies suggests that it may not be of much benefit.[28] Indeed, levodopa has been reported to produce only modest improvement of parkinsonian features.[2] Other medications such as trihexiphenidyl show no clinical benefit.[2,3] For patients with seizures phenytoin, phenobarbital, carbamazepine, valproic acid and clonazepam have been found to be effective.[3,4,24,29,36,52,53,55]

Botulinum toxin injections are useful for treating limb dystonia and injection under the tongue has been reported to provide benefit in patients with feeding dystonia.[44] One must, however, closely monitor response and repeat injections as needed, usually every three to four months. Side effects include local autonomic dysfunction, flu like reaction, and dysphagia if injected in the neck or tongue muscles. Surgical management for dystonia such as ramisectomy, rhizotomy, or transection of spinal accessory nerve (in case of cervical dystonia) and stereotactic procedures such as thalamotomy, pallidotomy and pallidal deep brain stimulation may be helpful in medically refractory cases.[82,87] Treatment of chorea with deep brain stimulation of the globus pallidus internum was unsuccessful in a single case but this has not been evaluated in patients with parkinsonism as a predominant feature.[87]

There are no reports of medical treatment of dementia associated with NA, although the acetylcholinesterases, such as donepezil, rivastigmine, and galantamine, may be tried. For behavioral problems such as depression, irritability, aggressiveness and depression, selective serotonin reuptake inhibitors (SSRIs) may be helpful. Clomipramine and SSRIs can also be helpful for the comorbid obsessive-compulsive disorder. If antipsychotics are needed for the treatment of delusions or hallucinations, atypical antipsychotics such as olanzapine or quetiapine are preferable because they are better tolerated and have a lower risk of tardive dyskinesia than the traditional typical neuroleptics.

Rehabilitation

Rehabilitation measures should include management of chorea, dysphagia and a regular exercise regimen.[88] Patients can benefit from trunk weights, positioning in semi-reclining chairs, and adequate padding in chairs. Adaptation at home and work place including precautions for falls must be undertaken. Patients should be provided with walkers as appropriate. Personal safety measures such as helmets, grab bars, padding on hard surfaces and appropriate floor textures would add to the quality of life of these patients. Swimming and stationary bikes are relatively safe methods of exercise. During the later stages of the disease, the aim must be to prevent contractures and a skin care program is essential to prevent skin breakdown.

Dysphagia should be evaluated early by a speech therapist, who can provide useful instructions for proper positioning during swallowing, consistency of food, and other techniques for efficient swallowing. Other helpful feeding adjustments include the use of thickeners, straws, and weighted cups. Built up rim for plates are helpful when patients with chorea feed themselves. Careful attention to dysphagia early in the disease helps prevent aspiration. Careful consideration should be given to enteric feeding by percutaneous gastrostomy as soon as patients show evidence of aspiration with the modified barium swallow test.

It is also important to provide patients and their families psychological support and counselling in order help them cope with the devastating effects of the disease. Genetic counselling should be provided to patients and family members. Recent genetic studies indicate that the spectrum of NA is broad as seen in a kindred with autosomal dominant inheritance with chorea, parkinsonism with acanthocytosis and presence of polyglutamine repeat in ubiquitinated intranuclear inclusions, and torsin A in the cerebral cortex on autopsy in one individual.[89] Future studies need to look more closely at the different mutations and possibility of gene therapy in such familial cases. Research into cellular and biochemical mechanisms of neurodegeneration in NA, including studies on neuronal membrane abnormalities may contribute to better understanding of the disease and lead to more effective treatments.

References

1. Yamamoto T, Hirose G, Shimazaki K, et al. Movement disorders of familial neuroacanthocytosis syndrome. Arch Neurol 1982;39:298–310
2. Spitz MC, Jankovic J, Killian JM. Familial tic disorder, parkinsonism, motor neuron disease and acanthocytosis: a new syndrome. Neurology 1985;35:366–377
3. Critchley EMR, Clark DB, Wikler A. Acanthocytosis and neurological disorder without abetalipoproteinemia. Arch Neurol 1968;18:134–140
4. Levine IM, Estes JW, Looney JM. Hereditary neurologic disease with acanthocytes: a new syndrome. Arch Neurol 1968;19:403–409
5. Estes JW, Morley T, Levine IM, et al. A new hereditary acanthocytosis syndrome. Am J Med 1967;42:868–881
6. Stevenson VL, Hardie RJ. Acanthocytosis and neurological disorders. J Neurol 2001;248(2):87–94
7. Kuroiwa Y, Ohnishi A, Sato Y, et al. Chorea acanthocytosis: clinical pathological and biochemical aspects. Intl J Neurol 1984;18:64–74
8. Hardie RJ, Pullon HWH, Harding AE, et al. Neuroacanthocytosis: a clinical, hematological and pathological study of 19 cases. Brain 1991;114:13–49
9. Quinn N, Schrag A. Huntington's disease and other choreas. J Neurol 1998;245(11):709–716
10. Rubio JP, Danek A, Stone C, et al. Chorea-acanthocytosis: genetic linkage to chromosome 9q21. Am J Hum Genet 1997;61:899–908
11. Requena CI, Arias GM, Lema DC, et al. Autosomal recessive chorea-acanthocytosis linked to 9q21. Neurologia 2000;15:132–135
12. Rubio JP, Levy ER, Dobson-Stone C, et al. Genomic organization of the human Gα14 and Gαq genes and mutation analysis in chorea-acanthocytosis (CHAC). Genomics 1999;57:84–93
13. Ueno S, Maruki Y, Nakamura M, et al. The gene encoding a newly discovered protein, chorein, is mutated in chorea-acanthocytosis. Nat Genet 2001;28:121–122
14. Rampoldi L, Dobson-Stone C, Rubio JP, et al. A conserved sorting-associated protein is mutant in chorea-acanthocytosis. Nat Genet 2001;28:119–120
15. Ho MF, Monaco AP, Blonden LA, et al. Fine mapping of the McLeod locus (XK) to a 150–380 kb region in Xp21. Am J Hum Genet 1992;50:317–330
16. Ho MF, Chelly J, Carter N, et al. Isolation of the gene for McLeod syndrome that encodes a novel membrane transport protein. Cell 1994;77(6):869–880
17. Ho MF, Chalmers DMB, Harding AE, et al. A novel point mutation in the McLeod syndrome gene in

neuroacanthocytosis. Ann of Neurol 1996;39(5):672–675

18. Hanaoka N, Yoshida K, Nakamura A, et al. A novel frameshift mutation in the McLeod syndrome gene in a Japanese family. J Neurol Sci 1999;165(1):6–9

19. Dotti MT, Battisti C, Malandrini A, et al. McLeod syndrome and neuroacanthocytosis with a novel mutation in the XK gene. Mov Disord 2000;15(6):1282–1284

20. El Nemer W, Colin Y, Collec E, et al. Analysis of deletions in three McLeod patients: exclusion of the XS locus from the Xp21.1–Xp21.2 region. Eur J Immunogenet 2000;27(1):29–33

21. Ueyama H, Kumamoto T, Nagao S, et al. A novel mutation of the McLeod syndrome gene in a Japanese family. J Neurol Sci 2000;176(2):151–154

22. Jung HH, Hergersberg M, Kneifel S, et al. McLeod syndrome: a novel mutation, predominant psychiatric manifestations, and distinct striatal imaging findings. Ann Neurol 2001;49(3):384–392

23. Sobue G, Mukai E, Fujii K, et al. Peripheral nerve involvement in familial chorea-acanthocytosis. J Neurol Sci 1986;76(2–3):347–356

24. Malandrini A, Fabrizi GM, Palmeri S, et al. Choreoacanthocytosis like phenotype without acanthocytes: clinicopathological case report. A contribution to the knowledge of the functional pathology of the caudate nucleus. Acta Neuropath (Berl) 1993;86:651–658

25. De Yebenes JG, Brin MF, Mena MA, et al. Neurochemical findings in neuroacanthocytosis. Mov Disord 1988;3:300–312

26. Alonso ME, Teixeira F, Jimenez G, et al. Chorea-acanthocytosis: report of a family and neuropathological study of two cases. Can J Neurol Sci 1989;16(4):426–431

27. Rinne JO, Daniel SE, Scaravilli F, et al. Neuropathological features of neuroacanthocytosis. Mov Disorders 1994;9(3):297–304

28. Rinne JO, Daniel SE, Scaravilli F, et al. Nigral degeneration in neuroacanthocytosis. Neurology 1994;44:1629–1632

29. Bird TD, Cederbaum S, Valey RW, Stahl WL. Familial degeneration of the basal ganglia with acanthocytosis: a clinical, neuropathological, and neurochemical study. Ann Neurol 1978;3(3):253–258

30. Kito S, Itoga E, Hiroshige Y, et al. A pedigree of amyotrophic chorea with acanthocytosis. Arch Neurol 1980;37(8):514–517

31. Sorrentino G, De Renzo A, Miniello S, et al. Late appearance of acanthocytes during the course of chorea-acanthocytosis. J Neurol Sci 1999;163(2):175–178

32. Ueno E, Oguchi K, Yanagisawa N. Morphological abnormalities of erythrocyte membrane in the hereditary neurological disease with chorea, areflexia and acanthocytosis. J Neurol Sci 1982;56(1):89–97

33. Oshima M, Osawa Y, Asano K, Saito T. Erythrocyte membrane abnormalities in patients with amyotrophic chorea with acanthocytosis. Part 1. Spin labeling studies and lipid analyses. J Neurol Sci 1985;68(2–3):147–160

34. Asano K, Osawa Y, Yanagisawa N, et al. Erythrocyte membrane abnormalities in patients with amyotrophic chorea with acanthocythosis. Part 2. Abnormal degradation of membrane proteins. J Neurol Sci 1985;68(2–3):161–173

35. Terada N, Fujii Y, Ueda H, et al. Ultrastructural changes of erythrocyte membrane skeletons in chorea-acanthocytosis and McLeod syndrome revealed by the quick-freezing and deep-etching method. Acta Haematol 1999;101(1):25–31

36. Freinberg TE, Cianci CD, Morrow JS, et al. Diagnostic tests for neuroacanthocytosis. Neurology 1991;41:1000–1006

37. Clark MR, Aminoff MJ, Chiu DT, et al. Red cell deformability and lipid composition in two forms of acanthocytosis: enrichment of acanthocytic populations by density gradient centrifugation. J Lab Clin Med 1989;113(4):469–481

38. Biemer JJ. Acanthocytosis: biochemical and physiological considerations. Ann Clin Lab Sci 1980;10(3):238–249

39. Bosman GJCGM, Bartholomeus IGP, DeGrip WJ, Horstink MWIM. Erythrocytic anion transporter and anti-brain immunoreactivity in chorea-acanthocytosis: a contribution to etiology, genetics and diagnosis. Brain Res Bull 1994;33(5):523–528

40. Kay MM, Goodman J, Goodman S, Lawrence C. Membrane protein band 3 alteration associated with neurologic disease and tissue-reactive antibodies. Exp Clin Immunogenet 1990;7(3):181–199

41. Olivieri O, De Franceschi L, Bordin L, et al. Increased membrane protein phosphorylation and anion transport activity in chorea-acanthocytosis. Haematologica 1997;82(6):648–653

42. Sakai T, Antoku Y, Iwashita H, et al. Chorea-acanthocytosis: abnormal composition of covalently bound fatty acids of erythrocyte membrane proteins. Ann Neurol 1991;29(6):664–669

43. Russo D, Redman C, Lee S. Association of XK and Kell blood group proteins. J Biol Chem 1998;273(22):13950–13956

44. Sakai T, Mawatari S, Iwashita H, et al. Choreoacanthocytosis. Clues to clinical diagnosis. Arch Neurol 1981;38(6):335–338

45. Sakai T, Iwashita H, Kakugawa M. Neuroacanthocytosis syndrome and chorea-acanthocytosis (Levine-Critchley syndrome). Neurology 1985;35(11):1679

46. Hardie RJ. Acanthocytosis and neurological impairment: a review. Q J Med 1989;71(264):291–306

47. Aasly J, Skansden T, Ro M. Neuroacanthocytosis: the variability of presenting symptoms in two siblings. Acta Neurol Scand 1999;100:322–325

48. Aguilar I, Bascompte JL, Berga L, et al. A further case of chorea-acanthocytosis. Acta Haematol 1988;80(3):175–176

49. Shibasaki H, Sakai T, Nishimura H, et al. Involuntary movements of chorea-acanthocytosis: a comparison with Huntington's chorea. Ann Neurol 1982;12(3):311–314

50. Bramanti P, Ricci RM, Candela L, et al. A polygraphic test for the diagnosis of amyotrophic choreo-acanthocytosis. Acta Neurol (Napoli) 1987;9(2):134–138

51. Bostantjopoulou S, Katsarou Z, Kazis A, Vadikolia C. Neuroacanthocytosis presenting as parkinsonism. Mov Disord 2000;15(6):1271–1273

52. Kazis A, Kimiskidis V, Georgiadis G, Voloudaki E. Neuroacanthocytosis presenting with epilepsy. J Neurol 1995;242(6):415–417

53. Schwartz MS, Monro PS, Leigh PN. Epilepsy as a presenting feature of neuroacanthocytosis in siblings. J Neurol 1992;239:261–262

54. Kartsounis LD, Hardie R. The pattern of cognitive impairments in neuroacanthocytosis: a frontal subcortical dementia. Arch Neurol 1996;53:77–80

55. Sotaniemi KA. Chorea-acanthocytosis. Neurological disease with acanthocytosis. Acta Neurol Scand 1983;68(1):53–56

56. Gross KB, Skrivanek JA, Carlson KC, Kaufman DM. Familial amyotrophic chorea with acanthocytosis. Arch Neurol 1985;42:753–757

57. Villegas A, Moscat J, Vazquez A, et al. A new family with hereditary chorea-acanthocytosis. Acta Haematol 1987;77(4):215–219

58. Vance JM, Pericak-Vance MA, Bowman MH, et al. Chorea-acanthocytosis: a report of three new families and implications for genetic counselling. Am J Med Genet 1987;28(2):403–410

59. Spencer SE, Walker FO, Moore SA. Chorea-amyotrophy with chronic hemolytic anemia: a variant of chorea-amyotrophy with acanthocytosis. Neurology 1987;37(4):645–649

60. Faillace RT, Kingston WJ, Nanda NC, Griggs RC. Cardiomyopathy associated with the syndrome of amyotrophic chorea and acanthocytosis. Ann Intern Med 1982;96(5):616–617

61. Barnett MH, Yang F, Iland H, Pollard JD. Unusual muscle pathology in McLeod syndrome. J Neurol Neurosurg Psychiatry 2000;69(5):655–657

62. Malandrini A, Fabrizi GM, Truschi F, et al. Atypical McLeod syndrome manifested as X-linked chorea-acanthocytosis, neuromyopathy and dilated cardiomyopathy: report of a family. J Neurol Sci 1994;124(1):89–94

63. Kawakami T, Takiyama Y, Sakoe K, et al. A case of McLeod syndrome with unusually severe myopathy. J Neurol Sci 1999;166(1):36–39

64. Takashima H, Sakai T, Iwashita H, Matsuda Y, et al. A family of McLeod syndrome, masquerading as chorea-acanthocytosis. J Neurol Sci 1994;124(1):56–60

65. Witt TN, Danek A, Reiter M, et al. McLeod syndrome: a distinct form of neuroacanthocytosis. Report of two cases and literature review with emphasis on neuromuscular manifestations. J Neurol 1992;239(6):302–306

66. Malandrini A, Fabrizi GM, Bartalucci P, et al. Clinicopathological study of familial late infantile Hallervorden-Spatz disease: a particular form of neuroacanthocytosis. Childs Nerv Syst 1996;12(3):155–160

67. Higgins JJ, Patterson MC, Pappadoupoulos NM, et al. Hypoprebetalipoproteinemia, acanthocytosis, retinitis pigmentosa, and pallidal degeneration (HARP syndrome). Neurology 1992;42(1):194–198

68. Orrell RW, Amrolia PJ, Heald A, et al. Acanthocytosis, retinitis pigmentosa, and pallidal degeneration: a report of three patients including the second reported case with hypoprebetalipoproteinemia (HARP syndrome). Neurology 1995;45(3 Pt 1):487–492

69. Jankovic J. Differential diagnosis and etiology of tics. In: Cohen DJ, Jankovic J, Goetz CG, eds. Tourette Syndrome, Adv Neurol. Vol 85. Philadelphia: Lippincott Williams and Wilkins, 2001:15–29

70. Gross KB, Skrivanek JA, Emeson EE. Ganglioside abnormality in amyotrophic chorea with acanthocytosis. Lancet 1982;2(8301):772

71. Hirayama M, Hamano T, Shiratori M, et al. Chorea-acanthocytosis with polyclonal antibodies to ganglioside GM1. J Neurol Sci 1997;151(1):23–24

72. Kutcher JS, Kahn MJ, Andersson HC, Foundas AL. Neuroacanthocytosis masquerading as Huntington's disease: CT/MRI findings. J Neuroimaging 1999;9(3):187–189

73. Okamoto K, Ito J, Furusawa T, et al. CT and MRI findings of neuroacanthocytosis. J Comput Assist Tomogr 1997;21(2):221–222

74. Serra S, Xerra A, Scribano E, et al. Computerized tomography in amyotrophic chorea-acanthocytosis. Neuroradiol 1987;29(5):480–482

75. Tanaka M, Hirai S, Kondo S, et al. Cerebral hypoperfusion and hypometabolism with altered striatal signal intensity in chorea-acanthocytosis: a combined PET and MRI study. Mov Disord 1998;13(1):100–107

76. Hardie R. Cerebral hypoperfusion and hypometabolism in chorea-acanthocytosis. Mov Disord 1998;13(5):853–854

77. Brooks DJ, Ibanez V, Playford ED, et al. Pre synaptic and post synaptic striatal dopaminergic function in neuroacanthocytosis: a positron emission tomographic study. Ann Neurol 1991;30:166–171

78. Danek A, Uttner I, Vogl T, et al. Cerebral involvement in McLeod syndrome. Neurology 1994;44(1):117–120

79. Vita G, Serra S, Dattola R, et al. Peripheral neuropathy in amyotrophic chorea-acanthocytosis. Ann Neurol 1989;26(4):583–587

80. Gross KB, Skrivanek JA, Carlson KC, Kaufman DM. Familial amyotrophic chorea with acanthocytosis. New clinical and laboratory investigations. Arch Neurol 1985;42(8):753–756

81. Aminoff MJ. Acanthocytosis and neurological disease. Brain 1972;95:749–760

82. Limos LC, Ohnishi A, Sakai T, et al. "Myopathic" changes in chorea-acanthocytosis. Clinical and histopathological studies. J Neurol Sci 1982;55(1):49–58

83. Ohnishi A, Sato Y, Nagara H, et al. Neurogenic muscular atrophy and low density of large myelinated fibres of sural nerve in chorea-acanthocytosis. J Neurol Neurosurg Psych 1981;44(7):645–648

84. Jankovic J, Orman J. Tetrabenazine therapy of dystonia, chorea, tics, and other dyskinesias. Neurology 1988;38(3):391–394

85. Jankovic J. Treatment of hyperkinetic movement disorders with tetrabenazine: a double-blind crossover study. Ann Neurol 1982;11(1):41–47

86. Kingston D. Tetrabenazine for involuntary movement disorders. Med J Aust 1979;1(13):628–630

87. Wihl G, Volkmann J, Allert N, et al. Deep brain stimulation of the internal pallidum did not improve chorea in a patient with neuro-acanthocytosis. Mov Disord 2001;16(3):572–575

88. Francis KD, Rubin AJ. Movement disorders including tremors. In: Grabois M, Garrison S, Hart KA, Lehmkuhl D, eds. Physical Medicine and Rehabilitation, the Complete Approach. Blackwell Sci. Inc. UK, 2000

89. Walker RH, Morgello S, Davidoff-Feldman B, et al. Autosomal dominant chorea-acanthocytosis with polyglutamine-containing neuronal inclusions. Neurology 2002; 58(7):1031–1037

241 Sydenham Chorea

Cathy Chuang and Blair Ford

Historical background

Sydenham chorea (also known as St. Vitus' dance, chorea minor, rheumatic chorea, and auto-immune chorea) was first described by Thomas Sydenham in 1686 as an acute chorea of childhood.[1] Its association with "rheumatism," first described in the 19th century by Bouteille, was later explained by an infection with group A beta hemolytic streptococcus.[2] However, since chorea can often be the sole manifestation of acute rheumatic fever (ARF) in the absence of any clinical or laboratory evidence of rheumatic inflammation, this relationship remained controversial for many years. It was not clarified until 1956 when Taranta and Stollerman demonstrated that chorea is a late manifestation of streptococcal infection which occurs when typical antibody titers are on a downward trend.[3]

Epidemiology

The incidence of Sydenham chorea (SC) has been steadily decreasing along with the decline in both the severity and incidence of acute rheumatic fever. In Eshel's recent 30 year survey (1960–1990), the incidence of chorea fell from 4.15 to 1.21 per 100 000 between the second and third decades.[4] However, there have been a few recent reports of a possible resurgence in the last decade.[5]

The age of onset ranges between three and 17 years, with a mean age of nine to ten. It is nearly twice as common in females than males, and has a seasonal predominance in the spring time following the peak occurrence of acute rheumatic fever.[2,6,7] The duration of chorea can range from one week to two years with an average duration of four months.[7] Recurrences occur in about 20–30% of cases.[2,6–8] "Pure chorea" in the absence of carditis or polyarthritis occurs in between 24–74% of case studies.[3,7–9] Family history of either rheumatic fever or chorea is present in 8.9–36% of cases.[2,6,7]

Clinical features

The main clinical feature, chorea, is often accompanied by dysarthria, ataxia, and personality changes including emotional lability, inattention, obsessive-compulsive behavior, and irritability.[2,6–8,10] Examination reveals hypotonia, hung-up reflexes, lack of coordination, and motor impersistence in the form of "milk-maid's grip," "darting tongue," and "pronator sign."[7] The chorea is usually bilateral but in 10–20% it is unilateral.[6,7] There is usually a benign, self-limited course without any neurological or psychological sequelae, but approximately 30% will develop cardiac complications of ARF.[2,6–8] There have been reports of minor abnormalities of coordination,[11] tremor and residual chorea,[12] and reappearance of chorea under stress later in life.[9] Patients with a history of SC are also more susceptible to drug-induced chorea and recurrence of chorea during pregnancy (chorea gravidarum).[12]

Neuroimaging is usually normal but recent studies have revealed basal ganglia lesions on magnetic resonance imaging (MRI)[13–15] and striatal hypermetabolism on fluorodeoxyglucose positron emission tomography (FDG-PET)[16,17] and single photon emission computed tomography (SPECT).[18,19] An abnormal electroencephalogram (EEG) is common with diffuse slowing occurring in between 29–85% of cases.[2,14] Laboratory evidence of recent streptococcal infection by erythrocyte sedimentation rate (ESR), throat culture, and antistreptolysin O (ASO) titer is variably present.[2,3,5,8,10] Husby found that 46% of patients with SC had anti-neuronal antibodies reacting to subthalamic nucleus and caudate nucleus antigens compared to 14% of patients with rheumatic carditis and 1.8–4% of normal controls. Positive antibodies correlated with disease severity.[20] The B-cell alloantigen, D8/17, has been found to be expressed in higher levels (>20%) in patients with rheumatic fever, as compared to controls (<7%). This antigen was recently reported to be present in two patients with isolated chorea as the initial manifestation of ARF.[21] This may be a more sensitive diagnostic test to support the diagnosis of SC. Neuropathological studies have been rare in this non-fatal disease but have usually shown widespread vascular, degenerative, or inflammatory lesions with some predilection for the striatum.[2,22–24]

Differential diagnosis of childhood chorea includes Wilson's disease, hyperthyroidism, systemic lupus erythematosus, antiphospholipid syndrome, stroke, Huntington's disease, benign hereditary chorea, neuroacanthocytosis, and drug-induced chorea secondary to anticholinergics, levodopa, neuroleptics, anticonvulsants, or oral contraceptives.[25]

Treatment

Historically, the treatment of SC, has been best described in the words of Schwartzmann: "of the therapies used in the past, there is no limit to the measures tried."[8] The gamut of remedies employed includes arsenic as a "general tonic" and appetite stimulant,[2] amidopyrine, chloretone, sulfanilamide, phenylethylhydantoin,[26,27] injections of milk or insulin, intravenous sodium salicylate or blood transfusions, intravenous or intraspinal magnesium, sulphur

Table 241.1	Therapy for Sydenham's chorea	
	Recommended dose	**Potential side effects**
First line agents		
Anticonvulsants:		
Valproic acid	15–20 mg/kg/day divided bid or tid	Nausea, ataxia, dizziness, sedation, tremor, hirsutism rash, bone marrow suppression, hepatitis, penerantitis
Carbamazepine	15–25 mg/kg/day divided tid	
Gabapentin	300 mg tid, maximum 1200–1600 mg tid	Rash, sedation, nausea, dry mouth, bone marrow suppression
Second line agents		
Dopamine depleters:		
Tetrabenazine	25 to 50 mg tid	Somnolence, fatigue, dizziness, nausea
Reserpine	0.5 mg bid, titrate dose as tolerated	Sedation, hypotension, depression, parkinsonism
Benzodiazepines:		
Clonazepam	0.5 mg bid or tid, titrate dose as tolerated	Sedation, ataxia, behavioral problems
Third line agents		
D2-receptor blocking agents:	0.5 mg to 5 mg bid or tid	Sedation, parkinsonism, tardive syndromes, dystonic reactions, hypotension
Haloperidol		
Prophylactic therapy		
Benzathine penicillin	10 days of IM injections followed by monthly injections of 1.2 million units of penicillin for 5 years	Allergic reactions, nausea, seizures

injections, intraspinal electrargol or serum, fever therapy, typhoid shock, ammonium chloride, triple bromides, quinine, calcium, diphenhydramine, ketogenic diet, vitamins such as pyridoxine and thiamine, and psychotherapy.[8,28] Most of these treatments were either ineffective or resulted in significant side effects.[8,26–29]

Fever therapy was once a standard treatment for SC with efficacy rates between 75–100%.[28,30–32] This consisted of raising the patient's temperature to 104–107°F for two hours using either a "hot-box" or injecting typhoid vaccine. Pyridoxine, vitamin E, and thiamine have also reported to be effective treatments.[8,29,31,33] When these were abandoned, bed rest, isolation, and sedation with bromides, barbiturates, or benzodiazepines became popular treatment modalities.[2,8,9,34]

Based on the presumed inflammatory nature of this disease, corticosteroids and ACTH have been used with variable results. Older reports did not find cortisone or adrenocorticotropic hormone (ACTH) treatment effective,[35,36] but subsequent studies have shown more favorable results.[37,38] Based on the more recent discovery of anti-neuronal antibodies in SC and the postulated autoimmune pathophysiological mechanism, the use of immunomodulatory therapies has been further studied in a controlled trial of plasmapheresis and intravenous immunoglobulin (IVIG), with good preliminary results.[10,39,40] Neuroleptics such as chlorpromazine and haloperidol have been demonstrated to be effective therapy for chorea.[41,42] However, given the risk of extrapyramidal side effects, specifically tardive dyskinesia and dystonia, these should be avoided.[43]

More recently, several reports have demonstrated that anticonvulsants, specifically valproic acid and car-bamazepine, are very effective at controlling chorea with a low risk of side effects. These agents have even helped in cases where haloperidol and benzodiazepines have failed.[44–48] Therefore, valproic acid and carbamazepine should be the first line of therapy for SC. The usual dosage for valproic acid is 15–20 mg/kg/day divided two or three times per day, and for carbamazepine is 15–25 mg/kg/day divided three times per day. Gabapentin was recently reported to be effective at treating a patient with delayed-onset hemichorea-hemiballism secondary to a stroke, and therefore may be effective at treating other secondary causes of chorea. The starting dose of gabapentin is 300 mg three times a day and can be gradually increased every week up to a maximum dose of 1200–1600 mg three times per day.[49] Alternative therapies for chorea resistant to anticonvulsants include reserpine and tetrabenazine (TBZ), which are depletors of presynaptic dopamine storage. Both have been found to be effective, and do not pose the added risk of tardive consequences that neuroleptics do.[50,51] Potential side effects, however, include sedation, hypotension, depression, and parkinsonism. The dosage of reserpine is 0.1 mg twice a day, increased to 0.5 mg per day by the end of three weeks. Tetrabenazine is not currently available in the United States. The usual dose is 25 mg three times per day (see Table).

Since all of these medications have potential side effects, it is important to comment on the necessity of symptomatic treatment for SC. Some cases of chorea may be mild and since the course is usually benign and self-limited, medical therapy is only warranted when the involuntary movements, dysarthria, ataxia, or behavioral changes become so disabling that they interfere with the normal functional abilities of the child. In mild, non-disabling, cases, children should not be treated merely for cosmetic or social reasons, and parents should be reassured of the benign nature of the condition. However, regardless of whether symptomatic therapy is required, all children with SC should be treated with prophylactic therapy to prevent recurrences or other potential complications of ARF. Most studies have recommended 10 days of intramuscular benzathine penicillin followed by monthly injections of 1.2 million units of penicillin for five years or until age 18 or 20.[2,8,52] However, it is not known whether five years is sufficient since recurrences of SC can occur after this period.[2]

References

1. Sydenham T. The whole works of that excellent practical physician, Dr. Thomas Sydenham. 10th ed. London: R. Wellington, 1734
2. Thiebaut F. Sydenham's chorea. In: Vinken PJ, Bruyn GW, eds. Handbook of Clinical Neurology. Vol 8. Amsterdam: North-Holland Publishing Company, 1968: 409–436
3. Taranta A, Stollerman GH. The relationship of Sydenham's chorea in infection with group A streptococci. Am J Med 1956;20:170–175
4. Eshel G, Lahat E, Azizi E, et al. Chorea as manifestation of rheumatic fever. A 30-year survey (1960–1990). Eur J Pediatr 1993;152:645–646
5. Ryan M, Antony JH, Grattan-Smith PJ. Sydenham's chorea: a resurgence in the 1990's? J Pediatr Child Health 2000;36:95–96
6. Nausieda PA, Grossman BJ, Koller WC, et al. Sydenham chorea: an update. Neurol 1980;30:331–334
7. Aron AM, Freeman JM, Carter S. The natural history of Sydenham's chorea. Am J M 1965;38:83–95
8. Schwartzman J. Chorea Minor. Review of 175 cases with reference to etiology, treatment, and sequelae. Rheumatism 1950;6:89–95
9. Lessof M. Sydenham's chorea. Guys Hosp Report 1958; 107:185–206
10. Swedo SE, Leonard HL, Schapiro MB, et al. Sydenham's chorea: physical and psychological symptoms of St. Vitus dance. Pediatr 1993;91:706–713
11. Bird MT, Palkes H, Prensky AL. A follow-up study of Sydenham's chorea. Neurol 1976;26:601–606
12. Nausieda PA, Bieliauskas LA, Bacon LD, et al. Chronic dopaminergic sensitivity after Sydenham's chorea. Neurol 1983;33:750–754
13. Kienzle GD, Breger RK, Chun RWM, et al. Sydenham chorea: MR manifestations in two cases. AJNR 1991; 12:73–76
14. Heye N, Jergas M, Hotzinger H, et al. Sydenham chorea: clinical, EEG, MRI, and SPECT findings in the early stage of the disease. J Neurol 1993;240:121–123
15. Emery ES, Vieco PT. Sydenham chorea: magnetic resonance imaging reveals permanent basal ganglia injury. Neurol 1997;48:531–533
16. Goldman S, Amrom D, Szliwowski HB, et al. Reversible striatal hypermetabolism in a case of Sydenham's chorea. Mov Dis 1993;8:355–358
17. Weindl A, Kuwert T, Leenders KL, et al. Increased striatal glucose consumption in Sydenham's chorea. Mov Dis 1993;8:437–444
18. Lee PH, Nam HS, Lee KY, et al. Serial brain SPECT images in a case of Sydenham chorea. Arch Neurol 1999;56:237–240
19. Dilenge ME, Shevell MI, Dinh L. Restricted unilateral Sydenham's chorea: reversible contralateral striatal hypermetabolism demonstrated on single photon emission computed tomographic scanning. J Child Neurol 1990;14:509–513
20. Husby G, van de Rijn I, Zabriske JB, et al. Antibodies reacting with cytoplasm of subthalamic and caudate nuclei neurons in chorea and acute rheumatic fever. J Exp Med 1976;144:1094–1110
21. Feldman BM, Zabriske JB, Silverman ED, Laxer RM. Diagnostic use of B-cell alloantigen D8/17 in rheumatic chorea. J Pediatr 1993;123:84–86
22. Colony HS, Malamud N. Sydenham's chorea. A clinicopathological study. Neurol 1956;6:672–676
23. Greenfield JG, Wolfsohn JM. The pathology of Sydenham's chorea. Lancet 1922;2:603–606
24. Ichikawa K, Kim RC, Givelber H, Collins H. Chorea gravidarum. Report of a fatal case with neuropathological observations. Arch Neurol 1980;37:429–432
25. Schrag A, Quinn N. Huntington's disease and other choreas. J Neurol 1998;245:709–716
26. Kirk TR. Phenyethylhydantoin in the treatment of Sydenham's chorea. New York State J Med 1948;48: 2165–2167
27. Greenwald HM, Greenberg B. Treatment of Sydenham's chorea with Nirvanol. Arch Pediatr 1941;58: 48–57
28. Schwartzman J, McDonald DH, Perillo L. Sydenham's chorea. Report of 140 cases and review of the literature. Arch Pediatr 1948;65:6–23
29. Graham S. Arsenic in the treatment of chorea. Arch Dis Child 1928;3:206–209
30. Bennett AE, Hoekstra CS. The pathogenesis, diagnosis, and management of infectious chorea. Dis Nerv System 1941;2:199–202
31. Stone S. Treatment of Sydenham's chorea by fever and vitamin B therapy. New Eng J Med 1940;223:489–496
32. Weisman DL. Treatment of Sydenham's chorea with typhoid paratyphoid vaccine. New York State J Med 1936;36:1587–1598
33. Dowd G. Alpha-tocopherol in the management of Sydenham's chorea. Ann New York Acad Sci 1949;52: 419–421
34. El-Ghalmi A, Aboul-Dahab YW. Hydroxyzine in the treatment of rheumatic chorea in children. Arch Pediatr 1961;78:478–482
35. Aronson N, Douglas H, Lewis JM. Cortisone in Sydenham's chorea. Report of two cases. JAMA 1951;145: 30–33
36. Dixon A St. J, Bywaters GL. Methods of assessing therapy in chorea with special reference to the use of ACTH. Arch Dis Child 1952;27:161–166
37. Ainger LE, Ely RS, Done AK, Kelley VC. Sydenham's chorea. Effects of hormone therapy. Am J Dis Child 1955;89:580–590
38. Green LN. Corticosteroids in the treatment of Sydenham's chorea. Arch Neurol 1978;35:53–54
39. Swedo SE. Sydenham's chorea. A model of childhood autoimmune neuropsychiatric disorders. JAMA 1994; 272:1788–1791
40. Garvey MA, Swedo SE, Shapiro MB, et al. Intravenous immunoglobulin (IVIG) and plasmapharesis as effective treatments of Sydenham's chorea (SC). Neurol 1996;46(Suppl 2):A147
41. Shenker DM, Grossman HJ, Klawans HL. Treatment of Sydenham's chorea with haloperidol. Develop Med Child Neurol 1973;15:19–24
42. Tierney RC, Kaplan S. Treatment of Sydenham's

chorea. Am J Dis Child 1965;109:408–411

43. Shields WD, Bray PF. A danger of haloperidol therapy in children. J Pediatr 1976;88:301–302

44. Alvarez LA, Novak G. Valproic acid in the treatment of Sydenham's chorea. Pediatr Neurol 1985;1:317–319

45. Daoud AS, Zaki M, Shakir R, Al-Saleh Q. Effectiveness of sodium valproate in the treatment of Sydenham's chorea. Neurol 1990;40:1140–1141

46. McLachlan RS. Valproic acid in Sydenham's chorea. Br Med J 1981;283:274–275

47. Dhanaraj M, Radhakrishnan AR, Srinivas K, Sayeed ZA. Sodium valproate in Sydenham's chorea. Neurol 1985;35:114–115

48. Roig M, Montserrat L, Gallarat A. Carbamazepine: an alternative drug for the treatment of nonhereditary chorea. Pediatr 1988;82:492–495

49. Kothare SV, Pollack P, Kulberg AG, Ravin PD. Gabapentin treatment in a child with delayed-onset hemichorea/hemiballismus. Pediatr Neurol 2000; 22:68–71

50. Naidu S, Narasimhachari N. Sydenham's chorea: a possible presynaptic dopaminergic dysfunction initially. Ann Neurol 1980;8:445–447

51. Hawkes CH, Nourse CH. Tetrabenazine in Sydenham's chorea. Br Med J 1977;1:1391–1392

242 Ballism and Chorea

Kapil Dev Sethi

Ballism, meaning "to throw" in Greek, refers to violent, irregular flinging movements of the limbs primarily due to contractions of the proximal muscles. "Hemiballism" refers to movements involving the upper and lower extremities on the same side with or without involvement of the face. "Monoballism" refers to ballism confined to one extremity. Paraballism is a term given to ballism affecting the lower extremities and bilateral ballism refers to ballism affecting both sides of the body.[1] The most common form of ballism seen in clinical practice is hemiballism.

Chorea consists of irregular, non-repetitive, brief, jerky, flowing movements that move randomly from one part of the body to another. The movements are brisk and abrupt in some cases (such as in Sydenham's chorea). While in others, they are slower and more flowing (as in Huntington's disease). The term "choreoathetosis" has been used in this latter situation where chorea may be combined with features of dystonia and athetosis.

It is generally accepted that ballism and chorea reflect a continuum of the same disorder and may coexist in the same patient, or ballism may evolve into chorea or dystonia. There is an overlap between chorea and ballism in regard to etiology, pathogenesis and treatment. Therefore, these two are discussed together in this chapter.

History

Kussmaul was the first to employ the term hemiballism in 1895.[2] Jakob, and then Martin, established the clinicopathological correlation of hemiballism with the lesion of the contralateral subthalamic nucleus of Luys.[3,4] Subsequently, experimental studies in the Rhesus monkey firmly linked lesions of the subthalamic nucleus with contralateral hemiballism.[5–7] There have been several descriptions of hemiballism in which the contralateral subthalamic nucleus was spared; in these instances the lesions involved the thalamus, neostriatum, or the cerebral cortex.[8,9] Crossman demonstrated that injections of gamma amino butyric acid (GABA) antagonists into the subthalamic nucleus or in different regions of the lenticular nucleus produced hemiballism in alert monkeys.[10,11]

The term chorea was used to describe a variety of movement disorders in the early literature. Some of these like Morvan's fibrillary chorea are now known to be fasciculations. The term St Vitus dance came into use in the seventeenth century to describe an epidemic dance psychosis. Sydenham was the first to isolate the nosological entity of "chorea minor" s. *infectiosa* from the heterogenous group of St Vitus dance. Sydenham's chorea was subsequently linked with rheumatism and endocarditis.[12]

On February 15th, 1872, George Huntington delivered a lecture on Sydenham's chorea and only in the last paragraph did he mention chronic progressive hereditary chorea as a curiosity.[13] This was soon recognized by many to be of autosomal dominant inheritance.[13] The gene for Huntington's disease (HD) was localized to chromosome 4 in 1983[14,15] and after a diligent search for over 10 years found to be an excessive number of CAG repeats.[16]

Epidemiology

Ballism is an infrequent movement disorder. The exact prevalence is unknown but in a large movement disorder clinic 21 cases of hemiballism were seen out of 3084 patients.[17] The exact frequency of choreic disorders other than HD is unclear. Huntington's disease occurs with a worldwide prevalence of 5–10 per 100 000 population.[18]

Etiology

Ballism and chorea may be seen in a variety of clinical situations. The reported causes of ballism are listed in Table 242.1. The causes of biballism appear in Table 242.2. The etiologic classification of chorea is given in Table 242.3.

Pathophysiology and pathogenesis

Classically, ballism has been associated with an ischemic or hemorrhagic lesion of the contralateral subthalamic nucleus of Luys. However, recent neuroimaging studies have shown that the lesions of areas outside of subthalamic nucleus (such as the caudate and putamen) are found more often than previously thought.[17] There seems to be a somatotopic organization within the subthalamic nucleus. In monoballism affecting the lower extremity, the posterior portion of the subthalamic nucleus is involved.[19] Whenever the globus pallidus is involved, the lesion is in the external segment. The classic studies of Carpenter established a sound, clinicopathological correlation between experimental lesions of the subthalamic nucleus and contralateral hemiballism. They showed that for the production of hemiballism the lesion had to involve at least 20% of the subthalamic nucleus.[7] Interestingly, by making a lesion in the globus pallidus they were able to abolish the hemiballism.

According to the current models of the basal ganglia circuitry the subthalamic nucleus is an integral part of the indirect pathway and it exerts an excitatory influence on the medial globus pallidus.

Table 242.1   The causes of hemiballism

1. Vascular causes
   Infarction affecting the subthalamic nucleus or its connections or the striatum
   Transient vascular insufficiency involving anterior circulation or the posterior circulation
   Arteriovenous malformation
   Venous angioma
   Subdural hematoma

2. Brain tumors
   Primary (i.e. cystic gliomas and other cysts)
   Metastatic brain tumors

3. Infectious and post-infectious
   Tuberculous meningitis with or without tuberculoma
   Sydenham's chorea
   AIDS with cerebral toxoplasmosis
   Cysticercosis

4. Autoimmune disorders
   Systemic lupus erythematosus

5. Iatrogenic
   Oral contraceptives
   Surgical complication of stereotactic thalamotomy and pallidotomy
   Transiently in deep brain stimulation of subthalamic area in Parkinson's disease

6. Metabolic causes
   Hyperglycemia

7. Degenerative diseases
   Multiple systems atrophy
   Tuberous sclerosis

8. Miscellaneous
   Multiple sclerosis
   Head trauma

Table 242.2   Causes of bilateral ballism

Bilateral striatal hemorrhagic infarctions
Multiple sclerosis
Phenytoin intoxication
Oral contraceptives
Disseminated intravascular dissemination of cancer
Systemic lupus erythematosus
Ventriculoperitoneal shunting
Nonketotic hyperglycemia
Dopaminergic drugs – induced dyskinesia in Parkinson's disease

Table 242.3   Etiological classification of chorea

1. Developmental choreas
   Physiological chorea of infancy

2. Cerebral palsy – anoxic, kernicterus

3. Hereditary choreas
   Huntington's disease
   Benign hereditary chorea
   Neuroacanthocytosis
   Spinocerebellar ataxias
   Ataxia telangiectasia
   Tuberous sclerosis
   Hallervorden-Spatz Syndrome
   Dentatorubral-pallidoluysian atrophy (DRPLA)
   Familial calcification of basal ganglia

4. Metabolic disorders
   Wilson's disease
   Mitochondrial disease e.g. Leigh's disease
   Porphyria
   Aminoacidopathies (propionic academia)

5. Drug induced chorea
   Dopamine blocking agents (tardive dyskinesia or withdrawal emergent syndrome)
   Antiparkinsonian drugs
   Anticonvulsants
   Amphetamines, cocaine
   Tricyclics
   Oral contraceptives
   Anticholinergics
   Lithium
   Digoxin

6. Systemic metabolic disorders
   Hyperthyroidism
   Hypoparathyroidism
   Chorea gravidarum
   Hyper and hyponatremia
   Hypomagnesemia, hypocalcemia
   Hypoglycemia
   Hyperglycemia
   Acquired hepatocerebral degeneration
   Polycythemia rubra vera

7. Infectious and post-infectious
   Sydenham's chorea
   Tuberculous meningitis
   AIDS

8. Immunological
   SLE and the primary antiphospholipid syndrome

9. Vascular (often hemichorea)
   Infarction
   Hemorrhage
   AVM

10. Tumors

11. Trauma – including subdural and epidural hematoma

SLE, systemic lupus erythematosis; AVM, arteriovenous malformation.
AVM, arteriovenous malformation

Normally the lateral globus pallidus is inhibited by an output from the striatum and in turn inhibits the subthalamic nucleus. Hemiballism is believed to be due to a lack of tonic inhibition of the lateral globus pallidus by the putamen, leading to a greater inhibition of subthalamic nucleus and lack of excitation of the medial globus pallidus, leading to disinhibition of the thalamus and the motor cortex.[20] This may not hold true for every case of ballism and does not explain why a lesion of the presumably under-excited or inactive medial globus pallidus would abolish hemiballism in experimental situations.[7] Also, this model does not explain the rare occurrence of hemiballism with a lesion of the lateral pallidal segment.

Chorea may have a similar mechanism but the disorders resulting in chorea are often subacute or chronic and there may have been complex adaptive changes as a result of the degenerative process.

The neurochemistry of Huntington's disease and neuroacanthocytosis has been studied well and the reader is referred to these chapters. The neurochemistry of hemiballism and chorea in other disorders is less clear. The existing evidence points to an overactivity of dopaminergic systems. The evidence includes a response to dopamine blocking agents and dopamine depleting agents and an elevation of cerebrospinal fluid homovanillic acid (HVA).[21,22] The role of other neurotransmitters like GABA may be important. This is supported by the induction of hemiballism/hemichorea by the injections of GABA antagonists into the subthalamic nucleus or in different regions of the lenticular nucleus in alert monkeys.[10,11]

Neurophysiological investigations of hemiballism are sparse. One study demonstrated that the electromyographic discharges due to the involuntary movements in hemiballism were more regular and rhythmic than those seen in Huntington's chorea. This suggests the activation of neural circuits involved in tremor in addition to those involved in chorea.[23] In chorea random discharges of agonist and antagonistic muscles are observed in bursts that are very variable in duration. Some bursts are short while longer bursts reminiscent of dystonia may be seen.[24]

Clinical manifestations

Typically, hemiballism has an acute onset but in some instances may evolve over several days to weeks. The patient may be awakened by the abrupt onset of violent flinging movements of the proximal parts of an arm and a leg on one side of the body. The movements can cause injury of the involved limbs and exhaustion. Less commonly, there may be involvement of the same side of the face, with facial and tongue movements. Distally, the choreic movements of the fingers may be apparent. The movements are said to disappear during sleep, but careful observations have revealed that hemiballism may persist during lighter stages of sleep. The involuntary movements may be improved with action but, more frequently, they are worsened by attempts to move.

Bilateral ballism is uncommon. It results in severe bilateral movements with dysarthria, dysphagia, and in rare cases, mutism.

Chorea is characterized by random, irregular, and non-repetitive jerky movements. The onset and evolution of these movements depends on the underlying etiology. Vascular chorea may be abrupt in onset while degenerative disorders like HD result in an insidious onset of movements that may be barely perceptible for years.

Differential diagnosis

Ballism and chorea need to be differentiated from tics, myoclonus, and other involuntary movements. Myoclonus refers to lightning jerks and is often action

and stimulus-sensitive. Tics result in more complex stereotyped movements that are often under the patient's voluntary control. In addition, the patient has an urge to execute these movements, an urge that is relieved by the actual movement. The movements wax and wane over time and may be associated with psychiatric manifestations like obsessive-compulsive features.

Laboratory investigations

In the setting of acute hemiballism, an imaging study—preferably computed tomography (CT) with contrast enhancement to look for hemorrhage and other lesions is advisable. A magnetic resonance imaging (MRI) scan with enhancement may be necessary to look for small lesions of the subthalamic nucleus or areas of abnormal enhancement consistent with tumor or abscess. Magnetic resonance imaging may also reveal multiple lacunes in vascular chorea or hemorrhagic infarctions in cases with non-ketotic hyperglycemia.[25]

Routine blood chemistry should include fasting and postprandial blood sugar determinations and measurement of serum calcium. In appropriate patients, anti-epileptic drug levels should be obtained. In young patients with hemiballism, one should look for evidence of acquired immune deficiency syndrome (AIDS). In a child with chorea or ballism one should always look for evidence of previous streptococcal infection and active carditis. In selected cases genetic testing for HD should be obtained and a fresh blood film examined for acanthocytes.

Serum antinuclear antibodies and anticardiolipin antibodies should be looked for in young women with chorea/ballism.

Treatment

The management should be aimed at the treatment of the underlying cause and the symptomatic treatment of chorea/ballism itself. Because of the diversity of underlying disorders resulting in chorea/ballism this review will focus on symptomatic therapy. However a brief mention will be made of approaches to the treatment of the underlying cause in certain situations.

Hemiballism due to destructive lesions is treated symptomatically. The natural history of hemiballism due to vascular causes is that of slow resolution over weeks to months.[26] In other instances a prolonged course with death due to exhaustion has been reported. Most reports of successful interventions in hemiballism have been open label studies or anecdotal experiences. In the absence of double-blind crossover studies it is difficult to assess the efficacy of a given drug in this disorder with such a variable course (Table 242.4, Evidence class III).

The general approach to symptomatic therapy for chorea and ballism is very similar. The aim is to block the postsynaptic dopamine D_2 receptors, to deplete dopamine, or to increase GABA-ergic neurotransmission. However, in the case of hemiballism that runs its

Table 242.4   Drug treatment of chorea/ballism

Drug class	Drug	Usual dose	Side effects	Evidence Class
1. Dopamine depleting agents	Reserpine	0.75 mg–4.0 mg per day	Sedation, depression, parkinsonism, hypotension	III
	Tetrabenazine	75 mg–200 mg per day	Sedation, parkinsonism, hypotension, sialorrhea	II
2. Dopamine blocking agents	Chlorpromazine	75 mg–300 mg	Akathisia, sedation, dysphoria, dyskinesia, hypotension	III
	Perphenazine	6 mg–32 mg	Akathisia, sedation, dysphoria, tardive dyskinesia, hypotension, dysphoria	III
	Haloperidol	3 mg–30 mg	Akathisia, sedation, dysphoria, dyskinesia, hypotension	III
IM	Fluphenazine	25 mg–62.5 mg IM every 2 weeks	Akathisia, sedation, dysphoria, dyskinesia, hypotension	II
3. Atypical neuroleptics	Olanzapine	5 mg–10 mg	Akathisia, sedation	III
	Risperidone	2 mg–12 mg	Hypotension, tardive dyskinesia	III
	Clozapine	50 mg–200 mg	Sedation, sialorrhea	III
4. Anticonvulsants	Sodium valproate	750 mg–1500 mg per day	Tremors, hair loss, weight gain	III
	Carbamazepine	15 mg–24 mg/kg in children	Ataxia, diplopia, sedation	III
5. GABA-generic drugs	Clonazepam	3 mg–5 mg	Sedation, dependence	III
	Progabide	900 mg		III
6. Miscellaneous	Ondansetron	24 mg per day		III
	Verapamil	240 mg per day	Constipation	

IM, intramuscular.

course over weeks, one is more liberal with the use of dopamine blocking agents (DBA). In the case of chorea that is usually chronic the DBA are avoided due to the risk of inducing tardive dyskinesia superimposed on the pre-existing chorea.

Dopamine depleting agents

Chorea/ballism is thought to result from a relative overactivity of the dopaminergic systems. Dopamine depleting agents have been used to treat chorea/ballism.[22,27,28] Two dopamine depleting drugs, tetrabenazine and reserpine, have been successfully. Most of the experience has been anecdotal and based on a series of cases. However, a double-blind study using tetrabenazine has been reported (Table 242.4, Evidence class II).[22]

The usual dose of reserpine is 0.25 mg started once daily and gradually escalated. The maximum dose employed in most patients is 1.0 mg 4 times daily. Patients may be able to tolerate even larger dosages if the titration is slow. In fact, a patient with progressive hemichorea received 6.75 mg per day.[27] The side effects include sedation, hypotension and the development or aggravation of depression. Drug-induced parkinsonism is another potential side effect. In fact, Carlsson's observation of reserpine-induced akinesia in the rodent led to the discovery of dopamine deficiency in idiopathic Parkinson's disease.

Tetrabenazine is a presynaptic monoamine-depleting drug with a weak postsynaptic dopamine blocking activity. It has been successfully employed in the treatment of various hyperkinetic movement disorders including dystonia and tics, and since Dalby's report, in chorea/ballism.[28,29] Jankovic reported a double-blind cross-over study of tetrabenazine in the treatment of hyperkinetic movement disorders.[22] Out of the 19 patients with hyperkinetic movement disorders there were four patients with tardive dyskinesia, one with Huntington's disease and two with dystonic choreoathetosis. The mean dose in these seven patients was 180 mg per day in divided dosages. Response was assessed using clinical scales and blinded videotape assessment. Improvement was seen in all patients with tardive dyskinesia. Marked improvement was seen in the patient with HD. The patients with congenital choreoathetosis improved to a lesser extent. Side effects were frequent and included daytime drowsiness, sialorrhea, insomnia, restlessness and anxiety, parkinsonism and mild postural hypotension. The long term efficacy and safety of this drug in the treatment of hyperkinetic movement disorders has been documented.[30] Another double-blind placebo controlled cross-over study looked at the efficacy and safety of tetrabenazine, and thioproazate (DBA) in patients with chorea.[31] Out of 10 patients studied nine had Huntington's disease and one had chorea in cerebral palsy. This patient remained unchanged on tetrabenazine but the response to thiopropazate was not well documented.

Tetrabenazine is not uniformly effective in the treatment of hemichorea/hemiballism. Failure to control movements with tetrabenazine using a dose of 75 mg per day has been reported.[32]

The usual starting dose is 12.5 mg gradually increasing to 25 mg 3 times a day. The maximum dose is 200 mg daily administered in divided dosages. Higher doses may be used in rare cases. Unfortunately this drug is not commercially available in the USA.

Dopamine blocking drugs

Neuroleptics, including chlorpromazine,[21] perphenazine 6–32 mg per day,[33] and haloperidol 3–30 mg per day[34] have been reported to improve hemiballism/hemichorea. In the case of perphenazine, escalating dosages resulted in drowsiness and elevation of liver enzymes. Tiapride has been reported to be efficacious in some patients,[35] and pimozide has proved useful in cases with prolonged hemiballism.[36]

These have all been open label studies (Table 242.4, Evidence class III). These drugs were discontinued subsequently and the results have been variable. In some cases, there was a re-emergence of hemiballism, suggesting that the movements had not stopped spontaneously. In others movements did not return making it likely that a spontaneous remission had occurred. However, the response to dopamine receptor blockers is not uniform, and several treatment failures have been reported.[37,38]

These agents have also been utilized in the treatment of chorea. A double-blind study of fluphenazine in the treatment of chorea has been reported (Table 242.4, Evidence class II).[39] Out of the nine patients with chorea there was one with senile chorea and the rest had HD. Flufenazine at 25 mg was administered intramuscularly and repeated every two weeks with dose escalation to 62.5 mg if necessary. The solitary patient with senile chorea improved significantly. The only side effect reported in this study was dry mouth.

Atypical neuroleptics

There are scattered reports of the use of newer atypical agents in the treatment of chorea/ballism. Olanzapine[40] and risperidone[41] have been reported effective in hemiballism. Clozapine in low dosages (50 mg per day) has been successful in two cases.[42]

Anticonvulsants

Anticonvulsants are mainly effective in the treatment of paroxysmal choreoathetosis.[43] In the setting of persistent chorea/ballism these drugs are used less often. Most reports concern the use of sodium valproate. This agent has been very efficacious in the treatment of Sydenham's chorea[44] and sometimes in the treatment of chorea in Huntington's disease. It has also been effective in post-traumatic choreoathetosis.[45] The response of hemichorea/hemiballism to valproate has been less consistent. Whereas, some found it effective;[32,46] others found the response to be highly variable.[47] Sodium valproate may be employed in patients with hemiballism who are intolerant or unresponsive to neuroleptics and dopamine depleting agents. In cases with chorea, where the course is more prolonged, DBA should be avoided and sodium valproate may be used earlier. The usual dose is 250 mg 3 times a day (tid) escalating to 500 mg tid. The usefulness of determining serum concentrations of the drug is not established in this setting. The side effects include increase in weight, hair loss and tremors.

Other anticonvulsants have rarely been used in the treatment of chorea/ballism. Carbamazepine has been reported to be effective in the treatment of Sydenham's chorea.[48] In one report of nonhereditary chorea five children aged 4–9 years were treated with carbamazepine 15–24 mg/kg with improvement in chorea. The blood level was in the range of 6.5–8.8 μg/ml. In one child the drug was discontinued because of a rash with re-emergence of chorea suggesting a true ameliorative effect and not a spontaneous resolution of chorea.[49]

GABA-ergic drugs

Gamma amino butyric acid (GABA) is a potent inhibitory transmitter in the striopallidal circuit. The mechanism of action of sodium valproate in chorea may involve its GABA-mimetic effects. Another GABA-ergic agent progabide in the dose of 900 mg per day has been reported to be of benefit in chorea/ballism.[38] In a limited study, clonazepam was found to be effective in suppressing choreiform movements in three patients with Huntington's chorea, three patients with non-familial chorea, and in one patient with senile chorea. In two patients with chorea of doubtful aetiology the response was not very satisfactory. The effective dose varied from 3–5 mg a day.[50]

Miscellaneous drugs

Ondensteron has been effective in the treatment of hemichorea in one patient[51] and dimethyl-aminoethenol (Deanol), which increases acetylcholine, has been reported to benefit patients with hemiballism.[52] Verapamil has been used in a patient with violent "choreic storm" superimposed on a preexisting cerebral palsy. This patient had failed with high doses of dopamine blocking agents.[53] Table 242.4 summarizes the drug treatment of chorea/ballism.

Surgical therapy

Surgical therapy is reserved for those patients who are unresponsive to medications or are sensitive to their side effects. Surgical treatments were more widely used prior to the introduction of effective drugs. In fact the surgery for hemiballism has a long history. Initially, drastic measures like peripheral denervation and lesioning of the spinal cord and the cerebral cortex were employed.[54] In one case the affected arm was amputated! More elegant approaches were employed after the introduction of stereotactic techniques by Spiegal in 1947. Hemiballism and hemichorea are more likely to be treated stereotactically whereas patients with bilateral chorea are less optimal candidates because of the risks of bilateral surgery. The preferred procedure is a stereotactic thalamotomy.[55,56] However, it has been known since the observations of Carpenter that a lesion of the globus pallidus may ameliorate experimental hemiballism/hemichorea.[7] Pallidotomy has been used in humans with hemiballism with good results.[57]

Deep brain stimulation (DBS) for movement disorders is most commonly performed in patients with dyskinesia and tremor associated with Parkinson's disease or in those with essential tremor. The role of DBS in patients with choreiform movements is poorly defined. There is one report of thalamic stimulation in two children with disabling choreiform disorders due to intracerebral hemorrhage or cerebral palsy.[58] Each patient displayed choreiform movements in the upper extremities both at rest and with intention, which interfered with daily activities and socialization. Following thalamic stimulation both children obtained significant improvement in their choreiform movements, and their upper extremity function improved. More studies are needed to study the safety and efficacy of DBS in chorea/ballism.

Gamma knife radiosurgery

Radiosurgery, first established by Leksell, using a collomated cobalt source, is now usually termed "the gamma knife". Its place as a non-operative modality to treat cerebral arteriovenous malformation is secure. It has also been used in the treatment of trigeminal neuralgia. The indications for gamma knife continue to expand and a limited literature exists about the use of gamma knife in the treatment of movement disorders. The main use has been in patients with essential tremor and Parkinson's disease. There is one report of a patient with progressive hemiballism due to arteriovenous malformation of the basal ganglia that improved with the use of gamma knife.[59] The lesion created by the gamma knife continues to expand for several months and complications are frequent. More studies are needed before gamma knife can be recommended for patients with chorea.

The treatment of chorea/ballism in special situations

Chorea in systemic lupus erythematosis (SLE) and the primary antiphospholipid antibody (APLA) syndrome

Chorea may occur in 2% of patients with SLE and may be the presenting manifestation. The mechanism is not fully understood but may involve vascular occlusions associated with APLA or it may be due to anti-neuronal antibodies.[60] Haloperidol has been employed in symptomatic therapy.[61] Chorea may also improve with corticosteroids.[62] The APLA syndrome is characterized by venous thromboses, strokes and recurrent miscarriages and the presence of APLA antibodies. Chorea may occur in the primary APLA syndrome and may respond to aspirin or warfarin.[63,64] The efficacy of all these measures is hard to assess as the chorea may resolve spontaneously in SLE and primarily APLA syndrome.[60]

Chorea in CNS infections

Chorea/ballism has been reported in tuberculous meningitis often with associated basal ganglia infarcts.[65] In addition to the symptomatic therapy anti-tuberculous drugs need to be employed. Hemiballism/hemichorea in AIDS patients is often due to toxoplasmosis affecting the basal ganglia.[66] In this setting DBA are often used in addition to treatment aimed at the offending organism.

Chorea gravidarum

Chorea may occur during pregnancy.[67] It may represent a hormonal change during pregnancy that may aggravate a chronic dopaminergic sensitivity after rheumatic chorea[68] or may herald an autoimmune disease.[69] The chorea invariably resolves with delivery. The symptomatic therapy is usually avoided because of the fear of teratogenic effects on the fetus. In a patient with chorea gravidarum associated with lupus anticoagulant, the treatment with prednisone and aspirin resulted in the resolution of chorea.[70]

Chorea in metabolic disorders

The underlying metabolic disorder needs to be treated. In case of recurrent chorea due to hypoglycemia the anti-diabetic drugs need to be modified. The chorea due to striatal hemorrhagic infarctions in non-ketotic hyperglycemia may persist for weeks or months after the correction of the metabolic abnormality.[25,71]

The chorea in hyperthyroidism may respond to anti-thyroid drugs or propranolol.[72] In hypoparathyroidism treatment with vitamin D and calcium may reduce the severity of the chora.[73] Chorea is rare in Wilson's disease but may be prominent in acquired hepatocerebral degeneration. In this setting the treatment of the underlying liver disease may help. Liver transplantation may result in a complete cure.[74]

Chorea due to drugs

Anticonvulsant drugs, usually in toxic range and many other drugs both prescribed and the drugs of abuse like cocaine and amphetamines may result in chorea.[75] In general the chorea due to drugs other than DBA will improve upon removal of the offending drug.

Chorea in multiple sclerosis (MS)

Paroxysmal dystonia (tonic seizures) in MS are more common[76] but persistent chorea may be seen in rare cases.[77,78] The chorea may disappear spontaneously. The paroxysmal dystonia may respond to anticonvulsants or acetazolamide.[79] The treatment of chorea is symptomatic.

Chorea in polycythemia vera

Rarely, chorea may occur in polycythemia. The chorea responds to reduction in hyperviscosity with venesection and may improve with DBA.[80,81]

Chorea in brain tumors

Both the primary brain tumors and metastatic tumors may result in ballism. The treatment includes surgery and radiation in addition to symptomatic therapy.[82]

Course and prognosis

The prognosis depends on the underlying cause. In general, the prognosis of vascular hemiballism is favorable. However, the prognosis of ballism due to other causes depends on the underlying condition (such as malignant disease and AIDS). It is unclear whether the site of the lesion influences the prognosis. Lang reported two patients with hemiballism of long duration in which the lesions were outside the subthalamic nucleus and suggested that the lesions outside the subthalamic nucleus, especially involving the striatum, may be associated with a worse prognosis.[36] However, others have suggested that lesions outside of subthalamic nucleus may be associated with a better chance of recovery.[26] In some patients, hemiballism may evolve into a hemidystonia. In others it transforms into hemichorea before a complete resolution. Complications include exhaustion, bronchopneumonia, and injuries to the involved limbs. The prognosis of chorea also depends on the underlying cause.

References

1. Buruma OJS, Lakke JPWF. Ballism. In: Vinken PJ, Bruyn GW, Klawans HL, eds. Handbook of Clinical Neurology. Extrapyramidal Disorders. Vol 49. Amsterdam: Elsevier Science, 1986:369–380
2. Barbeau A. History of movement disorders and their treatment. In: Barbeau A, ed. Disorders of Movement, Current Status of Modern Therapy. Vol 8. Lancaster: MTP Pr, 1981:1:28
3. Jakob A. Arteriosklerotische muskelstarre mit hinzutretendem hemiballismus. In: Foerster O, Wilmanns K, eds. Die extrapyramidalen erkrankungen. Berlin: Springer Verlag, 1923:13:225.
4. Martin JP. Hemichorea resulting from a local lesion of the brain (the syndrome of the body of Luys). Brain 1927;50:637–651
5. Whittier JR. Ballism and the subthalamic nucleus. Arch Neurol Psychiatr 1947;58:672–692
6. Whittier JR, Mettler FA. Studies on the subthalamic nucleus of the rhesus monkey. J Comp Neurol 1949;90:319–372
7. Carpenter MB, Whittier JR, Mettler FA. Analysis of choreoid hyperkinesia in the Rhesus monkey. J Comp Neurol 1950;92:293–332
8. Martin JP. Hemichorea (hemiballismus) without lesions in the corpus luysii. Brain 1957;80:1–11
9. Schwarz GA, Barrows LJ. Hemiballism without involvement of Luys' body. Arch Neurol 1960;2:420–434
10. Crossman AR, Sambrook MA, Jackson A. Experimental hemichorea/hemiballismus in the monkey. Brain 1984;107:579–596
11. Crossman AR, Mitchell IJ, Sambrook MA, Jackson A. Chorea and myoclonus in the monkey induced by gamma aminobutyric acid antagonism in the lentiform complex. Brain 1988;111:1211–1233
12. Eftychiadis AC, Chen TSN. St Vitus and his dance. J Neurol Neurosurg & Psych 2001;70:14–17
13. Conneally PM. Huntington's disease: genetics and epidemiology. Am J Hum Genet 1984;36:506–526
14. Gusella JF, Wexler NS, Conneally PM, et al. A polymorphic DNA marker genetically linked to Huntington's disease. Nature 1983;306:234–238
15. Zabel Bu, Naylor SI, Sakaguchi AY, Gusella JF. Mapping of the DNA locus D4s10 and the linked Huntington's disease gene to 4p 16–p15. Cytogenet Cell Genet 1986;42:187–190
16. Huntington's Disease Collaborative Research Group. A novel gene containing a trinucleotide repeat that is expanded and unstable on Huntington's disease chromosomes. Cell 1993;72:971–974
17. Dewey RB, Jankovic J. Hemiballism-hemichorea: clinical and pharmacologic findings in 21 patients. Arch Neurol 1989;46:862–867

18. Harper PS. The epidemiology of Huntington's disease. Hum Genet 1992;89:365–376

19. Nakano K, Kayahara T, Tsutsumi T, Ushiro H. Neural circuits and functional organization of the striatum. J Neurol 2000;247(Suppl 5):1–15

20. Guridi O, Obeso JA. Subthalamic nucleus, hemiballism and Parkinson's disease: a reappraisal of a neurosurgical dogma. Brain 2001;124:5–19

21. Tatlow WFT, Fischer CM, Dobkin AB. The clinical effects of chlorpromazine on dyskinesia. Can Med Assoc J 1954;71:380–381

22. Jankovic J. Treatment of hyperkinetic movement disorders with tetrabenazine: a double-blind, placebo-controlled study. Ann Neurol 1982;11:41–44

23. Hashimoto T, Yanagisawa N. A comparison of the regularity of involuntary muscle contractions in vascular chorea with that in Huntington's chorea, hemiballism and parkinsonian tremor. J Neurol Sci 1994;125:87–94

24. Berardelli A, Noth J, Thompson PD, et al. Pathophysiology of chorea and bradykinesia in Huntington's disease. Mov Disord 1999;14:398–403

25. Awad E, Figueroa RE, Sethi KD. Striatal hemorrhagic infarctions in hyperglycemia. Ann Neurol 1991;30(2):258–259

26. Hyland HH, Forman DM. Prognosis in hemiballismus. Neurology (Minneapolis) 1957;7:381–391

27. Friedman JH. A case of progressive hemichorea responsive to high dose reserpine. J Clin Psychiatry 1986;47:149–150

28. Jankovic J, Orman J. Tetrabenazine therapy of dystonia, chorea, tics, and other dyskinesias. Neurology 1988;38:391–394

29. Dalby MA. Effect of tetrabenazine on extrapyramidal movement disorders. BMJ 1969;654:422–423

30. Jankovic J, Beach J. Long term effects of tetrabenazine in hyperkinetic movement disorders. Neurology 1997;48(2):358–362

31. McLellan DL, Chalmers RJ, Johnson RH. A double-blind trial of tetrabenazine, thiopropazate, and placebo in patients with chorea. Lancet 1974;1:104–107

32. Lenton RJ, Cofti M, Smith RG. Hemiballism treated with sodium valproate. Br Med J 1981;283:17–18

33. Johnson WG, Fahn S. Treatment of vascular hemiballism and hemichorea. Neurology 1977;27:634–636

34. Klawans HL, Hamilton M, Nausieda PA, et al. Treatment and prognosis of hemiballismus. N Engl J Med 1976;295:1348–1350

35. Trillett M, Joyeux O, Masson R. Tiapride et mouementsanormaux. Sem Hop Paris 1977;53:21–27

36. Lang AE. Persistent hemiballism with lesions outside the subthalamic nucleus. Can J Neurol Sci 1985;12:125–128

37. Tegtmyer GF. No response of hemiballism to haloperidol. JAMA 1975;233:1223

38. Gonce M, Schoenen J, Charlier M, Delwaide P. Successful treatment of hemiballismus with progabide, a new GABA-mimetic agent. J Neurol 1983;229:121–124

39. Terrence CF. Fluphenazine decanoate in the treatment of chorea: a double-blind study. Curr Ther Res Clin & Exp 1976;20:177–182

40. Safirstein B, Shulman LM, Weiner WJ. Successful treatment of hemichorea with olanzapine. Mov Disord 1999;14(3):523–532

41. Evidente VG, Gwinn-Hardy K, Caviness JN, Alder CH. Risperidone is effective in severe hemichorea/hemiballismus. Movement Disorders 1999;14(2):377–379

42. Stojanovic M, Sternic N, Kostic VS. Clozapine in hemiballismus: report of two cases. Clinical Neuropharmacology 1997;20(2):171–174

43. Sethi KD. Paroxysmal dyskinesias. The Neurologist 2000;6(3):177–185.

44. Daoud AS, Zaki M, Shakir R, al-Saleh Q. Effectiveness of sodium valproate in the treatment of Sydenham's chorea. Neurology 1990;40:1140–1141

45. Chandra V, Spunt AL, Rusinowitz MS. Treatment of post-traumatic choreoathetosis with sodium valproate. J Neurol Neurosurgery & Psych 1983;46(10):963

46. Chandra V, Wharton S, Spunt AL. Amelioration of hemiballismus with sodium valproate. Ann Neurol 1982;12:407

47. Sethi KD, Patel BP. Inconsistent response to divalproex sodium in hemichorea/hemiballism. Neurology 1990;40:1630–1631

48. Harel L, Zecharia A, Straussberg R, et al. Successful treatment of rheumatic chorea with carbamazepine. Pediatric Neurology 2000;23(2):147–151

49. Roig M, Montserrat MD, Gallart A. Carbamazepine: an alternative drug for the treatment of nonhereditary chorea. Pediatrics 1988;82:492–495

50. Boralessa H, Lionel ND, Peiris JB. Clonazepam in the treatment of choreiform activity. Medical Journal of Australia 1976;1:225–227

51. Erdinc OO, Ozdemir G, Uysal S, et al. Improvement of hemichorea with ondansetron. Postgraduate Medical Journal 1997;73(856):127

52. Jameson HD, Blacker HM, Fuchs ME. Hemiballismus/hemichorea treated with dimethylaminoethanol. Dis Nerv Syst 1977;33:931–932

53. Ovesview F, Meador KJ, Sethi KD. Verapamil for hyperkinetic movement disorders. Movement Disorders 1998;13(2):341–344

54. Strain RE, Perlmutter I. Hemiballism relieved by ventral quadrant section of the cervical spinal cord without paralysis. J Neurosurg 1957;14:332–336

55. Bullard DE, Nashold BS Jr. Stereotactic thalamotomy for treatment of post-traumatic movement disorders. J Neurosurg 1984;61:316–321

56. Krauss JK, Mundinger F. Functional stereotactic surgery for hemiballism. J Neurosurg 1996;85:278–286

57. Suarez JI, Metman LV, Reich SG, et al. Pallidotomy for hemiballism: efficacy and characteristics of neuronal activity. Annals of Neurology 1997;42:807–811

58. Thompson P, Kondziolka D, Albright N. Thalamic stimulation for choreiform movement disorders in children. Report of two cases. J Neurosurg 2000;92(4):718–721

59. Kirino T. Relief of hemiballism from a basal ganglia arteriovenous malformation after radiosurgery. Neurology 1999;52(1):188–190

60. Khamashta MS, Gil A, Anciones B, et al. Chorea in systemic lupus erythematosus: association with antiphospholipid antibodies. Ann Rheum Dis 1988;47:681

61. Heilman KN, Kohler WC, LeMaster PC. Haloperidol treatment of chorea associated with systemic lupus erythematosus. Neurology 1971;21:963

62. Lahat E, Eshel G, Azizi E, et al. Chorea associated with systemic lupus erythermatosus in children. A case report. Isr J Med Sci 1989;25:568–570

63. Asherson RA, Derksen RH, Harris EN. Chorea in systemic lupus erythematosus and "lupus-like" disease: association with antiphospholipid antibodies. Semin Arthritis Rheumat 1987;16:253–259

64. Hodges JR. Chorea and the lupus anticoagulant. J Neurol Neurosurg Psych 1987;50:368–369

65. Udani PM, Parekh UC, Dastur DK. Neurological and

related syndromes in CNS tuberculosis. J Neurol Sci 1971;14:341–357

66. Nath A, Jankovic J, Pettigrew LC. Movement disorders and AIDS. Neurology 1987;37:37–41

67. Beresford OD, Graham AM. Chorea gravidarum. J Obstet Gynaecol Br Emp 1950;57:616–625

68. Nauseida PA, Beiliaukas LA, Bacon LA, et al. Chronic dopaminergic sensitivity after Sydenham's chorea. Neurology 1983;33:750–754

69. Agrawal BL, Foa RP. Collagen vascular disease appearing as chorea gravidarum. Arch Neurol 1982;39: 192–193

70. Lubbe WF, Walker EBN. Chorea gravidarum associated with circulating lupus anticoagulant: successful outcome of pregnancy with prednisone and aspirin therapy. Case report. Br J Obstet Gynaecol 1983; 90:487–490

71. Hashimoto T, Hanyu N, Yahikozawa H, Yanagisawa N. Persistent hemiballism with striatal hyperintensity on T_1-weighted MRI in a diabetic patient: a 6-year follow-up study. J Neurol Sci 1999;165:178–181

72. Dhar SK, Nair CP. Choreoathetosis and thyrotoxicosis. Ann Int Medicine 1974;80:426–428

73. Muenter MD, Whisnant JP. Basal ganglia calcifications, hypoparathyroidism and extrapyramidal motor manifestations. Neurology 1968;18:1075–1080

74. Stracciari A, Guarino M, Pazzaglia P, et al. Acquired hepatocerebral degeneration: full recovery after liver transplantation. J Neurol Neurosurg & Psych 2001; 70:136–137

75. Toru M, Matsuda O, Makiguchi K. Involuntary movements caused by diphenythydantoin intoxication in a patient. Psychiatr Neurol Jpn 1980;82:727–736

76. Berger J, Sheremata WA, Melamed E. Paroxysmal dystonia as the initial manifestation of multiple sclerosis. Arch Neurol 1984;41:747–750

77. Mao C-C, Gancher ST, Herndon RM. Movement disorders in multiple sclerosis. Mov Disord 1988; 3:109–116

78. Tranchant C, Bhatia KP, Marsden CD. Movement disorders in multiple sclerosis. Mov Disord 1995;10: 418–423

79. Sethi KD, Hess DC, Huffnagle VH, Adams RJ. Acetazolamide treatment of paroxysmal dystonia in central demyelinating disease. Neurology 1992;42:919–923

80. Bruyn GW, Padberg G. Chorea and polycythemia. Eur Neurol 1984;23:26–33

81. Rigon G, Baratti M, Quani F, Cazetti S. Polycythemia: description of a clinical case. Minerva Med 1987; 78:1325–1329

82. Glass JP, Jankovic J, Borit A. Hemiballism and metastatic brain tumor. Neurology 1984;34:204–207

243 Essential Tremor

Alireza Minagar and William C Koller

Man has long known tremor as a disorder of the elderly but tremor as an isolated manifestation affecting young individuals and with a familial basis has been reported within the last two centuries. Critchley[1] provided one of the most detailed reviews of essential tremor (ET) and mentioned one of the earlier references to tremor: "The keepers of the house shall tremble" (Ecclesiastes, XII.3). Galen in the second century differentiated tremor from other movements in his treatise, *On Tremor, Palpitation, Spasm, and Rigor*[2] and defined tremor as "an involuntary alternating up-and-down motion." James Parkinson was aware of the difference between the senile tremor and tremor of the paralysis agitans.[3] Later, Charcot[4] commented on the prominent clinical characteristics of familial and senile tremor. He also recognized the variability of clinical expression of ET.

In 1836 the first cases of familial tremor were reported.[1,5–7] However, in 1887, Dana[6] wrote the first detailed account of familial tremor and ET. He described three families with tremor, covering 45 patients with tremor within a single pedigree. Dana observed the affected body parts, variability in severity and age of onset, amelioration during sleep, and absence of increased mortality. He differentiated familial tremor from senile tremor and wrote that senile tremor "generally affects first and entirely the head and neck." He also believed that ET was associated with neuroses, psychoses, epilepsy, unique talents, and high intellect.

Other neurologists were also familiar with the unique characteristics of ET. In the early 1920s Minor proposed the concept of status macrobioticus multiparus—the triad of familial tremor, longevity, and fecundity.[1] Other traits that have been associated with ET by other authors include inebriety, nervousness, emotivity, and anxiety.[8] Raymond regarded "neuropathic shock" as the precipitating cause of ET.[9]

Definition and clinical manifestation

Tremor consists of rhythmic oscillations of a body part, usually an extremity, when held in a sustained position or during movement. Tremor results from simultaneous or alternating contraction of agonist and antagonist muscle groups. It is usually classified based on the behavioral conditions in which it happens. Tremor is categorized as rest, postural, kinetic, isometric, or action tremor according to whether it occurs during voluntary muscle activity, steady posture, or active movements. A summary of various categories of tremor is presented in Table 243.1.

Essential tremor is a combination of postural and kinetic tremors, although one may dominate the other. Rest tremor is a rare phenomenon in elderly individuals with advanced disease; therefore, coexisting Parkinson's disease or another cause of parkinsonism should be considered. Essential tremor is a rhythmic 4–12 Hz entrainment of motor unit activity that forces the upper limbs into oscillation. The frequency of the oscillation is independent of reflex arc length and mechanical characteristics of the body part. Older patients with ET demonstrate tremor frequencies in the lower range of 4–12 Hz, while tremor frequencies of younger patients frequently extend into the frequency range of 8–12 Hz. Qualitatively, this component of physiological tremor resembles the abnormal motor unit entrainment in mild ET and may be of the same origin. Indeed, electromyographic, amplitude, and frequency of mild ET share similarities with physiological tremor and pathological tremors such as dystonic tremor and Parkinson's action tremor.[10] These quantitative characteristics of tremor, as well as many laboratory studies, are not useful in the diagnosis of ET and differentiating it from other tremor categories. Generally ET has tremor as its unique manifestation and other neurological manifestations are absent. Muscular tone is normal, and there is no weakness or in-coordination except that due to tremor. Mild abnormalities of tone or gait are occasionally reported. Singer et al.[11] found that 50% of ET patients exhibited tandem gait abnormalities, as compared to 28% of age-matched controls.

Essential tremor affects different parts of body with various frequencies. It almost invariably involves the hands (95% of cases), but also involves the head (34%), face (5%), voice (12%), trunk (5%), and lower extremities (20%).[12] The majority of patients have tremor in the upper extremities in isolation. Tremor in the lower extremities is usually asymptomatic. Essential tremor is a disabling for many patients and activities of daily living such as writing and eating may be impaired. Recently, Lombardi and colleagues in a study of 18 patients with ET found that they have cognitive deficits on tests of verbal fluency, naming, mental set-shifting, verbal memory, and working

Table 243.1   Summary of various tremors
Rest tremor
Postural tremor
Kinetic tremor
Isometric tremor
Action tremor

memory; ET patients in this study also showed signs of depression.[13]

Essential tremor manifests insidiously and advances gradually at a variable rate, as determined by unknown factors. The progression of the disease can be defined as an increase in tremor amplitude or extension of tremor to previously unaffected body parts. It is the former that impairs the patient's voluntary movements and results in disability. Despite its progressive nature, ET is not associated with increased mortality.

A host of factors can affect the tremor and overall it tends to progress with age so that with advancing age tremor frequency declines and amplitude increases. Alcohol may produce a prominent ameliorative effect on ET. In many patients ingestion of small amounts of alcoholic beverages lessens the tremor. Essential tremor typically remits during sleep and the appearance of tremor in a given patient may vary, not only with passage of years, but even over the course of a single day.

The diagnosis of ET is made either incidentally or when the patient presents because of the mechanical or social disability resulting from the tremor. The core and secondary criteria for the diagnosis of ET are the following: (1) core criteria: bilateral action tremor of the hands and forearms (but not rest tremor), absence of other neurological signs, with the exception of the cogwheel phenomenon; (2) secondary criteria: long duration (> 3 years), positive family history, and beneficial response to alcohol. In general, tremor is scarcely confused with any other neurological movements. Its rhythmic, oscillating nature allows easy recognition.

Epidemiology

ET is perhaps the most frequent movement disorder with a prevalence ranging from 1% to 22% in an elderly population.[14,15] Even based on conservative and age-specific prevalence rates, 1.2% to 2% of individuals in their seventh decade of life or older have tremor.[16] These large differences in the prevalence rate may be explained by variations in the definition of ET and differences in the study methods. The 1990 United States consensus figures estimated that there were as many as 620 000 individuals with ET in the elderly population alone. Essential tremor is often described as familial, with 17.4% to 100% of patients showing a positive family history. Applying the prevalence rate of ET derived from a Finnish study to the US Census Bureau population statistics (1988), one can estimate that more than five million individuals over 40 years of age in the US are affected. Essential tremor affects all ethnic groups, with the apparent exception of some isolated populations in New Guinea. Age is a significant risk factor for the expression of ET and ET may be regarded as an age effect on the nervous system in vulnerable individuals. Larson and Sjogren[17] performed the earliest comprehensive community study in an isolated island in Northern Sweden. The prevalence of ET reached 3.73% in individuals older than age 40. There is no consensus about the sex distribution of ET, however, sex chromosome abnormalities have been reported in some patients.[18]

In 1981, Haerer et al.,[19] performed the first epidemiological study of ET in the US. This study was part of a survey of major neurological disorders in a biracial Mississippi county. The minimum prevalence rate of 0.33% occurred in African–American men. Essential tremor was more prevalent in women than men. The study demonstrated a 10-fold increase in ET among those aged between 70 and 79 compared to the group aged 40–49.

Rajput et al.,[20] performed the second epidemiological study in the US. This study was based on a retrospective review of medical records over a 45-year period in Rochester, Minnesota. The estimated prevalence rate was 0.31% and the incidence of ET increased sharply after age 49. Incidence rates among men and women were similar.

Louis et al.,[16] examined a random sample of 2117 Medicare recipients living in Washington Heights-Inwood in northern Manhattan, New York and after age adjustments, reported the prevalence rate of ET to be 4.02% in the elderly individuals. In this study the prevalence rate was more significantly increased in men than in women. The prevalence increased with age and was higher in Whites than in African–Americans. Hispanic Americans had an intermediate prevalence rate.

Genetics

The tendency of ET to run in families has been recognized for many years. In the American medical literature Dana[6] reported on three families with tremor in 1887. In the intervening years authors reviewing ET have reaffirmed its heritable nature.[8,9] Family history positivity varies from 17.4% to 100%. It is commonly presumed that the familial and sporadic forms of ET are phenotypically similar. However, the familial form appears to have a narrow phenotype. A comprehensive genetic population study was conducted in a region of northern Sweden by Larsson and Sjogren.[17] In this study, 210 cases of ET were traced to nine ancestral families in this geographically and ethnically restricted area. The pattern of occurrence of ET was consistent with autosomal dominant inheritance.

During a genome scan for familial ET in 16 Icelandic kindreds with 17 affected members, investigators, using an autosomal dominant model, identified linkage to chromosome 3q13.1. The gene on chromosome 3 with a LOD score of 3.71 was designated as *FET1*. A second study evaluated a large American kindred of Czech descent in whom ET affected 18 of 67 family members. In this kindred, a gene for ET (*ETM2*) was mapped to chromosome 2p22–p25 with a maximum LOD score of 5.92. Anticipation was identified in the family, and performance of repeat expansion detection analysis recommended that the ETM gene might be a triplicate repeat.

Diagnostic difficulties

Essential tremor may be misdiagnosed and mislabeled as incipient Parkinson's disease. Other neurological disorders that are associated with tremor include multiple sclerosis, Wilson's disease, Huntington's chorea, and cerebellar degenerative diseases. In addition, tremor can be precipitated by drugs, toxins, and systemic illnesses such as thyrotoxicosis. Occasionally ET may be misdiagnosed as an anxiety disorder.

Clinical variants

A number of atypical tremor disorders appear to be related to ET.[21] Their association with ET is based on a high occurrence of a positive family history of ET, frequent presence of a mild postural tremor, and improvement of tremor with alcohol ingestion. In the majority of patients with ET, various degrees of postural and kinetic tremor are observed; however, in the kinetic-dominant tremor a remarkable dissociation happens, with the postural component being minimal or absent.[22] Cerebellar manifestations do not exist and disability may be severe in these patients. Resting tremor is not a defined part of ET, however, it has been observed in severely affected or elderly individuals.[5] Koller and Rubino[23] described a group of patients with a mixture of resting and postural tremor with minimal kinetic tremor and no parkinsonian features despite a long duration of tremor. Tremor in these patients did not respond to anti-parkinsonian medications. A number of case reports of familial paroxysmal tremor with clinical manifestations similar to ET also exist.[24,25]

A task-specific or selective action tremor involving the hands is primary writing tremor, during which pronation of the forearm elicits a pronation/supination tremor that is not observed during other movements of the arm.[26–28] Usually the patient's major complaint is impaired handwriting. Tremor manifests for the duration of writing, making the task impossible. Electromyography (EMG) discloses an alteration of antagonistic muscles, and there is no significant increase of reflex excitability or cortical hyperexcitability.[26] Primary writing tremor should be differentiated from writer's cramp, which is a segmental dystonia of the hand.

Essential tremor can affect one body segment solely or predominantly. Isolated tremors of the tongue, chin, and voice may happen. Tongue tremor is frequently observed when the patient is examined in the postural position, although frequently the patient is unaware of any difficulty with the tongue. However, a tongue tremor may be a patient's main complaint, interfering with eating and speaking. Isolated chin spasm (geniospasm) not involving the lips may also happen. Isolated trembling of chin may also happen in families, transmitted as an autosomal dominant gene.[29,30] Speech involvement may occur in patients with ET and occasionally, may be the predominant manifestation.[31,32] Isolated tremor of the trunk and head, particularly when of slow frequency (2–3 Hz) may be the initial presentation of a focal dystonia.[33]

Truncal tremor is sometimes observed in ET patients with a long history of severe hand and head tremors, although truncal tremor as the manifesting symptom is rare. Heilman described three patients with the sole manifestation being orthostatic tremor of the trunk and the proximal legs.[34] Wee reported a family exhibiting both typical ET of the hands and orthostatic trunk tremor.[35]

Pathophysiology

Our knowledge about the anatomical localization of neurological abnormalities in ET is limited and pathophysiology of ET remains an enigma. Essential tremor is a central tremor, probably caused by an abnormal oscillation of a central nervous system "pacemaker," the location of which is currently unknown. One of the major barriers in understanding the mechanism(s) of ET is inducing ET in laboratory animals. The experimental tremor induced by harmaline in laboratory animals is phenotypically similar to human ET. Harmine, a β-carboline related to harmaline, is a known tremoroginic agent in humans. Harmaline induces a fine, generalized 8–12 Hz tremor in subprimates and primates. Harmaline-induced tremor is attenuated by ethanol, diazepam, and barbiturates,[36] similar to human ET. The pacemaker of harmaline tremor is in the inferior olive (IO). This abnormal neuronal function arises from increased electrotonic coupling among olivary neurons and from increased neuronal oscillation induced by membrane inhibition-rebound excitation. The electrotonic coupling is mediated through dendrodendritic gap junctions that are modulated by a calcium-activated, hyperpolarizing potassium current that rhythmically activates a low-threshold calcium spike. Harmaline intensifies these mechanisms of normal olivary oscillation and synchronization.[37–39] This increased olivary rhythmicity continues even after transection of the cerebral structures at various levels (cerebellar peduncles, C2–C3 spinal cord, cerebellectomy), implying that harmaline-induced tremor arises from the IO rather than from its connections.

Various postmortem examinations of patients with ET have reported nonspecific changes and gross anatomical changes in ET may not occur. However, detailed neurohistochemical and neurochemical studies of postmortem tissue specimens are lacking. Based on the available data, it may be concluded that ET is due to neuronal dysfunction, with no associated gross or histopathological abnormalities.

Electrophysiological studies generally confirm that a possible central oscillator causes ET. The possible central oscillator could be in the brain, the spinal cord, or both. This oscillator, depending on its neuroanatomic and functional connectivity, may be influenced by different sensory stimuli that can reset or entrain its rhythm. Therefore, application of a sudden muscle stretch reflex or electric nerve stimulus to a tremulous limb, will reset the tremor if there is enough sensory feedback to the tremor oscillator. This mechanical or electric stimulus must have sufficient strength compared to the strength of the oscillator to generate any alteration in the tremor rhythm.

Positron emission tomography (PET) studies of patients with ET have revealed a variety of inconclusive findings. One study of ET patients at rest demonstrated increased metabolic activity in the

---

Table 243.2   Treatment of essential tremor

1. Start with primidone, 50 mg at night time (warn patient of possible side effects but recommend continuation of drug even if side effects occur).

2. Increase primidone to 125 mg at night time, if necessary.

3. Increase primidone to 250 mg at night time, if necessary.

4. Add or switch to propranolol-LA, 80 mg in the morning.

5. Increase propranolol-LA to 160 mg in the morning, if necessary.

6. Increase propranolol-LA to 240 mg, if necessary.

7. Increase propranolol-LA to 320 mg in the morning, if necessary.

8. If medicine therapy fails, consider sterotaxic surgery, e.g., DBS of the thalamus

---

DBS, deep brain stimulation.

thalamus and medulla (probably IOs) but not in the cerebellum.[40] Blood flow measurements with $H_2^{15}O$ have revealed bilateral cerebellar activity at rest with further increases during visible tremor. Hyperactivity during involuntary trembling was detected in the thalamus, striatum, and motor cortex. Another study revealed elevated blood flow in the cerebellum and red nucleus but not in the medulla.[41] Therefore, ET is associated with bilateral hyperactivity in the cerebellar connections.[41,42] Also, PET studies have indicated that ethanol-suppression of ET may be mediated by a decline of cerebellar synaptic hyperactivity in the cerebellar cortex, causing increased afferent input to the IOs. However, it should be emphasized that cerebellar blood flow is increased in almost all categories of tremor. The observation of bilaterally increased cerebellar blood flow does not necessarily indicate that ET arises from the cerebellum.

Treatment

Propranolol (and other β-adrenergic blockers) and primidone are currently the only two medications that have been clearly shown to be effective in suppressing ET. It is unclear which should be the drug of first choice although it appears that marked tremor reduction is more often achieved with primidone than propranolol. As many as 20% of patients will suffer side effects for several days after the first dose of primidone, but if the patient is warned of these potential adverse reactions only a minority will discontinue taking the drug. Side effects with chronic therapy are uncommon with primidone but are more of a concern with propranolol. Many elderly patients cannot take β-adrenergic blockers. Some patients may require both propranolol and primidone therapy. The treatment schedule for ET is provided in Table 243.2. In cases of propranolol and primidone failure, alprazolam should be tried. Botulinum toxin type A is effective for a variety of movement disorders such as dystonia and hemifacial spasms. The drug appears to possess some efficacy for ET of the head and voice, but less so for the hand. Hopefully, future research will find new therapeutic agents for those who are not responding to the medications in current use.

Thalamotomy and deep brain stimulation

Stereotaxic thalamotomy is an effective procedure in the treatment of parkinsonian, cerebellar, and essential tremors. The technical aspects of the procedure have improved greatly in the last decade. The site of lesion selected is the ventral anterior or the ventral intermediate nucleus of thalamus. Stereotaxic thalamotomy can be performed with the use of mild sedation and local anesthesia. Temporary intellectual deficits and transitory hemiparesis may occur. A lasting weakness is unusual. Other infrequent adverse events include seizures, involuntary movements, and cerebellar signs. Bilateral thalamotomy is associated with much more serious complications. In particular, a severe, persistent dysarthria and permanent mental changes can occur. Therefore, bilateral operations cannot be recommended. Deep brain stimulation (DBS) of the thalamus is also highly effective in reducing ET and appears to have less adverse reactions than thalamotomy.[43,44] It appears that 90% of patients have significant tremor reduction with the tremor being totally abolished in 50% of patients. Bilateral procedures can also be performed without permanent deficits. The fact that stimulus parameters can be adjusted for increased efficacy or reduced adverse reactions, makes DBS of the thalamus more desirable than a destructive lesion. However long-term maintenance of DBS equipment often results in additional surgical procedures. Infections also represent a potential problem. Nonetheless DBS of the thalamus has proven to be an effective short-term and long-term treatment in the management of ET; even a unilateral DBS of the thalamus appears to improve hand and voice tremors. Therefore, currently DBS of the thalamus has become the surgical procedure of choice for ET.

References

1. Critchley M. Observations on essential (heredofamilial) tremor. Brain 1949;72:113–139
2. Sider D, McVaugh M. Galen on tremor, palpitation, spasm, and rigor. Trans Stud Coll Physicians Phila 1979;1:183–210
3. Parkinson J. An essay on the shaking palsy. London: Whittingham & Rowland, 1817
4. Charcot JM. Policlinique due Mardi. Paris: Lecons de Mardi, 1888:448–451
5. Larsen TA, Calne DB. Essential tremor. Clin Neuropharmacol 1983;6:185–206
6. Dana CL. Hereditary tremor, a hitherto undescribed form of motor neurosis. Am J Med Sci 1887;94:386–393
7. Most GF. Encyclopadie de Gesanten Medizinischen und Chirurgischen Praxis, Vol. 2. 1836;555
8. Flatau J. Le tremblement essentiel hereditaire (abstract). Rev Neurol 1909;17:417

9. Raymond F. Le tremblement essentiel hereditaire (abstract). Rev Neurol 1909;17:416

10. Deuschl G, Krack P, Lauk M, Timmer J. Clinical neurophysiology of tremor. J Clin Neurophysiol 1996;13: 110–121

11. Singer C, Sanchez-Ramos J, Weiner WJ. Gait abnormalities in essential tremor. Mov Disord 1994;9:193–196

12. Elble R, Koller WC. The diagnosis and pathophysiology of essential tremor. In: Elble R, Koller WC, eds. Tremor. Baltimore: John Hopkins University Press, 1990

13. Lombardi WJ, Woolston DJ, Roberts JW, Gross RE. Cognitive deficits in patients with essential tremor. Neurology 2001;57:785–790

14. Larsen TA, Calne DB. Essential tremor. Clin Neuropharmacol 1983;6:185–206

15. Rajput AH, Offord KP, Beard CM, Kurland LT. Essential tremor in Rochester, Minnesota: a 45-year study. J Neurol Neurosurg Psychiatry 1984;47:466–470

16. Louis ED, Marder K, Cole L, et al. Differences in prevalence of essential tremor among elderly African-Americans, Whites, and Hispanics in northern Manhattan, NY. Arch Neurol 1995;52:1201–1205

17. Larsson T, Sjogren T. Essential tremor: a clinical and genetic population study. Acta Psychiatry Neurol Scand 1960;36(Suppl 144):1–176

18. Baughman FA Jr, Higgins JV, Mann JD. Sex chromosome anomalies and essential tremor. Neurology 1973;23:623–625

19. Haerer AF, Schoenberg BS, Anderson DW. Prevalence of essential tremor in the biracial adult population of Copiah county, Mississippi. Ann Neurol 1981;10:93–94

20. Rajput AH, Offord KP, Beard CM, et al. Essential tremor in Rochester, Minnesota: a 45-year study. J Neurol Neurosurg Psychiatry 1984;47:466–470

21. Koller WC, Glatt S, Biary N, Rubino FA. Essential tremor variants: effects of treatment. Clin Neuropharmacol 1987;10:342–350

22. Biary N, Koller WC. Kinetic predominant tremor: effect of clonazepam. Neurology 1987;37:471–474

23. Koller WC, Rubino FA. Combined resting-postural tremor. Arch Neurol 1985;42:683–684

24. Bain PG, Findley LJ. Familial paroxysmal tremor: an essential tremor variant (letter). J Neurol Neurosurg Psychiatry 1994;57:1019

25. Garcia-Albea E, Jimenez-Jimenez FJ, Ayuso-Peralta L, et al. Familial paroxysmal tremor: an essential tremor variant? (letter). J Neurol Neurosurg Psychiatry 1993; 56: 1329

26. Klawans HL, Glantz R, Tanner CM, Goetz CG. Primary writing tremor: selective action tremor. Neurology 1982;32:203–206

27. Rothwell JC, Traub MM, Marsden CD. Primary writing tremor. J Neurol Neurosurg Psychiatry 1979;42; 1106–1114

28. Ravits J, Hallett M, Baker M, Wilkins D. Primary writing tremor and myoclonic writer's cramp. Neurology 1985;35:1387–1391

29. Grossman BJ. Trembling of the chin: an inheritable dominant character. Pediatrics 1957;19:453–455

30. Lawrence BM, Matthews W, Diggle JA. Hereditary quivering of the chin. Arch Dis Child 1968;43:249–254

31. Brown JR, Simonson J. Organic voice tremor. Neurology 1967;17:520–527

32. Hachinski VC, Thomsen IV, Buch NH. The nature of primary vocal tremor. Can J Neurol Sci 1975;2:195–197

33. Riveat J, Marsden CD. Trunk and head tremor as isolated manifestations of dystonia. Mov Disord 1990;5: 60–65

34. Heilman KM. Orthostatic tremor. Arch Neurol 1984;4: 880–881

35. Wee AS, Subramony SH, Currier RD. Orthostatic tremor: a variant of essential tremor. Neurology 1986; 36:1241–1245

36. Lamarre Y, Mercier LA. Neurophysiological studies of harmaline-induced tremor in the cat. Can J Physiol Pharmacol 1971;49:1049–1058

37. Llinas R, Baker R, Sotelo C. Electrotonic coupling between neurons in cat inferior olive. J Neurophysiol 1974;37:560–571

38. Llinas R, Yarom Y. Electrophysiology of mammalian inferior olivary neurons in vitro. Different types of voltage-dependent ionic conductances. J Physiol (Lond) 1981;315:549–567

39. Llinas R, Yarom Y. Oscillatory properties of guinea-pig inferior olivary neurons and their pharmacological modulation: an in vitro study. J Physiol (Lond) 1986; 376:163–182

40. Hallett M, Dubinsky RM. Glucose metabolism in the brain of the patients with essential tremor. J Neurol Sci 1993;114:45–48

41. Wills AJ, Jenkins IH, Thompson PD, et al. Red nuclear and cerebellar but no olivary activation associated with essential tremor: a positron emission tomography study. Ann Neurol 1994;36:636–642

42. Wills AJ, Jenkins IH, Thompson PD, et al. A positron emission tomography study of cerebral activation associated with essential tremor and writing tremor. Arch Neurol 1995;52:299–305

43. Koller WC, Hristova A. Efficacy and safety of stereotaxic surgical treatment of tremor disorders. Eur J Neurol 1996;3:507–514

44. Koller WC, Pahwa R, Busenbark K, et al. High frequency unilateral thalamic stimulation in the treatment of essential and parkinsonian tremor. Ann Neurol 1997;42:292–299

244 Treatment of Orthostatic Tremor

Paul Greene

In 1984, Heilman reported three patients with shaking or quivering of the trunk and legs that appeared shortly after standing and disappeared with sitting or walking, calling this orthostatic tremor (OT).[1] Patients with similar characteristics had been noted before in movement disorder centers, and three such patients had actually been reported before in 1970 by Pazzaglia et al.[2] Shortly after Heilman's description, Thompson et al. reported the presence of a 16 Hz tremor in the legs of a patient with OT.[3] No tremor at this high frequency had been reported before, thus providing convincing evidence that this was indeed a unique condition. Although this condition has been reported with increasing frequency since Heilman's original report, it is still considered extremely uncommon, and there are no published estimates of the prevalence or incidence of OT. In one series of 200 consecutive patients from a tremor clinic, five (2.5%) had the clinical syndrome of OT.[4] This certainly overestimates the prevalence of OT relative to other tremors because patients with OT, being unusual, were more likely to be referred.

The etiology of OT is unknown. The tremor of OT was not reset by electrical stimulation of peripheral nerves, but was reset by transcranial magnetic stimulation in two of three reports, suggesting a central origin of the tremor.[5–7] A positron emission tomography (PET) study suggested increased blood flow in the cerebellum bilaterally and in the thalamus and lentiform nuclei contralateral to an arm with 16 Hz tremor in patients with OT compared to rest, suggesting cerebellar involvement in the origin of the tremor.[8] Several patients have also been identified with the clinical features of OT combined with cerebellar ataxia due to idiopathic cerebellar degeneration or pontine infarct.[9,10]

There is a continuing debate about the relationship between OT and essential tremor (ET). Some authors argue that OT is a task-specific form of ET because patients with OT often have upper extremity tremor consistent with ET and a family history of ET. In addition, some patients with typical ET of the arms and minimal symptoms in the legs may develop an intermediate 10 Hz–13 Hz tremor of the legs on standing.[11,12] Others, however, point out that patients with OT do not always have postural tremor or a family history of ET, rarely improve with beta-blockers or alcohol, and often improve with clonazepam (unlike patients with ET) and have other neurological features atypical for ET (maximum symptoms in the legs, muscle cramps in the legs, broad-based stance, and so forth).[13,14] This controversy is unlikely to be resolved until a specific test is developed for ET or

OT, such as identification of the genes responsible for ET.

The essential features of OT are high frequency tremor of the legs and trunk which appears on standing, usually after a delay of seconds to minutes, and is improved with sitting or walking. The disease usually starts late in the seventh decade (range third to eighth decades). Other features which are commonly present, but not essential for diagnosis, include: (1) sensation of imbalance when standing; (2) relief of symptoms by leaning against a wall or rocking from side to side; (3) broad-based stance with narrow-based gait and difficulty with tandem walking; (4) crescendo tremor with prolonged standing; (5) anxiety and autonomic symptoms, such as flushing, diaphoresis and tachycardia with prolonged standing; (6) muscle tightness or pain with prolonged standing; (7) difficulty writing while standing. When these clinical features are combined with a 14 Hz–16 Hz tremor of leg muscles, there is no differential diagnosis for OT, except for task-specific ET, as described above. However, occasional patients with this syndrome have had associated neurological conditions, including Parkinson's disease, diabetic neuropathy, stroke, hydrocephalus, head trauma, chronic relapsing polyradiculoneuropathy (CRP), and cerebellar disease. In some cases, treatment of the underlying parkinsonism, hydrocephalus or CRP induced resolution of the OT.[15,16]

There has been only one controlled study of a treatment for OT: a double-blind, crossover study with placebo control of gabapentin in four patients with OT.[17] Patients taking 1800 mg/day to 2400 mg/day of gabapentin improved significantly compared to placebo. Another open label report also found improvement from gabapentin (ranging from 60% to 80% improvement on a subjective scale) in seven of seven patients with OT.[18] Side effects were only seen in the open label study, and consisted of transient diplopia, drowsiness, unsteadiness, constipation, dry mouth and nausea.[18] Most of these patients had improved with clonazepam, but had not tolerated the side effects. Despite the lack of any controlled study, clonazepam is the medication most often cited as being effective in the treatment of OT. In two reviews published in 1991, approximately 23/34 patients treated with clonazepam were reported to improve.[11,19] Benefit was described as ranging from mild improvement to almost complete resolution of symptoms. Doses required were high: from 1 mg to 8 mg per day (2 mg–4 mg per day in most cases). Some patients reported to benefit from clonazepam had to stop the medication due to drowsiness or ataxia or

Table 244.1 Treatment of orthostatic tremor

Drug	Approach
Gabapentin	Titrate dose to 1800–2400 mg/day on a tid or qid regimen.
Clonazepam	Titrate dose to 2–4 mg/day on a tid or qid regimen; may go as high as 8 mg/day.
Primidone	Titrate dose to 125–625 mg/day on a tid regimen.
Combinations of Gabapentin, Clonazepam and Primidone	If partial benefit from Gabapentin, Clonazepam or Primidone, another drug can be added.
Carbidopa/levodopa	Carbidopa/levodopa, Phenobarbital or Valproic acid. Can be tried if other agents fail.
Phenobarbital	
Valproic acid	

tid, three times a day; qid, four times a day.

had loss of benefit. The other medication frequently reported to help OT is primidone, either alone or in combination with clonazepam.[20,21] Benefit has been described as ranging from modest to marked at doses ranging from about 125 mg–625 mg daily. Few side effects have been reported, perhaps because of the modest doses used. After successfully using levodopa to treat a patient with OT and Parkinson's disease, Wills et al. tested levodopa in patients with OT and no parkinsonism. They conducted an uncontrolled, open-label trial of eight patients with blinded video rating and found significant improvement in standing compared to the pre-treatment state, with patients taking 600 mg levodopa daily in a controlled-release preparation with benserazide.[16] Five patients continued taking levodopa, while three stopped due to nausea or insomnia. Other medications occasionally reported as beneficial include phenobarbital,[22] valproic acid,[14] and chlorazepate.[23]

References

1. Heilman KM. Orthostatic tremor. Arch Neurol 1984;41:880–881
2. Pazzaglia P, Sabattini L, Lugaresi E. Su di un singolare disturbo della stazione eretta (osservazione di 3 casi). Riv di Freniatria 1970;46:450–457
3. Thompson PD, Rothwell JC, Day BL, et al. The physiology of orthostatic tremor. Arch Neurol 1986;43:584–587
4. Martinelli P, Gabellini AS, Gulli MR, Lugaresi E. Different clinical features of essential tremor: a 200-patient study. Acta Neurol Scand 1987;75:106–111
5. Tsai CH, Semmler JG, Kimber TE, et al. Modulation of primary orthostatic tremor by magnetic stimulation over the motor cortex. J Neurol Neurosurg Psychiatry 1998;64:33–36
6. Pfeiffer G, Hinse P, Humbert T, Riemer G. Neurophysiology of orthostatic tremor. Influence of transcranial magnetic stimulation. Electromyogr Clin Neurophysiol 1999;39:49–53
7. Mills KR, Nithi KA. Motor cortex stimulation does not reset primary orthostatic tremor (letter). J Neurol Neurosurg Psychiatry 1997;63:553
8. Wills AJ, Thompson PD, Findley LJ, Brooks DJ. A positron emission tomography study of primary orthostatic tremor. Neurology 1996;46:747–752
9. Setta F, Jacquy J, Hildebrand J, Manto MU. Orthostatic tremor associated with cerebellar ataxia (letter). J Neurol 1998;245:299–302
10. Benito-Leon J, Rodriguez J. Orthostatic tremor with cerebellar ataxia (letter). J Neurol 1998;245:815
11. FitzGerald PM, Jankovic J. Orthostatic tremor: an association with essential tremor. Mov Disord 1991;6:60–64
12. Papa SM, Gershanik OS. Orthostatic tremor: an essential tremor variant? Mov Disord 1988;3:97–108
13. Walker FO, McCormick GM, Hunt VP. Isometric features of orthostatic tremor: an electromyographic analysis. Muscle Nerve 1990;13:918–922
14. McManis PG, Sharbrough FW. Orthostatic tremor: clinical and electrophysiologic characteristics. Muscle Nerve 1993;16:1254–1260
15. Gabellini AS, Martinelli P, Gulli MR, et al. Orthostatic tremor: essential and symptomatic cases. Acta Neurol Scand 1990;81:113–117
16. Wills AJ, Brusa L, Wang HC, et al. Levodopa may improve orthostatic tremor: case report and trial of treatment. J Neurol Neurosurg Psychiatry 1999;66:681–684
17. Onofrj M, Thomas A, Paci C, D'Andreamatteo G. Gabapentin in orthostatic tremor: results of a double-blind crossover with placebo in four patients. Neurology 1998;51:880–882
18. Evidente VG, Adler CH, Caviness JN, Gwinn KA. Effective treatment of orthostatic tremor with gabapentin. Mov Disord 1998;13:829–831
19. Britton TC, Thompson PD, van der Kamp W, et al. Primary orthostatic tremor: further observations in six cases. J Neurol 1992;239:209–217
20. Van der Zwan A, Verwey JC, van Gijn J. Relief of orthostatic tremor by primidone. Neurology 1988;38:1332
21. Poersch M. Orthostatic tremor: combined treatment with primidone and clonazepam (letter). Mov Disord 1994;9:467
22. Cabrera-Valdivia F, Jimenez-Jimenez FJ, Garcia Albea E, et al. Orthostatic tremor: successful treatment with phenobarbital. Clin Neuropharmacol 1991;14:438–441
23. Veilleux M, Sharbrough FW, Kelly JJ, et al. Shaky-legs syndrome. J Clin Neurophysiol 1987;4:304–305

245 Myoclonus

Steven J Frucht

The term myoclonus refers to rapid, shock-like movements arising from the peripheral or central nervous system. Myoclonus was first described in the latter part of the nineteenth century by a variety of terms, including myoclonus fibrillaris multiplex, fibrillary chorea, myokymia and convulsive tremor. The first person to use the term myoclonus in its current context was Friedrich, who coined the phrase "paramyoklonus multiplex" in 1881.[1] Several years later, Unverricht reported several families affected with myoclonus and epilepsy.[2] Further reports of familial myoclonus followed with Lafora and Glueck's description in 1911 of the disorder later known as Lafora's disease.[3] Ramsay-Hunt was the first to report myoclonus in patients with cerebellar degeneration, using the term "dyssynergia cerebellaris myoclonia" in 1921.[4]

In 1963, Lance and Adams focused attention on a previously unrecognized clinical entity, posthypoxic myoclonus. They called attention to myoclonus occurring with action and also highlighted the devastating impact of negative myoclonic jerks on functional performance.[5] In 1971, Lhermitte reported the effectiveness of L-5-hydroxytryptophan in patients with posthypoxic myoclonus, ushering in a new era of experimental therapeutics.[6] Later that decade, valproic acid and clonazepam were reported to be effective in reducing myoclonus. The first large symposium on myoclonus was held in 1979,[7] followed by another in 1986.[8] By this time, Fahn, Marsden and Van Woert had proposed a classification scheme for myoclonic disorders,[9] and neurophysiologists had defined the origins of several forms of myoclonus, including cortical reflex myoclonus,[10] reticular reflex myoclonus[11] and propriospinal myoclonus.[12] The last decade has witnessed significant progress in the unravelling of the genetics of inherited myoclonic disorders. Several new medications have also been developed that may be useful for patients with myoclonus.

The purpose of this chapter is to summarize the current state of knowledge of the etiology, pathophysiology and treatment of myoclonus.

Epidemiology

Myoclonus is not a diagnosis in itself, but rather a movement disorder that is found in a wide range of illnesses. It is easily overlooked, especially if it does not contribute to functional disability.

Only one study has evaluated the incidence and prevalence of myoclonus. Using the medical record linkage system of Olmsted County Minnesota, Caviness identified all patients with myoclonus or diseases known to exhibit myoclonus between 1976 and 1990.[13] He found that the average incidence of persistent pathologic myoclonus was 1.3 cases per 100 000 person-years. The lifetime prevalence of myoclonus was 8.6 cases per 100 000. The incidence of myoclonus increased with age, and men were disproportionately affected. Extrapolating to current population figures, between 10 000 and 45 000 people in the United States (US) may be currently affected with myoclonus. These estimates are similar to the number of people affected with Huntington's disease, an illness that has attracted far more public interest and research funding.

Etiology

Myoclonus may occur in a large number of neurological conditions. In 1982, Marsden, Hallet and Fahn proposed a classification system for myoclonic disorders based on their etiology,[14] and this scheme was later revised by Fahn in 1986.[8] As shown in Table 245.1, it is helpful to consider myoclonus in five major etiological categories.

Physiological myoclonus is common, affecting everyone at one time or another. Hypnic jerks, hiccups, normal startle and benign infantile myoclonus are examples of physiological myoclonus, and these conditions rarely require treatment. Essential myoclonus, also known as myoclonus dystonia, is a rare autosomal dominant disorder with incomplete penetrance. Myoclonus usually begins in the first or second decade of life, and seizures, dementia, ataxia and electroencephalographic (EEG) abnormalities are absent. Irregular, asymmetric myoclonic jerks typically affect the arms, neck and face in these patients. Dystonia may be present in individuals affected by myoclonus, or in other family members who do not have myoclonus (hence the term myoclonus dystonia). Obsessive-compulsive disorder, drug addiction and alcohol abuse are over-represented in these families. The latter may stem from the exquisite response of myoclonus in this disorder to alcohol, a response that is not replicated by available medications. The gene for this disorder has recently been linked to chromosome 7q21 in eight families.[15] It is unknown whether sporadic cases of myoclonus dystonia are also linked to this locus.

The third category of myoclonic disorders is epileptic myoclonus. These patients are usually managed by an epileptologist, and they will not be considered further in this chapter.

Symptomatic myoclonus accounts for the largest group of patients. They are best considered in two groups, symptomatic myoclonus *with* prominent seizures (the progressive myoclonic epilepsies), and

Table 245.1   Classification of myoclonus by etiology

Physiological myoclonus
Hypnic jerks
Anxiety-induced myoclonus
Exercise-induced myoclonus
Hiccups
Benign infantile myoclonus

Essential myoclonus
Autosomal dominant
Sporadic

Epileptic myoclonus
Epilepsia partialis continua
Photosensitive myoclonus
Myoclonic absence
Infantile spasms
Lennox–Gastaut
Cryptogenic myoclonic epilepsy
Myoclonic epilepsy of Janz

Symptomatic myoclonus
Progressive myoclonic epilepsies
Sialidoses type I and II
Gaucher's type 3
G_{M2} gangliosidoses
Myoclonus epilepsy with ragged red fibers (MERRF)
Ceroid lipofuscinoses
Unverricht-Lundborg disease
Dentatorubral-pallidoluysian atrophy (DRPLA)
Juvenile Huntington's disease
Juvenile neuroaxonal dystrophy

Symptomatic myoclonus without prominent seizures
Posthypoxic myoclonus (Lance-Adams syndrome)
Post-traumatic myoclonus
Myoclonic dementias (Alzheimer's disease,
    Creutzfeldt-Jakob disease)
Basal ganglia diseases (Corticobasal ganglionic
    degeneration, Parkinson's disease, Huntington's
    disease, olivopontocerebellar degeneration,
    Hallervorden-Spatz disease, Wilson's disease)
Drug-induced myoclonus
Metabolic-induced myoclonus
Viral infections

symptomatic myoclonus *without* prominent seizures. The progressive myoclonic epilepsies are a group of inherited, neurodegenerative disorders characterized by epilepsy, myoclonus, cognitive decline and ataxia. Sialidoses, myoclonus epilepsy with ragged red fibers syndrome (MERRF), Lafora's disease, the ceroid lipo-fuscinoses, Unverricht-Lundborg disease and den-torubral-pallidoluysian atrophy (DRPLA) are some of these illnesses; they will be discussed further in the genetics section of this chapter. Symptomatic myoclonus without prominent seizures includes the myoclonic dementias (Alzheimer's disease, Creutzfeldt-Jakob disease) and basal ganglia disorders (corticobasal ganglionic degeneration, Parkinson's disease, olivopontocerebellar atrophy). In these illnesses, myoclonus is rarely the most important source of disability. Metabolic and drug-induced myoclonus are common causes of myoclonus, usually resolved by correcting the metabolic abnormality or

stopping the offending drug. Posthypoxic myoclonus, also known as Lance-Adams syndrome, is an important cause of symptomatic myoclonus, and it will also be discussed in this chapter.

Pathophysiology

A full discussion of the neurophysiology of myoclonus is beyond the scope of this chapter. For the clinician faced with treating a patient with myoclonus, a critical distinction is whether or not the myoclonic jerks are positive (that is, associated with active contraction of a muscle or group of muscles) or negative (occurring during an interruption in muscle tone). Negative myoclonus may affect any part of the body. Asterixis refers to negative myoclonic jerks that affect the arms, typically producing a hand flap when the patient holds both arms forward with wrists in extension.[16] Negative myoclonus may also affect the trunk and legs, producing a bouncing gait that may be misinterpreted as psychogenic. Often, positive and negative myoclonic jerks are present in the same patient. The technique of back-averaged EEG is extremely helpful in differentiating positive from negative myoclonus, and also for localizing the source of the myoclonic jerks to a cortical or subcortical origin. However back-averaging is often not available, forcing the neurologist to rely on clinical features to help differentiate positive from negative myoclonic jerks, and cortical from subcortical myoclonus.

Although there are exceptions, the following rules apply to most patients with myoclonus. Negative myoclonus often occurs in the setting of metabolic dysfunction or drug intoxication. When encountering a patient with negative myoclonus, particular attention should be paid to serum electrolytes, blood urea nitrogen, ammonia, liver function tests, toxicology screen and medications. When negative myoclonus is not due to drugs or metabolic derangements, a structural origin should be considered, such as a thalamic[17] or cortical origin.[18] Negative myoclonus is common in posthypoxic myoclonus, and is often an important source of disability. Negative myoclonus is notoriously unresponsive to medications, with the exception of cortical negative myoclonus, which may respond to antiepileptic agents.

Positive myoclonic jerks may originate from cortical or subcortical foci. Cortical myoclonus often affects the hand or the foot, may be associated with giant somatosensory evoked potentials (SSEPs), and is often stimulus-sensitive. Brainstem myoclonus often preferentially affects proximal muscle groups and may be stimulus-sensitive. Myoclonus originating from the spinal cord is often rhythmic, and is not usually stimulus-sensitive. Again, these statements should be viewed only as a guide to localization as there are many exceptions.

Genetics

The last decade has witnessed dramatic advances in the identification of genes responsible for inherited myoclonic disorders. They are summarized in Table 245.2. Startle disease, also known as hyperekplexia, is

Table 245.2 The genetics of myoclonic disorders

Disorder	Locus	Inheritance	Gene
Hyperekplexia	5q	AD	Inhibitory glycine receptor
Essential myoclonus	7q	AD	Epsilon-sarcoglycan
Sialidoses I, II	6p	AR	Lysosomal sialidase
Gaucher's type III	1q	AR	Lysosomal glucocerebrosidase
G_{M2} gangliosidoses	5q	AR	β-hexosaminidase
Juvenile neuroaxonal dystrophy	20p	AR	?
MERRF	mtDNA	mitochondrial	tRNA-Lysine
DRPLA	12	AD	Atrophin-1
Lafora	6q	AR	Laforin
Unverricht-Lundborg	21q	AR	Cystatin B
Ceroid			
Infantile	1p	AR	Palmitoyl protein thioesterase
Late-infantile	11p	AR	Tripeptidyl peptidase 1
	13q	AR	CLN 5 gene
Juvenile	16p	AR	CLN 3 gene

AD, autosomal dominant; AR, autosomal recessive; MERRF, myoclonus epilepsy with ragged red fibers; DRPLA, dentatorubral-pallidoluysian atrophy; CLN, ceroid lipofuscinosis.

a rare condition in which unexpected auditory, somatosensory or visual stimuli produce exaggerated and often profound startle. This disorder may present in the newborn period with exaggerated startle and profound generalized muscular rigidity. Diagnosis and timely treatment are critical to prevent sudden death from apnea.[19] In childhood, patients may fall as the result of severe generalized tonic spasms. This autosomal dominant disorder is linked to mutations in the inhibitory glycine receptor GLRA1, located on chromosome 5q.[20] Essential myoclonus (also known as myoclonus dystonia) is an autosomal dominant form of myoclonus that has recently been mapped to a locus on chromosome 7q. Myoclonus may also occur in sialidoses types I and II, autosomal recessive disorders caused by mutations in lysosomal sialidase encoded on chromosome 6p.[21] Gaucher's type III, G_{M2} gangliosidoses and juvenile neuroaxonal dystrophy are three other autosomal recessive disorders in which myoclonus may be present. The genes for the first two are known (lysosomal glucocerebrosidase[22] and β-hexosaminidase[23]), and the last is linked to chromosome 20p.[24]

The genes for the five major forms of progressive myoclonic epilepsy have been identified. Myoclonus, epilepsy and ragged-red fibers, known as MERRF, is a multisystem mitochondrial disorder linked to mutations in the tRNA-Lysine gene of mitochondrial DNA.[25] Dentatorubral-pallidoluysian atrophy is an autosomal dominant neurodegenerative disease caused by expansion of CAG repeats in the DRPLA gene atrophin-1 on chromosome 12.[26] Lafora's disease and Unverricht-Lundborg are both autosomal recessive disorders with typical onset in late childhood. The former is linked to chromosome 6q (caused by

mutations in Laforin),[27] and the latter to chromosome 21q (caused by mutations in cystatin B).[28] Neuronal ceroid lipofuscinoses are a group of diseases with autosomal recessive inheritance linked by common pathology—the accumulation of lipopigment within neurons and other cells. At least four phenotypes have been described. Infantile ceroid is linked to chromosome 1p and has been mapped to mutations in palmitoyl protein thioesterase.[29] Two forms of late infantile ceroid have been mapped to chromosome 11p (mutations in tripeptidyl peptidase 1)[30] and chromosome 13q.[31] Juvenile onset ceroid, also known as Batten's disease, has been mapped to a protein encoded on chromosome 16p.[32] Genetic tests for many of the progressive myoclonic epilepsies are available on a commercial or research basis.

Clinical features and natural history

The clinical features and natural history of myoclonus varies with the underlying disorder. In general, physiological myoclonus is rarely severe enough to warrant treatment. Essential myoclonus, described above, does worsen over time, although most patients learn to accommodate for their myoclonic jerks. The natural history of the progressive myoclonic epilepsies, myoclonic dementias and basal ganglia diseases is one of continued neurological deterioration. Often, seizures, ataxia, cognitive decline or motor impairment dominate the clinical picture.

In contrast, patients afflicted with posthypoxic myoclonus (Lance-Adams syndrome) can persist with myoclonus in relative isolation for decades. The phenomenology and natural history of posthypoxic myoclonus have been characterized better than any other myoclonic disorder. After surviving a respiratory or cardiac arrest, patients with posthypoxic myoclonus are left with positive myoclonic jerks, which are specifically triggered by action. The severity of myoclonus increases with the precision of the task. Many patients also have negative myoclonus, which may affect the legs producing a characteristic bouncing gait. Dysarthria, dysmetria and ataxia are not uncommon in these patients.[5] Neurological deficits improve over time.[33]

Classification

As described above, the classification scheme of Fahn is very useful in organizing the various myoclonic syndromes. When approaching a patient with myoclonus, it is also helpful to define the phenomenology of the myoclonus. Myoclonus may be positive, due to active muscle contraction, or negative, arising from lapses in muscle tone. Stimulus-sensitive myoclonus is induced by sensory stimuli, including touch, pin, sound and threat. Myoclonus may be present at rest or only with action, and it may be rhythmic or irregular. Generalized myoclonus refers to jerks that involve the whole body at once, while multifocal myoclonus affects body regions randomly, one at a time. Focal myoclonus involves only one body part, typically an extremity.

It is also useful to classify myoclonus by the source of the myoclonic jerks within the nervous system. Myoclonus may originate from anywhere within the nervous system. Cortical myoclonus is perhaps the most common source of myoclonus, usually due to a hyperexcitable sensory or motor cortex. Cortical myoclonus may be positive or negative.[18] Thalamic lesions have been associated with contralateral negative myoclonus.[17] There are at least three forms of brainstem myoclonus; reticular reflex myoclonus (generalized, proximal flexor jerks), hyperekplexia (exaggerated startle) and palatal myoclonus (either essential or secondary to structural lesions). Spinal myoclonus may be segmental (usually rhythmic jerks affecting one segment of the cord), or propriospinal, with stimulus-sensitive long-latency axial flexion jerks.[12] Lesions in the nerve root, plexus and peripheral nerve may also cause myoclonus.

Diagnosis and work-up

Given the large number of conditions in which myoclonus may occur, it is not surprising that the work-up for a patient with myoclonus must be individualized. Clinical phenomenology is essential in evaluating these patients, and back-averaged EEG can be extremely helpful in defining the source of myoclonic jerks. If a diagnosis of progressive myoclonic epilepsy is entertained, genetic testing should be sent for the most likely candidate gene.

Magnetic resonance imaging is customary in patients with chronic myoclonus. This is particularly important when there is a possibility of a structural lesion causing myoclonus, such as that which occurs with focal cortical myoclonus, thalamic asterixis, secondary palatal myoclonus, segmental and propriospinal myoclonus, and myoclonus from root or plexus lesions. Contrast-enhanced scans should be performed when a structural lesion is suspected.

Differential diagnosis

Myoclonus is usually easily distinguished from other movement disorders by its speed. Most myoclonic jerks are between 10 and 50 milliseconds in length, and they rarely exceed 100 milliseconds. In contrast, tremor is rhythmic, oscillatory and slower than myoclonus. Tics may be brief, however they are intermittent and often under voluntary control. Paroxysmal dyskinesias are episodic and sometimes triggered by voluntary movement. While some forms of dystonia can have rapid clonic movements that mimic myoclonus, usually a sustained posture, sensory trick or null point is present that helps distinguish the two. Small choreic movements may appear myoclonic, however chorea usually flows from one body part to another. Psychogenic myoclonus is not uncommon in patients with conversion disorder, however it is virtually impossible to simulate the rapid jerks seen in organic myoclonus.[34] Myoclonus is one of the few movement disorders that can persist in sleep.

Treatment

The treatment of myoclonus poses a considerable challenge for the neurologist (Table 245.3). Only four placebo-controlled clinical trials of anti-myoclonic agents have been reported,[35-38] and only one of these was double-blind.[35] Only two drugs, Piracetam and L-5-hydroxytryptophan, have been subjected to controlled clinical trials, and neither is available in the US. In fact, the most commonly used anti-myoclonic drugs, valproic acid and clonazepam, have never been carefully tested in myoclonus patients. The treating physician is therefore forced to rely on the response of patients in published case series. Often the clinical rating of response to treatment is quite subjective ("mild improvement, marked improvement..."), preventing adequate comparisons between reports. Unlike epilepsy, multiple drugs often need to be used at the same time in order to obtain maximum benefit. Although isolated case reports of neurosurgical treatments for myoclonus exist, there is no evidence that these approaches are either safe or effective and they cannot be recommended.

The medications most commonly used to treat myoclonus are valproic acid, clonazepam, Piracetam, L-5-hydroxytryptophan and primidone. Piracetam, a nootropic agent with efficacy in cortical myoclonus, is not available in the US. L-5-hydroxytryptophan is also unavailable, and the risk of inducing a potentially lethal eosinophilia myalgia syndrome[39] has removed this drug from the available armamentarium. In the paragraphs that follow, the evidence supporting treatment of hyperekplexia, posthypoxic myoclonus, progressive myoclonic epilepsy, essential myoclonus, pathological hiccups, palatal myoclonus, spinal segmental myoclonus and propriospinal myoclonus will be reviewed.

Table 245.3 Treatment of myoclonus

A.

Drug	Total Dose	Common side effects	Rare serious adverse events
Valproic acid	10–15 mg/kg/day	Nausea, HA, tremor, alopecia	Liver failure, pancreatitis, thrombocytopenia
Clonazepam	1.5–15 mg/day	Somnolence, dizzyness, ataxia	
Levetiracetam	1000–3000 mg/day	Minimal	Psychosis
Piracetam	4.8–24 gm/day	Minimal	Seizure on rapid withdrawal
Primidone	250–750 mg/day	Ataxia, somnolence	
Acetazolamide	125–500 mg/day	Paresthesias, tinnitus, nausea	Stevens-Johnson, renal stones
Zonisamide	200–600 mg/day	Somnolence, anorexia, dizzyness	Stevens-Johnson, renal stones
L-5-HTP	100–400 mg/day	Nausea	Eosinophilia-myalgia

B.

Myoclonus type	First-line treatment	Second-line treatment
Cortical	Valproic acid	Zonisamide
	Clonazepam	Primidone
	Levetiracetam	Acetazolamide
	Piracetam	
Subcortical	Clonazepam	
		Valproic acid
		Tetrabenazine
		L-5-HTP

C.

Etiology	First-line treatment	Second-line treatment
Hyperekplexia	Clonazepam	Valproic acid
		Clobazam
Posthypoxic myoclonus	Clonazepam	L-5-HTP
	Valproic acid	
	Levetiracetam	
	Piracetam	
Progressive myoclonic epilepsy	Piracetam	Acetazolamide
	Valproic acid	Zonisamide
	Clonazepam	
Essential myoclonus	Clonazepam	Alcohol
	Benztropine	Gamma-hydroxy-butyric acid
Pathological hiccups	Valproic acid	Neuroleptics
	Baclofen	
	Amitryptyline	
Palatal myoclonus	Clonazepam	Carbamazepine
	Sumatriptan	L-5-HTP
	Botulinum toxin	Diazepam
Spinal myoclonus	Clonazepam	Valproic acid
	Tetrabenazine	L-5-HTP

Treatment options for patients with myoclonus appear above. Several caveats apply. First, this table should only be used as a rough guide to treatment, as each patient's medical and neurologic history will guide the appropriate choice of medications. Second, the dose of each drug is purposely presented as a range (A). Each medicine should be started individually at low dose, and the dose gradually increased until benefit is seen or side effects are encountered. Third, treatment of myoclonus usually requires polypharmacy; two or more first-line drugs are likely to be needed in most patients. Fourth, in this author's opinion all first-line drugs should be tried before second-line drugs are used (B,C). The drugs appear in each column in the order that the author uses them.

The author's choice of which drug to use first is based on experience and risk of side effects. Finally, drugs such as piracetam, tetrabenazine and L-5-HTP are not commercially available in the United States, and ideally they should be used only with informed consent and the approval of an institutional review board.

Hyperekplexia

Most families with autosomal dominant hyperekplexia due to mutations in the glycine receptor have been treated with clonazepam. Clonazepam effectively abolishes startle and falling episodes (Class III).[40,41] The importance of recognizing this condition in the neonatal period cannot be over emphasized. In 15 babies identified with hyperekplexia, untreated infants experienced recurring episodes of apnea until age 1 year. Three died unexpectedly in infancy. Treatment with clonazepam (0.1–0.2 mg/kg per day) reduced pathological startle and abolished apneic spells (Class III).[19] Valproic acid[42] and clobazam[43] have also shown to be effective in this condition in single case reports (Class III). A double-blind placebo-controlled cross-over study of four patients treated with either clonazepam or vigabatrin showed that clonazepam, but not vigabatrin, reduced startle (Class II).[44] Based on these studies, clonazepam appears to be the drug of choice for this disorder. Valproic acid and clobazam are possible alternative agents.

2594   XIII   Movement Disorders

Posthypoxic myoclonus

Frucht and Fahn reviewed the clinical features and response to treatment of 122 published cases of posthypoxic myoclonus.[45] Unfortunately, there are no placebo-controlled or double-blind therapeutic studies of posthypoxic patients. The authors identified patients who obtained a marked or full improvement from treatment with various medications, and also identified medications that had not produced such a response in any patient with posthypoxic myoclonus. Twenty-four patients obtained marked improvement with clonazepam, while 23 did not. Similarly, 10 were improved with valproic acid, while 12 were not. Seventeen patients treated with L-5-hydroxytryptophan improved, while 26 did not. Three patients received benefit from Piracetam, while three did not. Phenobarbital, phenytoin, nitrazepam and tetrabenazine were of no benefit in any patients, and diazepam was seldom helpful. Based on these results, the authors recommended that patients with posthypoxic myoclonus be treated with clonazepam and valproic acid, either alone or in combination. Piracetam may be helpful, particularly in patients with cortical myoclonus. A new agent, levetiracetam, may also be useful in these patients (Frucht, personal communication).

Progressive myoclonic epilepsy

In 1982, Iivanaine and Himberg reported their results treating patients with Unverricht-Lundborg disease.[46] Previously, these patients were routinely treated with phenytoin and carbamazepine. Twenty-six patients were switched to valproic acid and clonazepam in high doses of both drugs, with dramatic improvements in myoclonus, walking and functional performance. Acetazolamide has been shown to improve action myoclonus in two patients with Ramsay-Hunt syndrome (Class III).[47] Although single patients with progressive myoclonic epilepsy have been reported to benefit dramatically from L-5-hydroxytryptophan, a double-blind placebo-controlled study of six patients showed no improvement in myoclonus or ataxia and significant side effects (Class I).[36] In a large, multicenter, randomized, double-blind crossover study of patients with Unverricht-Lundborg, high-dose Piracetam (24 gm/day) was shown to improve myoclonus and functional performance (Class I).[35]

Based on these studies, patients with progressive myoclonic epilepsy should not receive phenytoin or other anticonvulsants with potential cerebellar toxicity. Valproic acid and clonazepam should be used to treat seizures in these patients. Piracetam is probably the drug of choice to treat myoclonus in these patients. A trial of zonisamide, a new epileptic agent, in Unverricht-Lundborg disease is currently in progress.

Essential myoclonus

Treatment of essential myoclonus is challenging. No medication currently available in the US provides the symptomatic benefit seen with alcohol. In isolated patients, clonazepam may be helpful (Class III).[48,49] Three patients in one family with essential myoclonus obtained benefit from benztropine mesylate at 4–9 mg/day (Class III).[50] In a recent report, γ-hydroxybutyric acid was shown to be dramatically effective in a single patient (Class III).[51]

Pathological hiccups

Only rarely do hiccups persist and require treatment. Neuroleptics are commonly used to treat hiccups in the hospital, however the small but real risk of inducing a tardive syndrome should temper this approach. Valproic acid controlled intractable hiccups in an open-label study of four patients (Class III).[52] Baclofen also improved hiccups in a double-blind, randomized, placebo-controlled crossover study (Class I).[53] One patient responded to amitriptyline even though treatment with dopamine receptor blockers had failed (Class III).[54]

Palatal myoclonus

Palatal myoclonus may occur after structural lesions of the Guillain-Mollaret triangle (secondary palatal myoclonus) or without known cause (essential palatal myoclonus). There are no placebo-controlled studies of treatments for palatal myoclonus, and therapy is therefore empiric. In patients with symptomatic palatal myoclonus, clonazepam, carbamazepine, L-5-hydroxytryptophan and trihexyphenidyl have proven effective in some patients (Class III).[55-57] Phenytoin, barbiturates, diazepam, carbamazepine, L-5-hydroxytryptophan and trihexiphenidyl were helpful in patients with essential palatal myoclonus (Class III).[55] Sumatriptan has recently been shown to improve essential palatal myoclonus (Class III).[58] Botulinum toxin injections to the tensor velum palatini may suppress palatal movements in both disorders (Class III).[59,60]

Spinal segmental myoclonus

There are no placebo-controlled studies of spinal myoclonus. Of 19 patients with spinal myoclonus, 16 reportedly improved with clonazepam (Class III).[61] Tetrabenazine has also been reported to be helpful in 10 of 12 patients treated (Class III).[62] Valproate and L-5-hydroxytryptophan have been reported to be effective in one patient (Class III).[63]

Propriospinal myoclonus

Few patients with proprospinal myoclonus have been reported. Clonazepam (Class III),[12] and valproic acid have been reported to be useful (Class III).[64]

Conclusion

Myoclonus is a complex neurological disorder, with varied etiology, neurophysiology and neuropharmacology. This chapter will hopefully provide a framework for the clinician to diagnose and manage patients with myoclonus.

References

1. Friedreich N. Neuropathologische Beobachtung beim paramyoklonus multiplex. Virchow's Arch Pathol Anat Physiol Klin Med 1881;86:421–434

2. Unverricht H. Die Myoclonie. Vienna: Fran Deuticke, 1891:1–128

3. Lafora GR. The presence of amyloid bodies in the protoplasm of the ganglion cells: a contribution to the study of the amyloid substance in the nervous system. Bull Gov Hosp Insane 1911;3:83–92

4. Hunt JR. Dyssynergia cerebellaris myoclonica-primary atrophy of the dentate system: a contribution to the pathology and symptomatology of the cerebellum. Brain 1921;44:490–538

5. Lance JW, Adams RD. The syndrome of intention or action myoclonus as a sequel to hypoxic encephalopathy. Brain 1963;86:111–136

6. Lhermitte F, Oeterfalvi M, Marteau R, et al. Analyse pharmacologique d'un cas de myoclonus d'intention et d'action postanoxique. Rev Neurol (Paris) 1971;124:21–31

7. Fahn S, Davis JN, Rowland LP, eds. Advances in Neurology. Vol 26. New York: Raven Press, 1979

8. Fahn S, ed. Advances in Neurology. Vol 43. New York: Raven Press, 1986

9. Fahn S, Marsden CD, Van Woert MH. Definition and classification of myoclonus. In: Fahn S, ed. Advances in Neurology. Vol 43. New York: Raven Press, 1986: 1–5

10. Hallett M, Chadwick D, Marsden CD. Cortical reflex myoclonus. Neurology 1979;29:1107–1125

11. Hallett M, Chadwick D, Adam J, Marsden CD. Reticular reflex myoclonus: a physiological type of human post-hypoxic myoclonus. J Neurol Neurosurg Psychiatry 1977;40:253–264

12. Brown P, Rothwell JC, Thompson PD, Marsden CD. Propriospinal myoclonus: evidence for spinal "pattern" generators in humans. Mov Disord 1994;9:571–576

13. Caviness JN, Alving LI, Maraganore DM, et al. The incidence and prevalence of myoclonus in Olmstead County, Minnesota. Mayo Clin Proc 1999;74:565–569

14. Marsden CD, Hallett M, Fahn S. The nosology and pathophysiology of myoclonus. In: Marsden CD, Fahn S, eds. Movement Disorders. London: Butterworth Scientific, 1982:196–248

15. Klein C, Schilling L, Saunders-Pullman RJ, et al. A major locus for myoclonus-dystonia maps to chromosome 7q in eight families. Am J Hum Genet 2000;67: 1314–1319

16. Shibasaki H. Overview and classification of myoclonus. Clin Neurosci 1996;3:189–192

17. Tatu L, Moulin T, Martin V, et al. Unilateral pure thalamic asterixis: clinical, electromyographic, and topographic patterns. Neurology 2000;54:2339–2342

18. Shibasaki H. Myoclonus. Curr Opin Neurol 1995;8:331–334

19. Nigro MA, Lim HC. Hyperekplexia and sudden neonatal death. Pediatr Neurol 1992;8:221–225

20. Ryan SG, Sherman SL, Terry JC, et al. Startle disease, or hyperekplexia: response to clonazepam and assignment of the gene (STHE) to chromosome 5q by linkage analysis. Ann Neurol 1992;31:663–668

21. Pshezhetsky AV, Richard C, Michaud L, et al. Cloning, expression and chromosomal mapping of human lysosomal sialidase and characterization of mutations in sialidosis. Nat Genet 1997;15:316–320

22. Verghese J, Goldberg RF, Desnick RJ, et al. Myoclonus from selective dentate nucleus degeneration in type 3 Gaucher disease. Arch Neurol 2000;57:389–395

23. Nakai H, Byers MG, Nowak NJ, Shows TB. Assignment of β-hexosaminidase A α-subunit to human chromosomal region 15q23–q24. Cytogenet Cell Genet 1991;56:164

24. Taylor TD, Litt M, Kramer P, et al. Homozygosity mapping of Hallervorden-Spatz syndrome to chromosome 20p12.3–p13. Nat Genet 1996;14:479–481

25. Shoffner JM, Lott MT, Lezza AM, et al. Myoclonic epilepsy and ragged-red fiber disease (MERRF) is associated with a mitochondrial DNA tRNA(Lys) mutation. Cell 1990;61:931–937

26. Kanazawa I. Dentatorubral-pallidoluysian atrophy or Naito-Oyanagi disease. Neurogenetics 1998;2:1–17

27. Serratosa JM, Delgado-Escueta AV, Posada I, et al. The gene for progressive myoclonus epilepsy of the Lafora type maps to chromosome 6q. Hum Molec Genet 1995; 4:1657–1663

28. Pennacchio LA, Lehesjoki A-E, Stone NE, et al. Mutations in the gene encoding cystatin B in progressive myoclonus epilepsy (EPM1). Science 1996;271: 1731–1733

29. Camp LA, Verkruyse LA, Afendis SJ, et al. Molecular cloning and expression of palmitoyl-protein thioesterase. J Biol Chem 1994;269:23212–23219

30. Sleat DE, Gin RM, Sohar I, et al. Mutational analysis of the defective protease in classic late-infantile neuronal ceroid lipofuscinosis, a neurodegenerative lysosomal storage disorder. Am J Hum Genet 1999;64:1511–1523

31. Savukoski M, Kestila M, Williams R, et al. Defined chromosomal assignment of CLN5 demonstrates that at least four genetic loci are involved in the pathogenesis of human ceroid lipofuscinoses. Am J Hum Genet 1994;55:695–701

32. The International Batten Disease Consortium. Isolation of a novel gene underlying Batten Disease, CLN3. Cell 1995;82:949–957

33. Werhahn KJ, Brown P, Thompson PD, Marsden CD. The clinical features and prognosis of chronic posthypoxic myoclonus. Mov Disord 1997;12:216–220

34. Thompson PD, Colebatch JG, Brown P, et al. Voluntary stimulus-sensitive jerks and jumps mimicking myoclonus or pathological startle syndromes. Mov Disord 1992;7:257–262

35. Koskiniemi M, Van Vleymen B, Hakamies L, et al. Piracetam relieves symptoms in progressive myoclonus epilepsy: a multicenter, randomized, double-blind, cross-over study comparing the efficacy and safety of three dosages of oral piracetam with placebo. J Neurol Neurosurg Psychiatry 1998;64:344–348

36. Pranzatelli MR, Tate E, Galvan I, Wheeler A. A controlled trial of 5-hydroxy-L-tryptophan for ataxia in progressive myoclonic epilepsy. Clin Neurol Neurosurg 1996;98:161–164

37. Brown P, Steiger MJ, Thompson PD, et al. Effectiveness of piracetam in cortical myoclonus. Mov Disord 1993;8: 63–68

38. Truong DD, Fahn S. Therapeutic trial with glycine in myoclonus. Mov Disord 1988;3:222–232

39. Sternberg EM, Van Woert MH, Young SN, et al. Development of a scleroderma-like illness during therapy with L-5-hydroxytryptophan and carbidopa. N Engl J Med 1980;303:782–787

40. Ryan SG, Sherman SL, Terry JC, et al. Startle disease, or hyperekplexia: response to clonazepam and assignment of the gene (STHE) to chromosome 5q by linkage analysis. Ann Neurol 1992;31:663–668

41. Hayashi T, Tachibana H, Kajii T. Hyperekplexia: pedigree studies in two families. Am J Med Genet 1991;40:138–143

42. Dooley JM, Andermann F. Startle disease or hyperekplexia: adolescent onset and response to valproate. Pediatr Neurol 1989;5:126–127

43. Scarcella A, Coppola G. Neonatal sporadic hyperekplexia: a rare and often unrecognized entity. Brain Dev 1997;19:226–228

44. Tijssen MA, Schoemaker HC, Edelbroeck PJ, et al. The effects of clonazepam and vigabatrin in hyperekplexia. J Neurol Sci 1997;149:63–67

45. Frucht S, Fahn S. The clinical spectrum of posthypoxic mycolonus. Mov Disord 2000;15(S1):2–7

46. Iivanainen M, Himberg J. Valproate and clonazepam in the treatment of severe progressive myoclonus epilepsy. Arch Neurol 1982;39:236–238

47. Vaamonde J, Legarda I, Jimenez-Jimenez J, Obeso JA. Acetazolamide improves action myoclonus in Ramsay Hunt syndrome. Clin Neuropharmacol 1992;15:392–396

48. Lundemo G, Persson HE. Hereditary essential myoclonus. Acta Neurol Scand 1985;72:176–179

49. Fahn S, Sjaastad O. Hereditary essential myoclonus in a large Norwegian family. Mov Disord 1991;6:237–247

50. Duvoisin R. Essential myoclonus: response to anticholinergic therapy. Clin Neuropharmacol 1984;7:141–147

51. Priori A, Bertolasi L, Pesenti A, et al. γ-hydroxybutyric acid for alcohol-sensitive myoclonus with dystonia. Neurology 2000;54:1706

52. Jacobson PL, Messenheimer JA, Farmer TW. Treatment of intractable hiccups with valproic acid. Neurology 1981;31:1458–1460

53. Ramirez FC, Graham DY. Treatment of intractable hiccup with baclofen: results of a double-blind randomized, controlled, cross-over study. Am J Gastroenterol 1992;87:1789–1791

54. Stalnikowicz R, Fich A, Troudart T. Amitriptyline for intractable hiccups. N Engl J Med 1986;315:64–65

55. Deuschl G, Mischke G, Schenck E, et al. Symptomatic and essential rhythmic palatal myoclonus. Brain 1990;113:1645–1672

56. Ferro JM, Castro-Caldas A. Palatal myoclonus and carbamazepine. Ann Neurol 1981;10:402

57. Jabbari B, Rosenberg M, Scherokman B, et al. Effectiveness of trihexyphenidyl against pendular nystagmus and palatal myoclonus: evidence of cholinergic dysfunction. Mov Disord 1987;2:93–98

58. Scott B, Evans RW, Jankovic J. Treatment of palatal myoclonus with sumatriptan. Mov Disord 1996;11:748–751

59. Varney SM, Demetroulakos JL, Fletcher MH, et al. Palatal myoclonus: treatment with Clostridium botulinum toxin injection. Otolaryngol Head Neck Surg 1996; 114:317–320

60. Bryce GE, Morrison MD. Botulinum toxin treatment of essential palatal myoclonus tinnitus. J Otol 1998;27:213–216

61. Jankovic J, Pardo R. Segmental myoclonus: clinical and pathological study. Arch Neurol 1986;43:1025–1031

62. Jankovic J, Beach J. Long-term effects of tetrabenazine in hyperkinetic movement disorders. Neurology 1997;48:358–362

63. Jimenez-Jimenez FJ, Roldan A, Zancada F, et al. Spinal myoclonus: successful treatment with the combination of sodium valproate and L-5-hydroxytryptophan. Clin Neuropharmacol 1991;14:186–190

64. Chokroverty S, Walters A, Zimmerman T, Picone M. Propriospinal myoclonus: a neurophysiologic analysis. Neurology 1992;42:1591–1595

Dentatorubral-pallidoluysian Atrophy (DRPLA)

Shoji Tsuji

Dentatorubral-pallidoluysian atrophy (DRPLA) is a rare autosomal dominant neurodegenerative disorder that causes various combinations of cerebellar ataxia, choreoathetosis, myoclonus, epilepsy, dementia and psychiatric symptoms.[1] The term DRPLA was coined by Smith to describe a neuropathological condition associated with severe neuronal loss, particularly in the dentatorubral and pallidoluysian systems of the central nervous system in a sporadic case.[2,3] The hereditary form of DRPLA was first described in 1972 by Naito and his colleagues.[4] Since then, a number of reports on Japanese pedigrees with similar clinical presentations have been published,[5-14] and DRPLA has been established as a distinct disease entity.

The gene for DRPLA was discovered in 1994 and an unstable CAG trinucleotide repeat expansion in the protein-coding region of this gene was found to be the causative mutation.[15,16] To date, several other diseases have been found to result from an abnormal expansion of CAG repeats coding for polyglutamine stretches, including spinal and bulbar muscular atrophy (SBMA),[17] Huntington's disease (HD),[18] spinocerebellar ataxia type 1 (SCA-1),[19] DRPLA,[15,16] Machado-Joseph disease (SCA-3),[20] spinocerebellar ataxia type 2 (SCA-2),[21-23] spinocerebellar ataxia type 6 (SCA-6)[24] and spinocerebellar ataxia type 7 (SCA-7).[25] In this chapter, the clinical and molecular genetic aspects of DRPLA are described. The treatment for DRPLA remains symptomatic and largely ineffective.

Clinical features and diagnosis

The clinical features of DRPLA depend upon the age at onset, which ranges from childhood to late adulthood. Juvenile patients, with disease onset before the age of 20, usually exhibit a phenotype of progressive myoclonus epilepsy (PME), characterized by ataxia, seizures, myoclonus, and progressive intellectual deterioration. Epileptic seizures are a feature in all patients with onset before the age of 20. The frequency of seizures decreases with age after 20, and occurrence of seizures in patients with onset after the age of 40 is rare. Various forms of generalized seizures including tonic, clonic or tonic-clonic seizures are observed in DRPLA.

The differential diagnosis of childhood-onset and juvenile-onset DRPLA comprises other disorders that cause progressive myoclonic epilepsy, including mitochondrial encephalopathies, Lafora disease, Unverricht-Lundborg syndrome, sialidosis, and other lipid storage disorders.

Patients with onset after the age of 20 tend to develop cerebellar ataxia, choreoathetosis and dementia, thereby making this disease occasionally difficult to differentiate from Huntington's disease (HD) and the hereditary spinocerebellar ataxias (SCAs).[26] The most common spinocerebellar atrophy syndrome, Machado-Joseph disease (SCA-3), can be differentiated from DRPLA because the clinical features of MJD include various combinations of external ophthalmoplegia, bulging eyes, facial and lingual fasciculations, pyramidal signs, and distal muscular atrophy.

Most cases of DRPLA have been described in the Japanese population. In one study of 248 patients from 116 Italian families with autosomal dominant ataxia, only 1% carried the DRPLA mutation.[27] Despite treatment, which is limited, the mean duration of illness until death is 11 years.[28]

The brain MRI findings of DRPLA include atrophy of the cerebellum and brainstem structures. Patients with adult-onset DRPLA occasionally show involvement of the cerebral white matter, detected as areas with high intensity signals on T2-weighted images. In adult-onset patients, the pathology consists mainly of neuronal loss and astrocytosis involving the dentate nucleus and globus pallidus, and their respective projections to the red and subthalamic nuclei. There is moderately severe atrophy of the brainstem. In patients presenting with severe ataxia, degenerative changes may be found in the posterior columns and gracile and cuneate nuclei.

Molecular genetics

Dentatorubral-pallidoluysian atrophy is caused by an expanded CAG repeat on chromosome 12p13.31. In DRPLA, the CAG region is expanded to 49 to 79 repeat units, as compared to 6 to 35 repeat units in normal individuals.[15,29-31] There does not appear to be an overlap in the number of triplicate repeats between normal and affected individuals, in contrast to Huntington's disease. The human DRPLA gene spans approximately 20 kbp and consists of 10 exons, with the CAG repeats located in exon 5.[32] The detailed structure of the full-length cDNA of the human DRPLA gene has been determined.[32,33] The DRPLA cDNA is predicted to code for a protein of 1185 amino acids. To date, the function of this protein remains unknown.

The mode of inheritance of DRPLA is autosomal dominant with a high penetrance. There is considerable phenotypic heterogeneity, even within families. The prevalence of DRPLA in the Japanese population has been estimated to be 0.2–0.7 per 100 000, which is comparable to that of Huntington's disease.[34]

Although DRPLA has been reported to occur predominantly in Japanese individuals, several cases with similar clinical features have been described in other ethnic groups.[35-43] The DRPLA mutation has been identified in an African-American kindred with Haw River syndrome.[42] As with other triplet repeat expansion disorders, there is an inverse correlation between the age at onset and the size of expanded CAG repeats in DRPLA. Dentatorubral-pallidoluysian atrophy is characterized by prominent anticipation,[15,16,29,44,45] with earlier onset and a larger triplicate repeat expansion in succeeding generations. Paternal transmission results in more prominent anticipation (26–29 years/generation) than does maternal transmission (14–15 years/generation).

Northern blot analysis reveals that the DRPLA gene is widely expressed in various tissues including the heart, lung, kidney, placenta, skeletal muscle and brain, without predilection for regions exhibiting neurodegeneration.[32,33] Reverse transcription-polymerase chain reaction (RT-PCR) analysis of mRNA extracted from various regions of autopsied brains of patients with DRPLA demonstrated that DRPLA mRNA from a mutant DRPLA gene with expanded CAG repeats is expressed at levels comparable to the wild-type DRPLA gene, suggesting that CAG repeat expansion does not alter the transcription efficiency of the DRPLA gene.[33,45] Therefore, it seems likely that mutant DRPLA proteins with expanded polyglutamine stretches are toxic to neuronal cells, suggesting a "toxic gain of function."

Treatment

Dentatorubral-pallidoluysian atrophy is a progressive neurological disease with no effective therapy. The principle of therapy for DRPLA is symptomatic. Antiepileptic drugs should be given for patients with epileptic seizures. No systematic data is available to guide therapy but agents with good anti-myoclonic effects, such as clonazepam, valproate, and levitiracetam, are reasonable first-line drugs. Dopamine depleting agents (reserpine, tetrabenazine) and dopamine receptor blocking agents (haloperidol and many others) are effective at suppressing chorea and choreathetosis. Unfortunately, little is available to help the ataxia and dementia in DRPLA.

Genetic counseling

Genetic counseling should be made available to patients with DRPLA and their families. Most individuals diagnosed with DRPLA have an affected parent. Possible causes of an apparently negative family history include: failure to recognize the disorder in family members, early death of a parent before the onset of symptoms, non-paternity and late onset of the disease in the affected parent. As a result of genetic anticipation, affected offspring may express symptoms 25 years earlier than their parents.[15,16,29-31] This phenomenon should be taken into account in genetic counseling. At-risk asymptomatic adult family members may seek testing in order to make personal decisions regarding reproduction, financial matters, and career planning. Testing of asymptomatic at-risk adult family members usually involves pre-test interviews in which the motives for requesting the test, the individual's knowledge of DRPLA, the possible impact of positive and negative test results, and neurological status are assessed.

References

1. Naito N, Oyanagi S. Familial myoclonus epilepsy and choreoathetosis; hereditary dentatorubral-pallidoluysian atrophy. Neurology 1982;32:798–807
2. Smith JK, Gonda VE, Malamud N. Unusual form of cerebellar alaxia: combined dentatorubral and pallidoluysian degeneration. Neurology 1958;8:205–209
3. Smith JK. Dentatorubropallidoluysian atrophy. In: Vinken PJ, Bruyn QW, eds. Handbook of Clinical Neurology. Elsevier, Amsterdam, 1975:519–534
4. Naito H, Izawa K, Kurosaki T, et al. Two families of progressive myoclonus epilepsy with Mendelian dominant heredity (in Japanese). Pyschiatr Neurol Jpn 1972;74:871–897
5. Naito H, Ohama E, Nagai H. A family of dentatorubropallidoluysian atrophy (DRPLA) including two cases with schizophrenic symptoms (in Japanese). Psychiatr Neurol Jpn 1987;89:144–158
6. Oyanagi S, Naito H. A clinico-neuropathological study on four autopsy cases of degenerative type of myoclonus epilepsy with Mendelian dominant heredity (in Japanese). Psychiatr Neurol Jpn 1977;79:113–129
7. Tanaka Y, Murobushi K, Ando S, et al. Combined degeneration of the globus pallidus and the cerebellar nuclei and their efferent systems in two siblings of one family. Primary system degeneration of the globus pallidus and the cerebellar nuclei (in Japanese). Brain Nerve 1977;29:95–104
8. Hirayama K, Iizuka R, Maehara K, Watanabe T. - Clinicopathological study of dentatorubropallidoluysian atrophy. Part I. Its clinical form and analysis of symptomatology (in Japanese). Adv Neurol 1981;25:725–736
9. Iizuka R, Hirayama K, Maehara KA. Dentatorubropallidoluysian atrophy: a clinicopathological study. J Neurol Neurosurg Psychiatry 1984;47:1288–1298
10. Suzuki S, Kamoshita S, Ninomura S. Ramsay Hunt syndrome in dentatorubralpallidoluysian atrophy. Pediatr Neurol 1985;1:298–301
11. Iizuka R, Hirayama K. Dentatorubropallidoluysian atrophy. In: Vinken PJ, Bruyn GW, Klawans HL, eds. Handbook of Clinical Neurology. Elsevier, Amsterdam, 1986:437–443
12. Iwabuchi K. Clinico-pathological studies on dentatorubropallidoluysian atrophy (DRPLA). Yokohama Igaku 1987;38:291–301
13. Iwabuchi K, Amano N, Yagishita S, et al. A clinicopathological study on familial cases of dentatorubropallidoluysian atrophy (DHPLft). Clin Neurol 1987;27:1002–1012
14. Akashi T, Ando S, Inose T, et al. Dentatorubropallidoluysian atrophy: a clinicopathological study (in Japanese). Rinsho Seishin Igaku 1987;29:523–531
15. Koide R, Ikeuchi T, Onodera O, et al. Unstable expansion of CAG repeat in hereditary dentatorubropallidoluysian atrophy (DRPLA). Nat Genet 1994;6:9–13
16. Nagafuchi S, Yanagisawa H, Sato K, et al. Expansion of an unstable CAG trinucleotide on chromosome 12p in dentatorubral and pallidoluysian atrophy. Nat Genet 1994;6:14–18

17. La Spada AR, Wilson EM, Lubahn DB, et al. Androgen receptor gene mutations in X-linked spinal and bulbar muscular atrophy. Nature 1991;352:77–79

18. The Huntington's disease collaborative research group. A novel gene containing a trinucleotide repeat that is expanded and unstable on Huntington's disease chromosomes. Cell 1993;72:971–983

19. Orr HT, Chung MY, Banfi S, et al. Expansion of an unstable trinucleotide CAG repeat in spinocerebellar ataxia type 1. Nat Genet 1993;4:221–226

20. Kawakami H, Maruyama H, Nakamura S, et al. Unique features of the CAG repeats in Machado-Joseph disease. Nat Genet 1995;9:344–345

21. Sanpei K, Takano H, Igarashi S, et al. Identification of the spinocerebellar ataxia type 2 gene using a direct identification of repeat expansion and cloning technique, DIRECT. Nat Genet 1996;14:277–284

22. Pulst SM, Nechiporuk A, Nechiporuk T, et al. Moderate expansion of a normally biallelic trinucleotide repeat in spinocerebellar ataxia type 2. Nat Genet 1996;14: 269–276

23. Imbert G, Saudou F, Yvert G, et al. Cloning of the gene for spinocerebellar ataxia 2 reveals a locus with high sensitivity to expanded CAG/glutamine repeats. Nat Genet 1996;14: 285–291

24. Zhuchenko O, Bailey J, Bonnen P, et al. Autosomal dominant cerebellar ataxia (SCAB) associated with small polyglutamine expansions in the alpha 1a-voltage-dependent calcium channel. Nat Genet 1997;15: 62–69

25. David G, Durr A, Stevanin G, et al. Cloning of the SCA7 gene reveals a highly unstable CAG repeat expansion. Nat Genet 1997;17:65–70

26. Naito H. Clinical picture of DRPLA. No To Shinkei 1995;47:931–938

27. Filla A, Mariotta C, Caruso G, et al. Relative frequencies of CAG expansions in spinocerebellar ataxia and dentatorubroluysian atrophy in 116 Italian families. Eur Neurol 2000;44:31–36

28. Warner TT, Williams LD, Walker RWH, et al. A clinical and molecular genetic study of dentatorubropallidoluysian atrophy in four European families. Ann Neurol 1995;37:452–459

29. Ikeuchi T, Koide R, Tanaka H, et al. Dentatorubral-pallidoluysian atrophy (DRPLA): clinical features are closely related to unstable expansions of trinucleotide (CAG) repeat. Ann Neurol 1995;37:769–775

30. Ikeuchi T, Onodera O, Oyake M, et al. Dentatorubral-pallidoluysian atrophy (DRPLA): close correlation of CAG repeat expansions with the wide spectrum of clinical presentations and prominent anticipation. Semin Cell Biol 1995;6:37–44

31. Ikeuchi T, Koide R, Onodera O, et al. Dentatorubral-pallidoluysian atrophy (DRPLA). Molecular basis for wide clinical features of DRPLA. Clin Neurosci 1995;3:23–27

32. Nagafuchi S, Yanagisawa H, Ohsaki E, et al. Structure and expression of the gene responsible for the triplet repeat disorder, dentatorubral and pallidoluysian atrophy (DRPLA). Nat Genet 1994;8:177–182

33. Onodera O, Oyake M, Takano H, et al. Molecular cloning of a full-length cDNA for dentatorubral-pallidoluysian atrophy and regional expressions of the expanded alleles in the CNS. Am J Hum Genet 1995;57:1050–1060

34. Inazuki G, Kumagai K, Naito H. Dentatorubral-pallidoluysian atrophy (DRPLA). Its distribution in Japan and prevalence rate in Niigata. Seishin Igaku 1990;32:1135–1138

35. Titica J, van Bogaert L. Heredo-degenerative hemiballismus: a contribution to the question of primary atrophy of the corpus luysii. Brain 1946;69:251–263

36. De Barsy TH, Myle G, Troch C, et al. La dyssynergie ce rebelleuse myoclonique (R. Hunt): affection autonome ou rariante du type degeneratif de l'epilepsie-myoclonie progressive (Unvericht-Lundborg) Appoche anatomo-alinique. J Neurol Sci 1968;8:111–127

37. Farmer TW, Wingfield MS, Lynch SA, et al. Ataxia, chorea, seizures, and dementia. Pathologic features of a newly defined familial disorder. Arch Neurol 1989;46: 774–779

38. Warner TT, Williams L, Harding AE. DRPLA in Europe. Nat Genet 1994;6:225

39. Warner TT, Lennox GG, Janota I, Harding AE. Autosomal-dominant dentatorubropallidoluysian atrophy in the United Kingdom. Mov Disord 1994;9:289–296

40. Norremolle A, Nielsen JE, Sorensen SA, Hasholt L. Elongated CAG repeats of the B37 gene in a Danish family with dentatorubropallidoluysian atrophy. Hum Genet 1995;95:313–318

41. Connarty M, Dennis NR, Patch C, et al. Molecular reinvestigation of patients with Huntington's disease in Wessex reveals a family with dentatorubral and pallidoluysian atrophy. Hum Genet 1996;97:76–78

42. Burke JR, Ikeuchi T, Koide R, et al. The Haw River syndrome: dentatorubropallidoluysian atrophy (DRPLA) in an African-American family. Nat Genet 1994; 7:521–524

43. Potter NT. The relationship between (CAG)n repeat number and age of onset in a family with dentatorubral-pallidoluysian atrophy (DRPLA): diagnostic implications of confirmatory and predictive testing. J Med Genet 1996;33:168–170

44. Ueno S, Kondoh K, Kotani Y, et al. Somatic mosaicism of CAG repeat in dentatorubral-pallidoluysian atrophy (DRPLA). Hum Mol Genet 1995;4:663–666

45. Yazawa I, Nukina N, Hashida H, et al. Abnormal gene product identified in hereditary dentatorubral-pallidoluysian atrophy (DRPLA) brain. Nat Genet 1995;10: 99–103

247 Tardive Dyskinesia and Related Disorders

Stanley Fahn

Tardive dyskinesia (TD) is an iatrogenic syndrome of persistent abnormal involuntary movements caused by drugs that competitively block dopamine receptors, particularly the D_2 receptor. These disorders tend to appear late in the course of treatment, hence the term *tardive*. The clinical appearance of tardive dyskinesia is varied, and encompasses a variety of abnormal movements: repetitive, stereotyped choreiform chewing movements and facial grimacing, known as classic tardive dyskinesia, sustained dystonic spasms of the body, or tardive dystonia, tardive tics, tardive myoclonus, as well as intolerable restlessness, or akathisia. Tardive syndromes can persist long after the inciting dopamine receptor-blocking agent (DRBA) is discontinued, causing chronic or even permanent disability.

Included among movement disorders caused by DRBAs are *acute* movement disorders, chiefly acute dystonia and akathisia, as well as reversible drug-induced parkinsonism. The entire category is sometimes lumped together as "extra-pyramidal symptoms" or "EPS" but the term oversimplifies a complex group of disorders, each with its own distinct clinical features and treatment. While tardive dyskinesia and related syndromes represent rare complications of DRBAs, it is important for all physicians to inform patients taking these agents of the potential risk for a permanent movement disorder. These syndromes are scientifically important for what they reveal about the biochemistry and pharmacology of the basal ganglia. In the future, with the anticipated development of effective antipsychotic agents that do not block dopamine receptors, it is hoped that the incidence tardive dyskinesia will decline.

This chapter will review the epidemiology, clinical manifestations, pathophysiology and treatment of tardive dyskinesia and related disorders caused by DRBAs. Included in this discussion are two syndromes caused by the abrupt discontinuation of DRBAs, the withdrawal-emergent syndrome, and neuroleptic malignant syndrome.

Historical background

The first use of dopamine receptor antagonists for psychiatric disorders was in the early 1950s. Credit for the first report of TD is attributed to Schonecker,[1] who reported four patients with TD induced by chlorpromazine. Sigwald et al.,[2] provided the first detailed descriptions of the syndrome, which he divided into acute, sub-acute, and chronic subtypes. Uhrbrand and Faurbye[3] published the first systematic review of the

complication among 500 psychiatric patients and noted 29 patients with the disorder. Despite numerous reports of the classical oro-buccal-lingual stereotypic movements of tardive dyskinesia, establishment of this disorder as a distinct clinical entity took decades of epidemiological studies.[4–6] Tardive dyskinesia has also been noted in patients without psychiatric disorders who were exposed to dopamine receptor antagonists, such as those with gastrointestinal complaints,[7] Gilles de la Tourette syndrome,[8] or dystonia.[9]

Definitions and terminology

The term *tardive syndromes* refers to a group of disorders that fit all of the following essential criteria: (1) phenomenologically, the clinical features are those of a movement disorder, i.e., abnormal involuntary movements, or of a sensation of needing to move combined with the appearance of restlessness; (2) the disorder is caused by the patient having been exposed to at least one dopamine receptor blocking agent (DRBA) within six months of the onset of symptoms (in exceptional cases, exposure could be within 12 months); and (3) the disorder persists for at least one month after stopping the offending drug.[10,11] In the sections that follow, each type of movement disorder syndrome produced by DRBAs will be discussed separately. A list of tardive syndromes and related disorders discussed in this chapter is provided in Table 247.1. Additional rare tardive neurological syndromes attributed to DRBAs include myoclonus, tremor, tics, chorea, parkinsonism, and a tardive pain syndrome.

Table 247.1 Neurological adverse effects of dopamine receptor antagonists

1. Acute reactions
   a. Acute dystonia
   b. Acute akathisia

2. Drug-induced parkinsonism

3. Tardive syndromes
   a. Withdrawal-emergent syndrome
   b. Classical tardive dyskinesia (TD)
   c. Tardive dystonia
   d. Tardive akathisia

4. Syndromes induced by the abrupt withdrawal of dopamine receptor blocking agent
   a. Withdrawal-emergent syndrome
   b. Neuroleptic malignant syndrome

Pathophysiology

Dopamine receptors

It is important to understand dopamine receptors and the nature of the drugs that produce TD. Dopamine receptors are classified into five subtypes, based on the genetics of the receptors. They are labeled D_1, D_2, D_3, D_4, and D_5.[12,13] The D_1 and D_5 receptors were both previously known as D_1 receptors; both are distinct in activating adenyl cyclase. The D_2, D_3, and D_4 receptors were all previously grouped together as the D_2 receptor, and are still considered in the D_2 family of receptors.

The D_1 and D_2 receptors are found mainly in striatum and nucleus accumbens, as well as in substantia nigra, amygdala, cingulate cortex and entorhinal area. The anterior lobe of the pituitary gland has only D_2 receptors, and thalamus and cerebral cortex outside of cingulate and entorhinal area contain D_1 receptors only.[14] D_2 receptor affinities of dopamine receptor antagonists correlate closely with antipsychotic and anti-emetic properties of the drugs.[15] Dopamine receptor antagonists are often referred to as neuroleptics or antipsychotics; the former indicates the effect of drugs in producing parkinsonism, and the latter indicates the effect of controlling psychosis.

The D_3 receptor, another target of neuroleptics, is found chiefly in the mesolimbic areas. Because it is involved with emotional behaviors, it may be involved with tardive akathisia. Clozapine, an atypical neuroleptic with the lowest potential to induce parkinsonism of all available antipsychotics, is primarily a D_4 receptor antagonist, with minimal D_2 antagonism.

Dopamine receptor blocking agents

Many drugs block the DA receptor. The classic DRBAs are antipsychotic medications, but certain drugs used for nausea, cardiac disease, hypertension, and depression also block DA receptors. A complete list of DRBAs is provided in Table 247.2. Metoclopramide[16] and clebopride[17] are used mainly for dyspepsia and as anti-emetic agents. Amoxapine has a tricyclic structure, and is marketed as an antidepressant drug, but a metabolite has dopamine receptor blocking activity and has been implicated in producing TD.[18] Veralipride is a substituted benzamide that is used for the treatment of menopausal hot flushes.[19] Pimozide is marketed for the treatment of Tourette syndrome.

Some commercial preparations contain dopamine receptor antagonists in combination with other drugs, and this may lead to inadvertent use of these drugs. A popular combination is that of perphenazine and amitriptyline, marketed as Triavil and Etrafon. Risperidone is commercially promoted with the suggestion that it may carry a lower risk of drug-induced complications, but this appears not to be the case. Parkinsonism and TD have been noted in association with the calcium channel antagonists, flunarizine and cinnarizine.[20] Both of these medications have mild dopamine receptor antagonist activity,

which is thought be the mechanism for their complications.[21]

The risk of a tardive syndrome is directly proportional to its D_2 receptor affinity. Seeman and Tallerico[22] found that "atypical" antipsychotic drugs, a group that includes clozapine, quetiapine, risperidone, olanzapine, ziprasidone and others, bind more loosely than classical antipsychotic drugs (neuroleptics) to the D_2 receptors. Kapur et al.,[23] measured D_2 and 5-HT_2 receptor occupancies by positron emission

Table 247.2 Drugs that can produce tardive syndromes	
Class of drug	**Examples of drugs in each class**
1. Phenothiazines	
a. Aliphatic	Chlorpromazine (e.g. Thorazine) Triflupromazine (e.g. Vesprin)
b. Piperidine	Thioridazine (e.g. Mellaril) Mesoridazine (e.g. Serentil)
c. Piperazine	Trifluoperazine (e.g. Stelazine) Prochlorperazine (e.g. Compazine) Perphenazine (e.g. Trilafon) Fluphenazine (e.g. Prolixin) Perazine
2. Thioxanthenes	
a. Aliphatic	Chlorprothixene (e.g. Tarctan)
b. Piperazine	Thiothixene (e.g. Navane)
3. Butyrophenones	Haloperidol (e.g. Haldol) Droperidol (e.g. Inapsine)
4. Diphenylbutylpiperidine	Pimozide (e.g. Orap)
5. Dibenzazepine	Loxapine (e.g. Loxitane)
6. Dibenzodiazepine	Clozapine (e.g. Clozaril) Quetiapine (e.g. Seroquel)
7. Thienobenzodiazepine	Olanzapine (e.g. Zyprexa)
8. Substituted benzamides	Metoclopramide (e.g. Reglan) Tiapride Sulpiride Clebopride Remoxipride Veralipride
9. Indolones	Molindone (e.g. Moban)
10. Pyrimidinone	Risperidone (e.g. Risperidal)
11. Benzisothiazole	Ziprasidone (e.g. Geodon)
12. Benzisoxazole	Iloperidone (e.g. Zomaril)
13. Tricyclic	Amoxapine (e.g. Asendin)
14. Calcium channel blockers	Flunarizine (e.g. Sibelium) Cinnarizine (e.g. Stugeron)
15. N-acetyl-4-methoxytryptamine	Melatonin

tomography (PET) scans for patients receiving clozapine, risperidone or olanzapine. Clozapine showed a much lower D_2 occupancy (16–68%) than risperidone (63–89%) and olanzapine (43–89%); all three showed greater 5-HT$_2$ than D_2 occupancy at all doses, although the difference was greatest for clozapine. These studies support the clinical observations that clozapine and quetiapine are the most "atypical," with the least propensity to cause parkinsonism, tardive syndromes or other neuroleptic drug reactions.

Clinical presentations

Acute syndromes

Acute dystonia   The earliest abnormal involuntary movement to appear after initiation of dopamine receptor antagonist therapy is an acute dystonic reaction. In about half of the cases this reaction occurs within 48 hours and in 90% by five days after starting the therapy.[24,25] The reaction may occur after the first dose.[26] Dystonic movements are sustained muscle contractions, frequently causing twisting and repetitive movements, or abnormal postures.[27] In one series of 3775 patients, Ayd[24] found that acute dystonia was the least frequent extra-pyramidal syndrome, affecting about 2–3% of patients, with males and younger patients being more susceptible. The incidence rate increases to beyond 50% with highly potent dopamine receptor blockers such as haloperidol.[28] In one prospective study, Aguilar et al.,[29] reported that 23 of 62 patients developed acute dystonia after introducing haloperidol, that anticholinergic pre-treatment significantly prevents these, and that younger age and severity of psychosis were risk factors. In the prospective study by Kondo et al.,[30] 20 (51.3%) of 39 patients placed on nemonapride had dystonic reactions, with onset occurring within three days after the initiation of treatment in 90%. All agents that block D_2 receptors can induce acute dystonic reactions, including risperidone[31,32] and clozapine.[33] Serotonergic agents have also been reported to induce acute dystonic reactions.[34–36] The mechanism could relate to inadequate dopamine being released from the nerve terminals in the striatum due to the inhibitory effect of serotonin on dopamine neurons in the substantia nigra pars compacta. The opioid sigma(1) and sigma(2) receptors have also been implicated.[37]

Acute dystonic reactions most often affect the ocular muscles (oculogyric crisis), face, jaw, tongue, neck and trunk, and less often limbs. Oculogyric crisis has previously been noted to occur as a common feature of post-encephalitic parkinsonism.[38] A typical acute dystonic reaction may consist of head tilt backwards or sideways with tongue protrusion and forced opening of the mouth, often with arching of trunk and ocular deviation upwards or laterally.[39] The forcefulness of the muscle contractions can be extremely severe, and led to auto-amputation of the tongue in one patient.[40]

In patients with acute dystonic reactions, symptoms can be relieved within minutes using parenteral anticholinergics or antihistaminics.[41–43] Diphenhydramine 50 mg, benztropine mesylate or biperiden 1–2 mg is given intravenously and can be repeated if the effect is not seen in 30 minutes. Intravenous diazepam has also been shown to be effective and can be used as an alternative therapy.[44–46] If untreated, the majority of cases still resolve spontaneously in 12–48 hours after the last dose of the dopamine receptor antagonist. Dopamine receptor antagonists with high anticholinergic activities have low incidence rates of acute dystonic reactions.[47] Therefore, prophylactic use of anticholinergics[48] and benztropine[49] has been advocated, especially in young patients on high potency DRBAs.

Acute akathisia   The term akathisia, from the Greek, meaning unable to sit down, was coined by Haskovec in 1902,[50] long before antipsychotic drugs were introduced. Akathisia refers to an abnormal state of excessive restlessness, a feeling of needing to move about, with relief of this symptom upon actually moving. Akathisia was first observed in patients with advanced parkinsonism. Today, it is most frequently encountered as a side effect of neuroleptic drugs. Two major issues of akathisia remain in confusion. First, there is no consensus on diagnostic criteria. Some authors consider akathisia as a purely subjective state of restlessness and do not regard the restless movements as a necessary feature for the diagnosis.[51] Others require only the appearance of restlessness as sufficient for the diagnosis, even when the patient does not give a history of feeling restless.[52–54] A second point of confusion is that akathisia occurs not only as an early onset, self-limited form (acute akathisia), but also as a late onset, persistent form (tardive akathisia). Much of the literature on akathisia does not distinguish between acute and tardive akathisia. The recognition of tardive akathisia as a distinct subcategory of tardive syndromes has been more recent.[55–58] The phenomenology of acute and tardive akathisia are identical, but the timing and course of the two syndromes are distinct. The subjective aspect of akathisia is characterized by inner tension and aversion to remaining still. Patients complain of vague inner tension, emotional unease, or anxiety with vivid phrases such as "jumping out of skin" or "about to explode." Subjective descriptions, however, can be nonspecific. Inner restlessness and inability to remain still can be present in a significant number of psychiatric patients without akathisia and in control subjects without psychiatric problems.[57] In an attempt to clarify the issue, Braude et al.,[57] systematically surveyed frequency of various complaints and found that inability to keep the legs still was the most characteristic complaint, present in over 90% of patients with akathisia in contrast to about 20% of those with other psychiatric disturbances. Others noted more conservative estimation of the frequency of complaints related to the legs ranging from 27%[53] to 57%.[59] Various authors also described atypical features such as "acting out," have suicidal ideation, disruptive behaviors, homicidal violence, sexual torment, terror, and exacerbation of psychosis as akathitic phenomena.[60] Evaluation of the subjective aspect also depends on patients' ability to describe their feelings. Those with psychosis, dementia, or mental retardation are often unable to provide useful descriptions for diagnosis. Although akathisia may manifest as a subjective feeling alone, lack of specific subjective feeling and variable expression by patients pose a diagnostic dilemma. Therefore, presence of the motor phenomenon is very helpful for the diagnosis. Some patients may moan as part of a generalized akathitic state and have other motor evidence of akathisia, such as marching in place, inability to sit still with walking about, inability to lie quietly with writhing and rolling movements, and stereotypic caressing or rocking movements. The differential diagnosis of moaning includes parkinsonism, akathisia, levodopa,[61] dementia, and pain; and other syndromes of phonations, such as tics, oromandibular dystonia, and Huntington's disease, as discussed by Fahn.[62] The motor aspect of akathisia ("akathitic movements") is generally described as excessive movements that are complex, semi-purposeful, stereotypic, and repetitive. Braude et al.,[57] found that rocking from foot to foot, walking-on-the-spot, and coarse tremor and myoclonic jerks of feet were characteristic of akathitic movements. Others agree that various leg and feet movements were more common in patients with akathisia than those with TD.[53,59] However, they also noted that these did not distinguish akathisia from the group that did not meet criteria for akathisia,[53] and movements involving other parts of the body such as trunk rocking, respiratory grunting, face rubbing, and shifting weight while sitting were also frequent.[59] Although there are not enough data and consensus on the diagnostic movements of akathisia, they seem to be characteristic enough to be recognized by different authors who independently document similar phenomena.

Akathisia is seen in patients with Parkinson's disease,[63] in patients abusing cocaine,[64] and as an adverse effect of select serotonin re-uptake inhibitors.[65] Acute akathisia occurs not only as an adverse effect of DRBAs, but also fairly commonly as an acute adverse effect of the dopamine depletors reserpine, tetrabenazine and alpha-methyl tyrosine.[66] In Ayd's review,[24] half of the cases of acute akathisia occurred within 25 days of drug treatment and 90% by 73 days. Acute akathisia was the most common side effect of the DRBAs, occurring in 21.2% of patients in that study.[24] In a more recent study by Sachdev and Kruk[67] of 100 consecutive patients placed on neuroleptics, mild akathisia developed in 41% and moderate-to-severe akathisia in 21%. In a literature review, Sachdev[68] reported that incidence rates for acute akathisia with conventional neuroleptics vary from 8–76%, with 20–30% being a conservative estimate. Sachdev stated that preliminary evidence suggests that the newer atypical antipsychotic drugs are less likely to produce acute akathisia. Using the criterion that both subjective and objective phenomena are required for the diagnosis of acute

akathisia, Miller et al.,[69] found an incidence rate of 22.4%, of which 75% occurred within the first three days of exposure to a neuroleptic. Muscettola and colleagues[70] found a prevalence rate of 9.4%. As noted above, akathisia needs to be distinguished from other conditions such as agitated depression, restless legs syndrome, in which similar subjective sensations may be, in which described by patients, but are mainly localized to legs and are present particularly at night,[71] or complex motor tics with preceding aura that show more variety of abnormal movements and complex vocal tics.[72] Akathisia can also be obscured by other psychiatric disorders, or it could be mistaken for a psychiatric disease. For example, when patients with psychosis develop akathisia after withdrawal from antipsychotic drugs, it may be mistaken for recurrence of psychosis. Paradoxical dystonia, in which dystonic movements are relieved by movement, can be mistaken for akathisia.

The pathophysiology of acute akathisia remains poorly understood. Based on the observation in rats that show increased locomotor activity after blockade of the mesocortical dopamine system,[73] reduction of this dopaminergic projection was suggested to be responsible for akathisia.[66] However, tardive akathisia cannot be explained by this hypothesis because dopamine depletors can ameliorate those symptoms. The observation that acute akathisia can occur with a serotonin uptake inhibitor[74] indicates that inhibiting dopamine neurons in the substantia nigra by such drugs could further link the dopamine system with akathisia. These types of drugs have been reported to increase parkinsonism in patients with Parkinson's disease.[75]

Ayd[24] noted that acute akathisia may be self-limited, disappearing upon discontinuation of neuroleptics, and may be well controlled by anticholinergics despite continuation of neuroleptics. Others have noted that only patients with concomitant parkinsonism improve significantly with anticholinergics.[57,76] Amantadine may also help, but patients can develop a tolerance.[77,78] Beta-blockers at relatively low doses below 80 mg of propranolol per day have been noted to be effective in many studies including one with a double-blind design.[77–81] Non-lipophilic beta-blockers that have poor penetration to the central nervous system (CNS) are not as effective.[80,81] Selective beta-blockers may not be as effective as non-selective ones.[77,78] When two equally lipophilic beta-blockers, propranolol and betaxolol, were compared, they were equally effective in treating acute akathisia[82] although the former is a beta-2 blocker, and the latter a beta-1 blocker. Clonidine reduces central noradrenergic activity by stimulating central alpha-2 receptors and has been noted to be effective in a small number of studies. Sedating effect is pronounced, however.[83] Nicotine patches have been reported to reduce akathisia.[84] Cyproheptadine, an antiserotonergic agent, was reported to be effective in ameliorating akathisia by Weiss et al.[85] In a small placebo-controlled trial, mianserin, a 5-HT$_2$ antagonist, was found to reduce the severity of acute akathisia.[86]

Neuroleptic-induced parkinsonism

Neuroleptic-induced parkinsonism is a dose-related side effect of the DRBAs and is indistinguishable phenomenologically from idiopathic Parkinson's disease. Like Parkinson's disease, drug-induced parkinsonism may include a typical rest tremor and asymmetric signs.[87] It develops with use of both DRBAs and dopamine depleting drugs such as reserpine and tetrabenazine. Some authors have noted perioral tremor and termed this as rabbit syndrome, which is a localized form of parkinsonian tremor.[88] The incidence of parkinsonism varies from 15–61%,[89] with 19.4% found by Muscettola and colleagues.[70] Women are almost twice as frequently affected as men, which is the reverse of the ratio in idiopathic Parkinson's disease. Neuroleptic-induced parkinsonism also occurs increasingly with advanced age[24,87] in parallel with the incidence of idiopathic Parkinson's disease.

Blockade of dopamine receptors by antagonists or depletion of presynaptic monoamines by drugs such as reserpine mimics the deficient dopamine state in Parkinson's disease. All DRBAs can induce parkinsonism, but clozapine does not.[90] Parkinsonism from neuroleptics is typically reversible when the medication is reduced or discontinued. Sometimes, the reversal may take many months; an interval of up to 18 months has been noted in the literature.[91]

Some patients show persisting parkinsonism despite prolonged discontinuation of neuroleptics,[87,92,98] giving rise to consideration of a proposed condition of tardive parkinsonism. A study of eight-week exposure of rats to haloperidol found a highly significant 32–46% loss of tyrosine hydroxylase (TH) immunoreactive neurons in the substantia nigra, and 20% contraction of the TH stained dendritic arbor.[93] Perhaps such pathological changes account for some cases of prolonged drug-induced parkinsonism in humans. However, there is always the possibility that the patient had preclinical Parkinson's disease prior to developing drug-induced parkinsonism. Several cases in the literature had initial resolution of parkinsonism and later had reappearance of the symptoms without re-exposure to neuroleptics.[87] Two cases that had complete resolution of drug-induced parkinsonism after withdrawal of neuroleptic showed evidence of mild Parkinson's disease at autopsy.[94] Although one assumes that these patients had subclinical Parkinson's disease, the effect of neuroleptics on the disease progression is unknown. The use of the term "tardive parkinsonism" to refer to cases of persistent parkinsonism remains debatable. One would need to show that there are no Lewy bodies or that the PET scan shows no loss of fluorodopa uptake in patients believed to have tardive parkinsonism. Some are due to concurrent development of progressive Parkinson's disease, and there are no autopsied proven examples of non-PD in any example. As such, there is no evidence to date that tardive parkinsonism exists.

With the introduction of selective serotonin reuptake inhibitors (SSRIs) to treat depression, it has been noticed that these drugs can sometimes worsen parkinsonism in patients with Parkinson's disease[75] and occasionally can induce parkinsonism in patients who never had symptoms of Parkinson's disease.[95,96] In an intensive monitoring program in New Zealand of the SSRI drug fluoxetine over a four-year period, there were 15 reports of parkinsonism in 5555 patients exposed to the drug.[95] Of these 15, four patients were also on a neuroleptic and one was on metoclopramide. The explanation for inducing or enhancing parkinsonism is that increased serotonergic activity in the substantia nigra will inhibit dopamine-containing neurons, thus causing functional dopamine deficiency in the nigrostriatal pathway.[97]

Anticholinergics can be effective in reducing the severity of the parkinsonism induced by DRBAs, whereas dopaminergic drugs (that activate the dopamine receptors) are ineffective, probably because they are not able to displace the DRBA from its binding to the receptor. L-dopa up to 1000 mg in combination with a peripheral dopa decarboxylase inhibitor had no significant effect,[87] nor did apomorphine, a dopamine receptor agonist.[99] On the other hand, levodopa can effectively reverse parkinsonism induced by dopamine depletors, such as reserpine. In fact, the discovery of the dopamine hypothesis for parkinsonism was based on this observation.[100,101] Treatment is usually initiated with anticholinergics or amantadine.[102–104]

Tardive syndromes

Classical tardive dyskinesia Dyskinesia is a general term meaning simply abnormal movements. Over the years, tardive dyskinesia has become synonymous with the first described complication of long-term dopamine receptor antagonist therapy: rapid, repetitive, stereotypic movements involving oral, buccal, and lingual areas. Sustained dystonic movements of the lower face must be distinguished from classical tardive dyskinesia. Often patients on anticholinergics or other medications develop oral dyskinesia with dryness of mouth. Other movements such as myokymia, myoclonus, and tics must also be distinguished. The clinical features of classical tardive dyskinesia (TD) are quite distinct from other movement disorders.[10] The principal site is the face, particularly around the mouth, typically called oral-buccal lingual (O-B-L) dyskinesias. The mouth tends to show a pattern of repetitive, complex chewing motions, occasionally with smacking and opening of the mouth, tongue protrusion (fly-catcher tongue), lip pursing, sucking movements, and fish-like lip puckering movements. The rhythmicity and coordinated pattern of movement is striking. This stereotypic pattern is in contrast to the dyskinesias seen in Huntington's disease, where the movements are random without a predictable pattern. Usually the limb involvement TD is limited to the distal part. Like the mouth region, the movements of the distal limbs show a repetitive pattern, earning the label of piano-playing fingers and toes. When the patient is sitting, the legs often move repeatedly, with flexion and extension movements of toes and foot tapping. When patient is lying down, flexion and extension of thighs may be seen. The respiratory pattern can be involved with dyskinesia, causing hyperventilation at times, and hypoventilation at other times.[105] In a study of the breathing pattern in patients with TD, patients had an irregular tidal breathing pattern, with a greater variability in both tidal volume and time of the total respiratory cycle.[106] The presence of respiratory dyskinesia never causes a medical problem, although it may look alarming. Esophageal (associated with lingual) dyskinesias have also been reported, resulting in increased intraesophageal pressure and death due to asphyxiation in one patient.[107] The involuntary movements of the mouth in classical tardive dyskinesia are readily suppressed by the patients when asked to do so. Furthermore, the movements cease as the patient is putting food in the mouth, when talking, or by placing a finger on the lips. Since the movements do not interfere with basic functions, patients are often unaware of their movements. When the patient is asked to keep the tongue at rest inside the mouth, the tongue tends to assume a continual writhing motion of athetoid side-to-side and coiling movements. The constant lingual movements may lead to tongue hypertrophy, and macroglossia is a common clinical sign. On command, however, most patients with TD can keep the tongue protruded without darting back into the mouth for more than half a minute; patients with the chorea of Huntington's disease typically cannot maintain a protruded tongue. This inability to sustain a voluntary contraction is called motor impersistence, which is not seen in TD.

Epidemiological studies looking into prevalence of TD have been confounded by the factors that affect the detection of the abnormal involuntary movements as well as the variables that affect the prognosis of the movements. Therefore, it is not surprising to find a wide range of prevalence estimate from 0.5–65% in the literature.[5,6] The prevalence of TD was noted to have increased from 5% before 1965 to 25% in the late 1970s.[5,6] Mean prevalence rates calculated by two different reviewers, however, agree well at around 20%.[5,6] Host and treatment factors affect the development, severity, and persistence of TD, thereby resulting in different prevalence rates. Age of the patient correlates with the incidence, poor prognosis, and increased severity of tardive dyskinesia.[5,6,108,109] Female sex has been associated with increased prevalence of TD, especially in the older population.[5,6,110] Several authors noted increased incidence and prevalence among patients with affective disorders as compared to schizophrenia or schizoaffective disorders.[111] Prospective studies have noted that the total cumulative drug exposure correlates with incidence of withdrawal tardive dyskinesia,[112] and development of TD five years later in patients who did not have TD initially.[113] Continued use of DRBAs after appearance of TD also adversely affects subsequent prognosis.[108] Drug holidays were once advocated to decrease the risk of TD, but increased number of drug free intervals was found to worsen the prognosis after withdrawal.[114] The risk of developing TD is three times as

great for patients with more than two neuroleptic interruptions as for patients with two or fewer interruptions.[115] Other than reduced risk with clozapine, olanzapine and quetiapine, no other particular type of neuroleptic, including depot preparations, has been clearly identified as risk factor.[116] Chronic dopamine receptor antagonist treatment in rats may cause cell loss in the ventrolateral striatum,[117] changes in synaptic patterns in the striatum at the electron microscopic level,[118] and increases in glutamatergic synapses in the striatum.[119] In the accumbens in rats that developed vacuous chewing movements, the dendritic surface area is reduced, and dynorphin-positive terminals contact more spines and form more asymmetrical specializations than do those in animals without the syndrome.[120] Since TD is etiologically related to DRBAs and since the clinical pharmacology is most consistent with dopaminergic hyperactivity, many studies have been directed to the dopamine system.[121] The best model of human tardive dyskinesia is that produced in non-human primates. Primates show delayed onset of dyskinesia during the course of treatment and only a fraction of the population treated is affected by dyskinesia. The behavioral effect is spontaneous and bears resemblance to human TD. The dyskinesia also persists after withdrawal of the DRBAs. Unfortunately, neuropathological and biochemical data from this model are limited. One group suggested that the best neurochemical correlate of dyskinesia induced by DRBAs has been a decrease in gamma amino butyric acid (GABA) and glutamic acid decarboxylase (GAD) activity in the substantia nigra, subthalamic nucleus, and medial globus pallidus as compared to control animals without drug treatment or animals with drug treatment but without dyskinesia.[122] This finding correlates with postmortem biochemical studies on humans with TD and with a recent 2-deoxyglucose study in primates with TD. In the latter study, Mitchell et al.,[123] reported that primates with TD had a reduced glucose metabolism in the medial globus pallidus and in the VA and VL nuclei of the thalamus. Additional studies and new approaches are needed to understand the pathophysiology of classical tardive dyskinesia. The treatment of TD is discussed later.

Tardive dystonia Dystonia is most often an idiopathic disorder and can occur at all ages. Persistent dystonic movement as a complication of DRBA therapy has long been noted.[124] However, it was not been studied systematically to show that this represents a distinct syndrome until reported by Burke et al.[125] Tardive dystonia has a different epidemiology and pharmacological response than classical tardive dyskinesia. Although secondary dystonia can be caused by many neurological disorders,[126] tardive dystonia is one of the most common causes.[18] The onset of tardive dystonia can be from days to years after exposure to a DRBA.[18] Kiriakakis et al.,[127] found the range to extend from four days to 23 years of exposure (median 5, mean 6.2 ± 5.1 years) in their series of 107 patients, with a mean ($\pm$ SD) age at onset of 38.3 ± 13.7 years (range 13–68 years). There is no safe period from developing tardive dystonia, with one patient in the series by Burke et al.,[125] developing it after a one-day exposure. Men are significantly younger than women at onset of dystonia, and it develops after shorter exposure in men.[127] Yassa et al.,[128] found that severe tardive dystonia was more common in young men while severe classical tardive dyskinesia was more common in older women. The phenomenology of tardive dystonia can be indistinguishable from that of idiopathic dystonia, including the improvement with sensory tricks (geste antagoniste), which can be taken advantage of by creating mechanical devices to reduce the severity of the dystonia.[129] Focal dystonias, such as tardive cervical dystonia[130] and tardive blepharospasm,[131] can resemble primary focal dystonias. There is one clinical presentation of tardive dystonia that is particularly more characteristic of tardive dystonia, namely, the combination of retrocollis, trunk arching backward, internal rotation of the arms, extension of the elbows and flexion of the wrists.[18] Patients with idiopathic dystonia more often have lateral torticollis and twisting of the trunk laterally. Reduction of dystonic movements with voluntary action such as walking is often seen in tardive dystonia. This is distinctly unusual in idiopathic dystonia, in which the dystonic movements are usually exacerbated by voluntary action. Tardive dystonia can be severe enough to jeopardize patients by causing life-threatening dysphagia.[132,133] Many patients with tardive dystonia also have classical tardive dyskinesia at some point in their course.[18,134] It is not clear why some develop dystonia whereas others develop classical tardive dyskinesia or why some develop both. When patients have both types, dystonic symptoms are usually much more pronounced and disabling.[18,135]

Tardive akathisia Originally akathisia was mainly thought of as acute to sub acute side effect of dopamine receptor antagonists. Various authors, however, noted different variants of akathisia that occurred late in the course of the neuroleptic therapy or persisted despite discontinuation of neuroleptic therapy.[56–58] The clinical phenomenology of tardive akathisia is thought to be same as that of acute akathisia. In the study by Burke et al.,[59] mean age at onset of tardive akathisia was 58 years, with a range from 21–82 years, similar to the age range of classical tardive dyskinesia. Mean duration of dopamine receptor antagonist exposure before the onset was 4.5 years with a range from two weeks to 22 years. Over half of the patients had onset within two years. Again, the risk of developing tardive akathisia seems to start at the initiation of the drug therapy as in other tardive syndromes. All of the patients in the study by Burke et al.,[59] with tardive akathisia also had either tardive dyskinesia (93%) or tardive dystonia (33%) or both (27%) at the same time. But isolated tardive akathisia can exist as well. The pathophysiology of akathisia is not understood.

Tardive pain syndrome An unusual syndrome of tardive pain has been described,[136] occurring in the context of tardive akathisia and dystonia. Affected individuals complain of a distressing and unrelenting sensation localized to a body part, often the mouth, abdomen or genitalia. The discomfort is often described as unusual tingling or burning sensations, and does not have a radicular distribution. An organic source for pain is not found, and the sensation is presumed to reflect a central pain syndrome. Sometimes the pain is described in bizarre terms, such as "my teeth feel sticky," or "I have a vibration inside my pelvis," suggesting the possibility that the patient has a somatic delusion. The depictions of discomfort are consistent from patient to patient, and resemble descriptions of central pain syndromes in Parkinson's disease. Tardive pain syndrome is a diagnosis of exclusion, requiring a careful search for an underlying physical abnormality. It is debated whether tardive pain syndrome is a localized form of akathisia that for some reason an affected patient describes in dysesthetic terms. However, in the absence of actual movement or a description of needing to move the affected body part, the term akathisia cannot be used as formally defined. The pathogenesis of tardive pain is not understood but presumably involves an alteration in dopaminergic processing that involves sensory pathways of the thalamus and its connections. Tardive pain syndromes may respond to the agents useful in treating tardive dystonia and tardive akathisia, namely, dopamine depleting agents, atypical neuroleptics, and neuropathic pain agents, such as tricyclic antidepressants and anticonvulsants.

Syndromes induced by sudden withdrawal of dopamine receptor blocking agents

Withdrawal emergent syndrome The withdrawal emergent syndrome was first described in children who have been on antipsychotic drugs for a long period of time and then were withdrawn abruptly from their medication.[137] The movements are choreic and resemble those of Sydenham's chorea. The abnormal movements are brief and flow from one muscle to another in a seemingly random way. They differ from the movements of classical tardive dyskinesia, which are brief, but stereotypic and repetitive. The movements in withdrawal emergent syndrome involve mainly the limbs, trunk, and neck, and rarely the oral region, which is the most prevalent site in classical tardive dyskinesia. The dyskinetic movements eventually disappear spontaneously within several weeks. For immediate suppression of movements, dopamine receptor antagonists can be reinstituted and withdrawn gradually, without recurrence of the withdrawal emergent syndrome.[10] A withdrawal reaction from melatonin with orobuccolingual movements and akathisia was reported by Giladi and Shabtai,[138] and is described in Table 247.3. The withdrawal emergent syndrome is analogous to classical tardive dyskinesia seen in adults, except that the course is more benign and the movements are more generalized resembling the choreic movements of Sydenham's chorea. In fact, most cases of tardive dyskinesia reported in children have a benign course and the phenomenology has

Table 247.3   General guidelines for the treatment of tardive syndromes

1. Taper and slowly eliminate causative agents, if clinically possible. Avoid sudden cessation of these drugs, which could exacerbate the tardive syndrome
2. Avoid drugs, if possible, i.e. wait for spontaneous recovery. This is possible only if the dyskinesia is not severe or there is no accompanying tardive akathisia or tardive dystonia. Akathisia and dystonia are more distressful and disabling than is classical tardive dyskinesia
3. If necessary to treat the symptoms, first use DA depleting drugs: reserpine, tetrabenazine, alpha-methylparatyrosine. Attempt to overcome the adverse effects of depression and parkinsonism with antidepressants and anti-Parkinson drugs, respectively
4. Next, consider the true atypical antipsychotic agents, clozapine and quetiapine
5. If these fail, consider small doses of a dopamine receptor agonist to activate only the presynaptic dopamine receptor and reduce the biosynthesis of dopamine
6. For tardive dystonia, consider anti-muscarinics
7. For tardive akathisia, consider ECT
8. Typical antipsychotic agents can be used to control the dyskinesias when all the above approaches fail. Combining this with a dopamine depletor may increase the potency of the antidyskinetic effect, and may theoretically protect against a worsening of the underlying tardive pathology
9. Thalamotomy and pallidotomy have been performed for tardive dyskinesia and dystonia. Deep brain stimulation of the pallidum may eventually become the preferred surgical procedure if the symptoms remain severe and all medication trials fail

been reported to be more generalized choreic movements rather than stereotypic repetitive movements of oral, buccal, and lingual distribution. Acute withdrawal of chronic antipsychotic drugs in adults can also lead to transient tardive dyskinesia, which disappears within three months. These types of movements have been labeled as withdrawal dyskinesia.[139,140]

Neuroleptic malignant syndrome   Neuroleptic malignant syndrome (NMS) is an idiosyncratic reaction that can sometimes be life-threatening. The clinical triad consists of (1) hyperthermia, usually with other autonomic dysfunctions such as tachycardia, diaphoresis, and labile blood pressure; (2) extrapyramidal signs, usually increased muscle tone of rigidity or dystonia, often with accompanying elevation of muscle enzymes; and (3) alteration of mental status, such as agitation, inattention, and confusion. Fever is not essential.[141] The syndrome begins abruptly while the patient is on therapeutic, not toxic, dosages of medication. In a review of 340 clinical reports of NMS in the literature,[142] changes in either mental status or rigidity were the initial manifestations of NMS in 82.3% of cases with a single presenting sign. All the symptoms are fully manifest within 24 hours and reach a maximum within 72 hours. There does not seem to be any relationship with the duration of therapy. It can develop soon after the first dose or at any time after prolonged treatment. Recovery usually occurs within one to several weeks, but can also be fatal in 20–30% of cases.[143,144] Muscle biopsies have shown swelling and edema, with 10–50% of fibers involved with vacuoles, but with scanty mononuclear infiltration.[145] All agents that block D_2 receptors can induce NMS, including risperidone[146–150] and clozapine.[151–153] Tetrabenazine has been reported to cause NMS; this seems likely to be due to its D_2 blocking activity[154] rather than to its dopamine depleting action (by blocking the vesicular dopamine transporter). Reserpine has no known dopamine receptor antago-

nism, only dopamine depleting activity (also by blocking the vesicular dopamine transporter), and has not been reported to cause NMS. In a Japanese study, 10 of 564 (1.8%) patients who received antipsychotics developed NMS,[155] much greater than the 12 of 9792 patients (0.1%) reported previously.[156] Risk factors were psychomotor excitement, refusal of food, weight loss, and oral administration of haloperidol at 15 mg/day or above.[155] Young males appear to be more predisposed to NMS,[157] but the reason for this is uncertain. In a case-control study searching for risk factors, Sachdev et al.,[158] found that patients with NMS were more likely to be agitated or dehydrated, often needed restraint or seclusion, had received larger doses of neuroleptics, and more often had previous treatment with ECT before the development of the syndrome. The pathophysiological mechanism of NMS is not well understood. Autopsies have revealed abnormalities in muscle.[159] A similar syndrome has been reported following abrupt withdrawal of levodopa,[160–162] suggesting a common mechanism of acute dopamine deficiency.[143] There is also a report of a patient who developed the NMS syndrome following abrupt withdrawal of the combination of a long-acting neuroleptic and an anticholinergic agent.[163] Because it responds to procyclidine administration, NMS implicates a muscarinic overactivity. The idiosyncratic nature and rarity of the syndrome remain unexplained. Ram et al.,[164] evaluated the structure of the D_2 receptor gene in 12 patients who had a history of NMS. One patient was found to have a nucleotide substitution of an exon of the D_2 gene. IBZM SPECT in one patient showed the DA receptor to be blocked in the acute phase of NMS, but the patient had been receiving a D_2 blocker, which would be expected to result in this finding.[165]

Treatment of NMS consists of discontinuing the antipsychotic drugs and providing supportive measures. Rapid relief of symptoms has been reported with the use of dantrolene, bromocriptine, or L-dopa.[144,166] Nisijima et al.,[167] found L-dopa to be more effective than dantrolene, but Tsujimoto et al.,[168] found intravenous dantrolene plus hemodialysis to be effective. Gratz and Simpson[157] recommended using anticholinergics in an attempt to reverse rigidity prior to utilizing bromocriptine. Carbamazepine was dramatically effective in two patients (with recurrence on withdrawal of the drug).[169] Re-exposure to dopamine receptor antagonists does not necessarily lead to recurrence of NMS.[170,171] Residual catatonias that can last weeks to months have been reported, with some responding to ECT.[172]

Treatment

The most important point to remember in management of tardive syndromes is that they are permanent neurological disorders caused by physicians. Dopamine receptor blocking agents should not be used unless absolutely necessary for the well-being of the patient. All patients prescribed DRBAs should be forewarned of the risk of a tardive dyskinesia syndrome before being placed on the drug.

In one survey of 520 psychiatrists, only 54% of them disclosed this risk.[173] A study of the impact of informed consent based on questionnaires showed that patients did retain the information both at four weeks and at two years.[174] Another study comparing patients' knowledge of TD by a questionnaire revealed that those who were educated about the disorder had more knowledge about it six months later.[175]

Once a tardive syndrome is encountered, gradual removal of the etiological agent must be seriously considered. A slow taper appears to be safer than sudden withdrawal because the latter may exacerbate the severity of the syndrome. In classical tardive dyskinesia, prospective data show 33% remission in two years following elimination of the DRBA.[108] In retrospective studies, the remission rates were 12% for tardive dystonia and 8% for tardive akathisia.[18,59] Younger age is associated with better chance of remission[109] and earlier detection and discontinuation of dopamine receptor antagonists were more favorable for remission.[176] In a study involving chronic schizophrenics, only one of 49 patients who discontinued the antipsychotic drugs had a lasting recovery, but 10 others had some improvement one year later.[177]

There are necessary indications for long-term use of DRBAs, such as chronic psychotic disorders.[4] When patients are not able to discontinue antipsychotic medications, the concern is whether their TD will inexorably get worse, requiring higher and higher doses of antipsychotics to suppress the symptoms. There are no data to settle this issue but it appears that continuing antipsychotics does not necessarily aggravate the symptoms of TD, once established.

Treatment of classical tardive dyskinesia (TD)

Dopamine depletors The rational for using dopamine-depleting drugs, such as reserpine and tetrabenazine (TBZ) (a synthetic benzoquinolizine), is that these agents effectively reduce dopaminergic synaptic activity, thereby reducing the TD symptoms, without exposing the brain to an offending DRBA. This allows the possibility that over time the brain will heal itself and completely eliminate the TD. In contrast, DRBAs can effectively decrease TD, but the brain continues to be exposed. Alpha-methylparatyrosine is not very effective when used alone, but can be a very powerful antidopaminergic drug when used with other presynaptically acting drugs. Tetrabenazine has a quicker onset and shorter duration of action and has fewer peripheral catecholamine-depleting effects than reserpine. Like reserpine, TBZ has also not been implicated in causing TD. However, in contrast to reserpine, TBZ does have some dopamine receptor blocking activity,[154] which probably accounts for the few cases reported of acute dystonic reactions that have been encountered clinically.[178] Tetrabenazine's major advantage is the quicker onset and fewer side effects compared to reserpine. Tetrabenazine is rapidly absorbed after oral administration and extensively metabolized during the first pass through the liver or the gut. One of the major metabolites, dihydrotetrabenazine, has similar pharmacological actions as tetrabenazine, although its ability to pass through the blood-brain barrier is unclear. Large individual variations are noted, and patients with hepatic dysfunction might expect alteration of pharmacokinetics.[179] The dose has to be clinically titrated for each patient. Improvement with TBZ was noted in 68% of 38 patients in the literature at a mean daily dose of 138 mg.[6] Fahn[180] reported improvement in five of six patients at doses of 75–300 mg/day in a long-term study. Kazamatsuri et al.,[181] noted that 54% of patients improved by at least 50% in a six-week trial of TBZ compared to placebo treatment. Jankovic and Beach[182] reported that 90% of patients had a marked improvement. Ondo and colleagues[183] blindly rated videotapes taken of patients before and after TBZ treatment (mean duration of 20 weeks) and showed improvement in their dyskinesias. A major problem with TBZ therapy is with long-duration exposure. Most patients dramatically improve initially; then while maintained on the original dose they begin to develop features of parkinsonism. Lowering the dose reduces this unwanted effect, but the TD is then less well controlled. Both reserpine and TBZ can induce acute akathisia and depression, so one needs to monitor for these adverse effects and treat them if they should occur. Antidepressants, including monoamine oxidase inhibitors, can be used effectively to treat the depression. The selective norepinephrine reuptake inhibitor, reboxetine, has been found to rapidly reverse TBZ-induced depression.[184]

Atypical neuroleptics By definition the atypical antipsychotics have a reduced propensity for inducing extrapyramidal adverse effects, tardive dyskinesia included. However, there is a range of the degree of adverse effects encountered by the variety of drugs that have at one time or other been labeled as atypical neuroleptics. Today, we have strong candidates for this labeling for the dibenzodiazepine (clozapine and quetiapine) and less so for the thienobenzodiazepine, olanzapine. But originally the "atypical" label was applied to the benzamine derivatives, such as sulpiride, metoclopramide, and tiapride. However, all three compounds have been reported to induce tardive dyskinesia or neuroleptic malignant syndrome.[7,185–187] Similarly, risperidone has been touted as "atypical," but it more resembles a "typical" antipsychotic, causing parkinsonism and inducing tardive dyskinesia.[188] The typical antipsychotics, including sulpiride, tiapride and risperidone, by blocking and occupying dopamine D_2 receptors, are effective in reducing the severity of tardive dyskinesia.[189] But so do even stronger DRBAs, such as phenothiazines and haloperidol. The problem with using typical antipsychotics to treat TD is that they are in the class of the offending drugs, and hence will prolong the exposure of the patient to the drugs that cause TD. The question is whether the true "atypical" antipsychotics, such as clozapine and quetiapine, can reduce the symptoms of TD and still allow the healing process in the brain to proceed to eventually eliminate the pathophysiological causation of the symptoms. There are reports of clozapine successfully reducing the abnormal movements of tardive dyskinesia and tardive akathisia[190–192] and in some patients with tardive dystonia.[192–200] But the response rate is lower than with typical antipsychotics such as haloperidol. Clozapine permits the dyskinesia to disappear in about half the cases in one report.[201] In another, eight of the 20 patients with TD improved after an average time of 261 ± 188 days of treatment.[202] With an average dose of approximately 400 mg/d, Bassitt and Neto[192] obtained a 50% lessening of dyskinesia. It is still not clear whether the reduction of dyskinesia is due to the small amount of D_2 blocking effect or if actual healing of the TD can take place in the presence of clozapine. The proof of the latter and preferred category would be the lack of reappearance when clozapine is withdrawn. We are still waiting for a report of such a case. Without that evidence, it is likely that the reductions of tardive dyskinesia and tardive dystonia are due to the small amount of D_2 blocking activity by clozapine. Olanzapine has successfully reduced the symptoms of TD.[203] But olanzapine is not a true "atypical," and the reduction of the symptoms and signs is probably by blocking D_2 receptors. This would convey no advantage over using the more classical and conventional typical antipsychotics.

Dopamine agonists Some investigators have tried to activate the presynaptic dopamine receptors by using low doses of a dopamine agonist, which in turn would reduce the biosynthesis and release of dopamine. Another approach by Alpert and Friedhoff[204] was the use of levodopa in an attempt to desensitize the post-synaptic dopamine receptors. This can cause initial worsening of symptoms before eventual improvement is expected after discontinuation of levodopa. Unfortunately, dopaminergic drugs can also lead to overt recurrence of underlying psychosis.[56] This approach has theoretical merit, but is very difficult to carry out in many patients and has not been widely used since the initial reports. Aman-

tadine has been reported to have some benefit,[205] but it may be due to its glutamate receptor blocking effect rather than its dopaminergic effect.

Non-dopaminergic medications Although neuroleptics are most effective in controlling the abnormal movements, some patients do not respond to this treatment. Non-dopaminergic treatments have been attempted by numerous investigators.[206,207] Agents that enhance GABA transmission have been tried because of GABA's inhibitory effect on the dopaminergic system and experimental data indicating changes in the GABA system in patients and animals treated with chronic neuroleptics. Use of benzodiazepines, baclofen, valproate, and gamma-vinyl GABA have met with limited success, partly due to tolerance and side effects such as worsening of psychosis. Some improvement was found with clonazepam.[208] Propranolol, fusaric acid, and clonidine decrease noradrenergic activity and have been reported to be useful but require further study to clarify their role in treating tardive dyskinesia. Use of cholinergic drugs was based on the reciprocal dopamine-acetylcholine balance in the basal ganglia. Despite a flurry of reports in the 1970s, this modality has been quite limited, and should be reconsidered now that some adequate cholinergic drugs are available. Anticholinergics, lithium, pyridoxine, tryptophan, cyproheptadine, vasopressin, naloxone, morphine, and estrogen were reported to be of no benefit. Buspirone has been reported to be beneficial,[209] but it is not clear that this drug doesn't have dopamine receptor blocking activity. Calcium channel blockers have been reported to reduce the severity of tardive dyskinesia,[210–212] but not in all studies.[213] A combination of acetazolamide and thiamine was found to reduce both TD and drug-induced parkinsonism.[214] A role for antioxidants has been raised.[215,216] Treatment with vitamin E has been found to reduce the severity of tardive dyskinesia[217–220] or have no effect.[221] The meta-analysis mentioned above showed effectiveness. However, the largest double-blind study was carried out by the Veterans Administration multi-center, placebo-controlled clinical trial,[219] which found vitamin E not to be effective. As a potential prophylactic agent, vitamin E (3200 IU/day) was found not to protect against developing drug-induced parkinsonism.[222] Nor was vitamin E treatment able to prevent neuroleptic-induced vacuous chewing movements in rats.[223] There continue to be reports of TD responding to open label trials. Gabapentin[224] and pyridoxine[225] were reported in 1999. Injections of botulinum toxin into the muscles causing oral dyskinesia have been reported to be effective in reducing the movements.[226] Sporadic reports noted efficacy of electroconvulsive therapy in refractory cases of TD,[227] but Yassa et al.,[228] reported success in only one of nine patients.

Conclusions on treating classical TD Neuroleptics, by blocking D_2 receptors or depleting dopamine from synaptic terminals, are effective in reducing the abnormal involuntary movements of TD. Depletors do not cause TD and are therefore preferred. Avoiding side effects, particularly drug-induced parkinsonism, is a major limiting factor. If one needs to utilize an antipsychotic, it seems safer to use one that is suspected of having less ability to induce tardive dyskinesia, such as clozapine and quetiapine. Olanzapine comes closer to being a typical, rather than an atypical, antipsychotic. When clozapine and quetiapine occasionally reduce dyskinesias, the doses used suggest the response is from their D_2 blocking activity. Figures 247.1 and 247.2 are flow charts providing algorithms for treating TD.

Tardive dystonia

Like with classical TD, the most effective medications for tardive dystonia are also antidopaminergic drugs,[18] but the percentage of patients who improve is smaller. Reserpine and TBZ each produce improvement in about 50% of patients. Some patients who do not respond or have intolerable side effects to one may respond to the other. Dopamine receptor blocking agents are more effective in suppressing the

movements (77%). Symptomatically, those who remained on DRBAs after the onset of tardive dystonia and those who were withdrawn from them did not have a significant difference in their improvement rate. This again is in agreement with the data in classical tardive dyskinesia where continued use of DRBAs does not necessarily lead to aggravation of their movements.[229,230] The atypical antipsychotic, clozapine, has been helpful in some patients with tardive dystonia.[193–200] It is likely that its effect on of tardive dystonia in some situations is due to its D_2 receptor blocking activity resulting in a masking of the symptoms, because withdrawal will exacerbate the dystonia.[231] The combination of clozapine and clonazepam has been effective in some patients where either drug alone was much less satisfactory.[232]

In tardive dystonia, antimuscarinics are almost as effective as antidopaminergic drugs. This is different from classical tardive dyskinesia, which may get worse with antimuscarinics.[233] Kang et al.,[18] reported 46% improvement rate using antimuscarinics such as trihexyphenidyl and ethopropazine. CNS side effects

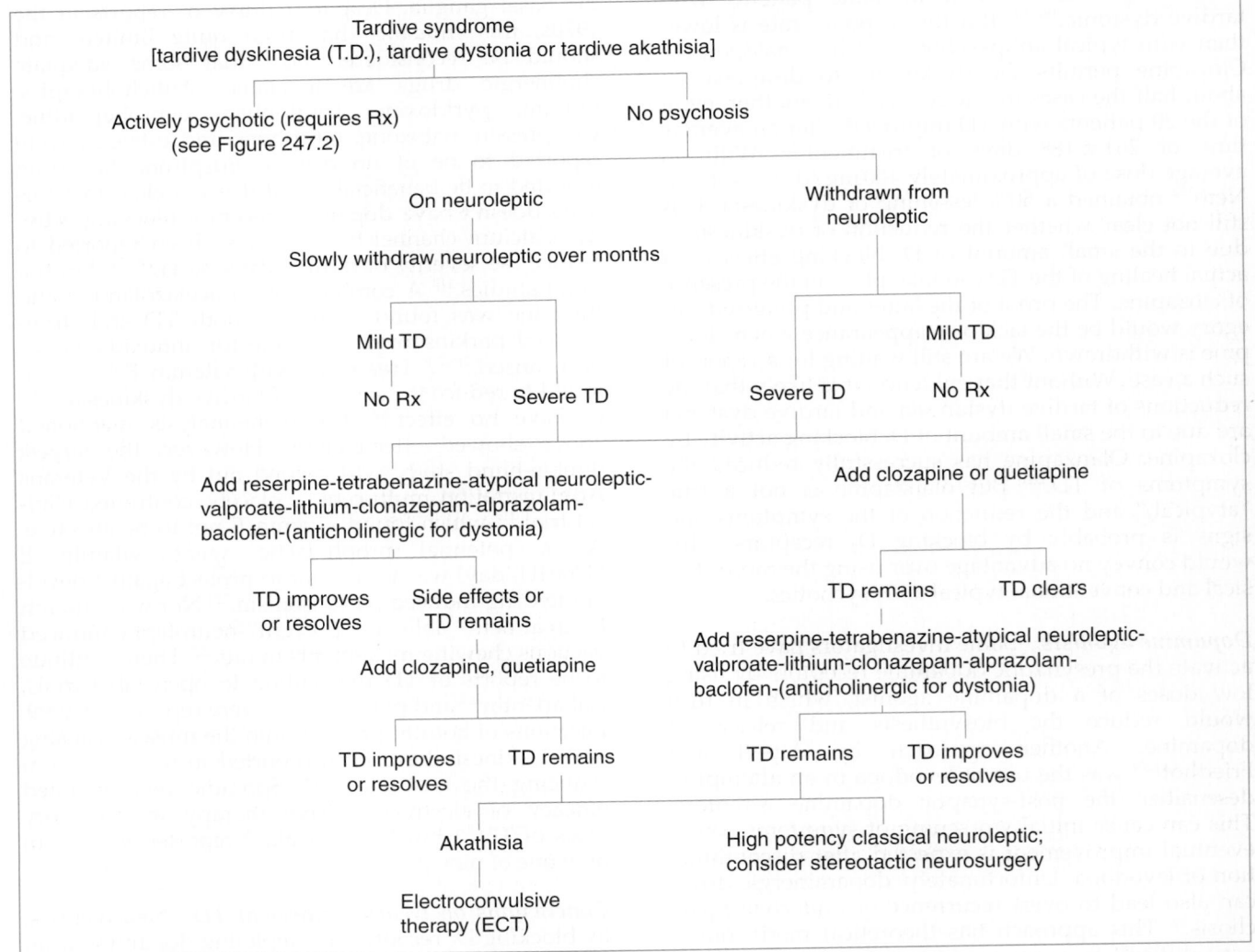

Figure 247.1   Treatment of tardive syndromes.

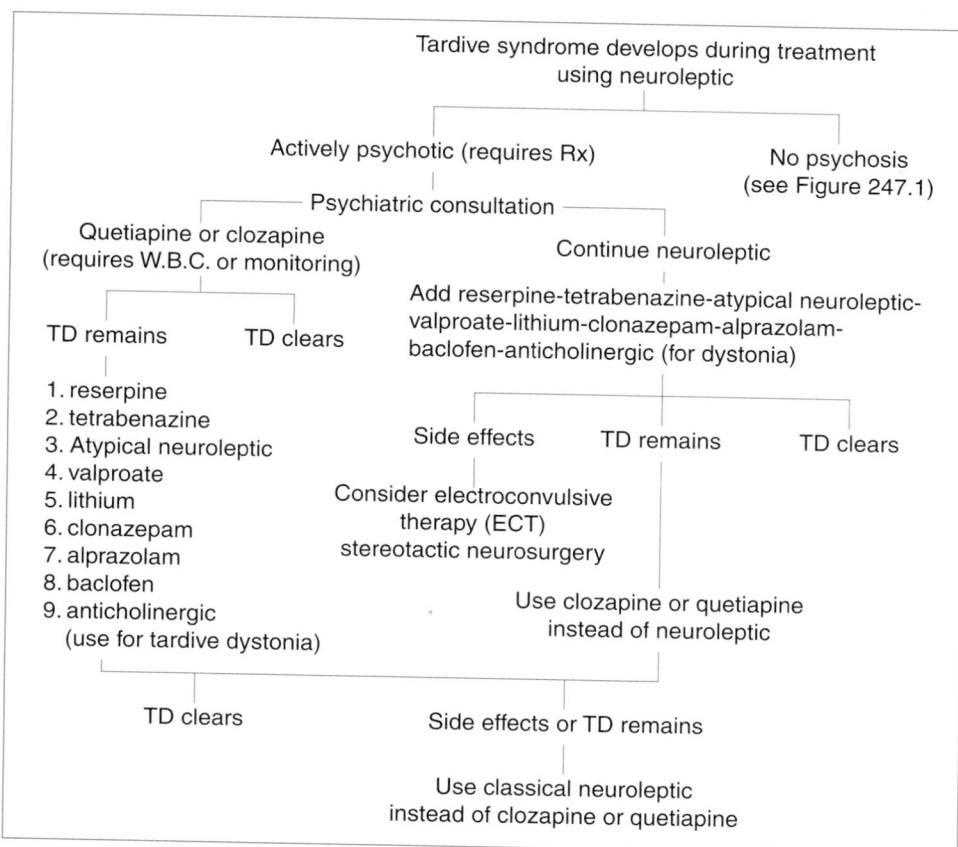

Figure 247.2 Treatment of tardive syndromes in the presence of psychosis.

of the antimuscarinics include forgetfulness, lethargy, psychosis, dysphoria, and personality changes; elderly patients are more susceptible to these. Peripheral side effects include blurred vision, dry mouth, constipation, urinary retention, and orthostatic dizziness. Those who develop side effects to one anticholinergic drug may tolerate another anticholinergic better. These medications are started at a low dose, 2.5 mg of trihexyphenidyl or 25 mg of ethopropazine, and increased slowly by 2.5 mg of trihexyphenidyl or 25 mg of ethopropazine weekly until sufficient control of dystonia or intolerable side effects are achieved. As in idiopathic dystonia, many patients respond only to a high dose of anticholinergics. Therefore every attempt must be made to control side effects so that high dose anticholinergics may be tried. Kang et al.,[18] reported use of maximum of 450 mg ethopropazine or 32 mg of trihexyphenidyl, and higher doses may be tolerated in young patients if judiciously used. Peripheral side effects are often controlled by peripheral cholinergic drugs such as oral pyridostigmine and pilocarpine eye drops.

The clinical pharmacology of tardive dystonia indicates two subtypes; one group that responds to antidopaminergic drugs like the other tardive syndromes, and one that responds to anticholinergics like idiopathic dystonia. Analysis of clinical characteristics of patients who respond to antidopaminergic drugs and those responding to anticholinergic drugs has not shown any significant difference.[18] However, the data from Kang et al.,[18] is retrospective and the treatment choice between

the two classes of drugs was rather arbitrary, partly based on anticipated side effects. For example, patients who were elderly or who had dementia were treated with dopamine-depleting drugs first, because these patients are at greater risk for anticholinergic side effects, such as memory loss and confusion.

Tardive akathisia

Tardive akathisia can be helped by reserpine up to 5 mg per day and TBZ up to 175 mg per day.[178] In this respect the clinical pharmacology is more like that of classical tardive dyskinesia than that of acute akathisia. Opioids were reported to be beneficial,[234] but the effect has not been persistent.[59] Electroconvulsive treatment can be effective in those patients whose akathisia has proven to be intractable.[235] Figures 247.1 and 247.2 depict flow charts on therapy that can also be applied to tardive akathisia.

Summary

In summary, since the initial description of tardive dyskinesia as an iatrogenic complication of dopamine receptor antagonists, considerable progress has been made in understanding the risks, epidemiology, and clinical subtypes of the condition. However, the precise pathogenesis remains poorly understood. Management of tardive syndromes must be based upon an appreciation of the pharmacology of the disorder. The only effective and safe antipsychotic agents that do not produce tardive dyskinesia appear to be clozapine and quetiapine, but their further long-term use must be observed before we can be certain of their true safety profile. Meanwhile, prevention is possible by avoiding indiscriminate use of DRBAs and limiting their use for disorders in which no other type of medication is available or effective. When prevention and withdrawal of the offending drugs for eventual remission fail, symptomatic suppression of abnormal movements can be achieved in many patients with pharmacological treatments. New approaches are needed, and prospective controlled clinical trials with particular attention to clinical subtypes are necessary for better management of this condition.

References

1. Schonecker VM. Ein eigentumliches Syndrom im oralen Bereich bei Megaphenapplikation. Nervenarzt 1957;28:35–43

2. Sigwald J, Bouttier D, Raymondeaud C, Piot C. Quatre cas de dyskinesie facio-bucco-linguo-masticatrice a l'evolution prolongee secondaire a un traitement par les neuroleptiques. Revue Neurologique 1959;100: 751–755

3. Uhrbrand L, Faurbye A. Reversible and irreversible dyskinesia after treatment with perphenazine, chlorpromazine, reserpine, and electroconvulsive therapy. Psychopharmacologia 1960;1:408–418

4. American Psychiatric Association Task force on late neurological effects of antipsychotics. Tardive dyskinesia. Washington, DC: The American Psychiatric Association, 1980

5. Kane JM, Smith JM. Tardive dyskinesia: prevalence and risk factors. Arch Gen Psychiatry 1982;39:473–481

6. Jeste DV, Wyatt RJ. Understanding and treating tardive dyskinesia. New York: Guilford Press, 1982

7. Casey DE. Metoclopramide side effects. Ann Intern Med 1983;98:673–674

8. Riddle MA, Hardie MT, Towbin KE, et al. Tardive dyskinesia following haloperidol treatment in Tourette's syndrome. Arch Gen Psychiatry 1987;44:98–99

9. Greene P, Shale H, Fahn S. Experience with high dosages of anticholinergic and other drugs in the treatment of torsion dystonia. Adv Neurol 1998;50:549–556

10. Fahn S. The tardive dyskinesias. In: Matthews WB, Glaser GH, eds. Recent advances in clinical neurology. Vol 4. Edinburgh: Churchill Livingstone, 1984:229–260

11. Stacy M, Jankovic J. Tardive dyskinesia. Curr Opin Neuro Neurosurg 1991;4:343–349

12. Kebabian JW, Calne DB. Multiple receptors for dopamine. Nature 1979;277:93–96

13. Sokoloff P, Giros B, Martres M, et al. Molecular cloning of a novel dopamine receptor (D_3) as a target for neuroleptics. Nature 1990;347:146–151

14. De Keyser J, Claeys A, De Backer J-P, et al. Autoradiographic localization of D_1 and D_2 dopamine receptors in the human brain. Neurosci Lett 1988;91:142–147

15. Creese I, Burt DR, Snyder SH. Dopamine receptor binding predicts clinical and pharmacological potencies of antischizophrenic drugs. Science 1976;192: 481–483

16. Ganzini L, Casey DE, Hoffman WF, McCall AL. The prevalence of metoclopramide-induced tardive dyskinesia and acute extrapyramidal movement disorders. Arch Intern Med 1993;153:1469–1475

17. Sempere AP, Duarte J, Palomares JM, Coira F, Claveria LE. Parkinsonism and tardive dyskinesia after chronic use of clebopride. Movement Disorder 1994;9:114–115

18. Kang UJ, Burke RE, Fahn S. Natural history and treatment of tardive dystonia. Mov Disord 1986;1:193–208

19. Masmoudi K, Decocq G, Chetaille E, et al. Extrapyramidal side effects of veralipride: Five cases. Therapie 1995;50:451–454

20. Micheli F, Fernandez Pardal M, Gatto M, et al. Flunarizine- and cinnarizine-induced extrapyramidal reactions. Neurology 1987;37:881–884

21. Micheli FE, Fernandez Pardal MMF, Giannaula R, et al. Movement disorders and depression due to flunarizine and cinnarizine. Mov Disord 1989;4:139–146

22. Seeman P, Tallerico T. Antipsychotic drugs which elicit little or no parkinsonism bind more loosely than dopamine to brain D_2 receptors, yet occupy high levels of these receptors. Mol Psychiatr 1998;3:123–134

23. Kapur S, Zipursky RB, Remington G. Clinical and theoretical implications of 5-HT_2 and D_2 receptor occupancy of clozapine, risperidone, and olanzapine in schizophrenia. Amer J Psychiat 1999;156:286–293

24. Ayd FJ. A survey of drug-induced extrapyramidal reactions. JAMA 1961;175:1054–1060

25. Garver DL, Davis JM, Dekermejian H, et al. Dystonic reactions following neuroleptics: time course and proposed mechanism. Psychopharmacology 1976;47: 199–201

26. Marsden CD, Tarsy D, Baldessarini RJ. Spontaneous and drug induced movement disorders in psychotic patients. In: Benson DF, Blumer D, eds. Psychiatric aspects of neurological disease. New York: Grune & Stratton, 1975:219–266

27. Fahn S. Concept and classification of dystonia. In: Fahn S, Marsden CD, Calne DB, eds. Dystonia 2. Advances in Neurology. Vol 50. New York: Raven Press, 1988:1–8

28. Boyer WF, Bakalar NH, Lake CR. Anticholinergic prophylaxis of acute haloperidol-induced acute dystonic reactions. J Clin Psychopharmacol 1987;7:164–166

29. Aguilar EJ, Keshavan MS, Martinez-Quiles MD, et al. Predictors of acute dystonia in first-episode psychotic patients. Am J Psychiatry 1994;151:1819–1821

30. Kondo T, Otani K, Tokinaga N, et al. Characteristics and risk factors of acute dystonia in schizophrenic patients treated with nemonapride, a selective dopamine antagonist. J Clin Psychopharmacol 1999;19: 45–50

31. Brody AL. Acute dystonia induced by rapid increase in risperidone dosage. J Clin Psychopharmacol 1996; 16:461–462

32. Simpson GM, Lindenmayer JP. Extrapyramidal symptoms in patients treated with risperidone. J Clin Psychopharmacol 1997;17:194–201

33. Kastrup O, Gastpar M, Schwarz M. Acute dystonia due to clozapine. J Neurol Neurosurg Psychiatry 1994; 57:119

34. Olivera AA. Sertraline and akathisia: spontaneous resolution. Biol Psychiatry 1997;41:241–242

35. Madhusoodanan S, Brenner R. Reversible choreiform dyskinesia and extrapyramidal symptoms associated with sertraline therapy. J Clin Psychopharmacol 1997; 17:138–139

36. Lopez-Alemany M, Ferrer-Tuset C, Bernacer-Alpera B. Akathisia and acute dystonia induced by sumatriptan. J Neurol 1997;244:131–132

37. Matsumoto RR, Pouw B. Correlation between neuroleptic binding to sigma(1) and sigma(2) receptors and acute dystonic reactions. Eur J Pharmacol 2000; 401:155–160

38. Duvoisin RC, Yahr MD. Encephalitis and parkinsonism. Arch Neurol 1965;12:227–239

39. Rupniak NMJ, Jenner P, Marsden CD. Acute dystonia induced by neuroleptic drugs. Psychopharmacology 1986;88:403–419

40. Pantanowitz L, Berk M. Auto-amputation of the tongue associated with flupenthixol induced extrapyramidal symptoms. Int Clin Psychopharmacol 1999; 14:129–131

41. Paulson G. Procyclidine for dystonia caused by phenothiazine derivatives. Dis Nerv Syst 1960;21:447–448

42. Waugh WH, Metts JC Jr. Severe extrapyramidal motor activity induced by prochlorperazine. New Eng J Med 1960;262:353–354

43. Smith MJ, Miller MM. Severe extrapyramidal reaction to perphenazine treated with diphenhydramine. New Eng J Med 264:396–397

44. Korczyn AD, Goldberg GJ. Intravenous diazepam in drug-induced dystonic reactions. Brit J Psychiatry 1972;121:75–77

45. Gagrat D, Hamilton J, Belmaker RH. Intravenous diazepam in the treatment of neuroleptics-induced acute dystonia and akathisia. Amer J Psychiatry 1978; 135:1232–1233

46. Rainer-Pope CR. Treatment with diazepam of children with drug-induced extrapyramidal symptoms. South Africa Med J 1979;55:328

47. Swett C. Drug-induced dystonia. Am J Psychiatry 1975;132:532–534

48. Arana GW, Goff DC, Baldessarini RJ, Keepers GA. Efficacy of anticholinergic prophylaxis for neuroleptics-induced acute dystonia. Am J Psychiatry 1988;145: 993–996

49. Goff DC, Arana GW, Greenblatt DJ, et al. The effect of benztropine on haloperidol-induced dystonia, clinical efficacy and pharmacokinetics: a prospective, double-blind trial. J Clin Psychopharmacol 1991;11:106–112

50. Haskovec L. Akathisia. Arch Bohemes Med Clin 1902; 3:193–200

51. Van Putten T. The many faces of akathisia. Compr Psychiatry 1975;16:43–47

52. Barnes TRE, Braude WM. Akathisia variants and tardive dyskinesia. Arch Gen Psychiatry 1985;42: 874–878

53. Gibb WRG, Lees AJ. The clinical phenomenon of akathisia. J Neurol Neurosurg Psychiatry 1986;49: 861–866

54. Munetz MR, Cornes CL. Akathisia, pseudoakathisia and tardive dyskinesia: clinical examples. Compr Psychiatry 1982;23:345–352

55. Fahn S. Tardive dyskinesia and akathisia. New Engl J Med 1978;299:202–203

56. Fahn S. Treatment of tardive dyskinesia: use of dopamine-depleting agents. Clin Neuropharmacol 1983;6:151–158

57. Braude WM, Barnes TRE. Late-onset akathisia—an indicant of covert dyskinesia: two case reports. Am J Psychiatry 1983;140:611–612

58. Weiner WJ, Luby ED. Persistent akathisia following neuroleptic withdrawal. Ann Neurol 1983;13:466–467

59. Burke RE, Kang UJ, Jankovic J, et al. Tardive akathisia: an analysis of clinical features and response to open therapeutic trials. Mov Disord 1989;4:157–175

60. Van Putten T, Marder SR. Behavioral toxicity of antipsychotic drugs. J Clin Psychiatry 1987;48(Suppl): 13–19

61. Fahn S, Brin MF, Dwork AJ, et al. Case 1, 1996: Rapidly progressive parkinsonism, incontinence, impotency, and levodopa-induced moaning in a patient with multiple myeloma. Mov Disord 1996;11:298–310

62. Fahn S. Discussion of differential diagnosis. In: Micheli F, Fernandez Pardal M, Giannaula R, Fahn S, eds. What Is It? Case 3, 1991: moaning in a man with parkinsonian signs. Mov Disord 1991;6:376–378

63. Lang AE, Johnson K. Akathisia in idiopathic Parkinson's disease. Neurology 1987;37:477–481

64. Daras M, Koppel BS, Atosradzion E. Cocaine-induced choreoathetoid movements (crack dancing). Neurology 1994;44:751–752

65. Poyurovsky M, Meerovich I, Weizman A. Beneficial effect of low-dose mianserin on fluvoxamine-induced akathisia in an obsessive-compulsive patient. Int Clin Psychopharmacol 1995;10:111–114

66. Marsden CD, Jenner P. The pathophysiology of extrapyramidal side-effects of neuroleptic drugs. Psychological Medicine 1980;10:55–72

67. Sachdev P, Kruk J. Clinical characteristics and predisposing factors in acute drug-induced akathisia. Arch Gen Psychiatry 1994;51:963–974

68. Sachdev P. The epidemiology of drug-induced akathisia. 1. Acute akathisia. Schizophrenia Bull 1995b; 21:431–449

69. Miller CH, Hummer M, Oberbauer H, et al. Risk factors for the development of neuroleptic induced akathisia. Eur Neuropsychopharmacol 1997;7:51–55

70. Muscettola G, Barbato G, Pampallona S, et al. Extrapyramidal syndromes in neuroleptic-treated patients: prevalence, risk factors, and association with tardive dyskinesia. J Clin Psychopharmacol 1999;19: 203–208

71. Blom S, Ekbom KA. Comparison between akathisia developing on treatment with phenothiazine derivatives and the restless leg syndrome. Acta Medica Scandinavica 1961;170:689–694

72. Jankovic J, Fahn S. The phenomenology of tics. Mov Disord 1986;1:17–26

73. Carter CJ, Pycock CJ. Studies on the role of catecholamines in the frontal cortex. Brit J Pharmacol 1978;42:402

74. Altshuler LL, Pierre JM, Wirshing WC, Ames D. Sertraline and akathisia. J Clin Psychopharmacol 1994;14: 278–279

75. Meco G, Bonifati V, Fabrizio E, Vanacore N. Worsening of parkinsonism with fluvoxamine—Two cases. Hum Psychopharmacol Clin Exp 1994;9:439–441

76. Kruse W. Treatment of drug-induced extrapyramidal symptoms. Dis Nerv Syst 1960;21:79–81

77. Zubenko GS, Barreira P, Lipinski JF. Development of tolerance to the therapeutic effect of amantadine on akathisia. J Clin Psychopharmacol 1984;4:218–219

78. Zubenko GS, Lipinski JF, Cohen BM, Barriera PJ. Comparison of metoprolol and propranolol in the treatment of akathisia. Psychiatr Res 1984;11:143–148

79. Adler L, Angrist B, Peselow E, et al. A controlled assessment of propranolol in the treatment of neuroleptics-induced akathisia. Br J Psychiatry 1986;149: 42–45

80. Lipinski JF, Zubenko GS, Cohen BM, Barriera PJ. Propranolol in the treatment of neuroleptics-induced akathisia. Am J Psychiatry 1984;141:412–415

81. Dupuis B, Catteau J, Dumon J-P, et al. Comparison of propranolol, sotalol, and betaxolol in the treatment of neuroleptics-induced akathisia. Am J Psychiatry 1987: 144:802–805

82. Dumon J-P, Catteau J, Lanvin F, Dupuis BA. Randomized, double-blind, crossover, placebo-controlled com-

parison of propranolol and betaxolol in the treatment of neuroleptics-induced akathisia. Am J Psychiatry 1992;149:647–650

83. Adler L, Angrist B, Peselow E, et al. Clonidine in neuroleptics-induced akathisia. Am J Psychiatry 1987;144:235–236

84. Anfang MK, Pope HG. Treatment of neuroleptics-induced akathisia with nicotine patches. Psychopharmacology 1997;134:153–156

85. Weiss D, Aizenberg D, Hermesh H, et al. Cyproheptadine treatment in neuroleptics-induced akathisia. Br J Psychiatry 1995;167:483–486

86. Poyurovsky M, Shardorodsky M, Fuchs C, et al. Treatment of neuroleptics-induced akathisia with the 5-HT$_2$ antagonist mianserin—double-blind, placebo-controlled study. Brit J Psychiat 1999;174:238–242

87. Hardie RJ, Lees AJ. Neuroleptic-induced Parkinson's syndrome: clinical features and results of treatment with levodopa. J Neurol Neurosurg Psychiatry 1988;51:850–854

88. Decina P, Caracci G, Scapicchio PL. The rabbit syndrome. Mov Disord 1990;5:263

89. Korczyn AD, Goldberg GJ. Extrapyramidal effects of neuroleptics. J Neurol Neurosurg Psychiatry 1976;39:866–869

90. Factor SA, Friedman JH. The emerging role of clozapine in the treatment of movement disorders. Mov Disord 1997;12:483–496

91. Fleming P, Makar H, Hunter FR. Levodopa in drug-induced extrapyramidal disorders. Lancet 1970;ii:1186

92. Stephen PJ, Williamson J. Drug-induced parkinsonism in the elderly. Lancet 1984;ii:1082–1083

93. Mazurek MF, Savedia SM, Bobba RS, et al. Persistent loss of tyrosine hydroxylase in immunoreactivity in the substantia nigra after neuroleptic withdrawal. J Neurol Neurosurg Psychiatry 1998;64:799–801

94. Rajput AH, Rozdilsky B, Hornykiewicz O, et al. Reversible drug-induced parkinsonism: clinical pathologic study of two cases. Arch Neurol 1982;39:644–646

95. Coulter DM, Pillans PI. Fluoxetine and extrapyramidal side effects. Am J Psychiatry 1995;152:122–125

96. DiRocco A, Brannan T, Prikhojan A, Yahr MD. Sertraline induced parkinsonism. A case report and an invivo study of the effect of sertraline on dopamine metabolism. J Neural Transm 1998;105:247–251

97. Baldessarini RJ, Marsh E. Fluoxetine and side effects. Arch Gen Psychiatry 1992;47:191–192

98. Melamed E, Achiron A, Shapira A, Davidovicz S. Persistent and progressive parkinsonism after discontinuation of chronic neuroleptic therapy—an additional tardive syndrome. Clin Neuropharmacol 1991;14:273–278

99. Merello M, Starkstein S, Petracca G, et al. Drug-induced parkinsonism in schizophrenic patients: motor response and psychiatric changes after acute challenge with L-dopa and apomorphine. Clin Neuropharmacol 1996;19:439–443

100. Carlsson A, Lindqvist M, Magnusson T. 3,4-Dihydroxyphenylalanine and 5-hydroxytryptophan as reserpine antagonists. Nature 1957;180:1200

101. Carlsson A. The occurrence, distribution and physiological role of catecholamines in the nervous system. Pharmacol Rev 1959;11:490–493

102. Mindham RHS, Gaind R, Anstee BH, Rimmer L. Comparison of amantadine, orphenadrine, and placebo in the control of phenothiazine-induced Parkinsonism. Psychol Med 1972;2:406–413

103. Johnson DAW. Prevalence and treatment of drug-induced extrapyramidal syndromes. Br J Psychiatry 1978;132:27–30

104. Konig P, Chwatal K, Havelec L, et al. Amantadine versus biperiden: a double-blind study of treatment efficacy in neuroleptic extrapyramidal movement disorders. Neuropsychobiology 1996;33:80–84

105. Yassa R, Lai S. Respiratory irregularity and tardive dyskinesia. Acta Psychiatr Scand 1986;73:506–510

106. Wilcox PG, Bassett A, Jones B, Fleetham JA. Respiratory dysrhythmias in patients with tardive dyskinesia. Chest 1994;105:203–207

107. Horiguchi J, Shingu T, Hayashi T, et al. Antipsychotic-induced life-threatening "esophageal dyskinesia." Int Clin Psychopharmacol 1999;14:123–127

108. Kane JM, Woerner M, Borenstein M, et al. Integrating incidence and prevalence of tardive dyskinesia. Psychopharmacol Bull 1986;22:254–258

109. Smith JM, Baldessarini RJ. Changes in prevalence, severity, and recovery in tardive dyskinesia with age. Arch Gen Psychiatry 1980;37:1368–1373

110. Kane JM, Woerner M, Lieberman J. Tardive dyskinesia: prevalence, incidence, and risk factors. J Clin Psychopharmacol 1988;8:52S–56S

111. Gardos G, Casey D, eds. Tardive dyskinesia and affective disorders. Washington, DC: American Psychiatric Press, 1983

112. Kane JM, Woerner MW, Lieberman JA, et al. The prevalence of tardive dyskinesia. Psychopharmacol Bull 1985;21:136–139

113. Chouinard G, Annable L, Mercier P, Ross-Couinard A. A five-year follow-up study of tardive dyskinesia. Psychopharmacol Bull 1986;22:259–263

114. Jeste DJ, Potkin SG, Sinha S, et al. Tardive dyskinesia: reversible and persistent. Arch Gen Psychiatry 1979;136:79–83

115. van Harten PN, Hoek HW, Matroos GE, et al. Intermittent neuroleptic treatment and risk for tardive dyskinesia: curacao extrapyramidal syndromes study. III. Am J Psychiatry 1998;155:565–567

116. Yassa R, Iskandar H, Ally J. The prevalence of tardive dyskinesia in fluphenazine-treated patients. J Clin Psychopharmacol 1988;8:17S–20S

117. Nielson EB, Lyon M. Evidence for cell loss in corpus striatum after long-term treatment with a neuroleptic drug (flupenthixol) in rats. Psychopharmacology 1978;59:85–89

118. Benes FM, Paskevich PA, Davidson J, Domesick VB. The effects of haloperidol on synaptic patterns in the rat striatum. Brain Res 1985;329:265–274

119. Meshul CK, Stallbaumer RK, Taylor B, Janowsky A. Haloperidol-induced morphological changes in striatum are associated with glutamate synapses. Brain Res 1994;648:181–195

120. Meredith GE, DeSouza IEJ, Hyde TM, et al. Persistent alterations in dendrites, spines, and dynorphinergic synapses in the nucleus accumbens shell of rats with neuroleptics-induced dyskinesias. J Neurosci 2000;20:7798–7806

121. Klawans HL. The pharmacology of tardive dyskinesia. Am J Psychiatry 1973;130:82–86

122. Gunne LM, Haggstrom JE, Sjoquist B. Association with persistent neuroleptics-induced dyskinesia of regional changes in brain GABA synthesis. Nature 1984;309:347–349

123. Mitchell IJ, Crossman AR, Liminga U, et al. Regional changes in 2-deoxyglucose uptake associated with neuroleptic-induced tardive dyskinesia in the Cebus monkey. Mov Disord 1992;7:32–37

124. Druckman R, Seelinger D, Thulin B. Chronic involuntary movements induced by phenothiazines. J Nerv Ment Dis 1962;135:69–76

125. Burke RE, Fahn S, Jankovic J, et al. Tardive dystonia: late-onset and persistent dystonia caused by antipsychotic drugs. Neurology 1982;32:1335–1346

126. Calne DB, Lang AE. Secondary dystonia. In: Fahn S, Marsden CD, Calne DB, eds. Dystonia 2. Advances in Neurology. Vol 50. New York: Raven Press, 1988:9–34

127. Kiriakakis V, Bhatia KP, Quinn NP, Marsden CD. The natural history of tardive dystonia—a long-term follow-up study of 107 cases. Brain 1998;121:2053–2066

128. Yassa R, Nair V, Iskandar H. A comparison of severe tardive dystonia and severe tardive dyskinesia. Acta Psychiatr Scand 1989;80:155–159

129. Krack P, Schneider S, Deuschl G. Geste device in tardive dystonia with retrocollis and opisthotonic posturing. Mov Disord 1998;13:155–157

130. Molho ES, Feustel PJ, Factor SA. Clinical comparison of tardive and idiopathic cervical dystonia. Mov Disord 1998;13:486–489

131. Sachdev P. Tardive blepharospasm. Mov Disord 1998; 13:947–951

132. Samie MR, Dannenhoffer MA, Rozek S. Life-threatening tardive dyskinesia caused by metoclopramide. Mov Disord 1987;2:125–129

133. Hayashi T, Nishikawa T, Koga I, et al. Life-threatening dysphagia following prolonged neuroleptic therapy. Clin Neuropharmacol 1997;20:77–81

134. van Harten PN, Hoek HW, Matroos GE, Koeter M, Kahn RS. The inter-relationships of tardive dyskinesia, parkinsonism, akathisia and tardive dystonia: the Curacao Extrapyramidal Syndromes Study. 2. Schizophr Res 1997;26:235–242

135. Gardos G, Cole JO, Salomon M, Schniebolk S. Clinical forms of severe tardive dyskinesia. Am J Psychiatry 1987;144:895–902

136. Ford B, Greene P, Fahn S. Oral and genital tardive pain syndromes. Neurology 1994;44:2115–2119

137. Polizos P, Engelhardt DM, Hoffman SP, Waizer J. Neurological consequences of psychotropic drug withdrawal in schizophrenic children. J Autism Child Schizo 1973;3:247–253

138. Giladi N, Shabtai H. Melatonin-induced withdrawal emergent dyskinesia and akathisia. Mov Disord 1999; 14:381–382

139. Gardos G, Cole JO, Tarsy D. Withdrawal syndromes associated with antipsychotic drugs. Am J Psychiatry 1978;135:1321–1324

140. Schooler NR, Kane JM. Research diagnoses for tardive dyskinesia. Arch Gen Psychiatry 1982;39:486–487

141. Peiris DTS, Kuruppuarachchi KALA, Weerasena LP, et al. Neuroleptic malignant syndrome without fever: a report of three cases. J Neurol Neurosurg Psychiat 2000;69:277–278

142. Velamoor VR, Norman RMG, Caroff SN, et al. Progression of symptoms in neuroleptic malignant syndrome. J Nerv Ment Dis 1994;182:168–173

143. Henderson VW, Wooten GF. Neuroleptic malignant syndrome: a pathogenetic role for dopamine receptor blockade. Neurology 1981;31:132–137

144. Gute BH, Baxter LR. Neuroleptic malignant syndrome. New Engl J Med 1985;313:163–166

145. Behan WMH, Madigan M, Clark BJ, et al. Muscle changes in the neuroleptic malignant syndrome. J Clin Pathol 2000;53:223–227

146. Webster P, Wijeratne C. Risperidone-induced neuroleptic malignant syndrome. Lancet 1994;344: 1228–1229

147. Raitasuo V, Vataja R, Elomaa E. Risperidone-induced neuroleptic malignant syndrome in young patient. Lancet 1994;344:1705

148. Dave M. Two cases of risperidone-induced neuroleptic malignant syndrome. Am J Psychiatry 1995;152: 1233–1234

149. Singer S, Richards C, Boland RJ. Two cases of risperidone-induced neuroleptic malignant syndrome. Am J Psychiatry 1995;152:1234

150. Levin GM, Lazowick AL, Powell HS. Neuroleptic malignant syndrome with risperidone. J Clin Psychopharmacol 1996;16:192–193

151. Miller DD, Sharafuddin MJA, Kathol RG. A case of clozapine-induced neuroleptic malignant syndrome. J Clin Psychiatry 1991;52:96–101

152. Dalkilic A, Grosch WN. Neuroleptic malignant syndrome following initiation of clozapine therapy. Am J Psychiatry 1997;154:881–882

153. Amore M, Zazzeri N, Berardi D. Atypical neuroleptic malignant syndrome associated with clozapine treatment. Neuropsychobiology 1997;35:197–199

154. Reches A, Burke RE, Kuhn CM, et al. Tetrabenazine, an amine-depleting drug, also blocks dopamine receptors in rat brain. J Pharmacol Exp Ther 1983;225: 515–521

155. Naganuma H, Fujii I. Incidence and risk factors in neuroleptic malignant syndrome. Acta Psychiatr Scand 1994;90:424–426

156. Deng MZ, Chen GQ, Phillips MR. Neuroleptic malignant syndrome in 12 of 9792 Chinese inpatients exposed to neuroleptics: a prospective study. Am J Psychiatry 1990 Oct;147:1149–1155

157. Gratz S, Simpson G. Neuroleptic malignant syndrome. Br J Psychiatry 1990;157:617–618

158. Sachdev P, Mason C, Hadzi-Pavlovic D. Case-control study of neuroleptic malignant syndrome. Am J Psychiatry 1997;154:1156–1158

159. Kubo S, Orihara Y, Kitamura O, Ikematsu K, Tsuda R, Nakasono I. An autopsy case of neuroleptic malignant syndrome (NMS) and its immunohistochemical findings of muscle-associated proteins and mitochondria Forensic Sci Int 2001 (Jan);115(1–2):155–158

160. Friedman JH, Feinberg SS, Feldman RG. A neuroleptic malignant-like syndrome due to levodopa therapy withdrawal. JAMA 1985;254:2792–2795

161. Hirschorn KA, Greenberg HS. Successful treatment of levodopa-induced myoclonus and levodopa withdrawal-induced neuroleptic malignant syndrome: a case report. Clin Neuropharmacol 1988;2:278–281

162. Keyser DL, Rodnitzky RL. Neuroleptic malignant syndrome in Parkinson's disease after withdrawal or alteration of dopaminergic therapy. Arch Intern Med 1991;151:794–796

163. Spivak B, Gonen N, Mester R, et al. Neuroleptic malignant syndrome associated with abrupt withdrawal of anticholinergic agents. Int Clin Psychopharmacol 1996;11:207–209

164. Ram A, Cao QH, Keck PE, et al. Structural change in dopamine D–2 receptor gene in a patient with neuroleptic malignant syndrome. Am J Med Genet 1995; 60:228–230

165. Jauss M, Krack P, Franz M, et al. Imaging of dopamine receptors with [I-123]iodobenzamide single-photon emission-computed tomography in neuroleptic malignant syndrome. Mov Disord 1996;11:726–728

166. Granato JE, Stern BJ, Ringel A, Karim AH, Krumholz A, Coyle J, Adler S. Neuroleptic malignant syndrome: successful treatment with dantrolene and bromocriptine. Ann Neurol 1983 July;14(1):89–90

167. Nisijima K, Noguti M, Ishiguro T. Intravenous injection of levodopa is more effective than dantrolene as therapy for neuroleptic malignant syndrome. Biol Psychiatry 1997;41:913–914

168. Tsujimoto S, Maeda K, Sugiyama T, et al. Efficacy of prolonged large-dose dantrolene for severe neuroleptic malignant syndrome. Anesth Analg 1998;86:1143–1144

169. Thomas P, Maron M, Rascle C, et al. Carbamazepine in the treatment of neuroleptic malignant syndrome. Biol Psychiatry 1998;43:303–305

170. Singh AN, Albaranzanchi AJ. Neuroleptic rechallenge after neuroleptic malignant syndrome in a 73-year-old woman with schizophrenia—four years' follow-up. J Drug Dev Clin Practice 1995;7:63–65

171. Singh AN, Hambidge DM. Successful use of risperidone after neuroleptic malignant syndrome (NMS): a 1-year follow-up. Hum Psychopharmacol Clin Exp 1998;13:65–66

172. Caroff SN, Mann SC, Keck PE, Francis A. Residual catatonic state following neuroleptic malignant syndrome. J Clin Psychopharmacol 2000;20:257–259

173. Kennedy NJ, Sanborn JS. Disclosure of tardive dyskinesia—effect of written policy on risk disclosure. Psychopharmacol Bull 1992;28:93–100

174. Kleinman I, Schachter D, Jeffries J, Goldhamer P. Informed consent and tardive dyskinesia. Long-term follow-up. J Nerv Ment Dis 1996 Sep;184(9):517–522

175. Chaplin R, Kent A. Informing patients about tardive dyskinesia—controlled trial of patient education. Br J Psychiatry 1998;172:78–81

176. Quitkin F, Rifkin A, Gochfeld L, Klein DF. Tardive dyskinesia: are first signs reversible? Am J Psychiatry 1977;134:84–87

177. Glazer WM, Morgenstern H, Schooler N, et al. Predictors of improvement in tardive dyskinesia following discontinuation of neuroleptic medication. Br J Psychiatry 1990;157:585–592

178. Burke RE, Reches A, Traub MM, et al. Tetrabenazine induces acute dystonic reactions. Ann Neurol 1985;17:200–202

179. Mehvar R, Jamali F, Watson MW, Skelton D. Pharmacokinetics of tetrabenazine and its major metabolite in man and rat: bioavailability and dose dependency studies. Drug Metab Dispos 1987;15:250–255

180. Fahn S. A therapeutic approach to tardive dyskinesia. J Clin Psychiatry 1985;46:19–24

181. Kazamatsuri H, Chien C, Cole JO. Treatment of tardive dyskinesia. Arch Gen Psychiatry 1972;27:95–99

182. Jankovic J, Beach J. Long-term effects of tetrabenazine in hyperkinetic movement disorders. Neurology 1997;48:358–362

183. Ondo WG, Hanna PA, Jankovic J. Tetrabenazine treatment for tardive dyskinesia: assessment by randomized videotape protocol. Amer J Psychiat 1999;156:1279–1281

184. Schreiber W, Krieg JC, Eichhorn T. Reversal of tetrabenazine induced depression by selective noradrenaline (norepinephrine) reuptake inhibition. J Neurol Neurosurg Psychiat 1999;67:550

185. Achiron A, Zoldan Y, Melamed E. Tardive dyskinesia induced by sulpiride. Clin Neuropharmacol 1990;13:248–252

186. Miller LG, Jankovic J. Sulpiride-induced tardive dystonia. Mov Disord 1990;5:83–84

187. Duarte J, Campos JM, Cabezas C, et al. Neuroleptic malignant syndrome while on tiapride treatment. Clin Neuropharmacol 1996;19:539–540

188. Buzan RD. Risperidone-induced tardive dyskinesia. Am J Psychiatry 1996;153:734–735

189. Chouinard G. Effects of risperidone in tardive dyskinesia: an analysis of the Canadian multicenter risperidone study. J Clin Psychopharmacol 1995;15:S36–S44

190. Huang CC, Wang RIH, Hasegawa A, Alverno L. Evaluation of reserpine and alpha-methyldopa in the treatment of tardive dyskinesia. Psychopharmacol Bull 1980;16:41–43

191. Wirshing WC, Phelan CK, Van Putten T, et al. Effects of clozapine on treatment-resistant akathisia and concomitant tardive dyskinesia. J Clin Psychopharmacol 1990;10:371–373

192. Bassitt DP, Neto MRL. Clozapine efficacy in tardive dyskinesia in schizophrenic patients. Eur Arch Psychiat Clin Neuros 1998;248:209–211

193. Lieberman J, Johns C, Cooper T, Pollack S, Kane J. Clozapine pharmacology and tardive dyskinesia. Psychopharmacology (Berlin) 1989;99(S):S54–S59

194. Lieberman JA, Saltz BL, Johns CA, et al. The effects of clozapine on tardive dyskinesia. Br J Psychiatry 1991;158:503–510

195. Van Putten T, Wirshing WC, Marder SR. Tardive Meige syndrome responsive to clozapine. J Clin Psychopharmacol 1990;10:381–382

196. Friedman JH. Clozapine treatment of psychosis in patients with tardive dystonia: report of three cases. Mov Disord 1994;9:321–324

197. Wolf ME, Mosnaim AD. Improvement of axial dystonia with the administration of clozapine. Int J Clin Pharm Therapeutics 1994;32:282–283

198. Trugman JM, Leadbetter R, Zalis ME, et al. Treatment of severe axial tardive dystonia with clozapine: case report and hypothesis. Mov Disord 1994;9:441–446

199. van Harten PN, Kamphuis DJ, Matroos GE. Use of clozapine in tardive dystonia. Prog Neuro-Psych Biol Psych 1996a;20:263–274

200. Raja M, Maisto G, Altavista MC, Albanese A. Tardive lingual dystonia treated with clozapine. Mov Disord 1996;11:585–586

201. Gerlach J, Peacock L. Motor and mental side effects of clozapine. J Clin Psychiatry 1994;55(Suppl B):107–109

202. Bunker MT, Sommi RW, Stoner SC, Switzer JL. Longitudinal analysis of abnormal involuntary movements in long-term clozapine-treated patients. Psychopharmacol Bull 1996;32:699–703

203. Littrell KH, Johnson CG, Littrell S, Peabody CD. Marked reduction of tardive dyskinesia with olanzapine. Arch Gen Psychiatry 1998;55:279–280

204. Alpert M, Friedhoff A. Clinical application of receptor modification treatment. In: Fann WE, Smith RC, Davis JM, Domino EF, eds. Tardive dyskinesia: research and treatment. New York: SP Medical and Scientific Books, 1980:471–474

205. Angus S, Sugars J, Boltezar R, et al. A controlled trial of amantadine hydrochloride and neuroleptics in the treatment of tardive dyskinesia. J Clin Psychopharmacol 1997;17:88–91

206. Jeste DV, Wyatt RJ. Therapeutic strategies against tardive dyskinesia: two decades of experience. Arch Gen Psychiatry 1982b;39:803–816

207. Jeste DV, Lohr JB, Clark K, Wyatt RJ. Pharmacological treatment of tardive dyskinesia in the 1980s. J Clin Psychopharmacol 1988;8:38S–48S

208. Thaker GK, Nguyen JA, Strauss ME, et al. Clonazepam treatment of tardive dyskinesia: a practical GABA-mimetic strategy. Am J Psychiatry 1990;147:445–451

209. Moss LE, Neppe VM, Drevets WC. Buspirone in the treatment of tardive dyskinesia. J Clin Psychopharmacol 1993;13:204–209

210. Kushnir SL, Ratner JT. Calcium-channel blockers for tardive dyskinesia in geriatric psychiatric patients. Am J Psychiatry 1989;146:1218–1219

211. Duncan E, Adler L, Angrist B, Rotrosen J. Nifedipine in the treatment of tardive dyskinesia. J Clin Psychopharmacol 1990;10:414–416

212. Suddath RL, Straw GM, Freed WJ, et al. A clinical trial of nifedipine in schizophrenia and tardive dyskinesia. Pharmacol Biochem Behav 1991;39:743–745

213. Loonen AJM, Verwey HA, Roels PR, et al. Is diltiazem effective in treating the symptoms of (tardive) dyskinesia in chronic psychiatric inpatients? A negative, double-blind, placebo-controlled trial. J Clin Psychopharmacol 1992;12:39–42

214. Cowen MA, Green M, Bertollo DN, Abbott K. A treatment for tardive dyskinesia and some other extrapyramidal symptoms. J Clin Psychopharmacol 1997;17:190–193

215. Cadet JL, Lohr BJ. Possible involvement of free radicals in neuroleptics-induced movement disorders: evidence from treatment of tardive dyskinesia with Vitamin E. Ann NY Acad Sci 1989;528:176–185

216. Behl C, Rupprecht R, Skutella T, Holsboer F. Haloperidol-induced cell death-mechanism and protection with vitamin E in vitro. NeuroReport 1995;7:360–364

217. Elkashef AM, Ruskin PE, Bacher N, Barrett D. Vitamin E in the treatment of tardive dyskinesia. Am J Psychiatry 1990;147:505–506

218. Dabiri LM, Pasta D, Darby JK, Mosbacher D. Effectiveness of vitamin E for treatment of long-term tardive dyskinesia. Am J Psychiatry 1994;151:925–926

219. Adler LA, Rotrosen J, Edson R, et al. Vitamin E treatment for tardive dyskinesia. Arch Gen Psychiat 1999;56:836–841

220. Sajjad SHA. Vitamin E in the treatment of tardive dyskinesia: a preliminary study over 7 months at different doses. Int Clin Psychopharmacol 1998;13: 147–155

221. Lam LC, Chiu HF, Hung SF. Vitamin E in the treatment of tardive dyskinesia: a replication study. J Nerv Ment Dis 1994 Feb;182(2):113–114

222. Eranti VS, Gangadhar BN, Janakiramaiah N. Haloperidol induced extrapyramidal reaction: lack of protective effect by vitamin E. Psychopharmacology 1998;140:418–420

223. Sachdev P, Saharov T, Cathcart S. The preventative role of antioxidants (selegiline and vitamin E) in a rat model of tardive dyskinesia. Biol Psychiat 1999;46:1672–1681

224. Hardoy MC, Hardoy MJ, Carta MG, Cabras PL. Gabapentin as a promising treatment for antipsychotic-induced movement disorders in schizoaffective and bipolar patients. J Affect Disorders 1999;54: 315–317

225. Lerner V, Kaptsan A, Miodownik C, Kotler M. Vitamin B6 in treatment of tardive dyskinesia: a preliminary case series study. Clin Neuropharmacol 1999;22:241–243

226. Rapaport A, Sadeh M, Stein D, et al. Botulinum toxin for the treatment of oro-facial-lingual-masticatory tardive dyskinesia. Mov Disord 2000 Mar;15(2):352–355

227. Price TRP, Levin R. The effects of electroconvulsive therapy on tardive dyskinesia. Am J Psychiatry 1978;112:983–987

228. Yassa R, Hoffman H, Canakis M. The effect of electroconvulsive therapy on tardive dyskinesia: a prospective study. Convulsive Therapy 1990;6:194–198

229. Gardos G, Cole JO, Haskell D, et al. The natural history of tardive dyskinesia. J Clin Psychopharmacol 1988;8:31S–37S

230. Casey DE, Povlsen UJ, Meidahl B, Gerlach J. Neuroleptic-induced tardive dyskinesia and parkinsonism: changes during several years of continuing treatment. Psychopharmacol Bull 1986;22:250–253

231. Krack P, Teschendorf W, Dorndorf W. Clozapine treatment of psychosis can worsen preexisting tardive dystonia. Mov Disord 1994;9(Suppl 1):54

232. Shapleske J, McKay AP, McKenna PJ. Successful treatment of tardive dystonia with clozapine and clonazepam. Br J Psychiatry 1996;168:516–518

233. Yassa R. Tardive dyskinesia and anticholinergic drugs. L'Encephale 1988;XIV:233–239

234. Walters A, Hening W, Chokroverty S, Fahn S. Opioid responsiveness in patients with neuroleptics-induced akathisia. Movement Disorders 1986;1:119–127

235. Hermesh H, Aizenberg D, Friedberg G, et al. Electroconvulsive therapy for persistent neuroleptics-induced akathisia and parkinsonism—a case report. Biol Psychiatry 1992;31:407–411

Further reading

Abad V, Ovsiew F. Treatment of persistent myoclonic tardive dystonia with verapamil. Br J Psychiatry 1993; 162:554–556

Ananth JHJ, Burgoyne K, Aquino S. Meige's syndrome associated with risperidone therapy. Amer J Psychiat 2000;157:149

Andersson U, Haggstrom J-E, Levin ED, et al. Reduced glutamate decarboxylase activity in the subthalamic nucleus in patients with tardive dyskinesia. Mov Disord 1989;4:37–46

Andreassen OA, Aamo TO, Jorgensen HA. Inhibition by memantine of the development of persistent oral dyskinesias induced by long-term haloperidol treatment of rats. Br J Pharmacol 1996;119:751–757

Andreassen OA, Finsen B, Ostergaard K, et al. The relationship between oral dyskinesias produced by long-term haloperidol treatment, the density of striatal preproenkephalin messenger RNA and enkephalin peptide, and the number of striatal neurons expressing preproenkephalin messenger RNA in rats. Neuroscience 1999a;88:27–35

Andreassen OA, Jorgensen HA. Neurotoxicity associated with neuroleptics-induced oral dyskinesias in rats—implications for tardive dyskinesia? Prog Neurobiol 2000;61:525–541

Andreassen OA, MacEwan T, Gulbrandsen AK, et al. Nonfunctional CYP2D6 alleles and risk for neuroleptics-induced movement disorders in schizophrenic patients. Psychopharmacology 1997;131:174–179

Andreassen OA, Weber C, Jorgensen HA. Coenzyme Q_{10} does not prevent oral dyskinesias induced by long-term haloperidol treatment of rats. Pharmacol Biochem Behav 1999b;64:637–642

Arnt J, Skarsfeldt T. Do novel antipsychotics have similar pharmacological characteristics? A review of the evidence. Neuropsychopharmacology 1998;18: 63–101

Asper H, Baggiolini M, Burke HR, et al. Tolerance phenomena with neuroleptics: catalepsy, apomorphine stereotypies and striatal dopamine metabolism in the rat after single and repeated administration of loxapine and haloperidol. Eur J Pharmacol 1973;22:287–294

Bailey L, Maxwell S, Brandabur MM. Substance abuse as a risk factor for tardive dyskinesia: a retrospective analysis of 1027 patients. Psychopharmacol Bull 1997; 33:177–181

Barnes TRE, Kidger T, Gore SM. Tardive dyskinesia: a 3-year follow-up study. Psychol Med 1983;13:71–81

Bassitt DP, Garcia LDL. Risperidone-induced tardive dyskinesia. Pharmacopsychiatry 2000;33:155–156

Beasley CM Jr, Tollefson GD, Tran PV. Safety of olanzapine. J Clin Psychiatry 1997;58(Suppl 10):13–17

Beasley CM, Dellva MA, Tamura RN, et al. Randomised double-blind comparison of the incidence of tardive dyskinesia in patients with schizophrenia during long-term treatment with olanzapine or haloperidol. Brit J Psychiat 1999;174:23–30

Benazzi F. Clozapine-induced neuroleptic malignant syndrome not recurring with olanzapine, a structurally and pharmacologically similar antipsychotic. Hum Psychopharmacol Clin Exp 1999;14:511–512

Bench CJ, Lammertsma AA, Dolan RJ, et al. Dose dependent occupancy of central dopamine D_2 receptors by the novel neuroleptic CP-88,059-01: a study using positron emission tomography and ^{11}C-raclopride. Psychopharmacology (Berl) 1993;112:308–314

Bench CJ, Lammertsma AA, Grasby PM, et al. The time course of binding to striatal dopamine D_2 receptors by the neuroleptic ziprasidone (CP-88,059-01) determined by positron emission tomography. Psychopharmacology (Berl) 1996;124:141–147

Benedetti F, Cavallaro R, Smeraldi E. Olanzapine-induced neutropenia after clozapine-induced neutropenia. Lancet 1999;354:567

Bharucha KJ, Sethi KD. Tardive tourettism after exposure to neuroleptic therapy. Mov Disord 1995;10: 791–793

Blin J, Baron JC, Cambon H, et al. Striatal dopamine D_2 receptors in tardive dyskinesia: PET study. J Neurol Neurosurg Psychiatry 1989;52:1248–1252

Bowers MB, Moore D, Tarsy D. Tardive dyskinesia: a clinical test of the supersensitivity hypothesis. Psychopharmacology 1979;61:137–141

258. Brandon S, McClelland HA, Protheroe C. A study of facial dyskinesia in a mental hospital population. Br J Psychiatry 1971;118:171–184

259. Broich K, Grunwald F, Kasper S, et al. D_2-dopamine receptor occupancy measured by IBZM-SPECT in relation to extrapyramidal side effects. Pharmacopsychiatry 1998;31:159–162

Brown K, Reid A, White T, et al. Vitamin E, lipids, and lipid peroxidation products in tardive dyskinesia. Biol Psychiatry 1998;43:863–867

Brown KW, White T, Wardlaw JM, et al. Caudate nucleus morphology in tardive dyskinesia. Br J Psychiatry 1996;169:631–636

Bruneau MA, Stip E. Metronome or alternating Pisa syndrome: a form of tardive dystonia under clozapine treatment. Int Clin Psychopharmacol 1998;13:229–232

Buchanan RW, Gellad F, Munson RC, Breier A. Basal ganglia pathology in schizophrenia and tardive dyskinesia—an MRI quantitative study. Am J Psychiatry 1994;151:752–755

Burkhard PR, Vingerhoets FJG, Alberque C, et al. Olanzapine induced neuroleptic malignant syndrome. Arch Gen Psychiat 1999;56:101–102

Bymaster F, Perry KW, Nelson DL, et al. Olanzapine: a basic science update. Brit J Psychiat 1999;174:36–40

Calabresi P, De Murtas M, Mercuri NB, Bernardi G. Chronic neuroleptic treatment: D_2 dopamine receptor supersensitivity and striatal glutamatergic transmission. Ann Neurol 1992;31:366–373

Caligiuri MP, Lacro JP, Rockwell E, et al. Incidence and risk factors for severe tardive dyskinesia in older patients. Br J Psychiatry 1997;171:148–153

Casteels-Van Daele M, Jaeken J, Van Der Schueren P, et al. Dystonic reactions in children caused by metoclopramide. Arch Dis Child 1970;45:130–133

Chakos MH, Alvir JMJ, Woerner MG, et al. Incidence and correlates of tardive dyskinesia in first episode of schizophrenia. Arch Gen Psychiatry 1996;53:313–319

Chatterjee A, Gordon MF, Giladi N, Trosch R. Botulinum toxin in the treatment of tardive dystonia. J Clin Psychopharmacol 1997;17:497–498

Chong SA. Fluvoxamine and akathisia. J Clin Psychopharmacol 1996;16:334–335

Christensen E, Moller JE, Faurbye A. Neuropathological investigation of 28 brains from patients with dyskinesia. Acta Psychiatr Scand 1970;46:14–23

Clow A, Theodorou A, Jenner P, Marsden CD. Cerebral dopamine function in rats following withdrawal from one year of continuous neuroleptic administration. Eur J Pharmacol 1980;63:145–157

Conley RR, Tamminga CA, Bartko JJ, et al. Olanzapine compared with chlorpromazine in treatment-resistant schizophrenia. Am J Psychiatry 1998;155:914–920

Corson PW, Nopoulos P, Miller DD, et al. Change in basal ganglia volume over 2 years in patients with schizophrenia: typical versus atypical neuroleptics. Amer J Psychiat 1999;156:1200–1204

Cross AJ, Crow TJ, Ferrier IN, et al. Chemical and structural changes in the brain in patients with movement disorder. In: Casey DE, Chase TN, Chritine AV, Gerlach J, eds. Dyskinesia: research and treatment. New York: Springer-Verlag, 1985:104–110

D'Alessandro R, Benassi G, Cristina E, et al. The prevalence of lingual-facial-buccal dyskinesia in the elderly. Neurology 1986;36:1350–1351

Dalgalarrondo P, Gattaz WF. Basal ganglia abnormalities in tardive dyskinesia—possible relationship with duration of neuroleptic treatment. Eur Arch Psychiat Clin Neuros 1994;244:272–277

Dave M. Clozapine-related tardive dyskinesia. Biol Psychiatry 1994;35:886–887

David WS, Sharif AA. Clozapine-induced myokymia. Muscle Nerve 1998;21:827–831

de la Fuente-Fernandez R. Tardive dyskinesia in dopa-responsive dystonia: a reappraisal of the dopamine hypothesis of tardive dyskinesia. Neurology 1998;50: 1134–1135

Delfs JM, Ellison GD, Mercugliano M, Chesselet MF. Expression of glutamic acid decarboxylase mRNA in striatum and palladium in an animal model of tardive dyskinesia. Exp Neurol 1995;133:175–188

Dresel S, Tatsch K, Dahne I, et al. Iodine-123-iodobenzamide SPECT assessment of dopamine D_2 receptor occupancy in risperidone-treated schizophrenic patients. J Nucl Med 1998;39:1138–1142

Dressler D, Oeljeschlager RO, Ruther E. Severe tardive dystonia: treatment with continuous intrathecal baclofen administration. Mov Disord 1997;12:585–587

Dunayevich E, Strakowski SM. Olanzapine-induced tardive dystonia. Amer J Psychiat 1999;156:1662

Durst R, Katz G, Zislin J, et al. Rabbit syndrome treated with olanzapine. Brit J Psychiat 2000;176:19

Duvoisin RC. Reserpine for tardive dyskinesia. N Engl J Med 1972;286:611

Elkashef AM, Egan MF, Frank JA, et al. Basal ganglia iron in tardive dyskinesia—an MRI study. Biol Psychiatry 1994;35:16–21

Eyles DW, Pond SM, Vander-Scyf CJ, Halliday GM. Mitochondrial ultrastructure and density in a primate model of persistent tardive dyskinesia. Life Sci 2000; 66:1345–1350

Fahn S, Burke RE. Tardive dyskinesia and other neuroleptics-induced syndromes. In: Rowland LP, ed. Merritt's textbook of neurology. 10th ed. Philadelphia: Lippincott Williams & Wilkins, 2000;696–699

Fahn S, Jankovic J, Lang AE. What Is It? Case 5, 1986. A man with oral-buccal-lingual dyskinesia. Mov Disord 1986;1:309–318

Fahn S, Mayeux R. Unilateral Parkinson's disease and contralateral tardive dyskinesia: a unique case with successful therapy that may explain the pathophysiology of these two disorders. J Neural Transm Suppl 1980;16:179–185

Fahn S. The medical treatment of movement disorders. In: Crossman A, Sambrook MA, eds. Neural mechanism in disorders of movement. London: John Libbey and Co., 1989:249–267

Fahn S. The varied clinical expressions of dystonia. Neurologic clinics 1984b;2:541–554

Faurbye A, Rasch PJ, Peterson PB, et al. Neurological symptoms in pharmacotherapy of psychoses. Acta Psychiatrica Scand 1964;40:10–27

Fenn DS, Moussaoui D, Hoffman WF, et al. Movements in never-medicated schizophrenics: a preliminary study. Psychopharmacology 1996;123:206–210

Fenton WS, Blyler CR, Wyatt RJ, McGlashan TH. Prevalence of spontaneous dyskinesia in schizophrenic and non-schizophrenic psychiatric patients. Br J Psychiatry 1997;171:265–268

Fibiger HC, Lloyd KG. Neurobiological biological substrates of tardive dyskinesia: the GABA hypothesis. Trends NeuroSci 1984;7:462–464

Filice GA, McDougall BC, Ercan Fang N, et al. Neuroleptic malignant syndrome associated with olanzapine. Ann Pharmacotherapy 1998;32:1158–1159

Friedman J, Lannon M, Comella C, et al. Low-dose clozapine for the treatment of drug-induced psychosis in Parkinson's disease. N Engl J Med 1999;340:757–763

Friedman JH, Kucharski LT, Wagner RL. Tardive dystonia in a psychiatric hospital. J Neurol Neurosurg Psychiatry 1986;50:801–803

Fukuoka T, Nakano M, Kohda A, et al. The common marmoset (Callithrix jacchus) as a model for neuroleptics-induced acute dystonia. Pharmacol Biochem Behav 1997;58:947–953

Galili-Mosberg R, Gilad I, Weizman A, et al. Haloperidol-induced neurotoxicity—possible implications for tardive dyskinesia. J Neural Transm 2000;107:479–490

Gatrad AR. Dystonic reactions to metoclopramide. Develop Med Child Neurol 1976;18:767–769

Gattaz WF, Emrich A, Behrens S. Vitamin E attenuates the development of haloperidol-induced dopaminergic hypersensitivity in rats—possible implications for tardive dyskinesia. J Neural Transm-Gen Sect 1993;92:197–201

Gerlach J. Current views on tardive dyskinesia. Pharmacopsychiatry 1991;24:47–48

Gervin M, Browne S, Lane A, et al. Spontaneous abnormal involuntary movements in first-episode schizophrenia and schizophreniform disorder: baseline rate in a group of patients from an Irish catchment area. Am J Psychiatry 1998;155:1202–1206

Granger AS, Hanger HC. Olanzapine: extrapyramidal side effects in the elderly. Aust NZ J Med 1999;29: 371–372

Graudins A, Fern RP. Acute dystonia in a child associated with therapeutic ingestion of a dextromethorphan containing cough and cold syrup. J Toxicol-Clin Toxicol 1996;34:351–352

Gunne LM, Growdon J, Glaaeser B. Oral dyskinesia in rats following brain lesions and neuroleptic drug administration. Psychopharmacology 1982;77:134–139

Gunne LM, Haggstrom J-E. Reduction of nigral glutamic acid decarboxylase in rats with neuroleptics-induced oral dyskinesia. Psychopharmacology 1983; 81:191–194

Gutierrez-Esteinou R, Grebb JA. Risperidone: an analysis of the first three years in general use. Int Clin Psychopharmacol 1997;12:S3–S10

Gwinn KA, Caviness JN. Risperidone-induced tardive dyskinesia and parkinsonism. Mov Disord 1997;12: 119–121

Haberfellner EM. Tardive dyskinesia during treatment with risperidone. Pharmacopsychiatry 1997;30:271

Harrison PJ. The neuropathological effects of antipsychotic drugs. Schizophr Res 1999;40:87–99

Hayashi T, Nishikawa T, Koga I, et al. Prevalence of and risk factors for respiratory dyskinesia. Clin Neuropharmacol 1996;19:390–398

Herran A, Vazquez-Barquero JL. Tardive dyskinesia associated with olanzapine. Ann Intern Med 1999;131:72

Hoffman WF, Casey DE. Computed tomographic evaluation of patients with tardive dyskinesia. Schizophr Res 1991;5:1–12

Hong KS, Cheong SS, Woo JM, Kim E. Risperidone induced tardive dyskinesia. Amer J Psychiat 1999;156: 1290

Ikeda H, Adachi K, Hasegawa M, et al. Effects of chronic haloperidol and clozapine on vacuous chewing and dopamine-mediated jaw movements in rats: evaluation of a revised animal model of tardive dyskinesia. J Neural Transm 1999;106:1205–1216

Inada T, Ohnishi K, Kamisada M, et al. A prospective study of tardive dyskinesia in Japan. Eur Arch Psychiatry Clin Neurosci 1991;240:250–254

Jain KK. An assessment of iloperidone for the treatment of schizophrenia. Expert Opin Investig Drugs 2000;9:2935–2943

Jankovic J. Stereotypies. In: Marsden CD, Fahn S, eds. Movement disorders 3. Oxford: Butterworth-Heinemann, 1994:503–517

Jauss M, Schroder J, Pantel J, et al. Severe akathisia during olanzapine treatment of acute schizophrenia. Pharmacopsychiatry 1998;31:146–148

Jeanjean AP, Laterre EC, Maloteaux JM. Neuroleptic binding to sigma receptors: possible involvement in neuroleptics-induced acute dystonia. Biol Psychiatry 1997;41:1010–1019

Jellinger K. Neuropathological findings after neuroleptic long-term therapy. In: Roizin L, Shiraki H, Grcevic N, eds. Neurotoxicology. New York: Raven Press, 1977:25–42

Jeste DV, Caligiuri MP, Paulsen JS, et al. Risk of tardive dyskinesia in older patients—a prospective longitudinal study of 266 outpatients. Arch Gen Psychiatry 1995;52:756–765

Jeste DV, Lacro JP, Palmer B, et al. Incidence of tardive dyskinesia in early stages of low-dose treatment with typical neuroleptics in older patients. Amer J Psychiat 1999;156:309–311

Jeste DV, Okamoto A, Napolitano J, et al. Low incidence of persistent tardive dyskinesia in elderly patients with dementia treated with risperidone. Amer J Psychiat 2000;157:1150–1155

Jeste DV, Wyatt RJ. Dogma disputed: is tardive dyskinesia due to postsynaptic dopamine receptor supersensitivity? J Clin Psychiatry 1981;42:455–457

Jimenez-Jimenez FJ, Tallon-Barranco A, Ortipareja M, et al. Olanzapine can worsen parkinsonism. Neurology 1998;50:1183–1184

Jonnalagada JR, Norton JW. Acute dystonia with quetiapine. Clin Neuropharmacol 2000;23:229–230

Kaneko K, Yuasa T, Miyatake T, Tsuji S. Stereotyped hand clasping: an unusual tardive movement disorder. Mov Disord 1993;8:230–231

Kanovsky P, Streitova H, Bares M, Hortova H. Treatment of facial and orolinguomandibular tardive dystonia by botulinum toxin A: evidence of a long-lasting effect. Mov Disord 1999;14:886–888

Kapitany T, Meszaros K, Lenzinger E, et al. Genetic polymorphisms for drug metabolism (CYP2D6) and tardive dyskinesia in schizophrenia. Schiz Res 1998;32: 101–106

Kapur S, Zipursky RB, Remington G, et al. 5-HT$_2$ and D$_2$ receptor occupancy of olanzapine in schizophrenia: a PET investigation. Am J Psychiatry 1998;155:921–928

Kelley JJ, Gao XM, Tamminga CA, Roberts RC. The effect of chronic haloperidol treatment on dendritic spines in the rat striatum. Exp Neurol 1997;146:471–478

Klawans HL, Barr A. Prevalence of spontaneous lingual-facial-buccal dyskinesia in the elderly. Neurology 1982;39:473–481

Klawans HL, Falk DK, Nausieda PA, Weiner WJ. Gilles de la Tourette syndrome after long-term chlorpromazine therapy. Neurology 1978;28:1064–8106

Klawans HL, Tanner CM. The reversibility of "permanent" tardive dyskinesia. Neurology 1983;33(Suppl 2): 163

Knable MB, Heinz A, Raedler T, Weinberger DR. Extrapyramidal side effects with risperidone and haloperidol at comparable D$_2$ receptor occupancy levels. Psychiat Res-Neuroimag 1997;75:91–101

Kraus T, Schuld A, Pollmacher T. Periodic leg movements in sleep and restless legs syndrome probably caused by olanzapine. J Clin Psychopharmacol 1999; 19:478–479

Kris MG, Tyson LB, Gralla RJ, et al. N Engl J Med 1983;309:433

Kurlan R, Shoulson I. Differential diagnosis of facial chorea. In: Jankovic J, Tolosa E, eds. Facial dyskinesias. Advances in Neurology. Vol 49. New York: Raven Press, 1988:225–238

Kurz M, Hummer M, Oberbauer H, Fleischhacker WW. Extrapyramidal side effects of clozapine and haloperidol. Psychopharmacology 1995;118:52–56

Kurzthaler I, Hummer M, Kohl C, et al. Propranolol treatment of olanzapine-induced akathisia. Am J Psychiatry 1997;154:1316

Labbate LA, Lande RG, Jones F, Oleshansky MA. Tardive dyskinesia in older out-patients: a follow-up study. Acta Psychiatr Scand 1997;96:195–198

Landry P, Cournoyer J. Acute dystonia with olanzapine. J Clin Psychiatry 1998;59:384

Lang AE. Clinical differences between metoclopramide- and antipsychotic-induced tardive dyskinesias. Can J Neurol Sci 1990;17:137–139

Lang AE. Withdrawal akathisia: case reports and a proposed classification of chronic akathisia. Mov Disord 1994;9:188–192

Lara DR, Wolf AL, Lobato MI, et al. Clozapine-induced neuroleptic malignant syndrome: an interaction between dopaminergic and purinergic systems? J Psychopharmacol 1999;13:318–319

Levenson JL. Neuroleptic malignant syndrome after the initiation of olanzapine. J Clin Psychopharmacol 1999;19:477–478

Levin T, Heresco-Levy U. Risperidone-induced rabbit syndrome: an unusual movement disorder caused by an atypical antipsychotic. Eur Neuropsychopharmacol 1999;9:137–139

LeWitt PA, Walters A, Hening W, McHale D. Persistent movement disorders induced by buspirone. Mov Disord 1993;8:331–334

Lieberman J, Kane JM, Woerner M. Prevalence of tardive dyskinesia in elderly samples. Psychopharmacol Bull 1984;20:22–26

Little JT, Jankovic J. Tardive myoclonus. Mov Disord 1987;2:307–311

Lohr JB. Oxygen radicals and neuropsychiatric illness—some speculations. Arch Gen Psychiatry 1991; 48:1097–1106

Margolese HC, Chouinard G. Olanzapine-induced neuroleptic malignant syndrome with mental retardation. Amer J Psychiat 1999;156:1115–1116

Marin C, Engber TM, Bonastre M, et al. Effect of long-term haloperidol treatment on striatal neuropeptides: relation to stereotyped behavior. Brain Res 1996;731:57–62

Maurer I, Moller HJ. Inhibition of complex I by neuroleptics in normal human brain cortex parallels the extrapyramidal toxicity of neuroleptics. Mol Cell Biochem 1997;174:255–259

Mazurek MF, Rosebush PI. Circadian pattern of acute, neuroleptics-induced dystonic reactions. Am J Psychiatry 1996;153:708–710

McCreadie RG, Thara R, Kamath S, et al. Abnormal movements in never-medicated Indian patients with schizophrenia. Br J Psychiatry 1996;168:221–226

Meissner W, Schmidt T, Kupsch A, et al. Reversible leucopenia related to olanzapine. Mov Disord 1999; 14:872–873

Meldrum BS, Anlezark GM, Marsden CD. Acute dystonia as an idiosyncratic response to neuroleptic drugs in baboons. Brain 1977;100:313–326

Meltzer HY. The role of serotonin in antipsychotic drug action. Neuropsychopharmacology 1999;21: S106–S115

Meyer-Lindenberg A, Krausnick B. Tardive dyskinesia in a neuroleptics-naive patient with bipolar-I disorder: persistent exacerbation after lithium intoxication. Mov Disord 1997;12:1108–1109

Miller CH, Simioni I, Oberbauer H, et al. Tardive dyskinesia prevalence rates during a ten-year follow-up. J Nerv Ment Dis 1995;183:404–407

Miller LG, Jankovic J. Metoclopramide-induced movement disorders—clinical findings with a review of the literature. Arch Intern Med 1989;149:2486–2492

Miller LG, Jankovic J. Persistent dystonia possibly induced by flecainide. Mov Disord 1992;7:62–63

Mion CC, Andreasen NC, Arndt S, et al. MRI abnormalities in tardive dyskinesia. Psychiat Res-Neuroimag 1991;40:157–166

Mithani S, Atmadja S, Baimbridge KG, Fibiger HC. Neuroleptic-induced oral dyskinesia: effects of progabide and lack of correlation with regional changes in glutamic acid decarboxylase and choline acetyltransferase activities. Psychopharmacology 1987;93:94–100

Modestin J, Stephan PL, Erni T, Umari T. Prevalence of extrapyramidal syndromes in psychiatric inpatients and the relationship of clozapine treatment to tardive dyskinesia. Schizophr Res 2000;42:223–230

Molho ES, Factor SA. Possible tardive dystonia resulting from clozapine therapy. Mov Disord 1999a;14: 873–874

Molho ES, Factor SA. Worsening of motor features of Parkinsonism with olanzapine. Mov Disord 1999b;14: 1014–1016

Moltz DA, Coeytaux RR. Case report: possible neuroleptic malignant syndrome associated with olanzapine. J Clin Psychopharmacol 1998;18:485–486

Mosnik DM, Spring B, Rogers K, Baruah S. Tardive dyskinesia exacerbated after ingestion of phenylalanine by schizophrenic patients. Neuropsychopharmacology 1997;16:136–146

Muller P, Seeman P. Brain neurotransmitter receptors after long-term haloperidol. Life Sci 1977;21: 1751–1758

Nagao T, Ohshimo T, Mitsunobu K, et al. Cerebrospinal fluid monoamine metabolites and cyclic nucleotides in chronic schizophrenic patients with tardive dyskinesia or drug-induced tremor. Biol Psychiatry 1979;14:509–523

Naumann R, Felber W, Heilemann H, Reuster T. Olanzapine-induced agranulocytosis. Lancet 1999;354: 566–567

Newman M, Anjee A, Jampala C. Atypical neuroleptic malignant syndrome associated with risperidone treatment. Am J Psychiatry 1997;154:1475

Nisijima K, Shimizu M, Ishiguro T. Treatment of tardive dystonia with an antispastic agent. Acta Psychiatr Scand 1998;98:341–343

Nutt JG, Muenter MD, Aronson A, et al. Epidemiology of focal and generalized dystonia in Rochester, Minnesota. Mov Disord 1988;3:188–194

O'Keefe R, Sharman DF, Vogt M. Effect of drugs used in psychoses on cerebral dopamine metabolism. Brit J Pharmacol 1970;38:287–304

Ohashi K, Hamamura T, Lee Y, et al. Propranolol attenuates haloperidol-induced Fos expression in discrete regions of rat brain: possible brain regions responsible for akathisia. Brain Res 1998;802:134–140

Ohmori O, Suzuki T, Kojima H, et al. Tardiveiveive dyskinesia and debrisoquine 4-hydroxylase (CYP2D6) genotype in Japanese schizophrenics. Schizophr Res 1998;32:107–113

Ornadel D, Barnes EA, Dick DJ. Acute dystonia due to amitriptyline. J Neurol Neurosurg Psychiatry 1992;55: 414

Petersen R, Finsen B, Andreassen OA, et al. No changes in dopamine D_1 receptor mRNA expressing neurons in the dorsal striatum of rats with oral movements induced by long-term haloperidol administration. Brain Res 2000;859:394–397

Pinder RM, Brogden RF, Sawyer PR, et al. Metoclopramide: a review of its pharmacological properties and clinical use. Drugs 1976;12:81–131

Poyurovsky M, Hermesh H, Weizman A. Severe withdrawal akathisia following neuroleptic discontinuation successfully controlled by clozapine. Int Clin Psychopharmacol 1996;11:283–286

Raedler TJ, Knable MB, Lafargue T, et al. In vivo determination of striatal dopamine D_2 receptor occupancy in patients treated with olanzapine. Psychiat Res Neuroimag 1999;90:81–90

Reasbeck PG, Hossenbocus A. Death following dystonic reaction to oral metoclopramide. Br J Clin Practice 1979;33:31–33

Richardson MA, Reilly MA, Read LL, et al. Phenylalanine kinetics are associated with tardive dyskinesia in men but not in women. Psychopharmacology 1999a; 143:347–357

Rollema H, Lu Y, Schmidt AW, et al. 5-HT$_{(1A)}$ receptor activation contributes to ziprasidone-induced dopamine release in the rat prefrontal cortex. Biol Psychiatry 2000;48:229–237

Rosebush PI, Kennedy K, Dalton B, Mazurek MF. Protracted akathisia after risperidone withdrawal. Am J Psychiatry 1997;154:437–438

Rosebush PI, Mazurek MF. Neurologic side effects in neuroleptics-naive patients treated with haloperidol or risperidone. Neurology 1999;52:782–785

Rupniak NMJ, Tye SJ, Steventon MJ, et al. Spontaneous orofacial dyskinesias in a captive Cynomolgus monkey: implications for tardive dyskinesia. Mov Disord 1990;5:314–318

Sachdev P, Kruk J, Kneebone M, Kissane D. Clozapine-induced neuroleptic malignant syndrome: review and report of new cases. J Clin Psychopharmacol 1995;15: 365–371

Sachdev P. The classification of akathisia. Mov Disord 1995a;10:235

Sachdev PS, Saharov T. The effects of beta-adrenoceptor antagonists on a rat model of neuroleptics-induced akathisia. Psychiatry Res 1997;72:133–140

Safferman AZ, Lieberman JA, Pollack S, Kane JM. Akathisia and clozapine treatment. J Clin Psychopharmacol 1993;13:286–287

Sagara Y. Induction of reactive oxygen species in neurons by haloperidol. J Neurochem 1998;71: 1002–1012

Saltz BL, Woerner MG, Kane JM, et al. Prospective study of tardive dyskinesia incidence in the elderly. J Am Med Assoc 1991;266:2402–2406

Sato S, Daly R, Peters H. Reserpine therapy of phenothiazine induced dyskinesia. Dis Nerv Syst 1971;32:680–685

Seeger TF, Seymour PA, Schmidt AW, et al. Ziprasidone (CP-88,059): a new antipsychotic with combined dopamine and serotonin receptor antagonist activity. J Pharmacol Exp Ther 1995;275:101–113

Segman R, Neeman T, Heresco-Levy U, et al. Genotypic association between the dopamine D_3 receptor and tardive dyskinesia in chronic schizophrenia. Mol Psychiatr 1999;4:247–253

Sethi KD, Hess DC, Harp RJ. Prevalence of dystonia in veterans on chronic antipsychotic therapy. Mov Disord 1990;5:319–321

Shirakawa O, Tamminga CA. Basal ganglia GABA$_{(A)}$ and dopamine D_1 binding site correlates of haloperidol-induced oral dyskinesias in rat. Exp Neurol 1994; 127:62–69

Sierra-Biddle D, Herran A, Diez-Aja S, et al. Neuroleptic malignant syndrome and olanzapine. J Clin Psychopharmacol 2000;20:704–705

Silberbauer C. Risperidone-induced tardive dyskinesia. Pharmacopsychiatry 1998;31:68–69

Soares KVS, McGrath JJ. The treatment of tardive dyskinesia—a systematic review and meta-analysis. Schizophr Res 1999;39:1–16

Sperner-Unterweger B, Czeipek I, Gaggl S, et al. Treatment of severe clozapine-induced neutropenia with granulocyte colony-stimulating factor (G-CSF)—remission despite continuous treatment with clozapine. Br J Psychiatry 1998;172:82–84

Sprouse JS, Reynolds LS, Braselton JP, et al. Comparison of the novel antipsychotic ziprasidone with clozapine and olanzapine: inhibition of dorsal raphe cell firing and the role of 5-HT$_{1A}$ receptor activation. Neuropsychopharmacology 1999;21:622–631

Stacy M, Jankovic J. Tardive tremor. Mov Disord 1992;7: 53–57

Stanley AK, Hunter J. Possible neuroleptic malignant syndrome with quetiapine. Brit J Psychiat 2000;176:497

Steen VM, Lovlie R, Macewan T, McCreadie RG. Dopamine D_3-receptor gene variant and susceptibility to tardive dyskinesia in schizophrenic patients. Mol Psychiatr 1997;2:139–145

Stephenson CME, Bigliani V, Jones HM, et al. Striatal and extra-striatal D_2/D_3 dopamine receptor occupancy by quetiapine in vivo-[I-123]-epidepride single photon emission tomography (SPET) study. Brit J Psychiat 2000;177:408–415

Stoessl AJ, Rajakumar N. Effects of subthalamic nucleus lesions in a putative model of tardive dyskinesia in the rat. Synapse 1996;24:256–261

Szymanski S, Gur RC, Gallacher F, et al. Vulnerability to tardive dyskinesia development in schizophrenia: an FDG-PET study of cerebral metabolism. Neuropsychopharmacology 1996;15:567–575

Tamminga CA, Smith RC, Pandey G, et al. A neuroendocrine study of supersensitivity in tardive dyskinesia. Arch Gen Psychiatry 1977;34:1199–1203

Tan EK, Jankovic J. Tardive and idiopathic oromandibular dystonia: a clinical comparison. J Neurol Neurosurg Psychiat 2000;68:186–190

Tarsy D, Kaufman D, Sethi KD, et al. An open-label study of botulinum toxin A for treatment of tardive dystonia. Clin Neuropharmacol 1997;20:90–93

Terland O, Flatmark T. Drug-induced parkinsonism: cinnarizine and flunarizine are potent uncouplers of the vacuolar H+-ATPase in catecholamine storage vesicles. Neuropharmacology 1999;38:879–882

Thaker GK, Tamminga CA, Alps LD, et al. Brain gamma-aminobutyric acid abnormality in tardive dyskinesia. Arch Gen Psychiatry 1987;44:522–529

Thomas P, Lalaux N, Vaiva G, Goudemand M. Dose-dependent stuttering and dystonia in a patient taking clozapine. Am J Psychiatry 1994;151:1096

Tollefson GD, Beasley CM, Tamura RN, et al. Blind, controlled, long-term study of the comparative incidence of treatment-emergent tardive dyskinesia with olanzapine or haloperidol. Am J Psychiatry 1997;154:1248–1254

Tominaga H, Fukuzako H, Izumi K, et al. Tardive myoclonus. Lancet 1987:322

Tsai GC, Goff DC, Chang RW, et al. Markers of glutamatergic neurotransmission and oxidative stress associated with tardive dyskinesia. Am J Psychiatry 1998;155:1207–1213

van Harten PN, Matroos GE, Hoek HW, Kahn RS. The prevalence of tardive dystonia, tardive dyskinesia, parkinsonism and akathisia—The Curacao Extrapyramidal Syndromes Study. 1. Schizophr Res 1996b;19:195–203

van Os J, Walsh E, van Horn E, et al. Tardive dyskinesia in psychosis: are women really more at risk? Acta Psychiat Scand 1999;99:288–293

Van Putten T, May PRA, Marder SR. Akathisia with haloperidol and thiothixene. Arch Gen Psychiatry 1984; 41:1036–1039

Vandel P, Haffen E, Vandel S, et al. Drug extrapyramidal side effects. CYP2D6 genotypes and phenotypes. Eur J Clin Pharmacol 1999;55:659–665

Vesely C, Kufferle B, Brucke T, Kasper S. Remission of severe tardive dyskinesia in a schizophrenic patient treated with the atypical antipsychotic substance quetiapine. Int Clin Psychopharmacol 2000;15:57–60

Waddington JL, Cross AJ, Gamble SJ, Bourne RC. Spontaneous orofacial dyskinesia and dopaminergic function in rats after six months of neuroleptic treatment. Science 1983;220:530–532

Walinder J, Skott A, Carlsson A, Roos B-E. Potentiation by metyrosine of thioridazine effects in chronic schizopherenics. Arch Gen Psychiatry 1976;33:501–505

Woerner MG, Alvir JMJ, Saltz BL, et al. Prospective study of tardive dyskinesia in the elderly: rates and risk factors. Am J Psychiatry 1998;155:1521–1528

Woerner MG, Kane JM, Lieberman JA, et al. The prevalence of tardive dyskinesia. J Clin Psychopharmacol 1991;11:34–42

Wojcik JD, Falk WE, Fink JS, et al. A review of 32 cases of tardive dystonia. Am J Psychiatry 1991;148: 1055–1059

Wolf SM. Reserpine: cause and treatment of oral-facial dyskinesia. Bull Los Angeles Neurol Soc 1973;38:80–84

Wood A. Clinical experience with olanzapine, a new atypical antipsychotic. Int Clin Psychopharmacol 1998; 13:S59–S62

Worrel JA, Marken PA, Beckman SE, Ruehter VL. Atypical antipsychotic agents: a critical review. Amer J Health Syst Pharm 2000;57:238–255

Yamada K, Kanba S, Anamizu S, et al. Low superoxide dismutase activity in schizophrenic patients with tardive dyskinesia. Psychol Med 1997;27:1223–1225

Yassa R, Nair V, Dimitry R. Prevalence of tardive dystonia. Acta Psychiatr Scan 1986;73:629–633

Yoshida K, Hasebe T, Higuchi H, et al. Marked improvement of tardive dystonia in a schizophrenic patient after electroconvulsive therapy. Hum Psychopharmacol Clin Exp 1996;11:421–423

Tourette's Syndrome and Tic Disorders

Roger Kurlan

Under the encouragement of his mentor Charcot, George Gilles de la Tourette set out to clarify conditions characterized by involuntary movements. Following the publication of Beard's 1880 American journal article on "The Jumping Frenchmen of Maine," a disorder comprising excessive startle, echolalia and echopraxia, Tourette surmised that if jumping Frenchmen existed in Maine, they should be found in Paris as well. He searched for similar cases at the Neurological Institute of the Salpetriere, but failed to identify any. Rather, he reported nine patients who had echophenomena, but were characterized mainly by the presence of motor and vocal tics, including coprolalia. In his now-classic publication of 1885 where he described the condition that bears his name, Gilles de la Tourette considered the disorder to be closely related to a group of startle diseases that included the jumping Frenchmen.[1]

Although Tourette himself indicated that the disorder was hereditary in nature, for many years the cause of Tourette's syndrome (TS) was ascribed to psychogenic causes and the importance of genetic factors was overlooked. The successful treatment of TS with neuroleptic drugs in the 1960s refocused attention from a psychological to an organic central nervous system cause. In the 1970s, researchers demonstrated a familial concentration for TS. Analysis of transmission patterns in families suggested involvement of a major gene. Studies indicate that TS may have variable clinical expression, involving a spectrum of tics and behavioral disturbances that include obsessive-compulsive disorder (OCD), attention deficit hyperactivity disorder (ADHD) and perhaps other psychopathology. Recognition of the heterogeneous expression and variable severity of TS has suggested that, rather than being a rare condition characterized by severe and bizarre symptoms, TS is often a mild condition that is much more common than generally appreciated.[2]

Epidemiology

The clinical characteristics of TS contribute to specific problems in epidemiological studies. First, in social situations such as during an interview, subjects commonly suppress their tics so they may not be observable. Second, because of the typical waxing and waning of symptoms, a single examination may not be adequate to identify the condition. Third, because the condition characteristically improves or resolves in adulthood, the tics may have been present only years prior to an evaluation. Fourth, many cases may be missed when relying solely on historical information since affected persons or their relatives may be unaware of the presence of tics. For example, in a study of a single large family affected by TS, 30% of 54 subjects with tics identified by examiners were not aware of their own tics.[3] Fifth, tics are more common in males, so the gender distribution of a studied population is of great importance. Finally, the full spectrum of the TS phenotype has not been accurately delineated so the nature of symptoms that should be included in defining an affected individual is open to different interpretations.[4]

Many of the past estimates for the lifetime prevalence rate for TS, ranging from 0.45 to 13/10 000, have been based largely on a review of medical records, case series of patients referred for medical evaluation or on data obtained from questionnaires without direct clinical examination.[3] Based on the clinical characteristics of TS noted above, these approaches are likely to be inaccurate, giving gross underestimates of disease prevalence. A recent community-based epidemiological study involving direct interviews and examinations of school children found that 0.8–3.8% were diagnosed with TS, using different set of diagnostic criteria [R. Kurlan, personal communication]. In this study, up to 19.7% of children either had a history of tics or were observed to have them, suggesting that tic disorders are much more common than generally described. Studies have consistently demonstrated that tics are particularly common, occurring in about 25% of cases, in children who have school problems and are receiving special education.[5–7] This finding raises the possibility that tics might be an observable sign of an underlying brain developmental disorder that contributes to academic difficulties.[8]

Tourette's syndrome appears to be worldwide in distribution, with clinical series and case reports being published from many countries.[9] Little information is available regarding whether there are differences in prevalence rates across ethnic groups. The principle risk factors for TS are male gender and hereditary. Both clinical and community-based studies agree that TS is more common in males than females, with a ratio of approximately 3:1.[9] Gender may be a risk factor for comorbid conditions, as there appears to be an association between female gender and OCD, and male gender and ADHD.[10]

Pathophysiology and pathogenesis

Although it is now largely accepted that most cases of TS occur on a genetic basis (see below), the pathogenetic mechanisms for the disorder remain unknown. Several lines of evidence support the hypothesis that striatal dopamine receptor super-sensitivity is present.

The observations of tic suppression by dopamine receptor antagonists, reduced levels of the dopamine metabolite homovanillic acid in the cerebrospinal fluid,[11] and the phenomenon of tardive tics following chronic dopamine antagonist therapy contribute to this notion. Disturbances of other brain neurochemical systems have also been implicated, including the endogenous opioid system[13–16] and cyclic adenosine monophosphate (AMP).[17] A promising line of investigation raises the possibility that sex hormones may mediate abnormal development of specific brain regions, particularly the basal ganglia and limbic system, resulting in TS.[18,19] An interesting lead is the consistent finding from a variety of neuroimaging techniques that there is an abnormality in structural and functional relationships between the left and right sides of the brain, particularly in the region of the basal ganglia.[20–23] A recent hypothesis suggests that some cases of TS arise as a post-streptococcal, autoimmune process, although clear evidence to support this concept is lacking.[24]

Genetics

Studies investigating the hereditary transmission pattern of TS in families have indicated major gene involvement. Although initial results supported an autosomal dominant mode of inheritance,[10] recent information suggests that the transmission pattern may be more complicated.[25] It has been observed, for example, that bilineal transmission, involving both the maternal and paternal sides, is common in TS families and may be related to the severity of symptoms.[26,27] Thus, polygenic influences may be important, with clinical expression being determined by the number of "susceptibility loci" that are inherited from either mother or father.

Clinical features

Tics are brief movements (motor tics) or sounds produced by the movement of air through the nose, mouth, or throat (vocal tics).[28] Compared to other involuntary movements, tics are not constantly present (except when very severe) and occur out of a background of normal motor activity. Motor and vocal tics may include virtually any movement or sound and are divided conceptually into simple and complex types. Simple motor tics are abrupt, sudden, brief, isolated movements such as an eye-blink, a facial grimace, a head jerk or a shoulder shrug. Some simple motor tics are slower, sustained, tonic movements (e.g., neck twisting, abdominal tightening) that resemble dystonia and are, therefore, termed dystonic tics.[29] Complex motor tics are more coordinated and complicated movements that may appear purposeful, as if performing a voluntary motor action. Examples include touching, tapping, hopping, smelling, copropraxia (obscene gestures), and echopraxia (mimicking movements performed by others). Motor tics usually recur in the same part of the body and multiple body regions are often involved. Over time, tics tend to recede from one body part and evolve elsewhere.

Simple vocal tics are inarticulate noises and single sounds, such as throat clearing, grunting, humming, or sniffing. Complex vocal tics have linguistic meaning and consist of full or truncated words, such as palilalia (repeating the individuals own words), echolalia (repeating the words of others), and coprolalia (obscene words). Although coprolalia has been the symptom perhaps most responsible for the notoriety of TS, this symptom may be mild, transient, may occur in thought only without verbal expression (mental coprolalia) and occurs in only a minority of cases.

Almost half of patients with TS experience patterns of uncomfortable somatic sensations, such as pressure, tickle, or warmth, that are localized to specific body regions, such as eyes, face, or neck. Patients attempt to relieve the uncomfortable sensations with movements often interpreted as voluntary, usually tonic stretching or tightening of muscles. Relief is temporary, however, and the movements are repeated. Some patients produce vocalizations in response to sensory stimuli in the larynx or throat. These premonitory sensations have been referred to as "sensory tics" and may represent a fairly specific clinical feature that distinguishes tics from other involuntary movements.[30]

Although chronic multiple motor and vocal tics represent the signs upon which the diagnosis of TS is currently based, tics are often accompanied by a variety of behavioral disturbances. About 50% of TS patients demonstrate symptoms of obsessive-compulsive disorder (OCD), such as compulsive checking, counting and perfectionism and obsessive fears or worries.[31] The notion that OCD is an alternative expression of the TS genetic trait is supported by family studies and segregation analyses.[10,32] About half of patients with TS show evidence of attention deficit hyperactivity disorder (ADHD), manifested by inattention, distractibility, impulsivity, and hyperactivity.[2] Recent evidence indicates that there is also an etiological relationship between TS and ADHD,[33] particularly when the ADHD symptoms appear after the onset of tics.[34] Other information suggests that the behavioral spectrum of TS includes other conditions, such as generalized anxiety disorder, panic attacks, phobias, and mood disorder, but the boundaries of the TS behavioral spectrum remain to be accurately delineated.[2,4,35–37]

Classification

Tourette's syndrome can be considered to represent one member of a family of primary tic disorders. As presented in the Diagnostic and Statistical Manual of Psychiatry (4th edition), diagnostic criteria for TS include: (1) the presence of multiple motor tics, (2) the presence of one or more vocal tics, (3) age at onset before 18 years, (4) duration of more than one year, and (5) the disturbance causes marked distress or significant impairment in daily functioning.[38] Chronic tic disorder (CTD) differs from TS in that motor or vocal tics, but not both, are present. Transient tic disorder (TTD) differs from TS and CTD by having a duration of less than one year.[38] Both CTD and TTD are generally viewed as variants of TS and possible expressions of the same genetic defect.[2,39] The severity of tics is variable in each of the primary tic disorders, and is not necessarily most severe in TS.

Some aspects of the diagnostic criteria for tic disorders have been questioned. Since vocal tics result from air moved by the action of pharyngeal, laryngeal, facial and respiratory muscles, the conceptual distinction between motor and vocal tics may not have a true neurobiological basis. Thus, diagnostic classification based on the presence of a single vocal tic may be scientifically invalid. Secondly, the TS diagnostic criterion that tics must be functionally disabling is controversial since it runs contrary to genetic and epidemiological information that indicates that the majority of individuals with TS have mild symptoms.

Diagnostic process

The diagnosis of TS or a related tic disorder will often be obvious to an experienced clinician after obtaining historical information and simple observation. Given the characteristic waxing and waning quality and the voluntary suppressibility of tics, they may be absent at the time of an examination. Clinicians should remember that for most affected individuals with TS, tics are mild and severe symptoms are not required for diagnosis. Neuroimaging or other diagnostic studies are generally not required. The presence of a family history of tics, OCD, or ADHD may be useful for establishing the diagnosis of TS. Since the clinical manifestations of TS may be quite variable, including both motor and behavioral dysfunction, each patient should be carefully evaluated to determine which aspects of the illness are most disabling. For most patients, one or two clinical problems (e.g., tics, OCD) will predominate and can serve as specific target symptoms for therapy.[40] Neurological and psychiatric assessments and testing with standardized neuropsychological measures of attention and psychopathology are often helpful in sorting out the relative contributions of motor and behavioral disturbances for an individual patient.

Differential diagnosis

Tics can usually be readily differentiated from other involuntary movements.[28] Simple motor tics can resemble the rapid muscle jerks of myoclonus. However, even when most tics are simple jerks, more complex forms of motor tics or more sustained dystonic tics may be present, allowing one to establish the diagnosis by association with these other forms of motor tics. Additionally, simple motor tics tend to have a less random, more predictable body distribution and a wider range of amplitude and forcefulness when compared to myoclonus. The characteristic voluntary suppressibility and premonitory sensory phenomena of tics and a tendency of myoclonus to increase with intentional actions may also help distinguish between the two movement disorders. It should be recognized, however, that voluntary suppressibility is not specific for tics, but can be seen to at least

some degree for virtually the whole range of hyperkinetic involuntary movements.

Repetitive eye blinking from tics can be distinguished from blepharospasm, a form of focal cranial dystonia, by the presence of tics at other sites. Furthermore, while tics typically begin in childhood, blepharospasm is largely a disorder with onset in adult life. Dystonic tics can be differentiated from torsion dystonia in that the latter is a continual movement that can result in a sustained abnormal posture whereas dystonic tics usually cause an abnormal posture that is present for only a short period of time. The presence of more typical abrupt, brief simple motor tics in other body regions would favor the diagnosis of dystonic tics rather than torsion dystonia. Dystonic tics are often preceded by localized premonitory sensations (sensory tics) that may be relieved by the movement[3] and such sensory phenomena are characteristically absent in dystonia.

Tics may be difficult to distinguish on phenomenological grounds from the repetitive, stereotyped complex motor acts designated "stereotypies."[41] Stereotypies tend to be defined by their occurrence in characteristic clinical settings, such as mental retardation, autism, pervasive developmental disorder, psychosis, and congenital blindness or deafness. Compared to tics, stereotypies are longer in duration, more restricted in repertoire, and tend to remain in the same body region.

Although they often co-exist, it may be difficult to differentiate complex motor tics and compulsions.[41] Compulsions are repetitive, stereotyped, purposeless motor acts performed in response to an obsession, often according to certain rules (rituals). Compulsive motor acts are often carried out in order to neutralize an unpleasant obsession, and may be repeated a specified number of times, in a specified order, or at a particular time of day (e.g., bedtime rituals). Compulsive rituals may be performed with the thought of preventing a future dreaded event, a feature that is absent in pure tics. Response to drug therapy (see below) may be useful in distinguishing tics and compulsions. While tics usually respond predictably to dopamine antagonist medications, compulsions do not, but rather benefit from antidepressant drugs that preferentially inhibit serotonin reuptake.

Tourette's syndrome and the other primary tic disorders must be distinguished from other medical conditions that can cause secondary tics. Tics may be seen in a variety of neurological disorders, including Huntington's disease, neuroacanthocytosis, Parkinson's disease, progressive supranuclear palsy, Meige syndrome, and startle disorders.[42] Occasional cases of chronic tics have been described following head trauma,[43,44] viral encephalitis,[44] and carbon monoxide intoxication.[45] Chronic neuroleptic therapy can also induce a chronic tic disorder (tardive TS).[46] As mentioned earlier, it has been proposed that tics might occur as a result of streptococcal infection in a postinfectious autoimmune process analogous to Sydenham's chorea. It has also been proposed that a variety of insults in the perinatal period can interfere with normal brain developmental processes, particularly in the region of the basal ganglia and its connections, leading to a symptom complex that resembles TS. This has been referred to as the "developmental basal ganglia syndrome,"[47] and can include tics, other involuntary movements (chorea, dystonia, stereotypies), obsessive-compulsive symptoms, inattention, and aggressive behaviors. All of these secondary tic disorders can usually be identified on the basis of the neurological history and the presence of additional movement disorders (e.g., with chorea in Huntington's disease and neuroacanthocytosis) and other signs of neurological dysfunction.

Treatment

General approach

The first step in the management of TS is to determine whether treatment is even required. The goal of treatment is not to achieve complete tic suppression but to allow a patient to function and live normally. It is always important to consider the treatment of tics in the context of the associated psychopathology (ADHD, OCD, anxiety, depression), which, if present, can be more disabling than the tic disorder. In these cases, psychiatric evaluation and treatment is advisable. Patients with mild tics who have made a good adaptation in their lives can generally avoid the use of any medications.[40] Educating patients, family members, and school personnel about TS, restructuring the school environment (e.g., small group teaching, one-on-one tutoring, allowing TS students to work at their own pace, extra time to complete exams, and strategies to reduce stress), and providing supportive counseling are measures that may be sufficient to avoid the use of medications.

Medication therapy should only be considered if the symptoms of TS are functionally disabling and not remediable by non-pharmacological interventions.[40] A number of therapeutic agents are now available to treat the symptoms of TS and each medication should be chosen on the basis of specific target symptoms and potential side effects. For example, tic-suppression may be the most important goal for one patient, while treatment of OCD may take precedence in another. Drug dosages should be titrated slowly ("start low, go slow") in order to achieve the lowest satisfactory dosage and to avoid side effects. The maximum dosage utilized depends on achieving a tolerable suppression of symptoms. It is critical that the patient, family members and school personnel understand the ever-changing nature of TS, so that medications can be adjusted in a rational fashion, increasing when the symptoms upsurge and decreasing during periods of relative remission. In the long run, a reasonable goal is to use as little medication as possible (i.e., "less is best").

Many agents are available for treating TS, and there is no clear consensus on which approach is best. Only a minority of the agents available for treating TS have been tested in a large, randomized clinical trial, and few agents have been compared to each other.

The choice of medication depends on the severity of symptoms, side-effect profile, presence of comorbid psychopathology, and the physician's experience. Some experts use neuroleptics early on in the treatment while others consider this class to be the treatment of last resort. Often, the ideal agent for a given patient is found only through trial and error. In the sections that follow, medications for tic disorders and the common associated psychiatric symptoms are described in detail.

Tic suppression

Alpha agonists It appears that drugs acting as alpha agonists are often beneficial for treating tics. Although a few small-scale controlled clinical trials failed to confirm efficacy,[48,49] the beneficial effect on clonidine in suppressing tics was established in a recent large-scale, multicenter controlled clinical trial.[50] Alpha agonists are often considered first-choice medications for suppressing tics since their long-term side effects are usually more benign than alternative drugs. Also, the alpha agonists have the added advantage of helping to improve associated symptoms of ADHD. Clonidine (Catapres) is initially prescribed at a dosage of 0.05 mg (half of a 0.1 mg tablet) per day (usually at bedtime), which is gradually increased to achieve the lowest effective three times a day (before school, after school, bedtime) dosage. Some younger children may require four daily doses (adding a lunch time dose) due to a short duration of action in this age group. The total daily dosage of clonidine usually does not exceed 0.5 mg. The drug is also supplied as a transdermal one-week patch (Catapres-TTS) in sizes of 3.5, 7.0, and 10.5 cm², which are equivalent to 0.1, 0.2, and 0.3 mg per day, respectively. This formulation may be particularly useful for young children who cannot swallow pills, although the transdermal system can cause itching and skin rash. The optimal benefit of clonidine may not occur for several weeks on an adequate dosage. The dosage titration of clonidine is often limited by drug-induced sedation. The "start low, go slow" titration approach is usually effective in minimizing sedation and avoiding other common side effects, including irritability, dizziness, headache, dry mouth and insomnia. Since clonidine can cause hypotension, blood pressure and pulse should be monitored during dose titration. Acute withdrawal of clonidine should be avoided since hypertension, tachycardia, agitation and profuse sweating have been reported following abrupt discontinuation of the drug. Guanfacine (Tenex) has pharmacological properties similar to clonidine. It has advantages over clonidine that include single daily dosing and being less sedating. For these reasons, guanfacine has become the tic-suppressant of first-choice for many clinicians. To date, only open-label studies of guanfacine have been reported.[51-53] Guanfacine therapy is initiated at a dosage of 0.5 mg (half of a 1 mg tablet) at bedtime and is gradually titrated to a maximum of 4 mg/day. It is usually administered as a single bedtime dose, but it can be divided into two doses per day. Like clonidine, it appears that prolonged therapy (up to three months) with guanfacine may be required in order to achieve optimal clinical benefit.

Neuroleptics Neuroleptic drugs, which act as dopamine receptor antagonists, are the most predictably effective tic-suppressing medications. The efficacy of neuroleptics has been established in a number of controlled clinical trials [see reference 54 for a review]. Pharmacological blockade of dopamine receptors is rational, given the existing evidence that heightened dopamine receptor sensitivity underlies tic disorders.[11] Although neuroleptics probably remain the most commonly prescribed medications for TS, clinicians should avoid "reflex prescribing" following the diagnosis of TS since many patients may not require pharmacotherapy and a different medication may be more appropriate depending on the specific target symptoms identified. Neuroleptics have a side-effect profile that is generally worse than the alpha agonists. For tics that are acute, severe or painful, immediate tic-suppression therapy with a neuroleptic drug may be considered. Virtually any dopamine antagonist drug can be used to treat tics, and the tic-suppressing potency is directly proportional to D_2 receptor blocking ability. Recently, clinicians have moved toward the atypical antipsychotic agents, which have a lower affinity for the D_2 receptor than the traditional high potency D_2-receptor antagonist haloperidol. The best examples of this class are the antipsychotics clozapine and quetiapine, drugs that do not cause parkinsonism or tardive dyskinesias but are not especially effective for treating tics. Two recently marketed agents, risperidone and olanzapine, possess intermediate D_2 receptor blocking ability,[55] and have somewhat loosely been described as "atypical" antipsychotics. Like classical neuroleptic antipsychotics, these agents are effective for suppressing tics but can also cause parkinsonism and tardive dyskinesia. Tardive dyskinesia has been reported in patients with Tourette syndrome treated using neuroleptics.[56] As such, it is important for clinicians prescribing these "atypical" antipsychotics for Tourette's syndrome to warn their patients of this possible permanent complication. For tic suppression, risperidone (Risperdal) is started at a dosage of 0.5 mg (half of a 1 mg tablet) at bedtime and the dosage is gradually titrated as needed up to a maximum of 16 mg per day.[57] The drug can be administered as a single bedtime dose or divided into two daily doses. An oral solution of risperidone is available and may be useful for children who have difficulty swallowing pills. Olanzapine (Zyprexa) is another atypical neuroleptic with reported efficacy in suppressing tics.[58] Most recently, ziprasidone (Geodon), a potent blocker of D_2, D_3, as well as serotonin and α_2 receptors, was found to decrease tic severity by 35% in a group of patients.[59] If the atypical antipsychotics are ineffective or not tolerated, a classical high potency neuroleptic antipsychotic can be prescribed. These agents have a high binding affinity for D_2 receptors, and a higher propensity to cause parkinsonism or tardive dyskinesia. Some clinicians prefer fluphenazine (Prolixin;

0.5–20 mg/day) since the drug tends to produce less sedation and depression than some other drugs in this class. Haloperidol (Haldol; 0.25–20 mg/day) is also commonly used. Pimozide (Orap) is the only neuroleptic drug specifically promoted for the treatment of TS. It is equally as effective as other neuroleptics for tic suppression, but may be better tolerated since it tends to produce less sedation. Pimozide is initiated at 0.5 mg (half of a 1 mg tablet) at bedtime and the dosage is slowly titrated upwards in order to achieve a satisfactory reduction in tics. The maximum recommended dosage is 0.2 mg/kg/day (usually 10 mg or less). Pimozide therapy has led to prolongation of the Q-T interval or other changes on the electrocardiogram (ECG) and has rarely been associated with sudden death at high doses (60–70 mg), which are generally not employed in the treatment of TS. It is recommended that an ECG be obtained prior to prescribing pimozide and that the medication should be avoided if the Q-T interval is prolonged. Electrocardiogram monitoring is also recommended during the period of dosage adjustment and significant prolongation of the Q-T interval should be considered a basis for stopping further dose increases. A variety of acute and chronic motor side effects may accompany the use of neuroleptic drugs. At the low dosages employed to treat tics, acute dystonia is rarely encountered so that the standard use of prophylactic anticholinergic medications is not warranted. It is however, appropriate to discuss this potential adverse reaction with patients and parents. At the low dosages utilized for TS patients, drug-induced parkinsonism is also relatively uncommon. The appearance of parkinsonian features should prompt attempts to reduce neuroleptic drug dosage. Alternatively, the addition of anticholinergic medications for this problem can be considered. It has been reported that combined treatment with a neuroleptic drug and a serotonin reuptake inhibitor (see below) can result in acute, severe drug-induced parkinsonism in treated patients with TS.[57] Akathisia may improve with drug dosage reduction, although discontinuation of therapy may be required. Tardive dyskinesia is a potentially disabling complication of chronic neuroleptic therapy. Fortunately, although a real concern, tardive dyskinesia seems to develop only rarely in treated patients with TS, possibly related to the underlying state of dopamine receptor sensitivity. Drowsiness is a common unwanted effect of neuroleptic therapy. This side effect can often be avoided by using a single daily bedtime dose. The use of caffeine-containing beverages in the morning may provide a sufficient counteracting stimulant effect, if necessary. Dividing the dose and administering it in the late afternoon and at bedtime can sometimes lessen drowsiness. Sedation is sometimes accompanied by an irritable disposition, which may improve following dosage reduction. Persistent sedation or intellectual dulling may interfere with school and job performance and require discontinuation of neuroleptic therapy. Clinicians should monitor patients for dose-related depression that can occur during

Generic name	Brand name	How supplied	Daily dose
Clonidine	Alpha agonists Catapres	Tablets: 0.1 mg, 0.2 mg, 0.3 mg Transdermal System: TTS-1 (0.1 mg/day), TTS-2 (0.2 mg/day), TTS-3 (0.3 mg/day)	0.05–0.5 mg
Guanfacine	Tenex	Tablets: 1 mg, 2 mg	0.5–4 mg
Risperidone	Antipsychotics Risperdal	Tablets: 1 mg, 2 mg, 3 mg, 4 mg Oral Solution: 1 mg/ml	0.5–16 mg
Olanzapine	Zyprexa	Tablets: 2.5 mg, 5 mg, 7.5 mg, 10 mg	2.5–15 mg
Ziprasidone	Geodon	Capsules: 20 mg, 40 mg, 60 mg, 80 mg	20–160 mg
Haloperidol	Haldol	Tablets: 0.5 mg, 1 mg, 2 mg, 5 mg, 10 mg, 20 mg Oral Solution: 2 mg/ml, 50 mg/5 ml	0.5–20 mg
Pimozide	Orap	Tablets: 1 mg, 2 mg	0.5–10 mg
Fluphenazine	Prolixin	Tablets: 1 mg, 2.5 mg, 5 mg, 10 mg	0.5–20 mg
Tetrabenazine	Dopamine depletors Nitoman	Tablets: 25 mg	25–300 mg
Reserpine	Reserpine	Tablets: 0.25 mg	0.25–3 mg

Table 248.1   Tic-suppressing medications

neuroleptic therapy. Symptoms include tearfulness, sadness, decreased energy, loss of joy, irritability, and other signs of a depressive disorder. Depression may be particularly difficult to diagnose in children. Neuroleptic therapy may also lead to school and social phobias, requiring dosage reduction or discontinuation of therapy. Neuroleptics often result in an increased appetite, leading to significant weight gain. A strong dietary regimen and a vigorous daily exercise routine may be needed.

Catecholamine depletors   The catecholamine depleting agents tetrabenazine and reserpine are effective tic suppressing agents that do not carry a risk of inducing tardive dyskinesia. At some academic movement disorder centers, dopamine depletors are employed as a second line treatment, before antipsychotics.[60] These agents may produce unwanted dose-dependent sedation, hypotension, depression, akathisia, and parkinsonism. Unlike neuroleptics, they have never been associated with tardive dyskinesia. Neither drug has been tested in large groups of patients or subjected to a multicenter randomized controlled trial. Regrettably, tetrabenazine is not available in the USA, and must be imported from Canada or Europe. The drug comes in a 25 mg tablet that is started with one or one-half tablet at bedtime, gradually building up over weeks to a dose of 75–300 mg/d, given three times daily (tid) as a small dose in the morning and afternoon and a large dose before bed. Reserpine, at one time used to treat hypertension, is more difficult titrate in patients with Tourette's syndrome than tetrabenazine. This agent comes in 0.25 mg tablets, and is prescribed in a schedule similar to that of tetrabenazine, beginning with a night time dose of 0.25 mg, and gradually building up to four to 12 tablets daily, given mainly at bedtime. For both agents, during the initial weeks of therapy, it is especially important to monitor blood pressure.

Drowsiness is most severe at the onset of therapy but often resolves with tolerance. Clinicians should look for the development of parkinsonism, including masked facial expression, stooped posture, micrographia, generalized bradykinesia and rigidity, and postural instability, and reduce the dose accordingly if these signs develop. Histories of depression, or signs of depression on examination, are absolute contraindications to the use of these agents.

Other agents for tics   The alpha agonists, neuroleptics, and dopamine depleting agents are summarized in Table 248.1. For patients who do not tolerate or who have an insufficient response to these drugs, there is anecdotal evidence that other medications can reduce tics. Included are clonazepam (Klonopin),[61] baclofen and calcium channel blockers.[54] Given the ability of dopamine receptor blocking agents to suppress tics, it is surprising that dopamine agonists can also suppress tics. The dopamine agonist pergolide (Permax) has been reported to suppress tics in children and adults.[62] Selected patients with isolated facial tics or painful dystonic tics may improve following local intramuscular injections of botulinum toxin.[63] Botulinum toxin injections into the vocal cords have been described as effective for severe phonic tics.[64] Based on the hypothesis that some cases of TS result from a post-streptococcal, autoimmune process, it has been suggested that children with the onset or exacerbation of TS temporally related to streptococcal infection should be treated with antibiotics, immune globulin or plasma exchange. At present, however, there appears to be insufficient evidence to justify the routine use of such immune-modulating treatments.[24]

Agents for obsessive-compulsive disorder

For some patients with TS, co-morbid OCD may be more disabling than the tics themselves. A recent major advance in the pharmacotherapy of TS is the

Table 248.2 Serotonin reuptake inhibitors

Generic name	Brand name	How supplied	Daily dose
Clomipramine	Anafranil	Capsules: 25 mg, 50 mg, 75 mg	25–250 mg
Citalopram	Celexa	Tablets: 20 mg, 40 mg	10–40 mg
Fluvoxamine	Luvox	Tablets: 25 mg, 50 mg, 100 mg	25–300 mg
Paroxetine	Paxil	Tablets: 10 mg, 20 mg, 30 mg, 40 mg	10–60 mg
		Oral suspension: 10 mg/5 ml	
Fluoxetine	Prozac	Capsules: 10 mg, 20 mg	10–60 mg
		Oral solution: 20 mg/5 ml	
Sertraline	Zoloft	Tablets: 25 mg, 50 mg, 100 mg	25–200 mg

Table 248.3 Stimulants

Generic name	Brand name	How supplied	Daily dose	Dose per day
Methylphenidate	Ritalin	Tablets: 5 mg, 10 mg, 20 mg	2.5–60 mg	2–4
Dexmethylphenidate	Focalin	Tablets: 2.5 mg, 5 mg, 10 mg	2.5–20 mg	2–3
Methylphenidate-OROS	Concerta	Capsules: 18 mg, 36 mg, 54 mg	18–72 mg	1
Methylphenidate-extended release	Metadate CD	Capsules: 20 mg	20–60 mg	1
D-L-amphetamine	Adderall	Tablets: 5 mg, 10 mg, 20 mg, 30 mg	2.5–60 mg	1–2
Dextroamphetamine	Dexedrine	Tablets: 5 mg	2.5–40 mg	2–4
Dextroamphetamine-sustained release	Dexedrine spansule	Capsules: 5 mg, 10 mg, 15 mg	5–40 mg	1
Pemoline	Cylert	Tablets: 18.75 mg, 37.5 mg, 75 mg	18.75–112.5 mg	1
		Chewable Tablets: 37.5 mg		

availability of effective medications for treating associated OCD. Antidepressant medications that selectively inhibit serotonin reuptake (SSRIs) have shown the greatest clinical efficacy. Several controlled clinical trials have confirmed superior efficacy of SSRIs over other tricyclic antidepressants in patients with OCD. Clinical responses may be delayed by several weeks. Side effects of SSRI therapy tend to be less than those of traditional tricyclic antidepressants, and include sedation, nausea, dry mouth, dizziness, tremor, constipation, skin rash, increased appetite, weight gain and sexual dysfunction. As mentioned, the combined use of a SSRI and a neuroleptic can result in acute, severe, drug-induced parkinsonism.[65] A number of SSRIs are now available and are summarized in Table 248.2. Clinicians often select an SSRI medication based on its side-effect profile. Patients whose symptoms include insomnia or prominent anxiety often respond best to a more sedating drug, such as paroxetine (Paxil; 10–60 mg/day), fluvoxamine (Luvox; 25–300 mg/day), or clomipramine (Anafranil; 25–250 mg/day) given at bedtime. For those patients who are withdrawn, morning dosing of a more activating agent such as fluoxetine (Prozac; 10–60 mg/day) is often helpful. Sertraline (Zoloft; 25–200 mg/day) and citalopram (Celexa; 10–40 mg/day) are more intermediate on the sedation-activation spectrum. If one SSRI drug is not tolerated or is ineffective, others can be tried serially. Cognitive-behavioral therapy by a skilled clinician can also be of benefit for the symptoms of OCD.

Agents for attention deficit hyperactivity disorder

Drug therapy for ADHD should be integrated into a multifaceted treatment approach that includes educational accommodations and behavioral therapy. Alpha agonists are often used as first-line therapy for children with TS who have impaired school performance due to ADHD since these medications may also be useful in suppressing tics. If these drugs are insufficient, the use of stimulants can be considered. Prior recommendations to avoid stimulant drugs (particularly methylphenidate) in children with tics, because these drugs have been reported to exacerbate and even precipitate tics in some patients, are probably inaccurate.[50,66] Any worsening of tics is often mild, transient and tolerable when the medications are effective in alleviating the symptoms of ADHD. There have been rare reports of sudden death in children receiving both clonidine and a stimulant so ECG screening and monitoring should be considered if this treatment combination is employed.[67–70] Available stimulant medications are summarized in Table 248.3. Methylphenidate (Ritalin; 2.5–60 mg/day) is the most commonly used stimulant. New sustained-release preparations of the drug are now available and allow single morning dosing. Adderall (2.5–60 mg/day) is a racemic mixture of D-L amphetamine that can be prescribed in a single daily dose. Dextroamphetamine (2.5–40 mg/day) and the extended-release form of the drug (Dexedrine Spansules; 5–40 mg/day) can also be used, but are less commonly prescribed in the USA.

Pemoline (Cylert; 18.75–112.5 mg/day) has an intrinsically long duration of action, but the drug is usually avoided due to potential hepatic toxicity. The most common adverse effects of stimulant therapy include insomnia, nervousness, anorexia and headaches. For patients experiencing an unacceptable worsening of tics during stimulant therapy, a tic-suppressing drug can be added. The monoamine oxidase B inhibitor deprenyl, which is metabolized to amphetamine compounds, has been reported to improve ADHD in children with tics.[71]

Tricyclic antidepressants, such as desipramine (Norpramin; 25–100 mg/day) and nortriptyline (Pamelor; 10–50 mg/day), can be effective for ADHD in children with TS. Rare reports of sudden death in children treated with tricyclics have raised concerns about potential cardiotoxicity and the risks of this class of medications.[72,73] Electrocardiogram monitoring is recommended before and during treatment with tricyclic antidepressants.

Other associated behavioral disorders

Growing evidence supports the notion that in addition to OCD and ADHD, other behavioral disorders commonly accompany TS. For some patients, associated behavioral symptoms of anxiety, phobia, depression and conduct disorder may represent the primary complaints. It remains unclear whether this category of psychopathology is specific for TS or reflects the peculiar social and emotional difficulties associated with living with the illness. Disturbed interpersonal relationships with parents, siblings, peers, teachers and others may contribute to some of the observed problems. Supportive counseling or family therapy may be required. Pharmacotherapy directed at the specific behavioral target symptoms may be effective.

References

1. Gilles de la Tourette G (CG Goetz & HL Klawans [Trans.]). Étude sur une affection nerveuse caractérisée par de l'incoordination motrice accompagnée d'echolalie et de coprolalie [Study of a neurologic condition characterized by motor incoordination accompanied by echolalia and coprolalia]. In: Friedhoff AJ, Chase TN, eds. Advances in neurology. Vol 35. Gilles de la Tourette Syndrome. New York: Raven Press, 1982:1–16
2. Kurlan R. Tourette's syndrome: current concepts. Neurology 1989;39:1625–1630
3. Kurlan R, Behr J, Medved L, et al. Severity of Tourette's syndrome in one large kindred: implication for determination of disease prevalence rate. Arch Neurol 1987;44:268–269
4. Kurlan R. What is the spectrum of Tourette's syndrome? Curr Opinion Neurol Neurosurg 1988;1:294–298
5. Comings DE, Hines JA, Comings BG. An epidemiologic study of Tourette's syndrome in a single school district. J Clin Psychiatry 1990;51:463–469
6. Kurlan R, Whitmore D, Irvine C, et al. Tourette's syndrome in a special education population: a pilot study involving a single school district. Neurology 1994;44:699–702
7. Eapen V, Robertson MM, Zeitlin H, Kurlan R. Gilles de la Tourette's syndrome in special education schools: a United Kingdom study. J Neurol 1997;244:378–382
8. Kurlan R. Tourette syndrome in a special education population: hypothesis. Adv Neurol 1992;58:75–81
9. Sohar AH, Apter A, King RA, et al. Epidemiological studies. In: Leckman JF, Cohen DJ, eds. Tourette's syndrome: tics, obsessions, compulsions. New York: John Wiley and Sons, 1999:177–193
10. Pauls DL, Leckman JF. The inheritance of Gilles de la Tourette's syndrome and associated behaviors: evidence for autosomal dominant transmission. N Engl J Med 1986;315:993–997
11. Singer HS, Butler IJ, Tune LE, et al. Dopaminergic dysfunction in Tourette's syndrome. Ann Neurol 1982;12:361–366
12. Gilbert DL, Sethuraman G, Sine L, et al. Tourette's syndrome improvement with pergolide in a randomized, double-blind, crossover trial. Neurology 2000;54:1310–1315
13. Haber SN, Kowell NW, Vonsattel JP, et al. Gilles de la Tourette's syndrome: a postmortem neuropathological and immunohistochemical study. J Neurol Sci 1986;75:225–241
14. Gilman MA, Sandyk R. The endogenous opioid system in Gilles de la Tourette syndrome: a postmortem neuropathological and immunohistochemical study. Med Hypotheses 1986;19:371–378
15. Lichter D, Majumdar L, Kurlan R. Opiate withdrawal unmasks Tourette's syndrome. Clin Neuropharmacol 1988;11:559–564
16. Kurlan R, Majumdar L, Deeley C, et al. A controlled trial of propoxyphene and naltrexone in Tourette's syndrome. Ann Neurol 1991;30:19–23
17. Singer HS, Hahn I-H, Krowiak E, et al. Tourette's syndrome: a neurochemical analysis of postmortem cortical brain tissue. Ann Neurol 1990;27:443–446
18. Kurlan R. The pathogenesis of Tourette's syndrome: a possible role for hormonal and excitatory neurotransmitter influences in brain development. Arch Neurol 1992;49:874–876
19. Peterson BS, Leckman JF, Scahill L, et al. Steroid hormones and CNS sexual dismorphisms modulate symptom expression in Tourette's syndrome. Psychoneuroendocrinology 1992;17:553–563
20. Braun AR, Stoetter B, Randolph C, et al. The functional neuroanatomy of Tourette's syndrome. An FDG-PET study. Neuropsychopharmacology 1993;9:277–291
21. Peterson B, Riddle MA, Cohen DJ, et al. Reduced basal ganglia volume in Tourette's syndrome using three-dimensional reconstruction techniques from magnetic resonance images. Neurology 1993;43:941–949
22. Singer HS, Reiss AL, Brown JE, et al. Volumetric MRI changes in basal ganglia of children with Tourette's syndrome. Neurology 1993;43:950–956
23. Klieger P, Fett KA, Dimitsopulos T, Kurlan RM. Asymmetry of basal ganglia perfusion in Tourette's syndrome as shown by Tc-99m-HMPAO SPECT. J Nuclear Med 1997;38:188–191
24. Kurlan R. Tourette's syndrome and PANDAS: will the relationship bear out? Neurology 1998;50:1530–1534
25. Walkup JT, LaBuda MC, Singer HS, et al. Family study and segregation analysis of Tourette syndrome: evidence for a mixed model of inheritance. Am J Hum Genet 1996;59:684–693
26. Kurlan R, Eapen V, Stern J, Robertson MM. Bilineal transmission in Tourette's syndrome families. Neurology 1994;44:2336–2342
27. McMahon WA, van de Wetering BJM, Filloux F, et al.

Bilineal transmission and phenotypic variation of Tourette's disorder in a large pedigree. J Am Acad Child Adolesc Psychiatry 1996;35:672–680

28. Tourette Syndrome Classification Study Group. Definitions and classification of tic disorders. Arch Neurol 1993;50:1013–1016

29. Jankovic J, Stone L. Dystonic tics in patients with Tourette's syndrome. Mov Disord 1991;6:248–252

30. Kurlan R, Lichter D, Hewitt D. Sensory tics in Tourette's syndrome. Neurology 1989;39:731–734

31. Frankel M, Cummings JL, Robertson MM, et al. Obsessions and compulsions in Gilles de la Tourette's syndrome. Neurology 1986;36:378–382

32. Pauls DL, Towbin KE, Leckman JF, et al. Gilles de la Tourette's syndrome and obsessive-compulsive disorder: evidence supporting a genetic relationship. Arch Gen Psychiatry 1986;43:1180–1182

33. Comings DE, Comings BG. Tourette's syndrome and attention deficit disorder with hyperactivity: are they genetically related? J Am Acad Child Psychiatry 1984;23:138–146

34. Pauls DL, Leckman JF, Cohen DJ. Familial relationship between Gilles de la Tourette syndrome, attention deficit disorder, learning disabilities, speech disorders and stuttering. J Am Acad Child Adolesc Psychiatry 1993;32:1044–1050

35. Comings DE. A controlled study of Tourette syndrome. VII. Summary: a common genetic disorder causing disinhibition of the limbic system. Am J Hum Genet 1987;41:839–886

36. Kerbeshian J, Burd L, Klug MG. Comorbid Tourette's disorder and bipolar disorders: an etiologic-perspective. Am J Psychiatry 1995;152:1646–1651

37. Pauls DL Cohen DJ, Kidd KK, Leckman JF. Tourette syndrome and neuropsychiatric disorders: is there a genetic relationship? (letter). Am J Hum Genet 1988;43:206–209

38. Diagnostic and Statistical Manual of Mental Disorders. 4th ed. Washington: American Psychiatric Association, 1994

39. Kurlan R, Behr J, Medved L, Como P. Transient tic disorder and the clinical spectrum of Tourette's syndrome. Arch Neurol 1988;45:1200–1201

40. Kurlan R. Tourette's syndrome. In: Rakel RE, Bope ET, eds. Conn's current therapy. 53rd ed. Philadelphia: WB Saunders, 2001; pp. 931–935

41. Kurlan R, O'Brien C. Spontaneous movement disorders in psychiatric patients. In: Lange AE, Weiner WJ, eds. Drug-induced movement disorders. Mt. Kisco, NY: Futura, 1992:257–280

42. Jankovic J. Tics in other neurologic disorders. In: Kurlan R, ed. The Handbook of Tourette's syndrome and related tic and behavioral disorders. New York: Marcel Dekker, 1993:167–182

43. Fahn S. A case of post-traumatic tic syndrome. In: Friedhoff AJ, Chase TN, eds. Gilles de la Tourette Syndrome. New York: Raven, 1982:349–350

44. Sacks OW. Acquired Touretttism in adult life. In: Friedhoff AJ, Chase TN, eds. Gilles de la Tourette Syndrome. New York: Raven, 1982:89–92

45. Pulst SM, Walshe TM, Romero JA. Carbon monoxide poisoning with features of Gilles de la Tourette syndrome. Arch Neurol 1983;40:443–444

46. Klawans HL, Falk DK, Nausieda PA, Weiner WJ. Gilles de la Tourette's syndrome after long-term chlorpromazine therapy. Neurology 1978;28:1064–1068

47. Palumbo D, Maughan A, Kurlan R. Hypothesis III: Tourette syndrome is only one of several causes of a developmental basal ganglia syndrome. Neurology 1997;54:475–483

48. Leckman JF, Hardin MT, Riddle MA, et al. Clonidine treatment of Gilles de la Tourette syndrome. Arch Gen Psychiatry 1991;48:324–328

49. Singer HS, Brown J, Quaskey S, et al. The treatment of attention-deficit hyperactivity disorder in Tourette syndrome: a double-blind placebo-controlled study with clonidine and desipramine. Pediatrics 1995;95:74–81

50. The Tourette's Syndrome Study Group. Treatment of ADHD in children with tics. Neurology 2002;58:527–536

51. Chappell PB, Riddle MA, Scahill L, et al. Guanfacine treatment of comorbid attention-deficit hyperactivity disorder in Tourette's syndrome: preliminary clinical experience. J Am Acad Child Adolesc Psychiatry 1995;34:1140–1146

52. Hunt RD, Arnsten AFT, Asbell MD. An open trial of guanfacine in the treatment of attention deficit hyperactivity disorder. J Am Acad Child Adolesc Psychiatry 1995;34:50–54

53. Harrigan JP, Barnhill LJ. Guanfacine for treatment of attention-deficit hyperactivity disorder in boys. J Child Adolesc Psychopharm 1995;5:215–223

54. Kurlan R, Trinidad KS. The treatment of tics. In: Kurlan R, ed. The treatment of movement disorders. Philadelphia: Lippincott, 1995:365–3406

55. Worrell JA, Marken PA, Beckman SE, Ruehter VL. Atypical antipsychotic agents: a critical review. Amer J Health System Pharm 2000;57:238–255

56. Riddle MA, Hardie MT, Towbin KE, et al. Tardive dyskinesia following haloperidol treatment in Tourette's syndrome. Arch Gen Psychiatr 1987;44:98–99

57. Bruun RD, Budman CL. Risperidone as a treatment for Tourette's syndrome. J Clin Psychiatry 1996;57:29–31

58. Stamenkovic M, Schindler SD, Aschauer HN, et al. Effective open-label treatment of Tourette's disorder with olanzapine. Int Clin Psychopharm 2000;15:23–28

59. Sallee FR, Kurlan R, Goetz CG, et al. Ziprasidone treatment of children and adolescents with Tourette's syndrome: a pilot study. J Amer Acad Child Adolesc Psychiatr 2000;39:292–299

60. Jankovic J, Beach J. Long-term effects of tetrabenazine in hyperkinetic movement disorders. Neurology 1997;48:358–362

61. Merikangas JR, Merikangas KR, Kopp U, Hanin I. Blood choline and response to clonazepam and haloperidol in Tourette's syndrome. Acta Psychiatr Scand 1985;72:395–399

62. Gilbert DL, Sethuraman G, Sine L, et al. Tourette's syndrome improvement with pergolide in a randomized, double-blind crossover trial. Neurology 2000;54:1310–1315

63. Jankovic J. Botulinum toxin in the treatment of tics associated with Tourette's syndrome. Neurology 1993;43(Suppl 2):A310 (Abstract)

64. Scott BL, Jankovic J, Donovan DT. Botulinum toxin into vocal cord in the treatment of coprolalia associated with Tourette's syndrome. Mov Disord 1996;11:431–433

65. Kurlan R. Acute parkinsonism induced by the combination of a serotonin reuptake inhibitor and a neuroleptic in adults with Tourette's syndrome. Mov Disord 1998;13:178–179

66. Robertson MM, Eapen V. Pharmacologic controversy of CNS stimulants in Gilles de la Tourette syndrome. Clin Neuropharm 1992;15:408–425

67. Fenichel RR. Combining methylphenidate and cloni-

dine: the role of post-marketing surveillance. J Child Adolesc Psychopharm 1995;5:155–156

68. Popper, CW. Combining methylphenidate and clonidine: pharmacologic questions and news reports about sudden death. J Child Adolesc Psychopharm 1995;5: 157–166

69. Wilens TE, Spencer TJ. Combining methylphenidate and clonidine: a clinically sound medication option. J Am Acad Child Adolesc Psychiatry 1999;38:614–616

70. Swanson JM, Connor DF, Cantwell D. Ill-advised. J Am Acad Child Adolesc Psychiatry 1999;38:617–622

71. Feigin A, Kurlan R, McDermott MP, et al. A controlled trial of deprenyl in children with Tourette's syndrome and attention deficit hyperactivity disorder. Neurology 1996;46:965–968

72. Riddle MA, Nelson JC, Kleinman CS, Rasmusson A, Leckman JF, King RA, et al. Sudden death in children receiving Norpramin: a review of three reported cases and commentary. J Am Acad Child Adolesc Psychiatry 1991;30:104–108

73. Riddle MA, Geller B, Ryan N. Another sudden death in a child treated with desipramine. J Am Acad Child Adolesc Psychiatry 1993;32:792–797

249 Paroxysmal Dyskinesias

Stanley Fahn

Introduction

The most common paroxysmal neurological disorders are epilepsy and migraine. It is very unusual for a movement disorder to appear suddenly "out of the blue" and then disappear until the next attack. This chapter discusses a category of abnormal movements called the paroxysmal dyskinesias. These disorders usually produce sudden brief attacks of dystonia or choreoathetosis, often triggered by movement or excitement. The clinical features vary, and are the basis for the current nosology and classification of the paroxysmal dyskinesias. The pathophysiology of paroxysmal dyskinesias is not understood. The classification of the paroxysmal dyskinesias is incomplete and still evolving[1] as variants of the well-described syndromes come to light. After decades of attempts to understand these disorders using careful clinical observation, molecular biology has begun to shed new light on the classification of paroxysmal disorders,[2] and the mechanisms of disease.[3]

Historical aspects

Although Gowers[4] is often credited with the first report of movement-induced seizures, it is possible that his cases actually represented paroxysmal dyskinesia. One of his patients was a boy who experienced attacks during which he remained awake. Another patient was a girl whose attacks, beginning at the age of 11, occurred on suddenly arising after prolonged sitting. Subsequent to Gowers, a number of reports of "movement-induced seizures" appeared in the literature, many published under the designations of "reflex epilepsy" and "tonic seizures induced by movement." However, unlike most motor convulsions, there was no alteration in the state of consciousness. Moreover, some of these patients had more than tonic contraction, namely sustained twisting, athetosis and chorea. The presence of choreoathetosis led the earliest observers of these brief attacks to consider them as a form of epilepsy, originating in the basal ganglia or in the subcortical region. These disorders are today referred to as paroxysmal dystonia and paroxysmal choreoathetosis, rather than convulsive seizures.

There were many subsequent reports of paroxysmal dystonia.[5–8] The concept that attacks of tonic spasms and choreoathetotic movements could represent a paroxysmal type of movement disorder, and not a form of subcortical epilepsy, is attributed to Mount and Reback. They described a family in which 27 members were affected by attacks of dystonic posturing and athetosis, lasting 5 to 10 minutes. The dis-

order was inherited in an apparently autosomal dominant pattern. Mount and Reback called this disorder "familial paroxysmal choreoathetosis."

In 1967 Kertesz[9] introduced the label "paroxysmal kinesigenic choreoathetosis" (PKC), underscoring the observation that many attacks are triggered by movement. Demirkiran and Jankovic[1] recommended that the term "paroxysmal kinesigenic dyskinesia" (PKD) replace PKC because the movements can be other than choreoathetotic. In addition to movement-triggered episodes, patients with non-kinesigenic paroxysmal dyskinesias have also been described,[10] initially termed "paroxysmal dystonic choreoathetosis" (PDC) but now referred to as paroxysmal non-kinesigenic dyskinesia (PNKD).

Classification of the paroxysmal dyskinesias

The phenomenology of the paroxysmal dyskinesias comprises a wide range of hyperkinetic movements, from the brief, random, jerky movements of chorea to the sustained contractions of dystonia. Paroxysmal dyskinesias can be primary idiopathic disorders, some of which have been linked to a specific genetic defect, or they may represent the result of a known insult to the nervous system. A brief summary of the major types is provided in Table 249.1.

Paroxysmal kinesigenic dyskinesia (PKD)
General clinical features

The attacks of PKD consist of any combination of dystonic postures, chorea, athetosis, and ballism. They can be unilateral—always on one side or on either side—or bilateral. Unilateral episodes can be followed by a bilateral one. The attacks are brief, usually lasting only seconds, but rarely can last up to 5 minutes. They are precipitated by a sudden movement or a startle, usually after the patient has been sitting quietly for some time. The attacks can be severe enough to cause a patient to fall down, and there can be as many as 100 per day. After an attack, there is usually a short refractory period before another attack can take place. Speech can sometimes be affected, with inability to speak due to dystonia, but there is never any alteration of consciousness. The attacks can sometimes be aborted if the patient stops moving or warms up slowly. Very often patients report variable sensations at the beginning of the paroxysms. These can consist of paresthesias, a feeling of stiffness, crawling sensations, or a tense feeling.

Equivalent to PKD are equally brief attacks that are *not* precipitated by sudden movement or startle. Because the duration and therapeutic response is the

Table 249.1   Major types of paroxysmal dyskinesias

1. *Paroxysmal kinesigenic dyskinesia (PKD)*
   Duration   Seconds to 5 minutes
   Precipitant   Sudden movement
                     Startle
                     Hyperventilation
   Treatment   Sensitive to anticonvulsants
   Etiology   Primary—familial, sporadic
                     Secondary
   Genetics   Syndrome of infantile convulsions
                     and PKD has been mapped to
                     chromosome 16p11.2-q12.1
                     Syndrome of PKD without infantile
                     convulsions has been mapped to
                     chromosome 16q13-q22.1

2. *Paroxysmal non-kinesigenic dyskinesia (PNKD)*
   (Mount–Reback type)
   Duration   2 minutes to 4 hours
   Precipitant   None
   Aggravating   Alcohol, caffeine, and fatigue
     factors   Not sensitive to anticonvulsants
   Treatment   Primary—familial, sporadic
   Etiology   Secondary
                     Alternating hemiplegia of childhood
                     Psychogenic
   Genetics of three FDP1 (familial paroxysmal
     familial types   dyskinesia type 1) on 2q34
                     CSE (choreoathetosis/spasticity
                     episodic) on 1p
                     Familial infantile convulsions on
                     chromosome 16

3. *Paroxysmal exertional dyskinesia (PED)*
   Duration   5 to 30 minutes
   Precipitant   Continued exertion
   Etiology   Idiopathic—familial, sporadic
                     Symptomatic
                     Psychogenic
   Genetics   PED and autosomal recessive
                     rolandic epilepsy, chromosome
                     16p12-11.2

4. *Paroxysmal hypnogenic dyskinesia*
   Duration   a. Brief attacks (many are due to
                        supplementary/frontal lobe
                        seizures)
                     b. Prolonged attacks
   Genetics   Chromosome 20q13.2
                     Chromosome 15q24
                     Chromosome 1

5. *Benign dyskinesias in infancy and childhood*
   a. Paroxysmal dystonia/torticollis in infancy
   b. Paroxysmal tonic upgaze or downgaze
   c. Paroxysmal myoclonus of infancy
   d. Shuddering attacks
   e. Spasmus nutans
   f. Sandifer's syndrome
   g. Sterotypies

6. *Paroxysmal dyskinesias and epilepsy*
   a. Hypnogenic paroxysmal dyskinesias as frontal
      lobe epilepsy (see above)
   b. Infantile convulsions and paroxysmal dyskinesias on
      chromosome 16p12-q12

7. *Paroxysmal ataxia and tremor*
   a. EA-1 With myokymia/neuromyotonia
      Attacks   Ataxia and dysarthria
      Duration   Brief; <2 min
      Precipitant   Sudden movement or startle
      Treatment   Sometimes sensitive to
                      acetazolamide and to
                      anticonvulsants
      Interictal   Persistent myokymia/
                      neuromyotonia
      Other features May be accompanied by PKD
      Genetics   Point mutations on chromosome
                      12p13, involving the ion gated
                      potassium channel

   b. EA-2 With nystagmus
      Attacks   Ataxia and dysarthria
      Duration   Hours
      Precipitant   Exercise, fatigue, stress, alcohol
      Treatment   Sensitive to acetazolamide
      Interictal   Nystagmus
      Other features Headache, malaise, may develop
                      persistent ataxia
      Genetics   Mapped to chromosome 19p

   c. With ocular motility dysfunction
      Attacks   Ataxia, diplopia, oscillopsia, vertigo,
                      nausea, tinnitus
      Duration   Minutes to hours
      Precipitants   Sudden change in head position,
                      fatigue, and an environment
                      where objects are moving past
                      the patient
      Treatment   Lying quietly with eyes closed for 15
                      to 30 minutes; no response to
                      acetazolamide
      Other features The episodes become more
                      frequent and then become
                      constant with progressive ataxia
      Genetics   Genetically distinct from other
                      episodic ataxias

same as for PKD, these are listed under the PKD rubric, rather than developing an entirely new category. Often these attacks, lasting only a few seconds, can be triggered by hyperventilation.

Primary paroxysmal kinesigenic dyskinesia

The etiology of most case reports of PKD has been idiopathic and predominantly hereditary, with inheritance being autosomal dominant. For some unexplained reason, males are more often affected than females by a ratio of 3.75:1 (75 males and 20 females reported in Fahn[11]). A large series of 150 cases was reported from a questionnaire in Japan. This gender imbalance was supported by the additional 26 cases reported by Houser et al.,[12] consisting of 23 men and 3 women, and another 150 cases from Japan.[13] Adding all these cases together brings the total to 218 men and 53 women, or a ratio of 4.1:1. Age at onset shows a wide range, usually starting in childhood between the ages of 6 and 16, but can range from 6 months to 40 years. Excluding the cases by Nagamitsu et al.,[13] the mean age at onset is 12 and the median, 12. Familial cases may be more common among the Japanese[14–16] and Chinese.[17] The survey reported by Nagamitsu et al.[13] found 53 sporadic cases and 97 familial ones.

There is one report of PKD developing in a patient who had essential tremor.[18] EEGs are generally normal, and CT scans are also normal[19–23] with a few exceptions, such as the case reported by Watson and Scott[24] with suggested brainstem atrophy, and the one by Gilroy[25] with an ill-defined unilateral hemispheric lesion. However, Hirata et al.[26] demonstrated an abnormal EEG with rhythmic 5-Hz discharges over the entire scalp during episodes of PKD, raising the possibility that the PKD may have an epileptogenic basis. A patient was reported who developed PKD shortly after initiation of therapy with methylphenidate for attention deficit hyperactivity disorder. Attacks persisted long after methylphenidate was discontinued, and responded to treatment with carbamazepine.[27] The authors believe that the patient had a hereditary susceptibility for PKD that was triggered by the drug.

The attacks tend to diminish with age. Fortunately, PKD responds dramatically to anticonvulsants, and the early literature indicates that phenytoin was the most popular, followed by phenobarbital and primidone. Recently, carbamazepine appears to be the drug most commonly used. Valproate has also been effective,[21] although Hwang et al.[28] report that both carbamazepine and phenytoin were superior to valproate. Other anticonvulsants are also effective, including oxcarbazepine[29] and lamotrigine.[30–31] There is one report of response to levodopa,[32] but another of lack of effect by this drug.[33] Analogously, there is one report of three patients with PKD worsening with haloperidol,[34] but Garello et al.[33] reported no effect from this drug (as well as levodopa) in two brothers. The calcium channel blocker, flunarizine, which is also a neuroleptic, was effective in a 7-year-old girl who did not respond to carbamazepine or methylphenidate.[23]

The pathophysiology of PKD is still unclear, and its relationship to epilepsy remains speculative. That movement-induced seizures can occur[35] and because PKD responds dramatically to anticonvulsants are not sufficient reasons to consider PKD a form of epilepsy. The retention of consciousness and lack of postictal phenomena, as well as the presence of dystonia and choreoathetosis, should be sufficient to disqualify PKD from the epilepsies.

The differential diagnosis of PKD is focal epilepsy, tetany, hyperekplexia, tics, stereotypies and hysteria, as noted in the misdiagnosis of the case reported by Waller.[36] The clinical features are so distinctive, particularly if triggered by sudden movement, that there is little likelihood of not diagnosing the condition correctly once aware of its existence. Similarly, the remarkable response to anticonvulsants sets PKD apart from the other disorders. There is one case of primary PKD that has been observed to be the result of a consistent ictal discharge arising focally from the supplementary sensorimotor cortex, with a concomitant discharge recorded from the ipsilateral caudate nucleus without spread to other neocortical areas,[37] which suggests that some primary PKDs could be epileptic in origin. The non-kinesigenic, brief attacks of hemidystonia, often precipitated by hyperventilation, and controlled with anticonvulsants, has been considered a sign of epilepsy.[38,39] Hence each case of such suspected non-kinesigenic paroxysmal dyskinesia needs to be evaluated for a convulsive disorder.

There have been reports of two autopsies in PKD. Case 4 of Kertesz[9] died, apparently by suicide, and a postmortem examination revealed no clear-cut abnormality in the brain, just the presence of some melanin pigment in macrophages in the locus ceruleus. Stevens[40] had earlier reported the postmortem findings of one of his patients, which was also essentially normal, showing only a slight asymmetry of the substantia nigra.

Three independent laboratories have mapped autosomal dominant disorder PKD with infantile convulsions to chromosome 16p11.2-q12.1.[41–43] A second locus on this chromosome at 16q13-q22.1 has been found in other families, referring the gene as EKD2.[44] This locus does not overlap with the other families. This family is distinct from the others by not having infantile convulsions.

Secondary paroxysmal kinesigenic dyskinesia

The overwhelming majority of reported cases of PKD are idiopathic or familial in etiology. Although not reported as often, symptomatic PKD is probably more common. Table 249.2 lists the most common causes of symptomatic PKD.

In symptomatic PKD, like primary PKD, attacks lasting seconds are sometimes induced by hyperventilation. These also usually respond to anticonvulsants, such as carbamazepine, and are also seen in multiple sclerosis.[45,46] The author has also encountered a patient with attacks lasting seconds, induced by hyperventilation and not sudden movement, and following a mild cerebral ischemic episode, that also

Table 249.2 Common causes of symptomatic paroxysmal kinesigenic dyskinesia

Multiple sclerosis
Head injury
Perinatal hypoxic encephalopathy
Idiopathic hypoparathyroidism
Basal ganglia calcifications
Hemiatrophy
Putaminal infarct
Thalamic infarct
Medullary lesion (hemorrhage, subarachnoid cyst)
HIV infection
Hyperglycemia in the presence of a lenticular vascular malformation
Progressive supranuclear palsy
Spinal cord lesion
Huntington's disease

responded to carbamazepine. These pharmacological responses suggest that the brevity of the attack is a more important element than is sudden movement to distinguish the classification of the paroxysmal dyskinesias. Sethi et al.[46] reported success in treating three patients with paroxysmal dystonia (not induced by movement but triggered by hyperventilation and lasting many seconds) with acetazolamide, with or without a combination of carbamazepine.

Multiple sclerosis Although most of the paroxysmal dyskinesias associated with multiple sclerosis are not triggered by sudden movement, an occasional patient with multiple sclerosis will manifest typical PKD.[47] In fact, the presenting symptom of multiple sclerosis can be paroxysmal kinesigenic dyskinesias, as in the case reported by Roos et al.[48] These attacks were associated with a lesion in the caudate nucleus and responded to phenytoin. Three of the eight patients reported by Berger et al.[49] with paroxysmal dyskinesia associated with multiple sclerosis had the attacks induced by sudden movement; they were relieved with anticonvulsants. The case of PKD with multiple sclerosis reported by Burguera et al.[50] had a lesion in the left thalamus demonstrated by MRI. The PKD was the presenting symptom, as in other cases of demyelinating disease. Medullary lesions in multiple sclerosis and bilateral paroxysmal dystonia were reported by Gatto et al.[51]

Head trauma Case 3 of Whitty et al.[7] was a 13-year-old boy with onset 9 months after mild head trauma. Robin[52] reported a 33-year-old man with severe head injury who developed PKD 8 months later. Two of the three cases of post-traumatic paroxysmal dyskinesias reported by Drake et al.[53] had the movements induced by sudden movement of the affected body part. Another post-traumatic case was reported by Richardson et al.[54] These post-traumatic cases of PKD responded to anticonvulsants, similar to idiopathic PKD. Attacks of dystonia lasting several seconds and induced by tactile stimulation were reported secondary to a head injury; they disappeared within 2

months without treatment.[55] Another case of tactile-induced dyskinesias was reported by Nijssen and Tijssen[56] as a result of a thalamic infarct.

Perinatal hypoxic encephalopathy Rosen,[53] in 1964, appears to have been the first to report a case of PKD associated with perinatal hypoxic encephalopathy, with the onset beginning at age 12. This boy's attacks were usually triggered by a combination of startle and body contact. Mushet and Dreifuss[58] described a 9-year-old boy who developed brief attacks of athetosis and dystonia. They usually occurred when he was startled, but could also occur following sudden movement. At age 6 months he had a febrile illness, retrospectively thought to be encephalitis. He had considerable motor regression and was not able to walk; nor did he gain syntactical speech. His dyskinetic attacks were not suppressed by anticonvulsants, but did respond to anticholinergics.

Basal ganglia calcifications PKD has been reported to occur with basal ganglia calcifications with or without hypoparathyroidism.[59] Subsequent cases of hypoparathyroidism were also reported.[60,61] The clinical syndrome resembles that of primary infantile convulsions and childhood PKD.[62] Calciferol was effective in controlling these attacks. The case reported by Soffer et al.[63] was not noted to have the attacks induced by sudden movement, but the briefness of the attack resembles PKD.

Hemiatrophy Case 2 of the five cases described by Kinast et al.[19] had attacks of left hemidystonia lasting 1 minute and occurring up to 50 times a day. The major precipitating factor was not sudden movement, but stress and the anticipation of movement (also reported in one patient by Franssen et al.[64] Technically, like Case 4 described above, this patient did not fulfill the criterion of attacks induced by sudden movement. Examination revealed left-sided hemiatrophy and hyperreflexia, with a normal CT scan. Because the hemiatrophy syndrome can be associated with a delayed onset movement disorder,[65] it seems reasonable to consider it an etiological factor in this particular case.

Gilroy[25] reported a 32-year-old man with an abnormal right hemisphere on CT scan who had suffered multiple daily brief attacks of left hemidystonia since the age of 5 that were typical of PKD. The speculation is that the PKD was secondary to pathology in the involved hemisphere, but an arteriogram and cortical biopsy did not shed further light on the pathology.

Cerebral infarcts and hemorrhages With the advent of magnetic resonance imaging, more cases of PKD have been reported as a result of cerebral infarcts—with putaminal infarct,[66] thalamic infarct,[56,67,68] an infarct probably in the cortex,[69] and medullary hemorrhage.[70] As mentioned above, the case of Nijssen and Tijssen[56] had attacks stimulated by touching the affected limb. The attacks secondary to infarcts,[66,69] or to multiple sclerosis[46] can be painful tonic spasms.

Riley[71] reported a case of paroxysmal attacks of tightening of the throat muscles and elevation of the tongue to the roof of the mouth associated with a remote hemorrhage in the medulla.

Other etiologies PKD has also been reported to occur in a patient with progressive supranuclear palsy,[72] hyperglycemia in the presence of a lenticular vascular malformation,[73] and a spinal cord lesion.[74] A case of PKD was reported in which it was the first symptom in a patient who developed Huntington's disease.[75] HIV infection has now been reported to be associated with PKD and PKND.[76] A lesion in the medulla has been associated with PKD.[77]

Paroxysmal non-kinesigenic dyskinesia (PNKD)

General clinical features

Like PKD, the attacks of PNKD consist of any combination of dystonic postures, chorea, athetosis, and ballism. They can be unilateral (always on one side or on either side) or bilateral, and unilateral episodes can be followed by a bilateral one. They can affect a single region of the body or be generalized. Involvement of the neck can be a combination of torticollis and head tremor.[78] The major distinctions from PKD are the longer duration of each attack, the reduced frequency of the attacks, and a host of different aggravating factors. The attacks last minutes to hours, sometimes longer than a day, but usually they range from 5 minutes to 4 hours. They are primed by consuming alcohol, coffee, or tea, and also by psychological stress, excitement and fatigue. There are usually no more than three attacks per day, and often attacks may be months apart. The attacks can be severe enough to cause a patient to fall down. Speech is often affected, with inability to speak due to dystonia, but there is never any alteration of consciousness. The attacks can sometimes be aborted if the patient goes to sleep. As with PKD, very often patients report variable sensations at the beginning of the paroxysms. These can consist of paresthesias, a feeling of stiffness, crawling sensations, or a tense feeling.

A form of paroxysmal non-kinesigenic dyskinesia, known as intermediate-PDC, and more recently as paroxysmal exertional dyskinesia, is triggered only by prolonged exercise and not by other precipitants. This was first described by Lance in 1977[79] and was subsequently reported in another family by Plant et al.[80] and in a sporadic case by Nardocci et al.[81] This form is discussed separately. Under the classification scheme of Demirkiran and Jankovic,[1] this form is called paroxysmal exertional dyskinesia (PED).

Primary paroxysmal non-kinesigenic dyskinesia (Mount–Reback syndrome)

The initial reports of PNKD were familial,[34,79,82–91] with hereditary transmission being autosomal dominant. In 1980 Kinast et al.[19] (Case 4) and in 1981 Dunn[92] each described a child with PNKD without a positive family history. Since then Bressman et al.[93] have described seven sporadic cases of PNKD, and recently Nardocci et al.[81] added another one. The familial cases of idiopathic PNKD still greatly outnumber sporadic cases according to the reports in the literature. However, the sporadic cases are much more difficult to diagnose, and there is the need to differentiate a psychogenic etiology.[93,94] Based on the experience of Bressman and her colleagues,[93] the sporadic form may actually be more common than the familial form but is just rarely reported.

Males are slightly more often affected than females by a ratio of 1.4 : 1 (32 males and 23 females reported in the reviewed English literature).[11] Age at onset shows a wide range, usually in childhood between the ages of 6 and 16, but can range from 2 months to 30 years. The mean age at onset is 12 and the median 12. CT scans are normal.[88,91]

The EEGs are generally normal, but the case of Jacome and Risko[91] is of interest. The patient had unilateral PNKD and normal interictal EEGs. Photic stimulation at low frequencies induced paroxysmal lateralized epileptiform discharges from the contralateral hemisphere, and from this it was suggested that the disorder may have some epileptogenic basis.

Sleep aborted the episodes in one family that had myokymia in addition to the PNKD.[95] The presence of myokymia links this particular family to several with paroxysmal ataxia, in which myokymia is a feature.[96,97]

A family reported by Kurlan et al.[98] had some atypical features for classical PNKD. The long duration attacks were painful dystonic spasms that were not precipitated by alcohol, caffeine or excitement, but could follow exposure to cold or heat or result from exertional cramping. Other members of the family had only exertional cramping without PNKD. The authors suggested that exertional cramping may be a *forme fruste* of PNKD. It is also possible that the PNKD in this family may fall into the category of the intermediate form of paroxysmal dyskinesia that was reported by Lance[79] and Plant et al.[80] Also unusual was the presence of some fixed dystonia, which had not been reported previously. Bressman et al.[93] also described some sporadic cases of PNKD who had some interictal dystonia.

Lance[79] mentioned that autopsies performed on two patients with PNKD revealed no pathology. His Case II.4 had normal macroscopic findings, while Case IV.2 died of crib death and both macroscopic and microscopic findings were normal.

The attacks may diminish spontaneously with age.[19,79,93] Unfortunately, most patients have persistence of their attacks and they are difficult to treat. As a general rule, PNKD does not respond to the same type of anticonvulsants that so effectively treat PKD. An occasional patient will respond to such agents as carbamazepine, valproate and gabapentin.[99] Clonazepam, as introduced for PNKD by Lance,[79] appears to be the most successful agent, both for primary PNKD and symptomatic PNKD. A number of other drugs have been tried, sometimes with success. These include antimuscarinics,[82] chlordiazepoxide,[90,100] acetazolamide,[88,93] oxazepam and other benzodi-azepines,[98,101] and L-tryptophan.[98]

Kurlan and Shoulson[101] treated one patient with familial PNKD on alternate-day oxazepam. He had marked benefit from diazepam, but only for 4 weeks. Clonazepam and oxazepam gave relief for 2 to 3 weeks each. Eventually he was placed on a regimen of 40 mg oxazepam given on alternate days, the concept being that the benzodiazepine receptors became desensitized on daily doses. Alternate-day administration prevented this desensitization.

Trials of the dopamine receptor antagonist, haloperidol, were carried out by Przuntek and Monninger[34] and Coulter and Donofrio[102] with benefit. Przuntek and Monninger found that levodopa worsened one patient.

In contrast to idiopathic PKD, which is so distinctive, the major difficulty in the diagnosis of sporadic PNKD is to differentiate it from a psychogenic movement disorder, particularly in sporadic cases. The problem is that the disappearance of the movements with placebo or psychotherapy could be coincidental, since the attacks disappear spontaneously. However, if the paroxysms are frequent and the attacks are prolonged, then repeated trials with placebo can be informative. If such trials consistently produce remissions, then the diagnosis is clearly a psychogenic disorder.

Three different genetic mappings have been made for PNKD. The first type, originally described by Mount and Reback,[82] is referred to genetically as familial paroxysmal dyskinesia type 1 (FDP1), which was mapped to 2q33-35.[103–106] One of these families[34,105] shows a fair response to diazepam. The second type of PNKD has additional clinical features, including perioral paresthesiae, double vision and headache during attacks, and some also have a constant spastic paraparesis; this type was mapped to chromosome 1p[107] and has been called choreoathetosis/spasticity episodic (CSE). The third type of PNKD has been seen in familial infantile convulsions in which the gene has been mapped to chromosome 16.[108]

Secondary paroxysmal non-kinesigenic dyskinesia

The overwhelming majority of reported cases of PNKD are idiopathic or familial in etiology, but a number of cases of symptomatic PNKD have been reported. Table 249.3 lists the most common causes of symptomatic PKD.

The most common cause of symptomatic PNKD, as with PKD, is multiple sclerosis.[45–47,49,84,109] In multiple sclerosis, the paroxysmal movements may only be ocular, lasting several minutes.[110]

The next two most common causes are perinatal encephalopathy[84,93,111] and psychogenic.[93,94,112] A longer discourse of psychogenic PNKD is presented in the syllabus on psychogenic movement disorders.

Other causes of PNKD are encephalitis,[58,93] cystinuria,[113] hypoparathyroidism,[63,114,115] basal ganglia calcifications without altered serum calcium,[116] thyrotoxicosis,[117] transient ischemic attacks,[118,119] infantile hemiplegia,[120] head trauma,[53,121] hypoglycemia,[122–124] AIDS,[125] diabetes,[126] anoxia,[93] brain

Table 249.3   Common causes of symptomatic paroxysmal non-kinesigenic dyskinesia

Multiple sclerosis
Perinatal hypoxic encephalopathy
Psychogenic
Encephalitis
Idiopathic hypoparathyroidism
Basal ganglia calcifications
Thyrotoxicosis
TIA
Infantile hemiplegia
Cystinuria
Head injury
Hypoglycemia
AIDS
Diabetes
Anoxia
Brain tumor
Tardive syndrome?
Alternating hemiplegia of childhood

tumor,[93] and hypoglycemia induced by an insulinoma.[127] The patient with AIDS[125] had two attacks of dystonia, but details are lacking in regard to duration or characteristics of the attacks. PNKD caused by endocrine disorders responds to appropriate treatment, but in general, treatment of symptomatic PNKD is not often effective.

The syndrome commonly known as "alternating hemiplegia of childhood" typically contains periods of prolonged dystonic attacks, along with other elements of the syndrome.[128] The syndrome begins before 18 months of age. In addition to prolonged periods of dystonia, there are attacks of nystagmus, dyspnea and autonomic phenomena. Episodes of quadriplegia appear either when a hemiplegia shifts from one side to the other or as an isolated manifestation. The episodes are often followed by developmental deterioration. Eventually there is cognitive impairment and a choreoathetotic movement disorder. Sleep relieves the weakness and other paroxysmal phenomena, but they can reappear after awakening. The attacks can last from a few minutes to several days. Flunarizine is partially effective. Some infants manifest paroxysmal dystonia before the classical features of alternating hemiplegia develop.[129] Magnetic resonance spectroscopy was normal in the case of Nezu et al.[130]

Paroxysmal exertional dyskinesia (PED)

Lance[79] was the first to describe what he called an intermediate form of PDC (now called PNKD). Today, this family would appear to have PED. The family had attacks that were briefer than classical PNKD, lasting from 5 to 30 minutes, and which were precipitated by prolonged exercise and not by cold, heat, stress, ethanol, excitement or anxiety. The spasms affected mainly the legs. A second family was reported by Plant et al.[80] In both families the inheritance pattern was that of autosomal dominant transmission, and in neither family did anyone derive any

Table 249.4 Clinical features of paroxysmal kinesigenic (PKD), non-kinesigenic (PNKD), and exertional dyskinesia (PED)

Feature	PKD	PNKD	PED
Male : female	4 : 1	1.4 : 1	13 : 13 ($n = 26$)
Inheritance	AD	AD	AD
Genetic mapping	16p11.2-q12.1	1) Mount–Reback syndrome 2q34 (FDP1)	With autosomal recessive rolandic epilepsy; 16p12-11.2
	16q13-q22.1	2) With diplopia and spasticity (CSE); chromosome 1p	
		3) With familial infantile convulsions; chromosome 16	
Age at onset:			
range	<1–40	<1–30	2–30
median	12	12	11.5
mean	12	12	12
Attacks:			
duration	<5 min	2 min–4 h	5 min–2 hr
frequency	100/d–1/month	3/d-2/year	1/d–2/month
Trigger	Sudden movement, startle, hyperventilation	Nil	Prolonged exercise
Precipitant	Stress	ETOH, stress, caffeine, fatigue	Stress
Movement pattern	Any combination of dystonic postures, chorea, athetosis, and ballism; unilateral or bilateral		
Treatment	Anticonvulsants	Clonazepam, benzodiazepines, acetazolamide, antimuscarinics	Acetazolamide, antimuscarinics, benzodiazepines

benefit from barbiturate, levodopa, or clonazepam. A sporadic case was reported by Nardocci et al.[81] (Case 3). This patient also had interictal chorea without any family history of a similar condition, and was helped by clonazepam. Another sporadic case was reported by Wali;[131] this was an 18-year-old man in whom attacks of right hemidystonia lasting about 10 minutes were precipitated by prolonged running (about 10 minutes) or by cold. The EEG and CT scan were normal, and anticonvulsants were not helpful. Demirkiran and Jankovic[1] mentioned seeing five patients, three being females. The largest series of sporadic cases is that by Bhatia et al.[132] Familial cases appear to be autosomal dominant.[133] A large family with PED with four affected members had an onset of 9–15 years and a male : female ratio of 3 : 1.[134]

Some patients labeled as PKD (e.g., cases 1 and 3 of Jung et al.[17] and PNKD (e.g. Kurlan et al.[98]) have attacks that occur after prolonged exercise. It is possible that such patients may have a variant of PNKD, or represent a combination of it and one of the other paroxysmal dyskinesias. However, if the attacks last only seconds and respond to anticonvulsants, they fit clinically with these features of PKD. The family reported by Schloesser et al.[135] supports the notion that PED is a variant of PNKD. The father of the proband was affected by exertional cramping, and two other men in the family had PED. Women in the family had more prolonged attacks, fitting PNKD.

Ictal and interictal cerebral perfusion SPECT studies have been conducted.[133] During the motor attacks, decreased perfusion of the frontal cortex and increased cerebellar perfusion was observed. The perfusion of the basal ganglia also decreased. No cortical hyperperfusion indicative of an epileptic nature was seen. The authors conclude that PED represents a paroxysmal movement disorder rather than epilepsy. Posteroventral pallidotomy has been reported to ameliorate attacks of PED.[136]

A family with PED and autosomal recessive rolandic epilepsy has been described, with the gene mapped to chromosome 16p12-11.2.[137]

Table 249.4 lists the major distinguishing features of non-epileptic PKD, PNKD, and PED.

Molecular genetics of paroxysmal dyskinesias and ataxias

PKD with infantile convulsions has been mapped to 16p11.2-q12.1[41–43] PKD without convulsions has been mapped to 16q13-q22.1 with the gene referred to as EKD2.[44]

Two papers independently reported the mapping of a gene for PNKD to chromosome 2q31-36,[103,104] and the region has been narrowed to 2q33-q35 by Fink et al.[138] Another family was mapped by Raskind et al.[139] who narrowed the region to 2q34. A cluster of sodium channel genes are near the PNKD locus, but the mutated gene has not yet been identified. However, Jarman et al.[140] mapped the gene to a large British family and suggest that the leading candidate is the gene for the chloride/bicarbonate exchanger.

A family with PNKD with associated spasticity was studied by Auburger et al.;[107] their mutated gene was mapped to another potassium channel gene cluster on chromosome 1p. The attacks were said to consist of dystonia of limbs, imbalance, dysarthria, diplopia, and sometimes headache. The attacks lasted about 20 minutes and could be precipitated by exercise, stress, lack of sleep, and alcohol consumption. Some affected members had persistent spastic paraparesis, which would make this family different from classical Mount–Reback syndrome. This condition has been called choreoathetosis-spasticity episodica (CSE).

A family with infantile convulsions has an associated PNKD, and the abnormal gene has been mapped to chromosome 16.[108] Perhaps this disorder with its genetic mapping has been referred to by others as PKD with infantile convulsions.

A large Australian family with autosomal dominant hypnogenic frontal lobe seizures/dystonia has been found to have a missense mutation in the second transmembrane domain of the nicotinic acetylcholine receptor alpha 4 subunit (CHRNA4) gene, located on chromosome 20q13.2-13.3.[141] A second locus has been found on chromosome 15q24 and a third locus on chromosome 1 in a large Italian family.[142]

The genes for two of the hereditary episodic ataxias have been determined. In one of them, EA-1 (the type associated with myokymia or neuromyotonia) has been found to be due to point mutations in the gene Kv1.1 for the voltage gated potassium channel (KCNA1).[143,144] The gene is located on chromosome 12p13.[145] Different mutations have been found in different families.[146–148] The attacks are brief, lasting seconds to minutes, and myokymia is present during and between attacks. The attacks can be triggered by sudden movement,[2] and these can respond to anticonvulsants. Some families have episodes of myokymia without ataxia.[148]

Another episodic ataxia, EA-2, is the type that has a vestibular component, and doesn't have myokymia as an associated feature. The attacks last between 15 minutes to a few days and respond to acetazolamide. The gene was mapped to chromosome 19p13[149,150] and found to be mutations in the gene for the calcium channel CACNL1A4. Spontaneous mutations[151] as well as familial cases have been described. There is clinical heterogeneity, with attacks varying from pure ataxia to combinations of symptoms suggesting involvement of the cerebellum, brainstem, and cortex. Oculographic findings localized to the vestibulocerebellum and posterior vermis. Some affected individuals exhibited a progressive ataxia syndrome phenotypically indistinguishable from the dominantly inherited spinocerebellar ataxia (SCA) syndromes. SCA6 has been found to be due to an expanded CAG repeat on the same gene.[152] About one-half of the affected individuals have migraine headaches and several have episodes typical of basilar migraine.[153] Both familial hemiplegic migraine and EA-2 are caused by mutations in the Ca^{2+} channel gene CACNL1A4, and can be considered as allelic channelopathies.[154] When progressive ataxia is present, there is cerebellar atrophy on MRI scans, and not all cases have a CAG expansion.[155] On the other

Table 249.5   Clinical and genetic features of episodic ataxias

Type	Age at onset	Clinical	Acetazolamide response	Precipitant	Frequency/ duration	Interictal	Gene
Myokymia, neuro-myotonia (EA-1)	2–15	Aura of weightless or weak, then ataxia, dysarthria, tremor, facial twitching	In some kindreds; anticonvulsants may help	Startle, movement, exercise, excitement, fatigue	Up to 15 per day; usually one or less per day; seconds to minutes, usually 2–10 min	Myokymia, shortened Achilles tendon; PKD	12p13, K+ channel, different point mutations in KCNA1
Vestibular (EA-2)	0–40, usually 5–15	Ataxia, vertigo, nystagmus, dysarthria, HA, ptosis, hemiplegic ocular palsy, vermis atrophy	Very effective	Stress, alcohol, fatigue exercise, caffeine	Daily to q 2 months; usually hours; 5 min to weeks	Nystagmus, mild ataxia, less common: dysarthria and progr. cerebellar migraine	19p13, Ca+ channel CACNL1A4 familial
Ocular	20–50	Ataxia, diplopia, vertigo, nausea	No response	Sudden change in head position	Daily to yearly; minutes to hours	Symptoms gradually become constant	Unknown

hand, cases with the CAG expansion and cerebellar atrophy can also have EA-2.[156]

Not all families with migraine and episodic vertigo could be linked to the EA-2 markers on chromosome 19p, indicating genetic heterogeneity for this type of episodic ataxia.[157]

The third type of paroxysmal ataxia with ocular motility problems can be precipitated by sudden head movement. The gene for this third type of EA has not yet been mapped, but is genetically distinct from EA-1 and EA-2. Some of the features of all three types of episodic ataxias are presented in Table 249.5.

Summary

The paroxysmal dyskinesias are a group of disorders that can be divided into kinesigenic dyskinesias (which are induced by sudden movement and are brief in duration, lasting seconds to 5 minutes), the non-kinesigenic dyskinesias (which are not induced by sudden movement), and the exertional dyskinesias. The duration of PNKD is usually prolonged (duration 2 minutes to 4 hours, up to 2 days), and PED is intermediate in duration (duration 5 to 30 minutes). PNKD is often induced by alcohol, cold, heat, fatigue, caffeine, and stress.

As a general rule, the kinesigenic variety responds extremely well to anticonvulsants whereas these drugs are usually not beneficial in the other two types. PNKD is sometimes sensitive to clonazepam, benzodiazepines, acetazolamide, anticholinergics, and neuroleptics. Variants of these disorders are the paroxysmal dyskinesias that occur during sleep (hypnogenic paroxysmal dyskinesias, which may be a form of epilepsy) and the transient paroxysmal dystonias (particularly torticollis) in infants.

For all of these disorders, it seems plausible that the underlying defect is a genetically determined aberration in the function of a neuron ion channel. As more insight into the pathophysiology and pharmacology of these conditions is obtained, it is hoped that more specific and effective therapeutic approaches will become available.

References

1. Demirkiran M, Jankovic J. Paroxysmal dyskinesias: clinical features and classification. Ann Neurol 1995;38:571–579
2. Nutt JG, Gancher ST. A 10-year follow up—genotypic analysis disproves phenotypic classification. Mov Disord 1997;12:472
3. Griggs RC, Nutt JG. Episodic ataxias as channelopathies. Ann Neurol 1995;37:285–287
4. Gowers WR. Epilepsy and Other Chronic Convulsive Diseases. Their Causes, Symptoms and Treatment. New York: Dover (reprint of 1885 edition), 1964:75–76
5. Spiller WG. Subcortical epilepsy. Brain 1927;50:171–187
6. Wilson SAK. The Morrison Lectures on nervous semeiology, with special reference to epilepsy. Lecture III. Symptoms indicating increase of neural function. Br Med J 1930;2:90–94
7. Whitty CWM, Lishman WA, FitzGibbon JP. Seizures induced by movement: a form of reflex epilepsy. Lancet 1964;1:1403–1406
8. Burger LJ, Lopez RI, Elliott FA. Tonic seizures induced by movement. Neurology 1972;22:656–659
9. Kertesz A. Paroxysmal kinesigenic choreoathetosis. An entity within the paroxysmal choreoathetosis syndrome. Description of 10 cases, including 1 autopsied. Neurology 1967;17:680–690
10. Barnett, 1968.
11. Fahn S. The paroxysmal dyskinesias. In: Marsden CD, Fahn S, eds. Movement Disorders 3. Oxford: Butterworth-Heinemann, 1994:310–345
12. Houser MK, Soland VL, Bhatia KP, et al. Paroxysmal kinesigenic choreoathetosis: a report of 26 patients. J Neurol 1999;246:120–126
13. Nagamitsu S, Matsuishi T, Hashimoto K, et al. Multicenter study of paroxysmal dyskinesias in Japan—clinical and pedigree analysis. Mov Disord 1999;14:658–663
14. Kishimoto K. A novel case of conditionally responsive extrapyramidal syndrome. Ann Rep Res Inst Environ Med Nagoya Univ 1957;6:91–101
15. Fukuyama S, Okada R. Hereditary kinesthetic reflex epilepsy. Report of five families of peculiar seizures induced by sudden movements. Adv Neurol Sci (Tokyo) 1967;11:168–197
16. Kato M, Araki S. Paroxysmal kinesigenic choreoathetosis. Report of a case relieved by carbamazepine. Arch Neurol 1969;20:508–513
17. Jung S-S, Chen K-M, Brody JA. Paroxysmal choreoathetosis: report of Chinese cases. Neurology 1973;23:749–755
18. Nair KR, Bhaskaran R, Marsden CD. Essential tremor associated with paroxysmal kinesigenic dystonia. Mov Disord 1991;6:92–93
19. Kinast M, Erenberg G, Rothner AD. Paroxysmal choreoathetosis: report of five cases and review of the literature. Pediatrics 1980;65:74–77
20. Goodenough DJ, Fariello RG, Annis BL, Chun RW. Familial and acquired paroxysmal dyskinesias. A proposed classification with delineation of clinical features. Arch Neurol 1978;35:827–831
21. Suber DA, Riley TL. Valproic acid and normal computerized tomographic scan in kinesigenic familial paroxysmal choreoathetosis (letter). Arch Neurol 1980;37:327
22. Bortolotti P, Schoenhuber R. Paroxysmal kinesigenic choreoathetosis (letter). Arch Neurol 1983;40:529
23. Lou HC. Flunarizine in paroxysmal choreoathetosis. Neuropediatrics 1989;20:112
24. Watson RT, Scott WR. Paroxysmal kinesigenic choreoathetosis and brain-stem atrophy (letter). Arch Neurol 1979;36:522
25. Gilroy J. Abnormal computed tomograms in paroxysmal kinesigenic choreoathetosis. Arch Neurol 1982;39:779–780
26. Hirata K, Katayama S, Saito T, et al. Paroxysmal kinesigenic choreoathetosis with abnormal electroencephalogram during attacks. Epilepsia 1991;32:492–494
27. Gay CT, Ryan SG. Paroxysmal kinesigenic dystonia after methylphenidate administration. J Child Neurol 1994;9:45–46
28. Hwang WJ, Lu CS, Tsai JJ. Clinical manifestations of 20 Taiwanese patients with paroxysmal kinesigenic dyskinesia. Acta Neurol Scand 1998;98:340–345
29. Gokcay A, Gokcay F. Oxcarbazepine therapy in paroxysmal kinesigenic choreoathetosis. Acta Neurol Scand 2000;101:344–345

30. Pereira AC, Loo WJ, Bamford M, Wroe SJ. Use of lamotrigine to treat paroxysmal kinesigenic choreoathetosis. J Neurol Neurosurg Psychiat 2000;68:796–797

31. Uberall MA, Wenzel D. Effectiveness of lamotrigine in children with paroxysmal kinesigenic choreoathetosis. Develop Med Child Neurol 2000;42:699–700

32. Loong SC, Ong YY. Paroxysmal kinesigenic choreoathetosis: report of a case relieved by L-dopa. J Neurol Neurosurg Psychiatry 1973;36:921–924

33. Garello L, Ottonello GA, Regesta G, Tanganelli P. Familial paroxysmal kinesigenic choreoathetosis: report of a pharmacological trial in 2 cases. Eur Neurol 1983;22:217–221

34. Przuntek H, Monninger P. Therapeutic aspects of kinesigenic paroxysmal choreoathetosis and familial paroxysmal choreoathetosis of the Mount and Reback type. J Neurol 1983;230:163–169

35. Falconer M, Driver M, Serafetinides E. Seizures induced by movement: report of a case relieved by operation. J Neurol Neurosurg Psychiat 1963;26:300–307

36. Waller DA. Paroxysmal kinesigenic choreoathetosis or hysteria? Am J Psychiatry 1977;134:1439–1440

37. Lombroso CT. Paroxysmal choreoathetosis: an epileptic or non-epileptic disorder. Ital J Neurol Sci 1995;16:271–277

38. Kotagal P, Luders H, Morris HH, et al. Dystonic posturing in complex partial seizures of temporal lobe onset: A new lateralizing sign. Neurology 1989;39:196–201

39. Newton MR, Berkovic SF, Austin MC, et al. Dystonia, clinical lateralization, and regional blood flow changes in temporal lobe seizures. Neurology 1992;42:371–377

40. Stevens H. Paroxysmal choreo-athetosis. Arch Neurol 1966;14:415–420

41. Tomita H, Nagamitsu S, Wakui K, et al. Paroxysmal kinesigenic choreoathetosis locus maps to chromosome 16p11.2-q12.1. Am J Hum Genet 1999;65:1688–1697

42. Bennett LB, Roach ES, Bowcock AM. A locus for paroxysmal kinesigenic dyskinesia maps to human chromosome 16. Neurology 2000;54:125–130

43. Swoboda KJ, Soong BW, McKenna C, et al. Paroxysmal kinesigenic dyskinesia and infantile convulsions—Clinical and linkage studies. Neurology 2000;55:224–230

44. Valente EM, Spacey SD, Wali GM, et al. A second paroxysmal kinesigenic choreoathetosis locus (EKD2) mapping on 16q13-q22.1 indicates a family of genes which give rise to paroxysmal disorders on human chromosome 16. Brain 2000;123:2040–2045

45. Verheul GAM, Tyssen CC. Multiple sclerosis occurring with paroxysmal unilateral dystonia. Mov Disord 1990;5:352–353

46. Sethi KD, Hess DC, Huffnagle VH, Adams RJ. Acetazolamide treatment of paroxysmal dystonia in central demyelinating disease. Neurology 1992;42:919–921

47. Matthews WB. Tonic seizures in disseminated sclerosis. Brain 1958;81:193–206

48. Roos R, Wintzen AR, Vielvoye G, Polder TW. Paroxysmal kinesiogenic choreoathetosis as presenting symptom of multiple sclerosis. J Neurol Neurosurg Psychiatry 1991;54:657–658

49. Berger JR, Sheremata WA, Melamed E. Paroxysmal dystonia as the initial manifestation of multiple sclerosis. Arch Neurol 1984;41:747–750

50. Burguera JA, Catala J, Casanova B. Thalamic demyelination and paroxysmal dystonia in multiple sclerosis. Mov Disord 1991;6:379–381

51. Gatto EM, Zurru MC, Rugilo C. Medullary lesions and unusual bilateral paroxysmal dystonia in multiple sclerosis. Neurology 1996;46:847–848

52. Robin JJ. Paroxysmal choreoathetosis following head injury. Ann Neurol 1977;2:447–448

53. Drake ME Jr, Jackson RD, Miller CA. Paroxysmal choreoathetosis after head injury (letter). J Neurol Neurosurg Psychiatry 1986;49:837–843

54. Richardson JC, Howes JL, Celinski MJ, Allman RG. Kinesigenic choreoathetosis due to brain injury. Can J Neurol Sci 1987;14:626–628

55. George MS, Pickett JB, Kohli H, et al. Paroxysmal dystonic reflex choreoathetosis after minor closed head injury. Lancet 1990;336:1134–1135

56. Nijssen PCG, Tijssen CC. Stimulus-sensitive paroxysmal dyskinesias associated with a thalamic infarct. Mov Disord 1992;7:364–366

57. Rosen JA. Paroxysmal choreoathetosis associated with perinatal hypoxic encephalopathy. Arch Neurol 1964;11:385–387

58. Mushet GR, Dreifuss FE. Paroxysmal dyskinesia. A case responsive to benztropine mesylate. Arch Dis Child 1967;42:654–656

59. Arden F. Idiopathic hypoparathyroidism. Med J Aust 1953;2:217–219

60. Tabaee-Zadeh MJ, Frame B, Kapphahn K. Kinesiogenic choreoathetosis and idiopathic hypoparathyroidism. N Engl J Med 1972;286:762–763

61. Barabas G, Tucker SM. Idiopathic hypoparathyroidism and paroxysmal dystonic choreoathetosis (letter). Ann Neurol 1988;24:585

62. Hattori H, Yorifuji T. Infantile convulsions and paroxysmal kinesigenic choreoathetosis in a patient with idiopathic hypoparathyroidism. Brain Dev 2000;22:449–450

63. Soffer D, Licht A, Yaar I, Abramsky O. Paroxysmal choreoathetosis as a presenting symptom in idiopathic hypoparathyroidism. J Neurol Neurosurg Psychiatry 1977;40:692–694

64. Franssen H, Fortgens C, Wattendorff AR, van Woerkom TCAM. Paroxysmal kinesigenic choreoathetosis and abnormal contingent negative variation. A case report. Arch Neurol 1983;40:381–385

65. Buchman AS, Goetz CG, Klawans HL. Hemiparkinsonism with hemiatrophy. Neurology 1988;38:527–530

66. Merchut MP, Brumlik J. Painful tonic spasms caused by putaminal infarction. Stroke 1986;17:1319–1321

67. Camac A, Greene P, Khandji A. Paroxysmal kinesigenic dystonic choreoathetosis associated with a thalamic infarct. Mov Disord 1990;5:235–238

68. Milandre L, Brosset C, Gabriel B, Khalil R. Mouvements involontaires transitoires et infarctus thalamiques. [Transient dyskinesias associated with thalamic infarcts—report of five cases.] Rev Neurol 1993;149:402–406

69. Fuh JL, Chang DB, Wang SJ, et al. Painful tonic spasms: an interesting phenomenon in cerebral ischemia. Acta Neurol Scand 1991;84:534–536

70. LeDoux MS. Paroxysmal kinesigenic dystonia associated with a medullary hemorrhage. Mov Disord 1997;12:819

71. Riley DE. Paroxysmal kinesigenic dystonia associated with a medullary lesion. Mov Disord 1996;11:738–740

72. Adam AM, Orinda D. Focal paroxysmal kinesigenic choreoathetosis preceding the development of Steele-Richardson-Olszewski syndrome (letter). J Neurol Neurosurg Psychiatry 1986;49:957–968

73. Vincent FM. Hyperglycemia-induced hemichoreoathetosis: the presenting manifestation of a vascular malformation of the lenticular nucleus. Neurosurgery 1986;18:787–790

74. Cosentino C, Torres L, Flores M, Cuba JM. Paroxysmal kinesigenic dystonia and spinal cord lesion. Mov Disord 1996;11:453–455

75. Scheidtmann K, Schwarz J, Holinski E, et al. Paroxysmal choreoathetosis a disorder related to Huntington's disease? J Neurol 1997;244:395–398

76. Mirsattari SM, Berry MER, Holden JK, et al. Paroxysmal dyskinesias in patients with HIV infection. Neurology 1999;52:109–114

77. Jabbari B, Khajevi K, Rao K. Medullary dystonia. Mov Disord 1999;14:698–700

78. Hughes AJ, Lees AJ, Marsden CD. Paroxysmal dystonic head tremor. Mov Disord 1991;6:85–86

79. Lance JW. Familial paroxysmal dystonic choreoathetosis and its differentiation from related syndromes. Ann Neurol 1977;2:285–293

80. Plant GT, Williams AC, Earl CJ, Marsden CD. Familial paroxysmal dystonia induced by exercise. J Neurol Neurosurg Psychiatry 1984;47:275–279

81. Nardocci N, Lamperti E, Rumi V, Angelini L. Typical and atypical forms of paroxysmal choreoathetosis. Dev Med Child Neurol 1989;31:670–674

82. Mount LA, Reback S. Familial paroxysmal choreoathetosis. Arch Neurol Psychiat 1940;44:841–847

83. Forssman H. Hereditary disorder characterized by attacks of muscular contractions, induced by alcohol amongst other factors. Acta Med Scand 1961;170:517–533

84. Lance JW. Sporadic and familial varieties of tonic seizures. J Neurol Neurosurg Psychiat 1963;26:51–59

85. Weber MB. Familial paroxysmal dystonia. J Nerv Ment Dis 1967;145:221–226

86. Richards RN, Barnett HJ. Paroxysmal dystonic choreoathetosis. A family study and review of the literature. Neurology 1968;18:461–469

87. Horner FH, Jackson LC. Familial paroxysmal choreoathetosis. In: Barbeau A, Brunette J-R, eds. Progress in Neuro-Genetics. Amsterdam: Excerpta Medica Foundation, 1969:745–751

88. Mayeux R, Fahn S. Paroxysmal dystonic choreoathetosis in a patient with familial ataxia. Neurology 1982;32:1184–1186

89. Tibbles JA, Barnes SE. Paroxysmal dystonic choreoathetosis of Mount and Reback. Pediatrics 1980;65:149–151

90. Walker ES. Familial paroxysmal dystonic choreoathetosis: a neurologic disorder simulating psychiatric illness. Johns Hopkins Med J 1981;148:108–113

91. Jacome DE, Risko M. Photic induced-driven PLEDs in paroxysmal dystonic choreoathetosis. Clin Electroencephalogr 1984;15:151–154

92. Dunn DW. Paroxysmal dystonia. Am J Dis Child 1981;135:381–382

93. Bressman SB, Fahn S, Burke RE. Paroxysmal non-kinesigenic dystonia. Adv Neurol 1988;50:403–413

94. Fahn S, Williams DT. Psychogenic dystonia. Adv Neurol 1988;50:431–455

95. Byrne E, White O, Cook M. Familial dystonic choreoathetosis with myokymia; a sleep responsive disorder. J Neurol Neurosurg Psychiatry 1991;54:1090–1092

96. Van Dyke DH, Griggs RC, Murphy MJ, Goldstein MN. Hereditary myokymia and periodic ataxia. J Neurol Sci 1975;25:109–118

97. Vaamonde J, Artieda J, Obeso JA. Hereditary paroxysmal ataxia with neuromyotonia. Mov Disord 1991;6:180–182

98. Kurlan R, Behr J, Medved L, Shoulson I. Familial paroxysmal dystonic choreoathetosis: a family study. Mov Disord 1987;2:187–192

99. Chudnow RS, Mimbela RA, Owen DB, Roach ES. Gabapentin for familial paroxysmal dystonic choreoathetosis. Neurology 1997;49:1441–1442

100. Perez-Borja C, Tassinari AC, Swanson AG. Paroxysmal choreoathetosis and seizure induced by movement (reflex epilepsy). Epilepsia 1967;8:260–270

101. Kurlan R, Shoulson I. Familial paroxysmal dystonic choreoathetosis and response to alternate-day oxazepam therapy. Ann Neurol 1983;13:456–457

102. Coulter DL, Donofrio P. Haloperidol for nonkinesiogenic paroxysmal dyskinesia (letter). Arch Neurol 1980;37:325–326

103. Fouad GT, Servidei S, Durcan S, et al. A gene for familial paroxysmal dyskinesia (FPD1) maps to chromosome 2q. Am J Hum Genet 1996;59:135–139

104. Fink JK, Rainier S, Wilkowski J, et al. Paroxysmal dystonic choreoathetosis: Tight linkage to chromosome 2q. Am J Hum Genet 1996;59:140–145

105. Hofele K, Benecke R, Auburger G. Gene locus FPD1 of the dystonic Mount–Reback type of autosomal-dominant paroxysmal choreoathetosis. Neurology 1997;49:1252–1257

106. Matsuo H, Kamakura K, Saito M, et al. Familial paroxysmal dystonic choreoathetosis—clinical findings in a large Japanese family and genetic linkage to 2q. Arch Neurol 1999;56:721–726

107. Auburger G, Ratzlaff T, Lunkes A, et al. A gene for autosomal dominant paroxysmal choreoathetosis spasticity (CSE) maps to the vicinity of a potassium channel gene cluster on chromosome 1p, probably within 2 cM between D1S443 and D1S197. Genomics 1996;31:90–94

108. Szepetowski P, Rochette J, Berquin P, et al. Familial infantile convulsions and paroxysmal choreoathetosis: a new neurological syndrome linked to the pericentromeric region of human chromosome 16. Am J Hum Genet 1997;61:889–898

109. Joynt RJ, Green D. Tonic seizures as a manifestation of multiple sclerosis. Arch Neurol 1962;6:293–299

110. MacLean JB, Sassin JF. Paroxysmal vertical ocular dyskinesia. Arch Neurol 1973;29(2):117–119

111. Erickson GR, Chun RW. Acquired paroxysmal movement disorders. Pediatr Neurol 1987;3:226–229

112. Lang AE. Psychogenic dystonia: a review of 18 cases. Can J Neurol Sci 1995;22:136–143

113. Cavanagh NP, Bicknell J, Howard F. Cystinuria with mental retardation and paroxysmal dyskinesia in 2 brothers. Arch Dis Child 1974;49:662–664

114. Yamamoto K, Kawazawa S. Basal ganglion calcification in paroxysmal dystonic choreoathetosis (letter). Ann Neurol 1987;22:556

115. Dragasevic N, Petkovic-Medved B, Svetel M, et al. Paroxysmal hemiballism and idiopathic hypoparathyroidism. J Neurol 1997;244:389–390

116. Micheli F, Fernandez Pardal MM, Casas Parera I, Giannaula R. Sporadic paroxysmal dystonic choreoathetosis associated with basal ganglia calcifications (letter). Ann Neurol 1986;20:750

117. Fischbeck KH, Layzer RB. Paroxysmal choreoathetosis associated with thyrotoxicosis. Ann Neurol 1979;6:453–454

118. Margolin DL, Marsden CD. Episodic dyskinesias and

transient cerebral ischemia. Neurology 1982;32:
1379–1380

119. Bennett DA, Fox JH. Paroxysmal dyskinesias secondary to cerebral vascular disease—reversal with aspirin. Clin Neuropharmacol 1989;12:215–216

120. Huffstutter WM, Myers GJ. Paroxysmal motor dysfunction. Ala J Med Sci 1983;20:311–313

121. Perlmutter JS, Raichle ME. Pure hemidystonia with basal ganglion abnormalities on positron emission tomography. Ann Neurol 1984;15:228–233

122. Newman RP, Kinkel WR. Paroxysmal choreoathetosis due to hypoglycemia. Arch Neurol 1984;41:341–342

123. Winer JB, Fish DR, Sawyers D, Marsden CD. A movement disorder as a presenting feature of recurrent hypoglycaemia. Mov Disord 1990;5:176–177

124. Schmidt BJ, Pillay N. Paroxysmal dyskinesia associated with hypoglycemia. Can J Neurol Sci 1993;20:151–153

125. Nath A, Jankovic J, Pettigrew LC. Movement disorders and AIDS. Neurology 1987;37:37–41

126. Haan J, Kremer HPH, Padberg G. Paroxysmal choreoathetosis as presenting symptom of diabetes mellitus. J Neurol Neurosurg Psychiatry 1988;52:133

127. Shaw C, Haas L, Miller D, Delahunt J. A case report of paroxysmal dystonic choreoathetosis due to hypoglycaemia induced by an insulinoma. J Neurol Neurosurg Psychiatry 1996;61:194–195

128. Bourgeois M, Aicardi J, Goutieres F. Alternating hemiplegia of childhood. J Pediatr 1993;122:673–679

129. Andermann F, Ohtahara S, Andermann E, et al. Infantile hypotonia and paroxysmal dystonia: a variant of alternating hemiplegia of childhood. Mov Disord 1994;9:227–229

130. Nezu A, Kimura S, Ohtsuki N, et al. Alternating hemiplegia of childhood: report of a case having a long history. Brain Dev 1997;19:217–221

131. Wali GM. Paroxysmal hemidystonia induced by prolonged exercise and cold. J Neurol Neurosurg Psychiatry 1992;55:236–237

132. Bhatia KP, Soland VL, Bhatt MH, et al. Paroxysmal exercise-induced dystonia: Eight new sporadic cases and a review of the literature. Mov Disord 1997;12:1007–1012

133. Kluge A, Kettner B, Zschenderlein R, et al. Changes in perfusion pattern using ECD-SPECT indicate frontal lobe and cerebellar involvement in exercise-induced paroxysmal dystonia. Mov Disord 1998;13:125–134

134. Munchau A, Valente EM, Shahidi GA, et al. A new family with paroxysmal exercise induced dystonia and migraine: a clinical and genetic study. J Neurol Neurosurg Psychiat 2000;68:609–614

135. Schloesser DT, Ward TN, Williamson PD. Familial paroxysmal dystonic choreoathetosis revisited. Mov Disord 1996;11:317–320

136. Bhatia KP, Marsden CD, Thomas DGT. Posteroventral pallidotomy can ameliorate attacks of paroxysmal dystonia induced by exercise. J Neurol Neurosurg Psychiatry 1998;65:604–605

137. Guerrini R, Bonanni P, Nardocci N, et al. Autosomal recessive rolandic epilepsy with paroxysmal exercise-induced dystonia and writer's cramp: delineation of the syndrome and gene mapping to chromosome 16p12-11.2. Ann Neurol 1999;45:344–352

138. Fink JK, Hedera P, Mathay JG, Albin RL. Paroxysmal dystonic choreoathetosis linked to chromosome 2q: clinical analysis and proposed pathophysiology. Neurology 1997;49:177–183

139. Raskind WH, Bolin T, Wolff J, et al. Further localiza-

tion of a gene for paroxysmal dystonic choreoathetosis to a 5-cM region on chromosome 2q34. Hum Genet 1998;102:93–97

140. Jarman PR, Davis MB, Hodgson SV, et al. Paroxysmal dystonic choreoathetosis—genetic linkage studies in a British family. Brain 1997;120:2125–2130

141. Oldani A, Zucconi M, Asselta R, et al. Autosomal dominant nocturnal frontal lobe epilepsy—a video-polysomnographic and genetic appraisal of 40 patients and delineation of the epileptic syndrome. Brain 1998;121:205–223

142. Gambardella A, Annesi G, DeFusco M, et al. A new locus for autosomal dominant nocturnal frontal lobe epilepsy maps to chromosome 1. Neurology 2000;55:1467–1471

143. Browne DL, Gancher ST, Nutt TG, et al. Episodic ataxia/myokymia syndrome is associated with point mutations in the human potassium channel gene, KCNA1. Nat Genet 1994;8:136–140

144. Comu S, Giuliani M, Narayanan V. Episodic ataxia and myokymia syndrome: a new mutation of potassium channel gene Kv1.1. Ann Neurol 1996;40:684–687

145. Litt M, Kramer P, Browne D, et al. A gene for episodic ataxia/myokymia maps to chromosome 12p13. Am J Hum Genet 1994;55:702–709

146. D'Adamo MC, Liu ZP, Adelman JP, et al. Episodic ataxia type-1 mutations in the hKv1.1 cytoplasmic pore region alter the gating properties of the channel. EMBO J 1998;17:1200–1207

147. Zerr P, Adelman JP, Maylie J. Episodic ataxia mutations in Kv1.1 alter potassium channel function by dominant negative effects or haploinsufficiency. J Neurosci 1998;18:2842–2848

148. Eunson LH, Rea R, Zuberi SM, et al. Clinical, genetic, and expression studies of mutations in the potassium channel gene KCNA1 reveal new phenotypic variability. Ann Neurol 2000;48:647–656

149. Vahedi K, Joutel A, van Bogaert P, et al. A gene for hereditary paroxysmal cerebellar ataxia maps to chromosome 19p. Ann Neurol 1995;37:289–293

150. von Brederlow B, Hahn A, Koopman WJ, et al. Mapping the gene for acetazolamide responsive hereditary paroxysmal cerebellar ataxia to chromosome 19p. Hum Mol Genet 1995;4:279–284

151. Yue Q, Jen JC, Thwe MM, et al. De novo mutation in CACNA1A caused acetazolamide-responsive episodic ataxia. Am J Med Genet 1998;77:298–301

152. Zhuchenko O, Bailey J, Bonnen P, et al. Autosomal dominant cerebellar ataxia (SCA6) associated with small polyglutamine expansions in the alpha 1A-voltage-dependent calcium channel. Nat Genet 1997;15:62–69

153. Baloh RW, Yue Q, Furman JM, Nelson SF. Familial episodic ataxia: Clinical heterogeneity in four families linked to chromosome 19p. Ann Neurol 1997;41:8–16

154. Ophoff RA, Terwindt GM, Vergouwe MN, et al. Familial hemiplegic migraine and episodic ataxia type-2 are caused by mutations in the Ca²⁺ channel gene CACNL1A4. Cell 1996;87:543–552

155. Yue Q, Jen JC, Nelson SF, Baloh RW. Progressive ataxia due to a missense mutation in a calcium-channel gene. Am J Hum Genet 1997;61:1078–1087

156. Jodice C, Mantuano E, Veneziano L, et al. Episodic ataxia type 2 (EA2) and spinocerebellar ataxia type 6 (SCA6) due to CAG repeat expansion in the CACNA1A gene on chromosome 19p. Hum Mol Genet 1997;6:1973–1978

157. Baloh RW, Foster CA, Yue Q, Nelson SF. Familial

migraine with vertigo and essential tremor. Neurology 1996;46:458–460

Further reading

Aimard G, Vighetto A, Trillet M, et al. Ataxie paroxystique familiale sensible a l'acetazolamide. Rev Neurol (Paris) 1983;139:251–257

Akmandemir FG, Eraksoy M, Gurvit IH, et al. Paroxysmal dysarthria and ataxia in a patient with Behcet's disease. J Neurol 1995;242:344–347

Andermann F, Andermann E. Excessive startle syndromes: startle disease, jumping, and startle epilepsy. Adv Neurol 1986;43:321–338

Andermann F, Cosgrove JBR, Lloyd-Smith D, et al. Paroxysmal dysarthria and ataxia in multiple sclerosis. Neurology 1959;9:211–215

Angelini L, Rumi V, Lamperti E, Nardocci N. Transient paroxysmal dystonia in infancy. Neuropediatrics 1988;19:171–174

Anthony JH, Ouvrier RA, Wise G. Spasmus nutans, a mistaken identity. Arch Neurol 1980;37:373–375

Bain PG, Larkin GBR, Calver DM, Obrien MD. Persistent superior oblique paresis as a manifestation of familial periodic cerebellar ataxia. Br J Ophthalmol 1991;75:619–621

Bain PG, O'Brien MD, Keevil SF, Porter DA. Familial periodic cerebellar ataxia: a problem of cerebellar intracellular pH homeostasis. Ann Neurol 1992;31:147–154

Baloh RW, Winder A. Acetazolamide-responsive vestibulo-cerebellar syndrome: clinical and oculographic features. Neurology 1991;41:429–433

Baron DN, Dent CE, Harris H, et al. Hereditary pellagra-like skin rash with temporary cerebellar ataxia, constant renal amino-aciduria and other bizarre biochemical features. Lancet 1956;2:421–428

Bass N, Wyllie E, Comair Y, et al. Supplementary sensorimotor area seizures in children and adolescents. J Pediatr 1995;126:537–544

Beaumanoir A, Mira L, van Lierde A. Epilepsy or paroxysmal kinesigenic choreoathetosis? Brain Dev 1996;18:139–141

Beltran RS, Coker SB. Transient dystonia of infancy, a result of intrauterine cocaine exposure? Pediat Neurol 1995;12:354–356

Bird TD, Carlson CB, Horning M. Ten-year follow-up of paroxysmal choreoathetosis: A sporadic case becomes familial. Epilepsia 1978;19:129–132

Blass JP, Avigan J, Uhlendorf BW. A defect in pyruvate decarboxylase in a child with an intermittent movement disorder. J Clin Invest 1970;49:423–432

Blass JP, Kark RAP, Engel WK. Clinical studies of a patient with pyruvate decarboxylase deficiency. Arch Neurol 1971;25:449–460

Boel M, Casaer P. Paroxysmal kinesigenic choreoathetosis. Neuropediatrics 1984;15:215–217

Bratt HD, Menelaus MB. Benign paroxysmal torticollis of infancy. J Bone Joint Surg 1992;74B:449–451

Brown P, Thompson PD, Rothwell JC, et al. Paroxysmal axial spasms of spinal origin. Mov Disord 1991;6:43–48

Brunt ERP, Van Weerden TW. Familial paroxysmal kinesigenic ataxia and continuous myokymia. Brain 1990;113:1361–1382

Burke RE, Fahn S, Jankovic J, et al. Tardive dystonia: late-onset and persistent dystonia caused by antipsychotic drugs. Neurology 1982;32:1335–1346

Campistol J, Prats JM, Garaizar C. Benign paroxysmal tonic upgaze of childhood with ataxia—a neuroophthalmological syndrome of familial origin. Dev Med Child Neurol 1993;35:436–439

Damji KF, Allingham RR, Pollock SC, et al. Periodic vestibulocerebellar ataxia, an autosomal dominant ataxia with defective smooth pursuit, is genetically distinct from other autosomal dominant ataxias. Arch Neurol 1996;53:338–344

Dancis J, Hutzler J, Rokkones T. Intermittent branched-chain ketonuria: variant of maple-syrup-urine disease. N Engl J Med 1967;276:84

DeCastro W, Campbell J. Periodic ataxia. JAMA 1967;200:892–894

Deonna T, Roulet E, Meyer HU. Benign paroxysmal tonic upgaze of childhood—a new syndrome. Neuropediatrics 1990;21:213–214

Donat JF, Wright FS. Episodic symptoms mistaken for seizures in the neurologically impaired child. Neurology 1990;40:156–157

Donat JR, Auger R. Familial periodic ataxia. Arch Neurol 1979;36:568–569

Duchowny MS, Resnick TJ, Deray MJ, Alvarez LA. Video EEG diagnosis of repetitive behavior in early childhood and its relationship to seizures. Pediatr Neurol 1988;4:162–164

Echenne B, Rivier F. Benign paroxysmal tonic upward gaze. Pediat Neurol 1992;8:154–155

Espir MLE, Watkins SM, Smith HV. Paroxysmal dysarthria and other transient neurological disturbances in disseminated sclerosis. J Neurol Neurosurg Psychiatry 1966;29:323–330

Factor SA, Coni RJ, Cowger M, Rosenblum EL. Paroxysmal tremor and orofacial dyskinesia secondary to a biopterin synthesis defect. Neurology 1991;41:930–932

Fahn S, Marsden CD, Van Woert MH. Definition and clinical classification of myoclonus. Adv Neurol 1986;43:1–5

Fahn S. Atypical tremors, rare tremors, and unclassified tremors. In: Findley LJ, Capildeo R, eds. Movement Disorders: Tremor. New York: Oxford University, 1984:431–443

Fahn S. Motor and vocal tics. In: Kurlan R, ed. Handbook of Tourette's Syndrome and Related Tic and Behavioral Disorders. New York: Marcel Dekker, 1993: 3–16

Fahn S. Paroxysmal tremor. Neurology 1983;33(Suppl 2):131

Farmer TW, Mustian VM. Vestibulocerebellar ataxia. Arch Neurol 1963;8:471–480

Fejerman N. Mioclonias benignas de la infancia temprana. An Esp Ped 1984;21:725–731

Fish DR, Marsden CD. Epilepsy masquerading as a movement disorder. In: Marsden CD, Fahn S, eds. Movement Disorders 3. Oxford: Butterworth-Heinemann, 1994:346–358

Fleisher DR, Morrison A. Masturbation mimicking abdominal pain or seizures in young girls. J Pediatr 1990;116:810–814

Fukuda M, Hashimoto O, Nagakubo S, Hata A. A family with an atonic variant of paroxysmal kinesigenic choreoathetosis and hypercalcitoninemia. Mov Disord 1999;14:342–344

Gancher ST, Nutt JG. Autosomal dominant episodic ataxia: A heterogeneous syndrome. Mov Disord 1986;1:239–253

Gorard DA, Gibberd FB. Paroxysmal dysarthria and ataxia—associated MRI abnormality. J Neurol Neurosurg Psychiatry 1989;52:1444–1445

Gourley IM. Paroxysmal torticollis in infancy. Can Med Assoc J 1971;105:504–505

Griggs RC, Moxley RT III, Lafrance RA, McQuillen J. Hereditary paroxysmal ataxia: response to acetazolamide. Neurology 1978;28:1259–1264

Guerrini R, Belmonte A, Carrozzo R. Paroxysmal tonic upgaze of childhood with ataxia: a benign transient dystonia with autosomal dominant inheritance. Brain Dev 1998;20:116–118

Hallett M, Marsden CD, Fahn S. Myoclonus. Handbook of Clinical Neurology, Vol. 49, Extrapyramidal Disorders. Amsterdam: Elsevier, 1987:609–625

Hanson PA, Martinez LB, Cassidy R. Contractures, continuous muscle discharges, and titubation. Ann Neurol 1977;1:120–124

Hawkes CH. Familial paroxysmal ataxia: report of a family. J Neurol Neurosurg Psychiatry 1992;55: 212–213

Hayman M, Harvey AS, Hopkins IJ, et al. Paroxysmal tonic upgaze: a reappraisal of outcome. Ann Neurol 1998;43:514–520

Hening W, Walters A, Kavey N, et al. Dyskinesias while awake and periodic movements in sleep in restless legs syndrome: Treatment with opioids. Neurology 1986;36:1363–1366

Hill W, Sherman H. Acute intermittent familial cerebellar ataxia. Arch Neurol 1968;18:350–357

Hishikawa Y, Furuya E, Yamamoto J, Nan'no H. Dystonic seizures induced by movement. Arch Psychiat Nervenkr 1973;217:113–138

Holmes GL, Russman BS. Shuddering attacks: evaluation using electroencephalographic frequency modulation radiotelemetry and videotape monitoring. Am J Dis Child 1986;140:72–73

Homan RW, Vasko MR, Blaw M. Phenytoin plasma concentrations in paroxysmal kinesigenic choreoathetosis. Neurology 1980;30:673–676

Jabbari B, Coker SB. Paroxysmal rhythmic lingua movements and chronic epilepsy. Neurology 1981;31: 1364–1367

Kanazawa O. Shuddering attacks—report of four children. Pediat Neurol 2000;23:421–424

Kang UJ, Burke RE, Fahn S. Natural history and treatment of tardive dystonia. Mov Disord 1986;1:193–208

Keane JR. Galloping tongue: post-traumatic, episodic, rhythmic movements. Neurology 1984;34:251–252

Koller W, Bahamon-Dussan J. Hereditary paroxysmal cerebellopathy: responsiveness to acetazolamide. Clin Neuropharmacol 1987;10:65–68

Koller WC, Biary NM. Volitional control of involuntary movements. Mov Disord 1989;4:153–156

Lagueny A, Ellie E, Burbaud P, et al. Paroxysmal stimulus-sensitive spasmodic torticollis. Mov Disord 1993; 8:241–242

Lang AE. Focal paroxysmal kinesigenic choreoathetosis (letter). J Neurol Neurosurg Psychiatry 1984;47: 1057–1060

Lee BI, Lesser RP, Pippenger CE, et al. Familial paroxysmal hypnogenic dystonia. Neurology 1985;35: 1357–1360

Lee WL, Tay A, Ong HT, et al. Association of infantile convulsions with paroxysmal dyskinesias (ICCA syndrome): confirmation of linkage to human chromosome 16p12-q12 in a Chinese family. Hum Genet 1998;103:608–612

Lipson EH, Robertson WC Jr. Paroxysmal torticollis of infancy: Familial occurrence. Am J Dis Child 1978;132: 422–423

Lonsdale D, Faulkner WR, Price JW, et al. Intermittent cerebellar ataxia associated with hyperpyruvic acidemia, hyperalaninemia, and hyperalaninuria. Pediatrics 1969;43:1025–1034

Lüders HO. Paroxysmal choreoathetosis. Eur Neurol 1996;36:20–23

Lugaresi E, Cirignotta F, Montagna P. Nocturnal paroxysmal dystonia. J Neurol Neurosurg Psychiatry 1986;49:375–380

Lugaresi E, Cirignotta F. Hypnogenic paroxysmal dystonia: epileptic seizure or a new syndrome? Sleep 1981;4: 129–138

Meierkord H, Fish DR, Smith SJM, et al. Is nocturnal paroxysmal dystonia a form of frontal lobe epilepsy? Mov Disord 1992;7: 38–42

Menkes JH, Ament ME. Neurologic disorders of gastroesophageal function. Adv Neurol 1988;49: 409–416

Micheli F, Fernandez Pardal M, de Arbelaiz R, et al. Paroxysmal dystonia responsive to anticholinergic drugs. Clin Neuropharmacol 1987;10:365–369

Miley CE, Forster FM. Paroxysmal signs and symptoms in multiple sclerosis. Neurology 1974;24:458–461

Miller VS, Packard AM. Paroxysmal downgaze in term newborn infants. J Child Neurol 1998;13:294–295

Mink JW, Neil JJ. Masturbation mimicking paroxysmal dystonia or dyskinesia in a young girl. Mov Disord 1995;10:518–520

Nakken KO, Magnusson A, Steinlein OK. Autosomal dominant nocturnal frontal lobe epilepsy: an electroclinical study of a Norwegian family with ten affected members. Epilepsia 1999;40:88–92

Nightingale S, Barton ME. Intermittent vertical supranuclear ophthalmoplegia and ataxia. Mov Disord 1991;6:76–78

Ouvrier RA, Billson MD. Benign paroxysmal tonic upgaze of childhood. J Child Neurol 1988;3:177–180

Parker HL. Periodic ataxia. Mayo Clin Proc 1946;38: 642–645

Plant G. Focal paroxysmal kinesigenic choreoathetosis. J Neurol Neurosurg Psychiatry 1983;46:345–348

Postert T, Amoiridis G, Pohlau D, et al. Episodic undulating hyperkinesias of the tongue associated with brainstem ischemia. Mov Disord 1997;12:619–621

Rowland LP. Familial Periodic Paralysis, 8th ed. Merritt's Textbook of Neurology. Philadelphia: Lea & Febiger, 1989:720–724

Sanner G, Bergstrom B. Benign paroxysmal torticollis in infancy. Acta Paediatr Scand 1979;68:219–223

Scheffer IE, Bhatia KP, Lopes-Cendes I, et al. Autosomal dominant nocturnal frontal lobe epilepsy—a distinctive clinical disorder. Brain 1995;118:61–73

Sellal F, Hirsch E, Maquet P, et al. Postures et mouvements anormaux paroxystiques au cours du sommeil: dystonie paroxystique hypnogenique ou epilepsie partielle? (Abnormal paroxysmal movements during sleep: hypnogenic paroxysmal dystonia or focal epilepsy?) Rev Neurol 1991;147:121–128

Snyder CH. Paroxysmal torticollis in infancy. Am J Dis Child 1969;117:458–460

Tan A, Salgado M, Fahn S. The characterization and outcome of stereotypic movements in nonautistic children. Mov Disord 1997;12:47–52

Terzano MG, Monge-Strauss MF, Mikol F, et al. Cyclic alternating pattern as a provocative factor in nocturnal paroxysmal dystonia. Epilepsia 1997;38:1015–1025

Tinuper P, Cerullo A, Cirignotta F, et al. Nocturnal paroxysmal dystonia with short-lasting attacks: three cases with evidence for an epileptic frontal lobe origin of seizures. Epilepsia 1990;31:549–556

Vighetto A, Froment JC, Trillet M, Aimard G. Magnetic resonance imaging in familial paroxysmal ataxia. Arch Neurol 1988;45:547–549

Walters AS, Hening WA, Chokroverty S. Review and videotape recognition of idiopathic restless legs syndrome. Mov Disord 1991;6:105–110

White JC. Familial periodic nystagmus, vertigo, and ataxia. Arch Neurol 1969;20:276–280

Yokochi K. Paroxysmal ocular downward deviation in neurologically impaired infants. Pediat Neurol 1991;7: 426–428

Zacchetti O, Sozzi G, Zampollo A. Paroxysmal kinesigenic choreoathetosis. Case report. Ital J Neurol Sci 1983; 3:345–347

Zasorin NL, Baloh RW, Myers LB. Acetazolamide-responsive episodic ataxia syndrome. Neurology 1983;33: 1212–1214

250 Painful Legs and Moving Toes

Anette V Nieves and Anthony E Lang

Painful legs and moving toes (PLMT), is the simple descriptive name applied by Spillane et al. in 1971 to a rare condition which they observed in patients who complained of pain in the leg(s) with unusual abnormal movements of the toes.[1] Of their six initial patients, two had bilateral symptoms, three had a history of lumbago and/or sciatica, four had associated depression, and electromyography (EMG) was normal in three of the four patients tested. In their discussion of this condition Spillane et al. did briefly describe a patient with similar movements involving the fingers of the right hand only and without pain, but they disregarded this case as part of the same syndrome. However, in 1985 Verhagen et al.[2] broadened the accepted spectrum of the disorder by describing a case of *painful arm and moving fingers* (PAMF) without leg involvement and it is now recognized that pain is not a mandatory component and one variant is referred to as *painless* legs and moving toes (P[-]LMT).[3]

Table 250.1 Etiologies associated with painful legs and moving toes

1. Trauma (including surgery) to:
    - Cauda equina
    - Spinal nerve root
    - Plexus
    - Peripheral nerve
    - Soft/bony tissue of leg/foot (arm/hand in PAMF)
2. Mass lesions in any of the areas mentioned for trauma. Some examples include:
    - Tumors
    - Vascular lesions
    - Herniated discs
    - Hypertrophic mononeuritis[17]
3. Infections
    - Herpes zoster
    - HIV[24,25]
4. Neuropathy
    - Peripheral neuropathy
    - Entrapment neuropathy
5. Drugs
    - Vincristine + metronidazole[23]
    - Cytarabine[4]
    - Molindone[26]
    - Almitrine[27]
6. Idiopathic

PAMF, painful arm and moving fingers.

Epidemiology and genetics

This syndrome does not discriminate by gender, race, or age. The reported age of onset has ranged from the second decade of life[4] up to the late 70s.

No familial cases have been reported to date making it unlikely that the disorder is genetically transmitted. However, this does not eliminate the possibility of genetic predisposition given that so many individuals have similar peripheral injuries or insults (see below), but so few develop the syndrome.

Etiology

A variety of etiologies have been associated with this condition (see Table 250.1). The most common etiologies in order of occurrence are root lesions and peripheral trauma, peripheral neuropathy, and idiopathic.[5] Given the nature of the common causes, PLMT is typically grouped with other disorders presumed to originate from dysfunction in the peripheral nervous system (for example hemifacial spasm and stump dyskinesias).

Pathophysiology and pathogenesis

Despite the common peripheral pathology, available evidence favors a central origin for the clinical features although a peripheral origin cannot be excluded in some cases.[6–8] Some authors believe that like causalgia, pain and later movements occur after peripheral insult gives rise to abnormal impulse transmission in the peripheral sensory and sympathetic nerves, leading to a reorganization of the central processing of sensory information. This would explain why the pain is not limited to a dermatomal distribution.[5]

Nathan proposed that the movements of the toes may have a spinal origin caused by input from the posterior root fibers, which are firing frequently and spontaneously, exciting local spinal interneurons.[9]

Schoenen et al. found distinct patterns on EMG recordings of six patients with PLMT before and after an anesthetic block of the posterior tibial nerve with 2% xylocaine.[7] Half of the patients showed erratic, short discharges of low amplitude at a frequency of 4–6 Hz, consistent with a peripheral origin. The other half had alternating bursts of longer duration and higher amplitude at a frequency of 1.5–3 Hz, consistent with a central origin. Electromyographic recordings of a further patient with a unilateral presentation showed semi-rhythmic activity of distinct frequencies in the hand and foot, 1.9 Hz and 2.44 Hz respectively, suggesting the presence of multiple central oscillators.[10]

Since the movements tend to increase at the time of greatest pain and decrease or stop when pain is minimal or absent, some patients believe that the movements are somehow triggering the pain. Spillane et al. disproved this hypothesis using an ischemic block test in two patients.[1] A blood pressure cuff placed around the mid-thigh and inflated to 200 mmHg for 30 minutes eliminated the abnormal movements (also volitional movements in one of the patients), however the pain persisted.

Clinical features

Pain is generally the most disabling feature of the condition. It usually precedes the onset of movements by days to years[1,5,9] (a further clinical argument against the possibility that the movements somehow cause the pain), although the opposite can occur.[1,5] It is variously described as a crushing, cramping, throbbing, bursting, sharp, or burning sensation, which ranges from mild to severe. Although usually constant, variations in the intensity can occur.

The pain may worsen with walking,[1] any pressure on the thigh or foot,[1,6] stress,[1,11,12] rest,[1,9] caffeine,[11,13] coughing, swallowing and chewing,[14] and changes in the weather.[11,12]

The movements occur in various combinations of flexion, extension, adduction, and abduction of the toes. They have been described as continuous sinuous clawing and re-straightening, fanning and circular movements of the toes,[1] which cannot be imitated by the patient or the observer. These usually start distally and may spread proximally. Rare patients develop the movements in isolation without ever experiencing the pain component.

Some patients are able to suppress the movements voluntarily for a few seconds, which may aggravate or decrease the pain and subsequently increase the movements temporarily.[9] Pain and stress can aggravate the movements as well.[1]

The onset of symptoms can be unilateral or bilateral and involve the lower extremities, upper extremities, or both. When it begins in one limb, symptoms may spread over the subsequent days to years on the same side or to the opposite side of the body.[1,5] If bilateral initially, symptoms may resolve on one side.[5]

Pain and movements are usually mild at onset and gradually increase in intensity over time. Subsequently the intensity of symptoms may decrease in some patients. Remissions have been described usually in the context of a therapeutic intervention (see treatment section). These, however, may be transient and symptoms may return over variable periods of time. One of the original patients described by Spillane and colleagues experienced a second remission following an initial relapse.[1]

Although the movements are commonly reported to cease during sleep, in some patients movements persist even in deep and REM sleep.[6] The sleep cycle may be disrupted, with preponderant light sleep stages, decreased REM and lack of stage 4 sleep resulting in a common complaint of insomnia.

Depression can also complicate the syndrome[1] and

the physician should be aware of this since some patients may have suicidal ideation.[6] This could be due to the combination of severe and constant pain, insomnia, and lack of appropriate pain management.

Diagnosis

In idiopathic cases, except for the movements, neurological examination is essentially normal. In definable symptomatic cases examination may demonstrate appropriate neurological abnormalities.

Laboratory work up, including cerebrospinal fluid (CSF) analysis, is usually normal. Magnetic resonance imaging (MRI) may be helpful in identifying the lesions or injuries in the spinal cord, roots, plexus, or nerves, which could potentially be treated.

Electromyography and nerve conduction studies may be helpful in identifying the site of a causative lesion. Electromyograms of the movements typically show long duration bursts of activity of up to 2 seconds that comprise normal motor units with a normal recruitment pattern.[7,5,10] As mentioned earlier the pattern of EMG activity may differ depending on the origin of the abnormal movements (for instance central vs peripheral).

Differential diagnosis

There are other syndromes that may present with both pain and movement in the limbs. Among these are restless legs syndrome (RLS), spinal segmental myoclonus, thalamic syndrome, peripheral nerve, plexus, or spinal root lesions, dystonia, myokymia and painful cramps.[5] The movements of these syndromes are not those typical of PLMT. In RLS the involuntary movements do not involve the toes to the same extent as PLMT. Several types of movements occur in RLS including a variety of volitional complex movements performed to relieve the restlessness (a response not seen in PLMT) and less complex periodic myoclonic or dystonic-like involuntary movements.

Injuries to peripheral nerves, plexus, or spinal roots may cause semi-rhythmic or rhythmic involuntary movements of the limbs but without the overwhelming pain that usually accompanies PLMT. Analysis of the movement with EMG may be helpful in differentiating conditions like myokymia, myoclonus, and the like from P[-]LMT.

Treatment

Treatment for this condition, especially pain, tends to be extremely frustrating for both patient and physician. In search of some relief, the patients will try many different remedies themselves. These include immersion of the limb in cold or hot water,[1,10,13] local pressure,[1] exercise,[1,12] going barefoot,[1] wearing arch supports,[1] lying down with the foot elevated,[1] standing,[9] and alcohol consumption.[12] In an attempt to stop the movements some patients have tried bandaging their toes, but once the bandage is removed the movements may increase.[9] The use of foot orthotics improved pain and decreased the movements in a patient with tarsal tunnel syndrome who refused surgery.[15]

Numerous drugs have been tried alone or in combination without good or long lasting benefit (see Table 250.2). All reported treatment trials, with one exception,[13] have been conducted in a non-blinded fashion.

There have been a few reports claiming complete resolution of this syndrome with medication therapy although long-term results are lacking. In one patient progabide, a GABA agonist, up to 40 mg/kg gradually diminished the movements after four weeks; subsequently clomipramine (150 mg/day) was added and within 6 months pain had decreased and the movements disappeared.[16]

Guieu et al. found that adenosine levels in two patients with PLMT were lower than in patients with sciatica and controls.[13] An infusion of adenosine triphosphate (ATP) (20 mg of Striadyne) versus placebo given in a double-blind cross-over fashion provided relief of spontaneous pain in one of their two patients. They proceeded to give ATP infusions (30 mg/day of Striadyne) for 7 days and then once every 6 weeks. After a year of follow-up, both patients remained pain free and were receiving no other treatments. Surprisingly, no further reports confirming or refuting these results have appeared in the literature since.

Schoenen et al.[7] found that two of their three patients classified by EMG as having a central origin for their PLMT obtained some benefit from baclofen 50 mg three times daily (tid), while no benefit was reported in three patients with a probable peripheral origin. They also noticed that in two of these latter patients local anesthetic nerve block (see below) did not abolish the abnormal EMG activity, whereas all the patients with a central origin responded to the block.

Besides the few reports previously mentioned, there has been no striking benefit from the use of individual drugs. When used in various combinations mild to moderate relief has been obtained with benzodiazepines, baclofen, carbamazepine, and antidepressants (although the exact type is often not specified in the reports). Some medications that have been reported to exacerbate the symptoms include levodopa,[14] amantadine,[14] propranolol in some patients,[9] adrenaline,[1] and milacemide.[17]

Spillane et al.[1] noticed that sympathetic blockade seemed to provide the best results but these would generally last only a few hours to weeks, sometimes requiring multiple doses. However, sympathectomy in one of their patients gave rather disappointing results, with benefits lasting no more than three days. The various locally applied medications (that is for nerve or sympathetic blocks) have included 0.25% bupivacaine hydrochloride,[1] 0.5% lignocine with 0.25% bupivacaine,[1] guanethidine,[1,5,6] phenol,[1,6,14,18] and 24% iotrolan with 2% lidocaine followed by 99.9% ethanol.[19] Different concentrations of mepivacaine have been used in epidural blocks[18,19] with 2% giving a good but transient reduction of both pain and movements.[18] Okuda et al.[18] reported a single patient treated with 5 ml of 2% mepivacaine on alter-

nate days who was symptom free for over 10 years of follow-up. They also described another patient treated successfully with a continuous epidural block using the same drug. Good relief persisted as long as the infusion was ongoing.

Intrathecal injections of phenol 7.5% in glycerine have been reported to provided complete resolution of pain and movement for up to three hours.[14] Other injections that have been described to provide transient relief include phenol around the posterior roots,[6] and nerve blocks to posterior tibial nerve and medial and lateral plantar nerves with 1–1.5% lidocaine.[1,15]

Neurectomies of digital nerves and injections with botulinum toxin type A to the digital muscles have been used to control the movements. In one patient neurectomy eliminated the movements for one week after which they recurred to the pretreatment level.[1] In a patient with P[-]LMT injections with botulinum toxin type A into the extensor, flexor, and abductor muscles of the toes provided good temporary relief of the movements (personal communication with MH Mark).[20] Since it is known that the movements are not the cause of pain and are generally a minor component of the disability in most patients, this treatment probably has little to offer in the typical case of PLMT.

Transcutaneous electrical nerve stimulation (TENS) with or without vibratory stimulation (VS) or VS alone were studied in detail in a single patient with PLMT by Guieu et al.[11] In this study TENS was set to deliver biphasic pulses with a duration of 0.26 msec at a frequency of 100 Hz with a current intensity set by the patient below pain threshold. Four electrodes were used: one on the dorsal surface of the second, third and fourth toes, one above the instep opposite to the tibial nerve, another one-third of the distance up the leg on the anterolateral side, and the last one over the peroneal nerve on the popliteal fossa. Vibratory stimulation was set at a frequency of 100 Hz with an amplitude of 0.5 mm and applied to the forefoot with a pressure of 10 g/cm^2. These were compared to placebo treatment in which the TENS electrodes were placed but stimulation was not turned on and the patient was told that the current intensity was set sufficiently low that he would not feel it. Transcutaneous electrical nerve stimulation combined with VS controlled pain and movements much better than VS alone, which was more effective than TENS alone, which in turn was much better than placebo. After four months of self-treatment consisting of 3–4 sessions per week of combined stimulation, both pain and involuntary movements disappeared.

Summary and conclusions

Painful legs and moving toes and its variants are typically classified with other peripherally induced movement disorders although the generator of the symptoms may be central. Pain is usually the most disabling symptom. The long list of treatments reported for this uncommon disorder speaks to the difficulty encountered in managing these patients. Frequently the symptoms are very resistant to mul-

Table 250.2 Treatments used for PLMT/PAMF/P(-)LMT

Class	Medication	Max. dose (where specified)	Benefit	Reference
Anticonvulsants	Carbamazepine	800 mg/day	None to moderate	4–6,10,11,19,25,27
	Gabapentin	2100 mg/day	None	25
	Milacemide	4800 mg/day	Worse	17
	Phenytoin		None	14
	Primidone		None	12,14
	Progabide	40 mg/kg	Good	16
	Vigabatrin		None	10
Anticholinergics	Benzhexol		None	1,14
	Benztropine		None	14
	Orphenadrine		None	14
	Trihexyphenidyl		None	10,12,26
Antidepressants	(type not specified)		None to mild	1,5,18
	TCA (amitriptyline)	150 mg/day	None to mild	7 (6,10,11,14,25,27)
Benzodiazepines	(type not specified)		None to mild	5,6,18,28
	Clonazepam	4 mg/day	Mild to moderate	11,26,29
	Diazepam	12 mg IV	None	1,12,14
	Nitrazepam		None	11,14
Beta-blockers	(type not specified)		Worse to none	7,9
	Propranolol		Worse to none	1,6,12,14
Dopamine antagonist	Alphamethyldopa		None	14
	Chlorpromazine	300 mg/day	None to mild	1,14
	Haloperidol		None	10
	Pimozide		None	21
	Reserpine		None	14
	Tetrabenazine		None	21
Dopaminergic	Levodopa	3 g/day	Worse	14
Serotonin antagonist	Methysergide		None	14
Others	ACTH		None	6
	Adenosine	30 mg/day	Good	13
	Adrenaline	0.5 micrograms intra-arterial	Worse	1
		1 mg SC	None	1
	Amantadine	200 mg/day	Worse	14
	Baclofen	100 mg/day	None to moderate	5–7,10,12–15,18,24–26, 29
	Conventional analgesics (including aspirin)		None	6,1,18
	Folic acid	5 mg/day	None	1,11
	Mexiletine	600 mg/day	None	25
	Morphine	37 mg/week IM 60 mg PO	Moderate to good	11
	Quinine sulphate		None	6
	Secobarbital	200 mg/day	Mild to moderate	11
	Steroids*		None	6
	Tramadol		None	10
	Thymoxamine	5 mg IV	None	1
	Vitamin B6		None	25
	Vitamin B12		None	6
	Acupuncture		None	6
	Transcutaneous ionization of vinblastinenone		None	7
	TENS		None	6
	TENS	If used in combination with VS	Good	11
	Vibratory stimulation		None to mild (transient)	6,11,13
Anesthetic blocks	Sympathetic ganglion blockades		Good (transient)	1,5,6,13,19
	Epidural blocks		Good (transient)	18,19
	Nerve blocks		Good (transient)	1,7,15,27
Other local injections	Botulinum toxin		Good (P[-]LMT)	20
	Corticosteroids		None	11
	Phentolamine	10 mg IV	None	19
	Sodium amytal		None	1
Surgery	Sympathectomy		Good (transient)	1
	Digital neurectomy		Good (transient)	1

TCA, tricyclic antidepressant; TENS, transcutaneous electrical nerve stimulation; VS, vibratory stimulation; *, mode of delivery not specified.

tiple interventions. If an etiology is found it should be treated. There have been some cases in which the offending lesion has been treated[1,15,21,22] or an offending drug[23] has been removed and the condition has improved or remitted. Several trials of different medications should be next in line followed by nerve or epidural anesthetic blocks. In a patient with P[-]LMT, if no etiology is found, botulinum toxin to digital muscles can be tried. The development of better, more reliable therapies will probably be dependent upon further advances in our understanding of the pathogenesis of this enigmatic disorder.

References

1. Spillane JD, Nathan PW, Kelly RE, Marsden CD. Painful legs and moving toes. Brain 1971;94:541–556

2. Verhagen WI, Horstink MW, Notermans SL. Painful arm and moving fingers (letter). J Neurol Neurosurg Psychiatry 1985;48:384–385

3. Walters AS, Hening WA, Shah SK, Chokroverty S. Painless legs and moving toes: a syndrome related to painful legs and moving toes? Mov Disord 1993; 8:377–379

4. Malapert D, Degos JD. Painful legs and moving toes. Neuropathy caused by cytarabine. Rev Neurol (Paris) 1989;145:869–871

5. Dressler D, Thompson PD, Gledhill RF, Marsden CD. The syndrome of painful legs and moving toes. Mov Disord 1994;9:13–21

6. Schott GD. Painful legs and moving toes: the role of trauma. J Neurol Neurosurg Psychiatry 1981;44: 344–346

7. Schoenen J, Gonce M, Delwaide PJ. Painful legs and moving toes: a syndrome with different physiopathologic mechanisms. Neurology 1984;34:1108–1112

8. Auger RG. The syndrome of painful legs and moving toes due to hyperexcitability of the lateral plantar nerve. Ann Neurol 2000;48:432

9. Nathan PW. Painful legs and moving toes: evidence on the site of the lesion. J Neurol Neurosurg Psychiatry 1978;41:934–939

10. Ebersbach G, Schelosky L, Schenkel A, et al. Unilateral painful legs and moving toes syndrome with moving fingers—evidence for distinct oscillators. Mov Disord 1998;13:965–968

11. Guieu R, Tardy-Gervet MF, Blin O, Pouget J. Pain relief achieved by transcutaneous electrical nerve stimulation and/or vibratory stimulation in a case of painful legs and moving toes. Pain 1990;42:43–48

12. Funakawa I, Mano Y, Takayanagi T. Painful hand and moving fingers. A case report. J Neurol 1987; 234:342–343

13. Guieu R, Sampieri F, Pouget J, et al. Adenosine in painful legs and moving toes syndrome. Clin Neuropharmacol 1994;17:460–469

14. Lance JW, Andrews C. Dysesthesia-dyskinesia: a syndrome of painful legs and moving toes. Proc Aust Assoc Neurol 1973;9:87–90

15. Pla ME, Dillingham TR, Spellman NT, et al. Painful legs and moving toes associates with tarsal tunnel syndrome and accessory soleus muscle. Mov Disord 1996;11:82–86

16. Bovier P, Hilleret H, Tissot R. Progabide treatment of a case of the syndrome of painful legs and moving toes. Rev Neurol (Paris) 1985;141:422–424

17. Gordon MF, Diaz-Olivo R, Hunt AL, Fahn S. Therapeutic trial of milacemide in patients with myoclonus and other intractable movement disorders. Mov Disord 1993;8:484–488

18. Okuda Y, Suzuki K, Kitajima T, et al. Lumbar epidural block for "painful legs and moving toes" syndrome: a report of three cases. Pain 1998;78:145–147

19. Shime N, Sugimoto E. Lumbar sympathetic ganglion block in a patient with painful legs and moving toes syndrome. Anesth Analg 1998;86:1056–1057

20. Mark MH. Other choreatic disorders. In: Watts RL, Koller WC, eds. Movement Disorders Neurologic Principles and Practice. New York: McGraw-Hill, 1997: 527–539

21. Wulff CH. Painful legs and moving toes. A report of 3 cases with neurophysiological studies. Acta Neurol Scand 1982;66:283–287

22. Mitsumoto H, Levin KH, Wilbourne AJ, Chou SM. Hypertrophic mononeuritis clinically presenting with painful legs and moving toes. Muscle & Nerve 1990; 13:215–221

23. Gastaut JL. Painful legs and moving toes. A drug-induced case. Rev Neurol (Paris) 1986;142:641–642

24. Scherokman B, Jabbari B, Ling G. Painful legs, moving toes: favourable response to lioresal and association with HIV infection. Neurology 1991;41:225

25. Pitagoras DM, Oliveira M, Andre C. Painful legs and moving toes associated with neuropathy in HIV-infected patients. Mov Disord 1999;14:1053–1054

26. Sandyk R. Neuroleptic-induced painful legs and moving toes syndrome: successful treatment with clonazepam and baclofen. Ital J Neurol Sci 1990;11: 573–576

27. Herman-Bert A, Stevanin G, Netter JC, et al. Mapping of spinocerebellar ataxia 13 to chromosome 19q13.3-q13.4 in a family with autosomal dominant cerebellar ataxia and mental retardation. Am J Hum Genet 2000;67:229–235

28. Sanders P, Waddy HM, Thompson PD. An "annoying" foot: unilateral painful legs and moving toes syndrome. Pain 1999;82:103–104

29. Tan AK, Tan CB. The syndrome of painful legs and moving toes: a case report. Singapore Med J 1996;37: 446–447

251 The Restless Legs Syndrome and Periodic Limb Movements

Wayne A Hening

The restless legs syndrome (RLS) (see Table 251.1 for abbreviations) may have first been recognized by the British physician and anatomist, Thomas Willis, who wrote (in an English translation)[1] about a condition whose sufferers, "...whilst they would indulge sleep, in their beds, immediately follow leapings up of the tendons, in their arms and legs, with cramps, and such unquietness and flying about of their members, that the sick can no more sleep, than those on the Rack." This describes five key features of RLS: sensory discomfort ("cramps"), motor restlessness ("unquietness"), involuntary movements ("flying about of their members"), and the aggravation by night and rest ("in their beds"). Many more features of RLS, including family aggregation and contributing disorders, were described in the 1940s by Karl Ekbom, a Swedish neurologist who collected a large case series and recognized both the common occurrence of the condition and its core features.[2,3] The condition was subsequently codified by the American Sleep Disorders Association (now American Academy of Sleep Medicine).[4] Its key diagnostic clinical features were further delineated based on a con-

sensus of an international group of RLS experts (International RLS Study Group).[5]

Restless leg syndrome has long been linked to periodic limb movements (PLM), a movement disorder initially noted in sleep. In a paper on sleep myoclonus,[6] Symonds described a variety of different involuntary movements, among them PLM. Lugaresi subsequently established that one form of nocturnal myoclonus with a highly periodic character was associated with RLS.[7] It was discovered by Weitzman's group in the 1970s that these movements were quite common in adults and occurred in a wide range of conditions during sleep.[8,9] Because of their obvious periodicity (Figure 251.1), the movements are termed periodic limb movements in sleep (PLMS). Similar movements may occur while awake, especially in RLS patients.[10]

The American Academy of Sleep Medicine (AASM) criteria for PLMS include a sequence of four movements, with an interval of 5–90 seconds, a duration of 0.5–5 seconds, and an amplitude on electromyographic (EMG) tracing that is one fourth of a maximal effort.[4,11] Movements associated with respiratory disturbance in sleep are not counted as PLMS.

Table 251.1	Abbreviations and definitions
NREM sleep	Non-REM sleep. The majority of sleep, characterized by quiet eye movements. Graded as to depth (from light, stage 1, to deep or slow-wave sleep (SWS), stages 3 and 4) by predominant frequency of EEG waves. Deeper sleep involves slowest (delta frequency) waves
PLM	Periodic limb movement(s). One or more of a series of movements (minimum: 4 in series) that occur at intervals of about 5 to 90 seconds. Have typical form (Figure 256.1), minimum amplitude (1/4 maximum as measured in tibialis anterior muscle), most pronounced in legs but may involve arms or include other muscle groups
PLMS	Periodic limb movement(s) in sleep. PLM occurring during a sleep stage (NREM, REM). Formerly called nocturnal myoclonus. Waking movements have been called dyskinesias while awake (DWA) or PLMW (PLM Wake state). Only PLMS, not PLMW, are typically reported in a sleep study
PLMD	Periodic limb movement disorder. Condition of disturbed sleep with symptoms attributable to sleep disruption by PLMS. Implies exclusions of other sources of sleep complaint (insomnia, excessive daytime somnolence [EDS])
REM sleep	Rapid Eye Movement sleep. Recurrent episodes (at about 90 minute intervals) associated with rapid eye movements and often-low amplitude flickering or myoclonic extremity movements. Associated with activated EEG and with maximal dream recall. Normally, first episode occurs after an hour or more of sleep; successive episodes during night tend to increase in duration
RLS	The restless legs syndrome, a neurological sensorimotor disorder involving leg discomfort and motor restlessness provoked by rest in a circadian pattern with symptoms most severe in the period before the core temperature nadir (i.e. the evening and first part of the night)

For further information, refer to references 1 and 2 of general references on sleep science and sleep medicine.

XIII Movement Disorders

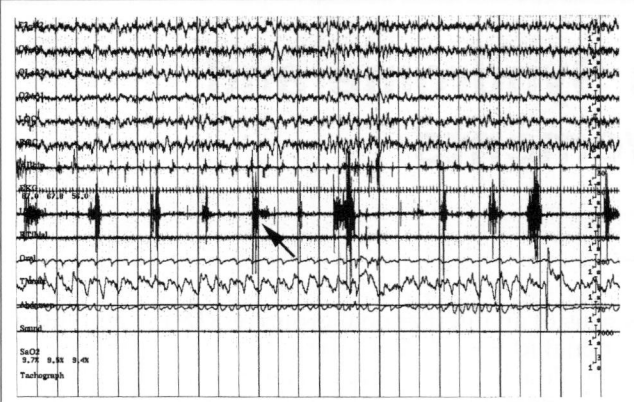

Figure 251.1 Series of Periodic Limb Movements. A series of periodic limb movements in a sleeping patient. These occur almost exclusively in the left leg. The burst indicated by the arrow shows several initial high amplitude brief components. The middle burst is prolonged, consistent with an arousal leading to prolonged movement. After this burst, there is an altered EEG rhythm and EMG activity spreading to chin and right leg, as well as altered respiratory rhythm. (Chin EMG has respiratory artifacts through tracing). Note approximate, but not exact periodicity. Top four traces—EEG from vertex (top two traces) and occiput (third and fourth traces) referenced to the opposite ear. Fifth and sixth traces, left and right EOG (electrooculograms). Seventh trace, chin EMG. Eighth trace, EKG. Ninth and tenth traces, left and right tibialis anterior EMGs. Eleventh trace, oral air flow. Twelve and thirteenth traces, thoracic and abdominal respiratory effort. Bottom trace, sound recording. Trace superimposed on abdominal effort is a displaced oximeter tracing indicating oxygen saturation. The entire record is 160 seconds long; thick vertical lines indicate 16-second divisions.

The AASM also defined a specific sleep disorder, periodic limb movement disorder (PLMD) that can be attributed to the effects of sleep disruption by PLMS. Recently, it has been questioned whether PLMS are ever more than an accompanying phenomena and whether they play any pathogenic role.[12,13]

Epidemiology

Restless leg syndrome

In the 1990s, a series of population studies and polls examining adults suggested that symptoms of RLS are extremely common, occurring in 10% or more of North American populations.[14-17] A similar figure of 11.4% was found in working-age women in Sweden.[18] These studies showed a higher prevalence of RLS in women, and increasing prevalence with age. In a more recent study of the elderly in Germany using a small set of diagnostic questions and clinician diagnosis, the investigators found that 10% could be diagnosed with RLS.[19] Another study in Chile, a South American country whose population is predominantly of European ancestry, found that 13% could be diagnosed with RLS.[20] Until very recently, all studies of RLS were conducted on populations of predominantly European origin. A lower prevalence of RLS has been reported in Japan[21] and Singapore.[22]

Periodic limb movements in sleep

Periodic limb movements are ascertained either by sleep studies, known as polysomnography (PSG),[11] or more recently by the use of movement measurements (actigraphy).[23-25] Periodic limb movements in sleep are relatively rare in younger individuals, but quite common in the elderly.[26]

Associated conditions

Several medical conditions are associated with an increased prevalence of RLS,[27] including iron deficiency, with or without actual anemia,[3] uremia,[28-30] peripheral neuropathy,[34-36] diabetes,[37] rheumatoid arthritis,[38] and fibromylagia syndrome.[38] There are also some specific inherited neurological disorders in which RLS has been reported, including familial amyloid neuropathy,[39] spinocerebellar ataxia,[40] especially type 3,[41,42] and Charcot-Marie-Tooth disease, type 2.[43] Patients with Parkinson's disease experience leg restlessness but the true prevalence of RLS is uncertain. Restless leg syndrome is also quite common in the pregnancy, especially in the third trimester,[31,32] usually resolving with delivery. Restless leg syndrome in pregnancy may, however, represent the first episode of a more chronic RLS that returns later in life.

Periodic limb movements occur in over 80% of patients with RLS,[44,45] as well as in other sleep disorders, including narcolepsy[46] and a disorder of REM sleep control called REM behavior disorder.[47] Periodic limb movements are common in conditions of dopamine deficiency, such as Parkinson's disease,[13,48] but uncommon in putative conditions of dopamine excess, such as schizophrenia.[49]

Etiology

The possible causes of RLS include genetic, degenerative, toxic, nutritional, and vascular. A major handicap in understanding the etiology or the pathogenesis of RLS is the lack of any core pathological lesion, such as the substantia nigral degeneration seen in Parkinson's disease. This is partly due to the lack of any pathological studies in RLS (although a brain bank has been established), but may also reflect the fact that the primary lesion in RLS is an abnormality of function.

Ekbom favored a vascular etiology for RLS, but this is no longer considered likely since many patients are quite young and unlikely to have significant vascular pathology. However, current research cannot exclude some altered vascular reactivity in RLS patients. Most experts favor the hypothesis that RLS arises from altered activity of neural systems, either directly through abnormal synaptic or axonal function or indirectly through effects on biosynthetic cofactors, such as iron.[50] Toxic factors are considered because of the high prevalence of RLS in uremia and possibly diabetes. Nutritional factors have been suggested by the association of RLS with iron deficiency[51,52] and possibly with certain vitamin deficiencies, such as folate[53] and B$_{12}$. It seems likely that genetic predisposition plays a significant role, but that expression of RLS may also be strongly related to environmental or biological factors such as toxins, nutrients, or metabolic state. The causes of PLM appear to be similar to RLS.

Early onset patients are more likely to have affected family members. These can be contrasted to later onset patients, who are more likely to have a clear precipitating cause for their RLS, such as a peripheral nerve disorder[87] or uremia.[85] It seems likely that most patients with age of onset under 40 belong to the group of those with an idiopathic, familial condition.

Pathophysiology

Currently, it is believed that RLS involves a dysfunction of the central dopaminergic system.[50,54] The main evidence for this is the notable response of RLS and PLM to dopaminergic medications, reactivation of symptoms by dopamine receptor blockers, and the presence of modest deficits in pre- and post-synaptic dopamine markers within the striatum, as measured using imaging studies.[55–57] A preliminary study of cerebral spinal fluid (CSF) did not find, however, alteration in the amount of the main dopamine metabolite, homovanillic acid (HVA).[58]

If the dopamine hypothesis is correct, RLS would appear to involve dopaminergic pathways other than the striatonigral pathways affected in Parkinson's disease, such as descending pathways to the spinal cord. The evidence for this is the absence of the typical motor findings of parkinsonism in RLS patients,[59] and the fact that most patients with RLS do not develop Parkinson's disease.

It is suggested that the putative dopamine dysfunction in RLS could be an inability to acquire or store sufficient amounts of iron in the central nervous system. Iron is a co-factor for tyrosine hydroxylase, the rate-limiting enzyme for the synthesis of dopamine. It has been shown that RLS patients have low iron stores, as measured by ferritin levels.[51,52] Spinal fluid ferritin[60] and brain iron in the substantia nigra[61] are low in RLS patients. It has been speculated that RLS patients cannot transport iron into the central nervous system (CNS) or that they have inappropriately increased elimination of iron from the body. Repleting iron can resolve symptoms in some patients.[51]

Opioid medications also benefit RLS and preliminary evidence suggests that blocking the opioid receptor with naloxone in treated patients can reactivate the symptoms.[64] The relationship between dopamine and opioid dysfunction in RLS remains uncertain. It has been suggested that the endogenous opiate system may act to modulate a relevant dopaminergic pathway.[65]

In one functional magnetic resonance imaging (fMRI) study, it was found that sensory symptoms in RLS were related to abnormal cerebellar and thalamic activation.[66] Periodic limb movements, in contrast to mimicked movements, also activated the red nucleus and pontine reticular structures.[66] Mimicked move-

ments showed basal ganglia and cortical activation not seen with PLM. It is uncertain whether these activated regions represent the abnormal loci of RLS and PLM or simply reflect reactive centers activated as a consequence of the abnormal sensory activity and movements.

It has been found that PLM can occur in patients with complete spinal cord transections.[67] This has led to the idea that a competent generator for PLM must be located within the spinal cord, even if some of its control elements are higher in the neuraxis. The precipitation of PLM, or occasionally RLS,[68] by spinal lesions and their amelioration by treatment supports this idea.[69,70] Recent studies have disagreed on how patterned the PLM are and how regular the sequence of muscle recruitment,[71,72] but these studies in general support a spinal origin and suggest an increased spinal excitability. Increased spinal flexor reflexes may be found in patients with PLM.[73] Perhaps consistent with the dopamine hypothesis of RLS and PLM, it is known that dopamine pathways descend to the spinal cord.[74,75] Furthermore, patients with cord transection can benefit from dopamine therapy,[76] suggesting a local effect on post-synaptic receptors.

One suggestion appreciated early on was that PLM might be related to periodic alternations of autonomic tone.[77] This association has been furthered by the finding that the sleeping electroencephalogram (EEG) can show cyclic alternation in its frequency and amplitude domains, a phenomena known as cyclic alternating pattern (CAP).[78] Cyclic alternating pattern is associated with autonomic alternations[79] and has been shown to be phase locked to PLMS, with the movements occurring during the more excitable phase (A) of the CAP cycle.[80] Other studies have demonstrated that PLMS are phase locked to changes in heart rate.[81]

Genetics

Familial clustering of RLS was first appreciated by Ekbom.[2,3] Large pedigrees with multiple affected members have been identified, supporting an autosomal dominant pattern of inheritance. Some families show anticipation, a lower age of onset in successive generations,[82,83] suggesting that, like Huntington's disease, RLS may be a disorder of unstable trinucleotide repeats. Concordance for RLS is very high (10 of 12 pairs) in a series of clinically ascertained monozygotic twins.[86] Recent advances have included a segregation analysis which found evidence of a dominant inheritance in early onset pedigrees,[88] the discovery of an initial linkage to chromosome 12q,[89] and the findings of an association with monoamine oxidase A.[90]

Classification

Restless leg syndrome and PLM are classified into two main categories: (1) primary, or idiopathic, and (2) secondary (see Table 251.2). The idiopathic condition is diagnosed when none of the typical associated conditions are present or when any such condition appears to have begun after the RLS or

Table 251.2	Restless legs syndrome classification

Primary	Secondary
"Idiopathic"	Iron deficiency
	Pregnancy
	Uremia
	Neuropathy
	Diabetes
	rheumatoid arthritis
	BIZ or folate deficiency
	?Parkinson's disease

PLM. Sometimes, the distinction is difficult to make. The phenomenology of RLS and the response to treatment does not differ between the two groups. The idiopathic category is favored by an early age of onset. Patients with an earlier age of onset appear to have a more slowly progressive disease and to lack the significant association of severity to low serum ferritin levels seen with later onset patients.[90]

Diagnosis

Diagnosis of RLS is made by determining the four diagnostic features as specified by the International RLS Study Group (IRLSSG; Table 251.3). The clear presence of all four features is usually adequate to exclude possible mimicking disorders (see differential diagnosis). A good history is critical for making the diagnosis. It is important to ascertain that the sensory discomfort and urge to move are specifically localized to the legs and not just a generalized discomfort or restlessness. That being said, it must be remembered that a significant fraction of more affected patients will also have symptoms in the arms[44,97] and more rarely other body parts (trunk, face, genitals). However, while these sites may be involved, it would be very rare for the legs not to be involved first and more severely. Some patients cannot designate a specific sensory discomfort, not even an "indescribable" one, but report that what they feel is simply a need or urge to move. The severity of RLS can vary over a wide range from an occasional discomfort to a severe, daily torture. What bothers patients can also vary:

while many complain of the classic insomnia due to exacerbation of symptoms at bedtime, others are more bothered by night time interruptions to sleep or by symptoms evoked by sustained periods of repose that may occur earlier in the day. Airplane travel, prolonged car trips, or long spectator events (such as an opera) can be particularly trying for some. Despite their degree of sleep disruption and sleep deprivation, RLS patients tend to complain of less daytime sleepiness than patients with disorders having a comparable impact on sleep. However, some patients will be bothered by sleepiness or by fatigue and mood changes related to sleep deficits.

Laboratory testing in RLS is generally brief unless co-morbid disorders are suspected on the basis of history of examination. It is mandatory to determine iron status, since low iron stores can precipitate or aggravate RLS.[51,52] The key measure is ferritin: patients with levels less than 50 mg/liter, which is within the normal range, should be considered for iron repletion. It is also important to be sure the patients do not have diabetes or kidney failure, so a blood chemistry, together with a determination of hematocrit, should be obtained if not already available. Electrodiagnostic testing should be performed in patients with symptoms of peripheral nerve dysfunction by history or exam. The neurological exam should pay particular attention to the peripheral nerves.

It has been suggested that a routine sleep study, or polysomnography (PSG), is not indicated for diagnosis of RLS,[98] although if there is a question of other sleep problems or some uncertainty as to diagnosis or therapeutic response, one should be considered. For this purpose, consultation with a sleep specialist would be helpful. On the sleep study, the findings suggestive of RLS include an increased amount of movement and wake periods, delayed sleep onset, abundant PLMS, often diminishing in the latter part of the sleep period, with abundant associated arousals and often frequent awakenings. However, no feature is pathognomonic.

A related procedure, the suggested immobilization test, has the patient sit quietly and try not to move for a period of an hour. During this period, sensory symptoms can be assessed and leg movement determined by EMG or actigraphy.[45,99] As with typical find-

Table 251.3	Key clinical features of RLS

Diagnostic Features	Desire or need to move the limbs usually associated with uncomfortable or unpleasant sensations
	Motor restlessness
	Symptoms are worse or exclusively present at rest (i.e., lying, sitting) with at least partial and temporary relief by activity
	Circadian pattern—symptoms maximal in evening/night
Typical Features	Involuntary movements: periodic limb movements (PLM; See Table 251.1 for definitions)
	Sleep disturbance and its consequences
	Normal neurological examination in idiopathic cases
	Generally chronic course, often progressive
	Positive family history

Modified from the International RLS Study group published consensus on clinical definition.[5]
A recent, May, 2002 NIH workshop revised the diagnostic criteria for RLS by deleting the requirement for motor restlessness and splitting the criteria on rest precipitation and activity relief into two separate criteria.

ings on PSG, this can support a clinical impression, but is not definitive. Imaging and pathology remain experimental in RLS and PLM and are probably clinically restricted to a search for potential co-morbid disorders.

For PLM, the diagnosis depends upon the determination of the number of PLM on polysomnography. Usually, only movements during sleep (PLMS) are counted. These must occur in a series of four movements, with individual movements of duration of 0.5–5 seconds separated by 5–90 seconds, and with an amplitude on PSG of 1/4 a maximal contraction of the anterior tibialis muscle.[11] Phenomenologically, these movements can be quite diverse[100] and include involvement of the arms and body shifts, but the prototypical movement is a leg flexion with ankle dorsiflexion and extension of the great toe. This movement resembles a Babinski[101] or flexor withdrawal reflex.[73] While the operational definition allows a wide variation in period of these movements, most movements in a typical patient will be spaced by 15–40 seconds. The EMG burst often shows a rapidly waxing and more slowly waning burst, often including an initial period of rapidly repeated brief (<200 ms) staccato bursts (Figure 251.1).

The PSG is usually scrutinized to be sure that the EMG potentials are not correlated to apneic episodes, since these should not be counted as PLMS. These EMG bursts usually occur in association with the relief of obstructive apnea by an exaggerated respiratory effort, which relieves the block to airflow. One deficiency of actigraphy as an alternate methodology for evaluating PLMs is that it doesn't provide clear evidence of sleep state or associated breathing difficulties.

The laboratory evaluation of PLMD generally requires a PSG to establish the presence of the movements, count their frequency, associate them with sleep and wake states, and determine if they cause arousals, although even PLMS without evident arousals[102] may impact on sleep.[81] Periodic limb movements in sleep are ubiquitous in many sleep disorders and the elderly, so when a diagnosis of PLMD is to be made, it is necessary to be certain that other disorders are not also present. In particular, in the upper airway resistance syndrome (UARS), patients may have movements as their need for increased airflow waxes and wanes, even without frank apneas or hypopneas.[103] Therefore, the PSG should be done with pressure monitoring, which can detect UARS.

It should also be clear that PLMS may vary from slight movements of the foot to widespread, even complex movements that involve the arms or other body parts.[97,100] If they cause an arousal, which is more disruptive of sleep, they can also lead to bodily shifts or other quasi-voluntary movements that can prolong the muscular activity.

Differential diagnosis

Restless leg syndrome needs to be distinguished primarily from akathitic and paresthetic or dysesthetic disorders that may be linked to an urge to move, and

also show greater prominence at rest and later in the day. Primary akathisia is not commonly encountered, but may occur in disorders such as Parkinson's disease (PD).[104–106] Much more common is drug-induced akathisisa (DIA), especially neuroleptic induced akathisia (NIA).[104,107,108] Drug-induced akathisisa is produced by dopamine blocking as well as other neuroactive medications, such as serotonin reuptake blockers. Neuroleptic induced akathisia and akathisia in PD may be present more prominently in the later parts of the day.[105,109] Patients can have PLMS as well as sleep disruption.[110] In most cases, the clinical setting helps to make a discrimination, but it remains unsettled whether RLS is increased in PD. In drug-induced cases, the same spectrum of drugs that provoke akithisia can also induce or aggravate RLS.

As clues to distinguish between RLS and akathisia, RLS patients tend to emphasize the provocative factors of rest and sleep, specify the sensory discomfort that induces restlessness, and find much greater relief with activity. Periodic limb movements are generally more prominent in RLS and repetitive, stereotypic movements (body rocking, marching in place) less common. Akathisia is usually evident as overt restlessness on exam, while RLS is not. In fact, akathitic motor restlessness can occur without subjective content, a condition sometimes called pseudo-akathisia.[111] A recently described condition, hypotensive akathisia[112] may mimic RLS, but is largely confined to the seated condition when orthostatic changes can cause dysphoric symptoms. Lying down relieves these discomforts, which would be atypical of RLS in which lying down would either cause similar symptoms or even more intense ones. The absence of symptoms when lying down generally excludes a firm diagnosis of RLS. This consideration also generally eliminates cases of nonspecific restlessness[113] or simple positional discomfort from prolonged sitting, which is quite common and can mimic some of the features of RLS. In this case, simple postural shifts generally produce relief.

The other conditions that can be confused with RLS are those involving some local pathology in the legs, either in peripheral nerves, blood vessels, joints, muscles, or other soft tissues. In most cases, these do not vary with activity and circadian time. For instance, small fiber diabetic neuropathy may cause symptoms similar to RLS. It has been suggested,[35] but never definitively confirmed, that peripheral neuropathy in general is associated with RLS. In some cases, the two will coexist and it may not be possible to further clarify the relationship. Whether RLS occurs in or can be caused by peripheral venous disease is also an unresolved issue.[114,115] It may be that related complaints in varicose veins are merely mimics similar to positional discomfort. Most cases of peripheral arterial disease, arthritis and bursitis, or muscular disorders can be readily distinguished on the basis of exam findings. Rarely will these disorders occur while lying down or have full relief with motor activity.

A history of muscle cramps[116–118] can be confused with RLS. Cramps present relatively discrete, often

Table 251.4   Major elements of good sleep hygiene

Sleep/wake/activity regulation	Regular sleep hours, especially for rising in morning Planned time in bed not to exceed time for sleep that is needed for daytime alertness Avoidance of naps or take only one brief nap (10–15 minutes) timed approximately 8 hours after rising Regular exercise, preferably daily, but not less than 6 hours before bedtime
Sleep setting and influences	Avoidance of bright light exposure late in evening or at night Exposure to bright light shortly after rising (unless wake before desired time) Avoidance of heavy eating or drinking within 3 hours of bedtime Quiet, dark room in which to sleep Suitable mattress and pillow for comfort and support Avoidance of non-sleep or intimacy-related activities in bedroom Avoidance of alerting or stressful activities or thoughts in hours before bedtime Avoidance of caffeine after midday meal Avoidance of tobacco smoking after dinner
Sleep promoting adjuvants	Light snack or hot bath before bedtime can be helpful Quiet activities, such as pleasurable, light reading, immediately before seeking sleep

Modified from Zarcone.[131]

short-lived, episodes of discomfort, and typically awaken patients from sleep. The diagnosis of cramps is made by finding a palpable, usually unilateral, active muscle contraction, with associated focal pain. Of course, cramps are very common in the general public[119,120] and so it is expected that many individuals will have both cramps and RLS.

Another possible confusing condition is painful legs and moving toes.[121] The dyskinetic movements in that condition, however, are usually at least semi-continuous and involve the toes with a writhing or tremor-like activity that can be readily observed. These movements are also much less dependent on activity than RLS symptoms.

The differential diagnosis for PLMS comprises a wide variety of normal and abnormal movements in sleep, including hypnic jerks, normal postural shifts, nocturnal seizures, parasomnias such as sleep walking and pathological arousals, and REM sleep behavior disorder.[27] Movements associated with abnormal respiratory events during sleep, such as respiratory apneas, hypopneas, and UARS, are also in the differential diagnosis.

The diagnostic situation is complicated by the fact that PLMS can co-exist with many of these disorders. Usually, a full PSG may be needed to discriminate PLMS from other disorders or to rule out other disorders as a necessity for a diagnosis of PLMD. However, it may be necessary to use a full head montage to rule out seizures, or a sustained video recording to fully assess an abnormal motor condition.[122]

Treatment

The first treatment for RLS was an opiate, laudanum, recommended by Willis.[1] While Ekbom was familiar with the efficacy of opiates and other sedative/hypnotic drugs, he felt that this was not a suitable treatment and recommended vasodilators,[2,3] basing this treatment on a presumed pathophysiology of

arterial insufficiency. The modern classes of therapeutic agents—including opioids, benzodiazepines, dopaminergic agents, and select anti-convulsants—were all first reported as successful by the middle 1980s. Since then, treatment advances have included: the recognition that particular iatrogenic exacerbations of RLS or PLMS, rebound and augmentation, are highly associated with more than minimal dose, sustained therapy with levodopa;[124,125] the introduction of dopamine agonists as alternative therapies of choice;[126–129] and the description of the first set of standards for management of RLS.[130] In all cases, treatment of RLS, unless aimed at alleviating an underlying disorder, is purely symptomatic.

General guidelines for treatment

Patients with mild RLS may not need medication if they can manage their discomfort and sleep loss with a variety of behavioral and lifestyle techniques. A moderate life style with minimal intake of caffeine, nicotine, and alcohol combined with regular exercise and avoidance of voluntary sleep deprivation may reduce symptoms. Good sleep hygiene[131] (Table 251.4), which includes regular bed and rise times, use of the bed only for intimacy and sleeping, and gradually reduced activity before bedtime, may be quite helpful. Patients also find that a hot bath (or more rarely, a cold shower), a massage, or a brief walk before bedtime can make sleep easier.

Patients with an underlying, treatable disorder may obtain relief by its treatment, including iron repletion for those with iron deficiency.[51] Patients with peripheral neuropathy or spinal cord lesions causing PLMS[70] or RLS may benefit from appropriate therapy. Renal transplantation has cured RLS in patients with end stage renal disease.[132]

It is important to review the patient's medications to be sure that these do not include medications likely to provoke RLS. Dopamine blocking agents and antidepressants are the most common medications that can aggravate RLS or PLM, but calcium channel blockers and anti-histamines have also been implicated. In some cases, RLS may be provoked by inadvertent reduction in some drugs, such as opioid medications (e.g. tramadol[133]). It is worth remembering that RLS may be an element of abstinence from narcotic drugs or cocaine formulations taken for recreational use.

Treatment should be tailored to the frequency and severity of RLS symptoms.[134] Patients with infrequent symptoms can be managed with prn medications. Opioids, benzodiazepines, and levodopa-carbidopa are among those medications that can be given in this manner. Patients with mild symptoms may also do well with levodopa/carbidopa, a mild opioid, or a benzodiazepine. However, patients with severe symptoms will generally need a dopamine agonist.

The quality of the leg discomfort may influence treatment. Patients whose limb discomfort is painful may do especially well with an anticonvulsant, especially gabapentin. The timing of symptoms can suggest which medications would be most helpful. Symptoms only at bedtime may respond well to clonidine. Patients with symptoms, including PLM throughout the night, may need a medication with a longer half-life, including sustained release levodopa/carbidopa or a dopamine agonist, which is preferable to routine middle of the night dosing.

Patients with symptoms during the day or even in the hours before bedtime may need coverage with multiple doses, unless they can be managed with very long-acting agents such as methadone. Patients with PLMD alone are generally managed similarly to RLS patients, although daytime or evening dosing is not needed. Such patients may do very well with clonazepam in low dose (0.5 to 2 mg nightly). If this is inadequate, use of dopaminergic agents is effective.

Co-morbid illness may dictate how medications should be managed. This may be true in Parkinson's disease (PD), hypertension, diabetes, respiratory disorder, or uremia. In PD, there may be a need to modulate therapy to avoid aggravating RLS. If RLS persists despite dopaminergic therapy well tailored to PD, agents of other classes (opioids, benzodiazepines, anticonvulsants, etc.), may be added to cover RLS symptoms or PLMS. Some RLS medications may help the associated disorders (e.g. clonidine in hypertension) or work against them (e.g. beta blockers in diabetes or sedatives in respiratory disorders). In cases of uremia, certain medications have already been shown to be helpful and tolerable (dopaminergic agents, clonidine, opioids).

It is generally useful to begin a new class of medications with very low doses and titrate up as needed. This also avoids side effects. Another consideration is that RLS patients who present for medical management generally follow a protracted course of years, if not decades. They also tend to become quite dependent on medication. As a result, it is pays to be cautious in initiating therapy, although there is no compelling reason to avoid treatment when quality of life is suffering from RLS or PLMD. This caution is most important for younger or middle aged patients.

Later in the course of RLS management, a history of previous response may guide therapy. Patients may become tolerant of medications after a while and dopaminergic agents, especially levodopa/carbidopa, may often cause iatrogenic increases in RLS symptoms (rebound and augmentation, see below under levodopa/carbidopa). This may be especially true of levodopa/carbidopa. A change in class of medication may be the first response to reduced responsiveness. Other responses include the use of medications from two or even three classes (e.g. a benzodiazepine and a dopaminergic agent or an opioid and an anti-convulsant). Finally, for highly refractory patients, strong opioids such as levodromoran or methadone can be administered. In some cases, rotating medications or even drug holidays (especially for dopaminergic agents and with coverage during a holiday from another class) have been used by some physicians. These may work, but require vigilance and care, since tapering RLS medications can lead to withdrawal re-emergence of symptoms or even other complications.

Treatment of children with RLS and pregnant women raises special issues. It seems prudent to reserve treatment in children for those whose RLS causes significant disruption of sleep or school activities. In many cases, caffeine restriction may be helpful. Children have been treated with clonidine or dopaminergic agents,[135] though only the latter has been subjected to any study. The intriguing connection between RLS and ADHD has opened the question of whether some cases of ADHD can be managed by treating RLS.[135] In pregnancy, anemia, iron deficiency, or folate deficiency[53] may contribute to RLS and these can often be alleviated with reduction of RLS symptoms. Most RLS agents have been subjected to relatively little study in pregnancy, but some dopaminergic agents and opioids may be less risky than other medications (see review,[136] for listing). None of the medications can be given a completely clear endorsement. In any case, the risks of treatment need to be balanced against the problems of RLS symptoms, including potential impact of these symptoms on the fetus.

Treatment with specific agents

Levodopa In general, dopaminergic agents have become the drugs of choice for primary treatment of most cases of RLS in the 1990s. While levodopa and dopamine agonists have dominated recent therapeutic trials in RLS and PLMD, even amantadine[139] and selegiline have been reported to be useful. The one class of medications used in PD that has not been reported to benefit RLS or PLMD are the anticholinergics. Indeed, antidepressants with anticholinergic effects may actually increase PLM[140] and RLS. Treatment with dopaminergic agents usually involves considerably lower doses than those typical of PD. Because of this (and perhaps because of the largely intact striato-nigral system in RLS patients), the long-term complications of PD treatment (dyskinesias, psychosis) seem to be rare in RLS and PLMD. More problematic for RLS and PLMD patients may be the short-term complications (GI disturbance, hypotension, headache). The first dopaminergic agent to achieve widespread use in RLS was levodopa combined with a decarboxylase inhibitor. After initial reports of benefit,[141,142] long-term studies found persistent usefulness.[143] It became apparent, however, that levodopa with its short half-life often did not offer all night symptom relief. End-of-dose rebound led to morning symptoms.[124] More seriously, levodopa also results in a worsening of symptoms when blood levels decline during the day. This phenomenon, called augmentation,[125] involves symptoms that begin earlier in the day, and are more severe, more easily provoked, and spread to previously uninvolved body parts (e.g. the arms). Augmentation occurs most often in more severe patients on higher doses. In patients with PLMD, augmentation could cause the emergence of initial RLS symptoms.[144] The problems of rebound and augmentation have led to certain limitations in treating patients with levodopa. First, where rebound is an issue, a sustained release levodopa formulation may work better than regular release.[145] Second, it is generally necessary to limit doses to 300 mg of levodopa per day or even 200 mg. Third, patients with daily RLS and symptoms that are especially severe are not candidates for levodopa monotherapy. Instead, dopamine agonists or other medications can be chosen. The rates of augmentation with dopamine agonists are lower and when augmentation occurs, it is more easily managed.[144,146] It is unclear whether non-dopaminergic medications can also cause augmentation.

Dopamine agonists A number of different dopamine agonists have been used in RLS. Bromocriptine, the earliest agonist approved in the United States, was first reported to be helpful.[126,147] As newer agonists have been introduced, they have also been tried in RLS. The most experience to date has been with pergolide, the second agonist approved, which has been studied in several double-blind trials.[148–150] A large scale multicenter international study of pergolide has now been completed in Europe and Australia.[151] Double-blind studies have either been completed or initiated with the newer agonists, pramipexole[128] and ropinirole. Other agonists not generally available in the United States have also been reported to be useful in RLS (cabergoline,[152] apomorphine,[153] talipexole,[154] DHEC (alpha-dihydroeryocryptine),[155] piribedil[156]). The general approach to treating RLS with agonists is common for each of the available agents. First, it is important to start with a low dose and gradually increase it. This both avoids the most severe side effects and ensures that an adequate dose level is not missed. Second, it is best to keep dose levels as low as is feasible. This will avoid high dose side effects and may also avoid the problem of augmentation. In Europe, dopamine agonist therapy is usually begun with domperidone, a peripheral blocker, which reduces the various systemic side effects of the agonists. In the United States, this medication is not approved, but it can be obtained from Canada by individual patients if needed. Third, dosage schedule may vary depending on the timing of symptoms and the half-life of the medication. While agonists may be administered as a single dose an hour or so before bedtime, patients with daytime or evening symptoms may need multiple doses. Selecting the most appropriate agonist poses as yet unresolved questions. Bromocriptine, which was the first agonist used,[126] has fallen out of favor. While there are no studies to show that it is not effective, the published information about bromocriptine is not as impressive as that for other agonists. The newer agonists, pramipexole and ropinirole, are non-ergot derived. This may give them a slight edge, compared to pergolide, in that their side effects may be somewhat less problematic. Pergolide, for example, has been reported to cause fibrosis in an RLS patient.[157] On the other hand, pergolide has been the best studied agonist[146,158,159] and has been used in both idiopathic and secondary RLS patients.[160,161] It has also been used in children.[135] Cabergoline is not marketed for RLS or PD in the United States and is quite expensive there; it is more readily available in Europe. Another factor in dopamine agonist treatment is the possibility of inducing excessive daytime sleepiness, including sleep attacks. This may be more common with pramapexole and ropinirole.[162,163] Restless legs syndrome patients have been noted clinically to have relatively little daytime sleepiness, despite their sometime severe sleep deprivation. However, they may develop sleepiness once their RLS is treated and higher dose dopamine agonist therapy can also lead to sleep attacks, although this has not been as common a problem as in PD. Typical daily doses of agonists for RLS therapy have been: bromocriptine 5–20 mg; pergolide, 0.1–1.0 mg; pramipexole 0.25–1.5 mg; and ropinirole 0.5–6 mg. As this indicates, there is a fairly wide range of doses that may be helpful, although not generally reaching into the higher ranges of PD doses.

Opioids Despite the long history of opioid use in RLS and its common use currently, there have been relatively few studies of opioids. In one double-blind study,[164] oxycodone was found to have statistically significant benefit relative to placebo in subjective ratings of RLS symptoms, PLM, and sleep efficiency. In another, smaller comparative study,[165] a much weaker opioid, propoxyphene, was not as effective as levodopa in reducing markers of RLS. Most recently, a mixed opioid/serotoninergic agent, tramadol,[166] was found in an open trial to have subjective benefit RLS. As most RLS studies, all of these were short-term trials, but a recent multicenter investigation[167] has found that RLS can in some cases be managed by opioid monotherapy. Given this paucity of published studies, the use of opioids must be governed by clinical experience. Among the basic uses of opioids are intermittent treatment manageable by prn treatment, patients for whom dopaminergic treatment is inadequate, Parkinson's disease patients whose RLS persists on dopaminergic treatment,[168] and patients refractory to other medications. It has been widely recognized that the stronger opioids often can offer relief to the most severe RLS patients not adequately managed by other medications. A strength of opioids is their alleviation of waking RLS symptoms; their benefits for PLM may be less impressive.[165,169] One advantage of the opioids is the wide range of potencies. Medications that have been used widely include milder agents such as codeine, propoxyphene, or tramadal, moderate strength agents such as hydrocodone and oxycodone, and stronger agents such as levorphanol or methadone. Typical doses are similar to those used for chronic pain, but dose timing should be adjusted to RLS symptoms. Other opioid agents, such as fentanyl patches, hydromorphone, and sustained release preparations have rarely been used, but might also be considered in appropriate contexts. Among the considerations in opioid therapy are patient acceptance and characteristics. While addiction is rarely a problem with opioids given for RLS, it may pose a risk to predisposed individuals. And although withdrawal is only rarely a major problem with RLS patients, sudden cessation of treatment can provoke a brisk reactivation of RLS symptoms and, even milder opioids can sometimes provoke a more typical opioid withdrawal.[133] Side effects can also constrain therapy. Constipation or urinary retention may be particularly troublesome for certain patients. Respiratory disturbance during sleep may also occur; perhaps exacerbated by long-term treatment.[167] Patients on long-term treatment need to be monitored for development of nocturnal respiratory disturbances. Augmentation, a major limitation on dopaminergic treatment, has not emerged as a significant problem with opioids. Other CNS problems associated with opioids such as sleepiness, confusion, and affective changes also need to be monitored. One drawback of using the opioids for those prescribing them, are the varied State rules for use of these largely controlled substances. However, many, if not most, physicians treating large populations of RLS patients find that the opioids are a valuable therapeutic resource, indispensable to some patients.

Benzodiazepines The benzodiazepines seem to be useful for treatment of both RLS and PLMD. Their greatest therapeutic strength is in improving the quality of sleep and reducing its fragmentation. The degree to which they benefit waking symptoms of RLS is not well established. Their impact on PLM is modest compared to dopaminergic agents and opioids, although some studies have shown significant decreases.[170,171] The greatest experience with the benzodiazepines is with clonazepam, which was introduced in the late 1970s as a treatment for both RLS[172] and PLMS.[173] This development emerged from its success as a treatment for myoclonus. Other benzodiazepines were introduced more recently.[174,175] There has been no systematic evaluation of different benzo-

diazepines in these conditions and, therefore, no clear-cut rationale for selecting one agent over another, except that there is the most experience with clonazepam. Despite its long half-life, some experts have found that patients can do well for years on low doses.[176] One additional benefit of clonazepam is that it may treat related motor sleep disorders, such as REM behavior disorder, which are more common in older patients and may coexist with RLS or PLMD. Clonazepam has also been reported as a suitable treatment for uremic patients with RLS.[177] For those who cannot tolerate clonazepam build-up, a shorter half-life benzodiazepine may be selected, but some (e.g. triazolam) may have too short a half-life to cover symptoms throughout the night. Benzodiazepines are generally used in single doses shortly before bedtime. Doses for daytime treatment of RLS are less well established. Diazepam has also been for daytime symptoms: a typical dose might be 5 mg twice a day. In general, where there is a need to cover daytime symptoms, another class of agents is probably preferred. Typically, clonazepam, in doses of 0.5–4 mg; temazepam, in doses of 15–30 mg; and triazolam,[175] in doses of 0.125–0.5 mg are taken at bedtime. Drawbacks include the potential for confusion or daytime sleepiness, especially in older patients. Respiratory depression may also be a problem, though in one series even patients with nocturnal respiratory disturbance tolerated benzodiazepines well.

Anti-convulsants The first anti-convulsant used in RLS was carbamazepine: it was shown to be beneficial in a large-scale double blind trial.[178] However, this study only used clinical monitoring. In a polysomnographic study, it was found to benefit subjective symptoms, sleep latency and sleep efficiency, but not PLMS.[179] However, one recent case study found carbamazepine useful in a severe case of PLMS.[180] This experience led to its use being endorsed by the AASM as a guideline in RLS therapy. Despite this, most experts currently feel that carbamazepine is not as useful as other agents and rarely resort to it.

In the last few years, gabapentin has been reported in open trials to be a successful medication for RLS.[181–185] It appears to be most useful in cases of RLS whose disturbing sensations seem truly painful and to work best in mild to moderate cases. It has also been reported to be helpful to uremic patients.[186] Other anti-convulsants such as valproic acid[187] or lamotrigine[188] have also been reported to be effective in some cases. Lamotrigine should be gradually titrated to avoid possible serious skin or systemic reactions.

Anticonvulsants can be used as monotherapy to cover all symptoms of RLS or in cases of PLMD. RLS patients are generally treated with divided doses, thereby covering daytime symptoms, while PLMD patients are given medications at night only. Patients may respond to doses lower than those commonly used to treat seizures; as is generally true in RLS, it is helpful to increase doses slowly so as not to miss a therapeutic window. However, doses in the usual therapeutic range for seizures are often reached in RLS.

Additional therapies Clonidine, a centrally active alpha adrenergic blocker, has been reported to be effective in both idiopathic[189] and uremic RLS patients.[190] A double-blind study reported that clonidine had a significant benefit in RLS, especially upon waking symptoms and sleep latency.[191] Clonidine seems useful mostly for patients whose symptoms are only prominent in the period just before sleep. Doses of 0.1–0.7 mg a day were used to obtain benefit in most cases. The newer sedatives, zolpidem, zopiclone, and zaleplon, may have a similar use in RLS and PLMD and they are currently prescribed to some patients. However, their benefits for RLS and PLMD have never been established in refereed publications. Zaleplon has a very short half-life and would most likely be useful only for those patients who have difficulty initiating sleep or when patients wake during the middle of the night. Another drug is baclofen, which was found in one small double-blind study to reduce arousal related to PLMS, primarily by decreasing the response to movements. It appeared to decrease the intensity, but not the frequency of movements:[192] indeed, frequency increased at all effective doses. Its effect on RLS waking symptoms is not clear. There have been a few cases in which either intrathecal morphine or spinal stimulators were found to assist RLS patients. Beyond these medications, a variety of sedatives and non-opioid analgesics have sometimes been used to reduce RLS symptoms. Melatonin, which has occasionally been used in RLS without report, has been reported to reduce PLMS.[193] Anti-depressants, while reported to increase RLS and PLMS, have also sometimes been used to treat them.[194,195] In one recent study, buproprion was found to reduce PLMS in depressed patients, perhaps because of its dopamine enhancing action.[196]

References

1. Willis T. Two discourses concerning the soul of brutes. London: Dring, Harper, and Leigh, 1683
2. Ekbom KA. Restless legs: a clinical study. Acta Med Scand (Suppl) 1945;158:1–122
3. Ekbom KA. Restless legs syndrome. Neurology 1960; 10:868–873
4. Diagnostic Classification Steering Committee of the American Sleep Disorders Association (MJ Thorpy, Chairperson). The international classification of sleep disorders: diagnostic and coding manual. Rochester, Minnesota: American Sleep Disorders Association, 1997:396
5. The International Restless Legs Syndrome Study Group (Arthur S. Walters MD, Group Organizer and Correspondent). Towards a better definition of the restless legs syndrome. Mov Disord 1995;10: 634–642
6. Symonds CP. Nocturnal myoclonus. J Neurol Neurosurg Psychiatr 1953;16:166–171
7. Lugaresi E, Coccagna G, Berti Ceroni G, Ambrosetto C. Restless legs syndrome and nocturnal myoclonus. *In:* Gastaut H, Lugaresi E, Berti Ceroni G, Coccagna G, eds. The abnormalities of sleep in man. Bologna: Aulo Gaggi Editore, 1968:285–294
8. Guilleminault C, Raynal D, Weitzman ED, Dement WC. Sleep-related periodic myoclonus in patients complaining of insomnia. Trans Am Neurol Assoc 1975;100:19–21
9. Coleman RM, Pollak CP, Weitzman ED. Periodic movements in sleep (nocturnal myoclonus): relation to sleep disorders. Ann Neurol 1980;8:416–421
10. Boghen D, Peyronnard JM. Myoclonus in familial restless legs syndrome. Arch Neurol 1976;33:368–370
11. Recording and scoring leg movements. The Atlas Task Force. Sleep 1993;16:748–759
12. Mendelson WB. Are periodic leg movements associated with clinical sleep disturbance? [See comments]. Sleep 1996;19:219–223
13. Montplaisir J, Michaud M, Denesle R, Gosselin A. Periodic leg movements are not more prevalent in insomnia or hypersomnia but are specifically associated with sleep disorders involving a dopaminergic impairment. Sleep Med 2000;1:163–167
14. Lavigne GJ, Montplaisir JY. Restless legs syndrome and sleep bruxism: prevalence and association among Canadians. Sleep 1994;17:739–743
15. National Sleep Foundation. Sleep in America 1995: National Sleep Foundation Gallup Poll. Washington, D.C., 1995
16. National Sleep Foundation. Sleep in America 2000: National Sleep Foundation Omnibus Poll. Washington, D.C.: National Sleep Foundation, 2000
17. Phillips B, Young T, Finn L, et al. Epidemiology of restless legs symptoms in adults. Arch Intern Med 2000;160:2137–2141
18. Ulfberg J, Nystrom B, Carter N, Edling C. Restless legs syndrome among working-aged women. Eur Neurol 2001;46:17–19
19. Rothdach AJ, Trenkwalder C, Haberstock J, et al. Prevalence and risk factors of RLS in an elderly population: the MEMO study. Memory and Morbidity in Augsburg Elderly. Neurology 2000;54:1064–1068
20. Miranda M, Araya F, Castillo JL, et al. Restless legs syndrome: a clinical study in adult general population and in uremic patients. Rev Med Chil 2001;129:179–186
21. Kageyama T, Kabuto M, Nitta H, et al. Prevalences of periodic limb movement-like and restless legs-like symptoms among Japanese adults. Psychiatry Clin Neurosci 2000;54:296–298
22. Tan EK, Seah A, See SJ, et al. Restless legs syndrome in an Asian population: a study in Singapore. Mov Disord 2001;16:577–579
23. Kazenwadel J, Pollmacher T, Trenkwalder C, et al. New actigraphic assessment method for periodic leg movements (PLM). Sleep 1995;18:689–697
24. Gorny S, Allen R, Krausman D, Earley C. Accuracy of the PAM-RL system for automated detection of periodic leg movements (Abstract). Sleep 1998;21:S183
25. Sforza E, Zamagni M, Petiav C, Krieger J. Actigraphy and leg movements during sleep: a validation study. J Clin Neurophysiol 1999;16:154–160
26. Ancoli-Israel S, Kripke DF, Klauber MR, et al. Periodic limb movements in sleep in community-dwelling elderly. Sleep 1991;14:496–500
27. Hening WA, Allen R, Walters AS, Chokroverty S. Motor functions and dysfunctions of sleep. *In:* Chokroverty S, ed. Sleep disorders medicine. Boston: Butterworth-Heinemann, 1999:441–507
28. Winkelman JW, Chertow GM, Lazarus JM. Restless legs syndrome in end-stage renal disease. Am J Kidney Dis 1996;28:372–378
29. Collado-Seidel V, Kohnen R, Samtleben W, et al. Clinical and biochemical findings in uremic patients with

and without restless legs syndrome. Am J Kidney Dis 1998;31:324–328

30. Hui DS, Wong TY, Ko FW, et al. Prevalence of sleep disturbances in Chinese patients with end-stage renal failure on continuous ambulatory peritoneal dialysis. Am J Kidney Dis 2000;36:783–788

31. McParland P, Pearce JM. Restless legs syndrome in pregnancy. Case reports. Clin Exp Obstet Gynecol 1990;17:5–6

32. Goodman JD, Brodie C, Ayida GA. Restless legs syndrome in pregnancy. Brit Med J 1988;297:1101–1102

33. Wetter TC, Stiasny K, Kohnen R, et al. Polysomnographic sleep measures in patients with uremic and idiopathic restless legs syndrome. Mov Disord 1998; 13:820–824

34. Gorman CA, Dyck PJ, Pearson JS. Symptoms of restless legs. Arch Intern Med 1965;115:155–160

35. Rutkove SB, Matheson JK, Logigian EL. Restless legs syndrome in patients with polyneuropathy. Muscle Nerve 1996;19:670–672

36. Gemignani F, Marbini A, Di Giovanni G, et al. Cryoglobulinaemic neuropathy manifesting with restless legs syndrome. J Neurol Sci 1997;152:218–223

37. O'Hare JA, Abuaisha F, Geoghegan M. Prevalence and forms of neuropathic morbidity in 800 diabetics. Ir J Med Sci 1994;163:132–135

38. Salih AM, Gray RE, Mills KR, Webley M. A clinical, serological and neurophysiological study of restless legs syndrome in rheumatoid arthritis. Br J Rheumatol 1994;33:60–63

39. Salvi F, Montagna P, Plasmati R, et al. Restless legs syndrome and nocturnal myoclonus: initial manifestation of familial amyloid polyneuropathy. J Neurol Neurosurg Psychiatry 1990;53:522–525

40. Abele M, Burk K, Laccone F, et al. Restless legs syndrome in spinocerebellar ataxia types 1, 2, and 3. J Neurol 2001;248:311–314

41. Schols L, Haan J, Riess O, et al. Sleep disturbance in spinocerebellar ataxias: is the SCA3 mutation a cause of restless legs syndrome? Neurology 1998;51: 1603–1607

42. van Alfen N, Sinke RJ, Zwarts MJ, et al. Intermediate CAG repeat lengths (53, 54) for MJD/SCA3 are associated with an abnormal phenotype. Ann Neurol 2001; 49:805–807

43. Gemignani F, Marbini A, Di Giovanni G, et al. Charcot-Marie-Tooth disease type 2 with restless legs syndrome. Neurology 1999;52:1064–1066

44. Montplaisir J, Boucher S, Poirier G, et al. Clinical, polysomnographic, and genetic characteristics of restless legs syndrome: a study of 133 patients diagnosed with new standard criteria. Mov Disord 1997;12: 61–65

45. Montplaisir J, Boucher S, Nicolas A, et al. Immobilization tests and periodic leg movements in sleep for the diagnosis of restless leg syndrome. Mov Disord 1998;13:324–329

46. Schenck CH, Mahowald MW. Motor dyscontrol in narcolepsy: rapid-eye-movement (REM) sleep without atonia and REM sleep behavior disorder. Ann Neurol 1992;32:3–10

47. Schenck CH, Mahowald MW. Polysomnographic, neurologic, psychiatric, and clinical outcome report on 70 consecutive cases with REM sleep behavior disorder (RBD): sustained clonazepam efficacy in 89.5% of 57 cases. Cleve Clin J Med 1990;57(Suppl):S9–S23

48. Wetter TC, Collado-Seidel V, Pollmacher T, et al. Sleep and periodic leg movement patterns in drug-free patients with Parkinson's disease and multiple system atrophy. Sleep 2000;23:361–367

49. Ancoli-Israel S, Martin J, Jones DW, et al. Sleep-disordered breathing and periodic limb movements in sleep in older patients with schizophrenia. Biol Psychiatry 1999;45:1426–1432

50. Earley CJ, Allen RP, Beard JL, Connor JR. Insight into the pathophysiology of restless legs syndrome. J Neurosci Res 2000;62:623–628

51. O'Keeffe ST, Gavin K, Lavan JN. Iron status and restless legs syndrome in the elderly. Age Ageing 1994;23: 200–233

52. Sun ER, Chen CA, Ho G, Earley CJ, Allen RP. Iron and the restless legs syndrome. Sleep 1998;21:371–377

53. Lee KA, Zaffke ME, Baratte-Beebe K. Restless legs syndrome and sleep disturbance during pregnancy: the role of folate and iron. J Womens Health Gend Based Med 2001;10:335–341

54. Winkelmann J, Trenkwalder C. Pathophysiology of restless-legs syndrome. Review of current research. Nervenarzt 2001;72:100–107

55. Staedt J, Stoppe G, Kogler A, et al. Nocturnal myoclonus syndrome (periodic movements in sleep) related to central dopamine D_2-receptor alteration. Eur Arch Psychiatry Clin Neurosci 1995;245:8–10

56. Turjanski N, Lees AJ, Brooks DJ. Striatal dopaminergic function in restless legs syndrome: ^{18}F-dopa and ^{11}C-raclopride PET studies. Neurology 1999;52:932–937

57. Ruottinen HM, Partinen M, Hublin C, et al. An F-dopa PET study in patients with periodic limb movement disorder and restless legs syndrome. Neurology 2000; 54:502–504

58. Earley CJ, Hyland K, Allen RP. CSF dopamine, serotonin, and biopterin metabolites in patients with restless legs syndrome. Mov Disord 2001;16:144–149

59. Alberts JL, Adler CH, Saling M, Stelmach GE. Prehension patterns in restless legs syndrome patients. Parkinsonism Relat Disord 2001;7:143–148

60. Earley CJ, Connor JR, Beard JL, et al. Abnormalities in CSF concentrations of ferritin and transferrin in restless legs syndrome. Neurology 2000;54:1698–1700

61. Allen RP, Barker PB, Wehrl F, et al. MRI measurement of brain iron in patients with restless legs syndrome. Neurology 2001;56:263–265

62. Iannaccone S, Zucconi M, Marchettini P, et al. Evidence of peripheral axonal neuropathy in primary restless legs syndrome. Mov Disord 1995;10:2–9

63. Polydefkis M, Allen RP, Hauer P, et al. Subclinical sensory neuropathy in late-onset restless legs syndrome. Neurology 2000;55:1115–1121

64. Walters A, Hening W, Cote L, Fahn S. Dominantly inherited restless legs with myoclonus and periodic movements of sleep: a syndrome related to the endogenous opiates? Adv Neurol 1986;43:309–319

65. Montplaisir J, Lorrain D, Godbout R. Restless legs syndrome and periodic leg movements in sleep: the primary role of dopaminergic mechanism. Eur Neurol 1991;31:41–43

66. Bucher SF, Seelos KC, Oertel WH, et al. Cerebral generators involved in the pathogenesis of the restless legs syndrome. Ann Neurol 1997;41:639–645

67. de Mello MT, Lauro FA, Silva AC, Tufik S. Incidence of periodic leg movements and of the restless legs syndrome during sleep following acute physical activity in spinal cord injury subjects. Spinal Cord 1996;34: 294–296

68. Hartmann M, Pfister R, Pfadenhauer K. Restless legs syndrome associated with spinal cord lesions

[letter]. J Neurol Neurosurg Psychiatry 1999;66: 688–689

69. Yokota T, Hirose K, Tanabe H, Tsukagoshi H. Sleep-related periodic leg movements (nocturnal myoclonus) due to spinal cord lesion. J Neurol Sci 1991;104:13–18

70. Lee MS, Choi YC, Lee SH, Lee SB. Sleep-related periodic leg movements associated with spinal cord lesions. Mov Disord 1996;11:719–722

71. Trenkwalder C, Bucher SF, Oertel WH. Electrophysiological pattern of involuntary limb movements in the restless legs syndrome. Muscle Nerve 1996;19:155–162

72. Provini F, Vetrugno R, Meletti S, et al. Motor pattern of periodic limb movements during sleep. Neurology 2001;57:300–304

73. Bara-Jimenez W, Aksu M, Graham B, et al. Periodic limb movements in sleep: state-dependent excitability of the spinal flexor reflex. Neurology 2000;54: 1609–1616

74. Lindvall O, Björklund A, Skagerberg G. Dopamine-containing neurons in the spinal cord: anatomy and some functional aspects. Ann Neurol 1983;14:255–260

75. Weil-Fugazza J, Godefroy F. Dorsal and ventral dopaminergic innervation of the spinal cord: functional implications. Brain Res Bull 1993;30:319–324

76. de Mello MT, Poyares DL, Tufik S. Treatment of periodic leg movements with a dopaminergic agonist in subjects with total spinal cord lesions. Spinal Cord 1999;37:634–637

77. Lugaresi E, Coccagna G, Montovani M, Lebrun R. Some periodic phenomena arising during drowsiness and sleep in man. Electroencephalogr Clin Neurophysiol 1972;32:701–705

78. Parrino L, Boselli M, Spaggiari MC, et al. Cyclic alternating pattern (CAP) in normal sleep: polysomnographic parameters in different age groups. Electroencephalogr Clin Neurophysiol 1998;107: 439–450

79. Ferri R, Parrino L, Smerieri A, et al. Cyclic alternating pattern and spectral analysis of heart rate variability during normal sleep. J Sleep Res 2000;9:13–18

80. Parrino L, Boselli M, Buccino GP, et al. The cyclic alternating pattern plays a gate-control on periodic limb movements during non-rapid eye movement sleep. J Clin Neurophysiol 1996;13:314–323

81. Winkelman JW. The evoked heart rate response to periodic leg movements of sleep. Sleep 1999;22: 575–580

82. Trenkwalder C, Seidel VC, Gasser T, Oertel WH. Clinical symptoms and possible anticipation in a large kindred of familial restless legs syndrome. Mov Disord 1996;11:389–394

83. Lazzarini A, Walters AS, Hickey K, et al. Studies of penetrance and anticipation in five autosomal-dominant restless legs syndrome pedigrees. Mov Disord 1999;14:111–116

84. Allen RP, LaBuda MC, Becker PM, Earley CJ. Family history study of RLS patients from two clinical populations (abstract). Sleep Res 1997;26

85. Winkelmann J, Wetter TC, Collado-Seidel V, et al. Clinical characteristics and frequency of the hereditary restless legs syndrome in a population of 300 patients. Sleep 2000;23:597–602

86. Ondo WG, Vuong KD, Wang Q. Restless legs syndrome in monozygotic twins: clinical correlates. Neurology 2000;55:1404–1406

87. Ondo W, Jankovic J. Restless legs syndrome: clinicoetiologic correlates. Neurology 1996;47:1435–1441

88. Winkelmann J, Muller-Myhsok B, Wittchen HU, et al. Complex segregation analysis of restless legs syndrome provides evidence for an autosomal dominant mode of inheritance in early age at onset families. Ann Neurol 2002;52(Suppl 3):297–302

89. Desautels A, Turecki G, Montplaisir J, et al. Identification of a major susceptibility locus for restless legs syndrome on chromosome 12q. Am J Hum Genet 2001;69(Suppl 6):1266–1270

90. Desautels A, Turecki G, Montplaisir J, et al. Evidence for genetic association between monoamine oxidase A and restless legs syndrome. Neurology 2002;59(Suppl 2):215–219

91. Tanner CM, Ottman R, Goldman SM, et al. Parkinson disease in twins: an etiologic study [see comments]. JAMA 1999;281:341–346

92. Picchietti DL, Underwood DJ, Farris WA, et al. Further studies on periodic limb movement disorder and restless legs syndrome in children with attention-deficit hyperactivity disorder. Mov Disord 1999;14:1000–1007

93. Allen RP, Earley CJ. Defining the phenotype of the restless legs syndrome (RLS) using age-of-symptom-onset. Sleep Med 2000;1:11–19

94. Nikkola E, Ekblad U, Ekholm E, et al. Sleep in multiple pregnancy: breathing patterns, oxygenation, and periodic leg movements. Am J Obstet Gynecol 1996;174: 1622–1625

95. Walters AS, Rosen R, Hening WA, et al. A test of the reliability and validity of a brief patient-completed severity questionnaire for the restless legs syndrome: the International RLS Study Group rating scale (abstract). Sleep 2001;24:In Press

96. Allen RP, Earley CJ. Validation of the Johns Hopkins restless legs severity scale. Sleep Med 2001;2:239–242

97. Chabli A, Michaud M, Montplaisir J. Periodic arm movements in patients with the restless legs syndrome. Eur Neurol 2000;44:133–138

98. Polysomnography Task Force: American Sleep Disorders Association Standards of Practice Committee. Practice parameters for the indications for polysomnography and related procedures. Sleep 1997;20: 406–422

99. Michaud M, Poirier G, Lavigne G, Montplaisir J. Restless legs syndrome: scoring criteria for leg movements recorded during the suggested immobilization test. Sleep Med 2001;2:317–321

100. Walters A, Hening W, Kavey N, et al. Restless legs syndrome: a pleomorphic sensorimotor disorder (abstract). Neurology 1984;34(Suppl 1):129

101. Smith RC. Relationship of periodic movements in sleep (nocturnal myoclonus) and the Babinski sign. Sleep 1985;8:239–243

102. Atlas Task Force. ASDA Report. EEG arousals: scoring rules and examples. Sleep 1992;15:173–184

103. Exar EN, Collop NA. The association of upper airway resistance with periodic limb movements. Sleep 2001;24:188–192

104. Sachdev P, Longragan C. The present status of akathisia. J Nerv Ment Dis 1991;179:381–391

105. Linazasoro G, Marti Masso JF, Suarez JA. Nocturnal akathisia in Parkinson's disease: treatment with clozapine. Mov Disord 1993;8:171–174

106. Comella CL, Goetz CG. Akathisia in Parkinson's disease. Mov Disord 1994;9:545–549

107. Sachdev P. Akathisia and restless legs. New York City: Cambridge University Press, 1995

108. Sachdev P. The development of the concept of akathisia: a historical overview. Schizophr Res 1995; 16:33–45

109. Poyurovsky M, Nave R, Epstein R, et al. Actigraphic monitoring (actigraphy) of circadian locomotor activity in schizophrenic patients with acute neuroleptic-induced akathisia. Eur Neuropsychopharmacol 2000; 10:171–176

110. Walters AS, Hening W, Rubinstein M, Chokroverty S. A clinical and polysomnographic comparison of neuroleptic-induced akathisia and the idiopathic restless legs syndrome. Sleep 1991;14:339–345

111. Havaki-Kontaxaki BJ, Kontaxakis VP, Christodoulou GN. Prevalence and characteristics of patients with pseudoakathisia. Eur Neuropsychopharmacol 2000;10: 333–336

112. Cheshire WP. Hypotensive akathisia: autonomic failure associated with leg fidgeting while sitting. Neurology 2000;55:1923–1926

113. Tan EK, Ondo WG. Motor restlessness. Int J Clin Pract 2001;55:320–322

114. Kanter AH. The effect of sclerotherapy on restless legs syndrome. Dermatol Surg 1995;21:328–332

115. Bradbury A, Evans C, Allan P, et al. What are the symptoms of varicose veins? Edinburgh vein study cross sectional population survey. BMJ 1999;318: 353–356

116. Layzer RB, Rowland LP. Cramps. N Engl J Med 1971; 285:31–40

117. Rowland LP. Cramps, spasms and muscle stiffness. Rev Neurol (Paris) 1985;141:261–273

118. Riley JD, Antony SJ. Leg cramps: differential diagnosis and management [see comments]. Am Fam Physician 1995;52:1794–1798

119. Abdulla AJ, Jones PW, Pearce VR. Leg cramps in the elderly: prevalence, drug and disease associations. Int J Clin Pract 1999;53:494–496

120. Leung AK, Wong BE, Chan PY, Cho HY. Nocturnal leg cramps in children: incidence and clinical characteristics. J Natl Med Assoc 1999;91:329–332

121. Dressler D, Thompson PD, Gledhill RF, Marsden CD. The syndrome of painful legs and moving toes. Mov Disord 1994;9:13–21

122. Aldrich MS, Jahnke B. Diagnostic value of video-EEG polysomnography. Neurology 1991;41:1060–1066

123. Guilleminault C, Philip P. Tiredness and somnolence despite initial treatment of obstructive sleep apnea syndrome (what to do when an OSAS patient stays hypersomnolent despite treatment). Sleep 1996;19:S117–S122

124. Guilleminault C, Cetel M, Philip P. Dopaminergic treatment of restless legs and rebound phenomenon. Neurology 1993;43:445

125. Allen RP, Earley CJ. Augmentation of the restless legs syndrome with carbidopa/levodopa. Sleep 1996;19: 205–213

126. Walters AS, Hening WA, Kavey N, et al. A double-blind randomized crossover trial of bromocriptine and placebo in restless legs syndrome. Ann Neurol 1988; 24:455–458

127. Wetter TC, Stiasny K, Winkelmann J, et al. A polysomnographic, controlled study of pergolide in the treatment of restless legs syndrome. Neurology 1998;50(Suppl):A69

128. Montplaisir J, Nicolas A, Denesle R, Gomez-Mancilla B. Restless legs syndrome improved by pramipexole: a double-blind randomized trial. Neurology 1999;52: 938–943

129. Ondo W. Ropinirole for restless legs syndrome [see comments]. Mov Disord 1999;14:138–140

130. Chesson AL Jr., Wise M, Davila D, et al. Practice parameters for the treatment of restless legs syndrome and periodic limb movement disorder. An American Academy of Sleep Medicine Report. Standards of Practice Committee of the American Academy of Sleep Medicine. Sleep 1999;22:961–968

131. Zarcone VP Jr. Sleep hygiene. In: Kryger MH, Roth T, Dement WC, eds. Principles and practice of sleep medicine. Philadelphia: W. B. Saunders, 2000:657–661

132. Yasuda T, Nishimura A, Katsuki Y, Tsuji Y. Restless legs syndrome treated successfully by kidney transplantation. A case report. Clin Transplants 1986:138

133. Freye E, Levy J. Acute abstinence syndrome following abrupt cessation of long-term use of tramadol (Ultram): a case study. Eur J Pain 2000;4:307–311

134. Hening WA. Restless legs syndrome: diagnosis and treatment. Hosp Med 1997;33:54–56, 61–66, 68, 73, 75

135. Walters AS, Mandelbaum DE, Lewin DS, et al. Dopaminergic therapy in children with restless legs/periodic limb movements in sleep and ADHD. Dopaminergic Therapy Study Group. Pediatr Neurol 2000;22:182–186

136. Hening W, Allen R, Earley C, et al. The treatment of restless legs syndrome and periodic limb movement disorder. An American Academy of Sleep Medicine Review. Sleep 1999;22:970–999

137. Earley CJ. Hemochromatosis and iron therapy of restless legs syndrome. Sleep Med 2001;2:181–183

138. Barton JC, Wooten VD, Acton RT. Hemochromatosis and iron therapy of restless legs syndrome. Sleep Med 2001;2:249–251

139. Evidente VG, Adler CH, Caviness JN, et al. Amantadine is beneficial in restless legs syndrome. Mov Disord 2000;15:324–327

140. Garvey MJ, Tollefson GD. Occurrence of myoclonus in patients treated with tricyclic antidepressants. Arch Gen Psychiatr 1987;44:269–272

141. Akpinar S. Treatment of restless legs syndrome with levodopa plus benserazide. Arch Neurol 1982;39:739

142. Montplaisir J, Godbout R, Poirier G, Bédard MA. Restless legs syndrome and periodic movements in sleep: Physiopathology and treatment with L-dopa. Clin Neuropharmacol 1986;9:456–463

143. Becker PM, Jamieson AO, Brown WD. Dopaminergic agents in restless legs syndrome and periodic limb movements of sleep: response and complications of extended treatment in 49 cases. Sleep 1993;16:713–716

144. Earley CJ, Allen RP. Pergolide and carbidopa/levodopa treatment of the restless legs syndrome and periodic leg movements in sleep in a consecutive series of patients. Sleep 1996;19:801–810

145. Collado-Seidel V, Kazenwadel J, Wetter TC, et al. A controlled study of additional sr-L-dopa in L-dopa-responsive restless legs syndrome with late-night symptoms. Neurology 1999;52:285–290

146. Silber MH, Shepard JW Jr., Wisbey JA. Pergolide in the management of restless legs syndrome: an extended study. Sleep 1997;20:878–882

147. Akpinar S. Restless legs syndrome treatment with dopaminergic drugs. Clin Neuropharmacol 1987;10: 69–79

148. Staedt J, Wassmuth F, Ziemann U, et al. Pergolide: treatment of choice in restless legs syndrome (RLS) and nocturnal myoclonus syndrome (NMS). A double-blind randomized crossover trial of pergolide versus L-dopa. J Neural Transm 1997;104:461–468

149. Earley CJ, Yaffee JB, Allen RP. Randomized, double-blind, placebo-controlled trial of pergolide in restless legs syndrome. Neurology 1998;51:1599–1602

150. Wetter TC, Stiasny K, Winkelmann J, et al. A random-

ized controlled study of pergolide in patients with restless legs syndrome [see comments]. Neurology 1999;52:944–950

151. Trenkwalder C, Brandenburg U, Hundemer H-P, et al. A randomized long-term placebo-controlled multicenter trial of pergolide in the treatment of RLS—the PEARLS-Study (abstract). Neurology 2001; 56(Suppl 3):A5

152. Stiasny K, Robbecke J, Schuler P, Oertel WH. Treatment of idiopathic restless legs syndrome (RLS) with the D$_2$-agonist cabergoline—an open clinical trial. Sleep 2000;23:349–354

153. Reuter I, Ellis CM, Ray Chaudhuri K. Nocturnal subcutaneous apomorphine infusion in Parkinson's disease and restless legs syndrome. Acta Neurol Scand 1999;100:163–167

154. Inoue Y, Mitani H, Nanba K, Kawahara R. Treatment of periodic leg movement disorder and restless leg syndrome with talipexole. Psychiatry Clin Neurosci 1999;53:283–285

155. Tergau F, Wischer S, Wolf C, Paulus W. Treatment of restless legs syndrome with the dopamine agonist alpha-dihydroergocryptine. Mov Disord 2001;16: 731–735

156. Evidente VG. Piribedil for restless legs syndrome: a pilot study. Mov Disord 2001;16:579–581

157. Danoff SK, Grasso ME, Terry PB, Flynn JA. Pleuropulmonary disease due to pergolide use for restless legs syndrome. Chest 2001;120:313–316

158. Winkelmann J, Wetter TC, Stiasny K, et al. Treatment of restless legs syndrome with pergolide—an open clinical trial. Mov Disord 1998;13:566–569

159. Stiasny K, Wetter TC, Winkelmann J, et al. Long-term effects of pergolide in the treatment of restless legs syndrome. Neurology 2001;56:1399–1402

160. Pieta J, Millar T, Zacharias J, et al. Effect of pergolide on restless legs and leg movements in sleep in uremic patients. Sleep 1998;21:617–622

161. Brown LK, Heffner JE, Obbens EA. Transverse myelitis associated with restless legs syndrome and periodic movements of sleep responsive to an oral dopaminergic agent but not to intrathecal baclofen. Sleep 2000;23:591–594

162. Frucht S, Rogers JD, Greene PE, et al. Falling asleep at the wheel: motor vehicle mishaps in persons taking pramipexole and ropinirole [see comments]. Neurology 1999;52:1908–1910

163. Hauser RA, Gauger L, Anderson WM, Zesiewicz TA. Pramipexole-induced somnolence and episodes of daytime sleep. Mov Disord 2000;15:658–663

164. Walters AS, Wagner ML, Hening WA, et al. Successful treatment of the idiopathic restless legs syndrome in a randomized double-blind trial of oxycodone versus placebo. Sleep 1993;16:327–332

165. Kaplan PW, Allen RP, Buchholz DW, Walters JK. A double-blind, placebo-controlled study of the treatment of periodic limb movements in sleep using carbidopa/levodopa and propoxyphene. Sleep 1993;16: 717–723

166. Lauerma H, Markkula J. Treatment of restless legs syndrome with tramadol: an open study. J Clin Psychiatry 1999;60:241–244

167. Walters AS, Winkelmann J, Trenkwalder C, et al. Long-term follow-up on restless legs syndrome patients treated with opioids. Mov Disord 2001;16: 1105–1109

168. Fazzini E, Diaz R, Fahn S. Restless leg in Parkinson's disease—clinical evidence for underactivity of catecholamine neurotransmission. Ann Neurol 1989;26:142

169. Kavey N, Walters AS, Hening W, Gidro-Frank S. Opioid treatment of periodic movements in sleep in patients without restless legs. Neuropeptides 1988;11: 181–184

170. Ohanna N, Peled R, Rubin AHE. Periodic leg movements in sleep: effect of clonazepam treatment. Neurology 1985;35:408–411

171. Horiguchi J, Inami Y, Sasaki A, et al. Periodic leg movements in sleep with restless legs syndrome: effect of clonazepam treatment. Jpn J Psychiatry Neurol 1992;46:727–732

172. Matthews WB. Treatment of restless legs syndrome with clonazepam. Br Med J 1979;1:751

173. Oshtory MA, Vijayan N. Clonazepam treatment of insomnia due to sleep myoclonus. Arch Neurol 1980; 37:119–120

174. Mitler MM, Browman CP, Menh SJ, et al. Nocturnal myoclonus: treatment efficacy of clonazepam and temazepam. Sleep 1986;9:385–392

175. Bonnet MH, Arand DL. The use of triazolam in older patients with periodic leg movements, fragmented sleep, and daytime sleepiness. J Gerontol: Med Sci 1990;45:139–144

176. Schenck CH, Mahowald MW. Long-term, nightly benzodiazepine treatment of injurious parasomnias and other disorders of disrupted nocturnal sleep in 170 adults. Am J Med 1996;100:333–337

177. Read D, Feest T, Nassim M. Clonazepam: effective treatment for restless legs syndrome in uremia. Br Med J 1981;283:885–886

178. Telstad W, Sørensen O, Larsen S, et al. Treatment of the restless legs syndrome with carbamazepine: a double blind study. Br Med J 1984;288:444–446

179. Zucconi M, Coccagna G, Petronelli R, et al. Nocturnal myoclonus in restless legs syndrome: effect of carbamazepine treatment. Funct Neurol 1989;4:263–271

180. Laschewski F, Sanner B, Konermann M, et al. Pronounced hypersomnia in a 13-year-old patient with periodic leg movements. Pneumologie 1997;51(Suppl 3):725–728

181. Mellick GA, Mellick LB. Management of restless legs syndrome with gabapentin (Neurontin) [letter]. Sleep 1996;19:224–226

182. Allen RP, Earley CJ. An open label clinical trial with structured subjective reports and objective leg activity measures comparing gabapentin with alternative treatment in the restless legs syndrome. Sleep Res 1996; 25:184

183. Adler CH. Treatment of restless legs syndrome with gabapentin. Clin Neuropharmacol 1997;20:148–151

184. Ehrenberg BL, Muller-Schwarze A, Frankel F. Open-label trial of gabapentin for periodic limb movement disorder of sleep. Neurology 1997;48:A278

185. Merren MD. Gabapentin for treatment of pain and tremor: a large case series. South Med J 1998;91: 739–744

186. Thorp ML, Morris CD, Bagby SP. A crossover study of gabapentin in treatment of restless legs syndrome among hemodialysis patients. Am J Kidney Dis 2001;38:104–108

187. Ehrenberg BL, Eisensehr I, Corbett KE, et al. Valproate for sleep consolidation in periodic limb movement disorder. J Clin Psychopharmacol 2000;20:574–578

188. Staedt J, Stoppe G, Riemann H, et al. Lamotrigine in the treatment of nocturnal myoclonus syndrome (NMS): two case reports. J Neural Transm 1996;103: 355–361

189. Handwerker JV, Palmer RF. Clonidine in the treatment

of restless legs syndrome. New Engl J Med 1985;313: 1228–1229

190. Cavatorta F, Vagge R, Solari P, Queirolo C. Risultati preliminari con clonidina nella sindrome delle gambe senza riposo in due pazienti uremici emodializzati. Min Urol Nefrol 1987;39:93

191. Wagner ML, Walters AS, Coleman RG, et al. Randomized, double-blind, placebo-controlled study of clonidine in restless legs syndrome. Sleep 1996;19:52–58

192. Guilleminault C, Flagg W. Effect of baclofen on sleep-related periodic leg movements. Ann Neurol 1984;15:234–239

193. Kunz D, Bes F. Exogenous melatonin in periodic limb movement disorder: an open clinical trial and a hypothesis. Sleep 2001;24:183–187

194. Sandyk R, Iacono RP, Bamford CR. Spinal cord mechanisms in amitriptyline responsive restless legs syndrome in Parkinson's disease. Int J Neurosci 1988; 38:121–124

195. Shaffer JI, Tallman JB, Boecker MR, et al. A report on the PLM suppressing properties of serotonin reuptake inhibitors. Sleep Res 1995;24:347

196. Nofzinger EA, Fasiczka A, Berman S, Thase ME. Bupropion SR reduces periodic limb movements associated with arousals from sleep in depressed patients with periodic limb movement disorder. J Clin Psychiatry 2000;61:858–862

252 Treatment of Hemifacial Spasm

Paul E Greene

Hemifacial spasm (HFS) is a disorder in which there are involuntary contractions on one side of the face in muscles innervated by the facial nerve (cranial nerve VII). According to Digre and Corbett, the condition was first described in 1875 by Schultze, but was first separated from other forms of facial twitching by Gowers in 1888.[1-3] According to Ehni and Woltman, the clue to the peripheral etiology of the condition came with the observation by Habel in 1898 of a woman whose HFS persisted after she developed an ipsilateral hemiparesis from a stroke, whereupon Babinski hypothesized that the spasms originated in the facial nucleus or facial nerve.[4-6] Hemifacial spasm is rare in this country. The incidence was 0.78 per 100 000 per year in Olmsted County, Minnesota between 1960 and 1984, which was 3% of the incidence of Bell's palsy (25.2 per 100 000).[7]

The etiology of HFS is thought to be compression of the facial nerve where it exits the brainstem (the root exit zone), usually by an aberrant artery, such as the anterior inferior cerebellar artery, posterior inferior cerebellar artery, or internal auditory artery.[1] Irritation of the nerve at this site is felt to generate spontaneous electrical activity, causing muscle contractions, and "cross-talk" or simultaneous activation of axons going to different parts of the face.[8] Rarely, HFS has been associated with compression of the facial nerve at the same location by arteriovenous malformations, aneurysms, tumors, bony overgrowths as in Paget's disease, or plaques of multiple sclerosis in the central myelin at the root exit zone.[1] Occasionally, HFS has been seen after Bell's palsy or other peripheral lesions of the facial nerve.[9] This has led to speculation that facial nerve compression induces a change in the facial nucleus, which is necessary for HFS to occur.[10] The likelihood of such a facial nucleus change would increase when the site of compression is closer to the nucleus. The majority of cases of HFS are sporadic, although there are occasional reports of familial cases.[11] However, HFS appears to be more common in the Orient, possibly because of a genetically based variation in vascular anatomy.[12]

The contractions in HFS take the form of individual muscle twitches, trains of twitches, and episodes of sustained muscle contraction produced by fusion of individual twitches.[13] These contractions diminish, but do not disappear, during sleep.[14] There are few other diseases that produce this picture. Facial dystonia is usually bilateral and does not produce muscle contractions which are synchronous in all involved muscles. The rippling movements of facial myokymia are often unilateral, but are not synchronous and are much slower than the twitching seen in HFS. Motor tics in the face may produce rapid twitching, but are usually suppressible and also do not produce synchronous muscle contractions. Synkinesis after Bell's palsy does produce synchronous contractions, but does not produce spontaneous contractions, except in patients developing HFS in addition to the synkinesis. Focal motor seizures are rarely limited to one side of the face, and would involve the masseter (cranial nerve V). All patients with HFS should have a magnetic resonance imaging (MRI) scan with attention to the posterior fossa, to identify patients with surgically accessible causes of facial nerve compression and the rare patients who develop tonic hemifacial contractions from brainstem multiple sclerosis or tumors.

Hemifacial spasm usually starts with twitching around the eye, but has spread to involve other seventh cranial nerve innervated muscles in most patients requesting treatment. As the disease progresses, trains of twitches become superimposed on individual twitches, and then episodes of sustained eyelid closure or tonic facial contraction may appear. A single large series concluded that HFS progressed very slowly, if at all, and had a benign outcome.[4] Although facial asymmetry is common, less than 15% of patients develop marked facial weakness, even when they have severe, sustained eyelid closure.[4]

Hemifacial spasm can be treated with medications, botulinum toxin (BTX) injections or by craniectomy and separation of an arterial loop from the root exit zone of the facial nerve (microvascular decompression). Medications are generally the least successful treatment. There is a single controlled study suggesting benefit from orphenadrine and dimethylaminoethanol,[15] but this treatment is rarely used today. Successful treatment of HFS in small numbers of patients has been reported with carbamazepine,[16-18] clonazepam,[19] baclofen,[20] gabapentin[21,22] and felbamate.[23] The success rate of these medications is low: improvement was "rare" in 218 patients treated with carbamazepine and 148 patients treated with phenytoin in one large series.[24] At our center, patients reported moderate to marked benefit in 19 of 87 trials with carbamazepine, clonazepam or baclofen, but benefit was not sustained in any of these cases (unpublished data). However, these series consisted of patients referred for BTX or surgery, presumably biased towards patients failing medical therapy.

Botulinum toxin blocks calcium mediated quantal release of acetylcholine, and BTX injections cause long lasting, but not permanent, muscle weakness. Botulinum toxin has proved useful in treating many forms of hyperkinetic movement disorders, including HFS.[25]

Table 252.1 Treatment of hemifacial spasm

Drug	Approach
Botulinum toxin injections	Titrate dose according to number of muscles requiring injection. Typical doses for the orbicularis oculi are 10–25 units. Doses for the face are more variable. Technique requires special training.
Microvascular decompression	Craniectomy
Anticonvulsants and baclofen	Rarely effective for long, but can be tried if botulinum toxin is ineffective and the patient does not wish to have surgery

In the largest published series, 546 of 592 patients (92.2%) reported moderate to excellent improvement after injection of 30 units around the eye and lower face (a unit is the LD_{50} for mice after intraperitoneal injection).[26] Benefit from BTX injections for HFS lasts 3–6 months, after which symptoms return and repeat injections are required. Botulinum toxin injections almost invariably eliminate spasms of the orbicularis oculi. However, significant facial weakness often limits benefit in lower facial muscles such as the zygomaticus major and risorius. The major side effects of BTX injections are ptosis and lower facial weakness, which may last from days to weeks. Other less common side effects include ecchymoses at the injection site, entropion of the lower lid, dry eye, excess tearing and bagginess under the eye. All side effects from BTX injections are transient. There is no evidence that chronic BTX injections induce any permanent change, and patients injected for HFS do not develop antibodies to BTX.

Microvascular decompression, first popularized by Janetta in the 1970s, appears to be the definitive treatment for HFS.[27] In the largest series published to date, 648 patients were followed for up to 20 years after the initial procedure.[24] Overall, 84% were felt to have an excellent response defined as over 98% absence of spasms. However, 61 of 648 patients (9.4%) required repeat operations, which were less likely to be successful. Serious complications (death, stroke or cerebellar hematoma) occurred in 0.9% of cases. Permanent facial weakness or hearing loss occurred in 7.4%. Other complications, including wound infection or hematoma, cerebrospinal fluid (CSF) leak, bacterial meningitis and pseudomeningocele occurred in 4.7% of cases. Other large series have reported similar results.[12,28] Vascular compression of the root exit zone of the facial nerve is not found in all cases, and some patients may have compression at more distal sites along the nerve.[29,30] Modern MRI techniques may allow preoperative identification of the site of compression and improve outcome.[31]

Despite the high success rate and relatively low complication rate of microvascular decompression, many patients prefer to avoid surgery if possible, and prefer periodic BTX injections as long as the results are satisfactory.

References

1. Digre K, Corbett JJ. Hemifacial spasm: differential diagnosis, mechanism, and treatment. Adv Neurol 1988; 49:151–176
2. Schultze F. Linksseitiger Facialiskrampf in folge eines Aneurysma der Arteria vertebralis sinsitra. Archiv f Pathol Anat 1875;65:385–391
3. Gowers WR. A Manual of Diseases of the Nervous System. Philadelphia: P Blakiston, 1888
4. Ehni G, Woltman HW. Hemifacial spasms: review of one hundred and six cases. Arch Neurol Psychiatry 1945;53:205–211
5. Habel A. Ueber Fortbestehen von Tic convulsif bei gleichseitiger Hemiplegie. Deutsche med Wchnschr 1898;24:189
6. Babinski. In: Gordon A. Convulsive movements of the face: their differential diagnosis; effect of alcohol injections. JAMA 1912;58:97–102
7. Auger RG, Whisnant JP. Hemifacial spasm in Rochester and Olmsted County, Minnesota, 1960 to 1984. Arch Neurol 1990;47:1233–1234
8. Nielsen VK. Pathophysiology of hemifacial spasm: I. Ephaptic transmission and ectopic excitation. Neurology 1984;34:418–426
9. Martinelli P, Giuliani S, Ippoliti M. Hemifacial spasm due to peripheral injury of facial nerve: a nuclear syndrome? Mov Disord 1992;7:181–184
10. Ferguson JH. Hemifacial spasm and the facial nucleus. Ann Neurol 1978;4:97–103
11. Micheli F, Scorticati MC, Gatto E, et al. Familial hemifacial spasm. Mov Disord 1994;9:330–332
12. Zhang K-W, Shun Z-T. Microvascular decompression by the retrosigmoid approach for idiopathic hemifacial spasm: experience with 300 cases. Ann Otol Rhinol Laryngol 1995;104:610–612
13. Elmqvist D, Toremalm NG, Elner A, Mercke U. Hemifacial spasm: electrophysiological findings and the therapeutic effect of facial nerve block. Muscle & Nerve 1982;5:S89–S94
14. Montagna P, Imbriaco A, Zucconi M, et al. Hemifacial spasm in sleep. Neurology 1986;36:270–273
15. Hughes EC, Brackmann DE, Weinstein RC. Seventh nerve spasm: effect of modification of cholinergic balance. Otolaryngol Head Neck Surg 1980;88:491–499
16. Shaywitz BA. Hemifacial spasm in childhood treated with carbamazepine. Arch Neurol 1974;31:63
17. Martinelli P. Primary hemifacial spasm and its treatment with carbamazepine. In: Birkmayer W, ed. Epileptic Seizures—Behaviour—Pain. Baltimore: University Park Press, 1976:342–352
18. Alexander GE, Moses H. Carbamazepine for hemifacial spasm. Neurology 1982;32:286–287

19. Herzberg L. Management of hemifacial spasm with clonazepam. Neurology 1985;35:1676–1767

20. Sandyk R, Gillman MA. Baclofen in hemifacial spasm. Int J Neurosci 1987;33:261–264

21. Patel J, Naritoku DK. Gabapentin for the treatment of hemifacial spasm. Clin Neuropharmacol 1996;19:185–188

22. Bandini F, Mazzella L. Gabapentin as treatment for hemifacial spasm. Eur Neurol 1999;42:49–51

23. Mellick GA. J Pain Symptom Manage 1995;10:392–395

24. Barker FG, Jannetta PJ, Bissonette DJ, et al. Microvascular decompression for hemifacial spasm. J Neurosurg 1995;82:201–210

25. Jankovic J, Brin MF. Therapeutic uses of botulinum toxin. N Engl J Med 1991;324:1186–1194

26. Poungvarin N, Devahastin V, Viriyavejakul A. Treatment of various movement disorders with botulinum A toxin: an experience of 900 patients. J Med Assoc Thai 1995;78:281–287

27. Janetta PJ, Abbasy M, Maroon JC, et al. Etiology and definitive microsurgical treatment of hemifacial spasm. J Neurosurg 1977;47:321–328

28. Fukushima T. Facial spasm and trigeminal neuralgia with operation of Jannetta. Operation 1983;37:1311–1315

29. Kaye AH, Adams CBT. Hemifacial spasm; a long term follow-up of patients treated by posterior fossa surgery and facial nerve wrapping. J Neurol Neurosurg Psychiatry 1981;44:1100–1103

30. Ryu H, Yamamoto S, Sugiyama K, et al. Hemifacial spasm caused by vascular compression of the distal portion of the facial nerve. Report of seven cases. J Neurosurg 1998;88:605–609

31. Mitsuoka H, Arai H, Tsunoda A, et al. Microanatomy of the cerebellopontine angle and internal auditory canal: study with new magnetic resonance imaging technique using three-dimensional fast spin echo. Neurosurg 1999;44:561–566

253 Wilson's Disease

Peter LeWitt

When hepatolenticular degeneration was described by Samuel Alexander Kinnier Wilson in 1912, this rare disorder caused by an inborn error of copper metabolism was fatal and incurable. Over the past nine decades, the molecular and biochemical pathogenesis of Wilson's disease (WD), as it is now known, has been described. Effective treatment can dramatically reverse the neurological and hepatic impairment of the disease, and prevent progression. Because it can produce a variety of clinical manifestation, WD is on the differential diagnosis of most movement disorders. It is essential for clinicians to recognize WD because it is one of the few curable causes of a movement disorder. Recent years have seen the discovery of the abnormal gene responsible for WD, a mutation in copper- and membrane-binding ATPase called ATP7B, which resides on chromosome 13 (13q14.3).[1] This chapter will review the pathophysiology, clinical manifestations, and treatment of WD.

Etiology

WD leads to impaired copper transport, a metabolic defect resulting in the accumulation of copper throughout the body, and causing widespread organ damage. Neurological symptoms of WD relate primarily to copper deposition in the brain, especially the basal ganglia. In the liver, copper deposition causes fatty infiltration, inflammation, and hepatocellular damage, leading to cirrhosis. Copper deposition in the kidney causes tubular and glomerular dysfunction. In the cornea, copper deposition in Descemet's membrane produces the pathognomonic green-brownish pigmentation, the Kayser-Fleischer ring, sometimes visible to unmagnified inspection and always seen on slit-lamp examination (Figure 253.1).

Copper is vital for life in trace amounts, but the body's tissues need protection against excess accumulation. Normally, ingested copper is excreted into the bile by a mechanism that is deficient in WD.[2] Intestinal absorption of copper is normal in WD, so the presence of defective copper excretion results in systemic copper overload and toxicity. The defective biliary copper excretion in WD results from a derangement of hepatic protein complexing whose specific pathophysiology have not been worked out. Wilson's disease does not result from defective production of ceruloplasmin, a liver-derived alpha-2-globulin copper-transporting glycoprotein that is often diminished in WD. A decreased ceruloplasmin concentration provides a useful diagnostic marker of the disease since the structural gene for ceruloplasmin resides on chromosome 8 and the WD genetic defect is on chromosome 13, defective synthesis of cerulo-

plasmin does not appear to be a key part of WD pathophysiology.[3]

Epidemiology

It is estimated that between 0.5 to 1% of the population harbors a single gene mutation for WD.[4] Heterozygotes do not develop WD but may exhibit minor abnormalities of copper metabolism. The prevalence of WD is about one out of 17 million, making this a very rare disorder.

Clinical manifestations

The initial signs and symptoms of WD are neurological, hepatic, and psychiatric in approximately 40%, 40% and 20% of cases, respectively. The hepatitis eventually gives rise to a nodular cirrhosis and liver failure. The psychiatric manifestations typically include depression, anxiety and psychosis. Why some patients present with hepatitis and others present with a neurological phenotype is not understood. Patients with the ApoE epsilon 3/3 genotype tend to have a delayed onset of symptoms.[5] Wilson's disease has developed during the sixth or seventh decade but such cases are extremely rare.[6]

Neurological abnormalities generally present during childhood or later. Three main phenotypes are recognized: (i) a parkinsonian syndrome, (ii) generalized dystonia, and (iii) postural and intention tremor with dysarthria and ataxia. The tremulous variant, sometimes referred to as "pseudosclerotic" WD, may produce the slow, high amplitude proximal tremor described as "wing beating." The speech may be dysarthric and irregular. The risus sardonicus, a grimacing facial expression, results from facial dystonia. Eye movements may show slowed saccades.

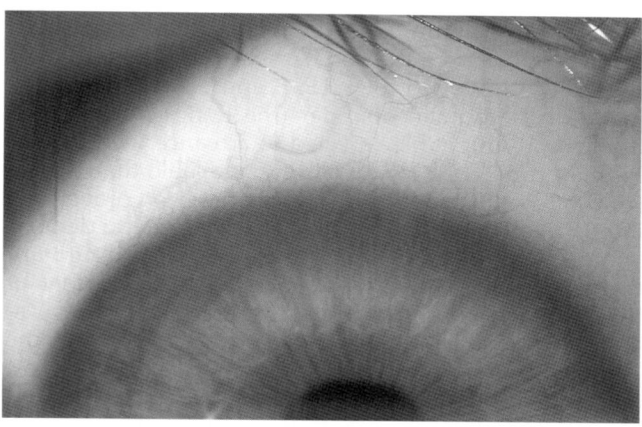

Figure 253.1 Wilson's disease Kayser-Fleischer ring. Courtesy of Dr Brian R Younge. (See color plate section.)

Cognitive deficits, behavioral disorders, and seizures may occur, but weakness and sensory problems are not typical of WD.

Diagnosis

In most cases, WD can be diagnosed by measuring serum ceruloplasmin; in 95% of affected patients, the ceruloplasmin level is low. However, the primary defect in WD does not relate to ceruloplasmin and the levels may be normal. In addition, other causes of low serum ceruloplasmin include low serum protein, liver failure, and heterozygosity. The Kayser-Fleischer ring is for recognition almost always present in affected individuals but may require a slit lamp examination, especially in an individual with brown eyes. Brain magnetic resonance imaging reveals increased T2 signals in the caudate, putamen, thalamus, midbrain, periaqueductal gray, and pontine tegmentum.[7,8]

Urinary copper excretion is usually elevated in WD, and diagnostic confirmation comes from a 24-hour copper excretion, which typically exceeds $100\,\mu g/24\,h$; the diagnosis is excluded by a reliable copper excretion less than $50\,\mu g/24\,h$.[9] The definitive test is a liver biopsy with measurement of copper concentration. Genetic linkage studies to chromosome 13 markers may be helpful within families, but there are so many different mutations causing WD that a definitive gene test has not been developed.

When WD is diagnosed in an individual, all siblings and cousins should be screened for the disease using clinical criteria, a slit lamp examination, tests of liver function and a serum ceruloplasmin. Asymptomatic or preclinical WD requires lifelong treatment to prevent the development of signs and symptoms, and organ damage.

Treatment

The importance of recognizing and treating WD is underscored by the fact that the untreated disease progresses inexorably to death, usually from severe neurological disease or liver failure, within a few years. The mainstay of treating symptomatic WD is removing the copper.

Successful treatment of WD began a half-century ago following discovery of massive copper deposition in tissues. This finding led to medications that could extract copper from the body, a search that continues to today. The discovery of ATP7B and an animal homologue of the human disorder (the Long-Evans Cinnamon rat)[10,11] might be expected to advance therapeutics in the future. For now, drugs are available that chelate copper to enhance its urinary excretion or prevent its intestinal absorption. The most effective way to demonstrate effective treatment is measurement of urinary copper excretion by decoppering agents. Reversal of liver damage, neurological impairments, and other systemic features are likely in cases treated early. Some patients have been fortunate enough to achieve almost complete recovery. The proper choice of treatments and good compliance are critical in achieving the best outcomes. In cases of rapid progression or severe hepatic disease, liver transplantation is curative.

Because of its rarity, most clinicians have little experience with WD. Several clinical programs devoted to WD have been active in evaluating treatment outcomes, including centers directed by Scheinberg,[12] Walshe,[13] Hoogenraad,[14] and Brewer.[15] Several aspects of WD treatment have attracted controversy. Among these is the importance of a low-copper diet, indications for hepatic transplantation and, most notably, the role of penicillamine as initial or maintenance therapy.[16] Wilson's disease patients can vary greatly in clinical manifestations and rate of progression, thus making clinical outcomes challenging to study in the context of therapeutic trials.

Dietary considerations

Content of copper varies among the various categories of food in the diet. Especially high concentrations of copper reside in shellfish and liver, and so these should be avoided. Some sources of water contain more copper than others, a situation that is enhanced by the use of water softeners.[17] For years, patients have been advised to avoid a long list of foods proposed to contain unacceptable quantities of copper. A copper-free diet is not feasible and probably offers no advantage over a low-copper diet, linked to lifelong use of medication, to assist in maintaining negative copper balance. Some foods previously thought to have a high copper content, including nuts, mushrooms, and chocolate, have more recently been shown not to contain increased quantities of this metal and so do not need to be avoided.[9]

Drugs for treating Wilson's disease

After the recognition in 1948 that WD resulted from systemic copper overload, there was a rapid search for treatments capable of binding this divalent metal ion. A compound developed to treat patients exposed to chemical warfare agents, dimercaptopropanol (also known as British anti-Lewisite, or BAL) was the first to be utilized for these purposes.[18,19] Though effective, this compound was toxic and required frequent painful intramuscular injections. Nonetheless, BAL proved the concept of decoppering by means of chelation and provided hope for the reversibility of WD.

The potent chelating agent dimethylcysteine (D-penicillamine), a metabolic byproduct of penicillin, proved to be a major advance.[20] Its mode of action is systemic in attaching to free copper, permitting removal of the bound metal via urinary excretion. Penicillamine is probably the most widely used treatment for initial treatment and chronic maintenance of WD.[21]

Penicillamine Penicillamine therapy began as a practical means for acute and long-term management of WD. Thousands of patients owe their lives to it, although the drug is associated with numerous problems limiting its safe use. Foremost of these is the rapid liberation of copper systemically when penicillamine therapy is started. One consequence of removing copper from the liver and other sites is its unintended transfer into the brain, thereby exacerbating the neurological consequences of brain copper deposition. Neurological deterioration occurs in up to half of patients treated with penicillamine, especially in the first few weeks of therapy.[21,22] This deterioration often causes an increase of motor impairment, especially tremors, dystonia, and parkinsonism. Fatal status dystonicus following the initiation of penicillamine has been reported.[23] In other instances, patients without prior neurological impairment have developed movement disorders, psychiatric and behavioral impairments, and other neurological problems following the start of penicillamine.[24,25] There does not seem to be a reliable means for predicting which patients might deteriorate in neurological status in the days and weeks following the start of penicillamine.

The worsening of neurological impairment at initiation of penicillamine therapy is a problem that has led to several alternative approaches, including decoppering by non-chelation strategies, such as zinc. The variability of outcomes from using any of the available anti-WD drugs and the relatively small number of patients available for careful study of treatments has compounded the difficulties of comparisons between penicillamine and other therapies.

The optimal dose of penicillamine (marketed as Cuprimine in the USA) is generally between 1–2 grams daily in divided doses and taken with meals. To lessen the risk for adverse outcomes, a starting dose of 250 mg/day has been advocated.[9] The dose can be gradually built up by 250 mg increments over several weeks, increasing the dose twice each week. Copper output in the urine is the best initial means for gauging the response to penicillamine. Months may pass before obvious milestones of neurological improvement have evolved. In addition to measurements of urinary copper output, other indicators include the abolition of ophthalmologic signs of copper deposition, corneal Kayser-Fleischer rings and sunflower cataracts.[26] Improvements of various abnormal findings on CT and MRI brain images can also confirm the benefits of decoppering with penicillamine.[7,13,27]

Beyond the neurological consequences resulting from rapid systemic liberation of copper, penicillamine therapy is limited by a number of toxicities. The most common adverse effect is urticaria, a problem that can limit use of the drug. Urticaria is one of the acute sensitization reactions that affect approximately one-third of patients treated with penicillamine.[12,28] Antihistamines, corticosteroid therapy, gradual build-up of penicillamine dosage, and other measures to achieve desensitization can help at controlling some of these problems.[29] Nevertheless, up to 20% of WD patients are unable to tolerate penicillamine.[9] Other more serious effects resulting from immunological activation can arise with prolonged use of this drug, including nephrotoxicity, Goodpasture's syndrome, systemic lupus erythematosus, thrombocytosis and myasthenia gravis. These conditions are listed in Table 253.1. Each of these problems appear to be a consequence of cumulative

exposure to the drug. Clinical experience has not yielded evidence as to how to avoid them. Some of the adverse effects from penicillamine may appear abruptly after years of stable dosage.

Pyridoxine supplementation was formerly thought to counteract some of the adverse effects of penicillamine but is probably not necessary. Penicillamine is teratogenic, and although decoppering therapy must be continued through pregnancy, use of this drug poses significant risks to a developing fetus.

Trientine Trientine (triethylene tetramine) was first investigated more than 30 years ago.[30] Its mode of action appears to be the same as penicillamine, although it is not as avid a binder of copper. This diminished potency as a chelator may be advantageous in attenuating the marked release of systemic copper that complicates the start of penicillamine treatment. Nonetheless, neurological deterioration can also occur with the start of trientine treatment, as shown by a single case report.[31] Its indication for use in the USA is restricted to patients who have become intolerant of penicillamine, and so there has been far less clinical experience with this agent.

The principles of therapy with trientine are similar to those applied to penicillamine, and close monitoring of urinary copper output is necessary to optimize results. Trientine, marketed as Syprine in the USA, is dosed in divided doses in the range of between 0.75–2 g/day, depending on benefits and adverse effects. Trientine should be separated from food intake to maximize its benefits. There has been only limited and somewhat inconclusive comparison of its effectiveness to that of penicillamine.[32]

Adverse effects associated with trientine tend to be less frequent and less severe than those developing with penicillamine. Although lupus nephritis can occur, adverse effects involving immunological activation are much less likely with trientine. Potential serious adverse effects include gastrointestinal

Table 253.1   Adverse effects of penicillamine [adapted from LeWitt and Pfeiffer, 1998][50]

Skin disorders ("penicillamine dermopathy")
  Urticaria and rash
  Epidermolysis bullosa
  Subcutaneous bleeding
  Impairment of dermal elastin and collagen synthesis
  Impaired wound healing
Systemic lupus erythematosis
Lymphadenopathy
Unexplained fever
Hematological disorders (thrombocytopenia, leucopoenia, eosinophilia, agranulocytosis)
Myasthenia gravis
Goodpasture's syndrome
Nephrotic syndrome
Immune complex nephritis
Retinal hemorrhage
Dysgeusia
Immunoglobulin-α deficiency
Acute polyarthritis

disturbances (colitis and duodenitis) and sideroblastic anemia. Proteinuria and iron deficiency have also been described.

Zinc The systemic handling of copper involves several transport proteins. Among these is metallothionein, a protein that binds to several metals, including zinc. In response to repeated exposure to zinc, metallothionein synthesis is greatly increased. Induction of supraphysiological levels of this protein within the intestinal mucosa is the basis by which metallothionein can help to achieve a negative copper balance in WD. Metallothionein produced within gut mucosal cells (enterocytes) binds avidly to the administered zinc as well as to copper in the gut. Dietary copper enters into mucosal cells and remains complexed with intracellular metallothionein. Copper secreted into digestive juices (saliva and gastric) is also removed from the gastrointestinal tract by this means. At the end of the enterocyte's six-day life cycle, this cell is sloughed and the bound copper exits from the body in the feces without opportunity for reabsorption.[9,33]

Therapy of WD with zinc has been under investigation for many years. Some of the earliest clinical experience was in WD patients not tolerating penicillamine. These studies provided evidence of its efficacy, although the regular use of zinc proved less effective at extracting copper than penicillamine.[17,34] Subsequent applications of zinc were aimed at maintaining a negative copper balance rather than as initial therapy for WD. In patients with neurological impairments, more aggressive decoppering therapy is generally needed[35,36] even though effective management of neurological WD has been claimed using zinc alone.[14] Failure of zinc to offer adequate management of progressive WD has also been reported.[34]

Clinical experience has indicated two roles for zinc: (1) to manage copper overload in diagnosed cases of WD that have not yet developed clinical signs,[33] and (2) for the symptomatic patient, as a chronic maintenance therapy started after the initial use of a more potent decoppering treatment. A third use for zinc is for patients unable to tolerate penicillamine, trientine, or ammonium tetrathiomolybdate.[17,34] Zinc monotherapy is the drug of choice in managing WD during pregnancy and in pediatric cases.[36]

While zinc therapy does not directly liberate copper from tissues, it gradually extracts systemic copper by means of secretion into digestive juices. This is a slow process, and the induction of metallothionein synthesis requires at least two weeks before increased fecal output of copper begins. The therapeutic benefit of zinc is diminished when it is combined with penicillamine, even when the two drugs are administered at different times of the day. Whether a similar reaction occurs with trientine remains unclear.

Zinc, administered as either the acetate or sulfate salt, has been given as 50 mg of elemental zinc three times per day. Half this daily dose may be sufficient for a maximal effect of zinc in managing WD but the larger dose provides an extra margin of safety.[35] There is very little toxicity from zinc, apart from gastric irritation. The acetate form is the marketed salt in the USA under the trade name Galzin. Zinc acetate is less likely than the sulfate salt to cause gastric irritation.[9] For optimal results, zinc needs to be taken at least one hour apart from meals. The reason for this is its binding to many dietary constituents, thereby preventing the occurrence of its metallothionein-stimulating action.[37]

Ammonium tetrathiomolybdate Ammonium tetrathiomolybdate (ATM) provides a novel concept for the treatment of copper overload in WD.[38] Its mode of action appears to be in the gut lumen, where it complexes with copper and albumin to prevent absorption of dietary copper. Taken with meals, ATM reduces the uptake of dietary copper. ATM is also absorbed into the bloodstream and so can act systemically to complex copper with albumin and limit entrance of copper into brain, liver, and other organs. With time, tissue stores become depleted of copper. While a dose range between 60–180 mg/day was used in initial studies, the latest experience has limited daily intake to 120 mg in divided doses.[39–43] ATM acts rapidly to increase copper output and experience to date in 55 studied patients has shown worsening of neurological status in only two of them. In each instance, the degree of worsening was quite mild.[42]

Adverse effects of ATM are much less frequent than with penicillamine. In the clinical trials to date, deterioration of neurological function has not been reported. Reversible bone marrow suppression has occurred, possibly from the much-lowered concentrations of copper.

Hepatic transplantation

An emerging option for managing malignant WD is liver transplantation. This procedure can normalize liver function and bring about a full recovery.[44] With a functioning liver transplant, dietary copper restriction and decoppering medications become unnecessary. While the first experience in treating WD with transplanted liver tissue was in the context of acute fulminant hepatic failure,[45] some patients with chronic hepatic insufficiency have also been treated with good results.[46] Intractable neurological WD has also been improved from liver transplantation.[47,48] The increased morbidity and mortality posed by transplantation and subsequent requirement for immunosuppression are reasons to restrict this therapy to patients failing adequate control by medication alone. The shortage of available cadaver material has made transplantation from living relatives a more practical approach in most instances.[49]

References

1. Tanzi RE, Petrukhin K, Chernov I, et al. The Wilson disease gene is a copper transporting ATPase with homology to the Menkes disease gene. Nature Genet 1993;5:344–350
2. Cartwright GE, Wintrobe MM. Copper metabolism in normal subjects. Am J Clin Nutr 1964;14:224–232
3. Iyengar V, Brewer GJ, Dick RD, Owyang C. Studies of cholecystokinin-stimulated biliary secretions reveal a high molecular weight copper-binding substance in normal subjects that is absent in patients with Wilson's disease. J Lab Clin Med 1988;111:267–274
4. Reilly M, Daly L, Hutchinson M. An epidemiological study of Wilson's disease in the Republic of Ireland. J Neurol Neurosurg Psychiatr 1993;56:298–300
5. Schiefermeier M, Kolleger H, Madic C, et al. The impact of apolipoprotein-E genotypic expression in Wilson's disease. Brain 2000;123:585–590
6. Walshe JM, Yealland M. Wilson's disease: the problem of delayed diagnosis. J Neurol Neurosurg Psychiatr 1992;55:692–696
7. Roh JK, Lee TG, Wie BA, et al. Initial and follow-up brain MRI findings and correlation with the clinical course in Wilson's disease. Neurology 1994;44:1064–1068
8. Saatci I, Topcu M, Baltaoglu FF, et al. Cranial MR findings in Wilson's disease. Acta Radiolog 1997;38:250–258
9. Brewer GJ, Yuzbasiyan-Gurkan V. Wilson disease. Medicine 1992;71:139–164
10. Sasaki N, Hayashizaki Y, Muramatsu M, et al. The gene responsible for LEC hepatitis, located on rat chromosome 16, is the homolog to the human Wilson disease gene. Biochem Biophys Res Commun 1994;202:512–518
11. Yamaguchi Y, Heiny ME, Shimizu N, et al. Expression of the Wilson disease gene is deficient in the Long-Evans Cinnamon rat. Biochem J 1994;301(part 1):1–4
12. Scheinberg IH, Sternlieb I. Wilson's Disease. In: Smith LH Jr, ed. Major Problems in Internal Medicine. Vol 23. Philadelphia: WB Saunders, 1984
13. Williams JFB, Walshe JM. Wilson's disease. An analysis of the cranial computerized tomographic appearances found in 60 patients and the changes in response to treatment with chelating agents. Brain 1981;104:735–752
14. Hoogenraad TU. Wilson's Disease. In: Warlow CP, van Gijn J, eds. Major Problems in Neurology. Vol 30. London: WB Saunders, 1996
15. Haggstrom GC, Hirschowitz BI, Flint A. Long-term therapy for Wilson's disease. South J Med 1980;73:530–531
16. LeWitt PA. Penicillamine as a controversial treatment for Wilson's disease. Mov Disord 1999;14:555–556
17. Yarze JC, Martin P, Munoz SJ, Friedman LS. Wilson's disease: current status. Am J Med 1992;92:643–654
18. Denny-Brown D, Porter H. The effect of BAL (2,3 dimercaptopropanol) on hepato-lenticular degeneration (Wilson's disease). N Engl J Med 1951;245:917–925
19. Cummings JN. The effects of BAL in hepatolenticular degeneration. Brain 1951;74:10–22
20. Walshe JM. Penicillamine. A new oral therapy for Wilson's disease. Am J Med 1956;21:487–495
21. Walshe JM, Yealland M. Chelation treatment of neurological Wilson's disease. Q J Med 1993;86:197–204
22. Brewer GH, Terry CA, Aisen AM, Hill GM. Worsening of neurological syndrome in patients with Wilson's disease with initial penicillamine therapy. Arch Neurol 1987;44:490–494
23. Svetel M, Sternic N, Pejovic S, Kostic VS. Penicillamine-induced lethal status dystonicus in a patient with Wilson's disease. Mov Disord 2001;16:568–569
24. Glass JD, Reich SG, DeLong MR. Wilson's disease. Development of neurological disease after beginning penicillamine therapy. Arch Neurol 1990;47:595–596
25. Brewer GJ, Turkay A, Yuzbasiyan-Gurkan V. Development of neurologic symptoms in a patient with asymptomatic Wilson's disease treated with penicillamine. Arch Neurol 1994;51:304–305
26. Walshe JM. Penicillamine: the treatment of first choice for patients with Wilson's disease. Mov Disord 1999;14:545–550
27. King AD, Walshe JM, Kendall BE, et al. Cranial MRI in Wilson's disease. Am J Roentgenol 1996;167:1579–1584
28. COPY TO COME
29. Chan CY, Baker AL. Penicillamine hypersensitivity: successful desensitization of a patient with severe hepatic Wilson's disease. Am J Gastroenterol 1994;89:442–443
30. Walshe JM. Treatment of Wilson's disease with trientine (triethylene triamine) dichloride. Lancet 1982;1:643–647
31. Dahlman T, Hartvig P, Lofholm M, et al. Long-term treatment of Wilson's disease with triethylene tetramine dihydrochloride (trientine). Q J Med 1995;88:609–616
32. Walshe JM. Copper chelation in patients with Wilson's disease. A comparison of penicillamine and triethylene tetramine hydrochloride. Q J Med 1973;42:441–452
33. Brewer GJ, Dick RD, Yuzbasiyan-Gurkan V, et al. Treatment of Wilson's disease with zinc: XII. Therapy with zinc in presymptomatic patients from the time of diagnosis. J Lab Clin Med 1994;123:849–858
34. Lipsky MA, Gollan JL. Treatment of Wilson's disease. In D-penicillamine we trust: what about zinc? Hepatology 1987;7:593–595
35. Brewer GJ, Dick RD, Johnson VD, et al. Treatment of Wilson's disease with zinc. XV: long-term follow-up studies. J Lab Clin Med 1998;132:264–278
36. Brewer GJ, Dick RD, Johnson VD, et al. Treatment of Wilson's disease with zinc. XVI: treatment during the pediatric years. J Lab Clin Med 2001;137:191–198
37. Yuzbasiyan-Gurkan V, Grider A, Nostrant T, et al. The treatment of Wilson's disease with zinc: X. Intestinal metallothionein induction. J Lab Clin Med 1992;120:380–386
38. Walshe J. Tetrathiomolybdate (MoS4) as an 'anti-copper' agent in man. In: Scheinberg IH, Walshe JM, eds. Orphan Disease, Orphan Drugs. Manchester: Manchester University Press, 1986:76–85
39. Brewer GJ, Dick RD, Yuzbasiyan-Gurkan V, et al. Initial therapy of Wilson's disease with tetrathiomolybdate. Arch Neurol 1991;48:42–47
40. Brewer GJ, Dick RD, Johnson V, et al. Treatment of Wilson's disease with tetrathiomolybdate. I: initial therapy in 17 neurologically affected patients. Arch Neurol 1994;51:545–554
41. Brewer GJ, Johnson V, Dick RD, et al. Treatment of Wilson's disease with ammonium tetrathiomolybdate. II: initial therapy in 33 neurologically affected patients and follow-up on zinc therapy. Arch Neurol 1996;53:1017–1025
42. Brewer GJ. Penicillamine should not be used as initial therapy in Wilson's disease. Mov Disord 1999;14:551–554
43. Brewer GJ. Recognition, diagnosis and management of Wilson's disease. Proc Soc Exp Biol 2000;223:39–46
44. Groth CG, Dubois RS, Corman J, et al. Hepatic trans-

plantation in Wilson's disease. Birth Defects 1973;9: 106–108

45. Rela M, Heaton ND, Vougas V, et al. Orthotopic liver transplantation for hepatic complications of Wilson's disease. Br J Surg 1993;80:909–911

46. Schilsky ML, Scheinberg IH, Sternlieb I. Liver transplantation for Wilson's Disease: indications and outcome. Hepatology 1994;19:583–587

47. Mason AL, Marsh W, Alpers DH. Intractable neurological Wilson's disease treated with orthotopic liver transplantation. Digest Dis Sci 1993;38:1746–1750

48. Schumacher G, Platz KP, Mueller AR, et al. Liver transplantation in neurologic Wilson's disease. Transplant Proc 2001;33:1518–1519

49. Tanaka K, Uemoto S, Inomata Y, et al. Living-related liver transplantation for fulminant hepatic failure in children. Transpl Int 1994;7(Suppl 1):S108–S110

50. LeWitt PA, Pfeiffer R. Neurological aspects of Wilson's disease: clinical and treatment considerations. *In:* Jankovic J, Tolosa E, eds. Parkinson's Disease and Related Movement Disorders. Third edition. Philadelphia: WB Saunders, 1998:377–399

254 Psychogenic Movement Disorders

Stanley Fahn, Daniel Williams and Blair Ford

Psychogenic movement disorders have been well-recognized since the division of neurology and psychiatry into separate disciplines over one hundred years ago. Charcot described patients with contractures and deformities who now would be considered to have psychogenic dystonia.[1] Gowers described "psychogenic laryngeal spasms" in his writings on epilepsy and hysteria[2] and used hypnosis to determine if these spasms could be altered during sleep, attempting to distinguish attacks due to hysteria from those due to organic disease.

Psychogenic movement disorders are abnormal movements that cannot be considered to result directly from organic disease, and which derive primarily from psychological and psychiatric causes. As commonly employed by movement disorder specialists, the term tends to exclude movements caused by certain types of psychiatric illness, such as the psychomotor retardation or parkinsonism that may accompany depression, the bizarre movements and postures of schizophrenia, or the stereotyped movements of autism.

The patient with a psychogenic movement disorder poses two central challenges to the clinician: (i) Establishing with certainty the origin of the movements as psychogenic, and (ii) Carrying out the appropriate psychiatric evaluation and treatment. Although psychogenic illness has long fascinated neurologists and psychiatrists alike, the pathogenesis remains obscure, and therapy for these disorders remains completely empiric.

Epidemiology

Psychogenic neurological symptoms have been estimated to account for between 1–9% of all neurological diagnoses.[3,4] Perhaps 10–15% of patients with a psychogenic movement disorder have an underlying organic movement disorder as well. This overlap between psychogenic movements and abnormal movements of organic origin is also observed in patients with psychogenic seizures ("non-epileptic seizures"), as well.[5,6]

Neurological diagnosis

Psychogenic disorders pose a daunting diagnostic and therapeutic challenge to physicians. Patients may be extremely disabled by their physical symptoms. In the field of movement disorders, it is typically the neurologist who must first recognize the syndrome as a psychiatric disorder. After making the diagnosis of a psychogenic movement disorder, it is the neurologist's task to ensure that the patient receives the appropriate psychiatric evaluation and treatment that is essential to a successful outcome.

Determining whether abnormal movements are produced by psychiatric disease or an organic disorder, or both, is one of the most difficult tasks in the movement disorder specialty. It is extremely important to be correct in the diagnosis because only then can the appropriate therapy be initiated. Failing to diagnose a psychogenic movement disorders invariably delays treatment and may perpetuate a patient's cycle of disability. In addition, some patients with unrecognized psychogenic symptoms have been subjected to inappropriate or dangerous testing and treatment, including stereotactic neurosurgery.

Movement disorder phenomenology

Psychogenic movement disorders are usually identified on the basis of (i) symptoms and signs that are incompatible with disease of organic origin, (ii) symptoms and signs that are inconsistent from moment to moment, and fluctuate throughout the evaluation, (iii) a discrepancy between the patient's disability and objective signs of motor deficit, and (iv) the presence of psychiatric abnormalities.

Although there is a modest neurological literature on psychogenic phenomenology, the published experience dealing specifically with psychogenic movement disorders is rather sparse. It is important to point out that no matter how much experience a clinician has had, encountering a new type of movement disorder for the first time does not automatically make it a psychogenic movement disorder. Clues that a psychogenic movement disorder may be present are summarized in Table 254.1.

The most common type of movements, whether isolated or in the presence of other types of movements, in patients with psychogenic movement disorders are shaking movements that resemble peculiar, atypical tremors. Bizarre gaits are a frequent feature of psychogenicity. The psychogenic gait can show posturing, excessive slowness, and hesitation. There can be sudden buckling of a leg, as if there is weakness,[7] but the failure to produce this dipping movement each time the patient steps on the leg is not consistent. There may be excessive swaying when tested for the Romberg sign, without actually falling. Excessive startle may mimic hyperekplexia, the excessive startle syndrome, the Jumping Frenchmen of Maine syndrome, or even reflex myoclonus.[8] Thompson et al.,[9] determined the physiological parameters that are typically seen in patients with psychogenic startles. There is a variable latency to the onset of the jerk and the latencies are greater than those seen in

Table 254.1   Clues relating to the movements that suggest a psychogenic movement disorder

1. Abrupt onset
2. Inconsistent movements (changing characteristics over time; pattern, body distribution, rapidly varying severity)
3. Incongruous movements and postures (movements don't fit with recognized patterns or with normal physiological patterns)
4. Presence of additional types of abnormal movements that are not consistent with the basic abnormal movement
    pattern or are not congruous with a known movement disorder, particularly:
        rhythmical shaking
        bizarre gait
        deliberate slowness carrying out requested voluntary movement
        bursts of verbal gibberish
        excessive startle (bizarre movements in response to a sudden, unexpected noise or threatening movement)
5. Entrainment of the psychogenic tremor to the rate of the requested rapid successive movement the patient is asked to
    perform
6. Spontaneous remissions
7. Movements decrease or disappear with distraction
8. Response to placebo, suggestion or psychotherapy
9. Paroxysmal disorder
10. Dystonia beginning as a fixed posture
11. Twisting facial movements that move the mouth to one side or the other (note: organic dystonia of the facial muscles
    usually do not move the mouth sidewise)

reflex myoclonus of cortical or brainstem origin. When a patient with psychogenic tremor is asked to carry out rapid successive movements, such as tapping the index finger on the thumb, the rate of the tremor becomes the same as the rapid successive movements, i.e. the tremor becomes entrained. In contrast, an organic tremor is the dominant rate; it will gradually force the voluntary movements to be the same rate as the tremor.

Idiopathic torsion dystonia usually begins with action dystonia,[10] but psychogenic dystonia often begins with a fixed posture. The posture may manifest so much rigidity that it is extremely difficult to move the limb about a joint. Often the psychogenic dystonia resembles reflex sympathetic dystrophy because there is accompanying pain and tenderness.[11–13] To make matters confusing, many cases of psychogenic dystonia of a limb follow a minor trauma to that limb, similar to the pattern of reflex sympathetic dystrophy. On the other hand, organic dystonia of a body part can be preceded by an injury to that body part,[14–18] so the diagnosis can be difficult to distinguish between organic and psychogenic dystonia. The clues in Tables 254.1 and 254.2 should help.

Table 254.2   Clues relating to other medical observations that suggest a psychogenic movement disorder

1. False weakness
2. False sensory complaints
3. Multiple somatizations or undiagnosed conditions
4. Self-inflicted injuries
5. Obvious psychiatric disturbances
6. Employed in the health profession, working with handicapped individuals or in health insurance claims
7. Presence of secondary gain, including continuing care by a "devoted" spouse
8. Litigation or compensation pending
9. Demonstrating exhaustion or fatigue during encounter

Diagnostic certainty

Fahn and Williams[19] categorized patients into four levels of certainty as to the likelihood of their having a psychogenic movement disorder (see Table 254.3). This classification has been used by subsequent authors.[20–22]

Just being suspicious that the signs and symptoms are psychogenic is insufficient for the diagnosis of documented psychogenic disorder. In order for the disorder to be documented as psychogenic, the symptoms must be completely relieved by psychotherapy, or by a clinician utilizing psychological suggestion, or by administration of placebos (again with suggestion being a part of this approach), or the patient must be witnessed as being free of symptoms when left alone, supposedly unobserved. This last feature would be a major factor in establishing malingering or a factitious disorder since such patients would not likely obtain relief of symptoms by manipulations of the examiner.

A movement disorder is proved to be psychogenic when it is completely resolved by psychotherapy, hypnotherapy, physical therapy or placebo. At times, the remission is sudden and dramatic. Spontaneous remissions in movement disorders that have an organic basis, like dystonia, essential tremors, myoclonic disorders, or parkinsonism, are extremely rare. Paroxysmal movement disorders present a special and difficult problem. The natural history of a paroxysmal movement disorder includes prolonged periods of remission, so the cessation of abnormal movements does not by itself establish the diagnosis of a psychogenic disorder. However, if the paroxysms are frequent and the attacks are prolonged, repeated trials with placebo can be informative. If such trials consistently produce remissions, then one can be convinced that the diagnosis is a documented psychogenic disorder.

Table 254.3	Guidelines for classifying diagnostic certainty in psychogenic movement disorders	
Certainty of diagnosis	**Clinical evidence**
A. Documented psychogenic disorder	1. Abnormal movements completely resolve using psychotherapy, or 2. Abnormal movements resolve when patient is unaware of being observed.

B. Clinically established psychogenic movement disorder	1. Abnormal movements that are incongruous with organic disease, and inconsistent during exam
	2. Presence of supporting features:
	   a. Neurological signs that are psychogenic, e.g. false weakness, false sensory.
	   b. Multiple somatizations are present.
	   c. An obvious psychiatric disturbance is present.
	   d. The movement disorder disappears with distraction.
	   e. Excessive (appearing deliberate) slowness of movement is present.

C. Probable psychogenic movement disorder	1. Abnormal movements are inconsistent or incongruent with an organic disease or support diagnosis of psychogenicity, or 2. Abnormal movements are consistent and congruent with an organic disorder but there are signs present that are definitely psychogenic, e.g. false weakness, false sensory.
D. Possible psychogenic movement disorder	Presence of obvious psychiatric disturbance in a patient with unusual movement abnormalities.

Psychiatric diagnosis

Definitions from DSM-IV-TR can be helpful regarding the psychiatric differential diagnosis of psychogenic movement disorders.[23] This is essential for appropriate psychiatric treatment. There are three categories into which most patients with psychogenic movement disorder can be subdivided: the somatoform disorders, the factitious disorders, and malingering.

Somatoform disorders

A somatoform disorder is one in which the physical symptoms are linked to psychological factors, yet the symptom production is not under voluntary control, i.e., not consciously produced. The two main types of somatoform disorders producing psychogenic neurological problems are conversion disorder and somatization disorder, the latter also known as hysteria or Briquet's syndrome. Other somatoform subsets are hypochondriasis, pain disorder, body dysmorphic disorder and undifferentiated somatoform disorder.

In conversion disorder, there are one or more symptoms affecting voluntary motor or sensory function that suggest a neurological or other medical condition. Psychological factors may be judged to play the primary etiological role in a variety of ways. There may be a temporal relationship between the onset or worsening of the symptoms and the presence of an environmental stimulus that activates a psychological conflict or need. Alternatively, the symptom may be noted to free the patient from a noxious activity or encounter. The symptom cannot, after appropriate investigation, be fully explained by a general medical condition, or by the direct effects of a substance, or as a culturally sanctioned behavior or experience.

A somatization disorder involves recurrent and multiple complaints of several years' duration for which medical care has been sought, but which are apparently not due to any physical disorder. The dynamics are presumably the same as those of conversion disorder and the symptoms may emerge from chronic, recurrent, untreated conversion disorder. There must be four pain symptoms, two gastrointestinal symptoms, one sexual symptom and one pseudoneurological symptom. Other requirements are age at onset under 30 years and severe enough symptomatology that the patient has taken medications, consulted a physician, or altered his or her lifestyle as a result of the symptoms.

Factitious disorder

A factitious disorder is one in which the physical symptoms are intentionally produced (hence under voluntary control) due to a pathological psychological need, such as a yearning to be cared for by assuming the role of a patient. External incentives for the behavior, such as economic gain or avoiding responsibility, are absent. This group includes Munchausen's syndrome. In contrast to malingering, factitious disorders are diagnosed as mental disorders. They are generally associated with severe dependent, masochistic or antisocial personality disorders. Consequently, treatment prognosis is generally less favorable than in cases of somatoform disorder.

Malingering

Malingering refers to voluntarily produced physical symptoms in pursuit of a goal such as financial compensation, avoidance of school or work, evasion of criminal prosecution, or acquisition of drugs. Malingering is not considered to be a mental disorder.

When faced with a patient having a psychogenic movement disorder, it is often not possible with certainty to distinguish among somatoform, factitious and malingering disorders. A patient's volitional intent is often impossible to determine with certainty, especially early in the course of assessment, though clarification will most often emerge in the course of treatment endeavor.

Comorbid psychiatric conditions

In addition to a primary Axis I diagnosis, most patients with psychogenic movement disorders have a co-existing Axis I diagnosis such as affective disorder, anxiety disorder, or adjustment disorder.[24] The lifetime incidence of major depression in somatization disorder is reportedly 80–90%.[25] Axis II diagnoses such a developmental disorder and personality disorder are also common.[24] The identification of specific stressors, sources of personal, familial, or marital conflict, possible symptom modeling, secondary gain (including financial compensation), and a global assessment of functioning all factor into the diagnostic process. A history of physical, sexual, or emotional abuse is often present in patients with conversion disorder.[24,26]

An assessment of the relevant psychodynamic and symbolic contributants to the physical symptoms aids the diagnosis. In conversion disorder, the movement disorder symptoms often arise in relation to a specific stressor. The patient is often unable to appreciate or articulate the relationship between inciting event and production of psychological symptoms, however obvious this may seem to the physician. Conversion symptomatology can occur in predisposed individuals who are unable to cope with the everyday demands of life, as well as healthy subjects subjected to unusually stressful situations such as medical illness.[25]

In a series of 24 patients with psychogenic movement disorders who underwent detailed psychiatric evaluation, the profile of a typical patient consisted of a young person (mean age 36 years, range 11–60), most often female (79%), of average or above average intelligence (96% combined), with a mean duration of symptoms of five years (range <1 month–23 years) unable to work and on disability (70% of patients).[24] The principal psychiatric diagnoses were conversion disorder (75%), followed by somatization (12.5%), factitious disorder (8%) and malingering (4%). Dysthymia, as a secondary psychiatric diagnosis, was present in 67% of patients. The rest included a variety of different psychiatric conditions such as major depression, adjustment disorder, organic mood or organic delusional disorders, obsessive-compulsive disorder, panic attacks, bipolar disorder and others.

Clinical features of psychogenic movement disorders

General features

Williams et al.[24] reviewed the records of 131 patients with psychogenic movement disorders and listed their motor disturbances. Dystonia, tremor, gait disturbances, paroxysmal dyskinesias, and myoclonus were the major motor types encountered. They found that 79% of patients had multiple types of abnormal movements, and that only 21% had a single definable type. Moreover, again in contrast to the vast majority of organic movement disorders, in 55% of the patients the movements were either intermittent or paroxysmal, while only 45% of the patients had only continuous movements. The onset was abrupt in 60%, and usually with a specific inciting event. In 43% of patients the movements spread beyond the initial site of involvement.

Factor et al.,[27] reviewed their 28 cases of psychogenic movement disorders. These represented 3.3% of all 842 consecutive movement disorder patients seen over a six year period. Tremor was most common (50%) followed by dystonia, myoclonus, and parkinsonism. Clinical clues included distractibility (86%) and abrupt onset (54%). Distractibility was more important in tremor and least important in dystonia. Other diagnostic clues included entrainment of tremor to the frequency of repetitive movements of another limb, fatigue of tremor, stimulus sensitivity, and a previous history of psychogenic illness.

An organic diagnosis was made originally in 75% of the patients with a psychogenic movement disorder, including three patients who carried a diagnosis of multiple sclerosis despite the lack of any positive laboratory data. A number of neurological findings presented as clues to psychogenicity. The most common was the presence of give-away weakness (37%). Next most common was a startle reaction that was non-physiological (29%). Pain and false sensory findings on examination were also encountered. Surprisingly, psychogenic seizures were concurrently present in 12% of the patients. The psychogenic movement disorder was disabling in 65% of the patients. A preceding history and inciting event of head trauma and peripheral trauma occurred in 25% and 12.5% of patients, respectively.

Williams et al.,[24] found that the most common psychiatric diagnosis was a somatoform disorder, particularly conversion disorder. Briquet's syndrome (somatization disorder) was diagnosed in 12.5%, and there were even fewer patients with a factitious disorder (8%) or malingering (4%). An accompanying depression or anxiety was found in 71% and 17% of patients, respectively.

Psychogenic dystonia

It is, in some ways, ironic that torsion dystonia can sometimes be due to psychogenic causation. From its earliest beginnings, idiopathic torsion dystonia was often mistaken as a manifestation of a psychiatric disturbance.[28] Soon after Schwalbe's description in 1908 however, Oppenheim[29] and Flatau and Sterling[30] set matters right by emphasizing the organic nature of this disorder. Although some early publications on dystonia mentioned the "functional" nature of the symptoms[31] or used the label, "neurosis",[32] these terms were employed in a manner different from today. "Functional" referred to a physiological activation of the abnormal movements with voluntary motor activity, which would otherwise disappear when the patient was quiet at rest. "Neurosis" was a term used to indicate a neurological, rather than a psychiatric, disorder, but one without a structural lesion. Today, it is common for the term "functional" to be equivalent to "psychogenic," and for "neurosis" not to be used at all in neurology, but to refer to certain type of psychiatric disorders.

Beginning in the 1950s, many patients with various forms of focal, segmental and generalized dystonia began to be misdiagnosed as having a conversion disorder. Among 44 patients with idiopathic dystonia reviewed by Eldridge et al.,[33] 23 (52%) had previously been referred for psychiatric treatment (without benefit). Marsden and Harrison[34] had a similar experience; 43% of their 42 patients were previously diagnosed as suffering from hysteria. Cooper and his colleagues reviewed their series of 226 patients and found that 56 (25%) had a diagnosis of psychogenic etiology at some time during their illness.[35] Lesser and Fahn[36] reviewed the records of 84 patients with idiopathic dystonia seen at Presbyterian Hospital in New York from 1969 to 1974 and found that 37 (44%) had been misdiagnosed previously with an emotional disorder. These 37 patients consisted of 11 with generalized dystonia, 14 with segmental dystonia, and 19 with focal dystonia (14 with torticollis, two with oro-mandibular dystonia, and three with blepharospasm).

Although some authors[37,38] suggested that an underlying psychiatric illness may exist in patients with torticollis, others[39–41] found no differences between dystonic patients and controls in regard to previous psychiatric history and current life adjustment or on psychiatric testing. Similarly, some authors[42,43] considered hand dystonia (writer's cramp, occupational cramp) to be psychogenic. But Sheehy and Marsden[44] studied 34 patients with writer's or other occupational cramps affecting the arm or arm. All patients underwent assessment by an psychiatric interview technique; these patients compared favorably with a control group, and the investigators concluded that their disorder was not psychiatric in origin. Another recent study involved psychiatric assessment in 20 subjects with focal hand dystonia and also concluded that none had any serious psychopathology.[45] Furthermore, patients with writer's cramp do not have increased anxiety.[46]

At the time of the first international symposium on dystonia held in 1975, Fahn and Eldridge[47] noted that no case of proven psychological dystonia had been reported. With the realization that patients with dystonia were being misdiagnosed as a psychiatric disorder, neurologists became sensitive to this problem and since then seemed to have to avoid a diagnosis of hysterical dystonia. However, at the annual meeting of the American Academy of Neurology in 1983, Fahn et al.,[48] described 10 patients as having documented psychogenic dystonia. Batshaw et al.,[49] had followed a patient who had been misdiagnosed as an organic dystonia and who had had a stereotactic thalamotomy based on that diagnosis; these authors eventually recognized that their patient had psychogenic dystonia and reported her as a case of Munchausen's syndrome. Fahn and Williams have described 22 cases of

documented or clinically established psychogenic dystonia, including a case of a young girl who underwent a stereotaxic thalamotomy.[19] Lang[22] reported on 18 patients with documented or clinically established psychogenic dystonia, 14 with a known precipitant. Involvement of the legs occurred in 12, despite onset in adulthood. Ten of Lang's patients had paroxysmal worsening of dystonia or other abnormal movements. Pain was a prominent feature in 14 of 16 patients with this complaint.

Psychogenic dystonia is difficult to diagnose since there are no laboratory tests to establish the diagnosis of organic idiopathic dystonia. The clues listed in Tables 254.1 and 254.2 should help alert the clinician to the possibility of a psychogenic etiology.

In a survey of 22 patients reported by Fahn[19] on documented and clinically established cases of psychogenic dystonia, he found that six had paroxysmal dystonia, and 16 had continual dystonia. Females outnumbered males by a ratio of 20:2. The youngest age at onset was eight years, and the oldest was 58 years. Those with paroxysmal dystonia were, as a general rule, older than patients with continual dystonia.

Psychogenic tumor

Koller et al.,[20] diagnosed 24 patients with psychogenic tremors. They described the tremors as complex; usually they were present at rest, with posture, and with action. The onset was abrupt, and in all but one the tremors lessened or were abolished with distraction. Psychogenic tremors are sometimes paroxysmal and not always continuous. Deuschl et al.,[50] reviewed 25 cases of psychogenic tremor. Sudden onset and rare remissions were typical. The "coactivation sign" and absent finger tremor were the most consistent criteria to separate them from organic tremors. Whereas most organic tremors show decreasing amplitudes when the extremity is loaded with additional weights, most psychogenic tremors show an increase of tremor amplitude, i.e. "coactivation sign." Overall, psychogenic tremor in their series had a poor outcome. Kim and colleagues[51] reviewed their series of 70 cases of pyschogenic tremor. They emphasized the abrupt onset (73%), often with the maximal disability at onset (46%), and then took static (46%) or fluctuating (17%) courses. Tremor usually started in one limb and spread rapidly to a generalized or mixed distribution. Other features were spontaneous resolution and recurrence, easy distractibility together with entrainment and response to suggestion.

Psychogenic gait

Keane[52] described 60 cases with a psychogenic gait abnormality out of 228 patients with psychogenic neurological problems. Among these abnormal gaits were 24 with "ataxia" (the most common gait abnormality), nine with trembling, two with "dystonia," two with truncal "myoclonus," and one with campto-cormia (markedly stooped posture). Among the myriad of associated psychogenic signs, knee giving-way, with recovery, was seen in five patients, and is a feature of a case presented recently as an unknown, unusual movement disorder.[7] In a video review of psychogenic gaits, Hayes and colleagues[53] emphasized certain features of the gait; exaggerated effort, extreme slowness, variability throughout the day, unusual or uneconomic postures, collapses, convulsive tremors, and distractibility.

Psychogenic myoclonus

Monday and Jankovic[54] reported 18 patients with psychogenic myoclonus (although no EMG observations were reported to indicate that myoclonus was the actual type of abnormal movement), and state that this is the most common form of psychogenic movement disorder encountered in their clinic. The myoclonus was segmental in 10, generalized in seven and focal in one. Psychogenic myoclonus accounted for 8.5% of the 212 patients with myoclonus in their clinic. Inconsistency, with continuously changing pattern anatomically and temporally, was common. The movements often increased with stress, anxiety, and exposure to noise or light. A Bereitschaftspotential preceding muscle jerks was found in five of six patients with a diagnosis of psychogenic myoclonus.[55] The authors suggest that this is a positive sign for the diagnosis of psychogenic myoclonus, but because one patient did not have a Bereitschaftspotential, its absence cannot be used to exclude the diagnosis.

Psychogenic tics

Psychogenic movements can sometimes resemble tics. It is more complicated when organic tics are also present. Dooley et al.,[56] described two children with Tourette syndrome who also had pseudo-tics, in whom the psychogenic movements resolved when the stressful issues in their lives were addressed.

Psychogenic parkinsonism

Psychogenic parkinsonism is relatively uncommon (Table 254.3). Lang et al.,[57] reported 14 patients with this disorder. Eleven patients had tremor at rest, but the tremor did not disappear with movement of the limb, and the frequency and rhythmicity varied. Rigidity was present in six patients, but without cogwheeling. All 14 patients had slowness of movement (bradykinesia) without the typical decrementing feature of organic bradykinesia. One patient had evidence of some organic parkinsonism as well, but required a fluorodopa PET scan to be certain.

Pathophysiology

The transformation of psychiatric disease into somatic symptoms is a poorly understood process. Freud and Breuer coined the term *conversion* to describe how certain individuals unconsciously repress feelings of extreme helplessness, distress, anger or conflict by the substitution of physical symptoms. According to psychodynamic theory, the development of a physical symptom binds unconscious feelings of conflict. This leads to a reduction of anxiety and psychological distress, termed *primary gain*. The specific physical symptom often embodies the unconscious conflict in symbolic terms.

Another hypothesis for symptom formation in conversion disorder is behavioral learning theory. In this model, conversion symptoms are viewed as sick role behaviors, learned in childhood and unconsciously brought forth as a means of coping with unbearable psychological stress. Sociocultural views of somatoform disorders postulate that unconsciously produced physical symptoms serve to communicate emotionally charged feelings or ideas that would otherwise be unacceptable in the cultural context. Patients may obtain *secondary gain* by using physical symptoms to manipulate their environments, or as a means to avoid unpleasant situations or responsibility.

Implicit in the idea of conversion symptoms is the concept of dissociation: a functional separation of aspects of identity, memory, experience, insight, self-perception and bodily function from the mainstream of conscious awareness.[58] The capacity for dissociation may be a precondition for the development of a somatoform disorder. Biologically-based studies are beginning to probe the neurological substrate of conversion and dissociation. Hypnosis, an inducible state of dissociation, can be studied using imaging techniques. PET activation studies reveal metabolic changes in the anterior cingulate gyrus during hypnosis, a brain region that may play a role in the perceptual and cognitive processing involved in dissociation.

Treatment
Psychotherapy

Therapeutic guidelines for psychogenic neurological symptoms have been described since Freud,[24,25,59–62] and encompass psychotherapy in all its forms, suggestion, hypnosis, physiotherapy, psychotropic medication, and other techniques. Treatment for psychogenic symptoms and conversion disorder has never been evaluated in controlled clinical trials. Consequently, while encouraging anecdotal reports of treatment successes abound, no therapeutic approach has proved superior to any other, and no consistently effective treatment has been established. There are few long-term outcome studies, and none in which a particular therapy is evaluated in a double-blind, placebo-controlled manner.

In one hospital-based treatment trial, patients suffering from conversion disorder were treated with suggestion, faradic stimulation, and medications. Symptom remission was achieved in all 61 participating subjects, and the 12-month relapse rate was 12 patients (20%).[63] In a study of 61 hospitalized patients with conversion disorder, the treatment consisted of reassurance and exercises. If symptom remission could be induced using these techniques by the end of the hospitalization, the eventual outcome was sustained benefit in 96%, at a median follow-up interval of 4.5 years.[64]

In a study of 24 hospitalized patients with psychogenic movement disorders at Columbia-Presbyterian Medical Center, treatment consisted of combined supportive psychotherapy, hypnosis, physical therapy, and pharmacotherapy. Among 22 individuals followed for almost two years, 19 (79%) continued out-patient psychotherapy after hospital discharge. Final clinical status at the follow-up interval included six patients (25%) with complete symptom remission and five patients (21%) with considerable symptom relief; the remainder had mild or no benefit. Final working status tended to correlate with the degree of symptom remission, as expected.[24] Among patients treated for psychogenic seizures, the outcome was similar.[5,65]

Patients with factitious disorder are generally more severely and chronically disabled than those with somatoform disorders. The treatment of choice in factitious disorder is probably psychotherapy, aimed at exploring the patient's underlying motives and modifying the self-injurious behavior.[25] The usual presence of a comorbid personality disorder involving dependent, masochistic or antisocial features will often render these individuals quite resistant to treatment, however. The danger of treatment termination by the patient is always present, and must be guarded against.

In one study of 24 patients with factitious disorder, none of whom had a movement disorder, individuals were offered a therapeutic program consisting of initial in-hospital psychotherapy, followed by long-term outpatient or interval in-patient analytically-oriented psychotherapy.[66] The complete course of treatment was four years or more, and patients underwent as many as 200 therapy sessions. Of 24 patients who were offered, and completed, the ambitious treatment program, only three (12.5%) individuals showed a sustained benefit, defined as the disappearance of the factitious symptomatology and improvements in social competence, whether returning to work or the establishment of successful relationships.[66] Additional guidelines regarding the problem of confrontation, setting limits, the establishment of a therapeutic relationship, and the eventual transition to an out-patient phase are described in this report.

Malingerers will not generally respond to any treatment modality but only give up their symptoms when the secondary gain is obtained, or is concluded to be unobtainable. Patients with malingering as well as factitious illness can be expected to confront the diagnosis of a psychogenic etiology with strong denial, hostility and departure from therapy.

Despite the lack of controlled trials for the many available treatment approaches, some therapeutic guidelines, based on experience and the literature, can be made. In order to establish and maintain an effective treatment relationship with the patient, psychogenic movement disorder symptomatology is best presumed, for purposes of maintaining therapeutic optimism, to be unconscious. For a fraction of cases, however, further assessment will prove this to be incorrect. Through a supportive enquiry into the contributing psychological elements, the therapist may gradually lead the patient towards a reduction, tolerance, or resolution of the conflicts responsible for con-

version symptoms. There are no specific guidelines about how to accomplish this and the therapy itself is highly individualized for each patient. Frequently, treatment of associated anxiety, depression, or other coexisting psychopathology with medication will be helpful. Behavioral programs that reward or reinforce the gradual abandonment of conversion symptoms may be beneficial. Implicitly, this concerns the secondary gain component relevant to symptom formation and retention. The long-term goal of psychotherapy for conversion disorder is to establish more effective coping strategies within the patient so that, after symptom resolution, stressful situations do not precipitate recurrent symptomatic regression.

Multidisciplinary hospital-based approach

In the experience at Columbia-Presbyterian Medical Center, a combined neurological and psychiatric approach to the patient with a psychogenic movement disorder, often conducted in the hospital setting in chronic cases, offers the greatest likelihood of therapeutic success. Hospitalization of the patient accomplishes several goals. It removes the patient from the environment that may be nurturing the psychogenic symptomatology. At the risk of legitimizing the patient's sick role, hospitalization assures the patient that the symptoms are being taken seriously. The confinement makes it difficult for the patient to reject psychiatric care. A therapeutic alliance is permitted to develop and the patient can be engaged. Multiple diagnostic and treatment strategies can be acted out simultaneously, assuring the patient that nothing has been missed, and providing a face-saving rationale for the inclusion of a psychiatric evaluation as part of the plan. If needed, the final supporting evidence for a definite diagnosis of psychogenic movement disorder is gathered. This may include video-EEG monitoring or special electrophysiological studies. Ideally, while in hospital, the patient can undergo a formal but supportive debriefing session, with neurologist and psychiatrist present, in which the diagnosis and its implications are presented, and a treatment plan is formulated. A formal transfer to psychiatry may be appropriate at this point.

Increasingly, however, it is more difficult to admit patients with suspected psychogenic movement disorders to the in-patient neurology service because this treatment is obstructed by third party payors. For patients who are reluctant to consider the possibility of underlying psychological contributants to their symptoms, the reluctance of insurers to approve a hospital admission can pose a barrier to treatment. Such patients may not accept the notion of psychogenesis at the initial office visit, and may not comply with a suggestion to arrange an out-patient psychiatric consultation. As such, the neurologist's resources for treatment may be limited. On the other hand, the recent experience at Columbia-Presbyterian Medical Center shows long-term favorable outcomes when patients are followed collaboratively by a movement disorder neurologist and the consulting psychiatrist on an out-patient basis. Patients with greater capacity for insight show the best response to combined ambulatory treatment.

Regardless of the setting, many patients who are initially unwilling to consider psychogenic factors in their illness may be engaged using a neurobiological explanation of pathogenesis. We emphasize the interplay of organic disease, neuropharmacology, and psychological influences in the production of physical symptoms. The contribution of psychological factors to organic conditions such as peptic ulcer disease, asthma, and coronary artery disease may be a useful analogy for patients.

Physical therapy

Physiotherapy and rehabilitation, providing both the expectation of recovery and encouragement for the patient's efforts in this regard, have improved chronic neurological conversion symptoms, even in the absence of other treatment.[67] The goal of physiotherapy is symptom reduction through gait training, passive range of motion, and an exercise program that enables the patient to assert conscious control over the abnormal movements. Physical therapy can also rationalize the return of physical function in patients who find it difficult to accept such restoration on the basis of psychiatric intervention alone. This is, of course, separate from the primary function of physical therapy in patients who have developed disuse atrophy or contractures secondary to psychogenic movement disorders.

Pharmacotherapy

Antidepressant and anxiolytic agents can contribute to symptom relief in somatoform disorders in patients experiencing depression or anxiety.[25] The use of psychotropic agents in patients with underlying affective disorder or schizophrenia is indicated.[26] The severity of an underlying depression should never be overlooked, as these patients are capable of committing suicide.[68] Psychiatric hospitalization may be necessary for some patients, especially with severe underlying psychopathology, depression, or suicidality. Patients with treatment-resistant major depressive disorder may require ECT.

For patients whose co-existing anxiety, depression, or other psychopathology has combined with physical symptoms into a somatizing disorder, the prospect of relief and redemption from a state of demoralization and disability, when presented in a supportive and integrated fashion, and enhanced by effective pharmacological relief, can generate a therapeutic "flight into health" reaction, sometimes with dramatic and even curative results.

Hypnosis

Hypnosis is a useful technique in selected patients, both diagnostically and therapeutically. The assessment of an individual's hypnotizability, quantified using the Hypnotic Induction Profile,[69] is recommended as a routine component of the approach to psychogenic movement disorder patients. In highly

hypnotizable individuals, conversion symptoms can be provoked, worsened, or ameliorated using hypnotic induction. Hypnotherapy as a primary treatment modality can directly influence conversion symptoms.[70] As an adjunct to psychotherapy, self-hypnosis is easily taught and can be helpful in enabling patients to gain symptom control. One valuable function of hypnosis is its ability to provide the patient exposure to the phenomenon of dissociation. Dissociation is generally regarded as an essential component of the psychopathological process of symptom formation in conversion disorder.[71] The trance state may enable the patient to more fully understand the dynamics of the conversion symptomatology. In some individuals with psychogenic movement disorders, the capacity for dissociation may be harnessed in the service of symptom resolution.

Use of placebo

Although physicians may be inclined to believe that a positive placebo response establishes a symptom as psychogenic,[72] complete diagnostic reliance on placebos is not advised. Administration of a placebo will improve organic symptoms such as pain in 30–40% of individuals.[73] The use of placebos has been described in patients with psychogenic dystonia[19] and psychogenic myoclonus,[55] but has not been rigorously evaluated. At a time when informed consent and patient autonomy represent ideals of patient care, the use of placebos has been equated by some as deceptive. Case 15 in a series of patients with psychogenic dystonia illustrates the potential risk to the patient-physician relationship and failure of therapy when the patient becomes aware that a placebo is being used.[19] No specific personality factors appear to correlate with susceptibility to placebo effect. Self-sufficient, highly educated persons, cooperative patients who tend not to use medication, and individuals who generally report few somatic symptoms tend to be responsive to placebo—profiles that appear the opposite of what one would expect to find in a population of psychogenic patients.

In a series of patients with psychogenic dystonia, 10 of 21 individuals received placebos as part of the diagnostic evaluation or treatment.[19] For diagnostic purposes, the use of placebo, whether a pill or injection, may be helpful. At Columbia-Presbyterian Medical Center, such a test is usually not performed to establish a definite diagnosis of psychogenic movement disorder. If used, the placebo should not be given on a single occasion to remove or induce a particular symptom, but rather be administered according to a protocol, preferably in a double-blind fashion after having obtained formal consent from the patient, much as would be done in a therapeutic trial. Over the past several years at Columbia-Presbyterian Medical Center, we have discarded the formal use of placebos in treating psychogenic movement disorders, but are not unaware that many other interventions, such as pharmacological treatment, physiotherapy, or hypnosis, may confer a placebo or symbolic effect that aids the therapeutic process.

Prognosis

Follow-up studies of patients with untreated somatoform disorders are in agreement that the overall outcome is poor, and the spontaneous resolution of symptoms is uncommon. In a recent follow-up study of 73 patients with presumed psychogenic motor symptoms ("unexplained medical symptoms") who were admitted to hospital, the index symptom was not improved, or was worse, in over half by the end of a six-year follow-up interval.[74] A similar outcome was described in a four-year follow-up study of 70 patients with conversion disorder and somatization disorder.[75]

The outcome of treatment would appear to depend greatly upon the underlying psychiatric disturbance. A good prognosis is associated with conversion disorder in patients aged less than 40 years who are admitted to hospital,[64] a short duration of symptoms, a change in marital status, symptom remission that occurs by the end of the hospital admission, and the presence of an underlying treatable psychiatric disorder, such as depression or anxiety.[24,64,74] Poorer prognoses attach to the presence of a personality disorder,[76] pending litigation and ongoing secondary gain in the form of financial compensation. One hopes that treatment itself is associated with a better prognosis, but in fact no controlled trial of treatment using an untreated control group has ever been done. A 10-year follow-up study of 73 patients with conversion disorder found that, in contrast to the most optimistic view of the effect of treatment, utilization of physician services may well be a marker for intractable disease.[76] In this series, patients with the most physician contact had the least likelihood of symptom remission.[76]

In the series of Columbia-Presbyterian Medical Center,[24] all treatment successes occurred in individuals with conversion disorder or somatoform disorder. No patient with malingering or factitious disorder improved. For patients with conversion disorder, response to treatment cannot be predicted in advance. There was no correlation between good outcome and such variables as age at onset, gender, IQ, or specific movement disorder phenomenology, but the population under study was small. The specific movement disorder phenomenology does not appear to relate to the prognosis. While the literature describes an inverse correlation between outcome and duration of illness, patients with chronic, disabling psychogenic movements of more than 10 years' duration will occasionally achieve complete symptom remission.[19]

Treatment by Williams et al.,[24] resulted in a long-term (>1 year) benefit in 52% of patients, with complete relief, considerable relief, and moderate relief in 25%, 21%, and 8%, respectively. Some relapse occurred in over 20%, and no improvement was seen in 12%. Of those who had been previously employed, 25% were able to resume full-time work, and 10%, part-time work, with 15% functioning at home.

In the series of 28 cases of psychogenic movement disorders reported by Factor et al.,[27] 35% resolved and this subgroup had a shorter duration of disease than those who did not resolve. Of 56 patients with any type of psychogenic neurological disorder other than pseudoseizures, Couprie et al.,[64] found that the long-term outcome was good in 96% of those who improved during a hospital stay, and that rapid improvement was related to recent onset of symptoms.

Conclusions

Psychogenic movement disorders occupy a border zone between neurology and psychiatry. The understanding and treatment of psychogenic movement disorders requires the sophistication and collaboration of both specialties. The physical symptoms bring the patient to the neurologist, but the etiological explanation for the symptoms comes only after careful psychiatric assessment. Despite the lack of controlled therapeutic trials in this field, clinical experience since the time of Charcot and Freud has revealed that a sustained, integrated, multimodal treatment approach, preferably in the hospital setting in chronic cases, offers the best chance of symptom remission for disabled patients. The treatment begins with a supportive explanation of the diagnosis, and may include a combination of several modalities, including psychotherapy, hypnotherapy, physical therapy, and pharmacological therapy. Further study is required to evaluate the specific efficacy or individual treatment approaches, prognostic factors, and long-term outcome.

References

1. Goetz CG. Charcot, the Clinician: The Tuesday Lessons. Excerpts from Nine Case Presentations on General Neurology Delivered at the Salpetriere Hospital in 1887–88 By Jean-Martin Charcot, translated with Commentary. New York: Raven Press, 1987:102–122

2. Gowers WR. A Manual of Diseases of the Nervous System, Vol. II, 2nd ed. Philadelphia: Blakiston, 1893; 984–1030

3. Marsden CD. Hysteria: a neurologist's view. Psychol Med 1986;16:277–288

4. Lempert T, Dietrich M, Huppert D, Brandt T. Psychogenic disorders in neurology: frequency and clinical spectrum. Acta Neurol Scand 1990;82:335–340

5. Krumholz A, Niedermeyer E. Psychogenic seizures: a clinical study with follow-up data. Neurology 1983;33: 498–502

6. Lesser RP, Leuders H, Dinner DS. Evidence for epilepsy is rare in patients with psychogenic seizures. Neurology 1983;33:502–504

7. Vecht CJ, Meerwaldt JD, Lees AJ, et al. Unusual Movement Disorder, Case 1, 1991. Unusual tremor, myoclonus and a limping gait. Mov Disord 1991;6: 371–375

8. Andermann F, Andermann E. Excessive startle syndromes: startle disease, jumping, and startle epilepsy. Adv Neurol 1986;43:321–338

9. Thompson PD, Colebatch JG, Brown P, et al. Voluntary stimulus-sensitive jerks and jumps mimicking myoclonus or pathological startle syndromes. Mov Disord 1992;7:257–262

10. Fahn S, Marsden CD, Calne DB. Classification and investigation of dystonia. *In:* Marsden CD, Fahn S, eds. Movement Disorders 2. London: Butterworths, 1987: 332–358

11. Schwartzman RJ, Kerrigan J. The movement disorder of reflex sympathetic dystrophy. Neurology 1990;40:57–61

12. Lang A, Fahn S. Movement disorder of RSD. Neurology 1990;40:1476–1477

13. Bhatia KP, Bhatt MH, Marsden CD. The causalgia-dystonia syndrome. Brain 1993;116:843–851

14. Schott GD. The relation of peripheral trauma and pain to dystonia. J Neurol Neurosurg Psychiat 1985;48: 698–701

15. Schott GD. Mechanisms of causalgia and related clinical conditions. The role of the central nervous and of the sympathetic nervous systems. Brain 1986;109: 717–738

16. Scherokman B, Husain F, Cuetter A, et al. Peripheral dystonia. Arch Neurol 1986;43:830–832

17. Gordon MF, Brin MF, Giladi N, et al. Dystonia precipitated by peripheral trauma. Mov Disord 1990;5(Suppl 1):67

18. Goldman S, Ahlskog JE. Post-traumatic cervical dystonia. Mayo Clin Proc 1993;68:443–448

19. Fahn S, Williams DT. Psychogenic dystonia. Adv Neurol 1988;50:431–455

20. Koller W, Lang A, Vetere-Overfield B, et al. Psychogenic tremors. Neurology 1989;39:1094–1099

21. Ranawaya R, Riley D, Lang A. Psychogenic dyskinesias in patients with organic movement disorders. Mov Disord 1990;5:127–133

22. Lang AE. Psychogenic dystonia: a review of 18 cases. Can J Neurol Sci 1995;22:136–143

23. American Psychiatric Association. Diagnostic and Statistical Manual of Mental Disorders, Fourth Edition, Text Revision. Washington DC: American Psychiatric Association, 2000

24. Williams DT, Ford B, Fahn S. Phenomenology and psychopathology related to psychogenic movement disorders. Adv Neurol 1994;65:231–257

25. Kellner R. Psychosomatic syndromes and somatic symptoms. Washington DC: American Psychiatric Press, 1991

26. Lazare A. Converson symptoms. NEJM 1981;745–748

27. Factor SA, Podskalny GD, Molho ES. Psychogenic movement disorders: frequency, clinical profile, and characteristics. J Neurol Neurosurg Psychiatry 1995;59: 406–412

28. Schwalbe W. Eine eigentumliche tonische Krampfform mit hysterischen Symptomen. Inaug Diss, Berlin: G. Schade, 1908

29. Oppenheim H. Uber eine eigenartige Krampfkrankheit des kindlichen und jugendlichen Alters (Dysbasia lordotica progressiva, Dystonia musculorum deformans). Neurol Centrabl 1911;30:1090–1107

30. Flatau, Sterling W. Progressiver Torsionspasms bie Kindern. Z Gesamte Neurol Psychiatr 1911;7:586–612

31. Destarac M. Torticolis spasmodique et spasmes fonctionnels. Rev Neurol 1901;9:591–597

32. Ziehen T. Ein fall von tonischer Torsionsneurose. Neurol Centrabl 1911;30:109–110

33. Eldridge R, Riklan M, Cooper IS. The limited role of psychotherapy in torsion dystonia. Experience with 44 cases. JAMA 1969;210:705–708

34. Marsden CD, Harrison MJG. Idiopathic torsion dystonia. Brain 1974;97:793–810

35. Cooper IS, Cullinan T, Riklan M. The natural history of dystonia. Adv Neurol 1976;14:157–169

36. Lesser RP, Fahn S. Dystonia: a disorder often misdiagnosed as a conversion reaction. Am J Psychiatry 1978;153:349–452

37. Meares R. Features which distinguish groups of spasmodic torticollis. J Psychosom Res 1971;15:1–11

38. Tibbets RW. Spasmodic torticollis. J Psychosom Res 1971;15:461–469

39. Cockburn JJ. Spasmodic torticollis: a psychogenic condition? J Psychosom Res 1971;15:471–477

40. Riklan M, Cullinan T, Cooper IS. Psychological studies in dystonia musculorum deformans. Adv Neurol 1976;14:189–200

41. Zeman W, Dyken P. Dystonia musculorum deformans. Handbook of Clinical Neurology. Amsterdam: North-Holland Publ. Co., 1968;6:517–543

42. Crisp AH, Moldofsky HA. A psychosomatic study of writer's cramp. Br J Psychiatry 1965;111:841–858

43. Bindman E, Tibbets RW. Writer's cramp, a rational approach to treatment? Br J Psychiatry 1977;131: 143–148

44. Sheehy MP, Marsden CD. Writer's cramp: a focal dystonia. Brain 1982;105:461–480

45. Grafman J, Cohen LG, Hallett M. Is focal hand dystonia associated with psychopathology? Mov Disord 1991;6: 29–35

46. Harrington RC, Wieck A, Marks IM, Marsden CD. Writer's cramp: not associated with anxiety. Mov Disord 1988;3:195–200

47. Fahn S, Eldridge R. Definition of dystonia and classification of the dystonic states. Adv Neurol 1976;14: 1–5

48. Fahn S, Williams D, Reches A, et al. Hysterical dystonia, a rare disorder: report of five documented cases. Neurology 1983;33(Suppl 2):161

49. Batshaw ML, Wachtel RC, Deckel AW, et al. Munchausen's syndrome simulating torsion dystonia. N Engl J Med 1985;312:1437–1439

50. Deuschl G, Koster B, Lucking CH, Scheidt C. Diagnostic and pathophysiological aspects of psychogenic tremors. Mov Disord 1998;13:294–302

51. Kim YJ, Pakiam ASI, Lang AE. Historical and clinical features of psychogenic tremor: a review of 70 cases. Can J Neurol Sci 1999;26:190–195

52. Keane JR. Hysterical gait disorders: 60 cases. Neurology 1989;39:586–589

53. Hayes MW, Graham S, Heldorf P, et al. A video review of the diagnosis of psychogenic gait: appendix and commentary. Mov Disord 1999;14:914–921

54. Monday K, Jankovic J. Psychogenic myoclonus. Neurology 1993;43:349–352

55. Terada K, Ikeda A, Van Ness PC, et al. Presence of Bereitschaftspotential preceding psychogenic myoclonus: clinical application of jerk-locked back averaging. J Neurol Neurosurg Psychiatry 1995;58:745–747

56. Dooley JM, Stokes A, Gordon KE. Pseudo-tics in Tourette syndrome. J Child Neurol 1994;9:50–51

57. Lang AE, Koller WG, Fahn S. Psychogenic parkinsonism. Arch Neurol 1995;52:802–810

58. Spiegel D, Hunt T, Dondershine HE. Dissociation and hypnotizability in post-traumatic stress disorder. Am J Psychiatr 1988;145:301

59. Oppenheim H. Section on Hysteria. *In:* Textbook of Nervous Diseases for Physicians and Students, fifth edition, translated by Bruce H., Edinburgh: Otto Schulzle, 1911:1053–1111

60. Kellner R. Somatoform and factitious disorders. *In:* American Psychiatric Association Task Force, ed., Treatment of Psychiatric Disorders, vol. 3. Washington DC: American Psychiatric Press, 1989:2119–2184

61. Krull F, Schifferdecker M. Inpatient treatment of conversion disorder: a clinical investigation of outcome. Psychother Psychosom 1990;53:161–165

62. Ford B, Williams DT, Fahn S. Treatment of psychogenic movement disorders. In: Kurlan R, ed. Treatment of Movement Disorders. Philadelphia: J.B. Lippincott, 1995:475–485

63. Hafeiz HB. Hysterical conversion: a prognostic study. Br J Psychiatr 1980;136:548–551

64. Couprie W, Wijdicks EFM, Rooijmans HGM, van Gijn J. Outcome in conversion disorder: a follow up study. J Neurol Neurosurg Psychiatry 1995;58:750–752

65. Walczak TS, Papacostas S, Williams DT, et al. Outcome after diagnosis of psychogenic nonepileptic seizures. Epilepsia 1995;36:1131–1137

66. Plassman R. Inpatient and outpatient long-term psychotherapy of patients suffering from fractitious disorders. Psychother Psychosom 1994;62:96–107

67. Delargy MA, Peatfield RC, Burt AA. Successful rehabilitation in conversion paralysis. Br Med J 1986;292:1730–1731

68. Slater ETO, Glithero E. A follow-up of patients diagnosed as suffering from hysteria. J Psychosom Res 1965;9:9–13

69. Spiegel D, Spira J. Hypnosis for psychiatric disorders. In: Dunner DL, ed. Current Psychiatric Therapy. Philadelphia: WB Saunders, 1993:517–523

70. Spiegel H, Spiegel D. Trance and treatment: the clinical uses of hypnosis. Washington DC: American Psychiatric Press, 1987

71. Williams DT, Hypnosis. In: Weiner J, ed. Textbook of Child and Adolescent Psychiatry, Second Ed. Washington DC: American Psychiatric Press 1996:937–949

72. Goodwin JS, Goodwin JM, Vogel AV. Knowledge and use of placebos by house officers and nurses. Ann Int Med 1979:91:106–110

73. Beecher HK. The powerful placebo. JAMA 1955;159:1602–1606

74. Crimlisk HL, Bhatia K, Cope H, David A, Marsden CD, Ron MA. Slater revisited: 6 year follow-up study of patients with medically unexplained symptoms. Br Med J 1998;316:582–586

75. Kent DA, Tomasson K, Corvell W. Course and outcome of conversion and somatization disorders: a four-year follow-up. Psychosomatics 1995;36:138–144

76. Mace CJ, Trimble MR. Ten-year prognosis of conversion disorder. Br J Psychiatr 1996;169:282–288

255 Hereditary Ataxias and other Cerebellar Degenerations

Thomas Klockgether

Introduction

The hereditary ataxias and cerebellar degenerations comprise a wide spectrum of disorders with ataxia as the leading symptom. In most of these disorders, ataxia is due to degeneration of the cerebellar cortex and its afferent or efferent fiber connections. A classification of ataxia that distinguishes between hereditary and non-hereditary ataxias is given in Table 255.1. The underlying genetic defects have been identified in most hereditary ataxias.

Historical perspective

The history of ataxia research started in 1863, when Friedreich, a German Professor of Medicine, was the first to describe patients with hereditary ataxia. Numerous subsequent clinical and neuropathological studies presented cases that were similar to Friedreich's ataxia (FRDA) and others with distinct features causing considerable confusion and uncertainty about diagnostic entities and proper classification. The first classification system that found wide acceptance was a neuropathological classification proposed by Holmes. He distinguished between spinocerebellar degeneration, degeneration of the cerebellar cortex, and olivopontocerebellar atrophy.[1] More recently, Harding used clinical and genetic criteria to diagnose and classify hereditary ataxias.[2] Starting in the nineties of the 20th century, the gene mutations underlying most types of hereditary ataxia were identified allowing first insights into the molecular pathogenesis of hereditary ataxias.[3]

General principles of therapy

Although the genetic defects of most hereditary ataxias are known, rational treatment approaches are available only in some rare forms of ataxia, such as ataxia with isolated vitamin E deficiency (AVED) or Refsum's disease. In most other types of ataxia only supportive treatment is possible.

In general, it is assumed that physiotherapy and speech therapy are helpful in ataxia disorders. The goal should be to maintain the highest possible level of autonomy, to cope with physical disability and to prevent secondary complications. With progression of the disease many patients will require walking aids and a wheelchair.

It has been repeatedly claimed that drugs that increase neurotransmission at central 5-HT receptors temporarily improve cerebellar ataxia.[4] Three recent studies investigated the anti-ataxic effect of the anxi-

Table 255.1 Classification of ataxias

Hereditary ataxias
  Autosomal recessive ataxias
    Friedreich's ataxia (FRDA)
    Ataxia telangiectasia (AT)
    Autosomal recessive spastic ataxia of Charlevoix-Saguenay (ARSACS)
    Abetalipoproteinemia
    Ataxia with isolated vitamin E deficiency (AVED)
    Refsum's disease
    Cerebrotendinous xanthomatosis
    Other autosomal recessive ataxias with known chromosomal localization
    Early onset cerebellar ataxia (EOCA)
  Autosomal dominant ataxias
    Spinocerebellar ataxias (SCA)
    Episodic ataxias (EA)
Non-hereditary ataxias
  Multiple system atrophy, cerebellar type (MSA-C)
  Sporadic adult-onset ataxia of unknown origin
Symptomatic ataxias
  Alcoholic cerebellar degeneration
  Ataxia due to other toxic reasons
  Ataxia caused by acquired vitamin deficiency or metabolic disorders
  Paraneoplastic cerebellar degeneration
  Immune-mediated ataxias

olytic 5-HT$_{1A}$ receptor agonist buspirone. Results of an open-label study of 20 patients with different forms of degenerative suggested an anti-ataxic action of buspirone at a dose of 30–60 mg per day.[5] Efficacy of buspirone was confirmed in a randomized, placebo-controlled study of 19 patients with ataxia due to cerebellar cortical atrophy.[6] In contrast, another study did not report a favorable effect of buspirone in ataxia.[7] The N-methyl-D-aspartate receptor antagonist amantadine was reported to have an anti-ataxic action in patients with olivopontocerebellar atrophy, but not in FRDA.[8] It is not clear, however, whether improvement was due to a specific effect on cerebellar ataxia or rather on accompanying parkinsonian symptoms. In our own experience, the efficacy of anti-ataxic drugs is low, and only very few patients really benefit from them.

There are numerous neurological and non-neurological symptoms that may occur in association with certain ataxia disorders. Well-known examples are cardiomyopathy and diabetes mellitus in FRDA. These accompanying symptoms require conventional medical and neurological treatment if not otherwise stated.

Friedreich's ataxia (FRDA)

With a prevalence of 2–3:100 000, FRDA is the most frequent recessively inherited ataxia. Mean age at onset is 15 years ranging from 2–51 years.[9] FRDA is a progressive disease leading to disability and premature death. Median latency to become wheelchair-bound after disease onset is 11 years. Life expectancy after disease onset is estimated 35 to 40 years.[10] Clinically, FRDA is characterized by gait and limb ataxia, dysarthria, lower limb areflexia, loss of proprioception and cardiomyopathy. A minority of FRDA patients develop diabetes mellitus.[9]

In 1996, a homozygous, intronic GAA repeat expansion in a novel gene named X25 was identified as the causative mutation.[11] Due to the mutation, tissue levels of its gene product, frataxin, are severely reduced. Frataxin is a mitochondrial protein the loss of which leads to mitochondrial iron overload, decline of mitochondrial respiratory activity and increased production of free radicals.[12,13] These alterations lead to a degeneration starting in the dorsal root ganglion cells and spreading to ascending and descending spinal pathways.

Improved understanding of the pathogenesis of FRDA prompted therapeutic trials with orally administered iron chelators and free radical-scavengers. Since these trials have not been completed it remains unknown whether these new therapeutic approaches are effective. Rustin et al., recently reported that idebenone (5 mg/kg per day), a short-chain quinone analogue acting as a free radical-scavenger given over 4–9 months decreased the left ventricular mass index in three FRDA patients.[14] Although these preliminary results obtained in an open, uncontrolled trial in only three patients are encouraging they do not justify a routine treatment of FRDA patients with idebenone.

Ataxia telangiectasia (AT)

Ataxia telangiectasia is an autosomal recessively inherited multisystem disorder with an estimated incidence of 0.2–2:100 000 live births. Ataxia telangiectasia starts in early childhood and leads to premature death, often around the age of 20 years. Clinically, AT is characterized by cerebellar ataxia, oculocutaneous telangiectasias, a high incidence of neoplasia, radiosensitivity and recurrent infections. Almost all patients have increased serum levels of α-fetoprotein. The gene affected in AT, ATM (ataxia telangiectasia mutated), encodes a member of the phosphoinositol-3 kinase family involved in cell cycle checkpoint control and DNA repair.[15] More than 200 distinct mutations distributed over the entire gene have been reported suggesting that most patients carry private mutations. In the central nervous system the mutations result in degeneration of the cerebellar cortex.

There is no effective treatment for AT. Treatment of infections should be initiated early and maintained over prolonged time. Administration of immunoglobulins can be considered in patients with repeated infections. Treatment of malignant neoplasias is a particular problem because AT patients have increased sensitivity to radiation and chemotherapy. Therefore, conventional radiotherapy should be avoided, and chemotherapy should be administered only on an individual basis.[16]

Autosomal recessive spastic ataxia of Charlevoix-Saguenay (ARSACS)

Autosomal recessive spastic ataxia of Charlevoix-Saguenay (ARSACS) is a rare autosomal recessive disorder clinically characterized by progressive ataxia and spasticity. Molecular genetic studies in an isolated population in Quebec, Canada, identified causative mutations in a novel gene encoding a large protein with a heat-shock domain.[17] Linkage to the same locus was established in a large Tunisian family with a similar phenotype.[18]

There is no effective therapy for ARSACS. A minority of patients with pronounced spasticity may benefit from antispastic drugs.

Abetalipoproteinemia

Abetalipoproteinemia is a rare autosomal recessively inherited disorder characterized by onset of diarrhea soon after birth and slow development of a neurological syndrome thereafter. The neurological syndrome consists of ataxia, weakness of the limbs with loss of tendon reflexes, disturbed sensation and retinal degeneration. Abetalipoproteinemia is caused by mutations in the gene encoding a subunit of a microsomal triglyceride transfer protein.[19] As a consequence, circulating apoprotein B-containing lipoproteins are almost completely missing, and the patients are unable to absorb and transport fat and fat-soluble vitamins. The neurological symptoms are due to vitamin E deficiency.

Management of abetalipoproteinemia consists of a diet with reduced fat intake and vitamin E supplementation. Intake of dietary fat should be restricted to 25% of the total daily calories. One third of daily fat should stem from food sources, two thirds should be given as medium-chain triglycerides. Patients should receive an adequate supply of essential fatty acids.[20]

Despite the principal absorption defect, vitamin E is supplemented orally since patients are able to secrete very small amounts of apoprotein B-containing lipoproteins. Recommended doses are 50–100 mg/kg per day. In addition, vitamin A (200–400 IU/kg per day) and vitamin K (5 mg every two weeks) are given. Levels of vitamin E and A should be closely monitored. Vitamin supplementation should be started as early as possible. Restoration of vitamin E levels will lead to clinical improvement or arrest of further deterioration.[20]

Ataxia with isolated vitamin E deficiency (AVED)

Ataxia with isolated vitamin E deficiency (AVED) is a rare autosomal recessively inherited disorder with a phenotype resembling FRDA. Patients with AVED carry homozygous mutations of the gene encoding α-tocopherol transport protein, a liver-specific protein that incorporates vitamin E into very low-density lipoproteins.[21] As a consequence, vitamin E is rapidly eliminated.

Since there is no absorption deficit, oral supplementation of vitamin E at a dose of 800–2000 mg per day is recommended.[22] Levels of vitamin E should be closely monitored.

Refsum's disease

Refsum's disease is a rare autosomal recessively inherited disorder due to mutations in the gene encoding phytanoyl-CoA hydroxylase that is involved in the α-oxidation of phytanic acid.[23] The clinical phenotype of Refsum's disease is caused by accumulation of phytanic acid in body tissues. Clinically, Refsum's disease is characterized by ataxia, demyelinating sensorimotor neuropathy, pigmentary retinal degeneration, deafness, cardiac arrhythmias and ichthyosis-like skin changes. Whereas ocular and hearing problems are usually slowly progressive, there may be acute exacerbations which are precipitated by low caloric intake and mobilization of phytanic acid from adipose tissue.

Refsum's disease is treated by dietary restriction of phytanic acid from 50–100 mg contained in a normal Western diet to less than 10 mg per day. The diet should provide adaequate caloric intake to prevent mobilization of phytanic acid from adipose stores. Details of the dietary management are given by Gibberd et al.[24] With good dietary supervision ataxia and neuropathy may improve. In contrast, the progressive loss of vision and hearing cannot be prevented.

In acute exacerbations, plasma exchange (four sessions over a period of 7–21 days) is effective in lowering phytanic acid levels and improving neurological and cardiac function. Plasmapheresis may be also considered in patients in whom dietary control is insufficient.[25]

Cerebrotendinous xanthomatosis

Cerebrotendinous xanthomatosis is a rare autosomal recessive lipid storage disorder with accumulation of cholestanol and cholesterin in various tissues. The disorder is due to mutations of the gene encoding 27-hydroxylase.[26] The clinical syndrome includes xanthomatous swelling of the tendons, cataracts and slowly progressive neurological symptoms including ataxia, pyramidal signs and cognitive decline.

Cerebrotendinous xanthomatosis is treated by oral administration of chenodeoxycholate (750 mg per day).[27] This treatment results in a marked drop of plasma cholestanol levels and prevents further progression of the neurological syndrome. In the early stages of the disease, clinical improvement may be achieved. Cataracts and xanthomatous swelling of the tendons are not affected by this treatment. Treatment can be further improved by addition of 3-hydroxy-3-methylglutaryl coenzyme A (HMG CoA) reductase inhibitors.[28]

Other autosomal recessive ataxias with known chromosomal localization

Recently, genes causing three different types of rare autosomal recessively inherited ataxia have been mapped to chromosomal gene loci. Portuguese and Japanese families suffering from ataxia with oculomotor apraxia (AOA) showed linkage to a 2 cM region on chromosome 9p13.[29] The neurological presentation of this disorder is similar to AT; however, telangiectasias, neoplasias and immunodeficiency are absent. Onset is usually in early childhood. In Japanese patients with ataxia and elevated levels of creatine kinase, γ-globulines and α-fetoprotein linkage at 9q34 was established.[30] In contrast to AOA, this disorder usually starts in late adolescence. An Israeli family with ataxia, optic atrophy and hearing impairment was mapped to 6p21-23.[30] Rational treatment approaches for these disorders are not available.

Early onset cerebellar ataxia (EOCA)

EOCA is used to denote those ataxias with an onset before the age of 20 years in which the genetic basis and aetiology are unknown. Apart from cerebellar ataxia patients may present with a variety of additional symptoms including retinal degeneration (Hallgren syndrome), hypogonadism (Holmes syndrome), optic atrophy (Behr syndrome), cataracts and mental retardation (Marinesco-Sjögren syndrome) and myoclonus (Ramsay Hunt syndrome). Since the aetiology of none of these disorders is unknown, rational treatment approaches are not available.

Spinocerebellar ataxias (SCAs)

The SCAs are a genetically heterogeneous group of autosomal dominantly inherited progressive ataxia disorders. Up to now, 15 different gene loci (SCA-1–8, 10–14, 16,17) have been found to be associated with SCA. All mutations that have been identified so far (SCA-1–3, 6, 8, 10, 12, 17) are expanded repeats, in six (SCA-1–3, 6, 7, 17) the mutation is an expanded CAG repeat localized in a coding region of the respective gene (Table 255.2). It is assumed the abnormal polyglutamine-containing proteins encoded by the mutated genes acquire a novel toxic function and exert deleterious effects on specific neuronal populations. In this respect, these disorders resemble other CAG repeat disorders, such as Huntington's disease and spinobulbar muscular atrophy.[31] The neuropathology of the SCAs is diverse. Many forms have widespread degeneration involving the cerebellum, brainstem, spinal cord and parts of the basal ganglia. A characteristic ultrastructural hallmark of the SCAs caused by translated CAG repeat mutations is the occurrence of neuronal intranuclear inclusions.

The prevalence of the dominant ataxias is estimated 0.9–1.3:100 000.[32] Mean age of onset of most SCAs is 30 to 40 years with considerable variation between and within families. SCA-6 has a later disease onset with an average of 50 years.[33] Patients who develop additional non-cerebellar symptoms die prematurely 20 to 25 years after disease onset, while

Table 255.2   Mutations and clinical phenotypes of spinocerebellar ataxias (SCA)

Disorder	Mutation	Gene product	Clinical phenotype
SCA-1	Translated CAG repeat expansion	Ataxin-1	Ataxia, pyramidal signs, neuropathy, dysphagia, restless legs syndrome
SCA-2	Translated CAG repeat expansion	Ataxin-2	Ataxia, slow saccades, neuropathy, restless legs syndrome
SCA-3 (Machado-Joseph disease)	Translated CAG repeat expansion	Ataxin-3	Ataxia, pyramidal signs, ophthalmoplegia, neuropathy, dystonia, restless legs syndrome
SCA-4	Unknown	Unknown	Ataxia, neuropathy
SCA-5	Unknown	Unknown	Almost pure cerebellar ataxia
SCA-6	Translated CAG repeat expansion	Calcium channel subunit (CACNA1A)	Almost pure cerebellar ataxia
SCA-7	Translated CAG repeat expansion	Ataxin-7	Ataxia, ophthalmoplegia, visual loss
SCA-8	Untranslated CTG repeat expansion	Unknown	Almost pure cerebellar ataxia
SCA-10	Intronic ATTCT repeat expansion	Unknown	Ataxia, epilepsy
SCA-11	Unknown	Unknown	Almost pure cerebellar ataxia
SCA-12	Untranslated CAG repeat expansion	Phosphatase subunit (PP2A–PR55β)	Ataxia, tremor
SCA-13	Unknown	Unknown	Ataxia, mental retardation
SCA-14	Unknown	Unknown	Ataxia, myoclonus
SCA-16	Unknown	Unknown	Almost pure cerebellar ataxia
SCA-17	Translated CAG repeat expansion	TATA binding protein	

life expectancy is not significantly reduced in patients with a pure cerebellar syndrome.[10]

Clinically the SCAs fall into three major groups which have been originally defined by Harding.[34] The majority of SCAs are characterized by progressive ataxia associated with a variety of additional extracerebellar symptoms including pyramidal signs, dysphagia, ophthalmoplegia and neuropathy. Many SCA-1, 2 and 3 patients have a restless legs syndrome. In SCA-5, 6, 8 and 11, clinical presentation is almost pure cerebellar. The SCA-7 condition is unique in that the ataxia is associated with progressive visual loss due to retinal degeneration (Table 255.2).

Despite the progress that has been made in elucidating the genetic basis of the various forms of SCA the pathogenesis of these disorders is not completely understood. Hence, there are no rational treatment approaches. Accompanying symptoms, such as restless legs syndrome are treated in standard manner.

Episodic ataxias (EAs)

Episodic ataxias are rare autosomal dominant disorders characterized by intermittent attacks of ataxia. To date, two different genetic and clinical variants are known. Missense mutations in a brain potassium channel gene, KCNA1 result in EA-1.[35] Episodic ataxia-1 is characterized by brief attacks of ataxia and dysarthria often provoked by movements and startle with onset in early childhood.

Truncating mutations of the CACNA$_{1A}$ gene encoding the α_{1A} voltage-dependent calcium channel subunit have been found in families with EA-2.[36] Compared with EA-1, attacks in EA-2 start later, last longer and are precipitated by emotional stress and exercise but not by startle. Some individuals who may or may not suffer from episodic ataxia have slowly progressive ataxia and cerebellar atrophy.

In both disorders acetazolamide is used to prevent attacks. The effect of acetazolamide is more reliable in EA-2 than in EA-1. If treatment is necessary, patients are typically started on a low dose (125 mg per day) which is then gradually increased (500–700 mg per day) until a satisfactory suppression of attacks is achieved.[37] Paraesthesias which frequently occur under acetazolamide may be reduced by oral potassium supplementation. As a second line treatment carbamazepine and phenytoin can be tried.

Multiple system atrophy (MSA)

MSA is a sporadic, adult-onset disease encompassing the former disease categories striatonigral degeneration, sporadic olivopontocerebellar atrophy and Shy-Drager syndrome. The prevalence of MSA is 4.4:100 000.[38] Mean age at disease onset is 55 years. Multiple system atrophy takes a unrelentlessly progressive course. After a median latency of six years, MSA patients become wheelchair-bound. The median life expectancy after disease onset is nine years.[10] Clinically, MSA patients present with various combinations of parkinsonism, cerebellar ataxia and autonomic failure (orthostatic hypotension, urinary incontinence).[39]

The aetiology of MSA is unknown. To date, no genetic or environmental risk factors have been found. The MSA brains show widespread degeneration encompassing the basal ganglia, brainstem, cerebellum and intermediolateral cell columns of the spinal cord. The ultrastructural hallmark of MSA is the presence of ubiquitinated oligodendroglial cytoplasmic inclusions.

There is no curative or preventive treatment for MSA. Parkinsonian symptoms respond to dopaminergic medication although the response is less robust than in idiopathic Parkinson's disease.[40] Autonomic symptoms are treated in standard manner. In our experience, there is no effective symptomatic treatment for ataxia. Amantadine (3 × 100 mg per day) may be considered because it has been suggested that this compound combines antiparkinsonian and anti-ataxic effects.[8]

Sporadic adult-onset ataxia of unknown origin

In many patients with sporadic adult-onset progressive ataxia, the underlying cause remains unknown. It is estimated that these patients are twice as frequent as patients with the cerebellar type of MSA.[41,42] Age of onset is around 55 years, and life expectancy is almost normal. Most of the patients have isolated cerebellar atrophy with little or no involvement of the brainstem.

In most patients of this group, cerebellar ataxia is the prominent symptom. However, pyramidal signs and sensory disturbances may occur. Sporadic adult-onset ataxia can be differentiated from MSA by the lasting absence of severe autonomic failure. In contrast, the clinical phenotype of sporadic adult-onset ataxia may resemble that of SCA patients. There are no specific treatment approaches for sporadic adult-onset ataxia.

Alcoholic cerebellar degeneration

Alcoholic cerebellar degeneration is probably the most common form of chronic cerebellar ataxia, although reliable estimates of prevalence are not available. Clinically, ataxia due to alcoholism is characterized by ataxic gait and stance without major involvement of the upper extremities. Ataxia occurs subacutely in heavy drinkers, and may then stabilize for years. Symptoms may progress particularly in those who continue to drink. The pathological changes consist of a loss of the Purkinje cell layer of the vermis and the anterior parts of the cerebellar hemispheres.

It is not entirely clear whether alcoholic cerebellar degeneration is due to nutritional deficiency of vitamin B_1 (thiamine), as in Wernicke's encephalopathy, or whether it is due to the toxic actions of alcohol or both.[43] Strict abstinence improves ataxia, whereas ataxia progresses in patients who continue to drink.[44] It is therefore essential that patients undergo an alcoholism cure. In addition, vitamin B_1 is supplemented. Initially, 50 mg are given intravenously and intramuscularly. Intramuscular injections are repeated for several days until supplementation is continued with an oral vitamin B_1 preparation. In addition to vitamin B_1 a multivitamin preparation is recommended.

Ataxia due to other toxic reasons

There are a number of compounds which may lead to cerebellar degeneration and persistent ataxia after chronic intake. These compounds include phenytoin, anti-cancer drugs (5-fluouracil, cytosin arabinosid) and solvents. Anticonvulsants other than phenytoin are generally considered safe although many of them cause reversible ataxia at higher doses. Intoxication with lithium salts my lead to irreversible ataxia. It is essential to stop further exposition. In epileptic patients, phenytoin should be replaced by an anticonvulsant drug that is less prone to damage the cerebellum.

Ataxia caused by acquired vitamin deficiency and metabolic disorders

Vitamin B_1   Wernicke's encephalopathy is an acute or subacute encephalopathy caused by deficiency of vitamin B_1 (thiamine) typically occurring in chronic alcoholics. Wernicke's encephalopathy may also result from excessive fasting, repeated vomiting and prolonged parenteral nutrition without adaequate vitamin supplementation. In addition to ataxia, the clinical syndrome includes eye muscle paresis, peripheral neuropathy, seizures and mental confusion. If not treated adequately, Wernicke's encephalopathy may result in a chronic amnesic state, Korsakow's psychosis. There is close relationship of Wernicke's encephalopathy and alcoholic cerebellar degeneration, since vitamin B_1 plays a prominent role in both disorders. Immediate parenteral application of high doses of vitamin B_1 is necessary. Initially, 50 mg are given intravenously and intramuscularly. Intramuscular injections are repeated for several days until supplementation is continued with an oral vitamin B_1 preparation. In addition to vitamin B_1 a multivitamin preparation is recommended.

Vitamin B_{12}   Vitamin B_{12} deficiency causes a macrocytic anemia, an axonal form of sensorimotor polyneuropathy and subacute combined degeneration of the spinal cord. Ataxia is often a prominent symptom of vitamin B_{12} deficiency. The most frequent cause is lack of intrinsic factor due to gastric disease. Vitamin B_{12} (hydroxycobalamin) is given intramuscularly at a dose of 1000 µg per day until neurological symptoms improve. Subsequently, the interval between applications is expanded to 3–4 days for a year, followed by life-long application of 1000 µg per month.

Vitamin E   Acquired vitamin E deficiency may occur as a consequence of malabsorption in gastrointestinal diseases such as coeliac disease, cystic fibrosis, short-bowel syndrome, biliary atresia and intrahepatic cholestasis. Patients present with ataxia of gait and stance, dysarthria and sensory neuropathy with loss of tendon reflexes.[45] To stop further progression, intramuscular application of vitamin E at a dose of 100–200 mg per day should be initiated as early as possible. Most patients are also deficient of other vitamins which should be supplemented together with vitamin E.

Hypothyrodism   Cerebellar ataxia is a rare neurological complication of hypothyrodism. The pathogenesis of this syndrome is unclear. Ataxia is completely relieved after adaequate substitution of thyroid hormone.

Paraneoplastic cerebellar degeneration (PCD)

Paraneoplastic cerebellar degeneration is an immune-mediated disorder that may occur in association with almost every tumor. Most frequently, however, small-cell lung cancer, cancer of the breast and ovary and lymphoma are involved. Paraneoplastic encephalomyelitis/sensory neuronopathy (PEM/SN) is another paraneoplastic syndrome. In contrast to PCD, PEM/SN affects multiple areas of the central nervous system, dorsal root ganglia and autonomic nerves. In 20% of the patients with PEM/SN, however, cerebellar ataxia is the presenting symptom.

In many, but not all patients with PCD, antibodies are found in the serum and cerebrospinal fluid (CSF) that react with antigens expressed by the nervous system and the tumor. These antibodies do not cause cerebellar degeneration. Rather, they are disease markers. Anti-Hu antibodies are found in association with small-cell lung cancer, anti-Yo antibodies mainly with ovarian cancer, anti-Tr with lymphoma and anti-Ri antibodies with various malignancies.

Ataxia in PCD has a subacute onset and rapidly progresses to severe disability. In most cases, ataxia precedes the detection of the underlying tumor. Ataxia involves upper and lower extremities and is accompanied by dysarthria and variable degrees of dysphagia. The clinical syndrome is similar in all types of PCD with the exception of PCD associated with anti-Ri antibodies. A highly characteristic feature of this disorder is the presence of opsoclonus leading to oscillopsia.

At disease onset, CT or MRI do not show major cerebellar atrophy. However, cerebellar atrophy usually develops as the disease progresses. A suspected diagnosis of PCD is confirmed by demonstration of specific antibodies. However, absence of antibodies does not rule out a diagnosis of PCD. In cases with suspected or proven PCD, a careful search for the underlying tumor is required. If this search is negative it has to be repeated every six months for 3 years.

In general PCD neither responds to treatment of the underlying tumor nor to immunosuppressive therapy. However, exceptions from this rule have been observed in individual cases.[46,47]

Immune-mediated ataxias

Recently, it has been recognized that there are immune-mediated cerebellar degenerations other than PCD. Ataxia may occur in patients with cryptic gluten sensitivity and circulating antigliadin antibodies. These patients do not necessarily have manifest coeliac disease with diarrhea, although half of them have mucosal changes in distal duodenal biopsies compatible with coeliac disease. It has been proposed to label this disorder "gluten ataxia".[48] Clinically, patients present with cerebellar ataxia and signs of sensory neuropathy. A gluten-free diet is recommended for patients with gluten ataxia, although controlled, prospective trials have not yet been completed.

Very rarely, ataxia is part of a polyglandular endocrine autoimmune syndrome in patients with circulating anti-glutamic acid decarboxylase antibodies. Improvement of ataxia after intravenous application of immunoglobulins has been reported in a single case.[49]

References

1. Holmes G. An attempt to classify cerebellar disease, with a note on Marie's hereditary cerebellar ataxia. Brain 1907;30:545–567
2. Harding AE. Classification of the hereditary ataxias and paraplegias. Lancet 1983;1:1151–1155
3. Klockgether T, Evert B. Genes involved in hereditary ataxias. Trends Neurosci 1998;21:413–418
4. Trouillas P, Serratrice G, Laplane D, et al. Levorotatory form of 5-hydroxytryptophan in Friedreich's ataxia: results of a double-blind drug-placebo cooperative study. Arch Neurol 1995;52:456–460
5. Lou JS, Goldfarb L, McShane L, et al. Use of buspirone for treatment of cerebellar ataxia. An open-label study. Arch Neurol 1995;52:982–988
6. Trouillas P, Xie J, Adeleine P, et al. Buspirone, a 5-hydroxytryptamine$_{1A}$ agonist, is active in cerebellar ataxia. Results of a double-blind drug placebo study in patients with cerebellar cortical atrophy. Arch Neurol 1997;54:749–752
7. Hassin-Baer S, Korczyn AD, Giladi N. An open trial of amantadine and buspirone for cerebellar ataxia: a disappointment. J Neural Transm 2000;107:1187–1189
8. Botez MI, Botez-Marquard T, Elie R, et al. Amantadine hydrochloride treatment in heredodegenerative ataxias: a double blind study. J Neurol Neurosurg Psychiatry 1996;61:259–264
9. Dürr A, Cossee M, Agid Y, et al. Clinical and genetic abnormalities in patients with Friedreich's ataxia. N Engl J Med 1996;335:1169–1175
10. Klockgether T, Lüdtke R, Kramer B, et al. The natural history of degenerative ataxia: a retrospective study in 466 patients. Brain 1998;121:589–600
11. Campuzano V, Montermini L, Moltò MD, et al. Friedreich's ataxia: autosomal recessive disease caused by an intronic GAA triplet repeat expansion. Science 1996; 271:1423–1427
12. Babcock M, De Silva D, Oaks R, et al. Regulation of mitochondrial iron accumulation by Yfh1p, a putative homolog of frataxin. Science 1997;276:1709–1712
13. Puccio H, Simon D, Cossee M, et al. Mouse models for Friedreich ataxia exhibit cardiomyopathy, sensory nerve defect and Fe-S enzyme deficiency followed by intramitochondrial iron deposits. Nat Genet 2001;27: 181–186
14. Rustin P, vonKleist-Retzow JC, Chantrel-Groussard K, et al. Effect of idebenone on cardiomyopathy in Friedreich's ataxia: a preliminary study. Lancet 1999;354: 477–479
15. Savitsky K, Bar-Shira A, Gilad S, et al. A single ataxia telangiectasia gene with a product similar to PI-3 kinase. Science 1995;268:1749–1753
16. Sandoval C, Swift M. Treatment of lymphoid malignancies in patients with ataxia-telangiectasia [see comments]. Med Pediatr Oncol 1998;31:491–497
17. Engert JC, Berube P, Mercier J, et al. ARSACS, a spastic ataxia common in northeastern Quebec, is caused by

mutations in a new gene encoding an 11.5kb ORF. Nat Genet 2000;24:120–125

18. Mrissa N, Belal S, Hamida CB, et al. Linkage to chromosome 13q11-12 of an autosomal recessive cerebellar ataxia in a Tunisian family. Neurology 2000;54:1408–1414

19. Sharp D, Blinderman L, Combs KA, et al. Cloning and gene defects in microsomal triglyceride transfer protein associated with abetalipoproteinaemia. Nature 1993;365:65–69

20. Kohlschuetter A. Abetalipoproteinemia. In: Klockgether T, ed. Handbook of Ataxia Disorders. New York: M. Dekker, 2000:205–221

21. Ouahchi K, Arita M, Kayden H, et al. Ataxia with isolated vitamin E deficiency is caused by mutations in the α-tocopherol transfer protein. Nature Genet 1995;9:141–145

22. Martinello F, Fardin P, Ottina M, et al. Supplemental therapy in isolated vitamin E deficiency improves the peripheral neuropathy and prevents the progression of ataxia. J Neurol Sci 1998;156:177–179

23. Jansen GA, Ofman R, Ferdinandusse S, et al. Refsum disease is caused by mutations in the phytanoyl-CoA hydroxylase gene. Nat Genet 1997;17:190–193

24. Gibberd FB, Billimoria JD, Goldman JM, et al. Heredopathia atactica polyneuritiformis: Refsum's disease. Acta Neurol Scand 1985;72:1–17

25. Harari D, Gibberd FB, Dick JP, Sidey MC. Plasma exchange in the treatment of Refsum's disease (heredopathia atactica polyneuritiformis). J Neurol Neurosurg Psychiatry 1991;54:614–617

26. Leitersdorf E, Reshef A, Meiner V, et al. Frameshift and splice-junction mutations in the sterol 27-hydroxylase gene cause cerebrotendinous xanthomatosis in Jews or Moroccan origin. J Clin Invest 1993;91:2488–2496

27. Berginer VM, Salen G, Shefer S. Long-term treatment of cerebrotendinous xanthomatosis with chenodeoxycholic acid. N Engl J Med 1984;311:1649–1652

28. Peynet J, Laurent A, De Liege P, et al. Cerebrotendinous xanthomatosis: treatments with simvastatin, lovastatin, and chenodeoxycholic acid in three siblings. Neurology 1991;41:434–436

29. Moreira MD, Barbot C, Tachi N, et al. Homozygosity mapping of Portuguese and Japanese forms of ataxiaoculomotor apraxia to 9p13, and evidence for genetic heterogeneity. Am J Hum Genet 2001;68:501–508

30. Bomont P, Watanabe M, Gershoni-Barush R, et al. Homozygosity mapping of spinocerebellar ataxia with cerebellar atrophy and peripheral neuropathy to 9q33-34, and with hearing impairment and optic atrophy to 6p21-23. Eur J Human Genet 2000;8:986–990

31. Klockgether T. Recent advances in degenerative ataxias. Curr Opin Neurol 2000;13:451–455

32. Polo JM, Calleja J, Combarros O, Berciano J. Hereditary ataxias and paraplegias in Cantabria, Spain. An epidemiological and clinical study. Brain 1991;114:855–866

33. Schöls L, Krüger R, Amoiridis G, et al. Spinocerebellar ataxia type 6: genotype and phenotype in German kindreds. J Neurol Neurosurg Psychiatry 1998;64:67–73

34. Harding AE. The clinical features and classification of the late onset autosomal dominant cerebellar ataxias. A study of 11 families including descendants of "the Drew family of Walworth". Brain 1982;105:1–28

35. Browne DL, Gancher ST, Nutt JG, et al. Episodic ataxia/myokymia syndrome is associated with point mutations in the human potassium channel gene, KCNA1. Nature Genet 1994;8:136–140

36. Ophoff RA, Terwindt GM, Vergouwe MN, et al. Familial hemiplegic migraine and episodic ataxia type-2 are caused by mutations in the Ca^{2+} channel gene CACNL1A4. Cell 1996;87:543–552

37. Griggs RC, Nutt JG. Episodic ataxias as channelopathies. Ann Neurol 1995;37:285–287

38. Schrag A, Ben Shlomo Y, Quinn NP. Prevalence of progressive supranuclear palsy and multiple system atrophy: a cross-sectional study. Lancet 1999;354:1771–1775

39. Gilman S, Low PA, Quinn N, et al. Consensus statement on the diagnosis of multiple system atrophy. J Neurol Sci 1999;163:94–98

40. Colosimo C, Albanese A, Hughes AJ, et al. Some specific clinical features differentiate multiple system atrophy (striatonigral variety) from Parkinson's disease. Arch Neurol 1995;52:294–298

41. Klockgether T, Schroth G, Diener HC, Dichgans J. Idiopathic cerebellar ataxia of late onset: natural history and MRI morphology. J Neurol Neurosurg Psychiatry 1990;53:297–305

42. Gilman S, Little R, Johanns J, et al. Evolution of sporadic olivopontocerebellar atrophy into multiple system atrophy. Neurology 2000;55:527–532

43. Butterworth RF. Pathophysiology of alcoholic brain damage: synergistic effects of ethanol, thiamine deficiency and alcoholic liver disease. Metab Brain Dis 1995;10:1–8

44. Diener HC, Dichgans J, Bacher M, Guschlbauer B. Improvement of ataxia in alcoholic cerebellar atrophy through alcohol abstinence. J Neurol 1984;231:258–262

45. Harding AE, Muller DP, Thomas PK, Willison HJ. Spinocerebellar degeneration secondary to chronic intestinal malabsorption: a vitamin E deficiency syndrome. Ann Neurol 1982;12:419–424

46. Paone JF, Jeyasingham K. Remission of cerebellar dysfunction after pneumonectomy for bronchogenic carcinoma. N Engl J Med 1980;302:156

47. David YB, Warner E, Levitan M, et al. Autoimmune paraneoplastic cerebellar degeneration in ovarian carcinoma patients treated with plasmapheresis and immunoglobulin. A case report. Cancer 1996;78:2153–2156

48. Hadjivassiliou M, Grunewald RA, Chattopadhyay AK, et al. Clinical, radiological, neurophysiological, and neuropathological characteristics of gluten ataxia. Lancet 1998;352:1582–1585

49. Abele M, Weller M, Mescheriakov S, et al. Cerebellar ataxia with glutamic acid decarboxylase autoantibodies. Neurology 1999;52:857–859

256 Therapy of Human Prion Diseases

Amos D Korczyn and Puiu Nisipeanu

Prion diseases are unusual human and animal conditions (Table 256.1), which involve the central nervous system and always lead to a fatal outcome. The uniqueness of prion diseases includes their pathogenesis, mode of transmission, and neuropathology. The "prion hypothesis," advanced by Stanley Prusiner and recently reviewed by him[1] and by others,[2,3] is now widely accepted. It maintains that the "infectious" agent is an abnormal conformation of a naturally occurring protein. The term "prion," as coined by Prusiner, refers to the proteinaceous infectious agent. The harmless naturally occurring prion protein (PrP^c) may transform into a protease-resistant form (PrP^{Sc} or PrP^{res}), which is strongly linked to disease pathogenesis, although by some dissenting scientists present data which they interpret as demonstrating that nucleic acids, or another unidentified agent, are also involved in the transmission of these diseases.[4–6]

The terminology of the diseases is still changing. The term "spongiform encephalopathy" has been coined to describe the typical pathology in the brain of humans or animals that manifest these diseases. However, it may be inadequate since in patients with fatal familial insomnia (FFI) and other disease types,[7,8] spongiosis is not typically seen. "Transmissible encephalopathies" is also problematic since it is not always easy to demonstrate transmissibility. The term "prion diseases" is preferable because it concentrates on the distinctive features of these diseases and the central role that is played by prions in the pathogenesis (which may, however, be different in sporadic, transmitted and genetic cases). Nevertheless, staining for prion proteins using specific antibodies may occasionally be negative in brain regions presumably affected by the disease.

Historically, several variants have been described (Table 256.2) although it is now clear that these are clinically different syndromes which result from the deposition of PrP^{Sc} in different parts of the brain, with a possible random foci of onset.

The majority of human prion diseases are sporadic, without any known aetiology. A sizeable group are inherited cases, and these always result from mutations in the gene of the prion protein, PRNP. A small number of cases can be attributed to exposure to known sources of PrP^{Sc}.

Clinical features

There is a wide scope of clinical phenomenology in human prion diseases regarding the age of onset, presenting symptoms, rate of progression, and the appearance of other neurological manifestations. The recent description of mental illness without neurological signs[8,9] extends the clinical heterogeneity of prion diseases even further.

Creutzfeldt-Jakob disease (CJD) Creutzfeldt-Jakob disease is frequently heralded by non-specific affective and other psychiatric symptoms, as well as sleep disturbances. It usually starts with *cortical manifestations*, mainly sub-acute cognitive decline, and memory loss is an early complaint, but cases have been reported which presented with focal manifestations imitating strokes,[10] such as hemisensory deficit,[11] hemianopia,[12] aphasia,[13] alien hand,[14,15] or with epileptic seizures, including status epilepticus. In the *Heidenhain variant*, CJD presents with cortical blindness. *Movement disorders* are common (Table 256.3). They may include parkinsonian features, mainly bradykinesia and rigidity. Cerebellar ataxia is a frequent initial manifestation and it may be very disabling.[16] Most patients eventually develop myoclonic jerks, initially driven by auditory (sometimes visual or tactile) stimuli (stimulus-sensitive myoclonus), later becoming spontaneous, at a rate of about 1 Hz, which may or may not be symmetrical.

Diagnostic criteria have been formulated for CJD (Table 256.4). While these criteria are important for epidemiological studies, they are less useful for clinical decisions of individual cases, particularly early on in the course of the disease. Myoclonus and akinetic mutism usually appear late in the disease, and the EEG may also not show typical features initially. Finally, the duration of the disease is unknown in a living patient, and can exceed two years in some cases.

Originally it was assumed that inherited prion diseases that were a result of different mutations of the PRNP gene would each result in a unique clinical phenotype. Remarkably, recent descriptions of patients with the E200K mutation of the PRNP gene showed marked phenotypic heterogeneity even within this single point mutation.[17–22] Although prion diseases are essentially limited to the central nervous system, a notable exception is demyelinating peripheral neuropathy in patients with CJD associated with the E200K mutation.[18,22] The pathogenesis of the neuropathy is unclear.

New variant CJD (nvCJD) New variant CJD (nvCJD) was first described in the UK.[23–25] It affects mainly young adults (15–51 years at onset) with initial psychiatric symptomatology comprising mainly depression and disturbing dysesthesias and pain, followed by a progressive cerebellar syndrome. Dementia and myoclonus then develop, leading to

Table 256.1   Prion diseases

Human Diseases
Creutzfeldt-Jakob disease (CJD)   Sporadic, Genetic, Iatrogenic, Transmitted
Gerstmann-Sträussler-Scheinker disease (GSS)   Genetic
Fatal Familial Insomnia (FFI)   Genetic, sporadic
Kuru   Transmitted

Animal Diseases
Scrapie
Transmissible mink encephalopathy
Chronic wasting disease of mule-deer and elk
Bovine spongiform encephalopathy
   (BSE, mad cow disease)
Spongiform encephalopathy in feline and captive wild cats

death within a few months. The pathological picture of nvCJD includes spongiform changes in the basal ganglia and thalamus. "Kuru type" amyloid plaques are widely distributed, which may have features distinguishing them from other prion diseases.

Gerstmann-Sträussler-Scheinker syndrome (GSS)
Gerstmann-Sträussler-Scheinker syndrome is an autosomal dominantly inherited disease that is much less common than CJD. Its onset is in the third to sixth decades of life and the presenting symptom is usually cerebellar ataxia, with the gradual appearance of cognitive impairment and occasionally spastic paraparesis, but it may present with dementia. The evolution of GSS is typically longer than that of CJD and death occurs in 5–10 years. All cases of GSS described to date were associated with specific mutations of the

PRNP gene. The pathological phenotype of GSS is defined as the occurrence of multicentric amyloid plaques in the central nervous system (CNS) composed largely of prion protein and spongiform changes.

Fatal familial insomnia (FFI) Hypersomnia or insomnia are well known to occur in CJD, and were reported by Heidenhain in one of his original cases. Nevertheless, a new familial disease was described recently, in which the insomnia was very severe.[26] These patients also had autonomic symptoms such as hypertension, tachycardia, hyperhydrosis and hyperthermia. Dysarthria, dysphagia, ataxia, and myoclonus developed later. Because of the predominance of the sleep abnormalities, this variant of prion disease was termed fatal familial insomnia. The pathological features include severe destruction of the thalamic nuclei with astrogliosis, but without spongiform changes or amyloid deposits.

Fatal familial insomnia is transmitted as a dominantly inherited disorder and was linked to a mutation at codon 178 of the *PRNP*. Interestingly, the same mutation may cause CJD, and which phenotype develops depends on a polymorphism at codon 129 of the *PRNP* gene, with homozygosity leading to FFI and heterozygosity to CJD.[27] It was suggested that in both cases the disease is initiated by a conversion, in

Table 256.2   Variants of Creutzfeldt-Jakob disease

- Occipital (Heidenhain)
- Thalamic
- Ataxic
- Oculomotor
- New variant CJD
- Dementia without characteristic pathology
- Dementia with spastic paraparesis
- Amyotrophic

Table 256.3   Movement disorders in prion disease

- Cerebellar ataxia
- Myoclonic jerks
- Parkinsonism (rigidity and hypokinesia)
- Tremor, chorea, athetosis, dyskinesias
- Dystonic postures
- Alien hand
- Akinetic mutism
- Terminal flexor rigidity
- Hemiparesis, dysarthria, dysphagia

Table 256.4   Diagnostic criteria for sporadic Creutzfeldt-Jakob disease

I   Rapidly progressive dementia

II A Pyramidal or extrapyramidal features
    B Visual or cerebellar problems
    C Myoclonus
    D Akinetic mutism

III A Typical EEG
    B Positive 14-3-3 protein in CSF

DEFINITE	Neuropathological/immunocytochemically confirmed
PROBABLE	I + 2 of II + III A or III B
POSSIBLE	I + 2 of II and duration <2 years

the thalamus, of the cellular form of PrP (PrP^c) into a β-pleated, protease resistant, isoform (PrP^{res}). If the patients are homozygous at codon 129, further local rapid transformation occurs, leading to the clinical picture of FFI, whereas in patients who are heterozygous at 129, a more widespread distribution of PrP^{res} throughout the brain will occur, with the consequence being the development of CJD rather than FFI.[26] Lately, cases with an apparent sporadic form of familial insomnia have also been described.[28]

Kuru The clinical features of kuru included, in many cases, childhood onset of ataxia and spasticity, which progressed and led to death within a few years. The disease was transmitted by ritualistic cannibalism and it is now mainly of historic interest. Kuru is perhaps the most stereotypic of the human prion diseases, and the elucidation of the transmitted nature of the disease by Gajdusek was the breakthrough leading to the understanding of basic mechanisms related to prion diseases. It is of scientific interest, however, that although 30 years or more may have passed since the practice of ritualistic cannibalism is thought to have ceased, a few new cases still occur in the region. None of these new cases occur in children (who had been most frequently affected in the past when kuru was prevalent), pointing to the very long incubation period that may occur in kuru and other prion diseases.

Movement disorders in prion diseases

Movement disorders of various kinds have been described in prion diseases (Tables 256.3 and 256.5). Some of these are very common either in the initial stages of CJD (e.g. cerebellar manifestations) or terminally (e.g. myoclonus). Cerebellar manifestations are also common in GSS and kuru.

The occurrence of variable involuntary movements in "psychiatric" patients exposed to antidepressant drugs may raise the suspicion of iatrogenic origin; conversely, some lithium-treated patients who developed myoclonus and paroxysmal electroencephalogram (EEG) abnormalities may be suspected of having CJD.

The heterogeneity in the site of pathology of prion diseases accounts for the variety of clinical manifestations, ranging from hemiparesis[29] to extrapyramidal dysfunction, cerebellar syndromes,[30] oculomotor deficits, and so forth. Since the pathology is rarely limited to a small anatomical area, there is also a large

Table 256.5 Clinical characteristics of Creutzfeldt-Jakob disease

- Presenile/senile dementia
- Cerebellar manifestations
- Extrapyramidal rigidity
- Myoclonic jerks
- Visual deterioration
- Epileptic seizures
- Muscle atrophy

overlap between these manifestations making an attempt to differentiate these entities difficult. Obviously, it is the rapid evolution of movement disorders (frequently with coexistent dementia, visual deficits, etc.,) that should direct attention to the possible diagnosis of CJD.

Cerebellar syndrome, occurring as the presenting symptom, is not rare in sporadic or genetic forms of CJD, or in kuru. Ataxia may be present at CJD onset in a high proportion of patients, as Brown et al. found cerebellar signs in 33% of patients.[31] In nvCJD virtually every patient became ataxic.[29] It manifests usually as a bilateral disease with a wide-based gait, with subsequent development of limb ataxia, nystagmus and later, dysarthria. These same manifestations can also appear, in other cases, subsequent to other features such as cognitive impairment. The ataxia may at times be so severe as to make the patient wheelchairbound; although by that stage other neural systems are usually clearly affected as well.

The cerebellar (ataxic) variant of CJD has been described by Brownell and Oppenheimer[32] in about 20% of patients. However, cerebellar dysfunction appears in the majority of subjects as the disease advances.[33] Interestingly, in CJD iatrogenically-induced by contaminated growth hormone or gonadotropin, the disease usually takes a predominant cerebellar course.[34] An ataxic variant of CJD was associated with valine homozygosity at codon 129 in the *PRPN*. It occurred in 16% of patients, who generally developed late dementia and had non-typical EEG.[35]

Myoclonus is probably the best-known movement disorder in prion diseases. Both Creutzfeldt[36] and Jakob[37] described it and indeed the appearance of myoclonus in the setting of rapidly progressing dementia is very suggestive of CJD. However alternative diagnoses such as Alzheimer's disease, dementia with Lewy bodies[38] and AIDS should be considered.

The frequency of myoclonic jerks is about 80%,[31,33] in either sporadic or familial cases of CJD.[39] It typically appears after months of the disease, although it can occur early.[31,35,40] The onset is usually in the limbs but it spreads to involve the whole body. The persistence of reflex-triggered myoclonus in the terminal stage of the disease may sometimes convey the false impression of responsiveness in an already comatose patient. The presence of myoclonus is strongly associated (78%) with characteristic EEG abnormalities, that is, periodic or pseudo-periodic sharp-wave complexes.[28]

The origin of myoclonus—as suggested by using jerk-locked averaging of scalp EEG[41–43]—may be cortical or subcortical, and its pattern differs from the pattern recorded in Alzheimer's myoclonic patients. Considering the *PRPN* genotype and types of PrP^{Sc},[35,39] it has been found that almost all patients with at least one methionine allele at codon 129 and PrP^{Sc} type 1 (about 70% of patients) have had myoclonus, which typically appeared during the first two months of the disease.

Other extrapyramidal signs, such as parkinsonism, dystonia, dyskinesias, tremors and choreo-athetosis, were described in about 50% of patients.[31,33] An exception was noted for patients with a longer duration of CJD (more than two years), where 93% had extrapyramidal features.[44] Of particular interest is chorea, which seems to be very frequent in nvCJD.[45] Will[29,45] found chorea in 20 out of 33 confirmed patients, in some preceding and later being replaced by myoclonus.

Recently, MacGowan et al.,[14] reported two CJD-pathologically proven patients who presented with a rare and striking phenomenon, namely "alien hand." Both exhibited uncontrolled, seemingly purposeful movements and myoclonus of the left hand, which they regarded as not intended, conducive to interference in some activities such as dressing or eating, and forcing them to try to restrain the movements by using the healthy hand. Additionally to myoclonus and ensuing cognitive decline and ataxia, both had severe proprioception loss of the left limbs, which may have contributed to the occurrence of "unawareness" of the limb movements.

There have been two other patients in whom "alien hand" has been observed early after CJD onset.[15] Interestingly, the patient reported by Rabinstein et al.,[46] had a right-dominant "alien hand." In other contexts, an "alien hand" was found to occur following lesions involving the corpus callosum (tumours, surgery, infarcts).[47] An alien non-dominant hand may also occur in posterior lesions of the right hemisphere. The dominant hand is affected in infarction of the left medial frontal cortex. Indeed a pathological signal was observed in the left mesial frontal cortex on magnetic resonance imaging (MRI) examination.[46] In the remaining subjects the spongiform changes were too widespread to allow clinical-pathological correlation.[14]

Patients with prion diseases may develop rapidly evolving hemiparesis (frequently being mistaken as a result of a stroke)[23] and can also exhibit pseudobulbar palsy, dysarthria and dysphagia, as well as akinetic mutism.

The pathophysiology and pathogenesis of prion diseases

While most patients with CJD are sporadic, a significant minority (perhaps as many as 10%) result from specific mutations in the *PRNP* gene. Others develop diseases following exposure to PrP^{Sc} in its various forms (Kuru, nvCJD and iatrogenically). How can a unifying hypothesis be formed to account for these various etiologies? The assumption is that prion diseases result, somehow, from deranged metabolism of the prion protein, which leads to neuronal loss and prion deposition in the neuropil, frequently in the form of amyloid plaques. According to this theory, a "seed" of PrP^{Sc} is needed which will induce the conversion of PrP^c to PrP^{Sc}. With each step, therefore, the number of PrP^{Sc} molecules will double, leading to the severe neuronal loss. This theory can explain relatively easily the iatrogenic cases, in which PrP^{Sc} gets

access into the brain;[48,49] in fact, this process can be replicated in experimental animals. However, in sporadic CJD no such exposure could be demonstrated. It is appealing to assume that a spontaneous conversion occurs which transforms PrP^c to PrP^{Sc} starting the chain of events and mutations of the prion protein gene may make this spontaneous conversion more likely to happen. The principal pathogenetic hypotheses recently reviewed by Collinge[3] include:

(i) Neurotoxic effects from a PrP fragment encompassing residues 106–126.
(ii) Neuronal death as a result of increased oxidative stress induced by PrP depletion (loss of function), as it is assumed that PrP may have antioxidant properties.
(iii) Apoptotic death, assuming that a certain level of PrP is indispensable for regulating apoptosis.
(iv) PrP^{Sc}, or even prions, may not be by themselves neurotoxic, and the neurodegeneration may be mediated by intermediate species, appearing during the conversion from PrP^c to PrP^{Sc}; PrP^{Sc} being only a relatively inert end product.
(v) Spongiform vacuolation can be induced in vitro by copper chelators. As PrP^c is thought to act as a copper transport protein, this function may be perturbed when PrP^c transforms to PrP^{Sc}.

Diagnostic methods

Pathology Firm diagnosis of prion diseases was traditionally based on pathological examination of the brain. The typical pathology of prion diseases, in humans and in animals, consists of spongiform changes, neuronal loss, and remarkable gliosis. The distribution of these changes in the brain differs in the various diseases. For example in CJD, the "status spongiosus" is mainly cortical. In GSS, the degenerative changes occur mainly in the cerebellum and amyloid plaques are abundant. Prion protein deposition is the only truly specific verification for prion disease, and possibly the earliest.[50,51] Intracerebral inoculation of brain tissue removed from a diseased individual into an experimental animal is another specific method to demonstrate the existence of prion disease.

Neuroimaging The main abnormalities observed in computed tomography (CT) and MRI in CJD reflect the atrophic changes, although these appear relatively late in the course of the disease. Because of their non-specific nature, these will not assist in the diagnosis except when atrophy progresses within a few months, since this is unlikely to be seen in other degenerative brain diseases.[52,53] The occurrence of hyperdense lesions in brain CT and of symmetric high signals in the basal ganglia (and sometimes cortically) on T2-weighted images on the MRI was observed in iatrogenic, genetic and sporadic CJD as well as in nvCJD.[54]

EEG Early in the course of the disease the EEG shows non-specific slowing consistent with the cognitive impairment. As the disease progresses, triphasic waves appear, as well as periodic 1 Hz spikes. Similar

EEG changes may occur in various metabolic encephalopathies or as a consequence to the toxic effects of drugs. In the right context, their occurrence provides strong evidence favoring the diagnosis of CJD.[55,56] Occasionally, the complexes appear as periodic lateralized epileptiform discharges (PLEDs). In GSS and FFI, EEG slowing typically occurs but periodic sharp wave discharges were only exceptionally reported.

Cerebrospinal fluid (CSF) The CSF is usually normal, except for a mild to moderate hyperproteinorrhachia in some cases, with no evidence of an inflammatory reaction. The CSF of CJD patients contains high concentrations of specific proteins, such as 14-3-3 and neuron-specific enolase (NSE).[57-60] A simple rapid radioimmunoassay proved these proteins to be a sensitive and relatively specific marker for prion diseases in humans and animals. These proteins probably reflect tissue destruction, and therefore may also be elevated in other brain disorders, such as encephalitis or a recent stroke. The reliability of the test in the early detection of prion disease remains to be established.

Serum levels of glial proteins such as S-100 may be increased,[61] but the relevance in the early diagnosis of CJD is unknown. A combination of all these markers together may be more specific (but probably less sensitive) for the diagnosis of CJD than either alone.

Treatment of prion diseases

Prion diseases are currently incurable, fatal diseases. The difficulties involved in their treatment may be at least threefold. Their aetiology is still uncertain; the diagnosis is established too late when neuronal loss is too extensive to be reversed or inhibited and the rarity of these diseases hinders controlled studies. Because of these difficulties, researchers have developed experimental models, the main one being by intracerebral or intraperitoneal injections of brain material derived from a diseased person or animal into recipient animals, particularly mice or hamsters. In most studies the drugs were used prophylactically, that is, prior to inoculation or after inoculation but before the onset of clinical disease. The relevance of these methods to human disease is thus open to question. An alternative method is the employment of cell lines, particularly engineered neuroblastoma or Chinese hamster ovary cells, which produce PrP^c and, when exposed to extrinsic PrP^{Sc}, convert the host PrP^c into PrP^{Sc}.

By the time the diagnosis of prion diseases is made, a significant amount of brain destruction has already accumulated. Because of the rarity of these diseases this situation is unlikely to change even if an early marker of the disease becomes available. However, early diagnosis will be possible in those cases with a high likelihood to develop prion diseases, namely those carrying *PRNP* mutations, who are identified through an affected family member. The exponential transformation of PrP^c to PrP^{Sc} during the disease course[19] dictates that early treatment should be the most effective.

Although the pathogenesis of prion diseases is still clouded, two main possibilities exist: either PrP^{Sc} is toxic, or the deficiency of PrP^c (created by its forced conversion to PrP^{Sc}) is pathogenic. The latter, "loss of function" theory is less popular because transgenic mice lacking the *PRNP* gene do not suffer from prion diseases. Therefore therapeutic attempts are directed at PrP^{Sc}. Whether the actual concentration of PrP^{Sc} is important is debatable, since several examples are available where even in the terminal stages of some prion diseases little or no accumulation of PrP^{Sc} can be demonstrated, such as FFI or other thalamic forms of prion diseases. Also, PrP^{Sc} concentration does not equal infectivity.[62] In fact it can be postulated that the insoluble, deposited, β-sheet conformation of PrP^{Sc} is so inert that it cannot cause cellular damage. Nevertheless PrP^{Sc} can be noxious without being deposited. The final answer to this question is critically important in order to determine the right approach for the treatment of prion diseases, since, if the amyloid deposit is not causing damage, then attempts to dissolve it in vivo may well increase the infectivity by releasing a noxious form of PrP^{Sc}.

Methods to treat prion diseases, which have been experimented so far, are based on the following principles:

(i) Attempts to reduce conversion of PrP^c to PrP^{Sc}.
(ii) Attempts to reduce the load of PrP^{Sc} by dissolving it, converting it back to PrP^c or otherwise accelerating its disposal.
(iii) Other methods are based on alternate presumptions, for example that PrP^{Sc} deposition is an epiphenomenon and other factors are responsible for cell death—viruses, viroids or other molecules.

Stabilization of PrP^c and prevention of PrP^{Sc} formation and accumulation in the brain represents an important target for experimental therapy trials.[63,64] As mentioned, PrP^{Sc} is a pathological conformer derived by a post-translational process from the normal host PrP^c; PrP^{Sc} has a high content of β-sheet and a lower α-helical content as compared with PrP^c. As with Alzheimer's disease, the deposited protein is β-pleated and insoluble. Whether this protein, once deposited, is involved in the disease process or is only a marker of the process is still unknown. In fact, the answer to this question might be critical to the development of therapies for prion diseases, since agents which stabilize or dissolve deposited PrP^{Sc} might each have opposite effects on the course of the disease in the two theoretical mechanisms.

Synthetic peptides as conversion inhibitors

Certain peptides from the central part (106–141) of the hamster PrP sequence were capable of inhibiting the conversion of PrP^c to PrP^{res} in a cell-free in vitro model. Recently, Chabry et al.,[65,66] have shown that a shorter peptide, similar to hamster PrP residues 119–136 (PrP119–136 is highly conserved in most species), also inhibited PrP^{Sc} formation independent of species, suggesting that this peptide may be useful in a diversity of prion diseases. Notably, this peptide encompasses the region of the codon 129 in the human *PRNP* gene, implicated as mentioned above in susceptibility to CJD. However, short peptides are easily degraded, have a poor permeability through the blood-brain barrier, and generate immune responses. Thus, their clinical utility is still doubtful.[65,66]

Dominant-negative inhibitors of PrP^Sc formation

Attempts to limit the conversion of PrP^c into PrP^Sc are hindered because the basic mechanisms of these processes are still speculative. For example, it may be that another protein, dubbed "protein X" is involved, which facilitates the reaction. The identity of this protein is unknown, and its existence is even in doubt. However, some data suggest that it acts by interacting with a specific sequence of PrP^Sc. If this is the case, then other molecules could be designed which would block this sequence, or perhaps otherwise inhibit "protein X."

Nuclear magnetic resonance of PrP^Sc and PrP^c mutant studies suggest that substitutions at four C-terminal residues (C-terminal domain folding consists of three α-helices and a short β-sheet) may act as dominant-negative inhibitors of PrP^Sc formation.[67] The strategy based on these results is to prevent the accumulation of PrP^Sc by blocking the interaction between a hypothetical Protein X, an auxiliary protein and PrP^c.[68] Protein X presumably binds to PrP^c in a small area involving four residues on the PrP^c molecule surface, which greatly contributes to the Protein X/PrP^c complex stability.

If PrP^Sc is indeed the culprit, then it would be possible, theoretically, to eliminate it by converting PrP^Sc back to PrP^c. Development of drugs to facilitate this conversion requires a better understanding of the mechanisms of the reaction governing the conversion of PrP^c to PrP^Sc and backwards.

Once formed, PrP^Sc assumes a β-pleated sheet confirmation, which is less soluble and then deposited as a prion plaque in the neuropil. It is possible that the deposition is in fact protective, since it is difficult to understand how an insoluble molecule could interact with neurons and cause their death. Therefore, one possible approach will be to accelerate the deposition of already formed PrP^Sc. Alternatively, PrP^Sc could be manipulated before it is deposited. Recently, Soto et al.,[69,70] discovered that β-pleated sheet formation can be prevented if proline molecules can be inserted in strategic sites along the amino-acid sequence of the protein. They synthesized a 13 amino-acid sequence containing three prolines (iPrP13), which is analogous to a critical portion sequence of the PrP^Sc. In their experiments iPrP13 induced the back-conversion of PrP^Sc into PrP^c in vitro, and also delayed the appearance of experimental scrapie in mice which have been inoculated with scrapie.[69,70]

Several agents were found to delay the conversion of PrP^c into PrP^Sc in vitro, as well as the appearance of scrapie in experimental animals. One such group is composed of dextran sulphate 500,[71] pentosan poly-

sulphate[72] and heteropolyanion,[23] as well as several related poly-anions. However, the efficacy of these agents is limited, since they do not prevent but only delay the onset of clinical symptoms, and most importantly they should be administered before or with the injection of the infectious material. Since they are not active if initiated after the clinical symptoms appear, their relevance to human disease is questionable.

When experimental scrapie is induced by intraperitoneal injection (as well as with nvCJD), PrP^Sc probably appears in the brain after being absorbed by reticuloendothelial cells, including follicular dendritic cells. Although the exact role of these cells is unknown, it is remarkable that the lymphotoxin-β receptor (which inhibits follicular dendritic cells) can delay experimental scrapie.[73]

Flupirtine, a centrally active non-opiate analgesic with a protective action against apoptosis, has been shown to reduce the neurotoxicity of the prion protein fragment PrP 106–126, in an *in vitro* model for prion diseases.[74]

Congo red is a classical amyloid-binding drug, used for staining amyloids in pathological preparations. Therefore it was hypothesized that if used in prion diseases it will bind the amyloid and perhaps prevent its assumed toxicity. Several studies have indeed confirmed the usefulness of this agent in scrapie-infected neuroblastoma cells and in rodents. In the latter, Congo red prolonged, in a dose-dependent way, the incubation period until disease onset, but again in order to achieve this goal the drug had to be given well in advance of the first symptoms becoming apparent. It is worth noting that the effect was similar if PRP^Sc was induced by intracerebral or intraperitoneal administration of scrapie (although intracerebral inoculation resulted in shorter incubation periods).

The mechanisms by which Congo red and the poly-anions are effective, while still unknown, are thought to be related to the prevention of the binding of glycosaminoglycans to PrP. It was recently suggested that Congo red acts by over-stabilizing PrP^Sc conformation, preventing its partial denaturation which may be required for PrP^Sc to function as a template in the PrP^c to PrP^Sc conversion.[75] None of these compounds readily crosses the blood-brain barrier, and this of course could theoretically reduce their efficacy in the *in vivo* studies. Interestingly, Congo red embedded in slow-release polymers in the brain does not prolong experimental scrapie.[76] Some Congo red analogues are currently under trial, including Sirius red F_3B, trypan blue and Evans blue. Only Sirius red F_3B seems to be as effective as Congo red.[77]

Antibiotics

Pocchiari et al.,[78] have demonstrated that the anti-fungal agent amphotericin B is able to delay the onset of experimental scrapie (263K scrapie) in hamsters inoculated intracerebrally or intraperitoneally. The effect was dose-dependent and time-dependent as amphotericin B was effective only when the treatment was initiated shortly after the infection and before the onset of the clinical disease. The less toxic derivative of amphotericin B, MS-8209, allowed for longer-term treatment with higher doses (10–25 mg/kg as compared with 1–2 mg/kg for amphotericin B) and significantly prolonged the survival of infected animals, even when the treatment was initiated at a later stage of incubation.[79] Both were found to delay the accumulation of PrP[Sc], of glial fibrillary acidic protein, and the appearance of astrocytic gliosis and spongiotic changes, although it was suggested that neurons constitute important sites of amphotericin B and MS-8209 action.[80,81]

The mechanism of action for amphotericin B is unknown, and several possibilities have been proposed.[78] Interestingly, after peripheral scrapie inoculation, amphotericin B is much more effective in reducing PrP[Sc] accumulation in the spleen than it is in the brain. This is significant because of the very poor penetration of the drug through the blood-brain barrier. Perhaps intrathecal administration, or more penetrating analogues, will be more effective.

Antineoplastic agents

Iododoxorubicine, a derivative of doxorubicin, has been shown to bind to amyloid fibrils. Tagliavini et al.,[82] have recently demonstrated the effectiveness of this compound in delaying the onset of scrapie and extending the survival of hamsters infected intracerebrally with an inoculum of the 263K scrapie agent. The finding that doxorubicin can be delivered into the brain via a peptide vector[83] may stimulate future trials.

Chemical chaperones

Cellular osmolytes (glycerol, trimethylamine N-oxide and dimethyl sulfoxide [DMSO]) were found to interfere with the formation of PrP[Sc] from newly synthesized PrP in a ScN2a cell line. Since these compounds are known to stabilize protein conformation, they may provide another strategy to prevent PrP conformational changes.[84]

Branched polyamines ("dendrimers," e.g. polypropyleneimine) were found to remove PrP[Sc] from ScN2a cells in culture, in a manner dependent on concentration and duration of exposure and were able to eradicate prion infectivity.[85]

Porphyrins and phthalocyanines

Some cyclic tetrapyrroles bind to proteins and impact on protein conformation. Recently cyclic tetrapyrroles (porphyrin and several phthalocyanine compounds) have been identified as having a marked effect against experimental scrapie.[86] In those experiments, only peripheral inoculation was used. A possible mechanism of the effect was assumed to be direct interaction of the compounds with PrP[Sc] (it was speculated that this mechanism also accounted for the activity of Congo red, amphotericin B and other related compounds).[86]

Phthalocyanine tetrasulfonate, TMPP-Fe^{3+} and DPG$_2$ Fe^{3+} which were previously found to inhibit PrP[Sc] formation in vitro, were recently tested *in vivo* in transgenic mice over-expressing hamster PrP^c infected with hamster 263K scrapie.[86]

As is the case with almost every other compound, the efficacy of tetrapyrroles such as phthalocyamine, depends on their early administration. This may be due to the fact that none of these tetrapyrroles is able to penetrate the blood-brain barrier. Their action seems to be related to a reaction with the infectious agent in peripheral tissues such as the spleen.

Basic fibroblast growth factor (bFGF)

The anti-apoptotic effect of sheet breaker peptides was sought by Fraser et al.,[49] in a murine-scrapie model of experimental retinopathy characterized by severe neuronal (photoreceptor) loss. Intravitreal injection of bFGF at a late stage of the disease was followed by a considerable increase in the number of surviving photoreceptors.

Dapsone

Dapsone, an anti-inflammatory drug which crosses the blood-brain barrier quite readily, was reported to be more effective against experimental scrapie, although the mechanism is still obscure.[76]

Antisense nucleotides

The exact function of prion proteins in humans is unknown. Knockout mice were created that lacked prion protein (PrP0/0), yet developed and functioned normally in most or all aspects.[87] It is therefore theoretically possible that humans may not have an obligatorily need for prion proteins. If this is the case, antisense oligonucleotides can be produced which will block prion protein synthesis. The main candidates for such a technology would be subjects at high risk of developing CJD or other prion diseases, such as those carrying a mutation of the prion protein gene with a high penetrance.

Immunologic strategies

A different theoretical approach is to attack the deposited amyloid. This approach is based on the assumption that the amyloid may be toxic. As with Alzheimer's disease, an attack on the amyloid, for example by immune mechanisms, could be envisaged. This approach has been employed successfully by Peretz et al.,[88] who employed a number of recombinant antibody antigen-binding fragments using in vitro systems, and showed inhibition of PrP[Sc] formation and even clearing of pre-existing PrP[Sc]. It was speculated that the effect was mediated by antibody binding to PrP^c on the membrane, thus preventing its exposure to PrP[Sc], which is presumably necessary for the conversion of PrP^c into PrP[Sc]. It is still unknown how these methods will affect humans or animals harboring prion diseases.

Tricyclic compounds

Tricyclic compounds such as chlorpromazine and particularly quinacrine were recently reported to protect cells against PrP[Sc].[89] Only *in vitro* studies were reported so far, and the critical experiments related to the usefulness in whole animal experiments is of utmost importance, particularly regarding the question as to whether the drugs will still be active if started after the clinical symptoms have appeared. The special attractiveness of these compounds lies in the fact that they are widely used and safe for humans and that they readily cross the blood-brain barrier.

Symptomatic therapies

Symptomatic therapy is commonly used in CJD, with some success. These drugs are completely non-specific. Anxiolytic and antidepressants are frequently used in the initial stages of the disease, anticonvulsants when seizures occur with clonazepam being particularly useful against the myoclonic jerks. However, relatively high doses of the latter drug are required which frequently induces sedation. Levodopa is helpful against the parkinsonian manifestations.

Prevention of prion diseases

As in other fields of medicine, and particularly neurology, prevention is desired. The abolition of ritual cannibalism, which was practiced in New Guinea, led to the virtual disappearance of Kuru.[90] Other examples of human transmission included children who had been treated with growth hormone or women treated with follicle-stimulating hormone (FSH). New cases have not appeared since the pituitary derived hormones were replaced by biologically engineered agents. Transplantation of tissues removed from cadavers who have died of CJD can also result in transmission of prion disease, such as following corneal and (in particular) dura mater. Attention to the source of donors is of prime importance, and other precautionary measures have been recommended and implemented.

Secure disinfection procedures of instruments used, particularly in neurosurgery, must be ensured. Inactivation by high-temperature (134°C) moist-heat sterilization has been suggested.[87] The high concentration of PrP^{Sc} in the tonsils of nvCJD victims demands the use of disposable instruments for tonsillectomy. The practical issues involved in handling the tissues of patients with established or suspected prion diseases have been addressed in a consensus report by Budka et al.[87] When following the recommended guidelines, autopsy or biopsy can be safely performed.

A potential source of transmission is blood donation by people who are harboring a prion disease. The causative agent can potentially be transmitted not only by whole blood but also by plasma or its derivatives, such as albumin, globulin, or coagulation factors. Although such cases have not been identified as yet, there is a potential risk because the preclinical stage may be quite long. This risk may be particularly high when considering people with nvCJD, because in their case the infective agent reaches the brain by the systemic route, and resides there in the lymphoreticular tissue.[91,92] Importantly, nvCJD occurs in young individuals, who are the most common

donors. Blood banks usually ask potential donors about any relevant disorder that the donor or members of their families may be aware of (in order to identify genetic cases) but this method is insensitive. Of late, several countries have excluded blood donations from people who have lived in the UK for extensive periods of time (usually six months or more), however this arbitrary decision is probably politically motivated as it is not based on any solid scientific data.

Recently Shaked et al. have showed that adding valproic acid, an antiepileptic drug extensively used for decades, to cultures resulted in significant increase in PrP^c in normal neuroblastoma cells lines (N2a) and of both PrP^c and PrP^{Sc} in NZa cells infected with scrapie. This may suggest careful consideration of valproic acid use in people at risk of developing CJD.[93]

References

1. Prusiner SB. Neurodegenerative disease and prions. N Engl J Med 2001;344:1516–1526
2. Korczyn AD. Prion diseases. Current Opinions in Neurology. 1997;10:273–281
3. Collinge J. Prion diseases of humans and animals: their causes and molecular basis. Ann Rev Neurosci 2001;24:519–550
4. Manuelidis L, Sklaviadis, Akowitz A, Fritch W. Viral particles are required for infection in neurodegenerative Creutzfeldt-Jakob disease. Proc Natl Acad Sci USA 1995;92:5124–5128
5. Manuelidis L, Fritch W. Infectivity, and host responses in Creutzfeldt-Jakob disease. Virology 1996;216:46–59
6. Lasmezas CI, Deslys J-P, Robain O, Jaegly A, et al. Transmission of the BSE agent to mice in the absence of detectable abnormal prion protein. Science 1997;275:402–406
7. Collinge J, Owen F, Poulter M, et al. Prion dementia without characteristic pathology. Lancet 1990;336:7–9
8. Kitamoto T, Amano N, Terao Y, et al. A new inherited prion disease (PrP-P105L mutation) showing spastic paraparesis. Ann Neurol 1993;34:808–813
9. Samaia HB, Mari JDJ, Vallada HP, Moura RP, et al. Prions linked to mental illness. Nature 1997;390:241
10. McNaughton HK, Will RG. Creutzfeldt-Jakob disease presenting acutely as stroke; an analysis of 30 cases. Neurol Infect Epidemiol 1997;2:19–24
11. Kothbauer-Margreiter I, Baumgartner RW, Bassetti C, Mathis J. Hemisensory deficit in a patient with Creutzfeldt-Jakob disease. Eur Neurol 1996;36:108–109
12. Vargas ME, Kupersmith MJ, Savino PJ, Frohman LP, et al. Homonymous field defect as the first manifestation of Creutzfeldt-Jakob disease. Am J Ophthalmol 1995;119:497–504
13. Mandell M, Alexander MP, Carpenter S. Creutzfeldt-Jakob disease presenting as isolated aphasia. Neurology 1989;39:55–58
14. MacGowan DJL, Delanty N, Petito F, et al. Isolated myoclonic alien hand as the sole presentation of pathologically established Creutzfeldt-Jakob disease: a report of two patients. J Neurol Neurosurg Psychiatry 1997;63:404–407
15. Inzelberg R, Nisipeanu P, Blumen SC, Carasso RL. Alien hand sign in Creutzfeldt-Jakob disease. J Neurol Neurosurg Psychiatry 2000;68:103–104
16. Kott E, Bornstein B, Sandbank U. Ataxic form of

Creutzfeldt-Jakob disease: its relation to sub-acute spongiform encephalopathy. J Neurol Sci 1967;5: 107–113
17. Bertoni M, Brown P, Goldfarb LG, et al. Familial Creutzfeldt-Jakob disease (codon 200 mutation) with supranuclear palsy. JAMA 1992;268:2413–2415
18. Neufeld MY, Josiphov J, Korczyn AD. Demyelinating peripheral neuropathy in Creutzfeldt-Jakob disease. Muscle Nerve 1992;15:1234–1239
19. Chapman J, Brown P, Goldfarb LG, et al. Clinical heterogeneity and unusual presentations of Creutzfeldt-Jakob disease in Jewish patients with PRNP codon 200 mutation. J Neurol Neurosurg Psychiatry 1993;56: 1109–1112
20. Shabtai H, Nisipeanu P, Chapman J, Korczyn AD. Pruritus in Creutzfeldt-Jakob disease. Neurology 1996;46: 940–941
21. Chapman J, Arlazoroff A, Goldfarb LG, et al. Fatal insomnia in a case of familial Creutzfeldt-Jakob disease with the codon 200 (Lys) mutation. Neurology 1996;46: 758–761
22. Antoine JC, Laplanche JL, Mosnier JF, et al. Demyelinating peripheral neuropathy with Creutzfeldt-Jakob disease and mutation at codon 200 of the prion protein gene. Neurology 1996;46:1123–1126
23. Will RG, Ironside JW, Zeidler M, et al. A new variant of Creutzfeldt-Jakob disease in the UK. Lancet 1996;347: 921–925
24. Zeidler M, Stewart GE, Barraclough CR, et al. New variant Creutzfeldt-Jakob disease: neurological features and diagnostic tests. Lancet 1997;350:903–907
25. Zeidler M, Johnstone EC, Bamber RWK, et al. New variant Creutzfeldt-Jakob disease: psychiatric features. Lancet 1997;350:908–910
26. Medori R, Tritschler HY, LeBlanc A, et al. Fatal familial insomnia, a prion disease with a mutation at codon 178 of the prion protein gene. N Engl J Med 1992;326: 444–449
27. Gambetti P. Fatal familial insomnia and familial Creutzfeldt-Jakob disease: a tale of two diseases with the same genetic mutation. Current Topics Microbiol Immunol 1996;207:19–25
28. Parchi P, Giese A, Capellari S, et al. Classification of sporadic Creutzfeldt-Jakob disease based on molecular and phenotypic analysis of 300 subjects. Ann Neurol 1999;46:224–233
29. Will RG, Zeidler M, Stewart GE, et al. Diagnosis of new variant Creutzfeldt-Jakob disease. Ann Neurol 2000;47: 575–582
30. Sethi KD, Hess DC. Creutzfeldt-Jakob's disease presenting with ataxia and a movement disorder. Mov Disord 1991;6:157–162
31. Brown P, Gibbs CJ, Rodgers-Johnson P, et al. Human spongiform encephalopathy: the National Institutes of Health Series of 300 cases of experimentally transmitted disease. Ann Neurol 1994;35:513–529
32. Brownell B, Oppenheimer DR. An ataxic form of subacute presenile polioencephalopathy (Creutzfeldt-Jakob disease). J Neurol Neurosurg Psychiat 1965;28: 350–361
33. Johnson RT, Gibbs CJ. Creutzfeldt-Jakob disease and related transmissible spongiform encephalopathies. N Engl J Med 1998;339:1994–2006
34. Goldfarb LG, Brown P. The transmissible spongiform encephalopathies. Ann Rev Med 1995;46:57–65
35. Parchi P, Capellari S, Chin S, et al. A subtype of sporadic prion disease mimicking fatal familial insomnia. Neurology 1999;52:1757–1763
36. Creutzfeldt HG. Uber eine eigenartige herdformige

Erkrankung des Zentralnerveusystems. Z Neurol Psychiatr 1920;57:1–18
37. Jakob A. Uber eigenartige Erkrankung des Zentralnerveusystems mit bemerkenswertem anatomischen Befunde (Spastische Pseudo-sklerose—Encephalomyelopathie mit disseminiek ten Degenerationsherden). Z Neurol Psychiatr 1921;64:147–228
38. Tschampa HJ, Neumann M, Zerr I, et al. Patients with Alzheimer's disease and dementia with Lewy bodies mistaken for Creutzfeldt-Jakob disease. J Neurol Neurosurg Psychiatry 2001;71:33–39
39. Brown P. The phenotypic expression of different mutations in transmissible human spongiform encephalopathy. Rev Neurol 1992;148:317–327
40. Zerr I, Schulz-Schaeffer WJ, Giese A, et al. Current clinical diagnosis in Creutzfeldt-Jakob disease: identification of uncommon variants. Ann Neurol 2000;48: 323–329
41. Shibasaki H, Neshige R, Hashiba Y. Cortical excitability after myoclonus: jerk-locked somatosensory evoked potentials. Neurology 1985;35:36–41
42. Matsunaga K, Uozumi T, Akamatsu N, et al. Negative myoclonus in Creutzfeldt-Jakob disease. Clin Neurophysiol 2000;111:471–476
43. Wilkins DE, Hallett M, Berardelli A, et al. Physiologic analysis of the myoclonus of Alzheimer's disease. Neurology 1984;34:898–903
44. Brown P, Rodgers-Johnson P, Cathala F, et al. Creutzfeldt-Jakob disease of long duration: clinicopathological characteristics, transmissibility, and differential diagnosis. Ann Neurol 1984;16:295–304
45. Bowen J, Mitchell T, Pearce R, Quinn N. Chorea in new variant Creutzfeldt-Jakob disease. Mov Disord 2000;15: 1284–1285
46. Rabinstein AA, Whiteman ML, Shebert RT. Abnormal diffusion-weighted magnetic resonance imaging in Creutzfeldt-Jakob disease following corneal transplantations. Arch Neurol 2002;59:637–639
47. Levine DN. The alien hand. In: Movements Disorders in Neurology and Neuropsychiatry. AB Joseph, RR Young (eds) second edition. Oxford: Blackwell Science, 1999:645–649
48. Collins SJ, Masters CL. Transmissibility of Creutzfeldt-Jakob disease and related disorders. Sci Prog 1995;78: 217–227
49. Brown P. The risk of bovine spongiform encephalopathy ("Mad Cow Disease") to human health. JAMA 1997;278:1008–1011
50. Castellani R, Parchi P, Stahl J, et al. Early pathologic and biochemical changes in Creutzfeldt-Jakob disease: study of brain biopsies. Neurology 1996;46:1690–1693
51. Budka H, Aguzzi A, Brown P, et al. Neuropathological diagnostic criteria for Creutzfeldt-Jakob disease (CJD) and other human spongiform encephalopathies (prion diseases). Brain Pathology 1995;5:459–466
52. Garcia Santos JM, Lopez Corbalan JA, Martinez-Lage JF, Sicilia Guillen J. CT and MRI in iatrogenic and sporadic Creutzfeldt-Jakob disease: as far as imaging perceives. Neuroradiology 1996;38:226–231
53. Hunter R, Gordon A, McLuskie R, et al. Gross regional cerebral hypofunction with normal CT scan in Creutzfeldt-Jakob disease. Lancet 1989;333:214–215
54. Almond JW, Brown P, Gore SM, et al. Creutzfeldt-Jakob disease and bovine spongiform encephalopathy: magnetic resonance imaging may have a role in diagnosing Creutzfeldt-Jakob disease. BMJ 1996;312: 180–181
55. Becker S, Herrendorf G, Poser S, et al. Accuracy and reliability of periodic sharp wave complexes in

Creutzfeldt-Jakob disease. Arch Neurol 1996;53: 162–166

56. Neufeld MY, Korczyn AD. Topographic distribution of the periodic discharges in Creutzfeldt-Jakob disease (CJD). Brain Topography 1992;4:201–206

57. Hsich G, Kenney K, Gibbs CJ, et al. The 14-3-3 brain protein in cerebrospinal fluid as a marker for transmissible spongiform encephalopathies. N Engl J Med 1996;335:924–930

58. Zerr I, Bodemer M, Gefeller O, et al. Detection of 14-3-3 protein in the cerebrospinal fluid supports the diagnosis of Creutzfeldt-Jakob disease. Ann Neurol 1998;43: 32–40

59. Rosenmann H, Meiner Z, Kahana E, et al. Detection of 14-3-3 protein in the CSF of genetic Creutzfeldt-Jakob disease. Neurology 1997;49:593–595

60. Aksamit AJ, Preissner CM, Homburger HA. Quantitation of 14-3-3 and neuron-specific enolase proteins in CSF in Creutzfeldt-Jakob disease. Neurology 2001;57: 728–730

61. Otto M, Wiltfang J, Schutz E, et al. Diagnosis of Creutzfeldt-Jakob disease by measurement of S100 protein in serum: prospective case-control study. BMJ 1998;316:577–582

62. Shaked GM, Fridlander G, Meinert Z, et al. Protease-resistant and detergent-insoluble prion protein is not necessarily associated with prion infectivity. The Journal of Biological Chemistry 1999;25:17981–17986

63. Head MW, Ironside JW. Inhibition of prion-protein conversion: a therapeutic tool? Trends Microbiol 2000; 8:6–8

64. Adjou KT, Deslys J-P, Demaimay R, et al. Prospects for the pharmacological treatment of human prion diseases. CNS Drugs 1998;2:83–89

65. Chabry J, Caughey B, Chesebro B. Specific inhibition of in vitro formation of protease-resistant prion protein by synthetic peptides. J Biol Chem 1998;273:13203–13207

66. Chabry J, Priola SA, Wehrly K, et al. Species-independent inhibition of prion protein (PrP) formation by a peptide containing conserved PrP sequence. J Virol 1999;73:6245–6250

67. Perrier V, Wallace AC, Kaneko K, et al. Mimicking dominant negative inhibition of prion replication through structure-based drug design. Proc Natl Acad Sci USA 2000;97:6073–6078

68. Zulianello L, Kaneko K, Scott M, et al. Dominant-negative inhibition of prion formation diminished by deletion mutagenesis of the prion protein. J Virol 2000;74: 4351–4360

69. Soto C. β-amyloid disrupting drugs. CNS Drugs 1999; 12:347–356

70. Soto C, Kascsak RJ, Saborio GP, et al. Reversion of prion protein conformational changes by synthetic β-sheet breaker peptides. Lancet 2000;355:192–197

71. Farquar CT, Dickinson AG. Prolongation of scrapie incubation period by an injection of dextran sulphate 500 with the month before or after injection. J Gen Virol 1986;67:463–473

72. Farquhar C, Dickinson A, Bruce M. Prophylactic potential of pentosan polysulphate in transmissible spongiform encephalopathies. Lancet 1999;353:117

73. Montrasio F, Frigg R, Glatzel R, et al. Impaired prion replication in spleens of mice lacking functional follicular dendritic cells. Science 2000;288:1257–1259

74. Perovic S, Schroder HC, Pergande G, et al. Effect of flupirtine on Bcl-2 and glutathione level in neuronal cells treated in vitro with the prion protein fragment (PrP106–126). Exp Neurol 1997;147:518–524

75. Caspi S, Halimi M, Yanai A, et al. The anti-prion activity of Congo red. Putative mechanism. J Biol Chem 1998;273:3484–3489

76. Manuelidis L, Fritch W, Zaitsev I. Dapsone to delay symptoms in Creutzfeldt-Jakob disease. Lancet 1998; 352:456

77. Rudyk H, Vasijevic S, Hennion RM, et al. Screening Congo red and its analogues for their ability to prevent the formation of PrP^{res} in scrapie-infected cells. J Gen Virol 2000;81:1155–1164

78. Pocchiari M, Casaccia P, Ladogana A. Amphotericin B: a novel class of anti-scrapie drugs. The Journal of Infectious Diseases 1989;160:795–802

79. Adjou KT, Demaimay R, Deslys JP, et al. MS-8209, a water-soluble amphotericin B derivative, affects both scrapie agent replication and PrP^{res} accumulation in Syrian hamster scrapie. J Gen Virol 1999;80:1079–1085

80. Beringue V, Adjou KT, Lamoury F, et al. Opposite effects of dextran sulfate 500, the polyene antibiotic MS-8209, and Congo red on accumulation of the protease-resistant isoform of PrP in the spleens of mice inoculated intraperitoneally with the scrapie agent. J Virol 2000;74:5432–5440

81. Adjou KT, Privat N, Demart S, et al. MS-8209, an amphotericin B analogue, delays the appearance of spongiosis, astrogliosis and PrP^{res} accumulation in the brain of scrapie-injected hamsters. J Comp Pathol 2000; 122:3–8

82. Tagliavini F, McArthur RA, Canciani B, et al. Effectiveness of anthracycline against experimental prion disease in Syrian hamsters. Science 1997;276:1119–1122

83. Rouselle C, Smirnova M, Clair P, et al. Enhanced delivery of doxorubicin into the brain via a peptide-vector-mediated strategy: saturation kinetics and specificity. J Pharmacol Exp Ther 2001;296:124–131

84. Tatzelt J, Prusiner SB, Welch WY. Chemical chaperones interfere with the formation of scrapie prion protein. Embo J 1996;15:6563–6573

85. Supattapone S, Nguyen HO, Cohen FE, et al. Elimination of prions by branched polyamines and implications for therapeutics. Proc Natl Acad Sci USA 1999;96: 14529–14534

86. Priola SA, Raines A, Caughey WS. Porphyrin and phthalocyanine antiscrapie compounds. Science 2000; 287:1503–1506

87. Budka H, Aguzzi A, Brown P, et al. Tissue handling in suspected Creutzfeldt-Jakob disease (CJD) and other human spongiform encephalopathies (prion diseases). Brain Pathology 1995;5:319–322

88. Peretz D, Williamson RA, Kaneko K, et al. Antibodies inhibit prion propagation and clear cell cultures of prion infectivity. Nature 2001;412:739–743

89. Korth C, May BCH, Cohen FE, Prusiner SB. Acridine and phenothiazine derivatives as pharmacotherapeutics for prion disease. PNAS 2001;98:9836–9841

90. Gajdusek DC. Unconventional viruses and the origin and disappearance of Kuru. Science 1977;197:943–960

91. Vamvakas EC. Risk of transmission of Creutzfeldt-Jakob disease by transfusion of blood, plasma, and plasma derivatives. J Clin Apheresis 1999;14:135–143

92. Wilson K, Code C, Ricketts MN. Risk of acquiring Creutzfeldt-Jakob disease from blood transfusions: systematic review of case-control studies. BMJ 2000;321: 17–19

93. Shaked GM, Engelstein R, Avraham I, et al. Valproic acid treatment results in increased accumulation of prion proteins. Ann Neurol 2002;52: 416–420

257 Hereditary Spastic Paraplegia

John K Fink

The Hereditary spastic paraplegias (HSPs) are a group of disorders in which the predominant symptom is insidiously progressive lower extremity weakness and spasticity. Hereditary spastic paraplegia is also referred to as familial spastic paraplegia (FSP), hereditary (or familial) spastic *paraparesis*, and Strümpell-Lorrain syndrome. Estimates of HSP's prevalence (1.3 to 9.6 per 100 000)[1–3] are similar to that of amyotrophic lateral sclerosis.[4,5] This review summarizes HSP's classification, clinical features, differential diagnosis, treatment, and genetic counseling; and advances in the genetic analysis of HSP. There are also plenty of previous reviews of HSP in the literature.[6–32]

Clinical classification

Harding classified HSP as "uncomplicated and "complicated".[33] In "uncomplicated" (referred to as "pure" HSP), neurological deficits are limited to progressive lower extremity spastic weakness, hypertonic urinary bladder disturbance, and often, but not always, mild diminution of lower extremity vibration sensation. "Complicated HSP" refers to those inherited syndromes in which progressive spastic paraparesis is accompanied by additional neurological abnormalities that are not attributable to other, co-existing disorders. For example, "complicated HSP" syndromes include those in which progressive lower extremity spastic weakness is accompanied by seizures, dementia, cataracts, amyotrophy, extrapyramidal disturbance, cutaneous abnormalities, or peripheral neuropathy. With several notable exceptions, discussed below, complicated and uncomplicated forms of HSP do not co-exist in the same families.

Harding further classified uncomplicated HSP as type I (symptom onset before age 35 years, greater lower extremity spasticity than weakness, and slow progression); and type II (symptom onset after age 35, significant lower extremity weakness in addition to spasticity, mild distal sensory loss, urinary bladder disturbance, and faster progression).[21–33] Classification of HSP by age-of-symptom onset alone is problematic because "early" and "late" age of symptom onset may occur within a given HSP family. This is particularly true for autosomal dominant HSP linked to chromosome 2p (the most common type of dominantly inherited HSP). It is true, however that different genetic types of HSP vary in the *average* age at which symptoms begin. (Although the *range* of ages of symptom onset may overlap between different genetic types of HSP.[9]

Symptoms of uncomplicated HSP

Insidiously progressive gait disturbance

Subjects with uncomplicated HSP experience slowly progressive gait disturbance due to insidiously progressive weakness and increased muscle tone in their legs. These symptoms may begin at any age from early childhood until late adulthood (see Table 257.1). Although gait disturbance typically progresses slowly over many years, it is noteworthy that individuals with symptom-onset in early childhood may not have obvious progressive worsening. Canes, walkers, or wheelchairs are often required.

Functional worsening during cold weather

It is very common for subjects with uncomplicated HSP to report increased lower extremity spasticity and functional gait worsening during cold winter months. Such seasonal variation should be distinguished from true exacerbations and remissions which do not occur in HSP.

Muscle cramps

Muscle cramps, particularly affecting the calves at night are common in subjects with uncomplicated HSP.

Urinary urgency and lower extremity paresthesiae

Urinary urgency and lower extremity paresthesiae often occur but are usually late features of HSP.

Mild upper extremity muscle tightness

Mild upper extremity muscle tightness is occasionally reported by subjects with uncomplicated HSP. Nonetheless, implicit in the diagnosis of uncomplicated HSP is the prediction that upper extremity strength and dexterity will be preserved and that dysphagia and dysarthria will not occur.

Subclinical cognitive disturbance and late-onset dementia

Subclinical cognitive disturbance and late-onset dementia have been described in some families with otherwise uncomplicated HSP. This has been reported in the most common form of uncomplicated autosomal dominant HSP (linked to the SPG4 locus on chromosome 2p);[34–37] and in several otherwise uncomplicated HSP kindreds in which the genetic locus was not known.[38] It is uncertain whether dementia in these HSP kindreds represents co-segregation of a separate disease processes such as senile dementia of the Alzheimer's type; or represents an extra-spinal manifestation of HSP. It is further

Table 257.1   Genetic loci (SPG) for hereditary spastic paraplegia

Spastic gait (SPG) locus	Chromosome (protein)	HSP syndrome
Autosomal dominant HSP		
SPG4	2p22 (Spastin)	Uncomplicated
SPG13	2q24-34	Uncomplicated
SPG8	8q23-q24	Uncomplicated
SPG17	11q12-q14	Complicated: spastic paraplegia associated with amyotrophy of hand muscles (Silver Syndrome)
SPG10	12q13	Uncomplicated
SPG9	10q23.3-q24.2	Complicated: spastic paraplegia associated with cataracts and gastroesophageal reflux, and motor neuronopathy
SPG3	14q11-q21 (Atlastin)	Uncomplicated
SPG6	15q11.1	Uncomplicated
SPG12	19q13	Uncomplicated
Autosomal recessive HSP		
SPG5	8p11-8q13	Uncomplicated
SPG11	15q13-q15	Uncomplicated or complicated: variably associated with HSP associated with thin corpus callosum, mental retardation, upper extremity weakness, dysarthria, and nystagmus
SPG7	16q.24.3 (Paraplegin)	Uncomplicated or complicated: variably associated with mitochondrial abnormalities on skeletal muscle biopsy and dysarthria, dysphagia, optic disc pallor, axonal neuropathy, and evidence of "vascular lesions," cerebellar atrophy, or cerebral atrophy on cranial MRI
SPG14	3q27-28	Complicated: spastic paraplegia associated with mental retardation and distal motor neuropathy
SPG15	14q	Complicated: spastic paraplegia associated with pigmented maculopathy, distal amyotrophy, dysarthria, mental retardation, and further intellectual deterioration
X-linked HSP		
SPG1	Xq28 (L1CAM)	Complicated: associated with mental retardation, and variably, hydrocephalus, aphasia, and adducted thumbs
SPG2	Xq28 (Proteolipid protein)	Complicated: variably associated with MRI evidence of CNS white matter abnormality
SPG16	Xq11.2	Uncomplicated
		Complicated: associated with motor aphasia, reduced vision, mild mental retardation, and dysfunction of the bowel and bladder

Table modified from references 69 and 77.

unknown whether cognitive disturbance is a feature of all or only some autosomal dominant chromosome 2p (SPG4) linked HSP kindreds; and whether cognitive disturbance is also present in other genetic types of autosomal dominant HSP.

Neurological findings in uncomplicated HSP

Lower extremity weakness, spasticity, and hyperreflexia

Neurological examination of subjects with uncomplicated HSP reveals bilateral lower extremity weakness and increased muscle tone that is maximal in iliopsoas, hamstrings, and tibialis anterior muscles; bilateral lower extremity hyperreflexia and bilateral extensor plantar responses. The majority of subjects have approximately equal degrees of weakness and spasticity. However, in some subjects spasticity predominates and only slight weakness occurs. In other subjects, weakness rather than spasticity is the major feature. As noted above, Harding's type I HSP

subjects had greater spasticity than weakness; type II HSP subjects had greater weakness than spasticity.[33] It has not been shown, however, whether such differences are associated with specific genetic types of HSP or variable within a given family. Determining the relative contribution of spasticity versus weakness to overall gait disturbance helps select subjects for whom spasticity reducing medications would be most appropriate.

Symmetry

Although subjects commonly describe symptoms beginning in one leg and often identify one leg as stronger and more flexible, they soon note symptoms in both legs. Side-to-side differences on neurological examination are generally within the range of normal physiological symmetry. Finding markedly asymmetric or unilateral leg weakness, spasticity, hyperreflexia, and extensor plantar response should prompt careful exclusion of alternative disorders including amyotrophic lateral sclerosis, multiple sclerosis, and focal structural abnormality of the spinal cord or brain.

Upper extremity hyperreflexia

Upper extremity deep tendon reflexes are often brisk (grades two to three on a zero to four scale) and occasionally, there may be slight spastic catch on rapid passive movements. Nonetheless, upper extremity strength and dexterity remain normal. Significant upper extremity weakness is not consistent with the diagnosis of uncomplicated HSP and suggests alternative disorders such as motor neuron disorders, primary lateral sclerosis, multiple sclerosis, or structural abnormality involving the brain or cervical spinal cord.

Dorsal column impairment

Most subjects with uncomplicated HSP eventually develop diminished vibration sensation in distal lower extremities. Decreased vibration sensation is usually mild and is not an early feature of HSP. Proprioception typically is preserved. When not attributable to other disorders (such as co-existent peripheral neuropathy), decreased vibratory sensation helps distinguish HSP from amyotrophic lateral sclerosis in which spastic weakness may precede amyotrophy; and from primary lateral sclerosis which may progress to involve upper extremities, speech, and swallowing.[39]

Muscle bulk

Muscle bulk is usually normal in subjects with uncomplicated HSP although some subjects have decreased muscle mass in distal lower extremities (particularly the shins). This is generally attributed to disuse atrophy although could reflect subtle loss of anterior horn cells which have been observed in postmortem examination of some HSP subjects.[25] Electromyography does not show motor neuron involvement in uncomplicated HSP, however. Significant distal muscle wasting suggests an alternative disorder (such as amyotrophic lateral sclerosis), co-existent peripheral neuropathy, or a "complicated" form of HSP. Silver syndrome (autosomal dominant), Troyer syndrome (autosomal recessive), and SPG15 (autosomal recessive) and are types of complicated HSP in which insidiously progressive lower extremity spastic weakness is associated with distal amyotrophy.[40–44] In addition, there are a number of complicated HSP syndromes that include peripheral neuropathy or motor neuronopathy.[45–53]

Pes cavus

Pes cavus is often but not invariably present in uncomplicated HSP. Pes cavus may be absent in definitely affected subjects. Neither the presence nor absence of pes cavus can be used in the absence of other neurological findings to predict whether an at-risk subject will develop HSP.

Neurodiagnostic testing

Electromyographic and nerve conduction studies

Electromyography (EMG) and nerve conduction studies (NCS) are useful in evaluating subjects with possible HSP because of their role in excluding alternative disorders (particularly those affecting the motor neuron). Electromyography and NCS typically are normal in uncomplicated HSP[54–56] although Schady and Scheard[57] and Schady and Smith[58] reported subclinical sensory neuropathy in otherwise uncomplicated HSP.

Somatosensory evoked potentials

Somatosensory evoked potentials (SSEP) recorded from the lower extremities often show conduction delay in dorsal column fibers.[56,59–62] Somatosensory evoked potentials recorded from the upper extremities are typically normal. Abnormal lower extremity SSEP is a helpful diagnostic finding. When abnormal, this finding helps distinguish HSP from primary lateral sclerosis and amyotrophic lateral sclerosis which do not involve sensory fibers.

Cortical evoked potentials

Though not widely available, cortical evoked potentials are helpful in demonstrating impaired corticospinal tract conduction to the lower extremities. Cortical evoked potentials recorded from the lower extremities typically become abnormal in HSP subjects and show reduced conduction velocity and amplitude of the evoked potential. In contrast, cortical evoked potentials to the upper extremities are usually normal or show only mildly reduced conduction velocity.[26,59,63–65]

Neuroimaging

Neuroimaging is important in evaluating HSP subjects to exclude other disorders such as multiple sclerosis, leukodystrophies, and structural abnormalities involving the brain or spinal cord. Magnetic resonance imaging (MRI) of the brain is normal in uncomplicated HSP. Spinal cord MRI is generally normal[66] although may show mild to marked atrophy of cervical and thoracic segments.[67,68]

Diagnostic criteria of uncomplicated HSP[8]

Clinical symptoms

Clinical symptoms of insidiously progressive gait disturbance due to bilateral lower extremity spastic weakness, often accompanied by urinary urgency and occurring in the *absence* of symptomatic involvement of the upper extremities, speech, and swallowing are the hallmarks of uncomplicated HSP.

Neurological examination

Neurological examination shows bilateral lower extremity spastic weakness, hyperreflexia and almost always, extensor plantar responses. Mildly impaired vibration sensation in the distal lower extremities is usually present but is typically a later feature. Pes cavus is often present. Important "negative findings" in the neurological examination of subjects with uncomplicated HSP include the absence of spinal sensory level, peripheral neuropathy, marked amyotrophy, fasciculations, upper extremity weakness, dysarthria, dysphagia, or cranial nerve impairment.

Family history

Family history consistent with inheritance of autosomal dominant, autosomal recessive or X-linked spastic paraplegia is an essential element in the diagnosis of HSP. Subjects with all the signs and symptoms of HSP but for whom family history is negative or unavailable are diagnosed as having "apparently sporadic" spastic paraplegia. Use of the term "hereditary" in such patients overstates the knowledge of their disorder and indicates that some of their relatives are at risk of developing this disorder.

Exclusion of other diagnoses

Exclusion of other diagnoses is of paramount importance. The emerging availability of laboratory tests for some forms of HSP not withstanding, HSP is a diagnosis of exclusion for the majority of subjects. The differential diagnosis of uncomplicated HSP[8,69] includes structural abnormalities involving the brain or spinal cord (such as tethered cord syndrome and spinal cord compression); leukodystrophies such as B_{12} deficiency, Pelizaeus-Merzbacher disease (X-linked), Krabbe disease (autosomal recessive), metachromatic leukodystrophy (autosomal recessive), adrenomyeloneuropathy (X-linked);[70–72] and other disorders such as Machado-Joseph disease (spinocerebellar ataxia type 3,[73,74] steadily progressive multiple sclerosis; motor neuron disease,[75] primary lateral sclerosis,[76,77] and tropical spastic paraplegia (human T-cell leukemia virus 1 [HTLV1]-associated myelopathy).[74] It is important to consider dopa-responsive dystonia in all subjects, particularly children with progressive gait disturbance and increased lower extremity tone.[78,79] We often recommend a two-week trial of levodopa-carbidopa, increasing to 25/100 bid. Although rare, dopa-responsive dystonia is treatable with low-dose levodopa-carbidopa. Note that the differential diagnosis of HSP includes familial clustering of non-genetic disorders (tropical spastic paraparesis);[80–83] disorders for which specific treatments are available (e.g. B_{12} deficiency, dopa-responsive dystonia, cervical spondylosis); and those whose prognosis differs significantly from HSP (e.g. familial amyotrophic lateral sclerosis and primary lateral sclerosis).

Neuropathology

The major neuropathological[21,25] features of autosomal dominant, uncomplicated HSP are axonal degeneration in the terminal portions of the corticospinal tracts and dorsal column fibers. Spinocerebellar fibers are involved to a lesser extent. Demyelination, if present, is consistent with the degree of axonal degeneration. In contrast to amyotrophic lateral sclerosis (ALS) and primary lateral sclerosis (PLS), axonal degeneration in uncomplicated HSP involves both motor (cortico-

spinal tracts) and sensory (dorsal column) fibers. Corticospinal tract degeneration is maximal in the thoracic region (affecting those fibers to the legs); corticospinal tracts terminating in the cervical region are much less affected. Dorsal column degeneration is maximal in the fasiculus gracilus fibers in the cervicomedullary region; fasciculus cuneatus axons are much less affected. Axonal degeneration is thus maximal at the terminal portions of the longest descending and ascending tracts.[12] There is usually no significant degeneration of cortical motor neurons or anterior horn cells although decreased numbers of such cells have been observed in some cases.[12,21] Dorsal root ganglia, posterior roots and peripheral nerves typically are normal in uncomplicated HSP.[21]

The primary pathology of HSP, axonopathy involving the distal ends of long motor and sensory fibers in the *central nervous system*, can be viewed as a central nervous system homologue of Charcot-Marie-Tooth type II which is characterized by distal axonal degeneration involving motor and sensory neurons of the *peripheral nervous system*.[84] It will be interesting to discover whether the molecular mechanisms underlying distal axonopathy are similar in these two clinically disparate groups of diseases.

Genetic analysis

There are autosomal dominant, autosomal recessive, and X-linked forms of HSP, each of which is genetically heterogeneous. The locations of HSP genes are designated "spastic paraplegia" (SPG) loci 1 through 15 in order of their discovery (Table 257.1).

Autosomal dominant HSP

Seven loci for autosomal dominant *uncomplicated* HSP and one locus for autosomal dominant *complicated* HSP have been identified (Table 257.1). Linkage to chromosome 2p (SPG4) is the most common type of uncomplicated autosomal dominant HSP and represents approximately 45% of such kindreds.[8,85,86] Each of the other genetic types of autosomal dominant HSP have been reported as only one to several kindreds. The "uncomplicated HSP phenotype" is very similar for each genetic type of uncomplicated HSP. Thus far, the average age of symptom onset and extent of clinical progression are the only clinical parameters by which genetic types of uncomplicated autosomal dominant HSP can be distinguished. Gait disturbance for autosomal dominant uncomplicated HSP linked to chromosomes 12 (SPG10), 14 (SPG3), and 19 (SPG12) begins on average before age 11. In contrast, gait disturbance for autosomal dominant uncomplicated HSP linked to chromosomes 2p (SPG4), 2q (SPG13) 8 (SPG8), and 15 (SPG6) begins after age 20.[9] As noted above, however, the range of ages at which symptoms first appear varies widely and may overlap between different genetic forms of HSP. This is particularly true for the most common form of autosomal dominant, uncomplicated HSP (linked to chromosome 2p) in which symptom onset has ranged from two to 75 years.[87]

We have observed several SPG3 (chromosome

14q11) linked HSP families in which symptoms began in early childhood, following which there was very little evident worsening. This contrasts with the slow, steady worsening that typically occurs in SPG4, for example. It is not known whether the lack of obvious worsening is unique to SPG3 HSP or is also a characteristic of other childhood onset autosomal dominant forms of uncomplicated HSP.

Spastin gene mutations cause the most common form of autosomal dominant HSP (linked to the SPG4 locus on chromosome 2p).[85,88] In 1999, Hazan et al.,[88] discovered mutations in a novel gene ("spastin") as the cause SPG4 linked HSP. Although spastin's function is not known, computer analysis predicts that spastin is an ATPase that may be involved in assembly or function of nuclear protein complexes.[88] More than 40 different spastin gene mutations have been identified, none of which are particularly common.[88]

Recently, Zhao et al., discovered mutations in a novel gene (SPG3) as the basis of chromosome 14q-linked autosomal dominant HSP.[89] Alvarado et al.,[90] identified SPG3A mutations in 25% of childhood onset, dominantly inherited HSP. The SPG3A mutation encodes a GTPase (designated "atlastin") that is homologous to the dyanmin family of large GTPases. Dynamins are important factors in synaptic vessicle recycling, uptake of activated receptor/ligand complexes, and the division and distribution of mitochondria.[91–96]

Autosomal recessive HSP

Autosomal recessive HSP is also genetically heterogeneous with four loci having been identified (Table 257.1). Among autosomal recessive HSP, linkage to chromosome 15q is the most common type, representing approximately 50% of such kindreds.[97]

Mutations in the paraplegin gene cause a rare form of autosomal recessive HSP (linked to chromosome 16q). In 1998 DiMichele et al.,[98] analyzed an autosomal recessive HSP kindred in which some subjects had abnormal mitochondria (ragged red fibers and cytochrome C oxidase negative fibers) on skeletal muscle biopsy. While some subjects had uncomplicated HSP, others had additional neurological abnormalities including dysarthria, dysphagia, optic disc pallor, axonal neuropathy, and evidence of "vascular lesions," cerebellar atrophy, or cerebral atrophy on cranial MRI.[98] Genetic linkage analysis identified linkage to a novel locus on chromosome 16p (SPG7). Casari et al.,[99] subsequently identified mutations in a novel gene ("paraplegin") at this locus in affected subjects from these kindreds.

Paraplegin contains an ATPase Associated with diverse cellular Activities (AAA motif) (as does spastin, mutations in which cause autosomal dominant HSP linked to chromosome 2p); is homologous to several yeast mitochondrial metalloproteases (AFG3, RCA1 and YME1), which have both proteolytic and chaperone activities;[99,100] and is localized to exclusively to mitochondria.[99] Mitochondrial abnormalities, evident in some chromosome 16p (SPG7)-linked autosomal recessive HSP due to paraplegin gene mutations were not found in subjects with autosomal dominant

HSP linked to chromosome 2p),[88,101–103] 8q,[103] 14q,[104] or 15q.[104] Thus, mitochondrial abnormalities are not common features of all types of HSP.

Additional loci for autosomal recessive HSP have been identified on chromosome 8p11-8q13 (SPG5: "uncomplicated" HSP); and chromosome 3q27-28 (SPG14: "complicated" HSP associated with mental retardation and distal motor neuropathy.

X-linked HSP

Three loci for X-linked forms of complicated HSP[99] have been discovered (Table 257.1). Proteolipid protein (PLP) gene mutations cause both childhood onset slowly progressive X-linked HSP and Pelizaeus-Merzbacher disease, an infantile-onset severe neurological disorder due to abnormal myelin formation. The PLP gene encodes an intrinsic myelin protein.[105] Mutations in the PLP gene cause X-linked Pelizaeus-Merzbacher disease, and slowly progressive, childhood-onset spastic paraplegia. This phenotypic variability has been attributed to the nature of the specific PLP gene mutations associated with each disorder.[106] Other mechanisms must also contribute, however, because both the early-onset, severe form (Pelizaeus-Merzbacher type) and the more slowly progressive, relatively mild form (HSP type) may occur in the same family (JK Fink, unpublished observation). Often, subjects with X-linked HSP due to PLP gene mutation have MRI evidence of central white matter disturbance.[66,107,108]

Neural cell adhesion molecule (L1CAM) gene mutations cause several developmental neurological disorders including X-linked spastic paraplegia,[109] X-linked hydrocephalus; and mental retardation, aphasia, shuffling gait, adducted thumbs (MASA) syndrome; and CRASH syndrome (corpus callosum hypoplasia, retardation, adducted thumbs, spastic paraparesis and hydrocephalus).[109–111]

A third locus (SPG16) for X-linked HSP has been identified on Xq11.2. Subjects linked to this locus exhibit either uncomplicated HSP; or HSP associated with motor aphasia, reduced vision, mild mental retardation, and bladder and bowel disturbance.

Laboratory testing for HSP gene mutations

Spastin gene testing is available through Athena Diagnostics (Boston, MA). This information will be useful to confirm the clinical diagnosis of HSP; and to improve genetic counseling and prenatal diagnosis. At present, testing for atlastin, paraplegin, and L1-cell adhesion molecule gene mutation is available in several research laboratories. Proteolipid protein gene analysis is available commercially. Even with the emerging availability of laboratory based testing to confirm the diagnosis of HSP, it is still important that subjects with progressive spastic paraparesis undergo evaluation, including neuroimaging as indicated, to exclude alternative or co-existent disorders.

Treatment

Presently, there is no treatment to reverse or prevent progressive axonal degeneration in HSP. Nonetheless, symptomatic treatment is available to reduce muscle spasticity (oral or intrathecal Lioresal or oral Dantrolene or Tizanidine;[112,113] and to reduce urinary urgency (with Oxybutynin for example). Note however, that the degree of spasticity is variable between HSP subjects and that excessive reduction of spasticity may cause functional gait worsening. It is advisable for HSP subjects to participate in regular physical therapy in order to improve range of motion, maintain and increase lower extremity strength, and increase cardiovascular conditioning.

Genetic counseling

The probability of inheriting or transmitting an autosomal dominant HSP gene mutation can be determined either by knowing the pattern of inheritance or by laboratory testing (genetic linkage analysis for families linked to known HSP loci or detection of mutations in the HSP genes identified thus far). Genetic penetrance, the frequency with which subjects who have an HSP gene mutation will exhibit symptoms of the disorder, is age-dependent, high, but incomplete. It is estimated that 85% of subjects with spastin gene mutation will exhibit signs of the disorder by age 45.[97] It is important to recognize that the degree of symptoms may be quite variable within a given family and between families with the same genetic type of HSP; some individuals may be markedly affected while others have only mild gait disturbance. Also, the age at which symptoms first appears may be variable within a given family. This is particularly true for the most common form of autosomal dominant HSP in which age of symptom onset has ranged from age two to age 75.

Caution must be exercised in providing genetic counseling in families in which HSP affects only siblings. This could be an autosomal recessive disorder (in which case, there is low risk that affected subjects will transmit the disorder through non-consanguineous matings). Alternatively, the disorder could be dominantly inherited with incomplete genetic penetrance; or late age of symptom onset (unaffected parents may still be at risk of developing symptoms).

Conclusions

Hereditary spastic paraplegia shows extreme genetic heterogeneity. To date, 17 different genetic types of HSP have been identified. Hereditary spastic paraplegia is similar in this regard to other inherited neurological disorders including spinocerebellar ataxias and hereditary motor sensory neuropathies which show similar degrees of genetic heterogeneity.

"Complicated HSP" and "uncomplicated HSP syndromes usually do not occur in the same family. The exceptions to this generalization are subjects with autosomal recessive HSP linked to chromosome 15q (SPG11, the most common form of autosomal recessive HSP); and those with chromosome 16q-linked autosomal recessive HSP (SPG7) due to paraplegin gene mutation. In these families, some subjects may exhibit uncomplicated HSP and others have HSP

associated with additional neurological impairments. Cognitive disturbance and dementia have been described in some affected subjects with autosomal dominant HSP linked to chromosome 2p (due to spastin gene mutation). It is uncertain whether this is a common finding for which many chromosome 2p-linked autosomal dominant HSP subjects are at risk, or represents co-occurrence of "complicated" and "uncomplicated" HSP in the same kindred. With these exceptions, "uncomplicated" and "complicated" HSP syndromes do not usually occur in the same families. Affected individuals from large families with "uncomplicated" HSP are not considered at risk of developing upper extremity involvement, dysphagia, dysarthria, or other neurological impairments of "complicated" HSP syndromes.

"Uncomplicated" HSP is due to axonal degeneration involving the distal axons of descending corticospinal tracts and ascending dorsal column fibers. HSP therefore, affects both motor and sensory fibers within the central nervous system. Degeneration is maximal at the distal ends of the longest CNS axons.

Genetic testing for HSP gene mutations is becoming available. Analysis of the spastin gene, mutations in which are the most common cause of autosomal dominant HSP, is available through Athena Diagnostics (Boston, MA). This will permit accurate diagnosis and counseling for nearly half of the subjects with autosomal dominant HSP. Analysis of atlastin, paraplegin, and PLP genes, mutations which cause, respectively, a rare form of recessively inherited HSP and a form of X-linked HSP, is available only on a research basis in several laboratories.

For most subjects, HSP is a diagnosis of exclusion. The differential diagnosis[8] includes treatable disorders (for example, B_{12} deficiency, dopa-responsive dystonia, cervical spondylosis); and those whose prognosis differs significantly from HSP (e.g. familial amyotrophic lateral sclerosis and primary lateral sclerosis). It is important that alternative disorders be considered carefully by appropriate diagnostic testing.

Treatment for HSP is symptomatic and includes physical therapy and medications to reduce spasticity (such as Lioresal) and urinary urgency (such as Oxybutynin).

Diverse HSP genes have been discovered (spastin, paraplegin, proteolipid protein, and L1-cell adhesion molecule). This diversity suggests that the phenotype of progressive spastic parapelgia can be caused by disruption of diverse molecular pathways. Discovery of additional HSP genes will further define these pathways and reveal whether common biochemical cascades are involved. Such an insight will permit the design of therapeutic interventions for this group of disorders.

Acknowledgments

This research is supported by grants from the Veterans Affairs Merit Review and the National Institutes of Health (NINDS). The author gratefully acknowledges the expert secretarial assistance of Ms. Lynette Girbach; and the participation of HSP subjects and their families without whom such investigations of HSP would not be possible.

References

1. McMonagle P, Webb S, Hutchinson M. The prevalence of "pure" autosomal dominant hereditary spastic paraparesis in the island of Ireland. J Neurol Neurosurg Psych 2002;72:43–46

2. Filla A, DeMichele G, Marconi R, et al. Prevalence of hereditary ataxias and spastic paraplegias in Molise, a region of Italy. J Neurol 1992;239:351–353

3. Polo AE, Calleja J, Combarros O, Bericiano J. Hereditary ataxias and paraplegias in Cantabria, Spain: an epidemiological and clinical study. Brain 1991;114: 855–856

4. Kondo K. Motor neuron disease: changing population patterns and clues for etiology. In: Schoenberg BS, ed. Advances in Neurology. New York: Raven Press, 1978: 509

5. Gunnarsson LG, Palm R. Motor neuron disease and heavy manual labor: an epidemiologic survey of Varmland County, Sweden. Neuroepidemiology 1984; 3:195

6. Kjellin KG. Hereditary spastic paraplegia and retinal degeneration (Kjellin syndrome and Barard-Scholz syndrome). In: Vinken PJ, Bruyn GW, eds. Handbook of Clinical Neurology. Vol 22, System Disorders and Atrophies, Part II. Amsterdam: North Holland, 1975: 467–473

7. Fink JK. Hereditary spastic paraplegia. Neuromuscular Disorders in Clinical Practice. In: Katirji B, Kaminski HJ, Preston DC, Ruff RL, Shapiro BE, eds. Butterworth-Heinemann, 2002:1290–1297

8. Fink JK, Heiman-Patterson T, Bird T, et al. Hereditary spastic paraplegia: advances in genetic research. Neurology 1996;46:1507–1514

9. Fink JK, Hedera P. Hereditary spastic paraplegia: genetic heterogeneity and genotype-phenotype correlation. Semin Neurol 1999;19:301–310

10. Fink JK. Hereditary spastic paraplegia. In: Adelman G, Smith BH, eds. The Encyclopedia of Neuroscience. 2nd ed. (CD-ROM). Amsterdam: Elsevier Science, 1997: 871–874

11. Fink JK. Advances in hereditary spastic paraplegia. Current Opinion in Neurology 1997;10:313–318

12. Behan W, Maia M. Strumpell's familial spastic paraplegia: genetics and neuropathology. J Neurol Neurosurg Psychiatry 1974;37:8–20

13. Skre H. Hereditary spastic paraplegia in Western Norway. Clin Gen 1993;6:165–183

14. Rhein J. Family spastic paralysis. J Nerv Ment Dis 1914;44:115–144

15. Philipp E. Hereditary (familial) spastic paraplegia: report of six cases in one family. New Zeal Med J 1949;48:22–25

16. Cartlidge N, Bone G. Sphincter involvement in hereditary spastic paraplegia. Neurology 1973;23:1160–1163

17. Roe P. Hereditary spastic paraplegia. J Neurol Neurosurg Psychiatry 1963;26:516–519

18. Boustany R-MN, Fleischnick E, Alper CA, et al. The autosomal dominant form of "pure" familial spastic paraplegia. Neurology 1987;37:910–915

19. Holmes G, Shaywitz B. Strumpell's pure familial spastic paraplegia: case study and review of the literature. J Neurol Neurosurg Psychiatry 1977;40: 1003–1008

20. Sutherland JM. Familial spastic paraplegia. In: Vinken

PJ, Bruyn GW, eds. Handbook of Clinical Neurology. Vol 22, System Disorders and Atrophies, Part II. Amsterdam: North Holland, 1975:420–431

21. Harding AE. Hereditary spastic paraplegias. Semin Neurol 1993;13:333–336

22. Baraitser M. Spastic paraplegia/HSP. In: Motulsky AG, Bobrow M, Harper PS, Scriver C, eds. The Genetics of Neurological Disorders. 2nd ed. New York: Oxford University Press, 1990:275–290

23. McKusick VA. Spastic Paraplegia, Hereditary. In: McKusick VA, ed. Mendelian Inheritance in Man. 8th ed. Baltimore: Johns Hopkins University Press, 1988: 1189

24. Bell GJ, Karam JH, Rutter WJ. Polymorphic DNA region adjacent to the 5′ end of the human insulin gene. Proc Natl Acad Sci (USA) 1981;78:5759–5763

25. Schwarz GA, Liu C-N. Hereditary (familial) spastic paraplegia. Further clinical and pathologic observations. AMA Arch Neurol Psychiatry 1956;75:144–162

26. Polo JM, Calleja J, Combarris O, Berciano J. Hereditary "pure" spastic paraplegia: a study of nine families. J Neurol Neurosurg Psychiatry 1993;56:175–181

27. Scheltens P, Bruyn RPM, Hazenberg GJ. A Dutch family with autosomal dominant pure spastic paraparesis (Strumpell's disease). Acta Neurol Scand 1990; 82:169–173

28. Holmes GL, Shaywitz BA. Strumpell's pure familial spastic paraplegia: case study and review of the literature. J Neurol Neurosurg Psychiatry 1977;40: 1003–1008

29. Reid E. The hereditary spastic paraplegias. J Neurol 1999;246:995–1003

30. Schwarz GA. Hereditary (familial) spastic paraplegia. AMA Arch Neurol Psychiatry 1952;68:655–682

31. Paskind HA, Stone TT. Family spastic paralysis: report of three cases in one family and observations at necropsy. Arch Neurol Psychiat 1933;30:481–500

32. Price GE. Familial lateral sclerosis (spastic paralysis). J Nerv Ment Dis 1939;90:51–55

33. Harding AE. Classification of the Hereditary Ataxias and Paraplegias. Lancet 1983;1:1151–1155

34. Heinzlef O, Paternotte C, Mahieux F, et al. Mapping of a complicated familial spastic paraplegia to locus SPG4 on chromosome 2p. J Med Genet 1998;35:89–93

35. Webb S, Coleman D, Byrne P, et al. Autosomal dominant hereditary spastic paraparesis with cognitive loss linked to chromosome 2p. Brain 1998;121:601–609

36. Byrne PC, Webb S, McSweeney F, et al. Linkage of AD HSP and cognitive impairment to chromosome 2p: haplotype and phenotype analysis indicates variable expression and low or delayed penetrance. Eur J Human Genet 1998;6:275–282

37. Reid E, Grayson C, Rubinsztein DC, et al. Subclinical cognitive impairment in autosomal dominant "pure" hereditary spastic paraplegia. J Med Genet 1999;36: 797–798

38. Tedeschi G, Allocca S, DiCostanzo A, et al. Multisystem involvement of the central nervous system in Strumpell's disease. A neurophysiological and neuropsychological study. J Neurol Sci 1991;103:55–60

39. Bruyn RP, Koelman JH, Troost D, deJong JM. Motor neuron disease (amyotrophic lateral sclerosis) arising from longstanding primary lateral sclerosis. J Neurol Neurosurg Psych 1995;58:742–744

40. Cross HE, McKusick VA. The Troyer syndrome. A recessive form of spastic paraplegia with distal muscle wasting. Arch Neurol 1967;16:473–485

41. Hughes CA, Byrne PC, Webb S, et al. SPG15, a new

locus for autosomal recessive complicated HSP on chromosome 14q. Neurology 2001;56:1230–1233

42. Patel H, Hart PE, Warner TT, et al. The silver syndrome variant of hereditary spastic paraplegia maps to chromosome 11q12-q14, with evidence for genetic heterogeneity within this subtype. Am J Hum Genet 2001; 69:209–215

43. Farag TI, El-badramany MH, Al-Sharkawy S. Troyer Syndrome: report of the first "non-Amish" sibship and review. Am J Med Genet 1994;52:383–385

44. Silver JR. Familial spastic paraplegia with amyotrophy of the hands. Ann Hum Genet, London 1966;30:69–73

45. Antinolo G, Nieto M, Borrego S, et al. Familial spastic paraplegia with neuropathy and poikiloderma. A new syndrome? Clin Genet 1992;41:281–284

46. Matthys JH. De la-araplegie spasmodique de Strumpell-Lorrain a l'amyotrophie de Charcot-Marie-Tooth. J Genet Hum 2000;10:326–337

47. McKusick VA. Catalogs of Autosomal Dominant, Autosomal Recessive, and X-Linked Phenotypes. In: Mendelian Inheritance in Man, 8th edition, Johns Hopkins University Press, 1988:677

48. Thomas PK, Misra VP, King RHM, et al. Autosomal recessive hereditary sensory neuropathy with spastic paraplegia. Brain 1994;117:651–659

49. Cavanagh NPC, Eames RA, Galvin RJ, et al. Hereditary sensory neuropathy with spastic paraplegia. Brain 1979;102:79–84

50. Stewart RM, Tunell G, Ehle A. Familial spastic paraplegia, peroneal neuropathy, and crural hypopigmentation: a new neurocutaneous syndrome. Neurology 1981;31:754–757

51. Vazza GZM, Boaretto F, Micaglio GF, et al. A new locus for autosomal recessive spastic paraplegia associated with mental retardation and distal motor neuropathy SPG14, maps to chromosome 3q27-q28. Am J Hum Genet 2000;67:504–509

52. Serena M, Rizzuto N, Moretto G, Arrigoni G. Familial spastic paraplegia with peroneal amyotrophy. A family with hypersensitivity to pyrexia. Ital J Neurol Sci 1989;11:583–588

53. Neuhauser G, Wiffler C, Opitz JM. Familial spastic paraplegia with distal muscle wasting in the Old Order Amish; atypical Troyer syndrome or "new" syndrome. Clin Genet 1976;9:315–323

54. Mcleod JG, Morgan JA, Reye C. Electrophysiological studies in familial spastic paraplegia. Neurol Neurosurg Psychiatry 1993;40:611–615

55. Owens LA, Peterson CR. Familial spastic paraplegia: a clinical and electrodiagnostic evaluation. Arch Phys Med Rehabil 1982;63:357–361

56. Dimitrijevic MR, Lenman JAR, Prevec T, Wheatly K. A study of posterior column function in familial spastic paraplegia. J Neurol Neurosurg Psych 1982;45:46–49

57. Schady W, Scheard A. A qualitative study of sensory functions in hereditary spastic paraplegia. Brain 1990;113:709–720

58. Schady W, Smith DI. Sensory neuropathy in hereditary spastic paraplegia. J Neurol Neurosurg Psychiatr 1994;57:693–698

59. Pelosi L, Lanzillo B, Perretti A. Motor and somatosensory evoked potentials in hereditary spastic paraplegia. J Neurol Neurosurg Psychiatry 1991;54:1099–1102

60. Pedersen L, Trojaborg W. Visual, auditory and somatosensory pathway involvement in hereditary cerebellar ataxia, Friedreich's ataxia and familial spastic paraplegia. Electroencephalogr Clin Neurophys 1981;52:283–297

61. Uncini A, Treviso M, Basciani M, Gambi D. Strumpell's familial spastic paraplegia: an electrophysiological demonstration of selective central distal axonopathy. Electroencephalogr Clin Neurophys 1987; 66:132–136

62. Battistella PA, Suppiej A, Mandara V. Evoked potentials in familial spastic paraplegia: description of three brothers and review of the literature. Giorn Neuropsi Evol 1997;17:201–212

63. Claus D, Waddy HM, Harding AE. Hereditary motor and sensory neuropathies and hereditary spastic paraplegia: a magnetic stimulation study. Ann Neurol 1990;28:43–49

64. Claus D, Jaspert A. Central motor conduction in hereditary spastic paraparesis (Strumpell's disease) and tropical spastic paraparesis. Neurol Croatica 1995; 44:23–31

65. Schady W, Dick JP, Sheard A, Crampton S. Central motor conduction studies in hereditary spastic paraplegia. J Neurol Neurosurg Psychiatry 1991;54:775–779

66. Cambi F, Tartaglino L, Lublin FD, McCarren D. X-linked pure familial spastic paraparesis: characterization of a large kindred with magnetic resonance imaging studies. Arch Neurol 1995;52:665–669

67. Durr A, Brice A, Serdaru M, et al. The phenotype of "pure" autosomal dominant spastic paraplegia. Neurology 1994;44:1274–1277

68. Krabbe K, Nielsen JE, Fallentin E, et al. MRI of autosomal dominant pure spastic paraplegia. Neuroradiology 1997;39:724–727

69. Fink JK. Hereditary spastic paraplegia. Emery and Rimoin's Principles and Practice of Medical Genetics, fourth edition. In: Rimoin DL, Pyeritz RE, Connor JM, Korf BR, eds. London: Churchill Livingston, 2001: 3124–3145

70. O'Neill BP, Swanson JW, Brown IFR, Griffin JW, Moser HW. Familial spastic paraparesis: an adrenoleukodystrophy phenotype? Neurology 1985;35: 1233–1235

71. Maris T, Androulidakis EJ, Tzagournissakis M, et al. X-linked adrenoleukodystrophy presenting as neurologically pure familial spastic paraparesis. Neurology 1994;45:1101–1104

72. Gudesblatt M, Moser H, Plaitakis A. Dominantly inherited familial spastic paraplegia through three generations as a manifestation due to adrenoleukodystrophy. Neurology 1995;45:A440 (Abstract)

73. Schols L, Amoiridis G, Epplen JT, et al. Relations between genotype and phenotype in German patients with the Machado-Joseph disease mutation. J Neurol Neurosurg Psychiat 1996;61:466–470

74. Matsumura R, Takayanagi T, Fujimoto Y, et al. The relationship between trinucleotide repeat length and phenotypic variation in Machado-Joseph disease. J Neurol Sci 1996;139:52–57

75. Rabin BA, Griffin JW, Crain BJ, et al. Autosomal dominant juvenile amyotrophic lateral sclerosis. Brain 1999;122:1539–1550

76. Fisher CM. Pure spastic paralysis of corticospinal origin. Can J Neurol Sci 1977;4:251–258

77. Younger DS, Chou SC, Hays AP, et al. Primary lateral sclerosis: a clinical diagnosis reemerges. Arch Neurol 1988;45:1304–1307

78. Nygaard TG. Dopa-responsive dystonia: clinical, pathological, and genetic distinction from juvenile parkinsonism. In: Segawa M, Nomura Y, eds. Age-related dopamine-dependent disorders. Monogr Neural Sci. Vol 14. 1st ed. Basel: Karger, 1995:109–119

79. Fink JK, Barton N, Cohen W, et al. Dystonia with marked diurnal variation associated with biopterin deficiency. Neurology 1988;38:707–711

80. Salazar-Grueso EF, Roos RP, Wollmann R, et al. HTLV-I infection associated with a familial spastic paraparesis syndrome. Ann Neurol 1989;26:152 (Abstract)

81. Araki S, Mochizuki M, Yamaguchi K, et al. Familial clustering of human T lymphotropic virus type 1 uveitis. British Journal of Ophthalmology 1993;77: 747–748

82. Renjifo B, Osterman J, Borrero I, Essex M. Nucleotide sequences of human T-lymphotropic virus type I (HTLV-I) from a family cluster with tropical spastic paraparesis/HTLV-I-associated myelopathy. Res Virol 1994;146:93–99

83. Cartier L, Ramirez E, Galeno H. Familial form of tropical spastic paraparesis. Report of four families. Rev Med Chile 1998;126:419–426

84. Chance PF, Pleasure D. Charcot-Marie-Tooth syndrome. Arch Neurol 1993;50:1180–1184

85. Fonknecten J, Mavel D, Byrne P, et al. Spectrum of SPG4 mutations in autosomal dominant spastic paraplegia. Hum Mol Genet 2000;9:637–644

86. Durr A, Davoine C-S, Paternotte C, et al. Phenotype of autosomal dominant spastic paraplegia linked to chromosome 2. Brain 1996;119:1487–1496

87. Hentati A, Pericak-Vance MA, Lennon F, et al. Linkage of the late onset autosomal dominant familial spastic paraplegia to chromosome 2p markers. Hum Molec Genet 1994;3:1867–1871

88. Hazan J, Fonknechten N, Mavel D, et al. Spastin, a new AAA protein, is altered in the most frequent form of autosomal dominant spastic paraplegia. Nat Genet 1999;23:296–303

89. Zhao X, Alvarado D, Rainer S, et al. Mutations in a novel GTPase cause autosomal dominant hereditary spastic paraplegia. Am J Hum Genet 2001;69:195

90. Alvarado DM, Ming L, Hedera P, et al. Atlastin gene analysis in early onset hereditary spastic paraplegia. Am J Hum Genet 2001;69:597 (Abstract)

91. Lindsey JC, Lusher ME, McDermott CJ, et al. Mutation analysis of the spastin gene (SPG4) in patients with hereditary spastic paraparesis. J Med Genet 2000; 37:759–765

92. White KD, Ince PG, Lusher M, et al. Clinical and pathologic findings in hereditary spastic paraparesis with spastin mutation. Neurology 2000;55:89–94

93. Santorelli FM, Patrono C, Fortini D, et al. Intrafamilial variability in hereditary spastic paraplegia associated with an SPG4 gene mutation. Neurology 2000;55: 702–705

94. Svenson IK, Ashley-Koch AE, Gaskell PC, et al. Mutation analysis of the spastin gene in hereditary spastic paraplegia type 4—evidence of aberrant transcript splicing caused by mutations in concanionical splice site sequences. Am J Hum Genet 2000;67(Suppl 2):375

95. Martinez-Murillo F, Choudhn A, Devaney J, et al. Genotype/phenotype correlations in 60 spastic paraparesis families. Am J Hum Genet 2000;67(Suppl 2):351 (Abstract)

96. Burger JJ, Fonknechten N, Hoeltzenbein M, et al. Hereditary spastic paraplegia caused by mutations in the SPG4 gene. Am J Hum 2000;67:372 (Abstract)

97. Martinez-Murillo FM, Kobayashi H, Pegoraro E, et al. Genetic localization of a new locus for recessive familial spastic paraparesis to 15q13-15. Neurology 1999;53: 50–56

98. DeMichele G, DeFusco M, Cavalcanti F, et al. A new locus for autosomal recessive hereditary spastic paraplegia maps to chromosome 16q24.3. Am J Hum Genet 1998;63:135–139

99. Casari G, Fusco M, Ciarmatori S, et al. Spastic paraplegia and OXPHOS impairment caused by mutations in paraplegin, a nuclear-encoded mitochondrial metalloprotease. Cell 1998;93:973–983

100. Settasatian C, Whitmore SA, Crawford J, et al. Genomic structure and expression analysis of the spastic paraplegia gene, SPG7. Hum Genet 2000;105: 139–144

101. Zelnik N, Leshinsky E., Kolodny EH. Familial spastic paraparesis. Is it mitochondrial disorder? Pediatric Neurosurgery 1995;23:225–226

102. Nance MA, Raabe WA, Midani H, et al. Clinical heterogeneity of familial spastic paraplegia linked to chromosome 2p21. Hum Hered 1998;48:169–178

103. Hedera P, DiMauro S, Bonilla E, et al. Phenotypic analysis of autosomal dominant hereditary spastic paraplegia linked to chromosome 8q. Neurology 1999; 53:44–50

104. Hedera P, DiMauro S, Bonilla E, et al. Mitochondrial analysis in autosomal dominant hereditary spastic paraplegia. Neurology 2000;55:1591–1592

105. Willard HF, Riordan JR. Assignment of the gene for myelin proteolipid protein to the X chromosome: implications for X-linked myelin disorders. Science 1985;230:940–942

106. Hodes ME, Zimmerman AW, Aydanian A, et al. Different mutations in the same codon of the proteolipid protein gene, PLP, may help in correlating genotype with phenotype in Pelizaeus-Merzbacher disease/X-linked spastic paraplegia (PMD/SPG2). Am J Med Genet 1999;82:132–139

107. Woodward K, Kendall E, Vetrie D, Malcolm S. Pelizaeus-Merzbacher disease: identification of Xq22 proteolipid-protein duplications and characterization of breakpoints by interphase FISH. Am J Hum Genet 1998;63:207–217

108. Hentati A. Contribution á l'étude des paraplegies spasmodiques et familiales pures (Strumpell-Lorrain) et associ'ed en Tunisie. Thesis for doctorate in Medicine. Faculté de Medicine de sfax (Tunisia) 1989

109. Jouet M, Rosenthal A, Armstrong G, et al. X-linked spastic paraplegia (SPG1), MASA syndrome and X-linked hydrocephalus result from mutations in the L1 gene. Nat Genet 1994;7:402–407

110. Fryns JP, Spaepen A, Cassiman J-J, van den Boorn N. X-linked complicated spastic paraplegia, MASA syndrome, and X-linked hydrocephaly due to congenital stenosis of the aqueduct of Sylvius: a variable expression of the same mutation at Xq28. J Med Genet 1991;28:429–431

111. Fransen E, Lemmon V, Van Camp G, et al. Crash syndrome: clinical spectrum of corpus callosum hypoplasia, retardation, adducted thumbs, spastic paraparesis and hydrocephalus due to mutations in one single gene, L1. Eur J Human Genet 1995;3:273–284

112. Dan B, Bouillot E, Bengoetxea A, Cheron G. Effect of intrathecal baclofen on gait control in human hereditary spastic paraparesis. Neuro Lett 2000;280:176–178

113. Meythaler JM, Steers WD, Tuel SM, et al. Intrathecal Baclofen in hereditary spastic paraparesis. Arc Phys Med Rehabil 1992;73:794–797

XIV Neurobehavioral Disorders: Cognitive Rehabilitation Behavioral Management and Pharmacologic Therapies

Section editor: Kenneth M Heilman

Treatment of Disorders of Cognition: An Introduction

Kenneth M Heilman and Leslie J Gonzalez Rothi

In this section, we discuss the treatment of disorders of cognition, which we define as the abilities to attend, perceive, and comprehend information; to manipulate, integrate, and maintain information; to intend to act or communicate; and to act or communicate. Although motor disorders such as weakness or ataxia may be considered neurobehavioral disorders and are the subject of treatment research, this section is concerned with treatments of disorders of higher forms of behavior we refer to as "cognition," as defined above. Specifically, we focus on the rehabilitation of aphasia, attentional, conative (intentional), memory, and emotional disorders. Although many people think of cognitive rehabilitation as exclusively behavioral therapies, we use the term more broadly to include any intervention designed to alleviate the functional effect of disorders of cognition. Thus, we discuss not only behavioral therapies/environmental enrichments but also somatic and physiological interventions such a pharmacotherapy.

Overall, the goal of cognitive rehabilitation is to promote maximal adaptive functioning in patients with neurobehavioral disorders. Many neurologists believe that other than treating a patient's underlying disease little can be done to rehabilitate cognitive-behavioral disorders. This pessimistic assumption is incorrect. It is the rare patient who cannot be helped. However, successful treatment of neurobehavioral disorders must involve a team of skilled clinicians from various professions, including neurologists, neuropsychiatrists, physiatrists, speech pathologists, occupational therapists, neuropsychologists, and educators, among others.

Relevance

Motor and sensory disorders can produce disabilities; however, many of the most disabling disorders are cognitive. Almost any disease that affects the central nervous system, including trauma, vascular-stroke, degenerative metabolic, deficiency states, infections, autoimmune, and tumor-neoplastic diseases, can cause neurobehavioral cognitive disorders. Perhaps the three most common causes of cognitive dysfunction are traumatic brain injury (more than 600 new cases per 100 000 persons annually),[1] stroke (300 to 500 new cases per 100 000 persons cases annually),[2] and degenerative dementia (more than 300 new cases per 100 000 persons annually).[3] Generally, patients with neurobehavioral or cognitive deficits require more restrictive living environments (that are also

more costly) than do other types of chronically ill neurological patients. For example, after rehabilitation for acute stroke, 82% of patients are able to walk independently, whereas only 58% are able to regain the ability to independently perform activities of daily living.[4] Cognitive disorders have been shown to be more enduring[5] and, most importantly, to have a greater negative effect on quality of life than all other forms of residual dysfunction resulting from neurological causes.[6,7]

After almost any form of brain injury, some spontaneous recovery may occur; however, many are skeptical that neurobehavioral treatments can be effective in providing a significant functional effect. This nihilism finds its beginnings in antiquity, but more recently, it can be traced to the work of Ramón y Cajal, who at the turn of the 20th century proposed the notion that the mature brain is unable to change—that its structure is immutable and, thus, cannot recover from injury or damage, especially not in response to treatment.[8] However, more recently, pessimism has been replaced by optimism, best displayed by work in basic neuroscience of cortical regeneration in chronic injury, such as that reported by Kilgard and Merzenich.[9] Specifically, it would appear that the cerebrum is capable of considerable plasticity—not only in normal structures (new learning in maturity) but also in the recovery from injury (functional recovery resulting from changes of neural structures). We hope that in the brief chapters that follow this introduction we will provide evidence that many effective therapies are available. We also hope to instill an optimism about the potential of emerging therapies.

Therapy goals

Neurobehavioral treatments may have one of several non-exclusive goals, including restitution, substitution, and compensation (also called "behavioral substitution"). Many of the treatments discussed in the following chapters have one or more of these processes as their goal. Each is defined briefly below.

Restitution

"Restitution" is defined as a recovery of the dysfunctional neural system that mediates certain behaviors in a manner that mimics its original format. Many behaviors are mediated by anatomically distributed networks, and, in the presence of damaged neurons, undamaged portions of networks may also become capable of mediating the lost behavior. That is, in almost all forms of brain injury not all the neurons that support a cognitive activity are damaged. Although some cells in the core of the lesion may be dead, there is often a "penumbra" of cells that may be dysfunctional but living. Many functional brain imaging studies suggest that often with the recovery of function, the penumbra mediates the recovered behavior.[10]

"Diaschisis" is a term used to describe the loss of function in neuronal systems that are remote from a lesion site.[11] It is usually thought to be a transient phenomenon, but the physiological down regulation may be chronic and the restitution of function may occur only when diaschisis ends. Without afferent input, neurons remote from the lesion may eventually die. This process is called "trans-synaptic degeneration."[12] Restitutive strategies may help reverse diaschisis and prevent trans-synaptic degeneration.

Injury to the nervous system may not kill all the cells in the region but rather injure the axons of some cells that mediate a behavior. Synaptogenesis, including axonal regeneration and collateral sprouting, may be important for recovery. However, synaptogenesis may result in aberrant connections that have negative functional consequences.[13] Restitutive therapies may have the potential to encourage synaptogenesis and to prevent aberrant connections.

Neurons in the nervous systems communicate with other neurons by releasing neurotransmitters. With cell injury or death, there may be a decrease in critical neurotransmitter levels. However, the cells that have receptors for these neurotransmitters may undergo up-regulation, referred to as "dennervation supersensitivity," thereby allowing a neuronal system to again mediate a cognitive activity. When up-regulation is inadequate, pharmacotherapy may offer the boost needed for these damaged system to regain functions.

Substitution

In contrast to restitutive processes of recovery, other undamaged portions of the brain not premorbidly involved in a function possibly may assume the lost function ("vicariation"). Such include (1) homologous cytoarchitectonic areas in the opposite hemisphere (for example when the left posterior temporal lobe is damaged and speech comprehension is lost, the right temporal lobe may assume this function),[14] (2) subcortical portions of the visual system analyze visual stimuli, such as emotional facial expressions, that prior to injury were analyzed by the calcarine cortex,[15] or (3) unrelated cytoarchitectonic areas in the same or opposite hemisphere.

Some neurotransmitters or neuromodulators such as acetylcholine possibly may enhance plasticity, and when these are given together with behavioral therapy, uninjured portions of the brain may be able to learn to mediate behaviors that were lost with brain injury.[16]

Compensation

"Compensation" is defined as using an alternative behavioral strategy to perform a lost function. With this treatment, the patient is encouraged to use behavioral strategies that can be mediated by intact portions of the brain rather than using strategies that were mediated by the parts of the brain that are dysfunctional. One of many examples of this is having a patient unable to tell the time using a digital clock instead of an analog clock with hands. Other examples include memory books for patients with various forms of amnesia, alarm clocks for patients with executive function deficits, and computerized communication systems for aphasia.

Conclusions

In the chapters that follow, various neurocognitive disorders and their treatments are discussed. There is now clear evidence that neurocognitive therapies work;[17,18] however, this is still an infant science, with much growth anticipated. Although we attempt to describe the most current therapies for various cognitive disorders, our hope is that these chapters will rapidly become obsolete because of the development of new and effective treatments.

References

1. Levin HS, Benton AL, Grossman RG, et al. Neurobehavioural consequences of closed head injury. New York: Oxford University Press, 1982
2. Sudlow CL, Warlow CP. Comparing stroke incidence worldwide. What makes studies comparable. Stroke 1996;27:550–558
3. Bachman DL, Wolf PA, Linn RT, et al. Incidence of dementia and probable Alzhiemer's disease in a general population: the Framingham study. Neurology 1993;43:515–519
4. Herman B. Tilburg epidemiological study of stroke: TESS. Tilburg: Dutch Heart Foundation, 1981
5. Gresham GE, Phillips TF, Wolf PA, et al. Epidemiological profile of long-term stroke disability: the Framingham study. Archives of Physical Medicine and Rehabilitation 1979;60:487–491
6. Ponsford JL, Olver JH, Curran C. A profile of outcome, two years after traumatic brain injury. Brain Injury 1995;9:1–10
7. Ponsford JL, Olver JH, Curran C, Ng K. Prediction of employment status, two years after traumatic brain injury. Brain Injury 1995;9:11–20
8. Cajal RY. Degeneration and regeneration of the nervous system. Oxford UK: Oxford University Press, 1928
9. Kilgard MP, Merzenich MM. Cortical map reorganization enabled by nuclkeus basalis activity. Science 1998;279:1714–1718
10. Warburton E, Price CJ, Swinburn K, Wise RJ. Mechanisms of recovery from aphasia: evidence from positron emission tomography studies. Journal of Neurology, Neurosurgery and Psychiatry 1999;66:155–161
11. Monakow CV. Die lokalisation im grosshirn. Wiesbaden, Germany: Bergmann, 1914
12. Chang CW. Evident trans-synaptic degeneration of motor neurons after spinal cord injury: a study of neuromuscular jitter by axonal microstimulation. American Journal of Physical Medicine Rehabilitation 1998;77:118–121
13. Finger S, Almli CR. Brain damage and neuroplasticity: mechanisms of recovery or development? Brain Research 1985;357:177–186

14. Musso M, Weiller C, Kiebel S, et al. Training-induced brain plasticity in aphasia. Brain 1999;122:1781–1790
15. De-Gelder B, Vroomen J, Pourtois G, Weiskrantz L. Non-conscious recognition of affect in the absence of striate cortex. NeuroReport 1999;10:3759–3763
16. Hughes JD, Jacobs DH, Heilman KM. Neuropharmacology and linguistic neuroplasticity. Brain and Language 2000;279:1714–1718
17. Malec JF, Basford JS. Post-acute brain injury rehabilitation. Archives of Physical Medicine and Rehabilitation 1996;77:198–207
18. Robey RR. A meta-analysis of clinical outcomes in the treatment of aphasia. Journal of Speech and Hearing Research 1998;41:172–187

259 Aphasia

Anastasia M Raymer and Lynn M Maher

Aphasia is an impairment of comprehension and production of verbal language caused by acquired brain damage.[1] The language disturbance may affect grammatical (word order and word endings), lexical (words), semantic (meaning), and phonological (sounds) aspects of language. Alexia and agraphia often co-occur with aphasia as reading and writing functions draw upon some of the same symbolic language mechanisms used in spoken language. Neurological disorders such as stroke, trauma, tumor, and degenerative conditions that damage left cortical and subcortical regions may cause aphasia. Thereby, it is difficult to estimate the incidence and prevalence of aphasia. In stroke alone, 30% of patients develop aphasia, leading to 80 000 new cases of aphasia each year.[2] Considering all etiologies, there are as many as one million Americans currently living with aphasia.[3]

The study of aphasia has a rich history.[1,4] Broca in the 1860s is usually credited with recognizing that loss of spoken language is associated with lesions of the left inferior frontal cortex, though Dax may have written similar ideas in the 1830s. Later in the 1800s, Wernicke and Lichtheim expanded notions about language loss and developed a model in which "centers" for different auditory, motor, and conceptual aspects of language processing are localized and interconnected in the left hemisphere (Figure 259.1). On the basis of their model, they distinguished different forms that aphasia may take. For a lengthy period of the 20th century, the localizationist approach was superceded by the writings of Jackson, Freud and their contemporaries who espoused a holistic view of language and aphasia. However, a resurgence of interest in the localizationist approach occurred in the 1960s with the influential writings of Norman Geschwind,[5] who proposed a connectionist account for a variety of cognitive disorders, including aphasia.

Modern psycholinguistic studies in normal and brain impaired individuals have led to more elaborated language processing models (Figure 259.2).[6,7] An array of interactive mechanisms allows for comprehension and production of phonologic, semantic, and grammatical aspects of words and sentences. As understanding of the language system has advanced, so too has our characterization of the aphasia syndromes.

Aphasia syndromes

The classification of aphasia, following the Wernicke-Lichtheim scheme, considers four areas of language functioning: auditory comprehension, repetition, fluency of verbal expression, and confrontation naming (Table 259.1). Aphasia syndromes vary in relation to the regions of the left hemisphere that are damaged. In general, lesions affecting pre-Rolandic regions lead to non-fluent aphasias, and lesions

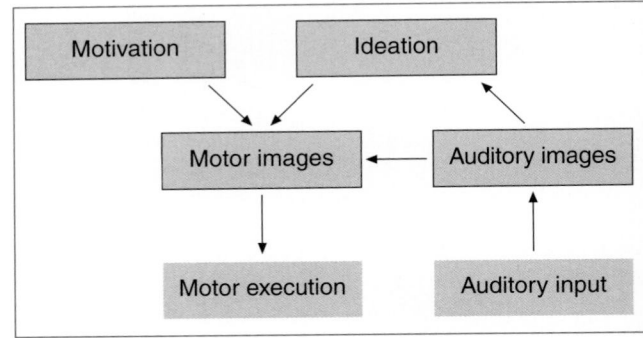

Figure 259.1 Wernicke-Lichtheim Language Model.[1,7]

Table 259.1 Aphasia syndromes

Aphasia syndrome	Fluency	Auditory comprehension	Repetition	Naming
Broca's	Non-fluent	+	−	−
Transcortical motor	Non-fluent	+	+	−/+
Global	Non-fluent	−	−	−
Mixed transcortical	Non-fluent	−	+	−
Wernicke's	Fluent	−	−	−
Transcortical Sensory	Fluent	−	+	−/+
Conduction	Fluent	+	−	−
Anomic	Fluent	+	+	−

+ Relatively intact; − significantly impaired.

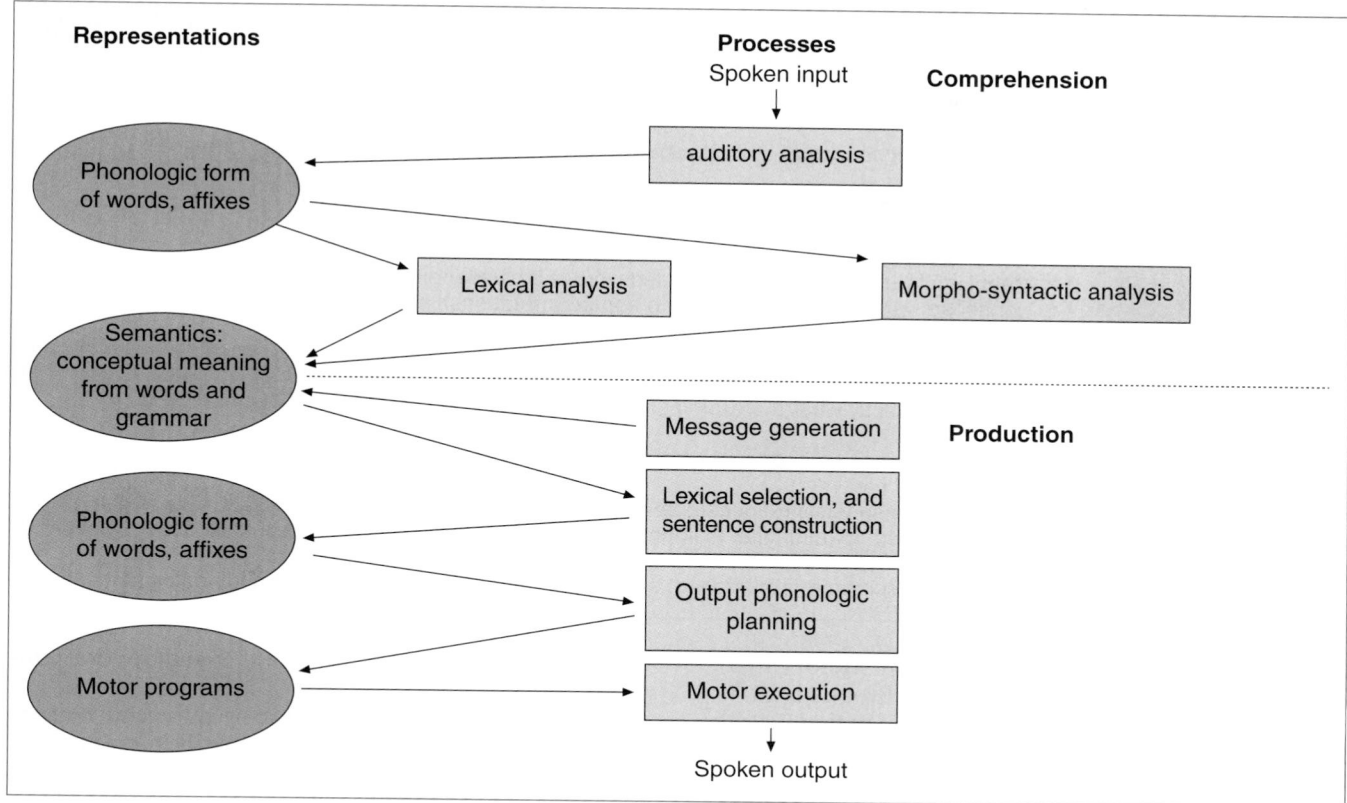

Figure 259.2   Language model (after Caplan[6]).

involving post-Rolandic structures lead to fluent aphasias. At least five different aspects of verbal expression contribute to the clinical impression of verbal fluency (Table 259.2).[8] A serious disturbance of any one or more of these domains may render the clinical impression of non-fluent verbal output. Anomia or word retrieval difficulty, often assessed in picture confrontation naming tasks, is typically apparent in all aphasia syndromes. In some individuals, anomia preferentially affects words from selective grammatical (e.g., nouns, verbs) or semantic categories (e.g., fruits, vegetables, animals, proper names).[9] Word retrieval errors vary across syndromes (Table 259.3). Some errors resemble the intended word in meaning or sound, whereas others have no apparent relationship.

Table 259.2	**Dimensions contributing to non-fluent verbal output[8]**
Amount/sentence length	≤4 words/utterance; <100 words/minute
Grammar	Omission of grammatical words and word endings
Prosody	Flattened contours
Articulation	Struggle initiating, sequencing articulatory movements
Initiation/elaboration	Lack spontaneous utterances; concise verbal responses

Non-fluent aphasias

In *Broca's aphasia* verbal expression and repetition are non-fluent and *agrammatic* as these individuals omit grammatical words (e.g., auxiliaries, articles) and word endings (e.g., plurals, verb tense). They speak *telegraphically*, using mostly nouns and verbs. Prosody may be flattened and difficulty initiating and sequencing articulatory movements for speech, sometimes referred to as *apraxia of speech*, may be present.[10] Individuals with Broca's aphasia may have *asyntactic* auditory comprehension leading to difficulty understanding the grammar or word order of sentences. Word retrieval difficulties particularly affect verbs[11–13] and semantic paraphasias may be noted. Deep dyslexia and deep dysgraphia may be evident in reading and writing. Acutely, Broca's aphasia may be associated with a large left frontal lesion, encompassing Broca's area and the surrounding frontal, opercular, and deep subcortical regions.[14–16] Chronically, Broca's aphasia may be seen as patients recover from large left hemisphere lesions.[15]

In *transcortical motor aphasia* (TCMA), verbal expression is non-fluent due to reduced amount of output, lack of initiation, and poorly elaborated verbal output.[17] Repetition abilities are preserved, sometimes leading to *echolalia*. Whereas picture naming may be normal, some may demonstrate perseverations in naming.[1] Auditory comprehension is relatively intact. Transcortical motor aphasia has been described acutely with left hemisphere lesions of the

Table 259.3   Terms for verbal production errors

Error type	Description
Semantic paraphasia (also verbal)	Words bearing meaningful relationship to target, e.g., apple: "fruit," "pie," "orange"
Phonemic paraphasia (also literal)	Phonologically similar words or non words, e.g., table: "pable," "stable"
Unrelated word	Words bearing no apparent relationship to target, e.g., car: "computer"
Circumlocution	Meaningful description of the intended word, e.g., baseball: "you throw it and hit it with a bat"
Neologism	Nonsense word or phrase bearing no apparent relationship to target, e.g., robot: "but key," "miss mosey"
Perseveration	Repeated aberrant response, e.g., oven: "barrel"; shirt: "barrel"
No response	Failure to give any response, e.g., pie: "I don't know"
Echolalia	Mimicking exactly what the examiner says, e.g., What do you call this?: "What do you call this?"
Automatisms	Verbal responses limited to common phrases or expletives, e.g., "That one here, I guess." "Shucks, I can't."
Stereotypies	Recurrent nonsensical response; perhaps with retained prosody, e.g., "Wada wada wada?"
Agrammatism	Utterances with grammatical elements omitted, e.g., The boy is eating cookies: "boy . . . eat . . . cookie"
Logorrhea	Press of speech, normally intoned, sometimes disrupted by paraphasias and neologisms

mesial frontal cortex (supplementary motor area), dorsolateral frontal cortex superior to Broca's area, or the thalamus.[16,18–20] Chronically, some patients with Broca's aphasia recover sufficient repetition abilities to be considered a TCMA.[15,21]

In *global aphasia*, patients are severely non-fluent, with verbal output limited to *automatisms* and *stereotypies*, which at times convey meaningful prosodic information.[8] Repetition, word retrieval and auditory comprehension are severely impaired. Patients may only respond to personal questions, midline commands, and prosodic aspects of utterances.[22] Global aphasia is associated with extensive left pre- and post-Rolandic damage.[14,15] Better recovery of auditory comprehension and verbal fluency is seen when lesions spare portions of Wernicke's area[23] and periventricular white matter,[24] respectively.

Mixed transcortical aphasia is the counterpart to global aphasia in which repetition is relatively spared. Echolalia may be evident in the verbal responses of these individuals. This infrequent syndrome occurs with damage to cortical watershed regions or multiple lesions that preserve left perisylvian cortex.[17]

Fluent aphasias

Wernicke's aphasia is characterized by fluent verbal expression in which there is an excessive press of speech or *logorrhea*. Spontaneous language, repetition, and naming are disrupted by numerous semantic, phonemic, and unrelated paraphasias and *neologisms* (Table 259.3), sometimes leading to *jargon aphasia*. Auditory comprehension is typically severely undermined. However, some patients have fairly preserved auditory comprehension and seem *anosognosic* or unaware of their nonsensical verbal output.[25,26] Whereas reading and auditory comprehension disturbances are typically commensurate, some individuals may demonstrate preserved reading comprehension.[27] Wernicke's aphasia is associated with lesions

affecting the posterior portion of the left superior temporal gyrus.[14–16]

Transcortical sensory aphasia (TSA) is the counterpart to Wernicke's aphasia in which repetition is spared.[17] Verbal expression is fluent and marked by numerous semantic and phonemic paraphasias and *circumlocutions* (Table 259.3). Naming, though typically impaired, may be spared in some individuals.[28,29] Oral reading may also be remarkably preserved.[30] Lesions affect the left angular gyrus,[31,32] thus TSA may be associated with Gerstmann syndrome.[17] Transcortical sensory aphasia may also be a manifestation of degenerative diseases affecting posterior cortex.[33,34]

Individuals with *conduction aphasia* have inordinate difficulty with repetition in relation to other language abilities.[35] In "repetition" conduction aphasia, selective repetition difficulty appears related to a verbal short term memory deficit.[36] In "reproduction" conduction aphasia, repetition difficulty occurs in conjunction with phonemic paraphasias in word production tasks. Patients exhibit *conduit d'approche*, successive attempts to self-correct their mispronunciations. As in Broca's aphasia, individuals with conduction aphasia may display asyntactic comprehension.[37,38] Phonologic dyslexia and dysgraphia may also be present. The lesion associated with conduction aphasia is in the region of the supramarginal gyrus, insula, and underlying white matter.[15,39]

Anomic aphasia is observed in individuals with fluent verbal output and intact repetition and comprehension.[40] Anomia is the selective symptom in anomic aphasia, in contrast to the anomia that is a symptom seen in most other aphasia syndromes. Nouns may be more affected than verbs.[13] Errors in conversation or picture naming may include circumlocutions, semantic paraphasias, or no response. While rare, anomic aphasia may occur acutely with lesions in the left temporo-occipital junction or thalamus.[41–43] More often anomic aphasia is observed chronically as

Table 259.4   Standardized aphasia assessment procedures

General aphasia batteries	Aphasia Diagnostic Profiles (ADP)[47]
	Boston Assessment of Severe Aphasia (BASA)[48]
	Boston Diagnostic Aphasia Examination (BDAE)[8]
	Examining for Aphasia[49]
	Multilingual Aphasia Examination[50]
	Porch Index of Communicative Ability (PICA)[51]
	Psycholinguistic Assessments of Language Processing in Aphasia (PALPA)[45]
	Western Aphasia Battery (WAB)[52]
Tests for specific language domains	Boston Naming Test[53]
	Action Naming Test[54]
	Object and Action Naming Battery[55]
	Peabody Picture Vocabulary Test (PPVT)[56]
	Revised Token Test[57]
	Auditory Comprehension Test for Sentences[58]
	Controlled Oral Word Association Test[59]
	Quantitative Production Analysis[60]
	Reading Comprehension Battery for Aphasia[61]
Functional aphasia tests	Communicative Activities of Daily Living (CADL-2)[62]
	Functional Assessment of Communication Skills for Adults (ASHA-FACS)[63]
	Communicative Effectiveness Index (CETI)[64]

patients recover from other aphasia syndromes.[15] Anomic aphasia also may be evident in early stages of language deterioration in degenerative diseases.[33]

Aphasia assessment and prognosis

A number of standardized aphasia tests have been developed for clinical use to identify patterns of language symptoms (Table 259.4). General aphasia assessment batteries include subtests that assess the domains of fluency, repetition, auditory comprehension and naming. Aphasia batteries assist clinicians in proposing a differential diagnosis of aphasia syndrome and/or a statement of the overall severity of impairment. Other supplemental tests allow assessment of specific domains of language (e.g., naming, auditory comprehension, reading), or types of impairment (e.g., severe aphasia). A recently developed test allows clinicians to characterize lexical, semantic, and syntactic impairments with respect to the cognitive model in Figure 259.2.[45] Finally, in keeping with the World Health Organization classification of consequences of diseases,[46] some *functional* aphasia tests assess the overall communication disability posed by the language impairments.

The clinician analyzes test results to develop an appropriate plan for management of the consequences of the aphasia in keeping with the prognosis for recovery.[1] Although aphasia is likely to persist, some recovery is likely. In general, a positive prognosis may be anticipated when the aphasia results from a recovering neurological disease, is in the first 6–12 months of recovery, and results from a lesion that is smaller, spares subcortical white matter, and is unilateral. Psychosocial factors such as age, gender, premorbid abilities, handedness, emotional state, and family support contribute to aphasia recovery but have a less potent impact. For most individuals, treat-ment may be beneficial for helping them to improve their language and communication abilities.[3,65]

Aphasia treatment

Efficacy of aphasia treatment

Aphasia treatment research is a challenging endeavor.[66] First, the assumption of group homogeneity is greatly undermined in this condition as aphasia comprises a number of heterogeneous syndromes. What may work in treatment of one form of aphasia or one individual with aphasia may not be effective for another. Second, it is difficult to complete a well-designed study of aphasia treatment. An ethical paradox occurs in aphasia treatment research when researchers attempt to randomize subjects and withhold treatment from a no-treatment control group. A number of subject selection characteristics must be controlled. Treatment needs to be specifically described and administered for a sufficient period of time. Despite these challenges, a number of studies have addressed the question of aphasia treatment efficacy.

Holland and colleagues[67] reviewed more than 200 English studies of aphasia treatment, 20 of which were group studies of more than 60 subjects with aphasia. In considering classes of experimental evidence delineated by the American Academy of Neurology (AAN), only three studies met the Class I designation as randomized controlled trials, and two others were Class II randomized observational studies. All others were considered Class III evidence, typically due to lack of subject randomization. Holland and colleagues[67] concluded that findings of the large group studies suggest that the effects of aphasia treatment for individuals with a single hemisphere stroke significantly surpass the effects of spontaneous recovery alone, particularly if individuals receive three hours of treatment per week for at least five months.

Meta-analyses are Class I evidence for treatment efficacy that assess the aggregate results of multiple group treatment studies. In three different meta-analyses examining 45,[68] 21,[69] and 55[70] different aphasia treatment studies, the results uniformly support the contention that aphasia treatment provided by a speech-language pathologist leads to greater language improvements than spontaneous recovery alone. Effects vary as to time post onset, amount and type of treatment provided, and type and severity of aphasia.

The majority of aphasia treatment studies have implemented single subject experimental treatment designs (SSDs), which are designated Class III evidence. These time series designs are well-suited to address the heterogeneous factors involved in aphasia treatment.[71] Recent statistical advances have allowed for meta-analysis of treatment effect sizes reported in SSDs. In one recent meta-analysis,[72] researchers calculated one metric of effect size for 12 aphasia treatment SSDs. In a subsequent meta-analysis of 53 different aphasia treatment SSDs,[73] researchers compared seven different estimators of treatment effect size. Although most experimental subjects were in the chronic stages of aphasia, all estimators indicated large effects associated with a variety of aphasia treatments.

Meta-analyses of aphasia treatment research in SSDs and group studies consistently support the view that aphasia treatment has a medium to large effect on language recovery in comparison to spontaneous recovery alone. However, this conclusion relates to aphasia treatment in general, merging the effects of a variety of aphasia treatment methods. Future analyses must evaluate the effects of specific aphasia treatments targeting particular aspects of aphasia. For example, Melodic Intonation Therapy (MIT)[74] is a technique to improve verbal expression in patients with aphasia. However, a review by the Therapeutics and Technology Assessment Subcommittee of AAN[75] considered the results of MIT studies to be Class III evidence of treatment effectiveness. Because of variations in research methodology, MIT studies could not be included in the SSD meta-analyses.[72,73] New statistical techniques for meta-analysis may allow for better assessment of effectiveness of selected aphasia treatments, such as MIT, in future studies.

Aphasia treatment rationale

Although pharmacological interventions have been attempted to support aphasia recovery,[76] the primary emphasis in aphasia treatment is on behavioral methods to improve language and communication skills.[74,77,78] Behavioral methods chosen vary in relation to a number of medical, neurological, cognitive and psychosocial factors. Foremost is the patient's constellation of aphasic symptoms. Some methods focus on auditory comprehension skills and others on verbal expression, as the patient's pattern of impairment warrants. Within modalities, some methods

Table 259.5   Factors clinicians manipulate in auditory comprehension stimulation training

Number of choices in array
Relatedness of foil pictures (semantic, phonological, visual)
Length of input
Paralinguistic information (rate, pause, delay, stress, pitch)
Redundancy, multiple repetitions; alternative ways to state the same concept
Stimulus word factors:
    Familiarity and relevance
    Frequency
    Semantic category
    Manipulability
    Emotionality
    Concreteness

target single-word semantic and phonological processing, and others stress sentence-level grammatical skills.

A second crucial factor influencing the choice of aphasia treatment is the patient's physiological stage of recovery.[79] *Restitutive* treatments, which help patients to relearn or reactivate language in a means compatible with normal functioning, are likely to be most effective in initial stages of aphasia recovery up to six months post injury, and less effective as physiological processes of recovery are maximized. In contrast, *substitutive* approaches invoke alternative cognitive and neural systems to assist in the communication process, and are less wedded to time of recovery from aphasia. *Vicariative* approaches engage other systems (e.g., prosody, right hemisphere) to mediate aspects of language processing. This perspective is based on Luria's[80] notion of intersystemic reorganization, use of a different cognitive system to support an impaired system. *Compensatory* treatments promote the use of alternative means to communicate, substituting for impaired language skills.

Auditory comprehension treatments

Lexical processing   Restitutive treatment for lexical processing has its roots in the work of Schuell[81] who advocated systematic auditory stimulation to facilitate recovery from aphasia.[82] Training incorporates auditory-verbal tasks such as answering questions, and following commands. Clinicians systematically manipulate aspects of the auditory-verbal signal or conditions of the tasks to increase difficulty over time (Table 259.5). Auditory stimulation approaches were implemented in a number of group studies of aphasia therapy.[83,84] Recent studies of word comprehension treatments have used auditory tasks to target the phonological or semantic aspects of auditory processing in keeping with the stages involved in lexical processing.[85,86] Computerized training programs are useful for practice in auditory comprehension skills.[87,88] Substitutive methods to support or circumvent severe auditory comprehension impairments summon alternative sensory modalities such as visual

Table 259.6 Examples of types of sentences used on auditory comprehension training

Active-reversible	The boy is chasing the girl
Active-non reversible	The boy is chasing the ball
Negatives	The boy is not chasing the girl
Passive-reversible	The girl is chased by the boy
Passive-non reversible	The ball is chased by the boy
Subject-relative-reversible	The boy that is chasing the girl is crying
Object-relative-reversible	The boy that the girl is chasing is crying
Subject cleft-reversible	It is the boy that is chasing the girl
Object cleft-non reversible	It is the ball that the boy is chasing

processes (e.g., lip-reading,[89] reading[90]). Visual Action Therapy, a systematic program whose ultimate goal is to train patients to pantomime, may vicariatively improve auditory comprehension skills in some patients.[74]

Sentence comprehension Recognizing the complexity of the grammatical system, restitutive sentence comprehension treatments often incorporate a linguistic approach to sentence training.[91–94] In question and pointing tasks, patients practice comprehension given repetitions and feedback for sentences in which clinicians manipulate aspects of grammar such as type of sentence and reversibility of sentence ele-

ments (Table 259.6). Some studies have shown improvements in comprehension of sentence grammar following this type of treatment.[91–93] An alternative vicariative approach to sentence comprehension treatment is *mapping therapy* which incorporates the visual modality in training.[95,96] Patients are taught to translate from grammatical word order (e.g., subject noun, verb, object noun) to the semantic roles played by words (e.g., agent, action, object). Patients have difficulty understanding reversible sentences where there is no one-to-one relationship between word order and semantic roles (e.g., reversible passives). Patients read the written sentence and answer questions about the verb, agent, and action, underlining each with a different colored pen. Over time, some patients improve comprehension of sentence structures that they practice.[95,96]

Compensatory strategies for auditory comprehension impairments Patients and family members are often counseled to use simple strategies when auditory comprehension impairments disrupt communication (Table 259.7). The listener with aphasia uses strategies to indicate instances when misunderstanding occurs. Because of unreliability in the use of "yes-no" responses during conversation, it is often helpful to establish a non-verbal signal (e.g. thumbs up/down, point to happy/sad face) to indicate agreement or non-agreement. Speakers who talk to individuals with aphasia can use strategies to simplify verbal messages, increase redundancy of messages, and enhance messages with alternative, non-verbal information (e.g., gestures).

Table 259.7 Functional strategies to support auditory comprehension and verbal expression for an individual with aphasia

Strategies for the listener with aphasia	Signal when misunderstanding or missing part of the message Use nonverbal gesture to indicate agreement/disagreement (e.g., thumbs up/down, point to happy/sad face) Remind speaker to speak slower Ask speaker to repeat
When speaking to the individual with aphasia	Speak directly to the individual Use short sentences Use simple, directly stated grammar Speak at a slower rate by using pauses Maintain a natural prosody It is not necessary to speak louder Repeat sentences Talk about familiar topics Signal a change of topics Embellish messages with alternative communication channels (writing, drawing, gestures, facial expression)

When listening to the speaker with aphasia	Gently provide missing words or multiple-choice options
	Encourage circumlocution to get a message across
	Encourage use of alternative modes to communicate messages
	Reiterate messages; speaker can confirm messages were understood
	  as intended
	Encourage speaker to disregard errors that don't disrupt intent of
	  messages
	Write down concepts already communicated to refer to at a later time
	Write down ideas when breakdown occurs and return to them later

Table 259.8   Word retrieval treatments for patients with different levels of word retrieval difficulties

Severe word retrieval deficits	(e.g., global, Broca's, Wernicke's aphasia) Voluntary Control of Involuntary Utterances[74] Treatment of Aphasic Perseveration[74] Verbal + Gestural Reorganization[117–121]
Mild-to-moderate deficits	(e.g., Broca's, Transcortical sensory, Wernicke's, anomic aphasia) Semantic Comprehension Treatment[103,106] Semantic Features Treatment[99,105] Semantic Feature Matrix Training[102,104] Phonological Comprehension Treatment[107,109] Phonological Cueing Hierarchies[108] Verbal + Gestural Reorganization[117–121] Self-generated Cues during Reading and Writing [99,115,116]

Verbal production treatments

Word retrieval treatments   Many studies have been devoted to identifying techniques to remediate word retrieval impairments, a common symptom in aphasia.[97,98] Clinicians often use a "cueing hierarchy" approach in treatment. When a patient fails to name a picture, the clinician provides a series of cues that have more and more potent influence on word retrieval. Sentence completion (e.g., Take a drink of…), initial phoneme ("w"), written words, or rhyming word cues may help a person to retrieve a word. With practice over time, word retrieval skills may be facilitated or the individual may learn to self-cue.[99–101] A cueing hierarchy is an inherent part of an approach devised for patients who make many perseverations—treatment of aphasic perseveration (TAP).[74] The clinician manipulates the time interval between naming responses and provides systematic cues to elicit a correct response rather than a perseverative response.

Recent investigations have examined restitutive techniques influenced by models such as that in Figure 259.2 that delineate semantic and phonological stages required for word retrieval. A number of treatments that target semantic processing have resulted in improvements in picture naming in some patients with aphasia (Table 259.8). The common theme of semantic treatments is that, during picture naming exercises, the patient acts upon the meanings of target words, features of words such as function, visual properties, locations, associated items, and category membership. Other restitutive treatments focus on the phonological stage of word retrieval and have reported some success for selected patients (Table 259.8). In phonological treatments, patients think about how words sound, considering numbers of syllables, initial phoneme, and rhyming words, and rehearse the words during picture naming, reading, or repetition activities. Studies that have contrasted semantic and phonological treatments suggest that semantic treatment may have a more potent influence on word retrieval than phonological treatment.[111,112] Treatments that combine semantic plus phonological processing (e.g., comprehension practice plus repetition practice) are more beneficial for improving word retrieval abilities.[113,114] Substitutive treatments promote means to circumvent anomia or to vicariatively mediate word retrieval (Table 259.8). For example, preserved phonological reading and writing abilities may be used to assist word retrieval in some patients. Patients can be trained to think of spellings of words and sound out or generate computerized phonemic cues to facilitate the production of spoken words.[99,115,116] Gesture is an alternative method to vicariatively mediate word retrieval. Patients may be trained to combine pantomimes with spoken words to facilitate word retrieval.[117–121] Because some patients with severe aphasia may not respond to these techniques,[108] an alternative method may be needed. One technique useful for some patients rendered virtually non-verbal by aphasia is voluntary control of involuntary utterances (VCIU).[74] Consistent with Luria's[80] concept of intra-systemic reorganization, clinicians train patients to modify their retained automatic verbal responses to voluntary, meaningful use of the same words.

Sentence production   Studies have examined a number of restitutive techniques to remediate sentence production deficits, particularly as they relate to individuals with Broca's aphasia (Table 259.9). As in sentence comprehension treatments, the premise of sentence production treatments is to systematically practice sentences of varied grammatical complexity. As patients experience difficulty, clinicians model target sentences, and patients then rehearse sentences to facilitate correct production. The methods vary in the context used for sentence practice, including story

Table 259.9   Treatments for sentence production deficits

Sentence Production Program for Aphasia[122] (formerly the Helm Elicited Language Program for Syntax Stimulation)
Syntactic Priming[124]
Thematic Mapping Treatment[91,93]
Linguistic-Specific Training[125,126]
Melodic Intonation Therapy[74,127]
Mapping Therapy[95,96]

Table 259.10 Compensatory methods for severe impairments of expression

Pantomime
Gestural codes (Amer-Ind, American Sign Language)
Facial expression
Writing
Drawing
Pointing boards/books
Augmentative Communication Devices
Computer systems (e.g., C-VIC)

Table 259.11 Functional treatments for aphasia

Promoting Aphasics' Communicative Effectiveness[144]
Conversational Coaching[145]
Supported Conversation[146]
Conversational Partner Training[139]
Group Therapy[140–143]

completion activities,[122,123] picture description,[91,93,124,125] or sentence reading.[126,127] One vicariative method for improving sentence production is mapping therapy, described earlier, which uses visual information to mediate language processing. Patients who participate in mapping therapy may improve both sentence comprehension and production.[95,96] Another vicariative approach to sentence production treatment is melodic intonation therapy, a treatment designed to invoke the right hemisphere's rhythmic capacity to support sentence production.[74,75] In this systematic program, patients produce sentences while tapping and using highly intoned, sing-song patterns. Over time the melody is reduced to a more natural prosodic pattern. The method is effective for some patients with Broca's aphasia.[128] A recent imaging study[129] demonstrated that following training with MIT, patients showed increased left frontal activation and right posterior deactivation, contrary to what might be predicted and suggesting that tapping may be an important element of the MIT procedure.

Compensatory methods for verbal expression impairments   As individuals with mild-to-moderate forms of aphasia attempt verbal communication, listeners may invoke strategies to support communication (Table 259.7). Some strategies help the speaker to facilitate the resolution of communication breakdowns. Others allow the speaker to confirm that the listener interpreted the message as the speaker intended. For some patients with severe aphasia, clinicians institute compensatory modes of communication (Table 259.10). "Unaided" compensatory techniques are accomplished without special equipment in contrast to "aided" strategies that use some external devise to support communication.[130] A primary unaided means of communication is the use of gestures. Patients learn to use pantomimes, body signals, facial expressions, referential pointing, or more formal gesturing systems such as Amer-Ind[131] or sign language.[132] Unfortunately, limb apraxia often co-occurs with severe aphasia, potentially interfering with the ability to use gestural communication.[133,134] Visual action therapy (VAT)[74] was devised to help patients with severe aphasia and limb apraxia to learn to pantomime as they are systematically trained to use manual gestures to represent pictured objects. Aided compensatory communication strategies can vary in sophistication. Paper and pencil can allow

some patients to draw[74] or write messages. Picture pointing boards or booklets help some patients communicate basic needs. Augmentative and alternative communication (AAC) devices or computers outfitted with appropriate hardware and software allow some patients to communicate using spelling or touch. Patients with aphasia may have difficulty manipulating some AAC systems as sufficient language capability is necessary for their successful operation.[130] Nevertheless, Weinrich and his colleagues have been successful in training patients with severe aphasia to use computer-aided visual communication (C-VIC).[135–137] In C-VIC, clinicians train patients to use the computer to generate visual depictions of sentence-like messages. Some patients trained with C-VIC have displayed improved spoken language abilities as well.[137]

Pragmatic/functional treatments in aphasia

Some "functional" treatments for aphasia target the disability that aphasia poses for a patient's communication rather than the language impairments that aphasia causes.[138] These treatments promote the exchange of information within the aphasia communication dyad using any means possible (Table 259.11). Patients are encouraged to use residual verbal language abilities. Emphasis is also placed on use of non-verbal signals or modalities to communicate messages. Conversational partners are often included in treatment sessions to be counseled and trained in the use of more effective communication strategies.[139] Finally, an efficient setting to implement and rehearse communication strategies and techniques is in group aphasia therapy.[140–142] One recent study showed significant improvements on language and communication measures in patients who participated in group aphasia therapy.[143]

Pharmacological intervention in aphasia

Aphasia results from disruption of the neurobiological substrate subserving language functions. Thus physicians have long been interested in pharmacological methods to modify the impaired neural system and maximize recovery from aphasia. Although some express skepticism as to the results of treatment efforts thus far,[76,147] some studies have suggested that pharmacological intervention may enhance recovery. Unfortunately, flaws in the research design of most of these studies preclude definitive statements.

The dopaminergic agonist bromocriptine has been administered to a number of patients with frontal lesions and non-fluent aphasias as frontal regions depend upon dopaminergic projections. Studies have documented improvements restricted to verbal fluency measures in selected patients.[148–151] However, other studies with bromocriptine, including one double-blind, placebo-controlled investigation, reported no significant benefits on language measures.[152–154]

Because the cholingergic system seems to play a role in left hemisphere temporal and thalamic functioning, some studies have investigated treatments with cholinergic drugs.[152,155] Administration of physostigmine[155] and bifemelane[156] led to improved word retrieval skills in patients with fluent aphasia. Treatment with donepizil improved verbal fluency in one patient with non-fluent aphasia.[152] All of these studies were lacking sufficient experimental control, however.

Finally, some studies have concentrated on the role of norepinephrine in aphasia recovery as it may generally increase cortical excitability.[157] Treatment with the noradrenergic agonist amphetamine hastened aphasia recovery in one clinical trial.[157,158] However, a double-blind, placebo-controlled comparison of amphetamine and behavioral treatment indicated no effect for the drug independent of behavioral treatment for improving word retrieval in two patients with aphasia.[159]

Summary

Speech-language pathologists provide a number of behavioral treatments to patients in an effort to ameliorate the effects of aphasia. Some methods are restitutive and attempt to recreate the language system in a means compatible with normal language functioning. Others provide substitutive methods to circumvent the impaired language system, sometimes vicariatively mediating language abilities. Although few randomized controlled experimental trials of aphasia treatment have been completed,[67] meta-analyses have shown that aphasia treatment has a significant effect on language functioning beyond what would be expected from spontaneous recovery alone.[68–70,72,73] In contrast, the effects of pharmacological interventions in aphasia treatment have often been less fruitful.[76]

Numerous questions remain unanswered in aphasia treatment research. Although some behavioral treatments are effective, greater efforts are underway to delineate the patient variables associated with maximum benefit from specific aphasia treatments. Some studies are contrasting treatments within experimental subjects to identify the optimum treatment for a particular aspect of aphasia. The neurobiology of treatment effects is being explored in imaging studies examining changes in neural activation patterns after treatment. Studies are now beginning to apply the new generation of statistical methods to analyze results of single subject treatment designs, rather than relying on basic descriptive methods. Although many treatments are effective in generating improvements for selected trained language behaviors, studies are underway to learn more about the

functional outcomes of those treatments in less-structured real-life communication settings. Finally, the relationship between pharmacology and behavioral intervention is only beginning to be explored.[157,160]

References

1. Benson DF, Ardila A. Aphasia: a clinical perspective. New York: Oxford University Press, 1996
2. Post-Stroke Rehabilitation Guideline Panel. Post-stroke rehabilitation: clinical practice guideline. Gaithersburg, MD: Aspen Publication, 1996
3. Albert ML. Treatment of aphasia. Arch Neurol 1998; 55:1417–1419
4. Heilman KM, Valenstein E. Introduction. In: Heilman KM, Valenstein E, eds. Clinical neuropsychology. 3rd ed. New York: Oxford University Press, 1993:3–16
5. Geschwind N. Disconnexion syndromes in animals and man (Part I). Brain 1965;88:237–294
6. Caplan D. Language: structure, processing, and disorders. Cambridge, MA: MIT Press, 1993
7. Ellis AW, Young AW. Human cognitive neuropsychology. East Sussex, UK: Erlbaum, 1988
8. Goodglass H, Kaplan E. The assessment of aphasia and related disorders. 2nd ed. Philadelphia, PA: Lea & Febiger, 1983
9. Caramazza A, Hillis A, Leek EC, Miozzo M. The organization of lexical knowledge in the brain: evidence from category- and modality-specific deficits. In: Hirschfeld L, Gelman S, eds. Mapping the mind: domain specificity in cognition and culture. Cambridge: Cambridge University Press, 1994:68–84
10. Kearns KP. Broca's aphasia. In: LaPointe LL, ed. Aphasia and related neurogenic language disorders. New York: Thieme, 1997:1–40
11. Damasio AR, Tranel D. Nouns and verbs are retrieved with differently distributed neural systems. Proc Natl Acad Sci, USA, 1993;90:4957–4960
12. Miceli G, Silveri MC, Villa G, Caramazza A. On the basis for the agrammatic's difficulty in producing main verbs. Cortex 1984;20:207–220
13. Zingeser LB, Berndt RS. Retrieval of nouns and verbs in agrammatism and anomia. Brain Lang 1990;39: 14–32
14. Damasio H, Damasio AR. Lesion analysis in neuropsychology. New York: Oxford University Press, 1989
15. Kertesz A. Aphasia and associated disorders. Orlando: Grune & Stratton, 1979
16. Kreisler A, Godefroy O, Delmaire C, et al. The anatomy of aphasia revisited. Neurology 2000;54: 1117–1122
17. Rothi LJG. Transcortical motor, sensory, and mixed aphasias. In: LaPointe LL, ed. Aphasia and related neurogenic language disorders. 2nd ed. New York: Thieme, 1997:91–110
18. Albert ML, Helm-Estabrooks N. Diagnosis and treatment of aphasia (Part I). JAMA 1988;259:1043–1045
19. Crosson B. Subcortical functions in language and memory. New York: Guilford Press, 1992
20. Freedman M, Alexander MP, Naeser MA. Anatomic basis of transcortical motor aphasia. Neurology 1984; 34:409–417
21. Taubner RW, Raymer AM, Heilman KM. Frontal-opercular aphasia. Brain Lang 1999;70:240–261
22. Barrett AM, Crucian GP, Raymer AM, Heilman KM. Spared comprehension of emotional prosody in a patient with global aphasia. Neuropsychiatry, Neuropsychol, Behav Neurol 1999;12:117–120

23. Naeser MA, Gaddie A, Palumbo CL, Stiassny-Eder D. Late recovery of auditory comprehension in global aphasia. Improved recovery observed with subcortical temporal isthmus lesion *vs*. Wernicke's cortical area lesion. Arch Neurol 1990;47:425–432

24. Naeser MA, Palumbo CL, Helm-Estabrooks N, et al. Severe non-fluency in aphasia. Role of the medial subcallosal fasciculus and other white matter pathways in recovery of spontaneous speech. Brain 1989;112:1–38

25. Maher LM, Rothi LJ, Heilman KM. Lack of error awareness in an aphasic patient with relatively preserved auditory comprehension. Brain Lang 1994;46: 402–418

26. Kinsbourne M, Warrington EK. Jargon aphasia. Neuropsychologia 1963;1:27–37

27. Ellis AW, Miller D, Sin G. Wernicke's aphasia and normal language processing: a case study in cognitive neuropsychology. Cognition 1983;15:111–144

28. Hart J, Gordon B. Delineation of single-word semantic comprehension deficits in aphasia, with anatomical correlation. Annals of Neurology 1990;27:226–231

29. Heilman KM, Rothi L, McFarling D, Rottmann AL. Transcortical sensory aphasia with relatively spared spontaneous speech and naming. Arch Neurol 1981;38: 236–239

30. Coslett HB, Roeltgen DP, Rothi LJG, Heilman KM. Transcortical sensory aphasia: evidence for subtypes. Brain Lang 1987;32:362–378

31. Alexander MP, Hiltbrunner B, Fischer RS. Distributed anatomy of transcortical sensory aphasia. Arch Neurol 1989;46:885–892

32. Kertesz A, Sheppard A, MacKenzie R. Localization in transcortical sensory aphasia. Arch Neurol 1982;39: 475–478

33. Cummings JL, Benson F, Hill MA, Read S. Aphasia in dementia of the Alzheimer type. Neurology 1985;35: 394–397

34. Kertesz A, Davidson W, McCabe P. Primary progressive semantic aphasia: a case study. J Int Neuropsychol Soc 1998;4:388–398

35. Kohn S, ed. Conduction aphasia. Hillsdale, NJ: Erlbaum, 1992

36. Shallice T, Warrington EK. Auditory-verbal short-term memory impairment and conduction aphasia. Brain Lang 1977;4:479–491

37. Caramazza A, Zurif EB. Dissociation of algorithmic and heuristic processes in language comprehension: evidence from aphasia. Brain Lang 1976;3:572–582

38. Heilman KM, Scholes RJ. The nature of comprehension errors in Broca's, conduction and Wernicke's aphasics. Cortex 1976;12:258–265

39. Anderson JM, Gilmore R, Roper S, et al. Conduction aphasia and the arcuate fasciculus: a re-examination of the Wernicke-Geschwind model. Brain Lang 1999;70: 1–12

40. Goodglass H, Wingfield A, eds. Anomia: neuroanatomical and cognitive correlates. San Diego, CA: Academic Press, 1997

41. Foundas AL, Daniels SK, Vasterling JJ. Anomia: case studies with lesion localization. Neurocase 1998;4:35–43

42. Raymer AM, Foundas AL, Maher LM, et al. Cognitive neuropsychological analysis and neuroanatomic correlates in a case of acute anomia. Brain Lang 1997;58: 137–156

43. Tranel D, Damasio H, Damasio AR. On the neurology of naming. *In*: Goodglass H, Wingfield A, eds. Anomia: neuroanatomical and cognitive correlates.

San Diego, CA: Academic Press, 1997:65–90

44. Raymer AM, Moberg P, Crosson B, et al. Lexical-semantic deficits in two patients with dominant thalamic infarction. Neuropsychologia 1997;35:211–219

45. Kay J, Lesser R, Coltheart M. PALPA: Psycholinguistic Assessments of Language Processing in Aphasia. Hove: Erlbaum, 1992

46. World Health Organization. ICIDH-2: International Classification of Functioning, Disability and Health. Geneva, Switzerland: World Health Organization, 2001.

47. Helm-Estabrooks N. Aphasia diagnostic profiles. Austin, TX: Pro-Ed, 1992

48. Helm-Estabrooks N, Ramsberger G, Morgan AR, Nicholas M. Boston assessment of severe aphasia. Austin, TX: Pro-Ed, 1989

49. Eisenson J. Examining for Aphasia. 3rd ed. Austin, TX: Pro-Ed, 1994

50. Benton AL, Hamsher K, Sivan AB. Multilingual aphasia examination. 3rd ed. San Antonio, TX: Psychological Corporation, 1994

51. Porch BE. Porch index of communicative ability. Austin, TX: Pro-Ed, 1981

52. Kertesz A. Western aphasia battery. New York: Grune & Stratton, 1982

53. Kaplan E, Goodglass H, Weintraub S. Boston naming test 2nd ed. Philadelphia: Lea & Febiger, 2001

54. Nicholas M, Obler L, Albert M, Goodglass H. Lexical retrieval in healthy aging. Cortex 1985;21:595–606

55. Druks J, Masterson J. An object and action naming battery. Austin, TX: Pro-Ed, 2000

56. Dunn LM, Dunn LM. Peabody picture vocabulary test. 3rd ed. Circle Pines, MN: American Guidance Service, 1997

57. McNeil M, Prescott T. Revised token test. Austin, TX: Pro-Ed, 1978

58. Shewan C. Auditory comprehension test for sentences. Chicago: Biolinguistic Clinical Institute, 1981

59. Borkowski JG, Benton AL, Spreen O. Word fluency and brain damage. Neuropsychologia 1967;5:135–140

60. Berndt RS, Wayland S, Rochon E, et al. Quantitative production analysis. Austin, TX: Pro-Ed, 2000

61. LaPointe LL, Horner J. Reading comprehension battery for aphasia. 2nd ed. Austin, TX: Pro-Ed, 1998

62. Holland AL, Frattali CM, Fromm D. Communication activities of daily living. 2nd ed. Austin, TX: Pro-Ed, 1998

63. Frattali CM, Thompson CK, Holland AL, et al. Functional assessment of communication skills for adults: ASHA FACS. Rockville, MD: American Speech-Language-Hearing Association, 1995

64. Lomas J, Pickard L, Bester S, et al. The communicative effectiveness index: development and psychometric evaluation of a functional communication measure for adult aphasia. J Speech Hear Dis 1989;54:113–124

65. Damasio AR. Aphasia. N Engl J Med 1992;326:531–539

66. Holland AL, Wertz RT. Measuring aphasia treatment effects: large-group, small-group, and single-subject studies. *In*: Plum F, ed. Language, communication and the brain. New York: Raven Press, 1988

67. Holland AL, Fromm DS, DeRuyter F, Stein M. Treatment efficacy: aphasia. J Speech Hear Res 1996;39: S27–S36

68. Whurr R, Lorch MP, Nye C. A meta-analysis of studies carried out between 1946 and 1988 concerned with the efficacy of speech and language therapy treatment for aphasic patients. Eur J Disord Commun 1992;27: 1–17

69. Robey RR. The efficacy of treatment for aphasic persons: a meta-analysis. Brain Lang 1994;47:582–608

70. Robey RR. A meta-analysis of clinical outcomes in the treatment of aphasia. J Speech Lang Hear Res 1998;41:172–187

71. McReynolds LV, Thompson CK. Flexibility of single-subject experimental designs: Part I. Review of the basics of single-subject designs. J Speech Hear Dis 1986;51:194–203

72. Robey RR, Schultz MC, Crawford AB, Sinner CA. Single-subject clinical-outcome research: designs, data, effect sizes, and analyses. Aphasiol 1999;13:445–473

73. Robey RR, McCallum AF, Francois LK. A meta-analysis of single-subject research on treatments for aphasia. Clinical Aphasiology Conference, Key West, FL, 1999

74. Helm-Estabrooks N, Albert ML. Manual of aphasia therapy. Austin, TX: Pro-Ed, 1991

75. Therapeutics and Technology Assessment Subcommittee of the American Academy of Neurology. Assessment: melodic intonation therapy. Neurology 1994;44:566–568

76. Small SL. Pharmacotherapy of aphasia: a critical review. Stroke 1994;25:1282–1289

77. Chapey R, ed. Language intervention strategies in adult aphasia. 3rd ed. Baltimore: Williams & Wilkins, 1994

78. Helm-Estabrooks N, Holland AL. Approaches to the treatment of aphasia. San Diego, CA: Singular Publishing Group, 1998

79. Rothi LJG. Behavioral compensation in the case of treatment of acquired language disorders resulting from brain damage. In: Dixon RA, Mackman L, eds. Compensating for psychological deficits and declines: managing losses and promoting gains. Mahwah, NJ: Erlbaum, 1995:219–230

80. Luria AR. Traumatic aphasia. Hague: Mouton, 1970

81. Schuell H, Jenkins JJ, Jimenez-Pabon E. Aphasia in adults. New York: Harper & Row, 1964

82. Duffy JR. Schuell's stimulation approach to rehabilitation. In: Chapey R, ed. Language intervention strategies in adult aphasia. 3rd ed. Baltimore: Williams & Wilkins, 1994:146–174

83. Wertz RT, Collins MJ, Weiss D, et al. Veterans administration cooperative study on aphasia: a comparison of individual and group treatment. J Speech Hear Res 1981;24:580–594

84. Wertz RT, Weiss DG, Aten JL, et al. Comparison of clinic, home and deferred language treatment for aphasia. Arch Neurol 1986;43:653–658

85. Grayson E, Hilton R, Franklin S. Early intervention in a case of jargon aphasia: efficacy of language comprehension therapy. Eur J Disord Commun 1997;32:257–276

86. Morris J, Franklin S, Ellis AW, et al. Remediating a speech perception deficit in an aphasic patient. Aphasiology 1996;10:137–158

87. Aftonomos LB, Appelbaum JS, Steele RD. Improving outcomes for persons with aphasia in advanced community-based treatment programs. Stroke 1999;30:1370–1379

88. Katz RC. Computer applications in aphasia treatment. In: Chapey RC, ed. Language intervention strategies in adult aphasia. 3rd ed. Baltimore: Williams & Wilkins, 1994:322–337

89. Shindo M, Kaga K, Tanaka Y. Speech discrimination and lip reading in patients with word deafness or auditory agnosia. Brain Lang 1991;40:153–161

90. Hough M. Treatment of Wernicke's aphasia with jargon: a case study. J Commun Disord 1993;26:101–111

91. Haendiges AN, Berndt RS, Mitchum CC. Assessing the elements contributing to a "mapping" deficit: a targeted treatment study. Brain Lang 1997;52:276–302

92. Jacobs BJ, Thompson CK. Cross-modal generalization effects of training non-canonical sentence comprehension and production in agrammatic aphasia. J Speech Lang Hear Res 2000;43:5–20

93. Mitchum CC, Haendiges AN, Berndt RS. Treatment of thematic mapping in sentence comprehension: implications for normal processing. Cogn Neuropsychol 1995;12:503–547

94. Shewan CM, Bandur DL. Language-oriented treatment: a psycholinguistic approach to aphasia. In: Chapey R, ed. Language intervention strategies in adult aphasia. 3rd ed. Baltimore: Williams & Wilkins, 1994:184–201

95. Byng S. Sentence processing deficits: Theory and therapy. Cogn Neuropsychol 1988;5:629–676

96. Saffran EM, Schwartz MF, Fink R, et al. Mapping therapy: an approach to remediating agrammatic sentence comprehension and production. In: Aphasia treatment: current approaches and research opportunities. NIH Publication No. 93-3424, 1992:77–90

97. Helm-Estabrooks N. Treatment of aphasic naming problems. In: Goodglass H, Wingfield A, eds. Anomia: neuroanatomical and cognitive correlates. San Diego, CA: Academic Press, 1997:189–202

98. Linebaugh CW. Lexical retrieval problems: Anomia. In: LaPointe LL, ed. Aphasia and related neurogenic language disorders. 2nd ed. New York: Thieme, 1997:112–132

99. Hillis AE. Treatment of naming disorders: new issues regarding old therapies. J Int Neuropsychol Soc 1998;4:648–660

100. Thompson CK, Kearns KP. An experimental analysis of acquisition, generalization and maintenance of naming behavior in a patient with anomia. In: Brookshire RH, ed. Clinical aphasiology: conference proceedings, 1981. Minneapolis: BRK Publishers, 1981:35–45

101. Greenwald ML, Raymer AM, Richardson ME, Rothi LJG. Contrasting treatments for severe impairments of picture naming. Neuropsychol Rehabil 1995;5:17–49

102. Boyle M, Coelho CA. Application of semantic feature analysis as a treatment for aphasic dysnomia. Am J Speech Lang Path 1995;4:94–98

103. Marshall J, Pound C, White-Thomson M, Pring T. The use of picture/word matching tasks to assist word retrieval in aphasic patients. Aphasiology 1990;4:167–184

104. Lowell S, Beeson PM, Holland AL. The efficacy of a semantic cueing procedure on naming performance of adults with aphasia. Am J Speech Lang Path 1995;4:109–114

105. Ochipa C, Maher LM, Raymer AM. One approach to the treatment of anomia. ASHA Div 2. Neurophysiol Neuro Speech Lang Disord 1998;15(3):18–23

106. Nickels L, Best W. Therapy for naming disorders (Part II). Specifics, surprises, and suggestions. Aphasiology 1996;10:109–136

107. Robson J, Marshall J, Pring T, Chiat S. Phonologic naming therapy in jargon aphasia: positive but paradoxical effects. J Int Neuropsychol Soc 1998;4:675–686

108. Raymer AM, Thompson CK, Jacobs B, leGrand HR. Phonologic treatment of naming deficits in aphasia: model-based generalization analysis. Aphasiology 1993;7:27–53

109. Raymer AM, Ellsworth TA. Response to contrasting verb retrieval treatments: A case study. Aphasiology, in press

110. Hillis AE. The role of models of language processing in rehabilitation of language impairments. Aphasiology 1993;7:5–26

111. Ennis MR, Raymer AM, Burks DW, et al. Contrasting treatments for phonological anomia: unexpected findings. J Int Neuropsychol Soc 2000;6:240 (abstract)

112. Howard D, Patterson K, Franklin S, et al. Treatment of word retrieval deficits in aphasia. Brain 1985;108: 817–829

113. Drew RL, Thompson CK. Model-based semantic treatment for naming deficits in aphasia. J Speech Lang Hear Res 1999;42:972–989

114. Le Dorze G, Boulay N, Gaudreau J, Brassard C. The contrasting effects of a semantic versus a formal-semantic technique for the facilitation of naming in a case of anomia. Aphasiology 1994;8:127–141

115. Bruce C, Howard D. Computer-generated phonemic cues: an effective aid for naming in aphasia. Br J Disord Commun 1987;22:191–201

116. Nickels L. The autocue? Self-generated phonemic cues in the treatment of a disorder of reading and naming. Cogn Neuropsychol 1992;9:155–182

117. Hoodin RB, Thompson CK. Facilitation of verbal labeling in adult aphasia by gestural, verbal or verbal plus gestural training. In: Brookshire RH, ed. Clinical aphasiology conference proceedings. Minneapolis: BRK Publishers, 1983:62–64

118. Kearns KP, Simmons NN, Sisterhen C. Gestural sign (Amer-Ind) as a facilitator of verbalization in patients with aphasia. In: Brookshire RH, ed. Clinical aphasiology conference proceedings. Minneapolis: BRK Publishers, 1982:183–191

119. Pashek GV. A case study of gesturally cued naming in aphasia: dominant versus non-dominant hand training. J Commun Disord 1997;30:349–366

120. Pashek GV. Gestural facilitation of noun and verb retrieval in aphasia: a case study. Brain Lang 1998;65: 177–180

121. Raymer AM, Thompson CK. Effects of verbal plus gestural treatment in a patient with aphasia and severe apraxia of speech. In: Prescott TE, ed. Clinical aphasiology. Vol 12. Austin, TX: Pro-Ed, 1991:285–297

122. Helm-Estabrooks N, Nicholas M. Sentence production program for aphasia. Austin, TX: Pro-Ed, 1999

123. Wambaugh JL, Thompson CK. Training and generalization of agrammatic aphasic adults' wh-interrogative productions. J Speech Hear Disord 1989;54:509–525

124. Fink R, Schwartz M. Syntactic priming as a treatment strategy for sentence processing deficits in aphasia. Presented at Clinical Aphasiology Conference, Asheville, NC, June 1998

125. Kearns KP. Response elaboration training for patient initiated utterances. In: Brookshire RH, ed. Clinical aphasiology. Minneapolis: BRK Publishers, 1985:196–204

126. Thompson CK, Shapiro LP, Roberts MM. Treatment of sentence production deficits in aphasia: a linguistic-specific approach to wh-interrogative training and generalization. Aphasiology 1993;7:111–133

127. Thompson CK, Ballard KJ, Shapiro LP. The role of syntactic complexity in training wh-movement structures in agrammatic aphasia: optimal order for promoting generalization. J Int Neuropsych Soc 1998;4:661–674

128. Naeser MA, Helm-Estabrooks N. CT scan lesion localization and response to melodic intonation therapy. Cortex 1985;21:203–223

129. Belin P, Van Eeckhout Ph, Zilbovicius M, et al. Recovery from non-fluent aphasia after melodic intonation therapy: a PET study. Neurology 1996;47:1504–1511

130. Hux K, Beukelman DR, Garrett KL. Augmentative and alternative communication for persons with aphasia. In: Chapey R, ed. Language intervention strategies in adult aphasia. Baltimore: Williams & Wilkins, 1994: 338–357

131. Skelly M. Amer-Ind gestural code based on universal American Indian hand talk. New York: Elsevier, 1979

132. Anderson SW, Damasio H, Damasio AR, et al. Acquisition of signs from American sign language in hearing individuals following left hemisphere damage and aphasia. Neuropsychologia 1992;30:329–340

133. Rothi LJG, Heilman KM. Ideomotor apraxia: gestural learning and memory. In: Roy EA, ed. Neuropsychological studies in apraxia and related disorders. New York: Oxford University Press, 1985:65–74

134. Maher LM, Ochipa C. Management and treatment of limb apraxia. In: Rothi LJG, Heilman KM, eds. Apraxia: the neuropsychology of action. Hove: Psychology Press, 1997:75–91

135. Weinrich M, Boser KI, McCall D. Representation of linguistic rules in the brain: evidence from training an aphasic patient to produce past tense verb morphology. Brain Lang 1999;70:144–158

136. Weinrich M, Steele RD, Carlson GS, et al. Processing of visual syntax in a globally aphasic patient. Brain Lang 1989;36:391–405

137. Weinrich M, Shelton JR, Cox DM, McCall D. Remediating production of tense morphology improves verb retrieval in chronic aphasia. Brain Lang 1997;58:23–45

138. Aten JL. Functional communication treatment. In: Chapey R, ed. Language intervention strategies in adult aphasia. Baltimore: Williams & Wilkins, 1994: 292–303

139. Lyon J. Volunteers and partners: moving intervention outside the treatment room. In: Shadden B, Toner MA, eds. Aging and communication. Austin, TX: Pro-Ed, 1997:299–323

140. Avent J. Manual for cooperative group treatment for aphasia. Boston: Butterworth-Heinemann, 1997

141. Elman RJ. Group treatment of neurogenic communication disorders. Woburn, MA: Butterworth-Heinemann, 1999

142. Marshall RC. Introduction to group treatment for aphasia: design and management. Woburn, MA: Butterworth-Heinemann, 1999

143. Elman RJ, Bernstein-Ellis E. The efficacy of group communication treatment in adults with chronic aphasia. J Speech Lang Hear Res 1999;42:411–419

144. Davis G, Wilcox M. Incorporating parameters of natural conversation in aphasia treatment. In: Chapey R, ed. Language intervention strategies in adult aphasia. Baltimore: Williams & Wilkins, 1981:169–194

145. Holland AL. Pragmatic assessment and treatment for aphasia. In: Wallace GL, ed. Adult aphasia rehabilitation. Boston: Butterworth-Heinemann, 1996: 161–173

146. Kagan A. Supported conversation for adults with aphasia: Methods and resources for training conversation partners. Aphasiology 1998;12:851–864

147. Small SL. The future of aphasia treatment. Brain Lang 2000;71:227–232

148. Albert ML, Bachman DL, Morgan A, Helm-Estabrooks N. Pharmacotherapy for aphasia. Neurology 1988;38: 877–879

149. Gupta SR, Mlcoch AG, Scolaro C, Moritz T. Bromo-

criptine treatment of non-fluent aphasia. Neurology 1995;45:2170–2173

150. Raymer AM, Bandy D, Schwartz RL, et al. Effects of bromocriptine in a patient with crossed aphasia. Arch Phys Med Rehabil, 2001;82:139–144

151. Sabe L, Leiguarda R, Starkstein SE. An open-label trial of bromocriptine in non-fluent aphasia. Neurology 1992;42:1637–1638

152. Hughes JD, Jacobs DH, Heilman KM. Neuropharmacology and linguistic neuroplasticity. Brain Lang 2000; 71:96–101

153. MacLennan DL, Nicholas LE, Morley GK, Brookshire RH. The effects of bromocriptine on speech and language function in a man with transcortical motor aphasia. *In:* Prescott TE, ed. Clinical aphasiology. Vol 20. Austin, TX: Pro-Ed, 1991:145–155

154. Sabe L, Salvarezza F, Garcia Cuerva A, et al. A randomized, double-blind, placebo-controlled study of bromocriptine in non-fluent aphasia. Neurology 1995; 45:2272–2274

155. Jacobs DH, Shuren J, Gold M, et al. Physostigmine pharmacotherapy for anomia. Neurocase 1996;2:83–91

156. Tanaka Y, Miyazaki M, Albert ML. Effects of increased cholingergic activity on naming in aphasia. Lancet 1997;350:116–167

157. Walker-Batson D, Curtis S, Natarajan R, et al. A double-blind, placebo-controlled study of the use of amphetamine in the treatment of aphasia. Stroke 2001;32:2093–2098

158. Walker-Batson D, Devous MD, Curtis SS, et al. Response to amphetamine to facilitate recovery from aphasia subsequent to stroke. *In:* Prescott TE. Clinical aphasiology, Vol 20. Austin, TX: Pro-Ed, 1991:137–143

159. McNeil MR, Doyle PJ, Spencer KA, et al. A double-blind, placebo-controlled study of pharmacological and behavioural treatment of lexical-semantic deficits in aphasia. Aphasiology 1997;11:385–400

160. Rothi LJG, Nadeau SE, Ennis MR. Aphasia treatment: a key issue for research into the twenty-first century. Brain Lang 2000;71:78–81

Treatment of Alexia and Agraphia

Pelagie M Beeson and Steven Z Rapcsak

The neuropsychological study of alexia and agraphia originated with the work of nineteenth-century European neurologists. Although the leading figures of German, French, and English neurology all made important contributions to this area of research, it seems fair to say that the elegant clinico-anatomical investigations of Jules Déjerine had the most profound and enduring influence on contemporary thinking about acquired disorders of reading and writing.

In 1891, Déjerine[1] described a patient who developed a sudden inability to read or write without significant aphasia. Postmortem examination of the brain demonstrated an infarction involving the left angular gyrus. Déjerine concluded that the left parietal lesion caused alexia and agraphia by destroying the cortical center for visual word images. Thus, according to Déjerine, orthographic memory representations for familiar words stored within the dominant angular gyrus played a critical role both in the comprehension and the production of written language. A year later, Déjerine[2] reported another patient who acutely lost his ability to read without any additional impairment of spoken language. Neurological examination revealed a right visual field defect, but was otherwise unremarkable. Importantly, and in contrast to Déjerine's first case, the patient had no obvious disturbance of written expression. The clinical condition remained essentially unchanged for another four years, at which time the patient suffered another stroke that resulted in total alexia and agraphia. At autopsy, there was evidence of a recent infarction in the region of the left angular gyrus, corresponding to the patient's second cerebrovascular accident that rendered him completely illiterate. An older lesion occupying the left ventro-medial occipital region was also seen and another small area of remote infarction was identified in the splenium of the corpus callosum. To explain the clinical syndrome of alexia without agraphia, Déjerine proposed that, in addition to producing right visual field loss, the left occipital lesion interrupted connections between right-hemisphere visual areas and left-hemisphere language centers. As the patient was only able to see within his intact left visual field, which projected information to the right occipital cortex, the destruction of interhemispheric white matter pathways produced a complete isolation of the left-hemisphere language areas from visual input. Since the left angular gyrus was not damaged by the first stroke, orthographic knowledge was initially preserved and therefore the patient was able to spell correctly. Destruction of the angular gyrus by the second stroke

resulted in alexia with agraphia, similar to what was observed in Déjerine's first patient.

Déjerine's neuroanatomical model of reading and writing was accepted by the major authorities of the day and his clinical observations have been replicated many times since. In fact, it was not until the 1970s that the application of a new theoretical approach, motivated by cognitive information-processing models of normal reading and writing, began to produce fresh insights into the neuropsychological mechanisms of alexia and agraphia. In the next section we briefly review the basic functional components of the cognitive model of written language processing that will serve as the conceptual framework for interpreting the various alexia and agraphia syndromes discussed in this chapter. A glossary of relevant terms is included in Table 260.1.

A cognitive model of reading and writing

The model of written word comprehension and production presented in Figure 260.1 makes a fundamental distinction between the procedures involved in reading or spelling familiar words and those used primarily for processing unfamiliar words or pronounceable non-words (e.g., chulf). It should be pointed out that some models also postulate the existence of lexical-non-semantic routes by which familiar words can be read or spelled without comprehension of the word's meaning. We have elected not to discuss these linguistic procedures in detail because there are no clinical alexia or agraphia syndromes that are attributable to selective damage to the proposed lexical-non-semantic reading or spelling routes and, consequently, these routes have not been specifically targeted in rehabilitation efforts.

According to the model, reading begins with the visual analysis of the written word. During this initial perceptual stage, the position and identity of the letters that comprise the word are determined. Under normal circumstances, the visual analysis system can process several letters simultaneously and therefore word length has only a negligible effect on reading speed and accuracy. Information about letter identity is transmitted to the orthographic input lexicon which functions as the internal memory store of familiar visual word forms. The activation of representations within the orthographic input lexicon indicates that the word is familiar, but comprehension of the word's meaning requires the activation of semantic memory representations. Although connections between the orthographic input lexicon and the semantic system are sufficient for written word comprehension, reading aloud also requires the retrieval of the

Table 260.1   Glossary of terms

Term	Definition
Allograph	Different physical forms of a letter (e.g. upper- *vs.* lower-case; print *vs.* script)
Allographic conversion	The process by which abstract orthographic representations are converted into the appropriate physical letter shapes
Content words	Words that carry semantic meaning, such as nouns, adjectives, and verbs
Functors	Words that serve grammatical functions within sentences, such as prepositions and articles
Grapheme	A letter or letter cluster that corresponds to a single phoneme in the language
Grapheme-to-phoneme conversion (a.k.a. letter-to-sound conversion)	The process of reading by converting letters to the corresponding sounds
Graphemic buffer	Working memory system that temporarily stores abstract orthographic representations while they are being converted into codes appropriate for various output modalities (i.e., writing, oral spelling, typing, spelling with anagram letters)
Graphic innervatory patterns	Motor commands to specific muscle effector systems involved in the production of handwriting
Graphic motor programs	Abstract spatiotemporal codes for writing movements, which contain information about the sequence, position, direction, and relative size of the strokes necessary to create different letters
Orthographic input lexicon	The memory store of familiar visual word forms
Orthographic output lexicon	The memory store of learned spellings
Orthography	The written form of words in a language
Phoneme	The smallest unit of meaningful sound in a language
Phoneme-to-grapheme conversion (a.k.a. sound-to-letter conversion)	The process of spelling by converting units of sound to the corresponding letters
Phonological input lexicon	The memory store of acoustic representations for familiar words used in auditory comprehension
Phonological output lexicon	The memory store of sound patterns for familiar words used in speech production
Semantic system	A component of long-term memory that contains knowledge of word meanings

phonological representation of the word from the phonological output lexicon. This pathway for processing written words via the semantic system is known as the lexical-semantic reading route (Figure 260.1).

Normal individuals can also read novel words or pronounceable non-words without difficulty. Since these items have not been encountered before, they have no pre-existing representation within the orthographic input lexicon. Consequently, unfamiliar orthographic patterns are read by a strategy that presumably relies on letter-to-sound (i.e., grapheme-to-phoneme) conversion rules. This approach involves segmenting novel letter strings into individual graphemes (e.g., ch-u-l-f), converting each grapheme into the corresponding phoneme, followed by the blending of phonemes to produce the appropriate spoken response. Because this reading procedure does not rely on the activation of familiar visual word forms, it is referred to as the non-lexical reading route.

According to the model, the written production of familiar words depends on the activation of representations within the orthographic output lexicon. The orthographic output lexicon functions as the memory store of learned spellings. In conceptually mediated writing tasks, such as spontaneous writing and written naming, entries in the orthographic output lexicon are activated by input from the semantic system. Connections between the semantic system and the orthographic output lexicon are referred to as the lexical-semantic spelling route. Writing to dictation can also be accomplished by a lexical-semantic strategy, relying on connections between the phonological input and the orthographic output lexicons via the semantic system (Figure 260.1).

In contrast to the lexical-semantic procedures used for spelling familiar words, novel words or non-words are spelled by a non-lexical strategy based on sound-to-letter (i.e., phoneme-to-grapheme) conversion rules. Non-lexical spelling involves segmenting the novel auditory stimulus into its component sounds, following which each phoneme is translated into the corresponding grapheme.

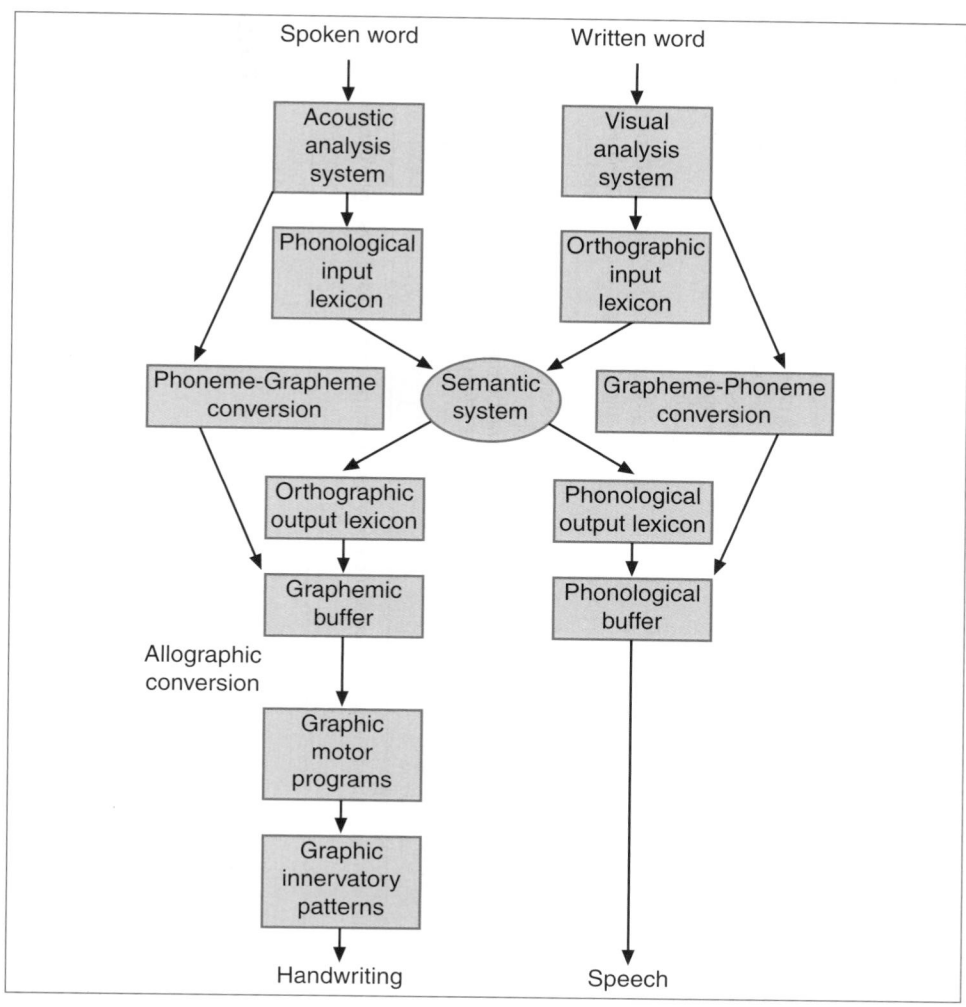

Figure 260.1 Simplified cognitive model of reading and writing.

Spellings generated by the lexical-semantic and non-lexical spelling routes are subsequently processed in the graphemic buffer—a working memory system that temporarily stores orthographic representations while they are being converted into motor output. As shown in Figure 260.1, the production of handwriting is accomplished through a series of hierarchically organized processing stages that include allographic conversion, motor programming, and the generation of graphic innervatory patterns. Allographic conversion refers to the activation and selection of motor programs required for producing different physical letter shapes (e.g., upper *vs.* lower case; print *vs.* script). Graphic motor programs contain abstract spatio-temporal information relevant to the sequence, position, direction, and relative size of the strokes necessary for writing specific letters.[3,4] Graphic innervatory patterns correspond to motor commands to muscle effector systems, specifying concrete kinematic parameters such as absolute stroke size, duration, and force.

Neuropsychological disorders of reading and writing

Acquired disorders of reading can be subdivided into peripheral and central types.[5] In the peripheral alexias, the reading disturbance is attributable to functional impairment at the stage of visual analysis. The most extensively investigated peripheral alexia syndrome is known as "pure alexia" or "letter-by-letter reading." As the name of the syndrome suggests, patients read in a sequential left-to-right fashion naming each letter in the word. As a result, there is a monotonic relationship between reading speed and word length (Table 260.2). Although the exact neuropsychological mechanisms of letter-by-letter reading remain to be elucidated,[6] in many cases there is evidence of early visual dysfunction affecting the perceptual identification of letters. Alternatively, the reading impairment may be caused by a disconnection between the visual analysis system and the orthographic input lexicon, leading to an inability to transmit information about multiple letter identities in parallel.[7] Letter-by-letter reading may represent a compensatory strategy in which the serial naming of letters provides the patient with an alternative access route to the orthographic input lexicon. Letter-by-letter reading is typically seen following damage to the left inferior occipito-temporal region.[8,9] Interestingly, some letter-by-letter readers can derive implicit lexical-semantic information about words they cannot identify explicitly.[10] Implicit recognition of written

Table 260.2 Summary of the primary features of various alexia syndromes

Alexia Syndrome	Effect							Locus of damage	
	Word length Short > Long	Spelling regularity Reg > Irreg	Word freq HF > LF	Concrete Con > Abstr	Word class Cont > Func	Inability to read non-words	Semantic errors	Cognitive processes impaired	Neurological lesion location
Pure alexia (letter-by-letter reading)	✓							Visual identification of letters and/or access to orthographic input lexicon	Left inferior occipito-temporal region
Surface dyslexia		✓	✓					Lexical-semantic reading route	Left posterior temporo-parietal cortex
Phonological/ deep dyslexia			✓	✓	✓	✓	✓ (Deep dyslexia)	Non-lexical reading route and lexical-semantic reading route (deep)	Left perisylvian region (Broca's area, Wernicke's area, and supramarginal gyrus)

✓, Significant effect; Reg, regular spelling; Irreg, irregular spelling; HF, high frequency words; LF, low frequency words; Concrete, concreteness; Con, concrete; Abstr, abstract word; Cont, content words; Func, functors.

words in these patients may be mediated by the right hemisphere.

In the central alexias, the perceptual processing of letter strings is preserved, and the disorder is attributable to the breakdown of the various linguistic procedures by which words and non-words are normally read. Three major central alexia syndromes have been identified: surface dyslexia,[11] phonological dyslexia,[12] and deep dyslexia.[13] Surface dyslexia reflects dysfunction of the lexical-semantic reading route with relative preservation of the non-lexical route (Table 260.2). As a result, reading success is strongly influenced by orthographic regularity. Words that contain regular grapheme-phoneme correspondences (e.g., mint) and non-words are read correctly. However, attempts to read words with irregular grapheme-phoneme mappings by relying on a non-lexical strategy result in regularization errors (e.g., steak–steek). Regularization errors are especially common when reading low frequency irregular words. Surface dyslexia is most often associated with damage to the left posterior temporo-parietal region.[14,15] The reading disorder is also frequently encountered in neurodegenerative syndromes characterized by prominent lexical-semantic impairment, including Alzheimer's disease (AD)[16] and semantic dementia.[17]

In phonological dyslexia, reading success is influenced by the lexical status of the letter string. Patients are unable to read non-words, but the reading of familiar words (both regular and irregular) is relatively preserved. Phonological dyslexia is caused by damage to the non-lexical reading route, so that word reading is accomplished primarily via a lexical-semantic strategy. As a result, reading accuracy is influenced by lexical-semantic features including concreteness (i.e., concrete words such as "apple" are read better than abstract words such as "pride"), grammatical word class (i.e., content words, such as nouns and verbs, are read better than functors, such as prepositions and pronouns), and word frequency (i.e., high frequency words are read better than low frequency words). Deep dyslexia incorporates all the major features of phonological dyslexia, but it is distinguishable from the latter by the presence of numerous semantic errors in reading (e.g., boy–man). Semantic errors indicate dysfunction within the lexical-semantic reading route in conjunction with an impairment of the non-lexical route.[18] Although phonological and deep dyslexia initially were considered to be distinct syndromes, more recent evidence suggests that they may be characterized as points on a continuum reflecting quantitative rather than qualitative differences. For that reason, a combined syndrome classification of phonological/deep dyslexia may be more appropriate (Table 260.2). Phonological and deep dyslexia are typically seen following damage to the perisylvian language zone which includes Broca's area, Wernicke's area, and the supramarginal gyrus.[9,19] Since deep dyslexia is usually associated with extensive left-hemisphere lesions, it has been proposed that reading in these patients may be mediated by the right hemisphere.[20]

Similar to the alexias, acquired disorders of writing can be subdivided into central and peripheral types.[4] Central agraphias reflect damage to the various linguistic spelling routes or the graphemic buffer and are manifested by similar impairments across different modalities of output (e.g., written spelling, oral spelling, typing). By contrast, in the peripheral agraphias the location of the damage is distal to the graphemic buffer and the dysfunction primarily affects the selection or production of letters in handwriting.

Central agraphia syndromes include lexical (or surface) agraphia,[21] phonological agraphia,[22] deep agraphia,[23] and agraphia due to dysfunction of the graphemic buffer.[24] Lexical agraphia reflects damage to the lexical-semantic spelling route (Table 260.3). Due to the loss or unavailability of word-specific orthographic information, patients are forced to rely on spelling by a non-lexical strategy (i.e., phoneme-to-grapheme conversion) so that words are simply spelled as they sound. As a result, spelling accuracy is strongly influenced by orthographic regularity. Regular words and non-words are spelled correctly, but attempts to spell words with irregular sound-to-spelling relationships result in phonologically plausible errors (e.g., tomb–toom). Low frequency irregular words are especially vulnerable to error. Lexical agraphia is typically seen following damage to left posterior temporo-parietal cortex.[25,26] The syndrome has also been described in patients with AD[27,28] and in semantic dementia.[29]

Phonological agraphia is attributable to dysfunction of the non-lexical spelling route. Patients have difficulty spelling non-words, but the spelling of familiar words (both regular and irregular) is relatively spared. Spelling accuracy is influenced by lexical-semantic variables (concreteness, word class, frequency), consistent with reliance on a lexical-semantic strategy. Deep agraphia shares all the linguistic features of phonological agraphia, but patients with the former syndrome also produce semantic errors indicating additional impairment of the lexical-semantic spelling route. As in the case of phonological and deep dyslexia, a combined syndrome of phonological/deep agraphia seems most appropriate to capture the overlapping features of these two disorders (Table 260.3). Phonological and deep agraphia are associated with damage to the perisylvian language areas.[25,26] Deep agraphia in patients with extensive left-hemisphere lesions may reflect right-hemisphere writing.[30]

Damage to the putative graphemic buffer leads to abnormally rapid decay of information relevant to the serial order and identity of stored graphemes. Characteristic spelling errors include letter substitutions, additions, deletions, and transpositions (e.g., guitar–guilat). These errors are observed in all spelling tasks and across all modalities of output. Spelling accuracy is not significantly influenced by lexical status (words vs. non-words), lexical-semantic features (concreteness, word class, frequency), or orthographic regularity. Stimulus length, however, has a strong effect on

Table 260.3   Summary of the primary features of various central agraphia syndromes

Central agraphia syndrome	Effect							Locus of damage	
	Word length Short > Long	Spelling regularity Reg > Irreg	Word freq HF > LF	Concrete Con > Abstr	Word class Cont > Func	Inability to read non-words	Semantic errors	Cognitive processes impaired	Neurological lesion location
Lexical (surface) agraphia		✓	✓					Lexical-semantic spelling route	Left posterior temporo-parietal cortex
Phonological/ deep dysgraphia			✓	✓	✓	✓	✓ (Deep dysgraphia)	Non-lexical spelling route and lexical-semantic route (deep dysgraphia)	Left perisylvian region (Broca's area, Wernicke's area, and supramarginal gyrus)
Graphemic buffer agraphia	✓							Graphemic buffer	Left parietal or frontal cortical regions

✓, Significant effect; Reg, regular spelling; Irreg, irregular spelling; HF, high frequency words; LF, low frequency words; Concrete, concreteness; Con, concrete; Abstr, abstract word; Cont, content words; Func, functors.

performance because each additional grapheme introduces a potential error by increasing the demand on limited memory storage capacity (Table 260.3). Lesion sites in patients with graphemic buffer agraphia have been variable, but left parietal and frontal cortical involvement is common.[26]

Peripheral agraphia syndromes include allographic disorders, apraxic agraphia, and non-apraxic disorders of neuromuscular execution[31] (Table 260.4). Allographic disorders are characterized by an inability to activate or select the letter shapes appropriate for the orthographic representations held in the graphemic buffer. Patients may have selective difficulty in writing upper- or lower-case letters, or they may produce case-mixing errors (e.g., tAblE). Other patients produce well-formed letter substitution errors that usually bear physical similarity to the target. According to our model, allographic disorders reflect the breakdown of the procedures by which orthographic representations are directly mapped onto letter-specific graphic motor programs (i.e., the allographic conversion process in Figure 260.1). Allographic disorders are usually associated with damage to the left parieto-occipital region.[26]

Apraxic agraphia is a writing disorder characterized by poor letter formation that cannot be attributed to sensorimotor (i.e., weakness, deafferentation), basal ganglia (i.e., tremor, rigidity) or cerebellar (i.e., ataxia, dysmetria) dysfunction affecting the writing limb. Errors of letter morphology include spatial distortions, stroke additions or deletions, frequently resulting in the production of illegible handwriting.

Apraxia agraphia is caused by damage to graphic motor programs, or it may reflect an inability to translate the information contained in these programs into specific motor commands. In right-handers, apraxic agraphia is associated with damage to a left-hemisphere cortical network dedicated to the motor programming of handwriting movements. The major functional components of this neural network include posterior-superior parietal cortex (i.e., the region of the intraparietal sulcus), dorsolateral premotor cortex, and the supplementary motor area (SMA).[26,31,32] Callosal lesions in right-handers may be accompanied by unilateral apraxic agraphia of the left hand.[33]

Damage to motor systems involved in generating graphic innervatory patterns results in defective control of writing force, speed, and amplitude. Typical examples include the micrographia of patients with Parkinson's disease and the disjointed and erratic handwriting produced by patients with cerebellar dysfunction. The breakdown of graphomotor control in these neurological conditions suggests that the basal ganglia and the cerebellum, working in concert with dorsolateral premotor cortex and the SMA, are critically involved in the selection and implementation of kinematic parameters for writing movements.[31]

Clinical assessment of alexia and agraphia

The initial goal of clinical assessment of reading and writing is to determine whether an individual can meet daily demands for written language use, including reading paragraph-level text and composing

Table 260.4   Summary of the primary features of various peripheral agraphia syndromes

Peripheral agraphia syndrome	Distinctive features	Characteristic errors	Cognitive processes impaired	Neurological lesion location
Allographic disorders	Inability to generate or select correct letter shapes in handwriting with spared oral spelling	Substitution of physically similar letter forms; case mixing errors. Impairment may be specific to case (upper *vs.* lower) or style (print *vs.* cursive)	Defective assignment of letter shapes to abstract orthographic representations held in the graphemic buffer	Left parieto-occipital region
Apraxic agraphia	Poor letter formation not attributable to allographic disorder, sensorimotor, cerebellar, or extrapyramidal dysfunction. Sparing of oral spelling, typing, spelling with anagram letters	Gross errors of letter morphology, spatial distortions, stroke insertions and deletions, writing may be completely illegible	Destruction or disconnection of graphic motor programs, or damage to systems responsible for translating these programs into graphic innervatory patterns	Left posterior-superior parietal lobe, dorsolateral premotor cortex, SMA
Non-apraxic disorders of motor function	Defective regulation of movement force, speed, and amplitude in handwriting	Micrographia (Parkinson's disease); disjointed and irregular writing movements (cerebellar disorders)	Dysfunction of motor systems involved in controlling the kinematic parameters of writing	Basal ganglia, cerebellum

written narratives. Reading and writing abilities can be screened using the appropriate portions of standardized aphasia tests,[34,35] and performance should be considered relative to premorbid language abilities. When alexia or agraphia is evident, careful assessment should provide information about the functional integrity of the various processing components involved in reading and writing. As depicted in Figure 260.1, some processing components are specific to written language, whereas others are shared with oral language tasks. By contrasting performance for single-word comprehension and production in written and spoken modalities, the hypothesized locus (or loci) of impairment may be identified.

In addition to examining performance across language modalities, it is also informative to determine the influence of different linguistic variables on reading and writing. This can be accomplished by using published tests containing word lists specifically designed to vary along a number of lexical-semantic dimensions (e.g., frequency, concreteness, grammatical class, orthographic regularity, length, morphological complexity), as well as stimuli for assessing non-word reading and spelling.[36,37] Clues regarding the location of damage can be obtained by examining what types of linguistic items pose the greatest difficulty, and what types of reading and writing errors are made. Ideally, the assessment should allow the examiner to determine whether the patient's performance fits the diagnostic criteria for the different alexia and agraphia syndromes discussed above and summarized in Tables 260.2, 260.3, and 260.4. In many instances, however, damage to multiple functional components results in alexia or agraphia profiles that do not conform to one of the identified syndromes. In those cases, it is still useful to characterize the status of impaired and preserved processes which will help guide the selection or design of the treatment approach. Some of the specific assessment tasks will be briefly reviewed below, followed by examples of clinically tested treatment approaches for the various alexia and agraphia syndromes.

Reading assessment

An assessment of reading includes measures of single word comprehension and oral reading, as well as reading accuracy, rate, and comprehension of sentence and paragraph-level material. Additional assessments are implemented as questions arise regarding the status of the component processes elaborated in Figure 260.1. Visual analysis of letters may be tested by having the patient match letters (both same-case and cross-case). Letter identification can be confirmed by naming visually presented letters (when oral production is adequate to do so). Next, the integrity of the orthographic input lexicon can be tested by lexical decision tasks in which patients are asked to discriminate between familiar and unfamiliar orthographic patterns by simply indicating whether the letter string is a real word or a non-word. Reading comprehension at the single-word level can

be assessed by word-picture matching tasks or by asking the patient to provide a definition of the written word. Reading aloud is evaluated with specifically designed word lists that allow examination of the influence of linguistic variables on performance, as mentioned above. Reading comprehension and speed at the sentence and paragraph level can be assessed using standardized tests.[38,39]

Writing assessment

A comprehensive evaluation of writing includes tests of spontaneous writing, written naming, writing to dictation, and copying. Spontaneous writing can be tested by asking the patient to compose a written narrative on a specific topic or by using picture description tasks from standardized tests.[34,35] Written naming is also assessed by using pictured stimuli from standardized tests.[34,36,40] Writing to dictation gives the experimenter control over the various linguistic features known to affect spelling, and is best accomplished by using one of the published word lists alluded to earlier. The evaluation of patients with agraphia should also include oral spelling, typing, and spelling with anagram letters in order to identify potential dissociations between the various output modalities. In testing for peripheral agraphia, the allographic conversion process can be assessed by asking patients to write in different case or style and to transcribe from upper to lower case and vice versa. In analyzing the motor components of writing, attention is paid to overall legibility, letter size, and morphology. Poor control of movement speed, force, and amplitude may be readily apparent from observing the patient in the act of writing. Any sensorimotor, basal ganglia, or cerebellar dysfunction affecting the writing limb is carefully noted and patients should be examined for limb apraxia (i.e., the ability to perform skilled limb movements with the extremities). Assessment of copying should include letters, words, and nonlinguistic visual patterns as stimuli.

Treatment of alexia

Treatment approaches for acquired alexia may be directed toward strengthening peripheral or central reading processes (or both), depending on the nature of the reading impairment. We will review examples of treatment for specific alexia syndromes that were shown to be effective in well-controlled, single-subject research studies. (See Table 260.5 for overview.) These case studies serve to illustrate how an understanding of the cognitive model of reading helps to guide treatment. It should be apparent from these clinical examples that behavioral treatment can improve different functional components of the reading process, and that the therapeutic principles outlined here are also applicable for treating patients with reading disorders that do not strictly conform to the alexia syndromes described earlier.

Treatment for peripheral alexia

Treatments for pure alexia are directed toward improving access to the orthographic input lexicon

Table 260.5 Selected treatment goals, approaches, and tasks for peripheral and central alexia syndromes

Alexia syndrome	Reading procedures impaired	Reading procedures utilized	Treatment		
			Potential goals	Example approaches	Example tasks
Pure alexia	Visual identification of letters or access to orthographic input lexicon	Serial processing of component letters	Improve letter recognition	Cross modality cueing (e.g. tactile input)	Trace letters with finger to decode words
			Improve word recognition	Multiple oral re-reading	Read selected passage repeatedly to increase reading rate
Surface dyslexia	Lexical-semantic reading route	Non-lexical reading route	Strengthen lexical-semantic reading route	Restore damaged orthographic representations and links to semantics	Repeated drill on association between written word and meaning
			Improve function of non-lexical reading route	Train specific letter-to-sound correspondences	Establish key word for each letter to facilitate correct sound association
Phonological/ deep dyslexia	Non-lexical reading route and lexical-semantic reading route (deep dyslexia)	Lexical-semantic reading route	Improve function of non-lexical reading route	Train use of letter-to-sound correspondences	Establish key word for each letter to assist in deriving sound from letter
			Strengthen lexical-semantic reading route	Strengthen link between written word and semantics	Repeated drill to re-establish link from word to meaning
				Strengthen semantic processing	Semantic treatment to clarify word meanings
				Improve access to phonology	Hierarchical cueing to elicit correct oral reading

and/or compensating for the impaired visual identifi-cation of letters. As mentioned above, a letter-by-letter reading approach is often spontaneously adopted by patients with this disorder and provides a useful compensatory strategy despite the fact that it results in a slow reading rate. Nevertheless, in the relatively acute stage of pure alexia, it may be neces-sary to guide the patient to employ the letter-by-letter reading strategy in order to provide an immediate means to decode written information. This can be accomplished by asking the patient to name the component letters of a word in sequence and attempt to identify the orally spelled word. Subsequent treat-ment plans are made on an individual basis, taking into account the nature of the underlying deficit. Treatment approaches that have been shown to be effective for improving reading speed and accuracy in pure alexia are summarized below.

Cross modality cueing   In some instances, letter identification is significantly impaired so that letter-by-letter decoding is ineffective. In such cases, pro-viding letter shape information via a non-visual modality may facilitate letter identification. For example, some patients can recognize letters when they are traced on their palm, or when they trace or copy the letters themselves.[41] It is assumed that letter recognition based on tactile/kinesthetic information allows access to the orthographic input lexicon that substitutes for activation of the lexicon via visual input. Maher et al.,[42] reported on the effectiveness of this type of cross-modality cueing for a patient with chronic pure alexia. Although the patient could not visually recognize letters or words, she was able to name letters in sequence after she traced each with her finger. A treatment protocol designed to take advantage of this residual skill resulted in improved word recognition and increased reading rate. Ulti-mately the patient showed improved letter recogni-tion so that every letter did not need to be traced, but simply tracing the first letter or two was sufficient to cue word identification.

Multiple oral re-reading   As indicated, letter-by-letter reading provides a serviceable, albeit slow, reading approach for patients with pure alexia so that improvement in reading rate is typically desired. Several researchers have documented the efficacy of an approach to improve reading rate in letter-by-letter readers using a strategy that employs repeated oral reading of text.[43–45] The treatment procedure, referred to as multiple oral re-reading (MOR), is intended to facilitate whole-word rather than letter-by-letter reading. The protocol is heavily dependent upon the patient's accomplishment of daily repeated oral reading as homework, which should result in signific-antly increased reading rate for the practiced text. Repeated reading of the same text appears to facilitate a shift from letter-by-letter reading to whole-word recognition because of clues provided by sentence context and familiarity with the text. Multiple oral re-reading is effective when the improvement in prac-ticed text facilitates reading rate for new (i.e. previ-ously unread) text. However, in some cases a word-length effect persists despite improved reading rate, suggesting that the serial letter identification strategy has not been completely abandoned.[43]

Brief exposure procedure   Another treatment approach for pure alexia involves the presentation of written words for brief exposures so that explicit letter-by-letter reading is not possible. The motivation for this treatment came from the observation that some individuals with pure alexia retain an ability to derive some implicit lexical-semantic information from words that they cannot explicitly identify.[10] Over-reliance on a letter-by-letter reading strategy in these patients may actually be counterproductive as it may interfere with implicit word recognition. Based on these findings, Rothi and Moss[46] devised a treat-ment protocol in which single words were presented on a computer screen for brief exposures (e.g., 500 msec) and the patient was asked to make a decision about the word, for example, "Is it an animal?" Although the patient often indicated that he had not actually read the word, he was encouraged to guess. Response accuracy was above chance indicat-ing some ability to apprehend the whole word at an implicit level. This brief exposure procedure resulted in improved reading rate in Rothi and Moss's patient, suggesting that it facilitated recovery of explicit whole-word reading. However, Rothi and col-leagues[42,47] reported failure of this treatment approach with two other patients, suggesting that it may be useful only for a subset of individuals with pure alexia.

Treatment for central alexias

Treatment approaches for central alexias can be dichotomized into those directed toward strengthen-ing the lexical-semantic route and those intended to improve compensatory use of the non-lexical reading route. Treatments designed to improve reading by the lexical-semantic route may focus on restoring damaged orthographic representations, reinforcing the link between orthographic representations and semantics, strengthening semantic representations themselves, or improving access to the phonological output lexicon. The lexical-semantic reading route may be supplemented by non-lexical reading strat-egies that employ grapheme-phoneme conversion. We will review some of the documented treatment approaches in the context of the major central alexia syndromes discussed earlier: surface dyslexia and phonological/deep dyslexia.

Treatment for surface dyslexia   Surface dyslexia is characterized by damage to the lexical-semantic reading route with over-reliance on the non-lexical route. It follows that treatment for surface dyslexia should be directed toward the restoration of lexical-semantic reading procedures to more closely approxi-mate a normal reading pattern. There may be a need to provide item-specific treatment to resolve difficulties that result from the use of a non-lexical reading strategy, such as homophone comprehension errors. In some cases, it may also be appropriate to facilitate better use of the non-lexical reading route as a compensatory strategy for the lexical-semantic impairment. Each of these approaches has been shown to benefit individuals with surface dyslexia.

- *Restoring damaged orthographic representations*
  Surface dyslexic reading in some patients is attributable to damage to the orthographic input lexicon. Due to the degradation of orthographic memory, words that were once familiar now appear unfamiliar and are therefore read by a non-lexical strategy. Patients with dysfunction at the level of the orthographic input lexicon may benefit from treatment approaches designed to strengthen damaged orthographic representations. An adaptation of the brief exposure procedure described by Rothi and Moss[46] for pure alexia treatment was used by Hillis[48] to facilitate processing at the level of the orthographic input lexicon rather than reliance on the non-lexical reading route in a patient with surface dyslexia. The treatment protocol involved presentation of words and non-words for 200 msec durations and required oral reading of real words only, with corrective feedback provided. The procedure resulted in improved oral reading of targeted words, as well as improved accuracy in rapidly distinguishing trained words from non-words, suggesting a strengthening of specific orthographic representations.

- *Strengthening orthographic-semantic associations*
  In some patients with surface dyslexia, the difficulty involves gaining access to semantic representations from visual input. Alternatively, the reading disorder may be attributable to the degradation of semantic representations themselves. In these cases, the activation of representations in the orthographic input lexicon does not result in access to meaning, and treatment should be directed toward strengthening links between orthography and semantics. Several treatment approaches have shown that repeated pairing of target words and their semantic representations (with corrective feedback) serves to improve reading of those words in individuals with surface dyslexia. For example, Coltheart and Byng[49] documented an effective treatment in which irregularly spelled words were presented in association with pictures or symbolic cues to denote their correct meaning (e.g., a tree branch associated with "bough," or a picture of "Big Ben" as a mnemonic for [British] "government"). Treatment resulted in improved reading of targeted words as well as some generalization to untrained words.[49,50] This generalization was thought to reflect an overall improvement of the lexical-semantic reading route in addition to item-specific learning.

- *Homophone training*
  Treatment for surface dyslexia may also be directed toward specific difficulties that arise from

over-reliance on the non-lexical reading route. For instance, treatment may be designed to tackle the problem with comprehension of homophonic words (e.g., "dear" and "deer"). Homophones have identical sound but they are spelled differently and have different meanings. In surface dyslexia, reading comprehension is based on the oral reading response (i.e., the phonological representation derived from the written word by the application of grapheme-phoneme conversion rules) rather than on direct access to semantics from the orthographic input lexicon. As a result of this sound-based reading strategy, patients cannot distinguish the meaning of homophonic words reliably and may define the written word "dear" as "an animal that lives in the forest." Homophones may be specifically targeted for treatment via the lexical-semantic reading route. For instance, Scott and Byng[51] demonstrated improved comprehension of homophonic words in surface dyslexia using a treatment protocol that required selection of the appropriate written homophone to complete a sentence with feedback provided about the correctness of the patient's response. A similar approach was described by Hillis.[48] The treatment protocol included the presentation of target words in print along with their written definition, and the patient was required to write the target word in a sentence. Hillis showed that the repeated pairing of the orthographic word form with semantic information provided by the sentence context served to strengthen the ability to read via the lexical-semantic route. Generalization occurred so that training one word of a homophonic pair resulted in mastery of the other member of the pair, thus improving the patient's ability to disambiguate homophones.

- *Enhancing use of the non-lexical reading route*
  In addition to treatments directed toward the lexical-semantic reading route, some individuals with surface dyslexia may benefit from treatment to enhance compensatory use of non-lexical reading procedures. Although reliance on the non-lexical reading route is expected to result in regularization errors for irregularly spelled words, the strategy is useful for decoding regularly spelled words and may provide partial phonological information to assist reading via the lexical-semantic route. Hillis[48] documented the value of such an approach to facilitate more consistent application of grapheme-phoneme conversion rules in a surface dyslexic. The procedure, similar to that used by dePartz[52] with a deep dyslexic patient (see below), employed the use of "key words" that were mastered by the patient and served to cue pronunciation of graphemes and grapheme combinations. For example, pronunciation of the digraph *oa* was cued by the key word "boat." The treatment program resulted in improved reading accuracy for trained words and also for untrained regular and irregular words. The improvement for irregular words suggests that partial phonological

information generated by grapheme-phoneme conversion may be sufficient to cue word recognition and facilitate reading via the lexical-semantic route.

Treatment for phonological/deep dyslexia Phonological and deep dyslexia are characterized by severe impairment of the non-lexical reading route, so that reading is accomplished via a lexical-semantic strategy. Although the lexical-semantic route is relatively preserved in phonological dyslexia, in deep dyslexia there is additional damage to the lexical-semantic reading procedure resulting in frequent semantic errors. Treatments directed toward strengthening the non-lexical reading route have been shown to be effective in both phonological and deep dyslexia. Additional treatments to stabilize the lexical-semantic route are indicated in patients with deep dyslexia in order to reduce or eliminate semantic errors. Semantic errors in oral reading may arise from damage to any of the components of the lexical-semantic reading route,[18] so that treatment may need to be directed specifically toward facilitating the transmission of information between the orthographic input lexicon and the semantic system, strengthening semantic representations, or improving access to the phonological output lexicon.

- *Strengthening the non-lexical reading route*
  Treatment directed toward improving the use of grapheme-phoneme correspondence rules in reading has the potential to provide the patient with a compensatory strategy that has general applicability rather than being limited to the specific set of words targeted during treatment. The ability to derive phonology from print by a non-lexical procedure may also assist reading via the lexical-semantic route and may play an especially important role in processing linguistic items that have relatively impoverished semantic representations (e.g., abstract words, functors). Finally, phonological information generated via the non-lexical reading route may be sufficient to block semantic errors in oral reading. Several case reports document success in retraining grapheme-phoneme correspondence rules to increase the availability and effectiveness of the non-lexical reading route in patients with phonological/deep dyslexia.[52,53] Given the severe impairment of the non-lexical route in these individuals, it may be necessary to establish a corpus of key words that the patient can read successfully and use to self-cue grapheme-phoneme conversion. For example, if the patient can consistently read the name "Kim" then this may be the key word to cue the retrieval of phoneme /k/ from the grapheme *k*. The key word can then be used to self-cue /k/ in words the patient has difficulty reading. Because the predictability of grapheme-phoneme correspondences is stronger for consonants than vowels, it is typically most effective to first establish key words for consonants. Treatment directed toward mastery of grapheme-phoneme correspondences and sub-

sequent phonemic blending has been shown to improve reading for non-words as well as real words in a patient with deep dyslexia.[52] In a similar vein, Nickels[53] showed that even though her patient was not able to perform phonemic blending to sound out words fully, retrieval of the initial phoneme was sufficient to self-cue oral reading. These observations suggest that the benefits of treatment to strengthen the non-lexical reading procedure are maximized by interaction with residual lexical-semantic reading abilities.[54] There is evidence that patients with phonological/deep dyslexia may benefit from treatments designed to improve phonological skills. Using a procedure shown to be effective with developmental reading disorders, Conway et al.,[55] implemented a treatment program in an individual with acquired phonological dyslexia that included a sequence of tasks progressing from oral awareness training to reading and spelling of multisyllabic words. The oral awareness training focused on knowledge of the placement and manner of articulation for phonemes and syllables. This treatment protocol served to strengthen their patient's general phonological abilities in addition to improving his reading (and spelling) for trained and untrained non-words and real words. The favorable response to this comprehensive treatment approach appears consistent with the view that phonological dyslexia reflects a general impairment of phonological processing rather than a phonological deficit that is specific to reading.[56]

- *Strengthening semantic processing*
  In cases of deep dyslexia, treatment may be warranted to reinforce the link between orthographic and semantic representations, or to strengthen semantic representations themselves. Hillis and Caramazza[57] described a treatment hierarchy that served to clarify semantic representations for a patient who made semantic errors on reading comprehension as well as spoken and written naming tasks. The treatment procedure involved selecting the appropriate picture to correspond to written words, along with correction of incorrect responses. The treatment resulted in improved reading comprehension of words that were trained, as well as improved oral and written naming for treated items. The general improvement across modalities confirmed the central semantic locus of the impairment and suggested that the treatment served to restore damaged semantic representations in addition to strengthening the link between the orthographic input lexicon and the semantic system. Similar generalization has been observed in cases where semantic treatment for written naming resulted in improved oral naming and reading comprehension.[58]

- *Improving access to the phonological output lexicon*
  In some patients, semantic errors in oral reading reflect a failure to activate the correct representation in the phonological output lexicon. Central semantic processing in these patients may be

preserved, as evidenced by good auditory and written word comprehension and by the absence of semantic errors in writing. Hillis and Caramazza[57] reported on the treatment for such a patient using a cued oral reading procedure. Treatment involved oral reading of target words with a phonemic cueing hierarchy to achieve correct production, and word repetition to stabilize correct productions. Treatment was successful in improving oral reading, as well as oral naming, for target words. The fact that oral naming improved as oral reading was treated confirmed the locus of damage to the phonological output lexicon that is common to both tasks. Hillis and Caramazza[57] suggested that the oral reading treatment lowered the activation threshold for targeted items in the phonological output lexicon as a consequence of the increased frequency of production in the training context.

Treatment of agraphia

Agraphia treatment is somewhat analogous to that described for the treatment of acquired alexia in that it may target the central or peripheral components of the writing process. Treatments for central agraphias may be directed toward the lexical-semantic or non-lexical spelling routes, or the graphemic buffer (as summarized in Table 260.6). In contrast, treatments for peripheral agraphias are designed to improve the selection and implementation of graphic motor programs for handwriting.

Treatment for central agraphias

Central agraphia syndromes include lexical (or surface) agraphia, phonological/deep agraphia, and graphemic buffer agraphia. In the following sections we will illustrate treatment approaches for each of these syndromes, with the understanding that clinical practice may require modifying the treatment protocol to suit the needs of the individual patient.

Treatment for lexical agraphia Lexical agraphia reflects damage to the lexical-semantic spelling route with over-reliance on non-lexical spelling procedures (i.e., phoneme-grapheme conversion). Spelling words as they sound is a useful compensatory strategy, but it results in phonologically plausible errors for irregular words. In addition, the loss of semantic influence on spelling creates difficulties in writing homophonic words that cannot be spelled correctly by direct phonological-to-orthographic conversion (i.e., without reference to the word's meaning). Therefore, treatment for lexical agraphia may be directed toward improving the spelling of irregular words and homophones by strengthening word-specific links between the semantic system and the orthographic output lexicon. Treatments may also be directed toward restoring damaged orthographic representations.

- *Strengthening semantic-orthographic associations*
  Patients with lexical agraphia can re-learn irregular spellings in an item-specific manner. For example, Behrmann and Byng[59] described a treatment

approach that employed a word-to-picture matching task supplemented by repeated copying and writing to dictation to improve spelling for targeted words. They also included homework that involved looking up target words in the dictionary and copying their spelling and definitions—a task designed to reinforce the link between semantic and orthographic representations. This treatment resulted in stabilized improvement in spelling trained words, as well as some generalization to untrained irregularly spelled words. The generalization appeared to reflect use of a lexical checking strategy to assess spelling accuracy and self-correct errors. The protocol was also effective for strengthening semantic-orthographic links for targeted homophones, so that spelling improved for trained and untrained members of homophonic pairs.[60]

- *Restoring damaged orthographic representations*
  Patients with lexical agraphia may be able to abandon non-lexical spelling strategies as representations in the orthographic output lexicon are restored. Numerous case reports demonstrate the value of treatments designed to strengthen specific orthographic representations for writing.[61–64] These treatments typically include hierarchically ordered tasks such as arrangement of component letters (i.e., anagram task) as well as direct and delayed copying of target words. The critical component of these treatment protocols is repeated, corrected spelling of the targeted words, resulting in item-specific mastery of spelling. The re-training of orthography usually takes place in the presence of pictured stimuli or in response to semantic information about the word, so that the link between semantics and restored orthographic representations is also strengthened.

Treatment for phonological/deep agraphia In phonological and deep agraphia, the non-lexical spelling route is severely impaired and spelling is accomplished primarily via a lexical-semantic strategy. Therefore, treatment in these disorders may be directed toward improving the availability and use of non-lexical spelling procedures. In deep agraphia, additional treatment is required to restore the dysfunctional lexical-semantic spelling route in order to eliminate semantic errors.

- *Strengthening the non-lexical spelling route*
  Re-establishing phoneme-to-grapheme conversion skills allows patients to generate plausible spellings for a variety of words. Partial orthographic information derived by the application of sound-to-letter correspondences can also serve to cue the retrieval of word-specific spellings from the orthographic output lexicon.[54] Finally, non-lexical spelling procedures may help constrain the output of the unstable lexical-semantic spelling route thus reducing the potential for semantic errors. Several case reports have documented success in retraining sound-to-letter correspondences to facilitate spelling via the non-lexical route in individuals

Table 260.6   Selected treatment goals, approaches, and tasks for central agraphia syndromes

Agraphia syndrome	Spelling procedures impaired	Spelling procedures utilized	Treatment Potential goals	Example approaches	Example tasks
Lexical (or surface) agraphia	Lexical-semantic spelling route	Non-lexical spelling route (phoneme-grapheme conversion)	Strengthen semantic-orthographic associations	Item-specific training	Word-to-picture matching followed by copy and writing to dictation
			Restore damaged orthographic representations	Item-specific training	Arrange component letters of word followed by direct and delayed copy
Phonological/ deep agraphia	Non-lexical spelling route & lexical-semantic spelling route (deep agraphia)	Lexical-semantic spelling route	Strengthen non-lexical spelling route	Retrain sound-to-letter correspondences	Establish key words to derive orthography from phonology
			Strengthen semantic processing	Semantic specification treatment for errors	Clarify semantic distinctions between target words and semantically related errors
			Improve access to orthographic output lexicon	Cueing hierarchy for written naming	Arrangement of component letters, repeated copy, and delayed recall of spellings
Graphemic buffer agraphia	Graphemic buffer	Lexical-semantic and non-lexical spelling route	Strengthen lexical-semantic spelling route	Cueing hierarchy for written naming	Arrangement of component letters, repeated copy, and delayed recall of spellings
				Error detection training	Visual inspection of spelling and sounding out of words to detect errors

with phonological/deep agraphia.[57,65,66] The treatments are analogous to the procedures used for strengthening the non-lexical route for reading in phonological/deep dyslexia.[48,52,53] That is, just as "key words" can be used to derive phonology from orthography, a corpus of key words can be used to derive orthography from phonology. Using this key word procedure, a deep agraphic patient reported by Hillis and Caramazza[57] was able to derive the first letter or two of words that could not be spelled via the lexical-semantic route; this information served to cue her retrieval of word-specific spellings and to block semantic errors in writing. Another deep agraphic patient who received treatment to strengthen phoneme-grapheme associations was subsequently able to type phonologically plausible spellings into a portable computer that provided synthesized speech for communication.[66] A variation of the key word procedure was described by Carlomagno and Parlato[67] who trained a patient with severe impairment of the non-lexical spelling route to use a corpus of preserved proper nouns to retrieve the spelling of consonant-vowel syllables. Using this lexical relay strategy, the patient was able to derive the spelling of untrained words, one syllable at a time. The lexical relay procedure has also been used to improve the spelling of items from grammatical categories that typically pose difficulties for patients with phonological/deep agraphia. For instance, Hatfield[68] used content words that could be spelled correctly by her deep agraphic patient to cue the spelling of orthographically similar function words (e.g., bean–been).

- *Strengthening semantic processing*
  When semantic errors in writing result from damage to the semantic system, patients may benefit from treatment programs designed to restore semantic representations. For example, Hillis[58] reported a patient who had a persistent impairment of her semantic system so that semantic errors were prominent in written naming and writing to dictation, as well as in oral naming, repetition, and spoken and written word comprehension. A treatment procedure was implemented to clarify the semantic distinctions between target words and semantically-related errors. When semantic errors were made on a written naming task, corrective feedback was offered that highlighted distinctive features of the target in contrast to other members of the semantic category. Treatment served to reduce semantic errors in written naming and writing to dictation, and it also resulted in improved oral naming and written and spoken comprehension of trained items. Generalization was also observed for untrained items in the same semantic category, suggesting that treatment served to enrich semantic representations and allow for more accurate distinctions among items in the treated categories.

- *Improving access to the orthographic output lexicon*
  In some patients with deep agraphia, semantic

errors reflect faulty transmission of information between the semantic system and the orthographic output lexicon. Treatment to strengthen the link between semantic and orthographic representations in these patients may serve to eliminate semantic errors. Hillis[69] demonstrated the efficacy of a cueing hierarchy for written naming of pictured stimuli that included tasks such as arrangement of component letters (i.e., anagram task) and delayed copying of target words. This procedure resulted in improved written naming of targeted items, as well as generalization to untrained items in the same semantic category, suggesting that the orthographic treatment served to strengthen semantic representations in addition to reinforcing functional links between the semantic system and the orthographic output lexicon. Similar procedures have been shown to be effective for rebuilding or strengthening the orthographic representations themselves.[62]

Treatment for graphemic buffer agraphia When orthographic representations are not adequately retained in the graphemic buffer, spelling accuracy notably declines as word length increases. Several treatment reports indicate that as specific orthographic representations are strengthened, the word-length effect dissipates for trained words.[65,69] It appears that improved spelling results from strengthening central spelling processes so that representations are less subject to decay, thus allowing adequate time for peripheral writing processes to be accomplished. Therefore, the approaches for strengthening orthographic representations that were described above are considered appropriate for the treatment of graphemic buffer agraphia. Another approach to compensate for the apparent decay of orthographic representations employs the training of self-directed strategies to detect and correct spelling errors. Such an approach was shown to be effective for a patient with agraphia due to impairment of the graphemic buffer.[63] The patient was trained to use a search strategy to detect errors (which mostly occurred at the ends of words), and to sound out each word as it was written to call attention to phonologically implausible misspellings. The patient was responsive to this treatment so that he ultimately improved his ability to self-correct his spelling in written narratives.

Treatment for peripheral agraphias

Peripheral agraphia syndromes include allographic disorders, apraxic agraphia, and non-apraxic disorders of neuromuscular execution. When central spelling processes are intact, it may be possible to circumvent handwriting difficulties by using a keyboard for written communication. In other patients, treatments may be specifically directed toward the various functional components involved in the motor control of handwriting movements (Figure 260.1).

Treatment for allographic disorders Damage to the allographic conversion process may result in impaired selection or production of letter shapes in handwriting in the presence of preserved oral spelling. A strategy whereby the patient self-dictates each letter has been shown to be effective to overcome the writing deficit.[70,71] An alphabet card may be used to assist the patient when a model is needed for letter shapes, and spelling may be checked one letter at a time as the word is orally spelled several times. Use of the self-dictation strategy has the potential of generalization so that written spelling improved for both trained and untrained words.[70,71]

Treatment for impaired graphomotor control   Treatments for apraxic agraphia have not been well documented in the literature. Given that copying skills may be relatively preserved, we suggest that treatment should include repeated direct and delayed copy tasks to re-establish the ability to write letters and words. A task hierarchy should initially include slow, deliberate, and feedback-dependent writing to regain graphomotor control, followed by repeated tasks to improve the automaticity of motor execution.

There has been some work reported relative to treatment for micrographia in patients with Parkinson's disease.[72] An increase in letter size was accomplished by the provision of parallel lines or a template to facilitate the re-calibration of the range and force of movements necessary to implement handwriting. The fading of external cues requires continuous monitoring of writing movements in order to maintain normal letter size, which can be accomplished by the verbal reminder to "write big."[72]

Many individuals with acquired agraphia also have hemiparesis affecting their ability to write with the dominant hand, so they must shift to writing with the non-dominant hand. Writing with the non-dominant hand can be mastered with practice, however, several investigators have reported on the use of various prosthetic devices to support the paralyzed right hand during writing. A particularly intriguing finding has been that writing produced with the aided hemiparetic right hand was linguistically superior to that written with the non-dominant left hand.[73–75] The writing prostheses have not gained widespread use to date, and the mechanisms underlying this phenomenon have been a matter of discussion and debate.[76,77]

Conclusions

In this chapter, we sought to present a theoretical framework for understanding neurological disorders of reading and writing, to suggest procedures for diagnostic assessment, and to provide a sample of clinically proven treatments for specific alexia and agraphia syndromes. In general, the treatment approaches considered here have focused on strengthening damaged components of the reading or writing process (i.e., restitution), as well as developing alternative or compensatory strategies to circumvent the impairment (i.e., substitution). It should be apparent from our review that some treatments may be effective for patients with different clinical profiles.

For example, treatment directed toward restoring the use of the lexical-semantic reading route may benefit both patients with surface and deep dyslexia. In addition, research has shown that patients who appear to have similar functional deficits may respond differently to the same treatment.[57] Therefore, although we advocate the use of a cognitive approach to determine the locus of impairment and direct treatment planning, we acknowledge that current understanding of cognitive processes and the effects of rehabilitation are inadequate for alexia and agraphia treatment to be prescriptive in any strict sense. In clinical practice, a patient's response to treatment may further clarify the nature of the reading or writing impairment and serves to guide the next stage of treatment.

We have not provided specific guidelines regarding the optimal time for intervention, the frequency or duration of treatment, or specific prognostic factors. These issues are highly dependent upon the individual patient, but we can offer some guidance based upon our review of the literature and our own clinical experience. First, it is noteworthy that most treatment studies for acquired alexia or agraphia were implemented with individuals who were considered to be neurologically stable and were a year or more post onset of the disorder. This argues against the notion that significant changes can only be accomplished during acute or sub-acute stages of recovery. In fact, it is our experience that even chronic patients can continue to achieve functional gains in reading and writing, given the proper guidance to take advantage of residual skills and develop new strategies. Such services are typically available from speech-language pathologists who specialize in neurological communication disorders.

With regard to the frequency of treatment, there appears to be considerable variability in treatment schedules—ranging from twice daily to once-a-week or even biweekly. We suggest that daily practice is essential for bringing about enduring changes in reading or writing; however, the implementation of treatment protocols with well-prescribed homework may require only weekly oversight by the therapist once they are established. Treatment sessions are necessary to determine the patient's responsiveness to a given protocol, to make adjustments as needed, and to plan subsequent phases of treatment. It is not uncommon for several treatment phases to be implemented in sequence so that improved skills are incorporated into successive treatment stages. In this way, progressive approximation of normal reading and writing processes is maximized, and appropriate strategic compensations are established. When a patient fails to respond to treatment, the therapist must determine if an alternative treatment approach is warranted, or whether further gains are not likely to be achieved. In most cases, responsiveness to treatment is typically discernable within several weeks.

Finally, the likelihood that a patient will respond to a given treatment is based upon a number of factors including the severity of the deficit, the status of the impaired and residual abilities, the nature of the neurological illness, as well as the patient's motivation. However, such information is far from adequate to truly predict treatment outcomes. For that reason, prognostic statements should be regarded as testable hypotheses that should be continually re-evaluated based upon a patient's actual response to treatment.

In closing, we wish to emphasize that our current understanding of acquired alexia and agraphia is likely to be informed and modified by future advances in areas such as neuroimaging, pharmacotherapy, and computational modeling. We anticipate that continued refinement of treatment approaches will result as we gain better insights into the cognitive processes that support reading and writing, as well as the neurobiological mechanisms of recovery following brain damage.

Acknowledgments

This work was supported in part by National Multipurpose Research & Training Center Grant DC-01409 from the National Institute on Deafness and Other Communication Disorders to The University of Arizona, and by the Cummings Foundation Endowment to the Department of Neurology at the University of Arizona.

References

1. Déjerine J. Sur un cas de cécité verbale avec agraphie, suivi d'autopsie. Mém Soc Biol 1891;3:197–201
2. Déjerine J. Contribution a l'etude anatomo-pathologique et clinique des differentes varietes de cecite verbale. Mém Soc Biol 1892;4:61–90
3. Ellis AW. Spelling and writing (and reading and speaking). In: Ellis AW, ed. Normality and pathology in cognitive functions. London: Academic Press, 1982:113–146
4. Ellis AW. Normal writing processes and peripheral acquired dysgraphias. Language and Cognitive Processes 1988;3:99–127
5. Shallice T, Warrington EK. Single and multiple component central dyslexic syndromes. In: Coltheart M, Patterson, K, Marshall JC, eds. Deep dyslexia. London: Routledge & Kegan Paul, 1980:119–145
6. Coltheart M, ed. Pure alexia: letter-by-letter reading. Hove, UK: Psychology Press, 1998
7. Patterson K, Kay K. Letter-by-letter reading: psychological descriptions of a neurological syndrome. Quarterly Journal of Experimental Psychology 1982;34A:411–441
8. Damasio AR, Damasio H. The anatomic basis of pure alexia. Neurology 1983;33:1573–1583
9. Black SE, Behrmann M. Localization in alexia. In: Kertesz A, ed. Localization and neuroimaging in neuropsychology. San Diego: Academic Press, 1994: 331–376
10. Saffran, EM, Coslett, HB. Implicit vs. letter-by-letter reading: a tale of two systems. Cognitive Neuropsychology 1998;15:141–165
11. Patterson KE, Marshall JC, Coltheart M. Surface dyslexia: neuropsychological and cognitive studies of phonological reading. London: Lawrence Erlbaum, 1985
12. Beauvois MF, Dérousné J. Phonological alexia: three dissociations. Journal of Neurology, Neurosurgery, and Psychiatry 1979;42:1115–1124
13. Coltheart M, Patterson K, Marshall JC, eds. Deep dyslexia. London: Routledge & Kegan Paul, 1980
14. Vanier M, Caplan, D. CT correlates of surface dyslexia. In: Patterson KE, Marshall JC, Coltheart M, eds. Surface dyslexia: neuropsychological and cognitive studies of phonological reading. London: Lawrence Erlbaum, 1985:511–525
15. Friedman RF, Ween JE, Albert ML. Alexia. In: Heilman KM, Valenstein E, eds. Clinical neuropsychology. 3rd ed. New York: Oxford University Press, 1993:37–62
16. Patterson KE, Graham N, Hodges JR. Reading in dementia of the Alzheimer type: a preserved ability? Neuropsychology 1994;8:395–407
17. Patterson K, Hodges JR. Deterioration of word meaning: implications for reading. Neuropsychologia 1992;30:1025–1040
18. Hillis AE, Caramazza A. Where do semantic errors come from? Cortex 1990;26:95–122
19. Marin OSM. CAT scans of five deep dyslexic patients. In: Coltheart M, Patterson, K, Marshall JC, eds. Deep dyslexia. London: Routledge & Kegan Paul, 1980:407–411
20. Coltheart M. Deep dyslexia: a right-hemisphere hypothesis. In: Coltheart M, Patterson, K, Marshall JC, eds. Deep dyslexia. London: Routledge & Kegan Paul, 1980:326–380
21. Beauvois M-F, Derousné J. Lexical or orthographic agraphia. Brain 1981;104:21–49
22. Shallice T. Phonological agraphia and the lexical route in writing. Brain 1981;104:413–429
23. Bub D, Kertesz A. Deep agraphia. Brain and Language 1982;17:146–165
24. Caramazza A, Miceli G, Villa G, Romani C. The role of the graphemic buffer in spelling: evidence from a case of acquired dysgraphia. Cognition 1987;26:59–85
25. Roeltgen DP. Agraphia. In: Heilman KM, Valenstein E, eds. Clinical neuropsychology. 3rd ed. New York: Oxford University Press, 1993:63–89
26. Rapcsak SZ, Beeson PM. Neuroanatomical correlates of spelling and writing. In: Hillis AE, ed. Handbook on adult language disorders: integrating cognitive neuropsychology, neurology, and rehabilitation. Philadelphia: Psychology Press, 2002:71–99
27. Rapcsak SZ, Arthur SA, Bliklen DA, Rubens AB. Lexical agraphia in Alzheimer's disease. Archives of Neurology 1989;46:65–68
28. Peniello MJ, Lambert J, Eustache F, et al. A PET study of the functional neuroanatomy of writing impairment in Alzheimer's disease: the role of the left supramarginal and angular gyri. Brain 1995;118:697–707
29. Graham NL, Patterson K, Hodges JR. The impact of semantic memory impairment on spelling: evidence from semantic dementia. Neuropsychologia 2000;38:143–163
30. Rapcsak SZ, Beeson PM, Rubens AB. Writing with the right hemisphere. Brain and Language 1991;41:510–530
31. Rapcsak SZ. Disorders of writing. In: Rothi LJ Gonzalez, Heilman KM, eds. Apraxia: the neuropsychology of action. Hove, UK: Psychology Press, 1997:149–172
32. Alexander MP, Fischer RS, Friedman R. Lesion localization in apractic agraphia. Archives of Neurology 1992;49:246–251
33. Watson RT, Heilman KM. Callosal apraxia. Brain 1983;106:391–403
34. Kertesz A. Western aphasia battery. New York: Grune & Stratton, 1982
35. Goodglass H, Kaplan E. Boston diagnostic examination for aphasia. 2nd ed. Philadelphia: Lea & Febiger, 2000
36. Kay J, Lesser R, Coltheart M. Psycholinguistic assessments of language processing in aphasia (PALPA). Hove, UK: Lawrence Erlbaum Associates, 1992
37. Goodman RA, Caramazza A. The Johns Hopkins University dyslexia and dysgraphia batteries. Published in Beeson PM, Hillis AE, Comprehension and production of written words. In: Chapey R ed. Language inter-

vention strategies in adult aphasia. 4th ed. Baltimore, MD: Lippincott, Williams & Wilkins, 2001:575–595

38. LaPointe LL, Horner J. Reading comprehension battery for aphasia. 2nd ed. Austin: Pro-Ed, 1998

39. Wiederholt JL, Bryant BR. Gray oral reading tests. 3rd ed. (GORT-3). Austin: Pro-Ed, 1992

40. Goodglass H, Kaplan E, Weintraub S. Boston naming test. 2nd ed. Philadelphia: Lea & Febiger, 2000

41. Seki K, Yajima M, Sugishita M. The efficacy of kinesthetic reading treatment for pure alexia. Neuropsychologia 1995;33:595–609

42. Maher LM, Clayton MC, Barrett AM, et al. Rehabilitation of a case of pure alexia: exploiting residual abilities. Journal of the International Neuropsychological Society 1998;4:636–647

43. Beeson PM. Treatment for letter-by-letter reading: a case study. In: Helm-Estabrooks N, Holland AL, eds. Approaches to the treatment of aphasia. San Diego: Singular Press, 1998:153–177

44. Moyer SB. Rehabilitation of alexia: a case study. Cortex 1979;15:139–144

45. Tuomainen J, Lain M. Multiple oral rereading technique on rehabilitation of pure alexia. Aphasiology 1991;5:401–409

46. Rothi LJG, Moss S. Alexia without agraphia: potential for model assisted therapy. Clinical Communication Disorders 1992;2:11–18

47. Rothi LJG, Greenwald M, Maher LM, Ochipa C. Alexia without agraphia: lessons from a treatment failure. In: Helm-Estabrooks N, Holland AL, eds. Approaches to the treatment of aphasia. San Diego: Singular Publishing Group, 1998:179–202

48. Hillis AE. The role of models of language processing in rehabilitation of language impairments. Aphasiology 1993;7:5–26

49. Coltheart M, Byng S. A treatment for surface dyslexia. In: Seron X, Deloche G, eds. Cognitive approaches in neuropsychological rehabilitation. Hillsdale, NJ: Lawrence Erlbaum Associates, 1989:159–174

50. Weekes B, Coltheart M. Surface dyslexia and surface dysgraphia: treatment studies and their theoretical implications. Cognitive Neuropsychology 1996;13:277–315

51. Scott C, Byng S. Computer assisted remediation of a homophone comprehension disorder in surface dyslexia. Aphasiology 1989;3:301–320

52. DePartz MP. Re-education of a deep dyslexic patient: rationale of the method and results. Cognitive Neuropsychology 1986;3:147–177

53. Nickels L. The autocue? Self-generated phonemic cues in the treatment of a disorder of reading and naming. Cognitive Neuropsychology 1992;9:155–182

54. Hillis AE, Caramazza A. Mechanisms for accessing lexical representations for output: evidence from category-specific semantic deficit. Brain & Language 1991;40:106–144

55. Conway TW, Heilman P, Rothi LJG, et al. Treatment of a case of phonological alexia with agraphia using the auditory discrimination in depth (ADD) program. Journal of the International Neuropsychological Society 1998;4:608–620

56. Patterson K, Lambon Ralph, MA. Selective disorders of reading? Current Opinions in Neurobiology 1999;9:235–339

57. Hillis AE, Caramazza A. Theories of lexical processing and rehabilitation of lexical deficits. In: Riddoch MJ, Humphreys GW, eds. Cognitive neuropsychology and cognitive rehabilitation. Hillsdale, NJ: Lawrence Erlbaum Associates, 1994:1–30

58. Hillis AE. Effects of separate treatments for distinct impairments within the naming process. Clinical Aphasiology 1991;19:255–265

59. Behrmann M, Byng S. A cognitive approach to the neuro-rehabilitation of acquired language disorders. In: Margolin DI, ed. Cognitive neuropsychology in clinical practice. New York: Oxford University Press, 1992:327–350

60. Behrmann M. The rites of righting writing: homophone mediation in acquired dysgraphia. Cognitive Neuropsychology 1987;4:365–384

61. Aliminosa D, McCloskey M, Goodman-Schulman R., Sokol, S. Remediation of acquired dysgraphia as a technique for testing interpretations of deficits. Aphasiology 1993;7:55–69

62. Beeson PM. Treating acquired writing impairment. Aphasiology 1999;13:367–386

63. Hillis AE, Caramazza A. Model-driven treatment of dysgraphia. In: Brookshire RH, ed. Clinical aphasiology. Minneapolis: BRK Publishers, 1987;17:84–105

64. Carlomagno S, Iavarone A, Colombo A. Cognitive approaches to writing rehabilitation: from single case to group studies. In Riddoch MJ, Humphreys GW, eds. Cognitive neuropsychology and cognitive rehabilitation. Hillsdale, NJ: Lawrence Erlbaum Associates, 1994:485–502

65. Cardell EA, Cheney HJ. A cognitive neuropsychological approach to the assessment and remediation of acquired dysgraphia. Language Testing 1999;16:353–388

66. Hillis Trupe AE. Effectiveness of retraining phoneme to grapheme conversion. In: Brookshire RH, ed. Clinical aphasiology. Minneapolis: BRK Publishers, 1986;16:163–171

67. Carlomagno S, Parlato V. Writing rehabilitation in brain damaged adult patients: a cognitive approach. In: Seron X, Deloche G, ed. Cognitive approaches in neuropsychological rehabilitation. Hillsdale, NJ: Lawrence Erlbaum Associates, 1989:175–209

68. Hatfield FM. Aspects of acquired dysgraphia and implication for re-education. In: Code C, Muller DJ, eds. Aphasia therapy. London: Edward Arnold, 1983

69. Hillis AE. Efficacy and generalization of treatment for aphasic naming errors. Archives of Physical Medicine and Rehabilitation 1989;70:632–636

70. Pound C. Writing remediation using preserved oral spelling: a case for separate output buffers. Aphasiology 1996;10:283–296

71. Ramage A, Beeson PM, Rapcsak SZ. Dissociation between oral and written spelling: clinical characteristics and possible mechanisms. Presentation at the Clinical Aphasiology Conference, Ashville, NC, June 1998

72. Oliveira RM, Gurd JM, Nixon P, Marshall JC, Passingham RE. Micrographia in Parkinson's disease: the effect of providing external cues. Journal of Neurology, Neurosurgery and Psychiatry 1997;63:429–433

73. Leischner A. Side differences in writing to dictation of aphasics with agraphia: a graphic disconnection syndrome. Brain and Language 1983;18:1–19

74. Brown JW, Leader BJ, Blum CS. Hemiplegic writing in severe aphasia. Brain and Language 1983;19:204–215

75. Lorch MP. Laterality and rehabilitation: differences in left and right hand productions in aphasic agraphic hemiplegics. Aphasiology 1995;9:257–271

76. Goldberg G, Porcelli J. The functional benefits: how much and for whom? Aphasiology 1995;9:274–277

77. Rothi LJ. Are we clarifying or contributing to the confusion? Aphasiology 1995;9:271–273

Treatment of Developmental Language Disorders

Kenneth M Heilman and Ann W Alexander

Introduction

Developmental language disorders are characterized by difficulty in the acquisition of spoken and/or written language in children and adults who hear normally, have normal cognitive ability, have no evidence of neurological damage of the vocal organ, and have adequate language exposure and education.[1]

As early as 1822,[2] Gall described children who had isolated language disorders. Vaisse introduced the term "congenital aphasia" and Liebman in 1898 discussed subtypes of congenital aphasia. According to Leonard,[2] descriptions of linguistic characteristics resulted in a myriad of labels such as "developmental language disorder," "developmental language impairment," "specific language deficit" and "language impairment," "language/learning disabled" or "language/learning impaired."[3] At the present time, the most widely adopted term, especially in the research literature, is "specific language impairment" or "SLI" according to Fey and Leonard.[4] In this chapter SLI will be used to refer to this disorder.

The recognition that developmental dyslexia (DD) was a form of SLI due to a core linguistic deficit in phonological processing has only come to light in the past 25 years. Dyslexia had been described as early as 1896 by Morgan[5] and was thought to be a visual deficit resulting in "word blindness." Morgan also noted a familial aggregation to the disorder. By 1925 Orton[6] was proposing a neural substrate deficit and prescribed multisensory interventions. In the 1970s, the work of Shankweiler, Liberman and Liberman,[7] as well as Vellutino,[8] described the core deficit in phonological processing. Recent findings by Wolf[9–11] suggest that a second core deficit is responsible for inefficient word and text reading—a deficit of time and fluency-related processes operating separately or in tandem with phonological processing.

Judging by the number of labels given to this disorder, it is no wonder the official diagnostic manuals do not even agree (DSM IV, ICD 9CM, and ASHA). In 1992, the American Speech-Language-Hearing Association (ASHA)[12] classified the disorder as "developmental language disorder," placing it in the category of *Communication Disorder*, which describes an impairment in the ability to receive, process, comprehend and send concepts of nonverbal, verbal and/or graphic symbol systems. It may be evident in the processes of hearing, language and/or speech and may range in severity. It may be developmental or acquired. Individuals may demonstrate one or any combination of communication disorders. A communication disorder may result in a primary disability or it may be secondary to other disabilities.

Under this definition there are subcategories of communication disorders: 1) speech disorders (articulation fluency and voice); and 2) language disorders involving at least one of the four subsystems of language (phonology, morphosyntax, semantics, and pragmatics). Phonology, morphology and syntax comprise the *form*, semantics comprises and *content* and pragmatics comprises the communicative *function* of language.

This chapter will review the development of spoken and written language and factors impacting it, as well as the assessments and treatment needed to develop a comprehensive and individualized intervention program for the individual with SLI and DD.

Epidemiology and demographics

Cantwell[13] summarizes studies giving estimates of the prevalence of specific language impairment (SLI) in the general population as ranging from 3% to more than 20%. Shaywitz[14] cites the prevalence rates of developmental dyslexia (DD) as being from 5% to 10% to 17.5%. The literature on SLI reports a predominance in males of 2–3:1, which was felt to be true for DD, but Shaywitz[14] reports that more recent studies are showing equal incidence in both sexes. Longitudinal studies of children with these disorders of spoken or written language reveal a persistent condition that impacts the individual in differing degrees as developmental demands change.[15–17] Once development is complete, however, their measured ability remains relatively constant.[14] Children with these disorders frequently have a strong family history of spoken and/or written language difficulties in parents and siblings, ranging from 24% to as high as 70%.[3,18–20] Histories obtained from questionnaires revealed considerable underreporting in contrast to the findings with direct examination of the family.

Clinical features

The child with SLI presents with the history of delayed emergence and a slower course in the acquisition of language skills. There is a "clumsiness" to language—a concreteness, with less diversity and less flexibility. The systems of language presenting the most difficulty are usually those requiring precise analysis and synthesis of linguistic input, of temporal sequences, of rapidly presented, often low contrast stimuli—the *form* of language: *phonology* and *morphosyntax*.[3] The child has less difficulty with the areas of language in which learning can occur with an associative or more "gestalt" approach—the *meaning* and *use* of language: *semantics* and *pragmatics*. Receptive ability (comprehension) is typically stronger than expressive ability (production) in all the systems.

The course of language development is very dynamic. The child with SLI lags behind with new skill acquisition; he finally acquires it, albeit with compromised quality, only to be challenged once more with a new developmental task. Snowling and colleagues[15] illustrated this in their longitudinal study of 87 4-year-olds with SLI. At 5½ approximately half of the children appeared to have developed normal speech. At age 8½ this group wrote, spelled and read well. However, at age 15 this group was impaired in phonological awareness, performing at the 10-year-old level in non word reading tasks and slightly below the age controls for real word reading and spelling. The group with persistent language difficulties at 5½ continued to have significant spoken language deficits and did not acquire appropriate word reading skills. A third group of children was diagnosed as dyslexic after entering school. While they performed as well as the resolved SLI group on vocabulary and grammar tasks (no discrepancy), and as poorly with phonological awareness and non word reading, they deviated from this group in their ability to read real words (an orthographic task). Thus, when language development is compromised, children seem to take different forks in the road.

Children with SLI often present with nonlinguistic difficulties. Comorbid neuropsychiatric disorders are common, especially attention deficit hyperactivity disorder (ADHD),[21–23] anxiety, depression and conduct disorders.[13] They also may evidence impaired sensory processing of rapidly presented sequential input in auditory, visual, and somatosensory domains;[24] slow reaction times;[25] poor sensorimotor coordination requiring bimanual and/or rhythmic output;[26] poor postural stability and low tone in the upper body, and labored acquisition of skilled motor tasks such as shoe tying and handwriting;[27] difficulty with temporal sequential ordering in short term auditory memory and working memory as well;[28,29] slight impairment in visual function such as binocular vergence control, with inefficient fixation on near targets, and less accurate localization of small dots on a screen; difficulty with recognizing several visual items presented simultaneously; trouble with words "swimming" or jumping around on the page; and trouble with left–right discrimination.[30–33] Badian et al.[34] reported that not only slow color naming, but also finger agnosia were the strongest predictors of DD in kindergarten boys. While not the etiology of the language deficits, these impairments may compound them, further impacting new, more complex skill development.

Diagnosis

The DSM IV[35] (American Psychiatric Association, 1994) of SLI relies on *discrepancy criteria*—there must be a measurable gap between an individual's performance on tests of speech and/or language relative to performance in other areas of cognition.

Problems with this system are the exclusion of written language disorders and the use of discrepancy criteria since there is no evidence that a language-processing deficit presents differently or responds differently in a child with or without a significant discrepancy between IQ and achievement.[36] The DSM IV classification does not describe the language system that is impaired.

The diagnosis of SLI/DD is based on the exclusion of substantial mental retardation, autism, hearing impairment, structural anomalies of the vocal organs, or gross neurological abnormality. Exposure to the child's primary language should be normal. To date there are no diagnostic laboratory tests. Diagnosis is clinical, but periodic assessments are useful since the child's abilities may vary as development progresses.

The diagnosis of SLI might be difficult in the toddler because of the wide variations in development. Toddlers with good comprehension and delayed expressive language have a good chance of developing normal language, but half of them will not.[16] To date there are no definitive determining criteria, but Olswang et al.[37] report that there are factors present in the toddler which would indicate immediate intervention, rather than close monitoring. These factors include: 1) a history of a paucity of babbling with less diversity, fewer consonants, many vowel errors and restricted syllable structure; 2) a six-month language delay and/or a large gap between comprehension and production with a delay in comprehension; 3) a paucity of expressive language and few verbs, mainly transitive; 4) limited use of gestures, especially those that are sequential in nature; 5) limited spontaneous imitation; 6) problems with play and social skills; 7) history of otitis media; 8) extreme parent distress.

Standardized assessments of spoken and written language, cognition, attention, and sensorimotor function including audition and vision are indicated if screening measures are positive and/or spoken or written language impairment is evident. If a phonological processing disorder is discovered, an audiological and otological exam are especially important because recurrent otitis media has been implicated in delaying language development. Phonological processing disorders, however, can be also associated with a central auditory processing disorder. If there is a decline in previously normal language function, an EEG should be obtained to rule out a seizure disorder (Landau–Kleffner Syndrome). Other health disorders such as anemia and exposure to toxin can negatively impact development, although typically in a more global fashion.

When evaluating children with language delays there are symptoms and signs that are suggestive of SLI/DD and not just a maturational lag. These symptoms and signs are listed in Table 261.1.

The preschool child at risk for dyslexia may appear stronger with spoken language skills and is easy to

Table 261.1 Suggestive symptoms and signs

History
Unusual language development
0–2 years: • babbled less with less diversity
• later with words, less diverse, mispronunciations rather than misarticulations
3–5 years: • late with word combinations; tendency to use phrases rather than sentences; particular difficulty with verbs and tenses
• avoids word games, rhymes, books; slow word retrieval for common objects, colors
5–7 years: • continued mispronunciations, especially multisyllable and novel words
• word-finding difficulties; hesitations, circumlocutions
• difficulty with verbal memory, sentence repetition, and story recall
• poor narrative temporo-sequential organization—telling the beginning, middle, end
• trouble acquiring alphabetic code and letter names; learning to read/spell is difficult
8–adult: • reading is slow and inaccurate, despite relatively stronger comprehension
• comprehension is concrete; trouble with inference and abstract concepts
• difficulty with writing—putting thoughts into words, weak mechanics/poor spelling
• test taking difficulties are due to less flexibility with language—ambiguities
• trouble with word problems in math, trouble retrieving math facts

Family history: • spoken or written language deficits/school problems/attention or behavioral problems
Environment: • impoverished language environment/dialect/bilingual home/noisy
Other developmental domains: • behavior is notably inattentive, impulsive, hyperactive or hypoaroused, anxious, oppositional, or depressed
• fine motor difficulties with learning new skills—tying his shoes, writing
• complains that words swim/blur on the page
• mouths objects, stuffs his mouth with food, messy eater/unaware

Physical findings (with the presence of language impairment)
Sensorimotor: • low muscle tone in the upper body, postural instability, mild tremor
• weak somatosensory maps—articulatory, finger
• oral and fine motor sequencing difficulties—awkward pencil grip, graphomotor problems
Speech quality: • hesitations, circumlocutions, mispronunciations, amount is limited
• temporal sequential disorganization on narrative discourse
Attention/behavior: • decreased alertness and arousal, decreased ability to sustain attention and control impulses; slow processing speed

miss. However, the child may evidence phonological processing weaknesses such as trouble with rhyming, learning names of letters, and rapid color naming. These phonological processing weaknesses often go hand and hand with sensorimotor deficits such as poor fine motor sequencing, postural instability, finger agnosia (inability to appreciate where fingers are in relation to each other without visual cues, i.e. weak somatosensory maps of individual fingers). Fawcett and Nicholson have developed two helpful screening instruments, the Dyslexia Early Screening Test (for use with children from 4:6 to 6:5 years of age) and the Dyslexia Screening Test (for use with children from 6:6 to 16 years).[38,39] These screening batteries measure acquisition of knowledge about letter and digit names, as well as sensorimotor measures and phonological processing measures. They are helpful when the child is at risk for dyslexia and exhibits no obvious language delays.

Pathophysiology and pathogenesis

Research in the field of developmental language disorders, particularly dyslexia, over the past 25 years has begun to provide information about the neurobiology of SLI/DD. Zeffiro and Eden[40] summarized this research at both macroscopic and microscopic levels.

Structural abnormalities, seen at a macroscopic level on both MRI and post-mortem studies, involved the perisylvian cortical regions, the thalamus, the corpus callosum and the occipital cortex.

At a microscopic level, Galaburda and colleagues[41,42] described multiple cerebrocortical microdysgeneses, primarily in the left perisylvian regions, including small ectopias and microgyria. While the etiology is felt to be genetic, the type of damage resembles that caused by an autoimmune process.[43] Galaburda and Eidelberg[44] found that magnocellular cells in the lateral medial geniculate nucleus (visual processing) and in the medial geniculate nucleus (auditory processing) were underdeveloped, either in number or structure. No differences were seen in the parvocellular system. The magno system is heavily myelinated. In the visual system it processes transient, low contrast information, in contrast to the parvocellular system which processes sustained, high contrast information. From the thalamus the magno system projects to primary visual cortex and from there to the visual motion area (V5/MT) and then on to the posterior parietal cortex areas, known to be important in detecting position and motion and directing spatial attention. The role of this system in language, however, is unclear.

The majority of functional imaging studies have been conducted in adults with DD and have focused on phonological processing and reading. According to Zeffiro and Eden,[40] their results are consistent with a localization of the principal pathophysiological process to perisylvian cortex, predominantly in the left hemisphere.

Evoked potentials studies demonstrate perceptual processing differences which are present even in the newborn child born to dyslexic families.[45-47] Leppanen and colleagues[45] showed that these infants had slower response to phonetic stimuli and activated the right rather than the left hemisphere, as the controls did. Breznitz[48] reports that ERP studies in adults and children with dyslexia have shown an asynchrony with processing of phonological and orthographic information as well as with auditory and visual information. Less sensitivity (or higher thresholds) for detection of changes in visual and auditory stimuli have also been reported in DD children in contrast to controls.[49]

These studies have demonstrated differences between SLI/DD and normal subjects; however, there is no simple explanation for the various clinical manifestations of the individual with SLI/DD. Whereas the brain is impacted by experience, the structure of the brain is under genetic influence. In the next section we will discuss the genetics of SLI/DD.

Genetics

It would seem that the etiology of SLI is a combination of nature and nurture. It is indeed familial and heritable but, as noted above, almost half of the children have a negative family history. Lahey and Edwards[50] found that the linguistic characteristics do not vary greatly when children with SLI are divided into groups based on the presence or absence of a family history. However, when children are divided by different linguistic characteristics, the family history becomes a differing factor. They found that a positive family history was twice as common in children with only production problems, in contrast to those with both production and comprehension problems (a more severe problem). Byrne, Willermann and Ashmore[51] also noted a stronger family history in the children with less severe language problems.

In 1929, Ley showed evidence of a hereditary basis in a twin study[2]. Subsequent twin studies have reported that 60% of the variance for reading ability can be accounted for on the basis of genetics.[52] Environmental influences are clearly important, but much harder to factor in. Cantwell et al.[13] report that over half of the children with the most severe language difficulties come from families who are disadvantaged. In these cases, there are many increased risk factors to take into account, such as prematurity, as well as impoverished language environments. To date, no research has been able to clarify which factors in the language environment have the greatest impact.

The use of concordance studies of monozygotic (MZ) and dizygotic (DZ) twins has allowed researchers to separate genetic and environmental influences on SLI/DD. More recent studies have also found a significant genetic influence.[20,53,54]

Establishing the chromosomal location of a gene or quantitative trait locus (QTL) for susceptibility to spoken and/or written language difficulties has been made possible with genetic linkage studies. For example, Varga-Khadem et al.[55] studied a family with a history of severe verbal and orofacial dyspraxia with evidence of structural and functional anomalies in both the cortical and subcortical motor-related areas of the frontal lobe and found an abnormal gene in the chromosomal band 7q31. While some studies have reported findings on chromosomes 15 and 1, the most replicated finding is on chromosome 6. The short arm of chromosome 6 has been found to be the site for a susceptibility locus for word reading, phonological awareness, rapid automatized naming, and orthographic coding.[56,57]

The course of spoken language development

As previously stated, language is comprised of four major subsystems. Two are rule governed and deal with the *form* of language (*phonology* and *morphosyntax*), and two are more associative in nature, dealing with the *content/meaning* of language (*semantic*) and with the *communicative function* of language (*pragmatics*). They have a hierarchical order of development, with a specific time line. Each subsystem is linked with and depends on the other for the normal acquisition of language skills. The phonological and pragmatic subsystems begin to develop during the first month of life and are the building blocks that serve as scaffolding for future development. The four subsystems are in place by the age of 3, but continue to grow and become more sophisticated throughout childhood and into adulthood.

While each subsystem is felt to be the result of weighted synaptic connections, forming neural networks unique to its task, there are features common to all: 1) the process of learning and cortical mapping; and 2) the linguistic and nonlinguistic factors which help or hinder these processes.

According to Merzenich et al.,[58] learning is thought to occur in a Hebbian[59] fashion such that inputs occurring nearly simultaneously are linked. This linkage is strengthened with repetition. According to connectionist models, learning alters the strength between synaptic connections and representations are instantiated by the patterns of activation of neuronal networks. Thus, representations are mapped into functional modules in a distinct, fine-grained fashion. Mapping is stronger and more distinct if input is perceptually salient, frequent, predictable, involves multiple sensory processes and is emotionally reinforcing. The more distinct or fine-grained the representation, the more easily it can be accessed and held in working memory for processing the form of language.[60,61] The neural networks have been conceptualized as being more constrained and rule-driven, but the subsystems dealing with concepts might be more associative. Snowling and Nation[62] propose that this perspective could explain the wide variation in the clinical presentations of individuals with SLI/DD.

Language perception and production develop in a

predictable pattern. The child progresses from an associative and global ability to a more specified approach.[63,64] At each level of acquisition, perception–comprehension precedes production–expression. Comprehension might be achieved in a more associative manner, but expression must be more precise. The child with SLI/DD typically experiences more difficulties with language expression, especially in those domains which require the most precision such as phonology and morphosyntax.

Language development requires the interaction between neural structures and environment stimuli. Pinker[65] noted that across languages the components with strong and regular phonology, strong semantic correlates, and high frequency are acquired more easily. The linguistic features without these attributes are acquired more slowly, and the child with SLI has most difficulty learning these features.[2]

Other nonlinguistic factors present "roadblocks" to the development of strong cortical representations. For example, impaired processing of brief, rapidly presented temporal sequences in the auditory, visual and tactile/kinesthetic modalities is thought to result in imperfect representations. Children with auditory processing deficits also have greater difficulty perceiving speech embedded in noise.[66] Similarly, subtle visual perceptual difficulties may compound the core linguistic deficit responsible for most reading difficulties.[31,33] Weak somatosensory representations would be expected to result from the impaired perception of tactile/kinesthetic input. Montgomery[67] reports a lack of awareness of the tactile/kinesthetic features of the articulatory gesture in adult dyslexics. This lack of awareness might weaken the acquisition of precise phonemic representations and interfere with the development of phonological awareness critical in the acquisition of phonological reading skills.[68] Children with SLI/DD have been reported to show slowed response times in all domains, which could create a problem with the time-limited capacity of working memory.[25]

Other important systems integral to the acquisition of new skills are the attention/arousal, working memory and executive function systems, which also have their own developmental course.[61,69] Attention/arousal is necessary to triage sensory input, such that the critical stimuli are fully processed. Working memory is a system for temporarily storing and manipulating the information important in decoding. These temporary holding systems can be either verbal or visual–spatial. The executive system is important in allocating resources needed to develop strategies, organize information and plan action. Executive functions include self-monitoring, intentional control and response inhibition. Finally, long-term goal orientation is an essential executive function.

The development of the phonological system

The phonological system analyzes the speech sounds of the language and develops rules for isolating, selecting, and combining these sounds.

Phonological processing is the core of language function, the building block that provides representations necessary for the normal development of the semantic and syntactic systems. It develops early in infancy. The newborn has been shown to detect the phonetic difference between syllables[70] and by 4 to 6 months infants have demonstrated the ability to accurately link the acoustic with the visual–kinesthetic features of articulatory gestures.[71,72]

Phonemic representations specific to a language require connections between four processes occurring nearly simultaneously: the acoustic components of the sound; the motor components producing the sound (articulatory gesture); the somatosensory component of the articulatory gesture; and the visual component of the articulatory gesture producing the sound.[68,73] They "fire together and wire together" to create a unit, a specific phonemic representation for each sound in the child's language. The bond between the auditory, visual, somatosensory and kinesthetic systems serves as a tool for precise analysis of phonemic patterns and sequences in words, essential to perception and production. Stackhouse and Wells[63] report that between the ages of 6 and 9 months, the baby's first phonological and semantic representations are perceptual "gestalts," with no segmentation. The prosodic (accented syllables/melodic content) features of these bundles are linked with the phonological features. First words are produced as a whole word "gestalt" with only the most salient phonemic and prosodic features. With continued use, the coarticulated features become grouped into phonemes and these phonological representations become more precise and distinct.[63,74]

Distinct phonological representations facilitate the processing of words and groups of words in working memory. The less ambiguous, more fine-grained the representation, the more easily the phonological information can be perceived, retrieved, held in working memory for processing, and produced. Similarly, stronger phonemic representations facilitate the encoding of accurate phonological representations of word parts and whole words.

These distinct and discrete phonemic representations also facilitate the growth of phonological sensitivity and the acquisition of phonological processing abilities such as phonological awareness, phonological short-term memory and rapid naming of known visual stimuli.[75,76] Phonological awareness is defined as the explicit awareness of the individual phonemes (sounds) in a spoken word. Phonological memory involves the ability to represent phonological information in short-term memory. The phonological units may vary in size from individual phonemes, morphemes, syllables, words, to groups of words. Rapid naming involves the efficient access of phonological information in long-term memory stores. Efficient word retrieval is thought to require multiple components that are interconnected. Not only is there a strong phonological factor, but efficient naming requires attention, executive functions for response preparation and a search/retrieval process, and a visual–verbal connection.[77,78] These phonological processing abilities have been found to be important factors for the optimal acquisition of reading and spelling.[7,79]

Children with SLI evidence differing degrees of difficulty with phonological perception, processing, retrieval and production. Psychophysical studies in infants of dyslexic families reveal abnormal speech perception.[45,46] The young child has difficulty perceiving differences between similar sounding words and rhymes. Learning new vocabulary requires many repetitions. Phonological awareness is often impaired, predicting reading and spelling disabilities. The processing of phonological information is inefficient with short-term memory tasks, such as nonword repetition and digit memory. The linking of sounds and letters is impaired, resulting in poor reading acquisition.

Efficient retrieval of phonological information from long-term memory is often impaired, resulting in word-finding deficits. Production deficits may be noted as early as infancy with less babbling, fewer consonants, and misarticulation of consonants. If articulation is less fluent, it may require more conscious resources, robbing resources needed for processing the sensory feedback, instrumental in "fine tuning" the phonemic representations. Verbal dexterity continues to be a problem. Difficulty with multisyllabic production may be evident and is also predictive of future reading ability.[80] These multisyllabic production difficulties may continue into adulthood. Elbro et al.[60] also noted that words are produced less distinctly even as late as adulthood.

If the assessment reveals that the individual with SLI/DD has difficulty in the phonological system, one should consider all the possible bottlenecks hindering learning—the linguistic and the nonlinguistic—that we have discussed.

The development of the pragmatic system

The pragmatic system integrates verbal and non-verbal language for social communications.

The pragmatic system, like the phonological system, develops early in infancy. The infant acquires early the ability to analyze and synthesize gestures, intonations and facial expressions for nonverbal communication and "social" interactions. With an innate attraction to the human face, the infant maintains eye contact and demonstrates ability to imitate facial expressions. Vocalizations are nonverbal, but interactive cooing and the appreciation of the melody, rhythm and inflections of speech (prosody) are evident in early infancy[81,82] At this early stage of development the inputs that must be represented and linked together (in an associative rather than a rule-governed fashion) for nonverbal communication are affective, prosodic, visual, nonspeech acoustic, and motor/kinesthetic (e.g. gestures). Once phonological, semantic and syntactic systems are developed, these nonverbal communicative attributes must also be linked in order for the child to communicate effectively in social situations.

There is less evidence for significant pragmatic development deficits in children with SLI, and the infant with SLI is usually social and communicative using nonverbal methods. Prosodic perception and production is typically not impaired. Unfortunately, complex linguistic demands may exceed the children's limited processing capacity and in these situations affective messages might be misperceived.[83]

Individuals with SLI typically understand language better than they can express it. During the preschool years, gestures serve as a substitute for compromised oral production, but SLI children may evidence fewer sequential gestures in toddlerhood.[37] These children are less likely to initiate conversations, have difficulty with keeping up with the topic, especially in group conversations, and have been noted to have difficulties resolving conflicts verbally. If they have a comorbid attention deficit disorder with a reduced processing capacity they might exhibit a pragmatic deficit, because while processing language they may be less aware of nonverbal cues and lack the executive function needed for self-monitoring.[2]

When a child evidences signs of pragmatic difficulties, it would be helpful to explore the attributes that might be hindering linguistic skills, including phonological representations and complex syntax. Sensorimotor and attention deficits (e.g. ADHD) might hinder his social interactions. Deficits in executive function could result in poor social interactions due to poor impulse control or a lack of self-monitoring. While social skills training is often recommended as a compensatory strategy for children with pragmatic difficulties, it may not generalize if the underlying linguistic and nonlinguistic deficits are not remediated.

The development of the semantic system

The semantic or lexical system specifies the meaningful vocabulary and word groupings of the language.

The semantic system (the content/meaning of language) is acquired when the infant has learned to segment the stream of sound into communicatively meaningful "chunks"—a whole word.[63] These whole word chunks or lexical entries become associated with an array of other afferent information when these co-occur. For example, on hearing the word "cat" while seeing a cat, touching a cat, smelling a cat, listening to a cat or being scratched by a cat, the child's brain is encoding these "cat" attributes into semantic–conceptual representations.[84] With repetition of these co-occurrences, synaptic connections are strengthened and the semantic/lexical representations become solidified. Not all the attributes of a lexical representation may be acquired at first, but will be acquired as the child's experience allows. The greater the number of associated attributes in a network, the stronger the semantic representation, increasing the ease of retrieval for processing and production.

Lexical semantic development is often somewhat below average, but usually a relative strength for individuals with SLI. Characteristically, children with SLI have been noted to have a delay in acquiring their first words—23 months in contrast to 11 months for normally developing children.[85] Storing a new word requires more exposures than is normally required.[2] Concrete nouns are more easily learned than action verbs. Children with SLI have a less diverse vocabulary and during the school years their vocabulary may become even more deficient if they have developed a reading disability and cannot acquire the vocabulary found in literature. These individuals often exhibit word-finding problems, which are felt to be due to problems of retrieval and/or storage.[2]

When the individual evidences difficulty with comprehension, it is essential to clarify whether it is at the word level or sentence level. Learning at the word level requires experiences with the word and accurate phonological representation for that word. If retrieval is a problem, the clinician must ascertain if this deficit is related to phonological factors and/or weak semantic representations. Environmental factors are strong contributors to vocabulary development and must be considered. With its weaknesses in selective attention, sustaining attention and working memory, ADHD may be a contributing factor.

The development of the syntactic system

The grammatical system analyzes word parts (morphemes) and word order (syntax) to provide structure/rules for organizing meaningful units.

With the acquisition of semantic lexical representations, the child is ready to learn how word order, function words (e.g. articles, prepositions), and inflectional endings can modify meaning. The development of the syntactic system further integrates the form of language with the content of language.

Once the child begins to make two-word combinations and change word forms (e.g. using plurals), it is evident that he has begun to develop this system of knowledge. Children with SLI often demonstrate a delay in these first word combinations. Trauner, Wulfeck, Tallal and Hessilink's[85] study found that the average age for these first word combinations in children with SLI was 37 months, in contrast to 17 months for the normally developing child. Productions are limited, with the use of phrases rather than sentences, few modifiers, and particular trouble with morphology, especially verbs.[37]

Working memory has been noted by Hulme and Tordoff[86] to be time limited and children with SLI have been found to have a slowed processing time.[25] Add to this the fact that syntactic analysis requires the processing of many operations: the analysis of the first word must be complete before it fades from memory and the next item is in line for processing. These demands are especially evident when the child is reading for comprehension. The more complex the syntax, the greater the demands on working memory.

Thus, ADHD with its weaknesses in selective attention, sustaining attention and working memory may be a contributing factor to poor syntactic development. Weak phonological and semantic systems would also present as bottlenecks in normal develop-

ment. These factors should be considered carefully in designing treatment.

The course of written language development

By age 3, all the spoken language subsystems are working together and complementing each other. Now, spoken language evolves into the development of written language (reading, spelling and writing), but this process is not innate and education is required to first link visual–graphemic with phonemic representations, and subsequently orthographic with phonemic lexical (whole word) representations.

The development of reading

A combination of well-defined phonological, orthographic and semantic representations is optimal for normal reading development. Reading comprehension also depends on syntax and working memory. Snyder and Downey[87] found that 8 to 9-year-old children's reading comprehension scores were best accounted for by their syntactic knowledge, followed by their ability to retell a story. The reading comprehension of older children (11 to 14 years) was found to rely on bottom-up (grapheme to phoneme transcoding) and top-down (whole word or orthographic strategies), depending on the material being read: for example, when having to decode isolated unfamiliar words in less familiar text, bottom-up processes are utilized; when given stories/text that contain familiar words, top-down strategies are used.

Children with SLI typically demonstrate impaired phonological awareness, thought to be the core deficit in developmental dyslexia.[8,28] In kindergarten they often have trouble associating letters with their sounds. Thus, they might depend more on whole word acquisition. Orthographic representations, however, are acquired more efficiently if there is an appreciation of the phonological components of the word.

Some children with strong cognitive and conceptual semantic abilities can offset decoding deficits in text reading by making use of context. Unfortunately, this strategy alone is less efficient than in combination with phonological decoding.

As content becomes more syntactically complex, the child requires an understanding of syntactic relationships to understand the material, especially if its content is not familiar. Syntactic deficits are often associated with dyslexia, and their impoverished vocabulary also impairs their reading comprehension.

Impaired attention, working memory and executive functions can also contribute to inefficient acquisition of reading from both a bottom-up and top-down approach.

The development of spelling and writing

The development of spelling mirrors that of reading but has an additional demand—writing, a motor skill requiring precise timing and coordination. A distinct visual–motor–somatosensory bond must be formed for each graphemic (letter) representation. The child must first develop the fine motor skills for printing.

Later, this skill will be refined and progress to cursive writing, in which letters are connected in a smooth and accurate fashion. Children with SLI/DD, however, often have trouble acquiring the fine motor skills required for writing. Spelling also places a greater demand on knowledge of phonemic sequences and phonics rules than reading does. When reading, the whole word form that comprises words may be recognized without having knowledge of phoneme sequence. Thus, the child with developmental dyslexia may acquire reading skills, but will continue to demonstrate spelling deficits. Written expression, like text reading, places high demands on working memory and executive functions. It also requires the additional demand of spelling and handwriting. It is not surprising that this ability remains problematic for the dyslexic even in adulthood.

Treatment

Historical overview

Leonard's[2] review of the history of treatment in individuals with specific language impairment reveals that while treatment approaches have varied widely both in the language areas being targeted and in the techniques used, they share common features. He cites Muma,[88] who pointed out that the natural techniques used by adults for normally developing children are applied—only more saliently and more frequently. Historically, the first treatment studies addressed the more common deficits found in SLI: phonological production (articulation) and morphosyntactic production. Treatment studies in the 1960s focused on morphosyntax and used operant conditioning. A gradual change through the 1970s and 1980s led to the application of the current linguistic theory with appropriate reinforcement strategies. Treatment for phonological production difficulties followed a similar course.

Studies on the treatment of semantic difficulties appeared in the 1980s, with the focus in the younger child on vocabulary acquisition and, in the older child, word finding. In the mid 1980s, a few studies were reported addressing pragmatic deficits, particularly with topic initiation, requests for additional information, and use of language for pretending.

By the 1990s, different techniques were used for helping the child address weaknesses and/or acquire compensatory skills. Prior to this, imitation-based approaches had been the principal technique. While still employed when working on a morphosyntactic concept, other approaches such as modeling, expansion of the child's production or conversational recasting, and implementing a language-stimulating milieu became mainstays.

The efficacy of intervention for phonological production difficulties was found to be significant in a review of 73 studies by Sommers, Logsdon and Wright.[89] Nye, Foster and Seaman[90] conducted a meta-analysis of 73 treatment studies designed to address language deficits, receptive and/or expressive in nature, and included reading deficits as well.

They found that there was large mean effect size (ES = 1.041, range of −0.677 to 2.90) for treatment groups collapsed across the type of approach. No one approach was significantly better than another, although modeling had a somewhat stronger effect size. Gains were greater in the interventions for the language/learning impaired (38 percentile points), followed by language delayed (22 percentile points), and least in the reading disabled (13 percentile points). Pragmatic function was the least responsive. Most studies were conducted in schools. Those conducted in clinics were more effective. Younger children showed more gains.

There were, however, substantial methodological weaknesses: the use of percentiles and/or age equivalents instead of standard scores did not permit comparison with peers and accurate measure of progress. The absence of descriptions of linguistic characteristics and few longitudinal studies were also deficiencies. Thirty-three of the studies had to be excluded due to weaknesses in design.

Leonard[2] concludes that there is evidence for significant gain in the acquisition of the targeted linguistic structures over those expected from maturation. However, 40% to 75% of these children do not achieve normal functioning despite years of treatment.[2,91] School interventions have been ineffective for 30% of children noted to be at risk for reading disabilities according to Snow et al.[92] Well-designed randomized controlled trials to address these treatment needs are essential, yet they are scarce.

There are many factors that make well-designed treatment studies difficult to perform. Developmental language disorder consists of a variety of deficits with various levels of ability in the language subsystems of phonology, semantics, syntax and pragmatics. It may affect receptive and/or expressive function and be on a continuum of severity. The child's neurological status is not static; it is constantly changing. That variability is a crucial factor because the child's language status appears to be normal at one point, only to fall out of range at another. To increase the confounding factors, there is heterogeneity in the nonlinguistic factors including environmental (home and school), deficits of attention, working memory and/or executive function, behavior disorders, and sensorimotor deficits. Finding the appropriate intervention would require an appreciation of each variable, and evaluating effectiveness requires controlling for as many of these variables as possible to ensure that gains could be attributed to the intervention.

Plasticity

Neuroplasticity has been studied extensively over the past 10 to 15 years. It is now recognized that this plasticity is not confined to early childhood and that adults can change their cortical maps (anatomical distribution of representations) with specific behavioral treatments.[58,93] The features that are important for reorganization include: intensity of the input (salient, frequent); task fractionation; repetition of the initial steps until they are mastered, followed by scaffolding of the subsequent, more complex steps; directed attention to the task; positive reinforcement.[94]

Liepert et al.[93] were able to demonstrate the acquisition of skilled movement in the paretic hands of 13 stroke patients using constraint therapy. Cortical mapping demonstrated enlargement of the hand representation after treatment, suggesting recruitment of adjacent brain areas.

Conway et al.[95] and Adair et al.[96] demonstrated similar findings in an adult with a mild acquired phonological alexia. He was treated with a systematic, intensive language treatment program designed to map phonemic representations that had been lost and to "re-develop" phonological processing. Both behavioral and brain activation changes resulted, with the right-sided homolog becoming activated for language processing along with increased activation of the left frontal and parietal opercular regions.

The knowledge that behavioral therapy can induce brain reorganization without a critical window allows us to be optimistic about the effects of language therapy. The essential factor for improving function in an impaired system seems to be the immersion of the patient in activities requiring its use. With this in mind, a closer look at treatment studies may guide us in choosing the most effective "immersion" techniques for the patient.

Treatment studies: Young children

The clinician who is planning language treatment must ask the following questions: 1) What type of intervention is most effective? Should the treatment be directed at lower level sensory representations or higher level semantic/cognitive systems? 2) Does a combination of bottom-up and top-down intervention result in greater gains than either one alone? 3) How intense must the intervention be to effect change? 4) Is there generalization to untreated stimuli/function? 5) What is the optimal age for treatment? 6) What is the impact of other factors such as ADHD, IQ, executive function, memory, rate/fluency ability, and sensorimotor deficits?

There is a need for well-controlled, randomized longitudinal treatment studies that address these issues. Unfortunately, to date there have been few, and most of the treatment studies have been in the preschool period. Fey, Catts and Larrivie[97] report that preschool language treatment addressing problems in spoken language and not lower level deficits in phonological processing may have yielded improvement in verbal ability, but yielded no gains in phonological sensitivity or reading development. Whitehurst and colleagues[98] demonstrated excellent gains in preschool oral language with daily dialogic reading techniques, but these gains did not generalize to improvements in phonological sensitivity or reading outcome. In the same vein, Snow[92] reported that 75% of preschoolers with language impairment develop reading disabilities despite speech/language therapy during the preschool years.

Preschool prevention studies reinforcing phonological awareness in children, even in those who were severely impaired, have yielded gains in the prevention of reading disabilities in the first and second grades with a minimal amount of intervention time.[99,100] However, there were many children who did not respond. The early prevention studies in phonological awareness have also been able to demonstrate that the combination of blending and segmenting approaches is more effective than either one alone.

Torgesen et al.[101] studied kindergartners identified as being at risk for dyslexia because they were in the bottom 12% in phonological awareness and letter name knowledge. One group received the Lindamoods' *Auditory Discrimination in Depth* Program[102] (LADD), providing extensive multisensory instruction in phonemic awareness and phonemic decoding skills, with minimal sight word training and text reading. Another group received Embedded Phonic Therapy (EP) which contains more sight word training with explicit phonics instruction embedded in the sight word practice and in the context of meaningful text reading and spelling. In EP, the time spent in the phonics training is minimal in contrast to the LADD group. The "equal time and attention" group received tutoring to support classroom instruction, and another group received no treatment. Treatment occurred for 20 minutes per day, 4 days a week from mid kindergarten until the end of second grade (a total of 87 hours). With treatment, the children in the LADD group were significantly better in phonemic awareness tasks than all other groups. They were also superior in the accuracy and fluency of decoding, evidencing normal (grade level) ability on the *Woodcock Reading Mastery Test—Revised*[103] (WRMT-R) Word Attack and Word Identification subtests. Thus, the less explicit and more global, semantic and associative interventions focusing on sight word reading and comprehension did not yield the necessary improvement in the phonological processing system and in word reading skills to perform at grade level in second grade.

Treatment studies: Older children

To date, the only large, well-controlled, randomized longitudinal treatment study of older school-aged children with severe reading disabilities to address gains both in spoken language and in reading is that of Torgesen et al.[23] Sixty children with a mean age of 9 years, 9 months, and a verbal IQ of 92 (*WISC-R*[104]), were randomly assigned to two treatment groups. One group received the Embedded Phonics (EP) treatment and the other the Lindamoods' *Auditory Discrimination in Depth* Program (LADD). Treatment was intensive—100 minutes daily for 8 to 9 weeks on a one-to-one basis for 67.5 hours. Follow-up measures were obtained annually for two years. At the two-year follow-up there were 26 children remaining in the LADD group and 24 in the EP.

Neurological assessments revealed a high incidence of comorbid ADHD, primarily the inattentive type. Treatment was managed by the children's private physicians and was not controlled. Poor

Table 261.2   Immediate and long-term outcomes for reading and spoken language and their effect sizes

Measure	LADD					EP				
	Pre	Post	Effect size	2-year	Effect size	Pre	Post	Effect size	2-year	Effect size
WISC-R Verbal IQ	92.2					93.0				
Language										
CELF Total	76.3	85.9*		89.7*		81.0	86.6*		89.9*	
SD	9.0	11.8		14.0		12.0	10.7		19.3	
CELF Exp. Lang.	76.2	83.1*		87.4*		78.5	83.8*		86.2*	
SD	9.1	10.0	0.72	13.3	1.0	11.5	10.8	0.48	10.5	0.7
CELF Rec. Lang.	79.7	90.7*		93.8*		85.0	91.5*		95.2*	
SD	11.0	15.1	0.84	16.2	1.04	13.9	12.2	0.5	11.2	0.8
Phonological measures										
LAC	56.3	89.2*		82.2*		49.4	69.0*		76.2*	
SD	13.5	10.1		14.1		15.3	17.3		13.4	
Nonword Rep.	88.2	100.8*		112.9*		89.6	103.0*		112.8*	
SD	15.3	16.1	0.80	13.7	1.7	18.0	19.0	0.7	14.0	1.45
RAN Digits	86.9	90.2*		91.3*		84.2	87.9*		87.9*	
SD	10.7	10.3	0.31	13.2	0.36	9.3	11.9	0.34	13.0	0.33
Reading measures										
WRMT-R Word Attack	68.5	96.4*		91.8*		70.1	90.3*		89.9*	
SD	11.8	7.0	2.97	12.5	1.92	9.2	8.3	2.31	10.4	2.02
WRMT-R Word Id	68.9	82.4*		87.0*		66.4	80.5*		83.9*	
SD	8.3	11.2	1.38	12.1	1.77	8.7	9.6	1.54	12.2	1.67
WRMT-R Passage Comp.	83.0	91.0*		94.7*		82.2	92.0*		96.9*	
SD	19.4	9.0	0.56	8.9	0.83	11.0	19.8	0.64	11.5	1.31
Gray Comp	73.3	85.6*		87.9*		79.4	86.0*		87.2*	
SD	10.8	10.0	1.18	11.8	1.29	12.3	10.4	0.58	15.1	0.57

CELF, *Clinical Evaluation of Language Fundamentals*, 3rd edn. (CELF-3), PRO-ED; LAC, *Lindamood Auditory Conceptualization Test*, The Riverside Publishing Co.; CTOPP, *Comprehensive Test of Phonological Processing*, PRO-ED; EP, Embedded Phonics; LADD, Lindamood Auditory Discrimination in Depth; WRMT-R, *Woodcock Reading Mastery Test—Revised*, American Guidance Service, Inc.; GORT-3, *Gray Oral Reading Tests*, 3rd edn., PRO-ED. Wisc-R, *Wechsler Intelligence Scale for Children*, Psychological Corp.
*$P = <0.01$.

attention was felt to be a significant problem during this study.

Table 261.2 summarizes the response to treatment in spoken language and reading with pre-treatment, immediately post-treatment, and two years post-treatment measures. To measure the magnitude of the gain, effect sizes (ES) were calculated. Effect sizes between 0.5 and 0.79 are moderate; ES of 0.8 or greater is large, corresponding with the correlation of 0.5 and higher.[105]

Both groups manifested significant gains in word reading on the WRMT-R[103] and in passage comprehension on the WRMT-R[103] and the GORT-3[106] (*Gray Oral Reading Test—3rd Edition*) immediately after treatment. Most gains were maintained or improved during the two years of follow-up. The LADD group's phonological processing ability as measured on the *Lindamood Auditory Conceptualization Test*[107] (LAC) began at early first grade level, rose to the fifth grade level immediately post treatment and fell to the beginning fourth grade level (the subjects were then in sixth to seventh grade). The EP group were functioning at the beginning first grade level, progressed to beginning second grade immediately after treatment, and gradually improved to beginning third

grade level during the two year follow-up. While these gains are significant, phonemic awareness still lagged behind normal for both groups. The Nonword Repetition phonological memory measure as measured on the *Comprehensive Test of Phonological Processing*[108] (CTOPP) evidenced greater improvement immediately after treatment with continued gains during follow-up. Naming measures (CTOPP) demonstrated significant treatment effects immediately after treatment, but no growth during follow-up. Both groups also evidenced robust gains on the *Clinical Evaluation of Language Fundamentals—3*[109] (CELF-3) in both receptive and expressive language skills, with comprehension showing somewhat greater gains. Growth continued for both receptive and expressive language during the follow-up period. The effect sizes were greater for the group treated with LADD.

Despite the overall improvements associated with the treatment groups, Torgesen and colleagues found that the interventions were not sufficient for a significant number of children. For example, in regard to reading nonwords (Work Attack) they found at the two-year measure that the LADD treatment moved 69% of the group into the average range and the EP moved 54%. The improvement for decoding of real words, both irregular and regular, was less effective, with only 39% of the LADD and 33% of the EP group moving to the average range.

Forty-six percent of the LADD group were able to move out of special education classes, in contrast to 33% of the EP group. The children who were able to return to general education were found to be older, have fewer attention/behavior difficulties, higher verbal abilities and higher socioeconomic status (SES). The most consistent predictors for rate of growth during treatment, as well as ultimate skill levels, were attention and receptive language scores.

Other studies have been reported that address the effectiveness of treatment for SLI/DD. Most were controlled studies,[110–113] one was not.[114] Some targeted language,[114] others targeted reading[108,112,113] and some targeted both.[23,110] Some monitored maintenance of the improvements for one to two years, others only the immediate improvements. Some targeted lower level sensory systems; others used metacognitive strategies; some combined the two in differing sequences. An overview of each study is presented in Table 261.3. The immediate and long-term outcomes for the treatment groups are presented in Table 261.4. To simplify the table, the control group outcomes are not presented, but will be mentioned in the text when necessary.

The groups differed in their overall intellectual ability, with Lovett and Torgesen's groups falling in the low average range in contrast to the average ability in other groups. The groups also differed in the severity of the subjects' deficits in spoken and written language. The Deutsch group's word reading skills (average of WA + WId) were only 1 SD below the mean; the Hook and Wise groups were 1.5 SD below; the Oakland, Lovett, and Torgesen groups were 2 SD below average. The Lovett group was severely impaired in reading comprehension (2 SD below the mean), while the others were approximately $1-1\frac{1}{3}$ SD below the mean. Spoken language ability (receptive and expressive) was normal in the Hook study, 1 SD below average for Tallal's TOLD and Torgesen's EP groups, and 1.5 SD below the mean for Tallal's CELF and Torgesen's LADD groups. They also differ in the severity of the reading disability, with the Lovett and Torgesen groups being severely impaired. Measures for pre treatment, immediately post treatment and one- to two-year follow-up are presented.

In order to further compare the results of the interventions immediately after treatment and after one to two years, Table 261.4 provides a summary of the effect sizes, when available, and a second measure used by Torgesen.[23] This measure reports effects in terms of the number of standard score points gained per hour of instruction, requiring the use of standardized measures with the same standard deviations. Table 261.4 provides these comparisons for measures of receptive language, expressive language, nonword repetition, phonological awareness, rapid naming of digits, phonemic decoding, word identification, and passage comprehension. The Oakland study did not provide standard deviations for ES calculations. The

group's word reading ability was measured by the *Wide Range Achievement Test—Revised*[120] (WRAT-R); the group mean improved from a Standard Score (SS72 to SS82) after 350 hours of treatment, in contrast to the No Treatment Control (NTC) group (SS76–SS79).

The data summarized in Table 261.4 suggest that the rates of growth (as measured by standard score/hour) for phonemic (nonword) decoding skills, word-reading ability, and reading comprehension are very similar for the phonological interventions employed by Wise, Lovett and Torgesen. The effect size for both non and real word reading is greater for Torgesen's LADD and EP interventions than for the interventions used by the Wise and Lovett groups. This may be due to the greater intensity afforded by one-to-one instruction. The Wise, Lovett and Torgesen interventions are similar in that all three used explicit phonics training, with a mastery-oriented progression. The growth per hour of treatment and the effect size for word-reading skills was notably less with the other studies.

In Hook et al.'s study, the FastForWord (FFW) program did not result in immediate reading gains, in contrast to the Orton Gillingham (OG) group. However, FFW did have moderate effect sizes for reading at the two-year follow-up, suggesting that it was ultimately helpful in effecting reading growth. Hook et al. found no statistical difference between the outcomes of the FFW and the longitudinal control (LC) groups treated with multisensory instruction over two years. However, the LC group's effect size lagged behind in word identification (ES = 0.3 vs. 0.76). There was less gain per hour with the use of the computerized Step4Word program than with the Wise, Lovett and Torgesen interventions. This training, however, was on a computer and did not entail the one-to-one contact used in the Torgesen intervention, but could be compared to the manpower requirement of the small group interventions of Wise and Lovett.

The Tallal field trial's FFW intervention, designed to address language deficits using a very bottom-up approach, was noted to be very effective for children with spoken language impairment immediately after treatment. The Hook FFW study did not demonstrate a similar effect on non-language-impaired children with normal receptive language and low average expressive language. Torgesen's LADD and EP groups were language impaired and demonstrated significant gains immediately post treatment with continued growth during the two-year follow-up. The LADD intervention was the more effective, further supporting a more bottom-up approach as more appropriate for remediating spoken language deficits.

To summarize, the younger child seems to need a bottom-up approach to learn to read. The older child responds to both bottom-up and top-down approaches for reading if explicit phonics instruction is included. The intervention aimed specifically at spoken language (FFW) did not result in immediate gains in reading. This would support previous findings that improving phonological processing without

Table 261.3   Treatment studies

Author	Treatment design	Time	n	Age	VIQ
1. Deutsch et al.[110]	1) Step4Word[116] (computerized to include Letter/Sound, decoding, Vocab, Grammar Syntax, early word reading) followed by 67 hours intensive training with FastForWord[117] (FFW → Step4W)	90 mins/day × 30 days = 45 hours	25	8.8	>80 TONI
	2) Matched controls—no treatment	None	25	8.5	>80 TONI
2. Hook et al.[111]	1) FastForWord[117] computerized intervention including: a) Discrimination of complex auditory information in a pre-word format with differing frequencies, time duration, phonemes (follow for 2 years, classroom multisensory reading) b) Exercises using modified speech to enhance rapidly changing acoustic components while working in words alone or in increasingly more complex sentences Compared to:	100 mins/day × 30–40 days = 67 hours, follow-up at 1 & 2 years	11	9.8	103
	1) Orton Gillingham multisensory approach to teach reading, spelling and writing (1:4) for short term and	100 mins/day × 25 days = 41.6 hours	11	11	100
	2) Longitudinal control (LC) group matched to FastForWord for 2-year follow-up (both groups received multisensory reading instruction in classroom)	No treatment/followed for 2 years	11	9.8	107
3. Tallal et al.[112]	FastForWord[117] Field Trial (see Hook re description)—no controls, varied subject selection, varied assessments	100 mins/day × 6–8 weeks = 67 hours		4–14	NA
	a) Reports language scores for some of group using TOLD-P:2[118]	100 mins/day × 6–8 weeks = 67 hours	77	NA	NA
	b) Reports language scores for CELF-3, Receptive Language	100 mins/day × 6–8 weeks = 67 hours	90	NA	NA
	c) Reports language scores for CELF-3, Expressive Language	100 mins/day × 6–8 weeks = 67 hours	60	NA	NA
4. Oakland et al.[114]	1) Alphabetic Phonics, a derivation of Orton Gillingham multisensory approach to teach reading, writing, spelling (12 received video-directed, 10 teacher directed—no group difference, groups were collapsed for analysis)	1 hour/day × 2 school years = 350 hours	24	9.9	96
	2) Matched Reading Disabled control group with classroom intervention and school special services	None	26	11	99
5. Wise et al.[113]	1) Phonological interventions include manipulation and attention to articulation + spelling and text reading (1:1 and small group 1:3). (The authors also had groups using other manipulation or attention to articulation—all 3 groups performed similarly. The combination group is used for comparison)	½ hour/day × 80 days = 40 hours with 1 year follow-up	37	9.1	104
	2) No treatment control followed for 1 year	None	31	8.7	Not done
6. Lovett et al.[115]	1) PHAB/WIST or WIST/PHAB (½ group) in sequence for 35 hours each (1:3). PHAB involves direct phonics and phonological awareness intervention using special orthographic techniques providing mnemonic support for visual cues. WIST teaches different word identification strategies—analogy, word parts, flexing vowel pronunciations.	½ hour/day × 70 days = 70 hours (14 weeks)	49	9.7	91
	2) Control group received classroom strategies and math in sequence for 35 hours each (1:3)	½ hour/day × 70 days = 70 hours (14 weeks)	22	9.7	91
7. Torgesen et al.[23]	1) ADD—the Lindamood Auditory Discrimination in Depth, with intensive multisensory intervention at the phonemic and with decoding/spelling of nonwords (85%). Reading decodable text (5%), sight words (10%) (1:1)	100 mins/day × 40 days = 67 hours (2 months) + follow-up at 1 and 2 years	26	9.7	92
	2) EP—Embedded Phonics—explicit instruction in word reading in text with writing, writing—50%, 30% with sight words, 20% with phonics instruction with reading and spelling (1:1)	100 mins/day × 40 days = 67 hours (2 months) + follow-up at 1 and 2 years	24	9.7	93

N, number of subjects; VIQ, verbal IQ; TOLD-P:2, Test of Language Development, primary Level; CELF-3, Clinical Evaluation of Language Development, 3rd ed.; NA, not available; TONI, Test of Nonverbal Intelligence; PHAB, Phonological Analysis and Blending/Direct Instruction; WIST, Word Identification Strategy Training.

Table 261.4 Summary of intervention studies: effect size and gains in standard scores per hour of treatment

Author	RLS Post/2 yrs	ELS Post/2 yrs	NWR Post/2 yrs	PA Post/2 yrs	RAN Post/2 yrs	Word Attack Post/2 yrs	Word ID Post/2 yrs	Passage Comp Post/2 yrs
Deutsch/Step FW 45 hours* (1:3)						0.18/NA† ES = 1.34	0.09/NA† ES = 0.39	0.18/NA† ES = 0.60
Hook/FFW 50–67 hours/ avg 58 hours (1:3)	0.04/–0.02† ES = 0.24/–0.1 TOLD	0.06/–0.04† ES = 0.33/–0.2 TOLD				–0.02/0.12† ES = –0.16/0.65	–0.05/0.12† ES = –0.19/0.65	0.02/0.17† ES = 0.05/0.72
Hook/OG 42 hours (1:3)						0.14/NA† ES = 0.97	0.02/NA† ES = 0.17	NA/NA†
Tallal/FFW 67 hours (1:1–3)	0.19/NA† CELF-3 0.19/NA TOLD	0.13/NA† CELF-3 0.13/NA TOLD						
Oakland/OG 350 hours (1:4)						NA/NA	0.03/NA†	NA/NA†
Wise/Phonol/Manip: Artic 40 hours (1:3–1:1)						0.33/NA† ES = 1.28	0.2/0.2 (1 yr)† ES = 0.96/0.92	0.13/NA† ES = 0.63
Lovett/Phab/Di + WIST 70 hours (1:3)						0.27/NA†	0.06/NA†	0.11/NA†
Torgesen/ADD 67.5 hours (1:1)	0.16/0.21† ES = 0.84/1.04	0.10/0.17† ES = 0.72/1.0	0.29/0.37† ES = 0.8/1.7	0.18/0.14†	0.05/0.07† ES = 0.31/0.37	0.41/0.35† ES = 2.97/1.92	0.2/0.27† ES = 1.38/1.77	0.12/0.17† ES = 0.56/0.83
Torgesen/EP 67.5 hours (1:1)	0.096/0.15† ES = 0.5/0.8	0.08/0.11† ES = 0.48/0.7	0.2/0.34† ES = 0.7/1.45	0.2/0.2†	0.05/0.05† ES = 0.34/0.33	0.30/0.29† ES = 2.31/2.02	0.21/0.26† ES = 1.4/1.67	0.15/0.21† ES = 0.64/1.31

Step FW, Step4Word; FFW, FastForWord; OG, Orton Gillingham; Phonol/Manip:Artic, Phonological Manipulation with Articulatory Awareness & Phonics; WIST, Word Identification Strategy Training; PhabDi, Phonological Analysis and Blending/Direct Instruction; ADD, Auditory Discrimination in Depth; EP, Embedded Phonics; RLS, Receptive Language Score; ELS, Expressive Language Score; NWR, Non Word Repetition; PA, Phonological Awareness; RAN, RAN Digits; Post/2 yrs, Immediately following treatment/2 yr follow-up test; NA, not available.

*Calculations made on gains from end of FFW to completion of Step FFW.

†Standard score change per treatment hour.

direct instruction in the alphabetic code is not effective in remedial treatment of reading disabilities. In contrast, the intensive interventions designed to address reading deficits did result in spoken language gains, especially if a bottom-up approach was used. Intensity of training seems to be the crucial factor for successful intervention.

While appropriate language intervention is the cornerstone of a treatment plan for the child with language impairments resulting from a faulty foundation in language subsystems, there are other factors which must be considered for optimal outcome. Torgesen's studies have implicated attention and behavioral control as significant obstacles to gains in reading. The child's attention, working memory and executive functions must be considered and treated accordingly. Sensorimotor deficits that have an impact on skill acquisition, most especially handwriting, should also be remedied. The linguistic environments at home and school must be investigated and, if deficient, measures for improving them should be considered. Working with the family and the school to facilitate a child's growth in all areas is essential.

Above all, the child's ability to persevere in the face of frustration is his most valuable asset. Some children come "packaged" with it, others have to be encouraged to develop it. The reinforcement of the appropriate work ethic will allow him or her to succeed despite being less dexterous with language, fine motor skill and organizational abilities.

Children's language development is a dynamic process, and thus, the clinician must continue to monitor progress even once intensive treatment has moved the child into the average range. Following treatment, the newly strengthened language systems may continue to have subtle weaknesses that will impede the child's ability to acquire the next level of skill. Thus, further intervention might be needed. These treatments should follow the tenets for optimal results:

1. The deficient skill must be broken into small steps, progressing from the simple to the complex. It must be "do-able." Mastery must be obtained at each level before it can serve as a scaffold for the next level.
2. Repetition, repetition, repetition. Each skill must be practised repetitively until it can be mastered.
3. Intensity of the intervention—daily intervention yields greater gains. With salient and frequent activation, cortical organization can be accomplished in fewer hours than the traditional therapy approaches of one to two sessions per week.
4. Attention is crucial. The child should be concretely reinforced for good attention and for trying. Mastery itself is reinforcing, but the extras increase the affective state and arousal, further enhancing learning. If ADHD is present, it must be treated appropriately.
5. Once the new skill has been acquired, ensure that it is practised in order to refine it, solidify it and automatize it. Practise, practise, practise.

With the advent of more rigorous intervention research, the outlook for the child with SLI/DD is much more optimistic. The reading deficits, which have resulted in the most significant functional impairments for so many, can be prevented and remedied for a larger number of children. Spoken language deficits have shown similar gains. As the science of intervention grows, even more refined techniques will become available, allowing the individuals with these disorders to be able to function more efficiently, at home, at school and in the workplace.

References

1. American Speech-Language-Hearing Association, Committee on Language Speech and Hearing Service in Schools. Definitions: communicative disorders and variations. ASHA 1982;24(11):949–950
2. Leonard LB. Children with Specific Language Impairment. Cambridge MA: MIT Press, 1998
3. Tallal P, Ross R, Curtiss S. Unexpected sex-ratios in families of language/learning-impaired children. Neuropsychologia 1989;27:987–998
4. Fey M, Leonard L. Pragmatic skills of children with specific language impairment. In: Gallagher T, Prutting C, eds. Pragmatic Assessment and Intervention Issues in Language. San Diego, CA: College-Hill Press, 1983:65–82
5. Morgan WP. A case of congenital word-blindness. BMJ 1896;2:1378
6. Orton ST. "Word-blindness" in school children. Arch Neurol Psychiatry 1925:581–615
7. Liberman IY, Shankweiler D, Liberman AM. The alphabetic principle in learning to read. In: Shankweiler D, Liberman I, eds. Phonology and Reading Disability. Ann Arbor, MI: University of Michigan Press, 1989:1–33
8. Vellutino F. Dyslexia: Theory and Research. Cambridge, MA: MIT Press, 1979
9. Wolf M. The word-retrieval process and reading in children and aphasics. In: Nelson KE, ed. Children's Language. Hillsdale, NJ: Lawrence Erlbaum, 1982: 437–493
10. Wolf M. Naming speed and reading: The contribution of the cognitive neurosciences. Reading Research Quarterly 1991;26:123–141
11. Wolf M, Obregon M. Early naming deficits, developmental dyslexia, and a specific deficit hypothesis. Brain Lang 1992;42(3):219–247
12. American Speech-Language-Hearing Association. Definitions of communication disorders and variations. ASHA 1993;35(Suppl 10):40–41
13. Cantwell DP, State MW, Voeller KKS. Speech and language disorders. Textbook of Pediatric Neuropsychiatry. Washington, DC: American Psychiatric Press, 1998:801–819
14. Shaywitz SE. Dyslexia. N Engl J Med 1998;338(5):307–312
15. Snowling M, Bishop DV, Stothard SE. Is preschool language impairment a risk factor for dyslexia in adolescence? J Child Psychol Psychiatry 2000;41(5):587–600
16. Rescorla L. Do late talking toddlers turn out to have reading difficulties a decade later? Ann Dyslex 2000;50:67–102
17. Scarborough HS, Dobrich W. Development of children with early language delay. J Speech Hear Res 1990;33(1):70–83
18. Lewis B, Thompson L. A study of developmental

speech and language disorders in twins. J Speech Hear Res 1992;35:1086–1094

19. Plante E. Phenotypic variability in brain-behavior studies of specific language impairment. *In:* Rice M, ed. Toward a Genetics of Language. Hillsdale, NJ: Lawrence Erlbaum, 1996:317–335

20. Tomblin JB, Buckwalter P. Studies of genetics of specific language impairment. *In:* Watkins R, Rice M, eds. Specific Language Impairments in Children. Baltimore, MD: Paul H Brookes, 1994:17–35

21. Johnson CJ, Beitchman JH, Young A, et al. Fourteen year follow-up of children with and without speech/language impairments; Speech/language stability outcomes. J Speech Lang Hear Res 1999;42(3):744–758

22. Tannock R, Brown E. Attention deficit disorder with learning disability. *In:* Brown TE, ed. Subtypes of Attention Disorders in Children, Adolescents and Adults. Washington, DC: American Psychiatric Press, 1999

23. Torgesen JK, Alexander AW, Wagner RK, et al. Intensive remedial instruction for children with severe reading disability: immediate and long-term outcomes from two intensive approaches. J Learn Disabil 2001;34(1):33–58

24. Tallal P, Stark RE, Mellits ED. Identification of language-impaired children on the basis of perception and production skills. Brain Lang 1985;25:314–322

25. Kail R. A method of studying the generalized slowing hypothesis in children with specific language impairment. J Speech Hear Res 1994;37:418–421

26. Wolff P, Michel G, Ovrut M. Rate variables and automatized naming in developmental dyslexia. Brain Lang 1990;39:556–575

27. Fawcett AJ, Nicolson RJ, Dean P. Impaired performance of children with dyslexia on a range of cerebellar tasks. Ann Dyslex 1996;46:259–283

28. Torgesen JK, Wagner RK, Rashotte CA. Longitudinal studies of phonological processing and reading. J Learn Disabil 1994;27(5):276–286

29. Torgesen JK. Studies of children with learning disabilities who perform poorly on memory span tasks. J Learn Disabil 1988;21:605–612

30. Eden GF, Stein JF, Wood HM, Wood FB. Differences in visual spatial judgement in reading-disabled and normal children. Percept Mot Skills 1996;82(1):155–177

31. Stein J, Walsh V. To see but not to read; the magnocellular theory of dyslexia. Trends Neurosci 1997;20(4):147–152

32. Stein JF, Talcott JB. The magnocellular theory of developmental dyslexia. Dyslexia 1999;5:59–78

33. Livingstone M. The magnocellular/parietal system and visual symptoms in dyslexia. *In:* Duane DD, ed. Reading and Attention Disorders: Neurobiological Correlates. Timonium, MD: York Press, 1999:81–92

34. Badian NA, McAnulty CB, Duffy FH, Als H. Prediction of dyslexia in kindergarten boys. Ann Dyslex 1990;40:152–169

35. American Psychiatric Association. Diagnostic and statistical manual of mental disorders IV. Washington, DC: American Psychiatric Association, 1994

36. Fletcher JM, Francis DJ, Rourke BP, et al. The validity of discrepancy-based definitions of reading disabilities. J Learn Disabil 1992;25(9):555–561, 573

37. Olswang LB, Rodriguez B, Timber G. Recommending intervention for toddlers with speech and language learning difficulties: we may not have all the answers, but we know a lot. Am J Speech Lang Path 1997; 7(1):23–32

38. Fawcett AJ, Nicolson RI. The Dyslexia Early Screening Test. London: The Psychological Corporation, 1996

39. Nicolson RI, Fawcett AJ. The Dyslexia Screening Test. London: The Psychological Corporation, 1996

40. Zeffiro T, Eden G. The neural basis of developmental dyslexia. Ann Dyslex 2000;50:3–30

41. Galaburda AM, Sanides F, Geschwind N. Human brain, cytoarchitectonic left-right asymmetries in the temporal speech region. Arch Neurol 1978;35(12): 812–817

42. Galaburda AM. The pathogenesis of childhood dyslexia. Res Publ Assoc Res Nerv Ment Dis 1988;66: 127–137

43. Rosen GD, Fitch RH, Clark MG, et al. Animal models of developmental dyslexia: Is there a link between neocortical malformations and defects in fast auditory processing. *In:* Wolf M, ed. Dyslexia, Fluency, and the Brain. Timonium, MD: York Press, 2001:129–158

44. Galaburda AM, Eidelberg D. Symmetry and asymmetry in the human posterior thalamus, II. Thalamic lesions in a case of developmental dyslexia. Arch Neurol 1982;39(6):333–336

45. Leppanen PH, Pihko E, Eklund KM, Lyytinen H. Cortical responses of infants with and without a genetic risk for dyslexia: II. Group effects. Neuroreport 1999; 10(5):969–973

46. Benasich A, Tallal P. Assessing auditory temporal processing in 5- to 9-month-old infants. Paper presented at the Meeting of the Society for Research in Child Development, New Orleans, 1993

47. Molfese DL. Predicting dyslexia at 8 years of age using neonatal perceptual responses. Brain Lang 2000;72: 238–245

48. Breznitz Z. The determinants of reading fluency; a comparison of dyslexic and average readers. *In:* Wolf M, ed. Dyslexia, Fluency, and the Brain. Timonium, MD: York Press, 2001:245–276

49. Talcott JB, Witton C, McClean M, et al. Dynamic sensory sensitivity and children's word decoding skills. Proc Natl Acad Sci 2000;97(6):2952–2957

50. Lahey M, Edwards J. Specific language impairment: Preliminary investigation of factors associated with family history and with patterns of language performance. J Speech Hear Res 1995;38:643–657

51. Byrne B, Willerman L, Ashmore L. Severe and moderate language impairment: Evidence for distinctive etiologies. Behav Genet 1974;4:331–345

52. Pennington BF. Genetics of learning disabilities. J Child Neurol 1995;10(Suppl 1):S69–S77

53. Bishop D. The biological basis of specific language impairment. *In:* Fletcher P, Hall D, eds. Specific Speech and Language Disorders in Children. London: Whurr Publishers, 1992:2–17

54. DeFries JC, Alarcon MS. Genetics of specific reading disabilities. Ment Retard Dev Dis Res Rev 1996;2:39–49

55. Vargha-Khadem F, Watkins K, Alcock K, et al. Praxic and nonverbal cognitive deficits in a large family with a genetically transmitted speech and language disorder. Proc Natl Acad Sci USA 1995;92:930–933

56. Cardon LR, Smith SD, Fulker DW, et al. Quantitative trait locus for reading disability on chromosome 6. Science 1994;266:276–279

57. Compton DL, Davis CJ, DeFries JC, et al. Genetic and environmental influences on reading and RAN: an overview of results from the Colorado twin study. *In:* Wolf M, ed. Dyslexia, Fluency, and the Brain. Timonium, MD: York Press, 2001:277–306

58. Merzenich M, Wright B, Jenkins W, et al. Cortical plas-

ticity underlying perceptual, motor, and cognitive skill development: implications for neurorehabilitation. Cold Spring Harb Symp Quant Biol 1996;61:1–8

59. Hebb DO. The Organization of Behavior: A Neuropsychological Theory. New York: Wiley, 1949

60. Elbro C, Nielsen I, Petersen DK. Dyslexia in adults; Evidence for deficits in non-word reading and in phonological representation of lexical items. Ann Dyslex 1994;44:205–226

61. Baddeley AD. Working Memory. New York: Oxford University Press, 1986

62. Snowling MJ, Nation KA. Language, phonology and learning to read. In: Hulme C, Snowling M, eds. Dyslexia: Biology, Cognition and Intervention. London: Whurr Publishers, 1997:155–156

63. Stackhouse J, Wells B. How do speech and language problems affect literacy development? In: Hulme C, Snowling M, eds. Dyslexia: Biology, Cognition and Intervention. London: Whurr Publishers, 1997:182–211

64. Frith U. Beneath the surface of developmental dyslexia. In: Patterson KE, Marshall JC, Coltheart M, eds. Surface Dyslexia. London: Routledge & Kegan Paul, 1985

65. Pinker S. The rules of language. Science 1991;253:530–535

66. Tallal P. Rapid auditory processing in normal and disordered language development. J Speech Hear Res 1976;19:561–571

67. Montgomery D. Do dyslexics have difficulty accessing articulatory information? Psychol Res 1981;43(2):235–243

68. Heilman KM, Voeller K, Alexander AW. Developmental dyslexia: a motor-articulatory feedback hypothesis. Ann Neurol 1996;39(3):407–412

69. Denckla MB. Research Findings: Reading Disability (RD) and ADHD Interactions. Washington, DC: International Dyslexia Association Conference 2000, Nov 10

70. Eimas P, Siqueland E, Jusczyk P, Vigorito J. Speech perception in infants. Science 1971;171:303–306

71. MacKain K, Studdert-Kennedy M, Spieker CS, Stern D. Infant intermodal speech perception is a left-hemisphere function. Science 1983;219:1347–1349

72. Kuhl PK, Meltzoff AN. The bimodal perception of speech in infancy. Science 1982;218:1138–1141

73. Liberman AM, Mattingly JG. The motor theory of speech perception revised. Cognition 1985;21:1–36

74. Studdert-Kennedy M. Imitation and the emergence of segments. Phonetica 2000;57(2–4):275–283

75. Wagner RK, Torgesen JK, Laughon P, et al. The development of young readers' phonological processing abilities. J Ed Psych 1993;35:1–20

76. Wagner RK, Torgesen JK, Rashotte CA, et al. Changing relations between phonological processing abilities and word-level reading as children develop from beginning to skilled readers: a 5-year longitudinal study. Dev Psychol 1997;33(3):468–479

77. Denckla MB, Rudel RG. "Rapid automatized naming" of pictured objects, colors, letters and numbers by normal children. Cortex 1974;10:186–202

78. Denckla MB, Rudel RG. Rapid "automatized" naming (RAN): Dyslexia differentiated from other learning disabilities. Neuropsychol 1976;14:471–479

79. Torgesen JK, Wagner RK. The nature of phonological processing and its causal role in acquisition of reading skills. Psychol Bull 1987;101:192–212

80. Larrivee L, Catts HW. Early reading achievement in children with expressive phonological disorders. Am J Speech Lang Path 1999;8:128–188

81. Trevarthen C. Facial expressions of emotion in mother-infant interaction. Hum Neurobiol 1985;4(1):21–32

82. Meltzoff AN, Moore MK. Imitation of facial and manual gestures by human neonates. Science 1977;198:74–78

83. Trauner D, Ballantyne A, Chase C, Tallal P. Comprehension and Expression of Affect in Language Impaired Children. J Psycholinguistic Res 1993;22(4):445–452

84. Rumelhart DE, Smolensky P, McClelland JL, Hinton GE. Schemata and sequential thought processes in PDP models. In: McClelland JL, Rumelhart DE, The PDP Research Group, eds. Parallel Distributive Processing. Cambridge, MA: MIT Press, 1986:Vol 2:7–57

85. Trauner D, Wulfeck B, Tallal P, Hesselink T. Neurological and MRI profiles of language impaired children. Technical Report CMD-9513, 1995. UC San Diego: Center for Research in Language

86. Hulme C, Tordoff V. Working memory development: The effects of speech rate, word length, and acoustic similarity on serial recall. J Exp Child Psych 1989;47:72–87

87. Snyder LS, Downey DM. The language-reading relationship in normal and reading-disabled children. J Speech Hear Res 1991;34(1):129–140

88. Muma J. Language intervention: Ten techniques. Language, Speech, and Hearing Services in Schools 1971;5:7–17

89. Sommers R, Logsdon B, Wright J. A review and critical analysis of treatment research related to articulation and phonological disorders. J Communication Disorders 1992;25:3–22

90. Nye C, Foster S, Seaman D. The effectiveness of language intervention with the language and learning disabled. J Speech Hear Dis 1987;52:348–357

91. Huntley R, Hold K, Butterfill A, Latham C. A follow-up study of a language intervention programme. Br J Disord Commun 1988;23:127–140

92. Snow CE, Burns MF, Griffin P. Preventing Reading Difficulties in Young Children. Washington, DC: National Academy Press, 1998

93. Liepert J, Bauder H, Wolfgang HR, et al. Treatment-induced cortical reorganization after stroke in humans. Stroke 2000;31(6):1210–1216

94. Tallal P, Merznich MS, Jenkings WM, Millers SL. Moving research from the laboratory to clinics and classrooms. In: Duane DD, ed. Reading and Attention Disorders: Neurobiological Correlates. Timonium, MD: York Press, 1999:93–112

95. Conway TW, Heilman P, Rothi LJ, et al. Treatment of a case of phonological alexia with agraphia using the Auditory Discrimination in Depth (ADD) program. J Int Neuropsychol Soc 1998;4(6):608–620

96. Adair JC, Nadeau SE, Conway TW, et al. Alterations in the functional anatomy of reading induced by rehabilitation of an alexic patient. Neuropsychiatry Neuropsychol Behav Neurol 2000;13(4):303–311

97. Fey ME, Catts HW, Larrivie L. Preparing preschoolers with language impairments for academic and social challenges of school. In: Fey ME, Windsor J, Warren SK, eds. Language Intervention: Preschool through Elementary Years. Baltimore, MD: Paul H Brooks, 1995:3–37

98. Whitehurst GJ, Falco FL, Lonigan CG, et al. Accelerating language development through picture book reading. Dev Psychol 1988;24(1):552–557

99. Warrick N, Rubin H, Rowe-Walsh S. Phoneme awareness in language delayed children: Comparative studies and intervention. Ann Dyslex 1993;43:153–173

100. Byrne B, Fielding-Barnsley R. Evaluation of a program to teach phonological awareness to young children; a one year follow up. J Ed Psych 1995;85:104–111

101. Torgesen JK, Wagner RK, Rashotte CA, et al. Preventing reading failure in young children with phonological processing disabilities: Group and individual responses to instruction. J Ed Psych 1999;4:579–593

102. Lindamood CH, Lindamood PC. Auditory Discrimination in Depth. Austin, TX: PRO-ED, 1984

103. Woodcock RW. Woodcock Reading Mastery Test-Revised. Circle Pines, MN: AGS, 1987

104. Wechsler D. Wechsler Intelligence Scale for Children-Revised. San Antonio, TX: Psychological Corporation, 1974

105. Cohen J. Statistical Power Analysis for the Behavioral Sciences. 2nd edn. Hillsdale, NJ: Lawrence Erlbaum, 1988

106. Wiederholt JL, Bryant BR. Gray Oral Reading Test—3rd edn. Austin, TX: PRO-ED, 1992

107. Lindamood CH, Lindamood PC. Lindamood Auditory Conceptualization Test. Austin, TX: PRO-ED, 1979

108. Wagner RK, Torgesen JK, Rashotte CA. Comprehensive Test of Phonological Processes. Austin, TX: PRO-ED, 1999

109. Semel E, Wiig EH, Secord W. Clinical Evaluation of Language Fundamentals—3. San Antonio, TX: Psychological Corporation, 1995

110. Deutsch G, Devivo K, Linn N, Noah SL. Classification of children with reading and language problems. Poster session, presented at the annual meeting of the International Neuropsychological Society, Denver, CO, Feb 2000

111. Hook PE, Jones SD, Macaruzo P. The efficacy of Fast-ForWord training on facilitating acquisition of reading skills in with specific reading disabilities—a longitudinal study. Ann Dyslex 2001;51:75–96

112. Scientific Learning Research. National Field Trials Research Findings [online] 1999 (accessed June 12, 2001). Available from URL: http://www.scilearn.com/scie/index.php3?main=nft/scienational2

113. Oakland T, Lack JL, Stanford G, et al. An evaluation of the dyslexia training program in a multisensory method for promoting reading in students with reading disabilities. J Learn Disabil 1998;31(2):140–147

114. Wise BW, Ring J, Olson RK. Training phonological awareness with and without explicit attention to articulation. J Exp Child Psychol 1999;72(4):271–304

115. Lovett MW, Lacerenza L, Borden SL, et al. Components of effective remediation for developmental reading disabilities: combining phonological and strategy-based instruction to improve outcomes. J Ed Psych 2000;92:263–288

116. Scientific Learning Corporation. Step4word. Berkley, CA: Scientific Learning Corporation, 1999

117. Scientific Learning Corporation. FastForWord. Berkley, CA: Scientific Learning Corporation, 1996

118. Newcomer PL, Hammill DD. Test of Language Development Primary Level—2nd edn. Austin, TX: PRO-ED, 1991

119. Cox AR. Alphabetic Phonics, an organized expression of the Orton Gillingham method. Ann Dyslex 1985;36:187–198

120. Jastak S, Wilkinson GS. Wide Range Achievement Test—Revised. Wilmington, DE: Jastak Associates, 1984

262 Treatment of Neglect

H Branch Coslett and Laurel J Buxbaum

Neglect is a disorder characterized by a failure to report, orient toward, or respond to stimuli on the contralesional side of space that cannot be attributed to sensory or motor dysfunction.[1] Neglect is not a unitary disorder, but a complex constellation of symptoms with different manifestations across patients. For example, patients may neglect the contralesional side of near (peripersonal) and not far (extrapersonal) space, or vice versa.[2] Some patients with neglect are predominantly deficient in moving attention and action into and toward contralesional space while others have primary deficits in attending to or perceiving contralesional stimuli.[3] The "personal" subtype of neglect may also dissociate from neglect of peripersonal space.[4] Some patients exhibit neglect in all sensory modalities (for example vision, audition, touch, proprioception, and so forth) whereas in other patients the deficits may be modality-specific. Anosognosia or unawareness of deficit is present in 20% to 58% of patients with neglect.[5,6]

Several accounts of neglect have been proposed. These theories are not mutually exclusive and, given the variability in the syndrome, it is possible that no single account accommodates all the features of the syndrome. Duncan and colleagues have argued that neglect is attributable to a combination of two deficits: decreased arousal and a lateralized attentional and/or perceptual deficit.[7] We have also suggested that reduced attentional resources or "cognitive activation" may represent an important component of neglect.[8]

A second account attributes neglect to damaged right-hemisphere dominant attentional mechanisms with a resulting failure to direct attention to the contralesional hemispace.[9] Another group of accounts suggests that neglect is caused by a failure to construct or maintain an internal representation of the contralesional side of space.[10] Neglect of contralesional limbs (personal neglect) has been attributed to an impaired representation of the left side of an internal body schema.[11]

Finally, Heilman and colleagues have emphasized that for both man and monkeys, neglect may be attributable to a deficit in intention.[12,13] According to this theory, the fundamental impairment in neglect is a failure to direct movements or attention into or toward the neglected hemispace.

In the following sections we briefly review current treatments of neglect. To facilitate exposition we have sorted the therapies according to putative mechanism (for example hemispheric activation). We recognize that the therapies may have implications for processing at multiple levels.

Treatments of decreased arousal

Pharmacologic treatments

Several lines of evidence suggest that a reduction in dopaminergic activity may, at least in part, cause neglect.[14,15] In light of these data, Fleet and colleagues administered 15 mg/day of the dopamine agonist bromocriptine to two patients with neglect.[16] Both patients exhibited significant improvement on a battery of tests; one subject deteriorated after the medication was discontinued. Subsequently, Geminiani, Bottini and Sterzi showed that 2 mg of apomorphine significantly improved neglect in four patients.[17] Three patients demonstrated relative improvement in motor as compared to perceptual tasks. Recently, Hurford, Bottini and Sterzi compared the efficacy of 20 mg/day of methylphenidate, which also has dopaminergic properties, and 30 mg/day of bromocriptine, and found them equally effective in a patient with chronic neglect due to middle cerebral artery (MCA) stroke.[18] Improvements with both medications were maintained once they were discontinued. Other dopaminergic agents such as amantidine are also under investigation.

While these studies are encouraging, other investigations have yielded conflicting findings. A recent study examined the performance of seven neglect patients on a computerized target search paradigm and found increased exploration of *ipsilesional* (right) hemispace with just 2.5 mg of bromocriptine.[19] One potential explanation for these data is that bromocriptine may inhibit dopamine receptors at low doses. Barrett, Crucian and Schwartz, however, reported a patient with motor neglect due to right MCA stroke whose performance on a line bisection task declined on a dose (20 mg/day) at which inhibitory effects are not expected.[20]

Phasic alerting treatments

Another group of treatments targeted at improving arousal uses external sources of stimulation to periodically alert patients. Robertson et al. reported data from eight chronic neglect patients with right hemisphere lesions who were taught a self-alerting paradigm.[21] Subjects were then taught to provide their own auditory feedback, and the ratio of subject feedback to examiner feedback was gradually increased. Patients significantly improved on several measures of neglect and attention immediately following training and these improvements were maintained for two weeks. In a related study, Robertson et al. demonstrated that an auditory tone prior to a left visual stimulus improved awareness of the left visual field in

Table 262.1 Activation treatments

Author	Experimental design	Intervention	Duration of treatment	Number of subjects	Time post injury	Outcomes measured	Results	Follow-up
Joanette, Brouchon, Gauthier & Samson, 1986[27]	Case study	Left vs. right active pointing	1 session	3 RCVAneg	1–7 months	Visual stimuli detection	Increased detection of stimuli with left hand pointing only	—
Robertson & North, 1992[28]	Single subject design	Left active finger movements in left and right space with or without visual input; right active finger movements in left space	1 session	1 RCVAneg	3 months	Letter cancellation	Left finger movements in left space improved performance with or without vision	—
Robertson, North & Geggie, 1992[25]	Single subject design	Scan to left arm; scan to left arm with active movements and alerting device; left active movements with alerting device	10–44 hours	2 RCVAneg; 1 RTBIneg	1–2 months	Letter cancellation; telephone dialing; reading; star cancellation; mobility scale; line orientation	Improvements with all treatments	Gains maintained at 6 weeks (scan to left arm with active movement and alerting device); partially maintained at 3 weeks (left active movements with scanning device)
Robertson & North, 1993[31]	Single subject design	Active vs. passive hand and leg movement	1 session	1 RCVAneg	3 months	Letter cancellation; tactile extinction	Active movements in left hemispace improved letter cancellation, not tactile extinction; no effect with passive motion	

Table 262.1   *Continued*

Author	Experimental design	Intervention	Duration of treatment	Number of subjects	Time post injury	Outcomes measured	Results	Follow-up
Robertson, Tegner, Goodrich & Wilson, 1994[23]	Quasi-experimental	Active left hand movement versus no movement during ambulation	1 session	5 RCVAneg; 1 RTBIneg	5–5 months post CVA/TBI	Deviation from center of door frame	Improvement with hand movement in 4 RCVAneg subjects	—
Robertson & North, 1994[29]	Single subject design	Active left hand movement versus bilateral active hand movement	1 session	2 RCVAneg	3 months	Reading task	Improvements with left hand movement only	—
Worthington, 1996[24]	Case study	Active left hand movement in left space with hand visible (visuomotor cueing) vs. active movement on lap	10 sessions; 1 per week	1 RCVAneg	4 months	Reading	Both treatments improved performance	Only visuomotor cueing gains maintained at 3 and 18 months
Cubelli, Paganelli, Achilli & Pedrizzi, 1999[34]	Quasi-experimental	Left, right, and bilateral active hand movements	1 session	10 RCVAneg	1–11 months	Letter cancellation	No improvements in 9 patients; 1 patient improved with left hand movement	—

RCVAneg, right hemisphere stroke with neglect; RTBIneg, right hemisphere traumatic brain injury with neglect.

Table 262.2 Caloric stimulation

Study	Experimental design	Intervention	Duration of treatment	Number of subjects	Time post injury	Outcomes measured	Results	Follow-up
Rubens, 1985[44]	Case study	Left or right ear with warm or cold water	2 sessions	18 RCVAneg	4–7 days	Line cancellation, reading, extrapersonal neglect	Improved performance with cold left/warm right stimulation	—
Cappa, Sterzi, Vallar & Bisiach, 1987[53]	Case study	Left ear cold or right ear warm caloric	1 session	4 RCVAneg	1–2 days	Line cancellation, circle cancellation, anosognosia scale, personal neglect test	Improved cancellation and personal neglect for all patients; improved anosognosia for 2 patients	Return to baseline after 15 minutes
Vallar, Sterzi, Bottini, Cappa, & Rusconi, 1990[51]	Single subject design	Left ear cold or right ear warm water	1 or 2 sessions	3 RCVAneg	2–12 days	Extra-personal neglect, personal neglect, anosognosia testing scale, sensory testing	Improvements in extrapersonal neglect, anosognosia, hemianesthesia with both cold and warm stimuli; greater impairment with cold stimuli	Return to baseline after 30–60 minutes
Bisiach, Rusconi, Vallar 1991[55]	Case study	Left ear cold caloric	1 session	1 RCVAneg	11 days	Verbal report of delusion	Decreased somato-paraphrenic delusions	—
Rode, Charles, Perenin, Vighetto, Trillet, Aimard, 1992[49]	Case study	Left ear cold caloric	2 sessions	1 RCVAneg	6 months	Extra-personal neglect, line crossing, personal neglect, anosognosia scale, visual-sensory-motor clinical exam	Improvements in extrapersonal neglect, anosognosia, and hemiplegia; no changes in hemianopia or sensation	Informal observation showed return to baseline

Table 262.2 *Continued*

Study	Experimental design	Intervention	Duration of treatment	Number of subjects	Time post injury	Outcomes measured	Results	Follow-up
Geminiani, Bottini, 1992[54]	Case study	Left ear cold caloric	1 session	5 RCVAneg	1 month	Line cancellation, anosognosia scale, personal neglect	Improved performance in line crossing, anosognosia, and mental representation	—
Vallar, Bottini, Rusconi, Sterzi, 1993[46]	Quasi-experimental	Cold caloric contralateral to lesion	1 session	19 RCVAneg; 10 LCVA; 1 R neoplasm; 1 L neoplasm	Minimum 14 days post CVA; no data on neoplasms	Sensory testing	R group better than L group immediately post stimulation; improved extinction in a subgroup of R patients	No difference between groups after 30 minutes
Vallar, Papagano, Rusconi, Bisiach, 1995[47]	Case study	Right ear cold caloric	3 sessions	1 LTBIneg	6 weeks	Line cancellation, Token test, object naming, digit span, sentence repetition	Improvements in line cancellation only	Return to baseline after 30 minute delay
Bottini, Paulesu, Sterzi, Warburton, Wise, Vallar, et al, 1995[50]	Single subject design	Left ear cold caloric	6 sessions	1 RCVAneg	4 weeks	Tactile stimulation during PET scan	Improved sensation post stimulation; PET showed interaction between touch and vestibular stimulation	—
Rode, Perenin, Honore, Boisson, 1998[52]	Quasi-experimental	Cold caloric contralateral to lesion	1 session	9 RCVAneg; 9 LCVA	Minimum 2.5 months	Motor function, personal neglect, and anosognosia	Improved performance all measures RCVA only	—

RCVAneg, right hemisphere stroke with neglect; LCVA, left hemisphere stroke; LTBIneg, left hemisphere traumatic brain injury with neglect.

eight neglect patients, the majority of whom had suffered right MCA strokes.[22] Maintenance of the treatment effect was not assessed.

These studies provide class III evidence that dopamine agonists and interventions to improve alertness ameliorate neglect. Treatment with dopamine agonists must be undertaken with caution in light of data demonstrating that the performance of some patients may be adversely affected by this therapy. The effects of therapy with these agents should be carefully monitored by serial administration of tasks on which the treated patient was impaired in order to demonstrate that the treatment is not deleterious.

Hemispheric activation approaches

Hemispheric activation with limb movements

Several studies have demonstrated that even small movements of the left hand on the left side of space may result in significant reductions in neglect. As can be seen in Table 262.1, active movements of the contralesional upper or lower extremity have significantly improved walking trajectory,[23] reading,[24] and cancellation performance[25] in patients with neglect. A meta-analysis of the activation literature found large effect sizes for both group and single subject studies of contralesional limb activation that support their therapeutic effectiveness.[26]

In contrast, several investigations indicate that neglect does not improve with movements of the ipsilesional extremity, or of bilateral extremities, possibly due to competition from the intact left hemisphere.[27–29] The results of passive range of motion (PROM) of the left extremity have been inconclusive, with some authors reporting improvements with PROM, and others finding no effects.[30,31]

Robertson has proposed that limb activation exerts its benefit by virtue of its effects on overlapping neural systems representing "personal" (body surface) and "peripersonal" (near body) space.[32] When the left limb is used, there is enhancement of the left portion of the representation of personal space. When the left limb is used in the left hemispace, this enhancement is accompanied by corresponding activation of the left portion of the peripersonal representation. It is this reciprocal activation in multiple corresponding spatial sectors that is putatively critical to the beneficial effect.[33]

While the activation approach to treatment of hemispatial neglect appears promising, replication of limb activation effects has been unsuccessful by some authors, who have suggested that the effects may be patient-specific.[34] Additionally, since bilateral limb movements appear to mitigate positive treatment effects, it is not clear whether traditional therapeutic activities, many of which are bimanual, may actually diminish the effects of limb activation treatment.

These studies provide class II and III evidence that moving the contralesional hand in the contralesional hemispace improves neglect. The clinical utility of the therapy is limited by the fact that it requires active motion of the contralesional extremity, a capacity that is absent in many patients with neglect.[35]

Eye patching/hemispatial glasses

Therapies designed to selectively activate right brain structures by manipulating visual input have also been investigated. Work in animals indicates that the superior colliculus plays an important role in the control of attention.[36–38] As the superior colliculus (SC) receives input from the contralateral eye and the colliculi have inhibitory connections with each other, one might predict that patching the right eye would decrease the activation of the left SC and reduce inhibitory influences on the right SC.

Other investigators have employed "hemispatial" glasses, a standard eyeglass frame with the ipsilesional (right) hemifields of both lenses blocked, to control the processing of visual information. Arai and colleagues reported 10 patients with neglect (1–31 months post cerebrovascular accident [CVA]) who wore hemispatial glasses during testing with line bisection, line cancellation, and figure copying tasks.[39] The glasses resulted in apparent improvements in some patients, and no effects or exacerbation of neglect in others. No data were reported enabling distinctions between patients who did or did not profit from the treatment.

Another recent study compared half-eye and full eye patching.[40] Twenty-two acute neglect patients were randomly assigned to control, half-patch, or full-patch groups. Both treatment groups wore their respective devices continuously for a three-month period. Outcome measures included change in scores on the functional independence measure (FIM) and left-sided performance on a computerized visual task.[41] There were significant improvements in attention to the left visual field in the half-patch compared to the other groups. The FIM results were difficult to interpret, however, because the half-patch group had lower FIM scores at baseline; thus, effects of "regression to the mean" cannot be ruled out.

Treatment with prisms

Several investigators have attempted to remediate neglect by employing lenses that shift the apparent site of a relevant stimulus into or toward the "good" right hemispace. For example, Rossi, Kheyfets, and Reding used fresnel prisms in a heterogeneous population of acute stroke patients with either visual extinction or homonymous hemianopia.[42] Patients were randomly assigned to control or treatment groups. The latter group wore prisms over their affected hemifield during all daily activities for four weeks. Subjects also wore prisms during outcome testing (measures of neglect, visual fields, and functional performance). The treatment group showed significant improvements on neglect tests as compared to controls, but there were no differences on measures of visual fields or functional performance.

Relatively impressive results were reported by Rossetti and colleagues in a randomized study of the effect of prisms on 12 neglect patients.[43] Subjects wore prisms for only approximately five minutes while they performed a repetitive reaching-to-target task, and then performed a battery of clinical neglect tests (such as line bisection and reading) without the prisms. The treatment group showed significant improvement that was maintained for at least two hours after the prisms were removed.

Thus, although there are few data and many unanswered questions there is class III evidence supporting the use of prisms in the treatment of neglect. This treatment shows significant promise.

Caloric and optokenetic stimulation

One possible interpretation of the dramatic effects observed in patients with neglect is that for these patients the egocentric representation of their bodies and space is rotated or shifted to the left. Vestibular and the intimately related systems mediating ocular motility appear to be critical to the genesis of this egocentric representation. Rubens assessed the possible influence of vestibular systems on neglect by delivering cold water caloric stimulation to the left ear of patients with neglect.[44] He reported, and many subsequent investigators have confirmed, that irrigation of the left external auditory canal with cold water (or right with warm water) often dramatically improves neglect and related disorders.

Caloric stimulation has been demonstrated to reduce personal and extrapersonal neglect.[45–49] Improvements in tactile sensitivity[46,50,51] and motor function[45,52] have also been observed. Finally, caloric stimulation has been successful in ameliorating anosognosia,[45,48,49,51,53] spatial representation deficits,[54] and somatoparaphrenic delusions, such as the conviction that the patient's arm belongs to a stranger.[55] Most investigators believe that cold contralesional caloric stimulation improves neglect by influencing an egocentric representation of space rather than by altering eye movements *per se*.[51,53]

Exposure to stimuli moving from right to left at a rate of approximately 30–45 degrees per second induces a slow phase-left, fast phase-right nystagmus.[56,57] Neglect outcome measures are typically administered while the subject is receiving the optokinetic stimulation. For example, subjects might be asked to denote the center of a line presented against a right-left moving background on a video monitor. Optokinetic stimulation has been reported to improve several aspects of neglect. Deficits in position sense,[57–59] motor skills,[60] body orientation,[56] and perceptual neglect[60,61] have temporarily improved during optokinetic stimulation. A recent functional magnetic resonance imaging (fMRI) study of optokinetic stimulation demonstrated bilateral activations in subcortical and cortical sensorimotor circuits.[62]

There is class III evidence demonstrating the efficacy of both caloric and optokinetic stimulation for the treatment of neglect. The clinical utility of these interventions is limited by several considerations. First, the beneficial effects appear to be short-lived; improvement typically lasts for 10–20 minutes for caloric stimulation and the utility of repeated caloric

stimulation has not, to our knowledge, been assessed. Additionally, most studies have involved acute patients, and the potential benefit for patients with chronic neglect has not been established. Optokinetic stimulation therapy is subject to similar criticisms. The duration of the effects of optokinetic stimulation has not been well investigated, but appears to be limited to when the stimuli are being applied.[60] In addition, as with caloric stimulation, the effect of repeated treatments has not been investigated, so it is not clear whether habituation or more permanent improvement may occur.

Additional therapies for neglect

Several additional therapies have been reported to be beneficial in the treatment of neglect. For example, Karnath, Christ and Hartje have demonstrated that vibration of neck muscles and rotation of the trunk may ameliorate neglect.[63] Smania et al. demonstrated that two patients with neglect improved after extensive practice with motor imagery.[64] These and other therapies are not discussed in detail because of space limitations and, in some instances, the paucity of data.[65,66]

References

1. Heilman KM, Watson RT, Valenstein E. Neglect and related disorders. *In:* Heilman KM, Valenstein E, eds. Clinical Neuropyschology. 2nd ed. New York: Oxford University Press, 1985:279–336
2. Mennemeier M, Wertman E, Heilman KM. Neglect of near personal space. Brain 1992;115:37–50
3. Coslett HB, Bowers D, Fitzpatrick E, et al. Directional akinesia and hemispatial inattention in neglect. Brain 1990;113:475–486
4. Zoccolotti P, Judica A. Functional evaluation of hemineglect by means of a semi-structured scale: personal vs. extra-personal differentiation. Neuropsychol Rehab 1991;1:33–44
5. Berti A, Ladavas E, Corte MD. Anosognosia for hemiplegia, neglect dyslexia, and drawing neglect: clinical findings and theoretical considerations. J Int Neuropsychol Soc 1996;2:426–440
6. Cutting J. Study of anosognosia. J Neurol Neurosurg Psychiatry 1978;41:548–555
7. Duncan J, Bundesen C, Olson A, et al. Systematic analysis of deficits in visual attention. JEP: General 1999;128:450–478
8. Coslett HB, Bowers D, Heilman KM. Reduction in cognitive activation after right hemisphere stroke. Neurology 1987;37:957–962
9. Heilman KM, Van Den Abell T. Right hemisphere dominance for attention: the mechanism underlying hemispheric asymmetries of inattention (neglect). Neurology 1980;30:327–330
10. Bisiach E, Luzzatti C. Unilateral neglect of representational space. Cortex 1978;14:129–133
11. Coslett HB. Evidence for a disturbance of the body schema in neglect. Brain Cogn 1998;37:527–544
12. Heilman KM, Bowers D, Coslett HB, et al. Directional hypokinesia: prolonged reaction times for leftward movements in patients with right hemisphere lesions and neglect. Neurology 1985;35(6):855–859
13. Watson RT, Miller BD, Heilman KM. Nonsensory neglect. Ann Neurol 1978;3:505–508

14. Marshall JF, Gotthelf T. Sensory inattention in rats with 6-hydroxydopamine-induced degeneration of ascending dopaminergic neurons: apomorphine-induced reversal of deficits. Exp Neurol 1979;65:733–748

15. Corwin JV, Kanter SL, Watson RT, et al. Apomorphine has a therapeutic effect on neglect produced by unilateral dorsomedial prefrontal cortex lesions in rats. Exp Neurol 1986;94:683–689

16. Fleet WS, Valenstein E, Watson RT, Heilman KM. Dopamine agonist therapy for neglect in humans. Neurology 1987;37:1765–1770

17. Geminiani G, Bottini G, Sterzi R. Dopaminergic stimulation in unilateral neglect. J Neurol Neurosurg Psychiatry 1998;65(3):344–347

18. Hurford P, Stringer AY, Jann B. Neuropharmacologic treatment of hemineglect: a case report comparing bromocriptine and methylphenidate. Arch Phys Med Rehabil 1998;79:346–349

19. Grujic Z, Mapstone MA, Gitelman DR, et al. Dopamine agonists reorient visual exploration away from the neglected hemispace. Neurology 1998;51:1395–1398

20. Barrett AM, Crucian GP, Schwartz RL. Adverse effect of dopamine agonist therapy in a patient with motor-intentional neglect. Arch Phys Med Rehabil 1999;80:600–603

21. Robertson IH, Tegner R, Tham K, et al. Sustained attention training for unilateral neglect: theoretical and rehabilitation implications. J Clin Exp Neuropsychol 1995;17:416–430

22. Robertson IH, Mattingley JB, Rorden C, Driver J. Phasic alerting of neglect patients overcomes their spatial deficit in visual awareness. Nature 1998;395:169–172

23. Robertson IH, Tegner R, Goodrich SJ, Wilson C. Walking trajectory and hand movements during walking in unilateral neglect: a vestibular hypothesis. Neuropsychologia 1994;32:1495–1502

24. Worthington AD. Cueing strategies in neglect dyslexia. Neuropsychol Rehabil 1996;6:1–17

25. Robertson IH, North N, Geggie C. Spatio-motor cueing in unilateral neglect: three case studies of its therapeutic effectiveness. J Neurol Neurosurg Psychiatry 1992;55:799–805

26. Lin K. Right hemisphere activation approaches to neglect rehabilitation post-stroke. Am J Occup Ther 1996;50(7):504–515

27. Joanette Y, Brouchon M, Gauthier L, Samson M. Pointing with left vs right hand in left visual field neglect. Neuropsychologia 1986;24(3):391–396

28. Robertson IH, North N. Spatiomotor cueing in unilateral left neglect: the role of hemispace, hand, and motor activation. Neuropsychologia 1992;30:553–563

29. Robertson IH, North N. One hand is better than two: motor extinction of left hand advantage in unilateral neglect. Neuropsychologia 1994;32:1–11

30. Ladavas E, Berti A, Ruozzi E, Barboni F. Neglect as a deficit determined by an imbalance between multiple spatial representations. Exp Brain Res 1997;116(3):493–500

31. Robertson IH, North N. Active and passive activation of left limbs: influence on visual and sensory neglect. Neuropsychologia 1993;31(3):293–300

32. Robertson IH. Cognitive rehabilitation: attention and neglect. Trends in Cogn Sci 1999;3:885–893

33. Rizzolatti G, Camarda R. Neural circuits for spatial attention and unilateral neglect. In: Jeannerod M, ed. Neurophysiological and Neuropsychological Aspects of Spatial Neglect. Holland: Elsevier Science Publishers, 1987:289–313

34. Cubelli R, Paganelli N, Achilli D, Pedrizzi S. Is one hand always better than two? A replication study. Neurocase 1999;5:143–151

35. Sterzi R, Bottini G, Celani MG, et al. Hemianopia, hemianaesthesia, and hemiplegia after right and left hemisphere damage. A hemispheric difference. J Neurol Neurosurg Psychiatry 1993;56:308–310

36. Sprague JM. Interaction of cortex and superior colliculus in mediation of visually guided behavior in the cat. Science 1966;153:1544–1547

37. Spark DL. Translation of sensory signals into commands for control of saccadic eye movements: role of the primate superior colliculus. Physiol Rev 1986;66:118–171

38. Hubel DH, Levay S, Wiesel TN. Mode of termination of retinotectal fibers in macaque monkey: an autoradiographic analysis. Brain Res 1975;96:125–140

39. Arai T, Ohi H, Sasaki H, et al. Hemispatial sunglasses: effect on unilateral spatial neglect. Arch Phys Med Rehabil 1997;78:230–232

40. Beis J-M, Andre J-M, Baumgarten A, Challier B. Eye patching in unilateral spatial neglect: efficacy of two methods. Arch Phys Med Rehabil 1999;80:71–76

41. Guide for the Uniform Data System for Medical Rehabilitation, Version 5.0. Buffalo: State University of New York at Buffalo, 1996

42. Rossi PW, Kheyfets S, Reding MJ. Frensel prisms improve visual perception in stroke patients with homonymous hemianopia or unilateral visual neglect. Neurology 1990;40(10):1597–1599

43. Rosetti Y, Rode G, Pisella L, et al. Prism adaptation to a rightward optical deviation rehabilitates left hemispatial neglect. Nature 1998;396:166–169

44. Rubens AB. Caloric stimulation and unilateral visual neglect. Neurology 1985;35:1019–1024

45. Rode G, Charles N, Perenin MT, et al. Partial remission of hemiplegia and somatoparaphrenia through vestibular stimulation in a case of unilateral neglect. Cortex 1992;28:203–208

46. Vallar G, Bottini G, Rusconi ML, Sterzi R. Exploring somatosensory hemineglect by vestibular stimulation. Brain 1993;116(1):71–76

47. Vallar G, Papagno C, Rusconi ML, Bisiach E. Vestibular stimulation, spatial hemineglect and dysphasia. Selective effects? Cortex 1995;31:589–593

48. Geminiani G, Bottini G. Mental representation and temporary recovery from unilateral neglect after vestibular stimulation. J Neurol Neurosurg Psychiatry 1992;55:332–333

49. Rode G, Charles N, Perenin MT, et al. Partial remission of hemiplegia and somatoparaphrenia through vestibular stimulation in a case of unilateral neglect. Cortex 1992;28:203–208

50. Bottini G, Paulesu E, Sterzi R, et al. Modulation of conscious experience by peripheral sensory stimuli. Nature 1995;376:778–781

51. Vallar G, Sterzi R, Bottini G, et al. Temporary remission of left hemianethesia after vestibular stimulation: a sensory neglect phenomenon. Cortex 1990;26:123–131

52. Rode G, Perenin MT, Honore J, Boisson D. Improvement of the motor deficit of neglect patients through vestibular stimulation: evidence for a motor neglect component. Cortex 1998;34:253–261

53. Cappa S, Sterzi S, Vallar G, Bisiach E. Remission of hemineglect and anosognosia during vestibular stimulation. Neuropsychologia 1987;25:775–782

54. Geminiani G, Bottini G. Mental representation and tem-

porary recovery from unilateral neglect after vestibular stimulation. J Neurol Neurosurg Psychiatry 1992;55: 332–333

55. Bisiach E, Rusconi ML, Vallar G. Remission of somatoparaphrenic delusion through vestibular stimulation. Neuropsychologia 1991;10:1029–1031

56. Karnath HO. Optokinetic stimulation influences the disturbed perception of body orientation in spatial neglect. J Neurol Neurosurg Psychiatry 1996;60(2): 217–220

57. Vallar G, Antonucci G, Guariglia C, Pizzamiglio L. Deficits of position sense, unilateral neglect and optokinetic stimulation. Neuropsychologia 1993;31:1191–1200

58. Vallar G, Guariglia C, Magnotti L, Pizzamiglio L. Optokinetic stimulation affects both vertical and horizontal deficits of position sense in unilateral neglect. Cortex 1995;31(4):669–683

59. Vallar G, Guariglia C, Magnotti L, Pizzamiglio L. Dissociation between position sense and visual-spatial components of hemineglect through a specific rehabilitation treatment. J Clin Exp Neuropsychol 1997;19: 763–771

60. Vallar G, Guariglia C, Nico D, Pizzamiglio L. Motor deficits and optokinetic stimulation in patients with left

hemineglect. Neurology 1997;49(5):1364–1370

61. Pizzamiglio L, Frasca R, Guariglia C, et al. Effect of optokinetic stimulation in patients with visual neglect. Cortex 1990;26:535–540

62. Bucher SF, Dieterich M, Seelos KC, Brandt T. Sensorimotor cerebral activation during optokinetic nystagmus: a functional MRI study. Neurology 1997;49: 1370–1377

63. Karnath HO, Christ K, Hartje W. Decrease of contralateral neglect by neck muscle vibration and spatial orientation of trunk midline. Brain 1993;116:383–396

64. Smania N, Bazoli F, Piva D, Guidetti G. Visuomotor imagery and rehabilitation of neglect. Arch Phys Med Rehabil 1997;78:430–436

65. Karnath HO, Schenkel P, Fischer B. Trunk orientation as the determining factor of the contralateral deficit in the neglect syndrome and as the physical anchor of the internal representation of body orientation in space. Brain 1991;114:1997–2014

66. Diller L, Weinberg J. Hemi-attention in rehabilitation: the evolution of a rational remediation program. In: Weinstein EA, Friedland RP, eds. Hemi-inattention and Hemispheric Specialization, Advances in Neurology. Vol 18. New York: Raven Press, 1977:63–82

263 Management of Attention-Deficit/Hyperactivity Disorder and Dyslexia (Specific Reading Disability)

Bennett A Shaywitz and Sally E Shaywitz

Attention-deficit/hyperactivity disorder (ADHD) and developmental dyslexia represent the most common neurobehavioral disorder of childhood; though prevalence rates vary enormously, a reasonable estimate for ADHD from samples in pediatric populations is 11%[1] with boys affected more commonly than girls and with male:female ratios varying between 2:1 and 4:1. Dyslexia is even more common, with prevalence rates ranging from 5% to 17.5%.[2] Good evidence based on sample surveys of randomly selected populations of children now indicate that dyslexia affects boys and girls equally; the long-held belief that only boys suffer from dyslexia reflected sampling bias in school-identified samples.[3] This chapter focuses on the management of these two very common disorders.

Attention-deficit/hyperactivity disorder (ADHD)

The diagnosis of ADHD is established on the basis of a history of symptoms of the cardinal constructs of ADHD—inattention, impulsivity and hyperactivity. The fourth edition of the Diagnostic and Statistical Manual of Mental Disorders (DSM-IV) criteria form the basis of the most widely recognized diagnostic schema; diagnosis depends on the endorsement of items on two nine-item symptom lists, one list for "inattention," the other for "hyperactive-impulsive" behavior. Current DSM-IV criteria[4] recognize three subtypes of ADHD: ADHD primarily of the inattentive type (ADHD/I, endorsement of 6/9 "inattention" items); ADHD primarily of the hyperactive-impulsive type (ADHD/HI, endorsement of 6/9 "hyperactive-impulsive" items) and ADHD combined type (ADHD/C, endorsement of 6/9 items on each of the "inattention" and "hyperactive-impulsive" lists). DSM-IV criteria require that the symptoms of ADHD be present in two or more settings (e.g., at home and in school) and the diagnosis is made from a synthesis of information obtained from both parents and from school reports. The symptoms of ADHD may be assessed systematically and expeditiously by using symptom rating scales for parents and teachers (e.g., Conners Rating Scales—revised for parents, teachers and adolescent self-report) and reviewed recently in pediatric clinical practice guidelines.[5] Teachers' perceptions of childrens' behavior differs significantly for boys and girls[6] and relative degrees of deficits and strengths may differ in boys and girls. Laboratory measures are generally not helpful in ADHD. Neuroimaging studies have been used in a number of research studies but routine computed tomography (CT) or magnetic resonance imaging (MRI) are not indicated in the evaluation. While the differential diagnosis of a child with symptoms of inattention, impulsivity and hyperactivity is extremely limited, a number of conditions are often associated with (co-occur with) ADHD. Of the co-occurring conditions, the most important is learning disability, primarily dyslexia. Thus, in evaluating the child with school problems, the examiner should consider ADHD and dyslexia each as diagnostic possibilities and reliable and valid measures to assess each problem should be employed. The diagnosis and management of dyslexia is discussed later in this chapter.

Management of ADHD encompasses two general domains: (a) pharmacological therapies and (b) non-pharmacological including educational, cognitive-behavioral and other psychological and psychiatric approaches. Within the last few years there have been two seminal developments in treatment. The first is that the evidence-based practice center at McMaster University, under contract with the Agency for Health Care Policy and Research (AHCPR), produced an evidence-based report on the treatment of ADHD;[7] the topic was proposed to the AHCPR by the American Academy of Pediatrics and American Psychiatric Association who served as partners to the Center. The second is the completion of the multimodal treatment study of children with ADHD (MTA) multimodal treatment of ADHD study by the National Institute of Mental Health (NIMH), a 14-month double-blind placebo trial of medication and behavioral therapy in ADHD (Table 263.1).[8]

The results of these investigations form the core of the clinical practice guidelines for the treatment of the school-aged child with ADHD published in Pediatrics, October, 2001.[9]

Table 263.1 MTA study design
Treatment arms 1) Medication management 2) Behavioral treatment 3) Combined treatment 4) Community care

In general, the results of the evidence-based review and the MTA study are that stimulants (methylphenidate and amphetamine) are the most effective agents for the treatment of ADHD. Results from the MTA study indicate that MPH (methylphenidate and MPH combined with behavioral therapy are superior to behavioral therapy alone and all are superior to the typical therapy available in the community. The evidence-based review indicates that each of the stimulants are superior to placebo and the stimulants (methylphenidate and amphetamine) are comparable to one another. Regular and sustained release MPH are comparable and D and L isomers of amphetamine are comparable. As for other agents, tricyclics, specifically desipramine, are superior to placebo. Few studies reviewed by the McMaster group[7] compared stimulants directly to tricyclics and these were technically inadequate, leading to the conclusion that more rigorous studies are required. Only five studies reviewed by the McMaster group were found which examined non-pharmacological treatment and all contained major limitations in methodology. Despite the limitations, all showed that stimulants were more effective than the non-pharmacological therapies, in agreement with the results of the MTA study. There was lack of evidence to support the superiority of combination, multimodal treatment over stimulant therapy alone, again similar with the MTA study. Finally, most studies are relatively short-term. Even the MTA study, at 14 months, is relatively short-term and the longer term effects of medication are unclear.[9]

Clinical approach to stimulant administration

Central to the management program is the recognition that ADHD is a chronic disorder, and while the symptoms may change as the child matures, in many children the disorder extends throughout childhood and into adult life. This means that management will need to be modified as the child progresses from primary school to middle school to high school and beyond. Both the evidence-based review and the MTA study examined ADHD in middle childhood. Thus, the evidence base is strongest for ADHD in the early school years, with few studies examining older children and adults with the disorder. Furthermore, to date few randomized clinical trials have been performed in adults[10] and while recent reports of the efficacy of amphetamine in adults are promising[11,12] more studies are clearly indicated. Difficulties with diagnostic criteria for ADHD in adults further complicate the problem of assessing therapy in adults, though a commentary on the recent report noted above[12] notes "...that ADHD exists in adults, is not an uncommon disorder, can be reliably diagnosed and, perhaps most important, can be effectively treated."[13]

Before beginning any pharmacotherapy, the physician, in collaboration with school personnel, should specify appropriate target outcomes to guide management. For example, is it the child's inattention in school that is the target of treatment, or his hyperactive, impulsive behavior? Once this has been decided upon, treatment with stimulants should be initiated.

The following approach describes the use of methylphenidate; doses will need to be modified for dexedrine or racemic amphetamine. We typically begin with MPH at an initial dosage of 0.3 mg/kg (rounded to nearest 5 mg) given in the morning immediately before the child leaves for school. This will provide enough time for the MPH to be absorbed and positive effects observed for at least two to three hours. Both the pharmacokinetics and the behavioral effects of the drug are indistinguishable whether it is given with breakfast or 30 minutes before breakfast. The school should be encouraged to place the child in academic subjects during these morning hours so that the effects of the drug on attentional processes will be maximal when the child needs the most help. Thus, though the effects of the medication will be waning by lunchtime, and in afternoon classes, if these are non-academic subjects, then the need for the medication will not be as great. Clinical response is monitored by periodic feedback about the child's school performance. This may be accomplished indirectly by reports from the parents or more directly from the child's teachers with a particular focus on monitoring target outcomes and adverse effects.

If the child is not responding satisfactorily after two weeks of treatment MPH dosage should be increased to 0.6–0.8 mg/kg. If there is no response after two weeks at this dose, consider switching to another stimulant. On many occasions the child will do well in the morning at the 0.3 mg/kg dose but the effects appear to wear off by early afternoon. In this situation it is reasonable to add another 0.3 mg/kg dose in the morning (for a total morning dose of 0.6 mg/kg). If afternoon function is still problematic, a second 0.3 mg/kg dose may be given three hours later. Another option would be to use a stimulant with a longer duration of action, such as sustained release MPH or amphetamine.

Another important issue that must be considered is whether medication should be administered daily, or just on school days, with drug holidays when the child is away from school. Administration solely during school offers the advantage of limiting potential toxicity while maximizing the effect of MPH when it is most needed i.e., during the school day. Our routine is to prescribe MPH each school day but omit the drug on weekends, school holidays, during the summer and for the first four to six weeks of the new school year. Discontinuing MPH at the end of one school year enables us to evaluate how the child will do off medication and offers a regular opportunity to discontinue medication permanently. Thus, if it appears that the child is doing well without medication during the initial portion of the new school year we do not resume pharmacotherapy. However, careful follow-up is critical since as the school year continues and academic pressures increase, initial sanguine assumptions about the lack of a need for medication may prove to be overly optimistic. Clearly such a procedure may need to be modified in particular situations. Thus, on occasions when a particular child's impulsivity and activity are preventing optimum peer and family interaction we have continued MPH on weekends. Furthermore, if the physician believes that the child's response to medication has been so dramatic and that starting a new school year without medication would be detrimental to the best interests of the child, he may decide that medication should be initiated as soon as school begins.

If one stimulant does not work at the highest feasible dose, it is reasonable to try another, for example, if methylphenidate proves ineffective, dexedrine or racemic amphetamine should be tried. If stimulants prove ineffective, the physician should re-evaluate the original diagnosis as well as review whether the child has been compliant with the treatment plan. Re-evaluation should also consider whether there are any co-occurring disorders that might influence the effectiveness of therapy.

Stimulant use in special situations

Pharmacotherapy for the child who has both dyslexia and ADHD presents a particular challenge. In practice, it makes intuitive sense to try to titrate the dose of stimulant in an effort to improve the child's inattention when he is receiving tutoring for dyslexia. This often means that the intervention program for dyslexia be coordinated with the time of maximal effect of the stimulant. We frequently suggest that the individual tutoring component of the reading program be scheduled for the morning when the dose of MPH is at its peak.

While the positive effects of stimulants in ADHD have been described, for the most part, in school-age children, stimulants may also be effective in younger (pre-school) children, though "...no definitive study supports the efficacy and safety of these medications in this age group."[14] At least two studies now document the effectiveness of stimulants in adolescents as well as in school-age children.[15,16] Studies have not demonstrated an increase in seizure frequency or severity when stimulants are administered to children with epilepsy, assuming appropriate anticonvulsant medications are administered as well.[17,18]

Details of stimulant administration

Methylphenidate (Ritalin) is supplied as tablets of 5, 10 and 20 mg. It is also supplied as a sustained release 20 mg tablet. A still longer acting preparation, Concerta, is supplied as an 18 mg tablet that uses osmotic pressure to effect delivery at a slow, sustained rate. Dexedrine (D-amphetamine) is supplied as capsules of 5 and 10 mg and 15 mg. The usual rule of thumb is that the standard dose of amphetamine is two thirds of the dose of the methylphenidate dose (0.2–0.5 mg/kg). Racemic amphetamine (Adderall) comes as tablets of 5, 10, 20 and 30 mg, composed of equal parts of four amphetamine salts (D-amphetamine saccharate, D-amphetamine sulfate, D,L-amphetamine sulfate, and D,L-amphetamine aspartate), resulting in a 75:25 ratio of the dextro- and levo-isomers of amphetamine. The standard dosage is about three quarters the dose of methylphenidate. Pemoline (Cylert), a third stimulant type, may

adversely affect liver function and periodic monitoring of liver function tests is required when the drug is used, and this necessity has limited the clinical usefulness of pemoline. For this reason, pediatric practice guidelines do not recommend use of this agent.

There are few contraindications to stimulants and side effects tend to be relatively mild and transient. Most common side effects are stomach ache, headache, and decreased appetite. Motor tics are noted in 15% to 30% of children; for the most part, these are relatively mild and disappear when medication is stopped. The issue is confounded because approximately half of children with Tourette syndrome have ADHD, and in these children the effects of medication on tics are unpredictable. The recent pediatric practice guidelines state that "...the presence of tics before or during medical management of ADHD is not an absolute contraindication to the use of stimulant medications."[9] In fact, the McMaster review indicated that there was no increase in tics in children treated with stimulants in seven studies comparing stimulants with placebo or with other medications.[7]

Mood changes, characterized by reports that the child "is not himself" may be reported in some children receiving stimulants. Often the symptom can be minimized by lowering the dose of medication. A commonly reported symptom is behavioral rebound as the medication wears off, though this symptom is not well documented in clinical trials. Small doses of stimulant in the late afternoon and evening are often effective in reducing the problem. Stimulants are often used therapeutically as appetite suppressants and it is not surprising that appetite suppression and weight loss are common side effects of stimulants. Clinical lore has it that methylphenidate produces less of an anorexic effect, though there are no clinical trials data to support significant differences between methylphenidate and dextro-amphetamine. While two decades ago there was a concern about the effects of stimulants on growth, a prospective follow-up study into adult life has found no significant effect on ultimate adult height.[19]

Other pharmacological agents

The tricyclics desipramine and imipramine are considered as second line medications and are administered only after stimulants have not been successful.[16,20,21] Reports of sudden deaths, presumably from cardiac arrhythmias, in children taking desipramine mandate caution in using these agents.[22] The standard dose of desipramine is 3 mg/kg and it is supplied in tablets of 10–150 mg. Clonidine and the closely related guanfacine, both α_2 agonists, are sometimes used in children with ADHD and tic disorder, particularly in those patients in whom stimulants have exacerbated the tics. The main side effects are syncope, electrocardiogram (ECG) abnormalities, confusion, and rarely, sudden death.[23] The standard dose of clonidine is 0.5–0.10 mg three times daily (tid) or as a 0.2 mg patch and it is supplied as tablets of 0.1, 0.2 and 0.3 mg and extended release patches of

0.1 mg/24 hr, 0.2 mg/24 hr and 0.3 mg/24 hr. Guanfacine, which may be less sedating and less hyptotensive than clonidine, is used in a standard dose of 0.5 mg tid and is supplied in tablets of 1 and 2 mg.

Non-pharmacological therapies

Educational management Educational approaches reviewed elsewhere[24] include: minimizing distracting stimuli by preferential seating, in carrels or in a self-contained classroom; providing a 1:1 tutorial by increasing teacher availability through the use of aides or in a resource room; assuring structure and predictable routines; monitoring and, if necessary, modifying non-academic structured times such as in the lunchroom, recess or physical education; teaching organizational and work-study skills, such as organizing materials and time.

Behavioral therapies Behavioral therapies include a wide variety of strategies; enthusiasm for these treatments comes from the recognition that while stimulant medications are often effective, their actions may be circumscribed. Thus, medications are effective in at most 70% of children, and many others may either refuse medication or discontinue it shortly after initiation.[25] Cognitive and behavioral strategies (CBT) encourage the active participation of the child in the learning and monitoring process; training addresses such issues as: problem definition, problem approach, focusing of attention, choosing an answer and self-enforcement and coping.[26] With its focus on self-guidance and problem solving, CBT offers an attractive long-term coping strategy for the child with ADHD that is both durable and generalizable. However, it has been difficult to document that CBT is effective in ADHD and, in fact, as noted above, the MTA study indicates that pharmacotherapy alone is superior to behavioral therapy and the combined pharmacotherapy and behavioral therapy is no better than pharmacotherapy alone. Some studies suggest that CBT may be a useful adjunct to pharmacotherapy and may be particularly helpful in treating the more internalizing symptoms of ADHD.[9] In addition, CBT may be helpful when children are tapered off medication.

Dyslexia

Dyslexia[27] is characterized by an unexpected difficulty in reading in children and adults who otherwise possess the intelligence, motivation, and schooling considered necessary for accurate and fluent reading. Since physicians are frequently asked about various reading programs for dyslexia, they should understand the principal elements of an effective training program. These elements reflect an understanding of the reading process and why it is so difficult for children and adults with dyslexia to learn to read. There is now a strong consensus among investigators in the field that the central difficulty in dyslexia reflects a deficit within the language system, and more specifically, within a particular component of the language system, phonology, which refers to getting to the sound structure of words.[2,28,30] To learn to read,

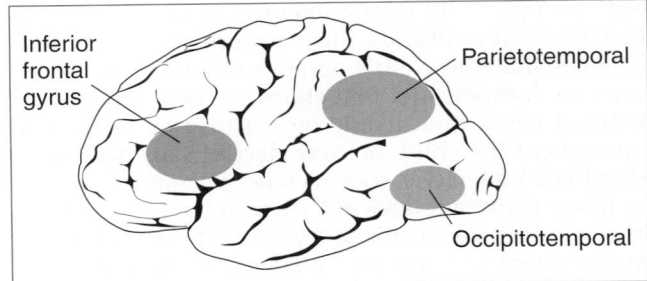

Figure 263.1   Neural systems for reading. Converging evidence indicates three important systems in reading, all primarily in the left hemisphere. These include an anterior system and two posterior systems: (1) anterior system in the left inferior frontal region; (2) parieto-temporal system involving angular gyrus, supramarginal gyrus and posterior portions of the superior temporal gyrus; (3) occipito-temporal system involving portions of the middle temporal gyrus and middle occipital gyrus. For details, please see text.

children must discover that spoken words can be broken down into elemental units of sound (phonemes), that the letters on the page represent these sounds, and that written words have the same number and sequence of sounds heard in the spoken word. This ability, termed phonemic awareness, is largely missing in dyslexic children and adults.

Converging evidence from a range of neurobiological investigations now demonstrate unequivocally the neurobiological basis of dyslexia. Studies using postmortem brain specimens,[31] brain morphometry,[32] and diffusion tensor MRI imaging[33] suggests that there are differences in the left temporo-parieto-occipital brain regions between dyslexic and non-impaired readers. Perhaps the most convincing evidence comes from studies using functional brain imaging. Such studies demonstrate a disruption in left hemisphere posterior reading systems in dyslexic readers.[34-44] In addition, some functional brain imaging studies show a relative increase in brain activation in frontal regions and right hemisphere systems in dyslexic compared to non-impaired readers (see Figure 263.1).[34,40,42,43,45,46]

Logan[47,48] has proposed two systems critical in the development of skilled, automatic processing, one involving word analysis, operating on individual units of words such as phonemes, requiring attentional resources and relatively slow processing and the second system operating on the whole word (word form), an obligatory system that does not require attention and processes very rapidly, on the order of 150 ms after a word is read. Converging evidence from a number of lines of investigation indicate that Logan's word analysis system is localized within the parieto-temporal region while the automatic, rapidly responding system is localized within the occipito-temporal area, functioning as a visual word form area,[49,50] which appears to respond preferentially to rapidly presented stimuli.[51] Still another reading related neural circuit involves an anterior system in the inferior frontal gyrus (Broca's area), a region that has long been associated with articulation and also serves an important function in silent reading and naming.[52,53]

Logan's model also helps to understand the strategies used in reading interventions. The first step in teaching is getting the beginning reader to analyze the word, to understand that the printed word corresponds to speech and is made up of individual units (phonemes). The system for word analysis is localized to the parieto-temporal system. As the reader becomes more skilled he learns that the spelling, phonology and meaning of the word become unitized, a process that appears to be localized to the occipito-temporal reading system.

Recognition of these systems allows us to suggest an explanation for the brain activation patterns observed in dyslexic children. We suppose that rather than the smoothly functioning and integrated reading systems observed in non-impaired children, disruption of the posterior reading systems results in dyslexic children attempting to compensate by shifting to other, ancillary systems, for example, anterior sites such as the inferior frontal gyrus. The anterior sites, critical in articulation,[34,52,53] may help the child with dyslexia develop an awareness of the sound structure of the word by forming the word with his lips, tongue and vocal apparatus and thus allow the child to read, albeit more slowly and less efficiently than if the fast occipito-temporal word identification system were functioning. A number of studies of young adults with childhood histories of dyslexia indicate that although they may develop some accuracy in reading words, they remain slow, non-automatic readers.[54,55] Thus, in dyslexic readers disruption of both dorsal and ventral posterior reading systems underlies the failure of skilled reading to develop, while a shift to ancillary systems supports accurate, but not automatic word reading.

Dyslexia in the school-age child

The management of dyslexia demands a life-span perspective; early on, the focus is on remediation of the reading problem. As a child matures and enters the more time-demanding setting of secondary school, the emphasis shifts to the important role of providing accommodations. The goal of effective intervention programs is to remediate this underlying problem in phonemic awareness but all too frequently the standard instruction provided through remediation is frequently too little, too general, and too unsystematic. Most recently, based on the work of the National Reading Panel,[56] evidence-based reading intervention programs have been identified that provide instruction in the most important elements in reading: phonemic awareness, phonics, reading fluency, vocabulary, and reading comprehension strategies. In identifying these programs, the National Reading Panel used the same methodology that has been recognized as the scientific standard and that has been used so successfully in providing evidence-based treatments for many other disorders affecting children, ranging from asthma to bacterial infections. Taking each component of the reading process in

turn, the intervention used with younger children and even with older children are programs to improve phonemic awareness (PA): the ability to focus on and manipulate phonemes (speech sounds) in spoken syllables and words. The elements found to be most effective in enhancing PA, reading, and spelling skills include: teaching children to manipulate phonemes with letters; focusing the instruction on one or two types of phoneme manipulations rather than multiple types; teaching children in small groups; and providing explicit instruction rather than incidental instruction in PA. The next step in teaching reading is to teach phonics, that is, to make sure that the beginner reader understands how letters are linked to sounds (phonemes) to form letter-sound correspondences and spelling patterns. Critical to teaching phonics is to make sure that the instruction is explicit and systematic; phonics instruction enhances children's success in learning to read and systematic phonics instruction is more effective than instruction that teaches little or no phonics or teaches phonics haphazardly or in a "by-the-way" approach. Furthermore, the effects of phonics instruction are substantial in kindergarten and first grade, indicating that systematic phonics programs should be implemented in these early grades. The evidence indicates that very young children who receive systematic phonics instruction benefit in their ability to read and spell words and first graders taught phonics are better able to decode and spell, and show significant improvement in their ability to comprehend text. In contrast, older children receiving phonics instruction are better able to decode and spell words and to read text orally, but their comprehension of text is not significantly improved.[54,57,58] This is understandable since, in higher grades, words are more unusual and unfamiliar, so that comprehension also depends on and reflects vocabulary and background knowledge.

Fluency refers to the ability to read orally with speed, accuracy and proper expression. Although it is generally recognized that fluency is an important component of skilled reading, it is often neglected in the classroom. The most effective method to build reading fluency is guided repeated oral reading, that is reading aloud repeatedly to a teacher, an adult, or a peer, and receiving feedback. The evidence indicates that guided oral reading has a clear and positive impact on word recognition, fluency and comprehension at a variety of grade levels and applies to all students—for good readers as well as those experiencing reading difficulties. Where the evidence is less secure is for programs for struggling readers that encourage large amounts of independent reading, that is, silent reading without any feedback to the student. Thus, even though independent silent reading is intuitively appealing, at this time the evidence does not support the notion that reading fluency improves. No doubt there is a correlation between being a good reader and reading large amounts; however, there is a paucity of evidence indicating that there is a *causal relationship* that is, if poor readers read more they will become more fluent. Fluency is of critical importance because it allows for the automatic, attention-free recognition of words, thus permitting these attentional resources to be directed to comprehension. In contrast to teaching phonemic awareness, phonics and fluency, interventions for reading comprehension are not as well established. In large measure this reflects the nature of the very complex processes influencing reading comprehension. The limited evidence indicates that the most effective methods to teach reading comprehension involve teaching vocabulary and teaching strategies that encourage an active interaction between reader and text. Such strategies which increase the reader's engagement in the reading process include: generating (and answering) questions during reading; summarizing as he reads; predicting what may occur and using graphic organizers, that is, systematically organizing the ideas in the text in a visual format. The available evidence supports multiple strategy instruction as an effective approach to improving reading comprehension.

One of the most exciting developments in reading and dyslexia is the converging evidence that, in many cases, and if recognized very early (at ages four and five years) the phonological difficulties associated with dyslexia may be significantly ameliorated or, perhaps, even prevented. As early as kindergarten, and perhaps even in pre-school, it is now possible to identify children "at-risk" for word reading difficulties on the basis of their performance on tasks that assess phonemic awareness and naming abilities. For example, measures most predictive of later reading ability involve the child's knowledge of letter sounds, the ability to blend sounds into words (done orally), and at the end of kindergarten, the ability to name letters rapidly. There is growing evidence that early identification and intervention in kindergarten and Grade 1 may substantially reduce the number of children requiring special services for reading disability. These early identification procedures are very sensitive but not very specific and so tend to over-identify children with dyslexia and this is reasonable given that the costs of delaying intervention are too great to wait. Even with the early identification and interventions designed to prevent reading disability, there will remain a substantial number of children who will need the interventions discussed above.

Dyslexia in adolescents, young adults and adults

The developmental course of dyslexia has now been characterized. Epidemiological, behavioral and, most recently, neurobiological (functional brain imaging) evidence indicate that dyslexia is persistent, it does not go away; on a practical level, this means that once a person is diagnosed as dyslexic there is no need for re-examination following high school to confirm the diagnosis. Second, over the course of development, skilled readers become more accurate and more automatic in decoding; they do not need to rely on context for word identification. Dyslexic readers, too, become more accurate over time, but they do not become automatic in their reading. Residua of the phonological deficit persist so that reading remains effortful and slow, even

for the brightest of individuals with childhood histories of dyslexia. Failure to either recognize (or measure) the lack of automaticity in reading represents, perhaps, the most common error in the diagnosis of dyslexia in accomplished young adults. It is often not appreciated that tests measuring word accuracy are inadequate for the diagnosis of dyslexia in young adults at the level of college, graduate or professional school and that, for these individuals, timed measures of reading or listening to the person read connected text aloud must be employed in making the diagnosis.

At all ages, and especially in young adults, dyslexia is a clinical diagnosis. Dyslexia is diagnosed by evidence of difficulties in reading that are unexpected for the person's cognitive capacity as shown by his/her education or professional status. In an accomplished adult, the level of education or professional status provides the best indication of cognitive capacity and graduation from a competitive college and completion of medical school and a residency indicates a superior cognitive capacity. Overwhelming evidence indicates that the history represents the most sensitive and accurate indicator of a reading disability. In bright young adults, a history of phonologically-based reading difficulties, requirements for extra time on tests and current slow and effortful reading, such as, signs of a lack of automaticity in reading, are the *sine qua non* of a diagnosis of dyslexia. A history of phonologically-based language difficulties, of laborious reading and writing, of poor spelling, of requiring additional time in reading and in taking tests, provide indisputable evidence of a deficiency in phonological processing which, in turn, serves as the basis for, and the signature of, a reading disability.

The most consistent and telling sign of a reading disability in an accomplished adult is slow and laborious reading and writing. It must be emphasized that the failure either to recognize or to measure the lack of automaticity in reading is perhaps the most common error in the diagnosis of dyslexia in accomplished young adults. Simple word identification tasks will not detect a dyslexic accomplished enough to graduate from college and attend law, medical or any other graduate degree school. Tests relying on the accuracy of word identification are inappropriate in diagnosing dyslexia in accomplished young adults; tests of word identification reveal little to nothing of his struggles to read. It is important to recognize that, since they assess reading accuracy but not automaticity (speed), the kinds of reading tests commonly used for school-age children may provide misleading data on bright adolescents and young adults. The most critical tests are those that are timed; they are the most sensitive to a phonological deficit in a bright adult. However, there are very few standardized tests for adult readers that are administered under timed and untimed conditions; the Nelson-Denny Reading Test represents an exception. Reading measures commonly used for school-age children may provide misleading data in some adolescents and young adults since they assess reading accuracy, but not automaticity (speed). Any scores obtained on testing must be considered relative to peers with the same degree of education or professional training.

Large-scale studies to date have focused on younger children; as yet, there are few or no data available on the effect of these training programs on older children. The management of dyslexia in students in secondary school, and especially college and graduate school, is primarily based on accommodation rather than remediation. College students with a history of childhood dyslexia often present a paradoxical picture; they are similar to their unimpaired peers on measures of word recognition yet continue to suffer from the phonological deficit that makes reading less automatic, more effortful, and slow. For these readers with dyslexia the provision of extra time is an essential accommodation; it allows them the time to decode each word and to apply their unimpaired higher-order cognitive and linguistic skills to the surrounding context to get at the meaning of words that they cannot entirely or rapidly decode. Although providing extra time for reading is by far the most common accommodation for people with dyslexia, other helpful accommodations include allowing the use of lap-top computers with spelling checkers, tape recorders in the classroom, and recorded books and providing access to syllabi and lecture notes, tutors to "talk through" and review the content of reading material, alternatives to multiple-choice tests (e.g., reports or orally administered tests), and a separate, quiet room for taking tests. With such accommodations, many students with dyslexia are now successfully completing studies in a range of disciplines, including medicine.

People with dyslexia and their families frequently consult their physicians about unconventional approaches to the remediation of reading difficulties; in general, there are very few credible data to support the claims made for these treatments (e.g., optometric training, medication for vestibular dysfunction, chiropractic manipulation, and dietary supplementation).

References

1. Wolraich ML, Hannah JN, Pinnock TY, et al. Comparison of diagnostic criteria for attention-deficit hyperactivity disorder in a country-wide sample. Journal of the American Academy of Child and Adult Psychiatry 1996;35:319–324
2. Shaywitz S. Current concepts: dyslexia. The New England Journal of Medicine 1998;338(5):307–312
3. Shaywitz SE, Shaywitz BA, Fletcher JM, Escobar MD. Prevalence of reading disability in boys and girls: results of the Connecticut Longitudinal Study. Journal of the American Medical Association 1990;264(8):998–1002
4. APA. Diagnostic and statistical manual of mental disorders, (DSM IV). Washington, DC: American Psychiatric Association, 1994
5. American Academy of Pediatrics, Committee on Quality Improvement, Subcommittee on Attention-Deficit/Hyperactivity Disorder. Clinical practice guideline: diagnosis and evaluation of the child with attention-deficit/hyperactivity disorder. Pediatrics 2000;105:1158–1170
6. Holahan J, Shaywitz B, Chhabra V, et al. Developmental trends in teacher perceptions of student cognitive and behavioral status as measured by the Multi-grade Inventory for Teachers: evidence from a longitudinal study. In: Molfese DM, Molfese V, eds. Developmental variations in language and learning. Mahwah, NJ: Lawrence Erlbaum, 2001:23–55
7. Jadad AR, Boyle M, Cunningham C, et al. Treatment of attention-deficit/hyperactivity disorder (AHRQ Publ. No. 00-E005). Rockville, MD: Agency for Healthcare Research and Quality, 1999
8. MTA, Multimodal treatment of ADHD. A 14-month randomized clinical trial of treatment strategies for attention-deficit/hyperactivity disorder. The MTA Cooperative Group. Multimodal Treatment Study of Children with ADHD. Archives of General Psychiatry 1999;56(12):1073–1086
9. American Academy of Pediatrics, Subcommittee on Attention-Deficit/Hyperactivity Disorder, Committee on Quality Improvement. Clinical practice guideline: treatment of the school-aged child with attention-deficit/hyperactivity disorder. Pediatrics 2001;108:1033–1044
10. Wilens T, Biederman J, Spencer T. Pharmacotherapy of attention deficit hyperactivity disorder in adults. CNS Drugs 1998;9:347–356
11. Paterson R, Douglas C, Hallmayer J, et al. A randomised, double-blind, placebo-controlled trial of dexamphetamine in adults with attention deficit hyperactivity disorder. Aust NZ J Psychiatry 1999;33:494–502
12. Spencer T, Biederman J, Wilens T, et al. Efficacy of a mixed amphetamine salts compound in adults with attention-deficit/hyperactivity disorder. Archives of General Psychiatry 2001;58:775–782
13. Gadow KD, Weiss M. Attention-deficit/hyperactivity disorder in adults: beyond controversy. Archives of General Psychiatry 2001;58:784–785
14. Vitiello B. Psychopharmacology for young children: clinical needs and research opportunities. Pediatrics 2001;108:983–989
15. Klorman R, Brumaghim J, Fitzpatrick P, Borgstedt A. Clinical effects of a controlled trial of methylphenidate on adolescents with attention deficit disorder. J Am Acad Child Adolesc Psychiatry 1990;29:702–709
16. Spencer T, Biederman J, Wilens T, et al. Pharmacotherapy of attention-deficit hyperactivity disorder across the life cycle. J Am Acad Child Adolesc Psychiatry 1996;35:409–432
17. Feldman H, Crumrine P, Handen B, et al. Methylphenidate in children with seizures and attention-deficit disorder. Am J Dis Child 1989;143:081–1086
18. Gross-Tsur V, Manor O, van der Meere J, et al. Epilepsy and attention deficit hyperactivity disorder: is methylphenidate safe and effective? J Pediatrics 1997;130:670–674
19. Mannuzza S, Klein RG, Bonagura N, et al. Hyperactive boys almost grown up. Archives of General Psychiatry 1991;48:77–83
20. Biederman J, Baldessarini RJ, Wright V, et al. A double-blind placebo controlled study of desipramine in the treatment of ADD: II. Serum drug levels and cardiovascular findings. Journal of the American Academy of Child and Adolescent Psychiatry 1989;28(6):903–911
21. Biederman J, Spencer T. Non-stimulant treatments for ADHD. European Child & Adolescent Psychiatry 2000;9(Suppl 1):I51–I59
22. Riddle MA, Nelson JC, Kleinman CS, et al. Sudden

death in children receiving norpramin: a review of three reported cases and commentary. Journal of the American Academy of Child and Adolescent Psychiatry 1991;30(1):104–108

23. Cantwell DP, Swanson J, Connor DF. Case study: adverse response to clonidine. Journal of the American Academy of Child Adolescent Psychiatry 1997;36(4): 539–544

24. Shaywitz SE, Shaywitz BA. Evaluation and treatment of children with attention deficit disorders. Pediatrics in Review 1984;6(4):99–109

25. Firestone P. Factors associated with children's adherence to stimulant medication. American Journal of Orthopsychiatry 1982;52(3):447–457

26. Kendall PC, Braswell L. Cognitive-behavior therapy for impulsive children. New York: Guilford Press, 1985

27. Shaywitz, SE. Overcoming dyslexia: a new and complete science-based program for overcoming reading problems at any level. New York: Alfred A Knopf, 2003

28. Shaywitz SE. Dyslexia. Scientific American 1996;275(5): 98–104

29. Torgesen JK. Phonological awareness: a critical factor in dyslexia. Orton Dyslexia Society, 1995

30. Wagner R, Torgesen J. The nature of phonological processes and its causal role in the acquisition of reading skills. Psychological Bulletin 1987;101:192–212

31. Galaburda AM, Sherman GF, Rosen GD, et al. Developmental dyslexia: four consecutive patients with cortical anomalies. Annals of Neurology 1985;18(2):222–233

32. Filipek P. Structural variations in measures in the developmental disorders. In: Thatcher R, Lyon G, Rumsey J, Krasnegor N, eds. Developmental neuro-imaging: mapping the development of brain and behavior. San Diego, CA: Academic Press, 1996:169–186

33. Klingberg T, Hedehus M, Temple E, et al. Microstructure of temporo-parietal white matter as a basis for reading ability: evidence from diffusion tensor magnetic resonance imaging. Neuron 2000;25:493–500

34. Brunswick N, McCrory E, Price CJ, et al. Explicit and implicit processing of words and pseudowords by adult developmental dyslexics: a search for Wernicke's Wortschatz. Brain 1999;122:1901–1917

35. Helenius P, Tarkiainen A, Cornelissen P, et al. Dissociation of normal feature analysis and deficient processing of letter-strings in dyslexic adults. Cerebral Cortex 1999;4:476–483

36. Horwitz B, Rumsey JM, Donohue BC. Functional connectivity of the angular gyrus in normal reading and dyslexia. Proc Natl Acad Sci USA 1998;95:8939–8944

37. Paulesu E, Demonet J-F, Fazio F, et al. Dyslexia-cultural diversity and biological unity. Science 2001;291: 2165–2167

38. Pugh K, Mencl EW, Shaywitz BA, et al. The angular gyrus in developmental dyslexia: task-specific differences in functional connectivity in posterior cortex. Psychological Science 2000;11:51–56

39. Rumsey JM, Andreason P, Zametkin AJ, et al. Failure to activate the left temporoparietal cortex in dyslexia. Archives of Neurology 1992;49:527–534

40. Rumsey JM, Nace K, Donohue B, et al. A positron emission tomographic study of impaired word recognition and phonological processing in dyslexic men. Archives of Neurology 1997;54:562–573

41. Salmelin R, Service E, Kiesila P, et al. Impaired visual word processing in dyslexia revealed with magneto-encephalography. Annals of Neurology 1996;40: 157–162

42. Shaywitz BA, Shaywitz SE, Pugh KR, et al. Disruption of posterior brain systems for reading in children with developmental dyslexia. Biological Psychiatry 2002;52: 101–110

43. Shaywitz SE, Shaywitz BA, Pugh KR, et al. Functional disruption in the organization of the brain for reading in dyslexia. Proc Natl Acad Sci USA 1998;95:2636–2641

44. Simos P, Breier J, Fletcher J, et al. Cerebral mechanisms involved in word reading in dyslexic children: a magnetic source imaging approach. Cerebral Cortex 2000; 10: 809–816

45. Georgiewa P, Rzanny R, Hopf J, et al. fMRI during word processing in dyslexic and normal reading children. NeuroReport 1999;10:3459–3465

46. Paulesu E, Frith U, Snowling M, et al. Is developmental dyslexia a disconnection syndrome? Evidence from PET scanning. Brain 1996;119:143–157

47. Logan G. Toward an instance theory of automatization. Psychological Review 1988;95:492–527

48. Logan G. Automaticity and reading: perspectives from the instance theory of automatization. Reading and Writing Quarterly: Overcoming Learning Disabilities 1997;13:123–146

49. Cohen L, Dehaene S, Naccache L, et al. The visual word form area: spatial and temporal characterization of an initial stage of reading in normal subjects and posterior split-brain patients. Brain 2000;123:291–307

50. Moore C, Price C. Three distinct ventral occiptotemporal regions for reading and object naming. NeuroImage 1999;10:181–192

51. Price C, Moore C, Frackowiak RSJ. The effect of varying stimulus rate and duration on brain activity during reading. Neuroimage 1996;3(1):40–52

52. Fiez JA, Peterson SE. Neuroimaging studies of word reading. Proc Nat Acad Sci USA 1998;95(3):914–921

53. Frackowiak R, Friston K, Frith C, et al. Human Brain Function. New York: Academic Press, 1997

54. Bruck M. Persistence of dyslexics' phonological awareness deficits. Developmental Psychology 1992;28(5): 874–886

55. Felton RH, Naylor CE, Wood FB. Neuropsychological profile of adult dyslexics. Brain and Language 1990; 39:485–497

56. Report of the National Reading Panel. Teaching children to read: an evidence based assessment of the scientific research literature on reading and its implications for reading instruction (Vol. NIH Pub. No. 00-4754): U.S. Department of Health and Human Services, Public Health Service, National Institutes of Health, National Institute of Child Health and Human Development, 2000

57. Bruck M. Outcomes of adults with childhood histories of dyslexia. In: Hulme C, Joshi RM (eds) Reading and spelling: development and disorders. Mahwah, NJ: Lawrence Erlbaum, 1998:179–200

58. Shaywitz SE, Fletcher JM, Holahan JM, et al. Persistence of dyslexia: The Connecticut Longitudinal Study at adolescence. Pediatrics 1999;104:1351–1359

264 Limb Apraxia

Cynthia Ochipa

Limb apraxia is the impaired ability to perform skilled, purposeful limb movements as a result of neurological dysfunction. In identifying limb apraxia, we exclude other neurological conditions that may cause impaired skilled motor performance such as weakness, akinesia, abnormalities of tone or posture, and movement disorders such as tremor or chorea.[1] The spatial, temporal, or conceptual errors observed in the gestural performance of individuals with limb apraxia are thought to reflect a disruption in the praxis system which is responsible for storing skilled motor information about purposeful movement. The neural substrate for praxis is represented in the left hemisphere of most right-handed individuals.[2-4]

Reports of the incidence of limb apraxia among individuals with left hemisphere lesions range from 50%[5] to 80%,[6] with variability likely due to subject selection and testing differences across investigators. Nevertheless, apraxia appears to be a common and enduring consequence of left hemisphere brain damage. Kertesz, Ferro, and Shewan[7] reported that 40% of 118 patients still had apraxia three or more months after the onset of a left hemisphere stroke. While some improvement in limb praxis performance may occur over time (such as improvements in gesture recognizability), significant impairments in the spatial and temporal aspects of gesture production often persist.[8]

Clinical subtypes

Ideomotor apraxia

Individuals with ideomotor apraxia commonly make spatial errors when performing skilled, purposeful limb movements.[9] These spatial errors may involve the failure to position the hand in an appropriate posture, the failure to properly orient the gestural movement through space, or the failure to coordinate joint movement. Another common error in ideomotor apraxia involves the use of a body part as if it were the imagined tool/object. Errors in movement speed or sequencing may also be seen.[10]

Ideomotor limb apraxia has been attributed to the destruction or disconnection of "movement formulas," or representations for skilled movements, thought to be located in the posterior portion of the left hemisphere,[3] specifically in the left inferior parietal lobe.[2] These representations guide both arms in the production of skilled movements. Posterior left hemisphere lesions, which presumably destroy these representations, result in deficits in both producing and understanding gestures.[2] Anterior left hemisphere lesions not involving the parietal lobe result in

gesture production difficulty in the context of spared gesture comprehension, presumably because the movement memories can no longer interact with anterior areas responsible for motor implementation.[2] Unilateral left hand apraxia has been described in patients with lesions of the corpus callosum which may disrupt the left hemisphere's ability to guide the ipsilateral left hand in the performance of skilled movements.[11-13]

Ideational and conceptual apraxia

The term ideational apraxia has been used to describe both impairments of actual tool use due to a conceptual disorder and the failure to perform a sequence of acts using tools and objects to achieve an intended goal.[4] The term conceptual apraxia is preferred for those individuals who demonstrate deficits related to impaired conceptual knowledge of tool use. In contrast to patients with ideomotor apraxia who make spatial or temporal errors in gestural performance, individuals with conceptual apraxia may make content errors such as gesturing a hammering motion for a spoon.[3,14] They also may fail to recognize the mechanical advantages afforded by tools or choose inappropriate tools to complete common tasks.[14] Individuals with ideational or conceptual apraxia often have diffuse or bilateral, posterior cerebral involvement.[15] However, the syndrome may result from focal damage to the posterior left hemisphere.[4,16]

Assessment of limb apraxia

When assessing limb praxis, the patient should be instructed to produce gestures as if they are actually holding the imagined tool (for example a hammer) and imagine the object they are acting upon (such as a nail). When the dominant hand cannot be tested due to hemiparesis, the non-dominant hand should be tested. The following tasks are useful in identifying apraxia at bedside or in the clinical setting. However, the importance of observation of tool/object use in natural contexts should not be overlooked. Task modifications may be necessary for patients with concomitant language impairment.

Gesture production and imitation

Gesture production tasks may include gesture to verbal command (for example "Show me how to use a knife to carve a turkey."), and gesture to visual presentation (for example the examiner shows the subject a tool and asks, "Show me how you use this."). Testing different input modalities (verbal command versus visual presentation) allows one to determine if deficits are related to sensory-specific input process-

Table 264.1 Summary of limb apraxia subtypes, clinical features, assessment tasks and presumed anatomical locations

Limb apraxia type	Clinical features	Assessment tasks	Typical anatomical location
Ideomotor	• Gesture production errors (e.g. spatial, temporal, body-part-as-tool) • Gesture comprehension may be spared or impaired	• Gesture to command • Gesture imitation • Actual tool use • Gesture comprehension	• Posterior left hemisphere (impaired production and comprehension) • Anterior left hemisphere (impaired production and spared comprehension)
Ideational	• Impaired sequencing of tool use	• Serial acts (e.g. fold letter, place in envelope, seal, stamp)	• Diffuse injury • Bilateral posterior cerebral • Posterior left hemisphere
Conceptual	• Content errors in tool use • Errors in tool selection	• Gesture to command • Tool-object matching (e.g. select hammer from field of choices when presented with nail) • Observation of tool use in natural environment	• Diffuse injury • Bilateral posterior cerebral • Posterior left hemisphere

ing mechanisms.[17,18] Gesture imitation may be tested by having the subject view the examiner during the performance of a gesture and duplicating that performance. Often imitation of gestures will be superior to gesture production to verbal command. However, it is possible for imitation performance to be worse.[19]

Gesture reception

Reception tasks may include discrimination between correct and incorrect pantomimes (for example "Is this the correct way to use a hammer?"), gesture naming (for example "What tool am I using?"), and gesture comprehension (for instance where the examiner pantomimes, and the patient selects the correct tool from an array of choices). Impaired gesture reception in the absence of gesture production difficulty may indicate a problem in accessing the movement representations through the visual modality.[18] Combined production and reception deficits may indicate destruction of the movement representations, implicating damage to the left inferior parietal lobe. Spared gesture comprehension in the context of impaired gesture production may suggest an anterior left hemisphere lesion.

Treatment and management of limb apraxia

Very little has been written about the rehabilitation of limb praxis. One reason this area has not been well-studied may be that many clinicians believe that limb apraxia is generally limited to the clinical examination of pantomime, and has a negligible impact on activities of daily living. However, recent studies have shown that individuals with limb apraxia make the same types of errors in actual tool use as they do in pantomime to command.[20,21] Additional studies have reported that the presence of apraxia is highly correlated with levels of dependency estimated by caregivers[22] and with low subjective well-being at one year post-stroke.[23]

The few studies reporting the direct treatment of apraxic deficits have indicated that apraxia responds to treatment (that is individuals with apraxia are able to learn gestures).[24–26] However, researchers have found poor generalization of gestural improvement to other gestures or contexts not specifically targeted in treatment.[25–27] This finding would suggest that if direct treatment of limb apraxia is attempted, the items targeted for treatment and the environmental context of treatment should be carefully selected for functional salience to the individual.[28]

When the direct treatment of limb apraxia cannot be accomplished, management of the functional disability should be attempted. In general, management of the deficit involves altering the environment to reduce the risk of personal injury and reducing the negative impact of the deficit on activities of daily living.[28] Specific strategies may include limiting access to potentially dangerous implements, limiting the available selection of implements to be used for a particular task, replacing tasks that may require tools with those that may be performed without tools, and avoiding tool use in novel contexts. Individuals with limb apraxia may be referred to rehabilitation specialists for training in alternative strategies for task performance.

References

1. Heilman KM, Rothi LJG, Apraxia. In: Heilman KM, Valenstein E, eds. Clinical Neuropsychology. New York: Oxford University Press, 1993:141–163
2. Heilman KM, Rothi LJG, Valenstein E. Two forms of ideomotor apraxia. Neurology 1980;32:342–346
3. Liepmann H. The left hemisphere and action (a translation from Munchener Medizinische Wochenschrift, 1905:48–49). Translations from Liepmann's essays on apraxia. Research Bulletin #506. Department of Psychology, University of Western Ontario, 1980
4. Liepmann H, Apraxia. In: Brown JW, ed. Agnosia and apraxia. Selected papers of Liepmann, Lange and Potzl.

New Jersey: Lawrence Erlbaum Associates, 1988:3–39.
(Original work published in 1920)

5. De Renzi E, Motti F, Nichelli P. Imitating gestures: a quantitative approach to ideomotor apraxia. Arch Neurol 1980;37:6–10

6. Poeck K. The clinical examination for motor apraxia. Neuropsychologia 1986;24:129–134

7. Kertesz A, Ferro JM, Shewan CM. Apraxia and aphasia. The functional-anatomical basis for their dissociation. Neurology 1984;34:40–47

8. Maher LM, Raymer AM, Foundas A, et al. Patterns of recovery in ideomotor apraxia. Paper presented at the annual meeting of the International Neuropsychological Society 1994, Cincinnati

9. Rothi LJG, Mack L, Verfaellie M, et al. Ideomotor apraxia. Error pattern analysis. Aphasiology 1988;2:381–388

10. Poizner H, Mack L, Verfaellie M, et al. Three dimensional computer graphic analysis of apraxia. Brain 1980;113:85–101

11. Leipmann H, Maas O. Fall von linksseitiger Agraphie und Apraxie bei rechsseitiger Lahmung. Zeitschrift fur Psychologie und Neurologie 1907;10:214–227

12. Watson RT, Heilman KM. Callosal apraxia, Brain 1983;106:391–403

13. Graff-Radford NR, Welsh K, Godersky J. Callosal apraxia. Neurology 1987;37:100–105

14. Ochipa C, Rothi LJG, Heilman KM. Ideational apraxia. A deficit in tool selection and use. Ann Neurol 1989;25:190–193

15. Ochipa C, Rothi LJG, Heilman KM. Conceptual apraxia in Alzheimer's disease. Brain 1992;115:1061–1071

16. De Renzi E, Lucchelli F. Ideational apraxia. Brain 1988;3:1173–1185

17. De Renzi E, Faglioni P, Sorgato P. Modality-specific and supramodal mechanisms of apraxia. Brain 1982;105:310–312

18. Rothi LJG, Mack L, Heilman KM. Pantomime agnosia. J Neurol Neurosurg Psychiatry 1986;49:451–454

19. Ochipa C, Rothi LJG, Heilman KM. Conduction apraxia. J Neurol Neurosurg Psychiatry 1994;57:1241–1244

20. McDonald S, Tate RC, Rigby J. Error types in ideomotor apraxia: a qualitative analysis. Brain Cogn 1994;25:250–270

21. Poizner H, Merians AS, Clark MA, et al. Kinematic approaches to the study of apraxic disorders. In: Rothi LJG, Heilman KM, eds. Apraxia. The Neuropsychology of Action. East Sussex: Psychology Press, 1997:93–109

22. Sundet K, Finset A, Reinvang, I. Neuropsychological predictors in stroke rehabilitation. J Clin Exp Neuropsychol 1988;10:363–379

23. Wyller TB, Sveen U, Sodring KM, et al. Subjective well-being one year after stroke. Clinical Rehabilitation 1997;11:139–145

24. Maher LM, Rothi LJG, Greenwald ML. Treatment of gesture impairment. A single case. ASHA 1991;33:195 (Abstract)

25. Ochipa C, Maher LM, Rothi LJG. Treatment of ideomotor apraxia. JINS 1995;2:149 (Abstract)

26. Pilgrim E, Humphreys GW. Rehabilitation of a case of ideomotor apraxia. In: Riddoch MJ, Humphreys GW, eds. Cognitive Neuropsychology and Cognitive Rehabilitation. Hove: Lawrence Erlbaum Associates, 1994:271–285

27. Coelho CA. Acquisition and generalization of simple manual sign grammars by aphasic subjects. J Commun Dis 1990;23:383–400

28. Maher LM, Ochipa C. Management and treatment of limb apraxia. In: Rothi LJG, Heilman KM, eds. Apraxia. The Neuropsychology of Action. East Sussex: Psychology Press, 1997:75–91

265 Intentional Disorders

Stephen E Nadeau

Intentional disorders reflect impairment in the function of systems that incorporate the prefrontal cortex. The role of these systems is to formulate or choose plans and to execute them. Plans may be translated into behavior, or they may remain invisible, as thinking. Prefrontal function is most essential in the context of novel situations, in which responses that have not already been formulated (as memories or reflexes) must be generated, *de novo*, to deal with the specific demands of the particular situation.

There is a paucity of experimental work on the treatment of intentional disorders. We believe the future in this field lies in reasoned and hypothesis-driven approaches based upon what we understand about the function of prefrontal systems. Therefore, we will begin with a brief analysis of these systems and some proposals regarding potential avenues of treatment that are based upon known principles of system function.

Prefrontal systems

Any systematic treatment-oriented approach to prefrontal systems must take into account: (1) the division of prefrontal function into several domains; (2) the relationship of prefrontal function to that of more posterior systems; and (3) the relationship of prefrontal and limbic systems to the basal ganglia.

Prefrontal domains

Prefrontal systems can logically be divided into three domains represented in dorsolateral, orbitofrontal, and midline prefrontal cortex, respectively. The dorsolateral prefrontal cortex is principally involved in the formulation of plans in which ongoing sensory feedback regarding environmental constraints is crucial. This, the domain of task performance, is readily probed with neuropsychological tests. Dorsolateral prefrontal cortex is well equipped for this role by virtue of its extensive connectivity with sensory association cortices in the temporal and parietal lobes. Orbitofrontal cortex is principally involved in the formulation of plans according to internal criteria for value. These criteria, operationally defined through extensive orbitofrontal connectivity with the limbic system, include traditional values, such as ethics, morals, and altruism, the gamut of "emotional feelings" including love, empathy, compassion, resentment, jealously, hate and bigotry, and "fundamental drives" such as hunger, thirst and sex. Dorsolateral and orbitofrontal cortices are extensively interconnected in a complex and as yet poorly defined manner. Midline prefrontal cortex is primarily implicated in initiating and sustaining plans. Patients with extensive, acute lesions of this region, for example from anterior cerebral artery vasospasm related to subarachnoid hemorrhage from anterior communicating artery aneurysms, exhibit akinetic mutism. Patients with disorders, such as Binswanger's disease, that cause more insidious damage to this region by injuring afferent and efferent connections, exhibit lack of spontaneity, inability to carry out multi-component tasks, and a tendency to be taciturn and respond to questions with single words or very short sentences.

The relationship of prefrontal function to that of more posterior systems

Two key dimensions can be defined in the relationship of prefrontal function to that of more posterior systems, which include premotor cortex, temporal and parietal cortices, and subcortical systems within the cerebrum and brainstem. First, whereas prefrontal cortex provides the substrate for the development of plans custom designed to fit novel situations, posterior systems provide the substrate for the generation of plans in situations in which pre-formulated approaches (memories) or reflexes will at least suffice and may be optimal. Second, whereas prefrontal cortex supports plans that are deliberate and willed, that is *intentional*, posterior systems support plans that are elicited automatically, that is, are *reactive*. This second dimension subsumes a concept proposed decades ago by Derek Denny-Brown, in which he linked prefrontal cortex with avoidance behavior and parietal cortex with approach behavior. Thus utilization behavior, the tendency exhibited by many patients with extensive prefrontal lesions to use objects in their environment in a correct way but in inappropriate contexts, can be viewed as an imbalance between intentional and reactive planning, in which reactive planning is disinhibited or released, or as an excess of approach over avoidance behavior.

The relationship of prefrontal and limbic systems to the basal ganglia

The role of the basal ganglia in brain function is scarcely clearer now than it was 30 years ago when the modern era of intensive study of these systems began. However, there is evidence that some of the effects of lesions of the prefrontal and limbic systems may be mediated via the basal ganglia and therefore may be susceptible to treatment aimed at the basal ganglia. The most dramatic evidence of this is provided by experiments in which hemispatial neglect induced in rats by unilateral ablation of the dorsomedial "shoulder" region of the prefrontal cortex (roughly the homologue of Brodmann's area 8 in primates) has been effectively treated using dopaminergic agents.[1] Although such treatment clearly cannot fully compensate for the loss of cortex, it may correct the dysfunctional hemispatial bias that results from the cortical lesion. Commensurate data are not available for other prefrontal systems or the limbic system. However, all of these systems have a precise relationship with the basal ganglia, dorsolateral prefrontal cortex with the head of the caudate nucleus, medial prefrontal/premotor cortex with the putamen, and orbitofrontal cortex and the limbic system with the ventral head of caudate and the nucleus accumbens.[2] Thus, there is the potential for at least partial compensation of some deficits resulting from damage to the cortical structures through dopaminergic treatment aimed at connected basal ganglia structures. It is also possible that enhancement of mesocortical dopaminergic input could normalize partially damaged cortical systems, particularly to the degree that dysfunction results from shearing of ascending dopaminergic projections in traumatic brain injury or mechanical disruption in the course of basal forebrain surgery. Human studies provide incipient support for these concepts.

Aberrant behaviors stemming from prefrontal dysfunction, their relationship to disorders of prefrontal systems, and potential avenues of treatment

Pharmacological approaches to the treatment of disorders stemming from prefrontal dysfunction are most likely to be beneficial when these disorders reflect, at least in part, imbalance between systems (e.g., motor impersistence, utilization behavior, Witzelsucht, distractibility, perseveration, obsessive-compulsive and ruminative behavior, indecisiveness (see Table 265.1, Figure 265.1), or cortical dysfunction that is potentially compensable through alteration of basal ganglia function. For example, utilization behavior, Witzelsucht (joking in socially inappropriate circumstances) and distractibility may reflect an imbalance between intentional and reactive components of plan formulation with release of reactive components. This is reminiscent of the disorder observed in attention deficit hyperactivity disorder (ADHD), which responds well to methylphenidate and D-amphetamine.[3] There are no ecological studies that define the impact of most of the behaviors listed in Table 265.1 and Figure 265.1 on the daily lives of patients with prefrontal disorders. However, distractibility is a "gatekeeper" dysfunction because it prevents patients with prefrontal lesions, no less than patients with ADHD, from sustaining an intentional plan to completion.

In principle, any disorder of prefrontal or limbic function is susceptible to alteration by adjustment of dopaminergic activity in the basal ganglia. Two functions, akinesia (reflecting dorsomedial prefrontal dysfunction) and apathy (reflecting limbic dysfunction or orbitofrontal-limbic disconnection) are particularly important because they are also "gate-keeper" functions. That is, no behavior is possible unless one is

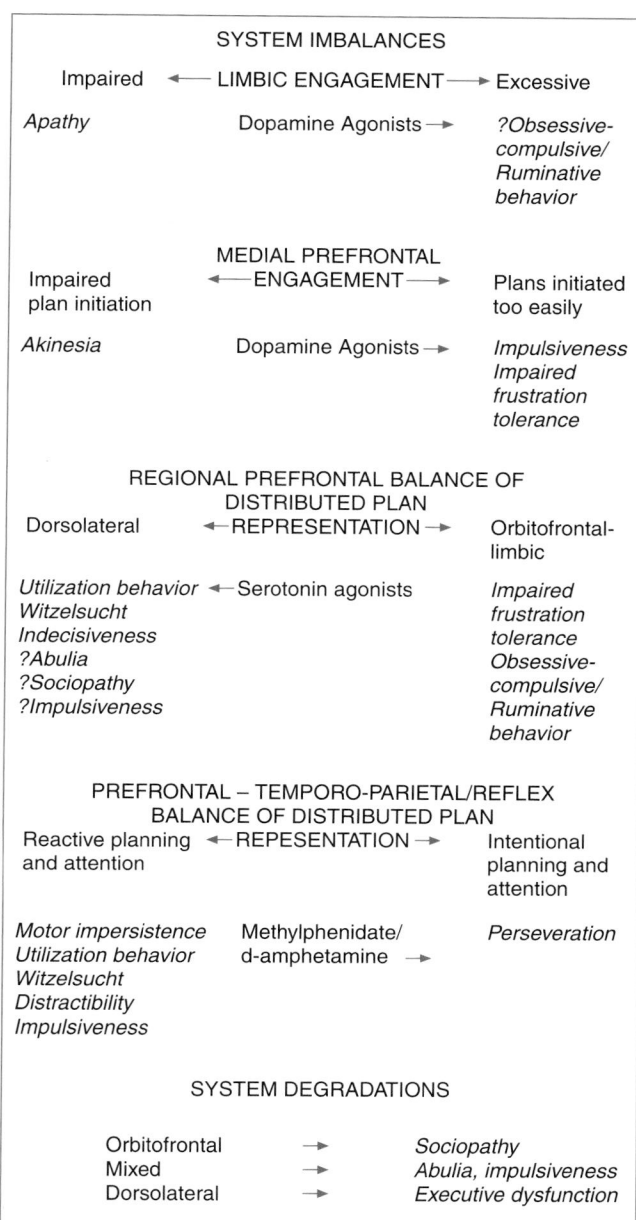

Figure 265.1 Disorders of cognitive systems potentially underlying intentional disorders. Along each dimension of the system imbalances, the behaviors resulting from imbalances in a particular direction are indicated in italics. The hypothetical impact of pharmacological agents on these imbalances is indicated by the direction of the arrow preceding or following the agent, e.g., dopamine agonists would tend to shift limbic and midline systems away from behavioral states associated with apathy and akinesia, whereas dopamine receptor antagonists might be used to shift limbic and midline systems away from states associated with obsessive-compulsive or ruminative behavior, impulsiveness and impaired frustration tolerance. Aberrant behaviors resulting from system degradations will only benefit from pharmacological agents to the extent that they also involve system imbalances.

Table 265.1   Aberrant behaviors stemming from prefrontal dysfunction and their relationship to disorders of prefrontal systems

Behavior	Posited locus of lesion	Prefrontal system disorder	Potential treatment
Akinesia	ML	Failure of task initiation	Dopaminergic agents
Motor impersistence	DL and OF-limbic	Imbalance between intentional and reactive planning with failure to sustain intentional movement or position; release of reflexive or reactive responses	Methylphenidate/ D-amphetamine
Utilization behavior	DL and OF-limbic	Imbalance between intentional and reactive planning with inappropriate release of reactive plans and often particularly inadequate inhibition by orbitofrontal-limbic systems	Methylphenidate/ D-amphetamine; possibly serotonin receptor blockers/ serotonin depletion
Witzelsucht	DL and OF-limbic	Utilization behavior involving humorous or quasi-humorous commentary	Methylphenidate/ D-amphetamine; possibly serotonin receptor blockers/serotonin depletion
Distractibility	DL and OF-limbic	Imbalance between intentional and reactive attention with release of reactive attention and associated reactive behavior	Methylphenidate/ D-amphetamine
Perseveration	DL	Imbalance between intentional and reactive systems causing failure of repeated plan execution to be inhibited by evidence from posterior sensory systems of plan completion	Dopamine/ norepinephrine blockers
Abulia	DL and OF-limbic	Failure to link each component of a complex plan to the motivational basis for the entire plan due to simplification of distributed plan representations	Behavioral; possibly serotonin receptor blockers/serotonin depletion
Apathy	OF-limbic	Failure of prefrontal distributed plan representations to elicit the limbic distributed representations that will drive behavior, as a result of OF-limbic disconnection or limbic dysfunction	Dopaminergic agents
Sociopathy	OF-limbic	Simplification or distortion of OF-limbic distributed plan representations, sometimes with inappropriate dominance by fundamental drives; may be the OF-limbic analog of simplification of executive function in the dorsolateral prefrontal domain	Behavioral; serotonin receptor blockers/ serotonin depletion
Impairment of executive function	DL	Simplification of distributed concept and plan representations and loss of capacity for manipulation of concept or plan component representations relative to one another, particularly involving the dorsolateral prefrontal domain	Behavioral
Simplification of syntax	DL	One of the defining features of Broca's aphasia: impairment of executive function within the domain of language, with loss of ability to maintain multiple simultaneous distributed concept representations and manipulate them preparatory to speaking	Behavioral
Adynamic aphasia	DL	A subtype of transcortical motor aphasia: inability to intentionally engage distributed concept representations preparatory to speaking with sparing of reactive engagement of such representations, e.g., during picture description	Dopaminergic agents/behavioral

continued

Table 265.1 *continued*

Behavior	Posited locus of lesion	Prefrontal system disorder	Potential treatment
Impulsiveness	DL, OF-limbic, ML	Initiation of behavior without adequate constraint by DL and OF-limbic systems, in many cases because of simplification of distributed plan representations in those systems (i.e., a mix of impairment of executive function and sociopathy), in some cases because of excessive bias toward reactive plan formation	Dopamine antagonists; possibly serotonin receptor blockers/serotonin epletion; methylphenidate/ D-amphetamine; behavioral
Impaired frustration tolerance	DL, OF-limbic, ML	A form of impulsiveness in which constraints of DL system often fail to impede initiation of behavior driven by OF-limbic system	SSRIs; dopamine antagonists
Obsessive-compulsive and ruminative behavior	DL and OF-limbic	Imbalance in the utilization of OF-limbic and DL distributed plan representations in conjunction with a disorder of OF-limbic plan generation; OF-limbic defined plans dominate despite catastrophic behavioral consequences	SSRIs
Indecisiveness	DL and OF-limbic	Imbalance between OF-limbic and DL distributed plan representations such that DL defined plans dominate even in situations in which OF-limbic components are essential, e.g., choosing a restaurant[78]	Serotonin receptor blockers/serotonin depletion

DL, dorsolateral; OF, orbitofrontal; ML, midline.

able to initiate behavior, and no behavior will occur if there is no motivation to behave. The fact that akinesia and apathy can be characterized, at least in part, as impairment in a degree of function, rather than disruption of a complex pattern of function (e.g., sociopathy, abulia, executive dysfunction), suggests that altering dopaminergic input could be of benefit. If dopamine agonists are capable of improving akinesia and apathy, dopamine antagonists might be capable of reducing impulsiveness, which in a sense is opposite to akinesia.

Obsessive compulsive disorder (OCD) and ruminative depression respond to serotonin-selective reuptake inhibitors (SSRIs). Indecisiveness as result of prefrontal damage, to the degree that it can be viewed as a complementary disorder to OCD and ruminative depression (see Table 265.1), might respond to depletion of serotonin systems, for example, with reserpine, or to the use of serotonin receptor antagonists (e.g., clozapine, risperidone, olanzapine, quetiapine, methysergide, or cyproheptadine). Apathy and akinesia caused by the effect of these drugs on dopaminergic systems might require co-treatment with dopamine agonists. Abulia, sociopathy, impulsiveness, utilization behavior, and Witzelsucht may, to some degree, reflect an imbalance in the function of prefrontal systems, rather than simplified function, or an imbalance between intentional and reactive systems. This may result in relatively greater impairment of the orbitofrontal-limbic contribution to plan formation. Thus, these behaviors might also benefit from serotonin depletion or serotonin receptor antagonism.

To the extent that aberrant behaviors stemming from prefrontal dysfunction are related to simplified or disordered distributed plan representations (e.g., abulia, sociopathy, impulsiveness, and impairment of executive function and its linguistic equivalent, simplification of syntax) (see Table 265.1), it is unlikely that pharmacological approaches will be beneficial. Behavioral approaches (to induce the learning of more adaptive plans) and compensatory approaches (employment of surrogate decision makers to the degree possible, increase in environmental constraints, reduction in degrees of freedom for action, increased tolerance for aberrant behaviors, family therapy) are likely to play a greater role in these circumstances.[4,5] Since behavioral approaches involve learning, their effectiveness can theoretically be potentiated by enhancing acetylcholinergic input to the cortex.[6] For Hebbian learning to occur, not only do connected neurons need to be simultaneously active, but they also need to be informed that the activity in which they are engaged is important. The orbitofrontal-limbic imprimatur of importance is conveyed through cholinergic projections to the hippocampal system from the medial septal nuclei (declarative memory formation) and via cholinergic projections to the cortical mantle from the nucleus basalis of Meynert (both declarative and procedural memory formation).[7] The efficacy of cholinomimetic therapy has now been well demonstrated in patients with Alzheimer's disease, but no definitive studies are available on its value in patients with other types of brain injury.

2792 XIV Neurobehavioral Disorders: Cognitive Rehabilitation, Behavioral Managment and Pharmacologic Therapies

Table 265.2 Dopaminergic agents

References	Nature of study	Drug	Dose range	N	Type of patient	Outcome	Regression with drug cessation
8–12	Open	Carbidopa-levodopa	Up to 25/250 mg qid	52	TBI*	Global improvement	Some
13–29‡	Open	Bromocriptine	7.5–120 mg/day	50	TBI (21), hydrocephalus (5), stroke (3), aneurysmal rupture (5), hypoxia (4), misc (11)	Improvement in apathy/akinesia/abulia in 40	Some
30	Open	Bromocriptine	10 mg/day	8	Dementia: vascular (5), AD* (2), FTD* (1)	Improvement in recurrent and stuck in set perseverations	Some
31	8 month double blind, placebo controlled, cross-over	Bromocriptine	30 mg/day	7	Vascular dementia	No improvement in kinesis, letter fluency, category fluency, reaction time, continuous performance, UPDRS†, alternating sequences, WCS†	NA
32	Single dose, double-blind, placebo controlled cross-over	Bromocriptine	2.5 mg	24	TBI with mild deficits	Improvement in complex reaction time, Stroop, WCS, Trailmaking Test, letter fluency	NA
27, 29, 33–40	Open	Amantadine	Up to 400 mg/day	57	TBI	Improvement in 39§	Some

*TBI, traumatic brain injury; AD, Alzheimer's disease; FTD, frontotemporal dementia; †WCS, Wisconsin Card Sort; UPDRS, United Parkinson's Disease Rating Scale; ‡Two studies (24, 25) involving 12 patients, employed a formal N of 1 treatment design; §In three studies (n = 35), improvement in agitation, violence assaultiveness (33, 34, 39), improvement in akinesia/apathy (27, 29, 34, 35, 39, 40); and in one (n = 7) improvement on Trailmaking Test and letter fluency (36).

Reports of pharmacological treatment of prefrontal dysfunction in humans

Dopaminergic agents

The limitations of the experimental design and the non-specificity of the endpoints in trials of levodopa/carbidopa (Table 265.2) preclude firm conclusions on the impact of this drug on any specific dimension of prefrontal function. To the extent that dopaminergic fibers have been destroyed, agents that act by more direct means might theoretically be more effective. These include bromocriptine and other D_2 receptor agonists, and agents that alter basal ganglia function by a non-dopaminergic mechanism, for example, amantadine, a low potency N-methyl-D-aspartate (NMDA) receptor antagonist thought to emulate the effects of dopamine by inhibiting cortical input to the subthalamic nucleus and subthalamic input to the globus pallidus interna. Beneficial effects of these drugs on behaviors suggestive of prefrontal dysfunction have been reported in many studies (Table 265.2), providing some support for the hypotheses elaborated earlier in this chapter. However, in some studies, there was no regression following cessation of the drug, raising questions about mechanisms of drug effect.

Methylphenidate and D-amphetamine

Both methylphenidate and D-amphetamine act to potentiate the release of the neurotransmitters dopamine and norepinephrine. Thus, their actions are potentially broader than those of dopaminergic agents, but their effects are also potentially limited to the degree that there is destruction of ascending catecholamine pathways. To the extent that they emulate the actions of dopaminergic drugs, they might alleviate akinesia, motor impersistence, and apathy via their impact on the basal ganglia. To the extent that they reproduce their effect on ADHD, they might be expected to benefit utilization behavior, Witzelsucht and distractibility (Table 265.1). The results of published studies (Table 265.3) provide some support for these concepts, although the magnitude of benefit observed has been far less in controlled trials than in open trials. Furthermore, the discovery of carry-over effects in cross-over studies suggests permanent effects on brain function that are not easily reconciled with our current understanding of the mechanism of action of these drugs.

Beta-blockers

Our theoretical schema does not posit a major role for β-blockers, α_1-blockers, or α_2-agonists in the treatment of intentional disorders, with the possible exception of perseveration. Clinical studies have focused exclusively on β-blockers and only on the target symptoms of restlessness, irritability, agitation, aggressiveness and provoked or unprovoked violence. Because the mechanisms underlying these complex behaviors are poorly understood, it is not possible to provide a cogent explanation for the beneficial effects of β-blockers that have been observed (Table 265.4). The beneficial effects of propranolol on violent behavior may not be linked to beta blockade, as in rats made irritable by expectancy of electroshock or by septal lesions, the same beneficial effects can be achieved with the dextro isomer, which has little beta blocking activity.[64] There is also evidence from animal studies that propranolol may retard neurological recovery.[65,66]

Antidepressants

Tricyclic antidepressants variously inhibit the re-uptake of norepinephrine and serotonin and therefore, might be expected to achieve effects similar to those of SSRIs, methylphenidate and D-amphetamine (Table 265.1). Trazodone is a weak serotonin re-uptake inhibitor and $5HT_1$ receptor agonist with possible indirect facilitatory effects on norepinephrine transmission. In open trials, tricyclic antidepressants have been beneficial for such motor intentional disorders as restlessness, distractibility, akinesia and apathy, as predicted in our theoretical scheme (Table 265.5). Both tricyclic antidepressants and trazodone have also been reported to alleviate more complex and poorly understood behaviors such as restlessness, agitation and violent or threatening behavior (Table 265.5).

Other

Other drugs, most notably anticonvulsants (carbamazepine, valproate), and neuroleptics have been used to control aberrant behaviors in brain injured patients. Because these drugs have been used exclusively to treat agitation, aggressiveness, and violent outbursts (see Fava[76] for a comprehensive review), which are complex behaviors of multi-factorial origin, they will not be reviewed here. Furthermore, the mechanism of action of anticonvulsants in curbing such behavior is unknown, and therefore cannot be placed in our theoretical scheme. Neuroleptics, although dramatically effective in treating psychosis, may do so at the expense of potentiating akinesia and apathy and may interfere with processes involved in neural recovery.[65,66]

Conclusions

The theoretical framework discussed earlier and the results of the clinical studies reviewed provide only the most tentative guidance for future investigations. A number of specific problems can be identified:

- Prefrontal systems are complex and pathological processes impact these systems in myriad combinations.
- The ecological importance of most of the behaviors identified in this review is unclear.
- The relationships we have posited between various pathological behaviors and dysfunction of specific systems are largely theoretical and not yet well substantiated by experimental evidence.
- Operational measures of the behaviors discussed here (Table 265.1) are substantially lacking, and it is likely that many will be very difficult to distinguish in practice (e.g., akinesia, apathy, and abulia).

Table 265.3   Methylphenidate and D-amphetamine

References	Nature of study	Drug	Dose range	N	Type of patient	Outcome	Change at cross-over
29, 41–49	Open†	Methylphenidate or D-Amphetamine			TBI, hydrocephalus, striatocapsular stroke	Moderate to marked improvement in akinesia/apathy, distractibility, impulsiveness, response inconsistency	NA
50	Double blind, placebo controlled, cross-over	Methylphenidate	0.3 mg/kg bid	10 responders in study of 15	TBI	Trend toward improvement in clinical ratings of distractibility, impulsiveness; neuropsychological probes of attention, letter and pattern fluency	Carry-over effects
51	Double blind, placebo controlled, cross-over	Methylphenidate	0.3 mg/kg bid	12	TBI: attempted replication of preceding study (50)	None	
52	Double blind, placebo controlled cross-over	Methylphenidate	0.3 mg/kg bid	10 children	TBI	None	
53	Single blind, placebo controlled, parallel group	Methylphenidate	Up to 30 mg/day	38	TBI	Improvement in anger, verbal learning, not attention	
54	Double blind, placebo controlled, cross-over	Methylphenidate	0.25 mg/kg bid; brief trials	19	TBI	Improvement in cognitive processing speed; no effect on distractibility or impulsiveness	
55	Double blind, placebo controlled, parallel group	Methylphenidate	0.3 mg/kg bid	12	Acute TBI	Rate of recovery: better on measures of disability, attention, vigilance, motor learning	Differences not apparent 2 months later
56	N of 1 case design	Methylphenidate		10	Acute TBI	Rate of recovery: better on digit span, counting backwards, symbol search subtest of WISC*	

TBI, Traumatic brain injury.
*WISC, Wechsler Intelligence Scale for Children; †Some case studies utilized formal n of 1 case design.

Table 265.4 β-blockers

References	Nature of study	Drug	Dose range	N	Type of patient	Outcome
57–60	Open	Propranolol	Up to 520 mg/day	14	TBI	Improvement
61	Open	Propranolol		3	AD	Improvement in wandering, pacing, deficits in impulse control, agitation and destructive behavior
62	Double blind, placebo controlled, parallel group	Propranolol	Up to 420 mg/day	21	TBI	Reduced intensity of episodic agitation
63	Double blind, placebo controlled, cross-over	Propranolol	Up to 520 mg/day	9	Dementia (4 TBI, 2 alcoholic	Improvement in 7 in frequency and intensity of episodes of violent and assaultive behavior
67	Double blind, placebo controlled, cross-over	Pindolol*	Up to 100 mg/day	11	5 TBI, 3 alcoholic dementia	Reduction in hostility, fewer attempted assaults, improved cooperation, greater communication
68	Double blind, placebo controlled, cross-over	Pindolol	Up to 100 mg/day	13	3 TBI, 7 alcoholic dementia	Trend to less aggressive behavior

AD, Alzheimer disease; TBI, traumatic brain injury.
*Mixed β-adrenergic agonist/antagonist with some activity at 5-hydroxytriptamine-2 receptor.

Table 265.5   Antidepressants

References	Nature of study	Drug	Dose range	N	Type of patient	Outcome	Regression with drug cessation
69–72	Open	Amitriptyline, protriptyline, desipramine		32	TBI	Reduced agitation, restlessness, violent or threatening behavior, distractibility; improved arousal, akinesia/apathy	Some
73–75	Open	Trazodone	Up to 400 mg/day	24	AD or alcoholic dementia	Improvement in irritability, agitation, restlessness, aggressive behavior, violent outbursts	

AD, Alzheimer disease; TBI, traumatic brain injury.

- Most of the pharmacological studies that have been reported have serious methodological shortcomings. There is strong reason to question the validity of N of 1 and crossover designs, both because the most crucial treatment periods are often during times of spontaneous recovery, and because there is suggestive evidence of permanent effects of a number of drugs on the brain, manifested as "carry-over" effects and failure of behavior to regress when drugs are discontinued. In short, parallel group studies are strongly preferred. It is unlikely that the effects of brief exposures to drugs, for example, one day, are the same as the effects of more chronic exposure. Evidence of this is most clear cut in the psychiatric literature, in which it is well established that weeks of treatment are necessary to significantly ameliorate depression and obsessive compulsive disorder. Thus, for example, the implications for long-term care of the otherwise methodologically excellent study of Whyte et al.,[54] in which patients were studied during one day of drug treatment, are unclear.

- The actions of most of the drugs reviewed are complex and as yet incompletely defined and the mechanism of their therapeutic effects poorly understood. This makes theoretically based predictions regarding drug actions hazardous. This is most dramatically exemplified by the SSRIs. We have drawn a parallel between OCD and ruminative depression, theorizing that both conditions reflect, in part, over-dominance of planning by orbitofrontal limbic systems. However, although both conditions improve with SSRI treatment, tryptophan depletion will rapidly reinstate symptoms in SSRI-treated depressed patients, but it will not reinstate symptoms in SSRI-treated OCD patients.[77] Clearly, the mechanisms by which SSRIs benefit patients with these two disorders have some fundamental differences. The mechanisms of action of other drugs reviewed here, including propranolol and valproate, are even less clear.

- The endpoints in drug studies are generally not adequately defined. In particular, some behaviors, most notably irritability, restlessness, agitation, aggressiveness, and violent outbursts, may stem from any of a variety of causes including but not limited to pain, anxiety, depression, impulsiveness, poor frustration tolerance, akathisia, and situational psychosis (related to sleep deprivation and intensive care unit environments). Of these, only impulsiveness, restlessness, akathisia and poor frustration tolerance can be directly related to disorders of prefrontal systems.

- Even looked at optimistically, the results of published clinical pharmacological studies are not easy to interpret. Arguably the most consistent and cogent results have been those achieved with bromocriptine in the treatment of akinesia/apathy/abulia. The substantial open trial evidence of efficacy of amantadine for this same endpoint is also theoretically plausible, but the reported beneficial effects of amantadine for agitation, violence and assaultiveness are difficult to account for. Open trials suggesting beneficial effects of methylphenidate and D-amphetamine for akinesia, distractibility, impulsiveness and response consistency are consistent with the concepts elucidated at the beginning of this chapter. However, the results of controlled studies of these drugs (mainly methylphenidate) are more difficult to interpret, for a number of reasons: complex endpoints (e.g., anger); carryover effects in crossover studies; in some studies, very brief treatment; and in acute studies, potential confounding of direct effects of the drug on behavior with effects of the drug on brain plasticity. The reported effects of propranolol, tricyclic antidepressants, and valproate are even more difficult to interpret.

We conclude where we started: that further progress in this field will depend substantially on well reasoned, hypothesis driven approaches to the modulation of disordered prefrontal function.

References

1. Corwin JV, Kanter S, Watson RT, et al. Apomorphine has a therapeutic effect on neglect produced by unilateral dorsomedial prefrontal cortex lesions in rats. Exp Neurol 1986;94:683–698
2. Alexander GE, DeLong MR, Strick PL. Parallel organization of functionally segregated circuits linking basal ganglia and cortex. Ann Rev Neurosci 1986;9:357–381
3. Heilman KM, Voeller KS, Nadeau SE. A possible pathophysiological substrate of attention-deficit-hyperactivity disorder. J Child Neurol 1991;6(Suppl):S76–S78
4. Dobkin BH. Neurologic Rehabilitation. Philadelphia: F.A. Davis Company, 1996
5. Campbell JJ, Duffy JD, Salloway SP. Treatment strategies for patients with dysexecutive syndromes. J Neuropsychiatry Clin Neurosci 1994;6:411–418
6. Kilgard MP, Merzenich MM. Cortical map reorganization enabled by nucleus basalis activity. Science 1998;279:1714–1718
7. Mesulam M-M, Mufson EJ. Neural inputs into the nucleus basalis of the substantia innominata (Ch4) in the rhesus monkey. Brain 1984;107:253–274
8. van Woerkom TCAM, Minderhoud JM, Gottschal T, Nicolai G. Neurotransmitters in the treatment of patients with severe head injuries. Eur Neurol 1982;21:227–234
9. Lal S, Merbtiz CP, Grip JC. Modification of function in head-injured patients with Sinemet. Brain Injury 1988;2:225–233
10. Haig AJ, Ruess JM. Recovery from vegetative state of six months duration associated with Sinemet (Levodopa/Carbidopa). Arch Phys Med Rehab 1990;71:1081–1083
11. Wolf AP, Gleckman AD. Sinemet and brain injury: functional versus statistical change and suggestions for future research designs. Brain Injury 1995;9:487–493
12. Kraus MF, Maki P. Case report. The combined use of L-dopa/carbidopa in the treatment of chronic brain injury. Brain Injury 1997;11:455–460
13. Ross ED, Stewart RM. Akinetic mutism from hypothalamic damage: successful treatment with dopamine agonists. Neurology 1981;31:1435–1439
14. Devinsky O, Lemann W, Evans AC, et al. Akinetic mutism in a bone marrow transplant recipient following

total-body irradiation and amphotericin B chemoprophylaxis. A positron emission tomographic and neuropathologic study. Arch Neurol 1987;44: 414–417

15. Echiverri HC, Tatum WO, Merens TA, Coker SB. Akinetic mutism: pharmacologic probe of the dopaminergic mesencephalofrontal activating system. Pediatric Neurology 1988;4:228–230

16. Catsman-Berrevoets CE, Harskamp FV. Compulsive pre-sleep behavior and apathy due to bilateral thalamic stroke: response to bromocriptine. Neurology 1988;38: 647–649

17. Crismon ML, Childs A, Wilcox RE, Barrow N. The effect of bromocriptine on speech dysfunction in patients with diffuse brain injury (akinetic mutism). Clin Neuropharmacol 1988;11:462–466

18. Stewart JT, Leadon M, Gonzalez-Rothi LJ. Treatment of a case of akinetic mutism with bromocriptine. J Neuropsychiatry 1990;2:462–463

19. Watali Y, Narita S, Kurahashi K, et al. Akinetic mutism from recurrent hydrocephalus: successful treatment with levodopa, bromocriptine and trihexyphenidyl. No To Shinkei 1987;39:377–382

20. Barrett K. Treating organic abulia with bromocriptine and lisuride: four case studies. J Neurol Neurosurg Psychiatry 1991;54:718–721

21. Anderson B. Relief of akinetic mutism from obstructive hydrocephalus using bromocriptine and ephedrine. J Neurosurg 1992;76:152–155

22. Parks RW, Crockett DJ, Manji HK, Ammann W. Assessment of bromocriptine intervention for the treatment of frontallobe syndrome: a case study. J Neuropsychiatry 1992;4:109–111

23. Müller U, von Cramon DY. The therapeutic potential of bromocriptine in neuropsychological rehabilitation of patients with acquired brain damage. Prog Neuro-Psychopharmacol Biol Psychiatry 1994;18:1103–1120

24. Pulaski KH, Emmett L. The combined intervention of therapy and bromocriptine mesylate to improve functional performance after brain injury. Am J Occupat Ther 1994;48:263–270

25. Powell JH, Al-Adawi S, Morgan J, Greenwood RJ. Motivational deficits after brain injury: effects of bromocriptine in 11 patients. J Neurol Neurosurg Psychiatry 1996;60:416–421

26. Caner H, Altinörs N, Benli S, et al. Akinetic mutism after fourth ventricular choroid plexus papilloma: treatment with a dopamine agonist. Surg Neurol 1999;51: 181–184

27. Karli DC, Burke DT, Kim HJ, et al. Case study. Effects of dopaminergic combination therapy for frontal lobe dysfunction in traumatic brain injury rehabilitation. Brain Injury 1999;13:63–68

28. Starkstein SE, Berthier ML, Leiguarda R. Psychic akinesia following bilateral pallidal lesions. Int J Psychiatry Med 1989;19:155–164

29. Marin RS, Fogel BS, Hawkins J, et al. Apathy: a treatable syndrome. J Neuropsychiatry Clin Neurosci 1995; 7:23–30

30. Imamura T, Takanashi M, Hattori N, et al. Bromocriptine treatment for perseveration in demented patients. Alzheimer Dis Assoc Dis 1998;12:109–113

31. Nadeau SE, Malloy PF, Andrew ME. A crossover trial of bromocriptine in the treatment of vascular dementia. Ann Neurol 1988;24:270–272

32. McDowell S, Whyte J, D'Esposito M. Differential effect of a dopaminergic agonist on prefrontal function in traumatic brain injury patients. Brain 1998;121: 1155–1164

33. Chandler MC, Barnhill JL, Gualtieri CT. Case studies. Amantadine for the agitated head-injury patient. Brain Injury 1988;2:309–311

34. Gualtieri T, Chandler M, Coons TB, Brown LT. Amantadine: a new clinical profile for traumatic brain injury. Clin Neuropharmacol 1989;12:258–270

35. Edby K, Larsson J, Eek M, et al. Amantadine treatment of a patient with anoxic brain injury. Child Nervous System 1995;11:607–609

36. Kraus MF, Maki PM. Effect of amantadine hydrochloride on symptoms of frontal lobe dysfunction in brain injury: case studies and review. J Neuropsychiatry Clin Neurosci 1997;9:222–230

37. Zafonte RD, Watanabe T, Mann NR. Case study. A potential treatment for the minimally conscious state. Brain Injury 1998;12:617–621

38. Shiller AD, Burke DT, Kim HJ, et al. Treatment with amantadine potentiated motor learning in a patient with traumatic brain injury of 15 years duration. Brain Injury 1999;13:715–721

39. Nickels JL, Schneider WN, Dombovy ML, Wong TM. Clinical use of amantadine in brain injury rehabilitation. Brain Injury 1994;8:709–718

40. Van Reekum R, Bayley M, Barner S, et al. N of 1 study: amantadine for the amotivational syndrome in a patient with traumatic brain injury. Brain Injury 1995;9:49–53

41. Stern JM. Cranio-cerebral injured patients. Scan J Rehab Med 1978;10:7–10

42. Daly DD, Love JG. Akinetic mutism. Neurology 1958;8: 238–242

43. Lipper S, Tuchman MM. Treatment of chronic posttraumatic organic brain syndrome with dextroamphetamine: first reported case. J Nerv Ment Dis 1976;162: 366–371

44. Weinberg RM, Auerbach SH, Moore S. Pharmacologic treatment of cognitive deficits: a case study. Brain Injury 1987;1:57–59

45. Watanabe MD, Martin EM, De Leon OA, et al. Successful methylphenidate treatment of apathy after subcortical infarcts. J Neuropsychiatry Clin Neurosci 1995;7: 502–504

46. Hornyak JE, Nelson VS, Hurvitz EA. The use of methylphenidate in paediatric traumatic brain injury. Pediatr Rehabil 1997;1:15–17

47. Weinstein GS, Wells CE. Case studies in neuropsychiatry: post-traumatic psychiatric dysfunction—diagnosis and treatment. J Clin Psychiatry 1981;42:120–122

48. Evans RW, Gualtieri CT, Patterson D. Treatment of chronic closed head injury with psychostimulant drugs: a controlled case study and an appropriate evaluation procedure. J Nerv Ment Dis 1987;175:106–110

49. Bleiberg J, Garmoe W, Cederquist J, et al. Effects of dexedrine on performance consistency following brain injury. Neuropsychiatry Neuropsychol Behav Neurol 1993;6:245–248

50. Gualtieri CT, Evans RW. Stimulant treatment for the neurobehavioural sequelae of traumatic brain injury. Brain Injury 1988;2:273–290

51. Speech TJ, Rao SM, Osmon DC, Sperry LT. A double-blind controlled study of methylphenidate treatment in closed head injury. Brain Injury 1993;7:333–338

52. Williams SE, Ris MD, Ayyangar R, et al. Recovery in pediatric brain injury: is psychostimulant medication beneficial? J Head Trauma Rehabil 1998;13(3):73–81

53. Mooney GF, Haas LJ. Effect of methylphenidate on brain injury-related anger. Arch Phys Med Rehabil 1993;74:153–160

54. Whyte J, Hart T, Schuster K, et al. Effects of methylphenidate on attentional function after traumatic brain injury. A randomized, placebo-controlled trial. Am J Phys Med Rehabil 1997;76:440–450

55. Plenger PM, Dixon CE, Castillo RM, et al. Subacute methylphenidate treatment for moderate to moderately severe traumatic brain injury: a preliminary double-blind placebo-controlled study. Arch Phys Med Rehabil 1996;77:536–540

56. Kaelin DL, Cifu DX, Matthies B. Methylphenidate effect on attention deficit in the acutely brain-injured adult. Arch Phys Med Rehabil 1996;77:6–9

57. Elliott FA. Propranolol for the control of belligerent behavior following acute brain damage. Ann Neurol 1977;1:489–491

58. Yudofsky S, Williams D, Gorman J. Propranolol in the treatment of rage and violent behavior in patients with chronic brain syndromes. Am J Psychiatry 1981;138:218–220

59. Mansheim P. Treatment with propranolol of the behavioral sequelae of brain damage. J Clin Psychiatry 1981;42:132

60. Ratey JJ, Morrill R, Oxenkrug G. Use of propranolol for provoked and unprovoked episodes of rage. Am J Psychiatry 1983;140:1356–1357

61. Petrie WM, Ban TA. Propranolol in organic agitation. Lancet 1981;1:324

62. Brooke MM, Patterson DR, Questad KA, et al. The treatment of agitation during initial hospitalization after traumatic brain injury. Arch Phys Med Rehabil 1992;73:917–921

63. Greendyke RM, Kanter DR, Schuster DB, et al. Propranolol treatment of assaultive patients with organic brain disease. A double-blind crossover, placebo-controlled study. J Nerv Ment Dis 1986;174:290–294

64. Bainbridge JF, Greenwood DT. The tranquilizing effects of propranolol demonstrated in rats. Neuropharmacology 1971;10:453–458

65. Feeney DM. Mechanisms of noradrenergic modulation of physical therapy: effects on functional recovery after cortical injury. In: Goldstein LB, ed. Restorative Neurology: Advances in Pharmacotherapy for Recovery After Stroke. Armonk, N.Y.: Futura Publishing Co., 1998:35–78

66. Feeney DM. Rehabilitation pharmacology. Noradrenergic enhancement of physical therapy. In: Ginsberg MD, Bogousslavsky J, eds. Cerebrovascular Disease: Pathophysiology, Diagnosis and Management, Vol. 1. Cambridge: Blackwell Scientific Press, 1998:620–636

67. Greendyke RM, Kanter DR. Therapeutic effects of pindolol on behavioral disturbances associated with organic brain disease: a double-blind study. J Clin Psychiatry 1986;47:423–426

68. Greendyke RM, Berkner JP, Webster JC, Gulya A. Treatment of behavioral problems with pindolol. Psychosomatics 1989;30:161–165

69. Jackson RD, Corrigan JD, Arnett JA. Amitriptyline for agitation in head injury. Arch Phys Med Rehab 1985;66:180–181

70. Mysiw WJ, Jackson RD, Corrigan JD. Amitriptyline for post-traumatic agitation. Am J Phys Med Rehabil 1988;67:29–33

71. Wroblewski B, Glenn MB, Cornblatt R, et al. Protriptylline as an alternative stimulant medication in patients with brain injury: a series of case reports. Brain Injury 1993;7:353–362

72. Reinhard DL, Whyte J, Sandel ME. Improved arousal and initiation following tricyclic antidepressant use in severe brain injury. Arch Phys Med Rehabil 1996;77:80–83

73. Simpson DM, Foster D. Improvement in organically disturbed behavior with trazodone treatment. J Clin Psychiatry 1986;47:191–193

74. Pinner E, Rich CL. Effects of trazodone on aggressive behavior in seven patients with organic mental disorders. Am J Psychiatry 1988;145:1295–1296

75. Lebert F, Pasquier F, Petit H. Behavioral effects of trazodone in Alzheimer's disease. J Clin Psychiatry 1994;55:536–538

76. Fava M. Psychopharmacologic treatment of pathologic aggression. Psychiatr Clin North Am 1997;20:427–451

77. Delgado PL, Moreno FA. Different roles for serotonin in anti-obsessional drug actin and the pathophysiology of obsessive-compulsive disorder. Br J Psychiatry 1998;35(Suppl):21–25

78. Eslinger PJ, Damasio AR. Severe disturbance of higher cognition following bilateral frontal lobe ablation. Neurology 1985;35:1731–1741

Evaluation and Management of Amnesic Disorders

Margaret G O'Connor and Mieke Verfaellie

Historical overview

Current understanding of amnesia has grown out of clinical descriptions and lesion analytic investigations of patients such as H.M., who became amnesic in the aftermath of bilateral temporal lobectomies for treatment of refractory seizures.[1,2] H.M.'s dense amnesia underscored the importance of the hippocampus and adjacent cortices in new learning. Cognitive studies of H.M., demonstrating dissociations in his processing abilities, were critical in establishing the psychological parameters of different memory processes.[3]

Over the last four decades, many other patients with amnesia have been studied. Initially, rival models regarding the nature of the memory deficit in amnesia were formulated, but disagreements may have stemmed largely from differences between patient groups in terms of underlying neuropathology and associated cognitive deficits. Researchers working with Korsakoff patients (who often have frontal network damage) suggested that amnesia was due to inadequate *encoding* or analysis of new information,[4,5] Amnesia was viewed a consequence of disrupted *consolidation* (or retention) by those working with H.M. and other patients with isolated medial temporal damage.[6] A third group of investigators, working with a variety of amnesic patients, emphasized the role of *retrieval* as critical in the amnesic syndrome.[7] Over time, studies indicated that various aspects of information processing are intrinsically linked and that amnesia could not be explained by selective disruption in a particular stage of memory.[8]

A major change in focus in amnesia research occurred in the 1970s and 1980s with the realization that not all aspects of memory are equally disrupted in patients with amnesia. Clinical analyses of premorbid memory revealed that remote *semantic memory* (knowledge of generic facts and concepts) is intact in amnesia whereas remote *episodic memory* (recall of experiental aspects of events) is impaired.[9] This classification dovetailed on proposals regarding memory subdivisions that arose within cognitive psychology.[10] The finding of selective disruption in the retrieval of episodic memories suggested that the storage and retrieval of semantic and episodic memory have different brain bases.

Similar dissociations were obtained in the domain of new learning. Studies of H.M.,[11,12] and subsequently of patients with Korsakoff syndrome and encephalitis,[13] established that patients with amnesia demonstrate intact *procedural memory*: they are able to learn and retain new habits and skills (e.g., riding a bicycle or playing a piano), despite the fact that their *declarative memory* (i.e., their knowledge of having been exposed to the information) is severely impaired.[14] Procedural memory is typically acquired gradually, across multiple presentations, but other forms of *implicit memory* (memory without awareness) that require only a single study exposure are also preserved in amnesia. Amnesics' performance is fully intact on a variety of priming tasks in which learning is expressed as a bias or facilitation in performance due to previous exposure to task stimuli.[15] Such learning occurs despite the fact that amnesics' *explicit memory* (i.e., conscious recollection) for the same stimuli is severely impaired.

The finding of dissociations in amnesics' performance, both in the retrieval of premorbid memories and the acquisition of new postmorbid memories reinforced the notion that memory is not a unitary phenomenon. It led to the development of models of memory that incorporate a number of dissociable memory processes thought to be mediated by distinct neural systems.[16–18]

Clinically oriented studies focused on the relationship between distribution of neural damage and various profiles of neuropsychological impairment in amnesic patients. This work led to the proposal that amnesics could be categorized according to site of neural damage.[19,20] Patients with hippocampal damage (related to cerebrovascular accidents, anoxia, and encephalitis) were described as having accelerated forgetting, preserved insight, and limited remote memory loss. Patients with diencephalic amnesia (due to Wernicke Korsakoff syndrome as well as diencephalic strokes or tumors) were seen as having tendencies towards confabulation, diminished insight, less accelerated forgetting, and extensive loss of information from remote memory. The distinction between diencephalic and medial temporal amnesics, however, has been called into question because both groups have damage to the same functional limbic-diencephalic system and because extraneous factors (e.g., associated frontal pathology) may have contributed to observed group differences.[21,22] More recent attempts to examine the relationship between the profile of amnesia and specific sites of neuropathology have concentrated upon the extent and location of lesion within the medial temporal lobe.[22,23]

Clinical features and assessment of amnesia

By definition, amnesia refers to a dense memory deficit in the context of normal intelligence and intact working memory (i.e., the ability to hold and manipulate information "on line"). *Anterograde amnesia* (AA) refers to an inability to learn new information from the period of time following the onset of amnesia. *Retrograde amnesia* (RA) refers to deficient recall of past events antedating the onset of amnesia. Patients with anterograde amnesia typically have some degree of retrograde memory deficit as well, although the extent may vary greatly. Isolated disorders of retrograde memory, although rare, have also been described.[24]

Evaluation of memory problems should take place in the context of a comprehensive evaluation geared towards ruling out associated deficits that may contribute to memory loss. Damage in brain regions other than those directly causing the amnesia (e.g., frontal networks) increases the likelihood of problems such as confabulation, diminished insight, attention and working memory impairment. If the patient has significant deficits affecting a broad spectrum of cognitive and perceptual abilities, a diagnosis of dementia or delirium should be considered.

The clinical evaluation of anterograde memory should survey a variety of memory processes including encoding, rate of forgetting, and retrieval. Information about these processes is inferred from a comparison of patients' performance on tasks of recall and recognition, both immediately and after a delay.[25] A comparison of performance on verbal and non-verbal tasks provides important information about material-specific memory deficits. Assessment of retrograde memory should examine memory for events (episodic memory) as well facts and concepts (semantic memory). A further distinction can be made between memory for personally relevant (autobiographical) information and memory for public events and facts. Of importance is also the temporal extent of amnesia, as retrograde amnesia can vary from being time-limited (a few months or years prior to illness) to being extremely extensive, covering up to 20 or 30 years before the onset of amnesia.

One goal of memory evaluations pertains to differential diagnosis. As noted, memory problems vary in relation to the location of lesion which, in turn, is of diagnostic value. A more common goal of memory evaluation is that of obtaining information about the patient's functional status relevant to the questions of safety awareness, capacity for work, and possible interventions.

Etiology of amnesia

Neurologically-based amnesia has been associated with a wide variety of medical conditions including cerebrovascular accidents, anoxia, herpes simplex encephalitis, tumors, and Wernicke Korsakoff's Syndrome, all of which may result in dysfunction in hippocampal and thalamic circuitry essential for learning (Table 266.1). Among the many conditions that have been associated with circumscribed amnesia are the following:

Cerebrovascular accidents Bilateral posterior cerebral artery (PCA) infarction is a well-recognized cause of global amnesia. Lesions in the posterior parahippocampus or collateral isthmus (a pathway connecting the posterior parahippocampus to association cortex) are viewed as critical in the memory disturbance in this patient group.[26] Amnesia has also been described in association with unilateral (primarily left) PCA infarction.[26–28] Deficits beyond amnesia (e.g., hemianopic alexia, pure alexia, color agonosia, and object agnosia) may affect the clinical presentation of these patients.[29] Thalamic strokes, related to infarction of the tuberothalamic and paramedian arteries, have also been associated with severe memory loss.[30] Material-specific memory deficits are seen following unilateral thalamic damage.[31,32]

Herpes simplex encephalitis (HSE) Patients with memory loss secondary to HSE are heterogeneous with respect to both clinical presentation and distribution of lesion. In the initial stages, patients may present with confusion, aphasia, and agnosia. Over time, these difficulties may resolve so that the patient is left with a dense and circumscribed amnesia. Herpes simplex encephalitis typically affects mesial temporal brain regions including the hippocampus and adjacent entorhinal, perirhinal and parahippocampal cortices. Associated damage in lateral aspects of the temporal lobe may exert deleterious effects on language and semantic memory, accounting for persistent aphasia and agnosia in some patients. Lesions may be asymmetrical, with greater involvement of left temporal regions associated with primarily verbal memory problems and involvement of right temporal regions affecting primarily non-verbal memory.[33] In addition to anterograde amnesia, patients may demonstrate dense retrograde amnesia in association with more extensive lateral lesions.[34,35]

Paraneoplastic limbic encephalitis (PLE) In general, PLE involves an autoimmune reaction to cancer elsewhere in the body and has been associated with lesions in limbic regions.[36] Patients with PLE-induced amnesia are relatively rare and, at the same time, heterogeneous. One patient with amnesia secondary to PLE had severe anterograde memory deficits, confabulation, and a dense retrograde amnesia of 25 years.[37] Another patient displayed a dense amnesia with an atypical rate of forgetting.[38] He demonstrated normal retention of new material for several days after exposure but dense and persistent loss thereafter.

Anoxic encephalopathy Memory problems may occur as a result of a number of events associated with oxygen depletion such as cardiac arrest, respiratory distress, and carbon monoxide poisoning. Because the medial temporal lobes are particularly sensitive to oxygen deprivation, anoxia may lead to

Table 266.1   Neurological conditions associated with amnesia

Condition	Herpes simplex encephalitis	Anoxia	Wernicke Korsakoff syndrome	Stroke	AcoA aneurysm
Etiology of brain damage	Viral infection	Oxygen deprivation due to cardiac or respiratory distress	Chronic thiamine deficiency associated with alcoholism	Bilateral infarction of PCA or thalamic infarction	Aneurysm associated with hemorrhage, vasospasm, hemotoma formation
Onset	Acute onset of flu-like illness	Acute but deficits may evolve over several days	Acute Wernicke stage followed by chronic Korsakoff stage	Acute	Acute
Pathology	Medial temporal, occasionally extending to lateral temporal and frontal brain regions	Medial temporal with more diffuse damage depending on length of coma	Diencephalic	Medial temporal, diencephalic and/or frontal depending on affected vasculature	Basal forebrain, frontal, striatum
Prominent features	Acute: generalized confusion Chronic: anterograde amnesia associated deficits dependent upon extent of lesion	Anterograde amnesia with associated deficits dependent upon extent of lesion	Wernicke's stage: confusion, ataxia, occulomotor palsies Korsakoff's stage: anterograde amnesia, limited insight, confabulation, temporally graded retrograde amnesia	Anterograde amnesia with associated deficits dependent upon extent of lesion	Anterograde amnesia characterized by impairment in strategic retrieval, limited insight, and confabulation
Prognosis	Some deficits resolve following acute stage but permanent amnesia in a subgroup of patients	Limited recovery over the first year	Poor prognosis	Limited recovery over first year	Substantial recovery in some patients over the first year; limited recovery in others

selective damage to medial temporal areas, resulting in circumscribed amnesia. The severity of amnesia depends on the extent of lesion: selective lesions of the CA1 field of the hippocampus result in a mild to moderately severe amnesia,[39] whereas more severe memory loss occurs with more extensive damage in the medial temporal lobes.[40] In cases of more diffuse cortical and subcortical brain damage, other cognitive and perceptual abilities may be affected.

Wernicke Korsakoff syndrome (WKS) Wernicke Korsakoff syndrome patients develop amnesia as a result of chronic alcohol abuse and thiamine deficiency.[41] In the acute phase of WKS, patients exhibit oculomotor palsies, ataxia and confabulation. The chronic phase is characterized by severe and persistent memory deficits due to damage in dorsomedial thalamic nuclei and mamillary bodies.[42,43] Additional

frontal dysfunction may be responsible for some of the unique characteristics of the WKS amnesia profile, which includes superficial and deficient encoding strategies, confabulation and source memory errors. Remote memory loss is common, but its interpretation is complicated by the fact that patients' premorbid lifestyle may have interfered with the establishment of salient remote memories that can serve as a framework for retrieval. Frontal damage also likely interferes with the strategic search of episodic information from the past.

Anterior communicating artery (ACoA) aneurysms Memory deficits associated with ACoA aneurysms result from damage to the basal forebrain, striatum and frontal brain regions.[44,45] Patients with ACoA aneurysm demonstrate memory problems characterized by sensitivity to proactive interference (i.e., prior learning interferes with subsequent acquisition), impaired temporal discrimination, source forgetting, and failure on tasks of semantic clustering. Because of the associated frontal damage, many patients exhibit confabulation and diminished insight. The group is heterogeneous with respect to density of amnesia but common to many patients with ACoA aneurysm is their normal performance on tasks of immediate recognition (versus impaired immediate recall). The discrepancy between normal recognition versus impaired recall is due to problems in the strategic search of memory.[46]

Transient global amnesia (TGA) Transient global amnesia refers to a circumscribed memory deficit of limited duration (<24 hours) that is reversible. Patients with TGA demonstrate profound antero-grade memory problems and variable profiles of ret-rograde amnesia, perhaps due to retrieval problems.[47,48] Memory problems may completely resolve in the weeks or months after the episode. Several studies, however, have shown that residual memory deficits may be detected.[49,50] Episodes of TGA may be precipitated by a variety of physical and/or emotional factors.[51] Common causes include migraine, temporal lobe epilepsy and vascular dys-function. Decreased perfusion to medial temporal structures is thought to be the underlying mechanism.[52]

Neuropathology of amnesia

Amnesia can result from damage to a variety of brain structures, most notably, the medial temporal lobe, diencephalon and basal forebrain. These structures form part of the extended limbic system, a system thought to be critical for new episodic learning. The limbic system has two interacting memory circuits: the Papez circuit, consisting of the hippocampus, fornix, mamillary bodies, anterior thalamus and pos-terior cingulate (with additional connections to the basal forebrain via the fornix); and the basolateral circuit, consisting of the amygdala and surrounding perirhinal cortex, dorsomedial thalamus and pre-frontal cortex. Memory deficits can arise from disrup-tions anywhere in these circuits, although profound amnesia typically results from damage to both circuits.

At present, it remains a matter of debate whether these two circuits make distinct contributions to memory. Focusing on the temporal lobe, some inves-tigators have suggested that more extensive lesions (involving the hippocampus as well as surrounding entorhinal and perirhinal cortex) simply cause more severe deficits that are qualitatively similar to those seen by selective hippocampal lesions.[53] Others suggest that the hippocampus and perirhinal cortices make qualitatively different contributions to memory, the former being critical for recall of episodic informa-tion and the latter being critical for stimulus familiar-ity or recognition.[22] Patients with selective lesions to the hippocampus or surrounding cortices will be crit-ical in evaluating these proposals.

The creation of durable memory traces requires interactions between the limbic system and neocortex.[54] The limbic system receives convergent input from neocortical areas and forms a compressed representation that links together the different cortical sites that process features of an experience. Over time, permanent cortico-cortical connections are established that can be retrieved without mediation of the limbic system. Limbic lesions therefore typically lead to a time-limited retrograde amnesia, whereas cortical damage can lead to a severe and extensive remote memory deficit, secondary to a loss of cortical representations. Critical cortical regions include posterior association areas that store featural informa-tion[55] as well as higher order convergence zones that trigger posterior cortical representations.[56] There is evidence in favor of hemispheric specialization, with right hemisphere areas more important for the storage of episodic (autobiographical) information, and left hemisphere areas more critical for the storage of semantic information.[57]

Frontal lobe damage or lesions in pathways con-necting the frontal and anterior temporal lobes can also lead to remote memory loss. Such loss is not due to a disruption or degradation of the memory traces itself, but rather, to a disruption of the retrieval processes that are necessary to contact stored representations.[58,59]

Treatment and management of memory disorders

Treatment of memory problems encompasses cogni-tive remediation techniques, psychosocial support and pharmacological intervention. Remediation goals should be identified on the basis of the patient's clini-cal presentation, which includes his/her medical status, level of insight, motivation, and neuropsycho-logical strengths and weaknesses. Historical informa-tion (e.g., family situation, previous occupation and educational attainment) may also influence the long-term goals of the rehabilitation plan.[60]

Cognitive remediation

Cognitive remediation is typically aimed at enhancing day-to-day episodic memory functions.[61] This is done by using "internal" and "external" memory aids to compensate for impaired memory abilities. A second goal may be to teach patients new generic knowledge about the world that is not tied to a particular episodic encounter. There is some suggestion that preserved memory abilities can be successfully used to support such learning.

Internal memory aids refer to the use of psycholog-ical strategies as a way of strengthening day-to-day memories. These strategies include increased organ-ization, repetition, and use of elaboration. These aids are best suited for individuals with mild, attention-ally-based, memory problems. Patients with dense amnesia due to damage in hippocampal circuitry are not good candidates for this type of intervention.[62] Such patients may be unaware of their memory deficits and unmotivated to use these techniques spontaneously, or they may forget to apply these strategies outside a training context.

Many psychological strategies focus on increasing the organizational structure of incoming information to enhance encoding and facilitate retrieval. List learning is facilitated by "chunking" techniques (e.g., coding a phone number according to groups of numbers rather than seven individual digits) and thematic organization (e.g., categorizing one's grocery list according to aisles in the supermarket). In more naturalistic situations involving conversational speech, the memory-impaired individual is encouraged to ask questions or re-frame what the speaker is saying as a way of "parsing" an extended exchange. Other remediation techniques focus on using previously established memories as a way of organizing new information. Spaced repetition (across different time intervals and different spatial locations) increases the likelihood that a "free standing" memory will be conceptually integrated with preexisting memories. Elaboration techniques such as verbal mnemonics or visual imagery may have similar effects in that the new memory becomes conceptually (or perceptually) linked to older memories that are resistant to decay. In a sense, elaboration provides the learner with alternative "addresses" to enhance retrieval.

External aids include augmentative technologies (e.g., electronic organizers such as the Palm Pilot) that serve as memory "prostheses."[63] Electronic assistants are often programmed to remind the patient about important events (e.g., medications). With adequate practice, even dense amnesics can use these aids as a way of mitigating the impact of memory loss on daily life.[64] Other, more conventional, external aids include notebooks, wall calendars, medication organizers and use of photographic material. In order to use external aids effectively the patient must have insight into his/her memory problem and he/she must be motivated. Occupational therapists work closely with patients to develop appropriate external memory aids that, otherwise, could be overwhelming to the individual with memory impairment.

Techniques that capitalize on amnesics' preserved implicit memory abilities may be useful to teach amnesic patients domain-specific facts or concepts.[65] One training method that has been used quite extensively is the vanishing-cues technique.[66,67] This technique takes advantage of patients' ability to produce previously studied items in response to word fragment cues. At the beginning of training, patients are given a definition and are presented with as many letters as necessary to produce the target word. With training, the letter cues are gradually reduced until the patient can spontaneously generate the desired information. This approach has been used to teach patients computer-related vocabulary, business-related terms and novel concepts. Although learning is typically slow and laborious, retention can be remarkably good. This method is most likely to be beneficial if information needs to be used in situations similar to that in which learning occurred.

One factor that may be critical in the efficacy of implicit learning methods is the use of training contexts that prevent patients from making errors.[68] Patients with memory deficits have great difficulty eliminating errors because they fail to remember whether a previously provided answer is correct or incorrect. Regardless of its accuracy, a previously generated answer is likely to be primed, and thus continues to be strengthened across subsequent learning trials. If this answer is incorrect, it may greatly interfere with acquisition of the correct response.

Psychopharmacology

The extent of pathological and behavioral heterogeneity across amnesics makes it unlikely that a single medication targeting a specific neurotransmitter system will be identified as the panacea for memory problems.[69] Even when the pathology of a particular form of amnesia is clearly understood, there is no guarantee that pharmacological intervention will be successful as severe damage to the neural substrates of memory may render the problem refractory to medications.

There have only been a few studies investigating pharmacological intervention in patients with circumscribed memory deficits. In two studies, clonindine, an alpha noradrenergic agonist, had significant beneficial effects on the memory problems of Korsakoff patients.[70,71] However, this effect was not replicated in a third study.[72] Studies of cholinergic agonists have yielded mixed results with respect to memory facilitation. Cholinergic medications did not enhance the memory abilities of a patient with memory loss due to a basal forebrain lesion,[73] whereas they were more effective in two other patients with memory loss related to encephalitis[74] and brain trauma.[75]

In light of the prevalence of Alzheimer's disease (AD) in our society, it is not surprising that most studies on the pharmacological management of memory disorders have concentrated on patients with AD. Previous studies demonstrated that cholinergic innervation of the hippocampus and neocortex is critical to new learning and that cholinergic depletion in AD corresponds to severity of dementia.[76–78] As a result, many studies have used cholinergic agonists for remediation of the memory problems of AD patients. To date, two such medications (tacrine and donepezil) have been approved by the FDA for treatment of AD. Both medications have been found to be only modestly beneficial in slowing the cognitive demise of AD patients and neither has resulted in significant recovery of function.[79,80] A number of other cholinomimetic agents, such as muscarinic and nicotinic agonists, are still under development and may be more promising in terms of future treatment.

In addition, hormonal supplements and herbal compounds have been investigated as possible treatments of memory deficits. Estrogens may stimulate cholinergic markers, increase blood flow, and prevent neuronal atrophy in the brain.[81] There have been several studies indicating that estrogen has a beneficial effect on cognitive abilities,[82,83] but other studies have not demonstrated similar efficacy.[84] The cognitive enhancing properties of Gingko biloba have been demonstrated in several investigations but the magnitude of the effect has been small.[85]

The limited success in remediation of the memory deficits of AD patients may, in part, be due to the pathological and behavioral heterogeneity in this patient group. The use of single medications that target neurotransmitters is not ideal. A more effective approach would include combinations of different neurotransmitters that affect different aspects of memory.[86]

Conclusions

Over the last few decades research in neuropsychology and cognitive psychology has provided important information regarding the psychological and neural organization of memory. While controversy remains regarding the precise roles of specific brain regions in certain aspects of memory, there is consensus that memory is composed of a variety of convergent processes that contribute to the analysis and integration of new information.

New ideas about memory have led to advances in the clinical evaluation of patients with memory disorders. It is now clear that memory breaks down differentially in association with different neurological illnesses. The specific pattern of deficits and residual learning abilities are considered alongside other neurodiagnostic information in the differential diagnosis of the memory impaired patient. Diagnostic clarity is important in order to provide the patient and family with information regarding prognosis and expected psychosocial consequences.

Less information is available regarding effective treatment of memory disorders. Most psychological interventions aimed at improving day to day memory have resulted in only modest generalization to contexts other than the one in which training occurred. Pharmacological studies have focused primarily on the use of cholinergic agonists in the remediation of the memory problems seen in association with Alzheimer's disease. To date, studies in this area have been disappointing. Medications have not been identified that have a clear and unequivocal effect on memory. Clearly, there is a need for further work in this area using pharmacological interventions that target multiple neurotransmitter systems in patients with well-defined memory problems.

Acknowledgments

Preparation of this chapter was supported by grants NS26985 and MH57681 and the Medical Research Service of the US Department of Veterans Affairs.

References

1. Scoville WB, Milner B. Loss of recent memory after bilateral hippocampal lesions. Journal of Neurology, Neurosurgery and Psychiatry 1957;20:11–12
2. Milner B. Amnesia following operation on the temporal lobes. In: Whitty CWM, Zangwill OL, eds. Amnesia. London: Butterworths, 1966:109–133
3. Corkin S. Lasting consequences of bilateral medial temporal lobectomy: clinical course and experimental findings in HM. Seminars in Neurology 1984;4:249–259
4. Butters N, Cermak LS. Alcoholic Korsakoff's syndrome: an information processing approach. New York: Academic Press, 1980
5. Cermak LS. Information processing deficits of alcoholic Korsakoff patients. Quarterly Journal of Studies on Alcohol 1973;34:1110–1132
6. Milner B. Disorders of learning and memory after temporal lobe lesions in man. Clinical Neurosurgery 1972;19:421–446
7. Warrington EK, Weiskrantz L. Amnesic syndrome: consolidation or retrieval? Nature 1970;228:628–630
8. Cermak LS. Amnesia as a processing deficit. In: Goldstein G, Tarter RE, eds. Advances in Clinical Neuropsychology. Vol 3. New York: Plenum, 1986:265–290
9. Kinsbourne M, Wood F. Theoretical considerations regarding the episodic-semantic distinction. In: Cermak LS, ed. Human memory and amnesia. Hillsdale, NJ: Erlbaum, 1982:195–217
10. Tulving E. Episodic and semantic memory. In: Tulving E, Donaldson W, eds. Organization of memory. New York: Academic Press, 1972:381–403
11. Milner B, Teuber HL. Alteration in perception and memory in man: reflections on methods. In: Weiskrantz L, ed. Analysis of Behavioral Change. New York: Harper and Row, 1968
12. Corkin S. Acquisition of motor skill after bilateral medial temporal lobe excision. Neuropsychologia 1968; 6:255–265
13. Brooks DN, Baddeley A. What can amnesic patients learn? Neuropsychologia 1976;14:111–122
14. Cohen NJ, Squire LR. Preserved learning and retention of pattern-analyzing skill in amnesia: dissociation of knowing how and knowing that. Science 1980;210: 207–210
15. Moscovitch M, Vriezen E, Gottstein J. Implicit tests of memory in patients with focal lesions or degenerative brain disorders. In: Spinnler H, Boller F, eds. Handbook of Neuropsychology. Amsterdam: Elsevier, 1993:133–173
16. Gabrieli JDE. Disorders of memory in humans. Current Opinion in Neurology and Neurosurgery 1993;6:93–97
17. Squire LR. Declarative and nondeclarative memory: multiple brain systems supporting learning and memory. Journal of Cognitive Neuroscience 1992;4: 195–231
18. Schacter DL. Priming and multiple memory systems: perceptual mechanisms of implicit memory. In: Schacter DL, Tulving E, eds. Memory Systems 1994. Cambridge, MA: MIT press, 1994:233–268
19. Butters N, Miliotis P, Albert M, Sax D. Memory assessment: evidence of the heterogeneity of amnesic symptoms. Advances in Clinical Neuropsychology 1984;1: 127–159
20. Lhermitte F, Signoret JL. Analyse neuropsychologique et differentiation des syndromes amnesiques. Revue Neurologique 1972;126:161–178
21. Weiskrantz L. On issues and theories of the human amnesic syndrome. In: Weinberger N, McGaugh J, Lynch G, eds. Memory systems of the brain. New York, NY: Guilford Press, 1985:380–415
22. Aggleton JP, Brown MW. Episodic memory, amnesia, and the hippocampal-anterior thalamic axis. Behavioral and Brain Sciences 1999;425–489
23. Squire LR, Knowlton BJ. Memory, hippocampus and brain systems. In: Gazzaniga MS, ed. The Cognitive Neurosciences. Cambridge, MA: MIT Press, 1995:825–837
24. Kapur N. Focal retrograde amnesia in neurological

disease: a critical review. Cortex 1993;29:217–234

25. Verfaellie M, O'Connor M. A neuropsychological analysis of memory and amnesia. Seminars in Neurology 2000;20:455–462

26. von Cramon D, Hebel N, Schuri U. Verbal memory and learning in unilateral posterior cerebral infarction. Brain 1988;111:1061–1077

27. Ott BR, Saver JL. Unilateral amnesic stroke: six new cases and a review of the literature. Stroke 1993;24:1033–1042

28. Benson D, Marsden C, Meadows J. The amnesic syndrome of posterior cerebral artery occlusion. Acta Neurologica Scandinavia 1974;50:133–145

29. DeRenzi E, Zambolin A, Crisi G. The pattern of neuropsychological impairment associated with left posterior cerebral artery infarcts. Brain 1987;110:1099–1116

30. von Cramon D, Hebel N, Schuri U. A contribution to the anatomical basis of thalamic amnesia. Brain 1985;108:993–1008

31. Speedie LJ, Heilman KM. Anterograde memory deficits for visuospatial material after infarction of the right thalamus. Archives of Neurology 1983;40:183–186

32. Speedie LJ, Heilman KM. Amnestic disturbance following infarction of the left dorsomedial nucleus of the thalamus. Neuropsychologia 1982;20:597–604

33. Eslinger PJ, Damasio H, Damasio AR, Butters N. Nonverbal amnesia and asymmetric cerebral lesions following encephalitis. Brain and Cognition 1993;21:140–152

34. Damasio AR, Van Hoesen GW. The limbic system and the localisation of herpes simplex encephalitis. Journal of Neurology, Neurosurgery and Psychiatry 1985;48:297–301

35. O'Connor MG, Butters N, Miliotis P, et al. The dissociation of anterograde and retrograde amnesia in a patient with herpes encephalitis. Journal of Clinical and Experimental Neuropsychology 1992;14:159–178

36. Newman NJ, Bell IR, McKee AC. Paraneoplastic limbic encephalitis: neuropsychiatric presentation. Biological Psychiatry 1990;27:529–542

37. Parkin AJ, Leng RC. Neuropsychology of the Amnesic Syndrome. Hillsdale: Lawrence Erlbaum Associates, 1993

38. O'Connor MG, Sieggreen MA, Ahern G, et al. Accelerated forgetting in association with temporal lobe epilepsy and paraneoplastic limbic encephalitis. Brain and Cognition 1997;35:71–84

39. Zola-Morgan S, Squire L, Amaral D. Human amnesia and the medial temporal region: enduring memory impairment following a bilateral lesion limited to field CA1 of the hippocampus. Journal of Neuroscience 1986;6:2950–2967

40. Rempel-Clower NL, Zola SM, Squire LR, Amaral DG. Three cases of enduring memory impairment after bilateral damage limited to the hippocampal formation. Journal of Neuroscience 1996;16:5233–5255

41. Verfaellie M, Cermak LS. Wernicke Korsakoff and related nutritional disorders of the nervous system. In: Feinberg TE, Farah MJ, eds. Behavioral neurology and neuropsychology. New York: McGraw Hill, 1996:609–619

42. Mair W, Warrington E, Weiskrantz L. Memory disorder in Korsakoff's psychosis: a neuropathological and neuropsychological investigation of two cases. Brain 1979;102:749–783

43. Victor M, Adams RD, Collins GH. The Wernicke-Korsakoff Syndrome and related neurologic disorders due to alcoholism and malnutrition. 2nd ed. Philadelphia: Davis, 1989

44. Damasio AR, Graff-Radford NR, Eslinger PJ, et al.

Amnesia following basal forebrain lesions. Archives of Neurology 1985;42:263–271

45. Irle E, Wowra B, Kunert HJ, et al. Memory disturbance following anterior communicating artery rupture. Annals of Neurology 1992;31:473–480

46. DeLuca J. Cognitive dysfunction after aneurysm of the anterior communicating artery. Journal of Clinical and Experimental Neuropsychology 1992;14:924–934

47. Harting C, Markowitsch AJ. Different degrees of impairment in irecall/recognition and anterograde/retrograde memory performance in a transient global amnesic case. Neurocase 1996;2:45–49

48. Hodges JR, Ward CD. Observations during transient global amnesia. Brain 1989;112:595–620

49. Mazzucchi A, Moretti G, Caffarra P, Parma M. Neuropsychological functions in the follow-up of transient global amnesia. Brain 1980;103:161–178

50. Gallassi R, Lorusso S, Stracciari A. Neuropsychological findings during a transient global amnesia attack and its follow-up. Italian Journal of Neurological Sciences 1986;7:45–49

51. Caplan LR. Transient global amnesia: characteristic features and overview. Toronto: Hogrefe, 1990

52. Goldenberg F, Podreka I, Pfaffelmeyer N, et al. Thalamic ischemia in transient global amnesia: a SPECT study. Neurology 1991;41:1748–1752

53. Zola SM, Squire LR. The medial temporal lobe and the hippocampus. In: Tulving E, Craik FIM, eds. The Oxford handbook of memory. Oxford: Oxford University Press, 2000:485–500

54. Squire LR, Alvarez P. Retrograde amnesia and memory consolidation: a neurobiological perspective. Current Opinion in Neurobiology 1995;5:169–177

55. Rubin DC, Greenberg DL. Visual memory-deficit amnesia: a distinct amnesic presentation and etiology. Proceedings of the National Academy of Sciences 1998;95:5413–5416

56. Damasio S, Eslinger P, Damasio H, et al. Multimodal amnesic syndrome following bilateral temporal and frontal damage: the case of patient DRB. Archives of Neurology 1985;42:252–259

57. Markowitsch HJ. Which brain regions are critically involved in the retrieval of old episodic memory? Brain Research Review 1995;21:117–127

58. Levine B, Black SE, Cabeza R, et al. Episodic memory and the self in a case of isolated retrograde amnesia. Brain 1998;121:1951–1973

59. Kroll NEA, Markowitsch HJ, Knight RT, von Cramon DY. Retrieval of old memories: the temporofrontal hypothesis. Brain 1997;120:1377–1399

60. Wilson B. Rehabilitation of Memory. London: Guilford Press, 1987

61. O'Connor M, Cermak LS. Rehabilitation of organic memory disorders. In: Meier M, Benton A, Diller L, eds. Neuropsychological Rehabilitation. New York: Guilford Press, 1987:260–279

62. Cermak LS. Imagery as an aid to retrieval for Korsakoff patients. Cortex 1975;11:163–169

63. Kapur N. Memory aids in the rehabilitation of memory disordered patients. In: Baddeley AD, Wilson BA, Watts FN, eds. Handbook of Memory Disorders. West Sussex: Wiley, 1995:533–556

64. Wilson B, Evans JJ, Emslie H, Malinek V. Evaluation of NeuroPage: a new memory aid. Journal of Neurology, Neurosurgery and Psychiatry 1997;63:113–115

65. Verfaellie M. Semantic learning in amnesia. In: Boller F, Grafman J, eds. Handbook of Neuropsychology 2nd revd. ed. Amsterdam: Elsevier, 2000;4:335–354

66. Glisky EL, Schacter DL, Tulving E. Learning and retention of computer-related vocabulary in memory-impaired patients: method of vanishing cues. Journal of Clinical and Experimental Neuropsychology 1986;8: 292–312

67. Glisky EL, Schacter DL. Acquisition of domain-specific knowledge in patients with organic memory disorders. Journal of Learning Disabilities 1988;21:333–339

68. Baddeley A, Wilson B. When implicit learning fails: amnesia and the problem of error elimination. Neuropsychologia 1994;32:53–68

69. Lombardi WJ, Weingartner H. Pharmacological treatment of impaired memory function. In: Baddeley AD, Wilson BA, Watts FN, eds. Handbook of Memory Disorders. West Sussex: Wiley & Sons, 1995:577–601

70. McEntee WJ, Mair RG. Memory enhancement in Korsakoff's psychosis by clonidine: further evidence for a noradrenergic deficit. Annals of Neurology 1980;7: 466–470

71. Mair RG, McEntee WJ. Cognitive enhancement in Korsakoff's psychosis by clonodine: a comparison with L-dopa and ephedrine. Psychopharmacology 1986;88: 374–380

72. O'Carroll RE, Moffoot A, Ebmeier KB, et al. Korsakoff's syndrome, cognition and clonidine. Psychological Medicine 1993;23:341–347

73. Chatterjee A, Morris M, Bowers D, et al. Cholinergic treatment of an amnestic man with a basal forebrain lesion: theoretical implications. Journal of Neurology, Neurosurgery and Psychiatry 1993;56:1282–1289

74. Peters B, Levin H. Memory enhancement after physostigmine treatment in the amnesic syndrome. Archives of Neurology 1977;34:215–219

75. Goldberg E, Gerstman L, Mattis S, et al. Effects of cholinergic treatment on post-traumatic anterograde amnesia. Archives of Neurology 1982;39:581

76. Perry ED, Tomlinson BE, Blessed G, et al. Correlation of cholinergic abnormalities with senile plaques and mental test scores in senile dementia. British Medical Journal 1978;2:1457–1459

77. Coyle JT, Price DL, DeLong MR. Alzheimer's disease: a disorder of cholinergic innervation. Science 1983;219: 1184–1190

78. Whitehouse P, Price D, Strubble R. Alzheimer's disease and senile dementia: loss of neurons in the basal forebrain. Science 1982;215:1237–1239

79. Frautschy S. Alzheimer disease: current research and future therapy. Primary Psychiatry 1999;6:46–68

80. Doody R. Clinical profile of donezepil in treatment of Alzheimer's disease. Gerontology 1999;45:23–32

81. Burns A, Murphy D. Protection against Alzheimer's disease? Lancet 1996;348:420–421

82. Henderson VW, Paganini-Hill A, Emanuel CK, et al. Estrogen replacement therapy in older women. Archives of Neurology 1994;51:896–900

83. Robinson D, Friedman L, Marcus R, et al. Estrogen replacement therapy and memory in older women. Journal of the American Geriatric Society 1994;42: 919–922

84. Barrett-Connor E, Silverstein E. Estrogen replacement therapy and memory in older women. Journal of the American Medical Association 1993;269:2637–2641

85. Oken BS, Storzbach DM, Kaye JA. The efficacy of Ginkgo biloba on cognitive functions in Alzheimer's disease. Archives of Neurology 1998;55:1409–1415

86. D'Esposito M, Alexander M. The clinical profiles, recovery, and rehabilitation of memory disorders. NeuroRehabilitation 1995;5:141–159

267 Executive Disorders

Michael P Alexander and Donald T Stuss

Executive disorders are impairments of implementation, control and modulation of basic cognitive functions such as language, memory, perception, and learned movement. Executive functions are characterized as initiation, intention, planning, sequencing, inhibition, flexibility, monitoring, and various complex aspects of attention. Since the most unambiguous executive impairments are caused by damage to the frontal lobes, "executive dysfunction" and "frontal lobe dysfunction" are often used interchangeably. This usage can cause confusion because executive impairments are also found in patients with no discrete frontal pathology, such as the diffuse axonal injury of trauma, and even in patients with depression, anxiety, sleep deprivation, or chronic pain. It is reasonable to characterize a patient's deficits as executive dysfunction only if it is clearly understood that the label does not necessarily imply a definite frontal lesion.

Anatomy

The frontal lobes comprise approximately 30% of the human cortex. The frontal lobes have substantial functional subdivisions, and executive impairments are not simply due to the size of frontal lesions wherever they may be. Understanding executive impairments requires understanding the functional anatomy of the frontal lobes. Frontal cortex is commonly considered to have six coarse functional regions: posterior (Brodmann's areas 4, 6, 44 and perhaps 8), ventrolateral (VL: areas 45 and 47), dorsolateral (DL: areas 9, 46 and perhaps 8), polar (area 10), orbital (area 11, 12 and 14), superior medial (SM) including supplementary motor (area 6) and anterior cingulate (ACG: area 24), and paracingulate (areas 32 and 25). The posterior region is motor and premotor cortex, and it is the only region not overtly involved in executive function. The frontal regions have different connection profiles with the posterior cortex, the thalamus, and with the limbic structures and different, but parallel, subcortical circuits to the striatum and the cerebellum.[1-4] Damage to cortical or subcortical connections may produce executive impairments more pervasive than suggested by cortical extent of lesion alone.

Pathology

There are a variety of diseases that affect frontal lobes and projections. Infarction is most common. Ischemic cerebral infarctions are usually unilateral and lesion boundaries are sharp, making this the ideal pathology for exploring the effects of focal lesions. Hemorrhages, tumors, and some traumatic contusions are also unilateral. Most traumatic contusions, particularly orbital ones, some multifocal infarctions, particularly after subarachnoid hemorrhage, and herpes simplex encephalitis are bilateral. Hydrocephalus, multiple sclerosis and diffuse axonal injury affect frontal function through bilateral white matter damage. Among degenerative disorders, frontotemporal dementia may be quite focally unilateral or bilateral frontal. Parkinson's disease, Huntington's disease and progressive supranuclear palsy all affect subcortical structures that are intrinsic to frontal functions. Some cerebellar disorders, particularly the degenerative ones, produce executive deficits through disruption of frontal circuits.

Assessment

The neurological examination of patients with frontal injury is often unrevealing.[5] Posterior frontal lesions (cortical or subcortical) may cause contralateral weakness, mild clumsiness or ataxia. Damage to premotor regions can produce a contralateral grasp reflex, resistive rigidity and bradyhypokinesia. Bilateral lesions cause postural abnormalities and even a parkinsonian gait disorder. Orbital damage causes anosmia.

Neuroimaging may be essential because frontal lesions often produce no or only subtle elemental signs. Computed tomography (CT) and magnetic resonance imaging (MRI) define structural lesions. Single photon emission computed tomography (SPECT) or positron emission tomography (PET) may be a valuable probe of regional functional impairments in degenerative diseases without focal atrophy.

It may be difficult to properly define executive deficits in patients with simple clinical tests. Thus, neuropsychological assessment may be required. There is no test that uniquely specifies frontal impairment. Many clinicians have the impression that all so-called frontal tests have high specificity for frontal injury and are generally sensitive to damage in all areas or functional regions of the frontal lobe. Neither impression is correct. All classical frontal lobe tests can be impaired due to even subtle impairments in language, memory, perception, attention, motivation, or effort. However, several tests do have high specificity for frontal impairments when these functions are intact.

Word list generation (verbal fluency) is particularly sensitive to damage throughout the left DL and VL regions and to right or left SM areas and their outflow projections including left dorsal caudate.[6] Complex list learning is sensitive to damage throughout the frontal lobes, but the profiles of impairment are based on different regional functions.[7] Recall and recognition are impaired with left lateral lesions (defective semantic encoding) and with posterior inferior medial lesions (poor episodic memory). Monitoring of performance is impaired after right frontal lesions, producing intrusions and repetitions. All frontal lesions appear to reduce the capacity for organizing a strategy to learn a long list of words, although standard test measures may not capture this. The Wisconsin Card Sorting Test is generally sensitive to frontal damage except to orbital-frontal injury.[8] The Stroop Test is particularly sensitive to SM damage (at least the superior medial area, perhaps the ACG). Many patients with frontal injury are impaired at regulation of attention, and thus demonstrate perseveration, loss of set, and impersistence. Right lateral lesions may produce clinically detectable impairments on sustained attention tasks, but most frontal attentional deficits require specialized probes not commonly utilized in clinical settings. These probes reveal specific patterns of deficit depending upon the frontal region injured. The most illuminating tests of prefrontal impairment demand that the patient generate rules of response and behavior without guidance from the examiner.[9] These are largely restricted to research settings at present. Frontal lesions often impair appreciation and usage of humor, reduce self-awareness, and cause loss of empathy and abnormal social behavior.[10] None of these is yet adequately measured with standard clinical assessment.

Rehabilitation

There are two reasons why there are no Class I randomized controlled trials of executive rehabilitation. First, it has been difficult to establish an operational definition of exactly which "executive disorders" are to be treated. Second, most treatments developed in clinical settings are aimed at the disability level of rehabilitation, not a specified executive impairment. Until the processes are discretely defined, specific rehabilitation procedures cannot be developed. Three types of treatments have been utilized, often together.

Drugs Methylphenidate and various dopaminergic (DA) agents have been tried on the assumption that some lesions damage ascending monoamine pathways. Patients with low arousal states or with poor attention are treated with stimulants. Patients with poor activation and intention are treated with DA agents. There are case reports of favorable response. Use is empirical.

Cognitive Programs have been developed that attempt to improve executive dysfunction through drills or training of defective functions such as planning, sequencing or problem solving. A few theoretically sound programs have demonstrated some possible efficacy,[11] but in others the treatment goals are vague, the target is disability, and sound guide-

lines for matching treatments to patients are unspecified.

Compensatory Explicitly focusing on a limiting disability or handicap, it is often possible to construct an environmental compensation that allows greater functional independence. These programs make, appropriately, no claims for directly treating executive dysfunction.

Summary

Frontal lobe damage produces impairments in executive functions. These impairments may be invisible to routine examination and even to most neuropsychological tests. Understanding the regional functional subdivisions of the frontal lobes and the relationship of that regional architecture to specific patterns of cognitive impairment will illuminate diagnosis and treatment.

References

1. Alexander GE, DeLong MR, Strick PL. Parallel organization of functionally segregated circuits linking basal ganglia and cortex. Annu Rev Neurosci 1986;9:357–381
2. Cummings JL. Frontal-subcortical circuits and human behavior. Arch Neurol 1993;50:873–880
3. Nauta WJH. The problem of the frontal lobe: a reinterpretation. J Psychiatr Res 1971;8:167–187
4. Petrides M, Pandya DM. Comparative architectonic analysis of the human and macaque frontal cortex. *In:* Boller F, Grafman J, eds. Handbook of Neuropsychology. Amsterdam: Elsevier, 1994:17–57
5. Alexander MP, Stuss DT. Disorders of frontal lobe functioning. Semin Neurol, 2000;20:427–437
6. Stuss DT, Alexander MP, Sayer L, et al. The effects of focal anterior and posterior brain lesions on verbal fluency. J Int Neuropsych Soc 1998;4:265–278
7. Stuss DT, Alexander MP, Palumbo CL, et al. Organizational strategies of patients with unilateral or bilateral frontal lobe injury in word list learning tasks. Neuropsychology 1994;8:355–373
8. Stuss DT, Levine B, Alexander MP, et al. Wisconsin Card Sorting Test performance in patients with focal frontal and posterior brain damage: effects of lesion location and test structure on separable cognitive processes. Neuropsychologia 2000;38:388–402
9. Levine B, Stuss DT, Milberg WP, et al. The effects of focal and diffuse brain damage on strategy application: evidence from focal lesions, traumatic brain injury and normal aging. J Int Neuropsych Soc 1998;4:247–264
10. Stuss DT, Alexander MP. The anatomical basis of affective behavior, emotion and self-awareness: a specific role of the right frontal lobe. *In:* Hatano G, Okada N, Tanabe H. eds. Proceedings of the 13th Toyota Conference of Affective Minds. Amsterdam: Elsevier, 2000:13–25
11. Levine B, Robertson I, Clare L, et al. Rehabilitation of executive functioning: an experimental-clinical validation of Goal Management Training. J Int Neuropsych Soc 2000;6:299–312

268 Alzheimer Disease and Mild Cognitive Impairment

Ronald C Petersen

Overview

As longevity increases, diseases of aging become more prominent. Disorders of cognition are particularly important as the number of elderly in our society increases, and dementia is a primary concern for many elderly persons. Among the dementias, Alzheimer disease (AD) is the most common cause of dementia of aging. Although AD is not an inevitable consequence of aging, its frequency increases dramatically as people enter into their 70s and beyond.

In 1990, it was estimated that approximately 4 million persons in the United States had AD, and this number has been projected to increase to 14 million by 2050.[1] In recent years, considerable attention has been paid to the milder forms of cognitive impairment that may precede the clinical diagnosis of probable AD, such as mild cognitive impairment (MCI).[2] This chapter discusses AD and MCI, and other forms of dementia are discussed elsewhere in the book.

In a person in whom AD ultimately develops, there presumably is a gradual progression of the pathological process that begins with normal aging and evolves to clinically probable AD and ultimately to neuropathologically proven AD.[3] As shown in Figure 268.1, these individuals likely pass through a transitional stage between normal aging and clinically probable AD. This phase of MCI has been documented in persons who typically have a memory impairment but are functionally impaired only

mildly. These persons do not meet the criteria for clinically probable AD yet are worthy of identification and monitoring.

In 2001, the American Academy of Neurology published three practice parameter papers that resulted from evidence-based medicine analyses of the extant literature on dementia.[4–6] The first paper considered MCI and reviewed the literature.[4] The second considered diagnostic issues concerning AD and other dementias,[5] and the third paper reviewed treatment recommendations for AD and other dementias.[6] These documents provide current assessments of diagnostic and management issues regarding AD.

Normal aging

Implicit in a discussion of AD and MCI is knowledge about cognitive changes in normal aging. Although considerable research has characterized cognitive changes with aging, there is no agreement on the nature or degree of impairment or the pathophysiological substrate for that clinical picture. Consequently, lack of precise knowledge of cognitive changes in normal aging makes the characterization of very early changes of MCI difficult.[7] Normative data have been published on various neuropsychological tests for persons up to 100 years old, but these data have been criticized.[8,9] In particular, some investigators have argued that normative data are contaminated by the inclusion of persons with incipient cognitive impairment, and consequently, the norms incorporate more of an impairment than would be the case had these subjects not been included.[8] These investigators argue for the elimination of these people from the norms, but this can be difficult on a practical basis.

As research on normal aging progresses, we will learn more about precise cognitive changes and this will allow a more precise evaluation of very early changes of incipient pathological processes. Currently, clinical judgment provides the best means of assessing early changes in MCI.

Dementia

Dementia refers to a change in cognitive function that is of sufficient severity to compromise a person's daily function. Although the specific definition of dementia can vary depending on a given subtype, features such as those listed in the *Diagnostic and Statistical Manual of Mental Disorders* (Third Edition-Revised) (DSM-III-R) are useful.[10] In general, they indicate that a person has a memory impairment

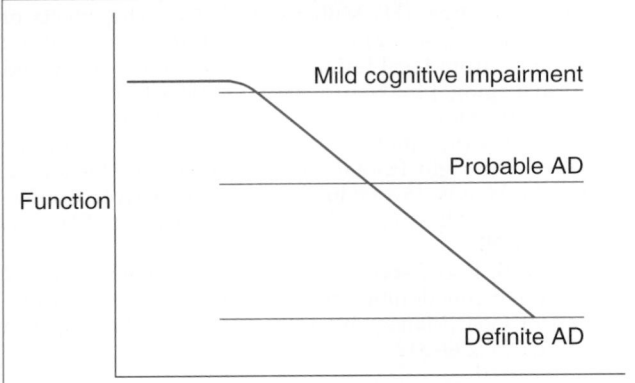

Figure 268.1 Theoretical progression of cognitive function from normal through mild cognitive impairment to probable and definite Alzheimer disease (AD) in persons who develop AD. (From Petersen.[2] By permission of Elsevier Science.)

beyond what would be expected for aging and at least one other cognitive domain such as attention, language, visuospatial skills, or problem solving is involved. These deficits are of sufficient severity to compromise a person's functional activities. The other primary feature requires that the cognitive deficit cannot be present in the setting of an altered sensorium such as in delirium or an acute confusional state. Once this type of cognitive impairment has been determined, the clinician must then decipher the underlying nature of the dementia. One problem with the DSM-III-R definition is that memory impairment is an essential feature. Whereas this is common in most dementias, it is conceivable that dementias other than AD, such as a frontotemporal dementia or Lewy body dementia, may present with a nonmemory cognitive domain being impaired early in the disorder. Nevertheless, the DSM-III-R criteria are generally useful.

If an elderly person presents with a gradually progressive amnestic disorder that has advanced to involve other nonmemory cognitive domains and these changes have affected daily functioning, AD is the most likely diagnosis. If the initial presentation is a change in comportment, personality, or behavior rather than memory, a frontotemporal dementia may be a reasonable alternative diagnosis. If the person has some features of parkinsonism, hallucinations, and wide fluctuations in behavior, dementia with Lewy bodies may be more likely than AD. Vascular dementia can involve abrupt changes in function because of large-vessel or embolic disease or it can present insidiously if subcortical ischemia is responsible for the changes in function. A prominent anomia with other features of language impairment can signal a primary progressive aphasia. If the time course of the dementia is relatively rapid over months and the clinical features include psychiatric symptoms and motor function abnormalities, a prion disorder such as Creutzfeldt-Jakob disease should be considered. These issues are discussed more completely elsewhere in this book.

Alzheimer disease

AD is the most common dementia in many countries throughout the world. It is slowly progressive, with a prominent memory disorder appearing early in the clinical presentation.[11] As the disease progresses, other cognitive domains become involved and behavioral alterations ensue.[12–15] AD is a degenerative disorder, and the definitive diagnosis can be made only at postmortem examination of the brain. The classic neuropathological features are neuritic plaques and neurofibrillary tangles.[16]

Epidemiology

AD is an age-related phenomenon. The incidence increases dramatically with increasing age and doubles every 5 years after age 65.[17] The prevalence of AD also increases dramatically with age and becomes quite common in the 70s and more so into the 80s. It is uncertain whether the actual incidence of AD con-

tinues to increase into the 90s, but clearly, the incidence of *dementia* increases rapidly in that age range. The prevalence of AD also doubles every 5 years, and the prevalence of AD is greater among women than men and likely reflects the greater longevity of women.[18–24]

Clinical diagnosis

The most commonly used criteria for the clinical diagnosis of AD include those in the *Diagnostic and Statistical Manual of Mental Disorders*, Fourth Edition (DSM-IV)[25] or the criteria of the National Institute of Neurologic, Communicative Disorders, and Stroke/Alzheimer's Disease and Related Disorders Association (NINCDS-ADRDA) work group.[26] The DSM-IV criteria are outlined in Table 268.1. The criteria for dementia of the Alzheimer type involve the development of multiple cognitive deficits with a memory impairment (inability to learn new information or to recall previously learned information) and one or more other cognitive domains, including aphasia (language disturbance), apraxia (inability to carry out a learned motor act), agnosia (difficulty recognizing objects), or disturbance in executive functioning (planning, organizing, sequencing, and abstracting). These cognitive impairments are sufficiently severe to impair one's functional abilities, and the onset and progression of the disorder needs to be gradual. These deficits cannot be accounted for by other neurological or psychiatric disturbances. The American Academy of Neurology practice parameter paper evaluated these criteria and determined that they were reliable.[5]

The history is an essential element in establishing the diagnosis of dementia. It is important to take the history not only from the patient but also from someone who knows the patient quite well. Several instruments can be used to obtain historical information, or an astute clinician can inquire about typical activities of daily living and any temporal changes in

Table 268.1 Diagnostic criteria for dementia of the Alzheimer type

Memory impairment
    Learning or recall
One or more
    Aphasia
    Apraxia
    Agnosia
    Executive dysfunction (planning, organizing,
        sequencing, abstracting)
Cognitive deficits of sufficient severity to affect social or
    occupational functioning and representing a change
    from previous level
Clinical course is gradual onset and progressive decline
Not due to delirium
No other central nervous system explanation,
    e.g., cerebrovascular disease, Parkinson disease

Modified from American Psychiatric Association.[25] By permission of the American Psychiatric Association.

Table 268.2	Dementia evaluation

History
Neurological examination
Medical examination
Neuroimaging study
Laboratory studies
Neuropsychological testing

the patient's ability to carry out these activities. The data available in the literature are not sufficient to establish the superiority of any of these instruments.

In addition to the history, a cognitive assessment with an instrument designed for assessing mental function can be quite useful. Instruments designed for this purpose include the Mini-Mental State Examination (MMSE),[27] the modified Mini-Mental State (3MS),[28] the Blessed Orientation Memory Concentration Test,[29] the Kokmen Short Test of Mental Status,[30] and the Clinical Dementia Rating scale (CDR).[31] These can be useful, but none is superior to the others. The components of a dementia evaluation are listed in Table 268.2.

General neurological examination

A person being evaluated for dementia should also have a general neurological examination. Typically in early AD, the examination findings are normal except for the mental status evaluation. However, in the course of the examination, features suggesting other contributing factors to the dementia can be elucidated. For example, if the person has increased tone, decreased rapid alternating motions, or bradykinesia, a Lewy body component can be suspected. If the person has asymmetric reflexes or a visual field defect or other lateralizing signs, a vascular component may be suspected. Similarly, other neurological features such as a peripheral neuropathy may suggest a toxic or metabolic problem. It is important to assess sensory function because sensory deprivation can affect the mental status and neurological examination. Finally, the neurological examination should be complemented by a general medical examination to search for other systemic contributions to the cognitive impairment.

Laboratory tests

The usefulness of various laboratory tests in evaluating a patient with dementia was assessed by the American Academy of Neurology practice parameter paper,[5] which concluded that vitamin B_{12} levels and thyroid function should be assessed because vitamin B_{12} deficiencies and thyroid diseases are common comorbidities that appear in the elderly. They can influence cognitive function, and although the treatment of these disorders may not completely reverse the dementia, their recognition and assessment are important.

It has been common practice, however, to perform various tests to determine if there are other contributing factors. Tests suggested for a dementia evaluation

Table 268.3	Laboratory evaluation of patients with dementia
Routine	**Optional**
Chemistry group	Erythrocyte sedimentation rate
Complete blood count	Chest radiography
Vitamin B_{12} level*	Electrocardiography
Thyroid function studies*	Urinalysis
Syphilis serology	Drug levels
CT/MRI*	HIV testing
	Lyme serology
	24-Hour urine for heavy metals
	Electroencephalography
	Cerebrospinal fluid analysis
	PET/SPECT

CT, computed tomography; HIV, human immunodeficiency virus; MRI, magnetic resonance imaging; PET, positron emission tomography; SPECT, single photon emission computed tomography.
*Suggested by the American Academy of Neurology.[5]

are listed in Table 268.3. However, it should be emphasized that a few of these have been demonstrated to actually have an effect on treating the dementia; nevertheless, because other medical conditions can present with alterations in cognitive function, these tests should be considered in the appropriate clinical setting.

Neuroimaging

Neuroimaging techniques such as computed tomography (CT) or magnetic resonance imaging (MRI) can be useful in excluding reversible and treatable causes of dementia, such as subdural hematoma, neoplasm, or infarction. The American Academy of Neurology practice parameter paper[5] recommended that a neuroimaging examination, either CT or MRI, be done in most circumstances at the time of the initial dementia assessment to consider these issues.

Recently, considerable research has been conducted on quantitative structural neuroimaging in aging and dementia.[32,33] In particular, atrophy of medial temporal lobe structures (e.g., the hippocampus) has been found in patients with AD.[32] However, this atrophy may be nonspecific, and although it is consistent with AD, it may occur in other conditions. Recent data on longitudinal volumetric measurements of the hippocampal formation have also indicated that the rate of progression of atrophy of persons with AD exceeds that of normal controls.[33] Investigations assessing the usefulness of volumetric measurements of the entorhinal cortex have been controversial.[34,35] Some investigators think that volumetric measurements of the entorhinal cortex are superior in assessing early changes in the AD process, whereas others argue that volumetric measurements of the hippocampus and entorhinal cortex are equally efficacious.[35] Nevertheless, a structural imaging test of the brain should be done early in the assessment of persons with suspected AD.

Functional neuroimaging has also been used in

assessing patients with AD. Single photon emission computed tomography (SPECT) and positron emission tomography (PET) have been evaluated for their usefulness in diagnosing AD. Although several SPECT studies have suggested the value of functional imaging in augmenting clinical acumen,[36–40] the added discriminability has not been demonstrated. Similarly, PET scanning has shown promise in its ability to distinguish among dementias,[41] and there is evidence that FDG-PET may be useful in assessing persons at risk for the development of AD, but the longitudinal outcome of these persons is not known.[42]

Functional imaging tests may be particularly useful in the differential diagnosis of dementia. Specifically, the ability of SPECT and PET to differentiate frontotemporal dementia from AD can be useful. In frontotemporal dementia, the frontal lobes show predominant hypoperfusion and hypometabolism, with relative sparing of posterior structures.[43–46]

Despite the potential of functional imaging tests, the American Academy of Neurology practice parameter paper[5] does not recommend that either SPECT or PET be used routinely in the initial or differential diagnosis of dementias.

Neuropsychological testing

Neuropsychological testing can be particularly useful in evaluating cognitive function in suspected dementia. Neuropsychological testing can help determine whether the person is experiencing cognitive changes of normal aging or the earliest signs of AD or possibly MCI. The particular profile of cognitive function can also be useful in differential diagnosis. For example, in a typical case of early AD, the subject will likely have difficulties in delayed verbal recall, learning, and perhaps naming. However, a subject with a frontotemporal dementia may have profound difficulties with executive function, sustained attention, and speed of processing, with relative preservation of naming and memory. Alternatively, a subject with depression may have a relatively flat learning curve in trying to learn a list of words over multiple trials but will be able to retain the amount learned after a delay. Although not diagnostic, the various clinical profiles can be helpful in distinguishing among various dementias. Neuropsychological testing can also be useful in providing a baseline for a person who may be reevaluated in the future. Consequently, depending on the clinical situation, neuropsychological testing can be an important adjunct.

Lumbar puncture

Several retrospective studies have found little evidence to recommend the routine use of a lumbar puncture in the evaluation of dementia.[47] However, in certain clinical circumstances in which the dementia is characterized by a subacute change in mental status, fever, nuchal rigidity, or systemic cancer or collagen vascular disease, the clinician may suspect an alternative contributing process. In an immunocompromised host, syphilis and fungal infections also need to be considered. Circumstances under which lumbar

Table 268.4 Indications for cerebrospinal fluid analysis in evaluation of dementia*
Rapidly progressive course
Unusual clinical presentation
Age younger than 60 years
Cancer
Central nervous system infection
Systemic infection
Reactive syphilis serology
Immunosuppression
Central nervous system vasculitis
Connective tissue diseases
*If lumbar puncture is not contraindicated.

puncture could be considered are listed in Table 268.4. As always, one has to be certain there are no contraindications to performing the examination.

Genetic testing

Genetic testing can be considered in young-onset, suspected familial AD. In persons in their 30s, 40s, or 50s who have a strong family history suggestive of an autosomal dominant disease, mutations on chromosome 1, 14, or 21 can be considered.[48] Genetic testing should be undertaken only in the setting of appropriate genetic counseling because the implications of the testing can have a substantial effect on the patient and family members. The type of genetic counseling should be similar to that recommended for Huntington disease.

In the more typical variety of late-onset AD, genetic testing for specific mutations is not useful. However, susceptibility polymorphisms for AD have been evaluated. The most popular polymorphism concerns the lipid-carrying protein apolipoprotein E (apo E).[49,50] A large neuropathologically based study of apo E4 showed an increased specificity of the AD diagnosis.[51] According to this study, 90% of the patients positive for $APOE \in 4$ had AD neuropathologically and suggested that apo E testing can increase diagnostic accuracy for AD by about 4%, and if $APOE \in 4$ is absent, it can increase the likelihood of something other than AD. These percentages augmented the clinician's diagnostic accuracy. However, current recommendations are that apo E testing not be performed routinely in asymptomatic persons.[50,52] That is, apo E testing is not recommended for persons who think they may be at risk because of a positive family history. Currently, the American Academy of Neurology does not recommend any other genetic markers for AD.[5]

Biomarkers

Considerable research has been conducted recently on cerebrospinal fluid (CSF) biomarkers for AD. Several studies have shown that CSF levels of β-amyloid 1–42 are reduced relative to those of normal control subjects,[53–56] but it is unclear whether these levels are useful in the early diagnosis. Similarly, CSF tau levels have been shown to be increased in AD patients relative to the levels in controls.[57–60] However, no study has compared CSF β-amyloid or tau levels with a clinical diagnosis. The combination of CSF β-amyloid 1–42 and tau may be useful, and studies have indicated the sensitivity and specificity are 85% and 87%, respectively.[54–56] However, it is not known if these biomarkers augment the diagnostic accuracy of the clinician. Another CSF marker, AD 7CNTP, has shown high sensitivity and specificity, but the patient populations in the studies have not been delineated carefully, and the usefulness of this marker is unknown.[61–63]

In summary, the American Academy of Neurology states that no biomarker has emerged as being appropriate for routine use in the clinical evaluation of suspected AD. Currently, quantitative neuroimaging, genotyping, and biomarkers have not achieved sufficient stature to replace or substantially augment the ability of the clinician to use the standard DSM IV or NINCDS-ADRDA criteria to diagnose AD.

Pathophysiology

Most investigators believe that AD is due entirely or partly to abnormal processing or deposition of amyloid. The pathogenic form of amyloid is the β-amyloid 1–42 fragment of the larger amyloid precursor protein (APP) and is generated by abnormal cleavage of APP. Typically, APP is cleaved by the protease α-secretase (Figure 268.2). However, when APP is cleaved by β- and γ-secretases, β-amyloid 1–42 is formed and deposited in the brain as an insoluble aggregate. This deposition presumably initiates a cascade of events resulting in inflammatory responses and cell destruction. This may not be the only pathological process, but it is believed to be an important component of the degenerative cascade. As discussed below, newer treatment strategies focus on intervening in the amyloid cascade.

The other primary pathological feature of AD is the abnormal processing of tau and the formation of neurofibrillary tangles. Great strides are being made in understanding the role of neurofibrillary tangles in the pathogenesis of AD. The recent development of animal models harboring both β-amyloid deposition and neurofibrillary tangles has generated excitement about a closer simulation of the actual pathological elements involved in human AD.

Mild cognitive impairment

Conceptual framework

Many clinicians are faced with the dilemma of determining the importance of the symptom of forgetfulness. It is not uncommon to encounter elderly subjects who believe that their memory has changed from a previous level of functioning and are concerned about the development of AD. MCI refers to the clinical state in which a subject is typically memory-impaired but not demented.[64]

The American Academy of Neurology has endorsed the concept of MCI recently in a practice parameter paper that stated that clinicians should

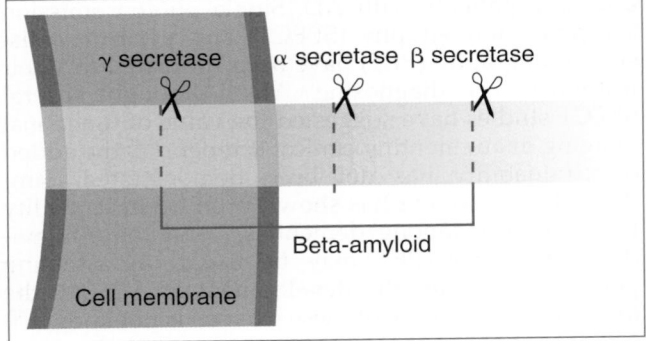

Figure 268.2   Cleavage of the β-amyloid 1–42 fragment of the larger amyloid precursor protein by normal α and abnormal β and γ secretases.

evaluate persons who have suspected memory impairment, and, if they meet the criteria for MCI, they should be counseled and followed closely because of the increased risk of progressing to clinically probable AD.[4] Ultimately, the clinician would like to intervene with an effective treatment, but no treatment is known to slow the progressive development of the symptoms of clinically probable AD. However, several international drug trials are being conducted for MCI and one or more may have positive results. Candidate treatments include cholinesterase inhibitors, antioxidants, anti-inflammatory agents, and nootropics.[65]

Clinical criteria

Although no criteria have been accepted for the diagnosis of MCI, most investigators have used a variation of those presented in Table 268.5. The drug trials mentioned above are using a variation of these criteria, and longitudinal clinical studies have indicated that when subjects are classified with the *amnestic* form of MCI, they have an accelerated rate of progression to clinically probable AD.[66] It should be emphasized that the criteria for MCI are *clinical*. That is, although neuropsychological testing can be helpful in differentiating these subjects from those experiencing normal aging, MCI is not a neuropsychological diagnosis. A recent study from France demonstrated the unreliability of the retrospective application of a form of MCI criteria using neuropsychological tests.[67] According to this study, if arbitrary neuropsychological cutoffs are applied in the absence of clinical judgment, the concept loses its predictive ability. However, when neuropsychological data are used in

Table 268.5   Clinical criteria for diagnosis of mild cognitive impairment

Memory complaint—preferably corroborated by an informant
Memory impairment for age and education
Essentially normal general cognitive function
Activities of daily living largely preserved
Not demented

conjunction with the criteria given in Table 268.5, the diagnosis can be quite reliable and predictive of eventual progression.[68]

The first criterion is a memory complaint (Table 268.5). Typically, the symptoms are mild and the subjects are aware of their deficit, and when this is corroborated by an informant, it can be particularly useful.[69] The second criterion refers to an objective memory impairment. That is, when these subjects are evaluated by a clinician and neuropsychologist, they have significant memory impairment usually defined by difficulties with learning and delayed recall relative to their age- and education-mates.[70,71] As mentioned above, no particular reference point for normal aging is entirely accurate, but normative data on subjects with similar demographic characteristics seem to be most useful. When these subjects are described clinically, they tend to fall 1.5 standard deviations below their age- and education-matched mates on measures of learning and recall. However, it must be emphasized that these are only *guidelines* and not cutoff scores for assisting in the diagnosis of MCI. Some subjects may fall within the normal range of memory function for their age mates, but if the clinician suspects that this represents a decline from the person's previous level of function, it may be adequate to support the diagnosis of MCI.

The third criterion refers to relatively normal general cognition. This implies that other cognitive domains such as language, executive function, attention, visuospatial skills, and problem solving are *relatively* preserved. Although close inspection of these subjects reveals that they have subtle deficits in some other cognitive domains, the deficits are not severe enough to suggest that the person is demented.[68] Because the criteria for dementia and AD described above require significant impairments in other nonmemory cognitive domains, these subjects do not meet the definition. This, of course, is a clinical judgment. Also with respect to the preservation of activities of daily living, most subjects do well; however, they may experience minor inefficiencies because of their memory deficits, so technically their activities of daily living are slightly impaired. The clinician, however, does not feel that this degree of impairment is sufficient to constitute dementia.

The last criterion is perhaps the most important. The clinician who evaluates these patients does not think that they meet the criteria for dementia or clinically probable AD. In essence, these subjects are functioning independently in the community and carrying out their routine daily activities. Because most clinicians believe that it would be a disservice to label these patients with the diagnosis of AD at this very mild stage of impairment, the concept of MCI has been developed to characterize them.

Evaluation

The clinical evaluation for persons with suspected MCI is virtually identical to that described above for clinically probable AD.[72] The history is particularly important, and the clinician should also perform a mental status examination and a general neurological examination. The performance on the mental status exam will likely appear normal. Most of the commonly used instruments, for example, MMSE, 3MS, and the Kokmen Short Test of Mental Status,[27,28,30] are relatively insensitive in this range of cognitive function. Consequently, persons with MCI typically score in the 26 to 28 point range on the MMSE (maximum = 30), which typically is in the normal range. However, these subjects have primarily a relatively isolated memory impairment, and if the mental status exam instrument does not have a significant memory component, it will not differentiate these subjects from those who are aging normally. Consequently, the clinician must be particularly attentive to memory function and perhaps augment the clinical examination with a memory test.[73,74]

The laboratory tests are similar to those described above for clinically probable AD (Table 268.3). Special attention should be paid to subtle medical issues that could affect only memory function. For example, in the appropriate clinical setting, Lyme disease serological testing may be useful because a memory impairment could be the only central nervous system manifestation of Lyme disease. Subtle thyroid or medication issues should also be considered.

Often, depression can be differentiated from clinically probable AD, but in its early stages, it could present with a subtle memory impairment. Consequently, the clinician should be attuned to the possibility of a psychiatric explanation of a subtle memory impairment.

Neuroimaging

Recently, several volumetric assessments of the medial temporal lobe with MRI have been informative.[32–35,75] As mentioned above, there is discussion about the relative utility of volumetric measurements of the hippocampal formation versus the entorhinal cortex.[34,35] Measurements of progressive whole brain atrophy are likely to be useful in assessing MCI also, although they may not manifest change until the degenerative condition has progressed to mild AD. Whether whole-brain volume changes will be important in assessing the early stages of AD remains to be determined, but they may be.[76]

Functional imaging measures, including magnetic resonance spectroscopy, SPECT, and PET, also hold promise but their value has not been demonstrated in this population.[77] Nevertheless, in selected instances, particularly if the structural imaging scan is normal, functional imaging modalities may provide additional useful information.[78]

Neuropsychological testing

Neuropsychological testing can be quite useful in differentiating persons with MCI from those with normal aging. The neuropsychological battery must involve sufficiently difficult learning and recall tasks to be able to tease apart the subtle deficits. As emphasized above, the neuropsychological test

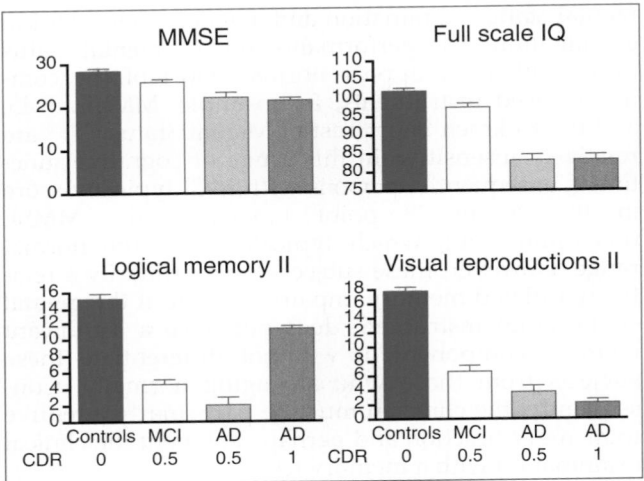

Figure 268.3   Comparison of cognitive profile of controls and persons with mild cognitive impairment (MCI), very mild clinically probable AD (CDR 0.5), or mild clinically probable AD (CDR 1). *Top*, Mini-Mental State Exam (MMSE) and Full Scale IQ represent measures of general intellectual function. *Bottom*, Memory function for verbal memory (Logical Memory II) and nonverbal memory (Visual Reproductions II). AD, Alzheimer disease; CDR, Clinical Dementia Rating scale. (From Petersen et al.[68] By permission of the American Medical Association.)

profile will not make the diagnosis of MCI, but it can be suggestive in the appropriate clinical context.[79] A typical neurocognitive profile of subjects with MCI is shown in Figure 268.3 and compared with that of appropriate control subjects and persons with very mild clinically probable AD (CDR 0.5). As seen in Figure 268.3, persons with MCI appear to be functioning more like normal elderly subjects in measures of general cognitive function (the MMSE and full scale IQ), whereas their memory function appears more similar to that of persons with very mild AD (delayed verbal recall [Logical Memory II] and nonverbal delayed recall [Visual Reproductions II]).[68]

Biomarkers

As with clinically probable AD, biomarkers for MCI are in the early stages of development; however, considerable work is in progress and the results are pending. There are some indications that the CSF measures of β-amyloid and tau may be useful in distinguishing between persons with MCI and those with normal aging.[54,58,80] These markers also may be useful for predicting progression, but the data are preliminary.[81] Currently, the data are insufficient to recommend measuring CSF levels of β-amyloid and tau in diagnosing MCI.

Genetics

The genetic features of MCI are similar to those of clinically probable AD. There appears to be a higher representation of *APOE* ∈ 4 carriers in MCI, and some studies indicate that the presence of an E4 allele may predict progression.[82,83] However, these data are only

mildly positive, and currently use of apo E is not recommended as either a diagnostic tool for MCI or an indicator of progression.

Heterogeneity of mild cognitive impairment

The issue of the heterogeneity of the concept of MCI has been recognized recently.[66] Thus far, the first or *amnestic* form of MCI has been discussed because it is the most common presentation of MCI and likely represents the preclinical features of probable AD. It is characterized by a prominent memory impairment in the setting of relatively preserved general cognitive function. However, other types of mild impairment of cognition may progress to AD. Other possible outcomes for intermediate stages of cognitive impairment are shown in Figure 268.4. A second form of MCI is a condition characterized by mild impairment of multiple cognitive domains,[66] that is, a mild impairment in memory and perhaps executive function. This could also be the incipient form of clinically probable AD; however, if sufficiently mild, it could also represent a variation of normal aging. In addition, vascular dementia could present with mild impairment in multiple cognitive domains without accentuating memory dysfunction.

A third form of MCI is referred to as single nonmemory domain MCI. As the name implies, other nonmemory cognitive domains may be impaired out of proportion to general cognition. For example, if a person presents with a prominent deficit in executive function, it may be the earliest stage of a frontotemporal dementia. A subject could present with prominent visuospatial deficits and some cognitive slowing, which may represent the early form of Lewy body dementia. Other presentations of forms of non-AD cognitive impairment are given in Figure 268.4. Although this is currently hypothetical, it is important for clinicians to recognize that eventually multiple incipient forms of cognitive impairment may be identified.

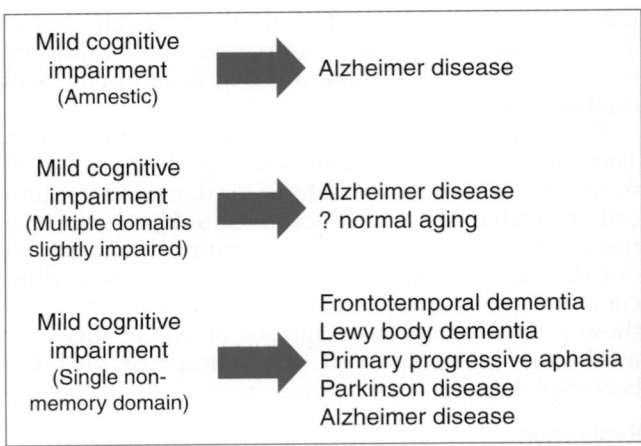

Figure 268.4   Theoretical heterogeneity of the clinical diagnosis of mild cognitive impairment with the suspected outcome. (From Petersen et al.[66] By permission of the American Medical Association.)

Summary

MCI is an important clinical entity to recognize. The field of AD research is moving toward early identification of clinical impairments. The concept of MCI has moved diagnosis back to include more subtle changes of cognitive impairment. In all likelihood, most persons with the amnestic form of MCI will ultimately have probable AD. However, at this point in their clinical progression, they appear to be functioning more normally than not and it would be a disservice to label them with the diagnosis of dementia or AD. Clinical research is progressing at a rapid rate in characterizing the clinical features of these subjects and documenting their outcome.

Treatment

Alzheimer disease

Symptomatic treatment Currently, four drugs have been approved by the United States Food and Drug Administration (FDA) for the treatment of clinically probable AD. All of them are cholinesterase inhibitors. The rationale for their use is from research indicating that patients with AD have a cholinergic deficit.[84] Acetylcholine is involved in many aspects of cognition, including memory and attention. Cholinergic neurons with cell bodies in the basal forebrain project to many regions of the neocortex and to the medial temporal lobe, including the hippocampus. It has been observed for many years that anticholinergic drugs such as scopolamine can produce a learning and recall deficit in normal subjects reminiscent of the cognitive changes in AD.[85] Furthermore, the level of the synthetic enzyme for acetylcholine, choline acetyltransferase, has been found to be decreased in the brains of persons with AD.[86,87] On the basis of these findings, a long-standing effort has been made to augment cholinergic functioning in the brains of patients with AD. In the past decade, acetylcholinesterase inhibitors have been shown to be effective in modulating the symptoms of AD.

The four FDA-approved drugs for AD have similar clinical profiles (Table 268.6). The first compound approved was tacrine (Cognex). However, it had several features that made its use difficult. It required dosing four times daily, and it caused liver toxicity, which necessitated regular monitoring of liver function. Newer drugs without these limiting features have been introduced, and tacrine is rarely used to treat AD.

Donepezil (Aricept), the next acetylcholinesterase inhibitor approved by the FDA, became available in the mid-1990s. It can be administered as a single dose daily and does not require any laboratory monitoring. It is heavily bound to plasma proteins and has a plasma half-life of approximately 70 hours. The typical starting dose is 5 mg daily, and if this is well tolerated, the dose can be increased, after 4 to 6 weeks, to 10 mg daily. The most common side effects include an increase in bowel frequency and nausea and vomiting. Theoretically, cholinesterase inhibitors can influence cardiac rhythm but this is not commonly encountered unless the patient has an underlying disturbance in cardiac conduction. Cholinesterase inhibitors may also have an effect on respiratory conditions such as chronic obstructive pulmonary disease and asthma. Occasionally, patients experience vivid dreaming, and theoretically cholinesterase inhibitors can interfere with the administration of anesthesia. The absorption of donepezil is not influenced by food intake.

Most studies on the efficacy of donepezil have shown a modest improvement in cognitive function as measured by scales such as the Alzheimer's

Table 268.6 Pharmacological treatment of Alzheimer disease

Drug	Mechanism	Dose		Titration interval	Side effects
		Initial	Target		
Symptomatic treatment					
Donepezil (Aricept)	AchI	5 mg daily	10 mg daily	4–6 wk	Nausea, vomiting, diarrhea, muscle cramps, anorexia, vivid dreaming
Rivastigmine (Exelon)	AchI	1.5 mg twice daily	6 mg twice daily	2–4 wk	Nausea, vomiting, diarrhea, weight loss, dizziness
Galantamine (Reminyl)	AchI	4 mg twice daily	12 mg twice daily	4 wk	Nausea, vomiting, diarrhea, anorexia, dizziness
Tacrine* (Cognex)	AchI	10 mg 4 times daily	40 mg 4 times daily	4 wk	Liver function testing required, diarrhea, anorexia, nausea, vomiting, myalgia
Disease-modifying treatment					
Vitamin E	Antioxidant	1000 IU daily	1000 IU twice daily	2–4 wk	Liver function, hemorrhage

AchI, acetylcholinesterase inhibitor.
*Seldom used currently.

Disease Assessment Scale–Cognitive Subscale (ADAS-Cog) and the Clinician's Interview-Based Impression of Change (CIBIC Plus).[6] It has been approved for treatment of mild to moderate AD, and the length of the response has been documented up to 52 weeks. It is uncertain if the actual degree of benefit persists longer than this, but the initial studies of 24 weeks have been extended to 52 weeks.

Studies have indicated that when donepezil therapy is discontinued, a patient's performance returns to the same level as in the untreated state, indicating that donepezil probably has a symptomatic effect on the disease but does not affect the underlying pathophysiological process.

Rivastigmine (Exelon), also approved by the FDA, is a pseudo-irreversible cholinesterase inhibitor and dissociates from the enzyme slowly.[88] It is also an inhibitor of butyrylcholinesterase, and this may have implications for its side-effect profile. The dosing of rivastigmine begins at 1.5 mg twice daily and increases in increments of 1.5 mg per dose to a maximum of 6 mg twice daily. Rivastigmine affords greater dosing flexibility, but it may be somewhat more difficult than donepezil for the patients because of the twice-daily dosing schedule. The side-effect profile of rivastigmine is similar to that of donepezil, with a higher incidence of gastrointestinal side effects.[88] To minimize the incidence of side effects, the dosing schedule is recommended to be advanced on a 2- to 4-week basis. The effect size of rivastigmine on ADAS-Cog and CIBIC Plus is approximately the same as for donepezil.[6]

Most recently, galantamine (Reminyl) has been approved by the FDA. This is a reversible inhibitor of acetylcholinesterase, but it also has some nicotinic receptor activity, which may provide an additional benefit over the other acetylcholinesterase inhibitors. The starting dose of galantamine is 4 mg twice daily. This is increased to 8 mg twice daily and, if tolerated, to 12 mg twice daily. The dose escalation should be done on a 4-week basis to minimize side effects. The side-effect profile is similar to that of the other acetylcholinesterase inhibitors, that is, potential gastrointestinal, cardiac, and pulmonary effects. The effect size of galantamine on ADAS-Cog and CIBIC Plus is similar to that of donepezil and rivastigmine. In one study, galantamine was shown to have an effect on activities of daily living and behavior.[89]

In summary, of the four drugs approved by the FDA for the treatment of AD, donepezil, rivastigmine, and galantamine are the most commonly used. In general, their effects on cognition and behavior appear to be equally efficacious, and they have a similar side-effect profile. There are slight differences in dosing schedules, side-effect profiles, and effects, but these are not marked (Table 268.6). The daily cost of these medications is approximately the same. Although their effects are modest, they appear to enhance the cognitive function of patients with AD, and they are the recommended treatment for mild to moderate AD.[6] These medications may also affect noncognitive symptoms, and this may be of substan-

tial value to patients and families. Most of the evidence indicates that these acetylcholinesterase inhibitors have an effect on cognition but not on the underlying nature of the disease. Nevertheless, the quality of life of the patients and the impact on their caregivers appear to be significant. Because so few studies have compared these drugs with one another, there is little to recommend one over the other. The most common side effects are gastrointestinal effects, but they can be minimized with slow titration of the drug when initiating therapy. The American Academy of Neurology's practice parameter paper on treatment of dementia has recommended that cholinesterase inhibitors be considered for mild to moderate AD, although the effect size is moderate.[6]

Disease-modifying treatment Vitamin E—Considerable research has indicated that oxidative damage occurs in the brains of AD patients. Consequently, the use of antioxidants in the treatment of AD has gained popularity. Epidemiological data have suggested that antioxidants may be associated with a lower incidence of AD.[90–94] In a large clinical trial of vitamin E (1000 IU twice daily) and selegiline (10 mg daily) in patients with moderate AD, both agents were effective in delaying the progression from moderate AD to a more severe state.[95] In this study, the progression to one of four end points—death, institutionalization, loss of basic activities of daily living, or progression on the CDR from 2 to 3—indicated that both vitamin E and selegiline were effective in decreasing the rate of progression. However, the results for selegiline were less convincing, and consequently because of its drug interactions and other potential toxicities, vitamin E was thought to be the preferred treatment. There are theoretical concerns about gastrointestinal toxicity and bleeding complications with vitamin E, but it generally is well tolerated. This finding has not been replicated nor has the optimal dose of vitamin E been determined by additional studies. On the basis of this one investigation, the American Academy of Neurology has indicated that vitamin E (1000 IU orally twice daily) can be considered in an attempt to slow the progression of AD.[6] The risk-to-benefit ratio for selegiline was thought to be less favorable.

Under investigation Anti-inflammatory medications—Research on the pathophysiology of AD has indicated that inflammation is involved to some extent in the degenerative process.[96,97] Because inflammation may influence the progression of the disease and, hence, the symptoms, several studies have attempted to determine the possible efficacy of anti-inflammatory medications in treating AD.[98–100] Epidemiological studies have indicated that nonsteroidal anti-inflammatory drugs (NSAIDs) may protect against the development of AD.[101–105] Certain NSAIDs such as indomethacin have been suggested to be beneficial, but the dropout rate in some of these studies has been high because of side effects.[98]

Thus far, the results of studies on treating AD with either glucocorticoids (e.g., prednisone) or NSAIDs have been mainly negative.[100] In a year-long study of patients with mild to moderate AD, no significant difference was found in performance on the ADAS-Cog.[100] In fact, the prednisone-treated group demonstrated a greater behavioral decline than those in the placebo group.

Recently, treatment with cyclooxygenase (COX)-2 inhibitors has been considered because they may be better tolerated than nonsteroidal anti-inflammatory agents.[106,107] However, the benefit of COX-2 inhibitors has not been demonstrated. Consequently few studies on the use of anti-inflammatory agents in the treatment of AD have had positive results.[108] Currently, a large multicenter trial is under way to assess an NSAID and a COX-2 inhibitor in preventing the onset of AD; the results will be forthcoming.

Estrogen replacement therapy—Some epidemiological evidence has indicated that postmenopausal women who receive estrogen replacement therapy may be protected from the development of AD.[109–113] Possibly, estrogen may have a neuroprotective role in delaying the onset of the disease, but the data for the use of estrogen as a treatment for AD are not positive.

A large randomized, double-blind, placebo-controlled trial of estrogen replacement therapy in patients with mild to moderate AD failed to demonstrate any benefit over the course of 12 months.[114] There was no change in the primary outcome measures of the study, and there was concern about deep venous thrombosis as a possible side effect. An additional, smaller 16-week trial also failed to find a beneficial effect for treatment of AD with estrogen.[115] Consequently, no available data suggest that estrogen is useful as a treatment for AD; currently, estrogen is not recommended for this purpose. Longitudinal studies are under way on the possible prophylactic effect of estrogen in decreasing the risk of developing dementia, but the data from these studies are pending.[116]

Amyloid treatments—Because the role of β-amyloid is considered paramount in the development of AD, several research strategies have been developed to alter the deposition of β-amyloid in the brain. Because β-amyloid is a major component of the neuritic plaques seen in AD and fibrillar β-amyloid is toxic to neurons, this potential treatment strategy has received much attention. β-Amyloid is processed by several proteases in various amylogenic and nonamylogenic pathways.[117] The protease α-secretase produces the nonamylogenic fragments and is the preferred pathway. However, the activity of two other proteases, β-secretase and γ-secretase, results in the generation of β-amyloid, and strategies have been developed to inhibit the activities of both these proteases.[118–121] The β-secretase enzyme, called BACE, is one target and γ-secretase is another. Clinical trials are being designed to assess the viability of these approaches, but no data are available.

In 1999, another therapeutic approach involving immunotherapy was advanced. Schenk et al.[122] demonstrated that transgenic mice that overexpressed

Table 268.7   Noncognitive symptoms in Alzheimer disease

Depression
Psychosis (delusions, hallucinations)
Apathy
Agitation
Sleep disorders

a human mutant form of APP had many of the pathological features of AD. When these mice were immunized against β-amyloid at birth, they showed significantly reduced β-amyloid plaque formation later in life. In addition, mice immunized in mid-life showed a reduction in further progression of the disease, with suggestion of regression of the underlying pathological process. Initial human safety trials on the immunization therapy approach have been completed, and a clinical trial was under way but has recently been halted because of side effects. The potential side effects from chronic immunization against β-amyloid in humans is a concern, and these potential effects will be monitored. Also, although β-amyloid is deposited in the brain during AD, it may not be central to the clinical manifestation of symptoms. Still, β-amyloid appears to be an attractive therapeutic target.

Noncognitive symptoms   Although most attention is focused on the cognitive symptoms of AD, noncognitive symptoms can be most bothersome to the patient and family. Relatively little work has been done on the noncognitive symptoms, but this is changing.[123] Noncognitive symptoms such as anxiety, depression, and psychosis can be worrisome and often constitute a major role in management by the physician (Table 268.7). These aspects of the disease are commonly the motivating factor for many telephone calls. These symptoms can also be the source of considerable stress, which may affect the health of both the patient and the caregiver. Consequently, noncognitive symptoms deserve considerable attention on the part of the treating physician.

Frequency of symptoms—The frequency of noncognitive symptoms in AD is elusive and estimates vary from virtually absent to more than 80% (Table 268.8).[124–128] In a study using the Neuropsychiatric Inventory, apathy was the most common noncognitive symptom, followed by agitation, anxiety, irritability, dysphoria, disinhibition, delusions, hallucinations, and euphoria.[127] The co-occurrence of noncognitive symptoms is also common, and the symptoms and symptom complexes tend to fluctuate. Consequently, the treatment strategies need to be reassessed regularly.

Assessment—When the treating physician is faced with a noncognitive symptom in a patient with AD, possible causes of the symptoms other than progres-

Table 268.8 Frequency of behavioral changes in Alzheimer disease

Behavioral change	Frequency, %
Depression	25–50
Disinhibition	20–35
Delusions	15–50
Hallucinations	10–25
Agitation	50–70
Anxiety	30–50
Aggression	25
Sexual disinhibition	5–10

Data from Cummings et al.[131]

sion of the underlying degenerative process should be considered. Intercurrent medical problems may manifest as a behavioral change in persons who may be unable to express their symptoms. Screening medical tests for urinary tract infection, pneumonia, congestive heart failure, and electrolyte abnormality need to be considered. If any of these conditions is present, treatment is imperative and may improve or eliminate the problematic behavior.

Behavioral management—Although the first reaction to treating a behavioral disorder is to prescribe medications, nonpharmacological methods occasionally can be useful, thereby avoiding potential side effects of the medication.[15] Assessment of the environment can be useful, with attention to changes in personnel, family crises, altered surroundings, or combinations of these. Often, simple attention to strategies of distraction, shifting attention, or exercise can ameliorate the behavior.[129]

Pharmacological treatments—When the behavior is sufficiently disruptive to the patient's quality of life or to those around the patient, pharmacological treatment may be necessary. The first step involves an accurate assessment of the underlying condition.[127] Several scales that may help the clinician assess the behavior are the BEHAVE-AD,[128] the Cohen-Mansfield Agitation Inventory (CMAI),[130] and the Neuropsychiatric Inventory (NPI).[131] The NPI is one of the most commonly used instruments in the field. It assesses 10 commonly encountered behaviors: delusions, hallucinations, agitation, dysphoria, anxiety, apathy, irritability, euphoria, disinhibition, and aberrant motor behavior. The frequency and severity of the symptoms are assessed, and a final index is derived for each behavior. The effect on the caregiver is also assessed. An abbreviated version (NPI-Q) is available for rapid clinical assessment in the office setting.[132] The frequency of noncognitive behaviors in AD is listed in Table 268.8.

Depression—Depression or dysphoria is common in AD. Depression can herald the onset of the disorder[133]

or it can develop as the dementia worsens.[127] In most instances, it worsens the symptoms and places a greater stress on the caregiver; thus, treatment of this component of the dementia is worthwhile. Generally, selective serotonin reuptake inhibitors (SSRIs) are preferred treatment for depression in AD; although tricyclic antidepressants may also be effective, their anticholinergic side effects may worsen the underlying dementia (Table 268.9).[134]

Psychosis—Forms of delusions are also common in AD, occasionally with paranoia.[135] Hallucinations can occur in AD, especially if Lewy bodies are present, and misidentification syndromes can occur, particularly if the right hemisphere is predominantly involved. The presence of psychosis can also indicate a more rapid decline in function.[14,136]

Atypical antipsychotic medications generally are preferred in the treatment of psychosis in AD because of a better side-effect profile. Risperidone has been shown to improve symptoms of psychosis and aggression but also to produce somnolence and extrapyramidal symptoms.[137] Studies of quetiapine have shown that it can reduce psychotic symptoms with relatively few side effects;[138] olanzapine has also been shown to be effective.[139] Atypical antipsychotic agents can be very expensive; however, they generally are preferable to typical antipsychotic agents such as haloperidol (Table 268.9).

Apathy—Apathy is among the most common noncognitive symptoms in AD.[123,127] Although it is not bothersome to the caregiver, it causes a decline in the quality of life for both the patient and caregiver. Pharmacological treatment for apathy is not well developed, but cholinesterase inhibitors (donepezil, rivastigmine, or galantamine) can be considered. Other medications include methylphenidate; dopaminergic agents such as bromocriptine, pramipexole, or ropinerole; or activating antidepressants such as fluoxetine.[140] However, the basis for their use is mainly theoretical, and their benefits have not been well documented.

Agitation—Agitation can be quite common in AD and bothersome to the caregivers because the patient appears to be in considerable distress.[141] This symptom may correlate with a decline in executive function. Initiating treatment with trazodone can be considered because it has a better side-effect profile than haloperidol.[142] Other antipsychotic agents, risperidone, olanzapine, and quetiapine, can be considered in conjunction with anticonvulsants such as carbamazepine and valproic acid.[143,144]

Summary—Noncognitive symptoms of AD are being studied more intensely. Treatment of these symptoms behaviorally and pharmacologically can have a substantial effect on the qualities of the lives of the patient and caregivers.

Table 268.9 Pharmacological treatment recommendations for noncognitive symptoms in dementia

Class	Agent	Usual mean daily dose (range), mg
Delusions	Risperidone (Risperdal)	1 (0.05–2)
	Olanzapine (Zyprexa)	5 (5–10)
	Quetiapine (Seroquel)	400 (50–400)
	Haloperidol (Haldol)	1 (0.5–3)
Agitation/aggression	Risperidone (Risperdal)	1 (0.05–2)
	Olanzapine (Zyprexa)	5 (5–10)
	Quetiapine (Seroquel)	400 (50–400)
	Haloperidol (Haldol)	1 (0.5–3)
	Trazodone (Desyrel)	100 (100–400)
	Buspirone (BuSpar)	15 (15–30)
	Propranolol (Inderal)	120 (80–240)
	Carbamazepine (Tegretol)	400 (200–1200)
	Divalproex (Depakote)	500 (250–2000)
	Lorazepam (Ativan)	1 (0.5–6)
Depression	Fluoxetine (Prozac)	20 (20–40)
	Sertraline (Zoloft)	50 (50–200)
	Paroxetine (Paxil)	20 (10–50)
	Citalopram (Celexa)	20 (10–30)
	Venlafaxine (Effexor)	100 (50–225)
	Nefazodone (Serzone)	400 (200–600)
	Mirtazapine (Remeron)	15 (7.5–30)
	Nortriptyline (Pamelor)	50 (50–100)
	Trazodone (Desyrel)	50 (100–400)
Anxiety	Oxazepam (Serax)	30 (20–60)
	Lorazepam (Ativan)	1 (0.5–6)
	Buspirone (BuSpar)	30 (15–45)
	Propranolol (Inderal)	120 (80–240)
Insomnia	Trazodone (Desyrel)	50 (50–200)
	Zolpidem (Ambien)	10 (5–10)
	Temazepam (Restoril)	15 (15–30)
	Zaleplon (Sonata)	10
Apathy	Donepezil (Aricept)	10 (5–10)
	Rivastigmine (Exelon)	9 (6–12)

From Cummings.[134] By permission of the American Academy of Neurology.

References

1. Brookmeyer R, Gray S, Kawas C. Projections of Alzheimer's disease in the United States and the public health impact of delaying disease onset. Am J Public Health 1998;88:1337–1342

2. Petersen RC. Aging, mild cognitive impairment, and Alzheimer's disease. Neurol Clin 2000;18:789–806

3. Petersen RC. Mild cognitive impairment: transition from aging to Alzheimer's disease. In: Iqbal K, Sisodia SS, Winblad B, eds. Alzheimer's Disease: Advances in Etiology, Pathogenesis and Therapeutics. Chichester, England: John Wiley & Sons, 2001:141–151

4. Petersen RC, Stevens JC, Ganguli M, et al. Practice parameter: early detection of dementia: mild cognitive impairment (an evidence-based review). Report of the Quality Standards Subcommittee of the American Academy of Neurology. Neurology 2001;56:1133–1142

5. Knopman DS, DeKosky ST, Cummings JL, et al. Practice parameter: diagnosis of dementia (an evidence-based review). Report of the Quality Standards Subcommittee of the American Academy of Neurology. Neurology 2001;56:1143–1153

6. Doody RS, Stevens JC, Beck C, et al. Practice parameter: management of dementia (an evidence-based review). Report of the Quality Standards Subcommittee of the American Academy of Neurology. Neurology 2001;56:1154–1166

7. Ivnik RJ, Smith GE, Lucas JA, et al. Testing normal older people three or four times at 1- to 2-year intervals: defining normal variance. Neuropsychology 1999;13:121–127

8. Sliwinski M, Lipton RB, Buschke H, Stewart W. The effects of preclinical dementia on estimates of normal cognitive functioning in aging. J Gerontol B Psychol Sci Soc Sci 1996;51:P217–P225

9. Sliwinski M, Lipton R, Buschke H, Wasylyshyn C. Optimizing cognitive test norms for detection. In: Petersen RC, ed. Mild Cognitive Impairment: Aging to Alzheimer's Disease. New York: Oxford, 2003:89–104

10. American Psychiatric Association: Diagnostic and Statistical Manual of Mental Disorders, Third Edition, Revised. Washington, DC: American Psychiatric Association, 1987

11. Fleming KC, Adams AC, Petersen RC. Dementia: diagnosis and evaluation. Mayo Clin Proc 1995;70:1093–1107

12. Burns A, Jacoby R, Levy R. Psychiatric phenomena in Alzheimer's disease. IV: Disorders of behaviour. Br J Psychiatry 1990;157:86–94

13. Drevets WC, Rubin EH. Psychotic symptoms and the longitudinal course of senile dementia of the Alzheimer type. Biol Psychiatry 1989;25:39–48

14. Rosen J, Zubenko GS. Emergence of psychosis and depression in the longitudinal evaluation of Alzheimer's disease. Biol Psychiatry 1991;29:224–232

15. Teri L, Larson EB, Reifler BV. Behavioral disturbance in dementia of the Alzheimer's type. J Am Geriatr Soc 1988;36:1–6

16. The National Institute on Aging and Reagan Institute Working Group on Diagnostic Criteria for the Neuropathological Assessment of Alzheimer's Disease. Consensus recommendations for the postmortem diagnosis of Alzheimer's disease. Neurobiol Aging 1997;18(Suppl 1):S1–S2

17. Kukull WA, Ganguli M. Epidemiology of dementia: concepts and overview. Neurol Clin 2000;18:923–950

18. Bachman DL, Wolf PA, Linn R, et al. Prevalence of dementia and probable senile dementia of the Alzheimer type in the Framingham Study. Neurology 1992;42:115–119

19. Canadian study of health and aging: study methods and prevalence of dementia. CMAJ 1994;150:899–913

20. Evans DA, Funkenstein HH, Albert MS, et al. Prevalence of Alzheimer's disease in a community population of older persons: higher than previously reported. JAMA 1989;262:2551–2556

21. Hendrie HC, Osuntokun BO, Hall KS, et al. Prevalence of Alzheimer's disease and dementia in two communities: Nigerian Africans and African Americans. Am J Psychiatry 1995;152:1485–1492

22. Hofman A, Ott A, Breteler MM, et al. Atherosclerosis, apolipoprotein E, and prevalence of dementia and Alzheimer's disease in the Rotterdam Study. Lancet 1997;349:151–154

23. Kokmen E, Beard CM, Offord KP, Kurland LT. Prevalence of medically diagnosed dementia in a defined United States population: Rochester, Minnesota, January 1, 1975. Neurology 1989;39:773–776

24. White L, Petrovitch H, Ross GW, et al. Prevalence of dementia in older Japanese-American men in Hawaii: The Honolulu-Asia Aging Study. JAMA 1996;276:955–960

25. American Psychiatric Association. Diagnostic and Statistical Manual of Mental Disorders, Fourth Edition. Washington, DC: American Psychiatric Association, 1994

26. McKhann G, Drachman D, Folstein M, et al. Clinical diagnosis of Alzheimer's disease: report of the NINCDS-ADRDA Work Group under the auspices of Department of Health and Human Services Task Force on Alzheimer's Disease. Neurology 1984;34:939–944

27. Folstein MF, Folstein SE, McHugh PR. "Mini-Mental State": a practical method for grading the cognitive state of patients for the clinician. J Psychiatr Res 1975;12:189–198

28. Teng EL, Chui HC. The Modified Mini-Mental State (3MS) examination. J Clin Psychiatry 1987;48:314–318

29. Katzman R, Brown T, Fuld P, et al. Validation of a short Orientation-Memory-Concentration Test of cognitive impairment. Am J Psychiatry 1983;140:734–739

30. Kokmen E, Smith GE, Petersen RC, et al. The short test of mental status: correlations with standardized psychometric testing. Arch Neurol 1991;48:725–728

31. Morris JC. The Clinical Dementia Rating (CDR): current version and scoring rules. Neurology 1993;43:2412–2414

32. Jack CR Jr, Petersen RC, Xu YC, et al. Medial temporal atrophy on MRI in normal aging and very mild Alzheimer's disease. Neurology 1997;49:786–794

33. Jack CR Jr, Petersen RC, Xu YC, et al. Prediction of AD with MRI-based hippocampal volume in mild cognitive impairment. Neurology 1999;52:1397–1403

34. Killiany RJ, Gomez-Isla T, Moss M, et al. Use of structural magnetic resonance imaging to predict who will get Alzheimer's disease. Ann Neurol 2000;47:430–439

35. Xu Y, Jack CR Jr, O'Brien PC, et al. Usefulness of MRI measures of entorhinal cortex versus hippocampus in AD. Neurology 2000;54:1760–1767

36. Van Gool WA, Walstra GJ, Teunisse S, et al. Diagnosing Alzheimer's disease in elderly, mildly demented patients: the impact of routine single photon emission computed tomography. J Neurol 1995;242:401–405

37. Claus JJ, van Harskamp F, Breteler MM, et al. The diagnostic value of SPECT with Tc 99m HMPAO in Alzheimer's disease: a population-based study. Neurology 1994;44:454–461

38. Johnson KA, Holman BL, Rosen TJ, et al. Iofetamine I 123 single photon emission computed tomography is accurate in the diagnosis of Alzheimer's disease. Arch Intern Med 1990;150:752–756

39. Johnson KA, Kijewski MF, Becker JA, et al. Quantitative brain SPECT in Alzheimer's disease and normal aging. J Nucl Med 1993;34:2044–2048

40. Bartenstein P, Minoshima S, Hirsch C, et al. Quantitative assessment of cerebral blood flow in patients with Alzheimer's disease by SPECT. J Nucl Med 1997;38:1095–1101

41. Mielke R, Heiss WD. Positron emission tomography for diagnosis of Alzheimer's disease and vascular dementia. J Neural Transm Suppl 1998;53:237–250

42. Silverman DH, Small GW, Chang CY, et al. Positron emission tomography in evaluation of dementia: regional brain metabolism and long-term outcome. JAMA 2001;286:2120–2127

43. Pickut BA, Saerens J, Marien P, et al. Discriminative use of SPECT in frontal lobe-type dementia versus (senile) dementia of the Alzheimer's type. J Nucl Med 1997;38:929–934

44. Read SL, Miller BL, Mena I, et al. SPECT in dementia: clinical and pathological correlation. J Am Geriatr Soc 1995;43:1243–1247

45. Talbot PR, Lloyd JJ, Snowden JS, et al. A clinical role for 99mTc-HMPAO SPECT in the investigation of dementia? J Neurol Neurosurg Psychiatry 1998;64:306–313

46. Ishii K, Sakamoto S, Sasaki M, et al. Cerebral glucose metabolism in patients with frontotemporal dementia. J Nucl Med 1998;39:1875–1878

47. Becker PM, Feussner JR, Mulrow CD, et al. The role of lumbar puncture in the evaluation of dementia: the Durham Veterans Administration/Duke University Study. J Am Geriatr Soc 1985;33:392–396

48. Hardy J, Gwinn-Hardy K. Genetic classification of primary neurodegenerative disease. Science 1998;282:1075–1079

49. Roses AD. Apolipoprotein E and Alzheimer's disease. In: Rosenberg RN, Prusiner SB, DiMauro S, Barchi RL, eds. The Molecular and Genetic Basis of Neurological Disease. 2nd ed. Boston: Butterworth-Heinemann, 1997:1019–1035

50. Farrer LA, Cupples LA, Haines JL, et al. Effects of age, sex, and ethnicity on the association between

apolipoprotein E genotype and Alzheimer disease: a meta-analysis. APOE and Alzheimer Disease Meta Analysis Consortium. JAMA 1997;278:1349–1356

51. Mayeux R, Saunders AM, Shea S, et al. Utility of the apolipoprotein E genotype in the diagnosis of Alzheimer's disease. Alzheimer's Disease Centers Consortium on Apolipoprotein E and Alzheimer's Disease. N Engl J Med 1998;338:506–511

52. Roses AD. The predictive value of APOE genotyping in the early diagnosis of dementia of the Alzheimer type: data from three independent series. In: Iqbal K, Winblad B, Nishimura T, et al., eds. Alzheimer's Disease: Biology, Diagnosis and Therapeutics. Chichester, England: John Wiley & Sons, 1997;85–91

53. Andreasen N, Hesse C, Davidsson P, et al. Cerebrospinal fluid beta-amyloid(1–42) in Alzheimer disease: differences between early- and late-onset Alzheimer disease and stability during the course of disease. Arch Neurol 1999;56:673–680

54. Galasko D, Chang L, Motter R, et al. High cerebrospinal fluid tau and low amyloid beta42 levels in the clinical diagnosis of Alzheimer disease and relation to apolipoprotein E genotype. Arch Neurol 1998;55:937–945

55. Hulstaert F, Blennow K, Ivanoiu A, et al. Improved discrimination of AD patients using beta-amyloid(1–42) and tau levels in CSF. Neurology 1999; 52:1555–1562

56. Shoji M, Matsubara E, Kanai M, et al. Combination assay of CSF tau, A beta 1–40 and A beta 1–42(43) as a biochemical marker of Alzheimer's disease. J Neurol Sci 1998;158:134–140

57. Arai H, Higuchi S, Sasaki H. Apolipoprotein E genotyping and cerebrospinal fluid tau protein: implications for the clinical diagnosis of Alzheimer's disease. Gerontology 1997;43(Suppl 1):2–10

58. Galasko D, Clark C, Chang L, et al. Assessment of CSF levels of tau protein in mildly demented patients with Alzheimer's disease. Neurology 1997;48:632–635

59. Kurz A, Riemenschneider M, Buch K, et al. Tau protein in cerebrospinal fluid is significantly increased at the earliest clinical stage of Alzheimer disease. Alzheimer Dis Assoc Disord 1998;12:372–377

60. Andreasen N, Minthon L, Clarberg A, et al. Sensitivity, specificity, and stability of CSF-tau in AD in a community-based patient sample. Neurology 1999;53:1488–1494

61. Ghanbari K, Ghanbari HA. A sandwich enzyme immunoassay for measuring AD7C-NTP as an Alzheimer's disease marker: AD7C test. J Clin Lab Anal 1998;12:223–226

62. Monte SM, Ghanbari K, Frey WH, et al. Characterization of the AD7C-NTP cDNA expression in Alzheimer's disease and measurement of a 41-kD protein in cerebrospinal fluid. J Clin Invest 1997;100:3093–3104

63. de la Monte SM, Volicer L, Hauser SL, Wands JR. Increased levels of neuronal thread protein in cerebrospinal fluid of patients with Alzheimer's disease. Ann Neurol 1992;32:733–742

64. Petersen RC. Conceptual overview. In: Petersen RC, ed. Mild Cognitive Impairment: Aging to Alzheimer's Disease. New York: Oxford University Press, 2003:1–14

65. Geda YE, Petersen RC. Clinical trials in mild cognitive impairment. In: Gauthier S, Cummings JL, eds. Annual of Alzheimer's Disease and Related Disorders—2001. London: Martin Dunitz, 2001;69–83

66. Petersen RC, Doody R, Kurz A, et al. Current concepts in mild cognitive impairment. Arch Neurol 2001;58:1985–1992

67. Ritchie K, Artero S, Touchon J. Classification criteria for mild cognitive impairment: a population-based validation study. Neurology 2001;56:37–42

68. Petersen RC, Smith GE, Waring SC, et al. Mild cognitive impairment: clinical characterization and outcome. Arch Neurol 1999;56:303–308

69. Daly E, Zaitchik D, Copeland M, et al. Predicting conversion to Alzheimer disease using standardized clinical information. Arch Neurol 2000;57:675–680

70. Smith GE, Petersen RC, Parisi JE, Ivnik RJ. Definition, course, and outcome of mild cognitive impairment. Aging Neuropsychol Cogn 1996;3:141–147

71. Ivnik RJ, Malec JF, Smith GE, et al. Mayo's older Americans normative studies: WAIS-R, WMS-R and AVLT norms for ages 56 through 97. Clin Neuropsychol 1992;6(Suppl):1–104

72. Petersen RC. Clinical evaluation. In: Petersen RC, ed. Mild Cognitive Impairment: Aging to Alzheimer's Disease. New York: Oxford University Press, 2003:229–242

73. Knopman DS, Ryberg S. A verbal memory test with high predictive accuracy for dementia of the Alzheimer type. Arch Neurol 1989;46:141–145

74. Petersen RC. Memory assessment at the bedside. In: Yanagihara T, Petersen RC, eds. Memory Disorders: Research and Clinical Practice. New York: Marcel Dekker, 1991;137–152

75. Fox NC, Warrington EK, Freeborough PA, et al. Presymptomatic hippocampal atrophy in Alzheimer's disease: a longitudinal MRI study. Brain 1996;119:2001–2007

76. Fox NC, Crum WR, Scahill RI, et al. Imaging of onset and progression of Alzheimer's disease with voxel-compression mapping of serial magnetic resonance images. Lancet 2001;358:201–205

77. Small GW, Mazziotta JC, Collins MT, et al. Apolipoprotein E type 4 allele and cerebral glucose metabolism in relatives at risk for familial Alzheimer disease. JAMA 1995;273:942–947

78. Reiman EM, Caselli RJ, Yun LS, et al. Preclinical evidence of Alzheimer's disease in persons homozygous for the epsilon 4 allele for apolipoprotein E. N Engl J Med 1996;334:752–758

79. Petersen RC. Mild cognitive impairment: transition between aging and Alzheimer's disease. Neurologia 2000;15:93–101

80. Growdon JH. Biomarkers of Alzheimer disease. Arch Neurol 1999;56:281–283

81. Sunderland T, Wolozin B, Galasko D, et al. Longitudinal stability of CSF tau levels in Alzheimer patients. Biol Psychiatry 1999;46:750–755

82. Petersen RC, Smith GE, Ivnik RJ, et al. Apolipoprotein E status as a predictor of the development of Alzheimer's disease in memory-impaired individuals. JAMA 1995;273:1274–1278

83. Tierney MC, Szalai JP, Snow WG, et al. A prospective study of the clinical utility of ApoE genotype in the prediction of outcome in patients with memory impairment. Neurology 1996;46:149–154

84. Whitehouse PJ, Price DL, Clark AW, et al. Alzheimer disease: evidence for selective loss of cholinergic neurons in the nucleus basalis. Ann Neurol 1981;10:122–126

85. Petersen RC. Scopolamine induced learning failures in man. Psychopharmacology (Berl) 1977;52:283–289

86. Bowen DM, Smith CB, White P, Davison AN. Neuro-

transmitter-related enzymes and indices of hypoxia in senile dementia and other abiotrophies. Brain 1976;99: 459–496

87. Davies P, Maloney AJ. Selective loss of central cholinergic neurons in Alzheimer's disease (letter). Lancet 1976;2:1403

88. Rosler M, Anand R, Cicin-Sain A, et al. Efficacy and safety of rivastigmine in patients with Alzheimer's disease: international randomised controlled trial. BMJ 1999;318:633–638

89. Tariot PN, Solomon PR, Morris JC, et al. A 5-month, randomized, placebo-controlled trial of galantamine in AD. The Galantamine USA-10 Study Group. Neurology 2000;54:2269–2276

90. Gale CR, Martyn CN, Cooper C. Cognitive impairment and mortality in a cohort of elderly people. BMJ 1996; 312:608–611

91. Goodwin JS, Goodwin JM, Garry PJ. Association between nutritional status and cognitive functioning in a healthy elderly population. JAMA 1983;249:2917–2921

92. La Rue A, Koehler KM, Wayne SJ, et al. Nutritional status and cognitive functioning in a normally aging sample: a 6-y reassessment. Am J Clin Nutr 1997; 65:20–29

93. Morris MC, Beckett LA, Scherr PA, et al. Vitamin E and vitamin C supplement use and risk of incident Alzheimer disease. Alzheimer Dis Assoc Disord 1998; 12:121–126

94. Perrig WJ, Perrig P, Stahelin HB. The relation between antioxidants and memory performance in the old and very old. J Am Geriatr Soc 1997;45:718–724

95. Sano M, Ernesto C, Thomas RG, et al. A controlled trial of selegiline, alpha-tocopherol, or both as treatment for Alzheimer's disease. The Alzheimer's Disease Cooperative Study. N Engl J Med 1997;336:1216–1222

96. Aisen PS, Davis KL. Inflammatory mechanisms in Alzheimer's disease: implications for therapy. Am J Psychiatry 1994;151:1105–1113

97. McGeer PL, Rogers J. Anti-inflammatory agents as a therapeutic approach to Alzheimer's disease. Neurology 1992;42:447–449

98. Rogers J, Kirby LC, Hempelman SR, et al. Clinical trial of indomethacin in Alzheimer's disease. Neurology 1993;43:1609–1611

99. Scharf S, Mander A, Ugoni A, et al. A double-blind, placebo-controlled trial of diclofenac/misoprostol in Alzheimer's disease. Neurology 1999;53:197–201

100. Aisen PS, Davis KL, Berg JD, et al. A randomized controlled trial of prednisone in Alzheimer's disease. Alzheimer's Disease Cooperative Study. Neurology 2000;54:588–593

101. Andersen K, Launer LJ, Ott A, et al. Do nonsteroidal anti-inflammatory drugs decrease the risk for Alzheimer's disease? The Rotterdam Study. Neurology 1995;45:1441–1445

102. Breitner JC, Gau BA, Welsh KA, et al. Inverse association of anti-inflammatory treatments and Alzheimer's disease: initial results of a co-twin control study. Neurology 1994;44:227–232

103. Breitner JC, Welsh KA, Helms MJ, et al. Delayed onset of Alzheimer's disease with nonsteroidal anti-inflammatory and histamine H_2 blocking drugs. Neurobiol Aging 1995;16:523–530

104. The Canadian Study of Health and Aging: risk factors for Alzheimer's disease in Canada. Neurology 1994;44:2073–2080

105. Stewart WF, Kawas C, Corrada M, Metter EJ. Risk of Alzheimer's disease and duration of NSAID use. Neurology 1997;48:626–632

106. Ho L, Pieroni C, Winger D, et al. Regional distribution of cyclooxygenase-2 in the hippocampal formation in Alzheimer's disease. J Neurosci Res 1999;57:295–303

107. Pasinetti GM, Aisen PS. Cyclooxygenase-2 expression is increased in frontal cortex of Alzheimer's disease brain. Neuroscience 1998;87:319–324

108. Sainati SM, Ingram DM, Talwalker S, et al. Results of a double-blind, randomized, placebo-controlled study of celecoxib in the treatment of progression of Alzheimer's disease. Presented at the Sixth International Stockholm/Springfield Symposium on Advances in Alzheimer Therapy. Stockholm, Sweden, April 5 to 8, 2000

109. Henderson VW, Paganini-Hill A, Emanuel CK, et al. Estrogen replacement therapy in older women: comparisons between Alzheimer's disease cases and nondemented control subjects. Arch Neurol 1994;51: 896–900

110. Kawas C, Resnick S, Morrison A, et al. A prospective study of estrogen replacement therapy and the risk of developing Alzheimer's disease: the Baltimore Longitudinal Study of Aging. Neurology 1997;48:1517–1521

111. Paganini-Hill A, Henderson VW. Estrogen deficiency and risk of Alzheimer's disease in women. Am J Epidemiol 1994;140:256–261

112. Paganini-Hill A, Henderson VW. Estrogen replacement therapy and risk of Alzheimer's disease. Arch Intern Med 1996;156:2213–2217

113. Tang MX, Jacobs D, Stern Y, et al. Effect of oestrogen during menopause on risk and age at onset of Alzheimer's disease. Lancet 1996;348:429–432

114. Mulnard RA, Cotman CW, Kawas C, et al. Estrogen replacement therapy for treatment of mild to moderate Alzheimer disease: a randomized controlled trial. Alzheimer's Disease Cooperative Study. JAMA 2000; 283:1007–1015

115. Henderson VW, Paganini-Hill A, Miller BL, et al. Estrogen for Alzheimer's disease in women: randomized, double-blind, placebo-controlled trial. Neurology 2000;54:295–301

116. McBee WL, Dailey ME, Dugan E, Shumaker SA. Hormone replacement therapy and other potential treatments for dementias. Endocrinol Metab Clin North Am 1997;26:329–345

117. Selkoe DJ. The genetics and molecular pathology of Alzheimer's disease: roles of amyloid and the presenilins. Neurol Clin 2000;18:903–922

118. Hussain I, Powell D, Howlett DR, et al. Identification of a novel aspartic protease (Asp 2) as beta-secretase. Mol Cell Neurosci 1999;14:419–427

119. Sinha S, Anderson JP, Barbour R, et al. Purification and cloning of amyloid precursor protein beta-secretase from human brain. Nature 1999;402:537–540

120. Vassar R, Bennett BD, Babu-Khan S, et al. Beta-secretase cleavage of Alzheimer's amyloid precursor protein by the transmembrane aspartic protease BACE. Science 1999;286:735–741

121. Yan R, Bienkowski MJ, Shuck ME, et al. Membrane-anchored aspartyl protease with Alzheimer's disease beta-secretase activity. Nature 1999;402:533–537

122. Schenk D, Barbour R, Dunn W, et al. Immunization with amyloid-beta attenuates Alzheimer-disease-like pathology in the PDAPP mouse. Nature 1999;400: 173–177

123. Chung JA, Cummings JL. Neurobehavioral and neuropsychiatric symptoms in Alzheimer's disease:

characteristics and treatment. Neurol Clin 2000;18:829–846

124. Ballard C, Bannister C, Solis M, et al. The prevalence, associations and symptoms of depression amongst dementia sufferers. J Affect Disord 1996;36:135–144

125. Borson S, Raskind MA. Clinical features and pharmacologic treatment of behavioral symptoms of Alzheimer's disease. Neurology 1997;48(Suppl 6):S17–S24

126. Devanand DP, Jacobs DM, Tang MX, et al. The course of psychopathologic features in mild to moderate Alzheimer disease. Arch Gen Psychiatry 1997;54:257–263

127. Mega MS, Cummings JL, Fiorello T, Gornbein J. The spectrum of behavioral changes in Alzheimer's disease. Neurology 1996;46:130–135

128. Reisberg B, Borenstein J, Salob SP, et al. Behavioral symptoms in Alzheimer's disease: phenomenology and treatment. J Clin Psychiatry 1987;48(Suppl):9–15

129. Petersen RC (ed). Mayo Clinic on Alzheimer's Disease. Rochester, Minnesota: Mayo Clinic, 2002:95–198

130. Cohen-Mansfield J, Deutsch LH. Agitation: subtypes and their mechanisms. Semin Clin Neuropsychiatry 1996;1:325–339

131. Cummings JL, Mega M, Gray K, et al. The Neuropsychiatric Inventory: comprehensive assessment of psychopathology in dementia. Neurology 1994;44:2308–2314

132. Kaufer DI, Cummings JL, Ketchel P, et al. Validation of the NPI-Q, a brief clinical form of the Neuropsychiatric Inventory. J Neuropsychiatry Clin Neurosci 2000;12:233–239

133. Devanand DP, Sano M, Tang MX, et al. Depressed mood and the incidence of Alzheimer's disease in the elderly living in the community. Arch Gen Psychiatry 1996;53:175–182

134. Cummings JL. Management of neuropsychiatric disturbances in patients with Alzheimer's disease. In: DeKosky ST, ed. Dementia Update. Minneapolis: American Academy of Neurology, 2001:108–122

135. Rubin EH, Drevets WC, Burke WJ. The nature of psychotic symptoms in senile dementia of the Alzheimer type. J Geriatr Psychiatry Neurol 1988;1:16–20

136. Stern Y, Albert M, Brandt J, et al. Utility of extrapyramidal signs and psychosis as predictors of cognitive and functional decline, nursing home admission, and death in Alzheimer's disease: prospective analyses from the Predictors Study. Neurology 1994;44:2300–2307

137. Katz IR, Jeste DV, Mintzer JE, et al. Comparison of risperidone and placebo for psychosis and behavioral disturbances associated with dementia: a randomized, double-blind trial. Risperidone Study Group. J Clin Psychiatry 1999;60:107–115

138. McManus DQ, Arvanitis LA, Kowalcyk BB. Quetiapine, a novel antipsychotic: experience in elderly patients with psychotic disorders. Seroquel Trial 48 Study Group. J Clin Psychiatry 1999;60:292–298

139. Street JS, Clark WS, Gannon KS, et al. Olanzapine treatment of psychotic and behavioral symptoms in patients with Alzheimer disease in nursing care facilities: a double-blind, randomized, placebo-controlled trial. The HGEU Study Group. Arch Gen Psychiatry 2000;57:968–976

140. McAllister TW. Apathy. Semin Clin Neuropsychiatry 2000;5:275–282

141. Deutsch LH, Bylsma FW, Rovner BW, et al. Psychosis and physical aggression in probable Alzheimer's disease. Am J Psychiatry 1991;148:1159–1163

142. Sultzer DL, Gray KF, Gunay I, et al. A double-blind comparison of trazodone and haloperidol for treatment of agitation in patients with dementia. Am J Geriatr Psychiatry 1997;5:60–69

143. Tariot PN, Erb R, Podgorski CA, et al. Efficacy and tolerability of carbamazepine for agitation and aggression in dementia. Am J Psychiatry 1998;155:54–61

144. Porsteinsson AP, Tariot PN, Erb R, Gaile S. An open trial of valproate for agitation in geriatric neuropsychiatric disorders. Am J Geriatr Psychiatry 1997;5:344–351

269 Diagnosis and Management of the Non-Alzheimer Dementias

Bradley F Boeve

Introduction

Alzheimer disease (AD) is the most common incurable cause of dementia. Multi-infarct dementia, classically thought to be the second-most common untreatable cause, is now considered within the spectrum of vascular dementia; this category also includes Binswanger disease, cerebral autosomal dominant arteriopathy with subcortical infarcts and leukoencephalopathy (CADASIL), and hippocampal sclerosis. The prevalence of vascular dementia has been debated, and recent studies have suggested that pure vascular dementia probably accounts for fewer than 20% of cases with dementia. With the application of immunocytochemical techniques in neuropathological examinations over the past 10 to 15 years, new categories of illnesses have emerged. Dementia with Lewy bodies (DLB) is now considered the second-most common irreversible cause of dementia, accounting for approximately 15% to 25% of cases. Its relationship to Parkinson disease (PD)—another disorder with Lewy bodies—is still evolving. Because α-synuclein is a constituent of Lewy bodies and Lewy neurites and mutations in the synuclein gene are associated with Lewy body parkinsonism, DLB and PD are considered "synucleinopathies."

Frontotemporal dementia (FTD) is a clinical syndrome manifested by personality–behavioral changes or progressive aphasia (or both). The most common neuropathological substrates for FTD include Pick disease, corticobasal degeneration (CBD), and dementia lacking distinctive histology (DLDH). Less common substrates are AD and progressive supranuclear palsy (PSP). This category of disorders accounts for approximately 10% to 15% of cases of untreatable dementia. CBD and PSP are classically considered Parkinson-plus syndromes, but these disorders can present clinically as personality–behavioral changes or progressive aphasia. Abnormal accumulations of hyperphosphorylated tau in neurons or glia is characteristic of Pick disease, CBD, PSP, and progressive subcortical gliosis (PSG), and mutations in the tau gene are associated with dementia or parkinsonism. These disorders and AD are considered "tauopathies." Creutzfeldt-Jacob disease (CJD), Gerstmann-Strausser-Schenker (GSS), fatal familial insomnia (FFI) are rare; however, because prion protein dysfunction is common to them all, they can be considered "prionopathies."

The nomenclature for the vascular and non-Alzheimer dementing illnesses is confusing. Most of the literature includes terms for clinical syndromes (e.g., FTD, primary progressive aphasia [PPA] and so forth) as well as ones for presumably distinct histopathological disorders (e.g., DLDH and Pick disease). Importantly, each syndrome is associated with a spectrum of disorders, and each disorder can be manifested clinically as various syndromes. Although histopathological examination is required to establish a specific diagnosis in the vascular and degenerative dementing illnesses, several sets of clinical diagnostic criteria have been proposed, although none of them are entirely accurate. Because no currently available therapy targets any of the pathophysiological processes of these disorders, errors in the diagnosis of specific diseases generally do not affect management.

However, determining the neurochemical alterations or topographic distribution of brain dysfunction can influence management and prognosis. Many signs and symptoms are associated with known or presumed neurochemical alterations (e.g., impaired memory is associated with acetylcholine deficiency; psychomotor slowing and bradykinesia are associated with dopamine deficiency; and hallucinations and delusions are associated with dopamine excess) or with dysfunction in certain neuroanatomical regions (e.g., amnesia is associated with mesial temporal, midline diencephalic, or basal forebrain dysfunction; nonfluent aphasia is associated with dominant hemisphere frontal opercular dysfunction; and visuospatial dysfunction is associated with nondominant parietal, with or without occipital, dysfunction). Symptomatic therapy involving agents that target such signs and symptoms can improve daily functioning, and this is the mainstay of treatment for management of vascular and degenerative disorders. As therapies are developed that target specific pathophysiological processes, it will become increasingly important to establish the underlying disorder, particularly if these therapies have important side effects. It is too early to know whether brain biopsy will be required or whether biomarkers will identify the pathophysiological process.

This chapter reviews the diagnostic and management considerations for each disorder and clinical syndrome for which clinical or pathological diagnostic criteria exist. Therapies directed toward specific target symptoms are also discussed. Although controlled clinical trials are emphasized, few therapies are available for vascular dementia and non-AD dementias with demonstrated efficacy; thus, comments based on open label trials, case reports, and clinical experience are included.

Diagnosis and management of the non-Alzheimer degenerative disorders

Dementia with Lewy Bodies/Parkinson disease with dementia

Background   In 1961, Okazaki et al.[1] described Lewy bodies in the cerebral cortex of patients with dementia (Figure 269.1). Lewy bodies are difficult to identify in standard hematoxylin- and eosin-stained sections of cerebral cortex, and this may explain why so few reports were published during the following two decades. With the application of ubiquitin immunohistochemical staining techniques in the 1980s, Lewy bodies were easier to identify in the cortical and subcortical regions. With the advent of α-synuclein immunocytochemistry (Figure 269.2), neuropathologists can now identify relatively easily extranigral Lewy bodies.

Several terms have been used to describe the condition of patients with known or suspected Lewy body lesions, including Lewy body disease, Lewy body dementia, the Lewy body variant of AD, diffuse Lewy body disease, cortical Lewy body disease, and senile dementia of the Lewy type. The Consortium on Dementia With Lewy Bodies developed consensus criteria for the clinical and neuropathological diagnoses of what is now termed *dementia with Lewy bodies* (DLB).[2] Because the contribution of Alzheimer pathological process to the clinical features in DLB is not clear, the presence of Alzheimer's pathological features does not exclude the diagnosis of DLB. On the basis primarily of cases in hospital- and referral-based samples, the frequency of DLB is approximately 15% to 25% of cases with irreversible dementia. There is growing evidence that the cognitive decline and neuropsychiatric manifestations of PD with dementia are due to cortical Lewy bodies.[3,4] Thus, DLB and PD with dementia are considered similar for purposes of management.

Diagnosis   The criteria for the clinical diagnosis of DLB according to the Consortium on Dementia With Lewy Bodies were published originally in 1996[2] and were refined in 1999.[5] The clinical and pathological criteria are shown in Tables 269.1 and 269.2, respec-

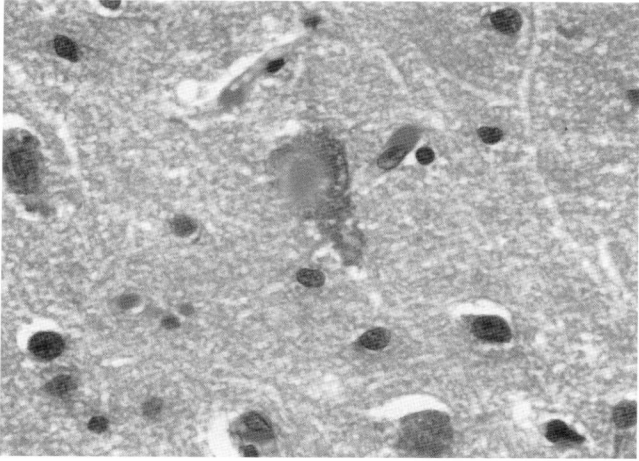

Figure 269.1   Lewy body (cingulate cortex) characteristic of Lewy body disease (H&E ×60). Courtesy Joseph E Parisi, MD. (See color plate section.)

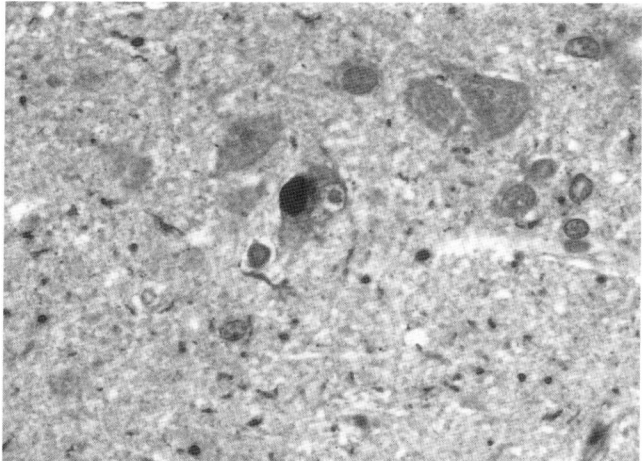

Figure 269.2   α-synuclein-positive Lewy body (cingulate cortex) characteristic of Lewy body disease (α-synuclein ×60). Courtesy Joseph E Parisi, MD. (See color plate section.)

Table 269.1   Clinical diagnosis of dementia with Lewy bodies (DLB): consortium on dementia with Lewy bodies or "McKeith" criteria

Core features
Progressive cognitive decline that interferes with normal social and occupational functioning
Deficits often prominent on tests of attention-concentration, verbal fluency, psychomotor speed, and visuospatial functioning
Prominent or persistent memory impairment may not be present early in course of illness
Two of the following core features are necessary for the diagnosis of *clinically probable* DLB, and one is necessary for the diagnosis of *clinically possible* DLB:
  Fluctuating cognition or alertness
  Recurrent visual hallucinations
  Spontaneous features of parkinsonism

Supportive features
Repeated falls
Syncope
Transient loss of consciousness
Neuroleptic sensitivity
Systematized delusions
Tactile or olfactory hallucinations
REM sleep behavior disorder
Depression

Features suggesting disorder other than DLB
Cerebrovascular disease evidenced by focal neurological signs or cerebral infarct(s) present on neuroimaging study
Findings on examination or ancillary testing that another medical, neurological, or psychiatric disorder sufficiently accounts for clinical features

Modified from McKeith et al.[2] By permission of the American Academy of Neurology. Data from McKeith et al.[5]

Table 269.2   Pathological diagnosis of dementia with Lewy bodies (DLB): consortium on dementia with Lewy bodies or "McKeith" criteria

Essential for diagnosis of DLB
Lewy bodies

Associated but not essential
Lewy-related neurites
Plaques
Neurofibrillary tangles
Regional neuronal loss, especially brainstem and nucleus basalis of Meynert
Spongiform change and loss of synapses
Neurochemical abnormalities and neurotransmitter deficits

From McKeith et al.[2] By permission of the American Academy of Neurology.

tively. A similar set of clinical criteria proposed by the Consortium to Establish a Registry in Alzheimer's Disease are shown in Table 269.3. Patients often describe "verbal blocking," in which they stop speaking in midsentence and seemingly lose what they intended to say. Increasingly, data indicate that the neuropsychological pattern of impairment—poor verbal fluency, attention-concentration, and visuospatial functioning—is distinct and different from that of AD, in which impairment is usually maximal in learning and memory and confrontational naming early in the course of the disease.[6] REM sleep behavior disorder—a parasomnia in which patients seemingly act out their dreams—has been associated with DLB, and the features of REM sleep behavior disorder can precede the development of dementia or parkinsonism (or both) by years or even decades.[7] Depression appears to be relatively common in DLB. Many patients have more of a postural than a rest tremor, and the parkinsonism can be more symmetrical than that typical of early PD. There appears to be less hippocampal atrophy on MRI scans in DLB than in AD

Table 269.3   Clinical diagnosis of dementia with Lewy bodies: consortium to establish a registry for Alzheimer's disease (CERAD) criteria

Core features
Clinical Dementia Rating score of 0.5 to 2
Two of the following:
    Delusions or hallucinations
    Extrapyramidal signs
    Unexplained falls or change of consciousness

Supportive features
Fluctuating course
Levodopa failure
Dementia > extrapyramidal signs
Weight loss, dysphagia, decreased mood

Reference: CERAD guide to the clinical assessment of Alzheimer's disease and other dementias (For information, contact Albert Heyman, MD., Box 3203, Duke University Medical Center, Durham, NC 27710).

and vascular dementia.[8] Recent clinicopathological analyses have shown that the accuracy of the clinical criteria has varied widely among investigators, and further refinement of the criteria will likely be necessary.

Management   Neuroleptic sensitivity, in which striking and irreversible parkinsonism can evolve shortly after use of neuroleptics, has led to the recommendation that conventional neuroleptics should be avoided in patients with DLB.[9] Neuroleptic sensitivity has been reported even with newer atypical neuroleptic agents, some of which have been minimally effective for psychotic features.[10] Therefore, if hallucinations, delusions, or agitation is a problem in a patient with DLB, clinicians should consider treatment with clozapine or quetiapine. Dramatic improvement has been reported in cognitive functioning and neuropsychiatric symptoms of patients with DLB treated with cholinesterase inhibitors, including tacrine, donepezil, rivastigmine, and galantamine.[11–14] For reasons that are not clear, increased parkinsonism occurs infrequently with the cholinesterase inhibitors; thus clinicians should consider prescribing one of these agents to patients with DLB who do not have a contraindication to its use. Carbidopa/levodopa can be used in the management of parkinsonism, but this can exacerbate psychotic symptoms or orthostatism. Psychotic symptoms in PD (with or without dementia) can improve with treatment with clozapine,[15–20] quetiapine,[20] risperidone,[21,22] olanzapine,[23,24] or cholinesterase inhibitors. Orthostatic hypotension, likely due to degenerative changes in the intermediolateral cell column of the spinal cord, can occur in DLB.[25] As in PD, management includes liberalizing salt in the diet, salt tablets, thigh-high compression stockings, fludrocortisone, and midodrine.

Depression is common in DLB, and although none of the newer antidepressant agents has been shown to be superior to the others, tricyclic antidepressants should be avoided in DLB because of their anticholinergic properties. The underlying cause for fluctuations in DLB is poorly understood, but this feature can improve with cholinesterase inhibitor therapy or, in some cases, following treatment of sleep disorders. There are anecdotal reports that modafinil or methylphenidate improves hypersomnia in patients with DLB. Violent dreams and dream enactment behavior as part of REM sleep behavior disorder, which often precedes or accompanies dementia or parkinsonism in Lewy body-associated disorders, typically improve with clonazepam or melatonin therapy.[7,26,27] Although some degree of neuronal loss occurs in DLB, it tends to be less severe than in AD and Pick disease, permitting pharmacological intervention. Patients with DLB who have pronounced parkinsonism, psychosis, and orthostatism are quite challenging to manage, but some clearly benefit from optimizing dosing of a cholinesterase inhibitor, carbidopa/levodopa, and an atypical neuroleptic, and treatment of orthostatism.[5,28–31] Specific treatment suggestions for the varying features in DLB-PD with dementia are shown in the Appendix.

Huntington disease

Background Huntington disease (HD) is an autosomal dominant neurodegenerative disorder that begins insidiously in middle adulthood and is characterized by progressive chorea, neuropsychiatric symptoms, and cognitive impairment. The genetic basis of HD has been identified on chromosome 4, in which an expansion of a trinucleotide repeat (CAG) increases polyglutamine, which in turn increases expression of the protein huntingtin. The neuropsychiatric features of HD include depression, hallucinations, delusions, disinhibition, and behavioral dyscontrol. Cognitive impairment reflects the predominantly frontostriatal distribution of neuropathological alterations, with dysfunction in psychomotor speed, attention-concentration, and motor greater than verbal learning and memory.

Diagnosis About one-fourth of patients exhibit cognitive impairment well before the onset of chorea, whereas others have chorea without marked cognitive impairment. Diagnosis is established through genetic testing; any person with suspected HD and the person's relatives should undergo genetic counseling before having genetic testing.

Management Trials with α-tocopherol,[32] the free radical scavenger OPC-14117,[33] and riluzole[34] have reported equivocal improvement in HD. Electroconvulsive therapy (ECT) has been effective for medically refractory depression,[35] and chorea reportedly has improved with ECT.[36] Some authors have suggested that clozapine is effective for managing psychotic features of HD.[37] Symptomatic therapy for target symptoms should be considered (Appendix).

Pick disease

Background Although Pick[38] first described focal cortical atrophy in a patient with progressive aphasia and rage attacks, other investigators 30 years later termed the ballooned cells as *Pick cells* and the silver stain-positive neuronal inclusions as *Pick bodies* (Figure 269.3). Debate continues about what should

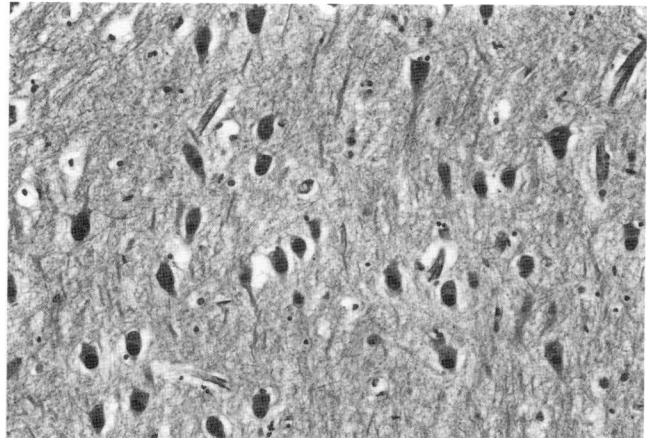

Figure 269.3 Pick bodies (hippocampus) characteristic of Pick disease (Bielschowsky ×20). Courtesy Joseph E Parisi, MD.

be considered Pick disease: some investigators require the presence of Pick bodies for the pathological diagnosis of Pick disease and others consider focal cortical atrophy as the defining feature. Most cases are sporadic, although familial cases have been reported.

Pick disease is characterized by the abnormal accumulation of hyperphosphorylated tau in neurons and glia;[39] thus, it is considered a "tauopathy." Unlike CBD and PSP—two other tauopathies that have about equal proportions of 3- and 4-repeat tau—Pick disease involves primarily 3-repeat tau (three exons on the tau gene on chromosome 17 undergo alternative splicing, resulting in three forms of 3-repeat tau and three forms of 4-repeat tau). A critical step in the pathophysiological mechanism of Pick disease and the other tauopathies appears to be hyperphosphorylation of tau, and some investigators speculate that intervention at this step may lead to effective treatment of the underlying disorder. Currently, however, no effective treatment exists.

Diagnosis Although there are cases with atypical clinical presentations such as primarily parietal lobe dysfunction, most cases have dysfunction maximal in the frontal or temporal (or both) cortical region. Thus, the clinical manifestations are typically behavior-personality change or aphasia or both. A clinical classification scheme has been proposed to identify persons who have underlying Pick disease (Table 269.4). Also, pathological criteria have been developed (Table 269.5).[40] Data about the accuracy of these criteria have not been published.

Management Treatment is based on target symptoms (Appendix). Because at the onset of symptoms patients are often younger than 65 years and are otherwise in good health, the time from the onset of symptoms to death can be more than 10 to 15 years.

Corticobasal degeneration

Background In 1967, Rebeiz et al.[41] identified three patients who had progressive asymmetrical akinetic-rigid syndrome and apraxia and distinctive histopathological features. In these patients, achromatic neurons and degeneration of the cerebral cortex, substantia nigra, and cerebellar dentate nucleus were found (leading to the term "corticodentatonigral degeneration"). Subsequently, findings in other patients were characterized by more basal ganglia than cerebellar degeneration (leading to such terms as "cortical-basal ganglionic degeneration," "corticobasal ganglionic degeneration," and "corticobasal degeneration"). Most cases appear to be sporadic, although familial cases exist.

Diagnosis The three sets of clinical criteria that have been published for making the diagnosis of CBD are given in Tables 269.6 to 269.8,[43–45] and the proposed pathological criteria are listed in Table 269.9[46] (Figures 269.4 and 269.5). Common to all three sets of clinical criteria is the combination of progressive

---

Table 269.4   Clinical diagnosis of Pick disease: ECAPD consortium criteria

Probable Pick disease

Core features
1. Progressive cognitive impairment sufficiently severe to interfere with social and occupational functioning
2. Onset before age 70 years
3. Evidence of
      Asymmetry on neuropsychological testing that persists beyond early stages
      and/or (to be tested prospectively)
      Asymmetry on structural neuroimaging

Features consistent with diagnosis of probable Pick disease
Progressive impairment of language skills (naming, comprehension, speech production)
Progressive impairment of praxic skills in the absence of additional motor signs
Progressive change in personality and behavior
Temporal atrophy as prominent as, or more so, than frontal atrophy; white matter changes in areas of atrophy

Features that make the diagnosis unlikely
Cognitive impairment in multiple domains early in the disease
Prominent visuospatial or visuoperceptual impairment
Prominent impairment of anterograde memory functions early in the disease
Global atrophy on imaging
Anterior horn cell disease
Strong family history of dementia

Possible Pick disease
Onset older than age 70 with core features 1 and 3
Progressive behavioral change in conjunction with core features 2 and 3
Core criteria with evidence of additional diseases known to cause cognitive impairment

---

Table 269.5   Pathological diagnosis of Pick disease: ECAPD consortium criteria

Definite Pick disease
Clinical criteria for probable or possible Pick disease
Histopathological confirmation of typical Pick disease characterized by a widespread occurrence of Pick inclusion bodies
In addition, there should be swollen achromatic Pick cells and neuronal loss astrocytosis in the setting of frontotemporal atrophy

From European Concerted Action on Pick's Disease (ECAPD) Consortium.[40] By permission of Blackwell Science.

Table 269.6   Clinical diagnosis of corticobasal degeneration (CBD)

Clinically possible CBD
No identifiable cause (e.g., tumor, infarct) and at least three of the following:
Progressive course }
Asymmetrical distribution } "PARA" syndrome
Rigidity }
Apraxia }

Clinically probable CBD
All four of the "clinically possible" criteria, no identifiable cause, and at least two of the following:
      Focal or asymmetrical appendicular dystonia
      Focal or asymmetrical appendicular myoclonus
      Focal or asymmetrical appendicular postural/action tremor
Lack of levodopa response

Clinically definite CBD
Meets criteria for clinically probable CBD, plus at least one of the following:
      Alien limb phenomenon
      Cortical sensory loss
      Mirror movements

Supportive findings
Asymmetrical amplitude on EEG
Focal or asymmetrical frontoparietal atrophy on CT or MRI
Focal or asymmetrical frontoparietal ± basal ganglia hypoperfusion on SPECT
Focal or asymmetrical frontoparietal ± basal ganglia hypometabolism on PET

CT, computed tomography; EEG, electroencephalography; MRI, magnetic resonance imaging; PET, positron emission tomography; SPECT, single photon emission computed tomography. Data from Boeve.[42]

---

asymmetrical rigidity and apraxia, known as the PARA syndrome. CBD is included in this chapter because neuropsychiatric morbidity occurs with the disorder,[47,48] and numerous patients have presented with progressive aphasia or dementia.[49,50] The patients with dementia typically present with features of frontotemporal dementia, although some have appeared clinically indistinguishable from those with AD.

Management   The only report to consider specifically the effect of various pharmacological interventions in CBD is that of Kompoliti et al.,[51] who found that no agent produced a consistent and prolonged benefit for any symptom or sign. Some patients have had some degree of improvement in parkinsonism with carbidopa/levodopa, but this has not been sustained. Valproic acid and clonazepam can improve myoclonus. Physical, occupational, and speech therapy can be worthwhile. Depression and sleep

Table 269.7   Clinical diagnosis of corticobasal degeneration: criteria of Lang et al.

Inclusion criteria
Rigidity plus one cortical sign (apraxia, cortical sensory
    loss, or alien limb phenomenon)
or
Asymmetrical rigidity, dystonia, and focal reflex
    myoclonus

Qualifications of clinical features
Rigidity: easily detectable without reinforcement
Apraxia: more than simple use of limb as object; clear
    absence of cognitive or motor deficit sufficient to
    explain disturbance
Cortical sensory loss: preserved primary sensation;
    asymmetrical
Alien limb phenomenon: more than simple levitation
Dystonia: focal in limb; present at rest at onset
Myoclonus: reflex myoclonus spreads beyond stimulated
    digits

Exclusion criteria
Early dementia
Early vertical gaze palsy
Rest tremor
Severe autonomic disturbances
Sustained responsiveness to levodopa
Lesions on imaging studies indicating another
    pathological process is responsible

Modified from Lang et al.[44] By permission of Elsevier Science.

Table 269.8   Clinical diagnosis of corticobasal degeneration: criteria of Kumar et al.

Core features
Chronic progressive course
Asymmetrical at onset (includes speech dyspraxia,
    dysphasia)
Presence of
"Higher" cortical dysfunction (apraxia, cortical sensory
    loss, or alien limb)
and
Movement disorders (akinetic-rigid syndrome resistant to
    levodopa, and limb dystonia or spontaneous and reflex
    focal myoclonus)

Qualifications of clinical features
Same as criteria of Lang et al. (Table 281.7)

Exclusion criteria
Same as criteria of Lang et al. (Table 281.7)

Modified from Kumar et al.[45] By permission of Lippincott
Williams & Wilkins.

Table 269.9   Pathological diagnosis of corticobasal degeneration: proposed criteria of Dickson et al.

Minimal essential features
Focal cortical neuronal loss
Substantia nigra neuronal loss
Cortical and striatal Gallyas/tau-positive neuronal and
    glial lesions, especially astrocytic plaques and
    threads, in both white and gray matter

Supportive features
Cortical atrophy, often with superficial spongiosis
Ballooned neurons, usually numerous in atrophic cortices

Data from Dickson et al.[46]

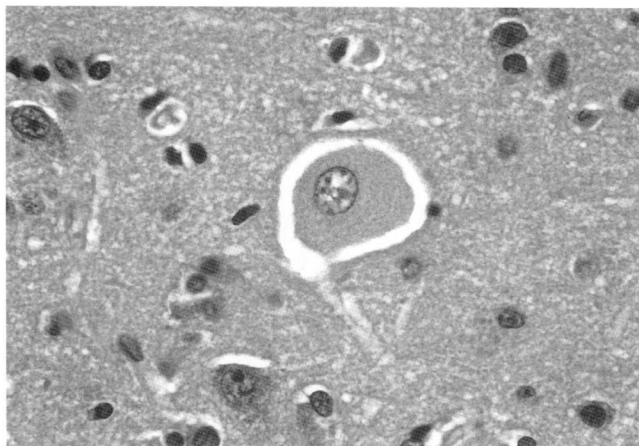

Figure 269.4   Ballooned, achromatic neuron (frontal
cortex) typical of corticobasal degeneration (H&E ×60).
Courtesy Joseph E Parisi, MD. (See color plate section.)

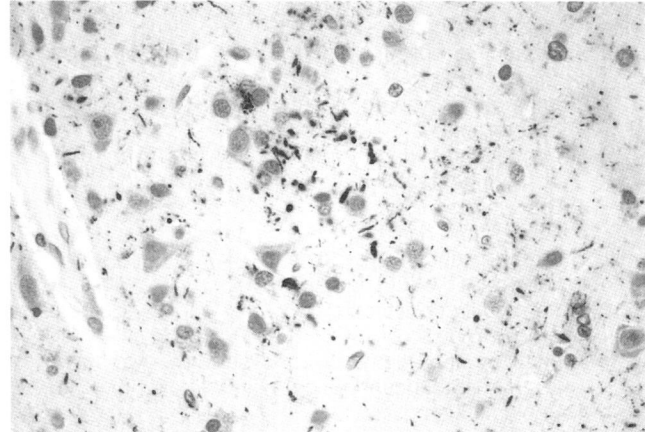

Figure 269.5   Tau-positive astrocytic plaque (parietal
cortex) typical of corticobasal degeneration (tau ×40).
Courtesy Joseph E Parisi, MD. (See color plate section.)

disorders are also treatable.[51] Other symptoms can
improve with therapy (Appendix).

Progressive supranuclear palsy

Background   In 1964, Steele et al.[52] described the clinical features of a syndrome (which still bears their
names) with degeneration of the brainstem, basal
ganglia, and cerebellum. Recent immunocytochemical
studies have demonstrated characteristic tau-positive
abnormalities (Figure 269.6).[53] Dementia occurs

frequently in PSP. Although most cases appear to be
sporadic, some are familial.

Diagnosis   The classic presentation of PSP is the constellation of supranuclear gaze palsy, postural instability and falls, and parkinsonism. These same

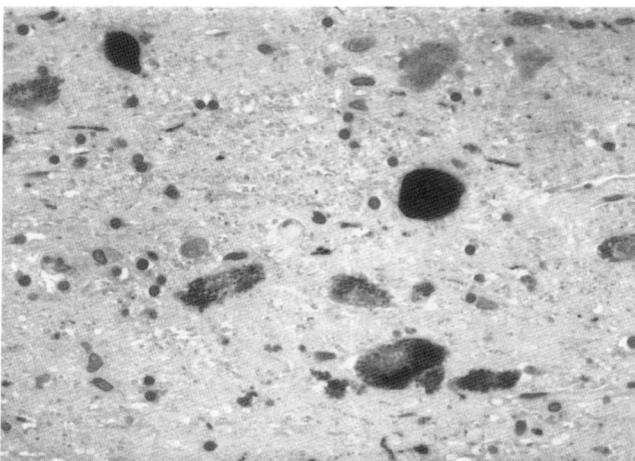

Figure 269.6   Tau-positive globose neurofibrillary tangle (substantia nigra) typical of progressive supranuclear palsy (tau ×40). Courtesy Joseph E Parisi, MD. (See color plate section.)

features form the core for the Mayo Clinic (Table 269.10)[54] and NINDS-SPSP (Table 269.11)[55] clinical criteria. The pathological criteria for the diagnosis of PSP are given in Table 269.12.[56] Numerous cases have had atypical features, including those mistaken for CBD; those with no gaze palsy, gait impairment, or parkinsonism; and those presenting with aphasia or having obsessive-compulsive features.[57]

Table 269.10   Clinical diagnosis of progressive supranuclear palsy: Mayo Clinic criteria

Core features
One of the following:
1. Supranuclear downgaze paresis plus three of a through i
2. Prominent early postural instability and falls plus five of a through i
3. Supranuclear downgaze paresis and prominent early postural instability plus two of the following:
    a) Bradykinesia
    b) Axial > limb rigidity
    c) Staring, nonblinking facies
    d) Wide-based shuffling gait
    e) Retrocollis or dystonic arm
    f) Sitting en bloc
    g) Pseudobulbar signs (two of dysarthria, dysphagia, emotional incontinence)
    h) Babinski sign
    i) Dementia or personality change

Exclusion criteria (none can be present)
1. Prominent and early dysautonomia
2. Prominent polyneuropathy
3. Pronounced rest tremor
4. Cortical sensory loss
5. Alien limb sign
6. Pronounced asymmetry

Modified from Collins et al.[54] By permission of the Journal of Neurology, Neurosurgery, and Psychiatry.

Table 269.11   Clinical diagnosis of progressive supranuclear palsy (PSP): National Institute of Neurological Disorders and Stroke–Society for Progressive Supranuclear Palsy criteria

Core features (mandatory inclusion criteria)
Possible *PSP*
Gradually progressive disorder
Onset at age 40 or later
Either vertical supranuclear palsy or both slowing of vertical saccades and prominent postural instability with falls in the first year of disease onset
No evidence of other diseases that could explain the foregoing features, as indicated by mandatory exclusion criteria

Probable PSP
Gradually progressive disorder
Onset at age 40 or later
Vertical supranuclear palsy and prominent postural instability with falls in the first year of disease onset
No evidence of other diseases that could explain the foregoing features, as indicated by mandatory exclusion criteria

Definite PSP
Clinically probable or possible PSP and histopathological evidence of typical PSP

Supportive features
Symmetrical akinesia or rigidity, proximal more than distal
Abnormal neck posture, especially retrocollis
Poor or absence of response of parkinsonism to levodopa therapy
Early dysphagia and dysarthria
Early onset of cognitive impairment including at least two of the following: apathy, impairment in abstract thought, decreased verbal fluency, utilization or imitation behavior, or frontal release signs

Exclusion criteria
Recent history of encephalitis
Alien limb syndrome, cortical sensory deficits, focal frontal or temporoparietal atrophy
Hallucinations or delusions unrelated to dopaminergic therapy
Cortical dementia of Alzheimer type
Prominent early cerebellar symptoms or prominent early unexplained dysautonomia
Severe, asymmetrical parkinsonian signs
Neuroradiological evidence of relevant structural abnormalities
Whipple disease, confirmed by polymerase chain reaction

From Litvan et al.[55] By permission of the American Academy of Neurology.

Management Management of the motor and gait aspects of PSP is challenging.[58–60] Parkinsonism responds poorly to carbidopa/levodopa, and gait assistance devices or confinement to a wheelchair is often necessary for management of gait impairment. The topography of cortical dysfunction tends to involve the frontal or frontosubcortical neural networks; thus, apathy and executive dysfunction are often present. Disinhibition, dysphoria, and anxiety

Table 269.12   Pathological diagnosis of progressive supranuclear palsy (PSP): National Institute of Neurological Disorders and Stroke criteria

Inclusion criteria
Typical PSP
Numerous NFTs or NTs or both in basal ganglia and brainstem
At approximately ×250 magnification:
    Two or more neurons with NFTs or NTs must be found in the same field in three of the following brain areas: pallidum, subthalamic nucleus, substantia nigra, or pons
    One or more neurons with NFTs or NTs must be found in the same field in at least three of the following brain areas: striatum, oculomotor complex, medulla, or dentate nucleus
    The presence of tau-positive astrocytes or processes in these areas supports the diagnosis

Atypical PSP
NFTs or NTs, or both, in the basal ganglia and brainstem is mandatory
At ×250 magnification:
    One or more neurons with NFTs or NTs must be found in the same field in at least five of the following brain areas: pallidum, subthalamic nucleus, substantia nigra, pons, medulla, or dentate nucleus
    The presence of tau-positive astrocytes or processes in these areas support the diagnosis

Combined PSP
    The presence of typical neuropathological changes of PSP together with findings that are diagnostic of another neurological disease

Exclusion criteria for PSP
Lewy body-associated diseases
Alzheimer disease
Multiple system atrophy
Pick disease
Corticobasal degeneration

NFT, neurofibrillary tangle; NT, neurophil thread. Data from Hauw et al.[56]

are also common,[61] but agitation and obsessive-compulsive features are less frequent. Treatment is directed toward target symptoms (Appendix). No improvement in cognition has been demonstrated with physostigmine,[62] and mixed results have been reported for donepezil.[63,64]

Progressive subcortical gliosis

Background   The term *progressive subcortical gliosis* was coined by Neumann and Cohn[65] to describe patients with dementia who had marked gliosis of subcortical white matter and no other distinctive histopathological feature. Decades later, two kindreds with varying degrees of dementia (most with features referable to frontotemporal dysfunction) with or without parkinsonism were identified with PSG-type lesions.[66] Subsequent analyses suggested the presence of prion protein deposits,[67] which later were found to be a contamination artifact.[68] Recent studies have shown prominent tau abnormalities in neurons and glia, and a tau mutation has been identified in one kindred.[69] Thus, there are sporadic and familial forms of PSG.

Diagnosis   Clinical features have varied from ones typical of frontotemporal dementia to those of PSP.[65–67,69–72] No clinical or radiographic features have been identified to be characteristic of PSG.

Management   Treatment is directed at problematic symptoms or behaviors (Appendix).

Argyrophilic grain disease

Background   Braak and Braak[73] have been instrumental in characterizing argyrophilic grains in the brains of patients who had a neurodegenerative disorder. If grains are present in patients who had dementia but there is no other marker of a neurodegenerative disorder, the term *argyrophilic grain disease* (AGD) or *Braak disease* is often used.[73] The grains are argyrophilic with standard stains and are immunoreactive to stains directed toward tau. Argyrophilic grains have been described in association with normal cognition, mild cognitive impairment, psychotic dementia, and several other neurodegenerative disorders.[74,75] Thus, the clinical significance and pathophysiological relevance of argyrophilic grains have not been defined entirely. No cases of familial AGD have been reported.

Diagnosis   No constellation of neurological signs or symptoms has been identified as characteristic of AGD.

Management   Treatment is directed at problematic symptoms or behaviors (Appendix).

"Frontotemporal dementia" with ubiquitin-positive inclusions

Background   Recent cases of FTD, with or without coexisting motor neuron disease, have been found to have intraneuronal inclusions that are ubiquitin-positive but tau-, amyloid-, synuclein-, and phos-

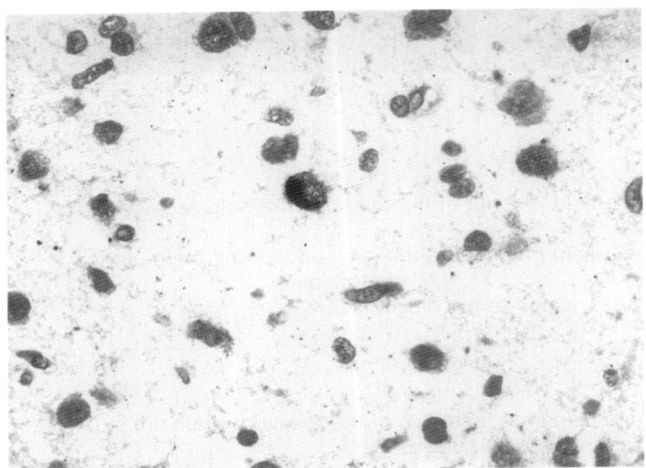

Figure 269.7   Intraneuronal inclusion (frontal cortex) that is positive for ubiquitin but negative for tau and α-synuclein associated with frontotemporal dementia (ubiquitin ×60). Courtesy Joseph E Parisi, MD. (See color plate section.)

phorylated neurofilament-negative[76] (Figure 269.7). Presumably, these immunocytochemical characteristics represent a pathophysiological process different from that of the tauopathies, amyloidopathies, and synucleinopathies.

Diagnosis   Most of the reported cases have had clinical features suggesting dysfunction of the frontotemporal neural networks, leading to the term *frontotemporal dementia*. However, some cases of ubiquitin-positive inclusions have clinical features maximally referable to posterior cerebral neural networks (Boeve et al., unpublished data). Therefore, the term *frontotemporal dementia* is not entirely accurate. Perhaps a more inclusive term such as *dementia with ubiquitin-positive inclusions* is more appropriate.

The clinical features are identical to those of some cases with dementia with tau-positive inclusions and those with no distinctive histopathological feature; thus, diagnosis can be established only by brain biopsy or autopsy.

Management   Treatment is directed at problematic symptoms or behaviors (Appendix).

Dementia lacking distinctive histopathology

Background   A small but important proportion of cases with degenerative dementia may not have any distinctive histopathological feature[77] (Figure 269.8). Although the application of immunocytochemistry (e.g., tau, phosphorylated neurofilament, and ubiquitin staining) over the past decade has permitted reclassification of some cases, many remain in this enigmatic category. Several terms have been applied to these cases, including *dementia lacking distinctive histopathology* (DLDH),[77,78] *nonspecific dementia*,[79] and *frontal lobe dementia of the non-Alzheimer type*.[80] Many cases have had coexisting motor neuron disease and a family history of dementia or motor neuron disease

(or both).[81,82] In one large family, DLDH has been linked to chromosome 3.[83]

Diagnosis   A wide spectrum of clinical syndromes has been been found to have DLDH, and no clinical criteria reliably predict nonspecific histopathological features.

Management   Treatment is directed at problematic symptoms or behaviors (Appendix).

Multiple system atrophy

Background   Striatonigral degeneration, olivopontocerebellar atrophy, and Shy-Drager syndrome variants form the multiple system atrophies (MSAs). The inclusions in oligodendroglia that are characteristic of

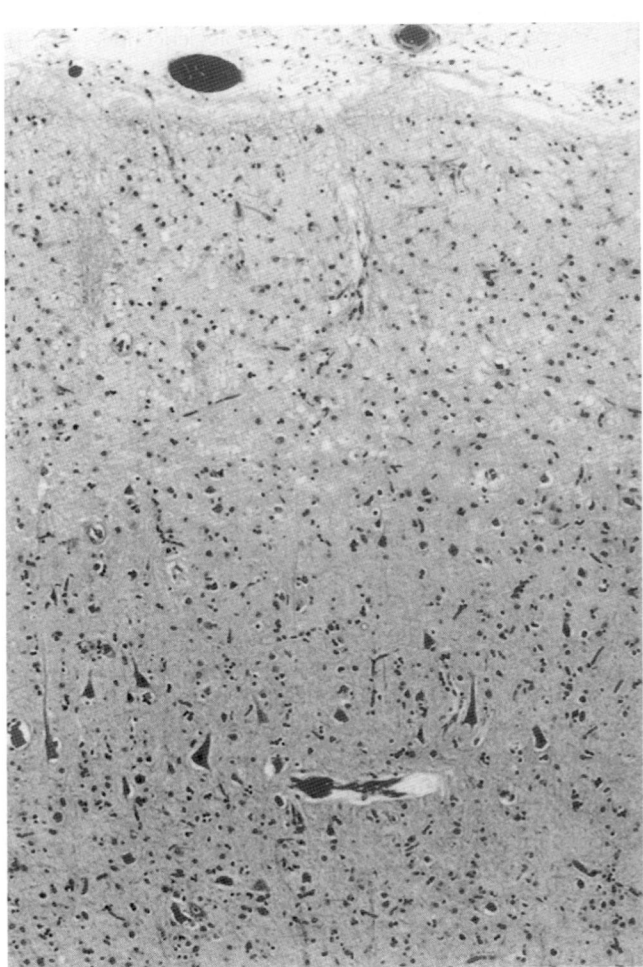

Figure 269.8   Marked neuronal loss, gliosis, and status spongiosis (frontal cortex) with no abnormalities revealed by tau, ubiquitin, α-synuclein, and prion immunocytochemistry, associated with parkinsonism and cognitive impairment— often termed "dementia lacking distinctive histopathology" (H&E ×25). From Boeve BF, Maraganore DM, Parisi JE, et al. Corticobasal degeneration and frontotemporal dementia presentations in a kindred with nonspecific histopathology. Dement Geriatr Cogn Disord 2002;13:80–90. By permission by S Karger AG, Basel. (See color plate section.)

MSA are immunoreactive to α-synuclein;[84] thus, MSA, PD, and DLB can be considered synucleinopathies.[85-87] Classically, functionally important cognitive impairment and cortical atrophy are not considered part of MSA, but rare cases of MSA have presented with progressive aphasia or frontal atrophy or both.[88,89]

Diagnosis For diagnosis of MSA, refer to Section XIII, on Movement Disorders. RBD is quite common in MSA[90] and the other two synucleinopathies, but it is rare or absent in the amyloidopathies and tauopathies (see below).[27] This may be relevant in understanding the pathophysiological mechanism of these disorders.

Management Treatment is directed at parkinsonism, orthostatism, and urinary incontinence. Nocturnal stridor is of concern whenever it develops in patients with MSA.[91] Because this high-pitched musical sound that occurs during inspiration represents dystonic closure of the vocal cords, patients are at risk of sudden death.[90,91] Thus, they should be referred for urgent polysomnography and a trial of nasal CPAP (continuous positive airway pressure) therapy (CPAP may maintain laryngeal patency) or for possible tracheostomy. For patients who have MSA with stridor and RBD, melatonin may be preferable to clonazepam.

Diagnosis and management of the human prion disorders

Creutzfeldt-Jakob disease

Background CJD has been applied to patients with rapidly progressive dementia who subsequently are found to have spongiform changes (Figure 269.9) and positive prion-protein immunostaining on neuropathological examination. The term *prion* was coined by Prusiner for *pro*teinaceous *in*fectious particles that appear to induce conformational changes in the prion protein that all humans have and ultimately cause neuronal death. There are sporadic, familial, and iatrogenic forms, and the so-called "new variant CJD" appears to be related to the ingestion of products from animals that previously had been fed contaminated food. GSS, FFI, and kuru are the three other prion disorders that affect humans.

Diagnosis The typical features of CJD include rapidly progressive dementia (time from onset of symptoms to death is often less than 1 year), myoclonus, and quasiperiodic sharp wave complexes on electroencephalography (Table 269.13).[92] Atypical presentations include clinical manifestations that reflect the topography of signal abnormalities on MRI or the distribution of spongiform changes on neuropathological examination, for example, progressive aphasia syndrome, frontal lobe dementia syndrome, progressive apraxia and rigidity (CBD syndrome), progressive visuoperceptual and visuospatial impairment syndrome (Heidenhain variant), and various neuropsychiatric presentations. Increased levels of

14-3-3 protein and neuron-specific enolase in the cerebrospinal fluid have been associated with CJD and may aid in diagnosis.[93] Increased signal changes on fluid attenuation inversion recovery (FLAIR) or diffusion-weighted magnetic resonance images may also

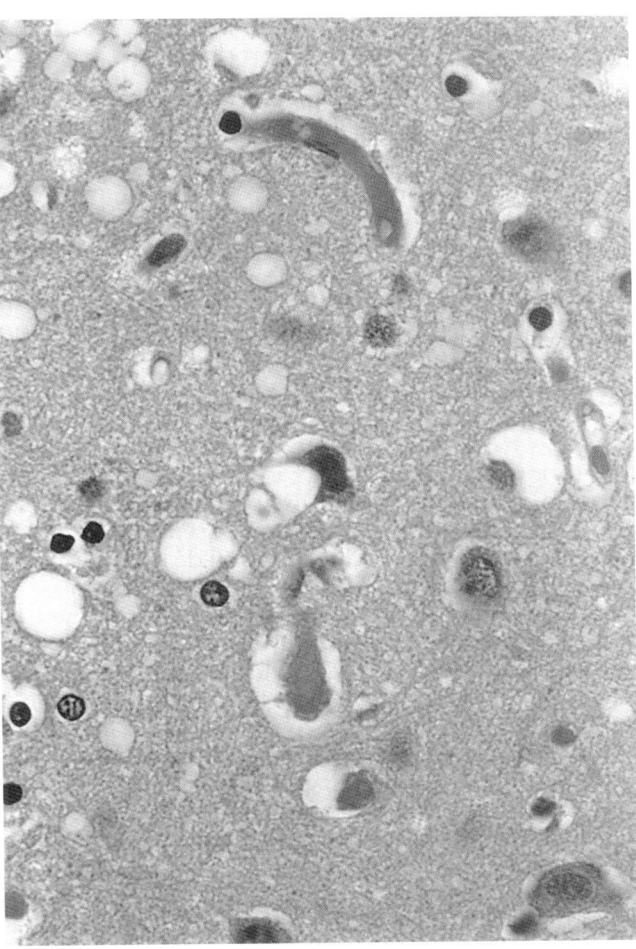

Figure 269.9 Marked spongiform changes characteristic of Creutzfeldt-Jakob disease (H&E ×150). Courtesy Joseph E Parisi, MD. (See color plate section.)

Table 269.13 Clinical diagnosis of Creutzfeldt-Jakob disease: World Health Organization criteria

Progressive dementia
At least two of the following findings:
  Myoclonus
  Visual or cerebral disturbance
  Pyramidal or extrapyramidal dysfunction
  Akinetic mutism
Characteristic electroencephalographic findings during an
  illness of any duration
  and/or
Positive assay for the 14-3-3 protein in cerebrospinal
  fluid and a fatal illness of less than 2 years' duration
Routine studies that do not suggest an alternative
  diagnosis

From World Health Organization.[92] By permission of the publisher.

be diagnostically relevant, particularly when the basal ganglia or cortical ribbon is involved.

Management No effective treatment directed against prion protein pathophysiology has been identified; thus, management is directed toward target symptoms or behaviors (Appendix). In many cases, involvement of a hospice is appropriate.

New variant Creutzfeldt-Jakob disease

Background Two cases of sporadic CJD in teenagers living in the United Kingdom (UK) were reported in 1995. Several additional cases with atypical clinical features were identified with most of the patients residing in the UK or France (none have been identified in the United States). The neuropathological findings of prion protein deposition in the cerebral and cerebellar cortices and the presence of so-called florid and multicentric plaques are atypical of sporadic CJD.[94] The clinical and histological features led to the term "new variant CJD" (nvCJD) for these cases. Analyses have established that the causative agent of the prion protein strain is bovine spongiform encephalopathy (BSE), also known as *mad cow disease*.[95] Cattle had been fed processed animal products that were unknowingly infected, and the cattle were then consumed by humans. This process of using animal products as cattle feed was banned in 1989, but because of the lengthy period from ingestion to clinical symptoms, nvCJD likely will continue to develop in humans for years to come.

Diagnosis Patients with nvCJD have tended to be younger than those with sporadic CJD, and the symptoms typically have been more "psychiatric," with depression, behavioral changes, apathy, delusions, and hallucinations.[96] Sensory symptoms have been common. Dementia usually evolves, as does myoclonus.[97] The duration of symptoms has generally been longer than for typical CJD, with some exceeding 3 years from onset to death.[98] Electroencephalographic findings are abnormal, but the quasiperiodic pattern of sharp wave complexes is rare. In several cases, signal changes in the posterior thalamus have been documented on MRI.[99] Examination of brain tissue or, more recently, tonsil tissue, establishes the diagnosis. The diagnostic criteria for nvCJD are listed in Table 269.14.[98]

Management No effective treatment is available for nvCJD; thus, management is directed toward target symptoms or behaviors (Appendix). In many cases, involvement of a hospice is appropriate.

Gerstmann-Straussler-Scheinker syndrome, fatal familial insomnia, and kuru

GSS and FFI are inherited prion disorders with an autosomal dominant pattern of inheritance. GSS typically presents with progressive cerebellar ataxia, pyramidal tract dysfunction, lower limb areflexia, and, later, dementia. In comparison, progressive insomnia dominates FFI. Progressive cerebellar ataxia

Table 269.14 Diagnostic criteria for new variant Creutzfeldt-Jakob disease (nvCJD): criteria of Will et al.

I   A. Progressive neuropsychiatric disorder
     B. Duration of illness >6 months
     C. Investigations do not suggest alternative diagnosis
     D. No history of potential iatrogenic exposure

II   A. Early psychiatric symptoms such as depression, anxiety, apathy, withdrawal, or delusions
     B. Persistent painful sensory symptoms such as frank pain or dysesthesia
     C. Ataxia
     D. Myoclonus or chorea or dystonia
     E. Dementia

III A. EEG does not show generalized triphasic periodic complexes at approximately 1/s or no EEG performed
     B. Bilateral pulvinar high signal on MRI
     Definite nvCJD: IA and neuropathological confirmation of nvCJD (i.e., spongiform change and extensive prion protein deposition with florid plaques throughout cerebrum and cerebellum)
     Probable nvCJD: I and 4/5 of II and IIIA and IIIB
     Possible nvCJD: I and 4/5 of II and IIIA

EEG, electroencephalography; MRI, magnetic resonance imaging.
From Will et al.[98] By permission of John Wiley & Sons.

is the principal manifestation of kuru, which now is nearly nonexistent since the canaballistic practices of the Fore people of New Guinea ceased. No disease-altering treatment exists for any of these disorders, and for GSS and FFI, management is symptomatic (Appendix).

Diagnosis and management of the focal or asymmetrical cortical degeneration syndromes

Many persons present with signs and symptoms that reflect focal or asymmetrical cortical dysfunction, and most of the degenerative and prion disorders can manifest in this manner. Various terms have been applied to these cases (Table 269.15). This classification scheme is adapted from Caselli.[100–103]

Although most patients have a preponderance of features that fit one of these syndromes, some have features that overlap two or more syndromes, and many have additional features that develop as their illness progresses. Also, parkinsonism or motor neuron disease (or both) can evolve in most of the syndromes. An intriguing and unexplained feature of focal and asymmetrical cortical degeneration syndromes is that the initial features reflect focal cortical dysfunction and, with time, additional features evolve that correspond to an expanding focus of ipsilateral cortical dysfunction or to cortical dysfunction involving the homologous region in the contralateral hemisphere. The manner in which cortical degeneration evolves varies, making counseling of patients and families difficult.

Table 269.15   Classification of clinical syndromes caused by neurodegenerative disorders

Mild cognitive impairment
Progressive amnesic syndrome

Frontotemporal dementia
Progressive neuropsychiatric syndrome
Progressive frontal network syndrome
Progressive dysexecutive syndrome

Primary progressive aphasia
Progressive aphasia syndrome
Progressive nonfluent aphasia
Semantic dementia
Associative agnosia

Corticobasal degeneration syndrome
Progressive perceptual-motor syndrome
Progressive apraxia and rigidity syndrome

Posterior cortical atrophy
Progressive visuoperceptual syndrome
Progressive posterior cortical syndrome
Progressive simultanagnosia or Balint syndrome

Mild cognitive impairment or progressive amnesic syndrome

Background   Patients with prominent forgetfulness but not frank dementia that has evolved insidiously and progressively worsened very likely have dysfunction in one or both mesial temporal lobes, and such patients often have features in keeping with the syndrome of mild cognitive impairment (MCI). While most individuals with MCI likely have evolving AD, argyrophilic grains and neurofibrillary tangles restricted in the mesial temporal lobes have been identified in MCI patients who have undergone autopsy.[104]

Diagnosis   The criteria for MCI are shown in Table 269.16; MCI is discussed in more detail in Chapter 268.

Management   Several therapeutic trials are currently in progress to test whether cholinesterase inhibitors or antioxidants can improve cognition or delay or prevent progression to dementia.

Table 269.16   Clinical diagnosis of mild cognitive impairment: Mayo Clinic criteria

Core features
A memory complaint
Normal activities of daily living
Normal general cognitive functioning
Abnormal memory functioning for age
   and
Patient is *not* demented by DSM-III-R criteria

DSM-III-R, Diagnostic and Statistical Manual of Mentol Disorders, III, Revised.
Data from Petersen RC, Smith GE, Waring SC, et al. Mild cognitive impairment: Clinical characterization and outcome. Arch Neurol 1999;56:303–308.

Progressive neuropsychiatric syndrome, progressive frontal network syndrome, progressive dysexecutive syndrome, frontotemporal dementia

Background   Several terms have been applied to a progressive neuropsychiatric syndrome indicative of frontal network dysfunction. These include *frontal lobe dementia, dementia of the frontal lobe type, dysexecutive syndrome*, and, the term used most often, *frontotemporal dementia* (FTD). Several disorders can present with features of FTD, especially disorders with tau-positive inclusions, ubiquitin-positive inclusions, and nonspecific histopathological features. A family history positive for dementia, parkinsonism, or motor neuron disease can often be elicited, parkinsonism or motor neuron disease can develop in patients with FTD. Several kindreds with familial FTD or parkinsonism (or both) have been found to have a mutation in the tau gene on chromosome 17,[105] and one large family has had dementia with nonspecific histological features linked to chromosome 3.[83] Numerous other kindreds with autosomal dominant FTD do not have tau mutations; thus there are likely to be mutations in yet-to-be identified genes that lead to FTD.

Diagnosis   In 1994, investigators in Sweden and England proposed clinical criteria for diagnosis of FTD.[106] These criteria were revised in 1998 with input from other clinicians (Table 269.17).[107]

Patients with marked degeneration in the nondominant (usually right) frontotemporal cortex tend to exhibit more behavioral problems and neuropsychiatric features.[108] For reasons unknown, some patients with FTD develop artistic talent beyond what they exhibited before the onset of cognitive or behavioral symptoms.[109] Also, appreciation of previously uninteresting or disliked forms of music has been reported.[110,111]

Management   No therapy has been developed that halts or delays the progression of neurodegeneration in the disorders that present with FTD. Management is tailored to address symptoms (Appendix). Various symptoms and behaviors can evolve and many can be difficult to manage. Support for caregivers is critical. The only trial specifically designed for FTD suggested that selective serotonin reuptake inhibitors can be beneficial for treating disinhibition, depressive symptoms, and compulsions.[112]

Progressive aphasia syndrome, primary progressive aphasia, progressive nonfluent aphasia, semantic dementia and associative agnosia

Background   In 1982, Mesulam[113] first described a series of patients who had aphasia without dementia, and later, he introduced the term *primary progressive aphasia* (PPA). Data have since been published on numerous other patients.[102,103,113,114] Although several subgroups have been described,[102,103] the clinical presentations fall into two main categories that are separable by fluency. Patients with nonfluent aphasia often have apraxia of speech and nonverbal oral apraxia and, in our experience, have a striking

Table 269.17   Clinical diagnosis of frontotemporal dementia: consensus criteria, 1998

Core features
Insidious onset and gradual progression
Early decline in social interpersonal conduct
Early impairment in regulation of personal conduct
Early emotional blunting
Early loss of insight
Instrumental functions of perception, spatial skills, praxis, and memory are intact or relatively well preserved

Supportive features
Behavioral disorder
Decline in personal hygiene and grooming
Mental rigidity and inflexibility
Distractibility and impersistence
Hyperorality and dietary changes
Perseverative and stereotyped behavior
Utilization behavior

Speech and language
Altered speech output
Aspontaneity and economy of speech
Press of speech
Stereotype of speech
Echolalia
Perseveration
Mutism

Physical signs
Primitive reflexes
Incontinence
Akinesia, rigidity, and tremor
Low and labile blood pressure

Investigations
Neuropsychology: significant impairment on frontal lobe tests in the absence of severe amnesia, aphasia, or perceptuospatial disorder
Electroencephalography: normal on conventional electroencephalogram despite clinically evident dementia
Brain imaging (structural and/or functional): predominant frontal and/or anterior temporal abnormality

From Neary et al.[107] By permission of the American Academy of Neurology.

tendency to say "yes" for "no" and vice versa. Structural or functional neuroimaging studies show abnormalities involving the frontal opercular area (area of Broca) or insula in the dominant hemisphere. The same spectrum of disorders that presents with FTD can manifest as progressive nonfluent aphasia-apraxia of speech. Patients with fluent aphasia typically have marked dysnomia, and imaging studies show that the dominant temporal lobe (often most evident in the inferolateral temporal cortex) can be involved anywhere from the anterior pole to the posterior perirolandic area. The phenomenology of the language disturbance in many patients with fluent aphasia includes the terms *semantic dementia* and *semantic aphasia*.

Some patients develop difficulties recognizing objects (visual agnosia) or faces (prosopagnosia), but auditory cues, for example, shaking a ring of keys or having a

person speak, allow the patient to recognize the object or person. It is important for clinicians to differentiate anomia from agnosia from visuoperceptual impairment in patients with impaired naming of objects or beings. Patients who cannot state the name of an object or a being but can demonstrate how the object is used or state identifying features of a being likely have anomia. Those who are unable to recognize an object or being but can describe the various aspects of an object or being likely have agnosia. Visual or associative agnosia refers to stimuli that are stripped of their meaning.

Controversy still exists about the minimal brain lesion necessary to cause prosopagnosia. For years, bilateral dysfunction of the inferior temporo-occipital cortex was considered necessary for prosopagnosia.[115] A detailed case report of a patient with prosopagnosia associated with right anterior temporal dysfunction (indicated by functional neuroimaging) suggests that this type of visual agnosia can occur with unilateral temporal lobe dysfunction.[116]

AD occurs more frequently in patients with fluent aphasia, and the tauopathies and nonspecific histopathology typically occur in those without AD. Some patients can have a protracted course, with features restricted to aphasia or agnosia, while others develop features of FTD or CBD or appear clinically indistinguishable from patients with AD in later stages. Parkinsonism or motor neuron disease can evolve; the latter portends a more rapid course.[117]

Diagnosis   The diagnostic criteria for PPA,[118] progressive nonfluent aphasia,[107] and semantic dementia and associative agnosia[107] are listed in Tables 269.18, 269.19, and 269.20, respectively.

Table 269.18   Diagnostic criteria for primary progressive aphasia

Core features
- Insidious onset and gradual progression of word finding, object-naming, or word-comprehension impairments as manifested during spontaneous conversation or as assessed through formal neuropsychological tests of language
- All limitations of daily living activities are attributable to the language impairment, for at least 2 years after onset
- Intact premorbid language function (except for developmental dyslexia)
- Absence of significant apathy, disinhibition, forgetfulless for recent events, visuospatial impairment, visual recognition deficits or sensory-motor dysfunction within the initial 2 years of the illness
- Acalculia and ideomotor apraxia may be present even in the first 2 years
- Other domains possibly affected after the first 2 years but with language remaining the most impaired function throughout the course of the illness and deteriorating faster than other affected domains
- Absence of "specific" causes such as stroke or tumor as ascertained by neuroimaging

From Mesulam.[118] By permission of John Wiley & Sons.

Table 269.19 Clinical diagnosis of progressive nonfluent aphasia: consensus criteria, 1998

Core features
Insidious onset and gradual progression
Disorder of expressive language is the dominant feature initially and throughout the disease course
Nonfluent spontaneous speech with at least one of the following: agrammatism, phonemic paraphasias, anomia
Other aspects of cognition are intact or relatively well preserved

Supportive features
Speech and language
Stuttering or oral apraxia
Impaired repetition
Alexia, agraphia
Early preservation of word meaning
Late mutism

Behavior
Early preservation of social skills
Late behavioral changes similar to those of frontotemporal dementia

Physical signs
Late contralateral primitive reflexes, akinesia, rigidity, and tremor

Investigations
Neuropsychology: nonfluent aphasia in the absence of severe amnesia or perceptuospatial disorder
Electroencephalography: normal or minor asymmetrical slowing
Brain imaging (structural and/or functional): asymmetrical abnormality predominantly affecting dominant (usually left) hemisphere

From Neary et al.[107] By permission of the American Academy of Neurology.

Table 269.20 Clinical diagnosis of semantic dementia and associative agnosia: consensus criteria, 1998

Core features
Insidious onset and gradual progression
Language disorder characterized by:
    Progressive, fluent, empty spontaneous speech
    Loss of word meaning, manifested by impaired naming and comprehension
    Semantic paraphasias
and/or
Perceptual disorder characterized by:
    Prosopagnosia—impaired recognition of identity of familiar faces
and/or
    Associative agnosia—impaired recognition of object identity
Preserved perceptual matching and drawing reproduction
Preserved single-word repetition
Preserved ability to read aloud and write to dictation orthographically regular words
Autobiographical memory is intact or relatively well-preserved

Supportive features
Speech and language
Press of speech
Idiosyncratic word usage
Absence of phonemic paraphasias
Surface dyslexia and dysgraphia
Preserved calculation

Behavior
Loss of sympathy and empathy
Narrowed preoccupations
Parsimony

Physical signs
Absent or late primitive reflexes
Akinesia, rigidity, and tremor

Investigations
Neuropsychology
Profound semantic loss, manifest in failure of word comprehension and naming and/or face and object recognition
Preserved phonology and syntax, and elementary perceptual processing, spatial skills, and day-to-day memorizing
Electroencephalography—normal
Brain imaging (structural and/or functional)—predominantly anterior temporal abnormality (symmetrical or asymmetrical)

From Neary et al.[107] By permission of the American Academy of Neurology.

Management Speech therapy can help many patients. For those with moderate to severe nonfluent aphasia, therapy with communication devices is warranted. No drug treatment has been shown to improve aphasia or agnosia.

Corticobasal degeneration syndrome, progressive perceptual-motor syndrome, progressive asymmetrical rigidity and apraxia syndrome

Background Although the core syndrome of progressive asymmetrical rigidity and apraxia has been considered characteristic of underlying CBD, about one-half of the patients with this syndrome in one series were found to have CBD, whereas the others had either AD, Pick disease, PSP, DLDH, or CJD.[119] Thus, it is presumptive and often incorrect to label these patients with the pathological diagnosis of CBD, and syndromic nomenclature would be more appropriate. The terms applied to these cases have included *progressive perceptual-motor syndrome, progressive asymmetrical rigidity and apraxia* (PARA syndrome), and *corticobasal degeneration* (CBD) syndrome.

Diagnosis Our original diagnostic criteria have been modified,[43] and the criteria given in Table 269.21

should be considered for the clinical diagnosis of the CBD syndrome.

Management Management is described above.

Posterior cortical atrophy, progressive visuoperceptual syndrome, progressive posterior cortical syndrome, progressive simultanagnosia, Balint syndrome

Background Visual agnosia is related to dysfunction in the ventral, or "What," pathway of complex visual

Table 269.21   Clinical diagnosis of corticobasal degeneration syndrome: proposed criteria

Core features
No identifiable cause (e.g., tumor, infarct) and at least three of the following:
Progressive course ⎫
Asymmetrical distribution ⎬ "PARA" syndrome
Rigidity ⎪
Apraxia ⎭

Supportive features
Cortical
Alien limb phenomenon
Cortical sensory loss
Constructional dyspraxia
Hemineglect
Focal or asymmetrical appendicular myoclonus
Mirror movements
    and/or

Extrapyramidal
Focal or asymmetrical appendicular dystonia
Focal or asymmetrical appendicular postural/action tremor
Lack of prominent and sustained levodopa response

Investigations
Impaired verbal fluency, visuospatial functioning, praxis on neuropsychometric testing
Focal or asymmetrical parietofrontal atrophy on CT or MRI
Focal or asymmetrical parietofrontal ± basal ganglia ± thalamic hypoperfusion on SPECT
Focal or asymmetrical parietofrontal ± basal ganglia ± thalamic hypometabolism on PET

CT, computed tomography; EEG, electroencephalography; MRI, magnetic resonance imaging; PET, positron emission tomography; SPECT, single photon emission computed tomography

progressive posterior cortical syndrome, posterior cortical atrophy, and *progressive simultanagnosia/Balint syndrome*.[102,103,121] The neuritic plaques and neurofibrillary tangles of AD rarely are most dense in the posterior cerebrum, but in patients with a progressive visuoperceptual-visuospatial syndrome, AD has been the most frequently identified histopathologic process. Nonspecific histopathology, progressive subcortical gliosis, CBD, and CJD have also been reported.[102,103,121]

Diagnosis   The criteria proposed for the diagnosis of posterior cortical atrophy (progressive visuoperceptual syndrome) are listed in Table 269.22.

Table 269.22   Clinical diagnosis of posterior cortical atrophy (progressive visuoperceptual syndrome): proposed criteria

Core features
Features are insidious in onset and course is progressive
Features cannot be accounted for by primary ocular abnormality (requires ophthalmological evaluation)
Two or more of the following symptoms:
    Unable to follow lines while reading
    Poor depth perception
    Often fails to appreciate objects in direction of gaze
    Unable to navigate in stores, while driving, in own home (spatial/geographic disorientation)
    Illusions
    Hallucinations
    Misidentification errors
    Micropsia
    Macropsia
    Metamorphopsia
Two or more of the following signs:
    Quadrant or hemifield defect
    Achromatopsia in quadrant or hemifield
    Hemispatial neglect
    Constructional dyspraxia
    Simultanagnosia
    Ocular apraxia
    Optic ataxia
    Cortical blindness

Supportive features
Relatively preserved visual acuity early
Preserved insight and expressive language functioning
No important behavioral abnormalities or memory impairment early in course
Absence of focal motor findings, parkinsonism, or frontal release signs early in course

Investigations
Neuropsychological deficits referable to parietal and/or occipital cortex dysfunction
No infarct, tumor, abscess, or other space-occupying lesion present on CT or MRI
Focal or asymmetrical atrophy in parietal and/or occipital cortex on CT or MRI
Focal or asymmetrical hypoperfusion/hypometabolism in parietal and/or occipital cortex on SPECT/PET

CT, computed tomography; MRI, magnetic resonance imaging; PET, positron emission tomography; SPECT, single photon emission computed tomography.

processing. All or parts of Balint syndrome correspond to dysfunction in the dorsal, or "Where," pathway. Overt visuoperceptual deficits are associated with abnormalities in the primary visual cortex or visual association cortex. Patients with simultanagnosia (the inability to grasp the gestalt of a visual image) or Balint syndrome (simultanagnosia, optic ataxia, and ocular apraxia) often present to ophthalmologists complaining of blurred vision, poor depth perception, inability to follow lines while reading, and so forth.[120] Those with frank visuoperceptual problems can experience micropsia (images appear smaller than they actually are), macropsia (images appear larger than they actually are), metmorphopsia (images appear to change shape or texture), illusions (objects appear to be images different from the actual objects, for example, perceiving a chair to be an animal), and hallucinations. Occasionally, delusional overtones develop and one's reflection in a mirror may be interpreted as an intruder in the house, or Capgras syndrome evolves (believing a person has been replaced by an identical-appearing impostor). Visual field defects or cortical blindness develops in some patients. Several terms have been used to describe these conditions, including *progressive visuoperceptual syndrome*,

Management Except for atypical neuroleptics to manage hallucinations and delusions and antidepressant agents to treat depression (which is common in this syndrome because insight is often preserved), no therapy has been shown to improve any of the features. Clinical experience indicates that some patients benefit from symptomatic therapy (Appendix).

Clinicopathological correlations in focal and asymmetrical cortical degeneration syndromes and implications for pathogenesis

The underlying theme in the syndromic classification schemes is that clinical manifestations reflect the topography of cerebral dysfunction more than specific neurodegenerative disorders do. That is, several neurodegenerative disorders can manifest as the same clinical syndrome, and each neurodegenerative disorder can present as various clinical syndromes. A summary of the clinicopathological correlations in the focal and asymmetrical cortical degeneration syndromes is shown in Figure 269.10. A few cases with PSG and AGD have also been identified (not shown in Figure 269.10). This clinicopathological heterogeneity has complicated the study of distinct neurodegenerative disorders and has given impetus to the identification of specific biomarkers.

Several interesting questions stem from this heterogeneity. If several patients can manifest the same clinical syndrome yet have different underlying histopathological processes, could there still be a common genetic or environmental factor that affects the topography of degeneration similarly? In the familial prion disorders, the genotype at codon 178 confers pathogenicity but the genotype at codon 129 seems to confer the topography of dysfunction, so that the genotype valine/valine leads to cerebral cortical dysfunction and, hence, cortical clinical findings of CJD; however, the genotype methionine/methionine leads to thalamic dysfunction and, thus, the features of fatal insomnia.[122] One could speculate that particular genotypes confer pathogenicity and that similar polymorphisms in the amyloidopathies, tauopathies, prionopathies, and nonspecific histopathological disorders are responsible for the varying clinical presentations of these disorders. Why do members of a kindred with the same pathological mutation exhibit widely varied clinical manifestations? Do polymorphisms or environmental factors or both influence the topography of neurodegeneration, leading to the varying clinical manifestations? These critical questions have not been answered.

Although most neurodegenerative disorders can present in a focal or asymmetrical fashion, synucleinopathies rarely do, and the course of CJD is often rapid enough to differentiate it from the other

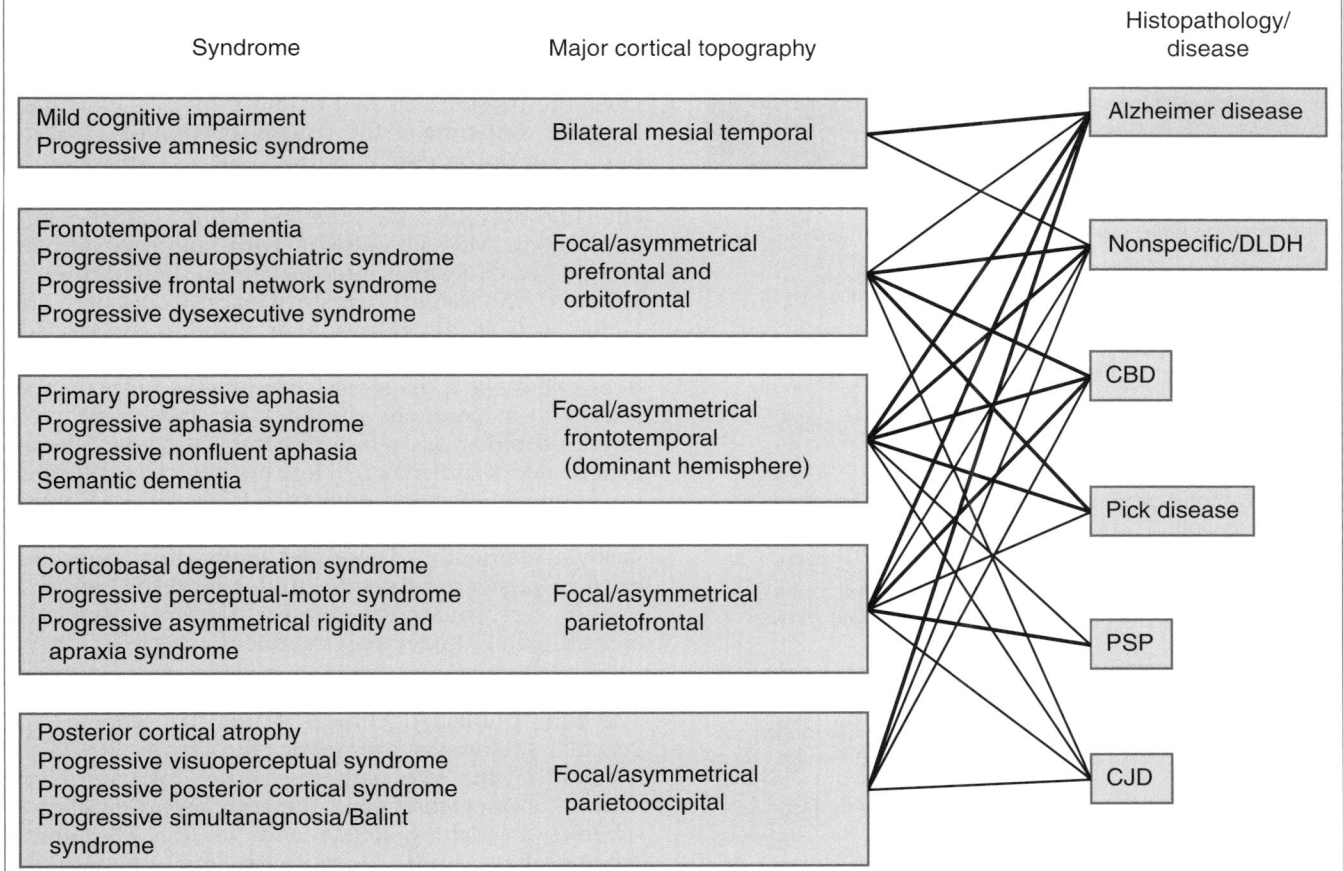

Figure 269.10 Associations between the focal and asymmetrical cortical degeneration syndromes and their corresponding cortical topographies and underlying histopathological features/diseases.

disorders. Thus, cases that present with focal and asymmetrical cortical dysfunction over several years typically represent an amyloidopathy or a tauopathy, or have nonspecific histopathological features. Furthermore, AD tends to underlie the syndromes associated with more posterior cerebral dysfunction, and non-AD tauopathies and nonspecific histopathological disorders occur in syndromes associated with anterior cerebral dysfunction.

Future directions in the management of the degenerative dementias and prion disease

The advances in molecular genetics and molecular biology have led to remarkable changes in our understanding of degenerative and prion-related dementing illnesses. A major shift is evolving in which the pathophysiological processes are becoming increasingly relevant for drug development rather than clinical characterization. One scheme is presented in Table 269.23.[86,87,123]

Immunological therapies, such as the ones currently directed against β-amyloid, represent exciting developments in the treatment of AD.[124,125] If a preventive or disease-altering therapy is developed against the cascade of events leading to tau dysfunction and neurodegeneration, it potentially could be helpful in most or all tauopathies. A similar approach may be key for the synucleinopathies and prionopathies. Because the tau protein abnormalities in AD are different from those in non-AD tauopathies, an effective treatment for AD or for non-AD tauopathies may not be helpful in the other. No genetic or biochemical abnormalities have been found in the nonspecific processes, but it is reasonable to assume that mutations in key genes may lead to immunocytochemical applications similar to what has happened in the amyloidopathies, tauopathies, and synucleinopathies, allowing reclassification of these cases into one or more categories. Of utmost importance is improving the accuracy in identifying the disease or pathophysiological process that underlies a degenerative disorder; reliance on clinical criteria, neuropsychometric findings, radiological findings, or some combination of these have been inadequate. It is hoped that the identification of certain markers of early or presymptomatic disease and refinements in biomarker technology eventually will allow clinicians to direct more effective therapies against these disorders.

Diagnosis and management of vascular dementia

Background

Vascular dementia is an enigmatic area in dementia care and research. Although it is clear that infarcts in important structures such as the thalamus and various cortical regions can cause cognitive impairment and impairment in the various cognitive domains correlates with the topographic distribution of infarcts, there are several lingering uncertainties. Does the presence of two or more infarcts constitute vascular dementia if the course of cognitive decline has been progressive rather than step-wise? If leukoariosis is so common in the cognitively normal elderly, how does one interpret white matter abnormalities on MRI in patients with cognitive impairment? How does one interpret severe leukoariosis in patients who have no history of any vascular risk factor such as hypertension or diabetes mellitus? Is Binswanger disease a discrete disorder, and if so, how does one make a diagnosis clinically? Is hippocampal sclerosis—a frequent finding in the cognitively impaired oldest old—due to cerebrovascular disease or repeated hypotension? How are clinicians expected to diagnose vascular dementia if there is so much debate about what does and what does not constitute vascular dementia? These and many other questions must be answered to better understand the contribution to cerebrovascular disease-associated dementia and ultimately to develop treatment.

Diagnosis

The four published clinical diagnostic schemes for vascular dementia are given in Tables 269.24 to 269.27;[126–129] the two pathological sets of criteria are shown in association with the corresponding clinical schemes in Tables 269.24 and 269.25. All clinical schemes have limited sensitivity, and although the Hachinski Ischemic Scale was developed (in 1975) long before the others, it was shown recently to have the highest sensitivity.[130]

Table 269.23 Classification of neurodegenerative and prion disorders based on presumed pathophysiological mechanism according to Hardy and Gwinn-Hardy[86,87,123]

Amyloidopathies
Alzheimer disease (sporadic and familial forms)

Tauopathies
Alzheimer disease (sporadic and familial forms)
Pick disease (sporadic and familial forms)
Corticobasal degeneration (sporadic and familial forms)
Progressive supranuclear palsy (sporadic and familial forms)
Progressive subcortical gliosis (sporadic and familial forms)
Argyrophilic grain disease
Frontotemporal dementia with parkinsonism linked to chromosome 17 (familial form)

Synucleinopathies
Parkinson disease (sporadic and some familial forms)
Dementia with Lewy bodies (sporadic and some familial forms)
Multiple system atrophy

Prionopathies
Creutzfeldt-Jakob disease (sporadic and familial forms)
Gerstmann-Strausser-Schenker (sporadic and familial forms)
Fatal familial insomnia (sporadic and familial forms)

Nonspecific undefined
Dementia lacking distinctive histopathology (sporadic and familial forms)
Frontotemporal dementia

Table 269.24   Clinical and pathological diagnosis of vascular dementia: NINDS-AIREN criteria

Probable vascular dementia
Dementia
Cerebrovascular disease present—defined as
    Presence of focal neurological signs
        (e.g., hemiparesis, lower facial weakness, Babinski
        sign, hemianopia, sensory deficit, dysarthria)
        consistent with stroke; history of stroke not necessary
        and
    CT or MRI evidence of infarcts, including multiple
        large-vessel infarcts, single strategically placed
        infarct, or multiple basal ganglia or white matter
        lacunes
Onset of dementia within 3 months after stroke or abrupt
    deterioration of cognitive function or functioning
    stepwise course

Alzheimer disease with vascular dementia
Possible Alzheimer disease by NINDS-ADRDA criteria
Clinical or imaging evidence for relevant cerebrovascular
    disease

Definite vascular dementia
Probable vascular dementia, according to core features
Cerebrovascular disease by histopathology
Absence of neurofibrillary tangles or neuritic plaques
    exceeding those expected for age
Absence of other clinical or pathological disorders
    capable of producing dementia

Data from Roman et al.[126]

Management

Management can be divided into strategies for 1) decreasing the risk of subsequent cerebrovascular disease, 2) improving cognition once vascular dementia is present, and 3) managing target symptoms. Hypertension, hyperlipidemia, and diabetes should be optimally treated to minimize the risk of cerebrovascular events. Patients with atrial fibrillation, congestive heart disease, patent foramen ovale, thoracic aortic debris or other risk factor should be given appropriate stroke prophylaxis. Tobacco use should be discouraged.[131] Although hypotension has been implicated in hippocampal sclerosis[132]—arguably a type of vascular dementia—no evidence suggests that maintaining or increasing blood pressure will delay or prevent progression of dementia or positively influence cognition. Ergoloids (Hydergine)—agents with vasodilatory effects—have been shown to modestly improve functional and neuropsychological status, particularly when prescribed at higher doses for patients with vascular dementia.[133] Modest improvement has also been demonstrated with *Ginko biloba*,[134–137] although clinicians should be aware of the rare occurrence of intracerebral hemorrhage with this agent.[138] Few reports have documented the efficacy of cholinesterase inhibitors in managing vascular dementia.[139] Other agents that have shown promise in treating vascular dementia include nimodipine (a calcium channel antagonist),[140,141] nicardipine (a calcium channel antagonist),[142] propentofylline (an agent that inhibits glutamate release and free radical production),[143–151] pentoxifylline (an agent that affects red blood cell deformability, platelet aggregation, and blood viscosity),[152–154] buflomedil (a vasodilating agent),[155] α-glycerylphosphorylcholine and cytosine diphosphocholine,[156] and memantine (an *N*-methyl-D-aspartate [NMDA] antagonist).[157,158] Clinicians can also consider therapy for management of target symptoms (Appendix).

Table 269.25   Clinical and pathological diagnosis of ischemic vascular dementia: ADDTC (California) criteria

Probable ischemic vascular dementia
Dementia by DSM-III-R criteria
Two or more strokes by history/examination and/or CT or
    T₁-weighted MRI
        or
Single stroke with clear temporal relationship to onset of
    dementia
Presence of at least one infarct outside cerebellum by CT
    or T₁-weighted MRI

Possible ischemic vascular dementia
Dementia by DSM-III-R criteria
Single stroke with temporal relationship to dementia
    or
Binswanger defined as all the following:
    Early onset incontinence or gait disturbance not
        explained by peripheral cause
    Vascular risk factors
    Extensive white matter changes on neuroimaging

Mixed dementia
Evidence of Alzheimer disease or other disease on
    pathology exam plus probable, possible, or definite
    ischemic vascular dementia
One or more systemic or brain diseases contributing to
    patient's dementia in the presence of probable,
    possible, or definite ischemic vascular dementia

Definite ischemic vascular dementia
Dementia
Multiple infarcts outside the cerebellum on
    neuropathology exam

DSM-III-R, Diagnostic and Statistical Manual of Mental
Disorders.
Modified from Chui et al.[127] By permission of the American
Academy of Neurology.

Table 269.26   Clinical diagnosis of vascular dementia: DSM-IV criteria

Core features
Impaired memory
At least 1 of
    Aphasia
    Apraxia
    Agnosia
    Impaired executive functioning
Symptoms impair work, social, or personal functioning
Symptoms do not occur solely during delirium
Cerebral vascular disease has probably caused the
    above deficits, as judged by laboratory data or by focal
    neurological signs and symptoms

Modified from American Psychiatric Association.[128] By
permission of the American Psychiatric Association.

Table 269.27   Clinical diagnosis of vascular dementia: Hachinski ischemia scale*

Feature	No. of points
Abrupt onset	2
Stepwise progression	1
Fluctuating course	2
Nocturnal confusion	1
Relative preservation of personality	1
Depression	1
Somatic complaints	1
Emotional incontinence	1
History of hypertension	1
History of strokes	2
Associated atherosclerosis	1
Focal neurological symptoms	2
Focal neurological signs	2

Score >7, multi-infarct dementia; score <4, Alzheimer disease. From Hachinski et al.[129] By permission of the American Medical Association.

Management of target symptoms in dementia

Since no currently available therapy directly and importantly alters the pathophysiological processes causing dementia, management of dementia, regardless of the cause, typically is tailored toward target symptoms. Although most reports on the available agents have involved patients with clinically suspected AD, many of these agents may be helpful in the management of non-AD disorders. Readers are encouraged to review some key articles and texts on the management of problematic symptoms and behaviors in dementia.[159–162]

In the office, a helpful exercise is to ask patients and their caregivers to cite and to rank by priority the symptoms or features they want most to alter. Initial therapy can be directed at the issue of top priority, and if this is better managed with therapy, then therapy can be directed toward the next most important issue, and so forth. Therapies for important symptoms and behaviors are described below; specific drugs and dosing suggestions are given in the Appendix.

Amnesia and forgetfulness

Cholinesterase inhibitors were developed to improve memory; however, because in AD and DLB the cholinergic neurons of the basal forebrain degenerate, progressively less and less acetylcholine is available to affect therapeutically as the illness worsens. Because neuronal death is comparatively less in DLB than in AD, the response to cholinesterase inhibitor therapy can be impressive in some patients with DLB.[11–14] Presumably, agents with nicotinic or muscarinic (or both) receptor agonist activity would be most likely to improve memory; however, preliminary studies have suggested that the systemic effects are too intolerable for many patients. Cholinergic agonists that are selective for the central nervous system may offer the most benefit for amnesia and forgetfulness. Some patients and their families have noticed improvement in forgetfulness with levodopa, modafinil, or methylphenidate therapy (Boeve, unpublished data).

Aphasia

Aphasia can result from dysfunction of the frontal, temporal, or parietal lobe of the dominant hemisphere as well as from lesions in the thalamus, basal ganglia, insula, and arcuate fasciculus. Aphasia is the core feature of the progressive aphasia syndromes, and aphasia can occur with AD, Pick disease, CBD, PSP, DLDH, CJD, and cerebrovascular insults. Speech therapy can improve communicability for some aphasic patients. When expressive language functions are severely compromised, specially designed devices can be helpful. No drug has been shown to improve aphasia.

Agnosia

Agnosia (the inability to recognize the meaning of stimuli) is characteristic of the associative agnosia syndrome, and it can occur in any of the cortical dementing disorders. No drug has been shown to improve agnosia.

Visuospatial and visuoperceptual dysfunction

Dysfunction in complex visual processing is characteristic of posterior cortical atrophy, and such dysfunction can occur in patients with DLB, CBD, AD, CJD, or DLDH. Ophthalmological consultation is reasonable for all patients with visuospatial and visuoperceptual dysfunction so that any potential ocular cause of visual impairment can be evaluated and treated. Otherwise, patients with marked impairment should not be allowed to drive or to operate machinery, and measures should be taken to minimize the potential for injury around the house. For patients who experience illusions, changing the illumination in rooms or removing problematic items from the house may minimize the illusions. Misidentification errors, particularly if they involve the spouse and children, can be troubling to family members; counseling the family on the dysfunction in complex visual processing may reduce the anxiety related to these errors. For those patients who are troubled by their own reflections in mirrors, covering the mirrors can suffice. Rarely, patients have shown improvement functionally and on neuropsychometric testing with cholinesterase inhibitor and levodopa therapy (Boeve, unpublished data). No drug has been shown in clinical studies to improve visuospatial and visuoperceptual dysfunction.

Dysexecutive syndrome and disinhibition

Inappropriate comments or gestures are the dread of many caregivers, particularly ones that have a sexual theme or are directed at children. Disinhibition is characteristic of FTD but can occur in other syndromes and diseases in which the frontal networks are dysfunctional. Atypical neuroleptics, antidepressants (particularly selective serotonin reuptake inhibitors), cholinesterase inhibitors, and anxiolytics can be effective.[14,112,163–167] If ineffective, avoidance of social settings may be the only way to minimize embarrassment due to inappropriate behavior.

Apathy

Apathy is common in FTD, but it also occurs with most dementing disorders. For example, a patient may look through a window or watch a monotonous TV channel for hours, or rarely initiate conversation or spontaneously perform activities around the house. Experience has shown that apathy can improve with treatment with psychostimulants, amantadine, levodopa, the dopamine agonists, buproprion, selegiline, or cholinesterase inhibitors as well as antidepressants when the apathy is part of depression.[14,163,168–171]

Hallucinations and delusions

Hallucinations and delusions are common in DLB and FTD, but they can occur in many other disorders and syndromes. Visual hallucinations are rarely present in CBD, and when they are associated with cognitive impairment and parkinsonism, their presence may suggest DLB rather than CBD.[48] If hallucinations or delusions are mild and visual and hearing impairment has been excluded as a cause, simple reassurance of the patient may be all that is necessary. When hallucinations or delusions are a problem, treatment with atypical neuroleptics and cholinesterase inhibitors can be beneficial.[13–19,21,22,168,172] Melatonin taken before bedtime has improved or eliminated visual hallucinations in some patients (Boeve, unpublished data). Levodopa, dopamine agonists, psychostimulants, amantadine, and selegiline should be used with caution, because each can aggravate psychotic features.

Agitation, aggression, and behavioral dyscontrol

Verbally and particularly physically aggressive behavior often leads to institutionalization. This behavior is also a problem in nursing homes. Behavioral dyscontrol can occur in all syndromes and disorders, particularly in the latter part of each illness. Traditionally, treatment has been with conventional neuroleptics and benzodiazepines, but atypical neuroleptics, cholinesterase inhibitors, carbamazepine, valproic acid, propranolol, or some combination of these is preferable.[13,23,24,168,173–202] If agitated depression is suspected, referral to a psychiatrist for consideration of electroconvulsive therapy is warranted.

Anxiety

Anxiety can occur in all the syndromes and disorders, and management can be challenging. Anxiolytics, antidepressants, cholinesterase inhibitors, and atypical neuroleptics, or some combination of these may be beneficial.[17,112,163,168,172,188]

Depression

Depression is common to all dementing disorders, and numerous effective antidepressant agents are available, although few have been studied in randomized, double-blind, placebo-controlled trials.[203–216] All these agents can have adverse cognitive or behavioral effects.[217,218] Agents with anticholinergic properties should be avoided, particularly tricyclic antidepressants. The presence of dementia should not preclude the use of electroconvulsive therapy if other therapies have not been effective.

Emotional lability and pseudobulbar affect

Frontosubcortical network dysfunction regardless of the underlying histopathological process can lead to emotional lability, with tearfulness induced by minimally emotional stimuli (pseudobulbar affect) being more common than excessive jocularity. If emotional lability is socially embarrassing, treatment with selective serotonin reuptake inhibitors can be effective; lithium therapy has also been suggested.[219–222] Although tricyclic antidepressants also minimize a pseudobulbar affect, the benefit must be weighed against the anticholinergic effects.

Urinary incontinence

The supratentorial control of continence has strong input from the frontal lobes; thus, incontinence often occurs in patients with frontal lobe dysfunction. Nearly all patients with dementia develop incontinence terminally. If urinary studies exclude an infection and urological evaluation does not reveal a treatable cause in the genitourinary structures, agents with anticholinergic properties can improve incontinence, but the improvement must be considered in the context of possible diminished cholinergic activity in the cerebral cortex.[223–225]

Insomnia

In patients, insomnia can result from primary insomnia (includes psychophysiological insomnia and inadequate sleep hygiene), restless legs syndrome, or central sleep apnea syndrome. In a caregiver, insomnia can be caused by the same spectrum of disorders in addition to disruptive snoring, obstructive sleep apnea/hypopnea syndrome, periodic limb movement disorder, or nocturnal wandering in their cognitively impaired bedpartner. Diagnosis requires a detailed sleep disorders interview, physical examination, and, in some cases, polysomnography. Primary insomnia can improve with treatment with trazodone, chloral hydrate, or melatonin.[162,226–231] Carbidopa-levodopa, dopamine agonists such as pergolide or pramipexole, gabapentin, or opiates are generally effective for restless legs syndrome and periodic limb movement disorder. Nasal CPAP, if calibrated to the correct pressure and used nightly, eliminates disruptive snoring and obstructive sleep apnea. Central sleep apnea syndrome can be difficult to treat, often requiring various combinations of CPAP, bilevel positive airway pressure, supplemental oxygen, and benzodiazepines. Referral to a sleep medicine specialist can be helpful.

Hypersomnia

Hypersomnia can result from restless legs syndrome, periodic limb movement disorder, central sleep apnea syndrome, obstructive sleep apnea, insufficient sleep, narcolepsy, or idiopathic hypersomnia. Consultation with a sleep disorders specialist and polysomnography with or without a multiple sleep latency test can be fruitful. Psychostimulants can be effective in elderly patients.[232]

Parasomnia

Parasomnias refer to unpleasant nocturnal experiences or behaviors. REM sleep behavior disorder—probably the most common parasomnia among the elderly—occurs in PD, DLB, and multiple system atrophy.[26,27] Patients seemingly "act out their dreams," and the dream content often involves a chasing or attacking theme. Polysomnography is often necessary to investigate nocturnal seizures or obstructive sleep apnea (a history identical to that of REM sleep behavior disorder can occur in severe obstructive sleep apnea). Treatment with a low dose of clonazepam or melatonin is often effective for reducing the chance of injury to patients and their bedpartners.[26,233,234] Quetiapine can improve REM sleep behavior disorder in some patients (Boeve, unpublished data). One also can counsel patients and bedpartners, for example, to move potentially injurious objects away from the bed and to place a mattress on the floor next to the bed.[26]

"Sundowning"

Delirium, confusion, disorganized thinking, impaired attention, wandering, agitation, insomnia, hypersomnia, hallucinations, illusions, delusions, anxiety, restlessness, hyperactivity, and anger have all been considered features of the *sundowning syndrome*.[235,236] The term implies that problem symptoms or behaviors develop during the evening or night, although few data support that this occurs.[236] The term is nebulous, and more descriptive terms such as "agitation" or "wandering" are more appropriate. Several therapies have been suggested to improve various elements of the sundowning syndrome (Appendix).[237] This author suggests that clinicians identify specifically which symptoms are a problem and treat them accordingly. Our clinical experience has shown that diagnosis and management of the primary sleep disorders with or without a scheduled nap after the noon meal can markedly improve symptoms or behaviors that are most bothersome in the afternoon or evening.

Appendix

See pages 2853–2854

References

1. Okazaki H, Lipkin LE, Aronson SM. Diffuse intracytoplasmic ganglionic inclusions (Lewy type) associated with progressive dementia and quadriparesis in flexion. J Neuropathol Exp Neurol 1961;20:237–244
2. McKeith IG, Galasko D, Kosaka K, et al. Consensus guidelines for the clinical and pathologic diagnosis of dementia with Lewy bodies (DLB): report of the consortium on DLB international workshop. Neurology 1996;47:1113–1124
3. Grace J, McKeith IG. Decline in cognitive function in Parkinson's disease may be due to dementia with Lewy bodies [letter]. BMJ 1998;316:1022
4. Apaydin H, Ahlskog JE, Parisi JE, et al. Parkinson disease neuropathology: Later-developing dementia and loss of the levodopa response. Arch Neurol 2002;59:102–112
5. McKeith IG, Perry EK, Perry RH. Report of the second dementia with Lewy body international workshop: diagnosis and treatment. Consortium on Dementia With Lewy Bodies. Neurology 1999;53:902–905
6. Ferman TJ, Boeve BF, Smith GE, et al. REM sleep behavior disorder and dementia: cognitive differences when compared with AD. Neurology 1999;52:951–957
7. Boeve BF, Silber MH, Ferman TJ, et al. REM sleep behavior disorder and degenerative dementia: an association likely reflecting Lewy body disease. Neurology 1998;51:363–370
8. Barber R, Ballard C, McKeith IG, et al. MRI volumetric study of dementia with Lewy bodies: a comparison with AD and vascular dementia. Neurology 2000;54:1304–1309
9. McKeith I, Fairbairn A, Perry R, et al. Neuroleptic sensitivity in patients with senile dementia of Lewy body type. BMJ 1992;305:673–678
10. Walker Z, Grace J, Overshot R, et al. Olanzapine in dementia with Lewy bodies: a clinical study. Int J Geriatr Psychiatry 1999;14:459–466
11. Shea C, MacKnight C, Rockwood K. Donepezil for treatment of dementia with Lewy bodies: a case series of nine patients. Int Psychogeriatr 1998;10:229–238
12. Fergusson E, Howard R. Donepezil for the treatment of psychosis in dementia with Lewy bodies. Int J Geriatr Psychiatry 2000;15:280–281
13. Lanctot KL, Herrmann N. Donepezil for behavioural disorders associated with Lewy bodies: a case series. Int J Geriatr Psychiatry 2000;15:338–345
14. McKeith IG, Grace JB, Walker Z, et al. Rivastigmine in the treatment of dementia with Lewy bodies: preliminary findings from an open trial. Int J Geriatr Psychiatry 2000;15:387–392
15. Factor SA, Brown D, Molho ES, Podskalny GD. Clozapine: a 2-year open trial in Parkinson's disease patients with psychosis. Neurology 1994;44:544–546
16. Greene P, Cote L, Fahn S. Treatment of drug-induced psychosis in Parkinson's disease with clozapine. Adv Neurol 1993;60:703–706
17. Valldeoriola F, Nobbe FA, Tolosa E. Treatment of behavioural disturbances in Parkinson's disease. J Neural Transm Suppl 1997;51:175–204
18. Musser WS, Akil M. Clozapine as a treatment for psychosis in Parkinson's disease: a review. J Neuropsychiatry Clin Neurosci 1996;8:1–9
19. Chacko RC, Hurley RA, Harper RG, et al. Clozapine for acute and maintenance treatment of psychosis in Parkinson's disease. J Neuropsychiatry Clin Neurosci 1995;7:471–475
20. Dewey RB Jr, O'Suilleabhain PE. Treatment of drug-induced psychosis with quetiapine and clozapine in Parkinson's disease. Neurology 2000;55:1753–1754
21. Leopold NA. Risperidone treatment of drug-related psychosis in patients with parkinsonism. Mov Disord 2000;15:301–304
22. Workman RH Jr, Orengo CA, Bakey AA, et al. The use of risperidone for psychosis and agitation in demented patients with Parkinson's disease. J Neuropsychiatry Clin Neurosci 1997;9:594–597
23. Aarsland D, Larsen JP, Lim NG, Tandberg E. Olanza-

pine for psychosis in patients with Parkinson's disease with and without dementia. J Neuropsychiatry Clin Neurosci 1999;11:392–394

24. Juncos JL. Management of psychotic aspects of Parkinson's disease. J Clin Psychiatry 1999;60(Suppl 8):42–53

25. Pakiam AS, Bergeron C, Lang AE. Diffuse Lewy body disease presenting as multiple system atrophy. Can J Neurol Sci 1999;26:127–131

26. Olson EJ, Boeve BF, Silber MH. Rapid eye movement sleep behaviour disorder: demographic, clinical and laboratory findings in 93 cases. Brain 2000;123:331–339

27. Boeve BF, Silber MH, Ferman TJ, et al. Association of REM sleep behavior disorder and neurodegenerative disease may reflect an underlying synucleinopathy. Mov Disord 2001;16:622–630

28. Geroldi C, Frisoni GB, Bianchetti A, Trabucchi M. Drug treatment in Lewy body dementia. Dement Geriatr Cogn Disord 1997;8:188–197

29. Cummings JL. Lewy body diseases with dementia: pathophysiology and treatment. Brain Cogn 1995;28:266–280

30. McKeith I, O'Brien J. Dementia with Lewy bodies. Aust N Z J Psychiatry 1999;33:800–808

31. McKeith IG, O'Brien JT, Ballard C. Diagnosing dementia with Lewy bodies. Lancet 1999;354:1227–1228

32. Peyser CE, Folstein M, Chase GA, et al. Trial of d-alpha-tocopherol in Huntington's disease. Am J Psychiatry 1995;152:1771–1775

33. Anonymous. Safety and tolerability of the free-radical scavenger OPC-14117 in Huntington's disease. The Huntington Study Group. Neurology 1998;50:1366–1373

34. Rosas HD, Koroshetz WJ, Jenkins BG, et al. Riluzole therapy in Huntington's disease (HD). Mov Disord 1999;14:326–330

35. Ranen NG, Peyser CE, Folstein SE. ECT as a treatment for depression in Huntington's disease. J Neuropsych Clin Neurosci 1994;6:154–159

36. Beale MD, Kellner CH, Gurecki P, Pritchett JT. ECT for the treatment of Huntington's disease: a case study. Convuls Ther 1997;13:108–112

37. Factor SA, Friedman JH. The emerging role of clozapine in the treatment of movement disorders. Mov Disord 1997;12:483–496

38. Pick A. Ueber die Bexiehungen der senilen Hirnatrophie zur Aphasie. Pragur Medicinische Wochenschrift 1892;17:165–167

39. Dickson DW. Pick's disease: a modern approach. Brain Pathol 1998;8:339–354

40. European Concerted Action on Pick's Disease (ECAPD) Consortium. Provisional clinical and neuroradiological criteria for the diagnosis of Pick's disease. Eur J Neurol 1998;5:519–520

41. Rebeiz JJ, Kolodny EH, Richardson EP Jr. Corticodentatonigral degeneration with neuronal achromasia: a progressive disorder of late adult life. Trans Amer Neurol Assoc 1967;92:23–26

42. Boeve B. Corticobasal degeneration. In: Adler CH, Ahlskog JE, eds. Parkinson's Disease and Movement Disorders: Diagnosis and Treatment Guidelines for the Practicing Physician. Totowa, New Jersey: Humana Press, 2000:253–261

43. Maraganore DM, Ahlskog JE, Petersen RC. Progressive asymmetric rigidity with apraxia: a distinctive clinical entity (abstract). Mov Disord 1992;7(Suppl 1):80

44. Lang AE, Riley DE, Bergeron C. Cortical-basal ganglionic degeneration. In: Calne DB, ed. Neurodegener-

ative Diseases. Philadelphia: WB Saunders Company, 1994;877–894

45. Kumar R, Bergeron C, Pollanen MS, Lang AE. Cortical-basal ganglionic degeneration. In: Jankovic J, Tolosa E, eds. Parkinson's Disease and Movement Disorders. 3rd ed. Baltimore: Williams & Wilkins, 1998;297–316

46. Dickson DW, Bergeron C, Chin SS, et al. Office of Rare Diseases neuropathologic criteria for corticobasal degeneration. J Neuropathol Exp Neurol 2002;61:935–946

47. Litvan I, Cummings JL, Mega M. Neuropsychiatric features of corticobasal degeneration. J Neurol Neurosurg Psychiat 1998;65:717–721

48. Geda Y, Boeve B, Parisi J, et al. Neuropsychiatric features in 20 cases of pathologically-confirmed corticobasal degeneration (abstract). Mov Disord 2000;15(Suppl 3):229

49. Grimes DA, Lang AE, Bergeron CB. Dementia as the most common presentation of cortical-basal ganglionic degeneration. Neurology 1999;53:1969–1974

50. Boeve B, Parisi J, Dickson D, et al. Demographic and clinical findings in 20 cases of pathologically-diagnosed corticobasal degeneration (abstract). Mov Disord 2000;15(Suppl 3):228

51. Kompoliti K, Goetz CG, Boeve BF, et al. Clinical presentation and pharmacological therapy in corticobasal degeneration. Arch Neurol 1998;55:957–961

52. Steele JC, Richardson JC, Olszewski J. Progressive supranuclear palsy: a heterogeneous degeneration involving the brain stem, basal ganglia and cerebellum with vertical gaze and pseudobulbar, nuclear dystonia and dementia. Arch Neurol 1964;10:333–359

53. Dickson DW. Neuropathologic differentiation of progressive supranuclear palsy and corticobasal degeneration. J Neurol 1999;246(Suppl 2):II6–15

54. Collins SJ, Ahlskog JE, Parisi JE, Maraganore DM. Progressive supranuclear palsy: neuropathologically based diagnostic clinical criteria. J Neurol Neurosurg Psychiatry 1995;58:167–173

55. Litvan I, Agid Y, Calne D, et al. Clinical research criteria for the diagnosis of progressive supranuclear palsy (Steele-Richardson-Olszewski syndrome): report of the NINDS-SPSP international workshop. Neurology 1996;47:1–9

56. Hauw JJ, Daniel SE, Dickson D, et al. Preliminary NINDS neuropathologic criteria for Steele-Richardson-Olszewski syndrome (progressive supranuclear palsy). Neurology 1994;44:2015–2019

57. Litvan I, Mangone CA, McKee A, et al. Natural history of progressive supranuclear palsy (Steele-Richardson-Olszewski syndrome) and clinical predictors of survival: a clinicopathological study. J Neurol Neurosurg Psychiatry 1996;60:615–620

58. Nieforth KA, Golbe LI. Retrospective study of drug response in 87 patients with progressive supranuclear palsy. Clin Neuropharmacol 1993;16:338–346

59. Cole DG, Growdon JH. Therapy for progressive supranuclear palsy: past and future. J Neural Transm Suppl 1994;42:283–290

60. Kompoliti K, Goetz CG, Litvan I, et al. Pharmacological therapy in progressive supranuclear palsy. Arch Neurol 1998;55:1099–1102

61. Litvan I, Mega MS, Cummings JL, Fairbanks L. Neuropsychiatric aspects of progressive supranuclear palsy. Neurology 1996;47:1184–1189

62. Litvan I. Cholinergic approaches to the treatment of progressive supranuclear palsy. J Neural Transm Suppl 1994;42:275–281

63. Perina M, Gomez Arevalo G, Garcia S, Gershanik O. Donepezil improves motor and cognitive function in patients with progressive supranuclear palsy (PSP) (abstract). Mov Disord 2000;15(Suppl 3):225

64. Fabbrini G, Barbanti P, Bonifati V, et al. Donepezil in the treatment of Progressive Supranuclear Palsy (abstract). Mov Disord 2000;15(Suppl 3):226–227

65. Neumann MA, Cohn R. Progressive subcortical gliosis, a rare form of presenile dementia. Brain 1967;90:405–418

66. Lanska DJ, Currier RD, Cohen M, et al. Familial progressive subcortical gliosis. Neurology 1994;44:1633–1643

67. Petersen RB, Tabaton M, Chen SG, et al. Familial progressive subcortical gliosis: presence of prions and linkage to chromosome 17. Neurology 1995;45:1062–1067

68. Gambetti P. Prion in progressive subcortical gliosis revisited [letter]. Neurology 1997;49:309–310

69. Goedert M, Spillantini MG, Crowther RA, et al. Tau gene mutation in familial progressive subcortical gliosis. Nat Med 1999;5:454–457

70. Will RG, Lees AJ, Gibb W, Barnard RO. A case of progressive subcortical gliosis presenting clinically as Steele-Richardson-Olszewski syndrome. J Neurol Neurosurg Psychiatry 1988;51:1224–1227

71. Foster NL, Gilman S, Berent S, et al. Progressive subcortical gliosis and progressive supranuclear palsy can have similar clinical and PET abnormalities. J Neurol Neurosurg Psychiatry 1992;55:707–713

72. Lanska DJ, Markesbery WR, Cochran E, et al. Late-onset sporadic progressive subcortical gliosis. J Neurol Sci 1998;157:143–147

73. Braak H, Braak E. Argyrophilic grain disease: frequency of occurrence in different age categories and neuropathological diagnostic criteria. J Neural Transm 1998;105:801–819

74. Jellinger KA. Dementia with grains (argyrophilic grain disease). Brain Pathol 1998;8:377–386

75. Botez G, Schultz C, Ghebremedhin E, et al. Clinical aspects of "argyrophilic grain disease" (German). Nervenarzt 2000;71:38–43

76. Kertesz A, Kawarai T, Rogaeva E, et al. Familial frontotemporal dementia with ubiquitin-positive, tau-negative inclusions. Neurology 2000;54:818–827

77. Knopman DS, Mastri AR, Frey WH II, et al. Dementia lacking distinctive histologic features: a common non-Alzheimer dementia. Neurology 1990;40:251–256

78. Knopman DS. Overview of dementia lacking distinctive histology: pathological designation of a progressive dementia. Dementia 1993;4:132–136

79. Kim RC, Collins GH, Parisi JE, et al. Familial dementia of adult onset with pathological findings of a "nonspecific" nature. Brain 1981;104:61–78

80. Brun A. Frontal lobe degeneration of non-Alzheimer type. I. Neuropathology. Arch Gerontol Geriatr 1987;6:193–208

81. Neary D, Snowden JS, Mann DM, et al. Frontal lobe dementia and motor neuron disease. J Neurol Neurosurg Psychiatry 1990;53:23–32

82. Neary D, Snowden JS, Mann DM. The clinical pathological correlates of lobar atrophy. Dementia 1993;4:154–159

83. Brown J, Ashworth A, Gydesen S, et al. Familial non-specific dementia maps to chromosome 3. Hum Mol Genet 1995;4:1625–1628

84. Dickson DW, Lin W, Liu WK, Yen SH. Multiple system atrophy: a sporadic synucleinopathy. Brain Pathol 1999;9:721–732

85. Dickson DW. Tau and synuclein and their role in neuropathology. Brain Pathol 1999;9:657–661

86. Hardy J, Gwinn-Hardy K. Neurodegenerative disease: a different view of diagnosis. Mol Med Today 1999;5:514–517

87. Hardy J. Pathways to primary neurodegenerative disease. Mayo Clin Proc 1999;74:835–837

88. Konagaya M, Konagaya Y, Miwa S, Matsuoka Y. Clinico-MRI study of hemispheric disorder in long-term follow-up cases of multiple system atrophy (Japanese). Rinsho Shinkeigaku 1998;38:1031–1036

89. Konagaya M, Sakai M, Matsuoka Y, et al. Multiple system atrophy with remarkable frontal lobe atrophy. Acta Neuropathol 1999;97:423–428

90. Plazzi G, Corsini R, Provini F, et al. REM sleep behavior disorders in multiple system atrophy. Neurology 1997;48:1094–1097

91. Isozaki E, Naito A, Horiguchi S, et al. Early diagnosis and stage classification of vocal cord abductor paralysis in patients with multiple system atrophy. J Neurol Neurosurg Psych 1996;60:399–402

92. World Health Organization. Human transmissible spongiform encephalopathies. Wkly Epidemiol Rec 1998;73:361–372

93. Collinge J. New diagnostic tests for prion diseases. N Engl J Med 1996;335:963–965

94. Ironside JW. Neuropathological findings in new variant CJD and experimental transmission of BSE. FEMS Immunol Med Microbiol 1998;21:91–95

95. Scott MR, Will R, Ironside J, et al. Compelling transgenetic evidence for transmission of bovine spongiform encephalopathy prions to humans. Proc Natl Acad Sci USA 1999;96:15137–15142

96. Zeidler M, Johnstone EC, Bamber RW, et al. New variant Creutzfeldt-Jakob disease: psychiatric features. Lancet 1997;350:908–910

97. Zeidler M, Stewart GE, Barraclough CR, et al. New variant Creutzfeldt-Jakob disease: neurological features and diagnostic tests. Lancet 1997;350:903–907

98. Will RG, Zeidler M, Stewart GE, et al. Diagnosis of new variant Creutzfeldt-Jakob disease. Ann Neurol 2000;47:575–582

99. Coulthard A, Hall K, English PT, et al. Quantitative analysis of MRI signal intensity in new variant Creutzfeldt-Jakob disease. Br J Radiol 1999;72:742–748

100. Caselli RJ, Jack CR Jr, Petersen RC, et al. Asymmetric cortical degenerative syndromes: clinical and radiologic correlations. Neurology 1992;42:1462–1468

101. Caselli RJ, Jack CR Jr. Asymmetric cortical degeneration syndromes: a proposed clinical classification. Arch Neurol 1992;49:770–780

102. Caselli RJ. Focal and asymmetric cortical degeneration syndromes. The Neurologist 1995;1:1–19

103. Caselli RJ. Asymmetric cortical degeneration syndromes. Curr Opin Neurol 1996;9:276–280

104. Petersen RC, Dickson DW, Parisi JE, et al. Neuropathological substrate of mild cognitive impairment. Neurobiol Aging 2000;21(Suppl 1):S198

105. Hutton M, Lendon CL, Rizzu P, et al. Association of missense and 5'-splice-site mutations in tau with the inherited dementia FTDP-17. Nature 1998;393:702–705

106. The Lund and Manchester Groups. Clinical and neuropathological criteria for frontotemporal dementia. J Neurol Neurosurg Psychiatry 1994;57:416–418

107. Neary D, Snowden JS, Gustafson L, et al. Frontotemporal lobar degeneration: a consensus on clinical diagnostic criteria. Neurology 1998;51:1546–1554

108. Miller BL, Chang L, Mena I, et al. Progressive right frontotemporal degeneration: clinical, neuropsychological and SPECT characteristics. Dementia 1993;4: 204–213

109. Miller BL, Cummings J, Mishkin F, et al. Emergence of artistic talent in frontotemporal dementia. Neurology 1998;51:978–982

110. Miller BL, Boone K, Cummings JL, et al. Functional correlates of musical and visual ability in frontotemporal dementia. Br J Psychiatr 2000;176:458–463

111. Boeve BF, Geda Y. Polka music and sematic dementia. Neurology 2001;57:1485

112. Swartz JR, Miller BL, Lesser IM, Darby AL. Frontotemporal dementia: treatment response to serotonin selective reuptake inhibitors. J Clin Psychiatry 1997;58: 212–216

113. Mesulam MM. Primary progressive aphasia without generalized dementia. Ann Neurol 1982;11:592–598

114. Duffy JR, Petersen RCN. Primary progressive aphasia. Aphasiology 1992;6:1–15

115. Damasio A. Disorders of complex visual processing: agnosias, achromatopsia, Balint's syndrome, and related difficulties of orientation and construction. In: Mesulam MM, ed. Principles of Behavioral Neurology. Philadelphia: F.A. Davis Company, 1985:259–288

116. Evans JJ, Heggs AJ, Antoun N, Hodges JR. Progressive prosopagnosia associated with selective right temporal lobe atrophy. A new syndrome? Brain 1995;118:1–13

117. Caselli RJ, Windebank AJ, Petersen RC, et al. Rapidly progressive aphasic dementia and motor neuron disease. Ann Neurol 1993;33:200–207

118. Mesulam MM. Primary progressive aphasia. Ann Neurol 2001;49:425–432

119. Boeve BF, Maraganore DM, Parisi JE, et al. Pathologic heterogeneity in clinically diagnosed corticobasal degeneration. Neurology 1999;53:795–800

120. Graff-Radford NR, Bolling JP, Earnest F IV, et al. Simultanagnosia as the initial sign of degenerative dementia. Mayo Clin Proc 1993;68:955–964

121. Benson DF, Davis RJ, Snyder BD. Posterior cortical atrophy. Arch Neurol 1988;45:789–793

122. Goldfarb LG, Petersen RB, Tabaton M, et al. Fatal familial insomnia and familial Creutzfeldt-Jakob disease: disease phenotype determined by a DNA polymorphism. Science 1992;258:806–808

123. Hardy J, Gwinn-Hardy K. Genetic classification of primary neurodegenerative disease. Science 1998;282: 1075–1079

124. Schenk DB, Seubert P, Lieberburg I, Wallace J. Beta-peptide immunization: a possible new treatment for Alzheimer disease. Arch Neurol 2000;57:934–936

125. Schenk D, Barbour R, Dunn W, et al. Immunization with amyloid-beta attenuates Alzheimer-disease-like pathology in the PDAPP mouse. Nature 1999;400: 173–177

126. Roman GC, Tatemichi TK, Erkinjuntti T, et al. Vascular dementia: diagnostic criteria for research studies. Report of the NINDS-AIREN International Workshop. Neurology 1993;43:250–260

127. Chui HC, Victoroff JI, Margolin D, et al. Criteria for the diagnosis of ischemic vascular dementia proposed by the State of California Alzheimer's Disease Diagnostic and Treatment Centers. Neurology 1992;42: 473–480

128. American Psychiatric Association. Diagnostic and Statistical Manual of Mental Disorders. 4th ed. Washington, DC: American Psychiatric Association, 1994

129. Hachinski VC, Iliff LD, Zilhka E, et al. Cerebral blood flow in dementia. Arch Neurol 1975;32:632–637

130. Chui HC, Mack W, Jackson JE, et al. Clinical criteria for the diagnosis of vascular dementia: a multicenter study of comparability and interrater reliability. Arch Neurol 2000;57:191–196

131. Anonymous. Vascular dementia: an updated approach to patient management. A roundtable discussion: part 3. Geriatrics 1994;49:39–40, 43–46

132. Dickson DW, Davies P, Bevona C, et al. Hippocampal sclerosis: a common pathological feature of dementia in very old (> or = 80 years of age) humans. Acta Neuropathol (Berl) 1994;88:212–221

133. Schneider LS, Olin JT. Overview of clinical trials of hydergine in dementia. Arch Neurol 1994;51:787–798

134. Gerhardt G, Rogalla K, Jaeger J. Drug therapy of disorders of cerebral performance. Randomized comparative study of dihydroergotoxine and Ginkgo biloba extract (German). Fortschr Med 1990;108:384–388

135. Stoppe G, Sandholzer H, Staedt J, et al. Prescribing practice with cognition enhancers in outpatient care: are there differences regarding type of dementia?—Results of a representative survey in lower Saxony, Germany. Pharmacopsychiatry 1996;29:150–155

136. Le Bars PL, Katz MM, Berman N, et al. A placebo-controlled, double-blind, randomized trial of an extract of Gingko biloba for dementia. North American EGb Study Group. JAMA 1997;278:1327–1332

137. Le Bars PL, Kieser M, Itil KZ. A 26-week analysis of a double-blind, placebo-controlled trial of the ginkgo biloba extract EGb 761 in dementia. Dement Geriatr Cogn Disord 2000;11:230–237

138. Matthews MK Jr. Association of Ginkgo biloba with intracerebral hemorrhage. Neurology 1998;50: 1933–1934

139. Mendez MF, Younesi FL, Perryman KM. Use of donepezil for vascular dementia: preliminary clinical experience. J Neuropsychiatry Clin Neurosci 1999;11: 268–270

140. Kanowski S. Aging, dementia and calcium metabolism. J Neural Transm Suppl 1998;54:195–200

141. Parnetti L, Senin U, Carosi M, Baasch H. Mental deterioration in old age: results of two multicenter, clinical trials with nimodipine. The Nimodipine Study Group. Clin Ther 1993;15:394–406

142. Anonymous: An experimental, randomized, double-blind, placebo-controlled clinical trial to investigate the effect of nicardipine on cognitive function in patients with vascular dementia. Spanish Group of Nicardipine Study in Vascular Dementia. Rev Neurol 1999;28:835–845

143. Kittner B. Clinical trials of propentofylline in vascular dementia. European/Canadian Propentofylline Study Group. Alzheimer Dis Assoc Disord 1999;13(Suppl 3):S166–S171

144. Kwon OS, Chung YB, Kim MH, et al. Pharmacokinetics of propentofylline and the quantitation of its metabolite hydroxypropentofylline in human volunteers. Arch Pharm Res 1998;21:698–702

145. Marcusson J, Rother M, Kittner B, et al. A 12-month, randomized, placebo-controlled trial of propentofylline (HWA 285) in patients with dementia according to DSM III-R. The European Propentofylline Study Group. Dement Geriatr Cogn Disord 1997;8:320–328

146. Mielke R, Moller HJ, Erkinjuntti T, et al. Propentofylline in the treatment of vascular dementia and Alzheimer-type dementia: overview of phase I and phase II clinical trials. Alzheimer Dis Assoc Disord 1998;12(Suppl 2):S29–S35

147. Plaschke K, Martin E, Bardenheuer HJ. Effect of

propentofylline on hippocampal brain energy state
and amyloid precursor protein concentration in a rat
model of cerebral hypoperfusion. J Neural Transm
1998;105:1065–1077

148. Rother M, Kittner B, Rudolphi K, et al. HWA 285
(propentofylline)—a new compound for the treatment
of both vascular dementia and dementia of the
Alzheimer type. Ann NY Acad Sci 1996;777:404–409

149. Rother M, Erkinjuntti T, Roessner M, et al. Propentofylline in the treatment of Alzheimer's disease and
vascular dementia: a review of phase III trials. Dement
Geriatr Cogn Disord 1998;9(Suppl 1):36–43

150. Saletu B, Moller HJ, Grunberger J, et al. Propentofylline in adult-onset cognitive disorders: double-
blind, placebo-controlled, clinical, psychometric and
brain mapping studies. Neuropsychobiology 1990;24:
173–184

151. Wimo A, Witthaus E, Rother M, Winblad B. Economic
impact of introducing propentofylline for the treatment of dementia in Sweden. Clin Ther 1998;20:
552–566

152. Black RS, Barclay LL, Nolan KA, et al. Pentoxifylline in
cerebrovascular dementia. J Am Geriatr Soc 1992;40:
237–244

153. Blume J, Ruhlmann KU, de la Haye R, et al. Treatment
of chronic cerebrovascular disease in elderly patients
with pentoxifylline. J Med 1992;23:417–432

154. Parnetti L, Mari D, Abate G, et al. Vascular Dementia
Italian Sulodexide Study (VA.D.I.S.S.): Clinical and
biological results. Thromb Res 1997;87:225–233

155. Cucinotta D, Aveni Casucci MA, Pedrazzi F, et al.
Multicentre clinical placebo-controlled study with
buflomedil in the treatment of mild dementia of vascular origin. J Int Med Res 1992;20:136–149

156. Di Perri R, Coppola G, Ambrosio LA, et al. A multicentre trial to evaluate the efficacy and tolerability of
alpha-glycerylphosphorylcholine versus cytosine
diphosphocholine in patients with vascular dementia.
J Int Med Res 1991;19:330–341

157. Ditzler K. Efficacy and tolerability of memantine in
patients with dementia syndrome. A double-blind,
placebo controlled trial. Arzneimittelforschung 1991;
41:773–780

158. Mobius HJ. Pharmacologic rationale for memantine in
chronic cerebral hypoperfusion, especially vascular
dementia. Alzheimer Dis Assoc Disord 1999;13(Suppl
3):S172–S178

159. Carlson DL, Fleming KC, Smith GE, Evans JM. Management of dementia-related behavioral disturbances:
a nonpharmacologic approach. Mayo Clin Proc 1995;
70:1108–1115

160. Robinson A, Spencer B, White L. Understanding difficult behaviors: some practical suggestions for coping
with Alzheimer's disease and related illnesses. Ypsi-
lanti, MI: Geriatric Education Center of Michigan,
Michigan State University, 1988

161. Knopman DS, Sawyer-DeMaris S. Practical approach
to managing behavioral problems in dementia
patients. Geriatrics 1990;45:27–30, 35

162. Boeve BF, Silber MH, Ferman TJ. Current management
of sleep disturbances in dementia. Curr Neurol Neurosci Rep 2002;2:169–177

163. Levy ML, Cummings JL, Kahn-Rose R. Neuropsychiatric symptoms and cholinergic therapy for Alzheimer's
disease. Gerontology 1999;45(Suppl 1):15–22

164. MacKnight C, Rojas-Fernandez C. Quetiapine for sexually inappropriate behavior in dementia [letter]. J Am
Geriatr Soc 2000;48:707

165. Stewart JT, Shin KJ. Paroxetine treatment of sexual disinhibition in dementia [letter]. Am J Psychiatry 1997;
154:1474

166. Leo RJ, Kim KY. Clomipramine treatment of paraphilias in elderly demented patients. J Geriatr Psychiatry
Neurol 1995;8:123–124

167. Tiller JW, Dakis JA, Shaw JM. Short-term buspirone
treatment in disinhibition with dementia [letter].
Lancet 1988;2:510

168. Kaufer DI, Cummings JL, Christine D. Effect of tacrine
on behavioral symptoms in Alzheimer's disease: an
open-label study. J Geriatr Psychiatry Neurol 1996;9:
1–6

169. Marin RS, Fogel BS, Hawkins J, et al. Apathy: a treatable syndrome. J Neuropsychiatry Clin Neurosci
1995;7:23–30

170. Katz IR. Diagnosis and treatment of depression in
patients with Alzheimer's disease and other dementias. J Clin Psychiatry 1998;59(Suppl 9):38–44

171. Kaufer D, Cummings JL, Christine D. Differential neu-
ropsychiatric symptom responses to tacrine in
Alzheimer's disease: relationship to dementia severity.
J Neuropsychiatry Clin Neurosci 1998;10:55–63

172. Stoppe G, Brandt CA, Staedt JH. Behavioural problems
associated with dementia: the role of newer antipsychotics. Drugs Aging 1999;14:41–54

173. De Deyn PP, Katz IR. Control of aggression and agitation in patients with dementia: efficacy and safety of
risperidone. Int J Geriatr Psychiatry 2000;15(Suppl 1):
S14–S22

174. Falsetti AE. Risperidone for control of agitation in
dementia patients. Am J Health Syst Pharm 2000;
57:862–870

175. Jeste DV, Okamoto A, Napolitano J, et al. Low incidence of persistent tardive dyskinesia in elderly
patients with dementia treated with risperidone. Am J
Psychiatry 2000;157:1150–1155

176. Irizarry MC, Ghaemi SN, Lee-Cherry ER, et al. Risperidone treatment of behavioral disturbances in outpatients with dementia. J Neuropsychiatry Clin
Neurosci 1999;11:336–342

177. Katz IR, Jeste DV, Mintzer JE, et al. Comparison of
risperidone and placebo for psychosis and behavioral
disturbances associated with dementia: a randomized,
double-blind trial. Risperidone Study Group. J Clin
Psychiatry 1999;60:107–115

178. De Deyn PP, Rabheru K, Rasmussen A, et al. A randomized trial of risperidone, placebo, and haloperidol
for behavioral symptoms of dementia. Neurology
1999;53:946–955

179. Lavretsky H, Sultzer D. A structured trial of risperidone for the treatment of agitation in dementia. Am J
Geriatr Psychiatry 1998;6:127–135

180. Herrmann N, Rivard MF, Flynn M, et al. Risperidone
for the treatment of behavioral disturbances in dementia: a case series. J Neuropsychiatry Clin Neurosci
1998;10:220–223

181. Fava M. Psychopharmacologic treatment of pathologic
aggression. Psychiatr Clin North Am 1997;20:427–451

182. Grossman F. A review of anticonvulsants in treating
agitated demented elderly patients. Pharmacotherapy
1998;18:600–606

183. Tariot PN, Erb R, Podgorski CA, et al. Efficacy and
tolerability of carbamazepine for agitation and
aggression in dementia. Am J Psychiatry 1998;155:
54–61

184. Lemke MR. Effect of carbamazepine on agitation in
Alzheimer's inpatients refractory to neuroleptics. J

Clin Psychiatry 1995;56:354–357

185. Leibovici A, Tariot PN. Carbamazepine treatment of agitation associated with dementia. J Geriatr Psychiatry Neurol 1988;1:110–112

186. Patterson JF. A preliminary study of carbamazepine in the treatment of assaultive patients with dementia. J Geriatr Psychiatry Neurol 1988;1:21–23

187. Lindenmayer JP, Kotsaftis A. Use of sodium valproate in violent and aggressive behaviors: a critical review. J Clin Psychiatry 2000;61:123–128

188. Davis LL, Ryan W, Adinoff B, Petty F. Comprehensive review of the psychiatric uses of valproate. J Clin Psychopharmacol 2000;20(Suppl 1):1S–17S

189. Raskind MA. Evaluation and management of aggressive behavior in the elderly demented patient. J Clin Psychiatry 1999;60(Suppl 15):45–49

190. Kunik ME, Puryear L, Orengo CA, et al. The efficacy and tolerability of divalproex sodium in elderly demented patients with behavioral disturbances. Int J Geriatr Psychiatry 1998;13:29–34

191. Herrmann N. Valproic acid treatment of agitation in dementia. Can J Psychiatry 1998;43:69–72

192. Narayan M, Nelson JC. Treatment of dementia with behavioral disturbance using divalproex or a combination of divalproex and a neuroleptic. J Clin Psychiatry 1997;58:351–354

193. Porsteinsson AP, Tariot PN, Erb R, Gaile S. An open trial of valproate for agitation in geriatric neuropsychiatric disorders. Am J Geriatr Psychiatry 1997;5:344–351

194. Haas S, Vincent K, Holt J, Lippmann S. Divalproex: a possible treatment alternative for demented, elderly aggressive patients. Ann Clin Psychiatry 1997;9:145–147

195. Lott AD, McElroy SL, Keys MA. Valproate in the treatment of behavioral agitation in elderly patients with dementia. J Neuropsychiatry Clin Neurosci 1995;7:314–319

196. Mellow AM, Solano-Lopez C, Davis S. Sodium valproate in the treatment of behavioral disturbance in dementia. J Geriatr Psychiatry Neurol 1993;6:205–209

197. Shankle WR, Nielson KA, Cotman CW. Low-dose propranolol reduces aggression and agitation resembling that associated with orbitofrontal dysfunction in elderly demented patients. Alzheimer Dis Assoc Disord 1995;9:233–237

198. Ott BR. Leuprolide treatment of sexual aggression in a patient with dementia and the Kluver-Bucy syndrome. Clin Neuropharmacol 1995;18:443–447

199. Pauszek ME. Propranolol for treatment of agitation in senile dementia. Indiana Med 1991;84:16–17

200. Gadbaw JJ. Use of propranolol for the control of disruptive behavior in senile dementia [letter]. J Geriatr Psychiatry Neurol 1989;2:116

201. Weiler PG, Mungas D, Bernick C. Propranolol for the control of disruptive behavior in senile dementia. J Geriatr Psychiatry Neurol 1988;1:226–230

202. Jenike MA. Treating the violent elderly patient with propranolol. Geriatrics 1983;38:29–30, 34

203. Anderson IM, Scott K, Harborne G. Serotonin and depression in frontal lobe dementia [letter]. Am J Psychiatry 1995;152:645

204. Orengo CA, Kunik ME, Molinari V, Workman RH. The use and tolerability of fluoxetine in geropsychiatric inpatients. J Clin Psychiatry 1996;57:12–16

205. Reynolds CF III. Depression: making the diagnosis and using SSRIs in the older patient. Geriatrics 1996;51:28–34

206. Magai C, Kennedy G, Cohen CI, Gomberg D. A controlled clinical trial of sertraline in the treatment of depression in nursing home patients with late-stage Alzheimer's disease. Am J Geriatr Psychiatry 2000;8:66–74

207. Meyers BS. Depression and dementia: comorbidities, identification, and treatment. J Geriatr Psychiatry Neurol 1998;11:201–205

208. Kaplan EW. Retrospective review of the effects of sertraline on 32 outpatients with dementia [letter]. Am J Geriatr Psychiatry 1998;6:184

209. Volicer L, Rheaume Y, Cyr D. Treatment of depression in advanced Alzheimer's disease using sertraline. J Geriatr Psychiatry Neurol 1994;7:227–229

210. Katona CL, Hunter BN, Bray J. A double-blind comparison of the efficacy and safety of paroxetine and imipramine in the treatment of depression with dementia. Int J Geriatr Psychiatry 1998;13:100–108

211. Karlsson I, Godderis J, Augusto De Mendonca Lima C, et al. A randomised, double-blind comparison of the efficacy and safety of citalopram compared to mianserin in elderly, depressed patients with or without mild to moderate dementia. Int J Geriatr Psychiatry 2000;15:295–305

212. Pollock BG, Mulsant BH, Sweet R, et al. An open pilot study of citalopram for behavioral disturbances of dementia. Plasma levels and real-time observations. Am J Geriatr Psychiatry 1997;5:70–78

213. Gottfries CG, Karlsson I, Nyth AL. Treatment of depression in elderly patients with and without dementia disorders. Int Clin Psychopharmacol 1992;6(Suppl 5):55–64

214. Nyth AL, Gottfries CG, Lyby K, et al. A controlled multicenter clinical study of citalopram and placebo in elderly depressed patients with and without concomitant dementia. Acta Psychiatr Scand 1992;86:138–145

215. Gottfries CG, Nyth AL. Effect of citalopram, a selective 5-HT reuptake blocker, in emotionally disturbed patients with dementia. Ann NY Acad Sci 1991;640:276–279

216. Nyth AL, Gottfries CG. The clinical efficacy of citalopram in treatment of emotional disturbances in dementia disorders. A Nordic multicentre study. Br J Psychiatry 1990;157:894–901

217. Geldmacher DS, Waldman AJ, Doty L, Heilman KM. Fluoxetine in dementia of the Alzheimer's type: prominent adverse effects and failure to improve cognition [letter]. J Clin Psychiatry 1994;55:161

218. Burke WJ, Dewan V, Wengel SP, et al. The use of selective serotonin reuptake inhibitors for depression and psychosis complicating dementia. Int J Geriatr Psychiatry 1997;12:519–525

219. Lauterbach EC, Schweri MM. Amelioration of pseudobulbar affect by fluoxetine: possible alteration of dopamine-related pathophysiology by a selective serotonin reuptake inhibitor [letter]. J Clin Psychopharmacol 1991;11:392–393

220. Messiha FS. Fluoxetine: a spectrum of clinical applications and postulates of underlying mechanisms. Neurosci Biobehav Rev 1993;17:385–396

221. Shader RI. Does lithium both cause and treat pseudobulbar affect? J Clin Psychopharmacol 1992;12:360

222. Seliger GM, Hornstein A. Serotonin, fluoxetine, and pseudobulbar affect. Neurology 1989;39:1400

223. Skelly J, Flint AJ. Urinary incontinence associated with dementia. J Am Geriatr Soc 1995;43:286–294

224. Ouslander JG, Zarit SH, Orr NK, Muira SA. Incontinence among elderly community-dwelling dementia patients. Characteristics, management, and impact on caregivers. J Am Geriatr Soc 1990;38:440–445

225. Ouslander JG, Uman GC, Urman HN, Rubenstein LZ. Incontinence among nursing home patients: clinical and functional correlates. J Am Geriatr Soc 1987;35: 324–330

226. Mishima K, Okawa M, Hozumi S, Hishikawa Y. Supplementary administration of artificial bright light and melatonin as potent treatment for disorganized circadian rest-activity and dysfunctional autonomic and neuroendocrine systems in institutionalized demented elderly persons. Chronobiol Int 2000;17: 419–432

227. Asplund R. Sleep disorders in the elderly. Drugs Aging 1999;14:91–103

228. Brusco LI, Fainstein I, Marquez M, Cardinali DP. Effect of melatonin in selected populations of sleep-disturbed patients. Biol Signal Recept 1999;8:126–131

229. Campbell SS, Terman M, Lewy AJ, et al. Light treatment for sleep disorders: consensus report. V. Age-related disturbances. J Biol Rhythms 1995;10:151–154

230. Gerner RH. Geriatric depression and treatment with trazodone. Psychopathology 1987;20(Suppl 1):82–91

231. Singer C, McArthur A, Hughes R, et al. High dose melatonin administration and sleep in the elderly (abstract). Sleep Research 1995;24A:151

232. Gurian B, Rosowsky E. Low-dose methylphenidate in the very old. J Geriatr Psychiatry Neurol 1990;3: 152–154

233. Schenck CH, Mahowald MW. REM sleep parasomnias. Neurologic Clinics 1996;14:697–720

234. Boeve BF. Melatonin for treatment of REM sleep behavior disorder: response in 8 patients [abstract]. Sleep 2001;24(Suppl):A35

235. Vitiello M, Bliwise D, Prinz P. Sleep in Alzheimer's disease and the sundown syndrome. Neurology 1992; 42(Suppl 6):83–94

236. Bliwise DL, Carroll JS, Lee KA, et al. Sleep and "sundowning" in nursing home patients with dementia. Psychiatry Res 1993;48:277–292

237. McGaffigan S, Bliwise DL. The treatment of sundowning: A selective review of pharmacological and non-pharmacological studies. Drugs Aging 1997;10:10–17

Appendix Table 269 Selected medications and suggested dosing schedules for treating symptoms, behaviors, and disorders in dementia*

Symptom, behavior, or disorder	Medication	Starting dose	Suggested titrating schedule	Typical therapeutic range
Apathy, psychomotor slowing, or subcortical dementia	Methylphenidate	2.5 mg qam	Increase in 2.5 to 5-mg increments q3–5 days in bid dosing (morning and noon)	5 mg qam–30 mg bid
	Amphetamine/dextroamphetamine	5 mg qam	Increase in 5-mg increments q7 days in qd–bid (morning and noon) dosing; maximum 25 mg bid	5 mg qam–20 mg bid
	Modafinil	100 mg qam	Increase in 100-mg increments each week; maximum 400 mg po qam	100–400 mg qam
	Carbidopa/levodopa	25/100 ½ tab tid	Increase in ½-tab increments over all 3 daily doses each week (take 1 hr before or after meals)	1–3 tabs tid
	Donepezil	5 mg qam	Increase to 10 mg qam 4 weeks later	5–10 mg qam
	Rivastigmine	1.5 mg bid	Increase in 1.5-mg increments for both doses every 2–4 weeks; maximum, 6 mg bid	1.5–6.0 mg bid
	Galantamine	4 mg bid	Increase in 4-mg increments for both doses every 4 weeks; maximum, 12 mg bid	4–12 mg bid
Forgetfullness	Donepezil	5 mg qam	Increase to 10 mg qam 4 weeks later	5–10 mg qam
	Rivastigmine	1.5 mg bid	Increase in 1.5-mg increments for both doses every 2–4 weeks; maximum, 6 mg bid	1.5–6.0 mg bid
	Galantamine	4 mg bid	Increase in 4-mg increments for both doses every 4 weeks; maximum 12 mg bid	4–12 mg bid
Depression or emotional lability/ pseudobulbar affect	Fluoxetine	10 mg qd	Increase to 20 mg 2–4 weeks later	10–40 mg qd
	Sertraline	25 mg qd	Increase to 50 mg 2 weeks later, titrate gradually up to maximum of 200 mg qd	50–100 mg qd
	Paroxetine	10 mg qd	Increase to 20 mg 2 weeks later, titrate gradually up to maximum of 60 mg/day	10–60 mg qd
	Citalopram	10 mg qd	Increase to 20 mg 2 weeks later, titrate gradually up to maximum of 60 mg/day	10–60 mg qd
Orthostatic hypotension	Fludrocortisone	0.1 mg qd	Increase in 0.1-mg increments q5–7 days; maximum, 1.0 mg/day	0.1–0.3 mg qd
	Midodrine	5 mg tid	Increase up to 10 mg tid if necessary	5–10 mg tid
Parkinsonism	Carbidopa/levodopa	25/100 ½ tab tid	Increase in ½-tab increments over all 3 daily doses each week (take 1 hr before or after meals)	1–3 tabs tid
Anxiety or obsessions/ compulsions	Sertraline	25 mg qd	Increase to 50 mg 2 weeks later, titrate gradually up to maximum of 200 mg qd	50–100 mg qd
	Paroxetine	10 mg qd	Increase to 20 mg 2 weeks later, titrate gradually up to maximum of 60 mg/day	10–60 mg qd
	Buspirone	5 mg bid	Increase in 5-mg increments in bid-tid dosing q3–5 days; maximum, 60 mg/day	5–10 mg tid
Insomnia	Trazodone	25 mg qhs	Increase in 25-mg increments q3–5 days	50–200 mg/night
	Chloral hydrate	500 mg qhs	Increase in 500-mg increments q5–7 days	500–1500 mg/night
	Melatonin	3 mg	Increase gradually up to 12 mg if necessary	3–12 mg/night

2854 XIV Neurobehavioral Disorders: Cognitive Rehabilitation, Behavioral Managment and Pharmacologic Therapies

Appendix *Continued*

Symptom, behavior, or disorder	Medication	Starting dose	Suggested titrating schedule	Typical therapeutic range
Restless legs syndrome/periodic limb movement disorder	Carbidopa/levodopa	25/100 or CR 25/100	1 tab qhs, increase to 2 tabs 1 week later if necessary	1-2 tabs qhs
	Pergolide	0.05 mg qhs	Increase in 0.05-mg increments q2-3 days	0.15-0.75 mg/night
	Pramipexole	0.125 mg qhs	Increase in 0.125-mg increments q2-3 days	0.25-0.75 mg/night
	Gabapentin	100 mg qhs	Increase in 100-mg increments q2-3 days	300-1200 mg/night
Excessive daytime somnolence	Methylphenidate	2.5 mg qam	Increase in 2.5 to 5-mg increments q3-5 days in bid dosing (morning and noon)	5 mg qam-30 mg bid
	Amphetamine/dextroamphetamine	5 mg qam	Increase in 5-mg increments q7 days in qd-bid (morning and noon) dosing; maximum, 25 mg bid	5 mg qam-20 mg bid
	Modafinil	100 mg qam	Increase in 100-mg increments each week; maximum 400 mg po qam	100-400 mg qam
REM sleep behavior disorder	Clonazepam	0.25 mg qhs	Increase in 0.25-mg increments q7 days	0.25-1.0 mg/night
	Melatonin	3 mg	Increase in 3-mg increments q3-5 days up to 12 mg if necessary	3-12 mg/night
Hallucinations, delusions, behavioral dyscontrol, agitation/aggression, nocturnal wandering, or disinhibition	Donepezil	5 mg qam	Increase to 10 mg qam 4 weeks later	5-10 mg qam
	Rivastigmine	1.5 mg bid	Increase in 1.5-mg increments for both doses every 4 weeks; maximum, 6 mg bid	1.5-6.0 mg bid
	Galantamine	4 mg bid	Increase in 4-mg increments for both doses every 4 weeks; maximum, 12 mg bid	4-12 mg bid
	Risperidone	0.5 mg qhs	Increase in 0.5-mg increments q7 days in bid dosing (morning and bedtime)	0.5 mg qhs-1.5 mg bid
	Olanzapine	5 mg qhs	Increase in 5-mg increments q7 days in bid dosing (morning and bedtime)	5 mg qhs-10 mg bid
	Clozapine†	12.5 mg qhs	Increase in 12.5-mg increments q2-3 days	25 mg qhs-50 mg tid
	Quetiapine	25 mg qhs	Increase in 25-mg increments q3 days. One dosing >100 mg qhs necessary, increase gradually with ~$\frac{1}{3}$ daily dose in am and $\frac{2}{3}$ in pm	25 mg qhs-100 mg qam/400 mg qpm
	Valproic acid†	125 mg qhs	Increase in 125-mg increments q3-7 days in bid to tid dosing	250 mg qhs-500 mg tid
	Carbamazepine†	100 mg qhs	Increase in 100-mg increments q3-7 days in bid to tid dosing	200 mg qhs-200 mg tid

bid, twice daily; po, orally; q, every; qam, every morning; qd, daily; qhs, at bedtime; tid, 3 times daily.
*Disclaimer: The choice of which agents to use and which dosing schedules to recommend must be individualized. It is the responsibility of the clinician to consider potential side effects, drug interactions, allergic response, life-threatening reactions (e.g., leukopenia with clozapine), dosing changes due to renal or hepatic dysfunction, etc., before administering any drug to any patient, including those listed above. Dr. Boeve, Mayo Foundation, the editors, and the publisher will not be responsible for any adverse reactions of any kind to any patient regarding the content of this information.
†Periodic laboratory monitoring necessary; refer to guidelines provided by manufacturer.

270 Behavioral and Emotional Complications of Neurological Disorders

Jonathan T Stewart

Our understanding of the behavioral and emotional manifestations of neurological illness has evolved for the most part over less than a century, beginning with psychiatric interest in treating the sequelae of encephalitis lethargica [Level of Evidence: III][1] and neurosyphilis [III].[2,3] Only in more recent years have we begun to appreciate the magnitude of psychiatric comorbidity associated with many common neurological illnesses, such as dementia, stroke and Parkinson's disease. With the advent of the specialty of geriatric psychiatry, our understanding of the evaluation and treatment of such patients continues to grow rapidly.

This chapter will focus on common psychiatric manifestations of the dementing illnesses, delirium, stroke, and Parkinson's disease. Although specific studies are not always available, it is reasonable to extrapolate much of this material to other diseases. For example, management of behavioral problems in frontal/subcortical dementias such as Pick's disease and vascular dementia will also pertain in a greater or lesser degree to certain patients with multiple sclerosis, head trauma or neoplasms. Issues specific to particular diseases are noted in the text, and the most common behavioral and pharmacological strategies are summarized below in Tables 270.1 and 270.2.

Further complicating the picture is the fact that neurological illnesses may partially or even completely mimic virtually any primary psychiatric illness. The principle of the so-called "therapeutic metaphor" has been brought forth in psychiatric literature [III].[4,5] This principle, briefly stated, asserts that the more closely a neurological illness resembles a primary psychiatric disorder, the more likely it is to respond to conventional treatment for that disorder. For example, patients with post-stroke depression respond quite well to antidepressant medications, and patients with obsessive-compulsive symptoms related to Sydenham's chorea reportedly respond to anti-obsessional agents. While this is a useful guiding principle, it is quite dependent upon a thorough understanding of typical behavioral manifestations of neurological illness. For example, it is quite common for abulia to be misdiagnosed as depression, or disinhibition as mania or a personality disorder, in the presence of a vascular dementia. In such a situation, the clinician unaware of these typical manifestations of frontal/subcortical disease will see only a "therapeutic metaphor" and not a better-fitting neurobehavioral diagnosis. Further complicating the picture is the fact that depression and abulia can indeed occur concurrently in a patient with a vascular dementia, and in fact frequently do. Proper treatment must always be predicated upon proper, and thorough, diagnosis.

Dementia

Up to 90% of demented patients manifest significant behavioral problems during the course of their illness [II].[6,7] These problems are a strong predictor of institutional placement [II],[8,9] and are a major source of caregiver stress [II].[10,11] Thus, diagnosis and management of these problems is a high priority in caring for demented patients.

There are few strong predictors of behavioral problems among demented individuals; premorbid psychopathology and personality style probably have some predictive value, however [II].[10,12–14] Also, the premorbid relationship between the patient and primary caregiver may be a predictor of behavioral problems specific to that relationship [II].[10] Behavioral problems may also be more common in dementias associated with executive dysfunction [II].[15,16] Behavioral problems become somewhat more prevalent in more severely demented individuals [II],[17,18] but this fact does not really capture qualitative differences. For example, depression is generally more common in mild dementia [II],[19–22] delusions are more common in moderate dementia [III][6,22,23] and screaming is more common in severe dementia [II].[24]

Certain specific behavioral problems may be more or less common in specific dementing illnesses. For example, sexual disinhibition is more common in vascular dementia than in Alzheimer's disease [III].[25] However, with a few exceptions, management strategies for a given behavioral problem will be similar regardless of diagnosis; that is, management of sexual disinhibition in vascular dementia is more or less the same as in Pick's disease or Huntington's disease. Important disease-specific issues are described in the text. Probably the most important such issue concerns patients with diffuse Lewy body disease. These patients have a high prevalence of psychotic symptoms [II],[26] but should generally not be treated with typical neuroleptic agents because of a very high incidence of serious neurotoxicity [II].[27,28]

Older patients in general, and demented individuals in particular, generally have a fairly high incidence of side effects from most psychotropic drugs [III].[29] Furthermore, in many instances the efficacy of these drugs for behavioral problems is not particularly robust. As such, the initial management of these problems should usually be non-pharmacological

Table 270.1   Overview of common behavioral interventions

Condition	Behavioral intervention
Dementia: Catastrophic reactions	Non-confrontive, "no-fail" environment
Dementia: Resistiveness	Slow, gentle approach Minimize goals of care
Dementia: Delusions	Reassurance, distraction Validation therapy
Dementia: Hallucinations	Benign neglect Reassurance, distraction Increase social contact
Dementia: Screaming	Assess, manage pain or discomfort Discontinue restraints Increase sensory stimulation
Dementia: Disinhibited aggression	Antecedent control
Dementia: Sexual disinhibition	Redirection Limit access to vulnerable females Restrictive garments
Dementia: Abulia	Limit goals
Dementia: Wandering	Provide purposeful activities, exercise Provide secure area, safety measures Visual barriers Manage sleep disturbance aggressively
Dementia: Sleep disturbance	Maximize exposure to sunlight Phototherapy Avoid excessive naps Provide exercise Keep room cool and quiet; provide nightlight Restrict caffeine, alcohol Manage pain, nocturia
Delirium: Agitation, fearfulness	Quiet environment Avoid conversations that can be misinterpreted Protective measures
Stroke: Depression	Supportive psychotherapy Aggressive rehabilitation
Stroke: Pathological laughing and crying	Patient education, benign neglect
Parkinson's disease: Dopaminergic psychosis	Patient education, benign neglect Increase social contact

[III].[5,30] While nurses, psychologists and others may be particularly adept at such measures, the physician must have a basic understanding of these techniques as well.

In the author's experience, probably the most important principle in managing the demented patient involves the creation of a "no-fail" environment. The majority of demented patients ultimately develop anosognosia [II].[31,32] A corollary of this is the fact that demented patients generally exhibit more behavioral problems when confronted with or made aware of their deficits [III].[30] Education of the family or professional caregiver about this principle, coupled with specific suggestions to create this "customer is always right" environment, can be surprisingly effective in minimizing behavioral problems [III].[33] Other important principles to teach include providing a

consistent routine and limiting goals and expectations of the patient [III].[33]

With non-institutionalized patients, most of the ongoing interventions will be with the family, and with the primary caregiver in particular [III].[33-35] An educational approach, coupled with concrete problem-solving is generally best. A very important part of this approach is the discussion of risks and benefits associated with psychotropic drugs. Often, the best intervention for certain behavioral problems may be "benign neglect," and families are generally much more amenable to this after a frank discussion of risk-benefit ratios [III].[36] Difficult decisions, such as institutionalization and advance directives, should be discussed early rather than at the last minute; often the patient can be involved in this discussion if initiated early enough. The family should also be referred

Table 270.2 Overview of common pharmacological interventions

Condition	Pharmacological intervention, common dosage	Common adverse reactions
Dementia: Resistiveness	Lorazepam 0.25–1 mg prior to care	Sedation, ataxia, falls
Dementia: Delusions, hallucinations	High-potency neuroleptics (haloperidol 0.25–3 mg/d, thiothixene 1–5 mg/d, others)	Extrapyramidal side-effects; contraindicated in Lewy body disease
	Atypical neuroleptics (risperidone 0.5–3 mg/d, olanzapine 2.5–10 mg/d, quetiapine 12.5–75 mg/d)	Sedation, orthostasis, some extrapyramidal side-effects (especially risperidone)
Dementia: Screaming	Consider empirical trial of an antidepressant	See below
Dementia: Disinhibited aggression	Propranolol 30–180 mg/d Consider strategies for non-specific agitation, below	Hypotension, bradycardia, bronchospasm See below
Dementia: Sexual disinhibition	Medroxyprogesterone acetate 100–500 mg/wk SSRI antidepressants (see below)	Venous thrombosis, hyperglycemia See below
Dementia: Non-specific agitation	Valproic acid 250–1500 mg/d	Sedation, tremor, elevated liver enzymes, thrombocytopenia
	Carbamazepine 200–600 mg/d	Sedation, ataxia, hyponatremia, agranulocytosis
	Trazodone 50–200 mg/d	Sedation, orthostasis, priapism
	Buspirone 15–60 mg/d	Occasional headache
	Lorazepam 0.5–2 mg/d	Sedation, ataxia, falls
	Atypical neuroleptics (risperidone 0.5–3 mg/d, olanzapine 2.5–10 mg/d, quetiapine 12.5–75 mg/d)	Sedation, orthostasis, some extrapyramidal side-effects (especially risperidone)
	High-potency neuroleptics (haloperidol 0.25–3 mg/d, thiothixene 1–5 mg/d, others)	Extrapyramidal side-effects; contraindicated in Lewy body disease
Dementia: Wandering	Dechallenge neuroleptic agents	
Dementia: Sleep disturbance	Hypnotics (temazepam 7.5–15 mg qhs, zolpidem 5–10 mg qhs)	Sedation, ataxia, falls
	Trazodone 50–100 mg qhs	Sedation, orthostasis, priapism
Dementia: Depression	SSRI's (sertraline 50–100 mg/d, citalopram 20–40 mg/d, paroxetine 10–40 mg/d)	Anorexia, diarrhea, sexual dysfunction, restlessness, hyponatremia, myoclonus
	Tricyclics (nortriptyline 25–100 mg/d, desipramine 50–150 mg/d)	Orthostasis, anticholinergic effects, sedation, exacerbation of bundle branch block
	Other agents (mirtazapine 15–30 mg/d, venlafaxine 75–225 mg/d, bupropion 100–300 mg/d, nefazodone 100–400 mg/d, others)	Various effects
	Electroconvulsive therapy (ECT)	Temporary memory loss, arrhythmias, anaesthesia risks
Delirium: Agitation, fearfulness	High-potency neuroleptics (haloperidol 0.5–8 mg/d, droperidol 0.625–7.5 mg/d IV, others)	Extrapyramidal side-effects; contraindicated in Lewy body disease or neuroleptic malignant syndrome
	Atypical neuroleptics (risperidone 0.5–3 mg/d, olanzapine 2.5–10 mg/d, quetiapine 12.5–75 mg/d)	Sedation, orthostasis, some extrapyramidal side-effects (especially risperidone)
Stroke: Depression	As for depression in dementia (see above)	See above

continued

Table 270.2 *continued*

Condition	Pharmacological intervention, common dosage	Common adverse reactions
Stroke: Mania	Valproic acid 500–2500 mg/d	Sedation, tremor, elevated liver enzymes, thrombocytopenia
	Carbamazepine 400–1000 mg/d	Sedation, ataxia, hyponatremia, agranulocytosis
	Lithium carbonate 300–1200 mg/d	Tremor, diarrhea, ataxia, nephrogenic diabetes insipidus
Stroke: Pathological laughing and crying	SSRI antidepressants (see above)	See above
Parkinson's disease: Depression	As for depression in dementia (see above)	See above
Parkinson's disease: Dopaminergic psychosis	Decrease polypharmacy, especially anticholinergic agents	Loss of motor control
	Decrease or eliminate evening or bed-time antiparkinsonian agents	Loss of motor control, nocturnal dystonias
	Atypical neuroleptics (risperidone 0.25–1.5 mg/d, olanzapine 2.5–7.5 mg/d, quetiapine 25–200 mg/d)	Sedation, orthostasis, some loss of motor control (especially with risperidone)
	Ondansetron 12–24 mg/d	Headache, constipation
Parkinson's disease: REM behavior disorder	Clonazepam 0.5–1 mg qhs	Sedation, ataxia, falls
Parkinson's disease: Nocturnal rigidity, restless legs syndrome	Increase antiparkinsonian agent at bed-time	May increase risk for hallucinations
Parkinson's disease: Nightmares, nocturnal hallucinations	Decrease or eliminate evening or bed-time antiparkinsonian agents	Loss of motor control, nocturnal dystonias
	Atypical neuroleptics (risperidone 0.25–1.5 mg/d, olanzapine 2.5–7.5 mg/d, quetiapine 25–200 mg/d)	Sedation, orthostasis, some loss of motor control (especially with risperidone)

to appropriate resources, such as support groups, respite programs and attorneys. Finally, the physician must maintain vigilance for excessive caregiver stress (an almost universal problem) and signs of elder abuse, and must intervene accordingly [III].[35]

Agitation and psychosis

Agitated behaviors are quite common among demented individuals, probably occurring in 50–80% of patients at some time during the illness [II].[6,7,17] These may range from relatively trivial, "nuisance" behaviors to serious combativeness. Of course, the former should generally not be treated pharmacologically [III].[36] Naturally, there are qualitative, as well as quantitative, differences in agitation; unfortunately, consideration of these qualitative differences is not prominent in the literature to date [III].[33,36–38] Numerous studies have addressed the efficacy of one medication or another for agitation in Alzheimer's disease patients, but they rarely reflect the fact that agitation in the context of refusing to bathe, for example, is probably different than agitation related to the belief that one's wallet has been stolen.

Most agitated behaviors in demented individuals are relatively chronic, evolving and progressing over a matter of months or even years [III].[22] Any acute agitation, or any acute behavioral change, should suggest either a superimposed delirium or a major environmental change (such as institutionalization, hospitalization or travel) [III].[22,33,36,39,40] In our experience, the most commonly identified causes of such acute decompensation are drug effects, infections and dehydration. Obviously, correction of the underlying problem is the treatment of choice; low doses of high-potency neuroleptics may also be helpful for truly problematic agitation or fearfulness [I],[6,36,41,42] but it is essential to discontinue these medications as soon as the underlying problem is corrected.

While a comprehensive, validated classification scheme for agitated behaviors in dementia is yet to be developed, numerous "themes" are commonly seen. Possibly the most common [II][43] is the so-called catastrophic reaction, which was defined by Goldstein as "a substantive emotional reaction precipitated by task failure" [III].[44] These patients appear to be quite defensive about their deficits, and only become agitated when unable to do something, or especially when corrected by the caregiver or others. It has been suggested that catastrophic reactions do not respond well to medications [III],[45] but rather to non-pharmacological interventions [III];[46] our experience suggests that conscientious application of the "no-fail environment" is probably the treatment of choice.

Many demented individuals only become agitated in the context of nursing care [II].[47] Such resistiveness is a major problem for both institutions and family caregivers; it may be more common in patients with frontal/subcortical diseases such as vascular dementia and Pick's disease [II].[16] The most important principle in management of resistiveness is limiting care to the minimum amount necessary [III].[33] A strict routine, preferably at the patient's best time of day and with their preferred caregiver, may also be helpful, as may reassuring the patient that, "as soon as we get this done, I'll leave you alone" [III].[33] We have also found that premedication with low-dose, short acting benzodiazepines such as lorazepam may also help [III].[48]

Psychotic symptoms are commonly seen, especially in moderately demented individuals; in the case of Alzheimer's disease, between one-third and two-thirds of patients develop delusions and/or hallucinations [II].[49,50] Delusions generally lead to more behavioral problems than hallucinations [II].[51] These psychotic symptoms are common in many dementing illnesses; they are an especially prominent feature (especially visual hallucinations) of diffuse Lewy body disease [II].[26,50,52]

The most common delusions in dementia are the belief that something has been stolen and delusions of infidelity or abandonment [III].[5,39] The belief that the patient must engage in some previous role, such as needing to care for a sick parent, pick up small children at school, or attend to customers at a previously-owned business, also seems common [III].[33] If these delusions are truly problematic, causing either significant emotional distress to the patient or management problems in spite of reassurance, redirection and other behavioral techniques, they generally respond to treatment with low-dose neuroleptics [II].[6,39,53] High-potency agents such as haloperidol or thiothixene are generally preferred in this population [III].[39,46] Doses between 0.5 and 3 mg per day of haloperidol are typical. The goal of neuroleptic treatment is to decrease the emotional and behavioral response to the delusional material; complete resolution of the delusion is unusual [III],[33] and treatment is often limited by extrapyramidal side-effects [I].[6,39] Atypical neuroleptics such as risperidone and quetiapine, also in low doses, are effective for delusions and are associated with less extrapyramidal side effects [I].[54–56] If extrapyramidal side effects are problematic, a reduction or change of neuroleptic is preferred over the addition of anticholinergics such as benztropine or diphenhydramine, since anticholinergic drugs may exacerbate the patient's cognitive deficits [I].[57] Neuroleptic agents should generally be dechallenged every three to six months, in order to minimize the risk of development of tardive dyskinesia [III].[33,39] Again, these agents should be avoided in diffuse Lewy body disease due to the high incidence

of serious extrapyramidal side effects [II],[27,28] even with the atypical agent, risperidone [II].[28,58]

Patients with Alzheimer's disease may also develop Capgras syndrome (the delusion that a family member or friend has been replaced by an impostor) or other forms of reduplicative paramnesia [III];[23,39,46,59,60] perhaps the most common delusion of this type is that the patient is not in his or her own home. Again, if truly problematic, these delusions may respond to neuroleptics; there is one case report of preferential response to the neuroleptic agent, pimozide [III].[61]

The most common type of hallucination seen in demented individuals is the so-called "phantom boarder syndrome," a visual hallucination in which people, children or animals are seen living in the home [II].[30,36,62] This is an especially prominent symptom in diffuse Lewy body disease [II].[26,63] Surprisingly, the majority of patients do not become upset by these hallucinations [III],[30,36,64] and in fact there is evidence that the hallucinations may actually be comforting to some patients [II].[62] The treatment of choice for these hallucinations is more often than not caregiver education and "benign neglect" [III].[33,36] These problems may be more common in socially isolated individuals; indeed, it is common for the hallucinations to improve dramatically or even resolve if the patient is placed in an environment with more interpersonal contact [III].[65] Hallucinations probably do not respond as well as delusions to neuroleptic agents [II].[65]

Occasionally, the hallucinations of a demented individual will be found to represent a misinterpretation of things seen on television, or even misrecognition of one's own reflection in a mirror. These symptoms are more accurately characterized as illusions, and are easily remedied by removing the offending object [III].[5,23,30]

Repetitive screaming is a fairly non-specific, generally multifactorial symptom, usually seen in severely demented individuals [II].[24] Physical restraint, pain, and social isolation are all prominent, remediable factors [II].[24] Some authors have suggested that non-specific screaming may represent a depressive equivalent in severely demented individuals [II];[24,66] thus, an empirical trial of an antidepressant agent may be a reasonable option [III].[36,66]

In reality, a great deal of agitation in this population defies simple classification. Furthermore, a significant proportion of patients will require more than the environmental measures described above. Numerous medications have been shown to have anti-agitation effects in demented individuals, although again, very few studies have attempted to address specific qualitative types of agitation. Neuroleptic agents have traditionally been used for many types of agitation in this population [II].[6,39,46,56,67] Unfortunately, neuroleptic treatment has a great deal of potential for neurological side effects, including disabling extrapyramidal symptoms, irreversible tardive dyskinesia [I][6,67,68] and possibly further cognitive decline [I].[69] Furthermore, the efficacy of neuroleptics for empirical treatment of agitation in dementia is rather poor; only about one-sixth to one-third of patients show even a modest response [I],[6,39,53,67] and many patients actually improve behaviorally when neuroleptics are withdrawn [I].[70] Not surprisingly, the best predictors of response to neuroleptic therapy are hallucinations, delusions and serious physical aggression [I].[6,67] The atypical neuroleptic agents, including clozapine, risperidone, olanzapine, and quetiapine, are reportedly effective for agitation and are associated with less extrapyramidal side effects than the typical neuroleptics [I].[55,56,64] No study to date has clearly demonstrated efficacy superior to typical neuroleptics, however.

Numerous other agents have been reported to be effective for agitation in demented individuals. The anticonvulsants, carbamazepine [I][71,72] and valproic acid [III],[73,74] generally with conventional blood levels, have both been demonstrated to have significant anti-agitation effects. The antidepressant agent trazodone has also demonstrated anti-agitation effects, and may also be useful as a hypnotic [I].[75] Orthostatic hypotension may be problematic, however. Other antidepressant agents have also been anecdotally reported to be effective for agitation, although there are no controlled studies to date [III].[22,56] Beta-blockers such as propranolol [II],[67,76,77] lithium salts [III],[67] and buspirone [III][78] have also been reported as effective for agitation. Short-acting benzodiazepines such as lorazepam and oxazepam are commonly used for agitation in this population [II],[46,67] although their efficacy has yet to be proven in controlled studies [I].[22] Side effects include sedation, ataxia, and probably some decrement in cognitive function [III];[67] disinhibition and paradoxical agitation are probably much less common than was once believed [II].[79] There is also one report of an anti-agitation effect of conjugated estrogens [III].[80] These were noted to be effective and well tolerated both by male and female patients. Finally, there have been several reports of successfully treating refractory agitation with electroconvulsive therapy (ECT), independent of any evidence of depression [III].[81,82]

Abulia and disinhibition

Dementing illnesses that affect the frontal lobes and associated subcortical structures are generally accompanied by prominent "personality changes" [III].[15,83,84] The most commonly observed "changes" are decreased drive and motivation (abulia), and disinhibition [II].[83–86] Abulia does not really respond to pharmacological interventions [I];[87] a caregiver-education approach is most important, emphasizing the neurological nature of the behavior (or lack thereof!) and the importance of setting modest expectations [III].[30] Probably the most important clinical issue in the abulic patient is differentiation from depression [III];[30] the presence of dysphoria, pessimism, worrying and anorexia are all suggestive of depression (or abulia with concurrent depression).

Disinhibition is usually the more problematic issue in patients with these illnesses. There is generally a "coarsening of the personality," with loss of manners, tactlessness, decreased concern with personal hygiene and undue familiarity with others [III].[85] Petty crimes such as vagrancy, shoplifting, and panhandling are also common and are unfortunately not amenable to pharmacological interventions. The only interventions that we have found to be effective for such patients involve antecedent control, for example keeping the patient away from more formal social gatherings or from retail stores.

Some patients with frontal or subcortical disease become irritable; in these cases, aggressive or "agitated" behavior may represent a disinhibition of the normal reaction to frustration [III].[85] Patients may become assaultive over relatively trivial annoyances, and may have no concept of the inappropriateness of their actions [II].[77] Again, antecedent control (for example, trying to keep other intrusive patients away from the patient) seems more effective than operant conditioning. Pharmacologically, a number of studies have demonstrated the efficacy of propranolol for aggression in a variety of dementias and other neurological illnesses [I];[67,77,88,89] the majority of subjects in these studies have had diagnoses of frontal lobe or subcortical pathology. The therapeutic range of propranolol for this indication is quite broad, with some demented patients responding to dosages as low as 10 mg per day and other patients, notably younger patients with head injury, requiring over 600 mg per day [II].[67,77,88] The dosage of propranolol should generally be titrated quite slowly, watching closely for symptomatic bradycardia or hypotension [III].[88,89] Relative contraindications to beta-blockers include bronchospasm, congestive heart failure and diabetes [III].[88,89] Beta-blockers must also be tapered very slowly if ineffective. Some of the other agents mentioned above, such as the anticonvulsants and lithium, may also be reasonable choices for this type irritability. We have found neuroleptic agents to be generally ineffective for this sort of aggression.

Another potentially serious problem with such patients is sexual disinhibition, which may range anywhere from inappropriate flirting to sexual assault [III].[36,85,90] Again, environmental changes, such as placing the patient in an environment with limited access to vulnerable females, is paramount. Special garments are also available that restrict the patient's ability to disrobe or expose himself/herself. Failing this, pharmacological therapy may be undertaken to inhibit the patient's sexual drive. The most commonly used agent for male patients is medroxyprogesterone acetate, given intramuscularly in dosages between 100 mg per month and 400 mg per week [III].[90,91] Side effects are minimal, generally including weight gain and increased risk of deep venous thrombosis. Feminization is uncommon. Leuprolide is also reportedly effective, but is much more expensive [III].[91–93] Finally, there is one report of using paroxetine, a selective serotonin uptake inhibitor (SSRI) antidepressant, to treat such sexual disinhibition [III].[94] These agents are also quite well tolerated. While there is no literature concerning pharmacological treatment of sexual disinhibition in women, it is probably reasonable to assume that the SSRI's might be effective, given their similar effect on libido in younger men and women treated for depression.

Wandering

Between one-third and two-thirds of demented individuals wander [III].[39] This is a potentially serious problem that may cause tremendous distress to loved ones, if not serious injury or death. A failure to effectively manage wandering often leads to institutionalization [III].[33]

Wandering does not generally respond to pharmacological interventions [III].[55] Moreover, several authors have hypothesized that at least some wandering may be related to neuroleptic-induced akathisia [III],[6,36,46,95] and there are anecdotal reports of wanderers improving with discontinuation of neuroleptics [III].[36,96]

There are a number of helpful interventions for wandering, including aggressive management of sleep problems (nocturnal wandering is obviously much more difficult to detect and prevent), increased activity and exercise during the day and provision of a secure area in which to wander. Other important precautions include complex locks and/or alarms on outside doors and windows, provision of an identifying bracelet and not allowing the patient to carry valuable items that might make them a target for thieves [III].[22,33,39,97,98]

Some patients, presumably those with a degree of visual agnosia [III],[99] may respond to visual barriers. The most common strategy is to make the outside door more difficult to recognize, either by painting it the same color or pattern as the surrounding wall, by concealing any windows or by hiding or camouflaging the doorknob [II].[39,99,100] Placing strips of colored tape on the floor in front of the doorway is also reportedly effective; in theory, the patient may misinterpret this as a barrier and not attempt to cross it [II].[101] Finally, an occasional stimulus-bound patient may respond to either a Stop sign or a Do Not Enter sign on the door [III].[33,102]

Certain demented patients spend a great deal of time exploring and manipulating the environment. Such patients will frequently try doors, going through them if they find them unlocked [II].[96,103] These patients may also manipulate other objects in the environment, for example pulling fire alarms or rearranging furniture and pictures; this is somewhat reminiscent of utilization behavior [III].[104] They may also become intrusive with other patients or go through their belongings, leading to their being assaulted. This does not seem to respond to pharmacological treatment, but probably does respond to provision of purposeful activities [III].[33,98] It is often helpful to provide relatively familiar activities to such patients, as for example providing PVC pipe fittings to a former plumber [III].[30]

Perhaps the most unpleasant wandering scenario occurs in a mildly to moderately demented individual who wishes to go home, seeing no purpose remaining in the institution and perhaps believing his children, his parents, or his customers are waiting for him [II].[96,103] These are difficult situations, since to confront the patient with the reality of the situation inherently violates the principle of maintaining a "no-fail" environment. Current literature does not address whether a "delusional" belief that there is something to be done at home predicts a response to neuroleptics; the author's experience is that it does not. Generally, we have found attempts at distraction, providing face-saving reasons to stay longer, stalling and blaming the "unjust" situation on someone else (generally the doctor or a judge) to be the best solutions to these situations.

Sleep disturbance

Between 40–70% of demented individuals exhibit sleep disturbances [III].[39] It is especially important to treat these aggressively, as they can lead to accidents, wandering and, perhaps most importantly, caregiver exhaustion and institutionalization [II].[105] Furthermore, demented individuals tend to become more confused and manifest more behavioral problems at night, when there are few orienting cues [III].[33]

Sleep architecture changes significantly in older individuals, with a decrease in stage III and stage IV (delta) sleep, a commensurate increase in nocturnal awakenings [II][106,107] and a tendency toward sleep phase advance ("early to bed, early to rise") [II].[107,108] Demented individuals manifest further disturbances of the circadian cycle, with even more nocturnal awakenings and fragmentation of the sleep-wake cycle [II].[106,107] The net result of these changes is that demented individuals are frequently awake at times when they either cannot be supervised adequately or when they might awaken other individuals.

Management of sleep disturbances in demented individuals should begin with efforts to restore the normal circadian rhythm. Avoidance of naps and keeping the patient awake until a predetermined bedtime are important first steps [III].[33,39,109] It has been demonstrated that phototherapy (bright light therapy) can normalize the circadian rhythm in demented individuals and improve sleep disturbances [III].[110,111] This is generally difficult to implement in this population, but it is probably reasonable to assume that liberal exposure to daylight might have similar effects.

Other important steps in a program of sleep hygiene include restriction of caffeine and alcohol, aggressive treatment of any painful condition that might awaken the patient at night, appropriate interventions to minimize nocturia (and uncomfortable wetness if the patient is incontinent), provision of exercise in the late afternoon and early evening and keeping the bedroom relatively cool and quiet. A small night-light is desirable as well, to decrease the likelihood of disorientation should the patient awaken [III].[33,39]

If non-pharmacological measures are ineffective, pharmacological treatment of sleep disturbance is certainly preferable to institutionalization or more restrictive measures. Short-acting hypnotics such as temazepam and zolpidem are effective and generally fairly well tolerated; some clinicians prefer trazodone, although this can cause orthostatic hypotension [III].[36,97,109] Alternatively, if the patient is already receiving a psychotropic drug, a more sedating agent can be substituted (for example, substituting mirtazapine for fluoxetine) [III].[36]

Depression

Depression is common in a number of dementing illnesses [II].[112] In the case of Alzheimer's disease, for example, between 10 and 30% of patients ultimately develop a concurrent treatable depression [III].[19,20,49,113,114] The incidence of depression in vascular dementia is probably similar [II].[115] AIDS dementia complex is also frequently associated with depression, but this is often confounded by the presence of abulia and apathy, as in any subcortical dementia [II].[116–118] It is clear that depression is a common treatable cause of excess disability in demented individuals [I].[119] Prompt detection of depression does not generally improve cognitive function, but will often result in dramatic improvements in quality of life, both for the patient and the caregiver [II].[20]

In the demented patient as in any elderly patient, depression may present atypically. It is common for mood symptoms such as sadness and crying to be absent [III];[97,120,121] instead, "attitude" symptoms such as pessimism, guilt, hopelessness and anhedonia (the inability to enjoy previously enjoyed activities) should be sought [III].[36] This can be especially challenging in demented patients with limited verbal abilities [III].[23] Depression should be strongly considered in patients with unexplained appetite or weight loss, decreased energy, loss of interest in previous activities, failure to thrive or unexpected difficulties with activities of daily living [III].[36] Irritability and possibly nonspecific agitation and screaming may also suggest a possible treatable depression [II].[24,36,66] So-called "secondary depressions," due to medications, thyroid dysfunction, remote effects of malignancy, stroke and chronic infections, must also be ruled out [III].[22,36]

Once detected, depression should be treated aggressively in any demented patient [III].[36,122] Treatment should be more or less identical to that prescribed for a non-demented individual [III];[112] it has been well demonstrated that demented patients with concurrent depression respond as well to antidepressants as non-demented elderly patients [II].[20,113,123] Most commonly, the SSRI's, including fluoxetine, sertraline, paroxetine, and citalopram, are used in this population, and are generally well tolerated [III].[22,36,121] Common side effects include activation, insomnia, nausea and anorexia, sexual dysfunction and occasionally myoclonus [I].[22] Several newer agents, including bupropion, nefazodone and mirtazapine, are also effective and well tolerated in this population [III].[22,36,121] Tricyclic antidepressants may also be used, but are associated with significant orthostatic hypotension, anticholinergic effects, and a quinidine-like effect on cardiac conduction [I].[22,121] Advantages of tricyclics

include well-validated therapeutic blood levels, potent appetite stimulation, and beneficial effects on pain and sleep [III].[121] Because of reports of increased monoamine oxidase levels in Alzheimer's disease, the use of monoamine oxidase inhibitors in this population has been advocated [III].[124] These agents are indeed effective, but their use is limited by orthostatic hypotension and necessary dietary restrictions [III].[22] Patients with AIDS dementia complex and depression reportedly respond well to psychostimulants such as methylphenidate [III],[116,118,125] but may have a high incidence of side effects from other antidepressant agents, especially tricyclics [III].[125] For more severe or refractory depression, ECT may also be an extremely useful option [II].[126,127] Antidepressant therapy should be maintained for at least six months, or possibly longer; some [II],[19,21,122] but not all [III],[66] authors have suggested that depressive symptoms in demented individuals are time-limited, improving as the dementia progresses.

Delirium

Delirium is commonly seen in acute medical settings, frequently presenting behavioral management problems. Delirium is quite common in acutely ill elderly patients; from one-sixth to one-third of older medical or surgical inpatients become delirious at some point during hospitalization [II].[41,128,129] Probably the strongest independent risk factor for development of delirium is pre-existing cognitive impairment [II].[41,128–131] Thus, delirium will commonly be seen in patients with a known history of dementia.

In addition to attentional deficits, distractibility and altered level of consciousness, delirious patients frequently present with agitation and other behavioral problems. Hallucinations and especially illusions are quite common, occurring in between 40 and 75% of patients [III].[129] Illusions are mostly visual, although they may be seen in other sensory modalities [III].[41,129] There is generally a prominent disturbance in the sleep/wake cycle, with increased confusion and behavioral problems at night [III].[41,129] Vivid dreams and nightmares may also seemingly merge with the illusions and hallucinations [III].[129,132]

Delirium is an extremely unpleasant, frightening condition for the patient [III].[133] Since delirium is always indicative of a serious medical problem, the highest priority in its management is determination and correction of the underlying etiology [III].[41,134] Concurrently, however, it is important to keep the patient as safe and comfortable as possible. Appropriate measures should be implemented to protect the patient from falls or other injuries, or from pulling out IV's, catheters, sutures, and the like; obviously, such devices should be kept to the minimum necessary [III].[41] Nursing interventions should be directed toward minimizing consequences of bedrest (pressure ulcers, deep venous thrombosis, deconditioning, and so forth). Delirious patients generally fare best in a relatively quiet, under-stimulating environment, with relatively subdued lighting and low noise levels [III].[41,133] Some patients may misinterpret what is being said, and may overhear conversations about other patients and believe that it refers to them [III].[133]

The goals of pharmacotherapy in delirium are to minimize unpleasant fearfulness and dangerous behavior. Low doses of high-potency neuroleptics such as haloperidol are most commonly used and are safe and effective in this population; these may be used either routinely or on a *pro re nata* (*prn*) basis [I].[129,134,135] If an intravenous agent is necessary, droperidol may also be used [III].[136,137] There have also been several reports of the utility of atypical neuroleptics for delirious patients [II],[138,139] although these agents are only available orally. Probably the only absolute contraindication to neuroleptic therapy is delirium due to neuroleptic malignant syndrome. Some clinicians prefer to use short-acting benzodiazepines such as lorazepam, but this may exacerbate the delirium or further confound the picture [III].[140] Physostigmine should be avoided in delirium due to its short half-life and serious side effects (bradyarrhythmias, seizures, bronchospasm) [III].[41,141,142]

In dosing neuroleptics or other agents, treatment is usually initiated with relatively low doses and gradually titrated as necessary to minimize the patient's discomfort and potentially dangerous behaviors. Neuroleptics are generally quite effective for the behavioral aspects of delirium, and in fact may give a false sense of security. It must be remembered that this treatment is symptomatic only, and must not substitute for definitive treatment of the underlying etiology of the delirium.

Stroke

Stroke is associated with a variety of psychiatric sequelae; since strokes are focal neurological lesions, many of these problems are also seen in other focal lesions, such as tumors or traumatic brain injury. By far, the most important psychiatric complication of stroke is depression. Between 25 and 50% of stroke victims develop a clinically significant depression [II];[143–147] depression is an extremely important cause of rehabilitation failure [II][145,148,149] and severe residual disability [II][150] following stroke. Unfortunately, this tremendously important complication is often overlooked; less than 20% of post-stroke depression will ever be treated [II].[144–146,151,152] This is probably due at least in part to the atypical presentation of depression in any older patient, as described in the section on depression in dementia.

Post-stroke depression is almost certainly multifactorial; psychological reactions to illness and disability are important factors, as are neurobiological factors [II].[143,146] Significant post-stroke depression is more commonly seen in left hemispheric infarcts, especially in lesions closer to the frontal pole or of the left basal ganglia [II].[143,153–156] It must be emphasized, however, that depression is quite common following right hemispheric lesions as well [II].[144,147,157–159] In fact, depression following a right hemispheric stroke may be more difficult to diagnose, as such lesions are more commonly associated with anosognosia and loss of the emotional prosody of speech [III].[159–161]

Post-stroke depression generally responds quite well to conventional treatment, which should include both a supportive psychological and rehabilitative approach and antidepressant medication. Most classes of antidepressants have been demonstrated to be effective in post-stroke depression [I];[162–164] choice of antidepressant agent is more or less the same as described in the section on depression in dementia, and is generally dictated by side effect profile. For more serious and refractory cases, ECT may also be safe and effective [III].[165,166] Post-stroke depression, especially more severe depression, often remits after one to two years [II];[167] it may therefore be reasonable to try to discontinue antidepressants after a period of time.

Mania is seen much less frequently than depression following stroke or other focal brain lesions [II]. The localization is more frequently in the right hemisphere [II],[168,169] but mania can be seen from left hemispheric lesions as well [II].[169–171] Often, the differential diagnosis between mania and disinhibition from frontal lobe or subcortical pathology can be difficult. Both types of patients may be hypersexual, unduly familiar, tactless, and impulsive; a truly manic patient may exhibit more overtly grandiose delusions, pressured speech and a decreased need for sleep. The psychiatric literature on secondary mania (i.e., related to neurological illness) is probably at least somewhat contaminated by patients who are only disinhibited and insightless (an example of the limitation of the "therapeutic metaphor") [III].[172]

True post-stroke mania responds to mood-stabilizing agents [III],[169,170] although perhaps not as readily as primary bipolar illness [III].[173,174] As in primary bipolar illness, compliance is often problematic. Some authors have suggested that secondary mania may respond better to anticonvulsant agents, especially valproic acid, than to lithium salts [III].[173]

The syndrome of pathological laughing and crying is quite common following stroke, affecting around 20% of patients [II].[175,176] Crying is somewhat more common than laughing, and occurs abruptly with any emotional stimulus (regardless of valence), or simply with asking the patient about the problem [III].[176] It is important to distinguish this syndrome from a true depression, although both conditions may occur together [II].[175,176]

The syndrome of pathological laughing and crying is mostly a cosmetic problem. Both the patient and his/her family should be educated about its nature, and about the fact that it is not necessarily indicative of depression. If the condition is truly problematic for the patient, pharmacological treatment can be initiated. It is believed that the condition is related to damage to ascending serotonergic fibers from the dorsal raphé [II].[176,177] This is the rationale for treatment with SSRI's, which are treatment of choice. Citalopram [I][178] or fluoxetine [III][179,180] in conventional dosages are rapidly effective, generally within a few days (in contrast to the three weeks that is generally necessary to achieve antidepressant effect). Nortriptyline [I][181] and low dose amitriptyline [I][182] are also effective, but are associated with more side effects.

Parkinson's disease

A number of psychiatric complications are commonly seen in patients with Parkinson's disease. Up to one-third of patients [II],[183,184] usually older patients [II],[183-185] ultimately develop a dementia, generally of the subcortical variety [II].[186-188] Behavioral management of this dementia is really no different than in any other dementing illness, although these patients may be more susceptible to medication-induced psychiatric problems [II].[185,189]

A more common problem in Parkinson's disease is depression. About 40% of patients develop a clinically significant depression that will benefit from treatment [II].[190,191] Significant depression may be more common in patients with an earlier age of onset [II][192] and with initial right-sided symptoms [II].[190,193] This depression is clearly not simply attributable to a psychological reaction to the diagnosis or disability, as it antedates any motor symptoms in up to 25% of patients [II],[191,194,195] its severity does not correlate with the severity of motor symptoms [II],[194,196] and it usually does not respond to treatment of the motor symptoms [II].[191,197]

Depression in Parkinson's disease responds quite favorably to antidepressant agents [I].[191,198] As in other illnesses, the selection of an antidepressant is mostly based on side effect profile. Tricyclic antidepressants are more difficult to use in this population, since they may exacerbate pre-existing orthostatic hypotension or constipation. Moreover, excessive anticholinergic load may predispose to drug-induced hallucinations, as described below [III].[198] The SSRI's are commonly used in this population; caution is advised if used concurrently with selegiline because of reports of mild central serotonin syndrome associated with this combination (delirium, hyperreflexia, myoclonus) [III].[199-201] Electroconvulsive therapy is also quite effective for depression in Parkinson's disease [II],[202,203] and has the added benefit of increasing dopamine turnover, thus improving bradykinesia and rigidity. This improvement in motor function is seen in about 50% of patients, and may last for weeks to months [II].[202,203] It is in fact often necessary to reduce the patient's antiparkinsonian medications for a period of time following a course of ECT.

Drug-induced psychotic symptoms are also exceedingly common in Parkinson's disease, generally occurring in about 30% of patients treated with either levodopa or dopamine agonists [II].[204-207] The most common symptoms are visual hallucinations, usually involving people, children or animals (much like the "phantom boarder" in dementia) [II].[196,205,207,208] They tend to be much more prominent at night [II].[205,208,209] Auditory hallucinations and delusions are less common [II].[205,210,211] The majority of patients who hallucinate are aware that the hallucinations are not real [II],[208,209,211,212] and in fact almost three-quarters of patients are not threatened by the hallucinations [II].[205,209] Major predictors of drug-induced psychosis

in Parkinson's disease include concurrent dementia [II],[198,207,212] advanced age [II][198,207,212] and especially treatment with multiple antiparkinsonian agents [II][204,205] (especially anticholinergic agents [II][198,204,205,207]). Psychotic symptoms may be somewhat more common with dopamine agonists than with levodopa [II].[205] It should also be remembered that prominent visual hallucinations and mild dementia in a patient with parkinsonian symptoms may also be indicative of diffuse Lewy body disease, regardless of whether or not the patient is already being treated with antiparkinsonian agents [II].[26,52]

In the majority of cases, the most appropriate initial management of antiparkinsonian-induced hallucinations is patient education and reassurance [III].[196,211,213] Many patients consider the hallucinations to be no more than an annoyance and appreciate the value of avoiding additional medications. For truly problematic psychotic symptoms, a number of strategies may be effective. The lowest effective dose of antiparkinsonian medication should be sought [II];[196,205] often the patient's dosage can be reduced with minimal deterioration of motor function. Evening and night time medication should be minimized, as motor control is less important when the patient is sleeping, and as later doses are more often associated with psychotic symptoms [III].[196] It is also helpful to avoid a multiple drug regimen, striving for monotherapy [III].[196,205,208] In some such cases, we have found sustained-release levodopa to be an effective strategy for managing end-of-dose failure, precluding the need for adding a dopamine agonist or other agent. It is especially important to try to eliminate anticholinergic agents from the regimen [II],[196,198,205,208,211] as they are quite frequently associated with psychotic symptoms [II].[198,204,205,207]

The above strategies are generally quite effective for drug-induced psychosis. If further interventions are necessary, several of the newer atypical antipsychotic agents, in very low doses, are quite effective [III].[196,198,211] Low doses of clozapine, generally between 12.5 and 75 mg per day, are quite effective and usually fairly well tolerated [I],[198,213-217] although there is still a 2% risk of agranulocytosis, even at this low dosage [III].[198,211] Olanzapine, generally in doses of 2.5 to 7.5 mg per day [III],[218,219] and quetiapine, in doses of 25 to 200 mg per day [III],[196,220] are also reportedly effective and quite well tolerated. Risperidone in very low doses (i.e., 0.25 to 1.5 mg per day) may also be helpful [III],[221,222] but is frequently associated with unacceptable increases in parkinsonian symptoms [III].[223,224] Finally, ondansetron, a $5HT_3$ serotonin receptor antagonist used for nausea associated with chemotherapy, is reportedly effective and well-tolerated for antiparkinsonian-induced psychosis, although its cost is currently prohibitive [III].[225,226]

A variety of sleep disturbances are common in Parkinson's disease, occurring in up to 74% of patients [II].[227] Depression is one obvious cause of sleep disturbance, and of course responds well to antidepressant medication as described above. Early in the course of the illness, REM behavior disorder is also quite common; this may even manifest before any motor dysfunction is apparent [II].[196,228] This REM behavior disorder is the result of failure of the flaccid paralysis that normally accompanies rapid eye movement (REM) sleep; as a result, the patient becomes very active and sometimes violent during REM sleep [II].[229] Often, the patient and the bed partner are able to describe the behavior in the context of a dream, for example, making grasping motions in response to a dream about falling from a tree. In general, REM behavior disorder responds quite well to clonazepam, usually 0.5 to 1 mg given at bed time [II],[229] although ataxia and daytime sedation may be problematic.

Patients with more advanced Parkinson's disease frequently complain of painful dystonias [II][230] or of disturbing rigidity and bradykinesia at night; complaints of difficulties turning over in bed or getting to the bathroom are common. Some patients also develop restless legs syndrome [III].[196] These problems generally respond well to a bed time dose of levodopa or a dopamine agonist, although as mentioned above, evening doses of antiparkinsonian agents increase the risk for development of psychotic symptoms [III].[196]

Sleep disturbance is often the earliest sign of incipient drug-induced psychosis. Indeed, sleep problems predict the development of hallucinations [II].[207,227] Patients frequently present with insomnia or fragmented sleep, which progresses to prominent, vivid dreams or nightmares and then to frank nocturnal hallucinations [II].[196,207,211,231] The appropriate approach to such patients is to reduce or eliminate evening or bed time antiparkinsonian medications; if this is ineffective, an atypical antipsychotic given at bedtime is generally effective [II].[196]

References

1. Ward CD. Encephalitis lethargica and the development of neuropsychiatry. Psychiatr Clin N Am 1986; 9:215–224
2. Kraepelin E. General Paresis. New York: The Journal of Nervous and Mental Disease Publishing Co, 1913
3. Duffy JD. General paralysis of the insane: neuropsychiatry's first challenge. J Neuropsychiatr Clin Neurosci 1995;7:243–249
4. Leibovici A, Tariot PN. Agitation associated with dementia: a systematic approach to treatment. Psychopharmacol Bull 1988;24:49–53
5. Tariot PN. Treatment strategies for agitation and psychosis in dementia. J Clin Psychiatry 1996;57(Suppl 14):21–29
6. Wragg RE, Jeste DV. Neuroleptics and alternative treatments: management of behavioral symptoms and psychosis in Alzheimer's disease and related conditions. Psychiatr Clin N Am 1988;11:195–213
7. Tariot PN, Blazina L. The psychopathology of dementia. In: Morris J, ed. Handbook of Dementing Illnesses. New York: Marcel Dekker, 1994:461–475
8. Cohen CA, Gold DP, Shulman KI. Factors determining the decision to institutionalize dementing individuals: a prospective study. Gerontologist 1993;33:714–720
9. Knopman DS, Berg JD, Thomas R, et al. Nursing home placement is related to dementia progression: experience from a clinical trial. Neurology 1999;52:714–718
10. Hamel M, Gold DP, Andres D, et al. Predictors and consequences of aggressive behavior by community-based dementia patients. Gerontologist 1990;30:206–211
11. Victoroff J, Mack WJ, Nielson KA. Psychiatric complications of dementia: impact on caregivers. Dementia Geriatr Cognit Dis 1998; 9:50–55
12. Shomaker D. Problematic behavior and the Alzheimer patient: retrospective as a method of understanding and counseling. Gerontologist 1987;27:370–375
13. Chatterjee A, Strauss M, Smyth K, Whitehouse P. Personality changes in Alzheimer's disease. Arch Neurol 1992;49:486–491
14. Magai C, Cohen CI, Culver C, et al. Relationship between premorbid personality and patterns of emotion expression in mid- to late-stage dementia. Int J Geriatr Psychiatry 1997;12:1092–1099
15. Royall DR, Mahurin RK, Gray KF. Bedside assessment of executive cognitive impairment: the Executive Interview. J Am Geriatr Soc 1992;40:1221–1226
16. Stewart JT, Gonzalez-Perez E, Zhu Y, Robinson BE. Cognitive predictors of resistiveness in dementia patients. Am J Geriatr Psychiatry 1999;7:259–263
17. Teri L, Larson EB, Reifler BV. Behavioral disturbance in dementia of the Alzheimer type. J Am Geriatr Soc 1988;36:1–6
18. O'Connor DW, Pollitt PA, Roth M, et al. Problems reported by relatives in a community study of dementia. Br J Psychiatry 1990;156:835–841
19. Reifler BV, Larson E, Hanley R. Coexistence of cognitive impairment and depression in geriatric outpatients. Am J Psychiatry 1982;139:623–626
20. Reifler BV, Larson E, Teri L, Poulsen M. Dementia of the Alzheimer's type and depression. J Am Geriatr Soc 1986;34:855–859
21. Zubenko GS, Rosen J, Sweet RA, et al. Impact of psychiatric hospitalization on behavioral complications of Alzheimer's disease. Am J Psychiatry 1992;149:1484–1491
22. American Psychiatric Association. Practice guidelines for the treatment of patients with Alzheimer's disease and other dementias of late life. Am J Psychiatry 1997;154(Suppl 5):1–39
23. Bolger JP, Carpenter BV, Strauss ME. Behavior and affect in Alzheimer's disease. Clin Geriatr Med 1994; 10:315–337
24. Cohen-Mansfield J, Werner P, Marx MS. Screaming in nursing home residents. J Am Geriatr Soc 1990;38:785–792
25. Leo RJ, Kim KY. Clomipramine treatment of paraphilias in elderly demented patients. J Geriatr Psychiatry Neurol 1995;8:123–124
26. Klatka LA, Louis ED, Schiffer RB. Psychiatric features in diffuse Lewy body disease: a clinicopathologic study using Alzheimer's disease and Parkinson's disease comparison groups. Neurology 1996;47:1148–1152
27. McKeith I, Fairbairn A, Perry R, et al. Neuroleptic sensitivity in patients with senile dementia of Lewy body type. Br Med J 1992;305:673–678
28. Ballard C, Grace J, McKeith I, Holmes C. Neuroleptic sensitivity in dementia with Lewy bodies and Alzheimer's disease. Lancet 1998;351:1032–1033
29. Hume AL, Owens NJ. Drugs and the elderly. In:

Reichel W, ed. Care of the Elderly. 4th ed. Baltimore: Williams and Wilkins, 1995:41–63

30. Weiner MF, Teri L, Williams BT. Psychological and behavioral management. *In:* Weiner MF, ed. The Dementias: Diagnosis, Management, and Research. 2nd ed. Washington: American Psychiatric Press, 1996: 139–173

31. Sevush S, Leve N. Denial of memory deficit in Alzheimer's disease. Am J Psychiatry 1993;150:748–751

32. Starkstein SE, Sabe L, Chemerinski E, et al. Two domains of anosognosia in Alzheimer's disease. J Neurol Neurosurg Psychiatry 1996;61:485–490

33. Stewart JT. Management of behavior problems in the demented patient. Am Fam Physician 1995;52: 2311–2322

34. Doty L, Heilman KM, Stewart JT, et al. Case management in Alzheimer's disease. J Case Mgmt 1993:2: 130–136

35. Weiner MF, Svetlik D. Dealing with family caregivers. *In:* Weiner MF, ed. The Dementias: Diagnosis, Management, and Research. 2nd ed. Washington: American Psychiatric Press, 1996:233–249

36. Lehninger FW, Ravindran VL, Stewart JT. Management strategies for problem behaviors in the patient with dementia. Geriatrics 1998;53(4):55–75

37. Cohen-Mansfield J. Agitated behaviors in the elderly—II. Preliminary results in the cognitively deteriorated. J Am Geriatr Soc 1986;34:722–727

38. Caine ED. Diagnostic classification of neuropsychiatric signs and symptoms in patients with dementia. Int Psychogeriatr 1996;8(Suppl 3):273–279

39. Alessi CA. Managing the behavioral problems of dementia in the home. Clin Geriatr Med 1991;7: 787–801

40. Luxenberg JS. Differentiating behavioral disturbances of dementia from symptoms of delirium. Int Psychogeriatr 1996:8(Suppl 3):425–427

41. Francis J. Delirium in older patients. J Am Geriatr Soc 1992;40:829–838

42. Cole MG, Primeau FJ, Elie LM. Delirium: prevention, treatment and outcome studies. J Geriatr Psychiatry Neurol 1998;11:126–137

43. Rabins PV, Mace NL, Lucas MJ. The impact of dementia on the family. JAMA 1982;248:333–335

44. Goldstein K. The effect of brain damage on the personality. Psychiatry 1952;15:245–260

45. Teasell R. Catastrophic reaction after stroke: a case study. Am J Phys Med Rehab 1993;72:151–153

46. Tueth MJ. Dementia: diagnosis and emergency behavioral complications. J Emerg Med 1995;13:519–525

47. Bridges-Parlet S, Knopman D, Thompson T. A descriptive study of physically aggressive behavior in dementia by direct observation. J Am Geriatr Soc 1994;42: 192–197

48. Fritz J, Stewart JT. Resistive aggression in dementia: treatment with lorazepam. Am J Psychiatry 1990;147: 1250

49. Wragg RE, Jeste DV. Overview of depression and psychosis in Alzheimer's disease. Am J Psychiatry 1989; 146:577–587

50. Ballard CG, Saad K, Patel A, Gahir M. The prevalence and phenomenology of psychotic symptoms in dementia sufferers. Int J Geriatr Psychiatry 1995;10: 477–485

51. Cohen-Mansfield J, Taylor L, Werner P. Delusions and hallucinations in an adult day care population: a longitudinal study. Am J Geriatr Psychiatry 1998;6:104–121

52. Ala TA, Yang KH, Sung JH, Frey WH. Hallucinations and signs of parkinsonism help distinguish patients with dementia and cortical Lewy bodies from patients with Alzheimer's disease at presentation: a clinicopathological study. J Neurol Neurosurg Psychiatry 1997;62:16–21

53. Schneider LS, Pollock VE, Lyness SA. A metaanalysis of controlled trials of neuroleptic treatment in dementia. J Am Geriatr Soc 1990;38:553–563

54. Katz IR, Jeste DV, Mintzer JE, et al. Comparison of risperidone and placebo for psychosis and behavioral disturbances associated with dementia: a randomized, double-blind trial. J Clin Psychiatry 1999;60:107–115

55. Stoppe G, Brandt CA, Staedt JH. Behavioral problems associated with dementia: the role of newer antipsychotics. Drugs Aging 1999;14:41–54

56. Tariot PN. Treatment of agitation in dementia. J Clin Psychiatry 1999;60(Suppl 8):11–20

57. Sunderland T, Tariot PN, Mueller EA, et al. Cognitive and behavioral sensitivity to scopolamine in Alzheimer patients and controls. Psychopharmacol Bull 1985;21:676–679

58. McKeith IG, Ballard CG, Harrison RWS. Neuroleptic sensitivity to risperidone in Lewy body dementia. Lancet 1995;346:699

59. Lipkin B. Capgras syndrome heralding the development of dementia. Br J Psychiatry 1988;153:117–118

60. Neitch SM, Zarraga A. A misidentification delusion in two Alzheimer's patients. J Am Geriatr Soc 1991;39: 513–515

61. Tueth MJ, Cheong JA. Successful treatment with pimozide of Capgras syndrome in an elderly male. J Geriatr Psychiatry Neurol 1992;5:217–219

62. Ballard CG, Bannister CL, Patel A, et al. Classification of psychotic symptoms in dementia sufferers. Acta Psychiatr Scand 1995;92:63–68

63. Gomez-Tortosa E, Ingraham AO, Irizarry MC, Hyman BJ. Dementia with Lewy bodies. J Am Geriatr Soc 1998;46:1449–1458

64. Schneider LS. Pharmacologic management of psychosis in dementia. J Clin Psychiatry 1999;60(Suppl 8): 54–60

65. Cole MG. Charles Bonnet hallucinations: a case series. Can J Psychiatry 1992;37:268–270

66. Greenwald BS, Marin DB, Silverman SM. Serotoninergic treatment of screaming and banging in dementia. Lancet 1986;2:1464–1465

67. Risse SC, Barnes R. Pharmacologic treatment of agitation associated with dementia. J Am Geriatr Soc 1986;34:368–376

68. Pollock BG, Mulsant BH. Antipsychotics in older patients: a safety perspective. Drugs Aging 1995;6: 312–323

69. Devanand DP, Sackeim HA, Brown RP, Mayeux R. A pilot study of haloperidol treatment of psychosis and behavioral disturbance in Alzheimer's disease. Arch Neurol 1989;46:854–857

70. Thapa PB, Meador KG, Gideon P, et al. Effects of antipsychotic withdrawal in elderly nursing home residents. J Am Geriatr Soc 1994;42:280–286

71. Tariot PN, Erb R, Leibovici A, et al. Carbamazepine treatment of agitation in nursing home patients with dementia: a preliminary study. J Am Geriatr Soc 1994; 42:1160–1166

72. Tariot PN, Erb R, Podgorski CA, et al. Efficacy and tolerability of carbamazepine for agitation and aggression in dementia. Am J Psychiatry 1998;155:54–61

73. Lott AD, McElroy SL, Keys MA. Valproate in the treatment of behavioral agitation in elderly patients

with dementia. J Neuropsychiatry Clin Neurosci 1995;7: 314–319

74. Porsteinsson AP, Tariot PN, Erb R, Gaile S. An open trial of valproate for agitation in geriatric neuropsychiatric disorders. Am J Geriatr Psychiatry 1997;5:344–351

75. Sultzer D, Gray KF, Gunay I, et al. A double-blind comparison of trazodone and haloperidol for treatment of agitation in patients with dementia. Am J Geriatr Psychiatry 1997;5:60–69

76. Weiler PG, Mungas D, Bernick C. Propranolol for the control of disruptive behavior in senile dementia. J Geriatr Psychiatry Neurol 1988;1:226–230

77. Shankle WR, Nielson KA, Cotman CW. Low-dose propranolol reduces aggression and agitation resembling that associated with orbitofrontal dysfunction in elderly demented patients. Alzheimer Dis Assoc Dis 1995;9:233–237

78. Sakauye KM, Camp CJ, Ford PA. Effects of buspirone on agitation associated with dementia. Am J Geriatr Psychiatry 1993;1:82–84

79. Dietch JT, Jennings RK. Aggressive dyscontrol in patients treated with benzodiazepines. J Clin Psychiatry 1988;49:184–188

80. Kyomen HH, Nobel KW, Wei JY. The use of estrogen to decrease aggressive physical behavior in elderly men with dementia. J Am Geriatr Soc 1991;39: 1110–1112

81. Carlyle W, Killick L, Ancill R. ECT: an effective treatment in the screaming demented patient. J Am Geriatr Soc 1991;39:637

82. Holmberg SK, Tariot PN, Challapalli R. Efficacy of ECT for agitation in dementia: a case report. Am J Geriatr Psychiatry 1996;4:330–334

83. Mesulam M-M. Frontal cortex and behavior. Ann Neurol 1986;19:320–325

84. Cummings JL. Frontal-subcortical circuits and human behavior. Arch Neurol 1993;50:873–880

85. Skuster DZ, Digre KB, Corbett JJ. Neurologic conditions presenting as psychiatric disorders. Psychiatr Clin N Am 1992;15:311–333

86. Levy ML, Miller BL, Cummings JL, et al. Alzheimer disease and frontotemporal dementias. Behavioral distinctions. Arch Neurol 1996;53:687–690

87. Nadeau SE, Malloy PF, Andrew ME. A crossover trial of bromocriptine in the treatment of vascular dementia. Ann Neurol 1988;24:270–272

88. Greendyke RM, Kanter DR, Schuster DB, et al. Propranolol treatment of assaultive patients with organic brain disease: a double-blind crossover, placebo-controlled study. J Nerv Ment Dis 1986;174:290–294

89. Stewart JT, Mounts ML, Clark RL. Aggressive behavior in Huntington's disease: treatment with propranolol. J Clin Psychiatry 1987;48:106–108

90. Cooper AJ. Medroxyprogesterone acetate (MPA) treatment of sexual acting out in men suffering from dementia. J Clin Psychiatry 1987;48:368–370

91. Amadeo M. Anti-androgen treatment of aggressivity in men suffering from dementia. J Geriatr Psychiatry Neurol 1996;9:142–145

92. Rich SS, Ovsiew F. Leuprolide acetate for exhibitionism in Huntington's disease. Movement Dis 1994;9: 353–357

93. Ott BR. Leuprolide treatment of sexual aggression in a patient with dementia and the Kluver-Bucy syndrome. Clin Neuropharmacol 1995;18:443–447

94. Stewart JT, Shin KJ. Paroxetine treatment of sexual disinhibition in dementia. Am J Psychiatry 1997;154:1474

95. Cohen-Mansfield J, Werner P, Marx MS, Freedman L. Two studies of pacing in the nursing home. J Gerontol 1991;46:M77–M83

96. Hussian RA. Wandering and disorientation. In: Carstensen LL, Edelstein BA, eds. Handbook of Clinical Gerontology. New York: Pergamon Press, 1987: 177–189

97. Winograd CH, Jarvik LF. Physician management of the demented patient. J Am Geriatr Soc 1986;34: 295–308

98. Rader J. A comprehensive staff approach to problem wandering. Gerontologist 1987;27:756–760

99. Namazi KH, Rosner TT, Calkins MP. Visual barriers to prevent ambulatory Alzheimer's patients from exiting through an emergency door. Gerontologist 1989;29: 699–702

100. Dickinson JI, McLain-Kark J, Marshall-Baker A. The effects of visual barriers on exiting behavior in a dementia care unit. Gerontologist 1995;35:127–130

101. Hussian RA, Brown DC. Use of two-dimensional grid patterns to limit hazardous ambulation in demented patients. J Gerontol 1987;5:558–560

102. Calkins MP, Chafetz PK. Structuring environments for patients with dementia. In: Weiner MF, ed. The Dementias: Diagnosis, Management, and Research. 2nd ed. Washington: American Psychiatric Press, 1996: 297–311

103. Hope RA, Fairburn CG. The nature of wandering in dementia: a community-based study. Int J Geriatr Psychiatry 1990;5:239–245

104. Lhermitte F. "Utilization behavior" and its relation to lesions of the frontal lobes. Brain 1983;106:237–255

105. Pollack CP, Perlick D. Sleep problems and institutionalization of the elderly. J Geriatr Psychiatry Neurol 1991;4:204–210

106. Prinz PN, Peskind ER, Vitaliano PP, et al. Changes in the sleep and waking EEGs of nondemented and demented elderly subjects. J Am Geriatr Soc 1982;30: 86–93

107. Culebras A. Update on disorders of sleep and the sleep-wake cycle. Psychiatr Clin N Am 1992;15: 467–489

108. Carrier J, Monk TH, Reynolds CF, et al. Are age differences in sleep due to phase differences in the output of the circadian timing system? Chronobiol Int 1999;16: 79–91

109. Weiner MF, Schneider LS, Gray KF, Stern RG. Pharmacological management and treatment of dementia and secondary symptoms. In: Weiner MF, ed. The Dementias: Diagnosis, Management, and Research. 2nd ed. Washington: American Psychiatric Press, 1996:175–210

110. Satlin A, Volicer L, Ross V, et al. Bright light treatment of behavioral and sleep disturbances in patients with Alzheimer's disease. Am J Psychiatry 1992;149: 1028–1032

111. Mishima K, Okawa M, Hishikawa Y, et al. Morning bright light therapy for sleep and behavior disorders in elderly patients with dementia. Acta Psychiatr Scand 1994;89:1–7

112. McAllister TW, Powers R. Approaches to the treatment of dementing illness. In: Emery VOB, Oxman TE, eds. Dementia: Presentations, Differential Diagnosis, and Nosology. Baltimore: Johns Hopkins University Press, 1994:355–383

113. Greenwald BS, Kramer-Ginsberg E, Marin DB, et al. Dementia with coexistent major depression. Am J Psychiatry 1989;146:1472–1478

114. Alexopoulis GS, Namabudiri DE. Depressive dementia: cognitive and biologic correlates and the course of illness. In: Emery VOB, Oxman TE, eds. Dementia:

Presentations, Differential Diagnosis, and Nosology. Baltimore: Johns Hopkins University Press, 1994: 321–335

115. Sultzer DL, Levin HS, Mahler ME, et al. A comparison of psychiatric symptoms in vascular dementia and Alzheimer's disease. Am J Psychiatry 1993;150: 1806–1812

116. Holmes VF, Fernandez F, Levy JK. Psychostimulant response in AIDS-related complex patients. J Clin Psychiatry 1989;50:5–8

117. Pajeau AK, Roman GC. HIV encephalopathy and dementia. Psychiatr Clin N Am 1992;15:455–466

118. Brown GR. The use of methylphenidate for cognitive decline associated with HIV disease. Int J Psychiatr Med 1995;25:21–37

119. Kramer SI, Reifler BV. Depression, dementia and reversible dementia. Clin Geriatr Med 1992;8:289–297

120. Charatan FB. Depression in the elderly: diagnosis and treatment. Psychiatr Ann 1985;15:313–316

121. Stewart JT. Diagnosing and treating depression in the hospitalized elderly. Geriatrics 1991;46(1):64–72

122. Tune LE. Depression and Alzheimer's disease. Depression Anxiety 1998;8(Suppl 1):91–95

123. Stoudemire A, Hill C, Gulley LR, Morris R. Neuropsychological and biomedical assessment of depression-dementia syndromes. J Neuropsychiatry Clin Neurosci 1989;1:347–361

124. Jenike MA. Monoamine oxidase inhibitors as treatment for depressed patients with primary degenerative dementia (Alzheimer's disease). Am J Psychiatry 1985;142:763–764

125. Melton SK, Kirkwood CK, Ghaemi SN. Pharmacotherapy of HIV dementia. Ann Pharmacother 1997;31: 457–473

126. Price TR, McAllister TW. Safety and efficacy of ECT in depressed patients with dementia: a review of clinical experience. Convuls Ther 1989;5:1–74

127. Zwil AS, Pelchat RJ. ECT in the treatment of patients with neurological and somatic disease. Int J Psychiatr Med 1994;24:1–29

128. Schor JD, Levkoff SE, Lipsitz LA, et al. Risk factors for delirium in hospitalized elderly. JAMA 1992;267: 827–831

129. Taylor D, Lewis S. Delirium. J Neurol Neurosurg Psychiatry 1993;56:742–751

130. Inouye SK, Viscoli CM, Horwitz RI, et al. A predictive model for delirium in hospitalized elderly medical patients based on admission characteristics. Ann Int Med 1993;119:474–481

131. Pompei P, Foreman M, Rudberg MA, et al. Delirium in hospitalized older persons: outcomes and predictors. J Am Geriatr Soc 1994;42:809–815

132. Lipowski ZJ. Update on delirium. Psychiatr Clin N Am 1992;15:335–346

133. Easton C, MacKenzie F. Sensory-perceptual alterations: delirium in the intensive care unit. Heart Lung 1988;17:229–237

134. Trzepacz PT. Delirium: advances in diagnosis, pathophysiology, and treatment. Psychiatr Clin N Am 1996;19:429–448

135. Breitbart W, Marotta R, Platt MM, et al. A double-blind trial of haloperidol, chlorpromazine, and lorazepam in the treatment of delirium in hospitalized AIDS patients. Am J Psychiatry 1996;153:231–237

136. Frye MA, Coudreaut MF, Hakeman SM, et al. Continuous droperidol infusion for management of agitated delirium in an intensive care unit. Psychosomatics 1995;36:301–305

137. Lawrence KR, Nasraway SA. Conduction disturbances associated with administration of butyrophenone antipsychotics in the critically ill: a review of the literature. Pharmacother 1997;17:531–537

138. Sipahimalani A, Masand PS. Use of risperidone in delirium: case reports. Ann Clin Psychiatry 1997;9: 105–107

139. Sipahimalani A, Masand PS. Olanzapine in the treatment of delirium. Psychosomatics 1998;39:422–430

140. Patkar AA, Kunkel EJS. Treating delirium among elderly patients. Psychiatr Serv 1997;48:46–48

141. Baldessarini RJ, Gelenberg AJ. Using physostigmine safely. Am J Psychiatry 1979;136:1608–1609

142. Smilkstein MJ. As the pendulum swings: the saga of physostigmine. J Emerg Med 1991;9:275–277

143. Robinson RG, Starr LB, Kubos KL, Price TR. A two-year longitudinal study of post-stroke mood disorders: findings during the initial evaluation. Stroke 1983;14: 736–741

144. Ebrahim S, Barer D, Nouri F. Affective illness after stroke. Br J Psychiatry 1987;151:52–56

145. Wade DT, Legh-Smith J, Hewer RA. Depressed mood after stroke: a community study of its frequency. Br J Psychiatry 1987;151:200–205

146. Gustafson Y, Nilsson I, Mattsson M, et al. Epidemiology and treatment of post-stroke depression. Drugs Aging 1995;7:298–309

147. Pohjasvaara T, Leppavuori A, Siira I, et al. Frequency and clinical determinants of poststroke depression. Stroke 1998;29:2311–2317

148. Sinyor D, Amato P, Kaloupek DG, et al. Post-stroke depression: relationships to functional impairment, coping strategies, and rehabilitation outcome. Stroke 1986;17:1102–1107

149. Morris PL, Raphael N, Robinson RG. Clinical depression is associated with impaired recovery from stroke. Med J Australia 1992;157:239–242

150. Bond J, Gregson B, Smith M, et al. Outcomes following acute hospital care for stroke or hip fracture: how useful is an assessment of anxiety or depression for older people? Int J Geriatr Psychiatry 1998;13: 601–610

151. Feibel JH, Springer CJ. Depression and failure to resume social activities after stroke. Arch Phys Med Rehabil 1982;63:276–278

152. Ramasubbu R, Kennedy SH. Factors complicating the diagnosis of depression in cerebrovascular disease. Part I: phenomenological and nosological issues. Can J Psychiatry 1994;39:596–600

153. Robinson RG, Kubos KL, Starr LB, et al. Mood disorders in stroke patients: importance of location of lesion. Brain 1984;107:81–93

154. Starkstein SE, Robinson RG, Price TR. Comparison of cortical and subcortical lesions in the production of post-stroke mood disorders. Brain 1987;110:1045–1059

155. Stern RA, Bachman DL. Depressive symptoms following stroke. Am J Psychiatry 1991;148:351–356

156. Herrmann M, Bartels C, Schumacher M, Wallesch CW. Post-stroke depression: is there a patho-anatomic correlate for depression in the post-acute stage of stroke? Stroke 1995;26:850–856

157. Sinyor D, Jacques P, Kaloupek DG, et al. Post-stroke depression and lesion location: an attempted replication. Brain 1986;109:537–546

158. Agrell B, Dehlin O. Depression in stroke patients with left and right hemisphere lesions: a study in geriatric rehabilitation in-patients. Aging 1994;6:49–56

159. Gordon WA, Hibbard MR. Post-stroke depression: an

examination of the literature. Arch Phys Med Rehabil 1997;78:658–663

160. Ross ED, Rush AJ. Diagnosis and neuroanatomical correlates of depression in brain-damaged patients. Arch Gen Psychiatry 1981;38:1344–1354

161. Ramasubbu R, Kennedy SH. Factors complicating the diagnosis of depression in cerebrovascular disease. Part II: neurological deficits and various assessment methods. Can J Psychiatry 1994;39:601–607

162. Lipsey JR, Robinson RG, Pearlson GD, et al. Nortriptyline treatment of post-stroke depression: a double-blind study. Lancet 1984;1:297–302

163. Reding MJ, Orto LA, Winter SW, et al. Antidepressant therapy after stroke: a double-blind trial. Arch Neurol 1986;43:763–765

164. Andersen G, Vestergaard K, Lauritzen L. Effective treatment of post-stroke depression with the selective serotonin reuptake inhibitor citalopram. Stroke 1994; 25:1099–1104

165. Murray GB, Shea V, Conn DK. Electroconvulsive therapy for post-stroke depression. J Clin Psychiatry 1986;47:258–260

166. Currier MB, Murray GB, Welch CC. Electroconvulsive therapy for post-stroke depressed geriatric patients. J Neuropsychiatry Clin Neurosci 1992;4:140–144

167. Robinson RG, Bolduc P, Price TR. A two-year longitudinal study of post-stroke depression: diagnosis and outcome at one and two year follow-up. Stroke 1987; 18:837–843

168. Robinson RG, Boston JD, Starkstein SE, Price TR. Comparison of mania and depression after brain injury: causal factors. Am J Psychiatry 1988;145:172–178

169. Cummings JL, Mendez MF. Secondary mania with focal cerebrovascular lesions. Am J Psychiatry 1984; 141:1084–1087

170. Jampala VC, Abrams R. Mania secondary to left and right hemisphere damage. Am J Psychiatry 1983;140: 1197–1199

171. Liu CY, Wang SJ, Fuh JL, et al. Bipolar disorder following a stroke involving the left hemisphere. Aust NZ J Psychiatry 1996;30:688–691

172. Stewart JT, Hemsath RH. Bipolar illness following traumatic brain injury: treatment with lithium and carbamazepine. J Clin Psychiatry 1988;49:74–75

173. Evans DL, Byerly MJ, Greer RA. Secondary mania: diagnosis and treatment. J Clin Psychiatry 1995; 56(Suppl 3):31–37

174. Robinson RG. Neuropsychiatric consequences of stroke. Ann Rev Med 1997;48:217–229

175. House A, Dennis M, Molyneux A, et al. Emotionalism after stroke. Br Med J 1989;298:991–994

176. Andersen G. Treatment of uncontrolled crying after stroke. Drugs Aging 1995;6:105–111

177. Andersen G, Ingeman-Nielsen M, Vestergaard K, Riis JO. Patho-anatomic correlation between post-stroke pathologic crying and damage to brain areas involved in serotonergic neurotransmission. Stroke 1994;25: 1050–1052

178. Andersen G, Vestergaard K, Riis JO. Citalopram for post-stroke pathological crying. Lancet 1993;342: 837–839

179. Seliger GM, Hornstein A, Flax J, et al. Fluoxetine improves emotional incontinence. Brain Inj 1992;6: 267–270

180. Sloan RL, Brown KW, Pentland B. Fluoxetine as a treatment for emotional lability after brain injury. Brain Inj 1992;6:315–319

181. Robinson RG, Parikh RM, Lipsey JR, et al. Pathological laughing and crying following stroke: validation of a measurement scale and a double-blind treatment study. Am J Psychiatry 1993;150:286–293

182. Schiffer RB, Herndon RM, Rudick RA. Treatment of pathologic laughing and weeping with amitriptyline. N Eng J Med 1985;312:1480–1482

183. Aarsland D, Tandberg E, Larsen JP, Cummings JL. Frequency of dementia in Parkinson's disease. Arch Neurol 1996;53:538–542

184. Hobson P, Meara J. The detection of dementia and cognitive impairment in a community population of elderly people with Parkinson's disease by use of the CAMCOG neuropsychological test. Age Aging 1999; 28:39–43

185. Gibb WRG. Dementia and Parkinson's disease. Br J Psychiatry 1989;154:596–614

186. Levin BE, Llabre MM, Weiner WJ. Cognitive impairments associated with early Parkinson's disease. Neurology 1989;39:557–561

187. Owen AM, James M, Leigh PN, et al. Fronto-striatal cognitive deficits at different stages of Parkinson's disease. Brain 1992;115:1727–1751

188. Tamaru F. Disturbances in higher function in Parkinson's disease. Eur Neurol 1997;38(Suppl 2):33–36

189. Pondal M, Del Ser T, Bermejo F. Anticholinergic therapy and dementia in patients with Parkinson's disease. J Neurol 1996;243:543–546

190. Starkstein SE, Preziosi TJ, Bolduc PL, Robinson RG. Depression in Parkinson's disease. J Nerv Ment Dis 1990;178:27–31

191. Cummings JL. Depression and Parkinson's disease: a review. Am J Psychiatry 1992;149:443–454

192. Starkstein SE, Berthier ML, Bolduc MS, et al. Depression in patients with early versus late onset of Parkinson's disease. Neurology 1989;39:1441–1445

193. Direnfeld LK, Albert ML, Volicer L, et al. Parkinson's disease: the possible relationship of laterality to dementia and neurochemical findings. Arch Neurol 1984;41:935–941

194. Santamaria J, Tolosa E, Valles A. Parkinson's disease with depression: a possible subgroup of idiopathic parkinsonism. Neurology 1986;36:1130–1133

195. Guze BH, Barrio JC. The etiology of depression in Parkinson's disease patients. Pscyhosomatics 1991;32: 390–395

196. Juncos JL. Management of psychotic aspects of Parkinson's disease. J Clin Psychiatry 1999;60(Suppl 8):42–53

197. Shaw KM, Lees AJ, Stern GM. The impact of treatment with levodopa on Parkinson's disease. Q J Med 1980; 49:283–293

198. Lieberman A. Managing the neuropsychiatric symptoms of Parkinson's disease. Neurology 1998;50(Suppl 6):S33–S38

199. Suchowersky O, deVries JD. Interaction of fluoxetine and selegiline. Can J Psychiatry 1990;35:571–572

200. Jermain DM, Hughes PL, Follender AB. Potential fluoxetine-selegiline interaction. Ann Pharmacother 1992; 26:1300

201. Ritter JL, Alexander B. Retrospective study of selegiline-antidepressant drug interactions and a review of the literature. Ann Clin Psychiatry 1997;9:7–13

202. Faber R, Trimble MR. Electroconvulsive therapy in Parkinson's disease and other movement disorders. Move Dis 1991;6:293–303

203. Moellentine C, Rummans T, Ahlskog JE, et al. Effectiveness of ECT in patients with parkinsonism. J Neuropsychiatry Clin Neurosci 1998;10:187–193

204. Tanner CM, Vogel C, Goetz CG, Klawans HL.

Hallucinations in Parkinson's disease: a population study. Ann Neurol 1983;14:136

205. Cummings JL. Behavioral complications of drug treatment of Parkinson's disease. J Am Geriatr Soc 1991;39: 708–716

206. Naimark D, Jackson E, Rockwell E, Jeste DV. Psychotic symptoms in Parkinson's disease patients with dementia. J Am Geriatr Soc 1996;44:296–299

207. Sanchez-Ramos JR, Ortoll R, Paulson GW. Visual hallucinations associated with Parkinson disease. Arch Neurol 1996;53:1265–1268

208. Comella CL, Tanner CM. The side effects of chronic treatment in Parkinson's disease. In: Joseph AB, Young RR, eds. Movement Disorders in Neurology and Neuropsychiatry. Boston: Blackwell Scientific Publications, 1992:236–246

209. Moskovitz C, Moses H, Klawans HL. Levodopa-induced psychosis: a kindling phenomenon. Am J Psychiatry 1978;135:669–675

210. Inzelberg R, Kipervasser S, Korczyn AD. Auditory hallucinations in Parkinson's disease. J Neurol Neurosurg Psychiatry 1998;64:533–535

211. Wolters EC. Dopaminomimetic psychosis in Parkinson's disease patients: diagnosis and treatment. Neurology 1999; 52(Suppl 3):S10–S13

212. Aarsland D, Larsen JP, Cummings JL, Laake K. Prevalence and clinical correlates of psychotic symptoms in Parkinson disease: a community-based study. Arch Neurol 1999;56:595–601

213. Pfeiffer R. Optimization of levodopa therapy. Neurology 1992;42(Suppl 1):39–43

214. Factor SA, Brown D, Molho ES, Podskalny GD. Clozapine: a two-year open trial in Parkinson's disease patients with psychosis. Neurology 1994;44:544–546

215. Wagner ML, Defilippi JL, Menza MA, Sage JI. Clozapine for the treatment of psychosis in Parkinson's disease: chart review of 49 patients. J Neuropsychiatry Clin Neurosci 1996;8:276–280

216. Factor SA, Friedman JH. The emerging role of clozapine in the treatment of movement disorders. Move Dis 1997;12:483–496

217. The Parkinson Study Group. Low-dose clozapine for the treatment of drug-induced psychosis in Parkinson's disease. N Eng J Med 1999;340:757–763

218. Wolters EC, Jansen EN, Tuynman-Qua HG, Bergmans PL. Olanzapine in the treatment of dopaminomimetic psychosis in patients with Parkinson's disease. Neu-

rology 1996;47:1085–1087

219. Graham JM, Sussman JD, Ford KS, Sagar HJ. Olanzapine in the treatment of hallucinosis in idiopathic Parkinson's disease: a cautionary note. J Neurol Neurosurg Psychiatry 1998;65:774–777

220. Parsa MA, Bastani B. Quetiapine (Seroquel) in the treatment of psychosis in patients with Parkinson's disease. J Neuropsychiatry Clin Neurosci 1998;10: 216–219

221. Meco G, Alessandria A, Bonifati V, Giustini P. Risperidone for hallucinations in levodopa-treated Parkinson's disease patients. Lancet 1994;343:1370–1371

222. Workman RH, Orengo CA, Bakey AA, et al. The use of risperidone for psychosis and agitation in demented patients with Parkinson's disease. J Neuropsychiatry Clin Neurosci 1997;9:594–597

223. Ford B, Lynch T, Greene P. Risperidone in Parkinson's disease. Lancet 1994;344:681

224. Rich SS, Friedman JH, Ott BR. Risperidone versus clozapine in the treatment of psychosis in six patients with Parkinson's disease and other akinetic-rigid syndromes. J Clin Psychiatry 1995;56:556–559

225. Zoldan J, Friedberg G, Goldberg-Stern H, Melamed E. Ondansetron for hallucinosis in advanced Parkinson's disease. Lancet 1993;341:562–563

226. Zoldan J, Friedberg G, Livneh M, Melamed E. Psychosis in advanced Parkinson's disease: treatment with ondansetron, a 5-HT$_3$ receptor antagonist. Neurology 1995;45:1305–1308

227. Nausieda PA, Weiner WJ, Kaplan LR, et al. Sleep disruption in the course of chronic levodopa therapy: an early feature of the levodopa psychosis. Clin Neuropharmacol 1982;5:183–194

228. Trenkwalder C. Sleep dysfunction in Parkinson's disease. Clin Neurosci 1998;5:107–114

229. Schenck CH, Hurwitz TD, Mahowald MW. REM sleep behaviour disorder: an update on a series of 96 patients and a review of the world literature. J Sleep Res 1993;2:224–231

230. Goetz CG, Wilson RS, Tanner CM, Garron DC. Relationships among pain, depression, and sleep alterations in Parkinson's disease. Adv Neurol 1987;45: 345–347

231. Comella CL, Tanner CM, Ristanovic RK. Polysomnographic sleep measures in Parkinson's disease patients with treatment-induced hallucinations. Ann Neurol 1993;34:710–714

271 Treatment of Emotional Communication Disorders

Jeffrey M Anderson and Kenneth M Heilman

Introduction

The inability to communicate emotion is a disability that may interfere with the quality of life and socially isolate a person. Emotions can be communicated by spoken or written words, but are often communicated by gestures such as facial expressions, tone of voice, or prosody (the tone of voice induced by changes in pitch, amplitude, stress and timing that are used to express emotion or syntax that allow the listener to know if a sentence is a statement, question or command). In this chapter we will first briefly discuss the types of emotional communication deficits that one can see in the clinic and then discuss how some of these can be managed and treated.

Background

Left hemisphere damage

Comprehension Many social interactions depend upon communicating an appropriate emotion. The two most important types of communication are speech and gestures, including facial expressions. Using speech, emotion can be conveyed by either words (propositional language) or by prosody (non-propositional language). This propositional or linguistic content is conveyed by a complex code that requires auditory or visual analysis, phonemic or orthographic decoding, and a lexical-semantic analysis. [Spoken words are formed by a series of speech sounds. These sounds are called phonemes. In order to comprehend or repeat speech a person must be able to recognize (decode) these speech sounds—this is phonemic decoding. Written words are formed by a series of letters. In order to read words a person has to recognize (decode) these letters—this is orthographic decoding. Peoples brains contain memories of words that were previously heard or seen. After a person decodes the phonemes or letters of a spoken or written word he or she search their stores of word memories (phonological lexicon or orthographic lexicon)—this is lexical analysis and semantic analysis is the term used to describe how a person determines the meaning of a spoken or written word.]

In the vast majority of people, including left-handers, the left hemisphere mediates most aspects of propositional language (the speech or writing used to express ideas). Injury to the posterior portions of the left hemisphere, from stroke, trauma, tumor, infection or degenerative processes may impair the comprehension of propositional speech. Patients with word deafness, Wernicke's, transcortical sensory, global or mixed transcortical aphasia have difficulties in comprehending propositional speech. These aphasic syndromes are often associated with reading disorders, but alexia with or without aphasia may impair the comprehension of written material that has emotional content.

Although patients with left hemisphere cerebral damage may be unable to understand propositional speech, many of these patients are still able to understand emotional intonations or prosody and emotional faces.[1,2] When the propositional and prosodic messages are congruent, the addition of emotional prosody may help aphasic patients understand the message.[3,4]

Expression Almost all patients with aphasia have problems expressing verbal-propositional messages. Many patients with aphasia also have difficulty writing their messages (agraphia). However, agraphia, even in the absence of aphasia may also impair written expression of language. Therefore, if the communication of emotion is dependent upon propositional language, individuals with aphasia and agraphia may be impaired.

Hughlings Jackson[5] noted that even severely aphasic patients, that were non-fluent after left hemisphere injury could express emotion by intoning simple recurrent utterances with prosodic emotional intonations. In addition, when non-fluent aphasic patients become angry or frustrated he noted that it was not unusual for them to express their emotional feelings by using explicatives. Hughlings Jackson posited that perhaps it was the right hemisphere that was mediating these activities. The role of the right hemisphere in expressing emotional intonations will be discussed in a subsequent section. Roeltgen, Sevush and Heilman[6] demonstrated that patients with aphasia and agraphia could write emotional words with a greater degree of accuracy than they could write non-emotional words.

Right hemisphere damage

Perceptual and comprehension disorders As was discussed in the prior section, it appears that the left hemisphere mediates these lexical-semantic processes important for speech for most right and left-handers. However, Borod et al.[7] presented right and left hemisphere-damaged patients, as well as controls, with emotional and non-emotional tasks that included word identification, sentence identification, and word discrimination. Borod and her co-workers[7] found that the right hemisphere-damaged subjects were more impaired than left hemisphere-damaged or controls in the emotional condition.

Speech, however, can convey another message which, unlike the message transmitted by words, is conveyed by changes in prosody including the amplitude, pitch, timbre, and tonal contours of speech. During the last two to three decades there have been multiple studies which suggest that patients with right temporal parietal damage have difficulty comprehending emotional prosody.[3,8,9] In addition, as previously discussed, there have also been reports of patients with severe word comprehension deficits associated with disorders such as pure word deafness[2] and global aphasia,[1] who maintained the ability to comprehend prosody, providing further support for the postulate that the right hemisphere has a dominant role in the comprehension of emotional prosody.

The mechanism underlying this prosodic hemispheric asymmetry is not entirely known. Patients with right hemisphere lesions, especially in the temporal parietal regions, may be unable to discriminate (i.e., same or different choice) between different emotional prosodies, suggesting that the deficit is not one of denotation or verbal-lexical labeling.[10] These findings also suggest that the right hemisphere contains emotional prosodic representations, that these representations are stored in the right temporal parietal region and that injury to these representations may impair the comprehension of emotional prosody.

When involved in an emotional discussion with a significant other, we may have been told, "It is not what you said, but you how you said it." In these cases the propositional word message and the emotional prosodic message may be incongruent. When emotionally intoned sentences were presented to right and left hemisphere-damaged patients, the comprehension of emotional prosody was more disrupted by incongruent propositional content with right hemisphere-damage patients. In contrast comprehension of the propositional content was more disrupted by incongruent emotional prosody for left hemisphere-damaged subjects.[4]

Gestures such as facial expressions are also an important aspect of emotional communication and the appropriate development of an emotional state. Repeated studies have demonstrated that right hemisphere-damaged patients are impaired in comprehending emotional facial expressions.[11–14] It has also been demonstrated that this deficit cannot be accounted for a purely lower-level perceptual disorder[4,15] or a higher order semantic-conceptual deficit.[16] It is also not directly related to a face-processing deficit, and perhaps the best explanation of this deficit is that they have degraded emotional facial representations. Support for this postulate comes from the observation that right hemisphere-damaged subjects have a defect in imaging emotional faces, but not for imaging objects. In contrast, subjects with left hemisphere disease have impaired imagery for objects, but not for emotional faces.[17] Stimulation

studies of epileptic patients suggest that these emotional facial representations are stored in the posterior portion of the temporal lobe.[18]

Expressive deficits   Bloom et al.,[19] studied emotional and non-emotional discourse production, and the ability to use words to convey emotion, with normal controls and patients with right and left hemisphere disease. In the non-emotional condition, subjects with left hemisphere damage were particularly impaired, while in the emotional condition patients with right hemisphere injury demonstrated deficits. Therefore, this emotional content appeared to facilitate the pragmatic performance of the left hemisphere damaged subjects.

The speech of patients with right hemisphere disease often lacks emotional prosody.[9,10] This prosodic expressive deficit can be formally tested by asking patients to express neutral sentences with different emotional prosodies. Expressive deficits can exist with and without prosodic comprehension deficits.[20] The patients who appear to have expressive, but no comprehension deficits often have lesions in the anterior portions of the right hemisphere. Ross[9] has suggested that expressive-receptive dichotomy of emotional prosody associated with right hemisphere lesions may be parallel to the manner in which the left hemisphere lesions disrupt the comprehension and expression of propositional speech.

Patients with right hemisphere dysfunction may not only have problems comprehending facial expressions, but they may also have problems in expressing emotions using facial gestures. This has been demonstrated both in the laboratory[21] and by viewing these patients in a natural situation.[16]

Treatment

Disorders of emotional communication have a significant impact on quality of life. This disorder often induces discord in that patient's family and increases the burden of care. Yet few treatment studies have addressed this issue in a systematic fashion. The treatment of propositional language speech disorders is discussed in another section of this text and will not be discussed here. While a handful of studies have documented the treatment of prosodic deficits, no studies are available in which treatment was attempted for deficits in the expression of facial emotions.

In reference to aprosodia treatment, an approach utilizing a non-auditory modality was attempted by Stringer[22] who utilized visual feedback to treat a patient with an expressive prosodic deficit. Stringer[22] documented that by monitoring their fundamental frequency, which is a measure of emotional prosody that can be quantified, the patient was able to improve the accuracy of their expression of emotional prosody.[22] Additionally, Staum[23] utilized a visual cue provided by musical notation to improve the speech prosody of hearing impaired children.

A modality specific technique was developed by Miller and Toca[24] in which they utilized an adapted version of Melodic Intonation Therapy to treat an autistic child with a deficit in prosodic production. In this study the child was first provided with a sample sentence that was produced with a "prosodic line" that matched that of a well known song (e.g. Happy Birthday). The child repeated this sentence along with the therapist and then produced it on their own. With additional trials this prosodic line was then shaped to match that of the target emotional prosody. In this process the child was provided with multiple models of emotional prosody to mimic and then to produce independently.

None of these studies compared the relative effectiveness of different treatment approaches. It could be conjectured that one plausible explanation for the effectiveness of the above studies was that either they helped to restitute partially dysfunctional cortical networks or that they engaged intact cortical regions that had not been involved in this task before treatment.

From a cognitive neuropsychological model, there are at least two major reasons why a patient might have a deficit in the production of emotional speech prosody or facial expressions. They might have a degraded representation of this target prosody or facial gesture, or they might be unable to access or engage the motor sequences related to those representations.

If a patient has a degraded emotional echoic (sound memories) or iconic (picture memories) representations this could lead to an inability to express a target emotional prosody or face because of a deficit in the ability to retrieve the critical prosodic or facial features of that emotion. A treatment strategy that solely focuses on the repetition of that emotional expression would likely fail because it lacked a credible representation to begin with. In this situation a treatment strategy that might be effective is to utilize an intact emotional representation from another modality. For example, patients with expressive aprosodia due to a loss of their echoic-prosodic representations, could possibly be trained by using verbal explicit instructions of how to produce a target prosody. A similar approach could also be used for emotional facial expressions.

In contrast, other patients might have intact representations for specific emotional prosodies or facial gestures, but they may be unable to access or engage the motor sequences that are needed to express that emotion. In this situation, providing these patients with explicit cognitive instructions may not help because they already have intact representations for emotions. Instead they would likely profit from relearning the motor skills needed to express those emotional faces or prosody through an imitative strategy. In this case, providing the patient with a prosodically correct auditory model of a target emotional prosody during therapy, theoretically might help them to reconstruct the motor sequences related to producing happy prosody. In a like fashion, providing the patient with a correct model of a smiling face during therapy, might help them to reconstruct the motor sequences associated with producing a happy face.

Based on this cognitive neuropsychological model, a study by Anderson et al.,[25] explored the effectiveness of three different strategies with a patient with a specific deficit in prosody expression after a large right hemisphere injury. The *Prosodic Imitation Strategy* used in that study provided a prosodically correct auditory model of the target prosody during treatment sessions. The *Explicit Verbal Instruction Strategy* provided only cognitive instructions (e.g., When you want to express happiness raise the pitch at the end of the sentence). Finally, during the *Facial Imitation Strategy* the patient was provided with a picture of a face correctly displaying the target emotion and on-line, video monitoring of their own face. Anderson and colleagues[25] noted that while each of the three strategies improved the production of this patient's prosody, the patient's production of emotional prosody was most improved after treatment with the Prosodic Imitation Strategy. Such a finding supports the conclusion that this patient had intact prosodic representations after his injury, but had a more prominent problem when attempting to access the motor sequences associated with those representations. Studies which explore these relationships from a cognitive neuropsychological perspective may provide the basis for more specific and efficacious treatment regimes in the future.

References

1. Barrett AM, Crucian GP, Raymer AM, Heilman KM. Spared comprehension of emotional prosody in a patient with global aphasia. Neuropsychiatry, Neuropsychology & Behavioral Neurology 1999;12:117–120
2. Kanter SL, Day AL, Heilman KM, Gonzalez-Rothi LJ. Pure word deafness: a possible explanation of transient deterioration following EC-IC bypass. Neurosurgery 1986;18:186–189
3. Heilman KM, Scholes R, Watson RT. Auditory affective agnosia: disturbed comprehension of affective speech. Journal of Neurology, Neurosurgery, & Psychiatry 1975;38:69–72
4. Bowers D, Coslett HB, Speedie LJ, Heilman KM. Comprehension of emotional prosody following unilateral hemispheric lesions; processing defects *vs.* distraction defects. Neuropsychologia 1987;25:317–328
5. Jackson JH. *In:* Taylor J, ed. Selected writings of John Hughlings-Jackson. London: Hodder and Stoughton, 1932
6. Roeltgen DP, Sevush S, Heilman KM. Phonological agraphia: writing by the lexical semantic route. Neurology 1983;33:755–765
7. Borod JC, Andelman F, Obler LK, et al. Right hemisphere specialization for the identification of emotional words and sentences: evidence from stroke patients. Neuropsychologia 1992;30:827–844
8. Heilman KM, Bowers D, Speedie L, Coslett HB. Comprehension of affective and non-affective prosody. Neurology 1984;34:917–921
9. Ross ED. The aprosodias: functional-anatomic organization of the affective components of language in the right hemisphere. Archives of Neurology 1981;38:561–569
10. Tucker DM, Watson RT, Heilman KM. Affective discrimination and evocation in patients with right parietal disease. Neurology 1977;17:947–950

11. DeKosky ST, Heilman KM, Bowers D, Valenstein E. Recognition and discrimination of emotional faces and pictures. Brain & Language 1980;9:206–214

12. Cicone M, Wapner W, Gardner H. Sensitivity to emotional expressions and situations in organic patients. Cortex 1980;16:145–158

13. Bowers D, Bauer RM, Coslett HB, Heilman KM. Processing of faces by patients with unilateral hemispheric lesions. I. Dissociation between judgments of facial affect and facial identity. Brain & Cognition 1985;4:258–272

14. Borod JC, Koff E, Perlman-Lorch M, Nicholas M. The expression and perception of facial emotion in brain-damaged patients. Neuropsychologia 1986;24:169–180

15. Blonder LX, Bowers D, Heilman KM. The role of the right hemisphere in emotional communication. Brain 1991;114:1115–1127

16. Blonder LX, Burns AF, Bowers D, et al. Right hemisphere facial expressivity during natural conversation. Brain & Cognition 1993;21:44–56

17. Bowers D, Blonder LX, Feinberg T, Heilman KM. Differential impact of right and left hemisphere lesions on facial emotion and object imagery. Brain 1991;114:2593–2609

18. Fried I, Mateer C, Ojemann G, et al. Organization of visuospatial functions in human cortex. Evidence from electrical stimulation. Brain 1982;105:349–371

19. Bloom RL, Borod JC, Obler LK, Gerstman LJ. Impact of emotional content on discourse production in patients with unilateral brain damage. Brain & Language 1992;42:153–164

20. Ross ED, Mesulam MM. Dominant language functions of the right hemisphere? Prosody and emotional gesturing. Archives of Neurology 1979;36:144–148

21. Buck R, Duffy R. Nonverbal communication of affect in brain-damaged patients. Cortex 1980;16:351–362

22. Stringer AY, Hodnett C. Transcortical motor aprosodia: functional and anatomical correlates. Archives of Clinical Neuropsychology 1991;6:89–99

23. Staum MJ. Music notation to improve the speech prosody of hearing impaired children. Journal of Music Therapy 1987;24:146–159

24. Miller SB, Toca JM. Adapted melodic intonation therapy: a case study of an experimental language program for an autistic child. Journal of Clinical Psychiatry 1979;40:201–203

25. Anderson JM, Beversdorf DQ, Heilman KM, Gonzalez Rothi LJ. Treatment of expressive aprosodia associated with right hemisphere injury. Journal of the International Neuropsychological Society 1999;5:157

Index

Page numbers in bold italics indicate information in **figures**

cyclophosphamide *continued*
  dosages 1409, 1410
  hearing loss 1914
  monoclonal gammopathy of undetermined
    significance 1364
  multifocal motor neuropathy with conduction
    block 2112, 2113, 2114, 2115
  myasthenia gravis 2383
    ocular 1819
  myopathies, inflammatory 2329, 2331, 2333–4,
    2335
  non-Hodgkin lymphoma 2149
  paraneoplastic neurological syndromes 2161,
    2163
  PNET/medulloblastoma of childhood 760
  pulse, as steroid-sparing agent 155
  sarcoid neuropathy 1436, 1437, 2121, 2122
  sensory ganglionopathies 2076
  side effects 1377, 1409, 2087, 2098, 2113, 2122,
    2123, 2331, 2334
    management 588, 2096–7, 2098
    monitoring 2122
    prevention 1412
  stiff person syndrome 838
  use in pregnancy 1554
  vasculitic neuropathy 2088, 2089, 2090, 2091, 2094
  vasculitis 585, 586, 587, 1409, 1410, 1411, 1412,
    1413
  see also CHOD; CHOP; CVP; MACOB-B; VBMCP
cyclophosphamide and prednisone, vasculitis 585,
    586, 588
cycloserine 10
cyclosporine
  Behçet disease 1091
  chronic inflammatory demyelinating
    polyradiculoneuropathy 2053
  cryoglobulinemia 1379
  inflammatory myopathies 2329, 2331, 2333, 2334,
    2335
  Lambert–Eaton myasthenic syndrome 839
  myasthenia gravis 2383, 2385
    ocular 1819
  neurosarcoidosis 1436, 1437
  neurotoxic effects 855
  neurotoxicity 2150, 2154
  sarcoid neuropathy 2121, 2122
  side effects 1089, 1091, 1358, 1377, 1819, 2122,
    2123, 2331, 2334, 2383
    monitoring 2122
    neurological 1384–5, 1392
    transplant recipients 1201, 1203, 1204
  Takayasu's arteritis 1411
  transplant recipients 1384–5, 1392
  vasculitis/vasculitic neuropathy 1410, 1412,
    2091, 2093
cyclothiazide 9
cyproheptadine
  akathisia 2603
  autonomic hyperactivity 2287, 2288
  Cushing disease 729
  migraine, childhood 160
cystathionine β synthase deficiency, childhood
    stroke and 621
cystatin C amyloid angiopathy, hereditary 2144
cysticercosis 1021–3, *1024, 1025*
  calcification 1025, *1025*
  myositis 2338
  treatment 1024–6
cystinosis 1487
cystopathy, neurogenic 2248
  treatment 2248, 2252–3
cysts, ventricular, surgery 1026
cytarabine (ara-C) 667
  leptomeningeal metastasis 826, 827
  leukemia 1356, 1357, 1358
  lymphoma of central nervous system 776, 777,
    1355, 1356
  progressive multifocal leukoencephalopathy,
    HIV/AIDS 959
  side effects 1358, 1393
    neurotoxic 849, 851
    peripheral neuropathy 2150, 2154
  see also DHAP
cytochrome P-450 (CYP) enzymes, drug
  metabolism 19–20

cytokines 1097
  effects in severe illness 1238–9
cytomegalovirus (CMV) infection
  diagnosis 1078
  encephalitis 953, 958, 959, 1076
  HIV/AIDS 951, 952, 953, 1391
    treatment 958, 959–60
  immunocompromised hosts 1395
    see also HIV/AIDS *above*; transplant recipients
      below
  perinatal 1056–8
    calcification 1056, *1057*, 1058
    clinical features 1056
    diagnosis 1056–7
    epidemiology 1056
    prevention and treatment 1057–8
  progressive polyradiculopathy, HIV-associated
    1982
  prophylaxis 1395
  transplant recipients 1072, 1073, 1074, 1076, 1078,
    1386
    treatment 1080, 1081
cytosine arabinoside *see* cytarabine
cytotoxic therapy
  monoclonal gammopathy of undetermined
    significance 1364
  side effects 2182–3
    gonadal dysfunction 2123
    vasculitic neuropathy 2089–92, 2094
cytoxan, lymphoma of CNS 1357

D 0870 (antifungal) 994
dacarbazine, neurotoxic effects 849
Dactylaria constricta 977, 984
daieparin 1181, 1182
Dalrymple sign 1457
dalteparin 400, 402, 530
danaparoid 400, 401, 402
  stroke 443, 455–6
Dandy–Walker syndrome 1606, 1609
Danon disease 1484, 1487, 1491, 2346, 2347–8
  cardiomyopathy 1280
dantrolene
  cramps 2414
  malignant hyperthermia 2395, 2397
  neurogenic bladder 2284
  neuroleptic malignant syndrome 2290, 2608
  side effects 2397
  spasticity
    after central nervous system injury 1692
    in cerebral palsy 1621
  spider bites 1040
  tetanus 931
dapsone
  hypersensitivity vasculitis 1411
  leprosy 1989
  prion diseases 2701
  side effects 1411
  as steroid-sparing agent 155
DDAVP *see* desmopressin
DDT 1531
De Basry syndrome 1647
De Sanctis–Cacchione syndrome 1671
deafness
  gentamicin-induced, mitochondrial disease 1564
  lysosomal storage disease 1489
  mitochondrial disease 1564
  psychogenic 1948
  see also hearing loss
deafness–dystonia–optic atrophy 2426
deamino-D-arginine vasopressin (DDAVP) *see*
  desmopressin
decision making, shared 56
Declaration of Helsinki 56, 57, 61
decompression surgery
  back pain 199, 204
  Bell's palsy 1970
  brain swelling 1135
  cerebral spine disease 1418–19
  cervical spondylosis 1427
  compression neuropathies 1421
  facial nerve 1863
  hemifacial spasm 1865
  intracranial hypertension 1164

  idiopathic 1736
  optic nerve sheath 1722, 1723–4
  spinal cord
    lymphoma 1357
    metastatic disease 816–17, *817*
    stroke patients 445
    syringomyelia 2522–3, *2524*
    traumatic head injury 1227–8
    trigeminal neuralgia 1852
    venous sinus thrombosis 552–3
deep brain stimulation (DBS)
  central pain 216–17, 218
  chorea/ballism 2578
  dystonia 2542–3
  essential tremor 2585
  neuroacanthocytosis 2566
  pallidal
    dystonia 2542–3
    Parkinson's disease 2510–11
  Parkinson's disease 2506, 2507–8, *2508*, 2509,
    2510–11, 2511–12
    gaze disorders 1811
  subthalamic nucleus 2511–12
  thalamic, Parkinson's disease 2509
deep vein thrombosis (DVT)
  prophylaxis 1184, *1185*
  spinal cord injury 1233–4
defibrillators, implantable, cardiomyopathy 1282
deflazacort, Duchenne muscular dystrophy 2320
degenerative diseases 1639–45
  general treatment 1636–8
dehydration
  alcohol withdrawal syndromes 1503, 1504
  hypernatremic, intracerebral hemorrhage and
    629
  and venous thrombosis 544
dehydroemetine, *Entamoeba histolytica* brain abscess
    1014
delaviridine
  HIV infection 955, 956
  side effects 955
delirium, behavioral and emotional complications
    2856, 2857, 2862–3
delirium tremens 1502–4, 2290
  Clinical Institute Withdrawal Assessment 2289,
    2290
delivery (birth) history, in infant/childhood
    diagnosis 1578
Delleman (oculocerebrocutaneous) syndrome 1667
delusions
  Alzheimer disease 2820, 2821
  dementia 2855, 2859
    management 2845, 2854, 2856, 2857, 2859
demeclocycline, hyponatremia of malignancy 844
dementia(s) 2810–11, 2826–54
  alcoholics 1506
  antiphospholipid-associated 576–7
  behavioral and emotional complications 2855–62
  catastrophic reactions 2858–9
    management 2856, 2858–9
  dementia paralytica 914
  frontotemporal 2826, 2837, 2838
    genetics 2423
    management 2837, 2844, 2845
    with ubiquitin-positive inclusions 2833–4, *2834*
  hereditary spastic paraplegia 2710
  HIV-associated 951, 952, 953, 956, 1389–90, *1390*
  hormonal factors 1466–8
  lacking distinctive histopathology 2826, 2834,
    2834, 2841
  late-onset, hereditary spastic paraplegia 2705–6
  with Lewy bodies 2811, 2826, 2827–8
    behavioral and emotional complications 2855,
      2859
    management 2827, 2844, 2845
    Parkinson's disease 2470
  lysosomal storage diseases 1489
  management of target symptoms 2844–6, 2853–4
  myoclonic 2590, 2591
  myxedematous 1460
  neuroacanthocytosis 2564, 2566
  Parkinson's disease 2453, 2454, 2470–1, 2827,
    2828
  resistiveness 2859
    management 2856, 2857

hypoxic 458
  perinatal, paroxysmal dyskinesias 2637, 2639
hypoxic-ischemic 458, 470–80, *473*
  cardiac surgery patients 461
  neonates 1578, 1588, 1589
Lyme disease 919
mitochondrial, childhood stroke and 622
multiple myeloma 1365
neonates 1584
post-operative 1249, 1250, 1252
radiation-induced 856–7
sodium disorders 1313–14
subacute necrotizing 2173
toxemia of pregnancy 1540–1
transmissible spongiform *see* prion diseases
transplant recipients 1383, 1384
uremic, transplant patients 1197
Wernicke's 1504–5, 2692
  in cancer anorexia–cachexia syndrome 845
  gaze palsy 1810–11
  pregnancy 1548–9
enchondromatosis, multiple 1672
endarteritis, Nissl–Alzheimer 914
endocarditis 1258–66
  culture-negative 1261
  Libman–Sacks 454, 615
  marantic 615
  stroke and 615
    prevention 454
  thrombotic 615
  verrucous 615
endocarditis, infective 1258
  Bartonella sp. 942
  diagnosis 1260–1, 1264
  epidemiology 1258
  etiology 1258–9
  fungal 1263
  intracerebral hemorrhage and 628
  neurological complications 613, 1258, 1259–60, 1261
    treatment 1261–5, *1265*
  pathophysiology and pathogenesis 1259
  Q fever 938–9, 940, 941–2
  Staphylococcus aureus 1258, 1259, 1260, 1261
    treatment 1262
  streptococcal 1259, 1261
    treatment 1262
  stroke and 613
    pregnancy 642
    prevention 454, 615
endocrinology, reproductive, neurological disorders and 1464–72
endodermal sinus (yolk sac) tumors 770, 771
  biomarkers 757
endolymphatic hydrops, delayed 1899
endoscopic procedures, pituitary tumor surgery 730
endothelial cells
  cerebral 20
  growth inhibition 669–70, 671
endothelial growth factor, vascular
  inhibitors 669
  tumor cells 663
endotracheal intubation 1139–42
  Guillain–Barré syndrome 2044
  intracerebral hemorrhage 481, 482
  sedation for 1169–70
  toxic gas exposure 1527, 1529
endovascular procedures
  arteriovenous malformations 651
  cerebral aneurysms 500–1, 509, *516*
    unruptured 521
  cervicocephalic arterial dissection 531–2
  critically ill patients 1136
  neurological complications 1249
  use in pregnancy 644, 651
  vascular malformations 511, 514
endozepine stupor 12
enemas
  constipation 2264
  fecal incontinence 2265
enolase, neuron specific *see* neuron specific enolase
enoxaparin 400, 402, 1181, 1182
  cervicocephalic arterial dissection 530
entacapone, Parkinson's disease 2451, 2452, 2458, 2462
Entamoeba histolytica infection 1003, 1004

brain abscess 1014
  clinical features 1006
  pathogenetic and pathological features 1005
enteric nervous system 2255, *2255*, *2256*
enteric neuropathy, paraneoplastic 2162
enterobacteriaceae
  brain abscess 875, 876
  Gram-negative, meningitis 863, 867, 868, 869
Enterococcus faecalis endocarditis 1259
enteroviruses
  encephalitis 894, 901
  meningitis 889, 890, 891, 893, 894
  non-polio, perinatal infections 1061, 1062
  transplant recipients 1072
Entomophthoraceae 984
  clinical features 983
  diagnosis 985
  epidemiology 974
  mycology 978
  outside CNS 988
  pathophysiology and pathogenesis 980
  treatment 991
entrapment neuropathy 1956
  acromegaly 2011, 2014, 2015
  chronic 1957
  hereditary neuropathy with liability to pressure palsy 2198–9
  hypothyroidism 1461, 2011, 2012–13
  pregnancy 1545–8
  rheumatoid arthritis 1420–1
enuresis, nocturnal 1311
envenomations 1039–49
enzyme replacement
  carbohydrate metabolism disorders 2349
  lysosomal storage disease 1495–6
enzyme-linked immunosorbent assay *see* ELISA
eosinophilia–myalgia syndrome 2336
eosinophilic meningitis 1022, 1028–9
  treatment 1023, 1029–30
eosinophilic myositis 2328, 2336
ependymoblastomas, radiotherapy 683
ependymomas
  association with heritable syndromes 755
  childhood 756
    distribution 756
    treatment 763
  myxopapillary, cauda equina **795**
  radiotherapy 682, 683, 685, 798
    children 763
  spinal cord
    epidemiology 793
    filum terminale 801
    pathology and molecular genetics 795
    treatment 797, 798
ephedrine
  multiple system atrophy 2490
  pharmacology 16
  side effects 2490
epidermal growth factor receptor (EGFR) 663
  inhibitors 663–4
  gliomas 747
epidermoid cysts
  brain 704–6
  spinal cord 800
epidermoid tumors
  hypothalamic dysfunction 1442
  treatment 1442
epidermolysis bullosa simplex with muscular dystrophy 2314
epidural abscess 884
epidural block
  painful legs and moving toes 2650, 2651
  varicella zoster pain management 187, 188
epidural empyema, fungal infection 977
epidural opioid infusion, cancer pain 238
epilepsy
  absence
    childhood 332, 334
     treatment 332, 334
    juvenile 332, 334
     treatment 332, 334
  aphasia 1630
  autonomic, gastrointestinal symptoms 2256
  benign occipital 335, 340
  benign rolandic

  of childhood (benign epilepsy with central-temporal spikes) 335, 339
    women 350
  catamenial 1464–5, *1465*
  cerebral palsy 1619
  children and infants 330–49
    classification 330–1, 333–6
    epidemiology 331
    treatment 342–6
    see also individual syndromes
  classification 262–5
    children 330–1, 333–6
    therapeutic importance 265–6
  cryptogenic 263, 264
  diagnosis 286–92
    electroencephalography 288–91, *290*, *291–2*, *293*, *294*
    neuroimaging 288, *289*
  diencephalic 1444
  elderly 358–63
    treatment 358–60, 361–3
  epidemiology
    children 331
    incidence 266–7, *267*
    prevalence 268, *268*
    therapeutic implications 268
  federal disability benefits, USA 378–9
  focal *see* epilepsy, localization-related
  generalized 263, 264, 268, 331
    children and infants 332–5, 337–9
  genetics 281
  glutamate in 11–12
  hormonal factors 1464–6
  hyperthyroidism 1455–6
  identification of epileptogenic region 308–10
  idiopathic 263, 264
  imitators 364–71
  legal and regulatory issues 372–81
    blood donation 380
    driving 372–4, 375–7
    employment 374, 375–9
    insurance 379
    legal resources 380
    violence and diminished responsibility 379–80
  localization-related (focal; partial; local) 263, 264, 279
    benign epilepsies of infancy 340
    children 331, 335, 339–41
    with mesial temporal sclerosis 340
  myoclonic (myoclonus) 2589, 2590
    early infantile 333, 339
    familial 2426
    juvenile 332, 335, 1465
    progressive myoclonic epilepsies 2426, 2590, 2591, 2592, 2593, 2594
    with ragged-red fibers (MERRF) 1562, 1563, 1565, 2353, 2354, 2590, 2591
    severe myoclonic epilepsy of Dravet 334
    women 350
  myoclonic-astatic, of Doose 331, 334, 338–9
  neurocysticercosis 1021
    treatment 1024, 1025
  with occipital calcifications 1667
  partial
    use of term 264
    otherwise see epilepsy, localization-related
  pathophysiology 270–82
    cell–cell interactions 273–9
    genetic and developmental considerations 281
    intrinsic cell properties and 270–3
    network properties and ictogenesis 279–81, *280*
  photosensitive, women 350
  post-traumatic 1691
  postanoxic 471
  pregnancy and 305, 352–4
    antiepileptic drugs and 352–4
  progressive myoclonic 1641
  reproductive dysfunction 1465–6
  risk factors 287
  seizures 261–2
    classification 262–5
  Sturge–Weber syndrome 1664, *1665*
  temporal lobe
    epileptogenic region 309–10
    mesial 341

headache *continued*
  transplant recipients 1073
  Valsalva-induced 142, 144
    clinical features 144–5
    indomethacin treatment 148
  vascular, sickle cell disease 1348–9
  see also migraine
hearing aids
  air conduction 1915, 1919
  analog *1919*
    method of function 1915–16, *1916*
  binaural 1915
  bone anchored (BAHA) 1915, 1920
  bone conduction 1915, 1919
  characteristics of gain 1916–17, *1917*
  CROS fitting 1917
  digital, method of function 1916–17, *1917*
  earmolds 1918–19, *1918*
  evaluation of performance 1921
  implantable 1915, 1919–20, *1920*
  monaural 1915
  prescription characteristics 1921
  provision relative to auditory deficit 1917–18
  selection and fitting 1915–19
  tinnitus 1922
  types 1915, 1919–21
hearing disorders
  muscle disease 2298
  temporomandibular disorders 172
hearing loss 1904
  acoustic neuroma 698
  central auditory dysfunction 1904, 1906
  clinical presentation 1908
  conductive 1904, 1908
    causes 1906
    management 1912–13, 1915
  congenital 1908
  etiology 1906–8
  head trauma 1880
  hereditary sensory and autonomic neuropathy
    2190
  hypothyroidism 2012
  investigation 1908–12
  labyrinthitis 1896
  management 1912–22
  Meniere's syndrome 1899
  mixed 1904, *1906*
  muscular dystrophies 2323
  neurofibromatosis-2 1652
  Paget disease 1475, 1476
  prelingual 1908
  progressive 1908
    management 1914–15
  sensorineural 1904, 1906
    causes 1906
    congenital 1908
    immune-mediated 1914
    management 1914–15
    progressive, antiphospholipid syndrome 577
  sickle cell disease 1350
  simulated 1948
  sudden 1908
    management 1914–15
  trauma-induced 1883
  see also deafness
heart, *see also* cardiac ...
heart block, cardiac embolism/stroke and 614
heart disease
  childhood stroke and 608, 610–15
  congenital, stroke prevention 454–5
  congenital cyanotic, brain abscess and 875, 876,
    882
  interventions, neurological complications
    1249–54
  Q fever endocarditis 938–9, 941–2
heart failure, congestive, amyloidosis 2138, *2139*,
  2142
Heart Outcomes Prevention Evaluation Study
  (HOPE) 388, 1290–1
heart surgery, infective endocarditis and 1262, 1263
heart transplantation
  cardiomyopathy 1282
  complications 1199, 1200
    neurological 1385
    preoperative conditions and 1197

Kearns–Sayre–Shy syndrome 1564–5
heart valves
  prosthetic
    anticoagulation therapy 646
      in pregnancy 645
    endocarditis 1259, 1260–1, 1262
    stroke prevention 453–4
    thromboembolism/stroke 613
  replacement, infective endocarditis patients 1262,
    1263
  see also valvular heart disease
heart–lung transplantation, neurological
  complications 1383, 1384
heat-shock proteins 2353
  deficiency 2355
height index of Klaus *1604*
Helicephalobus deletrix 1022
HELLP syndrome 1539, 1540, 1544
  stroke 639, *641*
    hemorrhagic 647, 651
helminthic infections, central nervous system
  1021–38
  see also specific infections and agents
Helminthosporium see Bipolaris sp.
hemangioblastomas 706–8, *707*
  association with heritable syndromes 755
  spinal cord *796*
    epidemiology 793
    pathology and molecular genetics 795–6
  von Hippel–Lindau disease 1658, 1659
hemangioma, cavernous (cavernoma) 1828–31
hematological malignancies
  peripheral neuropathy 2147–57
  see also leukemias
hematomas
  epidural 1227, *1227*
    radicular pain 189
  intracerebral 1227–8
  subdural 1226, *1226*
heme, intravenous (hematin), porphyria 2185–6
heme synthesis 2182
  metabolic pathway *2181*
hemianopsia
  bitemporal 1744, *1744*, *1745*
  homonymous 1746, *1746*, 1747, *1747*, 1748, *1748*,
    1749
  hysteria *1946*, 1947
  treatment 1808–10
hemiatrophy, paroxysmal kinesigenic dyskinesia
  2637
hemiballism 2573
  causes 2574
  clinical manifestations 2575
  diagnosis 2575
  pathophysiology and pathogenesis 2573–5
  prognosis 2579
  treatment 2575–9
Hemibase syndrome 1930
hemicrania
  continuous (hemicrania continua) 142
    clinical features 144
    treatment 146–7
  paroxysmal 142, 164
    chronic 93, 146
    clinical features 144
    diagnosis 146
    episodic 93, 146
    treatment 146–7
hemifacial spasm 1863–5, 2435–6, 2668–9
  prevalence 2422
  treatment 1864–5
hemiplegia of childhood, alternating 161, 2639
hemispherectomy
  epilepsy 294, 346
  Rasmussen syndrome 341
hemispheric activation, neglect patients 2769–72,
  2773–4
hemodilution, stroke 443
hemoglobinopathies, neurological complications
  1342–53
hemoglobinuria, paroxysmal nocturnal, thrombotic
  disease/stroke 543, 619
hemolytic uremic syndrome 1540, 1541
  transplant recipients 1385
hemophilia 564

intracerebral hemorrhage and 628–9
hemorrhage
  cavernous malformation 512
  central nervous system, coagulation disorders
    and 564
  into brain abscess 881
  intracerebral *see* intracerebral hemorrhage
  neonatal, infants of epileptic mothers 354
  periventricular–intraventricular 1585–6
    management 1586–7
  spontaneous subdural and epidural, pregnancy
    651
  subarachnoid *see* subarachnoid hemorrhage
hemostasis testing, stroke patients 568–9
Henoch–Schönlein purpura 1411, 2079, 2080, 2084
  childhood stroke and 617
  intracerebral hemorrhage/stroke and 629
  treatment 2093
heparin 400–2, 1180–1
  action 1180
  Behçet disease 1090, 1091–2
  cervicocephalic arterial dissection 530, 615
  clinical indications 401
  contraindications 1180
  deep vein thrombosis prevention 1184, *1185*
  low molecular weight 401, 402, 1181–2
    antiphospholipid antibody syndrome and 645
    Behçet disease 1091–2
    cervicocephalic arterial dissection 530
    pharmacology 399, 400–1
    prosthetic heart valve patients 646
    stroke treatment 443, 445
    venous sinus thrombosis 551
  pharmacology 399, 400–1
  prosthetic heart valve patients 645, 646
  protamine sulfate infusion and 483–4
  side effects 1180–1, 1182
  stroke prevention 401–2, 428, 432, 1184
    cardioembolic stroke 453, 454
  stroke treatment 443, 445, 455, 456, *1186*
  toxicity 401
  use in pregnancy 645
  venous thrombosis 415, 550, 551–2
    in pregnancy 652
heparin cofactor II (HCII) 565
heparinoids 399, 400, 401
hepatic dysfunction, cancer patients 845–6
hepatic encephalopathy 1294–301
  cancer patients 845–6
  chronic liver disease and 1294–7
    management 1296–7
  fulminant liver failure and 1298–300
  grading system 1294
  transplant patients 1197
hepatitis, viral, neuropathy 2022
hepatitis B-associated polyarteritis nodosa (PAN)
  586, 2081, 2094
hepatitis C virus infection
  cryoglobulinemia and 1374, 1375, 2022–4, *2023*
    treatment 1376–7, 1378–9
  vasculitic neuropathy 2081
    treatment 2088–9
hepatocerebral degeneration, chorea 2579
herbicide toxicity 1531
hereditary ataxias 2688–94
hereditary cerebral hemorrhage with amyloidosis
  2144
hereditary cystatin C amyloid angiopathy 2144
hereditary hemorrhagic telangiectasia 1660
  cardiac embolism/stroke and 612
  cerebrovascular malformations 626
hereditary motor neuropathies 2194–7
  bulbar 2195, 2196
  classification 2195
  distal 2194, 2195
  Jerash 2195
  proximal 2194, 2195
  scapuloperoneal 2194, 2195
hereditary neuralgic amyotrophy 2065–6, *2066*,
  2067
  differential diagnosis versus hereditary
    neuropathy with liability to pressure palsy
    2201, 2202
hereditary neuropathy with liability to pressure
  palsy (HNPP) 2198–204

Marburg multiple sclerosis variant 1119, *1119*
Marchiafava–Bignami disease 1505–6
Marchiafava–Micheli syndrome *see* paroxysmal
nocturnal hemoglobinuria
Marfan syndrome, childhood stroke and 622–3
marimastat 669, 671
Maroteaux–Lamy syndrome 1486, 1488, *1492*, 1493,
1644
Marshall Stickler syndrome, hearing impairment
1908
massage, tension-type headache 116
matrix metalloproteinase inhibitors 669, 671
cerebral hemorrhage 1136
gliomas 747
May–Thurner syndrome 614, 643
Mayo Asymptomatic Carotid Endarterectomy
(MACE) trials 420
measles, encephalitis 894, 895
mebendazole
eosinophilic meningitis 1030
hydatid disease 1023, 1028
trichinosis 1023, 1033
mecamylamine 14
mechlorethamine *see* MOP regimen
Meckel–Gruber syndrome 1600, 1670
meclizine
labyrinthitis/vertigo 1898
vertigo, trauma-induced 1884
median neuropathy, wrist *see* carpal tunnel
syndrome
Medical Subject Headings (MeSH) 51
meditation, pain disorder 256
Mediterranean spotted fever 935, 936
MEDLINE 50, 51–2
medroxyprogesterone acetate, sexual disinhibition
in dementia 2857, 2860
medulloblastoma
association with heritable syndromes 755
childhood 756
distribution 756
staging 759
treatment 758–60, 764
radiotherapy 682, 683, 759–60
mefloquine 1008, 1009, 1011
side effects 1012
use in pregnancy 1011
megacolon 2257
Chagas disease 1994, 1995, *1995*
megaesophagus, Chagas disease 1994, 1995, *1995*
megalencephaly 1595
megalocephaly 1595
megazol 1015
megestrol acetate, cancer anorexia–cachexia
syndrome 845
Meige's syndrome 2527, 2528
melanoma-associated retinopathy 834
melanosis, neurocutaneous 1667
melarsoprol
African trypanosomiasis 1015
side effects 1016
MELAS 622, 1562, 1563, 1565, 1640, 1642, 2353, 2354
Parkinson's 2423
treatment 1565, 1566, 1567
melatonin
cluster headache prevention 98
restless legs syndrome/periodic limb movement
disorder 2662
side effects 2601
sleep disorders, dementias 2853, 2854
dementia with Lewy bodies 2828
Melkersson–Rosenthal syndrome 1860
Melodic Intonation Therapy (MIT)
aphasia 2724, 2727
emotional communication disorders 2873
melphalan
amyloidosis 1369, 2141
gliomas 745
recurrent 746
monoclonal gammopathy-associated neuropathy
2130
POEMS syndrome 2133–4
side effects, peripheral neuropathy 2152
see also VBMCP
memantine
neuroleptic malignant syndrome 2290

nystagmus 1792
memory aids 2804
memory impairment/deficits
dementia/Alzheimer disease 2810–11
mild cognitive impairment 2814, 2815
traumatic brain injury 1693
treatment 2803–5
see also amnesia
MEN *see* multiple endocrine neoplasia
menadione, mitochondrial disorders 1566, 2174
Ménière's disease 1876, 1899–900
treatment 1900–1, 1914–15
meningioangiomatosis 1652
sporadic 1653
meningiomas 688–97
association with heritable syndromes 755
atypical 694
cavernous sinus 690, 1823, 1826–8, *1827*, *1828*,
1829
treatment 1827–8
cerebellopontine angle *692*
classification 693
clinical presentation 689–90
diagnostic imaging 690–3
effect on surrounding tissue 694
epidemiology 688
etiology 688–9
familial 1653
fibrous (fibroblastic) 693–4
foramen magnum 690
genetics and molecular biology 689
hormonal factors 1470
hyperostosis 694, *694*
hypothalamic dysfunction 1442
malignant 694, *694*
meningothelial (syncytial) 693, *693*
neurofibromatosis-2 1652, 1653
olfactory groove 690, *690*
pathology 693–4
psammomatous 693, *693*
radiation-induced 857
recurrence 696–7
spinal cord *800*
clinical features 801
diagnosis 801
epidemiology 799
neurofibromatosis-2 1653
pathology and molecular genetics 800–1
treatment 802
transitional 694, *694*
treatment/management 695–6, 1442
radiotherapy 684
tuberculum sellae 690, *691*
meningitis
aseptic
after brain tumor surgery 759
Behçet disease 1087, 1089, 1092
induction by antineoplastic agents 848, 851
medication-induced 892
nonviral causes 891–3
see also meningitis, viral
bacterial 863–73, *866*
brain abscess and 881
chemoprophylaxis 871, 872
Citrobacter meningitis in neonates 1065
clinical features 865
complications 865, 866
diagnosis 866–7, 1077
epidemiology 863
etiology 863–4
mortality rates in adults 865
neonates 867, 1063–6, 1590
pathophysiology and pathogenesis 864–5
sickle cell disease 1348
treatment 867–71, 1079, 1080, 1082
neonates 1590
vaccination 871–2
see also under names of specific organisms
carcinomatous 1717
cranial nerve palsies 1938, 1940
eosinophilic 1022, 1028–9
treatment 1023, 1029–30
fungal 891, 972, 977, 980–4
candidal meningitis in neonates 1067
diagnosis 987, 988, 989, 1077

HIV/AIDS 951, 952, 954
immunocompromised patients 1398–9
treatment 957, 958
HIV 1389
Mollaret's 705
Mycoplasma hominis **1064**
neonatal 867, 1063–6, *1064*, 1590
neurosarcoidosis 1435–6, 1438
non-infectious causes 989
non-tuberculous mycobacteria 910
occult spinal dysraphism 1595
Paragonimus sp. 1030
stroke and 617
strongyloidiasis 1022, 1023, 1032
syphilitic 914
transplant recipients 1072, 1073, 1074, 1076, 1204
treatment 1079–81
tuberculous 892, 905–6, 1398
chorea/ballism 2578
treatment 906–9
children 906, 908
resistance 908–9
viral 889–93
clinical features 890
diagnosis 890–1
differential 891–3
pathophysiology and pathogenesis 889–90
treatment 893, 894
meningocele 1594, 1596, *1596*
meningococcal meningitis 863, 865
chemoprophylaxis 871, 872
penicillin-resistant 863
treatment 867, 868, 869, 870
vaccination 871–2
meningoencephalitis
amebic
granulomatous 1007, 1014
primary 1007, 1013–14
Chagas disease 1992, 1994
Q fever 939
syphilitic 914
transplant recipients 1072, 1073
clinical features 1076
treatment 1079
trypanosomiasis 1014–15
meningomyelocele, lumbosacral 1594
Menkes disease 1640, 1641, 1644, 1647
childhood stroke and 621–2
menopause
epilepsy and 350
mood disorders 1469
menstrual disorders, epileptics 1465
mental disorders, clinical trials and 59–60
mental retardation 1617–18
psychiatric disorders in 1625–6
school and community services 1626
meperidine
contraindications 82, 83
cancer patients 846
migraine 82, 83
in pregnancy 86–7
porphyria 2185
side effects 82
spider bites 1040
use in intensive care unit 1168
mephenesin, trigeminal neuralgia 1851, 1852
meprobamate, tension-type headache 109, 111,
113
meralgia paresthetica 1546
merbendazole, trichinosis 2338
mercury toxicity 2224, 2227
diagnosis 2226
treatment 2226
merocraniam 1595
meropenem
bacterial meningitis 868, 869, 1079
brain abscess 875, 879, 880
MERRF 1562, 1563, 1565, 1640, 1642, 2353, 2354,
2590, 2591
mescaline 18
mesencepahlic cells, fetal transplantation,
Parkinson's disease 2512
mesencephalic tractotomy, central pain 216, 218
MeSH 51
mesoridazine 2601

metabolic acidosis 1321–5, 1526
  alcoholic 1323–4
    status epilepticus 317
    toxic gas exposure 1527, 1528, 1529
    treatment 1322
metabolic alkalosis 1325–6, 1526
  posthypercapnic 1326
  treatment 1326
metabolic disorders
  childhood stroke and 620–2
  intracererbal hemorrhage and 629
  seizures 365, 366–8
metabolic myopathies 2296, 2342–64
  diagnosis 2342–5
  inherited 2342–3
metabolism, effect of illness and injury 1238
metabolism of drugs 19–20
metabotropic receptors 6
  glutamate 9, 11
metachlorophenylpiperazine (MCPP) 18
metachromatic leukodystrophy 1485, 1486, 1488,
    1489, 1640, 1641, 1643, 1644, 2167, 2170–1
  diagnosis 1491, 1492
metalloproteinases, matrix 1098, 1100
metalloproteinases, matrix degrading
  tumor cells 662–3, 668–9
  see also matrix metalloprotein inhibitors
metals, neurotoxicity 2223–8
  diagnosis 2225–6
  screening, prevention and occupational
    monitoring 2226–7
metastat 669
metaxalone, cervical spondylosis 1426
methadone
  cancer pain 235
  neuropathic pain 184, 185, 225, 228, 2244, 2245
  opioid addiction treatment 1513, 1514
  restless legs syndrome 2659, 2661
  side effects 2245
methamphetamine misuse 1516
methemoglobin, toxic gas exposure 1527, 1529
methicillin-resistant Staphylococcus aureus (MRSA)
  epidural abscess 884
  transplant recipients 1079, 1080, 1081
methionine, nitrogen oxide poisoning 1530
methiothepin 18
methocarbamol, spider bites 1040
methotrexate
  hearing loss 1914
  inflammatory myopathies 2329, 2330, 2332, 2333,
    2335, 2336
  leptomeningeal metastasis 826, 827
    side effects 828
  leukemia 1356, 1357, 1358
  lymphoma of central nervous system 776, 777,
    1355, 1356, 1357
    radiotherapy and 777
  neuro-Behçet syndrome 1091
  sarcoid neuropathy 1436, 1437, 2121, 2122
  side effects 1358, 1377, 1393, 2099, 2122, 2123
    management 2099
    monitoring 2122
    neurotoxic 848–50
  as steroid-sparing agent 155
  use in pregnancy 1554
  vasculitis/vasculitic neuropathy 585, 586, 588,
    1409, 1410–11, 2090–1, 2094
methotrimeprazine, pain disorder 256
methyl-G, neurotoxic effects 849
methylcellulose, gastrointestinal motility disorders
    2285
methylene blue, poisoning by nitrogen oxide gases
    1529
methylergonovine, chronic daily headache 129
methylmalonic acidemia 622, 1671
methylmalonic aciduria 1643, 1644
methylmercury, toxicity 2224, 2225
α-methylparatyrosine, tardive dyskinesia 2608
methylphenidate
  attention deficit hyperactivity disorder 1634,
    2778–9
    and Tourette's syndrome 2629
  dementia patients 2844, 2853, 2854
    dementia with Lewy bodies 2828
  executive disorders 2809

fragile X syndrome 1637, 1639
intentional disorders/prefrontal dysfunction
    2790, 2793, 2794, 2797
multiple system atrophy 2490
narcolepsy 1307
neglect 2768
Parkinson's disease 2468
methylphenidate hydrochloride, opioid-induced
    sedation 846
methylprednisolone 587, 1450
  Behçet disease 1090, 1091
  contraindications 82
  cryoglobulinemia 1376, 1378
    mixed, hepatitis C virus-related 2023
  giant cell arteritis 154, 154
  Guillain–Barré syndrome 2044
  Hymenoptera stings 1046
  inflammatory myopathies 2330, 2332, 2335
  mitochondrial disease 1567
  multiple sclerosis 1112–13
    pregnancy 1554
  myasthenia gravis 2382, 2385
  neuroprotective effects, cardiac surgery 463
  optic neuritis 1720–1
  optic neuropathy, anterior ischemic 1724
  pain management
    complex regional pain syndrome 210
    giant cell arteritis 154
    severe migraine 82, 83
  radiculoplexus neuropathy
    diabetic 2009
    non diabetic 2068
  sarcoid neuropathy 1438, 2122
  sensory ganglionopathies 2074, 2076
  side effects 2330
  spinal cord infarction 561–2
  spinal cord injury 1231, 1233
    children 1689
  stiff person syndrome 838
  vasculitic neuropathy 2090, 2094
  vestibular neuritis 1873
methysergide
  contraindications 84
  headache
    chronic daily 131
    cluster 96, 97
    migraine 84, 85
    progressive supranuclear palsy 2486
  side effects 84, 85
metoclopramide 2601
  cancer anorexia–cachexia syndrome 845
  contraindications 79
  gastrointestinal motility disorders 2262, 2285
  labyrinthitis/vertigo 1898
  migraine/severe headache 79, 82
    childhood 159, 160
    in pregnancy 87
  multiple system atrophy 2490
  pharmacology 18
  side effects 79, 2601, 2602
metoprolol
  autonomic hyperactivity 2286, 2287
  contraindications 84
  migraine prophylaxis 84, 85
    children 160
  postural tachycardia syndrome 2280
  side effects 84
metronidazole
  bacterial meningitis 868, 869
  brain abscess 875, 879, 880
    Entamoeba histolytica 1014
    prophylaxis 882
  cobalamin metabolism disorder 1642
  hepatic encephalopathy 1297
  intestinal pseudo-obstruction 2263
  neurotoxic effects 849
  septic venous sinus thrombosis 550
  tetanus 931, 932
metyrapone
  Cushing disease 729
  glucocorticoid excess 1452
  side effects 729
metyrosine, pheochromocytoma 1452–3
Meuse fever 942
mexiletine

cancer pain 237
cramps 2414
multiple sclerosis 1124
myotonia 2368, 2369, 2372
neuropathic pain 184, 224, 226, 227, 2241, 2244
side effects 2241, 2244
MGUS see monoclonal gammopathy of
    undetermined significance
mianserin
  akathisia 2603
  multiple system atrophy 2490
  tension-type headache prevention 114
miconazole 991, 994
  amebic meningoencephalitis 1014
  contraindications 998
  drug interactions 999
  side effects 998
microangiopathy and Susac's syndrome 1869,
    1870
microcephaly 1579
  maternal substance abuse and 1591
microdeletion syndromes 1639
microglia 1097
  multiple sclerosis 1102
micronemesiasis 1022
microscopic polyangiitis (MPA) 2079, 2080, 2081,
    2084
  treatment 2090, 2091, 2092, 2094, 2095
Microsporum audouninii 977, 984
microsurgery, vascular malformations 511, 514
micturition syncope 1268
MIDAS syndrome 1661
midazolam 1167, 1168
  scorpion bite 1042
  sedation in intensive care unit 1167, 1170
  seizures
    brain abscess 880
    post-transplant 1203
  status epilepticus 325, 326–7
  tetanus 931
midodrine
  multiple system atrophy 2490–1
  orthostatic hypotension 1453, 2284, 2285
    dementia patients 2853
    neurogenic 2272, 2273
    Parkinson's disease 2465, 2466
  Parkinson's disease 2454
  pharmacology 19
  side effects 2284, 2285
  syncope 1272–3, 1274
mifepristone (RU486)
  hypercortisolism 729
  meningiomas 696, 1470
migraine 73–88
  abdominal 76, 163
  acephalgic 75
  auras 74, 75, 76, 427–8
    CADASIL 597, 599
  basilar (basilar artery; vertebrobasilar;
    Bickerstaff) 76, 160–1, 1875, 1876
  cerebral infarction/stroke 617–18
  cheiro-oral 75
  children and adolescents 158–62
  classification 76
  clinical features 74–5
  confusional 162
  cyclic 93
  diagnosis 76, 77
    differential 76–7
  epidemiology 73
  etiology 73
  footballer's 137, 162
  gastrointestinal symptoms 2256
  genetics 74, 1875
  hemiplegic 76
    familial 74, 161, 618, 1875
  historical aspects 73
  hormonal factors 1466
  menstrual 86, 1466
  nature of 71
  neuro-otological disorders 1875–6
    vertigo 1872, 1874–7, 1878–9
  ophthalmoplegic 76, 161–2, 1825
  oral contraceptives and 86
  pathophysiology 73

peripheral nervous system 1648–9
segmental 1651–2
spine and spinal cord 1651
tumors 799, 801, 802, 804
variant forms 1651–2
vestibular schwannoma 1884
visual system 1650
neurofibromatosis-2 (NF2) 803, 1646, 1647, 1648,
1652–3
brain tumors 697, 755
diagnostic criteria 1652
Gardner variant 1652
hearing impairment 1908
management 1653
spinal cord tumors 800, 801
vestibular schwannoma 1884
Whishart variant 1652
neurofibromatosis–Noonan syndrome 1652
neurofibromin 804
neurogenic weakness, ataxia and retinitis
pigmentosa (NARP) 1562, 1563, 1565, 1640,
2353, 2354
neuroimaging
antiphospholipid syndrome 578
cerebral venous/dural sinus disorders 546–9
cysticercosis 1021–2
epilepsy 309–10
fungal infections 979, 982, 985–7
HIV dementia 1390, *1390*
HIV/AIDS 953
hypertensive encephalopathy 593
Lyme disease 921
malignant brain tumors, childhood 757, 758
neurosarcoidosis 1436
stroke 445
transient ischemic attacks 427
tuberculosis 905
see also specific techniques
neurolabyrinthitis, vestibular *see* labyrinthitis
neuroleptic malignant syndrome 1443, 2290, 2432,
2471, 2607–8
neuroleptics
agitation
delirium 2857, 2863
dementia 2857, 2859–60
atypical
agitation, delirium 2857, 2863
Alzheimer disease 2820, 2821
antiparkinsonian-induced psychosis 2858, 2864
chorea/ballism 2576
chronic daily headache 132
Huntington's disease 2557
Parkinson's disease patients 2858
tardive dyskinesia 2609
basal ganglia disorders 1642
chorea/ballism 2576, 2577
contraindications, dementia with Lewy bodies
2828, 2857, 2859
dementia with Lewy bodies 2828
dopamine blocking activity 2601–2
Huntington's disease 2557
intravenous
contraindications 82
migraine/severe headache 82, 83
side effects 82, 83
neuroacanthocytosis 2565, 2566
Parkinson's disease patients 2471
side effects 2627–8, 2857, 2859
acute reactions 2602–3
parkinsonism 2604
sexual dysfunction 2249
tardive syndromes 2604–7
tic suppression/Tourette's syndrome 2627–8
withdrawal emergent syndrome 2606–7
see also specific drugs
neurolymphomatosis 1354, 1357, 2151
neurolysis
external 1963
internal 1964
neuromas
acoustic 697–701, *699*, *700*
injury 2008
plexiform 1649, 1651
ocular 1649, 1650
syndrome of bilateral acoustic neuroma *see*

neurofibromatosis-2
neurometabolic disorders, gene transfer studies 29
neuromodulation 6
neuromodulators 297, 306
neuromuscular blocking agents (NMBAs) 1189,
1190, 1193, 1194
neurological effects, critical illness
polyneuropathy 2231
neuromuscular disorders
chronic immune-mediated 2160
HTLV-I-associated 963–4
hyperthyroidism 1456–7
respiratory failure in 1303
rheumatoid arthritis 1422
neuromuscular junction blockade, prolonged
1189–90, 1191
treatment 1193–4
neuromuscular junction disorders, pregnancy 1550
neuromuscular ventilatory failure
endotracheal intubation 1140, 1141–2
mechanical ventilation 1145
neuromuscular weakness, intensive care unit
patients 1189–95
treatment 1192–4
neuromyelitis optica (Devic syndrome) 1120, *1121*
neuromyotonia 2432, 2642
clinical *see* Isaacs syndrome
paraneoplastic 840, 2162, 2164–5
neuron specific enolase (NSE)
biochemical marker for cerebral injury 461
status epilepticus 317, *317*, 319–20
complex partial 322
neuronal intranuclear inclusion, Huntington's
disease 2552, 2553–4
neuronitis
interstitial 2433
vestibular *see* labyrinthitis
neurons
electrotonic coupling 279
epileptogenesis
cell–cell interactions and 273–9
intrinsic properties and 270–3
network properties and 279–81, *280*
GABAergic 275–8
inhibitory circuits 277–8, *277*
membrane conductances
passive 270–1
voltage-dependent 271–3
neuro-oncology 659–60
see also brain tumors; tumors; *names of specific
tumors*
neuropathic pain *see* pain, neuropathic
neuropathy
alcoholic 1506
amyloid 1363, 1364, 1365, 1367–9
anti-MAG 1363–4, 1370
autoimmune 1102
autonomic, rheumatoid arthritis 1422
axonal *see* axonal neuropathy
brachial plexus *see* brachial plexus neuropathy
chronic renal failure 2025–6
combined sensorimotor 1421
compression *see* compression neuropathy
cranial
localized 1937–9
neurosarcoidosis 1437
non-localized 1937, 1938, 1940–2
diabetic *see* diabetic neuropathy; diabetic
polyneuropathy
diphtheric 1976–8
distal sensory, rheumatoid arthritis 1421
drug-induced, antineoplastic agents 850–1, 853,
854, 855
entrapment *see* entrapment neuropathy
facial 1860–6
giant axonal 1641
hereditary *see* hereditary ...
hyperthyroidism 1458
hypothyroidism 1461
IgA-associated 1363, 1364–5
IgG-associated 1363, 1364–5
IgM-associated 1330–1, 1362, 1363–4
ischemic momomelic 2026
length-dependent 2277
leprosy 1986–91

liver disease 2022–5
motor *see* motor ...
optic 1709–29
for detailed entry see optic neuropathies
painful 222–9
cancer 230, 231
classification 223
clinical features 222–3
mechanisms 222
treatment 223–8, 234, 235, 236–7
see also pain, neuropathic
paraneoplastic syndromes 2158–65
peripheral *see* peripheral neuropathy
pregnancy 1545–9
sensorimotor
possible paraneoplastic origin 840
rheumatoid arthritis 1421
sensory *see* sensory neuropathies
tomaculous *see* hereditary neuropathy with
liability to pressure palsy
trigeminal 1849–59
anatomical considerations 1849
see also trigeminal neuralgia
vasculitic 2078, 2079–80
clinical features 2085–6
diagnosis 2086–7
treatment 2087–100
xanthomatous 2024
see also polyneuropathy
neuropathy, ataxia, retinitis pigmentosa (NARP)
1562, 1563, 1565, 1640, 2353, 2354
neuropathy target esterase (NTE) 1532
neuropeptides, epileptogenesis 278–9
neuropharmacology 3–24
bioavailability of drugs 18–20
neurophysiological studies, corticobasal
degeneration 2494
neurophysiology 3–5
neuroplasticity, substance misuse and 1512
Neuropsychiatric Inventory (NPI) 2820
neuropsychiatric syndrome, progressive 2837
neuropsychological dysfunction, after cardiac
surgery 458–9
neuropsychological testing
Alzheimer disease 2813
mild cognitive impairment 2815–16, *2816*
neuroreaction 1944
neuroretinitis 1716, *1717*
cat-scratch disease 943, 944
neurosarcoidosis *see* sarcoidosis
neurosyphilis *see* syphilis
neurotization, nerve injury 1965–6
neurotmesis 1955, 1958, 1963
neurotoxicants 1519–20
neurotoxicity, peripheral neuropathy, grading 2147
neurotoxins
Isaacs syndrome 2415
scorpion bites 1041
spider bites 1039
ticks 1042–3
see also specific toxins
neurotransmission, principles 5–8
neurotransmitters 5
acetylcholine (cholinergic) 12–14
aspartate 8–9, 10
catecholamines 14–17
epilepsy 275–9
GABA 12
glutamate 7, 8–12
glycine 12
mechanisms of action 5–8
role in fibromyalgia 247
saccadic premotor neurons 1787
serotonin 17–18
vestibulo-ocular reflex 1785
neurotransplantation, Parkinson's disease 2512–13
neurotrophic factors
brain-derived, spinocerebellar degeneration 2211
traumatic central nervous system injury 1685
neutral lipid storage (Dorfman–Chanarin) disease
1670
nevirapine
HIV infection 955, 956
side effects 955
nevoid basal cell carcinoma syndrome 755, 1660

retinal (amaurosis fugax) 426, 428
spinal 560
treatment 428–33
crescendo transient ischemic attacks 428–9
during evaluation 428
vertigo 1869
transjugular intrahepatic portosystemic shunts
(TIPS), hepatic encephalopathy 1295, 1296,
1297
transmissible spongiform encephalopathies *see*
prion diseases
transplantation
Fabry disease 1662
mitochondrial disease 1564–5
neurological aspects 1383–7
neurological evaluation 1196–7
Parkinson's disease 2512–13
postoperative management 1196
pretransplantation conditions and 1197–8
primary central nervous system lymphoma 774
procedures 1199
see also bone marrow/heart/kidney/liver
transplantation
transplantation complications 1196–207, 1383–7
drug-related 1383, 1386–7
evaluation in ICU 1196–7
infection 1072–83, 1200, 1201, 1202, 1203–4,
1204–5, 1391–3
brain abscess in 875, 877, 882
clinical features 1076
diagnosis 1077–9
etiology 1072–3
pathophysiology and pathogenesis 1073–6
treatment 1079–82
myopathy 2232, 2234
postoperative 1199–206
early 1383, 1384–6
effects of drugs 1200–1, 1202, 1203
graft nonfunction and 1201
immunosuppression and 1201, 1203, 1204
infection 1200, 1201, 1202, 1203–4, 1204–5
late 1383, 1386–7
management 1201–3
repeat surgery 1206
transthyretin, amyloidosis 2137, 2140, 2141, 2142,
2143, 2144
tranylcypromine 16
tranylcypromine phenelzine, Parkinson's disease
2451
trauma/traumatic injury
cerebral aneurysms *497*, 502
children *1684*
epidemiology 1681–3
mild 1693
pathophysiology 1683–5
prognosis 1693–4
treatment
acute 1685–90
subacute 1690–3
head *see* head injury; traumatic brain injury
headache following 136–41
meningioma and 688–9
metabolic response 1238
nerve roots, radicular pain 189
ocular nerve palsies 1773, 1774, 1776, 1778
seizures following 1882
and venous thrombosis 543
see also spinal cord injury; traumatic brain injury
traumatic brain injury
athletes 1223–4, 1225
blood pressure management 1153, 1155
children *1684*
acute treatment 1685–90
epidemiology 1681–3
mild injury 1693
pathophysiology 1683–5
prognosis 1693
rehabilitation 1690–3, 1694
epidemiology 1221
hypertension 1153
hyperventilation 1135
management 1221–30
intensive care unit 1228–30
prehospital and emergency department
1221–3, 1224

surgical 1224, 1226–8
pathophysiology 1221
penetrating injuries 1228
primary 1221
prognosis 1230
rotational 1221
secondary 1221
translational 1221
trazodone
dementia/Alzheimer disease patients 2821, 2853,
2857, 2860, 2862
intentional disorders/prefrontal dysfunction
2793, 2796
parkinsonism plus disorders 2497
postherpetic neuralgia 1855
sonambulism 1311
trematodes 1021, 1022
tremor(s) 2440
cog-tremor 2448
corticobasal degeneration 2493, 2495
essential 2582–6
clinical manifestations 2582–3
clinical variants 2584
definition 2582
diagnosis 2583–4
epidemiology 2583
familial 2428
gender factors 1469
genetics 2583
pathophysiology 2584–5
pregnancy 1556
prevalence 2422
treatment 2585
pregnancy 1556
flapping *see* asterixis
genetics 2428
midbrain (rubral) 2440
multiple sclerosis 1123, 1124
oculopalatal 1787, 1788–9, 1791
origins/localization 2421
orthostatic 2587–8
Parkinson's disease 2464
psychogenic 2678, 2680, 2681
rest 2448, 2582
thyrotoxic 1458
toluene exposure 1522
tongue 2584
writing 2584
trench fever 942
trench foot 1959
Treponema pallidum 913
microhemagglutination assay 914, 915
Trial of Org 10172 in Acute Stroke Treatment
(TOAST) 439–40, 443, 455–6
triamcinolone 1450
Behçet disease 1090
triamterene, hypokalemic periodic paralysis 2374
triarylphosphates 1531
triazolam, restless legs syndrome/periodic limb
movement disorder 2661
tricarboxylic acid cycle defects 2353, 2354
Trichinella spiralis/trichinosis (trichinellosis) 1022,
1033
myositis 2338
treatment 1023, 1033–4
trichloroethylene, exposure and toxic effects 1519,
1520–1
Trichophyton sp. 977
Trichosporon sp. 984
Trichosporon beigelii 975, 984
Trichosporon cutaneum 984
tricyclic antidepressants
attention deficit hyperactivity disorder 2778,
2779
Tourette's syndrome 2630
cardiac contraindications 2242
cataplexy 1307
contraindications, dementia with Lewy bodies
2828
dementia/Alzheimer disease patients 2820, 2821,
2857, 2862
Huntington's disease 2557
intentional disorders/prefrontal dysfunction
2793, 2796
motor neuron disease 2218

multiple sclerosis 1123, 1124, 1126
pain management
back pain 203
cancer 236, 237
complex regional pain syndrome 211
fibromyalgia 248
headache
chronic daily 131
tension-type 111, 114, 115
traumatic 138
migraine prophylaxis 84, 85
neuropathic pain 184, 223–4, 226, 227, 2241,
2242
parasomnias 1311
parkinsonism plus disorders 2495, 2497
Parkinson's disease 2453, 2454, 2469
pharmacology 15
side effects 2241, 2242, 2857, 2862
sexual dysfunction 2249
tridihexethyl chloride, nystagmus 1792
trientine (triethylene tetramine)
side effects 1557, 2673–4
use in pregnancy 1557
Wilson's disease 2673
pregnancy 1557
trifluoperazine 2601
triflupromazine 2601
trigeminal-autonomic cephalgias 93, 142–4
clinical features 144
treatment 146–7, 149
trigeminal (5th cranial) nerve
cavernous sinus 1822
disorders 1822–3, 1826, 1831, 1839, 1840–1
decompression, cluster headache 100
trigeminal neuralgia 1849, 1850–2, 1856–7
pain 93
paroxysmal, multiple sclerosis 1124
progressive systemic sclerosis 1433
treatment 1851–2, 1856–7
trigeminal neuropathies 1849–59
anatomical considerations 1849
trigeminal rhizotomy, cluster headache 99, 100
trigeminal schwannomas 701–2, *702*
trigeminovascular parasympathetic pathway 143,
143
trigeminovascular system, migraine 74
trigonocephaly 1611
trihexyphenidyl
dystonia 2538, 2539, 2540–1
dopa-responsive 2547
tardive 2611
nystagmus 1792
palatal myoclonus 2594
Parkinson's disease 2452, 2456
side effects 1557
use in pregnancy 1557
writer's cramp 2532
trimethadione, epilepsy 272
trimethobenzamide
gastroparesis 2262
migraine, childhood 159
trimethoprim 1009
trimethoprim–sulfamethoxazole
bacterial meningitis 868, 869
brain abscess 875, 880
prophylaxis 882
Citrobacter infection, neonates 1590
fungal infection 991
neurotoxic effects 849
Nocardia infection, transplant recipients 1080,
1082
Pneumocystis carinii pneumonia prevention
1451
toxoplasma encephalitis, HIV/AIDS 957
vasculitis 585
Wegener's granulomatosis 2091–2
Whipple disease 1501
triorthocresyl phosphate 1531, 1533
triphyllocephaly 1611
triptans
chronic daily headache 129
contraindications 80, 81
migraine 79–80, 81
rebound headache 125, 128
side effects 80, 80–1